ACS(I)
Textbook of
Cutaneous and Aesthetic Surgery

Under the Aegis of Association of Cutaneous Surgeons (I)

ACS(I)
Textbook of
Cutaneous and Aesthetic Surgery

Third Edition

Volume 1

Editor-in-Chief
Manas Chatterjee
MD DNB (Dermatology and Venereology)
Brigadier
Armed Forces Medical Services and
Consultant Dermatologist
Base Hospital Delhi Cantt
New Delhi, India

Associate Editor
Biju Vasudevan MD
Professor and Head
Department of Dermatology
Armed Forces Medical College
Pune, Maharashtra, India

Emeritus Editor
Mysore Venkataram
DVD MD DNB DipRCPath (London) FRCP (Glasgow) FISHRS
Consultant Dermatologist and
Hair Transplant Surgeon
Director
Venkat Charmalaya—Centre for
Advanced Dermatology and
Postgraduate Teaching Centre
Bengaluru, Karnataka, India

JAYPEE

JAYPEE BROTHERS MEDICAL PUBLISHERS
The Health Sciences Publisher
New Delhi | London

Editorial Board

Editorial Advisory Editors

Jaypee Brothers Medical Publishers (P) Ltd

Headquarters
Jaypee Brothers Medical Publishers (P) Ltd
EMCA House, 23/23-B
Ansari Road, Daryaganj
New Delhi 110 002, India
Landline: +91-11-23272143, +91-11-23272703
+91-11-23282021, +91-11-23245672
Email: jaypee@jaypeebrothers.com

Corporate Office
Jaypee Brothers Medical Publishers (P) Ltd
4838/24, Ansari Road, Daryaganj
New Delhi 110 002, India
Phone: +91-11-43574357
Fax: +91-11-43574314
Email: jaypee@jaypeebrothers.com

Overseas Office
JP Medical Ltd
83 Victoria Street, London
SW1H 0HW (UK)
Phone: +44 20 3170 8910
Fax: +44 (0)20 3008 6180
Email: info@jpmedpub.com

Website: www.jaypeebrothers.com
Website: www.jaypeedigital.com

ACS(I) Textbook of Cutaneous and Aesthetic Surgery (Volume 1)

First Edition: 2012

Reprint: 2013

Second Edition: 2017

Third Edition: **2024**

ISBN: 978-93-90595-83-9

Printed at: Samrat Offset Pvt. Ltd.

Contributors

Aakash Gupta
MD DNB FRGUHS (Dermatosurgery)
Consultant Dermatologist and Dermatosurgeon
Leelawanti Skin and Laser Institute
New Delhi, India

Aarti Sarda MD FAGE SCE (Dermatology)
Consultant Dermatologist
Wizderm—Specialty Skin and Hair Clinic
Kolkata, West Bengal, India

Abdul Latheef EN
DVD MD MSc (Psychology) FRCP (Glasgow)
Professor
Department of Dermatology and Venereology
Government Medical College
Kozhikode, Kerala, India

Abhishek De
MD FAGE SCE (Dermatology) FRCP (Edinburgh)
Consultant Dermatologist, Aesthetician and Laser Surgeon
Associate Professor
Calcutta National Medical College
Kolkata, West Bengal, India

Adit Mohan Garg MD (DVL)
Consultant Dermatosurgeon
Divya Alok Hospital
Kota, Rajasthan, India

Afreen Ayub MD DNB MRCP (SCE)
Assistant Professor
Department of Dermatology
INHS Kalyani
Visakhapatnam, Andhra Pradesh, India

Alka Goel MD DNB MNAMS
Consultant Dermatologist
Dr Alka Goel's Skin and Laser Clinic
New Delhi, India

Aman Dua MD (Dermatology)
Managing Director
AK Clinics Pvt Ltd
Ludhiana, Punjab, India

Ameet Dandale DNB
Consultant, DNB Teacher Gr-1, and Head
Department of Dermatology
Bharat Ratna Dr Babasaheb Ambedkar General Hospital
Mumbai, Maharashtra, India

Amit Kerure MD (DVL)
Consultant Dermatologist and Hair Transplant Surgeon
Dr Amit Kerure Skin Clinic
Navi Mumbai, Maharashtra, India

Amit Luthra DNB
Consultant Dermatologist
Ishira Skin Clinic
New Delhi, India

Aneesh Kunnath Parambath
MD (DVL)
Specialist Dermatology
Aster DM Healthcare
Dubai, UAE

Aniketh Venkataram
MS (General Surgery) MCH (Plastic Surgery)
Consultant Plastic Surgeon
The Venkat Center for Skin ENT and Plastic Surgery
Bengaluru, Karnataka, India

Anil Ganjoo MD
Founder Director and Consultant Dermatologist
Skinnovation Clinics
New Delhi, India

Anil K Garg
MS MCh MA (Yoga) FISHRS ABHRS
Plastic Surgeon and CEO
Rejuvenate Plastic and Hair Transplant Centre
Indore, Madhya Pradesh, India

Anirudha Gulanikar
MBBS DVD DNB (Skin and VD)
Professor
Department of Dermatology
MGM Medical College
Aurangabad, Maharashtra, India

Anjali Pal
MD (Dermatology, Venereology and Leprology)
Consultant Dermatologist
Navpreet Hospital
Amritsar, Punjab, India

Ankan Gupta MD MNAMS EBDVD
Associate Professor
Christian Medical College
Vellore, Tamil Nadu, India

Ankur Talwar MD
Professor and Head
Department of Dermatology
Hind Institute of Medical Sciences
Lucknow
Consultant Dermatologist
Talwar Skin Centre
Lucknow, Uttar Pradesh, India

Anuj Pall MD PhD FISD (USA)
Chief Director
Escallent Institute of Lasers and Aesthetic Medicine (EILAM)
Gurugram, Haryana, India

Anurag Tiwari DVD DNB
Director and Consultant Dermatologist
Center for Skin Disease and Laser Treatment
Bhopal, Madhya Pradesh, India

Anusha H Pai MD (Dermatology)
Consultant Dermatologist
Derma-Care
Mangaluru, Karnataka, India

AP Balaji MD (DVL)
Consultant Dermatologist and Dermatosurgeon
Bhairavi Skin and Hair Clinic
Chennai, Tamil Nadu, India

Apratim Goel MD DNB FAGE
Medical Director
Cutis Skin Solution
Mumbai, Maharashtra, India

Arpita Arghya MBBS DDVL
Consultant Dermatologist and Cosmetologist
Skinchime—Skin, Hair, and Cosmetic Clinic
Bengaluru, Karnataka, India

Arvind Poswal MBBS
Director
Dr A's Clinic Pvt Ltd
New Delhi, India

(Sqn Ldr) Aseem Sharma
MD DNB MBA FAGE IFAAD
Chief Dermatologist
Skin Saga Centre for Dermatology
Mumbai, Maharashtra, India

Ashique KT
MBBS DDVL PGDHS FRCP (London)
Medical Director and Senior Consultant Dermatologist
Amanza Skin Clinic
Malappuram, Kerala, India

Atul Bothra
MD (Dermatology, Venereology and Leprosy)
Fellow
Department of Dermatosurgery
CUTIS Academy of Cutaneous Sciences
Bengaluru, Karnataka, India

Avitus John Raakesh Prasad DDVL
Managing Director
SP Derma Center
Madurai, Tamil Nadu, India

Ayushi Bothra MD (Dermatology)
Consultant Dermatologist
Skinvest
Mumbai, Maharashtra, India

Banani Choudhury
MD DNB MNAMS
Consultant Dermatologist
Jaslok Hospital and Research Centre
Sir HN Reliance Foundation Hospital and Research Centre
Mumbai, Maharashtra, India

Bhanu Prakash MD DHM PGDMLE
Professor
Department of Dermatology
Vydehi Institute of Medical Sciences and Research Center
Bengaluru, Karnataka, India

Biju Vasudevan MD
Professor and Head
Department of Dermatology
Armed Forces Medical College
Pune, Maharashtra, India

Bipin Deshpande MBBS DVD IFAAD
Dermatologist, Dermatosurgeon
Cosmetic Dermatologist
Chaitanya Clinic
Pune, Maharashtra, India

BS Chandrashekar MD DNB
Chief Dermatologist and Medical Director
CUTIS Academy of Cutaneous Sciences
Bengaluru, Karnataka, India

C Shanmuga Sekar MD
Associate Professor
Department of Dermatology
PSG Hospitals
Coimbatore, Tamil Nadu, India

Chander Grover
MD DNB MNAMS
Professor
Department of Dermatology and STD
University College of Medical Sciences and GTB Hospital
New Delhi, India

Chintan Subhash Gujarathi
MS (General Surgery) MCh (Plastic and Reconstructive Surgery) DNB (Plastic and Reconstructive Surgery)
Consultant Plastic, Cosmetic and Reconstructive Surgeon
Ruby Hall Clinic
Pune, Maharashtra, India

CR Srinivas MD (DVL)
Professor
Department of Dermatology
Kalinga Institute of Medical Sciences
Bhubaneswar, Odisha, India

D Dinesh Kumar
MD FRCP (Glasgow, London)
Consultant Dermatologist and Head
Dr Dinesh's Skin and Hair Clinic
Chennai, Tamil Nadu, India

Davinder Parsad MD
Professor
Department of Dermatology
Postgraduate Institute of Medical Education and Research
Chandigarh, India

Debdeep Mitra
MD DNB (Dermatology)
Professor
Department of Dermatology
Command Hospital Air Force
Bengaluru, Karnataka, India

Deepak Jakhar MD
Consultant Dermatologist
Dermosphere Clinic
New Delhi, India

Dhanashree S Bhide MD DNB
Dermatologist, Venereologist and Leprologist
KEM Hospital
Deenanath Mangeshkar Hospital
Pune, Maharashtra, India

Dilip Kachhawa
MD (Dermatology, STD, and Leprosy)
Principal and Controller
Senior Professor
Dr SN Medical College
Jodhpur, Rajasthan, India

Dinkar Sreekumar
DrNB (Plastic and Reconstructive Surgery)
Associate Consultant
Baby Memorial Hospital
Kozhikode, Kerala, India

Dipali Rathod
DNB DDVL FIDD FIADVL (Dermatopathology) MNAMS
Assistant Professor
Seth GS Medical College and KEM Hospital
Mumbai, Maharashtra, India

Divya Gorur
MD (Dermatology) FRGUHS (Dermatosurgery)
Consultant Dermatology
Cosme Skin and Hair Clinic
Bengaluru, Karnataka, India

Eswari L
MDDVL FRGUHS (Dermatosurgery) FAADV (Dermatopathology)
Associate Professor
Bangalore Medical College and Research Institute
Bengaluru, Karnataka, India

Feroze Kaliyadan
MD DNB MNAMS FRCP (London)
Professor
Sree Narayana Institute of Medical Sciences
Ernakulam, Kerala, India

Ganesh S Pai MD DVD FAAD
Medical Director
Department of Dermatology
Derma-Care
Mangaluru, Karnataka, India

Gautam K Singh MD (Dermatology)
Professor
Base Hospital Delhi Cantt
Army College of Medical Sciences
New Delhi, India

Gillian Roga
MD DNB (Dermatology) Fellowship in Hair Transplantation and Cosmetology
Consultant Dermatology, Cosmetologist and Hair Transplant Surgeon
Dr Gillian's Skin, Hair, Laser and Cosmetology Clinic
Chikmagalur, Karnataka, India

Govind S Mittal
MD DVL FRGUHS (Dermatosurgery)
Consultant Dermatologist and Dermatosurgeon
Therapeia Skin Hair and ENT Centre
Bengaluru, Karnataka, India

Garehatty Rudrappa Kanthraj MD
Professor and Head
Department of Dermatology, Venereology and Leprosy
JSS Medical College and Hospital
JSS Academy of Higher Education
(Deemed To Be University)
Mysuru, Karnataka, India

GR Rajput
MD (Dermatology, Venereology, and Leprosy)
Assistant Professor
Institute of Naval Medicine
INHS Asvini
Mumbai, Maharashtra, India

Gulhima Arora DNB MNAMS
Senior Consultant and Dermatologist
Mehektagul Dermaclinic
New Delhi, India

Gulshant Panesar
MD (Dermatology)
Associate Professor
Department of Dermatology
Santosh Medical College and Hospital
Ghaziabad, Uttar Pradesh, India

Gunjan Shah DDV
Director
iBrow Academy
Ahmedabad, Gujarat, India

Harish Prasad BR
MD (Dermatology) FRGUHS (Dermatosurgery)
Consultant Dermatosurgeon
Vitals Skin, Hair, Laser, Vitiligo Klinic
Bengaluru, Karnataka, India

Harsh Tahiliani
MD (Dermatology)
Consultant Dermatologist
Dr Tahiliani's Clinic
Visiting Consultant Dermatologist
Bhartiya Arogya Nidhi Hospital
Mumbai, Maharashtra, India

Harvinder S Marwah
MD DVD DDV MCPS
Consultant Dermatologist and Head
Dr Marwah's Skin, Hair, Laser, and Cosmetic Centre
Mumbai, Maharashtra, India

HM Omprakash MBBS DVD
Consulting Dermatologist
Department of Dermatology
Samastha Skin Clinic
Mysuru, Karnataka, India

Imran Majid
MD FRCP (Edinburgh)
Director
CUTIS Institute of Dermatology
Srinagar, Jammu and Kashmir, India

Indrashis Podder MD DNB MNAMS
Assistant Professor
Department of Dermatology
College of Medicine and Sagore Dutta Hospital
Kolkata, West Bengal, India

Ishmeet Kaur MD (Dermatology)
Assistant Professor
Department of Dermatology
NDMC Medical College and Hindu Rao Hospital
New Delhi, India

Jaishree Sharad MBBS DDV
Dermatologist
Skinfinitii Aesthetic Skin and Laser Clinic
Mumbai, Maharashtra, India

Jayadev B Betkerur MD
Professor
Department of Dermatology
Venereology, and Leprosy
JSS Medical College and Hospital
JSS Academy of Higher Education
(Deemed to be University)
Mysuru, Karnataka, India

Jayashree Venkataram FRCOG
Director
Venkat Charmalaya—Centre for Advanced Dermatology
Bengaluru, Karnataka, India

Jyoti Gupta MD
Consultant Dermatologist and Hair Transplant Surgeon
Dr Jyoti Gupta Dermatology Clinic
New Delhi, India

Kabir Sardana
MD DNB MNAMS
Director, Professor and Head
Department of Dermatology
Atal Bihari Vajpayee Institute of Medical Sciences and Dr Ram Manohar Lohia Hospital (PGIMER)
New Delhi, India

Kanika Sahni MD
Additional Professor
Department of Dermatology and Venereology
All India Institute of Medical Sciences
New Delhi, India

Kapil Dua
MS (ENT) Dip (ABHRS, USA) Diplomate of American Board of Hair Restoration Surgery
Chairman and Chief Hair Transplant Surgeon
AK Clinics
Ludhiana, Punjab, India
Imm Past President, ISHRS (USA)
Past President, AHRS (India)
Board Member
AAHRS Asia and ABHRS (USA)

Kavish Chouhan
MD (Dermatology)
Director
DermaClinix, KSK Surgicals, Expertified
New Delhi, India
Co-Founder, FUE Asia

KC Nischal
MD (Dermatology)
Chief Dermatologist and Director
Nirmal Skin and Hair Clinic
Bengaluru, Karnataka, India

KH Satyanarayana Rao
MD PGDMLE PGDHHM
Consultant Dermatologist
Central Health Service
Bengaluru, Karnataka, India

Koushik Lahiri
DVD (CAL) FIAD iFAAD FFAADV FRCP (Glasgow, Edinburgh, London)
Professor and Senior Consultant Dermatologist
Apollo Multispecialty Hospital
Honorary Medical Director
Wizderm Speciality Skin and Hair Clinic
Kolkata, West Bengal, India

Krishna Talukdar MD (Dermatology)
Professor and Head
Department of Dermatology
Jorhat Medical College and Hospital
Jorhat, Assam, India

Kshama Talwar MD
Associate Professor
Department of Dermatology
Hind Institute of Medical Sciences
Consultant Dermatologist
Talwar Skin Centre
Lucknow, Uttar Pradesh, India

Kumaresan M
MD FISHRS Diplomate American Board of Hair Restoration Surgery
Consultant Dermatologist
Cutis Skin Clinic and Hair Transplant Center
Coimbatore, Tamil Nadu, India

Kumudhini S
MD FAGE DNB FRGUHS
Chief Dermatologist
Deep Skin Dialogues
Chennai, Tamil Nadu, India

Laila Arif MBBS DVD
Consultant Dermatologist
Cutis Institute of Dermatology and Aesthetic Sciences
Kozhikode, Kerala, India

Lakshyajit D Dhami
MS (Gen Surg) MCh (Plastic Surg)
Consultant Cosmetic, Laser, and Plastic Surgeon
Mumbai, Maharashtra, India

(Late) Sanjeev Mulekar MD
Senior Consultant and Dermatologist
Mulekar Vitiligo Clinic
Mumbai, Maharashtra, India

Madhulika Mhatre MD FRGUHS
Director
Skin Saga Centre for Dermatology
Mumbai, Maharashtra, India

Madhuri Agarwal MD (Skin & VD) DDV
Consultant Dermatologist
Yavana Aesthetics Clinic
Mumbai, Maharashtra, India

Madura C
MD FRGUHS (Dermatosurgery)
Consultant Dermatologist and Dermatosurgeon
CUTIS Academy of Cutaneous Sciences
Bengaluru, Karnataka, India

Malavika Kohli MD DVD DNB
Director and Founder
Skin Secrets
Consultant Dermatologist
Jaslok Hospital and Research Centre
Breach Candy Hospital Trust
Mumbai, Maharashtra, India

Manas Chatterjee
MD DNB (Dermatology and Venereology)
Brigadier
Armed Forces Medical Services
Consultant Dermatologist
Base Hospital Delhi Cantt
New Delhi, India

Manish Gautam DVD DNB (Dermatology)
Chief Dermatologist
Skin Solutions, Vashi
Consultant Dermatologist
Apollo Hospitals
Navi Mumbai, Maharashtra, India

Manjit Sandhu Tahiliani DDVL
Consultant Dermatologist
Dr Tahiliani's Clinic
Mumbai, Maharashtra, India

Manjot Marwah
MD (Dermatology)
Consultant Dermatologist and Director
Dr Manjot's Clinic and LHR Clinic
Jalandhar, Punjab, India

Maya Vedamurthy
MD DD MAMS FRCP (Edinburgh, Glasgow)
Consultant Dermatologist
RSV Skin and Research Centre
Apollo Hospitals
Chennai, Tamil Nadu, India

Milind N Naik
MS (Ophthalmology)
Consultant Ophthalmologist
LV Prasad Eye Institute
Hyderabad, Telangana, India
Adjunct Professor
Department of Ophthalmology
University of Rochester
New York, USA

Milind S Wagh
MS (Gen Surg) MCh (Plastic Surg)
Consultant Plastic and Aesthetic Surgeon
Make A Change—A Centre for Cosmetic Surgery
Mumbai, Maharashtra, India

Mukta Sachdev
MD FAAD DpD(UK) DD (UK) FAAD (USA)
Head
Department of Dermatology
Manipal Hospital, Bengaluru
Medical Director
MS Skin Centre
MS Clinical Research Pvt Ltd
Bengaluru, Karnataka, India

Munish Paul
MD (Dermatology)
Consultant Dermatologist
Skin Laser Centre
Manipal Hospital
New Delhi, India

Murali Chakravarthy MD DA DNB
Director
Department of Anesthesia, Critical Care and Pain Relief
Director
Clinical Affairs
Fortis Hospitals
Bengaluru, Karnataka, India

Mysore Venkataram
DVD MD DNB DipRCPath (London) FRCP (Glasgow) FISHRS
Consultant Dermatologist and Hair Transplant Surgeon
Director
Venkat Charmalaya—Centre for Advanced Dermatology and Postgraduate Teaching Centre
Bengaluru, Karnataka, India

Nagendra Singh Beniwal
DNB (Dermatology)
Associate Professor
Department of Dermatology
Military Hospital
Jalandhar, Punjab, India

Naina Jain MD DVL
Assistant Professor
SGT Medical College
Gurugram, Haryana, India

Narendra Patwardhan
MD DV (London) DVD
Consultant Dermatologist
Joshi Hospital, Deenanath Mangeshkar Hospital
Pune, Maharashtra, India

Nazneen Arsiwala MD DVD
Co-Founder
Renewderm Skin, Hair, Laser and Aesthetics Centre, Mumbai
Consultant Dermatologist
Masina Hospital
Mumbai, Maharashtra, India

Neha Taneja MD DNB MRCP (SCE)
Consultant Dermatologist
DermaClinix—Hair Transplant and Skin Clinic
New Delhi, India

Nicholas J Collier
BM BS MSc MMedSci MD
Consultant Dermatologist and Mohs Surgeon
Mohs Unit
Department of Dermatology
Salford Royal Hospital NHS Foundation Trust
Northern Care Alliance NHS Group
Salford, England
Manchester, UK

Nikhil Mehta MD
Senior Resident
Department of Dermatology and Venereology
All India Institute of Medical Sciences
New Delhi, India

Nilesh N Goyal
MRCP UK DNB (Dermatology and Venereology) DVD SCS Dip IFAAD
Consultant Dermatosurgeon
Juvenis Clinic
Lilavati Hospital and Bombay Hospital
Mumbai, Maharashtra, India

Nirav V Desai DNB (Dermatology)
Dermatologist and Hair Transplant Surgeon
NISH (National Institute of Skin and Hair)
Skin Clinic and Hair Transplant Centre
Surat, Gujarat, India

Niteen V Dhepe
MD FAAD Fellow ASDS ASLMS EADV ISHRS IADVL ACSI
Medical Director
Skin City
The Postgraduate Institute of Dermatology Camp
Pune, Maharashtra, India

Niti Khunger MD DDV DNB
Head, Professor and Consultant Dermatologist
Department of Dermatology and STD
Vardhman Mahavir Medical College and Safdarjung Hospital
New Delhi, India

Nitika Deshmukh MD DNB
Consultant Dermatologist
Deenanath Mangeshkar Hospital
Pune, Maharashtra, India

Nitika Nijhara MD (Dermatology)
Consultant Dermatologist
BLK-Max Multi-Specialty Hospital
New Delhi, India

Pallavi Ailawadi MD DNB
Consultant Dermatologist
Skinacea Clinic
Faridabad, Haryana, India

Pankaj Das MD (Dermatology)
Assistant Professor
Armed Forces Medical College
Pune, Maharashtra, India

Pradeep Kumari MBBS DVD FCPS DNB
Dermatologist
Skin and Surgery International and Asia Institute of Hair Transplant
Pune, Maharashtra, India

Pradeep Sethi MD
Co-Founder
Eugenix Hair Sciences
Mumbai, Maharashtra, India

Pradyumna Vaidya MBBS DVD DNB
Consultant Dermatologist
Deenanath Mangeshkar Hospital and Jehangir Hospital
Pune, Maharashtra, India

R Jayashree DDVL
Consultant Dermatologist
Skin Hair and Nail Laser Clinic
Coimbatore, Tamil Nadu, India

R Raghunatha Reddy
MD DNB FRGUHS (Dermatosurgery)
Professor and Medical Director
Roots Institute of Dermatological Sciences
Bengaluru, Karnataka, India

Rachana Shilpakar MD
Consultant Dermatologist
Rainbow Children's Hospital
Bengaluru, Karnataka, India

Rachita Dhurat MD (Skin)
Professor and Head
Department of Dermatology
LTM Medical College and Hospital
Mumbai, Maharashtra, India

Rachita Talwar MD
Consultant Dermatologist
NMC Specialty Hospital
Al-Ain, UAE

Ragini Ghiya MD
Dermatologist and Hair Transplant Surgeon
Siddharth Hair Transplant Centre
Surat, Gujarat, India

Ragunatha S MD
Associate Professor
Department of Dermatology, Venereology and Leprosy
Sri Siddhartha Medical College
Tumkur, Karnataka, India

Rajat Kandhari MD MSc
Consultant Dermatologist
Dr Kandhari's Skin and Dental Clinic and Veya Aesthetics
New Delhi, India

Rajetha Damisetty MD (Dermatology)
Additional Medical Director
Oliva Hair and Skin Clinic
Hyderabad, Telangana, India

Rashi Pangti MD (Dermatology)
Assistant Professor
Lady Hardinge Medical College
New Delhi, India

Rashmi Sarkar MD FAMS IFAAD
Director Professor
Department of Dermatology
LHMC and Associated KSCH and SSK Hospital
New Delhi, India

Rasya Dixit MD (Dermatology)
Medical Director
Dr Dixit Clinic
Bengaluru, Karnataka, India

Ravina Surve MD (DVL) DNB (DVL)
Senior Resident
Kanachur Institute of Medical Sciences
Mangaluru, Karnataka, India

Reena Rai MD (DVL)
Professor and Head
Department of Dermatology
PSG Institute of Medical Sciences and Research
Coimbatore, Tamil Nadu, India

(Surg Cdr) Reetu Agarwal
DVD MD (Dermatology)
Professor
Base Hospital Delhi Cantt
New Delhi, India

Richa Kumar MD DNB (Dermatology)
Assistant Professor
Military Hospital
Pune, Maharashtra, India

Ridhima Lakhani MD DNB (Dermatology)
Consultant Dermatologist
Fortis Hospital
New Delhi, India

Rohit Batra MD
Consultant Dermatologist
Sir Ganga Ram Hospital
New Delhi, India

Roshni Singh MD
Senior Resident
Assam Medical College and Hospital
Dibrugarh, Assam, India

Ruchi Hemdani MD
Assistant Professor
Himalayan Institute of Medical Sciences
Dehradun, Uttarakhand, India

S Sacchidanand
MD (DVL) DVD DHA FRCP (Glasgow)
Executive Director
Siddaganga Medical College and Research Institute
Bengaluru, Karnataka, India
Vice Chancellor, RGUHS (2018–2021)

Sachin Dhawan MD DVD
Senior Consultant Dermatologist
Fortis Hospital, Gurugram
Director, Skin 'n Smiles
Gurugram, Haryana, India

Sadhana Deshmukh
DNB FCPS DDV (Dermatology and Venereology)
Founder and Medical Director
Dr Sadhana Deshmukh's Forever Young Skin Hair Laser Clinics, Bandra
PD Hinduja Hospital and Medical Research Centre, Khar
Mumbai, Maharashtra, India

Sandeep Arora MD
Professor and Head
Department of Dermatology
Army College of Medical Sciences and Base Hospital Delhi Cantt
New Delhi, India

Sanjay Bhalchandra Sane
MS (General Surgery)
Consulting Foot Surgeon
Joshi Hospital
Pune, Maharashtra, India

Sanjay Singh MD (Dermatology)
Consultant Dermatologist
Gorakhpur, Uttar Pradesh, India

Sanjeev Gupta MD DNB
Professor and Head
Department of Dermatology
MM Institute of Medical Sciences and Research
MMDU, Ambala, Haryana, India

Sanjeev J Aurangabadkar MD
Consultant Dermatologist
Dr Aurangabadkar's Skin and Laser Clinic
Hyderabad, Telangana, India

Satish S Savant MD FAMS FCPS DVD DDV
Director
The Humanitarian Clinic Skin Hair and Laser Center
Dr Savant's Institute of Dermatosurgery Cosmetology, Trichology and Laser Medicine
Mumbai, Maharashtra, India

Savita Yadav MD (Dermatology)
Consultant Dermatologist
Gurugram, Haryana, India

Savitha AS MD DNB FRGUHS
Professor
Sapthagiri Institute of Medical Sciences and Research Centre
Bengaluru, Karnataka, India

Seema Garg MBBS MSc FISHRS ABHRS
CEO, Rejuvenate Plastic and Hair Transplant Centre
Indore, Madhya Pradesh, India

Senkadhir Vendhan MD (Dermatology)
Specialist
Department of Dermatology
Dr Babasaheb Ambedkar Memorial Hospital (Central Railway)
Mumbai, Maharashtra, India

Seujee Das MD
Consultant Dermatologist
Apollo Clinic
Guwahati, Assam, India

Shashikumar BM
MD (DVL) FRGUHS (Dermatosurgery)
Associate Professor
Department of Dermatology
Mandya Institute of Medical Sciences
Mandya, Karnataka, India

Shehnaz Arsiwala MD DDV
Founder, Renewderm Skin, Hair, Laser, and Aesthetics Centre, Mumbai
Consultant Dermatologist
Saifee Hospital, Masina Hospital
Mumbai, Maharashtra, India

Shekhar Neema MD
Associate Professor
Department of Dermatology
Base Hospital
Lucknow, Uttar Pradesh, India

Shilpa K MD (Dermatology) DVL
Professor and Head
Bangalore Medical College and Research Institute
Bengaluru, Karnataka, India

Shital Poojary MD DNB
Professor and Head
Department of Dermatology
KJ Somaiya Medical College
Mumbai, Maharashtra, India

Shrenik Balegar MD (Dermatology)
Director
Cutibless—Skin and Hair Treatment Clinic
Former Consultant and Hair Transplant Surgeon
AK Clinics
Mumbai, Maharashtra, India

Shyamanta Barua MD (Dermatology)
Professor and Head
Department of Dermatology
Assam Medical College and Hospital
Dibrugarh, Assam, India

Siddharth Mani
MD (Dermatology)
Assistant Professor
Department of Dermatology
Indian Naval Hospital Ship (INHS)
Kochi, Kerala, India

Silonie Sachdeva MD FISD (USA)
Senior Consultant Dermatologist
Dr Silonie Skin and Laser Clinic
Amritsar, Punjab, India

Sindhuja T MD MRCP (SCE)
Consultant Dermatologist
Ankura Hospitals
Hyderabad, Telangana, India

Smriti Naswa MD (Skin VD)
Observer (IADVL)—Pediatric Dermatology
Consultant Dermatologist
Fortis Hospital
Mumbai, Maharashtra, India

Somesh Gupta MD
Professor
Department of Dermatology and Venereology
All India Institute of Medical Sciences
New Delhi, India

Somodyuti Chandra
MD (Gold Medalist) DNB MNAMS MRCP-SCE (UK) FRGUHS
Consultant Dermatologist
Medica Superspecialty Hospital
Kolkata, West Bengal, India

Sonal Bansal
MD (Dermatology, Venereology and Leprosy)
Dermatologist, Aesthetic Dermatologist
Dermaspace Skin Clinic
Gurugram, Haryana, India

Sonal Jain
MD DNB (Skin & VD) FRGUHS (Dermatosurgery)
Assistant Professor
Department of Skin and VD
ICARE Institute of Medical Science and Research
and Dr BC Roy Hospital, Haldia
Consultant Dermatologist and Hair Transplant Surgeon
Narayana Hospital
Kolkata, West Bengal, India

Soni Nanda
MD (Dermatology)
Founder and Director
Ojas Skin Care, New Delhi
Consultant
Max Hospitals
New Delhi, India

Shristi Shrestha
MD FRUGHS
Fellowship Student
Venkat Charmalaya—Centre for Advanced Dermatology
Bengaluru, Karnataka, India

Subodh Jane MD FRGUHS
Consultant Dermatologist
Skintotal Clinic
Amravati, Maharashtra, India

Sudarshan R
MD (Dermatology)
Assistant Professor
Department of Dermatology
SSPM Medical College and Lifetime Hospital
Sindhudurg, Maharashtra, India

Sujala S Aradhya MD
Consultant Dermatologist and Dermatosurgeon
Sujala Polyclinic and Laboratory
Bengaluru, Karnataka, India

Sujay Khandpur
MD DNB MNAMS
Professor
Department of Dermatology and Venereology
All India Institute of Medical Sciences
New Delhi, India

Sujit Shanshanwal MD
Consultant
SkinAmour Clinic
Mumbai, Maharashtra, India

Sunmeet Sandhu MD
Assistant Professor
Command Hospital
Bengaluru, Karnataka, India

Suraj Sachidanand MD MSEd
Specialist
Department of Dermatology
Manipal Hospital
Bengaluru, Karnataka, India

Surbhi Rajput
MD DNB (Dermatology and Venereology)
Graded Specialist Dermatology
Military Hospital
Meerut, Uttar Pradesh, India

Suresh Talwar MD
Medical Director and Consultant Dermatologist
Talwar Skin Centre
Lucknow, Uttar Pradesh, India

Sushil S Savant MD (Gold Medalist)
Assistant Director
The Humanitarian Clinic—Skin Hair and Laser Center
Dr Savant's Institute of Dermatosurgery Cosmetology, Trichology, and Laser Medicine, Mumbai, Maharashtra, India

Sushil Tahiliani MD (Dermatology) DVD
Director and Consultant Dermatologist
Dr Tahiliani's Clinic
Visiting Consultant Dermatologist
Hinduja Hospital
Mumbai, Maharashtra, India

Suvarna Samudrala MD
Consultant Dermatologist
Citrine Clinic
Gurugram, Haryana, India

Swapnil Shah MD (Dermatology)
Consultant Dermatologist
Private Clinic
Solapur, Maharashtra, India

T Salim MD DNB
Medical Director and Clinical Head
Cutis Institute of Dermatology and Aesthetic Sciences
Kozhikode, Kerala, India

Tanvi Dev MD DNB MRCP (SCE)
Assistant Professor
Department of Dermatology
Maulana Azad Medical College
New Delhi, India

Trupti Agrawal MD
Associate Dermatologist
Kokilaben Dhirubhai Ambani Hospital
Mumbai, Maharashtra, India

TS Nagesh MD
Professor and Head
Department of Dermatology, STD, and Leprosy
Sapthagiri Institute of Medical Sciences and Research Centre
Bengaluru, Karnataka, India

TS Vidya
MD FRGUHS (Aesthetic Dermatology)
Consultant Dermatologist and Cosmetologist
Sagar Hospitals and Skin and Cosmetic Clinic, Bengaluru, Karnataka, India

Tushar D Kshirsagar DNB (Dermatology)
Dermatologist and Hair Transplant Surgeon
Nuleaf Skin Clinic and Hair Transplant Centre
Pune, Maharashtra, India

Uday Kelkar
DIM MD (Microbiology)
Senior Chief Medical Officer
Senior Administrative Grade
In-Charge, Laboratories
Central Government Health Scheme
Pune, Maharashtra, India
Ministry of Health and Family Welfare
Government of India

Vaishalee Kirane
DVD DNB (Dermatology)
Dermatologist and Trichologist
Dr Vaishalee's Skin and Hair Clinic
Pune, Maharashtra, India

Venura Samarasinghe
MBChB MRCP (Dermatology)
Consultant Dermatologist and Mohs Surgeon
Department of Dermatology
St George's Hospital NHS Foundation Trust
London, UK

(Col) Vikas Pathania MD (Dermatology)
Professor and Head
Base Hospital
Lucknow, Uttar Pradesh, India

Vinay Saraf MD DVD
Senior Consulting Dermatologist
Dr Balabhai Nanavati Hospital and Research Centre
Mumbai, Maharashtra, India

Vishal Madan MD FRCP
Consultant Dermatologist, Laser, and Mohs Surgeon
Northern Care Alliance, Stott Lane
Salford, UK

Vishwanath Jigjinni MS FRCS
Head
Department of Plastic Surgery
Ruby Hall Clinic, Pune
Head
Department of Plastic Surgery
Indrayani Hospital and Cancer Institute
Pune, Maharashtra, India

Yogesh S Marfatia MD (Skin-VD)
Professor (Skin-VD)
SBKS Medical Institute and Research Centre
Vadodara, Gujarat, India

Zeba Chhapra DDVL
Consultant Dermatologist
CUTIS Skin Solution
Mumbai, Maharashtra, India

Message from President ACS(I)

The composite subspecialty of surgical, laser and aesthetic dermatology has grown by leaps and bounds in recent years. It is imperative for all concerned to keep abreast of the exponential expansion in new concepts and keep pace with the innovations in the subspecialty.

The third edition of this textbook is a comprehensive compendium that is well-illustrated with excellent clinical images and extensively covers the latest developments in the specified fields. It is hoped that this treatise will further embellish the composite subspecialty and be a handy reference for both practicing dermatosurgeons and residents in training.

I, on behalf of the Association of Cutaneous Surgeons (I) National Executive, thank all those who were involved in bringing out this edition of the textbook. My deepest appreciation for the hard work and sustained commitment of our Editor-in-Chief, Dr (Brig) Manas Chatterjee and Associate Editor, Dr (Col) Biju Vasudevan. I am grateful to all members of the Editorial Board and each and every author for their valuable contributions. My sincere thanks to M/s Jaypee Brothers Medical Publishers (P) Ltd, New Delhi, India, for their help in bringing out this edition.

Shyamanta Barua
Professor and Head
Department of Dermatology
Assam Medical College and Hospital
Dibrugarh, Assam, India
President, Association of Cutaneous Surgeons (I)

Preface to the Third Edition

The third edition of the *ACS(I) Textbook of Cutaneous and Aesthetic Surgery* was on the table very early after the second edition, since the sale of both the first and the second editions have been unprecedented. The progress made by the ACS(I) Textbook from the first to the second has been attempted to be maintained in the third edition. From 2020 when the project was envisioned and we were asked to chaperone the preparation of the third edition, it has been a roller-coaster journey, not in small measure impacted by the COVID-19 pandemic during which time, editorial assistance suffered due to obvious reasons. As happens during such a time, a large number of authors were impacted in various ways which affected their submission of chapters. Another thing that happened during that time was the slowing down of the reviewing process as reviewers were saddled with other responsibilities. With the loss of continuity, it became an uphill task getting everyone on board once we saw the back of the pandemic's worst phase and getting them to submit their material. However, at last we are ready with the book, which has now been rationalized to 140 chapters in 18 sections of two volumes for ease of navigation. A number of chapters, which were either felt to be superfluous at the current time or could be clubbed to avoid duplication of material, were reorganized to ensure a better experience for the reader. Most of the chapters have been revised by the original authors while some have been rewritten. A few new chapters have been added to keep-up with the recent advances in the field of procedural dermatology. A chapter format was prepared to attempt uniformity of all the chapters, which has been achieved to an extent.

With this textbook coming to its logical conclusion of publication, it has been a pleasure working with Dr (Colonel) Biju Vasudevan as always, for he has been the workhorse of this effort. The Emeritus Editor Dr Mysore Venkataram has always been at our side guiding and directing us in the right path. The Deputy and Assistant Editors have been tireless ensuring that the final product has the desired quality. I would fail in my duty if I do not sincerely appreciate the efforts of Dr (Lt Col) Shekhar Neema, already a star in the field of dermatologic surgery, who has been the backbone of the editorial effort. The members of the editorial board have been ever-ready to pitch in with their contribution.

I would sincerely thank the ACS(I) executive from 2020 till date who has been my pillars of strength and most understanding of the delays that this project has had to suffer due to unforeseen circumstances.

All at M/s Jaypee Publishers Medical Publishers (P) Ltd, New Delhi, India, from Shri Jitendar P Vij (Group Chairman), Mr Ankit Vij (Managing Director), Mr MS Mani (Group President), Ms Chetna Malhotra (Senior Director—Professional Publishing, Marketing, and Business Development), and Ms Nedup Denka Bhutia Pillai (Senior Development Editor), and the production team have been most tolerant of my schedules and have dovetailed their efforts to ensure a quality product.

I wish that this book is of benefit to those for whom it is intended, which is the budding dermatologic surgeons and procedural dermatologists of this country and elsewhere.

Jai Hind!

Manas Chatterjee

Preface to the First Edition

Dermatosurgery has been passing through interesting times, as disease dermatology paves the way for desire dermatology, as illness gets replaced by wellness and patients are replaced by clients—today's interventional dermatology seeks to dominate over armchair dermatology of yesterday. What we now have is a youthful, vibrant, fast-changing subspecialty. Change has been so striking over the last decade that, in some ways, dermatosurgery represents a Theseus' paradox, *"This is my grandfather's axe. My father replaced the shaft, and I put a new head on it. It is my grandfather's axe."*

Despite rapid progress, there have been few books in this field, especially focusing on brown skin, and the need for a comprehensive book, encompassing all the aspects of cutaneous surgery, lasers and aesthetics, has long been felt. Sensing this need, the Association of Cutaneous Surgeons (I) decided to bring out this book.

The rapidly changing profile, range, and scope of the subject, with multitudes of procedures being performed, necessitated a multi-authored book. Fortunately, our association is blessed with the talent that was needed for authoring the chapters—the result is what you see; an exhaustive compilation with 66 chapters, including nearly 33 subchapters, by as many as 105 authors. Every aspect of cutaneous surgery has been comprehensively dealt with, keeping in mind the recent advances.

The brown skin has many peculiarities and variations—in fact, it defies any classification! Pigmentation response, healing and scarring reactions, aging changes are all different in the brown skin. Similarly, the epidemiological situations are also different; vitiligo surgery is more relevant than skin cancer surgery! The textbook aptly seeks to address these challenges and requirements.

Our effort has been to keep the book comprehensive, yet simple; to make the book all-inclusive, yet reader-friendly; exhaustive and yet relevant—to the beginner and the expert, the novice, and the connoisseur. We hope that we have succeeded in achieving this objective.

Writing a book is an experience, exhilarating at times, excruciating at others. And, in a multi-authored book, it is even more so, as deadlines are chased furiously and frenetically. Despite the highs and the lows, I must say the experience has been something to cherish—it has been my privilege to have been the Editor-in-Chief for this effort—and on behalf of the editorial board, I thank each author for his contribution. It truly has been a **great work done by a number of smaller things together!**

I was indeed fortunate to have an experienced editorial board of senior dermatosurgeons, available at all times for counsel and advice. My heartfelt gratitude to each one of them. And I record with a touch of pride and happiness the splendid work done by my young team of Deputy and Assistant editors, who toiled for long hours in correcting proofs, and drafts. The book would not have been possible without their long endeavors.

Lastly, an effort of this size is never possible without the support and understanding from the family—my wife Dr Jayashree, my son Aniketh (both of whom contributed as authors) and daughter Ankitha (who supported silently)—my heartfelt thanks to them.

M/s Jaypee Brothers Medical Publishers (P) Ltd have done an outstanding work in bringing it out on time—in particular, my thanks to Shri Jitendar P Vij (CEO), Ms Sunita Katla (PA to CEO), Ms Shagufta Khan (Executive Assistant to MD), Mr Sumit Kumar and Mr Ram Murti (Graphic Designers), Ms Geeta Srivastava and Laxmidhar Padhiary (Proofreaders) and Mr Venugopal (Branch Manager). My gratitude to them.

I earnestly hope that the book will be appreciated by the readers, and welcome comments and feedback. My earnest hope is that the book will serve as an instrument in furthering progress in the field, and *the grandfather's axe shall improve further!*

Mysore Venkataram

Contents

Volume 1

Section 1: Basic Principles of Cutaneous Surgery

Section 2: Standard Surgical Techniques

Section 3: Heat and Cold Energy-based Procedures

Section 4: Needle-based Basic Procedures

Section 5: Vitiligo Surgery

Section 9: Miscellaneous Surgical Procedures

Volume 2

Section 10: Hair Transplantation Surgery

Section 14: Liposuction

Section 15: Lasers

SECTION 1

Basic Principles of Cutaneous Surgery

CHAPTER 1 Skin: Basic Aspects

Shashikumar BM, Savitha AS

KEY MESSAGES

- Knowledge of basic anatomy is important to understand further applied anatomy.
- Understanding physiology and anatomy of melanocyte helps to understand pigmentation response.
- Epidermal layers and their turnover, dermis and its responses, play vital role in explaining resurfacing techniques.

INTRODUCTION

Skin is the largest organ of body and it ensheathes all other organs. It plays a major role in defense (immunity), synthesis (vitamin D), homeostasis (temperature regulation and water and electrolyte balance) and aesthetics (complexion, wrinkles, and baldness). Dermatosurgery and aesthetic surgery deal with the surgical aspects of skin and its appendages. However, this subject is now driven by aesthetics, the wellness component rather than diseases, the illnesses. Better understanding of basic features gives an edge with regard to safety and efficacy while performing dermatosurgical procedures. While detailed anatomy can be found in a textbook of dermatology, this chapter briefly presents structural and embryological aspects of skin and its appendages. Applied anatomy of head and neck is considered in detail in the next chapter and details of each region are elaborated in respective chapters on different dermatosurgical procedures.

EMBRYOLOGY

Skin is made up of three layers, namely—(1) epidermis, (2) dermis, and (3) hypodermis or subcutis **(Fig. 1 and Table 1)**. It consists of cells, connective tissues, and special appendages, which are derived from ectoderm, neuroectoderm, and mesoderm.

Development of skin goes through three phases—(1) specification (0–2 months), (2) morphogenesis (2–5 months), and (3) differentiation (5–9 months).[1] It is regulated by various signaling pathways such as Notch, Wnt, Sonic Hedgehog (Shh), bone morphogenetic proteins, and fibroblast growth factors, many of which play a vital role in aging later in life.[2] Skin starts developing by 3 weeks of intrauterine life with formation of a single layer of cells derived from ectoderm lateral to neuroectoderm. At 4 weeks, it is composed of two layers—outer periderm or epitrichial layer and inner, stratum germinativum. Tonofilaments (12–16 weeks) and keratohyalin

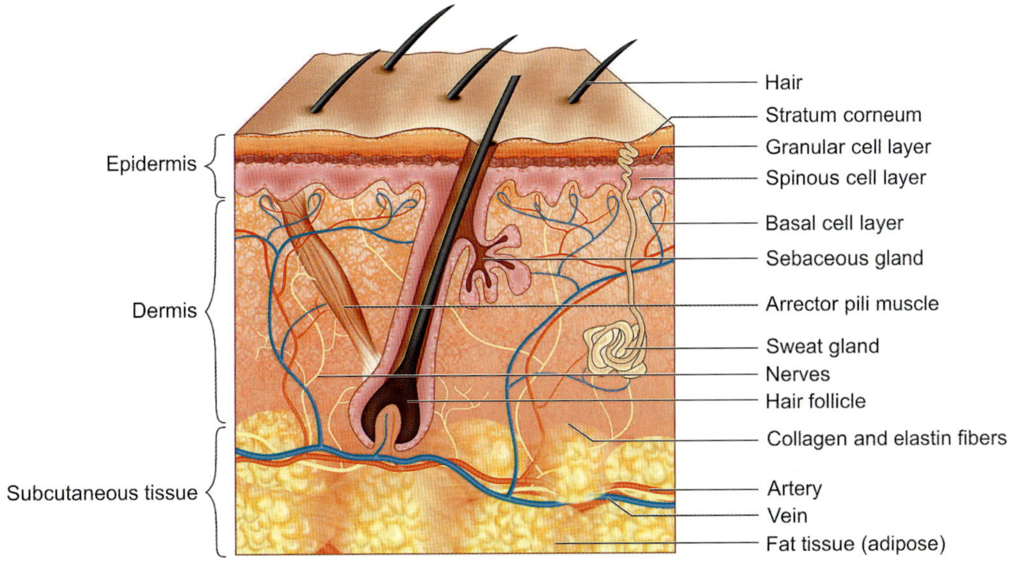

Fig. 1: Structure of skin.

TABLE 1: Layers of the skin.

Skin layer	*Description*
Epidermis	Outermost layer, serving as the barrier lined by stratified squamous epithelium
Dermis	Lies beneath epidermis separated by dermoepidermal junction. Consists of supporting matrix, cells, and vessels
Subcutis	Deeper layer consists of loose connective tissue and fat

granules (16–21 weeks) appear later with completion of cornification by 24 weeks. At 8–11 weeks, middle layer starts forming additional layers to skin. Basal lamina is secreted by basal cells and matures to form dermoepidermal junction as in adults by 12 weeks.[3]

Embryology of Hair

Early attempt to form hair follicle is seen at 9 weeks of intrauterine life at eyebrows, upper lip, and chin.

- There is aggregation of mesenchymal cells close to ectoderm leading to elongation of ectodermal cells (pregerm stage).
- These elongated cells also increase in number and start projecting down into mesenchyme.
- Simultaneously, the underlying collection of mesenchymal cells increases in number forming rudimentary hair papilla (hair germ stage).
- The short nubbins of ectodermal downgrowths form slanting columns of cells with basal cells reorienting themselves perpendicular to the long axis of growth (hair peg stage).
- The advancing tips of these downgrowths become bulbous and form a cup enclosing the aggregates of mesenchymal cells (bulbous hair peg stage).
- These cells in the lower layers of hair bulb are matrix cells, which form outer and inner sheaths and hair.
- As the matrical cells proliferate and cornify, they are pushed up to form hair. The junction of matrical cells and cornified cells is the Adamson's fringe.
- At 16 weeks, three bulges are seen on the posterior aspect of these columns. Arrector pilorum muscle attaches to lower most bulge, middle bulge differentiates into sebaceous glands, and upper most bulge forms apocrine gland. These apocrine glands persist in axilla, areola, periumbilical and anogenital areas, and regress to form anlage in other sites.
- Earliest hair emerges from follicular openings in eyebrow region at 17 weeks. By 20 weeks, entire body, except palms, soles, terminal phalanges, glans, and labia minora, is covered by hair. Under the influence of maternal hormones, sebum secretion starts by 15th week. Thus, hair follicle grows from a close interaction of ectoderm with mesenchyme—an interaction, which occurs through life during each hair cycle.[4]

Eccrine glands also develop as ectodermal downgrowths into dermis sans aggregation of mesenchymal cells. They first appear in palms and soles and start secreting by 6th month of intrauterine life.[4]

Nail development is earliest recognized in first trimester as a quadrangular area on tips of fingers and toes dorsally and is delineated by lateral and proximal shallow grooves. The primordial nail structure is made of three layers—(1) surface, (2) intermediate, and (3) germinative layers. Intermediate and germinative layers grow proximally and form nail matrix. Nail plate starts to form by 14 weeks and by 20 weeks, and it covers the nail bed completely. At the same time, granular layer is also lost from the nail matrix. Among all epithelial derivatives, nail plate is the first structure to cornify.

Dermis and nerves start developing by 5 weeks, vessels, both vascular and lymphatic by 12 weeks, delicate collagen by 12 weeks and mature collagen by 16 weeks, and elastic fibers by 24 weeks. Subcutis develops from aggregation of mesenchymal cells around blood vessels with accumulation of fat.

Summarizing the development, epidermis, pilosebaceous apocrine units, eccrine glands, and nails are derived from ectoderm; melanocytes, nerves and sensory receptors from neuroectoderm and dermis, blood vessels, lymphatic channels, cells such as Langerhans cells, fibrocytes, mast cells, macrophages, subcutis, and muscles are derived from mesoderm.

EPIDERMIS

Epidermis is the outermost layer of the skin and is composed of stratified squamous epithelium. From below upwards, it consists of four layers—(1) stratum basale, (2) stratum spinosum, (3) stratum granulosum, and (4) stratum corneum **(Figs. 2A and B)**. Stratum lucidum is an additional thin and homogeneous hyalinized layer that presents only in palms and soles. Total renewal time for epidermis is 39 days—13 days for proliferation, 12 days for migration, and 14 days for shedding.[4]

The epidermis is mainly composed of keratinocytes (80%). The "brick-like" shape of keratinocytes is provided by a cytoskeleton made of keratin intermediate filaments. As the epidermis differentiates, the keratinocytes become flattened. Other cells in the epidermis are the melanocytes, Langerhans cells, and Merkel cells. Melanocytes are found in the basal layer of the epidermis as well as in hair follicles. Melanocytes, derived from neural crest cells, primarily function to produce a pigment—melanin. Melanin accumulates in organelles called melanosomes that are incorporated into dendrites anchoring the melanosomes, which are transferred into the surrounding keratinocytes. The ratio of melanocytes to keratinocytes is approximately 1:36, and may vary in different regions such as hair and exposed skin. Absolute numbers of melanosomes

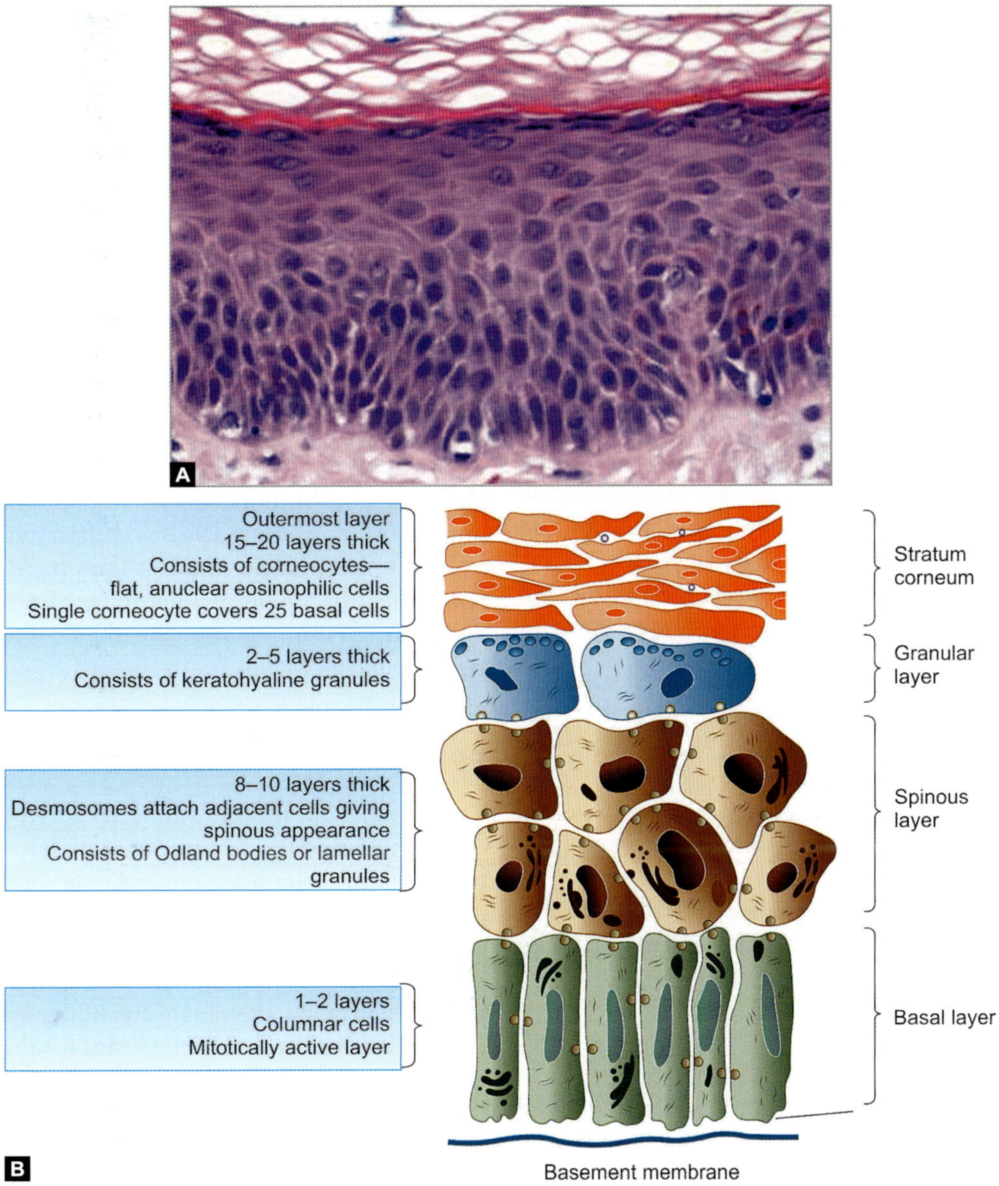

Figs. 2A and B: (A) Structure of epidermis: Uppermost layer—stratum corneum, stratum granulosum, stratum spinosum, and stratum basalis; (B) Layers of the epidermis.

are the same among the sexes and various races. Differing pigmentation among individuals is related to melanosome size, amount of melanin and its aggregation pattern, rather than cell number.[2]

Skin is thickest on the palms and soles of the feet (1.5 mm thick), while the thinnest skin is present on the eyelids and in the postauricular region (0.05 mm). Dermal thickness too varies in different parts of face—eyelid (5-6 mm), cheek (1.0-2.0 mm), and forehead 2.0 mm (nose 2.0 mm). Male skin is generally thicker than female skin in all anatomic locations. Children have relatively thin skin and likewise elderly people too have thin skin. This thinning with aging is primarily a dermal change, with the loss of elastic fibers, epithelial appendages, and ground substance, though epidermis too undergoes some thinning.[3]

Applied Anatomy

- Knowledge of cell turnover helps to understand the principle of several procedures, such as chemical peels and laser resurfacing.
- Knowledge of the barrier in skin is important for application of topical preparations.
- Cell adhesion and renewal play an important role in several treatments, such as resurfacing and post-resurfacing procedures.
- Knowledge of thickness of skin in different areas is vital in ensuring optimum choice of treatments and outcomes after such treatments. Levels of peels are determined by thickness and penetration of different ablative lasers too varies in depth.

TABLE 2: Fitzpatrick skin types.

Skin types	*I*	*II*	*III*	*IV*	*V*	*VI*
Skin color	Pale white or freckled skin	White skin	Olive skin	Light brown	Bark brown	Black
Tanning ability	Always burns and never tans	Burns easily and tans poorly	Mild burn and gradually tans	Burns minimally and tans easily	Rarely burns and tans easily	Never burns and always tans
Hair	Red and blonde	Blonde, red, and light brown	Dark blonde	Brown and dark brown	Dark brown	Black
Eyes	Blue, gray, and green	Blue, gray, green, and hazel	Brown, blue, gray, green, and hazel	Hazel and brown	Brown	Brown

SKIN TYPES

Depending on tanning and burning responses, six types of skin have been recognized by Fitzpatrick and Parrish scale **(Table 2)**. They also correlate roughly with skin color and have been used widely in assessing responses to resurfacing techniques. Indian and Asian skin varies greatly in color, presents in different shades, and does not always conform accurately to this classification. Most Indians and Asians belong to type 3–5 of Fitzpatrick scale.[5]

Applied Anatomy

Excessive stimulation of melanocytes in the process of wound healing can lead to increased melanin synthesis resulting in hyperpigmentation—a common complication of all resurfacing procedures in brown skin. Hence, it is important to prime the skin with sun protection and depigmenting creams before initiation of such procedures.

DERMIS

The dermis is composed of two layers—(1) the superficial papillary dermis and (2) the deeper reticular dermis. The papillary dermis is thinner, consisting of loose connective tissue containing capillaries. The reticular dermis consists of thicker collagen fibers, elastic fibers, larger blood vessels, and other appendages. There is a network of closely interlaced elastic fibers and coarse bundles of collagen fibers arranged in layers parallel to the surface. The reticular layer also contains resident cells, such as fibroblasts, nerve endings, lymphatics, and epidermal appendages.

Another important component of the dermis is the ground substance, an amorphous material that fills spaces between the fibrillar and cellular components of the dermis, imparting turgidity and resilience. The dermal matrix consists of glycosaminoglycans (mainly hyaluronic acid and dermatan sulfate) and glycoproteins. With aging, there is a decrease in these substances and the synthetic variant of hyaluronic acid is widely used as a filler in rejuvenation treatments.

The fibroblast is the major cell type of the dermis. These cells produce and secrete procollagen and elastic fibers. These collagen fibers provide tensile strength and are important in wound healing. Collagen constitutes 70% of the weight of the dermis. Elastic fibers constitute <1% of the weight of the dermis, but play an important functional role in defining elasticity of skin. Both tensile strength and elasticity are important concepts in excisions and wound healing.

Fibronectin, the major filamentous glycoprotein component of the dermal matrix, is also produced by the fibroblasts. Fibronectin ensheathes collagen and elastin bundles and also helps in attachment of keratinocytes to the basal lamina—a role, which is important in wound healing.[1]

EPIDERMAL APPENDAGES

Epidermal appendages are derived from ectoderm as epidermal downgrowths during embryonic stage. It includes eccrine and apocrine glands with their ducts and pilosebaceous unit comprising sebaceous gland and hair; they all act as reservoir of epidermis. The keratinocytes from the adnexa migrate to the skin surface and cause reepithelialization after an injury. Injury over the face heals faster when compared to back, vowing to the presence of more adnexal structures on the face.

Hair Follicle

Embryologically, hair is derived from both epidermis and dermis. They are distributed all over the body surface in varying density with most numerous on the scalp and face and absent on the palms, soles, dorsa of the terminal phalanges, labia minora, clitoris, and glans penis.

Types of Hair

- *Lanugo hair (Latin: Lana wool)*: Seen in fetus; they are soft, fine, and lightly pigmented.
- *Vellus hair (Latin: Vellus fleece)*: The fine hair that covers most of the body of youngsters and adults.
- *Terminal hair*: It is long coarse pigmented hair with larger diameters, distributed over the eyebrows, eyelashes, scalp, beard, axillae, and pubis. Terminal hair is the only hair to possess a medulla.

Human hair growth is cyclical and shedding is asynchronous. Hair cycle has three phases and is affected by various endogenous and exogenous factors **(Table 3)**.

TABLE 3: Three phases of hair cycle.

Phase	*Description*	*Duration*	*Percentage of hair*
Anagen	Active growth phase	3–5 years	84%
Catagen	Regression phase	3 weeks	2%
Telogen	Resting phase	3 months	14%

At any given point of time, follicles are found in all three phases of hair growth. This is extremely important for laser hair removal, because follicles in the anagen phase are susceptible to destruction, whereas resting follicles are more resistant. This explains why multiple treatments of an area may be necessary to ensure adequate hair removal. The intervals at which laser has to be performed depend on the length of the anagen phase, which would vary from area to area.[6]

Hair follicles show considerable morphological and functional heterogeneity. Hairs differ from site to site in shaft length, thickness, curl, color, and androgen sensitivity. Hair grows on an average 0.4 mm per day.[7] Terminal hairs grow longer and diameter exceeds 0.03 mm, whereas vellus hair's diameter is <0.003 mm. In androgenetic alopecia, there is miniaturization of hair with the formation of velluslike hair, which is depigmented, small, and measure <0.003 mm in diameter. The scalp hair of Caucasians is round whereas in dark skinned, it is oval and has curvature just above the bulb, which causes hair to curl. Caucasian hair follicles are oriented obliquely to the skin surface, whereas the hair follicles of dark skinned are oriented almost parallel to the skin surface. Asians have vertically-oriented follicles that produce straight hairs. These anatomic variations are an important consideration in avoiding alopecia when making incisions in the scalp. Hair color depends on the degree of melanization and distribution of melanosomes within the hair shaft. Melanosomes are large in dark skinned and small and aggregated in Caucasians. Red hair is characterized by spherical melanosomes. Melanocytes are decreased in gray hair.

Androgens are responsible for the follicular heterogeneity. Follicles over the body are either very sensitive (axilla and inguinal hair), mildly sensitive (beard hair), or insensitive to androgens (eyebrow).

Hair bulge is now known to be an important site for biotechnologist; stem cells are now produced from hair bulb and have great importance in future in organ transplant and artificial skin production.

Hair naturally grows in 1–4 hair follicular groupings called follicular units. The follicular unit is pyramidal and consists of 2–3 terminal hair, sebaceous gland, and single arborizing arrector pili muscle, which attaches circumferentially around the primary follicle with variable attachment to secondary follicles. This arrangement has become the basis of follicular unit transplantation, which is the redistribution of naturally occurring follicular groupings from the occipital donor region into the bald region of the recipient sites.[8,9] Loss of attachment of the arrector pili muscle is seen in miniaturized hair in androgenetic alopecia. Initially, the attachment of secondary follicles happens. When the arrector pili muscle is detached from the follicles along with miniaturization of primary follicle, hair loss is likely to be irreversible. This theory establishes the importance in early treatment androgenetic alopecia to halt balding.[10]

Sebaceous Glands

Sebaceous glands are derived embryologically from upper portion of hair follicle as an outgrowth. It is a lipid-producing gland that arises from the hair follicle at the junction of infundibulum and the isthmus. Sebaceous glands are associated with hair follicles all over the body. A sebaceous gland and the associated hair follicle are termed as pilosebaceous unit. The sebaceous glands exude lipids by disintegration of entire cells, a process known as holocrine secretion. Sebaceous glands of various sizes are distributed over the entire surface of the body with the exception of palms, soles, and the dorsa of the feet. The glands may also be found in certain nonhairy sites, including the eyelids (Meibomian glands), the nipples (Montgomery's glands), buccal mucosa and vermillion border of the lip (Fordyce spots), and around the genitals (Tyson's glands).[4]

Although sebaceous glands are well developed at birth, they regress soon and mature at puberty under the influence of androgens. Acne and acne form eruptions are common during this age. The hair and the sebaceous glands and the adipose cells are the site for the skin stem cells. This can be utilized for the development of stem cell therapy in dermatology.

Sweat Glands

There are thought to be over 2.5 million on the skin surface and they are present over the majority of the body. They are located within the dermis and are composed of coiled tubes, which secrete a watery substance. They are classified into two different types—(1) eccrine and (2) apocrine.

Eccrine Sweat Glands

They are the only true sweat glands. Eccrine sweat glands are composed of a secretory portion, an intradermal duct and an upper intraepidermal part, called acrosyringium. The acrosyringium has a unique symmetrical and helicoidal course. Eccrine glands are found all over the skin, especially on the palms, soles, axillae, and forehead with exception of oral lips, clitoris, labia minora, and external auditory canals.[4] Eccrine glands play a major role in thermoregulation and electrolyte balance. They are under psychological and thermal control. Sympathetic (cholinergic) nerve fibers innervate eccrine glands. A well-acclimatized person can perspire as much as several liters per hour and 10 L/day. In addition to secreting water and electrolytes, the sweat gland

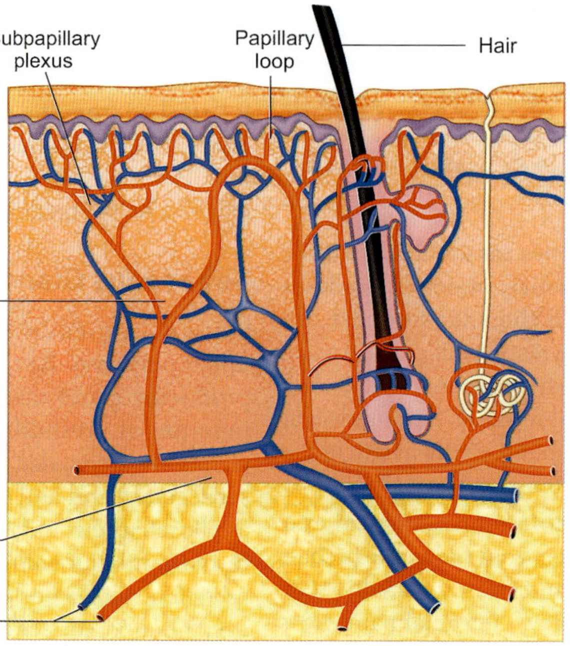

Fig. 3: Blood supply to skin.

excretes heavy metals, drugs and organic compounds, and macromolecules.

Apocrine Glands

Apocrine glands are larger, the ducts of which empty out into the hair follicles. They are present in the axillae, anogenital region, areolae, periumbilical region, external auditory canals (ceruminous glands), and on the eyelids (Moll's glands).[4] They become active at puberty, producing an odorless protein-rich secretion, which, when acted upon by skin bacteria, gives out a characteristic odor. These glands are under the control of sympathetic (adrenergic) nerve fibers.

BLOOD AND LYMPHATIC VESSELS

The dermis receives a rich blood supply through two intercommunicating plexuses **(Fig. 3)**. Branches from superficial artery plexus present at the junction of papillary and reticular dermis form capillary loops in the papillae of the dermis, each with a single loop of capillary vessels, one arterial and one venous. The veins drain into mid-dermal and subcutaneous venous networks. Dilatation or constriction of these capillary loops plays a direct role in thermoregulation of the skin. Lymphatic drainage of the skin occurs through abundant lymphatic meshes that originate in the papillae and feed into larger lymphatic vessels that drain into regional lymph nodes.[4]

NERVE SUPPLY

The skin has rich innervations, with the hands, face, and genitalia having the highest density of nerves. Pain, itch, and temperature sensation is detected by free sensory nerve ending. Pressure and vibration sensation is mediated by Pacinian corpuscles and touch sensation is by Meissner's corpuscles present in the dermis. The autonomic nervous system supplies the motor innervation of the skin—adrenergic fibers innervate blood vessels, hair erector muscles, and apocrine glands, while cholinergic fibers innervate eccrine sweat glands. Cutaneous nerves follow the route of blood vessels to the skin. The area supplied by a single spinal nerve, or single segment of the spinal cord, is termed as dermatome. Adjacent dermatomes may overlap considerably and are of importance to note when performing field blocks with local anesthesia.[4]

To have excellent cosmetic results, sound knowledge of surgical anatomy of skin is a must. It will also help in reducing complications during or after the dermatosurgery. Important anatomical landmarks, anatomical relations, and points are considered, which will help in excellent results and to minimize complications.

REFERENCES

1. Chu DH. Structure and development of skin. In: Wolff K, Goldsmith LA, Katz SI, Gilcrest BA, Paller AS, Leffell DJ (Eds). Fitzpatrick's Dermatology in General Medicine, 7th edition. NewYork: McGrawHill; 2007. pp. 5772.
2. McGrath JA, Uitto J. Structure and function of the skin. In: Griffiths C, Barker J, Bleiker T, Chalmers R, Creamer D (Eds). Rook's Textbook of Dermatology, 9th edition. Oxford: Blackwell Publishing; 2016. pp. 2.12.48.
3. McGrath JA, Eady RAJ, Pope FM. Anatomy and organization of human skin. In: Burns T, Breathnach S, Cox N, Griffiths C (Eds). Rook's Textbook of Dermatology, 7th edition. Oxford: Black well Publishing; 2004. pp. 3.13.84.

4. Jakubovic HR, Ackerman AB. Structure and function of skin: Development, morphology, and physiology. In: Moschella SL, Hurley HR (Eds). Dermatology, 3rd edition. Philadelphia: WB Saunders. 1992. pp. 387.
5. Sachdeva S. Fitzpatrick skin typing: applications in dermatology. Indian J Dermatol Venereol Leprol. 2009;75(1):936.
6. Prost-Squarcioni C. Histology of skin and hair follicle. Med Sci. 2006;22(2):1317.
7. Thappa DM. Structure and functions of the skin. In: Valia RG, Valia AR (Eds). Textbook and Atlas of Dermatology, 3rd edition. Mumbai: Bhalani Publishing House; 2008. pp. 740.
8. Savant SS, Gore D. Applied anatomy for dermatosurgeons. In: Savant SS, AtalShah R, Gore D (Eds). Textbook and Atlas of Dermatosurgery and Cosmetology, 1st edition. Mumbai: ASCAD; 1998. pp. 311.
9. Robinson JK. Anatomy for procedural dermatology. In: Robinson JK, Hanke CW, Siegel DM, Fratila A (Eds). Surgery of the Skin: Procedural Dermatology, 3rd edition. Philadelphia: Elsevier Mosby; 2015. pp. 227.
10. Sinclair R, Torkamani N, Jones L. Androgenetic alopecia: new insights into the pathogenesis and mechanism of hair loss [version 1; referees: 4 approved]. F1000 Research 2015;4(F1000 Faculty Rev):585.

CHAPTER 2

Applied Anatomy in Dermatosurgery

Madura C, AP Balaji, Aakash Gupta, Sonal Jain

PART A: REGIONAL ANATOMY

KEY MESSAGES

- The working knowledge on anatomy and its applied aspects are important in planning surgeries and to avoid complications.
- Knowing the surface anatomy, relaxed skin tension lines (RSTLs), blood and nerve supply, understanding the variations in soft tissue structures, and locating important danger zones at various regions are the highlights of this chapter.
- The knowledge on regional anatomy makes dermatosurgeon more confident and competent.

INTRODUCTION

The knowledge on regional anatomy makes a dermatosurgeon more competent in performing surgical procedures. The anatomy and its applied aspects are important in planning surgeries. There exists significant variation in the skin of each region and with relationship to underlying structures, expected functional alterations, and skin tension lines. The working knowledge of surface landmarks (to locate important structures), soft tissue planes and neurovascular distribution at various regions is equally important. Lastly, lymphatic drainage is critically important while treating cutaneous malignancy. This chapter describes brief anatomy pertaining to dermatologic surgery of scalp, ear, neck, torso, hand, feet, and external genitalia with more emphasis on applied aspects.

BASIC SKIN STRUCTURE

Skin has epidermis, dermis, and appendages. Each region has unique properties. The epidermis varies in thickness of 0.04 mm on the eyelids and genitalia to 1.5 mm on the palms and soles.[1] Understanding of the relative thickness of the skin in various regions helps the surgeon while planning a repair. The dermis is a connective tissue network of collagen and elastin fibers embedded in a ground substance. It is responsible for skin stretchability, a major factor in wound closure. The areas such as scalp and back are relatively inflexible and lack elasticity, even a small degree of skin rotation can cause protrusion at the pivot point unlike face which has significant elasticity. The stretchability is tested by lifting and stretching the skin between index and thumb to check the elasticity of the skin before wound closures. It is important to note that in anatomic sites, such as the back of the hand or elbow, the skin is easily movable but quite inelastic.

SKIN BIOMECHANICS

Skin possesses unique biomechanical properties which help in conforming and protecting the body. In depth knowledge of skin, biomechanics is important for the dermatosurgeon to understand skin response under mechanical stress and its applications in routine practice.

The properties of dermis mainly collagen, elastin, and ground substance determine biomechanical response of skin. Normally, collagen is arranged haphazardly but after stretching of the skin they orient themselves in a parallel fashion. This property of collagen imparts high tensile and low elastic strength. Elastin on the other hand maintains its ability to return to its original shape even after maximum strain and possesses low tensile strength. The relationship between elastin and collagen helps collagen to return to its original conformation after stretching. Ground substance is found between elastin and collagen and provides lubrication during stretching. It has minimal tensile and elastic strength.

The thickness of skin, age, sex, and location changes the biomechanical properties of skin. Younger skin is thicker than older skin due to more collagen and ground substance in the dermis. Also skin over the forearm is thinner, less tense and more elastic as compared to skin on the forehead.

To understand the biomechanical properties of skin, it is important to know the terminologies used to describe them **(Table 1)**.[2]

Stress is defined as force per unit area. Common example can be extraction of comedones due to pressure from a comedone extractor.

TABLE 1: Various terminologies used to understand biomechanics of skin.

Term	*Description*
Stress	Pressure in skin arising from externally applied force
Strain	Amount of deformation an object experiences in shape or size
Creep	Tendency of skin to slowly move or deform under stress
Elasticity	Ability of skin to return to its original shape when external forces are removed
Extensibility	Maximum strain skin can undergo before breakage
Viscosity	Ability to deform under stress and inability to return to its original shape
Anisotropy	Ability to exhibit different physical properties along different axis
Viscoelasticity	Stress causes temporary deformation is quickly removed (elastic) or permanent deformation if retained (viscous)
Hysteresis	Nonlinear relationship where force causes a change but when the force is removed the reversal in change is not as much as the initial

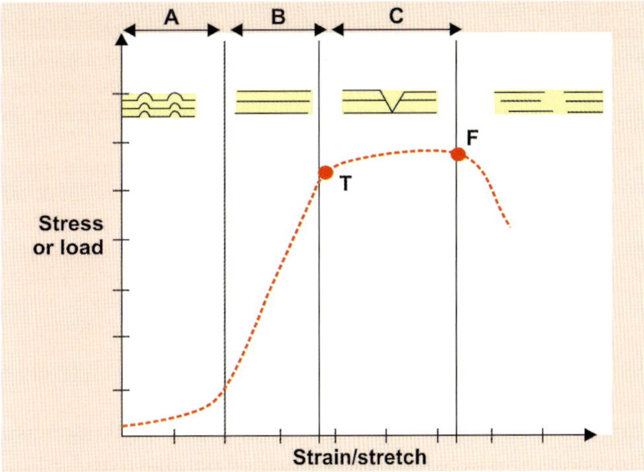

Fig. 1: Stress versus strain relationship of skin. (A) *Toe region:* Considerable extension occur with little force, there is initial deformation of randomly arranged collagen fibers; (B) *Elastic region:* Rapid extension with increasing force and collagen deformation occurs in direction of applied force; (C) *Plastic region:* Little extension with increased force and collagen brakes with further applied force.

Strain is defined as change in length divided by original length. For example, immediately postoperatively scar can be negligible but after sometime due to forces from muscle and joint, the scar may widen.

Creep is tendency to slowly deform under stress. After every excision with primary closure there is small increase in the length of skin along with straightened collagen fibers. This ability of skin helps to cover the site of previous defect. Mechanical creep occurs when the skin is stretched at a constant force beyond its inherent extensibility and it contributes to skin deformation. The stretching achieved during mechanical creep does not retract intraoperatively.

Stress relaxation occurs when skin is stretched for constant distance over time. The force required to maintain the stretch gradually decreases. This can explain why flap with edges tightly sutured immediately postoperatively appears viable after time and why the stress along incision decreases over time.

Elasticity is the ability of skin to return to its original shape when external forces are removed. Recoil of the skin after pinching is an example of elasticity. Elasticity can be determined by stretching the skin between thumb and index finger, known as "pinch test." Poor recoil of the lower eyelid after downward displacement shows loss of elasticity (snap test).

Viscosity is the inability of the object to return to its original shape once the stress is removed. A good example to understand can be hyaluronic acid filler which can be easily molded.

To understand the strength and limits of skin, dermatosurgeon must understand its stress-strain curve. An atypical stress-strain curve consists of three stages. During the initial stages, extension is characterized by the high compliance of the tissues where small loads produce large extensions. This occurs due to initial deformation of collagen bundles. In the second stage deformation is directly proportion to the stress which can be seen as straight line because elastin fibers dominate this behavior with little involvement of collagen. This relationship follows Hooke's law which can be expressed as $\sigma = E\varepsilon$ where σ is stress, E is constant (Young's modulus) and ε is strain. In the third stage as loading is continued further, increasing stress increases strain in a nonlinear fashion. The tissue continues to expand until a point is reached where it cannot adapt to support the load causing rupture. This occurs due to breakage of collagen fibers and results in almost complete relaxation of dermis called stress relaxation. After this point additional undermining will not reduce closure tension, but will make skin plastic and increase the risk of hematomas or nerve damage. The wounds closed under tension will stretch-back (with subsequent spreading of scars) at 12 weeks. Before planning any excision surgery, one must be aware of this phenomenon **(Fig. 1 and Box 1)**.[3-7]

Relaxed Skin Tension Lines

In 1881, Langer first described the concept of lines of minimal tension and called Langer's lines or lines of cleavage. His theory demonstrated that after applying round punches on cadavers the resultant defect had an oval shape. These lines of minimal tension are thought to correlate with the orientation of collagen bundles and elastic tissue in the dermis. Stretching of the collagen in the direction of the pull of the underlying muscles produces these lines. He considered the skin to be less extensible in the direction of the lines of tension than across them. The lines of skin tension result from the movement of underlying muscles. A correlation exists between skin crease lines and Langer's lines;[3,4] where skin crease lines are present,

BOX 1: Applied aspects.

- The stress versus strain relationship of skin explains intraoperative tissue expansion in closing the wound using the rule of halves.[2] Each suture progressively reduces the tension across the wound as the surgeon takes advantage of tissue creep
- This feature can be applied in closing a wound, intraoperative by placing temporary retention sutures (pulley stitch) for about 15 minutes for the mechanical creep to occur
- This load extension is maximum across Langer's lines
- Highly vascularized anatomical regions withstand tension better than poorly perfused ones, which may undergo necrosis
- On areas of less elasticity (scalp, upper back, and deltoid region), the results are aesthetically compromised by spreading scar

Langer's lines will generally run parallel to these skin creases. If incisions and excisions are performed parallel to these lines, the wound tension is decreased and scarring is minimized. The pattern of relaxed skin tension line (RSTL) is described separately for each region.

Kraissl's Lines

Kraissl's lines are a set of anatomical skin lines. They differ from Langer's lines in that unlike Langer's lines, which are defined in terms of collagen orientation, Kraissl's lines are oriented perpendicular to underlying muscle.

Whereas Langer's lines were defined in cadavers, Kraissl's lines have been defined in living individuals. Also, the method used to identify Kraissl's lines is not traumatic and coincides with wrinkle lines.

Biodynamic Excisional Skin Tension Lines

Recently, the concept of biodynamic excisional skin tension (BEST) lines has gained popularity which uses a computerized tensiometer to assess the direction of least tension across wounds[3] **(Fig. 2)**. There are many differences between Langer lines and BEST lines, a few of which have been described below.

Langer lines run in sagittal direction on the scalp whereas BEST lines run in a coronal direction. RSTL runs in horizontal-oblique direction on the lower limb, BEST lines run vertically down. Langer lines can be considered incisional lines whereas BEST lines are excisional lines which mean along them elliptical excision can be oriented. BEST lines are good for high load exceptional surgeries.

Dermatomes

Dermatome is the area of skin with sensory supply derived from specific spinal nerves **(Figs. 3A to C)**. It signifies the area anesthetized when specific nerves are blocked.

Anatomy of Scalp

Scalp

Scalp is a soft-tissue envelope of the cranial vault. It extends from the supraorbital margin anteriorly to occipital protuberance and nuchal lines posteriorly. Laterally it extends up to the temporal lines. Scalp is anatomically less complex but characteristics like rich blood supply and hair follicles make it imperative for the surgeon to have good understanding of the topic. A working knowledge of scalp anatomy is explained in this section.

Scalp is divided into five layers, from superficial to deep as skin, subcutaneous tissue, galea aponeurotica, loose connective tissue, and periosteum **(Fig. 4)**. The first three layers are bound together and glide as a single unit along the loose areolar tissue over the pericranium, which is adherent to the calvaria **(Box 2)**.[8-10]

Skin of the Scalp

Scalp is a hair-bearing structure covering the skull with numerous sebaceous and sweat glands. It has a relatively thin epidermis and thicker dermis. The dermis is of scalp ranges from 3 mm (forehead) to 8 mm (occiput). The dermis contains rich network of nerves, vascular, and lymphatic vessels. Langer's lines tend to be longitudinal on the scalp (*refer* **Figs. 12B and C)**.

Connective Tissue (Superficial Fascia)

This layer of scalp also referred to as dense connective tissue layer, contains subcutaneous fat and fibrous septa which attaches the skin to muscle and aponeurosis below making dissection in this plane difficult.

These fibrous septae are 4–7-mm thick being thickest at the vertex and divide the subcutaneous fat into smaller compartments. It is highly vascularized plane and contains nerves and blood vessels which supply other scalp layers.

There are multiple vertically oriented reticular fibers present that form strong attachments with the dermis above, and galea below. These vertical fibers bind the first three layers of the scalp together.

Galea Aponeurotica

Galea aponeurotica is a 1–2-mm thick fibrous layer also referred to as epicranial aponeurosis. It extends from occipitalis muscle posteriorly to frontalis muscle where it interdigitates with superficial musculoaponeurotic system (SMAS) anteriorly. Laterally, it continues as temporal fascia. There are blood vessels present in the galea which extends into superficial vascular plexus above and subgaleal layer below.

It is connected to the pericranium by loose areolar connective tissue, resulting in a largely avascular space which makes it an optimal site for undermining. It also provides mobility to the scalp and hair bearing areas with it.[8]

Subgaleal Layer or Loose Areolar Tissue

The subgaleal layer is a relatively avascular layer containing loose fibroareolar tissue. It connects the epicranial aponeurosis

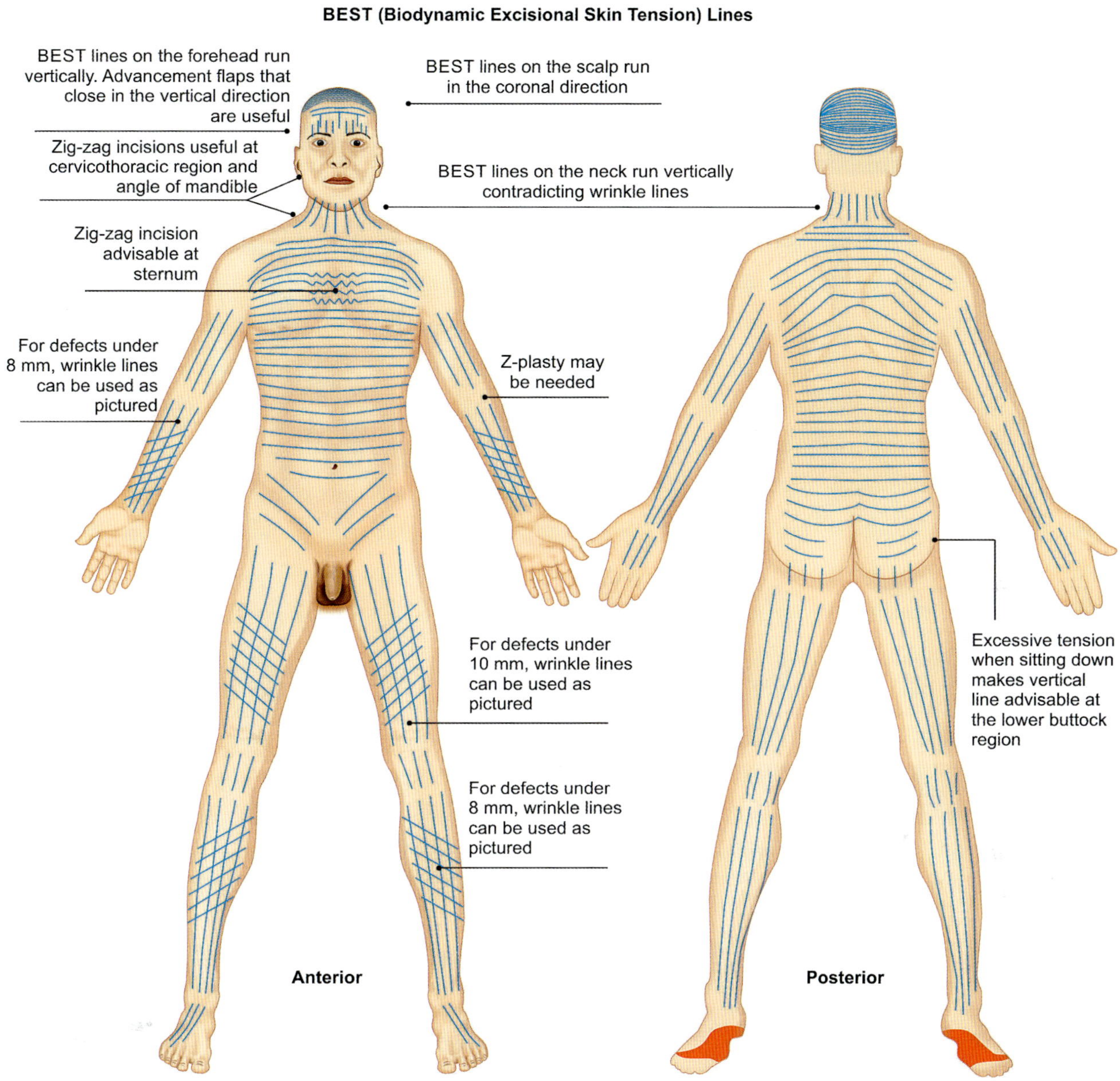

Fig. 2: Demonstration of biodynamic excisional skin tension (BEST) lines.
Source: Originally published in Paul SP. Biodynamic excisional skin tension lines for surgical excisions: untangling the science. Ann R Coll Surg Engl. 2018;100(4):330-7.

to the pericranium below and allows superficial three layers of the scalp to move over the pericranium.

Scalp flaps are elevated along this avascular plane but caution needs to be taken as certain emissary veins connecting scalp veins to diploic and intracranial venous sinuses traverse this layer. The easy glidability of scalp is due to property of subgaleal space that allows easy approximation of wide wounds, however in areas where this layer is absent closure can be difficult **(Boxes 3 and 4)**.[11,12]

Pericranium

Pericranium is a dense fibrous sheath which adheres to the coronal, sagittal, temporal and lamboid sutures of the skull and continues as endosteum. A subperiosteal hematoma, therefore, forms in the shape of the skull bones. This layer can be dissected from the outer table as an intact sheath.

Nerve Supply

Sensory Nerve Supply

The sensory supply to the scalp is located in the subcutaneous plane in a centripetal manner, i.e., from the periphery to the center. The nerve supply of the scalp is derived from the all the branches of trigeminal nerve (area of scalp anterior to the auricles) and cervical nerves C2 and C3 (area of scalp posterior to the auricles) **(Fig. 5 and Box 5)**.[14, 15] The sensory nerves include:

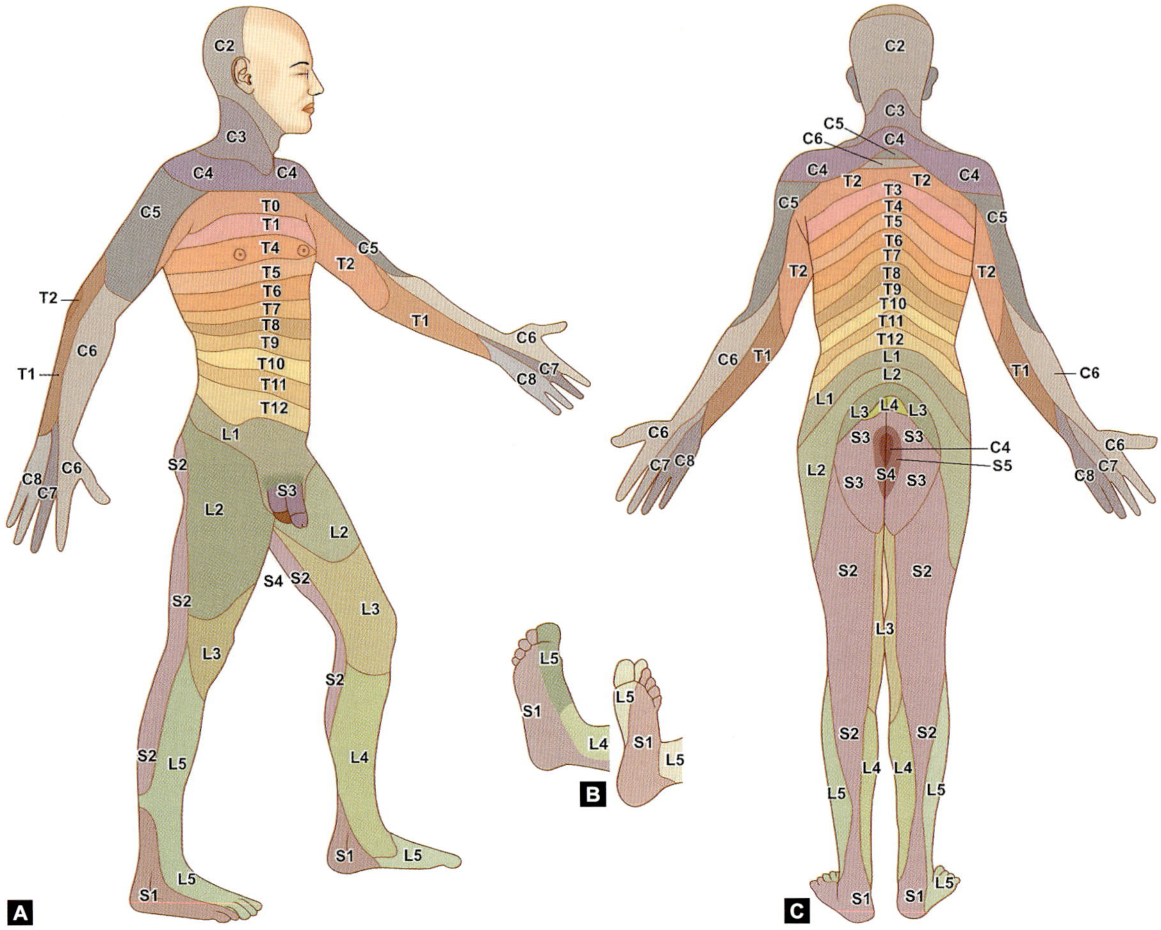

Figs. 3A to C: *Dermatomes:* (A) Anterolateral view; (B) Inferior view; (C) Posterior view.
Source: Drake RL, Vogl W, Mitchell AWM. Gray's Anatomy for Students, 1st edition. Churchill: Livingstone (Elsevier Science); 2005. pp. 898-936.

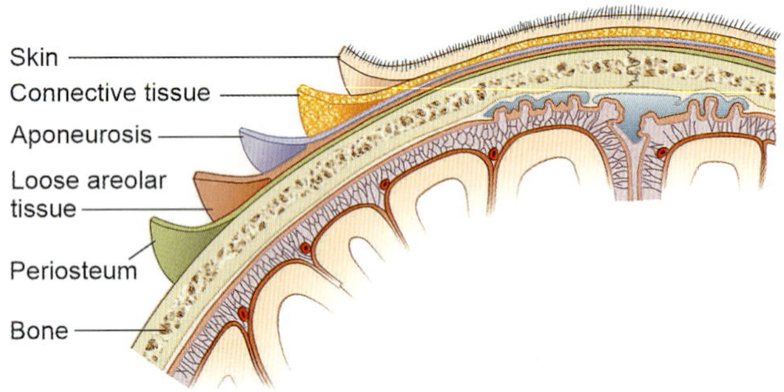

Fig. 4: Layers of scalp.
Source: Agur AMR, Lee MJ, Grant JC. Grant's Atlas of Anatomy, 13th edition. Baltimore, MD: Lippincott Williams and Wilkins; 2013.

- *Ophthalmic division of trigeminal nerve:* (1) Supratrochlear nerve and (2) Supraorbital nerve
- *Maxillary division of the trigeminal nerve:* (3) Zygomaticotemporal nerve
- *Mandibular division of the trigeminal nerve:* (4) Auriculotemporal nerve
- *The posterior ramus of the C2, C3:* (5) greater occipital nerve
- *Branch of the C2:* (6) lesser occipital
- *Branch of the C3:* (7) third occipital nerve

Motor Nerve Supply

Motor innervation of the scalp is done by the nerve supplying the adjacent muscles such as:

- Temporal branch of facial nerve
- Posterior auricular branch of facial nerve
- Anterior and posterior branches of mandibular branch of trigeminal nerve supplying temporalis muscle

Blood Supply

Arterial Supply

Scalp has a rich vascular supply. The blood supply of the scalp is from five paired arteries which are branches of external and internal carotid system. Bone perforators of the meningeal arteries also contribute minimally. The large arteries lie in subcutaneous layer, are held by the connective tissue bundles of the scalp, and sends penetrating branches superiorly into the skin. The arteries of the scalp run centripetally, that is the

BOX 2: Applied aspects of surgical layers of scalp (first three layers are called surgical layers of scalp).

- First three layers are called as surgical layers of scalp
- The incisions on the scalp should be closed vertically following relaxed skin tension lines, except for in the occipital area where incisions are best horizontal, paralleling the skin crease lines **(Fig. 12C)**
- Scalp incisions must be at an angle and parallel to the hair follicles to minimize their transection and to avoid localized scarring alopecia
- The sheets of connective tissue in second layer bind the blood vessels to the dermis and fibrous septa in such a way that vasoconstriction and vasospasms are prevented after venesection causing profuse bleed observed after scalp trauma. Also, after incision is made in the scalp retraction of vessels in fibrous septa makes it difficult to hold the vessel by artery forceps. Firm pressure for 5–10 minutes can achieve hemostasis
- The third layer galea is substantially stronger than the overlying skin and its site to secure retaining sutures which is anchored deep throughout this fascia. Also during artificial hair implantation, galea is the anchoring point
- Wounds superficial to the aponeurosis gape less because aponeurosis holds the skintight. Traumatic wounds that extend to the galea will tend to gape open widely and bleed profusely because the pull of the frontalis muscle anteriorly and occipitalis muscle posteriorly
- The galea is resistant to stretch; the top of the galea is adherent to the subcutaneous layer, making dissection between these two layers extremely difficult
- In deeper wounds, galea must be reapproximated properly by grabbing a large bite of galea with the suture needle; this minimizes tension on the overlying skin, and results in good scar[8]

BOX 3: Points to remember on subgaleal layer.

- The subgaleal layer is important from a surgical standpoint and lends itself to easy avascular dissection during surgical procedures.
- In addition, the blood supply to the scalp runs in the subcutaneous tissues, thus surgical dissection of the subgaleal space does not compromise the blood supply to scalp tissue
- The emissary veins connect the surface of scalp to the brain, therefore infections in the subgaleal space may dangerously communicate with the brain via this connection
- As this space extends beneath the orbicularis oculi and into the eyelids and root of the nose, injury/surgery on the scalp or forehead may result in the pooling of blood in the upper eyelids and sometimes lower eyelids, causing black eye
- Subcutaneous hemorrhage and inflammation in closed wound in second layer cause much pain with little swelling due to unyielding reticulum of fibrous tissue

larger trunks of the arteries start laterally, running in a central and medial fashion, becoming smaller as they enter a system of free anastomosis toward the medial aspect of the scalp. This makes a watershed area in the midline where perfusion may be less predictable. Therefore, any transaction of arteries on peripheral scalp may grossly limit blood supply to surrounding and distant areas.[15,16] The knowledge of centripetal blood supply and absence of musculocutaneous perforators in the scalp are important for surgical flap survival **(Figs. 6 and 7)** **(Box 5)**.

The arterial supply of the scalp is as follows:

- *Branches of internal carotid arteries:* Supraorbital and supratrochlear arteries

BOX 4: Anatomic surgical considerations.

- The scalp laxity determines the possible extent of scalp excisions. It depends on glidability and elasticity. The ability of the scalp to slide over the pericranium contributes to scalp laxity (determined by subgaleal space with loose fibroareolar tissue). The ability of the tissue to stretch (scalp can stretch maximally along Langer's lines) contributes to scalp elasticity
- Individual variations in loose fibroareolar tissue or in elastic tissue content explain why some scalps are tight and some are loose and stretch better. Excessive removal of tissue beyond the capacity of stretching will lead to plastic scalp
- Scalp undermining must be in proper plane. Extensive undermining can be associated with traumatized blood vessels and nerves which increase scaring in the undermined area, open up tissue planes, and increases risk of infection,[13] However, rich vascular plexus makes defects of the scalp to heal quickly, even by secondary intention
- Strips in hair transplantation (FUT method) should not be taken from below the occipital protuberance as chances of scar dehisence increases due to pull by neck muscles as well as chances of losing hair occipital protuberance in cases of retrograde alopecia.[59]

- *Branches of external carotid arteries:* Occipital, posterior auricular, and superficial temporal arteries

Venous Drainage

The venous drainage of scalp can be divided into superficial and deep venous system. The superficial venous system includes superficial temporal, occipital, posterior auricular, supraorbital and supratrochlear veins which follows the arteries **(Fig. 6)**. The deep venous system is drained by the pterygoid venous plexus. The veins of the scalp connect to the diploic veins of the skull via emissary veins. This establishes a connection between the scalp and the dural venous sinuses **(Box 5)**.

Lymphatic Drainage

There are no lymph nodes in the scalp, but multiple lymphatic vessels drain the scalp to local regional lymph node chains in centrifugal pattern. The region posterior to the auricle drain into the posterior auricular (mastoid) and occipital lymph nodes, which then drain into the superficial cervical nodal chains. The regions anterior to the auricle drain into the preauricular and parotid lymph nodes, which further drain into the submandibular and deep cervical nodes.[17]

Muscles of the Scalp

The occipitofrontalis muscle consists of two occipital bellies and two frontal bellies. The occipital bellies arise from the superior nuchal lines on the occipital bone. The frontal bellies originate from the skin and superficial fascia of the upper eyelids and help to raise the eyebrows. The occipital and frontal bellies insert into the epicranial aponeurosis. The galea connects the two muscles, and is referred as one structure, the occipitofrontalis muscle. Each occipital belly is innervated by the posterior auricular branch of the facial nerve, and each frontal belly is innervated by the frontal branch of the facial nerve **(Fig. 8)**.

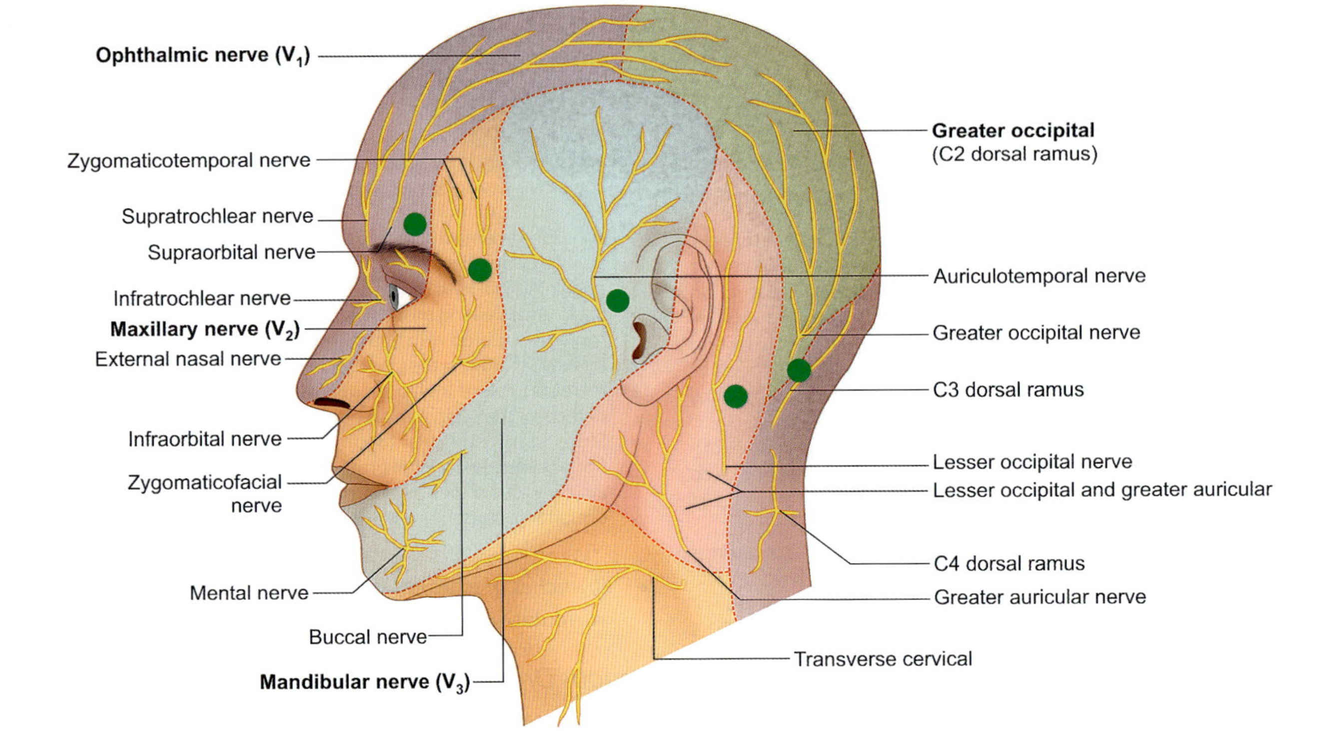

Fig. 5: *Sensory innervation of the scalp (lateral view):* Supratrochlear nerve supplies the scalp in the medial plane at the frontal region, up to the vertex. Supraorbital nerve supplies the scalp at the front, lateral to the supratrochlear nerve distribution up to the vertex. Zygomaticotemporal nerve supplies the scalp over the temple region. Auriculotemporal nerve supplies the skin over the temporal region of the scalp. Lesser occipital supplies the scalp over the lateral occipital region. Greater occipital nerve supplies the scalp in the median plane at the occipital region, up to the vertex.
Source: Drake RL, Vogl W, Mitchell AWM. Gray's Anatomy for Students, 1st edition. Churchill: Livingstone (Elsevier Science); 2005. pp. 898-936.

BOX 5: Applied aspects on neurovasculature of scalp.

- All nerves and vessels of the scalp originate below the level of the brow as it is extended circumferentially around the scalp following centripetal distribution. This anatomical location of the arteries and nerves of the scalp makes central scalp surgeries easy with minimal neurovascular trauma
- There is relative loss of vascular network and decrease in midline anastomoses with aging, that can affect wound healing, especially in deeper defects
- The incisions in the peripheral scalp can transect nerve trunks and result in large areas of permanent hypoesthesia, a complication that can be avoided or explained to the patient if one is familiar with the anatomical locations of these nerves
- Knowledge of anatomy of nerves is important during scalp blocks. Infiltrating local anesthetic around the scalp's periphery (through which all the sensory nerves traverse) can produce total scalp anesthesia
- The lymphatic drainage of scalp is diffuse, scalp lacks lymph nodes and there are no barriers to lymph flow contributing to the significant spread of pathology seen in this area

EAR

The external ear or auricle is organ of cosmesis **(Fig. 9)**. It is of both functional and cosmetic importance. It mainly protects the internal ear and localizes and directs the sound waves into the ear. The auricle or pinna is formed by complex cartilaginous framework with lot of depressions and elevations covered by skin. The important landmarks are helix, antihelix, tragus, antitragus, lobule, and concha. The skin is avidly attached to cartilage all over except on helix. The layers of ear are anterior surface of epidermis, dermis, perichondrium, cartilage, fat, posterior dermis, and epidermis (from anterior to posterior direction). The lobule does not contain cartilage and external ear is devoid of muscular attachment.

Ear has a rich blood supply from anterior and posterior auricular artery branch of superficial temporal artery. The occipital artery also contributes to blood supply of ear. Veins accompany the corresponding named arteries.

SENSORY SUPPLY

The sensory supply of the ear is as follows **(Figs. 10A and B):**

- The greater auricular nerve is a branch of the cervical plexus. It innervates posteromedial, posterolateral, and inferior auricle (lower two-thirds both anteriorly and posteriorly).
- The lesser occipital nerve innervates a small portion of the helix.
- The auricular branch of the vagus nerve innervates the concha and most of the area around the auditory meatus.
- The auriculotemporal nerve originates from the mandibular branch of trigeminal nerve and innervates anterosuperior and anteromedial parts of ear.

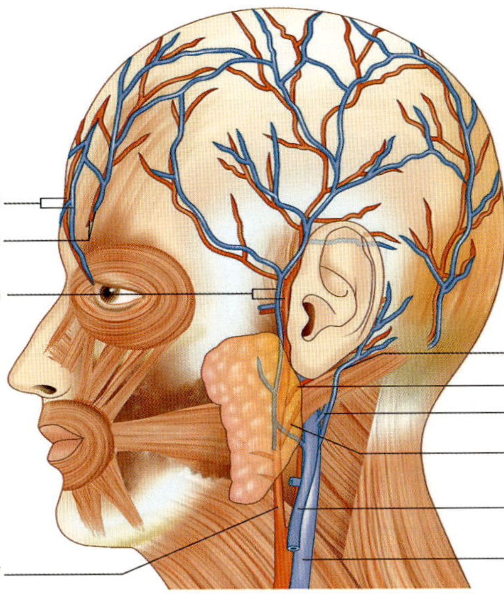

Fig. 6: Arterial and venous system of scalp in lateral view.
Source: Drake RL, Vogl W, Mitchell AWM. Gray's Anatomy for Students, 1st edition. Churchill: Livingstone (Elsevier Science); 2005. pp. 898-936.

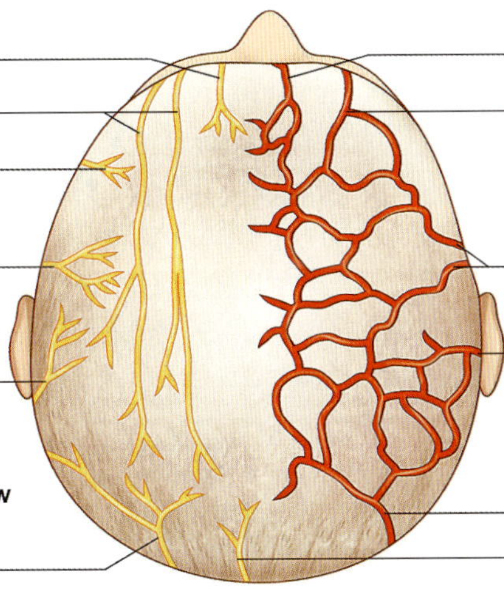

Fig. 7: Neurovascular supply of scalp in superior view from the midline anterior to posterior, the arteries are as follows: Supratrochlear artery, supraorbital artery, superficial temporal artery, posterior auricular artery, and occipital artery.
Note: Midline anastomoses are rare. Area anterior to the ear is trigeminal distribution and posterior to the ear is cervical distribution.
Source: Agur AMR, Lee MJ, Grant JC. Grant's Atlas of Anatomy, 13th edition. Baltimore, MD: Lippincott Williams and Wilkins; 2013.

The lymphatics of the ear drain to superficial, deep cervical, and mastoid lymph nodes **(Box 6)**.

NECK

The neck is the exposed part of body which extends between lower margin of mandible to upper margin of manubrium sterni.[10] It is long and supple structure and helps in movements of the body. It is a vulnerable region encompassing important vital structures.[14,15] The dermatologic surgeon must be familiar with the anatomy of the neck and be knowledgeable and cautious while operating on this area.

Surface Anatomy

The superficial landmarks of the neck are the hyoid, larynx, and trachea anteriorly, vertebral column posteriorly and the sternocleidomastoid muscle (SCM) laterally. SCM becomes more prominent on turning neck to one side. It divides neck into anterior and posterior triangles **(Figs. 11A and B)**. Adam's apple is the most prominent part on anterior neck. The thyroid cartilage is situated below hyoid bone and cricoid cartilage is below Adam's apple at the level of C6. Emergency laryngectomy is done between them.[19-22]

Skin and Subcutaneous Tissue

The skin covering the anterior and side of the neck is thin, elastic, and can readily be raised into folds, which contain the platysma muscle. On the contrary, skin over the nape of the neck is very dense, with thick dermis and adherent and richly supplied with nerves.

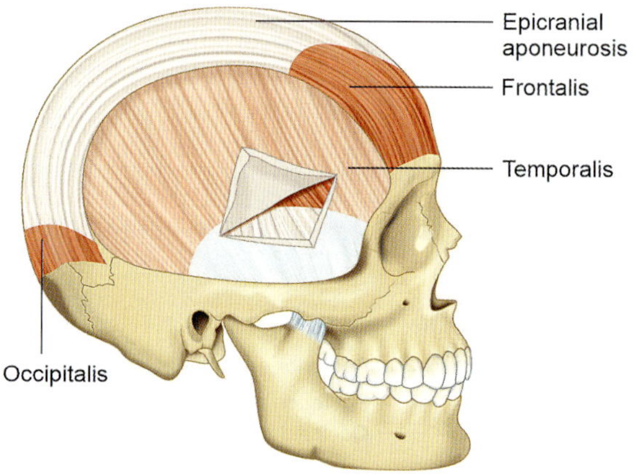

Fig. 8: Figure demonstrating the occipitalis, frontalis, and temporalis muscles of the scalp.
Source: Agur AMR, Lee MJ, Grant JC. Grant's Atlas of Anatomy, 13th edition. Baltimore, MD: Lippincott Williams and Wilkins; 2013.

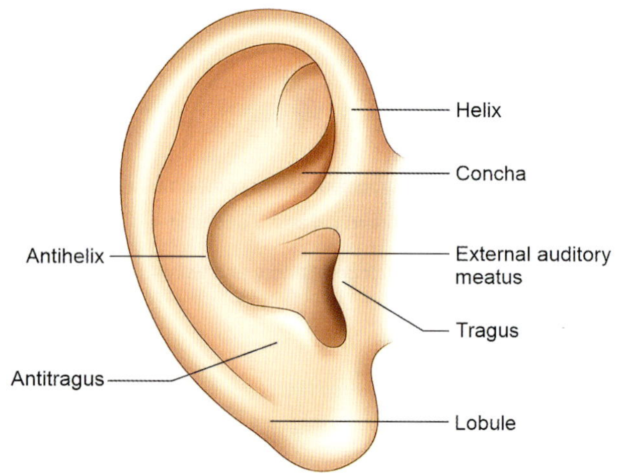

Fig. 9: Surface anatomy of the ear.

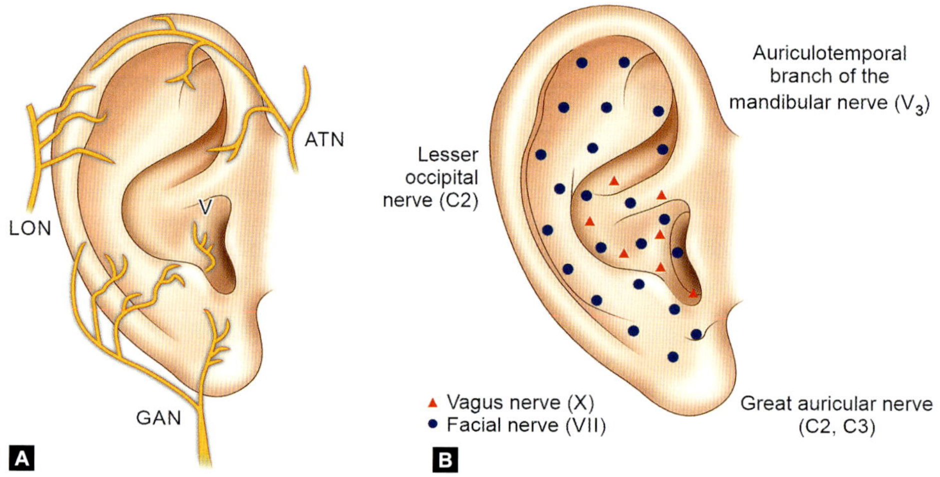

Figs. 10A and B: Sensory innervation of the external ear.
(ATN: auriculotemporal nerve; GAN: greater occipital nerve; LON: lesser occipital nerve; V: vagus nerve)
Source: Drake RL, Vogl W, Mitchell AWM. Gray's Anatomy for Students, 1st edition. Churchill: Livingstone (Elsevier Science); 2005. pp. 898-936.

BOX 6: Anatomic surgical considerations.

- As lobule has no underlying muscle, the wound closure is parallel to the force of gravity
- The level of undermining is subdermal in helix
- Excision surgeries around the ear with unopposed tension may affect the free margins (helices or lobule) of the ear and distort these structures. Wound closure in these locations often require flap and/or graft placement to lessen the risk[18]
- Simple excision and closure of skin lesions over edge of ear may distort the curvature of pinna, with a noticeable defect. Wedge excision or fillet flap for keloids are preferred
- Free grafts can be taken from retroauricular and preauricular area.

Skin Tension Lines

Relaxed skin tension lines typically lie in a transverse direction on the neck. The placement of excision lines in this orientation is essential, as vertical incisions have a tendency toward scar contractures **(Figs. 12A to C)**.

Muscles of the Neck

The main superficial muscles of the neck are platysma and SCM. The platysma is an extremely thin muscle. It originates inferiorly from the pectoralis and deltoid fascia. The fibers ascend upward and insert into under surface of mandible and modiolus and most fibers continue to ascend to get inserted into SMAS. In the midline, platysma is absent except when fibers from each side decussate with other side under the chin. It is innervated by the cervical branch of the facial nerve. It functions to depress the corner of mouth, to depress mandible during deep inspiration, and assists venous return. It can be made prominent by clenching the jaw and also acts as a mimetic muscle to express horror or disgust.

As part of aging, its medial fibers thicken to create platysmal bands. It is responsible for wrinkles of the neck. Superficial cervical fascia, a loose connective tissue separates

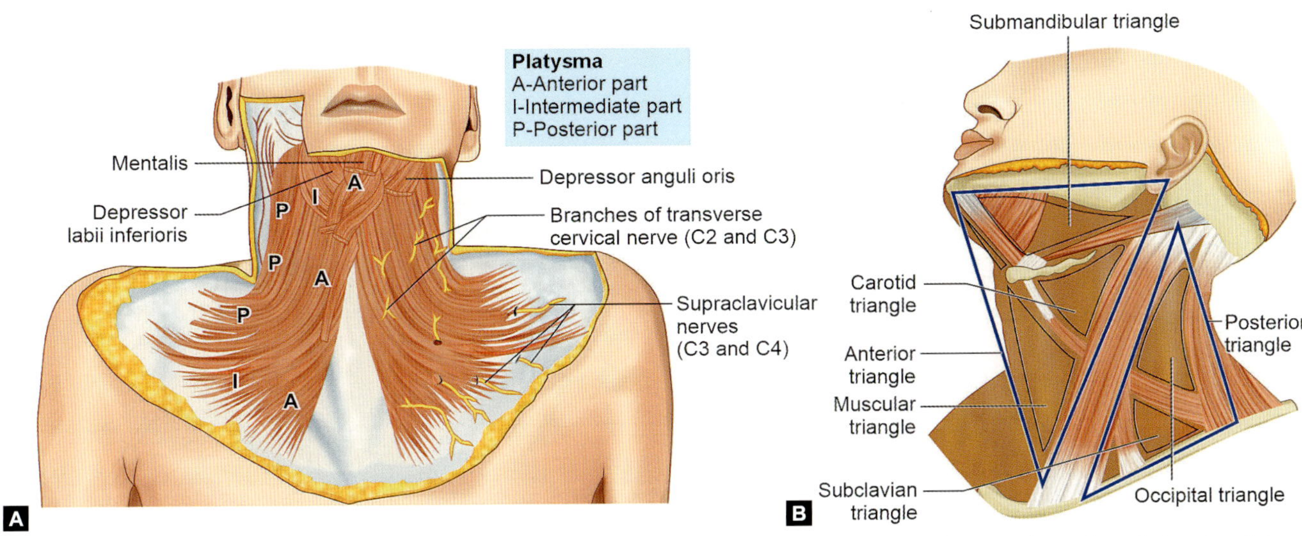

Figs. 11A and B: (A) Superficial muscles of neck anterior (platysma); (B) Lateral view (shows sternocleidomastoid muscle and triangles of the neck). Submental triangle (borders—hyoid bone, mandible, anterior belly of the digastric muscle, and midline); submandibular triangle (borders—anterior and posterior bellies of the digastric muscle, mandible); carotid triangle (borders—SCM, posterior belly of the digastric muscle, superior belly of the omohyoid muscle, stylohyoid muscle); muscular triangle (borders—hyoid bone, SCM, superior belly of the omohyoid muscle, midline posterior triangle); posterior triangle (borders—SCM, trapezius muscle, clavicle).
(SCM: sternocleidomastoid muscle)

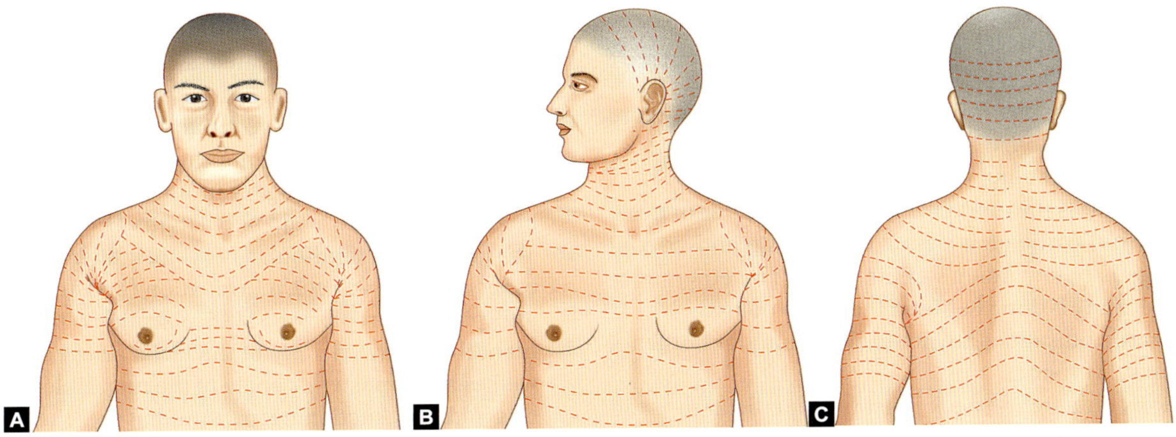

Figs. 12A to C: Relaxed skin tension line of the torso, neck, and head.

platysma and SCM from underlying structures and allows platysma to glide easily over SCM.[20] SCM is prominent landmark in neck which extends from the medial clavicle to the postauricular area and divide the neck into anterior and posterior triangles. It is supplied by spinal accessory nerve. The carotid pulsations are noted along anterior border of SCM at C6 vertebra.

Triangles of Neck

The anterior triangle is divided into four triangles by small muscles into submental, submandibular, carotid, and muscular triangles **(Figs. 11A and B)**. The submental triangle contains submental lymph nodes. Submandibular triangle is marking for danger zone for facial artery. The main content of the carotid triangle includes the internal and external carotid arteries, the internal jugular vein, vagus, and hypoglossal nerves.[21] The important structures in posterior triangle include spinal accessory nerve, greater auricular nerve, lesser occipital nerve, and transverse cervical nerve. The spinal accessory nerve [cranial nerve XI (CNXI)] innervates the sternocleidomastoid and trapezius muscles. It is located immediately below the SMAS fascia within the posterior triangle and emerges at the posterior border of the SCM at Erb's point. Erb's point is located by drawing an imaginary line connecting the middle of the angle of the mandible to the mastoid process, intersecting the posterior border of the SCM **(Fig. 13)**.[21,22] As spinal accessory nerve is covered only by skin and superficial cervical fascia, it is vulnerable to injury during surgery in the posterior triangle causing winging of scapula and difficulty with arm abduction.

The external carotid artery and the thyrocervical trunk provide blood supply to the face and neck. The venous system of the neck includes the internal jugular veins, the external jugular veins, and anterior jugular veins.

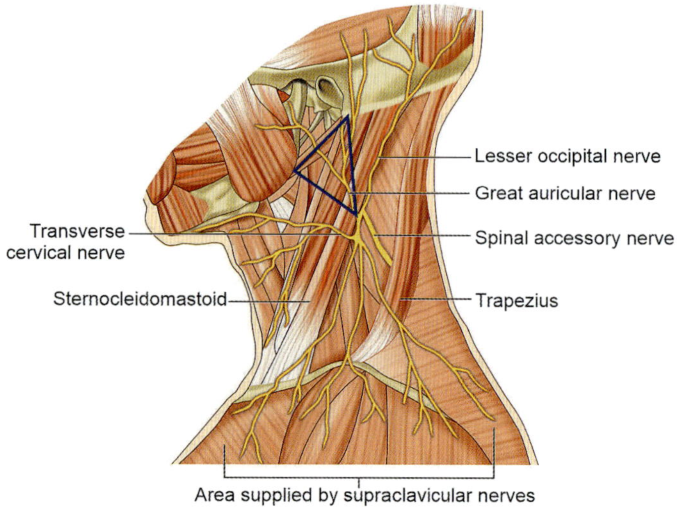

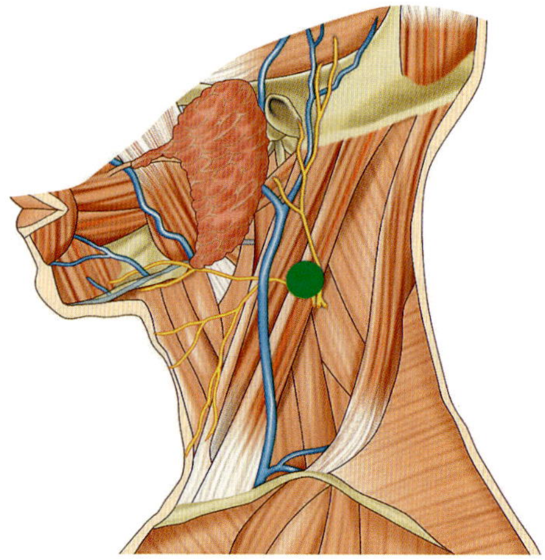

Fig. 13: Innervation of the neck and marking of Erb's point (lateral view). The spinal accessory nerve exits behind the sternocleidomastoid. Three important sensory nerves, the greater auricular, the transverse cervical, and the lesser occipital nerves, that supply sensation to the neck and ear emerge 2 cm above and 2 cm below Erb's point.

Applied Aspects

- The skin of the neck is relatively loose with transverse creases and wrinkles. Elective incisions are easily placed in these lines. Because of the concave shape of the neck, vertical incisions have a tendency toward scar contracture with web formation, which may have functional as well as cosmetic implications.
- Adam's apple is the most prominent part of anterior neck. The thyroid cartilage is below hyoid bone and cricoid cartilage is below Adam's apple at C6. The emergency laryngectomy is done between these two points.
- The carotid pulsations are noted along anterior border of SCM at C6 vertebra.
- Incisions on anterior neck must be superficial to avoid damage to the important underlying structures.
- Nape of neck is a common site for carbuncle. The skin is thick and dense, deeper incisions are required during excision. Wide unplanned excisions can lead to contractures.
- The botulinum toxin injections must be specifically injected into the platysmal bands, in the deep dermal layer. Transverse neck lines are injected more superficially as diffusion of toxin to the strap muscle or deeper muscles of the neck can cause dysphagia, dysphonia, dysarthria, or life-threatening breathing difficulties.[10,17]
- Platysma is the superficial muscle of the anterior neck. When performing surgery in this area, one should be mindful of suturing the platysma carefully as irregularities in this muscle may pull unevenly on a healing scar.
- Cervical branch of the facial nerve supplies motor innervation to the platysma muscle. This is important because skin incisions over the angle of the mandible can distort mouth, if careful observation to muscular innervation is not considered.
- Neck and face drain into submandibular, submental, occipital, and superficial cervical lymph nodes.
- Understanding the anatomy of lymphatic drainage of head and neck is crucial to locate a suspected malignancy or metastasis.
- Erb's point is the site where the accessory nerve exits from the SCM to cross the posterior triangle. Extreme care must be observed during surgery in the area 2 cm above and below this point to avoid nerve injury **(Fig. 13)**.
- The marginal mandibular nerve is vulnerable to injury especially during neck rejuvenation (liposuction of neck and platysma repair or SMAS placation). It crosses the mandible in the vicinity of the facial artery and vein, as well as at the posterior angle of the mandible. Injury can be avoided by suctioning in the midfat over the nerve, and avoiding dissection over mandibular rami.

TORSO

The regional anatomy of torso includes trunk and its extremities with special surgical considerations. The dermatosurgery is only restricted to skin and subcutaneous tissue in this area. We must be well-versed with the RSTLs, which are important in such areas and to understand surgical anatomy of axilla and breast.

Relaxed Skin Tension Lines

Relaxed skin tension lines are oriented transversely across the trunk and extremities, placing sutures along these lines reduce wound tension **(Figs. 13 and 14)**. Pinch test is a simple test to identify skin tension lines. Pinch the skin between thumb and index finger, if it produces straight lines it is parallel to skin tension lines on the contrary if S-shaped curve are seen lines are across skin tension lines. Pinch test can be difficult to evaluate on anterior chest, abdomen, upper arms, and back.[14]

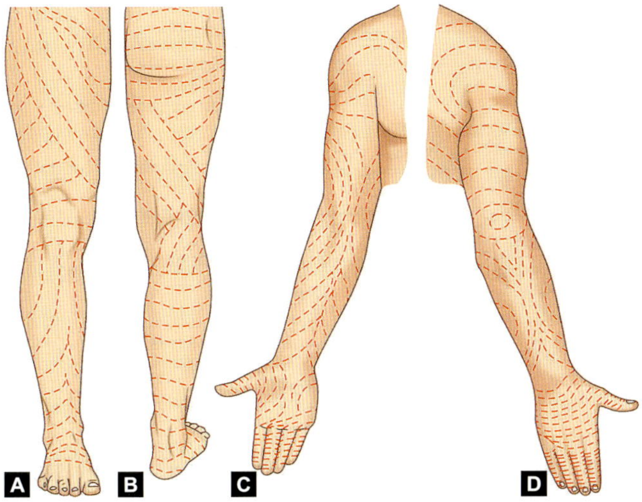

Figs. 14A to D: Relaxed skin tension line of the extremities.

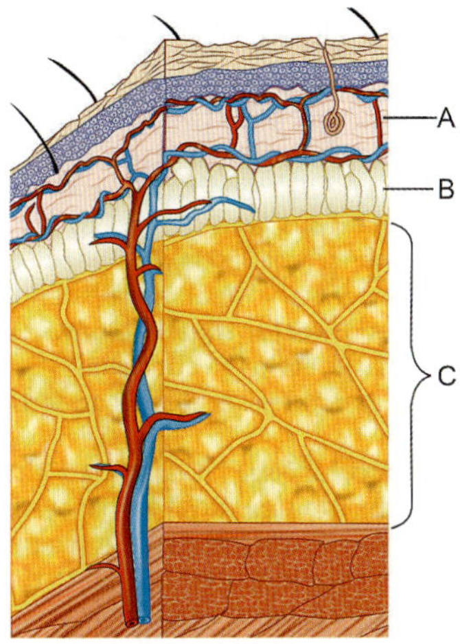

Fig. 15: Subcutaneous fat layers from dermis to muscle. (A: apical layer; B: mantle layer; C: deeper layer).

Pendulous structure like breast and abdomen where action of muscle is not important, closure should be done parallel to gravity.[15] Skin over joints such as nape of neck, elbow, wrist and ankle closure should be done perpendicular to action of underlying joint or muscle. This avoids wound contracture and therefore does not affect joint mobility.

Anatomic Surgical Considerations

The torso, arms, and legs are cylindrical structures and create varied forces unlike face. The mobile joints of limbs create added tensile forces. The wound closures are associated with large dog ears and also pose more tension during closure. Skin varies in thickness, being thickest on the back. The skin is slightly redundant on flexures compared to extensors. The shoulder, arm, and chest are high-risk area for keloid formation.[23-25] Thickness of the dermis varies from <0.5 mm to >5 mm. The dermal grafts can be harvested from areas of thick dermal tissue (lower back and thigh), for smaller harvest medial arm or postauricular regions are chosen. In some areas of limbs, superficial blunt dissection and undermining is recommended to avoid damage to vessels and nerves. Around joints, neurovascular bundles lie deep to the muscle fascia. The undermining must be in deep subcutaneous plane on the trunk. Remember, the blood supply is less in the trunk and extremities when compared to the face with varying amount of hair and appendages. Medial aspect of arm and groin forms uncommon but important donor sites for full thickness grafting as they are covered, more lax and provides easy closure.[26] Split thickness grafts are harvested from anterolateral thigh because of ease of harvesting and round contour. The yield over this area is more and even due to larger surface area.

Blood supply to the torso and limbs are less compared to face. Preserving a 1:1 length to base ratio will maximize the blood flow to the donor skin. Knowledge of lymphatic drainage is important; base of the flap should be planned inferiorly whenever possible.

Subcutaneous Fat

The apical, mantle, and deep layers are three layers of subcutaneous fat. Apical layer is a periadnexal (thecal) layer and it lies just beneath the reticular dermis, it is yellow in appearance **(Fig. 15)**. It surrounds sweat glands, hair follicles, vascular and lymphatic channels. Mantle layer is a superficial fat consisting organized layer of fat cells composed of more columnar-shaped lipocytes. It is separated from the deep layer of fat by a fascia-like layer of fibrous tissue. It acts as shock absorber and contributes to the skin's ability to resist trauma. Deep layer lies between mantle layer and muscle fascia. The thickness of this layer depends on the sex, genes, and diet of the individual. The fat cells are arranged in pearls and are gathered into globules. These globules are then packed together in lobules separated by fibrous septa and are then arranged between tangential and oblique fibrous planes. The tangential planes are much thicker and run parallel to the underlying muscle fascia and are of little consequence when performing liposuction. Oblique planes are thinner and interconnect with tangential fibrous layers. Though thinner, they are of a cosmetic importance because the vertical arrangement of subcutaneous fat from skin to muscle fascia causes cellulite.[27] The deep fat layer is the zone for liposculpture. The apical and mantle layers represent the "no-man's zone" of liposuction. Damage to these layers increases the risk of postoperative complications such as seroma or dermal necrosis **(Box 7)**.

Breast

Breast is a fibroglandular tissue with rich vascularity lying over the pectoral muscle. It extends from just below the clavicle to the axilla and across to the sternum. Breast contains mammary glands and abundant subcutaneous adipose tissue that gives the breast its size and shape which is encircled by dense connective tissue called fascia. The deep layer of this fascia lies

BOX 7: Applied aspects of subcutaneous fat.

- In the submental region, the fat immediately beneath the platysma must be removed and the fat between the digastric muscles and beneath superficial layer of deep fascia of neck should not be removed, as it can cause permanent depression
- In abdomen, subcutaneous fat is divided by superficial Camper's fascia and the deeper scarpa fascia. The deep fascia overlays the aponeurosis, and covers the small arteries and veins along the surface of the anterior rectus sheath. Liposuction is performed between these fascial layers in the abdomen
- The neurovascular structures are deeper to fascia and muscle in thigh and abdomen
- In buttocks, the subcutaneous fat is divided into superficial and deep compartments. The superficial fascial system (SFS) encases the superficial fat, is light yellow and dense, whereas the deeper fat is usually darker and less-structured
- Zones of adherence are sites where the SFS connects to the underlying muscle fascia which are different for men and women and responsible for the android and gynecoid appearance of hips. The gluteal crease represents another zone of adherence. The zones of adherence should not be violated with a liposuction cannula
- Fat can also be harvested from lower leg. The major vessel and nerves are beneath investing fascia of the superficial fat of the legs. Liposuction should not be performed on lateral knee due to insertion of thigh musculature.
- Owing to low vascularity of donor sites in lateral thigh and abdomen, these are preferred sites of fat harvest during autologous fat transfer[27]
- During superficial liposuction, liposuction of apical fat with dermal trauma does not produce contraction of the dermis. But widespread liposuction-induced trauma to the dermal–apical fat interface is injury to the dermal vasculature and possible dermal necrosis. Erythema ab lipoaspiration is a less extreme but more common consequence of excessively superficial liposuction
- Mantle layer fat has the teleologic duty to protect, cushion, and insulate
- Cellulite is probably the result of traction on the skin of subcutaneous fibrous septa. Both tangential and oblique planes can insert into the superficial apical and mantle layer septa and the deep fasciae that cover subjacent muscle. Any attempt to cut the fibrous attachments between skin and adipose tissue is unlikely to give satisfactory long-term results

on pectoralis muscle, and the superficial layer is just beneath the skin. Each breast comprises 15–20 radially arranged lobes each of which is comprised of many lobules. Nipple and areola are a part of pendulous structure and lack support. It differs from normal skin by being pigmented and rich in montgomery glands. A minimally invasive surgical technique for removing benign breast tissue mass involves using a single periareolar incision, dissection of the tumor free from the surrounding parenchyma, giving a cosmetically better scar. The epidermis and dermis are thin with fat layer beneath. The dermatosurgeon must be well-aware of this while performing vitiligo surgery especially during dermabrasion and while creating recipient sites for mini-punch grafting. The RSTL is curved, and wound closure must be planned accordingly. The vascularity of the breast is more and tumescence anesthesia must be given adequately. Implant and fillers are placed in retromammary space **(Fig. 16)**. The breast tissue lies on pectoralis major and minor muscle, which forms the basis for botulinum toxin injection for breast lift.

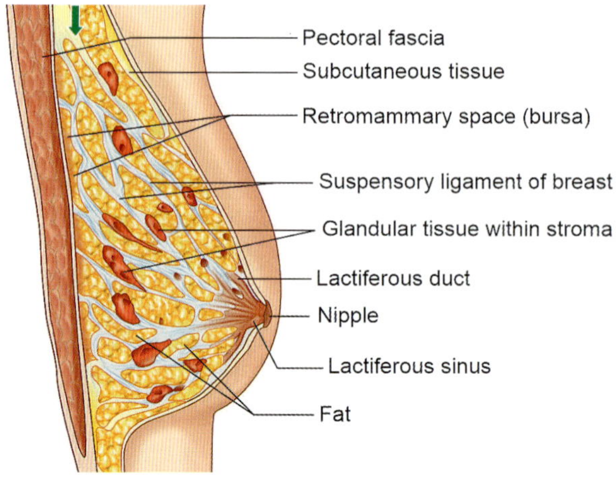

Fig. 16: Lateral section of the breast showing skin subcutaneous fat with glandular tissue retromammary and pectoral fascia. Implanters or fillers are placed in retromammary space during breast augmentation.

Axilla

It is a pyramidal-shaped structure between the arm and the chest wall. The anterior and posterior axillary folds are formed by pectoralis major and latissimus dorsi, respectively. It contains the axillary vessels and the brachial plexus, branches of the intercostal nerves and lymph nodes with fat and loose areolar tissue. The long thoracic nerve and intercostobrachial nerve are most superficial, damage to which must be avoided. The axilla is rich in sweat glands, they are concentrated most in the central elliptical area of approximately 4–5 cm. It is important to note that tail of breast tissue called "axillary tail of Spence" extends into the axilla. This is important clinically as it could be mistaken for abscess or excess fat accumulation, which does not require intervention. The axilla is more prone for hematoma and seroma after any surgical intervention, due to inability to compress the axillary cavity. This can increase the risk of postoperative infections, delayed healing and may lead to the formation of hypertrophic scars and irregularities on the skin surface. Compressive bandages avoid this complication.[28]

HAND

Hand is an important functional part with unique structure. Dermatologic surgery of the hand is generally limited to surgery of the skin and subcutaneous tissue. Vital structures such as nerve, arteries, veins, ligaments, and tendon sit superficially below a thin layer of skin and fat. Anatomy of the hand is complex, should be carefully considered to preserve function and cosmesis.

Surface Anatomy

The hand has a dorsal and ventral surface and a radial and ulnar aspect. The five digits are named or numbered from radial to ulnar side. The fingers are divided into distal, middle,

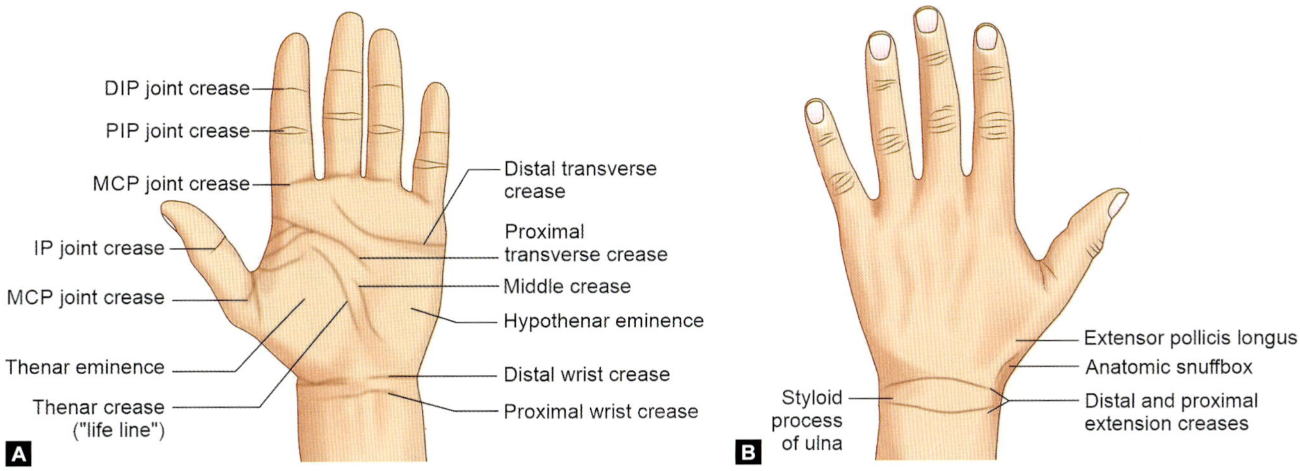

Figs. 17A and B: Surface anatomy of hand: (A) Left palm; (B) Left hand.
(DIP: distal interphalangeal; IP: interphalangeal; MCP: metacarpophalangeal; PIP: proximal interphalangeal).
Source: Drake RL, Vogl W, Mitchell AWM. Gray's Anatomy for Students, 1st edition. Churchill: Livingstone (Elsevier Science); 2005. pp. 898-936.

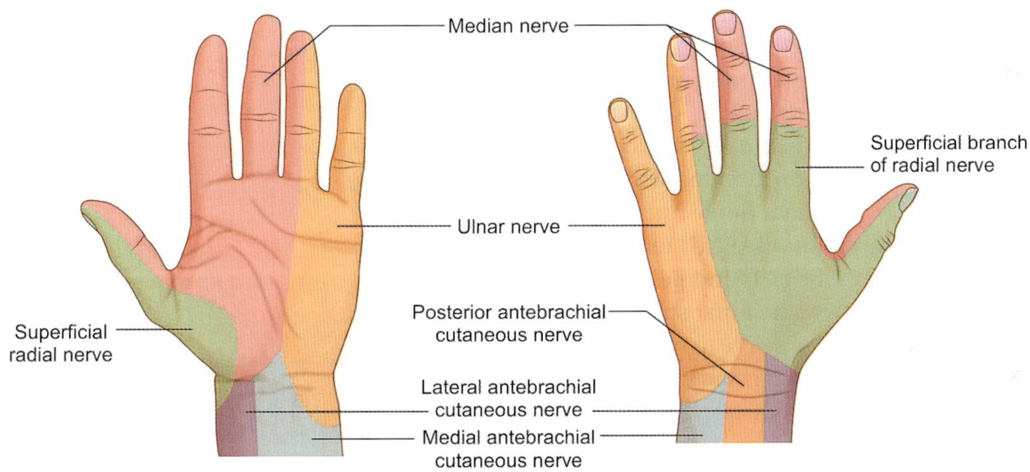

Fig. 18: Sensory distribution of hand. The radial nerve supplies the radial aspect of the dorsal two-thirds of the hand but notably not the distal aspects of the index, middle, or ring fingers. The ulnar third of the dorsal surface is supplied by the ulnar nerve, with the exception of the distal ring and little fingers. The ulnar nerve also supplies the palmar third to the hand on the ulnar aspect. The median nerve is responsible for the remainder of the sensation, most of which is on the palmar aspect of the hand.
Source: Drake RL, Vogl W, Mitchell AWM. Gray's Anatomy for Students, 1st edition. Churchill: Livingstone (Elsevier Science); 2005. pp. 898-936.

and proximal phalanges, thumb has two phalanges. The phalanges are attached to the metacarpals. There are two volar prominences, thenar eminence on the radial side and hypothenar eminence on the ulnar side **(Figs. 17 A and B)**.

Structure of Skin

There is a great disparity in the character of skin and soft-tissue envelope covering the dorsal and plantar surface of the hand. The dorsal skin is thin, pliable, and anchored to the investing fascia by loose areolar tissue. Palmar skin in contrast is characterized by a thick dermal layer and a heavily cornified epithelial surface. The skin of palm is laden with high concentration of sensory end organs and sweat glands. The skin is not as pliable as dorsal skin and it is held tightly by vertical fibers to the palmar fascia and palmar crease. Stability of palms is critical for functions of hands.

Deeper Anatomy

There are 20 intrinsic muscles of the hand that includes thenar muscles (action of thumb), hypothenar (action of little finger), lumbricals and interossei, responsible for dexterity of hand. The motor supply of intrinsic muscles of the hand and flexors are supplied by the ulnar nerve and median nerve and extensors are supplied by radial nerve **(Fig. 18)**.

Nerve Supply of Hand

Sensory innervation of the hand is by a combination of the ulnar, median, and radial nerves **(Fig. 18)**. Ulnar nerve supplies medial one-third of hand, median supplies lateral two-thirds and the radial nerve supplies the radial aspect of the dorsal two-thirds of the hand. Knowledge of sensory innervation is important when regional or digital anesthesia is being considered.

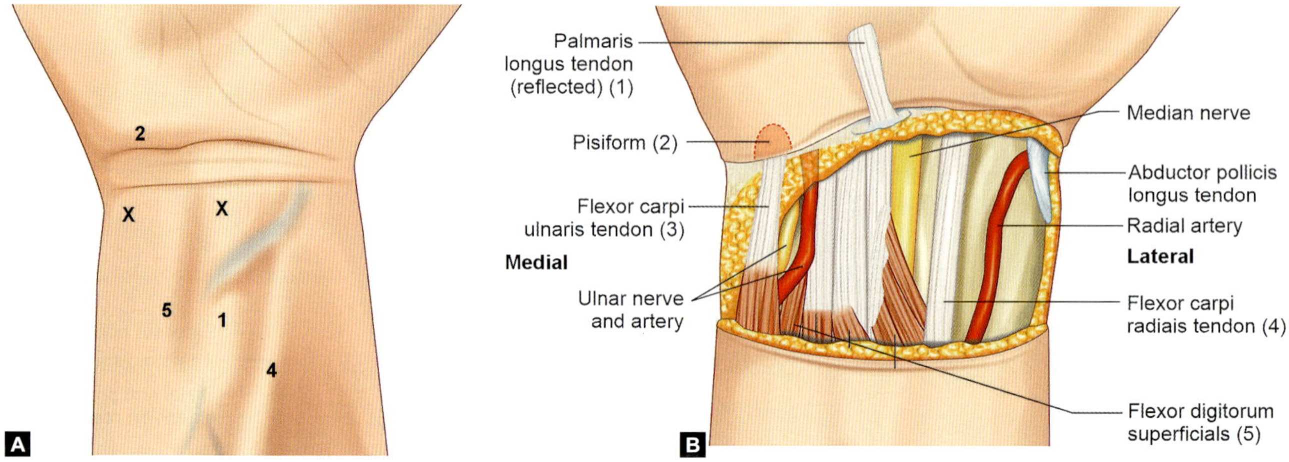

Figs. 19A and B: Surface anatomy of ulnar and median nerve. (A) The nerve can be accessed at the proximal crease of the wrist at the marked points; (B) Anterior view of right hand and wrist.

At the wrist, median nerve is located between the tendons of palmaris longus (PL) and the flexor carpi radialis (FCR) tendon. The PL tendon becomes more prominent on approximating thumb with ring finger with slight flexion at wrist, the median nerve passes just deep and lateral to PL tendon. It is located 2.5 cm proximal to the wrist crease between PL and FCR tendon. The ulnar nerve runs between the ulnar artery and flexor carpi ulnaris (FCU) tendon. The nerve is deeper to the tendon of the FCU and lies medial to the artery. It branches 1 cm distal to the ulnar styloid to give dorsal cutaneous branch of the ulnar nerve to supply skin of the back of the hand. The ulnar nerve is located under the tendon of the FCU muscle close to its distal attachment just above the styloid process of the ulna **(Figs. 19A and B)**.

The superficial branch of the radial nerve (SRN) runs along the medial aspect of the brachioradialis muscle, and then passes between its tendon and radius to pierce the fascia on the dorsal aspect. It branches to give digital branches just above the styloid process of the radius that pass superficially over the anatomic "snuff box". The nerve is located 3 cm proximal to the radial styloid, when wrist is slightly dorsiflexed. It is at this site the nerve can be easily accessed for biopsy.

Radial nerve block requires more extensive infiltration because of less predictable anatomic course and division into multiple, smaller cutaneous branches.[29]

Digital Nerve Supply

The sensory innervation of digits comes from palmar and dorsal digital nerves that run medially and laterally in the fingers. The palmar digital nerves are branches of ulnar and median nerves, they supply sensation to the volar skin, interphalangeal joints of all five digits and also the dorsal distal aspect of the finger, including the fingertip and nail bed. The ulnar side of the fourth finger receives innervation from the dorsal nerve. The dorsal nerves originate from the radial and ulnar nerves. They innervate the nail beds of the thumb and

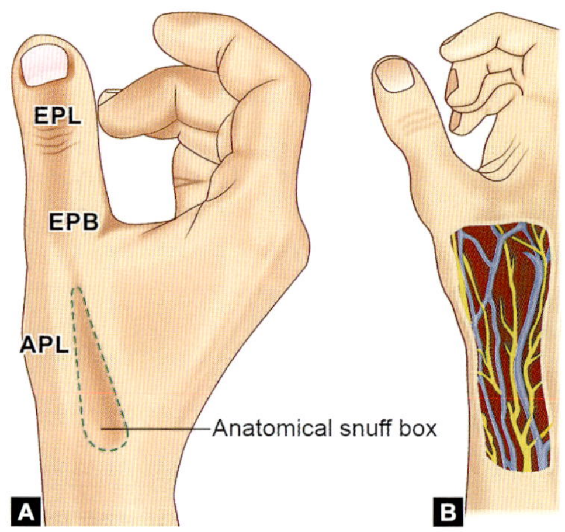

Figs. 20A and B: Location of radial nerve in anatomical snuff box at the level of radial styloid and location of radial cutaneous nerve that runs along the radial border of forearm (It is located 3 cm proximal to the radial styloid for nerve biopsy).
(APL: abductor pollicis longus; EPB: extensor pollicis brevis; EPL: extensor pollicis longus)

small fingers, as well as the dorsal aspect of all five fingers up to the distal interphalangeal joints **(Figs. 20 and 21)**.

The hand has rich blood supply, derived from superficial and deep palmar arch system formed by the radial and ulnar arteries. The superficial palmar arch lies directly deep to the palmar fascia. It gives rise to the volar common digital arteries and interosseous arteries. In distal palm common digital arteries bifurcate into the proper digital arteries. In the palm, the arteries lie volar to the corresponding nerves, a relation that is reversed in the digits. At the digits, the neurovascular bundle always lies volar to the ligament of Cleland. This pattern gives protection to the bundle and can serve as a guide for their surgical dissection. Common digital arteries arise from superficial palmar arch to form proper digital arteries at the webspaces. The palmar aspect of the digits receives arterial flow through these proper digital arteries. The dorsum of each

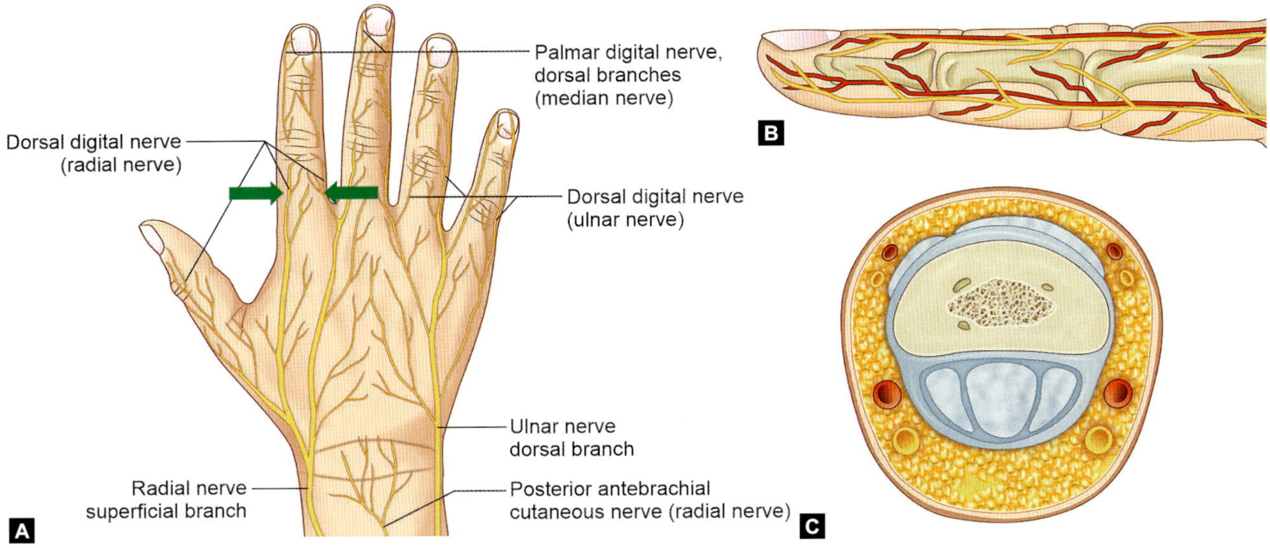

Figs. 21A to C: (A) Cutaneous nerve supply of dorsum of hands; (B) Dorsal and palmar digital arteries and nerves run together; (C) They are located alongside the phalanges at the 2, 4, 8, and 10 o'clock positions.

digit, distal to the proximal interphalangeal (PIP) joint, is vascularized by dorsal branches of the proper digital arteries. The deep palmar arch lies at the base of the metacarpals deep to the flexor tendons. It is the major blood supply to the thumb and radial half of the index finger by first metacarpal artery. Veins generally follow deep arterial systems as venae comitantes. A superficial venous system also exists at the dorsum of the hand and contributes to the cephalic and basilic vein in the upper extremity.

Applied Anatomy

Knowledge of anatomy is crucial for a dermatologic surgeon. Always assess the motor and sensory status prior to surgery on hand and note any deficit. As neurovascular bundles lie together, during digital anesthesia always withdraw the plunger of syringe to ensure that a vessel has not been entered. No vessel should be ligated in hand surgeries. During infiltration anesthesia, the dorsal approach is preferred because it is less painful than the palmar approach.[30] Tourniquet is the best way to achieve hemostasis in digits. Under no circumstance should hemostasis be achieved with ligature **(Box 8)**.

BOX 8: Surgical anatomic considerations of hand.

- Plan excisions, by keeping in mind the loose dorsal skin and fascia of the hand that becomes tight on full flexion. Avoid undue tension on wound edges or else it can cause wound dehiscence, unsightly scarring, and contractures
- The surgical incisions must be along relaxed skin tension lines and creases to minimize skin contractures. Palmar incisions must be parallel to flexion creases or at angle of 45° or less to avoid functionally bad, painful thick scars. Transverse dorsal incisions are preferred on the dorsum of the hand. Avoid longitudinal cuts on digits that may impair joint mobility. Curvilinear lazy "S" incisions over the dorsal surface of the digits not only prevents scar contracture but also minimizes the risk of injury to longitudinal structures of the digit[21]
- Dorsal surface of the hand has less fat and veins lie superficially, moreover extensor tendons run just under the thin skin and are therefore at risk from both scalpel and cryosurgery. Punch biopsies must be safely performed in this area by applying pressure to penetrate the skin and later on not to put too much downward pressure to reach the subcutaneous tissue and this minimizes injury to underlying vessels
- As the palmar skin is inelastic and is fixed to palmar fascia and positioned on the concave side, it is more prone for contractures. Hence excisions on palms may prove impossible to close, it must be handled only by a suitably trained specialist
- Biopsy should be deeper as the palmar skin is thick. Superficial biopsy reveals only thick stratum corneum. The flexor tendons are close to the skin of palm and also there is no laxity
- Deep dermal sutures are usually impossible to use as there is no depth to the dermis. In addition, although the epidermis may be very tough, the skin is actually torn very easily by a tightly pulled suture. Sutures need to be left for longer duration to ensure adequate healing making stitch marks more visible[31]
- Plane of neurotoxin injection is into deep dermis, and it should be avoided in subcutaneous tissue as it causes diffusion into intrinsic muscles of the hand causing weakness. The needle should be at an oblique angle as perpendicular injections can result in back flow from the injection tract because of thick skin

FOOT

The foot is a part of the body which is in regular contact with the ground and serves important function of locomotion. Plantar skin is unique in several ways. It is markedly thickened and glabrous with numerous eccrine glands and absent apocrine and pilosebaceous units. The only relevant anatomic landmark, pertaining to cutaneous surgery is highlighted.

Surface Anatomy

The foot has dorsal and the plantar aspects with five toes numbered from medial to lateral. Toes are subdivided into distal, middle, and proximal phalanges. The foot can be divided into the forefoot, midfoot, and hindfoot. The important joint landmarks are ankle joint, distal interphalangeal joints, PIP joints, and the metatarsal phalangeal (MP) **(Figs. 22A and B)**.

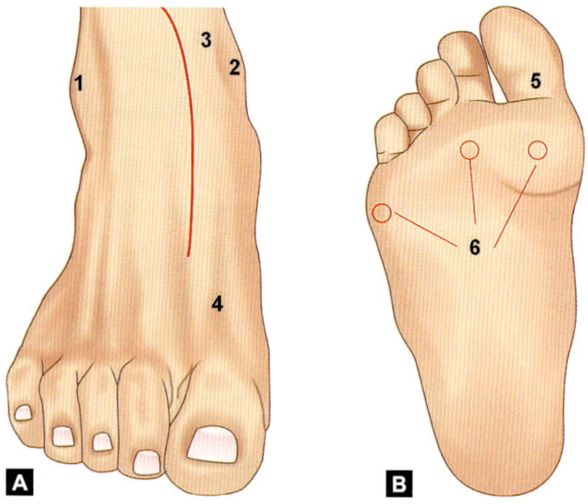

Figs. 22A and B: Surface anatomy of foot. (1) Lateral malleoli, (2) Medial malleoli, (3) Tibialis anterior, (4) Extensor hallucis longus tendon, (5) Ball of great toe. Red line indicates dorsalis pedis artery, (6) Head of metatarsal bone.

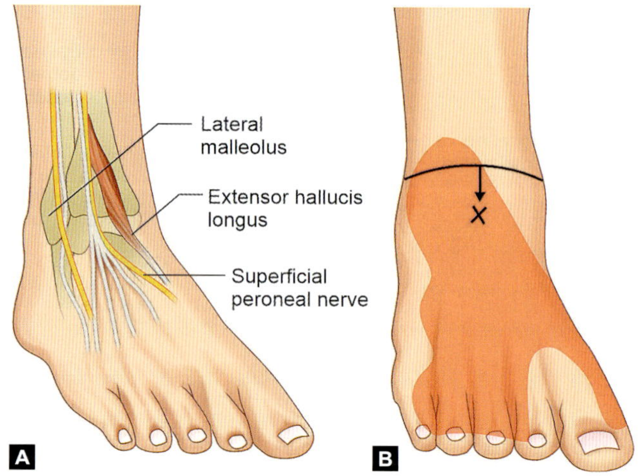

Figs. 23A and B: Location of superficial peroneal nerve and its sensory distribution, it lies in between the midpoint of medial malleolus and lateral malleolus. It is localized by palpating the extensor hallucis longus tendon and the lateral malleolus.

Skin of the plantar and the dorsal foot varies tremendously, in terms of thickness, and amount of subcutaneous fat. The plantar skin is thicker, tighter, and more fixed than the dorsal skin. It is particularly thick at ball of big toe and heel. The plantar skin has a well-developed stratum corneum with many sweat glands. The superficial fascia has abundant fibrous fatty tissue and is firmly attached to the underlying deep fascia by connective tissue septa. The cutaneous nerves and vessels lie within superficial fascia. The plantar aspect of the foot is well-vascularized.[32]

Musculature

In general, the muscles of the leg (and the foot and ankle) are divided into the anterior group of extensor muscles (dorsiflex ankle), posterior group of flexor muscles, and a lateral group of muscles (eversion of foot) derived from extensors. Plantar muscles of foot consist of intrinsic muscles of hallux and minimus, lumbricals, interossei, and short digital flexors. The tendons of the muscles are bound down by localized thickenings of the deep fascia, forming retinacular bands that prevent bowstringing of the tendons. The tendons that cross ankle joint are deflected from a straight course and held down by retinacula.

Vascular Supply

The dorsalis pedis and plantar arteries are main arterial supplies to the foot. The posterior tibial artery terminates as medial and lateral plantar arteries. The lateral plantar arteries continue as plantar arch, it gives off three perforating and four plantar metatarsal branches and numerous other branches that supply skin, fascia, and muscles of the sole. The blood supply to skin of feet is by perforating musculocutaneous arteries and direct cutaneous blood vessels. The perforating musculocutaneous arteries supply muscle and overlying skin whereas, the direct cutaneous vessels supply specific and larger areas of the skin and end in subdermal plexus. Thus, the subdermal arterial plexus forms the major blood supply to the skin, and it is important to know that any area of skin is not solely dependent on one artery. This is also responsible for tiny skin bleeders encountered during skin surgery. Venous blood drains the entire thickness of dermis into the subdermal venous plexus. Plantar and dorsal digital veins arise from plexuses and unite into four plantar veins. These connect by perforating veins with dorsal veins and continue to form the deep plantar venous arch, which accompanies the plantar arterial arch. From the venous arch, medial, and lateral plantar veins run with their corresponding arteries, communicate with the great and small saphenous veins and form the posterior tibial veins behind the medial malleolus.

Sensory Innervation

Motor and sensory innervation to the foot is supplied by five nerves. The dorsal aspect of the foot is innervated by three nerves (superficial peroneal, deep peroneal, and saphenous nerves) that run on the anterior side of lower leg and ankle. The volar aspect of the foot is innervated by two nerves (posterior tibial and sural nerves) that run on posterolateral aspect of ankle.

Superficial peroneal nerve innervates most of the dorsum of the foot and the dorsal aspect of each of the toes and web-spaces, with the exception of the lateral portion of the great toe and the medial side of the second toe, and corresponding webspace. The nerve passes subcutaneously on anterolateral side of ankle. The superficial peroneal nerve (L4-S1) is located lateral to the extensor digitorum longus **(Figs. 23A and B)**.

The deep peroneal nerve (L4-L5) is located deeper in the ankle, lateral and slightly behind the extensor hallucis longus, it extends the toes. It supplies lateral portion of the

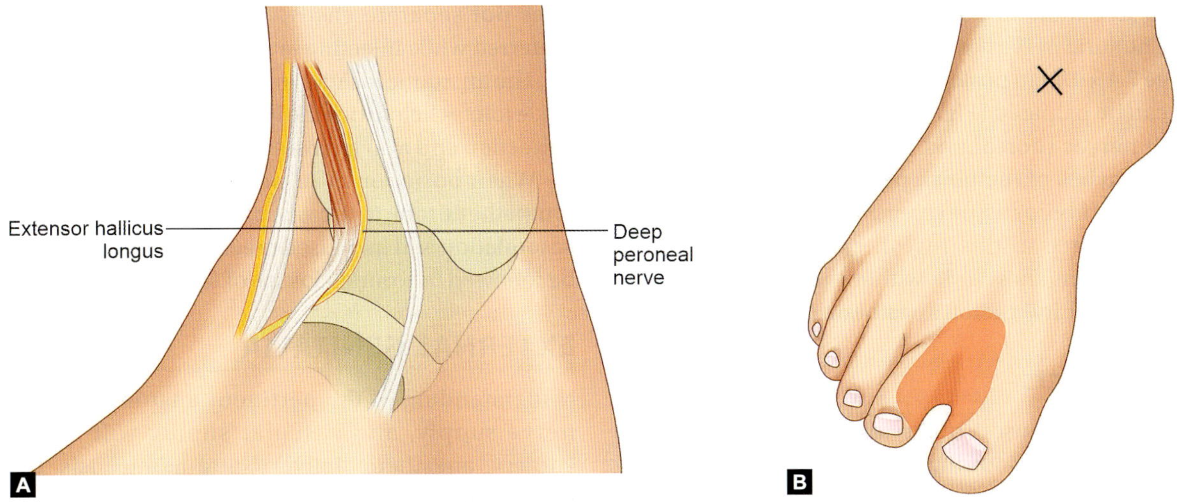

Figs. 24A and B: Location of deep peroneal nerve and its sensory distribution. It runs lateral to the dorsalis pedis artery.

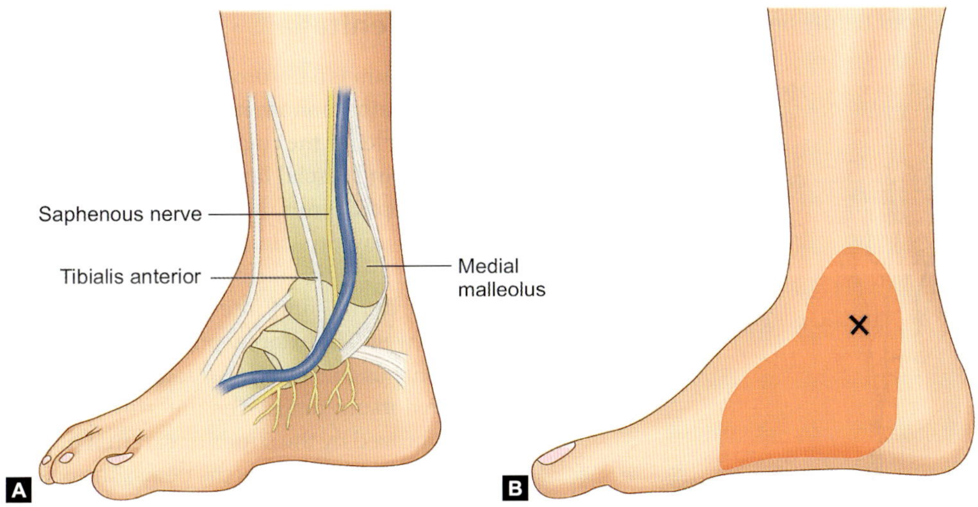

Figs. 25A and B: Location of saphenous nerve and its sensory distribution. It is located anterior to the medial malleolus.

great toe and medial side of second digit, as well as the first webspace. This area is referred as "flip-flop" region because it innervates the area surrounding the thong of a sandal. It can be located by dorsiflexing foot and great toe and it lies between anterior tibial tendon and the extensor hallucis longus tendon approximately 1 cm superior to the medial malleolus **(Figs. 24A and B)**.

The saphenous nerve (L3-L4) is just anterior to the medial malleolus alongside of the saphenous vein, provides sensation to the skin on anteromedial side of the leg and medial side of foot. It can be located between the medial malleolus and the anterior tibial tendon **(Figs. 25A and B)**.

The posterior tibial nerve is the largest in the ankle and branches into the medial and lateral plantar nerves in the foot, supplying sensation to the entire volar surface and providing motor innervation to the intrinsic muscles of foot. It runs deep to the posterior tibial artery. The nerve can be located posterolateral to the artery at the level of the medial malleolus **(Figs. 26 and 27)**.

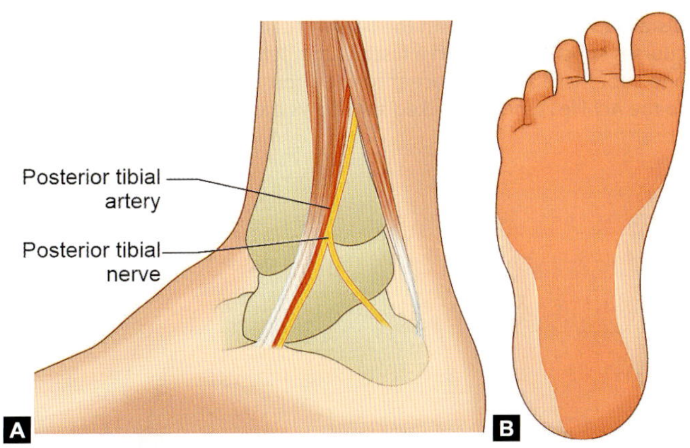

Figs. 26A and B: Location of posterior tibial nerve, it lies posterior to the artery and anterior to the Achilles tendon and its sensory distribution.

Sural Nerve

The sural nerve (S1-S2) is located superficially in subcutaneous plane between the lateral malleolus and the Achilles tendon.

It supplies sensation on posterolateral leg, lateral foot, and fifth toe. The sural nerve has relatively constant course and is on average 7.4 × 0.1 cm posterior to the distal tip of the fibula, where it can be palpated **(Fig. 27)**.[33,34]

Digital nerves (dorsal and ventral) of the toes are the terminal branches of the tibial, peroneal, and sural nerves. The presence of fibrous tissue (prevents spread of anesthetics) and limited space in this region cannot inject enough volume to achieve anesthesia within the toe, hence blocks are preferred over infiltration anesthesia **(Figs. 28A and B)**.

Applied Aspects

The knowledge on sensory innervations aids in giving ankle or digital anesthesia. Knowing vascular anatomy of the foot is important to avoid these vessels during administration of local anesthesia to avoid intravascular injections.

The injections on plantar region are painful and difficult due to thick, sensitive, and tightly bound skin to fascia that does not separate easily. Therefore, dorsal approach is preferred while injecting into plantar region.

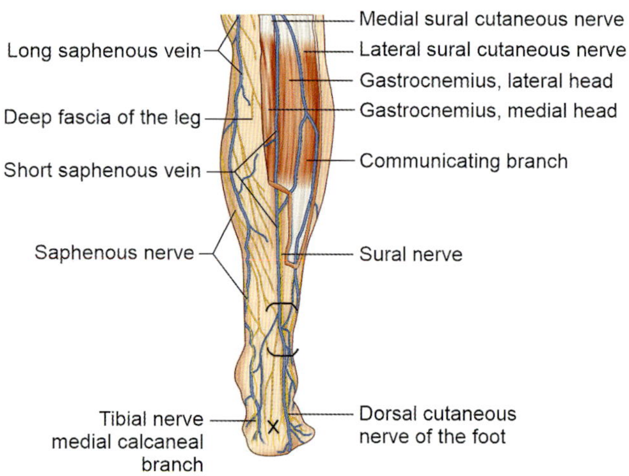

Fig. 27: The sural nerve pierces the deep (crural) fascia in the proximal calf distally to the junction with the lateral cutaneous sural nerve. Distally, it courses subcutaneously in a fascial sling between the deep crural fascia and superficial fascia adjacent to the short saphenous vein and lateral to the Achilles tendon. Marked site shows the site for sural nerve biopsy.

The anatomic location of the sural nerve at the level of the ankle joint is helpful for the incision placement and soft-tissue dissection and also to access it for biopsy.

When posterior tibial nerve is blocked, there is loss of sympathetic tone to the vascular supply of the foot leading to vasodilation and increased bleeding during surgery. Rules to be followed in wound closure of feet are given in **Box 9**.

EXTERNAL GENITALIA

Understanding of the pertinent anatomy of genital skin, nerve supply, and vascular supply will facilitate safe surgery, anesthetic delivery, and hemostasis. Knowledge of the lymphatic drainage of genitalia is also necessary for appropriate management of malignancies.

Male Genitalia

The scrotum is a fibromuscular pouch. Scrotal skin is unique as it contains smooth muscle called dartos muscle, which is responsible for the rugosity of scrotal skin. The skin, smooth muscle, and fascial layer cover the contents of the scrotum (testes, epididymis, and the cord). Its penile part does not contain any muscle **(Figs. 30A and B)**. The scrotal and perineal skin has a uniquely rich blood supply. Branches of the external and internal pudendal arteries supply the scrotal wall. The external pudendal arteries (two on each side) continue as the anterior scrotal arteries, and send branches to the dorsum penis. The anterior surface of the scrotum is vascularized by the superior external pudendal artery which also supplies the base of the penis. The posterior surface of the scrotum is arterialized by the superficial perineal artery which is a branch of the internal pudendal artery. If these vessels are occluded, the viability of the scrotal skin and perineum is jeopardized. The penile skin, which is vascularized by the dorsolateral and ventrolateral branches of the superficial external pudendal artery, has cross-connections with scrotal

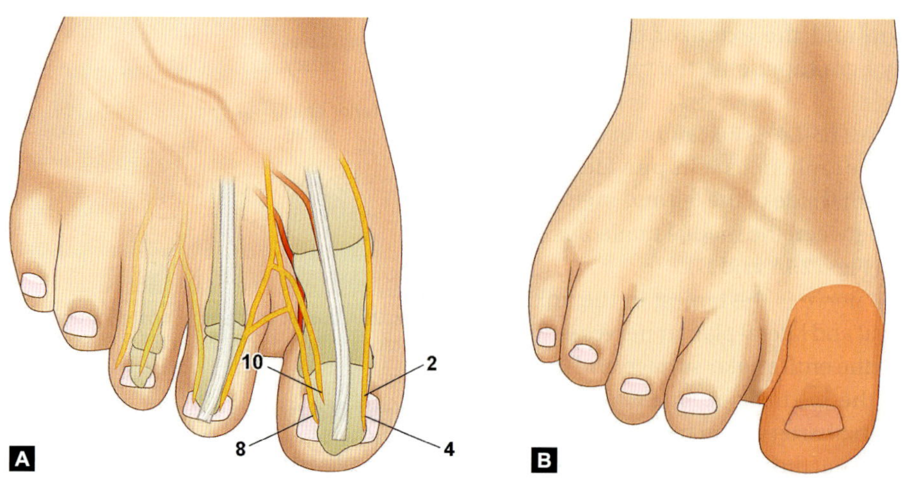

Figs. 28A and B: Dorsal and ventral digital nerves and sensory supply.

branches of the internal pudendal artery. General venous drainage of the scrotum is through pelvic venous plexuses that empty into the internal iliac vein and the anterior scrotal veins. Lymphatics of the scrotum drain into inguinal lymph nodes.

The scrotal skin and dartos muscle are supplied posteriorly by the posterior scrotal nerves and branches of pudendal nerve. Its anterior and upper part is supplied by ilioinguinal and genitor femoral nerves. The ilioinguinal nerve originates from the lumbar plexus and descends through the superficial inguinal ring to form the anterior scrotal nerves. The genitofemoral nerve supplies both the skin and the cremaster muscle.

The penis consists of a root and a body. The body is formed by the union of corpus cavernosa and corpus spongiosum. The two corpora are bounded by a thick fascia called the tunica albuginea. Buck's fascia, a tough sheath binds all the components. The skin surrounding the body of the penis is very loose and becomes redundant at prepuce but is immobile over corona and glans. The penis is innervated by somatic and autonomic nerves. The dorsal nerve of the penis is one of two terminal branches of pudendal nerve, other branch reaches the scrotum. The dorsal arteries of the penis lie lateral to the deep dorsal vein. All these components form the dorsal neurovascular bundle of penis.

BOX 9: Rules to be followed in wound closure in feet.

- Place incisions along relaxed skin tension lines and long flexion and extension creases and plantar crease lines **(Fig. 29)**. Do not injure neurovascular bundles of the foot as they are relatively superficial because of less subcutaneous fat
- Follow nerve pathways in the overlying skin to avoid damaging them. Curved or oblique incisions can compensate for the resulting scar contraction
- Avoid placing incisions along bony prominences or weight-bearing surfaces, as it causes more pain
- Adequate hemostasis is by means of tourniquet to keep a bloodless field. Ligation of vascular structures should be avoided as much as possible
- There should be little or no undermining or angled dissection until the subcutaneous layer is completely separated. This will preserve blood supply to the skin
- Avoid inadvertent trapping of underlying structures while suturing. Dog ear commonly occurs on the dorsal foot, and they remodel well, hence, these redundancies are not corrected

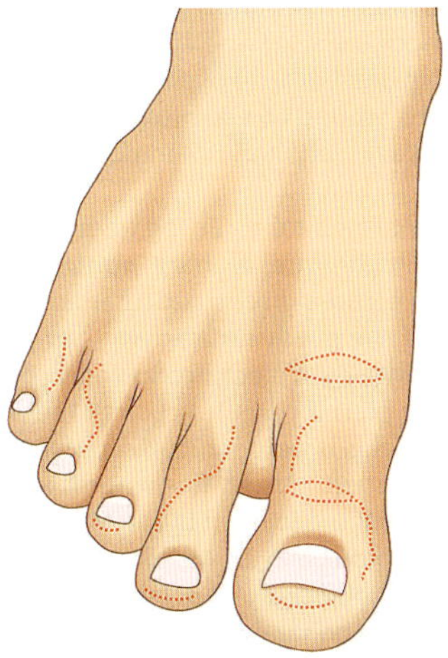

Fig. 29: Excision line planning on foot based on relaxed skin tension line and joints movements.

Female External Genitalia

The external genitalia consist of the mons pubis, labia majora and minora, vestibule, and clitoris. The mons pubis consists of skin and subcutaneous tissue overlying the pubic symphysis.[35,36] The labia majora are prominent longitudinal folds of skin supported by underlying fat. They are homologous to the male scrotum.[37] The skin overlying the outer aspect is pigmented and hair bearing.[38] The labia are united anteriorly and posteriorly at the commissures **(Figs. 31A and B)**.

The labia minora, smaller folds within the pudendal cleft of the labia majora, surround the vaginal vestibule. Posteriorly, the labia minora unite as the frenulum of the

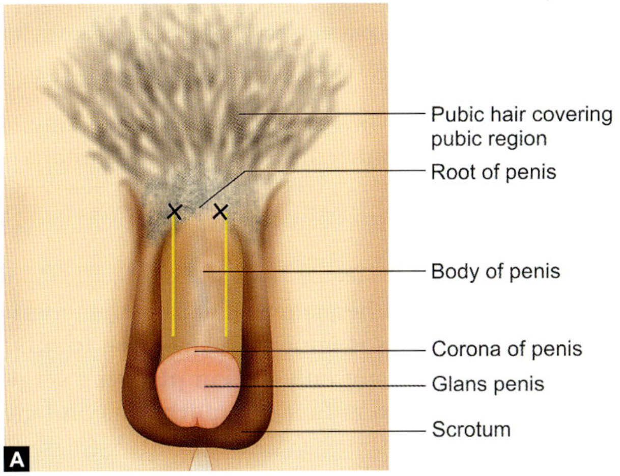

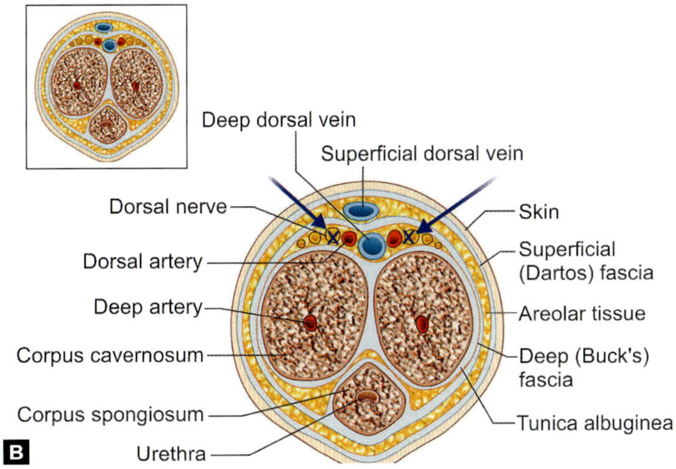

Figs. 30A and B: Male genital anatomy and applied aspects. It shows the location of dorsal penile nerves beneath Buck's fascia at the 1 and 11 o'clock positions.

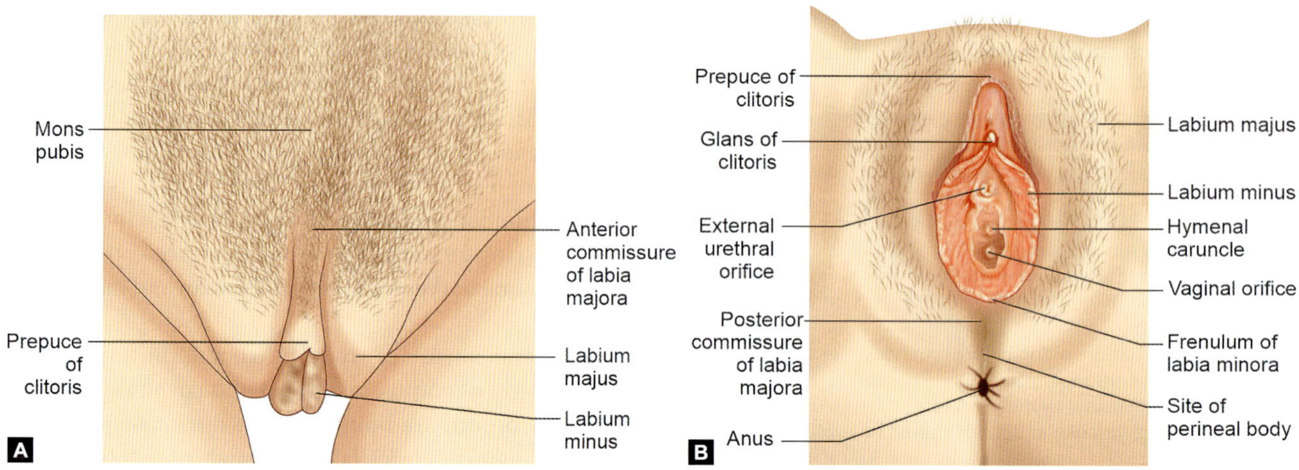

Figs. 31A and B: Female external genitalia. (A) Anterior view; (B) Anteroinferior view (lithotomy position).

labia (fourchette). Anteriorly, the labia split into the superior (lateral) and inferior (medial) portions. The superior portions pass above the clitoris to form the prepuce, and the inferior portions pass below the clitoris, forming the frenulum of the clitoris. The clitoris is the homologous of the male penis.

The labia majora are composed essentially of two layers: Skin and subcutaneous tissue. The skin that covers the lateral face is thick with hyperpigmentation and thick curly hair, with numerous sebaceous and sweat glands. The medial surface is instead covered by a thinner skin, translucent with a minor presence of hairs, of rosy color until it becomes a mucosa. The labia minora are two skinfolds, flattened, free of fat, medial in respect to the labia majora, and delimiting the vaginal vestibule, and they are separated from the interlabial grooves. The anterior extremity runs anteriorly toward the clitoris and the posterior extremity runs toward the perineum.

The blood supply and drainage of the external female genitalia occur mostly via branches of the internal iliac vessels. The majority of the venous drainage follows the same pattern, terminating in the internal iliac vein. Portions of anterolateral aspects of labia majora drain into external iliac vein. The lymphatics of the female genitalia drain to both superficial and deep nodes. The lymphatics from the lower portion of the vagina join those from the vestibule and labia to drain into the superficial inguinal lymph nodes. The perianal region, extending up the anal canal to the dentate line is drained by superficial femoral nodes. Proximal to the dentate line, drainage is by deeper pelvic lymph nodes.[39]

The nerve supply of the female external genitalia also comes from two distinct sources. The ilioinguinal (L1) and genitofemoral (L1, L2) nerves supply the skin and subcutaneous tissue overlying the mons pubis and anterolateral portions of the labia majora. The remainder of the female genitalia is supplied by the pudendal nerve (S2, S3, and S4).

BOX 10: Surgical anatomic considerations of genitalia.

- Small procedures on the external genitalia can be performed with local infiltration of anesthetic, larger procedures require blocks. As a rule, it is best to avoid the use of epinephrine when injecting the penis. Avoid direct infiltration of the foreskin, as this can rarely result in tissue necrosis
- Scrotal skin is thin and because of rich vascularity, bleeds profusely, always sutures the wounds on scrotum. It heals excellently. Always dress the wounds as reactionary bleeding can occur to avoid patient getting panic
- Biopsy on external genitalia can be adequately sampled using a punch or snip technique. A sharp punch tool combined with adequate tension on the skin and subcutaneous tissue helps ensure least distortion of the overlying epidermis or mucosa. Hemostasis can be achieved with light electrocoagulation or pressure
- Sutures should be placed perpendicular to the natural skin tension lines. In the penis, this is perpendicular to the long axis to prevent traction during erection. Absorbable sutures are preferred
- The Bartholin's glands are located bilaterally at the base of the labia minora and drain through 2–2.5 cm long ducts that empty into the vestibule at about 4 o'clock and 8 o'clock positions.[40] The glands are usually size of a pea and rarely exceed 1 cm. They are not palpable except in the presence of disease or infection
- The aging process and, more importantly, the endless variation in the anatomy of the labia minora, may generate concern in women when evaluating the appearance of their own external genitalia. An increasing number of women seek to improve the shape or size of their labia minora or majora and they should be approached with sensitivity and extreme professionalism

The surgical anatomic considerations of genitalia are summarized in **Box 10**.

CONCLUSION

A good understanding of the anatomy, circulation, innervation, function, and cosmesis is important before performing a surgical procedure. It not only aids in planning surgical procedures but also to reduce complications and gives optimum results.

PART B: ANATOMY OF FACE

KEY MESSAGES

- Knowledge of facial anatomy is particularly important for facial aesthetic surgeons for giving minimal scar to the patient.
- Danger ones of face should be dealt with utmost care while performing surgeries to prevent any complications.
- Periorificial areas should be operated without any tension to prevent any visible deformities.

INTRODUCTION

The shape and structure of face are formed by the underlying facial bones. The facial soft tissues have five layers—skin, subcutaneous layer, superficial musculoaponeurotic system (SMAS), retaining ligaments with spaces, and periosteum with deep fascia. This section of regional anatomy discusses the applied aspects of surgical anatomy.

FACIAL UNITS

Gonzales-Ulloa[41] first described the regional aesthetic units of the face and emphasized the need for restoring facial skin units in complete regions and to put an end to the "patch" work in order to give better aesthetic outcomes in facial reconstruction surgeries. The facial subunit principle divides the facial skin into subunits that are grouped by skin color, texture, thickness, mobility, quantity of subcutaneous fat, and hair distribution. Each subunit affects the aesthetics of surrounding units. So, creating cutaneous grafts of the same size, shape, and thickness as the region on where the repair is being done should be kept in mind while operating on face.[42]

Face is divided into seven subunits **(Fig. 32)**:

1. Forehead
2. Periocular unit
3. Nose unit
4. Cheek
5. Lips
6. Chin
7. Ear

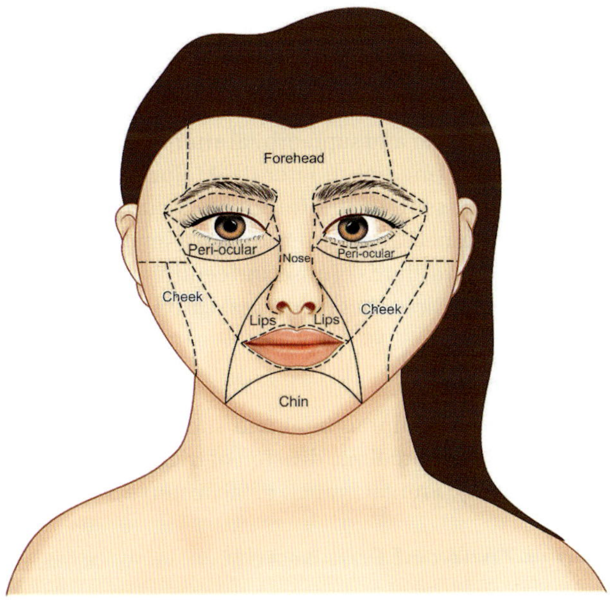

Fig. 32: Cosmetic units of face.

Contours

Convex in the center and concave on the sides.

Subunits of Forehead

- *Horizontal:* Upper and lower half subunits
- *Vertical:*
  - Central/median subunit (between medial ends of eyebrows)
  - Paramedian subunit (medial eyebrows to lateral orbital rim)
  - Lateral subunit (lateral orbital rim to zygomatic arch)

FOREHEAD

The forehead is the most visible and cosmetically prominent area of face. It is a unique elongated hairless continuation of the scalp, bounded superiorly by hairline and inferiorly by eyebrows.

Boundaries[43]

- Forehead is bounded by anterior hairline superiorly and nasion, the glabella, and the eyebrows inferiorly.
- The lateral ends of the eyebrows determine the lateral borders of the main forehead.
- Temple and temporal hairline forming the lateral most extent.

Layers of Forehead Skin[44] (Five Layers)

1. Skin—thickest at center (1.08 mm) and thins out superiorly and laterally
2. Subcutaneous layer
3. Galea aponeurotica
4. Frontalis muscle
5. Periosteum

The first three layers: skin, subcutaneous tissue, and galea aponeurotica are firmly attached and form a single thick rigid unit which freely glides over the pericranium. The galea aponeurotica splits to ensheathe the frontalis muscle.

Relaxed Skin Tension Lines[45]

The deep, horizontal forehead lines, relaxed skin tension lines (RSTLs) are result of tight attachment of subcutaneous fat, galea aponeurotica, and frontalis muscle by fibrous septa. The lines run horizontally curving down in a vertical direction laterally. At the glabellar region, they are vertically oriented **(Fig. 33)**.

Blood Supply

Highly vascular area: Supplied by a rich network of anastomoses by branches of external carotid artery—dorsal nasal, supratrochlear and supraorbital arteries and superficial temporal artery (medial to lateral). Majority of skin and subcutaneous tissue of the forehead is supplied by the branches of external carotid artery except a small area around the eyes, upper two-thirds of nose and central forehead which is supplied by the branches of internal carotid artery.

Nerve Supply

- *Sensory supply:* Supraorbital and supratrochlear nerves (branches of ophthalmic division of trigeminal nerve)
- *Motor supply:* Frontal branch of facial nerve

Danger Zones of Forehead[46]

- *Brow and glabella:* Supratrochlear artery is superficial and should be taken care of while injecting fillers in the glabellar area.
- *Temple area:* Frontotemporal branch is superficial and can be traced by Pitanguy line (from a point 0.5 cm inferior to the tragus to another point 2 cm superior to the lateral eyebrow). Alternatively, course of the temporal nerve can be traced by drawing a line from the lowest point of the earlobe to the lateral brow, with another line originating at the tragus and terminating at the lateral canthus bisecting the original line **(Fig. 34)**.

Applied Aspects

- The anatomical boundaries of forehead must be sought to disguise the resulting scars. Always aim at maintaining boundaries. Wound closure along RSTL will lessen tension and results in better scars.
- Forehead skin is minimally mobile expect high tension on wound closure.
- Multiple fibrous bands traverse connective tissue layer—breaking of these bands during surgery can lead to heavy bleed, hence undermining should be done at subgaleal level an avascular plane.
- Closure in two-layers with re-approximation of galea minimizes tension on transcutaneous sutures.
- Better healing and less risk of necrosis due to rich vasculature
- Forehead anesthesia is easily achieved via nerve blocks.
- Know the danger areas as superficial structures prone for damage.
- Avoid infection of subgaleal space.
- The skin, subcutaneous tissue, and galea aponeurotica glide as a single unit over the underlying pericranium by the layer of loose areolar connective tissue enabling it to be mobile.

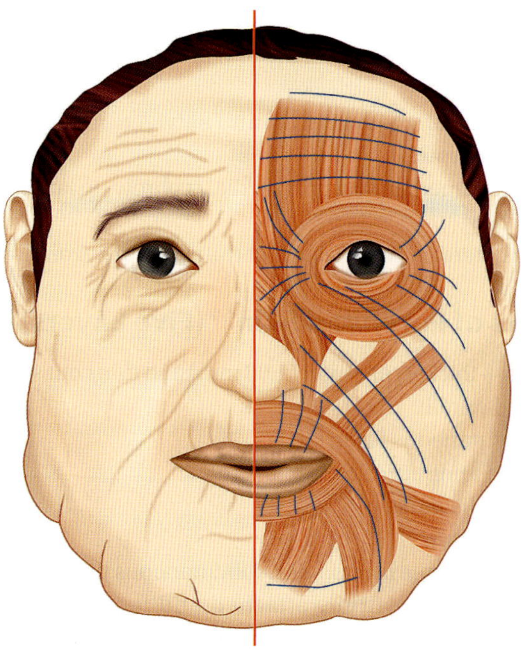

Fig. 33: Relaxed skin tension lines on face.

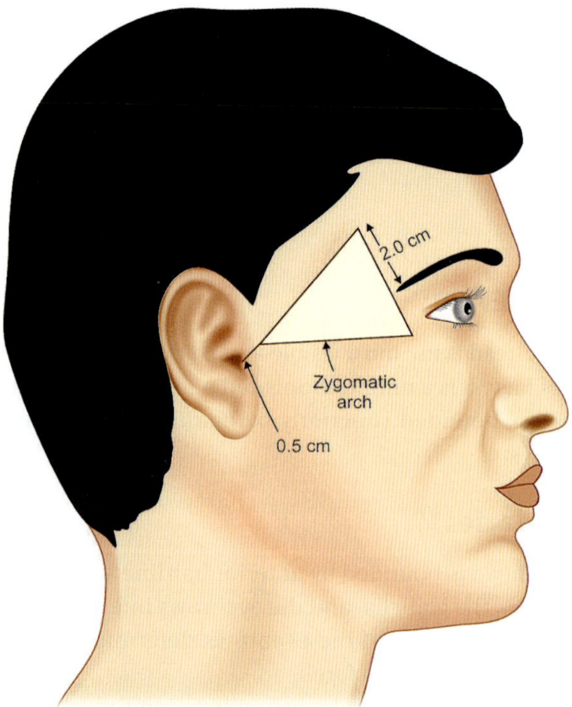

Fig. 34: Dangerous area where frontotemporal branch is at risk.

- In the temporal area, the loose connections with underlying temporalis fascia enhance skin mobility of lateral forehead and temporal region and helps as tissue reservoir for local flaps.
- As forehead skin is nonmalleable, risk of dog ear post-punch excision is common; planning elliptical excision along RSTL gives good results.

PERIOCULAR UNIT

The eyes are the most important aesthetic units of the face. If the eye region appears bright and fresh, the person has an aura of youth, health, and vitality. The palpebral aperture between the upper and lower eyelid margins measures 28–30 mm horizontally and 10–12 mm vertically.

Boundaries

- The upper eyelid is bounded superiorly by inferior aspect of the brow subunits, laterally by lateral orbital wall, medially by medial orbital walls, and inferiorly by gray line of the upper lid.
- The lower eyelid is bounded superiorly by gray line of the lower lid, laterally by lateral orbital wall, medially by medial orbital walls, and inferiorly by infraorbital rim.

Contours

- Upper eyelid—convex and skin is 0.38 mm thick.
- Lower eyelid—upper part is convex and lower part is concave, skin is 0.83 mm thick.

Subunits[47]

- *Upper eyelid:* Pretarsal and the upper lid fold or preseptal space
- *Lower eyelid:* Pretarsal, preseptal, and lid-cheek junction
- *Medial canthus*: Bounded by the medial orbital wall and the upper and lower lacrimal puncta
- *Lateral canthus:* It forms a triangle, beginning at the lateral palpebral angle and diverging laterally, ending at the lateral orbital rim. The limbs of this triangle are formed by the lateral orbital rim and two imaginary lines representing continuation of the ciliary margins.

The eyelids are broken down into three soft-tissue depressions at junction of the inferior orbital septum and tarsal plate, the inferior orbital rim, and the location over the zygomatic ligament.

Layers of Periorbital Skin

- Eyelid skin is the thinnest in the body (<1 mm) and contains sparse subcutaneous fat.
- Eyelid skin has a lamellar structure **(Tables 2 and 3)**.
- The periorbital fat pads are found posterior to the orbital septum.

TABLE 2: Lamellar structure of eyelid.

Anterior lamella	*Middle lamella*	*Posterior lamella*
• Skin • Orbicularis oculi muscle	• The orbital septum originates at the arcus marginalis along the orbital rim separating the two lamellae • Continuous with the periosteum of the orbit • Retains the periorbital fat within the orbit	• Tarsal plate • Lid retractors • Conjunctiva

TABLE 3: Anatomy of upper and lower eyelid.

Upper eyelid	*Lower eyelid*
Central and nasal fat pads	Central, nasal, and lateral fat pads
Orbital septum separates the central and nasal fat	• Inferior oblique muscle separates the nasal and central fat • Central and lateral fat by a septum and fascial extension from Lockwood's ligament (the arcuate expansion)

Relaxed Skin Tension Lines[45]

The RSTLs radiate around under the eye and then curve down around the cheek. They run horizontally along the upper and lower eyelids and lateral to the eye RSTLs run perpendicularly to each other. The classic "crow's feet" lines radiate out from the lateral canthus.

Blood Supply

Rich vascular supply and many anastomoses are present between the upper and lower eyelids. Eyelids are supplied from the facial system (external carotid artery) and the orbital system (internal carotid artery).

- Upper eyelid gets supply from superior marginal arcade derived from ophthalmic artery (internal carotid artery).
- Lower eyelid gets blood supply from inferior marginal artery derived from angular artery that is a branch of facial artery (external carotid artery).

Nerve Supply

Sensory supply of upper eyelid is from supraorbital, supratrochlear, and lacrimal nerve (ophthalmic division of trigeminal nerve). The medial aspect is supplied by infraorbital nerve. Lateral aspect and temple are supplied by zygomaticotemporal branch of maxillary nerve. Sensory supply of lower eyelid comes from central aspect is supplied by infraorbital nerve (maxillary division of trigeminal nerve). Lateral aspect is supplied by zygomaticotemporal branch of maxillary nerve.

Motor supply is from the superior division of facial nerve that innervates the upper eyelids via temporal (frontal) branches and lower lids via zygomatic and buccal branches.

Applied Aspects

- Eyelid skin is thin and continuous with conjunctiva at free margins so it is important to prevent asymmetry which can lead to ectropion.
- Lesions heal excellently owing to rich blood supply. Hence excision and secondary healing of small lesions like moles gives superior results.
- Owing to rich blood supply, bruises are common hence slow infiltration of anesthesia can prevent this complication.
- Sublesional infiltration with local anesthesia (ballooning), avoids danger to tarsal plate
- Use extremely thin grafts.
- Deep incisions can inadvertently injure the orbital septum due to highly vascular retro-orbital fat.
- Scleral shields after eutectic mixture of local anesthesia (EMLA) is applied prior to scleral shield application to prevent corneal damage.
- Defects of the medial canthus should prompt suspicion for lacrimal injury.
- Subdermal undermining is preferred wherever necessary, however small excisions do not require undermining.
- Important points to note during upper eye lid blepharoplasty:
  - The nasal fat pad is fibrous and pale (white color) must be differentiated from prolapsed lacrimal gland which is firm, pinkish-gray color, and glandular structure. Its injury can result in dry eye syndrome.
  - The medial palpebral artery is located in the medial fat pad can lead to significant bleeding intraoperatively.
  - Full-thickness defects that are <25% of the lid width can be converted to a wedge with primary closure.
  - Principles of upper blepharoplasty incision design should be followed to maintain the relationship of the 3 arcs of the upper eyelid–brow subunit.
- Important points to note during lower eyelid blepharoplasty:
  - Inferior oblique muscle should be identified as aggressive fat transposition techniques that suture the fat below the rim can lead to diplopia due to impaired inferior oblique function.
  - Preserve the arcuate expansion of Lockwood's ligament to maintain lateral lid support.

NOSE (NASAL UNIT)

Boundaries

- *Superior:* Nasion
- *Lateral:* Junction of the cheeks and nasal dorsal side walls
- *Inferior:* Alar groove and columella

Contours

Nasal unit has a convex contour.

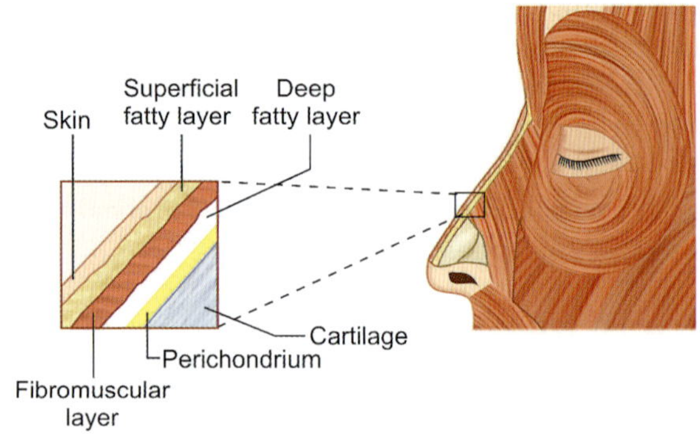

Fig. 35: Layers of skin of nasal subunit.

Subunits[48]

There are nine subunits of clinical significance in the nasal unit:

- The upper two-thirds include dorsum, right, and left dorsal side walls.
- The lower third includes tip, right and left alar side walls, right and left alar bases, and columella.

Layers of Skin of Nose[49] (Fig. 35)

The nasal envelope (SSTE—skin and soft tissue envelope) of nose is made up of five layers:

1. *Skin:* The nasal skin of proximal dorsum, nasal root, and side walls is the thinnest (0.77 mm), less sebaceous and more mobile. The nasal tip (1.25 mm) and alar lobules are thicker and has more sebaceous skin whereas nasal infratip, soft triangles, alar margins, and columella are thin, non-sebaceous, not pliable, and fixed to the underlying cartilage structure.
2. *Superficial fatty layer:* It consists of adipose tissue. This layer is tightly attached to the overlying skin with vertically oriented fibrous septae. It is thickest at the nasal radix and thinnest at the rhinion.
3. *Fibromuscular layer:* It forms the core part of nose and consists of nasal SMAS along with a superficial fatty layer. It allows movement of the nasal envelope to offer blood supply and to maintain the thickness of the skin. It also integrates and transmits the contractile force of nasal muscles.
4. *Deep fatty layer:* This layer lacks major vessels and fibrous septa.
5. *Periosteum or perichondrium (longitudinal fibrous sheath):* The fifth layer consists of fused perichondrium or periosteum with fibrous tissue.

Relaxed Skin Tension Lines[45]

Relaxed skin tension line is oriented horizontally on the nose.

Blood Supply

The superficial blood supply of the nose is originated from ophthalmic artery (internal carotid artery), facial artery (external carotid artery), and internal maxillary artery. These arteries form vascular arcades in different patterns as it reaches the nasal periphery. Blood is supplied as dual perfusion or split perfusion at the center of the nose.

The Kiesselbach's plexus (Little's area) refers to anastomoses of terminal branches of vessels at anterior portion of nasal septum. These are septal branches of anterior ethmoidal artery, sphenopalatine artery, and greater palatine artery.

Nerve Supply[50]

See **Table 4** for sensory supply of nose.

Danger Zones[46]

Dangerous triangle comprises the lower part of nose, upper lip, and adjacent area. Any infection or injury around nose can readily spread to cavernous sinus thrombosis due to absence of valves in the venous tributaries in this area **(Fig. 36)**.

TABLE 4: Sensory supply of nose.

Nerve	*Source*	*Site of innervation*
Supratrochlear and infratrochlear nerves	Ophthalmic division of trigeminal nerve	Base of nose and some parts of lateral walls
External nasal nerve	Anterior ethmoidal nerve	Nasal tip
Infraorbital nerve	Maxillary nerve	Lateral wall of lower nose, columella, and nasal vestibule

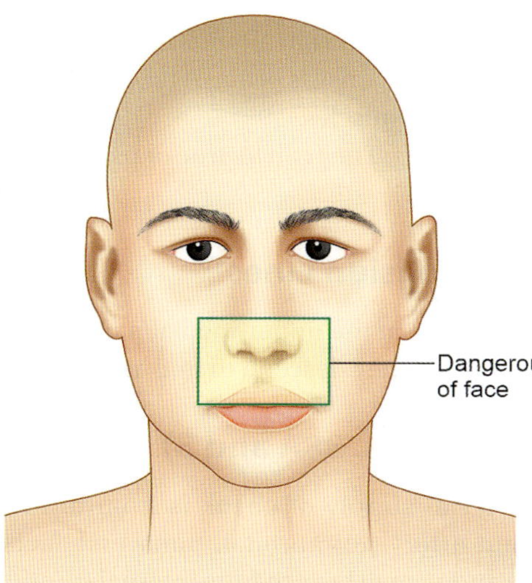

Fig. 36: Dangerous area of face.

Applied Aspects

- Damage to the nasal SMAS or deep dermis may result in irreversible complication due to formation of a severe and irregular scar at the nasal envelope.
- Dissection at the level of deep fatty layer helps to maintain the integrity of nasal envelope and reduces the risk of damaging the neurovascular bundle.
- Highly sebaceous skin is predisposed to inflammation, dehiscence, and more visible incision lines. Hence any reconstructive technique becomes less successful on highly sebaceous nose. It is good on less sebaceous areas of nose.
- Punch excisions on nose can be left to heal with secondary intention with good results.
- It is safe to dissect under nasal SMAS during the operation because nasal circulatory system runs within or above the SMAS.
- Skin over dorsum and lateral aspect is mobile and therefore forms the tissue reservoir for skin flap to cover a nasal tip wound.
- An incision on the bridge of nose should be horizontal/oblique and if placed vertically can lead to depression in nasal profile.
- Owing to variation in thickness and contour in nose, elliptical excisions often heal with standing cone deformity, hence 4:1 is preferred over 3:1. Reverse beveling during primary closure gives good flush approximation and superior cosmesis.
- Tip and ala—subcutaneous fat is interwoven with dense collagen network and so collection of fluid, infection or local anesthetic can lead to excruciating pain.
- Ala and tip—difficult to do primary excision and closure and therefore, grafts, flaps or secondary healing are preferred.
- Lesion at ala should be cut down to the very edge of nostril.
- The undermining plane is directly above the periosteum or perichondrium and below the nasal muscle and SMAS. This subnasalis avascular space permits good hemostasis and also preserves muscle pedicle.
- Always address the three nasal layers (the internal mucosal lining, the bony and cartilaginous framework, and the soft-tissue covering) and the three-dimensional nasal topography during reconstruction.

CHEEK

Boundaries

- *Superior:* Infraorbital rims and the superior aspects of the zygomatic arches (orbital-cheek crease)
- *Lateral:* Preauricular creases
- *Inferior*: Jaw line
- *Medial*: Nasolabial and melolabial (labiomandibular) grooves and the lateral aspects of nasal dorsal side walls.

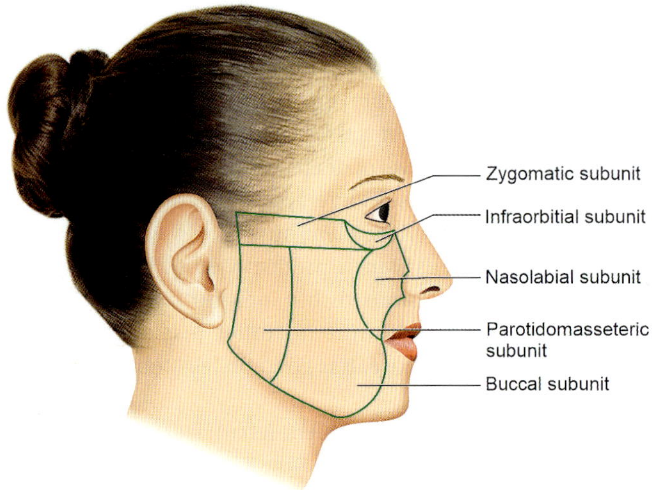

Fig. 37: Cosmetic units of cheek.

Contours

The cheek is a convex area of either side of the face constituting the largest anatomic unit of face.

Subunits (Fig. 37)

Divided into five subunits:

1. Infraorbital
2. Zygomatic
3. Nasolabial
4. Buccal subunit
5. Parotido masseteric

Zygomatic and buccal subunits are separated by the inferior border of the zygomatic arch and the anterior border of the masseter muscle.

The cheek unit encompasses the parotid gland and duct and major fat pads of the face, including the buccal and malar fat pads, and the suborbicularis oculi fat (SOOF) pads.

Layers of Skin[50]

The soft tissues and fascia are arranged in a concentric manner over the bony skeleton.

- *Skin:* It shows heterogeneity in thickness (0.6 mm—infraorbital subunit to 2.1 mm—nasolabial subunit), laxity, and quality in each of the subunits of cheek across genders.
- *Subcutaneous layer:* It consists of fat and connective tissue fibers running through it and connects SMAS with dermis. Vascular perforators run vertically as they come from deep arteries. It is very thick in the nasolabial area and thin/almost disappears at close to eyelids and lips. It is characterized by the way the fat of this layer is arranged and compartmentalized into multiple, distinct superficial fat pads (malar, nasolabial, and jowl fat pads).
- *Superficial musculoaponeurotic system and the superficial muscle layer:* It contains tendon fibers of mimic muscles attaching them to the skin and plays role in facial movement. Superficial mimic muscles of cheek consist of orbicularis oculi, levator labii superioris alaeque nasi, levator labii superioris, zygomaticus minor, zygomaticus major, risorius, platysma, and depressor anguli oris muscles.
- *Parotidomasseteric fascia:* Thin and glazed fascia lies over parotid gland posteriorly and overmasters muscle anteriorly. It is formed by continuation of deep cervical fascia. It covers the parotid duct, facial nerve branches, and transverses facial artery.
- *Buccal space:* This space is filled by buccal fat pad, the parotid duct, minor salivary glands, inconstant accessory parotid gland, motor buccal nerve (branch of facial nerve), sensory buccal nerve (mandibular branch of trigeminal nerve), facial artery and vein along with buccal artery.
- *Deep muscle layer:* It consists of masseter, buccinators, and levator anguli oris muscles.
- *Retaining ligaments:* They can be true or pseudo retaining ligaments (**Table 5**).

TABLE 5: Difference between pseudo and true retaining ligaments.

Pseudo retaining ligaments (originate from SMAS)	*True retaining ligaments (originate from periosteum)*
• Multiple and exist at sequential facial plane • Originates from dermis and attach to underlying SMAS • Strongest over forehead, eyes, nose, lips, and chin • Intermediate strength over lateral cheek and neck • Loose over medial cheek and temple	• Strongest ligament attachment • Originates from periosteum and attaches to overlying skin and muscle • Zygomaticus cutaneous ligament originates from periosteum of zygoma and mandible • Mandibular ligament arise from body of mandible and inserts inferior to depressor anguli oris (DAO)
Fasciocutaneous ligaments	*Osteocutaneous ligaments*
• Masseteric cutaneous ligament • Platysma-auricular fascia (PAF)	• Superior temporal septum • Zygomatic ligament • Zygomatic cutaneous ligament • Orbicularis retaining ligament • Lateral orbital thickening • Mandibular retaining ligament

Relaxed Skin Tension Lines[45]

They run horizontally at the upper-medial part and curve in a vertical direction as they descend to mid and lower third.

Blood Supply (Figs. 38A and B)

Majority of arterial supply of cheek is from branches of external carotid artery (infraorbital, transverse facial, and facial arteries) and a small branch from internal carotid artery (zygomaticofacial artery).

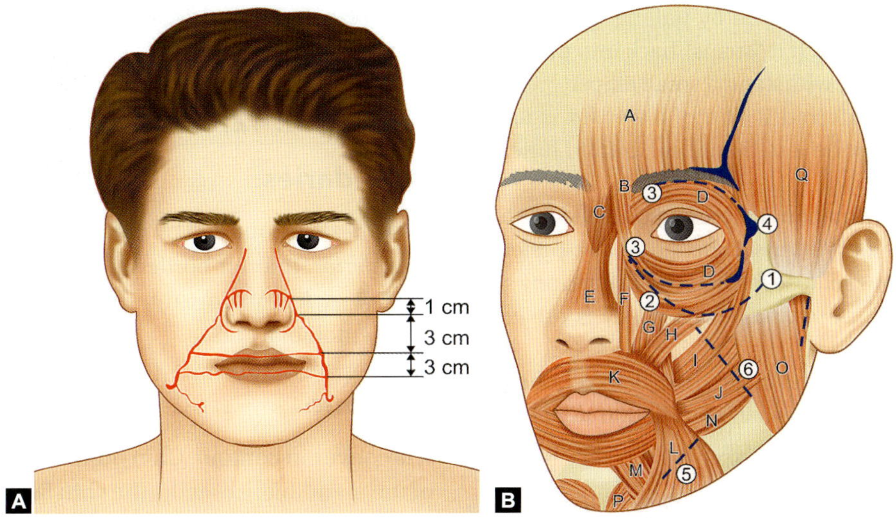

Figs. 38A and B: (A) Blood supply of cheek; (B) Muscles of face and retaining ligaments. A–frontalis; B and C–glabella complex; D–orbicularis oculi; E–nasalis; F–levator labii superioris alae nasi; G–levator labii superioris; H and I–zygomaticus minor and major; J–risorius; K–orbicularis oris; L–depressor anguli oris; M–depressor labii inferioris; N and O–masseter-mentalis; Q–temporalis; 1–zygomatic ligament; 2–zygomatic cutaneous ligament; 3–orbicularis retaining ligament; 4–lateral orbital thickening; 5–mandibular retaining ligament; 6–masseteric cutaneous ligament.

Nerve Supply

Sensory supply is from infraorbital nerve and zygomaticofacial nerve (branches of maxillary branch of trigeminal nerve), auriculotemporal nerve, mental nerve, and buccal nerve (mandibular branch of trigeminal nerve). The anterior branch of auriculotemporal nerve innervates the parotidomasseteric region.

Motor supply is from facial nerve and its branches.

Danger Zones of Cheek (Figs. 39 to 41)[46]

- *Marginal mandibular branch of facial nerve:* It emerges from the parotid gland at approximately two rami before coursing anteromedially, and courses parallel to the inferior border of the mandible. The remainder of the path is mostly anteromedial as the rami and advances to innervate muscles in the lower lip and chin. Injury can lead to unopposed lip elevation; loss of chin wrinkling may occur if mentalis function is impaired. Speech impairments, uncontrolled drooling, and cosmetic disfigurement may occur as well **(Fig. 39)**.
- *Zygomatic and buccal branch of facial nerve:* It emerges from the parotid gland and courses roughly parallel to the parotid duct before crossing the duct and innervating the target muscles. Zucker's point, which is the midpoint of a line drawn between the root of the helix to the oral commissure, may be used to find the starting point of the buccal and zygomatic branches of the facial nerve. Injury can cause upper lip and commissure of same side to sag **(Fig. 40)**.
- *Infraorbital nerve:* It can be easily injured when emerges from the infraorbital foramen in the cheek subunit. Injury can lead to loss of sensation of medial part of cheek, upper lip, and inferior eyelid **(Figs. 41A and B).**

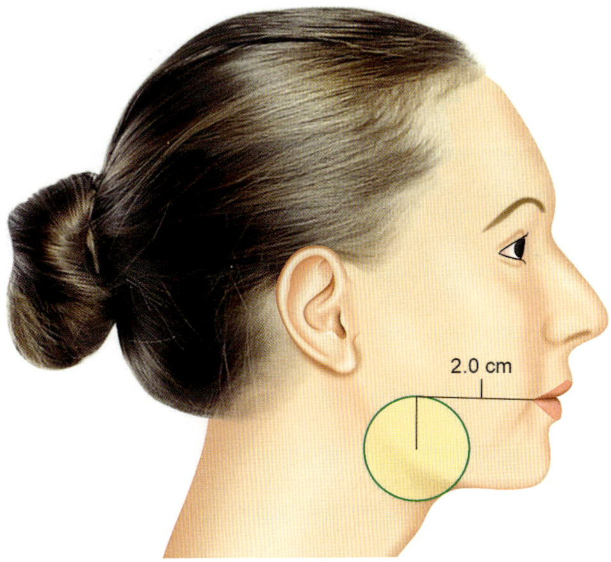

Fig. 39: Dangerous area where marginal mandibular nerve is at risk.

Applied Aspects

- Nasolabial subunit is in close proximity to the nasal ala, lip, and commissure so distortion is a possibility, which must be prevented during flap reconstruction.
- Cheek demands less symmetry as its counterpart is not comparable from the same point of view.
- Excision and closure close to lower eyelid along the curved RSTLs may cause excessive traction on the lower eyelid leading to ectropion.

- Eyelid tension can be assessed by pulling the lower lid down away from the eye. If it "snaps" back into place, the lower lid will probably withstand a small ellipse.
- A vertical ellipse preferred if skin of lower lid is under tension, the scar may be less than ideal, but lid function will be preserved.
- The risk of dog ear formation is more on nonmalleable area of cheek. The secondary intension healing is also preferred in such areas if proper ellipse formation will give long scar.
- Follow the RSTLs for excision, lazy S plasty is preferred on malar area.
- Liposuction and submental injection of deoxycholic acid can cause injury to the marginal mandibular nerve.
- Infraorbital nerve block can be given to block the medial part of cheek subunit.
- Undermining should be done at the level of superficial subcutaneous fat.

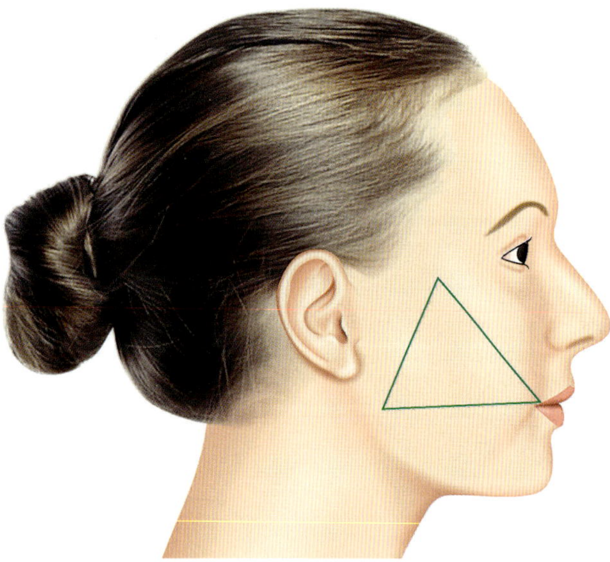

Fig. 40: Dangerous area where zygomatic and buccal branches of facial nerve are at risk.

- Infiltration anesthesia of cheek can result in temporary facial palsy.

CHIN (FIG. 42)

Boundaries

- *Superior:* Bounded by mentolabial crease.
- *Inferior:* Inferior border of osseous chin.
- *Lateral:* Round and shallow lateral extensions of mentolabial crease.

Contour

It is convex in contour. Chin button formed by the influences of the mandible, lower lip, the chin fat pads, and the mentalis muscles is a major part of this subunit.

Layers of Skin of Chin

It is structured by three layers:

1. *Skin:* It continues from the lower lip skin but is thicker than the lip skin. It is thickest skin of the face (1.19–2.6 mm).
2. *Subcutaneous layer:* It fills a distinct subcutaneous compartment, the chin fat compartment.
3. *Chin muscles:* Mentalis muscle is a paired muscle located at the tip of chin.

Relaxed Skin Tension Lines[45]

They run in a curved vertical direction as they descend to mandibular border.

Blood Supply

It is supplied by mental artery, labiomental artery and terminal part of submental artery and small branches of inferior labial artery.

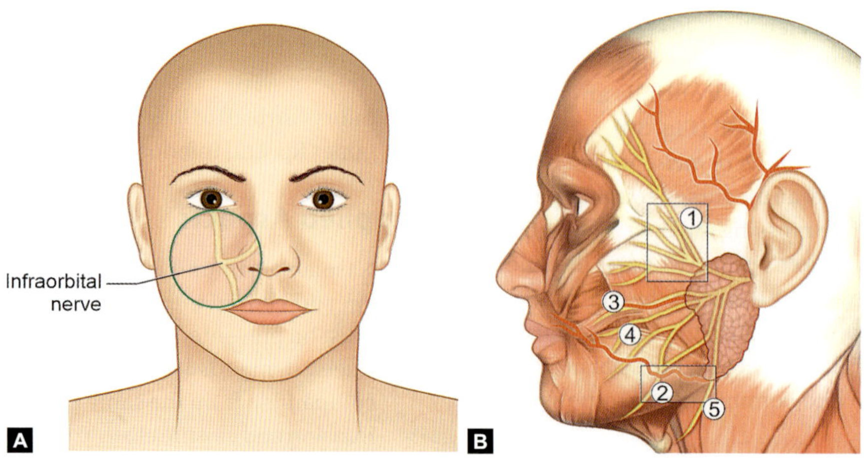

Figs. 41A and B: (A) Dangerous area where infraorbital nerve is at risk; (B) Dangerous area. 1–temporal branches of facial nerve; 2–facial artery and marginal mandibular nerve; 3–parotid duct; 4–buccal branches of facial nerve; 5–cervical branch of facial nerve.

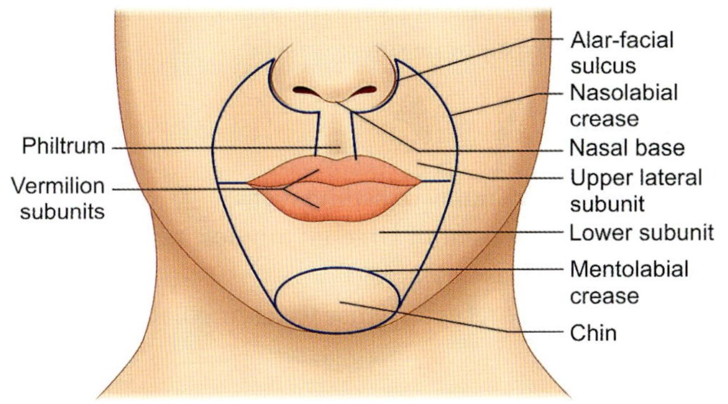

Fig. 42: Cosmetic units of perioral region.

Nerve Supply

- *Sensory:* Branches of mental nerve (mandibular branch of trigeminal nerve)
- *Motor:* Zygomatic, buccal, and marginal branches of facial nerve

Applied Aspects

- Muscles insert directly in skin so sharp undermining should be done.
- Mental nerve block can be used to anesthetize the chin and lower lip.
- Undermining is preferred at the level of superficial subcutaneous fat.
- Secondary intension healing gives acceptable results on chin.
- Always maintain the chin contour while planning excision surgeries.

LIPS AND PERIORAL AREA

Boundaries[45]

Upper Lip

- *Superior:* Alar grooves
- *Lateral:* Nasolabial groove
- *Inferior:* Interlabial gap

Lower Lip

- *Superior:* Interlabial gap
- *Inferior:* Mentolabial groove
- *Lateral:* Melolabial grooves

Contour

Convex throughout: However, normal shape of the lips varies with age, and is influenced by ethnicity.

Subunits[45]

Upper Lip

Mucosal, philtral, and lateral formed by the vermilion border and the philtrum ridges/columns; the cupid's bow is formed by the subunits of the upper lip.

Lower Lip

Central and mucosal units separated by the vermilion border.

The surface of the lip is comprised of four zones:

1. *Hairy skin:* Perioral skin measuring 0.86-mm thick.
2. *Vermilion border:* It is the rim of paler skin that demarcates the vermilion from the surrounding skin.
   Cupid's bow: The contour of the line formed by the vermilion border of the upper lip. In frontal view, it resembles an archer's bow, which curves medially and superiorly from the commissures to the paramedian peaks located at the bases of the pillars of the philtrum (crista philtrae) with an inferior convexity lying between those peaks. The philtrum is the vertical groove in the midline of the upper lip bordered by these lateral pillars (ridges).[51]
3. *Vermilion*: The red part of the lips. It is covered with a specialized stratified squamous epithelium, which is in continuity with the oral mucosa of the gingivolabial groove.
4. *Oral mucosa:* Stratified squamous nonkeratinized epithelium which covers the inner aspect of the oral cavity.[52]

Layers

Structurally, each lip is composed of orbicularis oris muscle (which forms the bulk of the lip) invested extraorally by the skin and subcutaneous tissue, intraorally by mucosa and submucosa, and over its free edge by the vermilion.

The skin surrounds the outer surface of the lip and mucosa its inner surface. The skin of lips is thinner (mean 1.9 mm) compared to adjoining cheek.

The subcutaneous tissue comprises of connective tissue and muscular fibers. Subcutaneous adipose tissue is almost absent in the lips.

The submucosa contains numerous minor salivary glands and is connected loosely to underlying muscle.

Relaxed Skin Tension Lines

The RSTL on the perioral area runs in a curved vertical direction as they descend to the mandibular border.

Blood Supply

Lips are supplied mainly by superior and inferior labial arteries with variable contribution of infraorbital, mental, labiomental, and submental arteries.

Nerve Supply

The motor innervation is by zygomatic, buccal, and marginal branches of facial nerve.
Lip elevators: Zygomatic and buccal branches
Lip depressors: Marginal mandibular branches
Lateral retractors: Buccal branches

Sensory Innervation

Upper lip: Superior labial branches of infraorbital nerve (V2)
Lower lip: Branches of mental nerve (V3).

Danger Zones

It consists of area from corners of mouth to the bridge of the nose including the nose. Any retrograde infection from the nasal area can spread to brain, causing cavernous sinus thrombosis, meningitis, and brain abscess **(Fig. 36)**.

Applied Aspects

- Orbicularis muscle provides elasticity allowing them to be stretched thus facilitating the closure of lip defects.
- Vermilion zone shows less keratinization and extensive anastomoses of inferior and superior labial arteries can cause excess bleed.
- Gingival sulci are convenient sites to insert gauze to promote eversion of lips to ease surgery on lips.
- Lip vermilion is free margin hence vectors of pull must be parallel to the free margins.
- Submucosa—muscle layer association provides a surgical plane that separates the mucosa from the muscle and can be used to raise an advancement flap.
- Thin vermilion mucosa with numerous underlying capillaries imparts its red color.
- Vermilion continuity should be ensured during lip reconstruction especially at vermilion-skin junction, and every asymmetry above 1 mm of this line.

SUPERFICIAL MUSCULOAPONEUROTIC SYSTEM

Superficial musculoaponeurotic system was first described by Mitz and Peyronie in 1974. It is a fibrous network which encloses muscles of facial expression, allowing their organized movement during contraction and also contributes to appearance of skin tension lines. It divides deep and superficial adipose tissue and has region-specific morphology. The fibrous septum of SMAS runs across the fat and attaches to the dermis thus acting as a distributor of force for the various facial muscles.

Boundaries[53]

- *Superior:* Zygomatic arch
- *Inferior:* Platysma muscle
- *Anterior:* Subcutaneous superficial fatty tissue
- *Posterior:* Parotidomasseteric fascia

Variation[54]

SMAS is classified into two distinct types:
1. Type 1—Composed of large fat lobules, relatively loose, lateral to the nasolabial fold.
2. Type 2—Scarce fat cells, dense tissue, medial to nasolabial fold.

Composition

Superficial musculoaponeurotic system consists of 1–3 muscle fiber layers and its composition varies depending on the location.

- *Scalp:* SMAS is represented by fibrous galea aponeurotica which splits to ensheathe frontalis, occipitalis, procerus, and few periauricular muscles.
- *Sternocleidomastoid region:* The sternocleidomastoid muscle is situated beneath the platysma and enclosed by superficial layer of cervical fascia.
- *Buccal region:* Muscle fibers of buccinator intermingle with orbicularis muscle. Adipose lobules are separated by strong connective tissue septa.
- *Oral region:* Deep fibers of orbicularis insert into the maxilla and mandible and into the skin of nasal septum. A broad layer consisting of muscle fibers and connective tissue fibers can be found adjacent to these deep muscle fibers.

Blood Supply

Superficial musculoaponeurotic system receives its blood supply from transverse facial artery and partially from musculocutaneous perforators of facial artery. Precaution should be taken while rhytidectomy and parotidectomy due to risk of transection of transverse facial artery as it traverses through the SMAS.[55]

Applied Aspects

- It serves as a guide to the depth of key neurovascular structures.
- It is helpful in reconstructive surgeries for facial palsy or face-lifting procedures.
- It prevents necrosis of the skin and subcutaneous tissue during dissection from the pre-auricular region.
- In aesthetic surgeries, superior elevation of SMAS is done to elevate superficial dermal and muscular structures in order to reverse age-related drooping of facial fat.
- Surgical plane[56] **(Figs. 43 and 44)**.

MUSCLES OF FACE (FIG. 38B)[57]

The muscles of face can be divided into two groups: (A) the muscles of facial expression, and (B) the muscles of mastication.

The muscles of facial expression are unique; in the sense they do not act in isolation but have complex anatomic and physiologic interactions. Most facial muscles insert directly into the skin and soft tissue, thereby facilitating "expression". Emotions and facial animations are conveyed and understood by the coordinated action of these muscles. The muscles of facial expression are connected to the overlying skin through a series of fibrous septae and an intervening fascial layer known as SMAS. Thus when the underlying muscle contracts, the overlying skin moves with it. The muscles of mastication, such as the masseter, pterygoids, and temporalis, have bony attachments and function to move the jaw in a way similar to muscles elsewhere on the body. Muscles of facial expression have been described in **Table 6**.

Applied Anatomy

- Muscles of face are temporarily paralyzed using botulinum toxin; this can be advocated post scar revisions surgeries for good cosmetic results.
- Injury to important neurovascular bundle near muscle should be avoided to preserve facial symmetry.
- Masseter and temporalis muscle flaps can be used to cover large facial defects.
- Clinching teeth with demarcate anterior border of masseter used as landmark.

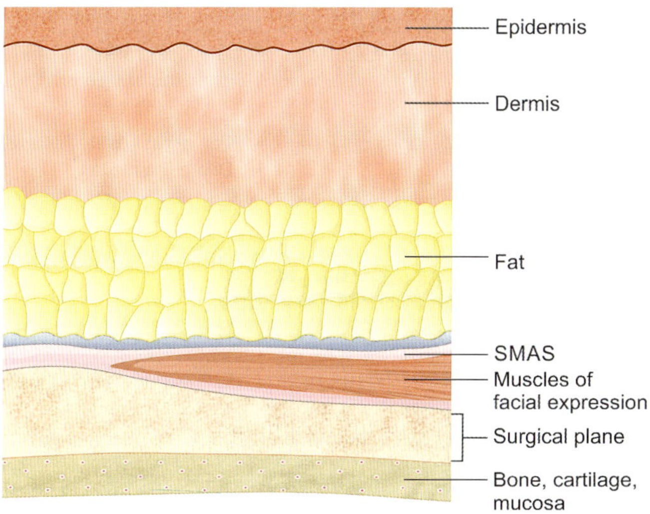

Fig. 43: Lateral face—a plane deep to superficial musculoaponeurotic system can be chosen.
(SMAS: superficial musculoaponeurotic system)

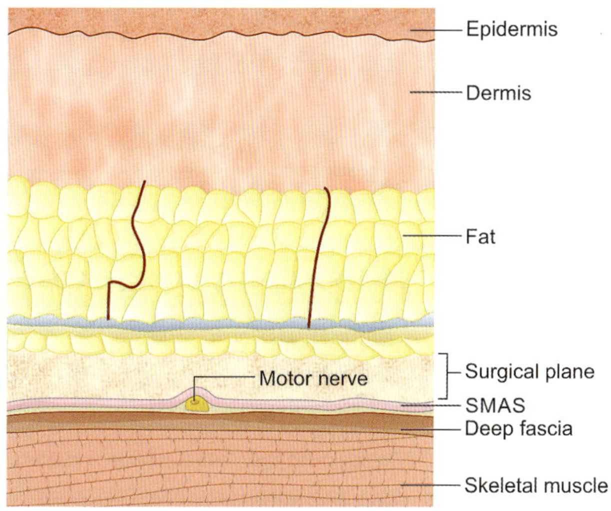

Fig. 44: Central face—for small procedures, plane superficial to the superficial musculoaponeurotic system can be chosen.
(SMAS: superficial musculoaponeurotic system)

TABLE 6 : Muscles of face with origin, insertion, nerve supply, and function.

Muscle	*Origin*	*Insertion*	*Nerve supply*	*Function*
Frontalis	Epicranial aponeurosis	Orbicularis oculi, corrugators, and dermis of brow	Temporal branch of facial nerve	• Brow elevator • Horizontal furrow
Orbicularis oculi	• Orbital part—nasal part of frontal bone, frontal process of maxilla, and medial canthus tendon • Preseptal and pretarsal parts—medial canthus tendon	Lateral palpebral raphe	Temporal and zygomatic branch of facial nerve	• Forceful closure of eyes • Superior fiber—depress the brow
Corrugators supercili	Superomedial aspect of orbital rim	Middle of brow	Temporal branch of facial nerve	Pulls brow inferomedially
Depressor supercili	Medial orbital rim near lacrimal bone	Medial brow	Facial nerve	Brow depressor
Procerus	Nasal bone	Glabella	Zygomatic branch	Depress lower forehead in midline to create crease at bridge of nose
Zygomaticus major	Body of zygoma	Corner of mouth	Zygomatic and buccal branch of facial nerve	Lifts corner of mouth

Contd...

Contd...

Muscle	*Origin*	*Insertion*	*Nerve supply*	*Function*
Zygomaticus minor	Body of zygoma	Lateral aspect of upper lip	Zygomatic and buccal branch of facial nerve	Lifts corner of mouth
Levator labii superioris	Maxilla just above infraorbital foramen	Upper lip and orbicularis oris	Zygomatic and buccal branch of facial nerve	Elevate upper lip
Levator labii superioris alae nasi	Frontal process of maxilla	Nasal cartilage and upper lip	Zygomatic and buccal branch of facial nerve	Elevate upper lip
Levator anguli oris	Canine fossa of maxilla	Upper lip	Zygomatic and buccal branch of facial nerve	Elevate corner of mouth
Risorius	Platysma over lateral cheek, parotid-masseteric fascia	Corner of mouth	Marginal mandibular nerve	Pulls corner of mouth laterally
Orbicularis oris	Maxilla and mandible	Skin around lips	Buccal and marginal mandibular nerve	Pursing, dilation and closure of lips
Depressor anguli oris	Mandible along oblique line lateral to depressor labii inferioris	Modiolus	Marginal mandibular nerve	Depress corner of mouth
Depressor labii inferioris	Mandible along oblique line in front of mental foramen	Skin and mucosa of lower lip	Marginal mandibular nerve	Lip depressor
Mentalis	Incisive fossa of mandible	Chin	Marginal mandibular nerve	Elevate and protrude lower lip, dimpling of chin
Nasalis • Transverse part • Alar part	 • Maxilla over canine tooth • Maxilla below and medial to compressor naris	 • Dorsum of nose • Alar cartilage	 Buccal branch of facial nerve	 • Compress nasal aperture • Dilate the nostril

TABLE 7: Fat compartments of face **(Figs. 45A and B).**

Superficial fat compartments	*Deep fat compartments*
Nasolabial fat	Suborbicularis oculi fat
Malar cheek fat (medial, middle, and lateral)	Deep cheek fat
Temporal fat pad (central, middle, and lateral)	Buccal fat
Orbital fat (superior, inferior, and lateral)	Galeal fat
Jowl	
Preplatysmal and premental fat	

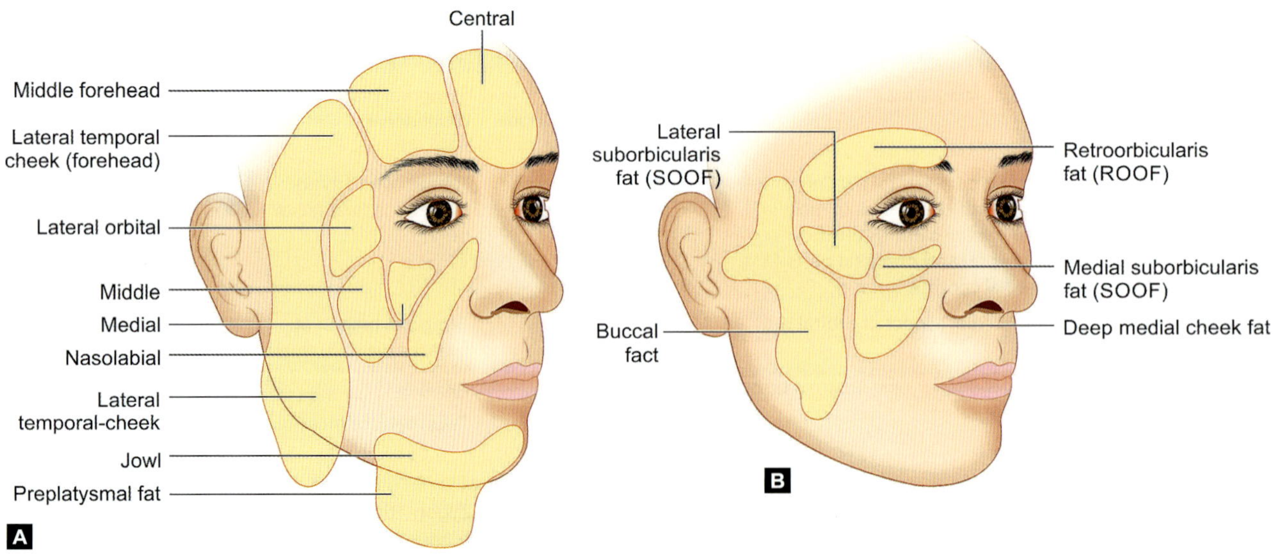

Figs. 45A and B: Fat compartments.

Fat Compartments of the Face[58]

Fat within the subcutaneous layer of face is not located in one layer but is actually compartmentalized. The borders of the compartments are formed by fascial septae that travel from deep fascia or periosteum and insert into the dermis. Fat compartments can be divided into superficial and deep compartments based on the depth. Various fat compartments are depicted in **Table 7** and are described elsewhere in the book.

Applied Aspects

- Volume loss in fat occurs with aging.
- In autologous fat transplant, fat is injected into the deep fat compartments for augmentation.
- Lateral temporal fat and postauricular fat compartment fuses beneath the ear. Greater auricular nerve may be transacted in this area.

CONCLUSION

Surgeons are constantly striving to produce the most aesthetically pleasing incision, most meticulous skin closure to create the best surgical scar. Surgical techniques of repairing facial deformities have social implications.

Patient's self-identity is largely influenced by a surgeon's manipulation and handling of facial tissues and one should have a thorough knowledge of anatomy for the same.

BEFORE YOU EVER OPERATE ON SKIN, RECALL WHAT LIES UNDERNEATH. IF YOU CAN'T RECALL, LOOK IT UP!!

REFERENCES

1. Farmer ER, Hood AF. Pathology of the skin. Norwalk, CT: Appleton and Lange; 1990. pp. 3-29.
2. Marcus J, Horan DB, Robinson JK. Tissue expansion: past, present and future. J Am Acad Dermatol. 1990;23:813-25.
3. Fung YC. Biomechanics in mechanical properties of living tissues. Springer-Verlag: New York; 1981.
4. Hussain SH, Limthongkul B, Humphreys TR. The biomechanical properties of the skin. Dermatol Surg. 2013;39(2): 193-203.
5. Paul SP. Biodynamic excisional skin tension lines for surgical excisions: untangling the science. Ann R Coll Surg Engl. 2018;100(4):33.
6. Barbenel JC. Skin biomechanics. In: Payne PA (Ed). Concise encyclopaedia of biological and biomedical measurement systems. Pergamon Press: Oxford; 1991. p. 347.
7. Wan Abas WAB, Barbenel JC. The response of human skin to small tensile loads in vitro. Eng Med.1982;11:43.
8. Gibson T, Stark HL, Evans JH. Directional variation in extensibility of human skin in vivo. J Biomech. 1969;2:201-4.
9. Larrabee WF Jr. A finite element model of skin deformation. In Biomechanics of skin and soft tissue: a review. Laryngoscope. 1986;96:399-412.
10. Agur AMR, Lee MJ, Grant JC. Grant's Atlas of Anatomy, 13th edition. Baltimore, MD: Lippincott Williams and Wilkins; 2013.
11. McMinn NH, Hutchings RT, Logan BM. Color Atlas of Head and Neck Anatomy, 2nd edition. Baltimore, MD: Mosby-Wolfe; 1995. pp. 161-3.
12. Snell RS. Clinical anatomy for medical students, 5th edition. Boston, MA: Little Brown and Co; 1990. pp. 659-61.
13. Seery GE. Surgical anatomy of the scalp. Dermatol Surg. 2002;28:581-7.
14. Dzubow LM. Facial flap: biomechanic and regional applications. Norwalk, CT: Appleton and Lange; 1989.
15. Chayen D, Nathan H. Anatomical observations on the subgaleotic fascia of the scalp. Acta Anat. 1974;87:427-8.
16. Drake RL, Vogl W, Mitchell AWM. Gray's Anatomy for Students, 1st edition. Churchill: Livingstone (Elsevier Science); 2005. pp. 898-936.
17. Roenigk HH, Ratz JL, Roenigk RK. Roenigk's Dermatologic Surgery. In: Roenigk RK, Ratz JL, Roenigk HH (Eds). Current techniques in procedural dermatology, 3rd edition. New York, London: Informa Healthcare; 2007.
18. Moore K. Clinically oriented anatomy, 2nd edition. Baltimore, MD: Williams and Wilkins; 1985. p. 855.
19. Nouri K. Complications in Dermatologic Surgery. Philadelphia, PA: Saunders Elsevier. 2008; pp. 16-65.
20. Tromovitch TA, Stegman SJ, Glogau RG. Flaps and Grafts in Dermatologic Surgery. Chicago, IL: Yearbook Medical Publishers; 1989.
21. Bernstein G. Surface landmarks for the identification of key anatomic structures for the face and neck. J Dermatol Surg Oncol. 1986;12:722-6.
22. Labbe D, Franco RG, Nicolas J. Platysma suspension and platysmaplasty during neck lift; anatomical study and analysis of 30 cases. Plast Reconstr Surg. 2006;117(6):2001-7.
23. Robinson JK. Basic cutaneous surgery concepts. In: Robinson JK, Arndt KA, Le Boit PE, Wintroub BU (Eds). Atlas of Cutaneous Surgery. Philadelphia: Saunders; 1996. pp. 1-4.
24. King RJ, Motta G. Iatrogenic spinal accessory nerve palsy. Ann R Coll Surg Engl. 1983;65:35-7.
25. Datubo-Brown DD. Keloids: a review of literature. Br J Plast Surg.1990;43(1):70-7.
26. Kim S, Chung SW, ChaI H. Full thickness skin grafts from the groin: donor site morbidity and graft survival rate from 50 cases. J Korean Assoc Oral Maxillo Fac Surg. 2013;39(1):21-6.
27. Salasche SJ, Bernstein G, Senkarik M. Surgical Anatomy of the Skin. Norwalk, CT: Appleton and Lange; 1988.
28. Swinehart JM. Treatment of axillary hyperhidrosis: combination of the starch-iodine test with the tumescent liposuction technique. Dermatol Surg. 2000;26:392-6.
29. Spektor M, Kelly J. Regional anesthesia of the thorax and extremities. In: Roberts Hedges (Ed). Clinical Procedures in Emergency Medicine, 5th edition. Philadelphia, PA: Saunders Elsevier; 2010. pp. 528-30.
30. Botting J, Schofield J. Anatomical hazards and pitfalls. In: Brown's Skin and Minor Surgery: a text and colour atlas, 5th edition. Taylor and Francis Group; 2015.
31. Swanson NA. Atlas of Cutaneous Surgery,1st edition. Boston, Massachusetts: Little Brown and Company; 1987.
32. McCurdy JA Jr. Five years of experience using fat for leg contouring (Commentary). Am J Cosmet Surg. 1995;12(3):228.
33. Dinehart SM. Topical, local, and regional anesthesia. In: Wheeland R (Ed). Cutaneous Surgery. Philadelphia: WB Saunders; 1994. pp.105-10.
34. Eastwood DM, Irgau I, Atkins RM. The distal course of the sural nerve and its significance for incisions around the lateral hindfoot. Foot Ankle. 1992;13(4):199-202.

35. Yavagal S, de Farias TF, Medina CA, Takacs P. Normal vulvovaginal, perineal, and pelvic anatomy with reconstructive considerations. Semin Plast Surg. 2011;25(2):121-9.
36. Neill S, Lewis F. Ridley's the vulva, 3rd edition. Hoboken: Wiley-Blackwell; 2009.
37. Puppo V. Embryology and anatomy of the vulva: the female orgasm and women's sexual health. Eur J Obstet Gynecol Reprod Biol. 2011;154(1):3-8.
38. Dickinson RL. Atlas of Human Sex Anatomy, 2nd edition. Baltimore: Williams and Wilkins; 1949.
39. Stenchever MA. Comprehensive Gynecology, 4th edition. St. Louis: Mosby; 2001. pp. 482-6, 645-6.
40. Hill DA, Lense JJ. Office management of Bartholin gland cysts and abscesses. Am Fam Physician. 1998;57:1611-6,1619-20.
41. Gonzales-Ulloa M. Restoration of the face covering by means of selected skin in regional aesthetic units. Br J Plast Surg. 1956;9:212-21.
42. Burget GC, Menick FJ. The subunit principle in nasal reconstruction. Plast Reconstr Surg. 1985;76:239-47.
43. Heffelfinger RN, Sanan A, Bryant LM. Management of forehead scars. Department of Otolaryngology—Head and Neck Surgery Faculty Papers. 2017. Paper 35.
44. Chopra K, Calva D, Sosin M, Tadisina KK, Banda A, Cruz CD, et al. A Comprehensive examination of topographic thickness of skin in the human face. Aesthet Surg J. 2015;35(8):1007-13.
45. Fattahi TT. An overview of facial aesthetic units. J Oral Maxillofac Surg. 2003;61:1207-12.
46. Talmor G, Trang A, Ahadiat O, Paskhover B, Wysong A. Anatomic danger zones of the head and neck. Dermatol Surg. 2020;46:1549-59.
47. Alghoul MS, Kearney AM, Pacella SJ, Purnell CA. Eyelid reconstruction. Plast Reconstr Surg Glob Open. 2019;7:e2520.
48. Cerci FB. Usefulness of the subunit principle in nasal reconstruction. An Bras Dermatol. 2017;92(5 Suppl 1):159-62.
49. Kim TK, Jeong JY. Surgical anatomy for Asian rhinoplasty. Arch Craniofac Surg. 2019;20(3):147-57.
50. Mendelson BC, Jacobson SR. Surgical anatomy of the mid-cheek: facial layers, spaces, and the midcheek segments. Clin Plast Surg. 2008;35(3):395-404.
51. Hennekam RCM, Cormier-Daire V, Hall J, Mehes K, Patton M, Stevenson R. Elements of morphology: standard terminology for the nose and philtrum. Am J Med Genet Part A. 2009;149A(1):61-76.
52. Standing S. 2005. Gray's anatomy: the anatomical basis of clinical practice. Edinburg: Elsevier.
53. Hwang K, Choi JH. Superficial fascia in the cheek and the superficial musculoaponeurotic system. J Craniofac Surg. 2018;29(5):1378-82.
54. Hunto JR, Vattoth S. A practical review of the muscles of facial mimicry with special emphasis on the superficial musculoaponeurotic system. Am J Roentenol. 2015;204(1):W19-26.
55. Guyuron B, Seyed Forooton NS, Katira K. The super-high SMAS facelift technique with tailor tack plication. Aesthetic Plast Surg. 2018;42(6):1531-9.
56. Miller CJ, Antunes MB, Sobanko JF. Surgical technique for optimal outcomes. J Am Acad Dermatol. 2015;72:388.
57. Vigilante CE. Anatomy and functions of the muscles of facial expression. Oral Maxillofacial Surg Clin N Am. 2005;17(1):1-15.
58. Rohrich, Rod J, Pessa, Joel E. The fat compartments of the face: anatomy and clinical implications for cosmetic surgery. Plast Reconstr Surg. 2007;119(7):2219-27.
59. Dua K, Uprety S, Dua A. Donor Harvesting: Strip Dissection. J Cutan Aesthet Surg. 2018;11(4):190-4.

CHAPTER 3

Applied Advanced Surgical Anatomy of Face

Mukta Sachdev, Suraj Sachidanand, Dinkar Sreekumar

KEY MESSAGES

- Facial anatomy is complex but can be understood better when resolved into a layered arrangement of planes.
- Aging is a combination of volume loss and tissue laxity contributing to descent of fat pads and development of rhytids.
- Layers of the face are continuous with the scalp and the neck, with discrete layers changing into different structures as they pass craniocaudally.
- Injection of fillers must respect the relative position of vasculature to avoid untoward complication.

INTRODUCTION

Aging is a multifactorial process. Physiological and morphological changes occur in both skeletal and soft tissue composites—the bones, ligaments, muscles, fascia, fat, and skin. The onset and rate of these structural changes varies between individuals of different genders and ethnicities. Due to the heterogeneity of the effects of each of the structures, it is difficult to ascertain which is the key player in the clinical changes that occur as the face ages. Thus, it is challenging to modify a specific structure with rejuvenation procedures, especially as limited treatment options are available to target bone, muscle, or ligaments.[1]

LAYERS OF THE FACE

With increasing interest in the anatomy of the face, surgeons and clinical anatomists have turned their attention toward the gross anatomy of the face. In the last decade, new findings and concepts regarding facial anatomy have been introduced, of which the most influential is probably the layered arrangement of the face.[1] These layers are arranged as follows: Layer 1—skin; layer 2—subcutaneous fat including the retinacula cutis, composed of fibrous connective tissue; layer 3—superficial musculoaponeurotic system (SMAS); layer 4—deep fat, and layer 5—periosteum or deep fascia. However, this general concept has to be adapted for each facial region, since there are regions where more layers (e.g., the temple with 10 layers) or fewer layers (e.g., the tear trough with three layers) can be identified. Moreover, the understanding of a parallel arrangement of layers has to be altered when considering the line of ligaments. The line of ligaments separates the medial mimetic face from the lateral face (predominantly static, concerned with mastication). In the medial midface there is no distinct parallel arrangement of the layers; here the muscles of facial expression course obliquely from bone to skin, whereas in the lateral midface the layers are in parallel and continuous with each other while extending from the neck to the scalp.[2]

THE LINE OF LIGAMENTS

Facial ligaments are well as they are released during face-lifting procedures to achieve the desired effects. Of the described ligaments, the zygomatic ligament (also called McGregor's patch) is the strongest, resisting the greatest force before ultimate failure during biomechanical testing. Interestingly, all major facial ligaments (irrespective of whether they are true or false) can be arranged into a single line located immediately lateral to the lateral orbital rim and extending from the temporal crest to the mandible.

From superior to inferior, the ligaments are the temporal ligamentous adhesions, lateral orbital thickening, zygomatic ligament, and mandibular ligament.[1]

In the medial midface (i.e., medial to the line of ligaments) are the midfacial deep fat compartments; surgically relevant spaces are found in the lateral midface, e.g., premasseteric spaces. It is of some clinical importance that injections medial to the line of ligaments will result in projection of the overlying soft tissues, whereas injections lateral to this line lead to a lifting effect in more inferiorly located regions. This is a result of the oblique arrangement of the medial midface versus the parallel arrangement of the lateral midface.[2]

DEEP AND SUPERFICIAL FAT COMPARTMENTS OF THE FOREHEAD

Therapeutic options for the forehead mostly include neuromodulator applications in order to temporarily reduce the contractile activity of the frontalis, corrugator supercilii, depressor supercilii, and orbicularis oculi muscles. The treatment approach has changed from rigid injection schemes to more individualized treatments based on each person's individual anatomy. A recent trend includes restoration of the volume loss of the frontal soft tissue. This is due to fact that the frontal bone undergoes age-related changes, similar to those of the midfacial bones. As the covering soft tissues are thinner than those of the midface and fat is redistributed from superficial to abdominal or ectopic locations (liver, bone marrow), frontal hollowing can result. This contributes significantly to a more skeletal appearance of the face. Volume can be restored in the superficial and deep compartments of the forehead using soft tissue filler. Three superficial fat compartments are present and located in layer 2 between the skin (layer 1) and the frontalis muscle. As the frontalis muscle is a continuation of the galea aponeurotica, it can be regarded as layer 4 (if the thin sheet covering the muscle is regarded as layer 3). Between the frontalis muscle (layer 4) and its underlying fascia (layer 6), a thin layer of fat can be identified—the subfrontal fat (layer 5). Inside this fat, the supraorbital and supratrochlear vessels travel superiorly after they emerge from their respective foramina. The subfrontal fat lies between the inferior and middle frontal septa, which are formed by the transition of the vasculature from deeper to superficial layers and extend from the periosteum to the fascia covering the underside of the frontalis muscle.[2]

Deep to the frontalis muscle and its fascia (layer 6) the three deep forehead compartments can be found. These compartments are located in layer 7 and are bounded inferiorly by the middle frontal septum and superiorly by the superior frontal septum and are located between the frontalis muscle complex and the periosteum.[2]

Located between the inferior frontal septum (superior boundary) and the orbicularis retaining ligament (inferior boundary) **(Fig. 1)** and lateral to the emergence of the supraorbital neurovascular bundle from the supraorbital foramen, the retro-orbicularis fat (ROOF) is located. This fat is located deep to the orbicularis oculi muscles (layer 3) and superficial to the periosteum of the frontal bone; it is connected with the lower temporal compartment via the superior interval.[2]

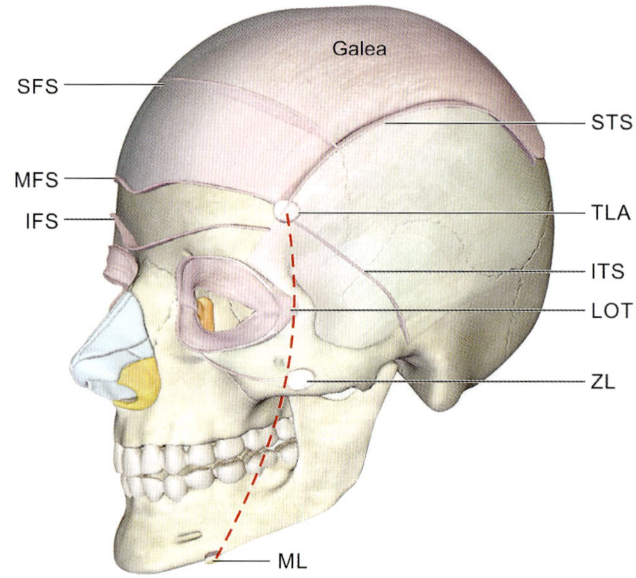

Fig. 1: Virtual model of the face showing the major facial ligaments. Note how the ligaments are arranged as a single line located immediately lateral to the lateral orbital rim and extending from the temporal crest to the mandible. (IFS: inferior frontal septum; ITS: inferior temporal septum; LOT: lateral orbital thickening; MFS: middle frontal septum; ML: mandibular ligament; SFS: superior frontal septum; STS: superior temporal septum; TLA: temporal ligamentous adhesion; ZL: zygomatic ligament)
Source: Cotofana S, Lachman N. Anatomy of the facial fat compartments and their relevance in aesthetic surgery. J Dtsch Dermatol Ges. 2019;17(4):399-413.

TEMPORAL FAT PADS

Volumizing procedures of the temple are used to restore volume loss, which may be due to changes of the bony skeleton and/or to reduce volume of the temporalis muscle or temporal fat pads. As the fat pads are related to the respective layers, the layered anatomy of the temple should be kept in mind. The layers of the temple are directly contiguous with the five layers of the SCALP: Skin; Connective tissue (here subcutaneous fat); Aponeurosis (here galea aponeurotica); Loose connective tissue, and Periosteum. These five layers are continuous into the temple, although they change their names after passing the superior temporal septum **(Fig. 1)**. The galea aponeurotica becomes superficial temporal fascia, while the periosteum is now the deep temporal fascia. The anterior and posterior branches of the superficial temporal artery can be found within the superficial temporal fascia. Application of soft tissue fillers using the superficial technique places the product into the subcutaneous fat, i.e., into layer 2, which is, thus, superficial to the superficial temporal artery. Two compartments are located between the superficial and deep temporal fascia in layer 4—the upper and lower temporal compartments. The upper temporal compartment is located between the superior and inferior temporal septa and contains no relevant neurovascular structures, whereas the lower temporal compartment is located between the inferior temporal septum and the adhesions of the zygomatic arch, and contains the frontal branches of the facial nerve (motor), the zygomaticotemporal branches (sensory), and the temporal part of the sentinel vein. Between 2–5 cm cranial to the zygomatic arch, the deep temporal fascia divides into a superficial lamina (layer 5) and a deep lamina (layer 7) of the deep temporal fascia, and encloses the superficial temporal fat pad and the proximal part of the sentinel vein (layer 6), which is here termed the medial zygomaticotemporal vein. The superficial lamina is continuous in the midface with the parotideomasseteric (PM) fascia (layer 5) and extends into the neck as the investing layer of the deep cervical fascia.[1] The deep lamina of the deep temporal fascia travels deep to the zygomatic arch into the masticatory space and is connected there to the parotido-temporal fascia.[1] Deep to the deep temporal fascia, the temporal extension of the buccal fat pad (of Bichat) is located; here it is referred to as the deep temporal fat pad and is located in layer 8. The temporalis muscle is located in layer 9 and receives its arterial blood supply from branches of the internal maxillary artery, the anterior and posterior deep temporal arteries, which travel superficial to the periosteum (layer 10). Soft tissue fillers applied with the deep technique are in contact with the bone and should be placed in proximity to the temporal crest in order to avoid contact with the deep temporal arteries.[1]

INFRAORBITAL REGION: TEAR TROUGH AND SUBORBICULARIS OCULI FAT

The infraorbital region is one of the most difficult areas to treat, although the layering is less complex than that of the temple or the forehead. Clinically, dark circles in the medial infraorbital area (i.e., tear troughs) as well as palpebromalar grooves (i.e., lateral depressions between the lower eye lid and the cheek eminence) are of concern. The depression immediately inferior to the tear trough is called the nasojugal groove and is continuous with the midcheek groove (also referred to as a mediojugal fold). Together, the nasojugal groove and the palpebromalar groove form the so called "V-frame" deformity, which is a sign of facial aging and can be related to the loss of subcutaneous fat from the superficial nasolabial, and superficial medial cheek fat compartments. The infraorbital area can be separated into medial and lateral parts by a vertical line through the medial margin of the pupil. In the medial part (area of the tear trough) only three layers can be identified—skin (layer 1), orbicularis oculi muscle (orbital part) (layer 2), and periosteum (layer 3). The angular artery is located in the groove between the cheek and the lateral aspect of the nose, running vertically deep to the orbicularis oculi muscle, whereas the angular vein is located in the depth of the nasojugal groove, 4.2 ± 0.7 mm inferior to the inferior orbital rim and running obliquely from inferolateral to superomedial deep to the orbital part of the orbicularis oculi muscle. Several layers are present in the lateral infraorbital part. Deep to the orbital part of the orbicularis oculi muscle (layer 3) the suborbicularis oculi fat (SOOF) is located; this usually has separate medial and lateral parts.[1] This fat is separated by the superficial lamina of the deep temporal fascia (layer 5) from the fat within the prezygomatic space (layer 6) overlying the periosteum (layer 7). The inferior boundary of both the SOOF and of the prezygomatic space is the zygomatico-cutaneous ligament and the superior boundary is the bilaminar orbicularis retaining ligament. The SOOF is connected via the temporal tunnel to the lower temporal compartment, since both are located in layer 4 and reside on top of the superficial lamina of the deep temporal fascia. Along the medial wall of the zygomatico-cutaneous ligament, the angular vein can be identified after it emerges deep to the zygomaticus major muscle; it has a variable course superficial or deep to the zygomaticus minor muscle. The zygomatico-cutaneous ligament fuses with the orbicularis retaining ligament where it crosses the vertical medial pupillary line just before reaching the tear trough—in other words, the tear trough is the superficial landmark for the medial end of the SOOF. Treatment of malar mounds can be challenging due to the multi-layered arrangement in the lateral infraorbital area.[2]

Midface: Parotideomasseteric (lateral midface), buccal (lateral midface), and central midface (medial midface) regions.

The midface has three craniocaudal subdivisions—upper, middle, and lower with reference to the horizontal. However, an additional subdivision of the midface should be made when incorporating functional anatomy and its relation to the line of ligaments 2.

PAROTIDEOMASSETERIC REGION LOCATED IN THE LATERAL MIDFACE

The PM region contains the masseter muscle and the parotid gland. It extends from the auricle to a vertical line at the lateral margin of the bony orbit (when viewed from lateral). Its layers are parallel and include the following structures: Skin (layer 1), subcutaneous fat, i.e., middle and lateral superficial fat compartments (layer 2), SMAS (layer 3), deep (sub-SMAS) spaces (layer 4), and PM fascia (layer 5). Deep to layer 5 are the branches of the facial nerve, the parotid gland, the parotid duct, and the variable accessory parotid gland. The marginal mandibular, buccal, and zygomatic branches of the facial nerve travel within fibrous connective tissue sheets that connect the PM fascia to the SMAS, which encloses surgical access spaces that are used in face-lifting procedures. These spaces are the lower, middle, and upper premasseter spaces. The transverse facial artery runs in the superior premasseter space and gives off a branch that runs within the zygomatic ligament (McGregor's patch) to provide axial blood supply to the overlying SMAS. Deep to the masseter muscle is the buccal fat pad with its four extensions, of which the temporal extension is called the deep temporal fat pad. The buccal fat pad is located in a separate spaces called the masticatory space, and is separated from the premasseter spaces by the masseter muscle, and from the buccal spaces by the facial vein within the facial vein canal.[1]

BUCCAL REGION OF THE LATERAL MIDFACE

The buccal region is less well defined as it can be assigned to both the medial and lateral midface. However, with respect to the underlying anatomy, this area covers the most mobile area of the face, specifically the cheek and its contents, which are dominated by the buccinator muscle in layer 6. The layers in this region are parallel, and it contains the following structures: Skin (layer 1); subcutaneous fat (i.e., jowls fat compartment) (layer 2); SMAS in its superior part and the horizontal, modiolar part of the platysma (layer 3); buccal space (layer 4); buccopharyngeal fascia (layer 5), and buccinator muscle (layer 6). The facial artery travels inside the buccal space, whereas the facial vein runs inside the facial vein canal, which forms the posterior boundary of the buccal space and is not considered as a content of the buccal space. The buccal fat pad is located in the masticatory space, which is posterior to the buccal space within the masticatory space.[1]

The jowl deformity is caused by the gliding of the platysma against the mandible, since between the mandibular ligament and the masseter muscle the facial artery and facial vein cross the mandible and are covered in deep fat here. This fat is not connected to the fat within the buccal space or to the buccal fat pad in the masticatory space. With age-related facial changes, the platysma glides and the overlying (subcutaneous) jowl fat compartment glides inferiorly and causes the appearance of jowls.[2]

CENTRAL MIDFACE LOCATED IN THE MEDIAL MIDFACE

The central midface is the facial region where the majority of minimally invasive aesthetic injections are performed. The deep and superficial midfacial fat compartments are located here and this area is prone to age-related changes as the underlying bone undergoes remodeling, with a corresponding change in the maxillary angle. If this angle changes, the position of the fat compartments changes too and the clinical signs of facial aging become visible.[2]

The layers are arranged differently because the deep fat compartments are bound by the muscles of facial expression; these originate from the bone and insert into the nasolabial sulcus, the orbicularis oris muscle complex or the modiolus. Thus, it is most important for a practitioner to understand the two- and three-dimensional anatomy of this region for safe and effective results following surgical and non-surgical procedures: Skin (layer 1); subcutaneous fat, i.e., the superficial nasolabial and the superficial medial cheek fat compartment (layer 2); SMAS and orbital part of orbicularis oculi muscle (layer 3); deep nasolabial fat compartment (located within the premaxillary space) (layer 4); levator labii superioris alaeque nasi muscle (layer 5); deep pyriform space (medial to the infraorbital foramen) (layer 6); and deep medial cheek fat compartment (between the infraorbital foramen and the angular vein) (layer 6) and deep lateral cheek fat compartment (between the angular vein and the zygomaticus major muscle (layer 4); and periosteum (layer 7 medial to the angular vein; layer 5 lateral to the angular vein). Next to the origin of the zygomaticus major muscle, the zygomatic ligament (McGregor's patch) is located; this is included in the line of ligaments and forms the boundary between the medial and lateral midface. The presence of the zygomaticus minor muscle is variable; it follows the course of the zygomatico-cutaneous ligament, which forms the superior boundary of the deep medial and lateral cheek fat compartments, whereas the constant zygomaticus major muscle is connected via a broad fascial membrane (the transverse facial septum) to the underlying maxilla. The transverse facial septum forms the inferior boundary of the deep lateral cheek fat and thus the superior boundary of the buccal space. It is the leading cause of "apple-cheeks" when smiling.[2]

FAT DISTRIBUTION AROUND THE PERIORAL REGION AND THE CHIN

The boundaries of the perioral region are the nasolabial sulci, the nose, the modiolus, the labiomandibular sulci, and inferiorly the submental septum. The major difference between this region and all other facial regions is that there is no clear layered arrangement and there are no subcutaneous fat compartments. The subcutaneous fat is dispersed, since the underlying muscles of facial expression and the collagenous fibers form a strong network that connects the skin firmly to the underlying muscular layer. This makes precise movements of the overlying skin possible; these are needed for various facial expressions and for food intake. The layers can be best summarized as follows: Skin (layer 1), subcutaneous fat (layer 2), musculature (e.g., orbicularis oris muscle) (layer 3), deep fat (deep chin fat in the midline and the (deep) labiomandibular fat located around the mental foramen), and periosteum (layer 5). The fat located between the periosteum and the musculature is an important gliding space that protects the neurovascular bundle as it emerges from the mental foramen.[2]

The change in subcutaneous arrangement between the firm perioral attachment and the loose and layered arrangement of the remainder of the facial regions where a clear subcutaneous layer is present underlies the formation of the nasolabial as well as the labiomandibular sulcus.[2]

CONCLUSION

The concept of the layered arrangement of the face is an effective way to understand the spatial relationship and the functional interplay of the soft tissues of the face. Understanding the layers, the compartments, and their contents is crucial for safe and effective minimally invasive rejuvenation procedures. Since each structure (bone, ligaments, fascia, muscles, fat compartments, and skin) exhibits specific contributions to the process of facial aging, it is important to determine which structure is the key player in the presenting clinical scenario. Injection of soft tissue fillers should thus be performed with caution and with a precise anatomical understanding of the facial fat compartments, as one must target a specific fat compartment in order to achieve the desired effect. Applying the product in the wrong fat compartment might yield an aesthetically undesirable result.[2]

ANATOMY OF THE FACIAL DANGER ZONES

Knowledge of the facial anatomy is essential. As evidenced by numerous studies, the facial vasculature has many variations and can be found in various tissue planes, depending on location within the face. Anticipating the depth and course of vessels allows practitioners to develop techniques to avoid intravascular injection, vascular injury, and/or compression.[3]

BROW AND GLABELLAR REGION

Pertinent Anatomy

The corrugators originate along the nasal process of the frontal bone, coursing superolateral under the frontalis, inserting dermally at the brow. Over time, contraction of this muscle creates vertical rhytides at the brow level. Likewise, procerus muscle activity leads to horizontal nasal rhytides, also referred to as "bunny lines".[3]

The supratrochlear artery, a branch of the ophthalmic artery, exits the superomedial orbit 17–22 mm lateral to midline, piercing or passing superficial to the corrugator, deep to the orbicularis and frontalis **(Fig. 2)**. Approximately 15–25 mm above the orbital rim, the artery traverses the frontalis and orbicularis to enter the subcutaneous plane. It continues running superiorly in the subcutaneous plane 15–20 mm from midline in a paramedian position.[3] At the level of the brow, the supratrochlear artery runs vertically in line with the medial canthus ± 3 mm. Another study demonstrated the artery within the glabellar frown line in 50% of cases and an average of 3.2 mm lateral in the remaining cases. The supratrochlear artery branches anastomose with the angular, supraorbital, and dorsal nasal arteries.[3]

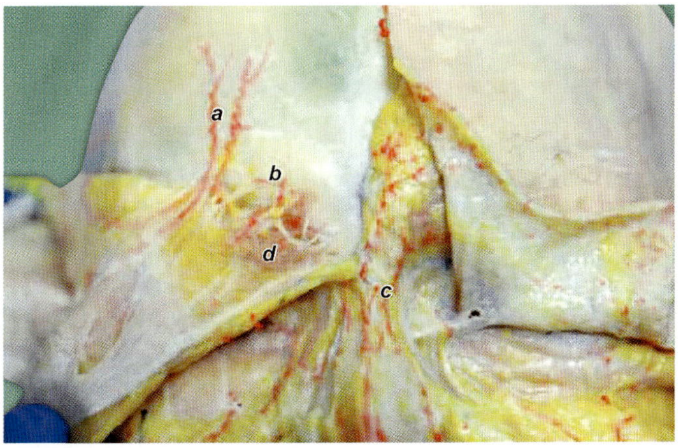

Fig. 2: The supraorbital artery (a) is shown exiting above the brow, ramifying a periosteal branch before traversing the subgaleal plane. The supratrochlear artery (b) lies medial, piercing the corrugator muscle (d), and anastomosing with the dorsal nasal artery (c) and the supraorbital artery (a).
Source: Scheuer JF 3rd, Sieber DA, Pezeshk RA, Campbell CF, Gassman AA, Rohrich RJ. Anatomy of the facial danger zones: maximizing safety during soft-tissue filler injections. Plast Reconstr Surg. 2017;139(1):50e-8e.

The supraorbital artery, also a branch of the ophthalmic artery, exits the orbit through the supraorbital notch approximately 32 mm lateral to midline, generally corresponding to a vertical line intersecting the medial limbus of the cornea. Erdogmus and Govsa found that the artery most commonly pierced the frontalis 20–40 mm above the orbital rim, and then surfaced in the subcutaneous tissue between 40 and 60 mm. However, Kleintjes observed the supraorbital artery sending vertical branches entering the subcutaneous tissue as low as 15–20 mm above the rim after a short intramuscular course. In addition to the dorsal nasal, supratrochlear, and angular arteries, the supraorbital artery sends branches that anastomose with the frontal branch of the superficial temporal artery most often at the junction of the transverse inferior and middle thirds of the forehead.[3]

Maximizing Safety

In the brow and glabella area, the vasculature is initially deep, quickly transitioning to the intramuscular and subcutaneous level. Therefore, we recommend using a low-G' filler injected intradermally to fill glabellar frown lines and bunny lines, in the brow and glabellar area. Apply digital pressure at the supraorbital rim during injection to occlude vessels. Intravascular injection at this level can travel retrograde through the anastomoses between the supraorbital, supratrochlear, and ophthalmic arteries, leading to blindness and tissue loss **(Fig. 3)**. In multiple reviews, the glabella was the most common filler injection site leading to visual loss.[3]

TEMPORAL REGION

Pertinent Anatomy

Within the temporal fossa, the frontal branch of the superficial temporal artery and temporal branch of the facial nerve run within the temporoparietal fascia. In a recently published cadaver study, the origin of the frontal branch from the superficial temporal artery was on average located 17.2 mm anterior and 36.9 mm superior to the tip of the tragus. Typically, the frontal branch of the superficial temporal artery can be located coursing over the frontalis 15.8 mm superior and 14.8 mm posterior to the peak of the brow. A line connecting these two points delineates the most common course of the artery, although variations do exist. In the study, the authors defined their danger zone as the area starting 2.5 mm lateral and 3.0 mm superior to the peak of the brow, and thus recommended digital pressure to this area when injecting the temporal hollow. Trussler et al. histologically observed the frontal branch artery running in the temporoparietal fascia in close proximity to the temporal branch of the facial nerve 2 cm above the zygomatic arch.

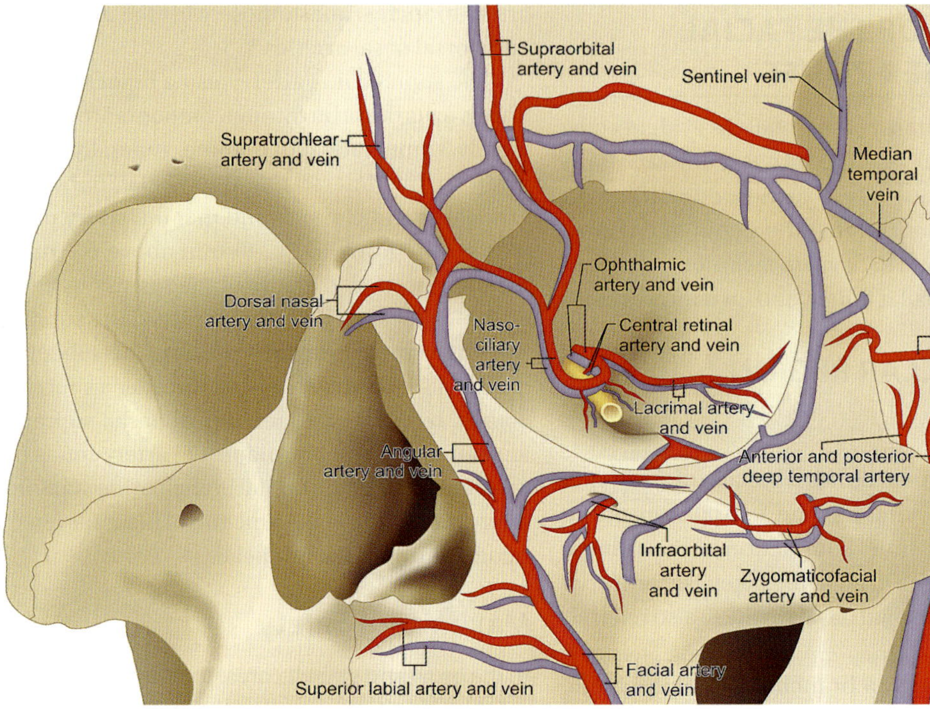

Fig. 3: Potential routes for retrograde embolization to the ophthalmic vessels.
Source: Carruthers JD, Fagien S, Rohrich RJ, Weinkle S, Carruthers A. Blindness caused by cosmetic filler injection: a review of cause and therapy. Plast Reconstr Surg. 2014;134:1197-1201.

In our dissection, we observed similar findings; the frontal branch of the superficial temporal artery ran within the temporoparietal fascia 2 cm above the arch, transitioning to become completely subcutaneous just superior to the brow near the border of the frontalis. The frontal branch of the superficial temporal artery arborized with the supraorbital arterial system in the deep and superficial planes **(Fig. 4)**. This presents another pathway of retrograde embolization to the arterial supply of the globe. In a cadaver study, dye injected into the superficial temporal artery was found within the ipsilateral globe, and even bilaterally in certain specimens.[3]

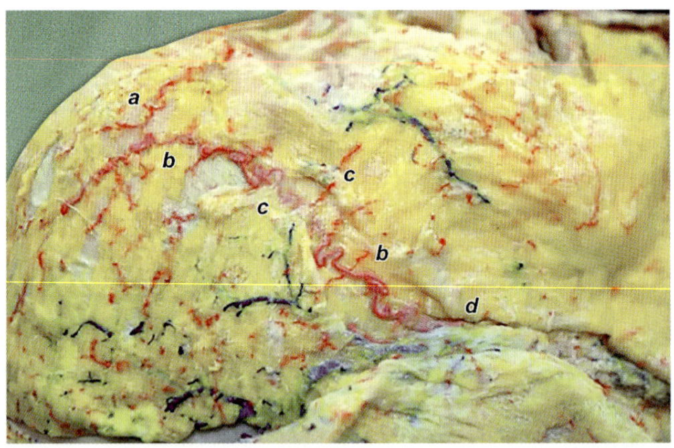

Fig. 4: The superficial temporal artery (d) is demonstrated ramifying its frontal branch (b). The subcutaneous tissue (c) has been reflected anteriorly and posteriorly to delineate the course of the frontal branch artery within the superficial temporal fascia. The frontal branch artery (b) can be clearly seen anastomosing with the supraorbital artery (a) superficial to the frontalis muscle after transitioning to the subcutaneous plane.
Source: Scheuer JF 3rd, Sieber DA, Pezeshk RA, Campbell CF, Gassman AA, Rohrich RJ. Anatomy of the facial danger zones: maximizing safety during soft-tissue filler injections. Plast Reconstr Surg. 2017;139(1):50e-8e.

Of additional concern, the middle temporal vein runs approximately 20 mm above and parallel to the zygomatic arch within the superficial temporal fat pad. Given its average size of 5.1 mm (range, 2.0–9.1 mm) and its connection to the cavernous sinus, Jung et al. recommended injecting within a fingerbreadth of the zygomatic arch in the preperiosteal plane. Although extremely rare, there have been reports of fatal nonthrombotic pulmonary embolism during fat injections when the middle temporal vein was cannulated. Hyaluronic acid (HA) facial injections have also been implicated as a cause of nonthrombotic pulmonary embolism. Tansatit et al. recommend pressing the pretragal area during filler injection to prevent a nonthrombotic pulmonary embolism through inadvertent cannulation of the middle temporal vein. In their cadaveric study, retrograde injections of the middle temporal vein did not fill the supraorbital, supratrochlear, or any of the medial orbital veins.[4] However, anterograde injections drained into the internal jugular vein. Thus, middle temporal vein injections are less likely a mechanism for ocular embolism, although it has been postulated.[3]

Despite efforts to place filler in the subcutaneous anatomical plane, cadaver studies have shown unintended deeper location of filler in the superficial temporal fascia, temporalis muscle, and encompassing a superficial muscular artery. In an attempt to obtain uniform results, some authors have heavily diluted the fillers, injecting them in the deep subcutaneous plane adjacent to the superficial temporal fascia.[3]

Maximizing Safety

In the temporal region, fillers should be injected deeply or superficially. Deep filler injections in the temporal fossa should be in the preperiosteal plane. They should be injected within a fingerbreadth of the arch and/or >25 mm above it to avoid the middle temporal vein. In the preperiosteal plane, a high-G′ filler in greater amounts will be needed to translate results superficially. Therefore, we choose to inject filler in the superficial subcutaneous tissue, staying just below the dermis while applying pressure just superior to the peak of the brow. The frontal branch of the superficial temporal artery runs one layer deeper in the temporoparietal fascia and therefore is at less risk. As the artery approaches the temporal fusion line, it transitions to the subcutaneous plane. Embolic phenomena occur when the cannulated artery propagates filler into the supraorbital system, or filler travels retrograde into the main superficial temporal artery system. Either can lead to blindness. We caution against injecting at intermediate depths because it becomes nearly impossible to discern which layer is being injected.[3]

INFRAORBITAL REGION

Pertinent Anatomy

Midface filler injections allow augmentation without the need for an alloplastic implant. Within this region, the infraorbital artery and nerve typically exit the infraorbital foramen. If the artery is inadvertently cannulated, this again provides another route for filler embolization. Likewise, injury to the nerve can lead to hyperesthesia/hypoesthesia and pain. Basic anatomical knowledge of the infraorbital foramen allows practitioners to better predict its location and avoid its contents.[3]

There is great variation in the literature regarding anatomical landmarks for the vertical plane of the infraorbital foramen. It has been documented in-line with the first premolar, second premolar, and the canine teeth. Likewise, a minority of patients have multiple foramina. The average distance between the infraorbital foramen and the inferior orbital rim is 6.3–10.9 mm. The average distance of the infraorbital foramen from facial midline is 25.7–27.1 mm in men and 24.2–26.8 mm in women. Other authors have described it being approximately 33–41% of the total distance when measuring from the medial to the lateral canthus. Approximately 50% of the time, Aziz et al. found the infraorbital foramen in the same vertical plane as the supraorbital foramen.[3]

Maximizing Safety

Overall, when injecting deep into the midface, the above measurements should be kept in mind to avoid intravascular cannulation or vascular injury. Generally, the infraorbital foramen will be located approximately one-third of the distance between the medial and lateral canthi up to 11 mm below the infraorbital rim. Clinically, the infraorbital foramen lies slightly less than a fingerbreadth below the infraorbital rim in the vertical plane of the medial limbus, or immediately lateral to it. We avoid direct deep injections into this area, choosing to inject just lateral. Injections more medial approaching the medial canthus should be avoided completely. If filler is needed in this area, it can be injected laterally and pushed medially.[3]

LIPS/COMMISSURE

Pertinent Anatomy (Upper Lip)

Perioral filler injections are becoming more common as patients frequently request more full and voluptuous lips. The goals for the patient must be determined before injection—volume versus vermilion-cutaneous enhancement, or both. Young patients generally have adequate volume but desire enhancement of the vermillion-cutaneous border. Volume is often required in older patients and those with thin lips, occasionally along with vermilion-cutaneous enhancement.[3]

Although many variations of the perioral vasculature are documented in the literature, a general concept of the most common anatomy increases the reproducibility of safe results. The takeoff of the superior labial artery off the facial artery is on average 10.4–12.1 mm lateral and approximately 43° superior to the corner of the mouth, or 5–9 mm above this landmark. However, the origin can at times be inferior to the commissure. The superior labial artery then usually runs superior to the vermillion border, then coursing inferior to the border just before approaching Cupid's bow. In the upper lip, the superior labial artery is 3–7.6 mm deep to skin, running usually between the orbicularis and the oral mucosa, or less often within the orbicularis. In two separate studies, the superior labial artery was found 4.5–7.6, 2.6–3.2, and 5.6–6.7 mm deep as measured from the skin, oral mucosa, and lower margin of the lip, respectively. Throughout its course, the superior labial artery gives off small-caliber deep (between the mucosa and muscle, or through the muscle), and superficial (between the skin and muscle) ascending branches. These can travel superiorly to anastomose with the inferior alar, columellar, and anterior septal branches.[3]

Maximizing Safety

Injections into the upper lip should be <3 mm deep, with an intermediate or low-G′ filler either at the vermillion-cutaneous border or within the dry vermillion. The superior labial artery is typically posterior at the mucosal-muscular interface and several millimeters above the inferior border of the lip. Intravascular injection can lead to tissue necrosis.[3]

Pertinent Anatomy (Commissure)

Along with other authors, we observed the facial artery lying deep to the risorius and zygomaticus major and 12–15.5 mm lateral to the commissure. However, there are cases where the artery can be running through separate muscle bands of the zygomaticus major. Clinically, the area encompassing the facial artery and the superior labial artery origin can be estimated by placing a thumb beside the corner of the mouth.[3]

Maximizing Safety

Because the facial artery and the origin of the superior labial artery generally lie deep to or within the muscle, superficial subcutaneous injections in a linear crosshatching fashion safely address volume deficiency and laxity in this area.[3]

Pertinent Anatomy (Lower Lip)

There have been attempts to categorize all of the origins and variants of the inferior labial artery. To recapitulate each is beyond the scope of this article. However, the inferior labial artery has been observed running horizontally at the level of the vermillion-cutaneous level, and at the height of the labiomental fold perfusing the lower lip with vertically oriented branches. At the level of the vermillion-cutaneous border, the inferior labial artery lies 6.4–7.1, 5.9–9.4, and 4.4–4.8 mm from the anterior, superior, and posterior borders of the lower lip, respectively **(Fig. 5)**. As the inferior labial artery branches from the facial artery, it enters the lower lip and travels between the mucosa and muscle. The numerous patterns of the inferior labial artery and its varied origins may lie in the fact that there are no universally accepted definitions distinguishing between the inferior labial artery and the labiomental artery. Although the inferior labial artery has numerous variations ranging from a common trunk with the superior labial artery to its complete absence, these patterns may overall not be as important as ascertaining the correct depth of the artery when injecting fillers. In an attempt to clarify, Lee et al. classified an artery traveling in the middle of the lower lip as a horizontal labiomental artery, regardless of the final trajectory toward the lower lip; an artery traveling along the level of the lower lip vermillion-cutaneous border with an origin near the commissure was called an inferior labial artery. When this distinction is not made, the origin of the inferior labial artery varies in the literature between just superior to the corner of the mouth, all the way to the lower margin of the mandible.[3]

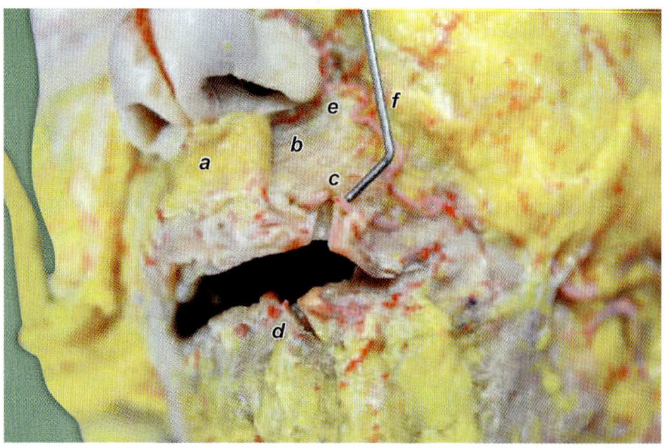

Fig. 5: The subcutaneous tissue (a) has been reflected, revealing the orbicularis oris muscle (b). The superior labial artery (c) can be seen running deep to the orbicularis on the labial mucosa, superior to the inferior lip border. The inferior labial artery (d) is demonstrated running in a similar fashion in the lower lip. The facial artery (f) is seen ramifying the inferior alar artery (e) in the upper third of the nasolabial fold.
Source: Scheuer JF 3rd, Sieber DA, Pezeshk RA, Campbell CF, Gassman AA, Rohrich RJ. Anatomy of the facial danger zones: maximizing safety during soft-tissue filler injections. Plast Reconstr Surg. 2017;139(1):50e-8e.

Maximizing Safety

Lower lip injections should be with an intermediate- or low-G' filler either at the vermillion-cutaneous border or within the dry vermillion, no >3 mm deep. The inferior labial artery is typically posterior at the mucosal-muscular interface and below the superior border of the lip. Intravascular injection in the area leads to tissue necrosis.[3]

NASOLABIAL FOLD

Pertinent Anatomy

Filling a deep nasolabial fold instantly gives the face a rejuvenated appearance. As for other areas of the face, the various naming schema and classification systems of the facial artery and its superior course have led to confusion in the literature. For our purposes, the arterial portion running from the cheilion to the alar base is referred to as the facial artery until the takeoff of the lateral nasal artery. Thereafter, it is referred to as the angular artery.[3]

After giving off the superior labial artery near the commissure, the facial artery continues superiorly adjacent to the nasolabial fold. In the cadaver study by Yang et al., the facial artery was observed in close proximity to the nasolabial fold, with its entire course being medial (42.9%), lateral (23.2%), or crossing the nasolabial fold (33.9%). At the transition between the upper middle third and the middle lower third of the nasolabial fold, the facial artery was on average 1.7 mm medial and 0.3 mm medial to the nasolabial fold, respectively. At the level of the ala, the facial artery branches to yield the inferior alar artery and the lateral nasal artery immediately above. It then continues as the angular artery when present. There are also “duplex” or “detouring” patterns, where an ipsilateral duplicate facial artery may branch low in the face, traveling to the infraorbital area and then crossing medially at the nasojugal groove to become the angular artery. Lastly, there are patterns where the angular artery is absent or arises in a retrograde fashion from the ophthalmic artery. This is not a comprehensive review of every branching pattern of the facial artery, but instead an illustration of the variability.[3]

When injecting in the region of the nasolabial fold, the depth of the artery becomes all the more pertinent to avoid an intravascular injury. Lee et al. described the relationship of the facial artery with regard to the facial muscles in a cadaver dissection series. In 85.2% of cadavers, the facial artery was superficial to the mimetic muscles at some point between the alar base and the modiolus **(Figs. 6 and 7)**. In 16.7%, the artery was completely subcutaneous from the modiolus to the alar base. In only 14.8% of cadavers did the facial artery remain completely beneath the mimetic muscle all the way to the alar base. In our dissection, the artery became very superficial in the upper third of the nasolabial fold as it ramified the inferior alar artery and the lateral nasal artery. It is in this area that it becomes most prone to injury during subcutaneous filler injections.[3]

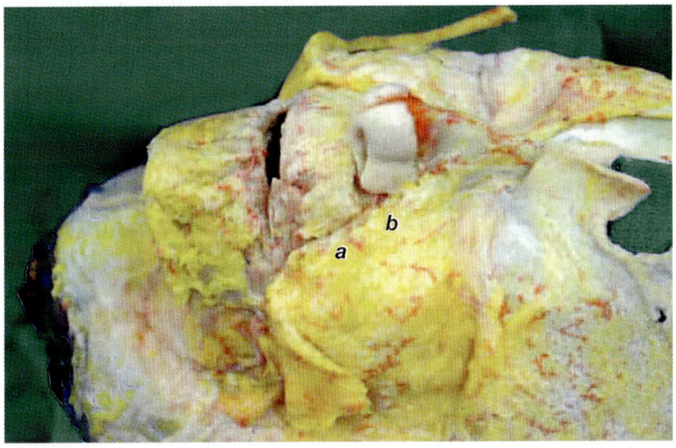

Fig. 6: The nasolabial portion of the facial artery is seen running beneath subcutaneous tissue (a) until its upper third, where it becomes more superficial (b) and at greater risk for injury during injections.
Source: Scheuer JF 3rd, Sieber DA, Pezeshk RA, Campbell CF, Gassman AA, Rohrich RJ. Anatomy of the facial danger zones: maximizing safety during soft-tissue filler injections. Plast Reconstr Surg. 2017;139(1):50e-8e.

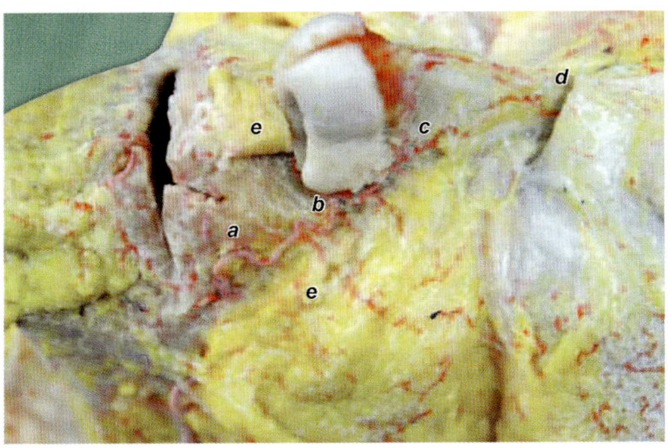

Fig. 7: With the subcutaneous tissue (e) reflected, the facial artery (a) is seen running in the nasolabial fold sporadically within the muscle but mostly in the plane between the subcutaneous tissue and muscle. The artery becomes superficial (b) in the upper third of the nasolabial fold and is at risk during superficial injections. The transition of the facial artery into the angular artery (c), and its anastomosis with the dorsal nasal artery (d) is demonstrated. Of note, the facial artery lies approximately 1.5 cm lateral to the commissure.
Source: Scheuer JF 3rd, Sieber DA, Pezeshk RA, Campbell CF, Gassman AA, Rohrich RJ. Anatomy of the facial danger zones: maximizing safety during soft-tissue filler injections. Plast Reconstr Surg. 2017;139(1):50e-8e.

Maximizing Safety

In the lower two-thirds of the nasolabial fold, injections into the deep dermal and superficial subcutaneous plane are generally safe because most of the facial artery course lies beneath muscle and/or above it but in deeper planes; however, in the upper one-third, the artery can become very superficial. Near the alar base, we recommend injecting either intradermally or in the preperiosteal plane. Subcutaneous injections in this area can lead to alar and cheek necrosis if the facial artery or its branches are cannulated or injured. This is also a pathway for ocular embolism through propagation in the angular artery and its anastomoses with dorsal nasal branches. In one review, the nasolabial fold was the second most common injection site leading to tissue necrosis, and, in another study, the third most common site leading to visual loss[3] **(Fig. 7)**.

NOSE

Pertinent Anatomy

In general, the layers of the nose are as follows—epidermis, dermis, subcutaneous fat, muscle and fascia (musculoaponeurotic layer), areolar tissue, perichondrium/periosteum, and cartilage/bone. As discussed previously, the facial artery gives rise to the lateral nasal artery and angular artery through a variety of patterns. The facial artery is on average 3.2 mm lateral to the most lateral point of the ala. More importantly, the facial artery gives rise to the inferior alar branch traveling along the inferior margin of the nostril and lateral nasal artery, which runs in the subdermal plexus 2–3 mm superior to the alar groove over the cephalic margin of the lower lateral cartilage. After this branching point, the facial artery now continues toward the medial canthus as the angular artery while anastomosing with the dorsal nasal arterial system running over the nasal dorsum **(Fig. 8)**. Toriumi et al. illustrated a subdermal vascular plexus that was most prominent in the nasal tip and a larger arterial and venous system of the nasal skin found superficial to the nasal musculature (superficial musculoaponeurotic system layer) in the subcutaneous plane. There is sparse vasculature within the areolar layer beneath the muscular layer aside from what they termed the "deep" or "lateral nasal veins" running cephalic to the lateral crura. Saban et al. described a "marginal artery" coursing over the lower lateral cartilage caudal border

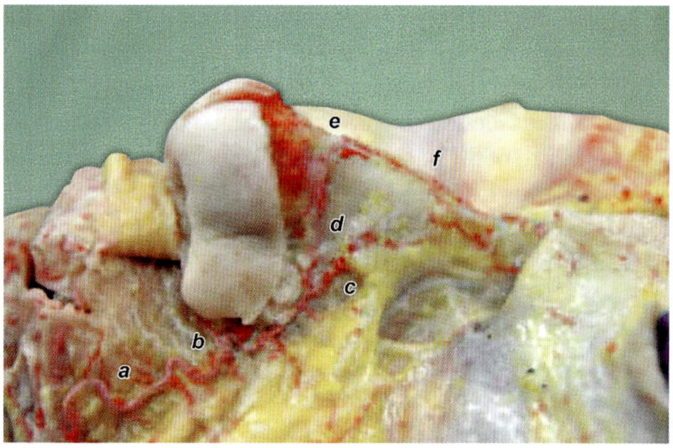

Fig. 8: The facial artery (a) ramifies the inferior alar branch (b) and the lateral nasal artery (d) before becoming the angular artery (c). The dorsal nasal artery (f), lateral nasal arteries (d), and columellar artery (not pictured) form a rich vascular network at the nasal tip in the subdermal layer (e). *Source:* Scheuer JF 3rd, Sieber DA, Pezeshk RA, Campbell CF, Gassman AA, Rohrich RJ. Anatomy of the facial danger zones: maximizing safety during soft-tissue filler injections. Plast Reconstr Surg. 2017;139(1):50e-8e.

toward the tip after branching from either the facial artery or the lateral nasal artery. The dorsal nasal artery (a terminal branch of the ophthalmic artery) emerges from the medial obit and courses over the dorsum above the muscular layer to contribute to the subdermal plexus at the tip.[3]

Maximizing Safety

Given the shallow nature of the vasculature located within the nose, a misplaced injection can lead to disastrous results. Superficial injections compressing or injuring the superficial vasculature in the tip and alar facial groove can lead to blood pressure (BP) and alar necrosis, respectively. Likewise, given the BP, dorsal, and sidewall vessel anastomoses with the ophthalmic artery, intravascular injections in these areas can cause retrograde propagation of filler, leading to ocular ischemia and blindness. Therefore, all lateral injections should be >3 mm above the alar groove and deep. Injections to the BP and dorsum should be deep in the preperichondrial and preperiosteal planes. In several reviews analyzing facial danger zones, nasal filler injections were documented as the leading cause of tissue necrosis and the second leading cause of visual loss after the glabella.[3]

Conclusion

Despite detailed published descriptions of the facial vasculature, the anatomy can be quite variable, and vascular injuries can occur even after the best precautions are taken. Likewise, actual needle depth can be difficult to track and at times unpredictable. Most importantly, practitioners need to recognize complications in a timely manner and take the appropriate measures to minimize what can be a devastating result.[3]

PERIORBITAL REGION

Looking bright and youthful in today's culture impacts quality of life in many patients. Facial aging is a complex and dynamic process. All people age differently as a result of imbalance, disharmony, and disproportion of the aging process between the overlying soft tissue and the underlying bony frameworks. The upper periorbital subunit is one of the first facial regions to show signs of aging, and even minor changes in its structure and volume can distort the perceived emotions and health of patients. An aesthetic and youthful upper periorbital subunit is characterized by a well-defined brow of appropriate height and shape, fullness of the upper periorbit, a crisp and well-defined upper eyelid crease, minimal skin excess, and good skin quality.[5]

In the aging process of this facial area, one group of patients displays signs of aging due predominantly to soft tissue ptosis of the upper eyelid, requiring surgical excision. Another group presents with volume depletion of the soft tissue and bony resorption of the orbit. The loss of septal support, leading to brow prolapse and an exacerbation of upper eyelid fullness and congestion, can also contribute to the aging process. This appearance is characterized by deflation of the upper eyelid as well as hollowing and visibility of the supraorbital bony rim, leading to a sunken, hollow, and skeletonized orbit, which can make the patient appear sickly, anorexic, and old. In recent years, modern facial rejuvenation surgery has evolved toward volume restoration in addition to tissue suspension.[5]

Comprehensive analysis of both soft tissue and bony structural changes is essential for the periorbital rejuvenation. Surgical procedures and office-based nonsurgical procedures form an important basis for periorbital rejuvenation, including cosmeceuticals, chemical peels, laser and light treatments, neurotoxins, and fillers. Improved understanding of the pathophysiology of aging and technical advancements in nonsurgical techniques has enabled us to achieve better and more comprehensive improvement for patients.[5]

The eyes are probably the most important aesthetic unit in the human body. When the eye region appears bright and fresh, the whole person has an aura of health, vitality, and youthfulness. There is a marked transition from the thin eyelid skin to the thicker skin of the eyebrow and cheek. Eyelid skin is the thinnest in the body, often <1 mm thick, and unique in having no subcutaneous fat.[5]

The orbicularis oculi muscle, the sphincter muscle of the eyelids, is arbitrarily divided into three portions—pretarsal, preseptal, and orbital. The pretarsal portion of the muscle is thin, overlies the tarsal plates, and is essential for eyelid position and reflexive blinking. Weakening this portion of the muscle will change the eyelid shape and contour. The preseptal portion courses in concentric curves, anterior to the orbital septum. The muscle is involved in involuntary and voluntary eyelid closure. The orbital orbicularis muscle fibers interdigitate with the frontalis and are primarily responsible for forced eyelid closure and depression of the eyebrow.[5]

The blood supply of the eyelids is derived from the facial system, which arises from the external carotid artery, and the orbital system, which originates from the internal carotid artery along branches of the ophthalmic artery. The superficial and deep plexuses of arteries provide a vast blood supply to the upper and lower eyelids. The venous drainage of the eyelids can be divided into two portions—a superficial, or preseptal, system that drains into the internal and external jugular veins, and a deep, or posttarsal, system that flows into the cavernous sinus.[5]

Branches of the ophthalmic and maxillary divisions of the trigeminal nerve provide the sensory innervations of the eyelids. The upper eyelid is innervated by the supraorbital, supratrochlear, and lacrimal nerves. The medial aspect of the upper and lower eyelids is supplied by the infratrochlear nerve. The lateral aspect of the upper eyelid and temple is supplied by the zygomaticotemporal branch of the maxillary nerve. The central aspect of the lower eyelid is supplied by infraorbital nerve, a branch of the maxillary nerve, and the lateral aspect of the lower eyelid is supplied by the zygomaticofacial branch of the maxillary nerve. Facial motor function is provided by the facial nerve and the oculomotor nerve. The superior division of the face innervates the upper eyelids via its temporal (frontal) branches and the lower lids via zygomatic and buccal branches.[5]

Hyaluronic Acid

The ideal substance to treat the periorbital region should be biocompatible, nonimmunogenic, stable, and secure, and should offer good cosmetic results, having long-term duration obtained with minimal complication. Of the available fillers, HA is the one that most approximates all of these characteristics. When used as an injectable filler agent, HA consists of repeating polymer chains of the polysaccharide with internal crosslinks of agents that bind the polymer together. By varying the type of cross-linking material and the amount, the characteristics of the gel can vary in the degree of hardness, amount of lift, duration of survival, and resistance of degradation by heat or enzymes. The use of hyaluronic acid with low viscosity, low concentrations, and high malleability is recommended for this area.[5]

Technique

When treating the periorbital region with HA, the authors perform asepsis and antisepsis with three passes of alcoholic chlorhexidine using sterile gloves and gauzes. They mark a point in the hemipupilar line in the upper eyelid crease and a lateral point at the end of the crease. The use of anesthetic lidocaine and an adrenaline button aims vasoconstriction in the area. The anesthetic effect is not necessary because the caliber of the needles and cannulas are extremely small. 27 G × 50 mm or 30 G × 25 mm cannulas are used. One orifice is made with a needle of the same gauge of the cannula with an inclination in the direction that will be introduced the cannula with an angle of approximately 45°. In this way, the entire dermis is transfixed, reaching the subcutaneous. The application is made by slow retroinjection. A small amount of HA with a concentration of 15 mg/mL (Juvederm Volbella, Allergan) with high flexibility is used, ranging from 0.1 to 0.2 mL per point.[5]

The filling technique for rejuvenation of the lower periorbicular region is held by the authors at deeper levels when compared to the upper region. For this reason, larger volumes of hyaluronic acid are often used. Tracing a point about 2 cm below the lower edge of the orbit in intersection with the lateral line of limbo, a micropuncture is made with the needle toward the lower corner of the eye up to the submuscular plane. An angle of approximately 60° is used for the insertion of the cannula below the orbicularis muscle of the eye. One application with the fanning technique is performed until the direction of hemipupillary line. Volumes ranging from 0.3 to 08 mL of AH are applied in this region. A fourth point is held at a distance of 1.5 cm from the horizontal line from the outer corner of the eye where it meets the malar groove. Strong pressure is applied toward the bone ground at the end of the procedure so that the product can be regularly distributed.[5]

AESTHETICS OF THE PERIORBITAL REGION

The periorbital region is an area where hyperfunction of muscles results in a tired and aged appearance and increased rhytids. Hyperdynamic glabellar musculature can create an angry appearance, while overuse of the lateral eyelid muscles can narrow the eyelid aperture.[6] Treatment with botulinum toxin can lessen the contraction of hyperdynamic periorbital muscles, improve the eyelid aperture and brow position, and decrease periorbital rhytids.[6]

The position and orientation of the eyebrow is related to the relative strength and contraction of the brow depressors versus the brow elevators. The main elevators of the eyebrow are the paired frontalis muscles. The temporoparietalis muscle is a rarely described and highly variable muscle. In conjunction with the frontalis, it raises the eyebrows, widens the eyes, and wrinkles the skin of the forehead. This muscle may display a greater mass in younger individuals. Depression of the eyebrow is accomplished by contraction of the midline procerus muscles and the paired corrugator and orbicularis oculi muscles.[6] Correct placement of appropriate amounts of toxin to minimize rhytids, without negatively affecting eyebrow position, is important.[6]

ANATOMY OF THE PERIORBITAL MUSCLES

Frontalis

The frontalis muscle is a large, vertically oriented, fan-shaped muscle that covers the majority of the forehead

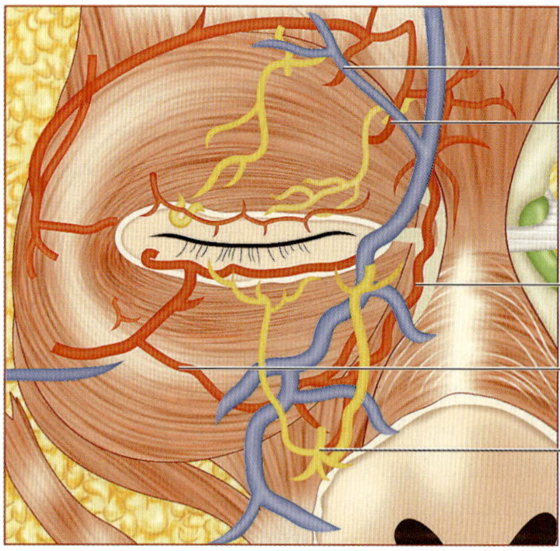

Fig. 9: Main branches of the blood supply of the periorbital region. *Source:* Bravo BS, Rocha CR, Bastos JT, Silva PM. Comprehensive treatment of periorbital region with hyaluronic acid. J Clin Aesthet Dermatol. 2015;8(6):30-5.

and is located within the sheaths of the galea aponeurosis **(Fig. 9)**. It originates from the galea aponeurosis near the anterior hairline and inserts into the forehead skin near the eyebrow. There is no bony origin or insertion for the frontalis muscles. The inferior fibers of the frontalis muscle interdigitate with the procerus and orbicularis muscles. Medially, the two halves of the frontalis muscle have a variable relationship, with some right and left frontalis muscles having no connection, while others interdigitate and even overlap in the lower half of the forehead. The motor innervation to the frontalis muscle is the temporal branch of the facial nerve. Contractions of the superior and inferior portions of the muscle have different actions, with the superior portion causing descent of the anterior hairline and the inferior portion causing elevation of the brow. For this reason, injection of toxin into the superior frontalis muscle can decrease forehead rhytids, without creating brow ptosis.[6]

Corrugator Supercilii

The paired corrugator supercilii muscles are obliquely oriented and are located in the inferomedial brow deep to the inferior portion of the frontalis muscles. These are the only periorbital muscles with a bony connection, with the medial head originating from the frontal bone at the superomedial orbit and the insertion being into the skin of the middle portion of the eyebrow and into the fascia on the deep surface of the frontalis muscle. As the muscle courses laterally, it becomes superficial, with its ending point being at a variable location in the eyebrow skin. The muscle is pierced by the supraorbital and supratrochlear neurovascular bundles. These nerves exit a notch or foramen in the supraorbital rim, pierce the corrugator muscles, and then pierce the frontalis muscles and branches of the nerve travel on the superficial aspect of the frontalis. The motor innervation to the corrugator muscles is from two separate branches of the facial nerve and may present a variable pattern of contralateral or cross-innervation. The medial head of the muscle is supplied by the zygomatic branch of the facial nerve, whereas the lateral portion is supplied by the temporal branch of the nerve. Contraction of the muscle causes vertical grooves in the glabellar skin and imparts an angry expression. Contraction also causes an inferomedial descent of the medial clubhead of the brow. Injection of toxin into the corrugators decreases the vertical glabellar rhytids and causes slight lateralization of the medial brow.[6]

Procerus

The procerus is a midline flat and pyramidally shaped muscle. It is located at the root of the nose and contributes to nasal contour of the upper half of the nose. The procerus originates from the periosteum and perichondrium of the nasal bones and upper lateral cartilages and from the fascia of the nasal superficial musculoaponeurotic system. It inserts into the midline skin overlying the nasal root and thus has no bony attachments. The procerus interdigitates superiorly with the frontalis muscle, inferiorly with the nasalis muscle, and laterally with the depressor supercilii, orbicularis oculi, and deeper corrugator muscles.[1] The motor innervation to the procerus muscle is supplied by the zygomatic branch of the facial nerve. Contraction of the midline muscle is responsible for horizontal glabellar rhytids, descent of the medial brow, and transverse midline nasal rhytids. These are different from the so called bunny lines or lateral nasal rhytids, which appear on the lateral aspect of the nasal dorsum and occur from contraction of the levator labii superioris alaeque nasi muscle. Injection of botulinum toxin into the procerus can decrease the transverse folds at the medial nasal root and can slightly elevate the medial brow.[6]

Orbicularis Oculi

The orbicularis oculi are paired sphincteric muscles that are protractors of the eyelids and depressors of the eyebrows. The muscles are located beneath the thin eyelid and thicker eyebrow skin. The muscles are separated into pretarsal (superficial to the tarsal plates), preseptal (superficial to the orbital septum), and orbital (more peripheral) portions. These designations are not true anatomic separations of muscle but rather names that identify the muscle location. In fact, there are no true separations or septa distinguishing these muscle segments.[6]

The origins and insertions of the orbicularis muscles as well as its anatomical relationships with adjacent structures are complex. The muscle primarily travels in the soft tissues of the eyelids but is fixed medially and laterally to the bony orbital wall by the orbital retaining ligaments.[1] The orbital retaining ligament medially to the midpupillary line is termed the tear trough ligament and is responsible in some individuals for adding to the concavity just inferior to the convex medial orbital fat, also known as the tear trough deformity. The orbicularis muscles interdigitate with the corrugator and frontalis superiorly.[6]

Laterally, the orbicularis muscles travel superficial to the temporalis fascia; medially, the muscle covers the depressor supercilii; and inferiorly, the muscles travel between the superficial and deep (suborbicularis oculi fat) fat pads of the cheek. The inferomedial extent of the lower eyelid orbicularis muscles covers the levator labii superioris and the levator labii superioris alaeque nasi muscles.[6]

The motor innervation of the orbicularis oculi muscles is innervated by multiple nerves and has multiple motor endplates. The medial and inferior portions of the muscle are innervated by the zygomatic branch, and the lateral and central portions of the muscle are innervated by the anterior portion of the temporal branch of the facial nerve.[1] Contraction of the orbicularis muscles causes closure of the eyelids and descent of the eyebrows. Contraction of the palpebral marginal portion of the orbicularis causes an involuntary weak eye closure (blink), and contraction of the orbital more peripheral component of the muscle creates a voluntary, sphincteric, and potentially stronger eye closure (squint). The orbital component is responsible for most eyelid wrinkles and for descent of the lateral brow. Injection of the orbicularis oris muscles can decrease dynamic lateral canthal lines, decrease rhytids of the lower eyelid, and elevate the lateral or tail of the brow.[6]

PERIORBITAL INJECTION OF BOTULINUM TOXIN (BOXES 1 AND 2)

Injection of botulinum toxin in the periorbital region can be performed to decrease rhytids, to increase the eyelid aperture, to change the eyebrow position or shape, or to create a combination of these effects. The injection of toxin should affect a diminished muscular contraction of the desired muscle, while not negatively decreasing adjacent muscle contraction.[6]

The relative contraction of the brow elevator (frontalis muscle) and the brow depressors (corrugators, procerus, and orbicularis oculi muscle) affects the position and shape of the eyebrow. The purpose of frontalis muscle injection is usually to diminish transverse forehead rhytids. Toxin injections are usually performed in the superior half of the muscle. Overinjection of toxin, especially in the inferior portion of the frontalis muscle, may result in brow ptosis.[6]

Injection of the corrugator and procerus muscle decreases the vertical and transverse folds at the root of the nose. These injections can also affect medial brow elevation. In that, the medial portion of the corrugator originates from the superomedial orbit, and injection in this region should be deep to treat this part of the muscle. As the muscle travels laterally, it becomes more superficial. For this reason, injection of the lateral portion of the muscle should be more superficial. If the injections are placed too inferiorly, if there is diffusion of toxin, or if there is an anatomical dehiscence in the septum orbitale, toxin can affect the levator aponeurosis of the upper eyelid, causing ptosis of the lid.[6]

Injection of the orbicularis oculi at the lateral canthus can decrease dynamic lateral canthal lines, elevate the lateral

BOX 1: Soft tissue landmarks used as anthropometric reference points.

Beginning superiorly:
- *Vertex (v):* The highest seen point on the head with the head in Frankfort horizontal
- *Trichion (tr):* The junction of the hairline and the forehead in the midline
- *Glabella (g):* The most prominent point of the forehead in the midline between the eyebrows
- *Nasion (n):* The midline point of the junction of the frontonasal suture and the superior nasal bones. Externally, nasion often corresponds to the point of greatest concavity of the nasal dorsum near a line level with the upper lid lash line
- *Orbitale (or):* The palpable point of the lowest margin of the inferior orbital rim
- *Porion (po):* The most superior point of the external auditory meatus.
- *Frankfurt horizontal:* The line connecting porion and orbitale. This line is parallel to the floor for horizontal (FH) anthropometric measurements. It is an approximation of neutral head position in straight gaze
- *Endocanthion (en):* The point of the medial canthus where the upper and lower lids join
- *Pronasale (prn):* The most prominent point of the nasal tip
- *Subnasale (sn):* The deepest point at the junction of the base of the columella and the upper lip in the midline
- *Stomion (sto):* The midline point where the upper lip touches the lower lip
- *Sublabial (sl):* The midline point at the junction of the lower border of the cutaneous lower lip and the superior border of the chin. It is the deepest point of the labiomental groove
- *Pogonion (pg):* The most prominent point of the chin in the midline
- *Gnathion (gn):* The most inferior point of the lower border of the mandible; also called menton (me). In cephalometric analysis, gnathion and menton are two different points on the mandible

Source: Grabb and Smith's Plastic Surgery, 6th edition.

BOX 2: The neoclassical canons frequently used for facial analysis.

- The height of vertex to endocanthion is equal to the height of endocanthion to gnathion (two-section canon)
- The heights of trichion to nasion, nasion to subnasale, and subnasale to gnathion are equal (three-section canon)
- The heights of vertex to trichion, trichion to glabella, glabella to subnasale, and subnasale to gnathion are equal (four-section canon).
- The width of the ala equals one-fourth the width of the distance between the zygomas (nasofacial proportion canon)
- The length of the nose is equal to the height of the ear (nasoaural proportion canon)
- The inclination of the nasal dorsum is equal to the inclination of the ear (nasoaural inclination canon)
- The distance between the medial canthi is equal to the width of the eye fissure (medial to lateral canthus of the eye) (orbital proportion canon)
- The distance between the medial canthi equals the width of the ala (orbitonasal proportion canon)
- The width of the mouth equals 1% the width of the ala (naso-oral proportion canon)

Source: Grabb and Smith's Plastic Surgery, 6th edition

brow, and increase the eyelid aperture. The orbicularis muscle near the lateral aspect of the lower eyelid is quite superficial, and injections should therefore approximate the superficial location of this muscle. Care should be taken to avoid superficial veins that course through the immediate subcutaneous tissue in the lateral canthal region. It is also important to avoid an injection in this region which is too inferior on the upper cheek. If toxin diffuses too inferiorly, the origin of the zygomaticus major muscle can be affected causing asymmetry of the smile.[6]

Injection of botulinum toxin in the periorbital muscles can significantly improve periorbital aging. The ability to modulate eyebrow position and eyelid aperture, as well as decrease periorbital rhytids and folds, provides an important adjunct to periorbital rejuvenation. A thorough knowledge of muscular anatomy and the position of important anatomical landmarks are necessary to assure efficient injection and minimize complications.[6,7]

CONCLUSION

Although there is heterogeneity of structural changes among individuals, facial anatomy and facial aging follow a regular pattern. This enables the clinician empowered with knowledge of facial anatomy to appropriately modify the effects in a safe manner, respecting any anatomical structures that traverse the region.

REFERENCES

1. Neligan PC. Plastic Surgery. Volume 3: Craniofacial and Pediatric Plastic Surgery, Anatomy of the Head & Neck, 4th edition; 2018. pp. 1,3,5,7,9,10,14.
2. Cotofana S, Lachman N. Anatomy of the facial fat compartments and their relevance in aesthetic surgery. J Dtsch Dermatol Gets. 2019;17(4):399-413.
3. Scheuer JF 3rd, Sieber DA, Pezeshk RA, Campbell CF, Gassman AA, Rohrich RJ. Anatomy of the facial danger zones: maximizing safety during soft-tissue filler injections. Plast Reconstr Surg. 2017;139(1):50e-8e.
4. Lee SH, Lee HJ, Kim YS, Tansatit T, Kim HJ. Novel Anatomic Description of the Course of the Inferior Palpebral Vein for Minimally Invasive Aesthetic Treatments. Dermatol Surg. 2016;42:618-23.
5. Bravo BS, Rocha CR, Bastos JT, Silva PM. Comprehensive treatment of periorbital region with hyaluronic acid. J Clin Aesthet Dermatol. 2015;8(6):30-5.
6. Sykes JM, Trevidic P, Suárez GA, Criollo-Lamilla G. Newer understanding of specific anatomic targets in the aging face as applied to injectables: facial muscles—identifying optimal targets for neuromodulators. Plast Reconstr Surg. 2015;136(5 Suppl):56S-61S.
7. Mathes SJ. Plastic Surgery: The Head and Neck. 2nd edition. W B Saunders Co Ltd; 2006. p. 1000.

CHAPTER 4

Wound Healing and Wound Management

Manas Chatterjee, GR Rajput, CR Srinivas, C Shanmuga Sekar

KEY MESSAGES

- Wound healing includes three phases: Inflammatory, proliferative, and remodeling.
- Neutrophils play a role in the initial inflammatory stage of the wound process.
- Macrophages function to remove residual bacteria, foreign bodies, and remaining necrotic tissue in the late inflammatory phase.
- Platelets, which are the initial cells in healing process, release several important mediators which are responsible for the initiation and progression of wounds through the subsequent phases of wound healing.
- Mast cells are increased in numbers in keloids and hypertrophic scars.
- Transforming growth factor-β (TGF-β) is the main inflammatory mediator responsible for the recruitment of neutrophils to start the inflammatory phase of wound healing.
- Vascular endothelial growth factor (VEGF) is responsible for the neoangiogenesis in the later stages of wound healing.
- Matrix metalloproteinases (MMPs) are zinc-dependent endopeptidases which degrade the extracellular matrix and help in wound remodeling.
- Proper wound management includes wound cleaning, dressings, and debridement.
- Management of wounds depends on the type of wound and is affected by general and local factors.
- Moist environment aids wound healing.
- Various types of dressings, such as occlusive, semiocclusive, and biological dressings such as grafts, are available.

WOUND HEALING

INTRODUCTION

Dorland's medical dictionary defines wound as "disruption in the normal continuity of the body structure." Even though the conventional definition specifies a wound as separation or discontinuity of the skin, mucous membrane or tissue caused by physical, biological, or chemical insult, the healing process depends on local wound factors, systemic mediators, the underlying disease, and the type of injury. Chronic wounds are the result of an inadequate repair process that is unable to restore anatomic and functional integrity in an appropriate length of time.[1]

PHASES IN WOUND HEALING

The three phases in wound healing are **(Figs. 1A to D)**:

1. Inflammatory phase
2. Proliferative phase
3. Remodeling phase

Inflammatory Phase

The initial phase after cutaneous injury is dominated by inflammatory reactions mediated by cytokines, chemokines, growth factors, and their actions on cellular receptors.

The first step in this phase is *vascular response and hemostasis*.[2] Hemostasis consists of two phases: (1) Formation of fibrin clot and (2) coagulation. Following tissue injury, hemostasis occurs to minimize hemorrhage. When the blood vessels constrict, platelets are activated by binding to the exposed collagen in the extracellular matrix (ECM). The platelets then release various factors, such as fibronectin (FN), thrombospondin, and von Willebrand factor, which promote further platelet activation and aggregation.[3] The activated factors result in the formation of a fibrin matrix which functions as a provisional matrix to stabilize the wound site. The aggregated platelets then become trapped in the fibrin matrix, thus forming a stable clot within the provisional matrix.

Platelets release several important mediators which are responsible for the initiation and progression of wounds through the subsequent phases of wound healing. The degranulation of alpha granules and dense bodies causes release of mediators such as platelet-derived growth factor (PDGF) and transforming growth factor (TGF)-β. TGF-α and PDGF recruit various cells, such as neutrophils and macrophages to enter the wound. PDGF also recruits fibroblasts to the wound and activates the production of collagen and glycosaminoglycans by fibroblasts, which are important for the repair of the ECM.[4,5]

The next step in this phase is *inflammation*, which begins within the first 24 hours after an injury. The vasoactive

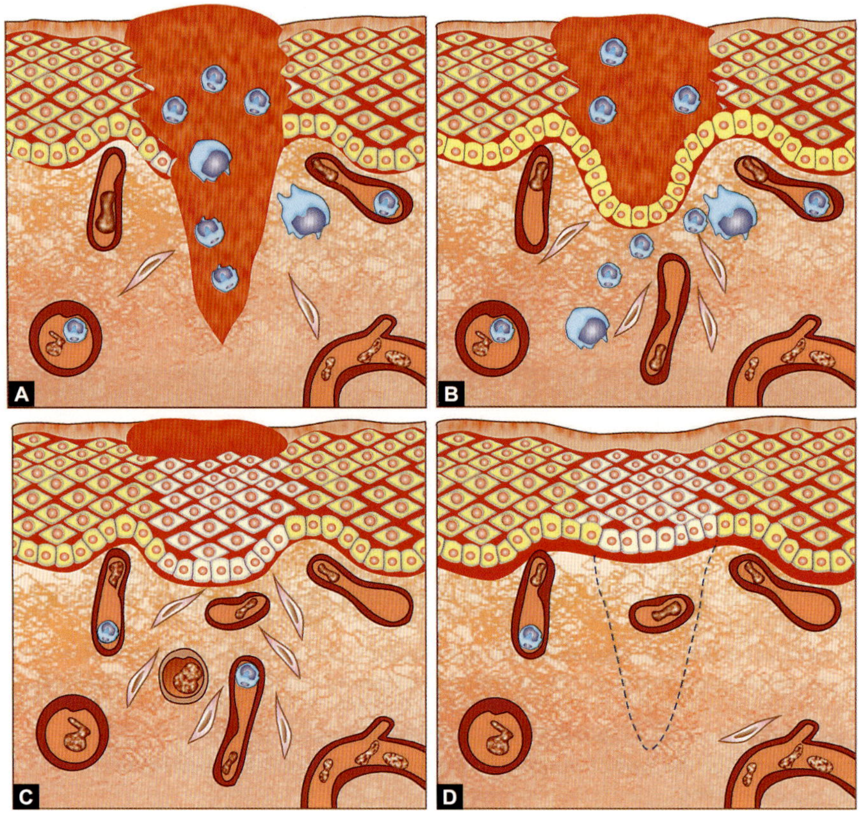

Figs. 1A to D: (A) Inflammatory phase—the wound is rinsed by blood and filled with blood–collagen and fibrin constituents; (B) Proliferative phase—resorption of blood–collagen and re-epithelialization; (C and D) Maturation and remodeling phase—growth of new epithelial cell.

substances released by the damaged cells and clot breakdown mediate this response. The dilated capillaries become leaky and thus allow the efficient movement of neutrophils from the vasculature to the site of injury. Leukocyte migration occurs by diapedesis and margination. As various chemical signals are released from the wound site, the endothelial cells in the nearby vessels are activated and begin to express specialized cell adhesion molecules (CAMs) called selectins. These CAMs cause the neutrophils to bind to the endothelial cell surface by a process called pavementing. The adherent neutrophils begin to roll along the endothelial cell lining and then by a process called diapedesis, they squeeze through the cell junctions that have been made leaky by the mast cell mediators.[6,7]

The primary function of the neutrophils is phagocytosis of any foreign materials and to kill bacteria by the powerful battery of enzymes and reactive oxygen species, which they can generate. The neutrophils actually initiate the first stage of the proliferative phase by releasing interleukin 1 (IL-1) and tumor necrosis factor alpha (TNF-α) to begin the activation of fibroblasts and epithelial cells.

During the inflammatory phase, activated macrophages also play a key role in the regulation of wound healing. Wound macrophages are derived from fixed tissue monocytes that originate from circulating monocytes. In this early phase of wound healing, the macrophage either from circulation or tissue resident pool differentiate themselves into M1 subtype which has predominant function of scavenging and removing residual bacteria, foreign bodies, and remaining necrotic tissue.[8] Macrophages also secrete a number of growth factors and cytokines, such as PDGF, TGF-β, TNF-α, fibroblast growth factor (FGF), insulin-like growth factor (IGF)-1, and IL-6, which then recruit fibroblasts and endothelial cells to the wound site for matrix deposition and neovascularization. The macrophages also produce tissue inhibitors of matrix metalloproteinases (TIMP) which inhibit the enzymatic destruction of tissues.[9] The result of the inflammatory phase is a clean wound bed. These M1 subset of macrophages are switched to M2 subset during remodeling phase with different role in wound healing as discussed subsequently.[10]

Proliferative Phase

The proliferative phase is characterized by fibroblast proliferation, myofibroblast synthesis, and collagen deposition to provide a stable ECM at the wound site. Myofibroblast differs from fibroblast as these cells have smoother muscle actin which is contractile in nature and hence supports wound closure. Within a few days after wounding, the fibroblasts start synthesizing collagen. Deposition of collagen gradually enables the skin integrity to be restored. The new ECM consists of collagen, proteoglycans, and FNs. In addition, angiogenesis occurs such that new blood vessels replace the previously damaged capillaries and provide nourishment for the matrix.

The hallmark of proliferation stage is formation of granulation tissue. Granulation tissue consists of a dense network of blood vessels and capillaries, elevated cellular density of fibroblasts and macrophages, and randomly organized collagen fibers. Fibroblasts migrate into the wound in response to mediators released from the platelets and macrophages and move through the ECM. The fibroblasts also secrete matrix metalloproteinases (MMPs), which facilitate their movement through the matrix and help with the removal of damaged matrix components. Once the fibroblasts and myofibroblasts have entered the wound, they produce collagen, proteoglycans, and other components which form the framework of ECM.

Neoangiogenesis is stimulated by angiogenic factors secreted by keratinocytes at the wound site. Endothelial cells are activated by TNF-α and basic FGF (bFGF) to initiate angiogenesis. The newly formed blood vessels invade the matrix and promote blood flow to support the high metabolic activity in the newly deposited tissue. Angiogenesis is regulated by a combination of local stimulatory factors, such as vascular endothelial cell growth factor (VEGF) and antiangiogenic factors, such as angiostatin, endostatin, thrombospondin, and pigment epithelium-derived growth factor.[11] Local factors that stimulate angiogenesis include low oxygen tension, low pH, and high lactate levels.[12] Initially, the neoangiogenesis occurs in a haphazard manner, but subsequently, this process becomes more organized under the influence of various chemokines and cytokines mentioned earlier. It is stated that initially a ring-like circular arrangement of vessels is formed at the center of the wound which get feed from radially arranged vessels, ultimately establishing connection to capillaries of normal skin surrounding the wound.[13]

Remodeling Phase

The last phase of wound healing is the remodeling phase in which granulation tissue matures to form a scar. The tissue remodeling phase starts as early as a few days after injury and lasts up to 2 years. The capillaries aggregate to form larger blood vessels and cell density and overall metabolic activity of the wound decreases. The collagen fibers become organized, resulting in increased tensile strength of the wound. Initially, there is an increased deposition of type III collagen, also referred to as reticular collagen, that is gradually replaced by type I collagen, the dominant fibrillar collagen in skin.[14] As the wound continues to remodel, changes in collagen organization increase the tensile strength to a maximum of about 80% of normal tissue.[11]

An important group of proteinases are MMPs which play a central role in wound healing as they degrade certain constituents of provisional wound tissue, such as collagen I, III, IV, and VII.[15] They also facilitate epithelial cell migration into the wound, angiogenesis, and overall tissue remodeling. MMPs are secreted by epidermal cells and modulate TIMPs as well as degrade other growth factors.[16,17] Similarly, a disruption in the balance between MMPs and their inhibitors has been reported in diabetic and venous stasis ulcers.[18] In addition, MMPs can be found in increased levels in chronic wounds.[19] MMP expression is regulated by TGF-β. TGF-β also minimizes matrix degradation by downregulating protease secretion and stimulating synthesis of TIMP.

The process of collagen synthesis and degradation usually continues for a long time as the matrix strives to achieve the original, highly organized structure that was present before the injury. The scar tissue is always weaker than the normal surrounding matrix and can only achieve about 80% of the tensile strength that was present initially. If matrix synthesis is greater than degradation, then a hypertrophic scar may form. Conversely, if matrix degradation is greater than synthesis or if synthesis is inhibited by pharmacologic agents such as steroids or cancer chemotherapeutic agents, the scar becomes too weak and wound dehiscence can occur.

Epithelialization of Skin Wound

Re-epithelialization accounts for 80% of wound closure in human beings, whereas in rodents, the contraction by muscle contributes majorly to wound closure.[20] Within few hours of injury, the re-epithelialization process starts wherein the cobblestone-like keratinocytes turn into flat migratory keratinocytes. The migration of keratinocyte occurs by leapfrogging over each other, thus migrating toward the center of the wound;[21,22] however, a few authors believe that the entire row drags itself toward the center of the wound.[23-26] In addition to these actions, three other mechanisms are described—epidermal tongue or extension membrane, lamellipodial crawling, and shuffling.[27,28] The keratinocyte situated in front row facing the wound forms the epidermal tongue by rearranging the cytoskeleton and this is followed by succeeding keratinocyte migrating over this arrangement known as leapfrogging; the leading cells make their way through fibrin, FN, and vitronectin toward the center of the wound (lamellipodial crawling). The leading cells loosen their contact with the adjacent cells and rearrange themselves and proceed toward the wound center (shuffling). Once a cell comes in contact with other cells migrating from different directions, the contact inhibition occurs, sending signal to stop the proliferation and further movement. The keratinocytes firmly attach with each other and reorganize themselves into natural cobblestone arrangement followed by stratification.[25,26]

Role of Fibronectin in Wound Healing

Fibronectin is related with all stages of wound healing. In the initial inflammatory stage, plasma FN interacts with platelets to speed up clot formation. Once at injury site, the platelets express binding site for FN, thus forming the scaffolding at wound site. Tissue FN helps in marking the microbiome, thus playing the role of opsonization and removing the pathogens from the site. A few isoforms of FN are degraded by macrophages and these FN fragments help in tagging the parenchymal cells which have potential to survive. During the proliferation stage, tissue FN is related with collagen III laying process.[29]

FACTORS RESULTING IN CHRONICITY OF WOUND

These include both local and systemic factors as shown in **Table 1**.

WOUND HEALING IN DERMATOLOGICAL AND AESTHETIC CONDITIONS AND PROCEDURES

Keloids and Hypertrophic Scars

The presence of TGF-β isoforms, receptors, and activity modulators, rather than the mere presence or absence of TGF-β, may have a major role in the development of both keloids and hypertrophic scarring.[30] Similar results were detected with coculturing of keloid-derived keratinocytes and fibroblasts,[31] suggesting that keratinocytes might have an important role in keloid and hypertrophic scar pathogenesis by producing signals that stimulate the fibroblasts in the underlying dermis to proliferate or produce more ECM. Increased number of mast cells have been reported during the active period of hypertrophic and keloid scar formation.[32] Clinically, the release of histamine by these cells contributes to the common patient complaint of itchiness. In addition, the vasodilatory effect of histamine may promote erythema and leakage of plasma proteins into the regional tissues.

The major effectors of ECM degradation and remodeling belong to a family of structurally related enzymes called MMPs. The levels of MMP expression in normal cells are low and allow healthy connective tissue remodeling. Several MMPs have been shown to mediate the breakdown of type I and III collagen, the most abundant types of collagen in the skin ECM.[33] Specifically, MMP-2 and MMP-9 activity persist after wound closure and seem to play a potent role in the remodeling process.[34] Interestingly, hypertrophic scars and keloids were found to have high levels of MMP-2 and low levels of MMP-9.

TABLE 1: Factors affecting wound healing and resulting in chronicity of wound.

Local factors	*Systemic factors*
Oxygenation	Age and gender
Infection	Sex hormones
Foreign body	Stress
Venous sufficiency	Ischemia
	Diseases: Diabetes, keloids, fibrosis, hereditary healing disorders, jaundice, uremia
	Obesity
	Medications: Glucocorticosteroids, nonsteroidal anti-inflammatory drugs, chemotherapy
	Alcoholism and smoking
	Immunocompromised conditions: Cancer, radiation therapy, human immunodeficiency virus/acquired immunodeficiency syndrome (HIV/AIDS), nutrition

Decorin, a small proteoglycan with one dermatan sulfate sugar chain, is normally prevalent in the dermal ECM. Decorin is able to bind and neutralize TGF-β, thus minimizing the stimulatory effects of this cytokine on collagen, FN, and glycosaminoglycan production.[35] The low levels of decorin found in hypertrophic scarring may thus account for their irregular collagen organization as well as increased ECM production.

Other abnormalities seen in keloids include delayed apoptosis of myofibroblasts and prolongation of scar maturation.

Acne Scars

The pathogenesis of acne is currently attributed to multiple factors such as increased sebum production, alteration of the quality of sebum lipids and androgen activity, proliferation of *Propionibacterium acnes* (*P. acnes*) within the follicle, and follicular hyperkeratinization.[36]

The inflammatory process occurs in the infundibular region which result in follicular rupture and perifollicular abscess formation. These initiate a cascade of wound healing events. Holland et al. found that the inflammatory reaction at the pilosebaceous gland was stronger and had a longer duration in patients with scars than those without; in addition, the inflammatory reaction was slower in those with scars than patients who did not develop scars. They showed a strong relationship between severity and duration of inflammation and the development of scarring, suggesting that treating early inflammation in acne lesions may be the best approach to prevent acne scarring.[37]

Fibroblasts and keratinocytes produce enzymes including those that determine the architecture of the MMPs and TIMPs. Therefore, an imbalance in the ratio of MMPs to tissue inhibitors of MMPs results in the development of atrophic or hypertrophic scars. Inadequate response results in diminished deposition of collagen factors and formation of an atrophic scar, while if the healing response is too exuberant, a raised nodule of fibrotic tissue forms hypertrophic scars.[38]

WOUND HEALING AFTER PROCEDURES

Cryosurgery

Freezing of tissue with liquid nitrogen results in blister formation in a span of 2–3 days. Rupture of the blister results in eschar formation. Postprocedural depigmentation can occur in dark-skinned patients as the melanocytes are sensitive to reduced temperature.

Chemical Peeling

Chemical peels are utilized to produce controlled damage to the epidermis and superficial dermis. Depending on depth of penetration of peeling agent, there occurs epidermal regeneration and neocollagen formation resulting in remodeling.

Dermabrasion

Dermabrasion creates a partial thickness wound to heal by secondary intention. In partial thickness wounds, the adnexal structures are preserved and act as a reservoir for epidermal proliferation. TGF-β, keratinocyte growth factor, and epidermal growth factor (EGF) stimulate reepithelization from both the appendageal structures and epithelial cells.

Fractional Lasers

The mechanisms of the action of laser resurfacing include tissue ablation, immediate collagen shrinkage, and dermal collagen remodeling.[39] Fractional laser may result in microscopic epidermal regeneration. Collagen contraction induced by fractional reticular dermal ablation was thought to be the underlying factor leading to clinically observed skin tightening.[40] The improvement resulting from the ablation process may be seen soon after the epidermal regeneration phase is complete, whereas the clinical benefit arising from the dermal remodeling process normally starts months after treatment and continues over years after the initiation of the cutaneous wound healing cascade. A recent in vivo study in human skin revealed that neocollagenesis was persistent for a minimum of 3 months after a CO_2 ablative fractional resurfacing treatment as confirmed by a constant upregulation of the heat shock protein 47 (HSP47) expression.[41]

WOUND MANAGEMENT

WOUNDS CLASSIFICATION

Types of Cutaneous Wounds[42]

- *Type I:* Those having superficial loss of tissue involving epidermis and superficial (papillary) dermis. These heal by epithelialization with negligible granulation and contraction.
- *Type II:* Involving full thickness of dermis up to subcutaneous tissue
  - *Type IIA:* Without significant tissue loss, heal with epidermization and minimal granulation tissue with some contracture
  - *Type IIB:* Substantial tissue loss, heal by granulation/contraction.

In addition, wounds can be classified in different ways. They may be *open* (incisions, lacerations, abrasions, puncture wounds, penetration wounds, and gunshot wounds) and *closed* (contusions and hematomas). Surgical wounds can be classified as *clean, clean contaminated* (a wound involving normal tissue colonized with microorganisms), *contaminated* (a wound containing foreign or infected material), and *infected* (a wound with presence of pus). In dermatosurgery, a more relevant classification is classification in to *acute* and *chronic wounds.*

- *Acute wounds:* These wounds of less than 4 weeks occur with incisional wounds, excisional surgical wounds, and traumatic skin injury including burns. These wounds are characterized by definite orderly progression of inflammation, granulation tissue formation, and healing through activation of mitogen-activated protein kinase pathways and activator protein-1. There is no underlying healing defect and when large, these wounds are best dealt within the hospital settings.
- *Chronic wounds:* Chronic wound is classified as one that fails to heal within 4 weeks and shows no sign of improvement within 8 weeks. These wounds suffer from impairment of inflammation, angiogenesis, re-epithelialization, and wound remodeling, leading to the apparent loss of capacity to heal. Leg ulcers and pressure sores are examples. These wounds are best dealt within the community rather than in hospitals to reduce cost of care and dependency.

The most common types of wound seen by a dermatosurgeon are chronic wounds (trophic ulcers due to leprosy, diabetes, and venous and arterial leg ulcers) in addition to postoperative wounds.

WOUND ASSESSMENT[44]

Proper wound assessment is the key to proper wound management; the factors that need to be assessed are shown in **Box 1**.

FACTORS THAT AFFECT WOUND HEALING AND THE POTENTIAL FOR INFECTION[45]

Factors affecting healing include general, local, and wound factors and are shown in **Box 2**. These have been dealt with and need to be carefully considered during management.

History of Wound Management and Use of Natural Products

In some ways, the early history of medicine is dominated by the care of wounds, especially those injuries caused in battles.

BOX 1: Wound assessment.

- Wound bed color or tissue type
- Exposed bone, tendon, or muscle
- *Exudate:* Color and amount
- Wound odor
- Clinical infection or spreading infection
- *Measurement:* Linear, tracing on grided acetate films and counting number of grids, photography, computerized planimetry in research settings
- Depth can be measured using sterile probe or spatula, volume of fluid under an occluding membrane
- Condition of surrounding skin for callus (tissue breakdown or ulceration underneath), cellulitis, eczema or maceration
- *Pain assessment:* Pain related to change of dressing or bathing or constant as in case of ischemia or neuropathy
- *Primary factor delaying healing:* Diabetes mellitus, malnutrition, systemic steroid use, and others
- *Investigation of primary pathology:* Doppler
- Research studies use laser Doppler assessment of blood flow, ultrasound measurement of depth, optical coherence tomography, wound pH, and direct measurement of arterial and venous pressures
- *Assessment of chronic wounds:* TIME system[43,44] [*T*issue (viability, as necrotic tissue, slough or eschar delay healing and need removal), *I*nfection/*I*nflammation (infection needs treatment), *M*oisture (balance important as too much and too little moisture are both bad), *E*dge (if nonprogressive or undermined may be debrided or grafted]

BOX 2: Factors affecting wound healing.

- *General factors:*
  - Age
  - *Underlying illnesses or disease:* Amino acid deficiencies (histidine and tryptophan), diabetes or immunocompromise (correction of iron, B-complex deficiencies in addition to others mentioned below to be considered for chronic wounds) (correction of anemia, malnutrition, and infections)
  - Medications such as corticosteroids, anticoagulants, non-steroidal anti-inflammatory, colchicine, and antineoplastic pharmacotherapy delay wound healing[47,48]
  - Conditions predisposing to ulceration such as varicose veins, hypertension, and leprosy
  - Effect of the injury on healing (e.g., devascularization)
  - Skin disorders such as epidermolysis bullosa require special care of wounds including of anemia, malnutrition, infection, and pruritus
- *Wound factors:*
  - Rest to injured organ
    - Adequate rest ensures faster healing
  - Organ or tissues injured
  - Extremity location due to lesser blood supply
  - Extent of injury
  - Nature of injury (for example, a laceration will be a less complicated wound than a crush injury)
  - Contamination or infection
  - Time between injury and treatment (sooner is better)
- *Local factors:*
  - Hemostasis and debridement
  - Use of electrosurgery
  - Timing of closure
  - Formation of biofilms (can lead to chronicity of wounds)

In Mesopotamia (2100 BC), after cleaning a wound with beer, a bandage with wine and turpentine was applied. In Ancient Egypt, a natural product such as honey became common in wound management; after irrigating a wound with wine, physicians would then cover the wound with fat and honey. In Greece, during the time of Homer, wounds were covered and treated with herbs, whereas infected wounds were healed by dropping scrapings from bronze spears into them.

400 years later, Hippocrates taught that wounds should be washed with wine, bandaged, and then saturated with more wine. Galen, of ancient Rome, cleaned wounds with vinegar but nevertheless believed that suppuration ("*pus bonum et laudabile*") was necessary for healing. This belief prevailed for many centuries.

When gunpowder was first used in battle, boiling oil was used as wound treatment, with the aim "to inactivate" the gunpowder effect within gunshot wounds. This practice was abandoned when, in 1542, Ambroise Paré performed one of the first cohort studies to demonstrate that egg yolk and turpentine were better than boiling oil for treatment of gunshot wounds.

In 1867, the first antiseptic dressings were introduced by Lister, who soaked lint and gauze in phenol and then applied them to wounds. In general, before 20th century, it was believed that wound heal best when left open and dry as advocated by Pasteur. However in 1958, Odland observed that a blister healed faster when left unbroken. In 1962, Winter showed in swine that superficial wounds kept moist healed faster by two times. Hinman and Maibach repeated this study in humans with similar results. These studies transmuted wound care by bespeaking importance of moist wound healing.

There are limited data on natural products, such as yogurt (which seems to help in controlling wound odor), tea tree oil, and potato peelings; however, there is a great interest in the use of honey for wound healing. Although science and technology march ever forward, we must not fail to exploit the potential of natural products because they may represent a hope for modern medicine.[46]

Techniques of Wound Management

Different techniques of wound management include wound cleaning, closure, dressings, use of antimicrobials, use of agents which promote wound healing, etc. The choice of technique may vary depending on the different wound and host factors as mentioned in **Box 2**.

Wound Cleansing[49]

Wound cleansing is done to remove foreign material or debris present in the wound. It includes wound irrigation and debridement.

Irrigation:[50] Irrigation helps in cleansing and removal of superficial debris. It should be noted that swabbing is not helpful. Solutions used for irrigation include potable tap water, saline, boiled and cooled water, or distilled water.[51] Solutions used should be at body temperature. Povidone-iodine solution can be used as it can maintain bactericidal activity even at low concentration. It should be used in low concentration, as high concentration is toxic for tissues. Its effect on wound healing is not clearly established, but there is some evidence to suggest a beneficial effect on chronic wounds.[52,53] As iodine can cause contact dermatitis, it should be used with caution.

However, due to their cytotoxic effects, higher concentration povidone-iodine-based antiseptics and hydrogen peroxide should no longer be used in any wound to prevent infection. Both solutions alter the migration and proliferation of skin fibroblasts, fundamental cells in the proliferative phase of wound healing and the MMP release by the dermal fibroblasts, thus making the wound bed a harsh environment for adequate healing. Chlorhexidine too is not without its own concerns. The required antibactericidal concentration varies widely among microorganisms. For example, methicillin-resistant *Staphylococcus aureus* (MRSA) only requires a concentration of 0.002%, while gram-negative organisms might require a bactericidal concentration of 1%. Hexachlorophene is tissue toxic and tends to be painful to apply on open wounds.

As a precaution, hands must be washed before changing dressings and irrigation. Equipment needed for irrigation is simple and consists of a 50-cc syringe with 18-G needle for wound irrigation which produces a pressure of 8–10 psi. Amount used should be at least 100–300 cc with continued irrigation until all visible particles are removed. A general rule of thumb is to use 50–100 cc per cm of wound length.

Debridement: If irrigation alone is ineffective in removing contaminants from a wound, the wound should be lightly scrubbed. Gentle scrubbing may be useful in wounds older than 3–4 hours, even if they are clean, as it removes a glycoprotein matrix that may cover the wound and allows bacterial colonization. Debridement of devitalized tissue is paramount to reducing risk of infection. Scalpel excision of wound margins can be used in grossly contaminated wounds. Debridement is more relevant for infected wounds and hence, more information is provided on debridement later in this chapter.

Management of Infected Wounds[54]

Infection is said to have occurred when bacterial numbers in wound overwhelm the immune response and clinical signs of infection appear. Risk of infection can be reduced by proper hand washing, infection control, wound cleansing, and debridement. Protection of wounds from exogenous sources of contamination is important. Prevention of infection can enhance wound healing and reduce hospital stay and cost. In presence of systemic and clinical signs of infection, systemic antimicrobial therapy should be considered. Culture swab is required only if clinical signs of spreading infection are present such as pyrexia, heat, redness, swelling, or pain. One must review antibiotic choice and duration when swab results are available. Changing of dressing daily or alternate days, depending on exudate, is important. If purulent material or foul odor is present, more frequent cleansing and possibly debridement are required.

Topical antimicrobials: Topical antiseptic agents are commonly used but suffer from certain disadvantages. They have been shown to retard wound healing.[55,56] Topical antibiotics, particularly neomycin and gentamicin are frequent causes of contact dermatitis. However, certain topical antimicrobial agents are useful and are mentioned further:

- *Silver dressings, e.g., silver sulfadiazine:* Silver compounds are widely used in burn care, being effective against *Staphylococcus aureus* and *Pseudomonas aeruginosa*, in a concentration as low as 10 mmol/L and possibly having an effect by enhancing epithelialization.[57]
- Povidone-iodine in low concentration as described earlier.
- Honey[58] stimulates tissue growth and epithelialization, as well as reducing inflammation and infection, debriding, and deodorizing wounds.[59] It is also effective against antibiotic resistant bacteria, including MRSA.[60]
- Cane sugar containing sucrose, which is not metabolized outside the gastrointestinal tract, prevents bacterial growth by decreasing available water and it has also been claimed to stimulate granulation tissue.[61]
- Metronidazole acts against anaerobes.
- Newer anti-infective biomaterials, antimicrobial biocides, and novel types of antimicrobial agents such as rapamycin are now available.[62]

Topical antibiotics in general should not be used for prolonged periods. Systemic antibiotics should be preferred where there is clinical sign of infection.

Wound closure:[1,43,52,63] Wound closure has definite role in management of clean wounds. Clean wounds should be closed immediately to allow healing by primary intention. A closed dressing exposes the wound continuously to proteinases, chemotactic, and complement and growth factors in the surrounding fluid, which may be otherwise lost in case the wound is left exposed. The electrical gradient required for stimulation of fibroblasts and epithelial cell migration is maintained and further trauma to the wound is avoided by this physical barrier. However, contaminated and infected wounds should not be closed but left open to heal by secondary intention. In treating clean contaminated wounds and clean wounds that are more than 6–8 hours old, one must manage with surgical toilet, the wound left open and then closed 48 hours later. This is called delayed primary (or tertiary) closure. **Table 2** shows different types of wound closure and their characteristics.

Negative-pressure Wound Therapy

Negative-pressure wound therapy (NPWT) or vacuum-assisted closure (VAC) has played a major role as a bridge to reconstruction. It is a significant, clinically proven advancement in wound care that promotes active wound

TABLE 2: Indications and key points to consider for each closure type.

Intention (closure)	*Unique characteristics*	*Key points*
Primary	Clean, minimal contaminated, mostly shearing forces 6–8 hours old	May close with tape, staplers, and sutures
Secondary	Noncosmetic animal bites, abscess cavities, ulcers	• No sutures • Delayed skin coverage, graft
Tertiary	Too contaminated to close	Clean, debride, and observe 4–6 days before suturing

healing at the cellular level through negative pressure. Pressure used is negative pressure or subatmospheric pressure (100–125 mm Hg) in a continuous or intermittent manner. The intermittent negative pressure is delivered at wound site through a porous dressing, which applies mechanical forces known as macrostrain (physical response) and microstrain (biological response) and subsequently removes exudates by an electromechanical pump.

PRIMARY WOUND REPAIR[45]

Primary closure requires that clean tissue is approximated without tension. Primary closure is done by suturing, wound adhesives, or staples. Injudicious closure of a contaminated wound will promote infection and delay healing. These have been dealt with in detail in the chapter on sutures.

Body hair entangled in sutures and staples or buried inside the wound can alter the healing process and increase the risk of infection. It is important to understand that routine hair removal by shaving before suturing can lead to poor outcomes. If hair has to be removed, scissors or clippers should be used. It has also been shown that use of clean nonsterile gloves are not inferior to sterile gloves in terms of infection control.

The hair apposition technique (HAT) for scalp wounds and lacerations should be considered for the repair of scalp lacerations that are noncrush injuries <10 cm long with regular wound edges, minimal contamination, without evidence of underlying skull fractures and with an intact galea in patients with hair strands longer than 3 cm. These techniques are associated with less scarring, fewer overall complications, shorter procedural time, lower pain scores, and substantially lower costs than standard suturing and stapler techniques. The HAT consists of twisting together three to seven strands of hair on either side of the wound. The two bundles of hair are then interlocked in a 360° revolution and a small drop of tissue adhesive can be applied. The hair is not tied. This same process is repeated as needed for the entire length of the wound. The glue will break down and the hair will unravel by itself after 7–10 days.[64]

BOX 3: Tips on technique of using 2-octyl cyanoacrylate.

- Maintaining everted skin apposition with fingers or forceps during application to improve apposition
- Using multiple thin applications, with the first layer protecting the skin from the exothermic reaction of the layers above it
- Allowing the adhesive to dry between applications
- Advising the patient not to scrub the site where the adhesive is applied so that the cyanoacrylate does not get rubbed off

TISSUE ADHESIVES (2-OCTYL CYANOACRYLATE)[65]

The commonly used wound adhesives include 2-butyl cyanoacrylate and 2-octyl cyanoacrylate.

2-octyl cyanoacrylate use is often correlated with laceration repair, which is certainly a popular application. However, it is also widely used for operative incision repair. Sutureless pediatric circumcisions, cleft lip repair, and upper eyelid blepharoplasties are a few innovative surgical incision closures that have been facilitated with the use of 2-octyl cyanoacrylate. It is most commonly used in dermatology to hold in place punch and suction blister grafts. Cosmetic results with 2-octyl cyanoacrylate equals those of sutures. Tips on use of 2-octyl cyanoacrylate are in **Box 3**. More details can be found in the chapter on wound and closure materials.

Contraindications for Use of Tissue Glue

- A person with a history of allergy to cyanoacrylates
- Animal bite wound
- Stellate crush injury
- Partial thickness facial laceration in a patient with diabetes
- Decubitus ulcers
- Nonsurgical puncture wounds.

In addition, 2-octyl cyanoacrylate should be used carefully on the oral mucosa, hands, feet, or joints, where repetitive movement and washing may cause the adhesives to slough prematurely.

Follow-up

Close attention should be paid when closing wounds near surrounding structures that could become encased in or stuck to the glue. In such a case, petroleum jelly or acetone can be used, which weakens the polymerization. Using water and alcohol, which speed up the exothermic reaction that polymerizes 2-octyl cyanoacrylate, is to be avoided.

Patients who have had 2-octyl cyanoacrylate applied to their wounds should be monitored for allergic-type reactions. Generally, it takes 7–14 days for 2-octyl cyanoacrylate to flake off and prolonged retention, either on the surface or within the edges of the wound, could lead to allergic reactions.

BOX 4: Recommendations for use of tissue glue.

- Useful in wounds with edges <5 mm apart, clean, sharp edges, nonmobile areas and laceration <5 cm in length
- Not useful in wounds near eye, on mucous membrane or mucosal surfaces, wet wounds or those exposed to body fluids, or in areas with dense hair, wounds under significant tension

Complications

Inflammation, tissue necrosis, granulation tissue formation, and wound breakdown can occur when cyanoacrylates are implanted subcutaneously. The process causing the toxicity is thought to be related to the byproducts of degradation, namely cyanoacetate and formaldehyde. Recommendations for use of tissue glue are in **Box 4**.

WOUND: SECONDARY HEALING[45]

To promote healing by secondary intention, perform wound toilet and surgical debridement.

- Surgical wound toilet involves cleaning the skin with antiseptics, irrigation of wounds with saline, and surgical debridement of all dead tissue and foreign matter. Dead tissue does not bleed when cut.
- Wound debridement involves removal of dead and devitalized tissues and debris to promote healing.

Types of Debridement

Debridement is the removal of necrotic debris which accumulates on the surface of or around a wound which may impair healing by forming a physical barrier to re-epithelialization, as well as acting as a focus for infection. Different types of debridement are described further:

Surgical debridement: It is a rapid and selective form of debridement used for wounds with a significant amount of necrotic tissue **(Box 5)**.

BOX 5: Tips for surgical wound debridement.

- Systematically perform wound toilet and surgical debridement, initially to the superficial layers of tissues and subsequently to the deeper layers
- After scrubbing the skin with soap and irrigating the wound with saline, prepare the skin with antiseptic keeping in mind what has been mentioned earlier in this chapter
- Do not use antiseptics within the wound
- Debride the wound meticulously to remove any loose foreign material such as dirt, grass, wood, glass, or clothing
- With a scalpel or dissecting scissors, remove all adherent foreign material along the wound edge with a thin margin of underlying tissue and then irrigate the wound again
- Continue the cycle of surgical debridement and saline irrigation until the wound is completely clean
- Leave the wound open after debridement to allow healing by secondary intention
- Pack it lightly with damp saline gauze and cover the packed wound with a dry dressing
- Change the packing and dressing daily or more often if the outer dressing becomes damp with blood or other body fluids
- Large defects will require closure with flaps or skin grafts but may be initially managed with saline packing
- During debridement, one must excise only a very thin margin of skin from the wound edge

Autolytic debridement: This involves debridement by autolysis of necrotic tissue by body enzymes and moisture. It occurs after the use of dressings that maintain fluid contact with necrotic tissue such as films, hydrogels, and hydrocolloid dressings in dry wounds, and foams, alginates, or hydrofibers in more sloughy wounds. These dressings exploit the presence of endogenous collagenases and proteases present in a wound to break down necrotic tissue. Care must be taken to protect surrounding normal tissue.

Mechanical debridement: Moist dressing is applied to a wound and then removed after drying. Hydrotherapy is another form of mechanical debridement. The latter can also be done under pressure in a whirlpool.

Enzymatic debridement: They enhance granulation tissue formation and epithelialization. Studies in animal models have shown the effectiveness of collagenase in wound debridement.[66] Streptokinase/streptodornase and proteolytic enzymes derived from Antarctic krill have also been shown to be effective in wound debridement;[67] papain is also used in some countries.

High-pressure water irrigation: Hydrocision or pressurized irrigation (Versajet, Smith and Nephew) is the new tool in surgical debridement and cleaning of the wound with either high or low pressure, razor thin stream of water, saline or antibiotic solution, and is serving as a better alternative compared to the above methods. High-pressure irrigation is effective in removing bacteria, particulate matter, and necrotic debris from the wounds, thus lowering the rate of infection compared to low pressure irrigation. The only concern is that there is a risk of bacteria being driven into soft tissue by the high pressure. It is particularly useful in concavities of pressure sores and joint spaces and in tight spaces. It is indicated for use in necrotic wounds and deep burns also. Since it preserves the viable dermal tissue, it allows rapid wound healing with better cosmetic outcome.

Maggot therapy (biosurgery): Maggots are used for treatment of chronic wounds refractory to conventional treatment. *Lucilia sericata* is a commonly used maggot. Up to 1,000 maggots are introduced into the wound and left for 1–3 days before a dressing change. They facilitate healing by secretion of proteolytic enzymes that liquefy necrotic tissue, maggot digestion of necrotic tissue, and MRSA and β-hemolytic streptococcus, increase in wound pH secondary to larval excretion of ammonia and calcium carbonate and secretion of allantoin and urea. Movement of maggots stimulate granulation tissue. Maggots effectively separate necrotic from living tissue, thereby making subsequent surgical debridement unnecessary or much easier.[68,69]

WOUND DRESSINGS

Wound dressings protect the surface of wounds and prevent bacterial, fungal, and viral (herpes group of viruses most commonly) contamination of healing wounds. Occlusive dressings help in creating a moist environment, which has a beneficial effect on wound healing through accumulation of endogenous growth factors and other biological effects on angiogenesis, generation of granulation tissue, and reepithelization. Though rate of tissue bacterial colonization are slightly higher, it has been shown to be nonsignificant in terms of prevention of reepithelization.[70,71]

Properties of an Ideal Dressing

- Able to maintain a good moisture balance at the wound bed but not too much to avoid maceration of surrounding tissue
- Easy to remove without damaging the wound or surrounding skin
- Impermeable to bacteria
- Prevents capillary loops penetrating into dressing material
- Capable of being sterilized
- Confer mechanical protection to the wound
- Nontoxic and nonallergenic
- Comfortable for the patient
- Conformability with patient lifestyle and requirements
- Cost-effective
- Have a long shelf life.

Wound dressings can help healing by different mechanisms. Functions of wound dressings are shown in **Table 3**.

Types of Dressings

Before a discussion on the various types of dressings is embarked upon, the conventional composite dressing needs to be understood as it has stood the test of time. It composes four or five layers:

1. A layer of antibiotic ointment in contact with wound surface
2. A contact layer of nonadhesive material, such as paraffin gauze, silver sulfadiazine, and framycetin/chlorhexidine tulle or iodine tulle. The last two if available obviates the need for the first layer
3. An absorbent layer of dry gauze
4. Outer securing layer of tape or roller bandage. Tackifiers such as tincture benzoin may be used to increase adhesion of dressing to the skin
5. Sometimes, a fifth layer of gauze or cotton padding may interpose before the layer of tape or roller bandage.

Adhesive bandages such as Band-Aid® are premade composite dressings **(Fig. 2)**.

Different types of dressings and their properties are shown in **Box 6**.

Dressings can also be classified into passive and interactive dressings. Passive dressings are simple products which only protect wound without interacting with them. Most modern dressing products are interactive dressings as they interact with the wound bed to provide optimum environment at the wound dressing interface.

TABLE 3: Functions of wound dressings.

Function	*Benefit*
Covering the wound	Protection from trauma and contamination from bacteria and foreign material and minimizes fluid and heat loss, provide contact with topical antibiotics, cosmetic acceptability of wound till it heals
Absorption of wound drainage	Keeps wound moist but not wet, minimizes maceration
Compression	Increases hemostasis, minimizes edema and hematoma formation, prevents dehiscence
Providing moist environment	Facilitates healing of acute wounds and reduces pain of chronic wounds
Immobilization	Assists re-epithelialization, reduces pain, promotes healing, improves resultant scar

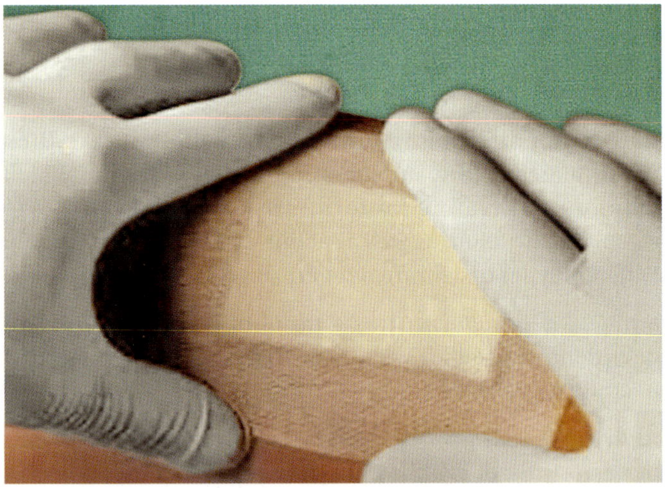

Fig. 2: Composite dressing.

BOX 6: Different types of dressings.

- *Nonadherent fabrics:*
  - *Absorptive:* Gauze, foams, alginates
- *Occlusive/moisture-retentive dressings:*
  - *Nonbiologic traditional:* Foams, polyurethane films, hydrocolloids, hydrogels, alginates
  - *Nonbiologic—new:* Hydrofiber dressings, collagen dressings, hyaluronic acid dressings
  - *Biologic grafts:* Split-thickness skin grafts, full-thickness skin grafts, composite grafts
  - *Biologic/biosynthetic—skin substitutes:* Cultured epidermal grafts, dermal replacements, biocomposite skin substitutes
- Odor-absorbing dressings
- Biosynthetic dressings

Appropriate Wound Dressings in Different Types of Wounds[72]

Each of the various types of dressing can be used in a specific setting and **Table 4** shows different types of dressings and their role in different types of wound. It has been proved that moist environment is beneficial for healing. The moisture vapor transmission rate (MVTR) measures the moisture retentive property of a dressing. A dressing is moisture retentive if its MVTR is <840 g/m^2/24 hours. The MVTR of hydrocolloids is <300 g/m^2/24 hours, in contrast to gauze whose MVTR is 1,200 g/m^2/24 hours. MVTR is a useful tool for choosing dressing according to the wound type.[73]

Different types of dressings are discussed in detail further.

Gauze

Gauze is one of the most commonly used absorptive dressing. It is excellent at drawing fluid and exudates away from wound surface but loses its efficacy when saturated. It is usually used to cover nonocclusive, nonadhering fabric dressing material and absorb discharge, which drains through them. It can also be used to cover occlusive dressing as secondary dressing to keep them in place. Wide mesh gauze is not to be placed in direct contact with wounds as it adheres to surface causing pain on removal; only exception is when mechanical debridement is warranted.

TABLE 4: Types of dressings and their role in different types of wound.

Types of wound	*Suitable dressings*
Acute wounds	
• Abrasions, lacerations • Catheter or cannula sites • Burns	• Films, hydrocolloids, foams • Films • Hydrocolloids, hydrogels, biosynthetic dressings
• Donor sites of grafts • Dermabrasion, chemical peels	• Films, hydrocolloids • Hydrogels
Surgical wounds	Films, hydrocolloids, hydrogels, alginates
Chronic wounds	
Venous ulcer: • Heavy exudates • Moderate exudates • Mild exudates • Malodorous	 • Foams, alginates, hydrofibers • Hydrocolloids, foams • Hydrogels, hydrocolloids • Foams, alginates, hydrocolloid charcoal
Arterial	Hydrogels
Neuropathic: • Moist • Dry	 • Hydrogels, alginates, hydrofibers • Hydrogels, hydrocolloids
Pressure ulcers: • Stage I • Stage II–III • Stage IV	 • Films, thin hydrocolloids • Hydrocolloids, foams, hydrogels, debriding agents • Alginates, hydrofibers, debriding agents
Fungating	Hydrocolloids, hydrogels, alginates, foams, charcoal

Semipermeable (Polyurethane) Films (Fig. 3)

For example, OpSite™, Tegaderm™, Bioclusive™, etc.

Semipermeable (polyurethane) films are often coated with adhesive to ease application. They are impermeable to bacteria and fluids but are permeable to air and water vapor. One can inspect the wound without need for removal of these dressings. They can be left in situ for days at a time. They provide a moist environment but are not good for large amounts of exudate. They provide however no mechanical protection of the wound. Care needs to be taken during removal as new epithelium can be stripped off during removal.

Low-adherence Dressings

For example, Bactigras **(Fig. 4)**, Jelonet, etc.

These provide a moist wound environment. They allow exudate to pass from wound to a secondary dressing and are low adherence and hence good for fragile skin.

Hydrogels (Fig. 5)

For example, Hizel™, Aquaform™, Nu-Gel™, and Sterigel.

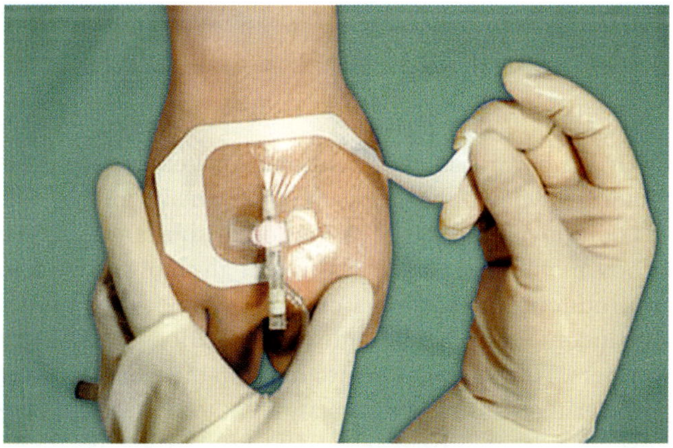

Fig. 3: Polyurethane films.

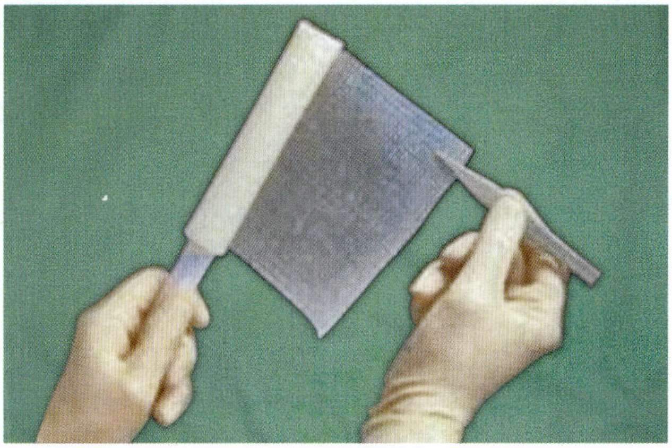

Fig. 4: Bactigras dressing.

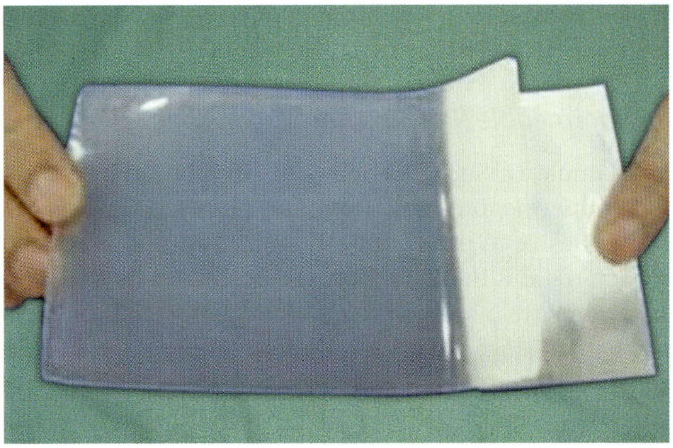

Fig. 5: Hydrogel wound dressing.

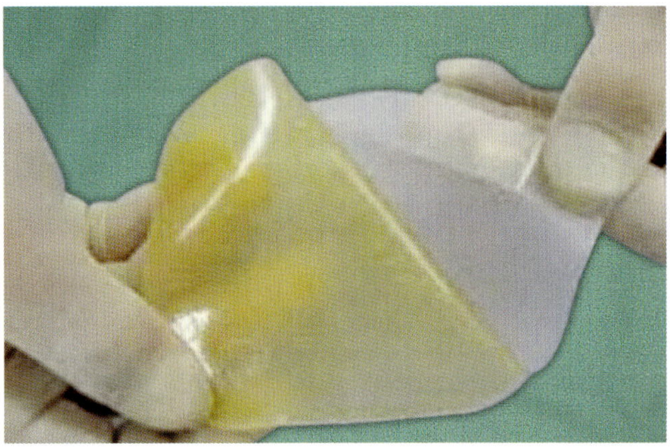

Fig. 6: Hydrocolloid dressing.

Hydrogel, an insoluble hydrophilic material, is produced by utilizing synthetic polymer such as polymethylmethacrylate and polyvinyl pyrrolidine. Various other substances such as carboxymethyl cellulose, pectin, and glycerol can be used for production of hydrogel dressing. They are formed of translucent, jelly-like nonadhesive matrices of insoluble polymers. They donate water to moisten the wound surface. However, their absorptive capacity is limited. These dressings are semipermeable to gas and water vapor and are used as gel, sheets, or impregnated in gauze. They require a secondary dressing to be applied over them. They have a cooling effect due to reduced temperature by about 5°C by water entrapment. Care needs to be taken to avoid maceration of surrounding skin. They are best suited for dry wounds or those with minimal exudates.

Hydrocolloids (Fig. 6)

For example, DuoDerm™, Tegasorb™, Comfeel™, Granuflex™.

Hydrocolloid is an interactive dressing with outer impermeable layer and inner colloidal layer. They are opaque mixture of adhesive absorbent polymers and gelling agents such as gelatin, pectin, and sodium carboxymethyl cellulose. They adhere to wound edges and hence allow the patient to bathe and shower. They have a polyurethane backing. Hydrophilic particles in the dressing interact with wound exudate to form a yellow gel. They provide an acidic environment, which is antibacterial and antiviral. Hydrocolloids help autolytic wound debridement and are good for difficult-to-dress areas such as heel, sacrum, etc. Care needs to be taken as they may cause increased amount of granulation tissue and maceration. They are not indicated for arterial/neuropathic ulcers and infected or heavily exuding wounds because of risk of maceration of wound edges. Another disadvantage is their tendency to produce malodorous exudates which can be mistaken for infection.

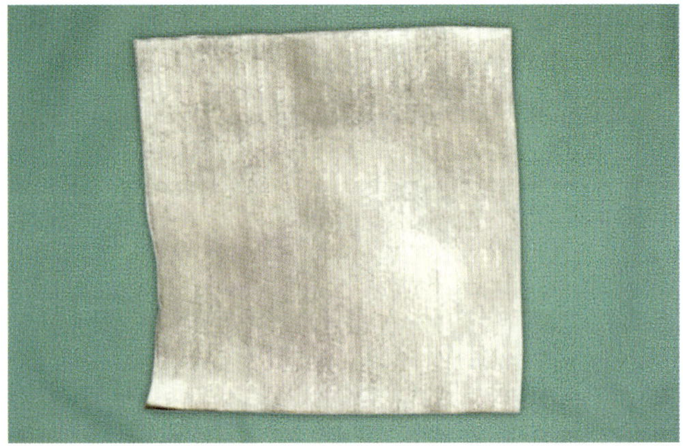

Fig. 7: Hydrofiber dressing.

Hydrofibers (Fig. 7)

For example, Aquacel™.

Hydrofibers are carboxymethyl cellulose fibers in a nonwoven sheet. They form a soft gel when exposed to heavily exudative wounds and are very highly absorptive. They require a secondary dressing as they absorb three times the amount of exudate than that of alginates, which are the highest in this class. These dressing can absorb up to 25 times its initial weight. They are indicated for pressure ulcers, lower limb ulcers, and surgical wounds. Silver-containing hydrofiber dressing is preferred in immunobullous disorders.

Alginates (Fig. 8)

For example, Kaltostat™, Sorbsan™, CarraSorb™, and Algisite™.

Alginates are derived from brown seaweed and are highly hydrophilic. They change from fibrous to gel form on absorbing water (up to 20 times their weight). Ingredients include calcium salts of alginic, mannuronic, and guluronic acids. In sodium-rich environment of wounds, calcium and sodium ions exchange and free calcium helps clotting. When placed over a moist wound, an ion exchange reaction occurs between calcium in the alginate and sodium in the wound fluid, producing soluble calcium-sodium alginate—a gelatinous mass, which helps in maintaining moist

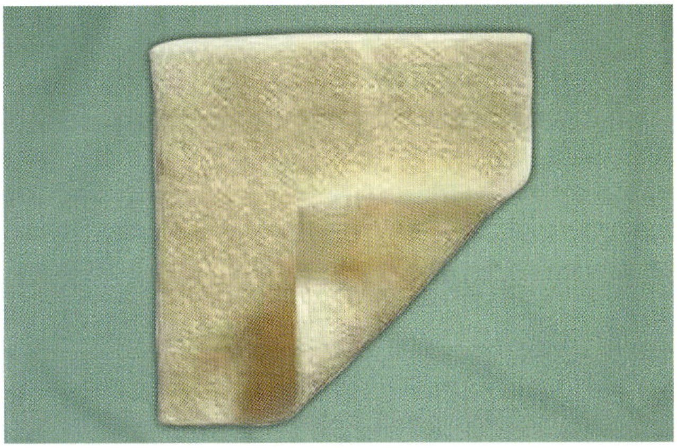

Fig. 8: Alginate dressing.

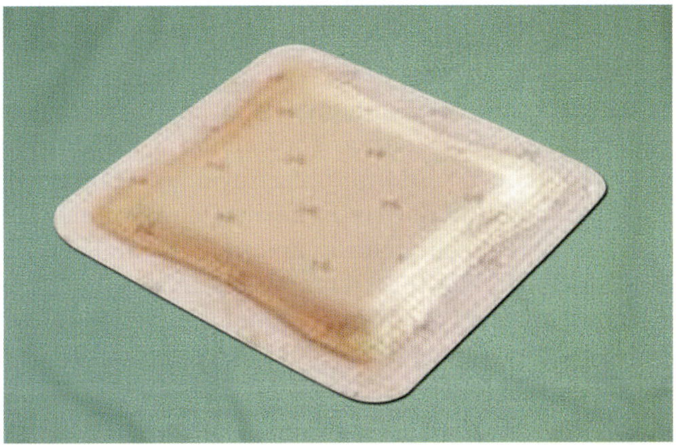

Fig. 9: Foam dressing.

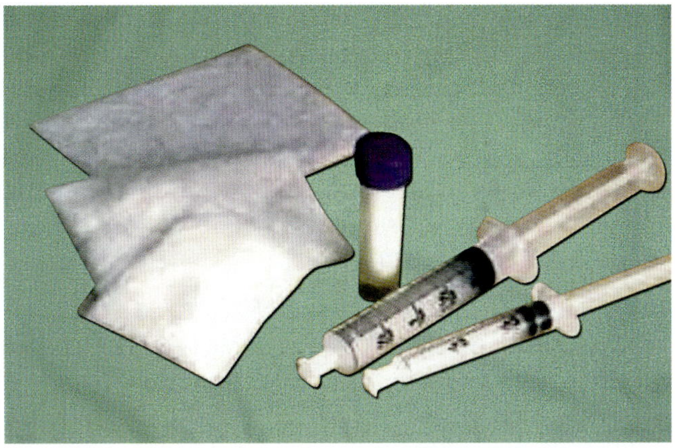

Fig. 10: Collagen sheets and particles.

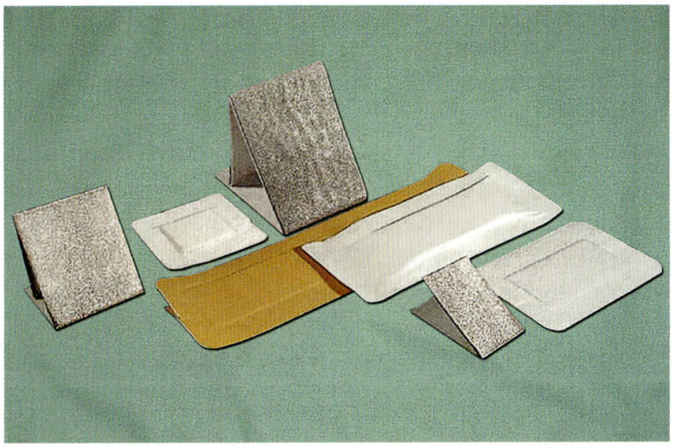

Fig. 11: Silver impregnated antimicrobial dressing.

environment and facilitates autolytic debridement. Secondary dressing is required to absorb exudates and this dressing needs to be changed daily. They conform to the shape of the wound and should be cut accordingly because if larger, they can cause periwound maceration because of their tendency to absorb fluid across entire surface (lateral wicking).[73]

Foams (Fig. 9)

For example, Silastic™ Allevyn, HyperFoam™, Mepilex, Lyofoam™, Allevyn™, and Tielle™.

Foams are absorbent, opaque polyurethane or silicone sheets. They are permeable to gas and water vapor and have a semipermeable backing. They create a moist environment and provide thermal insulation to the wound. They are nonadherent, easy to apply and remove, and are meant for highly exuding wounds. They can be layered in combination with other materials with overlying compression bandages. Their fluid absorption capacity varies with foam thickness; their MVTR ranges between 800 and 5,000 $g/m^2/24$ hours. They may be used for their cushioning effect, but they are not a substitute for pressure-relieving devices. Foams may produce excessive malodorous drainage necessitating frequent dressing change.[73]

Collagen Dressings (Fig. 10)

For example, Kollagen™ and Catrix™.

They are usually of human, porcine or bovine origin and are available as particle or sheet form. They accelerate wound healing by providing a collagenous matrix to enhance cell migration. Chemotaxis of fibroblasts and macrophages occurs providing a temporary scaffold to allow ingrowth of tissue. They absorb wound exudates to form a soft biodegradable gel over the wound surface, which maintains wound moisture.

Antimicrobial Dressings (Fig. 11)

For example, Inadine™ and Iodosorb™.

They counter the effect of bacterial colonization on delays in wound healing. They are slow release iodine preparations (cadexomer iodine) with concentrations of the range of 0.001%. These low concentrations do not adversely affect wound healing. Care needs to be taken since thyroid function may be affected on long-term iodine dressings. Other antimicrobial dressing compounds include silver compounds. Silver-impregnated dressings are bactericidal and maintain a moist environment to facilitate wound healing. They have broad spectrum action against bacteria such as vancomycin-resistant enterococci, MRSA, and fungi. Metronidazole gel in dressings is antibacterial for anaerobes. Silver nitrate and silver sulfadiazine release silver at concentration of 3,200 ppm. Most pathogenic organisms are killed in vitro at concentration of 10–40 ppm. The newer nanochemistry technique has produced microfine particles which increase silver's solubility and produces silver ions concentration of 70–100 ppm.[73]

Odor-Absorbing Dressings

For example, CliniSorb™.

These are based on activated charcoal **(Fig. 12)**. They are combined in other dressings for best effect.

Hyaluronic Acid Dressings

For example, Hyalofill.

They are made of biodegradable absorbent biopolymers that form a hydrophilic mesh. They accelerate granulation tissue formation and re-epithelialization. They also help to stabilize clot and attract inflammatory cells.

The latest types in dressings are those containing compounds or drugs. This could be local antiseptics (silver, other antiseptics, and honey) and pain-relieving drugs such as ibuprofen and morphine. They may be in the form of powders such as nanoflex powder dressings.

Biological Dressings—Skin Grafts

Skin grafts are biological dressings and are of different types:

Pinch and Split-thickness Grafts

Pinch grafts are small (2–3 mm^2), partial-thickness skin removed under local anesthesia and placed as islands on venous and arterial ulcers. Split thickness grafts are usually meshed before application for large wounds.

Other Skin Grafts

The possibility of expanding a small donor site up to 10,000-fold led to the application of cultured keratinocytes for grafting.[74] Autografts and allografts have been used clinically.

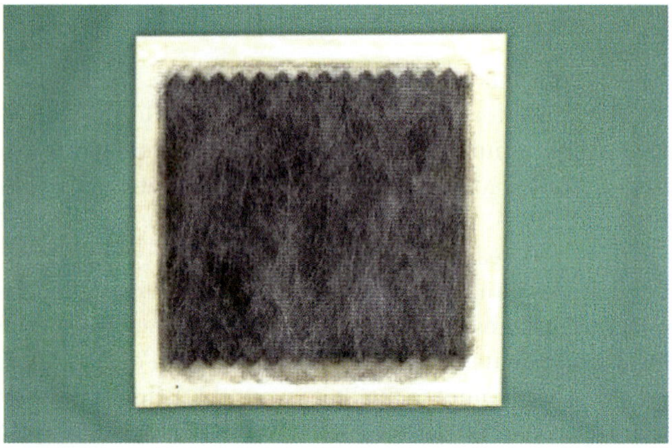

Fig. 12: Charcoal dressing.

Cultured epidermal autografts have also been used to treat epidermolysis bullosa wounds,[75] wound beds of shaved congenital naevi,[76] and chronic leg ulcers,[77] where repeated grafting from passaged cultures is a major advantage. Keratinocytes can also be suspended in fibrin. Use of allografts helps by producing growth factors and matrix proteins. Tissue engineered substitutes of epidermis, dermis, or combined epidermis–dermis are available. Use of bone marrow stem cells is an area of research.

Tissue engineered human skin substitute:

- *Epidermal substitute:* Epicell™, EpiDex™, MySkin™, CellSpray™, Bioseed-S **(Table 5)**
- *Dermoepidermal (composite) substitute:* Apligraf™, OrCel™, PolyActive™, Laserskin™, TISCOVER® **(Table 6)**
- *Dermal substitute:* Integra™, Biobrane™, Alloderm™, Dermagraft™, TransCyte™, Graftjacket™, MatriDerm™ **(Table 7)**.

There are two types of human skin substitute—cellular matrix and acellular matrix. The cellular matrix is made up of keratinocytes and fibroblast over collagen matrix, whereas acellular matrix is dermal component with fibroblast on collagen matrix. Apligraf™ is the Food and Drug Administration (FDA)-approved skin substitute used in venous ulcer and made up of keratinocyte and fibroblast-seeded collagen. Integra™ is an artificial skin made up of

TABLE 5: Epidermal substitute.[78-83]

EpiDex	Autologous keratinocytes of the outer root sheath of plucked anagen hair follicles
Bioseed-S	Autologous keratinocytes resuspended in an allogeneic fibrin sealant
MySkin™	Autologous keratinocytes seeded on a synthetic silicone polymer support layer
EpiCel®	Autologous keratinocytes Sheets attached to petrolatum gauze support
CellSpray	Suspension of noncultured autologous keratinocytes

TABLE 6: Dermospidermal (composite) substitute.[90-93]

PolyActive	Synthetic polyethylene oxide terephthalate/ polybutylene terephthalate (PEO/PBT) scaffold seeded with autologous keratinocytes and fibroblasts
Tiscover™ (A-Skin)	Autologous full-thickness cultured skin consisting of a pigmented epidermis on fibroblast proliferated dermis
Apligraf™	Bovine type I collagen seeded with allogeneic neonatal foreskin fibroblasts and keratinocytes
OrCel™	Bovine type I collagen sponge seeded with allogeneic neonatal foreskin fibroblasts and keratinocytes
TissueTech autograft system (Laserskin and Hyalograft 3D)	Recombinant hyaluronic acid (HA) membrane seeded with autologous fibroblasts and keratinocytes and is comprised of Hyalograft® as a dermal substitute and Laserskin as the epidermal substitute

TABLE 7: Dermal substitute.[84-89]

Matriderm®	Cell-free bovine type I collagen matrix and α-elastin hydrolysate lyophilized dermis
TransCyte	Porcine dermal type I collagen coated with bio-absorbable polyglactin and with a silicone film covered nylon mesh containing allogenic neonatal foreskin fibroblasts
Integra™	Cell-free dermal regeneration template composed of a dermal layer made of bovine type I collagen and shark chondroitin-6-sulfate GAG with a silicone polymer as an epidermal layer
Alloderm™	Cell-free dermal substitute composed of allogeneic lyophilized cadaveric collagen as the dermis analog
Biobrane®	Cell-free dermal substitute composed of an inner dermal analog 3D nylon fabric and porcine type I collagen peptides with outer ultrathin silicone film as epidermal analog
Dermagraft™	Synthetic PGA/PLA, ECM, and allogeneic neonatal foreskin fibroblasts

(3D: three dimensional; ECM: extracellular matrix; GAG: glycosaminoglycan; PGA/PLA: polyglycolic acid/polylactic acid)

chondroitin 6 sulfate and collagen matrix. Alloderm™ is fibroblast with all cellular component removed.

Bandaging

Bandaging is an important component of wound care. Bandaging is particularly important in the setting of leg ulcers and venous ulcers.[94,95] Techniques of bandaging, different types, in different anatomical settings, their advantages, and disadvantages are described separately.

The various wound dressings and their clinical applications are enlisted in **Table 8**.

WOUND MANAGEMENT IN SPECIAL SITUATIONS IN DERMATOSURGERY

Bleeding Control in Dermatosurgery

Bleeding must be controlled. If required, dermatosurgical wound hemostasis can be achieved by direct pressure, application of a tourniquet or blood pressure cuff inflated 20 mm Hg above the patient's systolic blood pressure, or with the use of topical or subcutaneous epinephrine. Epinephrine-moistened gauze (1:100,000) applied directly over the wound for 10 minutes helps to constrict small blood vessels and decrease the bleeding. Pressure should only be applied for 5 minutes when controlling bleeding over the nose tip, mucosa, penis, and earlobe. Hemostatic gelatin foam can also be used. Large nondigital vessels can be directly visualized and ligated with clamping or a figure-of-8 suture. The digital arteries should never be ligated or clamped as they run parallel and in very close proximity to the digital nerve and clamping both is almost inevitable. The blind clamping of any bleeding wound is strongly discouraged. Large extremity tourniquets are rarely needed, but when used, they must be properly placed. Cotton gauze should be placed on the limb to provide some protection to the skin and then an inflatable tourniquet or blood pressure cuff can be inflated to 20 mm Hg higher than the patient's systolic blood pressure, not to exceed 250 mm Hg, to control distal arterial blood flow. The tourniquet should be inflated for no longer than 20–30 minutes before it is deflated for 5 minutes. Total inflation time should not exceed 1 hour. For digital tourniquets, a stretched Penrose drain can be placed at the base of a previously exsanguinated digit or a commercial rubber ring tourniquet can be applied for a maximum of 30 minutes.

Dressings after Specific Dermatosurgical Procedures

While details can be found in individual chapters, a brief discussion is provided further.

- *Minor wounds after excisions:* Composite four-layer dressing after minor surgery may be removed after 1 day for wound inspection. The edges of the wound have to be palpated to look for induration/swelling and if so, relevant sutures are to be removed and the hematoma evacuated by pressure to prevent infection/dehiscence. This can be followed by secondary suturing and dressing. In case of infection as evidenced by features of inflammation and discharge from the wound, pus culture is appropriate and antibiotics should be started/changed and dressings changed daily. If wound is progressing well, it may be redressed and removed after 7–10 days.
- If the procedure is of minor nature such as a biopsy or electrosurgery, dressing may be dispensed with or done for a day or two. Thereafter, topical antibiotic ointment should be adequate.
- A pressure dressing is required on donor area after procedures such as hair transplant and skin grafting.
- A bimodal dressing for differential pressure is recommended for liposuction.
- Following resurfacing procedures (dermabrasion, laser, or radiofrequency), it is preferable to have an open dressing with zinc oxide paste and allow the wound to ooze out, wiping the wound with sterile wipes repeatedly for the first 24–48 hours till oozing stops.
- *Pressure sores:* Decubitus ulcers are best prevented. This is done by turning or shifting the susceptible patient every 2–3 hours, use of pressure-relieving bed such as water–air bed and education of relatives. Once ulcer develops, absorbent padding for incontinence, nutritional support, healing by secondary intention, or grafting in addition to management of infection are required. Pressure on the ulcer must be avoided at all times.

Adjuvants in Wound Management

Several agents have been promoted as wound-healing adjuvants. While evidence may be lacking for many of these agents, they are useful in special situations such as venous ulcers, nonhealing leg ulcers, etc.

TABLE 8: Topical antimicrobial agents, wound dressings and their clinical applications.

Product	*Indications and action*	*Advantages*	*Disadvantages*	*Use*	*Examples*
Antimicrobials Mupirocin	• Wounds infected with gram-positive organisms • Prevents bacterial protein and cell wall synthesis	• Very effective against *Staphylococcus*, especially methicillin-resistant *Staphylococcus aureus* (MRSA) • Do not damage healthy tissue	Costly	Can be applied daily	T-bact (Glaxo), Bactroban, Mupibact
Retapamulin	Effective against *Staphylococcus aureus* and pyogenes inhibit bacterial protein synthesis	Effective against mupirocin and fusidic acid resistant *Staphylococcus*	Costly		Retarel (Ajanta Pharma)
Silver-impregnated dressings	Deep burns and skin sloughing disorders (toxic epidermal necrolysis and Stevens–Johnson syndrome), donor sites and meshed skin grafts	Effective for wounds infected both with gram-negative and gram-positive organisms, especially MRSA and virus and fungi also	Argyria Costly	Change every 5–7 days	Acticoat (Smith and Nephew), Silvel (Datt Pharma), Biatain Ag (Coloplast), Actisorb (Johnson and Johnson), Aquacel Ag (ConvaTec)
Foams	Pressure ulcers and lower limb ulcers with minimum-to-moderate exudates	Absorbent occlusive thermal insulation	Opaque, malodorous discharge	Change every 3 days	Alleyn (Smith and Nephew), Lyofoam (ConvaTec), 3 m foam dressing (3 m Health Care), Biatain foam dressing (Coloplast)
Films	Partial thickness Wounds with minimal exudates, pressure ulcers, and grafts	• Transparent occlusive moisture-retentive protection from contamination • Easy to inspect wounds	No absorption, fluid-trapping, skin stripping, not for infected wounds	Leave on till 7 days or when fluid leaks or secretions collect underneath	Tegaderm (3 m Healthcare), Biocclusive (Johnson and Johnson), OpSite (Smith and Nephew), Dermasite (Dermasciences), Comfeel film (Coloplast)
Hydrogels	• Dry wounds • Painful wounds mainly pressure sores, lower limb ulcers, skin tears, and surgical wounds	Moisture retentive nontraumatic removal	May overhydrate	Change in 1–3 days	Intrasite gel (Smith and Nephew), Solosite (Smith and Nephew), Restore hydrogel (Hollister)
Hydrocolloids	Wounds with minimum-to-moderate exudates like pressure ulcers and venous stasis ulcers	Absorbent, occlusive, protection from contamination	Opaque, fluid trapping, maldorous discharge	Left on till 7 days	DuoDerm (Convatec), Comfeel (Coloplast), 3 m Tegasorb (3 m Health Care), Restore (Hollister), Nu-Derm (Johnson and Johnson)
Alginates	• Pressure sores, diabetic ulcers, infected wounds, lower extremity ulcers with moderate to heavy exudates • Mild hemostasis	Highly absorbent, hemostatic, nontoxic, nonallergenic	Fibrous debris	Left on till soaked with exudate	Kaltostat (Convatec), Algiderm (Bard), Kalginate (De Royal)
Enzymatic debridement	For necrotic sloughy wounds	Digest necrotic matter without harming normal tissue	• Papain is nonselective and may be painful • No absorbing action, so need a secondary dressing	Minimum daily use	• Collagenase • Santyl (Healthport), Accuzyme (Healthport), Salutyl (Elder Pharma), Debridace (Virchow Healthcare)
Growth factors	Useful in small nonhealing wounds	Accelerate healing of chronic wounds	Not indicated in necrotic wounds, cancerous growths, require a secondary dressing with gauze	To be applied daily	Plermin (Dr Reddy's Lab), Eugraf (Lupin), Epigrof (Marksons), Regen D (Bharat Biotech)

Platelet-rich Plasma and Platelet-rich Fibrin in Wound Healing

Platelet-rich plasma (PRP) is used in various clinical disciplines and is considered to improve tissue regeneration due to the presence of essential growth factors and cytokines. PRP is autologous form of concentrated platelets and growth factors occurring naturally in the body. PRP can be made either by centrifugation or filtering whole blood with anticoagulant to obtain a formulation of platelets and plasma with supraphysiologic concentrations of platelets.[96]

Platelet-rich plasma contains bioactive molecules which play an important role in wound healing. These include PDGF, TGF, platelet factor 4 (PF4), IL-1, platelet-derived angiogenesis factor (PDAF), vascular endothelial growth factor (VEGF), EGF, platelet-derived endothelial growth factor (PDEGF), epithelial cell growth factor (ECGF), and IGF. These molecules, along with other bioactive molecules, have diverse functions in the local regeneration environment, such as proliferation, migration, cell differentiation, and angiogenesis.[97]

In addition to platelets and their products, the natural wound response requires the presence of a fibrin matrix, which enhances the delivery of growth factors.[98] PRF is an immune and platelet concentrate that collects on a single fibrin membrane **(Fig. 13)**.[99] The PRF membranes simultaneously support the development of the three keys to healing and soft tissue maturation, namely angiogenesis, immunity, and epithelial cover.

Platelet-rich plasma is also used in the management of acne scars, facial rejuvenation in skin aging, and in the treatment of alopecia.

Pentoxifylline: It increases fibrinolysis, decreasing blood viscosity, increasing red cell deformability, and inhibiting platelet aggregation. The drug is useful in chronic venous leg ulcers.[100]

Prostaglandin E2 and I2, iloprost, and calcium channel blockers such as nifedipine: These have shown conflicting results in various studies. Some calcium channel blockers may help keratinocyte migration.[99] The serotonin antagonist, ketanserin has been shown to be of benefit when applied topically to diabetic foot and leg ulcers.[101,102]

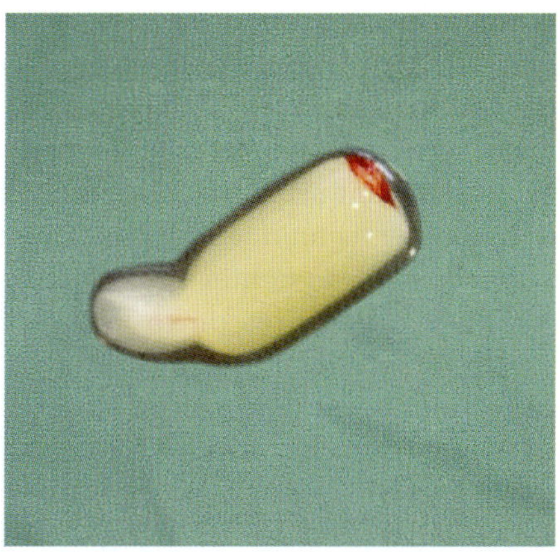

Fig. 13: Platelet-rich fibrin pellet ready to be transferred over wound.

Ascorbic acid: High-dose ascorbic acid has been beneficial in wound management.[103] It is a cofactor for proline hydroxylase necessary for collagen synthesis.

Zinc: Its precise role in wound healing is unclear at present. It has important antioxidant role in the skin. Systemic zinc is mainly useful in those who are zinc deficient. Topical zinc may be beneficial in wound healing through local actions, reducing infection and promoting epithelialization.[91,104]

Oxygen and nitric oxide: Nitric oxide has also been shown to regulate collagen synthesis, cell proliferation, and wound contraction.[105] The inducible form [inducible nitric oxide synthase (iNOS)] is synthesized in the early stages of normal wound healing. Hyperbaric oxygen therapy increases wound nitric oxide levels which is thought to promote healing of chronic wounds, particularly diabetic foot ulcers.

VAC: Negative pressure is used to assist wound closure, particularly deep wounds, chronic leg ulcers, and diabetic ulcers.[106-109] Removal of wound fluid helps the process of healing.

Ultrasound: Low-frequency, noncontact ultrasound has been shown to improve wound healing, though this method is still to be completely validated.

Electrical stimulation of skin: These promote wound healing by stimulating fibroblast function, increasing TGF-β expression, and facilitate wound contraction. Pulsed stimulation is better than continuous.

Low-level laser therapy: The effect of He–Ne laser on tissue regeneration by monitoring collagen synthesis in wound granulation tissues in Swiss albino mice has been evaluated using analysis of laser-induced fluorescence (LIF) and light microscopy techniques. There has been dose-dependent increase in wound collagen levels in addition to improvement in other wound-healing parameters. Low-level light therapy with blue LED light also impacts wound healing.[110]

Photodynamic therapy: Collagen-based scaffolding material embedded with a liposomal formulation of metatetra (hydroxyphenyl) chlorine and photodynamic therapy on wound healing in mice has shown rapid improvement.[111]

Extremely low-frequency electromagnetic fields (ELF-EMF): Data analysis supports three main effects of electromagnetic fields on the wound-healing pathways: (1) An anti-inflammatory effect by modulation of cytokine profile that induces the transition of the healing process from a chronic proinflammatory to an anti-inflammatory state; (2) a neoangiogenic effect by increased endothelial cells proliferation and tubulization and production of FGF-2; and (3) a re-epithelialization effect by stimulation of collagen formation.[112]

Growth factors to augment wound healing: The addition of exogenous growth factors in pharmacological amounts may have measurable effects in wound-healing models but can be disappointing in the clinical arena.[113] PDGF is the only growth factor which has been found useful clinically in diabetic ulcers.[114] Promising results of the first human gene therapy trial using PDGF have been reported.[115] There are reports on the role of EGF in animal models.[116] EGF, IL-1, and TGF-β have also shown encouraging results, though not replicated consistently. More recently, FGF receptor 1 oncogene partner 2 (FGFR1OP2), has been shown to significantly modulate fibroblast-driven wound closure in vitro and in vivo. The dynamic role of cytoskeleton in different experimental models may provide a novel platform for designing the therapeutic target of wound management.[117]

Topical insulin: Many experiments on animals as well as humans have been performed, but the usefulness of insulin in wound healing still remains speculative and safety issues still have to be addressed.

Topical insulin in combination with zinc in animal studies has been shown to heal wounds faster. It regulates wound inflammatory response by stimulating proliferation and migration of macrophages and keratinocytes in adjacent tissues.[102]

Wound healing promoters: Substances such as tretinoin, aloe vera extracts, benzoyl peroxide, chamomilla extracts promote granulation, epithelialization, alleviate pain and irritation, and are astringent and deodorant. Animal studies have proved beneficial effects of chamomilla being anti-inflammatory/antimutagenic. Human studies are lacking/warranted), dexpanthenol (converted to pantothenic acid forming coenzyme A), tetrachlorodecaoxide solution (TCDO combines with hemoglobin, myoglobin, and cytochromes releasing molecular oxygen), clostebol acetate (promotes protein synthesis), topical vitamin E, etc. have been shown to promote healing.

Others: Infrared radiation, ultraviolet C (UVC) radiation, and warming devices have been used, though evidence to support their use is not available.

Triage-based Wound Care

Triage is the process of prioritizing patient care based on need and available resources. Clinicians in wound clinics triage daily because time and resources never seem to be sufficient.

Creation of a Wound Care Service

It is important that a wound care service outside of operation theaters is created to reduce load and increase patient accessibility. This kind of a service would be helpful in reducing costs and increasing wound-healing rates, being manned by medical and paramedical personnel with a special interest and expertise in this important aspect of care. Specialists may be chosen depending on the major causes of wounds in the specific area but must include a dermatologist, surgeon, and wound care nurse, in addition to support staff. Interdisciplinary management of wounds is the new mantra. Home care wound management using telemedicine has also been possible.[118] In addition, self-care taught properly is highly important in the management of wounds such as in leprosy. It is sustainable and can be carried out as part of routine work.

Future of Wound Care

These include tissue engineering techniques such as stem cells and gene therapy for achieving wound closure. Stem cells have the ability to migrate to the site of injury or inflammation, participate in regeneration of damaged tissue, stimulate proliferation and differentiation of resident progenitor cells, secrete growth factors, remodel matrix, increase angiogenesis, inhibit scar formation, and improve tensile strength of the wound. Stem cells hold good hope for exploitation in the form of gene transfer.[119-125]

Nanotechnology in Wound Care[126]

Nanomaterial has at least one dimension in nanometer and holds prominent future in wound management. In wound care, this material has displayed potential to promote cell differentiation, migration, angiogenesis, and remodeling. Different types of nanomaterial has been studied till date including lipid nanoparticle, nanocomposite, polymeric nanoparticles, silver-based nanoparticle, and nanofibers to mention a few.

Three-dimensional Printing in Wound Care

The need for personalized, patient-specific, and wound-specific dressing with controlled spatial release of growth factors and antibacterials has been felt in management of chronic wounds. In this regard, three dimensional (3D) printing technology is proven to be an emerging option for creating tailormade wound dressings. Various technologies are in vogue to achieve the desired output. Traditional fused deposition modeling (FDM) also known as roller extrusion FDM fabricates 3D parts by feeding a filament through a heated element using a stepper motor fitted with a roller gear.[127] Another technique includes pneumatic FDM which uses air pressure to achieve the desired result.[128] Piston-based FDM utilizes piston to infuse bioink into the system, electrohydrodynamic jet printing (e-Jet) and micro-to-nano size liquid deposition (droplet creation) technique uses microcapillary nozzles to create fluid flows by electrohydrodynamic force.[129]

Three-dimensional printing technology combined with nanomaterial has a potential to revolutionize wound care in chronic nonhealing wounds and also paves a way for scarless wound healing in planned surgeries/interventions.

CONCLUSION

- A moist wound bed is needed for all stages of wound healing.
- Wound healing is affected by many factors—age, vascular state, nutritional state, comorbidity, drug therapy, debris, and infection.
- A systematic assessment of the wound is essential to evaluate healing and treatment efficacy.
- Regular wound reassessments are required.
- Infection control guidelines should be followed in the management of all wounds. Tetanus prophylaxis may be needed in contaminated wounds.
- Potable tap water may be used to wash and cleanse most chronic wounds.
- Cleansing solutions should be at body temperature to prevent wound cooling.
- There is insufficient evidence to determine if one type of dressing is superior to another.
- Clinical infection should be treated with systemic antibiotics and not topical antimicrobials.
- Routine wound swabs are not recommended.
- Topical antimicrobial dressings, where used, should be for short-term use only.
- The frequency of dressing changes, type, and location of wound and patient acceptability, including impact on comfort and odor control are important factors in the choice of dressing for a particular wound.
- In the treatment of wounds, the new trend in the wound device market is to produce dressings containing compounds or drugs. These could be local antiseptics (silver, other antiseptics, and honey) and pain-relieving drugs such as ibuprofen and morphine. New treatments such as anti-TNF-α and *Lactobacillus plantarum* cultures have also been successfully used in hard-to-heal, atypical wounds. Knowledge of influencing factors such as smoking and biofilms on the healing process has also improved. Smoking results in delayed healing and increased risk of postoperative infection, whereas the role of biofilm is being debated, with thoughts on them delaying wound healing. Organizing models for optimal wound management are constantly being developed and refined.[98]

REFERENCES

1. Schreml S, Szeimies RM, Prantl L, Landthaler M, Babilas P. Wound healing in the 21st century. J Am Acad Dermatol. 2010;63:866-81.
2. Kirsner RS, Eaqlstein WH. The wound healing process. Dermatol Clin. 1993;11:629-40.
3. Cho J, Mosher DF. Role of fibronectin assembly in platelet thrombus formation. J Thromb Haemost. 2006;4:1461-9.
4. Bennett NT, Schultz GS. Growth factors and wound healing: biochemical properties of growth factors and their receptors. Am J Surg. 1993;165:728-37.
5. Rumalla VK, Borah GL. Cytokines, growth factors, and plastic surgery. Plast Reconstr Surg. 2001;108:719-33.
6. Frenette PS, Wagner DD. Adhesion molecules—part 1. N Engl J Med. 1996;334:1526-9.
7. Frenette PS, Wagner DD. Adhesion molecules—part II: Blood vessels and blood cells. N Engl J Med. 1996;335:43-5.
8. Sindrilaru A, Scharffetter-Kochanek K. Disclosure of the culprits: macrophages-versatile regulators of wound healing. Adv Wound Care. 2013;2:357-68.
9. Cross KJ, Mustoe TA. Growth factors in wound healing. Surg Clin N Am. 2003;83:531-46.
10. Lucas T, Waisman A, Ranjan R, Roes J, Krieg T, Muller W, et al. Differential roles of macrophages in diverse phases of skin repair. J Immunol. 2010;184:3964-77.
11. Goldberg SR, Diegelmann RF. Wound healing primer. Surg Clin North Am. 2010;90:1133-46.
12. Bhushan M, Young HS, Brenchley PE, Griffiths CE. Recent advances in cutaneous angiogenesis. Br J Dermatol. 2002;147:418-25.
13. Demidova-Rice TN, Durham JT, Herman IM. Wound healing angiogenesis: innovations and challenges in acute and chronic wound healing. Adv Wound Care. 2012;1:17-22.
14. Clore JN, Cohen IK, Diegelmann RF. Quantitation of collagen types I and III during wound healing in rat skin. Proc Soc Exp Biol Med. 1979;161:337-40.
15. Baker EA, Leaper DJ. Proteinases, their inhibitors, and cytokine profiles in acute wound fluid. Wound Repair Regen. 2000;8:392-8.
16. Chen WY, Rogers AA, Lydon MJ. Characterization of biologic properties of wound fluid collected during early stages of wound healing. J Invest Dermatol. 1992;99:559-64.
17. Vaalamo M, Leivo T, Saarialho-Kere U. Differential expression of tissue inhibitors of metalloproteinases (TIMP-1, 2, 3, and 4) in normal and aberrant wound healing. Hum Pathol. 1999;30:795-802.
18. Cowin AJ, Hatzirodos N, Holding CA, Dunaiski V, Harries RH, Rayner TE, et al. Effect of healing on the expression of transforming growth factor beta(s) and their receptors in chronic venous leg ulcers. J Invest Dermatol. 2001;117:1282-9.
19. Wysocki AB. Fibronectin in acute and chronic wounds. JET Nurs. 1992;19:166-70.
20. Volk SW, Bohling MW. Comparative wound healing: are the small animal veterinarian's clinical patients an improved translational model for human wound healing research? Wound Repair Regen. 2013;21:372-81.
21. Krawczyk WS. A pattern of epidermal cell migration during wound healing. J Cell Biol. 1971;49:247-63.
22. Lambert WC, Cohen PJ, Lambert MW. Role of the epidermis and other epithelia in wound healing: selected concepts. Clin Dermatol. 1984;2:24-33.
23. Gov NS. Collective cell migration patterns: follow the leader. Proc Natl Acad Sci USA. 2007;104:15970-1.
24. Omelchenko T, Vasiliev JM, Gelfand IM, Feder HH, Bonder EM. Rho-dependent formation of epithelial "leader" cells during wound healing. Proc Natl Acad Sci USA. 2003;100:10788-93.
25. Farooqui R, Fenteany G. Multiple rows of cells behind an epithelial wound edge extend cryptic lamellipodia to collectively drive cell-sheet movement. J Cell Sci. 2004;118:51-63.
26. Matsubayashi Y, Razzell W, Martin P. "White wave" analysis of epithelial scratch wound healing reveals how cells mobilise

back from the leading edge in a myosin-II-dependent fashion. J Cell Sci. 2011;124:1017-21.
27. Jacinto A, Martinez-Arias A, Martin P. Mechanisms of epithelial fusion and repair. Nat Cell Biol. 2001;3:E117-23.
28. Stone RC, Pastar I, Ojeh N, Chen V, Liu S, Garzon KI, et al. Epithelial-mesenchymal transition in tissue repair and fibrosis. Cell Tissue Res. 2016;365:495-506.
29. Patten J, Wang K. Fibronectin in development and wound healing. Adv Drug Deliv Rev. 2021;170:353-68.
30. Lu L, Saulis AS, Liu WR, Roy NK, Chao JD, Ledbetter S, et al. The temporal effects of anti-TGF-beta1, 2, and 3 monoclonal antibody on wound healing and hypertrophic scar formation. J Am Coll Surg. 2005;201:391-7.
31. Lim IJ, Phan TT, Song C, Tan WT, Longaker MT. Investigation of the influence of keloid-derived keratinocytes on fibroblast growth and proliferation in vitro. Plast Reconstr Surg. 2001;107:797-808.
32. Smith CJ, Smith JC, Finn MC. The possible role of mast cells (allergy) in the production of keloid and hypertrophic scarring. J Burn Care Rehabil. 1987;8:126-31.
33. Ghahary A, Ghaffari A. Role of keratinocyte fibroblast cross-talk in development of hypertrophic scar. Wound Repair Regen. 2007;15:S46-53.
34. Fujiwara M, Muragaki Y, Ooshima A. Keloid-derived fibroblasts show increased secretion of factors involved in collagen turnover and depend on matrix metalloproteinase for migration. Br J Dermatol. 2005;153:295-300.
35. Armour A, Scott PG, Tredget EE. Cellular and molecular pathology of HTS: basis for treatment. Wound Repair Regen. 2007;15:S6-17.
36. Kurokawa I, Danby FW, Ju Q, Wang X, Xiang LF, Xia L, et al. New developments in our understanding of acne pathogenesis and treatment. Exp Dermatol. 2009;18:821-32.
37. Holland DB, Jeremy AH, Roberts SG, Seukeran DC, Layton AM, Cunliffe WJ. Inflammation in acne scarring: a comparison of the responses in lesions from patients prone and not prone to scar. Br J of Dermatol. 2004;150:72-81.
38. Chivot M, Pawin H, Beylot C, Chosidow O, Dreno B, Faure M, et al. Acne scars: epidemiology, physiopathology, clinical features and treatment. Ann Dermatol Et Venereol. 2006;133:813-24.
39. Ross EV, McKinlay JR, Anderson RR. Why does carbon dioxide resurfacing work? A review. Arch Dermatol. 1999;135:444-54.
40. Rahman Z, MacFalls H, Jiang K, Chan KF, Kelly K, Tournas J, et al. Fractional deep dermal ablation induces tissue tightening. Lasers Surg Med. 2009;41:78-86.
41. Hantash BM, Bedi VP, Kapadia B, Rahman Z, Jiang K, Tanner H, et al. In vivo histological evaluation of a novel ablative fractional resurfacing device. Lasers Surg Med. 2007;39:96-107.
42. Bennett RG. Fundamentals of cutaneous surgery, 1st edition. St Louis, MO: CV Mosby; 1988. p. 778.
43. NHSSB Wound Management Manual. (2005). [online] Available from https://www.bcpft.nhs.uk/about-us/our-policies-and-procedures/w/1444-wound-management-guidelines/file. [Last accessed in March 2024].
44. WHO Guidelines on Wound Management. Best practice guidelines in disaster situations. [online] Available from https://cdn.who.int/media/docs/default-source/integrated-health-services-(ihs)/csy/surgical-care/emergencysurgicalcareindisastersituations.pdf [Last accessed March 2024].
45. Falanga V. Classifications for wound bed preparation and stimulation of chronic wounds. Wound Repair Regen. 2000;8:347-52.
46. Howell JM. Current and future trends in wound healing. Emerg Med Clin North Am. 1992;10:655-63.
47. Schultz G, Sibbald RG, Falanga V, Ayello EA, Dowsett C, Harding K, et al. Wound bed preparation: a systematic approach to wound management. Wound Repair Regen. 2003;11:S1-28.
48. Singer AJ, Quinn JV, Thode HC Jr, Hollander JE; TraumaSeal Study Group. Determinants of poor outcome after laceration and surgical incision repair. Plast Reconstr Surg. 2002;110:429-35.
49. Marks JG Jr, Cano C, Leitzel K, Lipton A. Inhibition of wound healing by topical steroids. J Dermatol Surg Oncol. 1983;9:819-21.
50. Petrosillo N. Natural products and wound management: a never-ending story. Clin Infect Dis. 2008;47:730-1.
51. Cooper DD, Seupaul RA. Is water effective for wound cleansing? Ann Emerg Med. 2012;60(5):626-7. doi: 10.1016/j.annemergmed.2012.06.011. Epub 2012 Jul 28. PMID: 22841710.
52. Pronchik D, Barber C, Rittenhouse S. Low-versus high-pressure irrigation techniques in Staphylococcus aureus-inoculated wounds. Am J Emergency Med. 1999;17:121-4.
53. Fernandez R, Griffiths R. Water for wound cleansing. Cochrane Database Syst Rev. 2008;23:CD003861.
54. Kramer SA. Effect of povidon-iodine on wound healing: a review. J Vasc Nurs. 1999;17:17-23.
55. Eming SA, Smola-Hess S, Kurschat P, Hirche D, Krieg T, Smola H. A novel property of povidon-iodine: inhibition of excessive protease levels in chronic non-healing wounds. J Invest Dermatol. 2006;126:2731-3.
56. Brennan SS, Leaper DJ. The effect of antiseptics on the healing wound: a study using the rabbit ear chamber. Br J Surg. 1985;72:780-2.
57. Lineweaver W, Howard R, Soucy D, McMorris S, Freeman J, Crain C, et al. Topical antimicrobial toxicity. Arch Surg. 1985;120:267-70.
58. Geronomus RG, Mertz PM, Eaglstein W. Wound healing: the effects of topical antimicrobial agents. Arch Dermatol. 1979;115:1311-4.
59. Robinson JK, Hanke CW, Siegel DM, Fratila A. Surgery of the Skin: Procedural Dermatology, 2nd edition. St. Louis: Mosby–Elsevier; 2010. p. 120.
60. Molan PC. Re-introducing honey in the management of wounds and ulcers—theory and practice. Ostomy Wound Manage. 2002;48:28-40.
61. Blaser G, Santos K, Bode U, Vetter H, Simon A. Effect of medical honey on wounds colonized or infected with MRSA. J Wound Care. 2007;16:325-8.
62. Chirife J, Herszage L, Joseph A. Microbiological basis for the use of sugar in treating infected wounds. Antimicrob Agents Chemother. 1983;23:766-73.
63. Martin C. Recent Developments in Wound Management: intelligent biomaterials to novel antimicrobials. 24 September 2009, London, UK. IDrugs. 2009;12:695-8.
64. García-Gubern CF, Colon-Rolon L, Bond MC. Essential Concepts of wound management. Emerg Med Clin N Am. 2010;28:951-67.
65. Karaduman S, Yürüktümen A, Güryay SM, Bengi F, Fowler JR Jr. Modified hair apposition technique as the primary closure method for scalp lacerations. Am J Emerg Med. 2009;27:1050-5.
66. Goyal N, Benyo S, Patel VA, Goldenberg D, Talavera F, Toriumi D, et al. (2021). 2-Octyl Cyanoacrylate (Dermabond) Wound adhesives. [online] Available from http://emedicine.

medscape.com/article/874047-overview#showall [Last accessed March 2024].

67. Mekkes JR, Zeegelaar JE, Westerhof W. Quantitative and objective evaluation of wound debriding properties of collagenase and fibrinolysin/desoxyribonuclease in a necrotic ulcer animal model. Arch Dermatol Res. 1998;290:152-7.
68. Mekkes JR, Le Poole IC, Das PK, Kammeyer A, Westerhof W. In vitro tissue-digesting properties of krill enzymes compared with fibrinolysin/DNAse, papain and placebo. Int J Biochem Cell Biol. 1997;29:703-6.
69. Klein MB, Hunter S, Heimbach DM, Engrav LH, Honari S, Gallery E, et al. The versajet water dissection: a new tool for tangential excision. J Burn Care Rehabil. 2007;26:483-7.
70. Reames MK. The use of maggots in wound debridement. Ann Plast Surg. 1988;21:388-91.
71. Mumcuoglu KY. Clinical applications for maggots in wound care. Am J Clin Dermatol. 2001;2:219-27.
72. Winter GD, Scales JT. Effect of air drying and dressings on the surface of a wound. Nature. 1963;197:91-2.
73. Hutchinson JJ. Prevalence of wound infection under occlusive dressings: a collective survey of reported research. Wounds. 1990;1:23-33.
74. O'Toole EA, Mellerio JE. Wound healing. In: Burns DA, Breathnach SM, Cox N, Griffiths C (Eds). Rook's Textbook of Dermatology, 8th edition. Oxford: Wiley-Blackwell; 2010. pp. 1419-27.
75. Sarabahi S. Recent advances in topical wound care. Indian J Plast Surg. 2012;45:379-87.
76. Green H, Kehinde O, Thomas J. Growth of cultured human epidermal cells into multiple epithelia suitable for grafting. Proc Natl Acad Sci USA. 1979;76:5665-8.
77. Collin B, Balderson D, Papini R, Marsden J, Moss C. Cultured autologous keratinocyte grafting of chronic erosions in three patients with epidermolysis bullosa. Clin Exp Dermatol. 2006;31:718-9.
78. Gallico GG, O'Connor NE, Compton CC, Remensnyder JP, Kehinde O, Green H. Cultured epithelial autografts for giant congenital naevi. Plast Reconstr Surg. 1989;84:1-9.
79. Limova M, Mauro T. Treatment of leg ulcers with cultured epithelial autografts: clinical study and case reports. Osteotomy Wound Manage. 1995;41:54-60.
80. Hendricks WM, Swallow RT. Management of stasis ulcers with Unna's boots versus elastic support stockings. J Am Acad Dermatol. 1985;12:90-8.
81. Weibrich G, Hansen T, Kleis W, Buch R, Hitzler WE. Effect of platelet concentration in platelet-rich plasma on peri-implant bone regeneration. Bone. 2004;34:665-71.
82. Conde ME, Fernando SME, Suarez FR. Platelet rich plasma: applications in dermatology. Actos Dermosifiliogr. 2015;106:104-11.
83. Anitua E, Sanchez M, Nurden AT, Zalduendo M, de la Fuente M, Orive G, et al. Autologous fibrin matrices: a potential source of biological mediators that modulate tendon cell activities. J Biomed Mater Res A. 2006;77:285-93.
84. Choukroun J, Diss A, Simonpieri A, Girard MO, Schoeffler C, Dohan SL, et al. Platelet-rich fibrin (PRF): a second-generation platelet concentrate. Part IV: Clinical effects on tissue healing. Oral Surg Oral Med Oral Pathol Oral Radiol Endod. 2006;101:e56-60.
85. Gohel MS, Barwell JR, Tayler M, Chant T, Foy C, Earnshaw JJ, et al. Long term results of compression therapy alone versus compression plus surgery in chronic venous ulceration (ESCHAR): randomized controlled trial. BMJ. 2007;335(7610):83.
86. Jull A, Arroll B, Parag V, Waters J. Pentoxifylline for treating venous leg ulcers. Cochrane Database Syst Rev. 2012;12(12):CD001733.
87. Trollinger DR, Isseroff RR, Nuccitelli R. Calcium-channel blockers inhibit galvanotaxis in human keratinocytes. J Cell Physiol. 2002;193:1-9.
88. Martínez-de Jesús FR, Morales-Guzmán M, Castañeda M, Pérez-Morales A, García-Alonso J, Mendiola-Segura I. Randomized single-blind trial of topical ketanserin for healing acceleration of diabetic foot ulcers. Arch Med Res. 1997;28:95-9.
89. Quatresooz P, Kharfi M, Paquet P, Vroome V, Cauwenbergh G, Piérard GE. Healing effect of ketanserin on chronic leg ulcers in patients with diabetes. J Eur Acad Dermatol Venereol. 2006;20:277-81.
90. Taylor TV, Rimmer S, Day B. Ascorbic acid supplementation in pressure sores. Lancet. 1974;2:544-6.
91. Varkey M, Ding J, Tredget EE. Advances in skin substitutes—potential of tissue engineered skin for facilitating anti-fibrotic healing. J Funct Biomater. 2015;6(3):547-63.
92. Tausche AK, Skaria M, Bohlen L, Liebold K, Hafner J, Friedlein H, et al. An autologous epidermal equivalent tissue engineered from follicular outer root sheath keratinocytes is as effective as split-thickness skin autograft in recalcitrant vascular leg ulcers. Wound Repair Regen. 2003;11(4):248-52.
93. Groeber F, Holeiter M, Hampel M, Hinderer S, Schenke-Layland K. Skin tissue engineering—in vivo and in vitro applications. Adv Drug Deliv Rev. 2011;63(4-5):352-66.
94. Dixit S, Baganizi DR, Sahu R, Dosunmu E, Chaudhari A, Vig K, et al. Immunological challenges associated with artificial skin grafts: available solutions and stem cells in future design of synthetic skin. J Biol Eng. 2017;11:49.
95. Gómez C, Galán J, Torrero V, Ferreiro I, Pérez D, Palao R, et al. Use of an autologous bioengineered composite skin in extensive burns: clinical and functional outcomes. A multicentric study. Burns. 2011;37(4):580-9.
96. Shevchenko RV, James SL, James SE. A review of tissue-engineered skin bioconstructs available for skin reconstruction. J R Soc Interface. 2010;7(43):229-58.
97. Supp DM, Boyce ST. Engineered skin substitutes: practices and potentials. Clin Dermatol 2005;23(4):403-12.
98. Nathoo R, Howe N, Cohen G. Skin substitutes: an overview of the key players in wound management. J Clin Aesthet Dermatol. 2014;7(10):44-8.
99. Nicholas MN, Yeung J. Current status and future of skin substitutes for chronic wound healing. J Cutan Med Surg. 2017;21(1):23-30.
100. Kumar RJ, Kimble RM, Boots R, Pegg SP. Treatment of partial-thickness burns: a prospective, randomized trial using Transcyte. ANZ J Surg. 2004;74(8):622-6.
101. Halim AS, Khoo TL, Mohd Yussof SJ. Biologic and synthetic skin substitutes: An overview. Indian J Plast Surg. 2010;43(Suppl):S23-8.
102. Zaulyanov L, Kirsner RS. A review of a bi-layered living cell treatment (Apligraf®) in the treatment of venous leg ulcers and diabetic foot ulcers. Clin Interv Aging. 2007;2(1):93-8.
103. Nyame TT, Chiang HA, Orgill DP. Clinical applications of skin substitutes. Surg Clin. 2014;94(4):839-50.
104. Uccioli L; TissueTech Autograph System Italian Study Group. A clinical investigation on the characteristics and outcomes of treating chronic lower extremity wounds using the tissuetech autograft system. Int J Low Extrem Wounds. 2003;2(3):140-51.

105. Strömberg HE, Agren MS. Topical zinc oxide treatment improves arterial and venous leg ulcers. Br J Dermatol. 1984;111:461-8.
106. Rostan EF, DeBuys HV, Madey DL. Evidence supporting zinc as an important antioxidant for skin. Int J Dermatol. 2002;41:606-11.
107. Sen CK, Khanna S, Gordillo G, Bagchi D, Bagchi M, Roy S. Oxygen, oxidants, and antioxidants in wound healing: an emerging paradigm. Ann NY Acad Sci. 2002;957:239-49.
108. Eginton MT, Brown KR, Seabrook GR, Towne JB, Cambria RA. A prospective randomized evaluation of negative-pressure wound dressings for diabetic foot wounds. Ann Vasc Surg. 2003;17:645-9.
109. Vuerstaek JDD, Vainas T, Wuite J, Nelemans P, Neumann MH, Veraart JC. State-of-the-art treatment of chronic leg ulcers: a randomized controlled trial comparing vacuum-asssisted closure (V.A.C.) with modern wound dressings. J Vasc Surg. 2006;44:1029-38.
110. Prabhu V, Rao SB, Chandra S, Kumar P, Rao L, Guddattu V, et al. Spectroscopic and histological evaluation of wound healing progression following Low Level Laser Therapy (LLLT). J Biophotonics. 2012;5:168-84.
111. Adamskaya N, Dungel P, Mittermayr R, Hartinger J, Feichtinger G, Wassermann K, et al. Light therapy by blue LED improves wound healing in an excision model in rats. Injury. 2011;42: 917-21.
112. Garrier J, Bezdetnaya L, Barlier C, Gräfe S, Guillemin F, D'Hallewin MA. Foslip®-based photodynamic therapy as a means to improve wound healing. Photodiagnosis Photodyn Ther. 2011;8:321-7.
113. Costin GE, Birlea SA, Norris DA. Trends in wound repair: cellular and molecular basis of regenerative therapy using electromagnetic fields. Curr Mol Med. 2012;12:14-26.
114. Braund R, Hook S, Medlicott NJ. The role of topical growth factors in chronic wounds. Curr Drug Deliv. 2007;4:195-204.
115. Wieman TJ, Smiell JM, Su Y. Efficacy and safety of a topical gel formulation of recombinant platelet-derived growth factor-BB (becaplermin) in patients with chronic neuropathic diabetic ulcers: a phase III randomized placebo-controlled double-blind study. Diabetes Care. 1998;21:822-7.
116. Margolis DJ, Morris LM, Papadopoulos M, et al. Phase I study of H5.020CMV.PDGF-beta to treat venous leg ulcer disease. Mol Ther. 2009;17(10):1822-9.
117. Kalay Z, Cevher SC. Oxidant and antioxidant events during epidermal growth factor therapy to cutaneous wound healing in rats. Int Wound J. 2012;9(4):362-71.
118. Lin A, Hokugo A, Nishimura I. Wound closure and wound management: A new therapeutic molecular target. Cell Adh Migr. 2010;4:396-9.
119. Terry M, Halstead LS, O'Hare P, Gaskill C, Ho PS, Obecny J, et al. Feasibility study of home care wound management using telemedicine. Adv Skin Wound Care. 2009;22:358-64.
120. Hanson SE, Bentz ML, Hematti P. Mesenchymal stem cell therapy for nonhealing cutaneous wounds. Plast Reconstr Surg. 2010;125:510-6.
121. Cha J, Falanga V. Stem cells in cutaneous wound healing. Clin Dermatol. 2007;25:73-8.
122. Langer R. Biomaterials in drug delivery and tissue engineering: one laboratory's experience. Acc Chem Res. 2000;33:94-101.
123. Korbling M, Estron Z. Adult stem cells for tissue repair—a new therapeutic concept? N Eng J Med. 2003;349:570-82.
124. Eming SA, Kreig T, Davidson JM. Gene therapy and wound healing. Clin Dermatol. 2007;25:79-92.
125. Gottrup F, Jørgensen B, Karlsmark T. News in wound healing and management. Curr Opin Support Palliat Care. 2009;3: 300-4.
126. Ashwini T, Prabhu A, Baliga V, Bhat S, Thenkondar ST, Nayak Y, et al. Transforming Wound Management: Nanomaterials and Their Clinical Impact. Pharmaceutics. 2023;15(5):1560.
127. Dudek P. FDM 3D printing technology in manufacturing composite elements. Arch Metal Mater. 2013;58:1415-8.
128. Long J, Etxeberria AE, Nand AV, Bunt CR, Ray S, Seyfoddin A. A 3D printed chitosan-pectin hydrogel wound dressing for lidocaine hydrochloride delivery. Mater Sci Eng C. 2019;104:109873.
129. Shi G, Wang Y, Derakhshanfar S, Xu K, Zhong W, Luo G, et al. Biomimicry of oil infused layer on 3D printed poly(dimethylsiloxane): Non-fouling, antibacterial and promoting infected wound healing. Mater Sci Eng C. 2019;100:915-27.

CHAPTER 5

Bandages in Dermatosurgery

Harish Prasad BR, Ruchi Hemdani

KEY MESSAGES

- Bandage should be used only to hold in place the primary dressing, which covers a wound.
- It should not be applied so tightly that it stops circulation or so loosely that it allows the dressing to slip.
- Bandages are terminated by applying several overlying circular turns and fastening the ends securely.
- Compression bandage reduces effect of venous hypertension by reducing superficial venous pressure.

INTRODUCTION

Bandages are materials that are placed over dressing or splints primarily to secure them in place allowing minimal movement of surgical or injured site. They can also serve other important purposes including achieving hemostasis, provision of immobilization after a graft, and provision of support to surgical site **(Box 1)**. Therefore, a dermatosurgeon needs to be familiar with different types of bandages and their application techniques particularly in invasive surgeries involving different parts of body such as vitiligo surgery, which also requires adequate immobilization for proper graft uptake.

A bandage is any material that is used to secure a dressing over the wound and can serve many other additional purposes as well

Bandaging the wound is an art; a technique, which takes into consideration the site, size, shape, and mobility of the part of body where it is being applied. There can be no universal bandaging technique owing to the variety of shapes and body movements.

GENERAL PRINCIPLES OF BANDAGING

- Bandage should be used only to hold in place the dressing, which covers a wound
- It should never be applied directly over a wound
- A bandage should be applied firmly and fastened securely. It should not be applied so tightly that it stops circulation or so loosely that it allows the dressing to slip **(Box 2)**.

The materials commonly used for bandages are given in **Box 3**.

BANDAGE TECHNIQUES

Following body shapes should be considered while selecting bandaging technique:

- Body shapes with blunt ends such as fingers, hands, forefoot, or head
- Body parts with a tapered shape such as an arm, leg, or trunk, where the circumference of the body part either increases or decreases
- Joints, which allow a hinge movement, such as the knee, elbow, and ankle
- Body parts with an almost constant circumference such as the midfoot, middle of the hand, ankle, and wrist.

*Types of bandages (summarized in **Table 1**) and their basic application techniques to apply on nearly all parts of the body are as follows*:

Triangular and Cravat Bandages

These are easy to apply, quick, and stay well. Hence, they are valuable in dermatosurgeries to place temporary bandages

BOX 1: Uses of bandages in dermatosurgery.

- To prevent wound contamination by holding dressings in position
- To provide rest and to support the part that is injured/operated as in liposuction
- To prevent and control hemorrhage postinvasive surgeries
- To restrict movement/immobilize an operated site as in vitiligo surgeries for effective graft uptake
- To maintain pressure as in compression dressings for venous insufficiency and lymphedema

BOX 2: Quick assessment of circulation postapplication of bandages.

- Check the pulse distal to the injury
- Blanch the fingernail or toenail, if applicable
- Inspect the skin below the bandaging for discoloration
- Ask the patient, if any numbness or coldness to the bandaged part
- Remove and reapply the bandage, if necessary

BOX 3: Materials commonly used for bandages.

- Cotton
- Cotton gauze
- Jute
- Muslin
- Special materials such as crepe bandage, flannel, and rubber
- Elastic bandages

TABLE 1: Types of bandages.

S. No.	*Bandage*	*Body site where commonly used*	*Primary role*	*Additional role*	*Specific point*
1.	Roller 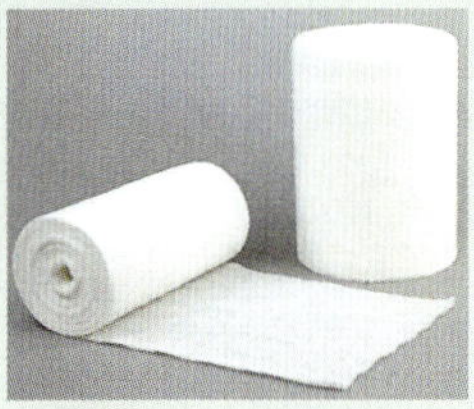 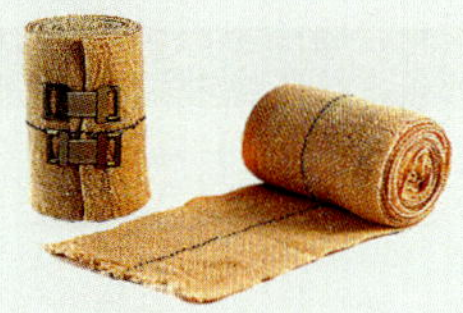	Strained or sprained joints and extremities	Supportive (elastic roller bandage) and cover gauze dressings (cotton roller bandage)	Wound compression (sterile cotton roller bandage)	These are held in place with tape, clips, or pins
2.	Tubular 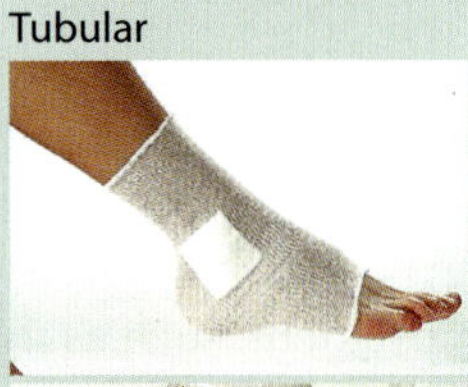 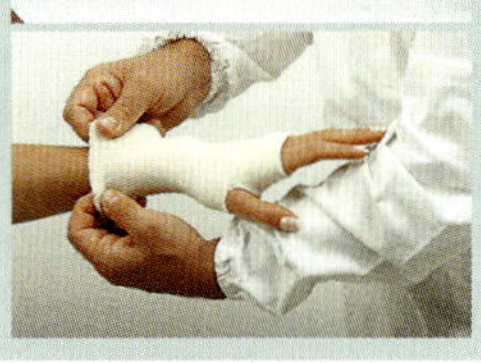	Difficult to bandage areas such as fingers and toes *Others:* Elbows and knees	Secure dressing	Provide support	
3.	Triangular and cravat 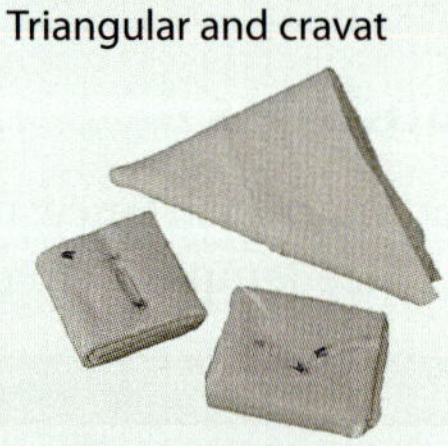	Upper limbs	Supportive as slings, immobilization, and elevation	Upon folding can be used as cold compresses and wound compression	Easy to apply, quick, and stay well
4.	Tailed 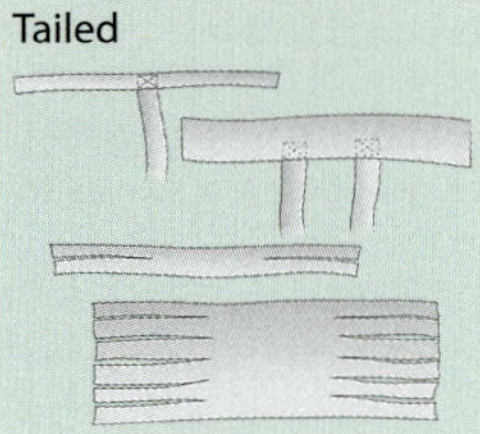	Parts not amenable to roller bandaging	Secure dressing		

till the completion of surgery, e.g., to cover the donor sites in vitiligo surgeries or hair transplantation. A square of sterile gauze material about 3 feet × 3 feet, or slightly more, is folded diagonally. The long side of the triangle is called the "base", the point opposite the base is called the "apex", and the points at each end of the base are called the "ends". This bandage may be used either as a triangle or as a cravat. Cravat (term derived from neck kerchief worn by boy scouts) is made from the triangle by bringing the apex to the base and folding it upon itself a sufficient number of times to obtain the desired width **(Fig. 1)**.

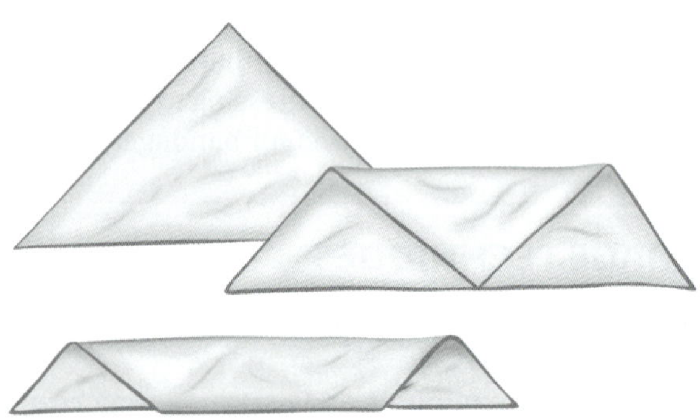

Fig. 1: Triangular and cravat bandages.

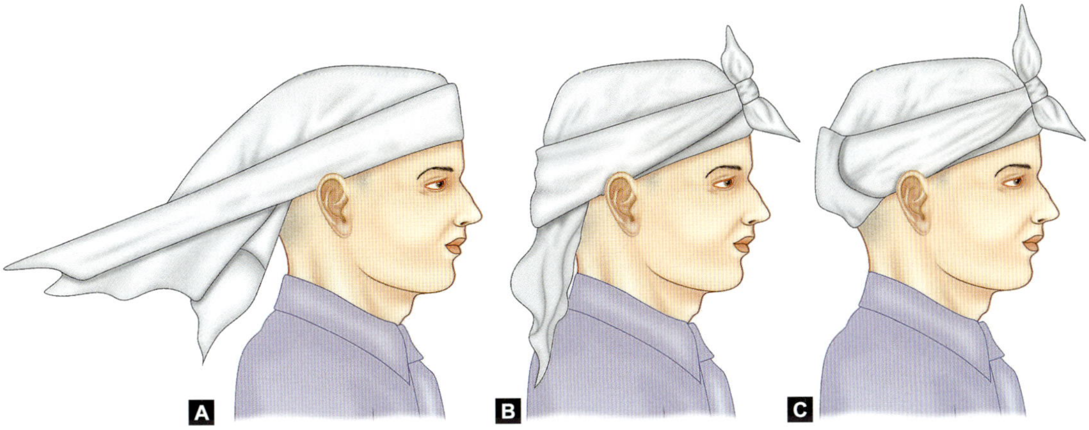

Figs. 2A to C: Triangle of forehead or scalp.

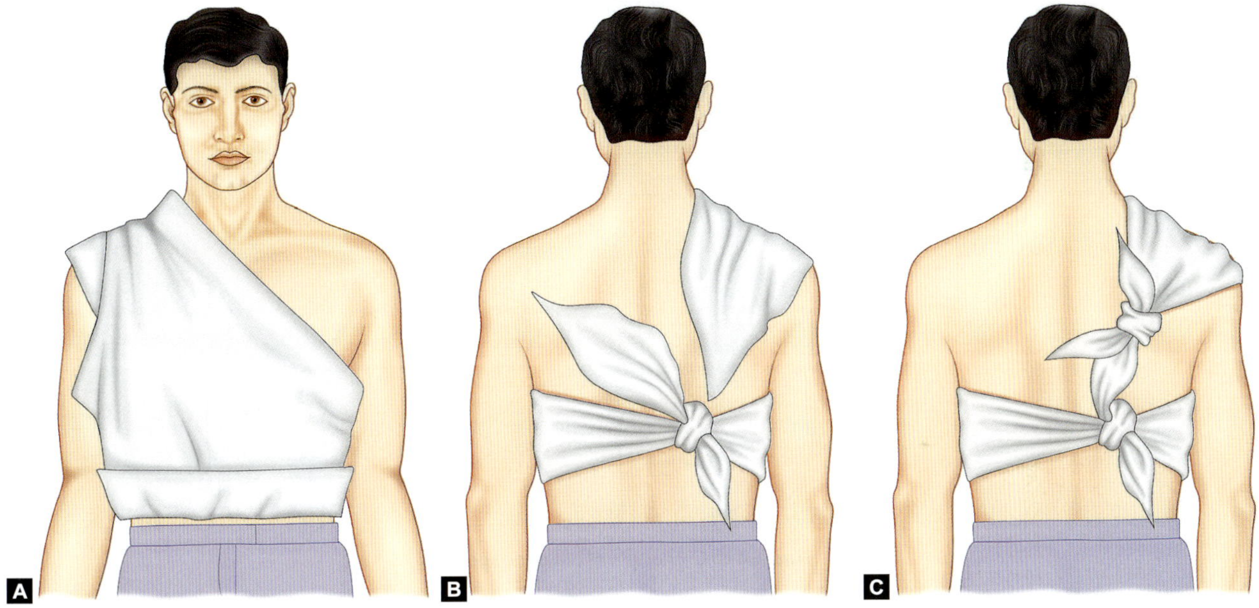

Figs. 3A to C: Triangle of chest bandage.

Triangle of Forehead or Scalp (Fronto-occipital) (Figs. 2A to C)

This is used to hold dressings on the forehead or scalp.

- Place middle of base of triangle, so that edge is just above the eyebrows and bring apex backward, allowing it to drop over back of head (occiput). Bring ends of triangle backward above ears.
- Cross ends over apex at occiput, carry ends around forehead, and tie them in a square knot.
- Turn up apex of bandage toward top of head. Tuck in behind crossed part of bandage.

Triangle of Chest or Back (Figs. 3A to C)

This bandage is used to hold dressings on burns or wounds of chest or back.

- Drop apex of triangle over shoulder on injured side. Bring bandage down over chest (or back) to cover dressing, so that middle of base of bandage is directly below injury. Turn up a cuff at base.
- Carry ends around and tie in a square knot, leaving one end longer than the other.
- Bring apex down and tie to long end of first knot.

Triangle of Shoulder (Figs. 4A to D)

The triangle of the shoulder is used to hold dressings on wounds of the shoulder. Two bandages are required, one a triangle and the other a cravat or roller bandage.

- Place center of cravat or roller bandage at base of neck on injured side and fasten just forward of opposite armpit.
- Slide apex of open triangle under cravat at base of neck and place over dressing on injured shoulder and upper arm. Turn up cuff at base.
- Bring ends around arm and tie.
- Secure apex to cravat at neck by fastening with adhesive tape.

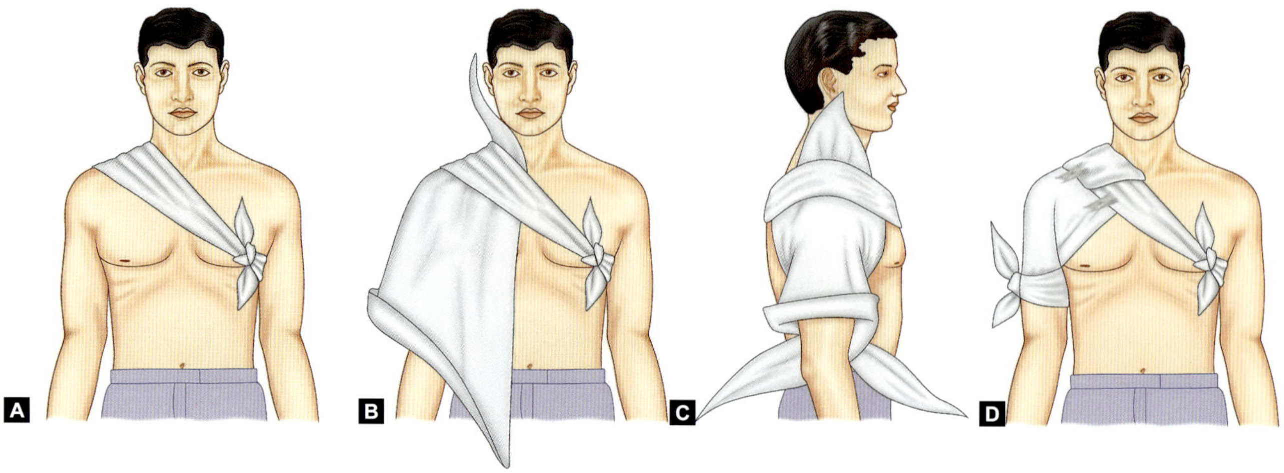

Figs. 4A to D: Triangle of shoulder bandage.

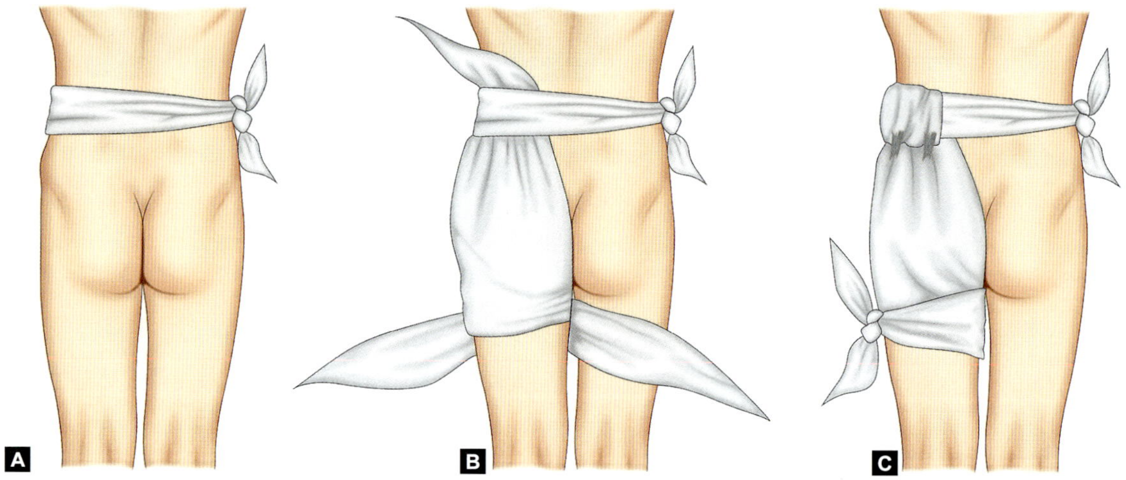

Figs. 5A to C: Triangle of hip bandage.

Triangle of Hip (Figs. 5A to C)

The triangle of the hip is used to hold dressings on the buttock or hip. It requires two bandages, one a triangle and the other a cravat or roller bandage.

- Fasten cravat or roller bandage around waist.
- Place base of triangle below buttock (gluteofemoral fold) and slide apex under cravat at waist. Fold base upward to form cuff and carry ends of base around thigh.
- Tie ends of base with square knot. Fasten apex to waist cravat by an adhesive tape.

Triangle of Foot (Figs. 6A to E)

Triangle of foot is used to hold dressings of considerable size on the foot.

- Center foot upon bandage at right angles to base with heel well forward of base.
- Carry apex of triangle over toes to ankle and tuck excess fullness of bandage into small pleats on each side of foot.
- Cross each half of bandage toward opposite side of ankle.
- Bring ends of triangle around ankle.
- Tie ends in square knot.

Triangle of Hand (Figs. 7A to E)

The triangle of the hand is used to hold dressings of considerable size on the hand.

- Place middle of base of triangle well up on palmar surface of wrist.
- Carry apex around ends of fingers. Cover back (dorsum) of hand to wrist and tuck excess fullness of bandage into small pleats on each side of hand.
- Cross each half of bandage toward opposite side of wrist.
- Bring ends of triangle around wrist.
- Tie ends in square knot.

Cravat of Head (Figs. 8A to C)

The purpose of this bandage is to apply pressure to control hemorrhage from wounds of lower scalp, e.g., bandaging donor site during hair transplantation.

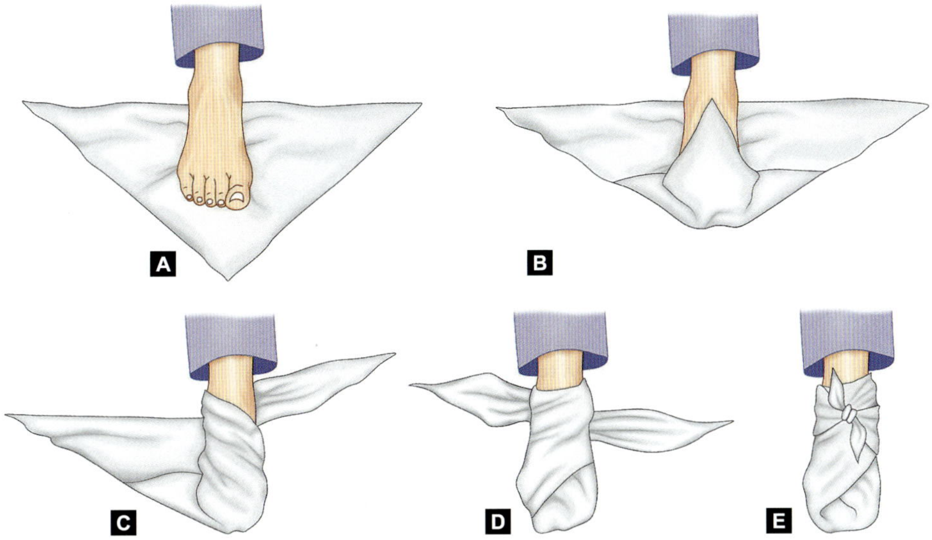

Figs. 6A to E: Triangle of foot bandage.

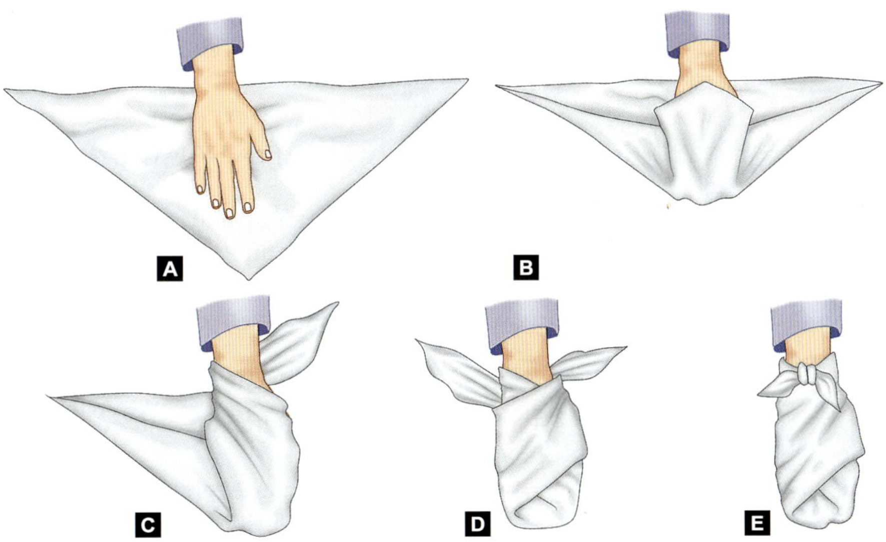

Figs. 7A to E: Triangle of hand.

- Place middle of cravat over dressing.
- Pass each end completely around head.
- Tie in square knot.

Cravat Bandage of Eye (Figs. 9A to D)

The cravat bandage of the eye is used to hold a dressing over the eye, e.g., following ptosis surgery. Two cravats are required.

- Lay center of first cravat over top of head with the front end falling over uninjured eye.
- Bring second cravat around head, over eyes, and over loose ends of first cravat. Tie in front.
- Bring ends of first cravat back over top of head, tying there and pulling second cravat up and away from uninjured eye.

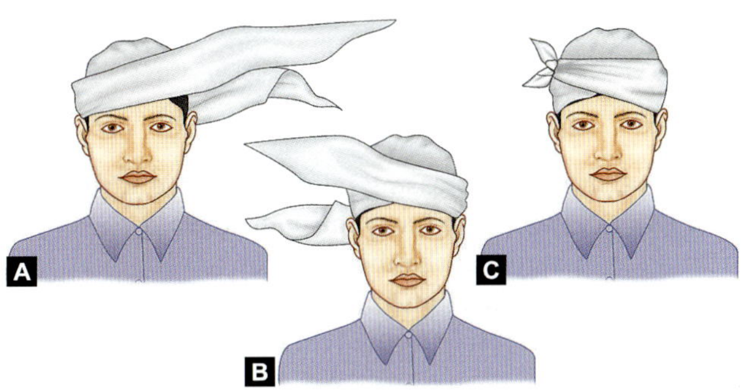

Figs. 8A to C: Cravat of head.

Shoulder–Armpit Cravat (Figs. 10A to C)

The shoulder-armpit cravat (bisaxillary) is used to hold dressings in the axilla or on the shoulder.

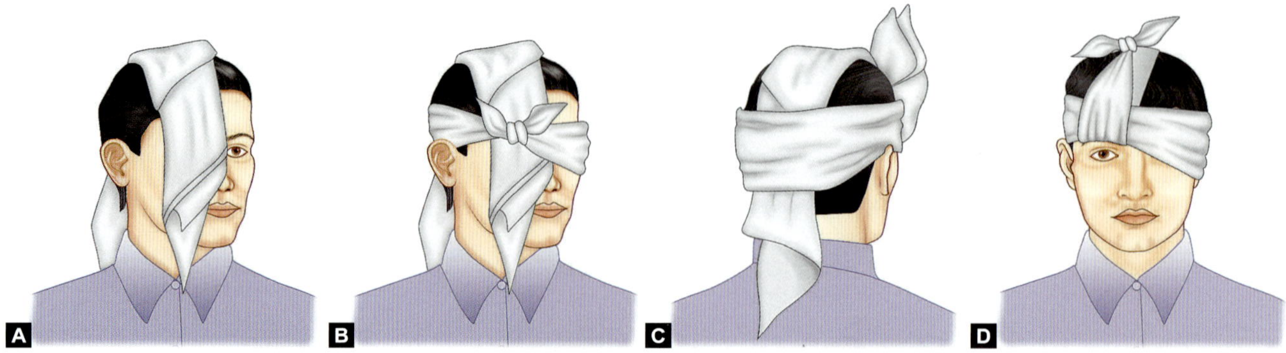

Figs. 9A to D: Cravat bandage of eye.

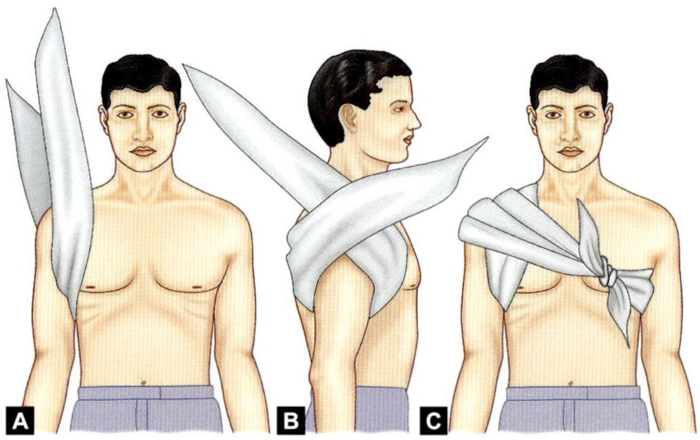

Figs. 10A to C: Shoulder–armpit cravat.

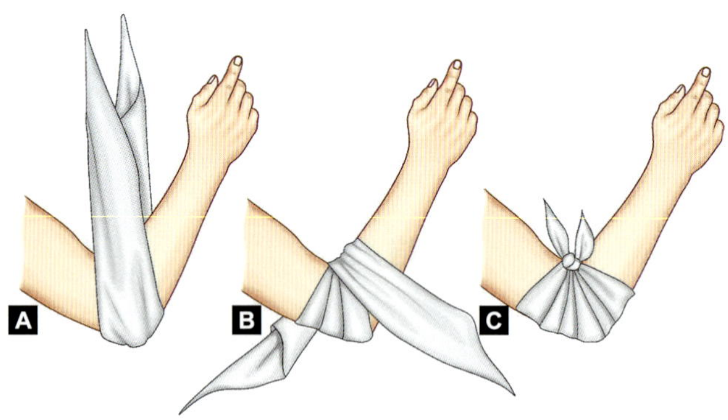

Figs. 11A to C: Cravat of elbow.

- Place cravat over dressing in axilla, so the front end is longer than the back. Carry the ends upward.
- Bring ends across each other over top of shoulder.
- Cross ends over back and chest, respectively, to opposite axilla. Tie ends just in front of uninjured axilla.

Cravat of Elbow (Figs. 11A to C)

The cravat of the elbow is used to hold dressings around the elbow.

- Bend arm at elbow and place center of cravat at point of elbow (olecranon).

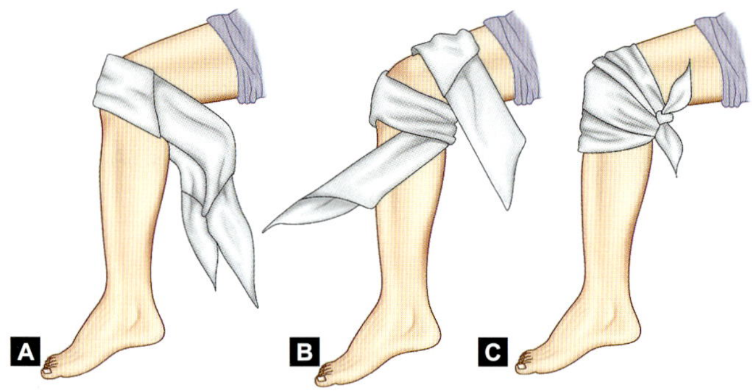

Figs. 12A to C: Cravat of knee bandage.

- Bring ends up and across each other in overlapping spiral turns. Continue one end up arm and the other end down forearm.
- Bring ends to front of elbow (antecubital fossa) and tie.

Cravat of Knee (Figs. 12A to C)

The cravat of the knee is used to hold dressings around the knee.

- Place center of cravat over knee cap and let ends hang down each side of knee.
- Cross ends underneath and continue several overlapping descending turns down calf and several overlapping ascending turns up thigh.
- Bring ends together and tie under knee.

Cravat of Leg (Figs. 13A to C)

The cravat of the leg is used to hold dressings on the leg, e.g., in leg ulcers.

- Place center of cravat over dressing.
- Begin ascending turns with upper end and descending turns with lower end with each turn covering two-thirds of preceding turn until dressing is covered.
- Terminate by tying both ends in square knot.

Cravat of Palms (Figs. 14A to F)

This bandage is used to hold dressings on the palm.

- Lay center of cravat over center of palm with ends hanging down each side.

- Bring the thumb end across back of hand, over palm, and through hollow between thumb and palm.
- Bring the other end across back of hand, toward base of thumb, and obliquely across palm to base of little finger.
- Cross both ends at back of hand.
- Continue procedure, ends crossing first at back of hand, and then over palm.
- Tie in square knot at wrist.

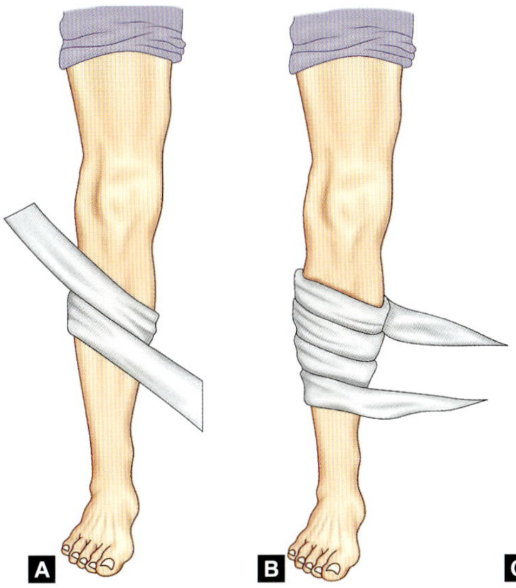

Figs. 13A to C: Cravat bandage of leg.

Roller Bandages

The roller bandages are used to hold dressings in place, to support surgery site, and to create pressure for control of hemorrhage. Roller bandages are made from gauze, flannel, muslin, rubber, or elastic webbing and the width and length depending upon the part to be bandaged.

Sizes Recommended (Fig. 15)

The sizes most frequently used are 2 inches width and 6 yards long for hand, finger, toe, and head bandages; 3 inches wide and 10 yards long for extremities; and 4 inches wide and 10 yards long for thigh, groin, and trunk.

Sizes of bandage: The size of the bandage varies according to the part it is supposed to bandage **(Table 2)**.

For convenience and ease of application, the strip of material is rolled into the form of a cylinder. Each bandage of this type should consist of only one piece, free from wrinkles, seams, selvage, and any imperfections that may cause discomfort to the patient.

Applying the Roller Bandage

When a roller bandage is to be applied to a part, the roll should be held in the right hand, so that the loose end is on the bottom.

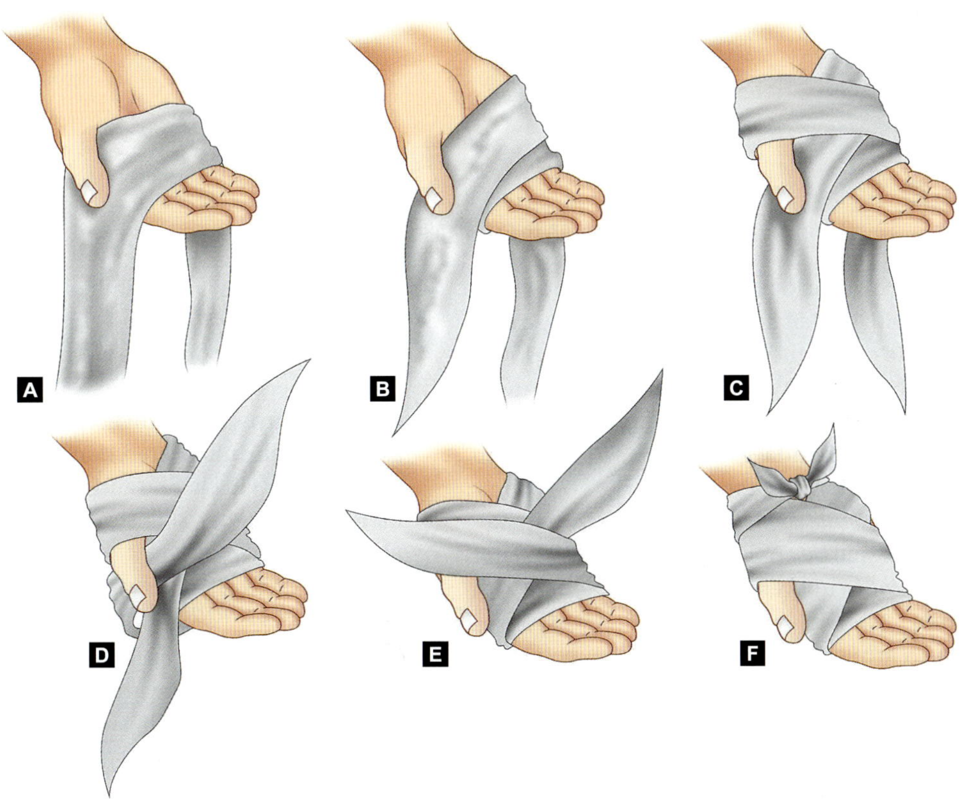

Figs. 14A to F: Cravat bandage of palm.

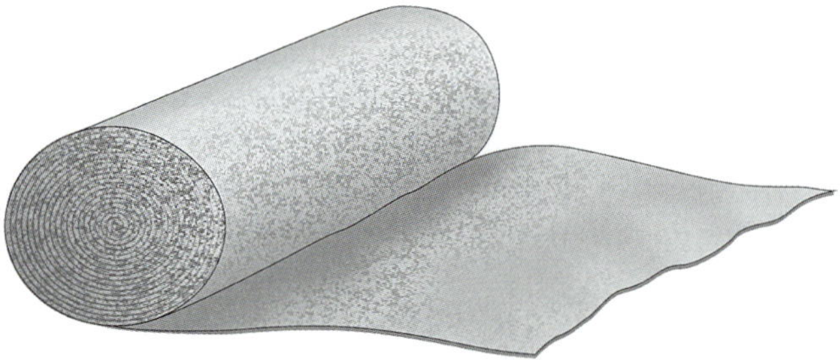

Fig. 15: Roller bandage.

TABLE 2: Size of the bandage in terms of width and length.

Parts to be bandaged	*Width (cm)*	*Length (m)*
Head	5	4–6
Trunk	10–15	6–8
Leg	6–8	4
Arm	5–6	3–4
Fingers	2.5	2
Hand	5	3
Wrist	5	3

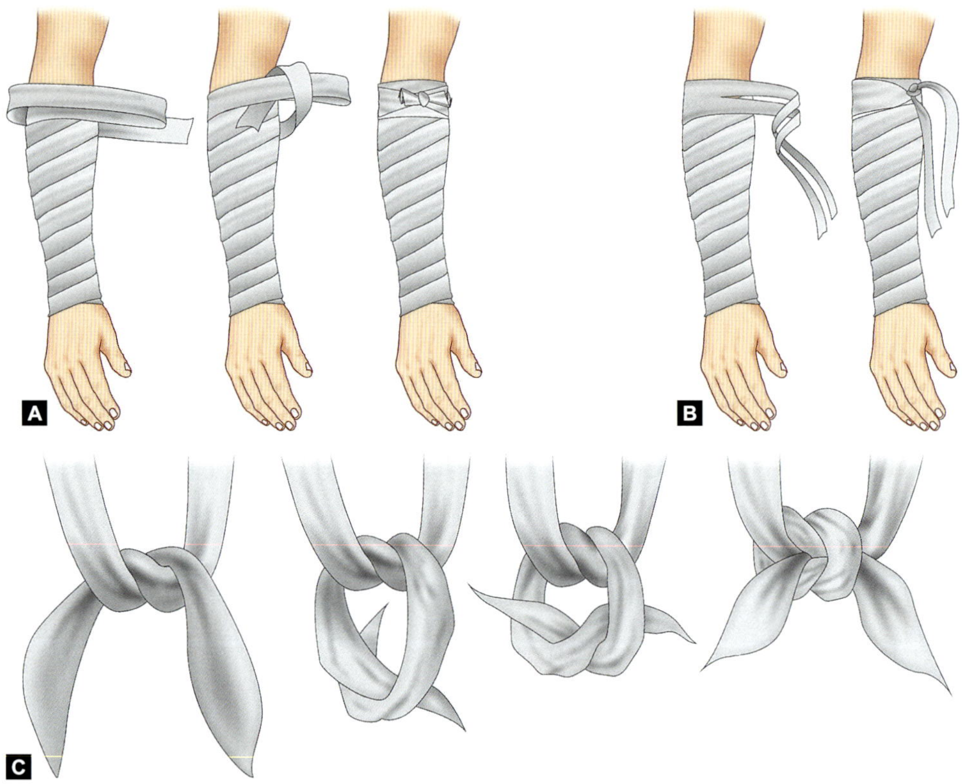

Figs. 16A to C: Fastening the bandage.

The outside surface of the loose end is next applied to the part and held there with the left hand. The roll is then passed around the part by the right hand, which controls the tension and direction of the bandage. Two or three of the initial turns of a roller bandage should overlie each other to secure the bandage. In applying the bandage, it is often necessary to transfer the roll from one hand to the other.

Precautions to be taken while applying roller bandages:

- Roller bandages should be applied evenly, firmly, and not too tightly. Excessive or uneven pressure will interfere with the circulation.
- In bandaging an arm or leg, the entire extremity (except the fingers or toes) should be covered to maintain uniform pressure. The fingers or toes should be left exposed, so the circulation in these parts can be checked.
- An extremity should be bandaged in its final position, since bending will change the pressure of parts of the bandage.
- It is safer to use a large number of turns rather than a few too firmly applied turns to secure splints or dressings. This is particularly important in applying a wet bandage or one that may become wet while securing a wet dressing.
- Bandage turns should overlap to completely cover the skin, since any uncovered skin may be pinched between turns. To prevent chafing and irritation when two parts are bandaged together, skin surfaces should be separated by absorbent material.

Fastening the Bandage

Bandages are terminated by applying several overlying circular turns and fastening the ends securely. The ends may be tied or fastened with adhesive tape. Two methods of tying are given in **Figures 16A to C**.

- The end of the bandage is folded back upon itself to form two ends, which can be tied.

- The end of the bandage is split lengthwise for a suitable distance and the split ends are then brought around in opposite directions and tied.
- The square knot is the best type of knot for tying bandages. It holds firmly and can be easily unfastened.

Removing the Bandage

Bandage scissors are preferable when the bandage is to be removed by cutting. Interference with the underlying dressing and wound should be carefully avoided. Folds should be gathered up when the bandage is merely unwound.

Types of Roller Bandages Based on Site of Application

Circular bandage: A circular bandage is used to cover cylindrical parts and to anchor bandages. As illustrated in **Figure 17**, a turn is made around the part and anchored. Similar succeeding turns are made overlying each other completely. The bandage is then terminated and secured.

Spiral bandage ***(Figs. 18A to C)****:* Spiral bandage covers a larger area than that covered by the circular bandage. It can be applied to the arm as well as to other cylindrical parts.

- Anchor at wrist.
- Apply succeeding spiral turns up the forearm with each turn overlapping one-third of preceding turn.
- Terminate and secure just below elbow.

Recurrent bandage of head with one bandage ***(Figs. 19A to D)****:* This bandage is used to hold a dressing on the scalp.

- Anchor bandage with several turns around the head terminating behind head. At this point, fold bandage upward with assistant holding fold in place with two fingers.
- Continue bandage over top of head to center of forehead. Fold bandage back at this point and hold it there with

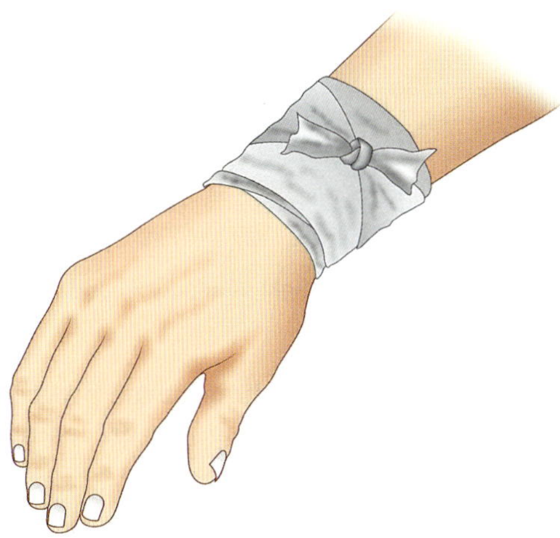

Fig. 17: Circular bandage.

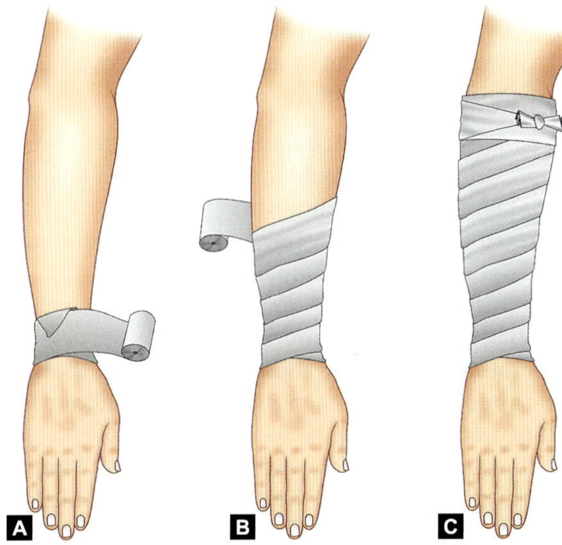

Figs. 18A to C: Spiral bandage.

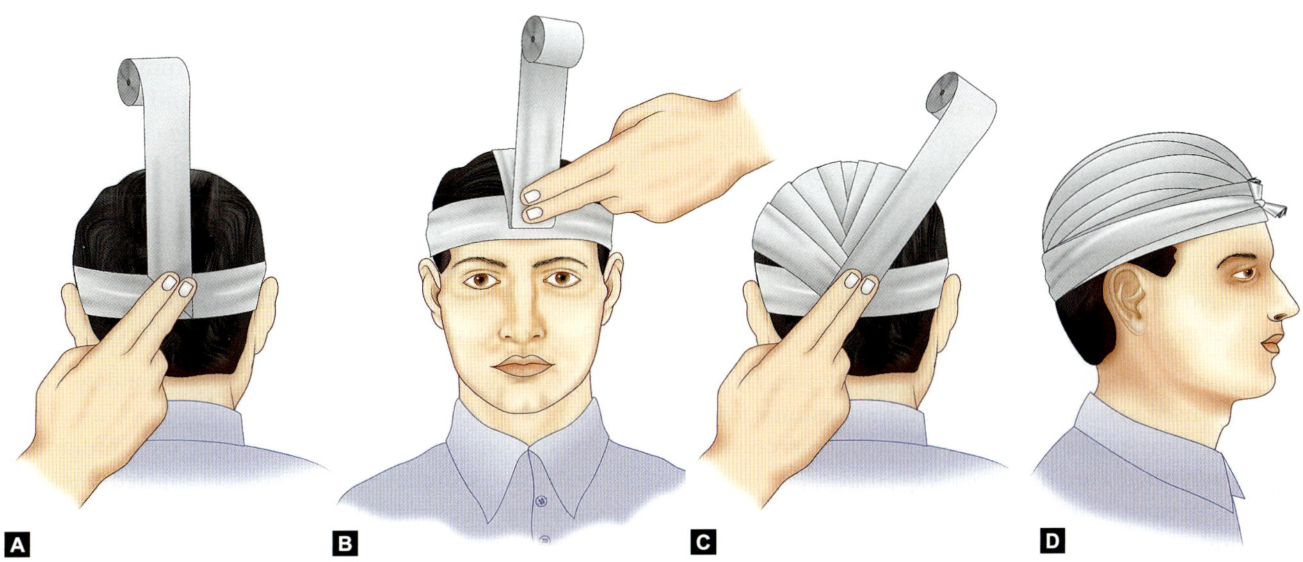

Figs. 19A to D: Recurrent bandage on head.

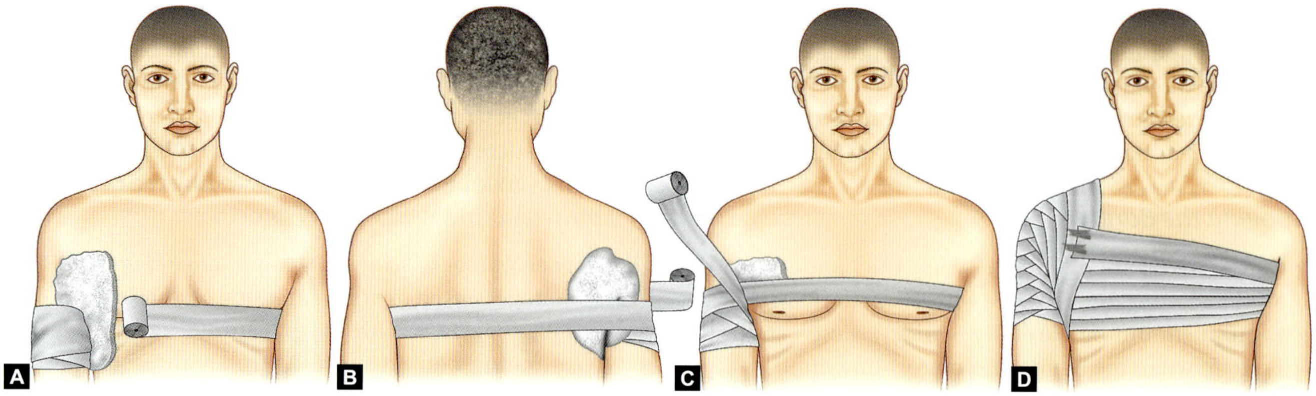

Figs. 20A to D: Shoulder bandage.

free hand. Carry bandage back to point held by assistant at rear of head.

- Continue procedure until entire head is covered, turns alternating to the left and right of the center line, and each turn overlying the outer half of the preceding turn.
- Apply several circular turns around head, covering the ends of the initial turns, and secure.

Shoulder bandage ***(Figs. 20A to D)****:* Shoulder bandage is used to retain dressings of the shoulder and axilla, e.g., following surgery for hidradenitis suppurativa.

- Pad the axilla well and anchor by several circular turns around upper arm where surgery is performed.
- Carry across back to axilla of opposite side; then across chest obliquely to top of primary turns.
- Carry around arm, axilla, and upward toward shoulder. Repeat procedure and each turn overlying about two-thirds of preceding turn.
- Continue until entire shoulder is covered. The line crossings on the shoulder be straight and should pass over the point of the shoulder. Secure with adhesive tape.

Figure of eight bandage for hand ***(Fig. 21)****:* This bandage is used to hold dressings on dorsum of hand or palm, e.g., flap rotation or tendon transfer.

- Anchor bandage on hand with circular turns near ends of fingers. Carry obliquely across back of hand to thumb. Bring under thumb and across palm to back of hand.
- Carry obliquely across back of hand to bottom of primary turn and across palm.
- Follow with several similar turns, each one overlying about two-thirds of preceding turn on back of hand. After sufficient turns, terminate with circular turns around wrist and secure.

Figure of eight bandage for elbow ***(Figs. 22A to D)****:* This bandage is used to hold a dressing in the antecubital fossa.

- Anchor with circular turn above elbow and carry bandage obliquely downward over hollow of elbow.
- Circle forearm below elbow to anchor, bring obliquely upward over hollow of elbow, and pass around upper arm at primary circle.

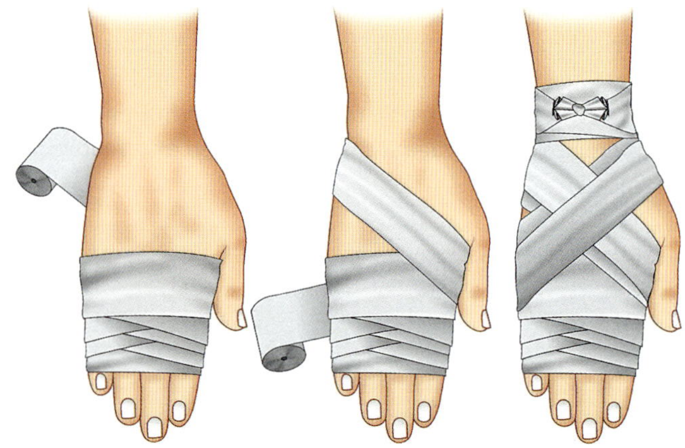

Fig. 21: Figure of eight bandage of hand.

- Repeat procedure with oblique turns progressing up forearm and each turn overlapping preceding turn by two-thirds.
- Terminate at starting point and secure.

Front of elbow bandage ***(Fig. 23)****:* This bandage is also used to hold dressings on the antecubital fossa. Unlike the figure of eight of the elbow, this bandage leaves back of elbow exposed. It allows movement of joint without disturbing the dressing. Anchor bandage with circular turns around forearm below elbow. Carry bandage obliquely upward over hollow of elbow and circle arm just above elbow. Bring obliquely downward over hollow of elbow and pass around forearm at primary circle. Repeat procedure until hollow of elbow is covered, each oblique turn overlapping preceding oblique by three-fourths, and each circular turn overlying each preceding circular turn. Terminate at circular turns above elbow and secure.

Finger bandage ***(Figs. 24A to C)****:* The finger bandage secures dressing on finger.

- Anchor bandage at wrist. Bring over back of hand and make one complete turn at base of injured finger over dressing. Make spiral turn to tip of finger to hold dressing while applying bandage.
- Make another spiral turn back to base of finger.

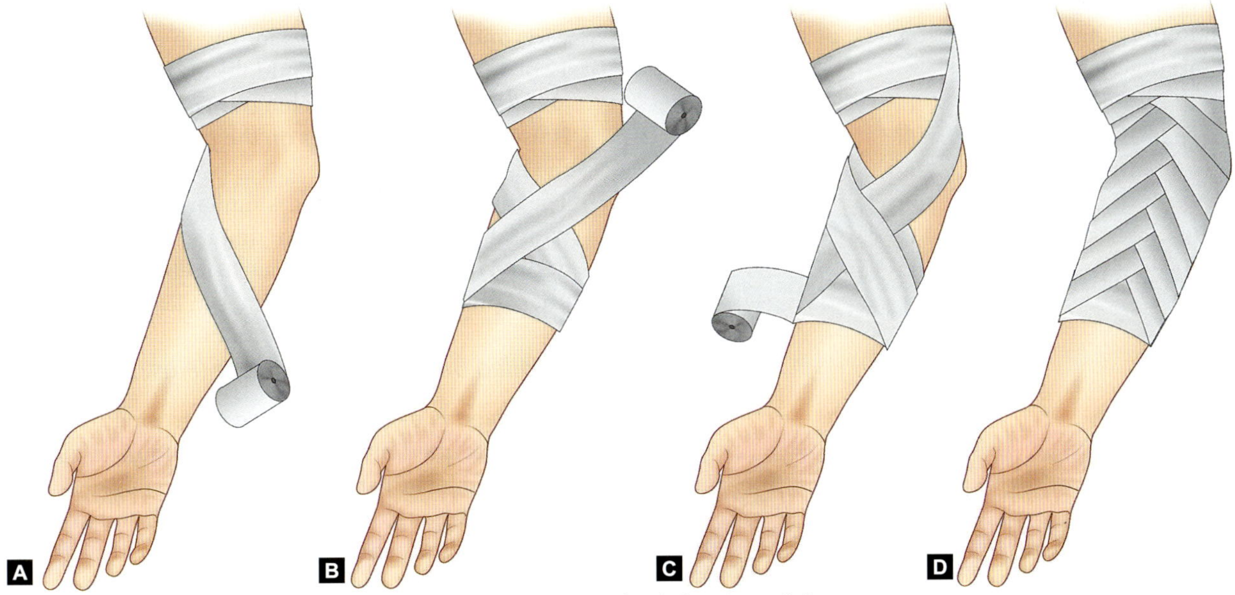

Figs. 22A to D: Figure of eight bandage of elbow.

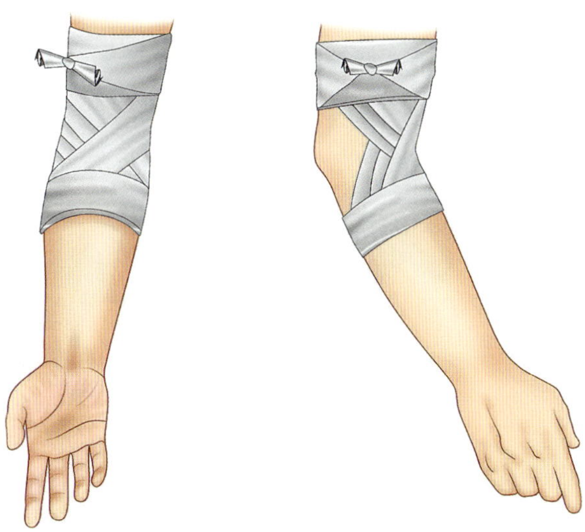

Fig. 23: Front of elbow bandage.

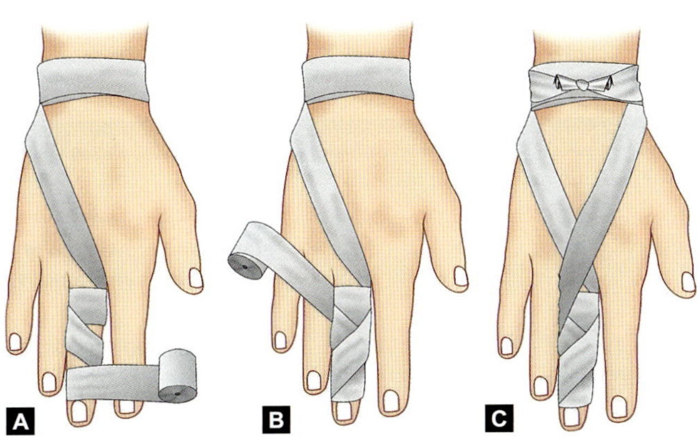

Figs. 24A to C: Finger bandage.

- Complete bandage with figure of eight progressing from tip to finger base. Terminate with circular turns around wrist and secure.

Foot roller bandage ***(Figs. 25A to D)****:* The foot roller bandage is used to hold dressings on foot, e.g., plantar ulcers or following flap rotation.

- Anchor around foot near base of toes. Carry obliquely across instep and around heel. Continue obliquely across instep, crossing preceding turn to base of large toe.
- Repeat procedure, turns gradually ascending on both foot and heel, and crossings being in line along middle of in-step.
- Continue procedure in above-step.
- Terminate above ankle and secure.

Figure of eight bandage of foot (with heel exposed) ***(Figs. 26A to C)****:* This bandage is used to hold dressings on foot, e.g., plantar ulcers, flap rotation, melanoma excision.

- Anchor just above ankle, bring bandage obliquely across instep to base of large toe, with turn around base of toes.
- Continue obliquely across in-step to point of beginning.
- Repeat procedure, leaving heel exposed, with turns ascending until arch and in-step are covered. Terminate at starting point and secure.

Tailed Bandages

Tailed bandages consist of the T-bandage, the double T-bandage, the four-tailed bandage, and the many-tailed bandages **(Figs. 27A to D)**. These bandages are used to secure dressings to parts, which do not lend themselves to roller bandage applications.

- The T-bandage is a T-shape bandage consisting of a vertical strip of material sewn or pinned to the center of a horizontal strip. This bandage may be used to secure dressing on scalp, ear, eye, or perineum.
- The double T-bandage may be made by sewing two vertical strips of material to the center of a horizontal strip and

about 4 inches apart. The double T-bandage may be used to hold dressings on the chest, back, or perineum, e.g., scrotal surgery, vitiligo grafts.

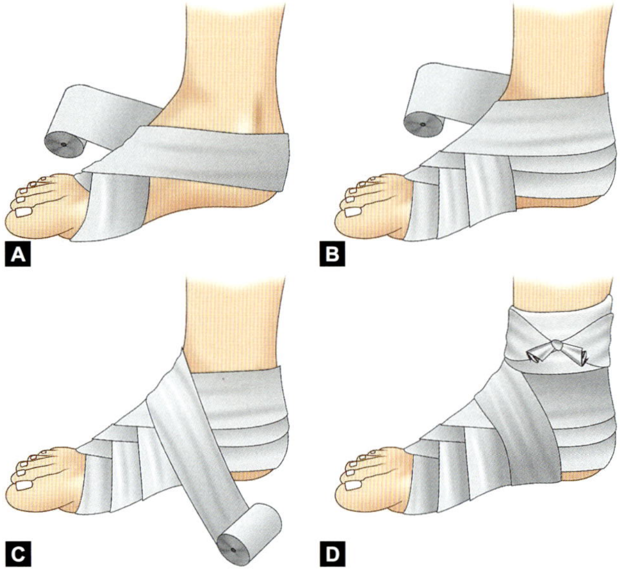

Figs. 25A to D: Foot roller bandage.

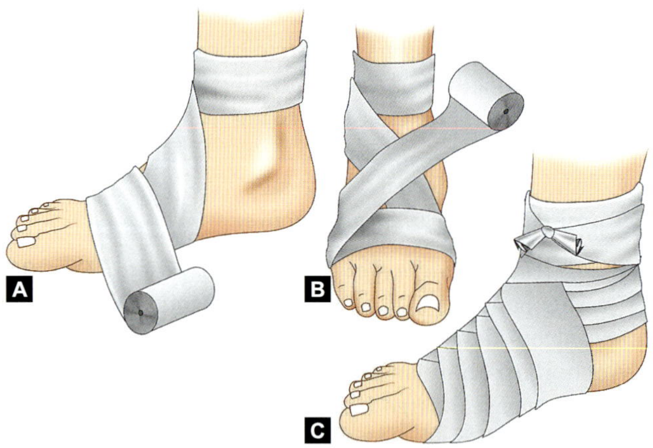

Figs. 26A to C: Figure of eight bandage of foot with heel exposed.

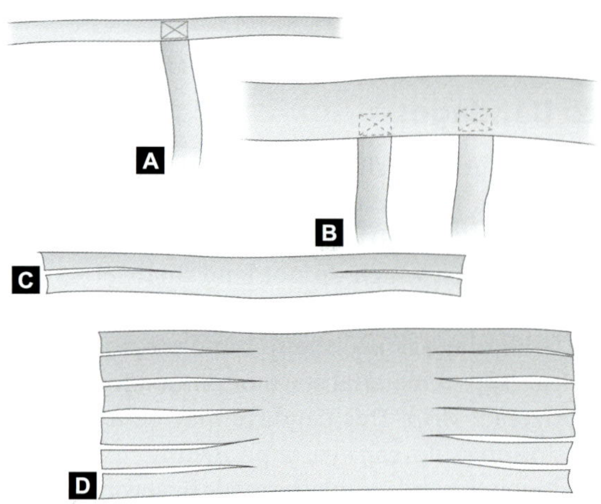

Figs. 27A to D: Tailed bandage.

- The four-tailed bandage is a piece of material 4–6 inches wide and about 30 inches long with each end cut about 12 or 14 inches down its middle, leaving the center piece about 12 or 14 inches in length. The four-tailed bandage is used to hold dressings on the jaw, nose, forehead, and the back of the head.
- The many-tailed bandage is similar in construction to the four-tailed bandage, except that the ends are cut into the desired number of tails about 16 inches in length and the uncut portion is about 20 inches in length.

Four-tailed Bandage of the Nose (Figs. 28A and B)

This bandage is used for holding a dressing following any surgery performed around the nose. A four-tailed bandage of the desired length and width is used.

- Split the bandage lengthwise from each end to within 3 or 5 inches of the center of the strip.
- Place the top of the center over nose and carry the two upper ends under ears and around to nape of neck and tie.

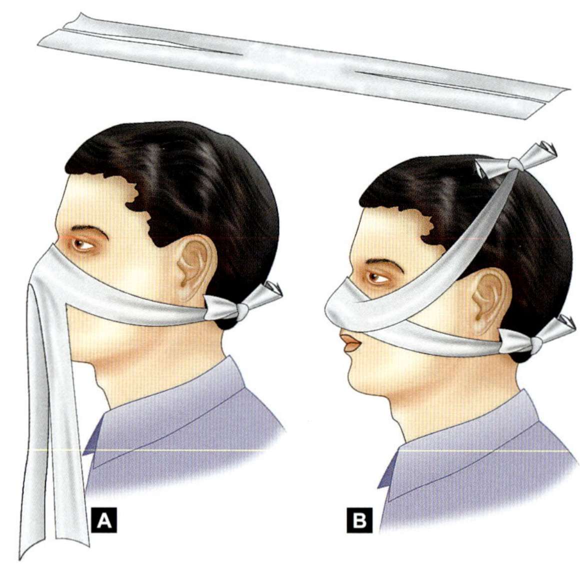

Figs. 28A and B: Four-tailed bandage of the nose.

TABLE 3: Different types of compression bandages and their indications.

Types of bandage	*Ankle pressure*	*Indication*
Compression hosiery	15–35 mm Hg	Varicose veins, mild edema and prevention of venous ulcers and venous insufficiency
Single layer bandages	15–50 mm Hg (depending on technique)	Uncomplicated venous leg ulcers with or without lymphedema and venous insufficiency following thrombosis
Multilayer bandages	35–50 mm Hg	Uncomplicated and complicated venous leg ulcers and ulcers secondary to lymphedema

- Fold the bottom of the center under nose and carry the two lower ends above ears to top of head and tie.

Special Bandages: Compression Bandaging

These reduce effect of venous hypertension by reducing superficial venous pressure. They increase the rate of wound healing, especially if multilayered. The optimal pressures are 35–40 mm Hg and it is essential not to deliver such high levels of pressure to an ischemic leg, as it may result in necrosis or gangrene. Doppler pressures should always be measured and compression dressings are only used, if the ankle brachial pressure index is >0.8. Traditional crepe bandages do not provide adequate compression. Newer short stretch high performance bandages are more effective in this regard. Combining compression therapy with surgery to correct superficial venous reflux does not lead to improved healing rates compared with compression alone, but reduces ulcer recurrence and increases ulcer-free time. **Table 3** lists different types of compression bandages and their indications.

RECOMMENDED READING

1. Mysore V. Bandaging and Splinting: Field Manual No. 8-50. Department of the Army: Washington DC; 1957. pp. 1-39.

CHAPTER 6

Dermatosurgical Instruments

Anirudha Gulanikar, Ankan Gupta

KEY MESSAGES

- Proper knowledge of instruments is important to ensure optimal safety and surgical outcome.
- High-quality instruments, even if they are of high cost, should be preferred—they have longer shelf life and greater precision.
- Proper maintenance, cleaning, and disinfection enhance safety.
- Proper training of staff is needed for proper care of instruments.
- Care should be taken to avoid injury to the surgeon during surgery.

INTRODUCTION

Surgery or Cheirourgia, which is a Greek word—"cheir" means "hand" + "ergon" means "work", is the branch of medicine that deals with the physical manipulation of a bodily structure to diagnose, prevent, or cure an ailment. The history of surgical instruments can go back to stone ages. *Sushruta* is considered as the "founding father of surgery". Sushruta is known for one of the oldest known surgical texts in Sanskrit—The *Sushruta Samhita* and the instruments for cosmetic surgery. The early modern era of surgery starts from Hippocrates, Celsus, and Galen. The scientific surgery starts from John Hunter (1728–93). Joseph Lister developed antiseptic in surgery.

As surgical technology evolves continuously, so does the type and complexity of surgical instruments. Surgical instruments require special care and handling to maintain proper function and longevity. This is dependent solely on knowledge of the instruments and how they are used. The names are difficult, the differences are minute, and the uses and handling for each instrument even more obscure. The surgeon and the staff in operating room must be well trained with instruments they are handling.

While some of these are specific for each surgery (such as those for vitiligo surgery, hair transplantation, liposuction, etc.), others are common and basic. Such basic and common instruments have been discussed in this chapter, while specific instruments have been mentioned in the corresponding chapters.

SURGICAL EQUIPMENT

Operating Table

The installation of a high-quality surgical table is preferred. The table makes the patient more comfortable and provides easy access for the surgeon. The adjustability and dimensions of the table are important parameters to be considered. Powered tables with foot-operated or fingertip controls are the most desirable. Adjustments in back and foot elevation are essential for the patient's comfort. The tilt positioning of the table is important, because it enables the physician to change the angle of the table **(Fig. 1)**. Both manual and automatic tables are available. Automatic tables are preferred for ease of maneuvering. Additional attachments to be considered include a U-shaped head armrest for hair transplantation.

Trolley and Stands

The trolleys and stands with their adjustable heights allow for easy access to the instruments. A table unit with 4–6 wheels is the most maneuverable and stable, and can be moved during the procedure as per requirement and convenience **(Figs. 2 and 3)**.

Waste Containers

Well-equipped surgical suites should include kick-bucket waste containers. These waste containers are made of either

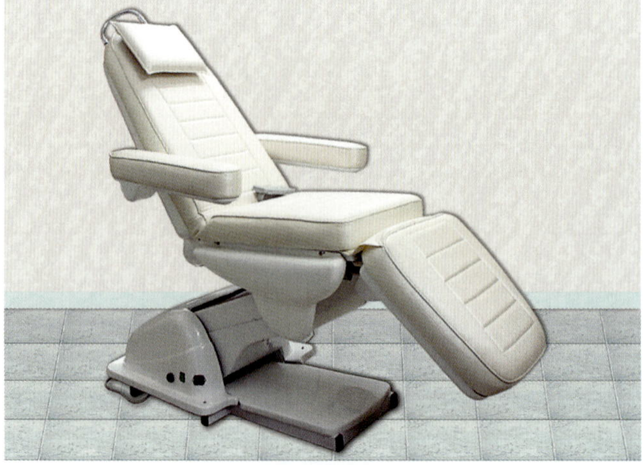

Fig. 1: Operating table.

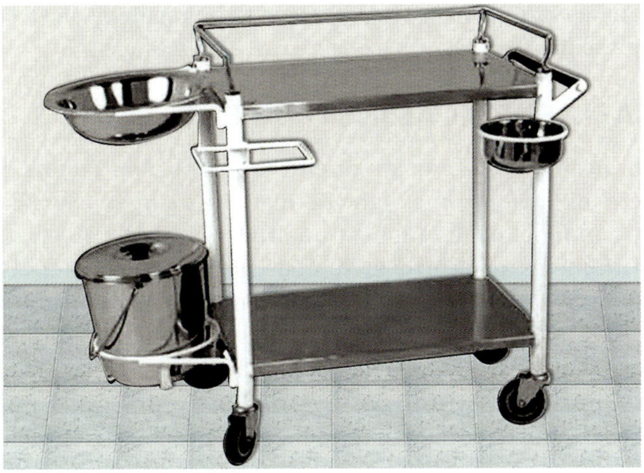

Fig. 2: Instrument trolley.

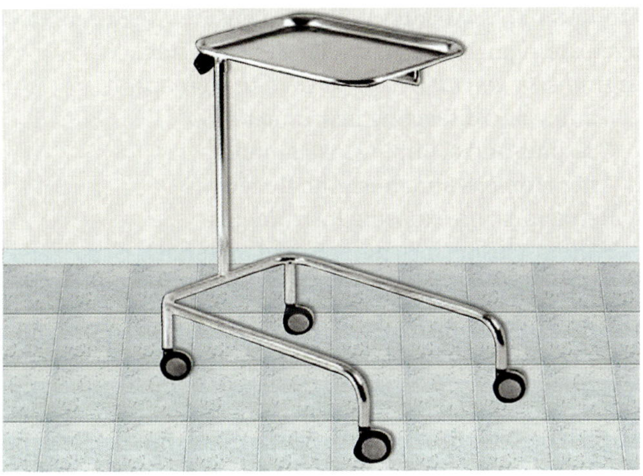

Fig. 3: Mayo's trolley.

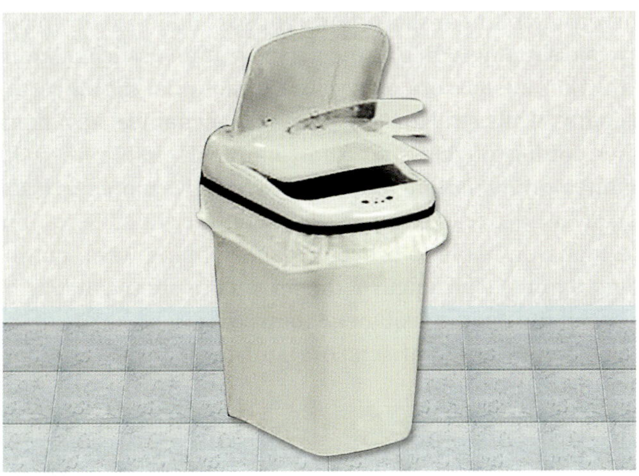

Fig. 4: Plastic waste disposal container.

plastic **(Fig. 4)** or stainless steel with rubber baskets. They can be mounted on wheels, have a protective hard rubber, and steel rim that the staff can use to move the bucket with their feet during the procedure.

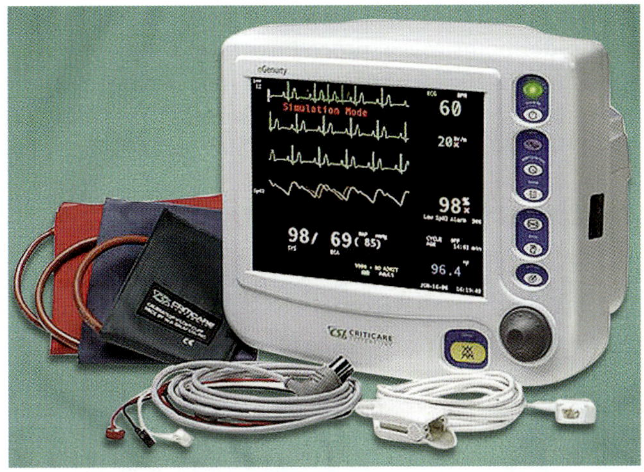

Fig. 5: Noninvasive blood pressure monitor (NIBP).

Monitoring Equipment

Monitoring equipment should be available, so that the staff can determine the patient's pulse, blood pressure, electrical cardiac activity, and blood oxygen saturation at a glance. Pulse oximeters of different types are available. Digital pulse oximeters are small, which are attached to the patient's finger and show only pulse rate and oxygen saturation. These are adequate for most skin surgeries. Larger pulse oximeters show other parameters such as blood pressure **(Fig. 5)** and may be used for extensive surgeries such as liposuction. The data should be recorded by the attending personnel.

Medical Gases

Oxygen cylinders should be available, preferably more than one. Nitrous oxide and compressed air are the gases that are necessary only in larger theaters.

Emergency Equipment

A major consideration in an office-based operating room should be the management of emergencies. All staff should be trained to use emergency equipment. The staff should also be trained in pediatric as well as adult basic and advanced life support. Adequate equipment must be immediately available. The following equipment is essential:

- Stethoscope
- Blood pressure apparatus
- Thermometer
- Cardiac monitor and pulse oximeter
- Defibrillator **(Fig. 6)**
- Laryngoscope with endotracheal tubes of various sizes **(Fig. 7)**
- Ambu bag with airways of various types and sizes
- Oxygen supply/cylinder
- Intravenous fluids and drugs for emergency treatment
- Availability of transportation from the operating room to an emergency facility.

Even though general anesthesia is not required to perform dermatosurgical procedures, availability of Boyle's apparatus **(Fig. 8)** can be of additional help in case of serious emergencies. An emergency kit with all necessary equipment should be available and all operating theater staff should be familiar with this kit. The kit needs to be regularly checked by a senior staff.

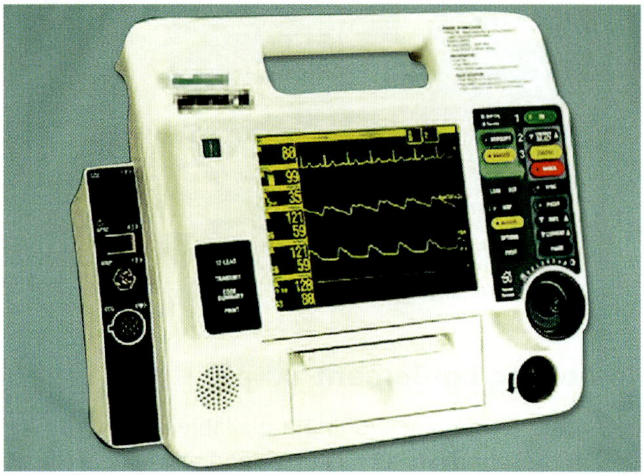

Fig. 6: Cardiac monitor and defibrillator.

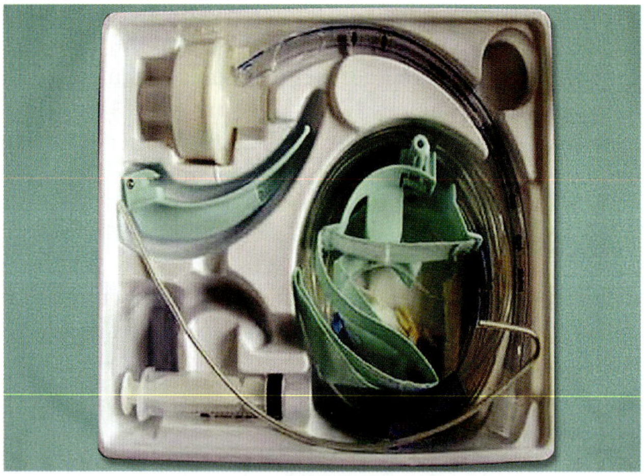

Fig. 7: Endotracheal intubation kit.

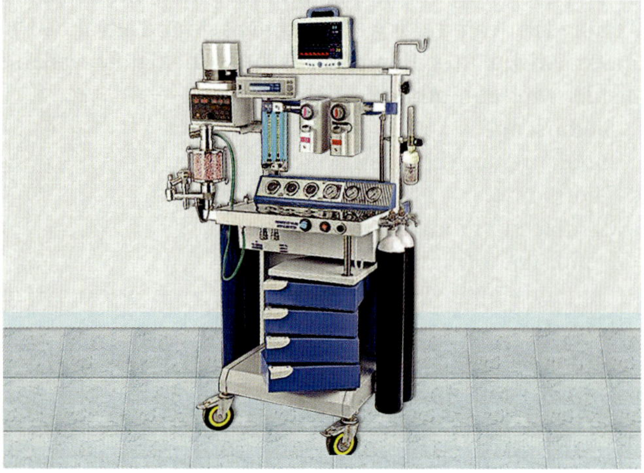

Fig. 8: Anesthesia Boyle's apparatus.

BASIC SURGICAL INSTRUMENTS

Surgical instruments are one of the important factors in determining outcome of the dermatologic surgery. Surgical instruments of the highest quality should be preferred. Instruments made up of high-grade stainless steel are costly, but have a long life. To make them more effective in use and to have a longer life, some instruments have tungsten carbide inserts in the jaws of needle holders and blades.

Surgical instruments are precisely designed and manufactured tool and may be either disposable or reusable. They must be resistant to physical and chemical effects, body fluids, secretions, cleaning agents and sterilization, and hence most of them are made of high-quality stainless steel; chromium and vanadium alloys to ensure the durability of edges, springiness, and resistance to corrosion.

Surgical instruments can be divided into groups:

- Cutting and dissecting instruments
- Grasping and clamping instruments
- Artery forceps and mosquito forceps
- Retractors and exposing instruments
- Wound-closing instruments and materials
- Special instruments used in nail surgery, vitiligo surgery, acne scar surgery, and hair transplant surgery.

Scissors

Surgical scissors are available in various sizes and shapes, each suited for specific purpose. Specialized scissors should not be used for cutting suture, as it may result in loss of sharpness of the scissors. The jaws of the scissors may be straight or curved and blunt or sharp. Serrations are added to one blade to avoid slipping, while trying to cut any thin tissue including skin. Curved scissors offer more directional mobility and visibility, while straight scissors have mechanical advantage when cutting tough tissues. Short-handled scissors are useful for fine work, while long-handled scissors give more reach and usually used to reach deeper areas such as cavities. Serrations are made on blade to prevent tissues lipping when cutting **(Figs. 9 to 14)**. The length of the scissor tips should match the depth of the incision you need to make.

Different types of scissors and their indications are mentioned in **Box 1**.

Forceps

Surgical forceps are the most utilized instruments in dermatosurgery. Surgical forceps may be broadly classified as ring forceps or hemostats and thumb forceps or dissecting and holding forceps. Thumb forceps are used by compression between thumb and forefinger and are used for grasping, holding, or manipulating body tissue. They have no ratchet in

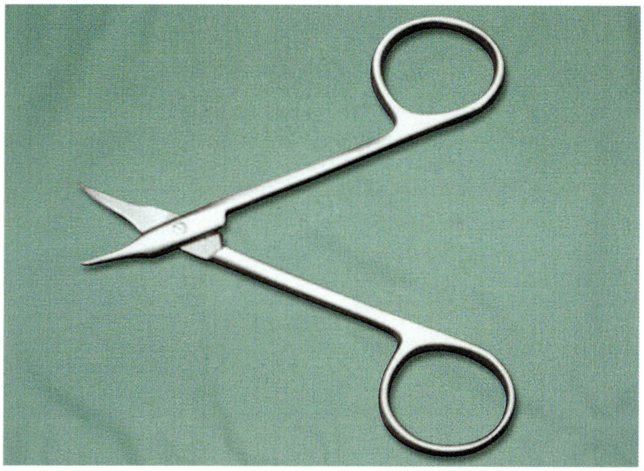

Fig. 9: Gradle scissor.

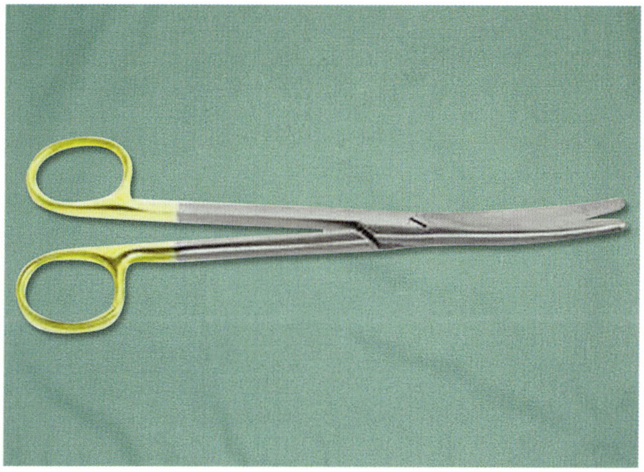

Fig. 10: Mayo's scissor.

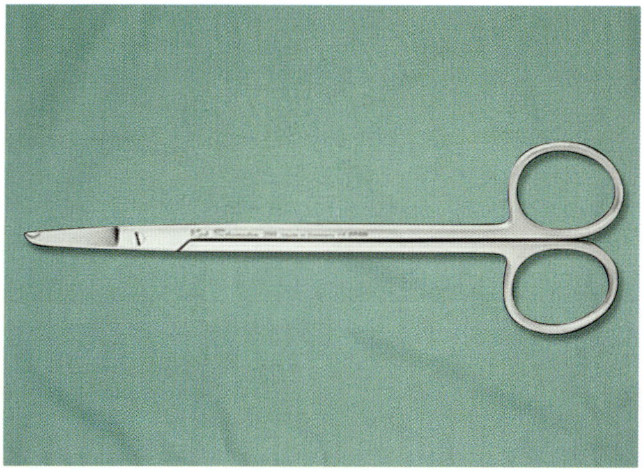

Fig. 11: Littures scissor.

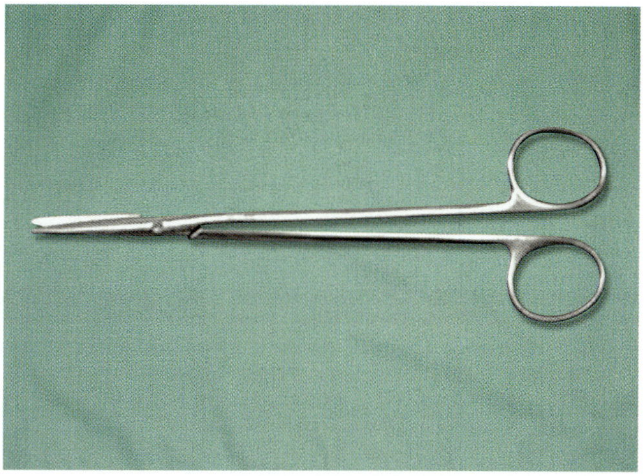

Fig. 12: Metzenbaum scissor.

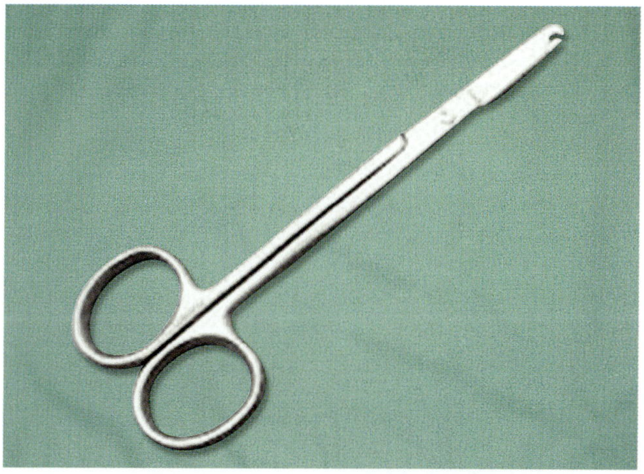

Fig. 13: Spencer's suture removal scissor.

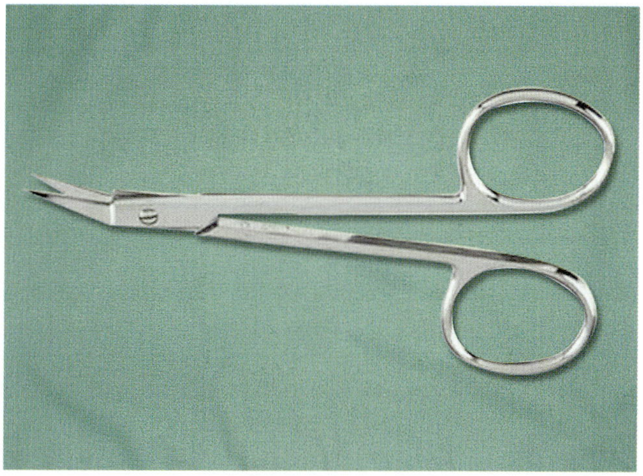

Fig. 14: O'Briens scissor.

the handle. Thumb forceps are of two types—dressing forceps and tissue forceps. Dressing forceps are used when dressing wounds and removing dressings. Tissue forceps generally have teeth, which offer a better grip on tissues while minimizing tissue damage.

They hold the tissue in place during an operation or during insertion of another surgical instrument into a cavity. A variety of forceps are available for various surgical procedures. The choice of forceps depends on individual surgeon and the purpose. Forceps are available in various sizes and shapes

(Figs. 15 to 29). Serrated forceps cause more tissue injury and, hence, nontoothed forceps are preferred by many surgeons to avoid crushing. Straight tips on forceps are used for general precision work, and slightly curved or fully curved tips provide more visibility.

Different types of forceps and their indications are mentioned in **Box 2**.

BOX 1: Types of scissors and their indications.

- Iris scissors are short tipped and are useful for dissection and cutting
- Castroviejo's spring scissor is also used for finework
- *Horizontally curved and blunt-tipped scissors*: For undermining example, Mayo's blunt tipped—undermining and blunt dissection
- *Straight sharp-tipped scissors*: For tough fibrotic tissues
- *Straight blade scissors*: For trimming flaps
- *Beveled or sharper outer-edged scissors*: For tissue dissection
- *Littauer, Northbent, Shortbent, and Spencer*: For suture removal, they have concavity, which helps in elevating and cutting sutures. O'Brien's suture cutting in delicate and tight areas
- *Gradle scissors*: Small scissors used for tiny dissection, have slightly curved and sharp blades, used for surgery around eye, and sharp cutting

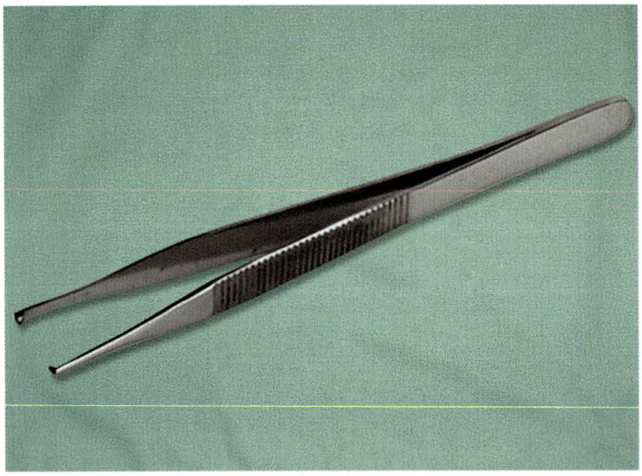

Fig. 15: Adson's forceps toothed.

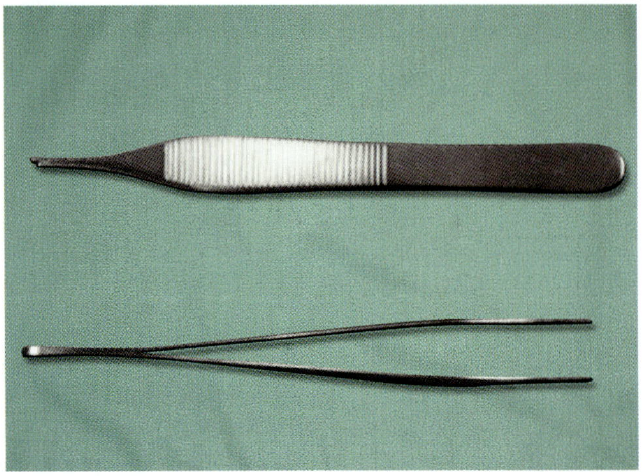

Fig. 16: Adson's forceps plain.

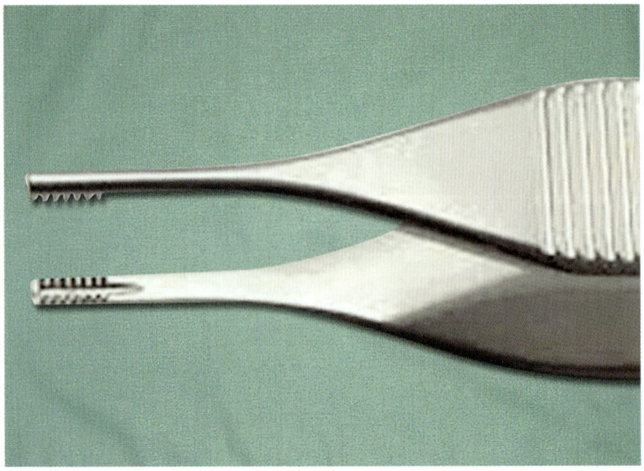

Fig. 17: Adson–Brown forceps.

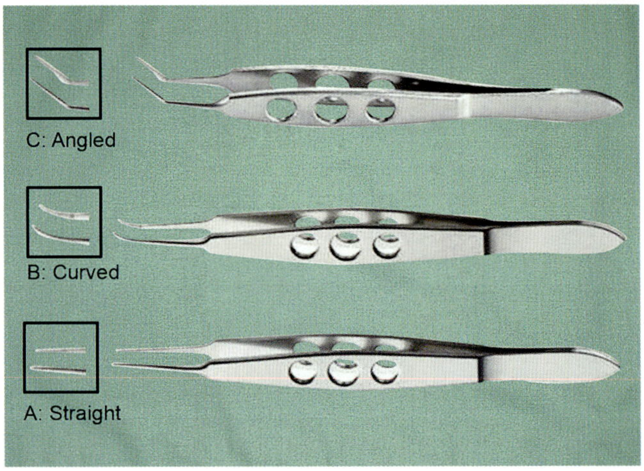

Fig. 18: Bishop–Harmon forceps.

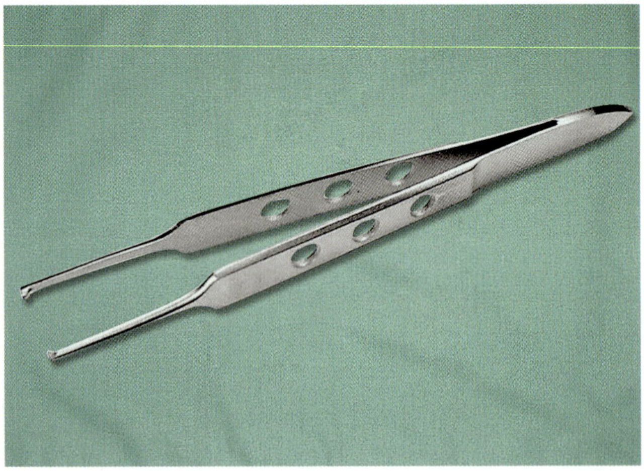

Fig. 19: Bishop–Harmon tissue forceps.

Scalpels and Blades

There are a wide variety of blades and handles available, but the commonly used by many surgeons is handle number 3. Handles are of two types—Bard-Parker and Beaver.

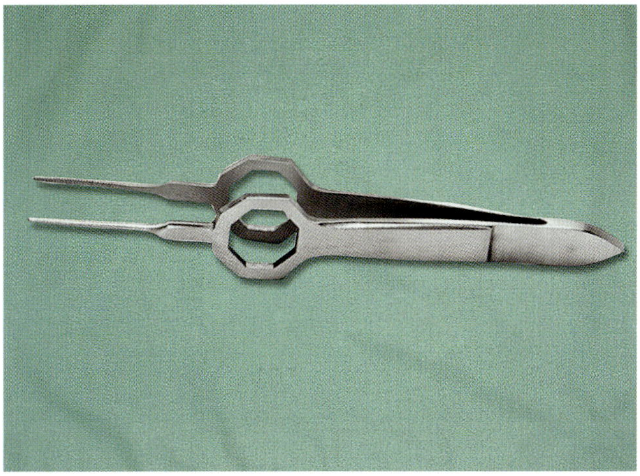

Fig. 20: Fosters tissue forceps.

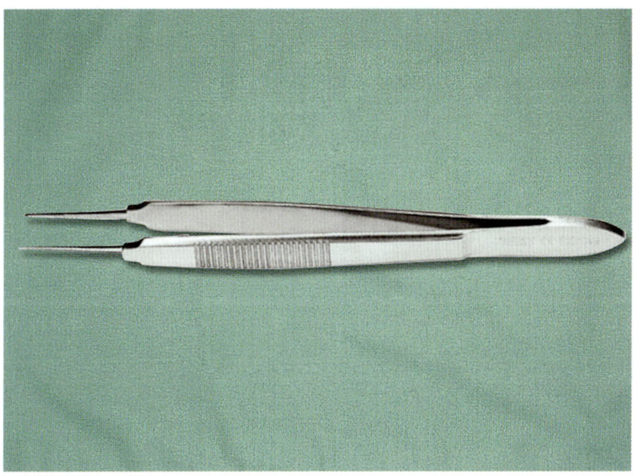

Fig. 21: Castroviejo forceps.

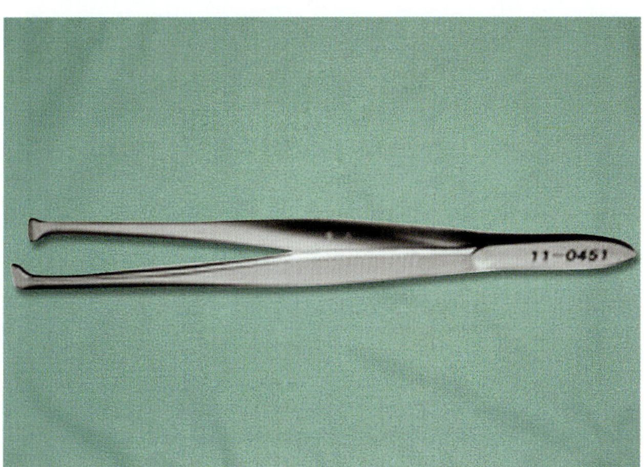

Fig. 22: Graefe's forceps.

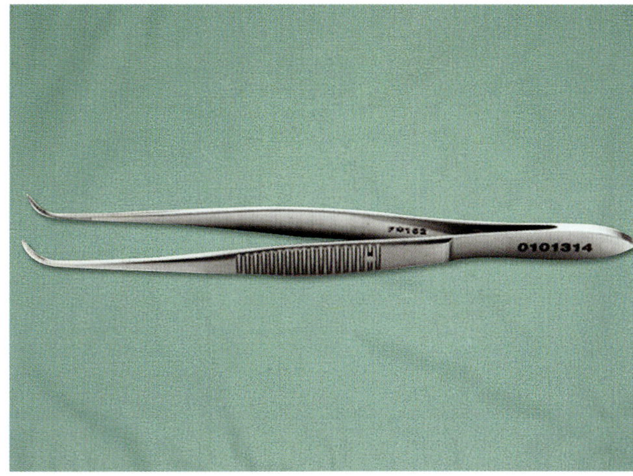

Fig. 23: Iris forceps.

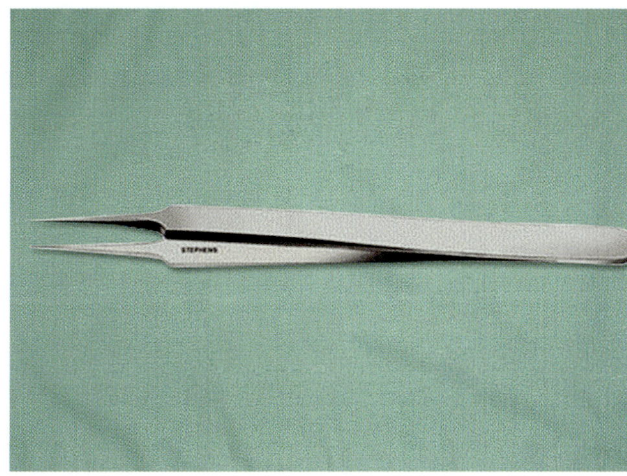

Fig. 24: Jewelers forceps (straight).

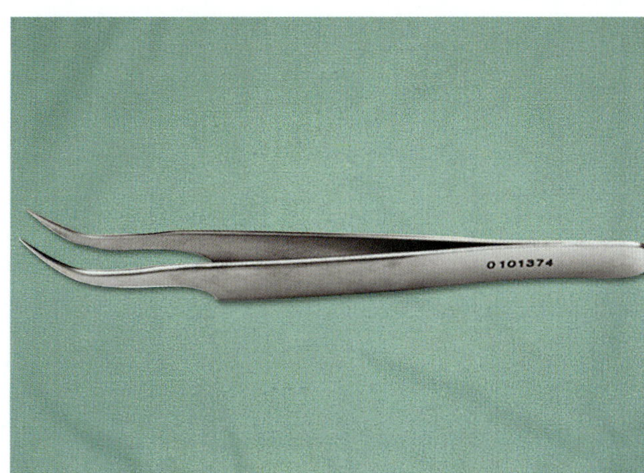

Fig. 25: Jewelers forceps (curved).

Bard–Parker handles are the ones, which are usually used in skin surgeries. Disposable plastic handles are also available. Different scalpel handles and their corresponding blades are shown in **Figures 30 to 32**. Blades are also available in various sizes and shapes. They are made from stainless steel, carbon steel, or Teflon-coated blades **(Box 3)**.

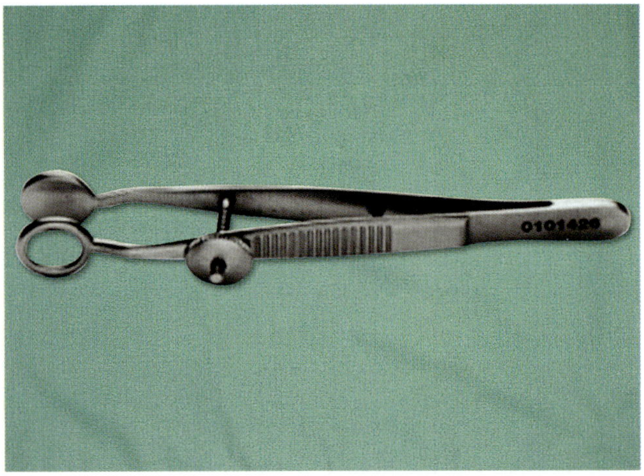

Fig. 26: Chalazion forceps/clamp.

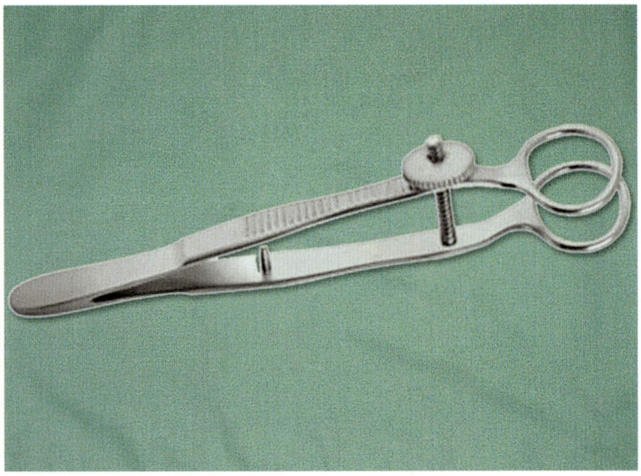

Fig. 27: Earlobe clamp.

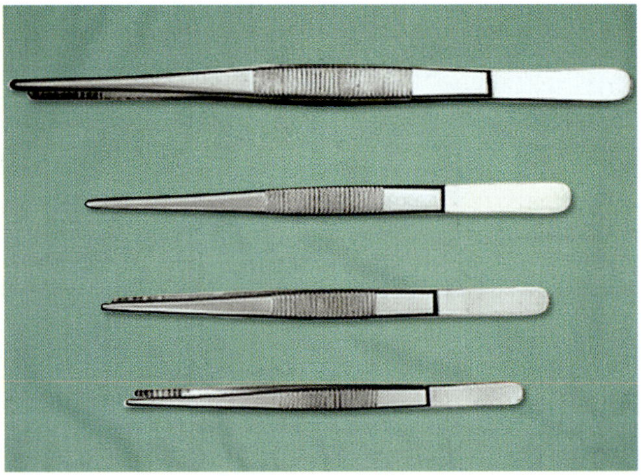

Fig. 28: Dressing forceps.

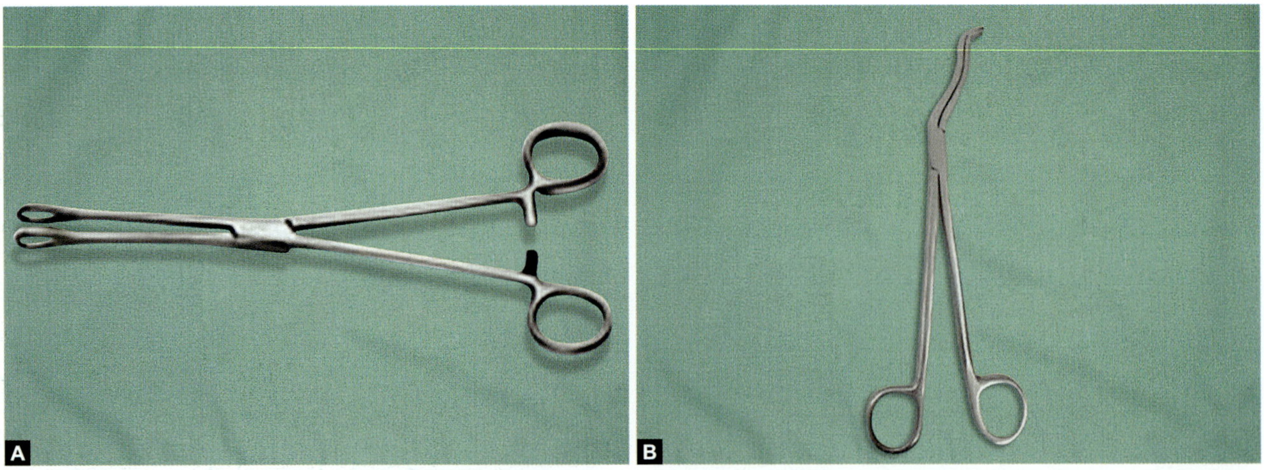

Figs. 29A and B: (A) Foster forceps; (B) Cheatle forceps.

Needle Holders

A needle holder is a surgical instrument to hold a suturing needle for closing wounds during suturing and surgical procedures. The parts of a simple needle holder are jaws, joint, and handles. Most needle holders also have a clamp mechanism that locks the needle in place, allowing the user to maneuver the needle through various tissues. To maintain a firm grip on the needle, jaws are often textured and are short as compared to handles. Jaws may be smooth or firm toothed.

The tips may also have a metal alloy for secure grasping. The beaks of a needle holder are stronger and different from the beaks of a hemostat. There are cross-hatches on the face of a beak of the needle holder to have a positive grasp of the suture needle. The hemostat has parallel grooves on the face of the beaks to hold tissue.

The selection of a needle holder usually depends on the needle used and the anatomic site **(Box 4)**.

Hemostats/Artery Forceps

Hemostat is a vital surgical tool used in almost every surgical procedure, usually to control bleeding. Ring forceps, also called hemostats or locking forceps, are an instrument for grasping or exerting traction upon tissue especially for delicate operations. The hemostat has handles that can be held in place by the locking mechanism **(Fig. 39)**. When they are used to control blood flow, they are called hemostats. Hemostats are typically used to compress blood vessels or other tubular structures to obstruct the flow of blood or fluids.

The locking mechanism is typically a series of interlocking teeth, a few on each handle that allows the user to adjust the clamping tension of the pliers. Mosquito forceps **(Figs. 40A and B)** are nontraumatic with straight or curved jaws, whereas Kocher type has teeth **(Fig. 41)**.

BOX 2: Types of forceps and their indications.

- *Adson's*: The most versatile type, with broad handle and narrow teeth suitable for facial surgery and wound closure
- *Adson's anatomical*: Useful for tissue undermining and wound closure
- *Bishop–Harmon and Castroviejo small forceps*: These are used for delicate work, microsurgery, eyelid surgery, and thin skin
- *Jewelers forceps*: They are small and used for delicate work
- *Graefe and Green forceps*: They are useful to hold eyelid skin or cartilage
- *Brown Adson forceps (like Adson but with 16 teeth)*: Tissue forceps are for holding and manipulating delicate tissues. These forceps have a wide, flat thumb grasp area that is commonly serrated. The jaws are short and the tips are narrow
- Foerster forceps, which may also be known as Foerster–Ballenger sponge forceps, are commonly used in surgical procedures to hold gauze squares that will absorb excess fluids and blood from the surgical site or hemostasis. The ratcheted locking mechanism of these finger ring forceps securely grip the gauze and hold it in place
- *Chalazion forceps*: Used for eyelid surgery and mucous cyst removal to achieve hemostasis
- *Earlobe clamp*: Surgery of ear and earlobe repair
- *Cheatle sterilizer forceps* are used to remove sterilized instruments from boilers and formalin cabinets. Both forceps and container would be sterilized in boiling water at the start of each operating session

Retractors

A retractor **(Fig. 42)** is a surgical instrument, by which a surgeon can either actively separate edges of a surgical incision or wound, or can hold back underlying organs and tissues, so that body parts under the incision may be accessed. Types of retractors include double- and single-hooked with blunt and curved prongs. They are used to move skin flaps, when extensive undermining is required, to remove deep lesion, and to displace vessels and nerves.

Skin Hooks

Skin hooks **(Figs. 43A and B)** are widely used in dermatologic surgery instead of forceps to avoid undue damage to skin edges, as they are less traumatic. Skin hooks with one, two, or multiple teeth are available. They are used in donor dissection in hair transplant surgery, flap surgery, grafts, etc. **(Box 5)**.

Dermal Curette (Fig. 44)

Curettage is the term used to describe surgical scraping. It is commonly used instrument for treatment and diagnosis in

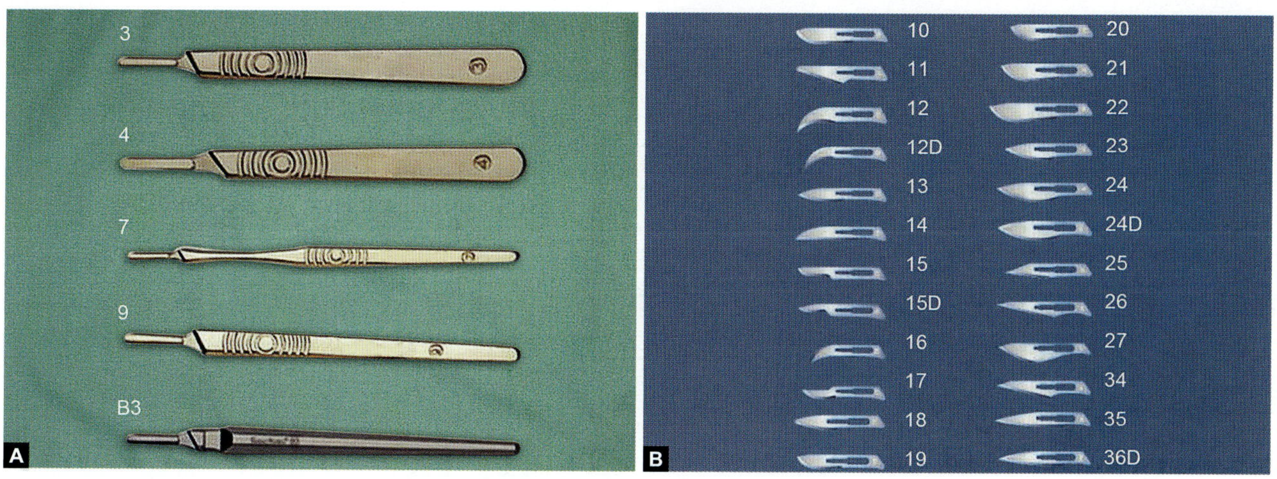

Figs. 30A and B: Scalpel blades and their handles.
- *Handle #3*: For use with scalpel blades #10, #11, #12, and #15
- *Handle #4*: For use with scalpel blades #20, #21, #22, #23, and #24
- *Handle #7*: For use with scalpel blades #10, #11, #12, and #15
- *Handle #9*: For use with scalpel blades #6, #9, #10, #11, #12, #15, and #16
- *Handle # B3*: For use with 6, 9, 10, 11, 12, 12D, 13, 14, 15, 15D, 15T, and 1

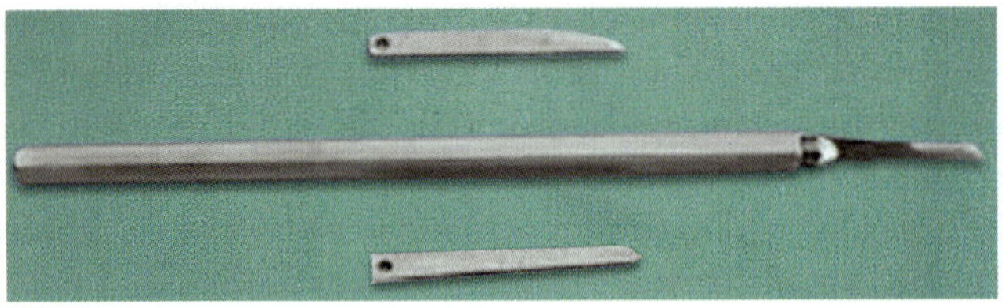

Fig. 31: Beaver scalpel handle with 64 and 67 number blades.

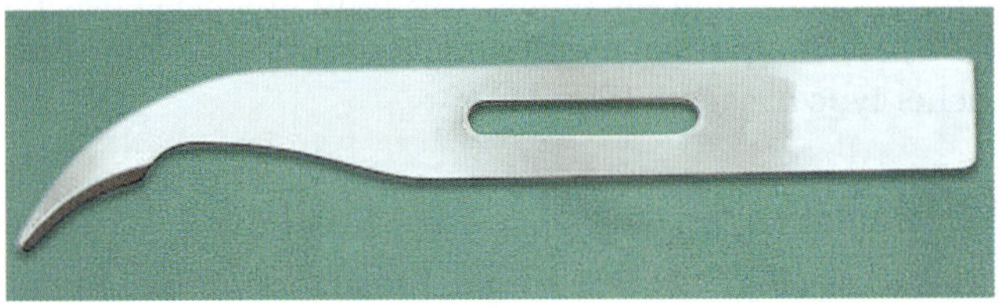

Fig. 32: Stich cutting blade.

BOX 3: Blade numbers and their uses.

- *Blade number 15*: It is the most commonly used blade in dermatosurgery and is ideal in performing skin biopsies where incision is <5 cm
- *Blade number 15D*: It is useful in procedures where incision is <5 cm involving delicate areas such as face
- *Blade number 11*: It has a tapered sharp point and allows precise, vertical, and acute angled incisions. It is useful to drain an abscess and to perform a shave biopsy
- *Blade number 10 and 21*: They have wide convex belly, and are useful during excision of large lesions, in surgeries involving thick skin, such as trunk and scalp, to make incisions longer than 5 cm and in wound debridement
- *Blade number 12*: Sometimes used for suture cutting
- Blade 64 and 67 are of small size and require Beaver handle. Number 64 blade has a round tip with sharp cutting edge and number 67 blade has a sharp tip used for fine cutting, near delicate areas such as near eye, ear, and ear canal surgery

BOX 4: Uses of different needle holders.

- Crile–Wood needle holders **(Fig. 33)** are long, have blunt tips, and are used for 3-0 or 2-0 suture needles
- Castroviejo needle holders **(Figs. 34A and B)** are small-jawed with a detachable spring handle and are used for 6-0 or 7-0 suture needles
- Ryder or Derf needle holders **(Figs. 35A and B)** are used for 4-0 or 5-0 suture needles
- Halsey needle holder—long delicate jaws for suture 5-0 or smaller **(Fig. 36)**
- Webster needle holder—for suture 6-0 or smaller **(Fig. 37)**
- Baumgartner needle holder and Collier needle holder—3-0–6-0 suture; has fenestrated jaws **(Figs. 38A and B)**

dermatology. Simple technique used for removal of lesion on surface such as warts, superficial benign and malignant lesions. Lesions where the disease margins are not well defined are also not usually suitable for this treatment. The instrument is available with a round loop tip. The loop is sharp on the inside and blunt on the outside so the lesion can be removed but surrounding skin is not damaged. Different sizes are available from 2–7 mm.

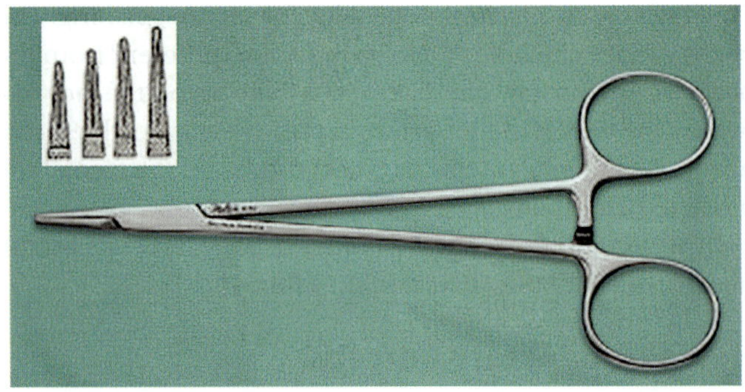

Fig. 33: Crile–Wood needle holder (curved and straight).

Comedone Extractors (Fig. 45)

Comedone extractors, popularly known as blackhead removers, are used to remove black and white heads from the skin. The use of this device has grown in demand due to the growing awareness of self-care techniques and products. They are available in different sizes and specifications. The loop of comedone extractor is smaller than curette and it does not have sharp cutting edges.

Biopsy Punches and Shave Blades (Fig. 46)

Shave and punch biopsies are essential procedures used in dermatology practice. These office-based procedures are easy to perform and can be used as a diagnostic, therapeutic, and cosmetic tool in dermatology.

Biopsy Punches (Fig. 47)

It is a circular hollow blade attached to a handle ranging in different sizes. It is available as disposable, reusable, with plunger, and as automated instrument.

Shave Blades

Shave biopsy is the most commonly used technique for biopsy. It is quick, simple, and effective method and has the simplicity of wound care, cosmesis, and cost-effectiveness. It is used predominantly in epidermal skin lesion such as warts, skin tags, or as saucerization biopsy where deep tissue up to deeper dermis is removed. These biopsies may be indicated in patients with wider lesions or in those with lesions that are difficult to remove with an elliptical excision because of cosmesis or anatomic location such as upper back, shoulder, and chest.

How to Hold Surgical Instruments (Figs. 48 to 51)

Scissors

When cutting the tissue, it is important to see that the tissue is correctly located between the two blades of the scissors.

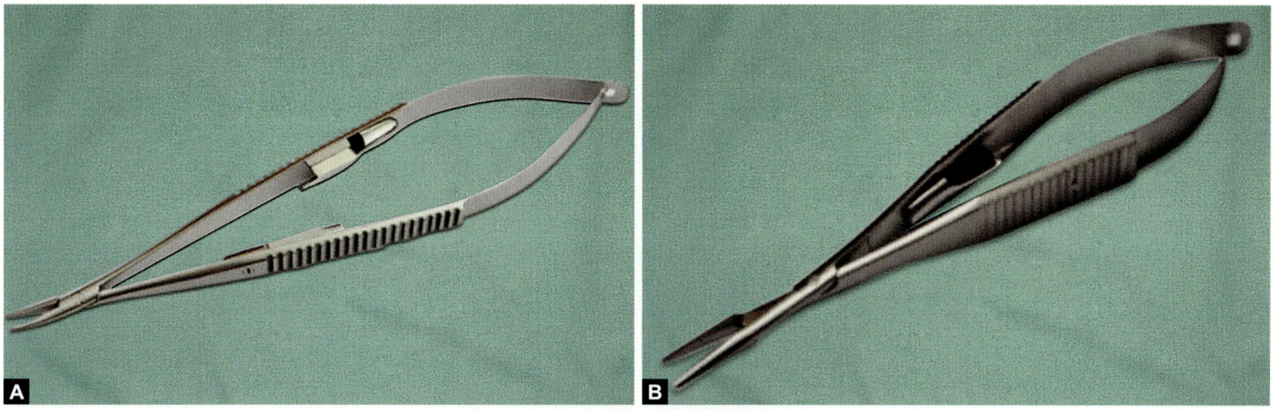

Figs. 34A and B: Castroviejo needle holders.

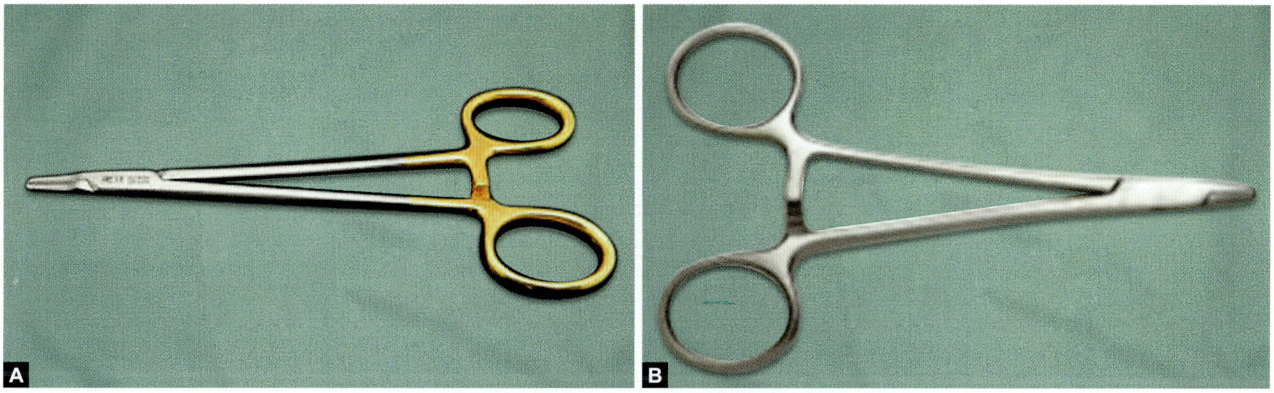

Figs. 35A and B: Ryder and Derf needle holders.

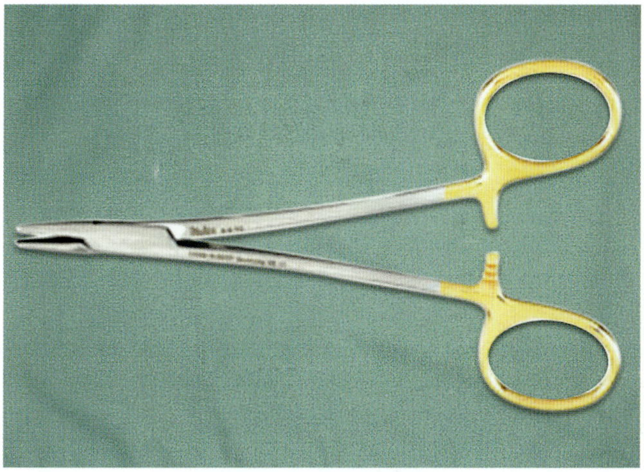

Fig. 36: Halsey needle holder.

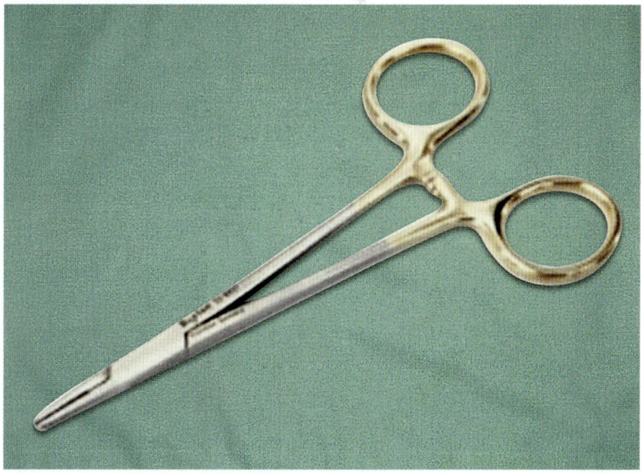

Fig. 37: Webster needle holder.

The surgeon's grip on the scissors must be proper. The grip is properly achieved by putting ring finger and thumb through the rings of the scissors and index finger placed near fulcrum on the shanks.

Forceps

The forceps should be held in the first three fingers as one would hold a pen, using the first three fingers. Grasp the forceps between thumb and middle finger and use index finger to stabilize. It is always advisable to grasp the dermis rather than epidermis to prevent injury to wound edge.

Needle Holder

The needle holder should be held in a way that is comfortable and affords maximum control. Grasp the needle holder by partially inserting the thumb and ring finger into the loops of the handle. The index finger provides additional control and stability.

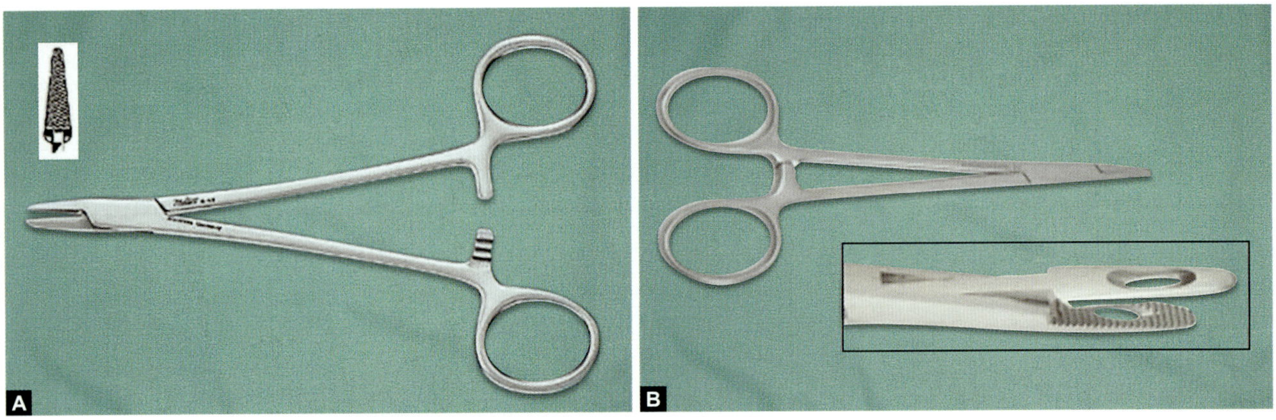

Figs. 38A and B: Baumgartner needle holder (A) and Collier needle holder (B).

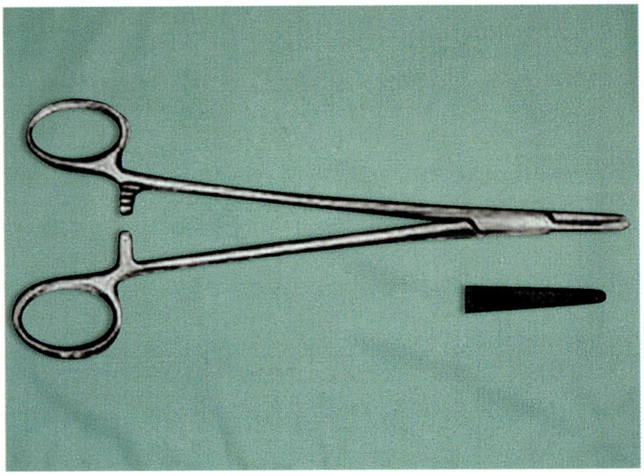

Fig. 39: Artery forceps.

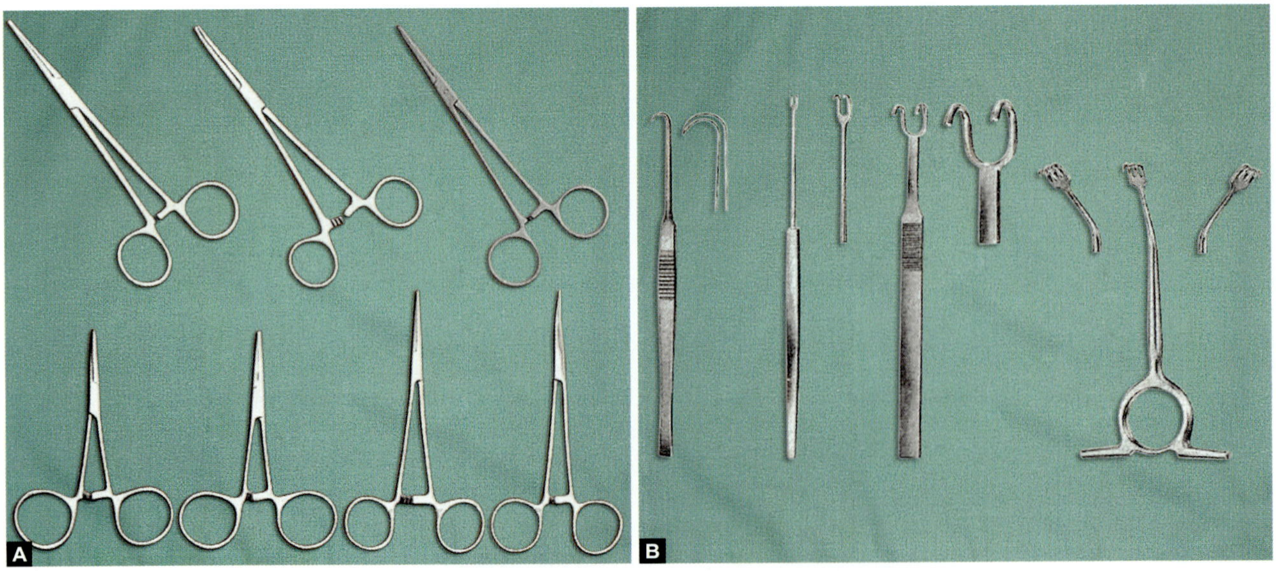

Figs. 40A and B: (A) Mosquito artery forceps; (B) Skin hook.

Needle

Needle should be held just behind its midpoint. If the needle is held near the tip, it will point downward. If the needle is held near the thread end, it will point upward. It is approximately held at junction of proximal 2/3 and distal 1/3 portion of the needle.

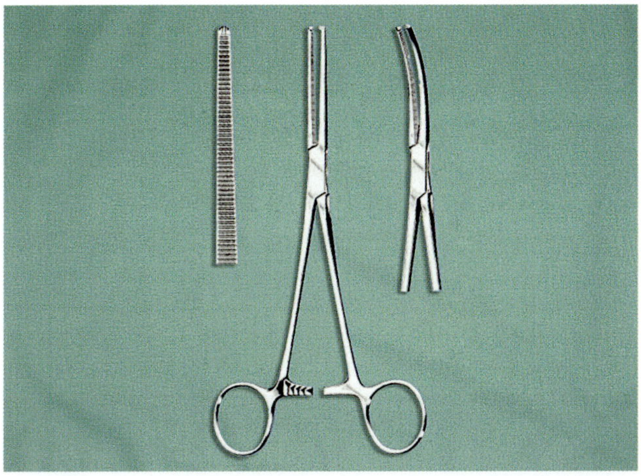

Fig. 41: Kocher artery forceps.

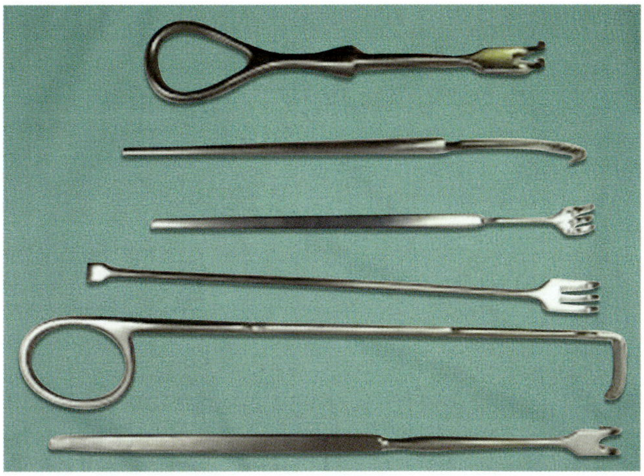

Fig. 42: Retractors—army navy and catspaw.

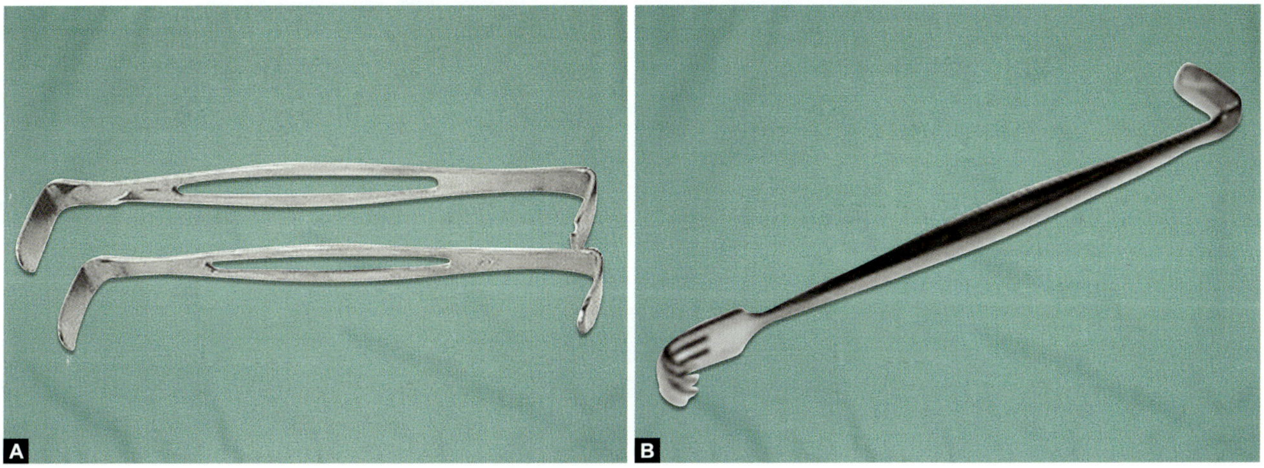

Figs. 43A and B: Skin hooks.

BOX 5: Skin hooks and their uses.

- Gillies skin hook—large hook with long shaft; good for retracting scar tissue
- Tyrell Iris skin hook—small hook for delicate procedures
- Frazier skin hook—holds tongue, lips, and cheeks away from surgical area; Shepherd's crook design

Scalpel

Scalpel should be held like pen with handle resting on anatomical snuffbox. Before taking incision, stabilize the skin with thumb on one side and fingers other side. Make incision with properly held scalpel.

Hemostat

Holding for hemostat is same as scissors. Use tips of the jaw to hold vessels and secure the lock. Learn to release hemostat with single hand.

Curette

The most commonly used method is the "fountain-pen technique". To do this, the curette is held between the thumb, index, and middle finger, while the skin should be stretched with the fingers of the other hand. Another commonly used method is the "potato-peeler technique", wherein the handle of the curette is held in the distal interdigital fold of the index finger, and supported by the other fingers of the curetting hand. The thumb serves to provide a stable base.

ARRANGEMENT OF INSTRUMENTS

The instruments should be arranged on a trolley, surgical stand, or surgical tray with pointed or sharp ends pointing away. The order of instruments should be predetermined and should be same every day for a particular surgery, so that the arrangement is familiar to the surgeon and assisting nurse. Separate specific trays may be prepared for each surgery. The height of the tray or trolley should be at a level comfortable to the surgeon/assisting nurse. Care should be taken to see that there is no admixture of clean and soiled instruments. Gauze or pads should be kept separately, so that they do not obscure sharp objects.

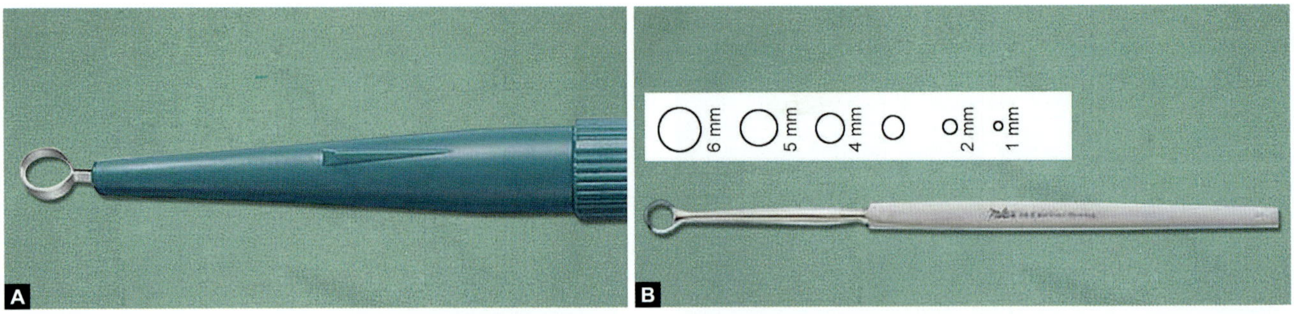

Figs. 44A and B: Dermal curette.

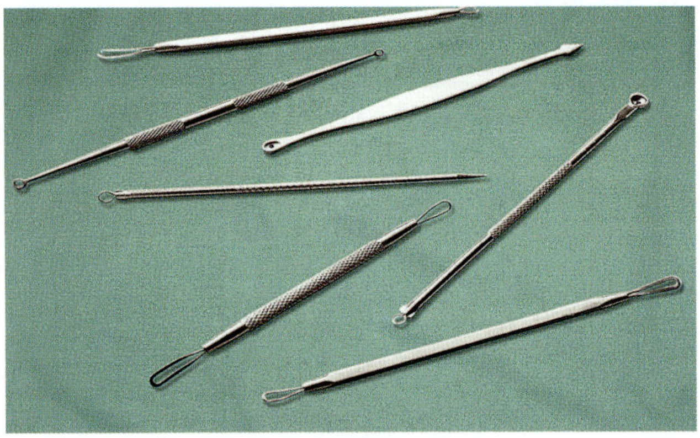

Fig. 45: Comedone extractors.

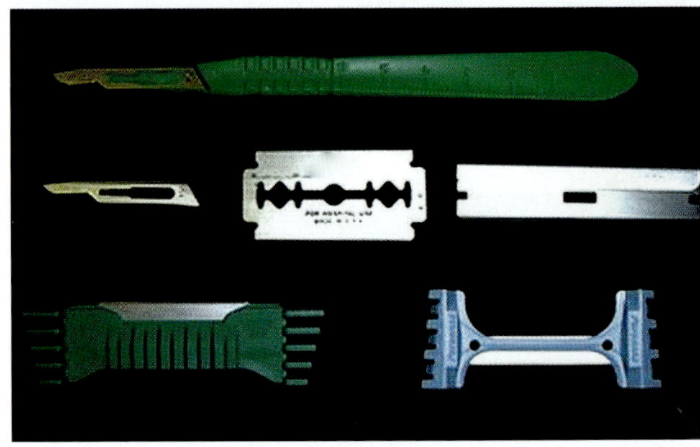

Fig. 46: Shave biopsy blades.

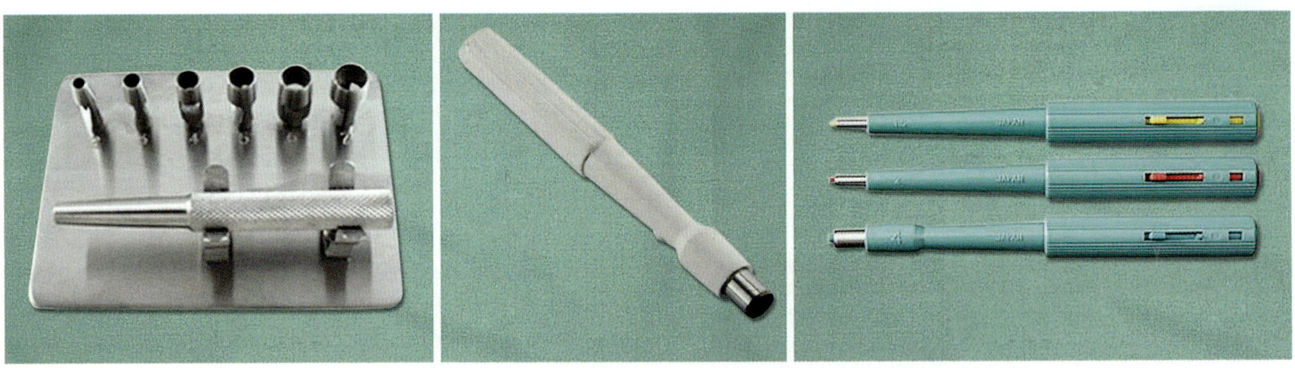

Fig. 47: Biopsy punches.

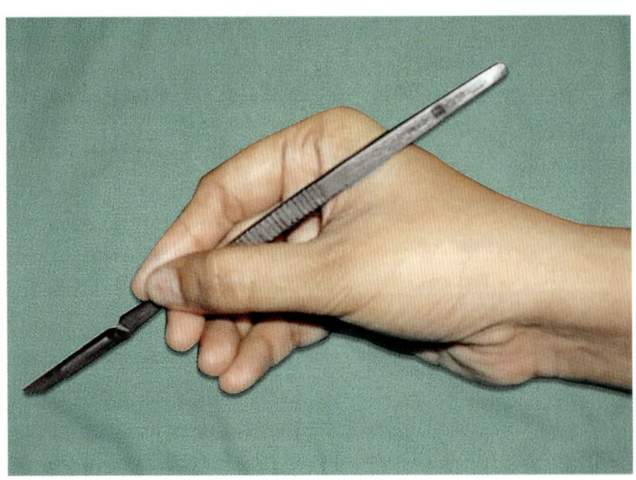

Fig. 48: Holding scalpel.

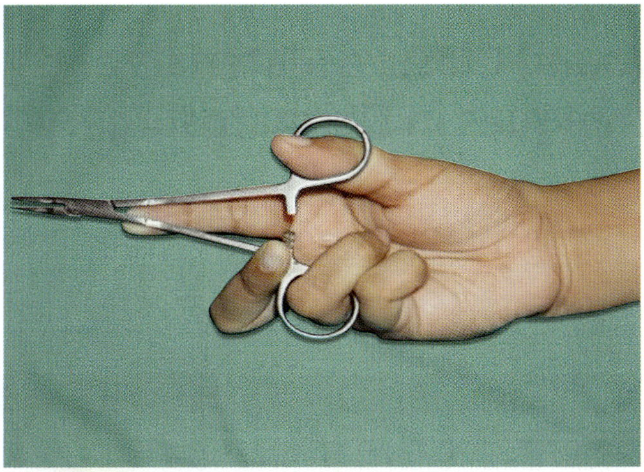

Fig. 49: Holding needle holder.

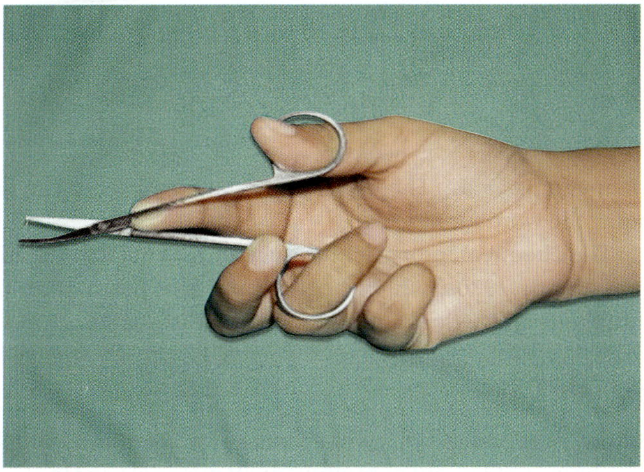

Fig. 50: Holding scissor.

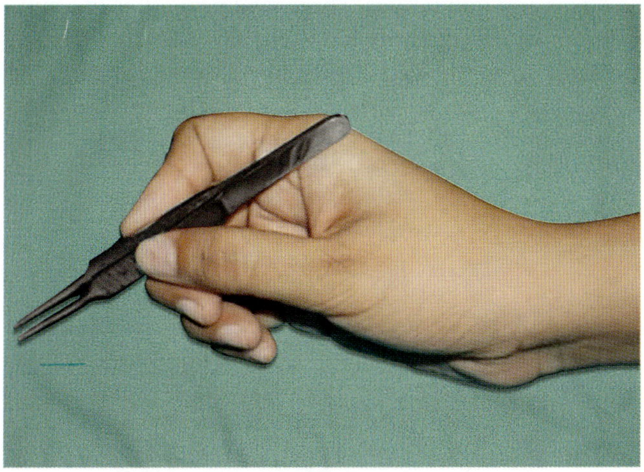

Fig. 51: Holding forceps.

MAINTENANCE OF INSTRUMENTS

Proper care and maintenance of instruments is important to enhance longevity. A trained nurse should clean the instruments. All instruments should be inspected daily during cleaning to check for any damage or wear and tear.

BOX 6: Quality of instruments.

- The instrument should sustain repeated use and sterilization
- They should be from reputed manufacturer and of high-quality stainless steel
- Instruments with high polished or brushed surface are available
- Black finished instruments are used in laser surgery, as black surface is not reflective
- Care must be taken of working and cutting surface of instruments
- Some instruments such as needle holder and scissors are available with special tungsten carbide alloy inserts. This material is hard and maintains precise cutting edge

BOX 7: Precautions during surgery.

- Always work away from the surgeon's field
- Keep instruments in an orderly manner with all instruments pointing in the same direction
- Use properly fitting gloves
- Always use instruments to handle tissue; avoid exposure of hands to the surgical field
- Sharp objects such as needles or blades should be handled after mounting on another instrument such as forceps or needle holder and never with hand
- If hand needs to be entered into the operating field, introduce only one hand, after withdrawing all sharp instruments from the field of surgery
- Do not recap needles

BOX 8: Cleaning of instruments.

- Wash with warm water to remove debris
- Use neutral PH detergent to soak the instruments, if debris are adherent
- Instruments must be dried before sending to sterilization
- Instrument should be inspected for proper functioning before sterilization

In particular, fine forceps and fine scissors are prone to get damaged frequently and need special care.

The tips for instrument selection, to avoid injury during use of surgical instruments, and cleaning are mentioned in the **Boxes 6 to 8**, respectively.

RECOMMENDED READING

1. Brown MD. Advanced surgical reconstructive techniques. Dermatol Clin. 2005;23(1):44-5.
2. Bishop WJ. The Early History of Surgery, 1st edition. London, UK: Robert Hale Limited; 1960.
3. Bogle MA, Fisher VT, Joseph AK. Instruments and materials. In: Robinson JK, Hanke CW, Siegel DM, Fratila A (Eds). Surgery of the Skin: Procedural Dermatology, 2nd edition. Edinburg: Mosby Elsevier; 2010. pp. 65-72.
4. Colleman W, Hanke CW, Thomas H, et.al. Cosmetic Surgery of the Skin: Principles and Techniques, 2nd edition. USA: Mosby Publishers; 2005. pp.7-17.
5. Roenigk RK, Roenigk HH Jr. Roenigk and Roenigk's Dermatologic Surgery: Principles and Practice, 2nd edition. New York: Marcel Dekker Publishers; 1996. pp. 192-205, 293-5, 313-5, 329-35.
6. Sawant S, Shan R, Gore D. Textbook and Atlas of Dermatologic Surgery and Cosmetology. Mumbai, India: ASCAD Publishers; 1998. pp. 3-23.

CHAPTER 7

Wound Closure Materials and Techniques in Dermatosurgery

Govind S Mittal, Mysore Venkataram, Aneesh Kunnath Parambath

KEY MESSAGES

- Knowledge of proper wound closure materials is essential for ensuring rapid wound healing.
- Choice of suture materials is based on its properties—memory, elasticity, knot strength, tensile strength, tissue reaction, and capability to be absorbed.
- A surgical wound attains progressively increasing cutaneous tensile strength after suturing: 3–5% of original strength 2 weeks after suturing, 20% of the ultimate wound strength by 3rd week, and 50% by 1 month.
- Important factors to be considered while choosing the suture material are the location of wound, static and dynamic wound tension, presence of wound infection, and cost of suture material.
- Skin tapes, staples, or wound adhesives are also useful in certain situations.

INTRODUCTION

The choice of an appropriate wound closure material and technique is important for the best functional and cosmetic results. Various methods for mechanical wound closure include sutures,[1] staples, tapes, and adhesives. All these promote primary wound healing.

HISTORY

Suture materials have undergone an evolutionary process over many decades. In golden era, sutures were made of plant materials (flax, hemp, and cotton) or animal materials (hair, tendons, arteries, muscle strips, nerves, silk, and catgut).[2] Interestingly, South Americans used large black ant sutures by coaxing insects to bite wound edges with their powerful jaws acting in a similar manner to Michel Clips. Subsequently, ant's body was twisted off leaving its head in place.[3,4] Needles were made of bone or metals such as silver, copper, and aluminum bronze wire (aluminum bronze is an alloy).

The earliest reports of surgical suture date back to 3,000 BC in ancient Egypt, and the oldest known suture is in a mummy from 1,100 BC. The first detailed description of a wound suture and the suture material used in it is by the Indian sage and physician Sushruta **(Fig. 1)**, written in 500 BC. Galen of Pergamon, AD 150 **(Fig. 2)**, commented for the first time on the use of catgut.[3] Catgut was not derived from cats but was made from the twisted intestine of herbivorous animals (usually sheep or goat) and even today it is widely used accounting for nearly half of all sutures used. The origin of the word "catgut" is not fully known, but it may have been an abbreviation of the word "cattlegut". Alternatively, it may have been derived from the word *kitgut* or *kitstring,* the word *kit,* meaning violin. The kit may have led to the word cat, *kit* being the word for little cat.

The chemical industry introduced the synthetic threads in the early 1930s, which began the era of production of numerous synthetic absorbable and nonabsorbable sutures.[3]

SUTURES

Suture is a foreign body either natural or synthetic, which may be monofilament or multifilament material used to close a surgical or accidental wound and to secure apposition of the edges and join tissues. Three vital properties of a suture material, which affect its handling are memory, elasticity, and knot strength. Tensile strength, tissue reaction, and

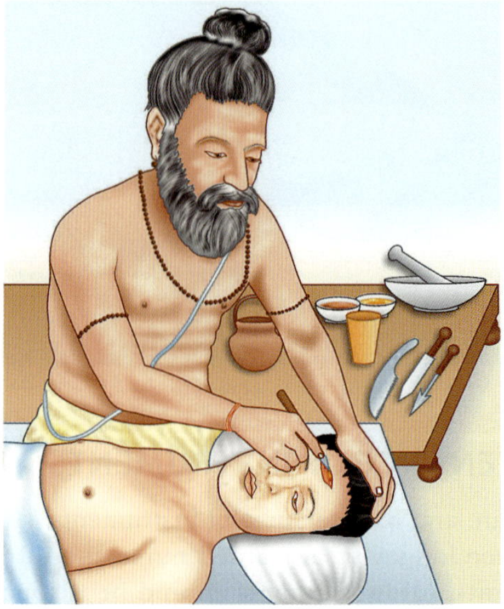

Fig. 1: Sushruta: Father of anesthesia and plastic surgery.

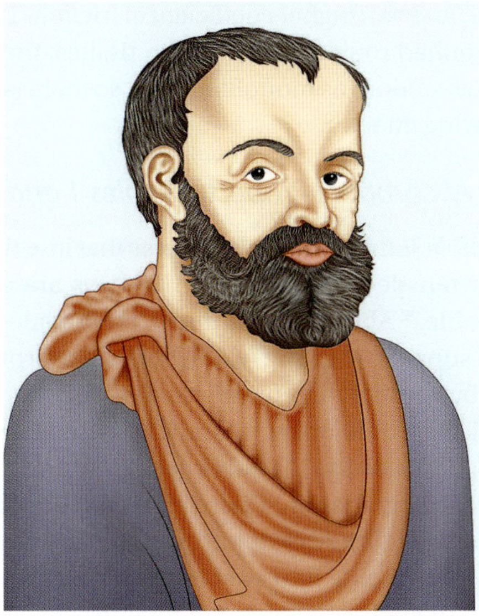

Fig. 2: Claudius Galen (129–200 AD).

capability to be absorbed are other important characteristics of the suture material. The selection of the type of suture to be used depends on tissue type and anatomical location. Several suture materials have been developed today over its millennia of history and each material presents advantages and disadvantages. An ideal suture material has great strength and knot security while remaining elastic with minimal tissue reactivity.[1]

Characteristics of an Ideal Suture

Ideal suture material should:[5,6]

- Be easy to handle
- Cause minimal tissue injury or tissue reaction (natural material elicits more tissue reaction than synthetic)
- Allow secure knots
- Have high tensile strength
- Not cut through tissue
- Be sterile and resistant to infection
- Have favorable absorption profile
- Be affordable.
  No single material can provide all of these characteristics.

Properties of a Suture to be Assessed before Selection[6-9]

- *Tensile strength*: It is a measure of the material's ability to resist breakage. It is the force required to break the suture material divided by the cross-sectional area. Sutures with larger diameter (thicker) have a higher tensile strength.
- *Elasticity*: It is ability of the material to regain its original form and length after stretching. This is important since tissues tend to swell due to the trauma and inflammation after surgery. Depending on its elasticity, a suture can stretch, as the tissue swells up and recoils to its original form when the edema subsides. Polybutester had high elasticity.
- *Plasticity*: It is ability to deform without breaking and to maintain a new form after the deforming or stretching force is gone. When a suture with high plasticity stretches due to tissue edema, the suture stretches and retains the new form even after the tissue edema subsides (as opposed to the property of sutures with high elasticity). This could influence or reduce wound apposition. However, suture with high plasticity ensures high knot security.
- *Capillarity*: Extent to which absorbed fluid is transferred along the suture.
- *Memory*: Inherent capability of suture to return or to maintain its original gross shape (related to elasticity, plasticity, and diameter). High memory sutures (such as polypropylene and nylon) are relatively stiffer and knots made with them have a greater tendency to untie themselves, and hence need additional throws while placing the knot to be secured.
- *Knot strength*: Amount of force necessary to cause a knot to slip (related to the coefficient of static friction and plasticity of a given material). The knot is the weakest section of the suture. In general, flat knots are more secure than sliding knots.
- *Pliability*: Ease of handling of suture material; ability to adjust knot tension and to secure knots.
- *Tissue reactivity*: This is an inflammatory response produced by implanted suture materials. In general, natural and multifilament sutures have greater tissue reaction when compared to synthetic materials.
- *Absorbable*: Progressive loss of mass and/or volume of suture material. By definition, absorbable sutures lose most of their tensile strength within 60 days of being implanted in the body.
- *Nonabsorbable*: Surgical suture material that is relatively unaffected by the biological activities of the body tissues and is therefore permanent unless removed.

Suture Size (as per the United States Pharmacopeia Classification System)[6]

Size refers to the diameter of the suture strand and is denoted as zeroes. Zero is the baseline average size suture. The more zeroes characterizing a suture size, the smaller the resultant strand diameter (e.g., 4-0 or 0000 is larger than 5-0 or 00000). The smaller the suture, the less tensile strength of the strand. Modern sutures range from #5 (heavy braided suture for orthopedic use) to #11-0 (fine monofilament suture for ophthalmic use).

Tissue Response to Suture Materials

All sutures are foreign bodies and produce an inflammatory response in the host dermis. Natural suture materials evoke more inflammatory reaction than synthetic materials.[10] Peak inflammatory response is seen between 2nd day and 7th day with abundance of polymorphonuclear leukocytes, lymphocytes, and large monocytes in dermis.[11] Epithelial cells deeply invade the suture tracts between the 3rd day and 8th day.

A surgical wound never attains the same cutaneous tensile strength as of normal uncut skin. 2 weeks after suturing, 3–5% of original strength will be achieved by a surgical wound. By the end of 3rd week, 20% of the ultimate wound strength is achieved and by 1 month, only 50% of wound strength is attained.[5]

Classification of Suture Materials

Suture materials can be classified in different ways:

- Based on type of filament as monofilament and multifilament sutures
- Based on absorbability as absorbable and nonabsorbable.

Based on Type of Filament

- *Monofilament suture* (***Table 1***): It is made of a single strand and is relatively more resistant to harboring microorganisms.[6] Great care must be taken in handling and tying monofilament suture because crushing or crimping of this suture can nick or weaken the suture and lead to undesirable and premature suture failure.
- *Multifilament suture* (***Table 2***): It is composed of several filaments twisted or braided together. It has increased capillarity and thus increases the absorption of fluid leading to form a tract for the entry of pathogens. Multifilament suture generally has greater tensile strength and better pliability and flexibility than monofilament suture.[6] This type of suture handles and knots well. It is less stiff but has a higher coefficient of friction. They should not be pulled roughly through the tissues; their surfaces are not as smooth as monofilaments, so there is a dragging and sawing effect.[10]

TABLE 1: Monofilament sutures.

Absorbable	*Nonabsorbable*
Surgical gut—plain and chromic	Nylon
Poly(glycolic acid)	Polypropylene (prolene)
Poliglecaprone 25	Hexafluoropropylene
Poly(trimethylene carbonate)	Polybutester
Polydioxanone (PDS II)	
Glycomer 631	
Polyglytone 6211	

TABLE 2: Multifilament sutures.

Absorbable	*Nonabsorbable*
Poly(glycolic acid)	Surgical silk
Polyglactin 910	Cotton
Polyglactin 910 Rapide	Polyamide braided
Polyglactin 910 coated with antibacterial agent triclosan	Polyester

Based on Absorbable Property (Tables 1 and 2)

- *Absorbable suture materials*: Sutures that lose the majority of their tensile strength within 60 days are considered absorbable.[12] Absorbable sutures[9,13,14] provide temporary wound support, until the wound heals. Absorption occurs either by proteolytic enzymatic degradation as seen in natural materials or by hydrolysis as seen in synthetic materials. Hydrolysis causes less tissue reaction than enzymatic degradation. Chemical treatments such as use of chromic salts increase the absorption time (e.g., chromic catgut). Absorbable sutures should be used as deep sutures and are placed into subcutaneous tissues to eliminate dead space and into the dermis to minimize tension during wound healing. Placing them too superficially may result in epithelization of the suture tunnels leading to permanent suture tracts and cyst formation. This can compromise the appearance of the scar.[5,6]

Factors influencing absorption:[6] Accelerated absorption may occur in patients with—

- Fever
- Infection
- Protein deficiency
- In a body cavity that is moist or filled with fluid or if sutures become wet during handling prior to implantation.

Different Suture Materials and their Properties

Absorbable Sutures (Table 3)

Absorbable sutures include natural and synthetic sutures.

Natural: These include—

- *Catgut*: Catgut, commonly known as surgical gut, is chiefly made of collagen derived from naturally occurring purified connective tissue of intestinal submucosa of sheep or the intestinal serosa of cattle.[12] Weak spots produced during manufacture may cause uneven absorption of suture and premature rupture. In comparison with the other absorbable sutures, surgical gut sutures tend to lose their tensile strength and knot security rapidly.[15] Approximately, 60% of the tensile strength of surgical gut is lost in 4–5 days postimplantation and knot security is retained only for 2 weeks. For this reason, it is not wise to use this suture in patients predisposed to delayed wound healing.[9]

Plain surgical gut is treated with an aldehyde solution to strengthen the suture and make it more resistant to enzymatic degradation. These are indicated in repairing rapidly healing tissues that require minimal support and for ligating superficial blood vessels.

TABLE 3: Absorbable sutures and their characteristics.[8]

Properties	*Catgut*	*Poly(glycolic acid)*	*Polyglactin*	*Polydioxanone*	*Poly(trimethylene carbonate)*	*Poliglecaprone*
Handling	Fair	Fair–good	Good	Poor	Good	Excellent
Knot security	Poor	Fair–good	Fair	Poor	Good	Good
Tensile strength	Low	High	High	Moderate	High	High
	Proteolysis by	Hydrolysis by	Hydrolysis by	Hydrolysis by	Hydrolysis by	Hydrolysis by
	60–90 days, unpredictable	90–120 days	60–90 days	180–210 days	180–210 days	90–120 days
Coefficient of friction	High	High	Medium	Low	Low	Low
Memory	Low	Low	Low	High	Low	Low
Tissue reactivity	High	Low–moderate	Low–moderate	Low	Low	Low
Uses	Mucosal tissues, vessel ligation	Buried	Commonly used in dermatological surgeries Buried; Vicryl Rapide (Ethicon) in wounds requiring short-term dermal support	Buried; in wounds requiring long-term dermal support	Buried; in wounds requiring long-term dermal support	Buried
Other		Low elasticity Beige, violet, or green	Low elasticity Clear or violet	Clear or violet	Clear or green	High elasticity Clear

Chromic surgical gut is a catgut soaked in chromic salts. This was introduced to enhance the tensile strength by increasing the resistance to degradation. Tensile strength varies depending on the chromic salt concentration.[12,15] Normally, tensile strength of chromic gut sutures is maintained for 10–14 days.

The tendency to fray during knot construction is the distinct disadvantage of surgical gut. Gut sutures have been banned in Europe and Japan owing to concerns regarding bovine spongiform encephalopathy. It is no more used in dermatologic surgery today.

Synthetic: These include—

- *Poly(glycolic acid) or dexon*: It was the first available synthetic absorbable suture, which was introduced in 1970.[1] This is an absorbable synthetic homopolymer of glycolic acid. It is available in both monofilamentous and braided forms. It is supplied as an uncoated or coated form. Coated poly(glycolic acid) suture is undyed or dyed green or violet, which provides easier visibility.[9,13,14] Being synthetic, it elicits less inflammatory response than surgical gut. It is degraded by hydrolysis. Poly(glycolic acid) possesses good tensile strength and excellent knot security. After 2 weeks of implantation, 65% of the initial tensile strength remains with poly(glycolic acid) suture, in contrast to 0% of surgical gut suture.[5]
- *Polyglactin 910 (vicryl)*: Polyglactin 910 is the most widely used absorbable suture material in dermatologic surgery resulting in excellent cosmetic outcome. It is a synthetic braided multifilament copolymer consisting of 90% of glycolide and 10% of lactide. The suture is coated with calcium stearate, which permits easy tissue passage and precise knot placement.[6] It is degraded by hydrolysis and therefore yields only minimal tissue reaction. Vicryl is completely hydrolyzed by 60 days postimplantation.[16] It is an excellent option for soft tissue approximation and vessel ligation. Greater residual tensile strength and a faster absorption rate render polyglactin 910 suture to be superior when compared to poly(glycolic acid) suture.[1,13]

Variants:[1,3]

- *Vicryl Rapide®* irradiated with gamma rays to speed absorption.
- *Vicryl Plus,* the only suture impregnated with triclosan for its antibiotic and anti-inflammatory effect
- *Poliglecaprone 25 (Monocryl)*: It is a synthetic monofilament suture that is a copolymer of glycolide and ecaprolactone.[6] High tensile strength (50–60%) is maintained for 7 days, which will be absorbed completely by 3 months. It offers better handling and knot security than most other monofilament sutures. Hence, it is useful for subcuticular closure and soft tissue approximations and ligations.
- *Poly(trimethylene carbonate) (Maxon)*: It is a synthetic monofilament absorbable suture. It retains 75% of original strength at 2 weeks of postimplantation. Complete absorption does not occur until 180–210 days.[15] Its advantages over other sutures are improved handling properties, lacks memory, passes easily through tissues, and demonstrates superior strength.[14]

Maxon has proved to be an excellent addition to the armamentarium of the surgeon and is considered to be one of the best absorbable suture materials available so far.

- *Polydioxanone*: Polydioxanone is a polyester monofilament suture made of p-dioxanone. Stiffness, which is one of the important disadvantages of monofilament, has been addressed in its updated version—PDS II thus making it more easy to handle.[1] Polydioxanone retains 74% of its tensile strength at 2 weeks postimplantation and takes 180 days to be completely absorbed.[15,17] Polydioxanone has also demonstrated minimal tissue reaction. Hence, it is a suture material of choice for wounds that require prolonged tensile strength.
- *Glycomer 631*: It is a synthetic absorbable monofilament similar to poliglecaprone 25 in characteristics but with prolonged strength akin to poly(trimethylene carbonate). It passes through the tissue more easily but the knot security is inferior.[5]
- *Polyglytone 6211*: Polyglytone 6211 is a recently developed monofilament, absorbable, and synthetic suture.[9,13] It is polyester of glycolide, caprolactone, trimethylene carbonate, and lactide. It loses its tensile strength rapidly, mimicking surgical gut. However, absorption occurs via hydrolysis. Knot strength decreases to 50–60% of original strength at 5 days postimplantation.

Nonabsorbable Sutures (Table 4)

Nonabsorbable sutures maintain most of their tensile strength for at least 60 days postimplantation.[12] These sutures should be just tight enough to approximate, but not strangulate tissues.[14] Nonabsorbable sutures often cause less scarring because they provoke less immune response and thus are used where cosmetic outcome is important. They require manual removal postoperatively after a certain time.

Nonabsorbable sutures include natural and synthetic suture materials.

Natural: These include—

- *Surgical silk*: Silk is a natural suture material extruded by silk worm larvae of *Bombycidae* family during their cocoon production.[1,14] It is braided and black dyed, thus allows for easy handling and greater visibility. However, due to its braided configuration, silk is prone to get infected and can be infiltrated by tissue ingrowth.[12,15] Coating with wax or silicone helps to reduce tissue friction and capillarity.[5,6] Silk is a naturally occurring organic substance and evokes a significant inflammatory response, second only to catgut.[11] A special quality of silk is its ease of handling. Unfortunately, its tensile strength is very low. Although classified as a nonabsorbable material, silk suture becomes absorbed by proteolysis and is often undetectable in the wound site by 2 years. Due to its property of reactivity, it is rarely used for cutaneous closures; however, it is commonly used on mucosal and intertriginous areas, as it is soft and pliable.
- *Surgical cotton*: It is made of twisted, long, and stable cotton fibers.[6] Tensile strength is 50% in 6 months and 30–40% by 2 years. Surgical cotton is nonabsorbable and becomes encapsulated within body tissues.

Synthetic: These include—

- *Nylon*: It was introduced in 1940 as the first synthetic suture material.[1] Nylon suture materials are available in

TABLE 4: Nonabsorbable sutures and their characteristics.[8]

Properties	*Silk*	*Nylon, monofilament*	*Nylon, multifilament*	*Polyester*	*Polypropylene*	*Polybutester*
Handling	Excellent	Poor	Fair—good	Good	Poor	Good
Knot security	Excellent	Poor	Fair—good	Good	Poor	Fair—good
Tensile strength	Low	High	High	High	Moderate	High
Coefficient of friction	High	Low	High	High	Very low	Very low
Memory	Low	High	Medium	Medium	High	Low
Tissue reactivity	High	Low	Moderate	Low–moderate	Low	Low
Uses	Mucosal tissues, conjunctiva or intertriginous zones; to elevate or retract tissues	Percutaneous; buried if prolonged dermal support is needed	Minimal use in dermatologic surgery	Minimal use in dermatologic surgery	Widely used in dermatological surgeries Percutaneous; buried, if prolonged dermal support is needed; running subcuticular closures	Percutaneous; running subcuticular closures
Other	Black	Black, green, or clear		Green or clear	High plasticity Blue or clear	High elasticity Blue or clear

both mono (Ethilon/Monosof) or braided multifilament (Nurolon/Surgilon) forms. It is a polyamide polymer fiber, which is chemically inert. Due to its property of elasticity, it is useful for surface (epidermal and superficial) closure. Monofilament nylon suture has a great deal of memory and its proclivity for knot slippage is known.[5] Multifilament braided nylon sutures exhibit decreased memory and they are associated with higher infection rate. The braided forms are coated with silicone. Nylon is quite pliable, especially when moist. Of note, a premoistened form is available for cosmetic plastic surgery. Nylon suture has good handling characteristics. It is hydrolyzed slowly, but remaining suture material is stable at two years, due to gradual encapsulation by fibrous connective tissue.[6]

- *Nylon monofilament (Ethilon)*: It remains one of the most popular nonabsorbable sutures in dermatological surgery as a result of its high tensile strength, low tissue reactivity, high elasticity, and low cost.[15]
- *Polypropylene (Prolene)*: It was developed in 1970 as a first synthetic nonabsorbable suture. It is a monofilament suture made of isostatic crystalline stereoisomer of a linear propylene polymer with few unsaturated bonds.[5,14] Its significant advantage is its high plasticity, which allows it to expand to accommodate the wound edema. This decreases the risk of the suture cutting the tissue.[1] However, it leaves the stitches loose once the swelling subsides, which is due to its properties of high memory and lack of elasticity. Polypropylene has a tensile strength more than nylon and can easily pass through tissues. This material is biologically inert and elicits minimal tissue reaction. It does not adhere to the tissues, which make it ideal for intradermal suture such as subcuticular closure. As a result of its smooth surface, prolene may be smoothly implanted and removed without tugging of the skin. It is available as dyed or undyed form. This material is useful in contaminated and infected wounds, as it minimizes sinus formation and suture extrusion.[6] Because of smooth surface, knot security is decreased and it should be compensated for with extra throws.[12,15]
- *Hexafluoropropylene*: It is a newly developed nonabsorbable monofilament suture made of polyvinylidene fluoride and poly(vinylidene fluoride-co-hexafluoropropylene).[14] It exhibits lack of adherence to tissues, which makes it a possible choice for "pullout" sutures. Like polypropylene, it resists infection and elicits minimal tissue response. It is dyed blue.
- *Polyester*: Polyester[5] sutures are nonabsorbable synthetic braided multifilament sutures composed of polyethylene terephthalate. Due to its unique properties, such as minimal tissue reactivity, high tensile strength, good handling, and lasting indefinitely in the body, it is ideal for face lifts. Other indications include prosthetic implantations and cardiovascular surgeries. Polyester sutures are available in both coated or uncoated forms.
- *Polybutester suture*: The newest advance in nonabsorbable sutures is polybutester suture, which is a block copolymer that contains butylene terephthalate (84%) and poly(tetramethylene ether glycol) terephthalate (16%).[18] It is the newest of the synthetic nonabsorbable sutures.[1] Being monofilamentous, it produces little inflammatory response and is less likely to harbor bacteria. High elasticity is one of its unique and advantageous characteristics. As previously discussed, high elasticity allows it to stretch with wound edema but return to its original length and form once swelling has subsided. Polybutester is able to stretch to 50% of its original length at a load of 25% of its knot breaking point.[15,19] This high degree of elasticity provides obvious clinical advantages, as it is less likely to cut through the skin during swelling and effectively approximates wound edges throughout the healing process.

CHOOSING THE RIGHT SUTURE MATERIAL

Important factors to be considered while choosing the suture material are the location of wound, static and dynamic wound tension, presence of wound infection or fever, and cost of suture material.

Following are the general principles to be considered for suture selection:

Based on Tensile Strength

The tensile strength of the suture should never exceed the tensile strength of the tissue. As the wound heals, the relative loss of suture strength over time should be slower than the gain of tissue tensile strength. Aesthetic concerns are at a premium in the anatomic regions of the head and neck.

- Eyelid, periorbital area, nose, pinna, lip, and vermillion—sutures with relatively less tensile strength and smaller sizes are preferred.
- The activity and mobility of the face, anterior and posterior neck, scalp, superior trunk, and nasal and oral mucosa require sutures with higher tensile strength.
- Major musculocutaneous flaps tend to be closed under significant tension and hence require maximal long-term tensile strength.

Based on Absorbable Property

Sutures are no longer needed when a wound has reached maximum strength. Therefore, consider nonabsorbable suture in skin, fascia, and tendons (slowly healing tissues), while mucosal wounds (rapidly healing tissues) may be closed with absorbable sutures.

Based on Type of Filament

Special consideration of suture selection in infected wounds is imperative. Multifilament sutures are more likely to

TABLE 5: The preferred size of suture materials.[12,20]

Site	*Suture size*
Thin-skinned areas of low tension (eyelids and scrotum)	6-0
Face	5-0 and 6-0 depending on other factors
Facial areas closed under some tension (forehead and other body areas)	4-0 and 5-0 depending on other factors
Thick-skinned areas (scalp, back, and scapular areas) closed under tension	3-0 or 2-0

harbor contaminants than monofilament sutures; thus, monofilament sutures are generally preferable in potentially contaminated tissues. Use the smallest inert monofilament suture materials, such as nylon or polypropylene, in this setting.

Based on Size of Suture Material (Table 5)

Optimal suture size is generally the smallest size necessary to achieve the desired tension-free closure. If wound tension is high, smaller diameter sutures may actually injure tissues by cutting through them. Therefore, closely match the tensile strength of the suture and tissue.

In general, monofilament nylon and polypropylene are most commonly used in epidermal/skin closure in dermatosurgery. In young children, sometime absorbable suture material such as Poliglecaprone 25 (Monocryl) is used in epidermal closure or subcuticular sutures since they may not cooperate for a session of suture removal. Similarly, in areas of dermatosurgical procedures involving the scrotum where suture removal is not planned or cosmesis is not of significant concern, absorbable material such as chromic catgut can be used. Polyglactin 910 (Vicryl and Vicryl Rapide) is the commonly used absorbable suture material for subcutaneous or intradermal buried sutures. Care must be taken to avoid the violet-colored sutures in very fair skinned individuals or in areas of thin skin where it may be sometimes visible through the closed wound.

To summarize, there can be no single guideline as to which universal suture material must be used in a given area or closure. The dermatosurgeon has to take the final call on case-to-case basis keeping in mind patient factors, size, and location of the surgical wound, intended timing of planned suture removal and individual suture characteristics as discussed above, and decide on the material to be used.

NEEDLES

Surgical needles are made of stainless steel alloys, which have excellent resistance to corrosion.[21] Scientists have successfully used the concept of high nickel maraging stainless steels

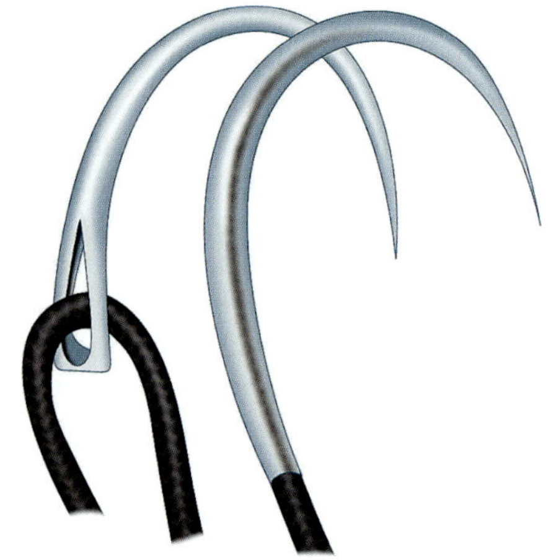

Fig. 3: Traumatic and atraumatic needles.

(S45500/SURGALLOY™) to develop stainless steel wires with superior strength, greater resistance to bending, and ductility for use as surgical needles.

Wound closure and healing are affected by the initial tissue injury caused by needle penetration along with subsequent suture passage. Hence, proper selection of needle is necessary.

Surgical needles may be classified as traumatic or atraumatic.[2] Traumatic needles are needles with eyes, which are available without suture thread; whereas, atraumatic needles comprise an eyeless needle swaged to a specific length of suture thread **(Fig. 3)**. Atraumatic needles are commonly preferred in dermatosurgical procedures.

Ideal Surgical Needle Characteristics[6]

- High-quality stainless steel
- Smallest diameter possible
- Stable in the grasp of the needle holder
- Capable of implanting suture material through tissue with minimal trauma
- Sharp enough to penetrate tissue with minimal resistance
- Sterile and corrosion-resistant to prevent introduction of microorganisms or foreign materials into the wound.

Anatomy of Needle

The swaged needle has three parts—the point (or the tip), body, and the swage (or shank) **(Figs. 4 and 5)**. The body of the needle is important for interaction with the needle holder and the ability to transmit the penetrating force to the point. Swage or the Shank forms the end where the suture attaches to the needle, creating a single and continuous unit of suture and needle.

Advantages of Eyeless or Swaged Needles

- It minimizes the trauma on the sutured tissue, as suture end of the swaged needle is smaller than the needle body. Moreover, in traumatic needle, the thread comes out of

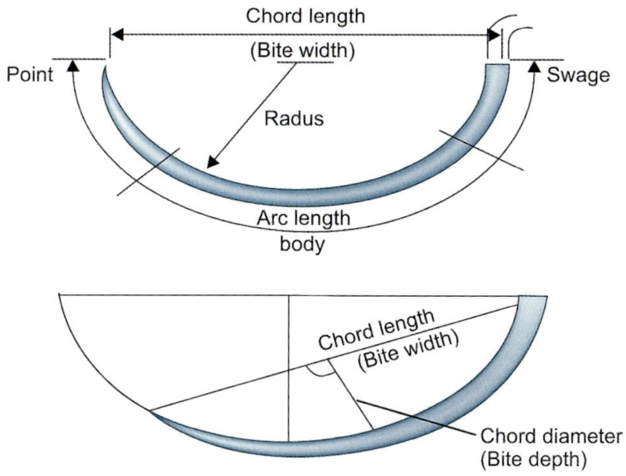

Fig. 4: Anatomy of needle.

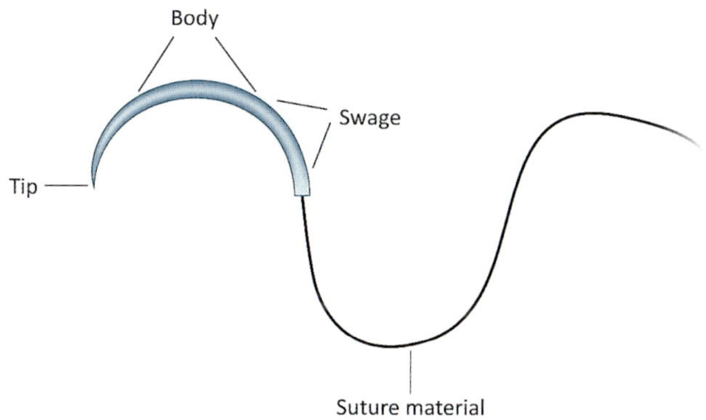

Fig. 5: Parts of swaged needle.

the needle's hole on both sides. When passing through the tissues, this suture may tear the skin to a certain extent, thus the name traumatic.[3,10]

- Unlike in eyed needle, suture is less likely to become unthreaded prematurely.
- Decreased handling helps to maintain suture integrity.
- Time spent on threading the suture on the needle is avoided in atraumatic needles.
- Sutures are supplied in sealed packets after gamma ray sterilization. Hence, each patient has the benefit of a new, sharp, and guaranteed sterile needle.
- Nearly all modern sutures feature swaged atraumatic needles.

Silicone Coating

Needles coated with silicone are available allowing easier tissue passage.[6]

Needle Measurements

Chord Length

This is the linear distance from the point of the curved needle to the swage (bite width) **(Fig. 4)**.[6]

Needle Length

The distance measured along the needle from the point to the swage is termed as needle length. It is the needle length and not the chord length (bite width), is the measurement supplied on suture packages.

Radius

This is the distance from the body of the needle to the center of the circle along which the needle curves (bite depth).

Diameter

The gauge or thickness of the needle wire is considered as the diameter.

Needle Types

Needles can be classified based on different criteria such as size, body type, and on cross section.

Based on Size

Different needle lengths are available for each suture size and the length required depends on the thickness of the tissue being sutured.[22] Always use the thinnest needle and the finest filament the wound can tolerate.

Based on Body Types

Surgical needles are available in various body shapes such as straight needle, curved, and compound curved of which curved needles are exclusively used in dermatosurgery.[6]

Curved needle has a predictable path through tissue and requires less space for maneuvering than a straight needle. Body curvature is commonly a quarter inch, three-eighth inch, half inch, or five-eighths inch circle **(Fig. 6)**. The three-eighths inch circle is used most commonly for skin closure. It is shaped like a fish hook in case of subcutaneous sutures.[5]

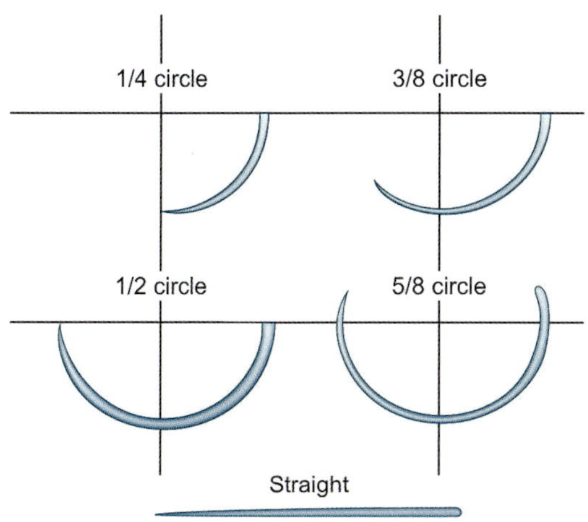

Fig. 6: Different shapes of curved needle.

It is important to rotate the wrist when passing the curved needle through the tissue.

Based on Cross-section

Needle may be either cutting or noncutting (round-bodied). Cutting needles are commonly used in dermatosurgery since they are designed for penetration through dense, irregular, and relatively thick tissues like skin.

Commonly Used Cutting Needles in Dermatosurgery

- *Conventional cutting*:[6] This type of needle has three cutting edges (triangular cross-section that changes to a flattened body). The third cutting edge is on the inner and concave curvature (surface seeking) and can cut through wound edge **(Figs. 7 and 8)**.
- *Reverse cutting*:[6] The third cutting edge is on the outer convex curvature of the needle (depth seeking). These needles are stronger than conventional cutting needles and have a reduced risk of cutting through the tissue. The needles are designed to penetrate tough tissues such as skin, tendon sheaths, and oral mucosa. Reverse cutting needles are commonly used in cosmetic surgery, causing minimal trauma.
- *SUB Q needles* **(Fig. 9)**:[3] These are the needles especially designed for cosmetic surgeons seeking excellence in skin closure. The cross-sectional geometry of the needle tip offers finer cutting edges for easier penetration of skin. Each cutting edge is sharpened by a special process for smooth and controlled passage through skin.

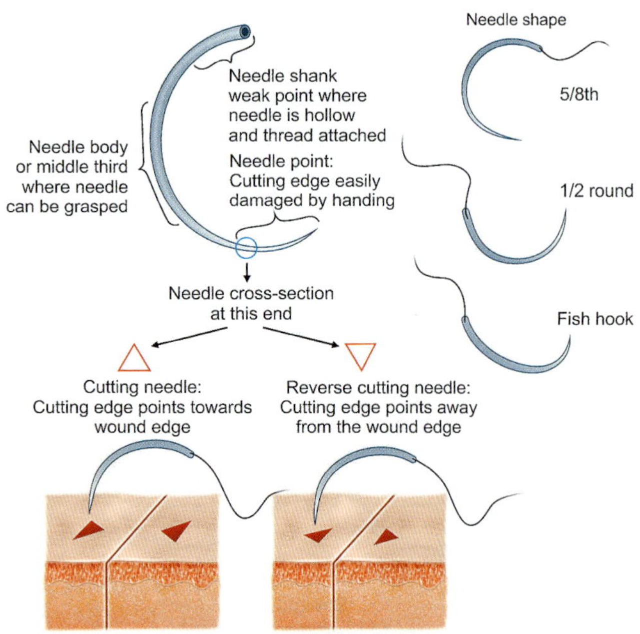

Fig. 7: Types of needles.

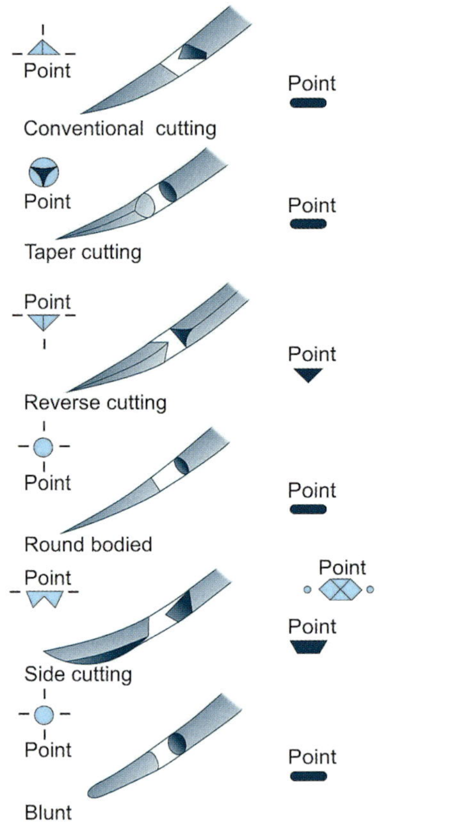

Fig. 8: Cross-section of different types of eyeless needle.

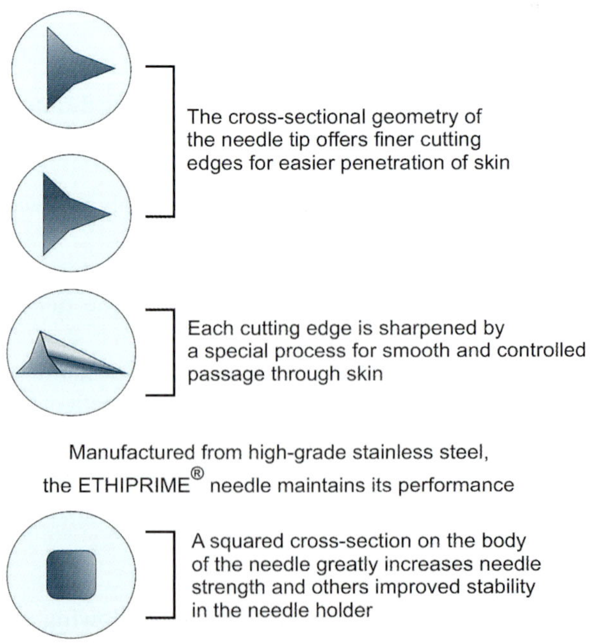

Fig. 9: SUB Q ethiprime® needle, special needle for cosmetic surgery.

Needle and Needle Holder Interaction

Suture needles should be handled carefully. Avoid blunting the cutting point or bending the weaker end of the suture needle.[23,24] The stability of the needle within the needle

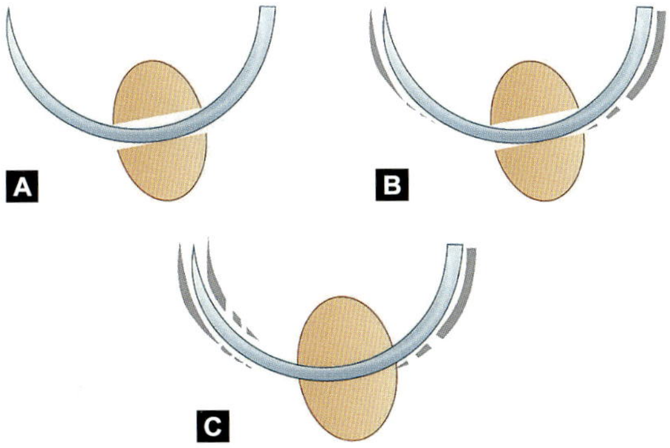

Figs. 10A to C: Interaction between the needle holder and suture needle.[6] (A) Needle holder of appropriate size for the needle; (B) Needle holder that is too large for the needle. Pressure applied by the needle holder leads to inadvertent straightening of the suture needle; (C) Needle holder that is too small for the needle. The needle rotates around the long axis of the needle holder.

holder affects needle control and performance. The jaws of the needle holder must be appropriate to the needle size to hold it securely and prevent rocking, turning, and twisting.[6] The difference between the length of the handle and the jaw creates a mechanical advantage for exerting force through the needle point. The jaws of the needle holder contact a curved needle at one point on the outer curvature and two points along the inner curvature as shown in **Figures 10A to C**. The force against the needle creates a moment arm, which may flatten the curvature of the needle. The needle holder clamping moment must be less than the surgical yield of the needle, which otherwise can bend and break the needle. Repetitive injury by the needle holder also may cause the needle to break. A bent needle further increases soft tissue injury affecting cosmetic outcome.

Surgical Glove Selection

Surgeons who use sutures and needles should wear sterile surgical gloves without cornstarch. Cornstarch has been documented to promote wound infection, to cause serious peritoneal adhesions and granulomatous peritonitis and to be a well-documented vector of the latex allergy epidemic.[25]

Holes allow the transmission of blood-borne viral infections between the patient and the surgeon. Food and Drug Administration (FDA) has laid down specific standards of criteria for surgical gloves. The use of the Biogel double-glove hole indication system is recommended to detect the location and presence of holes in the gloves, allowing the surgeon to change the gloves when a hole is detected.[26,27]

PRINCIPLES OF SUTURING

The technique of suturing cutaneous wounds is a millennium old. The goals of suturing are closing the dead space, supporting and strengthening wounds until healing increases their tensile strength, approximating skin edges for an aesthetically pleasing and functional result, and minimizing the risks of formation of hematoma and infection.

Selection of proper suturing technique is important to ensure best cosmetic results in dermatologic surgery. The choice of suture technique depends on the type and anatomic location of the wound (e.g., eyes and vermilion border of the lips), the thickness of the skin, the degree of tension, and the desired cosmetic result.[28] Wound eversion is essential to maximize the likelihood of good epidermal approximation. Eversion is desirable to minimize the risk of scar depression secondary to tissue contraction during healing. Usually, inversion is not desirable and it probably does not decrease the risk of hypertrophic scarring in an individual with a propensity for hypertrophic scars. Suture material elicits a foreign body tissue reaction. During wound closure, meticulous aseptic technique is critical to minimize the risk of wound infection. Gentle handling of the tissue is also important to optimize wound healing.

Often, two layers are sutured:

1. Deep sutures below the surface to maintain the closure until the wound has fully healed and can support itself without widening of the scar
2. Surface sutures to closely approximate the epidermal edges providing the best possible cosmetic result.

To obtain the best cosmetic results, it is important to have good quality instruments that are the correct size for the location and nature of the wounds being closed. The instruments also need to be correctly sterilized and handled carefully.

The basic suturing kit includes:

- Needle holder
- Fine suture cutting scissors
- Toothed tissue forceps or skin hook
- Appropriate suture material.

Techniques of Needle Holding and Suture Placement

The jaw of the appropriate needle holder is used to grasp the needle at its distal portion at the junction of anterior two-thirds and posterior one-third. The needle holder is tightened by squeezing it until the first ratchet catches. The needle holder should not be tightened excessively because damage to both the needle and the needle holder may result. The needle is held vertically and longitudinally perpendicular to the needle holder **(Figs. 11 to 16)**.[28]

- As described earlier, incorrect placement of the needle in the needle holder may result in a bent needle, difficult penetration of the skin, and/or an undesirable angle of entry into the tissue.
- The needle holder is held by placing the thumb and the fourth finger into the loops and by placing the index finger on the fulcrum of the needle holder to provide stability **(Fig. 12)**.

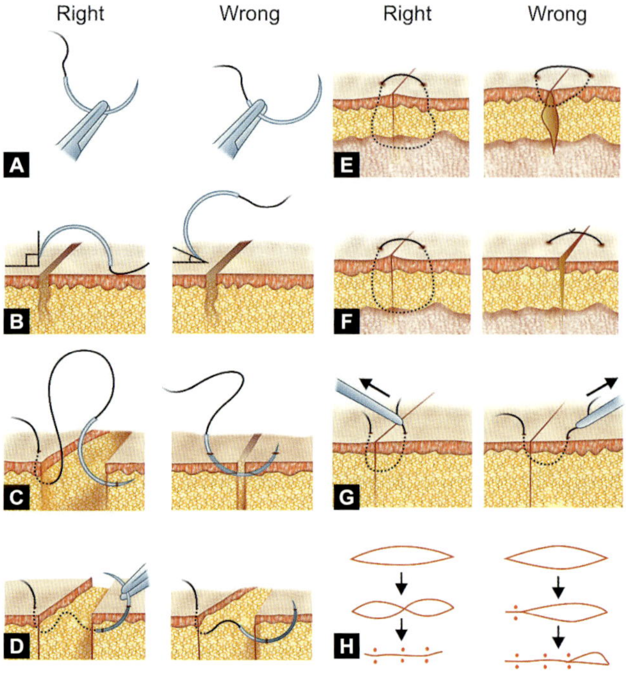

Figs. 11A to H: Techniques of needle holding and suturing.

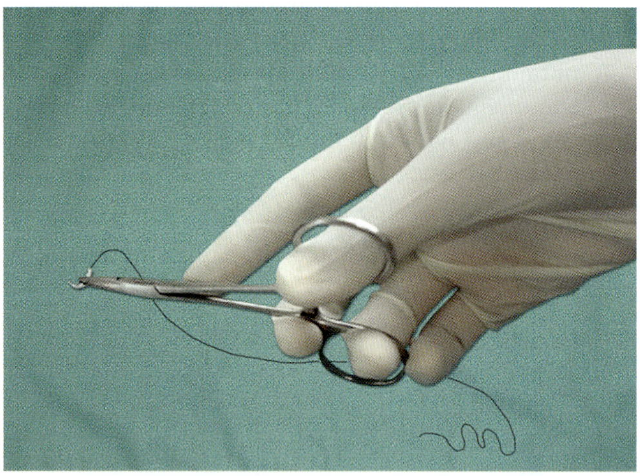

Fig. 12: Holding needle holder to provide stability.

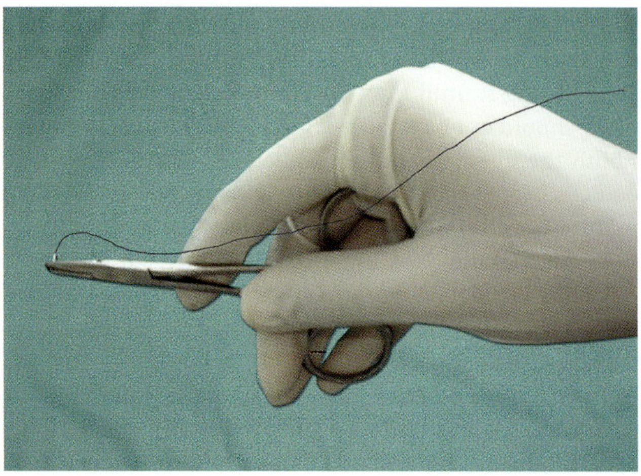

Fig. 13: Holding needle holder to increase dexterity.

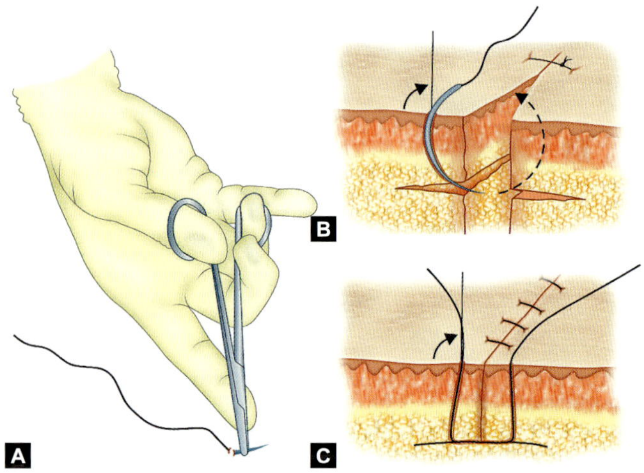

Figs. 14A to C: Basic suturing: (A) Proper grip; (B) Angle of entry; (C) Angle of exit.

Alternatively, the needle holder may be held in the palm to increase dexterity **(Fig. 13)**.

- The tissue must be stabilized to allow suture placement. Depending on the surgeon's preference, toothed or untoothed forceps or skin hooks may be used to gently grasp the tissue. Excessive trauma to the tissue being sutured should be avoided to reduce the possibility of tissue strangulation and necrosis.
- The needle should always penetrate the skin at a 90° angle, which minimizes the size of the entry wound and promotes eversion of the skin edges **(Figs. 14A to C)**.[29] The needle should be inserted 1–3 mm from the wound edge, depending on skin thickness. The depth and angle of the suture depend on the particular suturing technique. The needle should be driven in an arc that follows the curvature of the needle **(Figs. 15A to C)**.
- Fine forceps are necessary for grasping the needle, as it exits the tissue after a pass. Prior to removing the needle holder, grasping and stabilizing the needle are important. This maneuver decreases the risk of losing the needle in the dermis or subcutaneous fat and it is especially important, if small needles are used in areas such as the back, where large needle bites are necessary for proper tissue approximation **(Fig. 16)**.
- The needle tip is grasped with the needle holder and by rotating the needle holder in the same arc as the needle, the rest of the needle will emerge from the tissue and the attached suture material will follow.
- The needle must be repositioned in the jaws of the needle holder for penetrating the deep tissue of the opposing wound edge. The needle must penetrate the opposing side at precisely the same depth as the side from which it is emerged. The opposing wound edge is stabilized with forceps or skin hook prior to penetration with the needle.
- In general, the two sides of the suture should become mirror images, and the needle should also exit the skin perpendicular to the skin surface.[30]

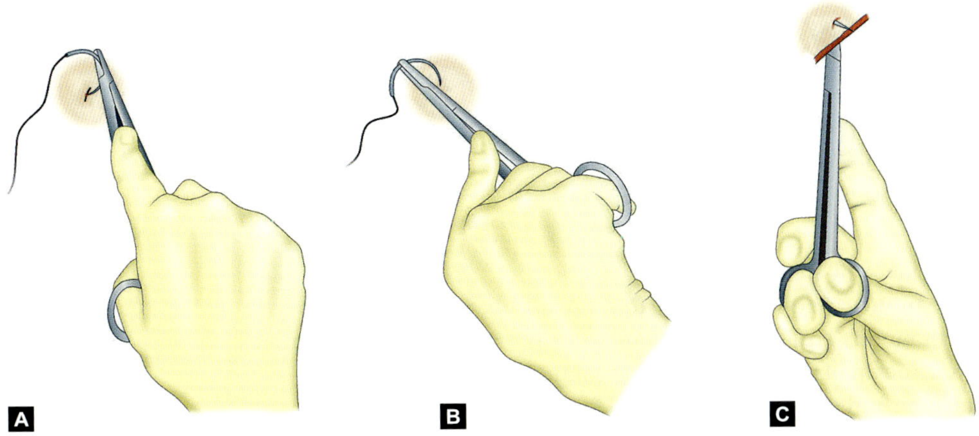

Figs. 15A to C: (A) Proper grip of the needle with hand—fully pronated; (B) Needle progressed along its arc by progressively supinating the hand; (C) Needle exits with fully supinated hand.

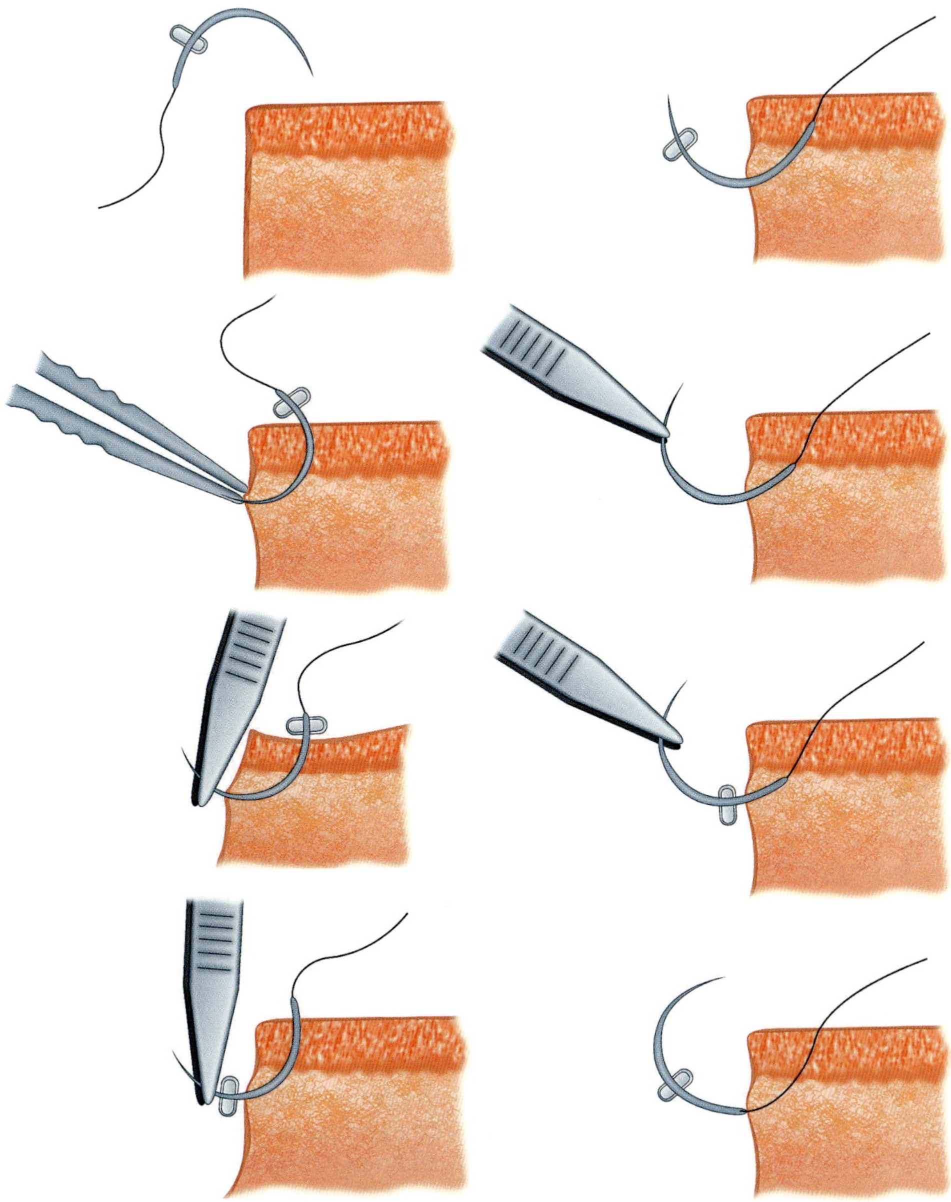

Fig. 16: Illustration showing exit of the needle with the help of fine forceps and needle holder.

Key Precautions

- Avoid picking up the needles with your fingers. Always use needle holder and forceps to control them.
- Place needles with other sharp instruments in a kidney tray when not in use. Never pass them hand-to-hand.

Knot Tying

Once the suture is satisfactorily placed, it must be secured with a knot **(Figs. 17 to 20)**. The instrument tie is used most commonly in cutaneous surgery. The square knot is traditionally used. First, the tip of the needle holder is rotated clockwise around the long end of the suture material for two complete turns. The tip of the needle holder is used to grasp the short end of the suture. The short end of the suture is pulled through the loops of the long end by crossing the hands, such that the two ends of the suture material are situated on opposite sides of the suture line. The needle holder is rotated counterclockwise once around the long end of the suture. The short end is grasped with the needle holder tip, and the short end is pulled through the loop again. First throw may get loosened while forming and tightening the second throw resulting in separation of skin edges. Rotate the threads clockwise or anticlockwise to lock them. As the second throw tightens, it unlocks the trapped first throw without giving it a chance to slacken. An effective method of preventing slippage is to ask your assistant to compress the tightened first throw with a finger or tip of the mosquito forceps, while you form and tighten the second throw, leading the tightening loop under the compressing finger or forceps **(Fig. 21)**.

- The suture should be tightened sufficiently to approximate the wound edges without constricting the tissue. Sometimes, leaving a small loop of suture after the second throw is helpful. This reserve loop allows the stitch to expand slightly and is helpful in preventing the strangulation of tissue because the tension exerted on the suture increases with increased wound edema.[10,31] Depending on the surgeon's preference, one to two additional throws may be added.
- Knot should be placed on one side of the wound for all sutures and not on the wound.

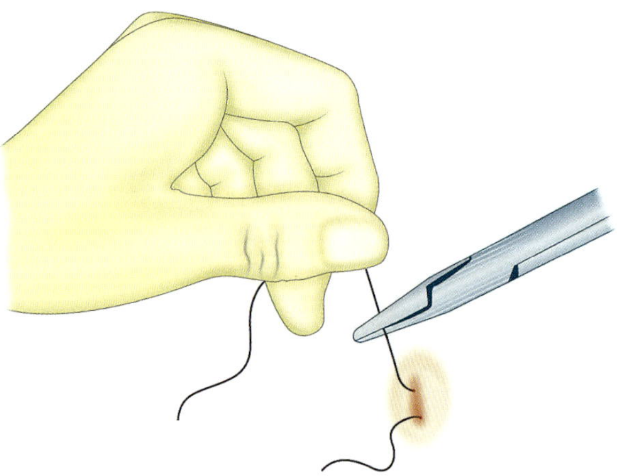

Fig. 17: Place the needle holder on the long thread.

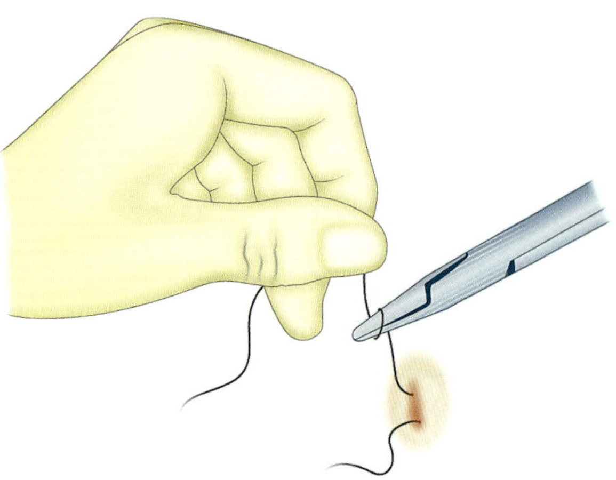

Fig. 18: Take a turn of the long thread around the needle holder.

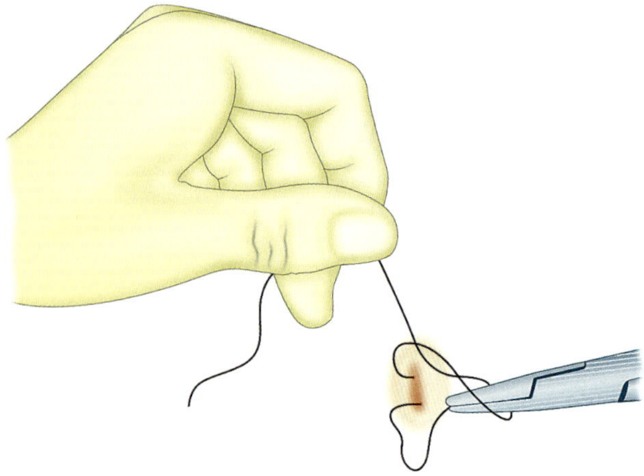

Fig. 19: Short end is grasped through the loop.

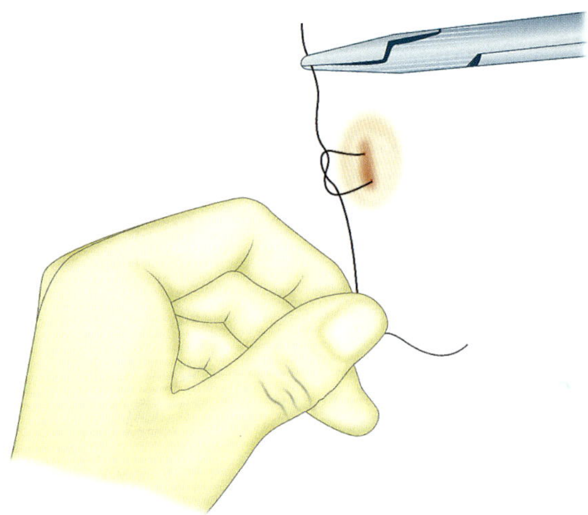

Fig. 20: Short end is pulled through the loop taking away from you while long end of the thread is drawn toward you.

- Properly squaring successive ties is important. That is, each tie must be laid down perfectly parallel to the previous tie. This procedure is important in preventing the creation of a granny knot, which tends to slip and is inherently weaker than a properly squared knot. When the desired number of throws is completed, the suture material may be cut off with scissors, leaving 0.5–1 cm of suture on either side of the knot (if interrupted stitches are used) or the next suture may be placed.

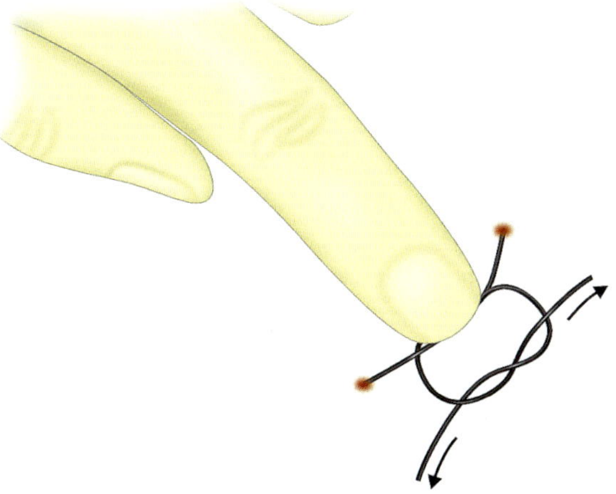

Fig. 21: Assistant compressing the tightened first throws with a finger while you form and tighten the second throw.

SUTURING TECHNIQUES

Different suturing techniques exist. It can be interrupted, continuous/running, or special sutures.

Tables 6 and 7 summarize the suturing patterns.

Interrupted Sutures

Simple Interrupted Sutures

The simple interrupted suture is the gold standard and the most commonly employed suture in cutaneous surgery.

Procedure: This suture is placed by inserting the needle perpendicular to the epidermis 1–2 mm from the skin edge, traversing the epidermis and the full thickness of the dermis, and exiting perpendicular to the epidermis on the opposite side of the wound. The two sides of the stitch should be symmetrically placed in terms of depth and width. This will minimize the possibility of mismatched wound-edge heights (i.e., stepping). In general, the final configuration of the suture should be flask shaped, that is, the stitch should be wider at its base (dermal side) than at its superficial portion (epidermal side) **(Fig. 22)**.[10] Such configuration prevents wound inversion.[32]

Distance between two sutures vary with the site of the wound and is approximately 3 mm on eyelid, 5 mm on face, and 1–2 cm at other sites.[33] Proper tension is important to

TABLE 6: Comparison of various interrupted sutures.

Properties	*Simple interrupted sutures*	*Vertical mattress sutures*	*Half-buried vertical mattress sutures*	*Pulley sutures*	*Far-near near-far modified vertical mattress sutures*	*Horizontal mattress suture*
Tensile strength	Moderate	High	Moderate	High	Moderate	High
Advantages	Less potential for wound edema and impaired circulation Allows expression of serum or blood from between sutures	Reduces dead space, maximizes wound eversion and minimizes wound tension	Eliminates two of four entry points of vertical mattress suture thus minimizes the scarring	Facilitates greater stretching of wound edges	Elevates the deeper tissue of the wound and evert the epidermis	Reduces dead space, everts wound edges, and reduces wound tension
Disadvantages	May leave a series of cross-hatched linear scars More time needed to tie individual knots	Greater risk of cross-hatching if not removed early	Risk of cross-hatching present but minimal	Risk of cross-hatching, if not removed early	Bites must be symmetrical or the wound will invariably misalign	Risk of strangulation of the dermal blood supply and edge necrosis is known, if tied too tightly
Uses	To approximate the wound edges of uneven thickness Most commonly employed suture in cutaneous surgery	In closing high-tension wounds	Used in cosmetically important areas such as face	Useful when additional wound closure strength is desired	Useful when tissue expansion is desired	Used as stay stich to temporarily approximate wound edges In thick glabrous skin (palms and soles)

TABLE 7: Comparison of various continuous and special sutures.

Properties	*Simple running sutures*	*Running horizontal mattress sutures*	*Running locked sutures*	*Dermal–subdermal sutures*	*Running subcuticular sutures*	*Running subcutaneous sutures*	*Half buried horizontal mattress sutures*	*Barbed sutures*
Tensile strength	Low	Moderate	High	Low	Low	Low	Low	Moderate
Advantages	Useful for long wounds in which wound tension has been minimized Allows rapid reapproximation of wound edges Less scarring compared to interrupted sutures	Allows good skin eversion Results in smoother and flatter scars as compared to simple running sutures	Useful in wounds under moderate tension and in those demanding additional hemostasis	Reduces dead space and wound tension	Provides best cosmetic outcome as it precisely approximates the wound edges	Used to close deep portion of surgical defects under moderate tension	Used primarily to position the corners and tips of flaps	Quicker wound closing time Reduces the amount of scar tissue
Disadvantages	Risk of dehiscence if the suture material ruptures Not as strong as interrupted sutures	Time consuming	Can cause tissue strangulation, if placed too tightly	Weaker than simple running sutures of skin	Does not provide significant wound strength Fails, if the suture is cut in just one place	Risk of suture breakage resulting in formation of dead space beneath the skin surface	May result in depressed scar	Skin dimpling around the suture placement
Uses	In split and full thickness skin graft Over eyelids, ears, dorsa of hands and scalp wounds especially when good hemostasis is expected	In areas with a high tendency for inversion, such as face and neck	In areas with good vascularization such as scalp	In wound closure following lipoma/large epidermal cyst excision	Valuable in areas where best cosmetic result is desired Useful in children when absorbable suture material is used	Subcutaneous closures	In M-plasties and V-Y closures	For face lift, breast reduction

ensure precise wound approximation while preventing tissue strangulation. Tight sutures cause ischemia, delay healing, and increase scarring.[29]

Advantages

- Interrupted sutures are easy to place and have greater tensile strength.
- They have less potential for causing wound edema and impaired cutaneous circulation when compared to running sutures.
- By altering the depth or angle of the needle, this technique can also be used to approximate the wound edges of uneven thickness.[5] While taking the simple interrupted sutures on the thicker tissue such as scalp, the needle is passed deep into the subcutaneous tissue and is curved slightly away from the wound edge so that a large chunk of tissue deep in the wound is encompassed. This helps in controlling bleeding too.
- It allows expression of serum or blood from between sutures.

Disadvantage: The major disadvantage of this technique is that they tend to leave a series of cross-hatched linear scars resembling railroad tracks.[34] The risk of cross-hatching can be minimized by removing sutures early to prevent the development of suture tracks.

Vertical Mattress Sutures

This is an excellent suturing method, which provides effective wound support.

Procedure: The vertical mattress suture is a variation of the simple interrupted suture. The needle is introduced 5–10 mm from the wound edge and a deep bite of tissue is taken before exiting the skin in the same position on the opposite wound edge. The needle is then reversed on the needle holder, and the needle is reintroduced 1–3 mm from the second side of the wound and a smaller bite of tissue is taken before exiting on the first side of the wound. A knot can then be secured as shown in **Figure 23**. The width of the stitch should be

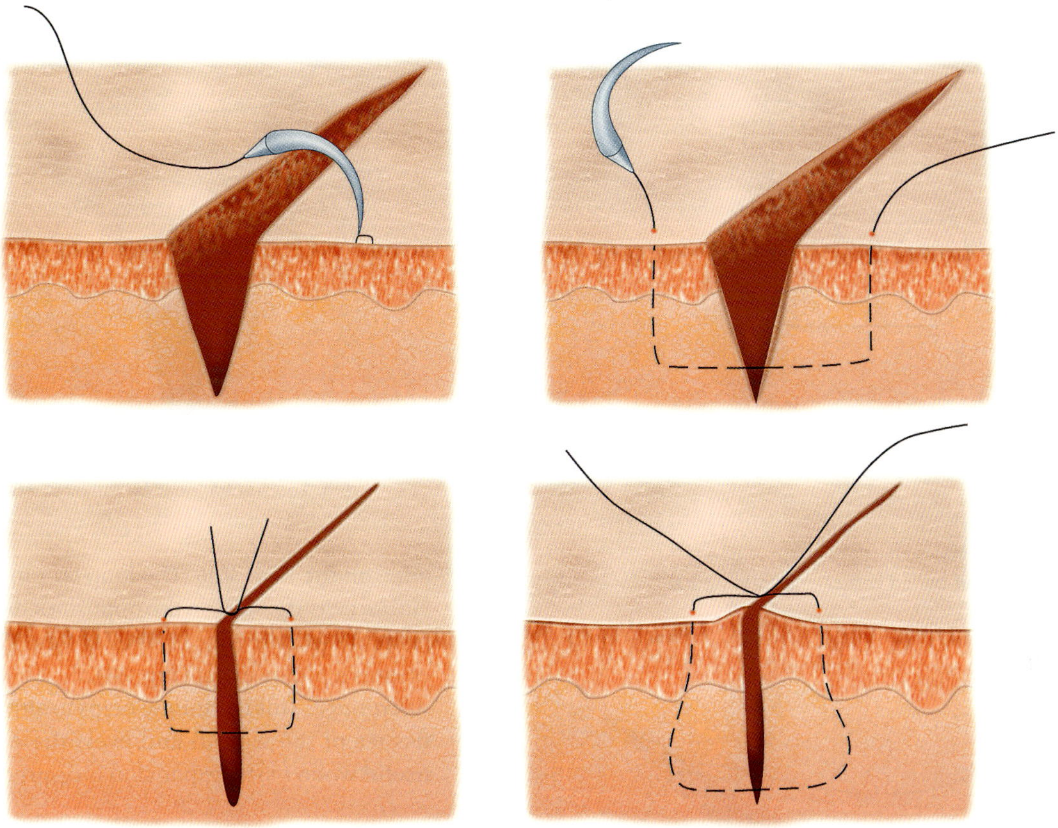

Fig. 22: Simple interrupted suture showing a flask-shaped stitch maximizing wound eversion.

increased in proportion to the amount of tension on the wound. That is, the higher the tension, the wider the stitch. Simple interrupted sutures may be placed in-between the vertical mattress sutures. Placing each stitch precisely and taking symmetric bites are especially important with this suture.[34-36]

Advantage: A vertical mattress suture is especially useful in maximizing wound eversion, reducing dead space, and minimizing tension across the wound.

Disadvantage: This suture tends to leave the most obvious and unsightly cross-hatching, if not removed early. The risk of cross-hatching is greater because of increased tension across the wound and the four entry and exit points of the stitch in the skin.

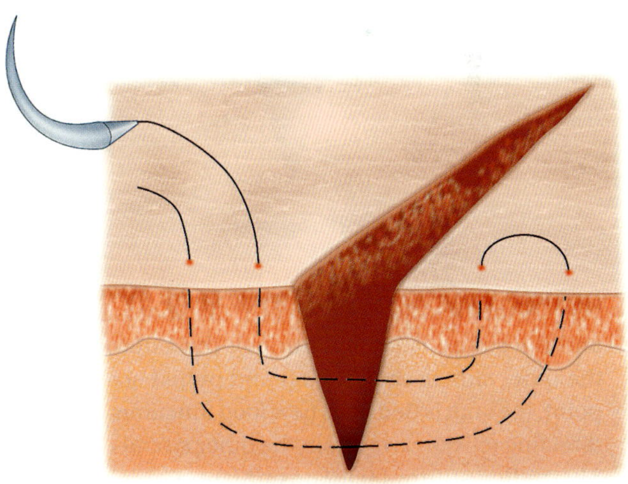

Fig. 23: Vertical mattress suture.

Modifications of the vertical mattress suture:

- *Half-buried vertical mattress sutures*: The half-buried vertical mattress suture is a modification of the vertical mattress suture and eliminates two of the four entry points, thereby reducing scarring **(Fig. 24)**. It helps in closing the dead space better than a simple interrupted suture. The half-buried vertical mattress suture is placed in the same manner as the vertical mattress suture, except that the needle penetrates the skin to the level of the deep part of the dermis on one side of the wound, takes a bite in the deep part of the dermis on the opposite side of the wound without exiting the skin, crosses back to the original side of the wound, and exits the skin. Entry and exit points therefore are kept on one side of the wound.[35,36]
  It is used in cosmetically important areas such as the face and along hairline where the suture marks on one side can be camouflaged by the hair.
- *Pulley sutures*: The pulley suture is a modification of the vertical mattress suture. When pulley sutures are used, a

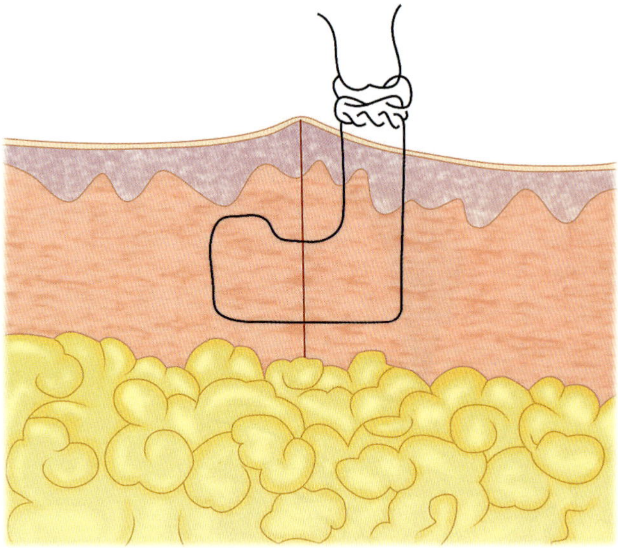

Fig. 24: Half-buried vertical mattress suture.

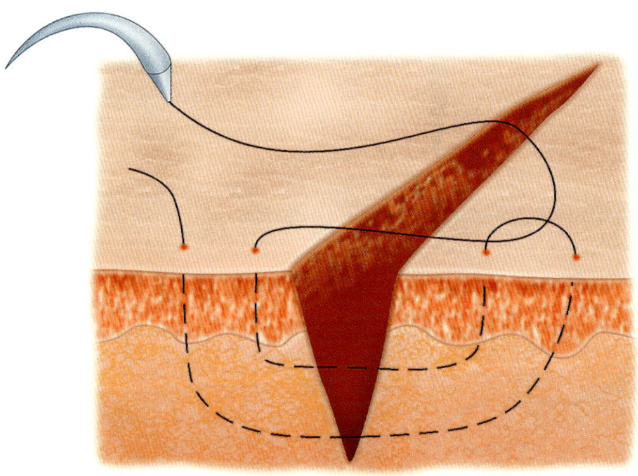

Fig. 25: Pulley stitch.

vertical mattress suture is placed, the knot is left untied, and the suture is looped through the external loop on the other side of the incision and pulled across. At this point, the knot is tied. This new loop functions as a pulley, directing tension away from the other strands **(Fig. 25)**. The pulley suture facilitates greater stretching of the wound edges and it is used when additional wound closure strength is desired.

- *Far-near near-far modified vertical mattress sutures*: Another stitch that serves the same function as the pulley suture is the far-near near-far modification of the vertical mattress suture **(Fig. 26)**.
  - *Procedure*: The first loop is placed approximately 4–6 mm from the wound edge on the far side and approximately 2 mm from the wound edge on the near side. The suture crosses the suture line and reenters the skin on the original side at 2 mm from the wound edge on the near side. The loop is completed and the suture exits the skin on the opposite side 4–6 mm away from the wound edge on the far side. This placement creates a pulley effect **(Fig. 26)**.[28]
  - *Advantage:* This technique helps to elevate the deeper tissues of the wound and evert the epidermis. It is useful when tissue expansion is desired.[34]

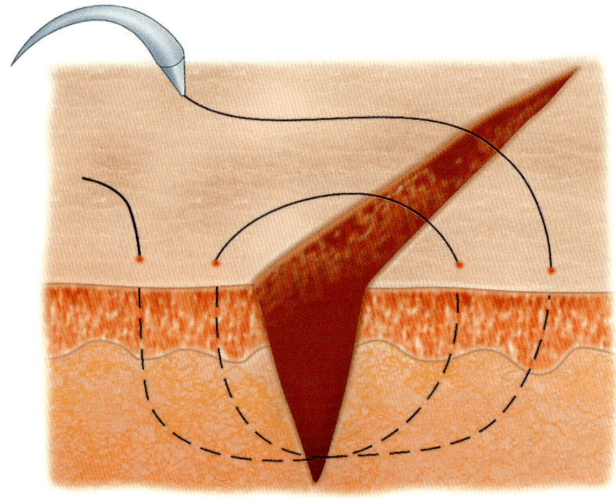

Fig. 26: Far-near near-far pulley stitch.

Horizontal Mattress Suture

This is used to reduce the dead space and evert wound edges and helps to reduce high wound tension.[24]

Procedure:[33,34] The horizontal mattress suture is placed by entering the skin 5–10 mm from the wound edge. A deep bite of tissue is taken before exiting the skin in the same position on the opposite wound edge. The needle re-enters the skin on the same side of the suture line 5–10 mm laterally. The needle is then passed dermally or subcutaneously to the side of initial penetration and the knot is tied on the surface **(Fig. 27)**.

Advantages:

- This is particularly useful in thick glabrous skin (palms and soles).[34]
- This may also be used as a stay stitch to temporarily approximate wound edges allowing placement of simple interrupted or subcuticular stitches. The temporary stitches are removed after the tension is evenly distributed across the wound. However, they have a high risk of producing suture marks, if left in place for longer than 7 days. According to few surgeons, horizontal mattress sutures are superior to their vertical counterparts.[33]

Disadvantage: Theoretical risk of strangulation of the dermal blood supply and subsequent edge necrosis, if tied too tightly, is its chief disadvantage.[33] Taking generous bites, using bolsters, tying knots only as tightly as necessary to approximate the wound edges and removing the sutures as early as possible may decrease the risk.

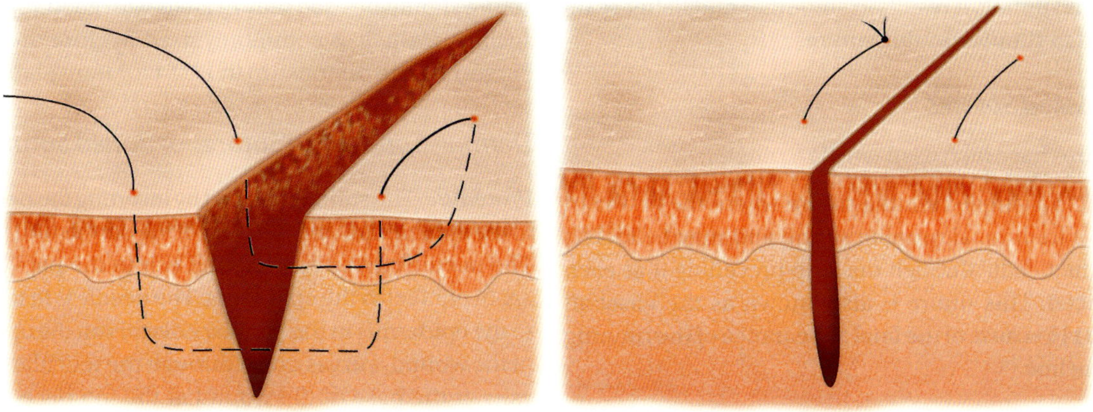

Fig. 27: Horizontal mattress suture.

Continuous (Running) Sutures

Simple Running Sutures

The simple running suture, otherwise also called as continuous over-and-over suture, is an uninterrupted series of simple interrupted sutures **(Fig. 28)**.[24]

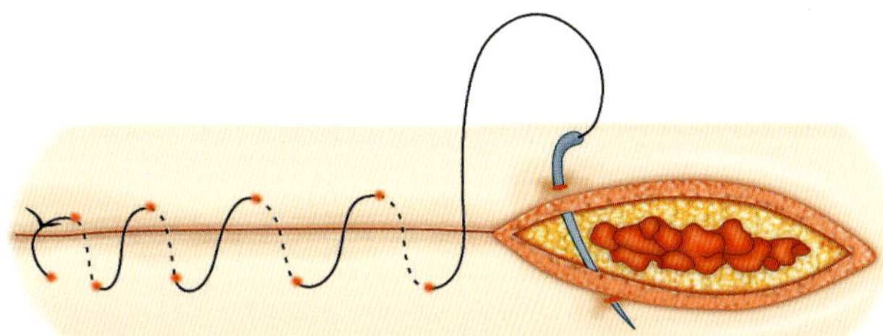

Fig. 28: Simple continuous suture.

Procedure: The suture is started by placing a simple interrupted stitch, which is tied but not cut. A series of simple sutures are placed in succession without tying or cutting the suture material after each pass. Sutures should be evenly spaced, and tension should be evenly distributed along the suture line. The line of stitches is completed by tying a knot after the last pass at the end of the suture line. The knot is tied between the tail end of the suture material where it exits the wound and the loop of the last suture placed **(Fig. 29)**.[33]

Advantages:

- Running sutures are useful for long wounds in which wound tension has been minimized with properly placed deep sutures and in which approximation of the wound edges is good.[34]
- Quicker placement and more rapid reapproximation of wound edges, compared with simple interrupted sutures.
- This type of suture may be used to secure a split or full-thickness skin graft. It is also useful over eyelids, ears, and the dorsa of hands.[33]
- Less scarring occurs with running sutures compared with interrupted sutures because fewer knots are made with simple running sutures; however, the number of needle insertions remains the same.
- Continuous sutures can also be placed in a locking fashion to provide hemostasis by compression of wound edges especially in scalp wound closures.

Disadvantages:

- Possible cross-hatching
- The risk of dehiscence, if the suture material ruptures
- Difficulty in making fine adjustments along the suture line
- Can strangulate the blood supply, if wounds tension is high
- It is not as strong as interrupted sutures.

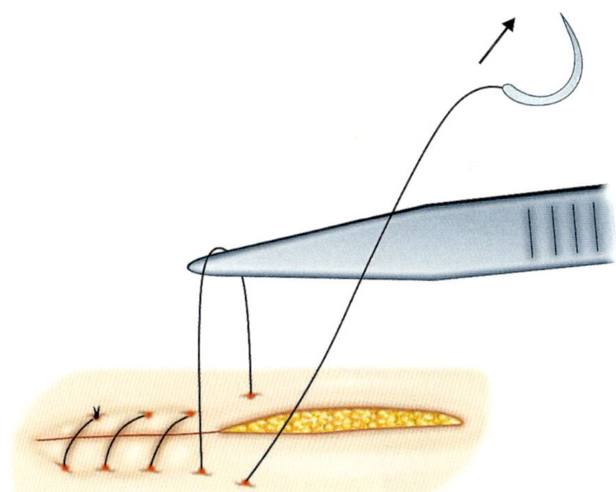

Fig. 29: Control the thread loop with fine forceps, as it is tightened to ensure that it sits perfectly without snagging on other structures.

Running Horizontal Mattress Sutures

Procedure: A simple suture is placed, and the knot is tied but not cut. Instead of crossing over the wound prior to reentering the skin, the running horizontal mattress suture is done by re-entering the skin on the same side through which the suture material is exited **(Fig. 30)**.[30,34] The final loop is tied to the free end of the suture material.

Advantages: The running horizontal mattress suture is used for skin eversion. It is useful in areas with a high tendency for inversion, such as the neck. It can also be useful for reducing the spread of facial scars. Although this technique is slightly more time consuming, it results in smoother and flatter scars as compared to simple running sutures.[30]

Running Locked Sutures

Locked sutures have increased tensile strength.

Procedure: It is a simple running suture where the first knot is tied as in a traditional running suture and may be locked by passing the needle through the loop preceding it as each stitch is placed. This suture is also known as the baseball stitch **(Fig. 31)** because of the final appearance of the running locked suture line.[28]

Advantage: They are useful in wounds under moderate tension or in those requiring additional hemostasis.

Disadvantage: They increase the risk of impairing the microcirculation surrounding the wound and thus can cause tissue strangulation, if placed too tightly. Therefore, this type of suture should be used only in areas with good vascularization such as scalp. It is commonly used to close the donor after harvesting the donor strip in FUT hair transplant surgery.

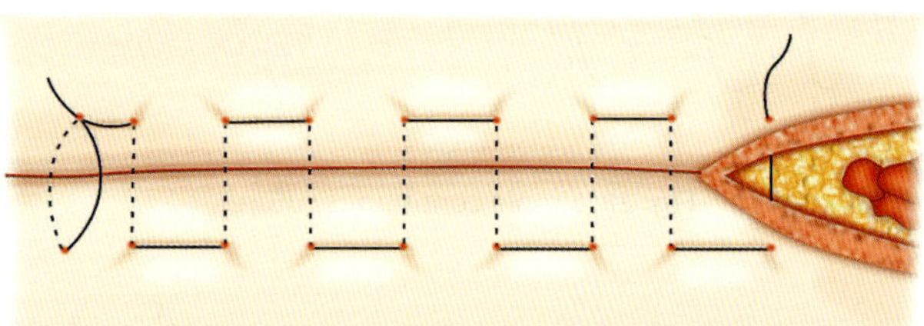

Fig. 30: Running horizontal mattress suture.

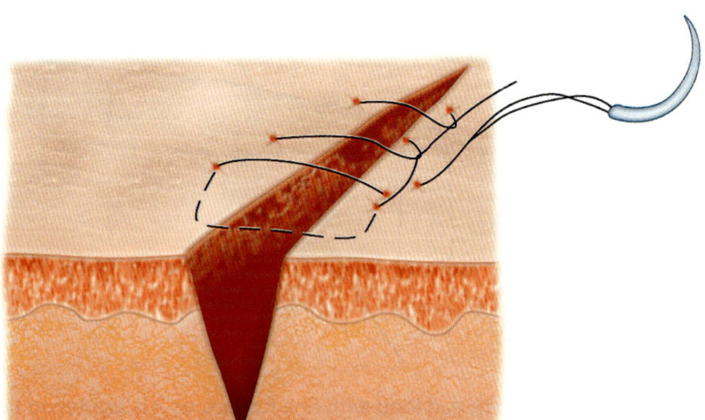

Fig. 31: Running locked suture.

Dermal–Subdermal Sutures or Buried Sutures

Procedure: The suture is placed by inserting the needle parallel to the epidermis at the junction of the dermis and the subcutis. The needle curves upward and exit in the papillary dermis, again parallel to the epidermis. The needle is inserted parallel to the epidermis in the papillary dermis on the opposing edge of the wound, curves down through the reticular dermis, and exits at the base of the wound at the interface between the dermis and the subcutis and parallel to the epidermis. The knot is tied at the base of the wound and the excess remnant of the suture tail is cut off. This will minimize the possibility of tissue reaction and extrusion of the knot. If the suture is placed more superficially in the dermis at 2–4 mm from the wound edge, eversion is increased.[28]

Advantages: It reduces dead space and redistributes wound tension. It provides prolonged dermal support reducing changes of wound dehiscence. It is used in closing the wound following excision of lipoma or any large epidermal cyst. These sutures are not cut in the postoperative period and thus absorbable suture material is used. If placed well, they reduce the need for multiple epidermal sutures and also can be combined with alternative methods such as adhesives and staples.

Possible pitfalls while placing buried sutures:

- Very superficial placement of buried sutures may cause extrusion of the suture material from the surface
- Unevenly placed sutures with vertical disparity may result in step-off deformity of the wound edges **(Fig. 32)**. To avoid this, the suture must be kept at the same vertical level on both edges of the wound.
  Proper undermining of the wound edges can ease the proper placement of the buried sutures.

Modifications of the buried suture:

- *Buried vertical mattress suture*: This suture is placed by entering in the subcutaneous tissue while arcing the needle along the curve upward toward the superficial

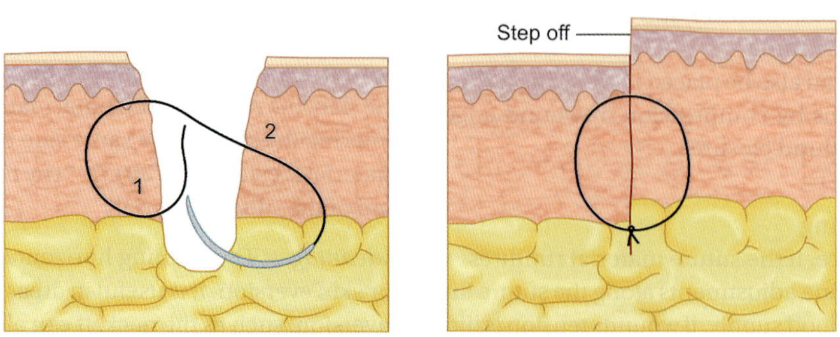

Fig. 32: Step-off deformity.

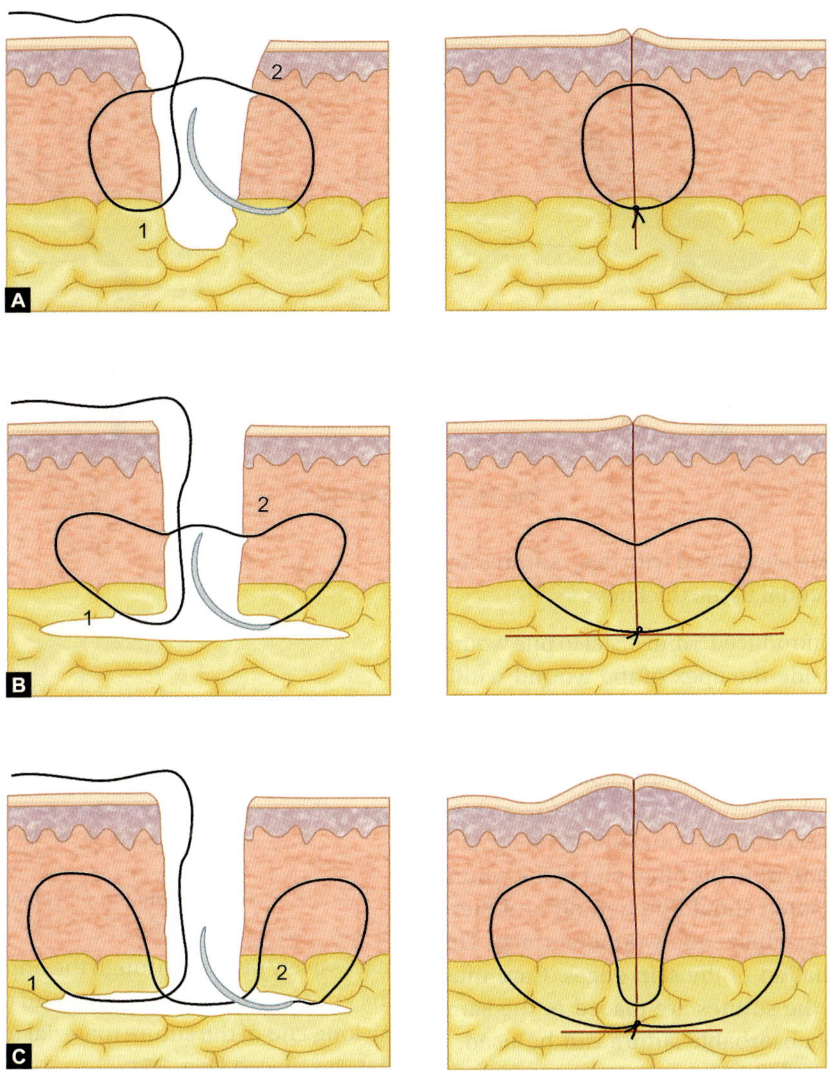

Figs. 33A to C: Buried mattress suture and its modifications. (A) Classical buried dermal suture with mild wound edge eversion; (B) Buried vertical mattress suture with more wound edge eversion; (C) Butterfly buried vertical mattress suture with greatest wound edge eversion. (1 and 2 are points of entry of the needle).

dermis and exiting along the mid-dermis along the wound edge **(Fig. 33)**. A mirror image of this done on the opposite wound edge as well—entering the mid dermis, arcing toward the upper reticular dermis, and exiting in the deeper subcutaneous tissue along the wound edge and the knot is tied deep as in the buried suture. This kind of "looping of the dermis" helps in prolonged wound eversion.

- *Buried butterfly suture:* Sufficient undermining is necessary before placing this stitch. This modification creates further wound eversion than the buried vertical mattress suture. In this suture, the needles enter the undersurface of the flap along the subcutaneous tissue, with the needle arcing upward toward the reticular dermis and exiting along the undersurface of the flap along the wound edge at the level of the subcutis. A similar "loop" is created on the opposite side, like the wing of a butterfly, entering proximally at the subcutis level on the wound edge, arcing upward through the dermis, and exiting distally away from the wound edge **(Fig. 33)**.

  When this suture is pulled and knot is tied, there is redistribution of the wound tension in the tissues surrounding the wound edge, which may cause temporary dimpling and irregularity of the skin surface, and eversion of the epidermal wound edges. This irregularity later resolves as the suture disintegrates over time and a thin line scar is obtained.

Running Subcuticular Sutures

The running subcuticular suture is a buried form of the running horizontal mattress suture.[5] It is valuable in areas in which the best possible cosmetic result is desired. The suture does not provide significant wound strength, although it does precisely approximate the wound edges. Therefore, the running subcuticular suture is best reserved for wounds in

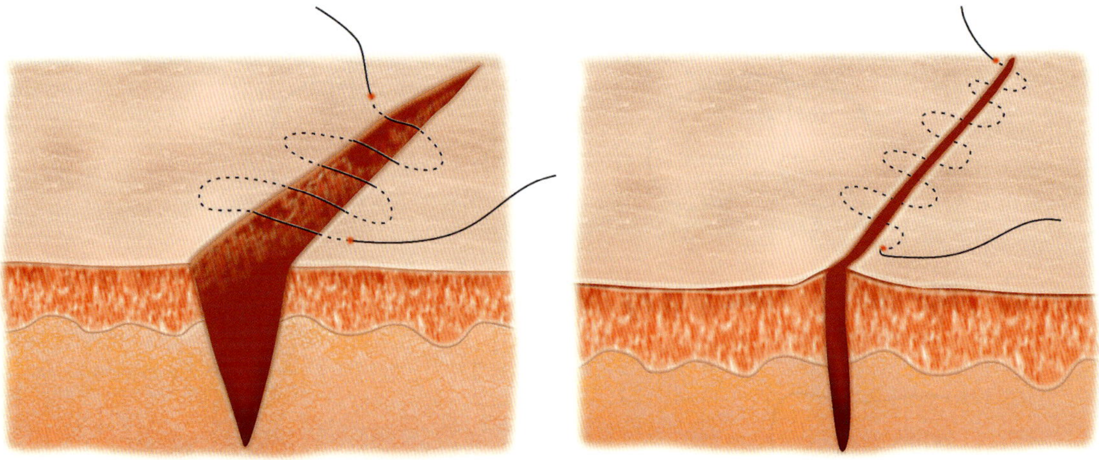

Fig. 34: Subcuticular stitch.

which the tension has been eliminated with deep sutures and for closing wounds with equal tissue thickness.[33,34]

Procedure: The needle is introduced 5 mm distal to one wound end and brought out inside the apex of the wound within the dermis. The free end of suture can be tied off on itself or secured with a bead or crimp. Horizontal bites through the papillary dermis parallel to the skin surface are then taken from alternating sides of the wound working toward the other wound apex. The second epidermal puncture is made when the needle exits 5 mm from the other end of the wound **(Fig. 34)**. Both ends of stitch should be tied off and Steri-Strips may be applied to stabilize the wound surface. This provides close approximation of the skin edges. Care must be taken to ensure that the sutures are placed at the same level. Absorbable or nonabsorbable suture can be used. If absorbable sutures are used, first subcutaneous interrupted sutures should be taken prior to running subcuticular suture. Among nonabsorbable sutures, polypropylene (prolene), which is a monofilament suture with minimal drag, is ideal, and it should be removed at 1–2 weeks after suturing.[33]

Advantages:

- It results in an excellent cosmetic outcome. Since the epidermis is penetrated only at the beginning and end of the suture line, the subcuticular suture effectively eliminates the risk of cross-hatching and no suture marks are visible.
- It is known to be a useful technique in children when absorbable suture is used so that suture removal is avoided.[34]

Disadvantage: Like any of the running sutures, it is quicker to perform but fails if the suture is cut in just one place.

Running Subcutaneous Sutures

The running subcutaneous suture begins with a simple interrupted subcutaneous suture, which is tied but not cut. The suture is looped through the subcutaneous tissue by successively passing through the opposite sides of the wound. The knot is tied at the opposite end of the wound by knotting the long end of the suture material to the loop of the last pass that was placed **(Fig. 35)**.[35]

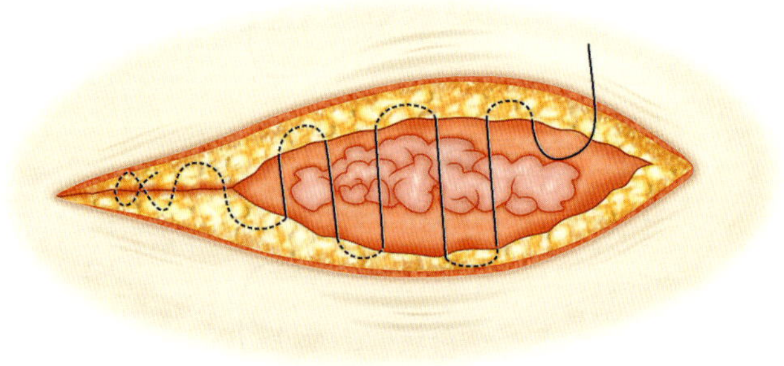

Fig. 35: Running subcutaneous sutures.

Advantage: It is used to close the deep portion of surgical defects under moderate tension.

Disadvantage: It has the risk of suture breakage and the formation of dead space beneath the skin surface.

Special Suturing Techniques

These include tips sutures, purse-string suture, and barbed sutures.

Tip Sutures

They are special sutures, which have a vital role in flap surgeries, as they can keep the flaps in place without causing much damage to flaps.

Commonly used tip sutures are described here:

- *Half-buried horizontal mattress sutures*:
  Procedure: The half-buried horizontal mattress suture or tip stitch begins on the side of the wound on which the flap is to be attached **(Fig. 36)**.[3] The suture is passed through the dermis of the wound edge to the dermis of the flap tip.

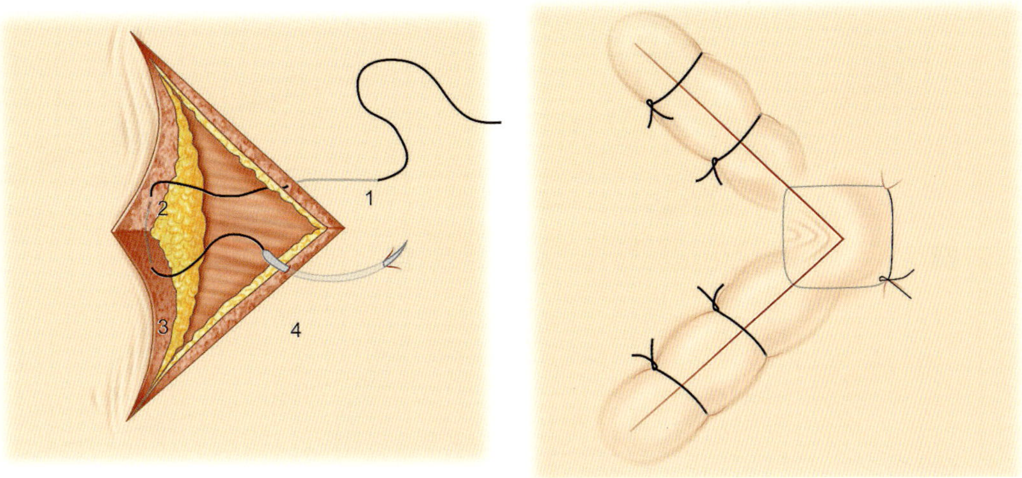

Fig. 36: Tip stitch.

The needle is passed laterally in the same dermal plane of the flap tip, exits the flap tip, and reenters the skin to which the flap is to be attached. The needle is directed perpendicularly and exits the skin; then, the knot is tied.[20]

Advantages:

- Tip stitch is used primarily to position the corners and tips of flaps and to perform M-plasties and V-Y closures.[33]
- It helps to have the knots on one side of the suture line with no suture marks on the other side. For example, when insetting the areola in breast reduction, this technique leaves the suture marks on the dark, pebbly areola instead of on the breast skin.

Disadvantage: In larger flaps with greater tension, this technique has been reported to position the flap tip deeper than the surrounding tissue, often resulting in a depressed scar.[33]

- *Modified half-buried horizontal mattress sutures*: This stitch places an additional vertical mattress suture superficial to the half-buried horizontal mattress suture.[37] A small skin hook instead of forceps is used to avoid trauma of the flap.
- *Deep tip stitch*: The deep tip stitch is essentially a full-buried form of the three corner stitch.[38] The suture is placed into the deep dermis of the wound edge to which the flap is to be attached, passed through the dermis of the flap tip, and inserted into the deep dermis of the opposite wound edge.

Purse–String Suture (Fig. 37)

It is a buried horizontal mattress suture, which is placed in the mid-to-deep part of the dermis to prevent the skin from tearing. This closure provides uniform tension to the wound, enhances hemostasis at the tissue edge, and significantly decreases the size of the defect thus offering excellent long-term cosmetic and functional results.[39]

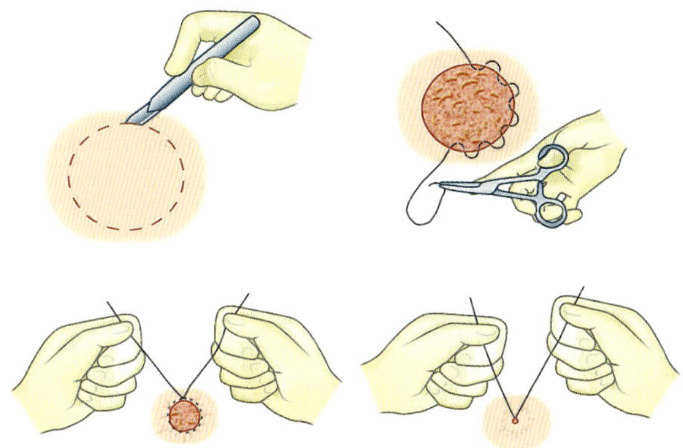

Fig. 37: Purse–string suture.

The purse–string suture may be most appropriate for primary closure for small skin defects or as a partial closure for larger round wounds. It is useful following the local excision of both melanoma and nonmelanoma skin cancer. In addition, this technique is especially suitable for patients who insist on maintaining an active lifestyle in the immediate postoperative period, individuals concurrently being treated with anticoagulants, antiplatelet agents, or both, and people with extensive postoperative defects that would otherwise require either a skin graft or a large cutaneous flap. However, if tied too tightly, the suture may strangulate the approximated tissue.[28]

Tape Buttress Technique

This is a simple yet interesting technique described by Davis et al.[40] in areas where the skin is thin, sun damaged, or atrophic, and there are chances of tissue tearing and the suture cutting through the wound edge. This can often happen along the upper extremities or near the shin.

In this technique, surgical strips or tapes are placed parallel to the axis of the wound bed along the edge and then simple interrupted sutures or mattress sutures are placed through the strips that act as a buttress.

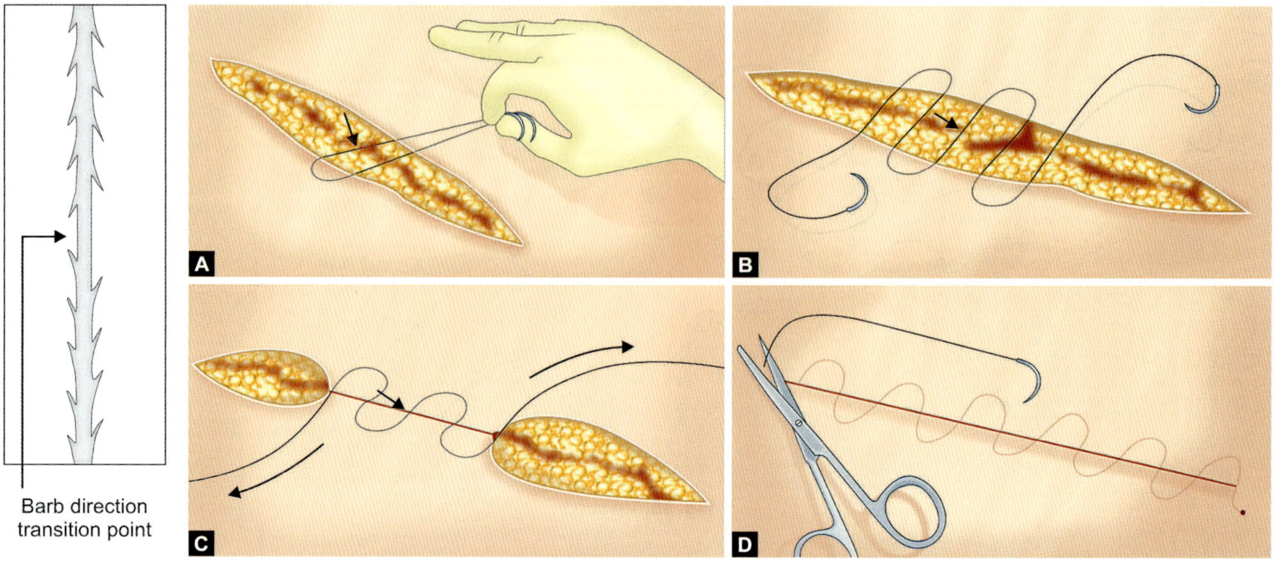

Figs. 38A to D: Simple wound closure with bidirectional barbed suture. (A) Start by taking one end of the suture and pull it through until the transition zone has reached the tissue; (B) Taking one end of the suture, we must complete at least two loose bites or arcs through the tissue. Then a few more bites are taken with the other end of the suture in similar fashion; (C) Each of the strands are then grasped and pulled and the tissue is approximated to the desired tension; (D) The bites are continued sinusoidally until the ends of the wounds are approximated. The last bite is taken about 1 cm beyond the wound exiting the skin and the suture cut flush with the skin.

Barbed Sutures

The use of self-retaining barbed sutures in wound closure is a relatively recent advance and is a particularly important evolutionary step in development of newer suture materials providing a technology that would avoid the need to tie knots. It was first adopted by plastic surgeons for use in various minimally invasive percutaneous rejuvenation procedures such as facial thread lifting and cosmetic breast surgeries. They can be either absorbable (polydioxanone) or nonabsorbable (polypropylene) variations with microscopic etching that creates the effect of many barbs. The barbes may be placed in a single direction as in unidirectional barbed sutures (used in rejuvenation procedures such as thread lifting) or they may change direction in the middle of the suture as in bidirectional barbed sutures (used in wound closure) **(Figs. 38A to D)**.[41]

The technique to place a barbed suture differs from that of a traditional suture. The thickness of the needle is kept smaller than the thickness of the suture material itself to give better grip inside the tissue through which it passes. When only the full thickness of the skin and subcutaneous fat is to be approximated, an absorbable bidirectional suture can be passed from the center of the wound to each end, exiting about 1 cm from the wound edge. The suture is cut flush with the skin at each end **(Figs. 38A to D)**.

Advantage: The chief advantage is the avoidance of suture knots, which facilitates improved blood supply to wound edges, resulting in quicker wound closing time.[42] The knotless configuration greatly reduces the amount of scar tissue that is created during healing in vivo.

Disadvantage: Barbed sutures may result in suture extrusion especially when sutures, 2.0 or greater, are placed too close to the superficial dermis.[41] They also carry an increased risk of infections. Barbed sutures are costlier than their regular counterparts and therefore are preferred predominantly for cosmetic surgeries. Most importantly, their placement demands experience and skill, as it would be difficult to correct a wrongly placed suture.

SUTURE REMOVAL (FIG. 39)

Proper suture removal technique is important to maintain good results after sutures are executed. Prompt removal reduces the risk of suture marks, infection, and tissue reaction.[5,34] To prevent dehiscence and spread of the scar, sutures should not be removed too soon. As a general rule, the greater the tension across a wound, the longer the sutures should remain in place. Sutures should be removed within 1–2 weeks of their placement, depending on the anatomic location as mentioned in **Table 8**.

Interrupted Suture

After cleansing the interrupted suture with antiseptic solution, one end of the suture should be grasped with forceps and pulled gently toward one side of the wound, elevating the knot. The opposite side of the suture should then be cut with fine suture scissors immediately under the knot **(Fig. 35)**.[5] Then, the suture is grasped by the knot and gently pulled toward the wound or suture line until the suture material is completely removed. If the suture is pulled away from the suture line, the wound edges may separate. Wound should be examined for

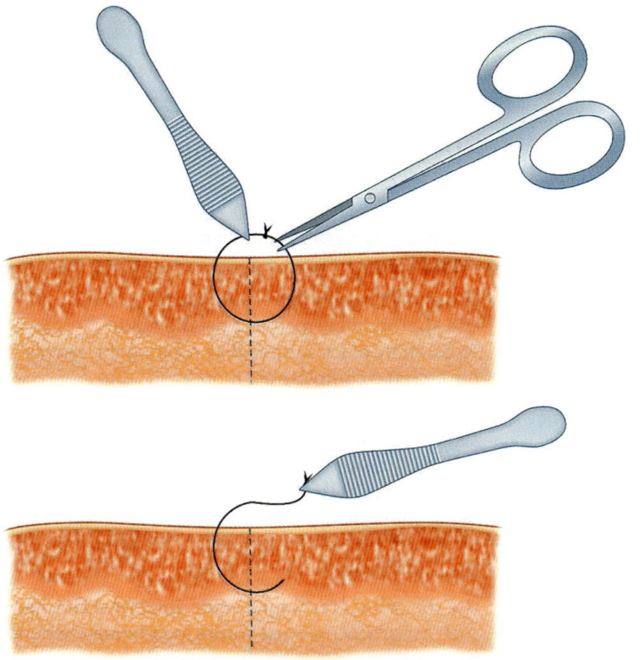

Fig. 39: Suture removal.

TABLE 8: Removal of suture as per anatomic location.

Anatomic location	*Days of suture removal postimplantation*
Face and ears	5–7
Eyelids	3–5
Neck	7
Scalp	10
Trunk and upper extremities	10–14
Lower extremities	14–21

any leftover sutures. Steri-Strips may be applied with a tissue adhesive to provide continued supplemental wound support after the sutures are removed.

When multiple sutures are taken, alternate sutures are removed and the wound should be examined for dehiscence. If the wound has healed completely, all sutures can be removed. If dehiscence is seen, remaining sutures are left intact, which have to be removed 4–7 days later.

Running Suture

A running suture is removed by cutting its every other loop and grasping the intervening loop with forceps and pulling it out.[5]

Running Subcuticular Suture

A running subcuticular suture is removed by cutting the knot at one end and pulling the suture out slowly from the other end to minimize the risk of suture breakage in the wound.[5,34]

CHOOSING THE RIGHT SUTURING TECHNIQUE(S)

The ideal skin closure technique should:[43]

- Precisely approximate the wound edges
- Provide adequate eversion
- Reduce tension along the skin edges
- Be relatively fast for the dermatosurgeon to complete the closure
- Leave minimal or no suture marks and provide maximum cosmetic outcome
- Be planned according to relaxed skin tension lines.

The best technique will vary depending on the size and location of the wound or defect and the intrinsic nature of the skin based on its site. One of the most standard techniques involves closure of the deeper dermis layer with buried sutures to approximate the skin edges and reduce the tension, followed by simple or vertical mattress interrupted or running sutures.

There are certain advanced techniques of closure of deep tissue, in order to relieve wound tension. These include suspension,[44] fascial plication,[45] imbrication,[46] ImPli stitch,[47] and corset plication[48] among others. The details of these are beyond the scope of this book and we encourage the readers to read the references indicated for further learning.

Beyond reducing the wound tension, it is important to ensure proper wound edge apposition to facilitate maximum contact between the adjacent wound edges and good wound edge eversion. Achieving wound edge eversion is of prime importance for improving overall scar cosmesis, especially in areas such as the face, than in the trunk. Whenever maximum wound eversion is desired, this can be done with the help of both buried sutures (and its modifications) and vertical or horizontal mattress sutures.

In areas such as the scalp, where excessive bleeding is anticipated, techniques such as running locking suture and horizontal mattress suture may help to ensure hemostasis. However, they must be executed with caution so as to prevent strangulation of wound edges and tissue necrosis.

COMMON COMPLICATIONS WHILE SUTURING

Surgical repair of a wound may be associated with certain snags or complications such as slippage of the knot, breaking of the suture thread, bending of the needle, postsurgical suture track marks on the wound, and so on. These can occur as a result of common errors of the dermatosurgeon with respect to selection of the appropriate suture material or suturing technique for a particular wound in question. These common pitfalls, the possible error, and how to prevent and/or manage the same have been mentioned in the **Table 9**. If the error or complication has been identified early, it is best that it is corrected at the earliest, preferably at the time of the

TABLE 9: Common complications while suturing.

Complication	*Possible error*	*How to prevent or correct*
Slippage of the knot	• High wound tension • Use of materials such as polypropylene or Nylon which have high friction coefficient	• Increase the number of throws while knotting to prevent slippage • An assistant could help holding the wound edges together while tying the knot
Breaking of suture while tying	• High wound tension • Selection of suture material with low tensile strength or fine caliber	• Adequate undermining to reduce the wound tension • Use suture with larger caliber or higher tensile strength
Bending of the needle	• Using too fine or small needle • Mismatched large size of needle holder with too much pressure • Insufficient "arc-motion" while suturing	• Use an adequately larger size needle • Use appropriately matched needle holder • To correctly place suture while rotating the needle through the complete arc motion
Suture track marks or Railroad marks	• Delayed removal of sutures • Sutures tied too tightly • High caliber suture or needle used	• Remove sutures at the earliest possible. If the "wound allows", can remove at least alternate sutures early • Use finest caliber needle and suture possible for epidermal closure • Avoid strangulation of the tissue while tying the knot. Knot must be tight enough to allow approximation of the wound edges.
Wound edge inversion	• Incorrectly placed buried sutures or epidermal sutures	• Use the correct technique while epidermal closure such as vertical mattress suture for adequate wound eversion • Arc the needle slightly away from the edge while placing the top stitch • Loop a good portion of the dermis while placing the buried suture
Incision step-off	• Unevenly placed sutures • Unequal distance of the point of entry and exit of either side of the wound edge • Wrongly placed dermal sutures	• Cut off the wrongly or unevenly placed suture on table and place corrective interrupted suture

surgery itself. This can improve the surgical and/or cosmetic outcome without having the need of a possible scar revision at a later date.

ALTERNATIVE WOUND CLOSURE METHODS

While the most common method of closing a wound is with sutures, other materials such as skin tapes, staples, or wound adhesives are also useful in certain situations.[33]

Skin Tapes

Wound closure tapes (e.g., Steri-Strips and CoverStrips) are reinforced microporous nonocclusive material (e.g., paper, plastic, and Rayon fabric) backed by a thin film of acrylic polymer adhesive **(Fig. 40)**.[7] Adhesive tapes are used most frequently as adjunctive wound support after staples or sutures are removed, in conjunction with buried dermal sutures, or with absorbable running subcuticular sutures in low-tension wounds.[49]

Procedure

It is important to first obtain good hemostasis and eversion of the wound edges before using the wound closure tapes. An adhesive solution such as tincture of Benzoin or Mastisol

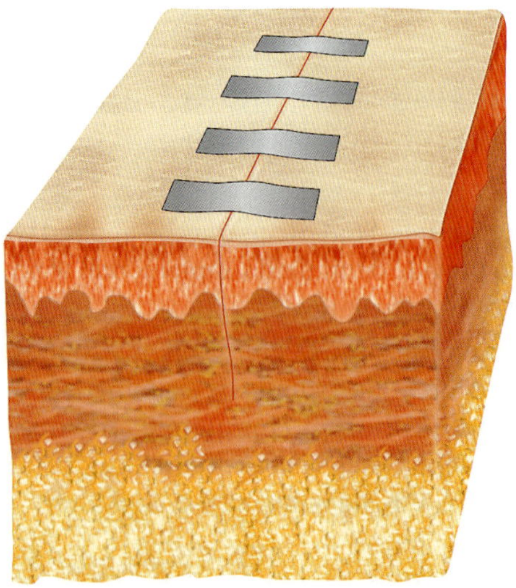

Fig. 40: Skin tapes.

(Ferndale Laboratories, Inc., Ferndale, MI) may be applied to the skin before using tapes to enhance its adhesive property.[7,8] Once the adhesive has dried to a tacky feel, strips of tapes should be placed perpendicularly across the wound without overlapping one another. Tapes that are kept dry and clean may remain adherent for up to 1–2 weeks. Tapes have little usefulness in hairy or highly mobile areas. Moisture, soap, and wound exudate decrease the duration of tape adhesion.

Advantages

- They can effectively approximate the low tension wound edges, relieve tension, and prevent inversion of the wound edges.[33]
- They provide extra support to a suture line, when running subcuticular sutures are used or following staples wound closure technique.
- They also provide added strength to the wound when used after suture removal and improve cosmetic outcome.

Disadvantage

They are rarely adequate for primary wound closure.

Staples

The principle of mechanical staplers in surgery is exactly the same as paper stapling machines.[3,33] Staples are formed from high-quality stainless steel and are easy to place. They are primarily used in the closure of wounds under high tension on the trunk, extremities, and scalp. In dermatological surgery, they are commonly used for closing scalp reductions or to close donor site during hair transplantation.[10] They are also useful to position a skin closure or flap temporarily before suturing and to secure split-thickness skin grafts.[8,10] A novel high purity magnesium alloy has been employed to produce biodegradable staples.[50]

Procedure

The central section of the "U"-shaped staple is held while the outer ends are pushed through the skin and then bent so that the ends meet, forming a closed ring **(Fig. 41)**.[33] They are removed by straightening the base of the "U" to open out the ends so that the staples can be withdrawn.

Advantages

- They are particularly useful for long incisions, as they may shorten the wound closure time by 70–80%
- Decreased risk of infection
- Improved wound eversion
- Minimal tissue reactivity.

Disadvantages[10,33]

- Less precise wound approximation and the need for a second operator to evert and reapproximate skin edges during staple placement.
- Staples must be removed early to prevent cross-hatch skin marks.
- They are contraindicated in finely contoured areas, over bony prominences, or in highly mobile areas.
- The cost is usually more than that of suture material.

Skin Clips

Skin clips are novel noninvasive, painless, needle-free, and easy-to-apply wound closure devices that neither require anesthesia injections nor create additional damage to the wound area (e.g., DermaClip and Medline™ Skin Closure Clips).

Procedure

The DermaClip device is applied to the approximated edges of a wound and is closed by pulling the polypropylene tabs in opposing directions until a "click" is heard, indicating that the device is locked **(Fig. 42)**. As the device closes, the angled faces of the polypropylene bridge encounter each other and

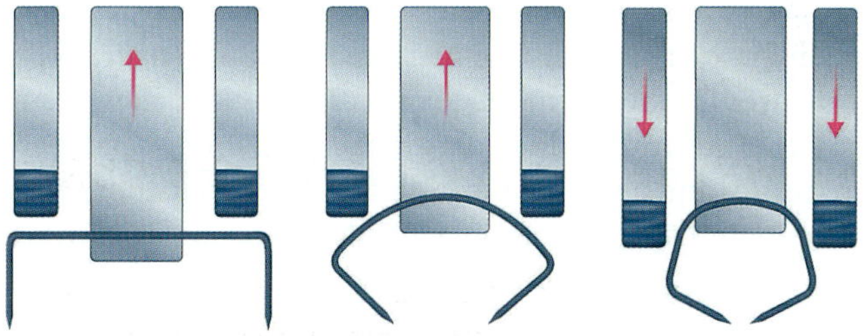

Fig. 41: Skin staples.

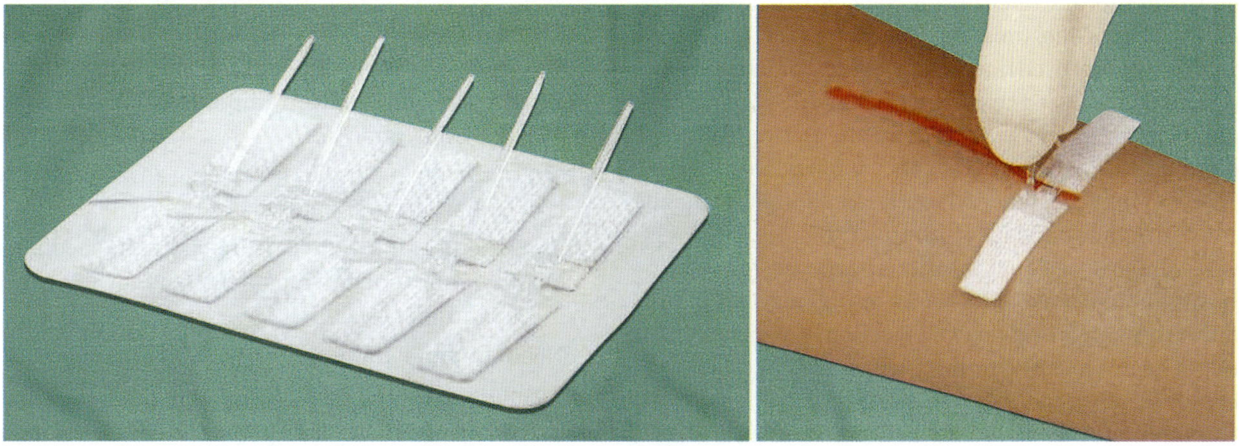

Fig. 42: DermaClip.

create a lifting action of the wound edges, putting the viable dermis on each side of the wound into contact.[51]

Advantages

- Unlike tissue adhesives, DermaClip can be used on large as well as small wounds.
- It is easy to use and handle than tissue glues.
- It does not cause burning sensation on unanesthetized wounds when compared to tissue glues.
- It can be easily used in emergency rooms or warfronts by even untrained personnel.

Disadvantages

- It cannot be reliably used in high-tension wounds and gaped wounds. They may require deeper application of absorbable sutures to reduce wound tension.
- Adhesive property of the clips may be compromised over a period, especially if the area becomes wet too often.

Surgical Adhesives

Skin adhesives have been developed and used widely for more than two decades. They have a role in wound closure, especially in wounds without tension. They do not evert the wound edges by themselves and hence eversion must be provided by deeper sutures. They can be classified into—(1) natural or biological tissue adhesives, (2) synthetic polymer-based tissue adhesives, and (3) biomimetic tissue adhesives.[52]

Use of natural or biological tissue adhesives in clinical medicine is a recent development and these are costlier when compared to their synthetic counterparts. But, they offer a variety of advantages including longer and stronger adhesive properties and better tissue flexibility after application. Many of them find applications in achieving adequate hemostasis especially in deeper surgical wounds and internal surgeries. Most of these commercially available products utilize the biological properties of human fibrinogen, human thrombin, human fibronectin, human factor XIII, calcium chloride, albumin, chitosan, and often bovine collagen (e.g., HemCon®, Progel, Tiseel, BioGlue, Crosseal, and TachoSil).[52]

Most commonly used materials in clinical practice are the synthetic polymer-based cyanoacrylate adhesives, which can be used in combination with, or as an alternative to sutures in wound closure. Two varieties of cyanoacrylates that are available are octyl2cyanoacrylate (Dermabond®; Ethicon) and Nbutyl2cyanoacrylate (Indermil®; Syneture).[3,8] The adhesive remains in liquid form until exposed to water or water-containing tissue, after which it polymerizes within 3 minutes through an exothermic reaction in which a small amount of heat is released forming a flexible film that bonds to the underlying surface.

Biomimetic adhesives found mainly in mussels are likely to become the next generation of tissue adhesives for clinical use.[52] They are basically naturally occurring hydrogels, which are soft materials that possess 3D network structure with tunable physical and chemical properties and provide ideal conditions to support the wound healing process. With the rapid development of processing technologies, such as 3D-bioprinting, stem cell, and nanoparticle-hydrogel composites, a new generation of hydrogel-based adhesives with high adhesion ability may be available in near future.[53]

Procedure

Wound should be completely reapproximated before applying cyanoacrylates as healing may be impaired, if the adhesive seeps into the wound bed and may result in foreign body reactions.[33]

Defat the closure site with alcohol or acetone. Octyl-2-cyanoacrylate, which is available in prefilled single use vials with various applicator tips, is applied in a thin layer over the entire wound and extending 5–10 mm beyond the wound edge. Once the layer is dried (10–30 seconds), another layer is applied. Three to four layers are necessary. *N*-butyl-2-cyanoacrylate requires only a single application by droplet that sets in 30 seconds. No additional bandaging is required, and the patient is advised to not perform wound care at home. By 7–14 days, most of the adhesive sloughs off with the epidermis. Topical ointments or creams should not be applied on the wound when adhesives are used, as they can weaken the polymerized film and result in wound gaping. Octyl-2-cyanoacrylate is preferred over N-butyl-2 cyanoacrylate, as it is three to four times stronger than latter, more flexible, and is easier to use.[3] Adhesive is originally sterilized by dry heat and ethylene oxide gas. It is meant for single use only and remaining opened material after each wound closure procedure should be discarded.

Advantages

- They are quick and easy to apply when compared to suturing. Moreover, it eliminates the trauma to tissues caused by needles and sutures.
- They act as waterproof coating and have antibacterial activity against common microbes like staphylococci, *Pseudomonas*, and *E. coli*.
- They promote moist wound healing environment, which is essential for faster epithelialization.
- They are useful for the closure of simple lacerations in children, uncooperative patients, and for the closure of incisions under casts.
- Needs minimal training.
- Cosmetic outcome is good.
- No postoperative visit is required for removal, as it sloughs off naturally over the course of 7–14 days.

Relative Contraindications[3]

- Avoid using near the eyes
- In areas that are highly mobile or subject to friction (e.g., over joints, hands, and feet)
- Any wound with evidence of active infection, gangrene, or bedsores
- On patients with known hypersensitivity to cyanoacrylate
- Patients with peripheral vascular disease.

BOX 1: Tips for proper wound closure.

- Do not place absorbable sutures superficially, as it can lead to permanent suture tracts and can result in suture extrusion. Absorbable sutures should always be placed deeper in subcutaneous tissue and lower dermis.
- Polyglactin 910 (Vicryl) is an excellent absorbable suture in soft tissue approximation particularly in areas such as face, anterior and posterior neck, scalp, superior trunk, and nasal and oral mucosa, which require sutures with higher tensile strength.
- Polypropylene (Prolene), a nonabsorbable suture material, is ideal for subcuticular closure in areas, such as eyelid, periorbital area, nose, pinna, lip, and vermillion, which require less tensile strength.
- Monofilament nylon (Ethilon) having its maximal long-term tensile strength property is useful in suturing major musculocutaneous flaps that need to be closed under significant tension.
- Avoid multifilament sutures in contaminated tissues. Monofilament sutures are preferred in infected tissues. However, great care must be taken in handling and tying monofilament suture because crushing or crimping of this suture can weaken the suture leading to premature suture failure.
- Smaller suture sizes of 5-0–6-0 are preferred on head and neck surgeries.
- Reverse cutting needles with three-eighths inch circle gives best cosmetic outcome, causing minimal trauma.
- Grasp the needle with the jaw of the needle holder at its distal portion at the junction of anterior two-thirds and posterior one-third. This can prevent blunting the cutting point or bending the weaker end of the suture needle.
- The jaws of the needle holder must be appropriate to the needle size to hold it securely and prevent rocking, turning, and twisting.
- Do not tighten the needle holder excessively. The needle should be held vertically and longitudinally perpendicular to the needle holder.
- Tissue bites in simple interrupted suture should be taken at the same level on either side of the wound edges to minimize the possibility of stepping. Simple interrupted sutures lead to cross-hatched linear scars, which can be minimized by removing them early.
- Use running subcuticular suture for closing wounds with equal tissue thickness. Eliminate the tension with deep sutures before placing running subcuticular suture to achieve the best possible cosmetic result.
- Running subcuticular suture is a useful technique in children when absorbable suture is used so that suture removal is avoided.
- Simple running suture may be used to secure a split or full-thickness skin graft. It is also useful over eyelids, ears, and the dorsa of hands.
- Excellent suturing method to provide effective wound support is vertical mattress suture. Placing each stitch precisely and taking symmetric bites are especially important.
- Purse-string sutures should not be tied too tightly, as it may strangulate the approximated tissue.
- Staples are particularly useful for long incisions, as they shorten the wound closure time.
- Surgical glues are useful for the closure of simple lacerations in children, uncooperative patients, and for the closure of incisions under casts.

Laser-assisted Tissue Bonding

Laser-assisted tissue bonding (LTB) is a fast and efficient method for wound closure; LTB was recently developed. This can be divided into two different systems—laser tissue welding (LTW) and laser tissue soldering (LTS).[54] Laser welding is an innovative technique where the bonding of wounds is achieved using laser energy.[8] Compared with previously mentioned closure materials, laser welding is faster, watertight, and avoids a foreign-body reaction. Although collateral thermal injury has prevented its regular clinical use, introduction of LTS has shown to minimize this injury. This process involves the application of a biologic "solder" (e.g., bovine serum albumin) prior to temperature-controlled laser welding. Additional studies are necessary to determine its use in dermatologic surgery.

CONCLUSION

Skillful wound closure requires not only knowledge of proper surgical techniques but also knowledge of the physical characteristics and properties of wound closure materials. Today, dermatosurgeon has a significantly increased number of wound closure materials to choose from. While choosing appropriate material, it is important to consider the risk of infection, closure speed, cost, cosmetic results, and wound location. The tips for proper wound closure are mentioned in **Box 1**.

Wound closure technology has kept its pace of advancement along with the latest techniques in surgery and provides the cosmetic surgical fraternity a wide range of wound closure methods.

REFERENCES

1. Bloom BS, Goldberg DJ. Suture material in cosmetic cutaneous surgery. J Cosm Laser Ther. 2007;9(1):415.
2. Chu CC, Greisler HP, von Fraunhofer JA. Wound Closure Biomaterials and Devices, 1st edition. Boca Raton, FL: CRC Press; 1997.
3. Doctor HG. Dermabond liquid stitches. Surgeons and Sutures, 3rd edition. Cincinnati, OH, United States: EthiconJohnson and Johnson; 2005. pp. 279.
4. Lejaren H. Sutures in Ancient Surgery. Brooklyn, NY: Davis and Geck; 1927. p. 38.
5. Kudur MH, Pai SB, Sripathi H, Prabhu S. Sutures and suturing techniques in skin closure. Indian J Dermatol Venereol Lerpol. 2009;75(4):42534.
6. Lai SY, Becker DG, Edlich RF. (2010). Sutures and Needles. [online] Available from: emedicine.medscape.com/article/884838. [Last accessed March, 2021].
7. Ammirati CT. Advances in wound closure materials. In: James WD, Cockerell CJ, Maloney ME (Eds). Advances in Dermatology. Philadelphia: Mosby; 2002. pp. 31338.
8. Terhune M. Materials for wound closure. [online] Available from: www.emedicine.com/derm/topic825.htm. [Last accessed March, 2021].
9. Moy RL, Lee A, Zalka A. Commonly used suture materials in skin surgery. Am Fam Physician. 1991;44:21238.

10. Kirk RM. Handling instruments. Basic Surgical Techniques, 6th edition. London, United Kingdom: Churchill, Livingstone; 2010. pp. 920.
11. Postlethwait RW, Willigan DA, Ulin AW. Human tissue reaction to sutures. Ann Surg. 1975;181(2):14450.
12. Bennet RG. Selection of wound closure materials. J Am Acad Dermatol. 1988;18(4 Pt 1):61937.
13. Watts GT. Sutures for skin closure. Lancet. 1975;1:581.
14. Lober CW, Fenske NA. Suture materials for closing the skin and subcutaneous tissues. Aesthetic Plast Surg. 1986;10:2458.
15. Madsen ET. An experimental and clinical evaluation of surgical suture materials. Surg Gynecol Obstet. 1953;97:7380.
16. Conn J, Oyasu R, Welsh M, Beal JM. Vicryl (polyglactin 910) synthetic absorbable sutures. Am J Surg. 1974;128(1):1923.
17. Ray JA, Doddi N, Regula D, Williams JA, Melveger A. Polydioxanone (PDS), a novel monofilament synthetic absorbable suture. Surg Gynecol Obstet. 1981;153(4):497507.
18. Edlich RF, Gubler K, Wallis AG, Clark JJ, Dahlstrom JJ, Long WB. Wound closure sutures and needles: a new perspective. J Environ Pathol Toxicol Oncol. 2010;29(4):33961.
19. Rodeheaver GT, Nesbit WS, Edlich RF. Novafil. A dynamic suture for wound closure. Ann Surg. 1986;204(2):1939.
20. Aston SJ. The choice of suture material for skin closure. J Dermatol Surg. 1976;2:5761.
21. Szarmach RR, Livingston J, Edlich RE. An expanded surgical and needle evaluation and selection program by a healthcare resource management group purchasing organization. J Long Term Eff Med Implants. 2003;13:15570.
22. Swanson NA, Tromovitch TA. Suture materials, 1980s: properties, uses, and abuses. Int J Dermatol. 1982;21:3738.
23. Borges AF. Techniques of wound suture. Elective Incisions and Scar Revision. Boston: Little Brown; 1973. pp. 6576.
24. Swanson NA. Basic Techniques. Atlas of Cutaneous Surgery. Boston: Little Brown; 1987. pp. 2649.
25. Edlich RF, Long WB, Gubler KD, Rodeheaver GT, Thacker JG, Borel L, et al. Citizen's Petition to Food and Drug Administration to ban cornstarch powder on medical gloves: Maltese cross birefringence. Am J Emerg Med. 2009;27(2):227-35.
26. Edlich RF, Wind TC, Heather CL, Thacker JG. Reliability and performance of innovative surgical double-glove hole puncture indication systems. J Long Term Eff Med Implants. 2003;13(2):6983.
27. Edlich RF, Gubler K, Wallis AG, Clark JJ, Dahlstrom JJ, Long WB. Scientific basis for the selection of skin closure techniques. J Environ Pathol Toxicol Oncol. 2010;29(4):36372.
28. Wiggan JM, Elston DM. (2010). Suturing Techniques. [online] Available from: http://emedicine.medscape.com/article/1824895. [Last accessed March, 2021].
29. Arnold H. Surgery of the skin and subcutaneous tissue. Farquharson's Textbook of Operative General Surgery, 9th edition. Boca Raton, Florida, United States: CRC Press; 2005. pp. 120.
30. Stegman SJ. Suturing techniques for dermatologic surgery. J Dermatol Surg Oncol. 1978;4:638.
31. Richey ML, Roe SC. Assessment of knot security in continuous intradermal wound closures. J Surg Res. 2005;123:2848.
32. Adams B, Levy R, Rademaker AE, Goldberg LH, Alam M. Frequency of use of suturing and repair techniques preferred by dermatologic surgeons. Dermatol Surg. 2006;32:6829.
33. Thorne CH. Techniques and principles in plastic surgery. Grabb & Smith's Plastic Surgery, 6th edition. Philadelphia, USA: Wolters Kluwer/Lippincott: Williams & Wilkins; 2007. pp. 314.
34. Popkin GL, Robins P. Closure of skin wounds. Workshop manual for basic dermatological surgery. Kenilworth: NJ: Schering, Inc; 1983. pp. 1836.
35. Zachary CB, Suture techniques. In: Zachary CB (Ed). Basic Cutaneous Surgery. New York: Churchill Livingstone; 1991. pp. 5375.
36. Odland PB, Murakuani CS. Simple suturing technique and knot tying. In: Wheeland RG (Ed). Cutaneous Surgery, 1st edition. Philadelphia: WB Saunders Co.; 1994. pp. 17888.
37. Bechara FG, AlMuhammadi R, Sand M, Nordwig TS, Peter A, Klaus H, et al. A modified corner stitch for fixation of flap tips. Dermatol Surg. 2007;33(10):12779.
38. Chan JL, Miller EK, Jou RM, Posten W. Novel surgical technique: placement of a deep tip stitch. Dermatol Surg. 2009;35(12):20013.
39. Cohen PR, Martinelli PT, Schulze KE, Nelson BR. The cuticular purse string suture: a modified purse string suture for the partial closure of round postoperative wounds. Int J Dermatol. 2007;46(7):74653.
40. Davis M, Nakhdjevani A, Lidder S. Suture/Steri-Strip combination for the management of lacerations in thin-skinned individuals. J Emerg Med. 2011;40(3):322-3.
41. Paul MD. Bidirectional barbed sutures for wound closure: evolution and applications. J Am Coll Certif Wound Spec. 2009;1(2):51-7.
42. Kaminer MS, Bogart M, Choi C, Wee SA. Long-term efficacy of anchored barbed sutures in the face and neck. Dermatol Surg. 2008;34(8):10417.
43. Regula CG, Yag-Howard C. Suture products and techniques: what to use, where, and why. Dermatol Surg Off Publ Am Soc Dermatol Surg Al. 2015;41 Suppl 10:S187-200.
44. Robinson JK. Suspension sutures in facial reconstruction. Dermatol Surg. 2003;29(4):386-93.
45. Kantor J. The fascial plication suture: an adjunct to layered wound closure. Arch Dermatol. 2009;145(12):1454-6.
46. Radonich MA, Bisaccia E, Scarborough D. Management of large surgical defects of the forehead and scalp by imbrication of deep tissues. Dermatol Surg. 2002;28(6):524-6.
47. Yag-Howard C. Novel approach to decreasing tension when approximating wound edges in advancement flaps: The ImPli stitch. Dermatol Surg. 2012;38(4):661-3.
48. Tierney E, Kouba DJ. A subcutaneous corset plication rapidly and effectively relieves tension on large linear closures. Dermatol Surg. 2009;35(11):1806-8.
49. Kolt JD. Use of adhesive surgical tape with the absorbable continuous subcuticular suture. ANZ J Surg. 2003;73(8):626-9.
50. Wu H, Zhao C, Ni J, Zhang S, Liu J, Yan J, et al. Research of a novel biodegradable surgical staple made of high purity magnesium. Bioact Mater. 2016;1(2):122-6.
51. Freed JS, Ko J. An innovative advance in non-invasive wound closure: a new paradigm. Mil Med. 2018;183(suppl_1):472-80.
52. Ge L, Chen S. Recent advances in tissue adhesives for clinical medicine. Polymers (Basel). 2020;12(4):939.
53. Zhang L, Liu M, Zhang Y, Pei R. Recent progress of highly adhesive hydrogels as wound dressings. Biomacromolecules. 2020;21(10):3966-83.
54. Al-Mubarak L, Al-Haddab M. Cutaneous wound closure materials: an overview and update. J Cutan Aesthetic Surg. 2013;6(4):178-88.

CHAPTER 8

Setting Up a Dermatosurgery Unit

HM Omprakash

KEY MESSAGES

- Before designing a dermatosurgery unit, one has to keep in mind the statutory standards and in the end tailor makes the facility to meet ones requirement.
- Dermatosurgery unit is viewed as a luxury—but in reality, it is a place of high standard of patient safety with most economical use of manpower and other resources.
- Dermatosurgery unit types could be—unrestricted type, restricted type or laser surgery unit.
- Dermatosurgery unit design should look into—location of unit, dimensions, power, water, lighting, instruments and waste disposal.
- Before commissioning a unit one has to look into—trained personnel, sterilization–disinfection services and basic, advanced cardiovascular life support system.

INTRODUCTION

Dermatologists are increasingly performing cutaneous surgery. The surgeries performed range from simple procedures such as electrosurgery, biopsies, chemical cauteries, sclerotherapy, soft tissue augmentation, botulinum toxin chemodenervation to more aggressive surgeries such as vitiligo surgery, nail surgeries and more complex labor intensive procedures such as hair restoration, liposuction, etc. Since patient's safety is the first concern, it is not only the dermatologist skill which matters but also the infrastructure. A well-equipped, well-designed surgical suite improves the experience for both patients and the dermatologist.[1]

NOMENCLATURE

The units where dermatosurgeries are performed have different nomenclature: the dermatosurgery unit, the operation theater, the ambulatory surgery facility, the office surgery and the free standing outpatient surgery center, outpatient surgical suite. But in this chapter, it shall be known as the *dermatosurgery unit.*

WHY THE NEED FOR SEPARATE DERMATOSURGERY UNIT?

The paucity of financial resources and high cost of leasing or owning separate dermatosurgery unit is forcing many dermatologists to operate on the patient in their consultation rooms. This is putting both the patient and dermatologist at the risk. The risks are infection, anaphylaxis or hemodynamic and airway compromise inherent to the use of topical or infiltration anesthetics, hence the rationale of having a separate dermatosurgery unit with clean if not sterile environment and back up of advanced life support.

Even though it may make sense to use the existing minor or major operation theater of an existing hospital, it has definite drawbacks.

Patients attending traditional major operation theater are sick, unlike dermatology patients. To get a slot for surgery at patients or dermatologists, convenience is often difficult. Also it would cost more to hire the operation theater on hourly basis.[1]

Patients prefer dermatosurgery unit to hospital-based operation theater because the environment is less threatening. If the dermatosurgery unit is located in the same premises as the consultation room, patients are already familiar with the surroundings, personnel and prefer this personalized care.[2]

Thus, the dermatosurgery unit may be housed in a major hospital or private clinic premises or in shared premises with common theater shared by different doctors: plastic surgeons, general surgeons or like-minded dermatologist willing to do group practice.[3]

REQUIREMENTS OF A DERMATOSURGERY UNIT

Each dermatologist will have his own likes and dislikes. So before embarking on designing, one has to keep in mind the statutory standards and in the end, tailor makes the facility to meet ones requirement.

The Indian standard—basic requirements for hospital planning,[4] the Medical Council of India guidelines,[5] the Indian Association of Dermatologist, Venereologist and Leprologist guidelines,[6] have issued guidelines which are of use to a dermatosurgeon.

The International guidelines include American Association for Accreditation of Ambulatory Surgery facilities,[7] Singapore Directives for Private Ambulatory surgical centers providing ambulatory surgery,[8] Netherlands Building Guidelines for a surgical department,[9] WHO guidelines.[10]

However, industry leaders whose publications are opinion makers: Satish S Savant,[11] Walter P Unger[12] should also be referred to before starting a dermatosurgery unit.

THE DERMATOSURGERY UNIT TYPES

There are three types of dermatosurgery zones:

1. Unrestricted zone
2. Restricted zone
3. Laser surgery unit.

Unrestricted Zone

Majority of dermatosurgeries are performed on intact skin, with only resident cutaneous flora. Only the site of surgery requires isolation. Hence, both the patient and dermatologist can enter the operation theater in routine clothes. This is where most procedures such as cryotherapy, electrosurgery, soft tissue augmentation, botulinum toxin chemodenervation, skin biopsies are carried out. Here only topical, infiltration anesthesia is permitted with oral and intramuscular sedation. Spinal, epidural, regional blocks and general anesthesia are not permitted **(Fig. 1)**.[13]

Restricted Zone

But invasive surgeries such as vitiligo surgeries, hair transplantation, laser resurfacing require a separate theater. This is the restricted zone **(Fig. 2)** or the traditional operation theater, wherein the patient, dermatologist must change their dress, don cap, mask and use separate operation theater footwear.[14] General anesthesia, intravenous anesthesia are permitted.[8]

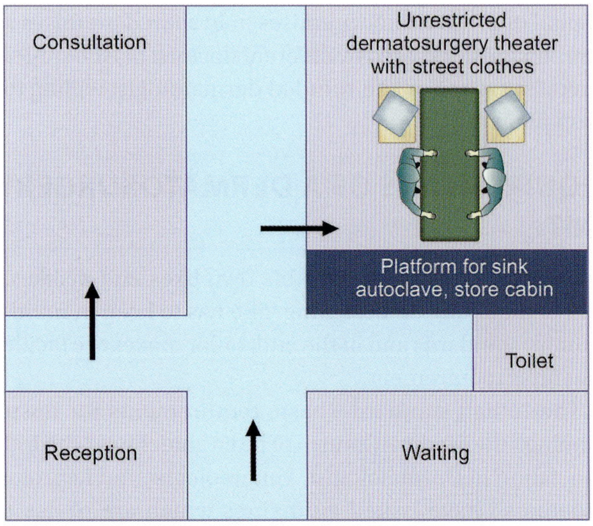

Fig. 1: Unrestricted type of dermatosurgery unit.

Laser Zone

It is dealt in a separate chapter.

A dermatosurgical theater can include all the zones in the same complex or may include one theater of unrestricted zone.

LOCATION OF THE DERMATOSURGERY UNIT IN THE OFFICE OR HOSPITAL

The Indian standard for hospital planning[4] clearly defines that where should be the traditional operation theater unit be located **(Box 1)**.

What follows is the layouts and requirements of the dermatosurgery unit. These are ideal requirements. Minimal requirements have already been laid out in IADVL taskforce recommendations.[6]

Layout of the Restricted Zone Type of Dermatosurgery Unit

There are four well-defined zones depending upon the degree of cleanliness. Zoning is done to keep the theater free from microorganisms.

1. *Protective zone*: This includes waiting area, preanesthetic examination room, changing rooms, and theater supply rooms.

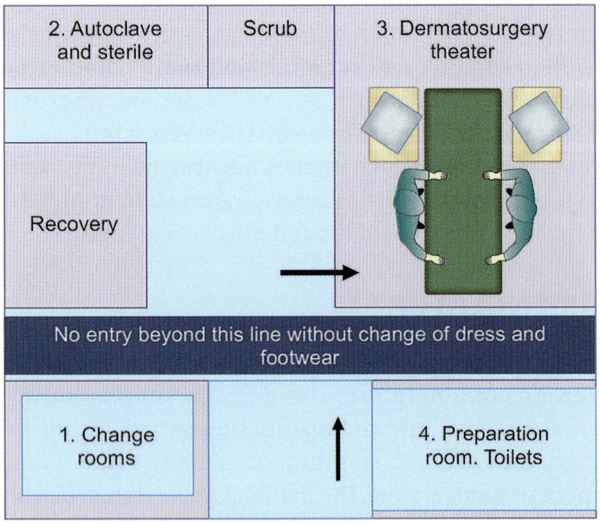

Fig. 2: Restricted type of dermatosurgery unit.

BOX 1: Location of the dermatosurgery unit.

- Quiet environment
- Freedom from noise and other disturbance
- Freedom from contamination and possible cross infection
- Maximum protection from solar radiation
- Convenient relationship with surgical ward, intensive care unit, central sterilization, blood bank, radiology, pathology and supply department
- Efficient lift service if located on upper floors
- Lastly the obvious electric supply, ventilation, fire extinguisher, and water supply

2. *Clean zone*: This includes theater pack preparation, preoperative room, and recovery room.
3. *Aseptic zone or sterile zone:* The sterilization room, operation theater.
4. *Disposal zone or dirty zone*: The soiled instruments and dressings are washed or disposed here.[4]

Guidelines for the Restricted Type of Dermatosurgery Unit Complex

- The door of the complex should be two leaf types with self-closing hinges. The door should be 1 meter wide.
- The floor and side of the passage in the complex should be tiled to withstand repeated washing or else the side walls can be just painted with washable paint and light color.
- The corridor of the complex should be adequate for ease of mobility of trolleys. The required dimensions may be 2 meters.[15]
- Suitable fire alarms and powder type fire extinguishers should be in place **(Fig. 3)**. Carbon dioxide type fire extinguishers are suitable for equipment in the theater, but foam type and water should be not used on lasers and other type equipment in theater.[16]
- Change room should have lockers.
- No window curtains or floor mats are permitted in the premises.
- Scrub zone should have elbow operated or foot operated taps and elbow operated hand disinfectant dispenser. Since water can harbor Pseudomonas and other microbes the water should be UV and heat treated.

Common Features of the Operation Theater of both Restricted and Unrestricted Type

- The operation theater should be dust proof and moisture proof.
- Corners and junctions of walls, floor and ceiling could be rounded to prevent accumulation of dust and to facilitate cleaning **(Fig. 4)**. The flooring of restricted type theater **(Fig. 5)** should be seamless and made of epoxy resin. But in the unrestricted type, it could be tiled **(Fig. 6)** or concrete able to withstand repeated washing.
- All doors should be 1.5 meters in width and half leaf type with self-closing devices in place. If laser is in use then the laser usage sign with the wavelength being used should be displayed on the door.
- The dimension of the theater could be 3 × 3 meters,[11] 4 × 4 meters[17] or 4 × 5 meters[12] minimum.
- The height of the wall should be 2.6 meters[15] or 3.0 meters.[4]

Lighting of Theater

- Natural light through windows should be provided. But windows should be sealed tight.

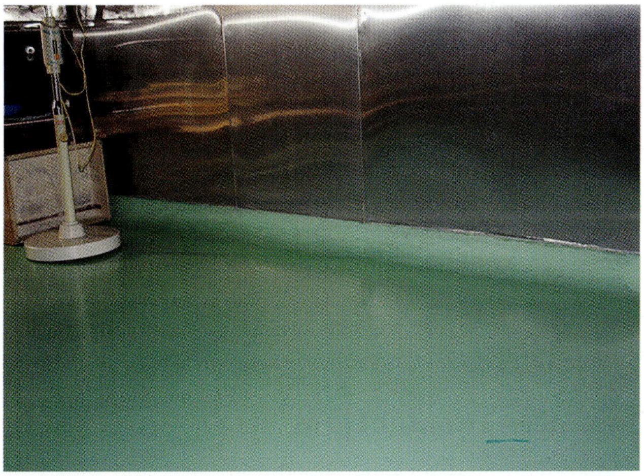

Fig. 4: Restricted theater with rounded corners and epoxy seamless flooring.

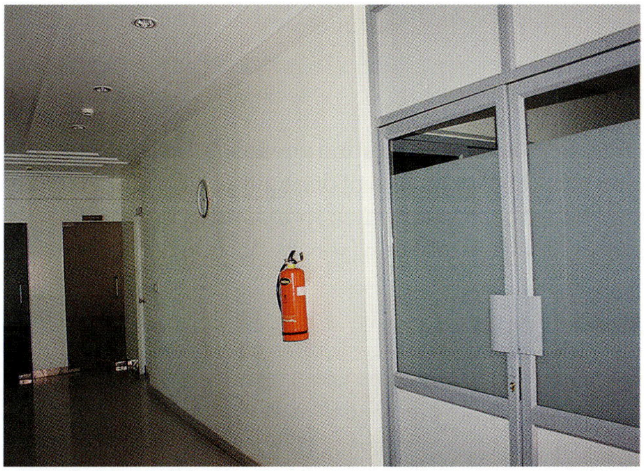

Fig. 3: Note the fire alarms in ceiling, powder type fire extinguishers, tiled floor, and washable walls.

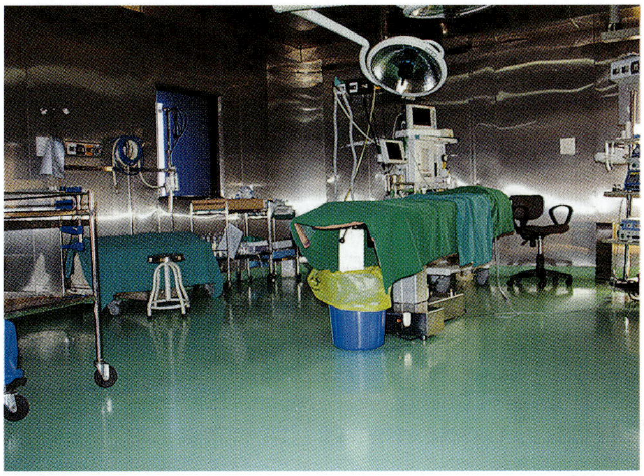

Fig. 5: Restricted theater–seamless epoxy flooring, natural closed window light with washable walls.
Courtesy: Vikram Hospital, Mysore.

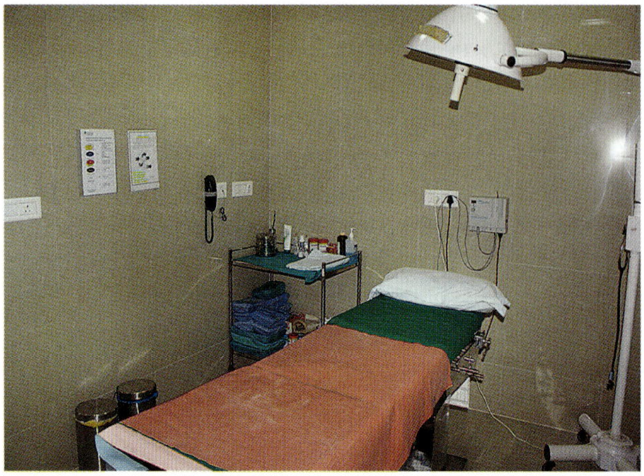

Fig. 6: Unrestricted theater with tiled walls and floors, electrical outlets, phone, OT light, table, trolley, kick bucket for waste.
Courtesy: Vikram Hospital, Mysore.

- General lighting by ceiling mounted fluorescent tubes at the rate of 1 W per square foot (i.e., for 120 square feet 120 W, 3 tubes of 40 W)[18] is sufficient.
- *The artificial light:* Fluorescent tubes, compact fluorescent lamps (CFL) or light emitting diodes (LED); should match the color of the objects, as they are seen in outdoor natural sunlight. This is called color rendering index (CRI). Sunlight CRI is 100. Tubes and CFL with CRI of 90–98 are available. Also ask for "Daylight" version of the lamps.
- Compact fluorescent lamps and cluster white LED lights can save power and last longer. Tubes have a life of 15,000 hours but LED lights last 50,000 hours. But for the long life, low power consumption and being mercury free; LED light requires further standardization as of today.

Operation Theater Light

- Before purchasing a light for the surgical field, check for: (1) intensity of light, (2) size of the illuminated field, (3) production of heat and shadows, (4) ease of changing the position of light and (5) ceiling mounted or floor movable.
- Shadow less lighting delivering 3,000–8,000 foot candles[19] is the basic operation theater light required (i.e., the dental chairs have halogen lamp of 50 W power. Each Watt of power will give 50 foot candle of illumination at the site of surgery. So a 50 W of halogen bulb can roughly give 2,500 foot candles of illumination on the site of surgery).
- For dermatologist looking for precise illumination, single bulb 100 W, 12 V halogen bulb giving 30,000 Lux illumination are available.
- Light-emitting diode operation theater light with long life, low heat are entering the market and may change halogen bulb in future.

Electrical Outlets

- All 3-pin outlets should be located about 1.5 meters above the floor. This is to prevent wires on the floor. There should be good earthing.
- No extension cords or boards are permitted.
- 5 ampere and 15 ampere sockets are required. The 5 ampere sockets, on an average 4 should be located on each wall.
- Online UPS are required for lasers and operation theater lights. Preferably, draw the current for costly devices through servo stabilizer which is a one-time investment.
- Standby generators should be planned.

Air Conditioning

- Air conditioning minimum requirement is of office type with 10 μm dust filter. In our country, this is basically for operators comfort rather than for clean air supply (applicable only to unrestricted type theater).
- The temperature of theater should be 21° and humidity 50–55%.
- But National Accreditation Board for Hospitals (NABH) does not recommend split and windows AC for restricted type operation theaters.[20]

Operation Table

- Stainless steel operation table, with adjustable head, foot end and arm rest is the heart of the theater. This could be manual or electric power controlled, with foot or fingertip controls.
- The dimension of the table could be a minimum of 1 meter length and 30 cm breadth.[19]
- Dental chairs with the same specification could be used in unrestricted theaters.

Instrument Trolley

Mayo stand with four wheels is the most preferred instrument trolley. An autoclaved rubber sheet/Mackintosh should be draped on the table over which a sterile pack is placed every time. If simple cloth is placed, moisture will percolate down and contaminate the instruments.

Surgeons Stool

Surgeons stool with wheels and pneumatic height adjustment, controlled by foot in case of dermatologist is already gloved and also with back rest which sometimes could double up as armrest is a good addition (*see* also section on ergonomics).

Waste Containers

Four main types of wastes are generated in the theater of a dermatologist: (1) blood soaked gauze, (2) latex gloves, (3) glove paper and plastic cover, (4) sharps, needle and syringes. These are segregated at source[21] into: (i) yellow plastic cover, (ii) blue plastic cover, (iii) white plastic cover, (iv) plastic container with disinfectant respectively with the biohazard logo **(Fig. 7)**. Each of the plastic covers is spread out in kick-bucket type steel containers with rubber baskets.

Surgical Instruments

- The surgical instruments depend upon the type of work and individual surgeon's preference.[11,12] The list of instruments given in **Table 1** is not comprehensive and consists of basic requirements for a functional theater.
- Specific instruments may be needed according to individual surgeries, for which the reader may consult individual chapters on procedures in respective chapters of this textbook.

ADVANCE CARDIOVASCULAR LIFE SUPPORT

As per government of India and Supreme Court verdict, all personnel in the operation theater should be familiar with basic and advanced life support.[22] Basic life support (BLS) does not require any devices or drugs, but advanced cardiovascular life support (ACLS) does. A standby anesthetist may be necessary for certain procedures. Also it is better to liaison with a local hospital with ICU facility and ambulance service. The reader is referred to the chapter on Dermatological Surgery and Resuscitation for more details.

Advanced cardiovascular life support is taught in batches at various institutes. One should register to these courses, get the precourse material and learn before going to course: (1) BLS and the usage of defibrillator; (2) drugs used in CPR; (3) ECG; (4) understand 10 core cases in ACLS-respiratory arrest case, VF treated with CPR and AED, VF/Pulseless VT case, pulseless electrical activity case, asystole case, acute coronary syndrome case, bradycardia case, unstable tachycardia case, stable tachycardia case and acute stroke case.

The ACLS training involves 3 days: day 1 BLS, day 2 and day 3 ACLS. The training involves—interactive lectures, videos and practice session using mannequin, defibrillator, Ambu bag, ET tubes and drugs. A candidate at the end will have written test and will have to perform BLS and ACLS both in children and adults to pass. Every 2 years, this course has to be repeated.[23]

The drugs and devices required for advanced life support are enlisted in **Table 2**.[24]

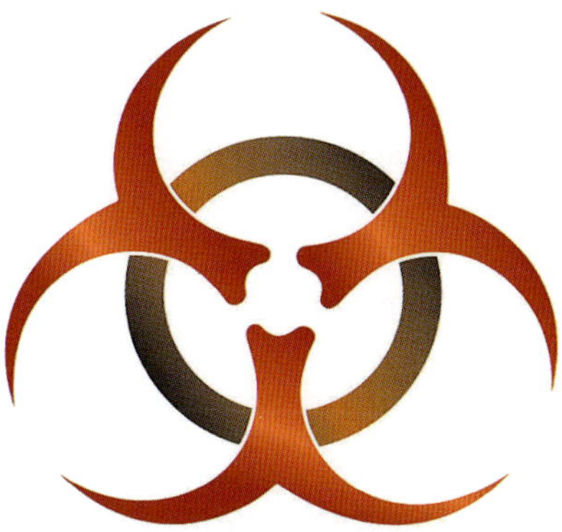

Fig. 7: Biohazard logo.

OPERATION ROOM RECORDS

A record containing: (1) patient identity, (2) diagnosis, (3) procedures performed, (4) persons involved in the procedures and (5) complications should be maintained.

This is not only a statutory requirement, but also helping auditing: procedures performed, complications and improvisation of ones' skills.

Surgical Drapes and Attires: Mask, Caps, Suits, Gowns, Gloves, Patient's Suits

Drapes for the operation field are available in different material: cotton and disposable paper or plastic. Cotton is porous and comfortable for the patient. But disposable paper and plastic avoids the need for washing and autoclaving.

Mask definitely protects the dermatologist from splash of blood, injectable anesthetics and most important viral particles during electrosurgery. Surgical wound is protected from operators and assistant secretions in the event of coughing and sneezing; since the aerosol can travel up to 3 meters. Mask should cover both nose and mouth. Cotton, paper and gauze masks should not be used. Paper with synthetic material offer effective barrier.[25] The pore size of the mask should be 1 micron.[26]

Surgical cap should cover the hair on scalp. This prevents contamination of the surgical suit and also the operation site by hair organism.

Surgical suits or theater suits or scrub suits are pants and shirts into which the theater personnel change from street clothes. This has to be cotton and clean but not sterile. These are required for restricted zone of theater.

TABLE 1: Basic requirements for a functional theater.

Forceps	*Sharp instruments*	*Scissors*	*Miscellaneous*
Cheatles Sponge holding Adson non-toothed Adson toothed Jewelers Mosquito artery Spencer suture removal	Bard parker handle no. 3, 4 and 5 Disposable surgical blades no. 11, 15 Disposable punch Comedone extractor Curette of 3–4 mm diameter	5 inch blunt and sharp (Lister) Iris scissors Castroviejo	Skin hooks Needle holder- Halsey and box type Nail splitter

TABLE 2: Drugs and devices for advanced life support.

Devices	*Quantity*	*Drugs*	*Quantity*
Ambu bag	1	Adrenaline 1:1,000	10
Laryngoscope with different size blades	1	Atropine 0.6 mg	10
Endotracheal tube of different size 6–8 (no.)	1	Sodium bicarbonate (7.5%) ampoules	12
IV cannula adult and pediatric	2	Chlorpheniramine maleate 22.75 mg/mL, 2 cc	10
Drip set	2	Hydrocortisone 100 mg/mL	2
Airway of all size	1	Injection furosemide	10
Stethoscope	1	Aminophylline 250 mg/2 mL ampoules	5
BP apparatus	1	Dopamine 200 mg/5 mL	2
Cardiac monitor with built in defibrillator	1	Normal saline 500 mL	2
Oxygen cylinder with connectors	1	5% Dextrose normal saline 500 mL	2
Suction device	1	Mephentermine 15 mg/mL	5
Disposable syringe	2	Dextrose 25%	2 ampoules

Gowns are sterile cotton material, full sleeve knee length attires to prevent contamination of the operation site, put on by dermatologist and nurses on surgical suits.

Sterile plastic apron could be donned on surgical suite during dermabrasion to prevent soiling of cotton suite.

Patient suits are required to prevent soiling of the clothes during surgery. They just have to be clean and not sterile.

Gloves can be of latex or nonlatex type of various sizes. Double gloving can be practiced when operating on high-risk cases (For hand hygiene, glove donning technique, refer chapter on Disinfection and Sterilization).

Cloth instrument packing is the traditional way of securing the instrument tray. They have to be 270 thread count Pima cotton fabric. The only drawback is the cloth has to be laundered every time. Hence, nowadays disposable paper crepe type or medical grade plastic paper reels are available **(Fig. 8)**.[27] The storage shelf life varies 1–12 months depending upon the material **(Fig. 9)** (refer the manufacturer guidelines).

Disinfection and Sterilization of Theater Equipment

The reader is referred to the chapter on Disinfection and Sterilization for detailed description. Specific features are mentioned. Disinfection in the operation theater can be referred to as given below:

- Cleaning working surface (category-a).
- Equipment which cannot be autoclaved or need not be autoclaved, e.g., electrosurgery tips, sharps, gloves, linen, OT dresses, stainless steel instruments comedone expressor, forceps, gallipots (category-b).
- Nondisposable items (category-c).
- Spillages of infectious material.

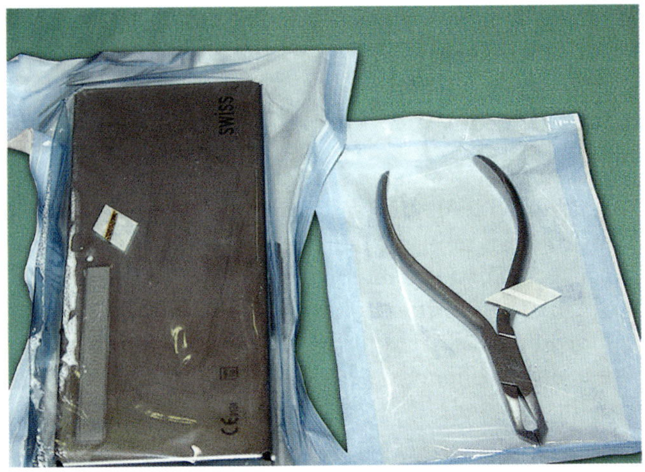

Fig. 8: Medical grade plastic paper pack with one side transparent and autoclave indicator, left autoclaved with black line and right not autoclaved with white line.

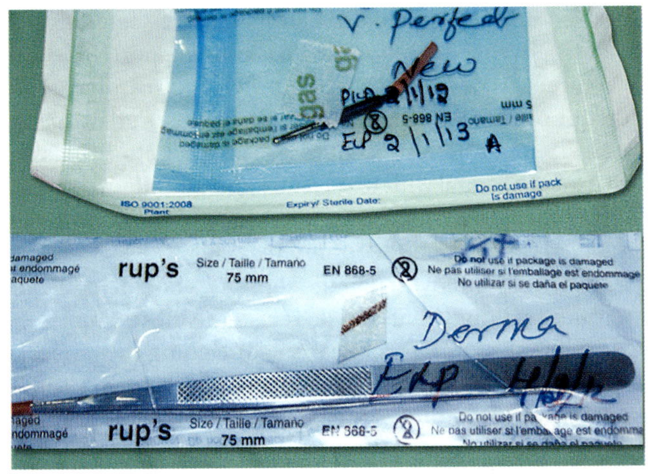

Fig. 9: Top: Medical grade plastic reel used to ETO gas sterilize electrosurgery tip expiry date 1 year. Bottom: Forceps autoclaved expiry 1 month.

Cleaning Working Surfaces

Before surgery

- Mop the floor using 0.5% chlorine solution.
- Using cloth wipes the operation table and trolley with 0.5% chlorine solution **(Box 2)**.

After surgery

- Repeat above steps. Keep it ready for next case.

Disinfection of Category "b" and "c" Items

- Items in category "b" and "c" should be collected in separate plastic buckets or basin or waste disposal leak-proof plastic container for sharps.

- About 0.5% chlorine solution should be poured and left in contact for minimum of 10 minutes to maximum of 30 minutes. The instruments and linen should be fully immersed in the solution.
- After the "contact" time, wearing mask and thick rubber gloves should be rinsed in tap water or lukewarm water. Do not use very hot water because it coagulates blood and makes it hard to clean.

1. Cleaning removes debris
2. Disinfection reduces the bacterial and viral load, but does not remove debris or sterilize
3. Sterilization kills microbes
4. Sterilization is not a method of cleaning[10]

- Using a tooth brush to scrub the instruments or brush the clothes.
- Use later, commercial detergents to further clean.
- Do not use soaps as it leaves a precipitate on the steel surface.
- Linen, drapes, suits, gowns, hand towels should be washed with household detergent at 71°C for 25 minutes. Later they can be sterilized or disinfected[10] (Note: Drapes, gowns and hand towels require later autoclaving, but not suits).
- After cleansing and disinfecting the instruments and clothes must be dried. Later sent for sterilization.

Steam Sterilization (Autoclave)

- Dry the equipment or clothes.
- Wrap the equipment in clothes or paper or medical grade plastic paper pack **(Figs. 8 and 9)**.
- Lay the instruments in the autoclave so that all the surface of the device will come in contact with heat.
- Before packing lay the instruments such as scissors in open position.

BOX 2: Preparation of 0.5% chlorine solution.

- Procure commercially available bleaching powder
- Add 150 gram in 10 liters of tap water (10 tablespoon or 30 teaspoon)
- First premix the required amount of powder in small quantity of tap water and later add remaining quantity of water
- Use the same day

- Refer the manufacturer's time recommendations for the duration of autoclave.
- Also buy a small autoclave which can be reused many times in a day than large one, once a day. Table top autoclave should be considered.
- Generally, it is 121°C for 15 minutes, pressure of 2.4 bar in porous stainless steel containers.
- The outside of the packs should not be wet, if so, the autoclave process has failed.
- Appropriate color indicators should be used on packs to know the adequacy of autoclaving.
- Date of autoclave should be mentioned. The expiry date varies. If polythene bags are used for biopsy trays before autoclaving, sterility is ensured for 8 weeks. If double packed and medical grade plastic paper packs are used the sterility is valid for 1 year.

Chemical Sterilization

- Cleaned, disinfected, dried instruments should be fully soaked in a steel or plastic container having 2% glutaraldehyde for 8–10 hours[10] (Note: For disinfection, the contact time is 20 minutes).
- Instruments like scissors should be in open position when soaked.
- After 10 hours, using autoclaved water (100 mL of water autoclaved for 20 minutes and not boiled water) the instruments should be washed, dried and packed, stored in a sterile tray. Note the contact time for high level disinfection **(Table 3)** is just 20 minutes compared to 10 hours required for sterilization.

OPERATION THEATER FUMIGATION AND/ OR SURFACE DISINFECTION

Three agents are currently available for theater fumigation or surface disinfection.

1. *40% formalin solution*: Formalin fumigation overnight either using a fumigator or formalin in a galipot is sufficient.[29] About 500 mL of 40% formalin in 1,000 mL of water, for 1,000 feet^3 of operation theater area in an electric

TABLE 3: Methods of high level disinfection.

Chemical used	*Quantity required*	*Time for disinfection*	*To be changed*	*Comment*
Formalin in chamber	7 g of formalin for 1 cubic meter area at 20°C (1 g tablet available)	12 hours	Daily	For disinfecting electrosurgery electrodes and cables. For disinfecting sharp instruments Note: It is an irritant and carcinogen
Glutaraldehyde	2.45% concentration	20 minutes	14 days	For disinfecting sharp instruments
Isopropyl alcohol	70%	2 minutes	Daily	Caution: Inflammable near lasers and electrosurgery units

Note: Safer alternatives to formalin chamber and glutaraldehyde should be explored like peracetic acid. Formalin chamber may not be effective in cold areas of the country and cooler nights. Newer agents for high level disinfection and sterilization such as glutaraldehyde + dioxahexane + rust inhibitors at 5% concentration is available for emergency disinfection of equipment within 5 minutes.[28]

boiler/fumigator is the ideal concentration. This requires sealing of windows and doors overnight while fumigating.

2. Glutaraldehyde 5 grams, benzalkonium chloride 5 gram, alkyl urea 3 grams and 1,6-dihydroxy-2, 5-dioxahexane 11.2 gram; all the above in 100 gram packing. Around 0.5% spray or mopping daily may be done. To be left on surface for 20 minutes and later wiped off.
3. Aldehyde free, quick acting ethanol 10 grams, 2-propanol 9 gram and 1-propanol 6 gram solution in 100 gram to be sprayed before 5 minutes of surgery on the floor, table, light and later wiped.[28] During spraying, no electrical switches to be operated since the sparks can ignite the fumigant.

House Keeping of the Operation Theater

The operation theater needs only be clean of dust and organic matter.

- Daily in the morning, the floor, the operation table, chair, light, shelves and sink should be wet mopped free of dust, with water. *Note*: Avoid using broom which could aerosolize the dust. Use of detergent or chemical disinfectant for floor is optional, unless one is planning dermabrasion, skin grafting, hair restoration or liposuction. The wet mop later should be put in a proper place to dry.
- Later, the operation theater trolley should be mopped with a chemical disinfectant or isopropyl alcohol before surgery and between two surgeries.
- The floor and other areas of blood spillage should be mopped with chemical disinfectant or chlorine bleach.
- Cleaning the walls, ceiling on a daily basis is not mandatory but periodic maintenance could be undertaken.
- Use of fan in the operation theater should be avoided as it causes aerosolization of dust.
- If there is an air conditioner, maintenance of the same is necessary. Legionnaires' disease should be a reminder. But however when invasive surgeries are being carried out: hair restoration, liposuction, complex closures, laser resurfacing; fumigation should be done daily or prior to each surgery.

Operation Theater Etiquettes

- The door of theater should be kept closed always.
- Unnecessary movement in and out of theater should be avoided.
- People with respiratory or skin infection should stay out.
- Staff must respect and maintain the dignity of the patient.
- Patients' privacy and modesty should be respected by all staff at all times.
- Patient must be explained in detail of the diagnosis, anesthesia planned, pain involved, and instrument being used like either laser or electrosurgery, postoperative care including the necessity of dressing, sunscreens or antibiotics, complications expected and their remedy. The next follow-up should be informed prior. If the patient is receiving oral sedation, the necessity of an attendant after surgery should be prior informed. The cost of the therapy should be explained.[30]
- Use of mobile in the operation theater should be restricted. Keep it in silent mode and in case you want to take the call, inform the patient and then proceed.[31]

WASTE DISPOSAL

Each dermatologist clinic and operation theater should be registered with the state health authorities. The waste collected in leak proof plastic bags or plastic cans have to be handed over to the local agents, authorized by health department, for either incineration or land fill on daily basis. No waste should be left overnight in the theater.

Dermatologist in remote area should look into two main options of waste management:

1. *Sharps, plastic syringes, needle*: These should be shred after treatment in chlorine bleach for 12 hours.
2. *Blood soaked gauze*: These should be incinerated after treating in chlorine bleach for 12 hours.[32]

ERGONOMICS

Ergon (work) + Nomo's (law) is the study focusing on worker's safety and productivity. In a well-designed work atmosphere, the workers should not be able to find any design or architectural deficiency but only concentrate on his/her work at hand.

In the theater during hair transplantation, large area Vitiligo punch grafting and large area electrosurgery, a dermatologist could experience strain in the following four segments: (1) lower limb, (2) back, (3) neck and shoulder and (4) arm, wrist and hand.

But unfortunately surgical training discourages about complaining of stress and fatigue. Surgeons till now were reluctant to have their unique work habits analyzed or criticized by others.[33] However, there is an increasing awareness about these aspects now.

What is the Best Posture during Standing or Sitting?

Standing: During standing, the head should be upright on torso, torso upright with the center of gravity over the hips, knees slightly bent and hands by the sides.

Sitting: During sitting, one thinks that 90° hip flexion, 90° knee flexion, 90° elbow flexion with back and neck erect is ideal posture which is a myth. The ideal position of hip flexion is 105° with the back supported by the back rest. This puts least pressure on the intervertebral disk.

BOX 3: Ergonomically designed chair.

- The seat height is adjustable with pneumatic pedestal (15–22 inches)
- Good lumbar support
- A seat pan with curved front
- Five pronged base support to prevent the chair from falling
- A good foot rest to prevent the stress of dangling thigh and leg on the hip **(Fig. 10)**.

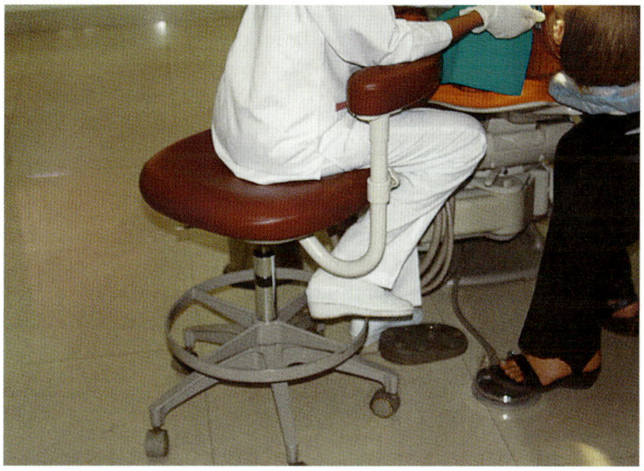

Fig. 10: An ideal chair with good base, foot rest, seat pan, lumbar seat support which can change to hand support and adjustable height.

Which Position is Better: Sitting or Standing?

Both are good depending on the surgery. During standing position, the pressure on the intervertebral disk is 33% lesser than that of sitting. So standing in upright posture is more disk-friendly. But sitting requires 20% less energy than standing. During sitting only a few muscle groups are active and receive oxygenation. The large muscles of lower limbs are inactive and under prolonged tension leading to CO_2 buildup and fatigue. The features of ergonomically designed chair have been mentioned in **Box 3**.

To reduce the effect of posture on the body, several rules should be kept in mind:

- Change the position frequently.
- All procedures require forward bending putting strain on neck and back so position the operation table in a high visual field range to keep head balanced on spine.
- Arms should be kept next to the body, lifting and moving away from trunk increases strain (this is the neutral position of the arm).
- Precise surgery requires proper visualization and arm support. Ideally the operation table should be at 5–10 cm above elbow height. Elbow height is measured from the floor to the olecranon process of the elbow of the operator.
- Take regular breaks during prolonged surgeries, even before pain or discomfort sets in.
- By this you are preventing injuries.
- A break of 30 seconds is as good as long breaks.[34]

CONCLUSION

A dermatosurgical procedure is deemed successful if there is aseptic wound healing, surgery was painless with minimal blood loss. To achieve this, one has to have a clean, unobstructed work place which is easy to disinfect and in some situations sterilize. This place should have good set of instruments, advanced life support with good lighting. To achieve this, World Health Organization calls for "sober down to earth planning and design" of theater. Operation theater should not be viewed as a luxury but in reality, it is a place of high standard of patient safety with most economical use of manpower and other resources.

REFERENCES

1. Geisse JK. The dermatologic surgical suite. Semin Dermatol. 1994;13:29.
2. MedScape. Outpatient Surgical Suite 16. [online] Available from: emedicine.medscape.com/article/1128609. [Last Accessed April, 2021].
3. Golberg LH, Peterson SR, Silaprint S. The incidence of major complications from mohs micrographic surgery performed in office-based and hospital-based settings. J Am Acad Dermatol. 2005;53:62834.
4. Indian Standard Bureau. Basic requirements for hospital planning. IS12433 (part 2). 2001Reaffirmed. Indian Standard Bureau. 2006;2639.
5. MCI. The minimum standard requirements for the medical college—Amended (November 2010). [online] Available from: www.mciindia.org. [Last Accessed April, 2021].
6. Rajendran SC, Omprakash HM. Standard guidelines for setting up a dermatosurgery theater. Indian J Dermatol Venereal Leprol. 2009;75:7682.
7. International Joint Commission. Accreditation for Ambulatory Care. [online] Available from: www.jointcommissioninternational.org/ambulatorycare. [Last Accessed April, 2021].
8. Ministry of Health. Directives for private ambulatory surgical centers providing ambulatory surgery. Singapore. 2007:16
9. Building guidelines for a surgical department. Netherlands Board for Hospital Facilities. 2004:116.
10. WHO. Surgical care at the district hospital. Geneva: WHO; 2003. pp. 213.
11. Savant SS, Gore D. Instruments, equipment and universal precautions. In: Savant SS (Ed). Textbook of Dermatosurgery and Cosmetology. Mumbai, India: Association of Scientific Cosmetologists and Dermatosurgeons; 2005. pp. 2634.
12. Unger WP. The surgical suite. In: Unger WP, Shapiro R (Eds). Hair Transplantation. New York: Marcel Dekker; 2004. pp. 8334.
13. Malkin J. Ambulatory surgical centers. In: Malkin J (Ed). Medical and Dental Space Planning: A Comprehensive Guide to Design, Equipment and Clinical Procedures, 3rd edition. New York: John Wiley and Sons; 2002. pp. 3346.
14. Malkin J. Ambulatory surgical centers. In: Malkin J (Ed). Medical and Dental Space Planning: A Comprehensive Guide to Design, Equipment and Clinical Procedures, 3rd edition. New York: John Wiley and Sons; 2002. pp. 3523.
15. Ministry of Health. Regulations governing private hospitals and unattached operating theater units. Government of South Africa. 1993. pp. 810.

16. Ridley SA, Parry G. Guidelines for Fire safety in Intensive Care Unit. NHS, UK: Intensive Care Society Publication; 1998. pp. 116.
17. Lawrence C. Equipment. In: Lawrence C (Ed). An Introduction to Dermatological Surgery, 2nd edition. London: Churchill Livingstone; 2002. pp. 910.
18. Malkin J. Construction methods and building systems. In: Malkin J (Ed). Medical and Dental Space planning: A comprehensive guide to design, equipment and clinical procedures, 3rd edition. New York: John Wiley and Sons; 2002. pp. 55661.
19. Perez M, Lodha R, Nouri K. Surgical equipment and instrumentation. In: Nouri K, Leal S(Eds). Khouri Techniques in Dermatologic Surgery. Missouri: Mosby; 2003. pp. 2531.
20. NABH. (2010). The revised guidelines for air conditioning system for operation theater. (2010). [online] Available from: https://nabh.co/Announcement/RevisedGuidelines_AirConditioning.pdf. [Last Accessed April, 2021].
21. BioMedical Waste Management and Handling Rules, Second Amendment, 2000. Ministry of Environment and Forests, Government of India. 2000.
22. Female sterilization operation. Ensuring right to safety, dignity and informed choice. Government of India standards. 2005. Order dated 01.03.2005 passed in writ petition {civil} no209/2003; Ramkant Rai v/s. Union of India and others. (Available from www.hrln.org).
23. Field JM, Soderberg ES, Gonzales L. Advanced Cardiovascular Life Support Provider Manual, Professional. Texas: Published on behalf of American Heart Association; 2006. pp. 1142.
24. Ministry of Health and Family Welfare. Emergency drugs for both tubectomy and vasectomy camps. In: Standard operating procedures for sterilization services in camps. Ministry of Health and Family Welfare, Government of India: Family planning division; 2008. pp. 301.
25. Pratt RJ, Pellowe C, Loveday HP, Robinson N, Smith GW, Barrett S, et al. The epic project: Developing national evidence-based guideline for preventing healthcare based guidelines for preventing healthcare associated infections. Phase I: Guideline for preventing hospitalacquired infections. J Hosp Infect. 2001;47 (Supplement): S34.
26. Sawchuk WS, Weber PJ, Lowy DR, Dzubow LM. Infectious papillomavirus in the vapor of warts treated with carbon dioxide laser or electrocoagulation: detection and protection. J Am Acad Dermatol. 1989;21:419.
27. Marra DE, Fincher EF, Moy RL. Surgical preparation, facilities and monitoring. In: Roenigk's Dermatologic Surgery. Current Techniques in Procedural Dermatology, 3rd edition. New York: Informa; 2007. pp. 19.
28. Korsolex. Baccillol agents. [online] Available from: www.Bodechemie.de. [Last Accessed April, 2021].
29. Savant SS, Gore D. Instruments, equipment and universal precautions. In: Savant SS (Ed). Textbook of Dermatosurgery and Cosmetology. Mumbai, India: Association of Scientific Cosmetologists and Dermatosurgeons; 2005. pp. 26.
30. Satyanarayana Rao KH. Informed consent: an ethical obligation or legal compulsion? J Cutan Aesthet Surg. 2008;1:335.
31. Operation Theater Standard No27, Theater Etiquette. Royal United Bath Hospital NHS Trust, Theater practice policy, Reference no. 742. Combe Park: Royal United Bath Hospital; 2006.
32. Categories of biomedical waste. Schedule I. Ministry of Environment and Forest, Government of India. [online] Available from: envfov.nic.in/legis/hsm/biomed.html. [Last Accessed April, 2021].
33. Burguer R. Surgery and Ergonomics. Arch Surg. 1999;134: 10116.
34. Jacobs K. Ergonomics for Therapists. Missouri: Mosby; 2008; 1460.

CHAPTER 9

Disinfection and Sterilization

Uday Kelkar, Somodyuti Chandra

KEY MESSAGES

- Dermatosurgeons should be familiar with different processes such as cleaning, disinfection, and sterilization.
- Dermatosurgical instruments used in hair transplantation, liposuction, vitiligo surgery, dermabrasion, nail surgery, and scar revisions belong to critical device category. Most other instruments are noncritical.
- Handwashing by healthcare personnel is the most important procedure for preventing nosocomial infections and is of two types—(1) typical surgical scrub and (2) routine hand scrub.
- Methodical cleaning before high-level disinfection and sterilization removes organic and inorganic materials on the surfaces of instruments and enhances the efficiency of these processes.
- Disinfectants are classified as high-level, intermediate-level, and low-level disinfectants.
- Sterilization, which is an absolute process, achieves destruction of all microbes including spores and can be carried out either by physical or chemical methods.

INTRODUCTION

Dermatosurgical practice involves procedures that are performed mostly in outpatient settings and some procedures performed exclusively in operation theater. In dermatological surgery, adverse events in the form of infections are not common, but the potential for nosocomial infections does exist. The rates of postoperative infections tend to be low, but have been documented to be ranging from 0.2–3.5%.[1-3] Superficial infections occur essentially as a result of breach in the laid down and advocated standard infection control practices. Disinfection and sterilization constitute the foundation and core of standard infection control practices. Maintenance of strict asepsis is essential to minimize postoperative infections and their consequences. Awareness about these practices and principles is of great importance as dermatosurgeons today perform increasing number of procedures. This is particularly so, since many of these procedures are aesthetic procedures with possible medicolegal implications.

The pandemic of severe acute respiratory syndrome coronavirus 2 (SARS-CoV-2) has necessitated the need to redefine the outpatient practices and importance of disinfection and sterilization in all healthcare facilities. The dermatology practice is not an exception but rather one of the fields where the healthcare worker and practitioner would be coming in close contact with the patient. The redefined practices not only aid in preventing transmission of this deadly pathogen but would also ensure reduced transmission of infections.

The reader is also suggested to read this chapter in conjunction with Chapter 10 on Universal Precautions.

BASIC PRINCIPLES OF DISINFECTION AND STERILIZATION

Infections can be either of endogenous or exogenous origin. Factors associated with transmission of infective material exogenously in hospitals and clinics include:

- Use of inadequately sterilized equipment
- Presence of shedders of pathogenic microorganisms among the hospital personnel
- Contaminated environment and contaminated surfaces[4,5]
- Poor standards in antiseptic precautions

Appropriate disinfection and sterilization policy is the mainstay of a successful infection control program to ensure that medical and surgical equipment does not transmit infectious pathogens to patients. It is important to appreciate that different practices are needed for different instruments and equipment, and practitioners must identify the right process such as cleaning, disinfection, or sterilization is needed, primarily on the basis of items intended for use.

IMPORTANT DEFINITIONS

- *Sterilization* is defined as a process that destroys or eliminates all forms of microbial life including bacterial endospores. Sterilization is carried out in hospitals and clinics by physical or chemical methods. Sterilization is intended to convey an absolute process.
- *Disinfection* is defined as a physical or chemical procedure performed on inanimate objects such as instruments and environmental surfaces that eliminate many pathogenic microorganisms. High-level disinfection is a procedure that destroys all microorganisms except high numbers

of bacterial endospores. Unlike sterilization, disinfection is not sporicidal. Few disinfectants will kill spores with prolonged exposure time, and these are called *chemical sterilants*.

- *Decontamination* is defined as removal of pathogenic organisms from objects in order to make them safe to handle.
- *Antisepsis* is defined as a procedure wherein a germicide is used on skin or living tissue with the intention of inhibiting or destroying microorganisms. The term is inappropriately used interchangeably with disinfection. Antiseptics are not designed to be used on medical devices, instruments, or environmental surfaces and should not be confused with disinfectants, which are too irritating to be used on skin or tissue.
- *Germicide* is a chemical agent that destroys microorganisms on either inanimate objects or living tissue.
- *Cleaning* is a prerequisite for disinfection or sterilization. It is the physical removal of organic material or soil from objects usually done by using water with or without detergents. Generally, cleaning is designed to remove rather than to kill microorganisms.

CLASSIFICATION OF MEDICAL DEVICES

The choice of a sterilization or disinfection procedure depends on the type of items to be processed. A helpful categorization devised by Spaulding stratifies medical equipment into critical, semi-critical, and noncritical devices on the basis of the risk of infections implicated with their use.[6]

Critical Devices

Instruments or equipment having a contact with the bloodstream or sterile areas of the body is classified as critical devices. Risk of acquiring infections is significant, if these devices are contaminated. Bloodstream catheters, implants, needles, scalpels, and surgical instruments are some of the examples of critical devices. Dermatosurgical instruments used in hair transplantation, liposuction, vitiligo surgery, dermabrasion, nail surgery, scar revisions, etc. belong to this category. Critical devices require sterilization prior to use on patients.

Semi-critical Devices

Equipment that comes in contact with mucous membrane is considered as semi-critical devices. Although these items come in contact with intact mucous membranes, they do not ordinarily penetrate body surface. Endoscopes, endotracheal tubes, anesthesia-breathing circuits, cystoscopes, respiratory care equipment, and urinary catheters are examples of semi-critical devices. Sterilization is the preferred method for processing these devices. However, sterilization is not absolutely essential and hence in situations where sterilization is not feasible, high-level disinfection after thorough cleaning is an acceptable alternative.

Noncritical Devices

Devices coming into contact with intact skin of patients are classified as noncritical. The risk of acquiring infections from these devices is minimal. Stethoscopes, cardiac electrodes, crutches, sphygmomanometer cuffs, surfaces of medical equipment, and environmental surfaces are grouped under this category. Most instruments used in aesthetic procedures such as microdermabrasion, lasers, and phototherapy glasses belong to this category. The cleaning and disinfection policy for these depend upon the physical characters of these items or surfaces. It ranges from simple detergent-based cleaning to low-level disinfection methods.

ANTISEPSIS AND NORMAL BACTERIAL SKIN FLORA

Antisepsis is defined as a procedure wherein a germicide is used on skin or living tissue with the intention of inhibiting or destroying microorganisms. It is important to understand the normal skin microorganisms to understand the antiseptics.

Normal human skin is colonized with bacteria; different areas of the body have varied total aerobic bacterial counts. Total bacterial counts on the hands of medical personnel have ranged from 3.9×10^4 to 4.6×10^6. Bacteria recovered from the hands are divided into two categories—transient and resident.[6] The hands of healthcare workers may become persistently colonized with pathogenic flora (e.g., *Staphylococcus aureus*), gram-negative bacilli, or yeast. Investigators have documented that, although the number of transient and resident flora varies considerably from person-to-person, it is often relatively constant for any specific person.[7,8]

Transient flora, which colonizes the superficial layers of the skin, is more common source of the organisms most frequently associated with healthcare-associated infections and is amenable to removal by routine handwashing. They are often acquired by healthcare workers during direct contact with patients or contact with contaminated environmental surfaces within close proximity of the patient. Resident flora (e.g., coagulase-negative staphylococci and diphtheroids) is found in deeper layers of the skin and is more resistant to removal. However, resident flora is less likely to cause infections.

Handwashing

Handwashing by healthcare personnel, the most commonly performed antiseptic procedure, is also the most important procedure for preventing nosocomial infections. When done with plain soap, it results in mechanical removal of microorganisms and if done with detergents containing antimicrobial agents, it results in chemical removal of microorganisms as well. In practice, handwashing is broadly of two types—(1) typical surgical scrub and (2) routine hand scrub after examining a patient. Surgical hand scrub is an elaborate detailed procedure performed for a minimum 2 minutes; while a casual hand scrub is advocated after patient examination (for details see chapter Universal Precautions). Different handwash antiseptics are discussed below.

Alcohol-based Hand Scrubs

The majority of alcohol-based hand antiseptics contain isopropanol, ethanol, n-propanol, or a combination of two of these products. Alcohols are usually used as a combination of two alcohols or along with other agents such as hexachlorophene, quaternary ammonium compounds, povidone-iodine, triclosan, or chlorhexidine gluconate. The antimicrobial activity of alcohols can be attributed to their ability to denature proteins. Alcohol solutions containing 60–95% alcohol are most effective and higher concentrations are less potent because proteins are not denatured easily in the absence of water.

Chlorhexidine: Chlorhexidine gluconate, a cationic biguanide, acts by disruption of cytoplasmic membranes, resulting in precipitation of cellular contents. Chlorhexidine has good activity against gram-positive bacteria, somewhat less activity against gram-negative bacteria and fungi and only minimal activity against tubercle bacilli. The antimicrobial activity of chlorhexidine is only minimally affected by the presence of organic material, including blood. Chlorhexidine has substantial residual activity; addition of low concentrations (0.5–1.0%) of chlorhexidine to alcohol-based preparations results in greater residual activity than alcohol alone.

Iodophors: Iodine molecules rapidly penetrate the cell wall of microorganisms and inactivate cells by forming complexes with amino acids and unsaturated fatty acids, resulting in impaired protein synthesis and alteration of cell membranes. The antimicrobial activity of iodophors can be affected by pH, temperature, exposure time, concentration of total available iodine, and the amount and type of organic and inorganic compounds present (e.g., alcohols and detergents). Iodine and iodophors have bactericidal activity against gram-positive, gram-negative, and certain spore forming bacteria (e.g., clostridia and *Bacillus* species) and are active against mycobacteria, viruses, and fungi. However, in concentrations used in antiseptics, iodophors are not usually sporicidal. Povidone-iodine 5–10% has been classified as a safe and effective agent for use as an antiseptic handwash. The majority of iodophor preparations used for hand hygiene contain 7.5–10% povidone-iodine.

FACTORS AFFECTING THE EFFICACY OF DISINFECTION AND STERILIZATION

The germicidal activity depends on a number of factors, based on intrinsic qualities of the organism and the chemical and external physical environment.[6,9-12]

Number and Location of Microorganisms

All other conditions remaining constant, the larger the number of microbes, the more time a germicide needs to destroy all of them. This emphasizes the need for scrupulous cleaning of medical instruments, before disinfection and sterilization. Meticulous cleaning reduces the number of microorganisms that must be inactivated, increasing the margin of safety when the germicide is used. The location of microorganisms also affects the efficacy of germicides. Medical instruments with multiple pieces need to be disassembled and equipment such as endoscopes that have crevices and channels needs more meticulous disinfection than flat surface equipment, because penetration of the disinfectant into all parts of the equipment is more difficult.

Innate Resistance of Microorganisms

Microorganisms differ greatly in their susceptibility to chemical germicides and sterilization processes. Spores are generally resistant to disinfectants, because the spore coat and cortex act as a barrier. *Mycobacteria* have a waxy cell wall that prevents disinfectant entry, and gram-negative bacteria possess an outer membrane that acts as a barrier to the uptake of disinfectants.[13,14] The sterilization or disinfection time is dependent upon the time required to destroy the most resistant forms. Prions possess the highest innate resistance to chemical germicides, followed by bacterial spores, coccidia (*Cryptosporidium*), mycobacteria (*M. tuberculosis*), non-lipid or small viruses (poliovirus and *Coxsackievirus*), fungi (*Aspergillus* and *Candida*), vegetative bacteria (e.g., *Staphylococcus* and *Pseudomonas*), and lipid or medium size viruses (herpes and HIV).[15-17]

Concentration and Potency of Disinfectants

With other variables constant and with one exception (iodophors), the more concentrated the disinfectant, the greater its efficacy and the shorter the time necessary to achieve microbial kill. However, all disinfectants are not similarly affected by concentration changes. For example, quaternary ammonium compounds and phenol have a concentration exponent of 1 and 6, respectively; thus, halving the concentration of a quaternary ammonium compound requires doubling its disinfecting time, but halving the concentration of a phenol solution requires a 64-fold increase in its disinfecting time.[12,18,19] Length of the contact time with disinfectant thus depends on the potency of the germicide.

Physical and Chemical Factors

Temperature, pH, relative humidity, and water hardness affect the disinfection time. The activity of most disinfectants increases as the temperature increases, but some exceptions exist. An increase in pH improves the antimicrobial activity of some disinfectants (e.g., glutaraldehyde and quaternary ammonium compounds) but decreases the antimicrobial activity of others (e.g., phenols, hypochlorites, and iodine).[12] Relative humidity is the single most important factor influencing the activity of gaseous disinfectants/sterilants such as ethylene oxide (ETO), chlorine dioxide, and formaldehyde. Water hardness (i.e., high concentration of divalent cations) reduces the rate of kill of certain disinfectants because divalent cations (e.g., magnesium and calcium) in the hard water interact with the disinfectant to form insoluble precipitates.[9,20]

Types of Matter: Organic and Inorganic

Presence of serum, blood, pus, or fecal or lubricant material interferes with the antimicrobial activity of disinfectants. Interference occurs by a chemical reaction between the germicide and the organic matter resulting in a complex that is less germicidal. Chlorine and iodine disinfectants, in particular, are prone to such interaction.[21] Inorganic contaminants such as salts have an effect of protecting microorganisms by interfering in the sterilization cycle. Meticulous cleaning of medical devices before any sterilization or disinfection procedure is therefore very important, as organic and inorganic soils can be easily removed by washing.[22]

Duration of Exposure

Items need exposure to the germicide for the appropriate contact time. All lumens and channels of endoscopic instruments must come in contact with the disinfectant. The disinfectant must be introduced reliably into the internal channels of the devices.

Cleaning

As emphasized above, methodical cleaning is necessary before high-level disinfection and sterilization, as the organic and inorganic materials that may persist on the surfaces of instruments interfere with the efficiency of these processes. Cleaning is the process of removing alien material (e.g., soil and organic material) from objects. Cleaning is important for several reasons:

- Instruments and materials used during a procedure are usually covered with blood and remains of tissues; they may have also been in touch with chemicals and fluids, dirt and dust. The tubing of hollow instruments may also be full of these soils. Cleaning plays an immensely important role in this process.
- A major requirement for critical devices is that they should be sterile. However, sterility alone is not sufficient for safe use. An instrument, which is covered with sterile dirt or with remains of chemicals or corrosion, still is a serious health hazard. Thus, all potentially dangerous soil or remains have to be removed by cleaning.
- In case the proteinaceous material dries on the device, the disinfection or sterilization process becomes less effective or ineffective. Surgical instruments should be presoaked or rinsed to prevent drying of blood and to soften or remove blood from the instruments. Ultrasonic cleaners are a useful addition to the available equipment to ensure that the material sticking to the instruments gets dislodged prior to cleaning.
- The process of cleaning reduces the bioburden (the population of microorganisms residing on the materials) considerably **(Fig. 1)**. Reduction of the bioburden ensures that the disinfection or sterilization process will be more effective, as much less organisms have to be killed.
- Cleaning also ensures that the pyrogens and endotoxins are effectively removed.

Methods of Cleaning

Cleaning is normally done by using water with detergents or enzymatic products. Cleaning can be either manual or automatic. Cleaning is done manually in most of healthcare settings. In manual cleaning, the two essential components are friction and use of fluids. Friction (e.g., rubbing/scrubbing the soiled area with a brush) is an old and dependable method. Fluids, usually water, under pressure are used to remove soil and debris from internal channels after brushing and when the design does not allow passage of a brush through a channel.[23] It is of vital importance that the instruments should be disassembled as much as possible.

The most common type of automatic cleaners is ultrasonic cleaner **(Fig. 2)**. Ultrasonic cleaning removes soil by cavitation and implosion in which waves of acoustic energy are propagated in aqueous solutions to disrupt the bonds that hold particulate matter to surfaces. The process of

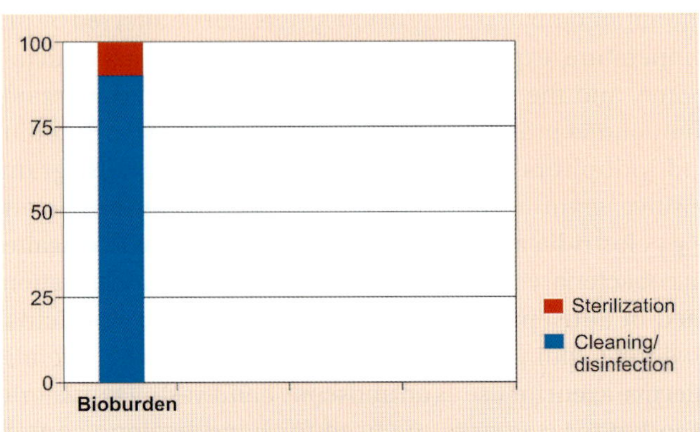

Fig. 1: Percentage reduction of bioburden.

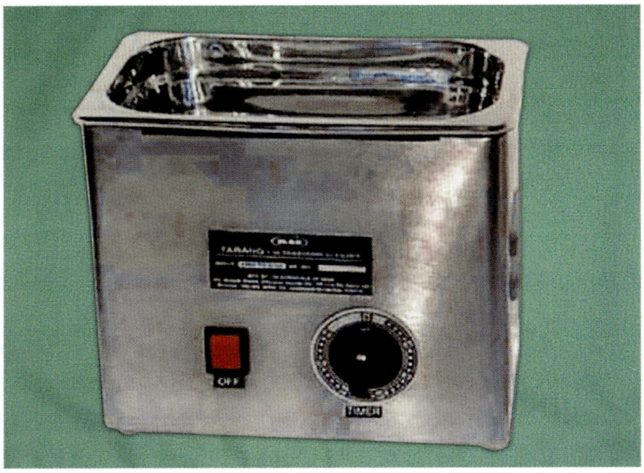

Fig. 2: Ultrasonic cleaner.

sonication can act synergistically to increase the cidal efficacy of a disinfectant.[24]

Washer sterilizers are modified steam sterilizers that clean by filling the chamber with water and detergent through which steam passes to provide agitation. Instruments are subsequently rinsed and subjected to a short steam sterilization cycle.[25] Washer decontaminators act like a dishwasher that uses a combination of water circulation and detergents to remove soil. Washer disinfectors are generally computer-controlled units for cleaning, disinfecting, and drying solid and hollow surgical and medical equipment. Studies have shown that manual and mechanical cleaning of endoscopes achieves approximately a $\log(10^4)$ reduction of contaminating organisms.[26]

Instrument cleaning requires a neutral or near neutral pH detergent solution because such solutions generally provide the best material compatibility profile and good soil removal. Enzymes, usually proteases, sometimes are added to neutral pH solutions to assist in removing organic material. Enzymes in these formulations attack proteins that make up a large portion of common soil (e.g., blood and pus). Cleaning solutions also can contain lipases (enzymes active on fats) and amylases (enzymes active on starches). Enzymatic cleaners are not disinfectants and proteinaceous enzymes can be inactivated by germicides. Enzyme solutions should be used in proper dilution of the enzymatic detergent and contact with equipment for the amount of time specified on the label.[27]

Validation of Cleaning Process

Although the effectiveness of high-level disinfection and sterilization mandates effective cleaning, it is rather difficult to validate the cleaning process. The ideal and foolproof method to ensure adequate cleaning is to conduct microbiologic sampling, but this is not practicable and hence not routinely recommended.[28] Visual inspection of the cleaned and dried gadgets is the commonly employed and acceptable method

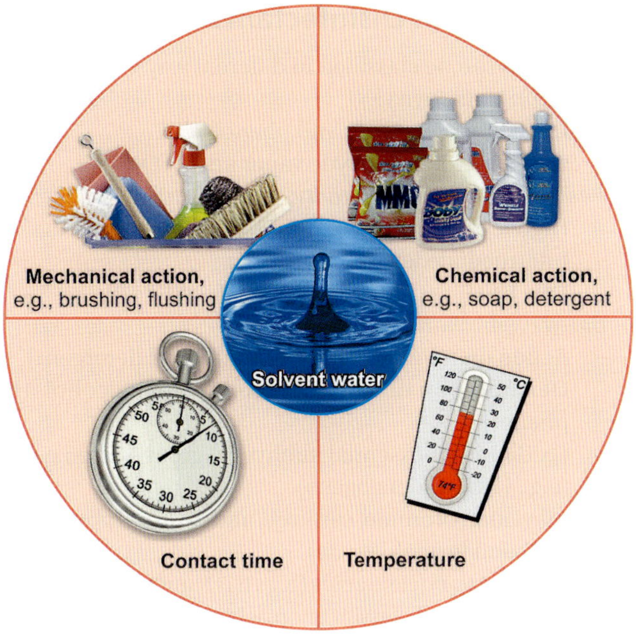

Fig. 3: Cleaning circle: all factors are essential.

employed in hospitals. Instruments must be individually inspected and be visibly clean **(Fig. 3)**.

DISINFECTION

Disinfection describes a process that eliminates most or all pathogenic microorganisms, except bacterial spores. Since disinfected products are not wrapped, they can be contaminated and do not remain germ-free. Disinfection decreases the population of microorganisms by a limited reduction factor (up to 10^5) in contrast to sterilization, which inactivates all varieties of microorganisms including spores, resulting in a very low probability of persistence. Some disinfectants can kill spores with prolonged exposure time and are called chemical sterilants. The required efficacy of the disinfection process is linked to the intended use and the microorganisms relevant for that use (e.g., bedpans require a lower level of disinfection than a flexible endoscope). For disinfectants, the level and intended spectrum of activity are specified in international standards.

In practice, instruments are usually disinfected by liquid chemicals. The choice of specific cleaning or disinfecting agents is largely a matter of judgment, guided by product label claims and instructions. A single liquid chemical germicide might not satisfy all disinfection requirements in a given practice or facility. Realistic use of liquid chemical germicides depends on consideration of multiple factors, including the degree of microbial killing required; the nature and composition of the surface, item, or device to be treated; and the cost, safety, and ease of use of the available agents.

The properties of an ideal antiseptic or disinfectant are given in **Box 1**.

Classification of Disinfectants

Disinfectants can be classified in different ways:

- *Based on consistency*:
  - Liquid (e.g., alcohols and phenols)
  - Gaseous (formaldehyde vapor and ETO)
- *Based on spectrum of activity*:
  - High level
  - Intermediate level
  - Low level
- *Based on mechanism of action*:
  - Action on membrane (e.g., alcohol and detergent)
  - Denaturation of cellular proteins (e.g., alcohol and phenol)
  - Oxidation of essential sulfhydryl groups of enzymes (e.g., H_2O_2 and halogens)
  - Alkylation of amino, carboxyl, and hydroxyl group (e.g., ETO and formaldehyde)
  - Damage to nucleic acids (e.g., ETO and formaldehyde)
- A commonly used classification, which is universally used, is as follows **(Table 1)**:
  - *High-level disinfectants*: Chemicals that kill all microorganisms and can act as sterilants, if applied for prolonged length of time. However, if spores are present in large numbers, they are not killed.
  - *Intermediate-level disinfectants*: They kill all mycobacteria, vegetative bacteria, most viruses, and most fungi, but not bacterial spores.
  - *Low-level disinfectants:* They can kill most vegetative bacteria, but only some fungi and some viruses.

Different Agents and Methods

Both chemical and nonchemical methods are available.

Chemical Disinfectants

A wide variety of germicides, which differ in their spectrum of activity against various forms of microorganisms, are available **(Fig. 4)**. Chemical composition and structure of the outer cell layers determine the uptake of germicide.

- *Alcohols:* Alcohols in healthcare refer to two water-soluble chemical compounds—(1) ethyl alcohol and (2) isopropyl alcohol. These alcohols are rapidly bactericidal against vegetative forms of bacteria; they also are tuberculocidal, fungicidal, and virucidal, but do not destroy bacterial spores. Their cidal activity drops sharply when diluted below 50% concentration, and the optimum bactericidal concentration is 60–90% solutions in water (volume/volume).[29] Alcohols act by denaturation of proteins. The mixtures of alcohol and water is more bactericidal because proteins are denatured more quickly in the presence of water than absolute alcohols, which have a dehydrating action.[29] Methyl alcohol (methanol) has the weakest bactericidal action of the alcohols. Ethyl alcohol, at concentrations of 60–80%, is a potent virucidal agent inactivating all of the lipophilic viruses (e.g., herpes, vaccinia, and influenza virus) and many hydrophilic viruses [e.g., adenovirus, enterovirus, rhinovirus, and rotaviruses but not hepatitis A virus (HAV) or poliovirus].[30] Isopropyl alcohol is not active against the nonlipid enteroviruses but is fully active against the lipid viruses. Ethyl and isopropyl alcohol have the ability to inactivate the hepatitis B virus (HBV)[31] and the herpes virus[32] and ethyl alcohol to inactivate human immunodeficiency virus (HIV).[33]
  Alcohols have been used effectively to disinfect noncritical devices and to disinfect external surfaces of equipment. However, alcohols are not recommended for sterilizing medical and surgical materials, as they lack sporicidal action and they cannot penetrate protein-rich materials. Disadvantages of alcohols are:
  - They damage the shellac mountings of lensed instruments.
  - Tend to swell and harden rubber and certain plastic tubing after prolonged and repeated use.
  - Bleach rubber and plastic tiles.[34]
  - Alcohols are flammable and consequently must be stored in a cool and well-ventilated area.
  - They also evaporate rapidly, making extended exposure time difficult to achieve unless the items are immersed.
- *Chlorine and chlorine compounds*: Hypochlorites, the most widely used of the chlorine disinfectants, are available as liquid (e.g., sodium hypochlorite) or solid (e.g., calcium hypochlorite). The most prevalent chlorine products is the

BOX 1: Characteristics of an ideal disinfectant.

- Wide spectrum of activity
- Ability to destroy microbes within reasonable period of time
- Activity in the presence of organic matter
- Activity over a wide range of pH
- Stability and shelf life
- Speedy action
- High penetrating power
- Nontoxic, nonallergenic, nonirritative, and noncorrosive
- Should not leave nonvolatile residue or stain
- Easily available and reasonable cost

TABLE 1: Spectrum of activity of disinfectants.

	Vegetative cells	*Mycobacteria*	*Spores*	*Fungi*	*Viruses*	*Examples*
High level	+	+	+	+	+	Ethylene oxide, glutaraldehyde, and formaldehyde
Intermediate level	+	+		+	+	Phenolics and halogens
Low level	+			+	+/-	Alcohols and quaternary ammonium compounds

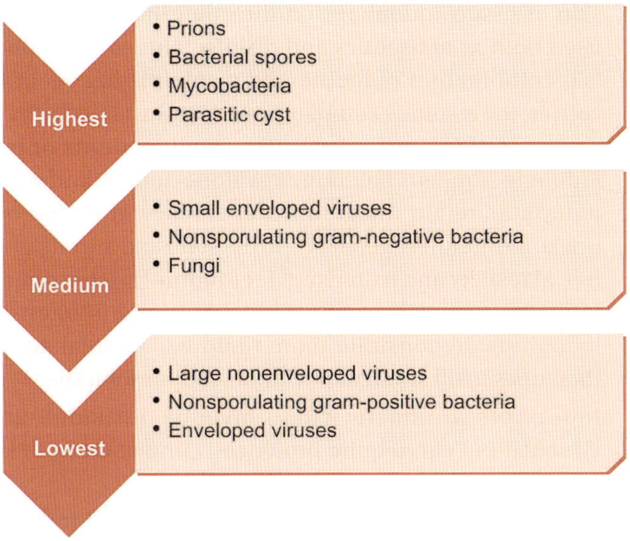

Fig. 4: Resistance of microorganisms to disinfectants in descending order.

aqueous solutions of 5–6% sodium hypochlorite, usually called household bleach. They have a broad spectrum of antimicrobial activity, do not leave toxic residues, are unaffected by water hardness, are inexpensive and fast acting,[35] remove dried or fixed organisms and biofilms from surfaces,[36] and have a low incidence of serious toxicity.[37] Sodium hypochlorite at the concentration used in household bleach can produce ocular irritation or oropharyngeal, esophageal, and gastric burns.[38] Hypochlorites are corrosive in nature specially to metals, are inactivated by organic matter, and lead to discoloration of fabrics and release of toxic chlorine gas when mixed with ammonia or acid.[39] The actual microbicidal mechanism of chlorine may be due to a combination of several factors such as oxidation of sulfhydryl enzymes and amino acids, ring chlorination of amino acids, loss of intracellular contents, decreased uptake of nutrients, inhibition of protein synthesis, decreased oxygen uptake, breaks in DNA, and depressed DNA synthesis. The microbicidal activity of chlorine is attributed largely to undissociated hypochlorous acid (HOCl). The dissociation of HOCI to the less microbicidal form (hypochlorite ion OCl) depends on the pH. The disinfecting efficacy of chlorine decreases with an increase in pH.[40] Chlorine dioxide, sodium dichloroisocyanurate, and chloramine T are the other compounds used as chlorine-releasing agents. The advantage of these compounds over the hypochlorites is that they retain chlorine longer and so exert a more prolonged bactericidal effect.[41] Chlorine solution is used for disinfecting countertops and floors. It has been recommended for decontaminating blood spills. For small spills of blood on noncritical surfaces, the area can be disinfected with a 1:100 dilution of 5–6% sodium hypochlorite. Hypochlorites and other germicides are substantially inactivated in the presence of blood.[42] Large spills of blood require that the surface be cleaned before a 1:10 (final concentration) solution of household bleach is applied.[43]

- *Superoxidized water*: Superoxidized water is a relatively new disinfectant with good microbicidal properties.[44] Saline is electrolyzed to create a disinfectant or antiseptics. The solution is nontoxic to biologic tissues. Superoxidized water is generally noncorrosive to equipment. The activity of this disinfectant decreases substantially in the presence of organic material.
- *Formaldehyde*: Formaldehyde is used as a disinfectant and sterilant in both its liquid and gaseous states. Formaldehyde inactivates microorganisms by alkylating the amino and sulfhydryl groups of proteins and ring nitrogen atoms of purine bases. Formaldehyde alcohol is a chemical sterilant and formaldehyde is a high-level disinfectant. Formaldehyde is sold and used principally as water-based solution called formalin, which is 37% formaldehyde by weight. The aqueous solution is a bactericidal, tuberculocidal, fungicidal, virucidal, and sporicidal. Formaldehyde, however, is a potential carcinogen and ingestion of formaldehyde can be fatal. Long-term exposure to low-levels in the air or on the skin can cause asthma-like respiratory problems and skin irritation such as dermatitis and itching. For these reasons, employees should have limited direct contact with formaldehyde and an employee exposure standard for formaldehyde that limits an 8-hour time weighted average exposure concentration of 0.75 ppm.[45] These considerations and its pungent odor and irritating fumes limit its role in sterilization and disinfection processes.
- *Glutaraldehyde:* Glutaraldehyde is a saturated dialdehyde, which is a high-level disinfectant and chemical sterilant. The biocidal activity of glutaraldehyde results from its alkylation of sulfhydryl, hydroxyl, carboxyl, and amino groups of microorganisms, which alters RNA, DNA, and protein synthesis. 2% alkaline glutaraldehyde has excellent cidal action against bacteria, fungi, viruses, and a relatively slow action (20 to >30 minutes) against *Mycobacterium tuberculosis*. Aqueous solutions of glutaraldehyde are acidic and generally in this state, these are not sporicidal. Only when the solution is "activated" (made alkaline) by the use of alkalinating agents to pH 7.5–8.5, then the solution becomes sporicidal. Once activated, these solutions have a limited shelf life of about 14 days, because of the polymerization of the glutaraldehyde molecules at alkaline pH levels. Newer glutaraldehyde formulations (e.g., glutaraldehyde-phenol-sodium phenate, potentiated acid glutaraldehyde, and stabilized alkaline glutaraldehyde) have a longer shelf life (e.g., use life 2,830 days). The use of glutaraldehyde-based solutions in healthcare facilities is widespread because of their advantages, including excellent biocidal properties, activity in the presence of organic matter (20% bovine serum), and noncorrosive

action to endoscopic equipment, thermometers, rubber, or plastic equipment.[46,47] *It is very suitable for most dermatosurgical equipment.*

Acute or chronic exposure to glutaraldehyde can result in skin irritation or dermatitis, mucous membrane irritation (eye, nose, and mouth), or pulmonary symptoms.[38] Measures that can be used to resolve these problems include ducted exhaust hoods, air systems that provide 7–15 air exchanges per hour, ductless fume hoods with absorbents for the glutaraldehyde vapor, tight-fitting lids on immersion baths, and personal protection (e.g., nitrile or butyl rubber gloves but not natural latex gloves, goggles) to minimize skin or mucous membrane contact. Sodium bisulfate can be used to neutralize the glutaraldehyde and make it safe for disposal.

- *Ortho-phthalaldehyde:* Ortho-phthalaldehyde (OPA) is a high-level disinfectant that contains 0.55% 1,2-benzenedicarboxaldehyde, with a pH of 7.5. OPA, such as glutaraldehyde, interacts with amino acids, proteins of microorganisms. OPA has excellent microbicidal activity. OPA is effective against a wide range of microorganisms, including glutaraldehyde-resistant mycobacteria. OPA kills spores by blocking the spore germination process.

  Ortho-phthalaldehyde has several potential advantages over glutaraldehyde. It has excellent stability over a wide range of pH 3–9, is not a known irritant to the eyes and nasal passages, does not require exposure monitoring, has barely perceptible odor, and requires no activation.[48] OPA, such as glutaraldehyde, has excellent material compatibility.

  A potential disadvantage of OPA is that it stains proteins gray including unprotected skin and thus must be handled with caution.[49] Personal protective equipment should be worn when contaminated instruments, equipment, and chemicals are handled. In addition, equipment must be thoroughly rinsed to prevent discoloration of patient's skin or mucous membrane.
- *Hydrogen peroxide*: Hydrogen peroxide has excellent bactericidal, virucidal, sporicidal, and fungicidal properties. Hydrogen peroxide works by producing destructive hydroxyl-free radicals that can attack membrane lipids, DNA, and other essential cell components and has shown promise as chemical sterilant in concentrations from 6 to 25%. The product marketed as a sterilant is a premixed, ready to use chemical that contains 7.5% hydrogen peroxide and 0.85% phosphoric acid (to maintain a low pH).[49] The effectiveness of 7.5% hydrogen peroxide at 10 minutes is at par with 2% alkaline glutaraldehyde at 20 minutes in manual disinfection of endoscopes.[50] Hydrogen peroxide should be stored in dark containers to remain stable. The decomposition or loss of potency in small containers is <2% per year at ambient temperatures.[51]
- *Iodophors*: Iodine solutions or tinctures have long been used by health professionals primarily as antiseptics on skin or tissue. Iodophors, on the other hand, have been used both as antiseptics and disinfectants. An iodophor is a combination of iodine and a solubilizing agent or carrier; the resulting complex provides a sustained release reservoir of iodine and releases small amounts of free iodine in aqueous solution. Povidone–iodine and other iodophors retain the germicidal efficacy of iodine but unlike iodine, these generally do not stain and are relatively free of toxicity and irritancy.[52] Free iodine (I_2) contributes to the bactericidal activity of iodophors and dilutions of iodophors demonstrate more rapid bactericidal action than does a full strength povidone–iodine solution.

  Iodophors are bactericidal, mycobactericidal, and virucidal but can require prolonged contact times to kill certain fungi and bacterial spores.[6,53]
- *Peracetic acid*: Peracetic acid is characterized by rapid action against all microorganisms. Special advantages of peracetic acid are that it lacks harmful decomposition products and enhances removal of organic material and leaves no residue. It remains effective in the presence of organic matter and is sporicidal even at low temperatures. Peracetic acid can corrode copper, brass, bronze, plain steel, and galvanized iron but these effects can be reduced by additives and pH modifications. Peracetic acid is believed to function similarly to other oxidizing agents, that is, it denatures proteins, disrupts the cell wall permeability, and oxidizes sulfhydryl and sulfur bonds in proteins, enzymes, and other metabolites.[54]

  Peracetic acid inactivates gram-positive and gram-negative bacteria, viruses, fungi, mycobacteria, and bacterial spores.

  Peracetic acid is available in combination with hydrogen peroxide (0.23% peracetic acid plus 7.35% hydrogen peroxide) for their synergistic action in inactivating all microorganisms except bacterial spores within 20 minutes.
- *Phenolic disinfectants*: Phenol has occupied a prominent place in the field of hospital disinfection since its initial use as a germicide by Lister in his pioneering work on antiseptic surgery. Phenol derivatives originate when a functional group (e.g., alkyl, phenyl, benzyl, and halogen) replaces one of the hydrogen atoms on the aromatic ring. Two phenol derivatives commonly found, as constituents of hospital disinfectants are ortho-phenylphenol and ortho-benzyl-para-chlorophenol. In high concentrations, phenol acts as a gross protoplasmic poison, penetrating and disrupting the cell wall and precipitating the cell proteins. Low concentrations of phenol and higher molecular weight phenol derivatives cause bacterial death by inactivation of essential enzyme systems and leakage of essential metabolites from the cell wall.[55] Commercially available phenolic disinfectants are not sporicidal, but are tuberculocidal, fungicidal, virucidal, and bactericidal at their recommended use dilution.

Phenolic germicides are disinfectants for use on environmental surfaces (e.g., bedside tables, bedrails, and laboratory surfaces) and noncritical medical devices. Phenolics are not high-level disinfectants for use with semicritical items but can be used to preclean or decontaminate critical and semicritical devices before terminal sterilization or high-level disinfection.

- *Quaternary ammonium compounds*: The quaternary ammonium compounds are widely used as disinfectants. The quaternaries are good cleaning agents. Each compound exhibits its own antimicrobial characteristics. Some of the chemical names of quaternary ammonium compounds used in healthcare are alkyldimethylbenzylammonium chloride, alkyl didecyl dimethyl ammonium chloride, and dialkyldimethylammonium chloride. The newer quaternary ammonium compounds (i.e., fourth generation), referred to as twin chain or dialkyl quaternaries (e.g., didecyldimethylammonium bromide and dioctyl dimethyl ammonium bromide), reportedly remain active in hard water and are tolerant of anionic residues.[56]

The bactericidal action of the quaternaries has been attributed to the inactivation of energy-producing enzymes, denaturation of essential cell proteins, and disruption of the cell membrane.[56]

Quaternaries available as hospital disinfectants are generally fungicidal, bactericidal, and virucidal against enveloped viruses. They are not sporicidal and generally not tuberculocidal. The quaternaries are commonly used in ordinary environmental sanitation of noncritical surfaces, such as floors, furniture, and walls.

- *Other germicides*: New disinfectants that require further evaluation include glucoprotamin, tertiary amines, and a light activated antimicrobial coating. In preliminary studies, nanoemulsions (composed of detergents and lipids in water) showed activity against vegetative bacteria, enveloped viruses, and *Candida*. This product represents potential agent for use as a topical biocidal agent.[57] Metals such as silver, iron, and copper can be used for environmental control, disinfection of water, or incorporated into medical devices (e.g., intravascular catheters).[58,59] Surfacine is a new persistent antimicrobial agent that may be used on animate or inanimate surfaces. It incorporates a water-insoluble antimicrobial compound (silver iodide) in a surface immobilized coating. Surfacine is applied to the animate or inanimate surfaces by spraying or coating without any prior surface treatment.
- *Ultraviolet radiation*: The wavelength of ultraviolet (UV) radiation ranges from 328 to 210 nm (3,280–2,100 A). Its maximum bactericidal effect occurs at 240–280 nm. Mercury vapor lamps emit >90% of their radiation at 253.7 nm, which is near the maximum microbicidal activity. Inactivation of microorganisms results from destruction of nucleic acid through induction of thymine dimers. Ultraviolet radiation has been employed in the disinfection of drinking water, air, titanium implants, and contact lenses.[60] Bacteria and viruses are more easily killed by UV light than are bacterial spores. Ultraviolet radiation has several potential applications, but unfortunately, its germicidal effectiveness and use are influenced by organic matter, wavelength, type of suspension, temperature, type of microorganism, and UV intensity, which is affected by distance and dirty tubes. The application of UV radiation in the healthcare environment operating rooms, isolation rooms, and biologic safety cabinets is limited to destruction of airborne organisms.

STERILIZATION

Sterilization is defined as a process that destroys or eliminates all forms of microbial life including bacterial endospores. Sterilization is intended to convey an absolute process. Sterilization is carried out in hospitals and clinics by various physical (such as heat) or chemical methods. Recently, a number of newer methods like low-temperature sterilization systems (e.g., hydrogen peroxide gas plasma, peracetic acid immersion, and ozone) have been developed and are being utilized to sterilize medical devices.[61,62]

Methods of Sterilization

Heat

Heat is considered as the most reliable methods of sterilization for articles that can withstand heat. Heat acts by oxidative effects as well as denaturation and coagulation of proteins. Factors affecting sterilization by heat are:

- *Nature of heat*: Moist heat is more effective than dry heat.
- *Temperature and time*: Temperature and time are inversely related. As the temperature increases, the time taken for sterilization decreases.
- *Number of microorganisms*: Direct relation with time
- *Nature of microorganisms*: Spores are relatively resistant to heat
- *Type of material and presence of organic matter*: In presence of organic matter such as proteins and fats, the time taken increases.

Dry heat: Dry heat acts by denaturation of proteins. Articles such as bacteriological loops and tips of forceps are sterilized by holding them in a Bunsen burner flame till they are red hot.

Incineration: Incineration is a method of terminal destruction of contaminated material. Incineration results in loss of material and hence used only when the article in question such as a soiled dressing and bedding is not to be reused.

Hot air oven: Articles to be sterilized are exposed to high temperature of about 160°C for about 1 hour in an electrically heated oven. Since air is a poor conductor of heat, even distribution of heat inside the oven is achieved by a fan. Heat is transferred to the articles by radiation, conduction, and convection.

Glassware, oils, petroleum jelly, and powders are materials, which are sterilized using hot air oven. Articles to be sterilized must be perfectly dry before placing them in oven. Articles must be placed with sufficient distance between them so that circulation of hot air is uniformly maintained inside the hot air oven. The holding time observed is 60 minutes at 160°C, 40 minutes at 170°C, and 20 minutes at 180°C. The hot air oven must not be opened till the temperature inside has not fallen below 60°C to prevent breakage of glassware.

Moist heat:

- *Steam sterilization*: Among the available methods for sterilization, moist heat in the form of saturated steam under pressure is the most widely used and the most dependable, as it is a nontoxic, inexpensive system requiring relatively shorter sterilization time **(Fig. 5)**. It is recommended that all equipment, which can withstand the effects of temperature, should be sterilized by steam sterilization.[63,64] Moist heat destroys microorganisms by the irreversible coagulation and denaturation of enzymes and structural proteins.

  The basic principle of steam sterilization, as accomplished in an autoclave, is to expose each item to direct steam contact at the required temperature and pressure for the specified time. Thus, there are four parameters of steam sterilization—steam, pressure, temperature, and time.[65,66] Pressure serves as a means to obtain the high temperatures necessary to quickly kill microorganisms. Specific temperatures must be obtained to ensure the microbicidal activity. The two common steam-sterilizing temperatures are 121°C and 132°C. Recognized minimum exposure periods for sterilization of wrapped healthcare supplies are 30 minutes at 121°C in a gravity displacement sterilizer or 4 minutes at 132°C in a prevacuum sterilizer. Sterilization time further varies depending on the type of item (e.g., metal versus rubber, plastic, and items with lumens), whether the item is wrapped or unwrapped, and the kind of sterilizer.

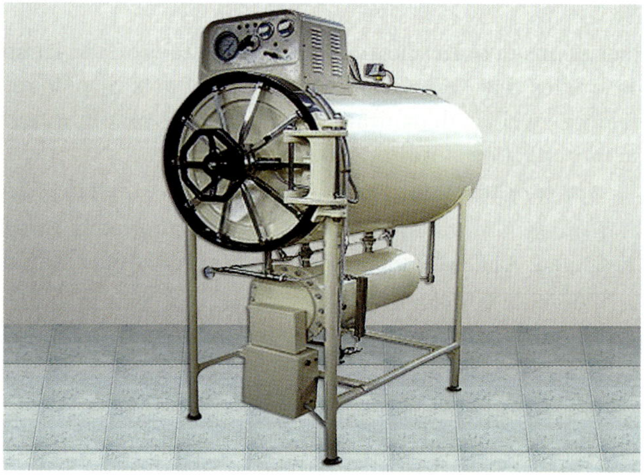

Fig. 5: Horizontal steam sterilizer.

- *Autoclaves*: The different types of steam sterilizers (autoclaves) include:
  - Simple "pressure cooker type" laboratory autoclave
  - Steam jacketed downward displacement laboratory autoclave
  - High-pressure prevacuum autoclave

  In the gravity displacement sterilizer, steam is admitted at the top or the sides of the sterilizing chamber and, because the steam is lighter than air, it forces air out from the bottom of the chamber through the drain vent. The gravity displacement autoclaves are primarily used to process laboratory media, water, pharmaceutical products, regulated medical waste, and nonporous articles whose surfaces have direct steam contact. The high-speed prevacuum sterilizers are similar to the gravity displacement sterilizers except they are fitted with a vacuum pump (or ejector) to ensure air removal from the sterilizing chamber and load before the steam is introduced. The advantage of using a vacuum pump is that there is nearly instantaneous steam penetration even into porous loads. The different cycle times to be followed are depicted in **Table 2**.
- *Flash sterilization*: Flash sterilization is a modification of conventional steam sterilization (either gravity, prevacuum, or steam flush pressure pulse) in which the item is placed in an open tray or is placed in a specially designed, covered, and rigid container to allow for rapid

TABLE 2: Minimum cycle times for steam sterilization cycles.

Type of sterilizer	*Item*	*Exposure time at 121°C*	*Exposure time at 132°C*	*Drying time*
Gravity displacement	Wrapped instruments	30 minutes	15 minutes	15–30 minutes
	Textile packs	30 minutes	25 minutes	15 minutes
	Wrapped utensils	30 minutes	15 minutes	15–30 minutes
Dynamic air removal (e.g., prevacuum)	Wrapped instruments		4 minutes	20–30 minutes
	Textile packs		4 minutes	5–20 minutes
	Wrapped utensils		4 minutes	20 minutes

Source: Modified from association for the advancement of medical instrumentation.[65,66]

penetration of steam. Typical sterilization temperatures and times are 132–135°C with 3–4 minutes exposure time for porous loads and instruments.[63,67] Flash sterilization has generally been used as a quick or last resort sterilization method when a unique instrument is urgently needed for a procedure or is dropped on the floor. The autoclaving process needs periodic monitoring. Chemical indicators are incorporated regularly with autoclaving cycles. Single parameter chemical indicators indicate attainment of a certain temperature by a visible color change. Multiparameter chemical indicators called as integrators indicating temperature, pressure, and time are also available. Biological indicators containing spores of:

- *Geobacillus stearothermophilus* (formerly *Bacillus stearothermophilus*) need to be used periodically to substantiate the process of sterilization,[10] especially in developing countries such as India.[68]

Low-temperature Sterilization Technologies

Ethylene oxide has been widely used as a low-temperature sterilant since the 1950s. Alternative technologies to ETO with chlorofluorocarbon, which are currently available, include 100% ETO, ETO with a different stabilizing gas such as carbon dioxide or hydrochlorofluorocarbons (HCFC); immersion in peracetic acid, hydrogen peroxide gas plasma, and ozone.

Ethylene oxide: It is a colorless gas that is flammable and explosive. Essential parameters for ETO sterilization are—adequate gas concentration, proper temperature between 37° and 63°C, relative humidity of 40–80%, and correct exposure time.[69] It has been the most commonly used process for sterilizing temperature and moisture-sensitive medical devices. Two types of ETO sterilizers are available—(1) mixed gas and (2) 100% ETO. ETO cycles are lengthy, costly, and potentially hazardous to patients and staff. The big advantage is that it can sterilize heat or moisture-sensitive medical equipment without deleterious effects. ETO is a potential human carcinogen.[70] The mode of action of ETO is considered by alkylation of protein, DNA, and RNA. ETO inactivates all microorganisms including bacterial spores.

The basic ETO sterilization cycle consists of five stages—(1) preconditioning and humidification, (2) gas introduction, (3) exposure, (4) evacuation, and (5) air washes, and takes approximately 2.5 hours excluding aeration time. Mechanical aeration for 8–12 hours at 50–60°C allows desorption of the toxic ETO residual contained in exposed absorbent materials. Most modern ETO sterilizers combine sterilization and aeration in the same chamber as a continuous process. ETO is absorbed by many materials. For this reason, following sterilization, the item must undergo aeration to remove residual ETO.

Ethylene oxide is highly useful to sterilize critical items and sometimes semicritical items, which are moisture or heat sensitive and cannot be sterilized by steam sterilization.

Hydrogen peroxide gas plasma: Gas plasmas are generated in an enclosed chamber under deep vacuum using radiofrequency or microwave energy to excite the gas molecules and produce charged particles, many of which are in the form of free radicals. The free radicals interact with essential cell components (e.g., enzymes and nucleic acids) and thereby disrupt the metabolism of microorganisms.

This process has the ability to inactivate a broad range of microorganisms, including resistant bacterial spores. Materials and devices that cannot tolerate high temperatures and humidity, such as some plastics, electrical devices, and corrosion-susceptible metal alloys, can be sterilized by hydrogen peroxide gas plasma.[71,72]

Peracetic acid sterilization: Peracetic acid is a unique cidal agent, which has the ability to maintain its efficacy in the presence of organic matter.[73,74] Peracetic acid, a 35% liquid solution, is thought to function by denaturing proteins, disrupting cell wall permeability, and oxidizing sulfhydryl and sulfur bonds in proteins.[54]

Other Sterilization Methods

Ionizing radiation: Sterilization by ionizing radiation, primarily by cobalt 60 gamma rays or electron accelerators, is a low-temperature sterilization method that has been used for a number of medical products (e.g., tissue for transplantation, pharmaceuticals, and medical devices). The method is suitable for large-scale sterilization because of high sterilization costs and is not suitable for healthcare facilities.

Liquid chemical sterilants: Sterilization processes based on liquid chemical sterilants have been used as pointed earlier, but in general, do not convey the same sterility assurance level (SAL) as sterilization achieved using thermal or physical methods. The use of liquids as sterilants is restricted to reprocessing critical devices that are heat sensitive and incompatible with other sterilization methods.

Filtration: Filtration does not kill microbes; it separates them out. Membrane filters with pore size between 0.2 and 0.45 μm are commonly used to remove particles from solutions or liquids, which are heat labile such as serum, antibiotic solutions, sugar solution, or urea solution. Filtration is aided by using vacuum pumps.

Air filters: Air can be filtered using HEPA (high-efficiency particle air) filters. They are usually used in biological safety cabinets, modern operation theaters, positive pressure, and negative pressure rooms. HEPA filters deliver air with a filtering efficacy of 99.97% for particle size of 0.3-μm diameter. The HEPA filters need frequent monitoring by particle counters or similar tests.

Vaporized hydrogen peroxide: Hydrogen peroxide solutions have been in use as chemical sterilants for many years. It is environmentally safe, compatible with all materials, and relative ease of operation, installation, and monitoring. Few limitations are that cellulose cannot be processed, nylon becomes brittle, and penetration capabilities are less than those of ETO.[75,76]

Ozone: Ozone has been used for years as a drinking water disinfectant. Ozone is produced when O_2 is energized, which then splits into two monatomic (O_1) molecules. The monatomic oxygen molecules then collide with O_2 molecules to form ozone, which is O_3. Thus, ozone consists of O_2 with a loosely bonded third oxygen atom that is readily available to attach to, and oxidize, other molecules. This additional oxygen atom makes ozone a powerful oxidant that destroys microorganisms but is highly unstable.

Formaldehyde steam: Low-temperature steam with formaldehyde is used as a low temperature sterilization method in many European countries. It has certain advantages; the cycle time for formaldehyde gas is faster than that for ETO and the cost per cycle is relatively low. However, ETO is more penetrating and operates at lower temperatures than do steam/formaldehyde sterilizers.

Sterilization Cycle Verification

The efficacy of the sterilization process is measured by the SAL of a product and is defined as the probability of a single viable microorganism persisting on a product after sterilization.[77,78] In short, SAL is an estimate of lethality of the entire sterilization process.

The sterilization procedure should be monitored at different intervals, routinely, on installation, and after repairs by using a combination of mechanical, chemical, and biological indicators to evaluate the sterilizing conditions and indirectly the microbiologic status of the processed items.[65,66,69,79] The mechanical monitors for steam sterilization include the daily assessment of cycle time and temperature by examining the temperature record chart and an assessment of pressure via the pressure gauge. The mechanical monitors for ETO include time, temperature, and pressure records.[69]

Both biological and chemical indicators can be used for verification. Chemical indicators are convenient and inexpensive. Biological indicator, on the other hand, can measure the microbial killing power of the sterilization process.[80] Chemical indicators are affixed on the outside of each pack to show that the package has been processed through a sterilization cycle, but these indicators do not prove sterilization has been achieved. Chemical indicators usually are either heat-sensitive or chemical-sensitive inks that change color when one or more sterilization parameters are achieved. If the internal and/or external indicator suggests inadequate processing, the item should not be used.[81]

Biological indicators are recognized by most authorities as being closest to the ideal monitors of the sterilization process,[82,83] because they measure the sterilization process directly by using the most resistant microorganisms (*Bacillus* spores), and not by merely testing the physical and chemical conditions necessary for sterilization. Since the *Bacillus* spores used in biological indicators are more resistant and present in greater numbers than are the common microbial contaminants found on patient care equipment, the demonstration that the biological indicator has been inactivated strongly implies that other potential pathogens in the load have been killed.[84] Steam and low-temperature sterilizers (e.g., hydrogen peroxide gas plasma and peracetic acid) should be monitored at least weekly with the appropriate commercial preparation of spores. If a sterilizer is used frequently (e.g., several loads per day), daily use of biological indicators allows earlier discovery of equipment malfunctions or procedural errors and thus minimizes the extent of patient surveillance and product recall needed in the event of a positive biological indicator.[79] Each load should be monitored, if it contains implantable objects. If feasible, implantable items should not be used until the results of spore tests are known to be negative.

HIGH-LEVEL DISINFECTION OF DERMATOSURGICAL OPERATION THEATERS

This has been dealt in more detail in the chapter on dermatosurgical theater and only relevant details are mentioned here. A dermatosurgical operation theater should adhere to the definition of a clean room, which is defined as—a room in which the concentration of airborne particles is controlled, and which is constructed and used in a manner to minimize the introduction, generation, and retention of particles inside the room and in which other relevant parameters, e.g., temperature, humidity, and pressure are controlled as necessary. As per available guidelines,[85] the ventilation requirements for operating rooms should have an outward air movement in relation to the adjacent area, a minimum of 15 total air changes per hour, a relative humidity of 30–60%, and a design temperature of 20–23°C. The use of laminar airflow systems is advised in operation theaters, but their value has not been fully documented for all types of theaters.[86]

Most of the operation theaters continue to use aldehydes for high-level disinfection of the theater environment. It has been observed that there is a general relationship between aerobic bacterial count and risk of infection. There is a significant risk of infection with counts in the range of 700–1,800 bacteria-carrying particles (BCPs) per cubic meter. However, the risk is slight when the BCP load is <180 per cubic meter.[87] Formaldehyde is the commonly used agent either as a gas utilizing potassium permanganate or as dispersed by a sprayer-like device. Other agents used as high-level disinfectants essentially through a fogger are hydrogen peroxide, hydrogen peroxide along with silver nitrate, peracetic acid, and other chemical compounds of aldehydes. The inanimate surfaces in the operation theater need proper periodic cleaning and disinfection. Grossly contaminated surfaces can be potential source of hospital-acquired infections. The operation theater should be thoroughly washed with water and detergent mixture so as to rid of all spills and proteinaceous materials before a disinfectant is used for mopping the surfaces.

Air Conditioning Units

Opportunistic fungi such as *Aspergillus*, *Rhizopus*, *Fusarium*, and *Penicillium* are capable of proliferating in air conditioning (AC) units. The filters utilized in these units can act as a suitable nidus for growth and proliferation of the pathogenic fungi, the spores of which can be discharged and carried through the theater air. Presence of fungi in AC units and subsequent dispersal of spores can be a potential hazard, especially for the immunocompromised patients. The operating room and clinic AC units should be meticulously maintained and frequently monitored to minimize the chances of growth and proliferation of potentially pathogenic fungi. Split AC units appear to be a safer option than the window mounted AC units.[88]

Staphylococcus aureus and β-hemolytic streptococci are important healthcare-associated pathogens and can persist in the environment. They can be shed and infections can occur when healthcare personnel are heavily colonized with these organisms. *S. aureus* and β-hemolytic streptococci have been linked to airborne transmission in operation theaters, burn units, and neonatal units.[89,90]

Surveillance of the AC units, the use of disinfectants and the personnel working in the close vicinity during operative procedures, needs to be incorporated as a periodic monitoring tool to be used judiciously. Periodic screening, treatment of shedders, and abstaining from operations till the treatment is completed would ensure that the risk of transmission of infections is minimized.[5]

The dermatological procedures routinely carried out in clinics and hospitals along with the recommended disinfection/sterilization methods advocated are summarized in **Table 3**.[91]

Automation

The disinfection process is getting automated with the use of foggers/mist producers wherein disinfectants such as hydrogen peroxide are applied in form of mist or vapor. Two new technologies are mercury vapor lamps, which produce ultraviolet radiation in spectrum around 253 nanometers which acts as a germicidal, and the second is pulsed xenon, which produces entire 200–280 nanometer spectrum of UV radiation. Both the techniques are sporicidal as well though the time of exposure for mercury vapor is 50 minutes and for pulsed xenon is about 15 minutes. The same germicidal effect is achieved by exposure to hydrogen peroxide mist for 2.5 hours.

PROTECTING MAXIMALLY FROM COVID-19 TRANSMISSION: OPD MANAGEMENT

The field of dermatology is a high-risk category, since the patient management often involves close contact with the patients. The potential of transmission and cross-infections is significant. In most of the clinics, the waiting space in the outpatient rooms is limited. The clinics can be crowded and there is need to manage the patients and the space effectively. The need is to manage in a way so that the space is effectively utilized maintaining the concept of distancing. It is crucial to risk assess the patients for their comorbidities as well.

The coronavirus responsible for the pandemic is a highly contagious pathogen, which is transmitted by direct airborne transmission and by fomites. The standard operating procedure (SOP) for preventing transmission in outpatient departments (OPDs) would essentially consist of:

- Hand hygiene
- PPEs—personal protective equipment

TABLE 3: Dermatological equipment requiring disinfection/sterilization.

Name of procedure	*Instruments used*	*Recommended disinfection/sterilization method*
Skin grafting for vitiligo	• Stainless punches • Disposable punches • Venesection tray with artery forceps, blades, forceps, and scissors	• Autoclaving • Not to be reused • ETO sterilization • Autoclaving
Hair transplant	Needles, forceps, cutting boards, blades, plastic blade holders, BP handle artery forceps, Adson's forceps needle holder, and plastic bottles for spraying saline	• All heat stable material to be autoclaved • Heat labile material ETO sterilization or prolonged exposure to chemical disinfectant such as glutaraldehyde, ortho-phthalaldehyde
Chemical peels	Brushes to apply chemicals on face from the bottle	ETO
Laser	Metal spacers, interchangeable hand pieces of metal or plastic, and dedicated goggles	• All heat stable material to be autoclaved • Heat labile material ETO sterilization or prolonged exposure to chemical disinfectant such as glutaraldehyde and ortho-phthalaldehyde

(ETO: ethylene oxide)

- Respiratory hygiene and cough etiquettes
- Injection safety
- Medication storage and handling
- Cleaning and disinfection of medical equipment
- Environmental cleaning and disinfection.

It is important to decide the order of treatment of patients in OPD (also referred to as triage). Triage of patients is essential for effective management and control of potential transmission of pathogens in OPD settings.

- To be done by receptionist—suitably trained so as not to annoy patients
- The patients and relatives (attendants)—should be screened for active fever with infrared body thermometers. They usually come with screening distance of 5 cm or less.
- Pulse oximeter—additional gadget—quite useful for patient and healthcare worker (HCW) monitoring.

The coronavirus disease-2019 (COVID-19) symptoms are not specific, they vary from being asymptomatic to fever, cough, dyspnea, myalgia, anosmia, or fatigue. Less frequently, productive cough, headache, hemoptysis, and diarrhea have also been documented. Some of these patients might have conjunctival congestion too.

A questionnaire should be prepared that is to be filled in by the patient and attendant—a self-declaration/consent—to state that they have not suffered from recent upper respiratory tract infection (URTI)/lower respiratory tract infection (LRTI)/diarrhea/conjunctivitis, or any other COVID related symptoms and have not travelled to/from COVID-infected area in last 15 days. They have no person in household who is similarly affected and no member of the family has travelled to/from COVID-infected area in last 15 days.

It would be prudent to identify patients suffering from fever or COVID-like symptoms based on the declaration given as—likely to be infective. These patients should be attended immediately, if possible, in a separate room, giving basic treatment with minimal interaction and examination. As far as possible, avoid checking of potentially infected patients, if there is no emergency.

Good Practice Guidelines

- If feasible, all OPD patients to visit with prior appointment
- In an hour, give appointments to patients in such a way that there is minimal or zero waiting time. If feasible, ask the patients to wait in their own cars and send an SMS 10 minutes prior to their appointment.
- Encourage follow-up consultation telephonically.
- Do not keep any magazines or reading material in the waiting room.
- All persons entering clinic to be asked to wear disposable three-ply mask properly.
- No shoes, socks to be allowed inside the clinic
- Encourage use of donning of disposable footwear—prior to entering clinic—saves on repeated cleaning and floor disinfection—effective and economical ultimately.
- Do not allow use of mobiles in clinics—potential source of fomites or ensure that the mobiles are also disinfected along with hands.
- Do not allow patients or attendants to handle remote devices for TVs in the clinics.
- All patients and attendants to compulsorily use sanitizer and ensure that the same is used in proper manner. Instructions be given not to touch surfaces, their own body parts, etc.
- All ophthalmologists/optometrists must use PPEs including N95 masks and eye shields/face shields while examining the patients.
- Maintain physical distance always apart from examination of patients.
- If possible, do not keep any chair for attendant or patient. As soon as patient comes, he/she can be made to sit in the examination chair. Attendant can stand—this would minimize contacts and potential fomites transmission.
- The door knobs/touch surfaces can be covered with plastic bag/disposable cap/antibacterial covers or some other innovative idea, prior to start of clinic. These should be disposed at the end and then surfaces wiped with sanitizer.

Cleaning and Disinfection Protocols for OPD

- The entire clinic should be cleaned with soap and water.
- After drying, the same should be disinfected with 1% sodium hypochlorite.
- Dilute the sodium hypochlorite solution received from supplier by about 5 times with water. 1 liter of solution + 5 liters of water are enough to mop all surfaces in a normal sized clinic.
- 28 grams of calcium hypochlorite (bleach) powder in each liter of water are used to make a 1% solution.
- Sodium hypochlorite should be stored in a cool dark place away from sunlight.
- Undiluted sodium hypochlorite has a shelf life of 6 months to 1 year from the date of manufacture, after which bleach degrades at a rate of 20% each year.
- A 1% sodium hypochlorite solution has a shelf life of 24 hours.
- It must be stored separately from corrosives, soaps, detergents, or other cleaning products.
- Surfaces such as TV screens, computer key pads, mouse, screens, all equipment with lenses, ultrasonic probes, scopes—*should not be disinfected with sodium hypochlorite*. They should be disinfected with alcohol-based solutions only.
- Disinfecting with sodium hypochlorite—at least thrice a day, prior to opening, after about 2 hours, and after end of OPD
- The ambient air in the clinic needs no disinfection routinely.
- Ideally, gloves are worn only in case of contact with body fluids or skin lesions.

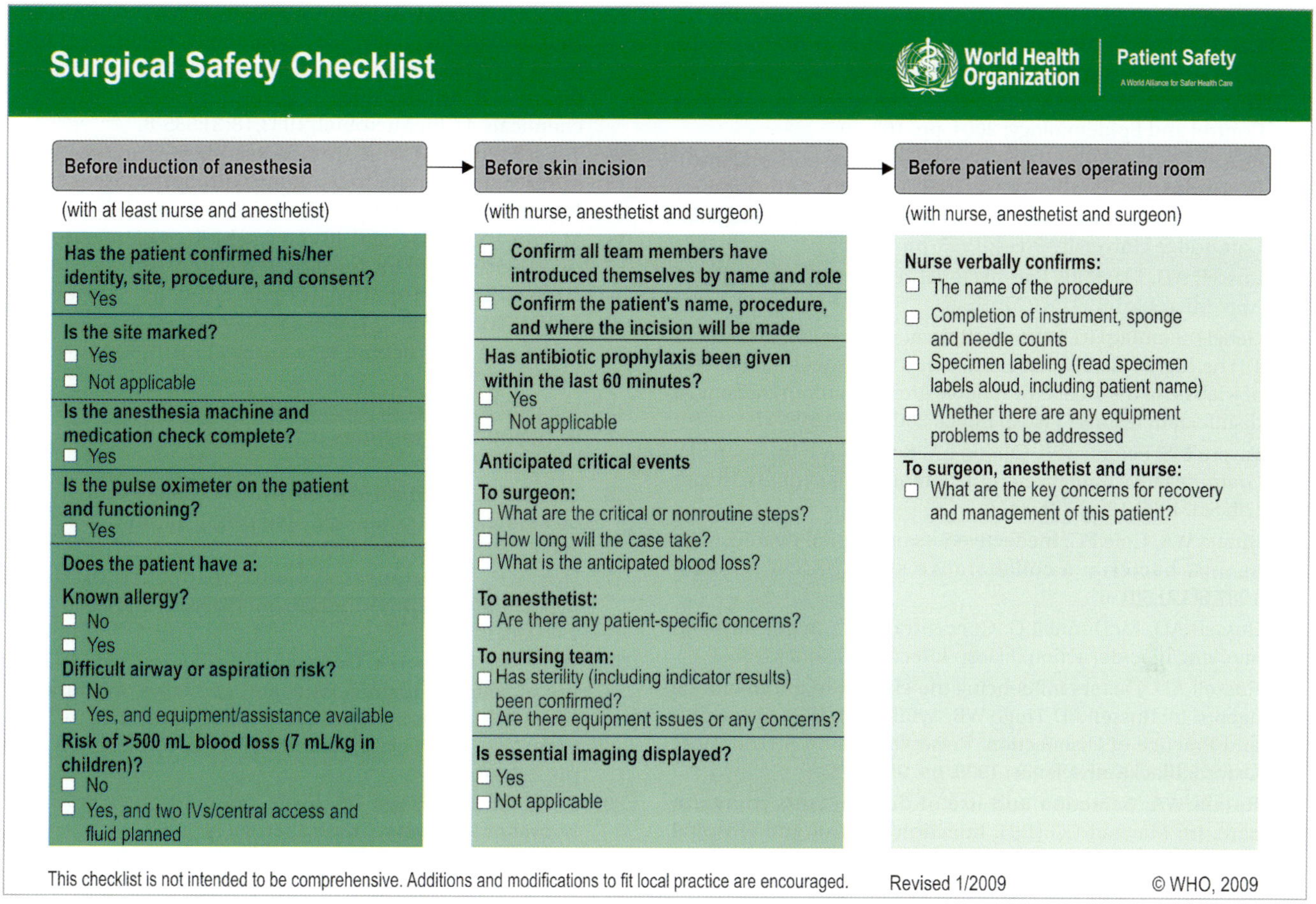

Surgical Safety Checklist

World Health Organization | Patient Safety
A World Alliance for Safer Health Care

Before induction of anesthesia	Before skin incision	Before patient leaves operating room
(with at least nurse and anesthetist)	(with nurse, anesthetist and surgeon)	(with nurse, anesthetist and surgeon)
Has the patient confirmed his/her identity, site, procedure, and consent? ☐ Yes **Is the site marked?** ☐ Yes ☐ Not applicable **Is the anesthesia machine and medication check complete?** ☐ Yes **Is the pulse oximeter on the patient and functioning?** ☐ Yes **Does the patient have a:** **Known allergy?** ☐ No ☐ Yes **Difficult airway or aspiration risk?** ☐ No ☐ Yes, and equipment/assistance available **Risk of >500 mL blood loss (7 mL/kg in children)?** ☐ No ☐ Yes, and two IVs/central access and fluid planned	☐ **Confirm all team members have introduced themselves by name and role** ☐ **Confirm the patient's name, procedure, and where the incision will be made** **Has antibiotic prophylaxis been given within the last 60 minutes?** ☐ Yes ☐ Not applicable **Anticipated critical events** **To surgeon:** ☐ What are the critical or nonroutine steps? ☐ How long will the case take? ☐ What is the anticipated blood loss? **To anesthetist:** ☐ Are there any patient-specific concerns? **To nursing team:** ☐ Has sterility (including indicator results) been confirmed? ☐ Are there equipment issues or any concerns? **Is essential imaging displayed?** ☐ Yes ☐ Not applicable	**Nurse verbally confirms:** ☐ The name of the procedure ☐ Completion of instrument, sponge and needle counts ☐ Specimen labeling (read specimen labels aloud, including patient name) ☐ Whether there are any equipment problems to be addressed **To surgeon, anesthetist and nurse:** ☐ What are the key concerns for recovery and management of this patient?

This checklist is not intended to be comprehensive. Additions and modifications to fit local practice are encouraged. Revised 1/2009 © WHO, 2009

Fig. 6: Surgical safety checklist.

CONCLUSION

Disinfection and sterilization are very important concepts in ensuring safe surgery. World Health Organization has recently commenced a "safe surgery" initiative to help reduce risks involved in surgeries around the world by adhering to proven standards of care. WHO advocates use of a "Surgical Safety Checklist" prior to operative procedure. That the use of checklists significantly reduces the surgical morbidity, and mortality has been documented after pilot studies conducted by WHO. The checklist **(Fig. 6)** is available for downloading at following web address:

http://whqlibdoc.who.int/publications/2009/9789241598590_eng_Checklist.pdf

REFERENCES

1. Amici JM, Roques AM, Lasheras A, Gachie JP, Guillot P, Beylot C, et al. A prospective study of the incidence of complications associated with dermatological surgery. Br J Dermatol. 2005;153(5):967-71.
2. Chan BC, Patel DC. Perioperative management and the associated rate of adverse events in dermatological procedures performed by dermatologists in New Zealand. Australas J Dermatol. 2009;50(1):23-8.
3. Salanitri S, Gonçalves A, Helene A, Helena F, Lopes J. Surgical complications in hair transplantation: a series of 533 procedures. Aesthet Surg J. 2009;29(1):72-6.
4. Ram J, Kaushik S, Brar GS, Taneja N, Gupta A. Prevention of postoperative infections in ophthalmic surgery. Indian J Ophthalmol. 2001;49(1):59-69.
5. Kelkar U, Kelkar S, Bal AM, Kulkarni S, Kulkarni S. Microbiological evaluation of various parameters in ophthalmic operating rooms. The need to establish guidelines. Indian J Ophthalmol. 2003;51(2):171-6.
6. Spaulding EH. Chemical disinfection of medical and surgical materials. In: Lawrence C, Block SS (Eds). Disinfection, Sterilization, and Preservation. Philadelphia: Lea & Fibiger; 1968. pp. 517-31.
7. Price PB. Bacteriology of normal skin: a new quantitative test applied to a study of the bacterial flora and the disinfectant action of mechanical cleansing. J Infect Dis. 1938;63(3):301-18.
8. Sprunt K, Redman W, Leidy G. Antibacterial effectiveness of routine hand washing. Pediatrics. 1973;52(2):264-71.
9. Favero MS, Bond WW. Chemical disinfection of medical and surgical materials. In: Block SS (Ed). Disinfection, Sterilization, and Preservation. Philadelphia: Lippincott Williams & Wilkins; 2001. pp. 881-917.
10. Bean HS. Types and characteristics of disinfectants. J Appl Bacteriol. 1967;30:616.
11. Russell AD, Hugo WB, Ayliffe GAJ. Principles and Practice of Disinfection, Preservation and Sterilization. England, Oxford: Blackwell Scientific Publications; 1999.

12. Russell AD. Factors influencing the efficacy of germicides. In: Rutala WA (Ed). Disinfection, Sterilization and Antisepsis: Principles, Practices, Challenges, and New Research. Washington, DC: Association for Professionals in Infection Control and Epidemiology; 2004. pp. 162-70.
13. Russell AD, Russell NJ. Biocides: activity, action and resistance. In: Hunter PA, Darby GK, Russell NJ (Eds). Fifty Years of Antimicrobials: Past Perspectives and Future Trends. England: Cambridge University Press; 1995. pp. 327-65.
14. Russell AD. Plasmids and bacterial resistance to biocides. J Appl Microbiol. 1997;83(2):155-65.
15. Gebel J, Sonntag HG, Werner HP, Vacata V, Exner M, Kistemann T. The higher disinfectant resistance of nosocomial isolates of Klebsiella oxytoca: how reliable are indicator organisms in disinfectant testing? J Hosp Infect. 2002;50(4):309-11.
16. Favero MS, Petersen NJ, Carson LA, Bond WW, Hindman SH. Gram-negative water bacteria in hemodialysis systems. Health Lab Sci. 1975;12(4):321-34.
17. Rutala WA, Cole EC. Ineffectiveness of hospital disinfectants against bacteria: a collaborative study. Infect Control. 1987;8(12):501-6.
18. Russell AD, McDonnell G. Concentration: a major factor in studying biocidal action. J Hosp Infect. 2000;44(1):1-3.
19. Russell AD. Factors influencing the efficacy of antimicrobial agents. In: Russell AD, Hugo WB, Ayliffe GAJ (Eds). Principles and Practice of Disinfection, Preservation and Sterilization. Oxford: Blackwell Science; 1999. pp. 951-1023.
20. Rutala WA. Selection and use of disinfectants in health care. In: Mayhall CG (Ed). Infection Control and Hospital Epidemiology. Philadelphia: Lippincott Williams & Wilkins; 1999. pp. 1161-87.
21. Lewis DL, Arens M. Resistance of microorganisms to disinfection in dental and medical devices. Nat Med. 1995;1(9):956-8.
22. Jacobs P. Cleaning: principles, methods and benefits. In: Rutala WA (Ed). Disinfection, Sterilization, and Antisepsis in Health Care. New York, Champlain: Polyscience Publications; 1998. pp. 165-81.
23. Reichert M. Preparation of supplies for terminal sterilization. In: Reichert M, Young JH (Eds). Sterilization Technology for the Health Care Facility. Gaithersburg: Aspen Publication; 1997. pp. 36-50.
24. Jatzwauk L, Schone H, Pietsch H. How to improve instrument disinfection by ultrasound. J Hosp Infect. 2001;48(Suppl A):S80-3.
25. Schultz JK. Decontamination alternative. Infect Control Hosp Epidemiol. 1990;11(1):8-9.
26. Roberts CG. Studies on the bioburden on medical devices and the importance of cleaning. In: Rutala WA (Ed). Disinfection, Sterilization and Antisepsis: Principles and Practices in Health-care Facilities. Washington, DC: Association for professional in infection control and epidemiology; 2001. pp. 63-9.
27. Hutchisson B, LeBlanc C. The truth and consequences of enzymatic detergents. Gastroenterol Nurs. 2005;28(5):372-6.
28. Dancer SJ. How do we assess hospital cleaning? A proposal for microbiological standards for surface hygiene in hospitals. J Hosp Infect. 2004;56(1):10-5.
29. Ali Y, Dolan MJ, Fendler EJ. Alcohols. In: Block SS (Ed). Disinfection, Sterilization, and Preservation. Philadelphia: Lippincott Williams & Wilkins; 2001. pp. 229-54.
30. Tyler R, Ayliffe GA, Bradley C. Virucidal activity of disinfectants: studies with the poliovirus. J Hosp Infect. 1990;15(4):339-45.
31. Bond WW, Favero MS, Petersen NJ, Ebert JW. Inactivation of hepatitis B virus by intermediate-to-high-level disinfectant chemicals. J Clin Microbiol. 1983;18(3):535-8.
32. Tyler R, Ayliffe GA. A surface test for virucidal activity of disinfectants: preliminary study with herpes virus. J Hosp Infect. 1987;9(1):22-9.
33. Martin LS, McDougal JS, Loskoski SL. Disinfection and inactivation of the human T-lymphotropic virus type III/Lymphadenopathy-associated virus. J Infect Dis. 1985;152(2):400-3.
34. Spaulding EH. Alcohol as a surgical disinfectant. AORNJ. 1964;2:67-71.
35. Rutala WA, Weber DJ. Uses of inorganic hypochlorite (bleach) in health-care facilities. Clin Microbiol Rev. 1997;10(4): 597-610.
36. Merritt K, Hitchins VM, Brown SA. Safety and cleaning of medical materials and devices. J Biomed Mater Res. 2000;53(2):131-6.
37. Hoy RH. Accidental systemic exposure to sodium hypochlorite (Clorox) during hemodialysis. Am J Hosp Pharm. 1981;38(10):1512-4.
38. Weber DJ, Rutala WA. Occupational risks associated with the use of selected disinfectants and sterilants. In: Rutala WA (Ed). Disinfection, Sterilization, and Antisepsis in Health Care. NewYork, Champlain: Polyscience Publications; 1998. pp. 211-26.
39. Reisz GR, Gammon RS. Toxic pneumonitis from mixing household cleaners. Chest. 1986;89(1):49-52.
40. Hoffman PN, Death JE, Coates D. The stability of sodium hypochlorite solutions. In: Collins CH, Allwood MC, Bloomfield SF, Fox A (Eds). Disinfectants: Their Use and Evaluation of Effectiveness. London: Academic Press; 1981. pp. 77-83.
41. Griffiths PA, Babb JR, Fraise AP. Mycobactericidal activity of selected disinfectants using a quantitative suspension test. J Hosp Infect. 1999;41(2):111-21.
42. Bloomfield SF, Miller EA. A comparison of hypochlorite and phenolic disinfectants for disinfection of clean and soiled surfaces and blood spillages. J Hosp Infect. 1989;13(3):231-9.
43. Chitnis V, Chitnis S, Patil S, Chitnis D. Practical limitations of disinfection of body fluid spills with 10,000 ppm sodium hypochlorite (NaOCl). Am J Infect Control. 2004;32(5):306-8.
44. Selkon JB, Babb JR, Morris R. Evaluation of the anti-microbial activity of a new super-oxidized water, Sterilox®, for the disinfection of endoscopes. J Hosp Infect. 1999;41(1):59-70 .
45. Occupational Health and Safety Administration, US Department of Labor. (2002). OSHA Fact Sheet: Formaldehyde. [online] Available from: https://www.osha.gov/OshDoc/data_General_Facts/formaldehyde-factsheet.html. [Last accessed March, 2021].
46. Scott EM, Gorman SP. Glutaraldehyde. In: Block SS (Ed). Disinfection, Sterilization, and Preservation. Philadelphia: Lippincott Williams & Wilkins; 2001. pp. 361-81.
47. Masferrer R, Marquez R. Comparison of two activated glutaraldehyde solutions: Cidex Solution and Sonacide. Respir Care. 1977;22:257-62.
48. Cooke RPD, Goddard SV, Whymant Morris A, Sherwood J, Chatterly R. An evaluation of Cidex OPA (0.55% ortho-phthalaldehyde) as an alternative to 2% glutaraldehyde for high-level disinfection of endoscopes. J Hosp Infect. 2003;54(3):226-31.

49. Rutala WA, Weber DJ. Disinfection of endoscopes: review of new chemical sterilants used for high level disinfection. Infect Control Hosp Epidemiol. 1999;20(1):69-76.
50. Sattar SA, Taylor YE, Paquette M, Rubino J. In-hospital evaluation of 7.5% hydrogen peroxide as a disinfectant for flexible endoscopes. Can J Infect Control. 1996;11(2):51-4.
51. Hobson DW, Seal LA. Evaluation of a novel, rapid acting, sterilizing solution at room temperature. Am J Infect Control. 2000;28(5):370-5.
52. Gottardi W. Iodine and iodine compounds. In: Block SS (Ed). Disinfection, Sterilization, and Preservation. Philadelphia: Lea & Febiger; 1991. pp. 152-66.
53. Chang SL. Modern concept of disinfection. J Sanit Eng Div Proc Am Soc Civ Eng. 1971;97(5):689-707.
54. Block SS. Peroxygen compounds. In: Block SS (Ed). Disinfection, Sterilization, and Preservation. Philadelphia: Lippincott Williams & Wilkins; 2001. pp. 185-204.
55. Prindle RF. Phenolic compounds. In: Block SS (Ed). Disinfection, Sterilization, and Preservation. Philadelphia: Lea & Febiger; 1983. pp. 197-224.
56. Merianos JJ. Surface active agents. In: Block SS (Ed). Disinfection, Sterilization, and Preservation. Philadelphia: Lippincott Williams & Wilkins; 2001. pp. 283-320.
57. Hamouda T, Hayes MM, Cao ZH, Tonda R, Johnson K, Wright DC, et al. A novel surfactant nanoemulsions with broad-spectrum sporicidal activity against Bacillus species. J Infect Dis. 1999;180(6):1939-49.
58. Weber DJ, Rutala WA. Use of metals and microbicides in the prevention of nosocomial infections. In: Rutala W (Ed). Disinfection, Sterilization, and Antisepsis in Health Care. Champlain, NewYork: Polyscience Publications; 1995. pp. 271-85.
59. Noyce JO, Michels H, Keevil CW. Potential use of copper surfaces to reduce survival of epidemic methicillin-resistant *Staphylococcus aureus* in the healthcare environment. J Hosp Infect. 2006;63(3):289-97.
60. Russell AD. Ultraviolet radiation. In: Russell AD, Hugo WB, Ayliffe GAJ (Eds). Principles and Practices of Disinfection, Preservation and Sterilization. Oxford: Blackwell Science; 1999. pp. 688-702.
61. Garner JS, Favero MS. CDC Guideline for hand washing and hospital environmental control, 1985. Infect Control. 1986;7(4):231-43.
62. Rutala WA. Disinfection, sterilization and waste disposal. In: Wenzel RP (Ed). Prevention and Control of Nosocomial Infections. Baltimore: Williams and Wilkins; 1997. pp. 539-93.
63. Joslyn L. Sterilization by heat. In: Block SS (Ed). Disinfection, Sterilization, and Preservation. Philadelphia: Lippincott Williams & Wilkins; 2001. pp. 695-728.
64. Bucx MJ, Veldman DJ, Beenhakker MM, Koster R. The effect of steam sterilization at 134 degrees C on light intensity provided by fibre light into laryngoscopes. Anaesthesia. 1999;54(9):875-8.
65. Association for the Advancement of Medical Instrumentation. (2002). Steam sterilization and sterility assurance in health care facilities. ANSI/AAMI ST46. [online] Available from: https://webstore.ansi.org/standards/aami/ansiaamist462002. [Last accessed March, 2021].
66. Association for the Advancement of Medical Instrumentation. (2006). Comprehensive guide to steam sterilization and sterility assurance in healthcare facilities, ANSI/AAMIST79. [online] Available from: https://webstore.ansi.org/standards/aami/ansiaamist792006. [Last accessed March, 2021].
67. Crow S. Steam sterilizers: an evolution in design. Infect Control Hosp Epidemiol. 1993;14(8):488-90.
68. Kelkar U, Bal AM, Kulkarni S. Monitoring of steam sterilization process by biological indicators a necessary surveillance tool for developing countries. Am J Infect Control. 2004;32(8):512-3.
69. Association for the Advancement of Medical Instrumentation. Ethylene oxide sterilization in health care facilities: Safety and effectiveness. Arlington, VA: AAMI; 1999.
70. US Department of Health and Human Services. (2021). National Toxicology Program. [online] Available from: https://ntp.niehs.nih.gov/. [Last accessed March, 2021].
71. Timm D, Gonzales D. Effect of sterilization on microstructure and function of microsurgical scissors. Surg Serv Management. 1997;3:479.
72. Feldman LA, Hui HK. Compatibility of medical devices and materials with low temperature hydrogen peroxide gas plasma. Med Dev Diag Indust. 1997;19:57-62.
73. Malchesky PS. Medical applications of peracetic acid. In: Block SS (Ed). Disinfection, Sterilization, and Preservation. Philadelphia: Lippincott Williams & Wilkins; 2001. pp. 979-96.
74. Bradley CR, Babb JR, Ayliffe GA. Evaluation of the Steris System 1. Peracetic acid endoscope processor. J Hosp Infect. 1995;29(2):143-51.
75. French GL, Otter JA, Shannon KP, Adams NMT, Watling D, Parks MJ. Tackling contamination of the hospital environment by methicillin resistant *Staphylococcus aureus* (MRSA): a comparison between conventional terminal cleaning and hydrogen peroxide vapour decontamination. J Hosp Infect. 2004;57(1):31-7.
76. Boyce JM, Havill NL, Otter JA, McDonald LC, Adams NMT, Cooper T, et al. Impact of hydrogen peroxide vapor room bio decontamination on environmental contamination and nosocomial transmission of *Clostridium difficile*. The Society of Healthcare Epidemiology of America. Infect Control Hosp Epidemiol. 2008;29(8):723-9.
77. Favero MS. Sterility assurance: concepts for patient safety. In: Rutala WA (Ed). Disinfection, Sterilization and Antisepsis: Principles and Practices in Healthcare Facilities. Washington, DC: Association for Professional in Infection Control and Epidemiology; 2001. pp. 110-9.
78. Oxborrow GS, Berube R. Sterility testing validation of sterilization processes, and sporicide testing. In: Block SS (Ed). Disinfection, Sterilization, and Preservation. Philadelphia: Lea & Febiger; 1991. pp. 1047-57.
79. Association for the advancement of medical instrumentation. Good hospital practice: steam sterilization and sterility assurance. Arlington, VA: AAMI; 1993.
80. Rutala WA, Gergen MF, Weber DJ. Evaluation of a rapid readout biological indicator for flash sterilization with three biological indicators and three chemical indicators. Infect Control Hosp Epidemiol. 1993;14(7):390-4.
81. Association of Operating Room Nurses. Recommended practices for sterilization in perioperative practice settings. Standards, Recommended Practices, and Guidelines. Denver, CO: AORN; 2000. pp. 347-58.
82. Schneider PM, Reich RR, Kirckof SS, Foltz WG. Performance of various steam sterilization indicators under optimum and suboptimum exposure conditions. In: Rutala WA (Ed). Disinfection, Sterilization and Antisepsis: Principles, Practices,

Challenges, and New Research. Washington, DC: Association for Professionals in Infection Control and Epidemiology; 2004. pp. 200-23.
83. Greene VW. Control of sterilization process. In: Russell AD, Hugo WB, Ayliffe GAJ (Eds). Principles and Practice of Disinfection, Preservation and Sterilization. Oxford, England: Blackwell Scientific Publications; 1992. pp. 605-24.
84. Maki DG, Hassemer CA. Flash sterilization: carefully measured haste. Infect Control. 1987;8(8):307-10.
85. Simmons BP. Guideline for hospital environmental control. Atlanta GA: U.S. Department of Health and Human Services, Public Health Service, Centers for Disease Control; 1981.
86. Centers for Disease Control and Prevention. Health care infection control practices advisory committee. Draft guideline for environmental infection control in health care facilities, Appendix G. Atlanta, Georgia, United States: CDC; 2001. pp. 197.
87. World Health Organization. Hospital acquired infections: guidelines to laboratory methods. WHO Regional Publications European Series No.4. Copenhagen: WHO; 1978. pp. 28-33.
88. Kelkar U, Bal AM, Kulkarni S. Fungal contamination of air conditioning units in operating theaters in India. J Hosp Infect. 2005;60(1):81-4.
89. Wenzel RP, Veazey JM, Townsend TR. Role of inanimate environment in hospital acquired infections. In: Cundy KR, Ball W (Eds). Infection Control in Healthcare Facilities: Microbiological Surveillance. Baltimore: University Park Press; 1977. pp. 71-98.
90. Mortimer EA, Wolinsky E, Gonzaga AJ, Rammelkamp CH. Role of airborne transmission in staphylococcal infections. Br Med J. 1966;1(5483):319-22.
91. Patwardhan N, Kelkar U. Disinfection, sterilization and operation theater guidelines for dermatological practitioners in India. Indian J Dermatol Venereol Leprol. 2011;77(1):83-93.

CHAPTER 10

Universal Precautions for a Dermatosurgeon

Yogesh S Marfatia, Smriti Naswa

KEY MESSAGES

- It is not possible to evaluate every patient undergoing dermatosurgery for all transmissible blood-borne, respiratory, and other pathogens; thus, universal precautions every time everywhere are the key to prevention of infection.
- Universal precautions encompass the following measures:
  - Hand hygiene breaks the chain of transmission of infection through person-to-person contact.
  - Personal protective equipment such as gloves, masks, and gowns creates a physical barrier to the source of microorganisms.
  - Safe handling and disposal of the sharps is of utmost importance; as most common form of occupational exposure to blood and the most likely to result in infection is needlestick injury.
  - Hospital waste should be properly collected and disposed off in respective colored bags.
  - Postexposure prophylaxis protocols for human immunodeficiency virus (HIV) and hepatitis B virus (HBV) must be followed in cases of accidental exposure.

INTRODUCTION

Definition of universal precautions:[1] Universal precautions are a simple set of effective practices designed to protect health workers and patients from infection with a range of pathogens including blood-borne viruses. These practices are used when caring for all patients regardless of diagnosis. They are applied universally.

Healthcare workers deal with blood every day. Blood is a very good culture medium and nidus for various pathogenic microorganisms, many of which are associated with high morbidity and mortality **(Box 1)**. The importance lies in the fact that most blood exposures in health settings are preventable. Dermatosurgeons must take stringent precautions to prevent occupational exposure to blood-borne pathogens. A thorough knowledge about strategies such as universal precautions, immunization against hepatitis B, provision of personal protection, and the management of exposures is a must for every healthcare physician.[1] Adherence to recommended practices decreases transmission of infectious agents. But, observed adherence to universal precautions is not universal and varies from 43 to 89%.[2] Universal precaution guidelines were developed in response to HIV/AIDS epidemic and several guidelines have been published[2-4] **(Box 2)**.

EPIDEMIOLOGY

Annual Infection of Healthcare Personnel with Blood-borne Pathogens

There are approximately 35 million health workers worldwide, of whom approximately 385,000[5] experience percutaneous exposures to blood-borne pathogens annually; two million of those to HBV, 0.9 million to hepatitis C virus (HCV), and 170,000 to HIV. These injuries may culminate into 15,000 HCV, 70,000 HBV, and 1,000 HIV infections. Of the estimated 385,000 needlestick injuries occurring in hospitals each year, 23% occur in surgical settings.[6] Moreover, about 90% of these infections occur in developing countries.[1] The most common cause of occupational exposure is needlestick injury.[5] Among NaSH (National Surveillance System for Health Care Workers) hospitals in US, the operating room is the second most common environment in which sharps injuries occur, accounting for 27% of injuries, following 40% injuries in in-patient units. It is interesting to note that majority of such exposures occur from medical floors.[5] **Table 1** lists the blood-borne pathogens against which universal precautions

BOX 1: Do dermatosurgical procedures require mandatory preprocedure testing of blood-borne pathogens such as human immunodeficiency virus (HIV), hepatitis B virus (HBV), and hepatitis C virus (HCV)?

- The answer lies in what is the *basis behind application of universal precautions* as quoted by the WHO:
  "It is not feasible, effective, or cost-effective to test all patients for all pathogens prior to giving care in order to identify those who are infected and take precautions only with them. Knowing a patient is infected does not prevent occupational exposure to blood. Thus, decisions regarding the level of precautions to use are based on the nature of the procedure and not on the actual or assumed serological status of the patient."
- Negative serology for infective pathogen does not rule out infection as the patient may be in *window period*.
- No test is 100% specific and sensitive.
  Adaptation of universal precautions is essential irrespective of serostatus of patient.

BOX 2: Key points about skin.

- Healthcare-associated pathogens frequently colonize areas of normal, intact patient skin, besides being recovered from infected or draining wounds.
- Normal skin sheds nearly 106 squamous cells per day, containing viable microorganisms (cutaneous microflora), which contaminate the patients' immediate environment including clothes, bed covers, furniture, and others.
- Many studies have shown that hands or gloves of HCWs can be contaminated with pathogens such as *C. difficile*, Gram-negative bacilli, enterococci, or *S. aureus* even by touching intact skin of patients or while performing "clean procedures" on them.
- Following contact with contaminated environment or patients, microorganisms can survive on hands from 2 to 60 minutes.
- After detergent action of soaps/handrubs, 50–60% of the normal barrier function [measured as recovery of transepidermal water loss (TEWL)] recovers rapidly within 6 hours, but complete normalization of the function requires 5–6 days.

(HCW: healthcare worker)

TABLE 1: List of blood-borne pathogens.[7]

Viral	*Bacterial*	*Parasitic*
Human immunodeficiency virus (HIV)		
Hepatitis B virus (HBV)	Syphilis	Malaria
	Brucella	Toxoplasma
Hepatitis C virus (HCV)		Microfilaria
Hepatitis G virus (HGV)		
Epstein–Barr virus (EBV)		
Cytomegalovirus (CMV)		
Human T lymphotropic viruses (HTLV-1 and HTLV-II)		
Ebola virus		
Zika virus (under investigation)		

are necessary.[7] Universal precautions apply to certain body fluids, which harbor potentially infectious pathogens,[8] which are listed in **Table 2**.

NEWER VIRUSES AFFECTING THE WORLD

SARS-CoV-2 Virus or COVID-19 Virus

The recent pandemic by severe acute respiratory syndrome coronavirus 2 (SARS-CoV-2), a respiratory pathogen causing highly contagious respiratory infection, has led to paradigm shift in the way healthcare setups practice worldwide. As the vaccination drives have started in 2021 all over the world, healthcare workers (HCWs) hope the pandemic gets over soon, but all experts agree that coronavirus disease 2019 (COVID-19) virus is going to remain endemic in the world. The Ministry of Health and Family Welfare (MOHFW), Government of India (GOI)[9,10] has laid down guidelines to be practiced for personal protective equipment (PPE) in COVID-19 scenario. Special interest group (SIG) of aesthetics (IADVL academy)[11] has also come up with their recommendations. The guidelines in nutshell are described in **Table 3**.

TABLE 2: Universal precautions and other potentially infectious materials (OPIMs).[8]

Universal precautions apply to:	*Universal precautions do not apply to:**
Semen	*If the following body fluids are not blood-stained:*
Vaginal secretions	Feces
Synovial fluid	Nasal secretions
Cerebrospinal fluid	Sputum
Pleural fluid	Sweat
Peritoneal fluid	Tears
Pericardial fluid	Urine
Amniotic fluid	Vomitus
	Saliva (except in the dental setting, where saliva is likely to be contaminated with blood)

*These are covered under "standard precautions" or "routine practices". These practices aim to protect against the transmission of all microorganisms through contact with all body fluids, excretions, mucous membranes, non-intact skin, and soiled items in addition to precautions for blood. An example in this chapter is Ebola virus disease (vide supra).[8] For further details, refer to the Glossary section.

Special points on procedures on face area:[11]

- Should be deferred, if the patient is coming from containment zone
- Double pair of gloves to be worn by doctor and assisting staff
- Povidone–iodine can be used to coat oral and nasal mucosa, as it has shown to be virucidal to COVID-19 virus for a period of 3 hours
- In case of cannula insertion, suitable skin dressing/ medical plaster to be used to seal entry ports for 48 hours.

Notes on procedure room:[11]

- Disposable instruments should be used wherever possible and in case of using reusable instruments, they should be immediately sent for proper and thorough sterilization.
- Good ventilation in the treatment area helps to prevent aerosol excess in the area; whenever possible, air conditioners can be put off and rooms can be kept open during consultations/procedures (protocol followed in hospital setup of Naswa, which is a COVID-19 designated hospital).
- SIG-aesthetics of IADVL (Indian Association of Dermatologists, Venereologists, and Leprologists) academy suggests use of smoke evacuators with triple filters close to procedure area.
- In operation theaters, negative pressure operation areas are recommended.

Nipah Virus[12]

As per Government of India latest reports, Nipah virus disease is not a major outbreak and is limited to only local occurrence in two districts in Kerala, i.e., Kozhikode and Malappuram.

TABLE 3: Area-wise safety and precaution guidelines in current coronavirus disease 2019 (COVID-19) pandemic in a dermatology clinic.[9-11] The dermatology and/or aesthetic dermatology clinic is considered as low-/medium-risk area for COVID-19.

Area	*Risk strata*	*Staff*	*Patient*	*Remarks*
Reception	Mild risk	Triple layer mask[#] with latex/nitrile gloves	Cloth mask/triple-layer mask	Proper physical distancing should be ensured
Consultation room	Mild	Triple-layer mask with latex/nitrile gloves	Patient should be continuously wearing mask unless examining face area, the examination should be kept brief	Physical distance (1 meter) should be maintained during the consultation except in the examination part No aerosol-generating procedures to be done in OPD
Procedure room	Moderate	See **Table 4**	Triple-layer mask—in case of procedures not involving face	Details in **Table 4**
Housekeeping staff	Mild (frequent touching of floor/surfaces)	Triple layer mask with latex/nitrile gloves	—	—
CSSD/Laundry	Mild	Triple-layer mask with latex/nitrile gloves	—	—

[#]Triple layer mask is synonymously called surgical triple-ply mask.

Notes:[9]

- The hand hygiene and basic respiratory etiquettes comprise the basic preventive measures to prevent COVID-19 spread in public and PPE alone is not a substitute to them, but should be followed in addition to them.
- Handwashing soap and water should be preferred mode of hand hygiene over sanitizers, wherever possible, because of increased chances of irritant/allergic contact dermatitis in the latter.
- A physical distance of 1 meter should always be followed from contacts/suspect/confirmed COVID-19 cases
- As per MOHFW guidelines, nitrile gloves should be preferred over latex gloves. Among latex, nonpowdered gloves should be preferred over powdered gloves. This is because
  - Nitrile gloves resist chemicals and disinfectants such as chlorine.
  - The latex gloves have high risk of irritant contact dermatitis.
- Teleconsultation should be preferred mode of follow-up consultation (wherever possible, postprocedure). Authors (Marfatia and Naswa) feel that going paperless with e-consent forms and e-prescriptions can be given a considerate thought considering the COVID-19 virus remains active in fomites for up to 3 days.

TABLE 4: Universal precaution guidelines in aesthetic/dermatologic/dermatosurgical procedures.[9-11]

Type of procedure		*Risk stratification (as per MOHFW guidelines)*	*Recommended PPE*
Noninvasive (chemical peels, electroporation, nonablative lasers, IPL, lipolysis by cryo-/radiofrequency/ultrasound/laser, light emitting diodes)		Mild	Triple layer/N95 mask* + Latex/nitrile gloves
Minimally invasive (botulinum toxin, filler injections, injection lipolysis, mesotherapy, microblading, thread lifts, microdermabrasion, medium depth peels, hair-removing lasers, radiofrequency procedures, sclerotherapy, and dermaroller)		Moderate	Triple-layer/N95 mask + gloves + gown + goggles (in aerosol-generating procedures/procedures involving face)
Invasive	*Dermatosurgeries/operation theater setup* Vitiligo surgery, mechanical dermabrasion, dermatosurgeries such as sebaceous cyst removal, platelet-rich plasma therapy, hair transplant, and deep chemical peels	Moderate	Triple-layer mask + Face shield + Sterile latex gloves + gown (or coveralls with/without aprons), head and shoe cover
	Aerosol-generating procedures Skin resurfacing ablative lasers, Q-switched Nd:YAG lasers		As above+ Goggles (in aerosol-generating procedures)

*In conjunction with recommendations by MOHFW and SIG-aesthetics IADVL academy with respect to mask usage, in resource restricted setup, the triple-layer mask should suffice in all cases pertaining to dermatology consultations/procedures, except if the patient is coming from containment zone, where being elective procedures, the procedures should be deferred and consultations be done through tele-medium unless an emergency. While where the procurement of N95 mask is not a difficulty, all cases should be considered as asymptomatic carriers (at least till the vaccination drive is over and till pandemic does not settle to endemic levels), doctors can wear N95 in all procedures.

For dermatologists, practicing in these areas, it is suggested they remain updated with prevailing guidelines by local authorities and defer all nonemergency/elective procedures in sick patients. Only procedures, which may be medical emergencies such as skin biopsy in a severe, life-threatening drug reactions, may be performed as per discretion of the doctor and recommendations by MOHFW should be followed which are essentially similar to other respiratory pathogens such as COVID-19 and H1N1 influenza. For further details, this Reference 12 can be looked into.

Bird Flu

The recent pandemic of avian influenza in north India had not seen an animal to human transmission. In case, such a possibility arises, being an influenza virus, the precaution for respiratory illness as mentioned in COVID-19 guidelines would work for flu as well.

This virus is easily disinfected with routine disinfectants such as alcohol hence the other precautions mentioned in the chapter should cover for this disease too.

Ebola Virus

Ebola virus disease (EVD), which was formerly known as Ebola hemorrhagic fever, is a severe illness with an average case fatality rate of 50%. The EVD outbreak in West Africa in 2014 has affected more than eight countries in the world and by March 22, 2015, 10,326 deaths have been reported by WHO worldwide.[13,14] Allaranga et al. had observed that almost one-tenth of all cases of EVD in Africa occurred in healthcare and laboratory workers. WHO reported that by October 27, 2014, a total of 521 healthcare workers had acquired EVD and 272 had died.[14]

The natural hosts of Ebola virus are the fruit bats of *Pteropodidae* family. Since India comes under the home range of these bats, there is a potential risk of Indian population being affected with the virus and its disease.[14]

In healthcare settings, Ebola is spread through direct contact with blood or body fluids of a person who is sick with Ebola or with objects (e.g., bathroom surfaces and medical equipment) that have been contaminated with infectious blood or body fluids (hence, the safe work practices to prevent Ebola spread come under standard precautions rather than universal precautions.[8] For details vide glossary section). The virus can enter a person's body through broken skin or unprotected mucous membranes. For all healthcare workers caring for patients with Ebola, PPE that fully covers skin and clothing and prevents any exposure of the eyes, nose, and mouth is recommended.[15]

Key safe work practices recommended by Centers for Disease Control and Prevention (CDC) include the following:

- Promptly isolate external ventricular drain (EVD) patient in a single room with a closed door and a private bathroom
- Restrict entry of nonessential healthcare workers or other visitors
- Monitor the patient care area at all times
- The healthcare workers should take sufficient time to don and doff PPE slowly and correctly without distraction, preferably in presence of a trained observer
- Reinforce the need to keep hands away from the face during any patient care and to limit touching surfaces and body fluids
- Frequently disinfect gloved hands by using an alcohol-based handrub (ABHR), particularly after contact with body fluids
- Prevent needlestick and sharps injuries by adhering to correct sharps handling practices
- Avoid unnecessary procedures involving sharps
- Use needleless IV systems whenever possible
- Immediately clean and disinfect any visibly contaminated PPE surfaces, equipment, or patient care area surfaces using a disinfectant wipe
- Footwear should be closed-toe, soft-soled, washable, and have a closed back
- Although airborne transmission of Ebola has not been documented to date, CDC recommends that all healthcare workers entering the room of a patient with Ebola wear respiratory protection, which includes an NIOSH-certified, fit-tested N-95 or higher respirator, or a powered air-purifying respirator (PAPR).
- Double-gloving is an easy way to remove gross contamination by changing an outer glove during patient care and when removing PPE.
- Regularly clean and disinfect surfaces in the patient care area even in the absence of visible contamination
  - Only nurses or physicians should clean and disinfect surfaces in the patient care areas to limit the number of additional healthcare workers who enter the room.

Doffing

- Removing used PPE is a high-risk process that requires a structured procedure, a trained observer, a doffing assistant in some situations, and a designated area for removal to ensure protection.
- PPE must be removed slowly and deliberately in the correct sequence to reduce the possibility of self-contamination or other exposure to Ebola.

For further details on Ebola virus see Reference 15.

Zika Virus

Zika virus disease (ZVD) is caused by a *Flavivirus*, the outbreaks of which have been recorded in Africa, the Americas, Asia, and the Pacific. People with ZVD can have symptoms including mild fever, skin rash, conjunctivitis, muscle and joint pain, malaise, or headache, lasting for 2–7 days. Zika virus is a cause of microcephaly and Guillain-Barré syndrome.[16]

Zika virus is primarily transmitted through the bite of an infected mosquito from *Aedes aegypti* in tropical regions. Sexual transmission of Zika virus is also possible. Blood transfusion as a mode is being investigated.[17]

Clinical symptoms and recent history of travel to an area with active Zika virus transmission can give a clue to the diagnosis, which can only be confirmed through laboratory tests on blood or other body fluids, such as urine, saliva, or semen.[17]

Till the possibility of spread of Zika by blood is confirmed, it is advised to follow all universal precautions in probable or confirmed case of Zika. Though Zika is not present in India yet, the breeding grounds including the vector has ample presence. Hence, any recent travel to the places or a pregnant woman or child with suspected symptoms should be thoroughly tested.

Multi-drug-resistant Bacteria

The Indian Network for Surveillance of Antimicrobial Resistance (INSAR) group, India, in a study conducted at 15 tertiary care centers on 26,310 isolates of *S. aureus*, found the prevalence of methicillin-resistant *Staphylococcus aureus* (MRSA) to be 41%. Along with this, MRSA had a high rate of resistance to ciprofloxacin, gentamicin, co-trimoxazole, erythromycin, and clindamycin.[18]

Healthcare workers frequently become contaminated with MDR bacteria. Hayden et al. found that 62% of HCWs, who entered the room of patients known to be colonized with VRE, contaminated their gloves or hands during care.[19]

Contaminated HCW hands, in turn, were capable of transmitting VRE to inanimate surfaces. In a study by Morgan et al. even after appropriate use of gloves and gown while caring for a patient on contact precautions, 1.7–4.2% of HCWs had an MDR bacterium on their hands without hand hygiene. This emphasizes the importance of hand hygiene after removal of gloves and gown.[20]

Overall, 8% of HCW room entries occurred with an HCW who had MDR bacteria on their hands. This highlights the importance of performing hand hygiene before room entry. A greater risk of contamination was observed when HCWs performed a physical examination or remained in the room longer. Hence, universal use of gown and gloves for all patient contact in the ICU may be an answer to this problem.[20]

Healthcare workers entering a room that had environmental contamination with MDR bacteria were over four times as likely to become contaminated with that organism, highlighting the importance of environmental cleaning.[20]

Although cosmetic surgeries are done in otherwise healthy individuals, basic procedures such as skin biopsy might be required to be done bedside in ICU patients. Hence, universal precautions are of equal importance to these procedures as any other major/minor surgeries. Moreover, it is safe to do the dermatosurgeries in OT specifically meant for these procedures (avoiding shared OTs). These measures assume more importance in public hospitals.

MODES OF OCCUPATIONAL EXPOSURE TO BLOOD

- Percutaneous injury (needlestick or other sharps injury)
- Mucocutaneous injury (splash of blood or other body fluids into the eyes, nose, or mouth)
- Blood contact with nonintact skin.

Factors Affecting Occupational Exposure[1]

The risk of infection for health workers depends on:

- Prevalence of disease in the patient population
- The nature and frequency of exposures—higher risk in:
  - Operating, delivery, and emergency rooms
  - Laboratories
  - Cleaners and waste collectors.

Risk of infection after exposure has been explained in **Table 5**.

WHO SUGGESTS FOLLOWING INTERVENTIONS UNDER THE UNIVERSAL PRECAUTIONS[1]

- Handwashing after any direct contact with patients
- Wearing gloves for contact with body fluids, nonintact skin, and mucous membranes
- Wearing a mask, eye protection, and a gown (and sometimes a plastic apron), if blood or other body fluids might splash
- Covering all cuts and abrasions with a waterproof dressing
- Preventing two-handed recapping of needles
- Safe collection and disposal of needles (hypodermic and suture) and sharps (scalpel blades, lancets, razors, and

TABLE 5: Risk of infection with human immunodeficiency virus (HIV), hepatitis B virus (HBV), and hepatitis C virus (HCV) after exposure by various modes.[1,21]

Virus	*Mode of exposure*	*Risk of infection*
HIV	Needlestick or cut exposure to HIV-infected blood	0.3%
	Exposure of the eye, nose, or mouth HIV-infected blood	0.1%
	Nonintact skin	<0.1%
	After a mucous membrane exposure	Approximately 0.09%
HBV	Single needlestick or cut exposure risk	6–30%
HCV	Needlestick or cut exposure risk	1.8% (*range*: 0–7%)
	After a mucous membrane exposure	Rare
	Intact/nonintact skin	None

scissors) with required puncture- and liquid-proof safety boxes in each patient care area
- Promptly and carefully cleaning up spills of blood and other body fluids
- Using a safe system for healthcare waste management and disposal.

Discussion of the steps included in universal precautions for a dermatosurgeon will be under following headings:
- Hand hygiene
- Personal protective equipment
- Safe practices to use sharps and their disposal
- Hospital waste management
- Postexposure prophylaxis (to HIV, HBV, and HCV)
- WHO promotes the slogan "*Clean Care, Safer Care*" highlighting the importance of hand hygiene.

Appropriate handwashing can minimize microorganisms acquired on the hands by contact with body fluids and contaminated surfaces. Handwashing breaks the chain of infection transmission from person-to-person contact.[22] But, adherence of healthcare personnel (HCPs) to recommended hand hygiene procedures has been poor, ranging from 5 to 81%.[23]

Hand Hygiene[22-24]

It is a general term that applies to handwashing, antiseptic handwash, antiseptic handrub, or surgical hand antisepsis. Detailed description of different handwash chemicals can be found in Chapter 9 (Sterilization and Disinfection).

Hand hygiene can be divided into three types according to the method and type of cutaneous microflora they affect **(Table 6)**.

Handrub versus Handwash

Contents of alcohol-based handrubs with optimal antimicrobial efficacy:[23,24]
- About 75–85% ethanol, isopropanol, or n-propanol, or a combination of these; WHO recommendation formulations containing either 75% v/v isopropanol or 80% v/v ethanol
- As per WHO, alcohol solutions containing 60–80% alcohol are considered to have efficacious microbicidal activity, with concentrations higher than 90% being less potent.[24]

Advantages of Handrub[24]

- Elimination of the majority of germs (including viruses)
- *Waterless procedure*: No need for any particular infrastructure (clean water supply network, washbasin, soap, and hand towel)
- Less time taken (20–30 seconds)
- Humectants are present in the handrub, thus no drying or irritation of skin
- Availability of the product at the point of care.

TABLE 6: Various types of hand hygiene.[22-24]

S. No.	*Type of hand hygiene*	*Cutaneous microflora affected*	*Duration*	*Method*	*Remarks*
1.	Routine/social handwash	Likely to reduce transient flora	10–15 seconds	Washing hands with plain (i.e., nonantimicrobial) soap and water	
2.	Hygienic hand antisepsis Antiseptic handwash Antiseptic handrub	Reduces transient microbial flora without necessarily affecting the resident skin flora	15–30 seconds	Treatment of hands with either an antiseptic handrub or antiseptic handwash *Antiseptic handwash*: It is broad spectrum, but is usually less efficacious and acts more slowly than the hygienic handrub *Antiseptic handrub*: These preparations are broad spectrum and fast acting, and persistent activity is not necessary	
3.	Surgical hand antisepsis Surgical hand scrub/wash Surgical handrub	Eliminates transient flora and reduces resident skin flora	Minimum 2–3 minutes	Surgical hand scrub/presurgical scrub refers to surgical hand preparation with antimicrobial soap and water Surgical handrub refers to surgical hand preparation with a waterless, alcohol-based handrub	Surgical hand antisepsis is required preoperatively by the surgical team before performing invasive procedures

Disadvantages of Handrub

Handrubs are not preferred over soaps and are less efficacious, especially if:[24]

- The hands are soiled/dirty
- When exposure to potential spore-forming organisms is strongly suspected or proven
- After using the lavatory.

Indications for Hand Hygiene[24]

- Before and after touching the patient
- Before handling an invasive device for patient care, regardless of whether or not gloves are used
- After contact with body fluids or excretions, mucous membranes, nonintact skin, or wound dressings
- If moving from a contaminated body site to another body site during care of the same patient
- After contact with inanimate surfaces and objects (including medical equipment) in the immediate vicinity of the patient
- After removing sterile or nonsterile gloves.

Notes:

- Use an alcohol-based handrub as the preferred means for routine hand antisepsis in all other clinical situations described above, *if hands are not visibly soiled* (in which case soap and water are advised)
- Soap and alcohol-based handrub should not be used concomitantly.

Routine/Social Handwashing[22]

It is usually limited to hands and wrists; the hands are washed with soap (plain or antimicrobial) and water.

- *Duration*: Minimum 10–15 seconds (of rubbing the hands); duration of entire procedure—40–60 seconds

Steps in Handwashing

- *Preparing for handwashing*:
  - Remove jewelry and watches before washing hands
  - Ensure that the nails are clipped short (do not wear artificial nails)
  - Roll the sleeves up to the elbow.
- Wet the hands and wrists, keeping hands and wrists lower than the elbows (permits the water to flow to the fingertips, avoiding arm contamination).
- Apply soap (plain or antimicrobial) and lather thoroughly.
- Use firm, circular motions to wash the hands and arms up to the wrists, covering all areas including palms, back of the hands, fingers, between fingers and lateral side of fifth finger, knuckles, and wrists. Rub for minimum of 10–15 seconds.
- Repeat the process, if the hands are very soiled.
- Clean under the fingernails.
- Rinse hands thoroughly, keeping the hands lower than the forearms.
- If running water is not available, use a bucket and pitcher.
- Do no dip your hands into a bowl to rinse, as this recontaminates them.
- Collect used water in a basin and discard in a sink, drain, or toilet.
- Dry hands thoroughly with disposable paper towel or napkins, clean dry towel, or air-dry them.
- Discard the towel, if used, in an appropriate container without touching the bin lids with hand.
- Use a paper towel, clean towel, or your elbow/foot to turn off the faucet to prevent recontamination. Routine handwashing is illustrated in **Figure 1**.

Hand Antisepsis/Decontamination[22,24]

Hand antisepsis removes or destroys transient microorganisms and confers a prolonged effect.

Specific antiseptics: Recommended for hand antisepsis—

- 2–4% chlorhexidine
- 5–7.5% povidone–iodine
- 1% triclosan
- 70% alcoholic handrubs.

  Duration is 15–30 seconds.

Immersion of hands in bowls of antiseptics is not recommended.

It may be carried out in one of the following two ways:

1. *Antiseptic handwash*: Wash hands and forearms with antimicrobial soap and water (details already discussed earlier).
2. *Antiseptic handrub*: Decontaminate hands with a waterless, alcohol-based hand gel or handrub. This is appropriate for hands that are not soiled with protein matter or fat **(Fig. 2)**.

Steps

1. Apply the product to the palm of one hand. The volume needed to apply varies by product.
2. Rub hands together, covering all surfaces of hands and fingers, until hands are dry.
3. Do not rinse.

Note

- When there is visible soiling of hands, they should first be washed with soap and water before using waterless handrubs gels or alcohol swabs.
- If soap and water are unavailable, hands should first be cleansed with detergent-containing towelettes, before using the alcohol-based handrub, gel, or swab.

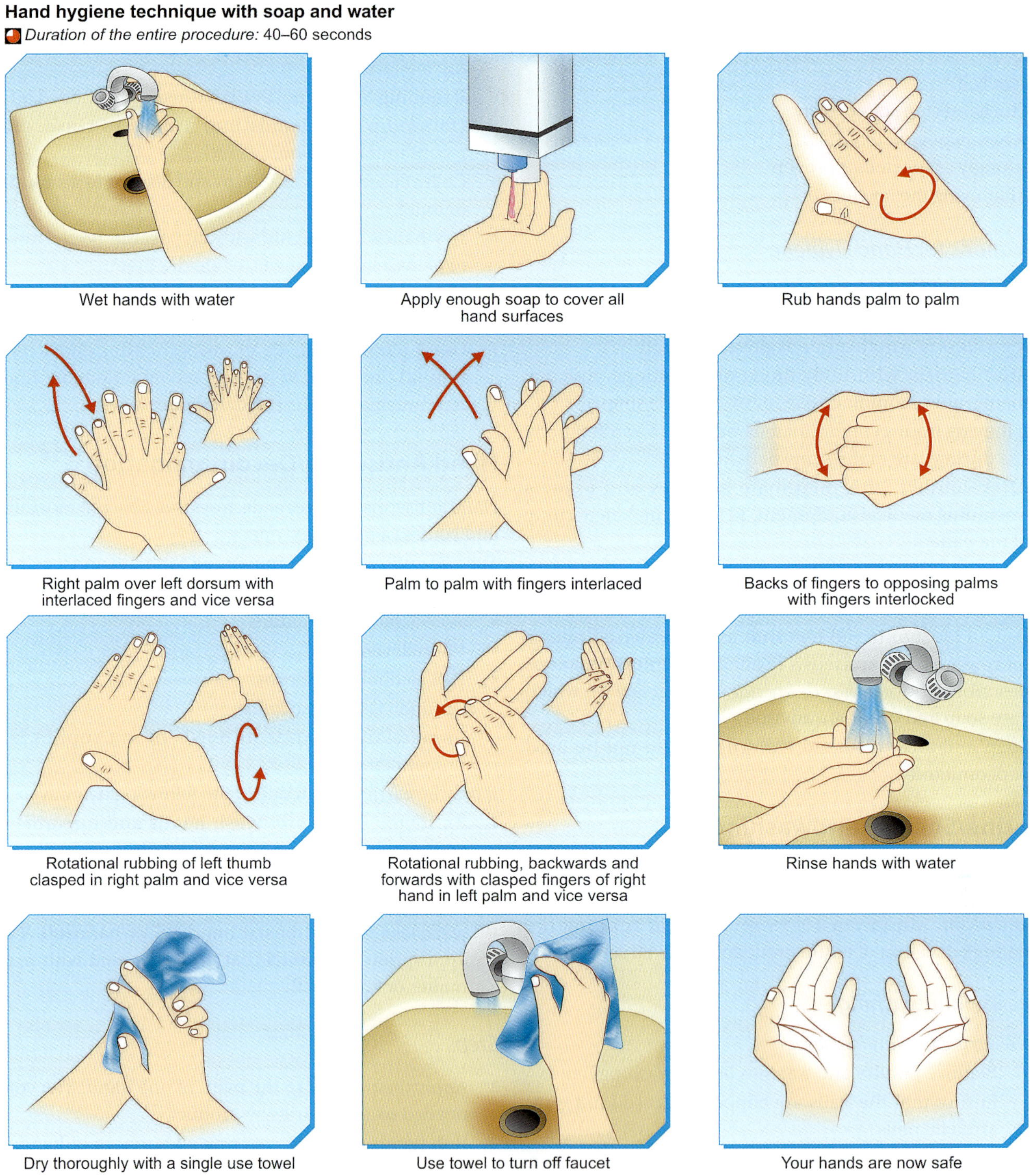

Fig. 1: Routine handwashing with soap and water.
Source: Reproduced with permission—WHO Guidelines on Hand Hygiene in Health Care. World Health Organization; 2009.[24]

Surgical Hand Antisepsis

Recommendations for Surgical Hand Preparation[24]

The hands and forearms are washed thoroughly with an antiseptic soap.

Duration is minimum 2–3 minutes [long scrub times (e.g., 10 minutes) are not necessary].

Steps (Fig. 3)

- Remove rings, wristwatch, and bracelets before beginning surgical hand preparation. Artificial nails are prohibited.
- Sinks should be designed to reduce the risk of splashes.
- If hands are visibly soiled, wash hands with plain soap before surgical hand preparation. Remove debris from

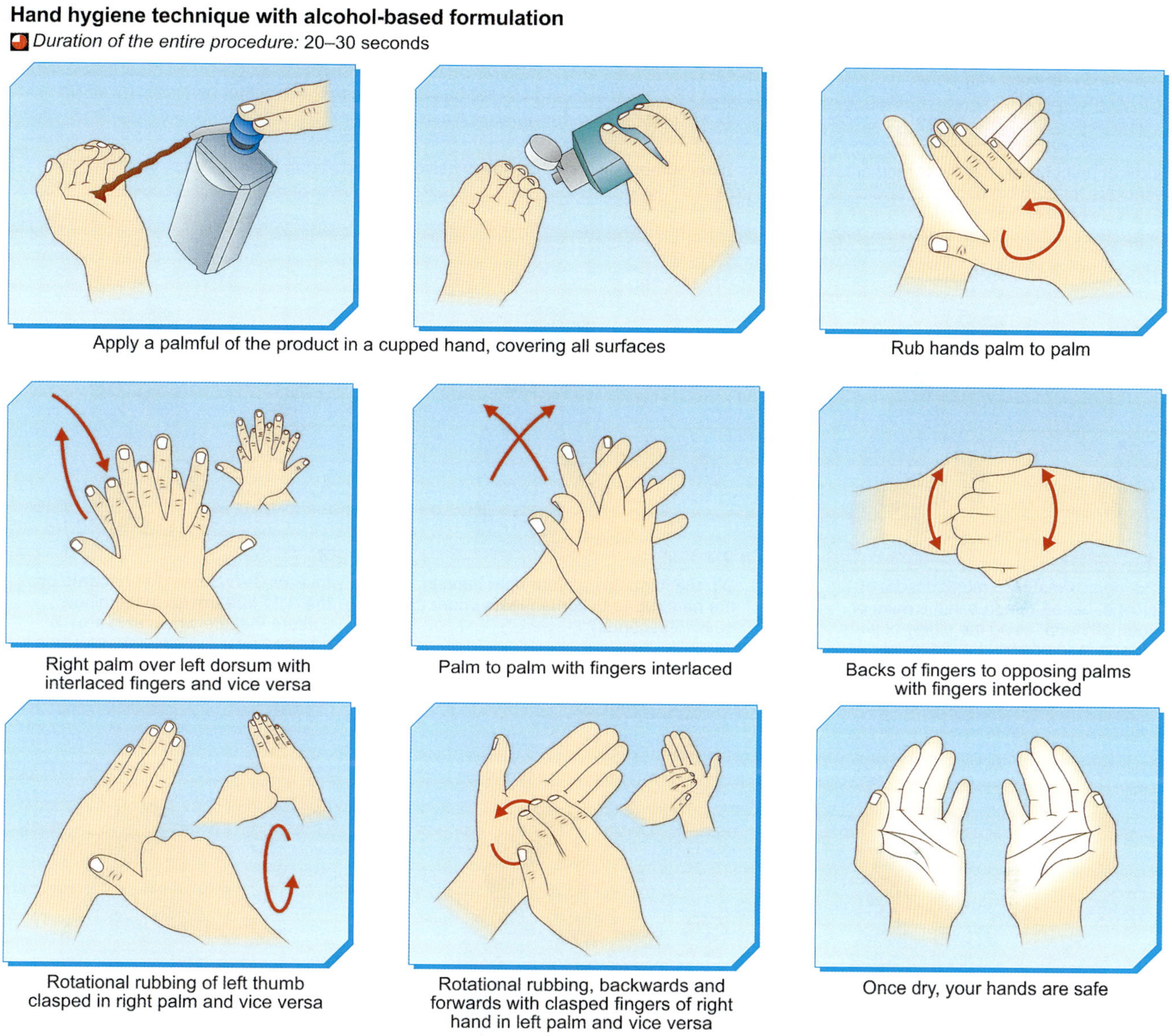

Fig. 2: Antiseptic hand hygienic technique with alcohol-based handrub.
Source: Reproduced with permission—WHO Guidelines on Hand Hygiene in Health Care. World Health Organization, 2009.[24]

underneath fingernails using a nail cleaner, preferably under running water.

- Brushes are not recommended for surgical hand preparation.
- Surgical hand antisepsis should be performed using either a suitable *antimicrobial soap or suitable alcohol-based handrub*, preferably with a product ensuring sustained activity, before donning sterile gloves (handrub is preferred, if quality of water is not assured in the operating theater).
- *Surgical hand scrub/wash*: Procedural steps for surgical scrub with a medicated soap—
  - Start timing. Scrub each side of each finger, between the fingers, and the back and front of the hand for 2 minutes
  - Proceed to scrub the arms, keeping the hand higher than the arm at all times. This helps to avoid recontamination of the hands by water from the elbows and prevents bacteria-laden soap and water from contaminating the hands.
  - Wash each side of the arm from wrist to the elbow for 1 minute.
  - Repeat the process on the other hand and arm, keeping hands above elbows at all times. If the hand touches anything at any time, the scrub must be lengthened by 1 minute for the area that has been contaminated.
  - Rinse hands and arms by passing them through the water in one direction only, from fingertips to elbow. Do not move the arm back and forth through the water.
  - Proceed to the operating theater holding hands above elbows.
  - At all times during the scrub procedure, care should be taken not to splash water onto surgical attire.

The handrubbing technique for surgical hand preparation must be performed on perfectly clean, dry hands.
On arrival in the operating theater and after having donned theater clothing (cap/hat/bonnet and mask), hands must be washed with soap and water.
After the operation when removing gloves, hands must be rubbed with and alcohol-based formulation or washed with soap and water if any residual talc or biological fluids are present (e.g. the glove is punctured).

Surgical procedures may be carried out one after the other without the need for handwashing, provided that the handrubbing technique for surgical hand preparation is followed (Images 1 to 17)

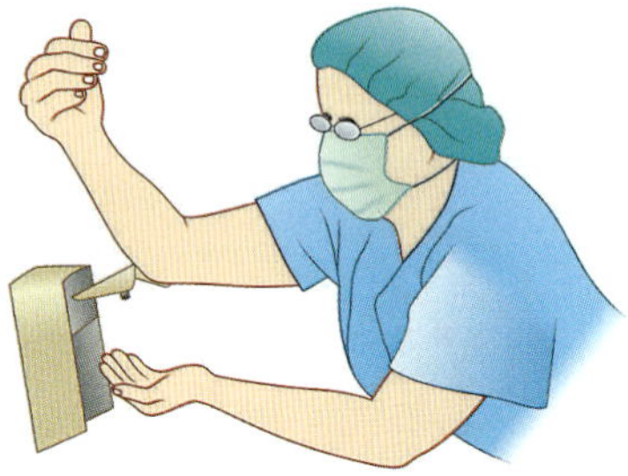

1
Put approximately 5 mL (3 doses) of alcohol-based handrub in the palm of your left hand, using the elbow of your other arm to operate the dispenser

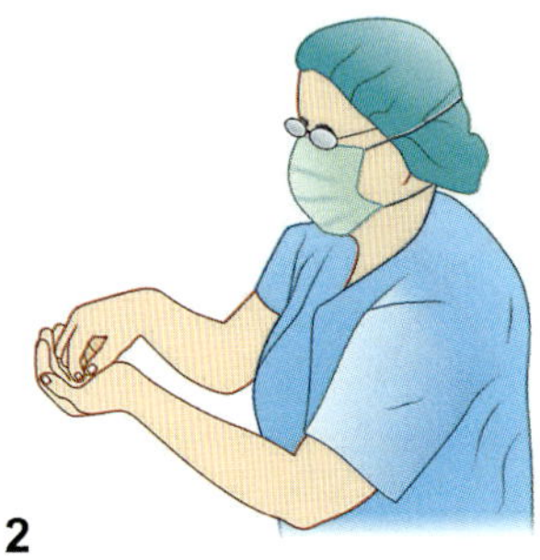

2
Dip the fingertips of your right hand in the handrub to decontaminate under the nails (5 seconds)

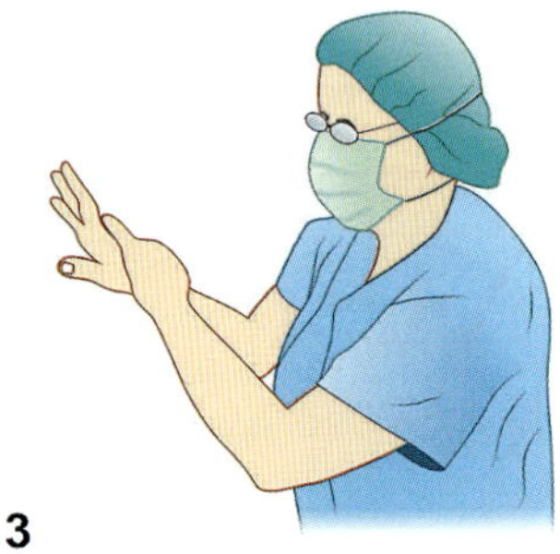

3
Images 3–7: Smear the handrub on the right forearm up to the elbow. Ensure that the whole skin area is covered by using circular movements around the forearm until the handrub has fully evaporated (10–15 seconds)

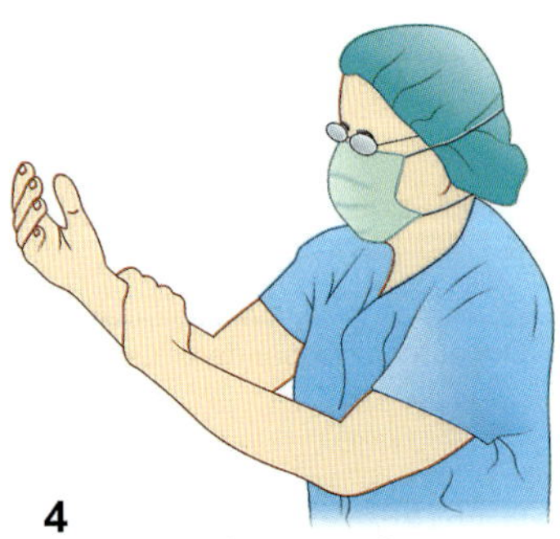

4
See legend for image 3

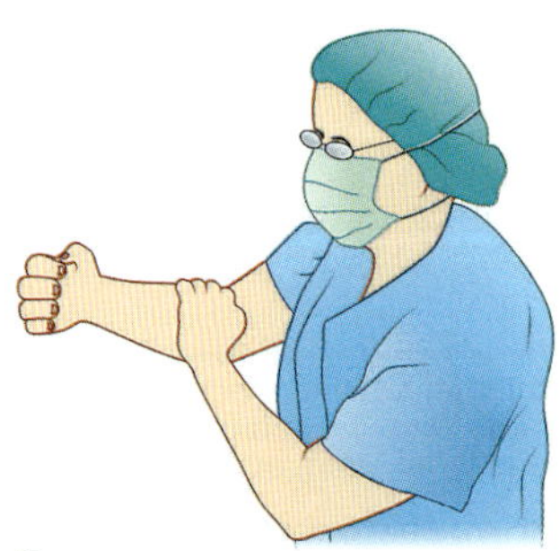

5
See legend for image 3

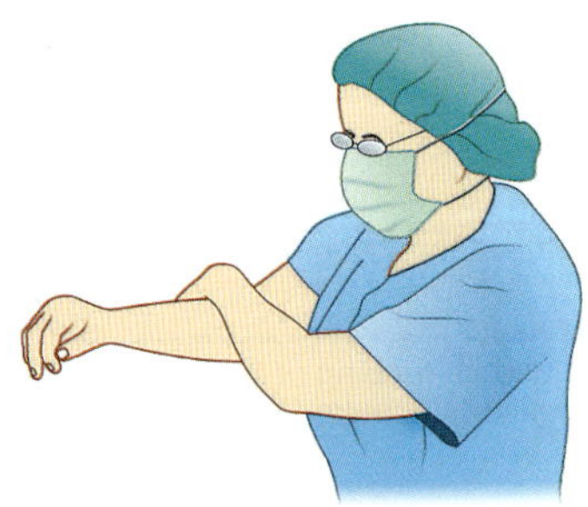

6
See legend for image 3

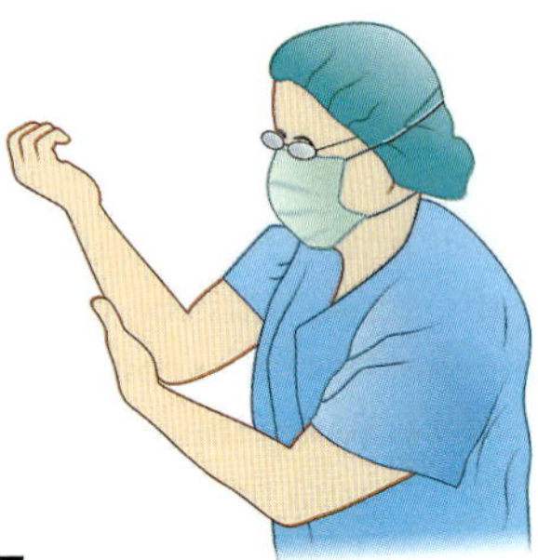

7
See legend for image 3

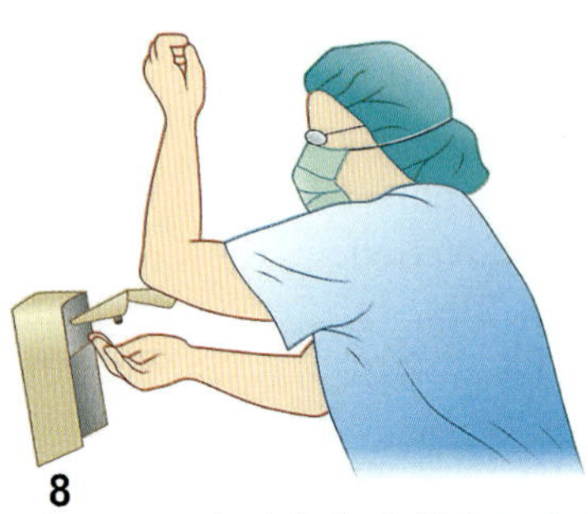

8
Put approximately 5 mL (3 doses) of alcohol-based handrub in the palm of your right hand, using the elbow of your other arm to operate the dispenser

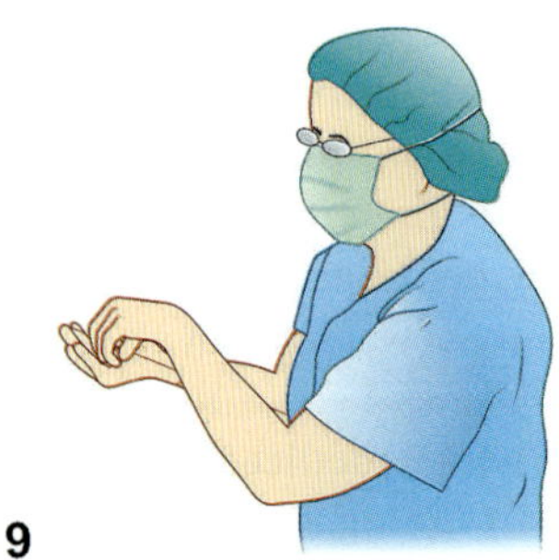

9
Dip the fingertips of your left hand in the handrub to decontaminate under the nails (5 seconds)

Contd...

Contd...

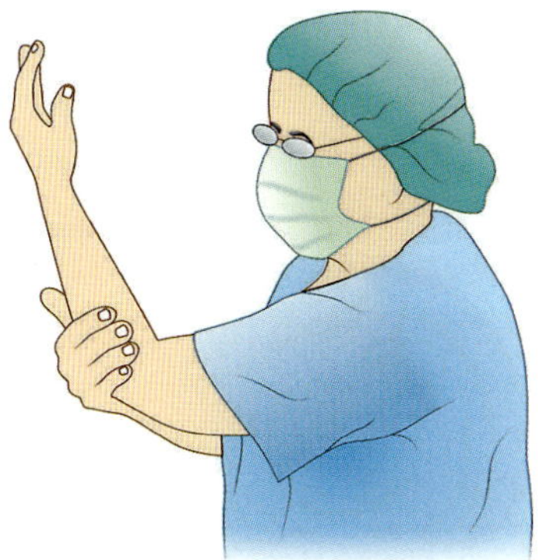

10

Smear the handrub on the left forearm up to the elbow. Ensure that the whole skin area is covered by using circular movements around the forearm until the handrub has fully evaporated (10–15 seconds)

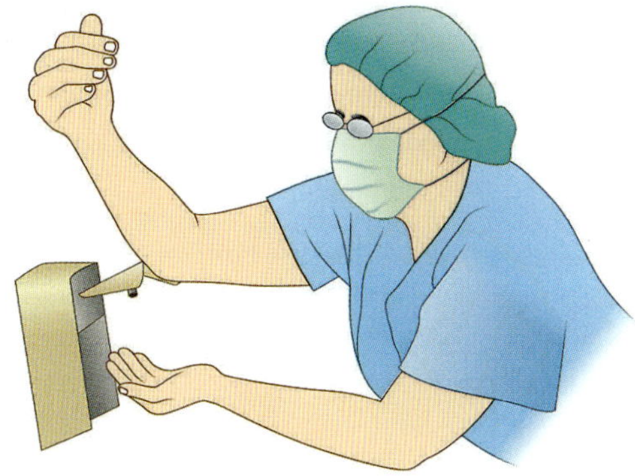

11

Put approximately 5 mL (3 doses) of alcohol-based handrub in the palm of your left hand, using the elbow of your other arm to operate the dispenser. Rub both hands at the same time up to the wrists, and ensure that all the steps represented in images 12–17 are followed (20–30 seconds)

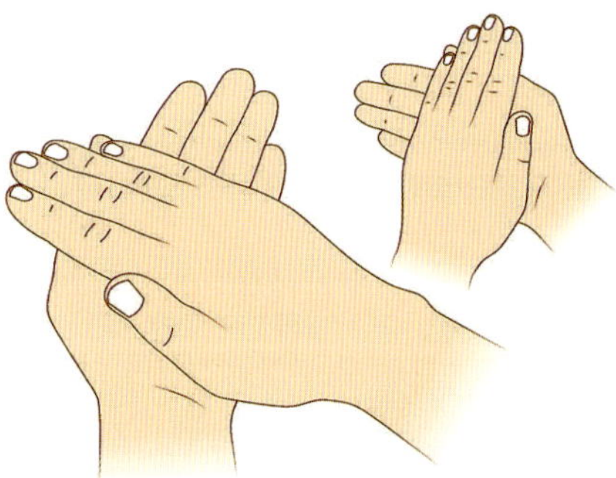

12

Cover the whole surface of the hands up to the wrist with alcohol-based handrub, rubbing palm against palm with a rotating movement

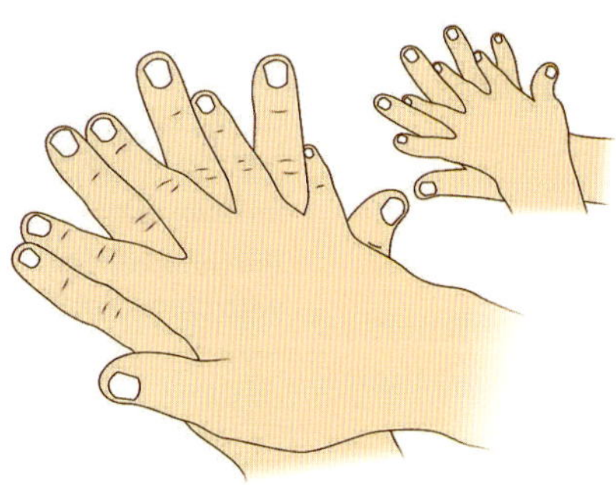

13

Rub the back of the left hand, including the wrist, moving the right palm back and forth and vice versa

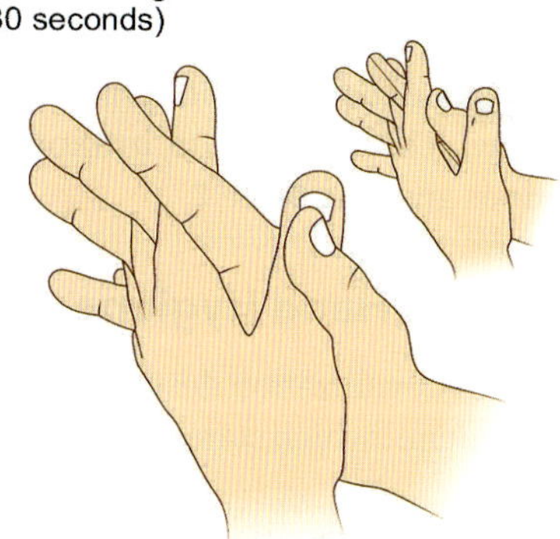

14

Rub palm against palm back and forth with fingers interlinked

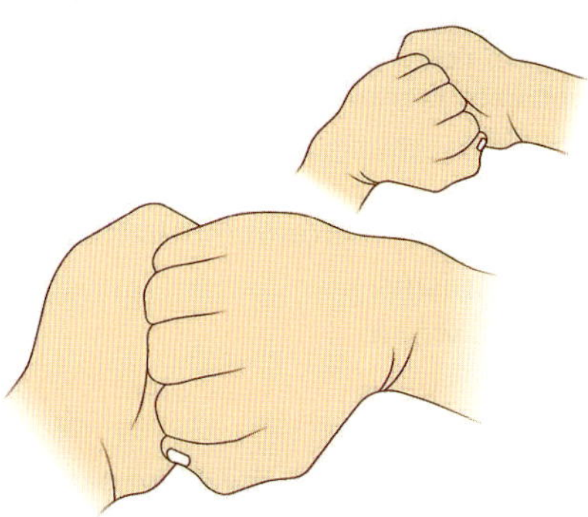

15

Rub the back of the fingers by holding them in the palm of the other hand with a sideways back-and-forth movement

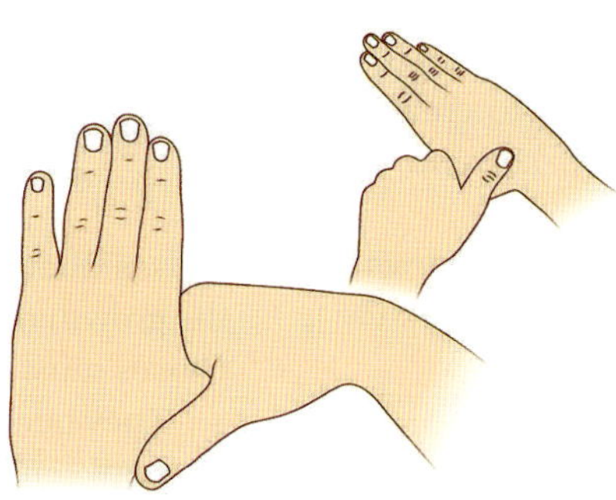

16

Rub the thumb of the left hand by rotating it in the clasped palm of the right hand and vice versa

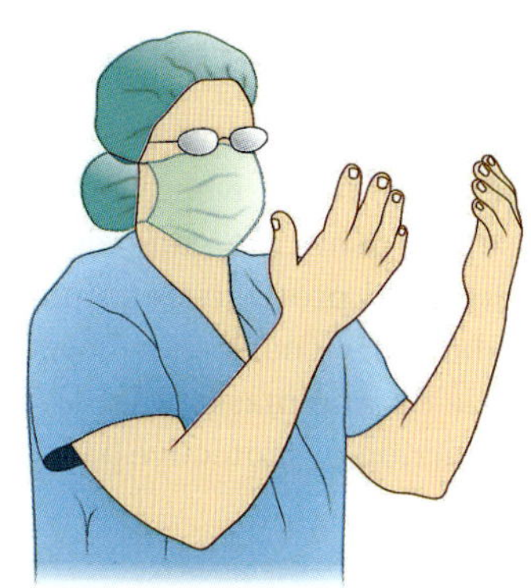

17

When the hands are dry, sterile surgical clothing and gloves can be donned

Repeat the above-illustrated sequence (average duration 60 seconds) according to the number of times corresponding to the total duration recommended by the manufacturer for surgical hand preparation with an alcohol-based handrub

Fig. 3: Illustration of surgical handwash.
Source: WHO Guidelines on Hand Hygiene in Health Care. World Health Organization; 2009.[24]

TABLE 7: Chemicals causing contact dermatitis.

Irritant contact dermatitis (ICD)	*Allergic contact dermatitis (ACD)*
In decreasing frequency	Quaternary ammonium compounds
Iodophors	Iodine or iodophors
Chlorhexidine	Chlorhexidine
Chloroxylenol	Triclosan
Triclosan	Chloroxylenol
Alcohol-based products	Alcohols
ICD and ACD due to alcohol-based handrubs are very rare	

- Once in the operating theater, hands and arms should be dried using a sterile towel and aseptic technique before donning gown and gloves.

- *Surgical handrub*: When using an alcohol-based surgical handrub product with sustained activity, follow the manufacturer's instructions for application times. Apply the product to dry hands only.

Chemicals used for hand hygiene may cause adverse reactions, which include both irritant and allergic contact dermatitis as given in **Table 7**.

Summary of Hand Hygiene

World Health Organization describes it as "My five moments for hand hygiene", which states that HCWs should clean their hands:[24]

- Before touching a patient
- Before clean/aseptic procedures
- After body fluid exposure/risk
- After touching a patient
- After touching patient's surroundings.

Personal Protective Equipment

- Personal protective equipment (PPE) helps to create a physical barrier between the exposed worker and the source of microorganisms.[8]
- Personal protective equipment includes gloves, gowns, laboratory coats, shoe covers, goggles, glasses with side shields, and masks **(Fig. 4)**.[8]
- Selection of protective barriers **(Table 8)**.

Gloves

Gloves are PPE for hands and may be made of materials such as vinyl, latex, and nitrile.[25]

Key points to be remembered about gloves

- Gloves are for single-patient and single-procedure use only.
- Technique for removing gloves should be a *glove-to-glove or skin-to-skin technique* to prevent contamination of hands.

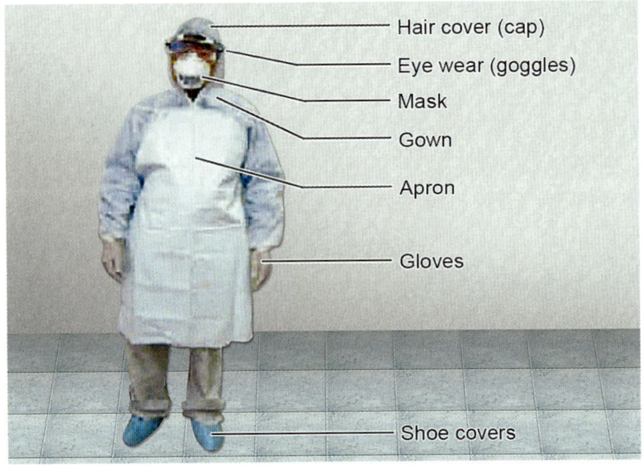

Fig. 4: Full personal protective equipment.[22]
Note: Do not combine surgical hand scrub and surgical handrub.

TABLE 8: Suggested personal protective equipment (PPE) as per type of exposure (NACO).[26]

Type of exposure	*Examples*	*Protective barriers*
Low risk		
Contact with skin with no visible blood	Injections; minor wound dressing	Gloves helpful but not essential
Medium risk		
Probable contact with blood; splash unlikely	Insertion or removal of intravenous cannula; Handling of laboratory specimens; Large open wounds dressing; Venepuncture, handling blood spills	Gloves, gowns, and aprons may be necessary
High risk		
High chances of contact with blood, infected body fluid as well as splashing; Uncontrolled bleeding	Major surgical procedures (e.g., oral surgery), endoscopy, vaginal delivery, and uncontrolled bleeding	Gloves Waterproof gown or apron Eye wear Mask

- Gloves often create a moist environment that facilitates the growth of microorganisms.
- Gloves must be changed when:
  - They become heavily soiled
  - Between two patients
  - Going from dirty to clean area in the same patient.
- Hand hygiene is of foremost importance in safe practices and the use of gloves does not replace the need for hand hygiene. Hands should be properly washed before the gloves are put on and after their removal.
- Heavy duty rubber gloves should be worn for cleanings instruments, handling soiled linen, or when dealing with spills.

World Health Organization describes method to don **(Fig. 5A)** and remove **(Fig. 5B)** gloves in a proper fashion.

The purpose of this technique is to ensure maximum asepsis for the patient and to protect the healthcare worker from patient's body fluid. To achieve this goal, the skin of the healthcare worker remains exclusively in contact with the inner surface of the glove and has no contact with the outer surface. Any error in the performance of this technique leads to back of asepsis requiring a change of gloves.

A. How to don sterile gloves

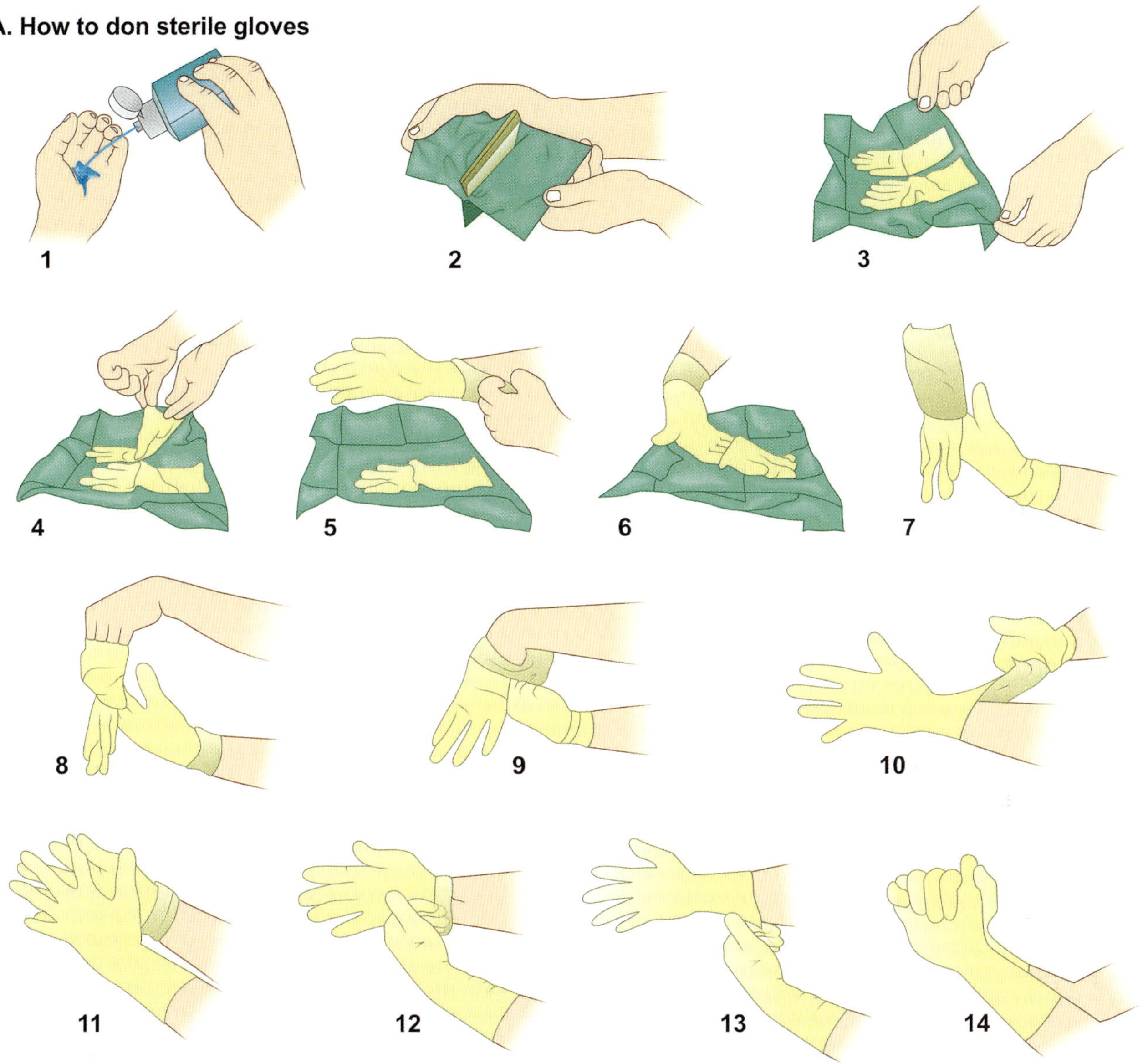

1. Perform hand hygiene before and "aseptic procedure" by hand rubbing or hand washing.
2. Check the package for integrity. Open the first non-sterile packaging by peeling it completely off the heat seal to expose the second sterile wrapper, but without touching it.
3. Place the second sterile package on a clean, dry surface without touching the surface. Open the package and fold it towards the bottom so as to unfold the paper and keep it open.
4. Using the thumb and index finger of one hand, carefully grasp the folded cuff edge of the glove.
5. Slip the other hand into the glove in a single movement, keeping the folded cuff at the wrist level.

6–7. Pick up the second glove by sliding the fingers of the gloved hand underneath the cuff of the glove.

8–10. In a single movement, slip the second glove on to the ungloved hand while avoiding any contact/resting of the gloved hand on surfaces other than the glove to be donned (contact/resting constitutes spaces until the gloves fit comfortably).

11. If necessary, after donning both gloves, adjust the fingers and interdigital spaces until the gloves fit comfortably.

12–13. Unfold the cuff of the first gloved hand by gently slipping the fingers of the other hand inside the fold, making sure to avoid any contact with a surface other than the outer surface of the glove (lack of asepsis requiring a change of glove).

14. The hands are gloved and must touch exclusively sterile devices or the previously disinfected patient's body area.

Contd...

Contd...

B. How to remove sterile gloves

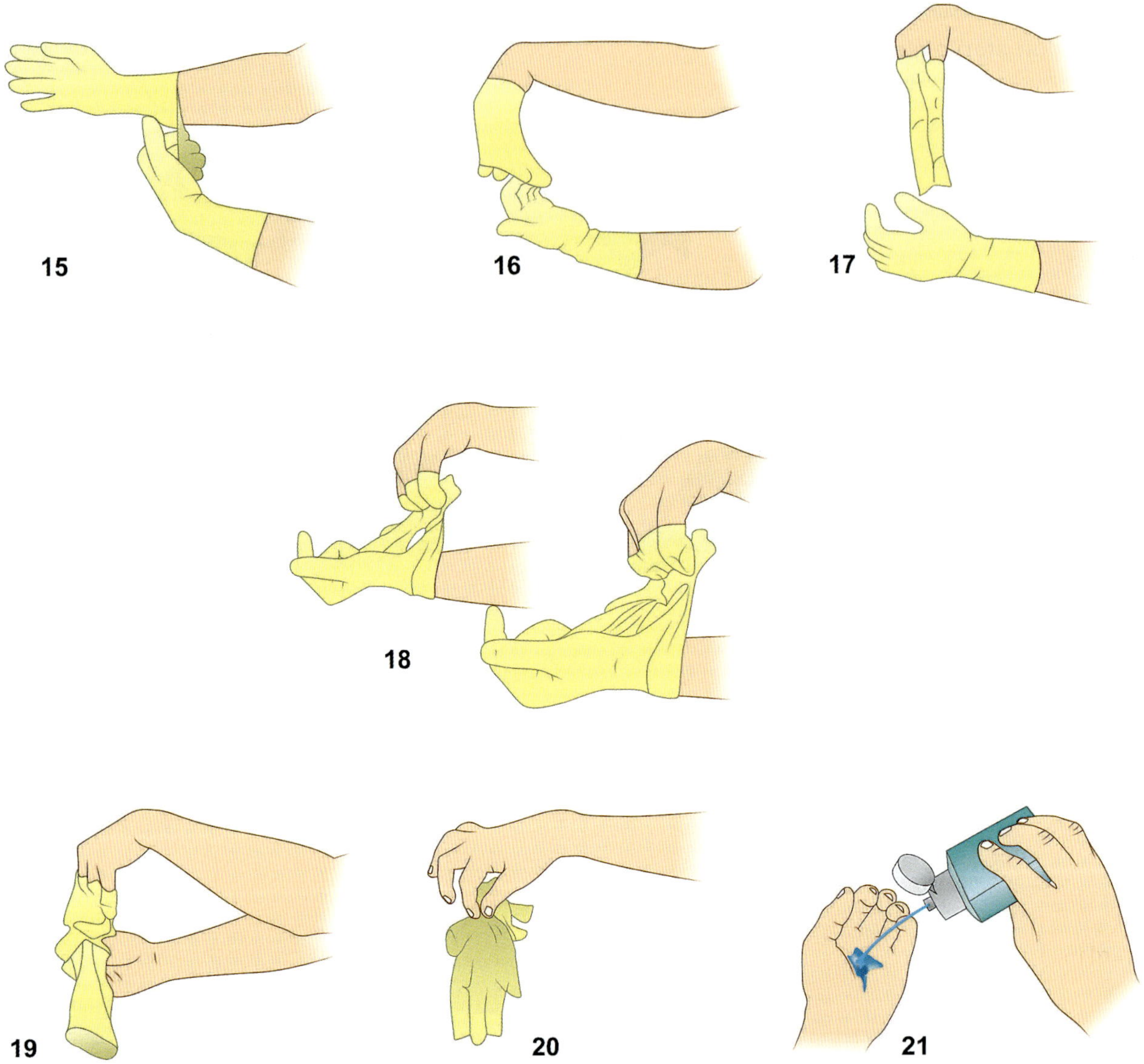

15–17. Remove the first glove by peeling it back with the fingers of the opposite hand. Remove the glove by rolling it inside out to the second finger joints (do not remove completely).

18. Remove the other glove by turning its outer edge on the fingers of the partially ungloved hand.

19. Remove the glove by turning it inside out entirely to ensure that the skin of the healthcare worker is always and exclusively in contact with the inner surface of the glove.

20. Discard gloves.

21. Perform hand hygiene after glove removal according to the recommended indications.

NB: Donning surgical sterile gloves at the time of a surgical intervention follows the same sequences except that:

- It is preceded by a surgical hand preparation;
- Donning gloves is performed after putting on the sterile surgical gown;
- The opening of the first packaging (non-sterile) is done by an assistant;
- The second packaging (sterile) is placed on a sterile surface other than that used for the intervention;
- Gloves should cover the wrists of the sterile gown.

Figs. 5A and B: (A) How to don sterile gloves; (B) How to remove sterile gloves.[24]
Source: WHO Guidelines on Hand Hygiene in Health Care. World Health Organization; 2009.[24]

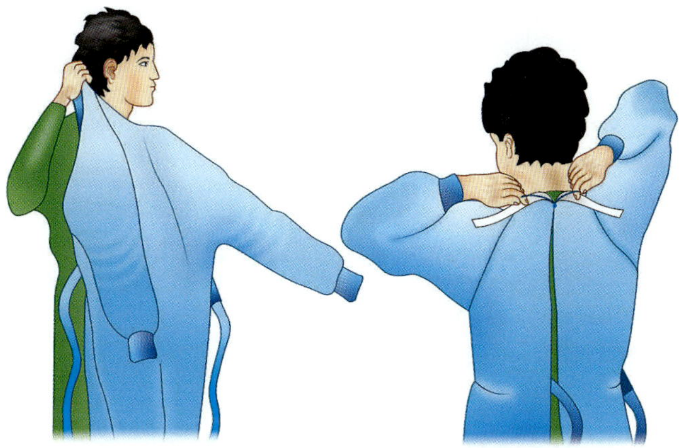

Fig. 6: Method to don gown.[25]

Gowns

Gowns must always be used especially when a splash of blood/body fluids is anticipated. Gowns can be either reusable or disposable.[22]

The steps of gown donning and removal are discussed here.

Gown donning[25] ***(Fig. 6)***

- Perform hand hygiene
- Put gown on, opening to the back
- Fasten both the neck and waist ties.

Gown removal[25]

- Unfasten ties and peel gown away from neck
- Slip fingers of one hand under the wrist cuff and pull hand inside
- With inside hand, push sleeve off with the other arm
- Fold dirty-to-dirty and roll into bundle (do not shake)
- Discard in hamper
- Perform hand hygiene.

Face Protection

Face protection is an effective barrier to protect a worker's eyes, nose, or mouth from splashes or aerosolized body fluids.[22]

Different types of face protection are a mask with safety glasses, a fall face shield, or a mask with an attached visor.[25]

Wearing a mask and safety goggles[25] ***(Fig. 7)***

- Place mask over nose, mouth, and chin
- Fit flexible nose piece of mask over nose bridge
- Secure on head with ties or elastic
- Adjust to fit
- Then position goggles over eyes and secure to the head using the ear pieces or head band
- Adjust to fit comfortably.

Boots/Shoe Covers

Boots/shoe covers are used to protect the wearer from splashes of blood, body fluids, secretions, and excretions over feet. If using personal shoes, shoe covers should be worn so as to cover the shoes adequately.[22]

Occlusive Bandage

All skin defects such as cuts and scratches must be covered with waterproof dressing before patient care.[7]

Overall, the steps given in **Box 3** should be followed while donning and removing PPE.

Adverse reactions to latex gloves are common; viz itching, erythema, eczema leading to allergic contact dermatitis of hands. Adverse reactions to latex gloves are common. The allergy to latex can be prevented by the following measures:[27,28]

- *Use of powder-free, low-protein latex, and/or nonlatex gloves*:
  - Nonlatex gloves include those containing neoprene (polychloroprene polymer), styrene butadiene block

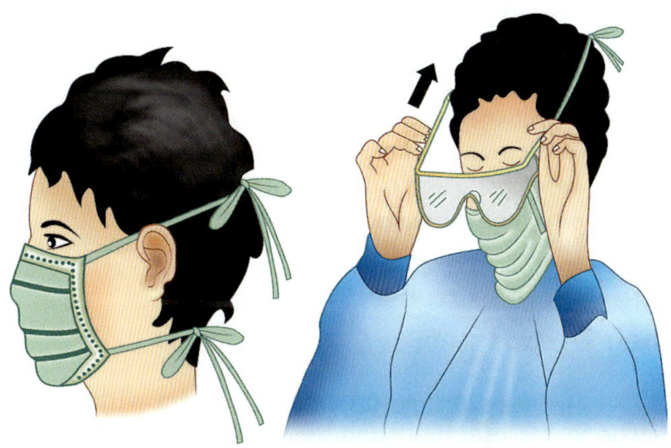

Fig. 7: How to wear face protection.[25]

BOX 3: Steps to wear and remove personal protective equipment (PPE).[22]

Steps to wear PPE:
- Wash hands
- Wear scrub suit or old set of thin clothes before entering the designated changing room or area
- Wear boots or shoe covers with trousers tucked inside
- Wash hands
- Wear cap
- Wear the mask
- Wear the gown
- Wear an impermeable apron, if splashes of blood or body fluids are expected
- Wear protective eyewear/goggles
- Wash hands and dry them
- Wear gloves with gown sleeve cuff tucked into glove

Steps to remove PPE:
Following the steps for removal of PPE in proper order is crucial, as it prevents the HCP to get infected with contaminated PPE. The steps are:
- Remove gloves
- Remove gown
- Perform hand hygiene
- Remove eye protection
- Remove mask
- Remove boots and place in appropriate container
- Perform hand hygiene

(HCP: healthcare personnel)

polymer, styrene ethylene butadiene co-polymer, nitrile (butadiene co-polymer), etc.
  - *Important to note*: Vinyl gloves are not as effective as latex gloves against viral penetration (hence should not be used by dermatosurgeon; can be used by hospital kitchen workers, etc.)
- Good housekeeping practices to remove latex-containing dust from the work place including:
  - Avoiding contact with eyes and face
  - Handwashing after glove removal
  - Use of high-efficiency particulate air (HEPA) vacuum cleaners
- Use of glove liners
- Attention to hand care and minimizing occlusion (prevents nonimmune irritant contact dermatitis)
- Occupational Safety and Health Administration (OSHA) guidelines suggest employers/hospitals to provide workers with education programs and periodic screening questionnaires related to latex allergy
- "Hypoallergenic" gloves are usually made from latex, so latex-sensitive workers should be careful while using them.
- Latex proteins are water soluble. Manufacturing processes such as washing and chlorination can reduce the burden of latex protein antigen.

Safe Practices to use Sharps and Their Disposal

A dermatosurgeon has to come in contact with various sharps in his practice such as disposable syringes and needles, scalpel, blade, hollow-bore needles of IV cannula, suture needles, and even instruments of electrosurgical/radiofrequency devices.

The most common form of occupational exposure to blood and the most likely to result in infection is needlestick injury. The most common causes of needlestick injury are two-handed recapping and the unsafe collection and disposal of sharps.[1]

Risk of Various Sharps Causing Injuries in a Hospital Set-up

About 7–50% of exposures during operative procedures have some type of blood exposure to HCP and in 2–15% of these exposures; the cause is a percutaneous injury, usually from a suture needle **(Table 9)**.[5]

Aggregate data from NaSH indicate that six devices are responsible for nearly 80% of all injuries.

Overall, hollow-bore needles are responsible for 56% of the injuries[5] **(Table 8)**.

Unpublished data by CDC suggests that likelihood of injuries from sharp devices is:[5]

- After use and before disposal of a sharp device—in 40%
- During use of a sharp device on a patient—41%
- During or after disposal—15%.

TABLE 9: Risk of various sharps causing percutaneous injuries in hospital set-up as per Centers for Disease Control and Prevention (CDC).[5]

Type of sharps/devices causing percutaneous injuries	*Contribution in injuries in hospital set-up as per NaSH (percentage)*
Disposable syringes	30%
Suture needles	20%
Winged steel needles	12%
Scalpel blades	8%
Intravenous (IV) catheter stylets	5%
Phlebotomy needles	3%

Hollow-bore Needle versus Solid Sharp Injuries[5]

Injuries from hollow-bore needles (e.g., needles used for blood collection or IV catheter insertion) are associated with an increased risk for HIV transmission because these devices are likely to contain residual blood. Solid sharps, such as suture needles and scalpels, generally deliver a smaller blood inoculum, especially if they first penetrate gloves or another barrier. Therefore, these may have lower risk for HIV transmission.

According to CDC, in December 2001, out of the documented percutaneous exposures to HCPs, which resulted in HIV seroconversion, 90% were due to hollow bore needles.[5]

Guidelines for Safe Practices by CDC

Measures of safe practices and safe handling of sharps are dually advantageous and help to protect both the healthcare provider and patient from exposure to the other's blood.

Work Practices to Prevent Sharp Injuries through the Use and Handling of a Device[5]

- *Before the beginning of a procedure that involves the use of a needle or other sharp device*:
  - Necessary equipment for performing a procedure available within arm's reach
  - Adequate lighting and space to perform the procedure
  - Sharps in a procedure tray should always point away from the operator
  - Place sharps disposal container as close to the point-of-use as appropriate for immediate disposal of the sharp
  - Obtain assistance from other staff or a family member to assist in calming or restraining the patient, if the patient is likely to be uncooperative, combative, or confused.
  - Inform the patient of what the procedure involves and explain the importance of avoiding any sudden movement that might dislodge the sharp.
- *During a procedure that involves the use of needles or other sharp devices*:
  - Double gloving
  - Maintain visual contact with the procedure site and location of the sharp device

- When handling an exposed sharp, take care to avoid injury to oneself and other staff
- Do not handpass exposed sharps from one person to another; use a predetermined neutral zone or tray for placing and retrieving used sharps. Verbally announce when sharps are being placed in a neutral zone.
- Use instruments, rather than fingers, to grasp needles, retract tissue, and load/unload needles and scalpels
- Use alternative cutting methods such as blunt electrocautery and laser devices when appropriate
- Use round-tipped scalpel blades instead of pointed sharp-tipped blades
- Use of blunt suture needles is preferred
- If the procedure necessitates reusing a needle multiple times on the same patient (e.g., giving local anesthesia), recap the needle between steps using techniques enumerated in next subsection.

▪ *During clean-up following a procedure*:
  - Visually inspect procedure trays and other surfaces such as patient beds containing waste materials and sharps left inadvertently after the procedure.
  - Transport reusable sharps in a closed container that has been secured to prevent the spillage of contents.

▪ *During disposal*:
  - Visually inspect the sharps container for hazards caused by overfilling.
  - Make sure the sharps container being used is large enough to accommodate the entire device.
  - Avoid bringing the hands close to the opening of a sharps container; never place hands or fingers into a container to facilitate disposal of advice.
  - Keep the hands behind the sharp tip when disposing the device.
  - If disposing of a sharp with attached tubing (e.g., winged steel needle), be aware that the tubing can recoil and lead to injury.

▪ *After disposal*:
  - Visually inspect sharps containers for evidence of overfilling before removal. If a sharps container is overfilled; take help of safety assistants, obtain a new container, and use forceps to remove protruding devices and place them in it.
  - Keep filled sharps containers in a secure area.

▪ *Improperly disposed sharps*:
  - If an improperly disposed sharp is encountered in the work environment, handle the device carefully, keeping the hands behind the sharp at all times.
  - Use a mechanical device to pick up the sharp, if it cannot be performed safely by hand.

Safe Recapping Procedures[29]

In situations where recapping is considered necessary, safe approaches are needed to be followed. The bottom line remains that the workers should never move an exposed needle tip toward an unprotected hand.

Following are some options (though they need to be further investigated for their safety potential):

▪ *Single-handed scooping*:
  - Recapping by laying the cap on a flat surface and scooping it on to the tip of a syringe held in one hand
  - Must keep the free hand away from the sheath and well behind the exposed needle.

▪ *Recapping devices*:
  - Some devices permit *single-handed recapping* by parking a needle cap on a flat surface
  - Some devices are designed to protect the hand that holds the cap during *two-handed recapping* procedures.

Other Sharps[7]

▪ *Safe handling of sharps*:
  - Extreme care should be used to avoid autoinoculation
  - All chipped or cracked glassware should be discarded in appropriate containers
  - Broken glass should be picked up with a brush and pan. Hands must never be used
  - The disposable needles should never be manipulated, bent, broken, recapped, or removed from syringes
  - The used sharps should never be passed directly from one person to another
  - One should always dispose of his/her own sharps
  - Used needles should be discarded in puncture-proof rigid containers (plastic or cardboard boxes) after disinfection in 0.5–1% freshly prepared sodium hypochlorite solution (common bleach)
  - If a needle shredder is available, only the needles or the needles along with syringe nozzle may be shredded depending upon the type of the shredder
  - Sharp disposal containers should be sent for disposal *when three-fourth full.*

▪ *Safe handling of specimens (blood, etc.)*:
  - Specimens, especially blood and body fluids, should be collected in presterilized screw-capped plastic containers properly sealed to prevent spillage or leakage.

▪ *Safe handling of blood/body fluid spills*:
  - In case of a spill of blood/body fluid in the OT, the area should be flooded with a disinfectant solution, e.g. freshly prepared 0.5–1% sodium hypochlorite solution and left for 30 minutes.
  - After wearing gloves, the area should be covered with paper towels or gauze sponges to absorb the liquid followed by a thorough wash with soap and water.
  - All contaminated materials should be disposed of as infectious waste.

TABLE 10: Categories of biomedical waste and color coding and type of container for their disposal [as per the Biomedical Wastes (Management and Handling) Rules, by Ministry of Environment and Forests, India].[30]

Category number	*Waste category*	*Color coding and type of container*	*Treatment and disposal*
1	Human anatomical waste (human tissues, organs, and body parts)	Yellow (plastic bag)	Incineration*/deep burial
3	Microbiology and biotechnology waste (wastes from laboratory cultures, vaccines, human, and animal cell culture used in research, toxins, dishes, and devices used for transfer of cultures)	Yellow (plastic bag) Red (disinfected container/plastic bag)	Yellow–incineration* Red–local autoclaving/microwaving
4	Waste sharps (needles, syringes, scalpels, blades, glass, etc. that may cause puncture and cuts. This includes both used and unused sharps)	Blue/white translucent (plastic bag/ puncture-proof container)	Disinfection (chemical treatment**/ autoclaving/microwaving and mutilation/ shredding)
5	Discarded medicines and cytotoxic drugs	Black (plastic bag)	Incineration*/destruction and drugs disposal in secured landfills
6	Soiled waste (items contaminated with blood, and body fluids including cotton, dressings, soiled plaster casts, lines, beddings, and other material contaminated with blood)	Yellow (plastic bag) Red (disinfected container/plastic bag)	Yellow–incineration* Red–local autoclaving/microwaving
7	Solid waste (wastes generated from disposable items other than the waste sharps, such as tubing, catheters, intravenous sets, etc.)	Red (disinfected container/plastic bag) Blue/white translucent (plastic bag/ puncture-proof container)	Red–disinfection by chemical treatment** autoclaving/microwaving Blue/white translucent–disinfection by chemical treatment** autoclaving/ microwaving and mutilation/shredding##
8	Liquid waste (waste generated from laboratory and washing, cleaning, house-keeping, and disinfecting activities)	—	Disinfection by chemical treatment** and discharge into drains.

#Only categories relevant to dermatosurgical practices are included.
**Chemicals treatment using at least 1% hypochlorite solution or any other equivalent chemical reagent. It must be ensured that chemical treatment ensures disinfection.
##Mutilation/shredding must be such so as to prevent unauthorized reuse.
*There will be no chemical pretreatment before incineration. Chlorinated plastics shall not be incinerated.

Healthcare Waste Management and Disposal[30]

"Biomedical waste" means any waste, which is generated during the diagnosis, treatment, or immunization of human beings or animals or in research activities pertaining thereto or in the production or testing of biologicals.

The waste disposal follows the rule of "*Decontaminate-Disinfect-Dispose*" **(Table 10)**.

Notes:

- Color coding of waste categories with multiple treatment options shall be selected depending on treatment option chosen.
- Waste collection bags for waste types needing incineration shall not be made of chlorinated plastics.
- Category 8 (liquid) does not require containers/bags.
- Category 3, if disinfected locally, needs not be put in containers/bags.

CHEMICAL DISINFECTANTS EFFECTIVE IN INACTIVATING HIV (TABLE 11)[31]

Postexposure Prophylaxis

Definition: Postexposure prophylaxis (PEP) is short-term antiretroviral treatment to reduce the likelihood of HIV infection after potential exposure, either occupationally or through sexual intercourse.[32]

Postexposure Prophylaxis of HIV

Six steps of PEP as advised by NACO are:[33,34]

Step 1: First aid in management of exposure ***(Table 12)***—
For the skin: If the skin is broken after a needle-stick or sharp instrument—

- Immediately wash the wound and surrounding skin with water and soap, and rinse. Do not scrub.
- Do not use antiseptics or skin washes (bleach, chlorine, alcohol, and betadine).

TABLE 11: Chemical disinfectants effective in inactivating human immunodeficiency virus (HIV).

Solution	*Strength of solution (in %)*	*Minimum time of contact for effective disinfection (in minutes)*
Sodium hypochlorite solution*	1%	30
Ethanol	70%	3–5
2-propanol (isopropyl alcohol)	70%	3–5
Povidone–iodine	2%	15
Formaline	4%	30
Glutaraldehyde (CIDEX)	2%	30
Hydrogen peroxide	6%	30

*Contains 10,000 ppm of chlorine. Household bleach contains 4–5% of available chlorine that may be diluted to form 1% available chlorine. Minimum contact time recommended is 30 minutes.

TABLE 12: Dos and Don'ts after exposure with human immunodeficiency virus (HIV)-infected blood/other potentially infectious materials (OPIM).

Dos	*Don'ts*
Remove gloves, if appropriate	Do not panic
Wash the exposed site thoroughly with running water	Do not put pricked finger in mouth
Irrigate with water or saline, if eyes or mouth have been exposed	Do not squeeze wound to bleed it
Wash the skin with soap and water	Do not use bleach, chlorine, alcohol, betadine, iodine, or any antiseptic or detergent
Do consult the designated physician immediately as per institutional guidelines for the management of the occupational exposure	

After a splash of blood or body fluids on unbroken skin:

- Wash the area immediately
- Do not use antiseptics.

For the eye:

- Sit in a chair, tilt head back, and irrigate exposed eye immediately with water or normal saline with the help of a colleague.
- If wearing contact lens, leave them in place while irrigating, as they form a barrier over the eye and will help to protect it. Once the eye is cleaned, remove the contact lens and clean them in the normal manner. This will make them safe to wear again.
- Do not use soap or disinfectant on the eye. For the mouth:
  - Spit fluid out immediately
- Rinse the mouth thoroughly, using water or saline and spit again. Repeat this process several times.
- Do not use soap or disinfectant in the mouth.
- Consult the designated physician of the institution for management of the exposure immediately.

Step 2: Establish eligibility for PEP—

- The risk of infection transmission is proportional to the amount of HIV transmitted, which depends on the nature of exposure (Exposure Code—EC) and the status of the source patient (Status Code—SC).
- A baseline rapid HIV testing of exposed and source person after informed consent must be done for PEP.
- However, initiation of PEP should not be delayed while waiting for the results of HIV testing of the source of exposure.

First PEP dose within 72 hours—window of opportunity:

- Start treatment, ideally within *2 hours*, but certainly within 72 hours; PEP is not effective after 72 hours of exposure.
- If the risk is in significant, PEP could be discontinued, if already commenced.

Assessing risk of transmission:

- Exposure is defined under three categories based on the amount of blood/fluid involved and the entry port **(Table 13)**.

Assess exposed individual:

- The exposed individual should be sent to experienced physician for assessment.

The wearing of gloves during any of these accidents constitutes a protective factor.

Note: In case of an accidental exposure to blood (AEB) with material such as discarded sharps/needles, contaminated for over 48 hours, the risk of infection is negligible for HIV, but still remains significant for HBV. HBV survives longer than HIV outside the body.

- Exposed individuals who are known or discovered to be HIV positive should not receive PEP.

TABLE 13: Exposure code (EC).

Categories of exposure	*Definition and example*
Mild exposure	Mucous membrane/nonintact skin with small volumes, e.g.: • A superficial wound (erosion of the epidermis) with a plain or low-caliber needle • Contact with the eyes or mucous membranes • Subcutaneous injections following small-bore needles
Moderate exposure	Mucous membrane/nonintact skin with large volumes *or* percutaneous superficial exposure with solid needle, e.g., a cut or needlestick injury penetrating gloves
Severe exposure	Percutaneous with large volume, e.g.: • An accident with a high-caliber needle (>18 G) visibly contaminated with blood • A deep wound (hemorrhagic wound and/ or very painful) transmission of a significant volume of blood • An accident with material that has previously been used intravenously or intra-arterially

Step 3:

- *Counseling for PEP*:
  - Exposed persons should be sent to experienced HIV care physician for appropriate counseling.

Note:

- Exposed person, known or discovered to be HIV positive, is not eligible for PEP and should be sent for assessment for initiation of ART
- It should be clear that PEP is not mandatory
- *Document exposure*:
  - Documentation of exposure is essential. Special leave from work should be considered for a period of 2 weeks.

Step 4:

- Prescribe PEP
- *Deciding on PEP regimen*:
  - There are two types of regimens:
    1. *Basic regimen*: 2-drug combination
    2. *Expanded regimen*: 3-drug combination

The decision to initiate the type of regimen depends on the type of exposure and HIV serostatus of the source person **(Table 14)**.

- Duration of PEP—4 weeks
- *Seek expert opinion in case of*:
  - Delay in reporting exposure (>72 hours)
  - Unknown source
  - Known or suspected pregnancy, but initiate PEP
  - Breastfeeding mothers, but initiate PEP
  - Source patient is on ART
  - Major toxicity of PEP regimen.

Step 5:

- HIV chemoprophylaxis **(Table 15)**[33-35]
- *Antiretroviral (ARV) drugs during pregnancy*:
  - None of the current ARV drug regimens recommended for PEP are contraindicated for pregnant women.[35]

ARV drugs during breastfeeding: Breastfeeding should not contraindicate PEP, but the risks and benefits of continuing breastfeeding while HIV transmission risk is unknown should be discussed with the mother.[35]

TABLE 14: Human immunodeficiency virus (HIV) postexposure prophylaxis (PEP) evaluation.

	Status of source (SC)		
Exposure code (EC)	*HIV+ and asymptomatic*	*HIV+ and clinically symptomatic*	*HIV status unknown*
Mild	Consider 2-drug PEP	Start 2-drug PEP	Usually no PEP or consider 2-drug PEP
Moderate	Start 2-drug PEP	Start 3-drug PEP	Usually no PEP or consider 2-drug PEP
Severe	Start 3-drug PEP	Start 3-drug PEP	Usually no PEP or consider 2-drug PEP

TABLE 15: Postexposure prophylaxis (PEP) regimens.[35]

	Preferred regimen	*Alternate regimen*
2-drug regimen (basic PEP regimen)	Tenofovir disoproxil fumarate (TDF) 300 mg once daily + lamivudine (3 TC) 150 mg twice daily or 300 mg once daily*	TDF 300 mg once daily + emtricitabine (FTC) 200 mg once daily*
3-drug regimen## (expanded PEP regimen) (consult expert opinion)	Lopinavir/ritonavir (LPV/r)** 400/100 mg twice a day or 800/200 mg once daily with meals atazanavir/ritonavir (ATV/r)** 300 mg + 100 mg once daily	Raltegravir (RAL) 400 mg twice daily Darunavir/ritonavir (DRV/r)** 800 mg + 100 mg once daily or 600 mg + 100 mg twice daily
(Basic regimen plus a protease inhibitor) (Conditional recommendation, very low-quality evidence)		Efavirenz (EFV)# 600 mg once daily
Not recommended	ddI + d4T combination NNRTI such as nevirapine should not be used in PEP because of ADR and hepatotoxicity in immunocompetent HCW	

*Strong recommendation, low quality evidence
#If protease inhibitor is not available and the 3rd drug is indicated, one can consider using efavirenz (EFV 600 mg once daily). Monitoring should be instituted for side effects of this drug, e.g., central nervous system (CNS) toxicity such as nightmares and insomnia.
##The latest guidelines recommend 3-drug regimen for everyone, for three reasons—simplified prescription, availability of less toxic and better-tolerated medications, and this removes the need to obtain information about drug resistance risk. The 2-drug regimen is now prescribed when there is nonavailability of third drug (in resource-restricted set-ups) and where the risk of additional toxicity outweighs the benefit.
**Ritonavir requires refrigeration.
(ADR: adverse drug reaction; ddI: didanosine; d4T: stavudine; HCW: healthcare worker)

- *Side effects and adherence to PEP*:
  - More side effects, most commonly nausea and fatigue, among HCP taking PEP than persons living with HIV/AIDS (PLHAs) taking ART.
  - These occur mainly at the beginning of the treatment and include nausea, diarrhea, muscular pain, and headache.
  - Most side effects are mild and transient.
  - Anemia and/or leukopenia and/or thrombocytopenia may occur during the month of treatment.
  - Side effects can be reduced through medications.
  - A complete blood count and liver function tests (transaminases) may be performed at the beginning of treatment (as baseline) and after 4 weeks.

- *Adherence*: More than 95% adherence is important in order to maximize the efficacy of the medication in PEP. Recent evidence shows PEP uptake has been insufficient—only 57% of the people who initiated PEP have completed the full course.[32] To improve uptake and completion of PEP, WHO recommends providing the full 28-day course at first visit, rather than requiring patients to return multiple times for prescriptions.[32]

Step 6:

- *Follow-up of an exposed person*:
  - Whether or not PEP is started, a follow-up is needed to monitor for possible infections and to provide psychological support.
  - Exposed persons should have post-PEP HIV tests. HIV test at 3 months and again at 6 months is recommended. If the test at 6 months is negative, no further testing is recommended.

Postexposure Prophylaxis of Hepatitis B

Routine hepatitis B immunization of all HCP:[1,21]

- Routine immunization of all HCP (including nursing staff and sweepers and cleaners) comes under universal precautions.
- They should be vaccinated against the hepatitis B virus. The vaccination for hepatitis B consists of three doses—initial, 1 month, and 6 months. Most (99%) seroconvert after completing the full course.

Efficacy of PEP for HBV:

Percutaneous exposure from hepatitis B surface antigen (HBsAg)-positive blood:

- Multiple doses of hepatitis B immunoglobulin (HBIg) initiated within 1 week offer 75% protection
- Combination of HBIg with hepatitis B vaccine series increases to 85–95% protection

Recommendations for HBV postexposure management **(Table 16)**:

- PEP for HBV during pregnancy and lactation
- HBIg and hepatitis B vaccine are not a contraindication to pregnancy and lactation.[21]

TABLE 16: Recommendations for hepatitis B virus (HBV) postexposure management.[21,36]

Vaccination and antibody response status of exposed workers	*Treatment*		
	Source HBsAg positive	*Source HBsAg negative*	*Source unknown or not available for testing*
Unvaccinated	HBIg (0.06 mL/kg IM) × 1 and hepatitis B vaccination series	Hepatitis B vaccination series	Hepatitis B vaccination series
Previously vaccinated:			
Responder [i.e., with adequate levels of serum antibody to HBsAg (i.e., anti-HBs > 10 mIU/mL)]	No treatment	No treatment	No treatment
Nonresponder (i.e., serum anti-HBs < 10 mIU/mL)	HBIg (0.06 mL/kg IM) × 1 and revaccinate Or HBIg (0.06 mL/kg IM) × 2 (at the time of exposure and 1 month after exposure)	No treatment	If known high-risk source, treat as if source is HBsAg (+)
Ab response unknown	Test-exposed person for anti-HBsAb: 1. If adequate, no PEP necessary 2. If inadequate, administer HBIg × 1 and vaccine booster	No treatment	*Test-exposed person for anti-HBs*: 1. If adequate, no PEP necessary 2. If inadequate, give vaccine booster and recheck titer in 1–2 months

(HBIg: hepatitis B immunoglobulin; HBsAg: hepatitis B surface antigen; PEP: postexposure prophylaxis)

Postexposure Prophylaxis of Hepatitis C

Immunoglobulin and antiviral agents (e.g., interferon with or without ribavirin) are not recommended for PEP of hepatitis C. Because 15–25% of patients with acute HCV infection spontaneously resolve their infection, treatment of these patients during the acute phase could expose them unnecessarily to the discomfort and side effects of antiviral therapy (interferon ± ribavirin).[17]

In the absence of PEP for HCV, recommendations for postexposure management are intended to achieve early identification of chronic disease and, if present, referral for evaluation of treatment options.[21]

Recommended investigations following occupational exposure to HCV:[36]

- For the source, perform testing for anti-HCV
- Perform baseline and follow-up testing for anti-HCV and alanine aminotransferase (ALT) 4–6 months after exposures
- Perform HCV RNA at 4–6 weeks, if earlier diagnosis of HCV infection desired
- Confirm repeatedly reactive anti-HCV enzyme immunoassays (EIAs) with supplemental tests
- When HCV infection is identified early, the person should be referred for medical management to a specialist.

Summary of Universal Precautions[37]

- *Handwashing*:
  - After touching blood, bodily fluids, secretions, excretions, and contaminated items

  - Immediately after removing gloves
  - Before contact with next patient
- *Gloves*:
  - For contact with blood, bodily fluids, secretions, and contaminated items
  - For contact with mucous membranes and nonintact skin
- *Mask, goggles, and face masks*:
  - Protect mucous membranes of eyes, nose, and mouth when contact with blood and bodily fluids is anticipated.
- *Gowns*:
  - Protect skin from blood or bodily fluid contact
  - Prevent soiling of clothing during procedures that may involve contact with blood or bodily fluids.
- *Linen*:
  - Handle soiled linens so that they do not touch skin/mucous membranes
  - Do not prerinse soiled linens.
- *Patient care equipment*:
  - Handle soiled equipment in a manner that prevents contact with skin or mucous membranes and to prevent contamination of clothing or the environment
  - Clean reusable equipment before reusing it.
- *Environmental cleaning*:
  - Routine care, cleaning, and disinfection of equipment and furnishings in patient care areas.
- *Sharps*:
  - Avoid recapping used needles
  - Avoid removing used needles from disposable syringes
  - Avoid bending, breaking, or manipulating used needles by hand
  - Place used sharps in puncture-resistant containers.
- *Patient resuscitation*:
  - Use mouthpieces, resuscitation bags, or other ventilation devices to avoid mouth-to-mouth resuscitation.
- *Patient placement*:
  - Place patients who contaminate the environment or cannot maintain appropriate hygiene in private rooms.

CONCLUSION

Universal precautions every time and everywhere are the key to prevention of infection with blood-borne pathogens and there is no substitute.

GLOSSARY

- *Blood-borne pathogens* means pathogenic microorganisms that are present in human blood and can cause disease in humans. These pathogens include, but are not limited to, HBV and HIV.[38]
- *Other potentially infectious materials (OPIMs)* mean: (1) The following human body fluids—semen, vaginal secretions, cerebrospinal fluid, synovial fluid, pleural fluid, pericardial fluid, peritoneal fluid, amniotic fluid, saliva in dental procedures, any body fluid that is visibly contaminated with blood, and all body fluids in situations where it is difficult or impossible to differentiate between body fluids; (2) any unfixed tissue or organ (other than intact skin) from a human (living or dead); and (3) HIV-containing cell or tissue cultures, organ cultures, and HIV- or HBV-containing culture medium or other solutions; and blood, organs, or other tissues from experimental animals infected with HIV or HBV.[38]
- *Occupational exposure* means reasonably anticipated skin, eye, mucous membrane, or parenteral contact with blood or OPIMs that may result from the performance of an employee's duty.[38]
- *Source individual* means any individual living or dead, whose blood or other potentially infectious materials may be a source of occupational exposure to the employee.[38]
- *Universal precautions* are an approach to infection control. According to the concept of universal precautions, all human blood and certain human body fluids are treated, as if known to be infectious for HIV, HBV, and other blood-borne pathogens.[38]
- *Routine practices/standard precautions* are a combination of universal precautions and body substance isolation (BSI), which includes guidelines for body secretions such as urine, vomitus, feces, or sputum are not controlled under universal precautions.[8] For further details, see Reference 39

Abbreviations:
AEB: Accidental exposure to blood
ALT: Alanine amino transferase
ACD: Allergic contact dermatitis
CMV: Cytomegalovirus
EIAs: Enzyme immunoassays
EBV: Epstein–Barr virus
EC: Exposure code
FDC: Fixed dose combination
HCW: Healthcare workers
HCP: Healthcare personnel
HEPA: High-efficiency particulate air
HBV: Hepatitis B virus
HCV: Hepatitis C virus
HGV: Hepatitis G virus
HTLV: Human T lymphotropic viruses
IV: Intravenous
ICD: Irritant contact dermatitis
MMWR: Morbidity and mortality weekly reports
NACO: National AIDS control organization
NaSH: National Surveillance System for HCWs
OSHA: Occupational Safety and Health Administration
OPIM: Other potentially infectious material
PPE: Personal protective equipment
PEP: Postexposure prophylaxis
TEWL: Transepidermal water loss

REFERENCES

1. World Health Organization. (2003). Aide-memoire for a strategy to protect health workers from infection with bloodborne viruses. World Health Organization. https://apps.who.int/iris/handle/10665/68354
2. Siegel JD, Rhinehart E, Jackson M, Chiarello L. Guideline for isolation precautions: preventing transmission of infectious agents in healthcare settings. Am J Infect Control. 2007;35(10):S65-S164.
3. Centers for Disease Control and Prevention. (2017). Perspectives in Disease Prevention and Health Promotion Update: Universal Precautions for Prevention of Transmission of Human Immunodeficiency Virus, Hepatitis B Virus, and Other Blood Borne Pathogens in Health-Care Settings. MMWR Recommendations and Reports 2017. [online] Available from: https://www.cdc.gov/mmwr/preview/mmwrhtml/00000039.htm [Last accessed April, 2017].
4. Last JM. (2002). Universal Precautions. Encyclopedia of Public Health. [online] Available from: www.encyclopedia.com/doc/1G2-3404000889.html. [Last accessed April, 2021].
5. Centers for Disease Control and Prevention. (2008). Workbook for designing, implementing, and evaluating a sharps injury prevention program. [online] Available from: www.cdc.gov/sharpssafety/pdf/sharpsworkbook_2008.pdf. [Last accessed April, 2021].
6. Food and Drug Administration. (2015). Blunt-Tip Surgical Suture Needles Reduce Needle stick Injuries and the Risk of Subsequent Blood borne Pathogen Transmission to Surgical Personnel: FDA, NIOSH and OSHA Joint Safety Communication. [online] Available from: https://www.fda.gov/media/83834/download [Last accessed April, 2021].
7. National Institute of Communicable Diseases and NACO. (1999). HIV Testing Manual: Laboratory Diagnosis, Biosafety, and Quality Control. [online] Available from: http://www.naco.gov.in/sites/default/files/National_Guidelines_for_HIV_Testing_21Apr2016.pdf. [Last accessed April, 2021].
8. Canadian Centre for Occupational Health and Safety. (2011). Routine Practices. [online] Available from: http://www.naco.gov.in/sites/default/files/National_Guidelines_for_HIV_Testing_21Apr2016.pdf. [Last accessed April, 2021].
9. Ministry of Health and Family Welfare Directorate General of Health Services [Emergency Medical Relief]. (2020). Novel Coronavirus Disease 2019 (COVID-19): Guidelines on rational use of Personal Protective Equipment. [online] Available from: https://www.mohfw.gov.in/pdf/GuidelinesonrationaluseofPersonalProtectiveEquipment.pdf. [Last accessed April, 2021]
10. Ministry of Health and Family Welfare Directorate General of Health Services [Emergency Medical Relief]. (2020). Novel Coronavirus Disease 2019 (COVID-19): Additional guidelines on rational use of Personal Protective Equipment (setting approach for Health functionaries working in non-COVID areas). [online] Available from: https://www.mohfw.gov.in/pdf/AdditionalguidelinesonrationaluseofPersonalProtectiveEquipmentsettingapproachforHealthfunctionariesworkinginnonCOVIDareas.pdf. [Last accessed April, 2021].
11. Arora G, Arora S, Talathi A, Kandhari R, Joshi V, Langar S, et al. Safer practice of aesthetic dermatology during the COVID-19 pandemic: recommendations by SIG aesthetics (IADVL Academy). Indian Dermatol Online J. 2020;11(4):534-9.
12. National Center for disease control Directorate general of health services, MOHFW, GOI. Nipah virus guidelines. [online] Available from: https://www.ncdc.gov.in/index4.php?lang=1&level=0&linkid=113&lid=228. [Last accessed April,2021]
13. World Health Organization. (2015). Ebola Situation Report. [online] Available from: apps.who.int/iris/bitstream/10665/159060/1/roadmapsitrep_25Mar2015_eng.pdf?ua=1&ua=1. [Last accessed April, 2021].
14. Dara S, Singh SK, Khokhar A. (2015). Ebola virus: Awareness about the disease and personal protective measures among junior doctors of a tertiary hospital in Delhi, India. [online] Available from: www.ijmedph.org/sites/default/files/IntJMedPublicHealth_2015_5_3_217_161524.pdf. [Last accessed April, 2021].
15. Centers for Disease Control and Prevention. (2015). Guidance on Personal Protective Equipment (PPE) To Be Used By Healthcare Workers during Management of Patients with Confirmed Ebola or Persons under Investigation (PUIs) for Ebola who are Clinically Unstable or Have Bleeding, Vomiting or Diarrhea in U.S. Hospitals, Including Procedures for Donning and Doffing PPE. [online] Available from: www.cdc.gov/vhf/ebola/healthcare-us/ppe/guidance.html. [Last accessed April, 2021].
16. National Health Portal India. (2016). Zika virus disease. [online] Available from: www.nhp.gov.in/disease/communicable-disease/zika-virus-disease. [Last accessed April, 2021].
17. World Health Organization. (2016). Zika virus. [online] Available from: www.who.int/mediacentre/factsheets/zika/en/. [Last accessed April, 2021].
18. Mathur P, Singh S. Multidrug resistance in bacteria: A serious patient safety challenge for India. J Lab Physicians. 2013;5(1):5-10.
19. Hayden MK, Bonten MJ, Blom DW, Lyle EA, van de Vijver DAMC, Weinstein RA. Reduction in acquisition of vancomycin-resistant Enterococcus after enforcement of routine environmental cleaning measures. Clin Infect Dis. 2006;42(11):1552-60.
20. Morgan DJ, Rogawski E, Thom KA, Johnson JK, Perencevich EN, Shardell M, et al. Transfer of multidrug-resistant bacteria to healthcare workers' gloves and gowns after patient contact increases with environmental contamination. Crit Care Med. 2012;40(4):1045-51.
21. Centers for Disease Control and Prevention; U.S. Public Health Service. Updated US Public Health Service Guidelines for the Management of Occupational Exposures to HBV, HCV, and HIV and Recommendations for Post exposure Prophylaxis. MMWR Recomm Rep. 2001;50(RR-11):1-52.
22. World Health Organization. (2017). Practical Guidelines for Infection Control in Health Care Facilities. WHO Regional Office for South East Asia/WHO Regional Office for the Western Pacific 2004; SEARO Regional Publication No. 41: pp. 76-101. [online] Available from: www.wpro.who.int/NR/rdonlyres/006EF250-6B11-42B4-BA17-C98D413BE8B8/0/practical guidelines infection_control.pdf. [Last accessed April, 2021].
23. Boyce JM, Pittet D, Centers for Disease Control and Prevention. (2002). Guideline for Hand Hygiene in Health-Care Settings: Recommendations of the Health care Infection Control Practices Advisory Committee and the HICPAC/SHEA/APIC/IDSA Hand Hygiene Task Force. MMWR Recomm Rep. 2002;51(RR-16):1-45, quiz CE1-4..
24. World Health Organization. (2009). WHO Guidelines on Hand Hygiene in Health Care. [online] Available from: https://apps.who.int/iris/bitstream/handle/10665/44102/9789241597906_eng.pdf?sequence=1. [Last accessed April, 2021].

25. Centers for Disease Control and Prevention. (2016). Guidance for the Selection and Use of Personal Protective Equipment (PPE) in Healthcare Settings. [online] Available from: https://www.cdc.gov/hai/pdfs/ppe/ppeslides6-29-04.pdf [Last accessed April, 2021].
26. National AIDS Control Organization, Indian Nursing Council. (2012). Training Manual for Auxiliary Nurse Midwives (ANM). [online] Available from: naco.gov.in/sites/default/files/Website%20file%20ANM%20English.pdf. [Last accessed April, 2021].
27. Reddy S. (2017). Latex Allergy. American Family Physician. [online] Available from: www.aafp.org/afp/980101ap/reddy.html. [Last accessed April, 2021].
28. Canadian Centre for Occupational Health and Safety. (2009). Latex Allergy. [online] Available from: www.ccohs.ca/oshanswers/diseases/latex.html. [Last accessed April, 2021].
29. Canadian Centre for Occupational Health and Safety. (2005). Needlestick and Sharp Injuries. [online] Available from: http://www.ccohs.ca/oshanswers/diseases/needlestick_injuries.html. [Last accessed April, 2021].
30. Ministry of Environment & Forests. (1998). The Biomedical Wastes (Management & Handling) Rules, Ministry Of Environment & Forests 1998/2000. [online] Available from: https://hspcb.gov.in/BMW%20Rules.pdf [Last accessed April, 2021].
31. Ministry of Health & Family Welfare. Manual for Control of Hospital Associated Infections, National AIDS Control Organization. New Delhi: Government of India: Ministry of Health & Family Welfare; 1999. pp. 47-8.
32. World Health Organization. (2014). Post-exposure prophylaxis to prevent HIV infection. Fact sheet. 1 December 2014. [online] Available from: https://www.ghdonline.org/uploads/HIV-WHO-PEP.pdf [Last accessed April, 2021].
33. UP State Aids Control Society. (2016). Post Exposure Prophylaxis (PEP)—NACO guidelines. [online] Available from: http://upsacs.in/pdf/GUIDELINES/PEP.pdf. [Last accessed April, 2021].
34. NACO, Ministry of Health and Family Welfare. (2007). Antiretroviral Therapy Guidelines for HIV-infected Adults and Adolescents including Post-exposure Prophylaxis, NACO, Ministry of Health and Family Welfare, Government of India. [online] Available from: https://lms.naco.gov.in/frontend/content/1.%20Antiretroviral%20Therapy%20Guidelines%20for%20HIV-Infected%20Adults%20and%20Adolescents%20Including%20Post-exposure.pdf. [Accessed April, 2021].
35. World Health Organization. (2014). Post-exposure prophylaxis for HIV. Supplementary section to the 2013 WHO consolidated guidelines on the use of antiretroviral drugs for treating and preventing HIV infection, Chapter 5: Clinical guidelines across the continuum of care: HIV diagnosis and ARV drugs for HIV prevention. pp. 15-21. [online] Available from: www.who.int/hiv/pub/guidelines/arv2013/December2014-ARVsupplement-chap5.pdf?ua=1. [Last accessed April, 2021].
36. Beal J, Deitrick L, Janelle J, Orrick JJ. (2015). Pre-Exposure Prophylaxis (PrEP), Non-Occupational Post-Exposure Prophylaxis (nPEP) and Occupational PEP (oPEP). Florida/Carribean AIDS education and training center (FCAETC). [online] Available from: https://npin.cdc.gov/publication/pre-exposure-prophylaxis-prep-non-occupational-post-exposure-prophylaxis-npep-and. [Last accessed April, 2021].
37. National AIDS Control Organization. (2007). Operational guidelines for programme managers and service providers for strengthening STI/RTI services. National AIDS Control Organization. Ministry of Health and Family Welfare Government of India. [online] Available from: http://www.naco.gov.in/sites/default/files/Operational%20Guidelines%20STI%20RTI.pdf. [Accessed April, 2021].
38. Occupational Safety and Health Administration. (2016). Blood borne pathogens, Appendix A. [Standard number: 1910.1030]. Part Title: Occupational Safety and Health Standards. [online] Available from: www.osha.gov/pls/oshaweb/owadisp.show_document?p_table=STANDARDS&p_id=10051#1910.1030(b). [Last accessed April, 2021].
39. World Health Organization. (2007). Aide Memoire. Standard precautions in health care. [online] Available from: www.who.int/csr/resources/publications/EPR_AM2_E7.pdf. [Last accessed April, 2021].

CHAPTER 11

Topical Anesthesia

Gautam K Singh

KEY MESSAGES

- Topical anesthesia is a method of pain relief in skin, conjunctiva, and mucous membranes.
- It is commonly used for dermatosurgical and aesthetic procedures.
- Users should be aware of pharmacology and potential adverse events.

INTRODUCTION

Topical anesthesia is defined as superficial loss of pain sensation in skin, conjunctiva, and mucous membranes, produced by direct application of local anesthetic creams, ointments, sprays, or gels.[1] Injection of local anesthesia can be painful and distressing on one hand, and on the other hand, it can cause a transient swelling due to tissue edema, which can distort the surface anatomy at the surgical site. Use of topical anesthesia can alleviate these unwanted side effects of local anesthesia and is one of the most frequently used modes of anesthesia for several dermatosurgical and aesthetic procedures. It was only by serendipity, that, in 1860, Albert Niemann discovered the anesthetic properties of cocaine. Cocaine was identified as the first local anesthetic when it was noted to cause transient numbness on the tongue.[2] Karl Koller, in 1884, used cocaine for ophthalmic procedures after he demonstrated its anesthetic properties on applying it over conjunctiva.[3] Since then, the discovery of various amide and ester local anesthetics have opened newer paradigms in this field of topical anesthesia.

MECHANISM OF ACTION

Topical anesthetics work by reversibly blocking free nerve endings in the dermis, thereby blocking nerve conduction temporarily in the area where it is applied. This nerve conduction is blocked, probably by competing reversibly with calcium-binding sites that control sodium permeability, thereby decreasing nerve cell membrane permeability of sodium ions. This change in nerve cell permeability decreases depolarization and increases excitability threshold until the ability to generate an action potential is lost.[1]

PHARMACOLOGY

All topical anesthetics are weak bases. They are made of three components:[4-7]

1. *Aromatic ring*: Primarily responsible for the lipid solubility and diffusion across the nerve cell membrane thus determining the intrinsic property of topical anesthetics
2. *Tertiary amine*: Responsible for protein-binding properties
3. Intermediate length ester or amide linkage.

The depth of anesthesia, and onset and duration of action depend on the site of application (faster onset at sites with thin stratum corneum and mucosa), vascularity of tissues in the area applied, and duration of contact and the surface area. Other important factors are lipid solubility, protein binding, pH level, pKa level, and vasodilatory effects of the specific topical anesthetic.

Amide-type topical anesthetics are metabolized via microsomal enzymes in the liver, while ester anesthetics are primarily metabolized by plasma cholinesterase and other nonspecific esterases. Ester anesthetics are known to cause allergic contact dermatitis, whereas amide topical anesthetics have lower incidence of contact dermatitis.[8-10] An ester hydrolysis metabolite, para-aminobenzoic acid (PABA), is known to be associated with allergic dermatitis.[11]

ROUTES OF SKIN PENETRATION

Stratum corneum is the main barrier for topical anesthetic drug delivery. There are three pathways to cross this barrier **(Fig. 1)**:

1. Transappendageal route or shunt pathway (through the openings of the sweat glands and hair follicles)
2. Para or transcellular route (through the cornified cells)
3. Intercellular route (through the intercellular spaces of the stratum corneum).

Through mucosal surfaces such as the oral mucosa, conjunctiva, and genitals, which lack stratum corneum, topical anesthetics are able to penetrate more easily than through a keratinized surface. The skin penetration and efficiency of the topical anesthetic can be increased by several measures as mentioned in **Table 1**.

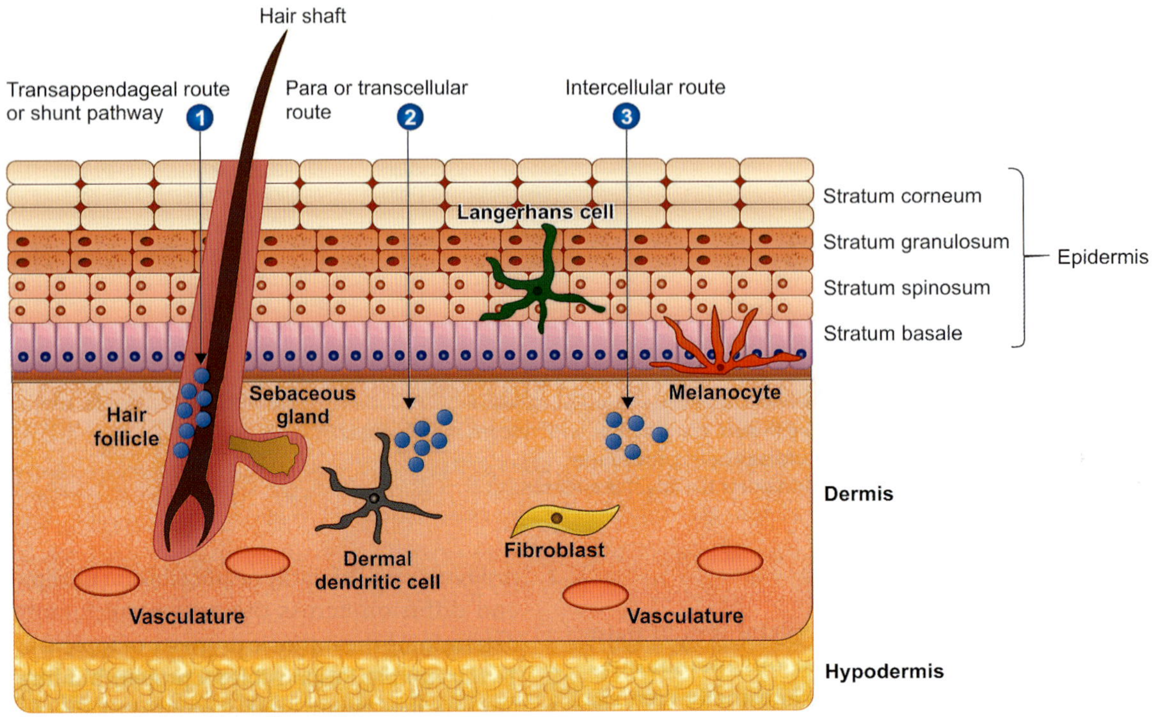

Fig. 1: Schematic diagram depicting the different routes of penetration of topical anesthesia in the skin.

TABLE 1: Factors determining the dermal drug delivery.

S. No.	*Mechanism*	*Comment*
1.	Drug form	Free bases are more lipophilic than salts hence have better penetration
2.	Melting point	The lower the melting point, the better the penetration is. Eutectic mixtures have a lower melting point, thus better penetration than either component by itself
3.	Drug concentration	Higher the concentration of drug in the vehicle, higher the rate of penetration
4.	Chemicals-enhancing skin permeation	Solvents (water, alcohols, glycerol, low molecular weight ethers, sucrose esters, silicone fluids), surfactants (bile salts), and chemicals (urea and anticholinergic drugs) promote skin permeability by increasing the permeability of the stratum corneum temporarily and reversibly
5.	Physical means of enhancing permeation	Exfoliation of the skin, degreasing by alcohol, by covering the application area with a dressing or patch of nonporous material such as Micropore and Tegaderm
6.	Energy-dependent active measures	• Iontophoresis (low-voltage current to drive charged drugs through skin): Lignocaine HCl 10%/ adrenaline 0.1% topical iontophoretic patch (LidoSite) is the first Food and Drug Administration (FDA) approved prefilled active anesthetic patch • Electroporation (uses short electrical impulses of high voltage to create transient pores in the skin) • Sonophoresis or phonophoresis (low frequency, ultrasonic energy to disrupt stratum corneum) • Magnetophoresis/magnetokinesis (application of magnetic field to enhance permeation) • Thermal energy (heat increases skin permeability) • Erbium:YAG laser pretreatment • Skin pretreatment with a hand-applied, plastic microneedle array, or radiofrequency microneedling
7.	Delivery from lipid vesicles	• Liposomes (microscopic vesicles, which are composed of one or more lipid bilayers arranged in concentric fashion enclosing an equal number of aqueous compartments capable of entrapping lipid soluble or water-soluble drugs): 5% liposome-encapsulated tetracaine produced better superficial local anesthesia than 5% eutectic mixture of local anesthetics (EMLA) • Niosomes (microvesicles similar to liposomes, but are prepared from nonionic surfactants and are more stable and may provide faster penetration to the stratum corneum than liposomes. They do not go deeper either) • Transfersomes (prepared using bile salt: *sodium cholate* and can penetrate through pores very easily)

VARIOUS TOPICAL ANESTHETICS

- *Eutectic mixture of local anesthetics (EMLA):* An "eutectic" mixture is a group of chemicals, which melt at lower temperatures than any of their individual components. This property permits higher concentrations of anesthetics to be used than any individual component. It is an emulsion of water in oil (5%) with a melting point of around

18°C and consists of 25 mg/mL of prilocaine, 25 mg/mL of lignocaine, an emulsifier, a thickener, and distilled water adjusted to a pH level of 9.4. EMLA is applied in a thick layer (1–2 g/10 cm^2, up to a maximal dose of 20 g/200 cm^2) to intact unbroken skin. After application to skin, this cream layer is occluded using clear plastic wrap to facilitate local penetration through stratum corneum. Depth of anesthesia is directly proportional to contact time with EMLA. Anesthesia effect has been shown to reach a maximal depth of 5 mm after 2 hours of application and 3 mm after 1 hour of contact time. Dermal analgesia can be expected after 3 hours of contact time and generally lasts about 1–2 hours after removal of the drug. Due to the variation of drug penetration and unpredictable outcomes, EMLA should be avoided over palms and soles. EMLA is pregnancy category B drug but caution should be exercised in lactating mothers, as it is secreted in breast milk (AstraZeneca insert). The pediatric dosing of EMLA is shown in **Table 2**.

- *Lignocaine, tetracaine, and epinephrine*: This contains 4% lignocaine with 0.5% tetracaine and 0.1% epinephrine. This can safely be used on bleeding surfaces along with surface pressure to achieve hemostasis and local analgesia. This is generally not effective on intact skin; however, 1–3 mL application using a cotton-tipped applicator directly on the wound can achieve hemostasis. It is a safe and cost-effective alternative than most of the other topical anesthetics; however, due to presence of epinephrine, caution needs to be exercised while using in parts containing end arteries. It should be used with caution when it is used in wounds >6 cm or contaminated or complex wounds. It is safe to use in children >2 years of age.
- *Tetracaine, epinephrine, and cocaine*: This consists of 11.8% cocaine, 0.5% tetracaine, and 0.05% epinephrine. A dose of 1 mL/cm^2 of laceration can be applied using a cotton-tipped applicator with firm pressure that is maintained for 30–40 minutes. It was the first topical anesthetic mixture to be used for lacerations and wounds; however, at present, it is not available due to concerns of toxicity with cocaine.[12]
- *Betacaine LA*: It contains lignocaine, phenylephrine, and prilocaine. This is a proprietary anesthetic and exact concentration of its ingredients is a trade secret. The pocket insert of the merchandise reports concentrations of prilocaine and lignocaine to be four times that of EMLA. It should not be applied to a wound >300 cm^2 in adults and is not advocated for use in children.[13]
- *Bupivanor*: It contains 1:26,000 norepinephrine and 0.48% bupivacaine. It is an effective topical anesthesia during laceration repair, especially on the face and scalp.[14]
- *4% tetracaine*: It is an ester anesthetic with a long duration of action in a lecithin gel base, with a recommended application time of 30 minutes under occlusive dressing and maximum dose limit of 50 mg.[13]
- *ELA-max*: It contains 4% in standard preparation or 5% (ELA-max 5) lignocaine cream in a liposomal matrix and is Food and Drug Administration (FDA) approved for the temporary relief of pain resulting from minor cuts and abrasions. ELA-max is applied to intact skin for 10–45 minutes with occlusion and provides an extended duration of anesthesia as compared to nonliposomal preparations. Maximum area of application is 500 cm^2.[13]
- *Lidoderm patch*: It is 5% lignocaine on an adhesive material containing. Each patch contains 700 mg of lignocaine (50 mg/g adhesive) in an aqueous base. It has been approved by the FDA for the treatment postherpetic neuralgia.
- *Benzocaine*: It is an ester local anesthetic mostly used as a topical pain reliever for oral mucosal ulcers and otalgia. It is available as an orabase, cream, lozenges, throat spray, aerosol, gel and toothache drops. It is generally well tolerated and nontoxic when applied topically and is safe in the pediatric population >2 years of age. Over dosage oral preparations can result in pulmonary aspiration due to relaxing the gag reflex.
- *Proxymetacaine or proparacaine*: 0.5% proparacaine solution is suitable for corneal anesthesia in ophthalmic use. With a single drop, the onset of anesthesia usually begins within 1 minute, the maximum anesthetic effect is achieved at 5 minutes, and duration of corneal anesthesia is about half an hour.
- *Miscellaneous agents with topical anesthetic potential*: Tetradotoxin,[15,16] 10% capsaicin[17] (acts on transient receptor potential vanilloid 1, i.e., the transient receptor potential channel of the vanilloid receptor family subtype 1), 0.8% nalbuphine,[18] etc.

TABLE 2: Pediatric dosing of eutectic mixtures of local anesthetics (EMLA).

S. No.	*Age and body weight (kg)*	*Maximum dose of EMLA cream (g)*	*Maximum area of application (cm^2)*	*Maximum application time (hours)*
1.	0–3 months (<5)	1	10	1
2.	3–12 months (5–10)	2	20	4
3.	1–6 years (10–20)	10	100	4
4.	7–12 years (>20)	20	200	4

CONTRAINDICATIONS

Topical anesthetics with an ester group are contraindicated in patients with known allergy to PABA, hair dyes, and sulfonamides.

TABLE 3: Systemic side effects of topical anesthetics.

S. No.	*System*	*Side effect*
1.	Central nervous system (CNS)	• High concentration of anesthetic in plasma can produce CNS depression (drowsiness, obtundation, coma, or respiratory arrest) or CNS excitation (confusion, agitation, muscle twitching, and seizures). Solutions containing epinephrine may add to the CNS stimulatory effect • Loss of gag reflex can occur with oral absorption from mucosal anesthetics
2.	Cardiovascular system	Tachycardia, increase in blood pressure, ventricular arrhythmias (torsades de pointes, ventricular tachycardia, ventricular fibrillation, conduction block, or asystole). Local anesthetics that contain epinephrine may cause angina, tachycardia, and hypertension
3.	Methemoglobinemia (with benzocaine and prilocaine): (methemoglobin >1%)	• Dyspnea, headache, cyanosis, exercise intolerance, fatigue, dizziness, and loss of consciousness. Elevated methemoglobin in arterial blood gives it a characteristic chocolate-brown color. Severe methemoglobinemia (methemoglobin >50%) manifests as seizures, dysrhythmias, coma, and death (>70%) • Treatment includes supplemental oxygen, hyperbaric oxygen therapy (HBOT), exchange transfusion, and intravenous administration 1% methylene blue
4.	Nonspecific	Circumoral numbness, metallic taste in mouth, diplopia, tinnitus, and dizziness

Adverse Effects

- *Local side effects*: Contact dermatitis due to the anesthetic or any of the components can cause stinging or burning sensation at the site of application. It can also lead to skin discoloration, swelling, neuritis, tissue necrosis, and sloughing in extremely rare cases.
- Systemic toxicity can manifest due to use on broken skin, repeated use, excess dosage particularly in infants or elderly patients or in patients with liver disease, etc. Systemic effects of absorbed topical anesthetics are shown in **Table 3**.[1,19-21] Treatment of systemic toxicity is decided as per local anesthetic systemic toxicity treatment guidelines[22] of the American Society of Regional Anesthesia and Pain Medicine (ASRA) and encompasses airway management, cardiovascular support, seizure suppression, and use of 20% intralipid. Thus, the risk of adverse events with topical anesthetics with improper application is real and physicians must exercise caution and good judgment while using them.

REFERENCES

1. Kumar M, Chawla R, Goyal M. Topical anesthesia. J Anaesthesiol Clin Pharmacol. 2015;31(4):450-6.
2. Biscoping J, Bachmann-Mennenga MB. Local anesthetics from ester to isomer. Anasthesiol Intensivmed Notfallmed Schmerzther. 2000;35(5):285-92.
3. Jackson T, McLure HA. Pharmacology of local anesthetics. Ophthalmol Clin North Am. 2006;19(2):155-61.
4. Covino BG. Local anesthesia 1. N Engl J Med. 1972;286(18):975-83.
5. Covino BG. Local anesthesia 2. N Engl J Med. 1972;286(19): 1035-42.
6. Covino BG. Local anesthetic agents for peripheral nerve blocks. Anaesthesist. 1980;29(7):33-7.
7. Covino BG. Physiology and pharmacology of local anesthetic agents. Anesth Prog. 1981;28(4):98-104.
8. Kluger N, Raison-Peyron N, Michot C, Guillot B, Bessis D. Acute bullous irritant contact dermatitis caused by EMLA® cream. Contact Dermatitis. 2011;65(3):181-3.
9. Fuzier R, Lapeyre-Mestre M, Mertes PM, Nicolas JF, Benoit Y, Didier A, et al. Immediate- and delayed-type allergic reactions to amide local anesthetics: clinical features and skin testing. Pharmacoepidemiol Drug Saf. 2009;18(7):595-601.
10. Suhonen R, Kanerva L. Contact allergy and cross-reactions caused by prilocaine. Am J Contact Dermat. 1997;8(4):231-5.
11. Mackie BS, Mackie LE. The PABA story. Australas J Dermatol. 1999;40(1):51-3.
12. Kundu S, Achar S. Principles of office anesthesia: Part II. Topical anesthesia. Am Fam Physician. 2002;66(1):99-102.
13. Friedman PM, Mafong EA, Friedman ES, Geronemus RG. Topical anesthetics update: EMLA and beyond. Dermatol Surg. 2001;27(12):1019-26.
14. Smith GA, Strausbaugh SD, Harbeck-Weber C, Shields BJ, Powers JD, Hackenberg D. Comparison of topical anesthetics without cocaine to tetracaine-adrenaline-cocaine and lignocaine infiltration during repair of lacerations: bupivacaine-norepinephrine is an effective new topical anesthetic agent. Pediatrics. 1996;97(3):301-7.
15. Wang L, Shankarappa SA, Tong R, Ciolino JB, Tsui JH, Chiang HH, et al. Topical drug formulations for prolonged corneal anesthesia. Cornea. 2013;32(7):1040-5.
16. Schwartz DM, Fields HL, Duncan KG, Duncan JL, Jones MR. Experimental study of tetrodotoxin, a long-acting topical anesthetic. Am J Ophthalmol. 1998;125(4):481-7.
17. Haanpää M, Treede RD. Capsaicin for neuropathic pain: Linking traditional medicine and molecular biology. Eur Neurol. 2012;68(5):264-75.
18. Lee CH, Lin SL, Chi TT, Chang SH, Wang HC. Effect of topical administration of 0.8% nalbuphine on the cornea in dogs after phacoemulsification. J Vet Med Sci. 2013;75(8):1041-7.
19. Vallurupalli S, Manchanda S. Risk of acquired methemoglobinemia with different topical anesthetics during endoscopic procedures. Local Reg Anesth. 2011;4:25-8.
20. Cortazzo JA, Lichtman AD. Methemoglobinemia: a review and recommendations for management. J Cardiothorac Vasc Anesth. 2014;28(4):1055-9.
21. Adams V, Marley J, McCarroll C. Prilocaine induced methaemoglobinaemia in a medically compromised patient. Was this an inevitable consequence of the dose administered? Br Dent J. 2007;203(10):585-7.
22. Neal JM, Bernards CM, Butterworth JF 4th, Di Gregorio G, Drasner K, Hejtmanek MR, et al. ASRA practice advisory on local anesthetic systemic toxicity. Reg Anesth Pain Med. 2010;35(2):152-61.

CHAPTER 12

Infiltration Anesthesia

Sudarshan R, KC Nischal

KEY MESSAGES

- Infiltration anesthesia aims at anesthetizing nerve ending in finite area by directly injecting into the tissue of interest.
- Technically easy to practice and requires minimal postoperative care.
- Useful in dermatosurgical and cosmetic procedures involving larger surface area for minimal local anesthetic concentration.

INTRODUCTION

In infiltration anesthesia, local anesthetics are injected directly into the tissue of interest without considering the course of the nerve supplying it. Lidocaine with or without adrenaline is the most commonly used local anesthetic for this indication. Other commonly used agent is bupivacaine. Onset and duration of action are delayed if injected into subcutaneous rather than into dermis. Bupivacaine acts for longer duration than lidocaine.[1] Adding adrenaline decreases blood loss, reduces the toxicity and increases the duration of action of local anesthetic. Disadvantages of infiltration anesthesia include need for larger volume of local anesthetic agent (LAA) for anesthetizing small areas and risk of distortion of morphologic features of the lesion. When larger surface areas have to be anesthetized, greater volumes with lower concentration (0.3–0.5% lidocaine) can be effectively used.[2]

Ring Block

Ring block is a modification of infiltration anesthesia where LAA is infiltrated all around the area of interest but not into it. This prevents distortion of tissues when histopathology of the tissue is contemplated and also prevents false-negative cultures from the interest area when infections are suspected. Preservatives in LAA preparations have antibacterial effects and thus this disadvantage arises.[3]

Field Block

Here, the LAA is injected subcutaneously to anesthetize area distal to the site of injection. By this technique, larger areas can be anesthetized with lesser quantity of LAA.[4]

Regional Block

Regional blocks can be achieved either by intravenous infusion of LAA (Bier block) or infiltration of LAA around a nerve or nerve plexus (peripheral nerve block). Peripheral nerve blocks are used for hands/foot, fingers/toes, and face.[5] Peripheral nerve blocks are classified as minor and major. When a single nerve is anesthetized, it is referred to as minor block. When two or more nerves, nerve plexus or large nerve fiber are blocked more proximally, it becomes a major nerve block. Onset of action is rapid and duration of action can be altered choosing an appropriate LAA or combining LAA with epinephrine.[2] Use of inadequate dose of LAA leads to blockage of peripherally placed and some small, sensitive central nerve fibers. Vasa nervorum is placed in the center; therefore central fibers regain function (sensation) earlier than peripheral nerve fibers.[4] There is a risk of laceration of nerve, transient motor paralysis, intravascular injection, and compartment syndrome during peripheral nerve blocks.

Cryoanesthesia

As cooling numbs the skin it can be used for achieving local analgesia and anesthesia. This technique has been aptly termed as cryoanesthesia. Cryoanesthesia can be employed for both diagnostic as well as therapeutic dermatosurgical procedures. When used for performing skin biopsies, Luck et al. have shown that it does not interfere with the histological interpretation.[6] Various modalities adopted include applying ice cubes, vapocoolant sprays, and cryosprays. Depending upon the pain sensitivity and tolerance, ice cubes alone can be used for numbing the skin before injecting LAA or used in addition to topical anesthesia. Reduction of temperature to 10°C is considered ideal for anesthetic effect. Application of ice for 10 seconds reduces skin temperature to 11.4°C from 18°C for 5 seconds. Ice wrapped in aluminum foil is better than latex wrapping if the duration of contact is more than 20 seconds and for less than 20 seconds, both are equivocal.[7] Vapocoolant sprays contain either ethyl chloride or dichlorotetrafluoroethane. Ethyl chloride has to be sprayed from a distance of 3–9 inches taking care so that, there is whitening and not frosting of skin (spray duration 3–7 seconds).[8] However, ethyl chloride sprayed twice for 5 seconds each time at a distance of 5 cm perpendicularly from skin efficiently reduced pain of venepuncture.[9] Ethyl chloride is inflammable and hence avoided during procedures such as cautery or lasers. Liquid nitrogen is used as cryosprays and care should be taken not to cause frosting. Sprays act fast and can be sprayed before injecting LAA or intralesional steroids into keloids or molluscum curettage in children. Forced cold air delivered at a distance of 1 cm for 30 seconds was found to augment the anesthetic effect of topical anesthetic for injecting botulinum toxin for palmar hyperhidrosis.[10] The mean beginning time of anesthesia with forced cold air for non-facial skin was found to be 54.61 seconds.[11] Analgesia was much better with ethylchloride spray than eutectic mixture of local anesthetics (EMLA).[12]

LOCAL ANESTHETICS DURING PREGNANCY

The use of local anesthetics during pregnancy is generally acceptable, but after careful consideration. Lidocaine, ropivacaine, and prilocaine are pregnancy risk category B LAA and bupivacaine, mepivacaine, articaine, and procaine are category C LAA.[7] Epinephrine and dexmedetomidine are category C.[3] Progesterone increases the risk of cardiotoxicity of bupivacaine and ropivacaine (ropivacaine is 3–5 times less potent cardiodepressive than bupivacaine) and hence these are to be used cautiously during pregnancy.[13] Pregnancy has a greater impact on spread and depth of epidural and spinal anesthesia rather than on infiltration or topical anesthesia (latter more commonly practiced by dermatologists and dermatosurgeons). Topical lidocaine is considered safe in comparison to other topical anesthetics during pregnancy; hence other LAAs have not been recommended during pregnancy or lactation.[14]

For the use of topical anesthesia in pregnant and nursing mothers, there is level of evidence III and strength of recommendation C.[14] Small quantities of lidocaine with epinephrine can be used in pregnant and nursing mothers (level of evidence II, strength of recommendation B).[14] However, following aspects need to be considered when administration of LAA is planned for a pregnant mother:

- Avoiding during organogenesis (15–56 days of gestation) when possible
- Reduce the dose of LAA[2]
- Be alert about vasovagal reactions, which may occur at a higher rate during pregnancy
- Position the patient on her left side to avoid vena caval and aortic compression.

LOCAL ANESTHETICS IN CHILDREN

Metabolism of LAA is reduced due to immature Cytochrome P 450 in neonates. CYP1A2 is completely functional only after 3 years of age. Ropivacaine clearance is maximal only by 8 years of age. Volume of distribution of LAA is larger for infants and hence single doses cause lesser peak serum concentration but not repeated doses. Basal heart rate is higher in children <2 years and hence LAA with cardiotoxicity should be used in lesser doses. There is greater and faster absorption of LAA from neonatal skin as well as children's mucosa. Hence appropriate dosing of LAA and close monitoring for any signs of toxicity are prudent. Topical anesthesia commonly used in children are EMLA, ELA-Max (4% liposomal lidocaine) and vapor coolants. Dose of medication, time of application, and maximal area applicable vary in children **(Table 1)**.[15-17]

TABLE 1: Dosage of topical anesthetic agents in children.

Topical anesthetic agent		*Maximum total dose and time*	*Maximum application area (cm^2) (body weight mentioned within brackets)*
EMLA	1–3 months or <5 kg	1 g (1 hour)	10
	4–12 months and >5 kg	2 g	20
	1–6 years and >10 kg	10 g	100
	7–12 years and >20 kg	20 g	200
ELA-max or max 5		–	100 (<10 kg); 600 (>10 kg)
Topicaine		–	100 (>10 kg)
Cocaine		1 mg/kg/dose (≥6 years) Not recommended in ≤6 years due to risk of toxicity	–
Liposomal lidocaine (LMX 4 or 5)		–	<100 (<20 kg)

(EMLA: eutectic mixture of local anesthetics)

Commonly used infiltrative LAA used in children are lidocaine, bupivacaine, ropivacaine, mepivacaine, prilocaine, and articaine.[18] In view of longer duration of action and low incidence of side effects (viz., bradycardia, hepatic dysfunction), ropivacaine is preferred over other LAA. Due to reduced concentration of α1-acid glycoprotein, the free LAA is more in circulation and hence there is greater risk of toxicity. Maximum dose of the infiltrative LAA is summarized in **Table 2**.

LOCAL ANESTHETICS IN GERIATRICS

Reduced plasma clearance due to poor circulation and organ dysfunction as well as neuronal degenerative changes necessitate reduction in the dose of LAA (10–20% for nerve blocks and repeated dosing, grade of evidence D).[7]

LOCAL ANESTHETICS IN COMORBIDITIES

Hepatic dysfunction: No dose changes for nerve blocks (grade of evidence C). However, if there is renal impairment, then dose may have to be reduced.

TABLE 2: Dosage and potency of infiltrative local anesthetic agents in children.

Local anesthetic agent	*Maximum dose without epinephrine*	*Maximum dose with epinephrine*	*Potency of LAA*
Lidocaine	1.5–3 mg/kg	4.5–7 mg/kg	1
Bupivacaine	0.5–2 mg/kg	2 mg/kg	4
Ropivacaine	3 mg/kg (maximum 225 mg from 12 years of age)	–	3.3
Mepivacaine	4–6 mg/kg (maximum 270 mg)	–	
Prilocaine	6 mg/kg	10 mg/kg	
Articaine	5 mg/kg (>4 years of age)	7 mg/kg (from 4 years of age)	
Procaine	Maximum 15 mg/kg	–	

(LAA: local anesthetic agent)

Renal dysfunction: A total of 10–20% reduction in dose recommended for nerve blocks. Clearance of bupivacaine and ropivacaine more affected than of lidocaine.[7]

Cardiac dysfunction: Absorption as well as clearance of LAA is affected in cardiac failure and hence dose adjustments not required (grade of evidence D). However, in case of renal or hepatic dysfunction, dosage should be reduced by 10–20% (grade of evidence C). Delayed clearance of LAA can increase risk of central nervous system (CNS) side effects.

MEASURES TO ALLEVIATE THE PAIN OF LAA INJECTION

Pain of local anesthetic injections can be alleviated by the following measures:[19,20] The reader is also referred to the chapter on analgesics for more details.

- Combining local anesthetic with 8.4% sodium bicarbonate (10:1) to render the pH neutral. Solutions of local anesthetics are acidic (pH 5.0–7.0) and hence cause pain and stinging sensation on infiltration. Solutions of lidocaine with adrenaline is more painful than plain lidocaine as the former is more acidic (pH 3.3–5.5) than latter.[21,22] Reconstituted buffered lidocaine with or without adrenaline can be kept at room temperature for 1 week.[23,24] Buffering the LAA is suggested only for lidocaine. Precipitation happens on buffering bupivacaine and hence it is not recommended.[14]
- Injection of freshly prepared LAA with epinephrine is less painful than a premixed combination. This is because latter is more acidic to improve stability of epinephrine. Solution can be prepared by mixing 0.3 mL of 1:1000 epinephrine with 30 mL of lidocaine.[25]
- 1:10 diluted 1% lidocaine with epinephrine (3 mL) in bacteriostatic normal saline (30 mL) (9 mg sodium chloride + 9 mg benzyl alcohol) was found to be less painful than buffered lidocaine with epinephrine.[26]
- Slow administration of only the required amount of the local anesthetic to prevent tissue distention, which may give rise to pain.
- Precool the concerned area with ice pack for 10 seconds. This gives anesthesia for 2 seconds sufficient for needle prick. Cold air cooling also reduces pain of injection.
- *Warming the anesthetic to 40°C:*[27] Systematic review and meta-analysis by Hogan et al. have revealed that the pain of injection of LAA can be reduced by warming the injection solution to body temperature.[28]
- Using vibration during injections.
- Infiltrating LAA into the lacerated wound edge is less painful than injecting through the intact skin[29,30]
- Addition of 0.5 M mannitol to lidocaine was found to reduce the pain of LAA injection.[31]

Slow rate of infiltration, precooling, using warm solution, and vibrating the skin have level of evidence II and strength of recommendation B.[14] Few other practical tips for making the injections relatively painless are:

- As soon as the needle is introduced into the skin, push some local anesthetic, wait for 1–2 minutes so that the area is anesthetized and then introduce the needle further ahead.
- When lesion on the palmar or plantar area is to be anesthetized, it is preferable to introduce the needle through the dorsal thin skin along with the above said technique for infiltration.
- Apply topical anesthesia cream if deep infiltration is desired for about 30–60 minutes under occlusion. Application of topical anesthesia before infiltrating LAA reduces not only the pain but also the dose of infiltrative LAA.[14]
- Repetitive pinching of skin while injecting local anesthetic.[32]
- Ethyl chloride spray can be used to reduce pain of LAA injection (level of evidence III, strength of recommendation C).[14]
- Although it has long been held that finer needles cause less pain, Palmon et al. did not find significant difference in pain when 25-guage and 30-gauge needle were used.[33] Playing music during infiltration of anesthesia was found to reduce and pain and allay the anxiety.[34]

MEASURES TO ACHIEVE RAPID ANESTHESIA AND ANALGESIA

Stratum corneum is a tough barrier which prevents transcutaneous permeation of various molecules. Occlusion of topical anesthetics and local heat application increases the penetration of LAA. Disruption of this barrier definitely enhances the penetration of topically applied agents.

Mechanical methods of disruption include exfoliating the skin such as microdermabrasion, degreasing the skin with alcohol or acetone, abrading the skin with lasers [fractional ablative viz., CO_2, erbium-doped yttrium-aluminum-garnet (Er:YAG)][35,36] or creating microchannels through dermaroller or fractional microneedling. Jetpeel™ consists of a high velocity spray which contains oxygen and normal saline. This causes gentle exfoliation of skin without dryness.[37] Jetpeel™-3 has been used efficaciously in delivering the local anesthetic but also reduced the dose of botulinum toxin to treat palmar hyperhidrosis.[38] Other methods include iontophoresis, electroporation, sonophoresis, and magnetophoresis. The charged molecules are pushed through the skin by low voltage current in iontophoresis and are dependent on the current intensity and duration of treatment. Transient pores are created by short pulses of high voltage current in electroporation. In electroporation, there is dielectric breakdown of stratum corneum due to the pulsed electric fields.[39] Depth of anesthesia was more with iontophoresis than electroporation or electroporation.[40] Ultrasound waves cause cavitation and steaming which facilitates movement of molecules through skin. Various frequencies are used 20–100 kHz or 0.7–16 MHz for this purpose.[41]

Investigational tools include poly L-lactide microneedle array and biodegradable microneedles which deliver lidocaine.[42,43]

Delivery of drugs through liposomes, niosomes, micelles, transferosomes, and lipid polymer hybrid nanoparticles has been investigated.[44] Lidocaine-loaded lipid polymer hybrid nanoparticles were more efficient in lidocaine delivery than liposomes.[45] Hair follicles are a major route of transcutaneous drug delivery; hence follicular penetration was found to be better with sebum like lipid material of liposomes and with liposomes less or equal to 640 nm diameter.[46] Liposomal tetracaine 5% anesthetized better than EMLA. Niosomes are similar to liposomes but produced from nonionic surfactants. They are smaller, more stable and penetrate faster than liposomes. Transferosomes are produced from bile salts and they can squeeze through pores of size five times lesser than them.[41] EMLA delivered in nanotechnology has shown >30% reduction in pain within 10 minutes of its application.[47]

Hyaluronidase has been used along with LAA as it facilitates the dispersion of the latter leading to faster and better analgesia.[48,49] It also reduced the quantity of LAA by 2.4 folds.[50] Nevarre et al. have noted increased pain on injection and reduced duration of action when LAA was combined with hyaluronidase. It may also elicit allergic reactions due to the preservative, thimerosal in it.[51] Due to cross-reactivity, individuals who are sensitive to bee venom should not be administered hyaluronidase. However, there was no evidence of any adverse effect of hyaluronidase on wound healing.[49]

Theoretically, alkalinization of local anesthetics results in reduced ionized to unionized proportion of LAA, thereby reducing the time for onset of action. However, clinical studies have showed inconsistent results and hence routine alkalinization of local anesthetics is not recommended for hastening the effect. Bupivacaine and etidocaine cannot be alkalinized as they tend to precipitate on mixing with sodium bicarbonate.[52] Nerve blocks are done by single, double or multiple injections. Multiple injection technique was found to produce better analgesia than any other method.[53]

Mixtures of LAAs such as lidocaine with bupivacaine, bupivacaine with mepivacaine and prilocaine with ropivacaine have been used with intent to achieve faster and long-lasting anesthesia. However, there is no sufficient evidence to prove their superiority over the use of single LAA.[14]

MEASURES TO PROLONG THE DURATION OF ACTION OF LAA

Duration of action of local anesthetics is prolonged by addition of adrenaline (1:2,00,000 dilution) or low molecular weight dextran 40 (1:1 dilution) to the local anesthetic. Both the agents delay the clearance of the drug from the site of administration (former by causing vasoconstriction and latter by delaying its systemic absorption) and hence prolong its action.[54] Fentanyl has been used with LAA to enhance the quality as well as the duration of action of LAA. This works on the principle that afferent nerve fibers contain opioid receptors and hence, opioid analgesics placed around the nerve augment the local anesthetic effects.[55]

Mannitol: Hyperosmolar solutions transiently increase the permeability of perineurium thereby increasing the efficacy of lidocaine and diphenhydramine. 0.5 M mannitol was found to significantly increase the duration of anesthesia. In comparison to 0.9 M mannitol, 0.5 M was well tolerated without any irritation.[56,57]

Magnesium sulfate: Magnesium antagonizes peripheral N-methyl-aspartate receptors which mediate pain. As an adjuvant to LAA, magnesium sulfate was found to reduce pain but reduced postprocedure opioid requirement more significantly. It also reduced postoperative shivering and nausea. It is used in a dose of 80 mg/kg or 500–6,000 mg.[58]

Clonidine: Clonidine is an alpha-2 adrenergic agonist. Along with lidocaine, it was found to reduce onset of anesthesia, improved as well as prolonged duration of anesthesia (by nearly 6 hours) and reduced the peak lidocaine levels (thereby reduces lidocaine toxicity). Dosage is 1–3 μg/kg (30–250 μg).[58] Epinephrine is contraindicated in patients with myocardial infarction, hypertensives, pheochromocytoma and those on tricyclic antidepressants, beta blockers, monoamine oxidase inhibitors, and phenothiazines. Clonidine reduces peripheral vascular resistance and hence is safe in patients with contraindications for epinephrine.[59]

Dexmedetomidine: It is a highly selective alpha-2 adrenoceptor agonist ($\alpha2:\alpha1 = 1{,}620:1$) and causes hyperpolarization of nerve membrane thereby retarding the action potentials.[60] Dexmedetomidine was better than fentanyl (opioid analgesic) and sufentanil (synthetic opioid, 5–10 times more potent than fentanyl) as local anesthesia adjuvant in prolonging the duration of anesthesia and efficacy.[61,62] Dexmedetomidine provided prolonged analgesia than clonidine and lacked the side effects of clonidine viz., hypotension, bradycardia. Dexmedetomidine can be used in children at minimal effective and safe dosage (evidence A1).[63]

Use of newer delivery technologies also impacts the action of LAAs and their adjuvants. Addition of dexmedetomidine to ropivacaine and use of ropivacaine loaded lipid hybrid nanoparticles were found to prolong the duration of analgesia significantly.[64,65] Dexmedetomidine and ropivacaine in nanostructured lipid carriers increased the depth and duration of analgesia.[66] Dexmedetomidine has also been used with levobupivacaine. Transactivated transcriptional activator (TAT) modified levobupivacaine and dexmedetomidine co-delivered lipid polymer hybrid nanoparticles were better than nanostructured lipid carriers.[67] The only extended release LAA approved by FDA is liposomal bupivacaine and has approval for infiltration use and interscalene brachial plexus infiltration.[68]

VASOCONSTRICTORS AND LOCAL ANESTHETIC AGENT

Vasoconstrictors when used with LAA control blood loss during procedure and retard local clearance of LAA. This increases efficacy and reduces the risk of systemic toxicity of LAA.[2-4,69] Various agents used are as follows:

Epinephrine

Epinephrine is the most common vasoconstrictor used with LAA. It has both alpha (vasoconstriction action) as well as beta adrenergic effect (increases blood pressure and pulse rate). Efficacy of lidocaine 1% with epinephrine has been found to be equivalent to lidocaine 2%.[70] Combination of epinephrine with lidocaine is more potent than when former is used with bupivacaine or etidocaine. This is due to high protein binding of latter LAA which itself decreases the clearance of these agents resulting in delayed onset of action. It takes about 7–15 minutes for achieving optimal hemostatic effect with epinephrine and its action last for approximately 60 minutes.[3] Dosage of epinephrine in cardiac patients is 40–200 μg (0.04–0.2 mg or 4–20 mL of 1:1,00,000 epinephrine) and in healthy adults is 500 μg (0.5 mg or 50 mL of 1:1,00,000 epinephrine). The hemostatic effect is dose dependent and 1:50,000 dilution worked better than 1:1,00,000 and 1:2,00,000.[71] However, vasoconstrictor effects were similar between 1:1,00,000, 1:2,00,000 and 1:4,00,000 dilutions. Dilutions beyond 1:4,00,000 showed delayed onset of anesthesia and reduced duration of action.[72] It has long been held that use of vasoconstrictors with LAA is contraindicated for areas with end arterial supply such as digits/toes, penis, ear lobes, and nose tip. Recent evidence suggests that lidocaine with adrenaline is safe for ears, digits, toes, and tip of nose.[73,74] Similarly, several studies have demonstrated the safety of lidocaine with adrenaline combination for digits and toes in patients with normal circulatory status.[75-78] Hence, lidocaine with adrenaline may be used with caution, particularly in an otherwise healthy young patient without any vascular insufficiency in injections to fingers and toes, if benefits outweigh the risk of such a combination. However, in people with suspected vascular insufficiency, elderly patients, and in patients with unreliable history of previous disease states, such combinations are contraindicated because of the risk of precipitating vascular complications such as gangrene. In such individuals, only plain lidocaine should be used. Based on various studies and reports, the recent guidelines on use of local anesthesia suggest that LAA with epinephrine can be safely used for regions such as ear, nose, and digits (level of evidence I, II and strength of recommendation A). However, for penis, it is level II with strength of recommendation of B.[14] Review by Schnabl revealed lack of casual relationship between use of epinephrine and necrosis of digits or penis. They opine that contraindication for its use is more for legal implications.[79]

Systemic side effects of epinephrine start after 5–10 minutes of injection and last for about 10–15 minutes.[80] Small quantities of epinephrine with lidocaine can be used in stable cardiovascular patients (level of evidence I, II, strength of recommendation B).[14] Systemic reactions to epinephrine for nontoxic doses of epinephrine containing LAA was 2% during Mohs and was in the form of subjective feeling of tremulousness. These reactions occurred in non-dose dependent manner. Due to age-related obtundation of nervous system, these side effects were less in geriatric patients.[81] Although, there has been debate over the use of vasoconstrictor with LAA for harvesting the split thickness and full thickness graft, there is no consensus on this and hence, it can be used in healthy patients without any vascular insufficiency.

Malignant hypertension can occur with epinephrine-LAA in patients on nonselective beta blockers such as propranolol, labetalol, timolol. This is due to unopposed alpha adrenergic activity as protective beta adrenergic effects are blocked by propranolol. However, in view of low doses of epinephrine used, there is no need to discontinue nonselective beta blockers before cutaneous surgeries.[3] Epinephrine also causes CNS side effects such as restlessness, tremors, headache, cerebral bleed and causes hypertension in pheochromocytoma and hyperthyroid patients. Being a stress hormone, it increases blood sugars.

Topical epinephrine fails to increase the duration of action of topical anesthetics due to poor penetration of intact skin or mucosa. However, phenylephrine 0.005% can be used for the same purpose.

Levonordefrin

Levonordefrin is an active isomer of nordefrin, which has alpha-1 adrenergic activity and minimal to absent beta adrenergic activity. Because of its latter action, variation in blood pressure and pulse rate is minimal.

Phenylephrine

Phenylephrine has only alpha-adrenergic activity and often used in subarachnoid blocks. This is used as an alternative to epinephrine for topical anesthesia.

COMPLICATIONS DURING LOCAL ANESTHESIA

Local Neural Toxicity

Local anesthesia infiltration can cause transient motor paresis. Extraneural deposition of LAA as in nerve blocks has been found to be cytotoxic to neuronal cells and Schwann cells through several mechanisms which are less understood. Perez-Castro et al. found that bupivacaine was more toxic than lidocaine, though latter causes more transient neurological symptoms.[82] Damage caused to Schwann cells differs with duration of exposure to LAA and the concentration used. Even at low concentration, bupivacaine caused significant cell death on prolonged exposure. On intermediate duration of exposure, both bupivacaine and ropivacaine were equally toxic. Higher concentration as with articaine 4% or prilocaine 4% carries higher risk of direct neurotxicity.[7] Prolonged extraneural exposure to bupivacaine resulted in significant demyelination and nerve inflammation.[83]

Syncope

Syncope secondary to vasovagal attack (presence of pallor, hyperhidrosis, hyperventilation, and hypotension) is common, particularly in anxious patients, and those with unstable autonomic nervous system. It is always advisable to ask about previous syncopal attacks before administration of anesthesia. Vasovagal syncopal attack can be treated by raising the foot end of the bed. For this reason, all procedures needing local anesthesia should be done in supine position. Injection atropine may be helpful in cases that develop bradycardia **(Table 3)**.[5] Hence it is preferable to keep a syringe filled with atropine ready before administration of local anesthesia.

Hypersensitivity Reactions

Hypersensitivity reactions are potentially serious and hence should always be recognized and treated early. However, it must be recognized that true allergic reactions to local anesthetics are rare.[84-86] Vasovagal syncopal attacks are often mistakenly considered as hypersensitivity reactions. Careful evaluation and skin testing are needed for proper diagnosis.[87-89] Sensitivity to local anesthetics may be either due to the anesthetic itself or the preservatives (parabens) or agents used to stabilize epinephrine (sulfites).[7,86,90]

Esters are metabolized to para-aminobenzoic acid (PABA) which is allergenic. Sensitivity to local anesthetics can be either of type I reaction (anaphylaxis) or type IV (delayed hypersensitivity). Anaphylaxis, though very rare, may be potentially fatal. Hypotension due to anaphylaxis should be differentiated from vasovagal syncope and dysrhythmias. There can be tachycardia in anaphylaxis, bradycardia in vasovagal and irregular pulse in dysrhythmias.[91] Ester group anesthetics are more prone to cause anaphylaxis than the amide group anesthetics.[90] Type IV reaction can be either due to amides or ester-based local anesthetics. Amides and ester groups of local anesthetics do not cross-react. However, within the group, there may be cross-reaction to other agents.[92] Rarely, hypersensitivity can exist in a patient, to both amide and ester group of local anesthetics.[93] Delayed type hypersensitivity reaction may rarely vary with the site of deposition of LAA.

TABLE 3: Common adverse reactions during administration of LAA and their management.

Signs and symptoms	*Cause*	*Corrective measures*
• *CNS excitation:* Headache, anxiety tinnitus, tingling of lips, and tongue, twitching, seizures • *Cardiac depression:* Hypotension respiratory depression	Lidocaine toxicity	• Stop further administration of LAA • Airway, breathing, and circulation management • Diazepam for convulsion, ephedrine for hypotension, atropine for bradycardia
• Tachycardia, palpitations, apprehension, anxiety, hypertension	Epinephrine	• Stop further administration, observe for 10–15 minutes, reassure patient • Esmolol, sotalol may be used for hypertension • Phentolamine may be needed
• Bradycardia, hypotension, nausea, pallor, dizziness/fainting	Vasovagal syncope	• Lower the head end • Elevate the leg end, monitor vitals, and intervene accordingly
• Edema, erythema, dyspnea • Bronchospasm, tachycardia, hypotension	Anaphylaxis	• Intravenous hydrocortisone, adrenaline subcutaneously, bronchodilator (nasal or oral spray) • Be prepared for emergency tracheotomy or cricothyroidotomy • Lidocaine sensitivity to be performed to prevent such an occurrence

(CNS: central nervous system; LAA: local anesthetic agent)

Source: Sanchez JP, Balingit JS, McCutcheon R. Local and Regional Anesthetic Blocks Made Simple. Philippines: Nazarene Printers; 2002.[5]

Wobser et al. reported "Compartment Allergy" a case of delayed hypersensitivity to prilocaine which occurred only on patch and superficial subcutaneous application but not on deep subcutaneous injection. He hypothesized that, this could be due to *"lower dendritic cell (DC) density in deeper cutaneous compartments and/or different DC subsets exhibiting distinct functional immunomodulatory properties in the various layers of the skin"*.[94]

Skin Testing

Skin testing is an important means of determining possible hypersensitivity. However, both false positives and false negatives may occur.

Skin testing for topical cream anesthesia: Contact hypersensitivity to topically applied anesthetics is infrequent.[86-88] Topical allergic reaction is usually mild, limited to development of dermatitis or contact urticaria. Hence a patch test is not recommended as a routine in all cases. However, where there is a suspicion of hypersensitivity, a patch testing may be performed. Apply about 1–2 mm thick layer of anesthetic preparation over about 1 cm^2 area for 30 minutes and check for history of itching or any erythema or maculopapular rash.

Intradermal testing: All anesthetic injections may be associated with systemic hypersensitivity which may be potentially fatal. Hence intradermal test is mandatory in all such cases. This is performed by injection of lidocaine or bupivacaine with 0.1 mL on flexural forearm about 1–2 inches below the antecubital fossa. If the patient complains of any itching with the development of urticarial rash in the form of erythema, edema, and induration at the site of intradermal test, it indicates a positive test, indicating that the patient is hypersensitive to it. In such a situation, it is not safe and ethical to administer/use the same local anesthetic.

Alternatives for Anesthesia in Patients with Lidocaine Hypersensitivity

In cases of hypersensitivity to lidocaine, anesthesia can be achieved by using an anesthetic from the ester group. If there is any allergy to the preservative, then preservative free lidocaine may be used, if such a preparation is available. If there is hypersensitivity to both amide and ester groups, then the alternative would include:[95]

- Diphenhydramine and chlorpheniramine are alternatives though they provided milder anesthesia.[51,96,97]
- Benzyl alcohol can also be used for anesthesia.[98]
- Intravenous sedation/general anesthesia can be used in a hypersensitive patient, if the circumstances of the case demand.
- Cryoanesthesia (discussed earlier)
- *Vibrational anesthesia:* Competitively inhibits Aδ and C fibers. Reduces pain in minor procedures (level of evidence IV)

Prilocaine has caused cross-sensitivity with bupivacaine and pramoxine.[82]

Systemic toxicities with EMLA are usually due to inappropriate technique (large quantities, large surface area of application, and long duration of application), inappropriate local factors (abraded skin, vascular malformations, and eczema), inappropriate demographics (prematurity, age <3 months), and drug inter-actions.[99]

Methemoglobinemia

Amide LAA undergoes N-dealkylation and then hydrolysis. However, prilocaine undergoes first hydrolysis which results in formation of orthotolidine. This product oxidizes ferrous ion (Fe^{2+}) in hemoglobin to ferric (Fe^{3+}) leading to impaired release of oxygen causing hypoxia termed methemoglobinemia. Patients appear cyanotic and their blood is chocolate colored when MetHb level is 3–5 mg%. Doses of prilocaine >10 mg/kg or >600 mg are required for producing this side effect. However, lower doses can cause same side effect in patients with congenital or idiopathic methemoglobinemia, infants <6 months (immature NADH reductase enzyme complex),[99,100] glucose-6-phosphate dehydrogenase enzyme deficiency and those on medications which cause methemoglobinemia (viz. dapsone, chloroquine, sulfonamides, primaquine, acetaminophen, phenobarbital, phenytoin, nitroglycerin, nitrofurantoin, nitroprusside, aniline dyes, para-aminosalicylic acid, and benzocaine). In mild cases, methemoglobinemia resolves spontaneously or with supportive care such as oxygen administration; if severe, intravenous administration of reducing agents such as methylene blue, vitamin C may be required. Methylene blue is contraindicated in G6PD deficient individuals and such patients should be treated with ascorbic acid, though latter works much slowly.

Guay in his study of patients of methemoglobinemia secondary to LAA found that maximum cases were due to benzocaine (77 out of 97). Benzoic esters are metabolized similar to anilides and it is hypothesized that, methemoglobinemia could be due to a variation in metabolism and/or elimination of benzocaine. In patients with methemoglobinemia due to benzocaine application on mucosa, there is a high-risk of development of rebound methemoglobinemia after administration of methylene blue for up to 18 hours. Hence, these patients should be carefully monitored after antidote therapy. Methemoglobinemia has also been reported with lidocaine and tetracaine; however, NADH deficiency was not evaluated in them.[100]

Local Anesthetic Systemic Toxicity

Local anesthetic systemic toxicity (LAST) is occurrence of systemic toxicity (cardiovascular and central nervous system) due to administration of local anesthesia. About 20% LAST cases occur outside hospital setting and up to 50% of cases are due to non-anesthetists.[101] In a retrospective study, it was found that large doses of lidocaine (>30 mL) were relatively safe with symptoms of early lidocaine toxicity in only two out of 563 patients. This cohort included patients with risk factors such as heart disease, diabetes, hypertension, and smoking.[102] Though not common, it can happen (2–2.8/10,000 peripheral nerve blocks).[103] Among all peripheral nerve blocks, intercostal nerve blocks have maximal rate of reabsorption of LAA, thereby having the highest risk for systemic toxicity.[63] More than body mass index other factors, viz., total local anesthetic dose, test dosing, and patient comorbidities are more predictive of high plasma LAA concentration.[101]

Causes, Mechanisms, and Clinical Features of LAST

Systemic toxicity can occur due to inadvertent intra-arterial or intravenous injection as well as systemic absorption. Symptoms due to intra-arterial injections often occur during nerve blocks in head and neck region. Because of proximity to brain, CNS side effects occur very fast and also recover fast due to rapid cerebral circulation. Even low doses may give this side effect. Symptoms due to inadvertent intravascular injection occur within 60 seconds due to immediate effect on brain and symptoms are delayed for 1–5 minutes in cases of intermittent intravascular injection and with regional blocks when large quantities of LAA (5–10 mL) are used. Symptoms due to systemic absorption are delayed and take about 20–30 minutes or more. It occurs if large quantities of LAA are used or with continuous LAA infusion or in the presence of risk factors viz., in infants <4 months and elderly, severe hepatic dysfunction, advanced cardiac failure, uremia, metabolic acidosis, and late pregnancy. Rapid systemic absorption can also occur when LAA is injected in highly vascular areas. Since LAST can have delayed manifestation from 15 minutes to more than an hour, it is advised that patients receiving higher or toxic doses of LAA be monitored closely for 30 minutes after injection (recommendation I, evidence B). The mechanism of toxicity and clinical features are summarized in **Table 4**. Even though there is initial CNS excitation followed by suppression, occasionally, CNS depression can occur directly without preluding excitation phase.[2,4] Seizures were five times more common with peripheral nerve block than epidural block.

All the LAAs are potential cardiovascular depressants, both central and peripheral. CNS side effects precede cardiac side effects and cardiac depression occurs at doses which cause CNS depression. However, this classical presentation is not seen in 40% of cases with LAST as they present with isolated cardiac features and/or delayed presentation (>5 minutes after injecting LAA).[101] Delay in presentation has been hypothesized to be due to fewer intravascular injections, due to use of ultrasound assistance for injection, use of local anesthesia infiltration techniques, and use of continuous local anesthetic infusion. Cardiotoxicity is more severe with bupivacaine and etidocaine in comparison to lidocaine. The increased toxicity of bupivacaine is attributed to slower dissociation of bupivacaine from sodium channels during diastole leading to cumulative blockage of channels and a more intense depression of rapid phase of depolarization in Purkinje fibers and ventricular muscles. This leads to ventricular arrhythmias and myocardial depression. Bupivacaine is a racemic mixture of R- and S-stereoisomers and R-isomers are more cardiotoxic. Hence, pure S-stereoisomers of bupivacaine, i.e., ropivacaine (single S-enantiomer) and levobupivacaine (levo-S-bupivacaine) have less cardiotoxicity.[2,4] It is difficult to resuscitate patients with bupivacaine-induced cardiac toxicity and hence great caution has to be exercised to prevent inadvertent intravascular injection.

As the symptoms of CNS toxicity are much easier to recognize than cardiovascular collapse, a new ratio encompassing these has been proposed to check potential of LAA to cause these side effects. Cardiovascular collapse/CNS (CC/CNS) ratio is the ratio of drug dose required to cause catastrophic cardiovascular collapse to drug dose required to cause seizures. Greater the cardiotoxicity, lower is the ratio. Ascending order of this ratio is racemic bupivacaine (lowest), levobupivacaine, ropivacaine, and lidocaine (highest). However, CVS toxicity can occur without preceding CNS toxicity irrespective of agent used.[104]

TABLE 4: Mechanism of toxicity and clinical features of LAST.

System involved	*Mechanism of toxicity*	*Clinical features*
CNS system	*Initial phase:* Inhibition of cerebral cortical inhibitory pathway	Sensory disturbances (perioral paresthesia, dysgeusia), tinnitus, visual disturbances, dysarthria, dizziness, muscle twitching, confusion, and convulsions
	Delayed phase: Inhibition of excitatory neurons	Mental obtundation, unconsciousness, coma, respiratory arrest
CVS system	Inhibition of Na channels lead to decreased rate of depolarization and propagation of action potentials	Hypertension, tachycardia (due early CNS excitation), dysrhythmia (bradycardia, tachycardia, ventricular ectopy), reentrant tachyarrhythmia
	Inhibition of calcium channel and sodium-calcium channel leads to reduced myocardial contraction; impairs mitochondrial oxidative phosphorylation; inhibits cAMP production	Myocardial depression, asystole
	Suppress baroreceptor reflex; reduce vascular tone	Hypotension

(CNS: central nervous system; CVS: cardiovascular system; LAST: local anesthetic systemic toxicity)

Risk factors for LAST are age (<16 and >60 years), sex (female > male), muscle mass (lean mass more prone viz., infants, debilitated elderly), comorbid cardiac, hepatic, neurological and metabolic (isovaleric acidemia, mitochondrial disease, carnitine deficiency, and diabetes mellitus) conditions, low plasma protein binding (liver disease, infants, and pregnancy), LAA used (bupivacaine is more riskier and difficult to resuscitate after LAST, most cases of LAST are due to ropivacaine and lidocaine), technique of anesthesia administration (local anesthetic infusions can present after 1–4 days especially in patients with lean body mass).[101]

Methods to Mitigate Risk of LAST

The American Society of Regional Anesthesia and Pain Medicine recommends following techniques to reduce the risk of LAST:[101,105]

- *Minimalistic approach:* Use of just adequate dose of LAA is better. Lean body mass is a better index for dose calculation than whole body weight in overweight/obese individuals. Whenever combination of LAAs is used, lesser doses of each should be used as the side effects can accrue.
- *Choosing right LAA:* LAA with higher CC/CNS ratios should be preferred.
- *Safe technique of administration:* Aspirate before injecting so as to confirm that needle is not intravascular. However, this has about 2% false negative possibility. Administer LAA as small boluses slowly rather than depositing large doses in a single shot. Maintaining a gap of one circulation time viz., 30–45 seconds between these boluses is a safe practice.
- *Use of marker of intravascular injection:* A test dose of epinephrine 5 μg/mL of LAA has been used to know the expected response and adverse reaction in case of intravascular injection. An intravascular injection of 3 mL of LAA with epinephrine (1:2,00,000), viz., 15 μg of epinephrine causes tachycardia (10 beats/minute) and rise in systolic pressure by 15 mm Hg. But this may not be appreciated in elderly patients and those on beta blockers, sedated or under general anesthesia.
- *Ultrasound-guided administration of peripheral nerve blocks:* This reduces but not completely avoids intravascular injection of LAA.[101]
- Level of vigilance when administering liposomal bupivacaine should be as same as local anesthetic (class of recommendation I, evidence C).
- Administering appropriate quantity of LAA reduces the risk of toxicity and can be easily calculated using the formula suggested by Walsh and Arya as follows,[106]

$$\text{Maximum allowable volume of LAA (mL)} = \frac{\text{Maximum allowable dose (mg/kg)} \times \text{Body weight (kg)}}{10 \times \text{Concentration of LAA (\%)}}$$

Management of LAST

Most important aspect of management is early recognition of LAST! Monitor the vitals for 30 minutes after administration of LAA and keep speaking to patient to recognize any early CNS side effects. Any alteration of mental function or variations of cardiac parameters is LAST. Like in any hypersensitivity or toxicity reactions, maintenance of airway, breathing, and circulation is critical for resuscitation of an individual with LAST. Seizures can be effectively treated with benzodiazepines and if refractory may require succinylcholine (*see* **Table 3**). However, these need anesthetist or an intensivist's intervention. CNS or cardiac complications necessitate advanced life support and appropriate timely intervention. Epinephrine <1 mg/kg has been suggested to improve cardiac contractility and maintain blood pressure. Amiodarone is preferred over calcium channel blockers and beta blockers to treat ventricular tachyarrhythmias as latter reduce vascular resistance and also suppress cardiac muscles. Intravenous lipid emulsion therapy, also called as lipid resuscitation has been considered a standard care for resuscitation of LAST.[105] Immediately after maintaining airway, lipid emulsion therapy should be started.[101] Lipid resuscitation is discussed in detail in separate section.

OTHER SIDE EFFECTS

Bruising

Bruising is common in elderly due to thin dermis. Bruise can be localized by immediate application of pressure or ice cubes at the site.

Vasoconstriction

In case of mild ischemia due to lidocaine with adrenaline, apply topical nitroglycerin; for severe cases, start phentolamine 2.5–5.0 mg which is diluted in 4.5–9.0 mL of normal saline.[77]

Myonecrosis

Intramuscular injection of LAA can cause variable muscle necrosis which is also LAA dependent (bupivacaine, chloroprocaine > ropivacaine, procaine, tetracaine).[107]

Drug Fever

Drug fever was noted with EMLA but not plain 2% lidocaine jelly. Drug fever correlated with increase in serum IL-6 levels.[108]

Pseudobullous Dermatosis

Both intraepidermal (subcorneal and suprabasal) as well as subepidermal clefting have been observed with EMLA application. Epidermal necrosis and multifocal clefting was more common with genital lesions secondary to EMLA application.[109,110]

Various adverse reactions noted with EMLA are erythema, edema, pain, allergic contact dermatitis, contact urticaria, purpura, post inflammatory hyperpigmentation, and skin necrosis when applied to leg ulcers in patients with disordered microcirculation.[111-114] Loss of vision has been documented during eyelid infiltration secondary to corneal perforation.[115]

Lipid Resuscitation

Intravenous lipids have long been used for parenteral nutrition. It is an emulsion composed of egg phospholipids or soyabean oil in water. It has also been used to treat systemic toxicity of LAA (LAST) and referred as intravenous lipid emulsion therapy and lipid rescue. Commonly 20% emulsions are used for this purpose. Among various preparations available, Intralipid™ has maximum studies.

Mechanism of Action of Intravenous Lipids

Various mechanisms have been hypothesized and include:[116,117]

- *Lipid sink:* Lipid soluble LAA agents in circulation or tissue binding sites are attracted and absorbed by the intravenous lipids.
- *Influence on cardiac myocyte fatty acid metabolism:* LAA inhibit fatty acid metabolism in heart and intravenous lipids counteract this by being an exogenous source of energy.
- Acts as a positive inotrope.
- Relieves the sodium channel (Nav 1.5) by the drug.
- Regulate carnitine transport, thereby improving fatty acid metabolism in cardiac muscles.

Method of Use

Initially a loading dose of 1.5 mL/kg (if <70 kg) or 100 mL (if >70 kg) is administered over 2–3 minutes and subsequently a slow infusion of 0.25 mL/kg/min (i.e., about 18 mL/min if patient is <70 kg) or 200–250 mL (if >70 kg) is administered over 15–20 minutes. If the hypotension persists, then one or two additional boluses are administered and the dose of continuous infusion is doubled (0.5 mL/kg/min). Continuous infusion is continued for 10 minutes after the CVS stability. Maximum recommended dose is 12 mL/kg for initial dosing (recommendation II b, evidence B).[101]

Adverse effects of lipid resuscitation include alteration of laboratory tests (renal and liver function test, electrolytes, creatine kinase, and total proteins; this tends to persist for 24 hours after administration of intravenous lipids), pancreatitis, pulmonary dysfunction, acute renal failure, and deep vein thrombosis.[118]

Positioning of Lipid Resuscitation for LAST

Rather than initiating lipid resuscitation after the onset of CVS and CNS adverse effects, it is now advised to start lipid emulsion treatment as soon as features of LAST recognized. The change in recommendation is based on following observations. LAAs have to be shuttled off by lipids when peak toxic concentrations are present. Maximum dose of intravenous lipid is 12 mL/kg. However, doses used for lipid resuscitation are <50% and hence are relatively safe.[101] It can be used for treating toxicity due to lipophilic drugs, viz., bupivacaine and can be considered for treating toxicity due to other LAAs, amitriptyline, and bupropion.[119,120]

TIPS

Safety tips when administering local anesthesia

- Ethyl chloride is more inflammable than alcohol; even though it vaporizes rapidly, it is safe to avoid it when electrocautery is planned.
- When injecting lidocaine or bupivacaine (especially latter) ensures that the needle is not within a vessel as it can precipitate arrhythmias.
- Avoid using lidocaine with adrenaline, in patients with hypertension, history of Raynaud's phenomenon, peripheral vascular disease, vasospasm, history of thromboembolism, and history of thromboangitis obliterans.
- On anesthetizing oral mucosa, ingestion of food has to be avoided for 1 hour as swallowing is impaired and hence can lead to aspiration. Also, there is a risk of tongue bite.
- Whenever mixture of LAA is used, it should be presumed that the toxicities are additive.[2,121,122]

OTHER USES OF LOCAL ANESTHETIC AGENT

Neuropathic Pain

Intravenous infusion of lidocaine alone or with oral sodium channel blockers has been used successfully in the treatment of neuropathic pain. Interestingly, even though they reduce the neuropathic pain, normal pain and other sensations are unaffected. This could be due to higher doses of anesthetic required to block the normal sensation in comparison to neuropathic pain. Often, the pain relief stays for duration much longer than the elimination half-life (t½) of that LAA. Lidocaine 5% plaster, bupivacaine, mepivacaine, and ambroxol 20% cream have been used to treat localized neuropathic pain with variable results. Topical clonidine 0.1% was found to reduce diabetic peripheral neuropathic pain.[123,124] High dose topical capsaicin 8% is better than low dose preparations (0.025%, 0.075%) in the treatment of postherpetic neuralgia (PHN). However, it is 2nd- or 3rd-line option for treating PHN.[125]

Premature Ejaculation

As penile hypersensitivity has been hypothesized to be a cause for premature ejaculation, topical anesthesia is used to reduce neuronal excitability thus delaying ejaculation.[88] Lidocaine spray, EMLA, topical eutectic mixture for premature ejaculation (TEMPE) containing lidocaine and prilocaine spray and dyclonine/alprostadil (latter is a vasodilator) cream have been used in its treatment.[126] The eutectic mixture of pure lidocaine 150 mg/mL and prilocaine 50 mg/mL without any excipient as metered aerosol spray (Fortacin™, TEMPE, PSD502) has been approved by European Union for treatment of premature ejaculation. It has a rapid onset of action (<5 minutes). Side effects noted were—genital hypoaesthesia in both partners, erectile dysfunction, and vulvovaginal discomfort or burning sensation.[127]

Assessment of Polyneuropathy

As small nerves are affected much earlier in diabetic neuropathy, EMLA which effectively inhibits these small fibers has been used to check for early polyneuropathy in diabetes mellitus. Stimulated skin wrinkling test is adopted for the same. Here the area to be tested is exposed to EMLA for 5–30 minutes and the wrinkling of skin noted. Wrinkling is due to vasoconstriction mediated by postganglionic sympathetic innervation. The advantage of EMLA over water immersion is that the response is more linear and sustained for 90 minutes with former. This test can be used to check the nerve function in leprosy as well.[128]

Antibacterial Property of Local Anesthetic Agent

It is interesting to know that some of the topical anesthetic agents have antibacterial properties. Lidocaine 2% showed significant reduction of colonies of *Staphylococcus aureus* and *Viridans streptococci* [90% ($p < 0.01$) and 92% ($p < 0.001$) respectively]. Clinically, there were no infections after intravitreal injections when subconjunctival lidocaine was infiltrated in comparison to other modalities of anesthesia used for same procedure.[129] Proparacaine and tetracaine also have shown inhibitory action on *Viridans streptococci* and proparacaine showed the lowest minimal inhibitory concentration (MIC) amongst itself, tetracaine, and lidocaine.[130]

Others

Continuous infusion of local anesthetic at the site of surgery is required for alleviation of postsurgical pain.[131] Topical anesthesia can be used for tuberculin skin testing without any risk of altered test result.[132] Pramoxine is used for its antipruritic property in many over-the-counter topical antipruritic and antihemorrhoids formulations.[133]

PREPROCEDURE PREPARATION

An anxiolytic administered before any procedure improves patient comfort and avoids occurrence of untoward reactions of patients such as restlessness, variations in blood pressure. Midazolam is an ultrashort acting sedative of benzodiazepine group and has anxiolytic, sedative, anticonvulsant, and muscle relaxant properties. Hence, it is extensively used in many day care procedures performed on children as well as adults. It is readily absorbed by any route of administration with peak plasma concentration occurring in 20–60 minutes. Midazolam is metabolized in liver and inhibits cytochrome P 250 3A4 enzyme complex potentiating lidocaine toxicity.[3] It has an elimination t½ of 2 hours. It is used in a dose of 0.25–0.5 mg/kg in infants <6 months and in children between 6 months and 6 years, up to 1 mg/kg stat dose. Toxicity leads to depression of cardiovascular system and CNS. Occasionally, paradoxical muscle excitation may occur. It should be cautiously used in patient with cardiac conditions, open angle glaucoma, myasthenia gravis, and elderly individuals.[134]

LOCAL ANESTHETIC FAILURE

Infrequently, there are situations where local anesthesia does not work. This could be due to following factors:[135]

- Increased local blood flow leading to rapid clearance of the LAA.
- Local tissue acidosis (due to conditions such as inflammation or infection) leading to enhanced ionization of LAA which retards diffusion of LAA across the axonal membrane.
- Local tissue edema, whereby, LAA has to traverse longer distance to diffuse into nerve membrane.
- Tachyphylaxis (discussed earlier).
- *Genetic:* Some patients with Ehlers–Danlos syndrome show poor response to topical anesthesia.[136]
- Excessive coffee consumption leads to increased alertness which adversely affects sleep leading to stress and anxiety. This could lead to failure of local anesthesia.[137]
- Genetic variation in gene coding voltage gated sodium channel Nav 1.5 present in peripheral nerves was observed (A572D mutation in SCN5A gene coding for Nav 1.5).[138]

CONCLUSION

Local anesthesia is an integral part of dermatosurgery and cosmetic surgery. However, LAA can give rise to some life-threatening side effects much graver than the risk of procedure itself. Hence, performing surgeons need to be vigilant of the same to render better care to patients and clients.

REFERENCES

1. Thomson CJ, Lalonde DH. Randomized double-blind comparison of duration of anesthesia among three commonly with lignocaine versus eutectic mixture of local anesthetics: used agents in digital nerve block. Plast Reconstr Surg. 2006;118:429-32.
2. Berde CB, Strichartz GR. Local anesthetics. In: Miller RD, Eriksson LI, Fleisher LA, Wiener-Kronish JP, Young WL (Eds). Miller's Anesthesia, 7th edition. Philadelphia: Churchill Livingstone Elsevier; 2010. pp. 913-39.
3. Huether MJ, Brodland DG. Local anesthetics. In: Wolverton SE (Ed). Comprehensive Dermatologic Drug Therapy, 2nd edition. Philadelphia: Saunders Elsevier; 2007. pp. 825-49.

4. Caterall WA, Mackie K. Local anesthetics. In: Brunton LL, Chabner BA, Knollman BC (Eds). Goodman & Gilman's The Pharmacological Basis of Therapeutics, 12th edition. USA: McGraw-Hill; 2011. pp. 565-82.
5. Sanchez JP, Balingit JS, McCutcheon R. Local and Regional Anesthetic Blocks Made Simple. Philippines: Nazarene Printers; 2002.
6. Luck L, Longley BJ. Cutaneous cryoanesthesia does not affect histopathology of biopsy specimens. Cutis. 1999;64:225-6.
7. Park KK, Sharon VR. A review of local anesthetics: minimizing risk and side effects in cutaneous surgery. Dermatol Surg. 2017;43(2):173-87.
8. Campbell JR, Maestrello CL, Campbell RL. Allergic response to metabisulfite in lidocaine anesthetic solution. Anesth Prog. 2001;48(1):21-6.
9. Rao PB, Mohanty CR, Singh N, Mund M, Patel A, Sahoo AK. Effectiveness of different techniques of ethyl chloride spray for venepuncture-induced pain: a randomised controlled trial. Anesth Essays Res. 2019;13(3):568-71.
10. Patel R, Halem M, Zaiac M. The combined use of forced cold air and topical anesthetic cream for analgesia during the treatment of palmar hyperhydrosis with botulinum toxin injections. J Drugs Dermatol. 2009;8:948-51.
11. Sari E, Sandikci MM, Bakar B, Tellioglu AT. Estimated beginning time of local anesthesia effectiveness in forced cold air application: a preliminary study. J Cosmet Laser Ther. 2016;18(1):22-4.
12. Irkoren S, Ozkan HS, Karaca H. A clinical comparison of EMLA cream and ethyl chloride spray application for pain relief of forehead botulinum toxin injection. Ann Plast Surg. 2015;75(3):272-4.
13. Moller RA, Covino BG. Effect of progesterone on the cardiac electrophysiologic alterations produced by ropivacaine and bupivacaine. Anesthesiology. 1992;77(4):735-41.
14. Kouba DJ, LoPiccolo MC, Alam M, Bordeaux JS, Cohen B, Hanke CW, et al. Guidelines for the use of local anesthesia in office-based dermatologic surgery. J Am Acad Dermatol. 2016;74(6):1201-19.
15. Mysore V, Nischal KC. Guidelines for administration of local anesthesia for dermatosurgery and cosmetic dermatology procedures. Indian J Dermatol Venereol Leprol. 2009;75:68-75.
16. Brodland DG, Huether MJ. Local anesthetics. In: Wolverton SE (Ed). Comprehensive Dermatologic Drug Therapy. Philadelphia: WB Saunders Company; 2001. pp. 736-66.
17. Package insert Prilox™. Neon Labs, India.
18. Crisan D, Scharffetter-Kochanek K, Kastler S, Crisan M, Manea A, Wagner K, et al. Dermatologic surgery in children: an update on indication, anesthesia, analgesia and potential perioperative complications. J Dtsch Dermatol Ges. 2018;16(3):268-76.
19. Mutalik S. How to make local anesthesia less painful? J Cut Aesth Surg. 2008;1:37-8.
20. Radha Atal-Shah. Anaesthesia in dermatosurgery. In: Satish S (Ed). Textbook of Dermatosurgery and Cosmetology, 2nd edition. Mumbai: ASCAD; 2005. pp. 53-64.
21. Christoph RA, Buchanan L, Begalla K, Schwartz S. Pain reduction in local anesthetic administration through pH buffering. Ann Emerg Med. 1988;17(2):117-20.
22. Hruza GJ. Anesthesia. In: Bolognia JL, Jorizzo FL, Rapini RP (Eds). Dermatology. New York: Elsevier Science; 2003. pp. 2233-42.
23. Stewart JH, Cole GW, Klein JA. Neutralized lidocaine with epinephrine for local anesthesia. J Dermatol Surg Oncol. 1989;66:572-4.
24. Stewart JH, Chinn SE, Cole GW, Klein JA. Neutralized lidocaine with epinephrine for local anesthesia. J Dermatol Surg Oncol. 1990;16(9):842-5.
25. Grekin RC, Auletta MJ. Local anesthesia in dermatologic surgery. J Am Acad Dermatol. 1988;19:599-614.
26. Zaiac M, Aguilera SB, Zaulyanov-Scanlan L, Caperton C, Chimento S. Virtually painless local anesthesia: diluted lidocaine proves to be superior to buffered lidocaine for subcutaneous infiltration. J Drugs Dermatol. 2012;11(10): e39-42.
27. Dinehart SM. Topical, local, regional anesthesia. In: Wheeland R (Ed). Cutaneous Surgery. Philadelphia: WB Saunders; 1994. pp. 102-12.
28. Hogan ME, Vandervaart S, Perampaladas K, Machado M. Systematic review and meta-analysis of the effect of warming local anesthetics on injection pain. Ann Emerg Med. 2011;58(1):86-98.e1.
29. Bartfield JM, Sokaris SJ, Raccio-Robak N. Local anesthesia for lacerations: pain of infiltration inside vs outside the wound. Acad Emerg Med. 1998;5(2):100-4.
30. Kelly AM, Cohen M, Richards D. Minimizing the pain of local infiltration anesthesia for wounds by injection into the wound edges. J Emerg Med. 1994;12(5):593-5.
31. Younkin K, Reader A, Drum M, Nusstein J, Beck M. Anesthetic efficacy of a combination of 0.5 M mannitol plus 36.8 mg of lidocaine with 18.4 μg epinephrine in maxillary infiltration: a prospective, randomized, single-blind study. Anesth Prog. 2014;61(2):63-8.
32. Fosko SW, Gibney MD, Harrison B. Repetitive pinching of the skin during lidocaine infiltration reduces patient discomfort. J Am Acad Dermatol. 1998;39:74-8.
33. Palmon SC, Lloyd AT, Kirsch JR. The effect of needle gauge and lidocaine pH on pain during intradermal injection. Anesth Analg. 1998;86:379-81.
34. Sorensen EP, Gu H, Tabacchi M, Council ML. Music reduces pain and anxiety associated with local anesthesia for dermatologic procedures: a randomized controlled trial. J Am Acad Dermatol. 2021;85(4):989-91.
35. Tian T, Luo Y, Jiang T, Dong Y, Yu A, Chen H, et al. Clinical effect of ablative fractional laser-assisted topical anesthesia on human skin: A randomized pilot study. J Cosmet Laser Ther. 2016;18(7):409-12.
36. Meesters AA, Bakker MM, de Rie MA, Wolkerstorfer A. Fractional CO_2 laser assisted delivery of topical anesthetics: A randomized controlled pilot study. Lasers Surg Med. 2016;48(2):208-11.
37. Golan J, Hai N. JetPeel: A new technology for facial rejuvenation. Ann Plast Surg. 2005;54(4):369-74.
38. Iannitti T, Palmieri B, Aspiro A, Di Cerbo A. A preliminary study of painless and effective transdermal botulinum toxin A delivery by jet nebulization for treatment of primary hyperhidrosis. Drug Des Devel Ther. 2014;8:931-5.
39. Hofmann GA, Rustrum WV, Suder KS. Electro-incorporation of microcarriers as a method for the transdermal delivery of large molecules. Bioelectrochem Bioenerg. 1995;38(1):209-22.
40. Wallace MS, Ridgeway B, Jun E, Schulteis G, Rabussay D, Zhang L. Topical delivery of lidocaine in healthy volunteers by electroporation, electroincorporation, or iontophoresis: an evaluation of skin anesthesia. Reg Anesth Pain Med. 2001;26(3):229-38.
41. Kumar M, Chawla R, Goyal M. Topical anesthesia. J Anaesthesiol Clin Pharmacol. 2015;31(4):450-6.

42. Nayak A, Das DB. Potential of biodegradable microneedles as a transdermal delivery vehicle for lidocaine. Biotechnol Lett. 2013;35(9):1351-63.
43. Baek SH, Shin JH, Kim YC. Drug-coated microneedles for rapid and painless local anesthesia. Biomed Microdevices. 2017;19(1):2.
44. Ji M, Liu G, Cui Y, Zhao P. Safety and efficacy concerns of modern strategies of local anesthetics delivery. 3 Biotech. 2020;10(8):333.
45. Wang J, Zhang L, Chi H, Wang S. An alternative choice of lidocaine-loaded liposomes: lidocaine-loaded lipid-polymer hybrid nanoparticles for local anesthetic therapy. Drug Deliv. 2016;23(4):1254-60.
46. Lauterbach A, Müller-Goymann CC. Applications and limitations of lipid nanoparticles in dermal and transdermal drug delivery via the follicular route. Eur J Pharm Biopharm. 2015;97(Pt A):152-63.
47. Gagliano-Jucá T, Castelli MR, Mendes GD, Arruda AM, Chen LS, de Oliveira MA, et al. Pharmacokinetic and pharmacodynamic evaluation of a nanotechnological topical formulation of lidocaine/prilocaine (nanorap) in healthy volunteers. Ther Drug Monit. 2015;37(3):362-8.
48. Remy M, Pinter F, Nentwich MM, Kampik A, Schönfeld CL. Efficacy and safety of hyaluronidase 75 IU as an adjuvant to mepivacaine for retrobulbar anesthesia in cataract surgery. J Cataract Refract Surg. 2008;34911):1966-9.
49. Wohlrab J, Finke R, Franke WG, Wohlrab A. Clinical trial for safety evaluation of hyaluronidase as diffusion enhancing adjuvant for infiltration analgesia of skin with lidocaine. Dermatol Surg. 2012;38(1):91-6.
50. Schulenburg HE, Sri-Chandana C, Lyons G, Columb MO, McLure HA. Hyaluronidase reduces local anaesthetic volumes for sub-Tenon's anaesthesia. Br J Anaesth. 2007;99(5):717-20.
51. Nevarre DR, Tzarnas CD. The effects of hyaluronidase on the efficacy and on the pain of administration of 1% lidocaine. Plast Reconstr Surg. 1998;101(2):365-9.
52. Chassard D, Berrada K, Boulétreau P. Alkalinization of local anesthetics: theoretically justified but clinically useless. Can J Anaesth. 1996;43:384-93.
53. Chin KJ, Handoll HH. Single, double or multiple-injection techniques for axillary brachial plexus block for hand, wrist or forearm surgery in adults. Cochrane Database Syst Rev. 2011;6:CD003842.
54. Kaplan JA, Miller ED, Gallagher EG. Postoperative analgesia for thoracotomy patients. Anaesth Analg. 1975;54:773-7.
55. Sindjelic RP, Vlajkovic GP, Davidovic LB, Markovic DZ, Markovic MD. The addition of fentanyl to local anesthetics affects the quality and duration of cervical plexus block: a randomized, controlled trial. Anesth Analg. 2010;111(1):234-7.
56. Son JY, Lim JS, Park JH, Park JH, Kim MS, Park JH, et al. Mannitol Enhances the Antinociceptive effects of diphenhydramine as an alternative local anesthetic. Pain Res Manag. 2020;2020:7934164.
57. Pathak PK, Singh AK, Agrawal S, Singh D, Mali DK, Kumar U. Role of 0.5 M mannitol as an adjuvant with lidocaine with or without epinephrine for inferior alveolar nerve block: a randomized control trial. J Clin Exp Dent. 2019;11(6):e500-5.
58. Bai JW, An D, Perlas A, Chan V. Adjuncts to local anesthetic wound infiltration for postoperative analgesia: a systematic review. Reg Anesth Pain Med. 2020;45(8):645-55.
59. Sivaramakrishnan G, Sridharan K. Effect of clonidine on the efficacy of lignocaine local anesthesia in dentistry: a systematic review and meta-analysis of randomized, controlled trials. J Investig Clin Dent. 2018;9(2):e12296.
60. Weerink MAS, Struys MMRF, Hannivoort LN, Barends CRM, Absalom AR, Colin P. Clinical pharmacokinetics and pharmacodynamics of dexmedetomidine. Clin Pharmacokinet. 2017;56(8):893-913.
61. Sun S, Wang J, Bao N, Chen Y, Wang J. Comparison of dexmedetomidine and fentanyl as local anesthetic adjuvants in spinal anesthesia: a systematic review and meta-analysis of randomized controlled trials. Drug Des Devel Ther. 2017; 11:3413-24.
62. Zhang T, Yu Y, Zhang W, Zhu J. Comparison of dexmedetomidine and sufentanil as adjuvants to local anesthetic for epidural labor analgesia: a randomized controlled trial. Drug Des Devel Ther. 2019;13:1171-5.
63. Suresh S, Ecoffey C, Bosenberg A, Lonnqvist PA, de Oliveira GS Jr, de Leon Casasola O, et al. The European Society of Regional Anaesthesia and Pain Therapy/American Society of Regional Anesthesia and Pain Medicine Recommendations on Local Anesthetics and Adjuvants Dosage in Pediatric Regional Anesthesia. Reg Anesth Pain Med. 2018;43(2):211-6.
64. Hao J, Wu Z, Luo Z, Dong B. Addition of dexmedetomidine to ropivacaine for local infiltration anaesthesia improves analgesic efficacy after tonsillectomy and adenoidectomy: a randomized controlled trial. Int J Pediatr Otorhinolaryngol. 2020;137:110168.
65. Li A, Yang F, Xin J, Bai X. An efficient and long-acting local anesthetic: ropivacaine-loaded lipid-polymer hybrid nanoparticles for the control of pain. Int J Nanomedicine. 2019;14:913-20.
66. Yang Y, Qiu D, Liu Y, Chao L. Topical anesthetic analgesic therapy using the combination of ropivacaine and dexmedetomidine: hyaluronic acid modified long-acting nanostructured lipid carriers containing a skin penetration enhancer. Drug Des Devel Ther. 2019;13:3307-19.
67. Li M, Feng S, Xing H, Sun Y. Dexmedetomidine and levobupivacaine co-loaded, transcriptional transactivator peptide modified nanostructured lipid carriers or lipid-polymer hybrid nanoparticles, which performed better for local anesthetic therapy? Drug Deliv. 2020;27(1):1452-60.
68. Coppens SJR, Zawodny Z, Dewinter G, Neyrinck A, Balocco AL, Rex S. In search of the Holy Grail: Poisons and extended release local anesthetics. Best Pract Res Clin Anaesthesiol. 2019;33(1):3-21.
69. Katzung BG, White PF. Local anesthetics. In: Katzung BG, Masters SB, Trevor AJ (Eds). Basic and Clinical Pharmacology, 11th edition. New Delhi: Tata McGraw Hill Education Private Limited; 2009. pp. 439-50.
70. Haddox JD, Baumann PL. Local Anesthetics. In: Craig CR, Stitzel RE (Eds). Modern Pharmacology with Clinical Applications, 5th edition. USA: Little, Brown and Company (Inc.); 1997. pp. 347-53.
71. Shoroghi M, Sadrolsadat SH, Razzaghi M, Farahbakhsh F, Sheikhvatan M, Sheikhfathollahi M, et al. Effect of different epinephrine concentrations on local bleeding and hemodynamics during dermatologic surgery. Acta Dermatovenerol Croat. 2008;16(4):209-14.
72. Kim H, Hwang K, Yun SM, Kim DJ. Usage of epinephrine mixed with lidocaine in plastic surgery. J Craniofac Surg. 2020;31(3):791-3.
73. Häfner HM, Röcken M, Breuninger H. Epinephrine-supplemented local anesthetics for ear and nose surgery: clinical use without complications in more than 10,000 surgical procedures. J Dtsch Dermatol Ges. 2005;3:195-9.
74. Häfner HM, Schmid U, Moehrle M, Strölin A, Breuninger H. Changes in acral blood flux under local application of

ropivacaine and lidocaine with and without an adrenaline additive: a double-blind, randomized, placebo-controlled study. Clin Hemorheol Microcirc. 2008;38(4):279-88.
75. Lalonde D, Bell M, Benoit P, Sparkes G, Denkler K, Chang P. A multicenter prospective study of 3,110 consecutive cases of elective epinephrine use in the fingers and hand: the Dalhousie Project clinical phase. J Hand Surg Am. 2005;30(5):1061-7.
76. Thomson CJ, Lalonde DH, Denkler KA, Feicht AJ. A critical look at the evidence for and against elective epinephrine use in the finger. Plast Reconstr Surg. 2007;119(1):260-6.
77. Krunic AL, Wang LC, Soltani K, Weitzul S, Taylor RS. Digital anesthesia with epinephrine: an old myth revisited. J Am Acad Dermatol. 2004;51(5):755-9.
78. Wilhelmi BJ, Blackwell SJ, Miller JH, Mancoll JS, Dardano T, Tran A, et al. Do not use epinephrine in digital blocks: myth or truth? Plast Reconstr Surg. 2001;107(2):393-7.
79. Schnabl SM, Ghoreschi FC, Scheu A, Kofler L, Häfner HM, Breuninger H. Use of local anesthetics with an epinephrine additive on fingers and penis-dogma and reality. J Dtsch Dermatol Ges. 2021;19(2):185-96.
80. Son HW, Park SH, Cho HO, Shin YJ, Son JH. Epinephrine-induced lactic acidosis in orthognathic surgery: a report of two cases. J Korean Assoc Oral Maxillofac Surg. 2016;42(5):295-300.
81. McLawhorn JM, Clark S, Lander S, Truong V, Aston CE, Collins L, et al. Incidence of epinephrine reactions with local anesthesia in mohs micrographic surgery. Dermatol Surg. 2020;46(5):581-5.
82. Perez-Castro R, Patel S, Garavito-Aguilar ZV, Rosenberg A, Recio-Pinto E, Zhang J, et al. Cytotoxicity of local anesthetics in human neuronal cells. Anesth Analg. 2009;108(3):997-1007.
83. Yang S, Abrahams MS, Hurn PD, Grafe MR, Kirsch JR. Local anesthetic Schwann cell toxicity is time and concentration dependent. Reg Anesth Pain Med. 2011;36(5):444-51.
84. Gall H, Kaufmann R, Kalveram CM. Adverse reactions to local anesthetics: analysis of 197 cases. J Allergy Clin Immunol. 1996;97:933-7.
85. Swanson JG. Assessment of allergy to local anesthetic. Ann Emerg Med. 1983;12:316-8.
86. Phillips JF, Yates AB, Deshazo RD. Approach to patients with suspected hypersensitivity to local anesthetics. Am J Med Sci. 2007;334:190-6.
87. Eggleston ST, Lush LW. Understanding allergic reactions to local anesthetics. Ann Pharmacother. 1996;30:851-7.
88. Boren E, Teuber SS, Naguwa SM, Gershwin ME. A critical review of local anesthetic sensitivity. Clin Rev Allergy Immunol. 2007;32(1):119-28.
89. Berkun Y, Ben-Zvi A, Levy Y, Galili D, Shalit M. Evaluation of adverse reactions to local anesthetics: experience with 236 patients. Ann Allergy Asthma Immunol. 2003;91(4):342-5.
90. Huang W, Vidimos A. Topical anesthetics in dermatology. J Am Acad Dermatol. 2000;43:286-98.
91. Lim GFS, Huether MJ, Brodland DG. Local anesthetics. In: Wolverton SE, Wu JJ (Eds). Comprehensive Dermatologic Drug Therapy. 4th edition. Philadelphia: Elsevier; 2021. pp. 631-49.
92. González-Delgado P, Antón R, Soriano V, Zapater P, Niveiro E. Cross-reactivity among local anesthetics in a case of allergy amide-type to mepivacaine. J Investig Allergol Clin Immunol. 2006;16(5):311-3.
93. Caron AB. Allergy to multiple local anesthetics. Allergy Asthma Proc. 2007;28:600-1.
94. Wobser M, Gaigl Z, Trautmann A. The concept of "compartment allergy": prilocaine injected into different skin layers. Allergy Asthma Clin Immunol. 2011;7:7.
95. Orhan ME, Yüksel U, Bilgin F, Doğrul A. Comparison of the local anesthetic effects of chlorpheniramine, midazolam, lidocaine, and normal saline after intradermal injection. Med Sci Monit. 2007;13(4):PI7-11.
96. Xia Y, Chen E, Tibbits DL, Reilley TE, McSweeney TD. Comparison of effects of lidocaine hydrochloride, buffered lidocaine, diphenhydramine, and normal saline after intradermal injection. J Clin Anesth. 2002;14(5):339-43.
97. Bartfield JM, Jandreau SW, Raccio-Robak N. Randomized trial of diphenhydramine versus benzyl alcohol with epinephrine as an alternative to lidocaine local anesthesia. Ann Emerg Med. 1998;32(6):650-4.
98. García F, Iparraguirre A, Blanco J, Alloza P, Vicente J, Báscones O, et al. Contact dermatitis from prilocaine with cross-sensitivity to pramocaine and bupivacaine. Contact Dermatitis. 2007;56(2):120-1.
99. Tran AN, Koo JY. Risk of systemic toxicity with topical lidocaine/prilocaine: a review. J Drugs Dermatol. 2014;13(9):1118-22.
100. Guay J. Methemoglobinemia related to local anesthetics: a summary of 242 episodes. Anesth Analg. 2009;108:837-45.
101. Neal JM, Barrington MJ, Fettiplace MR, Gitman M, Memtsoudis SG, Mörwald EE, et al. The Third American Society of Regional Anesthesia and Pain Medicine Practice Advisory on Local Anesthetic Systemic Toxicity: Executive Summary 2017. Reg Anesth Pain Med. 2018;43(2):113-23.
102. Patrinely JR Jr, Darragh C, Frank N, Danford BC, Wheless L, Clayton A. Risk of adverse events due to high volumes of local anesthesia during Mohs micrographic surgery. Arch Dermatol Res. 2021;313(8):679-84.
103. El-Boghdadly K, Chin KJ. Local anesthetic systemic toxicity: continuing professional development. Can J Anaesth. 2016; 63(3):330-49.
104. Di Gregorio G, Neal JM, Rosenquist RW, Weinberg GL. Clinical presentation of local anesthetic systemic toxicity: a review of published cases, 1979 to 2009. Reg Anesth Pain Med. 2010;35(2):181-7.
105. ASRA. (2011). Checklist for Treatment of Local Anesthetic Systemic Toxicity. [online] Available from: https://www.asra.com/content/documents/asra_last_checklist.2011.pdf [Last accessed August, 2023].
106. Walsh K, Arya R. A simple formula for quick and accurate calculation of maximum allowable volume of local anaesthetic agents. Br J Dermatol. 2015;172(3):825-6.
107. Tasch MD, Butterworth JF. Adverse reactions to local anesthetics. In: Lobata EB, Gravenstein N, Kirby RR (Eds). Complications in Anesthesiology. Philadelphia: Lippincott Williams and Wilkins; 2008. pp. 865-78.
108. Kamata M, Tada Y, Yazawa N, Watanabe T, Kikuchi K, Sato S. Drug fever caused by eutectic mixture of local anesthetic cream. J Investig Allergol Clin Immunol. 2011;21(5):421.
109. Kieliszak CR, Griffin JR, Pollinger TH, Junkins-Hopkins JM. Pseudo-bullous dermatosis induced by topical anesthetic agent-clues to this localized toxic reaction. Am J Dermatopathol. 2017;39(2):e19-e22.
110. Lewis FM, Agarwal A, Neill SM, Calonje JE, Stefanato CM. The spectrum of histopathologic patterns secondary to the topical application of EMLA® on vulvar epithelium: clinicopathological correlation in three cases. J Cutan Pathol. 2013;40(8):708-13.
111. Pérez-Pérez LC, Fernández-Redondo V, Ginarte-Val M, Paredes-Suárez C, Toribio J. Allergic contact dermatitis from EMLA cream in a hemo-dialyzed patient. Dermatitis. 2006;17(2):85-7.

112. Waton J, Boulanger A, Trechot PH, Schmutz JL, Barbaud A. Contact urticaria from Emla cream. Contact Dermatitis. 2004;51(5-6):284-7.
113. Cervigón I, Torres-Iglesias LM, Palomo A. Purpura after application of a eutectic mixture of local anesthetic. Actas Dermosifiliogr. 2008;99:499-500.
114. Stahl M, Meyer C, Haas E, Glaenz T, Zutt M. Leg ulcer progression caused by topical anesthesia with EMLA cream. J Dtsch Dermatol Ges. 2008;6(7):566-8.
115. Parikh M, Kwon YH. Vision loss after inadvertent corneal perforation during lid anesthesia. Ophthal Plast Reconstr Surg. 2011;27:e141-2.
116. Bartlett D. Intravenous lipids: antidotal therapy for drug overdose and toxic effects of local anesthetics. Crit Care Nurse. 2014;34(5):62-6; quiz 67.
117. Nadrowitz F, Stoetzer C, Foadi N, Ahrens J, Wegner F, Lampert A, et al. Leffler A. The distinct effects of lipid emulsions used for "lipid resuscitation" on gating and bupivacaine-induced inhibition of the cardiac sodium channel Nav1.5. Anesth Analg. 2013;117(5):1101-8.
118. Cao D, Heard K, Foran M, Koyfman A. Intravenous lipid emulsion in the emergency department: a systematic review of recent literature. J Emerg Med. 2015;48(3):387-97.
119. Gosselin S, Hoegberg LC, Hoffman RS, Graudins A, Stork CM, Thomas SH, et al. Evidence-based recommendations on the use of intravenous lipid emulsion therapy in poisoning. Clin Toxicol (Phila). 2016;54(10):899-923.
120. Levine M, Hoffman RS, Lavergne V, Stork CM, Graudins A, Chuang R, et al. Systematic review of the effect of intravenous lipid emulsion therapy for non-local anesthetics toxicity. Clin Toxicol (Phila). 2016;54(3):194-221.
121. Kyttä J, Heavner JE, Badgwell JM, Rosenberg PH. Cardiovascular and central nervous system effects of co-administered lidocaine and bupivacaine in piglets. Reg Anesth. 1991;16(2):89-94.
122. Munson ES, Paul WL, Embro WJ. Central nervous-system toxicity of local anesthetic mixtures in monkeys. Anesthesiol. 1977;46:179-83.
123. Oliveira JD, Ribeiro LNM, Rodrigues da Silva GH, Casadei BR, Couto VM, Martinez EF, et al. Sustained release from ionic-gradient liposomes significantly decreases ETIDOCAINE Cytotoxicity. Pharm Res. 2018;35(12):229.
124. Casale R, Symeonidou Z, Bartolo M. Topical Treatments for Localized Neuropathic Pain. Curr Pain Headache Rep. 2017;21(3):15.
125. Laklouk M, Baranidharan G. Profile of the capsaicin 8% patch for the management of neuropathic pain associated with postherpetic neuralgia: safety, efficacy, and patient acceptability. Patient Prefer Adherence. 2016;10:1913-8.
126. Linton KD, Wylie KR. Recent advances in the treatment of premature ejaculation. Drug Des Devel Ther. 2010;18:1-6.
127. Porst H, Burri A. Fortacin™ spray for the treatment of premature ejaculation. Urologia. 2017;84(2_suppl):1-10.
128. Ping Ng KW, Ong JJ, Nyein Nyein TD, Liang S, Chan YC, Lee KO, et al. EMLA-induced skin wrinkling for the detection of diabetic neuropathy. Front Neurol. 2013;4:126.
129. Tustin A, Kim SJ, Chomsky A, Hubbard GB 3rd, Sheng J. Antibacterial properties of 2% lidocaine and reduced rate of endophthalmitis after intravitreal injection. Retina. 2014; 34(5):935-42.
130. Reynolds MM, Greenwood-Quaintance KE, Patel R, Pulido JS. Selected antimicrobial activity of topical ophthalmic anesthetics. Transl Vis Sci Technol. 2016;5(4):2.
131. Fustran Guerrero N, Dalmau Llitjós A, Sabaté Pes A. Continuous infusion of local anesthetic at the site of the abdominal surgical wound for postoperative analgesia: a systematic review. Rev Esp Anestesiol Reanim. 2011;58:337-44.
132. Beydon N, Lebras MN, de Lauzanne A, Clavel A, Holvoet-Vermaut L, Houdouin V, et al. Randomized study of the effect of topical anesthesia on tuberculin skin test reaction size in children. Pediatr Infect Dis J. 2010;29:180-2.
133. MedlinePlus. (2017). Pramoxine. [online] Available from: https://medlineplus.gov/druginfo/meds/ a682429.html. [Last accessed August, 2023].
134. DrugsUpdate. (2017). Midazolam information from Drugs Update. [online] Available from: http://www.drugsupdate.com/generic/view/312. [Last accessed August, 2023].
135. Local anesthetics and other drugs affecting sodium channels. In: Rang HP, Dale MM, Ritter JM, Flower RJ (Eds). Rang and Dale's Pharmacology, 6th edition. Philadelphia: Churchill Livingstone Elsevier; 2007. pp. 638-44.
136. Arendt-Nielsen L, Kaalund S, Bjerring P, Høgsaa B. Insufficient effect of local analgesics in Ehlers Danlos type III patients (connective tissue disorder). Acta Anaesthesiol Scand. 1990; 34(5):358-61.
137. Premnath S, Alalshaikh G, Alfotawi R, Philip M. The association between coffee consumption and local anesthesia failure: social beliefs and scientific evidence. Cureus. 2020;12(4): e7820.
138. Clendenen N, Cannon AD, Porter S, Robards CB, Parker AS, Clendenen SR. Whole-exome sequencing of a family with local anesthetic resistance. Minerva Anestesiol. 2016;82(10): 1089-97.

CHAPTER 13 Tumescent Local Anesthesia

Mysore Venkataram, Aniketh Venkataram

KEY MESSAGES

- Tumescent anesthesia has allowed dermatological surgeries such as liposuction and hair transplantation to be performed under local anesthesia.
- It has allowed high doses such as 45 mg/kg to be administered safely.
- Proper knowledge of pharmacology of lignocaine is necessary for administration.
- It should not be combined with other types of anesthesia such as intravenous anesthesia.

INTRODUCTION

Tumescent local anesthesia (TLA) is a form of local anesthesia, which has been used for several dermatosurgical procedures, particularly liposuction. It uses very dilute solution of anesthetic agent such as lignocaine in large quantities. The word tumescent means tumid—firm and swollen **(Figs. 1 and 2)**. It has revolutionized the administration of anesthesia for a wide range of cutaneous procedures, particularly liposuction, and has made it possible for performing surgeries under local anesthesia, which were otherwise being done under general anesthesia. It has enhanced safety and comfort for the patient, avoided hospital admission, and reduced cost of surgery. In the authors' opinion, it is one of the most significant contributions by a dermatologist to dermatologic surgery in the last century.

PRINCIPLE

The procedure consists of using a local anesthetic—epinephrine-saline mixture (also called Klein's solution), over a wide area to provide anesthesia and analgesia, using sufficient quantity of lidocaine far in excess of the conventional dosage. The underlying principle here is that contrary to conventional thinking, larger doses of lidocaine, even up to 45–55 mg/kg body weight, can be administered safely with this modification called tumescent technique. Conventional teaching has widely regarded, without adequate pharmacological proof, that the safe upper limit for lidocaine administration is 4.5 mg/kg with adrenaline up to 7 mg/kg body weight. In a radical departure from this hitherto-accepted fact, Klein showed that, in tumescent anesthesia, much higher doses can safely be administered, because, in tumescent anesthesia, rate of absorption of lidocaine is slow, leading to smaller peak values and hence lesser toxicity.[1]

Subcutaneous infiltration of large volumes of this solution causes the targeted tissue to become temporarily

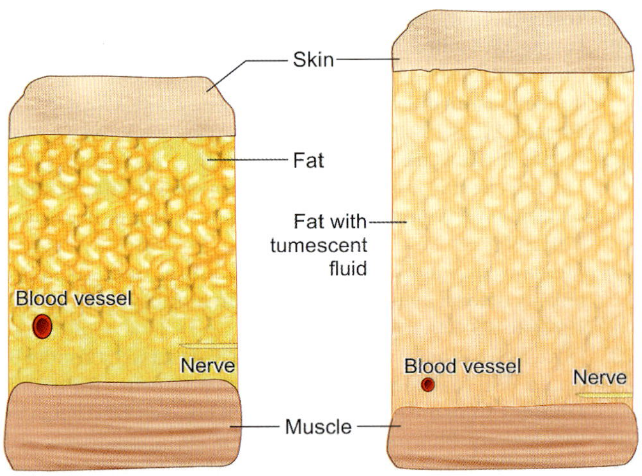

Fig. 1: Tissue before and after tumescent anesthesia—schematic diagram.

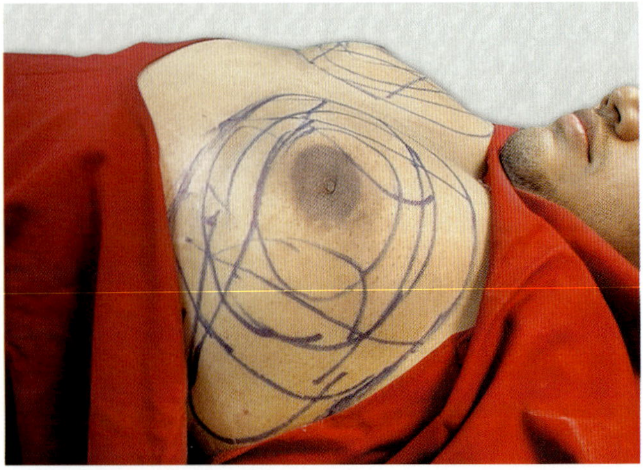

Fig. 2: Male breast after tumescence—swollen and firm.

BOX 1: The reasons for the slow absorption of lidocaine.[3]

- Subcutaneous fat has a low volume of blood flow
- Lidocaine is lipophilic and is easily sequestered in fat
- Diluted epinephrine in saline solution ensures vasoconstriction, thus minimizing systemic absorption and bleeding
- The large volume of tumescent solution itself compresses blood vessels by hydrostatic pressure
- The very low dilution of lidocaine in Klein's solution does not achieve the gradient required for systemic absorption
- Most of the solution is removed during aspiration, minimizing the quantity and duration available for absorption
- Thus, tumescent anesthesia is like a slow sustained release tablet

swollen and firm. The resulting increased subcutaneous interstitial pressure spreads the solution through adjacent tissues by bulk flow. Lidocaine toxicity is a function of serum lidocaine concentration and since concentration is low, the toxicity is less. Diluted epinephrine produces intense local vasoconstriction, slows systemic absorption of lidocaine, and thus reduces peak serum lidocaine concentrations, which reduce the risk of systemic lidocaine toxicity **(Box 1)**.[2,3]

CONCENTRATIONS

The usual tumescent solution concentration used by dermatologic surgeons is 0.05–0.1% lidocaine. The concentration of adrenaline or epinephrine is at 1:1,000,000–1.5:1,000,000. About 10 mEq of sodium bicarbonate is added to 1 liter of tumescent solution to raise pH and to prevent stinging (due to acidic pH of lidocaine). The recommended usual dose is 35 mg/kg body weight and maximum dose of lidocaine is 55 mg/kg body weight for most patients.[4,5] The recommended concentration of epinephrine in tumescent solutions is 0.5–1.5 mg/L. The total dosage of epinephrine should be minimized, within these limits, and usually should not exceed 50 µg/kg.[2,6]

Higher concentrations of lidocaine are commonly required in regions of body with more fibrous tissues like flank and abdomen.

PROCEDURE

Tumescent anesthesia is classically used in liposuction and it has made liposuction a safe and gold-standard method of surgery and hence is described in detail:

- Adits are small holes made for insertion of infiltration cannulae. These are done with 1.5–2-mm dermal punches at different locations of the area under infiltration anesthesia with 1 mL of 2% lignocaine.
- The preparation of tumescent fluid is discussed in **Table 1**. The required lidocaine dosages are dependent on appropriate epinephrine concentration in the tumescent solution. The concentration of lignocaine and epinephrine should be carefully calculated for each area, in relation to weight of the patient.[7,8]

TABLE 1: Tumescent anesthetic solution for liposuction: concentrations.

Lidocaine	*Epinephrine*
500 mg (0.05%)	With 0.5 mg (1:2 million) or
750 mg (0.75%)	With 0.75 mg (1:1.5 million) or
1,000 mg (1%)	With 1 mg (1:1.5 million)
Sodium bicarbonate	10 mEq (10 mL of 8.4% $NaHCO_3$)
Triamcinolone	10 mg (an optional ingredient)
Physiologic saline	1,000 mL of 0.9% NaCl

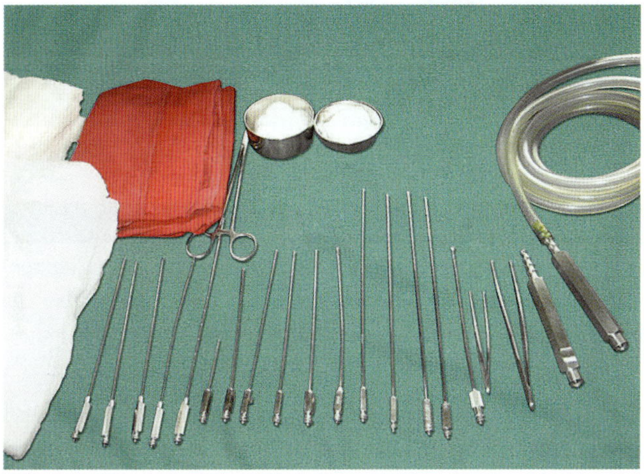

Fig. 3: Cannulae used for infiltration.

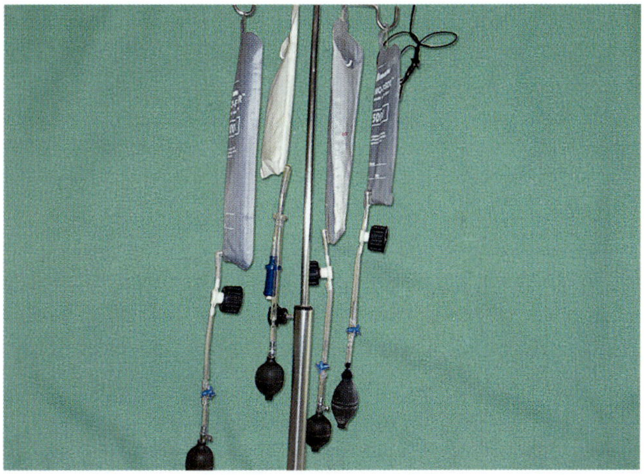

Fig. 4: Infiltration cuffs.

- *Infiltration of tumescent fluid*: The delivery system for tumescent solution consists of fluid, infiltration cannulae of size 0.5–1 mm **(Fig. 3)** infusion bags, infiltration pressure cuffs **(Fig. 4)**, and an infiltration pump **(Fig. 5)** to hasten delivery of the fluid. About 2–3 liters of fluid is infiltrated gradually, in different directions, first into deeper layers of fat and then into the superficial layers. The endpoint is a firm feel of the skin, which makes the skin swollen and difficult to grasp. It is important to be slow and to avoid jerky, sudden movements to avoid pain. Normally, it takes about 1–2 hours for proper anesthesia.

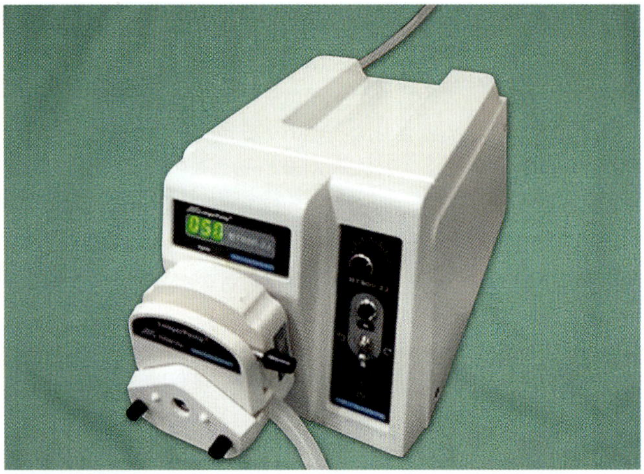

Fig. 5: Infiltration pump.

TABLE 2: Recommended area wise dosages of lidocaine.

Area	*Lidocaine dosage per liter*	*Lidocaine dosage in volume*
Abdomen—upper and lower	750–1,000 mg/L	800–2,000 mL
Hip (flank or love handle) each side	750–1,000 mg/L	400–1,000 mL
Lateral thigh—each side	600–750 mg/L	500–1,200 mL
Anterior thigh each side	600–750 mg/L	600–1,200 mL
Proximal medial thigh—each side	750–1,000 mg/L	250–700 mL
Knee	750–1,000 mg/L	200–500 mL
Male breast—each side	1,000–1,500 mg/L	300–800 mL
Submental area—chin	750–1,000 mg/L	100–200 mL

Table 2 shows formulation of tumescent solution for different areas.[9]

- *Detumescence*: It is important to wait for about 30 minutes after tumescence, for the infiltration fluid to percolate properly in all layers of fat and its full pharmacological effects to take effect. This is indicated by the slight decrease in firmness and the ability to grasp the skin.
  Using a warm (40°C) solution is associated with significantly less discomfort to the patient during infiltration; it also reduces the likelihood of hypothermia.[10]

Advantages of tumescent anesthesia in liposuction:[11,12]

- Profound local anesthesia
- Reduced surgical blood loss due to vasoconstriction
- The reduction of IV fluid requirements
- Enhanced aesthetic results—as tumescence reduces contours by swelling the tissue
- Enhanced postoperative pain relief caused by persistent fluid in the fat
- Enhanced overall safety—while deaths have been reported after liposuction in general anesthesia, tumescent liposuction has been remarkably safe

OTHER INDICATIONS FOR TUMESCENT ANESTHESIA

While liposuction was first designed and used in liposuction, since then it has been used in a number of dermatological surgeries, which have the following features in common:[13]

- They all involve large areas or multiple lesions.
- They need prolonged duration of anesthesia.
- Infiltration anesthesia would be needed in far excess of the upper limit of lignocaine and hence unsafe.
- Multiple punctures during infiltration would be painful and hence single or minimal number of entries is preferable.
- Many of these lesions/areas may bleed and vasoconstriction would therefore be necessary to ensure minimal bleeding.

As clear from the above-cited mechanisms, tumescent anesthesia is helpful in satisfying all these requirements.

Fat transfer: Fat transfer involves liposuction first and hence always needs tumescent anesthesia. It has been suggested that lignocaine may induce stem cell apoptosis and hence may have a negative impact on adipose derived stem cells.[14] Goldman et al. have suggested that tumescent liposuction without lignocaine may be used when fat transfer is planned and ropivacaine be used instead.

Hair transplantation: Bi-level (deep and superficial planes) tumescent anesthetic infiltration technique is a highly useful method of anesthesia for hair transplant harvesting and transplanting.[15] It has been used both in donor (both strip and excision techniques) and recipient areas to ensure prolonged anesthesia using minimal levels of lignocaine and also prevent bleeding by vasoconstriction.

Donor area: In strip technique, tumescence is used in two levels—

1. *Upper level in papillary dermis*: During strip excision, increasing the rigidity of donor area helps to decrease follicular transection during the harvest. This is achieved by the superficial tumescence. This superficial tumescence also causes blockage of fine nerve fibers in papillary dermis and the small blood vessels.
2. *Subcutis*: Deeper tumescence at subcutis and below acts by increasing the distance between the vascular plane and the plane of dissection, i.e., follicles residing in upper fat, thus reducing the chances of injury to nerves and large blood vessels.

Recipient area: It results in prolonged anesthesia, vasoconstriction, and thereby allows smooth implantation, dense packing of hair follicles, and prevents popping. *However, tumescence over recipient area has one disadvantage—it contributes to postoperative swelling.*

Role of tumescence in *follicular unit excision* (FUE) method is more controversial. Here, superficial tumescence can change the direction of emerging hair and this may increase the chances of transection. Hence, many authors have argued against using tumescence. However, deeper tumescence, which is below the level of hair follicle, can help in prolonging the duration of anesthesia and thereby reducing the amount of lidocaine used. This is particularly relevant in FUE mega sessions.

Tumescent anesthesia has been used in body hair transplantation also. Since large areas on chest are often used for donor extraction, neither infiltration nor nerve blocks are useful. Tumescent anesthesia helps in anesthetizing large areas with minimal amount of lidocaine. It also produces the necessary turgor, which facilitates extraction.[16]

Facial procedures: Tumescent anesthesia can be administered prior to extensive facial procedures such as laser resurfacing, subcision for acne scarring, microneedle radiofrequency, blepharoplasties, and face lifts.[17,18] The dermal tumescent technique of injection (into the dermis as opposed to the subcutaneous tissue layer) provides the skin surgeon with a temporarily bloodless dermal field and satisfactory anesthesia to perform these surgical procedures.[19] The formulation of 0.08% final concentration of lidocaine is generally used for facial procedures. Introduction of anesthetic fluid through infiltration cannulae adits at multiple sites is employed as shown in **Figure 6**.[20]

For laser resurfacing, the anesthesia achieved using TA is excellent, with added skin turgor, which stretches wrinkles for maximal exposure for the laser beam as well as provides added skin hydration. The postoperative period is less painful, as the burning sensation is minimized by the remaining anesthesia. This used to be relevant in the earlier days, when full face ablative CO_2 laser was done frequently. For face lift procedures, the anesthesia provides an excellent plane, allowing for safe and bloodless dissection.[17-20]

Vitiligo surgery: Harvesting of the graft from the donor area in vitiligo surgery can also be done by using tumescent anesthesia, particularly while harvesting large areas of donor skin for split thin skin grafting. In particular, mega vitiligo surgery sessions (150–400 cm^2) or Giga sessions (>400 cm^2) either by punch grafting or split skin grafting have been described and tumescent anesthesia would be particularly useful in these situations.[21]

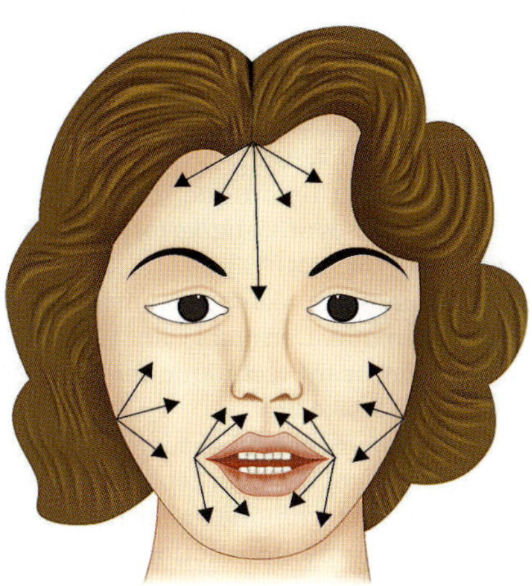

Fig. 6: Infiltrator insertion sites. Infiltration is made via entry sites to anesthetize the face.

BOX 2: Various applications of tumescent anesthesia.

- Liposuction
- Hair transplantation
- Facial procedures such as laser resurfacing, subcision for acne scarring, microneedle radiofrequency, blepharoplasties, and face lifts
- Dermatologic surgeries such as shave biopsy, lipoma excision, and Mohs micrographic surgery
- Vitiligo surgery
- Surgery for burns
- Anesthesia for zoster dermatitis
- Axillary hyperhidrosis
- Breast surgeries such as breast augmentation, breast reduction, and mastectomy
- Endovenous laser therapy
- Mini-abdominoplasty, brachioplasty, and medial thigh lifts
- Hand surgeries
- Repair of inguinal hernia
- Management of pilonidal cysts
- Endoscopic thyroid and parathyroid surgeries
- Lymph node dissection
- Serial excision of birthmarks and scars

Other Surgeries

Tumescent anesthesia has been used for a number of other surgeries such as venous surgeries (striping, endovenous laser ablation, and stab ligation),[22-26] acne scarring (subcision, resurfacing, and microneedle radiofrequency),[17] hand surgery,[27] lipomas,[28] breast augmentation,[29] axillary hyperhidrosis,[30] burn scar surgeries, excision of malignant tumors, and other procedures.[18,19,31-38]

Box 2 *lists the different surgeries that have been performed under tumescent anesthesia.*[13]

Other Anesthetics

Apart from lignocaine, other anesthetic agents such as prilocaine and ropivacaine have been used, though infrequently.[39,40] Mixed anesthetic solutions using local anesthetics prilocaine and ropivacaine diluted with original Ringer's solution with epinephrine (1:1,000,000) with concentration of mixture between 0.3 and 0.08% have also been used. The maximum dose of the local anesthetics was 4 mg/kg prilocaine and 2 mg/kg ropivacaine.

ADVERSE EVENTS WITH TUMESCENT ANESTHESIA

Over the last three decades, tumescent anesthesia has proved to be remarkably safe. The technique has stood its test of time and has established itself as a gold-standard method in liposuction and also useful in several other surgeries. Side

TABLE 3: Plasma lidocaine concentration and toxicity.

3–6 μg/mL	Subjective pharmacologic effects
5–9 μg/mL	Objective toxicity
8–12 μg/mL	Seizures and cardiac depression
12 μg/mL	Coma
20 μg/mL	Respiratory arrest
26 μg/mL	Cardiac arrest

effects have been few and nonserious. Several safety studies are available in liposuction[41,42] and these are dealt in detail in the chapters on liposuction.

Adverse events associated with TLA may be due to:[43]

- Lack of pharmacological awareness of this form of anesthesia
- Casual attitude and lack of protocols in calculation of dosage
- Clinician's error in calculation of dosages and fluids, such as inadvertent IV delivery of tumescent solution, miscommunication leading to excessive lidocaine in the tumescent lidocaine solution
- Drug interactions that reduce lidocaine metabolism by impairing cytochrome P450 1A2 and 3A4. The reader is referred to the Chapter 12 on local anesthesia for the list of drugs, which can affect lignocaine metabolism
- Combination formulations of tumescent solutions using bupivacaine, mepivacaine, or triamcinolone
- Pre-existing medical conditions.

Mild side effects include nausea, vomiting, drowsiness, lightheadedness, paresthesias, tinnitus, blurred vision, nystagmus, ataxia, slurred speech, confusion, etc. The threshold serum concentration for these signs of mild lidocaine toxicity is 6 μg/mL.[43] Respiratory depression, vasodilatation, and hypotension suggest serious toxicity. **Table 3** lists plasma lignocaine concentration and toxicity.

These side effects can be avoided by due diligence and adherence to standard dosages.[7]

USE OF OTHER FORMS OF ANESTHESIA WITH TUMESCENT ANESTHESIA

Oral anxiolytics, sedatives, or narcotic analgesics may be used with tumescent liposuction at dosages that are not associated with respiratory depression. Oral clonidine has been shown to have beneficial effects in reducing pulse rate, hypertension due to its sympatholytic effects, and reducing postoperative syncope due to its atropine-like effect.[8] Lorazepam or diazepam and paracetamol are recommended. Intramuscular anxiolytics, sedatives, or narcotic analgesics should be used with great caution with tumescent liposuction and only after full consultation with the anesthetist, as the dose-response relationships can vary widely and may be associated with respiratory depression. Intravascular anxiolytics, sedatives, or narcotic analgesics should be avoided, as they may be associated with increased risk of mortality and morbidity, if not used properly. They may, however, be used only if the procedure is performed by an experienced dermatosurgeon in a hospital setting with full intensive care unit (ICU) facilities and only if an anesthetist is present during the procedure and for postoperative care. The use of inhalational (general) anesthesia for tumescent, liposuction is not recommended.

SUMMARY

Tumescent anesthesia introduced by dermatologist Jeffrey Klein is one of the most significant inventions in cutaneous surgeries particularly liposuction. Dermatosurgeons need to learn this systematically, as it needs proper pharmacological knowledge and appreciation of anatomy of the region.

PEARLS

- Detailed history and physical examination to determine presence of hepatic or renal disease.
- Obtain a thorough medication history to detect cytochrome P450 inducers or inhibitors.
- Calculate the maximum allowable dose of local anesthetic in milligrams.
- Calculate the maximum allowable volume of diluted local anesthetic concentration for infiltration.
- Exercise great caution when administering additional local anesthetics for at least 12–18 hours after tumescent anesthesia.

ACKNOWLEDGMENT

Our thanks to Dr Shristi Shrestha and DR Monika Reddy.

REFERENCES

1. Klein JA. Anesthesia for liposuction in dermatologic surgery. J Dematol Surg Oncol. 1988;14(10):1124-32.
2. Lillis PJ. Liposuction surgery under local anesthesia: limited blood loss and minimal lidocaine absorption. J Dermatol Surg Oncol. 1988;14(10):1145-8.
3. Klein JA. The tumescent technique for liposuction. Am J Cosmetic Surg. 1987;4:263.
4. Klein JA. Tumescent technique for regional anaesthesia permits lidocaine doses of 35 mg/kg for liposuction. J Dermatol Surg Oncol. 1990;16(3):248-63.
5. Klein JA. The tumescent technique: anesthesia and modified liposuction technique. Dermatol Clin. 1990;8(3):425-37.
6. Lillis PJ. The tumescent technique for liposuction surgery. Dermatol Clin. 1990;8:439.
7. Venkataram M. Tumescent liposuction: standard guidelines of care. Indian J Dermatol Venereol Leprol. 2008;74 Suppl:S54-60.
8. Klein JA. Tumescent technique for local anesthesia improves safety in large-volume liposuction. Plast Reconstr Surg. 1993;92:1085-98.
9. Klein JA. Anesthetic formulation of tumescent solutions. Dermatol Clin. 1999;17:751-9.

10. Kaplan B, Moy RL. Comparison of room temperature and warmed local anesthetic solution for tumescent liposuction. A randomized double-blind study. Dermatol Surg. 1996;22: 707-9.
11. Ostad A, Kageyama N, Moy RL. Tumescent anesthesia with a lidocaine dose of 55 mg/kg is safe for liposuction. Dermatol Surg. 1996;22:921-7.
12. Habbema L. Safety of liposuction using exclusively tumescent local anesthesia in 3,240 consecutive cases. Dermatol Surg. 2009;35:1728-35.
13. Uttamani RR, Venkataram A, Venkataram J, Mysore V. Tumescent anesthesia for dermatosurgical procedures other than liposuction. J Cutan Aesthet Surg. 2020;13:275-82.
14. Goldman JJ, Wang WZ, Fang XH, Williams SJ, Baynosa RC. Tumescent liposuction without lidocaine. Plast Reconstr Surg Glob Open. 2016;4(8):e829.
15. Sattur S. Chapter 22: Anesthesia for hair transplantation. In: Venkataram Mysore (Ed). Hair Transplantation. New Delhi: Jaypee Brothers Medical Publishers (P) Ltd.; 2016. pp.138-45.
16. Mysore V. Body hair transplantation: case report of successful outcome. J Cutan Aesthet Surg. 2013;6(2):113.
17. Taylor MB, Zaleski-Larsen L, McGraw TA. Single session treatment of rolling acne scars using tumescent anaesthesia, 20% trichloracetic acid extensive subcision, and fractional CO_2 laser. Dermatol Surg. 2017;43 Suppl 1:S70-4.
18. Ramon Y, Barak Y, Ullmann Y, Hoffer E, Yarhi D, Bentur Y. Pharmacokinetics of high-dose diluted lidocaine in local anesthesia for facelift procedures. Ther Drug Monit 2007;29(5):644-7.
19. Behroozan DS, Goldberg LH. Dermal tumescent local anesthesia in cutaneous surgery. J Am Acad Dermatol. 2005;53(5):828-30.
20. Namias A, Kaplan B. Tumescent anesthesia for dermatologic surgery cosmetic and noncosmetic procedures. Dermatol Surg. 1998;24(7):755-8.
21. Paul M. Chapter 37B. ACSI Textbook of Cutaneous and Aesthetic Surgery, Volume 1, 2nd edition. 2017. pp. 442-50.
22. Cavallini A, Marcer D, Bernardini G, Ferrari Ruffino S. Endovenous laser ablation of great saphenous veins performed using tumescent cold saline solution without local anesthesia. Ann Vasc Surg. 2014;28(4):951-6.
23. Jibiki M, Miyata T, Futatsugi S, Iso M, Sakanushi Y. Effect of the wide-spread use of endovenous laser ablation on the treatment of varicose veins in Japan: a large-scale, single institute study. Laser Ther. 2016;25(3):171-7.
24. Cohn MS, Seiger E, Goldman S. Ambulatory phlebectomy using the tumescent technique for local anesthesia. Dermatol Surg. 1995;21(4):315-8.
25. Vuylsteke ME, Mordon SR. Endovenous laser ablation: a review of mechanisms of action. Ann Vasc Surg. 2012;26(3):424-33.
26. Bush RG, Hammond KA. Tumescent anesthetic technique for long saphenous stripping. J Am Coll Surg. 1999;189(6):626-8.
27. Prasetyono TO, Lestari PA. The onset and duration of action of 0.2% lidocaine in a one-per-mil tumescent solution for hand surgery. Arch Plast Surg. 2016;43(3):272-7.
28. Morioka D, Sato N, Ohkubo F. Excision of large lipomas using tumescent local anesthesia. J Cutan Med Surg. 2016;20(3): 263-5.
29. Rusciani A, Pietramaggiori G, Troccola A, Santoprete S, Rotondo A, Curinga G. The outcome of primary subglandular breast augmentation using tumescent local anesthesia. Ann Plast Surg. 2016;76(1):13-7.
30. Feldmeyer L, Bogdan I, Moser A, Specker R, Kamarashev J, French LE, et al. Short- and long-term efficacy and mechanism of action of tumescent suction curettage for axillary hyperhidrosis. J Eur Acad Dermatol Venereol. 2015;29(10):1933-7.
31. Bussolin L, Busoni P, Giorgi L, Crescioli M, Messeri A. Tumescent local anesthesia for the surgical treatment of burns and postburn sequelae in pediatric patients. Anesthesiology. 2003;99(6):1371-5.
32. Gümüs N. Tumescent infiltration of lidocaine and adrenaline for burn surgery. Ann Burns Fire Disasters. 2011;24(3):144-8.
33. Blome-Eberwein S, Abboud M, Lozano DD, Sharma R, Eid S, Gogal C. Effect of subcutaneous epinephrine/saline/local anesthetic versus saline-only injection on split-thickness skin graft donor site perfusion, healing, and pain. J Burn Care Res. 2013;34(2):80-6.
34. Girard C, Debu A, Bessis D, Blatière V, Dereure O, Guillot B. Treatment of Gorlin syndrome (nevoid basal cell carcinoma syndrome) with methylaminolevulinate photodynamic therapy in seven patients, including two children: interest of tumescent anesthesia for pain control in children. J Eur Acad Dermatol Venereol. 2013;27(2):e171-5.
35. Kendler M, Micheluzzi M, Wetzig T, Simon JC. Electrochemotherapy under tumescent local anesthesia for treatment of cutaneous metastases. Dermatolog Surg. 2013;39(7):1023-32.
36. Stoffels I, Dissemond J, Schulz A, Hillen U, Schadendorf D, Klode J. Reliability and cost- effectiveness of complete lymph node dissection under tumescent local anaesthesia vs. general anaesthesia: a retrospective analysis in patients with malignant melanoma AJCC stage III. J Eur Acad Dermatol Venereol. 2012;26(2):200-6.
37. Abramson DL. Tumescent abdominoplasty: an ambulatory office procedure. Aesthetic Plast Surg. 1998;22(6):404-7.
38. Kayaalp C, Olmez A, Aydin C, Piskin T. Tumescent local anesthesia for excision and flap procedures in treatment of pilonidal disease. Dis Colon Rectum. 2009;52(10):1780-3.
39. Kendler M, Simon JC, Wetzig T. Local anesthesia with lidocaine and prilocaine, using the tumescent technique, for the radiofrequency ablation of lower extremity varicose veins. Int J Dermatol. 2013;52(6):739-44.
40. Breuninger H, Hobbach PS, Schimek F. Ropivacaine: an important anesthetic agent for slow infusion and other forms of tumescent anesthesia. Dermatol Surg. 1999;25(10):799-802.
41. Coldiron BM, Healy C, Bene NI. Office surgery incidents: what seven years of Florida data show us. Dermatol Surg. 2008;34(3):285-91.
42. Hanke W, Cox SE, Kuznets N, Coleman WP 3rd. Tumescent liposuction report performance measurement initiative: national survey results. Dermatol Surg. 2004;30(7):967-78.
43. Klein JA, Kassarjdian N. Lidocaine toxicity with tumescent liposuction. A case report of probable drug interactions. Dermatol Surg. 1997;23(12):1169-74.

CHAPTER 14

Nerve Blocks in Dermatosurgery and Aesthetic Procedures

Savitha AS

KEY MESSAGES

- Nerve blocks are simple procedures with the advantage of not distorting the site of procedure.
- Large areas can be anesthetized with single injection and minimum quantity of anesthesia.
- Complications are vascular puncture bleeding, nerve damage, etc.

INTRODUCTION

As dermatologists are venturing to perform more procedures both aesthetic and surgical, patient comfort and pain avoidance during these procedures should also be given prime importance.

Nerve block is an important mode of anesthesia involving injection of anesthetic agent directly to the nerve or in its vicinity, and has several advantages. These blocks can be useful in procedures such as full-face dermabrasion, botulinum toxin injections to palms and soles, vitiligo surgery, nail surgery, surgery on nose, platelet-rich plasma therapy, hair transplantation, and fillers. Nerve blocks are ideal when a single nerve innervates the region of anesthesia.

ADVANTAGES OF NERVE BLOCKS

- Simple procedure carried out in day-care or outpatient setting
- Small quantities of drugs will anesthetize large areas, thus minimizing the risk of systemic toxicity
- There is no local distortion of tissues, thus preserving appearance
- Preferred option for areas such as digits, face, and ears
- Nerve blocks are better tolerated by the patient, as the number of injection pricks is less, this further reduces the risk of needlestick injury to the surgeon
- Acts longer.

DISADVANTAGES OF NERVE BLOCKS

The surgeon should be well versed with anatomy of the nerve and needs training:

- To cover large areas, sometimes multiple blocks have to be given
- Takes longer time to act
- Failure rate is high
- Local hemostasis due to adrenalin is not there
- Vascular puncture, bleeding, nerve damage, and local anesthetic systemic toxicity are general risks in peripheral nerve block regardless of technique or block location.

CONTRAINDICATIONS TO NERVE BLOCKS IN GENERAL

- Known allergy or sensitivity to the anesthetic agent
- Infection at the injection site
- Distorted anatomical landmarks
- Uncooperative patient
- Physician's lack of familiarity with nerve block.

INDICATIONS

Nerve blocks can be used in most places instead of local infiltration to the lesion. Few special dermatological indications will be mentioned along with the respective blocks.

ANESTHETIC AGENTS[1]

Lignocaine is the commonly used anesthetic agent. Other drugs, which are used as long-acting agents, are ropivacaine, bupivacaine, and mepivacaine. For routine dermatologic procedures, lignocaine is sufficient. The long-acting agents can be used in procedures, which take a long time and also in those which have some postoperative discomfort such as hair transplantation. Though epinephrine certainly has analgesic benefit when used with short- and intermediate-acting local anesthetics, studies with long-acting local anesthetics (e.g., ropivacaine) failed to show an increased duration of analgesia with coadministration of epinephrine. With increased use of ultrasound and potential concerns about neurotoxicity, its use with long-acting agents in nerve blocks is debated. Epinephrine is a valuable marker for intravascular injection. Recent recommendations are to use epinephrine for nerve blocks done without ultrasound guidance, or blocks in which

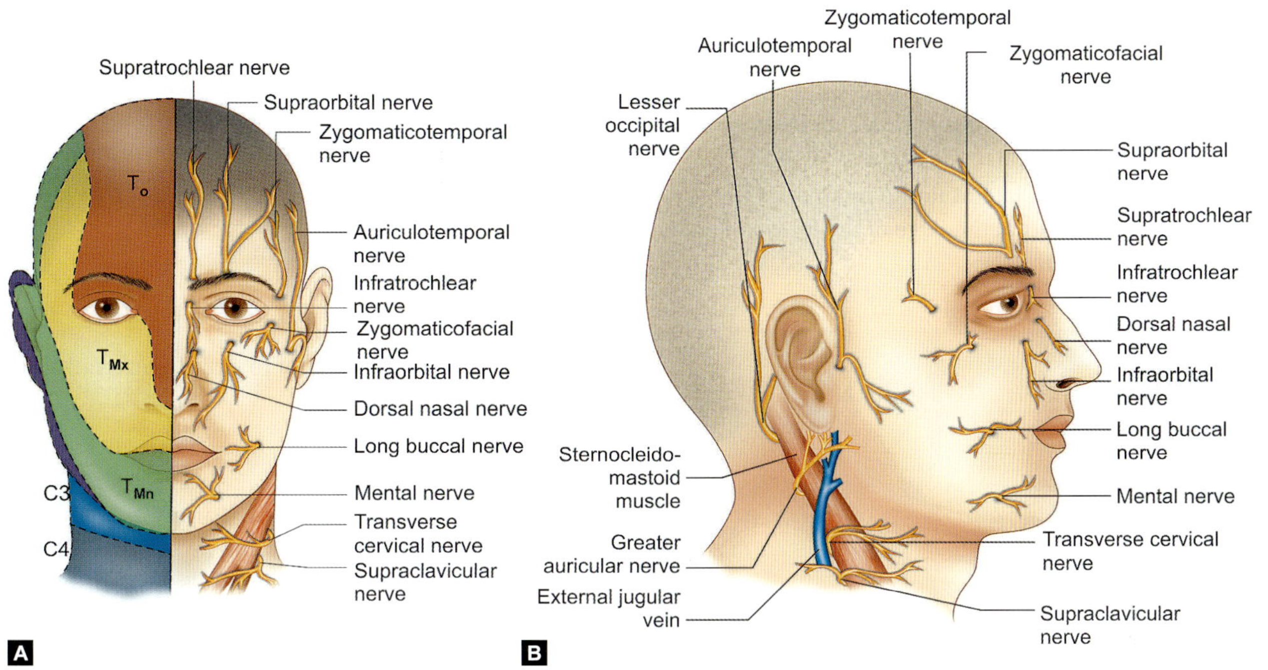

Figs. 1A and B: Sensory innervations of face.

the needle tip and local anesthetic spread are not adequately visualized, as a safety measure to detect intravascular injection.

PREPARATION

Before nerve block is given, the procedure, risks, and potential complications have to be explained to the patient, and consent obtained. A review of regional anatomy and the location of nerves and other important structures also are essential before the injection.

The area to be anesthetized is surgically prepared by cleaning with povidone-iodine prior to injection.

FACIAL NERVE BLOCKS

Dermatological Indications

Hair transplantation, platelet-rich plasma therapy, fat fillers, dermal grafts, dermabrasion, subcision, laser resurfacing, and blepharoplasty.

All the sensory innervations of the face are by the trigeminal nerve and the superficial cervical plexus **(Figs. 1A and B)**.

Supraorbital Nerve Block

The supraorbital nerve block is simple and easy with a very high success rate.

Anatomical Landmark[2]

Supraorbital nerve is a branch of frontal nerve. It exits the supraorbital foramen, and divides into medial and lateral branches, each branch accompanied by its artery to supply medial part of forehead and anterior scalp **(Fig. 2)**.

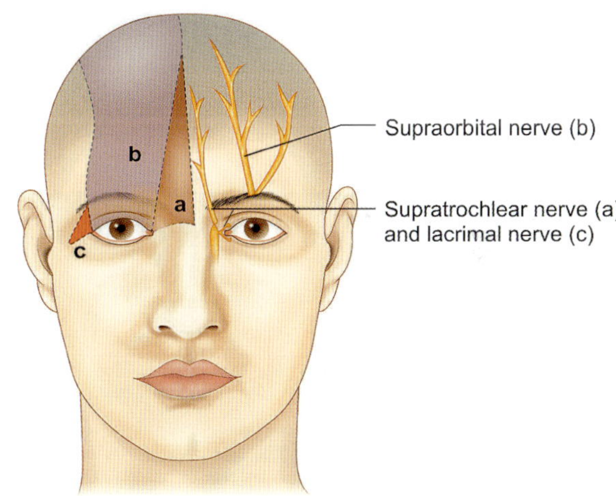

Fig. 2: Supraorbital and supratrochlear nerve and areas supplied by them.

Position

The patient is positioned supine in neutral position with the doctor at the head of the bed.

Procedure

- The supraorbital foramen is located with the pulp of the index finger of nondominant hand and marked with the pen. To locate the supraorbital foramen, the patient is asked to look straight ahead and imagine a line drawn vertically from the pupil up toward the inferior border of the supraorbital ridge. Then palpate along the supraorbital ridge until a subtle notch is felt; this is the supraorbital foramen.

- Another method is to place three fingers centered vertically over glabella, the major branches of supraorbital nerve emerge just lateral to the fingers **(Fig. 3)**.[3]
- Insert the needle just lateral to the foramen, the needle will seek bone contact at the edge of the foramen within 1 cm **(Figs. 4A to D)**.

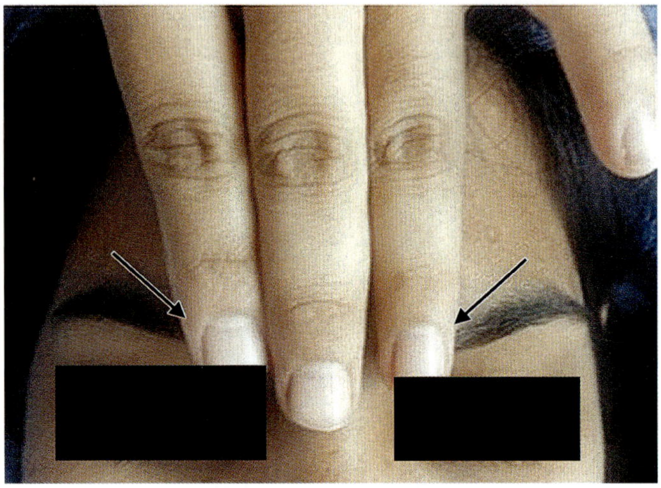

Fig. 3: Surface marking of supraorbital notch.

- Aspiration must be performed, as this area is very vascular. Inject very slowly 1.5–2 mL of anesthetic solution. The needle can be advanced medially to infiltrate the supratrochlear nerve also.
- A discrete massage supports the diffusion of the anesthesia.
- To prevent swelling of the anesthetic into the upper eyelid, it is recommended to firmly place either a finger or a roll of gauze under the orbital rim.[4]

Caution

Advance the needle medially to avoid penetration of the foramen.

Complications

- The puncture of the supraorbital artery
- A transitory palpebral ptosis can be seen, by diffusion of the product toward the elevator muscle of the eyelid
- Paresthesia sequels in the territory of the nerve may occur, because of an edema of the nerve, strangled in its foramen.[4]

Special Indications

Special indications are hair transplantation, upper lid blepharoplasty, and fillers in forehead.

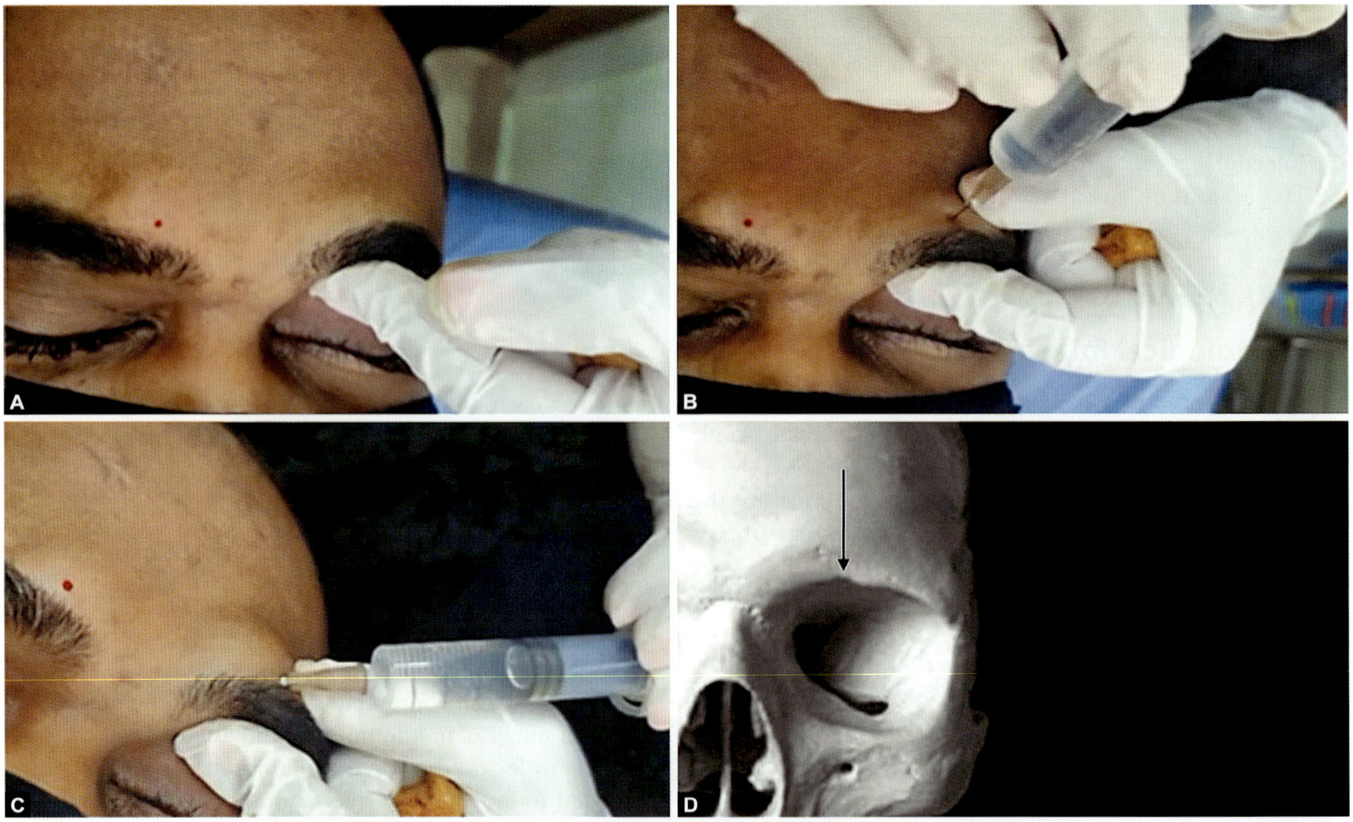

Figs. 4A to D: (A) Palpate the supraorbital notch with index finger of nondominant hand; (B) Insert the needle perpendicular at the lateral margin of the notch; (C) Deposit 1.5–2 mL of anesthetic solution with needle slowly advancing medially; (D) Supraorbital notch.

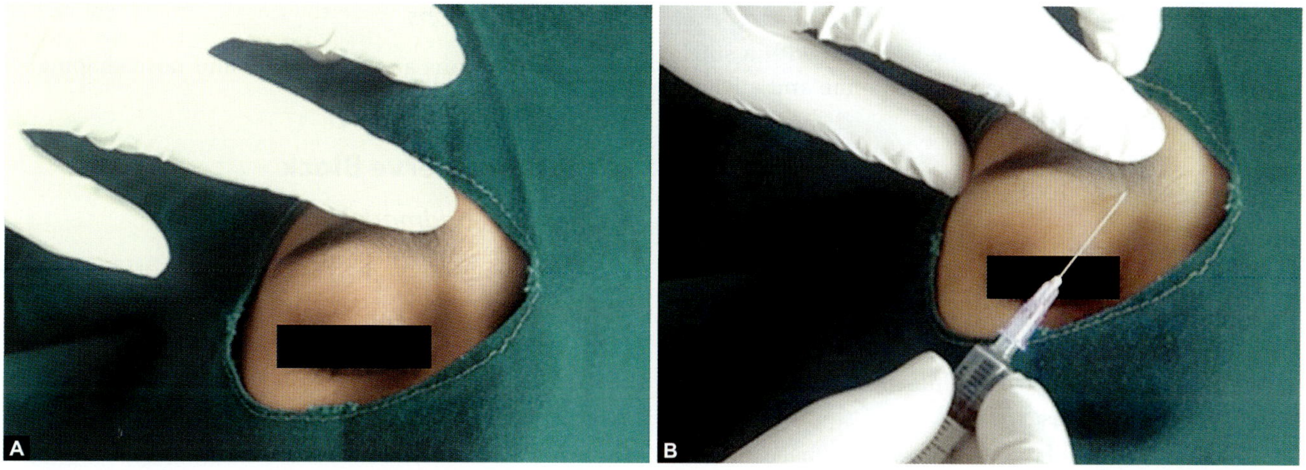

Figs. 5A and B: Supratrochlear nerve block: insertion is on the supraorbital ridge approximately 1 cm medial to the supraorbital notch.

Supratrochlear Nerve Block

The supratrochlear nerve block is often performed along with the supraorbital nerve block to achieve regional anesthesia over the ipsilateral forehead.

Anatomical Landmark

Supratrochlear nerve is also a branch of frontal nerve; it is smaller and exits the orbit 1 cm more medially than supraorbital nerve, above the trochlea (pulley) of the superior oblique muscle **(see Fig. 2)**. Some patients may have either a supratrochlear foramen or an absent supratrochlear notch instead.

Position

Position is same as that of supraorbital block.

Procedure

- As the supratrochlear foramen or notch can be hard to palpate (or even absent in some patients), the supraorbital foramen is often used as a landmark.
- The target area for insertion is on the supraorbital ridge approximately 1 cm medial to the supraorbital notch, between the notch and the bridge of the nose **(Figs. 5A and B)**.
- A discrete massage supports the diffusion of the product.

Complications

- Swelling or ecchymosis may result, if the anesthetic solution infiltrates into the loose areolar tissue of the eyelid.
- Puncture of the angular vein causing a hematoma (potentially obstructing the operative site) has also been described.[4]

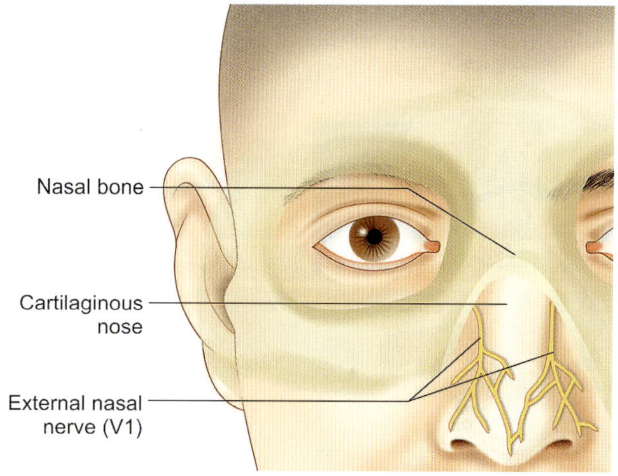

Fig. 6: Nasal nerves.

Special Indications

Special indications are hair transplantation, upper lid blepharoplasty, and filler injections.

Nasal Nerve Block

Dorsal nasal nerve is a branch of anterior ethmoidal nerve and provides sensory innervation to the skin of the lower half of the nose **(Figs. 6 and 7)**.[5]

Anatomical Landmark

The nasal nerve emerges at the lower border of the nasal bone 6–10 mm from the midline **(Fig. 6)**.

Procedure (Figs. 8A to C)

- With the nondominant hand, palpate the junction between the nasal bone and mobile cartilage.
- Insert the needle 5 mm lateral to midline and inject 1 mL of the anesthetic agent.

- Repeat the procedure on other side.
- Alternately, both nerves can be accessed with a single injection. Insert the needle in the midline and advance inferolateral on either side.

Regional Anesthesia to the Nose (Figs. 9A to C)

- Two injections will be necessary to block the area completely.
- First is at the root of the nose, at the level of the interior angle of the eye, an infiltration, closer to the nasal bone, with a direction toward the nasal base—blocks the infratrochlear and nasal nerve.
- Second, in the axis of nasal ala; toward its base and alar joint—blocks the area of infraorbital nerve.
- The injection must be particularly slow because the area is very sensitive: 1 mL on the first site and 1.5 mL of anesthetic solution, on the second site.[4]

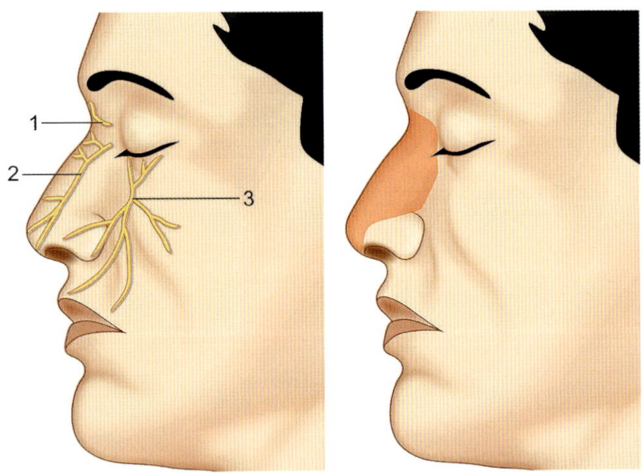

Fig. 7: Nerve supply to the nose (1—infratrochlear, 2—dorsal nasal, and 3—infraorbital; area in red is supplied by dorsal nasal nerve).

Special Indications

Special indications are rhinoplasty and nose shaping with fillers.

Infraorbital Nerve Block

Anatomical Landmark (Figs. 10A and B)

The infraorbital nerve leaves by the infraorbital foramen located at 4–7 mm below the infraorbital bone edge.

Procedure

Extraoral technique ***(Figs. 11A to D)****:*

- To locate the infraorbital foramen, the patient is asked to look straight ahead and imagine a line drawn vertically from the pupil down to the superior border of the infraorbital ridge. Then palpate along the ridge until a subtle notch is felt; this is the infraorbital notch. The infraorbital foramen is located about 4–7 mm below this notch.
- The point of puncture is done on the level of the lateral edge of the foramen.
- The needle will seek the bone contact (with <10 mm) at the edge of the foramen.
- The needle should be directed cephalic and medially and inject 1.5–2 mL of anesthetic solution after aspiration.
- The axis of the infraorbital foramen look toward the ala of the nose, so it is better to prick with a needle directed toward the root of the nose **(Figs. 11A to D)**.[6]

Caution: During the extraoral technique, the needle is in very close proximity to the facial artery. Because of this proximity, it is better to avoid adding vasoconstrictors to anesthetic solutions.

Complications

- Puncture of the infraorbital artery
- Paresthesia due to an edema of the nerve strangled in its foramen

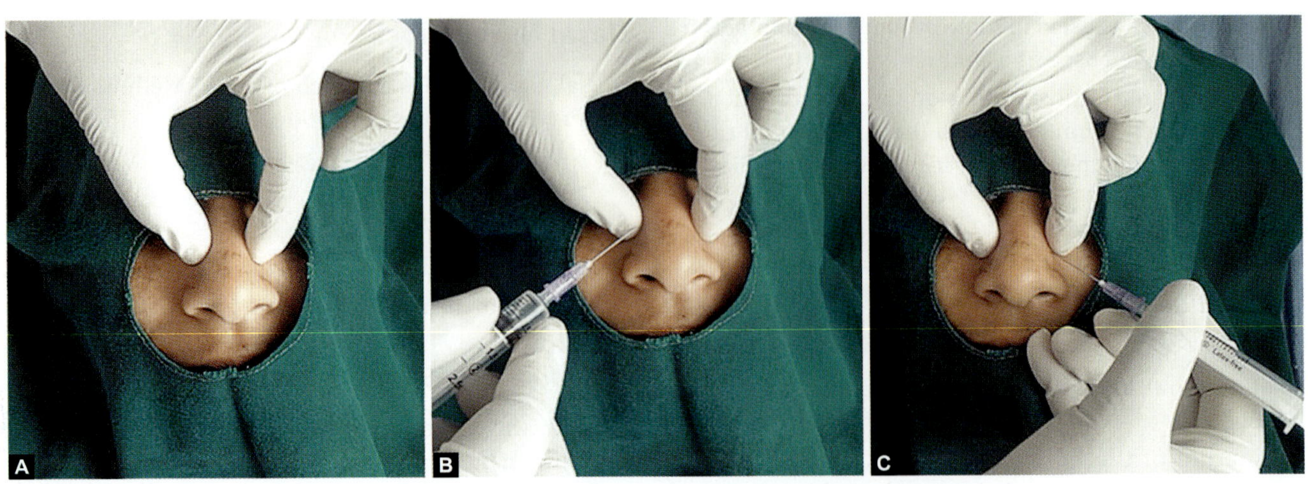

Figs 8A to C: (A) With your nondominant hand, palpate the junction between the firm nasal bone and mobile nasal cartilage; (B) Insert the needle 5 mm lateral to midline at the junction; (C) Repeat the procedure on the other side.

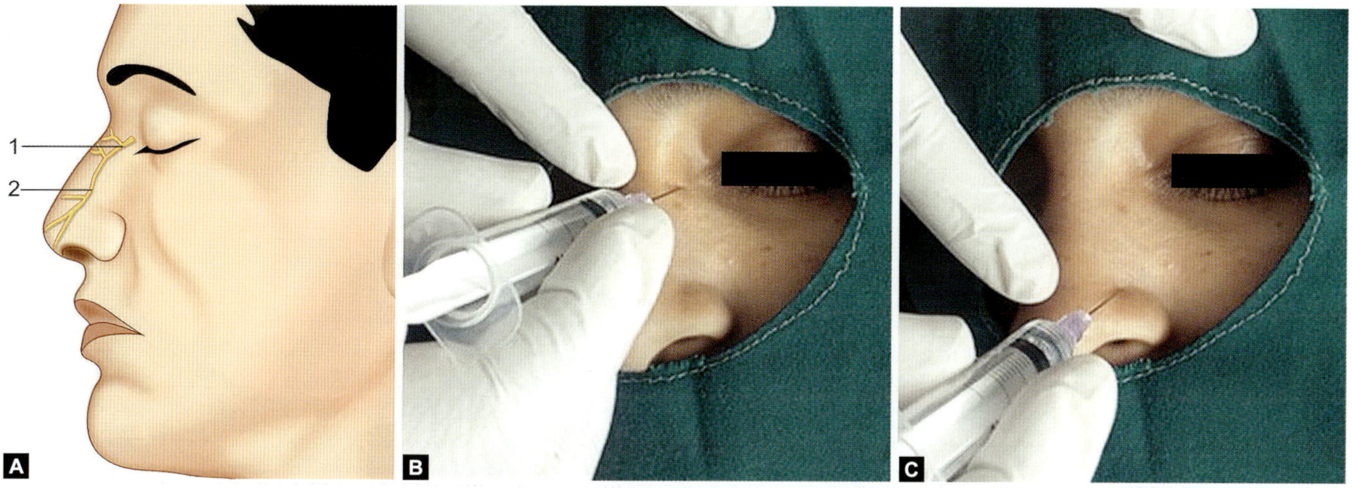

Figs. 9A to C: Regional block to nose. (A) 1—infratrochlear nerve and 2—nasal nerve; (B) Infiltration at root of nose 1 mL; (C) Infiltration at the ala—1.5 mL.

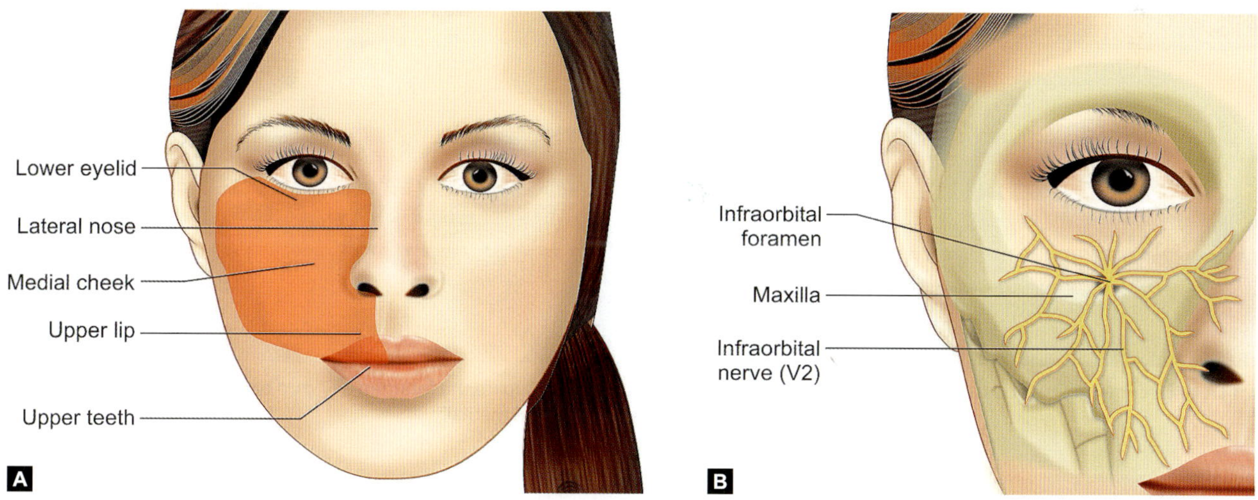

Figs. 10A and B: Infraorbital nerve sensory supply.

- Transitory paralysis of the extrinsic muscles of the ocular sphere by orbital passage of the anesthetic solution.

Endo-oral method (three and half method) ***(Figs. 12A to C)****:*[7]

- Palpate the infraorbital foramen with the middle finger of nondominant hand
- Hold the lip with the thumb and index finger
- Insert the needle at the upper canine tooth into the buccal recess directed toward the foramen. As the needle is inserted between the canine and first premolar, it is called the three and a half method
- Inject 2–3 mL of anesthetic solution after aspiration.

Caution: Difficult and more sensitive with risks of dysesthesias with injection in the infraorbital foramen.

Special Indications

These are acne scar surgeries, dermal fillers, fat transplants, dimple creation procedures, and upper lip surgeries.

Lacrimal Nerve

The lacrimal nerve is one of the terminal branches of the ophthalmic nerve. The nerve innervates the lacrimal gland and gives sensory supply to lateral part of upper eyelid and adjacent area of temple **(see Fig. 2)**.

Procedure

The needle is inserted at the lateral end of the eyebrow pointing upward toward the temple and 0.5 mL of solution is injected **(Fig. 13)**.

Long Buccal Nerve

The buccal nerve is situated just beneath the soft tissue and not within bone, so the success rate is very high. It is a pure sensory nerve and supplies the upper lip at the angle of the mouth **(Fig. 14)**.

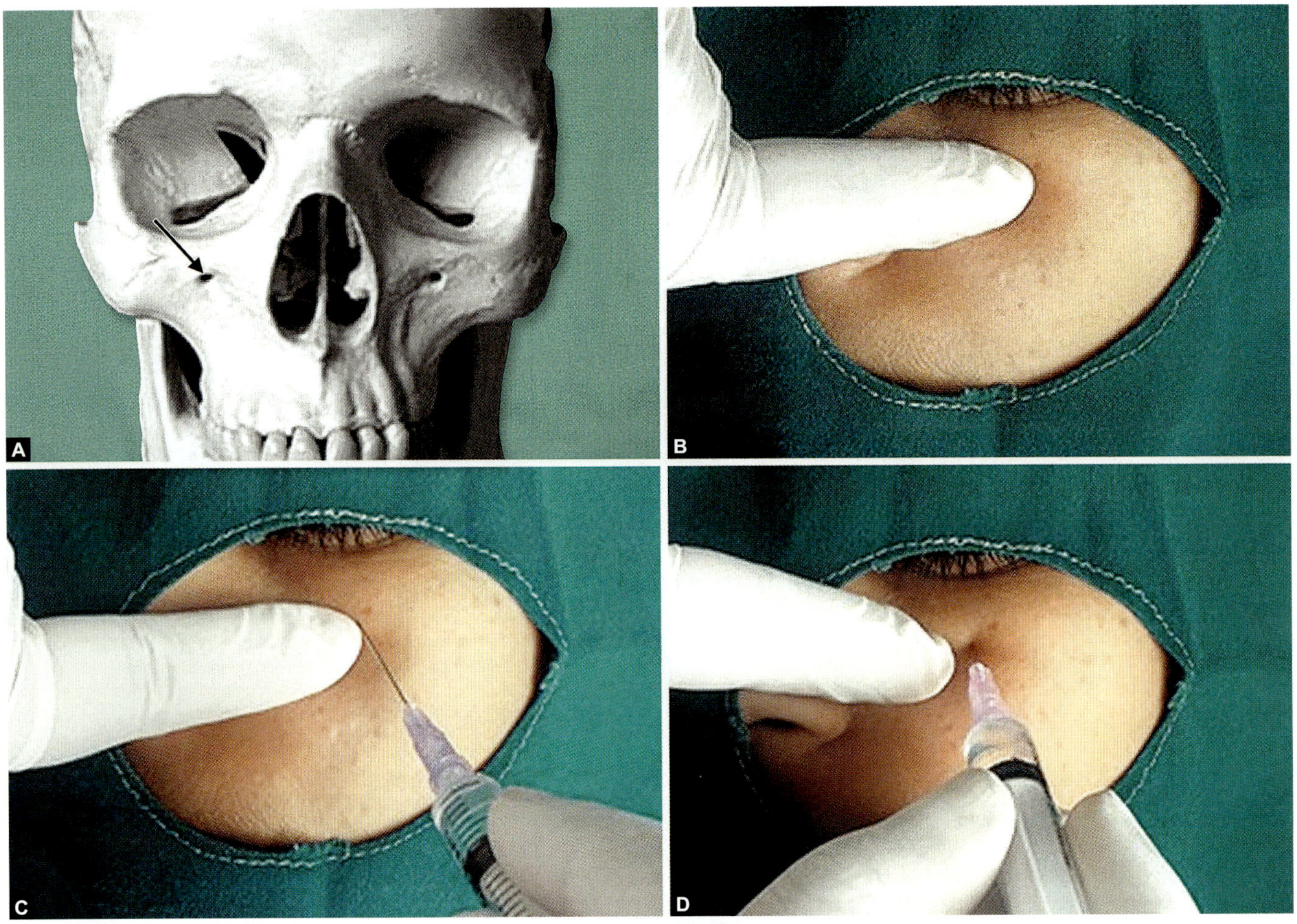

Figs. 11A to D: Extraoral method for infraorbital block. (A) Infraorbital foramen; (B) Palpate the foramen 5–7 mm below the infraorbital notch; and (C and D) Insert needle cephalic and medially.

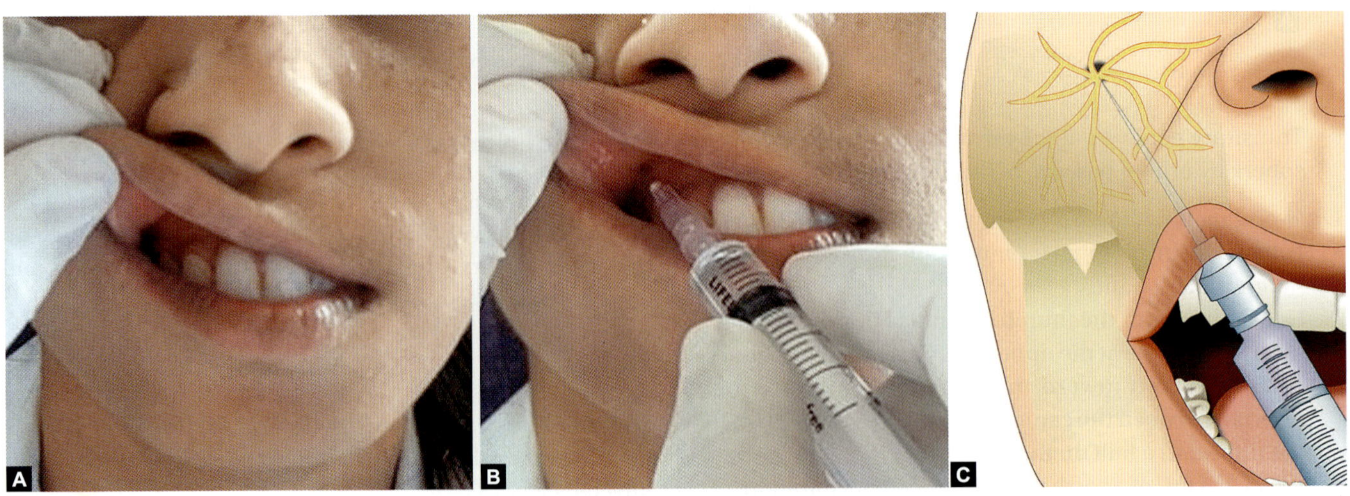

Figs. 12A to C: Intraoral method for infraorbital block. (A) Palpate infraorbital foramen; (B) Insert needle between incisor and first premolar into buccal recess; (C) Schematic diagram of the block.

Procedure

Intraoral method ***(Fig. 15)****:*[8,9]

- Injection site is located on the buccal mucosa distal to the third molar.
- The bevel of the needle should be toward the bone and inserted at a depth of 1–3 mm with the buccal soft tissue lateral and taut. The syringe should be parallel to the occlusal plane.

Transcutaneous method: Inject 2–3 cm lateral and superior to angle of mouth with needle pointing toward mouth **(Fig. 16)**.

Special Indications

Special indications are procedures at the angle of the mouth and lip augmentation.

Mental Nerve

Anatomical Landmark

The mental nerve is the terminal branch of the inferior alveolar nerve. It enters the face through the mental foramen and supplies the inferior lip and the chin **(Figs. 17A and B)**.

Procedure

Intraoral approach (four and a half method) ***(Fig. 18)****:*

- The intraoral approach to the mental nerve block with adjunctive topical anesthesia has been reported as subjectively and objectively less painful than the percutaneous approach.[10]
- The mental foramen is palpable between the two lower premolar teeth. Locate the mental foramen with the nondominant hand and insert the needle along the lower gum line into the buccal fold between the premolar teeth near the foramen. As the needle is inserted between two premolars, it is called four and half method.
- Do not place the needle directly into the foramen. Aspirate and inject 2–3 mL of anesthetic solution.

Transcutaneous route:

- Mental foramen is located 1 cm inferior and slightly anterior to the second premolar. It is in line with the mid-pupil on forward gaze. A line drawn through supraorbital and infraorbital foramen passes through the mental foramen **(Fig. 19)**.[11]
- Insert the needle at a point overlying the mental foramen
- Advance the needle perpendicular to bone until periosteum is reached, aspirate and inject 2–3 mL of

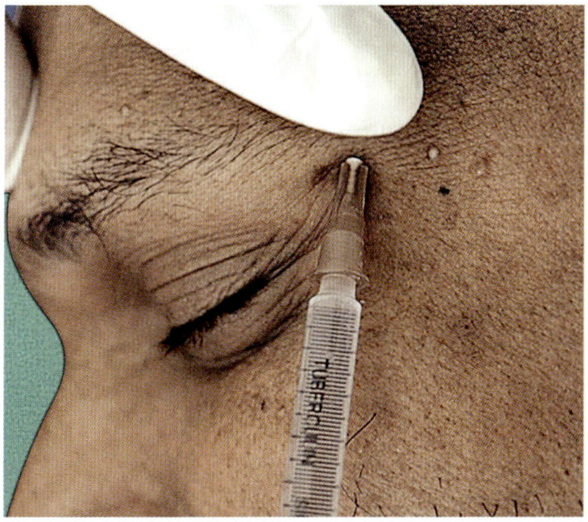

Fig. 13: Lacrimal nerve block.

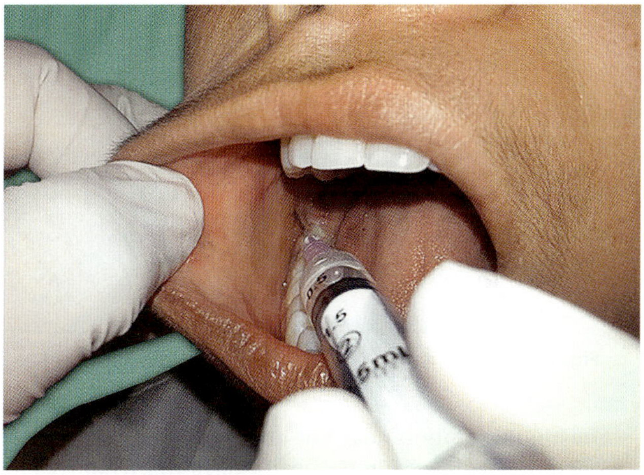

Fig. 15: Long buccal nerve block—intraoral method.

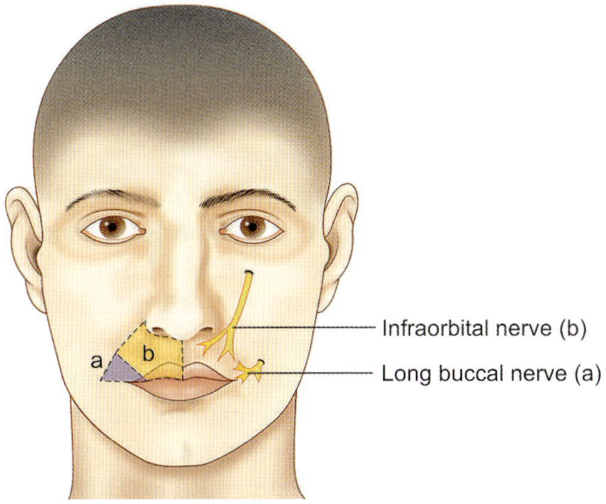

Fig. 14: Long buccal nerve and area supplied by it.

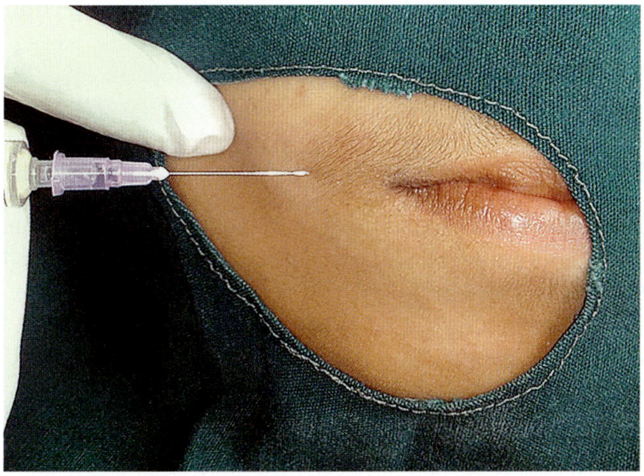

Fig. 16: Transcutaneous long buccal nerve block.

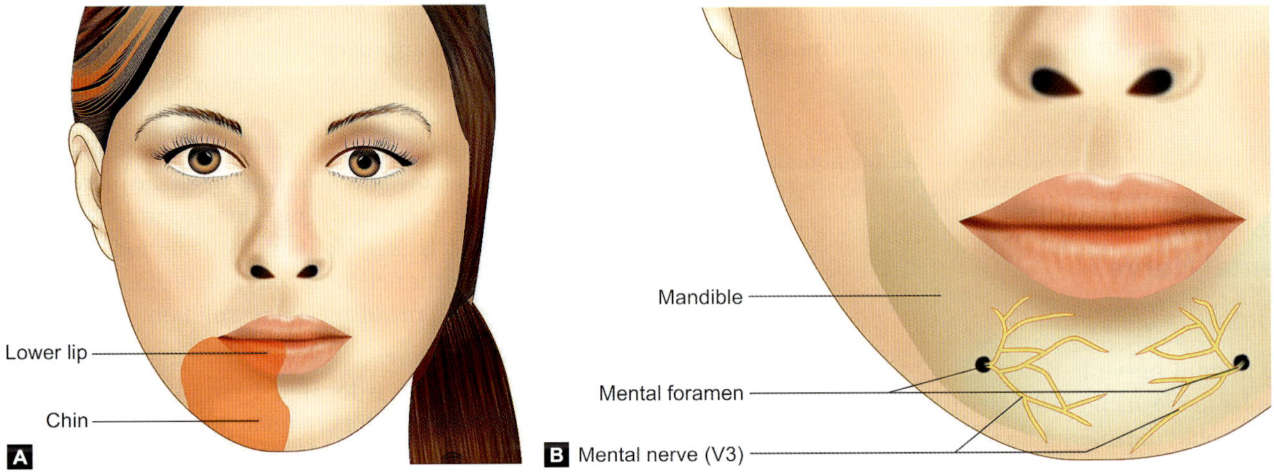

Figs. 17A and B: Mental nerve and area supplied by it.

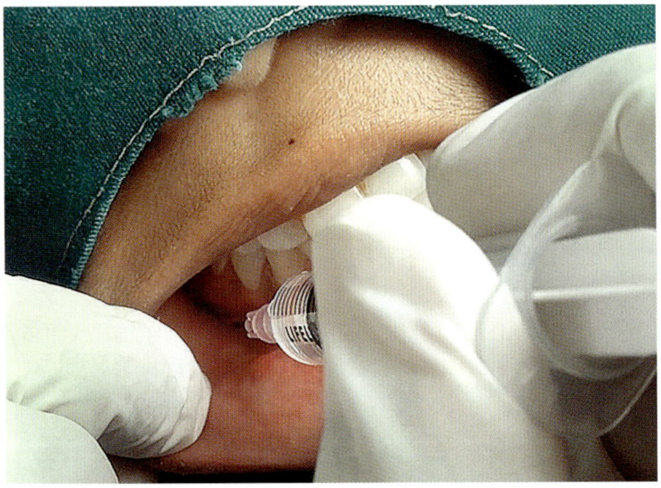

Fig. 18: Transoral mental nerve block—four and half method.

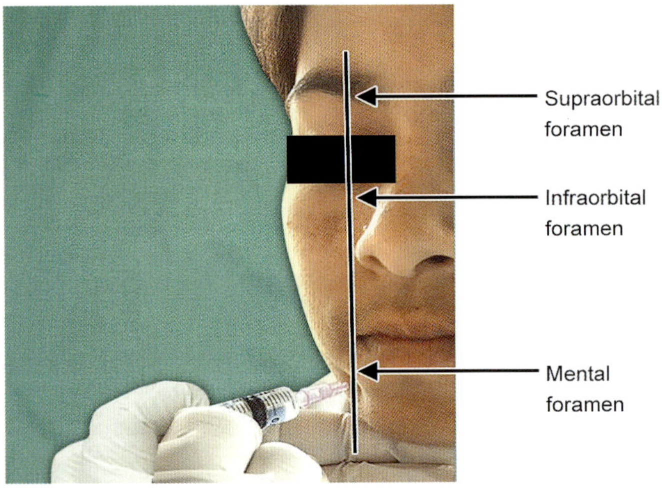

Fig. 19: Surface marking and mental nerve block.

anesthetic solution near but not in the mental foramen, and redirect the needle, if paresthesia or sharp pain occurs.

Special Indications

Special indications are lower lip surgery and filler injections.

NERVE BLOCKS FOR HAIR TRANSPLANTATION

Sensory Supply of Scalp[12]

The following six sensory nerve branches of the trigeminal nerve and the cervical nerve supply the scalp as shown in **Figures 20A and B**.

The common blocks used in hair transplantation are:[3]

- Greater occipital nerve block
- Supraorbital and supratrochlear nerve block
- Auriculotemporal block
- Zygomaticotemporal block

  With these blocks, most of the scalp can be anesthetized.

Greater Occipital Nerve Block

Anatomical Landmark

The greater occipital nerve runs on the lateral aspect of external occipital protuberance along with the occipital artery, which lies medial to it **(Figs. 21A to C)**.

Procedure

- The patient is in prone position
- Mark the mastoid process and the inion, which is the midline highest point on occipital protuberance.
- Injection point is at the proximal one-third of an imaginary line joining these two points. 2–2.5 mL of anesthetic solution is injected. The needle is inserted vertically at this point, and one-third of the anesthetic solution is injected. Then the needle is withdrawn up to subcutaneous plane, the angle of the needle changed by 30° to either side to inject the remaining anesthetic solution. This ensures the anesthetic is injected in a 60° arc around the nerve.

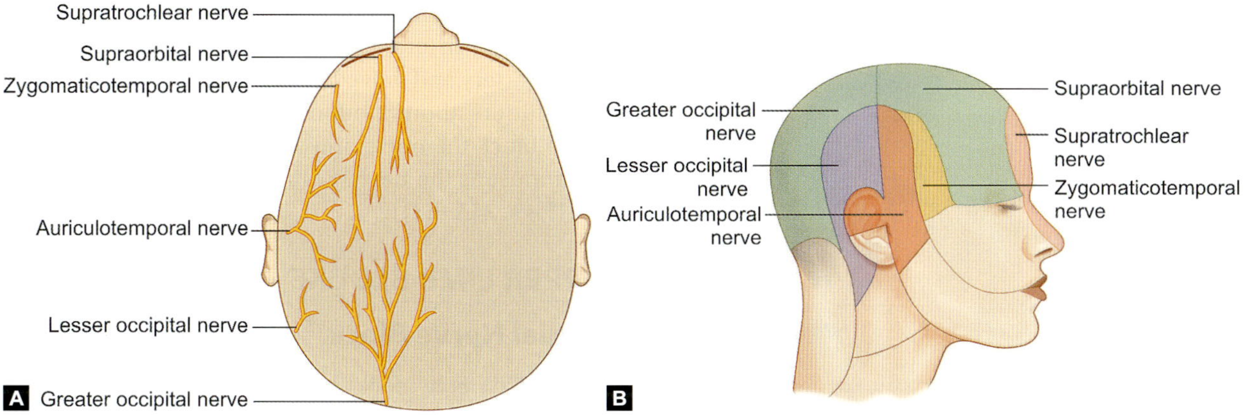

Figs. 20A and B: Sensory supply of the scalp.

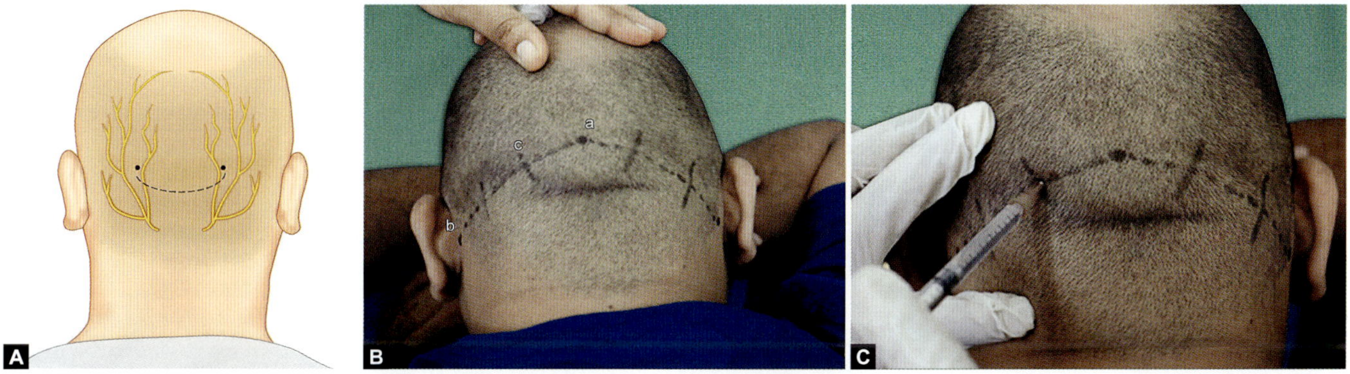

Figs. 21A to C: (A) The greater occipital nerve lies lateral to occipital protuberance; (B) a—inion, b—mastoid process, c—proximal one-third of the line joining the inion and mastoid process; (C) Injection point for greater occipital nerve block.

- To block the lesser occipital nerve, injection is given at the distal one-third of the line closer to mastoid process.

Zygomaticotemporal Nerve

Anatomical Landmark

The nerve lies 1.5 cm lateral to the outer canthus on the zygomatic arch. It emerges through a foramen located on the anterior wall of temporal fossa **(Fig. 22)**.

Procedure

- Palpate the lateral orbital rim at the level of frontozygomatic suture, which is usually palpable
- Place the index finger in the depression posterior to lateral orbital rim, insert the needle just behind the finger
- The needle is slowly advanced down along the posterior border of the lateral orbital rim. Aspirate and inject 1.5–2 mL of anesthetic agent **(Figs. 23)**.

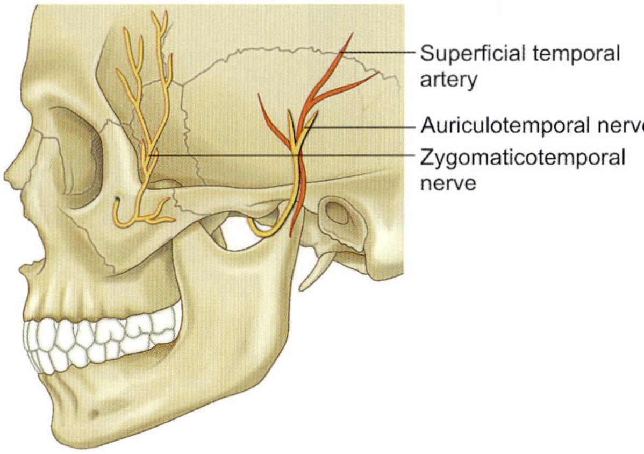

Fig. 22: Zygomaticotemporal and auriculotemporal nerve.

Auriculotemporal Nerve Block

Anatomical Landmark

This nerve originates from the posterior trunk of mandibular nerve, emerges from the superior border of parotid gland between the tragus and temporomandibular joint. It lies in close proximity to superficial temporal artery. It supplies part of the auricle, temporal, and temporoparietal area of scalp **(Fig. 22)**.

Procedure

- The patient is in supine position with the doctor on the side of the nerve to be injected and patient's head turned to contralateral side.

- Palpate the temporal artery, as it crosses the zygomatic arch near the root of the zygoma (just anterior to tragus).

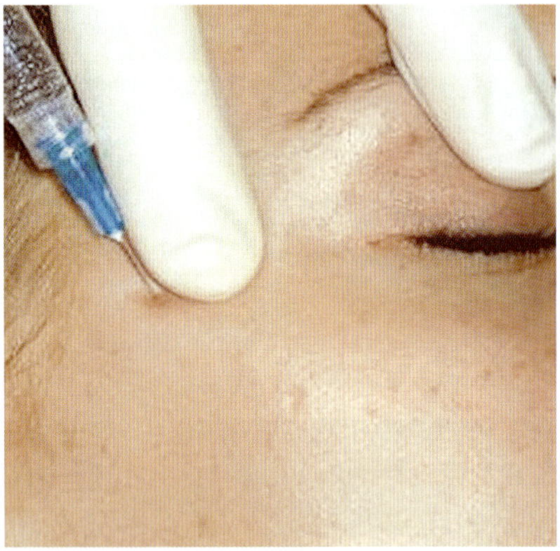

Fig. 23: Zygomaticotemporal nerve block.

This gives an approximate location of the nerve. The needle is inserted medial to the finger placed to palpate the artery and moved behind the artery.

- Infiltrate about 2 mL of anesthetic solution in the area to block the nerve and terminal branches. Aspiration is a must as the nerve lies in close proximity to the artery **(Figs. 24A to D)**.

UPPER LIMB BLOCKS

Radial Nerve Block[13]

The radial nerve block at the wrist level is essentially a field block and requires a more extensive infiltration because of its less predictable anatomic location and division into multiple, smaller cutaneous branches **(Figs. 24A to D)**.

Procedure (Figs. 25A and B)

- Palpate the radial styloid and radial artery to establish landmarks

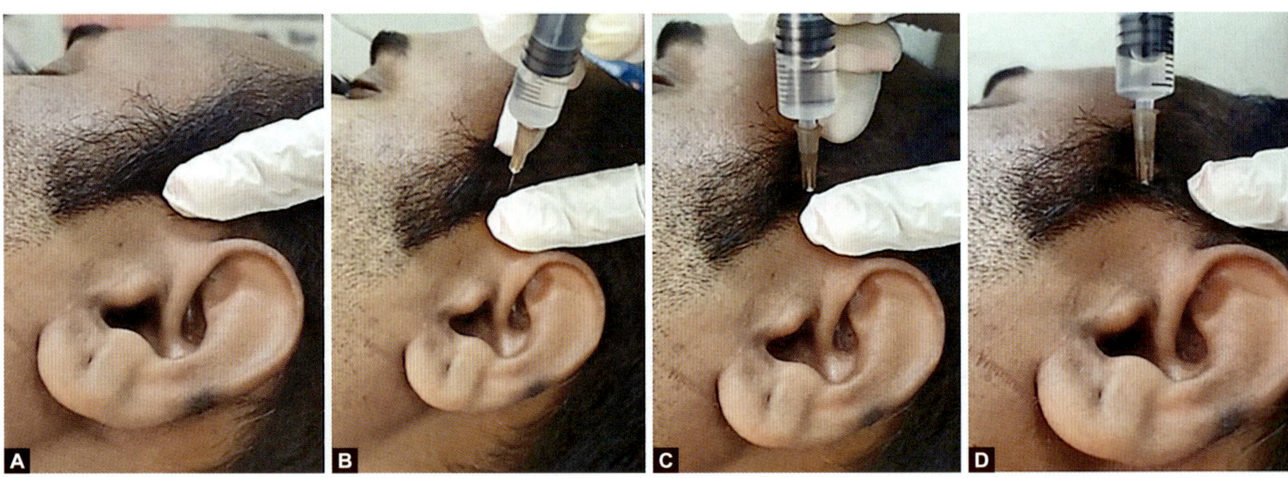

Figs. 24A to D: Auriculotemporal nerve block.

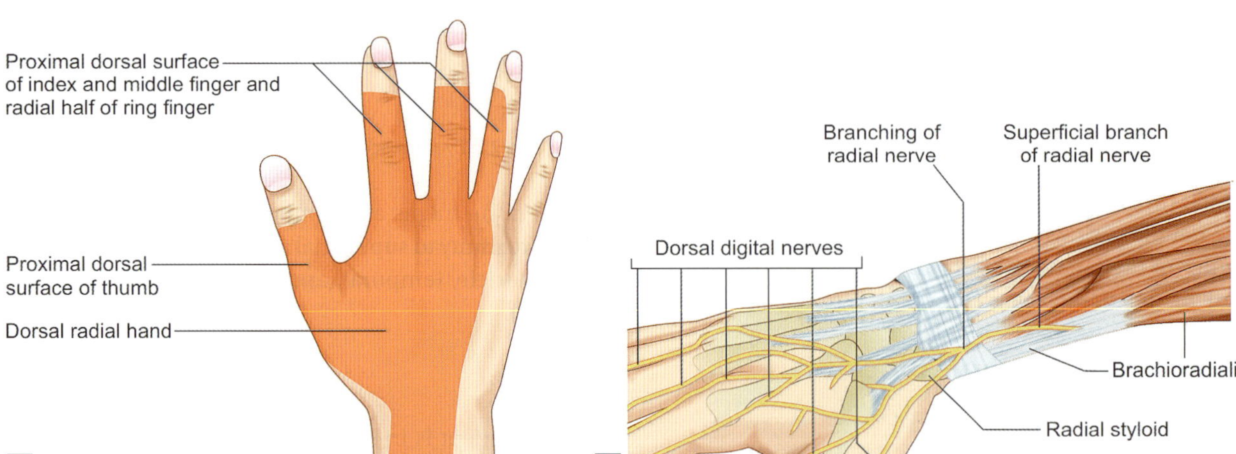

Figs. 25A and B: Branches of radial nerve and sensory supply.

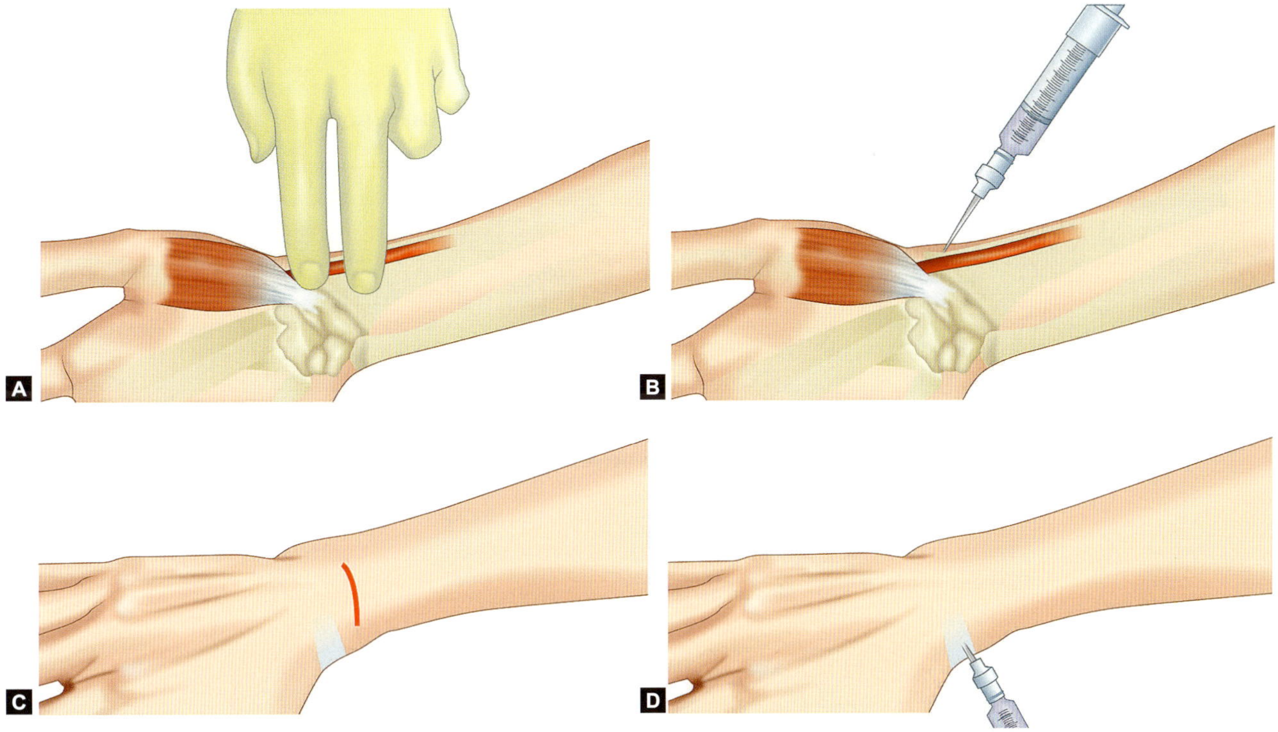

Figs. 26A to D: Radial nerve block. (A) Palpate the radial artery; (B) Inject 2 mL of anesthetic solution lateral to radial artery; (C and D) From point of entry, continue the block to dorsal aspect.

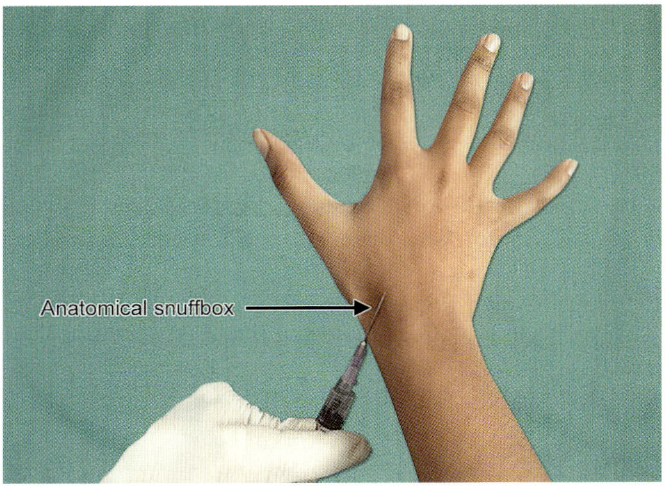

Fig. 27: Radial nerve block by injecting across anatomical snuffbox.

- Inject 2–3 mL of anesthetic solution lateral to the radial artery, at the junction of radial styloid and palmar crease
- From the point of entry, continue the field block till dorsal midpoint of the wrist.

Other method is to direct the needle from lateral to medial side of snuffbox **(Figs. 26 and 27)**.

Complications

Residual paresthesia due to an inadvertent intraneural injection

Median Nerve Block (Wrist Block)

Anatomical Landmark

At the wrist, the median nerve lies within the carpal tunnel, deep and radial to the palmaris longus (PL) tendon and medial to the flexor carpi radialis (FCR) tendon **(Fig. 28)**.

Procedure (Figs. 29A and B)

- The needle is inserted perpendicular to the skin between the PL and FCR tendons, angled such as to place the needle tip directly beneath the PL.
- The injection is made 2–3 cm proximal to the distal crease of the wrist to avoid injecting within the carpal tunnel.
- The location of the PL and FCR tendons can be highlighted by having the patient flex the middle finger against resistance or pinch the thumb and little finger together **(Fig. 29B)**.
- The needle is inserted to a depth of 1–2 cm. Passage through the fibrous flexor retinaculum may be felt. Injecting in a space too deep is better than in a space too shallow, as the retinaculum prevents anesthetic solution from reaching the nerve, if injected too superficially. An anesthetic volume of 3–5 mL is appropriate.
- To include the peripheral (palmar) branches, a small wheal of anesthetic solution is placed subcutaneously, as the needle is withdrawn and massaged gently over the volar wrist.

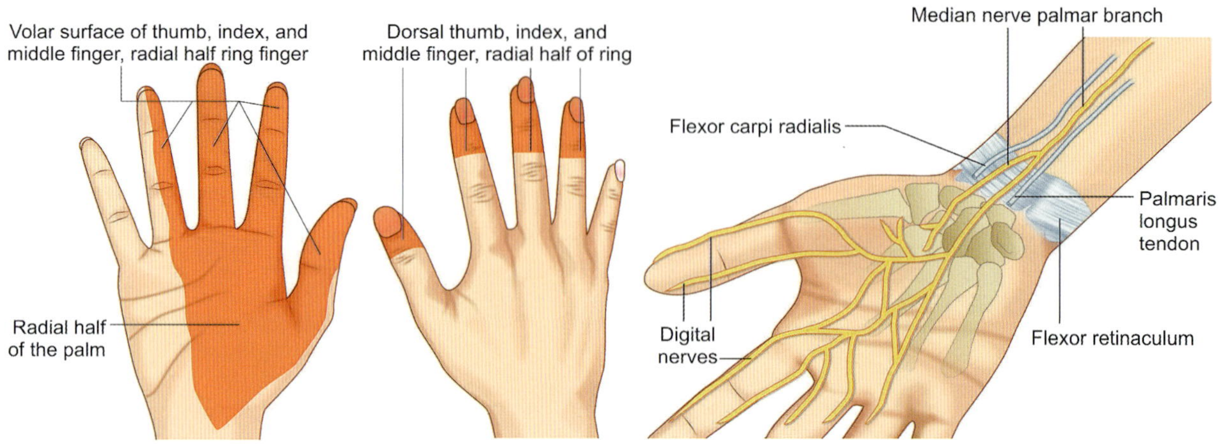

Fig. 28: Branches of median nerve and sensory supply.

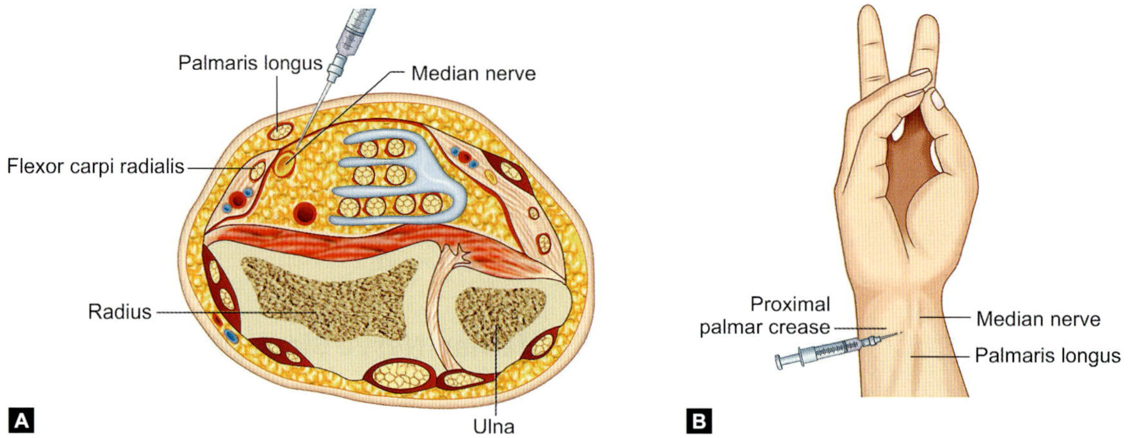

Figs. 29A and B: Median nerve block. (A) Anatomical location of nerve; (B) Schematic representation of median nerve block.

Special Indications

Median and radial nerve blocks can be utilized during botulinum toxin injections for palmar hyperhidrosis and removal of multiple corn or warts.

Ulnar Nerve Block

Anatomical Landmark

At the wrist, the ulnar nerve lies lateral to flexor carpi ulnaris tendon **(Fig. 30)**.

Procedure (Figs. 31A to D)

- Dorsiflexion at the wrist joint is the position for injection of anesthesia, this makes the flexor carpi ulnaris tendon prominent **(Fig. 31A)**
- Insert the needle beneath the tendon or just lateral to it, to a depth of 2–3 cm **(Fig. 31B)**, eliciting paresthesia indicates proper placement. Withdraw the needle several centimeters before infiltrating the nerve. About 2 mL of anesthetic agent needs to be deposited.
- To infiltrate the dorsal branches, insert the needle medial to the tendon and proceed medially for about 2 cm **(Fig. 31C)**.
- The pisiform bone also can be used as a landmark, infiltrating the agent lateral to it **(Fig. 31D)**.

Digital Nerve Blocks

Anatomy[14]

Each digit is innervated by four digital nerves. The two palmar digital nerves innervate the palmar aspect of the digit and the nail bed, whereas the dorsal nerves innervate the dorsum of the digit **(Fig. 32)**.

Proximal Digital Nerve Block (Fig. 33)

- Patient's hand should be placed flat on the table with palm down.
- The syringe is inserted perpendicularly into the web space, just distal to the metacarpophalangeal (MP) joint, lateral to extensor tendon
- The anesthetic solution is injected slowly through the dorsal aspect of the web space, advance the needle

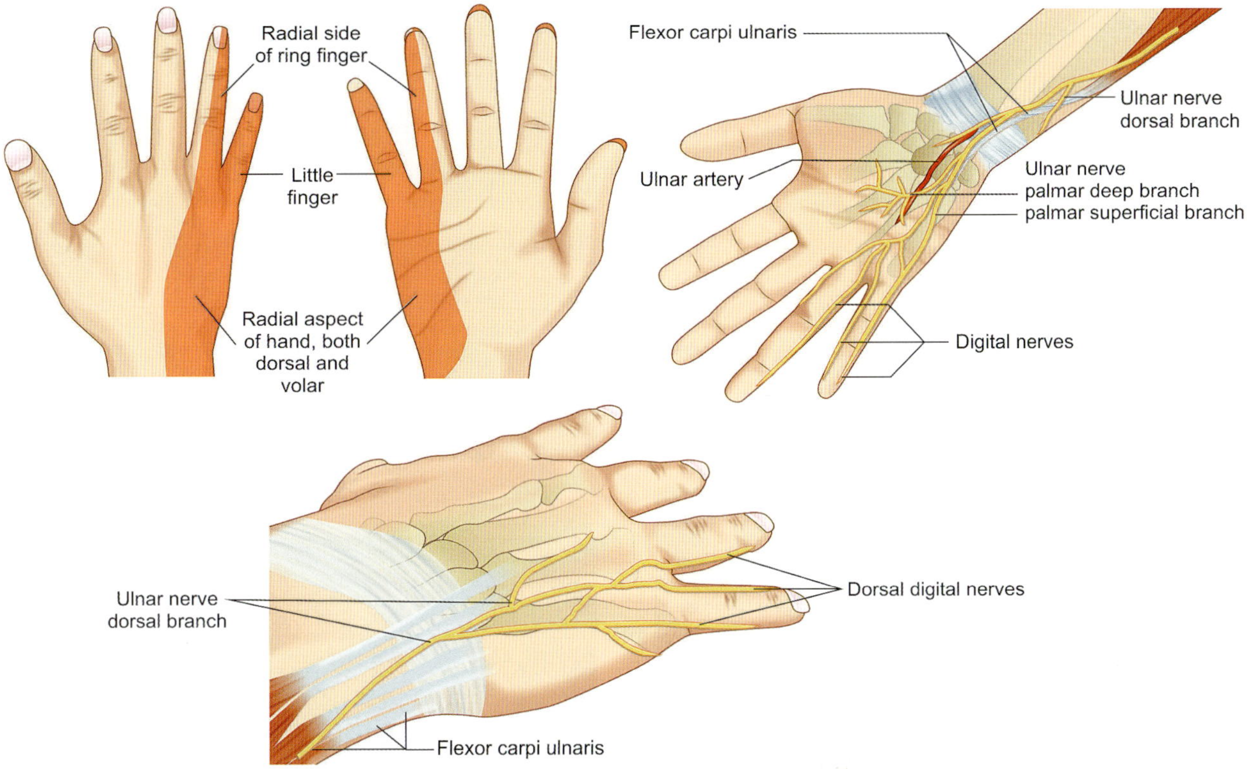

Fig. 30: Branches and sensory supply of ulnar nerve.

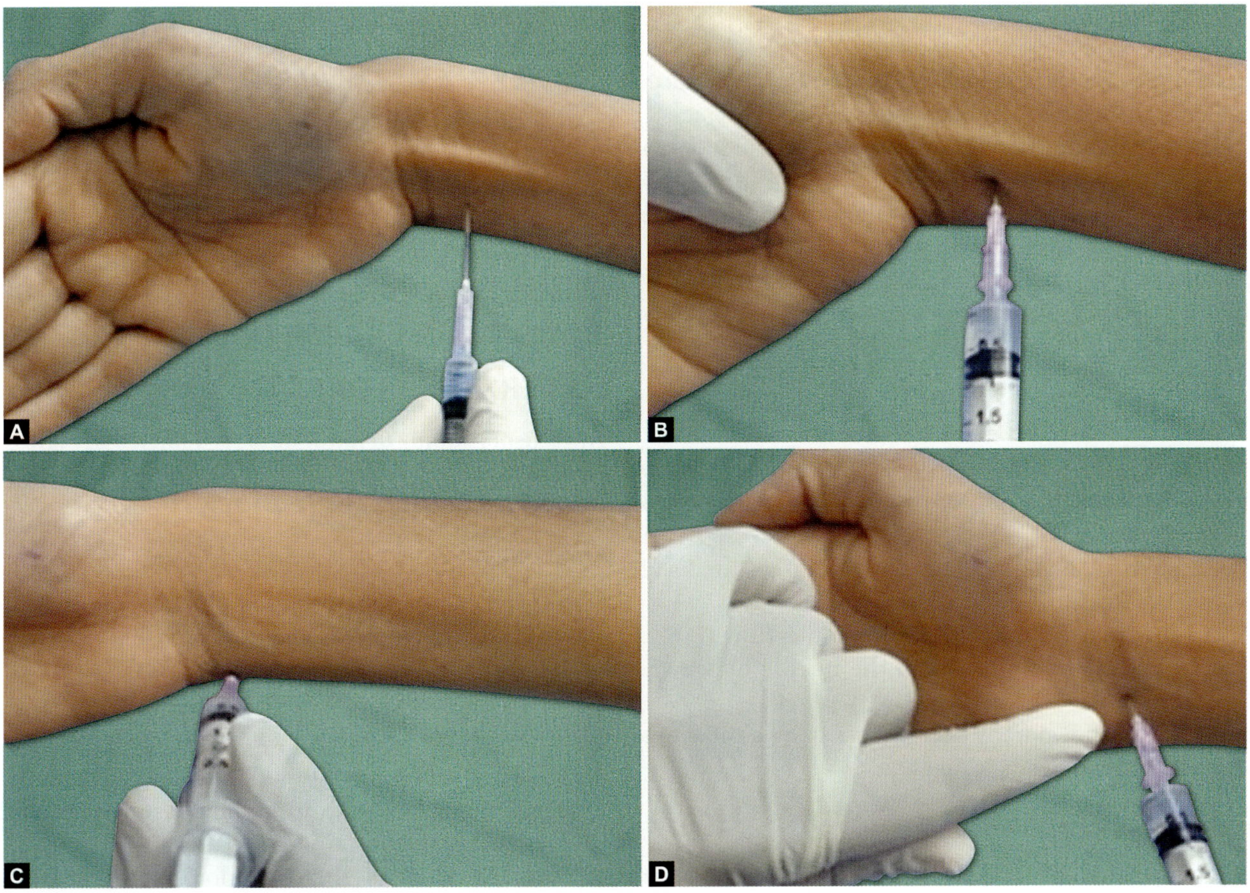

Figs. 31A to D: Ulnar nerve block.

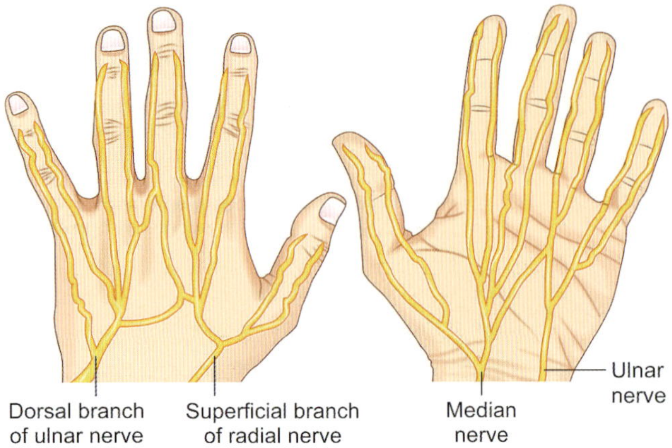

Fig. 32: Palmar and dorsal digital nerves.

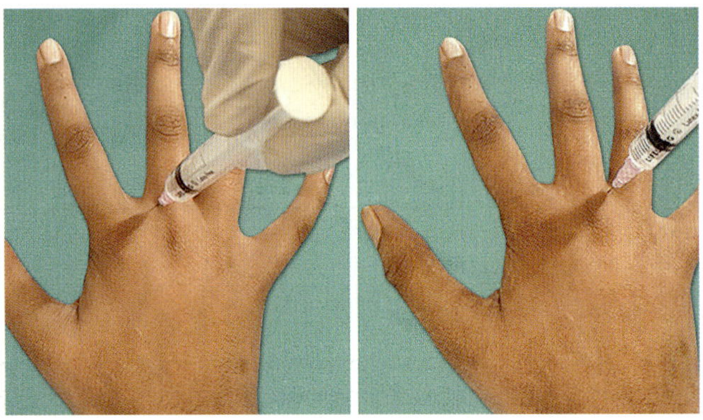

Fig. 33: Proximal digital nerve block.

straight down toward the volar aspect of the web space, and infiltrate the surrounding tissues of the web space

- The needle should not pierce the volar aspect of the web space
- Withdraw the needle and repeat the procedure on the other web space of the involved digit
- The toes (except the great toe) can be effectively anesthetized in the same manner.

Caution: Direct the needle inwards and downwards.

Transthecal Block (Fig. 34)[15]

- Place the patient's hand on the sterile field with the palm up
- Locate the flexor tendon sheath by palpating it at the distal palmar crease
- Insert the needle at a 45° angle just distal to the distal palmar crease
- Inject the anesthetic solution; it should flow freely. If resistance is met, reposition the needle by slowly withdrawing it
- Studies have shown transthecal blocks to be as effective as ring blocks for digital analgesia.

Distal Digital Block (Wing Block)[16]

Distal digital block offers total nail unit anesthesia. Here, the needle is inserted 2–3 mm proximal to the junction of proximal and lateral nailfold. Insert the needle vertically and advance toward ventral aspect injecting about 0.5–1 mL of anesthetic agent **(Fig. 35)**. Three types of distal digital blocks with areas covered are illustrated in **Figure 36**.

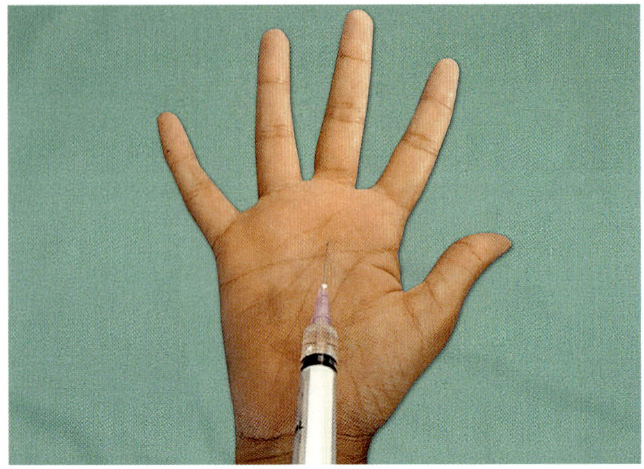

Fig. 34: Transthecal block.

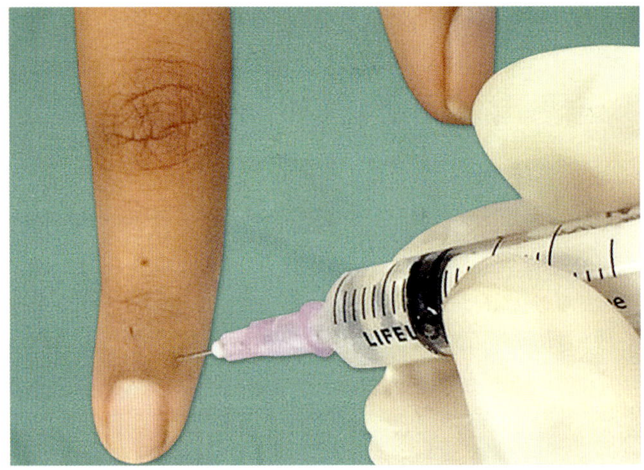

Fig. 35: Distal digital block.

LOWER LIMB BLOCKS

The sensory supply of lower limbs is depicted in **Figure 37**.

Posterior Tibial Nerve Block

Anatomical Landmark

At the level of ankle, the posterior tibial nerve can be found midway between the medial malleolus and the heel. The nerve lies beneath the flexor retinaculum **(Fig. 38)**.

Procedure (Figs. 39A to D)[17]

- Begin by palpating the medial malleolus and advance posteroinferiorly toward the Achilles tendon, until the pulsation of the posterior tibial artery is felt
- Mark the point 0.5–1 cm superior to the posterior tibial artery

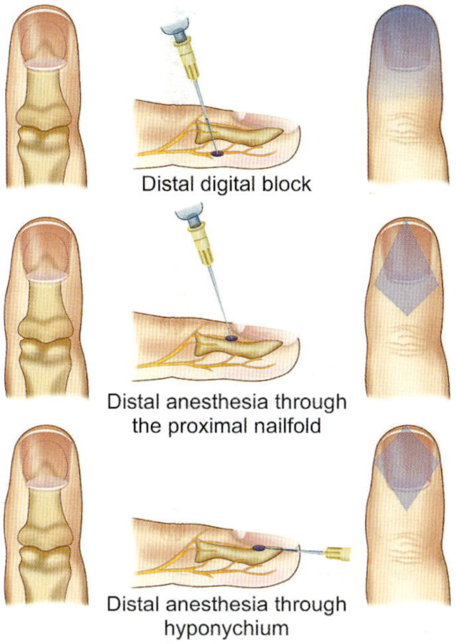

Fig. 36: Three types of distal digital blocks with areas covered.

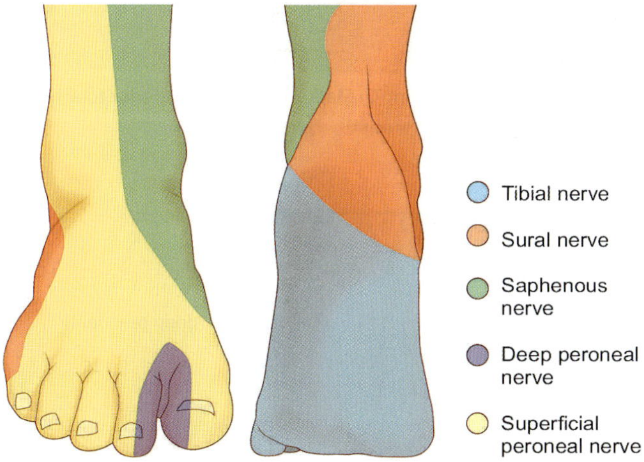

Fig. 37: Sensory supply of lower limb.

- If the artery is not palpable, mark a point 1 cm superior to the medial malleolus and slightly anterior to the Achilles tendon
- Advance the needle through the skin toward the tibia at a 45° angle in a mediolateral plane, just posterior to the artery
- Wiggle the needle slightly to induce paresthesia. If elicited, aspirate to make sure the needle is not in a vessel, wait for the paresthesia to resolve, and inject 3–5 mL
- If paresthesia is not elicited, advance the needle at a 45° angle until it meets the posterior tibia. Withdraw 1 cm and inject 5–7 mL of anesthetic solution while withdrawing needle another 1 cm.

Special Indications

Special indications are excision of multiple corn, or ablation of multiple warts, and plantar hyperhidrosis.

Deep Peroneal Nerve

Anatomical Landmark

In the distal one-third of the ankle, the deep peroneal nerve is between the tibialis anterior and extensor hallucis longus muscles and is superficial to the anterior tibial artery. The nerve crosses the ankle deep to the extensor hallucis longus tendon about 12.5 mm proximal to the ankle, and courses between the extensor hallucis longus and extensor digitorum longus tendons **(Fig. 40)**.

Procedure (Figs. 41A and B)[18]

- Identify the tendon of extensor hallucis longus by big toe dorsiflexion against resistance. A groove is felt just lateral to the tendon.
- The deep peroneal nerve lies lateral to the tendon and the dorsalis pedis artery. The needle entry site is about 2 cm

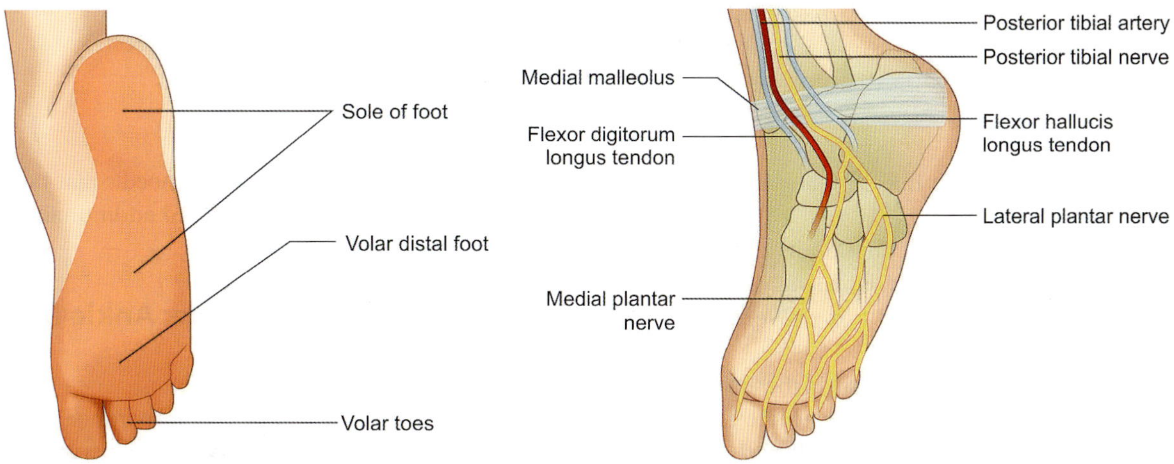

Fig. 38: Posterior tibial nerve and area supplied by it.

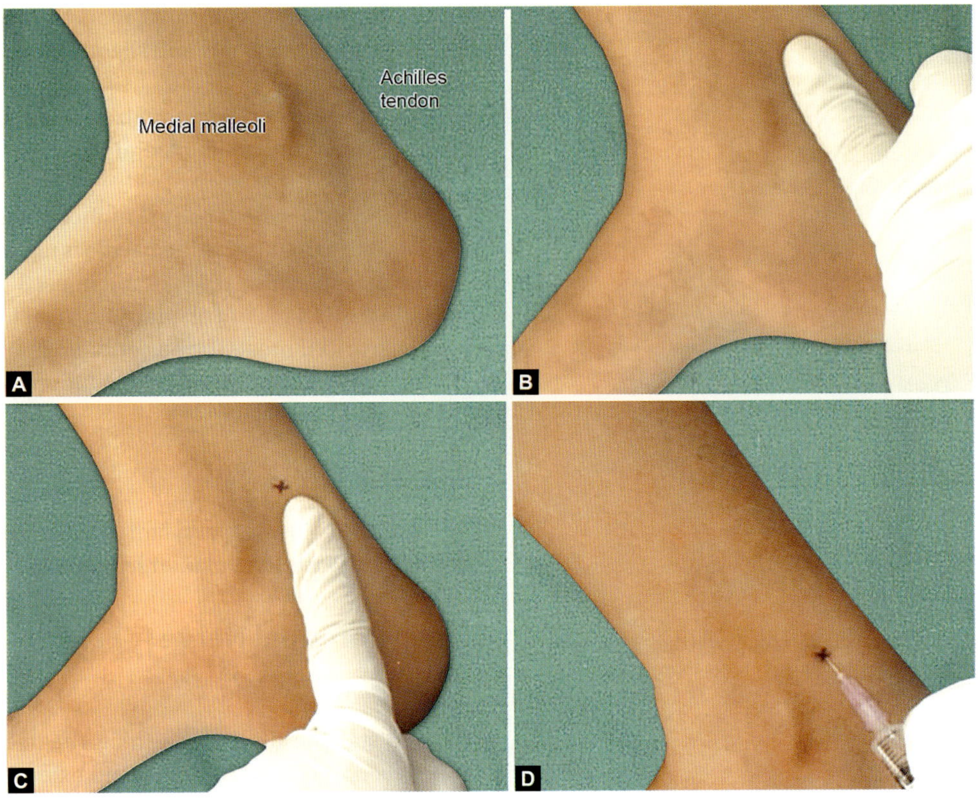

Figs. 39A to D: (A and B) Palpate posterior tibial artery between medial malleoli and Achilles tendon; (C) Mark a point 1 cm superior to artery; (D) Advance the needle toward tibia and inject 3 mL of anesthetic agent.

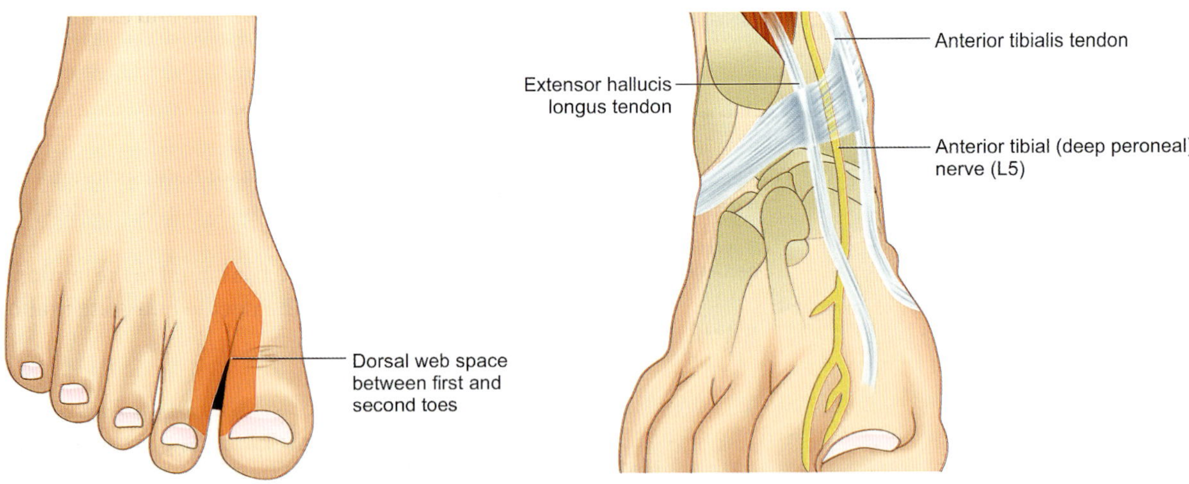

Fig. 40: Deep peroneal nerve and area supplied by it.

distal to the intermalleolar line, just lateral to the dorsalis pedis artery pulse.

- Advance the needle through the skin in a perpendicular manner until bone is encountered, usually within 2–3 cm.
- Withdraw the needle slightly to prevent periosteal injection.
- Patients may experience paresthesia in the first web space. If paresthesia occurs, withdraw the needle slightly until the paresthesia disappears and inject 2 mL of the local anesthetic solution.
- To increase the block success, the needle may be redirected 30° medially and laterally and an additional 2 mL of the anesthetic solution is injected.

Superficial Peroneal Nerve: Ankle Block

Anatomical Landmark

In the distal third of the leg, superficial peroneal nerve pierces the deep fascia to become superficial. The nerve splits into the medial dorsal cutaneous nerve and the intermediate dorsal cutaneous nerve, which give rise to the dorsal digital nerves. It lies lateral to extensor digitorum longus tendon at the level of lateral malleoli **(Fig. 42)**.

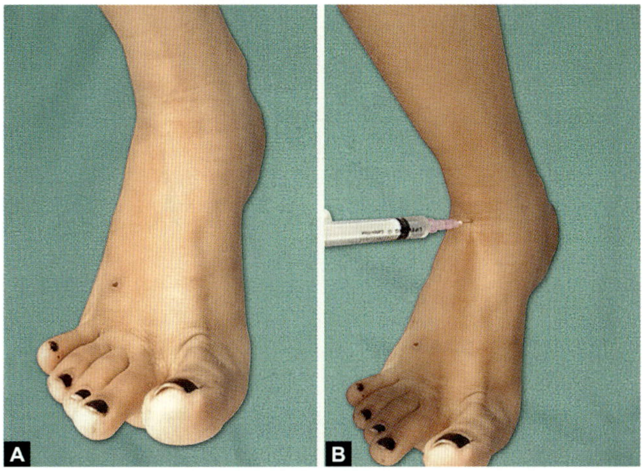

Figs. 41A and B: Deep peroneal nerve block. (A) Tendon of extensor hallucis longus made prominent by big toe dorsiflexion; (B) Inject lateral to the tendon.

Procedure (Figs. 43A and B)

- Draw a line from the distal anterior aspect of the lateral malleolus to the anterior border of the medial malleolus **(Fig. 43A)**
- Place an initial skin wheal of lidocaine anterior to the distal medial malleolus
- Insert the needle through the skin wheal and infiltrate 6–10 mL in a transverse fashion until the lateral malleolus is reached **(Fig. 43B)**

Saphenous Nerve Block[19]

Anatomical Landmark

At the level of ankle, the saphenous nerve is found between the medial malleolus and the anterior tibial tendon, just lateral to the saphenous vein **(Fig. 44)**.

Procedure

- Palpate the medial malleolus and the great saphenous vein at the ankle

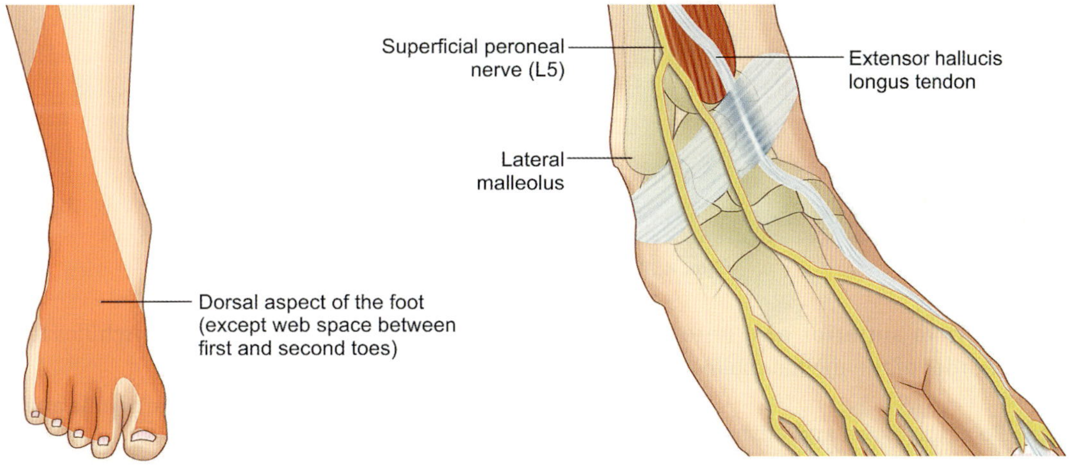

Fig. 42: Superficial peroneal nerve and area supplied by it.

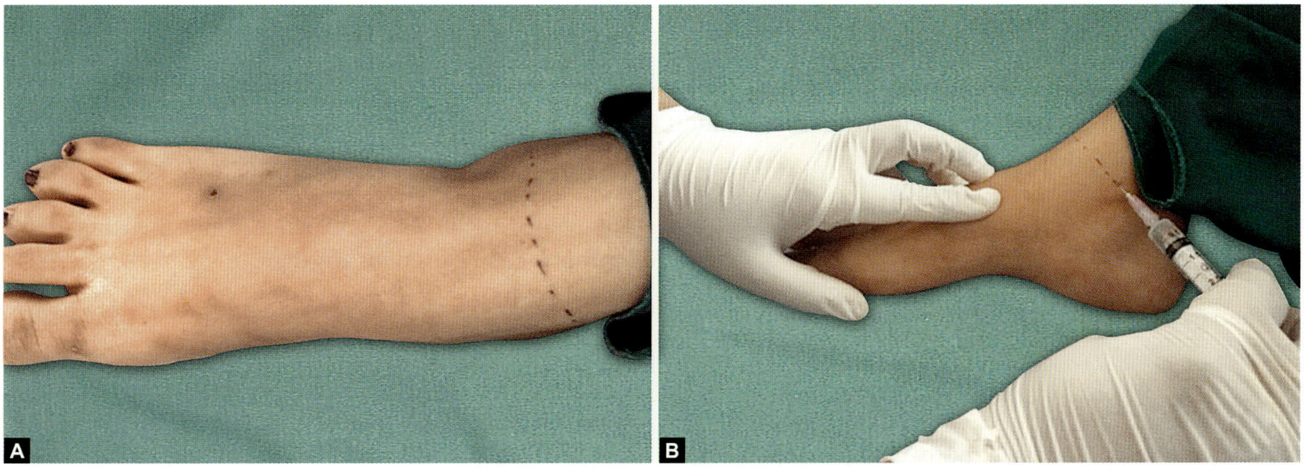

Figs. 43A and B: Superficial peroneal block.

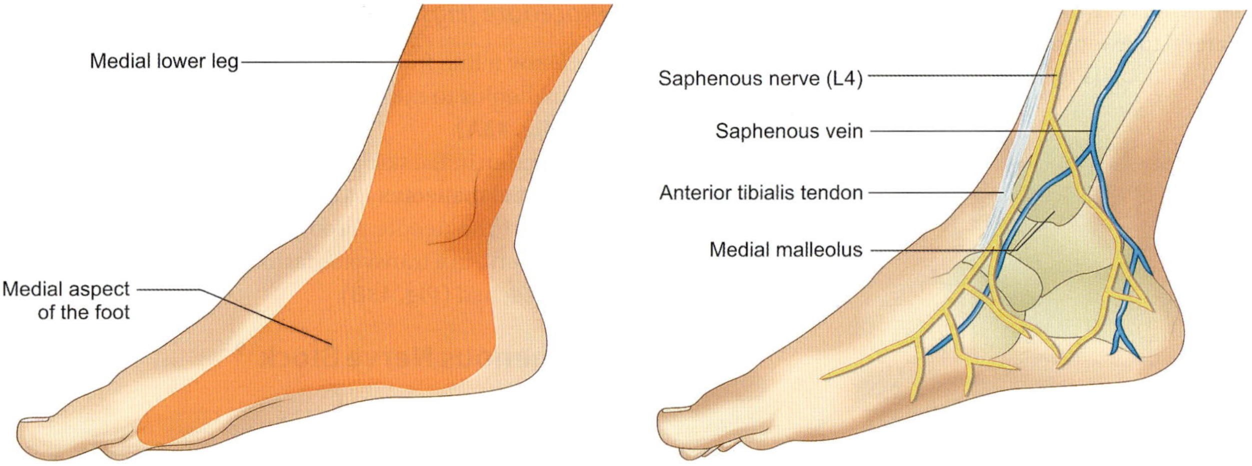

Fig. 44: Saphenous nerve and area supplied by it.

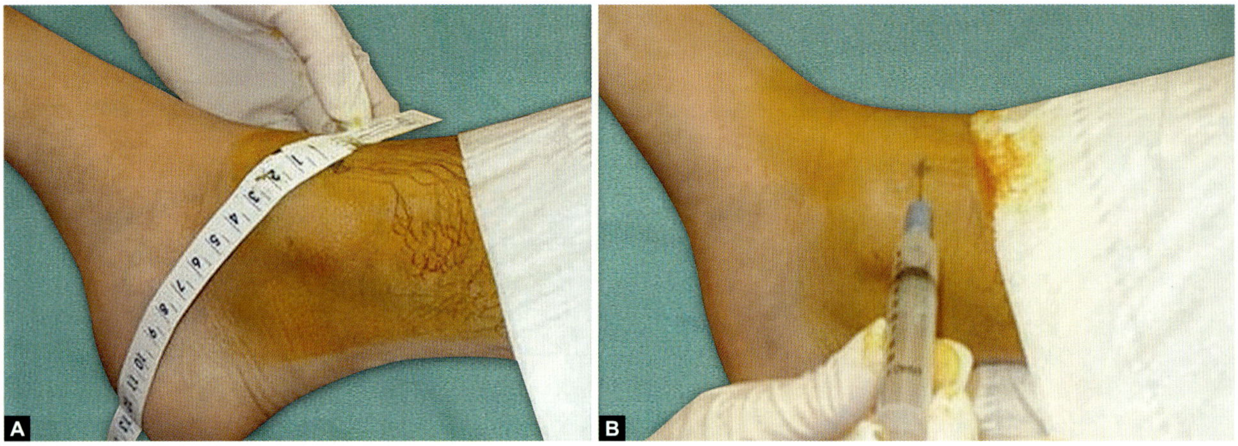

Figs. 45A and B: Saphenous nerve block.

- Mark the site 1.5 cm superior and anterior to the anterosuperior border of the medial malleolus **(Figs. 45 A and B)**
- Insert the needle at this point and advance laterally in a transverse line toward the lateral malleolus to identify the anterior tibial tendon while the foot is in dorsiflexion (dorsiflexion exaggerates the tendon)
- Also identify the anterior tibial ridge by advancing further in the transverse line while the foot is in plantar flexion
- Advance the needle through the skin toward the anterior tibial tendon in a superficial transverse line, without injecting the tendon itself

Sural Nerve[20]

Anatomical Landmark

Sural nerve enters the foot posterior to the lateral malleolus **(Fig. 46)**.

Procedure (Figs. 47A to C)

- Locate the posterior border of the lateral malleolus and the Achilles tendon **(Fig. 47A)**
- Mark the site just lateral to the Achilles tendon, between the two landmarks **(Fig. 47B)**
- Insert the needle and move the needle angling toward the lateral malleolus **(Fig. 47C)**
- Inject 5–7 mL of lidocaine in a transverse line until the lateral malleolus is reached.

DIGITAL BLOCKS (FIG. 48)

Web space block is similar to that in upper limb.

Three-sided Digital Block[21]

This type of digital block is effective in anesthetizing the great toe, but it can be used for any digit.

Procedure (Figs. 49A to C)

- Place the extremity with plantar side down
- Insert the needle at a 90° angle at the medial aspect of the digit, just distal to the metatarsophalangeal joint **(Fig. 49A)**

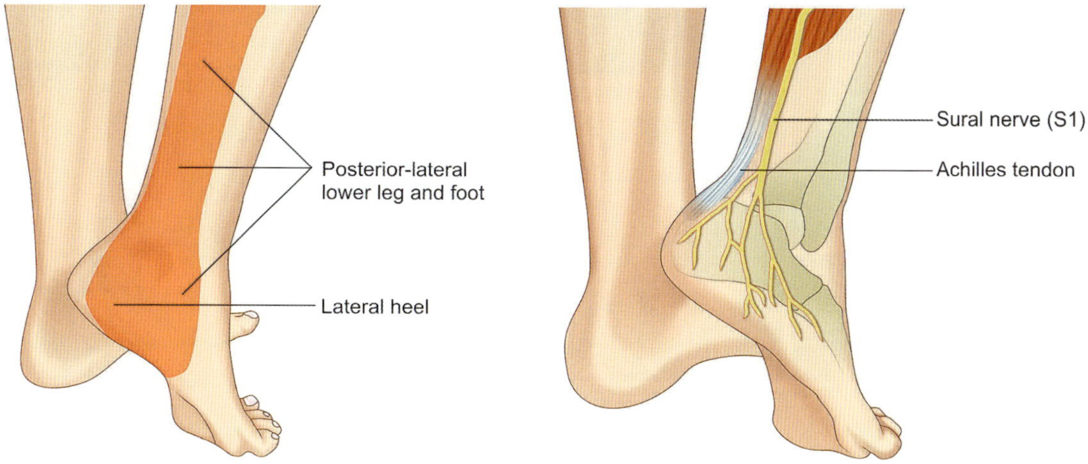

Fig. 46: Sural nerve and area supplied by it.

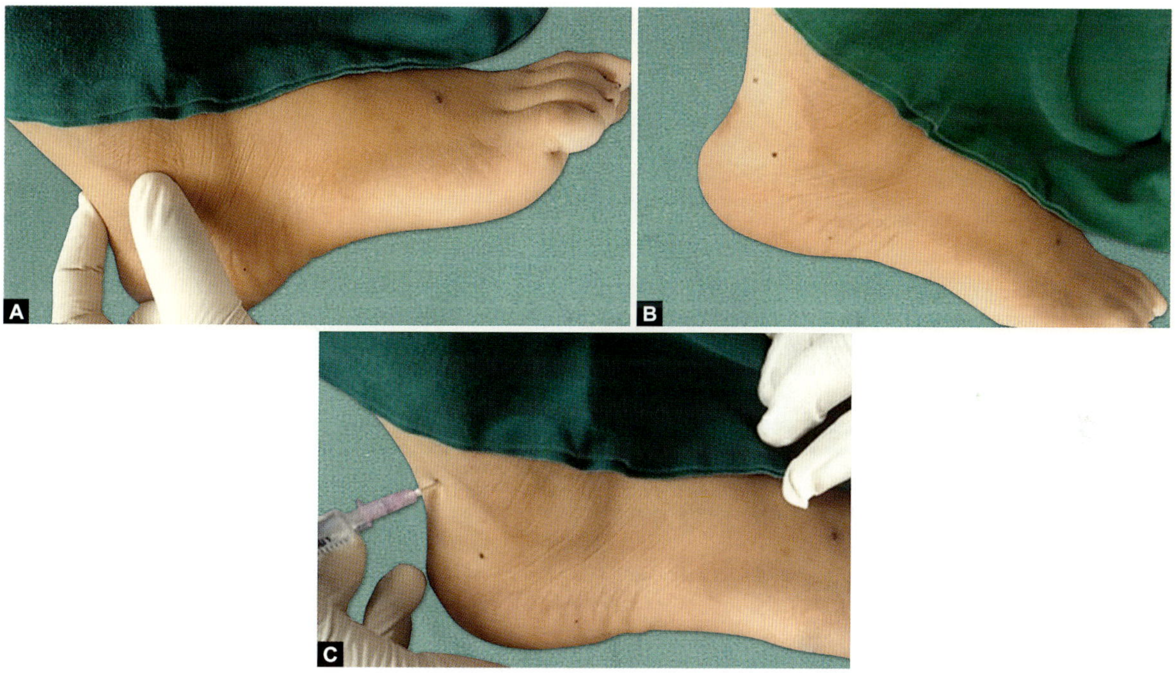

Figs. 47A to C: Sural nerve block.

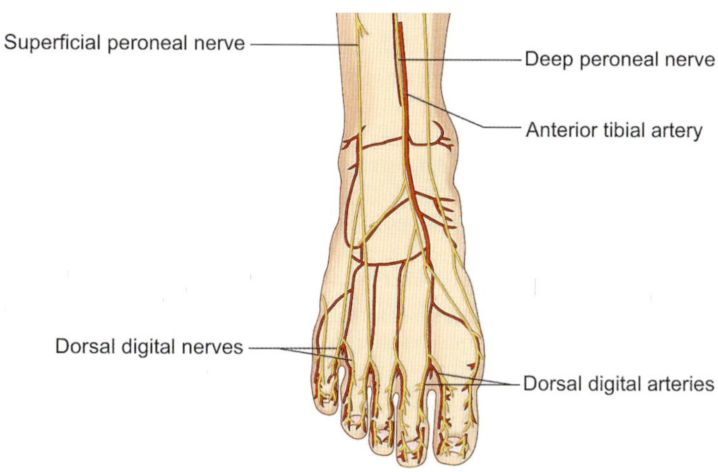

Fig. 48: Nerve supply to the digits of lower limbs.

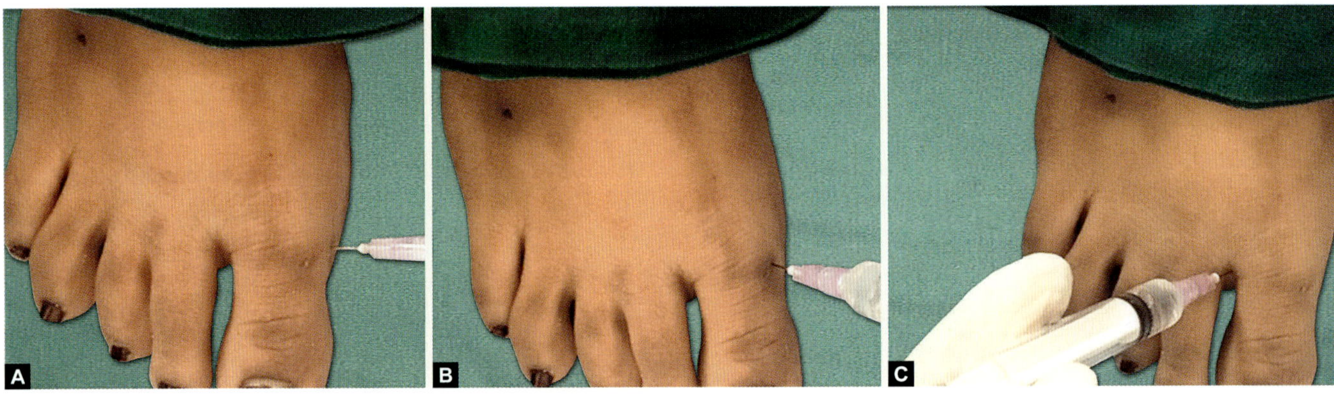

Figs. 49A to C: Three-sided digital block.

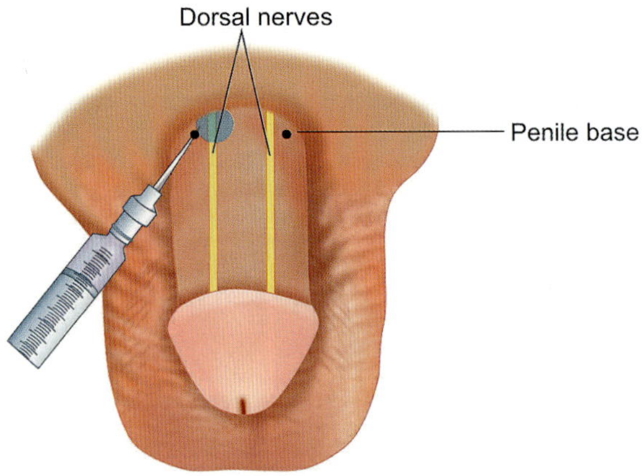

Fig. 50: Dorsal penile nerve block.

TABLE 1: Common peripheral nerve blocks practiced in dermatosurgery.

Nerve	*Anatomical landmark*	*Technique*
Supraorbital nerve	Exits through supraorbital notch	Insert needle just above the eyebrow along midpupillary line
Supratrochlear nerve	Present beneath the medial end of eyebrow	Insert needle 1 cm medial to supraorbital notch
Infraorbital nerve	Exits from infraorbital foramen present about 5 mm below the infraorbital margin in the midline	*Intraoral route*: Insert the needle vertically upwards with tip pointing toward the foramen in the gingivolabial sulcus between the 3rd and 4th teeth from midline (3½ method) *Extraoral route*: Insert needle at infraorbital foramen with the needle directed cephalic and medially
Long buccal nerve	Emerges 2–3 cm upper and lateral to the angle of mouth	Insert needle 2–3 cm lateral and superior to the angle of mouth with needle pointing toward mouth
Mental nerve	Emerges from the mental foramen	Insert needle in the gingivolabial sulcus in-between the 4th and 5th teeth from the midline (4½ method)
Median nerve	Situated deep to palmaris longus and medial to flexor carpi radialis	Ask the patient to slightly flex at wrist and appose thumb and little finger tightly. Now, insert the needle beneath the palmaris longus with needle pointing laterally and inferiorly
Ulnar nerve	Present beneath and lateral to flexor carpi ulnaris. It is also, proximal and lateral to pisiform	Insert needle proximal and lateral to pisiform bone. Alternatively, needle can be introduced between flexor carpi ulnaris and ulnar artery at the level of proximal wrist crease. Direct the needle below and outwards (lateral)
Radial nerve	Anatomical snuffbox at the radial side of wrist	Mark the anatomical snuffbox by asking the patient to abduct and hyperextend the thumb and all four fingers. Insert the needle just proximal and radial to the anatomic snuffbox with the needle directed across the snuffbox from lateral to medial
Dorsal digital nerve	Dorsolateral to extensor digital tendon and just beneath the superficial vein	At the level of web space, insert the needle at 20° angle or just into subcutis lateral to extensor tendon. Needle should be directed inward and downward

Contd...

Contd...

Nerve	*Anatomical landmark*	*Technique*
Palmar digital nerve	Lateral to flexor tendon	Insert the needle at 30° into subcutis lateral to flexor tendon. Needle should be directed medially and inferiorly
Posterior tibial nerve	Situated between Achilles tendon and medial malleolus, close to bone	Insert the needle anterior to Achilles tendon at the level of medial malleolus with needle directed toward posterior border of malleolus Hit the bone and slightly withdraw and inject
Deep peroneal nerve	Medial to extensor digitorum longus at the level of lateral malleolus	Ask the patient to dorsiflex the foot with slight eversion. Insert the needle just medial to extensor digitorum longus at the level of lateral malleolus. Needle should be inserted perpendicular to skin
Superficial peroneal nerve	Lateral to extensor digitorum longus tendon at the level of lateral malleolus	Ask the patient to dorsiflex the foot with slight eversion. Insert the needle just lateral to extensor digitorum longus at the level of lateral malleolus. Needle should be directed toward the lateral malleolus
Saphenous nerve	Situated anterior to medial malleolus and posteromedial to tibialis anterior tendon	Palpate the tibialis anterior tendon by asking the patient to dorsiflex and invert the foot. Introduce the needle slightly posteromedial to tibialis anterior tendon at the level of superior border of medial malleolus
Sural nerve	Anterior to Achilles tendon at the level of lateral malleolus	Insert the needle just anterior to Achilles tendon at the level of lateral malleolus with the needle directed toward the posterior border of lateral malleolus
Dorsal digital nerve of toes	Dorsolateral to extensor digital tendon	At the level of web space, insert the needle at 45° angle. Needle should be directed inward and downward toward the web space
Palmar digital nerve of toes	Lateral to flexor tendon	Insert the needle at 30° into subcutis lateral to flexor tendon. Needle should be directed medially and inferiorly
Penile nerve (at pubic symphysis)	Lower border of pubis symphysis	Place index and middle finger tips over the lower border of symphysis pubis at the base of penis on dorsal aspect in midline. Introduce the needle between the slightly spread index and middle finger. Needle should be directed perpendicular to skin and push it inferior to the lower margin of pubic symphysis
Dorsal penile nerves	They are paired and present 1 cm lateral to midline alongside dorsal penile artery or posterolateral to visible cutaneous dorsal vein in postpubertals	Hold the penis with thumb in midline just distal to penile base and introduce the needle perpendicular to skin and progress anterolaterally
Ventral ramus of penile nerve	Situated at the base of penis in midline on ventral side	Hold and lift the skin of ventral side with thumb and index finger at the base of penis. Insert the needle close to base of penis, lateral and just below the tip of the thumb

- Slowly inject the anesthetic solution, as the needle is advanced toward the volar or plantar side, without piercing the volar skin **(Fig. 49B)**
- Slowly withdraw the needle and redirect it medially
- Make another injection over the already anesthetized skin at the lateral aspect of the digit, with the needle at 90°, advancing it from the dorsal to ventral aspect, as was done medially **(Fig. 49C)**.

Distal Digital Block (Wing Block)

Wing block is similar to that of upper limb.

PENILE BLOCK

- The right and left dorsal penile nerves should be blocked as proximally to the base of the penis as possible
- Advance the needle slowly from medial to lateral side while the anesthetic solution is injected
- Withdraw the needle
- The point of injection is 2- and 10-O'clock positions at the base of penis **(Fig. 50)**
- The needle should be directed toward the center of the shaft, to a depth of about 0.5 cm or until loss of resistance is felt to suggest that the tip of the needle is within the Buck fascia
- Aspirate to ensure that the needle is not in a blood vessel, and slowly inject about 2 mL of local anesthetic on each side
- An alternative method is to inject 2 mL of local anesthetic solution on either side of the midline, avoiding injecting into the superficial dorsal penile vein.

CONCLUSION

Table 1 summarizes the different nerve blocks used in dermatosurgery.

TIPS AND PEARLS

- The key to successful regional anesthesia is familiarity with the local anatomy of the nerve and its associated landmarks.
- To help avoid injecting anesthetic into the nerve, the patient is told to signal if any paresthesia is felt in the region

of needle insertion. If paresthesia is elicited, the needle must be withdrawn 1–2 mm before the anesthetic solution is injected to avoid intraneural injection.

- To decrease the risk of directly injecting into an artery or vein, aspirate prior to injection.
- A few blocks are of easy and durable acquisition—supraorbital, infraorbital, mental, and nasal very safe from serious complications.
- On the other hand, the blocks carried out in the "plexus" beginning, such as the maxillary nerve and the mandibular nerve, are more delicate, with a rate of less raised success, even for accustomed, and with risks of complications raised in the literature. These are out of purview of dermatologists.

REFERENCES

1. Brummett CM, Williams BA. Additives to local anesthetics for peripheral nerve blockade. Int Anesthesiol Clin. 2011;49(4):104-16.
2. Shin KJ, Shin HJ, Lee SH, Song WC, Koh KS, Gil YC. Emerging points of the supraorbital and supratrochlear nerves in the supraorbital margin with reference to the lacrimal caruncle: implications for regional nerve block in upper eyelid and dermatologic surgery. Dermatol Surg. 2016;42(8):992-8.
3. Sattur S. Donor area strip harvesting. In: Mysore V (Ed). Hair Transplantation. New Delhi: Jaypee Brothers Medical Publishers (P) Ltd.; 2015. pp. 141-4.
4. Pulcini A, Gueri JP, European Society of Regional Anesthesia (ESRA). (2007). Regional blocks. [online] Available from: http://nesra.co.uk/files/training/education/Handbook%20of%20Regional%20Anesthesia%20ESRA.pdf. [Last accessed March, 2021].
5. Hornung DE. Nasal anatomy and the sense of smell. Adv Otorhinolaryngol. 2006;63:1-22.
6. Taleghani K, Sternbach G. Infraorbital nerve block. In: Rosen P, Chan TC, Vilke GM, Sternbach G (Eds). Atlas of Emergency Procedures. St Louis: Mosby Press; 2001. pp. 160-1.
7. Byrne KM, Hedges JR. Infraorbital nerve block: intraoral approach. In: Roberts JR, Hedges JR, Custalow C (Eds). Clinical Procedures in Emergency Medicine, 4th edition. Philadelphia: Elsevier; 2004.
8. Khoury JN, Mihailidis S, Ghabriel M, Townsend G. Applied anatomy of the pterygomandibular space: improving the success of inferior alveolar nerve blocks. Aust Dent J. 2011;56(2):112-21.
9. Dental Hygiene. (2017). Review of long buccal nerve block. [online] Available from: www.dentalhygiene411.com/administration-of-local-anesthetics/long-buccal-nerve-block. [Last accessed March, 2021].
10. Syverud SA, Jenkins JM, Schwab RA, Lynch MT, Knoop K, Trott A. A comparative study of the percutaneous versus intraoral technique for mental nerve block. Acad Emerg Med. 1994;1(6):509-13.
11. Ling Tan FF, Schiere S, Reidinga AC, Wit F, Veldman PH. Blockade of the mental nerve for lower lip surgery as a safe alternative to general anesthesia in two very old patients. Local Reg Anesth. 2015;8:11-4.
12. McMinn NH, Hutchings RT, Logan BM. Color Atlas of Head and Neck Anatomy, 2nd edition. Baltimore: Mosby-Wolfe; 1995. pp. 161-3.
13. The New York School of Regional Anesthesia (NYSORA). (2017). Wrist block. [online] Available from: www.nysora.com/posts/view/94. [Last accessed March, 2021].
14. Agur A, Ming L. Grant's Atlas of Anatomy, 10th edition. Lippincott: Williams & Wilkins; 2003. pp. 78-84.
15. Low CK, Wong HP, Low YP. Comparison between single injection transthecal and subcutaneous digital blocks. J Hand Surg Br. 1997;22(5):582-4.
16. Tahiliani S. Surgery of nails. In: Mysore V (Ed). ACSI Textbook on Cutaneous and Aesthetic Surgery. New Delhi: Jaypee Brothers Medical Publishers (P) Ltd; 2012. pp. 484-97.
17. Brown DL. Ankle block. In: Gray AT (Ed). Atlas of Ultrasound-Guided Regional Anesthesia, 2nd edition. Philadelphia: Elsevier Saunders; 2013. pp. 129-33.
18. Kelly JJ, Spektor M. Nerve blocks of the thorax and extremities. In: Roberts JR, Hedges JR, Custalow C (Eds). Clinical Procedures in Emergency Medicine, 4th edition. Philadelphia: Elsevier Saunders; 2004. pp. 584-9.
19. Myerson MS, Ruland CM, Allon SM. Regional anesthesia for foot and ankle surgery. Foot Ankle. 1992;13(5):282-8.
20. Russell DF, Pillai A, Kumar CS. Safety and efficacy of forefoot surgery under ankle block anaesthesia. Scott Med J. 2014;59(2):103-7.
21. Flarity-Reed K. Methods of digital block. J Emerg Nurs. 2002;28(4):351-4.

CHAPTER 15

Hemostasis in Dermatologic Surgery

T Salim

KEY MESSAGES

- Proper hemostasis is vital for ensuring proper postoperative results and preventing complications.
- Detailed history, particularly with reference to drug intake, should be sought in all cases posted for surgery.
- Electrocautery and suture techniques should be appropriately used to control intraoperative bleeding.

INTRODUCTION

Bleeding has always been a concern in all surgeries, including dermatologic surgery. Control of the bleeding process is essential for achieving an optimal surgical outcome. Methods to control bleeding and repair wounds have existed for many years. Dermatologic surgery is usually a mild form of surgery, and hence serious problems of hemostasis are rare. However, problems can be encountered in surgeries such as hair transplantation and other excisions on scalp, liposuction, flap surgeries on face, etc. Hence, dermatosurgeons should be familiar with all aspects of hemostasis.

HISTORY

Efforts have ranged from the use of raw meat by the ancient Egyptians[1] to the use of dried plasma in the World War I to achieve hemostasis.[2] The Egyptians used a mixture of wax, grease, and barley in an effort to stop bleeding.[3] In ancient Greece, hemostatic herbs were applied to wounds suffered in combat.[4] Native Americans are thought to have used scrapings of the inside of animal hides mixed with hot sand and eagle down as topical hemostatic agent.[5] More traditional techniques have included applying pressure, electrocautery, and suturing. In the last decade, however, advances in biotechnology have resulted in an explosive growth of topical hemostatic agents, which are available to the modern dermatologic surgeon.

DEFINITION

Hemostasis can be defined as a tightly regulated process that maintains the blood flow through the vasculature simultaneously as a thrombotic response to tissue damage occurs.[6] Hemostasis is blood clot formation at the site of vessel injury. It is a complex interaction between platelets, plasma proteins, and coagulation and fibrinolytic pathways. Hemostasis aims at reducing the amount of blood loss, as well as preventing rebleeding, hematoma formation, and need for repeated surgery.

MECHANISMS OF HEMOSTASIS

Understanding the mechanisms of hemostasis and thrombosis is critical to the management and stabilization of a patient undergoing any dermatologic surgical procedure. Maintaining hemostasis requires a complex interaction of the vessel wall, platelets, and the coagulation and fibrinolytic systems **(Flowchart 1)**.[7,8] There are two main phases of hemostasis: primary (i.e., the cellular phase) and secondary (i.e., the humoral phase). The clotting cascade involves the sequential activation of proenzymes in a stepwise response, which ultimately provides local generation of fibrin lattices that reinforce the platelet plug **(Fig. 1)**.

Primary Hemostasis

Primary hemostasis begins immediately after endothelial disruption and is characterized by vasoconstriction, platelet adhesion, and formation of a soft aggregate plug.[9] The first phase of hemostasis involves vasoconstriction at the site of injury and is elicited by the release of serotonin and thromboxane A2 (TXA2). The immediate vasoconstrictive period reduces blood flow through the injured tissue and

Flowchart 1: Factors that contribute to normal hemostasis.

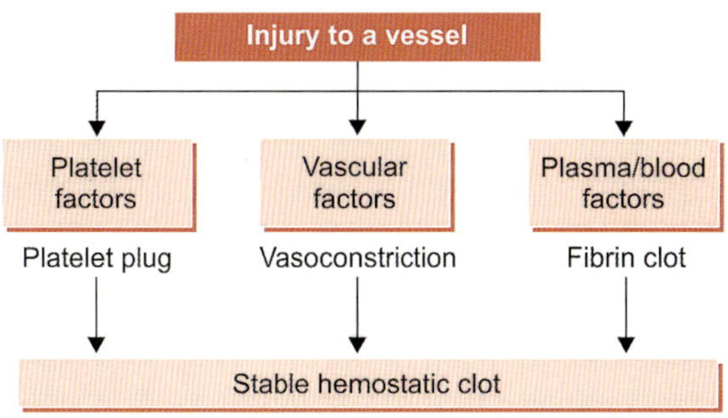

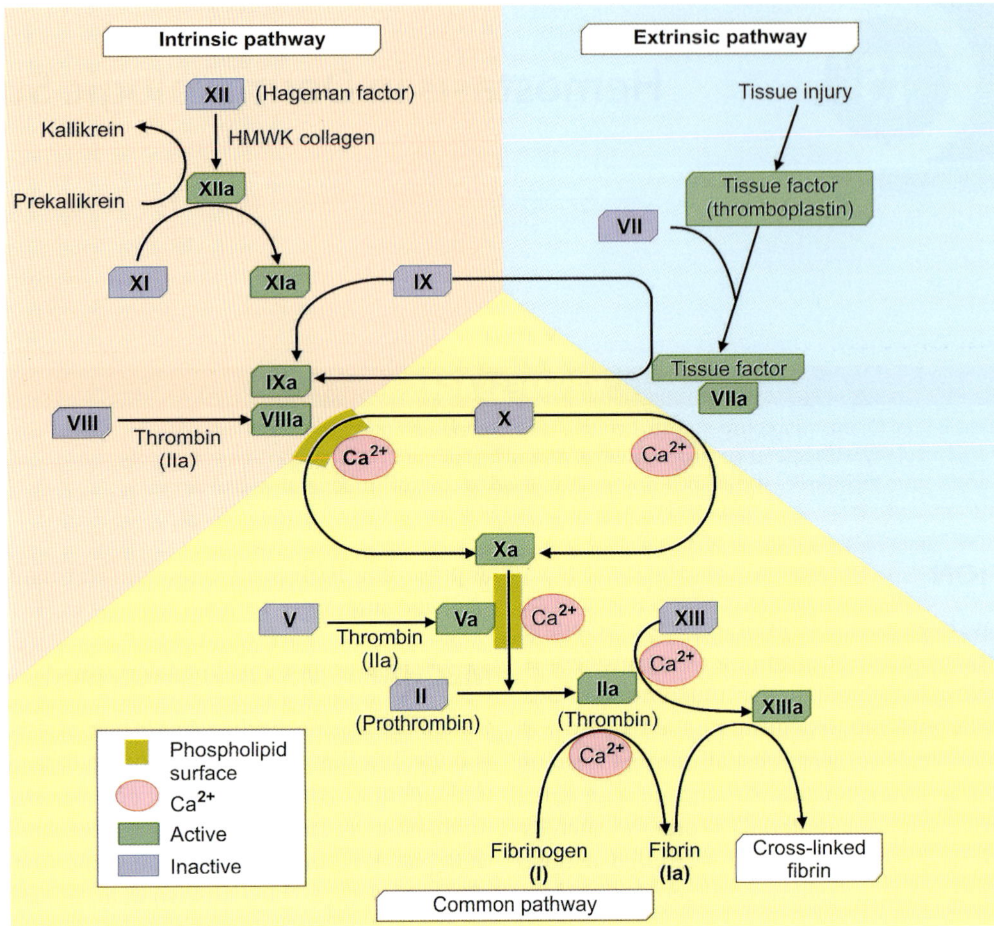

Fig. 1: The clotting cascade. (HMWK: high-molecular-weight kininogen)

provides some initial protection to the loss of circulating volume in the vascular compartment.

Circulating von Willebrand factor attaches to the subendothelium at the site of injury within few seconds after the injury and adheres to the glycoproteins on the surface of platelets. As platelets adhere to the injured surface, they are activated by contact with collagen-exposing receptors that bind circulating fibrinogen. A soft plug of aggregated platelets and fibrinogen is formed.[6-9] This phase of hemostasis is short lived, and the soft plug can easily be sheared from the injured surface.[9]

Secondary Hemostasis

The soft platelet plug is stabilized during secondary hemostasis to form a clot. Vasoconstriction and the resultant reduction in blood flow are maintained by platelet secretion of serotonin, prostaglandin, and thromboxane while the coagulation cascade is initiated. The coagulation cascade is a series of dependent reactions involving several plasma proteins, calcium ions, and blood platelets that lead to the conversion of fibrinogen to fibrin[9,10] **(Fig. 1)**. Coagulation factors are produced by the liver and circulate in an inactive form until the coagulation cascade is initiated. Then each step of the cascade is initiated and completed via a series of sequential and dependent coagulation factor activation reactions. In the final steps, thrombin converts the soluble plasma protein fibrinogen to the insoluble protein fibrin, while simultaneously converting factor XIII to factor XIIIa. This factor conversion stabilizes the fibrin and results in cross-linking of the fibrin monomers, producing a stable clot.[9,10]

TYPES OF BLEEDING IN DERMATOLOGIC SURGERY

Hemorrhage can be classified depending on the source of bleeding and the time of bleeding.[9]

Depending on the Time of Bleeding

- *Primary hemorrhage:* This is the most common form of bleeding occurring intraoperatively.
- *Reactionary hemorrhage:* This type of bleeding usually follows primary hemorrhage within 24 hours of surgery. Common causes for reactive hemorrhage in dermatologic surgery are slipping of ligature, clot dislodgement,

cessation of reflex vasospasm, and weaning of tumescence in tumescent anesthesia. This can result in hematoma formation with secondary infection and wound dehiscence.
- *Secondary hemorrhage:* This is a form of bleeding, which occurs between 7 and 14 days after surgery. Sloughing of a part of the vessels or infection of a surgical wound can lead to this type of bleeding. This is rarely encountered in dermatologic surgery.

Depending on the Source of Bleeding

- *Capillary hemorrhage:* Bright red blood, often associated with rapid ooze. This is the most common form of bleeding encountered.
- *Venous hemorrhage:* Bleeding secondary to venous injury presents as dark red, steady copious flow of blood.
- *Arterial hemorrhage:* Spurts of bright red blood, which rise and fall with the pulse are associated with arterial injury.

APPROACH TO EFFECTIVE HEMOSTASIS IN DERMATOLOGIC SURGERY

The approach should include the following steps:
- *Preoperative evaluation:*
  - History and examination
  - Laboratory investigations
- Intraoperative techniques
- Postoperative techniques.

Preoperative Evaluation

Evaluation of a patient preoperatively will identify patients at risk and effective hemostatic measures can be implemented. Several factors can contribute to the occurrence of intraoperative bleeding related to either the surgical procedure itself or the individual patient.[10,11]

A careful history will identify patients at risk for bleeding disorders **(Table 1)**. History should include detailed questions about factors of surgery **(Box 1)**. This will prove more beneficial than any test. Patients on medications for other ailments should be evaluated to identify drugs affecting hemostasis. Particularly, information should be sought about drug intake not only prescription drugs such as aspirin and warfarin but also herbals and food additives. All nonessential drugs and food additives should be stopped at least 2 weeks prior to surgery. If patent is on essential drugs, due consideration should be given as to whether it is safe to stop them and advice from physician sought. Anticoagulants are administered to prevent thrombotic episodes and such drugs need not be stopped for routine dermatologic surgery, as the likelihood of severe bleeding is minimal and the consequences of stopping the anticoagulant are potentially serious and life-threatening. Questions about any previous bleeding episodes, particularly during injury or dental extractions, should be asked. Proper physical examination should be done to detect any evidence of bleeding tendency such as ecchymoses and petechiae. The type of bleed and hemostatic techniques vary with site. Preoperative examination thus helps the surgeon to plan the most effective method of hemostasis according to the site. If any bleeding tendencies are suspected or detected during examination, they can be further evaluated and confirmed by proper laboratory screening. The laboratory screening should include bleeding time, platelet counts, prothrombin

TABLE 1: Common disorders of hemostasis.

Class	*Example*
Hypocoagulability	
Impaired platelet function	Drugs (e.g., aspirin and clopidogrel), radiation, splenomegaly, and autoimmune
Impaired clotting activity	• Impaired protein synthesis (e.g., vitamin K) • Classic hemophilia (factor VIII; ~80% of all hemophilias) • Hemophilia B (factor IX; ~15% of all hemophilias) • Hemophilia C (factor XI; ~5% of all hemophilias)
Hypercoagulability	
Increased platelet function	Atherosclerosis, diabetes, and smoking
Increased clotting	• Pregnancy • Oral contraceptives • Disseminated intravascular coagulation (DIC) activity

Source: Table adapted from: http://www.pathoplus.com/blood.htm

BOX 1: Preoperative evaluation.

History:
- *History of bleeding complications in the past procedures:* Dental extraction, teeth cleaning, and invasive surgery
- *History of spontaneous bleeding:* GI bleeding and epistaxis
- *History of large hematoma after a relatively small trauma:* Profuse bleeding after minor cuts and scratches

Conditions contributing to bleeding:
- Alcoholism
- Liver diseases

Inheritable coagulopathies:
- Hemophilia, VW disease

Use of anticoagulants:
- NSAIDs, vitamin E, and *Ginkgo biloba*

Examination:
- Site of the lesion to be operated
- Ecchymosis, petechiae, etc.

Laboratory investigations:
- Complete blood count with platelet count
- Bleeding time and clotting time
- Prothrombin time along with INR
- Partial thromboplastin time

(GI: gastrointestinal; INR: international normalized ratio; NSAIDs: nonsteroidal anti-inflammatory drugs; VW: von Willebrand)

time (PT), the international normalized ratio (INR), and partial thromboplastin time.

The *bleeding time* is a study of platelet function and will be prolonged in patients on aspirin, nonsteroidal anti-inflammatory drugs (NSAIDs), those with defective platelets and decreased platelet numbers. In contrast, *platelet count* is more specific and will only be abnormal if there is a quantitative deficiency of platelets.[12]

The *PT* detects abnormalities in extrinsic and common pathways of coagulation and will be increased by the use of warfarin and dicoumarin, but not heparin. Routine preoperative INR, bleeding time, and PT may not always be helpful in predicting operative and postoperative bleeding. A normal INR does not rule out the possibility of bleeding, but a high supratherapeutic INR (>5) indicates a significant risk of postoperative bleeding.[13] The *partial thromboplastin time* (PTT) reveals defect in intrinsic and common pathways and will be prolonged with both heparin and warfarin.

Hence, the coagulation of profile has to be studied in its entirety and in relation to history and circumstances of each patient.

Intraoperative Measures

There are several factors that may lead to intraoperative bleeding **(Box 2)**. Dermatologic surgeons have an array of options to control bleeding, including mechanical and thermal techniques and devices as well as pharmacotherapies and topical agents **(Box 3 and Table 2)**.

Rapid and effective hemostasis allows the surgeon to retain visualization of the surgical field. This can both reduce the procedure time and the risk of accidental injury.[7] Adequate lighting and wound retraction is essential to detect the source of bleeding. Suction can be used to increase visibility in case of increased intraoperative bleeding.[12]

An anxious patient is more likely to bleed more, due to increased sympathetic activity. It is therefore important to allay the anxiety of the patient, if necessary, by administering a tranquilizer. Likewise, preoperative hypertension too may lead to bleeding.

Role of Anesthesia in Preventing Intraoperative Bleeding

Adrenaline in concentration of 1:100,000, when given along with lignocaine, has significant vasoconstrictive effect, and thereby prevents bleeding. However, it takes 30 minutes after infiltration for this effect to set in. Tumescent anesthesia is the use of large quantity of saline mixed with adrenaline and lignocaine. It has the twin effects, producing anesthesia and also decreasing intraoperative bleeding due to the vasoconstrictive effect of adrenaline. A detailed discussion on this technique can be found in chapters on hair transplantation and liposuction.

BOX 2: Factors contributing to intraoperative bleeding.

- Surgical incisions
- Tissues not amenable to suturing
- Low-pressure suture lines
- Anticoagulant medications
- Diffuse capillaries (e.g., large surfaces)
- Unseen sources of bleeding
- Coagulopathies and platelet dysfunction

Measures to Reduce Blood Flow to the Site of Operation

Intraoperative measures to reduce the blood flow to the surgical field are of great use in routine dermatologic surgical procedures.

- *Direct pressure:* Application of direct pressure or compression at a bleeding site is often the surgeon's first choice to assist in the control of bleeding. It is often an underutilized tool for hemostasis. Constant pressure with surgical pad or mop for 10–20 minutes is effective in reducing capillary oozing and small venous hemorrhage.[12] Other mechanical methods, including sutures, staples, and ligating clips, are useful if the source of bleeding is easily identifiable and able to be sealed.
- *Tourniquet:* Use of tourniquet and pressure cuffs with intermittent release is of great value in surgeries of extremities. Tourniquet used in nail surgeries allows the surgeon to retain visualization of the surgical field.

BOX 3: Techniques for maintaining hemostasis in surgery.[14]

- *Mechanical techniques:*
  - Direct pressure
  - Sutures
  - Staples
  - Ligating clips
  - Fabric pads
  - Gauzes
  - Sponges
  - Blood component/replacement therapy
- *Thermal techniques:*
  - Electrocautery
  - Hemostatic scalpel
  - Laser
- *Chemical techniques:*
  - Pharmacotherapy
  - Hypotensive anesthesia
  - Epinephrine
  - Vitamin K
  - Protamine
  - Desmopressin
  - Aminocaproic acid
  - Tranexamic acid
- *Topical hemostats:*
  - Collagen
  - Cellulose
  - Gelatins
  - Thrombins
- *Topical sealants and adhesives:*
  - Fibrin sealants
  - Synthetic glues

TABLE 2: Mechanism of action, advantages/recommended use, and disadvantages/caution against the use of topical hemostatic agents.

Hemostatic agent	*Products*	*Mechanism of action*	*Advantages/recommended use*	*Disadvantages/caution against use*
Gelatin	Gelfoam, Gelfilm, Surgifoam, and Abgel	Provides physical matrix for clotting initiation	• Effectively controls small vessel bleeding • May be used to control bleeding from bone • Recommended as hemostatic plug wrapped in oxidized cellulose • Absorbed by the body within 4–6 weeks • Nonantigenic • Neutral pH allows its use with biological agents	• Should not be used in closed spaces as significant swelling may compress nerves • Use around brisk arterial bleeding can dislodge sponge. May embolize if in an intravascular compartment
Oxidized cellulose	Surgical	Provides physical matrix for clotting initiation, low pH contributes to coagulative necrosis	• Low pH has antimicrobial effect • Very good handling characteristics (cotton-like consistency, best when applied dry) • Does not stick to instruments • Typically dissolves in 2–6 weeks	• Must not be used with other biological hemostatic agents (e.g., thrombin) because of low pH • Low pH may increase inflammation of surrounding tissue
Microfibrillar collagen (MFC)	Avitene ultrafoam, Avitene ultrawrap, Helistat, Helitene, Instant, and Endo Avitene	Platelet adherence and activation	• No significant swelling • Absorbed in <8 weeks • Can control wide areas of parenchymal bleeding • Effective despite profound heparinization because of its mechanism of action	• Less effective in patients with thrombocytopenia • Sticks to operator's gloves
Thrombin	• Thrombin-JMI (bovine), Evithrom (human plasma-derived), and rh • Thrombin/ Recothrom (recombinant human)	Converts fibrinogen to fibrin to form clots, activation of clotting factors	• Effectively controls minor bleeding from capillaries and small venules when pressure or ligature is insufficient • Easy application • Fast acting	May bind to neural structures' immunologic response, and possibly increase in coagulopathy and thrombosis
Fibrin sealants	Tisseel, Evicel, and Crosseal	Thrombin and fibrinogen mixed at site of application; thrombin cleaves fibrinogen to fibrin that forms clots	• Effective in heparinized patients • Can be used for skin grafting Tisseel and Evicel are good for venous oozing from raw surface	Before application, wounds must be cleaned of antiseptics containing alcohol, iodine, or heavy metal ions that can denature applied thrombin and fibrinogen
Platelet sealants	Vitagel	MFC and thrombin combined with patient's plasma-derived fibrinogen and platelets	Platelets from patients strengthen clot while proteins in gel facilitate tissue regeneration	Need for centrifugation and preuse processing
Polyethylene glycol hydrogels	Coseal	Two synthetic polyethylene glycol polymers that mix and cross-link in wound site	• Good mechanical sealant for vascular reconstructions • Is not exothermic, does not cause inflammation, and does not potentiate bacterial infection	Swelling up to four times initial volume after 1 day, and can continue swelling
Cyanoacrylates	Dermabond	Liquid monomers form polymers in the presence of water and glue surfaces together	• Used as a replacement for sutures (5–0) for wounds on the face, extremities, and torso • Full binding strength within 2.5 minutes, attains strength of healed tissue after 7 days • Forms waterproof barrier	• Difficult to use in jagged lacerations • Must not be used for bites, punctures or crush wounds • Not recommended on mucosal surfaces, axilla, or perineum
Fibrin dressings	Dry fibrin sealant dressings	Freeze-dried (lyophilized) fibrinogen and thrombin on gauze dressing	• Initial success with US forces in Iraq and Afghanistan under FDA investigational drug protocol • Effectively stops bleeding from large surface abrasions • Longer shelf life than fibrin sealants and does not need mixing at site of application	• Not FDA approved • Needs strong packaging due to brittleness

Contd...

Contd...

Hemostatic agent	*Products*	*Mechanism of action*	*Advantages/recommended use*	*Disadvantages/caution against use*
Chitin dressings	Rapid deployment hemostat (RDH)	Vasoconstriction, mechanical sealing, mobilization of RBCs, clotting factors, and platelets	• Intended for emergency field use by first responders • Effective for minor wounds	Varied results for severe wounds like splenic lacerations in animal model
Chitosan dressings	HemCon	Deacylated form of chitin, similar mechanism	• Intended for emergency field use by first responders • Initial success with US forces in Iraq and Afghanistan • Has antimicrobial properties	• Animal testing yields inconsistent results • Contains chitosan from shellfish, so do not use it in patients with shellfish allergies
Mineral zeolite dressings	QuikClot	Molecular sieves absorb water at the site of wound to increase concentration of clotting factors, platelets, and RBCs	• Intended for emergency field use by first responders • Powdered form is effective for low-pressure bleeding, Zeolite embedded in mesh for high-pressure bleeding	Caution with high-pressure bleeds as they can force powdered form out of wound

(FDA: Food and Drug Administration; RBCs: red blood cells)

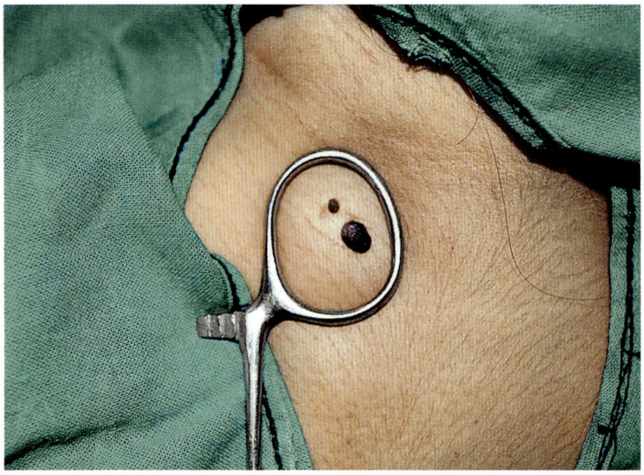

Fig. 2: Circumferential pressure hemostasis using ring of artery forceps.

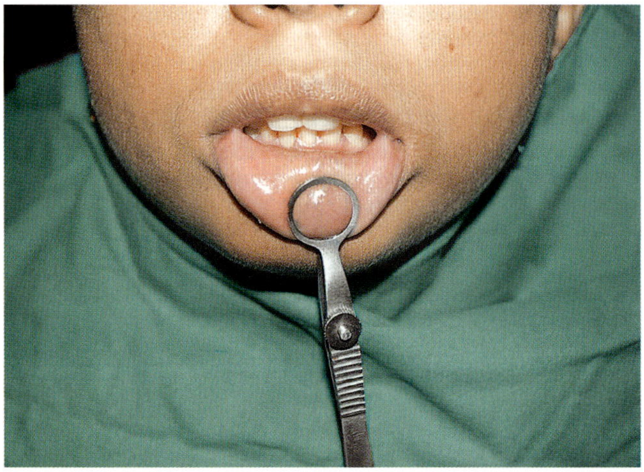

Fig. 3: Circumferential pressure hemostasis using chalazion ring forceps.

- *Circumferential pressure hemostasis:* Tourniquets and pressure cuffs cannot be used on areas such as trunk, scalp, tongue, lips, etc.

Circumferential pressure is a simple hemostatic method useful in these situations. Finger ring of an artery forceps or a needle holder pressed firmly around the lesion to be excised, exerts uniform circumferential pressure **(Fig. 2)**. This achieves effective hemostasis attaining a bloodless field in situations like scalp biopsy.[14]

For minor procedures on lips and tongue, circumferential pressure hemostasis can be achieved with the help of a simple device called chalazion ring forceps. Chalazion ring forceps are used in ophthalmologic surgery for incision and curettage of meibomian cyst. It has a flat plate on one of the handles and a ringed rim on the other handle, which can be clamped over the plate. The plate of the forceps can be pushed under lip or tongue in base position so that the ring is placed around the lesion to be excised. The screw is then tightened until the ring fits snugly so as to immobilize the lesion. This stabilizes the lesion as well as provides hemostasis **(Fig. 3)**. Circumferential pressure hemostasis using chalazion ring forceps is useful in procedures on lips, tongue, such as biopsy, excision of mucocele, pyogenic granuloma, etc.[15]

- *Sutures:* Larger vessels may need to be identified clamped and ligated. After ligation, vessel can be tied with suture or electrosurgical device can be used. An absorbable suture is used to tie off the vessel using a figure-of-eight suture or a simple suture.[12-16]
- *Presuturing technique:* This technique can be utilized in excision surgeries in order to prevent excessive blood loss during the surgery. Sutures are passed under the lesion to be excised. These are tied immediately after excising the lesion **(Figs. 4A to D)**. This technique is useful in treating vascular lesions like pyogenic granuloma and in biopsies on scalp **(Figs. 5A and B)**.

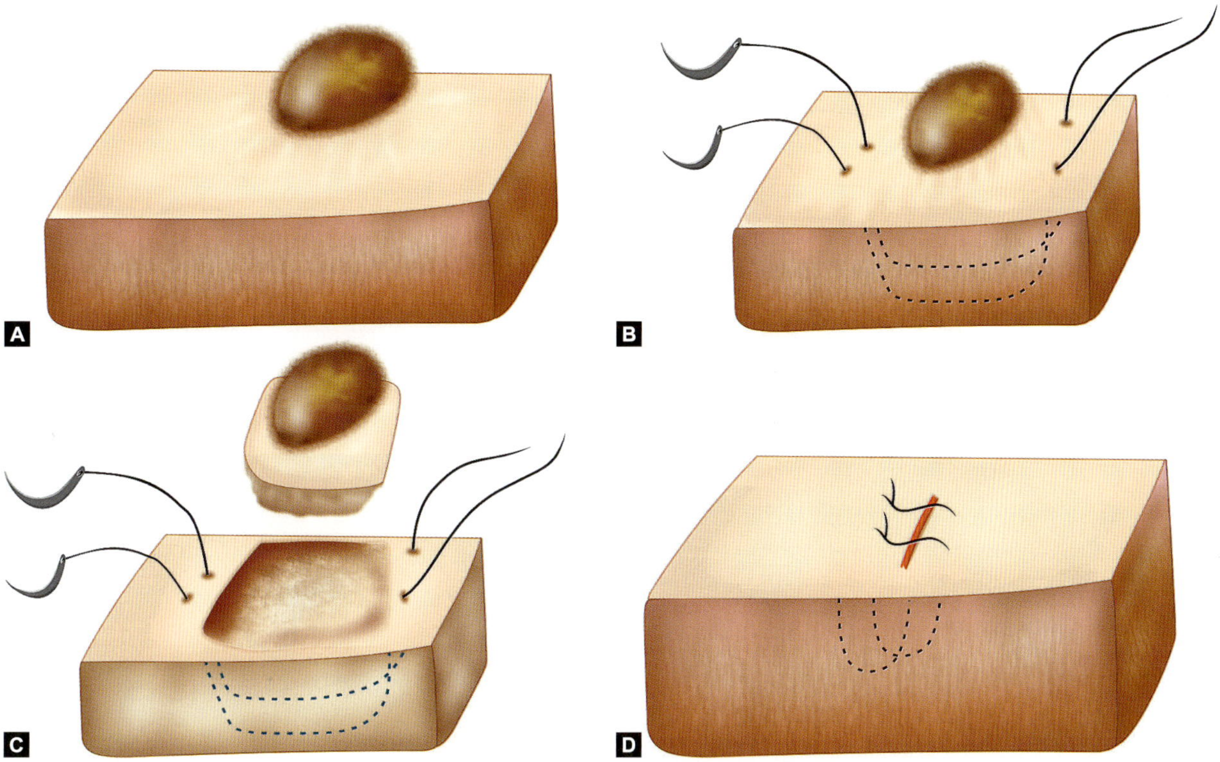

Figs. 4A to D: Presuturing technique.

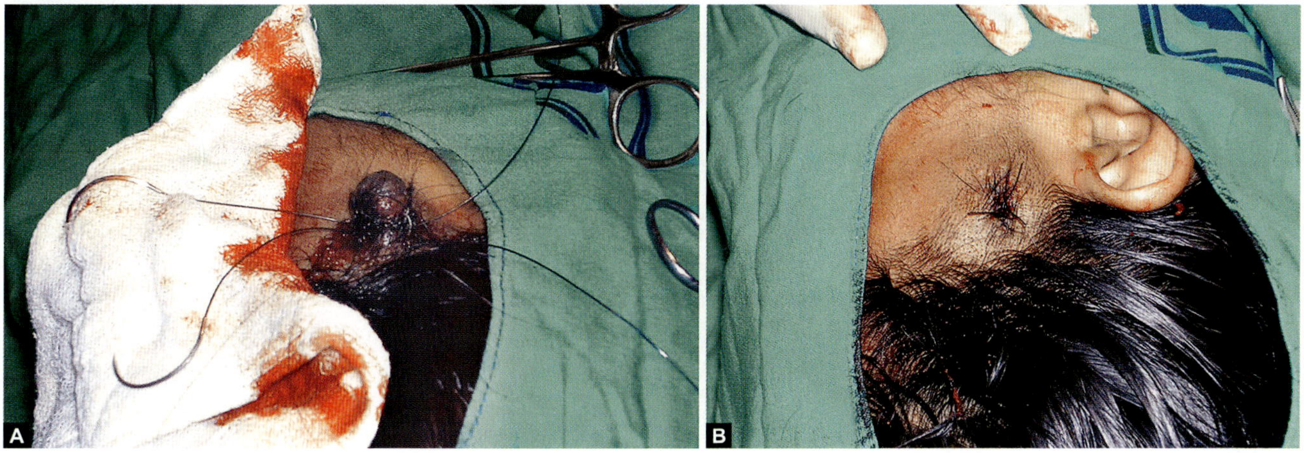

Figs. 5A and B: Presuturing technique for granuloma pyogenicum on face.

- *Figure-of-eight suture:* This is a suture technique to achieve effective hemostasis in area where there is diffuse bleeding and difficulty to pinpoint the source of bleeding. This suture technique is different from figure-of-eight suture used for ligating vessels. Suture is made as shown in **Figures 6A and B**. The circumferential pressure compresses the bleeding vessels so as to attain hemostasis **(Figs. 7A and B)**.
- *Thermal techniques:* Thermal techniques, such as hemostatic scalpels and lasers, also have become viable surgical options to reduce bleeding in dermatologic surgery. Much of the bleeding caused by cutaneous surgery can be controlled by electrocautery, electrocoagulation, or electrodesiccation. Bipolar electrocautery systems are simple devices useful in dermatologic surgical settings. However, care should be taken to minimize damage to surrounding tissue.[12] Too liberal use of electrocautery can contribute to a wider postoperative scar.

Bipolar radiofrequency paired with conductive saline is a new wound-sealing method effective in dermatologic surgery.[17] Bipolar radiofrequency paired with conductive saline effectively achieved hemostasis in patients undergoing

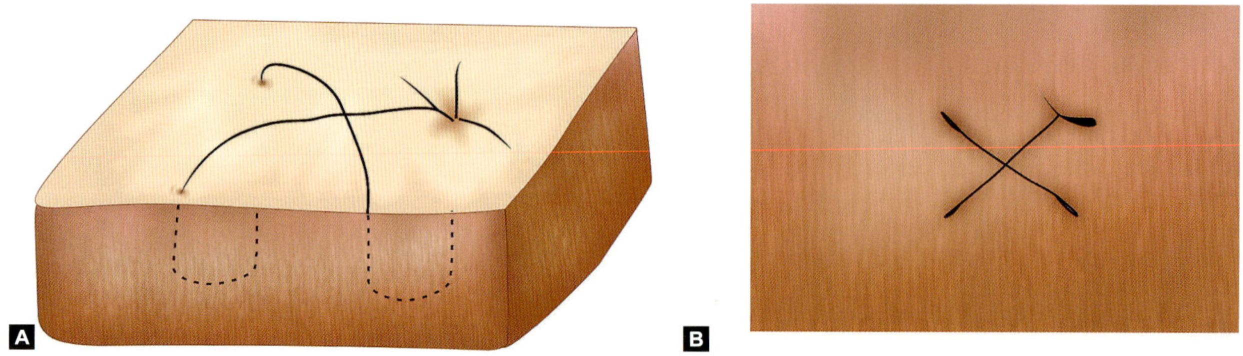

Figs. 6A and B: Figure-of-eight suturing.

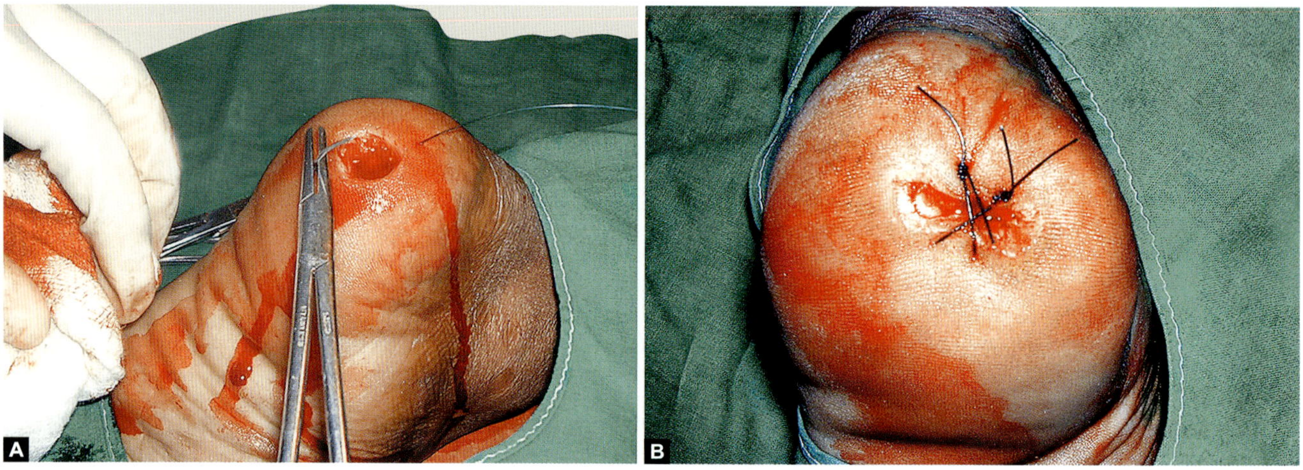

Figs. 7A and B: Figure-of-eight suturing.

dermatologic surgery and reduced problems associated with traditional bipolar electrosurgery. It is helpful in the setting of larger flaps and when patients are taking blood thinners. Better visualization of the field and less surgical time; creating a clean wound bed. This employs a bipolar mono terminal configuration and can be safely used in patients with implanted electronic devices, such as permanent pacemakers, automatic implantable cardioverter defibrillators (AICDs), and cochlear implants. All actively bleeding vessels, even actively pulsatile arterial bleeds, were controlled and sealed without the use of hemostats or other instruments. The investigators observed no char, burning, or collateral tissue destruction with saline-coupled bipolar electrosurgery.

Continuous wave CO_2 laser at 10,600 nm wavelength targets water as a chromophore and blocks small blood vessels. This is useful in laser blepharoplasty.

- *Hemostatic agents:* Topical hemostatic agents can be applied directly to the bleeding site and may prevent continuous unrelenting bleeding throughout the entire procedure and into the postoperative recovery period. Hemostasis using topical agents also can avoid the adverse effects of systemic hemostatic medications, such as "unwanted" blood clots. **Table 2** summarizes the currently available topical hemostatic agents useful in dermatologic surgery.[18] In surgical procedures where the amount of blood loss is unpredictable, topical hemostats can be used sparingly when blood loss is minimal and more liberally during severe bleeding. Furthermore, as hemostasis is attained and maintained at the bleeding site, there may be prolonged benefit with respect to postoperative blood loss.
- *Caustic hemostatic agents:* Topical caustic agents commonly used in dermatosurgical procedures include aluminum chloride, ferric subsulfate (Monsel's solution) silver nitrate, and zinc chloride paste **(Figs. 8A and B)**. These agents are effective, easy to use, and have made many surgeries cost-effective. They work by coagulating proteins leading to tissue necrosis and eschar formation enhancing thrombus formation and hemostasis.[19] Properties of caustic hemostatic agents are given in **Table 3**.

Aluminum chloride is the most widely used topical agent in dermatologic surgery as it is effective and does not lead to pigmentation of the skin. This solution can be applied with a cotton-tipped applicator after shave biopsies and has been shown to be very effective **(Figs. 9A to C)**.

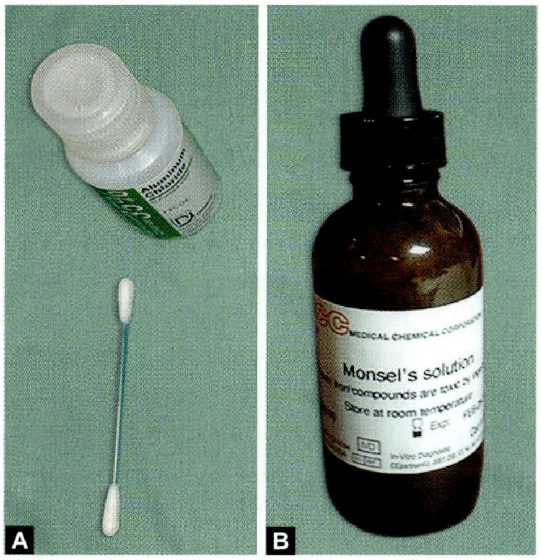

Figs. 8A and B: (A) Silver chloride solution with cotton-tipped applicator; (B) Monsel's solution.

Another topical agent that is still used in dermatologic procedures, but with decreased frequency, is Monsel's solution, which is composed of 20% ferric subsulfate. It has an acidic pH, which is thought to contribute to its hemostatic properties eliciting protein precipitation in vessels and oxidization.[19] It is effective after punch or shave biopsies but is used less frequently due to its tattooing effect on the skin. Less hyperpigmentation and tattooing of the skin occur with a 10% ferrous sulfate solution when applied to the skin for 1–2 hours postoperatively.

Silver nitrate is commonly used in the treatment of small wounds and is particularly effective in the cauterization of pyogenic granulomas of the hand. Application of the silver nitrate creates a thin eschar, which sloughs off within several days and may cause permanent skin pigmentation.[20] One of the oldest topical hemostatic agents known as "Moh's paste" was created by Frederic Mohs in 1941.[21] Zinc chloride is the

TABLE 3: Properties of caustic hemostatic agents.

Hemostatic agent	*Application*	*Mechanism of action*	*Advantages*	*Disadvantages*
Aluminum chloride 20–70% solution	Solution can be applied with a cotton-tipped applicator after shave excision	Precipitates proteins causing coagulation of vessels	• Inexpensive • Less likely to cause pigmentation	Can be used only on superficial wounds
	Aluminum chloride sticks are also available		Easily accessible and easy to apply	
Ferric subsulfate 20% solution (Monsel's solution)	Solution can be applied with a cotton-tipped applicator or gauze pad	Precipitates proteins intravascularly and oxidizes tissues	• Inexpensive • Excellent hemostasis • Easy to apply	Intradermal ferruginous deposits cause tattooing of the skin after use
Zinc chloride (Moh's paste)	Paste that can be applied topically. Left on for up to 48 hours	Precipitates proteins causing coagulation of small vessels	Effective in providing hemostasis to metastatic cutaneous wounds	Can be very painful and irritating to the patient
Silver nitrate	Solution can be applied with a cotton-tipped applicator	Precipitates proteins	• Used in the treatment of small wounds • Effective in the cauterization of pyogenic granulomas	May cause permanent skin pigmentation

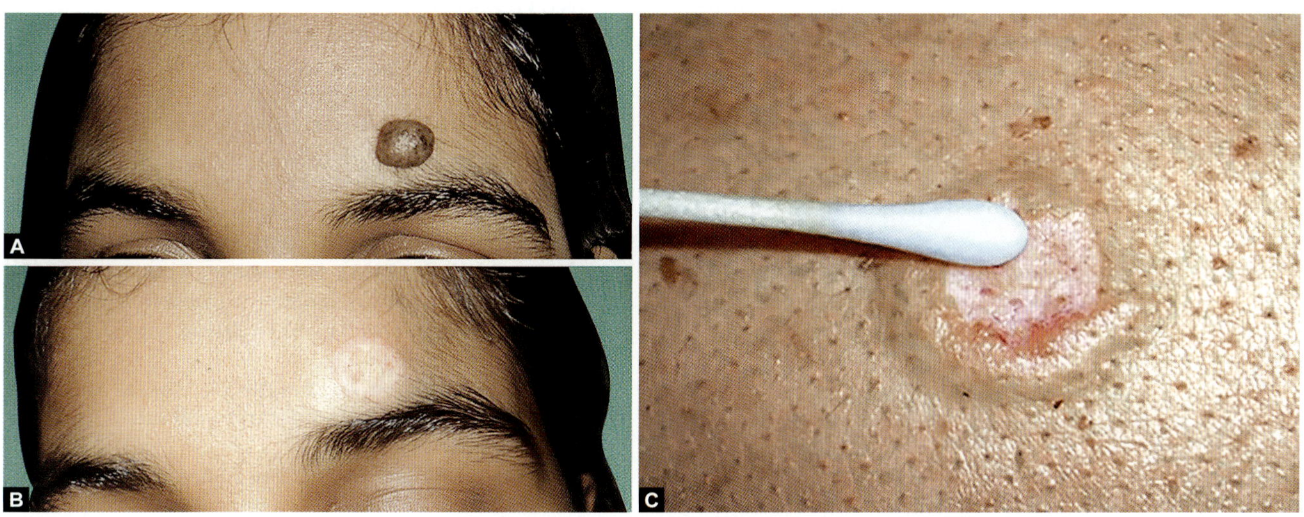

Figs. 9A to C: (A) Compound nevus before shave excision; (B) Application of silver chloride to achieve hemostasis; (C) After excision effective hemostasis achieved.

main component of the paste, and it can be applied with a tongue depressor, cotton-tipped applicator, or incorporated into gauze. It is effective in providing hemostasis to metastatic cutaneous wounds.[22]

Postoperative Care and Instructions

Pressure dressings are recommended for the first 24 hours postoperatively in almost all cases. A nonadherent dressing covering the wound or suture line followed by layers of gauze and then elastic dressing will provide adequate compression. Patients should be advised to limit their activities after surgery. Leg end elevation should be advised to patients with surgical wound over the legs in order to minimize the oozing.

Postoperative Bleeding

The most common time for the bleeding to occur is during the first few hours of surgery when the clots are quite fragile and vasodilatation can occur. If the bleeding is not controlled with direct pressure, it needs to be explored with attention for its cause, which is tackled accordingly. Usually, wound needs to be opened either partially or fully for exploration. Lidocaine without adrenaline can be used to avoid missing bleeding vessels with vasoconstriction. Cautery or suture can be used for ligation of bleeding vessels. Wound can be resutured after a period of observation.[12]

Ecchymoses are a result of blood lying within the tissue plains. Periorbital, perioral, and genital areas are more prone to ecchymoses. They usually resolve with time, ice packs, and elevation. Hematoma formation has to be ruled out.

Hematoma occurs when blood collects under closed wound. There is no visible bleeding but only swelling and tenderness of sudden onset. This can lead to wound dehiscence or necrosis. Early hematoma is a gelatinous mass that can be expressed partially by opening the wound and applying gentle pressure. In case of larger hematoma, complete evacuation has to be done followed by suturing the source of bleed. In case of doubt of further bleed, a drain should be placed for the next 24 hours.[12]

Seroma is a collection of transudative serum in a closed space. These can cause increased pressure and wound compromise. This is well managed by inserting a large-bore 18-gauge needle. Fenestrations are made on skin grafts to prevent seroma.

Postoperative bleeding can be highly daunting and threatening to patients, and hence, it is important to provide a checklist to patients in whom such bleeding is anticipated **(Box 4)**.

BOX 4: Postoperative instructions to patients.

- If there is any bleeding noted, do not be anxious
- Lie down, elevating the area of bleeding
- Apply firm pressure for 15 minutes with cotton pad
- If bleeding continues, call the telephone number provided

Anticoagulants and Blood Thinners during Cutaneous Surgery[13]

The risk of life-threatening thromboembolism associated with even brief cessation of blood thinners is significant. Unfortunately, primary care providers may be unaware of the bleeding risks associated with cutaneous procedures, such as Mohs excision and wound repair. The cutaneous surgeon should be aware of the various techniques and tools to reduce the risk of intraoperative and postoperative bleeding in patients taking blood thinners. Notwithstanding, bleeding complications carry far less morbidity and mortality than that of thromboembolism. Evidence continues to mount favoring blood thinner maintenance during cutaneous surgery, and hence, anticoagulants should be continued during the dermatosurgical procedures.

CONCLUSION

Control of the bleeding process is essential for achieving an optimal surgical outcome. Effective hemostasis simplifies many techniques in dermatologic surgery. Electrosurgical devices and newer topical agents and gels effectively tackle surgical bleeding. Anticoagulants and blood thinners should be continued during cutaneous surgery.

REFERENCES

1. Shekarriz B, Stoller ML. The use of fibrin sealant in urology. J Urol. 2002;167(3):1218-25.
2. Radosevich M, Goubran HI, Burnouf T. Fibrin sealant: scientific rationale, production methods, properties, and current clinical use. Vox Sang. 1997;72(3):133-43.
3. Sigerist H. A history of medicine. New York, NY: Oxford University Press; 1951.
4. Aris A. Hemostatic herbs. Ann Thorac Surg. 2002;74(4):1291.
5. Stone E. Medicine among the American Indians. New York, NY: PB Hoeber; 1932.
6. Lundblad RL, Bradshaw RA, Gabriel D, Ortel TL, Lawson J, Mann KG. A review of the therapeutic uses of thrombin. Thromb Haemost. 2004;91(5):851-60.
7. Gabay M. Absorbable hemostatic agents. Am J Health Syst Pharm. 2006;63(13):1244-53.
8. Adams GL, Manson RJ, Turner I, Sindram D, Lawson JH. The balance of thrombosis and hemorrhage in surgery. Hematol Oncol Clin North Am. 2007;21(1):13-24.
9. Porter RS (Ed). (2005). Hemostasis. The Merck Manuals Online Medical Library. [online] Available from: http://www.merck.com/mmpe/sec11/ch134/ch134a.html. [Last accessed February, 2012].
10. Oz MC, Rondinone JF, Shargill NS. FloSeal Matrix: new generation topical hemostatic sealant. J Card Surg. 2003;18(6):486-93.
11. Morikawa T. Tissue sealing. Am J Surg. 2001;182(Suppl 2): 29S-35S.
12. Nouri K, Khouri SL (Eds). Techniques in Dermatologic Surgery. Elsevier; 2003. pp. 85-91.

13. Schanbacher CF. Anticoagulants and blood thinners during cutaneous surgery: always, sometimes or never? Skin Therapy Lett. 2004;9(3):5-7.
14. Harahap M. Excision of small lesions on the scalp. In: Robins P (Ed). Surgical Gems in Dermatology, 1st edition. New York: Journal Publishing Group; 1988. pp. 73-4.
15. Ceiley R, Bodian E. Biopsy of oral lesions. In: Robins P (Ed). Surgical Gems in Dermatology, 1st edition. New York: Journal Publishing Group; 1988. pp. 15-7.
16. Samudrala S. Topical hemostatic agents in surgery: a surgeon's perspective. AORN J. 2008;88(3):S2-11.
17. Nelson A, Schanbacher C. New wound-sealing method effective in dermatologic surgery. American Society for Dermatologic Surgery (ASDS). 2011. Annual meeting. November 5, 2011.
18. Achneck HE, Sileshi B, Jamiolkowski RM, Albala DM, Shapiro ML, Lawson JH. A Comprehensive review of topical hemostatic agents: efficacy and recommendations for use. Ann Surg. 2010;251(2):217-28.
19. Palm MD, Altman JS. Topical hemostatic agents: a review. Dermatol Surg. 2008;34(4):431-45.
20. Quitkin HM, Rosenwasser MP, Strauch RJ. The efficacy of silver nitrate cauterization for pyogenic granuloma of the hand. J Hand Surg Am. 2003;28(3):435-8.
21. Mohs F. Chemosurgery: a microscopically controlled method of cancer excision. Arch Surg. 1941;42(2):279-96.
22. Kakimoto M, Tokita H, Okamura T, Yoshino K. A chemical hemostatic technique for bleeding from malignant wounds. J Palliat Med. 2010;13(1):11-3.

CHAPTER 16

Dermatosurgical Emergencies and Resuscitation

Murali Chakravarthy, Madura C

KEY MESSAGES

Though dermatological surgeries are daycare procedures performed in healthy individuals, despite that, surgical emergencies may occur, though rarely. Dermatosurgeons should be aware of procedures for resuscitation in such eventualities or may have qualified help to provide the same. Lack of it may be interpreted as deficiency of services, should a permanent harm occur to the patient. Syncope, bleeding, and issues concerning systemic toxicity of local anesthetic are the common events that might occur. Monitoring devices, basic resuscitation equipment, adequately trained staff are needed to manage an emergency. The adage "If you are prepared for an emergency, it ceases to exist" appears to be apt under these situations.

INTRODUCTION

Office-based dermatological procedures and cosmetic surgeries performed on a day care basis have become common. Excellent predictable outcome has encouraged individuals the choice of aesthetic dermatological surgeries. Such procedures are commonly supported by anesthesiologists at certain centers and by resident doctors or nurses at others. As long as the operator is not the one who will also provide the resuscitation, and the resuscitator is trained in providing airway and hemodynamic support, it is acceptable as per law. The support provided by the anesthesiologists in these situations is referred to as "Monitored Anesthesia Care".[1] Complications, though uncommon, have been reported in 6% of such procedures: bleeding or hematoma in 3%, infections in 2% and vasovagal reactions in 1%. Bleeding occurred more frequently in men; in patients taking anticoagulation, antiplatelet or immunosuppressive agents; in prolonged procedures. Vasovagal reactions were associated with age younger than 50 years.[2,3]

The preparedness of the dermatosurgeons in dealing with such crises affects the outcome of the situation. The emphasis is on the patient safety and adequate infrastructure to deal with the complications that may arise during the procedure. Availability of the monitoring devices, basic resuscitation equipment, adequately trained staff and the ability to manage an emergency should be always borne in mind prior to starting the scheduled procedure.[4,5] It may be misconceived by a few surgeons that complications are rare and therefore the contingency plan may not be required. Providing infrastructural support to deal with crises in day care surgery not only makes the day care procedures safer for the patient, but also avoids potential medicolegal complications. This chapter discusses the spectrum of emergencies that are commonly encountered by and the basic guidelines to manage these. Dermatological surgery is mostly cosmetic; therefore, the potential for medicolegal issues is high in the event of adverse outcome. In the author's view, the entire team in the dermatosurgeon's procedure room should be trained to provide at least basic life support (BLS), if not advanced cardiac life support (ACLS). Dermatosurgeons need to practice and adopt "safe surgery saves lives" campaign as proposed by World Health Organization.[6] The various emergency situations are given in **Box 1**. Patient safety checklist has been given in **Box 2**.

ANAPHYLAXIS

Anaphylaxis is a sudden violent manifestation of an acute immunological reaction, which might become life threatening at times. It is produced by a complex mechanism involving the immune system. The manifestation may vary from pruritus, urticarial in milder cases and inspiratory stridor, laryngeal edema, bronchospasm, hypotension, cardiac arrhythmias in more severe ones. Classic anaphylaxis manifests with a massive cardiovascular collapse within minutes of exposure to the offending antigen. The outcome in such events depends mainly on the preparedness of the team. It is a good practice

BOX 1: Various emergency issues.

- Anaphylaxis
- Syncope
- Lignocaine-related issues
- Breathlessness
- Chest pain
- Bleeding
- Acute stroke
- Status epilepticus
- Hypotension
- Hypoxia
- Cardiac arrest

BOX 2: Patient safety checklist to be practiced in dermatosurgical patients.

- Identify all the patients by name, check if the patient has consented to the procedure. All adult patients should consent themselves
- Ask the patient to show the site and side of the procedure
- Take history of allergies, if any
- Instruct the patient to continue all the medications that he has been prescribed
- Insert an intravenous cannula and maintain a running drip of ringer lactate. Other fluids such as dextrose and saline may be infused depending on the requirement
- In diabetic patients check the blood sugar by "glucostrip" method
- Connect electrocardiogram and pulse oximetry in all the patients. If access to chest is difficult to obtain, loose fitting clothes allowing access to chest may be worn
- Prepare the local anesthetic infiltration yourself. If you have a well-organized team, all medications should be loaded while a witness confirms the name of the medication
- It is author's practice to load 1:200,000 adrenaline in a 20-mL syringe for all cases (it is prepared by diluting 1 mg or 1 mL of adrenaline to 10 mL; discard 9 mL of this and dilute the remaining 1–20 mL). This solution may be used to treat several problems such as hypotension, bradycardia, bronchospasm, anaphylaxis, allergy among others

to start the monitoring devices prior to any interventions. It has been shown that presence of a professional watching the patient's vitals improves the detection of anaphylaxis and its treatment.[7,8]

Common causes of such anaphylaxis in a dermatological practice are adverse reactions to intravenous antibiotic agents, local anesthetic agents and other allergens such as latex rubber.

Anaphylactoid reactions are similar but are not immunologically mediated. They may be prevented by prior administration of corticosteroids and antihistaminic agents. These are common subsequent to administration of radiological ionic dyes and a few anesthetic agents such as atracurium and suxamethonium which are likely to release histamine.[9,10] However, these are not common in dermatosurgical practice. The management of anaphylaxis has been discussed in **Box 3**.

SYNCOPE

Syncope is a vagal mediated unconsciousness, commonly associated with extreme bradycardia and at times pulseless states. It is commonly encountered in anxious patients. It is often confused with anaphylaxis, if it occurs after an injection. Starting of an intravenous cannulation, surgical incision in inadequately anesthetized areas and even sight of blood might trigger it. An early sign of syncope, prior to loss of consciousness, is profuse sweating and cold skin. Vagal induced bradycardia in the setting of decreased systemic vascular resistance can initiate collapse. Pseudoseizure activity may occur, characterized by brief clonic activity. Blood pressure may initially decrease but is restored with supine position. The tips for avoiding syncopal attacks are mentioned in **Box 4**.

BOX 3: Management of anaphylaxis.[9]

- Place the patient supine on the examination table, preferably Trendelenburg position (head down)
- Loosen the clothing
- Assess the vital signs: Heart rate, blood pressure and oxygen saturation
- Maintain airway, breathing and circulation
- Start oxygen by face mask
- Efforts to minimize further antigen exposure should be made. Call for help. It is prudent to have a mechanism to call for help without having to leave the patient such as a call bell or "code blue"
- Secure an intravenous access if not already in place intramuscularly. Repeat dose at 5–10 minutes interval. In case intravenous access is available 5 mL adrenaline 1:10,000 can be administered and repeated after 10 min
- If the patient has severe hypotension, start intravenous fluids, preferably colloid if not improving, start inotropes such as dopamine
- Nebulized beta agonists such as albuterol with or without intravenous aminophylline may be considered in patients with severe bronchoconstriction. Simultaneously ranitidine 1 mg/kg IV, while a steroid may prevent a delayed reaction. Give hydrocortisone, 5 mg per kg, or approximately 250 mg intravenously (prednisone, 20 mg orally, can be given in mild cases)
- Monitor patients for 2–4 hours for a minor attack and in case of severe anaphylaxis, preferably admit the patient and monitor for 24 hours

BOX 4: Tips for avoiding syncopal attacks.

- Explaining the patient about the procedure and allaying anxiety often helps in reducing the incidence of syncope as also performing the procedures in a supine position
- Shielding the eyes and placing a surgical sheet to block the patient view from the operated area may help prevent the occurrence of syncope. A distracting conversation may be beneficial
- Following the procedure, the patient should slowly sit up and be observed for several minutes while postoperative instructions are being discussed. Sitting up suddenly and standing immediately after the procedure could also result in syncope after the completion of the procedure.[11]

Management of Syncope

Place the patient in supine and preferably in a head down (Trendelenburg) position. It is extremely important to lay the patient supine, should the patient be in sitting/recumbent position. Monitor vital parameters such as heart rate, blood pressure, and pulse oximetry. Reassure the patient; that may all be necessary in addition to the recumbent posture. Start intravenous access. Administer injection atropine 0.6 mg if heart rate is less than 40 per minute and intravenous fluids if blood pressure continues to be low. If alone, one should call for help and step up the monitoring only after minimal monitoring has been started to begin with.

LOCAL ANESTHETIC RELATED ISSUES

Patients with multiple allergies and atopy are more likely to develop local anesthetic allergy.[12] Most of the adverse reactions that are clinically seen are in fact manifestation of the over dosage of the local anesthetic by inadvertent intravascular injection in extremely vascular areas such as the scalp and face. It is prudent for the proceduralist to carry out a "negative aspiration" prior to injecting the local anesthetic. It can also occur in cases of tumescent liposuction when dosages over 55 mg/kg are used. In such cases, signs of over dosage are often delayed. A case of lignocaine over dosage leading to death late at mid night, after liposuction has recently been reported.[13] Toxic reactions to local anesthetic resulting from over dosage cause central nervous system or myocardial depression or excitation, perioral numbness, nausea, seizures or coma. Vasovagal syncope may be misdiagnosed as an allergic reaction and should be distinguished properly.

The preservatives added to local anesthetics to increase their shelf life. Some of the adverse reactions seen during administration of lignocaine may indeed be due to them.[14,15] Patients who are allergic to sulfa drugs may develop adverse reactions to "sulfites" which are added as preservatives to lignocaine. Anxiety regarding the use of needles, and/or the effects of epinephrine in lignocaine can lead to palpitations, panic attacks and vasovagal events that the patient may remember as an allergic reaction. Patients admitting to having had previous *syncopal or 'anaphylactic reaction'*.

Use of modern local anesthetics: Conventionally, most dermatological surgeons use lignocaine as the local anesthetic of choice. This choice is rather a habit than evidence based. There are several long-acting safer options available now. Ropivacaine, and bupivacaine are to mention a few. Levobupivacaine has recently entered the Indian market and has prolonged action and rarely causes systemic toxicity. This author urges dermatological surgeons to consider switching to safer local anesthetics such as levobupivacaine.

BREATHLESSNESS

The etiologies of breathlessness may be cardiac, respiratory or anxiety related. Patients with asthma and obstructive airway disease should be well investigated by a pulmonologist and rendered "dry" before scheduling for dermatologic surgery. Such patients should be advised to use the routine inhalers before arriving for surgery.[16] Dermatologic surgeons should also check the preoperative "basal" values of oxygen and carbon dioxide. In the absence of this knowledge, one may treat in vain to achieve magic numbers of partial pressures of more than 100 mm Hg and carbon dioxide of less than 40. Patients with "cardiac asthma" should be well prepared with diuretic and peripheral vasodilator therapy. At times, cardiac patients manifest with dyspnea when subjected to myocardial ischemia. Even young obese individuals might present with dyspnea of cardiac origin. Patients with respiratory compromise should not be operated without the guidance of pulse oximetry. If the oxygen saturation decreases during surgery, methods to administer the bronchodilator nebulization must be kept handy. Dyspnea, which does not abate with treatment, whether of cardiac or pulmonary origin is a reason to stop the scheduled procedure and to reschedule at a later convenient time. Dyspnea due to anxiety will respond well to a small intravenous dose (0.5–1 mg) of anxiolytic such as midazolam. Appropriate preoperative counseling is sufficient in most patients to avoid anxiety related problems.

CHEST PAIN

Chest pain may be a manifestation of not only coronary arterial ischemia but also anxiety. However, fear, stress of pain and procedure can also precipitate an acute myocardial infarction in any patient prone for ischemia. Although most dermatological surgical procedures are day care and performed in young healthy individuals, at times, if a high-risk patient is being subjected to aesthetic surgery, thorough evaluation would be mandatory. If a patient complains of chest pain during the procedure, place the patient supine and check the vitals.

Activate physician/emergency medical services (EMS). Record an electrocardiogram, which may be compared against the basal. If one is suspecting coronary ischemia, a tablet of nitroglycerin 5 mg should be placed immediately under the tongue. One must be aware of possible headache and hypotension following this measure. An IV cannula must be inserted immediately (if not already done) and a patent IV line is important for further management. If with these measures the chest pain settles and the patient is hemodynamically stable, one can proceed with the surgery. If the pain is unabated and electrocardiographic changes persist or worsen, the scheduled procedure should be deferred with. Patient may undergo the scheduled procedure after a consult with a cardiologist.

Patients at risk for myocardial ischemia should be thoroughly evaluated and medically optimized prior to the procedure. In the author's opinion, it may be wise to have "monitored anesthesia care" for all patients.

BLEEDING

A major surgical bleeder is rare in cutaneous surgeries. A patient receiving antiplatelet medications for concomitant comorbidities may pose special issues. Such patients may be better prepared by stopping the antiplatelet medication at least for 2 weeks prior to the planned procedure. Although the hemorrhage associated with cutaneous surgery may not be life threatening, its other effects such as causing a menacing hematoma and lifting of flaps compromising their viability may be of nuisance value.[17,18]

ACUTE STROKE

Patients on antiplatelet or antithrombotic therapy[19] and their sudden discontinuation, patients with carotid bruit, prior history of stroke, cardiovascular disease are all at potential risk for stroke.[18] Preprocedural evaluation by a physician or a neurologist has to be considered in such patients. During

BOX 5: Management of status epilepticus.

- Stop the ongoing procedure. First priority is always the maintenance of airway. Use an oral or nasopharyngeal airway as and when required (inserting these airways are out of the routine for dermatological surgeons, it is advisable for them to learn the insertion of these airways from their anesthesia or critical care colleagues)
- If available, oxygen can be delivered by face mask
- Monitor the vital signs
- Place the patient on a soft, flat surface away from sharp objects
- Look for and prevent tongue bite
- If seizures has stopped and the patient is breathing and has a pulse, place the patient in a recovery position (modified lateral position). It will allow the clearance of any pooled secretions
- Secure a peripheral intravenous line and send blood sample for blood glucose, serum electrolytes
- The benzodiazepine midazolam or lorazepam 1–2 mg or diazepam 5–10 mg intravenously will stop the seizures
- Call for physician and evaluate for seizures etiology and further management options

the procedure, the dermatosurgeon's role chiefly concerns the detection phase of a sudden neurologic deficit. This may include an alteration in consciousness (confusion, coma and seizures), aphasia, dysarthria, facial weakness or asymmetry, extremity weakness, paralysis, sensory loss, ataxia, visual loss or vertigo. Immediately activate the physician or EMS. A definitive hospital-based intervention must occur within 3 hours of the onset of the stroke symptoms to be beneficial. Meanwhile attend to the ABCs (airway, breathing, circulation) of resuscitation and monitor vitals and manage accordingly till the physician arrives.

STATUS EPILEPTICUS

Dermatosurgeons do encounter disease with potential epileptic manifestations in conditions such as tuberous sclerosis and systemic lupus erythematosus. It is wise to obtain any past history of seizures and antiseizure medications.[20] If the patients are epileptic on treatment, one should advise them to continue the treatment until the day of surgery. The management of status epilepticus has been discussed in **Box 5**.

COLLAPSE

Most commonly syncope, anaphylaxis, hypoglycemia, and cardiac arrest are reasons for collapse of a patient. These issues may be addressed as discussed in the chapter. However, associated with a vasomotor collapse are some of the key issues mentioned here which need attention.

HYPOTENSION

Low blood pressure may result from bleeding, syncope, anaphylaxis, acute myocardial infarction, and secondary to medications such as sedatives/anesthetic agents. Patient may complain of giddiness (or orthostatic hypotension).

Management

Place the patient in supine position and check vital signs such as, pulse rate and blood pressure. Treat the underlying cause. Tachycardia with low blood pressure indicates blood loss, start the patient on IV fluid crystalloids. Ringer's lactate 5–10 mL/kg bolus over 15 minutes can be administered and the blood pressure checked. If good response continues, IV fluid (Ringer's lactate) at the rate of 2–4 mL/kg/hour may be continued. If there is no response to the fluids, check for continued blood loss; send a sample of blood for checking the hemoglobin level. In the absence of matched donor blood, it is vital to maintain the circulating blood volume by administration of colloids such as starch solutions. More damage might be caused by allowing hypovolemia than anemia.[21,22] If hypotension persists, one should seek a physician's opinion and have a provision for starting an inotropic infusion such as injection dopamine 5 μg/kg/min should be commenced.

HYPERTENSION

Known hypertensives, elderly, female, anxious patients are prone for increased blood pressure during the procedure. Accelerated hypertensive patients can also present with giddiness, severe headache. Optimization of blood pressure for known hypertensives, reassuring the patients, premedication such as alprazolam, sedatives such as midazolam, lorazepam would help in the control of blood pressure. Involvement of a physician would be helpful if basic interventions do not reduce the blood pressure.

HYPOXEMIA

Patient developing desaturation during the procedure requires attention. Hypoxemia may be secondary to pain-induced hypoventilation, pulmonary embolism (during liposuction), cardiac failure, bronchospasm due to anaphylaxis.

Management

The management steps of hypoxemia are:

- Stop the procedure and start oxygen by face mask, 4 L/minute
- Talk to the patient and encourage them to breathe deeply
- Assess the vitals, talk to the patient. Reassure him. Determine the underlying cause
- Notify the physician
- Treat the underlying cause.

CARDIAC ARREST[7,23]

The most common cause of cardiac arrest is ventricular fibrillation, other arrhythmias such as pulseless ventricular tachycardia, pulseless electrical activity also can lead to cardiac arrest.

Cardiac arrest is confirmed when the patient is not responding, pulse is not felt, blood pressure is not recordable. Immediate measures to be taken are:

- Activate the emergency department/notify the physician or an anesthesiologist
- Start cardiopulmonary resuscitation as per American Heart Association (AHA) guidelines 2010[23]
- Start chest compression at the rate of 100/minute
- Get an automated external defibrillator device
- Diagnose ventricular fibrillation and defibrillate
- Continue chest compressions
- Begin ventilation
- Administer oxygen
- Obtain intravenous access
- Administer epinephrine or vasopressin
- Assess adequacy of clinical practice redesign efforts
- Intubate trachea
- Additional drug therapy
- Postresuscitation care and shift of the patient to a higher medical center for further management.

GENERAL RESUSCITATION PLAN IN DERMATOSURGERY

Training of each and every staff member in the dermatology OT with clearly defined roles for each staff is a must in managing an emergency scenario.

Preferably, an anesthetist should be available on the premises, particularly when surgeries such as liposuction are being performed. In his absence, a person trained in ACLS should be available. Various roles played by the staff members can be practiced several times so that they can act accordingly in an emergency situation. Cardiopulmonary resuscitation (CPR) training, which includes BLS and ACLS, are conducted by various health organizations in accordance with AHA. All the staff members should undergo the BLS course whereas the dermatosurgeon/team leader or the nursing staff should undergo both BLS and ACLS course. The resuscitation plan is detailed in **Box 6**.

List of Resuscitation Equipment

The basic resuscitation equipment in the form of crash cart should be made available in each dermatosurgeon's office **(Fig. 1)**.

Telephone remains the most important piece of emergency equipment in the dermatosurgeon's office; it provides the first link in the chain of initiating the EMS process.

Crash cart should comprise of:

- Portable oxygen cylinder with face mask or nasal prongs, oral or nasopharyngeal airways, intravenous cannulas, tubings, fluids and suction apparatus.
- *Medications:* Epinephrine 1:1,000, lorazepam, diazepam, diphenhydramine, dextrose 50%, nitroglycerin tablets, baby aspirin.

BOX 6: General resuscitation plan.

- Dermatologist or a physician should play role of team leader
- Patient is assessed by the team leader, and he assigns tasks to his team members
- Assigned staff member activates the emergency medical services or a physician or an anesthesiologist
- One staff member gets the automated external defibrillator and attaches it to the patient to analyze the rhythm and shock accordingly
- One staff member plays the role of chest compressor and other staff member takes care of airway
- Another staff member can serve as the recorder of the event times, serial vital signs measurements, securing intravenous access; administer medications and communication with the family members

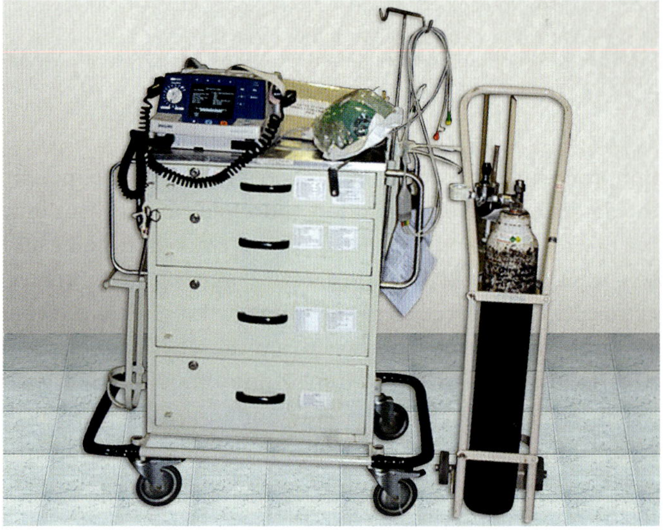

Fig. 1: Crash cart used by author.

- Automated external defibrillators (AEDs) are computerized devices consisting of adhesive electrodes which recognize cardiac rhythms and deliver an electrical shock across the chest wall to terminate the ventricular fibrillation. They are portable and user friendly. Adhesive electrodes are placed over the patient's cardiac apex and upper right chest to detect the cardiac rhythm. With audible and visual prompting, the device advises the operator to press the button and deliver a defibrillating shock.
- Laryngoscope, endotracheal tubes, AMBU bag.
- The crash cart inventory should be periodically reviewed and renewed as necessary **(Fig. 1)**.
- CPR is a life-saving measure which supports pumping of blood by the heart thus allowing oxygen to reach the brain. It is more effective when done as early as possible. The conduct of CPR is guided by AHA guidelines recently updated in 2015.[23]
- CPR includes recognition of cardiac arrest, activating EMS, and to get an AED, performing BLS and ACLS.
- *Components of BLS:* The primary survey "circulation airway breathing".
  - *Circulation:* Chest compression keeps the blood pumping to the vital organs. It is done at the rate of

100 compressions per minute, at an adequate depth of 2–2.5 inches, and allowing complete chest recoil.
   - *Airway and breathing:* Opening the patient's airway by performing the head tilt chin lift, and give breath by mask-mouth. Chest compression to ventilation ratio is 30:2.
- *Defibrillation:* Once the AED arrives, switch on the defibrillator; attach the adhesive electrodes to the patient's chest. Clear the patient and once the defibrillator analyzes the rhythm, follow the defibrillators instructions.

All the medic and paramedic staff members in the dermatology setup should be trained in performing the BLS, performing the chest compressions, maintaining the airway, handling the AED.

Components of ACLS: The Secondary Survey

- *Circulation:* Obtain IV access, attach ECG leads, and monitor for arrhythmias or cardiac arrest. Use of drugs/IV fluids to manage rhythm and blood pressure.
- *Airway:* Maintain the airway patency—use of airways, advanced airway management if needed using a laryngeal masks airway/endotracheal tube.
- *Breathing:* Give supplemental oxygen; assess the adequacy of ventilation by noting the chest rise, oxygen saturation, capnography (expired carbon dioxide measurement).
- *Differential diagnosis:* Find and treat the reversible causes for cardiac arrest, which is easily remembered in a mnemonic form as 5 Hs and 5 Ts.
   - *Hs:* Hypovolemia, hydrogen ion (acidosis), hyper/hypokalemia, hypoglycemia, hypothermia.
   - *Ts:* Toxins, tamponade, tension pneumothorax, thrombosis (coronary and pulmonary), trauma.
- General supportive care of the patient and specific pharmacologic therapy aimed at underlying event causing cardiac arrest should be initiated once the patient is successfully resuscitated.

Documentation of the Events

All adverse events and the measures taken are to be documented, discussed with the patient, and a discharge summary of the event to be issued to the patient. The exact time of the event may not be relevant but the flow of events and their management may be important. Such documentations are important from the medicolegal view point too.

There are certain tips given for the avoidance of complications in **Box 7**.

BOX 7: Tips for avoidance of complications.

- Thorough preoperative evaluation, optimal management of the coexisting medical illness[24]
- Preprocedural counseling, premedication to allay anxiety. Explanation in detail the procedure, postprocedural care
- Basic monitoring facilities: Pulse oximetry, noninvasive blood pressure, electrocardiogram should be made available
- Avoidance of drugs which has previously caused reactions
- Involvement of anesthesiologist (Standby anesthesiologists to provide monitored anesthesia care) as and when required, at the earliest and discussion of various anesthetic options available in the conduct of safe procedure
- Establishment of clear postprocedural instructions

DERMATOSURGICAL CONDITIONS THAT REQUIRE EMERGENCY INTERVENTIONS

Dermatosurgical emergencies are not only those faced during procedural intervention but also those that presents as emergencies to the dermatosurgery department for active intervention. They are enlisted in **Box 8**.

BOX 8: Dermatosurgical conditions that require emergency interventions.

- Hemorrhage
- Abscess
- Bleeding of varicose vein
- Blister drainage
- Burns and scalds
- Paraphimosis
- Fournier's gangrene
- Impacted finger ring
- Frenulum tear
- Traumatic nail avulsion
- Pyogenic granuloma
- Thrombophlebitis
- Cryoblister

TABLE 1: Types of hemorrhage.

Primary hemorrhage	It is the bleeding during intraoperative period
Reactionary hemorrhage	It is the bleeding which occurs within 24 hours postoperatively
Secondary hemorrhage	It usually occurs after 1 week of surgery which may be due to infection. This type of bleeding is rare in dermatosurgery

Hemorrhage

Bleeding is always a concern for dermatosurgeon as its better control results in optimal results. Postoperative bleeding can lead to the development of a hematoma, which subsequently can lead to surgical complications such as wound infection, dehiscence, and necrosis. Such adverse events not only cause anxiety and mental stress for the patient and the physician, but also may ultimately result in a poor outcome with suboptimal scar formation. There are multiple factors that can lead to bleeding during or after a surgical procedure. It includes age of the patient, medications, medical comorbidities, and poor knowledge of anatomy of vessels. Source of bleeding can be capillary, venous and arterial **(Table 1)**.

Preoperative evaluation of the patients: Preoperative evaluation of patients will help in recognizing patients at risk of bleeding. With regards to hemorrhage, there are four major categories, which need to be addressed in for bleeding risk: (1) anticoagulant drugs; (2) hypertension; (3) medical comorbidities; and (4) anatomy of blood vessels.

Drugs: The common drugs, which increase the risk of bleeding, are aspirin, non-steroidal anti-inflammatory drugs (NSAIDs), warfarin,[25] or other newer antiplatelet agents and anticoagulants.[26] Several herbal or over-the-counter (OTC) medications such as garlic, ginseng, ginger, feverfew, vitamin E, *Ginkgo biloba* and many can have intended or unintended effects on the coagulation pathway. Hence investigate the patients for risk of bleeding which include bleeding and clotting time, prothrombin time, and aPTT.

Hypertension[27]: Hypertension carries risk of intraoperative bleeding. The cutaneous surgery may be preceded in patients with a blood pressure 180 mm Hg systolic or 100 mm Hg diastolic or lower, and no other medical contraindications. For patients with blood pressure 181–200 mm Hg systolic or 101–110 mm Hg diastolic, cutaneous surgery may proceed depending on surgeon preference. If surgery does proceed, there may be a small risk of cardiovascular lability. For patients with blood pressure exceeding 200 mm Hg systolic or 110 mm Hg diastolic, it may be prudent to defer the surgical procedure until after his or her primary medical physician properly evaluates the patient.

Anatomy

The majority of operative cutaneous lesions are located on the head or neck. It is important to know the "danger zones" for arterial bleeding in procedural dermatology, all located on the head and neck:[28] (1) the frontal branch of the temporal artery located at the temple; (2) the facial artery at its crossing over the mandibular rim; (3) the angular artery adjacent to the nose. Knowing this anatomy makes the surgeon confident in putting incision of the proper depth and undermine in the correct plane to minimize bleeding complications.

Management of Hemorrhage

Intraoperative management: One of the first steps taken to help minimize intraoperative bleeding is the addition of epinephrine to the local anesthetic. The concentration of epinephrine added to the local anesthetic is usually either 1:100,000 or 1:200,000. The three major benefits are prolonging activity of the anesthetic agent, decreases volume of anesthetic required and controls bleeding.[29]

Goldman divides intraoperative hemorrhage into two major categories: "oozing" and "frank bleeding". He further subdivides "oozing" into superficial/dermal oozing and deep oozing, the latter more commonly seen due to muscular injury. Frank bleeding can be arterial/venous or arteriolar/venular. The superficial/dermal oozing is managed with 10 minutes of manual pressure. Electrosurgery and hemostatic agents such as aluminum chloride, 20% ferric sulfate (Monsel's solution), and 10–50% silver nitrate can also be used. If the oozing is deeper and more muscular, the same techniques of pressure and/or electro surgery may be used to control the hemorrhage. Arterial/venous hemorrhage is best managed using electro surgery (electrodessication and electrocoagulation) or heat cautery. Regardless, any electrosurgery should be precise to minimize excessive and unnecessary charring of surrounding tissue. Larger arterial or venous bleeding requires ligation of the vessels using absorbable sutures. The simplest and most commonly used stitch is the figure-of-eight stitch.

Occasionally, surgeon will encounter a surgical wound oozing to be continues and bleed despite multiple attempts at homeostasis. In such a case, it may be more practical to leave the wound partially open or consider placing a Penrose drain to allow for drainage. If a drain is used in the wound, it is important to remove it in a timely fashion (usually after 24 hours) to prevent infection.

Postoperative management: Once the cutaneous surgery is completed, the postoperative phase of patient care and instructions begins. There are two key components to the postoperative period which include:

i. *Bandaging the wound/surgical repair site:* A typical pressure dressing involves the placement of a nonadherent film followed by one or more layers of cotton gauze and finally, securing the dressing with adhesive tape. Pressure dressing is probably not effective beyond 24 hours henceforth patient had to come for follow-up after 2 days.
ii. *Educating the patient and any family member about proper care of the site while at home:* Patients should be provided with verbal and written instructions on wound care, what to do if there is bleeding (either oozing or frank bleeding), activity levels, alcohol use, signs and symptoms of infection or wound dehiscence or necrosis, and ultimately, when to call the surgeon. Avoiding any strenuous exercise, bending, lifting heavy objects, or physical activity that could potentially lead to direct trauma to the surgical site is important for healing and prevention of hemorrhagic complications. In addition, sites which are in constant motion due to daily activities such as lips or the perioral area require specific instructions such as minimizing talking/laughing, eating soft or well-cooked foods, avoiding sucking action via a straw, and taking care when inserting or removing dentures and also while brushing.

Abscess Drainage

The abscess requires emergency drainage to not only alleviate pain but also to prevent spread of infection. The most fearful abscesses faced in dermatosurgery department are palmar abscess, periungual abscess and abscess in danger zones. Cellulitis may precede or occur in conjunction with an abscess if not treated early. It is caused mainly by Staphylococcus and Streptococcus. Enteric organisms commonly cause

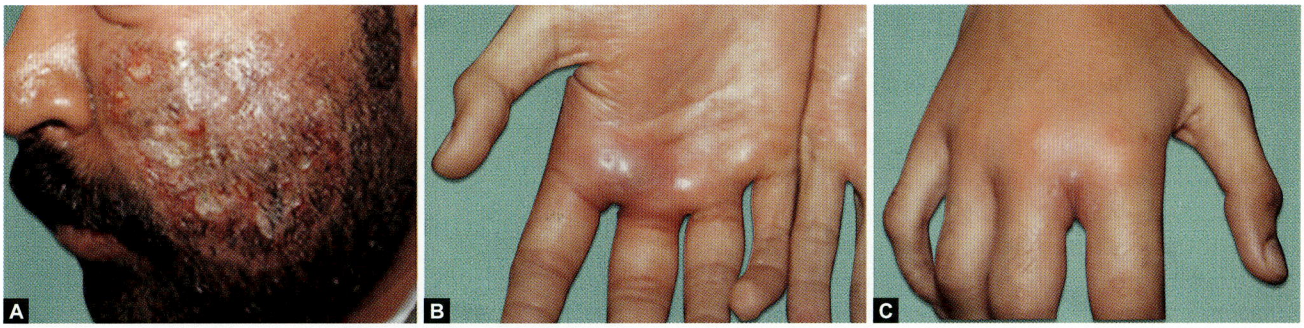

Figs. 2A to C: (A) Carbuncle over left check; (B and C) Palmar abscess.
Courtesy: CUTIS Academy of Cutaneous Sciences, Bengaluru.

perianal abscesses. Treatment is primarily through incision and drainage (I&D). Smaller abscesses (<5 mm) may resolve spontaneously with the application of warm compresses and topical antibiotic therapy. Larger abscesses require incision and drainage **(Figs. 2A to C)**.

Procedure: A Stab incision with 11 no. blade or 18 G needle is made at dependent point or at pus point. Pus sample is sent for culture and sensitivity. The cavity is explored by breaking loculations. Cavity is washed with the sterile saline or betadine solution using a syringe. Wound is secured with tight bandage.

Blister Drainage

Blister is a small pocket of fluid either serum or plasma within the upper layers of the skin, caused by friction, burning, freezing, chemical exposure or infection. It will be asymptomatic most of the time but if painful and if risk of infection is noticed then it has to be drained.

Procedure: Under aseptic precaution using a sterile needle the blister will be punctured to drain the fluid and the overlying skin is left in place so that it acts as biological dressing. Inspect the area for infection in the follow-up period.

Bleeding of Varicose Vein

It is one of the rare complications that present to dermatosurgery department. It is due to rupture of varicose vein. Varicose veins are enlarged veins, which are located under the skin surface usually on the leg **(Fig. 3)**. They are often easy to see, as they look thick and knobby. Varicose veins are asymptomatic and complications are less. Bleeding from varicose vein happens rarely. It can happen due to minor trauma to the skin or it can bleed spontaneously. If a varicose vein bleeds, then there is need to stop the bleeding by lying flat and raising the leg high and apply pressure with clean cloth or dressing on to the bleeding area for at least 10 minutes. Sclerotherapy has proven to be one of the best treatments to prevent repeat bleeding episodes. Wearing stocking of class II will act as preventive measure and avoids such complications.

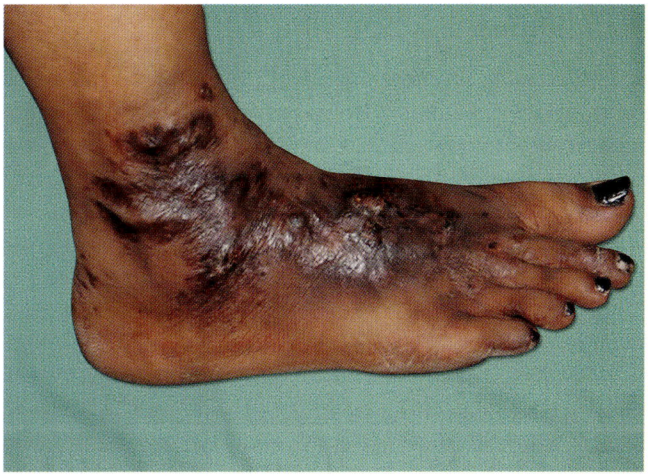

Fig. 3: Bleeding from varicose veins.
Courtesy: CUTIS Academy of Cutaneous Sciences, Bengaluru.

Burns and Scald

It is the damage to the skin caused mainly by heat. Burn is caused by dry heat (fire) whereas scald is caused by something wet, such as hot water or steam. It usually presents as red or peeling skin with pain, swelling, blister and charred skin. Acids or bases can cause burns when it comes in contact with tissue. Most acids produce a coagulation necrosis by denaturing proteins, forming a coagulum (e.g., eschar) that limits the penetration of the acid. Bases typically produce a more severe injury known as liquefaction necrosis. This involves denaturing of proteins as well as saponification of fats, which does not limit tissue penetration. So, bases produce more damage than acids. Chemical burns involving smaller body surface area and involving epidermis and superficial dermis will be handled by dermatosurgeon and for larger area involvement must be referred to higher center for management. Burns cases are treated in following manner:

- *Cool the burnt area* with cool or lukewarm running water for 20 minutes—do not use ice, iced water, or any creams or greasy substances such as butter
- *Remove any clothing or jeweler* that is near the burnt area of skin, including babies' nappies but do not move anything that is stuck to the skin

- *Make sure the person keeps warm* but take care not to rub it against the burnt area
- *Use painkillers* such as paracetamol or NSAID to treat any pain. *Systemic antibiotics prevents secondary infection*
- *If the face or eyes are burnt, sit up as much as possible,* rather than lying down, this helps to reduce swelling chemical and electrical burns, large or deep burns, burns on the face, hands, arms, feet, legs or genitals that cause blisters are usually admitted and treated under strict monitoring
- *Prefer regular closed dressings for deeper wounds and open dressings for superficial wounds with topical antibiotic creams.*

Paraphimosis

Paraphimosis is an uncommon medical emergency in which the foreskin of a penis becomes trapped behind the glans penis, and cannot be pulled back to cover the glans. If this condition persists for several hours, there will be signs of a lack of blood flow leading to gangrene. It is usually caused by medical professionals or parents who retract the foreskin during penile examination, urethral catheterization, or cystoscopy; if the foreskin is left retracted for a long period, some of the foreskin tissue may become edematous which makes subsequent reduction of the foreskin difficult. Paraphimosis can often be effectively treated by manual manipulation of the swollen foreskin tissue. This involves compressing the glans and moving the foreskin back to its normal position, perhaps with the aid of a lubricant, cold compression, and local anesthesia as necessary. If this fails, the tight edematous band of tissue can be relieved surgically with a dorsal slit or circumcision. An alternative method, the Dundee technique, entails placing multiple punctures in the swollen foreskin with a fine needle, and then expressing the edema fluid by manual pressure.

Fournier's gangrene: It is a type of necrotizing fasciitis affecting the external genitalia. It is a rare condition, which occurs, in older men, but it can also occur in women and children. It is more likely to occur in diabetics, alcoholics or those who are immune compromised. It presents as swelling or sudden pain in the scrotum associated with fever, pallor, generalized weakness, foul odor, and purulent discharge from the infected tissue. Fournier's gangrene is diagnosed clinically and sometime requires investigations. Fournier's gangrene is an emergency and treated with intravenous antibiotics and debridement (surgical removal) of necrotic (dead) tissue. In addition to surgery and antibiotics, hyperbaric oxygen therapy (HBOT) may be useful and acts to inhibit the growth of and kill the anaerobic bacteria.

Cryoblister

It is a temporary and expected side effect with cryotherapy. It usually occurs due the tissue damage caused by the cryogen, i.e., liquid nitrogen **(Fig. 4)**. It usually manifests 24–48 hours following cryotherapy. Patients are usually counseled about it and treatment include topical antibiotics with blister drainage.

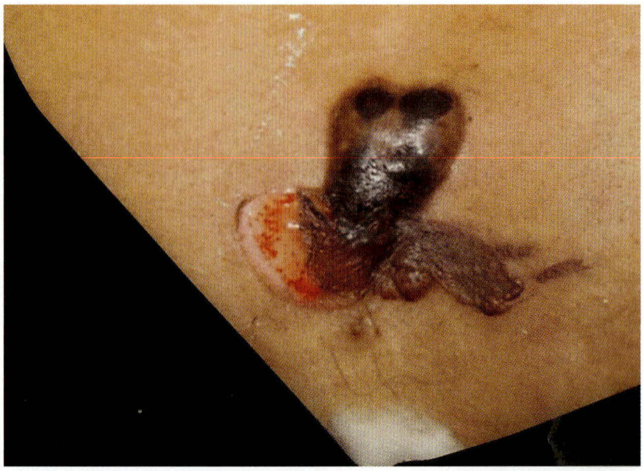

Fig. 4: Cryoblister following surface cryotherapy.
Courtesy: CUTIS Academy of Cutaneous Sciences, Bengaluru.

Traumatic Nail Avulsion

Most of the fingernail injuries are caused by crush trauma. It is common in children and young adults. Effective emergency treatment of traumatic nail injuries is important to prevent secondary deformities. If subungual hematoma is present involving more than 50% of the nail, then it has to be evacuated. It is done by making two small holes in the nail plate. If the avulsed nail plate is present intact, then it can be placed over the nail bed as a biological dressing. If it is too damaged, then nail substitutes can be used. If there are wounds or laceration present on the nail bed/matrix then it can be closed using absorbable sutures. In case of avulsion of the nail bed or matrix and the avulsed tissue is present, then it can be repositioned and sutured. If the avulsed tissue is not present, then conservative or reconstructive surgeries should be done.[30] If there is associated distal phalanx fracture, nail bed repair is done and a simple splint can be given in case of a non-displaced fracture. In case of a displaced fracture, K-wire is inserted and fixed.

CONCLUSION

Complications in dermatological surgery office-based procedures although rare, do occur, and the outcomes of such events are related to the initial diagnosis and early management. Well-equipped emergency OT, a good knowledge, training in emergency BLS and ACLS course makes dermatosurgeons get more confidence in identifying and managing emergencies. Thorough preprocedural evaluation and identification of high-risk patients,[24] optimization of coexisting medical illness with medications will go a long way in preventing adverse events during the procedure. Good communication and patient rapport are important. High-risk cases, technologically advanced procedures should be scheduled under monitored anesthesia care and in a hospital with full-fledged emergency backup facility. A well-planned and organized office setup under the leadership of a dermatologist proves to be beneficial to the patients and reduce the medicolegal complications too.

REFERENCES

1. Bing J, McAuliffe MS, Lupton JR. Regional anesthesia with monitored anesthesia care for dermatologic laser surgery. Dermatol Clin. 2002;20;123-34.
2. Amici JM, Rogues AM, Lasheras A, Gachie JP, Guillot P, Beylot C, et al. A prospective study of the incidence of complications associated with dermatological surgery. Br J Dermatol. 2005;153:967-71.
3. Esme P, Akoglu G, Erbil H. Medical and socioeconomic challenges of private dermatocosmetology clinics during COVID-19 pandemic: a survey from Turkey. J Cosmet Dermatol. 2020;19:3160-5.
4. Chan BC, Patel DC. Perioperative management and associated rate of adverse events in dermatological procedures performed by dermatologists in New Zealand. Australas J Dermatol. 2009;50:23-8.
5. Natalie LS. Dermatologic surgical complications. Medscape. 2009.
6. World Alliance for Patient Safety. Guideline 15: WHO guidelines for safe surgery. Geneva: World Health Organization; 2008.
7. Gloster HM. Acute emergencies in the dermatology office. In: Fader D (Ed). Complications in Cutaneous Surgery. London: Springer Science Publications; 2008.
8. Tang AW. A practical guide to anaphylaxis. Am Fam Physician. 2003;68:1325-33.
9. The diagnosis and management of anaphylaxis. Joint Task Force on Practice Parameters, American Academy of Allergy, Asthma and Immunology, American College of Allergy, Asthma and Immunology, and the Joint Council of Allergy, Asthma and Immunology. J Allergy Clin Immunol. 1998;101:S465-528.
10. Castells M. Diagnosis and management of anaphylaxis in precision medicine. J Allergy Clin Immunol. 2017;140:321-333.
11. Parry SW, Kenny RA. The management of vasovagal syncope: a review. Q J Med. 1999;92:697-705.
12. Gmyrek R. Local and regional anesthesia. Medscape. 2011.
13. Araujo LM, Amaral JL. Allergy to lidocaine: case report. Rev Bras Anesthesiol (online). 2004;54:672-6.
14. Cherobin ACFP, Tavares GT. Safety of local anesthetics. An Bras Dermatol. 2020;95(1):82-90.
15. Venkataram M, Nischal KC. Guidelines for administration of local anesthesia for dermatosurgery and cosmetic dermatology procedures. Ind J Dermatol Venereol Leprol. 2009;75:68-75.
16. Licker M, Schweizer A, Ellenberger C, Tschopp JM, Diaper J, Clergue F. Perioperative medical management of patients with COPD. Int J Chron Obstruct Pulmon Dis. 2007;2:493-515.
17. Alcalay J, Alkalay R. Controversies in perioperative management of blood thinners in dermatologic surgery: continue or discontinue? Dermatol Surg. 2004;30:1091-4.
18. Rausher EG. Overview preoperative evaluation and management. Medscape. 2011.
19. Kovich O, Otley CC. Thrombotic complications related to discontinuation of warfarin and aspirin therapy perioperatively for cutaneous operations. J Am Acad Dermatol. 2003;48:233-7.
20. Gloster HM. Acute emergencies in dermatology office. In: Fader D (Ed). Complications in Cutaneous Surgery. London: Springer publications; 2007. pp. 15.
21. Bacter CR, Canizaro PC, Shires GT. Fluid resuscitation of hemorrhagic shock. Postgrad Med. 1970;48:95-9.
22. Krausz MM. Initial resuscitation of hemorrhagic shock. World J Emerg Surg. 2006;1:14.
23. Executive Summary: 2015 American Heart Association Guidelines Update for Cardiopulmonary Resuscitation and Emergency Cardiovascular Care. Circulation. 2015;132: S315-67.
24. Leshin B, McCalmont TH. Preoperative evaluation of the surgical patient. Dermatol Clin. 1990;8:787-94.
25. Alcalay J. Cutaneous surgery in patients receiving warfarin therapy. DermatolSurg. 2001:27(8):756-8.
26. Kargi E, Babuccu O, Hosnuter M, Babuccu B, Altinyazar C. Complications of minor cutaneous surgery in patients under anticoagulant treatment. Aesthetic Plast Surg. 2002:26(6): 483-5.
27. Larson MJ, Taylor RS. Monitoring vital signs during outpatient Mohs and post-Mohs reconstructive surgery performed under local anesthesia. DermatolSurg. 2004:30 (5):777-83.
28. Robinson JK. Anatomy for procedural dermatology. In: Robinson JK, Hanke CW, Siegel DM, Fratila A (Eds). Surgery of the skin. New York: Moby Elsevier; 2010. pp. 3-27.
29. Hruza GJ. Anesthesia. In: Bolognia JL, Jorrizo JL, Rapini RP (Eds). Dermatology, 2nd edition. St Louis: Mosby Elsevier, 2008. pp. 2173-81.
30. Goldman G. Wound closure materials and instruments. In: Bolognia JL, Jorizzo JL, Rapini RP, (Eds). Dermatology, 2nd edition. St Louis: Mosby Elsevier; 2008. pp. 2183-93.

CHAPTER 17

Pharmacology of Analgesic and Anxiolytic Drugs Used in Dermatosurgery

Shyamanta Barua, Roshni Singh

KEY MESSAGES

- Prevention and treatment of pain is an important aspect of aesthetic surgery.
- Pain in dermatosurgical procedures is usually mild.
- Clonidine and midazolam are useful preoperative medications in dermatosurgery.
- Nonsteroidal anti-inflammatory drugs (NSAIDs) and opioids constitute first- and second-line analgesic agents in dermatosurgery.
- Many analgesics have drug interactions, which should be considered prior to surgery.

INTRODUCTION

Pain relief during and after surgery is an important aspect of intra- and postoperative management. This is particularly relevant in aesthetic surgeries, which are desired by the patient, where fear of pain is an important factor, which often dissuades prospective clients from undergoing the procedure. Proper pain management, therefore, contributes to greater patient satisfaction. Hence, proper understanding of analgesia is essential for dermatosurgeons.

This chapter presents a brief description of pharmacology of analgesics and anxiolytics used in dermatosurgery. The reader is referred to pharmacology books[1-5] for a detailed description of drugs; what is outlined here is an approach to the management of pain.

PATHOPHYSIOLOGY OF PAIN

Algesia or pain is an ill-defined, unpleasant sensation, usually evoked by an external or internal noxious stimulus. Analgesics are the drugs that relieve pain by acting on the central nervous system (CNS) or on the peripheral pain mechanisms, without significantly altering consciousness. There are two components in pathophysiology of pain:

1. The central component through which afferent inputs generate a pain sensation.
2. The peripheral component in which nociceptive afferent neurons are activated by noxious stimuli.[1,2]

There are two main categories of pain:

1. *Integumental pain:* Superficial, related to skin, muscle, and joints
2. *Visceral pain:* Deep-seated, related to heart, stomach, kidney, and gallbladder

Integumental pain is easier to manage and most dermatosurgeries do not involve the muscles, joints, and bones. The skin and the subcutaneous structures are relatively immobile, making the analgesic plan a fairly simple one. In contrast, the movement of the painful structure in thorax and upper abdomen renders the analgesic plan complex. Thus, the issue of pain relief in dermatosurgical practice is not as complex as in other dynamic areas of the body, such as thorax and upper abdomen. Integumental pain can be managed therefore with milder drugs.

ANALGESICS

Classification

Analgesics[2] are divided into two broad groups, viz:

1. *Opioid/narcotic/morphine-like analgesics:* These act primarily at the level of the spinal cord and brain.
2. *Nonopioid/nonnarcotic/nonsteroidal anti-inflammatory antipyretic analgesics:* These act primarily at peripheral sites to inhibit the synthesis or activity of pain-sensitizing substances such as prostaglandins (PGs).

Opioid Analgesics

Morphine is the prototype opioid analgesic. The sites of opioid analgesia include peripheral nervous system and both spinal and supraspinal brain areas, particularly the limbic system. They reduce both the sensory as well as the affective (emotional) components of pain. They are generally more effective against dull, continuous pain such as deep-seated visceral pain than a sharp intermittent integumentary pain.[1] Different opioid drugs and their dosages are shown in **Table 1**.

Adverse effects: These effects appear at parenteral doses of morphine higher than 15 mg and include respiratory depression, constipation, bronchospasm, postural hypotension, urinary retention, nausea and vomiting, and

TABLE 1: Distinctive features of opioid analgesics.

Drug	*Receptor activity* μ	κ	Δ	*Parenteral dose (mg)*	*Duration of analgesia (hours)*
Morphine	+++	+	+	10–15	4–6
Codeine	++	+	+	60	4–6
Fentanyl	+++	–	+	0.05–0.1	1–1.5
Methadone	+++	–	–	5–10	4–6
Meperidine	+++	+	+	50–100	2–4
Tramadol	+	–	–	50–100	4–6

Source: Adapted from Tripathi KD.[2]

urticaria and itching. Tolerance and dependence frequently develop on prolonged and repeated use. Serious toxicity is produced by 50 mg of morphine and the lethal dose in humans is estimated to be 250 mg.[1,2]

Contraindications:[2]

- Bronchial asthma
- Hypotension
- Hepatic damage
- Hypertrophy of prostate
- Head injury
- Hypothyroidism
- Biliary colic
- Extremes of age
- Undiagnosed acute abdominal pain.

Drug interactions: Phenothiazines, tricyclic antidepressants, monoamine oxidase (MAO) inhibitors, amphetamine, and neostigmine potentiate morphine and other opioids, either by retarding its metabolism or by a pharmacodynamic interaction at the level of central neurotransmitters. On the other hand, morphine retards the absorption of many orally administered drugs by delaying gastric emptying.[2]

Drugs used in dermatosurgery: As stated earlier, pain in dermatosurgical procedures is not very intense, and hence drugs such as morphine or pethidine are rarely needed. Commonly used drugs include tramadol and tapentadol.
Tramadol: It is a commonly used drug in dermatosurgery. It is a centrally acting analgesic that relieves pain by opioid effects (mediated almost exclusively through μ receptors) as well as additional mechanisms, such as its serotonergic and noradrenergic effects. It is indicated for mild-to-moderate short-lasting pain and can also be used to allay anxiety. The dose is 50–100 mg oral/intramuscular (IM)/slow intravenous (IV) infusion, 4–6 hourly. Maximum dosage is 400 mg/day orally, 600 mg/day parenterally, and 300 mg/day in patients >75 years old and for extended release. It is also available in combination with acetaminophen. It is not recommended for children. Analgesic action begins within an hour of ingestion, peaks within 2–3 hours, and lasts for 4–6 hours.[1,2]

Respiratory depression and sedation are very rarely associated with tramadol. Side effects include nausea, vomiting, sweating, itching, and constipation. Hence, it is often prescribed with domperidone to offset the onset of nausea and vomiting. Drowsiness has been reported. Seizures, though rare, may occur as a complication. It undergoes metabolism via cytochrome P450 system, and hence dosage may need to be reduced in patients with liver and renal function alterations (maximum dosage is 200 mg/day for patient with low creatinine clearance). Risk of serotonin syndrome is likely to increase when it is co-administrated with selective serotonin reuptake inhibitor (SSRI) therapy.[2]

The efficacy and relative safety make tramadol a commonly used drug to relieve severe pain in dermatosurgery, after procedures such as hair transplantation.

Tapentadol: It has similar structure and mechanism of action such as tramadol. It causes marked inhibition of norepinephrine (NE) transporter as compared to tramadol; thus, it mainly activates central noradrenergic pathway to allay pain. Side effects are also similar to tramadol, but nausea and vomiting are less pronounced. The dosage is 50–100 mg 2–4 times/day.[2]

Nonsteroidal Anti-inflammatory Drugs

All the drugs in this class have analgesic, antipyretic, and anti-inflammatory actions in different measures **(Table 2)**. In contrast to the opioid analgesics, they do not depress CNS, do not produce physical dependence, have no abuse liability, and are weaker analgesics. They not only act primarily on peripheral pain mechanisms, but also in the CNS to raise pain threshold.

Mechanism of action: Nonsteroidal anti-inflammatory drugs inhibit the cyclooxygenase (COX) enzyme in the arachidonic acid cascade to prevent the synthesis of prostanoids (prostaglandins), prostacyclin (PGI2), and thromboxane (TXA) **(Flowchart 1)**. There are two types of COX enzymes, namely COX-1 and COX-2. A third form, COX-3, has also been recently identified. The majority of traditional NSAIDs are nonselective inhibitors of both COX-1 and COX-2, although they vary in the degree of COX inhibition **(Table 3)**.[3]

Adverse effects: Nonsteroidal anti-inflammatory drugs[3] have several side effects, such as:

- *Gastrointestinal:* Gastric irritation, erosions, peptic ulceration, gastric bleeding/perforation, and esophagitis
- *Renal:* Sodium and water retention, chronic renal failure, interstitial nephritis, and papillary necrosis
- *Hepatic:* Raised transaminases and hepatic failure
- *Central nervous system:* Headache, mental confusion, behavioral disturbances, and seizure precipitation
- *Hematological:* Bleeding, thrombocytopenia, hemolytic anemia, and agranulocytosis
- *Others:* Asthma exacerbation, nasal polyposis, skin rashes, pruritus, and angioedema.

TABLE 2: Classification of nonsteroidal anti-inflammatory drugs and dosage.

Drug	Dosage
Nonselective cyclooxygenase (COX) inhibitors	
Salicylates: Aspirin	0.3–0.6 g, 6–8 hourly (maximum effect at 1,000 mg single dose)
Propionic acid derivatives: • Ibuprofen	• 400–600 mg (5–10 mg/kg) TDS
• Naproxen	• 250 mg BD-TDS
• Ketoprofen	• 50–100 mg BD-TDS
Fenamate: Mefenamic acid	250–500 mg TDS
Enolic acid derivatives: Piroxicam	20 mg BD for 2 days followed by 20 mg OD
Acetic acid derivatives: • Ketorolac	• 15–30 mg IM or IV every 4–6 hours, 10–20 mg 6 hourly oral
• Indomethacin	• 25–50 mg BD–QID
• Nabumetone	• 500–1,000 mg OD
Pyrazolone derivatives: Phenylbutazone	150 mg (+ paracetamol 250 mg + caffeine 30 mg)
Preferential COX-2 inhibitors	
Nimesulide	100 mg BD
Meloxicam	7.5–15 mg OD
Nabumetone	500 mg OD
Diclofenac	50–75 mg TDS oral, then BD oral, and 75 mg deep IM
Aceclofenac	100 mg BD
Selective COX-2 inhibitors	
Celecoxib	100–200 mg BD
Parecoxib	40 mg oral/IM/IV every 6–12 hours
Etoricoxib	60–120 mg OD
Analgesics–antipyretics with poor anti-inflammatory action	
p-aminophenol derivative: Paracetamol (acetaminophen)	325–650 mg (children 10–15 mg/kg) 3–4 times a day
Benzoxazocine derivative: Nefopam	30–60 mg TDS oral and 20 mg IM 6 hourly

(BD: twice a day; IM: intramuscular; IV: intravenous; OD: once a day; QID: four times a day; TDS: thrice a day)
Source: Adapted from Tripathi KD.[3]

Flowchart 1: Schematic representation of site of action of nonsteroidal anti-inflammatory drugs (NSAIDs).

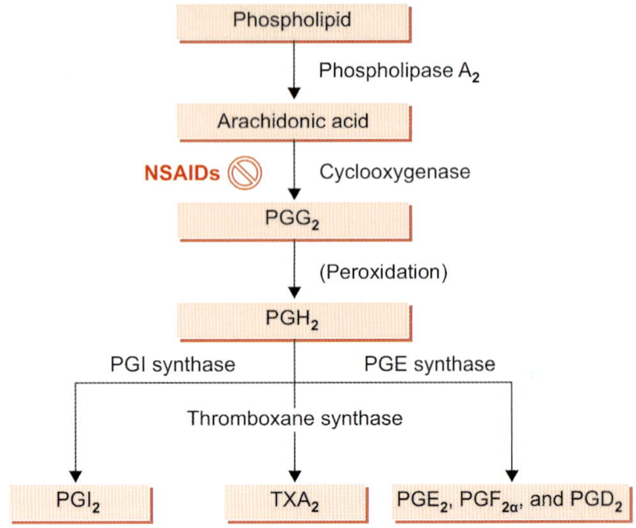

(PG: prostaglandin; TXA: tranexamic acid)

TABLE 3: Features of nonselective cyclooxygenase (COX) inhibitors and selective COX-2 inhibitors.

Action	*COX-1/COX-2 inhibitors*	*COX-2inhibitors*
Analgesic	+	+
Antipyretic	+	+
Anti-inflammatory	+	+
Antiplatelet aggregatory	+	–
Gastric mucosal damage	+	–
Renal salt/water depletion	+	+
Delay/prolongation of labor	+	+
Ductus arteriosus closure	+	?
Asthma precipitation	+	–

Source: Reprinted from Tripathi KD.[3]

Drug interactions: Drug interactions are frequent and may be potentially serious **(Table 4)**. Since patients often consume these drugs, without prescription or on long-term basis, proper history is important.[3]

NONSTEROIDAL ANTI-INFLAMMATORY DRUGS IN DERMATOLOGY

Acetaminophen (Paracetamol and N-acetyl-P-aminophenol)

Acetaminophen is an active metabolite of phenacetin with good analgesic, antipyretic action, and weak anti-inflammatory effects. It acts centrally and raises the pain threshold. Unlike aspirin, acetaminophen does not stimulate respiration or increase cellular metabolism. It has no effect on acid–base balance, cardiovascular system, or platelet function. It causes insignificant gastric irritation, mucosal erosion, and bleeding may occur in overdose. Other side effects include rash, hypersensitive reaction, and fatal hepatotoxicity (>150 mg/kg or >10 g in an adult). Its action lasts for 3–5 hours and peaks within 30–60 minutes. It can be used in all age groups, pregnancy, and lactation. It has least drug interaction and can be used in the presence of other diseases.[3]

Ibuprofen

Ibuprofen is a nonselective COX inhibitor. It can be used safely in children and adults, but its use is not recommended during pregnancy and should be avoided in peptic ulcer patient.[3] Inhibition of platelet aggregation and risk of intra- and postoperative bleeding have led to concerns about the use of NSAIDs. Studies have shown that aspirin increases bleeding time more significantly than ibuprofen. Therefore, aspirin should be stopped 1 week before elective surgery.

TABLE 4: Drug interactions with nonsteroidal anti-inflammatory drugs.

	Pharmacodynamic	*Pharmacokinetic*	
Diuretics	↓Diuresis	Oral anticoagulants	Metabolism inhibited
β-blocker	↓Antihypertensive effect	Sulfonylureas	Competes for plasma
Angiotensin-converting enzyme (ACE) inhibitors	↓Antihypertensive effect	Phenytoin	Protein binding
Anticoagulants	↑Risk of gastrointestinal bleed	Valproate	
Sulfonylureas	↑Risk of hypoglycemia	Digoxin	↓Renal excretion of interacting drug
Alcohol	↑Risk of bleed	Lithium	
Cyclosporine	↑Nephrotoxicity	Aminoglycosides	
Corticosteroids	↑Risk of gastrointestinal bleed	Methotrexate	

Source: Reprinted from Tripathi KD.[3]

Elevated bleeding times in patients on ibuprofen are in normal range and last for only hours, because it binds to platelet for a short duration.[6]

Diclofenac

Diclofenac is a preferential COX-2 inhibitor and is the most extensively used NSAIDs. It lacks antiplatelet action and can increase the risk of heart attack and stroke similar to the selective COX-2 inhibitors. It is available in tablet formulation, injection (IM), topical gel (1%, 3%), and transdermal patch.[3]

Selective COX-2 Inhibitors (Celecoxib, Etoricoxib, and Parecoxib)

Selective COX-2 inhibitors are usually used in patients at high risk of peptic ulcer, perforation, or bleeds. They should be avoided in patients with cardiac diseases. They should be started at the lowest dose for the shortest period.[3]

Analgesics for Children

Pain assessment can be difficult in children. Adequate pain management during and after dermatological procedures is imperative to improve patient's quality of life, to prevent long-term consequences, and to maintain good physician-patient relationship. Acetaminophen is commonly used first-line analgesic for mild pain. Ibuprofen is as effective as acetaminophen in children for mild-moderate pain. NSAIDs are used for mild-moderate pain and opioids are reserved for severe pain. The commonly used analgesics in children are listed in **Table 5**.[7]

ANXIOLYTICS

Most dermatosurgeries are performed under local anesthesia, and hence patient cooperation is vital.

An anxious patient is poorly cooperative; anxiety also leads to bleeding intraoperatively. Hence, relieving anxiety through pharmacological and nonpharmacological means is important.

Nonpharmacological methods include creating a pleasant ambiance, reassuring staff, music in the background, reading materials, and above all calm and assured presence of the dermatosurgeon. These are particularly important in children and in dermatosurgeries, such as vitiligo surgeries, tumor excisions, and hair transplantation.

Commonly used anxiolytics are benzodiazepines (BZDs—diazepam, lorazepam, and midazolam), clonidine, and propranolol.

Benzodiazepines

Benzodiazepines are one of the widely used class of drugs. They offer anxiolytic, hypnotic, muscle relaxant, anticonvulsant, and amnestic effects. They act by binding to a specific subunit on the gamma-aminobutyric acid A ($GABA_A$) receptor **(Fig. 1)** at a site that is distinct from the binding site of the endogenous GABA molecule. The $GABA_A$ receptor is an inhibitory channel which, when activated, decreases neuronal activity. They also increase the affinity of $GABA_A$ receptor for GABA, thereby increases the frequency of opening of $GABA_A$ receptor chloride channel. BZDs are the choice for anxiety due to their rapid action, relatively high therapeutic index, availability of flumazenil for treating overdosing, low risk of drug interaction, and having less effects on cardiovascular system and autonomic function.[6]

Diazepam

Diazepam[4,5] is a long-acting BZD. Peak blood levels after the IV and IM administration of diazepam injection are reached within 15–30 minutes, respectively, whereas it takes 1 hour after a single oral dosing. The acute half-life is 2–3 hours with a slower decline thereafter.

Required dose is 2–10 mg IM or IV. In children, dosage is 1 mg/4.5 kg.

TABLE 5: Most commonly used analgesics in children.

Route of administration	*Drug*	*Dose*	*Maximum dose per day*
Oral	Acetaminophen	10–15 mg/kg	30 mg/kg/day if <10 kg; 60 mg/kg/day if >10 kg
	Ibuprofen	5–10 mg/kg	40 mg/kg/day
	Diclofenac drops	0.5 mg/kg	1.5 mg/kg/day
	Metamizole	10 mg/kg	74 mg/kg/day
	Ketorolac	0.25 mg/kg	1 mg/kg/day
Intravenous	Acetaminophen	20 mg/kg	60 mg/kg
	Fentanyl	0.2–2 μg/kg	50–100 μg/kg
	Nalbuphine	0.1–0.2 mg/kg	160 mg

Source: Reprinted from Crisan D et al.[7]

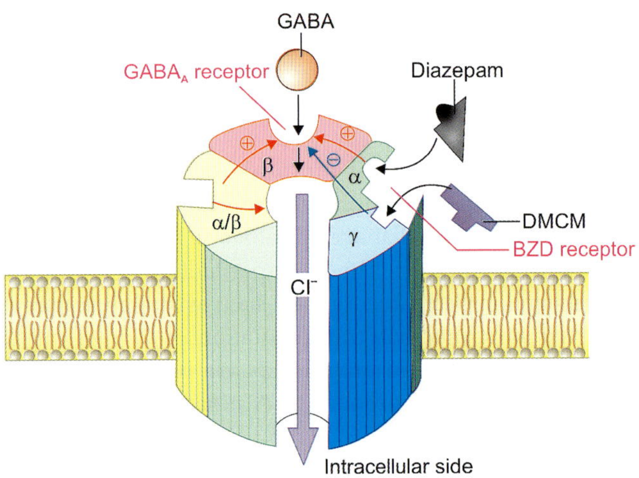

Fig. 1: Schematic depiction of GABA$_A$-BZD receptor-chloride channel complex.
Note: The chloride channel is gated by the primary ligand gamma-aminobutyric acid (GABA). The benzodiazepine (BZD) receptor modulates GABA$_A$ receptor in either direction: agonists like diazepam facilitate, while inverse agonists like DMCM hinder GABA-mediated Cl– channel opening.
Source: Reproduced with modification from Tripathi KD. Sedative-Hypnotics. In: Tripathi KD (Ed). Essentials of Medical Pharmacology, 6th edition. New Delhi: Jaypee Brothers Medical Publishers (P) Ltd; 2003. pp. 395.

Special precautions:

- *Intramuscular:* Diazepam injection should be injected deeply into the muscle.
- Rapid injection or the use of veins with a too small lumen carries the risk of thrombophlebitis. IV injection should be directed into a large lumen vessel, such as an antecubital vein, and the ampule solution should be administered slowly (e.g., 5 mg/min).
- Resuscitative facilities should be available as respiratory arrest is a possible complication.
- After parenteral administration, ambulation should be delayed at least 1 or 2 hours or until complete alertness is restored.
- *Pregnancy:* Being considered under the Food and Drug Administration (FDA) pregnancy category D, its usage in pregnancy and lactation should be limited only to emergencies.
- *Elderly:* The benefits of BZDs are least and the risks are greatest in the elderly. The elderly are at an increased risk of dependence and are more sensitive to the adverse effects such as memory problems, daytime sedation, impaired motor coordination, and increased risk of motor vehicle accidents and falls.[4,5]

Lorazepam

Lorazepam is a high-potency short-to-intermediate-acting 3-hydroxy BZD drug.

It is fast acting. Its relatively potent amnesic effect, with its anxiolytic and sedative effects, makes lorazepam a useful drug for premedication. Oral lorazepam is given 90–120 minutes before procedures and IV lorazepam as late as 10 minutes before procedures. It is given in the dosage as 1 mg tablet orally or 2 mg/mL intravenously. It has a relatively high addictive and abuse potential, a fact of importance, but not relevant in dermatosurgery.[4,5]

Midazolam

Midazolam[4,5] is an ultrashort-acting BZD derivative, with a rapid onset of action, high effectiveness, and low toxicity level. The drug is commonly used as a preanesthetic medication for inducing sedation and amnesia before dermatosurgical procedures. It is three times more potent than diazepam. The plasma levels peak in 20 minutes and $t_{½}$ is 1.5–3 hours.

Midazolam is water soluble and fat soluble in physiologic pH. It is freely soluble in alcohol and acetone.

Recommended Dosage

Oral:

- *Child:* ≥6 months: Single dose of 250–500 μg/kg, up to a maximum of 20 mg
- *Younger patients:* (6 months to <6 years) may require up to 1 mg/kg.

Intramuscular:

- *Adult:* 70–100 μg/kg (usual dose: 5 mg) given 20–60 minutes before surgery by deep IM injection

- *Child:* ≥1 year: 80–200 μg/kg given 20–60 minutes before surgery by deep IM injection
- *Elderly:* 20–50 μg/kg given 20–60 minutes before surgery by deep IM injection.

Intravenous:

- *Adult:* Initially, up to 2.5 mg given over at least 2–5 minutes and 5–10 minutes before procedure. Repeat after at least 2 minutes, if necessary. Usual total: 3.5–5 mg. Maximum total dose: 7.5 mg.
- *Child:* 6 months to 5 years: Initial: 50–100 μg/kg given over 2 minutes, increase slowly at 2 minutes interval up to a total of 600 μg/kg, maximum total dose: 6 mg.
- *Child:* 6–12 years: 25–50 μg/kg given over 2 minutes and increase slowly at 2 minutes interval up to a total of 400 μg/kg; maximum total dose: 10 mg.
- *Elderly:* Initially, 1–1.5 mg given over 2 minutes, increased by increments of 0.5–1 mg at 2 minutes intervals as needed.

Special precautions:

- Avoid midazolam in conjunction with opioids or other sedatives, as there is increased potential risk for respiratory depression, airway obstruction, or hypoventilation.
- Intravenous administration should be done only in the presence of adequate measures and trained staff for resuscitation.
- Concomitant use of grapefruit juice should be avoided as bioavailability of oral midazolam will be increased.
- It is in category D in pregnancy safety and hence is better avoided in pregnancy and lactation.

Clonidine

It is an alpha2 adrenergic agonist primarily used as an antihypertensive drug. As premedication, oral clonidine 5 μg/kg given 30 minutes prior to surgery reduces the requirement of lignocaine acid and prolongs the duration of analgesia without significant side effects and hence has found use in dermatosurgery, dental surgery, and other surgeries.[8-11] Clonidine is routinely administered by most liposuction surgeons as a preoperative medication, along with anxiolytics.[12] Clonidine has recently been used in several other surgical procedures, such as arthroscopy and in obstetric analgesia as an adjuvant, both preoperatively and postoperatively.

Clonidine[13] has been used as a preoperative medication for its antisympathetic, antihypertensive, anxiolytic, sedative, anesthetic, and analgesic effects. Effects of clonidine which can be beneficial in dermatosurgery patients include:

- *Antihypertensive effects:* Because of its central hypotensive effect as an alpha$_2$ adrenergic agent. Clonidine lowers intraoperative and postoperative responses to anesthetics and surgical stress.
- *Sedative effects:* Clonidine induces sedation because of its alpha$_2$ adrenergic effect. It also synergistically increases the potency of BZDs, such as lorazepam.
- *Anxiolytics:* Clonidine has an anxiolytic effect independent of its sedative effect.
- *Narcotic analgesic effects:* Clonidine both supplements and minimizes the need for narcotic analgesics and therefore prevents respiratory depression.
- Clonidine prolongs the action of lignocaine in peripheral blocks.
- Clonidine induces bradycardia and hypotension and also has antiarrhythmic effect. Thus, it effectively counteracts tachycardia induced by epinephrine in tumescent fluid.

Propranolol

Propranolol[14] is the prototype of beta blockers. It is a nonselective beta blocker with known cardiovascular effects. By inhibiting the peripheral sympathetic system, it helps to reduce anxiety. It has minimal sedation and least interference with psychomotor skills. It is avoided in those with cardiac disease (bradycardia and heart block), lung pathologies [chronic obstructive pulmonary disease (COPD) and bronchial asthma], peripheral vascular disease, and diabetes. The dose is 10 mg twice a day (BD) to 160 mg four times a day per orally (QID PO) (average 40–160 mg/day) and 2–5 mg IV over 10 minutes.

Anxiolytics for Children

Preoperative anxiety is associated with adverse outcomes, especially in children. It can lead to an increased requirement for analgesics, emergency delirium, and maladaptive behaviors, such as postoperative anxiety, nighttime crying, enuresis, decrease eating, apathy, withdrawal, and temper tantrums. Anxiety before surgery can be reduced by various preoperative modalities like behavioral preparation programs alone or combined with sedative premedications. The most commonly used anxiolytics in children are midazolam, clonidine, and triclofos **(Table 6)**.[15,16]

USE OF ANALGESICS AND ANXIOLYTICS IN DERMATOSURGERY PATIENTS

Dermatosurgeries are generally mild, and severe pain is not a feature in most surgeries. However, pain can occur after hair transplantation (strip excision), surgeries on scalp, scar revisions, flaps and grafts, etc. **(Box 1)**. Proper preoperative assessment, counseling about pain and its management should form an integral part of preprocedure consultation **(Table 7)**.

TABLE 6: Summary of the key characteristics of sedative premedication.

Drug, formulation, and route	*Mechanism of action*	*Age group*	*Suggested dose*	*Onset (minutes)*	*Duration*	*Advantages*	*Limitations and adverse effects*
Oral midazolam 2.5 mg/mL solution	Gamma-aminobutyric acid A ($GABA_A$) receptor agonist	1 month to 18 years	0.25–0.5 mg/kg (maximum 20 mg)	30–45	45–60 minutes	Reduced postoperative nausea and vomiting	Paradoxical agitation, postanesthetic excitation, and unpleasant taste
Buccal midazolam 10 mg/mL solution	$GABA_A$ receptor agonist	6 months to 18 years	0.3 mg/kg (maximum 10 mg)	20	30–45 minutes	Quick onset of action; better patient compliance	Paradoxical agitation, postanesthetic excitation, and dose limit 10 mg
Oral clonidine 100 µg tablets or 10 µg/mL solution	Central alpha (α_2) adrenoreceptor agonist	6 months to 18 years	4 µg/kg (maximum 200 µg)	45–60	45–90 minutes	Tasteless liquid and long window of action	Cautions in patients with cardiovascular disease/instability
Triclofos	Central nervous system (CNS) depressant (exact mechanism is not well understood)	1 month to 18 years	25–75 mg/kg	30–40	6–8 hours	Palatable than oral midazolam	• Less effective than midazolam • Avoided in patients with gastritis

Source: Adapted from Heikal S et al.[15]; Chaudhary S, et al.[16]

BOX 1: Dermatosurgeries which are associated with significant pain.

- Hair transplantation by strip method [e.g., follicular unit transplant (FUT)]
- Vitiligo surgery (split skin grafting) of large areas
- Some scar revisions and flaps
- Full face resurfacing by dermabrasion
- Ablative lasers
- Phenol peels

Pain and Patient Counseling

Pain perception is an extremely variable function and patients vary greatly in the amount of pain felt. In many, this is the main fear before surgery and "how much pain will I have?" is a frequently asked question during counseling. Hence, enough time should be spent on explaining to patients about this aspect; their anxiety should be allayed that pain, while it may occur, will be prevented/treated by appropriate drugs. Patient can be asked a direct question "are you a nervous person?", "how was the pain in your previous surgery?", and "would you prefer an anxiolytic before surgery?". Previous history of dental extractions serves as a useful guide and indicator.

Anxiolytics are preferred preoperatively, whereas analgesics are normally recommended postoperatively to relieve pain and inflammation.

Analgesics and Hemostasis

Some of the NSAIDs can adversely affect surgical outcome by interfering with the hemostasis and wound healing and hence necessitate discontinuation for an adequate duration prior to surgery or require constant patient monitoring.[11,12] This is definitely so for NSAIDs administered for nonlife-saving indications, which may need to be stopped before surgery.[17,18] Aspirin is commonly used by patients with ischemic heart disease and irreversibly inhibits the COX activity of platelets, resulting in anticoagulant effect.[17] Platelet recovery occurs in 2 weeks after stopping aspirin. However, in such instances, stopping the drug for better hemostasis needs to be assessed in the light of possible cardiovascular risk that the stoppage of drug may bring about. It is also well known that serious bleeding is rare in dermatosurgical procedures. Hence, it is generally not necessary to stop aspirin prior to surgery. Careful assessment should be done of the given situation and opinion of a physician sought before stopping the drug.

Choice of Analgesic

While choosing the analgesics in dermatosurgical patients, one should check the following preexisting comorbidities and the medications that the patient is consuming; as mentioned in the text earlier, drug interactions are quite common among analgesics and other medications. Most commonly used oral analgesic medications include diclofenac and tramadol. In addition to oral analgesics, the other modalities, such as suppositories of diclofenac sodium, transdermal patches of opioids, and nonopioids, could be tried. One should keep in mind that the multimodal analgesic plan is not only contemporary but will also decrease the side effect of any one drug. The drugs commonly used in multimodal therapy are:

- Intravenous paracetamol at a dose of 1 g administered once in 8 hours
- Transcutaneous diclofenac (NuPatch®) or fentanyl
- Rectal suppositories of paracetamol or diclofenac
- Oral analgesics, such as tramadol, paracetamol, diclofenac sodium, ketorolac, piroxicam, or nimesulide.

TABLE 7: Acute postsurgical pain management algorithm.

Preoperative	*Patient risk assessment:* • Higher risk • History of hyperalgesia • History of pain catastrophizing • Multiple same-day procedures • Female • Patient age <31 years • Regular opioid or anxiolytic use • Uncertain risk • Anatomic site • Anxiety disorder or depression • Body mass index • Sex • Size of defect • *Type of closure:* Linear repair, flap, or graft • Tension on wound edge	*Pain assessment scale* **(Fig. 2)**: • Wong-Baker Faces Pain Scale (≥3 years children and adults) • Numeric Pain Intensity Scale (NRSI), validated for adults • Visual Analog Scale (VAS) • Categorical Rating Scale	*Pain education:* • Pain physiology and management strategies • Preoperative information delivered by verbal instructions, multimedia content forms, such as videos and audio-augmented slides
Operative	*Low/medium risks:* • Injection pain reduction techniques (buffered lidocaine, vibration, site cooling, or distraction) • +/– intraoperative NSAID (ibuprofen 400 mg just after surgery)		*High risks:* • Additional injection pain reduction techniques • Regional anesthetic • Long-acting local anesthetic, such as bupivacaine or liposomal bupivacaine • Intraoperative analgesia (celecoxib 200 mg BD starting the night before or gabapentin 300–600 mg 1–2 hour prior to surgery. Ibuprofen 400 mg then q6h prn pain or acetaminophen 1,000 mg/ ibuprofen 400 mg then q6hr prn pain just after surgery) • Preoperative anxiolytics, as indicated
Post-operative	• NSAID +/– acetaminophen (ibuprofen 400 mg po 6h prn pain +/– acetaminophen 1 g po q6h prn pain or celecoxib 200 mg po q12h prn pain) • Cold analgesia (applied to the surgical site for 10–20 minutes every 1–4 waking hours as needed) • Rest +/– site elevation (as applicable)		• Pain assessment follow-up and counseling • Combination of NSAID and acetaminophen (Ibuprofen 400 mg po 6h prn pain +/– acetaminophen 1g po q6h prn pain or celecoxib 200 mg po q12h prn pain) or combination of opioid and nonopioid • Cold analgesia • Rest +/– site elevation (as applicable) • +/– o + stool softener and antiemetic

(BD: twice a day; NSAID: nonsteroidal anti-inflammatory drug; po: per orally; prn: as needed; q6h: every 6 hours)
Source: Adapted from Glass JS et al.[6]

Additional Modalities for Pain Relief

As mentioned earlier, the use of drugs, such as midazolam and clonidine preoperatively, can help in better management of pain. Infiltrating the incision with long-acting local anesthetic agents, such as bupivacaine, (0.06%) not only provides instant analgesia but also continues to provide it for about 5-6 hours. At a few centers, in hair transplant surgery, continuous infiltration of local anesthetic agents using an elastomeric pump has been used with good analgesic outcomes. Injection of triamcinolone acetate at the site of suture and recipient area in hair transplantation may reduce postoperative edema and hence reduce pain.

It is wise to practice a combination of one or more of the groups of medications/techniques mentioned above to get the maximum benefit from the components of the combinations.

CONCLUSION

- No single drug is superior to all others for every patient. Choice of drug is thus largely empirical. The nature of the surgical procedure along with consideration of risk factors in the given patient governs selection of the analgesic. Past experience of the patient, acceptability, and individual preference are also to be considered.
- For dermatological procedures and surgery, tramadol, acetaminophen, diclofenac, or ibuprofen may be suitable.
- For pediatric patients, only paracetamol, ibuprofen, and naproxen are to be used.
- Paracetamol is the safest analgesic in pregnancy while low-dose aspirin is probably the second-best drug.
- Midazolam is the preferred anxiolytic used before dermatosurgeries and clonidine is a better alternative.

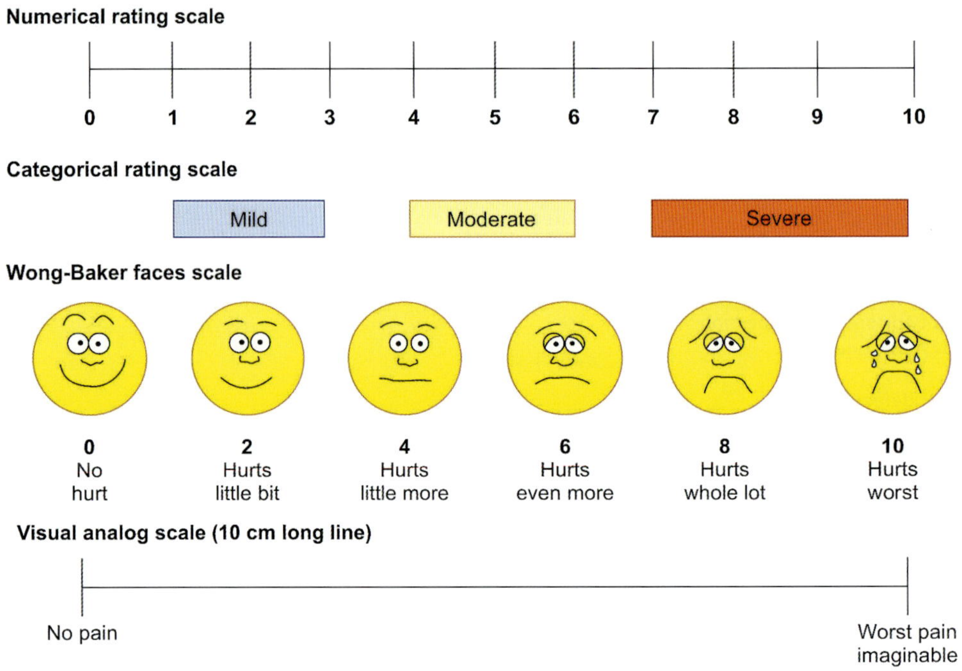

Fig. 2: Summary of pain scales.
Source: Adapted from Glass JS et al.[6]

- Avoid anxiolytics in pregnancy and lactation.
- Postoperative infiltration of bupivacaine and triamcinolone at the site of surgery can help reduce pain.

REFERENCES

1. Yaksh TL, Wallace MS. Opioids, analgesia, and pain Management. In: Brunton LL, Chabner BA, Knollmann BC (Eds). Goodman and Gilman's: The pharmacological basis of therapeutics, 13th edition. New York: McGraw-Hill Medical Publishing Division; 2018. pp. 355-86.
2. Tripathi KD. Opioid analgesics and antagonists. In: Tripathi KD (Ed). Essentials of Medical Pharmacology, 8th edition. New Delhi: Jaypee Brothers Medical Publishers (P) Ltd; 2019. pp. 497-514.
3. Tripathi KD. Nonsteroidal anti-inflammatory drugs and antipyretic-analgesics. In: Tripathi KD (Ed). Essentials of Medical Pharmacology, 8th edition. New Delhi: Jaypee Brothers Medical Publishers (P) Ltd; 2019. pp. 209-26.
4. Tripathi KD. Antidepressant and antianxiety drugs. In: Tripathi KD (Eds). Essentials of Medical Pharmacology, 8th edition. New Delhi: Jaypee Brothers Medical Publishers (P) Ltd; 2019. pp. 153-71.
5. Trevor AJ, Way WL. Sedative-hypnotic drugs. In: Katzung BG, Masters SB, Trevor AJ (Eds). Basic and Clinical pharmacology, 14th edition. New York: The McGraw- Hill Medical Publishing Division; 2018. pp. 381-95.
6. Glass JS, Hardy CL, Meeks NM, Carroll BT. Acute pain management in dermatology: risk assessment and treatment. J Am Acad Dermatol. 2015;73(4):543-60.
7. Crisan D, Scharffetter-Kochanek K, Kastler S, Crisan M, Manea A, Wagner K, et al. Dermatologic surgery in children: an update on indication, anesthesia, analgesia and potential perioperative complications. J Dtsch Dermatol Ges. 2018;16(3):268-76.
8. Pratap JN, Shankar RK, Goroszeniuk T. Co-injection of clonidine prolongs the anesthetic effect of lidocaine skin infiltration by a peripheral action. Anesth Analg. 2007;104(4): 982-3.
9. Ya Deau JT, La Sala VR, Paroli, Kahn RL , Jules-Elysée KM, Levine DS, et al. Clonidine and analgesic duration after popliteal fossa nerve blockade: randomized, double-blind, placebo-controlled study. Anesth Analg. 2008;106(6):1916-20.
10. Madan R, Bharti N, Shende D, Khokhar SK, Kaul HL. A dose response study of clonidine with local anesthetic mixture for peribulbar block: a comparison of three doses. Anesth Analg. 2001;93(6):1593-7.
11. Mishunin Yu V, Ostreikov IF, Nazarov NA, Bogdanova LE, Voĭkovskiĭ OV, Morozov IN, et al. Combined use of local anesthetic with clonidine in cases of tooth extraction. Stomatologiiâ. 2005;84(1):33-5.
12. Klein J (Ed). Tumescent Anesthesia and Microcannular Liposuction. Mosby Publications; 2000. pp. 201-4.
13. Venkataram M, Shivashankar, Venkataram J. Use of clonidine as a preoperative drug in hair transplantation. ISHRS meeting at Montreal; 2009.
14. Sedative-hypnotics. In: Tripathi KD (Eds). Essentials of Medical Pharmacology, 8th edition. New Delhi: Jaypee Brothers Medical Publishers (P) Ltd; 2019. pp. 441-54.
15. Heikal S, Stuart G. Anxiolytic premedication for children. BJA Educ. 2020;20(7):220-25.
16. Chaudhary S, Jindal R, Girotra G, Salhotra R, Rautela RS, Sethi AK. Is midazolam superior to triclofos and hydroxyzine as premedicant in children? J Anaesthesiol Clin Pharmacol. 2014;30(1):53-8.
17. Patrono C. Aspirin as an antiplatelet drug. N Engl J Med. 1994; 330(18):1287-94.
18. Proper SA, Fenske NA, Burnett SM, Luria LW. Compromised wound repair caused by perioperative use of Ibuprofen. J Am Acad Dermatol. 1998;18(5):1173-4.

SECTION 2

Standard Surgical Techniques

CHAPTER 18

Simple Excisions

Vinay Saraf, Ragunatha S

KEY MESSAGES

- Important steps in simple elliptical excision of lesion include planning the ellipse, incision, dissection of lesion, undermining of defect, and hemostasis.
- Undermining is essential to reduce the tension on wound margins. Undermining facilitates wound closure; avoids unnecessary vascular compromise; everts the wound margins; enhances the cosmetic outcome after scar contraction and prevents spread of scar at high wound tension areas.
- A good suture technique should ensure closure of dead space in subcutaneous tissue, decreased wound tension, and good approximation and eversion of wound margins.

INTRODUCTION

The elliptical (fusiform) excision is the mainstay and workhorse of cutaneous excisional and reconstructive surgery.[5] Majority of simple cutaneous excisions are done by performing the elliptical or fusiform excision. Proper planning and execution of this procedure needs good understanding of anatomy of skin, wound healing, tumor biology, resting skin tension lines (RSTLs), and functional considerations of head, neck, and face.[6] Thorough understanding of these basic principles will help the surgeon to execute the procedure meticulously, giving excellent cosmetic outcome.

HISTORY OF CUTANEOUS SURGERY

Surgery is a Greek word meaning "hand work". Excision means cutting out an organ, tumor, or other tissue. In 6th century BC, *Sushruta*, father of surgery in ancient India, wrote *Sushruta Samhita*, wherein he described 120 instruments, 300 surgical procedures, and eight categories of surgeries including plastic surgery. He used herbal juice which was similar to modern day anesthesia. His descriptions included excision surgery. In Egypt, China, and Arab countries, in 3,500 years ago, the surgeries being practiced were mainly excision and reconstructive surgery. The first description of skin tension lines (STLs) was made by Dupuytren in 1834. He demonstrated that circular incisions produced linear wounds. Langer is credited with major work on this subject. In 1973, Borges published drawings of RSTLs. He demonstrated that RSTLs were of more importance than wrinkle lines and indicated that they were identical for all individuals. He constructed detailed line maps which have been referred to as the correct direction for placement of incisions.[1-4]

INDICATIONS

The following are the indications for simple excisions:

- *Simple excision without suture (small benign lesions):*
  - Mucoceles
  - Hamartomas
  - Small epidermal inclusion cyst
- *Elliptical excision (moderate to large lesions):*
  - *Benign:*
    - Sebaceous cyst
    - Lipoma
    - Fibroma
    - Epidermoid cyst
    - Nevi
  - *Malignant:*
    - Basal cell carcinoma
    - Noninvasive squamous cell carcinoma
    - Bowen's disease
- *Modifications in simple excision:*
  - *Excision with full thickness graft or rotation flap:*
    - Large malignant lesions
  - *Punch incision:*
    - Sebaceous cyst
    - Lipoma.

CONTRAINDICATIONS

- Infected lesions
- Patients with history of keloidal tendency and bleeding tendency
- Patients on anticoagulants
- Recent isotretinoin use
- Uncontrolled diabetes and debilitating conditions
- Unreliable patients.

REQUIREMENTS: EQUIPMENT AND MATERIALS

Equipment and materials required during each step of excisional surgery should be kept ready for smooth conduction of procedure. The following is the checklist of requirements for cutaneous excisional surgery:

- *Counseling:*
  - Consent form
  - Patient instruction slip
- *Surgical preparation of the site:*
  - *Antiseptic solutions:* Surgical spirit and povidone-iodine
  - *Surgical drapes:* Hole cloth towel
- *Local anesthesia:*
  - Injection lignocaine (1 or 2%) with or without epinephrine (1:100,000)
  - Insulin syringe or syringe with 0.5 inch 30-gauge needle
- *Excision of the lesion:*
  - Sterile steel tray
  - Skin marking pen (to mark the lesion and ellipse)
  - Scalpel handle
  - Scalpel blade number 15
  - Cutting scissors straight and curved
  - Adson's serrated forceps, toothed, and plane
  - Skin hooks
  - Small mosquito artery forceps
- *Wound closure:*
  - Suture materials (absorbable/nonabsorbable sutures)
  - Cutting needles
  - Needle holder
- *Wound dressing:*
  - Spirit swabs
  - Gauze pieces
  - Dressing pads
  - Adhesive plaster or micropore
  - Antibiotic cream
- *Suture removal:*
  - Suture cutting scissor
- *Skin biopsy:*
  - 10% formalin
  - Histopathology requisition form
  - Empty clean vials with label to provide details of patient.

PREOPERATIVE PREPARATIONS

Patient education and counseling, assessment of risk factors for complications, and prophylactic antibiotics administration are important aspects of preoperative preparation.[3,7,8]

Counseling

As is true with all cosmetic dermatosurgery procedures, informed consent is a must. Information about the procedure, complications, postoperative care, and outcome of the surgery must be provided to the patient. All queries about the procedures should be duly addressed and expected results should be explained. Avoid patient with unrealistic expectation and suspicion about surgeon's credibility and charges.

Preoperative Evaluation of Patients

Thorough systemic examination and specific inquiries must be made to identify risk factors which may affect the surgical outcome **(Box 1)**.[2,3,9]

Prophylactic Antibiotics

The antibiotic prophylaxis is recommended only for patients with a high risk of endocarditis (e.g., prosthetic heart valves or systemic pulmonary shunts). Role of routine antibiotic prophylaxis in cutaneous surgery is not established. The prophylactic antibiotic therapy should cover both staphylococci and streptococci.

BOX 1: Preoperative evaluation of the patient.

Medical history and examination:
- *Bleeding disorders:*
  - Bleeding tendencies
  - Any current drug history, e.g., anticoagulants and antiplatelet agents
- *Hypersensitivity reactions:*
  - Drug hypersensitivity, including anesthetics
  - Allergic contact dermatitis to topical applications or adhesive tapes
- *Abnormal wound healing:*
  - Keloid formation
  - Delayed wound healing
- *Transmission of infections:*
  - HIV infection
  - Hepatitis B and hepatitis C infections
- *Postoperative infections:*
  - Damaged and infected skin
  - Diabetes
  - Debilitation
  - Hypogammaglobulinemia
  - Anemia
  - Severe malnutrition
  - Long-term antibiotic therapy
  - Corticosteroids therapy
  - Immunocompromised states
  - Emotional stress
  - Poor hygiene

Investigations:
- Complete blood count
- Bleeding time, clotting time, and prothrombin time
- Fasting blood sugar
- Blood venereal disease research laboratory (VDRL)
- Enzyme-linked immunosorbent assay (ELISA) for human immunodeficiency virus (HIV)
- Serology for hepatitis B and hepatitis C

Universal Precautions

The surgeon must prepare himself with universal precaution for patient's safety and for his own safety, never forgetting that we are practicing in human immunodeficiency virus (HIV) era. Universal precautions are strictly followed whenever there is potential risk of contact with blood or other body fluids. Masks and protective eyewear or face shield are worn if splatter of blood is anticipated.

SURGICAL PREPARATION OF SITE

The affected area, e.g., face, is washed with soap and water two to three times, and all make-up, contact lenses, and ornaments are removed, and handed over to a patient's relative. As far as possible see that one responsible person, preferably a relative, accompanies the patient. The operative area must be thoroughly cleansed with surgical scrub **(Fig. 1)**, preferably with povidone-iodine followed by methylated spirit, and then painted with povidone-iodine. The area must be isolated by sterile draping **(Fig. 2)**. Hole towels are a better choice for draping.

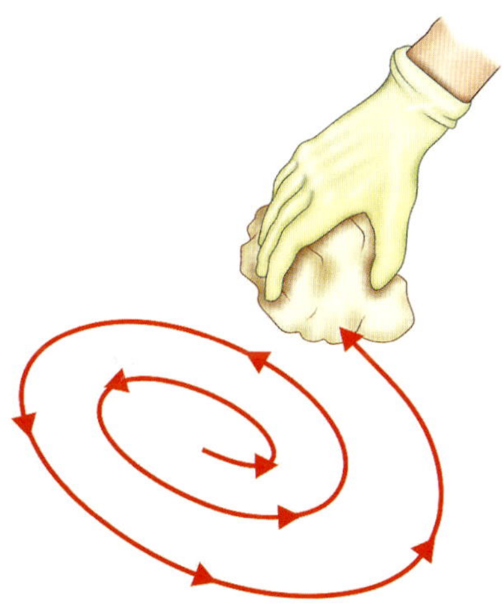

Fig. 1: Cleaning, surgical preparation should be started in the center going peripherally.

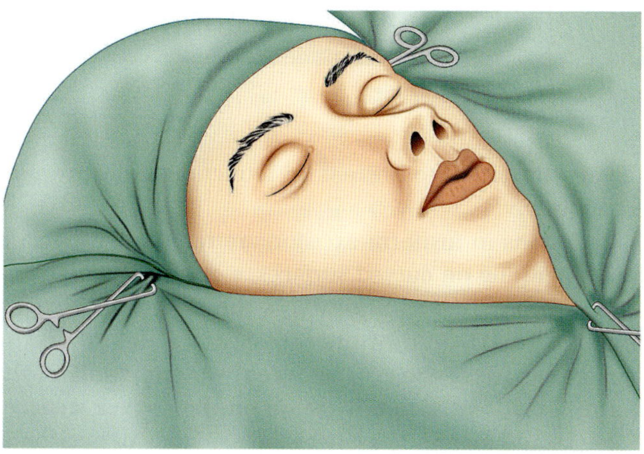

Fig. 2: Draping the surgical area is necessary for asepsis.

LOCAL ANESTHESIA

Always use xylocaine with adrenaline unless contraindicated. Addition of adrenaline provides bloodless surgical field; allows the use of greater volume of anesthetic agent; longer duration of anesthetic effect; and avoids reinjection if the procedure lasts for longer time. The recommended maximum safe dose of lignocaine in a 70 kg man with adrenaline is 7 mg/kg body weight (500 mg) and without adrenaline is 3 mg/kg body weight (200 mg).

TECHNIQUE OF ELLIPTICAL EXCISION

Small benign lesions, such as mucoceles, hamartomas, and small epidermal inclusion cysts, can be removed without suture under local infiltration anesthesia using a scalpel blade or small scissor. The lesion is held with small toothed forceps for precise removal of the lesion at the base. The hemostasis is maintained by pressure or Monsel's solution (ferric chloride) or electrodessication. The resulting wound, usually small, is left to heal by secondary intention under surgical dressing.[2,4,7] However, for larger lesions, elliptical excision is preferred. Important steps in elliptical excision of lesion include planning the ellipse, incision, dissection of lesion, undermining of defect, and hemostasis.

Planning the Ellipse

This is a very important step as it determines the outcome of procedure. Proper planning results in least noticeable scar without compromising the function. **Figures 3 to 5** show some of the instruments used. **Figure 6** demonstrates administration of local anesthesia. Well-planned incision line should run parallel to the favorable lines of closure, i.e., RSTLs or MSTLs. The incision line so planned not only makes the scar inconspicuous but it also heals faster, and gives a higher tensile strength. Maximum STL are usually, but not always, congruent with relaxed STL. These lines can be made obvious by pinching the skin in all directions. They can also be judged by asking the patient to smile or grimace. Incisions can also be taken along the wrinkle lines, or skin folds. Another option is to make a circular incision and wait for some time to allow it to turn into an oval shape after undermining the edges. Before final closure the oval shape can be converted into an ellipse. The length to width ratio of the ellipse or fusiform excision should be 3:1 or 4:1. The tips of the ellipse should meet at 30° angle **(Figs. 7 and 8)**.[2,3,7] For malignant lesions include 3–4 mm normal appearing margins **(Box 2)**.

Always consider the cosmetic units of the face because scars restricted to single cosmetic unit hide well as compared to the scars crossing multiple units. The cosmetic units of the face are chin, perioral region, cheek, periorbital region, nose, forehead, glabella, and temple. For further details, refer to the chapter on facial anatomy.

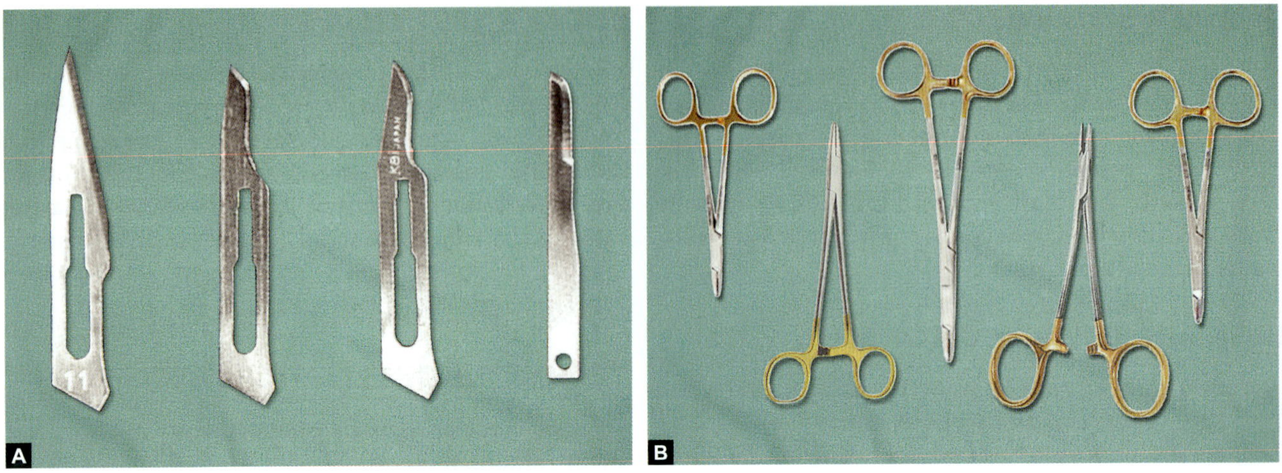

Figs. 3A and B: Scissors, needle holder, and scalpel blades.

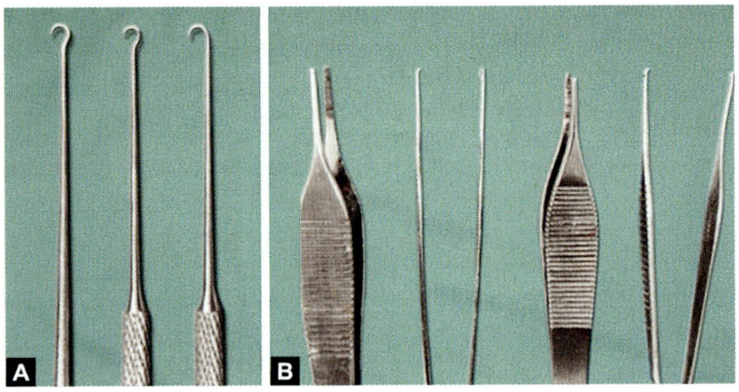

Figs. 4A and B: (A) Skin hooks; (B) Forceps.

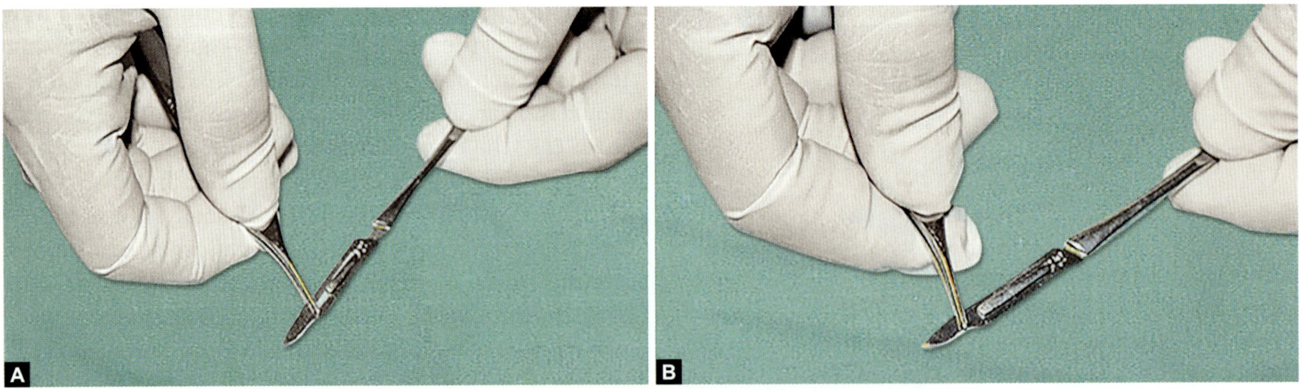

Figs. 5A and B: Mounting the 15 number blade on scalpel handle.

Nature of the lesion removed is also an important factor. For benign lesions, the surrounding normal skin excised is minimal, and on the other hand for malignant lesions, sufficient surrounding normal looking tissue is included in the excision to prevent recurrences.[5,10,11]

The shape of the lesion also plays an important role in deciding the excision line. For oval-shaped lesion, the long axis of the incision line must run parallel to the long axis of the lesion. This will shorten the length of the scar.[2,3] When taking incisions near lips or eyes, functional considerations are very important to prevent lip retraction and ectropion, respectively.[2,5,12]

Variations in fusiform excision are required, especially when operating on curved surfaces, e.g., cheeks and arms. Lazy S, also called as S plasty, is the preferred incision **(Figs. 9A to D)**. Aim of the S plasty is to lengthen the ultimate length of the scar between two endpoints of the wound. This is particularly useful on the convex surfaces of cheeks and extremities where the tendency of horizontal contraction of the scar is high. The horizontal and vertical

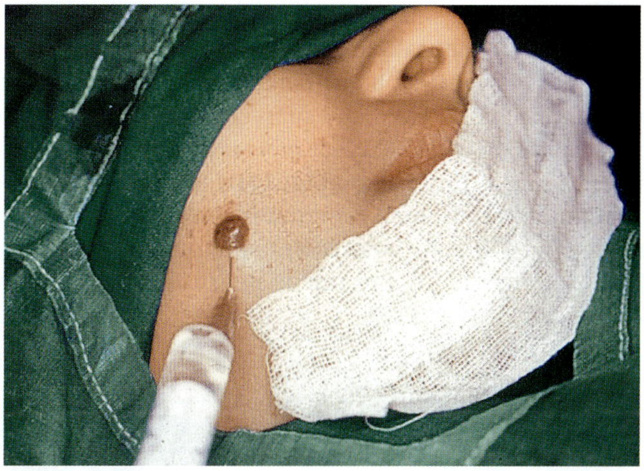

Fig. 6: Local field block is being given.

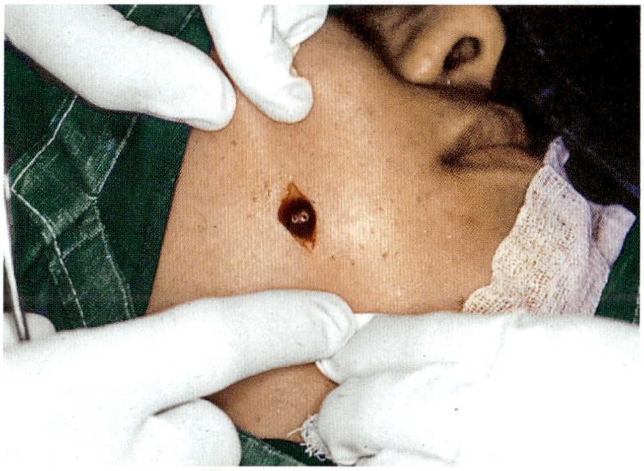

Fig. 7: The tips of the ellipse meet at 30° angle.

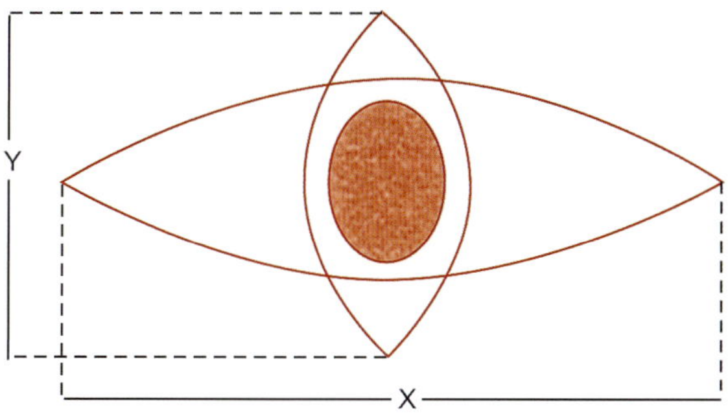

Fig. 8: Length to width ratio of the ellipse should be 3:1 or 4:1.

BOX 2: Planning the ellipse.

- Favorable lines of closure (MSTLs)
- Cosmetic units (face)
- Nature of lesion removed
- Functional consideration (lower eyelid)
- Dimensions
- Margins
- Fusiform excision variation
- Skin preparation and marking the ellipse

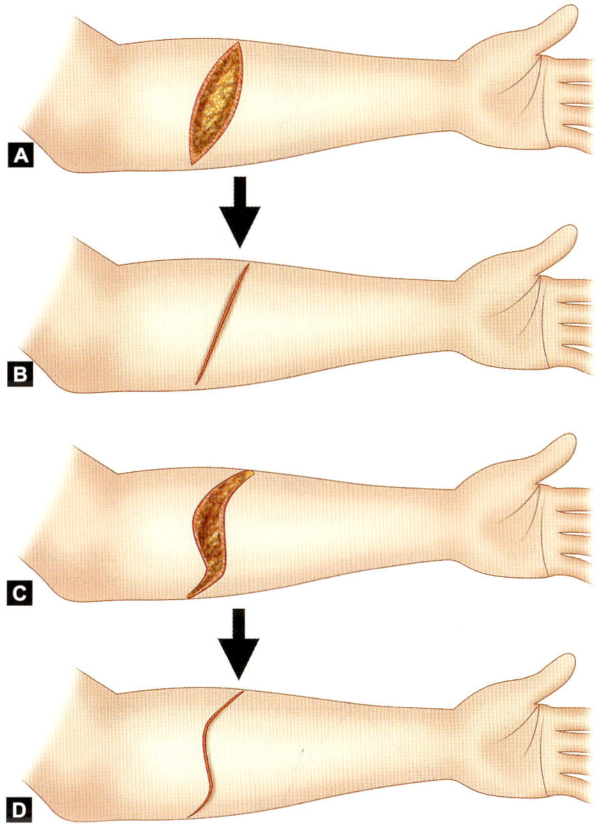

Figs. 9A to D: S-shaped incision. (A) Circumferential closure of a wound on a convex surface; (B) Will create tissue protrusions at the ends; (C) A S-plasty design; (D) Allows the terminal ends to remain in the same horizontal plane.

dimensions of the ellipse should be in 3:1 or 4:1 proportion. The long axis of the ellipse should run parallel to the long axis of the lesion otherwise it can result into depressed scar. By lengthening the scar, the horizontal forces of contraction will pull and straighten the "s", rather than resulting in depressed scar.[2,7] Marking the incision line of the ellipse before injecting local anesthesia is essential as the anesthetic will distort the tissue, and vasoconstriction may obscure the margins.[2,4] Alternately, a punch can be used to perform an elliptical excision **(Fig. 10)**.

Incision

Figures 11 to 19 show different steps of incision. To get the best cosmetic results, several aspects of incision need to be addressed. To avoid cross-hatching, the tips of the ellipse must meet at a fine point which prevents unnecessary injury and extension of the incision beyond that point **(Figs. 11 and 12)**. The scalpel handle must be held perpendicular to the skin at the initiation of the incision. Then tilt the scalpel at 45° angle **(Fig. 13A)** and incise through the margin till the other end is reached. Then turn the blade again perpendicular to the skin surface. For smaller incisions 15c or 11 number blade is used.[2,3] Incise perpendicularly **(Fig. 13B)** through the

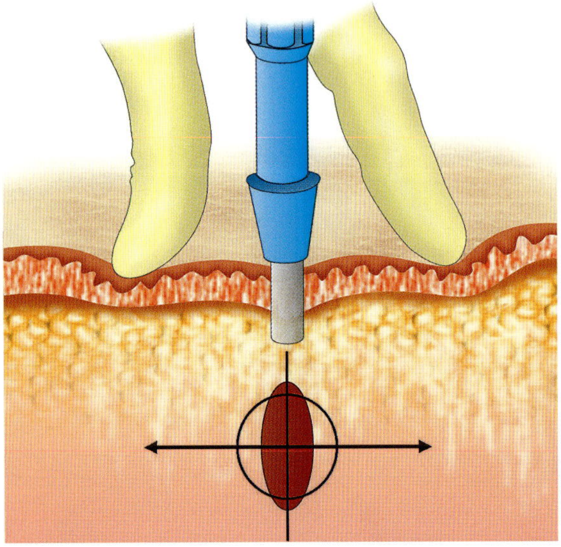

Fig. 10: Alternatively a punch excision can be done which can be converted to ellipse for final closure by stretching the punch wound.

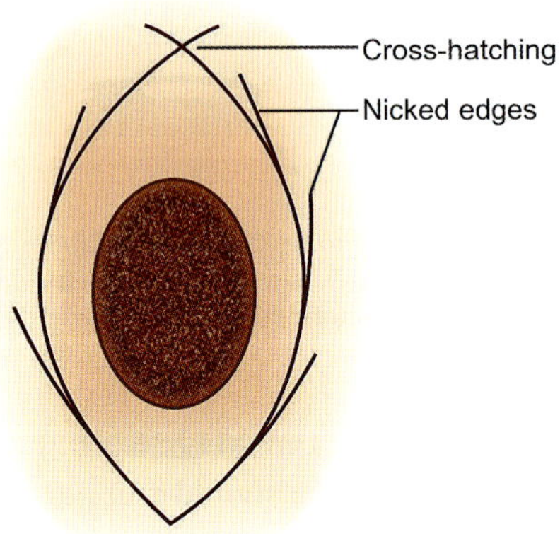

Fig. 11: Avoiding cross-hatching.

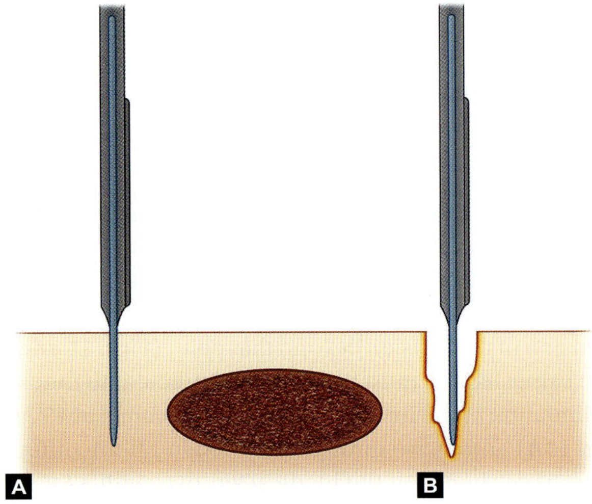

Figs. 12A and B: (A) Scalpel handle must be held perpendicular to the skin; (B) Avoid staircasing.

dermis up to the subcutaneous fat which everts the skin margins for cosmetically acceptable wound closure. In hairy areas, pass the scalpel blade parallel to the hair follicle to avoid follicle transection and subsequent bald area around the scar **(Fig. 13C)**.[2,7] Perfect movement of the scalpel in straight line is important **(Fig. 13D)**. Number of passes through the dermis should be minimum to avoid "staircasing" effect **(Fig. 11)** and compromise of approximation of the wound margins.[2,4] Right-angled incision helps in better wound closure **(Fig. 13E)**.

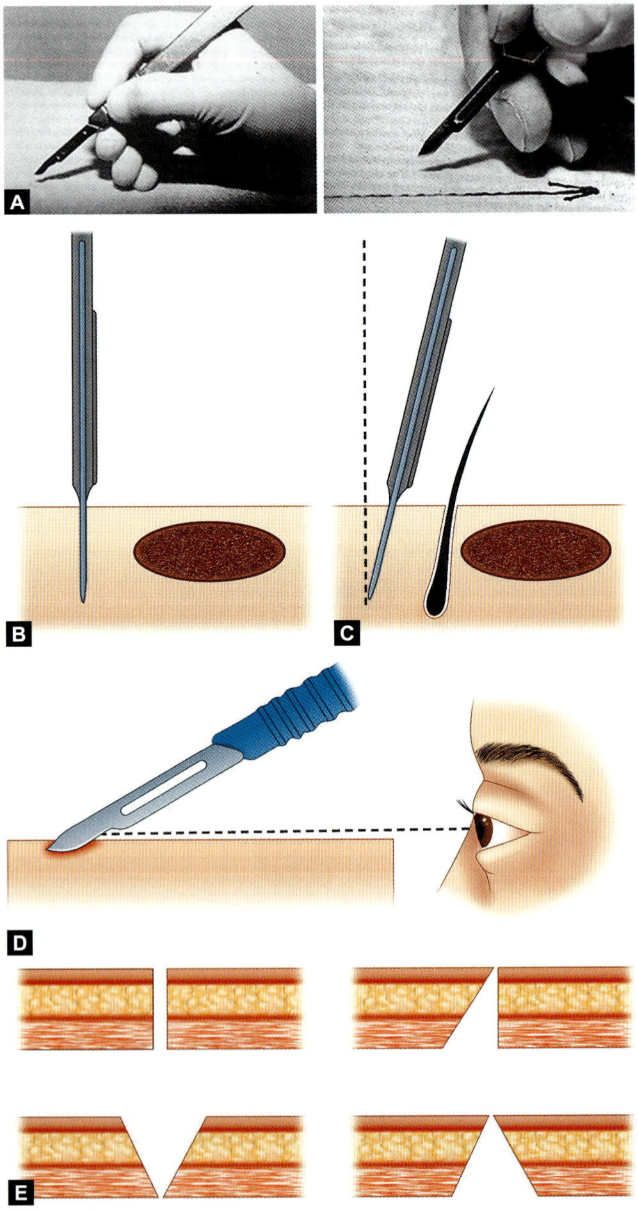

Figs. 13A to E: (A) Scalpel should always move toward the surgeon; (B) Incise perpendicularly through the dermis up to the subcutaneous fat; (C) In hairy areas, pass the scalpel blade parallel to the hair follicle to avoid follicle transection; (D) Perfect movement of the scalpel in straight line is important; (E) Right angle incision is must to get good alignment of the suture line.

Dissection of Lesion

Avoid boat-shaped excision by removing desired depth of tissue up to the depth of the incision at the two ends **(Figs. 15A and B)**. Removal of less amount of tissue at both ends causes protrusions at both ends resulting in pseudo-dog-ears **(Figs. 16A and B)**.[2,3,7]

Undermining the Defect

Undermining is essential to reduce the tension on wound margins. Undermining facilitates wound closure; avoids unnecessary vascular compromise; everts the wound margins; enhances the cosmetic outcome after scar contraction; and prevents spread of scar at high wound tension areas. Dead space can result from undermining that leads to seroma or hematoma. Obliteration of dead space can be done although this is not imperative **(Figs. 17 to 19)**.

Undermining must be done all around the wound including the two ends. After undermining there should be no tension on the wound margins and the edges of the wound should be everted without compromising vascularity.[2,3,7]

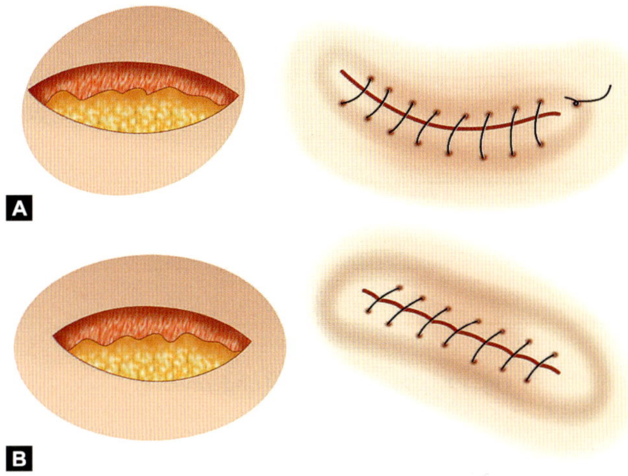

Figs. 16A and B: Depth of tissue removal should be uniform to avoid pseudo-dog-ears.

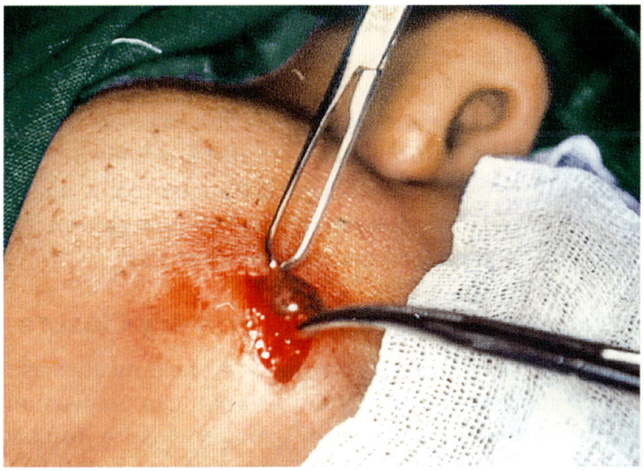

Fig. 14: Dissecting the lesion.

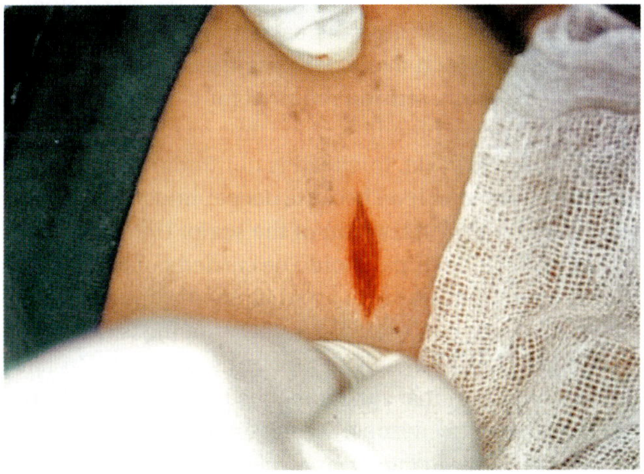

Fig. 17: Undermining completed after smooth incisions.

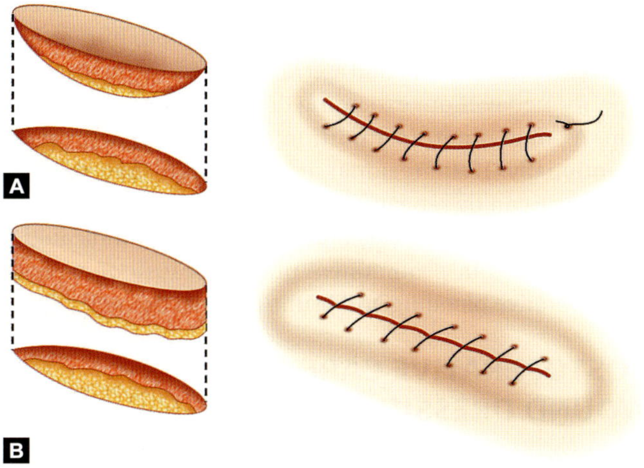

Figs. 15A and B: Avoid boat-shaped incisions.

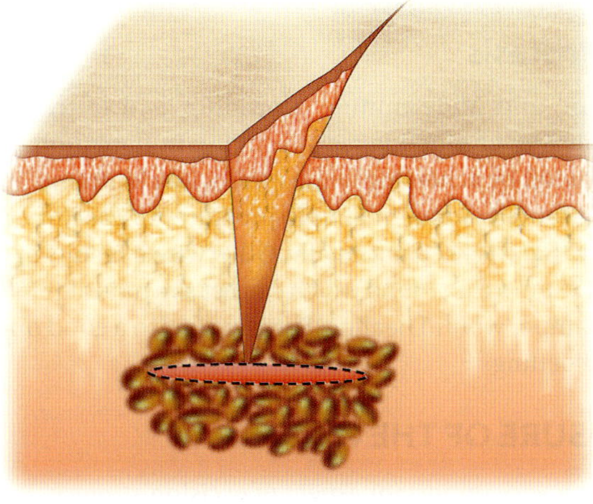

Fig. 18: Dead space can result from undermining.

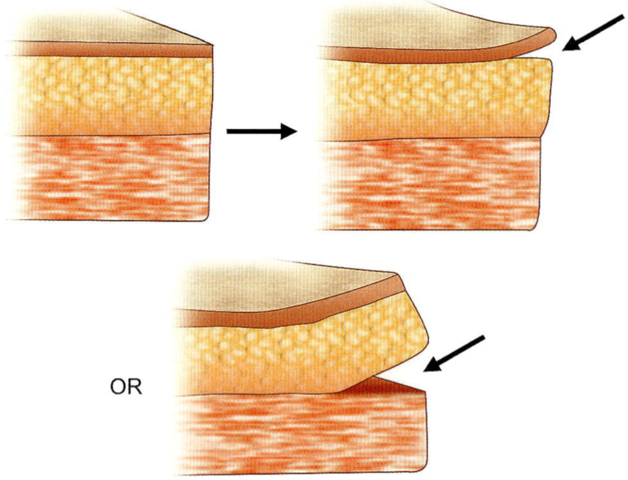

Fig. 19: Different depths of undermining.

Methods of Undermining

Basic rule of undermining is to do undermining as superficial as possible using blunt tipped scissors or small artery forceps. Author's choice is mosquito forceps; it is a smallest artery forceps. On scalp, it is carried out below the galea aponeurotica which avoids cutting the hair follicles, and supports the suture tension required for closure of the scalp wounds. It is also a bloodless plane thus results in minimal or no bleeding. However, forehead is not undermined at deep subcutaneous tissue level because deeper undermining might result in sensory denervation of the scalp. Undermining on cheeks, chin, and temple should be carried out at superficial subcutaneous tissue level to avoid injury to superficial motor nerves. On trunk and extremities undermining is done above muscle fascia at deep subcutaneous tissue level. On hands and feet with minimal subcutaneous tissue undermining is done just below the dermis. During undermining the wound margins are held very gently to avoid trauma to the margins. Another alternative method is to use skin hooks. This will help to give fine hairline scar with excellent cosmetic outcome which is the goal of elliptical excision.[2,3,7]

Hemostasis

Incision and undermining invariably lead to transection and nicking of blood vessels resulting in hematoma. It can be avoided by achieving hemostasis with clamping, ligation, electrocauterization, or simple pressure. In case of cautery, ensure that it is used minimally. Otherwise it results in a lot of dead tissue in the wound which can act as a nidus for infection and hamper wound healing. Suturing is also a good option to stop bleeding.[2,3]

CLOSURE OF THE WOUND

This is a very important aspect of excision surgery. By using correct suture material, suture technique and timing of suture removal, excellent cosmetic results can be obtained. A well-approximated, everted wound with minimal suture tracking is ideal outcome of simple excision surgery. Various modifications of suture techniques can be used in cutaneous surgery with each technique having its advantages and disadvantages to achieve best possible cosmetic results.[13]

OTHER SIMPLE EXCISION METHODS

The standard elliptical excision may not be suitable for excision of skin lesions in certain age groups and anatomical sites. In such situation, different excision techniques are utilized to give good cosmetic result with minimal scarring.

Circular Excision and Purse-string Closure

It is an effective technique used for excision of circular facial skin lesions in children. Apart from infantile hemangioma (at any stage of evolution), other skin lesions treated successfully with this technique include Spitz nevus, pyogenic granuloma, pilomatricoma, vascular malformations, and pigmented nevus.[14] In infantile hemangioma, circular excision and purse-string closure converts large circular lesion into a small ellipsoid scar by significantly reducing the transverse and longitudinal dimensions of the lesion. If required, the ellipsoid scar can be revised subsequently to a linear scar of same length. Hence, the smallest possible scar with minimal distortion of surrounding tissue can be achieved by this method.[15] However, to avoid pleat formation, this method is not indicated for lesions on the free margins such as periorbital region, or on the upper or lower lip.[16]

Intralesional Excision and Primary Closure

The long scar and dog-ear formation of elliptical excision and pleat formation of circular excision can be overcome by intralesional excision and primary closure. Infantile hemangiomas, involuting or involuted, are suitable for intralesional excision because of expanded dome-shaped tissue, and excess and redundant skin which permit easy scooping of fibrofatty tissue and closure of wound edge without tension, respectively. In this method, intralesional elliptical resection with dull apical angles and primary closure is performed without extending the incision into the normal skin. A small outermost portion of the lesion is preserved intentionally. If the residual lesion is large, then the same procedure can be repeated two to three times at the interval of 3 months each. Intralesional excision is not indicated for hemangiomas in proliferative phase because of excessive intraoperative bleeding and brittle residual tissue.[16]

POSTOPERATIVE CARE AND WOUND DRESSING

Postoperatively the wound is cleaned to remove blood and residual antiseptic. Dressing is applied in four layers

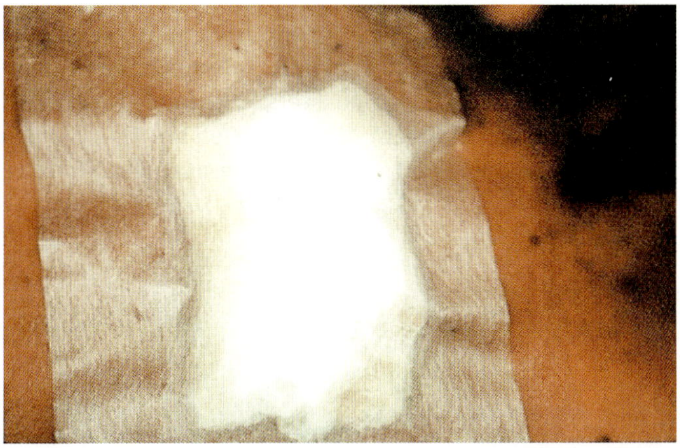

Fig. 20: Three-layered dressing.

comprising of occlusive ointment, a nonadherent gauze material, an absorbent cushion made of cotton covered with gauze material on both sides, and adhesive tape to secure the dressing **(Fig. 20)**. Dressing must kept dry all the time and the patient is instructed accordingly. If the dressing gets soiled it has to be replaced immediately. First redressing is to be done after 24 hours. The patient is trained to do subsequent dressings on his own till suture removal.

COMPLICATIONS AND THEIR MANAGEMENT[3]

With good planning technique and aseptic precautions, complications in cutaneous surgery are very rare. Patients should be warned and informed about them preoperatively. The surgeon should be able to recognize and manage them whenever they occur.

Hematoma

Hematomas are seen within 24–48 hours after surgery and they manifest as swelling, erythema, and tenderness at wound site. Hematomas are evacuated promptly by partially or completely opening the wound. Resuturing can be done if hematoma develops within early 24 hours provided the wound is not infected. Otherwise the wound is kept open and allowed to heal by second intention. Scar revision can be done at later date. Very small hematomas need not be opened; they can be managed with warm compresses till resolution.

Infection

Infection is a rare event in cutaneous surgery. The recorded incidence is <1%. If the wound is frankly infected, it is imperative that all the sutures be removed and patient is started on antibiotics. Author prefers to give tetanus toxoid injection and intravenous antibiotic preoperatively and to start the patient on an antibiotic course postoperatively for 1 week.

Dehiscence

The wound pulls apart in dehiscence usually as a result of underlying infection and/or hematoma. These causes should be promptly managed allowing the wound to heal by second intention. Delayed scar revision can be done at a later date.

Necrosis

Necrosis is a rare complication of simple excision surgery. It occurs only if the wound is closed under high tension thereby compromising the vascularity of the wound margins. The course of action should be suture removal, debridement of the necrotic tissue, and allowing the wound to heal by second intention. Corrective scar revision is undertaken at a later date.

Dog-ear

A skin protrusion present at the end of excision is commonly referred to as a dog-ear. These protrusions are caused by the presence of redundant skin at the ends or dressing sites of an excision. The amount of tissue protrusion formed in a given wound is fundamentally determined by the amount of rotation, advancement, and intrinsic tissue elasticity of the surrounding skin. The local surface contours also contribute to the final degree of tissue protrusion. Circumferential closures performed on highly convex surfaces, such as the arm, will result in tissue protrusions at the end of the closure. If excess subcutaneous fat is present at the apex of an excision, the resultant elevation of the angle of closure may mimic a tissue protrusion. Removal of excess fat with adequate undermining of the apex will invariably result in the dissolution of the pseudo-dog-ear.[3]

Methods of Dog-ear Correction

Before planning the removal of dog-ear, it is often beneficial to partially close the wound edges to determine whether a tissue protrusion will form.

Linear Repair

This is simple, easy to perform, and useful when it is desirable to extend the excision in a straight line. The apex of tissue protrusion is elevated with a skin-hook to define the geometry of tissue protrusion in the shape of a standing cone. The apex of the cone is drawn to one side so that the base of the tissue protrusion is in line with the long axis of the anticipated wound closure. The base is incised and undermined to free up a triangular wedge of tissue. The triangular section is then draped over the underlying wound edge with gentle tension and the base is incised over the line of closure. The wound is then repaired in a straight line.

Other methods of dog-ear repair are curved repair, hockey stick repair, L-shaped repair, T-shaped repair, and N-plasty repair.[3]

Summary of Dog-ear Repair

Closure of even the most carefully planned and executed excision may result in the development of tissue protrusions. Understanding the dynamics of tissue movement and elasticity allows anticipation and subsequent correction of dog-ears. An attempt should always be made to place the final incision lines parallel to the RSTLs. Proper design and execution of these techniques provides critical difference between an average and an excellent cosmetic outcome. **Figures 21 to 23** show the different steps of excision in different situations—scar excision, scrofuloderma, and neurofibroma, respectively.

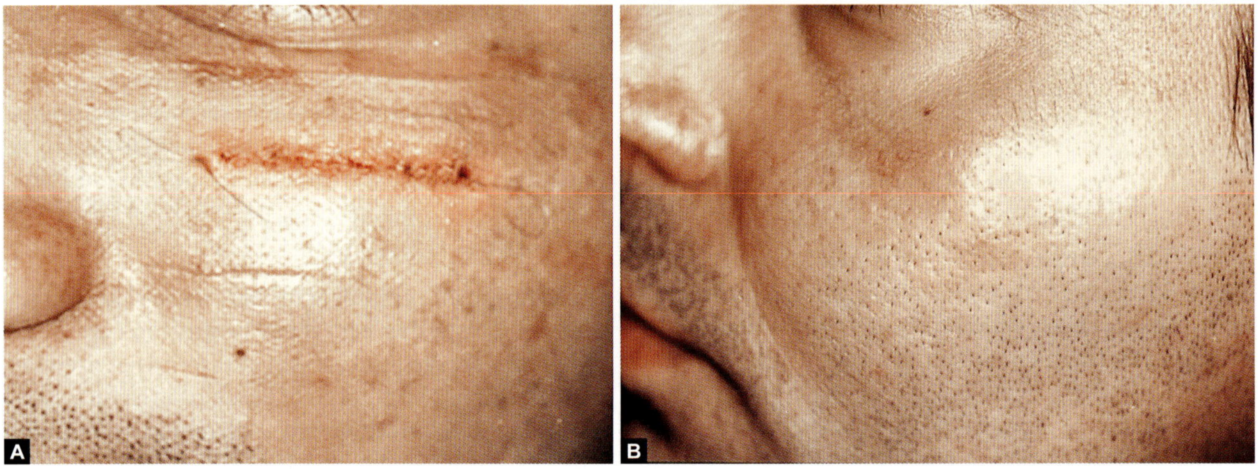

Figs. 21A and B: (A) Scar excision (before); (B) Scar excision (after).

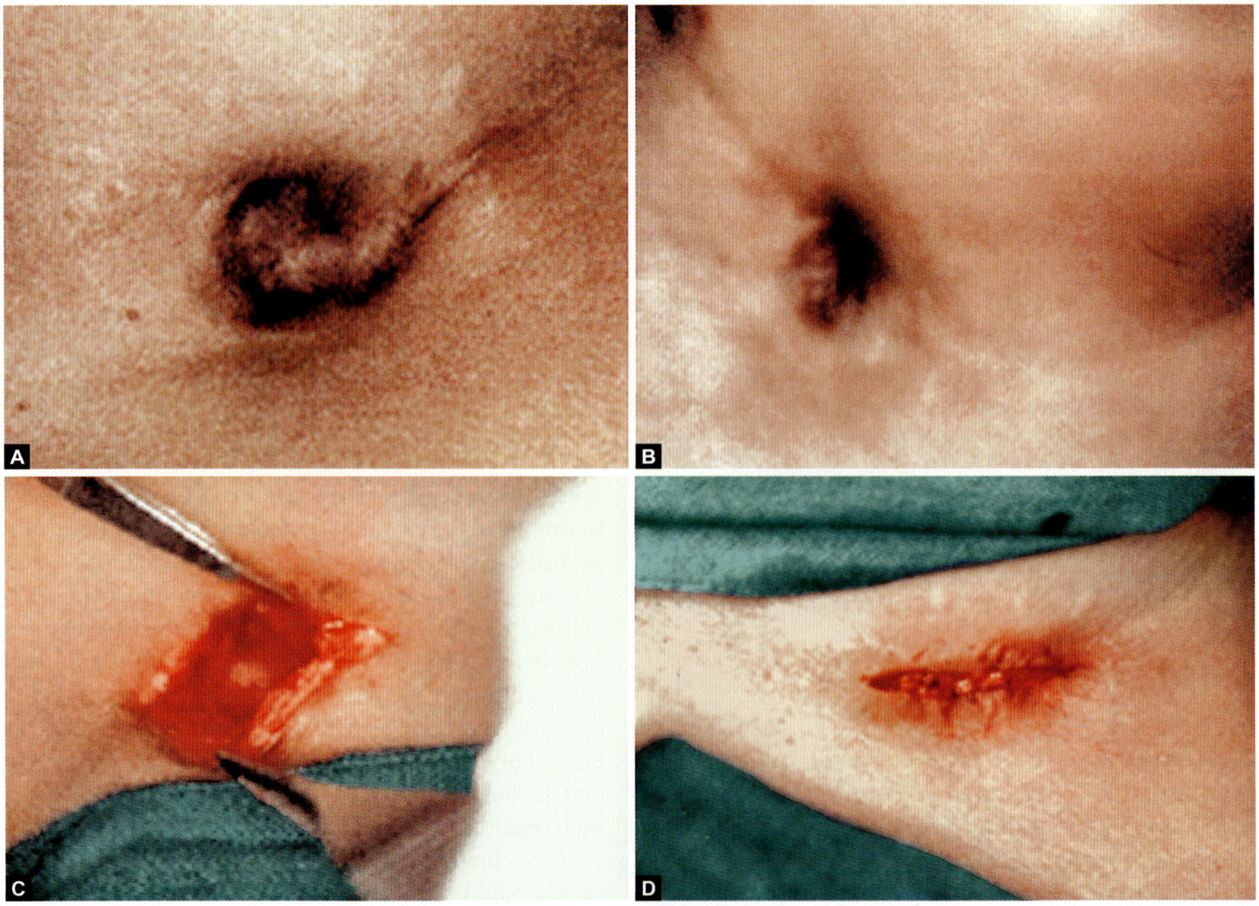

Figs. 22A to D

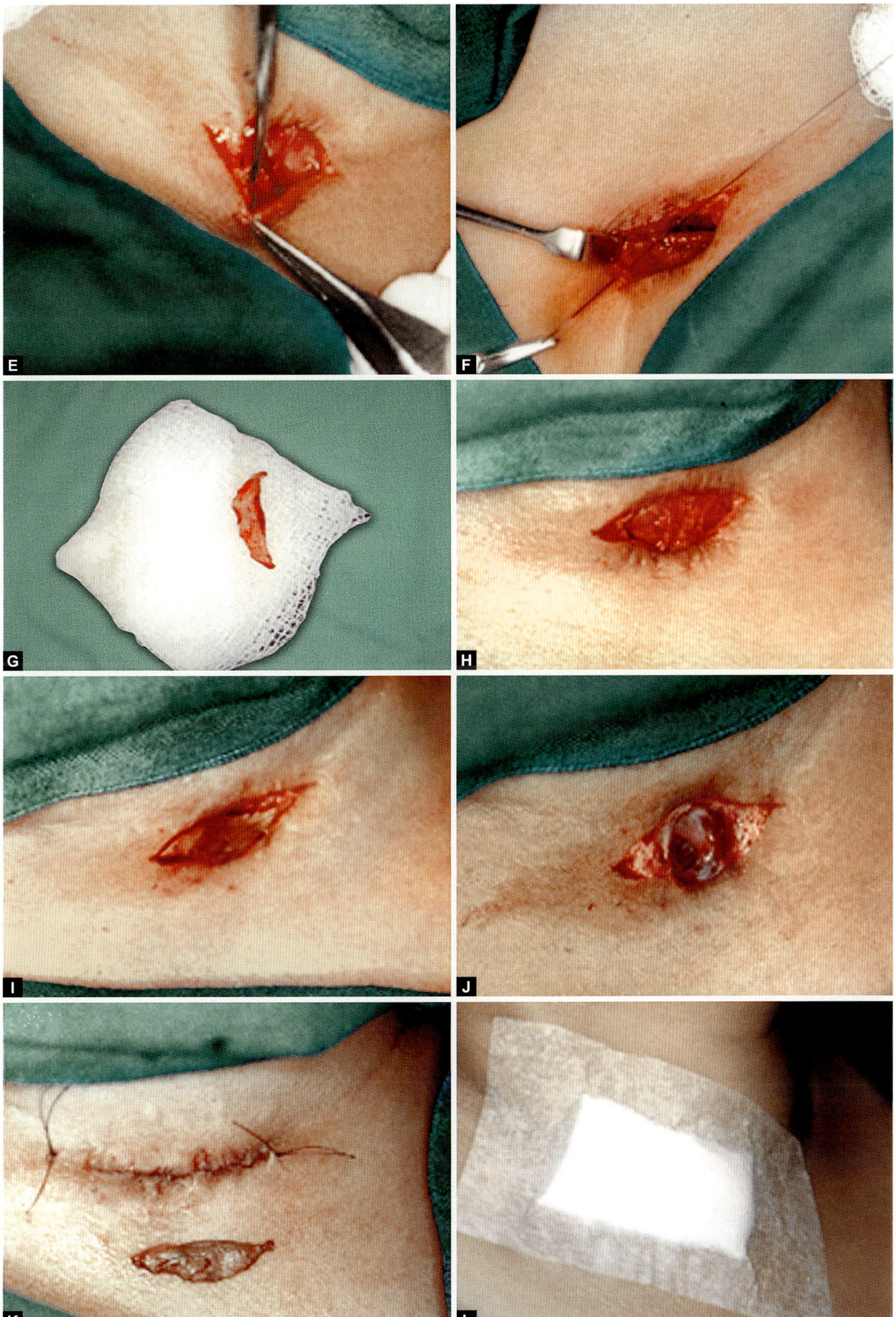

Figs. 22E to L

Figs. 22A to L: (A to H) Deep scar following scrofuloderma, with complete atrophy of subcutaneous tissue. Undermining the defect: scrofuloderma; (I to L) Excision and suturing done with occlusive dressing.

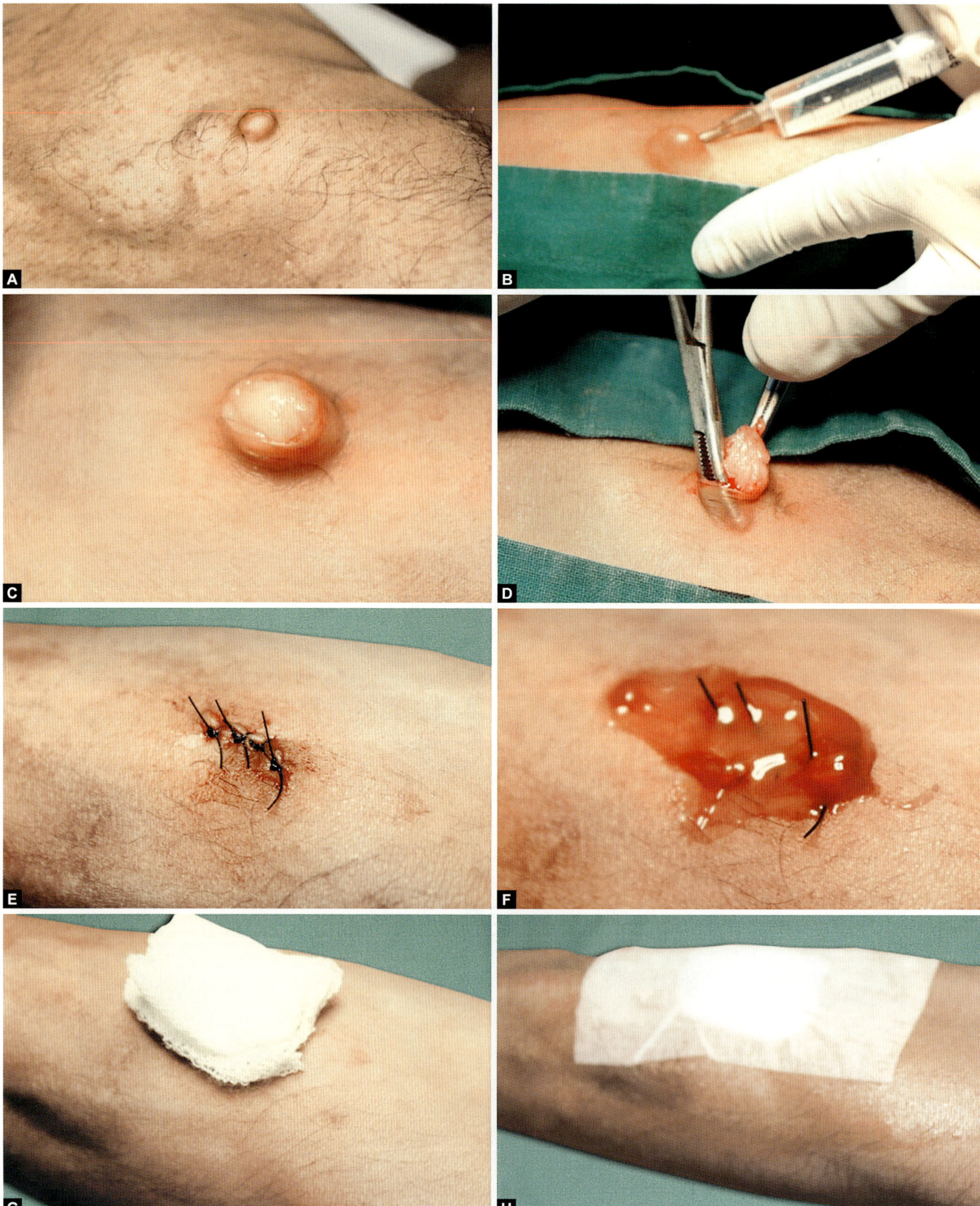

Figs. 23A to H: Excision of neurofibroma. (A) Neurofibroma; (B) Field block for neurofibroma; (C) After blunt dissection; (D) Blunt dissection in progress; (E) After suturing; (F) Povidone-iodine applied; (G) Nonocclusive gauze piece applied; (H) Dressing completed in three layers with micropore tape.

BOX 3: Advantages of elliptical excision.

- Inexpensive
- Costly equipment are not required
- Excellent cosmetic results
- No tissue destruction
- Not a blind procedure
- Good specimen can be obtained for histopathology

CONCLUSION

Elliptical excision is a cornerstone of cutaneous excisional surgeries because of several advantages **(Box 3)**. Understanding the basic principles of anatomy, wound healing, anesthesia, lines of closure, STL, tumor biology, surgical techniques of incision, suturing, and wound care are the prerequisites for cutaneous simple excision surgery. Mastery over these principles gives an excellent cosmetic result satisfying both the patient and the operating surgeon.

REFERENCES

1. Stegman SJ, Tromovitch TA, Glogau RG. Basics of Dermatologic Surgery. Chicago: Year Book Medical Publishers; 1982.
2. Leshin B. Proper planning and execution of surgical excisions. In: Wheeland RG (Ed). Cutaneous Surgery, 1st edition. Philadelphia: Saunders; 1994. pp. 171-7.
3. Goldberg LH. Cold steel surgery. In: Lask GP, Moy RL (Eds). The Ellipse, Principles and Techniques of Cutaneous Surgery, 1st edition. New Delhi: Jaypee Brothers Medical Publishers (P) Ltd.; 1996. pp. 165-70.
4. Perez M. Skin biopsy techniques. In: Nouri K, Leal-Khouri S (Eds). Techniques in Dermatologic Surgery. St. Louis: CV Mosby; 2003.
5. Webster RC, Smith RC. Cosmetic principles in surgery on the face. J Dermatol Surg Oncol. 1978;4:397-402.
6. Bennett RG. Fundamentals of Cutaneous Surgery. St. Louis: CV Mosby; 1988. pp. 353-444.
7. Leal-Khouri S. Suturing techniques. In: Nouri K, Leal-Khouri S (Eds). Techniques in Dermatologic Surgery. St. Louis: CV Mosby; 2003. pp. 71-3.
8. Hruza GJ. Suturing techniques. In: Lask GP, Moy RL (Eds). Principles and Techniques of Cutaneous surgery. New York: McGraw-Hill; 1996. pp. 171-85.
9. Chernosky ME. Scalpel and scissors as seen by the dermatologist. In: Epstein E, Epstein E Jr. (Eds). Skin Surgery, 6th edition, Philadelphia: Saunders; 1987. p. 88.
10. Stegman SJ. Planning closure of a surgical wound. J Dermatol Surg Oncol. 1978;4:390-3.
11. Zitelli JA. Tips for a better ellipse. J Am Acad Dermatol. 1990;22:101-3.
12. Spicer TE. Techniques of facial lesion excision and closure. J Dermatol Surg Oncol. 1982;8:551-6.
13. Stegman SJ. Suturing techniques for dermatologic surgery. J Dermatol Surg Oncol. 1978;4:63-8.
14. Hassanein AH, Couto JA, Greene AK. Circular excision and purse-string closure for pediatric facial skin lesions. J Craniofac Surg. 2015;26:1611-2.
15. Mulliken JB, Rogers GF, Marler JJ. Circular excision of hemangioma and purse-string closure: the smallest possible scar. Plast Reconstr Surg. 2002;109:1544-54.
16. Nomura T, Osaki T, Ishinagi H, Ejiri H, Terashi H. Simple and easy surgical technique for infantile hemangiomas: intralesional excision and primary closure. Eplasty. 2015;15:15:e3.

CHAPTER 19

Skin Biopsy and Mole Surgery

Dhanashree S Bhide

KEY MESSAGES

- Skin biopsy is an extremely important basic procedure for all the dermatologists. It helps to establish early and accurate diagnosis, which prompts the physician to start appropriate treatment on time and helps to prevent further complications of the disease due to delay in starting therapy.
- A dermatosurgeon should be familiar with different biopsy techniques (punch, excision, incision, and shave biopsies), the time and site of sampling as well as with special modifications needed in difficult areas such as scalp, mucosa, and nail.
- Benign moles are usually treated for cosmetic purposes and for functional reasons.
- Different commonly performed procedures for removing moles are excision and radiofrequency.
- Other procedures such as cryotherapy and lasers are less commonly performed because of their limitations in providing tissue sample for histopathology.

INTRODUCTION

This chapter describes easy-to-perform but common and useful procedures such as skin biopsy and mole surgery, which are necessary in day-to-day dermatosurgery office practice. A beginner with limited resources can master these techniques and treat a wide range of conditions with ease and in minimum budget. There is stepwise description of different biopsy techniques, the sites for performing biopsies, the time frame (early or late lesion), and the various bulbs necessary to collect the samples. This is important as the diagnostic yield depends on the site and time of collection (in vasculitis cases, it depends on whether early or late lesion is biopsied).

Mole surgery is a very commonly demanded procedure by patients for cosmetic reasons. The moles on face, if treated with skill and care, can give excellent results. Mastering different techniques and choosing the appropriate technique according to the type, size, and anatomical location of the mole are essential for good results. We have discussed various techniques for removing moles with illustrative diagrams and photographs. The pros and cons of each technique along with red flag signs is also discussed to help the dermatosurgeon to choose the appropriate technique.

SKIN BIOPSY

Skin biopsy is a very important and commonly performed office procedure in dermatology practice. This is an era of net savvy patients, evidence-based medicine, litigations, and demand for the proof of clinical judgment. Hence, biopsy becomes an important documentary evidence for supporting the diagnosis made and also the basis for starting the treatment.

BOX 1: Different types of biopsy.

- In excisional biopsy, entire lump or suspicious area is removed
- In incisional biopsy, only small sample from the affected area is removed by preserving the histological architecture of the cells
- In fine-needle aspiration biopsy, tissue sample is removed with the needle. In attempting this, the histological architecture of cells may not be preserved

In biopsy, cells or tissues are removed by using different techniques for examination. Biopsy "Bio" means life and "Opsia" means to view. Biopsy means to view life. It can be excisional, incisional, or a needle aspiration biopsy **(Box 1)**. The choice of biopsy technique depends on the size of lesion, anatomical location, and suspected diagnosis.

It is an art to choose correct site for perfect dermatological diagnosis. Everyone should master different techniques and apply the correct technique appropriate for that condition. The histopathological interpretation depends a lot on the technique and the morphology of the lesion.

History

One of the earliest diagnostic biopsies was developed as early as 1013–1107 AD by the Arab physician Abul Qasim. A needle was used to puncture a goiter and the material was examined.[1] Skin biopsy technique in modern times was introduced over 100 years ago. Before this, the histological diagnosis was done in connection with autopsies or necropsies. The term "biopsy" was coined by a dermatologist Ernest Besnier in 1879. As local anesthesia facilities were not available that time, it was not a commonly performed procedure. Local anesthesia was brought in use by an ophthalmologist Karl Koller in late1800[2] when he instilled cocaine solution to perform pain-free cataract surgery. A year after this, cocaine was injected in skin by William Halsted, an American surgeon. Around the end of 19th century, the infiltration anesthesia practice began and then the biopsy was performed on routine basis. Heinrich Auspitz and Hans von Hebra introduced sharp spoon in 1876. Punch instrument was originally used to trephine cut through skull bone. Its use was documented in abscess removal from tibia in 1852. A diskotome was created by Watson in 1877 to remove traumatic tattoos.[3] In 1878, Watson described punch use in correction of accidental gunpowder disfigurement[4] and Edward L Keyes in 1887 described punch for dermatology use.[3] He used the punch initially to remove powder crystals in the face of a youth due to firecracker injury. He devised serial sized punches. There was a difference in the diameter of half a millimeter between the two consecutive sizes.[3]

Various modifications in the design as well as the uses were considered.

Rotary drill by Urbach, disposable punch, punch for autograft experiments,[5] and use in hair transplant by Norman Orentreich[6] and Samuel Agres[6] were some of the modifications. The use of punch in acne scar surgery was suggested by Orentreich and Waine Johnson.[3]

Knowledge of Basic Anatomy

It is important to have the knowledge of relaxed skin tension lines (RSTLs) to determine the incision.[7] Properly taken incision, which is parallel to RSTL lines, gives a better and cosmetically acceptable scar, especially on the face. The RSTL lines can be made prominent by giving gentle lateral pressure in the area to be treated or by asking the patient to perform specific action **(Figs. 1A and B)**.

Indications[8,9]

Indications for skin biopsy are described in **Table 1**.

Contraindications

There are no absolute contraindications for diagnostic biopsies. However, the procedure should be performed with caution in following situations:

- Active infection at local site
- Bleeding tendencies or patients on anticoagulants (aspirin and warfarin)
- Allergies to local antiseptics or to local anesthetics
- Keloidal tendency
- Systemic conditions such as uncontrolled diabetes mellitus

Site Selection[8]

According to the Pathogenesis of the Lesion

- *For inflammatory lesions:* When the disease is in the process of evolution, choose a lesion with most

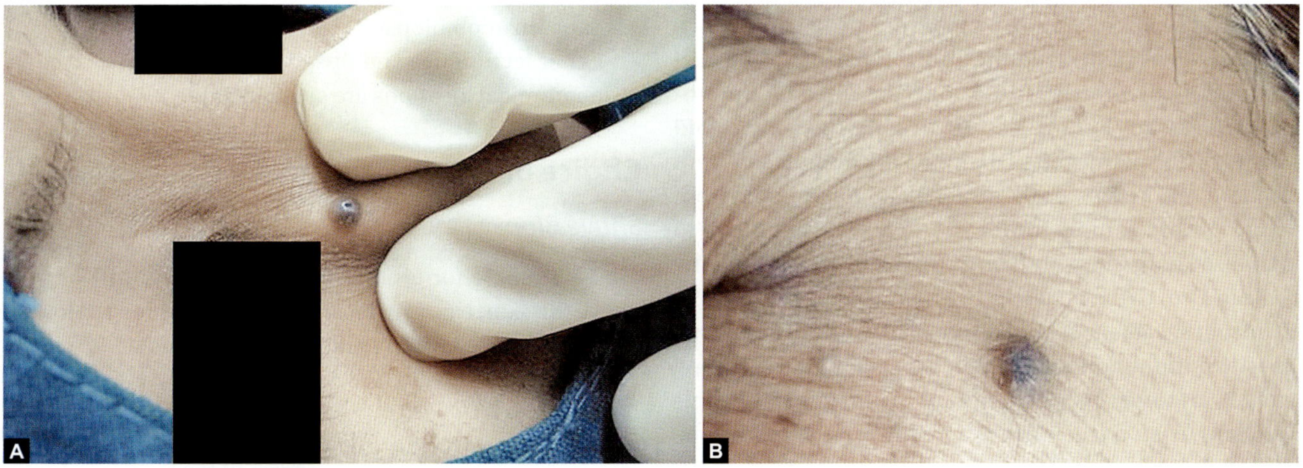

Figs. 1A and B: (A) Relaxed skin tension line (RSTL) lines made prominent by gentle lateral pressure; and (B) RSTL lines made prominent by tightly closing the eyes.

TABLE 1: Skin biopsy indications.

Diagnostic	*Prognostic*	*Therapeutic*	*Special tests*	*To evaluate effect of treatment*
• When clinical diagnosis not possible or doubtful • In all bullous and suspected neoplastic conditions • To confirm the clinical diagnosis	In lupus erythematosus to do lupus band test (clinically uninvolved skin sent for direct immunofluorescence study)	Excisional biopsy in conditions such as nevi, granuloma annulare, basal cell carcinoma, etc.	• Immunofluorescence • Special stains • Electron microscopy	For example, in leprosy before and after starting the treatment

advanced inflammatory change or from an active border. It is always good to include adjacent normal tissue for comparison.

- *For bullous diseases:* Early lesions should be biopsied to get more specific results. Lesions within 48 hours of their appearance give the best results.
- *Suspected malignancy*: If the lesion is small, excise it completely with adequate clearance on all sides.
- For diagnosis of rabies, biopsy should be taken from the nape of neck at the hairline. A deep punch biopsy with 5–6 mm in size punch should be taken. It should be deep enough to include nerves (virus is neurotropic) and should have at least 10 hair follicles. The specimen should be sent on sterile saline-moistened gauze for reverse transcriptase-polymerase chain reaction (RT-PCR) assay and immunofluorescent staining of frozen sections of the biopsy specimen.[10,11]

According to the Size of the Lesion

- Small lesions may be removed entirely
- Large lesions, central part, may be biopsied. Avoid crusted excoriated areas
- For larger bulla, a scooped shave biopsy may be taken

For Special Procedures[12-14]

- *Direct immunofluorescence in vesiculobullous disorders*: Perilesional skin.
  For diagnosis of bullous diseases, direct immunofluorescence (DIF) is found to be superior to indirect immunofluorescence (IIF) or enzyme-linked immunosorbent assay (ELISA) testing. In bullous pemphigoid patients, for performing DIF, sample can be taken from nonbullous lesions or perilesional skin preferable from trunk (avoid sample from extremities). If sample is to be taken from uninvolved perilesional skin, it should be within 1 cm of the bulla.
  The root sheath of plucked anagen hairs may demonstrate positive immunofluorescence, especially in the setting of BP, and may prove adequate for diagnosis. In this technique, an anagen hair is forcibly extracted from the scalp. The presence of a gelatinous follicular sheath above the hair bulb denotes an adequate specimen.
  Bullous scabies can give false-positive DIF.
- *Lupus band test in collagen vascular disease*: Clinically uninvolved skin.

Points to Remember while Choosing the Site for Biopsy[15]

- Avoid friction areas as there may be secondary changes.
- In case of polymorphic eruptions, more than one biopsy may be required.
- Normally, a well-formed lesion should be chosen for biopsy except in Henoch–Schönlein purpura, dermatitis herpetiformis, and suspected subepidermal blisters when very early lesions should be biopsied.
- In urticaria pigmentosa, instead of infiltration anesthesia, use of a field block to avoid mast cell degranulation is advised.

TIPS

For getting better results[8,12,16]

- Try to remove the vesicle intact. Smaller lesions—intact bulla can be biopsied.
- If the lesion is larger, bulla can be biopsied at the edge trying to keep the roof attached if it cannot be removed entirely.
- Try to avoid important cosmetic areas such as face, deltoid area, chest (chances of hypertrophic scarring), tibia (delayed healing), groins, and axillae (high incidence of secondary infection) as far as possible.
- Avoid biopsy in burnt-out lesions, lesions altered by trauma, or prior treatment.

Diagnostic accuracy of biopsy specimen can be increased if correct site, correct technique, and appropriate transport medium are chosen **(Tables 2 and 3)**.

Types of Skin Biopsy Techniques

- Shave biopsy
- Punch biopsy
- Incisional biopsy
- Excisional biopsy
- Saucerization biopsy
- Other techniques and tips to perform biopsies in special anatomical locations are given in **Table 2**.

Choice of Procedure

Shave Biopsy

This is suitable for lesions confined to epidermis or raised above the skin, e.g., skin tags, seborrheic keratoses. However, it cannot be used when malignancy is suspected.

Punch Biopsy

This is the most commonly performed biopsy procedure.

Excisional Biopsy

Excisional biopsy is suitable for lesions, which cannot be removed with punch because of their large size or due to their location or due to their depth.

Incisional Biopsy

Incisional biopsy can be used in large lesions to excise small portion of the tissue.

TABLE 2: Site, type of biopsy, and lesion selection.[12,16]

Disease	*Type of biopsy*	*Site and type of lesion*
Autoimmune bullous diseases	• Small vesicles and perilesional skin—punch biopsy • *Large bulla*: – Scooped shave biopsy extending up to reticular dermis – Incision biopsy from the edge involving the perilesional skin	• Preferred site is trunk • Extremities to be avoided
Epidermolysis bullosa	Saucerized removal of intact bulla is preferred	• Blisters <12 hours duration • Induce blister at a site where patient normally blisters can use pencil eraser, gloved finger, or cotton swab • Gentle traction given in downward direction • Twist given in each direction by 180° till erythema produces • Give lag period of 5 minutes before biopsy • Avoid topical anesthesia, which may induce artificial blisters
Vasculitis	Punch or deep shave biopsy	• For H and E, well-established purpuric lesion >72 hours • For DIF, fresh lesion <24 hours except in IgA vasculitis for which established lesion may be chosen
Panniculitis	• Deep incisional biopsy • Avoid punch biopsy, as it is likely to leave behind inflamed or necrotic fat • If at all punch is to be used, electric rotary power punch may be used	• Apply alcohol to skin surface and allow to evaporate • Take about 6 mm size biopsy • Divide and send for culture and special stains • The edge of necrotic focus ideal for this
Lupus and dermatomyositis	Punch biopsy—lesional, nonlesional sun exposed, and nonlesional sun protected	• Established but still active lesion • For long-standing disease, specimen from active lesion (disease persisting for >6 months)
SJS/TEN versus SSSS	Shave biopsy including entire epidermal thickness	Sheets of desquamating skin adequate sample
Scarring alopecia	Punch biopsy 4 mm and above	• Avoid active edge • Prefer established lesion
Nonscarring alopecia	Punch biopsy 4 mm and above	• Alopecia areata or syphilis—active lesion of recent onset is preferred • Patterned alopecia and TE—established area > 6 months

(DIF: direct immunofluorescence; IgA: immunoglobulin A; SJS: Stevens–Johnson syndrome; SSSS: staphylococcal scalded skin syndrome; TE: telogen effluvium; TEN: toxic epidermal necrosis)

Saucerization Biopsy[15]

This is a useful technique for vesiculobullous disorders and also for epidermal neoplasms such as seborrheic keratosis. It is performed with the help of razor blade, which is bent like an arc by holding between thumb and index finger. The plane of cleavage passes through the reticular dermis and sometimes through the subcutaneous tissue. The wound is allowed to heal by secondary intention.

Preprocedure Counseling

Obtain informed consent and counsel about possibility of a small scar, particularly when biopsy is planned on face or other cosmetically important areas.

Instruments necessary for different types of biopsies are shown in **Table 3**.

Chemical Hemostatic Agents

Chemicals which can be used to achieve hemostasis such as 20% aluminum chloride in absolute alcohol, Monsel's solution (ferric sulfate), trichloroacetic acid, and silver nitrate are useful, particularly for shave biopsy. A solution called BotroClot (sterile hemocoagulase solution) can also be used. The active ingredient is purified hemocoagulase enzyme complex isolated from *Bothrops atrox* or *Bothrops jararaca*,

TABLE 4: Transport medium according to type of study.

Type of study	*Transport medium*
Light microscopy H and E	Formalin
Direct immunofluorescence	• Normal saline, liquid nitrogen, Michel's medium, or Zeus medium • Normal saline gives highest yield and sends without freezing • Samples sent in liquid nitrogen require thawing
Immunohistochemistry	Formalin fixed paraffin embedded blocks
Electron microscopy	2.5% glutaraldehyde solution
Microorganism culture	Nonbacteriostatic saline

TABLE 3: Instruments for biopsy.

For shave biopsy	*For punch biopsy*	*For incisional and excisional biopsy*
• Blades No. 15 or 11, razor blade, or cutting scissors straight or curved • BP handle No. 3 • Chemical hemostatic agents or electrocautery for fulguration	• Biopsy punches 1–10 mm • Optimum size 4 mm • Cutting scissors • Forceps atraumatic • Skin hook	• Blades No. 15 or 11 • BP handle No. 3 • Atraumatic forceps—Adson forceps • Cutting scissors • Suture material—needle holder • Skin hook

species of South American snakes. It is a toxic and arrests the capillary bleeding by accelerating the physiological process of hemostasis. 5–10 drops of the solution can be used depending upon the severity of bleeding. It should be consumed within 1 month after opening the container. It is available as 10 mL solution in plastic container.

Transport Medium[12,16,17]

For hematoxylin and eosin staining, 10% buffered formalin is adequate. Commercially available formalin is 40%, which should be diluted 1 in 4 before use.

For immunofluorescence—Michel's solution if laboratory is located at a distance. Phosphate-buffered saline in a cold pack can be used, if laboratory is located within 4 hours **(Table 4)**.

Saline is superior to liquid nitrogen, Michel's medium, or Zeus medium, if it is possible to deliver the specimen in 48 hours.

Steps Common to All Minor Procedures

- Correct documentation with clinical photograph
- Informed written consent
- Universal precautions
- Proper sterilization of instruments
- Cleaning with betadine and spirit
- Marking the area before infiltration
- Infiltration of local anesthesia—1% xylocaine with or without adrenaline depending upon the site. While infiltrating, try to elevate the lesion by raising a wheal, which allows the lesion to prop up
- Postprocedure dressing, topical and oral antibiotic, and suture removal when indicated
- Carefully label the specimen including patient and physicians name, date, and location of the lesion

Procedure of Biopsy

Shave Biopsy[18,19]

Shave biopsy has the advantages of being quick, needs little training, does not require suturing for closure, faster healing, and good cosmetic result. However, its disadvantage is that deeper dermis and subcutaneous fat are not available for examination and, hence, the method is unsuitable for deeper pathologies.

Steps ***(Figs. 2A to H)****:* Steps involved in shave biopsy are as follows:

- Stabilize the lesion between the thumb and forefinger in a direction perpendicular to RSTL lines.
- A vertical cut is put at the periphery of the lesion using 11 or 15 No. scalpel blade attached to No. 3 BP handle.
- Blade is held parallel to the skin surface and then passed through the lesion through the cut that is already made at the periphery.
- The blade is advanced through the lesion by a smooth sweeping stroke rather than a sawing motion while grasping the lesion with forceps.
- Hemostasis is achieved by firm pressure or with the chemicals mentioned before the procedure can also be performed by using halved razor blade or curved scissors.
- Antibiotic cream is applied and a gauze dressing is given.

Alternative methods:

Scissor technique ***(Figs. 3A to E)****:* For pedunculated lesions, biopsy with scissors is simple and effective option. Operator's clinical judgment is important while sending the sample for histopathological examination.

Shave biopsy using a razor blade ***(Fig. 4A)****:* A razor blade can be broken into half and bent along its longitudinal axis. It is then held between the thumb and other fingers. Holding the blade without handle gives great flexibility. Horizontal sawing motion is used to the desired depth in the dermis. Superficial lesions can be easily removed by this technique. This blade has an advantage of being flexible and extremely sharp.[20,21]

Modification ***(Figs. 4B to D)****:* The plastic needle cover of a 22-gauge scalp vein set was cut to match the length of the blunt edges of the razor blade and then cut longitudinally on one side and slide along both the blunt edges. The tube latex of an intravenous infusion set was cut as per the length of the sharp edges and one sharp edge of the blade was inserted into a pocket made out of cutting the tube latex lengthwise. The cap over the nonsharp edges provides better grip and control to the surgeon and the flexible tube latex covers the unused sharp edge to prevent accidental cut injuries.[22]

Punch Biopsy[18,19]

Punch biopsy is indicated for routine histopathological examination as a therapy to remove small lesions such as nevi. If lesion is totally removed, it is excisional punch biopsy. If the lesion is partially removed, it is incisional punch biopsy. Its advantages are that it is simple and heals with minimal scar. However, it is unsuitable for lesions having pathologies deeper to subcutaneous tissue such as leiomyoma, dermatomyositis, and in difficult anatomical location, e.g., nasal cartilage.

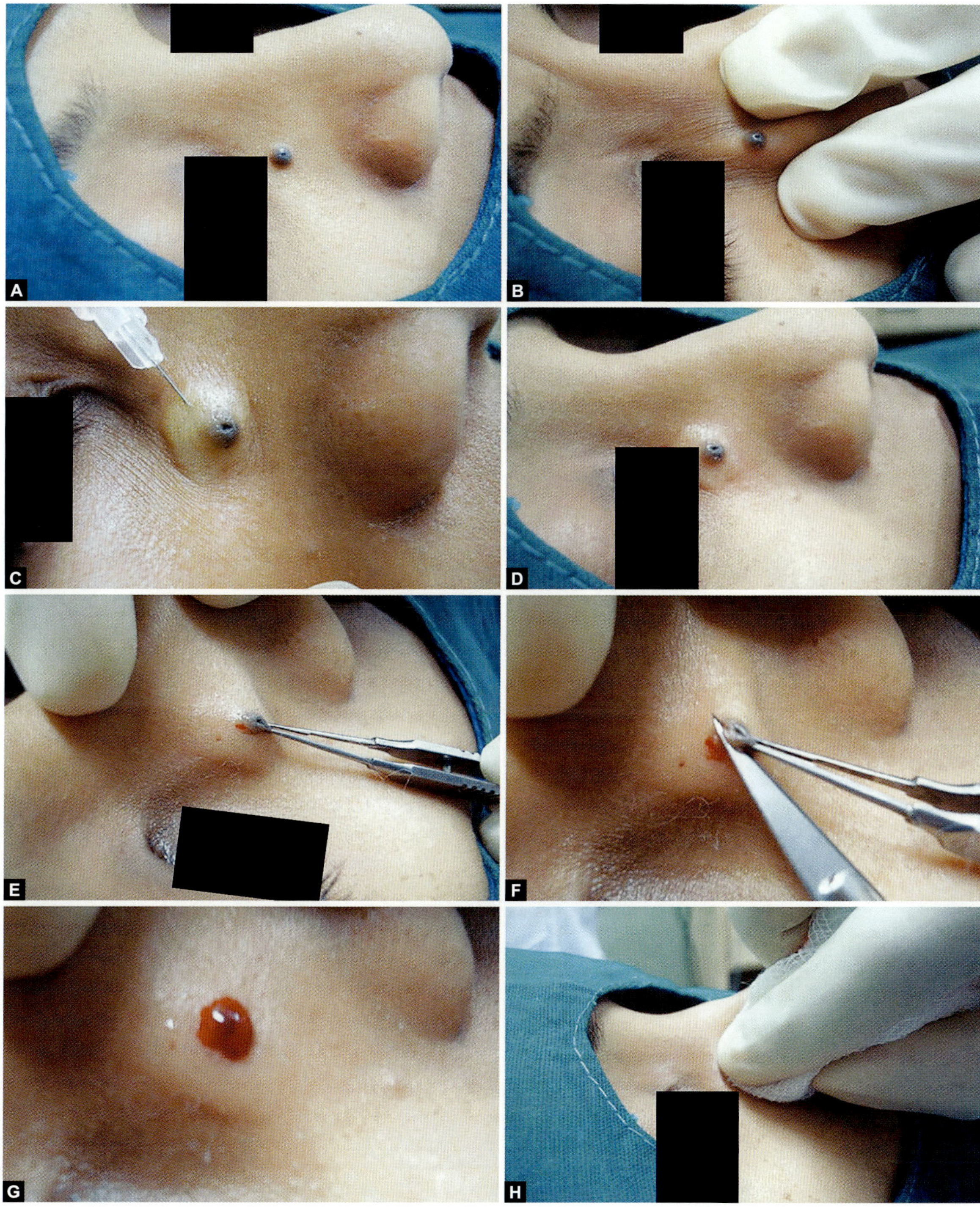

Figs. 2A to H: Steps of shave biopsy. (A) Mole on the nose; (B) Relaxed skin tension line (RSTL) lines made prominent; (C) Local anesthesia infiltration; (D) Lesion gets elevated; (E) Vertical cut at periphery; (F) Biopsy with blade parallel to surface; (G) Bleeding at site; and (H) Hemostasis by firm pressure.

Procedure of punch biopsy: Steps **(Figs. 5A to J)** of punch biopsy are as follows:

- Common steps are as mentioned above
- Routinely, a 4-mm punch is chosen
- Traction is given in a direction perpendicular to long axis of resting skin tension lines

While performing scalp biopsies, rim of the ring of a large artery forceps is pressed against the scalp surface

- Punch is held vertically and a steady pressure is applied
- Punch is rotated in a clockwise manner till tissue cast is completely separated from collagen fibers of reticular dermis and the punch reaches the subcutis. At this stage, there is feeling of giveaway

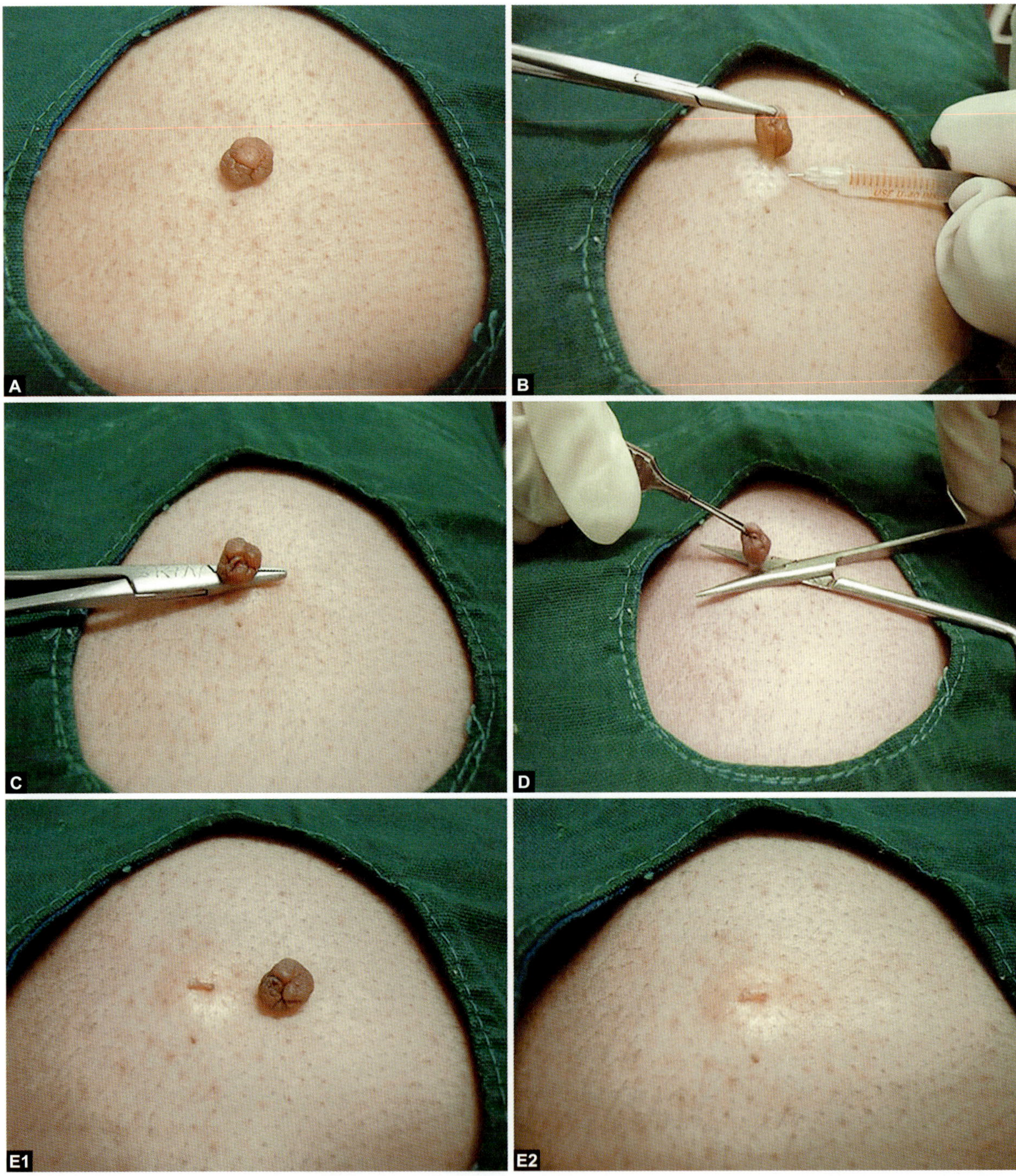

Figs. 3A to E: Shave biopsy (scissor technique). (A) Skin tag; (B) Local infiltration; (C) Base crushed with straight artery forceps; (D) Lesion excised with scissors; and (E1 and E2) Immediately after procedure.

- Punch is withdrawn
- Tissue cast is lifted with fine forceps or a needle to avoid crushing and damage. It is then cut at the base with scissors.
- On releasing the tension, the circular biopsy defect relaxes into ellipse.
- The wound is sutured for better healing with interrupted sutures by using 5-0 Prolene and dressing is given. For defects up to 3 mm, suture may not be taken in areas that are not important cosmetically.
- Sutures removed after 7–10 days.

Excisional Biopsy

Excisional biopsy is indicated for removing benign or malignant lesions, which can be removed and closed by primary closure. As entire lesion is removed, it is both

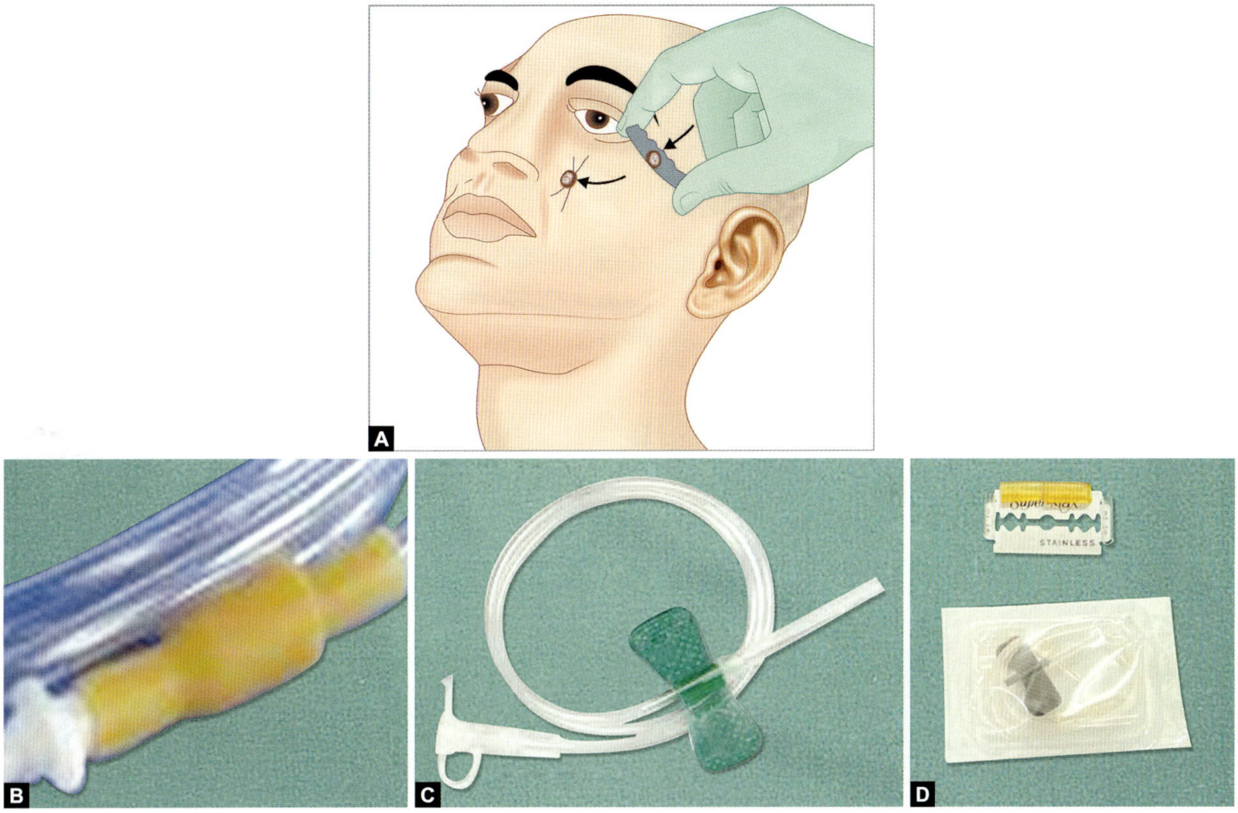

Figs. 4A to D: (A) Shave biopsy using a razor blade; (B) Rubber tubing of intravenous (IV) set; (C) 22-gauge scalp vein; and (D) Sharp edges of razor blade covered on one side.

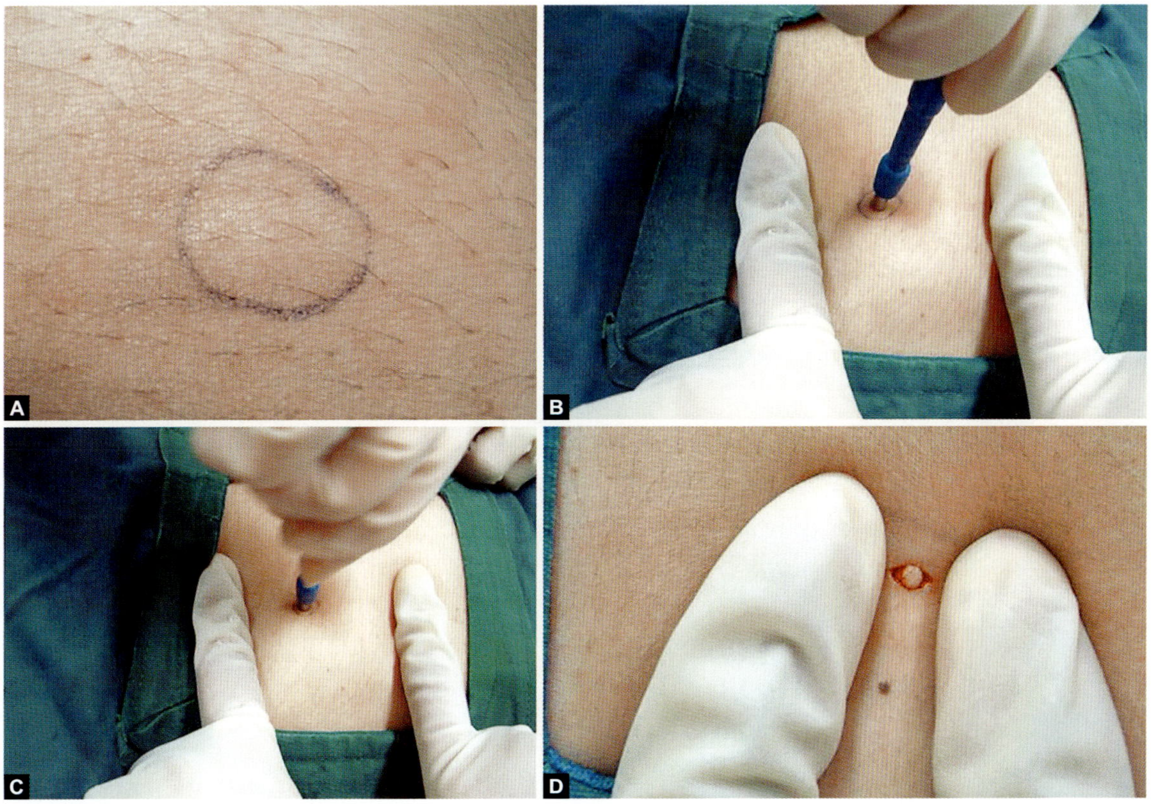

Figs. 5A to D: Steps in punch biopsy. (A) Site marked; (B) Punch held in vertical direction. Traction is given perpendicular to relaxed skin tension line (RSTL); (C) Punch rotated in clockwise manner; and (D) Circular defect relaxes into an ellipse.

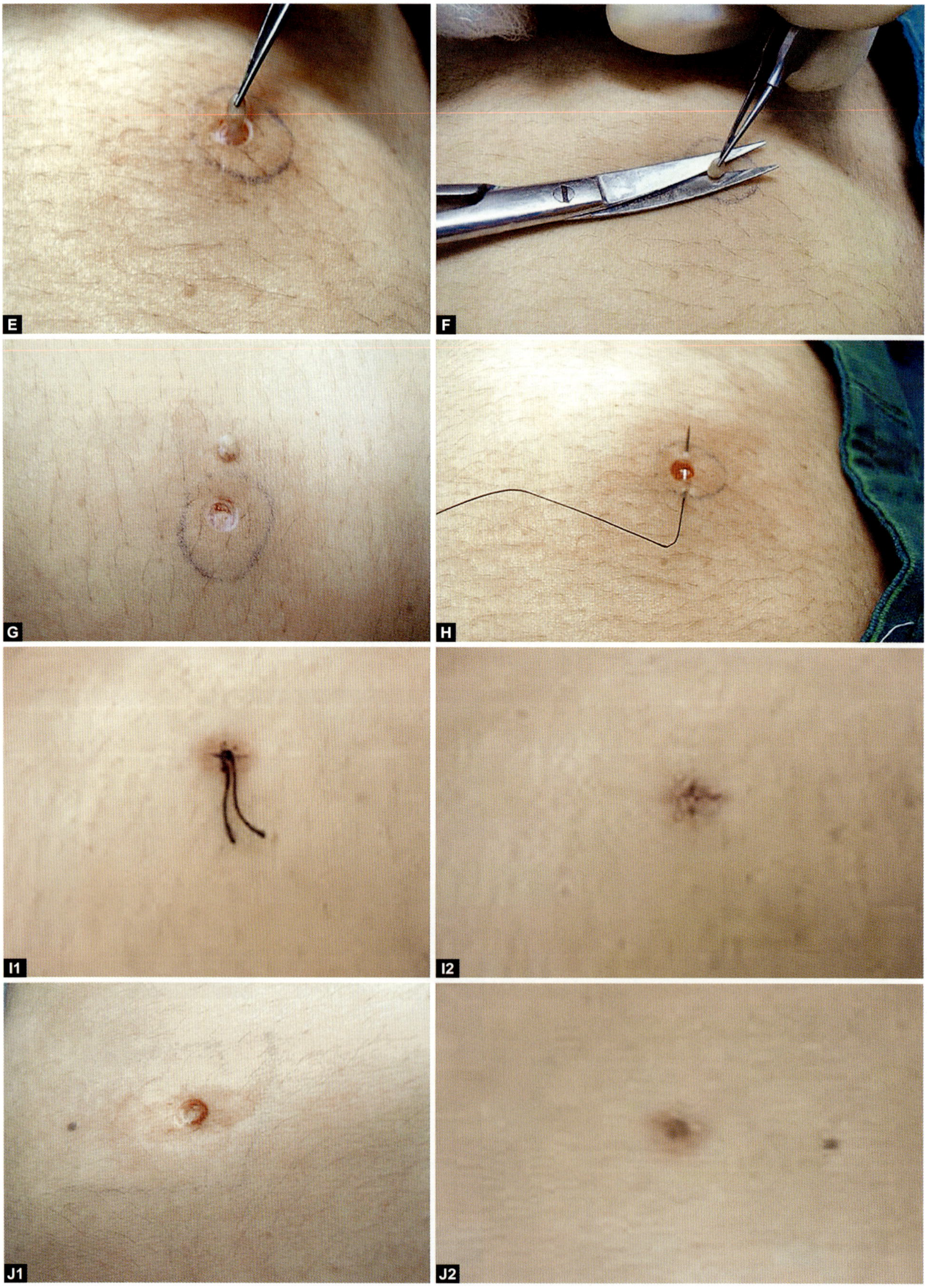

Figs. 5E to J: Procedure of punch biopsy. (E) Column of tissue grasped with forceps; (F) Tissue cut with scissors; (G) Biopsy specimen; (H) Suture taken; (I1 and I2) Healing after 1 week with suture; and (J1 and J2) Healing after 1 week without suture.

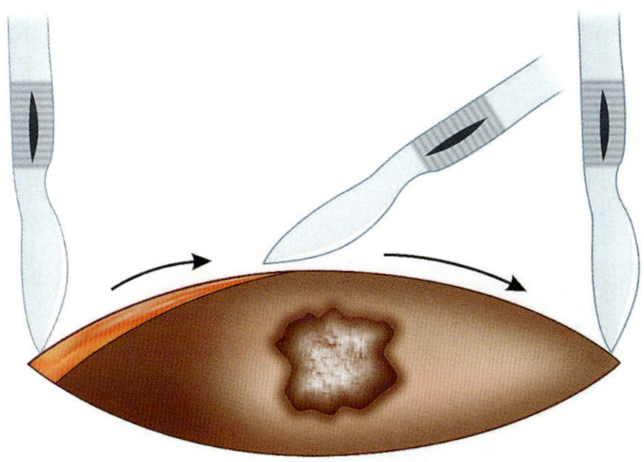

Fig. 6: Scalpel movement.

diagnostic and therapeutic modality. Its advantages are that entire specimen is available for histology and since the wound is sutured, it heals with good cosmetic result. However, training is needed for performing the procedure and skill needs to be acquired. If excision is incomplete, chances of recurrence are high.

Steps ***(Fig. 6)****:*

- Basic steps as mentioned
- While infiltration, give a field block
- Draw an ellipse using a surgical marker, methylene blue, or gentian violet. Apex of ellipse should have 30° angle on each side. The length should be three times of the width. 2–5 mm margin of normal skin, around the margin, should be included
- Area is kept taught and scalpel with No. 15 blade is held like a pencil
- Begin the incision at the apex holding the blade perpendicular to the skin
- As the incision progresses, blade is angled to 45° to cut the tissue with the belly of the blade
- At the end of the incision again, the scalpel is lifted vertically to prevent the excision from extending beyond the endpoint
- Same steps are repeated on other side
- Ellipse of tissue is separated from underlying tissue with scalpel or dissecting forceps
- Interrupted suture taken for larger and deeper defects suturing is done in two layers
- Dressing done after applying antibiotic cream
- Sutures are removed after 5–10 days depending on the area.

Incisional Biopsy (Wedge Biopsy)

Incisional biopsy is performed when tissue sample is required to perform special tests such as culture, microscopy, e.g., deep fungal infections, cutaneous tuberculosis, mycosis fungoides, and for diseases that can spread beyond the clinically visible margin, e.g., malignancies. By including the normal looking skin, exact extent of spread of malignancy can be determined.

Steps ***(Figs. 7A to D)****:*

- Basic steps as mentioned before
- In this type, biopsy is performed from active edge of the lesion in a wedge shape including the normal skin. Alternatively, it can be performed by using biopsy punches of size 5 mm and above
- Other steps are similar to excisional biopsy. The only difference is that in incisional biopsy, only part of the lesion is removed rather than the entire lesion **(Fig. 8)**.

Other Techniques[9]

Curette biopsy: This biopsy can be performed without local anesthesia using a sharp curette. Friable part of the lesion can be scraped off with the curette and sent for histological examination. This sample may be adequate for the diagnosis, but fails to determine the depth and lateral spread of the lesion and, hence, is not commonly performed.

Skin surface biopsy: This biopsy is done to inspect the stratum corneum. It is useful in detection of mites in scabies, dermatophytes, and other microorganisms. It can be useful for research purpose, e.g., sampling of follicular casts (microcomedones) to determine the density of sebaceous follicles in different areas of face.

Procedure:

- Cyanoacrylate gel is applied on the skin surface
- A glass slide is pressed on top for 1 minute
- Slide is then rolled off from the skin surface and examined under low power after staining
- As the glue is costly and not easily available, this procedure is not performed routinely

Oral biopsy:[12,23] Oral mucosal biopsy can be performed by the same technique as skin biopsy. However, there may be difficulties in performing the biopsy at this site due to various reasons:

- Area is vascular; hence, achieving hemostasis may be difficult
- Access is difficult due to enclosed cavity
- To achieve good illumination in the oral cavity can be difficult

The moist conditions due to saliva and extensive microflora make antiseptic scrub pointless. To achieve good hemostasis, wait for 10 minutes after infiltrating the anesthetic to have effect of epinephrine. *A chalazion clamp is useful for the biopsies on the lips, anterior buccal mucosa, or tongue to achieve hemostasis and to prevent slipping of tissue.* Another tool that can help to have better access is a plastic or metal cheek retractor. Grasping the tissues with dry cotton gauze allows firm grip. A punch biopsy can be easily performed for getting full-thickness specimen. For dome-shaped lesions, incisional or shave excision technique is useful. The area opposite to the second upper molar should be avoided,

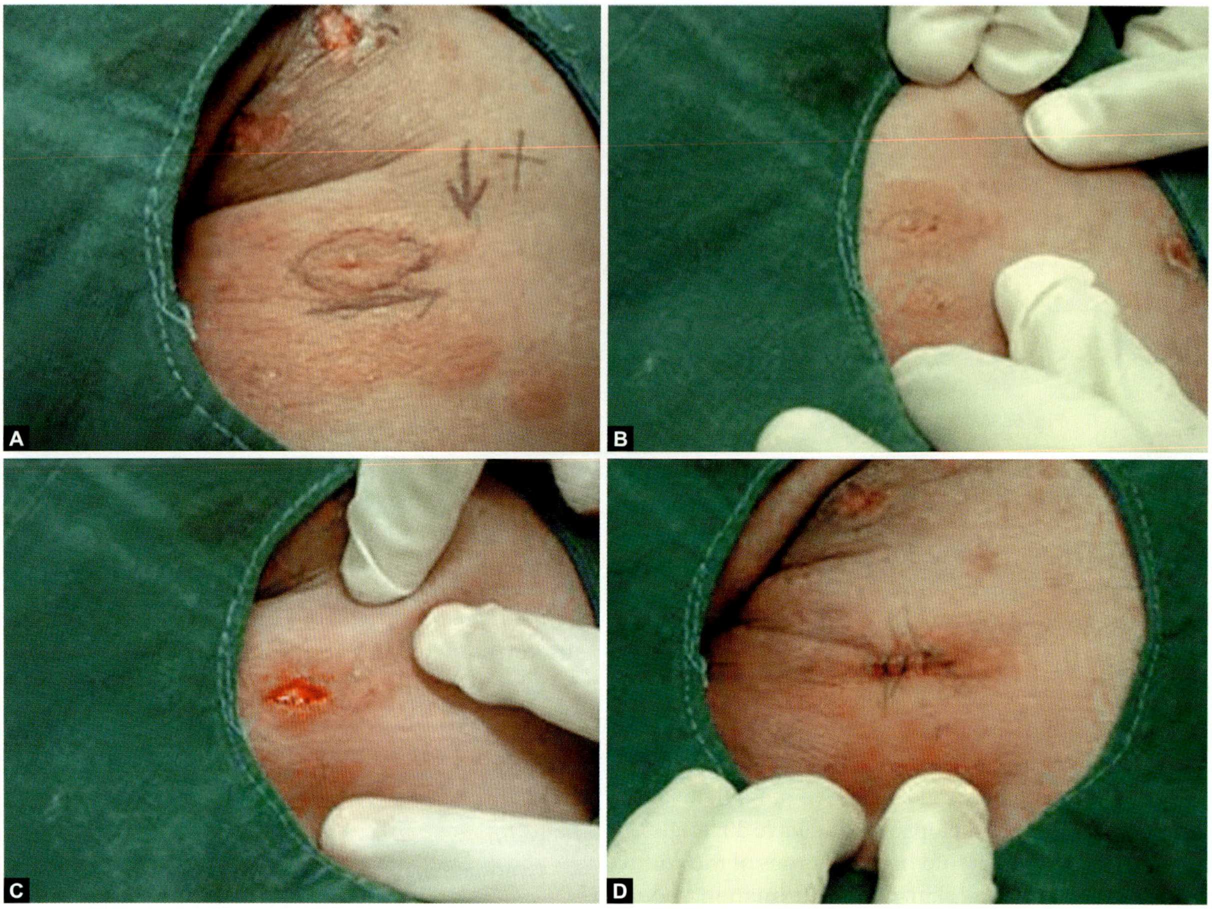

Figs. 7A to D: Incisional biopsy. (A) Ellipse marked parallel to relaxed skin tension line (RSTL); (B) Skin is made taut; (C) Elliptical incision is taken and tissue is removed; and (D) Closure with interrupted sutures.

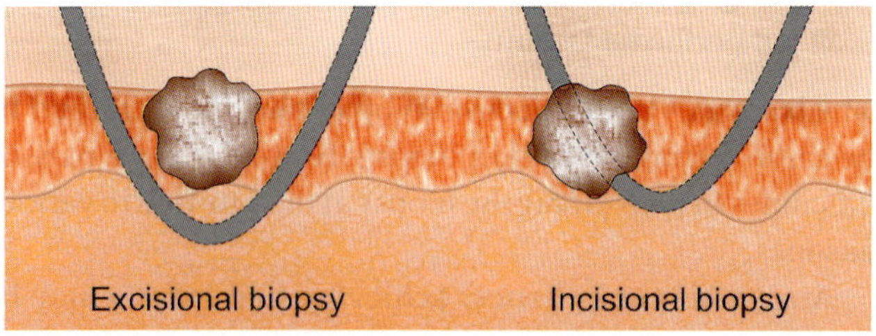

Fig. 8: Difference between incisional and excisional biopsy.

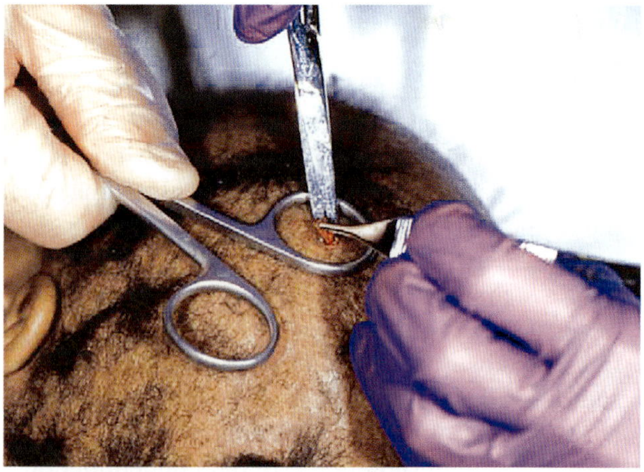

Fig. 9: Using the ring of the artery forceps for hemostasis.

as the duct of parotid gland opens there. While performing biopsies on the floor, area of sublingual salivary gland should be carefully approached. Suturing with silk is useful, as this type of suture is easy to work within a cramped space. This suture is nonirritating and remains soft. Wounds heal rapidly and with few complications.

For early detection of oral cancers and as a screening technique, cytologic testing (e.g., Oral CDx, OralCyte, ClearPrep OC) is recommended. It is a minimally invasive technique and can be performed without local anesthesia. With the commercially available brush, 10–20 rotations are performed to collect transepithelial cellular samples. These samples fixed onto a glass slide and cytological analysis is performed. In case of atypical cellular morphology, a scalpel biopsy should be carried out.[13]

Scalp biopsy:[9] As scalp is very vascular, achieving hemostasis is crucial. Xylocaine with adrenaline about 2–3 mL to tumescence the area is useful. The ring of the artery forceps can be used to give circumferential pressure to achieve bloodless field during surgery **(Fig. 9)**. A cotton tipped applicator is also very useful to control bleeding. Surrounding hairs need to be properly taped to prevent interference. KY jelly is useful to keep the hairs away from the biopsy field.

It is also important to do the biopsy in a direction parallel to hair growth to avoid transecting the follicles. This will prevent development of a patch of alopecia. Also, the biopsy should reach the subcutis, so that bulbs of terminal follicles are included. Always use at least 4 mm punch for biopsy. Two biopsies are preferred, one each for vertical and horizontal sectioning.

Nail biopsy:[20,24] It is performed for the diagnosis of tumors of nail apparatus and to diagnose a particular condition when the nails are dystrophic. Caution should be exercised in patients with diabetes, scleroderma, and peripheral vascular disease. It is performed by giving digital block at the base of the digit. The anesthetic used is xylocaine, preferably without adrenaline.

For nail bed biopsy, either a punch technique or a longitudinal elliptical biopsy technique is used. For punch biopsy, prior soaking in water helps to soften the nail plate. For elliptical biopsy, nail plate is separated from nail bed and cut away to expose the lesion.

For matrix biopsy, nail is avulsed and nail fold is reflected to expose the matrix. Then a transverse elliptical biopsy is performed. A longitudinal biopsy can be performed in nail dystrophies to obtain a specimen containing nail matrix, nail bed, and nail plate. More details can be found in the chapter on Nail Surgery.

Biopsy on palms and soles:[25] The skin in these areas is thick and inelastic. Hence, it is difficult to approximate the wound of biopsy. The incision should be taken parallel to the flexion creases or it should cross high tension areas at 45° angle. This prevents wound dehiscence. This area would require proper undermining and correct suture placement.

Complications of Biopsy

Though rare, the following complications may occur:

- Secondary infection
- Scarring
- Bleeding and hematoma formation
- Damage to underlying nerves and blood vessels in deep excisions
- Allergy to adhesive tape
- Rarely allergy to local anesthetic agent causing anaphylaxis

Tips for Better Procedural Outcome

The tips for better procedural outcome are given in **Figures 9 to 13**.

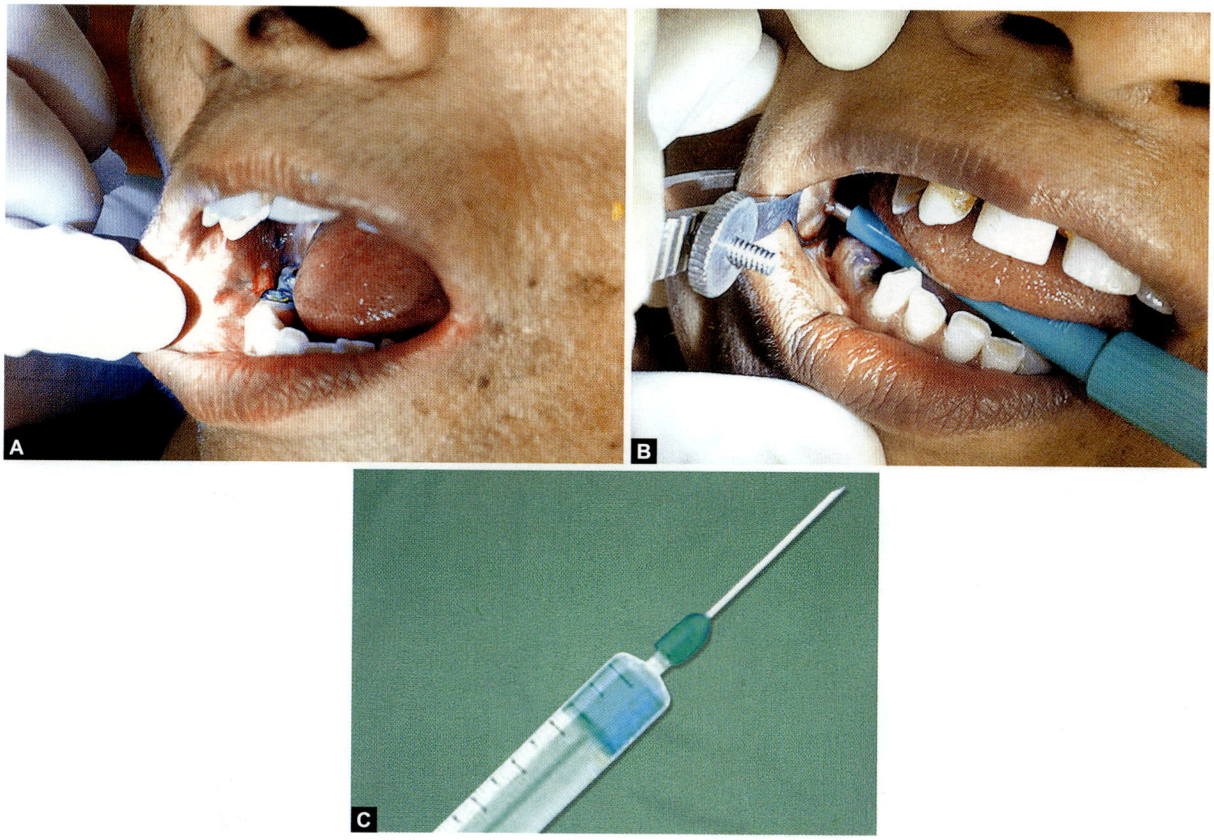

Figs. 10A to C: (A) Taking sample from oral mucosa; (B) Use of chalazion clamp; (C) Long spinal needle used for spinal anesthesia.

MOLE SURGERY[26,27]

Melanocytic nevi are benign proliferations of melanocytes. Melanocytic nevi include variety of congenital and acquired conditions. In this chapter, we will restrict to treatment options for common acquired melanocytic nevi.

Moles or melanocytic nevi presenting in cosmetically important areas affect the aesthetic perception of an individual. Hence, this seems to be one of the commonly demanded and performed procedures by dermatologists. Moles are removed for cosmetic and functional reasons. There are three types of nevi—(1) Junctional (flat), (2) Compound (raised but black in color), and (3) Intradermal (raised and skin colored). Ideally, all common acquired melanocytic nevi should be treated surgically and sent for histopathological analysis. Treatment with modalities such as cryotherapy, radiofrequency and laser, and light-based treatments do not provide adequate tissue for histopathological examination. However, it is observed that development of melanoma in skin of color is observed in areas not exposed to sunlight such as palms, soles, mucosa, and subungual areas. Hence, many of the abovementioned procedures are commonly practiced to treat nevi on face in Asian patients.

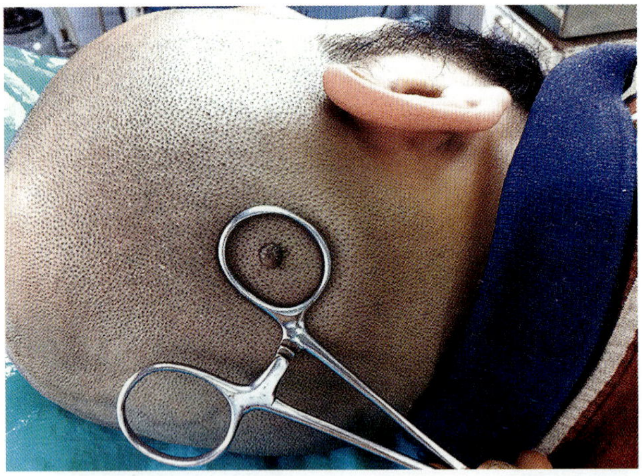

Fig. 11: Taking sample from scalp or from a vascular skin lesion. Use of eye of an artery forceps to give firm pressure.

Indications[28]

- Cosmetic
- Clinical atypia
- Enlargement
- Repeated trauma
- Congenital nevi >3 cm
- Nature uncertain
- Dysplastic nevi

Identification of Dysplastic Nevi[29]

Dysplastic nevus is suspected if the size is >5 mm, if the nevus is either flat or it is raised in the center and flat at the periphery, if the borders are irregular, and if there is pigment variegation.

Atypical moles are more common in fair-skinned individuals and those who have high sun exposure.

These are associated with increased risk of melanoma. Melanoma should be suspected if:[30]

- A—asymmetry
- B—border irregularity
- C—color unevenness
- D—diameter > 6 mm
- E—evolution

To differentiate benign melanocytic nevi from melanoma, following points are helpful:[31-36]

- *Presence or absence of maturation*: Benign nevi exhibit pattern of maturation with progressive depth in the dermis. Most melanomas lack pattern of maturation
- Positivity with HMB-45 and degree of labeling with MIB-1

Most of the times, these are benign lesions and melanoma is uncommon in common acquired melanocytic nevi.

Various Techniques for Treatment of Common Acquired Melanocytic Nevi[26,29]

- Shave excision
- Elliptical excision
- Round excision
- Punch excision

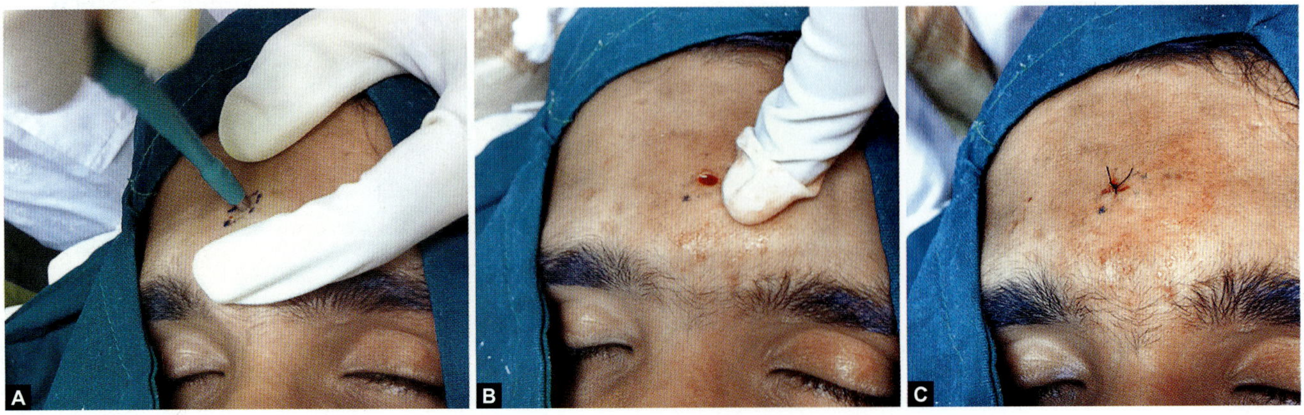

Figs. 12A to C: Taking sample from face. Even after punch biopsy, single stay suture can be taken to give cosmetically acceptable scar.

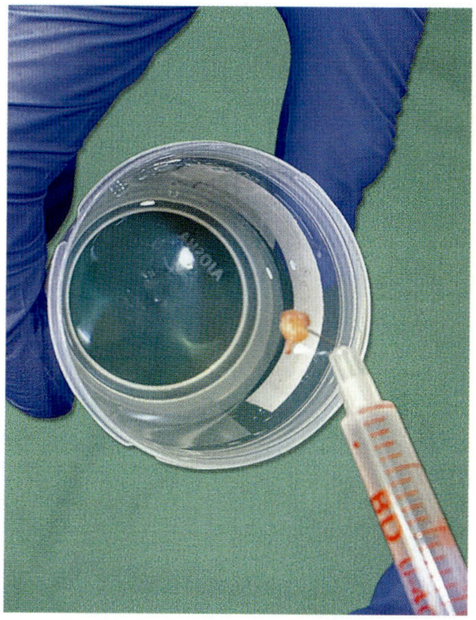

Fig. 13: Transferring the sample in a transport medium with bent needle attached to syringe to minimize the tissue trauma.

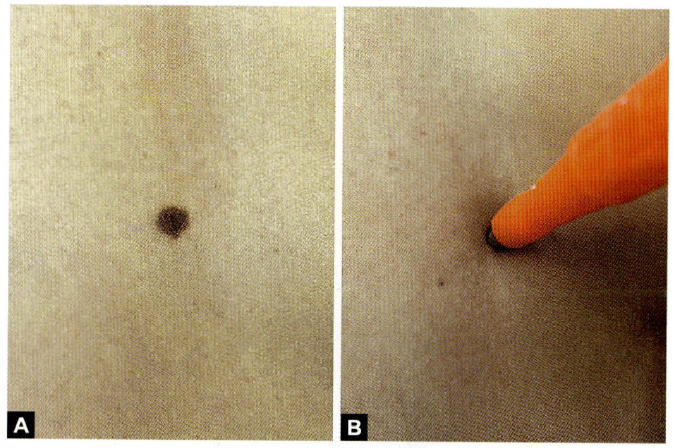

Figs. 14A and B: (A) Melanocytic nevus; (B) Excision with appropriate size punch

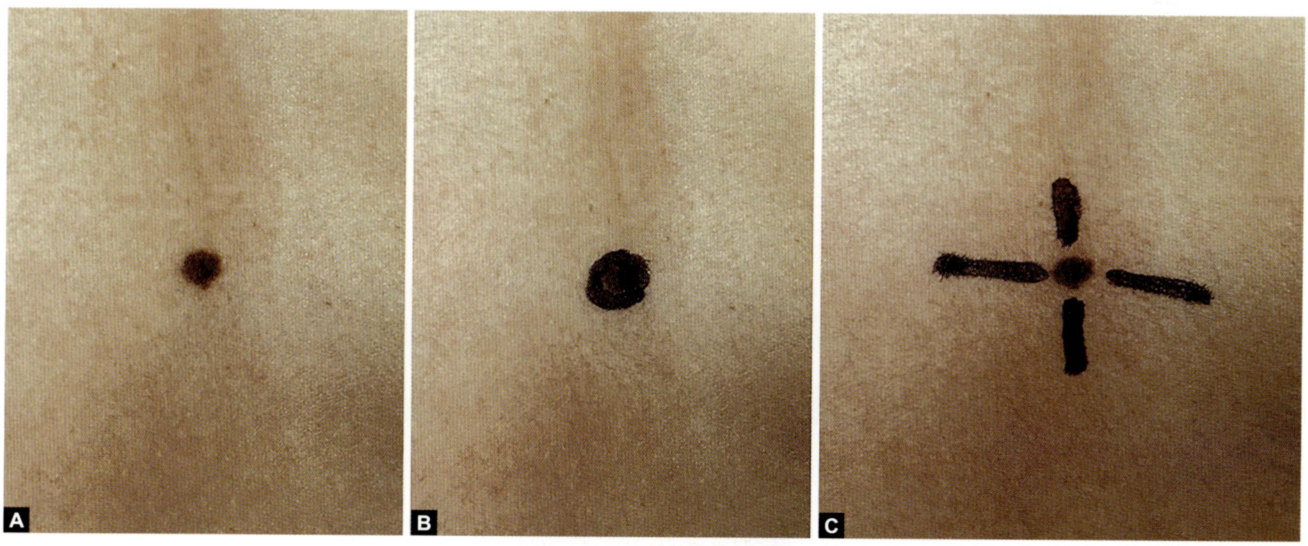

Figs. 15A to C: (A) Mole; (B) Circular marking; and (C) Marking with four lines.

- Radiofrequency
- Cryotherapy
- Lasers and light-based therapies

Surgical excision gives appropriate tissue sample for histopathological analysis. Hence, in suspicious moles, one must undertake surgery and not radiofrequency or cryotherapy. Flat junctional nevi are difficult to treat and have high chances of recurrence. The chances of recurrence, pigmentary changes, especially postinflammatory hyperpigmentation, are some of the side effects seen after mole surgery.

Though excision techniques are ideal, as they provide adequate tissue sample for HPE, the scar produced is not cosmetically acceptable. Hence, for better cosmetic outcome, other procedures are practiced.

Steps for Various Procedures

- Shave excision **(Figs. 2A to H)** is already mentioned in this chapter under the section of biopsy techniques.
- Elliptical excision **(Fig. 6)** is already mentioned in this chapter under the section of biopsy techniques.
- *Round excision:*[37,38] This technique can be used for papular and dome-shaped nevi on the face. This is carried out just outside the perimeter of the lesion. Stretching of skin would give elliptical defect and suturing of the elliptical wound will avoid dog ear formation and give better cosmetic results.

  The resultant wound of elliptical incision is larger as compared to round excision and, hence, the resultant scar is also smaller with round excision.

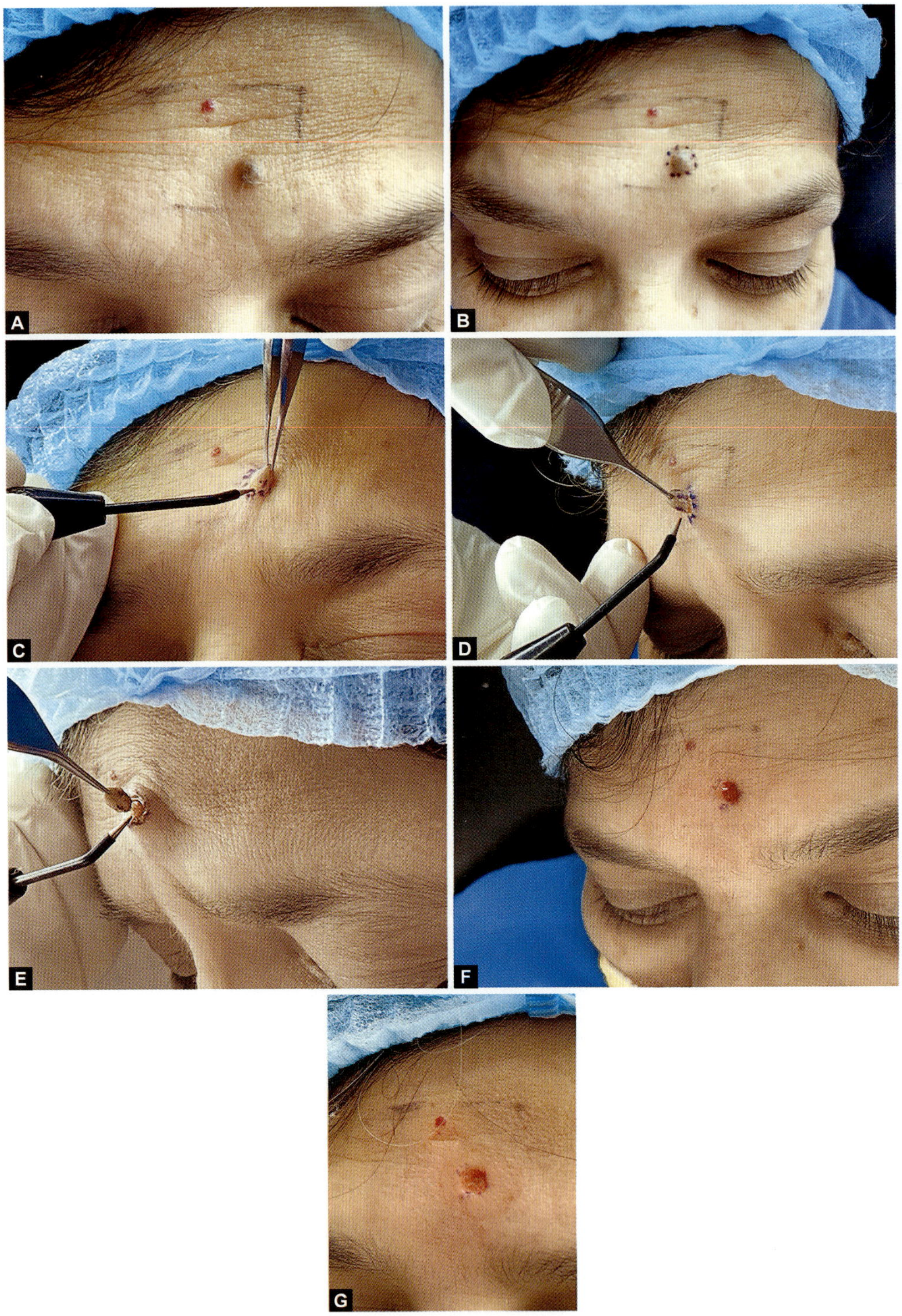

Figs. 16A to G: Mole surgery with radiofrequency device–steps. (A) Compound nevus on forehead; (B) Marking of outline; (C) Scoring of margins with pointed electrode; (D) Lifting with atraumatic forceps; (E) Separation all around in the same plane; (F) Immediately after procedure; and (G) Hemostasis achieved with ball point electrode and coagulation mode.

- *Punch excision* ***(Figs. 14A and B)****:*[39] Melanocytic nevi excision using appropriate size punch gives very good cosmetic outcome. Nevi up to 6 mm can be removed using punch with excellent cosmetic outcome. This leaves a smaller scar and the technique is very easy. It achieves complete removal of the lesion in trained hands.
- *Radiofrequency:*[40] The procedure of mole excision can also be performed by using radiofrequency device and gives excellent cosmetic results. However, in nevi where malignant change is suspected, this technique should be avoided as tissue sample may be inadequate.

- *Mark the outline before infiltration anesthesia* **(Figs. 15A to C)**:[41] Marking the outline in a circular fashion, which sometimes interfere with delineation of outline.
  We suggest a modification in the marking system suggested by Abdulaziz S Alroujayee et al. They suggested marking of a biopsy site with two crossed lines, which cross in the center of the lesion. For moles, we suggest to draw four lines, which end 1–2 mm away from the outer margin of the mole.
  Hence, when we are planning round excision or punch excision or excision using radiofrequency device, especially in suspected nevi that we can safely keep 2 mm free margin for excision.
- The area is anesthetized using injectable anesthesia or surface anesthesia under occlusion
- The further steps of the procedure for removing dome-shaped moles with radiofrequency are described in **Figures 16A to G**
- Pointed tip electrode is used to score the margins
- Cut coagulation mode is selected
- The lesion is lifted with atraumatic forceps and separated all around in the same plane

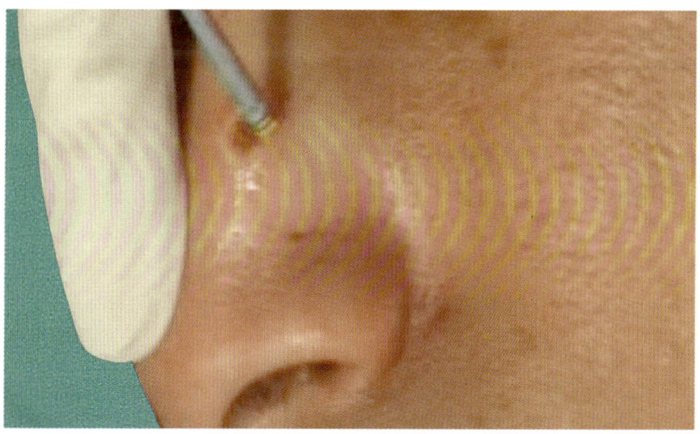

Fig. 17: Sculpting with ball point electrode (coagulation mode and touch-and-go technique for the inner edge).

- Hemostasis is achieved by using ball tip electrode and coagulation mode or by giving firm pressure
- As the wound is allowed to heal by secondary intention to make the defect shallow, sculpting of inner margin is carried out with the help of ball point electrode. The inner edge is treated, so as to make the defect shallow **(Fig. 17)**. Excellent postprocedure outcome **(Figs. 18A and B)**.

Alternative method: The loop electrode can be used to debulk the lesion. With the help of loop, the surface is shaved layer-by-layer till there is near complete removal. Tiny pinpoint bleeding spots are observed as endpoint. If any remnants of melanocytes are observed, they can be treated by using pointed electrode **(Figs. 19A and B)**.

Managing the hair on nevi **(Figs. 20A and B)**:[42] The CAMN that are hairy have a propensity for recurrence. This is because the nevus cells tend to extend along hair follicles deeply into skin. The hair follicles, therefore, harbor nevus cells beyond the depth for effective laser treatment. Techniques of hair removal, whether by laser devices, intense pulsed light (IPL), or electrolysis, may be needed for treating the hair in these lesions.

Laser hair removal (LHR) can be performed before undertaking the surgery or before performing radiofrequency treatment **(Figs. 19A and B)**.

It should be remembered that use of laser and light-based therapies in the treatment of melanocytic nevi is controversial issue. There may be changes suggestive of pseudomelanoma after such treatments.

- *Cryotherapy*:[31] Treatment of benign nevi with cryotherapy is usually not advocated. It was observed that benign nevi treated with cryotherapy show paradoxical loss of maturation and aberrant immunohistochemical findings. These changes mimic melanoma and pose diagnostic challenges.
- *Laser and light-based therapies*:[27,43,44] This treatment is controversial, as no tissue or margin is available for assessment.

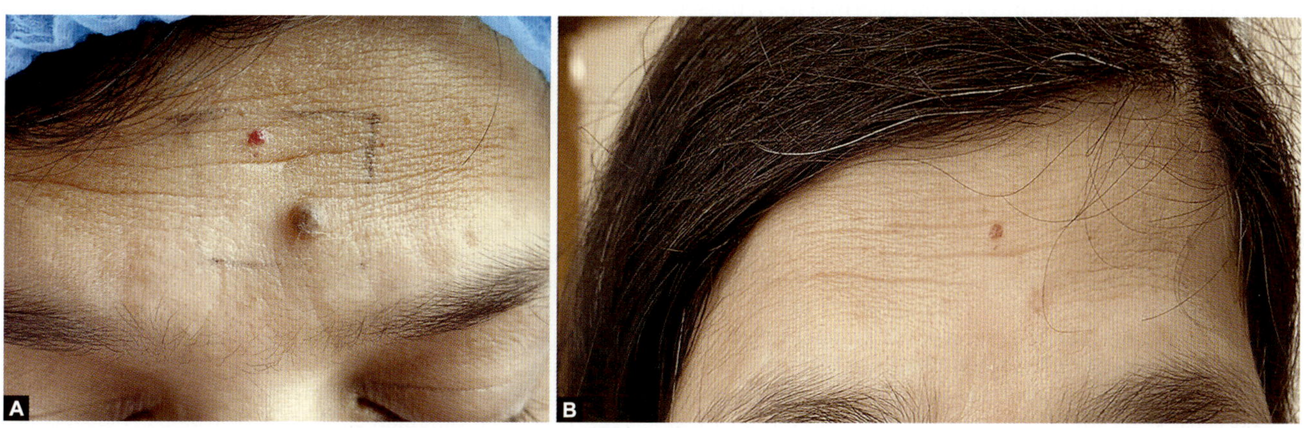

Figs. 18A and B: Pre- and postradiofrequency treatment of mole. (A) Pretreatment; and (B) Post-treatment.

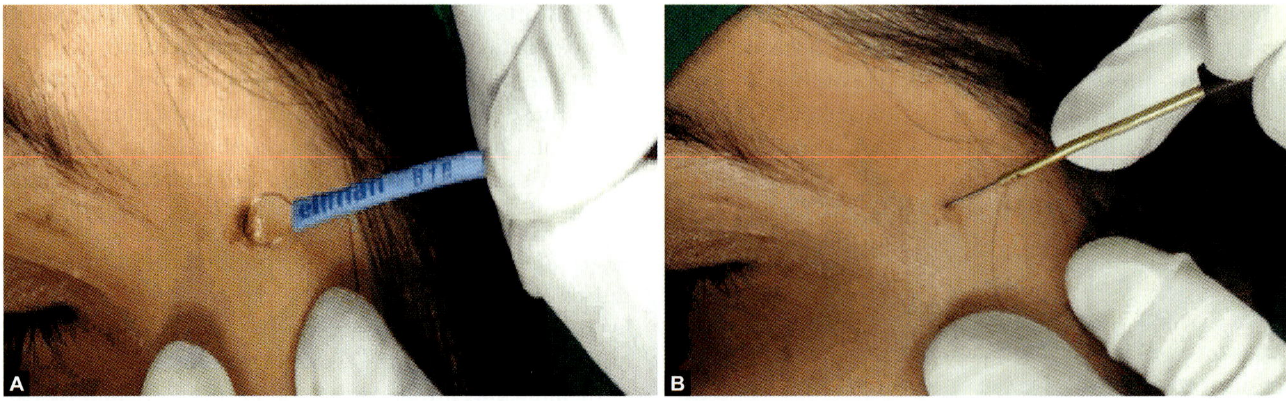

Figs. 19A and B: Alternative method using loop electrode. (A) Shaving of the lesion layer-by-layer using loop electrode; and (B) Use of pointed electrode to destroy the remnants of melanocytes.

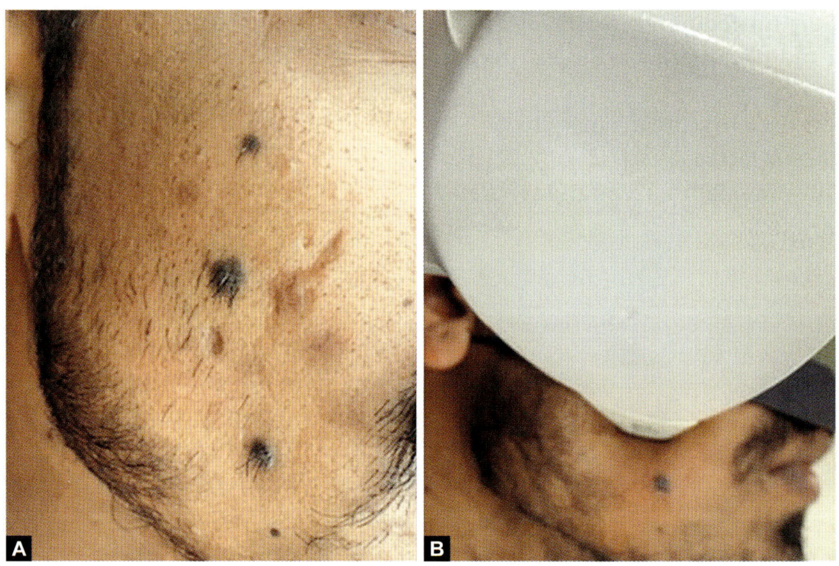

Figs. 20A and B: Treating the hair on mole. (A) Hairy compound nevus; and (B) Use of 810 diode laser for laser hair removal (LHR).

Junctional nevi are more sensitive to laser therapy. The lasers may not reach to the depth of intradermal and compound nevi. Usually, a combination of various lasers is necessary to get desired results in such situation. The junctional nevi can respond to Q-switched or normal mode pigment lasers. For compound and intradermal nevi, pulsed ablative lasers such as carbon dioxide (CO_2) or erbium-doped yttrium aluminum garnet (Er:YAG) may be required.

It is recommended to do lifelong follow-up for recurrence and development of melanoma after removal of benign common acquired melanocytic nevi.

REFERENCES

1. Anderson JB, Webb AJ. Fine needle aspiration biopsy and the diagnosis of thyroid cancer. Br J Surg. 1987;74:292-6.
2. Bobrow JC, Belcher MH. Surgery for cataract in lens and cataract section II. 2010;2011:91-162.
3. Parish LC. Historical aspects of cutaneous surgery. In: Parish LC (Ed). Wheeland Cutaneous Surgery, 1st edition; 1994. pp. 3-11.
4. Lahiri K. Evolution and evaluation of autologous mini punch grafts in vitiligo. Ind J Dermatol. 2009;54:159-67.
5. Lowenthal LJA. Punch biopsy with autograft. AMA Arch Dermatol Syphilol. 1953;67:629.
6. Orentreich N. Autografts in alopecias and other selected dermatological conditions. Ann N Y Acad Sci. 1959;83: 463-79.
7. Wilhelmi BJ, Blackwell SJ, Phillips LG. Langers lines: to use or not to use. Plast Reconstr Surg. 1999;104:208-14.
8. Algure PC, Mathes BM. Skin biopsy techniques for the internist. J Gen Intern Med. 1998;13:46-54.
9. Savant SS. Skin biopsy techniques. In: Savant SS (Ed). Textbook of Dermatosurgery and Cosmetology, 2nd edition. New York: Tata McGraw Hill; 2005. pp. 72-80.
10. Schupbach A, Zhang L, Thomas B, Ellerbroek J, Leone D. Fatal human rabies infection confirmed with skin biopsy specimen. J Am Acad Dermatol. 2012;67:321-3.
11. Macedo CI, Carnieli P, Brandao PE, Travassos da Rosa ES, Oliveira Rde N, Castilho JG, et al. Diagnosis of human rabies cases by polymerase chain reaction of neck-skin samples. Braz J Infect Dis. 2006;10:341-5.
12. Elston DM, Stratman EJ, Miller SJ. Skin biopsy: biopsy issues in specific diseases. J Am Acad Dermatol. 2016;74:1-16.

13. Seishima M, Izumi T, Kitajima Y. Antibody to bullous pemphigoid antigen 1 binds to the antigen at perilesional but not uninvolved skin in localized bullous pemphigoid. Eur J Dermatol. 1999;9:39-42.
14. Sladden C, Kirchhof MG, Crawford RI. Biopsy location for direct immunofluorescence in patients with suspected bullous pemphigoid impacts probability of a positive test result. J Cutan Med Surg. 2014;18:1-5.
15. Nischal U, Nischal KC, Uday K. Techniques of skin biopsy and practical consideration. J Cutan Aesthet Surg. 2008;1: 107-11.
16. Stratman EJ, Elston DM, Miller SJ. Skin biopsy: identifying and overcoming errors in the skin biopsy pathway. J Am Acad Dermatol. 2016;74:19-25.
17. Patel AN, Simpson RC, Cohen SN. In a patient with an immunobullous disorder, is transportation of the skin biopsy in normal saline adequate for direct immunofluorescence analysis? A critically appraised topic. Br J Dermatol. 2013; 169:6-10.
18. Pickett H, O'Callaghan M. Shave and punch biopsy for skin lesions. Am Fam Physician. 2011;84:995-1002.
19. Zuber TJ. Punch biopsy of the skin. Am Fam Physician. 2002; 65:1155-8.
20. Huerter CJ. Simple biopsy techniques. In: Huerter CJ (Ed). Wheeland Cutaneous Surgery, 1st edition. New York: McGraw Hill; 1994. pp. 159-70.
21. Shelley WB. The razor blade in dermatologic practice. Cutis. 1975;16:843-5.
22. Mushtaq S. Shave biopsy instrument: an ergonomic modification of razor blade. J Cutan Aesthet Surg. 2020;13:255-6.
23. Shanti RM, Tanaka T, Stanton DC. Oral biopsy techniques. Dermatol Clin. 2020;38:421-7.
24. Saraf V. Nail biopsy. In: Saraf V (Ed). Manual of Dermatologic Surgery. New York: McGraw Hill; 1999. pp. 108-12.
25. Savant SS, Gore D. Applied anatomy for the dermatosurgeon. In: Savant SS (Ed). Textbook of Dermatosurgery and Cosmetology, 2nd edition. New York: Elsevier; 2005. pp. 3-11.
26. Bandral MR, Gir PJ, Japatti SR. A comparative evaluation of surgical, electrosurgery and diode laser in the management of maxillofacial nevus. Maxillofac Oral Surg. 2018;17: 547-56.
27. Sardana K. The science, reality, and ethics of treating common acquired melanocytic nevi (moles) with lasers. J Cutan Aesthet Surg. 2013;6:27-9.
28. McGrouther DA. Skin burns. In: Mann CV, Russel RCG, Williams NJ (Eds). Bailey and Love's Short Practice of Surgery, 1st edition. London: Chapman & Hall; 1995. pp. 124-48.
29. Parkinson RW. What to do about moles? Postgrad Med. 1989;86:40-6.
30. Perkins A, Duffy RL. Atypical moles: diagnosis and management. Am Fam Physician. 2015;91:762-7.
31. Adeniran AJ, Prieto VJ, Chon S, Duvic M, Diwan AH. Atypical histologic and immunohistochemical findings in melanocytic nevi after liquid nitrogen cryotherapy. J Am Acad Dermatol. 2009;61:341-5.
32. Ruhoy SM, Prieto VG, Eliason SL, Grichnik JM, Burchette JL, Shea CR. Malignant melanoma with paradoxical maturation. Am J Surg Pathol. 2000;24:1600-14.
33. Gown AM, Vogel AM, Hoak D, Gough F, McNutt MA. Monoclonal antibodies specific for melanocytic tumors distinguish subpopulations of melanocytes. Am J Pathol. 1986;123:195-203.
34. Colombari R, Bonetti F, Zamboni G, Scarpa A, Marino F, Tomezzoli A, et al. Distribution of melanoma-specific antibody (HMB-45) in benign and malignant melanocytic tumors: a case reports of 345 immunohistochemical study on paraffin sections. Virch Arch A Pathol Anat Histopathol. 1988;413: 17-24.
35. Bergman R, Dromi R, Trau H, Cohen I, Lichtig C. The pattern of HMB-45 antibody staining in compound Spitz nevi. Am J Dermatopathol. 1995;17:542-6.
36. Li LX, Crotty KA, McCarthy SW, Palmer AA, Kril JJ. A zonal comparison of MIB1-Ki67 immunoreactivity in benign and malignant melanocytic lesions. Am J Dermatopathol. 2000;22:489-95.
37. Unis ME. Simplified surgery with surgical punches. J Dermatol Surg Oncol. 1987;13:906-8.
38. Tursen U, Kaya TI, Ikizoglu G. Papular and dome-shaped melanocytic nevi on face. Int J Dermatol. 2004;4:1-3.
39. Shilpa K, Somaiah S, Natraja HV. Scar evaluation in patients undergoing melanocytic nevi excision by punch excision technique: a pilot study. J Evol Med Dent Sci. 2015;4:6824-31.
40. Niamtu J. Nevus removal with 4.0-MHz radiowave surgery. J Oral Maxillofac Surg. 2014;34:1139-49.
41. Alroujayee AS. Skin biopsy: a better way to mark the skin before punch biopsy procedures. J Am Acad Dermatol. 2020; 82:e51-2.
42. Sardana K, Chakravarty P, Goel K. Optimal management of common acquired melanocytic nevi (moles): current perspectives. Clin Cosmet Investig Dermatol. 2014;7:89-103.
43. Suzuki H, Anderson RR. Treatment of melanocytic nevi. Dermatol Ther. 2005;18:217-26.
44. Drummer R, Kempf W, Burg TG. Pseudomelanoma after laser therapy. Dermatology. 1998;197:71-3.

CHAPTER 20

Surgical Management of Cutaneous Cysts and Lipomas

Vinay Saraf, Ragunatha S

KEY MESSAGES

- Cutaneous cysts and lipomas are most common benign tumors of skin and subcutaneous tissue.
- Depending on type, size, and location of the lesions appropriate surgical procedures are used.
- Minimal invasive techniques assisted with suction or laser punch result in complete removal of cysts with better cosmetic outcome compared to conventional surgical excision.
- Tumescent liposuction and lipolysis either by laser or injection of phosphatidylcholine/sodium deoxycholate followed by conventional excisions are the newer methods in surgical removal of lipomas.
- These procedures should be done by experienced dermatologists because of potential complications associated with lasers and injections.

SURGICAL MANAGEMENT OF CUTANEOUS CYSTS

INTRODUCTION

Cutaneous cysts are very common, and epidermoid cysts constitute 80% of the cutaneous cysts. Epidermoid cysts should always be subjected to histopathological examination, since it has been suggested that 1% of the epithelial cysts may have a basal or squamous cell carcinoma in their wall.[1]

Different surgical techniques for cutaneous cysts include punch removal, incisional excision, elliptical excision, and excision with secondary healing.

PUNCH REMOVAL TECHNIQUE

This is a rapid and easy technique **(Figs. 1A to D)** to remove cysts up to one centimeter in diameter using only 2–4 mm skin punch. The punch is held over the visible central punctum and the skin is held taut perpendicularly to the

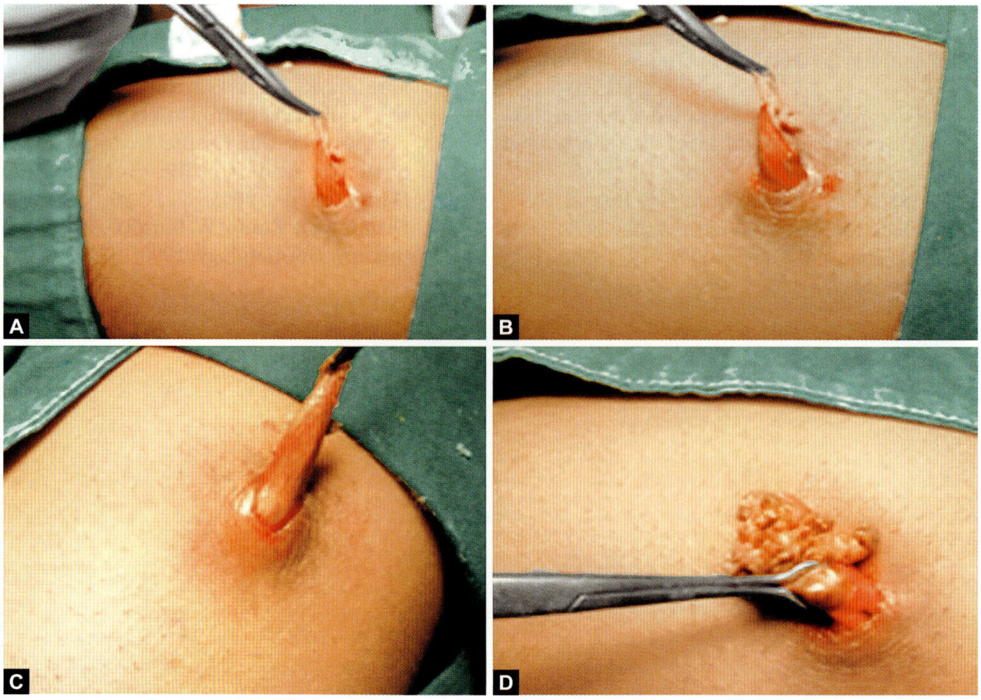

Figs. 1A to D: Cyst with avulsion of cyst wall through a small incision.

relaxed skin tension lines (RSTLs). The punch is advanced through the overlying skin into the cyst cavity. The contents are then evacuated with firm lateral pressure, carefully removing all the keratinous debris and the entire cyst wall. The edge of the wall usually presents itself at the wound margin, as the contents are evacuated. After evacuation of the cyst, a small 3–5 mm curette is used to curette and extract the cyst wall with gentle traction. Alternatively, small curved scissors can be used to dissect around the cyst wall and then gently pulling the cyst wall with Adson forceps till the base of the cyst is reached which is identified by observing its blood supply at the base. The base is clamped with artery forceps and cut with scissors. The wound is cleaned with hydrogen peroxide and closed with simple suture technique after achieving good hemostasis with pressure.[2]

INCISIONAL SURGICAL TECHNIQUE

In this technique **(Figs. 2A to J)**, a single linear incision aligned with the RSTLs or existing wrinkles over the cyst is made. The incision is stopped at the level of glistening white cyst wall. The cyst is then dissected out bluntly using mosquito forceps. The base is clamped and cut. After cleaning the wound with hydrogen peroxide, simple suturing technique is used to close the wound.[2-4]

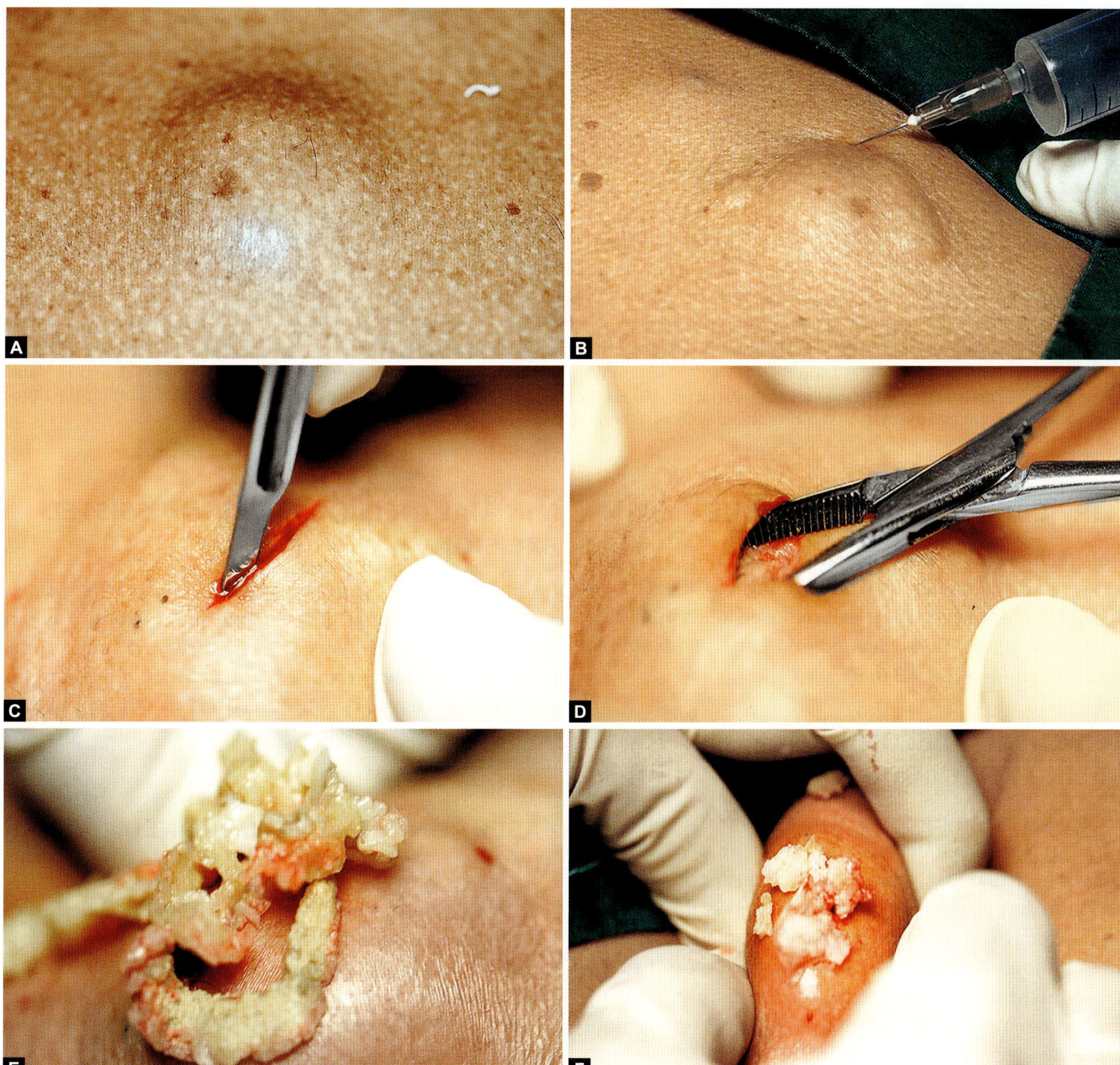

Figs. 2A to F

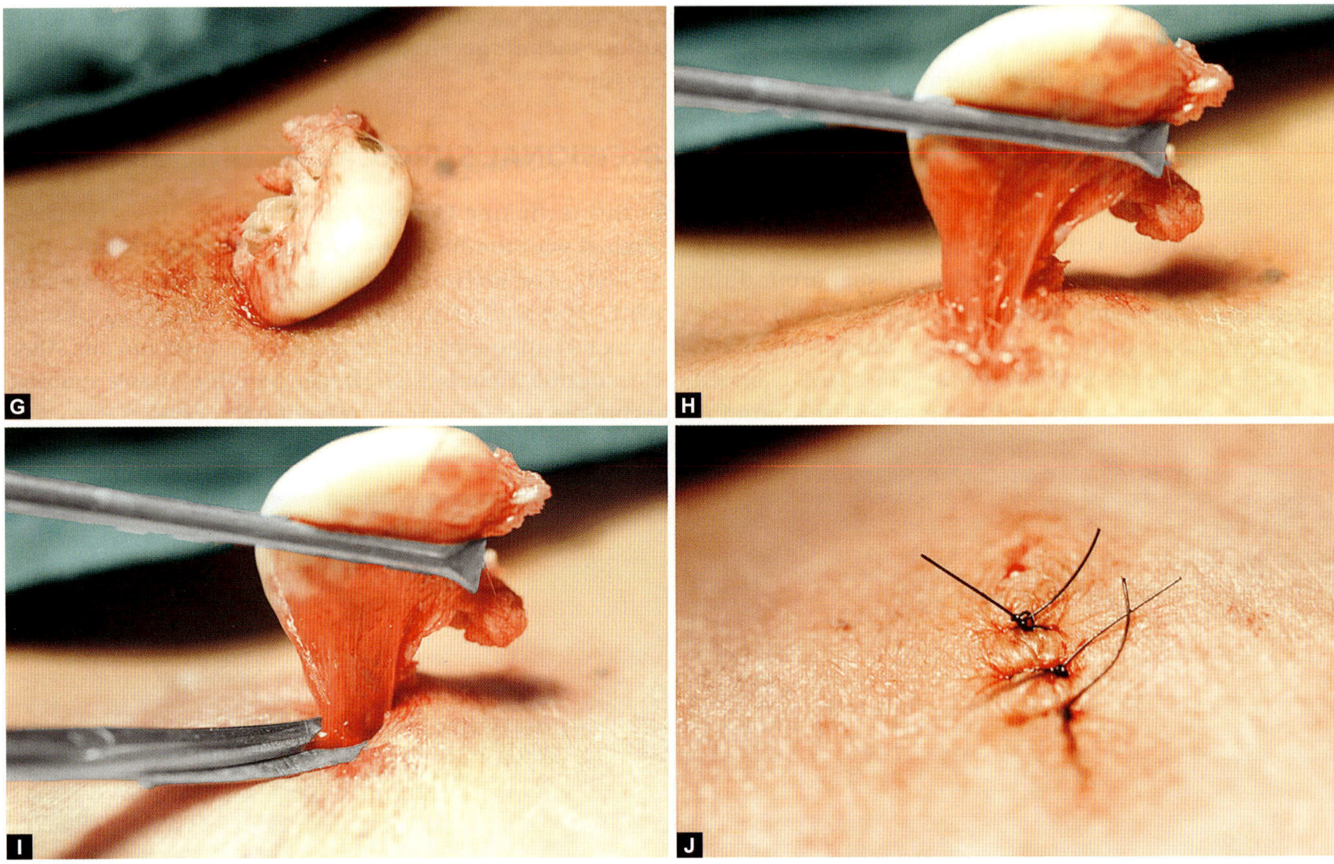

Figs. 2G to J

Figs. 2A to J: (A) Sebaceous cyst; (B) Giving field block; (C) Incision with 15 No. blade; (D) Blunt dissection with artery forceps; (E and F) Manual extraction of sebaceous material; (G) Cyst partially extracted; (H) Further extraction and clamping of the base of the cyst; (I) Cutting the fibrous strands and blood supply of the cyst; (J) Wound sutured with 3-0 Ethilon suture.

ELLIPTICAL EXCISION TECHNIQUE

In this technique, fusiform incision is done on overlying skin to include the punctum. Undermining and dissection is done all around the cyst. The cyst is removed intact by cutting at its base. The wound is cleaned and closed with simple suturing technique **(Figs. 3 to 6)**.[1]

EXCISION AND SECOND-INTENTION HEALING TECHNIQUE

This technique is used for numerous small epidermoid cysts commonly seen in male patients with acne on the lower posterior auricular skin, the earlobe, the posterior auricular sulcus, and the posterior auricular scalp skin over the mastoid. Simple selective incision and drainage, or isolated excisions is the method of choice. The wound is allowed to heal by second intention over the next 1–2 months period using daily hydrogen peroxide and topical antibiotic application. The cosmetic results are satisfactory.[2,3]

MINIMAL INCISION SUCTION-ASSISTED EXCISION

In minimal incision excisions, the contents of the cysts are squeezed out through incision site manually by applying lateral pressure. However, lateral pressure, sometimes, causes intracavitary rupture, fragmentation, infections, and recurrences. Hence, negative-pressure suction can be used instead of lateral pressure to completely remove the cysts measuring >2 cm.[5]

LASER PUNCH WITH POSTPONED MINIMAL EXCISION

It is a two-step procedure where carbon dioxide laser is used initially to make multiple punctures in the cyst to form a hole of 2–4 mm. The contents of the cysts are partially evacuated through hole with gentle pressure. Any remnants in the cyst are removed by washing with normal saline. The hole is sealed with a suture or glue and standard

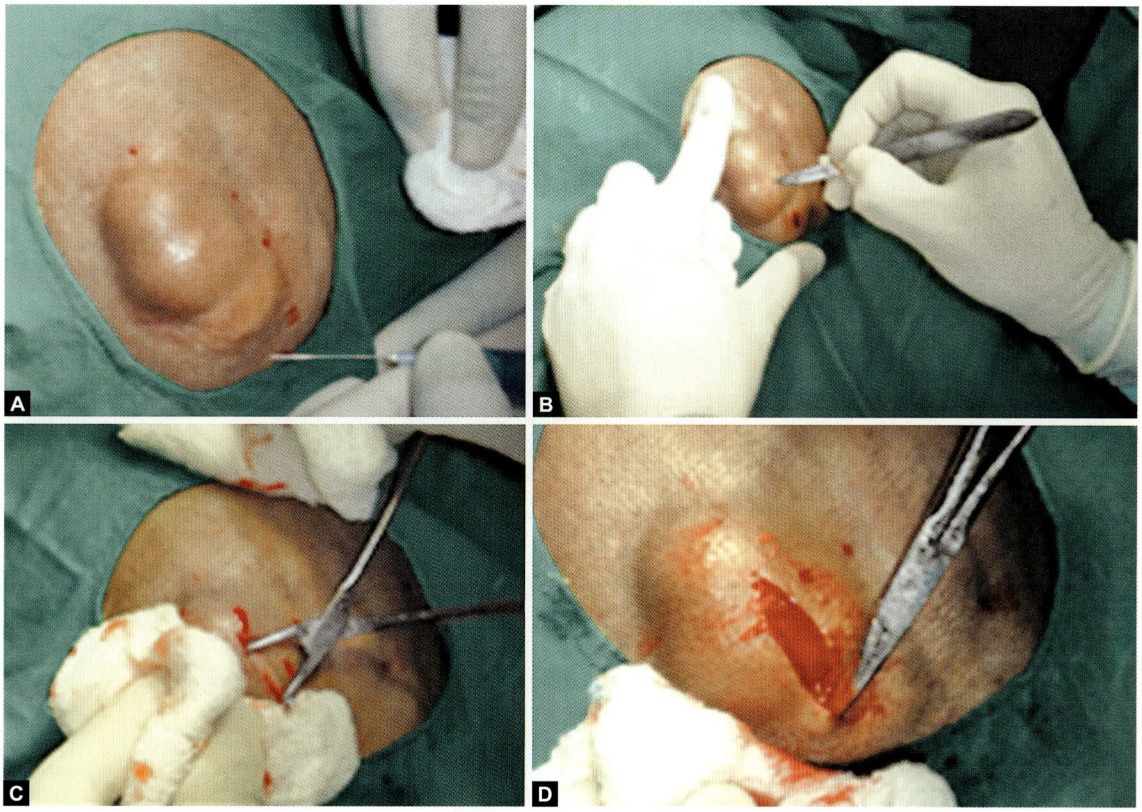

Figs. 3A to D: Excision of pilar cysts on scalp after undermining with blunt dissection incision over the cyst.

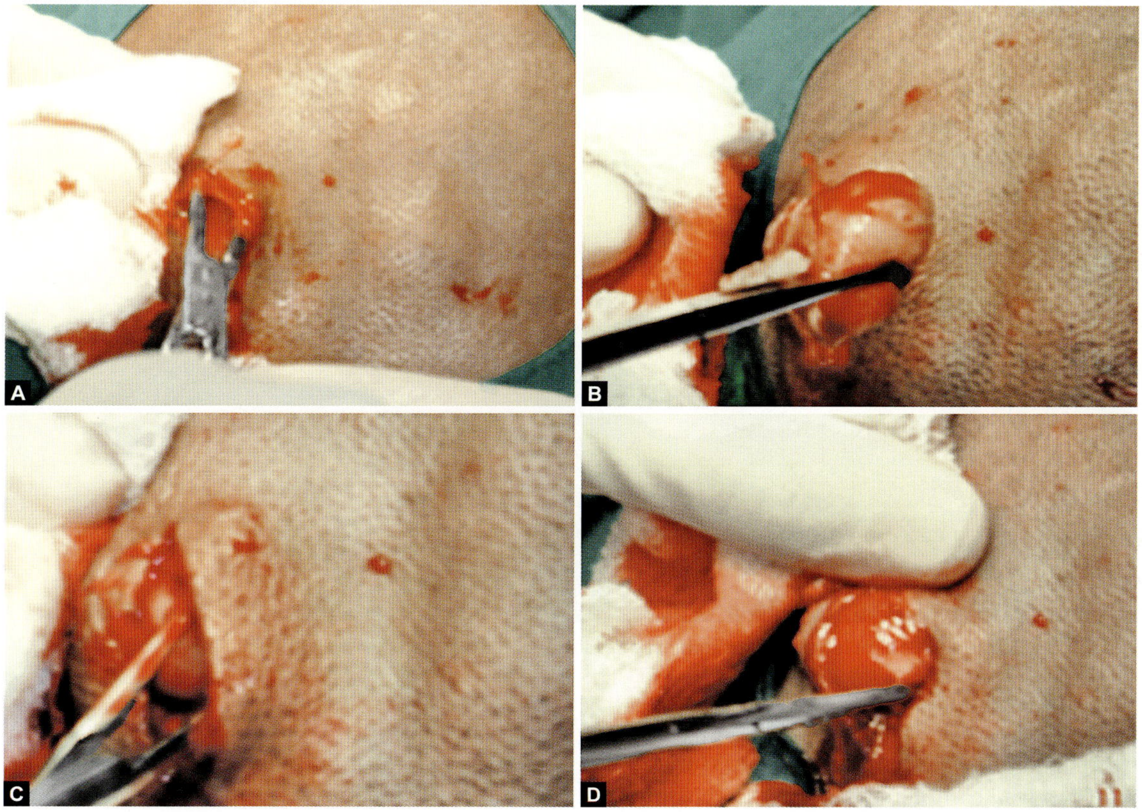

Figs. 4A to D: Undermining and extrusion of the cyst with intact cyst wall. (A) Multiple pilar cysts on scalp; (B) Removal with simple excision; (C) Blunt dissection with artery forceps; (D) Cysts removal with intact wall.

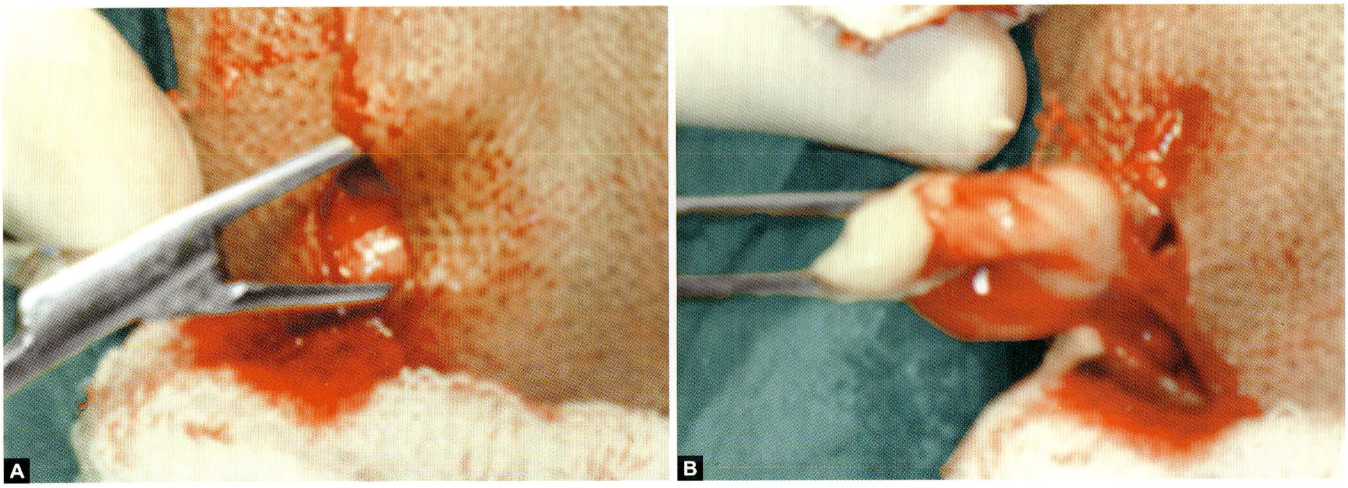

Figs. 5A and B: Excision of cyst—final step.

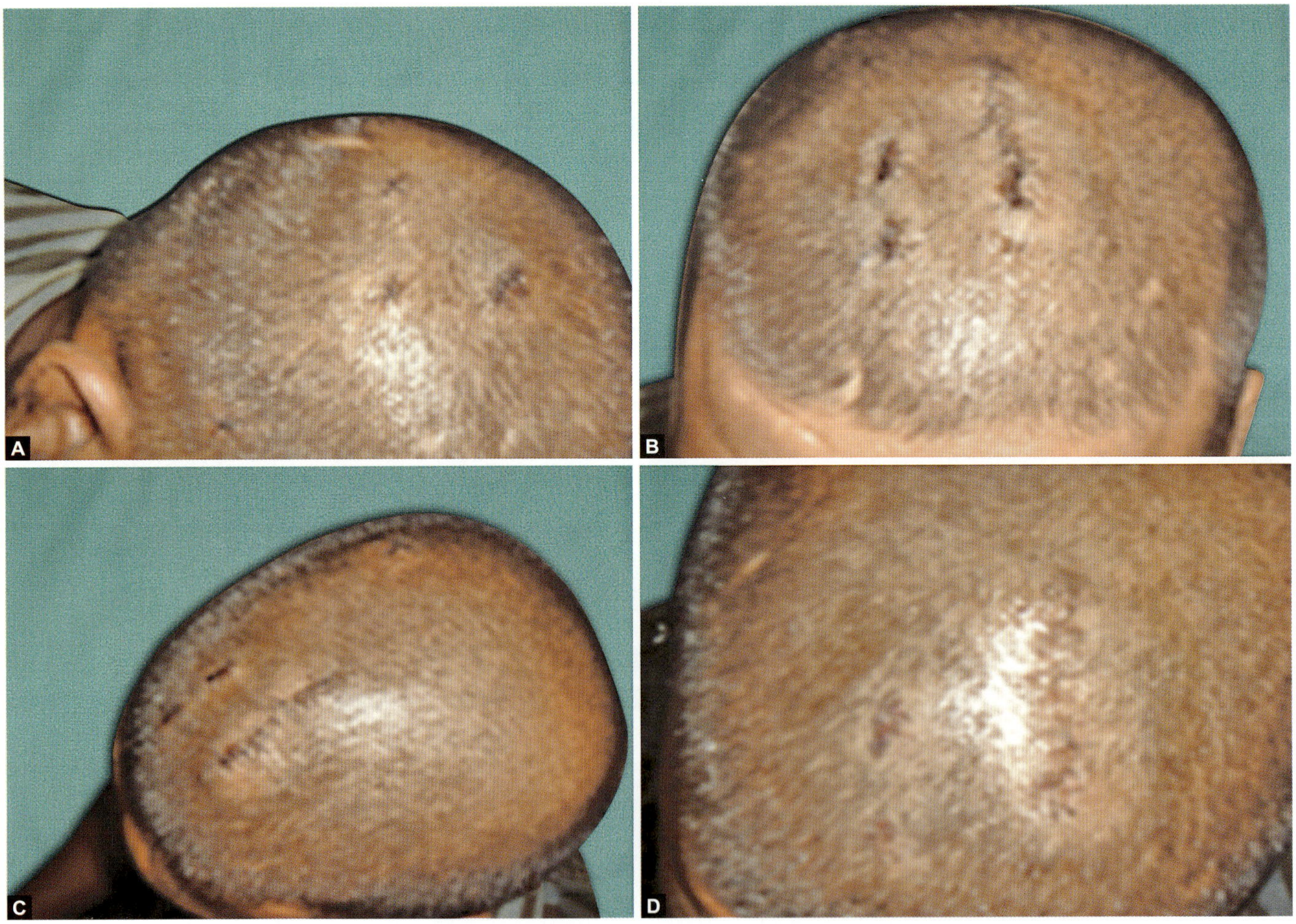

Figs. 6A to D: Simple interrupted suturing after suture removal good healing with minimal scarring.

postoperative care is advised. After 1 month, once the cyst has become small, minimal excision technique is performed to remove the cyst wall completely. This method is suitable for large cyst or cyst over thick skin where the cyst wall is more friable or expression of the contents is difficult.[6]

Carbon dioxide laser has also been used to make a small hole as a part of minimal invasive excision of epidermal cysts. Small, freely mobile, and noninflamed epidermal cysts measuring 0.5–1.5 cm have been treated successfully with this method.[7]

SPECIFIC TECHNIQUES FOR DIFFERENT TYPES OF CYSTS

Epidermoid Cysts

Epidermoid cysts can be managed by any of the earlier mentioned techniques.

Infected or Inflamed Cysts

These cysts are preferably treated with systemic antibiotics with small amount (5 mg/mL) of intralesional triamcinolone acetonide into the cyst cavity along with warm compresses. For fluctuant cysts, incision and drainage is best option. Finally, excision is done.[3,4]

Milia

Surgical evacuation is the best option using a number 11 blade with comedone extractor. A fine tip cautery with very low current electrodesiccation is another option. In both techniques, cosmetic results are good.[1]

Steatocystoma Multiplex

The therapeutic option is same as that for the treatment of epidermoid cysts.[2]

Mucous Cysts

Excision is the standard treatment approach. Care must be taken to orient the excision so as not to alter the appearance of the vermillion. Simple incising and draining the cyst is not enough to prevent recurrences. The underlying mucous or minor salivary glands must be removed down to the orbicularis oris muscle. The wound is closed with chromic catgut so no suture removal is required. Chalazion clamp can be used to fix the mucous cyst.[1,3]

Dermoid Cyst

Therapy consists of complete surgical excision. Skull films, CT scans, and MRI must be used to evaluate the dermoid and its potential intracranial extensions before surgery.[1,4]

CONCLUSION

A vast variety of cysts are encountered in the skin, and the dermatosurgeon must be well versed with both the common and uncommon types. With proper excision, evacuation, and closure techniques, good cosmetic results can be achieved.

SURGICAL MANAGEMENT OF LIPOMAS

INTRODUCTION

Lipomas are the benign tumors of mature adipocytes. Several types of lipoma are described. These include simple, fibrolipoma, angiolipoma, pleomorphic, spindle cell, and myolipoma. Lipoma can be a part of associated syndrome, e.g., Madelung syndrome, Gardner's syndrome, Cowden's syndrome, Bannayan-Riley-Ruvalcaba syndrome, and familial multiple lipomatosis.[8] Clinically, lipoma is a slow-growing, asymptomatic mobile swelling with characteristic doughy consistency. The lesion is usually located in the subcutaneous tissue but can be found in intermuscular septa, abdominal viscera, oral cavity, internal auditory canal, cerebellopontine angle and thorax.[9] However, subcutaneous lipoma is of concern for dermatologists. The size of lipoma may vary from a small swelling to a large tumor measuring >15 cm and can occur anywhere on the body.[10] Hence, appropriate lipoma removal techniques need to be used for better cosmetic result.

Depending on the size, type, and location of lipoma several lipoma removal techniques have been used successfully. These include conventional surgical excision, minimal invasive techniques such as stab incision squeeze technique (SIST) and distant incision technique, injection lipolysis, tumescent liposuction, and laser lipolysis.

Small lipomas can be easily excised surgically with good cosmetic outcome. However, excision of larger lesions measuring >10 cm can result in significant scarring. In such situation, tumescent local anesthesia (TLA) with liposuction has been used successfully. This technique may not be feasible for extensive fibrous lesions. Laser lipolysis, a minimally invasive and effective method of removal of such lesions has been proposed. It can be used alone or before liposuction.[11]

STAB INCISION SQUEEZE TECHNIQUE

The SIST is suitable for small, superficial, and encapsulated lipomas. Normal saline is injected preoperatively into the subcutaneous tissue immediately surrounding the lipoma to facilitate enucleation. A single linear stab incision, as short as one-fourth to one-third of the palpable diameter of the lipoma, is made. Blunt undermining and dissection with mosquito forceps is done to disrupt the fibrous tethers between the capsule and surrounding subcutaneous tissue. Pressure on the lateral aspects of the incision is exerted adequately to express the entire tumor (squeeze technique). The wound is closed with subcutaneous and surface sutures and pressure dressing **(Figs. 7A to F)**.[12]

DISTANT INCISION TECHNIQUE

This technique is used for lipomas of the forehead, lower eyelids, cheeks, lips, and sternal areas. Good cosmetic results are obtained by making the incision at a somewhat distant site. Incision may be hidden in the scalp, eyelids or nasolabial folds, preauricular skin, oral mucosa, or inframammary folds.[12-18]

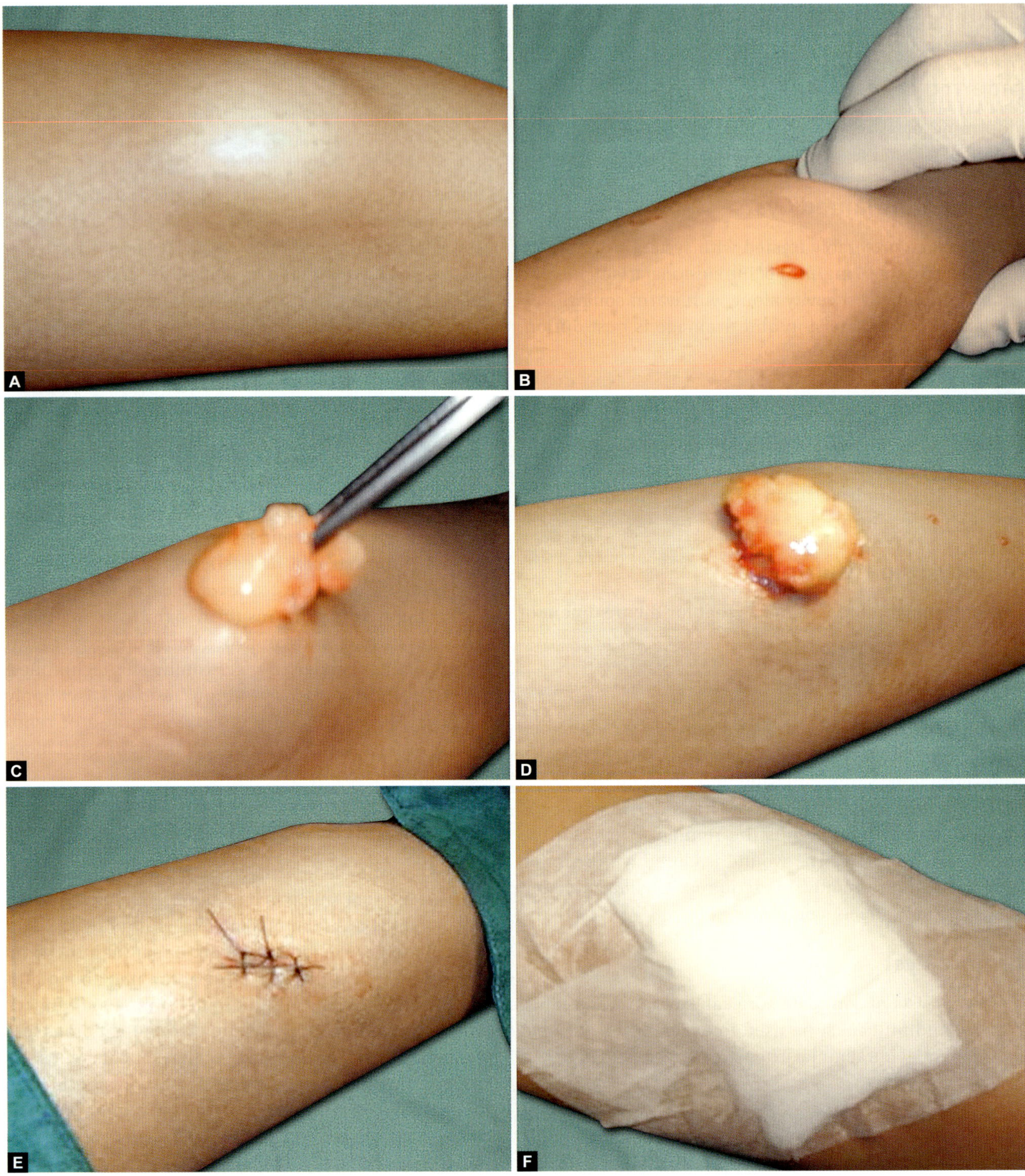

Figs. 7A to F: Lipoma removed through a small incision. (A) Large lipoma; (B) Small incision; (C and D) Fat removal with squeeze technique; (E) Wound closure with simple interrupted sutures; (F) Three layer dressing.

TUMESCENT LIPOSUCTION

Tumescent anesthesia is infused directly into the lesion and after 20 minutes, two to three small incisions are made for liposuction cannulas. One of the incisions is made at the dependent part of lipoma for drainage. A 3-mm diameter cannula with 10 mL Luer lock syringe is enough for liposuction. Complete removal of remaining stroma is done by a hemostat with blunt dissection. A Penrose drain is placed for 1 day and after 5–7 days wound is closed with suture. Tumescent liposuction is associated with ecchymosis, hematoma, and acute dimpling which resolve over a period of time.[10]

LASER LIPOLYSIS

In this technique, following TLA of lipoma and surrounding area, a small incision of 2 mm is made at the lateral edge of treatment area. Laser lipolysis is performed with continuous wave 980-nm diode laser delivered through a 600-µm fiberoptic cable, ensheathed, except for distal 2 mm, in a 1.2-mm diameter stainless steel cannula. The fiberoptic cannula is introduced into the lipoma through 2 mm incision and laser is delivered once the tip of the fiberoptic is localized inside the lesion. A total of 7,000 J of laser at 20 W power can be delivered in the deep, mid, and superficial planes of the lesion to ensure complete lipolysis and lysis of fibrous attachments and capsule. Adequate lipolysis is indicated by minimal resistance to the motion of cannula which is advanced approximately 2 mm/s. The laser is moved in a fan-like movement. The fragmented and partially liquefied contents of lipoma, fibrous tissue, and capsule are expressed through the incision site by applying lateral pressure. The incision site is left open for drainage and for prevention of formation of seroma or hematoma. Approximately 90% of lipomas can be removed completely with this technique. The retreatment of incompletely removed lipomas is generally well tolerated considering minimal invasive nature of the procedure.[11]

INJECTION LIPOLYSIS

Injection of detergents-like phosphatidylcholine (PDC)/sodium deoxycholate (DC) into the subcutaneous fat is usually done for nonsurgical contouring of body and removal of localized collection of excess fat. PDC/DC when injected into lipoma causes fat necrosis. Same technique and agents have been used successfully in the significant reduction of size of lipoma. However, there is lack of long-term efficacy, safety, and recurrences.[19-21]

Similarly, intralesional triamcinolone acetonide with equal amount of 1% lignocaine can be injected at the center of the lesion. Injection can be repeated several times every month for significant reduction in size of the lesion. It is used for the treatment of lipoma measuring <1 inch.[2]

Injection lipolysis is not an appropriate technique for complete removal of lipoma. But can be used preoperatively to reduce the size of the lesion.

CONCLUSION

Lipomas are benign tumors of mature adipocytes, with various types including simple, fibrolipoma, angiolipoma, pleomorphic, spindle cell, and myolipoma. They can be part of associated syndromes and can be found in various parts of the body. Lipoma size can range from small swellings to large tumors. Various lipoma removal techniques, including surgical excision, minimal invasive techniques, injection lipolysis, tumescent liposuction, and laser lipolysis, have been successfully used for cosmetic outcomes.

REFERENCES

1. Parlette HL III. Management of cutaneous cysts. In: Wheeland RG (Ed). Cutaneous Surgery. Philadelphia: WB Sanders. 1994; pp. 647-63.
2. Mevorah B, Bovet R. Treatment of retro-auricular keratinous cysts. J Dermatol Surg Oncol. 1984;10:40-4.
3. Danna J. A simple treatment for sebaceous cysts. N Orleans Med Sci J. 1994;98:528.
4. Robertson TM. Treatment of sebaceous cysts. Practitioner. 1989;233:700-1.
5. Park SW, Choi J, Lee HS, Kim J. Minimal incision suction-assisted excision of a large epidermal cyst. Aesthetic Plast Surg. 2015;39:570-3.
6. Wu H, Wang S, Wu L, Zheng S. A New Procedure for Treating a Sebaceous Cyst: Removal of the Cyst Content with a Laser Punch and the Cyst Wall with a Minimal Postponed Excision. Aesthetic Plast Surg. 2009;33:597-9.
7. Song SW, Burm JS, Yang WY, Kang SY. Minimally invasive excision of epidermal cysts through a small hole made by a CO_2 laser. Arch Plast Surg. 2014;41:85-8.
8. Pandya KA, Radke F. Benign skin lesions: lipomas, epidermal inclusion cysts, muscle and nerve biopsies. Surg Clin North Am. 2009;89:677-87.
9. Salam GA. Lipoma excision. Am Fam Physician. 2002;65:901-4.
10. Choi CW, Kim BJ, Moon SE, Youn SW, Park KC, Huh CH. Treatment of lipomas assisted with tumescent liposuction. J Eur Acad Dermatol Venereol. 2007;21:243-6.
11. Stebbins WG, Hanke W, Petersen J. Novel method of minimally invasive removal of a large lipoma after laser lipolysis with 980 nm diode laser. Dermatol Ther. 2011;24:125-30.
12. Shelley ED, Shelley WB. Piezosurgery: a conservative approach to encapsulated skin lesions. Cutis. 1986;38:123-6.
13. Vidimos AT. Management of lipomas. In: Wheeland RG (Ed). Cutaneous Surgery. Philadelphia: WB Sanders; 1994. pp. 675-83.
14. Fabri PJ, Adams JR. Simplified excision of lipomas. Surg Cynecol Obstet. 1987;165:173-4.
15. Hardin FF. A simple technique for removing lipomas. J Dermatol Surg Oncol. 1982;8:316-7.
16. Powell B, McLean NR. The treatment of lipomas by the "squeeze" technique. JR Coll Surg Edinb. 1985;30:391-2.
17. Harris WG. Treatment of lipomas by the squeeze technique. JR Coll Surg Edinb. 1986;31:258.
18. Peinert RA, Courtiss EH. Excision from a distance: a technique for removal of benign subcutaneous lesions. Plast Reconstr Surg. 1983;72:94-6.
19. Rotunda AM, Albon G, Kolodney MS. Lipomas treated with subcutaneous deoxycholate injections. J Am Acad Dermatol. 2005;53:973-8.
20. Nanda S. Treatment of lipomas by injection lipolysis. J Cut Aesthet Surg. 2011;4:135-7.
21. Amber KT, Ovadia S, Camacho I. Injection therapy for the management of superficial subcutaneous lipomas. J Clin Aesthet Dermatol. 2014;7(6):46-8.

CHAPTER 21

Keloids and Hypertrophic Scars

Somesh Gupta

KEY MESSAGES

- Keloids and hypertrophic scars are the result of an overgrowth of fibrous tissue following healing of a cutaneous injury and it causes significant morbidity.
- There are important differences between keloid and hypertrophic scar.
- There are several treatment modalities which are useful for the management of keloids, though no single modality is completely effective.
- The most commonly used modalities are pressure, silicone gel sheets, intralesional steroids, 5-fluorouracil (5-FU), cryotherapy, surgical excision, radiation therapy, and lasers.
- These may be used singly or more commonly in combination.
- Once established, however, keloids are difficult to treat, with a high recurrence rate regardless of therapy.
- One should realize that keloids will only improve and not disappear completely.
- Patients with a tendency for keloids should be advised about preventive measures.

INTRODUCTION

Keloids and hypertrophic scars are the result of an overgrowth of fibrous tissue following healing of a cutaneous injury. Keloids extend beyond the margins of the original wound, do not usually regress spontaneously and tend to recur after excision, while hypertrophic scars do not expand beyond the boundaries of the initial injury and may undergo partial spontaneous resolution.[1] Keloids have a tendency to grow symptomless, but pain and pruritus may be present.

Keloids and hypertrophic scars may cause functional impairment and cosmetic disfigurement and are often associated with morbidity, and significant psychosocial impact.[2]

HISTORY

The first description of keloids was given by Smith Papyrus in 3000 BC.[3] Subsequently, in 1806, Jean Louis Alibert used the term *"cheloide"*, derived from the Greek word *chele*, meaning *"crab's claw"*, to describe the lateral growth of tissue into unaffected skin and added—oid, meaning *"like"*.[4] In 1825, he wrote a chapter entitled *"Les cancroides ou Keloides"* which established the current term keloid. Unfortunately, in over 3,000 years history of keloids, there is no satisfactory treatment available for this troublesome disease. The research on keloids faces several hurdles including absence of animal models and lack of interest of funding agencies and industry.

EPIDEMIOLOGY

Keloids mostly arise at puberty with peak age of onset between 10 and 30 years of age.[3] In a cross-sectional study of 1,000 Indian patients, 65.2% of patients suffering from keloids were aged between 11 and 30 years, while 23.5% patients were in the age group of 31–50 years.[5] Keloids have been observed in infants and adults over the age of 70 years. Keloid was identified in 0.6% of the children aged between 6 and 11 years in Taiwan in a cross-sectional study. It was mostly seen following Bacillus Calmette-Guérin (BCG) vaccination.[6] BCG scar as a potential site of keloid formation during puberty has also been observed.[5]

There exists an equal risk between men and women. But female predominance may be due to the number of ear lobe keloids secondary to piercing among women.[7,8] It is mostly sporadic, though familial cases have been described. Spontaneous onset, i.e., onset of keloids without prior history of trauma has been reported to be rare, and are most often considered to arise due to microtrauma or minimal cutaneous inflammation in genetically susceptible individuals.[9] It is mostly autosomal dominant with incomplete penetrance and variable expression, though autosomal recessive cases have also been described.[10] The increased risk of developing keloids in identical twins strongly supports a role for genetics.[11]

The exact prevalence of keloids is not known and the data may be underestimation of its actual occurrence. According to various population-based data, it ranges from 4 to 16% in Black and Hispanic.[12] The prevalence in England is as low as 0.9%.[10] It is most common in darker racial ethnic group with reported incidence ratios ranging from 2 to 1 and from 19 to 1 between Blacks and Whites.[13] It is most prevalent in African American, Hispanic, and Asian population and least common in Caucasians and albinos.[14] In a 2019 study by Kouotou et al., prevalence in Black Africans was found to be 3.5%.[15] Its absence in albinos have led to speculation of role of melanocytes. Among the Asians, it is more common in Chinese population.[14] Why certain races are more susceptible is not known. Its predisposition has been associated with certain human leukocyte antigen (HLA) haplotypes; B4, B21, BW16, BW35, DR5, and DQW3 as well as blood group type A.[10] Recently, positive association of HLA DQA1*0104 and DQB1*0501 alleles with keloids in Chinese Han people have been demonstrated using PCR-SSP method, while a negative association was recorded with HLA DQA1*0501, DQB1*0201, and DQB1*0402.[16] HLA-DRB1*15 is associated with risk of developing keloid in Caucasians of Northern European origin.[17]

Some rare syndromes are associated with tendency to develop keloids which include Rubinstein–Taybi syndrome, Goeminne syndrome, Ehlers–Danlos syndrome, Leigh necrotizing encephalomyelopathy, Ullrich congenital muscular dystrophy, pachydermoperiostosis,[18,19] Bethlem myopathy, Dubowitz syndrome with atopic dermatitis, Noonan syndrome, and X-linked recessive polyfibromatosis.[9]

PATHOPHYSIOLOGY

Keloids are theorized to result from an imbalance of increased synthesis of collagen and extracellular matrix (ECM), and decreased degradation of these products. Overexpression of inflammatory mediators—namely, transforming growth factor beta (TGF-β), increase synthesis of ECM collagen via overactivation of keloid fibroblasts.[20] Overexpression of TGF-β1 and TGF-β2 with decreased expression of TGF-β3 production results in increased fibroblast activity and ECM collagen formation.[21] Keloid fibroblasts are increasingly sensitive to the effects of TGF-β1 due to the receptor's upregulation. TGF-β1 increases tissue inhibitors of metalloproteinase (TIMP) and decrease matrix metalloproteinase (MMP) production, resulting in reduced collagen degradation.[21] Other inflammatory proteins such as vascular endothelial growth factor (VEGF) and platelet-derived growth factor (PDGF) have also been implicated in the overproduction of collagen. Mechanotransduction pathways; stimulated by mechanical stress at certain areas of the body, such as the sternum, shoulder, and suprapubic areas; are activated by these molecules, resulting in hypertrophic scars and keloids.[21]

The exact pathophysiology of keloid is not fully understood. Multiple hypothesis has been postulated to explain the pathomechanism of keloids and hypertrophic scars. There are number of hypotheses which have been postulated as shown in the **Box 1**.

BOX 1: Various hypotheses of keloid formation.

- Sebum autoimmune hypothesis
- Hypoxia hypothesis
- Tension hypothesis
- Hormonal hypothesis
- Essential fatty acid hypothesis

According to the sebum autoimmune hypothesis, keloids are a result of immune reaction to sebum which acts as antigen after being secreted intradermally following trauma. This is supported by the clinical characteristics highlighted by some researchers.[22,23] Only humans develop true keloids and are the only animals with sebaceous glands. Keloids are common on seborrheic areas mostly. Interestingly, keloids are rarely described on volar skin which lacks sebaceous glands. Keloids are seen more frequently after puberty when the sebaceous glands are most active and its incidence decrease in the later decades of life when sebum production fall down. Also, after puberty, keloids can be activated from older wounds incurred during childhood, for example, earlobe keloids and keloids at vaccination sites.[24]

Hypoxia hypothesis asserts that hypoxia present in keloid and hypertrophic scar stimulate excessive collagen production. Transmission electron microscopy have demonstrated that the microvessels are occluded because of excessive endothelial tissue which leads to hypoxia.[25,26] Hypoxia/hypoxia inducible factor-1α has been found to provide a favorable microenvironment for keloidal keratinocytes to adopt a fibroblast-like appearance through epithelial-to-mesenchymal transition. This might lead to enhanced capacity of keloidal keratinocytes to invade in adjacent normal area beyond the wound margin.[27] According to tension hypothesis, keloids are caused and exacerbated by tension in wounds. This is supported by the occurrence of keloids and its recurrence in areas of highest tension on the body (chest wall, scapular region, and suprapubic regions) and lowest recurrence in areas of low tension (neck, earlobes, and lower limbs).[28,29]

Influence of hormones has been speculated due to its occurrence at puberty and pregnancy, worsening during pregnancy, and rarity in postmenopausal women.[14,30,31]

Acromegalics are highly susceptible to keloid formation.[14]

Keloid scars demonstrate a higher level of androgen binding than surrounding normal tissue or hypertrophic scars.[10] It is also interesting to note that circulating androgen concentrations rise during pregnancy. The chest, upper back and neck are areas predisposed to keloids and these areas have a higher rate of dihydrotestosterone metabolism.[32]

According to essential fatty acid hypothesis, an essential fatty acid deficiency of precursors and inflammatory competitors for arachidonic acid may be a factor in the multi-factorial etiology of keloid formations. Nutrition may also be a contributing factor in rural black South Africans.[33-35]

Irrespective of the earlier mentioned different hypotheses, the primary biochemical abnormality is the imbalance between matrix degradation and collagen synthesis, resulting in excess accumulation of collagen in the wound. One of the limiting factors in keloid research is the lack of a good laboratory model for study, though various animal models have been studied. Human skin graft on athymic mice and porcine model appear promising. These can probably help in better understanding of pathogenesis and thus helping in better treatment.[36]

In most patients, trauma is the main provoking factor which may occur in any form: abrasions, incisions, insect bites, chemical and thermal burns, acne, chickenpox, bacterial or viral infections, and vaccination. Many a times, patients do not recall an inciting event and these are known as *"spontaneous keloids"*. The most important risk factor for the development of keloids is a wound healing by secondary intention, especially if healing time is increased. It is widely accepted that keloids develop subsequent injury or inflammation of skin but the exact pathogenesis is unknown. Normal scars seem to have a negative feedback mechanism whereby fibroblasts are mobilized to repair a cutaneous defect and their activity is appropriately dampened to prevent excessive repair. Negative feedback mechanism is somehow defective in keloidal fibroblasts ultimately resulting in exuberant scar formation with the propensity to recur.[37]

The metabolic aberration which leads to keloid formation occurs in the final phase of wound healing when keloids fail to mature and become compact.[38] Aberrant expression of various growth factors and their receptors has been described for keloid-derived fibroblasts. For example, keloidal fibroblasts have been shown to over express the growth factors: VEGF, TGF-β1, TGF-β2, CTGF, as well as the PDGF-α receptor.[39-43] The key role of TGF-β has been extensively studied. It has been found that TGF-β1 and β2 are profibrotic and promote scar formation.[42] In one study, keloidal fibroblasts were found to have lower rates of apoptosis, thought to be related to a downregulation of apoptosis-related genes.[44]

Various polymorphisms of genes encoding TGF-β1, β2, β3 as well as the TGF-β receptor have been evaluated, but no statistically significant associations with keloids have been identified.[45-48] Thus, there is possibility of role of multiple genes that impart susceptibility to keloid development, with different genes contributing to keloid formation in different families. *Seifert et al.* studied the gene expression profiles of fibroblasts from different sites of the keloids; 105 genes were identified that were differentially regulated (79 genes were upregulated and 26 downregulated). The apoptosis inhibitor AVEN was found to be upregulated at the active margin of keloids, while apoptosis-inducing genes such as *ADAM12* and genes inducing ECM degradation such as *MMP-19* were upregulated in the regressing keloid center.[12] *p53* gene codon 72 polymorphism may play a role in susceptibility to keloid in Chinese population.[49]

At the initial stage, keloids possess cancer-like properties, with keloid fibroblast overproliferation. This leads to gradual invasion and migration into the surrounding tissue. There is increased angiogenesis and overexpression of cytokines such as TGF-β and plasminogen activator inhibitor-1 (PAI-1).[50]

Risk factors that increase the chances of keloids include:[51,52]

- African, American, Asian, or Hispanic ethnicity
- Between 10 and 30 years age
- Deep skin wounds such as those from burns or surgical scars
- Scars from acne, vaccination, or chicken pox
- Family history
- In darkly pigmented skin, the risk increases 15–20-folds
- People with blood group A
- Surgical intervention of preexisting keloid.

CLINICAL FEATURES

Keloids occur most commonly on the chest, shoulders, upper back, back of the neck, cheeks, and earlobes.[53,54] Unusual formation of keloid after recurrent episodes of herpes zoster can be seen.[55] Genital keloids have been reported to occur subsequent to circumcision or following trauma.[56,57] In addition, multiple cases of corneal keloids including giant ones following corneal trauma have been described.[58,59] Eyelids, mucous membranes, palms, and soles can also be affected.[54] Clinically, keloids range in consistency from soft and doughy to rubbery and firm nodules, which can be skin colored, hypopigmented, or erythematous secondary to telangiectasias. Lesions are usually devoid of hair follicles and other functioning adnexal glands. Earlobe keloid can assume several clinical forms: button-shaped keloid, dumbbell-shaped keloid, fibrotic intralobular type, and a more destructive lesion that involves the whole lobe.[14] *Park et al.* have classified ear lobe keloid in five types: (1) Pedunculated, (2) Sessile (single nodular), (3) Sessile (multinodular), (4) Buried, and (5) Mixed.[60]

By examining the keloid scars of 211 Afro-Caribbean patients in Jamaica, Bayat and colleagues described site-specific morphologies of keloid—trunk scars were geometrically-shaped with clear margins or irregular in outline, surface, and margin; back single scars were well-demarcated botryoid but multiple scars were butterfly-shaped, spheroidal, and irregular; chest scars were butterfly or non-butterfly-shaped, found most commonly in the midsternal line; upper limb scars mostly in the deltoid region (propeller-shaped) or elsewhere nodular, linear to irregular; on ear the most common site being the lobe, having reniform to bulbous shape; face and neck keloids were firm nodular to hard; posterior auricular keloids were either horizontal and oblong-shaped or vertical and reniform in outline; scalp keloids were most common in the occipital area varying from small papules to large plaques; and lower limb keloids varied from propeller, butterfly, and petaloid to dumbbell-shaped. Three plantar and eight pubic keloids were rare findings.[61]

Keloids are frequently symptomatic, with most patients reporting tenderness or pruritus. *Lee et al.*[62] evaluated 28 patients with keloids and found that >80% of patients experienced keloid associated pruritus and about half experienced pain.[62] Pruritus was found to affect 66.7% of black patients in a study, and was the most common complaint.[15] In the same study, 16.7% of patients were asymptomatic.[15] Most patients present with one or two keloids, but a few patients have multiple lesions such as in case of spontaneous keloids or keloids as a consequence of acne or chickenpox. Female sex, younger age at presentation, and the presence of a positive family history were associated with the development of keloid scars in multiple anatomical sites in Afro-Caribbean individuals in one study.[8] The presence of family history was found to be the single most important factor predicting keloid occurrence in Black Africans.[15] There are no well-documented cases of malignant degeneration of an unirradiated keloid except one recently reported case of basal cell carcinoma developing in the ear lobe keloid.[63] Keloids and hypertrophic scars are among the common cause of functional and aesthetic deformities leading to psychosocial stress to the patient and thus impairing the quality of life.[2] Interestingly, keloids, and hypertrophic scars can have severe negative psychosocial impact on the patients where keloids are not common as shown by Bock and associates in Germany, while a study by Olaitan did not show any negative impact in keloid endemic population of Nigeria.[45,64]

HISTOPATHOLOGY

Keloid is a clinical diagnosis and routine histological analysis is unnecessary.[65] However, several malignant tumors, i.e., dermatofibrosarcoma protuberans, trichilemmal carcinoma, and keloidal basal cell carcinoma and deep fungal infections such as lobomycosis resemble keloids. Hence, several authors recommend biopsy to rule out such cases.[66]

Keloids have a normal epidermal layer and thickened dermis. Collagen bundles are thicker, more eosinophilic, glassy, closely arranged and more abundant in keloids, yielding acellular, and node-like structures in the deep dermal region. In addition to collagen, proteoglycans are another major ECM component deposited in excess amounts in keloid scars. There is decreased concentration of adnexal structures.[67] The four histologic features that are considered pathognomonic for their diagnosis include (1) the presence of keloidal-hyalinized collagen, (2) a tongue-like advancing edge underneath normal-appearing epidermis and papillary dermis, (3) horizontal cellular fibrous bands in the upper reticular dermis, and (4) prominent fascia-like fibrous bands.[67,68]

Hypertrophic scar contains nodules of highly compact collagen, often with a capsule-like band at their periphery. Blood vessels are frequently observed at the periphery. In the early stage, bundles or tracts may be in curvilinear form demonstrating a whorl-like arrangement. By electron microscopy, the nodule is seen to contain highly stellate fibroblasts with dilated rough endoplasmic reticulum and few other organelles.[69]

Table 1 outlines the differentiating features of keloids and hypertrophic scars.

TREATMENT

It is difficult to eradicate keloids and hypertrophic scars, and most of the modalities used for treatment are associated with side effects. Counseling should be done regarding treatment options, side effects and cost, and the final decision to undertake treatment should lie with patients. As will be evident from subsequent reading, there is a vast armamentarium of treatment options. This suggests that none of the treatments is satisfactory in all patients and there is no universally accepted protocol. In general, keloids are more unresponsive, resistant, and have higher rate of recurrence as compared to hypertrophic scar. The treatment of hypertrophic scar and keloid is not very distinct and often overlap. Reported clinical trials suffer from lack of uniformity in case selection (no distinction of keloids and hypertrophic scars), subjective evaluation of treatment outcome and limited follow-up. Blinding is often difficult with many surgical procedures. It is important to realize that even keloids at different sites behave differently in response to treatment. For example, recurrence is less common after excision of an earlobe keloid **(Figs. 1 and 2)** while keloids in presternal region are resistant to most of the treatment modalities **(Figs. 3A and B)**.[70]

All the different treatments available for management of keloids and hypertrophic scars are listed in **Box 2**.

Several factors need to be assessed while choosing therapy in a given patient. These include size of keloid, its location, duration, previous treatments, and morphology. An international advisory panel on scar management recommended a combination of silicone gel sheet and intralesional corticosteroids as first-line therapy **(Figs. 4A and B)**. Second-line therapy for resistant cases included laser therapy followed by surgery with adjunctive silicone gel sheet, if required.[71] The treatment modalities have been used with variable success rates and recurrence rates. In general, there is approximately 70% chance of improvement with treatment; however, the mean amount of improvement to be expected was around 60%. There was no statistically significant difference between treatments.[72]

Corticosteroids

Corticosteroids are the most frequently used treatment modality, most commonly being triamcinolone acetonide (TAC). Besides triamcinolone, various other corticosteroids have been used for raised dermal scarring, such as dexamethasone, hydrocortisone acetate, and methylprednisolone. It is the first-line therapy for the treatment of keloids and second-line for hypertrophic scars.[11] The concentration of triamcinolone depends upon the amount of scar formation, the body area involved, and individual lesion. There is considerable

TABLE 1: Differentiating features between hypertrophic scars and keloids.

	Hypertrophic scars	*Keloids*
Clinical features	• Raised red or pink in color but do not extend beyond margins of original wound be it either traumatic or surgical • Generally appear within 4 weeks after trauma • Often observed in extensor surfaces such as knees and elbows • Rarely elevate >4 mm above skin surface • Regress after about 2 years	• Continue to evolve over time without a quiescent or regressive phase • Take up to 1 year to appear • Do not affect the joint areas of the body generally and affect sebaceous areas (upper part of body) • Grow larger into nodular appearances • May remain or continue to expand
Histopathological, biochemical, and molecular differences[53]		
Collagen bundles	Fine, well-organized, and wavy orientation parallel to epidermis	• Excessive deposition of collagen • Large, abundant, thick, and closely packed in random orientation to epidermis
Myofibroblast	Present	Absent
(α-smooth muscle actin expressing)	Nodular formation	Around blood vessel walls
Proliferating cell nuclear antigen (PCNA) expressing	Low expression	High expression
Mucin deposition	Negative	Focal expression in dermis
Adenosine triphosphate (ATP) level	Low expression	High expression
Hyaluronic acid localization	Major component papillary dermis	• Scanty in papillary dermis and abundant in reticular dermis • Thickened and granular/spinous layer with swollen keratinocytes • Shorter and less organized microfilaments
Desmosomes	Shorter cuboidal desmosomes	Shorter cuboidal desmosomes
Hemidesmosomes	Similar to normal skin	Lower density compared to normal skin
Amorphous substance on electron microscopy	Absent	Diffuse pattern
Apoptosis	Decreased	Increased/decreased
p53 level	Low	High

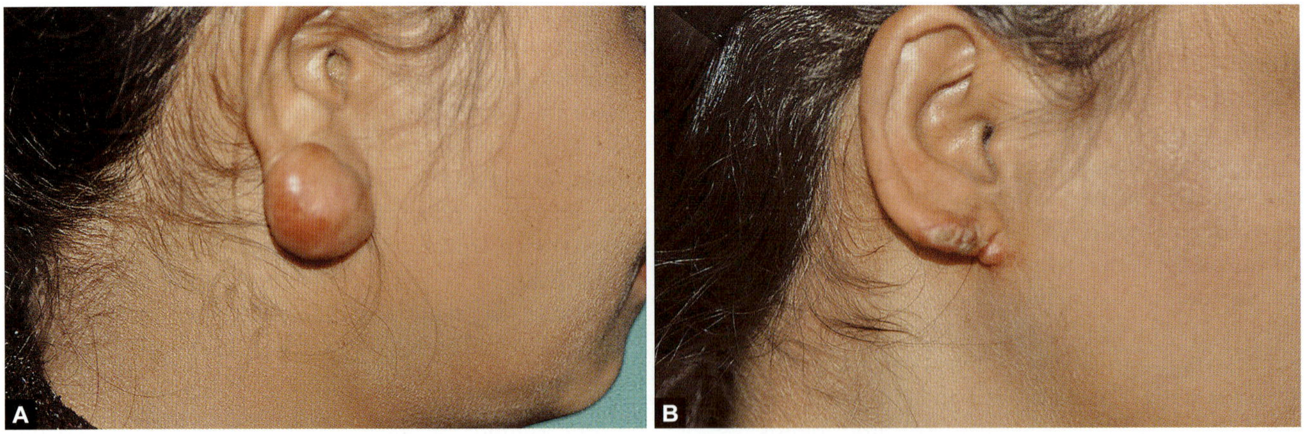

Figs. 1A and B: (A) Earlobe keloid before excision; (B) No recurrence 1 month later.

variation among practitioners regarding the protocol for therapy. Mostly, it is given at a dose of 5–10 mg/mL, injected into the upper dermis in hypertrophic scar every 3–6 weeks. In keloids, it can be given at a dose up to 40 mg/mL.[73] It also stimulates fibroblast degeneration.[74] It may also reduce plasma protease inhibitors so that collagenase degrades collagen. There is an increase in production of basic fibroblast growth factor (bFGF) and a decrease in the production of TGF-β1 by human dermal fibroblasts, endogenous VEGF, and insulin-like growth factor-1. There is 50–100% reduction and 9–50% recurrence in keloid.[71] Adverse effects of treatment include pain, skin and subcutaneous fat atrophy, telangiectasia,

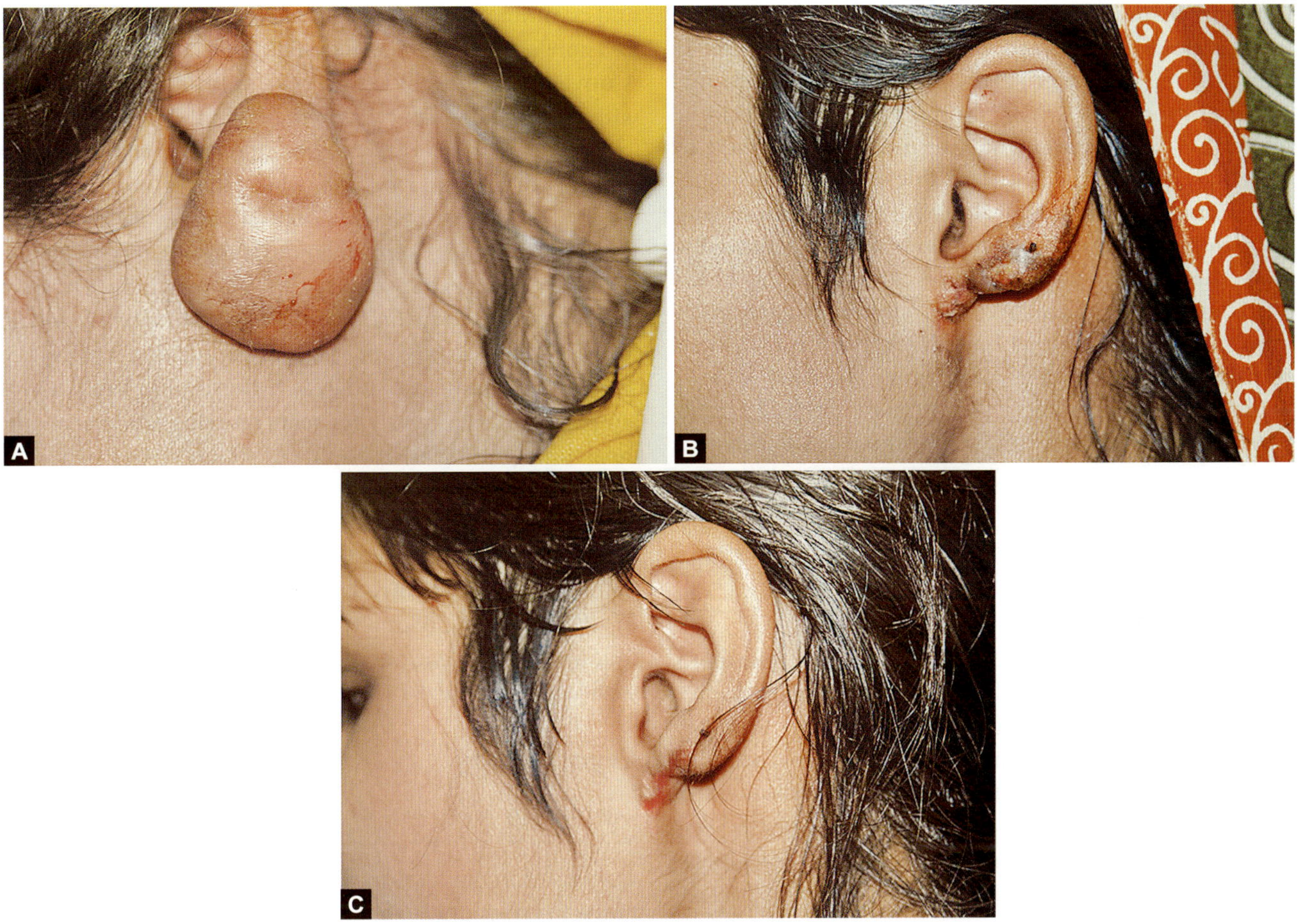

Figs. 2A to C: (A) A large earlobe keloid treated with excision and closure, (B) 1 week later; (C) 1 month later.

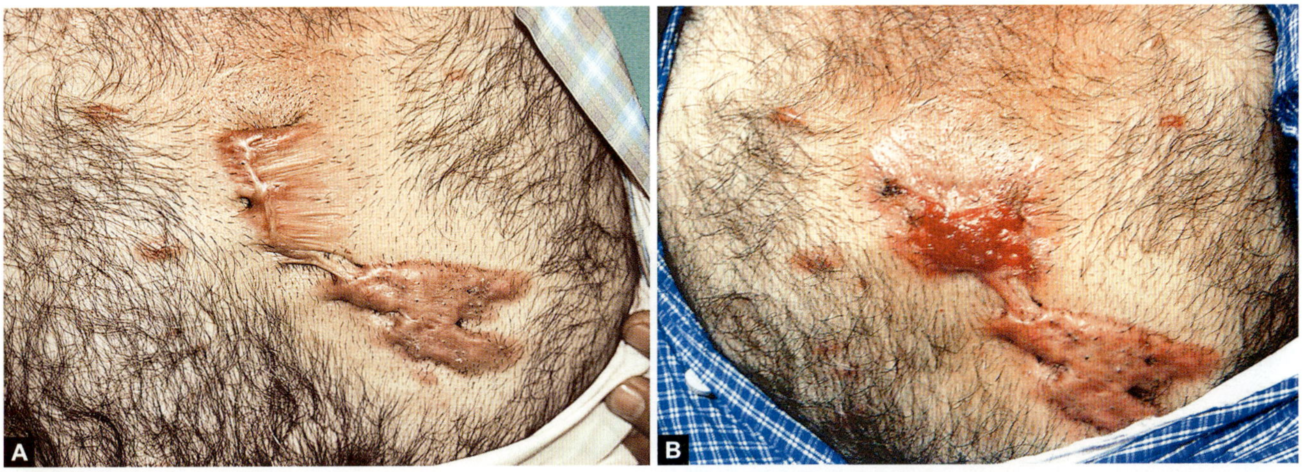

Figs. 3A and B: (A) Presternal keloid treated with different modalities including intralesional steroids, 5-fluorouracil (5-FU), pressure therapy, silicone gel sheet, and surgical and laser excision; (B) 1 year later—the lesion is worse than the baseline.

necrosis, ulcerations, and hypopigmentation. Cushing's syndrome resulting from intralesional triamcinolone has been reported in the literature. Most recent recommendations does not find adult patients at increased risk for developing Cushing's syndrome although children appear to be at risk for developing Cushing's syndrome.[75] Various measures have been used to reduce the pain due to intralesional injection. A mixture of 2% plain lignocaine and 0.5% bupivacaine in equal volumes injected subcutaneously, either beneath the keloid or around it as a field block leads to painless intralesional injection and prolongs postinjection analgesia.[76] Besides this, lidocaine tape has been found to significantly reduce the pain.[77] Results can be improved when intralesional steroid is combined with other therapies such as surgery, pulsed dye laser (PDL) irradiation, intralesional 5-FU, interferon (IFN)-α2b, cryotherapy, or intralesional bleomycin.[74,78,79] Intralesional steroids can be given by any syringe depending upon the thickness of the lesion. Use of a dental syringe is preferred by many physicians. Many treatments, once/twice a month may be followed to achieve the goals. A plastic syringe cap can be cut at the desired depth to act as a guard for intralesional injections.[80]

Topical steroid creams have been used but dermal absorption is limited. Hyaluronidase may be mixed with the steroids in some cases and given intralesional in 1:1 ratio. Recently, a study has used triple combination of 5-fluorouracil (5-FU), TAC, and hyaluronidase with good tolerability and result.[81] Steroids can be continued for prevention after remission unless side effects appear.

Surgical Excision

Surgical excision is one of the earliest forms of treatment, with the major limitation being very high recurrence rate. Cure rates for surgery alone ranged from 7 to 55%.[82] So, various other complementary modalities, such as intralesional corticosteroids, bleomycin, IFN, radiotherapy, and cryotherapy are used to avoid recurrence. Intramarginal excision is advised to prevent additional collagen synthesis.[82] A novel technique of keloid core extirpation was advised without any adjuvant by Lee et al.[83] In this technique, they excised the inner fibrous core from the keloid and covered the defect with a keloid rind flap, which was arterialized by the subcapsular vascular plexus. About 24 keloids of the ear, trunk, face, and genitalia were treated. Of these, 20 patients who healed primarily after surgery showed no evidence of keloid recurrence during the follow-up. Scars can also be excised and resurfaced with a skin graft, a flap, or normal skin that has been stretched by tissue expander. In hypertrophic scars, besides simple excision, Z-plasty for scars crossing joints or wrinkle creases at right angles, or W-plasty for facial scars can be done, so that the new scar is formed within the relaxed skin tension lines.[84] In general, earlobe keloids are less likely to recur **(Figs. 1 and 2)**.[85] Multimodal therapy in form of intramarginal keloid excision followed by intralesional corticosteroid injections and individually customized pressure splints for management of earlobe keloids have shown good results with less recurrences.[86]

BOX 2: Different treatments available for management of keloids and hypertrophic scars.

- *Local treatments:* Corticosteroids, retinoic acid, imiquimod, and silicone gel
- *Intralesional therapies:* Corticosteroids, bleomycin, 5-flurouracil, interferon, and verapamil
- *Surgical therapies:* Surgical excisions, radiofrequency debulking, and laser debulking
- *Physical therapies:* Cryotherapy, intralesional radiofrequency ablation, lasers (CO_2, Nd:YAG, and pulsed dye lasers), radiation, and silicone gel
- *Others:* Compression therapy and miscellaneous

(Nd:YAG: neodymium-doped yttrium aluminum garnet)

Cryotherapy

Cryotherapy is an easy, cheap, and safe mode of treatment, and is quickly becoming a popular modality. It induces vascular damage that may lead to hypoxia and ultimately tissue necrosis. It also leads to decreased inflammation and collagen reorganization.[87] Repeat sessions of cryotherapy is usually required for beneficial outcome and to prevent recurrences. Thaw cycles of 20–30 seconds is used and this should be repeated 1–12 times in total, depending on the size of the scar.[11] While many studies have documented the efficacy of contact or spray cryotherapy, the authors' found that the safety and efficacy of intralesional needle cryoprobe seems to be more than the contact or spray cryosurgery.[88,89]

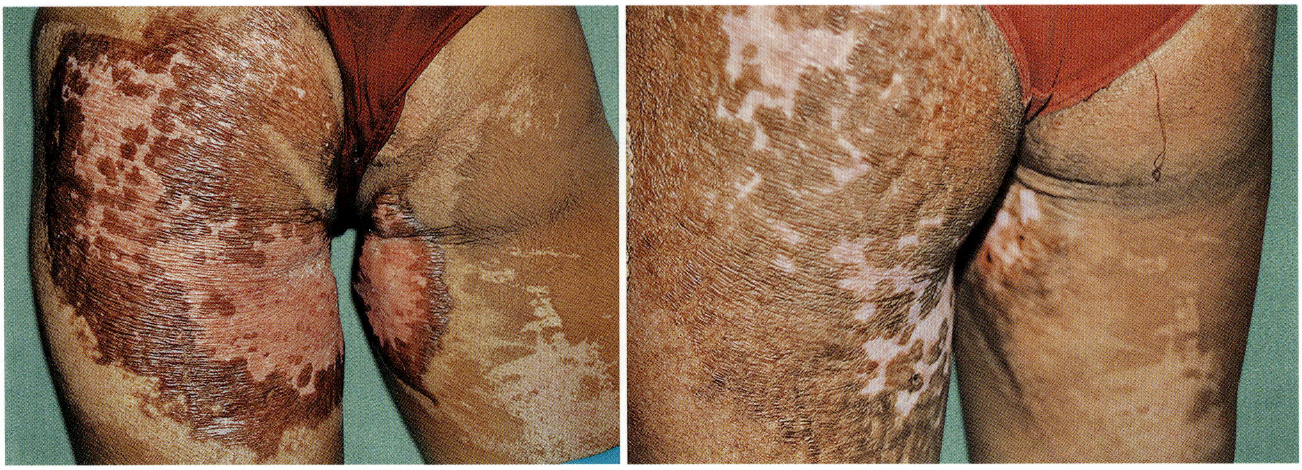

Figs. 4A and B: (A) Postburn keloid; (B) Good improvement in color, texture, and thickening with a combination of intralesional steroids, silicone gel sheet, and pressure garment.

A wide bore spinal needle or 18-gauge hypodermic needle is introduced into the lesion parallel to skin surface and the nozzle of cryogen is connected to this needle. Liquid nitrogen runs through the needle to freeze the deeper pathological tissue. When the scar becomes white, irrespective of the duration of the freezing process, the valve of the cryogun is closed and the needle is left to thaw for 2–3 minutes and is then withdrawn. With this, fewer treatment sessions are needed as compared to the contact/spray in which up to 20 sessions are required. The side effects are milder and include pain, local edema, epidermolysis, and transient hypopigmentation. Hypopigmentation is common and in dark-skinned patients may be striking and hence patients need to be properly counseled. Both hypopigmentation and recurrence after intralesional cryotherapy were significantly more likely in patients with Fitzpatrick type V–VI than I–II.[90] The re-epithelialization period is short, so the treatment intervals can be shortened to 2–3 weeks. The main advantage of intralesional therapy is that it causes minimal surface destruction and the volume of keloid can be frozen, increasing the success rate with less depigmentation, which makes it a useful technique in dark skinned individuals.[91] Comparing intralesional cryotherapy to spray cryotherapy, the former was found to be more effective, with both modalities achieving good results. Spray also required a larger number of sessions with smaller intervals (2 weeks apart) to achieve similar results and are better suited for thinner keloids.[87] In surface cryosurgery, the lethal zone also involves the surface epithelium which is not involved in keloids and deeper pathological tissue in the dermis may be spared. On histomorphometric analysis, the treated scars have more organized and parallel collagen fibers as compared to the pretreated scars. Better results are reported when cryosurgery is combined with intralesional triamcinolone than either of them alone.[74] Cryotherapy induces edema and cellular breakdown causing a decrease in density of fibrous tissue so that injection can be given easily. It may also provide anesthesia before infiltrating steroid, with studies reporting less poststeroid injection when combined with cryotherapy.[92] Response to treatment varies in different studies ranging from 32 to 80%.[93,94]

Laser Therapy

Lasers were introduced for hypertrophic scars and keloids in mid-80s. It is based on the principle of selective photothermolysis causing heat and coagulation necrosis. This leads to hypoxia, dissociation of disulfide bonds due to heating, and subsequent collagen fiber realignment.[95] There is also a hypothesis that laser causes regression of keloid due to induction of apoptosis and upregulation of extracellular signal regulated kinase and p38 mitogen-activated protein kinase activity. PDL causes decrease in fibroblast proliferation, collagen III deposition, downregulation of TGF-β1 expression, and decrease in the number of mast cells.[96,97] Side effects of laser treatment are postoperative purpura, hyperpigmentation or hypopigmentation, and blister formation. Argon laser was first to be used, but discontinued due to its poor response rate.[71] Carbon dioxide (CO_2) laser monotherapy also had recurrence rate as high as 90% or more.[98-100] Few authors have found CO_2 laser as effective and well-tolerable modality for managing keloid.[101,102] Recent literature support good efficacy of neodymium-doped yttrium aluminum garnet (Nd:YAG) laser in management of keloids[103,104] with significant improvement in pain associated with keloids.[105] Of all, PDL proved to be most effective in the improvement of scar texture, redness, size, reduction in itching and pain, and pliability,[106,107] frequently used with pulse duration of 0.45 ms and a fluence of 6.5–7.25 J/cm^2. However, a recent meta-analysis found fractionated CO_2 laser and Nd:YAG laser slightly better than PDL.[108] Lasers are effective not only in the treatment but also in the prevention of hypertrophic scars and early the intervention, better the results.[107,109] Other modalities such as steroids and silicone gel sheeting can be used along with the laser. Two laser combinations are also being tried by some people as combination of the CO_2 laser with erbium-doped yttrium aluminum garnet (Er:YAG) laser or PDL.[110-112] The combination of CO_2 laser and Nd:YAG laser has shown better improvement in keloids as compared to monotherapy with CO_2 laser, followed by least improvement with Nd:YAG laser. A comparative molecular study procollagen I yielded same results.[113] Ultrapulse CO_2 laser followed by topical application of TAC 40 mg/mL was used to treat keloids in 38 patients by Wang et al. Total of eight sessions a month apart were administered, with significant reduction in size of keloids as well as improvement in pain, itchiness, pliability, thickness, color, and stiffness.[114]

Pressure Therapy

Though, it has been popular for treatment and prevention of raised scars for past four decades, exact mechanism by which it works remains unknown, though several theories have been proposed. Various hypotheses include fibroblast degeneration due to localized hypoxia, reduced chondroitin-4-sulfate, and decreased activity of MMP-28.[115] Change in glycosaminoglycan levels due to mechanical pressure and capillary permeability during the early phase of wound healing decrease the scar formation time.[115,116] Role for prostaglandin E2 is also postulated.[117,118] Theoretically, pressure will be effective when it is above the arterial capillary closing pressure of 25 mm Hg. Thus, the recommendation is that pressure should be around 20–40 mm Hg, but not above 40 mm Hg, otherwise it will reduce the peripheral blood circulation.[107] The pressure should be applied 24 hours a day for a period of 20–25 weeks.[71] Custom-made garments is preferable as they apply uniform and controlled pressure to the scar only.[119-121] They are the preferred first-line treatment for hypertrophic burnt scars in many places as they mature rapidly with less erythema and thickness. Thus, pressure may alleviate itching and pain and may cause early scar maturation, decreasing contractures and avoiding the need for surgical intervention.[116,122] A meta-analysis has found no difference in the results after pressure therapy.[123] The pressure loss of the custom-made garments, discomfort from heat and sweating, swelling of limbs, rashes, eczema, excessive friction, blistering, breakdown of scar, and the compliance of the patient using the garment are other factors which can discourage the use of pressure therapy.[11,116] In literature, maximum use of pressure therapy has been in the context of treating earlobe keloids.

Silicone Material

Silicone is a popular method for prevention and treatment of raised scars. Silicone is available in the forms of gel sheets, gel cushion, liquid, creams, spray, vitamin-supplemented silicone silastic sheets, and orthosis garments.[11] It is suggested that silicone affects hydration of the skin by decreasing the water vapor transmission rate, which is responsible for decrease in capillary permeability, reduced hyperemia, and reduced collagen deposition.[124] Hydration also affects keratinocytes of the lesion to alter growth factor secretion which affects the fibroblasts.[125] Other mechanisms of action that has been postulated is the prevention of stretching of postoperative skin, interference with epidermal-mesenchymal interactions, and changes in the electric polarization and contraction properties of the scar skin.[126] A patient who is prone to form hypertrophic scars after surgical excisions should apply the sheets as soon as re-epithelialization is over. It is to be applied daily for at least 12 hours till the results achieved or for a minimum of 2 months. The time is hypothetical as the exact duration of application for the improvement of lesions is not known.[73] The sheet results in flattening of the lesion, increased malleability, and softening of the scar.[127-129] The side effects include itching, rash, bad smell from the sheet/gel, fragility of the sheet, skin maceration due to accumulation of water below the sheet, and poor compliance of the patient as it has to be used for long duration and for long hours.[130-132] Various combinations of therapies such as pressure therapy with silicone sheets have been applied, especially in anatomic areas that do not respond to sheet due to difficulty in maintaining the sheet in position as chin, breast, clavicle, neck, and face though complications increase with such combinations. Clobetasol propionate 0.05%, when applied under occlusion using silicone gel sheet, was found to be equally effective to intralesional TAC, with fewer side effects.[133] When silicone gel sheets were used impregnated with onion extract and aloe vera, it improved pliability of the scars, compared with silicone gel sheet alone.[134] In a review of 10 trials by *Hsu KC et al.*, silicone gel and silicone gel sheets led to significant improvement in scars as compared to placebo. However, with varied heterogeneity and inherent biases in studies, better controlled trials are needed.[135]

Radiotherapy

Radiation therapy can be used as monotherapy or as an adjunctive to surgical excision. It is an increasingly popular postsurgical excision therapy of keloids and hypertrophic scars due to low recurrence rates. The exact mechanism of its effect is still not known. Proposed mechanisms include effect on fibroblasts, including prevention of fibroblast repopulation after excision or modulation of humoral or cellular immunity leading to inhibition of fibroblasts, or by inhibiting angiogenesis.[136] Two type of modality has been used, i.e., external beam therapy or brachytherapy. *Shen et al.* in their retrospective study on 834 keloids that were treated with electron beam therapy over a 14-year period found a recurrence rate of 9.59%. Time to recurrence ranged from 6 to 28 months, and adverse effects were seen in 9.83% of subjects, most commonly with dyspigmentation.[136] *Berman et al.* conducted a retrospective analysis of 96 keloid scars treated with biologically effective dose (BED) of 30 Gy superficial radiation therapy (SRT) (given as three 6 Gy SRT treatment on day 1, 2, and 3 postsurgery). They found a recurrence rate of 10.4% at 12 months, which increased to 12.7% at 18 months. Recurrence was found to be more common in females, on chest, keloid scars that have previously recurred, and longer time for removal of sutures postsurgery.[137] No radiation therapy-induced malignancy was found in the patients.[137] *Wen et al.* retrospectively analyzed 151 keloids in 100 patients who received auxiliary postoperative radiotherapy 20 Gy in five fractions. Recurrence was seen in 14% with factors namely primary keloids, interval from surgery to radiotherapy, family history, and site significantly affecting the recurrence rate.[138] Van Leeuwen and colleagues conducted a systematic review including 33 studies using radiation therapy, as adjuvant treatment for postexcision keloids. They found lowest recurrence rates with high-dose radiation brachytherapy (10.5%) as compared with low-dose radiation brachytherapy (21.3%) and external beam radiation (22.2%). Also, lower recurrence rates were found with shorter time interval (<7 hours) between excision and radiation as compared with longer time intervals (>24 hours). It has been found that presternal keloids show higher recurrence rates with low irradiation dose in comparison to higher radiation dose.[136] However, another systemic review of 12 studies, including one randomized control trial showed the recurrence rate of 22%, with no effect for method of wound closure, type of radiotherapy, radiotherapy dose, and study type; on the recurrence rates.[139] External beam radiation reaches the border of the papillary layer and the reticular dermis, where the keloid is generated whereas the soft X-rays cannot reach to that level.[140] Postoperative radiation therapy has been found to be more effective than intralesional corticosteroid in a randomized study of ear lobe keloid.[141] The dosages according to *Ogawa et al.* are 20 Gy in four fractions over 4 days on anterior chest wall, scapular region, and suprapubic region;

10 Gy in two fractions over 2 days on earlobes; and 15 Gy in three fractions over 3 days on other sites.[142] Hyperpigmentation, hypopigmentation, and transient erythema are some of the side effects after irradiation. Risk of causation of malignant tumor by irradiation is an exaggeration; only few patients have reported to have developed the malignancy in several large series,[143] while other studies do not report development of malignancies postradiotherapy.[137] However, it is contraindicated in children and areas of breast and thyroid which are prone to malignancies.[54,136]

5-Fluorouracil

5-fluorouracil is a fluorinated pyrimidine, an antimetabolite, which inhibits thymidylate synthase and interferes with ribonucleic acid (RNA) synthesis and function.[144] It is used in malignancies as it affects rapidly proliferating cells. In keloids, it blocks collagen synthesis and has shown in tissue culture to inhibit fibroblast proliferation and increase fibroblast apoptosis. It also has an inhibitory effect on TGF-β-induced type I collagen gene expression in human fibroblasts.[144] Fibroblast regression depends on the duration of exposure to the drug and the dose given. It is usually given in the dose of 50 mg/mL. 5-FU given intralesionally once in a week or once in every 2 weeks is effective.[79] Symptomatic and inflamed lesions tend to respond most while the older, noninflamed, and asymptomatic scars respond less.[79] It has shown significant benefit in small and medium keloids as compared to larger ones.[145]

On an average, 5–10 injection sessions are required to achieve complete flattening of the lesions. A retrospective study found that 5-FU/steroid combination with excision had a 92% average reduction in lesion size compared with 73% in the group of patients who did not receive 5-FU and patients who received 5-FU/steroid without excision had an average lesion size reduction of 81%. Thus, it was concluded that combination of 5-FU/triamcinolone is superior to intralesional steroid therapy alone.[146] Similar result was seen by another group from Iran.[147] The risk associated with the 5-FU were pain, urticaria, skin breakdown, purpura, localized hair loss, pigment changes, and systemic absorption.[148]

Bleomycin

It was originally isolated from fungus, *Streptomyces verticillus* and has antitumor, antibacterial, and antiviral activity. It causes necrosis of keratinocytes. Mainly, it inhibits deoxyribonucleic acid (DNA) synthesis but can inhibit RNA and protein synthesis. It is known to induce apoptosis also.[79] The activity/concentration of enzyme TGF-β lysyl oxidase is increased in keloid and hypertrophic scars which is noticed to decrease after bleomycin injections.[79] It is administered either by intradermal injections or multiple punctures are made in the form of 40 punctures per 1 cm^2 with the help of 22 G needle or 0.1 mL (1.5 IU/mL) at a maximum dose of 6 mL is used.[149-152] In one study, there were four therapeutic sessions at 1-month intervals.[153] In another study, three applications were given at 15 days interval.[150] In short, the therapy can have two to six sessions for complete flattening of scars.[152] It is seen that the response of bleomycin is better if the lesion is >100 mm^2.[154] Bleomycin combined with triamcinolone injection was found to be effective in a study involving 35 keloids and two hypertrophic scars in 10 white patients. 4 mg of triamcinolone plus 0.375 IU bleomycin per cm^2 led to softening of 97.3% of lesions and flattening of 64.9% of lesions after one and two sessions, respectively. Dermal atrophy was originally noted in several lesions but was only present in one lesion at 24 months. Adverse effects of this method included ulceration. While neither hyper- nor hypopigmentation was noted, these participants had Fitzpatrick skin types II–IV.[78]

In a recent meta-analysis comparing bleomycin with other modalities such as TAC alone, 5-FU alone, TAC with 5-FU, and TAC with cryotherapy; found better improvement in scar thickness.[155] Bleomycin is easy to administer, high regression rate with less complications and low recurrence rate.[150] Caution is required in pregnant women and children. Complications can be hyperpigmentation, pain, ulceration, Raynaud's phenomenon, gangrene, fibrosis, neutrophilic eccrine hidradenitis, alopecia, edema, and nail changes but cutaneous toxicity occurs only when the dose is 200–300 units or above. It should not be combined with radiotherapy as both emit free radicals.[149]

Imiquimod

It is therapeutically safe and effective in the treatment of keloid.[156] It inhibits the collagen production by IFN release (IFN-α and IFN-γ) and alters expression of an apoptotic gene which is important for the progression of the disease.[79] It can be applied every night for 5 days a week, with 2 days off and can be continued for a total of 8 weeks. Common side effects are itching, burning, pain, blister/ulceration, localized hyperpigmentation, and flu-like symptoms—fever, headache, nausea, fatigue, muscle pain, and bone pain. The authors found that after excision, suppression of keloids with imiquimod is only temporary and the disease recur after discontinuation of imiquimod.[157] Similarly, a prospective, double blind, placebo-controlled did not find any significant reduction in recurrence rates when using imiquimod versus placebo after keloid excision.[158]

Chandawarkar et al.[159] carried out treatment of recurrent keloid in three steps:

- First step was excision of keloid, application of dermal replacement materials, and immobilization and dressing with a vacuum-assisted wound dressing.
- Second step was application of autologous split thickness skin graft.
- Third step was the local application of 5% imiquimod cream for 8 weeks. The patient was asymptomatic after 15 months of surgery.[159]

Although this is an interesting therapeutic approach, it is of a low-level evidence since it is based on one case report. As per a meta-analysis of seven studies by Klotz et al., recurrence rate of 39% was seen after application of imiquimod 5% cream postexcision of keloids. Recurrence rates varied from 5.4% for earlobe keloids to 76.8% for truncal keloids. Imiquimod was not recommended as a therapeutic option due to low certainty of its effect.[160]

Radiofrequency Device

By the use of ThermaCool® radiofrequency (RF) device, the changes in collagen fibril morphology and production changes were seen, but did not show any clinical improvement in hypertrophic scars and keloid.[161] In a study by *Teplyi et al.*, RF ablation has been shown to reduce keloid volume 63% faster when compared to verapamil or 5-FU, after 5 sessions.[162] In a study by *Kaushal et al.*, addition of intralesional RF ablation to intralesional TAC led to similar therapeutic response as compared to intralesional triamcinolone alone (80% patients vs. 73.4% patients with >75% improvement in keloids).[163] Side effects such as pain and hypopigmentation were less in the group with the combined treatment as compared to intralesional triamcinolone alone.[163] *Yadav et al.* used a combination device made up of a tuberculin syringe and intravenous (IV) cannula, for combined intralesional RF ablation and intralesional injection of corticosteroids, in one setting.[164] Creating a slit at the distal end of the cannula away from the skin after retracting the metallic needle further protects the epidermis from accidental thermal injury.[165]

Verapamil

It is a calcium channel antagonist used as an antiarrhythmic drug. In a study, it has shown to stimulate the synthesis of procollagenase increasing collagenase activity leading to reduction in fibrous tissue production.[136] Verapamil blocks the synthesis and secretion of ECM molecules and increase fibrinase.[166] It also reduces the basal interleukin-6 (IL-6) and VEGF production in the keloidal fibroblasts culture leading to inhibition of cell growth and proliferation by 29%.[167] It has been tried in combination with other modalities such as surgical excision alone or with W-plasty or skin grafting, pressure therapy, and topical silicone.[168-170] *Wang et al.* conducted a meta-analysis and found efficacy of intralesional verapamil similar to conventional corticosteroid injections with fewer side effects.[171]

Onion Extract and Heparin

The topical preparation (Contractubex®) containing onion extract, heparin, and allantoin are being used for many years to treat wounds and keloid. The exact mechanism of onion extract is unclear. In vitro studies have shown a dose-dependent inhibitory effect on fibroblasts proliferation. Besides this, it has been found to inhibit histamine and upregulate the expression of MMP-1.[172] Overall, it works by reducing inflammation and fibroblast proliferation. In an open randomized study comparing intralesional TAC and onion extract gel with intralesional triamcinolone alone, TAC with onion extract was more effective in terms of pain sensitiveness, itching and elevation but not in erythema and in duration. The gel was given three times daily for 3 months and intralesional triamcinolone every 4 weeks for a total of four treatments. All patients were treated for 3 months and followed up to 2 months.[173] There are contradictory reports in other studies. Combination of onion extract and petrolatum-based ointments found no improvement in scar, but onion extract and silicone sheet gel was found to be more effective.[174] Presently, there is no conclusive evidence of its efficacy in keloids.[172]

Botulinum Toxin

Various studies have assessed effect of botulinum toxin type A (BTA) on scar. BTA, when injected in the primary wound margins, is hypothesized to help in scar reduction by reducing the tensile force leading to decreased cell proliferation and collagen deposition.[175] Additionally, it reduces fibroblast proliferation by modulating the activity of TGF-β, and reducing transcription and expression of profibrotic cytokines in keloid-derived and hypertrophic scar-derived dermal fibroblasts. It is also postulated to modulate collagen deposition.[176] *Elhefnawy* in his prospective study have assessed effect of intralesional BTA in 20 patients with hypertrophic scars. It was given once a month for 3 months with a follow-up period of 6 month with significant improvement in all three parameters assessed, i.e., erythema, itching, and pliability.[177] Similarly, a randomized controlled trial has documented efficacy of BTA almost similar to intralesional steroid.[178] But *Pruksapong et al.* found steroids to be superior as compared to BTA.[179] In another meta-analysis, *Bi et al.* showed BTA as a superior modality.[180] *Ismail SA et al.* evaluated the efficacy of intralesional botulinum toxin A in 34 keloids. Botulinum toxin was injected at a dose of 2.5 U/cm^3, multiple injections 1 cm apart, maximum of 100 U in one session, at monthly intervals, till flattening or maximum six sessions, whichever is earlier. The authors found excellent flattening in 58.8% and good flattening in 20.6% of patients. There was significant decrease in itch and pain scores; with none of the lesions showing hyperpigmentation and 5.9% showing hypopigmentation. Recurrence reported 8.8%. Overall, the response was significantly better as compared to 5-FU 0.2–0.4 mL/cm^3 injected weekly for six sessions.[145] However, further randomized studies are still required to fully study the efficacy of botulinum toxin. Benefits of using BTA include avoiding steroid-associated side effects and greater improvement in symptoms. A recent study in mouse keloid model showed decreased Ki-67 (associated with decreased cell proliferation) with fewer and less haphazardly arranged collagen bundles. These findings were comparable with steroid injections.[181]

EMERGING DRUGS FOR SCAR REDUCTION

GROWTH FACTORS AND CYTOKINES

Basic Fibroblast Growth Factor

Delayed wound healing is a known risk factor for keloid formation and acceleration of wound healing should improve scarring. bFGF has been proven clinically to accelerate acute and chronic wound healing in pediatric burn scars. It activates the local macrophages up to the remodeling phase which occurs after several weeks of injury. There was a higher rate of developing hypertrophic scars in those who received conventional treatment than those who received bFGF which was evaluated by pigmentation, pliability, height, and vascularity of the lesion.[182]

Transforming Growth Factor-beta-3

Transforming growth factor-β3 is an antifibrotic and its administration may lead to the reduction in scars.[183-185] Mannose-6-phosphate inhibits the associated peptide, preventing the activation of TGF-β1 and 2, thus reducing scarring in both animal and human wounds. The efficacy can be increased by adding TGF-β3 isoform. Role of avotermin (recombinant and active human TGF-β3) as potential therapy for accelerating wound healing and improving scar appearance is well-documented in many studies.[186,187]

Interferon

Interferons compose a group of cytokines that mediate complex cellular interactions, including immunoregulatory, antifibrotic, and antiproliferative functions. IFN-α2b and IFN-γ have been evaluated as therapeutic treatment options for keloids. They act by suppressing collagen synthesis and scar contraction by fibroblasts. Currently, there is limited evidence regarding the efficacy of either IFN-α2b or IFN-γ compared to placebo.[188] One study reported 18.7% keloid recurrence after keloid excision with postoperative IFN at a mean follow-up of 7.9 months, while several studies reported either no significant difference in recurrence rates or a significant difference in scar volume compared to placebo.[21] Intralesional IFN-α2b in dose of 1.5 million IU, given twice over 4 days, reduced keloid to half its size by day 9.[189] The disadvantages include decreased wound strength, delayed re-epithelialization, and the pain associated. *Lee et al.* have assessed efficacy of intralesional IFN-α2b given along with intralesional TAC in the treatment of keloid. They found significant decrease in depth and volume of keloids with combination therapy of intralesional IFN-α2b and TAC when compared with intralesional TAC alone.[190] There is no consistent regimen of IFN-α2b that was used among published studies. Systemic side effects—namely, influenza like symptoms of fever and myalgias—have been reported.[21]

Interleukin-10

It has anti-inflammatory properties and decreases the levels of IL-6 and IL-8 which are thought to rise rapidly in wounds and have role in adult scar formation.[191]

Extracellular Matrix Modulators

- *Prolyl-4-hydroxylase inhibitors:* Prolyl-4-hydroxylase is an enzyme required for the formation of procollagen bundles. Its inhibition by agents such as FG-1648 (a topically active phenanthroline derivative), doxorubicin (commonly used chemotherapeutic agent), and mimosine (an analogue of catechol) can reduce collagen synthesis.[192-194]
- *Cis-hydroxyproline:* It can be given in a microsphere form with a magnetic field directed to the target tissue. It resulted in a 16% decrease in a collagen content in an animal model.
- *Tissue transglutaminase (TTG) inhibitors:* TTG has role in cross-linking of type III procollagen in hypertrophic scars and keloids.
- *Putrescine inhibits TTG:* In phase II clinical trials, it showed significant improvement in hypertrophic scars with minimal side effects.[195]

OTHER PRODUCTS AND THERAPIES

Topical Tamoxifen

It is a nonsteroidal antiestrogenic drug used in breast cancer. It decreases the expression of TGF-β which causes the proliferation of fibroblast and collagen production.[79]

Tranilast

The mechanism by which it inhibits the collagen is not known but in the dosage of 3–300 μM, it inhibits the collagen synthesis of fibroblasts and TGF-β1 in keloid. It is an antiallergic medicine which inhibits the release of histamine and prostaglandins from mast cells.[196]

Prostaglandin

Prostaglandin decreases keloid fibroblast migration and contraction through EP2/EP4—cyclic adenosine monophosphate (cAMP) mechanism.[197]

Tacrolimus

Tacrolimus is a potent immunosuppressive medication that acts on FKBP12 receptor. It suppresses production of IL-2 by inhibiting calcineurin. An open-label pilot study noticed decrease in erythema, induration, tenderness, and pruritus in most of the patients with keloid using tacrolimus 0.1% ointment twice daily for 12 weeks.[198] Concentration of 0.03% and 0.1% both have been found to decrease scar thickness in an experimental rabbit model.[199]

Rapamycin

At molecular level, rapamycin has been found to be dose- and time-dependent downregulating the expression of cytoplasmic proliferating cell nuclear antigen (PCNA), cyclin D1, fibronectin, collagen, and alpha-smooth muscle actin (SMA) leading to antiproliferative effect on fibroblast.[200]

Pentoxifylline

Pentoxifylline, a methylxanthine derivative, has been found to decrease fibrosis and recurrence rate by repressing wound contraction. In a study by *Berman and Duncan*, pentoxifylline was found to inhibit the fibroblasts and collagen, glycosaminoglycans, and fibronectin activity but had no effect on collagenase activity in the skin of patients with keloid, scleroderma, and morphea.[201] *Wong et al.* showed halting of progression of keloids, with reduction in pain and pruritus.[202] In a retrospective study by *Tan et al.*, addition of 6 months of postoperative pentoxifylline (400 mg, TID) to intralesional triamcinolone injections, led to significant decrease in high-risk patients who received the combination therapy versus those that did not (10.5% vs. 66.6%, respectively).[203]

Retinoic Acid

Tretinoin may improve chronic inflammation and prevent expansion of keloid tissues into the normal skin. They are potent inhibitors of MMPs and the study showed that significant upregulation if MMP-13 and significant downregulation of MMP-1 and MMP-8 in keloid derived fibroblasts at both messenger RNA (mRNA) and protein levels.[204] Retinoid (0.05% tretinoin) was applied locally on 11 patients of keloid for 12 weeks. About two patients developed contact dermatitis. At the end of the study, significant decrease in weight and size was found.[205] *Kwon et al.* in their study noticed similar efficacy of tretinoin to that of silicone gel in preventing development of hypertrophic scars and keloids and also improving appearance of scar after surgery.[206]

Dupilumab

Dupilumab (anti-IL-4, anti-IL-13) was found to reduce the size of two keloids in a single case report of an African American patient when administered for the treatment of atopic dermatitis. Increased IL-4R expression in keloids and increased IL-13 and CCL18 expression in both keloids and nonlesional skin have been shown previously with dupilumab acting against these cytokines.[207] However, further studies are imperative for any conclusive evidence to be drawn.

Collagenase

Intralesional injection of collagenase based on the principle of enzymic digestion resulted in temporary reduction in scar volume, returning to the same (or greater) levels after 6 months of follow-up. Side effects were numerous and severe including pain, swelling, blistering, ulceration, pyrexia, and ecchymosis at the site of injection.[208] However, collagenase injection in the management of keloids has limited evidence. Another study reported 50% reduction in volume of earlobe keloids after collagenase followed by compression modalities.[209] Compression and collagenase therapy may be beneficial in combination, by helping to break down aberrant collagen known to be pathogenic in keloids, and hence, maybe more suited for reduction in size before undergoing operative or other modalities.[209]

Collagenase D (derived from the larvae *Dermestes frischii*) was found to be more effective as compared to other types of collagenase such as *Clostridium histolyticum* collagenase and collagenase PC from *Paralithodes camtschatica* (red king crab).[210]

Hyaluronic Acid and Hyaluronidase

Hyaluronic acid can normalize hyperproliferation, growth factor production, and ECM deposition in keloid.[211] When used in high concentration, it has shown good results in reduction of scar thickness.[212]

Di Stadio A used a combination of cortisone and hyaluronic acid over two sessions leading to full clearance of the keloid with no recurrence seen at 1 year in a lesion previously refractory to cortisone injections alone.[213] However, in another study by *Nakamura H et al.*, a 1:1 combination of TAC 40 mg/mL with hyaluronidase 1,500 IU/mL reduced keloid height to at most 1 mm in 11/16 lesions [68.75%, similar to 12/16 lesions (75%) with 40 mg/mL intralesional administration of triamcinolone alone]. The synergistic effect of triamcinolone with hyaluronidase, as this mixture, was found to be as efficacious as triamcinolone 40 mg/mL alone.[214] Although, potential anti-inflammatory properties of hyaluronic acid has been shown previously in animal studies of tendons, why reduction in hyaluronic acid with hyaluronidase achieves a similar response, remains to be explained. It has also been hypothesized that hyaluronic acid or hyaluronidase may just potentiate the effect of cortisone, without directly affecting keloids or hypertrophic scars.

Tripterine

Tripterine is a bioactive pentacyclic triterpenoid compound which in in vivo studies has shown to possesses an anti-scarring function. Tripterine administration decreased expression of MMPs, VEGF, and bFGF, along with decreased phosphorylation of p65, inhibitor of nuclear factor kappa-B alpha (IκBα), and the downregulation of β-catenin; postulated in decreasing excessive scarring in keloids and hypertrophic scars.[215]

Extracorporeal Shockwave Therapy

Shockwave therapy for scar improvement led to no significant difference in improvement of keloids compared with intralesional steroids as determined by both the Patient and Observer Scar Assessment Scale (POSAS) and clinical features.[216] As of now, no strong conclusion can be drawn regarding this therapy.

Topical Mitomycin C

Topical mitomycin C, an antineoplastic derivative of *Streptomyces caespitosus,* has shown to reduce scarring after tracheal and laryngeal surgery. It is postulated to act by alkylating and cross-linking DNA, inhibiting cell proliferation. Regimens described in the literature include application of an absorbent material soaked in 1 mg/mL of mitomycin C for 3–5 minutes with reapplication at 3 weeks.[21] Adjunctive treatment with mitomycin C to surgical excision is reported to result in recurrence rates from 0–33% at 6 months, though some studies have demonstrated several patients with nonrecurrence at >12 months. Side effects include wound ulceration with intralesional mitomycin C, hypopigmentation, and posttreatment pain.[21]

Other Modalities

The list of treatment modalities tried is extensive and includes adhesive tape support, massage therapy, topical vitamin E, topical cyanoacrylates, allantoin-sulfomucopolysaccharide gel, glycosaminoglycan gel, moist exposed burn ointment, extracts from plants (madecassol from *Centella asiatica*, alpha Centella cream from *Bulbine frutescens*, leucocyanidin and ellagic from *Anogeissus latifolia*, extract of *Butea monosperma* bark), which may improve the wound epithelialization and increase wound tensile strength. Topical tocoretinate was reported to improve skin stiffness and glossy appearance of hypertrophic scars.[74] Although well-substantiated evidence is lacking for these modalities.

Catechins (Epicatechin gallate) resulted in improvement in quality of scar formation in a rat incisional wound model. Dermatography can be done in flat or slightly elevated scars, which includes microsurgical needle tattooing. This procedure can provide camouflage pigmentation along with the benefit of inducing atrophy of scars due to the cutting action of the needles.[74]

Flowcharts 1 to 4 depict suggested guidelines for management of keloids; however, it is important to note that management of keloids has to be individualized.

Flowchart 1: Management algorithm for small keloids.

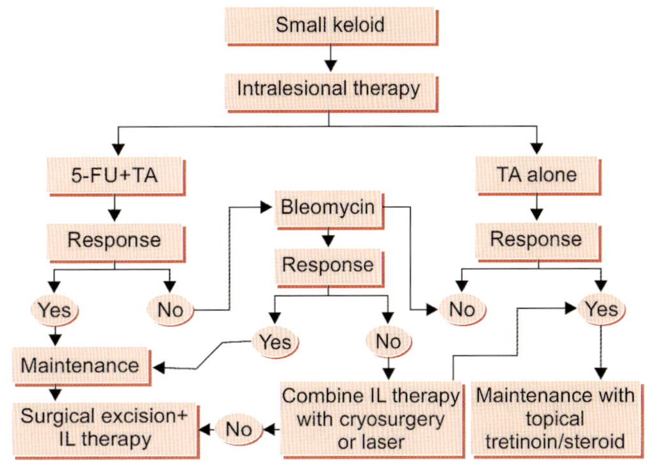

(5-FU: 5-fluorouracil; IL: interleukin)

Flowchart 2: Management algorithm for large and bulky keloids.

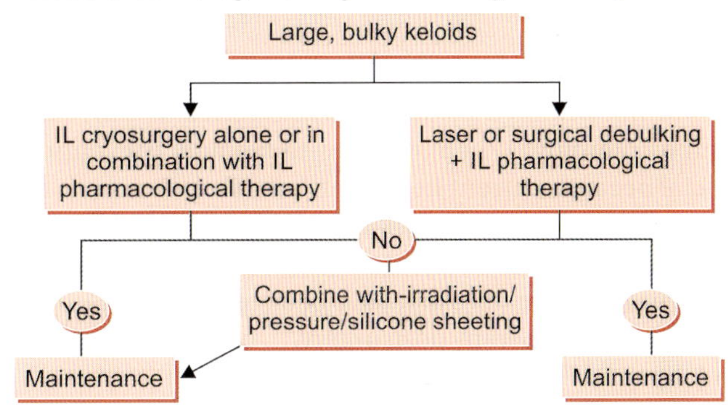

(IL: interleukin)

Flowchart 3: Management algorithm for extensive keloids.

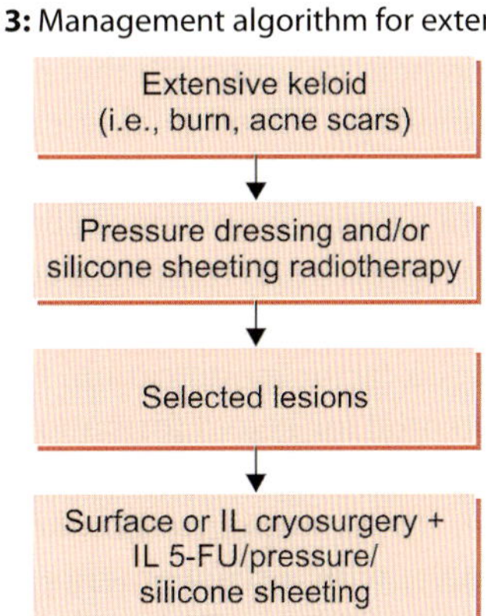

(5-FU: 5-fluorouracil; IL: interleukin)

PREVENTION

As is evident from the long list of treatment modalities, it is difficult to treat keloids. Also, the long duration of therapy, recurrence, and psychosocial aspect add to the cost of treatment. Associative side effects of various therapies must be kept in mind before deciding on any treatment modality. Thus, prevention is the optimal approach. Patients with a family history of keloids should consider not having ear piercings. If piercing is mandatory, it should be done in early childhood. Principles of prevention in keloid on the head and neck include withholding nonessential cosmetic surgery, closing

Flowchart 4: Management algorithm for earlobe keloids.

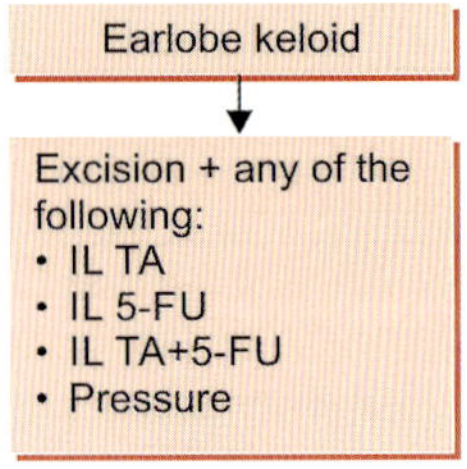

(5-FU: 5-fluorouracil; IL: interleukin)

all wounds with minimal tension (i.e., making incisions along Langer's lines), and the use of pressure garments for 4–6 months after injury. We should always aim for primary closure of wounds. Adequate debridement of contaminated wounds, good hemostasis, gentle handling of tissues, and limiting foreign bodies are other precautions to be taken. Adequate nutrition should be provided, so normal tissue substrates can be synthesized efficiently.[209] Foremost is the avoidance of all unnecessary procedures. The best way to deal with a keloid is not to get one. A person who has had keloid should not undergo elective skin surgeries or procedures such as piercing. When it comes to keloids, prevention is crucial because current treatments are often not completely successful and may not work at all. If any surgical modality is crucial, less tension on the closing margins is imperative. Other newer modalities that have been tried include external beam radiation therapy postsurgery,[217] botulinum toxin A,[218] and dipeptidyl peptidase-4.[218]

CONCLUSION

The management of keloids presents a multifaceted challenge requiring a comprehensive approach that integrates various therapeutic modalities. Through this chapter, we have explored the intricacies of keloid formation, risk factors, and the diverse array of treatment options available.

It is evident that prevention remains a cornerstone in the management of keloids, emphasizing the importance of early intervention and risk factor modification. Patient education regarding the potential for keloid formation, particularly in susceptible individuals, is paramount.

Furthermore, the therapeutic landscape for keloids continues to evolve, with advancements in both surgical and nonsurgical interventions offering promising outcomes. Dermatologists have a multitude of tools at their disposal.

However, it is essential to recognize that no single approach is universally effective, highlighting the necessity for personalized treatment plans tailored to the patient's unique characteristics and preferences.

In essence, the management of keloids necessitates a holistic approach encompassing prevention, patient education, and a diverse armamentarium of treatment modalities, all underpinned by a commitment to advancing scientific understanding and therapeutic innovation.

REFERENCES

1. Bayat A, McGrouther DA, Ferguson MWJ. Skin scarring. BMJ. 2003;326(7380):88-92.
2. Bock O, Schmid-Ott G, Malewski P, Mrowietz U. Quality of life of patients with keloid and hypertrophic scarring. Arch Dermatol Res. 2006;297(10):433-8.
3. Davidson S, Aziz N, Rashid RM, Khachemoune A. A primary care perspective on keloids. Medscape J Med. 2009;11(1):18.
4. Wittenberg GP, Fabian BG, Bogomilsky JL, Schultz LR, Rudner EJ, Chaffins ML, et al. Prospective, Single-blind, Randomized, Controlled Study to Assess the Efficacy of the 585-nm Flashlamp-Pumped Pulsed-Dye Laser and Silicone Gel Sheeting in Hypertrophic Scar Treatment. Arch Dermatol. 1999;135(9):1049-55.
5. Ramakrishnan KM, Thomas KP, Sundararajan CR. Study of 1,000 patients with keloids in South India: Plast Reconstr Surg. 1974;53(3):276-80.
6. Yang Y-C, Cheng Y-W, Lai C-S, Chen W. Prevalence of childhood acne, ephelides, warts, atopic dermatitis, psoriasis, alopecia areata and keloid in Kaohsiung County, Taiwan: a community-based clinical survey. J Eur Acad Dermatol Venerol. 2007;21(5):643-9.
7. Kelly AP. Medical and surgical therapies for keloids. Dermatol Ther. 2004;17(2):212-8.
8. Bayat A, Arscott G, Ollier WER, Mc Grouther DA, Ferguson MWJ. Keloid disease: clinical relevance of single versus multiple site scars. Br J Plast Surg. 2005;58(1):28-37.
9. Jfri A, Alajmi A. Spontaneous keloids: a literature review. Dermatology. 2018;234(3-4):127-30.
10. Marneros AG, Norris JEC, Olsen BR, Reichenberger E. Clinical genetics of familial keloids. Arch Dermatol. 2001;137(11):1429-34.
11. Ud-Din S, Bayat A. New insights on keloids, hypertrophic scars, and striae. Dermatologic Clinics. 2014;32(2):193-209.
12. Seifert O, Bayat A, Geffers R, Dienus K, Buer J, Löfgren S, et al. Identification of unique gene expression patterns within different lesional sites of keloids. Wound Repair Regen. 2008;16(2):254-65.
13. Kelly AP. Keloids. Dermatol Clin. 1988;6(3):413-24.
14. Maibach HI, Baran R. Textbook of Cosmetic Dermatology, 3rd edition. Oxfordshire, United Kingdom: Taylor & Francis; 2004.
15. Kouotou EA, Nansseu JR, Omona Guissana E, Menye CRM, Akpadjan F, Tounkara TM, et al. Epidemiology and clinical features of keloids in Black Africans: a nested case-control study from Yaoundé, Cameroon. Int J Dermatol. 2019;58(10):1135-40.
16. Lu W-S, Wang J-F, Yang S, Xiao FL, Quan C, Cheng H, et al. Association of HLA-DQA1 and DQB1 alleles with keloids in Chinese Hans. J Dermatol Sci. 2008;52(2):108-117.
17. Brown JJ, Ollier WER, Thomson W, Bayat A. Positive association of HLA-DRB1*15 with keloid disease in Caucasians. Int J Immunogenet. 2008;35(4-5):303-7.
18. Halim AS, Emami A, Salahshourifar I, Kannan TP. Keloid scarring: understanding the genetic basis, advances, and prospects. Arch Plast Surg. 2012;39(3):184-9.
19. Ghatnatti V, Sarma D, Saikia U. Enlarged hands and feet—Not always acromegaly. Indian J Endocrinol Metab. 2012;16(Suppl 2):S318-20.
20. Wang P-H, Huang B-S, Horng H-C, Yeh C-C, Chen Y-J. Wound healing. J Chin Med Assoc. 2018;81(2):94-101.

21. Betarbet U, Blalock TW. Keloids: a review of etiology, prevention, and treatment. J Clin Aesthet Dermatol. 2020; 13(2):33-43.
22. Fong EP, Chye LT, Tan WTL. Keloids: Time to dispel the myths? Plast Reconst Surg. 1999;104(4):1199-202.
23. Fong EP, Bay BH. Keloids—the sebum hypothesis revisited. Medical Hypotheses. 2002;58(4):264-9.
24. Coop CA, Schaefer S, England RW. Extensive Keloid Formation and Progression After Each Vaccination. Hum Vaccin. 2007;3(4):127-9.
25. Kischer CW, Shetlar MR, Chvapil M. Hypertrophic scars and keloids: a review and new concept concerning their origin. Scan Electron Microsc. 1982;(Pt 4):1699-713.
26. Kischer CW. The microvessels in hypertrophic scars, keloids and related lesions: a review. J Submicrosc Cytol Pathol. 1992;24(2):281-96.
27. Ma X, Chen J, Xu B, Long X, Qin H, Zhao RC, et al. Keloid-derived keratinocytes acquire a fibroblast-like appearance and an enhanced invasive capacity in a hypoxic microenvironment in vitro. Int J Mol Med. 2015;35(5): 1246-56.
28. Akaishi S, Akimoto M, Ogawa R, Hyakusoku H. The relationship between keloid growth pattern and stretching tension: visual analysis using the finite element method. Ann Plast Surg. 2008;60(4):445-51.
29. Viera MH, Amini S, Konda S, Berman B. Do postsurgical interventions optimize ultimate scar cosmesis. G Ital Dermatol Venereol. 2009;144(3):243-57.
30. Park TH, Chang CH. Keloid Recurrence in Pregnancy. Aesth Plast Surg. 2012;36(5):1271-2.
31. Kim H-D, Hwang S-M, Lim K-R, Jung Y-H, Ahn S-M, Kim Song J. Recurrent Auricular Keloids during Pregnancy. Arch Plast Surg. 2013;40(1):70.
32. Schierle HP, Scholz D, Lemperle G. Elevated levels of testosterone receptors in keloid tissue: an experimental investigation. Plast Reconstr Surg. 1997;100(2):390-5.
33. Louw L. Keloids in rural black South Africans. Part 1: general overview and essential fatty acid hypotheses for keloid formation and prevention. Prostaglandins Leukot Essent Fatty Acids. 2000;63(5):237-45.
34. Louw L, Dannhauser A. Keloids in rural black South Africans Part 2: dietary fatty acid intake and total phospholipid fatty acid profile in the blood of keloid patients. Prostaglandins Leukot Essent Fatty Acids. 2000;63(5): 247-53.
35. Louw L. Keloids in rural black South Africans. Part 3: a lipid model for the prevention and treatment of keloid formations. Prostaglandins Leukot Essent Fatty Acids. 2000;63(5):255-62.
36. Ramos MLC, Gragnani A, Ferreira LM. Is there an ideal animal model to study hypertrophic scarring? J Burn Care Res. 2008;29(2):363-8.
37. Robles DT, Moore E, Draznin M, Berg D. Keloids: pathophysiology and management. Dermatol Online J. 2007;13(3):9.
38. Wolfram D, Tzankov A, Pülzl P, Piza-Katzer H. Hypertrophic scars and keloids—a review of their pathophysiology, risk factors, and therapeutic management. Dermatologic Surg. 2009;35(2):171-81.
39. Marneros AG, Krieg T. Keloids—clinical diagnosis, pathogenesis, and treatment options. J Dtsch Dermatol Ges. 2004;2(11):905-13.
40. Khoo YT, Ong CT, Mukhopadhyay A, Han HC, Do DV, Lim IJ, et al. Upregulation of secretory connective tissue growth factor (CTGF) in keratinocyte-fibroblast coculture contributes to keloid pathogenesis. J Cell Physiol. 2006;208(2): 336-43.
41. Whitby DJ, Ferguson MW. Immunohistochemical localization of growth factors in fetal wound healing. Dev Biol. 1991; 147(1):207-15.
42. Haisa M, Okochi H, Grotendorst GR. Elevated levels of PDGF alpha receptors in keloid fibroblasts contribute to an enhanced response to PDGF. J Invest Dermatol. 1994; 103(4):560-3.
43. Chin GS, Liu W, Peled Z, Lee TY, Steinbrech DS, Hsu M, et al. Differential expression of transforming growth factor-beta receptors I and II and activation of Smad 3 in keloid fibroblasts. Plast Reconstr Surg. 2001;108(2):423-9.
44. Sayah DN, Soo C, Shaw WW, Watson J, Messadi D, Longaker MT, et al. Downregulation of apoptosis-related genes in keloid tissues. J Surg Res. 1999;87(2):209-16.
45. Bayat A, Bock O, Mrowietz U, Ollier WER, Ferguson MWJ. Genetic susceptibility to keloid disease and hypertrophic scarring: transforming growth factor beta1 common polymorphisms and plasma levels. Plast Reconstr Surg. 2003; 111(2):535-43.
46. Bayat A, Bock O, Mrowietz U, Ollier WER, Ferguson MWJ. Genetic susceptibility to keloid disease: transforming growth factor beta receptor gene polymorphisms are not associated with keloid disease. Exp Dermatol. 2004;13(2): 120-4.
47. Bayat A, Bock O, Mrowietz U, Ollier WER, Ferguson MWJ. Genetic susceptibility to keloid disease and transforming growth factor beta 2 polymorphisms. Br J Plast Surg. 2002; 55(4):283-6.
48. Bayat A, Walter JM, Bock O, Mrowietz U, Ollier WER, Ferguson MWJ. Genetic susceptibility to keloid disease: mutation screening of the TGFbeta3 gene. Br J Plast Surg. 2005;58(7):914-21.
49. Zhuo Y, Gao J, Luo S, Weisen Zeng, Zhiqi Hu, Feng Lu, et al. p53 gene codon 72 polymorphism and susceptibility to keloid in Chinese population. Zhongguo Xiu Fu Chong Jian Wai Ke Za Zhi. 2005;19(1):28-30.
50. Shih B, Bayat A. Genetics of keloid scarring. Arch Dermatol Res. 2010;302(5):319-39.
51. Shaheen A, Khaddam J, Kesh F. Risk factors of keloids in Syrians. BMC Dermatol. 2016;16(1):13.
52. Tirgan MH. Neck keloids: evaluation of risk factors and recommendation for keloid staging system. F1000Res. 2016;5:1528.
53. Köse O, Waseem A. Keloids and hypertrophic scars: are they two different sides of the same coin? Dermatol Surg. 2008;34(3):336-46.
54. Gauglitz GG, Korting HC, Pavicic T, Ruzicka T, Jeschke MG. Hypertrophic scarring and keloids: pathomechanisms and current and emerging treatment strategies. Mol Med. 2011;17(1-2):113-25.
55. Koley S, Saoji V, Salodkar A. Unusual formation of keloids after each episode of recurrent herpes zoster in an HIV positive patient. Indian J Sex Transm Dis AIDS. 2009;30(2): 109-11.
56. Xie L-H, Li S-K, Li Q. Combined treatment of penile keloid: a troublesome complication after circumcision. Asian J Androl. 2013;15(4):575-6.
57. Shrotriya R, Thorat T, Puri V, Kulkarni S. Labial keloid: rare presentation of a common malady. Indian J Burns 2015;23: 92-3.

58. Chawla B, Agarwal A, Kashyap S, Tandon R. Diagnosis and management of corneal keloid. Clin Exp Ophthalmol. 2007;35(9):855-7.
59. Jung JJ, Wojno TH, Grossniklaus HE. Giant corneal keloid: case report and review of the literature. Cornea. 2010;29(12): 1455-8.
60. Park TH, Seo SW, Kim JK, Chang CH. Earlobe keloids: classification according to gross morphology determines proper surgical approach. Dermatol Surg. 2012;38(3):406-12.
61. Bayat A, Arscott G, Ollier WER, Ferguson MWJ, Mc Grouther DA. Description of site-specific morphology of keloid phenotypes in an Afrocaribbean population. Br J Plast Surg. 2004;57(2):122-33.
62. Lee S-S, Yosipovitch G, Chan Y-H, Goh C-L. Pruritus, pain, and small nerve fiber function in keloids: a controlled study. J Am Acad Dermatol. 2004;51(6):1002-6.
63. Goder M, Kornhaber R, Bordoni D, Winkler E, Haik J, Tessone A. Cutaneous basal cell carcinoma arising within a keloid scar: a case report. Onco Targets Ther. 2016;9:4793-6.
64. Olaitan PB. Keloids: assessment of effects and psychosocial-impacts on subjects in a black African population. Indian J Dermatol Venereol Leprol. 2009;75(4):368-72.
65. Gulamhuseinwala N, Mackey S, Meagher P, Powell B. Should excised keloid scars be sent for routine histologic analysis? Ann Plast Surg. 2008;60(2):186-7.
66. Ogawa R, Akaishi S, Hyakusoku H. Differential and exclusive diagnosis of diseases that resemble keloids and hypertrophic scars. Ann Plast Surg. 2009;62(6):660-4.
67. Jumper N, Paus R, Bayat A. Functional histopathology of keloid disease. Histol Histopathol. 2015;30(9):1033-57.
68. Lee JY-Y, Yang C-C, Chao S-C, Wong T-W. Histopathological differential diagnosis of keloid and hypertrophic scar. Am J Dermatopathol. 2004;26(5):379-84.
69. Linares HA, Kischer CW, Dobrkovsky M, Larson DL. The histiotypic organization of the hypertrophic scar in humans. J Invest Dermatol. 1972;59(4):323-31.
70. Chuangsuwanich A, Gunjittisomram S. The efficacy of 5% imiquimod cream in the prevention of recurrence of excised keloids. J Med Assoc Thai. 2007;90(7):1363-7.
71. Mustoe TA, Cooter RD, Gold MH, Richard Hobbs FD, Ramelet AA, Shakespeare PG, et al. International clinical recommendations on scar management. Plast Reconstr Surg. 2002;110(2):560-71.
72. Leventhal D, Furr M, Reiter D. Treatment of keloids and hypertrophic scars: a meta-analysis and review of the literature. Arch Facial Plast Surg. 2006;8(6):362-8.
73. Brissett AE, Sherris DA. Scar contractures, hypertrophic scars, and keloids. Facial Plast Surg. 2001;17(4):263-72.
74. Atiyeh BS. Nonsurgical management of hypertrophic scars: evidence-based therapies, standard practices, and emerging methods. Aesthetic Plast Surg. 2007;31(5):468-92.
75. Fredman R, Tenenhaus M. Cushing's syndrome after intralesional triamcinolone acetonide: a systematic review of the literature and multinational survey. Burns. 2013;39(4): 549-57.
76. Mishra S. Safe and less painful injection of triamcenolone acetonide into a keloid—a technique. J Plast Reconstr Aesthet Surg. 2010;63(2):e205.
77. Tosa M, Murakami M, Hyakusoku H. Effect of lidocaine tape on pain during intralesional injection of triamcinolone acetonide for the treatment of keloid. J Nippon Med Sch. 2009;76(1):9-12.
78. Camacho-Martínez FM, Rey ER, Serrano FC, Wagner A. Results of a combination of bleomycin and triamcinolone acetonide in the treatment of keloids and hypertrophic scars. An Bras Dermatol. 2013;88(3):387-94.
79. Jones CD, Guiot L, Samy M, Gorman M, Tehrani H. The Use of chemotherapeutics for the treatment of keloid scars. Dermatol Reports. 2015;7(2):5880.
80. Gupta S, Jangra RS, Gupta S, Mahendra A, Gupta S. Creating a guard with a needle cover to control the depth of intra-lesional injections. J Am Acad Dermatol. 2016;75(2):e67-8.
81. Goyal NN, Gold MH. A novel triple medicine combination injection for the resolution of keloids and hypertrophic scars. J Clin Aesthet Dermatol. 2014;7(11):31-4.
82. Engrav LH, Gottlieb JR, Millard SP, Walkinshaw MD, Heimbach DM, Marvin JA. A comparison of intramarginal and extramarginal excision of hypertrophic burn scars. Plast Reconstr Surg. 1988;81(1):40-5.
83. Lee Y, Minn KW, Baek RM, Hong JJ. A new surgical treatment of keloid: keloid core excision. Ann Plast Surg. 2001;46(2): 135-40.
84. Arno AI, Gauglitz GG, Barret JP, Jeschke MG. Up-to-date approach to manage keloids and hypertrophic scars: a useful guide. Burns. 2014;40(7):1255-66.
85. Mutalik S. Treatment of keloids and hypertrophic scars. Indian J Dermatol Venereol Leprol. 2005;71(1):3-8.
86. Walliczek U, Engel S, Weiss C, Aderhold C, Lippert C, Wenzel A, et al. Clinical outcome and quality of life after a multimodal therapy approach to ear keloids. JAMA Facial Plast Surg. 2015;17(5):333-9.
87. Mourad B, Elfar N, Elsheikh S. Spray versus intralesional cryotherapy for keloids. J Dermatolog Treat. 2016;27(3):264-9.
88. Gupta S, Kumar B. Intralesional cryosurgery using lumbar puncture and/or hypodermic needles for large, bulky, recalcitrant keloids. Int J Dermatol. 2001;40(5):349-53.
89. Har-Shai Y, Dujovny E, Rohde E, Zouboulis CC. Effect of skin surface temperature on skin pigmentation during contact and intralesional cryosurgery of keloids. J Eur Acad Dermatol Venereol. 2007;21(2):191-8.
90. van Leeuwen MCE, van der Wal MBA, Bulstra AJ, Galindo-Garre F, Molier J, van Zuijlen PPM, et al. Intralesional cryotherapy for treatment of keloid scars: a prospective study. Plast Reconstr Surg. 2015;135(2):580-9.
91. Har-Shai Y, Amar M, Sabo E. Intralesional cryotherapy for enhancing the involution of hypertrophic scars and keloids. Plast Reconstr Surg. 2003;111(6):1841-52.
92. Wang X, Wu X, Liu K, Xia L, Lin X, Liu W, et al. Topical cryoanesthesia for the relief of pain caused by steroid injections used to treat hypertrophic scars and keloids. Medicine (Baltimore). 2017;96(43):e8353.
93. Zouboulis CC, Blume U, Büttner P, Orfanos CE. Outcomes of cryosurgery in keloids and hypertrophic scars. A prospective consecutive trial of case series. Arch Dermatol. 1993; 129(9):1146-51.
94. Rusciani L, Paradisi A, Alfano C, Chiummariello S, Rusciani A. Cryotherapy in the treatment of keloids. J Drugs Dermatol. 2006;5(7):591-5.
95. Alster TS, Williams CM. Treatment of keloid sternotomy scars with 585 nm flashlamp-pumped pulsed-dye laser. Lancet. 1995;345(8959):1198-200.
96. Kuo Y-R, Wu W-S, Jeng S-F, Huang H-C, Yang KD, Sacks JM, et al. Activation of ERK and p38 kinase mediated keloid fibroblast apoptosis after flashlamp pulsed-dye laser treatment. Lasers Surg Med. 2005;36(1):31-7.
97. Bettinger DA, Yager DR, Diegelmann RF, Cohen IK. The effect of TGF-beta on keloid fibroblast proliferation and collagen synthesis. Plast Reconstr Surg. 1996;98(5):827-33.

98. Apfelberg DB, Maser MR, White DN, Lash H. Failure of carbon dioxide laser excision of keloids. Lasers Surg Med. 1989;9(4):382-8.
99. Norris JE. The effect of carbon dioxide laser surgery on the recurrence of keloids. Plast Reconstr Surg. 1991;87(1):44-9.
100. Ang C-C, Tay Y-K, Kwok C. Retrospective analysis of earlobe keloids treated with the carbon dioxide laser ablation or cold steel debulking surgery. J Cosmet Laser Ther. 2013;15(5): 271-3.
101. Nicoletti G, De Francesco F, Mele CM, Chiara Cataldo, Roberto Grella, Sergio Brongo, et al. Clinical and histologic effects from CO_2 laser treatment of keloids. Lasers Med Sci. 2013;28(3):957-64.
102. Scrimali L, Lomeo G, Nolfo C, Pompili G, Tamburino S, Catalani A, et al. Treatment of hypertrophic scars and keloids with a fractional CO_2 laser: a personal experience. J Cosmet Laser Ther. 2010;12(5):218-21.
103. Al-Mohamady Ael-S, Ibrahim SM, Muhammad MM. Pulsed dye laser versus long-pulsed Nd:YAG laser in the treatment of hypertrophic scars and keloid: a comparative randomized split-scar trial. J Cosmet Laser Ther. 2016;18(4):208-12.
104. Rossi A, Lu R, Frey MK, Kubota T, Smith LA, Perez M. The use of the 300 microsecond 1064 nm Nd:YAG laser in the treatment of keloids. J Drugs Dermatol. 2013;12(11):1256-62.
105. Patel PM, Bakus AD, Garden BC, Lai O, Jones VA, Garden JM. Treatment of Pain in Keloids Using Only a Long-Pulsed 1064 nm Nd:YAG Laser. Lasers Surg Med. 2021;53(1):66-9.
106. Alster TS. Improvement of erythematous and hypertrophic scars by the 585-nm flashlamp-pumped pulsed dye laser. Ann Plast Surg. 1994;32(2):186-90.
107. de las Alas JMG, Siripunvarapon AH, Dofitas BL. Pulsed dye laser for the treatment of keloid and hypertrophic scars: a systematic review. Expert Rev Med Devices. 2012;9(6): 641-50.
108. Oosterhoff TCH, Beekman VK, van der List JP, Niessen FB. Laser treatment of specific scar characteristics in hypertrophic scars and keloid: a systematic review. J Plast Reconstr Aesthet Surg. 2021;74(1):48-64.
109. Gaston P, Humzah MD, Quaba AA. The pulsed tuneable dye laser as an aid in the management of postburn scarring. Burns. 1996;22(3):203-5.
110. Alster TS, Lewis AB, Rosenbach A. Laser scar revision: comparison of CO_2 laser vaporization with and without simultaneous pulsed dye laser treatment. Dermatol Surg. 1998;24(12):1299-302.
111. Cheng ET, Nowak KC, Koch RJ. Effect of blended carbon dioxide and erbium:YAG laser energy on preauricular and ear lobule keloid fibroblast secretion of growth factors: a serum-free study. Arch Facial Plast Surg. 2001;3(4):252-7.
112. Cheng ET, Pollard JD, Koch RJ. Effect of blended CO_2 and erbium:YAG laser irradiation on normal and keloid fibroblasts: a serum-free study. J Clin Laser Med Surg. 2003; 21(6):337-43.
113. Soliman M, Etman Y, AbdElhameed A, Elsharaby R, Tawfik A. Comparative Study between Nd-YAG laser, fractional CO_2 Laser, and combined Nd-YAG with fractional CO_2 Laser in the Management of keloid: clinical and molecular Study. J Cosmet Dermatol. 2021;20(4):1124-32.
114. Wang J, Wu J, Xu M, Gao Q, Chen B, Wang F, et al. Combination therapy of refractory keloid with ultrapulse fractional carbon dioxide (CO_2) laser and topical triamcinolone in Asians-long-term prevention of keloid recurrence. Dermatol Ther. 2020;33(6):e14359.
115. Hambleton J, Shakespeare PG, Pratt BJ. The progress of hypertrophic scars monitored by ultrasound measurements of thickness. Burns. 1992;18(4):301-7.
116. Macintyre L, Baird M. Pressure garments for use in the treatment of hypertrophic scars—a review of the problems associated with their use. Burns. 2006;32(1):10-5.
117. Renò F, Sabbatini M, Stella M, Magliacani G, Cannas M. Effect of in vitro mechanical compression on Epilysin (matrix metalloproteinase-28) expression in hypertrophic scars. Wound Repair Regen. 2005;13(3):255-61.
118. Renò F, Grazianetti P, Cannas M. Effects of mechanical compression on hypertrophic scars: prostaglandin E2 release. Burns. 2001;27(3):215-8.
119. Rayner K. The use of pressure therapy to treat hypertrophic scarring. J Wound Care. 2000;9(3):151-3.
120. Puzey G. The use of pressure garments on hypertrophic scars. J Tissue Viability. 2002;12(1):11-5.
121. Macintyre L. Designing pressure garments capable of exerting specific pressures on limbs. Burns. 2007;33(5): 579-86.
122. Leung PC, Ng M. Pressure treatment for hypertrophic scars resulting from burns. Burns. 1980;6(4):244-50.
123. Anzarut A, Olson J, Singh P, Rowe BH, Tredget EE. The effectiveness of pressure garment therapy for the prevention of abnormal scarring after burn injury: a meta-analysis. J Plast Reconstr Aesthet Surg. 2009;62(1):77-84.
124. Niessen FB, Spauwen PH, Robinson PH, Fidler V, Kon M. The use of silicone occlusive sheeting (Sil-K) and silicone occlusive gel (Epiderm) in the prevention of hypertrophic scar formation. Plast Reconstr Surg. 1998;102(6):1962-72.
125. McCarty M. An evaluation of evidence regarding application of silicone gel sheeting for the management of hypertrophic scars and keloids. J Clin Aesthet Dermatol. 2010;3(11): 39-43.
126. de Oliveira GV, Gold MH. Silicone sheets and new gels to treat hypertrophic scars and keloids: a short review. Dermatol Ther. 2020;33(4):e13705.
127. Carney SA, Cason CG, Gowar JP, Stevenson JH, McNee J, Groves AR, et al. Cica-Care gel sheeting in the management of hypertrophic scarring. Burns. 1994;20(2):163-7.
128. Chan KY, Lau CL, Adeeb SM, Somasundaram S, Nasir-Zahari M. A randomized, placebo-controlled, double-blind, prospective clinical trial of silicone gel in prevention of hypertrophic scar development in median sternotomy wound. Plast Reconstr Surg. 2005;116(4):1013-20.
129. Gold MH. A controlled clinical trial of topical silicone gel sheeting in the treatment of hypertrophic scars and keloids. J Am Acad Dermatol. 1994;30(3):506-7.
130. Musgrave MA, Umraw N, Fish JS, Gomez M, Cartotto RC. The effect of silicone gel sheets on perfusion of hypertrophic burn scars. J Burn Care Rehabil. 2002;23(3):208-14.
131. Nikkonen MM, Pitkanen JM, Al-Qattan MM. Problems associated with the use of silicone gel sheeting for hypertrophic scars in the hot climate of Saudi Arabia. Burns. 2001;27(5): 498-501.
132. Van den Kerckhove E, Stappaerts K, Boeckx W, den Hof BV, Monstrey S, der Kelen AV, et al. Silicones in the rehabilitation of burns: a review and overview. Burns. 2001;27(3):205-14.
133. Nor NM, Ismail R, Jamil A, Shah SA, Imran FH. A Randomized, Single-Blind Trial of Clobetasol Propionate 0.05% Cream Under Silicone Dressing Occlusion Versus Intra-Lesional Triamcinolone for Treatment of Keloid. Clin Drug Investig. 2017;37(3):295-301.

134. Pangkanon W, Yenbutra P, Kamanamool N, Tannirandorn A, Udompataikul M. A comparison of the efficacy of silicone gel containing onion extract and aloe vera to silicone gel sheets to prevent postoperative hypertrophic scars and keloids. J Cosmet Dermatol. 2021;20(4):1146-53.
135. Hsu K-C, Luan C-W, Tsai Y-W. Review of Silicone gel sheeting and silicone gel for the prevention of hypertrophic scars and keloids. Wounds. 2017;29(5):154-8.
136. Berman B, Maderal A, Raphael B. Keloids and hypertrophic scars: pathophysiology, classification, and treatment. dermatol surg. 2017;43 (Suppl 1):S3-S18.
137. Berman B, Nestor MS, Gold MH, Goldberg DJ, Weiss ET, Raymond I. A Retrospective Registry Study Evaluating the Long-Term Efficacy and Safety of Superficial Radiation Therapy Following Excision of Keloid Scars. J Clin Aesthet Dermatol. 2020;13(10):12-6.
138. Wen P, Wang T, Zhou Y, Yu Y, Wu C. A retrospective study of hypofractionated radiotherapy for keloids in 100 cases. Sci Rep. 2021;11(1):3598.
139. Miles OJ, Zhou J, Paleri S, Fua T, Ramakrishnan A. Chest keloids: effect of surgical excision and adjuvant radiotherapy on recurrence, a systematic review and meta-analysis. ANZ J Surg. 2021;91(6):1104-9.
140. Ogawa R, Mitsuhashi K, Hyakusoku H, Miyashita T. Postoperative electron-beam irradiation therapy for keloids and hypertrophic scars: retrospective study of 147 cases followed for more than 18 months. Plast Reconstr Surg. 2003;111(2):547-53.
141. Sclafani AP, Gordon L, Chadha M, Romo T. Prevention of earlobe keloid recurrence with postoperative corticosteroid injections versus radiation therapy: a randomized, prospective study and review of the literature. Dermatol Surg. 1996;22(6):569-74.
142. Ogawa R, Miyashita T, Hyakusoku H, Akaishi S, Kuribayashi S, Tateno A. Postoperative radiation protocol for keloids and hypertrophic scars: statistical analysis of 370 sites followed for over 18 months. Ann Plast Surg. 2007;59(6):688-91.
143. Ogawa R, Yoshitatsu S, Yoshida K, Miyashita T. Is radiation therapy for keloids acceptable? The risk of radiation-induced carcinogenesis. Plast Reconstr Surg. 2009;124(4): 1196-201.
144. Asilian A, Darougheh A, Shariati F. New combination of triamcinolone, 5-Fluorouracil, and pulsed-dye laser for treatment of keloid and hypertrophic scars. Dermatol Surg. 2006;32(7):907-15.
145. Ismail SA, Mohammed NHK, Sotohy M, Abou-Taleb DAE. Botulinum toxin type A versus 5-Fluorouracil in treatment of keloid. Arch Dermatol Res. 2021;313(7):549-56.
146. Davison SP, Dayan JH, Clemens MW, Sonni S, Wang A, Crane A. Efficacy of intralesional 5-fluorouracil and triamcinolone in the treatment of keloids. Aesthet Surg J. 2009;29(1):40-6.
147. Darougheh A, Asilian A, Shariati F. Intralesional triamcinolone alone or in combination with 5-fluorouracil for the treatment of keloid and hypertrophic scars. Clin Exp Dermatol. 2009;34(2):219-23.
148. Atiyeh BS, Costagliola M, Hayek SN. Keloid or hypertrophic scar: the controversy: review of the literature. Ann Plast Surg. 2005;54(6):676-80.
149. Yamamoto T. Bleomycin and the skin. Br J Dermatol. 2006;155(5):869-75.
150. Aggarwal H, Saxena A, Lubana PS, Mathur RK, Jain DK. Treatment of keloids and hypertrophic scars using bleom. J Cosmet Dermatol. 2008;7(1):43-9.
151. España A, Solano T, Quintanilla E. Bleomycin in the treatment of keloids and hypertrophic scars by multiple needle punctures. Dermatol Surg. 2001;27(1):23-7.
152. Saray Y, Güleç AT. Treatment of keloids and hypertrophic scars with dermojet injections of bleomycin: a preliminary study. Int J Dermatol. 2005;44(9):777-84.
153. Yeowell HN, Marshall MK, Walker LC, Ha V, Pinnell SR. Regulation of lysyl oxidase mrna in dermal fibroblasts from normal donors and patients with inherited connective tissue disorders. Arch Biochem Biophys. 1994;308(1):299-305.
154. Naeini FF, Najafian J, Ahmadpour K. Bleomycin tattooing as a promising therapeutic modality in large keloids and hypertrophic scars. Dermatol Surg. 2006;32(8):1023-9.
155. Kim WI, Kim S, Cho SW, Cho MK. The efficacy of bleomycin for treating keloid and hypertrophic scar: a systematic review and meta-analysis. J Cosmet Dermatol. 2020;19(12): 3357-66.
156. Berman B, Harrison-Balestra C, Perez OA, Viera M, Villa A, Zell D, et al. Treatment of keloid scars post-shave excision with imiquimod 5% cream: a prospective, double-blind, placebo-controlled pilot study. J Drugs Dermatol. 2009;8(5): 455-8.
157. Malhotra AK, Gupta S, Khaitan BK, Sharma VK. Imiquimod 5% cream for the prevention of recurrence after excision of presternal keloids. Dermatology. 2007;215(1):63-5.
158. Block L, Gosain A, King TW. Emerging Therapies for Scar Prevention. Adv Wound Care (New Rochelle). 2015;4(10): 607-14.
159. Chandawarkar RY, Piorkowski J, Amjad I, Deckers PJ. Combination therapy of a large, recurrent keloid. Dermatol Surg. 2007;33(2):229-35.
160. Klotz T, Munn Z, Aromataris EC, Greenwood JE. Imiquimod to prevent keloid recurrence postexcision: a systematic review and meta-analysis. Wound Repair Regen. 2020;28(1): 145-56.
161. Meshkinpour A, Ghasri P, Pope K, Lyubovitsky JG, Risteli J, Krasieva TB, et al. Treatment of hypertrophic scars and keloids with a radiofrequency device: a study of collagen effects. Lasers Surg Med. 2005;37(5):343-9.
162. Teplyi V, Grebchenko K. The usage of radiofrequency ablation for treatment of keloids and hypertrophic scars. Probl Radiac Med Radiobiol. 2019;24:561-73.
163. Kaushal V, Kumar S, Brar BK, Singh A. Comparative evaluation of therapeutic efficacy and safety of intralesional triamcinolone acetonide injection vs intralesional radiofrequency with intralesional triamcinolone acetonide in treatment of keloids. Dermatol Ther. 2020;33(6):e13919.
164. Yadav S, Gupta S. A simple device for ablation of keloidal tissue and serial deposition of intralesional drugs. J Am Acad Dermatol. 2018;78(5):e107-9.
165. Taneja N, Ahuja R, Gupta S. Modified technique of intralesional radiofrequency with drug deposition in keloids using customized intravenous cannulas. J Am Acad Dermatol. 2023;89(2):e89-90.
166. Xu S, Teng J, Xie J, Shen M, Chen D. Comparison of the mechanisms of intralesional steroid, interferon or verapamil injection in the treatment of proliferative scars. Zhonghua Zheng Xing Wai Ke Za Zhi. 2009;25(1):37-40.
167. Giugliano G, Pasquali D, Notaro A, Brongo S, Nicoletti G, D'Andrea F, et al. Verapamil inhibits interleukin-6 and vascular endothelial growth factor production in primary cultures of keloid fibroblasts. Br J Plast Surg. 2003;56(8): 804-9.

168. Copcu E, Sivrioglu N, Oztan Y. Combination of surgery and intralesional verapamil injection in the treatment of the keloid. J Burn Care Rehabil. 2004;25(1):1-7.
169. Lawrence WT. Treatment of earlobe keloids with surgery plus adjuvant intralesional verapamil and pressure earrings. Ann Plast Surg. 1996;37(2):167-9.
170. D'Andrea F, Brongo S, Ferraro G, Baroni A. Prevention and treatment of keloids with intralesional verapamil. Dermatology. 2002;204(1):60-2.
171. Wang R, Mao Y, Zhang Z, Li Z, Chen J, Cen Y. Role of verapamil in preventing and treating hypertrophic scars and keloids. Int Wound J. 2016;13(4):461-8.
172. Khansa I, Harrison B, Janis JE. Evidence-Based Scar Management: How to improve results with technique and technology. Plast Reconstr Surg. 2016;138(3 Suppl): 165S-78S.
173. Koc E, Arca E, Surucu B, Kurumlu Z. An open, randomized, controlled, comparative study of the combined effect of intralesional triamcinolone acetonide and onion extract gel and intralesional triamcinolone acetonide alone in the treatment of hypertrophic scars and keloids. Dermatol Surg. 2008;34(11):1507-14.
174. Hosnuter M, Payasli C, Isikdemir A, Tekerekoglu B. The effects of onion extract on hypertrophic and keloid scars. J Wound Care. 2007;16(6):251-4.
175. Heppt MV, Breuninger H, Reinholz M, Feller-Heppt G, Ruzicka T, Gauglitz GG. Current strategies in the treatment of scars and keloids. facial plast surg. 2015;31(4):386-95.
176. Austin E, Koo E, Jagdeo J. The cellular response of keloids and hypertrophic scars to botulinum toxin a: a comprehensive literature review. Dermatol Surg. 2018;44(2):149-57.
177. Elhefnawy AM. Assessment of intralesional injection of botulinum toxin type A injection for hypertrophic scars. Indian J Dermatol Venereol Leprol. 2016;82(3):279-83.
178. Shaarawy E, Hegazy RA, Abdel Hay RM. Intralesional botulinum toxin type A equally effective and better tolerated than intralesional steroid in the treatment of keloids: a randomized controlled trial. J Cosmet Dermatol. 2015;14(2): 161-6.
179. Pruksapong C, Yingtaweesittikul S, Burusapat C. Efficacy of botulinum toxin a in preventing recurrence keloids: double blinded randomized controlled trial study: intraindividual subject. J Med Assoc Thai. 2017;100(3):280-6.
180. Bi M, Sun P, Li D, Dong Z, Chen Z. Intralesional injection of botulinum toxin type a compared with intralesional injection of corticosteroid for the treatment of hypertrophic scar and keloid: a systematic review and meta-analysis. Med Sci Monit. 2019;25:2950-8.
181. Fanous A, Bezdjian A, Caglar D, Mlynarek A, Fanous N, Lenhart SF, et al. Treatment of keloid scars with botulinum toxin type a versus triamcinolone in an athymic nude mouse model. Plast Reconstr Surg. 2019;143(3):760-7.
182. Akita S, Akino K, Imaizumi T, Tanaka K, Anraku K, Yano H, et al. The quality of pediatric burn scars is improved by early administration of basic fibroblast growth factor. J Burn Care Res. 2006;27(3):333-8.
183. Rumalla VK, Borah GL. Cytokines, growth factors, and plastic surgery. Plast Reconstr Surg. 2001;108(3):719-33.
184. Border WA, Noble NA. Transforming growth factor beta in tissue fibrosis. N Engl J Med. 1994;331(19):1286-92.
185. Robson MC. Proliferative scarring. Surg Clin North Am. 2003;83(3):557-69.
186. Ferguson MWJ, Duncan J, Bond J, Bush J, Durani P, So K, et al. Prophylactic administration of avotermin for improvement of skin scarring: three double-blind, placebo-controlled, phase I/II studies. Lancet. 2009;373(9671):1264-74.
187. McCollum PT, Bush JA, James G, Mason T, O'Kane S, McCollum C, et al. Randomized phase II clinical trial of avotermin versus placebo for scar improvement. Br J Surg. 2011;98(7):925-34.
188. Tredget EE, Shankowsky HA, Pannu R, Nedelec B, Iwashina T, Ghahary A, et al. Transforming growth factor-beta in thermally injured patients with hypertrophic scars: effects of interferon alpha-2b. Plast Reconstr Surg. 1998;102(5): 1317-28.
189. Berman B, Duncan MR. Short-term keloid treatment in vivo with human interferon alfa-2b results in a selective and persistent normalization of keloidal fibroblast collagen, glycosaminoglycan, and collagenase production in vitro. J Am Acad Dermatol. 1989;21(4 Pt 1):694-702.
190. Lee JH, Kim SE, Lee A-Y. Effects of interferon-alpha2b on keloid treatment with triamcinolone acetonide intralesional injection. Int J Dermatol. 2008;47(2):183-6.
191. Yang GP, Lim IJ, Phan T-T, Lorenz HP, Longaker MT. From scarless fetal wounds to keloids: molecular studies in wound healing. Wound Repair Regen. 2003;11(6):411-18.
192. Kim I, Mogford JE, Witschi C, Nafissi M, Mustoe TA. Inhibition of prolyl 4-hydroxylase reduces scar hypertrophy in a rabbit model of cutaneous scarring. Wound Repair Regen. 2003;11(5):368-72.
193. Sasaki T, Majamaa K, Uitto J. Reduction of collagen production in keloid fibroblast cultures by ethyl-3,4-dihydroxybenzoate. Inhibition of prolyl hydroxylase activity as a mechanism of action. J Biol Chem. 1987;262(19):9397-403.
194. Ju H, Hao J, Zhao S, Dixon IM. Antiproliferative and antifibrotic effects of mimosine on adult cardiac fibroblasts. Biochim Biophys Acta. 1998;1448(1):51-60.
195. Dolynchuk KN, Ziesmann M, Serletti JM. Topical putrescine (Fibrostat) in treatment of hypertrophic scars: phase II study. Plast Reconstr Surg. 1996;97(1):117-23.
196. Suzawa H, Kikuchi S, Arai N, Koda A. The mechanism involved in the inhibitory action of tranilast on collagen biosynthesis of keloid fibroblasts. Jpn J Pharmacol. 1992;60(2):91-6.
197. Sandulache VC, Parekh A, Li-Korotky H, Dohar JE, Hebda PA. Prostaglandin E2 inhibition of keloid fibroblast migration, contraction, and transforming growth factor (TGF)-beta1-induced collagen synthesis. Wound Repair Regen. 2007;15(1):122-33.
198. Viera MH, Amini S, Valins W, Berman B. Innovative therapies in the treatment of keloids and hypertrophic scars. J Clin Aesthet Dermatol. 2010;3(5):20-6.
199. Menezes MCS, Vasconcellos L de S, Nunes CB, Alberti LR. Evaluation of the use of tacrolimus ointment for the prevention of hypertrophic scars in experimental model. An Bras Dermatol. 2019;94(2):164-71.
200. Ong CT, Khoo YT, Mukhopadhyay A, Do DV, Lim IJ, Aalami O, et al. mTOR as a potential therapeutic target for treatment of keloids and excessive scars. Exp Dermatol. 2007;16(5): 394-404.
201. Berman B, Duncan MR. Pentoxifylline inhibits the proliferation of human fibroblasts derived from keloid, scleroderma and morphoea skin and their production of collagen, glycosaminoglycans and fibronectin. Br J Dermatol. 1990; 123(3):339-46.
202. Wong TW, Lee JY, Sheu HM, Chao SC. Relief of pain and itch associated with keloids on treatment with oxpentifylline. Br J Dermatol. 1999;140(4):771-2.

203. Tan A, Martinez Luna O, Glass DA. Pentoxifylline for the prevention of postsurgical keloid recurrence. Dermatol Surg. 2020;46(10):1353-6.
204. Uchida G, Yoshimura K, Kitano Y, Okazaki M, Harii K. Tretinoin reverses upregulation of matrix metalloproteinase-13 in human keloid-derived fibroblasts. Exp Dermatol. 2003; 12(Suppl 2):35-42.
205. Panabiere-Castaings MH. Retinoic acid in the treatment of keloids. J Dermatol Surg Oncol. 1988;14(11):1275-6.
206. Kwon SY, Park SD, Park K. Comparative effect of topical silicone gel and topical tretinoin cream for the prevention of hypertrophic scar and keloid formation and the improvement of scars. J Eur Acad Dermatol Venereol. 2014;28(8): 1025-33.
207. Diaz A, Tan K, He H, Xu H, Cueto I, Pavel AB, et al. Keloid lesions show increased IL-4/IL-13 signaling and respond to Th2-targeting dupilumab therapy. J Eur Acad Dermatol Venereol. 2020;34(4):e161-4.
208. Kang N, Sivakumar B, Sanders R, Nduka C, Gault D. Intralesional injections of collagenase are ineffective in the treatment of keloid and hypertrophic scars. J Plast Reconstr Aesthet Surg. 2006;59(7):693-9.
209. Bae-Harboe Y-SC, Harboe-Schmidt JE, Graber E, Gilchrest BA. Collagenase followed by compression for the treatment of earlobe keloids. Dermatol Surg. 2014;40(5):519-24.
210. Shmoilov AM, Rudenskaya GN, Isaev VA, Baydakov AV, Zhantiev RD, Korsunovskaya OS, et al. A comparative study of collagenase complex and new homogeneous collagenase preparations for scar treatment. J Drug Deliv Sci Technol. 2006;16(4):285-92.
211. Hoffmann A, Hoing JL, Newman M, Simman R. Role of hyaluronic acid treatment in the prevention of keloid scarring. J Am Coll Clin Wound Spec. 2012;4(2):23-31.
212. Borgognoni L, Reali UM. Intralesional hyaluronic acid treatment of pathological scars. Ann Plast Surg. 1997;38(3): 308, 7A.
213. DI Stadio A. Ear Keloid treated with infiltrated non-cross-linked hyaluronic acid and cortisone therapy. In Vivo. 2016; 30(5):695-699.
214. Nakamura H, Gotoh M, Kanazawa T, Ohta K, Nakamura K, Honda H, et al. Effects of corticosteroids and hyaluronic acid on torn rotator cuff tendons in vitro and in rats. J Orthop Res. 2015;33(10):1523-30.
215. Jiang L, Sun J, Wang P. Tripterine emerges as a potential anti-scarring agent in NIH/3T3 cells by repressing ANRIL. Gen Physiol Biophys. 2020;39(4):355-62.
216. Wang C-J, Ko J-Y, Chou W-Y, Cheng J-H, Kuo Y-R. Extracorporeal shockwave therapy for treatment of keloid scars. Wound Repair Regen. 2018;26(1):69-76.
217. Zhang W, Li X, Li X. Efficacy and safety of botulinum toxin type a in preventing postoperative scars and improving the cosmetic appearance of scars: a systematic review and meta-analysis. J Cutan Med Surg. 2020;24(6):608-18.
218. Suwanai H, Watanabe R, Sato M, Odawara M, Matsumura H. Dipeptidyl peptidase-4 inhibitor reduces the risk of developing hypertrophic scars and keloids following median sternotomy in diabetic patients: a nationwide retrospective cohort study using the National Database of Health Insurance Claims of Japan. Plast Reconstr Surg. 2020;146(1): 83-9.

CHAPTER 22

Scar Revision

R Raghunatha Reddy, Shashikumar BM, Savitha AS

KEY MESSAGES

- The final appearance of scar depends on different factors—extent of injury and soft tissue loss, orientation and position of scar, age of the patient genetic factors affecting healing and scar formation, and techniques used in wound closure.
- Patient expectations have to be realistic; there is no perfect scar that can be designed.
- Proper knowledge of anatomic and cosmetic units is important in scar analysis.

INTRODUCTION

Scar formation is an inevitable result of surgery and trauma that results in full thickness epidermal loss. Scars especially those over facial and other exposed sites can be cosmetically, psychologically, and socially disturbing.[1] A preferred scar is one that has matured rapidly without contracture or increase in width or formation of more collagen than is necessary for its strength.[2] It is nearly impossible to have such an ideal scar despite adopting the best surgical technique and utmost wound care. The final appearance of the scar can vary greatly based on the extent of injury and soft tissue loss, orientation and position of the scar, age of the patient, genetic factors affecting healing and scar formation, and techniques used in wound closure.[3] Scars which are wide, raised, depressed, hyperpigmented and those that are against the relaxed skin tension lines (RSTLs) give poor cosmetic results.[1] Successful outcomes of scar revision surgery are reflected in matching the patient's expectations with technical achievability. Scar revision is one of the most commonly requested procedures particularly for the scars over the exposed and cosmetically important areas such as the face. A holistic approach to the patient undergoing scar revision is desirable and requires extensive preoperative assessment including that of patients' psychological state, technical skills and expertise, realistic expectations for achieving satisfactory outcome. As scars will have unique characteristics, therapeutic options should be tailored to the patient's requirements.[2]

DEFINITION

The Oxford English dictionary defines scar as "the trace of a healed wound, sore or burn, a fault or a blemish remaining as a trace of some former condition or resulting from some particular scar." Dorland's medical dictionary defines scar as "mark remaining after the healing of the wound or other morbid process". The lay population refers to scar as an unsightly healed wound. Conversely surgeons tend to think of surgical scar as an expected outcome of violation of the dermis. In etiopathological medical terminology, a scar is defined as "a nonregenerative wound healing as a result of surgery, laceration, burns, chronic wounds, acne, etc."[2]

PATIENT EXPECTATION

Individuals bearing scars deemed functionally or cosmetically undesirable often seek the services of a surgeon to eliminate the scars and to restore the tissue to its pre-injury state. In counseling patients about scar revision, it is important to emphasize that the procedure is designed to trade a poor scar for a better scar. Misconceptions about creating an invisible scar must be corrected.[4] The physician must educate the patient about the nature of scars and scar revision. It is equally important that the physician tries to understand what impact the scar has on the patient within his or her social context or from a functional standpoint. Only then can the physician adequately explore the different options and properly prepare the patient for a realistic outcome.[5]

IDEAL SCAR

An ideal scar is one that is nearly imperceptible and is level with the skin and blends in the RSTLs. Scar appearance can vary greatly due to surgical technique, final orientation of the scar, shape of the scar, and its location on the body.[1] A scar may be deemed cosmetically acceptable depending on its color, width, depth or height, location, and orientation.[5]

SCAR CLASSIFICATION[6]

For scar classification *see* **Table 1**.

FACTORS AFFECTING WOUND HEALING[2,7]

Table 2 showing factors affecting wound healing.

ASSESSMENT OF SCARS

Quantitative and qualitative measurement modalities are needed to effectively evaluate and monitor treatments of scars. Scar assessment is very important for the management and counseling purposes.

Objective Assessment of Scars

Scar-measuring devices should be noninvasive, accurate, reproducible, and easy-to-use to facilitate objective data collection and have clinical utility. Existing devices assess parameters such as pliability, firmness, color, perfusion, thickness, and three-dimensional topography.[8]

- *Pliability:* The pneumatonometer uses pressure to objectively measure skin pliability. It is composed of a sensor, a membrane, and an air-flow system that measures the amount of pressure needed to lock the system.[9] The cutometer is a noninvasive suction device that has been applied to the objective and quantitative measurement of skin elasticity. It measures the viscoelasticity of the skin by analyzing its vertical deformation in response to negative pressure.[10]
- *Firmness:* The durometer applies a vertically directed indentation load on the scar to measure tissue firmness.[11]
- *Color:* Spectrophotometric color analysis to calculate erythema and melanin index.
- *Thickness:* Tissue ultrasound palpation system (TUPS) has been used to quantify scar thickness.[10]
- *Perfusion:* Laser Doppler perfusion imaging is an established technique for the measurement of burn scar perfusion. It aids in early determination of burn depth and subsequent treatment course.[12]
- *Three-dimensional topography:* These can capture scar surface characteristics with high definition and reproducibility.

TABLE 1: Classification of scar.

Mature scar	*A light-colored flat scar*
Immature scar	A red, sometimes itchy or painful, and slightly elevated scar in the process of remodeling. Many of these will mature normally over time
Linear hypertrophic scar	A red, raised, sometimes itchy scar confined to the border of the original incision. These scars may increase in size rapidly for 3–6 months and then, after a static phase, begin to regress. After maturation, they may have an elevated, slightly rope-like appearance with the increased width
Widespread hypertrophic scar	A widespread red, raised, sometimes itchy scar that remains within the borders of the original injury
Minor keloid	A focally raised, itchy scar extending over normal tissue. This may develop up to 1 year after injury and does not regress on its own
Major keloid	A large raised (>0.5 cm) scar, possibly painful or pruritic and extending over normal tissue. This may result from minor trauma and can continue to spread over years

TABLE 2: Factors affecting wound healing.

Systemic factors	*Local factors*
• Malnutrition—protein, vitamin A, vitamin C deficiency • Drugs—steroids, penicillamine, nicotine, NSAIDs, and anticancer drugs • Chronic debilitating illness and infections • Endocrinological disorders • Systemic vascular disorders • Connective tissue disorders	• Poor surgical technique • Vascular disorders—arteriosclerosis, venous insufficiency • Tissue ischemia • Infections • Drugs • Foreign bodies

(NSAIDs: nonsteroidal anti-inflammatory drugs)

Subjective Assessment of Scars

Scar scales have been devised to quantify scar appearance in response to treatment.

- *The Vancouver Scar Scale (VSS):*[13] It is used mainly for burn scars.
- *Patient and Observer Scar Assessment Scale (POSAS):* The POSAS includes subjective symptoms of pain and pruritus and expands on the objective data captured in the VSS.[14]
- *Visual Analog Scale (VAS):* The multi-dimensional VAS is a photograph-based scale derived from evaluating standardized digital photographs in four dimensions (pigmentation, vascularity, acceptability, and observer comfort) plus contour.[15]
- *Manchester Scar Scale (MSS):* The Manchester Scar Scale, proposed by Beausang et al. in 1998, differs from the POSAS in that it includes an overall VAS that is added to the individual attribute scores.[16]
- *Stony Brook Scar Evaluation Scale (SBSES):* This is a six-item ordinal wound evaluation scale developed to measure short-term cosmetic outcome of wounds 5–10 days after injury up to the time of suture removal.[17]

These observer-dependent scales consider factors such as scar height or thickness, pliability, surface area, texture, pigmentation, and vascularity.[8]

TIMING OF THE SCAR REVISION SURGERY[1,2,4,5]

Scars tend to improve spontaneously as they mature. The timing of scar revision has traditionally been in the range of 6–12 months. However, some scars cause enough deformity that they should be considered for scar revision earlier. One rule of thumb is the "plateau phenomenon." That is, if the patient and the physician observe the scar over a 6- to 8-week period and there is no significant improvement, then a decision can be made as to whether scar revision is indicated. Typically, scar revision is not performed before 3 months following the injury. It is important to note resolution of the acute inflammatory changes in the tissues surrounding the scar. The skin should be soft, supple, and non-tender, demonstrating no significant residual erythema, edema, or induration. The necessity and timing of scar revision are a joint decision made by the patient and the physician. One of the roles of the physician is to inform and educate the patient about the available options and level of improvement that can be expected.

SCAR ANALYSIS AND PLANNING

A complete and proper examination of the scar and its surrounding tissue is essential to plan for an appropriate therapeutic modality. A thorough knowledge of vital anatomical structures such as vessels and nerves of significance and the implication of the procedure to the surrounding structures is also important. *"Surgery without the above knowledge and planning is like diving into water without the knowledge of depth".*

Factors which are to be considered are as follows:[7,18]

- *Physical examination:* Anatomical location and its proximity to vital structures, its directions with respect to local RSTL, length, width and shape, its contour (elevated, depressed, atrophic, hypertrophic or keloidal), color (hyper- or hypo- and depigmented), and total number of scars.
- Physical examination of the surrounding tissue is vital since local landmarks may be distorted, e.g., angle of eyes, around the lips, scalp margins. Care should be taken to avoid this complication.
- *Cosmetic units and cosmetic unit junctions* are two most important landmarks to be considered during the scar revision surgeries involving the face. An incision should be restricted to a cosmetic unit without crossing the cosmetic unit junction. The incision and ensuing suture lines and resultant scar should ideally be placed in a cosmetic unit junction wherever possible.
- For scars that are not oriented along the RSTL and are oriented at an angle of 30° or more, scar revision techniques like Z-plasty may be essential to orient the ensuing scar along the direction of RSTL or with a less acute angle.
- Psychological and cosmetic evaluation of the patient is of utmost importance. One must evaluate the patient's expectation which must be realistic and assess the psychological impact of the scar on the patient. If a scar is inducing a disproportionate psychological impact and if the expectation of the patient from the scar revision surgery is higher, it would be wiser to seek psychological assessment and proper counseling before proceeding with scar revision surgery. It should be stressed that *"no scar can ever be made to disappear, but it can only be altered or modified by scar revision procedures."*
- Invariably patients with scars over the face will have greater expectation and seek corrective measures with urgency. However, the results of scar revision surgery are at its best after 3–6 months with massage and other corrective invasive methods. Scar revision surgery should always be discouraged if the patient seeks the same with expectation of immediate results.

Preoperative Planning

As with any procedure, preoperative planning is of critical importance. Photographs should be taken, and the deformity carefully analyzed. There may be several reconstructive options, but after thoughtful planning one should choose the ideal procedure for an individual patient's scar. Appropriate knowledge of the local anatomy is essential to achieve the desired outcome and to avoid undesirable side-effects. Facial landmarks, such as cosmetic units and their junctions, free margins such as eyelids, lips, and nostrils, relation of the scar to the scalp and hairline and orientation of the scar to the RSTL is very essential. Limiting the incision within the cosmetic unit and placing the incision in the cosmetic unit junction are important for achieving satisfactory outcome. One should draw the planned incision lines prior to injecting local anesthesia.

Infiltrate local anesthetic agent such as 1–2% xylocaine with epinephrine 1:1,00,000 to 1:2,00,000 solutions into the mid-dermis at least 10 minutes prior to the procedure to create vasoconstriction and to enhance tissue turgor. This will aid in achieving a bloodless field and maximal anesthesia. If the requirement for the quantity of local anesthetic is more than the safe permissible limit, in such a situation it is ideal to use the tumescent anesthesia. Always identify the RSTLs and mark as well, since their directions over the face can be confusing to the best of the aesthetic surgeons. It is ideal to have a picture depicting RSTLs over the face pasted in the vicinity since the RSTLs run in multiple directions over the face. In a situation where it is difficult to identify RSTLs, one may perform pinch technique or make a punch biopsy and wait for few minutes as the long axis of the punched wound gets oriented along the RSTLs.

Preoperative Preparation

- Proper assessment and analysis of the scar.
- Planning for ideal procedure/surgery, shortlist two or three plans and list on priority.
- Counsel the patient by explaining in detail about the scar, planning. and the possible outcome by explaining the realistic outcome.
- Preoperative photographs of the scar from different angles.

- Obtain a proper history of any relevant illness and the medications the patient is taking, and which may have an influence on the outcome of the surgery.
- Elicit history of allergic reactions to drugs and history of vasovagal syncope.
- Perform appropriate routine investigation, and specific investigations if any required.
- Obtain informed consent for the surgery, anesthesia, and also for changing the plan of surgery on the operating table if the need arises.
- Advice to stop smoking a week before surgery.
- Advice to stop medications, which may interfere with healing and antiplatelets and anticoagulants at least a week prior to the surgery.
- Test dose of medications such as local anesthetic and antibiotics.
- Start appropriate antibiotic prophylaxis.
- Anxiolytics and if required mild sedation may be considered as per the patient assessment.

TECHNIQUES[2,7]

Nonsurgical: Several noninvasive procedures and medications have been described for the enhancement of healing process and to improve the outcome of resultant scar.

- Massage
- Silicone gel or sheeting
- Pressure dressings suitable to the scar and its anatomical location
- Vitamin E and A
- Herbal extract (Allium cepa, madecassol)
- Steroid injections
- Antimitotics
- Laser
- Soft tissue augmentation
- Radiotherapy
- Cryotherapy
- Interferon
- Makeup camouflage
- Electrical stimulation of skin (ESS) for depressed scars

Individually, the above-mentioned procedures and medications do not provide complete and satisfactory results and the available evidence to support their use is sparse. A combination of the above procedures and their appropriate utilization postoperatively can help achieve desirable results.

Topical silicone gel or sheeting has been reported to improve the scar contour, color, and texture.[19] The mechanism of action of silicone on scar improvement is not well understood. One theory is that hydration of subcutaneous tissue may have an effect on fibroblast activity.[19] Another theory postulates that there will be decreased fibroblastic activity due to the negatively charged static-electrical field is created under the silicone.[20] However, silicone gel or sheets have not been shown to be superior to massaging with lubricating gels or oils. Silicone sheets or gels have not been shown microscopically to penetrate the scar tissue to substantiate the therapeutic effect of scar remodeling or prevention of hypertrophic scars or keloids. Gels or self-adhesive sheets should be applied to the wound after suture removal and, ideally, continued for 3 months. The recommendation for silicone gel sheeting is a minimum 12-hour daily wear. The sheet should be snugly fit on the scar, a pressure garment be worn as per the suitability of the site. The heat generated while massaging has been postulated to be responsible for the scar remodeling by enhancing collagen synthesis. In the authors' own observations there was no significant difference with reference to remodeling between massaging with a drop of vegetable oil and that of silicone gel. However massaging along the direction of the scar either with a lubricating gel or oil or silicone gel, starting 2–3 weeks after the suture removal or wound healing twice daily for 30–60 seconds each time have shown to flatten the edges, smoothen the irregularities, remodel the scars faster, and prevents possibilities of hypertrophic scar formation.

Pressure dressing yielding constant pressure has been found useful in scar remodeling and preventing hypertrophic scaring and keloid. Ready to use pressure garments are available in various sizes and are ideal for use over the chest, trunk, and limbs and are particularly useful for post-burns scars.

Hyperpigmented scars can be treated with pigment lightening agents such as hydroquinone, kojic acid, retinoic acid, topical steroids, and alpha-hydroxy acids.[5] Improvement in the pigmentation is an important aspect of management of any scar.

There have been reports of herbal preparations and miscellaneous agents being useful for the above purposes but substantial evidence is lacking.[2]

Hair cover, makeup, and accessories can sometime offer excellent coverage for the scar. Newer makeup lines and techniques have improved and allow for more natural looking and for better coverage. Tattooing also has been used as a permanent camouflage technique that can be useful for hyperpigmented or abnormally pigmented scars especially those which cover a large area or are in an area less amenable to surgical revision.

A number of measures such as intralesional agents, soft tissue fillers, and pulsed dye lasers have been practiced for treating, camouflaging, and remodeling scars. Of these, intralesional injections of triamcinolone acetonide in strength of 10 mg/mL or 40 mg/mL diluted to 20 mg/mL alone or in combination with cryotherapy **(Figs. 1A and B)** have been most widely practiced with satisfactory results for both prevention and treatment of hypertrophic and keloid scars.

Soft tissue augmentation using injectable fillers is very effective for depressed or pitted scars. These agents include bovine collagen (collagen), homologous human collagen

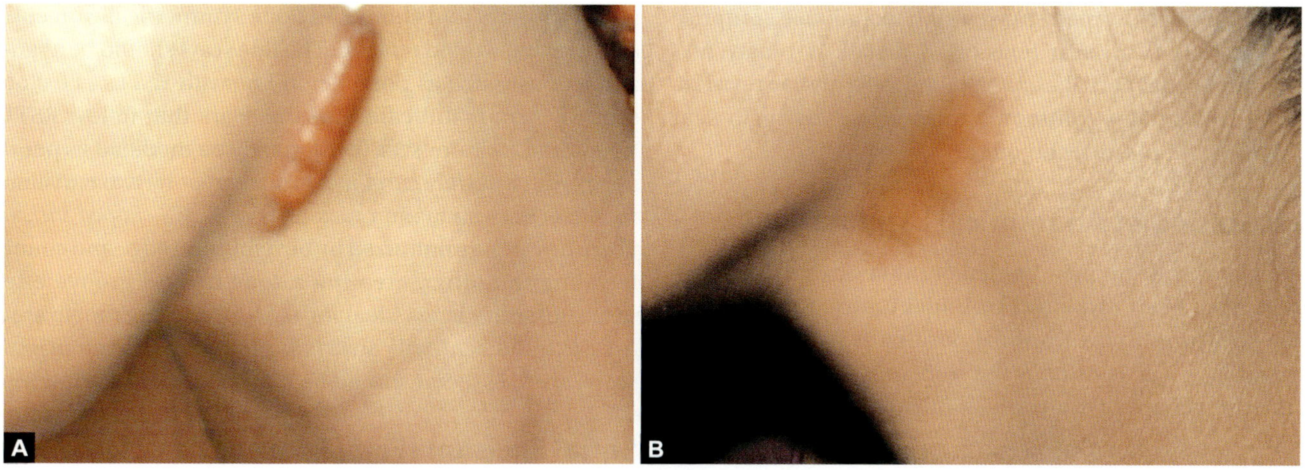

Figs. 1A and B: (A) Hypertrophic scar over the neck, treated with cryotherapy and intralesional steroid. Pretreatment; (B) After single treatment session.

(Dermologen), and autologous fat transplantation. Hyaluronic acid fillers are temporary and have been used successfully with good cosmetic acceptability but the disadvantage being their short-lived results and prohibitive cost. However they can be used with great satisfaction in situations warranting immediate cosmetic improvement of the depressed scars over cosmetically important areas.

MICRONEEDLING THERAPY

Microneedling therapy is also known as collagen induction therapy. The treatment is performed as an office procedure after application of a local anesthetic cream, by means of an instrument known as a dermaroller. A dermaroller is a simple, hand-held instrument consisting of a handle with a cylinder studded all around with fine, stainless steel needles 0.5–2 mm in length. This needle-studded cylinder is rolled on the skin in multiple directions to achieve a therapeutic benefit and hence the name "Dermaroller". These needles cause small pinpoint injuries on the treated skin, which apparently heal within 2–3 days with no posttreatment sequelae. Treatment with dermaroller is performed at 4–8 week intervals and multiple sittings are needed to achieve the desired effect on the skin.

There are certain advantages with dermaroller or microneedling therapy over laser resurfacing; former does not lead to any epidermal injury as is seen with lasers, there is minimal downtime associated with the procedure unlike ablative laser resurfacing and the treatment is far cheaper as compared to lasers. The treatment can be performed in an office setting and does not need any extensive special training or expensive instruments.[21]

Different lasers have been used for the treatment of hypertrophic scar and keloids, but only pulsed dye lasers are proven to be of significant benefit in both reducing the size and prevention of formation of hypertrophic scar and keloid scar. Early and more vascular the lesion, better the results with pulsed dye laser. Various other lasers such as carbon dioxide lasers and Erbium-doped yttrium-aluminum-garnet (Erbium:YAG) lasers have been used with varying success, but their benefits are limited due to the ablative nature and recurrences are common.

SURGICAL METHODS

Meticulous planning, atraumatic surgical technique, careful handling of the tissue, use of appropriate suture materials, and suturing techniques are essential components of surgical scar revision technique. Appropriate surgical instruments like fine needle holder with dissecting scissors, thumb forceps, and surgical hooks do play an important role in the surgical outcome. Accurate skin opposition and eversion should be achieved by giving importance to wound closure in multiple layers like buried intradermal suturing for achieving finely approximated wound edges. Skin opposition can be achieved with either interrupted percutaneous or subcuticular sutures with minimal skin tension to avoid suture indentation marks. Interrupted sutures are recommended as they can be used to correct the irregular wound margins and if a hematoma develops it is possible to drain the hematoma by removing individual sutures as required, whereas this advantage is lacking with continuous intradermal suturing. If intradermal suturing has been done with care with approximation of edges, skin opposition can also be achieved with tissue glues supported by steri-strip adhesive plaster over the intact sutures and to be continued for 3–4 weeks after suture removal. Buried vertical mattress sutures are ideal for wound edge eversion, especially for deep defects.[22] The placement of tension suture in the middle of the wound and then the others at each end allows redundancy to be worked out into the middle.[2] The sutures must be removed at an appropriate time to reduce the risk of permanent suture marks, it varies from 5 to 10 days depending on the site and inversely proportional to the tension on the wound edges.

The routinely formed scar revision techniques comprise fusiform (elliptical) scar revision, Z-plasty, W-plasty, VY-plasty, and serial partial excision with fusiform scar revision, of which the most commonly formed are fusiform scar revision and Z-plasty techniques.

Restoration of Anatomical Landmarks

If an eyebrow, vermillion border, or other anatomical landmarks have been displaced by initial injury, relocation of these structures to their normal position is more important than simple scar revision, even if this results in new scars or the use of flaps or grafts which might result in poor color match.[2]

Direct Excision (Simple Excision) (Figs. 2 to 4)

When possible, completely excise the scar tissue with an elliptical incision and close the wound primarily by advancement of the adjacent normal tissue. Undermining is very important and should be done symmetrically on either side to avoid wound tension. The fine scars should be aligned along or as much as possible; in line with RSTLs.[2] Fusiform scar revision is indicated for the scars that follow RSTLs. If required fusiform scar revision may be modified as per the needs with a *slightly curvilinear incision*[1] or by two curvilinear incisions in continuation making it as *lazy S-shaped incision*. Scarring can be minimized by beveling one edge and counter beveling the other, creating a tongue, and groove effect when sutured, this is ideal for scars over seborrhoeic areas. A re-excised scar will always be longer than the original scars, and this factor should be made clear to the patient.[1]

Serial Excision (Figs. 5A and B)

It is recommended when the scar is too large for a single fusiform excision without excessive tension on the skin closure.[2] It can be carried out in two or more stages as per the requirement related to the size and site of the scar, carries less risk and requires longer interval with minimal care between the stages. Serial partial excision when judicially executed

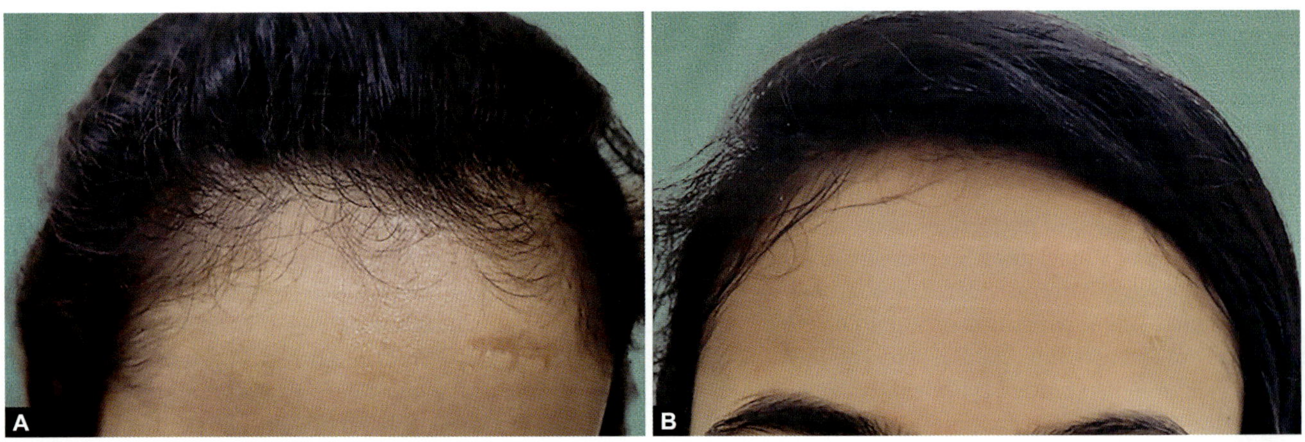

Figs. 2A and B: (A) Post-traumatic scar; (B) 3 months postelliptical excision.

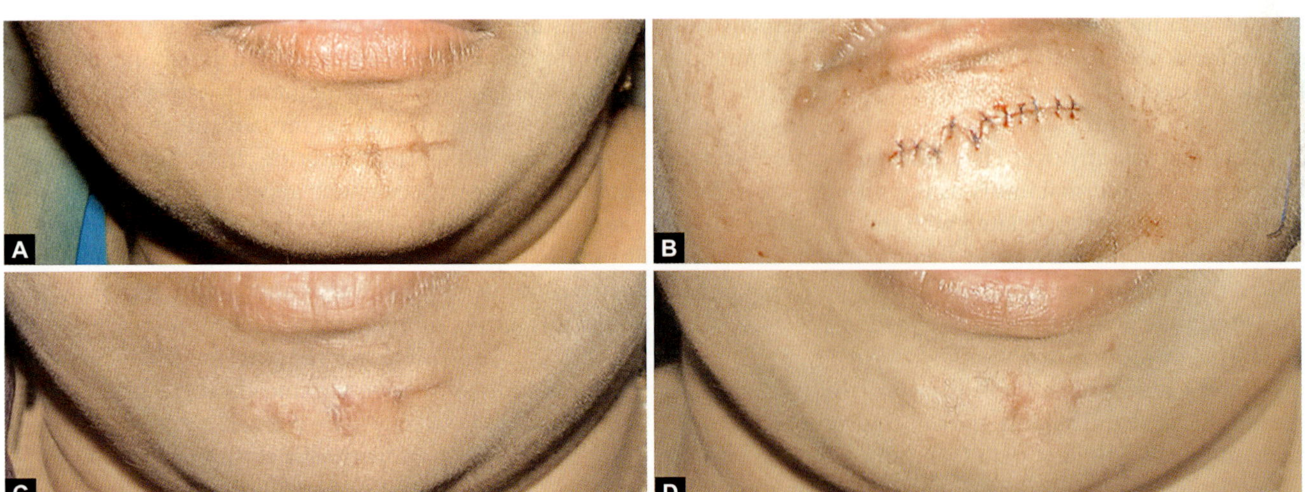

Figs. 3A to D: Scar revision by elliptical excision. (A) Postsurgical scar with suture indentation scars; (B) Elliptical excision with excision of vertical suture indentation scars, immediately after surgery; (C) Three months postsurgery; (D) Six months postsurgery.

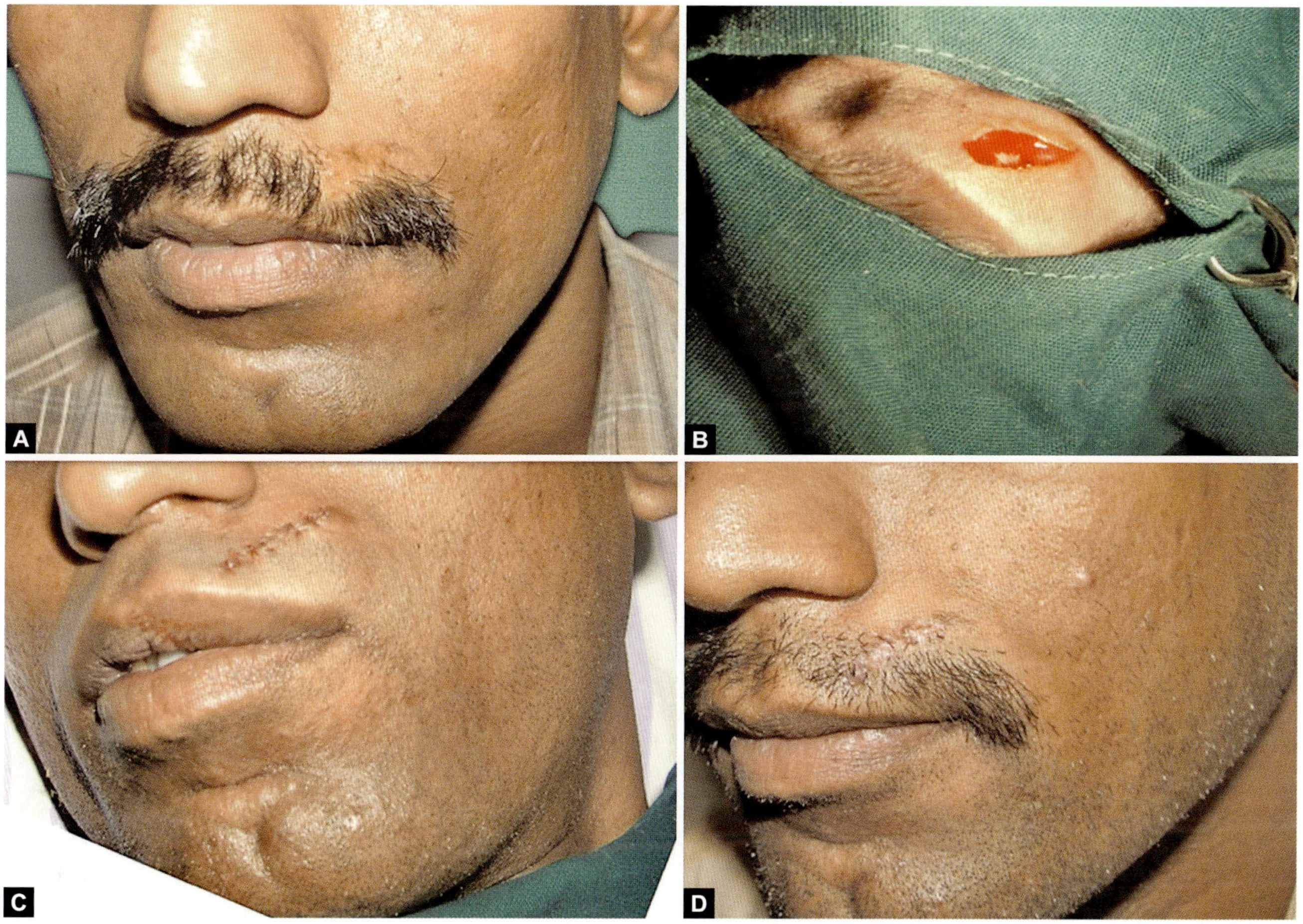

Figs. 4A to D: Scar revision by simple, elliptical excision. (A) Post-traumatic scar with cicatricial alopecia over mustache; (B) Elliptical excision, intraoperative; (C) Immediate postexcision and suturing; (D) Two months postsurgical, reduction in scar size, with few hairs over the scar.

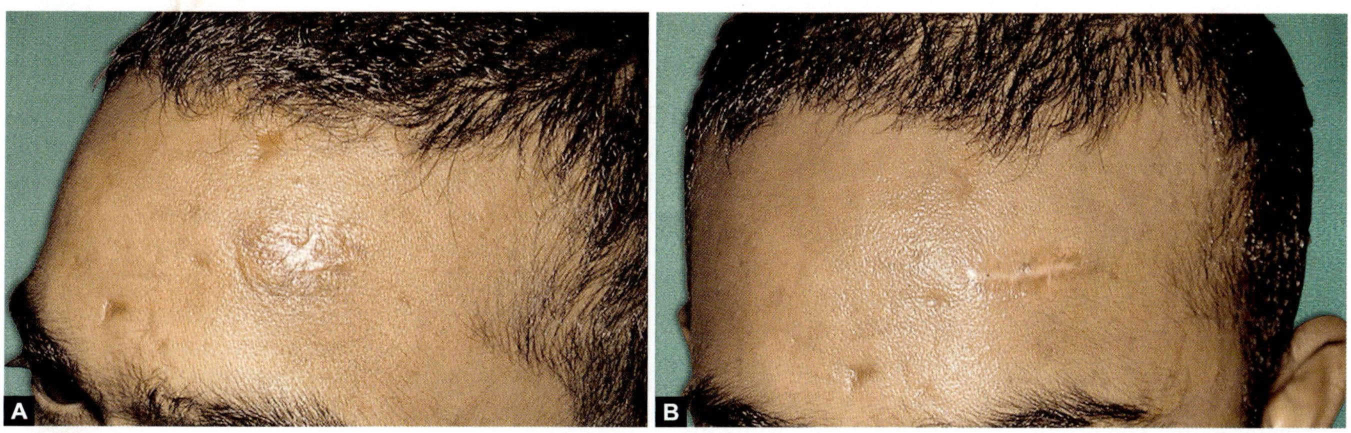

Figs. 5A and B: Scar revision by serial excision. (A) Post-traumatic scar for elliptical excision; (B) Post-traumatic scar 3 months after second session of elliptical excision by serial partial excision.

serves as an alternative to tissue expansion techniques with good results. Both tissue expansion and serial expansion make use of similar biochemical properties of the skin to make greater quantities of normal tissue. Tissue expansion techniques carry higher risks and complication rates. It needs weeks and months between operations, requires multiple visits to the surgeons, induces more discomfort during expansion, prone for infections, and in addition may lead to mechanical failure of the implants. As a result of this and prohibitive cost tissue expansion techniques are not ideal for routine scar revision except for certain sites like larger scars over scalp.

Reorientation Techniques for Scar Revision Surgeries

Z and W-plasties, geometric broken line closure, and VY-plasty are some of the scar revision surgeries which require reorientation of scars.

Optimal scar placement follows skin tension lines. On the face the margins of the cosmetic units (cosmetic unit junctions) generally follow RSTL. Where the orientation of the scar is unfavorable, the principle should be to reorient rather than to simply excise and resuture. The changes in local stress with facial muscle movements result increases making it difficult to assess optimal angle for scar placement over the face, for example labio-mental fold, necessitating to change the plan of action as against the original and an informed consent for the same should be obtained. Despite the expertise, it may be difficult to assess the exact direction of RSTLs over the face and it is advisable to always have a pictorial diagram of facial RSTLs, cosmetic units, and cosmetic unit junctions in the operation theater. In a difficult situation, alternative method is to excise the lesion circumferentially and to wait for few minutes for the defects to get oriented along the RSTLs.[18]

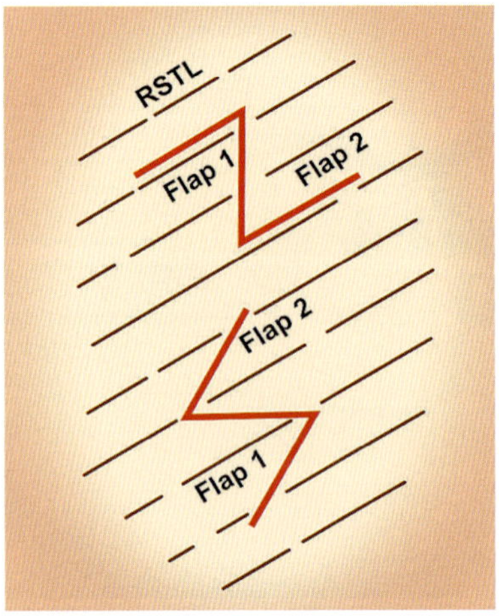

Fig. 6: Schematic diagram of Z-plasty. (RSTL: relaxed skin tension line)

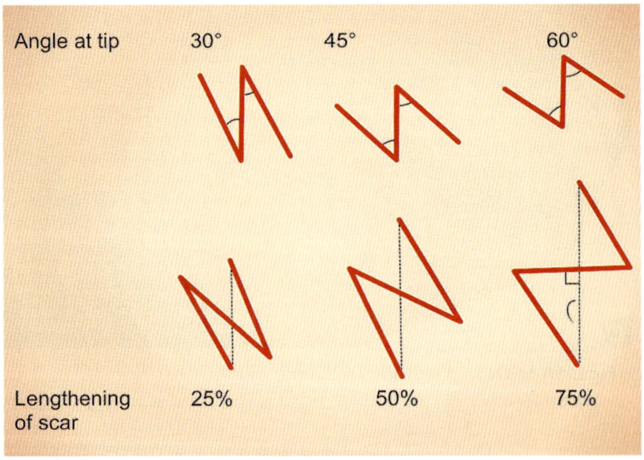

Fig. 7: Schematic representation of lengthening of scar according to the angle of Z-plasty.

Z-plasty

Z-plasty is one of the oldest yet most useful techniques for scar revision. Z-plasty creates irregular lines making the scar less visible. In addition to other benefits, it alters direction of prominent scar placed perpendicular to RSTLs by reorienting parallel to RSTLs. Furthermore, it has the advantage of lengthening a contracted scar which is ideal in situation of visible deformation of free margin, including the eyes, nasal ala, or lip.[1]

In principle, Z-plasty is two zigzag triangular flaps **(Fig. 6)** that are transposed into the shape of a "Z".

Two points in the construction of Z-plasty are critical to its understanding and performance—angle size and length of common diagonal (also referred to as common limb or the common member). The central diagonal refers to the scar, two arms that are of the same length as common diagonal are extended from the ends in opposite directions. The angle of designed triangle determines the degree of tissue lengthening, whereby greater angle results in greater gains. The classic 60° Z-plasty angle results in 90° change in scar direction and 75% gain in tissue length **(Fig. 7)**.

An incision is made along or around the scar and the outlined arms in opposite directions at each end but at the same length as that of the central limb. The skin is widely undermined and the flap is loosened. The tips of the triangular flaps are then transposed to change the direction of the common diagonal into the transverse diagonal **(Figs. 8 to 10)**. Thus a single Z-plasty effectively changes the direction of the scars and lengthens the scars simultaneously and the tension placed across the transverse diagonal critically increases. The resultant scars can be quite noticeable because of large "Z" configuration. 6–10 mm should be the length of the segment designed for Z-plasty. The longer the limbs, lengthier will be the resultant scar, thus diminishing the advantage of scar camouflage. In these cases, multiple Z-plasty has the advantage of better hiding the "Z" shape by using multiple smaller "Z" shapes along the scar lines, as well distributing the tension across the multiple smaller transverse diagonals.[1]

Multiple Z-plasties

Z-plasties can be combined in series to reduce tissue contraction **(Fig. 11)**.

Z-plasties are frequently used to correct contracted or asymmetrical anatomical landmark such as elevated or depressed oral commisure,[1] to reorient scars which are placed perpendicular to the RSTLs, to make the resultant

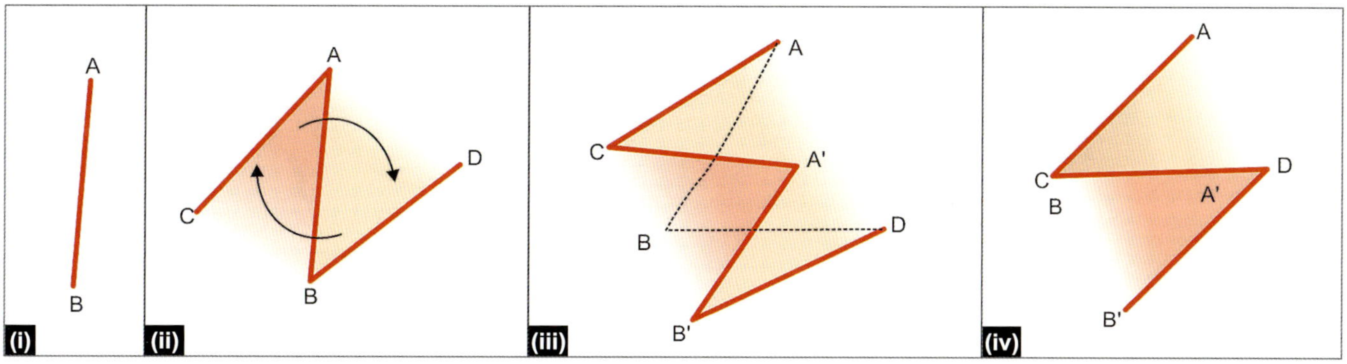

Fig. 8: Schematic representation of steps in Z-plasty. (i) A and B are ends of scar; (ii) AC and BD are two limbs of Z; (iii) CA'B' is flap one which is transposed to form CDB' in iv; (iv) DBA is flap two which is transposed to form DCA in iv.

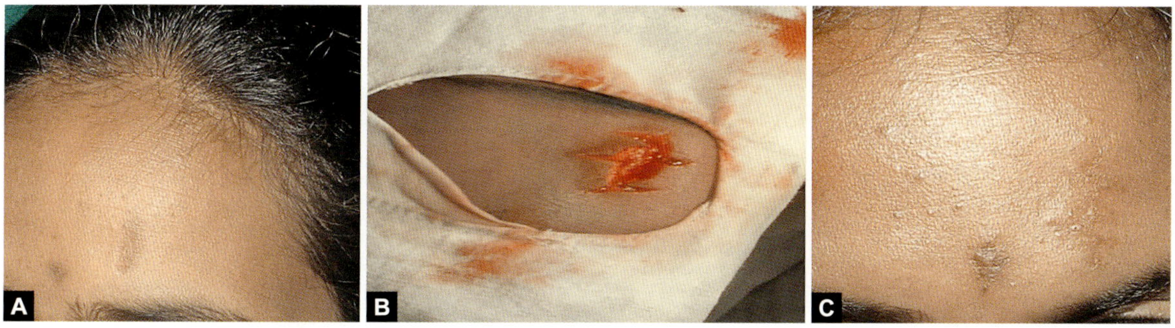

Figs. 9A to C: Z-plasty for vertical forehead scar. (A) Post-traumatic scar over the forehead; (B) Intraoperative, showing limbs of Z-plasty; (C) Postoperative after 3 months of surgery.

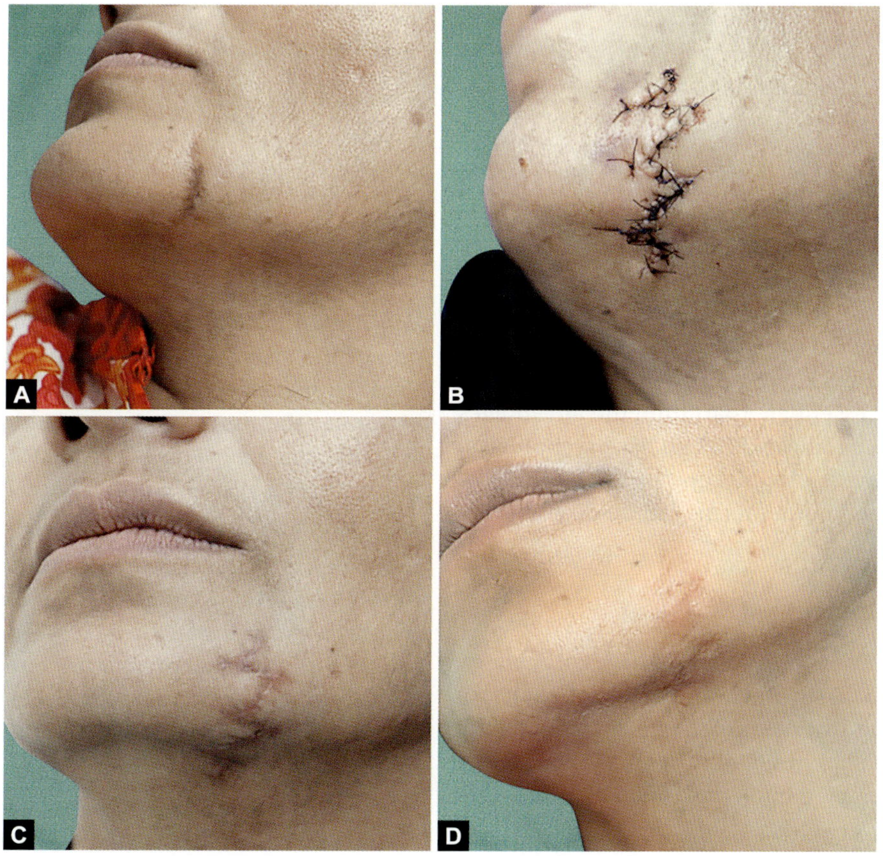

Figs. 10A to D: (A) Post-traumatic scar; (B) Immediate postoperative; (C) 2 weeks after surgery; (D) 3 months after surgery.

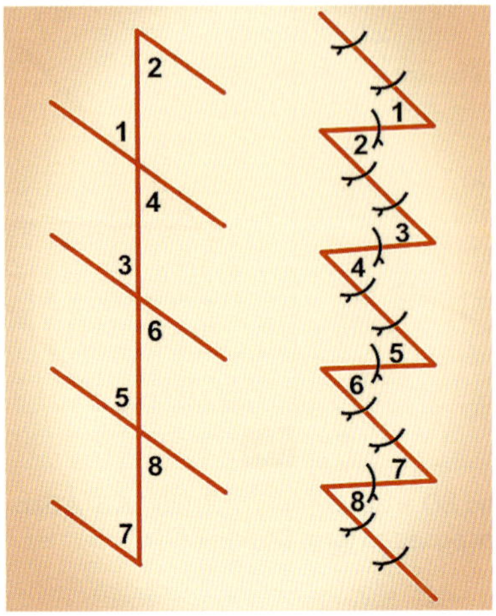

Fig. 11: Schematic diagram of multiple Z-plasties.

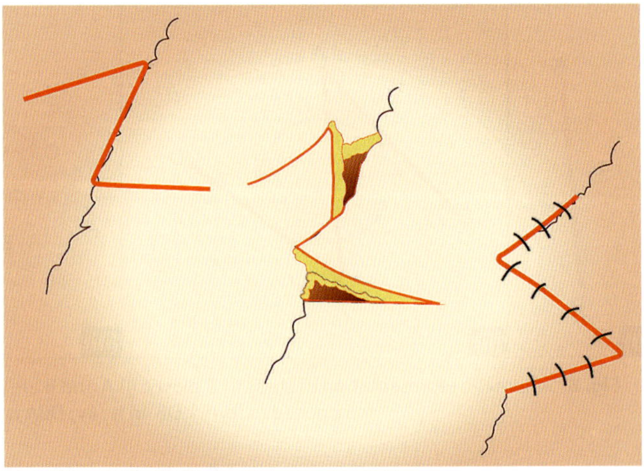

Fig. 13: Unequal triangle Z-plasty.

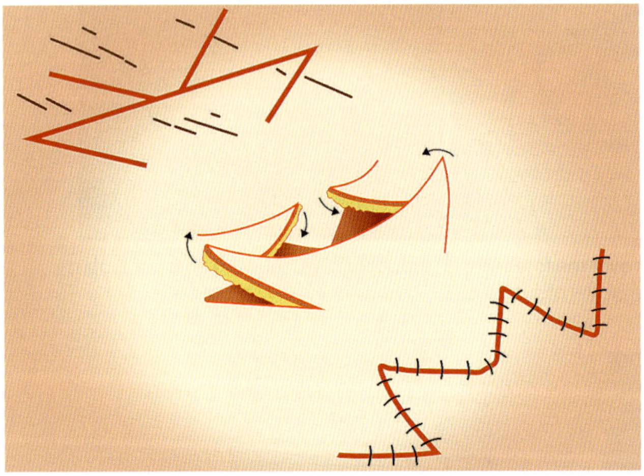

Fig. 12: Double opposing Z-plasty. Mirror images of Z-plasty incisions are drawn back-to-back. The flaps of each Z-plasty are interposed.

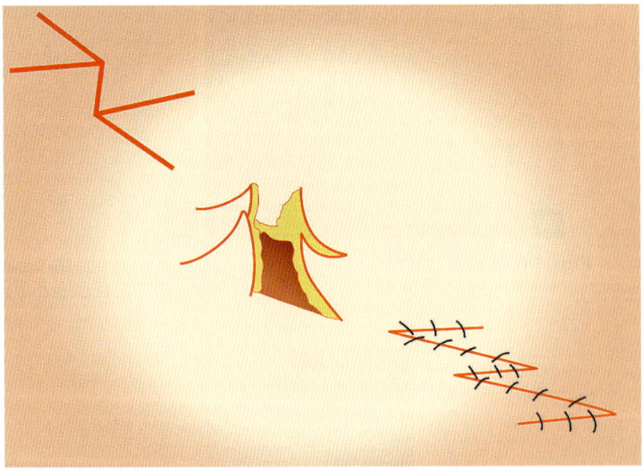

Fig. 14: Four flap Z-plasty.

scar more stronger at places where there are pulling forces on either sides like for example over the angle of the mandible. Z-plasties either single or multiple are practiced in releasing the contracted scars for releasing the contracture at places such as neck, axillae and other such places where movement are essential. Apart from the advantages of reorienting the scar parallel to RSTLs it has psychological advantage of breaking the monotony of appearance of preexisting scar, which in other terms can be described as *cheating the scar.*

Variations in Z-plasty[23]

Double opposing Z-plasties: In this mirror images of Z-plasty, incision are made back-to-back and flaps of each are interposed. It offers the advantage of significant lengthening in areas with limited skin availability such as release of a medial canthal web or scar contracture **(Fig. 12)**.

Unequal triangles (skew Z-plasty): Areas of varying skin elasticity such as the scar edges can be revised using unequal triangular flaps by changing the angle. The limb of "Z" on the less elastic side is kept longer than the other one **(Fig. 13)**.

Half Z-plasty: It is used when the surrounding skin on one side of the scar is elastic and the other side is inelastic. Here the inelastic side is incised to release the scar and a triangular flap from the normal side is transposed to fill the defect created. This is especially useful to release scar contractures at the burn-normal skin interface.

Four flap Z-plasty (Limberg flap): The angles of the "Z" at both ends of the scar are kept 90° and then each flap is subdivided into 45° angled flaps. This four flap Z-plasty gives an advantage of good gain in length and is particularly helpful for releasing severe scar contractures that tether or restrict normal flexion like first webspace contracture and post-burn axillary contractures **(Fig. 14)**.

Planimetric Z-plasty: In this, the central incision of the Z-plasty is extended. Redundant tissue is excised and rotation of tissue is minimized. It is used for scar interruption and elongation of skin on a planer surface **(Figs. 15A to C)**.

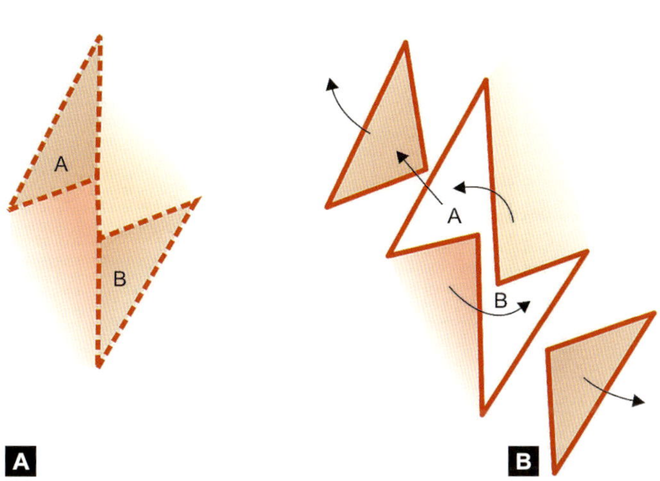

Figs. 15A to C: Planimetric Z-plasty.

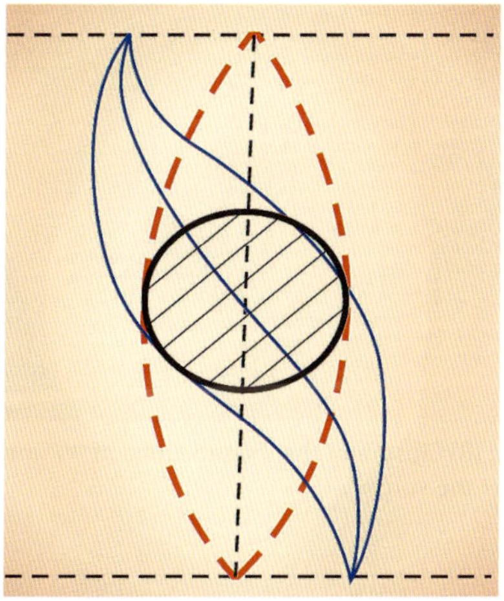

Fig. 16: Schematic S-plasty.

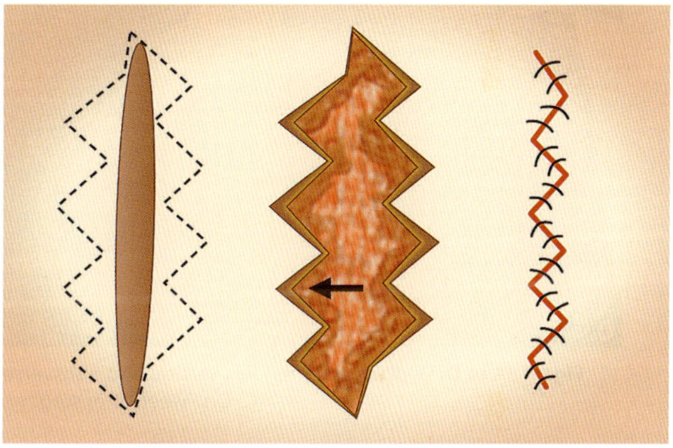

Fig. 17: Schematic diagram of W-plasty.

S-plasty (Fig. 16)

S-plasty is a modification of elliptical excision. It produces a more cosmetically acceptable scar on contour skin lesions and prevents dog ear formation. The S is marked around the lesion to be excised, with the length along the RSTL-like elliptical excision. Compared to elliptical excision the length to width ratio is increased, but the linear distance between the two apices of ellipse is maintained. The wound tension is distributed multidirectionally across the suture line, thus reducing the tension. Clinically it results in a less depressed wound, fewer dog-ear formations and thus better suited for contoured areas.

W-plasty and Geometric Broken Line Closure

Both W-plasty and geometric broken line closure techniques relay on similar principle that an irregular line is less visible then a straight line. This is especially advantageous when the scar is not along the RSTL, and therefore may be more visible. W-plasty is ideally indicated for scars which are perpendicular to RSTLs and those which are longer than 2 cm and located on the face. W-plasty **(Fig. 17)** consists of series of small triangular advancement flaps on either side of the scar.[24] W-plasty is performed by outlining a zig-zag line on one side of the scar and a mirror image of the same on the other side. The tips of the "W" should run parallel to RSTLs as the scar is running perpendicular to it. The scar is excised along the lines then approximated so that the mirror image is coinciding and forms a single zigzag line. The incision is carefully re-approximated by using a combination of dermal three-point tip suture (half buried intradermal suture) and interrupted percutaneous suture **(Figs. 18A to D)**. The advantage of W-plasty is reduced with longer scars because the resultant scar appears monotonous and noticeable. In such a situation, geometric broken line closure is more apt.[1]

Geometric broken line closure is designed to produce a randomly irregular scar. The irregularly irregular scar makes it more difficult for the eye to follow and gives better camouflage than W-plasty. The scar is outlined, another line is drawn at 3–6 mm perimeter around the scar. Random patterns are marked on one side and the mirror image is marked on the other. Each segment is at 3–7 mm, angles should be <30°. The rest of the steps are like those of W-plasty mentioned earlier **(Fig. 19)**.

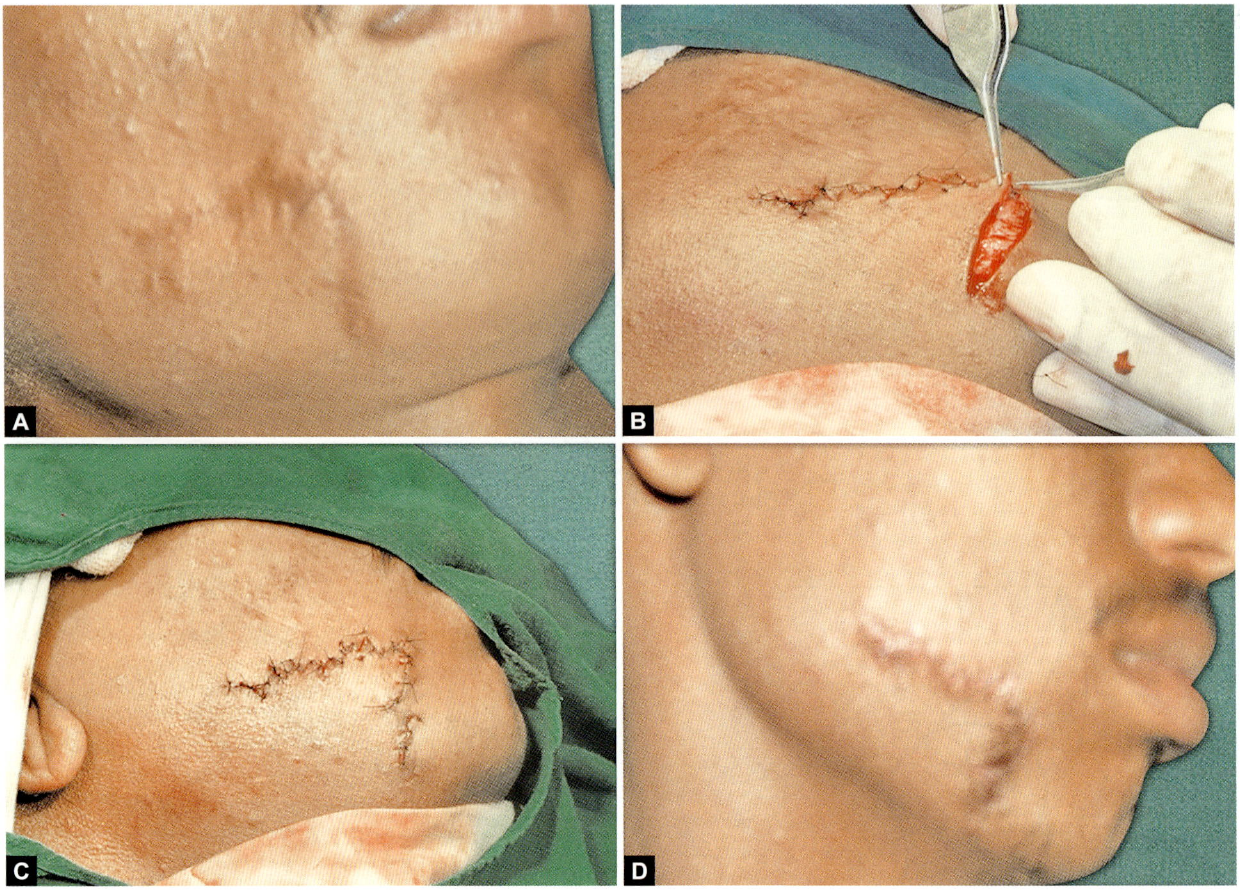

Figs. 18A to D: W-plasty. (A) Irregular, vertical and transverse, post-traumatic scar; (B) Closure of the incised limbs of "W" incision; (C) One week after surgery; (D) Two months after the surgery.

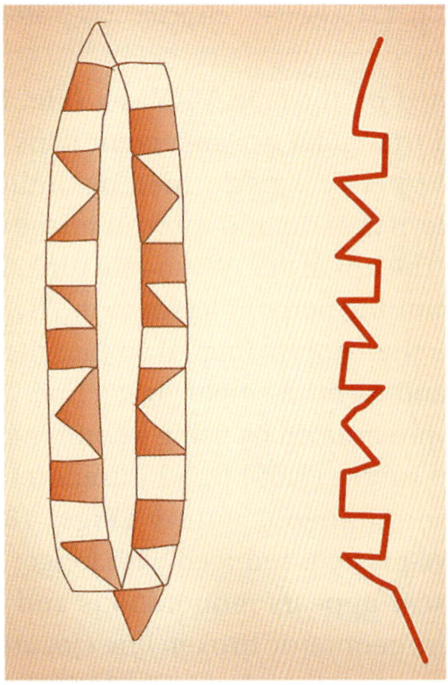

Fig. 19: Schematic representation of geometric broken line closure. The shaded portion is to be excised.

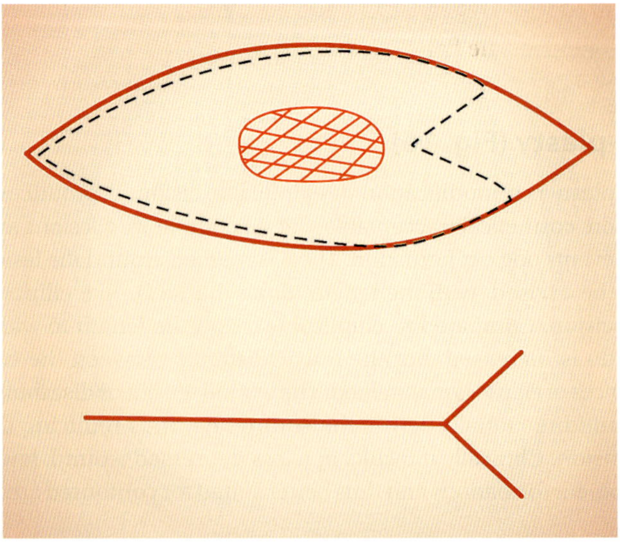

Fig. 20: M-plasty—continuous red line represents marking for elliptical excision; dotted line is marking for M-plasty.

M-plasty (Fig. 20)

M-plasty is modification of elliptical excision, which allows for more shortening of scar line. It can be performed either on one side or both sides of the ellipse considering the aesthetic boundaries. M-plasty also helps to reduce dog ear formation. The apical angle of M is ideally at 30°. Undermining the apex of M is not needed. The defect closure is started at the widest point, usually the middle.

V- to Y-repair and Y- to V-repair

In a situation of scars near the free margins such as around the eyes and mouth causing contracture and leading to ectropion or eclabion, V- to Y-repair is an ideal procedure to lengthen the scar and to relieve the contracture. This technique is ideal for small scars.

The technique involves making a V-shaped incision along the length of the contracted scar. The scar is released by undermining the wound sufficiently and pushing it up away from the incision. The newly created defect is then closed such that the two sides of the defect are brought together to form a straight line along the initial scar line and the resultant suture line resembles the letter Y. Just as the V- to Y-repair can raise an anatomic point, a Y- to V-repair can be used to lower it. The incision is made in a Y-shape and similarly to form a V[1] **(Figs. 21A to C)**.

Jumping Man Procedure[23]

It is a combination of Z-plasty with V-Y advancement described to manage epicanthal fold.

Trap Door Deformity Repair

A mild trapdoor deformity can usually be managed with intralesional steroids administered 4 weeks postoperatively. If the deformity is not corrected by the intralesional steroids, surgical revision may be required. An incision is made along the curvature of the flap to excise the most uneven or spread scar. The incised flap is then reflected back. The under surface is thinned and the base of the defect deepened. The flap can be thinned to a greater extent than it was. The excess flap tissue is trimmed. The wound edges are undermined sufficiently. The flap is then gently draped back and placed slightly inset to the surrounding skin and sutured appropriately.

Dermal Grafts

Autologous dermal grafts are used as fillers in the management of depressed scars. They have a long-term survival and are cost effective. The advantages of dermal graft over other techniques are no allergic reactions as it is autologous, readily available, easily contoured to fit the defect and is firm.

Procedure: The graft is harvested using skin biopsy punches from postauricular area as it relatively lacks appendages. The epidermis and excess fat is trimmed off. The epidermis can also be abraded either manually or using a motor before excision of graft. Subcision is carried out in the recipient area to create a pocket where the graft is placed. The donor graft should be 3–5 mm more than the recipient area dimensions. Trypsinization of the grafts helps in better handling. A method of insertion of dermal grafts for linear scars is railroading technique. Here the excised graft is trimmed to the required dimensions and one end is tied with 3-0 polyglactin 910. A 16-G needle with syringe attached for grip is inserted through one edge of the scar (recipient area). The sharp bevel of the needle exits from the other end of the scar. The needle is kept in the same position and moved side to side within the confines of the scar creating only one tunnel. The free end of the suture material tied to one end of the dermal graft is threaded into the bevel of the needle till the suture's free end exits through the hub of the needle. Sutured end of the dermal graft is at the level of bevel of the needle. The dermal graft is now railroaded through the tunnel till the other edge of the linear scar. Suture at one edge of the scar is cut and the graft is left in place. As only one tunnel is created, the possibility of graft losing track is less and pretrypsinization facilitates easy sliding of the graft in the tunnel. The edges of the scar can be secured with tapes or sutured with 5-0 polypropylene. The lift of the atrophic scar along with decrease in shadow effect can be visualized immediately. The sutures are removed after 5 days.[25]

Role of Botulinum Toxin[26]

Botulinum toxin has been utilized successfully in many facial and extra-facial regions to limit superfluous movement. In addition to botulinum toxin's well-known effect on reducing muscular activity there also appears to be an inhibitory effect of botulinum toxin itself on fibroblasts, thereby, offering another potential mechanism for producing a more satisfactory outcome for problematic scar revision and lesion removal.

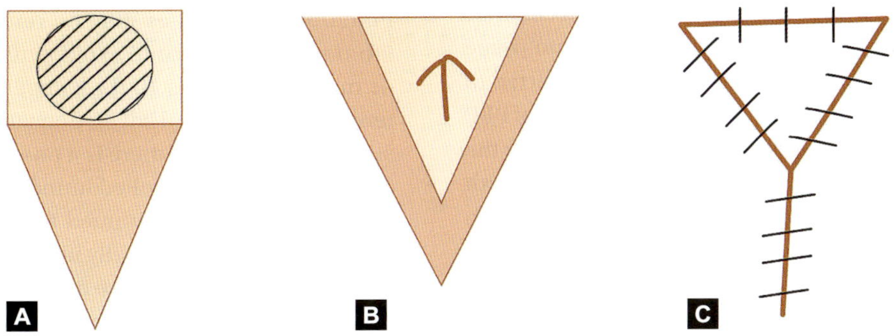

Figs. 21A to C: VY-plasty.

Prevention of Scars

A scar may not naturally conform to the best direction of the relaxed skin tension lines of the face or body. Although excision techniques such as Z- or W-plasty are useful in reorientation of scar direction, they are not always completely effective alternatives and may create extra scarring on the patient. In such situations, botulinum toxin may be used to eliminate the tension produced by muscular forces surrounding the scar. It would probably be the best practice in these circumstances to inject superficially at the time of the procedure or at suture removal and in a low dose.

In an Established Scar

Occasionally, scarring will appear in areas that are amplified by movement. This may be less obvious when one is young. However, as one ages, tissues become less supple and the skin diminishes in thickness allowing the underlying muscular activity to become more apparent as wrinkles and lines. In such areas, botulinum toxin may be employed to the cosmetic advantage of the patient.

Autologous Fat Graft

Adipose tissue has recently been identified as a source of processed lipoaspirate cells or adipose-derived stem cells (ADSCs).[27] Hence, fat grafts may not only serve as fillers, but also improve the quality of aged and scarred skin. Lipofilling with small cannulas (0.7–0.9 mm) is called micrografting. The microfat aspirate is further mechanically emulsified by shifting between two syringes and sieved through a filter to remove connective tissue remnants. This effluent is called nanofat. Nanofat does not contain lots of adipocytes, but the stem cell concentrate is comparable to microfat graft. Nanofat can be combined with microfat injections for scar filling and skin rejuvenation. The fat is harvested from the donor area preferably the thigh, processed and the injected into recipient area. The fat grafts can be combined with platelet-rich plasma (PRP) for better results.[28]

PLATELET-RICH PLASMA

It has been postulated that autologous PRP could be used for the treatment of depressed facial scars, because it can enhance wound healing, which has been shown to accelerate tissue repair.[29] PRP in combination with laser has been reported to work well in depressed scars. The possible mechanism of PRP in the reconstruction of a depressed scar is by promoting the recovery of laser-damaged skin through the numerous growth factors present in PRP, especially platelet-derived growth factor. This growth factor may help stimulate the production of other growth factors important in tissue remodeling, which promote connective tissue healing by upregulating collagen and protein synthesis.[30]

Platelet-rich plasma has been used in combination with microneedling for management of acne scars for better results.[31]

DERMABRASION AND ABLATIVE LASERS

If there are texture abnormalities and irregular elevated wound edges which could not be corrected by massaging for 2–3 months following the surgery, spot dermabrasion is an ideal technique either used alone or in combination with re-excision. Importance should be given to prevent post-inflammatory hyperpigmentation by sun avoidance and with topical depigmenting agents. Dermabrasion can be carried out by a motorized dermabrader with diamond fraises or with a dental micro motor apparatus attached with different shape and sizes of dental burs.

NONABLATIVE LASERS

Nonablative lasers such as long pulsed frequency doubled neodymium-doped yttrium aluminum garnet (Nd:YAG) laser and pulsed dye lasers are useful mainly in hyper-pigmented and hypervascular mature scars. They are effective in eliminating the unsightly vascular and pigmented components of the scar without compromising the integrity of the skin.[32]

POSTOPERATIVE CARE

- Immediate postoperatively look for appropriate hemostasis and possibility of hematoma if any.
- Appropriate and aesthetic dressings play an important role particularly overexposed areas.
- Keep the patient under observation for at least 1 hour or inpatient care may be considered as per the requirement of the individual patient.
- Restricting the mobility of the limb or part may be required, especially if the surgical site is in the vicinity of a joint.
- Appropriate antibiotics and anti-inflammatory drugs to be given for a required duration.
- Inspect the wound to look for any hematoma or early signs of infection and change the dressing ideally on the third postoperative day.
- Percutaneous sutures may be removed as early as the 5th day over the face to avoid suture indentation marks or may be as late as 10 days depending on the site and tension on the wound edges. Consider removal of alternate sutures on 5th day if there is a possibility of dehiscence.
- Steri-strips may be applied immediately following suture removal and to be continued for at least for 3–4 weeks, especially over cosmetically important areas.
- Avoidance of sun exposure and use of screens and other physical modes of sun protection should be advised to prevent postinflammatory hyperpigmentation.

- Mild pressure massage along the long axis of the scar with any lubricating agent like olive or mineral oil, twice or thrice daily for a period of 1–2 minutes each time for up to 1–3 months facilitates flattening of rough edges of the scar. This may also help in preventing hypertrophic scar formation.
- Therapeutic spot dermabrasion may be considered to flatten the edges.
- Procedures like Intralesional steroid injections and topical 5-fluorouracil may be considered in a patient prone to develop keloids and if there is any early indication for the same.
- Follow-up photographs should be taken ideally for at least 6 months postoperative period.

TIPS

For getting best results and pitfalls to be avoided

- Attempt scar revision on a mature scar—since the scars continue to remodel at least wait for 6 months before attempting any kind of surgical intervention.
- Do not attempt scar revision surgery in a patient who expects faster results, the best results of the scar revision surgery are obtained at least after 6 months.
- Counsel the patient thoroughly to make him/her understand possible results with best efforts, and it should be clear that no scar can be made to disappear, but can be made better, with reference to size, shape orientation, color, and anatomical function.
- Plan properly and apply the best possible procedure to the individual patient's requirements.
- Meticulously follow the principle of aesthetic surgery to give best possible results, with reference to marking, the incision, suturing techniques, suture removal, and application of steri-strips after suture removal.
- Informed consent and pre-, intra-, and postoperative photography should be obtained.
- Postoperative care with regular massaging and if required other interventions such as physiotherapy, dermabrasion, intralesional steroids are very essential for the best outcome.
- Do not overpromise the patient, always underpromise and deliver better results.
- Avoid wound infection and other possible causes for delayed wound healing.
- Do not compromise with the standard surgical prerequisites such as sterilization, proper operation theater setup, good instruments, good lighting, assistance, and resuscitation measures.
- Always seek the help of the plastic or aesthetic surgeons when required.

CONCLUSION

- Scars over the exposed and cosmetically important areas are commonly present to dermatologists.
- Scars that cause contractures and limitation of joint movement or cause distortion of vital anatomical structures like eyes, mouth, etc., usually present to plastic and reconstructive surgeons.
- Treatments such as chemical or surgical scar revisions may vary greatly as do the scars and patient characteristics. The treating physician should therefore be well versed in all procedures and should choose the procedure or combination of procedures best suited to the individual scar/patient.
- Examination and physical analysis of the scar, psychological assessment, and thorough counseling of the patient, with assessment of patient expectation are vital before scar revision surgery.
- Patients should be informed of the proposed plan and possible deviations from the proposed plan and informed consent should be sought. The patient should understand that *"no scar can ever made to disappear but can be significantly modified to look better cosmetically and or functionally."*
- Treatment options for scars vary from medical lines of management like trichloroacetic acid (TCA) chemical reconstruction of skin scars (CROSS), phenolization, topical and intralesional steroids to physical modalities like massage, pressure garments, augmentation by dermal fillers like collagen, silicone, fat, etc., to surgical interventions such as elliptical excision, "Z" plasty, "W" plasty, geometric broken line closure, V- to Y- or Y- to V-repair, or excision with either split or full thickness grafts, and complex closures involving flaps.
- Fractional and pixel lasers may play an important role in the treatment of post-acne scars. Scar resurfacing can be achieved with Er:YAG and CO_2 lasers and pulsed dye lasers can improve fresh and vascular scars and keloids.
- Selection of ideal suturing agent, suturing techniques, with removal of sutures at appropriate time and application of *steri-strips* for up to 4 weeks following suture removal and further management with pressure, massage or other interventions like dermabrasion or intralesional treatments all contribute to the final outcome of scar revision surgery.
- All patients seeking scar revision surgery should be explained that the results are not instantaneous and that it may take 6 months to 1 year to achieve best results.

REFERENCES

1. Lee KK, Gorman AK, Swanson NA. Scar revision. In: Robinson JK, Hanke CW, Sengelmann RD, Siegel DM (Eds). Surgery of the Skin: Procedural Dermatology, 1st edition. Philadelphia; Mosby; 2005. pp. 401-10.
2. Parkhouse N, Cubison TCS, Hmzah MD. Scar revision. In: Mathes SJ (Ed). Plastic Surgery, 2nd edition. Philadelphia: Saunders; 2006. pp. 235-67.
3. Kokoska MS, Thomas JR. Scar revision. In: Papel ID (Ed). Facial Plastic and Reconstructive Surgery, 3rd edition. New York: Thieme; 2009. pp. 59-65.
4. Shockley WW. Scar revision techniques. Oper Tech Otolayngol Head Neck Surg. 2011;22(1):84-93.
5. Moran ML. Scar revision: management of facial cutaneous defects. Otolaryngol Clin North Am. 2001;34:767-80.
6. Mustoe TA, Cooter RD, Gold MH, Hobbs FD, Ramelet AA, Shakespeare PG, et al. International clinical recommendations on scar management. Plast Reconstr Surg. 2002; 110(2):560-71.

7. Savant SS. Scar revision. In: Savant SS (Ed). Textbook of Dermatosurgery and Cosmetology, 2nd edition. Mumbai: ASCAD; 2005. pp. 202-7.
8. Fearmonti R, Bond J, Erdmann D, Levinson H. A review of scar scales and scar measuring devices. Eplasty. 2010; 10:e43.
9. Spann K, Mileski WJ, Atiles L, Purdue G, Hunt J. Use of a pneumatonometer in burn scar assessment. J Burn Care Rehabil. 1996;17(6 Pt 1):515-7.
10. Fong S, Hung L, Cheng J. The cutometer and ultrasonography in the assessment of postburn hypertrophic scar: a preliminary study. Burns. 1997;23(1):S12-18.
11. Falanga V, Bucalo B. Use of the durometer to assess skin hardness. J Am Acad Dermatol. 1993;29(1):47-51.
12. Bray R, Forrester K, Leonard C, McArthur R, Tulip J, Lindsay R. Laser Doppler imaging of burn scars: a comparison of wavelength and scanning methods. Burns. 2003; 29:199-206
13. Nedelec B, Shankowsky HA, Tredget EE. Rating the resolving hypertrophic scar: comparison of the Vancouver Scar Scale and scar volume. J Burn Care Rehabil. 2000;21(3): 205-12.
14. Draaijers LJ, Tempelman FR, Botman YA, Tuinebreijer WE, Middelkoop E, Kreis RW, et al. The patient and observer scar assessment scale: a reliable and feasible tool for scar evaluation. Plast Reconstr Surg. 2004;113(7):1960-5; discussion 1966-7.
15. Duncan JA, Bond JS, Mason T, Ludlow A, Cridland P, O'Kane S, et al. Visual analogue scale scoring and ranking: a suitable and sensitive method for assessing scar quality? Plast Reconstr Surg. 2006;118(4):909-18.
16. Beausang E, Floyd H, Dunn KW, Orton CI, Ferguson MW. A new quantitative scale for clinical scar assessment. Plast Reconstr Surg. 1998;102(6):1954-61.
17. Singer AJ, Arora B, Dagum A, Valentine S, Hollander JE. Development and validation of a novel scar evaluation scale. Plast Reconstr Surg. 2007;120(7):1892-7.
18. Borges AF. Relaxed skin tension lines. Dermatol Clin. 1989; 7:169-77.
19. Fulton VE. Silicone gel sheeting for the prevention and management of evolving hypertrophic and keloid scar. Dermatol Surg. 1995;21:947-51.
20. Hirshowitz B, Lindenbaum E, Har-Shai Y, Feitelberg L, Tendler M, Katz D. Static-electric field induction by a silicone cushion for the treatment of hypertrophic and keloid scars. Plast Reconstr Surg. 1998;101:1178-83.
21. Majid I. Microneedling therapy in atrophic facial scars: an objective assessment. J Cutan Aesthet Surg. 2009;2: 26-30.
22. Kaplan B, Potter T, Moy RL. Scar revision. Dermatol Surg. 1997;23:435-42.
23. Garg S, Dahiya N, Gupta S. Surgical scar revision: an overview. J Cutan Aesthet Surg. 2014;7:3-13.
24. Park SS. Scar revision through W-plasty. Fac Plast Surg Clin North Am. 1998;6:157-61.
25. Nirmal B, Somiah S, Sacchidanand SA. Railroading technique of dermal grafting for linear atrophic scarring. J Cutan Aesthet Surg. 2014;7:224-6.
26. Goodman GJ. The use of botulinum toxin as primary or adjunctive treatment for post acne and traumatic scarring. J Cutan Aesthet Surg. 2010;3:90-2.
27. Zuk PA, Zhu M, Mizuno H, Huang J, Futrell JW, Katz AJ, et al. Multilineage cells from human adipose tissue: implications for cell-based therapies. Tissue Eng. 2001;7:211-28.
28. Cervelli V, Nicoli F, Spallone D, Verardi S, Sorge R, Nicoli M, et al. Treatment of traumatic scars using fat grafts mixed with platelet-rich plasma, and resurfacing of skin with the 1540 nm nonablative laser. Clin Exp Dermatol. 2012;37(1): 55-61.
29. Ganio C, Tenewitz FE, Wilson RC, Moyles BG. The treatment of chronic nonhealing wounds using autologous platelet-derived growth factors. J Foot Ankle Surg. 1993;32(3): 263-8.
30. Oh IY, Kim BJ, Kim MN. Depressed facial scars successfully treated with autologous platelet-rich plasma and light-emitting diode phototherapy at 830 nm. Ann Dermatol. 2014; 26(3): 417-8.
31. Chawla S. Split face comparative study of microneedling with PRP versus microneedling with vitamin C in treating atrophic post acne scars. J Cutan Aesthet Surg. 2014;7: 209-12.
32. Cassuto DA, Emanuelli G. Non-ablative scar revision using a long pulsed frequency doubled Nd:YAG laser. J Cosmetic Laser Ther. 2003;5(3-4):135-9.

CHAPTER 23

Flap Surgeries: A Dermatologist's Perspective

Biju Vasudevan, Divya Gorur, Shilpa K

KEY MESSAGES

- Flap surgeries are considered to close large defect where primary closure creates tension.
- Plan in reverse.
- Size of the defect, site, and mobility of surrounding tissue are important factors to be considered while planning for the type of local flap surgery.
- The final lines of closure along the relaxed skin tension line (RSTL) ensure reduced wound tension and better cosmetic outcome.
- A thorough knowledge of the anatomy is essential for optimal outcome and to avoid complications.
- Aseptic precaution, intraoperative hemostasis, and minimal tissue-handling reduce complications.

INTRODUCTION

Closure of a large surgical defect is one of the most challenging hurdles which have to be overcome by any surgeon. The concept of flap surgery evolved to overcome this challenge. The history of flap surgery dates back to 600 BC, when Sushruta performed cheek flaps for nose and earlobe reconstruction. The forehead pedicle flap performed by him is even today referred to as "the Indian flap". During Roman times, Celsus (25 AD) and Oribasius (325–403 AD) described random circulation pedicled flaps and local tissue rearrangements for the lips, nose, ears, and forehead.[1,2]

DEFINITION

A flap is a unit of tissue that is transferred from one site (donor site) to another (recipient site) while maintaining its own blood supply.

The skin color and thickness, tissue composition, location, and subunits involved are the important factors that have to be considered while planning for the flap surgery. All layers absent must be reconstructed to receive optimal functional and aesthetic outcomes. Areas that provide a good source of tissue for recruitment include the forehead, cheek, chin, submenton, and neck.[3,4]

Flaps may range from simple advancements of skin to composite ones made up of different types of tissue. A local cutaneous flap is described as skin and subcutaneous tissue transferred from an area adjacent to the defect and having direct blood supply to cover the primary defect. A composite flap may include skin, muscle, bone, fat, or fascia and is more complex to deliver.

CLASSIFICATION OF FLAPS (FLOWCHART 1)

Flaps are classically categorized based on the following:

- Vascular supply
- Composition
- Method of transfer and design.

Based on blood supply, they are classified as random (no named blood vessel) and axial (named blood vessel) flaps.

Composite flaps include cutaneous, fasciocutaneous, musculocutaneous, and osteomusculocutaneous flaps.

Flaps based on method of transfer and design are:

- *Local:*
  - Rotational flap
  - Advancement flap
  - Transposition flap
- *Distant:*
  - Pedicle flap
  - Free flap.

Flowchart 1: Classification of flaps.

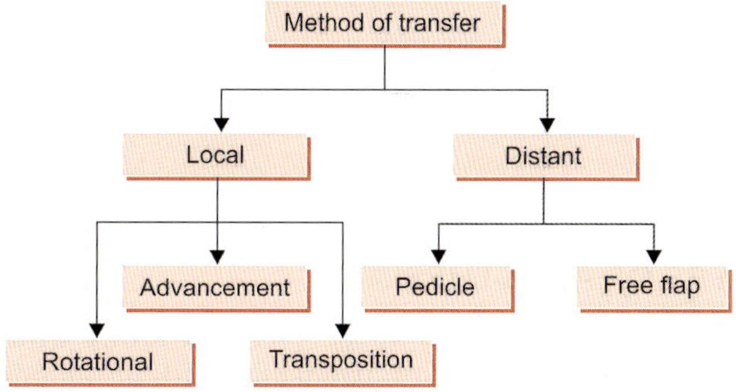

GENERAL PRINCIPLES WHILE PLANNING FOR FLAP SURGERY

- Ideal areas for tissue recruitment should be chosen, based on the size of defect and surrounding tissue mobility.
- Location of the defect is an important factor while designing the type of flap. Important facial landmarks to be considered to avoid distortion are angle of the mouth, philtrum, defects around the eyes, canthi, hairline, nasal ala, and tip of the nose.
- Incision is marked such that the scars rest within the relaxed skin tension lines (RSTLs) and should be closed parallel to the lines of maximal extensibility.[5] Incisions designed along subunit borders will fall within the RSTLs.
- If >50% of the cosmetic subunit is involved then consider resection of entire subunit.
- Ideal borders to camouflage scars include the nasolabial creases, supratarsal creases, mental crease, vermilion borders, and anterior hairline.
- Use of tumescent anesthesia reduces intraoperative bleeding and prolongs the duration of anesthesia, also at the same time increasing the safe upper limit of anesthetic agent, especially when large flaps are planned. A regional nerve block can be considered while operating on a large area.
- Once the defect is created, it is kept hydrated by placing wet saline gauze over the defect.
- Undermining reduces the tension during wound closure. This has to be done in avascular plane.
- A corner stitch is applied in most of the flap surgeries near the tip of flap which is usually angulated to close the defect with the flap tissue, a half-buried horizontal suture (corner suture) is placed, to secure the angled tip to the tissue. The needle enters vertically 5–6 mm away from wound margin; it is then passed horizontally from one side of flap tip to the other, at the level of deep dermis into the tip of flap. The needle exits the skin adjacent to the point of entry.

PREOPERATIVE EVALUATION

History of radiation, smoking, keloidal tendency, immunocompromised state, and diabetes are to be taken; since these factors may increase the risk of complications. Since one of the common indications for flap surgery is carcinoma, usually in elderly population, thorough investigation including complete hemogram, liver and renal function test, chest X-ray, and electrocardiogram (ECG) is essential for such patients, along with fitness certified by a physician.

TYPE OF ANESTHESIA

Most of the local flap surgery can be done under local anesthesia using 1% lignocaine with adrenaline. Sodium bicarbonate in the ratio of 1:4 can be used to reduce the burning sensation.

Tumescent anesthesia gives the added advantage of reduced bleeding and better undermining during the procedure. Nerve blocks also can be utilized while operating on large areas.

The composite flap and axial-pattern flap are complex procedures performed by plastic surgeons. Local flap surgeries are simpler as the tissue is recruited from the area surrounding the defect. These surgeries can be performed by a well-trained dermatosurgeon. Here we have described few simple local flap surgeries which can be done by dermatosurgeons with proper preoperative planning and thorough knowledge of anatomy.

ROTATIONAL FLAP

Indication

Rotation flaps are ideal to close spherical defects on the scalp. Other preferred sites are cheek defects 3–4 cm in diameter and defects <2 cm over lateral forehead and temple.

Technique

Rotational flaps are pivoted around a fixed point at the base of the flap and rotated along an arc toward the defect. Classically, rotation flaps are designed to move along an arc of 30° or less with the radius approximately two to three times the diameter of the defect and the length approximately four to five times the width of the defect **(Figs. 1A to C)**. Most rotational flaps may invariably possess a component of advancement in them and are termed rotation-advancement flaps.[6] Flaps that rotate or transpose around a cutaneous pedicle are restrained by the tethering effect of the base of that tissue. Flap design that fails to adjust for this force may end up with unwanted degrees of tension and/or surrounding tissue displacement.[6]

Variations of Rotation Flap

O-Z reconstruction is a double rotation flap, where two rotation flaps are designed in opposite orientation on both sides of the defect. The two flaps are opposed with a Z-shaped repair. The optimum design for wound closure is an acute angled-flap closure with length four times the radius of the defect. This type of double rotation is especially useful in scalp for recruitment of tissue from different locations. When two or more rotation flaps are designed together, the defect should preferably be located in the center of the scalp.[7]

Variations of O-Z plasty to close large scalp defect are triple rotation, pinwheel flap, and double hatchet flap, which have both rotational and advancement component.[8]

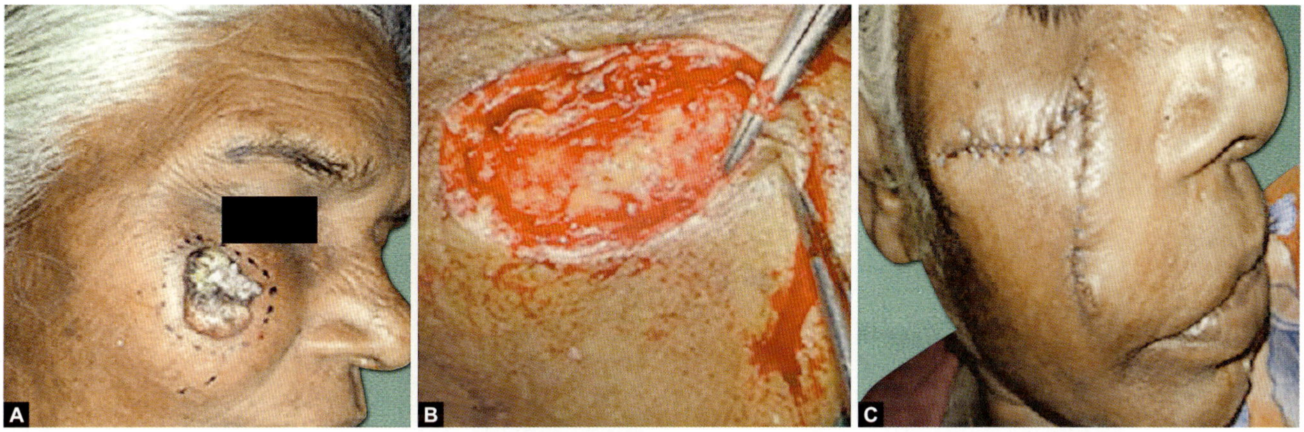

Figs. 1A to C: Classic rotation flap.

TIPS

- The angle of rotation should be 30° to prevent tip necrosis
- Width of the pedicle should be double the size of defect, length of the pedicle three to four times the size of defect
- Scalp incisions should be parallel to the hair shafts to avoid a linear hairless scar. The level of undermining in scalp is the galea aponeurotica

ADVANCEMENT FLAPS

Indications

Defects on forehead, medial cheek, eyebrows, lip margins, lower eyelid, and chin can be closed with this flap technique.

Types

The advancement flap can be following:

- Single pedicle
- Bipedicle which includes the H-plasty, A-T plasty, or V-Y plasty
- Subcutaneous tissue pedicle flap.

Defects on forehead, medial cheek, and eyebrows can be closed by unipedicle flap and H-plasty. O-T and A-T plasty are preferred on forehead, lip margins, lower eyelid, and chin.

Technique

Advancement flaps depend on the advancement of the surrounding tissue along a linear axis to close a defect. It is moved primarily in a straight line from the donor site to the recipient site. No rotational or lateral movement is applied. The advancement of two skin edges from a fusiform skin excision represents the simplest of advancement flap design **(Figs. 2A to D)**. Classically, advancement flaps have a length-to-width ratio of 1:1 or 2:1.[9] The defect can also be closed by a T- or H-plasty, where depending on the size of defect and incision taken, the line of closure will be T- or H-shaped.

Unipedicle Advancement Flap

Unipedicle advancement flaps have single cutaneous pedicle, incision is placed parallel to the defect, with movement of flap being unidirectional toward the defect. Thorough undermining of the flap and surrounding tissue is necessary to allow easy movement of the tissue. The thickness of the flap should be equivalent or proportional to that of the defect, ideally including a thin layer of fat to ensure adequate vascularity. Unipedicle advancement is designed with defect width to flap-width ratio of 1:3, which will ensure adequate flap perfusion.[10,11] Pinch in various directions around the defect to access the tissue reservoir for the flap. If the axis of greatest laxity lies along the short axis of the defect, then an advancement flap is appropriate. The standing cone deformities can be prevented by excising Burrow's triangle.

H-plasty Bipedicle Advancement Flap

H-plasty is a bipedicle advancement flap; here the incision is extended on both sides of the defect and advanced toward each other. Each portion of flap on both sides is responsible for covering a portion of the defect **(Figs. 3A to D)**. The flap length need not be equal on both sides; it can be altered based on elasticity and redundancy of adjacent tissue.[12,13]

A-T Plasty

In A-T plasty, a triangular defect is transformed into a T-shaped scar. Here instead of placing two incisions parallel to the defect, a single incision on the opposing side of defect is made. A standing cutaneous deformity develops at the defect site opposite the two incisions made, which can be excised and closed; the final suture line is in a T configuration. The advantage of this design is that it creates two small defects instead of a single large defect, which may be difficult to harvest in area of limited mobility.

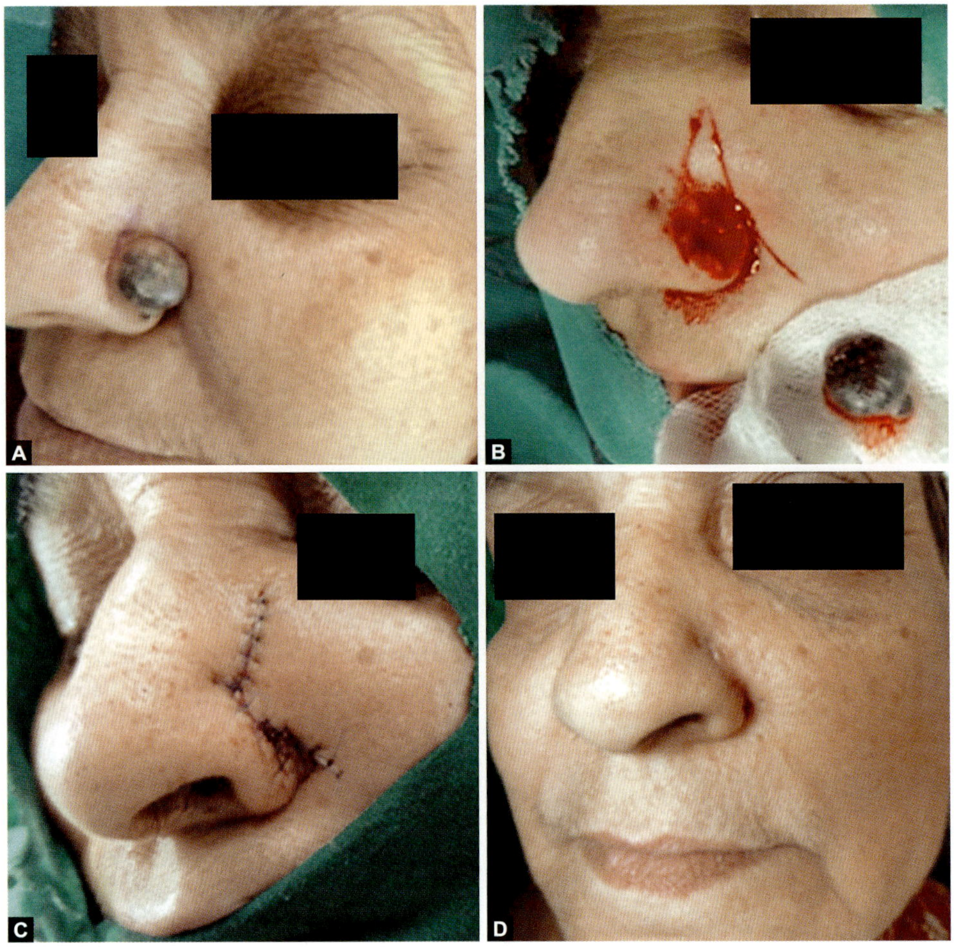

Figs. 2A to D: Advancement flap on the nose.

These flaps can also be performed above the eyebrow, vermilion border of the lip, and eyes.[14-16]

V-Y Plasty

The island pedicle flap is also called as V-Y plasty, owing to its final configuration of closure.[17,18] After the dermal margins are severed, the flap can be advanced as far as the deep pedicle allows **(Figs. 4A to C)**. The flap has a rich vascular supply from underlying vessels, hence chances of necrosis is minimal with this reconstruction. The island pedicle flap can be utilized to close defects on the upper lip and nose-lip-cheek junction.[19-22]

TRANSPOSITION FLAPS

Transposition flaps are versatile flaps whose design creates a second defect. The flap is raised from a donor site and rotated over an incomplete bridge of skin to be placed into the defect site. The donor site must also be closed as part of the design. The three classic transposition flaps include the (1) rhombic flap, (2) bilobed flap, and (3) Z-plasty. The other common configurations of transposition flap are triangle, rectangle, parabola, note, and island flap.

Rhombic Flap

The rhombus flap is a cutaneous random-pattern flap which is dependent on the dermal and subdermal plexus for its survival.

Indications

It is used for reconstruction of the defect on cheek, chin, nose, neck, and small defects on the trunk.

Technique

The classic Limberg flap is used to repair a defect which has a configuration of a rhombus with two opposing 60° angles and another two opposing 120° interior angles. The 60° and 120° rhombus can be taken as two equilateral triangle base to base. The short diagonal of the rhombus is equal to the sides of the rhombus. The flap is designed by extending the line of short diagonal to the length equal to that of diagonal, which is also the length of side of the defect. The majority of wound closure tension is at the donor site and has been calculated to be 20° to the

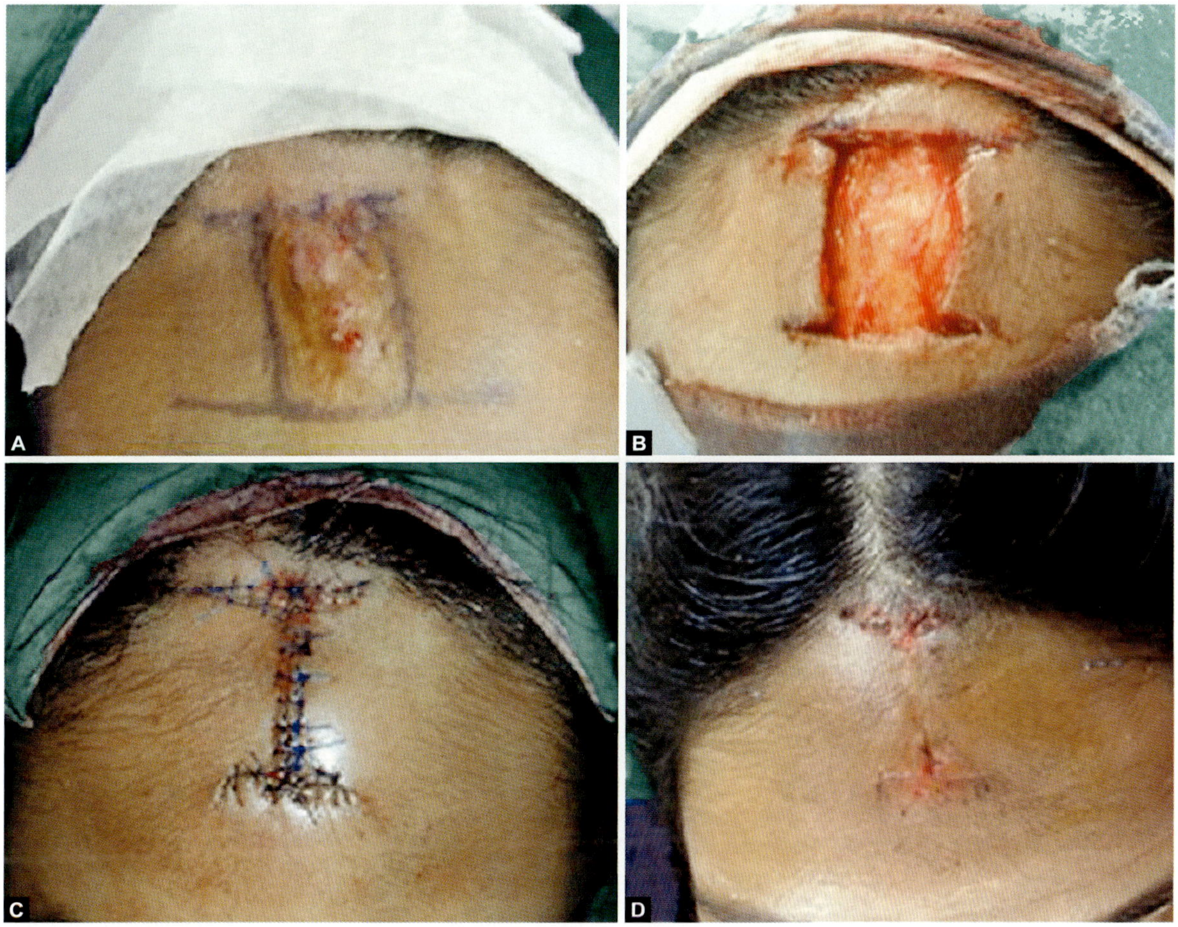

Figs. 3A to D: H-flap on forehead.

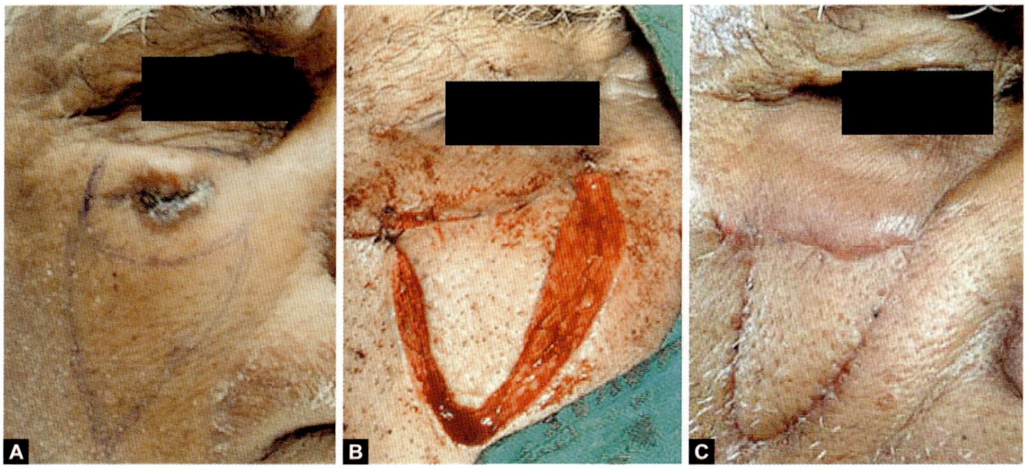

Figs. 4A to C: V-Y flap on the cheek.

short diagonal of the rhombus defect.[23] Skin mobility and extensibility are the important factors to be considered to minimize wound closure tension to avoid distortion of surrounding facial structures **(Figs. 5A to C)**. The rhomboid flap is a safe and versatile flap which can be used in every area of the human body and in various surgical specialties.[8,24,25]

The Dufourmentel modification of this flap design can be used for rhomboid shaped defects that have any combination of interior angles, not just those of 60° and 120°.

COMPLICATIONS

Bleeding, secondary infection, failure of flap, pincushioning, and flap necrosis are the common side effects encountered.

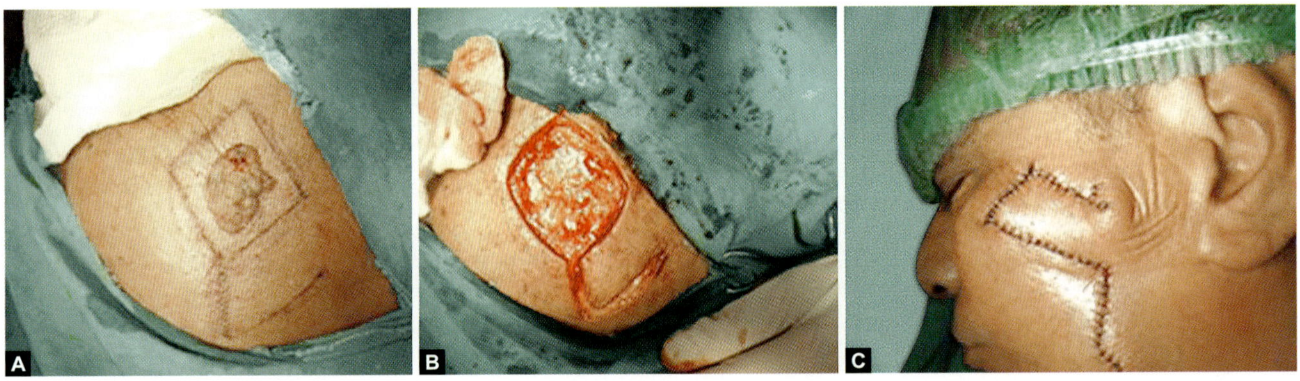

Figs. 5A to C: Classical rhomboid flap.

TABLE 1: Flap surgeries and their applications at various sites.

Rotation flap: Double rotation flap	Cheek defects in lower preauricular area and scalp
Advancement flap: • Unipedicle • H-plasty • O-T and A-T plasty • V-Y plasty	 • Forehead, medial cheek, and eyebrows • Forehead, lip margins, lower eyelid, and chin • Cheek and lateral canthus of eye • Sides of face
Transposition flap: • Rhombic • Island • Z-plasty	 • Cheeks, back, and buttocks • Forehead, cheeks, and upper nasal dorsum • Scars ≤2 cm against relaxed skin tension lines (RSTLs)

A well-designed flap with through undermining of the tissue before closing reduces wound tension and hence decreases chances of flap necrosis and failure. Intraoperative bleeding can be controlled by electrocautery or ligation. Placing of drains is usually not required in a local flap, a Penrose drain can be kept if there is significantly large dead space. Postoperative pressure dressing for 24–48 hours prevents formation of hematoma, which can compromise the local flap by inducing vasospasm and by creating a space between the flap and recipient bed. Strict aseptic precautions during surgery and giving postoperative systemic antibiotics reduces secondary infection.[26]

Late Complications

Pincushioning or trapdoor deformity is commonly seen after transposition flaps, which develops 2–3 months postoperatively. The flap appears bulky, protruding above the surface of surrounding normal skin. This can be due to curvilinear incision or failure to undermine the surrounding area during surgery. Hence, this complication can be avoided by overcoming these factors and also matching the depth of defect and the depth of donor flap. Once the trapdoor deformity does occur, it can be corrected by injecting 10 mg/mL of triamcinolone into the base of the flap two to three times in 4–6 weeks apart.

CONCLUSION

Table 1 depicts the application of flap surgeries at various sites.

REFERENCES

1. Champoneria MC, Workman AD, Gupta SC. Sushruta: father of plastic surgery. Ann Plast Surg. 2014;73(1):2-7.
2. Fang F, Chung KC. An evolutionary perspective on the history of flap reconstruction in the upper extremity. Hand Clin. 2014;30(2):109.
3. Burget GC, Menick FJ. The subunit principle in nasal reconstruction. Plast Reconstr Surg. 1985;76:239-47.
4. Larrabee WF Jr. Design of local skin flaps. Otolaryngol Clin North Am. 1990;23:899-923.
5. Murakami CS, Nishioka GJ. Essential concepts in the design of local skin flaps. Facial Plast Surg Clin North Am. 1996;4: 455-68.
6. Baker SA. Rotation flap. In: Baker SA (Ed). Local Flaps and Reconstruction, 2nd edition. Philadelphia: Elsevier; 2007. pp. 107-11.
7. Baker SA. Advancement flap. In: Baker SA (Ed). Local Flaps and Reconstruction, 2nd edition. Philadelphia: Elsevier; 2007. pp. 157-62.
8. Baker SA. Transposition flap. In: Baker SA (Ed). Local Flaps and Reconstruction, 2nd edition. Philadelphia: Elsevier; 2007. pp. 134-9.
9. Fernández-Calderón M, Casado-Sánchez C, Cabrera-Sánchez E, Casado-Pérez C. Versatility of hatchet flaps for the repair of scalp defects. Actas Dermosifiliogr. 2012; 103(7):629-31.
10. Redondo P. Repair of large defects in the forehead using a median forehead rotation flap and advancement lateral U-shaped flap. Dermatol Surg. 2006;32(6):843-6.
11. Krishnan R, Garman M, Nunez-Gussman J, Orengo I. Advancement flaps: a basic theme with many variations. Dermatol Surg. 2005;31(8 Pt 2):986-94.
12. Cook JL, Goldman GD. Random pattern cutaneous flap. Robinson JK (Ed.) Surgery of the skin: Procedural Dermatology, 2nd edition. Philadelphia: Elsevier; 2010. pp. 257-8.
13. Hirshowitz B, Mahler D. T-plasty technique for excisions in the face. Plast Reconstr Surg. 1966;37:453-8.
14. Moody BR, Sengelmann RD. Standing cone avoidance via advancement flap modification. Dermatol Surg. 2002;28: 632-5.

15. Stevens C, Tan L, Kassir R, Calhoun K. Biomechanics of A-TO-T flap design. Laryngoscope. 1999;109:113-7.
16. Jackson IT. Local flap reconstruction of defects after excision of nonmelanoma skin cancer. Clin Plast Surg. 1997; 24:747-67.
17. Gormley DE. Use of Burow's wedge principle for repair of wounds in or near the eyebrow. J Am Acad Dermatol. 1985;12:344-9.
18. O'Donnell M, Briggs C, Condon KC. The horn flap: a curved V-Y advancement flap with lateral pedicle. Br J Plast Surg. 1992;45:42-3.
19. Dini M, Innocenti A, Russo GL, Agostini V. The use of the V-Y fasciocutaneous island advancement flap in reconstructing postsurgical defects of the leg. Dermatol Surg. 2001;27:44-6.
20. Robbins TH. The "deep pedicle" V-Y advancement flap. Plast Reconstr Surg. 2004;113:463-4.
21. Zook EG, Van Beek AL, Russell RC, Moore JB. V-Y advancement flap for facial defects. Plast Reconstr Surg. 1980;65:786-97.
22. Cook J. Commentary on V–Y nasolabial advancement flaps in the repair of central facial defects. Dermatol Surg. 2001;27:659-60.
23. Lister GD, Gibson T. Closure of rhomboid skin defects: the flap of Limberg and Dufourmentel. Br J Plast Surg. 1972;25: 300-14.
24. Limberg A. Mathematical principles of local plastic procedures on the surface of the human body. Leningrad: Medgis; 1946.
25. Turan T, Kuran I, Ozcan H, Baş L. Geometric limit of multiple local Limberg flaps: a flap design. Plast Reconstr Surg. 1999;104(6):1675-8.
26. Jewett BS. Complications of flap surgery. In: Baker SA (Ed). Local Flaps and Reconstruction, 2nd edition. Philadelphia: Elsevier; 2007. pp. 691-9.

CHAPTER 24 Flaps for Facial Reconstruction

Chintan Subhash Gujarathi, Vishwanath Jigjinni

KEY MESSAGES

- Flaps include random pattern flaps and axial pattern flaps.
- Flaps are useful for closure of surgical wounds which cannot be closed by direct closure.
- The design of the flap is vital to ensure proper reconstruction.
- Axial pattern flaps are more advanced flaps, containing a specific vessel.
- Axial pattern flaps and local flaps are preferred for better aesthetic results on face.
- Proper knowledge of anatomy, aesthetic sense, and training are needed for proper results.

INTRODUCTION

The fundamental techniques of dermatosurgery are most applied in the treatment of the lesions of skin and soft tissues. These lesions are more commonly seen on the face due to its exposure to ultraviolet (UV) light, and a dermatosurgeon is frequently consulted for these facial lesions.

Patients are often concerned about facial lesions as the face is always the most exposed region of the body, barring few cultures. Facial expressions are the essential ingredients of social interaction. Patients with facial lesions are very anxious about scars and disfigurement following the treatment. It is important to understand that the central two fifths of the face is critical from the aesthetic point of view. Fortunately, in the facial region, due to an excellent blood supply, a dermatosurgeon has more reconstructive options than any other part of the body. The facial scars heal well with good aesthetic outcome. These facts should always be stressed by the surgeon to patients seeking consultation for facial lesions to alleviate their anxiety.

Understanding the anatomy of the facial skin, its aesthetic subunits, and blood supply as well as physiological and anatomical changes associated with aging is important for a dermatosurgeon treating facial lesions.

Comprehensive knowledge of skin flaps, in terms of anatomy, design, and blood supply, has evolved mainly due to their application in the reconstruction of facial defects. Hence, it is important to understand the basic concepts of skin flap surgery in order to treat facial lesions more comprehensively.

HISTORICAL BACKGROUND[1]

The application of flaps in reconstructive surgery is recorded in Sushrut Samhita, which dates back to 600 BC, wherein pedicled flaps for nasal reconstruction were described. In the 16th century, Tagliacozzi used an arm flap for nasal reconstruction. In 1794, a letter was published in a British magazine that described a potters' tribe in India, which was using forehead flap for nasal reconstruction.

Advancement flaps were first used by Celsius in the Roman era. Later, they were popularized by French surgeons.

Limberg in 1946[2] described a rhomboid transposition flap, while the bilobed flap was described by Esser in 1918. He also popularized rotation flaps with a back cut to increase the mobility of the flap.

All the flaps described above were random pattern flaps. But with the increased knowledge of cutaneous vascular anatomy, various axial pattern flaps (vide infra) were designed, such as forehead flap by McGregor (1963), delto-pectoral flap by Bakamjian (1965), groin flap by McGregor and Jackson (1972), and fasciocutaneous flaps in lower limbs by Pontén (1981).

The advances in anatomy and physiology led to the application of composite flaps such as muscle, musculo-cutaneous, osteocutaneous, and microvascular flaps, which are beyond the scope of this chapter. Furthermore, the introduction of tissue expander has made available larger segment local tissue for reconstruction.

Rhomboid flap is a transposition flap designed as a rhomboid (equilateral parallelogram).

It can be either of Limberg design (where transverse diagonal is also of the same length) or of Dufourmentel design (where transverse diagonal is of different lengths).

BASIC CONCEPTS OF FLAPS

Definition

The origin of the term *flap* is derived from the Dutch word *flappe*, which means a broad and loose structure hung and fastened only by one side. The flap in medical terms is defined as a unit of tissue of variable composition that is transferred from one site (donor) to another (recipient) while maintaining its blood supply **(Fig. 1)**.

Classification

- *Based on vascularity:* Flaps can be classified as random pattern or axial pattern **(Table 1)**.
  - *Random pattern flaps:* The blood supply of random pattern flaps is based on the unnamed microscopic vessels present in the subdermal and subcutaneous plexuses (subpapillary, subdermal, and interfascial). The three types of random pattern flaps are as follows:
    1. *Advancement flaps:* In this type of flap, a segment of tissue is moved in a linear axis to reconstruct the defect **(Fig. 2)**.
    2. *Transposition flap:* In this type of flap, a segment of tissue is transferred over an intervening area of normal skin to the defect **(*see* Fig. 1)**.
    3. *Rotation flap:* In this type of flap, the tissue is rotated around a pivot point to reconstruct the defect **(Fig. 3)**.
  - *Nonrandom flaps:*
    - *Axial pattern flaps:* In these flaps, there is a known constant blood vessel (which is larger than the subdermal plexus vessels and with a higher flow pressure), supplying a segment of tissue and making these flaps more reliable in terms of the blood supply. Hence, the length-to-breadth ratio, which in a random pattern flap is 1:1, can be extended much higher in axial pattern flaps up to 5:1 **(Fig. 4)**.
    - *Other nonrandom flaps:* Other nonrandom flaps such as fasciocutaneous, septocutaneous, and

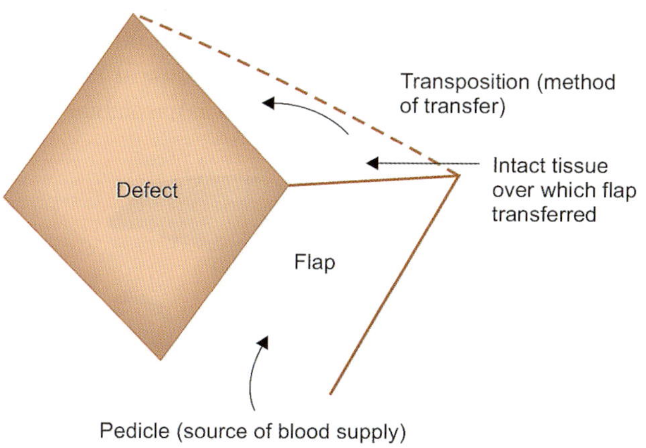

Fig. 1: Basics of flap.

TABLE 1: Classification of flaps.

Flap	*Defect design*	*Principle*	*Action imparted to pedicle in transfer*
Advancement	Quadrilateral	Sliding door	Linear
Rotation	Circular	Revolving door	Radial arc
Transposition	Quadrilateral	Hinged door	Lateral angular (jackknife)

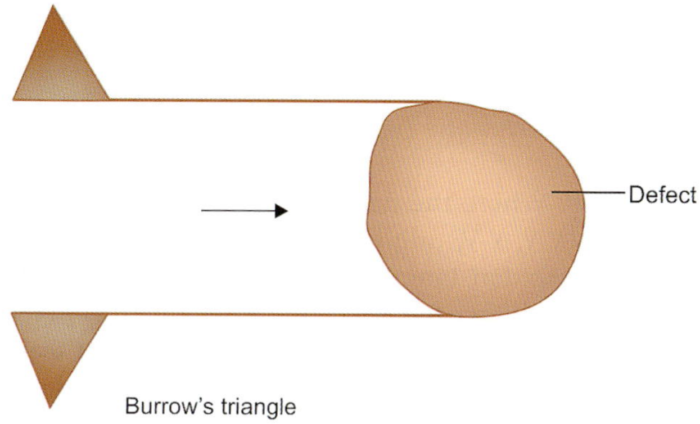

Fig. 2: Advancement flap.

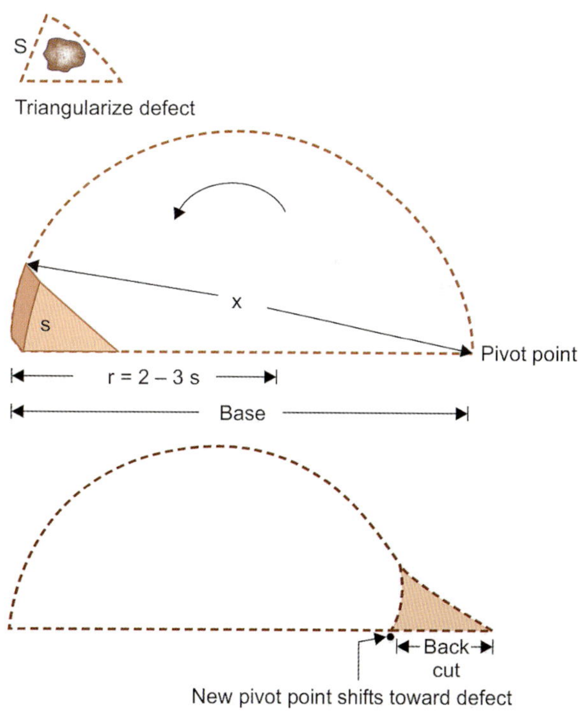

Fig. 3: Rotation flap.

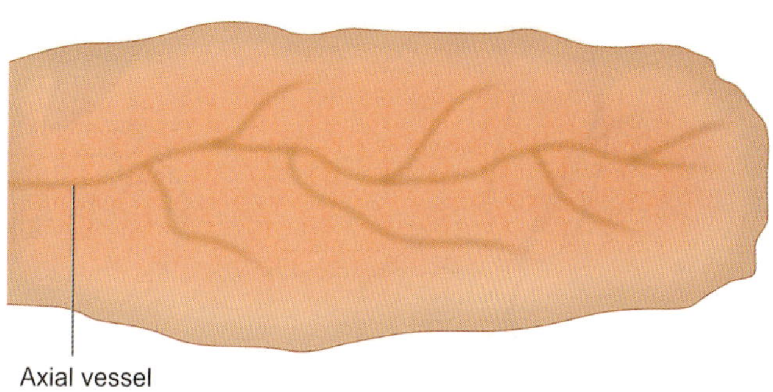

Fig. 4: Axial pattern flap.

perforator flaps are used in reconstruction of extremities and are beyond the scope of this textbook.

- *Based on tissue composition*: The flaps may be as follows:
  - *Simple:* Where a single type of tissue is transferred, for example, skin, muscle
  - *Composite:* Where a combination of tissue is transferred, for example, skin and muscle (e.g., myocutaneous)
- *Based on technique (movement):* The flap may be as follows:
  - *Local:* Where the defect is adjacent to the donor site (V-Y, Y-V, unipedicled, bipedicled, rotation, transposition, interpolation, and island)
  - *Distant:* Where the defect is in a different region than the donor site, for example, forehead, neck, or scalp.
  - *Free:* This microvascular technique of tissue transfer is beyond the scope of this chapter.

The distant flap may be *pedicled* where the blood supply is preserved through an intact tissue bridge or it may be *free flap* where the donor tissue is separated from the donor site along with the vascular pedicle and the blood supply is reestablished in the recipient area by anastomosis of vascular pedicle to the vessels in the recipient region.

FLAP ANATOMY AND DESIGN

As described earlier and shown in **Figure 1**, a flap is a segment of tissue harvested from a donor area and transferred into the defect, keeping its blood supply intact. This is the basis of flap design, which, in turn, forms the basis of good reconstruction. The important considerations in flap design are as follows:

- *Defect:* Always assess the defect carefully in terms of size, shape, tissues in the floor, and special tissue requirement, such as hair-bearing tissue.
- *Reconstructive options:* There are many reconstructive methods available to repair a defect. It is a good dictum to think of the simplest options first and go up the reconstructive ladder to more complex methods if the simpler options will not fulfill the reconstructive requirements. Also choosing the simplest option ensures availability of a lifeboat (backup plan).
- *Planning in reverse:* The surgeon should measure the defect carefully (or make a template of the defect with the help of a lint piece) and transfer these measurements (or the template) through all stages of its transfer in reverse fashion to the donor site to mark the flap outline, thus ensuring that flap dimensions are adequate **(Figs. 5A to C)**.
- *Donor site:* It is very important to choose the donor site carefully to get a good result in the flap reconstruction. The basic principle applied is "Stealing from Peter to pay Paul only if Peter can afford." Hence, the donor site should have relatively *excess tissue*, which can be transferred to the defect. This is best tested by pinching the skin and subcutaneous tissue in various areas and direction in the potential donor site.

In facial reconstruction, the *aesthetic appearance* is of prime importance. The tissue transferred should be optimum in terms of:

- Color match
- Texture

Special considerations are necessary in terms of sensation in some areas, hair-bearing skin in eyebrow and moustache area, and function in certain areas, such as eyelid and lips.

While designing a facial flap, a special consideration should be given to *aesthetic subunits* of the face as given by Burget and Menick **(Fig. 6)**. Such refinement improves the aesthetic results of flap reconstruction. It is also important to design flaps in such a way that the resulting donor scar falls in the line of junction of the aesthetic unit, such as nasolabial groove,

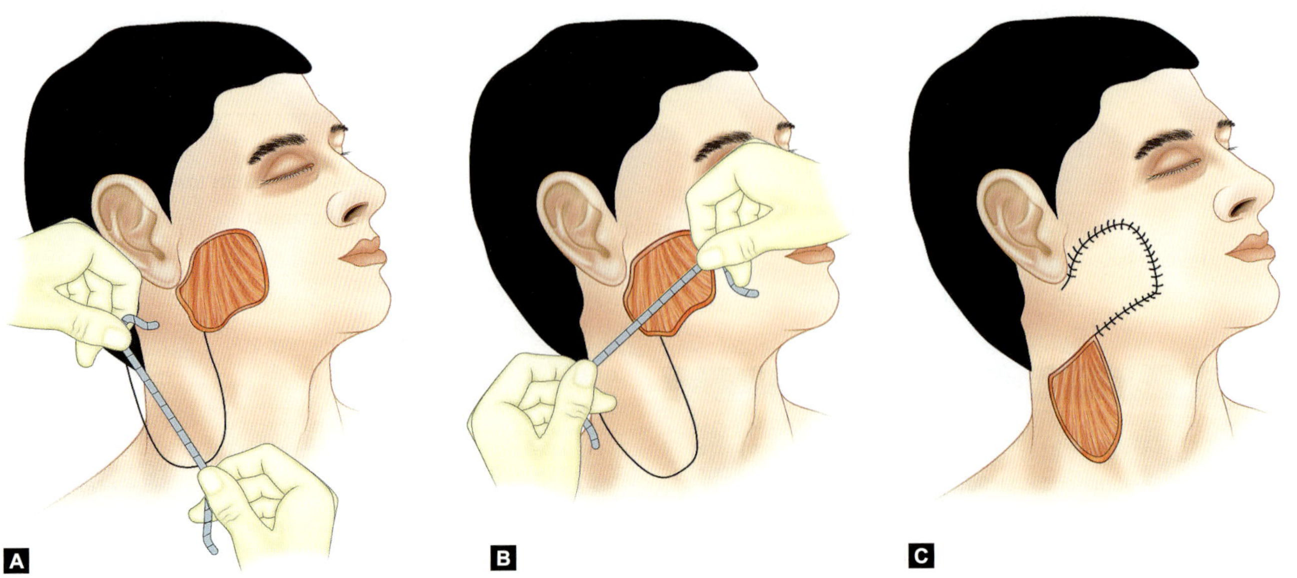

A B C

Figs. 5A to C: Planning in reverse.

or in the line of relaxed skin tension lines (RSTLs) **(Fig. 7)**. Older patients are good candidates for flap surgery due to laxity, inherently seen in aging skin, which is useful for flap harvesting. This age group also has very evident RSTL, which makes flap designing easier. Coincidently, this age group also has more prevalence of facial skin lesions.

- *Nose:* Eight subunits, namely dorsum, tip, two sidewalls, and two alae (if the root of the nose is also included—nine subunits.)
- *Periorbital subunits:* Eyebrow, orbital unit, supraeyebrow, and glabellar units (three units each side + one glabellar unit)
- *Forehead:* Paramedian, lateral, and lateral temporal subunit (lateral-to-anterior temporal line)

Blood Supply of Face

Blood supply of face is important in axial pattern flaps, such as lateral forehead flap (anterior branch of superficial temporal artery) and nasolabial flap (facial artery which terminates as angular artery). The length-to-breadth ratio of such flap is high and the flap can be designed to reach a defect farther away from the donor site. The facial skin gets its vascular supply through terminal branches of the external carotid artery, namely facial and superficial temporal arteries. The forehead gets its blood supply from branches of the ophthalmic artery, namely supratrochlear and supraorbital arteries.

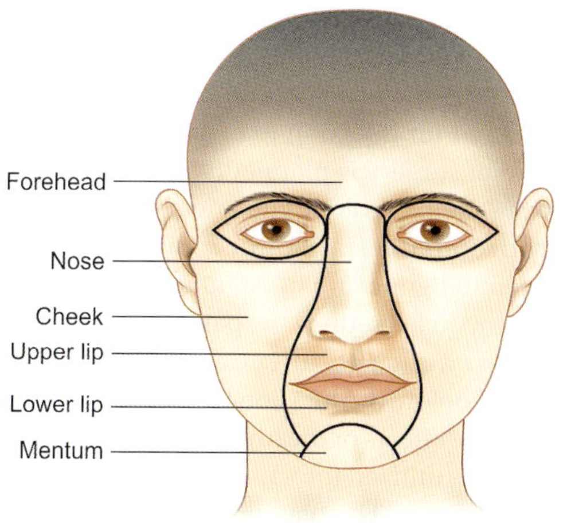

Fig. 6: Aesthetic subunits of face (Burget and Menick).

Nerve Supply of Face

Nerve supply of face is important as regards preserving sensation in areas such as lips and eyelids. It is also useful in giving nerve blocks **(Fig. 8)**. It is important to note that all three nerves, namely supraorbital, infraorbital, and mental nerves, emerge from bony canals, which lie in a vertical line that passes through the pupil on that side. All nerves mentioned are branches of three divisions of the trigeminal nerve, respectively. The ear is supplied in itslower half by the greater auricular nerve, which arises from the cervical plexus.

FLAP PHYSIOLOGY

The viability of a flap is based on the tissue perfusion, which is derived through an intact blood supply. This is possible through careful planning of the flap. Any segment of skin derives its blood supply from periphery and through deeper tissues. In a flap design, it is imperative to keep an intact tissue bridge, while other incisions are made to mobilize the flap and transfer it into the defect. The perfusion pressure in the capillaries has to be maintained above the critical capillary closure pressure to ensure that the tissue is adequately perfused and kept viable. This is related to the anatomy of local vasculature, i.e., axial or random pattern, and also to the density of the capillary network, which varies in different areas of the body. In any flap, this perfusion is insured by the following:

- *Length-to-breadth (L:B) ratio:* As described earlier, in a random pattern flap, this ratio is 1:1 but can be extended

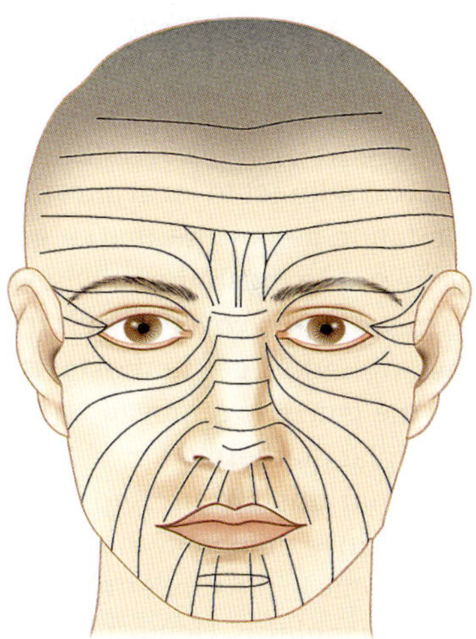

Fig. 7: Resting skin tension lines (RSTLs) of the face.

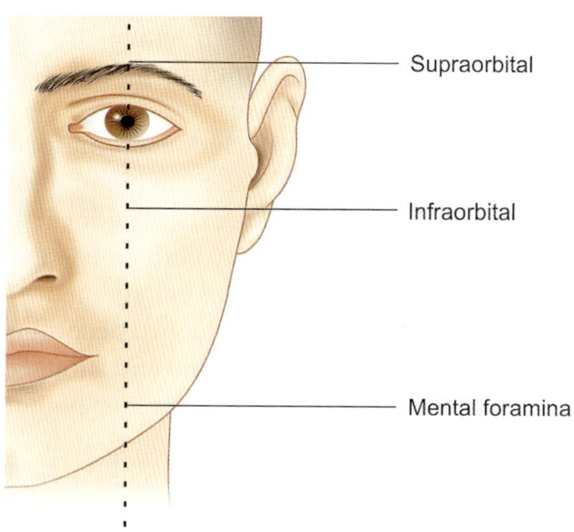

Fig. 8: Anatomy of foramina for nerve blocks.

in face to 4:1 or 5:1 due to its rich blood supply. But 3:1 ratio is a good safe limit in the face. In axial pattern flap, this ratio can be 6:1.

- *Delay phenomenon:* In some regions of the body where there is an inadequate blood supply, the length-to-breadth ratio can be increased by making partial incisions, for example, only lateral incisions. After a delay of 2 weeks, all incisions are made and the flap is transferred. The initial partial incisions help induct blood supply from nonincised tissues, thereby increasing the L:B ratio. This is applied mainly for the flaps in lower extremities and is rarely used in facial reconstruction.
- *Tissue tension:* The tissue tension reduces tissue perfusion by stretching and collapse of capillaries. Hence, the flaps should be designed such that there is no tissue tension when the flap is sutured into the defect. The common mistake is underestimating the size of the flap, which should ideally be larger (in length and breadth to account for dermal contraction) than the defect to avoid the tension.

Finally, *tissue handling* is also important for good results. The surgeon should familiarize with the use of skin hooks instead of handling the flap with tissue forceps which, if not used carefully, can damage the tissue. The *undermining* of edges should be limited. This procedure mobilizes a tissue at the expense of interrupting its blood supply. The importance of *hemostasis* cannot be overemphasized. A hematoma increases the tissue tension and interferes with blood supply of the flap, leading to flap necrosis and infection. The vitality of tissue is preserved by avoiding *desiccation* of tissues during surgery.

PREOPERATIVE CARE

When a patient is seen in a consulting room, a detailed history is noted and a comprehensive physical examination is done. It is important to note the history of hypertension, diabetes, and cardiac diseases. The history should include an enquiry about previous surgeries, dental procedures (especially under local anesthesia), regular medications including nonsteroidal anti-inflammatory drugs (NSAIDs), such as aspirin, and known allergies.

Physical examination should include checking for anemia, high blood pressure, and systematic examination of heart, lungs, abdomen, extremities, and neck. The local lesion is examined for its size, site, mobility, and consistency. The regional lymph nodes are checked for enlargement.

Preoperative investigations are planned according to the general health and the age of the patient and should include hemogram and routine urine test. The older patients may need more comprehensive investigations, such as blood sugar, urea, creatinine, electrolyte, liver function tests, chest X-ray, and electrocardiogram. Patients with poor health may require a consultation with the physician before the surgery is planned. Coagulation profile is checked in the patient suspected of bleeding diathesis.

Patients on antiplatelet drugs, such as aspirin, are instructed to stop their use 1 week before the scheduled date of surgery. Smokers are advised to stop smoking 4–6 weeks prior to the surgery. On the day of the surgery, appropriate instructions are given about starvation and taking essential medications, such as antihypertensive drugs. The diabetic patients are managed as per the planned anesthesia, for example, local or general. The patient is instructed about the shaving and shower and instructed to visit the hospital along with the results of investigations and a responsible accompanying person.

ANESTHESIA AND SURGICAL TECHNIQUES

Most of the small flaps can be done on an outpatient basis. As described earlier, the lesion should be marked with indelible ink. Then the proposed margin of resection is drawn around the lesion. The flap to be utilized for reconstruction is decided and its outline is marked using the planning in the reverse method **(*see* Figs. 5A to C)**.

Local anesthesia is sufficient in majority of cases. Lignocaine 2% with adrenaline in 1:200,000 is a commonly used local anesthetic agent. It can be diluted with an equal amount of water for injection to increase the volume where a larger field of surgery is planned. Addition of bupivacaine (0.25 or 0.5%) helps prolong the anesthesia and gives good postoperative analgesia. Sodium bicarbonate solution (7.5%) added to lignocaine in 1:5 dilution increases the pH of the latter and helps reduce the pain during the infiltration. It is a good practice to inject a local anesthetic drug 10–15 minutes before the incision to allow the anesthetic and vasoconstrictive effects of the injected solution to take place. This time can be utilized for hand scrub and the preparation of the operative part. The patient is made to lie comfortably on the operation table. It is a good practice to cover the eyes of the patient with a moist gauze to shield them from the bright operating lights unless the surgical field includes eyelids or eyebrows. For elderly patients and those with coexisting medical conditions, it is safe to have an anesthesiologist be present during the surgery, either to monitor the patient or to give sedation as an adjunct to local anesthesia.

Incisions are made as per the markings. The lesion is excised taking care not to crush the specimen with toothed forceps. The open wound is covered with moist gauze and firm pressure is applied to get hemostasis. After waiting for 2–3 minutes, the gauze is removed and the bleeding is controlled with bipolar diathermy.

Next, the flap margins are incised and the flap to be transposed is undermined minimally to allow it some mobility. The undermining is done in the subdermal fat layer, protecting the rich dermal vascular plexus. Hemostasis is achieved again, and the flap is ready to be transferred into the defect.

Always begin by closing the donor defect, which releases any tension on the flap. 4-0 or 5-0 absorbable sutures such as polyglactin (Vicryl) for deeper layers and 4-0 or 5-0 nylon (Ethilon) or polypropylene (Prolene) for skin are good suture materials. The subcutaneous tissue is approximated with interrupted and inverted sutures, taking a small bite of dermis to achieve good approximation of the wound edges and wound strength. The skin is approximated with interrupted sutures, either simple or vertical mattress, depending how easily the skin gets approximated. The most important point in skin closure is to ensure that the skin edges approximate well with eversion. The finer suture such as 6-0 polypropylene may be used for eyelid skin. With good hemostasis, there is rarely any need for wound drainage. Light dressing is applied after the wound closure without using excessive compression.

POSTOPERATIVE CARE

Most of the patients are treated on an outpatient basis. They should be given adequate pain relief. The use of NSAID should be minimal to prevent hematoma formation. Routine prophylactic antibiotics are not indicated. The patients are instructed to remove dressing on the first or second postoperative day and to wash the area with lukewarm water and soap. It helps to apply nonstaining ointment such as Neosporin or chloromycetin on the wound, which acts like a water-impermeable barrier and helps reassure patients. The patients are also warned that there is a possibility of some tissue swelling and ecchymosis, which will subside in 2–3 weeks. In the event of small bleeding, the patient is instructed to sit upright and told to apply firm pressure on the wound with a clean gauze piece for 15 minutes. The patient may be handed over a few of these at the time of discharge. The sutures are removed on the 5th to 7th postoperative day. The patient is instructed to massage the scar with vitamin E-based moisturizing cream or in some patients, silicone gel may be applied to facilitate the scar maturation. Patients are advised to use UV protection for a year after the surgery.

COMPLICATIONS OF FLAPS

- *Hematoma:* The face has excellent blood supply, which helps in better survival of flaps. But the disadvantage of a good blood supply is that there are more possibilities of hematoma formation. The hematoma increases tissue tension, jeopardizing the blood supply to the flap. Prevention is always better as in any other field of medicine. Meticulous hemostasis, withdrawal of drugs such as aspirin, vitamin E, and clopidogrel are important in prevention of the hematoma. The hematoma cannot be prevented by tight dressing; on the contrary, this excessive pressure may lead to flap necrosis. It is best to drain the wound in cases where there is a possibility of postoperative bleeding.
- *Flap necrosis:* A good flap design in terms of suitability of the donor site (adequate tissue), L:B ratio, and tissue tension is important in prevention of this complication. Smokers are advised to stop smoking 4–6 weeks prior to surgery.
- *Infection:* It is a relatively rare complication due to excellent blood supply in the face. Prophylactic antibiotics are not routinely used for such surgery. Meticulous design and planning and good tissue handling help prevent complications such as tissue necrosis, flap necrosis, and hematoma, which are precursors of infection. The infection manifests as pain, discharge, and the local signs of inflammation are evident. The treatment consists of wound drainage where possible and antibiotics.
- *Scars:* They are an inevitable sequel of any surgery. It is important to design the flaps carefully with due consideration of the aesthetic units, the borders between these units, and RSTLs as described earlier. Unacceptable scars may be revised 6–12 months after surgery once the scar maturation is complete.
- *Nerve damage:* This is a rare complication of cutaneous surgery, and any anesthesia or paresthesia due to division of terminal sensory branches usually resolves in 6–12 months. But care should be taken in the area lateral to the lateral end of eyebrow, where the temporal branch of the facial nerve is superficial and the damage to the nerve in this region will cause the paralysis of the frontalis muscle, leading to brow ptosis. (Surface anatomy of temporal branch is along Pitanguy's line, i.e., 0.5 cm below tragus to 1.5 cm above and lateral to the eyebrow.)

DETAILS OF BASIC FLAPS AND THEIR APPLICATION (TABLE 2)

Advancement Flaps

An advancement flap is one where a tissue is moved in a linear direction to fill a defect. In fact, undermining of the skin edges that is commonly done during wound closure is a type of advancement flap. Advancement flaps are useful in defects where closure with undermining will distort contours or hairline, for example, forehead, eyebrows, cheek close to eyelid, nasal dorsum, vermillion of lip, or ala of nose. A defect in these areas can be reconstructed with advancement flap from the adjacent area rather than by undermining the edges and direct closure of the wound which will cause distortion of hair line, eyebrow position, lid margin, and vermillion or alar rim. The advancement flap can be single pedicled, where tissue is moved from one side of the defect (U-plasty), or it can be bi-pedicled, where tissue is obtained from both sides of the defect (H-plasty). When advancement flaps are used, one creates discrepancy in the length of the two sides of the skin edges, which is corrected either by cutting out a tissue at the base as Burrow's triangle or by a Z-plasty in the trailing end of the wound **(*see* Fig. 2)**.

Key Points in Cheek Reconstruction

Cheeks represent the largest surface area of the face. Primary closure is the reconstructive method of choice if there is adequate laxity of tissues. However, if the flap surgery is planned, it is important to place incisions in established skin creases (RSTL) to camouflage resultant scars. Also, care is taken to avoid distortion of the sideburns and placement of hair-bearing skin into nonhair-bearing areas.

Transposition flaps: Banner flaps are the simplest form of transposition flaps that transfer skin from preauricular and nasolabial areas. However, the disadvantages include dog-ear formation and pincushioning effect.

Rhomboid flaps are useful for lateral lower cheek defects. The advantage over banner flaps is decreased propensity for trap dooming or pincushioning. Bilobed flaps are rarely required due to laxity in the cheeks.

Rotation flaps: Cervicofacial rotation flaps are useful in defects of upper medial cheeks. These flaps use loose preauricular and neck skin. Cervicopectoral rotation flaps are useful in lower and lateral cheek defects. These flaps use excess skin of neck and chest.

TABLE 2: Choice of flaps for regional defects.

Scalp	
Defect diameter ≤3 cm	Primary closure
3–6 cm	• *Pericranium intact:* Skin graft • *No pericranium:* Scalp rotation flaps with primary closure of donor site
6–9 cm	One large scalp flap based on major pedicle with skin graft of donor site
Larger defects	Tissue expansion (up to 50% scalp can be reconstructed by expanding the remaining scalp)
Forehead	Bilateral advancement flaps or Y- to T-shaped flaps
Cheek	
Medial	• Cheek advancement • Transposition flap • V-Y advancement flap, especially near alar base
Lateral	• Transposition flap and rhomboid flaps
Moderate-to-large defects	• Cheek-rotation flaps
Lip	
Central	Bilateral advancement flap
Lateral	Rotation
Nose	Advancement of dorsal nasal skin, bilobed flap or nasolabial flap, and forehead flap for large defects

Key Points in Lip Reconstruction

The general goals in lip reconstruction include:

- Maintaining a dynamic oral sphincter
- Sufficiently sized stoma
- Acceptable cosmetic results.

Up to 25% upper and 40% lower lip defects can be primarily closed.

Estlander flap: This flap is used to reconstruct the defect of the lateral lower lip where the upper lip is rotated into the lower lip. (An example of lip-sharing procedure is shown in **Figures 9A to C**.)

The classical examples of unipedicled advancement flaps are seen in the closure of defects near ala of the nose where the defect is cut as a crescent and the cheek skin is advanced to close the defect, giving an excellent result. The skin is undermined through a plane in the subcutaneous fat just below dermis, thus avoiding injury to deeper vessels and nerves while preserving the dermal vascular plexus, which is vital to its perfusion.

The mucosal advancement flap is used to resurface the vermillion of the lip, especially after excision of a lesion or after excision of segments affected by vitiligo. The undermining is done through submucosal plane and the approximation of the edges is done using an absorbable suture such as undyed polyglactin (Vicryl) or catgut (4-0 or 5-0). it is preferable not to use polyglecaprone (Monocryl) as it gives a troublesome pricking sensation, although the sutures are less visible because Monocryl is a transparent material.

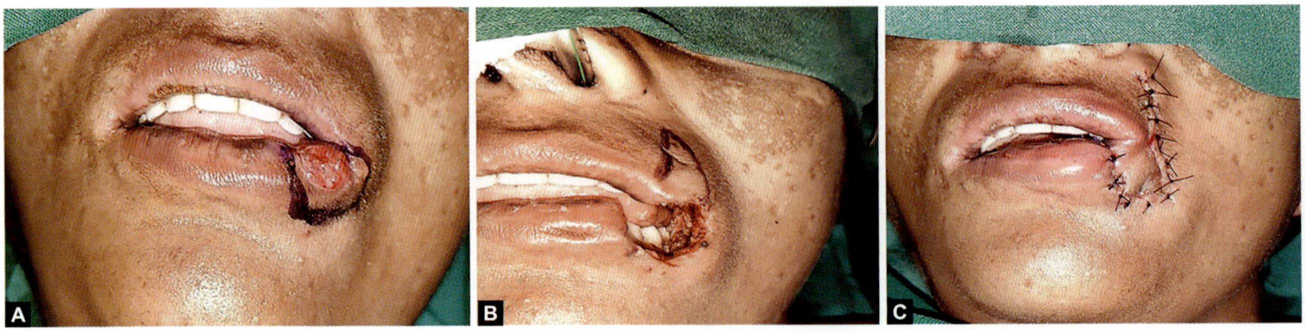

Figs. 9A to C: (A) Defect marking; (B) Postexcision defect with flap marking; (C) Flap inset and primary closure of donor defect.

Full thickness of tissue can also be advanced to reconstruct the defect, especially in lip or in helical rim. The advanced tissue unit is based on intact bridge of tissue, for example, posterior skin in case of helical advancement **(Figs. 10A and B)**.

V-Y Advancement Flap

Another useful advancement flap is V-Y advancement flap, which is versatile and uses matching tissue from the contiguous area **(Figs. 11A and B)**. Although more commonly used in hand surgery for fingertip reconstruction, this flap is useful for reconstruction in forehead, lower part of nose, and upper lip areas. This flap derives its perfusion through the intact bridge of subcutaneous tissue, which can be either deep to the flap or lateral to it. The advancement is obtained due to laxity in the subcutaneous plane and closure is helped by the tissue laxity on either side of the flap **(Fig. 12)**.

When V-Y advancement is done based on a deep pedicle, the flap is cut as per the markings. The flap is advanced into the defect. If there is lack of adequate mobility, then the leading edge and also the trailing edges can be undermined minimally to achieve a greater mobility.

In a lateral pedicle V-Y flap, the entire undersurface of the flap is undermined. Gentle dissection of the connective tissue septae in the lateral tissue achieves the desired advancement. The closure starts in the donor area, which helps to propel flap into the defect. It is useful in many regions of the face **(Figs. 11, 13 to 15)**.

The versatility of V-Y advancement is used even as an adjunct to other flaps, especially for closing the donor defect.

Transposition Flaps

The transposition flaps are more commonly used in the facial reconstruction due to availability of donor sites with adequate tissue laxity. They are used in forehead, cheek, temporal area, ear, and nasal tip. Many modifications have been done to suit a particular reconstructive requirement **(Fig. 16)**.[3]

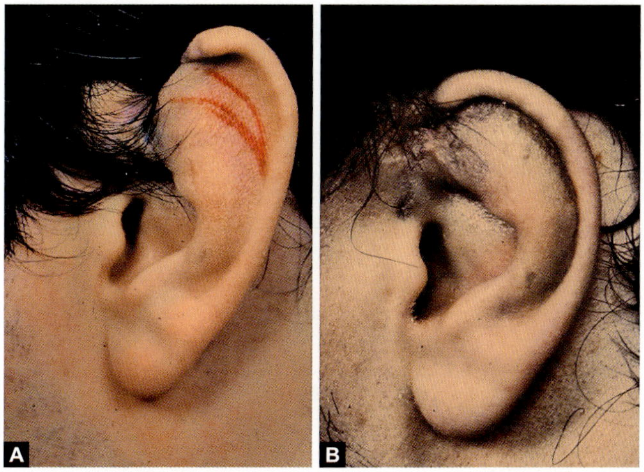

Figs. 10A and B: Helical advancement flap.

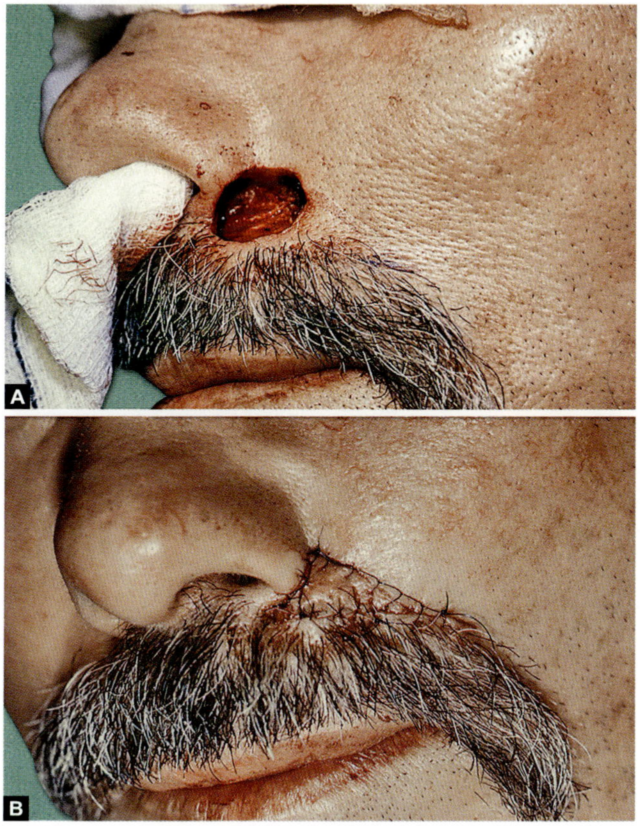

Figs. 11A and B: V-Y flap for upper lip.

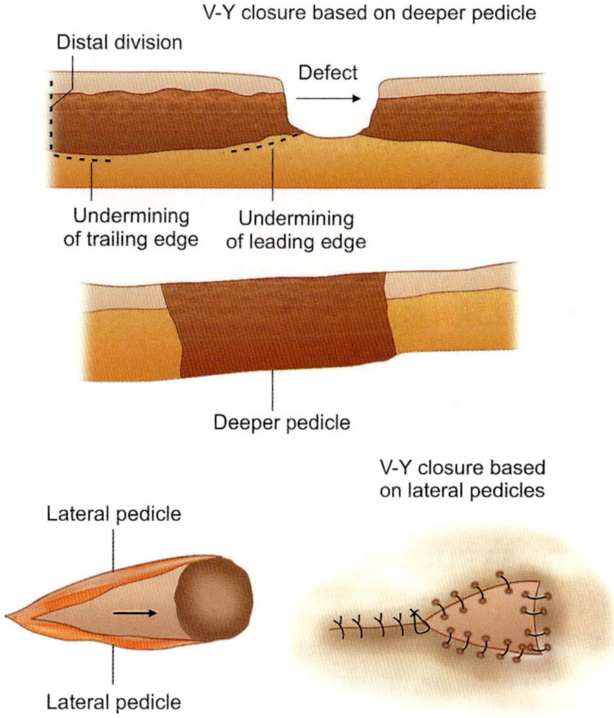

Fig. 12: V-Y advancement flap.

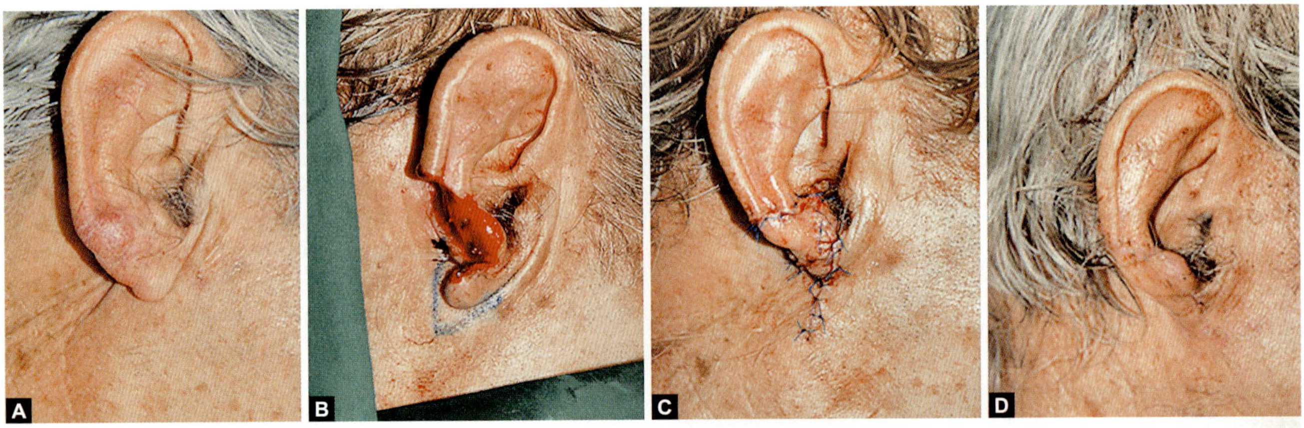

Figs. 13A to D: V-Y advancement flap for ear.

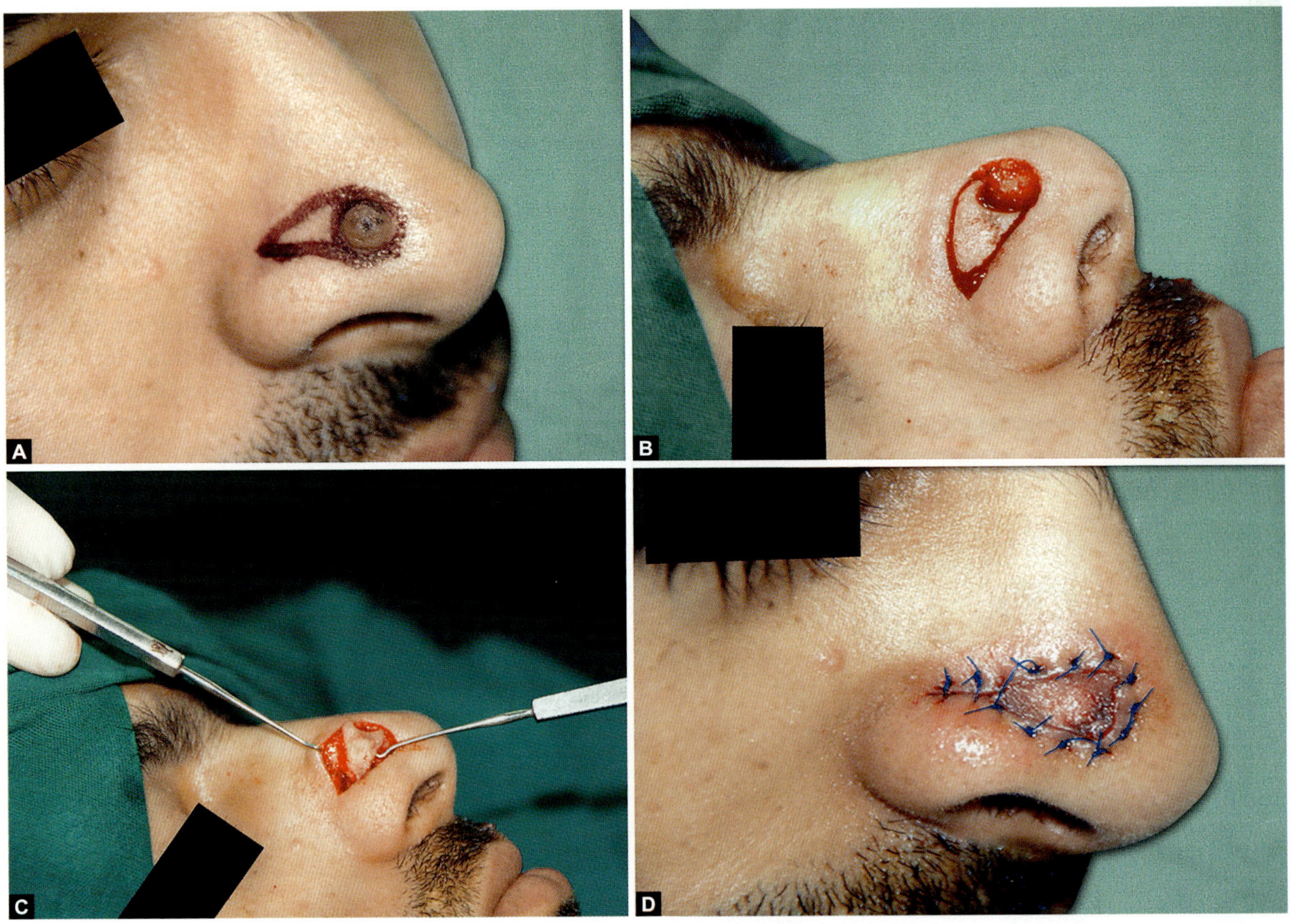

Figs. 14A to D: V-Y flap for nose.

DETAILS OF FLAP DESIGN AND RECONSTRUCTION

The lesion to be excised is demarcated with marking ink and the margin of excision is also marked. Then the direction of RSTLs or skin creases or maximum skin laxity is noted. The defect is now marked as a rhomboid with all sides equal and the angles as 60° and 120°. A V-shaped flap is marked starting from a point which is adjacent to the angle of 120°. Both the lines of V are of the same length as the rhomboid, and they form an angle of 60°. The lesion is excised, and the flap is undermined in the subcutaneous plane. The hemostasis, flap transfer, and the closure are done as described earlier.

Surgeons rarely excise the lesion to make a rhomboid-shaped defect. Hence, the rhomboid flap may be cut as

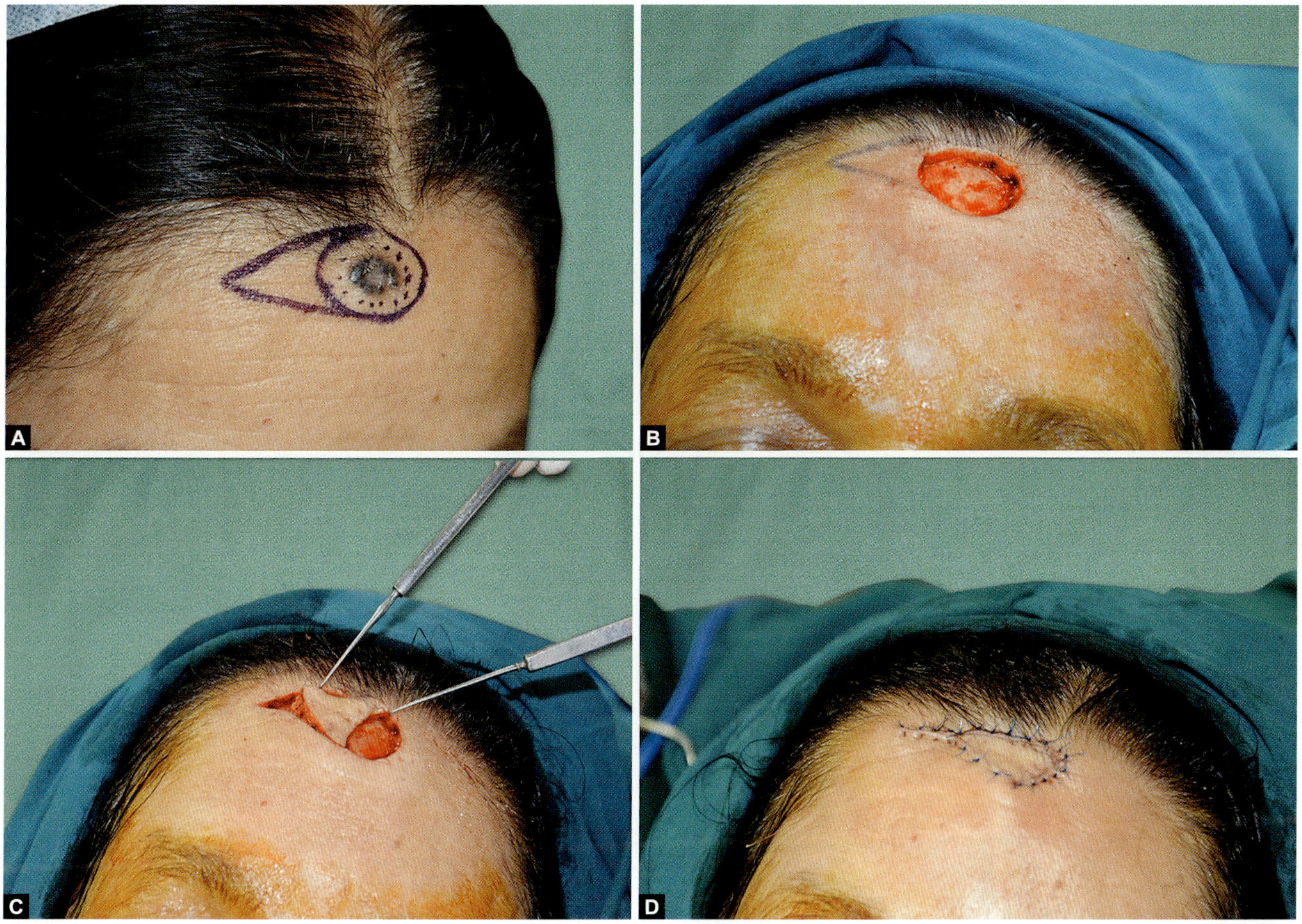

Figs. 15A to D: V-Y flap for forehead.

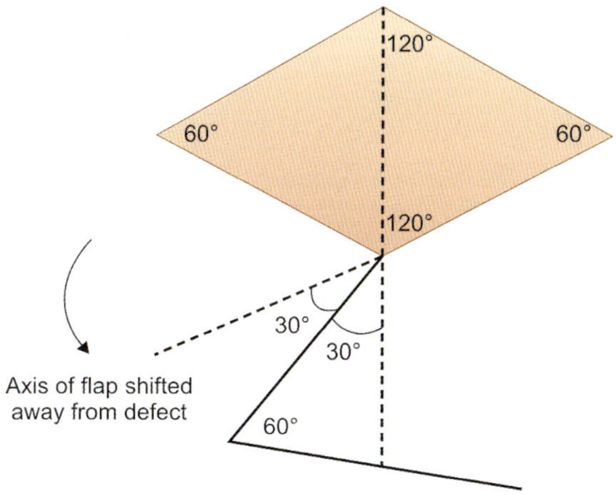

Fig. 16: Dufourmentel flap.

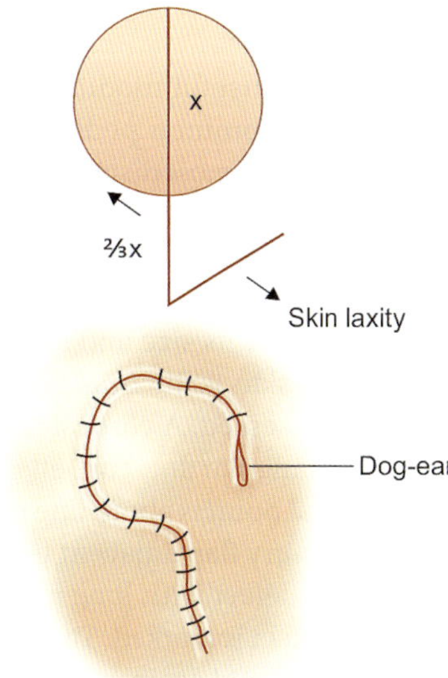

Fig. 17: Square peg in a round hole flap.

rhomboid or as an arc of circle or as a triangle to fit the defect with some adjustments.

A useful modification of the rhomboid flap is called "square peg in a round hole."[4] Most of the lesions are excised as a circle. The flap is then drawn from the periphery of the defect, noting the area of maximum skin laxity. A V-shaped flap is marked and cut to fit the defect, excising the angles of the flap when necessary. The main disadvantage of this flap is that it leaves a small dog-ear at the pivot point. This usually becomes less obvious with passage of time or may need a small revision surgery. But this flap certainly adds versatility to reconstruction of facial defects **(Figs. 17 to 19)**.

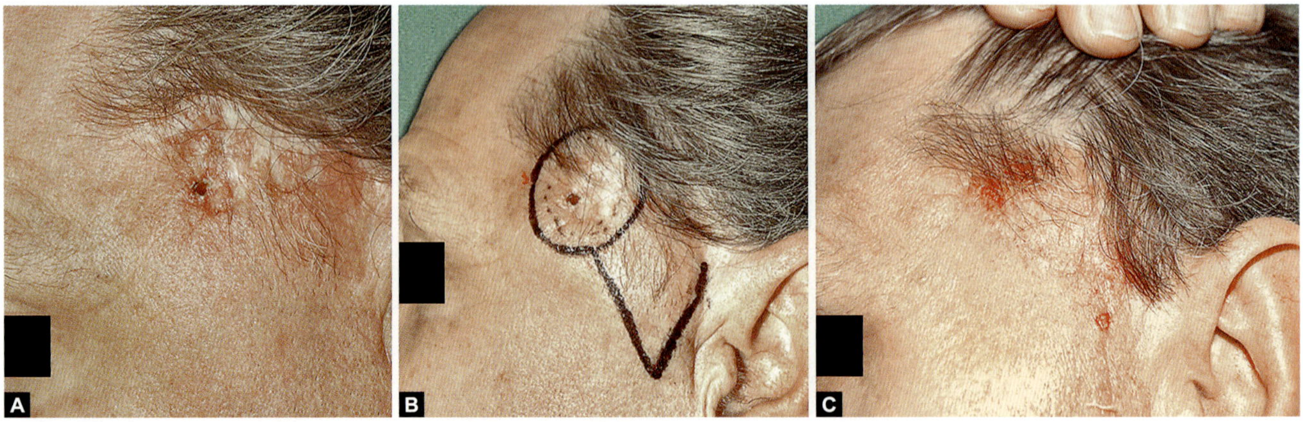

Figs. 18A to C: Square peg in a round hole flap.

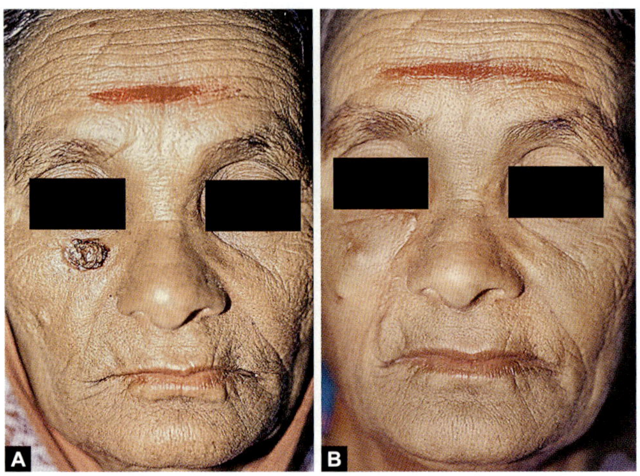

Figs. 19A and B: Transposition flap from nasolabial area.

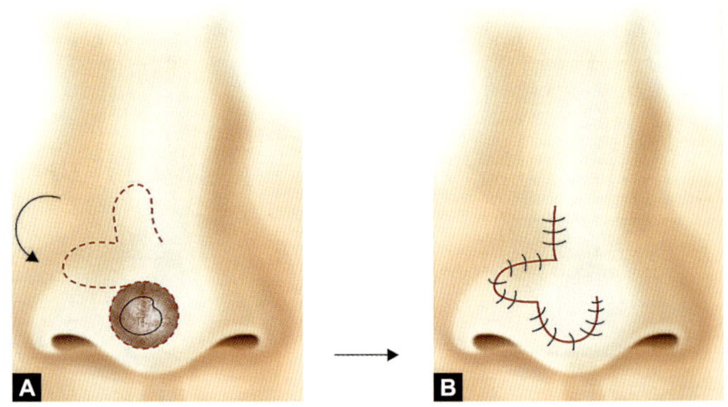

Figs. 20A and B: Bilobed flap.

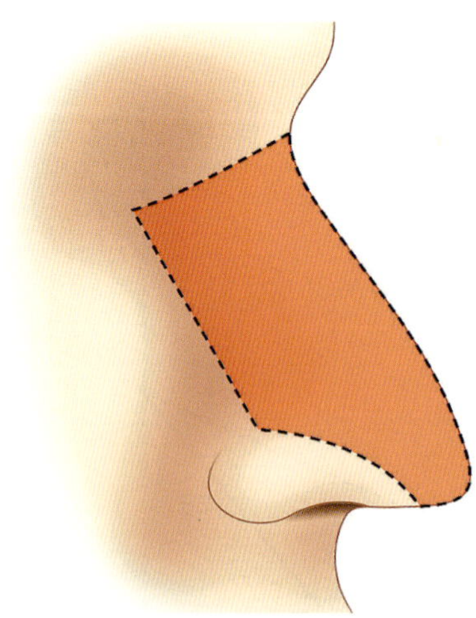

Fig. 21: Area for bilobed flap reconstruction.

Bilobed flap is another useful modification where two transposition flaps with a common pedicle are used to fill the successive defects and the most distal donor site is closed primarily.[4] It is useful for reconstruction of defects where tissue laxity in the contiguous area is deficient as to be closed primarily, for example, nasal tip and ala.[5]

The defect is assessed for its size and location. The area where there is maximum skin laxity from where the second flap will be designed is assessed. A vertical line through the defect is drawn. Excise triangular dog-ear between defect and rotation point. The pivotal point is about one radius distance from the defect. The primary flap adjacent to the defect and slightly smaller than the defect with long axis 30–45° to the line drawn through the defect is marked. Then the second flap adjacent to the primary flap and again smaller (about half the size of the first) than the primary at an angle 90–100° to the line through the defect is marked. The flaps are dissected through a *submuscular plane* (above the perichondrium), rotated into the successive defects. Allow no more than 50° of rotation per lobe. The defect of the second flap is closed primarily. It is important to base flaps on the lateral side while reconstructing defects of the nasal tip and base them on the medial side for the defects of the ala of nose. It is important not to cross the midline while designing the flaps **(Figs. 20 to 22)**.[6]

PLANNING OF BILOBED FLAP

Rotation Flaps

The rotation flaps are more useful in areas with uniform laxity that does not allow harvest of a flap and closure of the defect, for example, scalp **(Figs. 23A to C)**. The flaps are most

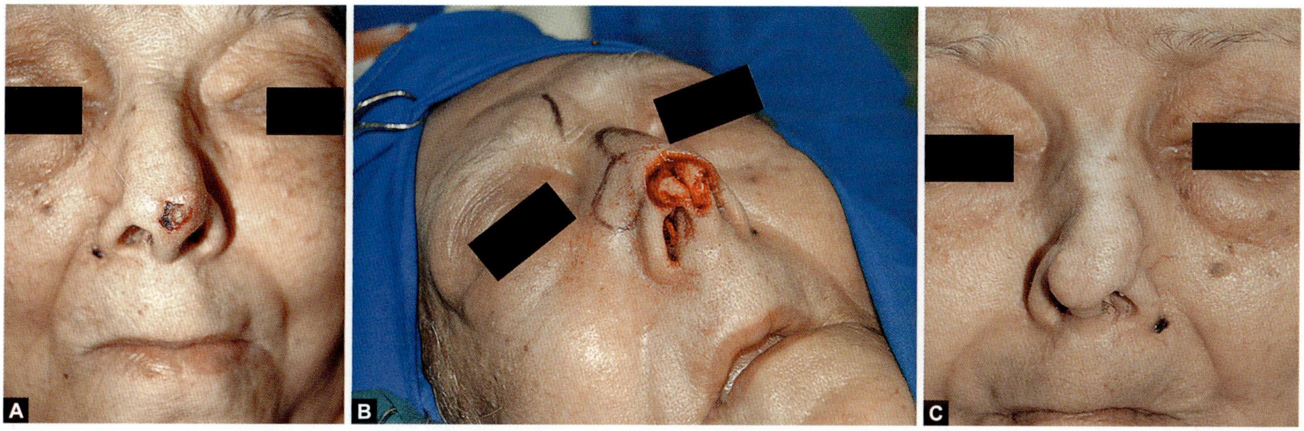

Figs. 22A to C: Bilobed flap.

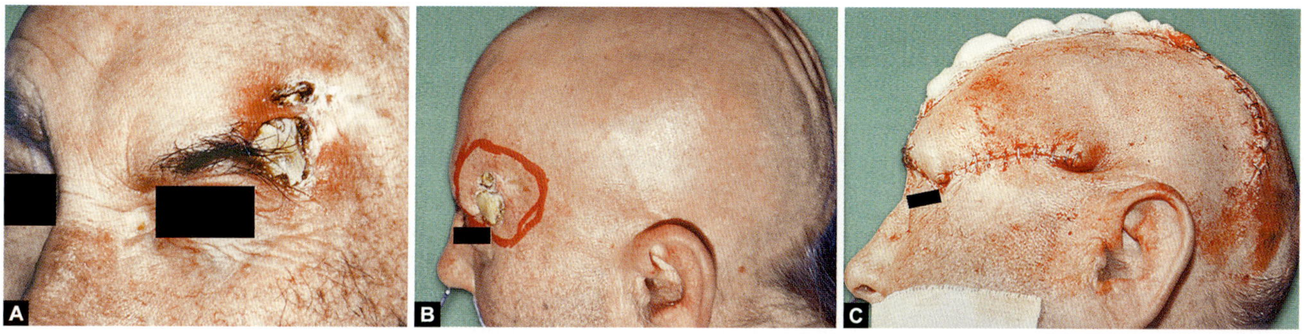

Figs. 23A to C: Rotation flap in scalp.

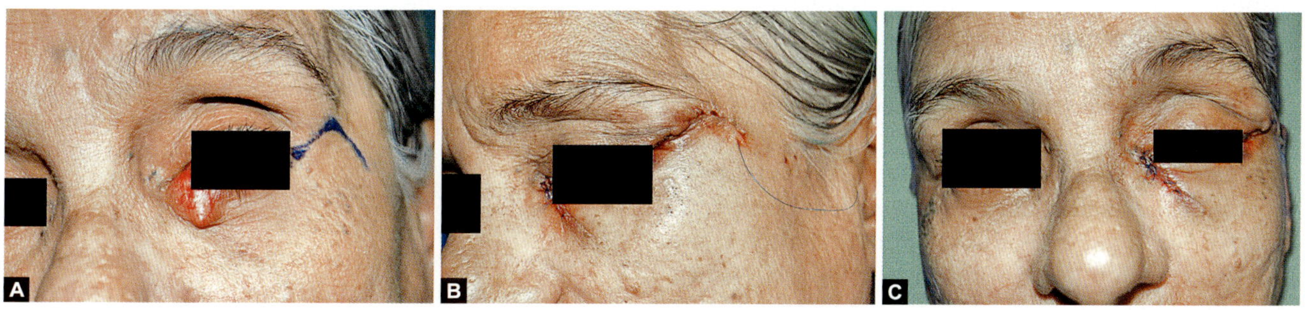

Figs. 24A to C: Tenzel flap for eyelid reconstruction.

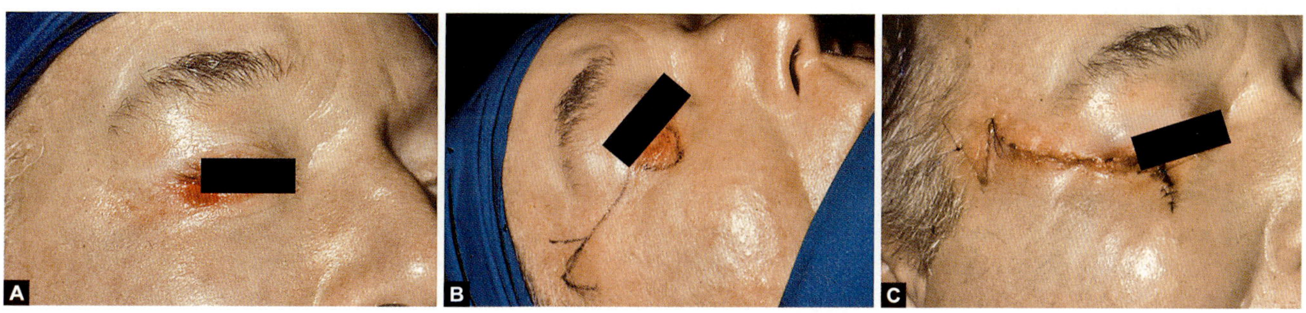

Figs. 25A to C: Mustardé flap for eyelid reconstruction.

useful in areas where there are no significant anatomical landmarks to obstruct the rotational movement of the flap. The large segment of tissue is rotated around a pivot point into the defect. The donor defect is usually repaired by direct closure (Tenzel flap) **(Figs. 24A to C)** or by local Z-plasty (Mustardé flap) **(Figs. 25A to C)** or by using a small skin graft. The mobility of this flap can be increased by a back cut or by cutting a Burrow's triangle near the pivot point;

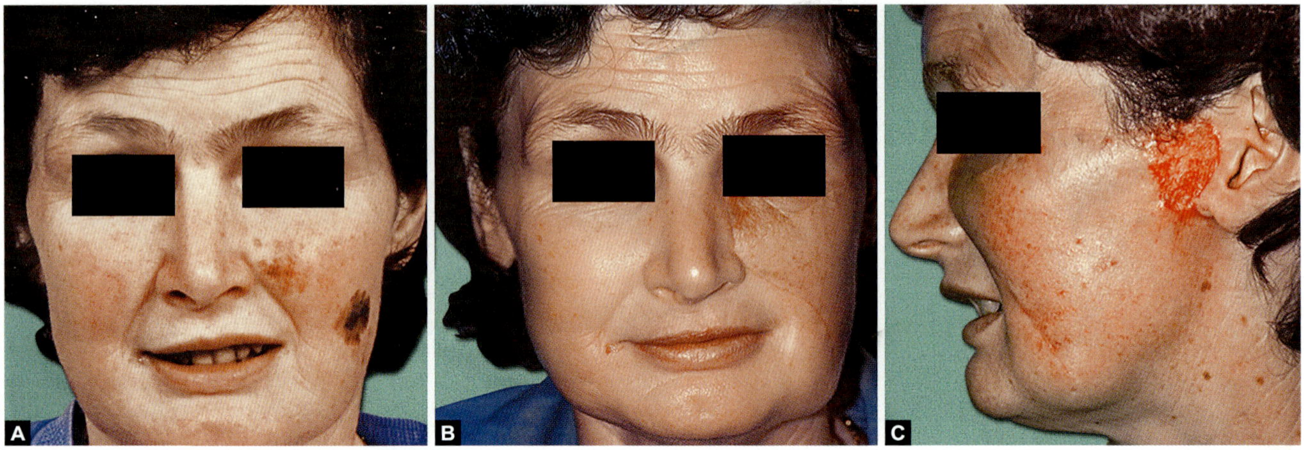

Figs. 26A to C: Cheek rotation flap.

the latter also helps reducing tension in the flap.[7] The long incisions are required to mobilize tissue sufficiently. The rotation flaps are generally inferiorly based to allow lymphatic drainage. These flaps are mainly used in scalp and cheeks where the long scars can be more easily concealed **(Figs. 26A to C)**.

It is important to triangularize the defect. The diameter of the semicircle should be three times the length of the defect and the circumference of the flap should be five to eight times the width of the defect. Always ensure that the length from the pivot point to the apex of the flap is greater than the distance to the apex of the defect so the flap can inset easily into it without excessive tension. Also note that the length of the leading edge of the flap is greater than the farthest point of the defect.

The flap is marked and incised. In the scalp, it is raised in the subgaleal plane and in cheek, it is raised in the subdermal plane. The flap is rotated and sutured into the defect. The donor defect is either closed primarily or grafted or repaired with another local flap.

AXIAL PATTERN FLAPS

Nasolabial Flap

The nasolabial flap is based on the perpendicular branches of the angular artery, which courses along the nasolabial groove. The flap can be harvested with the pedicle being proximal or distal. It is useful for the defects of lower part of nose, lower eyelid, upper cheek (distally based), and upper lip (proximally based). The distally based flap is perfused through anastomotic vessels between angular artery and the branches of ophthalmic artery near the medial orbital margin. The flap is marked with margins along the junction between aesthetic subunits or parallel to it, which ensures that the resulting scar lies in the junctional area, giving excellent aesthetic result **(Figs. 27A to F)**. The flap is dissected in a plane between subcutaneous fat and facial muscle, which ensures incorporation of the axial vessels in the flap. The flap is then transferred into the defect and sutured in two layers as described earlier. The donor site is too closed in two layers. A long flap can be used to reconstruct the full-thickness defects in the lower region of nose by folding the flap on itself. The disadvantage of this flap is that it may require further surgeries to divide the pedicle or to reduce the bulk of the flap **(Figs. 28A to C)**.

Median Forehead Flap

The median forehead flap is based on the terminal branches of angular artery and supratrochlear vessels. Being one of the earliest flaps that have been described, this is the most commonly utilized flap for the reconstruction of nose, upper eyelid, and inner canthus. In the midline, the frontalis muscle is absent and the flap is raised in the subcutaneous plane superficial to the periosteum. The donor site is closed in layers and the flap is inset into the defect. A central nasal defect can be reconstructed based on a pedicle from either side; however, a lateral nasal defect is better resurfaced by flap based on ipsilateral pedicle to decrease the distance between pivot point and defect. If the vertical height of the forehead is 7–8 cm, the flap is oriented vertically. If a longer flap is needed, then it can be oriented obliquely to get more length. It is important to note that the entire central third of forehead skin can survive on a single dominant pedicle.

In the design of the flap and the reconstruction of the primary defect, it is important to consider the aesthetic units of nose taking care not to transgress the boundaries **(Figs. 29 and 30)**. The disadvantage of this flap is that second surgery is needed to divide the pedicle which can be safely done after a delay of 3 weeks. The glabellar flap is a smaller flap and is useful for the smaller defects in the contiguous area **(Figs. 31A to C)**.

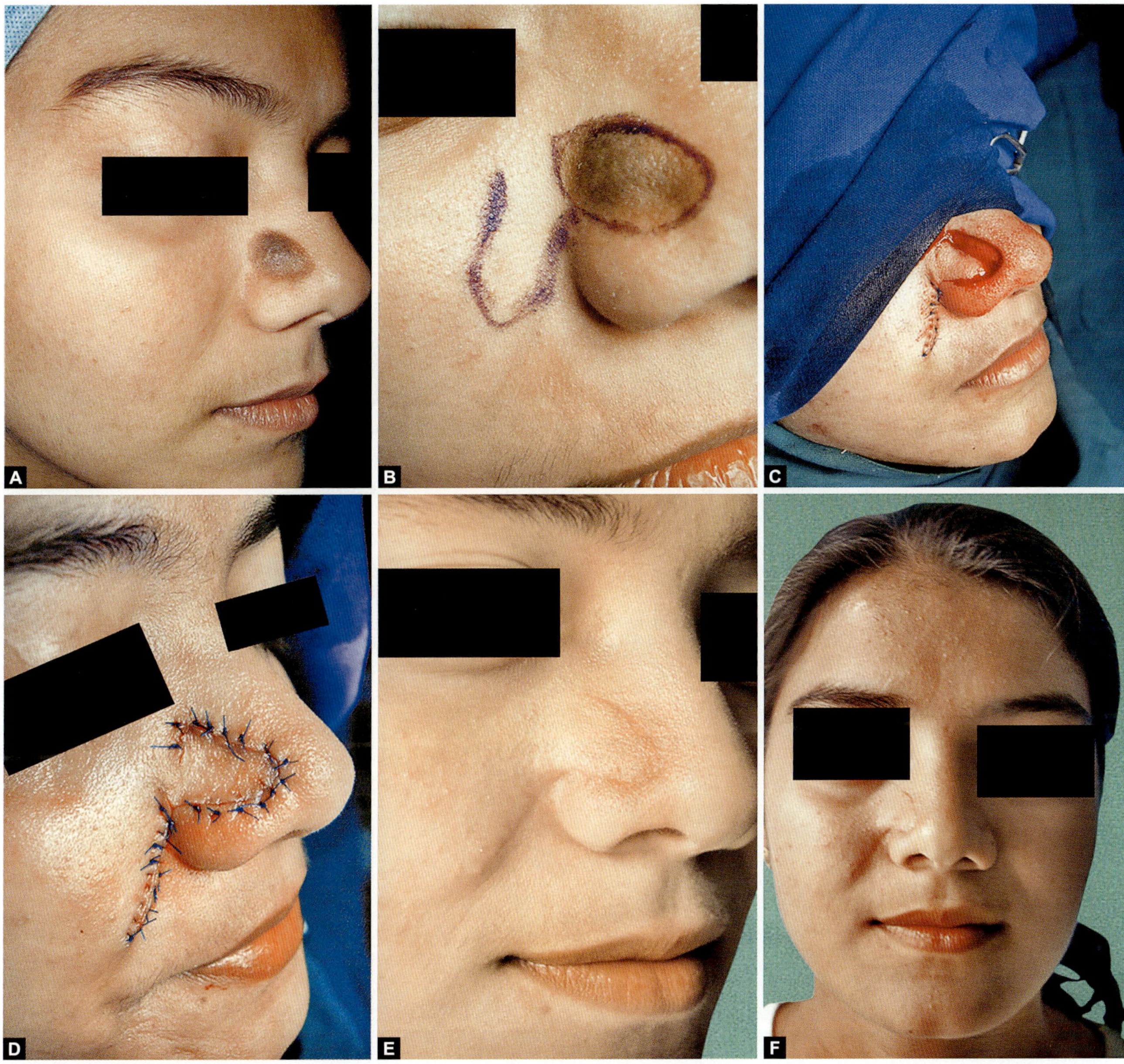

Figs. 27A to F: Nasolabial flap.

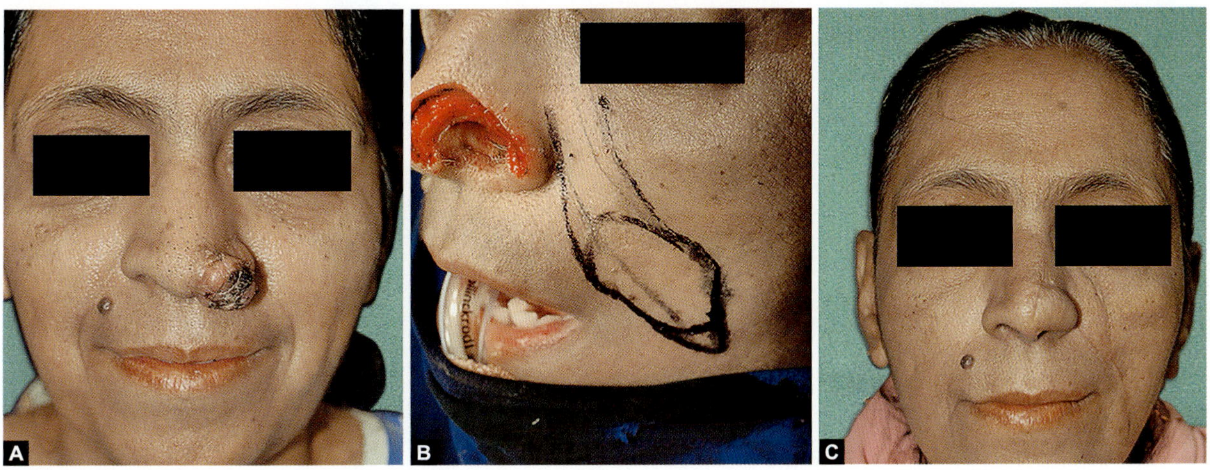

Figs. 28A to C: Alar reconstruction with nasolabial flap.

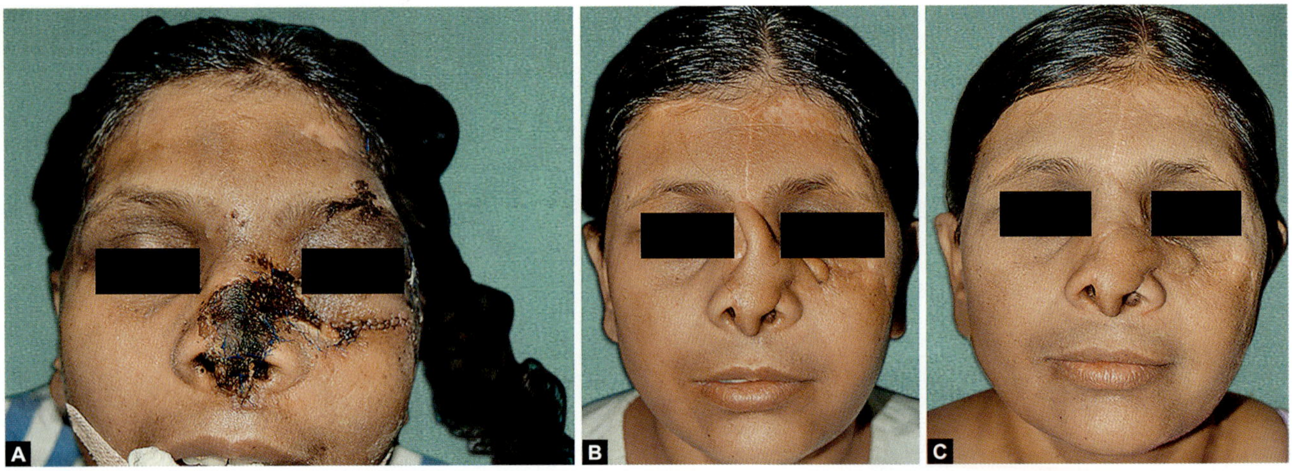

Figs. 29A to C: Median forehead flap for nasal reconstruction.

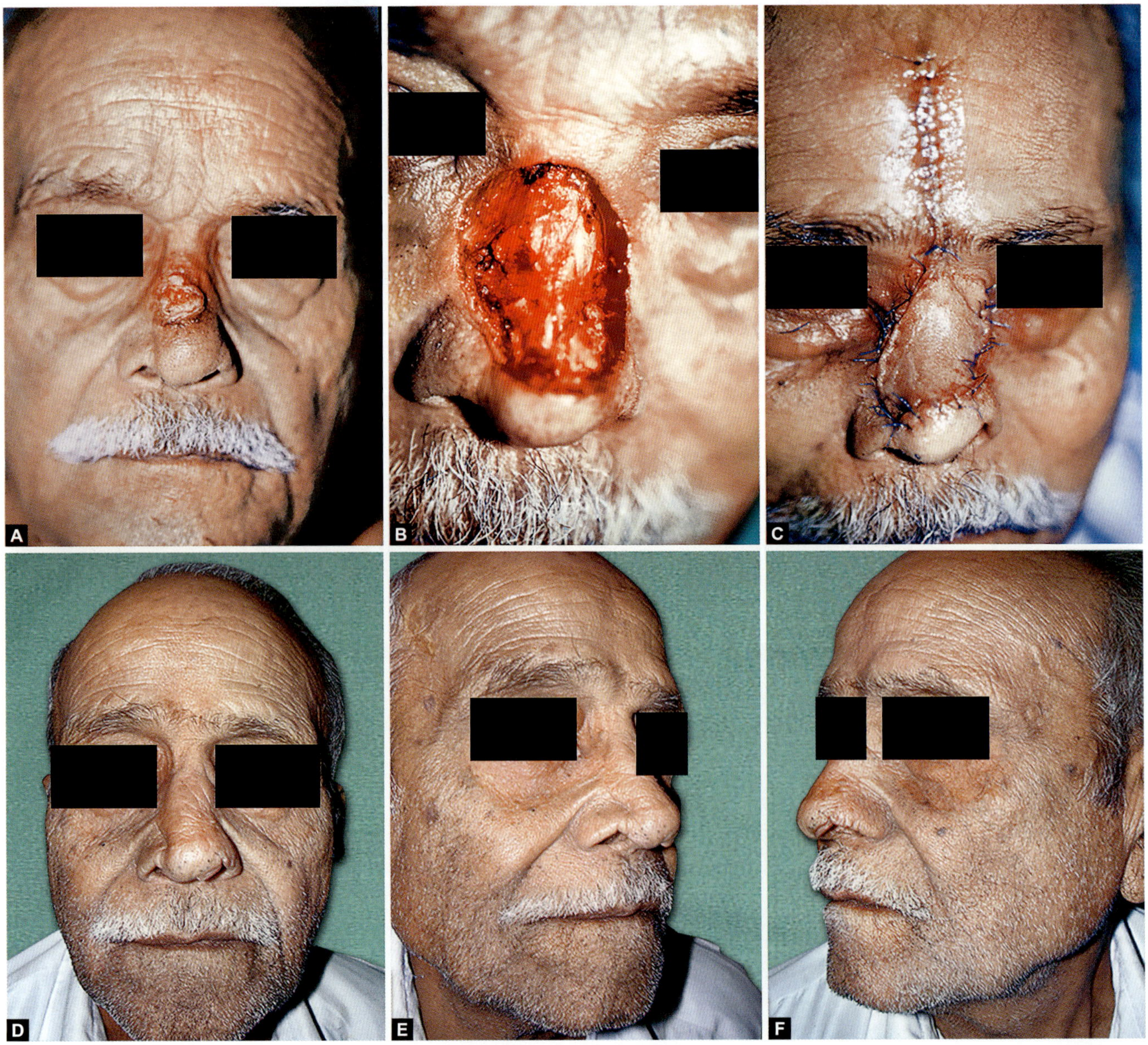

Figs. 30A to F: Forehead flap.

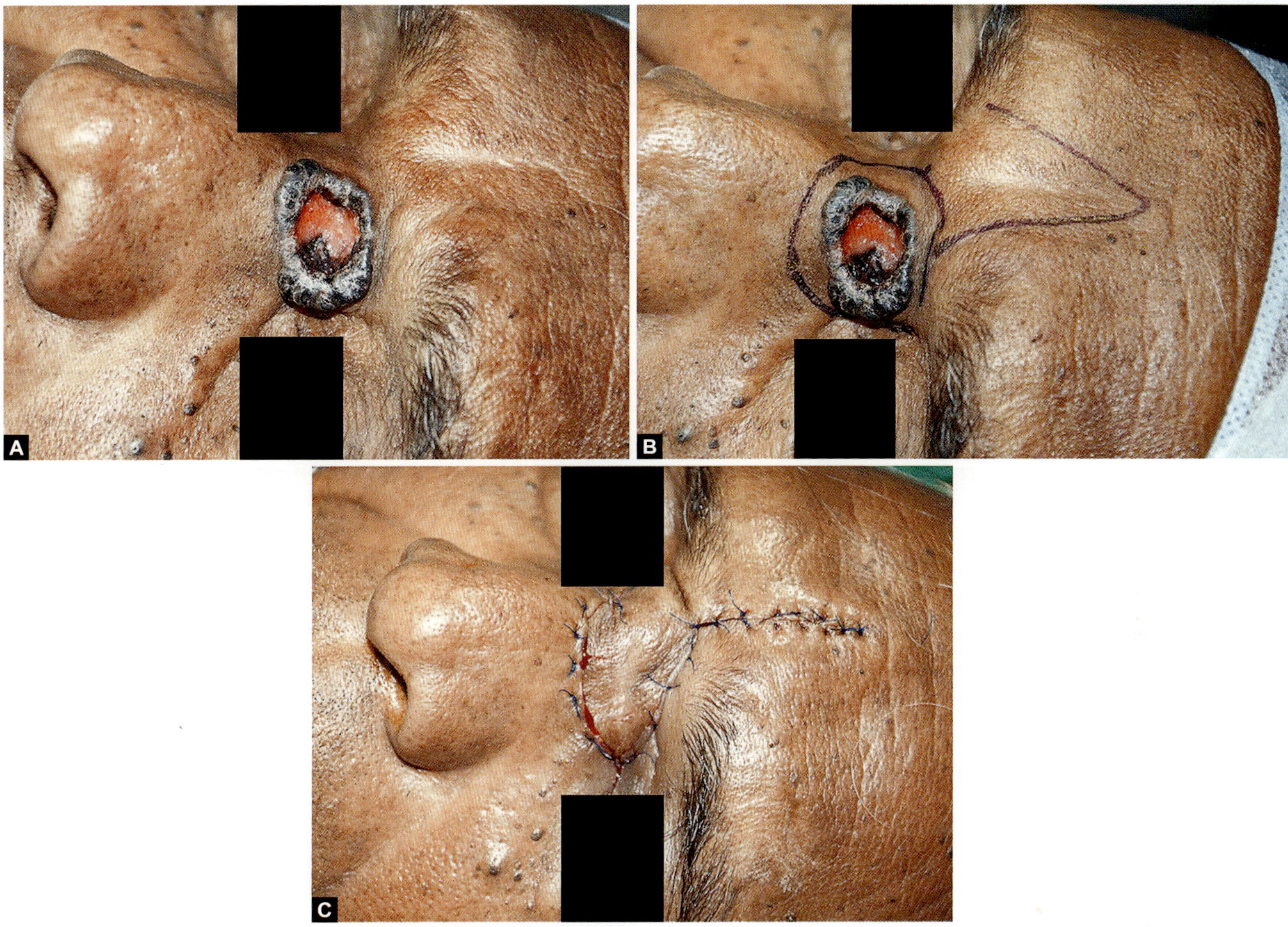

Figs. 31A to C: Glabellar flap for inner canthal defect.

PEARLS AND PITFALLS

Pearls:
- Always assess the defect before the flap design
- Consider the aesthetic units while designing the flap
- Design the flap slightly larger than the assessment
- Plan in reverse
- Meticulous hemostasis and gentle tissue handling

Pitfalls:
- Poor design in terms of *size*
- Tissue tension, poor hemostasis, and improper tissue handling, leading to flap necrosis
- Damage to facial nerve near lateral end of eyebrow and lower margin of mandible

CONCLUSION

- Advantage of local facial flaps is that the defect in facial skin is replaced with tissue with similar color and texture thus giving optimum results.
- Due to robust blood supply of facial skin many versatile local flaps can be done to fulfill the reconstructive needs.
- The surgeon should ensure that the scars of donor site of flap lie in the natural creases/wrinkes lines (RSTL's) without distortion of any facial landmarks or contours for superior outcome.

REFERENCES

1. Converse JM, McCarthy JG, Brauer RO, Ballantyne DL. Transplantation of skin: Grafts and flaps. In: Converse JM (Ed). Reconstructive Plastic Surgery, 2nd edition. Philadelphia: WB Saunders; 1977. pp. 152-239.
2. Limberg AA. Mathematical Principles of Local Plastic Procedures on the Surface of the Human Body. Leningrad: Medgriz; 1946.
3. Dufourmentel C. An L-shaped flap for lozenge-shaped defect. Transactions of the Third International Congress of Plastic Surgeons. Amsterdam: Excerpta Medical Foundation; 1963. p. 772.
4. Quaba AA, Sommerlad BC. A square peg into a round hole: a modified rhomboid flap and its clinical application. Br J Plast Surg. 1987;40(2):163-70.
5. Zimany A. The bilobed flap. Plast Reconstr Surg. 1953;11(6): 424-34.
6. Khouri R. Skin flaps. In: Nouri K, Leal-Khouri S (Eds). Techniques in Dermatologic Surgery. St Louis: Mosby; 2003. pp. 141-51.
7. Baker SR. Local Flaps in Facial Reconstruction, 2nd edition. Philadelphia: Mosby; 2007.

CHAPTER 25

Surgical Dermabrasion and Curettage

Satish S Savant, Sushil S Savant

SURGICAL DERMABRASION

KEY MESSAGES

- Dermabrasion is an effective way of resurfacing.
- It needs surgical skill and training.
- It can be used in both cosmetic and noncosmetic indications.
- Prolonged healing time and complications attributed to full face dermabrasion have increased the popularity of fractional lasers; however, multiple sessions of fractional lasers can never achieve the aesthetically superior results of full face dermabrasion.
- Spot dermabrasion is useful treatment modality in vitiligo surgeries and tumors of face including syringoma, trichoepithelioma, adenoma sebaceum, seborrheic keratosis, Darier's disease, etc.

INTRODUCTION

Dermabrasion is defined as sequential planning of the raised, altered, or otherwise normal skin from the epidermis through the papillary dermis to the desired level (up to the junction of upper and midreticular dermis) with either manual and/or electrical motorized abraders and further allowing this wound to heal by secondary intention, so as to achieve leveling (resurfacing) effect to make the cutaneous lesions and/or scars less conspicuous.

Dermabrasion involves mechanical removal of layers of skin. Dermabrasion restricted up to upper reticular to midreticular dermis creates a superficial wound and initiates a secondary intention wound healing process. The epidermis then regenerates from the epidermal appendages (hair follicles, pilosebaceous, and sweat glands) and from the margins. This process begins within 24 hours of dermabrasion and takes about 7–12 days to complete. The new epidermis shows greater organization and vertical polarity. Dermal regeneration is a slow process taking several months. The regenerated dermis demonstrates less elastosis and improved organization with compact horizontally arranged bundles of collagen interspersed with elastic fibers (collagen remodeling). Ground substance is decreased and telangiectasias are absent. The overall result is soft supple skin that appears more youthful and has fewer rhytids and dyschromias.

The objective of every dermabrasion should be to reorganize and restructure the collagen of the papillary dermis without causing injury beyond the upper reticular dermis, as any abrasion below this plane is likely to result in scarring.

Cryoanesthesia has been advocated to make the skin firmer as an aid to even dermabrasion. However, in India, cryoanesthesia is not available and, hence, facial dermabrasions are performed under general anesthesia (GA). Further, we have to dermabrade the skin in "as is where is condition" as per the pattern of various dermal layers. Hence, it is important to be aware of the markers for identification of the different layers, which are described in **Box 1**.

HISTORY[1-21]

Dermabrasion is a technique for skin resurfacing that has been in use for nearly 100 years. In 1905, Kromeyer, a German dermatologist, reported the use of power-driven abrading instruments on skin chilled with ether spray and CO_2 snow for the treatment of postacne scarring. He studied the effect of dermabrasion to various depths and established that the wounds healed without scars if the surgical injury did not penetrate through the reticular dermis, thus laying down the basic guideline for the depth of abrasion.

BOX 1: Guidelines for assessing depth of dermabrasion as one progresses through the skin (Author's original work).[3,10-14,42]

- Removal of skin pigment (epidermis)
- Appearance of multiple, tiny punctate bleeding points with high-field density (superficial papillary dermis)
- *Change in the pattern of bleeding:* Appearance of larger, rapidly bleeding points with low-field density and increased splattering (junction of mid to deep papillary dermis)
- Appearance of faintly visible pinkish or whitish to grayish parallel lines and ridges (junction of deep papillary to upper reticular dermis)
- *Excessive bleeding with fraying or appearance of breaks in the parallel lines and ridges with a feeling of resistance:* Optimal level and adequate depth of dermabrasion (junction of upper and midreticular dermis)
- *Herniation of tiny yellow bits of fat (lower reticular dermis ruptured at places):* Not a good sign, stop dermabrading at this level

Kurtin, a dermatologist at Mount Sinai Hospital in New York, was the first to present a series of patients who underwent dermabrasion with modified dental equipment in 1953. Various abrasive end pieces were described such as rasps, burrs, and wire brushes. Black coined the term "dermabrasion" in 1954. Alt and Yarborough further contributed to this field by advocating use of the diamond fraise and wire brush end pieces, respectively. Lowenthal reported that better results were obtained when ice pick scars were punch grafted prior to dermabrasion.

In India, Maneksha in 1955 used sandpaper for treating smallpox scars, acne scars, tattoos, and allied defects. The manual metallic dermabraders were introduced by him mainly to treat smallpox scars and till today, these form one of the essential instruments for performing controlled dermabrasion.

The authors introduced techniques to achieve safe dermabrasion at various levels of depth with therapeutic spot as well as regional and facial dermabrasion procedures for treating a variety of skin conditions such as papular lichen amyloidosis (PLA), stable vitiligo, acne scars, and genodermatoses such as adenoma sebaceum, multiple trichoepitheliomas, and Darier's disease. Dermabrasion has been used for treating many cutaneous conditions varying from acne scars to the removal of tattoos or tumors or scar revisions. It is possible to dermabrade skin in any area of the body by altering the methodology according to the anatomical features of the region.

The popularity of this procedure has diminished with the advent of newer procedures including chemical exfoliation, laser resurfacing, nonablative laser resurfacing, and microdermabrasion because of the invasiveness and longer downtime for dermabrasion. However, these procedures are useful for rectifying only superficial scars and pigmentary defects. In author's opinion, dermabrasion in hands of a skilled and experienced surgeon still remains an effective remedy for deep scars and rhytids.

INDICATIONS[9-35]

Conditions for which dermabrasion has been used are shown in **Table 1**.

CONTRAINDICATIONS[1-7,9,13-16,36-40]

Contraindications include keloidal tendency, atrophic hairless scars of burns and trauma, bleeding disorders, active infection, and history of taking isotretinoin (wait for 12–18 months). Patients with types 4–6 skin need special counseling.

PREOPERATIVE PROCEDURES[1-3,8,13,41-47]

The following techniques can be adopted 6–8 weeks before the planned date of dermabrasion, depending on the indication, for better end results:

- *Scar revision techniques:* Undermining (subcision), punch excision and closure, punch elevation, punch excision, and graft replacement **(Figs. 1 and 2)**
- *Electrocauterization and radiosurgery:* For raised lesions and borders

TABLE 1: Conditions for the use of dermabrasion.

Condition	Uses
1. Facial scars	Postacne scars, chickenpox, herpes zoster, smallpox, and traumatic scars
2. Acne	Chronic resistant acne (reduces size of sebaceous duct with better sebum drainage and prophylactic use), acne rosacea, and enlarged pores
3. Stable vitiligo	Therapeutic spot wounding, preparation of recipient area prior to grafting in all types of grafting methods: suction blister technique (SBT), ultrathin skin grafting, and melanocyte and keratinocyte suspension method
4. Hyperkeratotic lesions	Lichen simplex chronicus (LSC), hypertrophic lichen planus (HLP), papular lichen amyloidosis (PLA), porokeratosis, linear verrucous nevus (LVN), and prurigo nodularis
5. Pigmentation	Melasma, freckles, postinflammatory hyperpigmentation (PIH), tattoos, and periorbital hypermelanosis
6. Tumors	Syringoma, trichoepithelioma, adenoma sebaceum, seborrheic keratosis, Darier's disease, nevus depigmentosus, congenital nevi, neurofibromatosis, Bowen's disease, and basal cell carcinoma
7. Actinic	Actinic keratosis, actinic cheilitis, and photoaging
8. Miscellaneous	Pyogenic granuloma, fine wrinkling, rejuvenation, rhinophyma, and xeroderma pigmentosum (prophylactic)

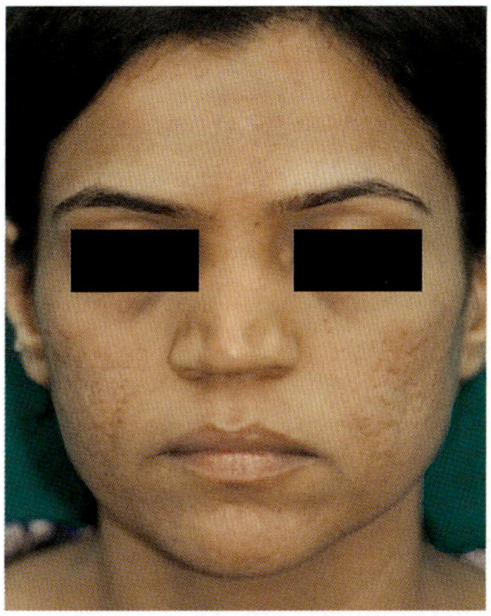

Fig. 1: Acne scar with PIH (Earlier treated with 10–12 sittings of fractional CO_2 laser ablation by previous treating doctors)
(CO_2: carbon dioxide; PIH: postinflammatory hyperpigmentation)
Courtesy: Dr Sushil S Savant, Mumbai.

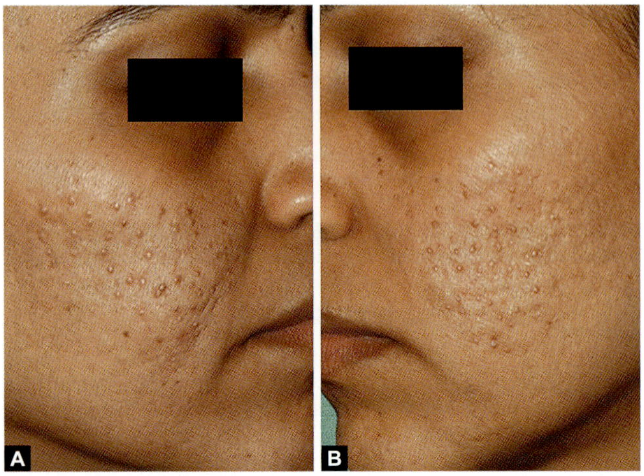

Figs. 2A and B: ASR—Punch replacement with take-up of grafts
Courtesy: Dr Sushil S Savant, Mumbai.

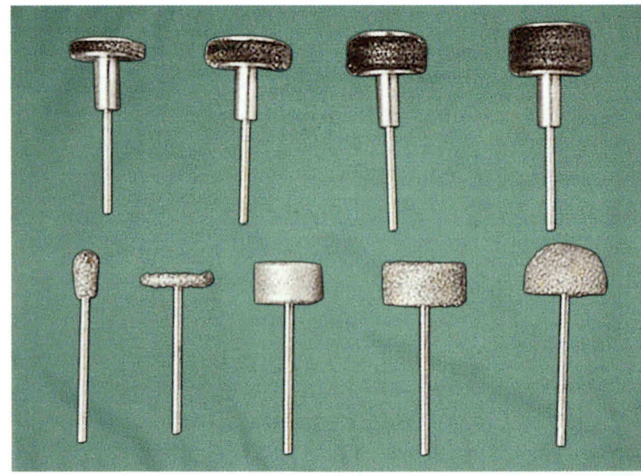

Fig. 4: Diamond fraises and wire brushes.

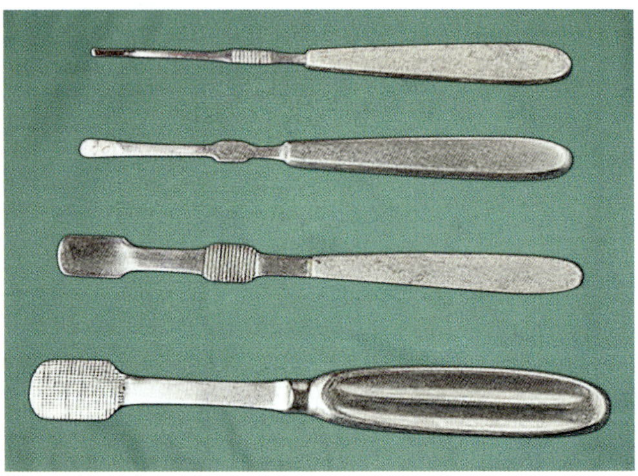

Fig. 3: Manual dermabraders.

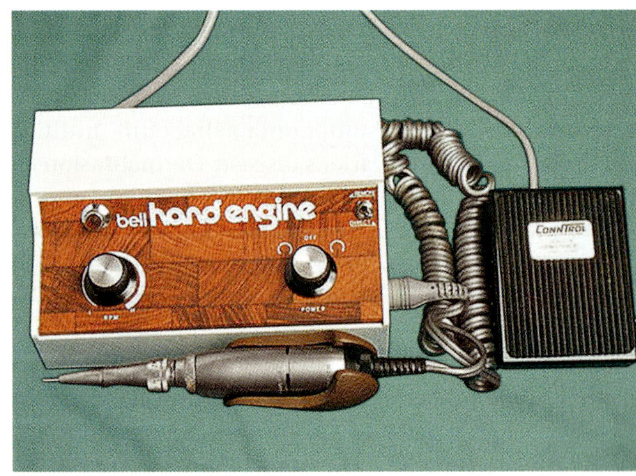

Fig. 5: Dermabrasion machine.

PATIENT INFORMATION

Patient counseling should include special emphasis on the following aspects:

- Realistic expectation of surgical outcome (50–70% improvement and not complete elimination)
- Multiple sittings may be required
- Postoperative sequelae, side effects, and complications. Postoperative sun avoidance and sun protection for 3 months
- If possible, the procedure should be deferred till beginning of monsoons [lesser chances of postinflammatory hyperpigmentation (PIH)] as per author's experience

EQUIPMENT

- *Mechanical (manual)* ***(Fig. 3)***:
  - Sandpapers (water paper No. 80 and 110)
  - Handheld metallic dermabraders (*Source*: Dr Maneksha's)
- *Electrical:*
  - Wire brushes, burrs, and diamond fraises (various sizes and shapes) **(Fig. 4)**
  - *Cable:* Unit or hand machine (average 15,000 rpm) **(Fig. 5)**

PREOPERATIVE WORKUP

This is performed as per any surgical procedure. Since facial dermabrasion is done under GA, preanesthetic checkup and clearance are needed. Informed consent and photographs are mandatory. In selected cases, particularly, full face dermabrasion, test spot dermabrasion at postauricular site may be done 4–6 weeks prior to planned date of surgery to study healing pattern and possibility of complications in a given case. Thus, it also carries medicolegal significance. Close shave and removal of excess hair are done just before operation. Injection of vitamin K (1 mL containing 10 mg) is given 1 day before surgery in cases of extensive dermabrasion.

If there is history suggestive of herpes labialis, prophylaxis with antivirals is indicated.

FACIAL DERMABRASION

Operative Procedure[1-3,5-7,9,17,20-22,24,26,29,32,33,41,42,45,48-54]

The important steps in this major procedure are as follows:

- *Use of protective gear by operating staff:* Cap, mask, gown, gloves, and face shield (universal precautions as splattering of blood often occurs during the procedure).
- *Mark the submandibular margin:* Just beneath and parallel to the inferior border of the mandibular ramus from infra-auricular area to the center of the chin on both the sides.
- Induction of GA with endotracheal intubation (infusing halothane), supine position with posterior tilting of head with head ring, hair taped with micropore tape and tucked under the cap, ears plugged with cotton, antibiotic ointment in eyes, roller gauze in mouth for cheek protrusion, and intravenous (IV) fluids as required.
- Surgical preparation and marking the pitted scars/lesions individually with marker pen.
- *Anesthesia:* The procedure can be done under different types of anesthesia—local, regional, or general. Spot dermabrasion can be done under local anesthesia (LA). Full face dermabrasion needs to be performed under GA. Tumescent anesthesia too has been used to perform dermabrasion.[45]
- *Technique:*
    a. Face is turned to one side and skin stretched by an assistant, so as to provide a flat and taut surface for planning.
    b. Using either wire brush or diamond fraise endpiece and hold the handpiece in safety razor grip **(Fig. 6)**. Direction of pull should be toward the handle of handpiece, i.e., perpendicular to the axis of the direction of rotating endpiece. First establishes the submandibular border by smooth strokes along the marked line from either ear to the chin. Ipsilateral sides are abraded from the temporal hairline to coalesce with the submandibular border. Feather the established inferior edge of the submandibular border by light perpendicular short strokes going 1 cm beneath it either with electrical or manual abraders. Establish the submandibular margin on the other side in a similar manner.
    c. Individual pitted marked out scar surface is moderately stretched. Using a pear-shaped diamond fraise endpiece and with pencil-like vertical grip of hand machine, gently rotate the handpiece clockwise in small circles to lightly abrade the base of the scar and firmly abrade its edges (shouldering). Smoothen out all the marked scars individually in a similar fashion.
    d. Raised lesions of trichoepitheliomas, adenoma sebaceum, Darier's disease, etc., are flattened out by abrading them individually with pear-shaped dermabraders or by sculpting with No. 15 blades or by radiosurgery to the level of the surrounding skin.
    e. *Segmental electrical cosmetic facial unit wise dermabrasion:* With wire brush or disk diamond fraise attached to handpiece held in a razor grip, head is turned to one side and skin is stretched **(Fig. 6)**. Establish the infraorbital margin by dermabrading downward on the cheeks and sideway on the temporal region along the bony margin in a curvilinear manner leaving 2–3 cm of normal skin around the eyes unabraded. Further, dermabrade segmentally in the following order of preference: right cheek, chin, left cheek, forehead, glabella, nose, and upper lip. Segmental abrasion should always either overlap or feather into the adjoining segments at the natural folds such as vermilion borders and nasolabial folds or peripheral regional boundaries such as the hairline and ear-to-ear submandibular line inferiorly. Abrade evenly up to adequate depth, i.e., up to the junction of mid and deep papillary dermis. This is followed by mechanical dermabrasion, which gives better control, thus, providing safety.
    f. *Manual dermabrasion (**Fig. 7**):* Manual metallic dermabraders yield better depth control. Large abraders are used for flatter surfaces and smaller ones are used for narrow surfaces and curvatures. Dermabrade till optimum depth is reached, i.e., up to the junction of upper and midreticular dermis or as per the requirement. It is better to underabrade to avoid complications. In between the procedure, hemostasis is achieved with ice-cold sponges. Manual dermabrader has the disadvantage of being more time-consuming.

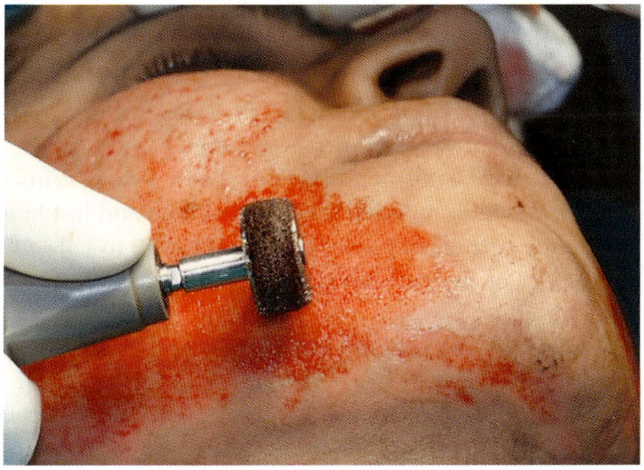

Fig. 6: Electrical dermabrasion
Courtesy: Dr Sushil S Savant, Mumbai.

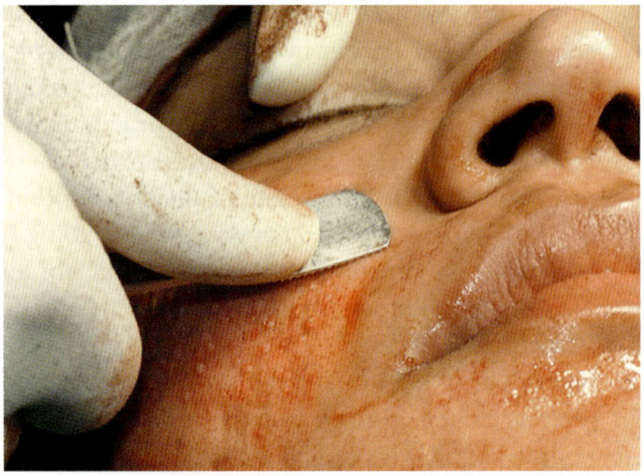

Fig. 7: Manual dermabrasion
Courtesy: Dr Sushil S Savant, Mumbai.

g. *Termination:* Finally, two quick face rubs with No. 80, followed by No. 110 sandpapers (waterpapers), are done in the same segmental, sequential order to smoothen out the surface. Hemostasis is achieved with ice-cold sponges.
h. For patients under GA with endotracheal intubation, abrade one side of the face fully in similar fashion going stepwise from steps (a) to (g). Other side is then abraded similarly after changing the direction of the endotracheal tube to the opposite side. Lastly, remove the tube and abrade the remaining area of chin and upper lip first electrically and then mechanically. Two quick rubs with sandpaper are given and hemostasis is achieved with ice-cold sponges.

Postoperative Management[3,13,51]

The guidelines for postoperative management are as follows:

- Intravenous fluids
- Admit the patient and discharge only when oozing stops (about 7 days)
- *Dressing:* Two methods are:
  1. Face is dressed only with double layer of framycetin tulle
  2. Face is not dressed at all allowing the serum to ooze continuously
- Towel is lightly wrapped around the neck to absorb the oozing serum. Two fans are placed across either cheek for faster drying of the secretions.
- *Medications:* Antibiotics, analgesics, and short course of tapering steroids (IV first day and changed to oral from day 2), usually 8 mg IV dexamethasone on day 1 and tapered fast. Injection of vitamin K (1 mL) should be continued from a day before surgery followed by on the day and the next day after dermabrasion (total of 3 consecutive days).
- Serous discharge oozes for 2–3 days and then dries to form crusts either directly on the face or on the stuck framycetin gauzes. Both fall off by 10–15 days.
- Emollients and sunscreens for next 3 months.
- Patient remains indoor for 4 weeks and avoids direct sunlight for further 2–3 months.

Figures 8 to 11 show pre- and postoperative results after dermabrasion in a patient with postacne scarring.

Side Effects

Side effects are many and include pain, edema, exudation, discomfort, crusting, erythema, milia, hyperpigmentation (reversible), persistent erythema, permanent hypopigmentation, and exacerbation of acne (reversible).

Complications[3,13,42,52,53]

Complications include bleeding, telangiectasia, gouging, infection, scarring, keloid, allergic contact dermatitis, and complications of LA or GA.

Advantages and Disadvantages

Relative advantages and disadvantages of the procedure are shown in **Table 2**.

REGIONAL/SPOT DERMABRASION[2-7,31-34,54]

Apart from face, dermabrasion can be done on any portion of the body (regional) or only the lesion (spot), according to the location and the clinical features of the lesion, after taking into consideration the side effects and complications.

The methodology for regional or spot dermabrasion is essentially the same; however, one may have to make a few modifications as described below:

- *Vitiligo:* Superficial spot dermabrasion till pinpoint bleeding (epidermabrasion) can be done for stable vitiligo in hairy area for faster repigmentation and as an adjuvant to medical line of treatment prior to grafting by SBT or ultrathin split-thickness skin graft (STSG) or application of melanocyte–keratinocyte suspension. Prior to grafting by thin Thiersch's STSG, slightly deeper dermabrasion is done till change in bleeding pattern (junction of mid to deep papillary dermis).
- *Hypertrophic lichen planus (HLP):* Two sittings of deep spot dermabrasion are usually required.
- *Papular lichen amyloidosis (PLA):* Leave island strips of normal skin in between the abraded area and lest large wounds created may delay healing **(Figs. 12 to 17)**.
- *Tattoo:* For deeper abrasion, multiple sittings may be required.
- *Striae and scars:* Abrade superficially and linearly along the lesion.
- *Lichen simplex chronicus (LSC), linear verrucous epidermal nevus, and prurigo nodularis:* Abrade deep and multiple sittings may be required depending on the depth and number of lesions.

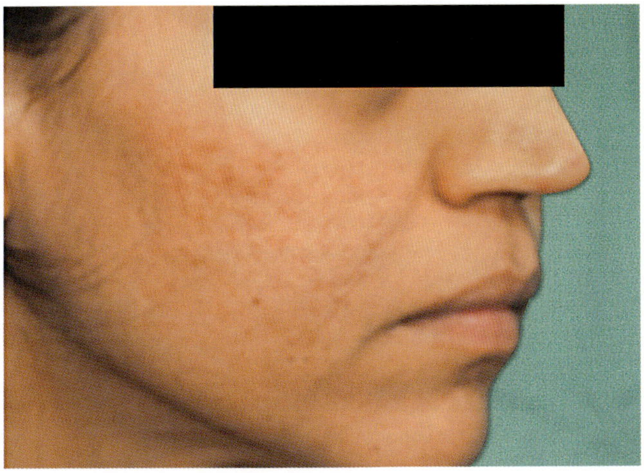

Fig. 8: Before (right cheek).

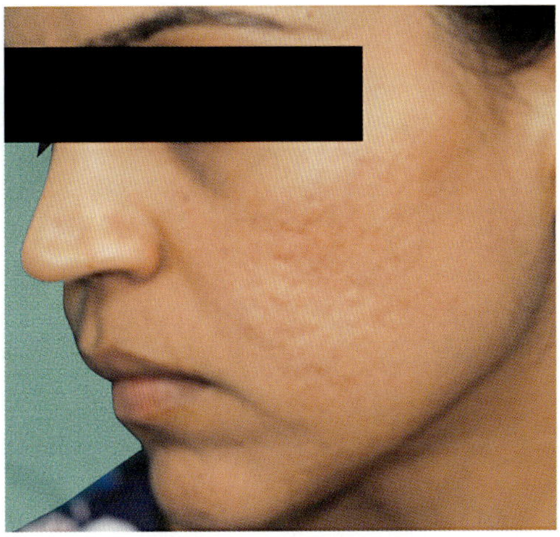

Fig. 10: Before (left cheek).

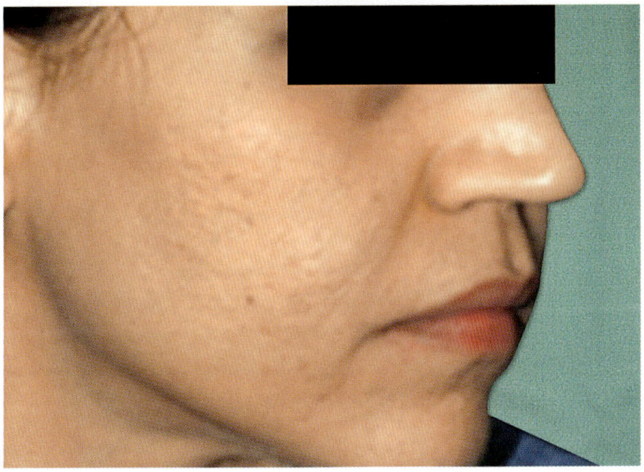

Fig. 9: Postoperative—1 year (right cheek).

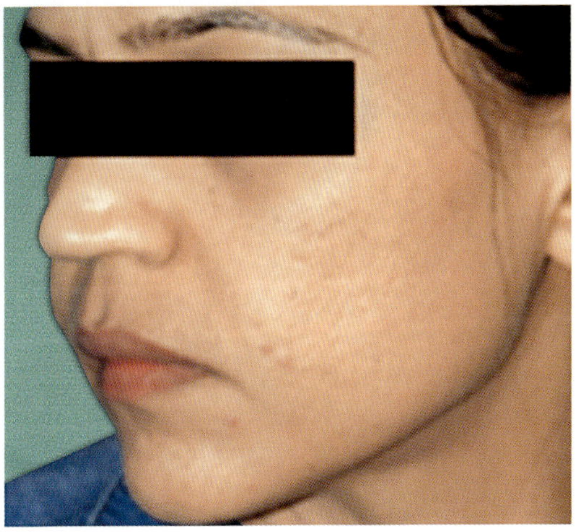

Fig. 11: Postoperative—1 year (left cheek).

Improvement in scars, PIH with rejuvenation.
(PIH: postinflammatory hyperpigmentation)
Courtesy: Dr Sushil S Savant, Mumbai.

TABLE 2: Full face dermabrasion: advantages and disadvantages.

Advantages	*Disadvantages*
• Excellent cosmetic improvement—50–80% even in cases of deep scars • *Multiple roles*: Cosmetic/Therapeutic/Prophylactic (for actinic keratoses/xeroderma pigmentosum to prevent malignancy) • All the scars and lesions are treated at one time • Can be combined with scar revision/electrocauterization, radiosurgery, chemical peeling, etc. • Better control over depth than other ablative procedures, as one can visually assess the various skin layers	• Hospital admission • Prolonged postoperative rest • Need for general anesthesia (GA) • Avoidance of sunlight for 3 months • Multiple sittings may be required for better cosmetic results • Deep ice pick scars cannot be corrected by dermabrasion alone • Permanent hypopigmentation may occur

Manual spot dermabrasion can also be performed with disposable presterilized scratch pads having roughened surfaces and commonly used to clean cautery tips.

Advantages

- Quick symptomatic relief in HLP, LSC, PLA, and prurigo nodularis
- Faster results compared to other modalities in LSC, PLA, HLP, and prurigo nodularis
- An adjuvant to medical treatment in vitiligo
- Inexpensive, simple office procedure
- Can be done under LA

Disadvantages

- It can be used only where cosmetic importance is secondary to functional importance: Patient acceptance is vital.

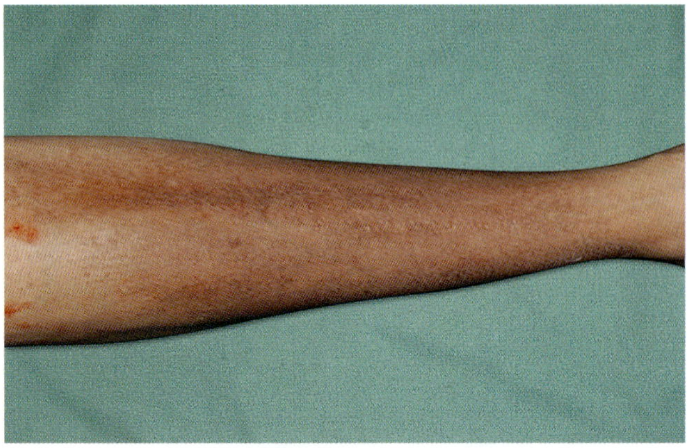

Fig. 12: Before.

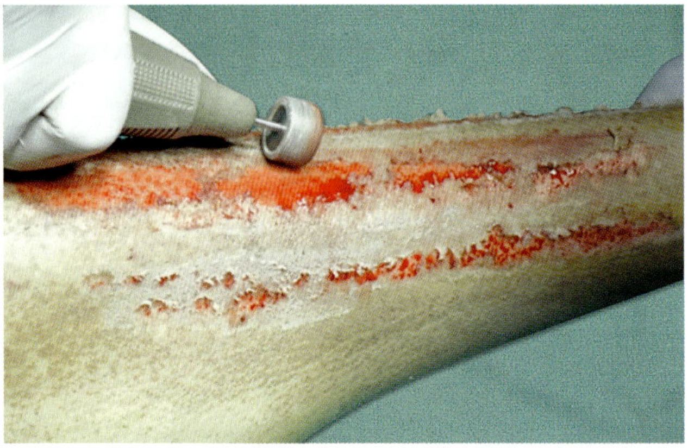

Fig. 13: Electrical dermabrasion.

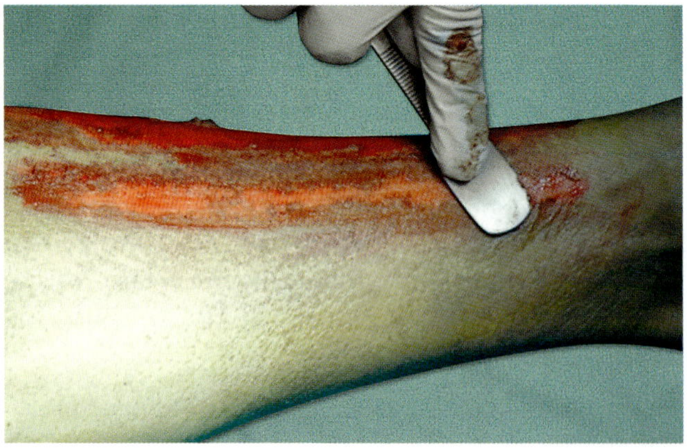

Fig. 14: Manual dermabrasion.

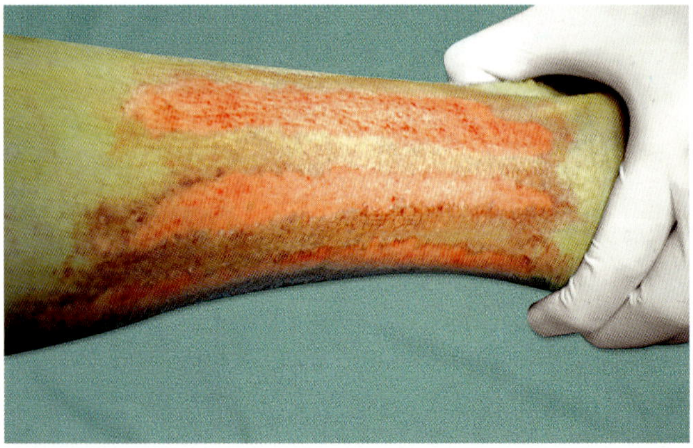

Fig. 15: Longitudinal dermabraded strip.

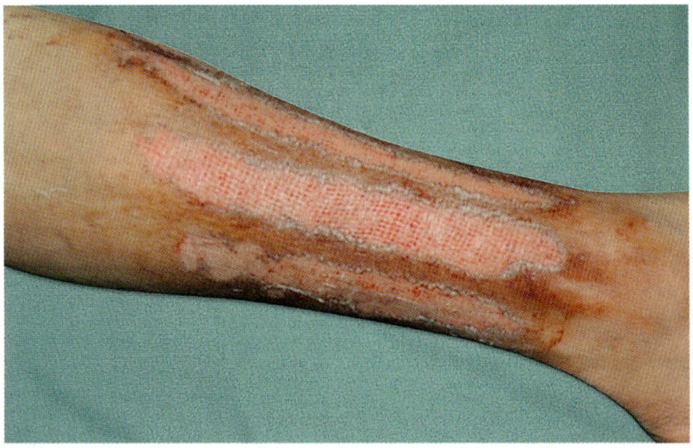

Fig. 16: Re-epithelialization.

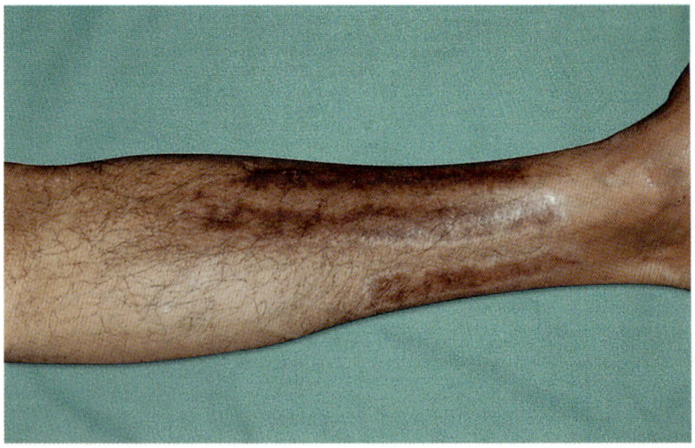

Fig. 17: Healing with superficial scarring and PIH.

Papular Lichen Amyloidosis: Therapeutic Spot/Regional Dermabrasion
(PIH: postinflammatory hyperpigmentation)
Courtesy: Dr Sushil S Savant, Mumbai.

- Abrasion may have to be carried to a deeper level for results and prevention of recurrence and may lead to scarring.
- Multiple sittings may be required.

COMBINATION TECHNIQUE (AUTHOR'S MODIFICATION)[55]

Dermabrasion can be combined with carbon dioxide (CO_2) laser for deep facial acne scars described as follows:

- First pass of CO_2 laser to abrade the epidermis after treating individual scars.
- Regular dermabrasion with diamond fraise/wire brush electrical and manual metallic dermabraders.
- Finally, one or two CO_2 laser passes for tightening effect.

However, the disadvantage is the persistent erythema and transient PIH, which can last up to 6 months postlaser procedure.

CONCLUSION

As stated earlier, dermabrasion is largely being replaced by lasers, particularly after the advent of fractional lasers. Facial dermabrasion is technically a difficult procedure and requires plenty of experience and training. Proper patient selection, recognition of planning depth, greater surgical skill and technique, and good postoperative care are all essential for its successful outcome. Despite recent publications that dermabrasion can be performed safely on patients taking systemic isotretinoin,[56,57] the author believes that it is prudent to stop isotretinoin at least 6–12 months prior to dermabrasion. The author is of the opinion that elective full face dermabrasion is a major invasive procedure where any preventable side effect should be avoided in the vital cosmetic facial area. It is useful to treat variety of conditions from acne scars to genodermatoses to facial rejuvenation. It can also be combined with other dermatosurgical modalities such as chemical peeling, soft-tissue augmentation, facelifts, and lasers. The author feels that it is still useful in the current scenario in the following situations:

- Therapeutic spot dermabrasion is a simple and useful modality to treat various skin conditions as an office procedure. It can be curative by itself or used as an adjuvant to medical line of treatment.
- It also gives faster results and since the technique is simple, many of the dermatologists can easily undertake it.
- As compared to fully ablative resurfacing with the CO_2 and erbium-doped yttrium aluminum garnet (Er:YAG) lasers, dermabrasion demonstrates similar or greater efficacy for the treatment of scars, rhytids, genodermatoses, etc., with less postoperative erythema and more rapid re-epithelialization. The most significant difference as compared to other modalities is that in dermabrasion, you know the exact depth which you have reached, whereas in other resurfacing modalities, it is a blind alley as you do not know how deep your chemical peel is going to sink or to what level your last laser pass is going to reach.

Although experience and skill are necessary in order to avoid complications with full face dermabrasion, its efficacy remains unmatched for the patient who is willing to endure the resultant recovery period. While new technologies continue to emerge, dermabrasion will likely remain an essential and unmatched modality for scar improvement.

TIPS

- In acne scars, it is mainly the surrounding skin which has to be abraded to the depth of the scar to obtain the leveling effect
- However, in case of elevated lesions such as benign tumors, lesions are abraded so as to bring them to the level of surrounding skin thus, achieving the contouring effect. This is far easier than that for acne scars and chances of scarring are less
- For facial dermabrasion, a test patch can be done 6 weeks prior to study healing patterns and complications
- Beginners can start with abrading lesions over trunk and extremities, which have lesser cosmetic significance to get a hang of the procedure before attempting facial abrasion
- Sterilized disposable scratch pads can be used for mild-to-moderate manual dermabrasion; however, authors have no personal experience using disposable scratch pads

CURETTAGE

KEY MESSAGES

- Curettage is a simple and effective dermatosurgical procedure to treat variety of superficial lesions with good end results.
- It is important for the surgeon to develop a tactile sense (feel) of the curette against normal skin as opposed to pathological skin conditions for successful outcome of the procedure.
- Therapeutic curettage and electrodesiccation, in combination, can be used to treat variety of benign, premalignant, or malignant conditions.

INTRODUCTION

It is a procedure where the skin lesion is removed in toto or partly by the act of physical scraping and scooping with a semi-sharp cutting edge of the ring of the tip of simple instrument called dermal curette. The procedure can be carried out under topical—surface/local infiltration anesthesia or no anesthesia depending upon the location and size of the lesion. Curettage can be used alone or combined with other surgical modalities for treating various benign, premalignant, or malignant lesions.

HISTORY[55,58-70]

Curettage is a simple and effective surgical technique for scrapping or scooping various skin lesions and is in use for last 150 years. Adapted from a uterine curette, the first dermal curette in the form of sharp scraping spoon was introduced as early as 1870 by a German Surgeon Richard von Volkmann for curettage of lupus vulgaris. The curette was then called Volkmann instrument (sharp spoon). This versatile instrument has also been used for scrapping scars and allows them to heal by secondary intention. Since then, curettage has been used by many dermatologists for treating various other dermal conditions. Louis A Duhring (1845–1913) considered it to be an important remedial procedure. Henrick Auspitz (1835–1886), Hans von Hebra (1847–1902), and George Fox (1846–1937) suggested and modified the curette from time to time and used it in various shapes (spoon/ring/cup) and of sizes (small, medium, and large) with or without central opening as per the condition to be treated. With passage of time, curettage has been used either alone or in combination with electrofulguration/desiccation, cryotherapy using liquid nitrogen, excisional surgery, laser ablation, or 5-fluorouracil to treat various superficial skin lesions with good results.

INSTRUMENTS[58-63]

Classical dermal curette has circular or oval, ring shaped, and fenestrated head with a semi-sharp inner surface (cutting edge), which is the critical operational portion with a pencil-like handle and a tapered neck. The fenestration in the center allows easy passage to soft tissue through the opening during the curettage. They may be single ended or double ended and are varying in sizes from 1 to 7 mm depending on the diameter of its inner ring. Most commonly used ones are the Fox or Piffard type 3–4 mm in size. Apart from these, they may be spoon or cup shaped with nonfenestrated ends serving the purpose of scraping or scooping the tissue. Disposable curettes (Acuderm) are also available **(Fig. 18)**.

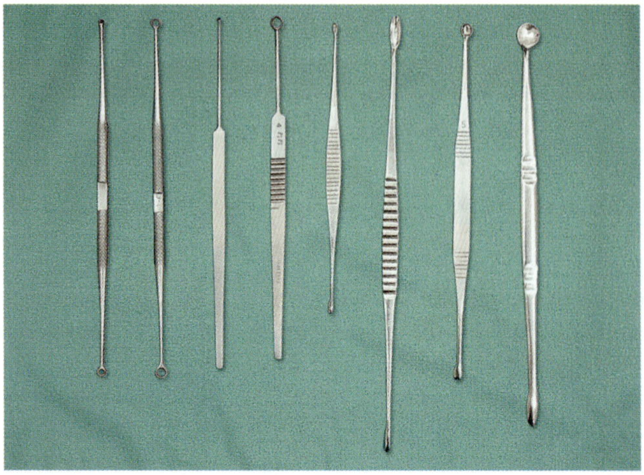

Fig. 18: Dermal curette.
Courtesy: Dr Sushil S Savant, Mumbai.

PRINCIPLES OF CURETTAGE[58-63,69-72]

The semi-sharp inner surface (cutting edge) of the ring of the curette imparts a soft feel to the operator while curetting various clinical lesions. This soft tactile sensation of the friable pathological tissue stands out in contrast to the firm feel of the surrounding normal dermal tissue. Once all the friable pathological tissue is curetted out, there is definite change in the feel of firmness when the surrounding normal tissue is reached. The operator has to learn to develop and appreciate this changing pattern of tactile sense while curetting for successful clinical outcome. Lesions present on areas with firm base and minimally mobile tissue, e.g., forehead, ear, nose, sole, palm can be easily curetted, whereas skin lesions located on nonfirm base or on mobile surfaces need to be supported by providing adequate traction and countertraction by the operator.

INDICATIONS[58-63,65-74]

Table 3 shows various conditions where curettage is performed.

CONTRAINDICATIONS (RELATIVE)

Large or deep-seated lesions located on cosmetically important areas and technically difficult sites (e.g., eyelid margins and medial canthi) as there can be scarring.

PROCEDURE[55,58-63,71-75]

- *Anesthesia:* The procedure is carried out under topical surface anesthesia with eutectic mixture of lignocaine and prilocaine (EMLA) or local infiltration using 2% lignocaine with adrenaline as per the size and extent of the lesion. Very small lesions may not require any anesthesia.
- *Instrument grip:*
  - *Pencil grip:* Instrument is held below the neck by the thumb, index, and middle finger of operating hand.
  - *Potato peel grip:* Instrument handle is held by the four flexed fingers of operating hand combined together and thumb is outstretched to stabilize the base.
- *Stabilization:* Stabilize the lesion by providing three-point traction to the skin surrounding the lesion to be curetted

TABLE 3: Various conditions where curettage is performed.

1. Diagnostic (curette biopsy)	• *Benign*: Fungal scraping, seborrheic keratoses, and molluscum contagiosum • *Premalignant*: Actinic keratoses, keratoacanthoma, and Bowen's disease • *Malignant*: Basal cell carcinoma and squamous cell carcinoma
2. Therapeutic	Molluscum contagiosum, filiform warts, dermatosis papulosa nigra, milia, seborrheic keratoses, small sebaceous cyst, pyogenic granuloma, hypertrophic granulation tissue in a nonhealing wound [debridement of nonhealing ulcer (NHU)], cutaneous horn, corn, giant congenital melanocytic nevi, etc.

by stretching it between the thumb and index finger of the nonoperating hand. At the same time, it provides countertraction to the base by the ulnar border of the operating hand.

- *Curettage technique* **(Fig. 19)**:
  Pencil grip: The cutting edge of the curette is applied to the center of the lesion and drawn to the periphery in all directions, so as to scrape the lesion completely or it can also be applied to one pole of the lesion and drawn through the lesion toward the operator's palm in downward movement, so as to scrape the lesion from normal surrounding skin. Multiple such movements adjacent to each other are made by alternately flexing and extending the fingers. One can also go from center to periphery in all directions.
  - *Potato peel grip technique:* Stabilize the lesion with thumb of the operating hand. The cutting edge is applied to the pole of the lesion and curette is moved through the lesion by repeatedly flexing the fingers till the lesion is removed entirely.
- Hemostasis is achieved with pressure or radiofrequency, wound is covered with antibiotic cream, and is either left open (small lesion) or dressed (large lesion).
- *Modifications:*
  - *Milia:* The surface epidermis is punctured with needle and lesion is extracted by giving pressure with the ring of the curette.
  - *Molluscum contagiosum (MC):* Puncture the lesion with angulated tip of electrocautery or radiofrequency and scoop out the MC with curette.
  - *Filiform wart/DPNs:* First electrofulgurate/dessicate the lesion followed by curettage of debris [electrodesiccation and curettage (ED&C)].
  - *Premalignant and malignant condition:* Multiple cycles (two to three) of curettage followed by electrodesiccation/laser ablation of the base.

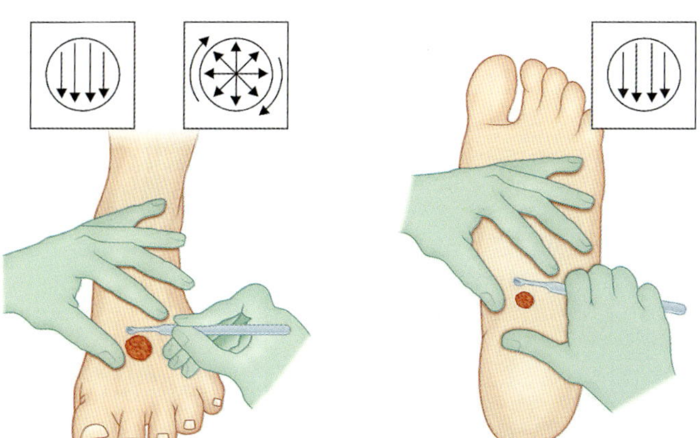

Fig. 19: Techniques of holding the curette.

Curettage can also be combined with cryo with liquid nitrogen (LN2), excisional 5-fluorouracil, or laser ablation.

POSTOPERATIVE CARE

Small superficial lesions—only topical application of antibiotic creams with no dressing.

Large deep lesions—topical antibiotic creams with dressings every 2–3 days for 1–2 weeks with oral antibiotics, anti-inflammatory drugs, and analgesics for 7–10 days wherever required.

COMPLICATIONS

Complications include postoperative bleeding, infection, hypo- or hyperpigmentation, scarring, and recurrence.

THERAPEUTIC CURETTAGE AND ELECTRODESICCATION[59,60,62,63,65,66,72-83]

This dual procedure consists of separating the skin lesion or tumor from its surrounding normal skin by scraping with curette (curettage) and alternating it with ED of the wound. It is a sequence of scraping and burning.

Role of curettage is to debulk the main tumor mass and to pursue subclinical (nonvisible) small tumor extensions.

Role of ED is to achieve destruction of residual tumor cells and hemostasis. Though termed as ED technically, it is electrocoagulation as it causes deeper destruction of remnant tumor cells at the base of the wound, which may have been missed out during curettage **(Table 4)**.

Indications

The indications are described in **Table 5**.

Contraindications

Large or deep-seated destructive premalignant and malignant lesions—basal cell carcinoma (BCC) (>2 years duration or >1 cm in diameter) and large size squamous cell carcinoma (SCC) located on cosmetically important areas and technically difficult sites (e.g., eyelid margins and medial canthi).

TABLE 4: Types of curettage (C) and electrodesiccation (ED) cycles.

Standard C and ED	Curettage followed by electrodesiccation, e.g., actinic keratoses, seborrheic keratoses
ED and C	Electrodesiccation is followed by curettage, e.g., warts, molluscum
Serial C and ED	Multiple cycles of C and ED are carried out alternately depending on premalignant and malignant conditions
C and ED combined	The standard or serial C and ED procedure is combined with biopsy, excisional surgery, Mohs surgery, etc.

Equipment

Curettes (1–7 mm), monopolar electrosurgical unit (cautery), or radiosurgical unit.

Procedure

This is carried out under local infiltrated anesthesia (1% xylocaine with adrenaline) followed by procedure of curettage (as mentioned earlier). In case of premalignant and malignant lesions, aggressive curettage is carried out initially with a large sized curette followed by further curettage of the base and edges with small size curette to scrape away the residual pieces of the tumor tissue till there is uniformly firm feel of the surrounding dermis ("gritty" feel and sound) along with pinpoint bleeding. Moderate-to-heavy ED&C coagulation of the base and edge is carried out with pointed or ball electrode of the electrocautery or radiofrequency, so as to destroy the tissue remnants. One can either do single cycle (benign) or repeat multiple cycles (premalignant and malignant) lesions **(Figs. 20 to 26)**.

TABLE 5: Indications of curettage.

1. Benign	Molluscum contagiosum, verruca vulgaris, verruca plana, dermatosis papulosa nigra, seborrheic keratoses, pyogenic granuloma, cutaneous horn, corn, adenoma sebaceum, giant congenital melanocytic nevi, etc.
2. Premalignant	Keratoacanthoma, actinic keratoses, and Bowen's disease
3. Malignant	Small basal cell or squamous cell carcinomas

Postoperative Care and Complications

As mentioned earlier, ED usually produces scarring and pigmentary changes.

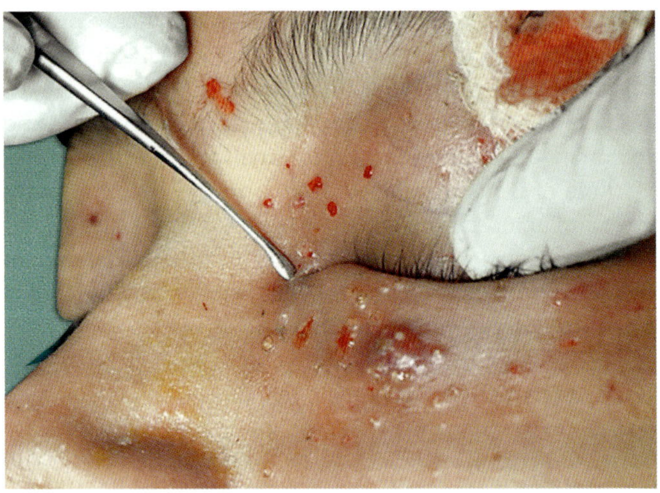

Fig. 20: Curettage in molluscum contagiosum.

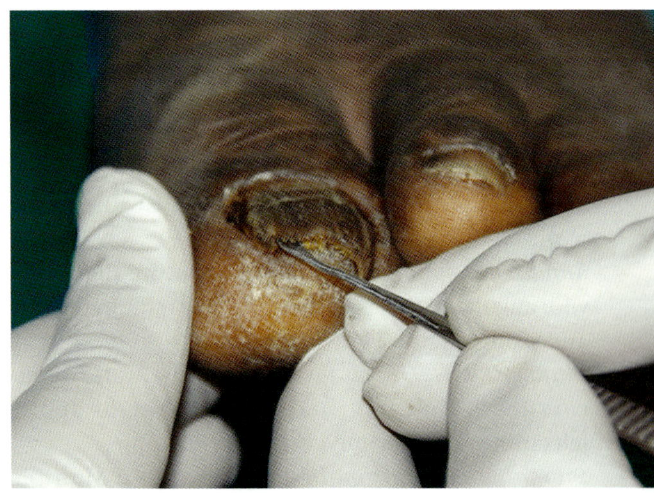

Fig. 22: Curettage for nail scrapping in onychomycosis.

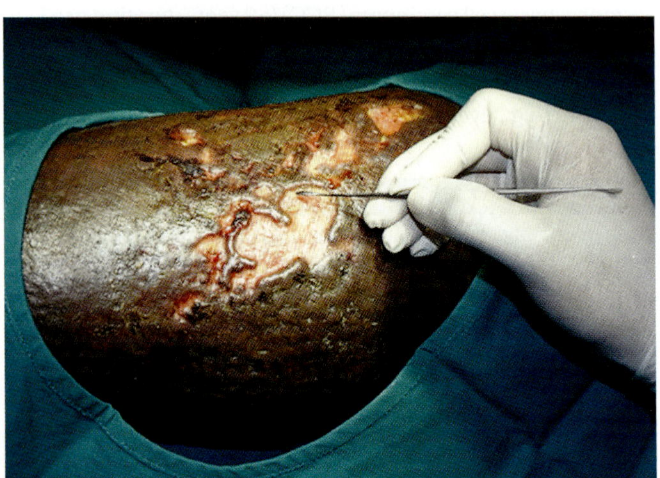

Fig. 21: Curettage of ulcer bed in livedoid vasculopathy.

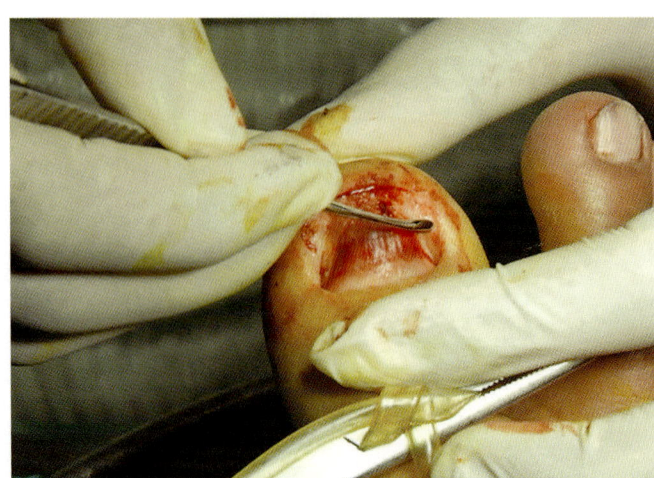

Fig. 23: Curettage following total nail avulsion for pincer nail.

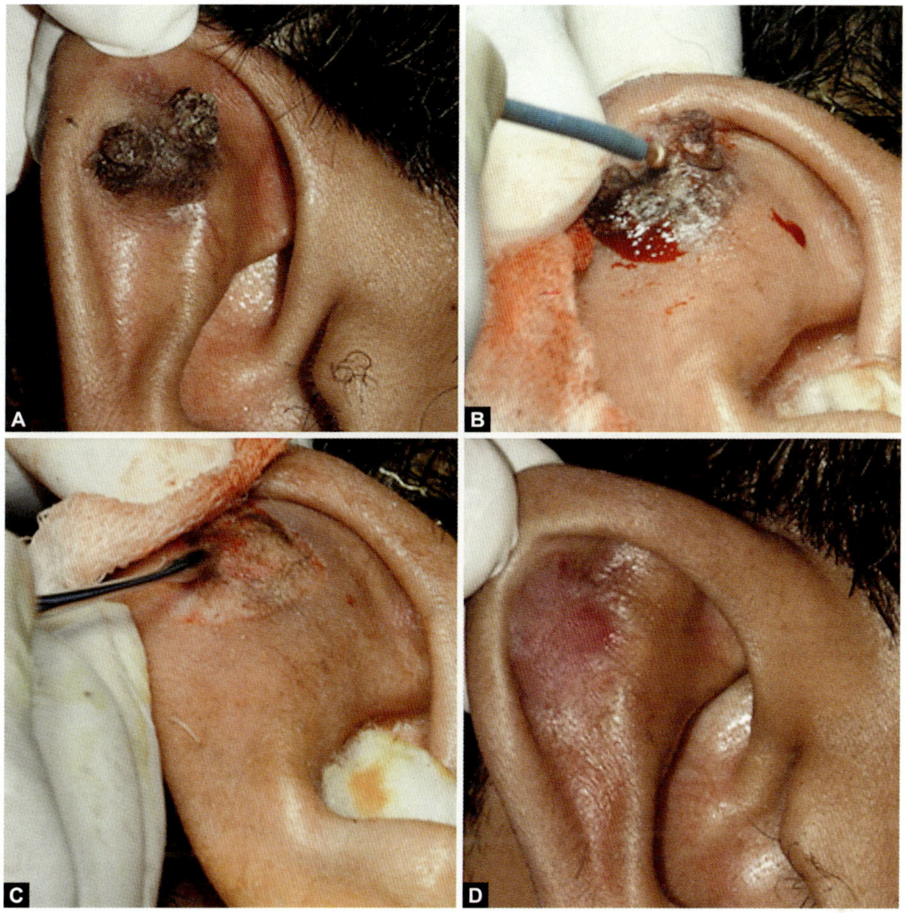

Figs. 24A to D: Electrocoagulation with ball electrode followed by curettage in Bowen's disease.
Courtesy: Sushil S Savant, Mumbai.

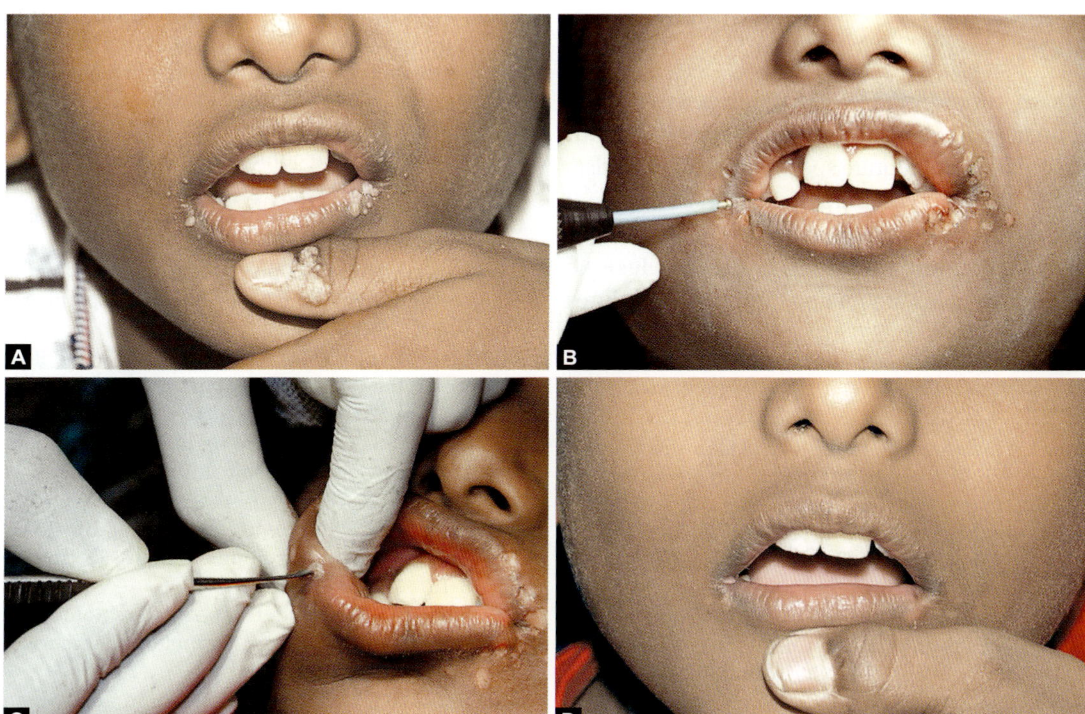

Figs. 25A to D: Electrodesiccation with needle electrode followed by curettage in verruca vulgaris.

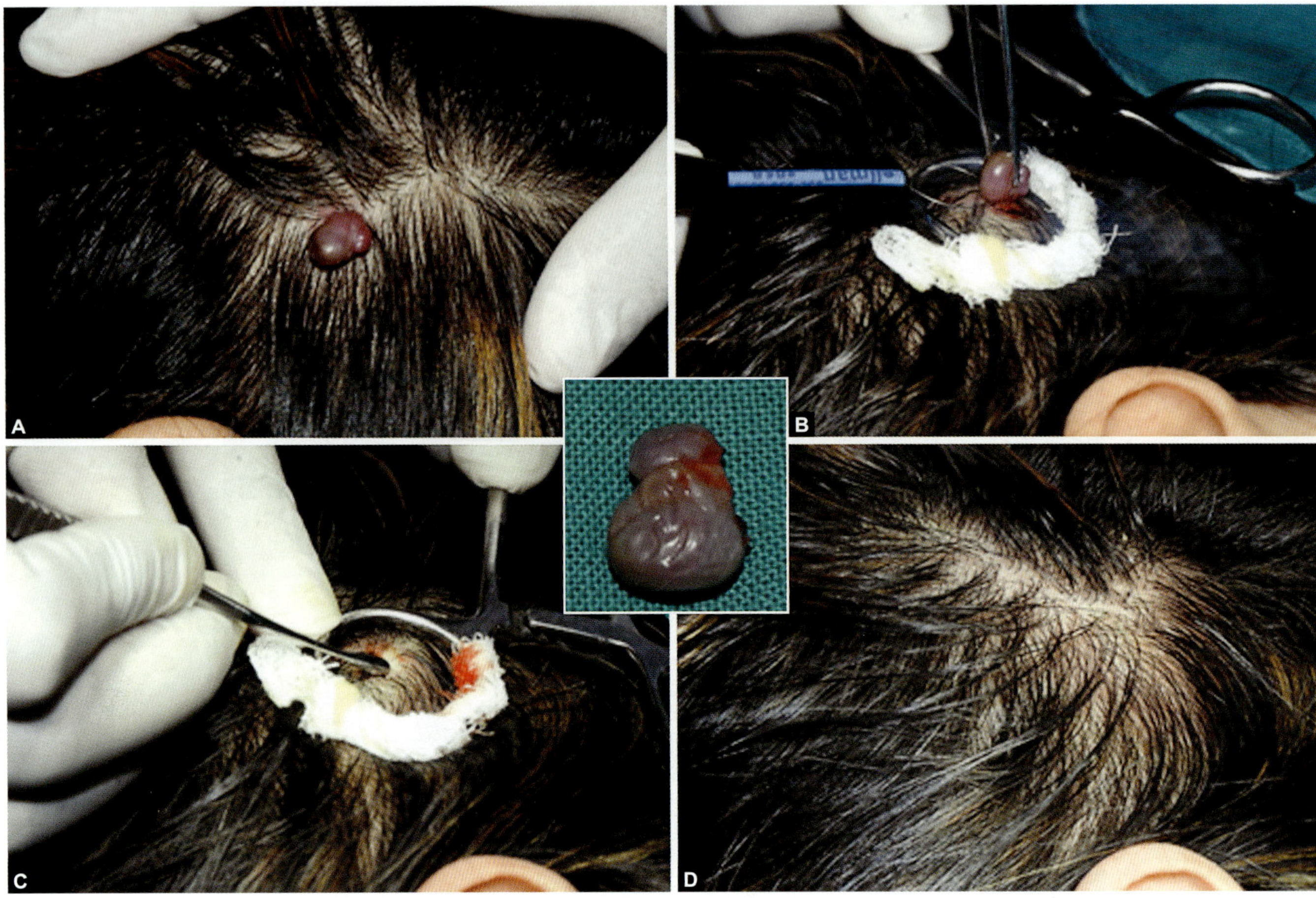

Figs. 26A to D: Electrosectioning with wire loop electrode followed by curettage in granuloma pyogenicum
Courtesy: Sushil S Savant, Mumbai.

CONCLUSION

Curettage is a safe, simple, effective, and inexpensive office procedure to treat variety of skin lesions successfully with good cosmesis and does not require special surgical expertise. If combined with ED or cryotherapy with LN2, excisional or laser surgery, or 5-fluorouracil, it can be also used to treat various premalignant and small malignant lesions successfully. Patient remains ambulatory and the procedures are easy to carry out.

REFERENCES

1. Coleman WP, Lawrence N. The history of skin resurfacing. In: Coleman WP, Lawrence N (Eds). Skin Resurfacing, 1st edition. Baltimore: Williams and Wilkins; 1998. pp. 3-6.
2. Padilla RS. Dermabrasion. In: Wheeland RG (Ed). Cutaneous Surgery, 1st edition. Philadelphia: WB Saunders Co.; 1994. pp. 470-90.
3. Savant SS, Savant SS. Dermabrasion. In: Savant SS (Ed). Textbook of Dermatosurgery and Cosmetology: Principles and Practice, 3rd edition. Mumbai: Bhalani Publishing House; 2018. pp. 346-67.
4. Iverson PC. Surgical removal of traumatic tattoos of face. Plast Reconstr Surg. 1947;2:427-30.
5. Kurtin A. Corrective surgical planning of skin: new technique for treatment of acne scars and other skin defects. AMA Arch Derm Syphil. 1953;68:389-94.
6. Mandy SH. Dermabrasion. In: Lask GP, Moy RL (Eds). Principles and Techniques of Cutaneous Surgery, 1st edition. New York: McGraw Hill; 1996. pp. 495-503.
7. Burks JW. Technique of surgical abrasion. In: Burks JW (Ed). Dermabrasion and Chemical Peeling, 1st edition. Springfield: McGraw Hill; 1956. pp. 94-103.
8. Lowenthal LJA. Punch biopsy with autografts. AMA Arch Derm Syphil. 1953;67:629.
9. Maneksha RJ. Scars. In: Maneksha RJ (Ed). Plastic Surgery in the Tropics, 1st edition. Mumbai: Bombay Popular Prakashan; 1965. pp. 20-31.
10. Savant SS. Therapeutic regional dermabrasion in papular lichen amyloidosis of shin. Indian J Dermatol Venereol Leprol. 1995;61:196-201.
11. Savant SS. Therapeutic spot dermabrasion: study of 197 sites in 11 skin conditions. Indian J Dermatol Surg. 1999;1: 5-15.
12. Savant SS. Therapeutic spot and regional dermabrasion in stable vitiligo. Indian J Dermatol Venereol Leprol. 1996;62: 139-45.
13. Savant SS. Facial dermabrasion in acne scar and genodermatoses—a study of 65 patients. Indian J Dermatol Venereol Leprol. 2000;66:79-84.

14. Roenigk HH. Dermabrasion for miscellaneous cutaneous lesions (exclusive of scarring for acne). J Dermatol Surg Oncol. 1977;3:322-8.
15. Epstein E. Dermabrasion for therapeutic purposes. In: Epstein E, Epstein E (Eds). Skin Surgery, 6th edition. Philadelphia: WB Saunders Co.; 1987. pp. 344-7.
16. Roenigk HH. Dermabrasion. In: Roenigk RK, Roenigk HH (Eds). Dermatologic Surgery: Principles and Practice, 1st edition. New York: Marcel Dekker Inc.; 1989. pp. 959-78.
17. Katz BE. Dermabrasion for scar revision. In: Roenigk RK, Roenigk HH (Eds). Surgical Dermatology, 1st edition. UK: Martin Dunitz; 1993. pp. 385-94.
18. Clabough W. Removal of tattoos by superficial dermabrasion. Arch Dermatol. 1968;98:515-21.
19. Matarasso SL. Indications for skin resurfacing. In: Coleman WP, Lawrence N (Eds). Skin Resurfacing, 1st edition. Baltimore: Williams and Wilkins; 1998. pp. 7-16.
20. Verheyden CN. Treatment of facial angiofibromas of tuberous sclerosis. Plast Reconstr Surg. 1996;98:777-83.
21. Yarborangh JM. Ablation of facial scars by programmed dermabrasion. J Dermatol Surg Oncol. 1988;12:292-4.
22. Hruza GJ. Dermabrasion. Facial Plast Surg Clin North Am. 2001;9:267-81.
23. Bohn J, Stevenson H, Aberg M. Dermabrasion of large congenital melanocytic nevi in neonates. Scand J Plast Reconstr Surg. 2000;34:321-6.
24. Aronsson A, Eriksson T, Jacobsson S, Salemark L. Effects of dermabrasion on acne scarring. A review and study of 25 cases. Acta Derm Venereol. 1977;77:39-42.
25. Kim EK, Hovsepian RV, Mathew P, Paul MD. Dermabrasion. Clin Plast Surg. 2011;38:391-5.
26. Surowitz JB, Shockley WW. Enhancement of facial scars with dermabrasion. Facial Plast Surg Clin North Am. 2011;19: 517-25.
27. Harmon CB, Zelickson BD, Roenigk RK, Wayner EA, Hoffstrom B, Pittelkow MR, et al. Dermabrasive scar revision. Immunohistochemical and ultrastructural evaluation. J Dermatol Surg. 1995;21:503-8.
28. Gold MH. Dermabrasion in dermatology. Am J Clin Dermatol. 2003;4:467-71.
29. Poulos E, Taylor C, Solish N. Effectiveness of dermasanding (manual dermabrasion) on the appearance of surgical scars: a prospective, randomized, blinded study. J Am Acad Dermatol. 2003;48:897-900.
30. Roxo RF, Sarmento DF, Kawalek AZ, Spencer JM. Successful treatment of a hypochromic scar with manual dermabrasion: a case report. J Dermatol Surg. 2003;29:189-91.
31. Gillard M, Wang TS, Boyd CM, Dunn RL, Fader DJ, Johnson TM. Conventional diamond fraise vs manual spot dermabrasion with dry well sanding screen for scars from skin cancer surgery. Arch Dermatol. 2002;138:1035-9.
32. Harmon CB. Dermabrasion. Derm Clin. 2001;19:439-42.
33. Jacob CI, Dover JS, Kaminer MS. Acne scarring: a classification system and review of treatment options. J Am Acad Dermatol. 2001;45:109-17.
34. Katz BE, Oca AG. A controlled study of the effectiveness of spot dermabrasion ("scar abrasion") on the appearance of surgical scars. J Am Acad Dermatol. 1991;24:462-6.
35. Robinson JK. Improvement of appearance of full thickness skin grafts with dermabrasion. Arch Dermatol. 1987;123: 1340-5.
36. McGregor IA. Free skin grafts. In: McGregor IA (Ed). Fundamental Techniques of Plastic Surgery and their Surgical Applications, 8th edition. Edinburgh: Churchill Livingstone; 1989. pp. 39-63.
37. Hung VC, Lee JY, Zitelli JA, Hebda PA. Topical tretinoin and epithelial wound healing. Arch Dermatol. 1989;125: 65-9.
38. Hevia O, Nemeth AJ, Taylor JR. Tretinoin accelerates healing after trichloroacetic acid chemical peel. Arch Dermatol. 1991;127:678-82.
39. Mandy SH. Tretinoin in the preoperative and postoperative management of dermabrasion. J Am Acad Dermatol. 1986;15:878-9.
40. Clark RA. Cutaneous tissue repair: basic biologic considerations. I. J Am Acad Dermatol. 1985;13:701-25.
41. Koranda FC. Treatment and modalities in facial acne scars. In: Thomas JR, Holt GR (Eds). Facial Scars Incision, Revision and Camouflage, 1st edition. St. Louis: CV Mosby Co.; 1989. pp. 278-89.
42. Savant SS, Gore D. Acne scar revision surgery. A study of 350 cases with pitted scars. Indian J Dermatol Surg. 1999;1: 11-2.
43. Johnson WC. Treatment of pitted scars: punch transport technique. J Dermatol Surg Oncol. 1976;2:337-9.
44. Orentreich DS, Orentriech N. Subcutaneous incision less (subcision) surgery for the correction of depressed scars and wrinkles. J Dermatol Surg Oncol. 1995;21:543-9.
45. Solotoff SA. Treatment for pitted acne scarring—postauricular punch grafts followed by dermabrasion. J Dermatol Surg Oncol. 1986;12:1079-84.
46. Mancuso A, Farber GA. The abraded punch graft for pitted facial scars. J Dermatol Surg Oncol. 1991;17:32-4.
47. Alam M, Omura N, Kaminer MS. Subcision for acne scarring: technique and outcome in 40 patients. Dermatol Surg. 2005;31:310-7.
48. Coleman WP, Klein JA. Use of tumescent technique for scalp surgery, dermabrasion and tissue augmentation. J Dermatol Surg Oncol. 1992;18:130-5.
49. Goodman G. Dermabrasion using tumescent anaesthesia. J Dermatol Surg Oncol. 1994;20:802-7.
50. Baker TM. Dermabrasion as a complement to aesthetic surgery. Clin Plast Surg. 1998;25:81-8.
51. Campbell RM, Harmon CB. Dermabrasion in our practice. J Drugs Dermatol. 2008;7:124-8.
52. Goldman MP, Fitzpatrick RE, Smith SR. Resurfacing complications and their management. In: Coleman WP, Lawrence N (Eds). Skin Resurfacing, 1st edition. Baltimore: Williams and Wilkins Co.; 1998. pp. 295-301s.
53. Branham GH, Thomas JR. Rejuvenation of the skin surface: chemical peel and dermabrasion. Facial Plast Surg. 1996; 12:125-33.
54. Ina Z, Romanzi A, Gherardini G. Tricks and tips for manual dermabrasion. Dermatol Surg. 2016;42:1393-4.
55. Savant SS. The carbon dioxide and erbium: YAG lasers. In: Savant SS (Ed). Textbook of Dermatosurgery and Cosmetology: Principles and Practice, 3rd edition. Mumbai: Bhalani Publishing House; 2018. pp. 743-65.
56. Bagatin E, Guadanhim LRS, Yarak S, Kamamoto CSL, de Almeida FA. Dermabrasion for acne scars during treatment with oral isotretinoin. Dermatol Surg. 2010;36:483-9.
57. Chandrashekar BS, Varsha DV, Vasanth V, Jagadish P, Madura C, Rajashekar L, et al. Safety of performing invasive acne scar treatment and laser hair removal in patients on oral isotretinoin: a retrospective study of 110 patients. Int J Dermatol. 2014;53:1281-5.

58. Mohs FE. The versatile curette. J Dermatol Surg Oncol. 1978;4:406.
59. Sturm HM, Leider M. An editorial on curettage. J Dermatol Surg Oncol. 1979;5:532-3.
60. Bennett RG. Curettage. In: Bennett RG (Ed). Fundamentals of Cutaneous Surgery, 1st edition. St. Louis: CV Mosby Co., 1988. pp. 532-52.
61. Krull EA. Surgical gems: the little curette. J Dermatol Surg Oncol. 1978;4:656-8.
62. Savant SS. Basics of cutaneous surgery. In: Sacchidanand S, Oberai C Inamdar AC (Eds). IADVL Textbook of Dermatology, 4th edition. Mumbai: Bhalani Publishing House; 2001. pp. 1326-56.
63. Savant SS. Curettage. In: Savant SS (Ed). Textbook of Dermatosurgery and Cosmetology: Principles and Practice, 3rd edition. Mumbai: Bhalani Publishing House; 2018. pp. 150-8.
64. Parish LC. Historical aspects of cutaneous surgery. In: Parish LC (Ed). Wheel and Cutaneous Surgery, 1st edition; 1994. pp. 3-11.
65. De Raeve LE, Roseuw DJ. Curettage of giant congenital melanocytic nevi in neonates: a decade later. Arch Dermatol. 2002;138:943-8.
66. Jackson R. Treatment of epitheliomas: electrodesiccation and curettage. In: Epstein E (Ed). Controversies in Dermatology, 1st edition. Philadelphia: WB Saunders Co., 1984. pp. 112-4.
67. Sebben JE. Electrosurgical management: Cutaneous malignancies. In: Sebben JE (Ed). Cutaneous Electrosurgery, 1st edition. Chicago: Year Book Medical Publishers; 1989. pp. 139-50.
68. Abadir DM. Combined curettage and cryosurgery for treatment of epithelial cancers of the skin. J Dermatol Surg Oncol. 1980;6:633-6.
69. Johnson TM, Tromovitch TA, Swanson NA. Combined curettage and excision: a treatment method for primary basal cell carcinoma. J Am Acad Dermatol. 1991;24:613-7.
70. Savant SS, Sarangi K. Curettage and 5-fluorouracil in the treatment of Bowen's disease with multiple cutaneous horns. Ind J Derm Surg. 2000;2:78-81.
71. Adam JE. The technique of curettage surgery. J Am Acad Dermatol. 1986;15:697-702.
72. Arndt KA. Operative procedures: Curettage. In: Arndt KA, Bowers KE, Chuttani AR (Eds). Manual of Dermatologic Therapeutics, 5th edition. Boston: Little Brown and Company; 1995. pp. 222-4.
73. Salasche SJ. Therapeutic curettage and electrodesiccation. In: Friedman RJ, Rigel DS, Kopf AW (Eds). Cancer of the Skin, 1st edition. Philadelphia: WB Saunders Company; 1991. pp. 434-50.
74. Leffeu DJ, Brown MD. Skin biopsy. In: Leffeu DJ, Brown MD (Eds). Manual of Skin Surgery, 1st edition. New York: Wiley-Liss; 1997. pp. 61-82.
75. Burge S, Graham C, Lester R. Curettage, cautery and diathermy. In: Burge S, Graham C, Lester R (Eds). Simple Skin Surgery, 2nd edition. Oxford: Blackwell Science Ltd., 1996. pp. 47-57.
76. Robinson JK. Electrosurgery. In: Robinson JK, Arndt KA, Leboit PE, Wintraub BU (Eds). Atlas of Cutaneous Surgery, 1st edition. Philadelphia: WB Saunders Co., 1996. pp. 61-5.
77. Pollack SV. Electrocoagulation. In: Pollack SV, Grekin RC (Eds). Electrosurgery of the Skin, 1st edition. New York: Churchill Livingstone Inc., 1991. pp. 37-50.
78. Nouri K, Spencer JM, Taylor JR, Hayag M, DeVoursney J, Shah N. Does wound healing contribute to the eradication of basal cell carcinoma following curettage and electrodessication? Dermatol Surg. 1999;25:183-7.
79. Spiller WF, Spiller RF. Treatment of basal cell epithelioma by curettage and electrodessication. J Am Acad Dermatol. 1984;11:808-12.
80. Kopf AW, Bart RS, Schrager D, Lazar M, Popkin GL. Curettage-electrodessication treatment of basal cell carcinoma. Arch Dermatol. 1977;113:439-43.
81. Kimyai-Asadi A, Jih MH. Curettage and electrodessication. In: Rusciani L, Robins P (Eds). Textbook of Dermatologic Surgery, 1st edition. Paclova: Piccin; 2008. pp. 473-8.
82. Crissey JT. Curettage and electrodesiccation as a method of treatment for epitheliomas of the skin. J Surg Oncol. 1971; 3:287-90.
83. Salasche SJ. Curettage and electrodesiccation in the treatment of mid-facial basal cell epitheliomas. J Am Acad Dermatol. 1983;8:496-503.

SECTION 3

Heat and Cold Energy-based Procedures

CHAPTER 26

Radiofrequency Surgery and Electrocautery

Bipin Deshpande

KEY MESSAGES

- Surgery has acquired a definite and permanent place in today's practice of dermatology.
- The contemporary dermatology has branched into clinical, cosmetic, and surgical dermatology.
- Surgical dermatology has further branched into contemporary methods of surgery and newer more advanced and refined modalities using electrical energy and electromagnetic waves.

INTRODUCTION

Dermatosurgery or cutaneous surgery is an ever-expanding field and has a definite place in the management of dermatological diseases. Dermatosurgery was commonly performed using scalpel or modalities such as chemical cautery, cryotherapy, and electrocautery.

Over the past two decades, due to technological advances, newer modalities of electrosurgery, radiofrequency (RF) surgery, and lasers have become available and these have expanded the applications in not only clinical dermatology but also provided superior results in aesthetic dermatology.

The goals of dermatosurgery are to remove the lesion completely with least effort and pain, with minimum intraoperative bleeding, faster healing, and minimal scarring with or without sutures. This surgery may be done in office (most commonly) or in operation theater.

Radiofrequency surgery and surgical lasers fulfills most of these goals. RF surgery is affordable and versatile.

FUNDAMENTALS[1,2]

Electric current is used in both electrocautery and RF surgery, but there are major differences how the equipment functions and uses electric current differently, treating skin lesions differently, with different outcome.

Table 1 explains the basic differentiating features between electrocautery and RF surgery. The only advantageous feature for both is affordability compared to lasers.

Research in electromagnetism has shown that radio waves occupy from 3 kHz to 300 GHz in the electromagnetic spectrum. In medicine, only spectrum from 200 kHz to 40 MHz is used and anything below 100 kHz stimulates nerve and muscle, causing fatal side effects.

Electrocautery destroys lesions with the hot electrode and the lesion is then removed without much bleeding as the hot electrode tip literally burns the lesion. Patient is not in the circuit. Here, the skill or the learning curve is minimal.

Radiofrequency surgery has a longer learning curve and one needs to develop skill for best results.

Before using RF surgery, one must be fully aware of its (1) physical characteristics, (2) biological characteristics, (3) equipment, and (4) functionality.

Physical characteristics of RF surgery[2,3] are related to:

- *Frequency of RF waves:* Any frequency above 500 kHz is good for skin; frequency from 500 kHz to 2 MHz is better termed *electrosurgery* as this equipment can be used to cut efficiently when the electrode tip is hot. *Electrosurgery* is the basic equipment developed using the concept of alternating current (AC) current and it has all the waveforms as well as electrodes and antenna plate which is also present in RF equipment.

TABLE 1: Basic differentiating features between electrocautery and radiofrequency surgery.

Parameter	*Electrocautery*	*Radiofrequency*
Electric current	Direct current (DC)	Alternating current (AC)
Treating electrode	Always hot	Always cold
Fine cutting	Inferior	Superior
Hemostasis	Very good	Good
Lateral tissue damage	Significant	Minimal
Postoperative healing	Slow	Fast
Cosmetic result	Inferior	Superior
Biopsy	Not possible	Possible
Applications	Limited	Many
Cost of equipment	Inexpensive	Affordable, cheaper than lasers

Source: Adapted from Savitha AS, Shilpa K, Chatterjee M, Vasudevan B, Neema S, Gorur D, et al (Eds). ACS(I) Procedural Dermatosurgery: A Step by Step Approach, 1st edition. New Delhi: Jaypee Brothers Medical Publishers; 2018. p. 485.

The application method of electrosurgery and RF is also similar, but due to the hot electrode, the lateral tissue damage is higher and the results are cosmetically inferior. Hence, the applications remain limited. Higher the RF above 2 MHz, colder the electrode **(Fig. 1)**. This makes cutting of the skin finer with least tissue damage proved at 3.8 MHz.[4]

- *Electrode size:* This is directly proportional to the heat dispersed while treating.
- *Tissue contact time:* This is directly proportional to the heat dispersed while treating.
- *Power:* This is directly proportional to the heat generated while treating.
- *Waveform:* The waveform and its heat dispersion effects need to be well understood beforehand. This is explained later.

Biological characteristics of RF surgery[4] help understand the actual tissue effects when using the equipment:

- All RF surgery units are monopolar and biterminal **(Fig. 2)**. Here, the equipment has an active electrode for treating and a return electrode or antenna plate that completes the circuit and patient remains part of this circuit. This is especially used in all applications where "cutting or incision" and "hemostasis or coagulation" is required **(Figs. 3 to 7)**.
- All RF surgery units can also function as monopolar monoterminal (without antenna plate) when patient is not part of the circuit. This function is useful for superficial epidermal lesions at optimum power, causing dehydration and destruction of lesions, helping them to clear off as seen in electrodesiccation and electrofulguration.

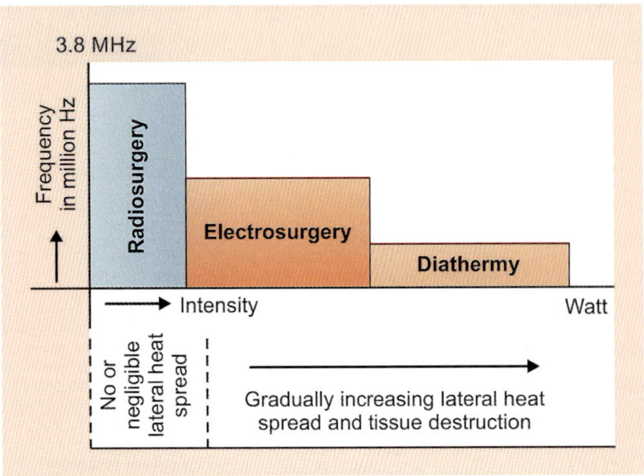

Fig. 1: Lateral dissipation principle.
Source: Adapted from Savitha AS, Shilpa K, Chatterjee M, Vasudevan B, Neema S, Gorur D, et al (Eds). ACS(I) Procedural Dermatosurgery: A Step by Step Approach, 1st edition. New Delhi: Jaypee Brothers Medical Publishers; 2018. p. 487.

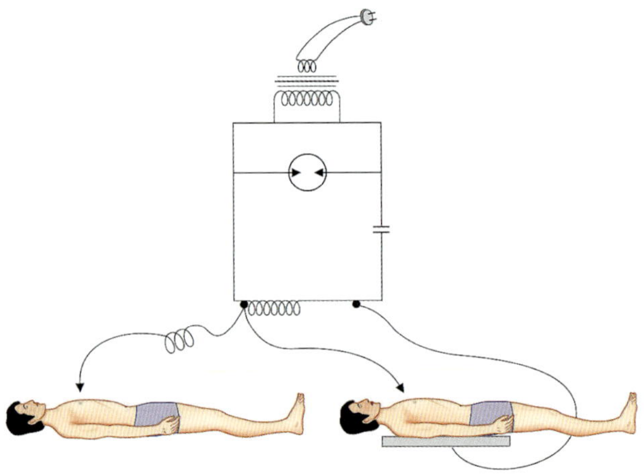

Fig. 2: Different waveforms of radiofrequency and their uses.
Source: Adapted from Savitha AS, Shilpa K, Chatterjee M, Vasudevan B, Neema S, Gorur D, et al. (Eds). ACS(I) Procedural Dermatosurgery: A Step by Step Approach, 1st edition. New Delhi: Jaypee Brothers Medical Publishers; 2018. p. 486.

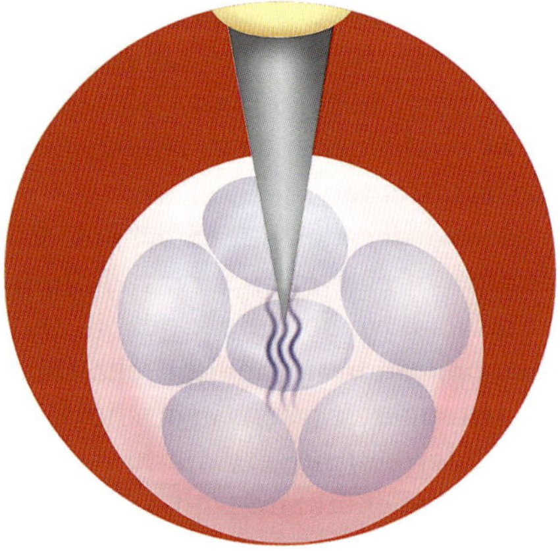

Fig. 3: Electrode touches skin.
Source: Adapted from Deshpande B (Ed). Dermatologic Surgery with Radiofrequency: Art of Successful Practice, 1st edition. Boca Raton: CRC Press; 2018. p. 25, Figure 7.2.

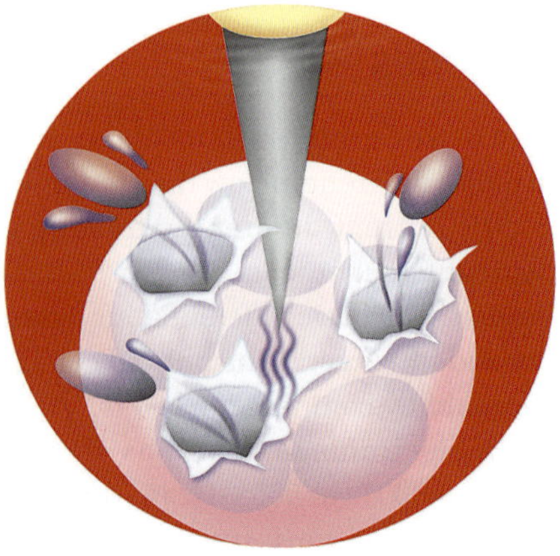

Fig. 4: Tissue resistance leads to boiling of intracellular and extracellular water molecules.
Source: Adapted from Deshpande B (Ed). Dermatologic Surgery with Radiofrequency: Art of Successful Practice, 1st edition. Boca Raton: CRC Press; 2018. p. 25, Figure 7.3.

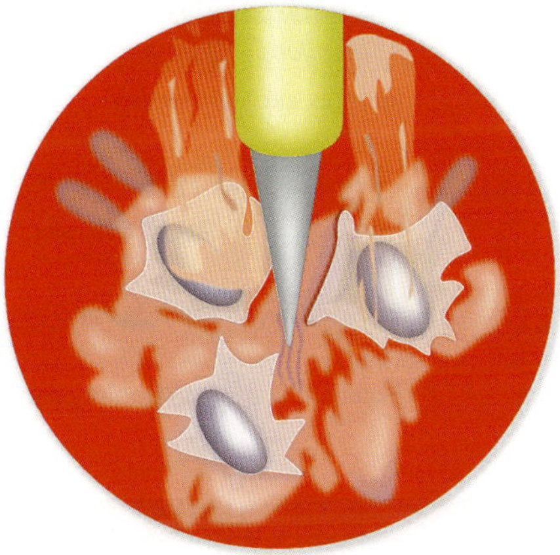

Fig. 5: Consequent heat generation causes tissue necrosis.
Source: Adapted from Deshpande B (Ed). Dermatologic Surgery with Radiofrequency: Art of Successful Practice, 1st edition. Boca Raton: CRC Press; 2018. p. 25, Figure 7.4.

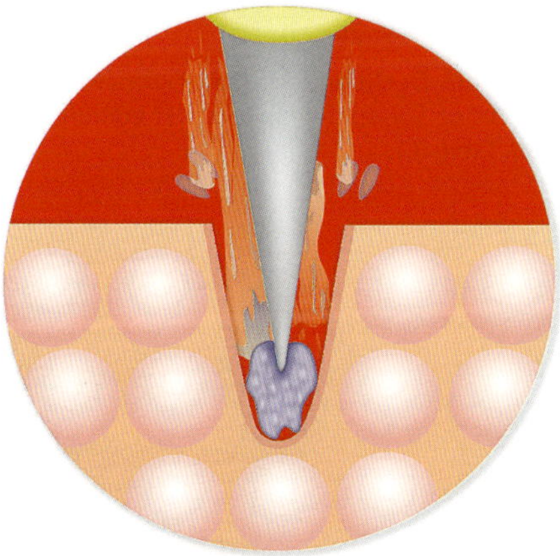

Fig. 6: Electrode cuts through causing very thin split (fine cut) in tissue.
Source: Adapted from Deshpande B (Ed). Dermatologic Surgery with Radiofrequency: Art of Successful Practice, 1st edition. Boca Raton: CRC Press; 2018. p. 25, Figure 7.5.

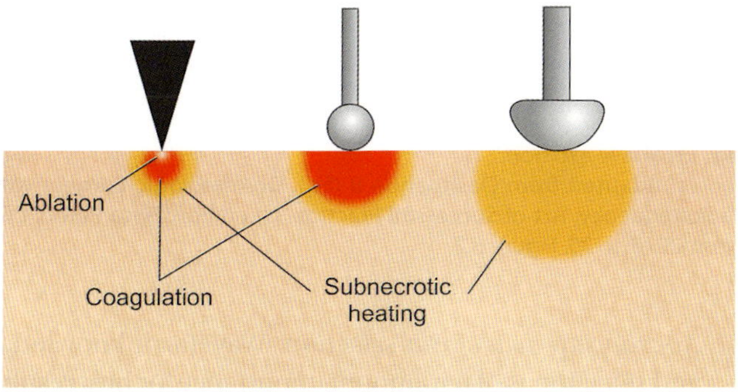

Fig. 7: Radiofrequency (RF) spot-size effects on tissues.
Source: Adapted from Deshpande B (Ed). Dermatologic Surgery with Radiofrequency: Art of Successful Practice, 1st edition. Boca Raton: CRC Press; 2018. p. 26, Figure 7.6.

Equipment

RF Surgery Unit[5]

All RF surgery units have common parts **(Fig. 8)**:

- RF unit or generator
- Handpiece (with or without activating switch)
- Antenna plate or ground plate (nonmetal)
- Foot pedal to activate unit
- Electrode of various shapes and sizes **(Fig. 9)**

Functionality

The knowledge of waveforms is of utmost importance. Kindly refer to **Table 2** for salient features of all the waveforms, their properties, and uses.

The schematic representation of the waveforms is shown in **Figure 10**.

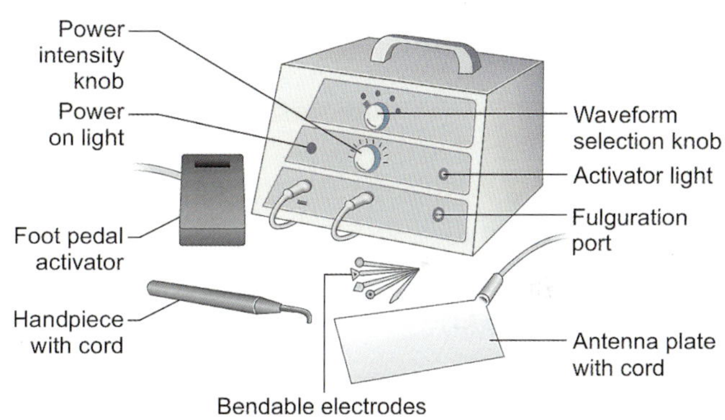

Fig. 8: Radiofrequency surgical unit.
Source: Adapted from Savitha AS, Shilpa K, Chatterjee M, Vasudevan B, Neema S, Gorur D, et al (Eds). ACS(I) Procedural Dermatosurgery: A Step by Step Approach, 1st edition. New Delhi: Jaypee Brothers Medical Publishers; 2018. p. 485.

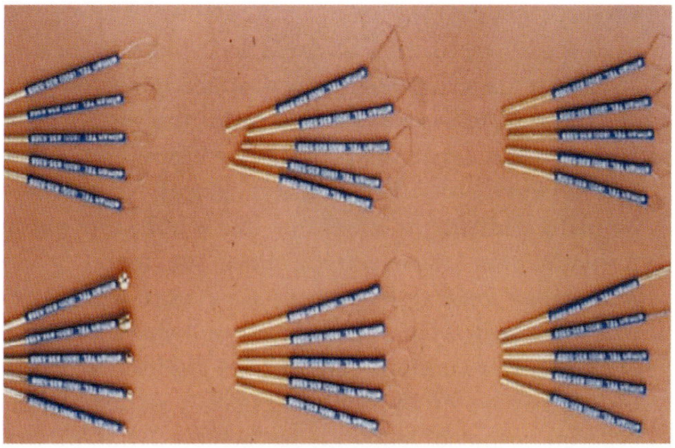

Fig. 9: Variety of radiofrequency (RF) surgery electrodes.
Source: Adapted from Savitha AS, Shilpa K, Chatterjee M, Vasudevan B, Neema S, Gorur D, et al (Eds). ACS(I) Procedural Dermatosurgery: A Step by Step Approach, 1st edition. New Delhi: Jaypee Brothers Medical Publishers; 2018. p. 485.

TABLE 2: Salient features of all the waveforms, their properties, and uses.

Waveform	*Electrode function and polarity*	*Lateral heat dissipation*	*Applications*
Fully filtered, fully rectified	*Electrosection:* 90% cut, 10% coagulated; bipolar	Minimum	Incision, excision, biopsy
Fully rectified	*Blend:* 50–50 cut-coagulated; bipolar	Medium	Incision, excision where bleeding is expected
Partially rectified	*Electrocoagulation:* 90% coagulated, 10% cut; bipolar	Maximum	Hemostasis, epilation, telangiectasia
Marked damped, spark gap	Electrodesiccation, electrofulguration; unipolar	Medium	Superficial epidermal lesions
Bipolar coagulation	Precise hemostasis using bipolar forceps	Medium	Excellent and precise point coagulation

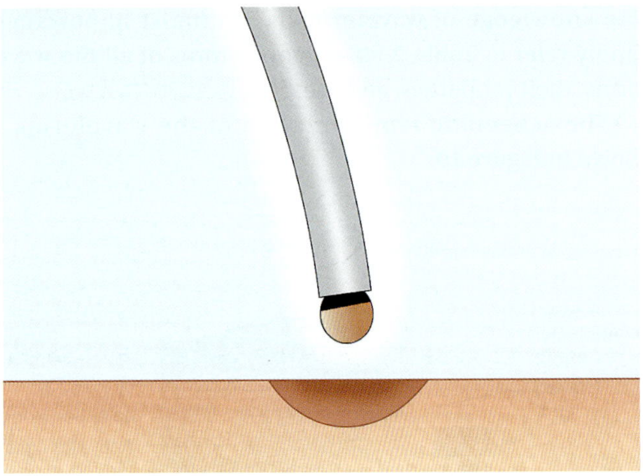

Fig. 10: Electrocoagulation.
Source: Adapted from Deshpande B (Ed). Dermatologic Surgery with Radiofrequency: Art of Successful Practice, 1st edition. Boca Raton: CRC Press; 2018. p. 28, Figure 7.11.

BOX 1: Tips to master radiofrequency surgery technique.

- Pressureless incision
- Fine and light strokes (feather touch or paintbrush like)
- Appropriate electrode size
- Appropriate waveform selection
- Appropriate power setting
- Antenna plate position
- Hydration of skin lesion
- Interval between two strokes

Source: Adapted from Deshpande B (Ed). Dermatologic Surgery with Radiofrequency: Art of Successful Practice, 1st edition. Boca Raton: CRC Press; 2018. p. 30, Table 8.1.

RADIOFREQUENCY SURGERY SKILLS[6] (TIPS AND TRICKS TO MASTER TECHNIQUE)

The hallmarks of RF surgery are:

- High RF, i.e., close to 4 MHz
- Cold electrodes, i.e., electrode remains cold throughout surgery

Both the above features assure a very fine skin incision. When these remain constant during the dermatosurgery, what are the other variables on which depends the superiority of the results? To understand this, please refer to **Box 1**.

- *Pressureless incision:* Skin incision using RF should never be using pressure; it should be like a hot knife gliding through butter (cold electrode cuts tissue finely)
- *Fine feather touch or paintbrush-like strokes:* It is prudent to excise lesions using method of "*shave excision*" **(Fig. 11)**. Here multiple fine strokes are used to cut the lesion, going step by step till it is fully removed. After excision, cosmetic blending is best achieved with "*portrait-shading strokes*" **(Fig. 12)**.
- *Appropriate electrode size and shape:* Thinner the electrode, finer the cut; electrode shape should match configuration of skin lesion.

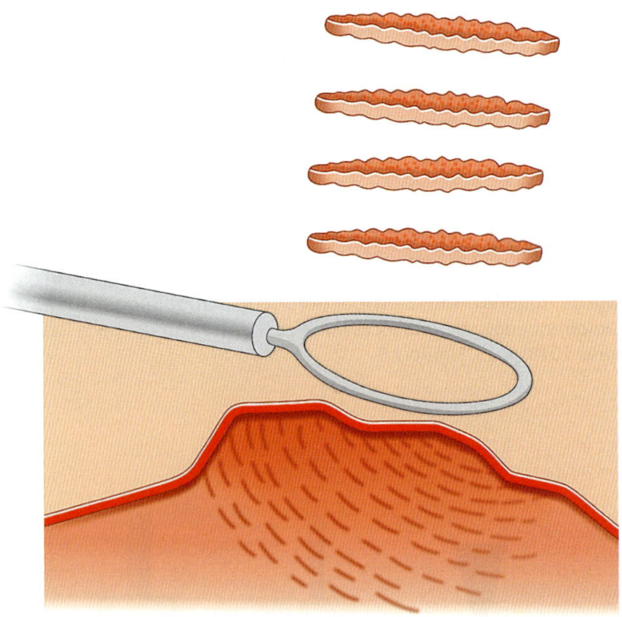

Fig. 11: Shave excision.
Source: Adapted from Deshpande B (Ed). Dermatologic Surgery with Radiofrequency: Art of Successful Practice, 1st edition. Boca Raton: CRC Press; 2018. p. 30, Figure 8.2.

- *Appropriate waveform selection:* Waveform knowledge and selection is of paramount importance for best results.
- *Appropriate power:* Lower power prevents smooth cutting, whereas higher power may damage by overzealous cutting.
- *Antenna plate position:* Position nearest to operative site gives best results.

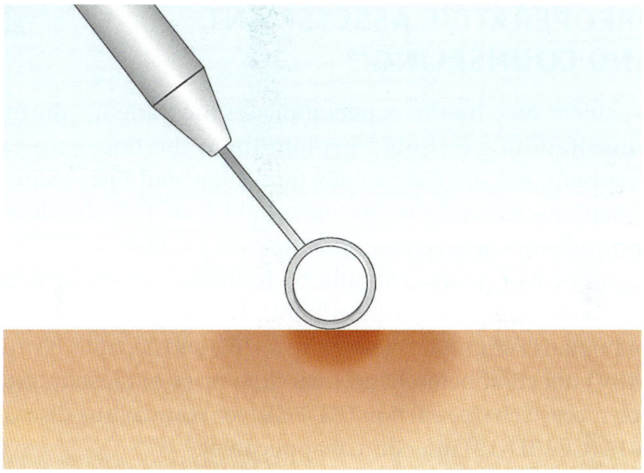

Fig. 12: Portrait-shading stroke, a radiofrequency (RF) masterstroke. *Source:* Adapted from Deshpande B (Ed). Dermatologic Surgery with Radiofrequency: Art of Successful Practice, 1st edition. Boca Raton: CRC Press; 2018. p. 30, Figure 8.3.

- *Hydration of lesions:* RF surgery always cuts due to vaporization; hence, lesion to be cut should be moist while cutting.
- *Interval between two strokes:* It is advisable to avoid hurried strokes to cut a lesion because of the possibility of scarring.

The above tips and tricks allow the dermatosurgeon to deliver better results compared to equipment which uses RF between 500 kHz and 3 MHz.

Furthermore, there are some gems and jewels which make RF surgery superior. I have worked upon these for more than a decade and they have helped me expand applications as well as made final result of all RF surgeries aesthetically superior. I have elaborated them as follows:

- *Radiovaporization:*[7] Tissue impedance to RF waves generates heat to explode cells, leading to necrosis and cut. When a straight needle electrode is inserted inside a protuberant lesion under local anesthesia, cut mode is selected with power on 3 or 4 (Ellman Surgitron) and treated; the soft tissues inside the lesion vaporize, causing the lesion to shrink (debulking) to more than half its size. This method was found to facilitate excision of certain lesions such as cysts, hypertrophic scars, keloids, submucous cysts, rhinophyma, and neurofibroma. Some practice will help reduce chances of scarring.
- *RF resurfacing:*[8] Depressed or deep punched out facial scars or atrophic chickenpox scars need resurfacing. In resurfacing, the sharpness of the punched out edges of the scars can be effectively blunted using RF at low power under local anesthesia. This helps alleviate sharp edges to soften their appearance. This is another artistic and skillful use of RF which can help many patients with acne, chickenpox, and traumatic scars. This method can be used to level hypertrophic scars as well.
- *RF blending technique:*[9] Whatever may be the lesion, patient remains unsatisfied if lesion leaves a prominent scar. It is mandatory to know the blending technique which assures an aesthetically pleasing scar. This technique must always be used after any RF surgery. It is simple and should be carried out using very low power of 1 or 2 to blend or merge the new postoperative skin with the adjacent normal skin. The circumferential blending done here with or without exfoliation is responsible for the aesthetically superior results of RF surgery.
- *Intralesional RF:*[10] Deep dermal and subcutaneous lesions can be effectively treated using insulated electrode under local anesthesia.

PRECAUTIONS, SAFETY MEASURES, AND PRACTICE SESSIONS

Electrocautery and RF surgery are done with electrical gadgets. Hence, all precautions and safety measures concerned with hazards of electric current should be taken care of. For both, it is advisable to have inverter backup in clinic.

For electrocautery specifically, one should be careful from burns due to hot electrode and shock from wire breaches.

For RF surgery,[11-14] there are two concerns:

1. *Patient safety issues:*
   a. *Cardiac pacemaker:* RF surgery is better avoided in patients having cardiac pacemaker or official permission should be obtained from the patient's cardiologist.
   b. *Electrical shock:* It is advisable for patients to remove their metal devices such as earrings, watches, and spectacles (theoretically), but in practice, I have not encountered any shock due to these devices or even dental metal implants.
   c. *Fire or burns:* This is possible in few instances such as if alcohol-based antiseptics are used for sterilizing or working in perianal, perineal, and genital areas when bowel gases (methane) which are inflammable are exposed to or accidentally to oxygen in operation theater.
2. *Practitioner safety issues:*
   a. *Electrical shock:* This can occur if the electrode is incompletely or loosely fitted in handpiece or there is accidental touch with bare electrode if its insulation is worn out. This is rare as during surgery as latex gloves give full protection.
   b. *Microorganism transmission:* Intact viral particles have been detected in smoke plume generated while excising warts or molluscum which exposes to infection. This can be best avoided using a smoke evacuator. Besides that, working with magnifying lens and surgical mask is better.

Practice Sessions (Radiofrequency Surgery)[15,16]

Radiofrequency surgery has a learning curve. Once we have understood thoroughly the fundamentals, it is recommended to have practice sessions or rehearsal on meat piece using all waveforms such as: (1) Straight needle, Vari-Tip, or thin wire, round loop electrodes with electrosection or blend current; (2) Ball-tip electrode with electrocoagulation; (3) Straight-needle electrode with electrodesiccation, and (4) Thick fulguration electrode with electrofulguration.

Some important points to remember during practice:

- Antenna plate is kept close to treatment site and one need not touch the skin.
- One should set power low and press foot pedal before touching meat piece.
- If the electrode sticks in tissue, the power set is low. Increase power gradually to a level when the electrode smoothly glides through tissue to make a fine and clean cut as if the tissue is split into two parts.
- If there is sparking while cutting, power is high. This can cause tissue charring.
- Cutting may not be smooth if the tissue dries, so moisten it.
- When electrocoagulating, keep ball-tip electrode a little away from tissue surface and retouch to give a pulsating effect due to partially rectified waveform.
- When electrodesiccating, lightly touch tissue at low power till it whitens due to dehydration.
- When electrofulgurating, keep electrode tip slightly away from tissue surface and increase power to above 4 till you see a spark jumping from electrode tip to tissue causing charring and necrosis.

OFFICE DERMATOSURGERY[17]

Electrocautery and RF surgery are commonly performed in office or clinic. We should devote sufficient time and space to achieve a successful office dermatosurgery setup.

Recommendations include:

- Minimum 10 × 10 feet room having two entrance doors (one for taking in patient and one connected to consulting room)
- Minimum requirements of minor operating theater such as patient bed fitted with magnifying lens, surgical trolley fully equipped with minimum requirements of minor surgery and emergencies, smoke evacuator, good illumination, electric fixtures (sufficient plugs and sockets, fans, air conditioner, extension boards, and exhaust fan), wash basin, two waste bins, wall-mounted mirror, handheld mirror, and music player (optional)
- Quiet and clean setup and surroundings

It goes without saying that a trained staff or nurse with or without assistant doctor is a must. This trained staff must be helpful in filling up informed consent forms, preoperative preparations, intraoperative assistance, postoperative dressings, and recordkeeping.

PREOPERATIVE ASSESSMENT AND COUNSELING[18]

Whatever may be the expectations of the patients, during consultation, we should explain them the best surgical treatment and discuss various modalities and their results, limitations, side effects, and treatment cost. This should be done with the help of photodocumentary evidence.

All posted patients should be routinely investigated for hemogram, blood sugar, bleeding and clotting time, and tests for human immunodeficiency virus (HIV) and hepatitis B virus (HBV) infection beforehand [real-time reverse transcriptase-polymerase chain reaction (RT-PCR) for coronavirus disease 2019 (COVID-19) infection, if applicable].

PREOPERATIVE REQUISITES[19]

Informed consent form must be duly filled and it should include statements regarding cardiac pacemaker (RF surgery) and local anesthesia test dose and whether patient has recovered from COVID-19 infection within past 2 weeks.

APPLICATIONS[20,21]

Electrocautery: This basic electrical equipment was and is still used for multiple common indications in clinical dermatology. This is commonly used by general practitioners in rural and urban areas and in many hospitals, as well as by many dermatologists even today.

The common applications of electrocautery are given in **Box 2**. The Steps of using electrocautery are mentioned in **Box 3**.

- *RF surgery:* Its applications are broadly classified into two categories:[22]
  1. *Therapeutic applications:* These are further classified into: (i) ablative and (ii) nonablative.

BOX 2: Common applications of electrocautery.

- Skin tags or acrochordons
- Papillomas
- Warts or Verrucae of all types
- Condylomata
- Vascular lesions such as capillary hemangioma and pyogenic granuloma
- Corns and calluses

BOX 3: Steps of using electrocautery.

- Local anesthesia is preferred in all as electrode is hot
- The machine power setting is according to individual experience
- The electrode touches the lesion to literally destroy it till its base
- The treated lesion first whitens due to dehydration and finally becomes brownish black due to charring and necrosis
- The heat also causes a sublesion separation blister which facilitates its easy peeling off or removal by just scrapping it with a moist gauze
- Usually, there is no bleeding as hot electrode coagulates the blood vessels

2. *Diagnostic applications:* The two basic techniques which are required in most applications are elaborated further.
   i. *Shave excision* ***(Fig. 11)****:*
      a. Electrodes used are round loop/triangular/diamond shaped
      b. Under infiltration anesthesia, the lesion is excised in a stepwise manner in thin slices till desired lesion is removed.
      c. Repeated delicate strokes at optimum power and appropriate waveform (electrosection or blend) gives best results.
      d. Hemostasis is achieved with pressure or electrocoagulation.
      e. RF blending technique is used to give finishing touches for superior cosmesis.
   ii. *Fine touch desiccation:*
      a. Electrodes used are Vari-Tip (thin wire)/straight needle/thick desiccation.
      b. Surface or infiltration anesthesia
      c. Surface of lesion is just finely touched with electrode at lowest power till it whitens.
      d. Instead of single long touch, multiple split-second touches are preferable.

Indications of RF can be classified as: (1) dermatological and (2) cosmetic **(Boxes 4 and 5)**.

BOX 4: Dermatological indications.

• Verrucae or warts	• Capillary hemangioma
• Condyloma acuminata	• Pyogenic granuloma
• Molluscum contagiosum	• Cherry angioma
• Corns and calluses	• Hypertrophic lichen planus
• Acrochordons or skin tags	• Prurigo nodularis
• Adenoma sebaceum	• Submucous cyst
• Papilloma	• Lymphangioma circumscriptum
• Dermatofibroma	• Keratosis (seborrheic)
• Keratoacanthoma	• Sebaceous hyperplasia
• Neurofibroma	• Xanthoma
• Histiocytoma	• Nail matrixectomies
• Steatocystoma multiplex	• Ingrown toenail
• Hypertrophic scars	• Lichen amyloidosis
• Keloids	• Chronic lichenified eczema
• Cutaneous horns	• Angiokeratoma
• Basal cell carcinoma	• Sebaceous cyst
• Squamous cell carcinoma	• Lipoma

BOX 5: Cosmetic dermatological indications.

• Melanocytic nevi (intradermal moles)	• Freckles
	• Lentigines
• Verruca plana (face)	• Rhinophyma
• Molluscum contagiosum (face)	• Seborrheic keratosis
• Milia	• Actinic keratosis
• Syringoma	• Cutaneous horns (face)
• Xanthelasma	• Epidermal nevus
• Trichoepithelioma	• Telangiectasia
• Senile comedones	• Resurfacing of depressed acne scars, chickenpox scars
• Closed comedones	
• Ear lobe repair	• Resurfacing of hypertrophic scars
• Gray hair epilation	

RADIOFREQUENCY SURGERY (STEPWISE)

Ablative Indications

Table 3 will give idea about the basic steps used in any RF ablative surgery, its corresponding electrode, the waveform selected, and power range according to Ellman Surgitron EMC equipment (this differs with the equipment used).

The most common indications which form the bulk of RF surgical practice are detailed out further as ready reckoner:

Warts, moles, larger skin tags, keratoses, corns, and calluses are the most common lesions which are excised using:

- Bulk excision is done using above-mentioned electrode with appropriate waveform and power setting **(Figs. 13 and 14)**.
- Shave excision is done using above-mentioned parameters in **Table 3 (Fig. 11)**.
- Blending technique mentioned earlier is the finishing step of immense importance for best cosmetic result.

Excision Tips for Various Lesions

- *Moles*[23] ***(Figs. 15A and B)****:* The best choice of moles for RF excision are the elevated dome-shaped moles which can be easily removed with negligible scarring. Prefer pressure hemostasis for facial moles as electrocoagulation may lead to scar. Flat moles should never be selected for removal with RF technique. It is possible that after excising the mole completely till skin surface level, one may find some remnants of mole tissue persisting and removing this will cause a depressed scar. Here, it is prudent to explain it to the patient immediately, showing him/her with the help of mirror. In this case, one should allow it to heal and follow-up the patient for recurrence in the next 4–6 weeks. In case of significant recurrence, one should redo deeper excision, informing patient of possibility of scar.
- *Warts*[23] ***(Figs. 16 and 17)****:* Always treat all visible warts. In case of more than 5–10 warts, treat in two to three separate sessions. In case of facial warts or multiple warts, avoid excision in all and treat small warts using electrodesiccation or electrofulguration. Plantar or palmar warts have more downtime and pain and hence if multiple, treat in more than one session. Warts on scalp, palms, soles, periungual areas, and in between webspaces are likely to bleed. Mucosal warts need careful and delicate handling. Patient must know about recurrence even after excision and agree to follow-up visits and recurrent treatments. Finish off excision with electrocoagulation whether required or not as it heats up floor of postoperative wound to prevent recurrence.
- *Corns/calluses:*[23] Always excise with wider margins. Prevent premature long-standing or excess walking for at least 4–6 weeks to prevent recurrence. In case of patients with sensory neuropathy or diabetes, postoperative wound

care is extremely important. Postoperatively, soft insole is very important. Barefoot walking must be avoided.

- *Keratoses on face*[23] ***(Figs. 18 and 19)***: Excising these on face is a very delicate job which requires full control over strokes and a very steady hand. Skill of RF surgery is tested in all flat keratoses where shave excision and blending technique decide the final result. Very delicate "portrait-shading strokes" for blending give the best result.
- *Sebaceous cyst*[23] ***(Figs. 20A to C)***: Here, the newer "small or tiny hole surgery" is best where a small superficial incision is made of 2–4 mm length. Cyst wall is identified and through lateral pressure, the cyst is expressed out and enucleated. Sometimes, cyst ruptures, then foul-smelling contents are expressed out, cyst wall is pulled out with help of forceps and cut. If it is difficult to pull out cyst wall,

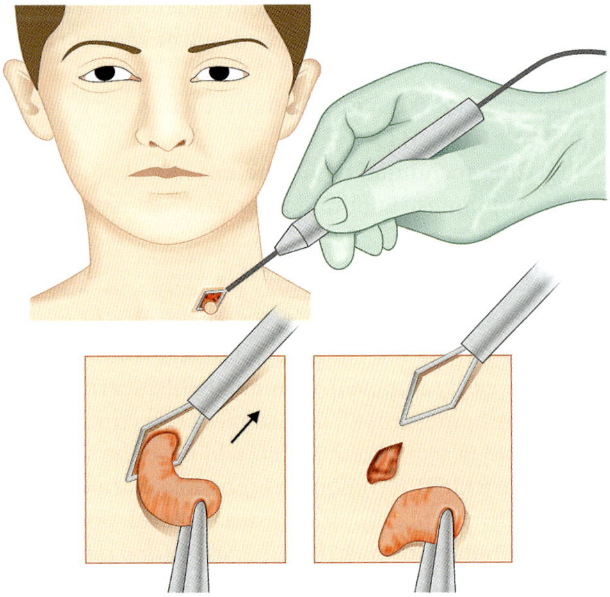

Fig. 13: Pedunculated lesion cut at base with loop electrode pushed over lesion.
Source: Adapted from Savitha AS, Shilpa K, Chatterjee M, Vasudevan B, Neema S, Gorur D, et al (Eds). ACS(I) Procedural Dermatosurgery: A Step by Step Approach, 1st edition. New Delhi: Jaypee Brothers Medical Publishers; 2018. p. 492.

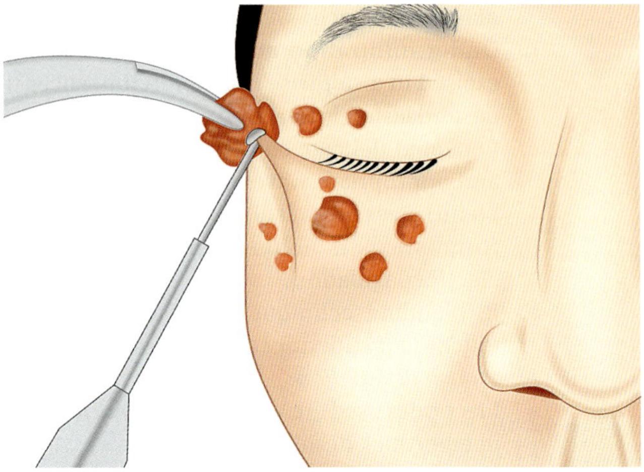

Fig. 14: Pedunculated lesion cut at base with straight needle electrode.
Source: Adapted from Savitha AS, Shilpa K, Chatterjee M, Vasudevan B, Neema S, Gorur D, et al (Eds). ACS(I) Procedural Dermatosurgery: A Step by Step Approach, 1st edition. New Delhi: Jaypee Brothers Medical Publishers; 2018. p. 492.

TABLE 3: Steps used in any RF ablative surgery.

Step	*Electrode*	*Waveform*	*Power*
Bulk excision	SN/VT/RL or T (of varied sizes)	Cut/blend	3–10 (according to lesion)
Shave excision	RL/T/D	Cut/blend	3–6 (according to lesion)
Coagulation	B	Coagulated	4–10
Blending	RL	Cut	1–3 (according to lesion)

(B: ball tipped; D: diamond; RF: radiofrequency; RL: round loop; SN: straight needle; T: triangular; VT: Vari-Tip)

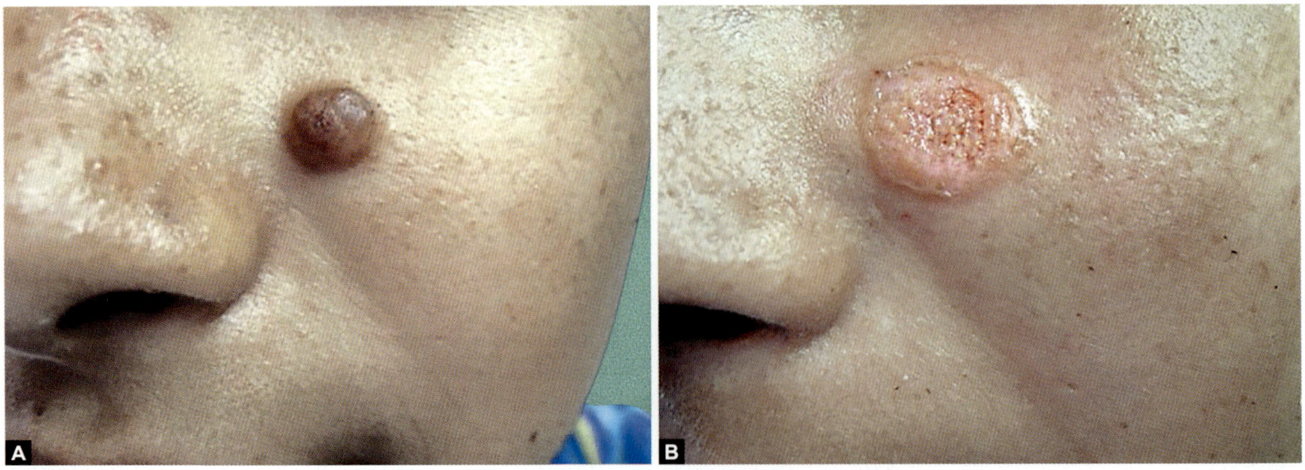

Figs. 15A and B: Mole excision, immediately after picture shows clean excision with edges blended into adjacent skin.
Source: Adapted from Savitha AS, Shilpa K, Chatterjee M, Vasudevan B, Neema S, Gorur D, et al (Eds). ACS(I) Procedural Dermatosurgery: A Step by Step Approach, 1st edition. New Delhi: Jaypee Brothers Medical Publishers; 2018. p. 500.

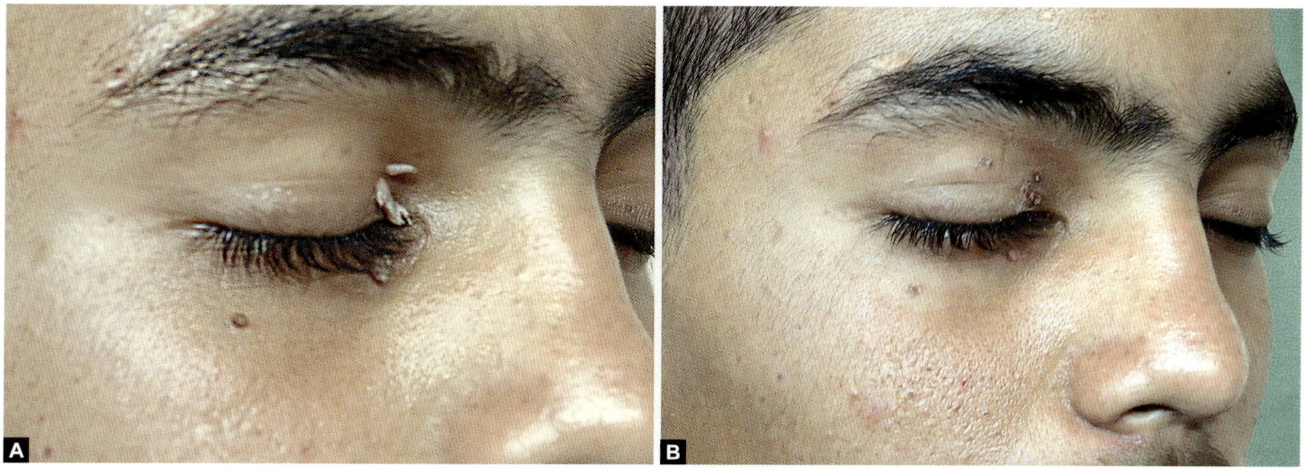

Figs. 16A and B: Warts on eyelid excised under local anesthesia, clean excision.

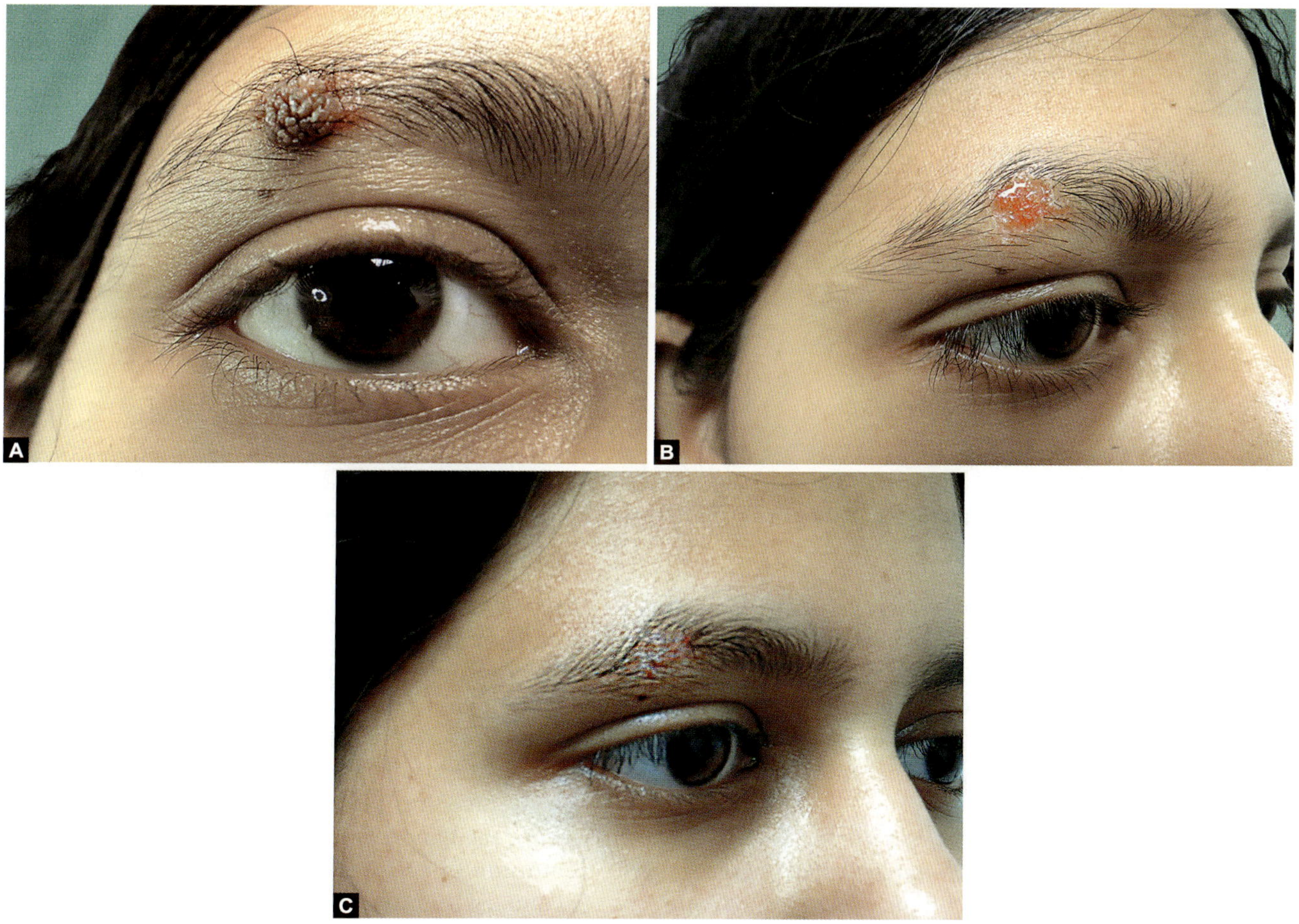

Figs. 17A to C: Warts on eyebrow excised under local anesthesia, clean excision, scarless healing.

insert Vari-Tip electrode inside and pass heat inside, which allows collapse of cyst wall at 2–3 power. This small wound heals on its own without suturing.

- *Submucous cysts and other mucosal lesions:*[24] These are commonly excised using round loop electrode on "blend waveform." Hemostasis is achieved with ball-tipped electrode and postoperative wound heals with secondary intention. Blending is unnecessary.
- *Vascular lesions (capillary hemangioma/pyogenic granuloma)*[24] ***(Figs. 21 and 22):*** Smaller lesions <0.5 cm can be electrocoagulated directly and scraped off. Larger lesions are first excised using "blend waveform."

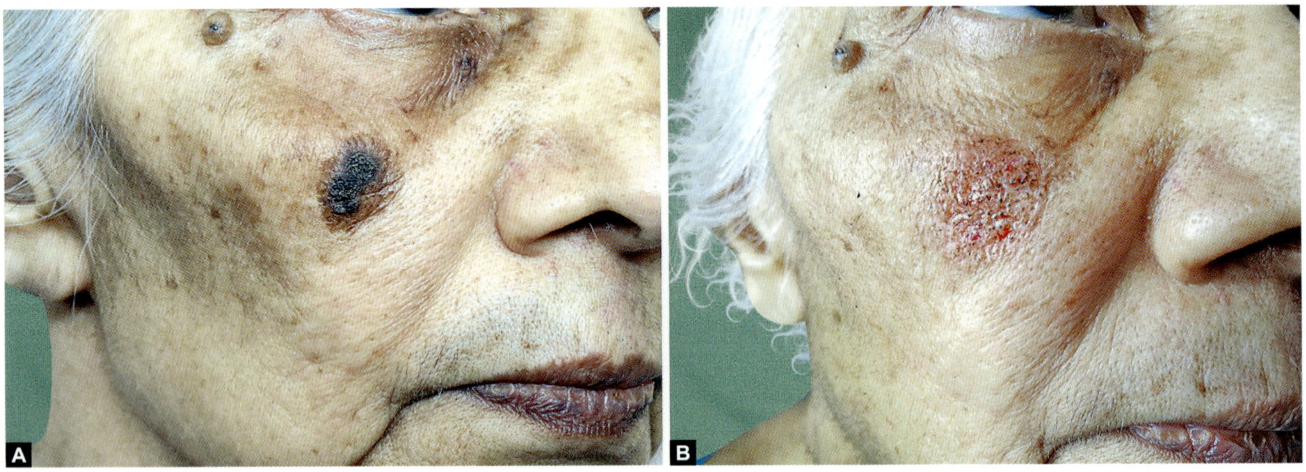

Figs. 18A and B: Seborrheic keratosis on cheek, clean and virtually bloodless excision under local anesthesia followed by fine blending of edges to allow scarless healing.

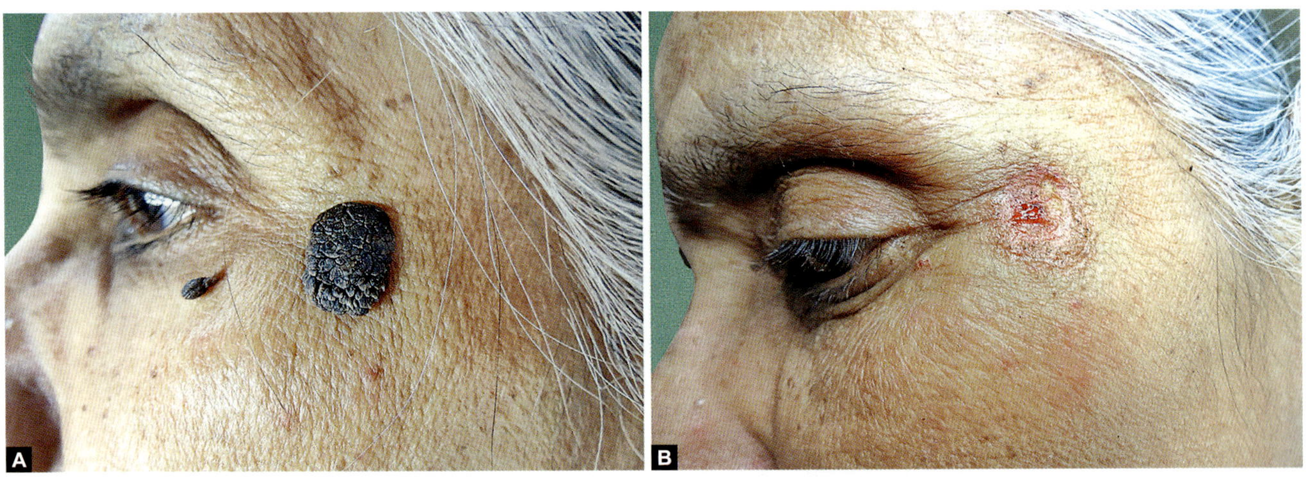

Figs. 19A and B: Seborrheic keratosis on temple area, clean and virtually bloodless excision.

Bleeding is arrested using "coagulated waveform." Finally, wound edges are blended for cosmesis. Postoperative wound heals with secondary intention. It is better to avoid direct electrocoagulation of larger lesion as if power used is less than optimum, the lesion will bleed more profusely and further excision will become more difficult and time-consuming.

- *Various papular and plaque-type lesions (trichoepithelioma/neurofibroma/keratoacanthoma/prurigo nodularis/hypertrophic lichen planus/chronic lichenified eczema/dermatofibroma/histiocytoma/angiokeratoma/lichen amyloidosis/giant molluscum/large skin tags)*[24] ***(Figs. 23 to 25)****:* Here, large single lesions are excised with straight needle electrode, whereas mostly the round loop or triangular electrode works best. "Blend waveform" is the choice but "cut waveform" is best on face. Shave excision method with higher power (up to 8–10) may be required for thicker lesions. "coagulation waveform" is used when required.
- *Hypertrophic scars and keloids:*[24] These are best excised using round loop electrode by shave method and blend waveform till all thickened tissue is planed down and removed. Larger lesions especially keloids are first excised using straight needle electrode (bulk excision) before shaving down to remove remnants. Usually, bleeding is less and can be easily stopped using electrocoagulation. On table, intralesional triamcinolone acetonide injection is given to prevent recurrence. Secondary intention healing is preferred. These have to be keenly followed up to prevent recurrence and all possible measures such as use of silicone topical gels, pressure bandages, and repeat intralesional triamcinolone injections are important. Keloids, especially on immobile areas such as ears, can be excised and effectively prevented from recurrence, but keloids on chest, back areas, and mandible are notorious for recurrence; hence, RF excision is best avoided in them.

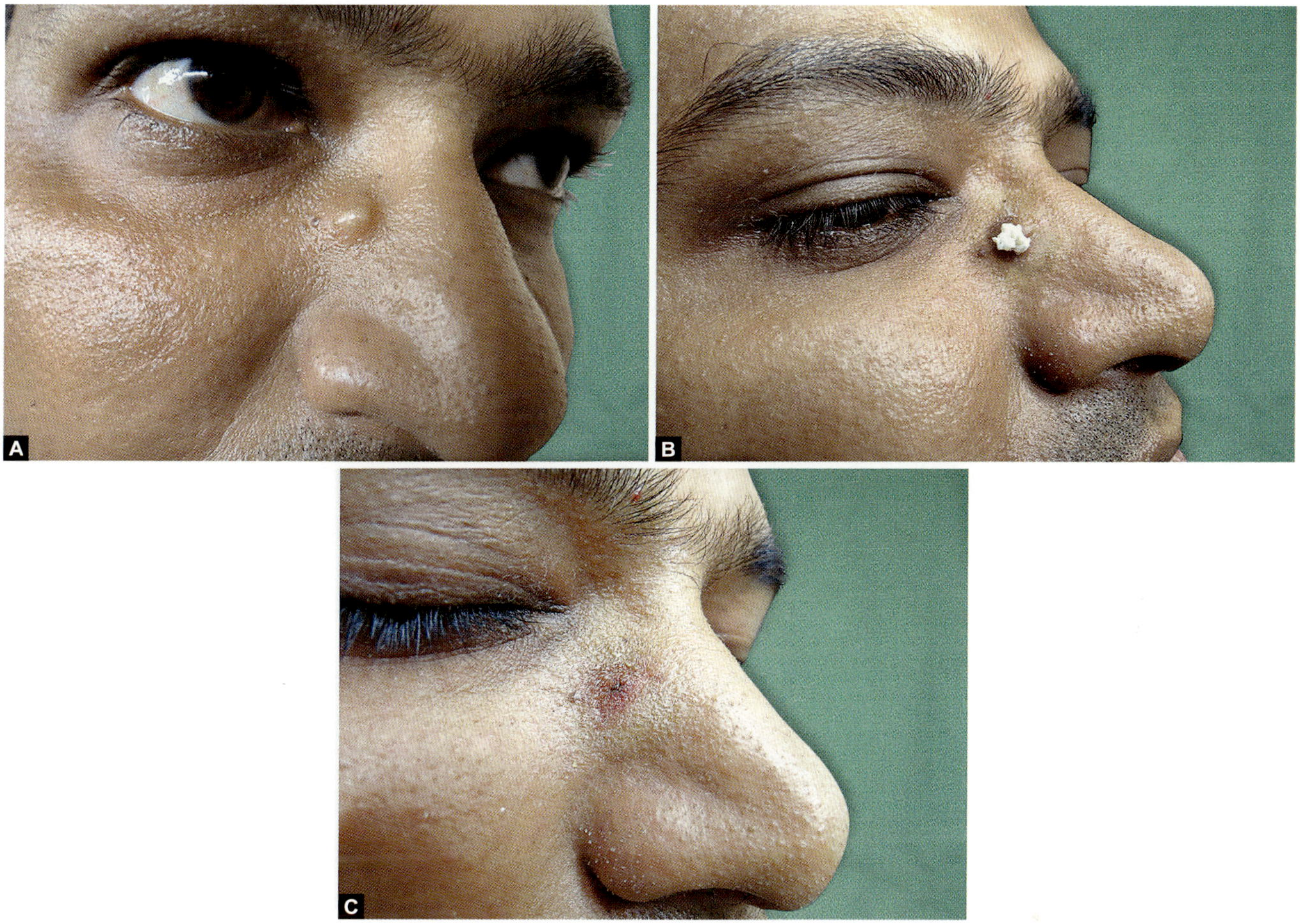

Figs. 20A to C: Sebaceous cyst on nose, excised under local anesthesia through small hole, sebum expressed out, wall pulled out and cut, virtually bloodless excision and scarless healing.

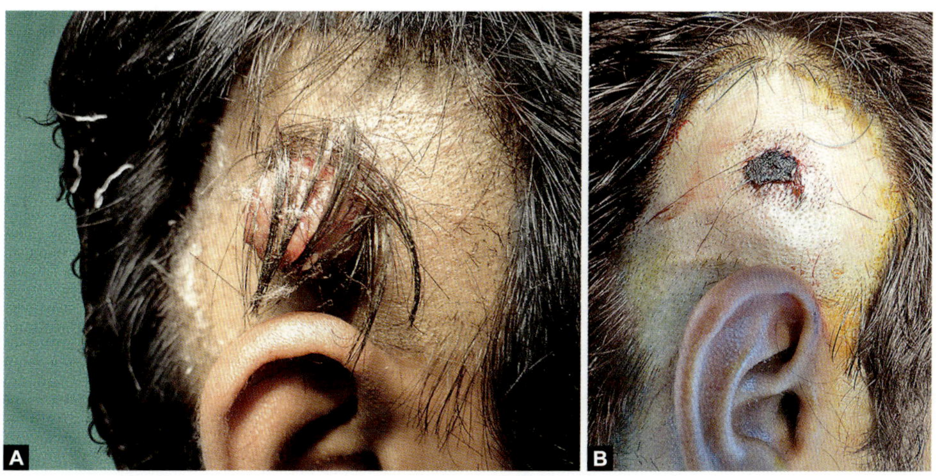

Figs. 21A and B: Pyogenic granuloma (large) on scalp, excised under local anesthesia, hemostasis achieved with electrocoagulation.

- *Digital lesions including periungual and subungual lesions*[24] ***(Figs. 26A and B)****:* For these, ring block is given as infiltration anesthesia with injection lignocaine (without adrenaline) and rest is as mentioned earlier.
- *Genital lesions (warts, condyloma acuminata, and molluscum):*[24] All steps are similar to those for mucosal lesions. Cut or blend waveform is used.
- *Freckles*[24] ***(Figs. 27A and B)****:* Multiple freckles are treated in one session. If they are plenty in number,

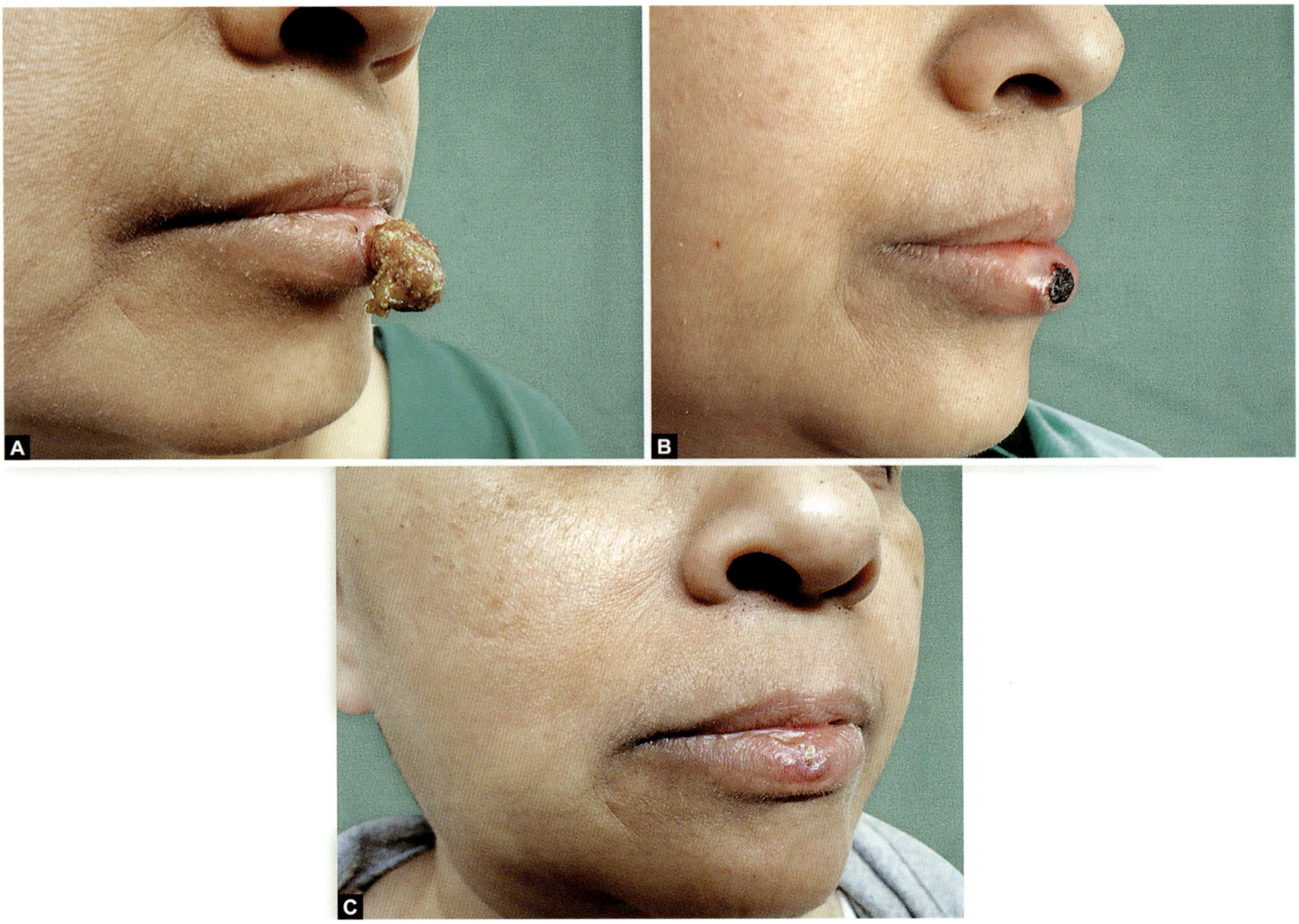

Figs. 22A to C: Pyogenic granuloma on lower lip, excised under local anesthesia followed by hemostasis using electrocoagulation, 1 month later with shallow scar.

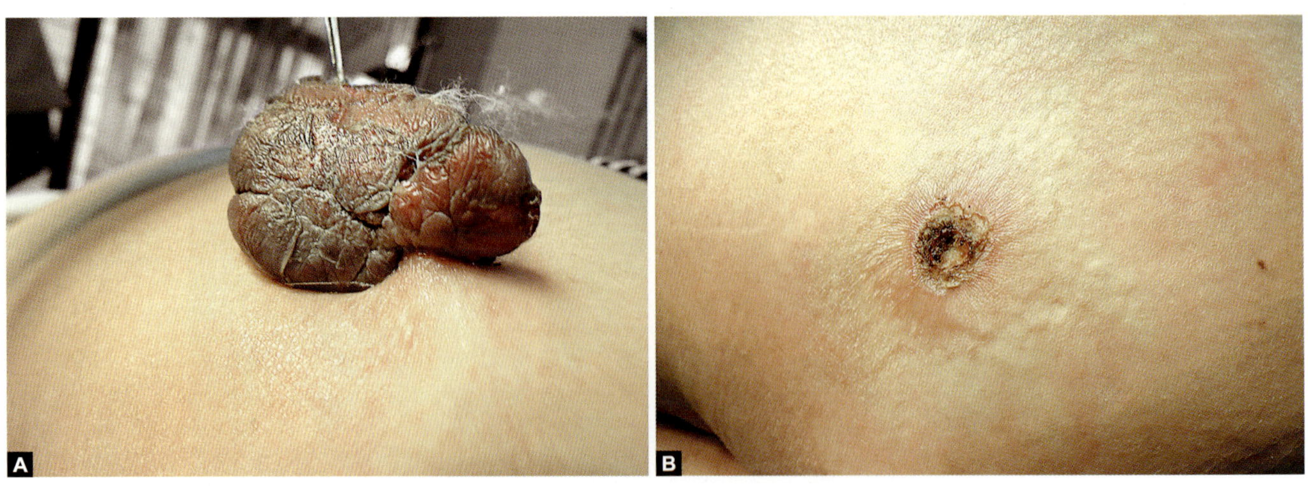

Figs. 23A and B: Large pedunculated skin tag, excised under local anesthesia with blend current.

it is best to treat all in two to three sessions at fortnightly intervals. Straight needle is held at angle of 60°–90° and each freckle is very finely and delicately ablated in one stroke at lowest power of "1." The removed freckles peel off automatically in 1 week with a stage of superficial scab formation before that. The treated area may develop postoperative dyschromia (hyperpigmentation) which finally clears with bleaching creams and face appears clear with even tone by 1–2 months after treatment.

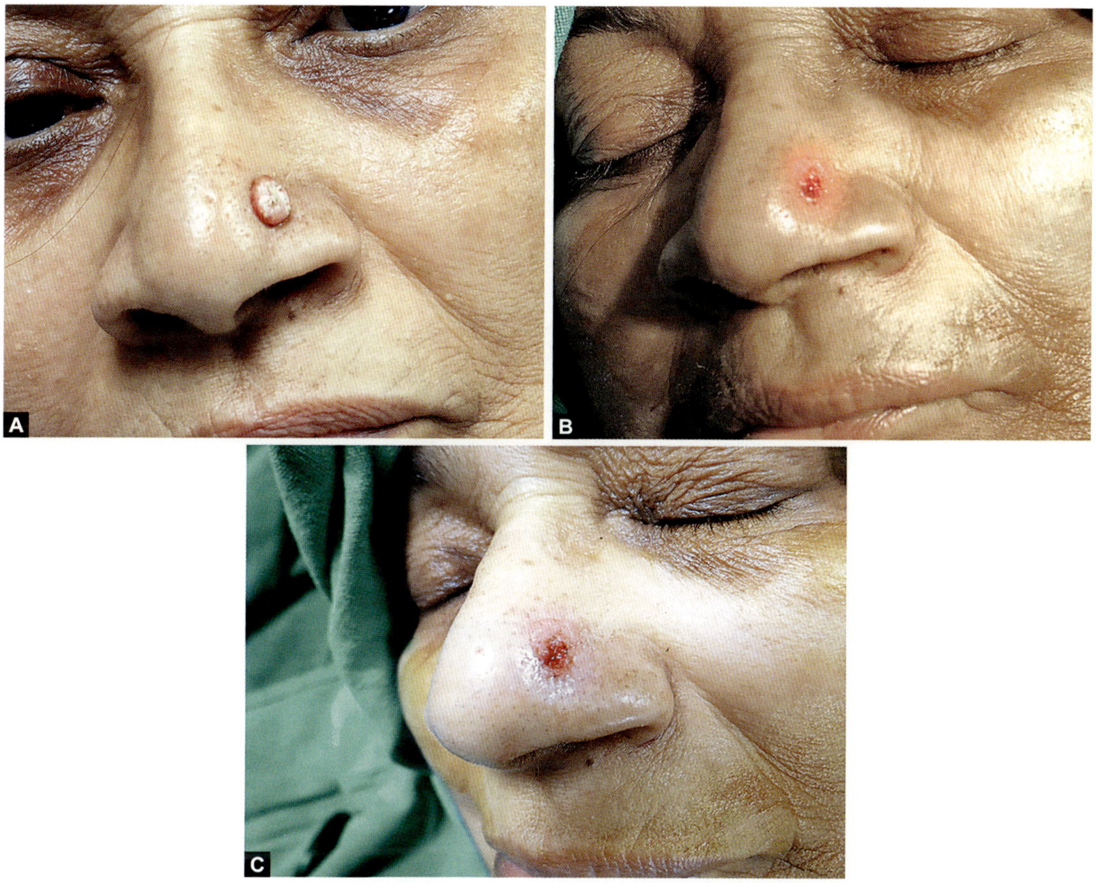

Figs. 24A to C: Calcinosis cutis, excised under local anesthesia, blending done, hemostasis achieved.

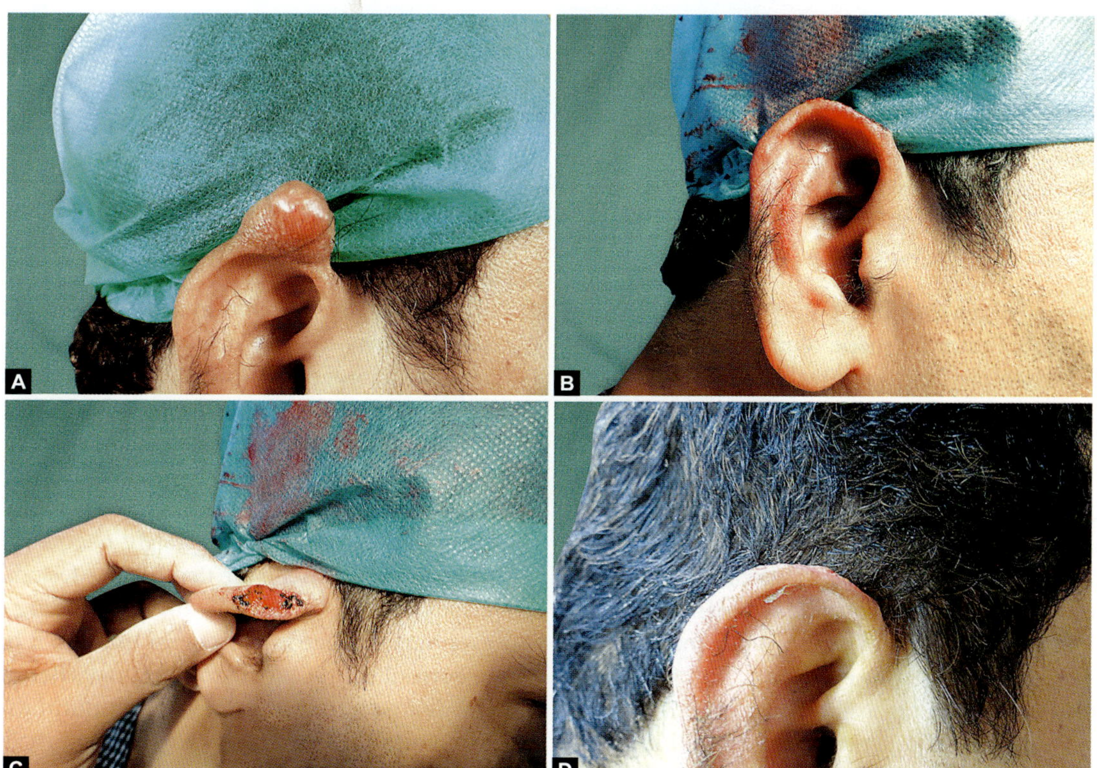

Figs. 25A to D: Benign cartilaginous tumor of external ear, excised in toto under local anesthesia, maintaining ear contour perfectly.

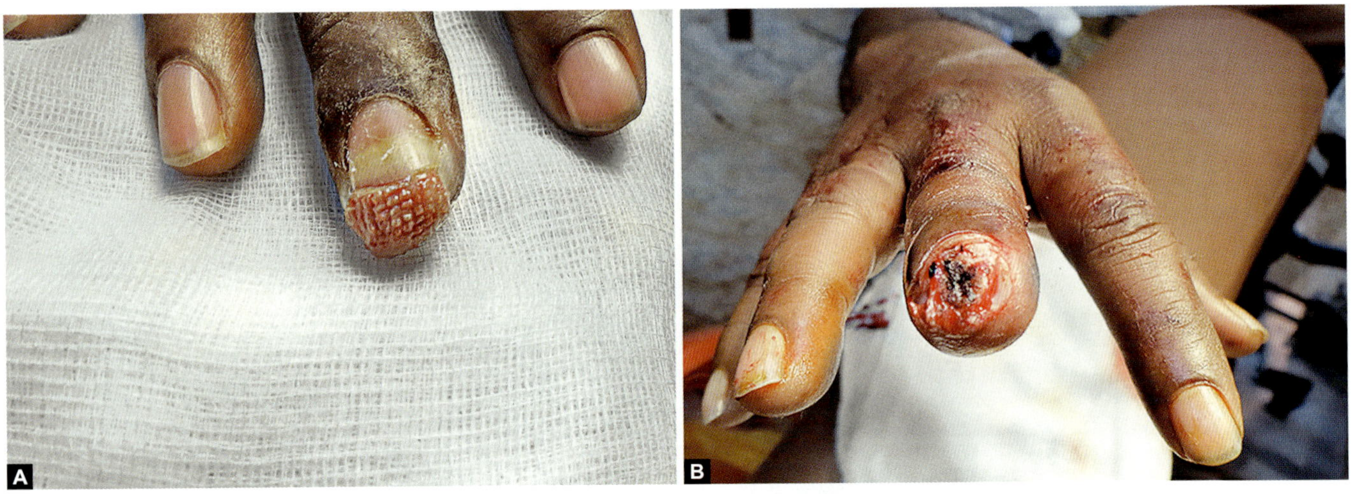

Figs. 26A and B: Pyogenic granuloma on fingertip, excised totally with its subungual portion under local anesthesia after tying Tourniquet at finger base, electrocoagulation done for hemostasis.

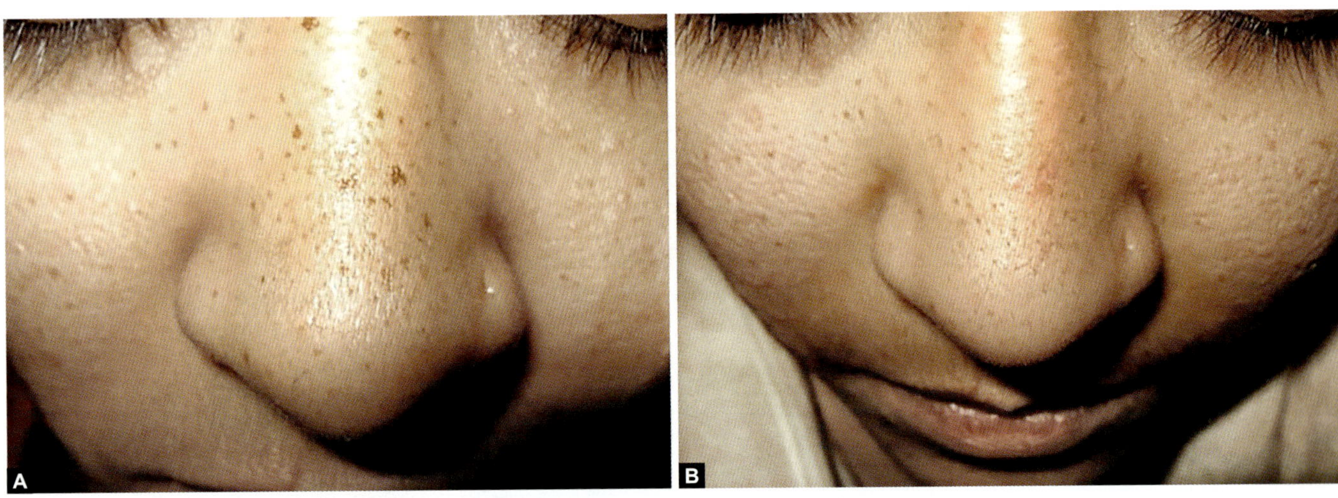

Figs. 27A and B: Freckles, fine ablation in single session.
Source: Adapted from Savitha AS, Shilpa K, Chatterjee M, Vasudevan B, Neema S, Gorur D, et al (Eds). ACS(I) Procedural Dermatosurgery: A Step by Step Approach, 1st edition. New Delhi: Jaypee Brothers Medical Publishers; 2018. p. 519.

- *Rhinophyma*[24] ***(Figs. 28A to C):*** Resecting rhinophyma is a skillful job. Restoring shape of nose by excising the overgrown sebaceous tissue requires careful shave excision with round loop electrode on "cut" waveform at power 3–6 depending on thickness. Infiltration anesthesia is given at various points around nose beforehand. I spend time studying the shape of nose from previous photos of the patient because nose shape matters a lot for face value and we should try to satisfy patient's expectations as much as possible. Nasal shape and symmetry should be restored. Intraoperative bleeding is usually manageable. Postoperative wound is allowed to heal with secondary intention. Complete wound healing may require 3–4 weeks. Color matching may require more than 2 months.
- *Basal cell carcinoma/squamous cell carcinoma*[24] ***(Figs. 29A to C):*** Clinically obvious basal cell carcinoma lesions on face can be excised and sent for histopathology. Lesions close to eyes, on nose, and large-sized lesions are best avoided for total excision; here, the rule is to do an incision biopsy using punch or scalpel or RF to confirm diagnosis and refer the case to oncosurgeon and cosmetic surgeon for complete excision. Use "cut" waveform for incisional or excision biopsy. Excision biopsy can be done using straight needle electrode with tooth forceps through the depth of the lesion. Round loop electrode may be used for this, depending on personal experience. Once bulk tissue is excised, it is transferred to formol saline for histopathology. Remnants of the lesion are excised with "blend" waveform using "shaving technique" and hemostasis achieved with ball electrode in electrocoagulation waveform. Healing is with secondary intention.

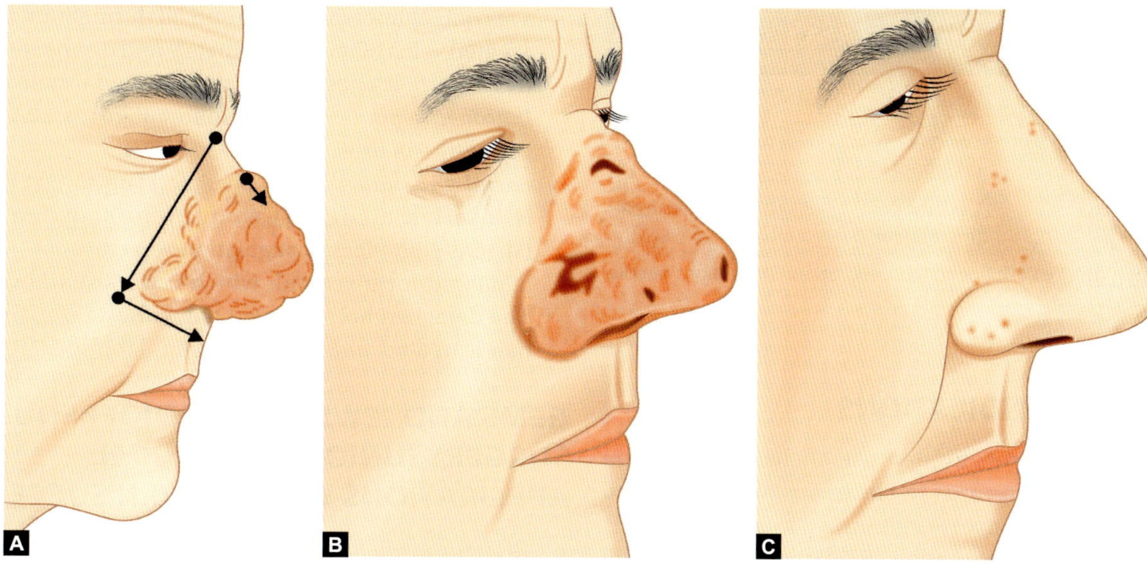

Figs. 28A to C: Rhinophyma, schematic diagrams for resection, plan of infiltrating local anesthetic, complete resection and final result.
Source: Adapted from Savitha AS, Shilpa K, Chatterjee M, Vasudevan B, Neema S, Gorur D, et al (Eds). ACS(I) Procedural Dermatosurgery: A Step by Step Approach, 1st edition. New Delhi: Jaypee Brothers Medical Publishers; 2018. p. 516.

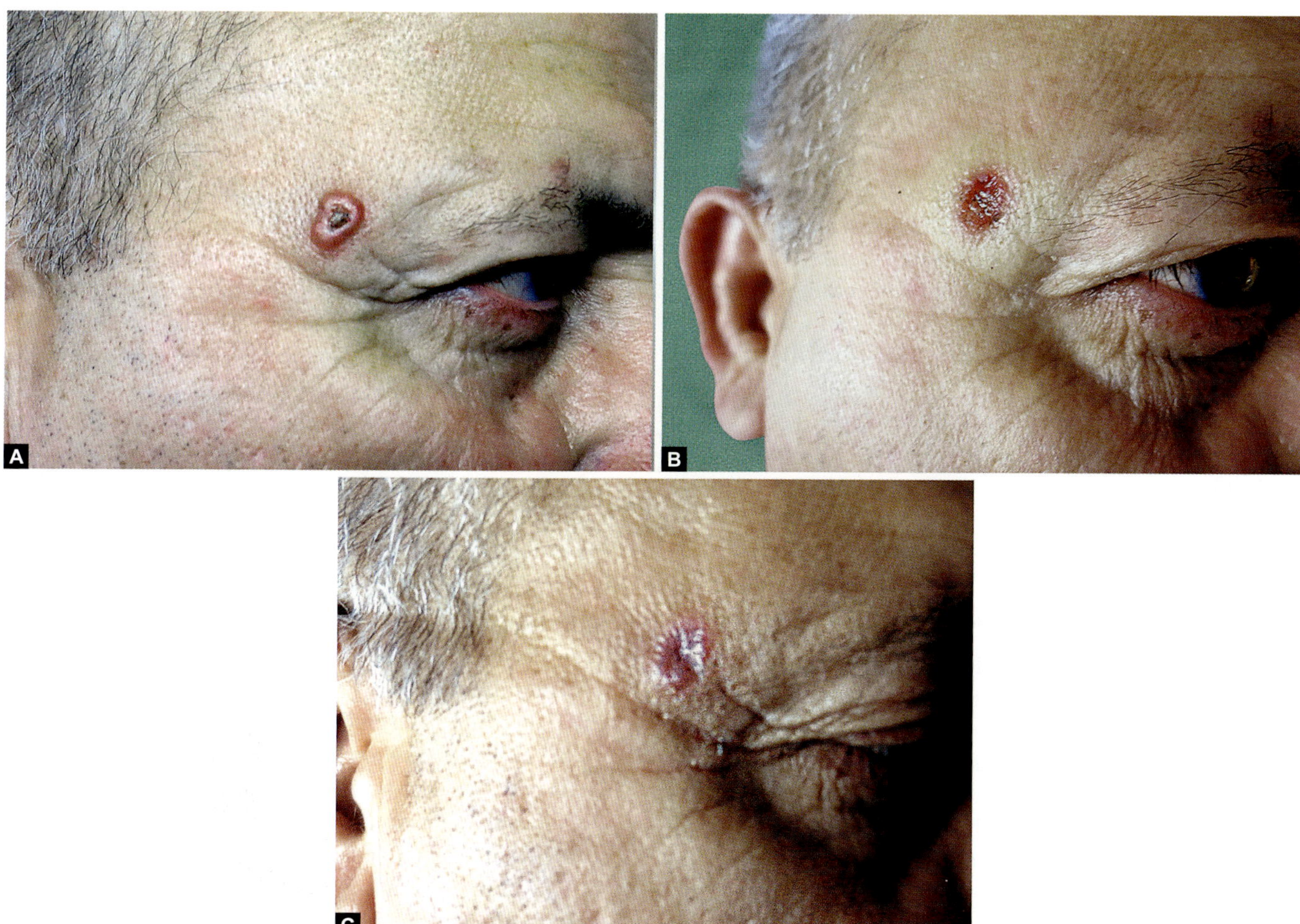

Figs. 29A to C: Well-differentiated squamous cell carcinoma, excision biopsy done under local anesthesia, complete healing (wide local excision was done later as final treatment).

TABLE 4: Desiccation/fulguration tips for various lesions[24] (performed under surface anesthesia).

Step	*Electrode*	*Waveform*	*Power*
FTD	VT/SN/DS	Desiccation (monopolar)	1–2 (lesion touched)
Fulguration	DS	Desiccation (monopolar)	4–8 (lesion not touched)

[DS: desiccation (thick); FTD: fine touch desiccation; SN: straight needle; VT: Vari-Tip]

NONABLATIVE INDICATIONS

Table 4 gives parameters for best use of electrodesiccation and fulguration with regards to electrodes, waveform, and power (according to Ellman Surgitron).

- *Milia:* Fine touch desiccation (FTD) for 1–2 seconds till lesion bursts open and whitens.
- *Molluscum contagiosum:* FTD till lesion bursts open or coagulates (indicated by whitening). When lesion bursts open, the contents are scrapped off with normal saline-moistened gauze. Larger molluscum (giant) are excised by the ablative method.
- *Verruca plana:* FTD till lesion whitens
- *Syringoma:* FTD till lesion whitens. Larger lesions are treated in two sessions because single session may not clear these lesions and prolonged single desiccation may cause scarring.
- *Closed comedones/senile comedones* ***(Figs. 30A to H)****:* FTD till whitening or appreciable shrinkage of lesion.
- *Dermatosis papulosa nigra:* FTD till whitening (here whitening as endpoint of desiccation is clearly noticed.)
- *Multiple seborrheic keratoses:* FTD till whitening or appreciable shrinkage
- *Skin tags:* FTD till whitening and shrinkage
- *Xanthelasma* ***(Figs. 31A and B)****:* FTD till appreciable shrinkage of lesion to almost fading
- *Cherry angioma:* FTD causes appreciable whitening and shrinkage; larger lesions are electrocoagulated.

MISCELLANEOUS APPLICATIONS

- *Earlobe repair:*[24] Incomplete or partial earlobe tear (diameter less than half the diameter of earlobe) can be best treated. The torn edges are refreshed on both sides with thin-wire electrode, hemostasis achieved, approximated perfectly and stuck with cyanoacrylate tissue glue. Aftercare includes avoiding pressure or traction on treated side and avoiding to sleep on that side for at least 1 week for best result.
- *Telangiectasia:*[24] Facial lesions are best treated using special, insulated telangiectasia electrode using electrocoagulation at "1" power at touching the veins hardly for a second at intervals of 2–3 mm all throughout its length. Treated veins blanch immediately and disappear within a week. Surface anesthesia is not required usually.
- *Ingrown toenails:*[24] Please follow **Figures 32A to F** for procedure in brief.
- *Facial gray hair:*[24] Thin, insulated (up to tip) electrode is inserted along hair shaft up to hair root and RF current with electrocoagulation waveform at power "1" is passed for a second, which causes sparking sound. The detached hair is pulled out with tweezer. Individual hair is treated and the procedure is laborious.

GEMS AND JEWELS OF RADIOFREQUENCY SURGERY (UNIQUE AND NOVEL APPLICATIONS WITH PROVEN SUCCESS)

- *RF resurfacing for depressed facial* scars:[25] Scars 5 mm to 1.5 cm wide with >1 mm deep can be effectively resurfaced under infiltration anesthesia in three steps—step 1 **(Fig. 33)**, step 2 **(Fig. 34)**, and step 3 **(Fig. 35)**. Refer to **Figures 36A and B** to appreciate the result.
- *Radiovaporization applications:*[25] Straight needle or Vari-Tip electrode is inserted inside the lesions (hypertrophic scars, keloids, sebaceous cyst, neurofibroma, submucous cyst, etc.) under local anesthesia and on "cut" waveform at 4–5 power (Ellman Surgitron), the lesions shrink appreciably and collapse. These lesions are then easily removed or allowed to heal as the debris inside is cleared automatically.
- *RF-assisted subcision for postacne scars:*[26] Here, RF current is passed using straight needle electrode to the trocar of the intravenous (IV) cannula through a window created beforehand in the plastic sheath. The IV cannula which is inserted into the scar tissue carries RF waves at the tip without damaging the adjacent skin and is moved to-and-fro to break the fibrotic bands.
- *Intralesional RF with a thin hypodermic needle in the management of papular acne scars:*[27] Thin hypodermic needle is inserted in the depth of papular acne scar and RF current is passed at the tip of this needle only for 1–2 seconds using electrocoagulation. This leads to shrinking and flattening of these scars.
- A simple and swift RF-based epilation technique for gray and blonde hair[28]
- *Efficacy and safety of a novel method of insulated intralesional RF ablation for deep dermal and subcutaneous lesions:* A 3-year institutional experience[29]
- *Intralesional RF ablation for nodular angiolymphoid hyperplasia on forehead:* A minimally invasive approach[30]
- Bipolar forceps of a high-power electrosurgical unit for precise removal of small benign skin lesions[31]
- *Biopsy using RF surgical technique*[32-34] ***(Fig. 37)****:* Histological tissue architecture is well preserved in most of

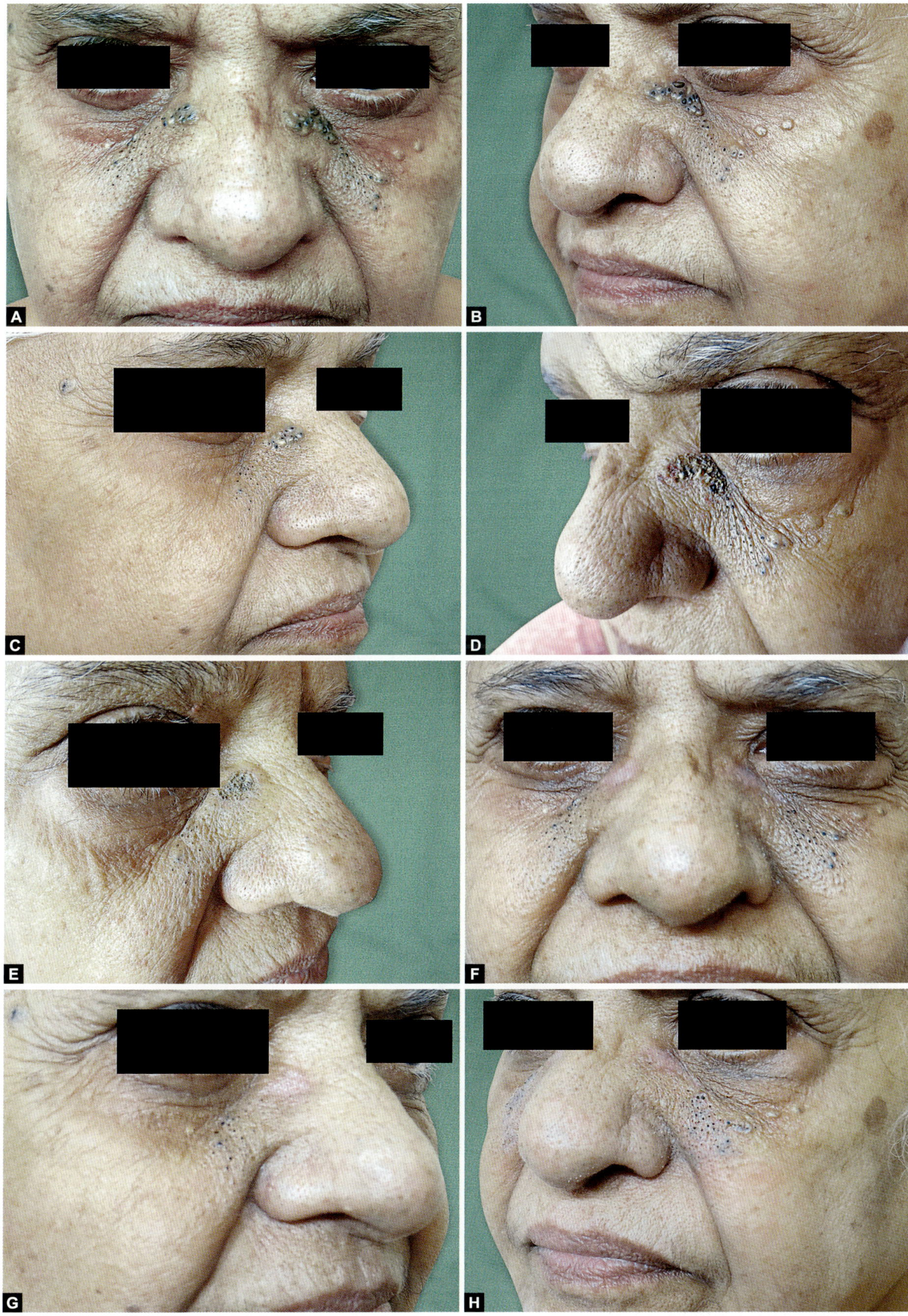

Figs. 30A to H: Senile comedones in large numbers bilaterally, electrodesiccated under local anesthesia, scabs form which peel off, heal without scarring, clears cosmetic disfigurement.

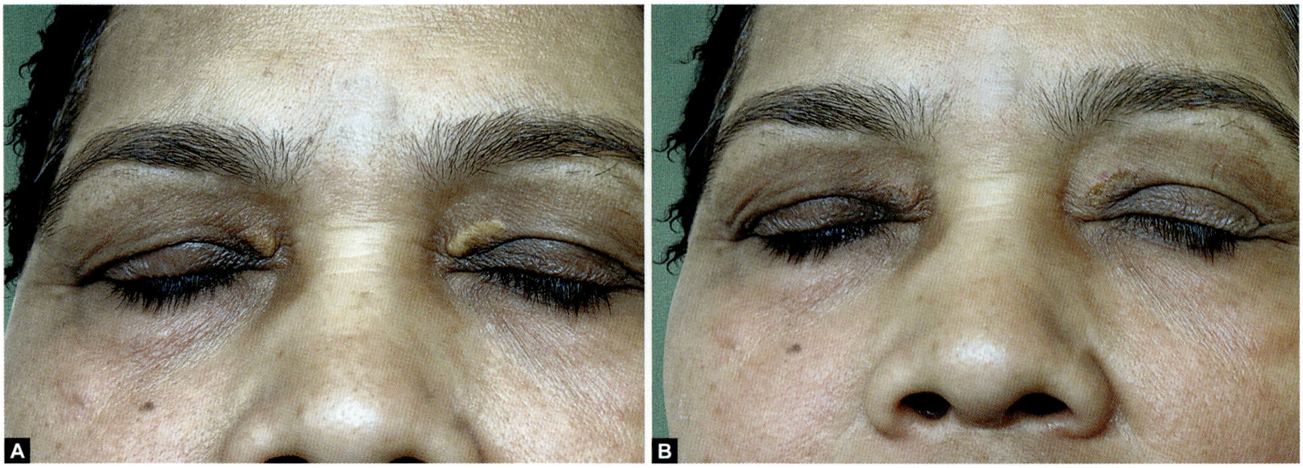

Figs. 31A and B: Xanthelasma, electrodesiccated under local anesthesia.

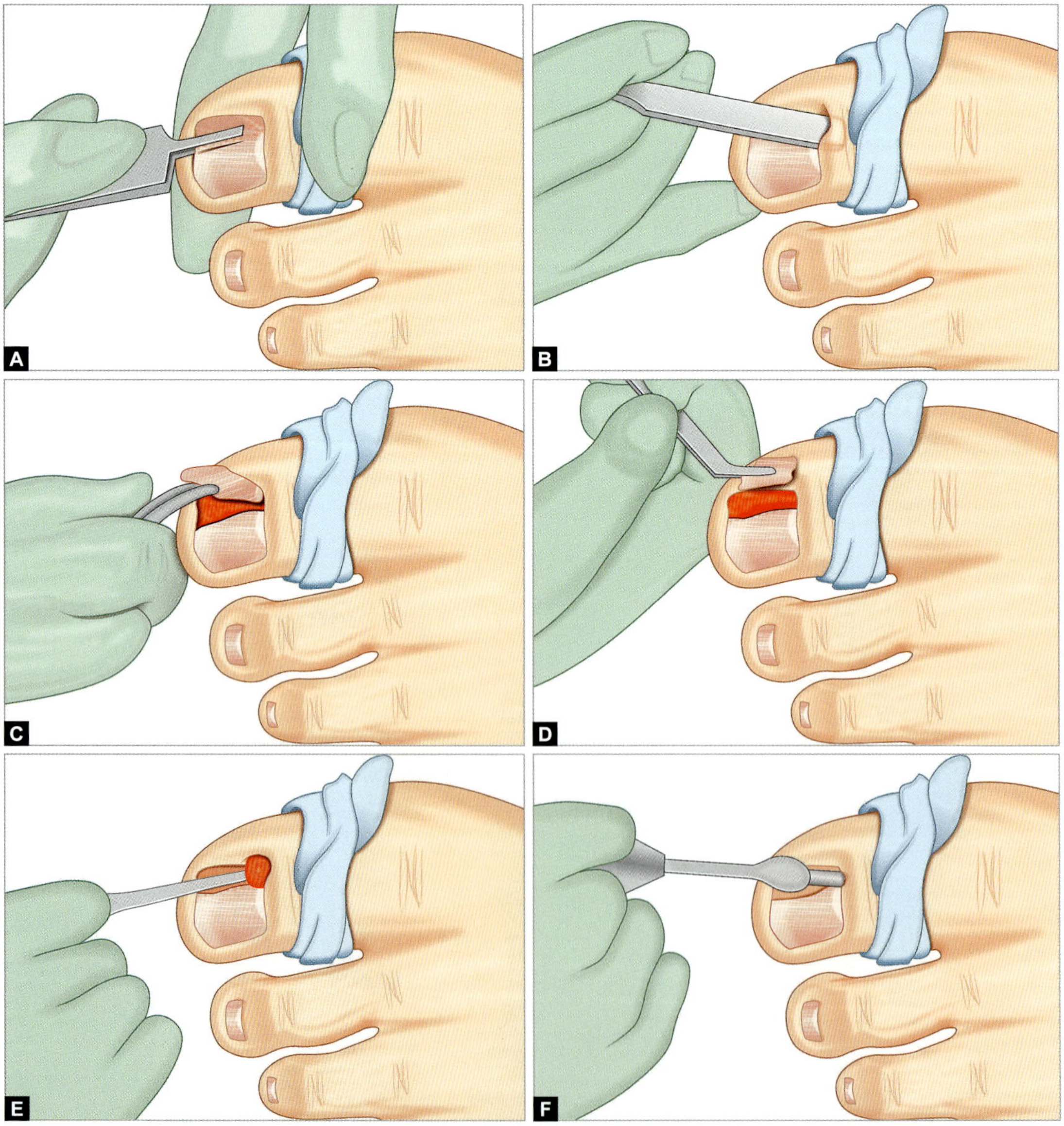

Figs. 32A to F: Ingrown toenail, stepwise procedure.
Source: Adapted from Savitha AS, Shilpa K, Chatterjee M, Vasudevan B, Neema S, Gorur D, et al (Eds). ACS(I) Procedural Dermatosurgery: A Step by Step Approach, 1st edition. New Delhi: Jaypee Brothers Medical Publishers; 2018. p. 515-6.

the biopsy sections done using RF. Thermal changes are reported by pathologist, but diagnostic challenges are rarely reported **(Figs. 38 and 39)**.

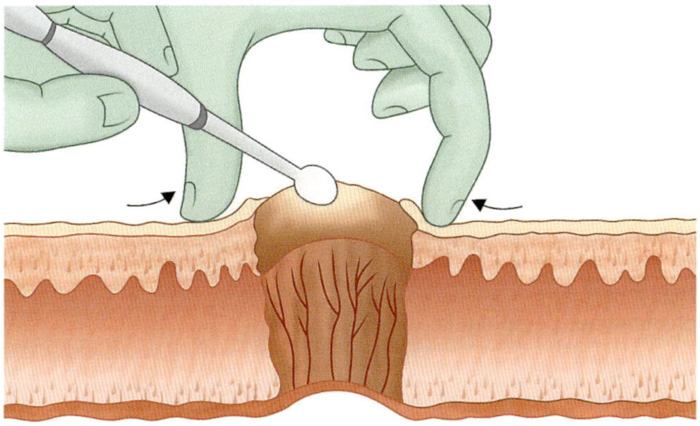

Figs. 33: Radiofrequency (RF) scar resurfacing step 1.
Source: Adapted from Deshpande B (Ed). Dermatologic Surgery with Radiofrequency: Art of Successful Practice, 1st edition. Boca Raton: CRC Press; 2018. p. 85, Figure 15.3.

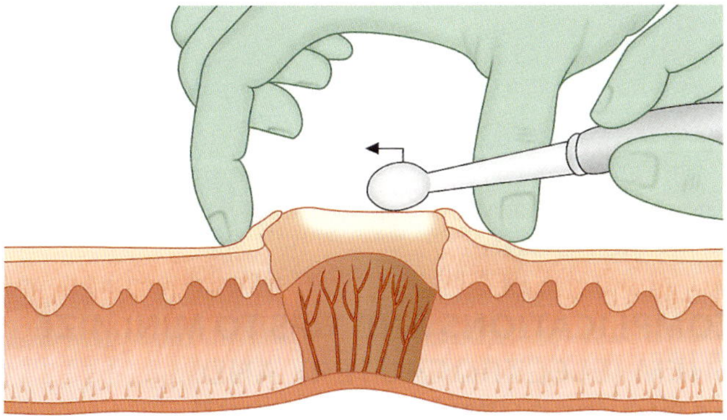

Fig. 34: Radiofrequency (RF) scar resurfacing step 2.
Source: Adapted from Deshpande B (Ed). Dermatologic Surgery with Radiofrequency: Art of Successful Practice, 1st edition. Boca Raton: CRC Press; 2018. p. 86, Figure 15.4.

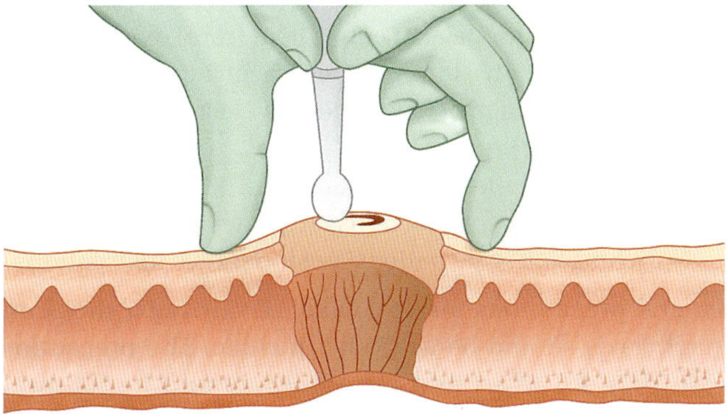

Fig. 35: Radiofrequency (RF) scar resurfacing step 3.
Source: Adapted from Deshpande B (Ed). Dermatologic Surgery with Radiofrequency: Art of Successful Practice, 1st edition. Boca Raton: CRC Press; 2018. p. 86, Figure 15.5.

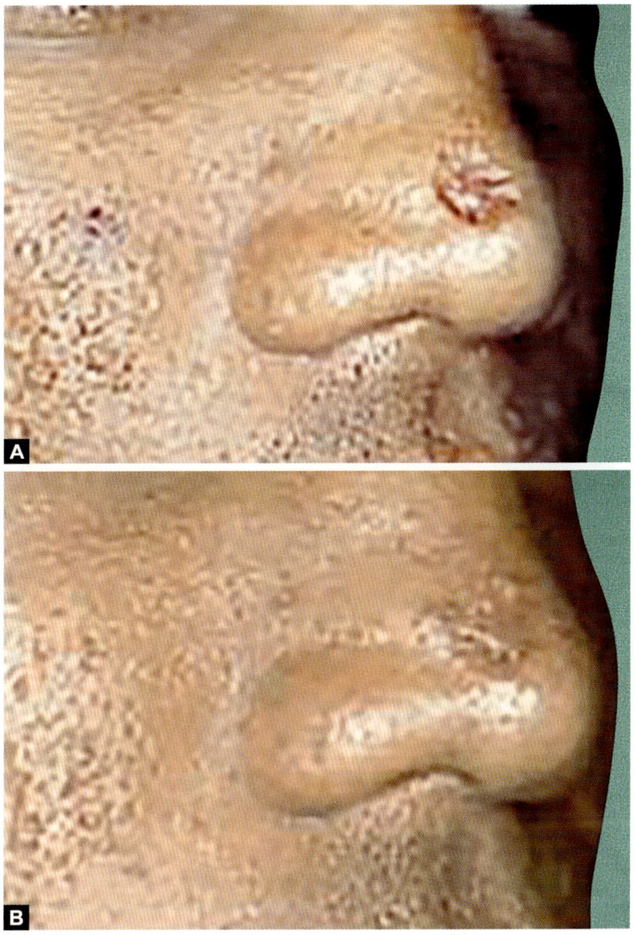

Figs. 36A and B: Nasal scar resurfacing.
Source: Adapted from Savitha AS, Shilpa K, Chatterjee M, Vasudevan B, Neema S, Gorur D, et al (Eds). ACS(I) Procedural Dermatosurgery: A Step by Step Approach, 1st edition. New Delhi: Jaypee Brothers Medical Publishers; 2018. p. 512.

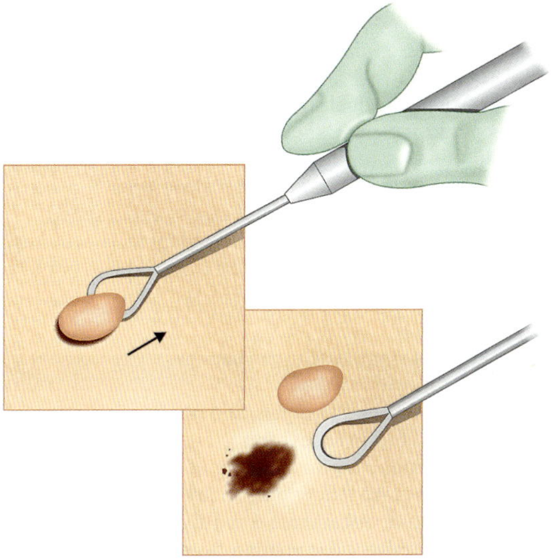

Fig. 37: Excision biopsy using radiofrequency (RF).
Source: Adapted from Savitha AS, Shilpa K, Chatterjee M, Vasudevan B, Neema S, Gorur D, et al (Eds). ACS(I) Procedural Dermatosurgery: A Step by Step Approach, 1st edition. New Delhi: Jaypee Brothers Medical Publishers; 2018. p. 517.

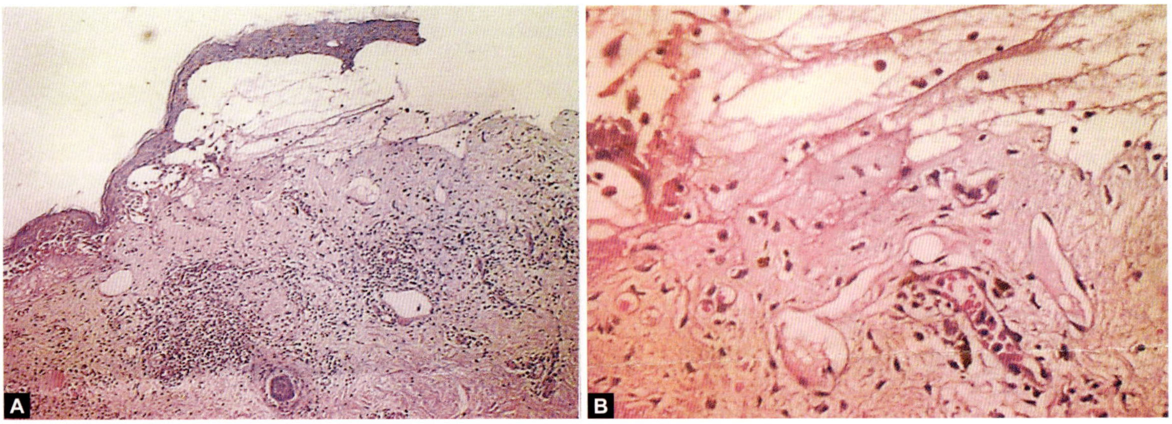

Figs. 38A and B: Photomicrograph of bullous pemphigoid.

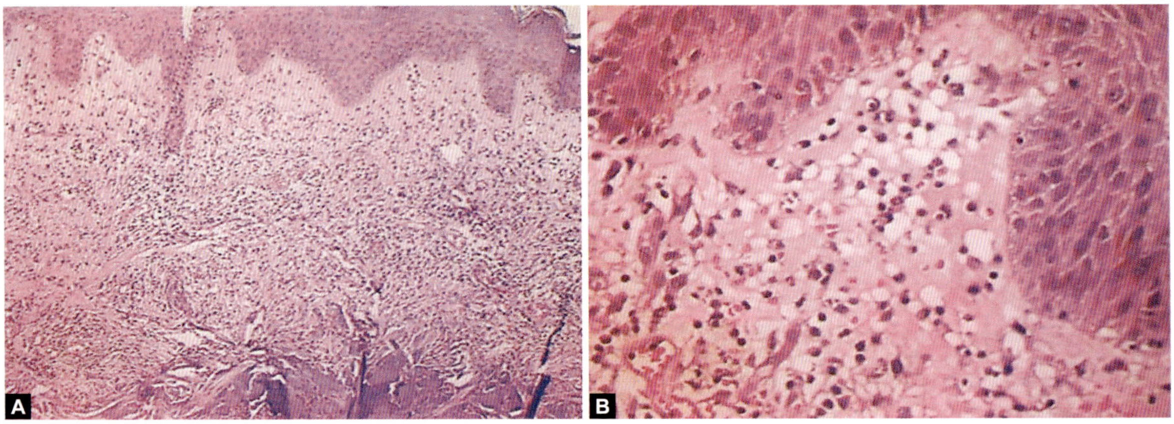

Figs. 39A and B: Photomicrograph of sweet syndromes.

POSTOPERATIVE CARE (ELECTROCAUTERY AND RF SURGERY) (BOXES 6 AND 7)

BOX 6: Excision wounds.

- Wounds are dressed daily except for that of ingrown toenail with topical antibiotic fusidic acid or mupirocin or nadifloxacin
- Oral antibiotic (individual choice) is given for 5–10 days
- Pain-relieving medicines (individual choice) are given depending on condition
- Head bath is avoided for 1 week for scalp lesions
- Foot and sole wounds require extra care to avoid sepsis
- Nonsoapy cleansing lotions are preferred for facial wounds
- Superficial postoperative abrasion like wounds need not be covered with dressing

BOX 7: Desiccation wounds.

- Lesions are applied soothing gels, and no dressing is required
- These lesions will form scabs, and these will fall off automatically in 5–10 days depending on the type of lesion, area, and weather conditions (scabs take longer time to fall off in humid weather)
- A short course oral deflazacort 6 mg twice daily for 3 days helps reduce postoperative inflammation faster, thus lessening chances of postoperative dyschromia and scars
- Topical antibiotic is enough usually; oral antibiotic is preferred in multiple or larger lesions, especially on face
- Nonsoapy cleansing lotion is preferred
- Facial lesions should be protected with sunscreen for outdoor work

COMPLICATIONS AND TIPS TO MINIMIZE THEM (ELECTROCAUTERY AND RADIOFREQUENCY SURGERY)[35]

Broadly speaking, complications can occur due to four factors as follows:

1. Anesthetics—surface (occasionally allergic contact dermatitis) or infiltration (vasovagal shock to frank anaphylaxis)
2. Unexpected stoppage of equipment (rare), electric power failure (common), improper electrical fittings or old wires (shock), breakage of electrode (old electrode, inadequate power setting)
3. Inappropriate electrode or setting of waveform or power or overzealous approach (tissue charring and scarring)
4. Noncompliance by patient (postoperative instructions)

General precautions for possibility of vasovagal shock and anaphylaxis should be available in clinic. The precautions regarding old wires and electrodes should be followed. There should be enough space in clinic for comfortable dermatosurgery. Overzealous approach should be avoided by all means. There is no substitute for precise operating protocol and this comes with proper understanding of the technology and practicing thoroughly beforehand.

Aftercare is equally important in all cases to prevent dyschromia and obvious scarring. This centers upon proper follow-up visits for 1–2 months after reepithelialization to achieve a negligible scar.

The "Say No List" for office RF dermatosurgery and Electrocautery should be always be followed to avoid complications.[11]

HOW TO ACHIEVE AESTHETICALLY SUPERIOR RESULTS?[36] (APPLIES TO RADIOFREQUENCY SURGERY)

To achieve aesthetically superior results has to be the foremost aim of today's dermatosurgeon. RF surgery allows you to achieve this in the best possible way. It does not have any preset protocols. Your experience and skill of using the equipment and electrodes assure aesthetically superior results in each and every RF surgery.

CONCLUSION

Electrocautery is perhaps the most basic equipment in a dermatologist's office and still occupies its place in many clinics of senior ones. However, RF surgical equipment remains an inseparable one in all clinics where office dermatosurgery is routinely performed. RF surgery thus occupies an uncompromised position in office dermatosurgery for the beginner and the established dermatologist as well and carries with it the advantage of portability for the hospital-based dermatosurgery.

REFERENCES

1. Brown JS (Ed). Radiosurgery. Minor Surgery: A Text and Atlas, 4th edition. London: Arnold Publishers; 2000. pp. 311-37.
2. Pollack SV (Ed). How electrosurgical devices work? Electrosurgery of the Skin, 1st edition. New York: Churchill Livingstone; 1991. pp. 7-13.
3. Deshpande B (Ed). Fundamentals features of radiofrequency surgery. Dermatologic Surgery with Radiofrequency: Art of Successful Practice, 1st edition. Boca Raton: CRC Press; 2018. p. 23.
4. Deshpande B (Ed). Fundamentals features of radiofrequency surgery. Dermatologic Surgery with Radiofrequency: Art of Successful Practice, 1st edition. Boca Raton: CRC Press; 2018. p. 24.
5. Pfenninger JS, Fowler GC (Eds). Radiofrequency Surgery (Modern Electrosurgery). Pfenninger and Fowler's Procedures for Primary Care, 2nd edition. United States: Mosby; 2003. pp. 213-24.
6. Deshpande B (Ed). Radiofrequency surgery operative skills. Dermatologic Surgery with Radiofrequency: Art of Successful Practice, 1st edition. Boca Raton: CRC Press; 2018. pp. 29-32.
7. Chiarello SE. Radiovaporization: Radiofrequency cutting current to vaporize and sculpt skin lesions. Dermatol Surg. 2003;29:755-8.
8. Deshpande B (Ed). Single step manoeuvre of radiofrequency resurfacing for selected deep and punched out scars on face. F056: Late-breaking Research: Surgical and Cosmetic. San Francisco, California: 73rd American Academy of Dermatology; 2015.
9. Deshpande B (Ed). Achieving aesthetically superior results: Tips and tricks. Dermatologic Surgery with Radiofrequency: Art of Successful Practice, 1st edition. Boca Raton; CRC Press; 2018. p. 104.
10. Subhadarshani S, Gupta V, Taneja N, Yadav S, Gupta S. Efficacy and safety of novel method of insulated intralesional radiofrequency ablation for deep dermal and subcutaneous lesions: a 3-year institutional experience. Dermatol Surg. 2018;44(5):714-20.
11. Sebben JE. The hazards of electrosurgery. J Am Acad Dermatol. 1987;16:869.
12. Sebben JE. Electrosurgery and Cardiac Pacemakers. J Am Acad Dermatol. 1983;9:457-63.
13. Pollack SV (Ed). Potential hazards of electrosurgery. Electrosurgery of the Skin, 1st edition. New York: Churchill Livingstone; 1991. pp. 71-2.
14. Deshpande B (Ed). Precautions and safety measures. Dermatologic Surgery with Radiofrequency: Art of Successful Practice, 1st edition. Boca Raton: CRC Press; 2018. pp. 33-4.
15. Pollack SV (Ed). Laboratory exercises. Electrosurgery of the Skin, 1st edition. New York: Churchill Livingstone; 1991. pp. 73-85.
16. Deshpande B (Ed). Radiofrequency surgery rehearsal or practice sessions. Dermatologic Surgery with Radiofrequency: Art of Successful Practice, 1st edition. Boca Raton: CRC Press; 2018. pp. 35-40.
17. Deshpande B (Ed). Office Dermatologic Surgery. Dermatologic Surgery with Radiofrequency: Art of Successful Practice, 1st edition. Boca Raton: CRC Press; 2018. pp. 5-7.
18. Deshpande B (Ed). Patient assessment and counselling. Dermatologic Surgery with Radiofrequency: Art of Successful Practice, 1st edition. Boca Raton: CRC Press; 2018. pp. 41-2.
19. Deshpande B (Ed). Prerequisites of office dermatologic surgery. Dermatologic Surgery with Radiofrequency: Art of Successful Practice, 1st edition. Boca Raton: CRC Press; 2018. pp. 9-10.
20. Brown JS (Ed). Electrocautery. Minor Surgery: A Text and Atlas, 4th edition. London: Arnold Publishers; 2000. pp. 111-20.
21. Vasudevan B, Chatterjee M, Shilpa K. Radiofrequency and electrocautery. In: Savitha AS, Shilpa K, Chatterjee M, Vasudevan B, Neema S, Gorur D, et al. (Eds). ACS(I) Procedural Dermatosurgery—A Step by Step Approach, 1st edition. New Delhi: Jaypee Brothers Medical Publishers (P) Ltd.; 2018. pp. 520-1.
22. Deshpande B (Ed). Applications. Dermatologic Surgery with Radiofrequency: Art of Successful Practice, 1st edition. Boca Raton: CRC Press; 2018. pp. 43-4.
23. Deshpande B (Ed). Specific applications: Radiofrequency Commonality. Dermatologic Surgery with Radiofrequency: Art of Successful Practice, 1st edition. Boca Raton: CRC Press; 2018. pp. 45-61.
24. Deshpande B (Ed). Expanding the applications of radiofrequency dermatologic surgery. Dermatologic Surgery with Radiofrequency: Art of Successful Practice, 1st edition. Boca Raton: CRC Press; 2018. pp. 63-82.
25. Deshpande B (Ed). Gems and jewels of radiofrequency surgery. Dermatologic Surgery with Radiofrequency: Art of Successful Practice, 1st edition. Boca Raton: CRC Press; 2018. pp. 83-7.
26. Yadav S, Gupta S. Radiofrequency-assisted subcision for postacne scars. J Am Acad Derm. 2018;78(1):e9-10.

27. Patra S, Kaur M, Gupta S. Intralesional radiofrequency with a thin hypodermic needle in the management of popular acne scars. J Am Acad Derm. 2019;84(6):e259-60.
28. Sanjeev G, Jagra RS, Gupta S. A simple and swift radiofrequency-based epilation technique for gray and blonde hair. J Am Acad Derm. 2020;82(1):e7-8.
29. Subhadarshani S, Gupta V, Taneja N, Yadav S, Gupta S. Efficacy and Safety of a Novel Method of Insulate Intralesional Radiofrequency Ablation for Deep Dermal and Subcutaneous Lesions: A 3 year Institutional Experience. Dermatol Surg. 2018;44(5):714-20.
30. Singh S, Dayal M, Walia R, Arava S, Sharma R, Gupta S. Intralesional Radiofrequency Ablation for Nodular Angiolymphoid Hyperplasia on forehead: A minimally invasive approach. Indian J Dermatol Venereol Leprol. 2014; 5:419-21.
31. Pangti R, Ambika D, Gupta S. Bipolar forceps of a high power electrosurgical unit for precise removal of small benign skin lesions. J Am Acad Dermatol. 2020;82(5):e155-6.
32. Turner RJ, Cohen RA, Voet RL, Stephens SR, Weinstein SA. Analysis of margins of cone biopsy specimen obtained with Cold Knife, CO2 and Nd:YAG Lasers and a Radiofrequency Surgical Unit. J Reprod Med. 1992;37(7):607-10.
33. Maness WL, Roeber FW, Clarke RE, Cataldo E, Riis D, Haddad AW. Histological evaluation of electrosurgery with varying frequency and waveform. J Prosthetic Dent. 1978; 40(3):304-8.
34. Deshpande B (Ed). Biopsy using radiofrequency surgery. Dermatologic Surgery with Radiofrequency: Art of Successful Practice, 1st edition. Boca Raton: CRC Press; 2018. pp. 89-92.
35. Deshpande B (Ed). Tips and tricks to minimize complications. Dermatologic Surgery with Radiofrequency: Art of Successful Practice, 1st edition. Boca Raton: CRC Press; 2018. pp. 95-8.
36. Deshpande B (Ed). Achieving aesthetically superior results: tips and tricks. Dermatologic Surgery with Radiofrequency: Art of Successful Practice, 1st edition. Boca Raton: CRC Press; 2018. pp. 103-4.

CHAPTER 27

Cryotherapy: In Noncosmetic Indications

Avitus John Raakesh Prasad

KEY MESSAGES

- Cryotherapy creates a controlled and targeted destruction of tissue by application of a cryogen.
- It is a simple, cost-effective treatment of various dermatoses giving acceptable and aesthetically acceptable outcome.
- It has a wide variety indications in which it can be used example viral infections, pigmented lesions like dermatosis papulosa nigra (DPN), Freckles, inflammatory dermatoses and various benign, premalignant and malignant tumors.
- It is a safe procedure in elderly patients and in pregnant women.
- Cryotherapy is done as an OPD procedure.

INTRODUCTION

Cryotherapy, also known as cryosurgery, is a controlled and targeted destruction of unwanted tissue by application of various cold substances. It has a variety of applications, most commonly in the treatment of a variety of benign lesions and well-circumscribed premalignant and malignant tumors, which present routinely in the dermatology. It is done as an in-office procedure. Cryotherapy is still one of the important therapeutic armamentariums in a dermatologist's hand, even though we are now in an age of lasers-based therapy. It has proven safe in patients with pacemakers in which electrocautery is contraindicated, in pregnancy, patients who are allergic to local anesthetics, and patients on blood thinners. The ease of use as an office-based procedure as no anesthesia is needed, more safety as compared to lasers, consistent reproducible results, and cost effectiveness as it does not require an elaborate operation theater (OT) setup make it the ideal procedure for a new dermatologist.

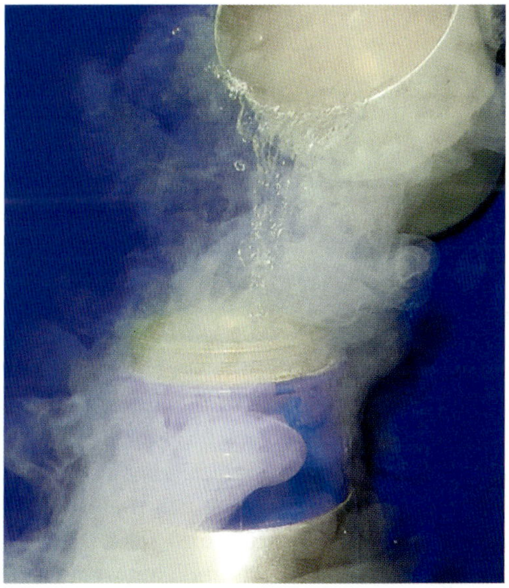

Fig. 1: Liquid state of nitrogen boiling and evaporating at room temperature.

HISTORY OF USE OF CRYOTHERAPY

The Egyptians in 2500 BC were the first to use the concept of using cold-based materials to treat injuries and inflammation. Salt solutions containing crushed ice at temperatures of –18° to –24°C was used by Arnott to freeze breast, cervical, and skin cancers in the 1840s. In 1892, James Dewar of Great Britain designed the first vacuum flask; this was one of the important inventions which enabled and helped in the storage and handling of liquefied gases. The first clinical application of cryotherapy using liquid air (–190°C) was in 1889 by a New York City physician, Campbell White, who used either a swab, a spray, or a brass roller device.[1] By the 1940s, following the World War II, liquid nitrogen (–196°C) became commercially available **(Fig. 1)**.

In 1950, this cryogen was introduced into clinical practice by Dr Ray Allington, who described the technique of using cotton swabs dipped in liquid nitrogen for the treatment of a variety of nonneoplastic skin diseases. Subsequently, this method became a common practice for the treatment of verrucae, keratoses, and diverse other nonneoplastic lesions.[2] In 1961, Cooper and Lee[3] introduced a closed system apparatus to spray liquid nitrogen. In the late 1960s, metal probes became available. In 1967, Setrag Zacarian introduced a handheld self-pressurized device, which is now used commonly after certain modifications. By 1990, 87% of dermatologists in the west used cryotherapy in their practice.[4]

Though most skin cancers are treated with excision or other destructive procedures, such as electrodessication and curettage, superficial basal cell skin cancers[5] and Bowen's disease can be treated with cryotherapy. The recurrence rates for primary basal cell carcinoma (BCC) vary with treatment modality. The 5-year recurrence rate for cryotherapy may be as low as 7.5%, if lesions are chosen judiciously.[6] Well-circumscribed lesions and tumors are most suitable for cryotherapy. The indolent local growth of these well-circumscribed tumors accounts for the high cure rates quoted in the literature.

MECHANISM OF ACTION

The mechanism of action in cryotherapy can be divided into three phases: (1) Heat transfer, (2) cell injury, and (3) inflammation.

Heat Transfer

The mechanism by which cryotherapy destroys the targeted cells is the quick transfer of heat from the skin to a heat sink, which in this case is liquid nitrogen, which has a boiling point of -196°C. The rate of heat transfer is dependent on the temperature difference between the skin and the liquid nitrogen.

When using the spray cryotherapy technique, the liquid nitrogen is applied directly on the skin, and evaporation (boiling heat transfer) occurs in which the heat in the skin is quickly transferred to the liquid nitrogen. This process results in the liquid nitrogen evaporating (boiling) almost immediately.

Cell Injury

Cell injury occurs during the thaw, after the cell is frozen. Because of the hyperosmotic intracellular conditions, ice crystals do not form until -5° to -10°C. The transformation of water to ice concentrates the extracellular solutes and results in an osmotic gradient across the cell membrane, causing further damage. Rapid freezing and slow thaw maximize tissue damage to epithelial cells and is most suitable for the treatment of malignancies. Fibroblasts produce less collagen after a rapid thaw.[7] Therefore, a rapid thaw may be more suitable for the treatment of keloids or benign lesions in areas prone to scarring.[8]

Keratinocytes need to be frozen to -50°C for optimum destruction. Melanocytes are more delicate and are destroyed by temperatures as low as 5°C, which often result in hypopigmentation following cryotherapy on darker-skinned individuals. Malignant skin cancers usually need a temperature of -50°C, while benign lesions only require a temperature of -20° to -25°C.

As the liquid nitrogen is sprayed, the temperature increases from -196° to 180°C when it touches the skin and there is drop in temperature of the skin or lesion being treated. Longer spray results in deeper freezing of tissue and more lateral spread occurs, which determines the depth reached **(Fig. 2)**.

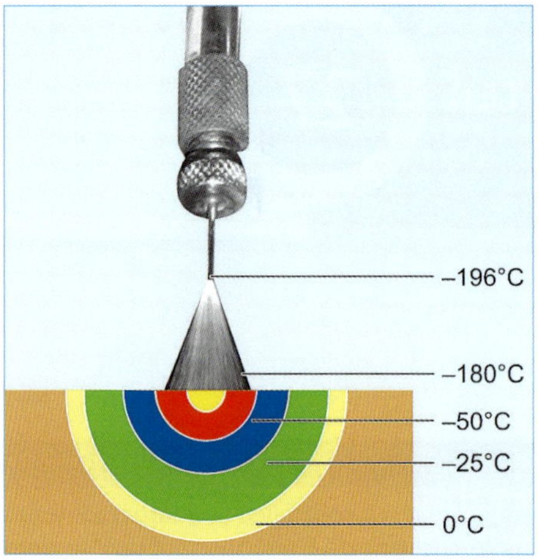

Fig. 2: Temperature changes as the liquid nitrogen is sprayed on the skin.

TABLE 1: Commonly used cryogens.

Cryogens which are used	*Boiling point*
Liquid nitrogen	–196°C
Nitrous oxide	-89°C
Solidified CO_2 (dry ice and CO_2 snow)	–78°C

Inflammation

The last response to cryotherapy is inflammation, which is usually observed as erythema and edema. Inflammation is the response to cell death and helps in local cell destruction.

A thorough cryotherapy treatment causes basement membrane separation, which may result in blister formation.

The commonly used cryogens and equipment are listed in **Table 1**.[9-11]

Out of these, liquid nitrogen is the commonly used cryogen in dermatology practice.

CRYOSURGERY EQUIPMENT[9-11]

- *Cryogun/cryogen spray canister:* It is a specially designed, portable, light weight, hand-held device to contain the liquid nitrogen. Liquid nitrogen is filled into the canister prior to treatment **(Fig. 3)**.
- *Attachments:* Cryospray nozzle and sprays tips with different size opening to allow specified amount of spray of cryogen through it. A roller is used for contact cooling in treating acne vulgaris **(Figs. 4 and 5)**.
- *Cryoprobes:* They are available in various shapes and sizes and get attached to the cryogen. As the cryogen is sprayed through it, it cools, and it is used in approximation to the lesion being treated. Cryoprobes are used as a conduit to transfer the temperature.
- *Cryogen storage device:* They are metal cylinders/containers that store gaseous cryogens as compressed gas and have an inbuilt internal pressure equalization mechanism, e.g., Dewar's gas container. The stored

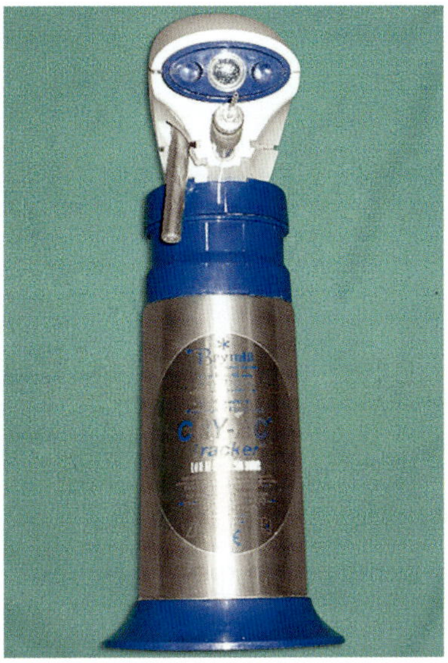

Fig. 3: Cryogun temperature sensing Brymill tracker AC.

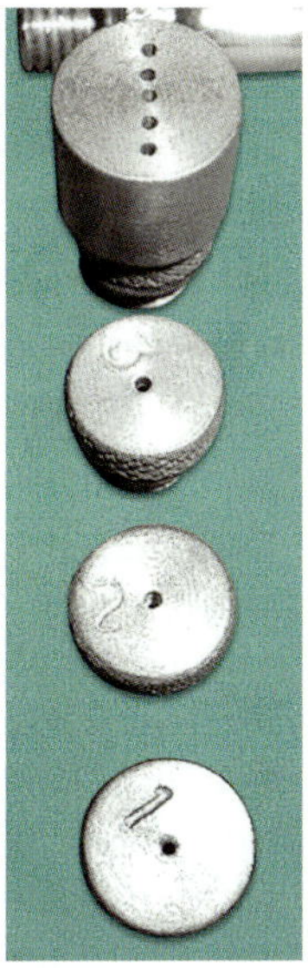

Fig. 4: Nozzle sizes available for precise spraying.

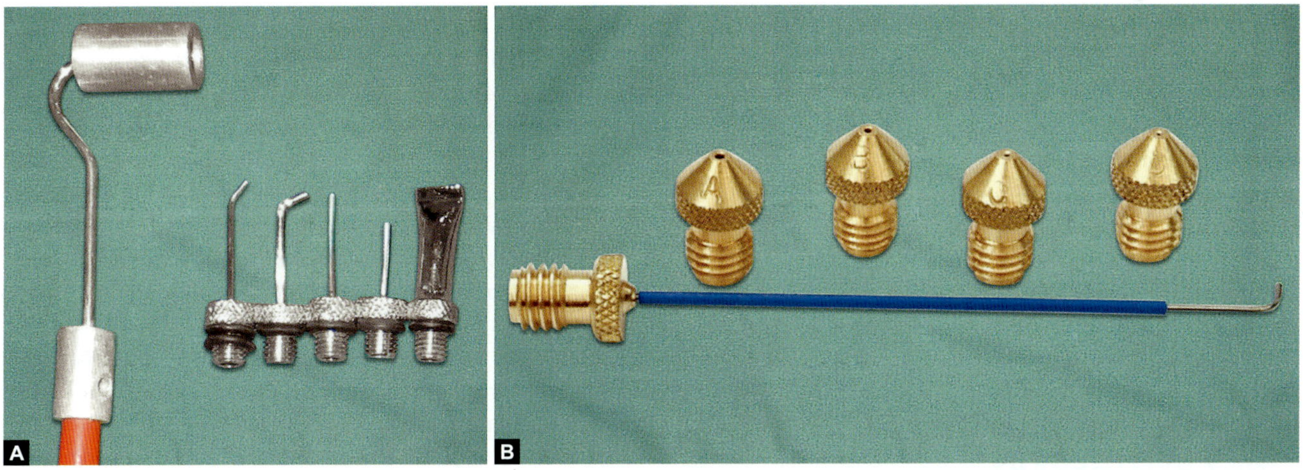

Figs. 5A and B: (A) Various nozzles and adaptors available for cryotherapy; (B) Brymill nozzles.

liquid nitrogen evaporates with time. The size of the tank determines how long it can contain the cryogen; usually a tank of 7–10 liters will hold liquid nitrogen for a week to 10 days before complete evaporation, but a 35-liters tank can hold for almost 100–120 days **(Fig. 6)**. The cryogen is transferred to the cryogun before the procedure by a siphon provided with the tank or by tilting the container to pour the cryogen into the gun via a funnel. Care must be taken by the operator while pouring the cryogen into the canister. Insulated gloves must be worn while transferring the cryogen.

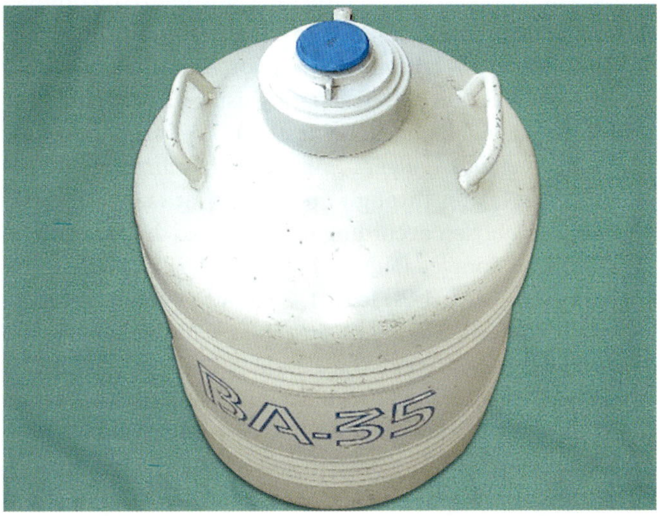

Fig. 6: Cryocan with 35 liters capacity given longer storage time for the cryogen.

CRYOTHERAPY PROTOCOL[12]

History taking and examination: A detailed history of the condition, its evolution, aggravating factors, and previous treatment history should be taken. Patients who are sensitive to cold, history of cold urticaria, and Raynaud's phenomenon or vascular insufficiency may be recorded. Physical examination taking into account the size, margin, location, depth of lesion, and history of keloidal tendencies should all be recorded.

Counseling and consent: A written informed consent is obtained from the patient after explaining the procedure, the achievable results, recurrence rate, and various complications of the procedure.

Preprocedure: Clean thoroughly with spirit or povidone iodine and prepare the area with drapes; see that it is adequately exposed. Particular areas such as the eyes must be protected with goggles, gauze, or padding. Anesthesia is not required as pain is an indicator to control the amount of cryospray. Intralesional anesthesia might be required when freezing larger lesions such as BCC or keloid. Vocal anesthesia is enough to assure the patient and minimize the discomfort.

COMMON INDICATIONS

- Idiopathic guttate hypomelanosis (IGH)
- Lentigo and freckles
- Dermatosis papulosa nigra, skin tags (acrochordons), and pedunculated lesions
- Molluscum contagiosum
- Verrucae plana, verrucae vulgaris, and plantar warts
- Seborrheic keratosis and actinic keratosis
- Cherry angioma and venous lake
- Fibromas
- Keloid
- BCC and squamous cell carcinoma (SCC).

TREATMENT MODALITIES USING CRYOTHERAPY

Various methods have been devised in the use of cryotherapy of lesions. They include the spray freeze technique, the applicator technique, and the cryoprobe method.

- *Spray freeze technique—timed freeze-thaw method:* Assess the lesion. Surgical paring using 15 or 11 blade or by curettage facilitates the destruction of certain lesions such as verrucae vulgaris. The cryogen is directly sprayed onto the lesion through an appropriate-sized nozzle, which is chosen according to the size of the lesion. The cryogen is sprayed in the center of the lesion, holding the spray tip or nozzle at least 1–2 cm away from the lesion until the desired margin is reached, which encircles the whole lesion. A freeze-thaw cycle is done by spraying for an adequate duration (holding time) after which the lesion is allowed to thaw to complete one freeze-thaw cycle. Complete thawing is suggested by the disappearance of the frozen-white surface. For larger lesions (>2 cm in diameter), treat separately with overlapping margins, covering different parts of the lesion in the same session.

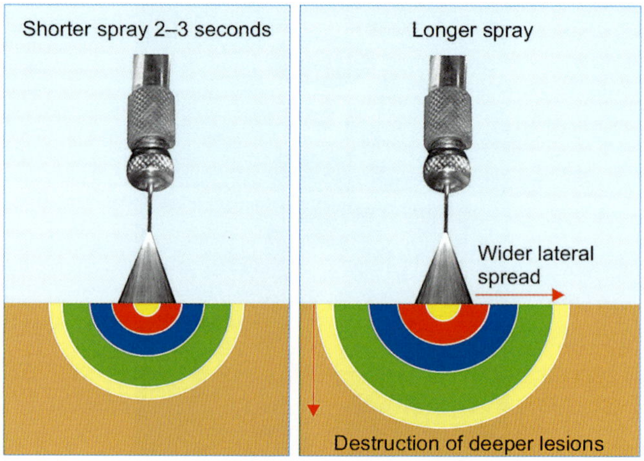

Fig. 7: Difference between shorter and longer sprays depending on lesion and depth which needs to be reached.

In case of malignant lesions, the lateral spread of freeze should extend at least 2 mm beyond the margin in a benign lesion and 5 mm or more for adequate results **(Fig. 7)**.

Freeze technique can be carried out in two ways:

1. *Open spray* **(Fig. 8)**: Used when treating larger lesions such as keloids, SCC, and BCC.
   a. *Direct-spray method:* The lesion is treated by a vertical spray technique without moving. This method is mostly used when treating well-circumscribed lesion.
   b. *Paintbrush method:* The lesion is treated by spraying from one side of the lesion and moving up and down across the lesion.
   c. *Spiral method:* The cryogen is sprayed initially in the center of the lesion and is then moved outward in concentric circles.
2. *Closed or confined spray:*[13] This technique is used in round, small, discrete lesions such as verrucae, fibroma, IGH, and cherry angiomas or those close to vital structures. For large, irregularly shaped lesions, sequential freezing is necessary. In this, the use of neoprene or polystyrene cones helps to confine the range of spray within the lesional area, preventing damage to surrounding areas.

   To concentrate the freezing and to prevent disease communication [especially in this era of conditions, such as human immunodeficiency virus (HIV) disease or hepatitis], disposable cones can be used to concentrate the liquid nitrogen. Disposable otoscope specula **(Fig. 9)**, which can be bought online, can be trimmed to make the aperture larger, or an angle can be cut to make a fusiform shape for oval lesions. Disposable specula come in a variety of sizes, ranging from 2.5 to 9 mm.[14]

   The nozzle tip of the spray gun is kept on the wide opening of the cone and the narrowed opening of the cone is kept on the lesion to be treated, and liquid nitrogen is sprayed on the lesion through the cone. The time for which the lesion is frozen is the freeze time, which is different for

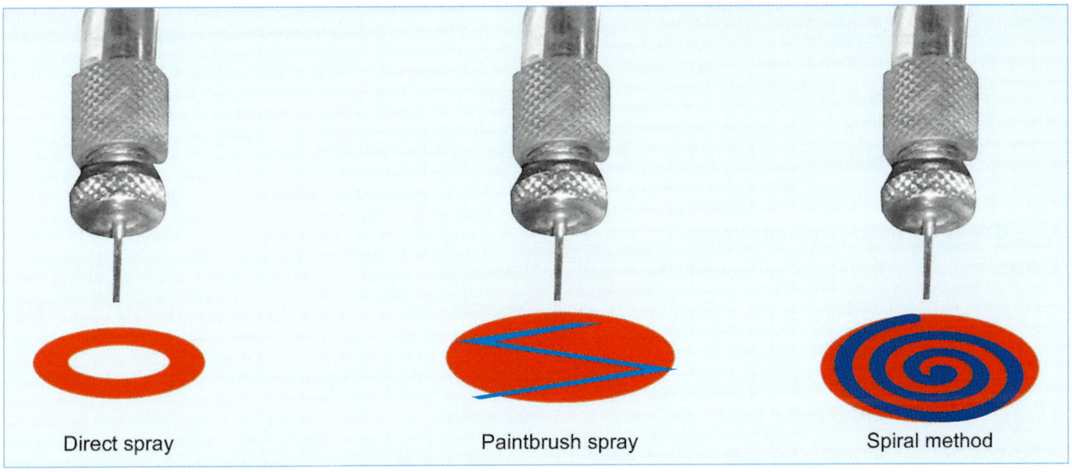

Fig. 8: Various open-spray techniques employed.

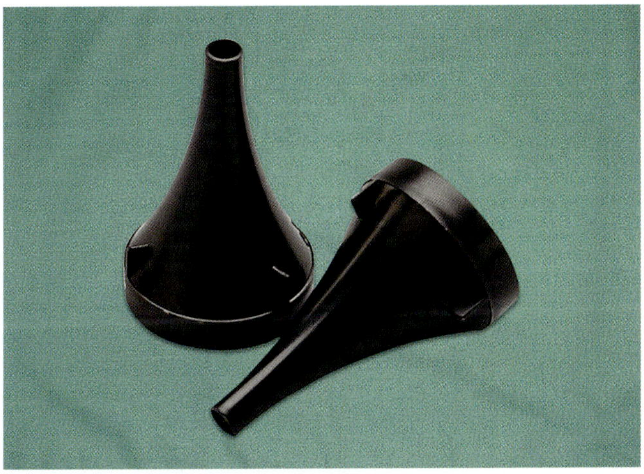

Fig. 9: Disposable otoscope specula.

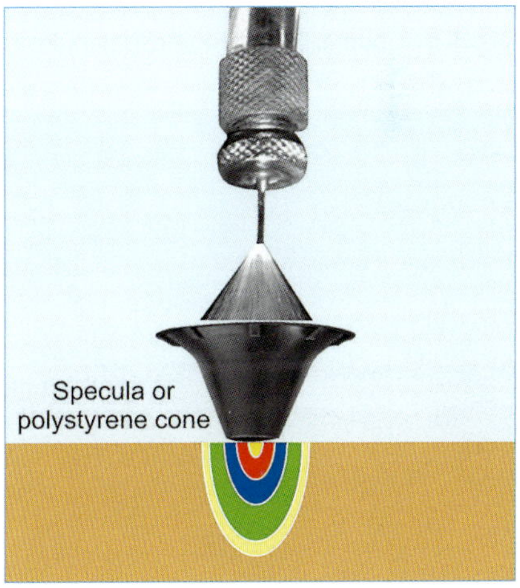

Fig. 10: Confined spray technique is used to prevent lateral spread.

different lesions. This freeze–thaw cycle can be repeated, depending on the type of lesion being treated **(Fig. 10)**.
Tip: The use of autoclavable cones, available with the microdermabrasion equipment, can be a good substitute.

- *Dipstick applicator method:*[15] This method is the original method used to apply liquid nitrogen to lesions. A cotton-tipped applicator is dipped into liquid nitrogen. The dipstick applicator is then firmly pressed against the lesion, delivering the cryo for the desired duration **(Fig. 11)**.

  The size of the bud should be smaller than the lesion. The depth of freeze can be increased by applying pressure on the lesion. Lower temperatures cannot be achieved in the dipstick applicator method as they are in the spray technique; therefore, this method is suitable only for benign and superficial lesions, e.g., freckles, verrucae plana, and IGH **(Table 2)**.
- *Forceps technique:*[16] The use of forceps or straight artery forceps to dip into liquid nitrogen and then clamp the lesion for 15 seconds will effectively deliver the cryo to achieve the temperature needed for the destruction of the treated lesion. Brymill has special cryo tweezers for the effective delivery of the cryogen **(Fig. 12A)**. It can be repeated twice for larger lesions. This technique is used mostly in pedunculated lesions.

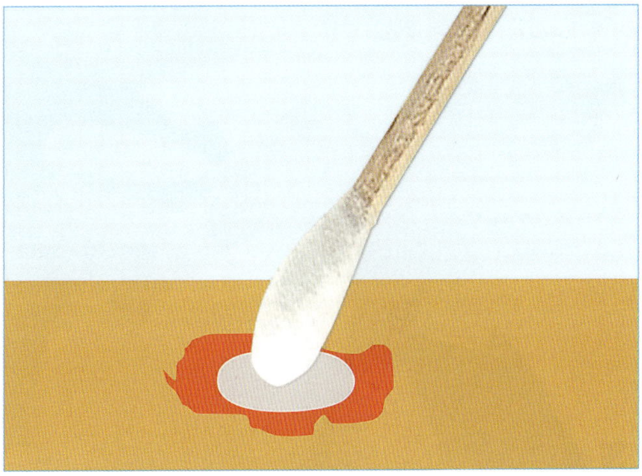

Fig. 11: Cotton-tipped applicator method.

TABLE 2: Common dermatological conditions in a dermatosurgery clinic where cryotherapy will be useful.

Dermatological conditions	*Techniques used*	*Freeze time*	*FT cycle*	*Number of sessions*
Verrucae plana and verrucae filiformis in mucosa	Dipstick	3–5 seconds	1–2	1–2
Verrucae filiformis	Forceps	5–6 seconds	1–2	1–2
Verrucae vulgaris	Cone-assisted spray	5–10 seconds, depending on size	2–3	2
Verrucae in palms and soles	Targeted cryotherapy	5–10 seconds, depending on size	2–3	2–3
Condyloma acuminata	Open-paint spray method	5–10 seconds	1–2	2–3
IGH	Dipstick	3–5 seconds	1	1–2
DPN	Dipstick	3–5 seconds	1	1–2
Cherry angioma	Cone-assisted spray	5–10 seconds, depending on size	1–2	1–2
Pedunculated lesions	Forceps/open spray	5–10 seconds	1–2	1–2
Keloids and large lesions	Targeted cryotherapy, paint-spray method, and intralesional	5–15 seconds, depending on method employed	3–5	4–6
BCC, superficial SCC, and Bowen's disease	Paint-spray method 5 mm beyond the margin in case of BCC	20–30 seconds	2–3	2–3

(BCC: basal cell carcinoma; DPN: dermatosis papulosa nigra; FT: freeze thaw; IGH: idiopathic guttate hypomelanosis; SCC: squamous cell carcinoma)

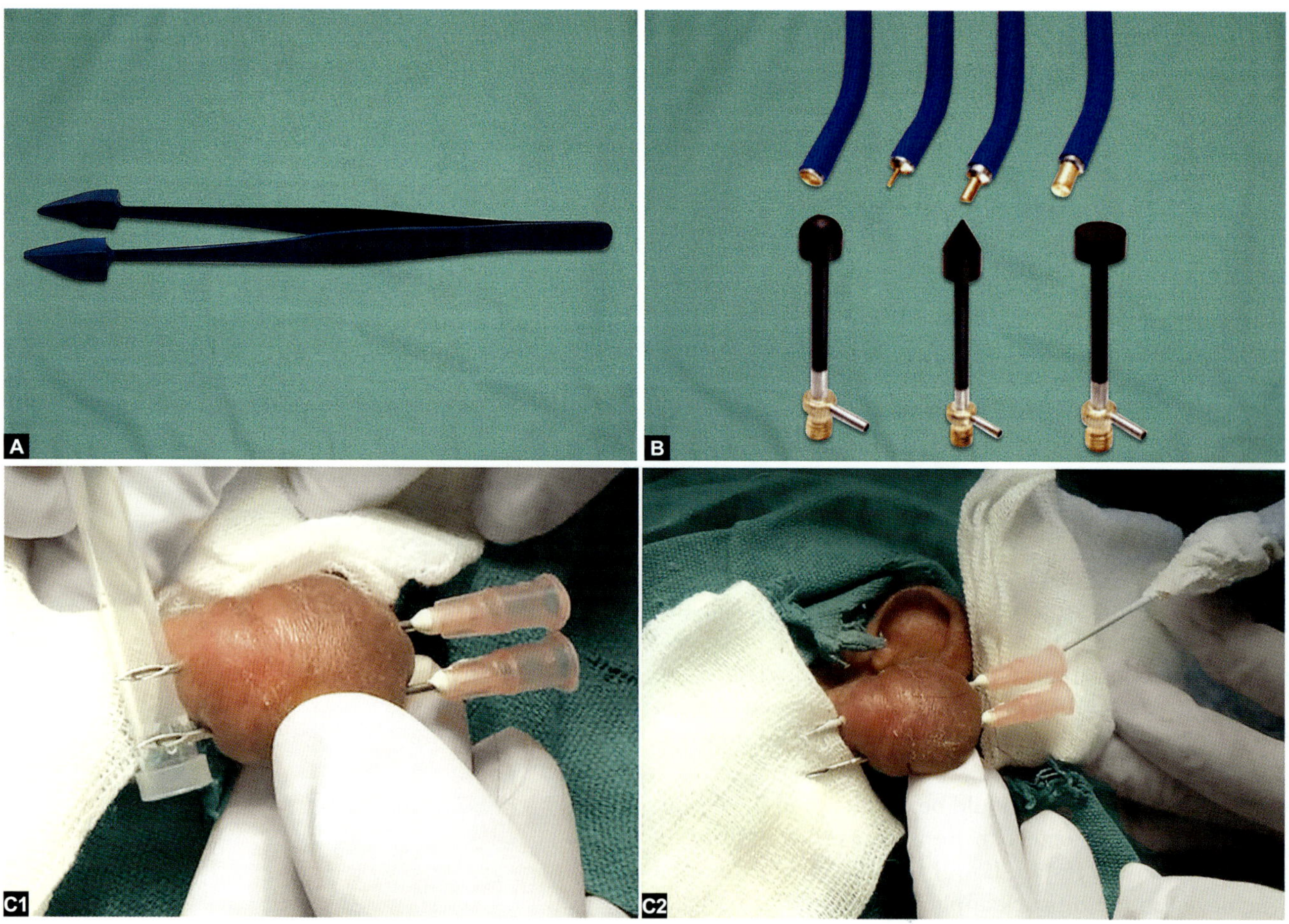

Figs. 12A to C: Forceps/special tweezers from Brymill.
Courtesy: Dr Kusuma MR.

- *Cryoprobe technique:* Manufacturers of cryo equipment have devised various metal attachments to serve as heat-conducting probes for cryotherapy. Copper, because of its high conductivity, is typically used **(Fig. 12B)**.

A thin film of white petrolatum can be applied to the treatment site, and the cryoprobe is attached to the cryogun nozzle and is firmly pressed against the lesion and the liquid nitrogen is passed.

While the cooling is occurring, the lesion gets attached to the probe, which should be raised above the surrounding normal skin by a few millimeters to prevent damage to the surrounding skin.[12] Once the lesion is frozen, it is allowed to thaw. The probe should be allowed to release spontaneously from the lesion during the thawing process and must not be pulled earlier. In this technique, a longer freezing time is required as compared to the open-spray technique. This technique is preferred in vascular lesions because direct application of the cryoprobe blanches the lesion and reduces the lesional temperature, thus increasing the depth of the freeze. Many practitioners do not use the probe because it is cumbersome and time consuming.

- *Intralesional cryotherapy:* This technique is used when treating larger lesions such as keloids. After obtaining adequate local anesthesia of the surgical site, the probe or large bore needle is inserted into the keloid scar by a gradual twisting motion until it penetrates the opposite end **(Fig. 12C)**. A liquid nitrogen source is attached to the proximal end of the probe or needle and the gas is passed through the needle until the keloid is sufficiently frozen by visual inspection, which typically takes 10–60 minutes, depending on the scar volume. After allowing the scar to thaw for approximately 60 seconds, the probe is gently removed, and the surgical site is dressed with an antibiotic ointment and sterile gauze.

INNOVATION IN CRYOTHERAPY

Use of Microdermabrasion Tips as a Substitute for Specula

Various nozzle sizes are available in the microderm tips **(Fig. 13)**. First, the size of the lesion is determined. In case of plantar warts, surgical paring of the wart helps to determine the actual size of the wart. The microderm tip is kept and firmly pressed against the lesion and the liquid nitrogen is sprayed into it with the use of the canister. Depending on the lesion, the freeze time is undertaken with two or three freeze–thaw cycles. The tip gets frozen and is attached to the lesion; wait till it falls off on its own. This is repeated for the other lesions **(Figs. 14 to 17)**. The cones are easily autoclavable, making it a good alternative to disposable cones.

Modification in the Treatment of Pedunculated Lesions

Freezing the pedicle rather than the whole lesion helps in lesser pain and faster healing **(Figs. 18A and B)**. In case the whole pedunculated lesions need to be done, use a toothed forceps and pull the lesion away from the normal skin and spray. This prevents unwanted exposure of normal skin to the cryogen leading to ulceration and longer healing time **(Figs. 19A and B)**.

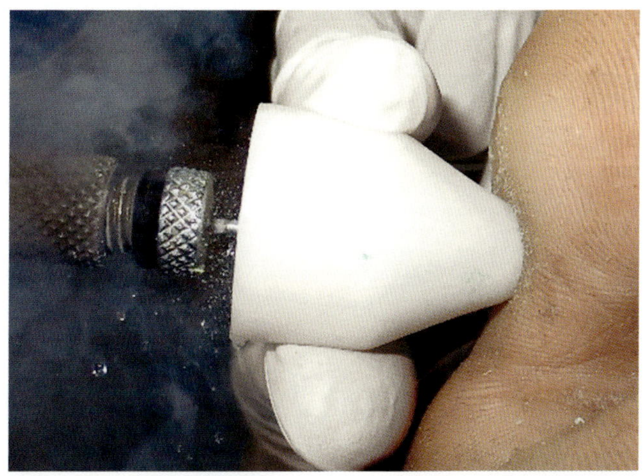

Fig. 14: Cryo is sprayed through the cone after paring of the wart and determining the diameter of lesion.

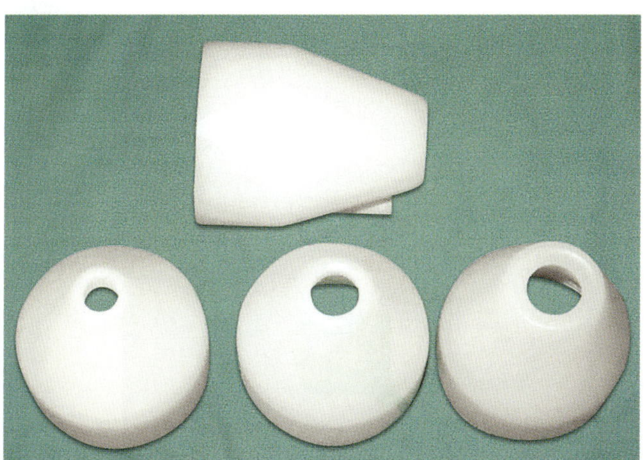

Fig. 13: Various sizes of microderm tips.

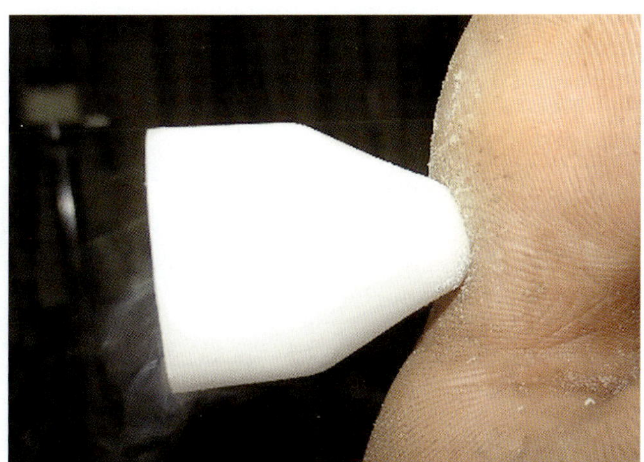

Fig. 15: The cone stays in place till complete thawing; note that there is no lateral spread beyond the margins of the cone.

Targeted Cryotherapy

An innovative technique devised by the author using biopsy punches ensures deeper delivery of cryo compared to the plastic cone method.

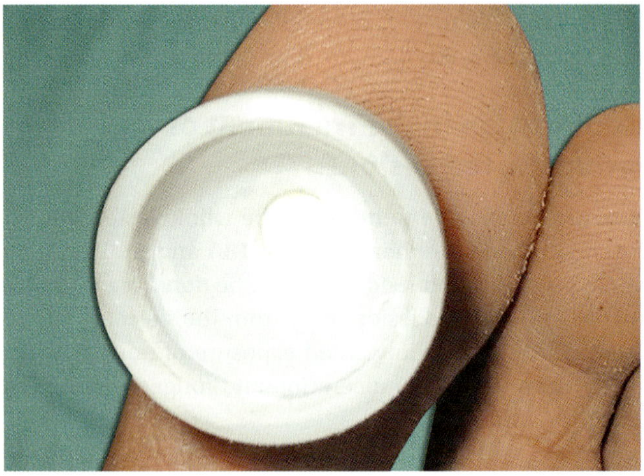

Fig. 16: The vertical look of the cone frozen with the lesion.

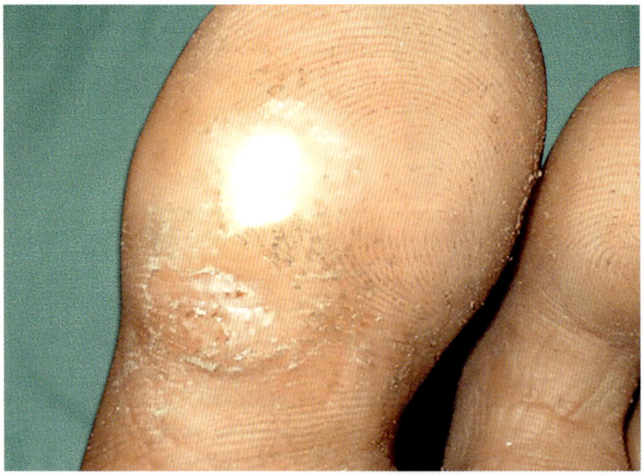

Fig. 17: Thawing of the lesion with very minimal lateral spread.

The metal cutting edge of the punch enters deeper into the lesions as the cryo is passed, sparing damage to surrounding skin.

What is unique about the use of punches is that it not only prevents lateral spread but as the cryo passes through the punch the punch starts to sink into the lesion delivering the cryo to deeper parts of the lesion, which is not possible with any other method.

Instruments

- Punches of different sizes cut to half their length **(Fig. 20)**
- Test-tube holder **(Fig. 21)**
- Cryo spray can and liquid nitrogen
- Gauze
- Surgical blade 15 with blade holder for paring in case of warts.

Procedure

In case of verrucae, paring is done to reduce the thickness of the lesion and determine the size of lesion, which in turn helps in deciding the size of punch which needs to be used. For all other cryo-treatable conditions, paring is not done. The punch is cut to half the length, the plastic part is covered with gauze, and a test-tube holder is used to grip it in case of smaller punches **(Figs. 22 and 23)**. Holding the punch with the fingers when cryo is being passed is not possible, it is very painful and can cause blisters in the fingers of the person performing the procedure.

The punch is kept on the lesion with slight pressure on the lesion so that there is no gap between the punch metal tip and the skin. If gap is present, then the cryo would seep into the normal skin, which would defeat the purpose of using the punch **(Fig. 24)**.

The cryocan filled with liquid nitrogen is used; the nozzle is kept on the top end of the punch. Note that when you cut the punch, make it smooth and flat so that the

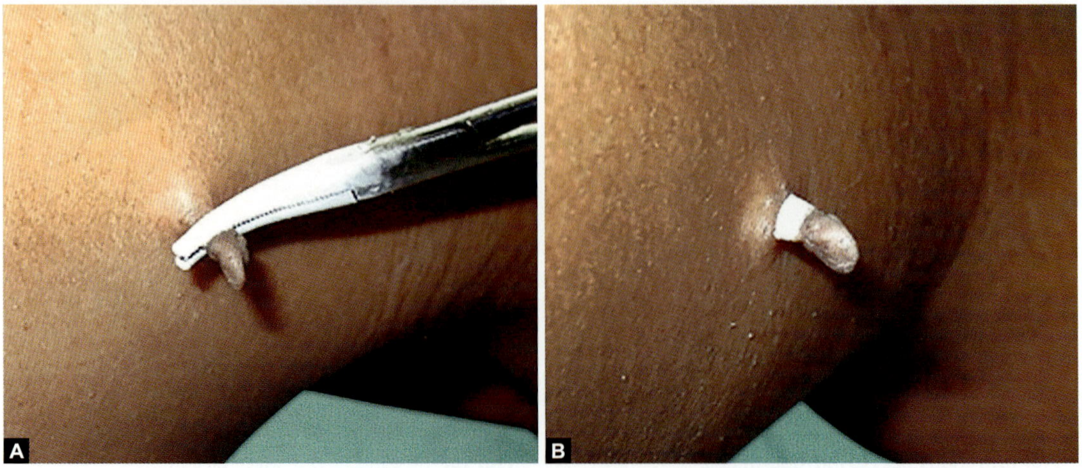

Figs. 18A and B: Only the pedicle of the lesion is clamped with the forceps.

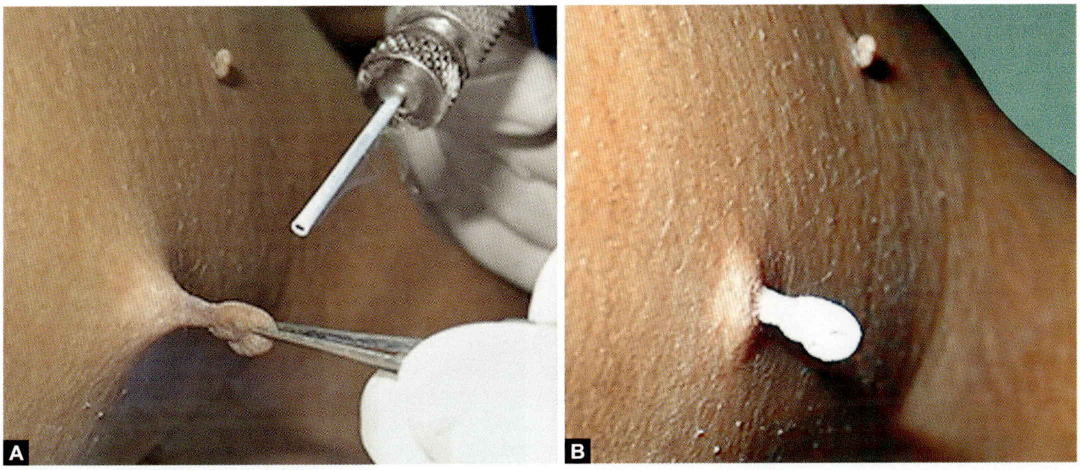

Figs. 19A and B: The lesion is pulled and the body of the lesion is sprayed leaving the base of the pedicle free from cryo damage.

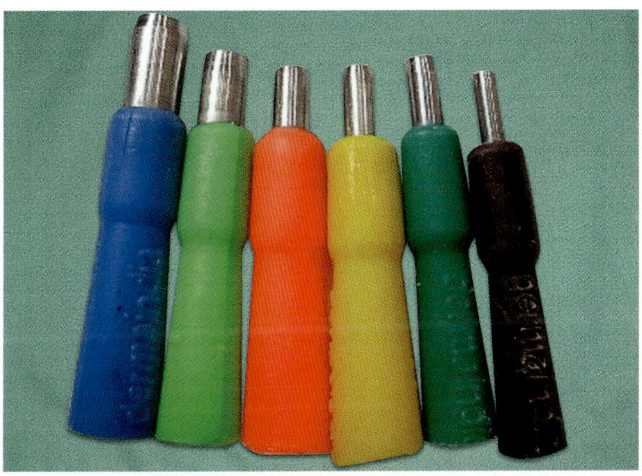

Fig. 20: Different sized punches are cut to half.

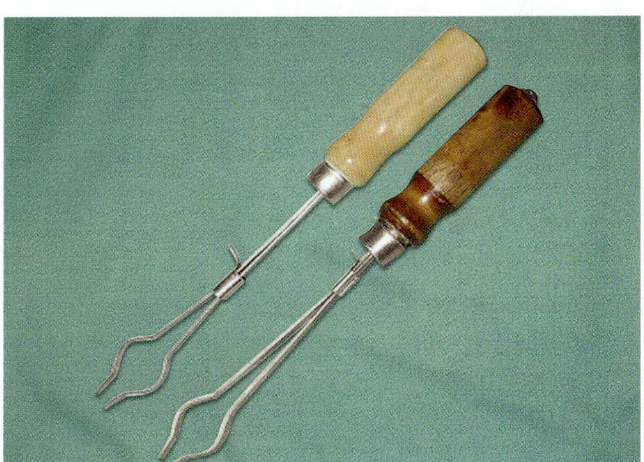

Fig. 21: Test-tube holder.

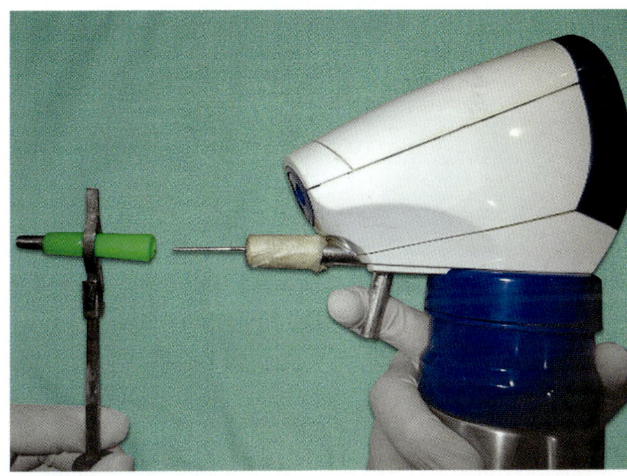

Fig. 22: Positioning of the cryo probe tip with the prepared punch.

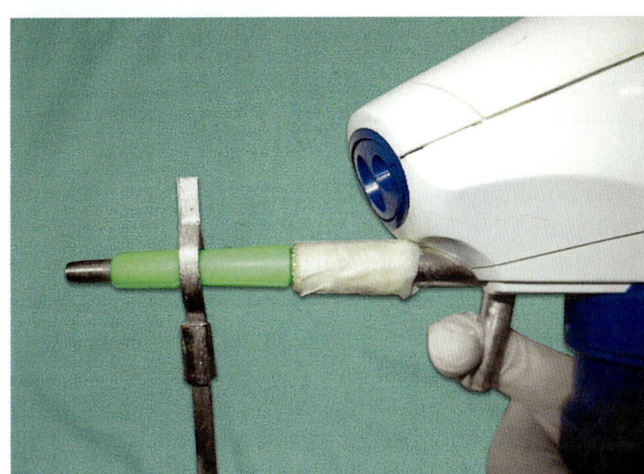

Fig. 23: Insertion of the cryo probe tip into the punch.

nozzle sits perfectly on it. The liquid nitrogen is passed and as the cryo touches the lesion through the punch, the metal tip of the punch also gets cooled, which starts to enter slowly, sinking into the lesion. Cryo is done till the beveled edge of the punch enters the skin in case of warts, since we need to reach up to the basal layer, whereas in other conditions, deeper cryo is needed. This helps in deeper delivery of the cryo and effective damage to the unwanted tissue. The punch need not be rotated to cut into the lesion, rather the effect of cooling itself makes the punch cold, cut into the lesion.

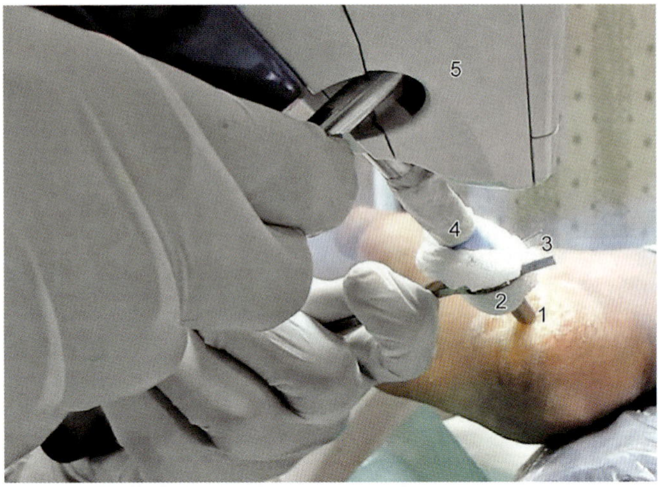

Fig. 24: The procedure being performed: 1. Metal tip of the punch in contact with the skin; 2. Gauze surrounding the punch for grip; 3. Test-tube holder to hold the punch firmly; 4. The nozzle of cryocan kept onto the top of the punch; 5. Cryocan.

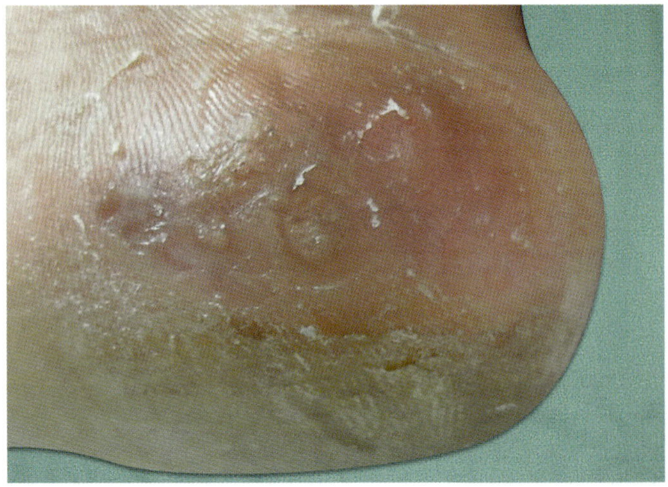

Fig. 26: Before cryo paring done.

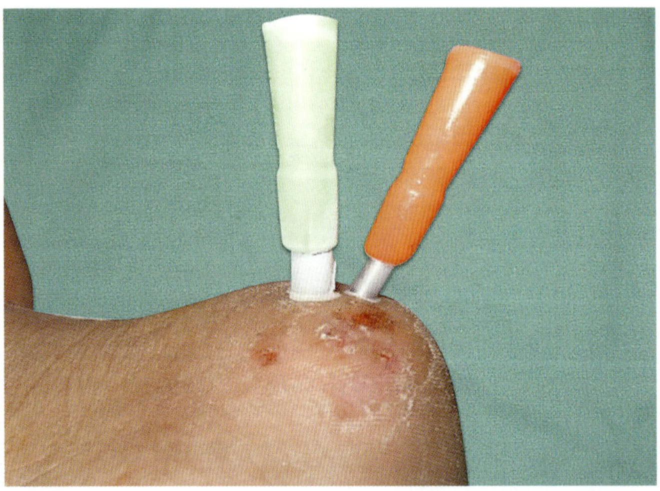

Fig. 25: The punches remain embedded; note the cryo surrounding the punch is minimal. Two punches are placed one beside the other.

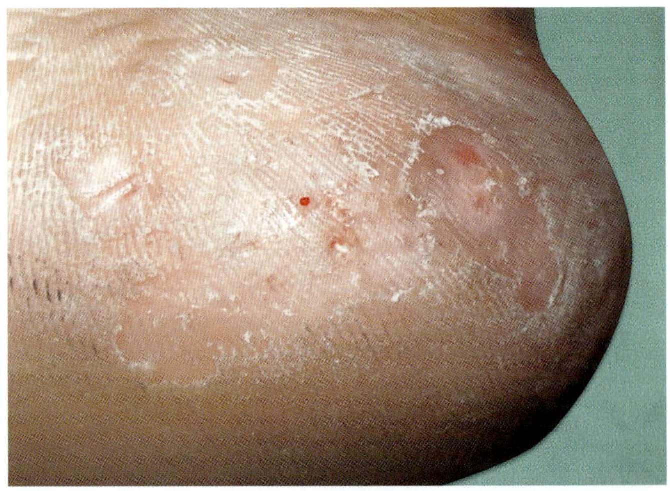

Fig. 27: 3 weeks after cryo, paring was done, revealing good clearance.

The punches remain embedded after the cryo **(Fig. 25)** and they are left to fall off on their own. The punches fall off in 10–20 seconds depending on the depth reached. The next punch can be placed adjacent to warts and the process is repeated. Depending on the lesions, the procedure can be performed two or three times on the same lesion.

The procedure is repeated after 3 weeks. Paring is done again before the next session of cryo to assess if there is any wart tissue remaining and this time smaller punches are used to treat **(Figs. 26 and 27)**.

Normally, if the depth has to be achieved, for example, in keloids,[17] the spray of cryo is done on a larger area surrounding the lesion and with longer duration of spray, but this results in severe collateral damage to normal skin, resulting in large blisters and pain. But with this method, the cryo can be sprayed longer, with no damage to surrounding normal tissue. This technique is useful even in larger lesions, such as keloids, where it can be sprayed into multiple areas but lessening the pain and damage to the tissue.

Indications in which targeted cryotherapy is used:

- Verrucae on plantar and palmar areas
- Dermatofibroma
- Pyogenic granuloma
- Keloid and hypertrophic scars
- Naevi

Advantages of targeted cryotherapy:

- Targeted damage to the unwanted tissue, sparing collateral damage to the surrounding skin
- Reduce the blistering reaction
- Lower incidence of hemorrhagic blisters
- Comparatively less pain due to reduction in area traumatized

- Deeper delivery of the cryo is possible by use of punches, which slides deeper into the lesions as the cryo is being performed.
- As the cryo reaches the depth, it loses optimal temperature in normal cryotherapy method, which is eliminated with this novel method.
- The chances of recurrence are much lesser as compared to normal cryotherapy technique because of the deeper delivery of cryotherapy to the lesion.

CASE SCENARIO

Case 1 (Figs. 28A to D)

A patient had visited a surgeon for a growth on the fifth toe of the left foot. The surgeon had excised the lesion, which turned out to be verrucae. But there was considerable damage to the periosteum of the distal phalange and reoccurrence of the verrucous lesion. On examination, it was diagnosed as verrucae, but a biopsy was sent to rule out any malignant change. As the biopsy report confirmed the diagnosis of verrucae vulgaris, cryotherapy was done using the spiral open-spray method. The patient improved after five sessions of cryo every 4 weeks. Once there was no evidence of verrucae, the patient was sent to an orthopedician because there was exposed, damaged periosteum.

Case 2 (Figs. 29A and B)

A 28-year-old male presented with verrucae filiformis of the glans penis since 6 months.

Cryotherapy was initiated after relevant blood tests. The dipstick method was employed in this case; three sessions of cryo were done once in 3 weeks. Complete clearance was seen.

It is best to treat mucosal lesions using the dipstick method because the freezing is quicker and prevents unwanted damage to normal mucosa (which can happen when using spray technique, which might lead to delayed healing).

Postprocedure Advice

The patient should be informed about the immediate skin reactions, which can follow after the procedure. 30 minutes post procedure, there is minimal perilesional erythema followed by edema setting in within a few minutes to few hours. Blister formation commonly occurs within 1–3 days, followed by crusting that lasts for up to 2 weeks. The crust falls off, leaving behind mild pinkish discoloration or erythematous atrophic scar. No dressing is required. Painkillers and anti-inflammatory drugs can be prescribed. In case if blisters occur (minimal chances), the fluid collected can be expressed out with a needle or syringe, leaving the blister roof intact as it is a natural dressing and prevents secondary infection.

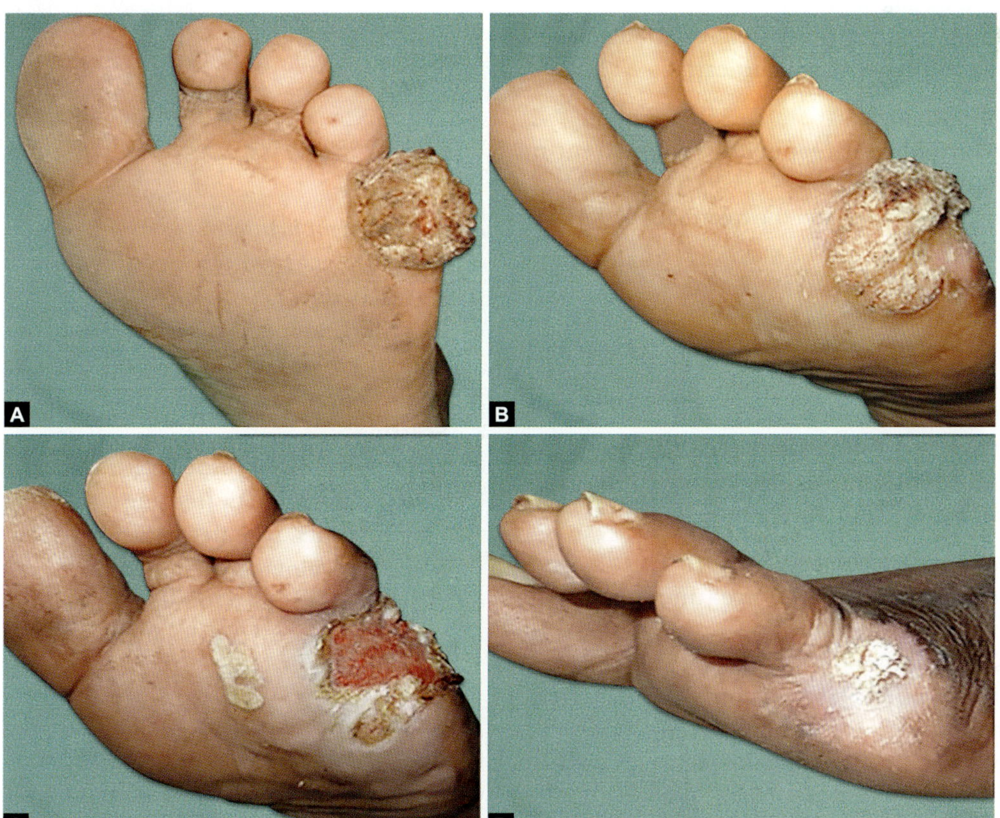

Figs. 28A to D: Treatment of large verrucae vulgaris.

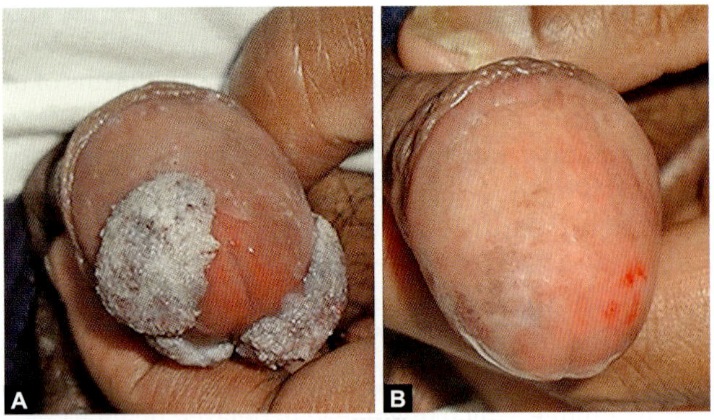

Figs. 29A and B: Treatment of verrucae filiformis on mucosal/glans penis.

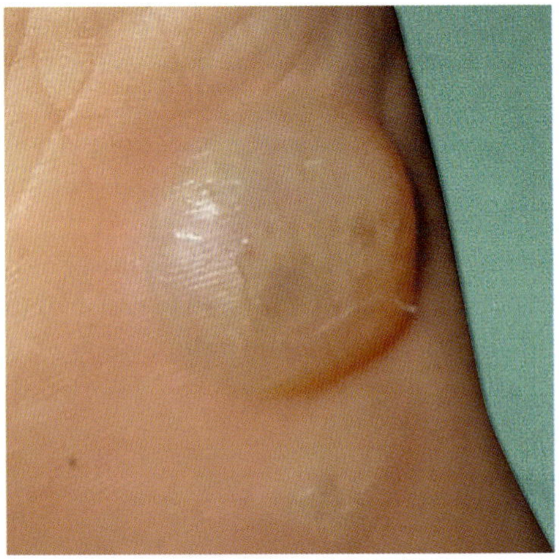

Fig. 30: Complication with cryoblister.

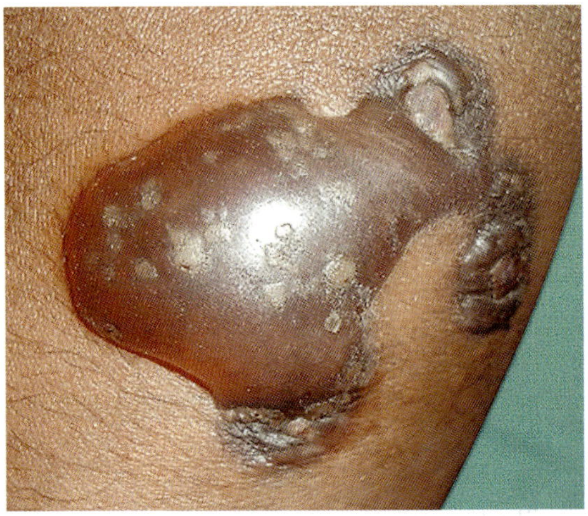

Fig. 31: Complication with hemorrhagic blister and necrosis.

COMPLICATIONS OF CRYOTHERAPY

There are common complications which are part of the treatment and there are complications associated with inappropriate patient selection, duration of freezing, and number of freeze-thaw cycles undertaken.[12,18,19]

Immediate complications:

- Local pain—more in the periungual area and when treating the face
- Edema, especially on the eyelids, lips, labia, and prepuce, more in infants and the elderly
- Syncope (vasovagal shock) in anxious patients, a very common occurrence in the OT, which the operator and assistant should be able to handle
- Urticaria, like wheals, can occur in few patients, which should not be confused with cold urticaria.

Temporary complications:

- Tingling and numbness, especially when treating verrucae on the fingers
- Headache (migraine-type) after the treatment of the head and neck area
- Cryoblister formation **(Fig. 30)**
- Hemorrhagic necrosis **(Fig. 31)**
- Subcutaneous emphysema—a rare complication seen in older patients with compromised skin or in patients with broken skin. Seen when treating venous lakes in the lip. It can follow intralesional cryotherapy when needles are used into the lesions such as keloids for deep cryotherapy.[20]

Prolonged temporary complications:

- Delayed wound healing after treatment over the extremities
- Temporary scar hypertrophy
- Excessive granulation tissue formation
- Milia formation
- Local hypoesthesia due to nerve damage, especially in areas where the nerves lie superficially, such as the sides of fingers, angle of jaw, postauricular area, sides of tongue, and ulnar fossa of elbow

Permanent complications:

- Atrophic scar, which occurs when freezing time is >30 seconds
- Cicatricial alopecia, when treating lesions in the scalp and when longer duration of freeze time in excess of 30 seconds is employed
- Scarring
- Hypopigmentation, especially in dark-skinned individuals, can be minimized by freezing for less than 30 seconds. In case it occurs, psoralen plus ultraviolet A (PUVA) soaks helps in regaining the pigmentation
- Damage to periosteum when treating lesions on bony prominences like the distal digits, mandible with longer freeze times.

Uncommon complications:

- Cartilage damage
- Pseudotumor recidiva
- Fibroxanthoma
- Traumatic neuroma.

CONTRAINDICATIONS TO CRYOTHERAPY

Absolute:
- Raynaud's disease
- Cold urticaria
- Cryoglobulinemia
- Cold intolerance
- Lesions in which tissue pathology is required before cryosurgery such as actinic/seborrheic keratosis, BCC, and SCC
- Lesions in areas of compromised circulation
- Skin tumors located in high-risk areas such as the temple or nasolabial folds.

Relative:
- Keloidal tendency
- Collagen vascular diseases
- Pyoderma gangrenosum
- Dark-skinned individuals due to the high risk of developing cosmetically inacceptable protracted hypopigmentation
- *Impaired sensation:* Patients cannot report when they become anesthetic from cold
- *Impaired circulation:* Tissue damage may result from vasoconstriction.
- Lesions over the nasolabial fold, eyelid margins, ala nasi, and hair-bearing areas (high risk of developing alopecia, especially cicatricial alopecia)
- Melanoma
- *Cardiac conditions:* Angina pectoris, arrhythmia, myocardial infarction (MI): For 6 months after MI, cryotherapy should be avoided. The initial shock of the ice application may cause a marked drop in blood pressure, thus causing an increase in heart attack rate.

NEWER ADVANCES

Thermosensors to monitor adequate freezing: A freezing tissue should be monitored to supplement clinical judgment and to standardize the procedure. Special thermosensors are attached to the delivery system to give accurate measure of the temperature at the target tissue **(Fig. 32)**. This negates the need of additional separate temperature-measuring devices to monitor the temperature.

Fractional cryotherapy: It is a technique described by Gupta et al. to reduce the complication rates and expand its indications. They employed the use of a thin plywood or transparent plastic plates, which are poor conductors of heat **(Fig. 33)**. Multiple uniform holes are made at specific distances using a drill machine. Depending on the site and indication for which fractionated cryosurgery has been planned for, the size and distance between holes can be customized. Larger holes template for the conditions which require aggressive treatment in conditions such as keloids and smaller holes template for cryoslush and rejuvenation.

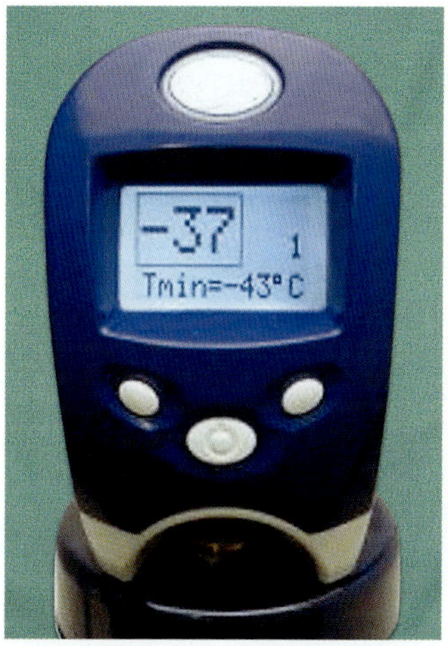

Fig. 32: Thermosensors to monitor adequate freezing.

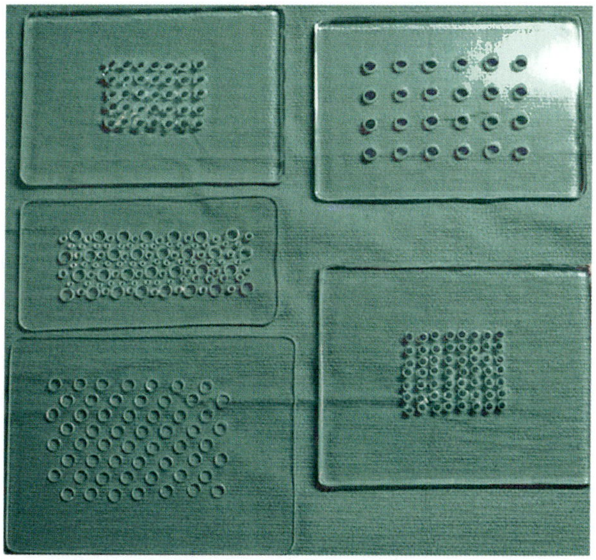

Fig. 33: Multiple transparent fractionated plastic plates.

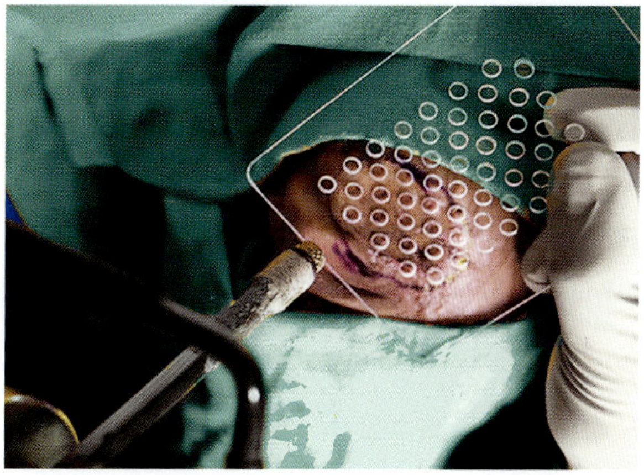

Fig. 34: Liquid nitrogen sprayed over the fractionated plate.

The plate is placed close to the skin and the liquid nitrogen is spared in spiral or painting fashion, covering the area which requires treatment **(Fig. 34)**. The time of freezing is slightly

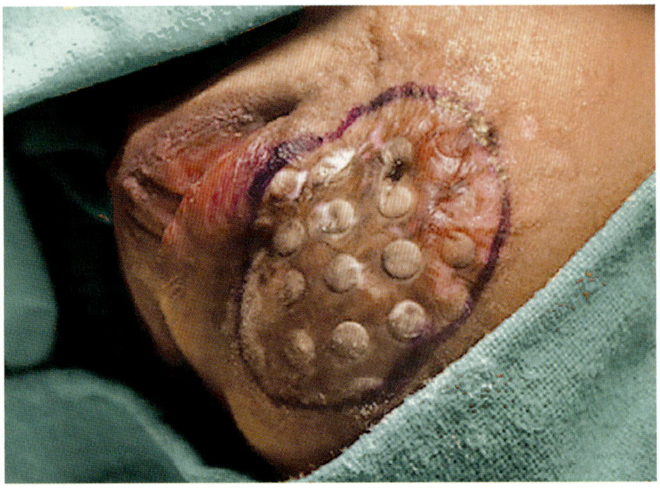

Fig. 35: Skin with frozen areas in a grid pattern with spared normal skin.

longer than conventional method. The conditions such as keloids require two to three freeze–thaw cycles of 30 seconds, with reposition if the lesion is nonuniform. Facial scars require one or two freeze–thaw cycles of 10–15 seconds **(Fig. 35)**.

The pain during procedure is much less compared to conventional uniform freezing. Multiple freeze–thaw cycles can be safely done in a single session and can be repeated at frequent intervals. For curved surfaces, special moldable plastic material is shaped according to the target tissue. Transparent plastic templates allow better visualization of the area to be treated under the template. Fractionating has the potential to expand the indications for cryotherapy in aesthetics and rejuvenation.[21]

CONCLUSION

Cryotherapy is a simple, safe, cost-effective office procedure for the treatment of various skin conditions where cryotherapy can give a cosmetically acceptable outcome even in benign, premalignant and well-circumscribed malignant tumors. It has minimal complications which can prevented or treated. Its important that care must be taken in patient selection and indication. Ideally should be performed only by a trained and experienced dermatologist or assistant.

REFERENCES

1. White AC. Liquid air: Its application in medicine and surgery. Med Rec. 1899;56:109-12.
2. Allington HV. Liquid Nitrogen in treatment of Skin Diseases. Calif Med. 1950;72:153-5.
3. Cooper IS, Lee AS. Cryostatic congelation: a system for producing a limited, controlled region of cooling or freezing of biologic tissues. J Nerv Ment Dis. 1961;133:259-63.
4. Freiman A, Bouganim N. History of cryotherapy. Dermatol Online J. 2005;11(2):9.
5. Menesi W, Buchel EW, Hayakawa TJ. A reliable frozen section technique for basal cell carcinomas of the head and neck. Can J Plast Surg. 2014;22(3):179-82.
6. Kuflik EG, Gage AA. The five-year cure rate achieved by cryosurgery for skin cancer. J Am Acad Dermatol. 1991;24 (6 Pt 1):1002-4.
7. Guan H, Zhao Z, He F, Zhou Q, Meng Q, Zhu X, et al. The effects of different thawing temperatures on morphology and collagen metabolism of -20 degrees C dealt normal human fibroblast. Cryobiology. 2007;55(1):52-9.
8. van Leeuwen MC, Bulstra AE, van Leeuwen PA, Niessen FB. A new argon gas-based device for the treatment of keloid scars with the use of intralesional cryotherapy. J Plast Reconstr Aesthet Surg. 2014;67(12):1703-10.
9. Drake LA, Ceilley RI, Cornelison RL. Guidelines for care for cryosurgery. J Am Acad Dermatol. 1994;31:648-53.
10. Kuflik EG. Cryosurgery updated. J Am Acad Dermatol. 1994;31:925-44.
11. Graham GF. Cryosurgery. Clin Plast Surg. 1993;20:131-47.
12. Sharma VK, Khandpur S. Guidelines for cryotherapy. Indian J Dermatol Venereol Leprol. 2009;75:90-100.
13. Torre D. Cryosurgical treatment of epitheliomas using the cone-spray technique. J Dermatol Surg Oncol. 1977;3(4):432-6.
14. Kuwahara RT, Rasberry RD, Amonette RA. Use of disposable otoscope specula in cryotherapy. Dermatol Surg. 2000;26(5): 493-4.
15. Orengo I, Salasche SJ. Surgical pearl: The cotton-tipped applicator—the ever-ready, multipurpose superstar. J Am Acad Dermatol. 1994;31(4):658-60.
16. Kuwahara RT, Huber JD, Ray SH. Surgical pearl: Forceps method for freezing benign lesion. J Am Acad Dermatol. 2000;43(2 Pt 1):306-7.
17. Zouboulis CC, Blume U, Buttner P, Orfanos CE. Outcomes of cryosurgery in keloids and hypertrophic scars. A prospective consecutive trial of case series. Arch Dermatol. 1993;129: 1146-51.
18. Elton RF. Complications of cutaneous cryosurgery. J Am Acad Dermatol. 1983;8:513-9.
19. Dawber RP. Cryosurgery: complications and contraindications. Clin Dermatol. 1991;8:96-100.
20. Martínez-Coronado J, Torres-Álvarez B, Castanedo-Cázares JP. Subcutaneous emphysema induced by cryotherapy: a complication due to previous punctures. Case Rep Dermatol Med. 2015:374817.
21. Gupta S, Yadav S, Patra S, Gupta S. Fractionated Cryotherapy. J Am Acad Dermatol. 2017;3:69-71.

SECTION 4 Needle-based Basic Procedures

CHAPTER 28 Microneedling

Pradeep Kumari

KEY MESSAGES

- Microneedling or percutaneous collagen induction is a technique aimed at minimal epidermal damage, creates nil lateral heat generation and provides good rejuvenation and scar reduction.
- Microneedling can be easily combined with other face rejuvenation procedures.
- Microneedling is now increasingly being used for drug penetration.

INTRODUCTION

Microneedling (MN) or percutaneous collagen induction (PCI) or dermaroller or skin needling therapy is a popular and simple skin resurfacing procedure. This minimally invasive procedure owes its popularity to producing non-confluent self-healing punctures in the skin without any surface ablation. This property of nonablative resurfacing makes it a viable, economical resurfacing option in skin of color with fewer adverse sequelae compared to other therapies.[1]

Traditionally, employed for acne scar reduction and face rejuvenation, microneedling today has widespread indications in focal diseases of inflammation, dyschromia, and photodamage, adjuvant therapy for enhanced drug delivery in the treatment of atrophic scars, alopecia, actinic keratoses, and disorders of pigmentation such as melasma and vaccines.

Repeatedly needling the skin for the purpose of improved healing by either individual needle or a bunch of needles was initially explored by many scientists. The first such attempt was made by Phillipe Simon in 1981 by performing what he labeled as "electrorhytidopuncture" by using galvanic currents and multiple needles and giving electrical stimulation for treatment of face wrinkles. The idea of creating controlled dermal injury for the purpose of regeneration in scars was tried in 1995 by doing "subcision" by Orentreich.[2] Later Desmond Fernandes developed the first MN product which became the modern-day Dermaroller® (Dermaroller Deutschland GmbH, Wolfenbüttel, Germany).

Camirand and Doucet had used a tattoo gun without any pigment—dry tattooing to treat scars when they noticed textural improvement in their tattooed scars. Desmond Fernandez later on found that dry tattooing was too superficial and cumbersome and better improvement can be achieved by causing controlled injury to reticular dermis. He designed the currently used dermaroller mounted on a rolling barrel to improve scars through neocollagenesis in 1999. Microneedling was named as per PCI as multiple micro wounds are induced in dermis which individually go through various wound healing phases and heal with new collagen and elastin regeneration along with collagen remodeling mainly in upper reticular dermis.

Later PCI was done using a 200-needle drum-shaped needling device making it faster as well as easy to do.[3]

Microneedling was reported as a valuable physical enhancer to transdermal drug delivery in 2011 by Escobar-Chavez and Bentilla Martinez.[4]

This led to usage of microneedling as an adjunct or pre-adjunct procedure in mesotherapy to deliver various growth factors, nutrients, platelet-rich plasma (PRP) therapy, cosmeceuticals and therapeutics in treatment of acne scars, rejuvenation, wrinkles, striae, alopecia, melasma, etc.

Over the years microneedling instrument has undergone various structural changes such as various barrel widths, needle lengths, detachable barrels, and addition of motor, LED light, etc.

INSTRUMENTS

Dermaroller is a handheld device and mainly there are two components **(Fig. 1)**:

1. Handle
2. Front portion having a barrel with attached needles—these needles usually are arranged on a cylindrical roller for easy movement or a static head which is spring loaded.

These devices can be operated manually, motorized as well as can have radiofrequency energy coupled with needle puncture/rolling. Static stamp type needling devices are more useful for localized scar.[5]

The standard medical dermaroller usually has a 12-cm handle with a 2 × 2 cm wide drum-shaped cylinder at one end.

A total of 192 stainless steel solid needles are inserted in eight rows with each row having 24 fine microneedles, the needle length can vary from 0.5 to 3 mm in length and 0.1 to 0.25 mm in diameter. This is a single use instrument sterilized by gamma ray irradiation. The needles are synthesized by reactive ion etching techniques on silicon or medical grade stainless steel. Rolling of this drum on skin leads to each needle penetrating the skin at angle, going through epidermis, deep into dermis (depth varying from 0.3 to 2.3 mm, corresponding to needle length of 0.5–2.5 mm) and finally gets extracted at a converse angle. Therefore, the tract formed by needle is straight, linear but vertically angulated conical microchannel. The tip is sharp and needles have a smooth circumference, the created microchannel is cylindrical cone with narrowing at its deeper end. During the process of rolling, skin gripping the needle temporarily curves and then snaps back into its resting position. This curving and snapping back can lead to entangles skin with poor quality equipment, too much pressure and/or blunt needles and can lead to scar worsening.[6]

Each pass produces 16 micropunctures in the stratum corneum per square centimeter without damaging the epidermis significantly.[7]

Rolling with a standard dermaroller containing 192 needles of 2 mm length and 0.07 mm diameter over an area of skin for 15 times results in approximately 250 holes/cm^2 up to the papillary dermis depending on the pressure applied.[8]

Five basic types of medical dermarollers, which are registered with the Food and Drug Administration (FDA), have been described in the dermaroller series by Anastassakis Konstantinos, and most dermarolling devices are adopted from these elementary types:[9,10]

1. C-8 (cosmetic type) is the basic dermaroller, has needle length 0.13 mm (130 µm). Mostly used for better penetration of topical agents. It is completely painless. These are homecare dermarollers. These can be used 2–3 times a week and a single dermaroller can be used up to 100 times. Postusage they should be washed in hot water and dried.

   Beauty mouse is a similar approved device intended for home use. Beauty mouse has 480 needles of 0.2 mm size placed on three drums inside a computer mouse shaped easy to hold device. This shape makes it easy to be used at home for application on large body areas such as arms, legs, and buttocks for treating cellulite and stretch marks.[11]
2. C-8HE (Cosmetic type for hair bearing surfaces, scalp) has a needle length of 0.2 mm (200 µm). Even this length is below the pain threshold.
3. CIT-8 (CIT: Collagen Induction Therapy, Medical type) has a needle length of 0.5 mm (500 µm) and helps in collagen induction and skin remodeling.
4. MF-8 type has a needle length of 1.5 mm (1,500 µm). This creates deeper microchannels on the whole epidermis and dermis and at the same time destroys scar collagen bundles.
5. MS-4 has a smaller cylinder, 1 cm length, 2 cm diameter, and only 4 circular arrays of needles (total 96 needles) that have 1.5 mm length. It is used on areas where better precision and deeper penetration are required. It is mostly used on facial acne scars. Devices similar to MS-4 are available with needle lengths of 0.5–0.75 mm, which are used for thin-skinned areas such as the periorbital and perioral regions.

VARIANTS OF DERMAROLLER

- *Dermastamp:* It is a miniature version of dermaroller and can be used for small isolated scars. The penetration of needles is vertical compared to dermaroller where needles enter skin at an angle. These are also available in different needle lengths (0.2–3 mm) and a diameter of 0.12 mm. This can be used for localized scars such as varicella scars.
- *Dermapen **(Fig. 2)**:* A spring-loaded MN device that is electricity powered and has a disposable needle cartridge

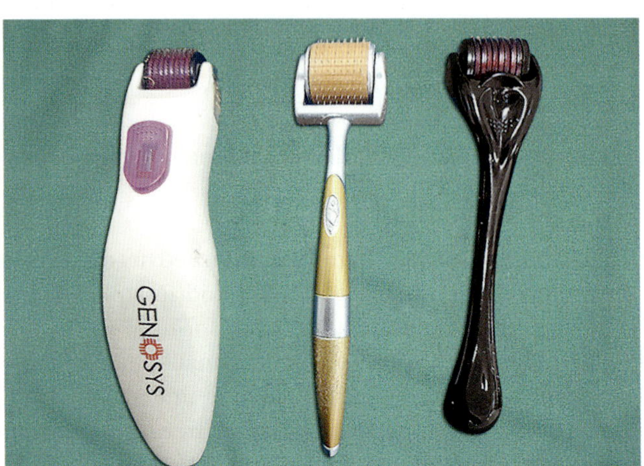

Fig. 1: Dermaroller instruments.
Courtesy: Horst Liebl, CEO Dermaroller Sarl, GmbH, Germany.

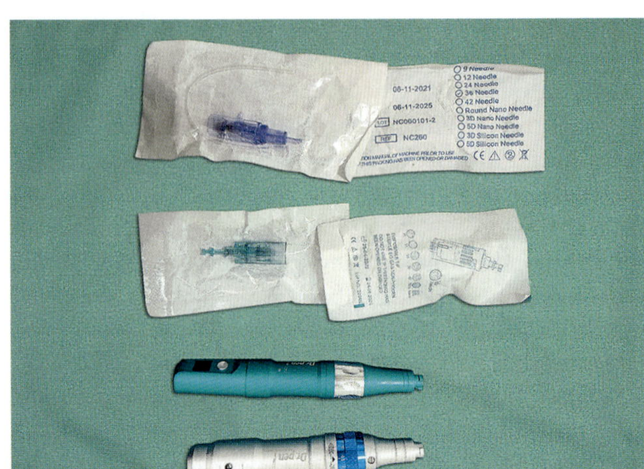

Fig. 2: Dermapen instrument.

can make the treatment faster and easier to conduct. This acts as an electrically powered pen, delivering stamp-like motions across the skin.[12]

The device is ergonomic, easy to use and needle length can be adjusted for different areas in same patient. Dermapen can operate at high-speed mode (700 cycles/min) and the low-speed mode (412 cycles/min) in a vibrating stamp-like manner. The needle tip can have 9–12 needles arranged in rows. The ease of operating in narrow areas such as nose corners, near eyes/lips, and changeability of needles makes it preferred and more economical microneedling device for many practitioners. Dermapen also overcomes the issue of varying angle of needle entry and varying depth of needle penetration based on pressure applied.

- *Dermafrac:* This treatment combines microdermabrasion, microneedling, simultaneous deep tissue serum infusion, and light emitting diode (LED) therapy. It is an instrument designed by DermaFrac™ (Genesis Biosystems, Lewisville, TX, USA) to target aging and sun-damaged skin, acne, enlarged pores, uneven skin tone, wrinkles fine lines, hyperpigmentation, and superficial scars. It is a 45-minute duration cycle for one session and takes the advantage of combining additive compatible therapies done together to produce better rejuvenation.
- *Microneedle delivery systems:* The various types of microneedles available for this purpose can be solid, drug coated, dissolving, hollow, and swellable polymer microneedles synthesized by microfabrication technique.
  - Solid microneedles can be used as a skin pretreatment. After inserting and removing the microneedles to form micron-scale pores in the skin surface, a drug formulation can be applied to the skin for slow diffusion of drug through the pores and into the body.[13]

    Of note, in 2011, Fluzone® Intradermal influenza virus vaccine (Sanofi Pasteur, Swiftwater, PA, USA) became the first and only microneedle-based product approved by the FDA for this process **(Fig. 3)**.
  - *Drug-coated microneedles:* Solid needle is coated with drug formulated with a water-soluble formulation. Needle can be removed after dissolution of drug into skin postinsertion into skin.
  - Dissolvable microneedles are made from made water-soluble or biodegradable polymer that encapsulates the drug within the microneedle matrix. In this way, no removal is needed afterward as both drug as well as needle completely dissolve or degrade in the skin.
  - Hollow microneedles are used for infusion of liquid formulations into the skin.
- Light-emitting dermaroller incorporates titanium microneedles and LED light emitted during treatment. No published data is available regarding its efficacy.

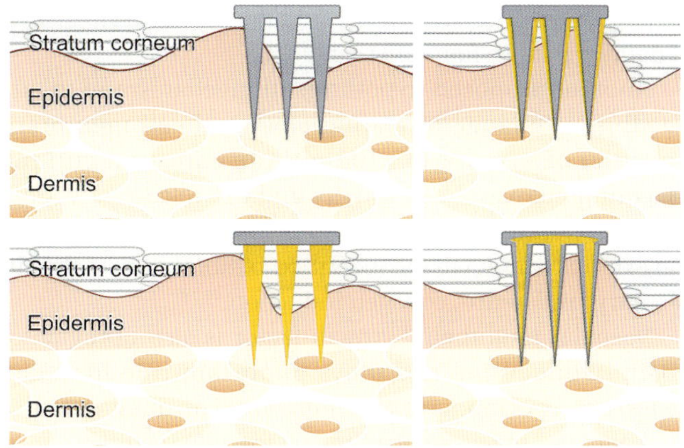

Fig. 3: Microneedle type illustration.

- Fractional radiofrequency microneedling—radiofrequency needling equipment works by creating radiofrequency thermal zones, hence imparting combined mechanical and thermal stimuli to the dermis.[14] The depth as well power of radiofrequency can be adjusted by operating person, thereby exercising good control over healing and intended effect.

PRINCIPLE AND MECHANISM OF ACTION OF MICRONEEDLING

The basis of microneedling relies on physical trauma created by repetitive application of device in the area to be treated in multiple directions (horizontal, vertical, and diagonal) with endpoint being uniform pinpoint capillary bleed. It has been proposed that the trauma generated by needle penetration in the skin induces regeneration of the dermis.[15,16]

Microconduits formed by needle on through epidermis to dermis with minimal damage to the epidermis lead to growth factor and wound healing cascade subsequently producing collagen and elastin in papillary dermis. These microchannels close within an hour and hence therapeutics should if delivered immediately. Healing starts immediately with sometimes superficial crusting observed for 2–3 days.[5]

Regeneration of dermis by controlled inflammatory/healing reaction and the remodeling of collagen is by secretion and participation of multiple growth factors such as by vascular endothelial growth factor (VEGF)/epidermal/fibroblast and platelet-derived growth factor, as well as transforming growth factor (TGF). The dermal injury causes localized breakage of old fibrotic tissue with some rupture of fine capillary-sized blood vessel rupture. Data on rat as animal model suggest a preferential stimulation of the antifibrogenic TGF-β_3 isoform production (as opposed to the pro-fibrogenic β_1 and 2) leading to regenerative effect of needling and support the formation of a physiological lattice pattern of collagen fibers found in normal skin instead of parallel pattern found in scars.[17]

Another proposed hypothesis of mechanism of microneedling is change of resting electrical cell membrane potential of –70 mV to –100 mV (demarcation current) triggering increased cell activity and the release of various proteins, potassium, and growth factors from the cells into the exterior leading to the migration of fibroblasts to the site of injury, and hence, collagen induction.[18,19]

Vascular endothelial growth factor is also upregulated postmicroneedling and plays important role in angiogenesis and keratinocyte function. Based on animal studies, the beneficial effects of needling on the skin include:

- Increased epidermal thickness by 112% over 8 weeks; histological findings are denser and more compact epidermis with more cellular layers and fewer gaps in the stratum corneum;
- Upregulation of type 1 collagen expression
- Increased expression of stromal glycosaminoglycans within the dermis
- Increased fibronectin expression which is important in collagen alignment during healing processes and a marker of fibroblast differentiation.[20]

The neocollagenosis is noticeable as early as 6 weeks and can continue up to 12 months. Appreciable changes are seen at 3 months onward in scars. The desired depth to achieve neocollagenosis is mid-reticular dermis; thus, the recommendation of at least 1.5-mm needle length dermaroller for it to reach 1.3 mm depth. Needle diameter also has an effect on the amount of neocollagenosis and maximal dermal injury without scarring is the desired thickness. A 0.25-mm diameter microneedle does this and is used and this is also the maximal limit for no scarring.

Needling has been shown to be able to regulate abnormal pigmentation by altering the secretion pattern of melanocyte-stimulating hormone (MSH) and interleukin (IL)-10. IL-10 is an anti-inflammatory cytokine and is upregulated at 2 weeks post microneedling. MSH appears to be downregulated 2 weeks probably because of IL-10 action.[21]

Microneedling has lower risk of postinflammatory hyperpigmentation and thus can be performed on all skin types. Topical anesthetic creams are often necessary as there is associated pain with microneedling.[22,23]

The summative conclusion of multiple studies comparing microneedling in atrophic acne scars to fractional laser, PRP, and TCA-CROSS is that needling can produce comparable clinical results to other mainstream adjuncts with explicit advantages relating to the lower risk of side effects especially hyperpigmentation risk.[24]

Multiple animal and human studies indicate preprocedure preparation by topical vitamin A and C for 3 weeks–3 months helps enhance microneedling results.[25-27]

INDICATIONS

- Skin rejuvenation of face—especially early changes like fine wrinkle and mild laxity.
- Atrophic acne scars—macular, rolling, linear, box car, and valley type.[28]
- Other atrophic nonacne scars—surgical, traumatic, and postburn scar (parchment such as hypo/hyper/depigmented scars)
- Open pores
- Androgenetic alopecia and alopecia areata—usually used as an adjunct to increase transdermal drug delivery of nutrient, PRP, etc. It has become recent focus as microneedle may stimulate stem cells in the dermal papilla, increase blood flow to hair follicles, and recruit growth factors and signaling pathways which induce hair restoration.[29]
- Pigmentation—melasma and periorbital hypermelanosis
- Miscellaneous conditions—stretch marks, axillary hyperhidrosis, and actinic keratosis in photo damaged skin.
- Rosacea and postacne erythema
- Skin laxity, wrinkle improvement in neck, chest, abdomen, and arms
- Introduction of nutrients, growth factors, PRP therapeutics—mesotherapy glutathione, tranexamic acid, ascorbic acid, minoxidil, finasteride, hyaluronic acid, peptides, etc., for indications of facial rejuvenation, periorbital hypermelanosis, melasma, and androgenetic alopecia (AGA), stretch marks.
- Stable vitiligo—as a therapeutic wounding modality
- Transdermal drug delivery[30]

CONTRAINDICATIONS

- Active acne
- Herpes labialis or any other local infection such as warts, molluscum, bacterial infection, etc.
- Moderate-to-severe chronic skin disease such as eczema, collagen vascular diseases, and psoriasis
- Blood dyscrasias, patients on anticoagulant therapy
- Extreme keloidal tendency
- Patient on chemo/radiotherapy
- Pregnancy and lactation
- Active disease with koebnerization potential—psoriasis, vitiligo, and lichen planus.
- Patients who have undergone facial surgery such as dermabrasion or permanent dermal fillers in preceding 6 months.

PREPROCEDURE WORKUP

- Counselling—explanation of steps of the procedure, expected outcomes and number of sessions required, postprocedure care, and complications to the patient.

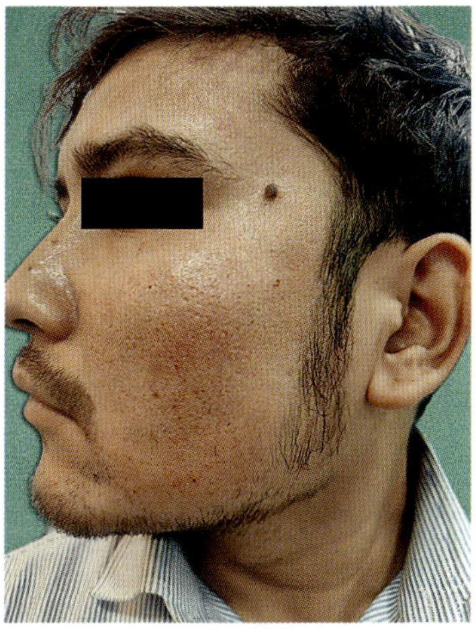

Fig. 4: Uniform capillary bleed.

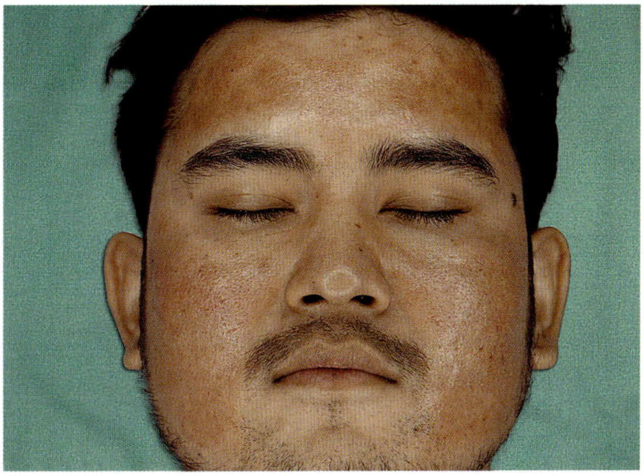

Fig. 5: Erythema postprocedure.

- Drugs to be withdrawn preprocedure—topical retinoid and hydroquinone 7 days prior. Rest are relative withdrawal indications such as aspirin, nonsteroidal anti-inflammatory drugs (NSAIDs), and blood thinners.
- Written informed consent and preprocedure photographs to be taken on the day of procedure and before topical anesthetic application.

PROCEDURE

Microneedling is a simple office-based procedure and requires 1–1:30 minutes of clinic time. Procedure should be undertaken only after patient is well aware of expected outcomes and an informed consent has been taken. Procedure is performed under topical anesthesia and a eutectic mixture of lignocaine and prilocaine/tetracaine is applied for 20–45 minutes. This can be applied under occlusion to achieve better depth of anesthesia. Once sufficient anesthesia is achieved, procedure is started.

- Skin should be prepared following aseptic precautions and using antiseptic solution and sterile normal saline. It is important to remove all residue of topical anesthetic as that tends be sticky and may get left out on surface if not removed with uniform gentle rubbing action.
- Procedure is done by rolling dermaroller on stretched skin in horizontal, vertical, and left and right diagonal directions. The rolling is to be done 5–10 times in each direction to achieve an endpoint of uniform pinpoint capillary bleeds which are easily controllable. Non-dominant hand should cover the vital structures such as eye and give a slight stretch to skin while dominant hand is for doing the rolling. This rolling should be done with gentle uniform pressure and not with traction or heavy pressure **(Fig. 4)**.
- Postprocedure cold saline soaks can be applied for few minutes before applying topical antibiotic cream and completing the procedure.
- The procedure is well tolerated and mild erythema is **(Fig. 5)** expected for 1–2 days. Patient can resume daily work from next day. Any friction, face pack, steam scrub on treated area should be avoided for 1 week.

TIPS AND TRICKS (TABLES 1 AND 2)

- Lateral movement and downward pressure should be avoided while doing rolling this can worsen scars.
- For more effect, increase the number of passes in an area and not pressure while doing procedure.
- Use smaller strokes of rolling when doing close to vital areas, bony areas.
- For Dermapen and dermastamp, repetitive puncture on same area without moving instrument laterally should be absolutely avoided in thin skin areas such as lids under eye areas. This can create a significant bleed/bruise and/or damage to a vital vessel in the area.
- For scalp use, smaller strokes and roller with thinner and longer microneedles.
- Perioral area gets better stabilized when patient clasps lips and pulls them in.
- Microneedling when being done for the purpose of transdermal drug delivery, application of active ingredients should be done immediately. Apply 1–3 layers of product and gently massage followed by gentle repeat dermarolling. Allow the treated area to dry by keeping open without any gauze or mask, etc.
- PRP when be combined with microneedling should be injected into treated area in addition to spray on the dermarolled area.
- Storage of dermarollers should not be done if not avoidable must follow full sterilization protocol for instrument and storage in a formalin chamber.
- One dermaroller is not to be used for >1 person under any circumstances.
- Priming of skin with vitamin A and C formulations starting 1 month prior to procedure can help maximize collagen formation and achieve better results.
- Checking for any erythema happening due to topical anesthetic cream after application is important step to avoid unwanted sequelae of postinflammatory hyperpigmentation postprocedure.
- An interval of 4–6 weeks in between session and 4–6 sessions is good.
- All active infections should be treated before doing microneedling procedure. Active acne phase should be over before initiating acne scar reduction microneedling. Occasional active acne can be avoided by skipping the active area.
- Dermaroller with needle size smaller than 1.5 mm may produce only gentle erythema and no significant capillary ooze.

- Procedures which can be done on same day as microneedling are subcision, TCA CROSS for some of the scars in microneedle area, and platelet-rich plasma therapy for entire treated area. Superficial to medium depth peels in the hands of expert can be combined with microneedling to increase the efficacy and depth of peel (the dermaroller to be used in this instance is 1.5 mm or lesser needle size).
- Fresh scars and scars <1 year old respond better with microneedling compared to ice-pick scars.

TABLE 1: Postmicroneedling changes.

Time scales	*Skin changes and improvement*
Day 1–2 (normally 24 hours)	Erythema and mild swelling
Day 2–7	Increased exfoliation and dryness
2nd week onward	Improvement in texture and tone begins
6th week onward	Improvement in fine lines and scars begins

TABLE 2: Interval between microneedling and other procedure in same area.

Treatment	*Approximate interval before or after microneedling treatment*
Botulinum toxin	2 weeks
Dermal fillers	• HA 2 weeks • Polylactic acidc/calcium hydroxylapatite 3 weeks
Skin peels	• Superficial 2 weeks • Medium 3 weeks • Deep 6 weeks
Laser and IPL • Resurfacing/fractional • IPL	6 weeks
Radiofrequency	3 weeks

(HA: hyaluronic acid; IPL: intense pulsed laser light)

POSTOPERATIVE CARE

- Topical and if needed oral antibiotic for extensive microneedling for first 3–5 days.
- Face wash with mild soap and water can be resumed after 2 days with application of topical antibiotic after very wash.
- Sun restriction and sun protection along with moisturizers for 7–10 days with physical cover while out in addition to using sunscreen even while indoors for 2 weeks.
- Avoidance of topical irritant applications such as retinoids, hydroquinone or other bleaching agents for 2–3 weeks postprocedure.

SCHEDULE OF REPEAT SESSIONS (FIGS. 6 TO 8)

Microneedling can be done in 4–6 weeks and 4–6 such sessions should be done. Some surgeons recommend doing first three sessions at 3-week intervals, followed by two sessions at 6-week intervals and 1–2 sessions at 8-week intervals.

For AGA usually more sessions are advised 8–12 sessions at monthly intervals.

ADVERSE EFFECTS

- Transient—mila, secondary bacterial infection, bruising, small hematoma, pain, bleeding (immediate), serous oozing (exudation—first 2 days), edema (last 5–10 days), discomfort, erythema, and exfoliation.
- Semitransient rail road track marks over bony areas or entire treatment area, retinoid dermatitis in combination with peels, dullness in response to extensive bruising, and transient postinflammatory hyperpigmentation.
- Long-term worsening of open pores and scars.

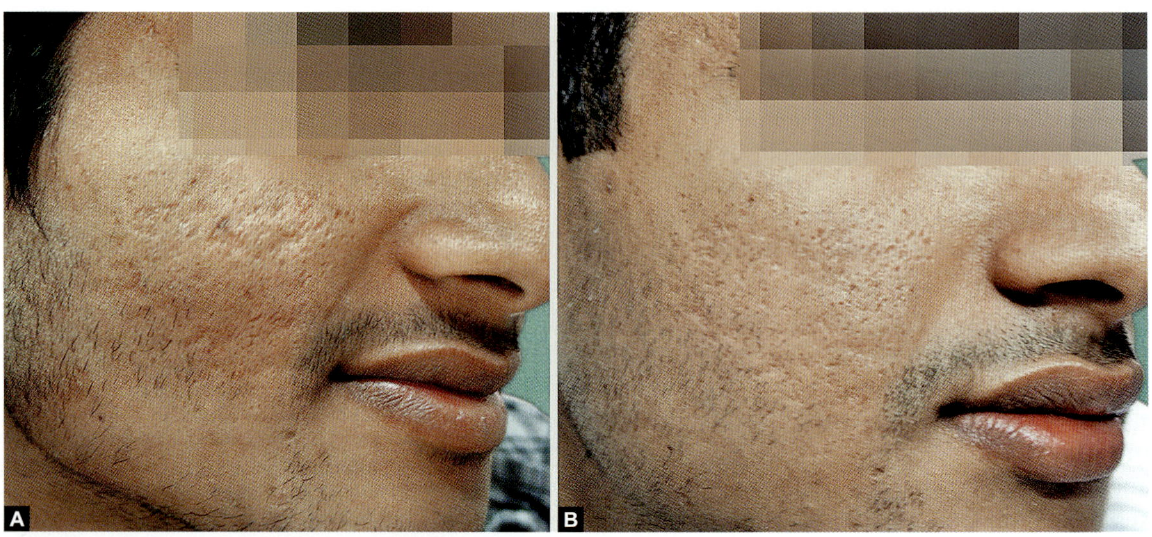

Figs. 6A and B: Acne scar before and after.

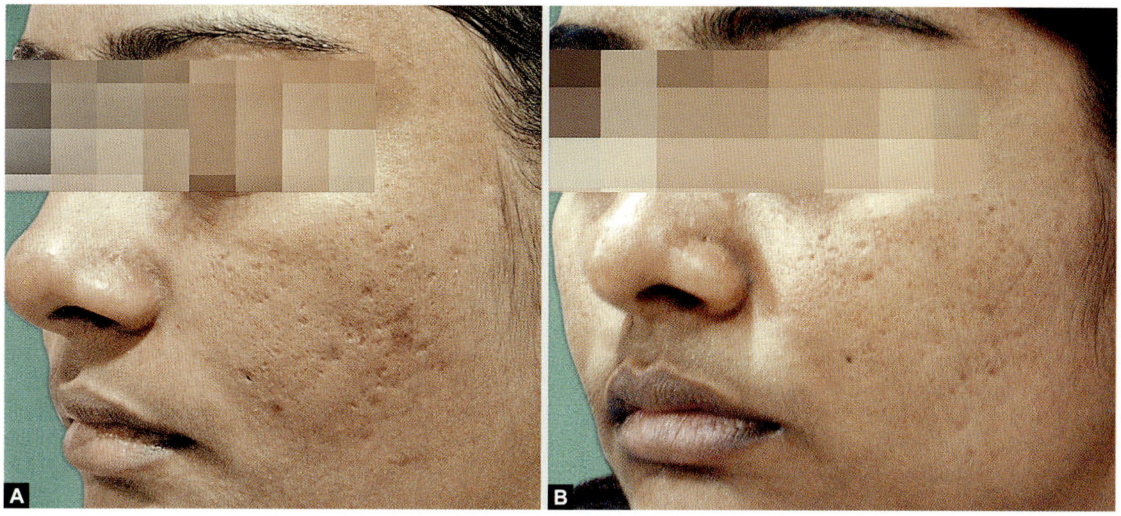

Figs. 7A and B: Acne scar before and after.

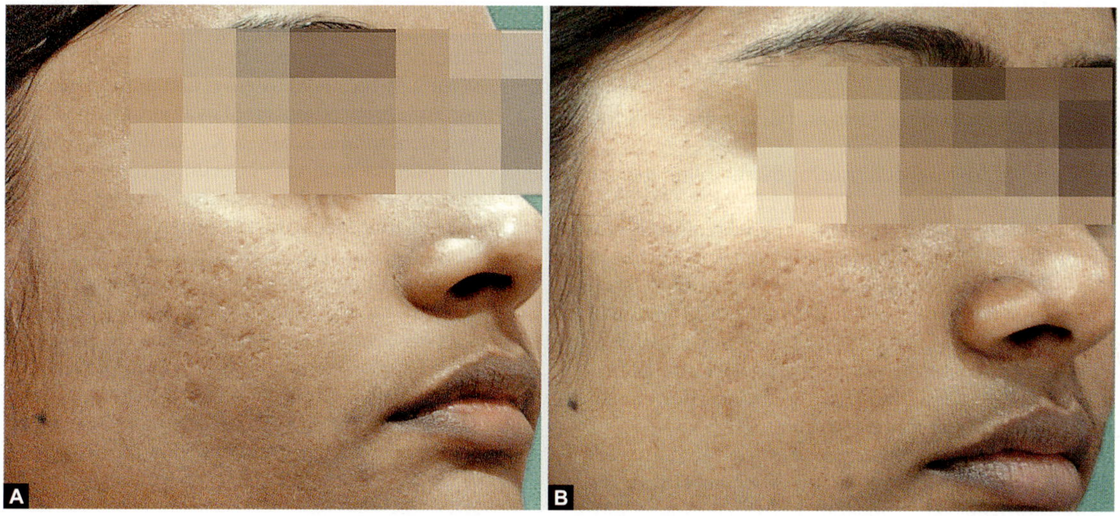

Figs. 8A and B: Acne scar before and after.

ADVANTAGES

- The main advantage of microneedling procedure is being an office-based procedure with very minimal downtime especially when done for scar reduction. All other scar reduction procedures have a significantly higher downtime. Microneedling devices are reasonable priced and require very less investment on the part of caregiver.
- Microneedling does not lead to any dermabrasive reduction in thickness of epidermis and thus safety of the procedure is very high. Risk of frosting, chemical burn, and postinflammatory hyperpigmentation is minimal in this procedure, if done in the right way.

DISADVANTAGES

- Old fibrosed scars, ice-pick scars, grade 4 acne scars respond less to mild and slow collagen generation compared to more intense treatments such as fractional CO_2 laser.
- For some patients pain of microneedling is a very big issue and they are not comfortable with needle-prick sensation even with local anesthesia.
- Microneedling involves capillary bleeds when done properly thus requires more aseptic care during the procedure to prevent infection.

CONCLUSION

In last 25 years of its existence, microneedling has established itself as a simple, economical as well as safe and effective treatment modality for multiple dermatological indications. Advantages of microneedling are good tolerability and practicality in Indian skin color.

Adverse events with microneedling are rare and have never resulted in any systemic toxicity.

Further larger studies are likely to provide more validation for newer indications and microneedle-based drug delivery, etc. Some further researches into elucidation of mechanism of action of microneedling in alopecia and pigmentation disorders are needed.

We thank the authors of the previous edition for their work.

REFERENCES

1. Fernandes D. Percutaneous collagen induction: an alternative to laser resurfacing. Aesthetic Surg J. 2002;22:307-9.
2. Orentreich D, Orentreich N. Subcutaneous incisionless (subcision) surgery for the correction of depressed scars and wrinkles. Dermatol Surg. 1995;21(6):543-9.
3. Liebl H. Device and method for applying an active ingredient to the skin. German; WO2001EP14747 20011214, 2002.
4. Escobar-Chávez JJ, Bonilla-Martinez D, Villegas-González MA, Molina-Trinidad E, Casas-Alancaster N, Revilla-Vázquez AL, et al. Microneedles: a valuable physical enhancer to increase transdermal drug delivery. J Clin Pharmacol. 2011:51(7): 964-77.
5. Doddaballapur S. Microneedling with dermaroller. J Cutan Aesthet Surg. 2009;2:110-11.
6. Bahuguna A. Microneedling: facts and fictions. Asian J Med Sci. 2013;4:14.
7. Nair PA, Arora TH. Microneedling using dermaroller: a means of collagen induction therapy. GMJ. 2014;69:247.
8. Bhardwaj D. Collagen induction therapy with dermaroller. Community Based Med J. 2013;1:35-7.
9. Singh A, Yadav S. Microneedling: advances and widening horizons. Indian Dermatol Online J. 2016;7(4):244-54.
10. Anastassakis K. (2014). The Dermaroller Series. [online] Available from http://www.mtoimportadora.com. br/site_novo/wp-content/uploads/2014/04/Dr.-Anastassakis-Kostas.pdf. [Last accessed September, 2023].
11. McCrudden MT, McAlister E, Courtenay AJ, González-Vázquez P, Singh TR, Donnelly RF. Microneedle applications in improving skin appearance. Exp Dermatol. 2015; 24:561-6.
12. Arora S, Gupta BP. Automated microneedling device—a new tool in dermatologist's kit: a review. J Pak Med Assoc. 2012;22:354-357.
13. Bariya SH, Gohel MC, Mehta TA, Sharma OP. Microneedles: an emerging transdermal drug delivery system. J Pharm Pharmacol. 2012;64(1):11-29.
14. Chandrashekar B, Sriram R, Mysore R, Bhaskar S, Shetty A. Evaluation of microneedling fractional radiofrequency device for treatment of acne scars. J Cutan Aesthet Surg. 2014;7(2):93-7.
15. Fernandes D, Signorini M. Combating photoaging with percutaneous collagen induction. Clin Dermatol. 2008; 26:192-9.
16. Alster T, Graham P. Microneedling: a review and practical guide. Dermatol Surg. 2017;44:397-404.
17. Bandyopadhyay B, Fan J, Guan S, Li Y, Chen M, Woodley DT, et al. A "traffic control" role for TGF-β3: orchestrating dermal and epidermal cell motility during wound healing. J Cell Biol. 2006;172(7):1093-105.
18. Liebl H, Kloth L. Skin cell proliferation stimulated by microneedles. J Am Coll Clin Wound Spec. 2012;4:2-6.
19. Zeitter S, Sikora Z, Jahn S, Stahl F, Strauß S, Lazaridis A, et al. Microneedling: matching the results of medical needling and repetitive treatments to maximize potential for skin regeneration. Burns. 2014;40(5):966-73.
20. Aust M, Reimers K, Kaplan H, Stahl F, Repenning C, Scheper T, et al. Percutaneous collagen induction–regeneration in place of cicatrisation. J Plast Reconstr Aesthet Surg. 2011;64(1): 97-107.
21. Aust M, Reimers K, Repenning C, Stahl F, Jahn S, Guggenheim M, et al. Percutaneous collagen induction: minimally invasive skin rejuvenation without risk of hyperpigmentation: fact or fiction? Plast Reconstr Surg. 2008;122(5):1553-63.
22. Fabbrocini G, Annunziata MC, D'Arco V, De Vita V, Lodi G, Mauriello MC, et al. Acne scars: pathogenesis, classification and treatment. Dermatol Res Pract. 2010;2010:893080.
23. Asif M, Kanodia S, Singh K. Combined autologous platelet-rich plasma with microneedling verses microneedling with distilled water in the treatment of atrophic acne scars: a concurrent split-face study. J Cosmet Dermatol. 2016;15:434-43.
24. Ramaut L, Hoeksema H, Pirayesh A, Stillaert F, Monstrey S. Microneedling: where do we stand now? A systematic review of the literature. J Plast Reconstr Aesthet Surg. 2018;71(1):1-14.
25. Aust M, Reimers K, Gohritz A, Jahn S, Stahl F, Repenning C, et al. Percutaneous collagen induction. Scarless skin rejuvenation: fact or fiction? Clin Exp Dermatol. 2010;35(4):437-9.
26. Kubiak R, Lange B. Percutaneous collagen induction as an additive treatment for scar formation following thermal injuries: preliminary experience in 47 children. Burns. 2017;43:1097-102.
27. Fernandes D. Minimally invasive percutaneous collagen induction. Oral Maxillofac Surg Clin North Am. 2005;17:51-63.
28. Fabbrocini G, Fardella N, Monfrecola A, Proietti I, Innocenzi D. Acne scarring treatment using skin needling. Clin Exp Dermatol. 2009;34(8):874-9.
29. Jeong K, Lee YJ, Kim JE, Park YM, Kim BJ, Kang H. Repeated microneedle stimulation induce the enhanced expression of hair-growth related genes. Int J Trichol. 2012;4(2):117-30.
30. McCrudden MT, McAlister E, Courtenay AJ, González-Vázquez P, Raj Singh TR, Donnelly RF. Microneedle applications in improving skin appearance. Exp Dermatol. 2015;24(8):561-6.

CHAPTER 29

Platelet-rich Plasma Therapy: Principles and Preparation

Gautam K Singh, Swapnil Shah, Pankaj Das

KEY MESSAGES

- Platelet-rich plasma (PRP) is an autologous blood product containing a high concentration of platelets in small volume of plasma.
- PRP is increasingly becoming popular amongst dermatologist because of its safety and efficacy.
- Variety of dermatological and aesthetic indications can be treated with judicious use of PRP.
- Each step in its preparation is important and is subjected to debate.
- The procedure is yet to be standardized and large double-blind studies are required to prove its efficacy in various indications.

INTRODUCTION

Platelet-rich plasma (PRP), also termed as autologous platelet gel, plasma rich in growth factors or platelet concentrate, is essentially an increased concentration of autologous platelets suspended in a small amount of plasma after centrifugation. There is no consensus definition of PRP; it is arbitrarily defined as a volume of the plasma fraction of autologous blood where platelet concentration is usually >10,00,000 platelets/μL or more than four folds from the baseline.[1] Platelets play an important role in hemostasis, wound healing, and tissue regeneration. Because of these properties, they are now being used in treatment of various disorders almost across all specialties of medicine including dermatology. However, even though PRP is widely used in dermatology clinics, its mechanism and effects are not completely understood. There is also a great debate in scientific community about methods of preparation. With numerous studies presenting contradictory results, the use of PRP remains controversial.

HISTORY

The first report of PRP used in medical science dates back to 1970, from Italy where it was used in open heart surgery.[2] The earlier reports in 1990s use large and expensive equipment, required a large volume of blood (450 cc), and therefore its use remains limited to large operating rooms. Initial interest of PRP was seen in oral surgery followed by sports medicine, thereafter it became an emerging therapeutic tools in many indications in dentistry, maxillofacial surgery, dermatology, and aesthetics. Since platelets contain growth factors in abundance, they are a logical option for replacement and renewal of cells, tissues, or part of organs. PRP is considered to be a growth factor cocktail, which promotes wound healing, angiogenesis, and tissue remodeling.[1]

Platelet-rich plasma is an autologous blood product. This means as long as the platelets are "minimally manipulated", PRP is not classified as a drug by the Food and Drug Administration (FDA). Because of this it is not subjected to federal regulations, PRP preparations and administration protocols are not specifically defined. FDA approves only the method of preparation of PRP looking at its safety for human injection.

PLATELET PHYSIOLOGY AND FUNCTION

Blood consists of 93% red blood cells (RBCs), 6% platelets, and 1% white blood cells (WBCs). These are small discoid cells with a lifespan of about 7–10 days. Humans have an average baseline blood platelet count of 200,000 (150,000–450,000 cells/μL of blood). Platelets lack nucleus, but possess an extensive cytoskeleton, mitochondria, lysosomes, ribosomes, and a modified version of smooth endoplasmic reticulum, as well as a number of unique organelles and membrane features. There are three types of platelet granules: (1) alpha, (2) dense, and (3) lysosomes. Alpha granules are the most numerous organelles in the platelet and contain over 300 different proteins; dense granules are relatively few in number and contain only a few small molecules, such as serotonin, adenosine diphosphate, adenosine triphosphate, guanosine 5'-diphosphate, guanosine 5'-triphosphate, histamine, calcium, magnesium, and polyphosphate. Platelet lysosomes may contribute to eventual clot lysis.[3]

MECHANISM OF ACTION

Subsequent to the injury platelets are activated and aggregate together to release their alpha granules containing growth factors that stimulate the inflammatory cascade and healing process.[4,5] All of these factors set the stage for tissue healing, which involves intricate overlapping processes that are often categorized into hemostasis, inflammation, proliferation, and remodeling. The various growth factors and their functions are described in **Table 1**. PRP offers multiple, synergistically working growth factors in an optimum concentration at the wound sites. These growth factors act on different stages of wound healing. PRP also contains adhesion molecules such as fibrin, fibronectin, and vitronectin. These proteins are capable of enhancing cell adhesion and act like a matrix for the formation connective tissue and epithelium. Thus, PRP not only accelerates but also modulates the wound-healing process resulting in better and faster wound healing.[6] The secreted growth factors (GFs) once released bind to their respective transmembrane receptors expressed over adult mesenchymal stem cells, osteoblasts, fibroblasts, endothelial cells, and epidermal cells.[7] This further induces an internal signal-transduction pathway, unlocking the expression of a normal gene sequence of a cell such as cellular proliferation, matrix formation, osteoid production, collagen synthesis, etc., thereby augmenting the natural wound-healing process.[8] PRP stimulates proliferation and differentiation of stem cells in the hair follicle bulge area via multiple molecular mechanisms which are as follows:[9]

- Upregulation of transcriptional activity of β-catenin which helps in differentiation of stem cells into hair follicle cells.
- Increased in B-cell lymphoma 2 (bcl-2) levels, being antiapoptotic it prolongs survival of dermal papilla cells.
- Activation of Akt and extracellular signal kinase (ERK) signaling pathways which prolongs survival of dermal papilla cells.
- Expression of fibroblast growth factor-7 (FGF-7) in dermal papilla cells which prolongs anagen phase of hair cycle.
- Increased in vascular endothelial growth factor (VEGF) and platelet-derived growth factor (PDGF) level increases perifollicular vascular plexus.

Another field of interest is aesthetic dermatology. PRP has been proposed to augment collagen remodeling by stimulating the removal of photodamaged extracellular matrix (ECM) components and inducing the synthesis of new collagen by dermal fibroblasts via various molecular mechanisms which are enumerated below:[10,11]

- Increased proliferation of human dermal fibroblasts.
- Increased expression of matrix metalloproteinase (MMP)-1 and MMP-3 and removal of photodamaged ECM.
- Increased production of procollagen type I peptide and expression of collagen type I, alpha-I which help in synthesis of new collagen.
- Increases expression of G1 cell cycle regulators which accelerates wound healing.

Another advantage of PRP is that it is depleted of RBCs. RBCs are known to inhibit the wound-healing response by inhibiting fibroblast functions.[12] The WBC composition of PRP is also important. An ideal PRP should have no or less neutrophils and optimum monocytes and T cells. Neutrophils in PRP result in delayed wound healing and result in bad scar formation.[13] Monocytes and T lymphocyte augment wound-healing responses.[14,15]

TABLE 1: Role of growth factors.

Growth factor	*Functions*
Transforming growth factor-β (TGF-β)	• Stimulates undifferentiated mesenchymal cell proliferation • Regulates endothelial, fibroblastic, and osteoblastic mitogenesis • Regulates collagen synthesis and collagenase secretion • Regulates mitogenic effects of other growth factors • Stimulates endothelial chemotaxis and angiogenesis • Inhibits macrophage and lymphocyte proliferation
Fibroblast growth factor (FGF)	• Promotes growth and differentiation of chondrocytes and osteoblasts • Mitogenic for mesenchymal cells, chondrocytes, and osteoblasts
Platelet-derived growth factor α and β (PDGF)	• Mitogenic for mesenchymal cells and osteoblasts. Stimulates chemotaxis and mitogenesis in fibroblast, glial, or smooth muscle cells • Regulates collagenase secretion and collagen synthesis. Stimulates macrophage and neutrophil chemotaxis
Epidermal growth factor (EGF)	• Stimulates endothelial chemotaxis or angiogenesis • Regulates collagenase secretion • Stimulates epithelial or mesenchymal mitogenesis
Vascular endothelial growth factor (VEGF)	• Increases angiogenesis and vessel permeability • Stimulates mitogenesis for endothelial cells
Connective tissue growth factor (CTGF)	Promotes angiogenesis, cartilage regeneration, fibrosis, and platelet adhesion
Insulin like growth factor (IGF-1 and -2)	• Chemotactic for fibroblasts • Stimulates protein synthesis • Enhances bone formation
Platelet factor 4 (PF-4)	Stimulate the initial influx of neutrophils into wounds. Chemoattractant for fibroblasts
Interleukin-8 (IL-8)	• Proinflammatory mediator • Recruitment of inflammatory cells
Keratinocyte growth factor (KGF)	• Promote endothelial cell growth, migration, adhesion, and survival • Angiogenesis

PREPARATION

Platelet-rich plasma is prepared by a process known as differential centrifugation. The centrifugation process separates blood components owing to their different specific gravities, i.e., RBCs being the heaviest, followed by WBCs, whereas platelets are the lightest. The ideology behind PRP treatment is the reversal of the RBC to platelet ratio by decreasing RBCs to 5% and more importantly concentrating platelets containing growth factors to 94%. It is a day care process performed under strict aseptic conditions as well as under optimum temperature regulations i.e., 20–22°C after taking patient consent. In order to inhibit platelet aggregation, it is prepared with an anticoagulant, commonly using anticoagulant citrate dextrose solution formula A (ACD-A) or sodium citrate.[16-18] The first centrifugation (soft spin) is slow to avoid spinning down platelets and to isolate plasma. Platelets are mostly concentrated right on top of the buffy coat layer. Subsequent centrifugation (hard spin) is faster, so that platelets are spun down and separate as a pellet at the bottom of the tube from platelet-poor plasma (PPP) above.

Depending on the equipment used to prepare PRP, the techniques are broadly divided into two types:[16-18]

1. *Open technique:* The system of preparation is open where the product is in contact with environment and carries a risk of bacterial contamination. The materials used are relatively inexpensive. Some of the open techniques are double spin method, buffy coat method, modified syringe technique, and turn-down turn-up technique.
2. *Closed technique:* Here the PRP is prepared in a closed system and the product till its final preparation is not exposed to the environment. There is minimal risk of contamination. The materials used are relatively expensive. Many commercially available PRP kits are designed to confirm to the closed technique.

Stepwise Procedures of Platelet-rich Plasma Preparation

- Informed consent
- Blood collection
- Centrifugation
- Platelet-rich plasma isolation
- Activation of PRP
- Injections.

Informed Consent

As with any dermatosurgical procedure, written informed consent along with photo documentation is a must. Patients should be explained about the procedure in detail. It should be ensured that patients should not have unrealistic outcome.

Blood Collection

Approximately 10–50 cc of blood is collected in a sterile syringe or directly into PRP tube using a wide-bore needle (19–21 G) depending upon the clinical indications. It is important to use a wide-bore needle to prevent the activation of platelets. One can also use commercially available as disposal kit for PRP preparation comprising of special BD Eclipse™ blood collection needle, BD Vacutainers, conical sterile 10 mL plastic tube, sterile pipette along with accessories **(Fig. 1A)** and commercial PRP kit **(Fig. 1B)**. The blood is mixed with anticoagulant by inverting the tubes 8–10 times. For 9 cc of blood collected 1 cc of anticoagulant is used. The common anticoagulants used in preparation of PRP are ACD-A, sodium citrate solution. These are chelating agents that bind to calcium and prevent coagulation proteins from initiating clotting cascade. The addition of citrate to the blood makes it more acidic and that is the reason for more pain or stinging while performing the injections. Few commercial kits recommend heparin (either as calcium or sodium salt) as an anticoagulant. It has been demonstrated that release of growth factors from platelets takes place more efficiently in presence of heparin. Ethylenediaminetetraacetic acid or lithium heparin should not be used as an anticoagulant as it deforms the platelet morphology.[16-18]

Platelet-rich plasma preparation by laboratory grade vacutainers containing ACD is easily available, cost effective, and sterile option. Commercial kits, although expensive offers a standardized option in PRP preparation. PRP tubes are FDA approved for preparation of PRP. These are sterile endotoxin free tube. There is no risk of environmental contamination as the tubes are closed systems. The chances of RBC contamination are virtually nil. Another advantage of these kits is there is approximately 11% WBC recovery with depletion of 96.5% granulocytes, which are proinflammatory in nature. One important note is the commercial PRP tubes are made up of medical grade glass and the inner surface of these tubes are not siliconized. Glass is an activator of platelet. This results in partial but reversible activation of platelets and platelets clumping. This is seen as sediments in the tube. It does not alter the effectiveness of PRP. Care must be taken

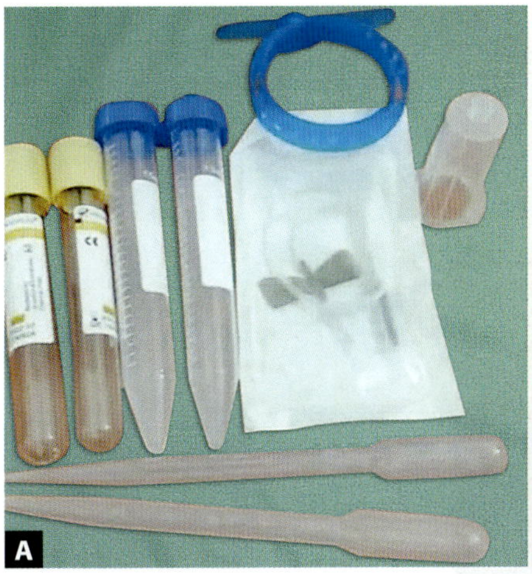
A

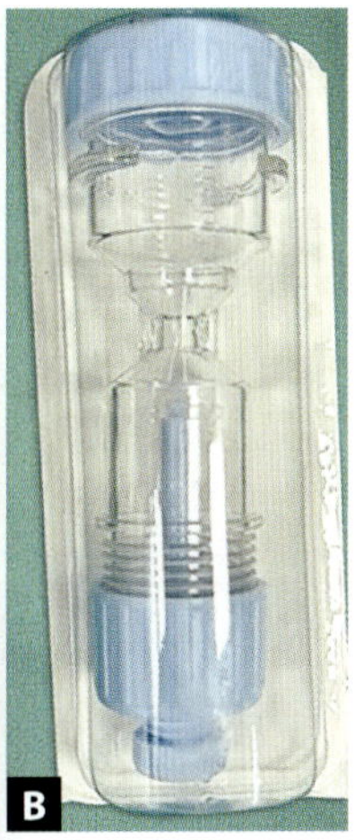
B

Figs. 1A and B: (A) Disposable set for collection of platelet-rich plasma comprising of acid citrate dextrose (ACD-A) 9-mL tube, 10-mL sterile tube, blood collection needle, vacutainer, transparent graduated sterile pipette; (B) Commercially available PRP kit.

to harvest these aggregates. Again because of these micro-clumps, cell counters often fail to show actual concentration of platelets. Various commercially available PRP kits may have different technology, concentration factors, blood volume use, and yield of PRP.

Centrifugation

It is the most controversial but most important step in preparation of PRP which has a critical impact on quality and quantity of PRP. Different protocols of centrifugations have been described with different variables such as number of spins, centrifugal acceleration, duration, and temperature of centrifugation. The centrifugation process for PRP preparation must be sterile and should result into maximum platelet separation from RBCs without causing any damage and lysis. When anticoagulated blood is centrifuged, three layers appear. This is due to differences in the density of the blood components—the deep layer consists of RBCs, the middle layer contains platelets and leukocytes, and the top layer is made up of PPP. The bottom part of the middle layer is also called buffy coat, which is rich in leukocytes **(Fig. 2)**. In the double-centrifugation protocol, the first spin (called the hard spin) separates the RBCs from the plasma, which contains the platelets, the WBCs, and the clotting factors. The second spin (called the soft spin) further separates the platelets, WBCs, and few remaining RBCs from the plasma. This is a very effective method of concentrating platelets. One can easily get concentration of almost 5–10 times of original. Based on this, one can follow either first soft and second hard spin protocol or vice versa. A single-spin protocol is a faster protocol in which whole blood is centrifuged at higher revolution per minute (RPM) for a shorter time (e.g., 1,500 g for 5 minutes). This is commonly used in most of the commercial kits. One can get low concentration of 1.7–5 times of original. The double-centrifugation protocol results in higher platelet concentrations than did the single-centrifugation protocol. However, the double-centrifugation protocol can cause alterations in platelet morphology, risk of damage to platelets is more because of more handling and is more sensitive to small processing errors.[19,20]

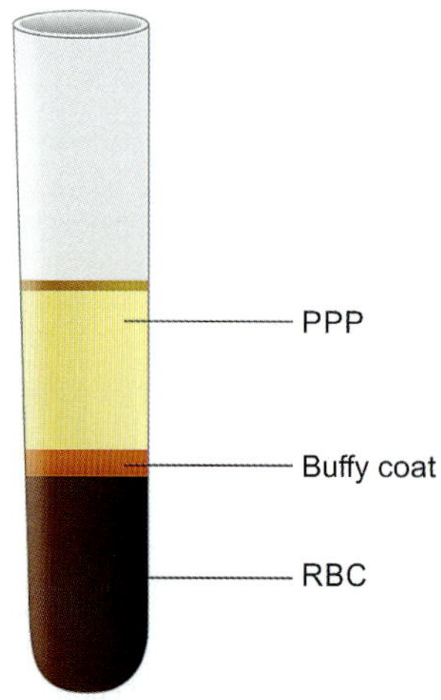

Fig. 2: Component of blood. Upper 1/3 is platelet-poor plasma, middle layer is buffy coat containing platelets and white blood cells. (PPP: platelet-poor plasma; RBC: red blood cell)

Double spin/double centrifugation method: Most commonly used technique for preparation of PRP.

Buffy coat method: It is a type of open technique where whole blood (WB) is centrifuged at a "high speed" with subsequent collection of the buffy coat. A buffy coat contains high concentration of leukocytes. From small volume of WB (10 mL), a very thin layer of a buffy coat can be produced. The difficulty lies in separating this thin buffy coat layer that contains mainly WBCs and platelets, from the underlying RBC layer. The steps of double spin and buffy coat methods are illustrated in **Table 2**.

Turn-down turn-up technique: This method needs only a 10-mL syringe and two vacutainers, preferably 8.5 mL. It is a double-spin method where vacutainers are placed in an inverted (cap-down) position for the first spin and the correct position for the second spin. Advantages include reduced handling and transferring and hence less chances of contamination and low-input cost. Machado et al.[21] were able to produce a 4.17-folds increase in platelet concentration in their PRP using this method as compared to a maximum of 3.19 folds by existing methods ($p = 0.063$).

Heat activates platelets. Room temperature should be around 20–22° while centrifugation. Hence, air conditioning of the room is a must while preparation of PRP. Few companies' market temperature-controlled centrifuges, which prevent

TABLE 2: Steps of double spin and buffy coat methods.

Steps of double spin/centrifugation method	*Steps of buffy coat method*
• Obtain whole blood by venipuncture in acid citrate dextrose (ACD) tubes • Do not chill the blood at any time before or during platelet separation • Centrifuge the blood using a "soft" spin • Transfer the supernatant plasma containing platelets into another sterile tube (without anticoagulant) • Centrifuge tube at a higher speed (a hard spin) to obtain a platelet concentrate • The lower one-thirds is PRP and upper two-thirds is platelet-poor plasma (PPP). At the bottom of the tube, platelet pellets are formed • Remove PPP and suspend the platelet pellets in a minimum quantity of plasma (2–4 mL) by gently shaking the tube	• Whole blood should be stored at 20°C to 24°C before centrifugation • Centrifuge whole blood at a "high" speed • Three layers are formed because of its density: The bottom layer consisting of RBCs, the middle layer consisting of platelets and WBCs, and the top PPP layer • Remove supernatant plasma from the top of the container • Transfer the buffy coat layer to another sterile tube • Centrifuge at low speed to separate WBCs or use leukocyte filtration filter

(PRP: platelet-rich plasma)

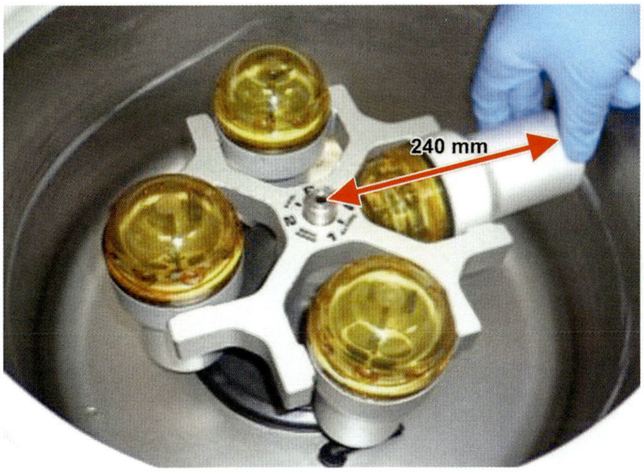

Fig. 3: Calculation of radius inside centrifuge machine.

the rise of temperature while making PRP. There is lot of debate on what is the optimum concentration of platelets in a PRP. According to Marx, 1×10^6 platelets/μL is considered as a therapeutic PRP (at least five times the normal).[1] Lower concentrations are reportedly unreliable in enhancing wound healing, while higher concentrations have not been shown to further enhance wound healing.[22] However Rappl et al.[23] noted that studies with one to three times concentrated PRP showed better results in wound healing than those with higher concentrations. A meta-analytical study by Martínez-Martines-Zapata et al.[24] revealed that the works with beneficial PRP treatment did indeed use protocols with lower platelet concentrations (i.e., one to three times the normal).

Most of the studies mention the centrifugation force in "g" value, which make it difficult in implementing in day-to-day practice. A formula is there to calculate RPM from given *g* force. $RPM = \sqrt{[RCF/(r \times 1.118)]} \times 1{,}000$; Where r is real radius of centrifugation in centimeter, RCF is relative centrifugal force expressed in "*g*" while RPM is revolution per minute. Once we know the radius of centrifugation RPM can be calculated by using calculation. R-max is the distance from the axis of rotation to the end of the tube which is most widely accepted radius of centrifuge machine. Many conversion sites are there, which convert *g* value to RPM. **Figure 3** illustrates the radius of centrifuge machine for calculation of RCF.

The experts from National IADVL PRP Taskforce recommend the use of double-spin manual method for the preparation of PRP. The recommended parameters for centrifuge are 100–300 *g* for 5–10 minutes for the first spin and 400–700 *g* for 10–17 minutes for the second spin. The recommended platelet concentration in PRP for the treatment of various dermatological conditions is 1–1.5 million platelets/μL. The activation of PRP is not required when it is injected into soft tissues.[18]

There are many innovative ways to prepare PRP, one such widely practiced is called modified syringe technique. Mototsugu Fukaya et al.[25] described a novel and low-cost method of PRP preparation using hypodermic syringes. Since hypodermic syringes are made for human injection, are sterile and endotoxin free and it is a closed system, they have all the advantages of commercial PRP kit with much less costs. The materials required for the procedure are: 5-cc Luer-lock hypodermic syringes, syringe tip caps, three-way connector, scalp vein set, and sterile ACD-A solution. The steps of modified syringe technique are illustrated in **Box 1** and **Figures 4A to F**.

BOX 1: Steps of modified syringe technique.

- Cut the finger guard of the syringes with sterile scissor, so as to convert syringe into a tube
- 0.5 cc of ACD-A is taken in two tubes
- 5 cc of blood is withdrawn into syringes using a 19 no. scalp vein set
- The tips of syringes are closed with sterile tip caps
- The syringes are directly kept into the centrifuge with tips facing upward
- Centrifuged with desired RPM. One can use single-spin or double-spin method
- After centrifugation, the blood is separated into lower RBC, buffy coat layer, and PPP
- Three-way connector is attached to the syringe tip. Upper end is closed. Another syringe is attached to the open end, and PPP is aspirated. Once the buffy coat is reached, tuberculin syringe is attached and the buffy coat is slowly aspirated, so as to obtain PRP
- For better control of aspiration, one can attach an intravenous (IV) line extension set to the three-way connector
- Using another three-way connector, one can mix PPP and PRP in a tuberculin syringe

(ACD-A: acid citrate dextrose A; PPP: platelet-poor plasma; PRP: platelet-rich plasma; RPM: revolution per minute)

CLASSIFICATION

According to the classification proposed by Ehrenfest et al.[26] four main families of preparations can be defined, depending on their cell content and fibrin architecture:

1. Pure platelet-rich plasma (P-PRP) or leukocyte poor PRP products are preparations without leukocytes and with a low-density fibrin network after activation. After the first spin, only the upper part of buffy coat is aspirated and the final concentrate has a large number of platelets with very few leukocytes.
2. Leukocyte- and PRP (L-PRP) products are preparations with leukocytes and with a low-density fibrin network after activation. The entire buffy coat and the superficial layer of RBCs are aspirated out and this gives a final solution which is rich in leukocytes and platelets.
3. Pure platelet-rich fibrin (P-PRF) or leukocyte poor platelet-rich fibrin preparations are without leukocytes and with a high-density fibrin network. These products only exist in a strongly activated gel form, and cannot be injected or used like traditional fibrin glues. This is derived from P-PRP. The P-PRP is mixed with activator and allowed to incubate for a small defined period of time. A stable P-PRF clot is obtained by this method.

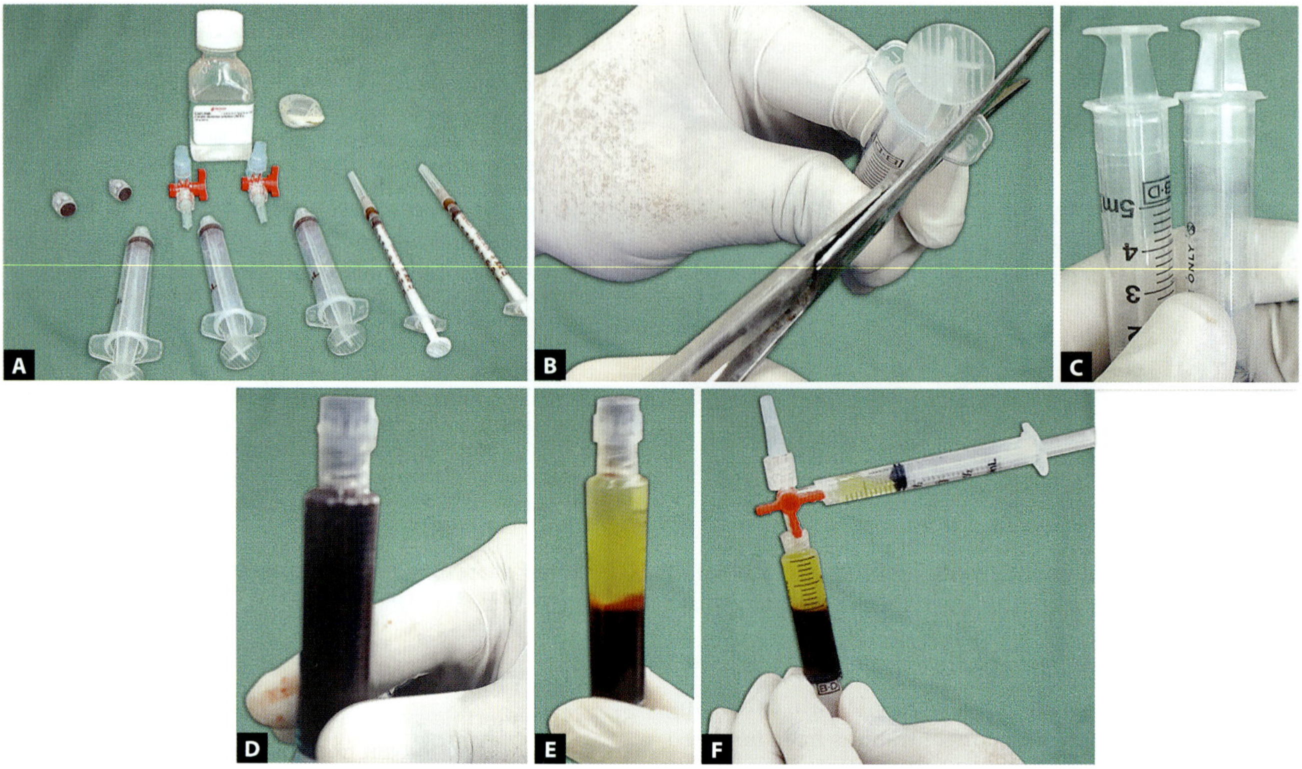

Figs. 4A to F: (A) Materials required for PRP preparation by modified syringe technique; (B) Cut the finger guard of syringes; (C) Syringes are converted to tubes; (D) Blood is collected, syringe cap applied and tube kept vertically in centrifuge; (E) After centrifugation, blood is separated in three layers; (F) After centrifugation, three-way connector applied and platelet-rich plasma is collected in tuberculin syringe.

4. Leukocyte- and platelet-rich fibrin (L-PRF) or second-generation PRP products are preparations with leukocytes and with a high-density fibrin network. Whole blood is centrifuged without adding anticoagulant. The three layers that are collected in this manner include a top layer of cellular plasma, a base layer of RBC, and an L-PRF clot in the middle.

Platelet-rich Plasma Activation

Platelets need to be activated for release of growth factors. Various factors activate platelets. These are calcium chloride, calcium gluconate, autologous thrombin, adrenaline, heat, motion, etc. Earlier protocol advocates mixing of $CaCl_2$ or autologous thrombin before injection of PRP. Collagen is a natural activator of platelets. Hence, recent protocols do not recommend activation of platelets before injection at least in dermatological use.[27] It has been recently shown that thrombin-activated PRP releases all growth factors at the same time in a bolus, while nonactivated PRP uses the platelets as a sustained drug delivery system,[28] which is more beneficial in aesthetic dermatology.

Platelet-rich Plasma Administration

Adequate anesthesia is necessary before injecting PRP. A topical anesthesia or nerve blocks are often used. Since, PRP is acidic in nature some authors advocate buffering of PRP before administration to reduce the stinging and pain. Platelet-rich plasma can be administered as an intradermal injection using insulin syringe or mesogun. It can also be sprayed or topically applied after dermaroller, ablative fractional lasers, or microneedle radiofrequency (RF). The frequency of administration also differs in different protocols. Few recommend once in a week and few once a month. Number of sessions varies usually from three to six.

Postprocedure Care

Adequate cooling is used after injections. Strict sun protection is advised. Patient is asked not to wash the face for at least 6 hours and advised not to rub, scratch, or prick the area.

CONCLUSION

The PRP has emerged as newer therapeutic tool in the field of dermatology and aesthetics. There are wide variations in the methods of preparation of PRP, in different studies and commercially available kits. In addition, there is lack of standardization in commercially available centrifuge machine which is being used for preparation PRP in routine clinical setting. Utmost care shall be taken to avoid contamination, proper biomedical waste disposal of tubes, and left over blood products during and post procedures. Tips and tricks of PRP are summarized in **Box 2**.

BOX 2: Tips and trick in preparation of platelet-rich plasma.

- Use wide-bore needle for withdrawing blood
- It is a good idea to use a scalp vein set while drawing blood
- Better to use commercial kits. If standard vacutainers are used, carry out the procedure under laminar flow hood
- Sterile ACD solution is available from Sigma-Aldrich or Fresenius Kabi. Anticoagulant and blood should be mixed well
- Air-conditioning of the room is a must
- Follow a centrifugation protocol, which gives optimum platelet concentration. Centrifugation protocol differs significantly withtype and make of centrifuge, length of tubes
- After preparation of PRP, allow it settle for 5–10 minutes
- Try not to take any RBCs in PRP
- Aspirate PRP using a wide-bore needle
- Use a good anesthesia. PRP is painful because of its acid nature

(ACD: acid citrate dextrose)

REFERENCES

1. Marx RE. Platelet-rich plasma (PRP): what is PRP and what is not PRP? Implant Dent. 2001;10:225-8.
2. Ross R, Glomset J, Kariya B, Harker L. A platelet-dependent serum factor that stimulates the proliferation of arterial smooth muscle cells in vitro. Proc Natl Acad Sci USA. 1974;71: 1207-10.
3. van der Meijden PEJ, Heemskerk JWM. Platelet biology and functions: new concepts and clinical perspectives. Nat Rev Cardiol. 2019;16(3):166-79.
4. Alves R, Grimalt R. A review of platelet-rich plasma: history, biology, mechanism of action, and classification. Skin Appendage Disord. 2018;4(1):18-24.
5. Coppinger JA, Cagney G, Toomey S, Kislinger T, Belton O, McRedmond JP, et al. Characterization of the proteins released from activated platelets leads to localization of novel platelet proteins in human atherosclerotic lesions. Blood. 2004;103(6):2096-104.
6. Fernandez-Moure JS, Van Eps JL, Cabrera FJ. Platelet-rich plasma: a biomimetic approach to enhancement of surgical wound healing. J Surg Res. 2017;207:33-44.
7. Marx RE, Carlson ER, Eichstaedt RM, Schimmele SR, Strauss JE, Georgeff KR. Platelet-rich plasma: Growth factor enhancement for bone grafts. Oral Surg Oral Med Oral Pathol Oral Radiol Endod. 1998;85:638-46.
8. Marx RE. Platelet-rich plasma: Evidence to support its use. J Oral Maxillofac Surg. 2004;62:489-96.
9. Li ZJ, Choi HI, Choi DK, Sohn KC, Im M, Seo YJ, et al. Autologous platelet-rich plasma: a potential therapeutic tool for promoting hair growth. Dermatol Surg. 2012;38: 1040-6.
10. Kim DH, Je YJ, Kim CD, Lee YH, Seo YJ, Lee JH, et al. Can platelet-rich plasma be used for skin rejuvenation? Evaluation of effects of platelet-rich plasma on human dermal fibroblast. Ann Dermatol. 2011;23:424-31.
11. Cho JW, Kim SA, Lee KS. Platelet-rich plasma induces increased expression of G1 cell cycle regulators, type I collagen, and matrix metalloproteinase-1 in human skin fibroblasts. Int J Mol Med. 2012;29:32-6.
12. Fredriksson K, Stridh H, Lundahl J, Rennard SI, Skold CM. Red blood cells inhibit proliferation and stimulate apoptosis in human lung fibroblasts in vitro. Scand J Immunol. 2004;59: 559-65.
13. Dovi JV, Szpaderska AM, DiPietro LA. Neutrophil function in the healing wound: adding insult to injury? Thromb Haemost. 2004;92(2):275-80.
14. Mirza R, DiPietro LA, Koh TJ. Selective and specific macrophage ablation is detrimental to wound healing in mice. Am J Pathol. 2009;175:2454-62.
15. Scott A, Khan KM, Roberts CR, Cook JL, Duronio V. What do we mean by the term "inflammation"? A contemporary basic science update for sports medicine. Br J Sports Med. 2004;38:372-80.
16. Arshdeep, Kumaran MS. Platelet-rich plasma in dermatology: Boon or a bane?. Indian J Dermatol Venereol Leprol. 2014;80:5-14.
17. Dhurat R, Sukesh M. Principles and methods of preparation of platelet-rich plasma: a review and author's perspective. J Cutan Aesthet Surg. 2014;7(4):189-97.
18. Dashore S, Chouhan K, Nanda S, Sharma A. Preparation of platelet-rich plasma: National IADVL PRP Taskforce Recommendations. Indian Dermatol Online J. 2021; 12(Suppl 1):S12-S23.
19. Marx RE. Platelet-rich plasma: evidence to support its use. J Oral Maxillofac Surg. 2004;62:489-96.
20. Nagata MJ, Messora MR, Furlaneto FA, Fucini SE, Bosco AF, Garcia VG, et al. Effectiveness of two methods for preparation of autologous platelet-rich plasma: an experimental study in rabbits. Eur J Dent. 2010;4:395-402.
21. Machado ES, Leite R, Dos Santos CC, Artuso GL, Gluszczak F, de Jesus LG, et al. Turn down-turn up: a simple and low-cost protocol for preparing platelet-rich plasma. Clin Sao Paulo Braz. 2019;74:e1132.
22. Fleming BC, Proffen BL, Vavken P, Shalvoy MR, Machan JT, Murray MM. Increased platelet concentration does not improve functional graft healing in bio-enhanced ACL reconstruction. Knee Surg Sports Traumatol Arthrosc. 2015; 23(4):1161-70..
23. Rappl LM. Effect of platelet-rich plasma gel in a physiologically relevant platelet concentration on wounds in persons with spinal cord injury. Int Wound J. 2011;8:187-95.
24. Martínez-Zapata MJ, Martí-Carvajal A, Solà I, Bolibar I, Angel Expósito J, Rodriguez L, et al. Efficacy and safety of the use of autologous plasma rich in platelets for tissue regeneration: a systematic review. Transfusion. 2009;49(1): 44-56.
25. Fukaya M, Ito A. A new economic method for preparing platelet-rich plasma. Plast Reconstr Surg Glob Open. 2014; 2:e162.
26. Dohan Ehrenfest DM, Rasmusson L, Albrektsson T. Classification of platelet concentrates: from pure platelet-rich plasma (P-PRP) to leucocyte- and platelet-rich fibrin (L-PRF). Trends Biotechnol. 2009;27(3):158-67.
27. Lee JW, Kwon OH, Kim TK, Cho YK, Choi KY, Chung HY, et al. Platelet-rich plasma: quantitative assessment of growth factor levels and comparative analysis of activated and inactivated groups. Arch Plast Surg. 2013;40(5):530-5.
28. Scherer SS, Tobalem M, Vigato E, Heit Y, Modarressi A, Hinz B, et al. Non-activated versus thrombin-activated platelets on wound healing and fibroblast-to-myofibroblast differentiation in vivo and in vitro. Plast Reconstr Surg. 2012;129(1):46e-54e.

CHAPTER 30

Platelet-rich Plasma Therapy: Indications and Procedures

Gautam K Singh, Nagendra Singh Beniwal, Swapnil Shah

KEY MESSAGES

- Platelet-rich plasma (PRP) is an autologous blood product containing a high concentration of platelets in small volume of plasma.
- PRP is increasingly becoming popular amongst dermatologists and aesthetician because of its safety, efficacy, and relatively inexpensive.
- Variety of dermatological and aesthetic indications does not have effective treatment, PRP and its variants provide ray of hope for such conditions.
- So far PRP has robust evidences for androgenetic alopecia, alopecia areata, acne scars, and chronic nonhealing ulcers.
- The PRP preparation, procedure, frequency of administration, and combinations with other aesthetic procedures are yet to be standardized and large double blind studies are required to prove its efficacy in various indications.

INTRODUCTION

Platelet-rich plasma (PRP) is an autologous blood product containing a high concentration of platelets in small volume of plasma.[1] Use of PRP in several medical disciplines such as dentistry, sports medicine, orthopedics is not new. Properties of PRP as an easy and inexpensive source of abundant growth factors have evolved its use in various dermatological and aesthetic indications such as alopecias (androgenetic alopecia, alopecia areata, telogen effluvium, and cicatricial alopecia), facial rejuvenation, acne scars, atrophic scars, facial ageing, wound healing, lipodermatosclerosis, morphea, lichen sclerosus, striae distensae, vitiligo, melasma, etc. PRP therapy when used for rejuvenation produces volumizing effect, improved skin texture as well as reduction in dyschromic pigmentation. Unlike laser or light-based therapies for various aesthetic and dermatological conditions PRP has an added advantage of almost minimal risk of postinflammatory hyperpigmentation. PRP can be safely and effectively combined with other dermatological procedures such as chemical peeling, dermabrasion, laser resurfacing, subcision, fractional microneedle radiofrequency, etc.[2,3] So far there is no FDA-approved indication in the field of dermatology or dermatosurgery but list of off label usage is ever increasing. The previous chapter has already focused on principles and methods of preparation of PRP. This chapter will describe the various indications of PRP and procedures involved in them. Overview of indications and contraindications of PRP is illustrated in **Table 1**.

TABLE 1: Indications and contraindications of PRP.[2,3]

Indications	*Contraindications*
• Hair growth—androgenetic alopecia, alopecia areata, hair transplantation • Skin rejuvenation • Tissue augmentation—contour defects, skin tightening, and lifting • Scar management—traumatic scars and acne scars • Chronic nonhealing ulcers • Lipodermatosclerosis • Striae distensae • Lichen sclerosus • *Pigmentary disorders:* Vitiligo, Melasma	*Absolute contraindications:* • Platelet dysfunction syndrome • Critical thrombocytopenia • Hemodynamic instability • Septicemia • Hypofibrinogenemia *Relative contraindications:* • Local infection at the site of the procedure • Anticoagulant use • Use of nonsteroidal anti-inflammatory drugs (NSAIDs) within 48 hours of the procedure • Corticosteroids injection in the area of treatment within a month before the procedure • Use of systemic corticosteroids • Hb <10 g/dL, or thrombocytopenia • Recent fever/flu • Chronic liver disease • Malignancies such as hematopoietic/bone

HAIR GROWTH

Platelet-rich plasma stimulates hair growth through the promotion of vascularization and angiogenesis. It also extends the duration of anagen and encourages hair follicles to enter in anagen. The process is accomplished through growth factor-mediated increased activation of wingless (Wnt)/β-catenin, extracellular signaling-regulated kinase (ERK), and protein kinase B (Akt) signaling pathways, which lead to the necessary cellular proliferation and differentiation.[4] PRP and its variants have been tried on androgenetic alopecia, alopecia areata, cicatricial alopecia, and telogen effluvium.[2,3]

Androgenetic Alopecia (Figs. 1 and 2)

Androgenetic alopecia (AGA) is a common hair loss disorder caused by genetic and hormonal factors that are characterized

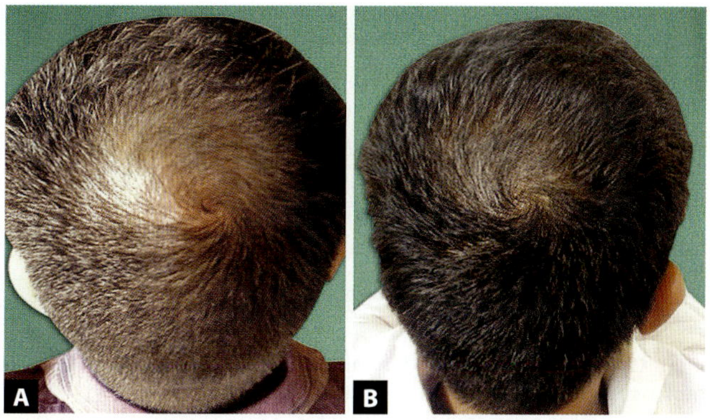

Figs. 1A and B: Platelet-rich plasma for androgenetic alopecia.
Courtesy: Dr Jagadish Gindodia.

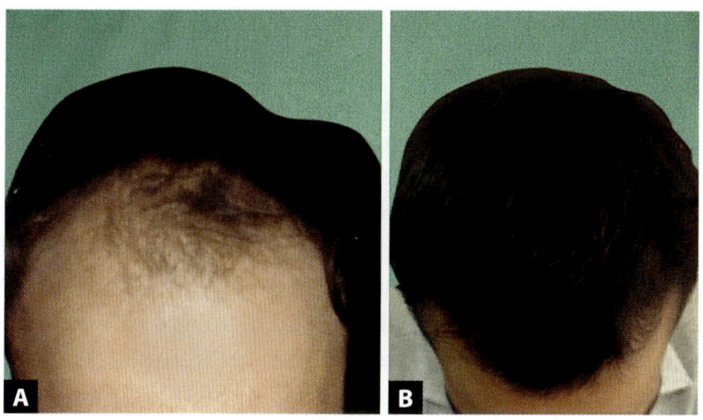

Figs. 2A and B: Platelet-rich plasma for androgenetic alopecia.
Courtesy: Dr Shankar Sawant.

by androgen-related progressive thinning of scalp hair in a defined pattern. By the age of 60 years, 45% of men and 35% of women develop AGA. Currently, US Food and Drug Administration-approved treatments for AGA include topical minoxidil lotion 5% for men, 2% for female, oral finasteride 1 mg, and light therapy. Due to the limited number of effective therapies for AGA, PRP has become an effective alternative treatment. Although, PRP does appear to be beneficial, the preparation, dosage, number, and interval of treatment sessions, as well as injection technique, vary between the studies due to a lack of standardization of PRP preparation.[5] PRP itself has undergone a generational change. PRP is the first-generation concentrate, whose growth factors (GFs) have a short life, ranging from minutes to an hour. The second-generation concentrates, whose prototype is platelet-rich fibrin (PRF) make use of the fact that platelets have a life of 7–10 days. Fibrin scaffolding helps in utilizing this property by causing a sustained release of GFs. And this scaffolding is achieved by not using an anticoagulant, but using a single-spin method in specialized tubes. This next generation PRP includes: (a) A-PRF (advanced) - Monocyte-rich PRF, (b) I-PRF (injectable), (c) CGF (concentrated GFs), (d) HAS - Hyperacute serum, and (e) T-PRF (titanium-activated).[6]

In a systemic review of PRP use in AGA compared with minoxidil, finasteride, and adult stem cell-based therapy where 12 trials were included, studies revealed total 84% of the studies reported a positive effect of PRP for AGA treatment. Among them, 50% of the studies demonstrated a statistically significant improvement using objective measures and 34% of the studies showed hair density and hair thickness improvement, although no *p* values or statistical analysis was described. In total, 17% of the studies reported greater improvement in lower-grade AGA, while 8% noted increased improvement in higher-grade AGA. Only 17% of the studies reported that PRP was not effective in treating AGA. The information analyzed highlights the positive effects of PRP on AGA, without major side effects and thus it be may considered as a safe and effective alternative procedure to treat hair loss compared with minoxidil and finasteride.[7] A study by Qu et al.[8] included patients with male and female pattern hair loss (FPHL) and concluded that PRP was effective in treating both conditions, while also improving hair texture, reducing seborrhea and inflammation, other pathomechanisms for progression of AGA. They also recommended that PRP worked best for lower grades of alopecia, namely, Grades II–III Norwood Hamilton for AGA, and Grades I–II Sinclair for FPHL. PRP has been used in hair transplantation in the following ways: (1) Adding PRP to the storage solution, (2) Bathing follicles in PRP before implantation, (3) Injecting PRP immediately after surgery, and (4) Putting PRP in the donor area. Recent studies have suggested that statistically significant improvements in hair density and stimulation of hair growth occur when follicular units are pretreated with platelet plasma GFs before implantation.[9]

Alopecia Areata

Trink et al.[10] conducted a randomized, double-blind, placebo-, and active-controlled, half-head parallel-group study to evaluate the efficacy and safety of PRP on alopecia areata (AA). A total of 45 subjects were randomized to one of three groups: PRP, triamcinolone acetonide (TAC, 2.5 mg/cm^3), or placebo. Three treatments with a 1-month interval were administered. All subjects were evaluated at baseline, 2 months, 6 months, and 12 months. The results of the study revealed that intralesional TAC and PRP resulted in significant hair regrowth in AA lesions compared with placebo or to baseline. Results were sustained at a 1-year follow-up. PRP and TAC decreased the number of dystrophic hairs as evaluated by dermoscopic findings and also minimized the itching or burning sensation of treatment. Nonetheless, PRP revealed significantly better dermoscopy results than having intralesional TAC. This study supports the use of PRP in AA to stimulate hair regrowth, especially of pigmented hairs, with a lower chance of relapse. Of note, the method of centrifugation that has been used in this study produced a platelet count that was, on average, 3.5 times higher than whole blood. No adverse effects were noted with PRP, TAC, or placebo administration.

TABLE 2: Procedure of PRP in different indications of hair growth.

Application and indications	*Anesthesia and analgesia*	*Delivery methods*	*Treatment schedule*
PRP in androgenetic alopecia and alopecia areata	Nerve block (supratrochlear/supraorbital), topical anesthesia (lidocaine cream 2% or lidocaine plus tetracaine combination cream), vibrating devices, cold compresses	Intradermal, 1 cm grid pattern (retrograde from deep to superficial	Every 4–6 weeks
PRP mesotherapy for AGA/ telogen effluvium	As above	1 mm dermaroller followed by intradermal PRP injection by mesogun, PRP spray over derma rolled area which is left overnight	3 monthly
PRP with hair transplantation	Nerve block for hair transplant or tumescent anesthesia	Follicular grafts dipped into PRP for 15 minutes before implantation—better graft survival rate; Intradermal PRP, before or after implantation for better graft uptake; PRP injection in around the donor site will help in minimizing bleeding, better wound healing, and reduce scarring	At the time of hair transplant

(AGA: androgenetic alopecia; PRP: platelet-rich plasma)

El Taieb MA et al.[11] conducted a randomized controlled study to investigate the efficacy of PRP in treating different types of alopecia areata. A total of 90 patients with patchy alopecia areata (AA) and/or alopecia totalis (AT) and/or alopecia universalis (AU) were included with ages between 10 and 40 years. The total volume of collected PRP was about 4 mL. Significant hair regrowth was noticed in patchy AA (70%) and AU (30%) after three sessions of PRP; however, AT did not respond to PRP. PRP led to significant, fully pigmented hair growth in AA lesions. Short vellus hair and yellow dots were significantly decreased after PRP treatment. Minoxidil group showed improvement of patchy AA (81%) more than AT and/or AU. Only 30% of patients in the control group experi- enced a significant hair growth of patchy AA type. Although both PRP and minoxidil 5% showed a significant increase in hair growth, subjects treated with PRP exhibited a significant decrease in short vellus hair, unlike patients treated with minoxidil and control who showed a significant increase in short vellus hair. Participants who underwent PRP treatments had better and an earlier response than participants treated with minoxidil 5% in terms of hair regrowth, reduction of short vellus hair, broken hairs, and yellow dots.

Procedure: There are various mean to use PRP to address hair growth as illustrated in **Table 2**.

AESTHETIC INDICATIONS (SKIN REJUVENATION AND TISSUE AUGMENTATION)

Platelet-rich plasma has revolutionized the aesthetic practice. Even though the evidences are not robust in various aesthetic indications but it gives opportunity to use in aesthetic conditions where the conventional methods are lacking or have unsatisfactory results. It has been marketed by various fancy names such as Vampire face lift, Kiss shot, etc. PRP has been proposed to augment collagen remodeling by stimulating the removal of photodamaged extracellular matrix (ECM) components and inducing the synthesis of new collagen by dermal fibroblasts. This is hypothesized by increased proliferation of human dermal fibroblasts, matrix metalloproteinase (MMP)-1, and MMP-3; increased removal of photodamaged ECM; increased production of procollagen type I peptide and expression of collagen type I, alpha-I which help in synthesis of new collagen and increased expression of G1 cell cycle regulators which accelerates wound healing.[12,13] Skin rejuvenation aims at defying signs of aging as well as improving skin texture, minimizing rhytides/wrinkles, volumizing effect, and reduction in dyschromic pigmentation.

Acne Scars

Currently, subcision, chemical peels, derma rollers, microneedling radiofrequency cautery (MNRF), fractional CO_2 laser, and fillers are being used extensively for treatment of acne scars either alone or in various combinations or sequentially. PRP as monotherapy is not good option. Pooja et al.[14] in a randomized controlled study compared the efficacy of fractional CO_2 monotherapy, microneedling monotherapy, and PRP intradermal injection monotherapy in post-acne scarring. Here, investigators concluded that CO_2 and microneedling monotherapy was significantly more efficacious than PRP monotherapy.

The current evidences of PRP on acne scars as an adjuvant to above procedures are quite encouraging. In a recent randomized trial for the treatment of acne scars; 90 patients separated into three treatment groups.[15] One group received microneedling, another group received intradermal PRP, and the third group was treated with alternating microneedling and intradermal PRP treatments. Though improvement was seen in all the groups, combination treatment was associated with the greatest mean improvement score, followed by microneedling, then PRP. Patient satisfaction was significantly greater in the combination group. On histology, the combination treatment yielded a thickened epidermis with more developed rete ridges compared to the single

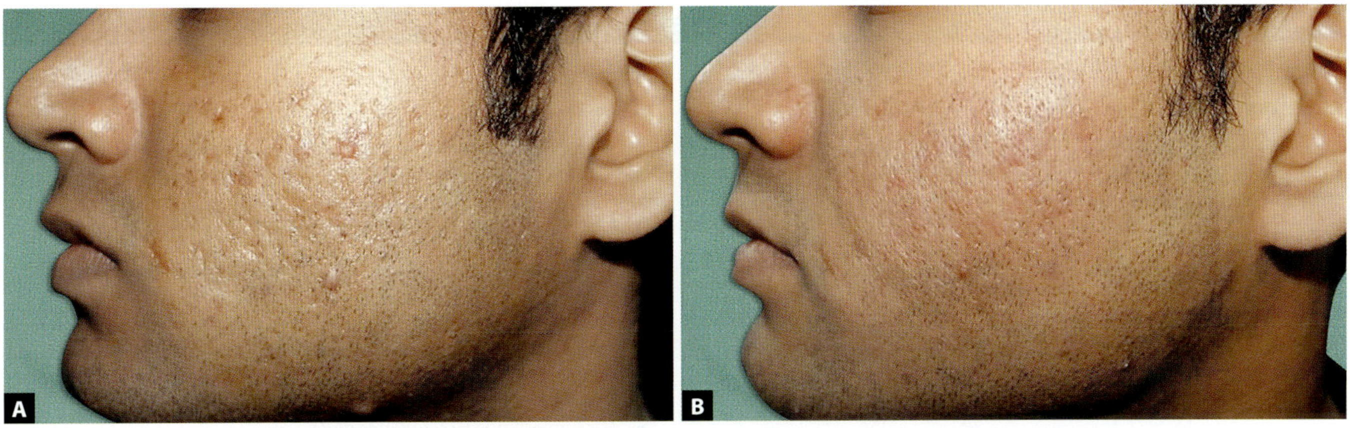

Figs. 3A and B: (A) Acne scars; (B) Post four sessions of intradermal platelet-rich plasma (PRP).

treatment modalities. In a recent meta-analysis evaluating combinations of microneedling and PRP therapy for acne scars; four randomized and 10 split-face non-randomized controlled studies with 472 patients were included. Compared to microneedling therapy without PRP, combination of microneedling and PRP was associated with increased odds of clinical improvement of >50% in Goodman's qualitative scale (GQS), and a significantly improved mean GQS score. Also, combined treatment was associated with a higher patient satisfying rate, while the incidence of severe adverse events such as severe erythema was not significantly different from each other.[16] It is recommended as an adjuvant treatment to fractional laser to decrease duration and intensity of laser associated side effects especially edema and erythema also addition to fat graft injection to avoid necrosis due to fat graft alone.[17] The result of intradermal PRP in acne scars is illustrated in **Figure 3A and B**.

Periorbital Rejuvenation

The current treatment options available for treating periorbital wrinkles, pigmentation, erythema, xerosis, loss of skin elasticity, and volume loss vary from topicals to resurfacing lasers. PRP is emerging as a promising safe and inexpensive option.[18] Kang et al.[19] reported improvement in both infraorbital wrinkles and skin tone in subjective and objective satisfaction scales in 20 Korean females when PRP was administered monthly for 3 months. Platelet-poor plasma (PPP) which is usually discarded in preparation of PRP when heated forms a gel like substance called biofiller. This biofiller is filled in glass vial of dental syringe which can be used like filler for indications like volume loss or periorbital rejuvenation. The current evidences of its use as biofiller are not encouraging, probably more reports may give us better knowledge[17] **(Table 3)**.

Striae distensae: The current evidence of PRP on striae distensae is poor. In a systemic review of 12 such studies it was observed that there was clinical and subjective improvements in patients of striae distensae without using validated scores or patient-reported outcome measures (PROMs). The main findings were that multiple treatments with platelet-rich plasma demonstrated increased epidermal thickness, rete ridges formation, and collagen/elastin formation, while decreasing the inflammatory cell infiltrate.[20]

WOUND HEALING

Platelet-rich plasma has high level of cytokines and growth factors essential for wound healing process such as platelet-derived growth factor (PDGF), epidermal growth factor (EGF), fibroblast growth factor (FGF), insulin-like growth factor (IGF_1, IGF_2), vascular endothelial growth factor (VEGF), transforming growth factor (TGF-β), and keratinocyte growth factor (KGF), etc. PRP or platelet rich fibrin (PRF) has been successfully employed for various wound healing applications, including diabetic ulcers, pressure ulcers, venous leg ulcers, refractory lipodermatosclerosis, necrobiosis lipoidica, scleroderma ulcers, trophic ulcerations of leprosy, resistant oral pemphigus vulgaris erosions, graft-versus-host disease oral ulcers, erosive oral lichen planus, pyoderma gangrenosum, ecthyma gangrenosum, ulcerated tophaceous gout, radiation dermatitis, acquired immunodeficiency syndrome-related crural ulcers, livedoid vasculopathy, and burns.[21] An evaluation by Cochrane meta-analysis on efficacy of PRP in chronic wound healing from 2016 concluded that PRP might improve healing in diabetic foot ulcers, but the evidence for other chronic wounds was not clear.[22] In a recent systematic review by Hesseler et al.[2] on PRP and chronic wounds; PRP was useful in variety of wounds. They proposed activated PRP or leukocyte-rich PRF topically applied 1–2 times weekly for 3–6 weeks for the treatment of chronic wound healing.

Procedures: Platelet-rich plasma is administered usually as leukocyte rich PRF topically applied weekly for 4–6 weeks. Leukocyte-rich PRF was used topically weekly in a traumatic nonhealing ulcer which recovered after 2 months **(Figs. 4A and B)**.

TABLE 3: Procedures of PRP in acne scars and skin rejuvenation.

Application and indications	*Anesthesia and analgesia*	*Delivery methods*	*Treatment schedule*
Acne scars			
Atrophic facial scars treated with PRP combined with fractional laser resurfacing	Topical anesthesia (lidocaine cream 2% or lidocaine plus tetracaine combination cream), vibrating devices, cold compresses	Fractional CO_2 laser/erbium YAG laser, followed by either intradermal or topical PRP; injection with 27–30 G needle, 0.02–0.3 mL per injection, 1–2 cm spacing	2–3 sessions with 3–4 weekly interval
Atrophic facial scars treated with PRP combined with microneedling and/or subcision	As above	• Intradermal/subcutaneous PRP or topical PRP before or after microneedling; 1–2 mL PRP injection administered 0.1–0.3 mL per injection with 1 cm spacing • Topical PRP approximately 0.5–2 mL; • Microneedling (192–600 needles), 1.5–2 mm size Subcision, then intradermal/subcutaneous PRP; total 1.5–3 mL PRP with 30 G needle, 0.1–0.2 mL per injection • Subcision, then microneedling, then topical PRP approximately 2 mL	2–3 sessions 3–4 weekly interval
Aesthetic indication (facial rejuvenation)			
PRP monotherapy	Topical anesthesia (lidocaine cream 2% or lidocaine plus tetracaine combination cream), vibrating devices, cold compresses, nerve block	• Intradermal/deep dermal/subdermal/ subcutaneous PRP to forehead lines, crow feet, tear troughs, marionette lines, nasolabial fold, midface, neck, or hands wrinkles • Insulin syringe or cannula, 2–6 mL total, 0.02–0.33 mL per injection, 1.5-mm to 1 cm spacing • Topical PRP serum to face	• Injectable is given 2–6 sessions every 3–4 weeks while • Topical PRP fortnightly
PRP combined with fractional laser resurfacing	As above	Intradermal PRP, then fractional CO_2 laser, then topical PPP × 20–30 minutes to cheek, periorbital area, and forehead; approximately 3 mL PRP	3 sessions every 4 weeks
PRP combined with microneedling	As above	Microneedling followed by topical PRP	3–6 sessions every 2–3 weeks
Striae distensae	Topical anesthesia	Intradermal PRP with insulin syringe, 2 mL total, 0.1 mL per injection, 1–2-cm spacing	3–6 sessions every 4 weeks

(YAG: yttrium aluminum garnet)

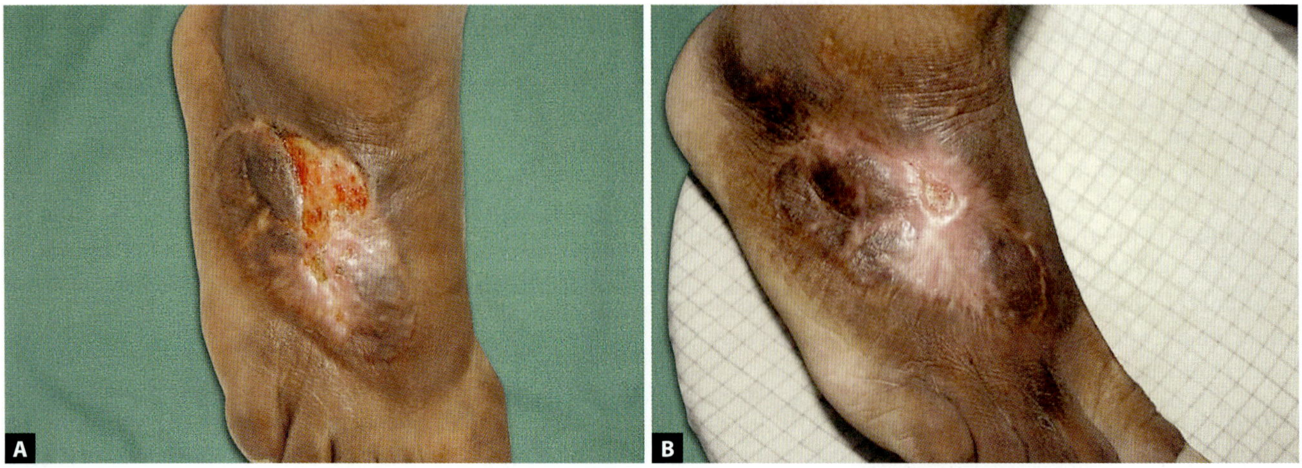

Figs. 4A and B: (A) Case of post-traumatic nonhealing ulcer; (B) Post-topical leukocyte-rich platelet-rich fibrin application after 2 months.

Lichen Sclerosus

In a five case series, intralesional PRP has been shown to alleviate symptoms, diminish lesions, reduce steroid use, and improve quality of life in patients with genital lichensclerosus.[23,24]

PIGMENTARY DISORDERS

Previous studies have shown that TGF-β1 in PRP can inhibit melanin synthesis by delaying activation of extracellular signal-regulated kinase. Concomitantly, PDGF in PRP has role to play in volumizing the skin by helping in angiogenesis, collagen synthesis, and extracellular matrix formation which results in reduced pigmentation and rejuvenation.[25]

Melasma

Currently, there are only few studies on PRP and their role in melasma. Intradermal PRP is being tried as an alternative or adjuvant therapy for melasma. In a meta-analysis and systemic review, intradermal PRP injections significantly improved chloasma as indicated by the significant decrease Melasma Area and Severity Index (MASI) and modified Melasma Area and Severity Index (mMASI) scores.[26]

In another meta-analysis on efficacy and safety of PRP in melasma which included 395 patients and compared pre- and posttreatment data from these studies revealed that the post-treatment mMASI score decreased by 1.18 (95% CI 0.89–1.47; p = 0.02). Subjective satisfaction evaluation of PRP treatment showed that melasma treated with the combination therapy of PRP + microneedling may have been the most efficacious treatment compared to PRP alone or in combination with intradermal injection.[27]

Vitiligo

Phototherapy treats vitiligo through melanocyte stimulation, migration, and increased melanin production and begins to affect the autoimmune pathway of the disease process over time. In addition to melanocytes, keratinocytes and fibroblasts as well as a multitude of inflammatory pathways are involved in vitiligo pathogenesis, and subsequent PRP stimulation of various factors may promote the differentiation, proliferation, and maturation of melanocytes and keratinocytes, leading to epidermal repigmentation.[28] PRP is a novel treatment option for vitiligo. PRP has been reported to be effective in combination with 308-nm excimer laser therapy. In a meta-analysis which included six studies involving 302 patients where phototherapy alone was compared with combination treatment with PRP and 308-nm excimer laser therapy. Combination therapy significantly improved the total response rate and reduced the no response rate. Additionally, the proportions of patients with repigmentation rates of ≥75%, ≥50%, and ≥25% were significantly higher in the combination group than in the monotherapy group. In addition, the rates of adverse events for combination therapy were comparable to those for laser therapy alone, and the recurrence rates were low.[29] In another meta-analysis where eleven studies with 670 cases were included which revealed compared with monotherapy, clinical improvement of repigmentation was significantly higher in 308-nm excimer laser combined with PRP (odds rate for response rate of 50–100% repigmentation, 4.47; 95% CI, 2.47–8.10; $p < .00001$) and in fractional carbon dioxide laser combined with PRP (mean difference for mean improvement grades of repigmentation, 1.61; 95% CI, 0.24–2.99; $p = .02$), respectively.[30] PRP is a promising treatment for stable vitiligo lesions in different body sites. The possible use of PRP in combination with traditional therapeutic options and the standardization of processing protocols represent a very fertile field for future research.

Procedure: In melasma PRP is usually administered as intradermal injection with 1 cm spacing, 2 weekly for 4–6 sessions; while in vitiligo intradermal can be combined with fractional CO_2 laser, excimer or NB-UVB D PRP with FCL, excimer, or NB-UVB 02–03 weekly for 4–6 sessions.

ANECDOTAL USAGE OF PLATELET-RICH PLASMA

There are many dermatological conditions where PRP has been used anecdotally. Single perineural injection of PRP significantly improved leprosy peripheral neuropathy in one RCT.[31] Intramatricial PRP injections showed improvement in two cases of nail dystrophy (lichen striatus and idiopathic trachyonychia) which were refractory to topical and/or intramatricial corticosteroids therapy.[32] A combination of intralesional PRP with methotrexate substantially improved PASI scores in patients of psoriasis in a prospective comparative trial.[33] Bolanča et al.[34] successfully treated a case of lichen planopilaris who has earlier failed to respond to conventional treatment.

ADVERSE EFFECTS

Platelet-rich plasmas being autologous in nature have an excellent safety profile but they are not without potential complications. Taking universal precaution, performing the procedure under total aseptic conditions is requisite of any good dermatosurgical procedures. There are always chances of mixing samples in busy center where stringent protocols are not being followed. Proper labeling of sample is mandatory to prevent interchanging of samples so to avoid exposure from harmful infective agents such as human immunodeficiency virus (HIV), hepatitis B and C infection, etc. This may invite even huge medicolegal issues on the doctors performing the PRP or related procedure. Dermatologist can use sample consent form attached as **Appendix** before starting PRP. It is always a good practice to

BOX 1: IADVL consensus statement for PRP.[17]

- P-PRP is the preferred type of PRP for facial rejuvenation while L-PRP is preferred for acne scars
- Moderate level of evidence is available in literature for PRP as a treatment modality for skin rejuvenation, acne scars, periorbital rejuvenation, lipofilling and as a combination therapy with ablative services such as fractional CO_2 laser and dermarollers
- Young patients with early signs of aging and those seeking an improvement in texture and tone by a natural, autologous treatment are the ideal patients
- PRP showed an improvement in all types of acne scars in terms of reduction in acne scar size. On visual analogue scale, rolling scars responded better to PRP as compared to boxcar and ice-pick scars
- PRP when combined with needling and subcision can be an effective treatment for even severe atrophic acne scars
- PRP in authors' experience is an excellent modality for temporary, modest improvement of periorbital area in terms of texture, pigmentation, and superficial wrinkles
- Addition of PRP to atrial flow regulator (AFR) significantly decreases the healing time, hence decreasing the chances of postinflammatory hyperpigmentation and increasing the patient satisfaction
- Bio-filler could prove to be a very cost-effective modality for treating superficial volume defects; further research is needed to establish the longevity and safety of this modality
- Intradermal PRP is the preferred mode to deliver PRP in all cases, as of today
- 3–6 sessions at monthly interval are recommended. Results are expected only after 4–6 weeks of treatment
- Topical anesthesia, nerve blocks, icing, and vibrators can be used to make the procedure comfortable for the patient
- The safety of the procedure has been established but the longevity of results is still questionable

(IADVL: Indian Association of Dermatologists, Venereologists and Leprologists; PRP: platelet-rich plasma; P-PRP: pure PRP; L-PRP: leukocyte PRP)

have baseline laboratory tests, viral markers [HIV, hepatitis B surface antigen (HBsAg), anti-hepatitis C virus antibody (HCV Ab)], venereal disease research laboratory (VDRL) test done to advise PRP session for the patients. Erythema, edema, injection site pain, bruising, scalp pruritus, transient hair shedding, cervical lymphadenopathy,[35] serum sickness[36] allergic reaction to calcium citrate preparation,[37] cutaneous sarcoidal lesions,[38] and one case of irreversible monocular blindness after glabellar injection[39] have been described as adverse effects following the PRP. Injection site pain can be minimized by usage of smaller-gauge needle, proper anesthesia (topical or regional) before the procedure or adding lidocaine, bicarbonate in PRP mixture. Anticoagulant such as ethylenediamine tetraacetic acid (EDTA), sodium citrate or ACD-A even the activator such as calcium chloride may alter the pH to acidic which may be the cause of burning or pain sensation following PRP infiltration. Bicarbonate buffer can be added to such solution to diminish the pain. But any addition or too much of handling of PRP is always associated with chances of contamination.

CONCLUSION

Platelet-rich plasma is emerging and evolving armamentarium in the hands of dermatologists. There are many dermatological disorders where nothing works, PRP has provided some hope for such situations. Lack of uniformity in preparation, machine, and procedures remains a challenge for evidence-based practice in longer run. Larger clinical trial with uniform set parameters in various dermatological conditions may provide us the actual efficacy of PRP or its variants. "IADVL consensus statement on PRP" as illustrated in **Box 1** is an attempt to highlight its indications and procedures.[17]

REFERENCES

1. Marx RE. Platelet-rich plasma (PRP): what is PRP and what is not PRP? Implant Dent. 2001;10:225-8.
2. Hesseler MJ, Shyam N. Platelet-rich plasma and its utility in medical dermatology: a systematic review. J Am Acad Dermatol. 2019;81(3):834-46.
3. Alves R, Grimalt R. A review of platelet-rich plasma: history, biology, mechanism of action, and classification. Skin Appendage Disord. 2018;4(1):18-24.
4. Li ZJ, Choi HI, Choi DK, Sohn KC, Im M, Seo YJ, et al. Autologous platelet-rich plasma: a potential therapeutic tool for promoting hair growth. Dermatol Surg. 2012;38:1040-6.
5. Stevens J, Khetarpal S. Platelet-rich plasma for androgenetic alopecia: a review of the literature and proposed treatment protocol. Int J Womens Dermatol. 2018;5(1):46-51.
6. Sharma A, Chouhan K, Bhatia S, Dashore S. Platelet-rich plasma in androgenetic alopecia. Indian Dermatol Online J. 2021;12(Suppl 1):S31-40.
7. Gentile P, Garcovich S. Systematic review of platelet-rich plasma use in androgenetic alopecia compared with Minoxidil®, Finasteride®, and adult stem cell-based therapy. Int J Mol Sci. 2020;21(8):2702.
8. Qu Q, Shi P, Yi Y, Fan Z, Liu X, Zhu D, et al. Efficacy of platelet-rich plasma for treating androgenic alopecia of varying grades. Clin Drug Investig. 2019;39:865-72.
9. Abdelkader R, Abdalbary S, Naguib I, Makarem K. Effect of platelet rich plasma versus saline solution as a preservation solution for hair transplantation. Plast Reconstr Surg Glob Open. 2020;8:e2875.
10. Trink A, Sorbellini E, Bezzola P, Rodella L, Rezzani R, Ramot Y, et al. A randomized, double-blind, placebo- and active-controlled, half-head study to evaluate the effects of platelet-rich plasma on alopecia areata. Br J Dermatol. 2013;169: 690e4.
11. El Taieb MA, Ibrahim H, Nada EA, Seif Al-Din M. Platelets rich plasma versus minoxidil 5% in treatment of alopecia areata: a trichoscopic evaluation. Dermatol Ther. 2017;30(1):e12437.
12. Kim DH, Je YJ, Kim CD, Lee YH, Seo YJ, Lee JH, et al. Can platelet-rich plasma be used for skin rejuvenation? Evaluation of effects of platelet-rich plasma on human dermal fibroblast. Ann Dermatol. 2011;23:424-31.
13. Cho JW, Kim SA, Lee KS. Platelet-rich plasma induces increased expression of G1 cell cycle regulators, type I collagen, and matrix metalloproteinase-1 in human skin fibroblasts. Int J Mol Med. 2012;29:32-6.
14. Pooja T, Gopal KV, Rao TN, Devi BG, Kumar SA. A randomized study to evaluate the efficacy fractional CO_2 laser, microneedling and platelet rich plasma in post-acne scarring. Indian Dermatol Online J. 2020;11:349-54.
15. Ibrahim ZA, EL-Ashmawy AA, Shora OA. Therapeutic effect of microneedling and autologous platelet rich plasma in

the treatment of acne scars: a randomized study. J Cosmet Dermatol. 2017;16:388-99.

16. Kang C, Lu D. Combined effect of microneedling and platelet-rich plasma for the treatment of acne scars: a meta-analysis. Front Med (Lausanne). 2022;8:788754.
17. Nanda S, Chauhan K, Shetty V, Dashore S, Bhatia S. Platelet-rich plasma in aesthetics. Indian Dermatol Online J. 2021; 12:S41-54.
18. Kassir M, Kroumpouzos G, Puja P, Katsambas A, Galadari H, Lotti T, et al. Update in minimally invasive periorbital rejuvenation with a focus on platelet rich plasma: a narrative review. J Cosmet Dermatol. 2020;19:1057-62.
19. Kang BK, Shin MK, Lee JH, Kim NI. Effects of platelet-rich plasma on wrinkles and skin tone in Asian lower eyelid skin: preliminary results from a prospective, randomised, split-face trial. Eur J Dermatol. 2014;24:100-1.
20. Sawetz I, Lebo PB, Nischwitz SP, Winter R, Schaunig C, Brinskelle P, et al. Platelet-rich plasma for striae distensae: what do we know about processed autologous blood contents for treating skin stretchmarks? A systematic review. Int Wound J. 2021;18(3):387-95.
21. White C, Brahs A, Dorton D, Witfill K. Platelet-rich plasma: a comprehensive review of emerging applications in medical and aesthetic dermatology. J Clin Aesthet Dermatol. 2021; 14(11):44-57.
22. Martinez-Zapata MJ, Martí-Carvajal AJ, Solà I, Expósito JA, Bolíbar I, Rodríguez L, et al. Autologous platelet-rich plasma for treating chronic wounds. Cochrane Database Syst Rev. 2016;2016(5):CD006899.
23. Goldstein AT, Mitchell L, Govind V, Heller D. A randomized double-blind placebo-controlled trial of autologous platelet-rich plasma intradermal injections for the treatment of vulvar lichen sclerosus. J Am Acad Dermatol. 2019;80(6): 1788-9.
24. Tedesco M, Pranteda G, Chichierchia G, Paolino G, Latini A, Orsini D, et al. The use of PRP (platelet-rich plasma) in patients affected by genital lichen sclerosus: clinical analysis and results. J Eur Acad Dermatol Venereol. 2019; 33(2):e58-9.
25. Cayirli M, Çalişkan E, Açikgoz G, Erbil AH, Erturk G. Regression of melasma with platelet-rich plasma treatment. Ann Dermatol. 2014;26:401-2.
26. Deng T, Cheng F, Guo S, Cheng H, Wu J. Application of PRP in chloasma: a meta-analysis and systematic review. Comput Intell Neurosci. 2022;2022:7487452.
27. Zhao L, Hu M, Xiao Q, Zhou R, Li Y, Xiong L, et al. Efficacy and safety of platelet-rich plasma in melasma: a systematic review and meta-analysis. Dermatol Ther (Heidelb). 2021;11(5): 1587-97.
28. Yin L, Adotama P, Svigos K, Gutierrez D, Lo Sicco K. Platelet-rich plasma, a promising adjunctive treatment for vitiligo: a case report. JAAD Case Rep. 2020;6(12):1320-22.
29. Chen J, Yu N, Li H, Tang Y, Zhu H. Meta-analysis of the efficacy of adding platelet-rich plasma to 308-nm excimer laser for patients with vitiligo. J Int Med Res. 2022; 50(9):3000605221119646.
30. Chen J, Wan Y, Lin Y, Jiang H. Current art of combination therapy with autologous platelet-rich plasma for stable vitiligo: a meta-analysis. Int Wound J. 2021;18(3):251-60.
31. Anjayani S, Wirohadidjojo YW, Adam AM, Suwandi D, Seweng A, Amiruddin MD, et al. Sensory improvement of leprosy peripheral neuropathy in patients treated with perineural injection of platelet-rich plasma. Int J Dermatol. 2014;53(1):109-13.
32. Kaur I, Jakhar D. Intramatricial platelet-rich plasma therapy: a novel treatment modality in refractory nail disorders. Dermatol Ther. 2019;32(2):e12831.
33. Chakravdhanula U, Anbarasu K, Verma VK, Beevi SS. Clinical efficacy of platelet rich plasma in combination with methotrexate in chronic plaque psoriatic patients. Dermatol Ther. 2016;29(6):446-50.
34. Bolanča Ž, Goren A, Getaldić B, Vučić M, Šitum M. Platelet-rich plasma as a novel treatment for lichen planopillaris. Dermatol Ther. 2016;29(4):233-5.
35. Stojadinovic O, Morrison B, Tosti A. Adverse effects of platelet-rich plasma and microneedling. J Am Acad Dermatol. 2020;82(2):501-2.
36. Owczarczyk-Saczonek A, Wygonowska E, Budkiewicz M, Placek W. Serum sickness disease in a patient with alopecia areata and Ménière's disease after PRP procedure. Dermatol Ther. 2019;32(2):e12798.
37. Latalski M, Walczyk A, Fatyga M, Rutz E, Szponder T, Bielecki T, et al. Allergic reaction to platelet-rich plasma (PRP): case report. Medicine (Baltimore). 2019;98(10): e14702.
38. Izhakoff N, Ojong O, Ilyas M, Guridi R, Lobos C, Druck PA, et al. Platelet-rich plasma injections and the development of cutaneous sarcoid lesions: a case report. JAAD Case Rep. 2020;6(4):348-50.
39. Kalyam K, Kavoussi SC, Ehrlich M, Teng CC, Chadha N, Khodadadeh S, et al. Irreversible blindness following periocular autologous platelet-rich plasma skin rejuvenation treatment. Ophthalmic Plast Reconstr Surg. 2017; 33(3S Suppl 1):S12-6.

APPENDIX

IADVL—Academy-Special Interest Group—Lasers and Aesthetics

Consent Form for Autologous Platelet-Rich Plasma (PRP)

Hospital/Clinic: ____________________

Patient's Name: ____________________ Age:__________

Contact No. ____________________

Address: ____________________

Indication for PRP--

I understand that PRP is an injection treatment whereby the patient's own blood is centrifuged to separate out the platelet portion that is then injected back into the skin to stimulate new collagen production and to energize the cells into rejuvenating themselves. The same process is also done for the hair to reduce hair loss and improve the hair growth.

I have been explained about maintenance treatments that may be required after completion of treatment.

The total number of treatment sessions may vary among individuals. Exact number of sessions cannot be predicted.

No guarantee, warranty, or assurance has been made to me as to the results that may be obtained. On rare occasion, there may be a patient who does not respond to treatment.

I was also informed about the other alternative methods as well as their benefits and disadvantages. I understand that for ideal results, this procedure can be combined with microneedling, laser and chemical peels, etc.

I understand the following side effects and complications may be experienced like pain, headache, stinging, mild-to-moderate swelling which may subside in 3–7 days, redness and heat, nausea, vomiting, dizziness, and transient increase in sugar levels.

I understand that variable results are seen due to the patients' lifestyle, medical profile, and age, the extent of wrinkling, extent of hair loss, smoking, sun damage, nutritional make-up, and genetic factors. The results depend on the platelet levels and the level of growth factors in these platelets which vary from person to person. I understand that the procedure is not FDA approved for cosmetic indications and approved for wound regeneration.

My medical history regarding herpes, allergy, acne, keloids, diabetes, and autoimmune disease, treatment with anticoagulants, NSAIDs, blood thinners or corticosteroids is disclosed correctly. I am not pregnant or breastfeeding.

Topical, local, or general anesthesia is required in few patients. I am ready to take the appropriate form of anesthesia.

I agree that any pictures taken of my treatment site may be used for publication or teaching purposes; however, my name or identity will not be disclosed, and complete confidentiality will be maintained.

By signing below, I acknowledge that I have read the adverse reactions as mentioned above and I feel that I have been adequately informed of the risks of platelet-rich plasma treatment.

Before each treatment, I will inform the doctor if I have taken any new medications since my last treatment.

I also agree to comply with the recommended aftercare instructions.

I hereby release Dr.................................... and its designated staff from liability associated with the above procedure.

My questions regarding the procedure have been answered satisfactorily.

I authorize Dr.................................... and his/her designated staff to perform platelet-rich plasma treatment on my body.

The payment and fee structure are informed to me. I am ready to pay per sitting or package basis. (Package if opted for includes minimum number of sittings and I have to pay accordingly if more sittings are required).

Signature of Patient/Thumb Impression

Signature of Parents/Guardian (For Minors) Date:......................................

______________________________________ Date:......................................

Name and Relationship if Signed by other than Parent

Witness:______________________________________

Name:______________________________ Signature_________________________ Date:......................................

Signature of Doctor:______________________________________ Date:......................................

Translated in Patients' Language by:______________________________________

CHAPTER 31

Microdermabrasion

Silonie Sachdeva

KEY MESSAGES

- Microdermabrasion (MDA) is a simple, safe, and commonly used treatment modality for treating photo damage, superficial acne scars, and dyschromias.
- Both aluminum oxide and diamond MDA methods are used.
- The treatment yields mild, but measurable improvement after repeated sessions.

INTRODUCTION

Microdermabrasion (MDA), also known as microresurfacing, is a dermatosurgical procedure used for mechanical exfoliation of skin. MDA is commonly referred to as skin polishing/body polishing and uses a mechanical medium as aluminum oxide crystals at high pressure to remove the outermost layer of stratum corneum from the epidermis. It is a painless and noninvasive procedure, performed in office by a dermatologist, which has become popular because of the ease of its technique, safety, and versatility of its application.

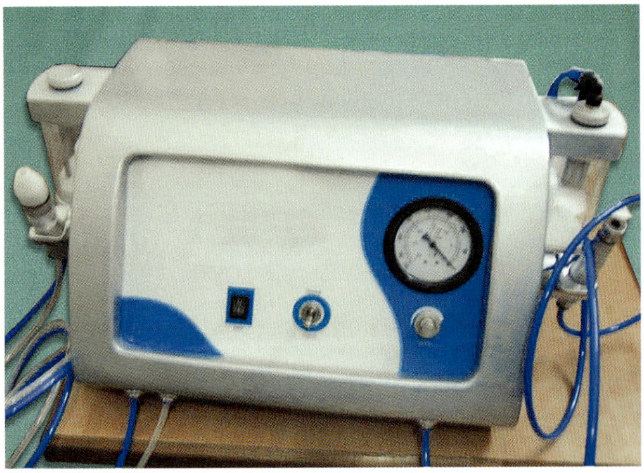

Fig. 1: Aluminum oxide microdermabrasion unit.

HISTORY OF MICRODERMABRASION

The history of MDA dates back to ancient Egyptian literature in which royal ladies used to sandblast their skin with various abrasive materials such as pumice stones, rocks, and shells to achieve skin resurfacing. This was the traditional way for facial rejuvenation. The first scientific use of MDA began in Europe in 1985 when Marini and Lo Brutto developed a close loop system with aluminum oxide crystals for exfoliation.[1] Since then MDA has become a popular dermatological procedure for noninvasive superficial skin resurfacing and has undergone many modifications in the machine and procedure **(Figs. 1 and 2)**.[2] Recent modifications in the machine included change in the medium for exfoliation. The first diamond tip MDA unit was introduced in 1999 and the bristle tip introduced in 2005.

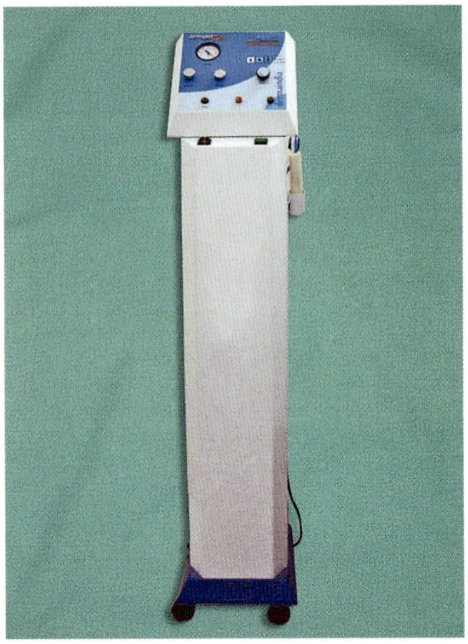

Fig. 2: Portable aluminum oxide microdermabrasion unit with wheels.

HISTOPATHOLOGICAL CHANGES IN MICRODERMABRASION

The changes in both epidermis and dermis after MDA are given in **Box 1**.

BOX 1: Histopathological changes after microdermabrasion.

- *Epidermis:*
  - Thinning of stratum corneum
  - Thickening of epidermis via stimulation of basal keratinocytes
  - Even and regular distribution of melanosomes with less melanization of epidermis
- *Dermis:*
  - Thickening of dermis
  - Focal compaction and homogenization of collagen
  - Formation of new collagen and elastin in dermis
  - Vascular ectasia

Histological Changes in Epidermis

The effects have been assessed ex-vivo on human abdominal skin. Early histological changes include thinning of stratum corneum. Retention of aluminum oxide crystals[3] has been observed on the surface of the stratum corneum. With repeated MDA sessions, thickening of the epidermis occurs due to stimulation of basal keratinocytes. There is more regular distribution of melanosomes, less melanization of the epidermis, and basal cell liquefaction.

There is decrease in transepidermal water loss (TEWL) due to improved epidermal barrier function.[4]

Histological Changes in Dermis

They include thickening of dermis with focal compaction and homogenization of collagen in papillary dermis, flattening of the rete pegs, vascular ectasia, and perivascular inflammation with deposition of new collagen and elastic fibers.[5,6] Coarse-grit crystal-free MDA induced a wound healing response characterized by rapid increase in induction of cytokeratin 16 and activation of the AP-1 transcription factor in the epidermis. AP-1 activation was followed by matrix metalloproteinase-mediated degradation of extracellular matrix. Consistent with this wound healing response, there was increased induction of Type I and Type III procollagen in dermis.[7] The skin's surface is disrupted; cell division occurs which stimulates fibroblast activity leading to increased collagen production. An improved lipid barrier functions through increased ceramide levels in the stratum corneum after MDA has been found after the second and third sessions.[8] The resulting change in the lipid barrier might be responsible for the improved texture and overall appearance of the skin following MDA.

MICRODERMABRASION UNIT AND ITS WORKING

Technical Aspects

The conventional MDA machine is based on use of aluminum oxide crystals for dermabrasion. These crystals are 100 µm in size, inert, nontoxic, and noncarcinogenic. They cause no adverse reaction on skin and are safe to use. Because of their smaller size, they do not carry any risk of inhalation. Besides, these crystals are insoluble in both water and organic solvents.

The unit consisted of the basic apparatus with a vacuum meter. Two plastic containers with closed flexible tubes are attached to the main body. These tubes open into the units hand piece and form a closed loop system. During the procedure, crystals are released through one tube on skin for micro-resurfacing and collected by the second tube. Other crystals used in MDA include sodium chloride, sodium bicarbonate, and magnesium oxide crystals.[9]

Diamond Tome Microdermabrasion

The next-generation MDA unit was the diamond tome MDA. This technique consists of treating the skin with a device that has rotating tips embedded with small diamonds. The tip is connected to a noiseless electric engine that generates suction for removing the dead skin cells through a flexible tube. The tips are interchangeable, with wands of different sizes (fine, medium, and coarse) so the dermatologist may choose the adequate grade for each case. The diamond tome MDA has several advantages over aluminum oxide MDA as natural diamond tips are easier to use, cause less irritation, and do not leave tiny crystal particles in the eyes, nose, or mouth. The skin barrier function of the forehead and cheek recovers within 2 days of diamond MDA.[10,11]

INDICATIONS FOR MICRODERMABRASION

- *Facial rejuvenation*: Microdermabrasion is useful in treating both aging and photoaging changes. Microscopic changes after MDA include increased hyalinization of the papillary dermis with newly deposited collagen fibers.
- *Acne scars*: Microdermabrasion is used in treatment of grade I acne associated with mild-to-moderate scarring.[12] However, the effects are mild and hence the technique should be used after proper counseling.
- *Dyschromias:* Hyperpigmentation includes melasma and postinflammatory hyperpigmentation. For best results, it is advocated that MDA is used in combination with topical bleaching agents.
- *Periorbital wrinkles:* Microdermabrasion improves the appearance of periorbital and perioral wrinkles caused due to repeated contractions of muscles.[13,14]
- *Striae:* It has been found that 10–20 sessions of MDA at an interval of not <1 month, with each session ending in bleeding points, results in some improvement in striae.[15]
- *To increase the rate of transepidermal delivery of drugs:* Microdermabrasion increases the transepidermal delivery of drugs. The flux and skin deposition of topical drugs as vitamin C increases 20-fold higher in MDA-treated skin than that across intact skin.[16]

- *Opening of blocked pores*: MDA is used widely to open blocked pores and improve the appearance of skin making it look smoother and of uniform texture.[3,5]

ANECDOTAL USES OF MICRODERMABRASION

Microdermabrasion has been used to create suction blisters for vitiligo grafting.[17] It has been tried with varying success in combination with pimecrolimus 1% cream to treat non-segmental childhood vitiligo[18] and on localized areas in adults **(Box 2)**.[19]

ADVANTAGES OF MICRODERMABRASION

- Conservative MDA (limited to papillary dermis) can be performed safely on all Fitzpatrick skin types.[3,5]
- No anesthesia is required.
- Microdermabrasion is a noninvasive and painless technique. Only, a mild pleasant tickling sensation is felt during the treatment. MDA does not irritate the skin.
- There is little or no downtime.
- It is well accepted by patients.
- It is safe to use during pregnancy and lactation.

BOX 2: Uses of microdermabrasion.

Well-established indications, known to yield satisfactory response:
- Facial rejuvenation
- Photoaging
- Transepidermal delivery of drugs

Useful in selected cases, known to yield moderate response:
- Acne and acne scarring **(Figs. 3 and 4)**
- Stretch marks **(Figs. 5 to 7)**
- Post-traumatic scars with duration <6 months
- Keratosis pilaris

Mild or doubtful response:
- Melasma
- Postinflammatory hyperpigmentation

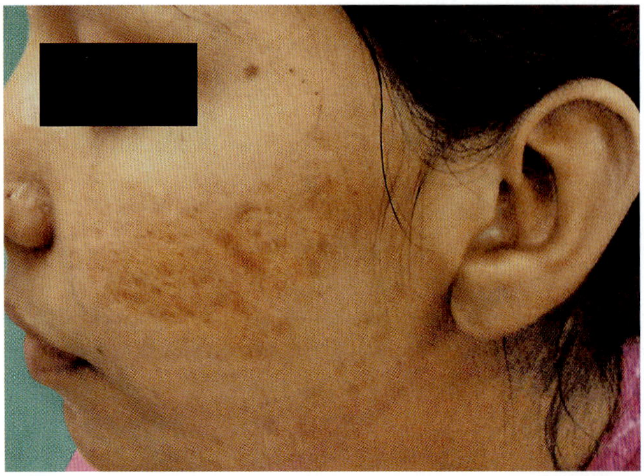

Fig. 3: Patient with acne scarring.

CONTRAINDICATIONS

There are very few contraindications.

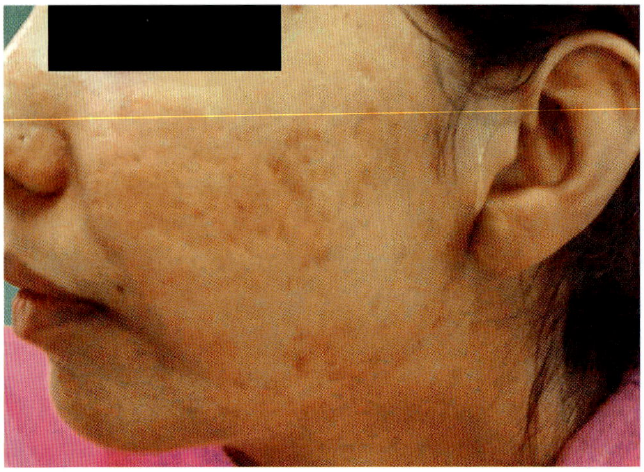

Fig. 4: Same patient showing improvement after two sessions with microdermabrasion.

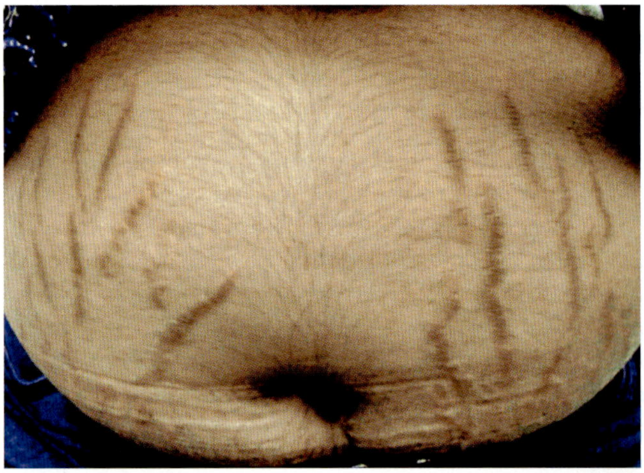

Fig. 5: A 20-year-old female patient with stretch marks on abdomen.

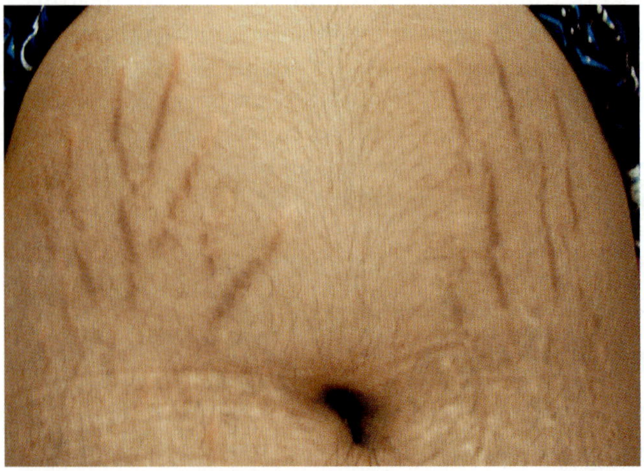

Fig. 6: Same patient immediately after microdermabrasion session showing mild erythematous changes.

Relative

Rosacea and telangiectasia.

Absolute

- Active infections, bacterial or viral including herpes simplex and verruca plana
- Skin ulcers and erosions
- Chronic skin diseases as lupus erythematosus, psoriasis, and eczema
- *Intake of oral isotretinoin*: For all resurfacing procedures, a waiting period of 6–12 months has been recommended in past.[20] However, several experts perform this procedure safely when the patient is being administered isotretinoin (personal communication). It has been suggested that abrasion of a small test area may be a useful predictor of wound healing, for earlier treatment using resurfacing[21]
- Pustular or cystic acne
- History of hypertrophic scarring or keloids
- History of radiation therapy to the head or facial surgery within 2 months
- Prophylaxis for herpes simplex should be given in case of known case of recurrent herpes simplex.

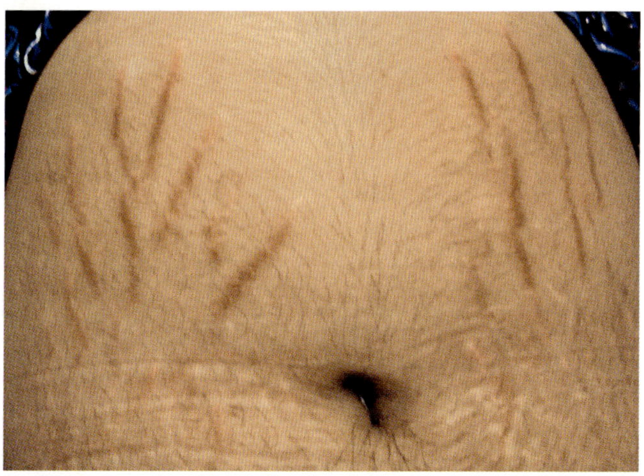

Fig. 7: Same patient with improvement in stretch marks after eight sessions.

PREOPERATIVE PREPARATION, PREPROCEDURE COUNSELING, CONSENT, AND PHOTOGRAPHY

Patient should be counseled for the number of sessions required, results expected, immediate effect on the skin after MDA, and what to expect while procedure is being done. Patient should be made to sign a consent form explaining the procedure and possible side effects. Preprocedure and postprocedure photographs should be taken at every session. It should be well emphasized that MDA is a mild procedure, aimed at giving only mild improvements and patients should have realistic expectations.

Patient Preparation

- Male patients should be asked to shave before MDA session of full face.
- No anesthesia is required as procedure is tolerated comfortably by most patients.
- Patient should be made to lie down on procedure table.
- Hair should be pulled back and covered with a head cap.
- Eyes should be closed during the procedure. They can also be covered with adhesive ocular shields.

Procedural Techniques

The first step is proper cleansing of the face with a mild gentle cleanser. Alternatively, patient can be instructed to thoroughly clean the face with a mild gentle cleanser before lying down on the table for the procedure. MDA should be started at a low vacuum and a moderate speed keeping in mind patient's comfort and required depth of treatment **(Table 1)**.

The hand piece should be properly sterilized to prevent any cross contamination. The power switch of the unit is switched on. The vacuum pressure is adjusted between 15 and 30 mm Hg. The skin to be treated is stretched between thumb and index finger of left hand of the operator and handpiece is held in right hand perpendicular to the skin surface. The handpiece is moved along specific lines of treatment on the area **(Figs. 8 and 9)**. Fresh aluminum oxide crystals or diamond

TABLE 1: Various parameters of microdermabrasion for each indication.

Indication	*Vacuum/pressure (in mm Hg)*	*Average no. of sessions required*	*Interval between two sessions (in weeks)*	*Level of ablation*
Facial rejuvenation	10–20	4	1–2	Epidermal
Acne scarring	15–25	6–8	1–2	Dermal
Fine lines, wrinkles	10–25	4–6	1–2	Epidermal
Pigmentation (epidermal) as melasma	15–25	6–8	2–4	Epidermal to superficial dermal
Stretch marks	15–30	8–10	2–4	Dermal

tips are used for dermabrasion. The skin is pulled in as the handpiece is moved and becomes little erythematous. During MDA, the used crystals, epidermal debris, and grime are collected by the second tube of the handpiece and brought back to second plastic container. The operator can adjust the intensity of the treatment by increasing or decreasing the suction pressure. Single or multiple pass may be used depending on the depth to be reached. For deep acne scars, dermabrasion is done at higher intensity with multiple passes till pinpoint bleeding points are seen. A standard session usually consists of one to three passes. The procedure may take between 15 and 30 minutes full for face. Repeat sessions may be done at weekly intervals till satisfactory results are achieved.

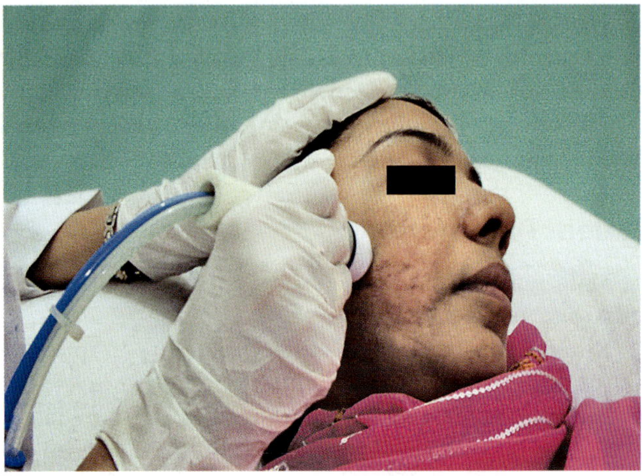

Fig. 8: Microdermabrasion procedure.

Postprocedure Instructions

- Patient should be advised to apply a sunscreen after the procedure and use a sunscreen regularly.
- For daily regimen, mild soap can be used on treated skin followed by a moisturizer.
- Facial bleach should be avoided on MDA-treated skin.
- Light make up can be done, if required. Harsh cosmetics should not be used on skin.

FACTORS AFFECTING THE LEVEL OF REMOVAL OF EPIDERMIS OR DERMIS DURING MICRODERMABRASION

The extent of stratum corneum removed during MDA depends strongly on the crystal flow rate and exposure time and weakly

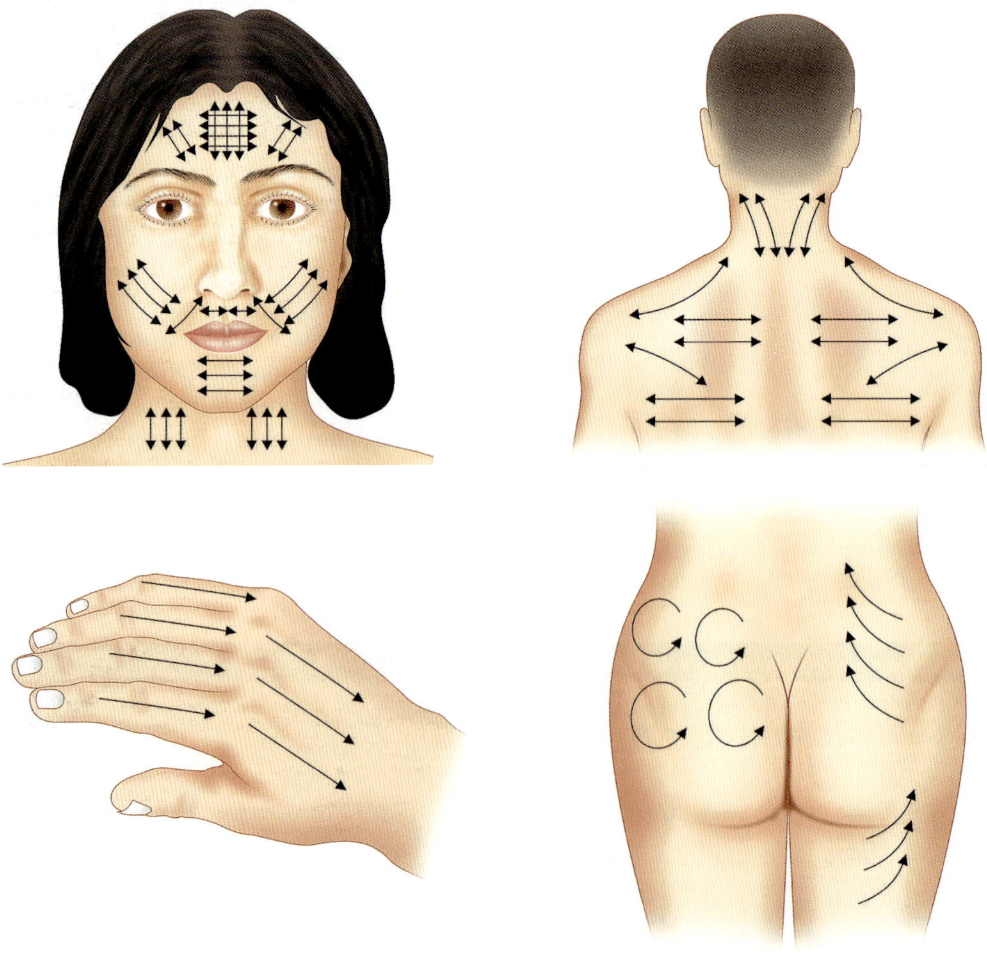

Fig. 9: Schematic representation of lines of movement while doing microdermabrasion.

on pressure. Slower movement of the handpiece (allowing longer contact of the abrasive crystals with the skin) and more passes achieve deeper abrasion.[5] Crystals are available in different sizes like 100, 130, and 180 μm. Though it is thought that the bigger the size of the crystal, greater is the depth of abrasion. This view, however, is not universally accepted.[5] Conservative MDA causes partial skin ablation. These effects are similar to superficial chemical peels.[3,5]

COMPLICATIONS

- Microdermabrasion is a relatively mild procedure with no significant on table or after procedure complications.[22]
- Mild transient erythema is common and does not need any treatment.
- Petechia or purpura may appear if vacuum pressure is too high and if there is history of severe sun damage.
- Streak lines may appear on face temporarily if handpiece is held too hard on the skin.[3,5]
- Postinflammatory pigmentation can occur after aggressive MDA session, particularly in skin of color.
- There is increased skin sensitivity, especially photosensitivity. Ultraviolet protective measures such as broad-spectrum sunscreens and topical bleaching agents can be used prophylactically.
- Ocular complications occur if proper eye shielding is not used and if aluminum crystals enter the eye, which include irritation, chemosis, photophobia, and punctate keratitis.[23]
- Superficial abrasions also called striping, due to characteristic lines or stripes seen in aggressive treatments.
- One case of unusual urticarial response in a patient has been reported so far.[24] However, this patient had a history of dermographism. Possible cause also included reaction to latex exposure from the MDA unit.
- *Eruptive self-resolving keratoacanthomas may develop after treatment with photodynamic therapy (PDT) and* MDA.[25]

Combination with Other Aesthetic Procedures

- Microdermabrasion is a versatile procedure and can be safely combined with several other aesthetic procedures.
- *Microdermabrasion with chemical peel:* Microdermabrasion has been combined with a trichloroacetic acid peel to improve the appearance of moderate deep rhytids, acne scars, and photodamaged skin.[26] MDA may be used prior to the superficial glycolic acid peel to increase the exfoliation and antiaging effects of both treatments within the same visit.[27] MDA followed by a 5% retinoid acid chemical peel has been used for the treatment of photoaging.[28]
- *Microdermabrasion and lasers:* Microdermabrasion has been combined with lasers in the same session for treatment of various types of skin including treatment of acne scars.[29] MDA has been used with the 1,450-nm diode laser for the treatment of inflammatory facial acne.[30,31]
- *Microdermabrasion preceding aminolevulinic acid-photodynamic therapy:* Topical 5-aminolevulinic acid (ALA) and PDT have been used to treat actinic keratoses and acne.[32] Consistent superior results have been obtained with the use of MDA prior to the application of ALA for 10 minutes. It appears that incubation of ALA with MDA for 10 minutes is as effective as, or more so than, ALA applied alone for 1 hour in producing erythema.
- *Application of topical antioxidant prior to microdermabrasion:* This maneuver enhances the effect of facial MDA.[33]
- *Microdermabrasion with botox and dermal fillers:* Microdermabrasion can be combined with botox injections for wrinkles and dermal fillers in the same session.
- *Transdermal delivery of drugs:* Microdermabrasion appears to enhance the absorption of hydrophilic substances across the lipophilic epidermal barrier.[34]
  - *Insulin in diabetes mellitus:*[35] Transdermal *insulin* delivery is an attractive needle-free alternative to subcutaneous injection conventionally used to treat diabetes
  - 2% kojic acid, vitamin C
  - 5-fluorouracil (5-FU), clobetasol17-propionate[36] in case of vitiligo
  - *5-aminolevulinic acid:* Microdermabrasion before application of 5-ALA also appears to speed up the acid's absorption, shortening incubation times from hours to potentially minutes
  - Pimecrolimus 1% in nonsegmental vitiligo[19]
  - Nicotinamide[37]
  - *Vaccine delivery across the skin:* More recently, human trials have addressed vaccination against traveler's diarrhea and influenza.[34]
- *Microdermabrasion with ultrasound-induced phonophoresis*: In photodamaged skin[38]
- *Light-emitting diodes (LED) and microcurrent with MDA*: Blue-light LED are used in inflammatory acne and red-light LED for photoaging to enhance collagen production.

CRYSTAL-FREE MICRODERMABRASION

Ultrasonic Microdermabrasion

These devices use a dull spatula blade with ultrasonic vibration to disrupt the stratum corneum.[39]

Ultrasound Phonophoration

Phonophoresis, also known as sonophoresis, relies on a quartz crystal within a transducer emitting acoustic ultrasonic pressure waves in response to an alternating current.

It has been postulated that the resulting waves impart on the stratum corneum, the principal biologic barrier to exogenous substances, certain chemical, thermal, and mechanical changes that are conducive to absorption. Some of these alterations are attributed to cavitation, a process that involves formation, growth, and collapse of gaseous cavities within the extracellular lipid component of the outermost skin layer. This phenomenon introduces channels of decreased resistance within the through stratum corneum for substances to penetrate through.[40] Ultrasound has also been shown to dilate and straighten the eccrine ducts and coils, promoting transepidermal transport. Sonophoresis has been shown to enhance cutaneous penetration of large molecules, such as erythropoietin, insulin, interferon-c, and topical steroids.[39]

Hydradermabrasion

Hydradermabrasion is also called as hydrafacial or jet peel or oxypeel. It works in the same manner as MDA but instead of exfoliating with propelled microcrystals, hydradermabrasion uses a combination of oxygen and aqueous solutions at supersonic speeds to remove debris and dead cells that are then suctioned away.[40-42] This new modality is novel as the treatment is exfoliating the epidermis, it is also hydrating the skin within the same treatment pass. This supersonic microdroplet jet results in a pressured widening of microcanals in the outer skin layers that facilitate greater hydration and cleansing of the skin. This moisturizing component allows for less irritation, reduced discomfort, and quicker recovery. Solutions and serums can also be formulated allowing better cleansing, extraction, and exfoliation while possessing antioxidant properties targeting specific skin types, textures, and conditions which cannot be delivered with traditional microdermabrasion.[43,44] Hydradermabrasion has the same indications for use as microdermabrasion making it an excellent choice for persons with darker skin tones, aging skin, sensitive skin areas, oily, and dry skin complexions. Histological examination revealed increased epidermal and papillary dermal thickness as well as greater antioxidant levels with replacement of elastic dermal tissue, collagen hyalinization, and fibroblast density correlating with a decrease in the appearance of fine lines, pore size, and hyperpigmentation in hydradermabrasion. Hydradermabrasion treatment is effective at improving skin quality by adding hydration, oxygen, and antioxidants to the exfoliated skin and thus should be considered an alternative to microdermabrasion **(Fig. 10)**.[45]

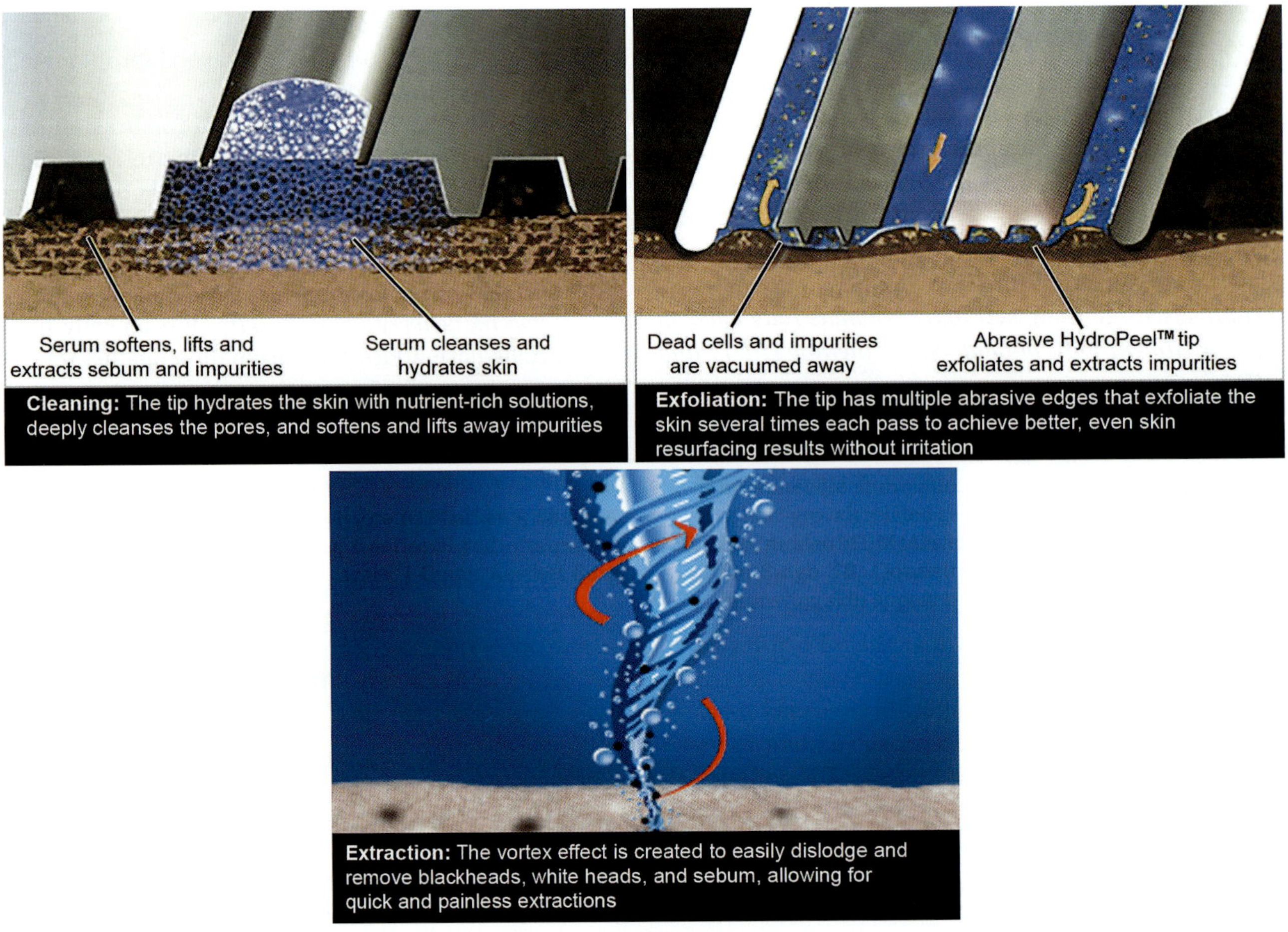

Fig. 10: Mechanism of hydradermabrasion on skin.

SILKPEEL DERMAINFUSION

SilkPeel is a unique dermal infusion process that combines microdermabrasion with two other processes to make it more effective. Dermal infusion combines gentle suction with a diamond-tipped wand to buff away damaged skin while also cleansing the skin of pore-clogging debris. During the same procedure, specialized topical medications are applied to this newly rejuvenated skin, amplifying the results. This three-in-one process is what makes dermal infusion the next step-up from a typical microdermabrasion.

SilkPeel dermal infusion has provided a gentle, painless, and convenient option for patients who want clearer, brighter, more youthful skin.

SUMMARY OF PEARLS

- MDA is a simple, noninvasive, painless in office procedure.
- It can be used for facial rejuvenation, photoaging, acne, fine wrinkles, transepidermal delivery of drugs, etc.
- It is a popular procedure because of its ease of techniques, safety, and less downtime.

REFERENCES

1. Spencer JM. Microdermabrasion. Am J Clin Dermatol. 2005;6:89-92.
2. Tsai RY, Wang CN, Chn HL. Aluminium oxide crystal microdermabrasion: a new technique for treating facial scarring. Dermatol Surg. 1995;21:539-42.
3. Whitaker E, Yarbourough JM. Microdermabrasion. [online] Available from: emedicine.medscape.com/article/843957-overview. [Last accessed July, 2022].
4. Freedman BM, Rueda-Pedraza E, Waddell SP. The epidermal and dermal changes associated with microdermabrasion. Dermatol Surg. 2001;27:1031-3.
5. Rajan P, Grimes P. Skin barrier changes induced by aluminium oxide and sodium chloride microdermabrasion. Dermatol Surg. 2002;28:390-3.
6. Shim EK, Barnette D, Hughes K, Greenway HT. Microdermabrasion: a clinicopathologic study. Dermatol Surg. 2001;27:524-30.
7. Hernandez-Perez E, Ibiett EV. Gross and microscopic findings in patients undergoing microdermabrasion for facial rejuvenation. Dermatol Surg. 2001;27:637-40.
8. Karimipour DJ, Rittié L, Hammerberg C, Min VK, Voorhees JJ, Orringer JS, et al. Molecular analysis of aggressive microdermabrasion in photoaged skin. Arch Dermatol. 2009; 145:1114-22.
9. Savardekar P. Microdermabrasion. Indian J Dermatol Venereol Leprol. 2007;73:277-9.
10. Lew BL, Cho Y, Lee MH. Effect of serial microdermabrasion on the ceramide level in the stratum corneum. Dermatol Surg. 2006;32:376-9.
11. Kim HS, Lim SH, Song JY, Kim MY, Lee JH, Park JG, et al. Skin barrier function recovery after diamond microdermabrasion. J Dermatol. 2009;36:529-33.
12. Llyod JR. The use of microdermabrasion for acne: a pilot study. Dermatol Surg. 2001;27:329-31.
13. Coimbra M, RohrichRJ, Chao J, Brown SA. A prospective controlled assessment of microdermabrasion for damaged skin and fine rhytides. Plast Reconstr Surg. 2004;113:143843.
14. Glaser DA, Patel U. Enhancing the eyes: use of minimally invasive techniques for periorbital rejuvenation. J Drugs Dermatol. 2010;9:118-28.
15. Tehrani R. Microdermabrasion for striae distensae. Indian J Dermatol Venereol Leprol. 2006;72:59.
16. Lee WR, Shen SC, Kuo-Hsien W, Hu CH, Fang JY. Lasers and microdermabrasion enhance and control topical delivery of vitamin C. J Invest Dermatol. 2003;121:1118-25.
17. Kaliyadan F, Manoj J, Venkitakrishnan S. Using a microdermabrasion machine as a suction blister device. Indian J Dermatol Venereol Leprol. 2008;74:392-3.
18. Farajzadeh S, Daraei Z, Esfandiarpour I, Hosseini SH. The efficacy of pimecrolimus 1% cream combined with microdermabrasion in the treatment of nonsegmental childhood vitiligo: a randomized placebo-controlled study. Pediatr Dermatol. 2009;26:286-91.
19. Hossani-Madani AR, Halder RM. Topical treatment and combination approaches for vitiligo: new insights, new developments. G Ital Dermatol Venereol. 2010;145:57-78.
20. Riveria AE. Acne scarring: A review and current treatment modalities. J Am Acad Dermatol. 2008;59:659-76.
21. Bagatin E, dos Santos Guandanhim LR, Yarak S, Kamamoto CSL, de Almeida FA. Dermabrasion for acne scars during treatment with oral isotretinoin. Dermatol Surg. 2010;36: 483-9.
22. Farris PK, Rietschel RL. An unusual acute urticarial response following microdermabrasion. Dermatol Surg. 2002;28: 606-8.
23. Spencer JM, Kurtz ES. Approaches to document the efficacy and safety of microdermabrasion procedure. Dermatol Surg. 2006;32:1353-7.
24. Gogia R, Grekin RC, Shinkai K. Eruptive self-resolving keratoacanthomas developing after treatment with photodynamic therapy and microdermabrasion. Dermatol Surg. 2013;39:1717-20.
25. Morgenstern KE, Foster JA. Advances in cosmetic oculoplastic surgery. Curr Opin Ophthalmol. 2002;13:324-30.
26. Kisner AM. Microdermabrasion with chemical peel. Aesthet J. 2001;21:191-3.
27. Briden E, Jacobsen E, Johnson C. Combining superficial glycolic acid (alpha-hydroxy acid) peels with microdermabrasion to maximize treatment results and patient satisfaction. Cutis. 2007;79:13-6.
28. Hexsel D, Mazzuco R, Dal'Forno T, Zechmeister D. Microdermabrasion followed by a 5% retinoid acid chemical peel vs. a 5% retinoid acid chemical peel for the treatment of photoaging—a pilot study. J Cosmet Dermatol. 2005;4:111-6.
29. Franz R. Laser therapy and microdermabrasion treat acne scars. Dermatol Nurs. 2001;13:396.
30. Wang SQ, Counters JT, Flor ME, Zelickson BD. Treatment of inflammatory facial acne with the 1,450 nm diode laser alone versus microdermabrasion plus the 1,450 nm laser: a randomized, split-face trial. Dermatol Surg. 2006;32:249-55.
31. Katz BE, Truong S, Maiwald DC, Frew KE, George D. Efficacy of microdermabrasion preceding ALA application in reducing the incubation time of ALA in laser PDT. J Drug Dermatol. 2007;6:140-2.
32. Freedman BM. Topical antioxidant application enhances the effects of facial microdermabrasion. J Dermatolog Treat. 2009;20:82-7
33. Glenn GM, Flyer DC, EllingsworthL R, Frech SA, Frerichs DM, Seid RC, et al. Transcutaneous immunization with heat-labile enterotoxin: development of a needle-free vaccine patch. Expert Rev Vaccines. 2007;6:809-19.

34. Andrews S, Lee JW, Choi SO, Prausnitz MR. Transdermal insulin delivery using microdermabrasion. Pharm Res. 2011;28:2110-8.
35. Lee WR, Tsai RY, Fang CL, Liu CJ, Hu CH, Fang JY. Microdermabrasion as a novel tool to enhance drug delivery via the skin: an animal study. Dermatol Surg. 2006;32:1013-22.
36. Yingcong ZBS, Banga AK. Enhanced delivery of cosmeceuticals by microdermabrasion. 2011;10:179-84.
37. DudelzakJ, Hussain M, Phelps RG, Gottlieb GJ, Goldberg DJ. Evaluation of histologic and electron microscopic changes after novel treatment using combined microdermabrasion and ultrasound induced phonophoresis of human skin. J Cosmet Laser Ther. 2008;10:187-92.
38. Tang H, Mitragotri S, Blankschtein D, Langer R. Theoretical description of transdermal transport of hydrophilic permeants: application to low-frequency sonophoresis. J Pharm Sci. 2001;90:545-68.
39. Ting WW, Vest CD, Sontheimer RD. Review of traditional and novel modalities that enhance the permeability of local therapeutics across the stratum corneum. Int J Dermatol. 2004;43:538-47.
40. Freedman BM. Hydradermabrasion: an innovative modality for nonablative facial rejuvenation. J Cosmet Dermatol. 2008;7:275-80.
41. Khalaj B, Khalaj BM. (2007). Hydrodermabrasion apparatus and method of use. United States patent US 20070239173 A1;2007. [online] Available from: https://www.freepatentsonline.com/y2007/0239173.html. [Last accessed July, 2022].
42. Rosso L, Lica SRL. Device for making hydro-microabrasions on human tissue. United States patent US 6432114 B1; 2002.
43. Waldron SH, Kent P; Altair Instruments Inc. Device for applying liquid skincare products in combination with vacuum and abrasion. United States patent US 8221437 B2.l;2012. [online] Available from: https://patents.google.com/patent/ US20110295273. [Last accessed July, 2022].
44. Burke KE. Photodamage of the skin: Protection and reversal with topical antioxidants. J Cosmetic Dermatol. 2004;3: 149-55.
45. Loesch MM, SomaniA, Kingsley MM, Travers JB, Spandau DF. Skin resurfacing procedures: new and emerging options. 2014;7:231-41

CHAPTER 32

Sclerotherapy

S Sacchidanand, TS Nagesh, Sujala S Aradhya

KEY MESSAGES

- Sclerotherapy refers to the introduction of a sclerosing solution into the lumen of a vessel producing endothelial damage and subsequent fibrosis.
- Sclerotherapy consists of liquid sclerotherapy and foam sclerotherapy.
- Indications include varicose veins, telangiectasia, and cysts.
- Smaller veins respond better to sclerotherapy.

INTRODUCTION

Sclerotherapy refers to the introduction of a foreign substance (sclerosing solution) into the lumen of a vessel producing endothelial damage, which leads to thrombosis and subsequent fibrosis. The extent of damage to the blood vessel wall determines the effectiveness of the solution. Sclerotherapy has been extensively used by dermatosurgeons in the management of superficial varicose veins and other venous abnormalities.[1,2]

HISTORY

Historical methods for causing venous endothelial damage include a slender rod of iron, reportedly used by Hippocrates himself; absolute alcohol, introduced by Monteggio and Leroy D'Etoilles in the 1840s; and ferric chloride, introduced by Charles Gabriel Pravaz in 1851.[3] The idea of injecting irritant substances into the vein for purpose of obliteration appears frequently in the French literature of last century. The injections were made with strong caustic and toxic substances. In 1908, Beniamino Schiassi in Bologna, first used iodine as sclerosant. Linser, started the use of 20% sodium chloride solution. The French school under the leadership of Sicard has used sodium salicylate in 20–40% solutions. Nobl has tried injections of 50% dextrose and a mixture containing equal parts of dextrose and levulose with 4% sucrose. Meisen uses equal parts of 25% sodium salicylate and 10% sodium chloride.[4]

Foam sclerotherapy was first described in 1939 by S McAusland. Subsequently, in 1949, Sigg reported that the injection of foam into a vein was beneficial because it washed away less rapidly, thus introducing the concept that foam with greater viscosity has advantages over other contemporary sclerotherapy techniques. The following year, Orbach compared the efficacy of sodium tetradecyl sulfate (STS) foam with that of an injection of an equal amount of STS in liquid form. He found that the STS foam had 3.5–4 times the thrombogenic property of the solution. In 1953, the Norwegian doctor Arve Ree injected pure ethamolin foam into varicose veins and reported excellent results in a series of 50 patients. In 1956, Peter Fluckiger was the first to notice that the foam could be directed into regions other than the site of injection by manual manipulation. This concept is now widely practiced with ultrasound-guided foam sclerotherapy.

OBJECTIVES AND MECHANISM

Varicose vein is one of the clinical manifestations of venous hypertension. It has been estimated that between 17 and 50% of persons with varicose veins have cutaneous findings. Patients with chronic venous insufficiency (CVI) and superficial venous insufficiency may benefit from sclerotherapy or surgical treatment of the superficial venous system.[5] The ultimate goal of sclerotherapy as an interventional procedure is to normalize venous physiology.

Sclerotherapy of incompetent perforators and/or varicose veins increases the efficacy of calf muscle pump, resulting in an improved clearance of extravascular fluid.[5] Sclerotherapy has shown to help in the healing of venous ulcers and stasis eczema.[6] Vascular fibrosis and obliteration occur in response to irreversible endothelial cellular damage and exposure of underlying subendothelial layer in a dose-dependent manner after sclerotherapy. If the sclerosant is too weak, it will not cause any endothelial injury; if little stronger, vessel is damaged but recanalization occurs forming an incompetent pathway; and if too strong, the endothelium is destroyed but the sclerosant flows into adjacent normal vessels causing extensive tissue necrosis. Hence, the key to successful outcome is to inject an appropriate amount and concentration of sclerosant which causes irreversible damage to the endothelium of the abnormal vessel, while leaving adjacent normal vessels untouched.[3] Injection of the sclerosant and its subsequent dilution with blood results in three zones. Zone 1 is the site of irreversible endothelial injury which scleroses completely and is replaced by fibrous tissue. Partial or complete thrombosis of the vessel takes place in Zone 2 which eventually recanalizes. In Zone 3, the sclerosant is diluted to below its injurious concentration, without causing any endothelial injury.[3] The extent of different zones depends on the concentration of the sclerosant used, vessel diameter, and the position of the patient.

INDICATIONS OF SCLEROTHERAPY IN VARICOSE VEINS[7,8]

Indications for sclerotherapy in varicose veins are shown in **Box 1**.

CONTRAINDICATIONS[8,9]

Contraindications for sclerotherapy are listed in **Table 1**.

SCLEROSING SOLUTIONS[7,10,11]

There are many sclerosing solutions available. Important parameters to be considered in selecting a sclerosant include:

- Vessel diameter
- Reflux considerations
- Patient allergy profile
- Pain tolerance
- Previous treatment response to a given agent
- Minimal sclerosing concentration
- Sclerosant complication profile

Sclerosing solutions are classified into three groups, based on their mechanisms of destruction of the endothelium; detergent agents, osmotic agents, and chemical irritants.

BOX 1: Indications of sclerotherapy in varicose veins.

- Pain
- Major tributaries of greater and lesser saphenous veins
- Major perforator reflux
- Lateral venous system varicosities
- Complications of varicose veins such as stasis dermatitis and venous ulcers
- Cosmetic—telangiectasias/spider webs

TABLE 1: Contraindications for sclerotherapy.

Absolute contraindications	*Relative contraindications*
• Acute superficial or deep vein thrombosis • Local infection in the area of sclerotherapy or severe generalized infection • Immobility, confinement to bed • Advanced peripheral arterial occlusive disease (stage 3 or 4) • Hyperthyroidism (in the case of sclerosants containing iodine) • Pregnancy in the first trimester and after the 36th week of gestation • Known allergy to the sclerosant • Severe systemic disease	• Leg edema • Saphenofemoral junction incompetence • Thrombophilia with history of deep vein thrombosis • Long-standing diabetes • Peripheral arterial occlusive disease stage II • Poor general health • Myocardial decompensation • Migraine • Bronchial asthma • Marked allergic diathesis • Known hypercoagulability

Detergent Agents

This group of sclerosants acts by protein theft mechanism; these agents cause vascular injury by altering the surface tension around the endothelial cells. Structurally, they contain one pole that is hydrophilic and one pole that is hydrophobic. Rapid endothelial cell wall damage occurs when over hydration results from the hydrophilic pole, attracting water into the cell, while the hydrophobic pole attaches to the vein wall. Examples of detergent agents include STS, polidocanol (POL), sodium morrhuate, and ethanolamine oleate.[3,11]

Osmotic Agents

This group of sclerosants causes endothelial cell damage through dehydration. Examples of osmotic agents include hypertonic saline and hypertonic saline dextrose.[11]

Chemical Irritants

This group of sclerosants causes endothelial cell damage by their direct corrosive action. After injection, the endothelium near the site of injection is destroyed within seconds. The corrosive action is limited because of rapid inactivation by blood proteins. At the site of endothelial destruction the chemical can penetrate further and diffuse into deeper layers of the vessel wall causing further destruction. Examples of chemical irritants include chromate glycerin and polyiodinated iodine. These agents are not approved by the US Food and Drug Administration (FDA).

The current FDA approved sclerosing agents include STS, POL, sodium morrhuate, and hypertonic saline and are dealt in greater detail.

Sodium Tetradecyl Sulfate

Sodium tetradecyl sulfate is a long chain fatty acid salt with strong detergent properties. It is a highly effective sclerosing solution used worldwide. Approved for use in the United States since 1946, it has been popular with vascular surgeons since the 1960s and was first described for use in telangiectasias in the 1970s. Appropriate concentrations for superficial telangiectasias are 0.1–0.2%. Other concentrations are 0.2–0.5% for reticular veins or small varicosities and 0.5–3% for larger varicosities related to major sites of valvular reflux. A relatively high incidence of postsclerosis pigmentation has been reported at high doses (1% STS).[11]

TABLE 2: Comparison of various sclerosants.[7,12-14]

Sclerosing solution	*Category*	*Advantages*	*Disadvantages*	*Vessels treated*	*Concentrations*	*Maximum volume/ dose of sclerosant*
Sodium tetradecyl sulfate	Detergent	• FDA approved • Painless unless injected extravascularly	May cause skin breakdown at higher concentrations	All sizes	• 0.1–0.2% telangiectasias • 0.2–0.5% reticular • 0.5–1.0% varicose • 1.0–3.0% axial varicose	10 cc of 3%
Polidocanol	Detergent	• FDA approved • Painless	Ulcerogenic	Small to medium	• 0.25–0.5% telangiectasias • 0.5–1.0% reticular • 1.0–3.0% varicose	20 cc of 3%, not to exceed 2 mg/kg
Hypertonic saline	Hyperosmolar	Low risk of allergic reactions	• Ulcerogenic • Painful	Small	• 23.4–11.7% telangiectasias • 23.4% reticular	Maximum 20 cc per session, restrict volume in salt restricted diets
Hypertonic saline + dextrose	Hyperosmolar	• Low risk of allergic reaction • Mild stinging • Low ulcerogenic potential	• Not FDA approved • Relatively weak sclerosant	Small	• Undiluted—telangiectasias • Undiluted—reticular	10 cc
Sodium morrhuate	Detergent	FDA approved	Allergic reactions highest	Small	• Undiluted—telangiectasias • Undiluted—reticular	2–5 cc of 5%, 50–250 mg depending on vein diameter
Chromated glycerin	Chemical irritant	Low skin ulcer potential	• Not FDA approved • Very weak sclerosant	Smallest	Undiluted to half strength—telangiectasias	
Polyiodinated iodine	Chemical irritant	Highly corrosive; allows treatment of largest veins	• Not FDA approved • Avoid in iodine allergic patients	Largest	• 1–2% for up to 5 mm veins • 2–6% for the largest veins	2–3 cc of 6%

(FDA: Food and Drug Administration)

Polidocanol

The detergent-based POL, a urethane compound, was originally developed as an anesthetic, but was found to have the property of sclerosing small diameter vessels after intradermal injection. POL contains hydroxyl polyethoxy dodecane dissolved in distilled water with 5% ethanol as a stabilizer.

Hypertonic Saline

Although approved by the FDA only for use as an abortifacient, it is a commonly employed solution in the United States of America. A theoretical advantage of hypertonic saline is its total lack of allergenicity when unadulterated.[11] It has been commonly used in various concentrations from 10 to 30%, with occasional addition of heparin, procaine, or lidocaine. However, evidence for benefits of the additional agents is lacking and hence hypertonic saline is used either unadulterated or diluted to 11.7% with sterile water for smaller telangiectasias. With hypertonic saline, damage of tissue adjacent to injection sites may easily occur. Skin necrosis may be produced by extravasation at the injection site particularly when injecting very close to the skin surface. Injection of hyaluronidase into sites of extravasation may significantly reduce the risks of skin necrosis with hypertonic saline.

Sodium Morrhuate

Sodium morrhuate is a 5% solution of salts of saturated and unsaturated fatty acids in cod liver oil. Approximately, 10% of its fatty acid composition is unknown. This agent is preferred primarily for sclerosis of esophageal varices. Although it is approved by the FDA for sclerosis of varicose veins, use in treatment of telangiectasias is not common because of its caustic qualities, with potential for cutaneous necrosis and higher risk of allergy. Its use is limited by reports of fatalities secondary to anaphylaxis.

Table 2 shows comparison of different sclerosing agents.[7,12-14]

PREPROCEDURE ASSESSMENT[9]

Case Selection

A reasonable approach for treating an individual with varicose veins should consider the likely benefits of a particular intervention in three areas, which are as follows:

1. Cosmetic benefit
2. Symptomatic benefit
3. Prevention of progression of venous insufficiency and venous ulceration

The correlation between symptoms and severity of varicose veins is so poor that it is very difficult to predict the likely outcome after intervention as far as symptoms are concerned. As a general observation, patients who obtain benefit from properly fitted graduated elastic hosiery are likely to benefit from intervention in appropriate cases. If the procedure is in a patient who has already developed signs of CVI, positive outcome is assured. If the purpose of the intervention is cosmetic, it is reasonable to go ahead after careful discussion with the patients about the risks and benefits, as with any other cosmetic procedure.

History

A detailed history including general medical conditions, smoking, physical activity, pregnancy and intake of estrogens, hormone replacement therapy, oral contraceptives, aspirin, and nonsteroidal anti-inflammatory drugs (NSAIDs) should be obtained. History of Raynaud's phenomenon, vascular insufficiency, and systemic diseases such as diabetes mellitus, hypertension, and ischemic heart disease should be recorded. Results of previous treatment received for the condition and whether it is a primary or recurrent lesion are also noted.

Examination

Physical examination to assess the skin for evidence of stasis dermatitis, stasis ulcer, examination of the venous system for varicosity, small vessels and large vessels, and status of perforators is essential. Examination should include looking for evidence of previous deep vein thrombosis. Arterial pulses should be checked properly. In case of vascular malformation, the extent of malformation, pulsations, and whether a bruit is present to rule out an arteriovenous fistula is important.

Investigations

General investigations such as complete blood counts, bleeding and clotting time, blood sugar, and electrocardiogram (ECG) may be carried out. The duplex ultrasound (Doppler test) is the most useful tool for workup and has replaced many of the physical examination maneuvers and physiological tests previously used for diagnosis.

Duplex Doppler Ultrasonography[15]

The advent of color flow duplex scanning has revolutionized the assessment of venous disease. It is a valuable noninvasive tool, simple in application. This technique combines B-mode real-time ultrasonography with pulsed Doppler ultrasonography. The B-mode image allows visualization of the underlying vessels so that a pulsed Doppler signal can then be specifically targeted to assess flow in a particular vessel.

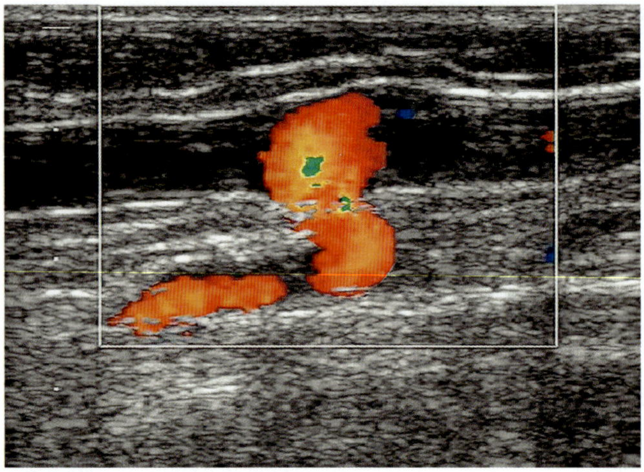

Fig. 1: Venous Doppler showing perforator incompetence.
Source: Dr HT Narayana, Professor and Head, Department of Radiodiagnosis, Sri Siddhartha Medical College, Tumkur.

Forward flow of venous blood toward the heart is augmented by a maneuver such as compression of the calf muscle; reverse flow of blood following this maneuver indicates that the vein is incompetent. The duplex scan provides the following information, which will have an effect on the decision to treat and the nature of the procedure.

- Patency and competence of the deep veins (obstruction and incompetence)
- Site and level of major incompetence (evaluation of perforator incompetence)
- Anatomy of the popliteal fossa can be identified accurately
- Anatomical abnormalities can be identified
- Duration and velocity of venous reflux

Duplex has become the modality of choice for the diagnosis before beginning a treatment protocol and allows to tailor treatment appropriately to individual cases. It has also been shown to be superior to venography **(Fig. 1)**.

PROCEDURE

Materials Required (Fig. 2)[16]

- Cotton balls soaked in spirit
- Protective gloves
- Disposable syringes of 1 cc or 3 cc with 30 gauge disposable transparent hub needles
- Elastocrepe for compression
- Hypoallergenic tape
- Topical nitroglycerin ointment (2%)
- Sclerosing solutions (stored separately from injectables) diluted with normal saline
- Magnifying loupes or lenses.

Sclerosant Concentrations[14]

Indications for different concentrations are shown in **Box 2**.

Principles of Varicose Vein Sclerotherapy[5]

- Always inject proximal to distal
- Inject the larger vein before smaller veins
- Vein must be emptied of blood by various maneuvers
- Exert direct finger pressure in spreading and compressing motion after injection
- Reflux points should be determined initially and treated specifically
- Immediate and adequate compression is important
- Ensure adequate ambulation immediately after treatment

Patient Preparation[16]

The patient should be in recumbent position that allows convenient access to the veins to be treated. Motorized table with height adjustment will facilitate easy access to all regions of the legs. Both the physician and the patient should be comfortable and proper lighting should be available. The area to be treated is exposed adequately and cleaned thoroughly with spirit or povidone-iodine. Usually anesthesia, intralesional or topical, is not required. An anxious patient is counseled and an analgesic or antianxiety drug may be administered. The sclerosant is diluted to the required concentration **(Table 2)** with distilled water or saline and loaded in a syringe.

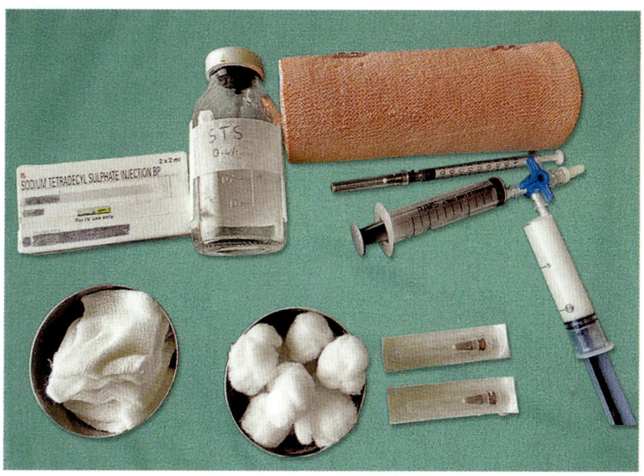

Fig. 2: Sclerotherapy tray.

BOX 2: Indications for different concentrations.

Higher concentrations:
- Younger patients
- Thick-walled vessels determined by palpation
- Hand/feet/pretibial veins
- Vessels >4 mm in diameter to compensate for dilution

Lower concentrations:
- Age >60 years
- 0.6–0.9 mm in diameter elevated spider veins
- Thin-walled vessels
- Easy bruisability
- History of spontaneous bleeding following minor trauma

TECHNIQUES

Techniques depend on the size of veins and are discussed here.

Sclerotherapy Techniques for Large Veins

There are two common techniques employed, i.e., Fegan's technique and Sigg's technique.[5]

Fegan's Technique

The classic technique presently employed with minor modifications is that of Fegan. The patient sits at end of the examining table with the leg to be treated dependent. The bulging varicosity is cannulized with a needle, butterfly, or angiocatheter **(Figs. 3 and 4)**. The leg is elevated and supported by the physician above cardiac level for 1–2 minutes to allow drainage of blood. Before injection, a small amount of blood is drawn into the syringe to ensure that the needle remains in the varicosity lumen. Too much blood may cause dilution of the sclerosant. As the injection of approximately

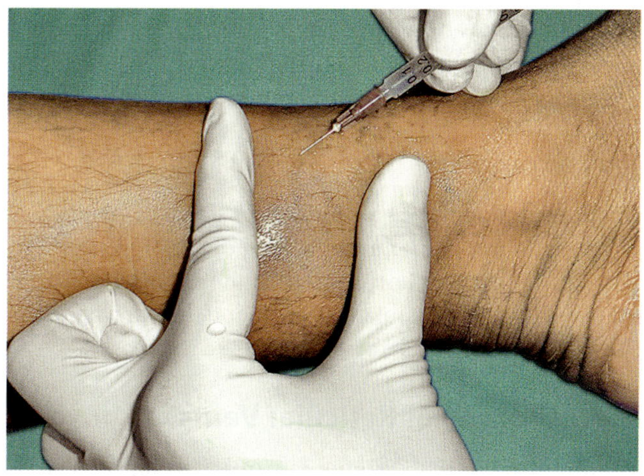

Fig. 3: Position of the hand while injecting.

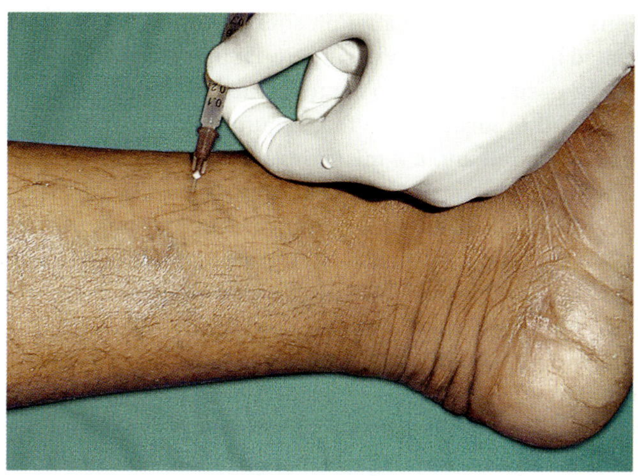

Fig. 4: Injection of sclerosant.

0.5–1.0 mL occurs, finger pressure several centimeters above and below the injection point is applied to confine the action of the sclerosing solution to the affected site. Finger pressure is maintained for 30–60 seconds followed by immediate application of compression with a foam pad. The pad is secured by foam elastic tape or relatively inelastic wrap around bandage to maintain compression immediately.

Fegan's method is particularly effective for incompetent perforators. The fascial defects through which perforators course may be palpated and serve as the site of needle entry. The site of perforators can also be marked during the venous Doppler study.

A widely used variation of Fegan's technique is the marking of varicosities with the patient standing while needle insertion is done with the patient recumbent or in slight reverse Trendelenburg position. This minimizes the movement of the leg and the inserted needle. Immediately after injection, the leg can be elevated and compression applied. Cannulation of previously marked varicosity is straight forward with the patient supine and may greatly hasten the procedure and minimize loss of proper needle positioning by patient movement. Direct finger pressure and lateral movement outward from the injection site is often useful not only to spread the sclerosant, but also to promote contact with greater surface area of the varicosity by emptying the vessel.

Sigg's Technique

A method frequently used in Europe for sclerosing saphenous junctions is the use of an open needle, called the Sigg's technique. A needle (not attached to the syringe) is inserted into the skin and manipulated until blood drips from the hub, following which the sclerosant is injected.

Sclerotherapy of Reticular Veins

Treatment of reticular veins is similar to large varicose veins; although the concentration, strength, and volume of sclerosing solution are decreased.[5] Subdermal reticular veins are treated only after all sources of reflux have been treated by sclerotherapy or surgery. Doppler ultrasound may also be used as a guide to demonstrate reflux in the reticular veins and to locate those that require treatment. With the patient recumbent, a 3 mL syringe with a 30-gauge needle is inserted into the reticular vein which is usually superficial and visibly blue. When the sensation of piercing the vein is felt, the plunger is pulled back gently until blood is seen. Usually a volume of no >0.5 mL per injection site is injected. The sclerosing solution most commonly used is STS in concentrations of 0.2–0.5%. The procedure may be done in multiple sittings. Treatment intervals may vary, but allowing 4–8 weeks between treatments helps to minimize the number of necessary sessions. **Figures 5 and 6** show the results after sclerotherapy.

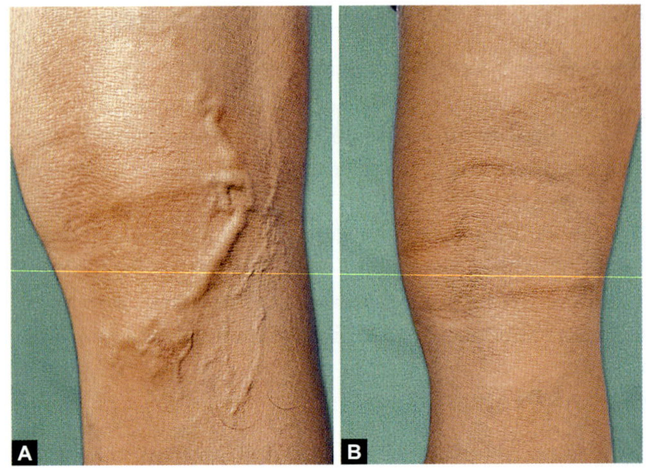

Figs. 5A and B: Before and after sclerotherapy.

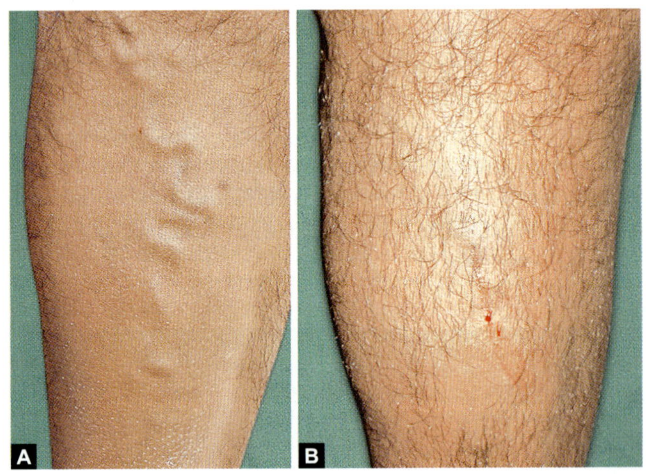

Figs. 6A and B: Before and after sclerotherapy.

POSTSCLEROTHERAPY COMPRESSION[5,17,18]

Rapid, immediate, and adequate compression after injection of the sclerosant is recommended. Graduated compression hoses (15–30 mm Hg) or cotton balls with Elastocrepe can be used for adequate compression.

Postsclerotherapy compression helps in:

- Limiting the flow of blood back into the varicosity, thereby decreasing both thrombus formation and the tendency for recanalization
- Improving the effectiveness with greater resolution of both small and large varicosities
- Complete mobility after treatment and enhances muscle pump function. This rapidly dilutes and removes any sclerosing solution that inadvertently entered deep system.

The duration of compression is still debated. Fegan recommended 6 weeks, but 3–5 days of compression has been suggested adequate. Walking may lessen the risk of deep vein thrombosis by avoiding stagnation of blood flow. Risks of deep vein thrombosis are also lessened by adhering to the principle of no >1.0 mL per injection site, with the usual volume being 0.5 mL.

SIDE EFFECTS AND COMPLICATIONS

Postsclerotherapy Hyperpigmentation

It is the appearance of increased visible pigmentation along the course of a treated vein of any size. Initially, pigmentation is due to the perivascular hemosiderin deposition, but over time, the hemosiderin is replaced by melanin. The incidence of pigmentation is related to the dilution and type of sclerosant as well as size of the treating vessel. Incidence ranges from 11 to 30% for hypertonic saline and POL and up to 30% with STS. Compression may help to prevent this side effect. Removal of postsclerotherapy coagula by a small incision using a 21-gauge needle and expressing it out may decrease the incidence of pigmentation. Pigmentation clears usually within 6 months and rarely persists for >1 year. A study has shown that weekly subcutaneous administration of desferrioxamine mesylate 500 mg reduces the time to depigmentation by 82% in patients with postsclerotherapy cutaneous hyperpigmentation treated for telangiectasias and reticular veins and prolonged postsclerotherapy hyperpigmentation in varicose veins.[19]

Matting

It is defined as the appearance of groups of new fine telangiectasias surrounding or replacing a previously treated area in blush-like manner. Resolution occurs spontaneously within a 3–12-month period with 70–80% spontaneous resolution within the first 6 months.

Cutaneous Necrosis

It may occur with all sclerosants if the solution spills outside the vessel into the skin. Studies have shown that extensive tissue necrosis following high concentration sclerotherapy may be rare, but its occurrence is serious and its treatment may be difficult.[20] In case of extravasation of the sclerosant, necrosis may be minimized by injecting normal saline in the ratio of 10:1 at the site. Application of 2% nitroglycerin paste at the extravasation site greatly reduces the risks of necrosis.

Superficial Thrombophlebitis

It is characterized by a very tender, indurated, and linear erythematous swelling. Incidence is 0.01–1% following sclerotherapy. Administered transdermally, glyceryl trinitrate speeds the resolution of venous inflammation in patients with sclerotherapy-related thrombophlebitis. Nitric oxide released from glyceryl trinitrate may exert a direct anti-inflammatory action on the inflamed veins and surrounding tissues.[21]

Pulmonary Embolism

It probably occurs from extension of a superficial thrombus into the deep venous system. It is usually associated with injection of large quantities of sclerosant at a single site. There are reports of acute massive pulmonary embolism following high ligation combined with compression sclerotherapy when both procedures were done simultaneously in a patient with hypercoagulable state.[22]

Arterial Injection

This dreaded complication is extremely rare and can lead to large areas of skin necrosis and damage to the subcutaneous tissue and muscle, which may take months to heal. Emergency treatment involves immediate application of ice, attempts to flush the inadvertently injected artery with normal saline and heparin, injection of procaine 3% to inactivate STS, and vascular surgery consultation for intravenous anticoagulation.

Allergic Reaction

Systemic allergic reactions to sclerotherapy treatment can occur rarely.[23] Anaphylaxis has been reported after sclerotherapy. However, very few reports of severe or fatal reaction have been reported. Hence, it is always recommended to make the patient stay in the hospital for about 30 minutes after the procedure before discharge. Also, emergency measures to manage anaphylaxis should be available at the place of treatment.

FOAM SCLEROTHERAPY

Foam sclerotherapy is often presented as a new method for the management of varicose veins. However, foam sclerotherapy was first described as early as 1939 by S McAusland. He injected froth, produced by shaking a rubber capped bottle filled with sodium morrhuate into spider veins. Further in 1944, Orbach demonstrated the use of air in sclerotherapy by air-block technique. In 1949, Sigg reported the benefit of foam as it washed away less rapidly, thus introducing the concept that foam with greater viscosity has advantages over other contemporary sclerotherapy techniques. Subsequently, in 1956, Peter Fluckiger was the first to notice that the foam could be directed into regions other than the site of injection by manual manipulation. Minor modifications in the way foam is produced, as well as the use of ultrasound to guide it to the sites of venous reflux, have resulted in a renewed interest in this technique.[24,25]

The detergent sclerosants such as STS and POL can only produce foam.[11] Sclerosing foam is a mixture of gas bubbles in a liquid solution that contains surface-active molecules. The gas must be well tolerated by patients, physiologic, and the bubble size should be preferably under 100 μ. According to the bubble diameter, foams can be classified as froth, macrofoam, minifoam, and microfoam. If the relative volume fraction of liquid is <5%, the foam is classified as dry, whereas if it is >5%, it is classified as wet. Wet foam (e.g., Tessari's foam) has the maximum stability. Uniform bubble diameter also provides more stability.[24]

Techniques[26]

- *Monfreux method:* Foam is produced in a glass syringe filled with 0.3–0.5 mL of sclerosant. Negative pressure is created by closing the tip of the syringe with sterile plug and holding tension on the piston until 2–3 mL of foam is generated. The consistency is low probably due to the large size of the bubbles and also this technique has a higher rate of side effects.
- *Cabrera method:* Juan Cabrera has used CO_2 for producing the foam.
- *Benigni–Sadoun method:* Plastic syringes are used with repeated and fast pulling and release of piston. The foam is very short lasting.
- *Lorenzo Tessari's Tourbillon technique:* Two plastic disposable syringes are connected by a three-way stopcock. The foam is formed by mixing the liquid sclerosant with four or five parts of air, through 20 passes between the two syringes with the hub at a 30° rotation. This rotation narrows the stopcock passage generating high turbulence, which produces high quality microfoam. This is one of the most frequently used technique.[27]
- *Modifications of Tessari:*
  - Two-way female connector[28]
  - Automated foaming device Turbofoam Kreussler Pharma, France[29]
- *Frullini method:* Mechanism of foam generation uses the same turbulence effect of Tessari method. Here a connecter is inserted in a vial of STS and the other end is connected to a syringe. The vial is positioned upside down and quick injection/aspiration of the solutions is performed.

Foam Stability

The stability of foam is affected by the injection technique, composition and volume of foam. The homogeneity of the bubble size, viscosity, and temperature all influence the quality and longevity of foam.[29]

The bubble size is inversely related to the difference in density between a liquid and gas as shown in the equation:[30]

D_p = bubble diameter
d_o = orifice diameter
σ = surface tension
$\Delta\rho$ = difference in density between a liquid and gas

The density of the air also determines the size of the bubbles in foam. Carbon dioxide being 1.5 times denser than room air produces smaller bubbles compared to room air. Also the foam bubbles produced by Tessari technique are smaller compared to other techniques. The smaller bubble size leads to increased surface area of the sclerosant as well as increased amount of sclerosant being delivered to the endothelial cells and hence more efficacious.[26,31]

Injection using ultrasound guidance and direct puncture technique are commonly used while performing foam sclerotherapy for large veins like great saphenous vein. Short and long catheters with balloon tips are used for the procedure. However, there is a possibility of deep vein thrombosis while using long catheters due to the passage through perforators.[32,33]

Advantages and Disadvantages

Foam preparations are considered to be three to four times more potent than equivalent concentrations and volumes of liquid sclerosants. The advantages of foam sclerosants compared to conventional liquid sclerotherapy are:[13,24]

- Increase in the effective surface area of foams compared with liquid
- Displacement of blood from the treated vein which produces prolonged undiluted intimal contact
- Increased vasospasm and sclerosis of veins at a greater distance from the injection site than can liquid preparations
- Smaller volumes and concentrations
- Enhanced visibility on duplex imaging due to echogenicity of foams and hence greater efficacy.

The main disadvantage of foam is the difficulty in standardization. In patients with patent ductus arteriosus, foam can lodge in the lungs and produce pulmonary fibrosis. There are reports of deep vein thrombosis and superficial thrombophlebitis following foam sclerotherapy. There are four case reports of transient ischemic attack and stroke following foam sclerotherapy for varicose veins in a patient, who later was found to have patent foramen ovale and atrial septal defects.[29,34] Also pain and pigmentation is relatively more in patients treated with foam.[24]

However, various randomized controlled studies comparing the incidence of adverse events with foam and liquid sclerotherapy of the saphenous vein have shown no statistical difference between these techniques.[29]

LASER TREATMENT OF TELANGIECTASIAS AND RETICULAR VEINS

Laser therapy is mainly indicated for telangiectasia/venulectasia or reticular veins <3 mm in diameter. It is mainly used for patients with areas of neovascularization with telangiectatic matting, veins resistant to sclerotherapy, and noncannulizable vessels. The concept of selective photothermolysis by laser with hemoglobin as the chromophore is the principle behind using lasers for leg veins.

Hemoglobin has an absorption spectrum which has broad peaks at 410 nm, 540 nm, and 577 nm and smaller peaks at 920 nm and 940 nm. The various lasers used include pulsed dye (585–605 nm), potassium titanyl phosphate (KTP) (532 nm), alexandrite (755 nm), diode (810 nm), neodymium-doped yttrium aluminum garnet (Nd:YAG) (1,064 nm), and intense pulse light (IPL). The important parameters which influence the treatment and management of individual vessels include the wavelength, pulse duration, and spot size. The larger vessels respond to longer wavelengths or the ratio of vessel to epidermal heating increases the probability of achieving complete vessel coagulation. However, lasers and IPL may not be replacements for sclerotherapy, mainly because hydrostatic pressure considerations are not addressed by light endothelial interactions and also it may be difficult to have sufficient penetration of photons safely through the thick epidermal-dermal wall surrounding the lower extremity vessels.[35]

Endovenous Ablation

Both radiofrequency and endovenous laser ablations have been used to treat varicose veins.[36,37]

CONCLUSION

Sclerotherapy is a simple and effective procedure for the treatment of varicose veins. With experience, larger veins can also be treated effectively with sclerotherapy. It can prevent the complications of varicose veins if done in the initial stages. Sclerotherapy being an outpatient procedure, when done with adequate precautions is associated with very minimal morbidity, mortality, and loss of work time compared to surgery. Sclerotherapy has emerged as a simple, safe and effective treatment modality for management of venous abnormalities, both therapeutically and aesthetically. The advent of foam sclerotherapy has carried the field further forward. New advances in laser ablation have opened new avenues for management of these common therapeutic and aesthetic problems.

TIPS AND TRICKS

- Using a bent needle to inject can help in keeping the injecting hand more stable.
- Always withdraw to look for blood in the syringe before injection and avoid the urge to inject till the needle is in the vein.
- Start with lower concentrations and lower volumes of injections in the initial days.
- Not >0.5–1 cc of the sclerosant to be injected at each site.
- Not >10 cc of the sclerosant injection per session.
- Vessel size is the best prognostic indicator of treatment response and complications.
- Patients can be asked to mark the vessels which they feel is most troublesome.
- Selection of sclerosant concentration can be done on an individual basis.

REFERENCES

1. Goldman MP. Treatment of varicose and telangiectatic leg veins: double-blind prospective comparative trial between aethoxysklerol and sotradecol. Dermatol Surg. 2002;28:52-5.
2. Lorenz MB, Gkogkolou P, Goerge T. Sclerotherapy of varicose veins in dermatology. J Dtsh Dermatol Ges. 2014;12(5): 391-3.
3. Feied C. Sclerosing solutions. In: Bergan JJ (Ed). The Vein Book. USA: Elsevier Academic Press; 2007. pp. 125-31.
4. De Takas G. Varicose veins and their sequelae. JAMA. 1929; 92:775-9.
5. Goldman MP, Weiss RA, Bergan JJ. Diagnosis and treatment of varicose veins: a review. J Am Acad Dermatol. 1994;31: 393-413.
6. Subbarao NT, Aradhya SS, Veerabhadrappa NH. Sclerotherapy in the management of varicose veins and its dermatological complications. Indian J Dermatol Venereol Leprol. 2013; 79:383-8.
7. Weiss RA, Weiss MA. Treatment of varicose and telangiectatic veins. In: Freedberg JM, Eisen AZ, Wolff K (Eds). Fitzpatrick's Dermatology in General Medicine, 6th edition. USA: McGraw Hill; 2003. pp. 2549-56.
8. Rabe E, Breu FX, Cavezzi A, Smith PC, Frullini A, Gillet JL, et al. European guidelines for sclerotherapy in chronic venous disorders. Phlebology. 2014;29:338-54.
9. Khunger N, Sacchidanand S. Standard guidelines for care: sclerotherapy in dermatology. Indian J Dermatol Venereol Leprol. 2011;77:222-30.
10. Sadick N, Li C. Small vessel sclerotherapy. Dermatol Clinics. 2001;19:475-81.
11. Weiss MA, Hsu JT, Neuhaus I, Sadick NS, Duffy DM. Consensus for sclerotherapy. Dermatol Surg. 2014;40(12): 1309-18.
12. Breadon J. Sclerotherapy. In: Burgess MC (Ed). Cosmetic Dermatology. Germany: Springer; 2005. pp. 147.
13. Weiss RA, Feied CF, Weiss MA. Treatment of large varicose veins. In: Weiss R, Feied C, Feied CF, Weiss M (Eds). Vein Diagnosis and Treatment: A Comprehensive Approach. USA: McGraw Hill; 2001. pp. 102.
14. Duffy DM. Sclerotherapy. In: Dover JS, Alam M, Nguyen TH (Eds). Treatment of Leg Veins. USA: Elsevier Saunders; 2006. pp. 71-105.
15. Labropoulos N, Landon P, Jay T. The impact of duplex scanning in phlebology. Dermatol Surg. 2002;28:1-5.
16. Weiss RA, Weiss MA. Sclerotherapy treatment of telangiectasias. In: Bergan JJ (Ed). The Vein Book. USA: Elsevier Academic Press; 2007. pp. 133-8.
17. Goldman MP. How to utilize compression after sclerotherapy. Dermatol Surg. 2002;28:860-2.
18. Nootheti P, Cadag KM, Magpantay A, Goldman MP. Efficacy of graduated compression stockings for an additional 3 weeks after sclerotherapy treatment of reticular and telangiectatic leg veins. Dermatol Surg. 2009;35:53-8.
19. Lopez L, Dilley RB, Henriquez JA. Cutaneous hyperpigmentation following venous sclerotherapy treated with desferrioxamine mesylate. Dermatol Surg. 2001;27: 795-8.
20. Bergan JJ, Weiss RA, Goldman MP. Extensive tissue necrosis following high concentration sclerotherapy for varicose veins. Dermatol Surg. 2000;26:535-42.
21. Berrazueta JR, Fleitas M, Salas E, Amado JA, Poveda JJ, Ochoteco A, et al. Local transdermal glyceryl trinitrate has

an anti-inflammatory action on thrombophlebitis induced by sclerosis of leg veins. Angiology. 1994;45:347-51.
22. Yamaki T, Nozaki M, Sasaki K. Acute massive pulmonary embolism following high ligation combined with compression sclerotherapy for varicose veins. Dermatol Surg. 1999;25:321-5.
23. Goldman MP. Complications and adverse sequelae of sclerotherapy. In: Bergan JJ (Ed). The Vein Book. USA: Elsevier Academic Press; 2007. pp. 149-53.
24. Geroulakos G. Foam sclerotherapy for the management of varicose veins: a critical reappraisal. Phlebolymphol. 2006; 13:202-6.
25. Orbach EJ. Sclerotherapy of varicose veins: utilization of an intravenous air block. Am J Surg. 1944;66:362-6.
26. Frullini A, Cavezzi A. Sclerosing foam in the treatment of varicose veins and telangiectases: history and analysis of safety and complications. Dermatol Surg. 2002;28:11-5.
27. Tessari L, Cavezzi A, Frullini A. Preliminary experience with a new sclerosing foam in the treatment of varicose veins. Dermatol Surg. 2001;27:58-60.
28. Hamel-Desnos C, Desnos P, Wollmann JC, Ouvry P, Mako S, Allaert FA. Evaluation of the efficacy of polidocanol in the form of foam compared with liquid foam in sclerotherapy of the greater saphenous vein: initial results. Dermatol Surg. 2003;29:1170-75.
29. Goldman MP, Jean-Jerome G, Weiss RA. Clinical methods for sclerotherapy of varicose veins. In: Goldman MP, Jean-Jerome G, Weiss RA (Eds). Sclerotherapy Treatment of Varicose and Telangiectatic Leg Veins, 5th edition. Edinburgh: Saunders Elsevier; 2011. pp. 242-7.
30. Hu WS. Oxygen Transfer in Cell Culture Bioreactors. Cellular Bioprocess Technology; 2004. pp. 1-14.
31. Redondo P, Cabrera J. Microfoam treatment of Klippel-Trénaunay syndrome and vascular malformations. J Am Acad Dermatol. 2008;59:355-6.
32. Breu FX, Guggenbichler S. European consensus meeting on foam sclerotherapy, April 4-6 2003, Tegernsee Germany. Dermatol Surg. 2004;30:709-17.
33. Cavezzi A, Tessari L. Foam sclerotherapy techniques: different gasses and methods of preparation, catheter versus direct injection. Phlebology. 2009;24:247-51.
34. Adatia S, Nambiar V, Kapadia R, Abuzinath A, Apel S, Alqarni M, et al. Acute ischemic stroke caused by paradoxical air embolism following injection sclerotherapy for varicose veins. Neurol India. 2013;61:431-3.
35. Sorhaindo SN. Laser treatment of telangiectasias and reticular veins. In: Bergan JJ (Ed). The Vein Book. USA: Elsevier Academic Press; 2007. pp. 157-65.
36. Weiss R, Elston DM. (2016). Varicose veins treated with radiofrequency ablation therapy. [Online] Available from https://emedicine.medscape.com/article/1085800-overview. [Last accessed August, 2023].
37. Khilnani NM, Elston DM. (2016). Varicose vein treatment with endovenous laser therapy. [Online] Available from: https://emedicine.medscape.com/article/1815850-overview. [Last accessed August, 2023].

CHAPTER 33

Sclerotherapy for Vascular Malformations

Sujay Khandpur, Tanvi Dev

KEY MESSAGES

- Sclerotherapy is an important simple, cheap, and easy minimally invasive technique for management of vascular malformation (VM).
- Indications include hemorrhage, lesions located at life- or limb-threatening sites, lesions threatening vital functions—seeing, hearing, eating, breathing, disabling pain, functional impairment secondary to swelling or pain, tissue loss or ulceration, and severe cosmetic deformity.
- In particular sclerotherapy is indicated for extratruncular diffuse infiltrative VM, extratruncular localized VM or as adjunct to surgery.
- The success of sclerotherapy procedure depends upon the concentration of the sclerosant used and its dwell time.
- Complications depend on VM morphology, extent and depth of the lesion (superficial or deep), and the type of sclerosant used.

INTRODUCTION

Sclerotherapy is a technique which induces local endothelial cell damage by selective intraluminal delivery of endothelial-cidal agent/sclerosant into chosen abnormal intravascular space that exerts its injurious effect on endothelial cell by direct contact in dose-dependent manner. It is an important therapeutic modality for treating venous malformations (VMs) that occur with an incidence of 1–2/10,000 births and a prevalence of 1%.[1] VMs not only produce a devastating cosmetic impact but may be associated with pain, bleeding, ulceration, secondary infection and even compress vital structures.[2]

Management of VM may be conservative or interventional. It requires a multidisciplinary approach with participation of a general surgeon, plastic surgeon, orthopedician, head and neck surgeon, dermatologist, pediatrician, interventional radiologist, physiotherapist, nurse, and a patient care coordinator.[3]

Conservative management is indicated when patient is either not wanting intervention or the symptoms are not meeting 'intervention threshold'.[4] Conservative therapy includes elevation of involved area during sleep, avoidance of activities producing symptoms, cessation of oral contraceptives, alleviation of paroxysmal pain due to localized intravascular coagulopathy with nonsteroidal anti-inflammatory drugs (NSAIDs) such as aspirin therapy, prophylactic administration of low molecular weight heparin for large VM in high-risk states, and use of pressure garments/stockings.

Interventional management includes sclerotherapy, lasers and other technologies, and surgery.[1] Of these, sclerotherapy is simple, cheap, and relatively noninvasive.

INDICATIONS FOR INTERVENTIONAL MANAGEMENT OF VENOUS MALFORMATIONS[5]

Absolute Indications

- Hemorrhage
- Lesions located at life- or limb-threatening sites
- Lesions threatening vital functions—seeing, hearing, eating, and breathing
- Disabling pain
- Functional impairment secondary to swelling or pain
- Tissue loss or ulceration
- Severe cosmetic deformity.

Relative Indications

- Vascular-bone syndrome
- Location at high risk of complications such as hemarthrosis, deep vein thrombosis (DVT)
- Recurrent infection
- Non-severe cosmetic deformity

Surgical excision is indicated when it can be completely removed without recurrence, the lesion is focal and well-defined, thrombosed, confined to a single or specialized muscle group, causing neurologic or compression symptoms, when there is good possibility of anatomic/functional restoration or for truncal VM.[1] However surgical excision is difficult to perform when VMs occupy multiple anatomic spaces, multiple muscle groups/fascial planes or encase critical structures.[6]

Laser therapy is preferred for multiple, focal, and well-defined mucocutaneous venous malformations.

Endovenous laser ablation can be used in large VMs to avoid using large volume of the sclerosant and its subsequent side effects.

SCLEROTHERAPY

This is indicated for extratruncular diffuse infiltrative VM, extratruncular localized VM or as adjunct to surgery.[6] The success of sclerotherapy procedure depends upon the concentration of the sclerosant used and its dwell time (time for which the sclerosing agent is in contact with endothelial cells).[7]

The commonly used sclerosing agents are:

- 100% ethanol
- 3% sodium tetradecyl sulfate (STS)
- 1% polidocanol (POL)
- 5% ethanolamine oleate alcoholic solution of zein (ethibloc)
- 5% sodium morrhuate
- Hypertonic 50% dextrose
- Hypertonic saline
- Acetic acid
- Methylmethacrylate
- Triamcinolone
- Bleomycin
- OK-432 (Picibanil)
- Tetracycline
- Doxycycline
- Pingyangmycin
- Aluminum potassium sulfate/tannic acid (used for internal hemorrhoids).

Sclerosing agents such as STS, POL, ethanolamine oleate, and ethanol are commonly used to treat vascular malformations.

Table 1 shows the properties and relative advantages and disadvantages of commonly used sclerosing agents for VM.

PROCEDURE

Preoperative preparation and counseling: Prior to the procedure a detailed history and a thorough physical examination is undertaken. This is followed by measurement of the lesion, a baseline photograph, and imaging studies (color Doppler/MRI) to estimate the location and extent of the lesion and flow velocity (low-flow or high-flow). A preoperative counseling is done in which the patient is explained about the specific indication for this procedure, technique to be employed, possible complications, postoperative pain and swelling etc.

Anesthesia: The procedure is performed under sedation or local, regional or general anesthesia in case of large and deep VM.[15] However for treatment of localized and relatively small VM, no anesthesia is required.

Sclerotherapy is performed in a room equipped with angiographic facilities, real-time ultrasonography, and facility to review previous images. The patient is positioned

TABLE 1: Advantages and disadvantages of commonly used sclerosing agents for venous malformation (VM).

Agent	*Mechanism of action*	*Advantages*	*Disadvantages*
Absolute ethanol[8,9]	• Dehydration of endothelial cells (EC) • Precipitation of cytoplasm • Sloughing and denudation of EC • Vessel wall fracture • Precipitation of blood proteins	• High response rate • Cheap • Easy to obtain • Long shelf life	• Very toxic—use with caution • Perilesional necrosis—skin necrosis • Very painful—indication for GA • Nerve impairment • Hemoglobinuria • Pulmonary artery vasospasm/ hypertension • Intoxication, bronchospasm, hyperthermia, cardiopulmonary collapse, death
5% Ethanolamine oleate[10,11]	Vascular fibrosis and sclerosis by: • Oleic portion- intimal and extravascular inflammation • Ethanolamine-suppresses fibrin clot formation	• Wide safety margin due to low penetrance beyond vessel wall • Low incidence of distal embolization—used in both HFL and LFL	• High dose—hemolysis, renal insufficiency, hepatotoxicity
3% sodium tetradecyl sulfate (anionic surfactant-injectable form is soapy in consistency)[12,13]	• Sludging of RBCs • Thrombosis • Intimal necrosis, adventitial fibrosis, luminal collapse	• Less toxic • Lower rates of skin necrosis, nerve impairment, systemic side-effects	• Less effective in permanent closure in high-flow lesion • Lower rate of permanent closure of VM
1% polidocanol (nonionic surfactant)[14]	• Endothelial cell overhydration • Effects intrinsic coagulation pathway	• Painless due to anesthetic effect • Low complications—skin necrosis, nerve impairment	• Systemic complications—hemolysis, hemoglobinuria, cardiac arrest

(HFL: high-flow lesions; LFL: low-flow lesions)

to allow best access of lesion, then draped, exposing all relevant access points. The instrument tray which includes labeled syringes, saline, iodinated contrast, sclerosants, 20- to 26-gauge needle with connector tubing or butterfly needle is kept ready. Some physicians perform a direct percutaneous phlebogram by injecting a contrast medium, prior to the procedure. In deep VM, butterfly needle is introduced into VM under real-time ultrasound, fluoroscopic or even MRI guidance, while in superficial lesions, it is entered by palpation alone. Syringe is gently aspirated until flashback of blood is observed signifying intraluminal position of needle followed by injecting of the sclerosing agent. The patient is continuously monitored to assess extravasation of the sclerosant, any resistance to injection, and signs of patient distress or skin blanching (which indicate chemical toxicity or ischemia to skin). The lesion is continuously palpated for induration and administration of the sclerosant is limited as it becomes firm. The procedure is terminated when maximum allowable sclerosant dose is reached.

For smaller lesions, sclerotherapy can be undertaken without any anesthesia as an OPD procedure. Under aseptic conditions and by fixing the lesion between the thumb and index finger, the agent is injected into each lesion with insulin syringe and 26-gauge needle, initially withdrawing blood to confirm appropriate entry of needle into the vascular space and then injecting the agent to reach appropriate induration of lesion and blanching.

Postprocedure, compression is applied to the lesion (for 3–4 hours for small lesions to 24 hours–3 to 7 days for large VM) to allow vascular wall apposition and reduce intralesional volume and dilution effects.[8,16-19]

Table 2 shows response to sclerotherapy in relation to morphology of VM.

IMMEDIATE POSTPROCEDURE MANAGEMENT

The patient is advised oral analgesics. Systemic steroids may be indicated after use of stronger sclerosants such as ethanol, following sclerotherapy on large areas, when VMs have proximity to vital structures or ethanol-treated head and neck lesions. Low-molecular-weight heparin may be administered if sclerotherapy is performed in conjunction with surgery. Doppler ultrasound is advised if there are concerns of DVT. Physiotherapy is indicated if the lesions are located on mobile regions as VM may form scars postsclerotherapy

Patient follow-up: A repeat session may be undertaken after 3 weeks–3 months. Lesion size is measured to look for shrinkage postsclerotherapy and also a repeat photograph is taken for comparison. A radiological review is also undertaken post therapy. Patient's disease status and expectations are also discussed and limitations of the procedure explained.

FOAM SCLEROTHERAPY

This modification of the sclerotherapy procedure has shown greater efficacy than liquid form since foam displaces blood from target vessel, remains undiluted, and persists in the vessel to maximize its action.

This technique was originally conceived in 1944 by Orbach.[16] Cabrera and co-workers (1990s) used therapeutic foam of sodium tetradecyl sulfate or polidocanol for varicose veins.[17]In 2003, they used sclerosant in microfoam form to treat VM. In this technique 0.25–4% POL-carbon dioxide mixture or 3–6:1 room air to sclerosant using STS or POL used.[18] It is a simple, easily available, cost-effective, and safe technique. Foam sclerotherapy results in exposure to

TABLE 2: Image-based classifications and treatment implications based on venous malformation morphology.[20]

	Grade of venous malformation	*Definition*	*Size*	*Response to sclerotherapy*
MR imaging	Grade 1	Well defined	<5 cm diameter	71% excellent result 29% good result 0% poor result
	Grade 2A	Well defined	>5 cm diameter	22% excellent result 44% good result 33% poor result
	Grade 2B	Ill defined	<5 cm diameter	26% excellent result 15% good result 60% poor result
	Grade 3	Ill defined	>5 cm diameter	0% excellent result 43% good result 57% poor result
	Tissue layer involved: • Skin • Subcutaneous • Muscle • Tendon • Bony cortex			Risk of skin or nerve injury Muscular involvement: Risk of contracture Bone or marrow involvement: Risk of fracture

larger endothelial cell surface, reduced volume of sclerosant required, more homogenous filling of vascular lumen, lower incidence of re-canalization, and lesser possibility of extravasation. The precision and safety can be further enhanced under ultrasound guidance. Excellent results were reported with foam POL sclerotherapy in low-flow vascular malformation of tongue, in 93.3% cases (14 out of 15 cases) in 1–6 sessions **(Table 3)**.[21]

RECENT ADVANCES IN FOAMING TECHNIQUES

Although the Tessari's Tourbillon technique and the double-syringe system technique of preparation of foam are in common clinical use, these are associated with significant limitations. Firstly, these are based on transmission of manual energy on the plunger of the syringe, hence there is lack of uniformity and standardization. Secondly, the size of microbubbles is variable and can be up to several millimeters, hence predisposing to emboli-related neurological and other ischemic effects.

Novel mechanical devices have been recently developed to circumvent the complications of manual preparation. Varithena is an FDA-approved device (2013) that consists of an aerosol canister [with 1% POL, gas (CO_2: O_2 in 35:65 ratio, nitrogen content <0.8%)] attached to a dispenser with a sieve of micrometer pore size. Other methods include mechanical devices using magnetic coupling and acoustic energy to generate foam. Hence, future techniques are expected to further increase the safety profile and therapeutic efficacy of foam sclerotherapy.[22]

COMPLICATIONS

They mainly occur due to extravasation of the sclerosant and depend on VM morphology, extent and depth of the lesion (superficial or deep) and the type of sclerosant used, e.g., ethanol is most toxic; complications are low with sodium tetradecyl sulfate, polidocanol, and ethanolamine oleate (**Table 3**).[19]

Complications include:

- *Minor local complications:*
  - Erythema, swelling, pain, and tenderness.
  - Skin blistering, hyperpigmentation, skin ulceration, and necrosis
- *Major local complications:*
  - Transient or permanent nerve impairment or paralysis
  - Thrombophlebitis, deep venous thrombosis
  - Muscular contracture
  - Compartment syndrome
- *Major systemic complications:*
  - Hemolysis
  - Renal toxicity
  - Pulmonary embolism
  - Ocular disturbances
  - Anaphylactic reactions
  - Hypotension, bradyarrhythmia, and cardiopulmonary collapse.

Tips on how to avoid complications and how to manage them **(Box 1)**[23]

- Avoid alcohol as primary sclerosing agent.
- Perform more number of sessions with lesser volume of sclerosant injected per session.

TABLE 3: Review of literature of sclerotherapy results.

S. No.	*Author*	*Type of lesions*	*Number of patients*	*Agent used*	*Result*	*Complications*
1.	Mahesh B et al. 2003[24]	Peripheral VM	40	Color Doppler ultrasound-guided 3% SDS	• HFLs—81.25% regression • LFLs—83.3% regression	–
2.	Jain R et al. 2002[25]	VM—9 Lymphangiomas—3 Venous pseudoaneurysm—1 AV malformation of pinna—1	15	USG-guided 1% polidocanol (1–20 injections)	*Complete response:* • VM—7 (77.8%) • Lymphangiomas—3 (100%) • AV malformation—1 (100%) *Partial response:* • VM—2 (22.2%) • Venous pseudoaneurysm (100%)	Minor complications
3.	Rimon U et al. 2004[26]	VM-face, neck, chest, extremities	21	95% ethanol ↓ GA	Complete to partial improvement in 17 cases (81%) after 1–9 sessions	• Five cases • Skin ulcer—2 • Skin blister—1 • Pulmonary embolism—1 • Pulmonary hypertension with CVS collapse—1

Contd...

Contd...

S. No.	*Author*	*Type of lesions*	*Number of patients*	*Agent used*	*Result*	*Complications*
4.	Berenguer B 1999[27]	Craniofacial VM	18	Ethanol or SDS ↓ GA	Cured or marked improvement- 76%	• Skin blisters—50% • Deep ulceration—13% • Nerve injury—7.5% • Hemoglobinuria—28%
5.	O'Donovan JC et al. 1997[7]	VM (15), Hemangioma (6)	• Sclerotherapy alone—13 • Sclerotherapy + surgery—8	3% SDS	Beneficial in 86%	Skin ulcers—14.28%
6.	Tan KT et al. 2007[28]	Peripheral VM	72	3% STS (mean—3.1 sessions)	• Patients became asymptomatic—15% • Good response—28% • Improved—24% unchanged-28% worsened—5.6%. Change in size by MRI • Decreased—54% • No change—31% • Increase—14%	• Skin necrosis—6.9% • Transient sensory deficit/ urticaria—1.4% • Venous thrombosis—one case
7.	Kuo HW et al. 2003[29]	Venous lake	2	1% polidocanol	Complete resolution after two sessions	Minimal scar
8.	Park CO et al. 2005[30]	• Lymphangioma • Acquired digital AVM	1 each	STS	Near complete clearance after several sessions	–
9.	Khandpur S et al. 2010[31] **(Figs. 1 to 8)**	VM-13	13	3% STS	90–100% subsidence in 11 cases (84.6%) after mean four injections	• Cutaneous blister formation, erosions, and crusting at injection site—seven cases (53.8%) • Atrophic scarring—four cases (30.8%)
10.	Jairath V, et al. 2014[32]	Cherry angiomas	100 lesions in 20 patients	3% sodium tetradecyl sulfate	42 lesions responded with single dose, 44 lesions required two sessions, remaining 14 lesions required four sessions	• Persistent crusting for >15 days in 17.2% of cherry angiomas. • Other side effects—postinflammatory hyperpigmentation, ulceration, which resolved with minimal scarring (n = 11), temporary scaring in 11 cases
11.	Wang Y, et al. 2014[33]	Angiolymphoid hyperplasia with eosinophilia	One patient	1% polidocanol solution	Bleeding and pruritus completely resolved after second treatment. Complete resolution after seven sessions, each injection given every 10 days	Mild pain, bleeding
12.	Kupetsky EA, et al. 2014[34]	Lymphangioma circumscriptum	One patient	1% sodium tetradecyl sulfate	After four treatment sessions (one every 4 weeks), 50% reduction in lesions	Not mentioned
13.	Deore GD, et al. 2014[35]	Recurrent oral pyogenic granulomas in a case of port-wine stain	One patient with multiple lesions	3% sodium tetradecyl sulfate		

Contd...

Contd...

S. No.	*Author*	*Type of lesions*	*Number of patients*	*Agent used*	*Result*	*Complications*
14.	Lee et al. 2017[36]	• VM-17 • Capillary malformation (CM)-4 • Lymphatic malformation (LM)-9	30	Percutaneous sclerotherapy using bleomycin (1 mg/mL; mean 3.2 sessions over 3 months)	• 100% improvement—four cases (13.3%); VM-3, CM-1 • >70% improvement—nine cases (30%); VM-5, CM-3, LM-1 • 40–70% improvement—10 cases (33.3%); VM-4, CM-4, LM-2 • <40% improvement—four cases (13.3%); VM-2, CM-2, LM-0 • No improvement—three cases (10%); VM-3, CM-0, LM-0	• Total cases—7 (23.3%) • Pain—6 (20%) • Headache—2 (6.6%) • Fever—1 (3.3%) • Ulceration—1 (3.3%) • Tingling—1 (3.3%)
15.	Song et al. 2019[37]	Oropharyngeal low-flow VM	27 children with 35 lesions: • *Group A:* n = 16 lesions (13 patients) • *Group B:* n = 19 lesions (14 patients)	Digital subtraction angiography (DSA) guided • Groups A (n = 13; 16 lesions, sclerosant: 3% polidocanol foam; mean 2.45 ± 0.6 sessions) • Group B (n = 14;19 lesions, sclerosant: Ping-yangmycin + dexamethasone; mean 2.07 ± 0.4 sessions)	*Group A:* 87.5% lesions improved (n = 16), • Cured (complete disappearance)—7 (43.7%) • Basic remission (>80% reduction in size)—5 (31.2%) • Effective (<80% reduction in size)—2 (12.5%) • Invalidation (no change)—2 (12.5%) • *Group B:* 84.21% lesions improved • Cured—9 (47.3%) • Basic remission—4 (21%) • Effective—2 (10.5%) • Invalidation—3 (15.8%)	• *Group A:* Fever (1; 7.7%), local swelling (3; 23.1%), necrosis (1; 7.7%) • *Group B:* Fever (1; 7.1%), digestive tract reaction (1; 7.1%)
16.	Vollherbst et al. 2020[38]	Head and neck VM	27 patients	Polidocanol ± Ethanol	• MRI based change in volume • >10% increase in size: Two cases (7.4%) • ≤10% increase up to <10% decrease in size: four cases (14.8%) • ≥10% decrease up to <25% decrease in size: Six cases (22.2%) • ≥25-50% decrease in size: 12 cases (44.4%) • ≥50% decrease in size: Three cases (11.1%)	• Swelling: 88.9% • Pain: 63% • Hemorrhage: 7.4% • Scarring: 3.7%

Contd...

Contd...

S. No.	*Author*	*Type of lesions*	*Number of patients*	*Agent used*	*Result*	*Complications*
17.	Tu et al. 2016[39]	Head and neck LM	41 patients • *Group A:* 10 cases • *Group B:* 19 cases • *Group C:* 12 cases	• *Group A:* Picibanil; mean 1.5 sessions • *Group B:* Doxycycline; mean 1.6 sessions • *Group C:* Ethanolamine; mean 1.4 sessions	• *Group A:* Excellent response (Resolution of tumid lesions, symmetrical appearance): Four cases (40%) Good response (<50% of original size): Four cases (40%) Lost to follow-up: Two cases (20%) • *Group B:* Excellent response:10 cases (52.6%); Good response: Five cases (26.3%); Fair response (>50% of original size): Two cases (10.5%) Lost to follow-up: Two cases (10.5%) • *Group C:* Excellent response: Five cases (41.7%); Good response: Three cases (25%); Fair response: One case (83%); Poor response (unchanged or worse): Two cases (18.2%); Lost to follow-up: One case (8.3%)	• Air compression: One case (2.4%) • Infection: One case (2.4%) • Hemorrhage: One case (2.4%)

(AV: arteriovenous; CVS: cardiovascular system; GA: gallic acid; HFLs: high-flow lesions; LFLs: low-flow lesions; SDS: sodium dodecyl sulfate; STS: sodium tetradecyl sulfate; VM: venous malformations)

- Examine local nerve function after sclerotherapy; in case of suspected nerve injury, treat with oral prednisolone (0.5 mg/kg/day for 5 days).
- In superficial VMs, use long, small-bore needles to create a tract between the VM and skin surface; withdraw the needle just outside the malformation after injection of the sclerosant and use autologous-clotted blood to seal the tract, to minimize the harmful effects of extravasation of the sclerosant.
- Perform ultrasound-guided injection wherever possible to ensure single vein wall entry of VM and correct needle positioning.
- Ensure free retrograde blood flow from the cannula before each injection.
- Improve visualization of sclerosant by mixing sclerosant with Lipiodol (oil-based contrast) and air
- For lower limb VM, use a tourniquet to prevent sclerosing agent from escaping and sclerosing deep veins.
- Nonsteroidal anti-inflammatory agents can be used for pain. Aspirin in low dose can be used to treat pain related to thrombosis of VM.

BOX 1: Specific tips for sclerotherapy according to type of venous malformation (VM).

- In cases of slow-flow VM, direct sclerotherapy into nidus is preferred
- In cases of intermediate-flow VM-flow, sclerotherapy controlled with balloon occlusion, tourniquet, and coil is preferred. Cyanoacrylate embolization prior to sclerotherapy may also be used
- In cases of high-flow VM, a multidisciplinary approach should be used since high rate of treatment failure, recurrence, and complications

CONCLUSION

Venous malformations are the commonest congenital vascular malformations. They can cause significant morbidity such as pain, tissue hypertrophy, hemorrhage, and cosmetic disfigurement. Radiographic imaging is a prerequisite to characterize the size, depth, and location of VM. The treatment modalities in addition to sclerotherapy include conservative approach and various medical, surgical, and ablative techniques. Sclerotherapy involves the injection of a special chemical called sclerosant into the VM to destroy the endothelial cell lining and finally reducing the size of the malformation.

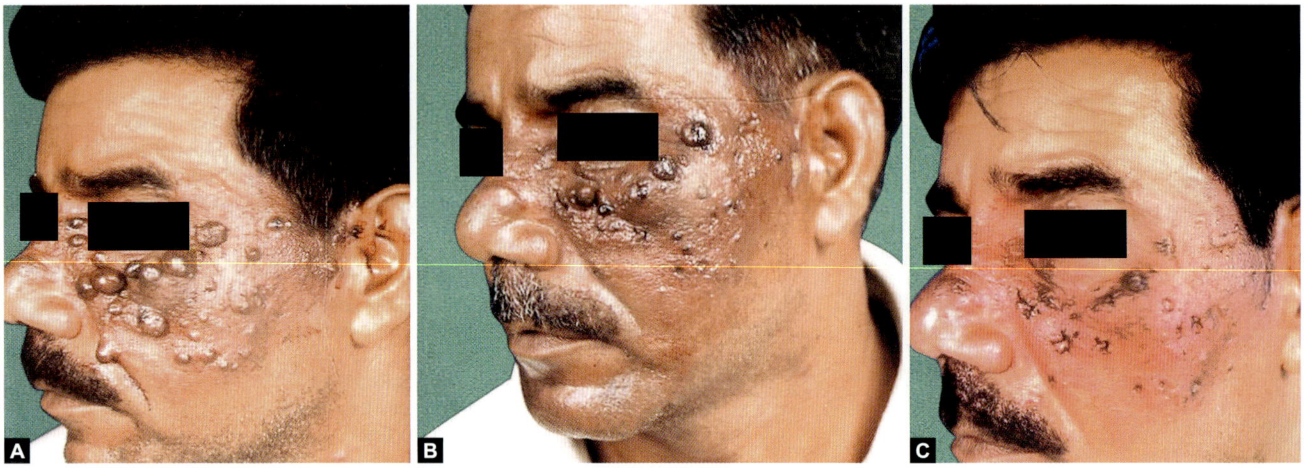

Figs. 1A to C: (A) Multiple nodules overlying port-wine stain left face; (B) Subsidence of majority of nodules after five sessions; (C) Resolution of all nodules after six sessions with atrophy at injection site.

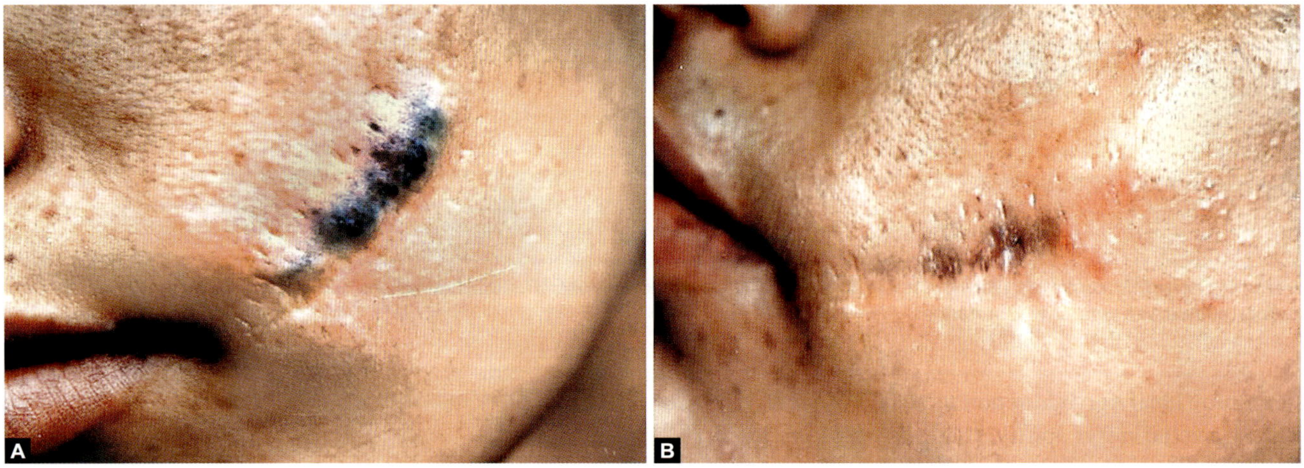

Figs. 2A and B: (A) Linear venous malformation left face with postexcision scar; (B) Subsidence of lesion after three sessions.

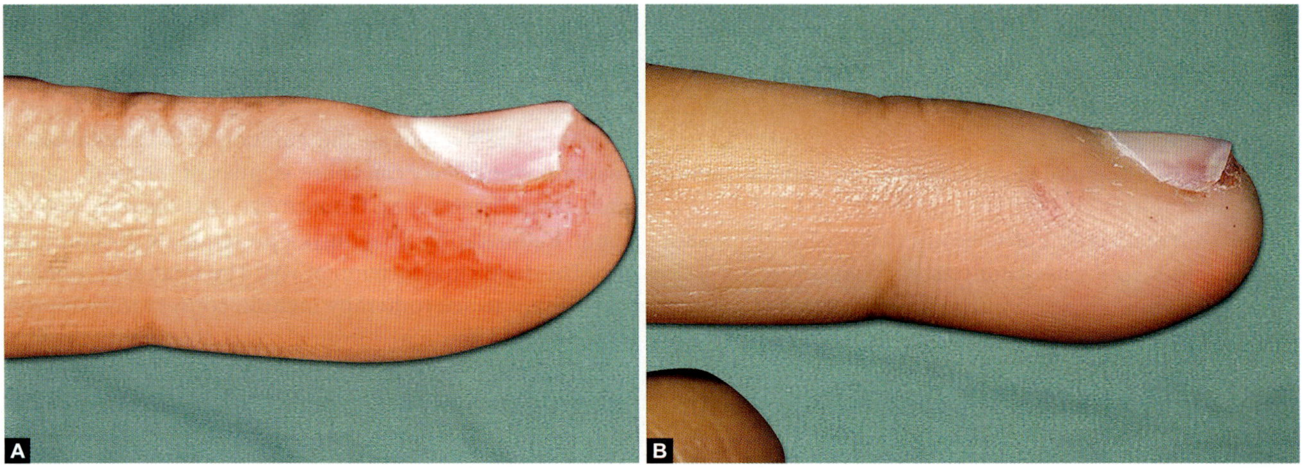

Figs. 3A and B: (A) Lesion over right middle finger; (B) >90% subsidence after one session.

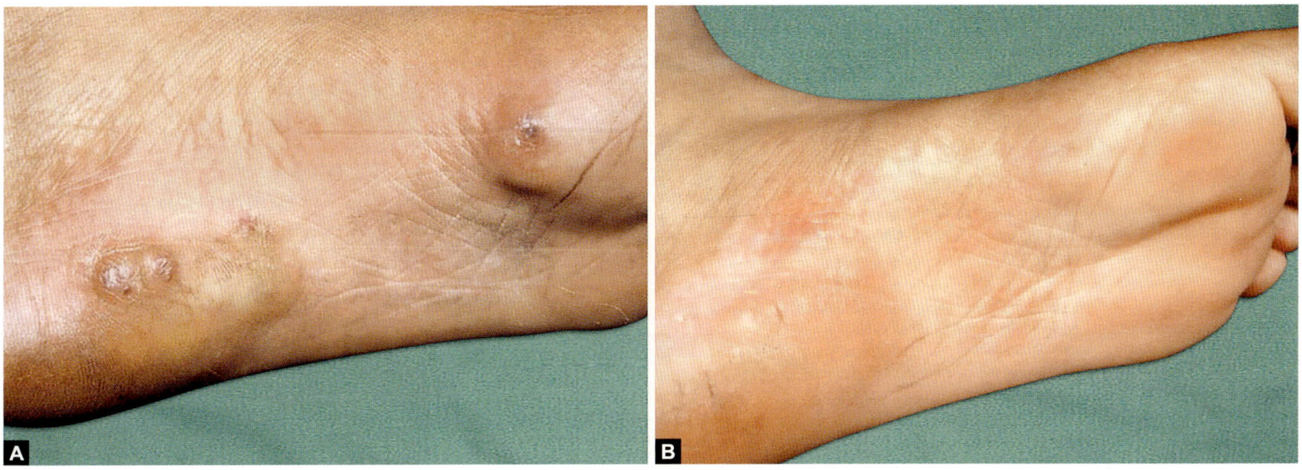

Figs. 4A and B: (A) Venous malformations—left sole; (B) Complete resolution after four sessions

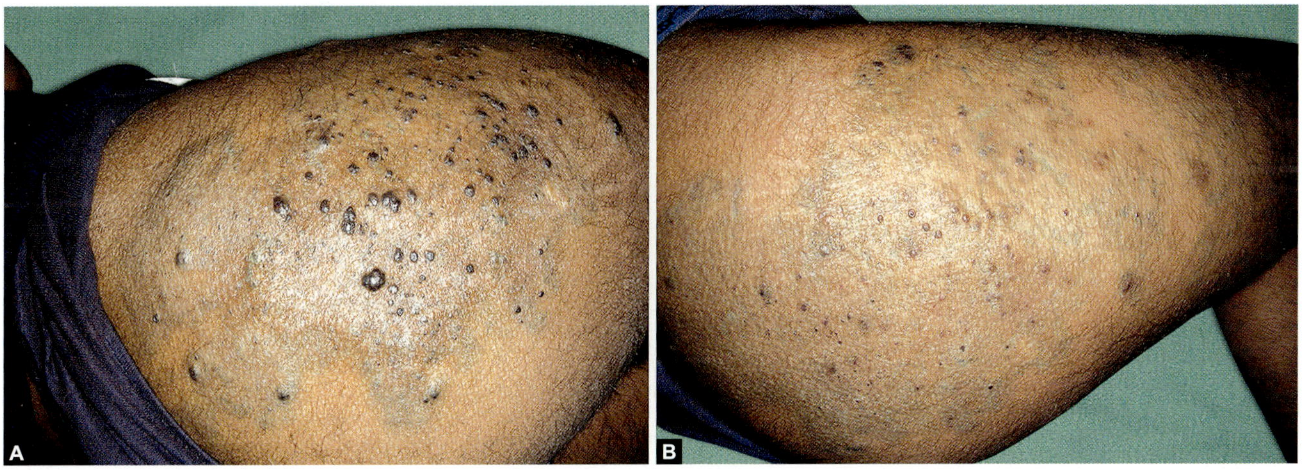

Figs. 5A and B: (A) Venous malformations right thigh; (B) >90% regression after four sessions.

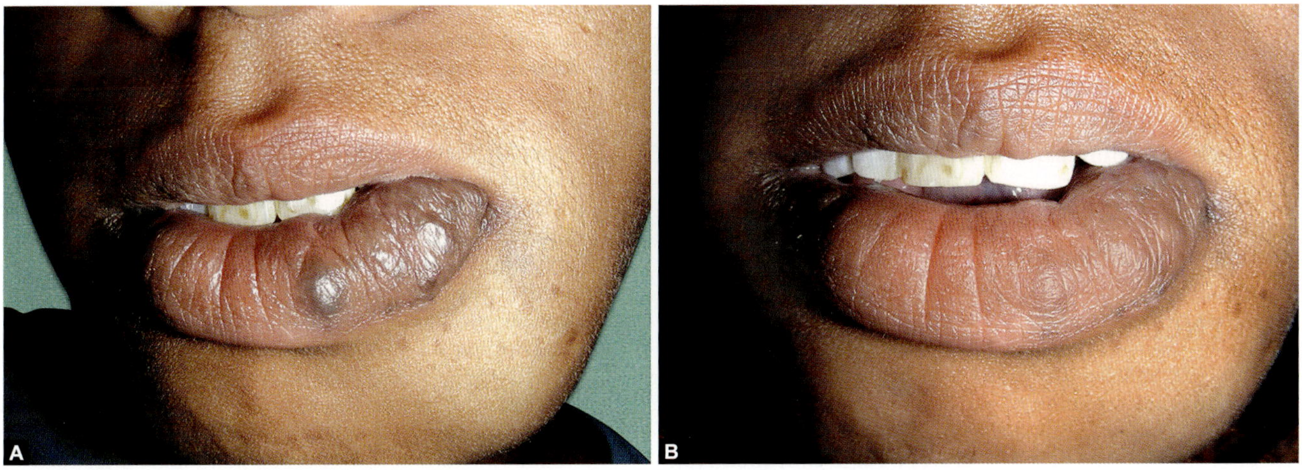

Figs. 6A and B: (A) Venous malformations lower lip; (B) >90% regression after two sessions.

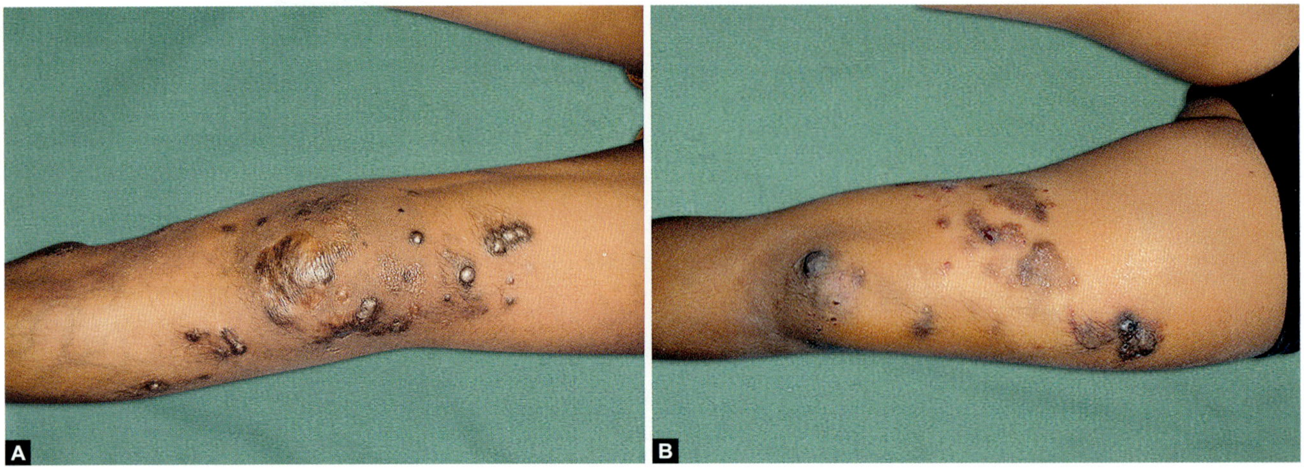

Figs. 7A and B: (A) Multiple venous malformations left lower limb; (B) Significant subsidence after three injections.

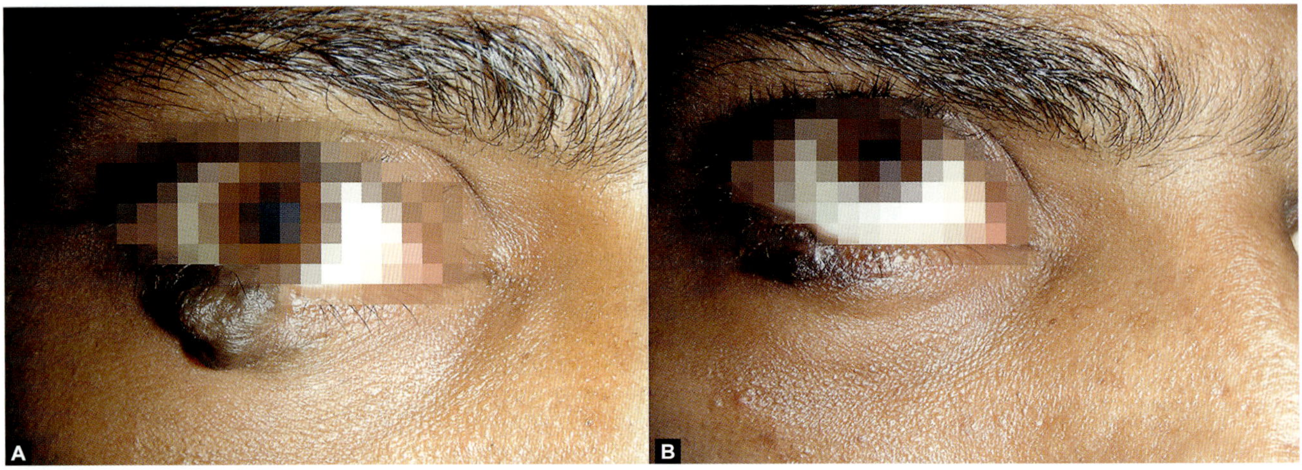

Figs. 8A and B: (A) Venous malformation right lower eyelid; (B) Near complete resolution after one injection.

Sclerosing agents such as sodium tetradecyl sulfate, polidocanol, ethanolamine oleate, and ethanol are commonly used to treat vascular malformations in multiple sessions over several months. Recent advances have been made in the techniques of foam sclerotherapy. Extravasation of the sclerosant (most commonly ethanol) can lead to complications. The minor complications include pain, tingling sensation, and cutaneous side effects such as blistering, necrosis, and scarring and major complications include localized nerve injury, deep vein thrombosis or systemic side effects such as pulmonary embolism and cardiopulmonary collapse. The adverse effects can be minimized by meticulous, image-guided injection techniques, prompt recognition, and treatment of the complications.

REFERENCES

1. Hein KD, Mulliken JB, Kozakewich HP, Upton J, Burrows PE. Venous malformation of skeletal muscle. Plast Reconstr Surg. 2002;110(7):1625-35.
2. Eifert S, Vyllavicencio JL, Kao TC, Taute BM, Rich NM. Prevalence of deep venous anomalies in congenital vascular malformations of venous redominance. J Vasc Surg 2000; 31(3):462-71.
3. Nagy M, Brodsky L. Multidisciplinary approach to management of hemangiomas and vascular malformations. Facial Plast Surg Clin Morth Am. 2001;9:551-9.
4. Buckmiller LM. Update on hemangiomas and vascular malformations. Curr Opin Otolaryngol Head Neck Surg. 2004;12:476-87.
5. Lee BB. New approaches to the treatment of congenital vascular malformations: a single center experience. Eur J Vasc Endovasc Surg. 2005;30:184-97.
6. Lee BB, Bergan JJ. Advanced management of congenital vascular malformations: a multidisciplinary approach. Cardiovasc Surg. 2002;10:523-33.
7. O'Donovan JC, Donaldson JS, Morello FP, Pensler JM, Vogelzang RL, Bauer B, et al. Symptomatic hemangiomas and venous malformations in infants, children and young adults: treatment with percutaneous injection of sodium tetradecylsulphate. Am J Roentgenol. 1997;169(3):723-9.
8. de Lorimier AA. Sclerotherapy for venous malformations. J Pediatr Surg. 1995;30:188-93.
9. Shin BS, Do YS, Lee BB, Kim DI, Chung IS, Cho HS, et al. Multistage ethanol sclerotherapy of soft-tissue arteriovenous malformations: effect on pulmonary artery pressure. Radiology. 2005;235(3):1072-7.

10. Johann AC, Aguiar MC, do Carmo MA, Gomez RS, Castro WH, Mesquita RA. Sclerotherapy of oral benign vascular lesion with ethanolamine oleate: an open clinical trial with 30 lesions. Oral Surg Oral Med Oral Pathol Oral Radiol Endod. 2005;100(5):579-84.
11. Hyodoh H, Fuita A, Hyodoh K, Furuse M, Kamisawa O, Hareyama M. High-flow arteriovenous malformation of the lower extremity: ethanolamine oleate sclerotherapy. Cardiovasc Intervent Radiol. 2001;24(5):348-51.
12. Siniluoto TM, Svendsen PA, Wikholm GM, Fogdestam I, Edström S. Percutaneous sclerotherapy of venous malformations of the head and neck using sodium tetradecylsulphate, Scand J Plast Reconstr Surg Hand Surg. 1997;31(2):145-50.
13. Anavi Y, Har-El G, Mintz S. The treatment of facial hemangioma by percutaneous injections of sodium tetradecylsulphate. J Laryngol Otol. 1988;102:87-90.
14. Guex JJ. Indications for the sclerosing agent polidocanol. J Dermatol Surg Oncol. 1994;19:959-61
15. Legiehn GM, Heran MKS. Venous malformations: classification, development, diagnosis and interventional radiological management. Radiol Clin North Am. 2008;46:545-97.
16. Orbach EJ. Sclerotherapy of varicose veins: utilization of intravenous air block. Am J Surg. 1944;66:362-6.
17. Cabrera Garrido JR, Cabrera Garcia-Olmedo JR, Garcia-Olmedo Dominguez MA. Elargissement des limites de la sclerotherapie nouveaux produits sclerosants. Phlebologie. 1997;50:181-8.
18. Pascarella L. Bergan JJ, Yamada C, Mekenas L. Venous angiomata treatment with sclerosant foam. Ann Vasc Surg. 2005;19(4):457-64.
19. Legiehn GM, Heran MKS. Classification, diagnosis and interventional radiological management of vascular malformations. Orthop Clin North Am. 2006;37:435-74.
20. Goyal M, Causer PA, Armstrong D. Venous vascular malformations in pediatric patients: comparison of results of alcohol sclerotherapy with proposed MR imaging classification. Radiology. 2002;223:639-44.
21. Mukul SK, Singh A, Kumar A, Pandey S, Singh S, Kumar A. Foam polidocanol sclerotherapy for low-flow vascular malformations of tongue. Ann Maxillofac Surg. 2019;9: 257-60.
22. Critello CD, Pullano SA, Matula TJ, De Franciscis S, Serra R, Fiorillo AS. Recent developments on foaming mechanical and electronic techniques for the management of varicose veins. Expert Rev Med Devices. 2019;16:931-40.
23. Odeyinde SO, Kangesu L, Badran M. Sclerotherapy for vascular malformations: complications and a review of techniques to avoid them. J Plast Reconstr Aesthet Surg. 2013;66:215-23.
24. Mahesh B, Thulkar S, Joseph G, Khazanchi RK, Srivastava A. Colour duplex ultrasound-guided sclerotherapy: a new approach to the management of patients with peripheral vascular malformations. Clin Imaging. 2003;27(3): 171-9.
25. Jain R, Bandhu S, Sawhney S, Mittal R. Sonographically guided percutaneous sclerosis using 1% polidocanol in the treatment of vascular malformations. J Clin Ultrasound. 2002;30(7):416-23.
26. Rimon U, Garniek A, Galili Y, Golan G, Bensaid P, Morag B. Ethanol sclerotherapy of peripheral venous malformations. Eur J Radiol. 2004;52(3):283-7.
27. Berenguer B, Burrows PE, Zurakowski D, Mulliken JB. Sclerotherapy of craniofacial venous malformations: complications and results. Plast Reconstr Surg. 1999;104(1): 1-11.
28. Tan KT, Kirby J, Rajan DK, Hayeems E, Beecroft JR, Simons ME. Percutaneous sodium tetradecyl sulfate sclerotherapy for peripheral venous vascular malformations: a single-center experience. J Vasc Interv Radiol. 2007;18(3):343-51.
29. Kuo HW, Yang CH. Venous lake of the lip treated with a sclerosing agent: report of two cases. Dermatol Surg. 2003; 29:425-8.
30. Park CO, Lee MJ, Chung KY. Treatment of unusual vascular lesions: usefulness of sclerotherapy in lymphangioma circumscriptum and acquired digital arteriovenous malformation. Dermatol Surg. 2005;31(11 Pt 1):1451-3.
31. Khandpur S, Sharma VK. Utility of intralesional sclerotherapy with 3% sodium tetradecyl sulphate in cutaneous vascular malformations. Dermatol Surg. 2010;36:340-6.
32. Jairath V, Dayal S, Jain VK, Jindal N, Gogna P, Sehrawat M, et al. Is sclerotherapy useful for cherry angiomas? Dermatol Surg. 2014;40(9):10227.
33. Wang Y, Tu Y, Tao J, Li Y. Angiolymphoid hyperplasia with eosinophilia responsive to sclerotherapy. Dermatol Surg. 2014;40(9):10423.
34. Kupetsky EA, PuglianoMauro M. Lymphangioma circumscriptum: sodium tetradecyl sulfate 0.1% versus hypertonic saline. Dermatol Surg. 2014;40:92830.
35. Deore GD, Gurav AN, Patil R, Shete AR, NaikTari RS, Khiste SV, et al. Sclerotherapy: a novel bloodless approach to treat recurrent oral pyogenic granuloma associated with portwine stain. Ann Vasc Surg. 2014;28(6):1564.e914.
36. Lee HJ, Kim TW, Kim JM, Kim GW, Ko HC, Kim BS, et al. Percutaneous sclerotherapy using bleomycin for the treatment of vascular malformations. Int J Dermatol. 2017; 56(11):1186-91.
37. Song D, Guo L, Sheng H, Li J, Wang L, Wu C, et al. DSA-guided percutaneous sclerotherapy for children with oropharyngeal low-flow venous malformation. Exp Ther Med. 2020;19: 3405-10.
38. Vollherbst DF, Gebhart P, Kargus S, Burger A, Kühle R, Günther P, et al. Image-guided percutaneous sclerotherapy of venous malformations of the head and neck: Clinical and MR-based volumetric mid-term outcome. PLoS One. 2020;15(10):e0241347.
39. Tu JH, Do HM, Patel V, Yeom KW, Teng JMC. Sclerotherapy for lymphatic malformations of the head and neck in the pediatric population. J Neurointerv Surg. 2017;9:1023-6.

SECTION 5 Vitiligo Surgery

CHAPTER 34

Overview of Vitiligo Surgery

Davinder Prasad

KEY MESSAGES

- Surgery for vitiligo is useful in resistant areas and residual lesions.
- The choice of surgical treatment depends on the type of vitiligo, extent and site of lesions, the availability of equipment, and expertise of the treating surgeon. Sometimes, more than one procedure may be required.
- Currently available methods are classified as grafting and nongrafting techniques. The grafting techniques, which are the more commonly used, include both tissue grafts and the more recent cellular methods.
- Methods of assessing stability include duration of stability by history, presence of Koebner's phenomenon, and test grafting; however, none of these methods are fully accurate.
- The Indian Association of Dermatologists, Venereologists and Leprologists (IADVL) Task Force recommends 1 year of absence of spread or absence of new lesions as the required duration of stability before surgery can be considered.

INTRODUCTION

Vitiligo is a common acquired depigmenting disorder, characterized clinically by white patches and histologically by an absence or near absence of functional melanocytes in the affected areas. Different clinical types of vitiligo include localized, generalized, and segmental patterns. The disease is of great cosmetic importance in brown or black skin and causes much social stigma. It runs a variable course, with many lesions achieving stability either with or without treatment. The pathogenesis of vitiligo is only partially understood; the destruction of melanocytes occurs due to a complex interaction of environmental, genetic, and immunologic factors. Conventional medical treatments (topical and systemic corticosteroids and immunomodulators) and physical therapies (phototherapy and lasers) are effective only in 50–60% of cases. Certain areas such as acral, bony, and nonhairy areas are resistant to these treatments. Surgical treatment is useful in such resistant areas and residual lesions. **Figure 1** shows an overview of current treatment modalities in vitiligo.

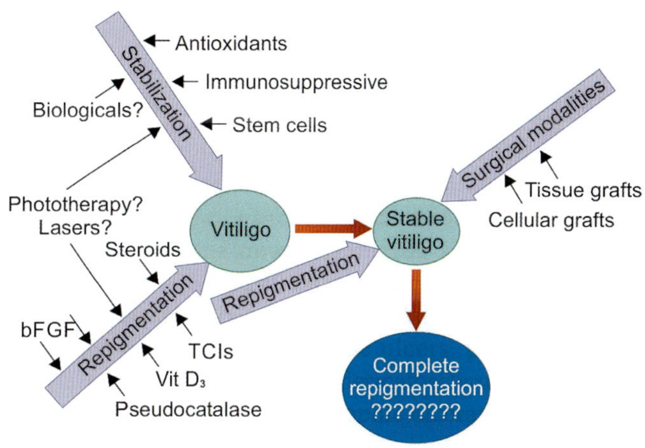

Fig. 1: Overview of management of vitiligo.
Courtesy: Dr Davinder Prasad, Chandigarh.

HISTORY

Different corrective surgical methods have evolved during the last four decades. Important milestones in the historical evolution of vitiligo surgery are thin Thiersch's graft,[1] epidermal grafting by suction blister,[2] punch grafting,[3] minipunch grafting,[4,5] cultured melanocytes grafting,[6,7] grafting of cultured epidermis,[8] autografting, psoralen plus ultraviolet A (PUVA),[9,10] transplantation of autologous cultured melanocytes,[11] single hair transplant,[12] ultrathin epidermal sheets and basal cell layer suspension,[13] minigrafting, and narrowband ultraviolet B (NB-UVB).[14]

PRINCIPLE OF SURGICAL TREATMENT

The basic objective of surgical treatment in vitiligo is to produce cosmetically acceptable repigmentation of the vitiliginous lesions. The basic principle is to introduce melanocytes into the lesional skin, which will then establish and function as epidermal melanin units. The cells survive and function if the stability has been achieved, and the disease is in a state of donor dominance. The melanocytes may be introduced through either tissue grafts or through cellular grafts.

METHODS OF SURGERY

The ideal surgical treatment modality for vitiligo should provide complete or near complete repigmentation, in the shortest possible time, with minimal discomfort to the patient, have no or minimal side effects, and is cheap. However, such an ideal treatment is not available. The choice of surgical treatment depends on the type of vitiligo, extent and site of lesions, the availability of equipment, and expertise of the treating cutaneous surgeon. Sometimes, more than one procedure may be required. Currently available methods are classified as grafting and nongrafting techniques. The grafting techniques, which are the more commonly used, include both tissue grafts and the more recent cellular methods **(Table 1)**.

Factors to be Considered for Patient Selection

For any surgical method to yield good results, proper selection of cases is of paramount importance. Stability of vitiligo is considered as the most important parameter while opting for any transplantation technique to treat vitiligo.

Concept of Stability in Vitiligo

Stability indicates absence of new lesions and absence of spread of existing lesions. An additional feature can be evidence of repigmentation and absence of Koebner's phenomenon (KP).[15] However, there are several aspects which need consideration while considering surgery:

- What should be the minimum duration of stability?
- Is stability patient specific or area specific or lesion specific?
- Validity of test grafting (TG).
- Importance of KP.
- How long does stability last?
- Induced versus spontaneous stability.
- Concept of cellular stability.

Each of these aspects is discussed here in detail.

TABLE 1: Techniques in vitiligo surgery.

Grafting techniques		*Nongrafting techniques*
Tissue grafts: Minipunch grafting	*Cellular grafts:* Noncultured cell suspensions—epidermal cell and follicular cell	Micropigmentation
Suction blister grafting	Cultured melanocytes/ keratinocytes grafts	Excision/closure
Thin split thickness grafting		Dermabrasion and chemabrasion
Hair follicle grafts, smash grafts, mesh grafts		Lasers and light therapy systems—excimer laser, excimer light, and targeted phototherapy

Duration of Stability

Despite the fact that surgery in vitiligo has been practiced for decades, it is important to note that consensus does not exist regarding the optimal required period of stability. The total lack of agreement among different workers can be striking, as seen in **Table 2**. Recently in their consensus recommendations, the IADVL Task Force for standard guidelines of care for dermatosurgical procedures attempted to provide a clear definition of stability—a patient reporting no new lesions, no progression of existing lesions and absence of Koebner phenomenon during the past 1 year.[16] Spontaneous repigmentation is also considered as favorable signs for vitiligo surgery.

Stability

Stability may be lesion-specific in many patients. Due to poorly understood reasons, simultaneous depigmentation and repigmentation have been noticed in different areas of the same patient.[17] Variable results have been obtained over the donor site and recipient site of the same patient.[17-20] A stable lesion has a well-defined, sometimes pigmented border, shows spotty pigmentation **(Fig. 2)**. An unstable vitiligo lesion has ill-defined border **(Fig. 3)**.

TABLE 2: Minimum period of stability in different studies.

Author	*Year*	*Period of stability*
Das SS and Pasricha JS	1992	4 months
Boersma BR and Westerhof W	1995	6 months
Jha AK, Pandey SS, and Shukla VK	1992	1 year
Savant SS	1992	2 years
Falabella R	2003	2 years
Falabella R	1995	2 years
Falabella R	1992	3 years

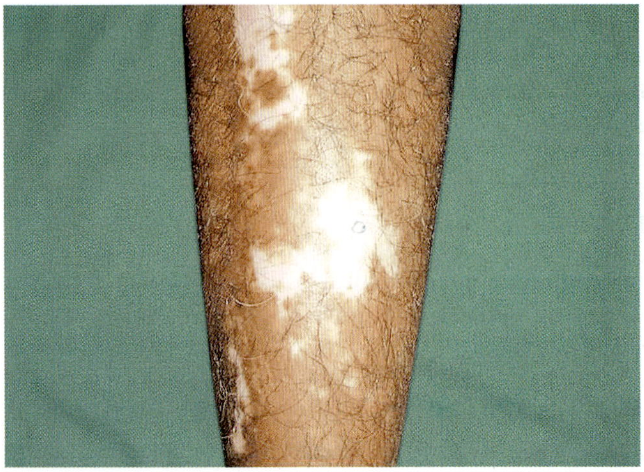

Fig. 2: Stable vitiligo.

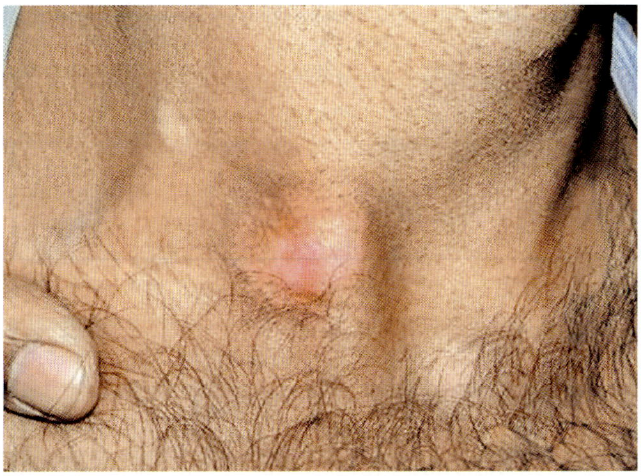

Fig. 3: Unstable vitiligo.

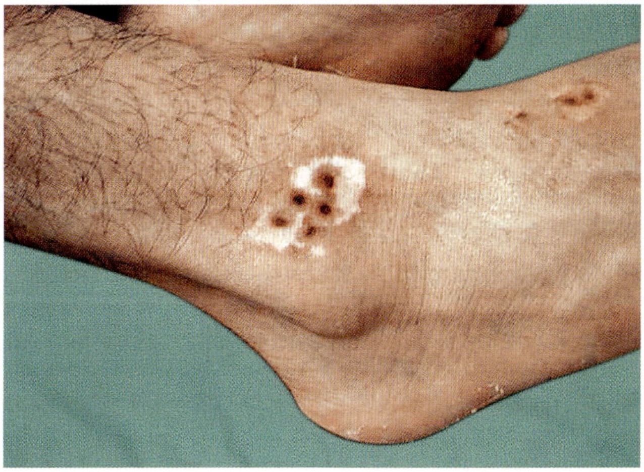

Fig. 4: Test grafting.

Test Grafting

In view of the earlier mentioned lack of consensus about the minimal period of stability, objective criteria are needed for defining stability. One such test was the introduction of TG or minigrafts test by Falabella in 1995.[19] TG consists of placing six to eight punch grafts within a vitiligo lesion and observing over the next 12 weeks (read the Chapter on punch grafting for details). Unequivocal repigmentation occurring beyond 1 mm from the border of the test graft indicates a positive test and therefore is an indicator of stability **(Fig. 4)**. This TG has been found to be a more reliable exercise than the arbitrarily defined period of stability alone.[21-23] However, the concept of TG too has been subjected to scrutiny.[17,21]

- It has been suggested that behavior of donor area, from where punches are taken, too should be taken into consideration, concurrently, in addition to the behavior of the minigrafts in the recipient site, while testing for stability. This is because donor area stability may be different from recipient area stability.
- TG positivity does not necessarily guarantee a favorable outcome in all cases even after perfect graft take up.

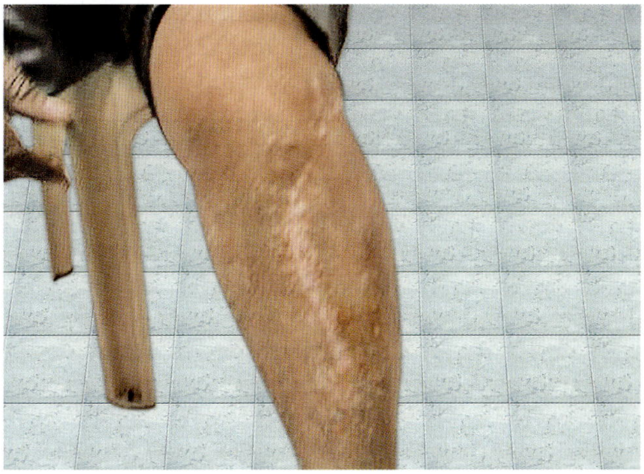

Fig. 5: Koebner's phenomenon.

- Encouraging results have been obtained even after grafting in some TG negative cases.
- Simultaneous donor site repigmentation and depigmentation of grafts at the recipient site or donor site depigmentation with complete repigmentation of the recipient area have been observed.

Juhlin emphasized and observed, neither the history nor test graft is a complete help to obtain good effect. It seems we have to wait until the method of identification and isolation of skin-homing melanocyte-specific cytotoxic T lymphocytes is available.[24] Falabella himself expressed his doubts about the comprehensiveness of minigraft test. He observed, even when the minigrafting test is positive, "depigmenting activity" may still be present and prevent satisfactory repigmentation.[8]

Koebner's Phenomenon

Koebner's phenomenon indicates active disease **(Fig. 5)**. More recently Njoo et al. explored the association between the experimentally-induced Koebner phenomenon (KP-e) and the Koebner phenomenon by history (KP-h), disease activity and therapeutic responsiveness in vitiligo vulgaris.[15] They proposed a scoring system to measure disease activity on a 6-point scale from 1 to +4 [vitiligo disease activity (VIDA) score **(Table 3)**]. It is suggested that surgery for vitiligo may be performed only in patients with VIDA scores of –1 or 0. The KP-e may function well as a clinical factor to assess present disease activity and may also predict the responsiveness to phototherapy. But despite the more comprehensive nature of the scoring system, VIDA scoring system was found lacking as VIDA score did not always predict a positive KP-e.

Hence, it can be concluded that, overdependence on KP or TG may be sometimes misleading in this enigmatic disease, because what these two reveal is the apparent clinical stability only and that may not be the true reflection of stability status of the disease at the cellular level.[21]

TABLE 3: Vitiligo disease activity (VIDA) score.

Disease activity	*VIDA score*
Active in past 6 weeks	+4
Active in past 3 months	+3
Active in past 6 months	+2
Active in past 1 year	+1
Stable for at least 1 year	0
Stable for at least 1 year and spontaneous repigmentation	–1

Longevity of Stability

Another important indicator is the longevity of stability status of vitiligo—how long would the disease remain stable, after achieving "stability"? When will it start to become unstable again in future? These are hard to predict as there are very few long-term follow-up studies to determine relapse after surgery. It is also known that the disease is extremely variable in behavior.

Induced versus Spontaneous Stability

Stability can be induced by treatment with steroids, PUVA, and narrowband phototherapy.[25,26] These treatments may stabilize the disease by promoting apoptosis of the perilesional and circulating melanocyte-specific cytotoxic CD8 cells.[26,27] However, relapse may occur after stopping treatment. There are no clear cut answers as to how long such induced stability would be maintained. A recent study proposed 1 year as the "period of stability of repigmentation" (as opposed to period of inactivity discussed so far)—suggesting that, to qualify as stable, the repigmentated status (not just absence of spread) must be maintained for a period of not <1 year.[28]

Cellular Stability

The earlier mentioned factors have focused on clinical stability. It is obvious that assessment of "cellular" stability is of paramount importance and the cellular parameters should also be taken into consideration, along with the clinical stability. Markers such as CD8 may prove useful in indicating stability of a lesion. Very recently a group of workers while determining the markers of the stability of vitiligo (CD8, CD45RO, and FOXP3) has observed that percentage of CD8 and CD45RO lymphocytes in lesional skin biopsy may provide objective indication of lesion or area based stability. They have also observed that a higher percentage of cytotoxic CD8 cells is associated with failure of melanocyte transplantation.[29-31] However, such markers are not available routinely.

The earlier mentioned discussion suggests that the subject is open to debate in several aspects. However, this does not mean that we should refrain from using the surgical option till those unexplored areas are charted and the cellular parameters become available; rather we should continue surgical intervention based on logical application of our clinical knowledge and after proper counseling. Clinical criteria based on different factors such as duration of stability, activity of disease, KP, and TG should all be the criteria to help us choose a suitable patient for surgery. As in any surgical procedure, situation of a given patient and his/her needs should always be paramount in our decision making.

Disease versus Lesional Stability (General vs. Local Stability)

There is no consensus regarding the minimum duration of stability or the relative importance of disease and lesional stability in selecting patients for vitiligo grafting. A recent publication studied 170 patients into two groups: Group A with lesional stability of >1 year but overall disease stability of only 6–11 months and Group B with overall disease stability of >1 year. Patients underwent either tissue or cellular vitiligo grafting on the selected lesions and the repigmentation achieved was scored from 0 (no repigmentation) to 6 (100% repigmentation). Average repigmentation achieved (on scale of 0–6) was 3.8 and 4.04 in Group A and Group B, respectively. In Group A, ≥90% repigmentation was achieved in 36.6% (30/82) patients, while 37.5% (33/88) achieved similar results in Group B. Additionally, 47.6% (39/82) and 53.4% (47/88) of cases achieved partial repigmentation in Group A and Group B, respectively. Statistical analysis revealed no significant differences between the two groups with respect to the repigmentation achieved or adverse effects observed. The study concluded that lesional stability seems to be as relevant as the overall disease stability in selecting patients for surgical intervention in vitiligo.[32]

CASE SELECTION

Surgery is indicated for patients with stable lesions of vitiligo vulgaris, localized or segmental vitiligo lesions, though it may be done for all types of vitiligo (including segmental, generalized, and acrofacial types), that do not respond to medical treatment and are stable. A test graft may be considered whenever there is a doubt about the stability or there is doubtful history. Acral lesions do not respond well to surgery and hence such patients should be counseled properly. Age of the patient is an important consideration, though there is no age limit for surgery. Younger patients respond better to surgery[33,34] but performing surgery in children may need general anesthesia, with its inherent risks and in whom the future course of the disease is extremely variable. Hence, it needs to be emphasized that each case should be considered individually on its merit.

PATIENT COUNSELING AND INFORMATION

Counseling should include detailed information about nature of the disease, the type and rationale of the surgical treatment chosen, expected outcome, need for proper immobilization after surgery, and possible complications. Concurrent need for concomitant medical therapy and phototherapy should all be emphasized. It should be stressed that surgical treatment only provides a cosmetic camouflage to the skin, but does not control disease activity; the objective is only cosmetic coverage, not perfect pigmentation. Areas such as lips and eyelids need special consideration in view of their special anatomical features. It is also important to assess psychological outlook and social problems of the patient.

PATIENT EXAMINATION

The stability of the disease should be assessed by a detailed history and examination of lesions. History taking should include questions about occurrence of recent lesions, increase in size of the existing lesions, occurrence of lesions at site of injury, and family history. Physical examination should include proper systemic and cutaneous examination to rule out any underlying conditions, presence of keloids, etc.

A detailed consent form describing the procedure and possible complications should be signed by the patient. The consent form should specifically state the limitations of the procedure, possibility of future disease progression, and the need for repeated procedures for satisfactory results. Preoperative photography is of vital importance, as in any surgical method of treatment and it also helps in medicolegal situations.

Preoperative Investigations

Routine investigations such as hemoglobin estimation, blood counts, bleeding and clotting time, and blood sugar estimation are adequate in most cases. In elderly patients, electrocardiogram (ECG) may be needed.

CHOICE OF METHOD OF SURGERY

The appropriate surgical method is chosen taking different factors into consideration: area affected, age of patient, patients' attitude and requirements, facility available, expertise of the surgeon, and cost of surgery. Each of the methods has its advantages and disadvantages. In general punch grafting is the easiest method, but is also associated with most side effects and least cosmetic acceptance. Suction blister grafting yields outstanding results both at donor and recipient areas, but has the limitation of limited yield of graft. Split thickness graft is quick and yield large grafts, but need surgical skill and the graft may be thicker. Cellular methods are safer, need less donor and hence are associated with more rapid healing, but are more expensive, need more training and specific infrastructure. An overview of different methods is shown in **Table 4 and Table 5** shows the choice of different methods for each area. The techniques are discussed in detail in subsequent chapters.

TABLE 4: Overview of surgical techniques in stable vitiligo.

Technique	*Indications*	*Advantages*	*Disadvantages*
Minipunch grafting	*Small irregular areas:* Acral areas, palms, and soles	Simple, easy, and inexpensive office procedure	• Scarring is frequent at the donor site • Cobblestoning is common. Least cosmetic acceptance • Results are not immediate as it needs follow-up phototherapy and takes 2–3 months for pigment spread
Suction blister grafting	*Small areas:* Lips and eyelids	• No scarring at the donor site • Good cosmetic results, particularly on the lips • Safe and inexpensive technique • Does not require special surgical skills	• Time consuming procedure • Yields only small size grafts
Thin split thickness skin grafting	Suitable for large areas	• Most commonly used technique • Covers large areas over a short period of time • Pigmentation is uniform • Systemic psoralen plus ultraviolet A (PUVA) therapy is not required routinely • Difficult areas such as eyelids, inner canthus of eyes, areola, nipples, and genitals can be treated	• Hyperpigmentation and hypertrophy is common, especially on exposed areas and dark-skinned patients • In extensive vitiligo there is a limitation of availability of the donor skin • Needs surgical skill • Donor healing may be delayed
Autologous noncultured epidermal cell suspension	All areas can be treated	• Larger areas can be treated at a single session with small donor skin • Repigmentation is uniform	• Laboratory facilities are required • Pigmentation takes up to 2–3 months • Expensive technique • Needs special training
Cultured melanocyte grafting	All areas can be treated	The melanocytes can be expanded up to 100 times by culture methods; hence large areas can be treated in a single session	• It is an expensive technique requiring a fully equipped tissue culture laboratory with experienced staff • The long-term safety of culture media and carcinogenic potential need further evaluation • Still experimental

TABLE 5: The choice of method for a given area.

Area	*Method of choice*	*Alternative methods*	*Comment*
Face	Suction blister and epidermal cell suspension	Split thickness grafts	Thin graft needed for good results; high degree of cosmesis expected
Lip, eyelids, and genitals	Suction blister and epidermal cell suspension	Split thickness grafts and punch grafting	Immobilization is difficult
Other areas such as abdomen and legs	Split thickness grafts and epidermal cell suspension	Punch grafts	
Acral areas, palms, and soles	Punch grafts		No method yields consistent results Results unsatisfactory

CONCLUSION

Vitiligo surgery has made major advances in techniques and it is now possible to cover large areas. However, the criteria for stability are yet to be defined clearly—perhaps this is because the etiology of vitiligo is yet to be understood fully. More follow-up studies and cellular marker studies are needed to define better criteria.

REFERENCES

1. Behl PN. Homologous thin Thiersch's grafts in treatment of vitiligo. Curr Med Pract. 1964;8:218-21.
2. Falabella R. Epidermal grafting: an original technique and its application in achromic and granulating areas. Arch Dermatol. 1971;104:592-600.
3. Orentriech N, Selmanwitz VJ. Autograft repigmentation of leucoderma. Arch Dermatol. 1972;105:784-6.
4. Falabella R. Repigmentation of leucoderma by minigrafts of normally pigmented, autologous skin. J Dermatol Surg Oncol. 1978;4:916-9.
5. Falabella R. Repigmentation of segmental vitiligo by autologous minigrafting. J Am Acad Dermatol. 1983;9:514-21.
6. Lerner AB, Halaban R, Klaus SN, Moellmann GE. Transplantation of human melanocytes. J Invest Dermatol. 1987;89:219-24.
7. Lerner AB. Repopulation of pigmented cells in patients with vitiligo. Arch Dermatol. 1988;124:1701-2.
8. Falabella R, Escobar C, Borrero I. Treatment of refractory and stable vitiligo by transplantation of in vitro cultured epidermal autografts bearing melanocytes. J Am Acad Dermatol. 1992;26:230-6.
9. Skouge JW, Morison WL, Diwan RV, Rotter S. Autografting and PUVA. A combination therapy for vitiligo. J Dermatol Surg Oncol. 1992;18:357-60.
10. Hann SK, Im S, Bong HW, Park YK. Treatment of stable vitiligo with autologous epidermal grafting and PUVA. J Am Acad Dermatol. 1995;32:943-8.
11. Olsson MJ, Juhlin L. Repigmentation of vitiligo by transplantation of cultured autologous melanocytes. Acta Derm Venereol (Stockh). 1993;73:49-51.
12. Malakar S, Dhar S. Repigmentation of vitiligo patches by transplantation of hair follicles. Int J Dermatol. 1999;38:237-8.
13. Olsson MJ, Juhlin L. Long-term follow-up of leucoderma patients treated with transplants of autologous cultured melanocytes, ultrathin epidermal sheets and basal cell layer suspension. Br J Dermatol. 2002;147:893-904.
14. Lahiri K, Malakar S, Sarma N, Banerjee U. Repigmentation of vitiligo with punch grafting and narrow-band UV-B (311 nm) a prospective study. Int J Dermatol. 2006;45:649-55.
15. Njoo MD, Das PK, Bos JD, Westerhof W. Association of the Koebner phenomen with disease activity and therapeutic responsiveness in vitiligo vulgaris. Arch Dermatol. 1999;135:407-13.
16. Parsad D, Gupta S. Standard guidelines of care for vitiligo surgery. Indian J Dermatol Venereol Leprol. 2008;74:S37-45.
17. Malakar S, Lahiri K, Malakar RS. How unstable is the concept of stability in surgical repigmentation of vitiligo? Dermatol. 2000;201:182-3.
18. Falabella R. Surgical treatment of vitiligo: why, when and how. J Eur Acad Dermatol Venereol. 2003;17:518-20.
19. Falabella R, Arrunategui A, Barona MI, Alzate A. The minigrafting test for vitiligo: detection of stable lesions for melanocyte transplantation. J Am Acad Dermatol. 1995;32:228-32.
20. Westerhof W, Boersma B. The minigrafting test for vitiligo: detection of stable lesions for melanocyte transplantation. J Am Acad Dermatol. 1995;33:1061.
21. Lahiri K, Malakar S, Banerjee U, Sarma N. Clinico-cellular stability of vitiligo in surgical repigmentation: an unexplored frontier. Dermatol. 2004;209:170-1.
22. Malakar S, Dhar S. Rejection of punch grafts in three cases of herpes labialis induced lip leucoderma, caution and precaution. Dermatol. 1997;195:414.
23. Malakar S, Dhar S. Acyclovir can abort rejection of punch grafts in herpes-simplex induced lip leucoderma. Dermatol. 1999;199:75.
24. Juhlin L. How unstable is the concept of stability in surgical repigmentation of vitiligo. Dermatol. 2000;201:183.
25. Lahiri K, Malakar S, Sarma N, Banerjee U. Inducing repigmentation by regrafting and phototherapy (311 nm) in punch failure cases of lip vitiligo-a pilot study. Indian J Dermatol Venereol Leprol. 2004;70:156-8.
26. JP Ortonne. Vitiligo pathogenesis: What's new? J Eur Acad Dermatol Venereol. 2003;17:30.
27. van den Wijngaard RM, Aten J, Scheepmaker A, Le Poole IC, Tigges AJ, Westerhof W, et al. Expression and modulation of apoptosis regulatory molecules in human melanocytes: significance in vitiligo. Br J Dermatol. 2000;143:573-81.
28. Parsad D, Pandhi R, Dogra S, Kumar B. Clinical study of repigmentation patterns with different treatment modalities and their correlation with speed and stability of repigmentation in 352 vitiliginous patches. J Am Acad Dermatol. 2004;50:63-7.
29. Rao A, Gupta S, Dinda AK, Sharma A, Sharma VK, Kumar G, et al. Study of clinical, biochemical and immunological factors

determining stability of disease in patients with generalized vitiligo undergoing melanocyte transplantation. Br J Dermatol. 2012;166(6):1230-6.

30. Kumar R, Parsad D. Melanocytorrhagy and apoptosis in vitiligo: Connecting jigsaw pieces. Indian J Dermatol Venereol Leprol. 2012;78:19-23.
31. Rao A, Gupta S, Sharma VK. Determinants of success of melanocyte transplantation in vitiligo: role of cytotoxic CD8 T cells. Pigment Cell Res. 2011;24:833.
32. Majid I, Mysore V, Salim T, Lahiri K, Chatterji M, Khunger N, et al. Is lesional stability in vitiligo more important than disease stability for performing surgical interventions? Results from a multicentric study. J Cutan Aesthet Surg. 2017;9:13-9.
33. Gupta S, Kumar B. Epidermal grafting in vitiligo: Influence of age, site of lesion, and type of disease on outcome. J Am Acad Dermatol. 2003;49:99-104.
34. Gupta S, Kumar B. Epidermal grafting for vitiligo in adolescents. Pediatr Dermatol. 2002;19:159-62.

CHAPTER 35

Minigrafting for Vitiligo

Koushik Lahiri

KEY MESSAGES

- Minigrafting in vitiligo remains the easiest, fastest, and cheapest of all surgical options in vitiligo.
- If deployed properly, it can produce excellent result.
- Stability must be assessed before opting for surgical options in vitiligo.
- Optimal punch sizes are 1, 1.2, and 1.5 mm. Punch sizes >1.5 mm are to be avoided.
- Cobblestoning and polka dotting remain the main complication if larger punches are used.
- Phototherapy, after minigrafting evokes encouraging results.

INTRODUCTION

Vitiligo is a result of disrupted epidermal melanization with an undecided etiology and incompletely understood pathogenesis. Various treatment options have resulted in various degrees of success. Various surgical modalities and transplantation techniques have evolved during the last few decades. Of them, miniature punch grafting (PG) has established its place as the easiest, fastest, and least expensive method. Various aspects of this particular procedure have been discussed here. The historical perspective, the instruments, evolution of mini grafting down the ages, and the methodology, advantages, and disadvantages have been discussed. A detailed discussion on the topic along with a review of relevant literature has been provided in this chapter.

HISTORICAL PERSPECTIVE

Vitiligo is the most significant form of cutaneous achromia which is an illusive, if not enigmatic problem down the ages. In all the ancient civilizations and religions, there is some reference to vitiligo. In the *Rigveda,* it was referred to as *"Kilas"* meaning a white spotted deer. It is interesting to note that as per the Vedic myth the anthropomorphic adoration of the sun, Bhagavantam, developed vitiligo after being gazed upon by his illegitimate son.[1] The disease was mentioned in *"Tarkh-e-Tibbl-e-Iran"* in the period of the *Aushooriyan*, as early as 2200 BC. In 1550 BC, information regarding vitiligo was noted in the Ebers Papyrus.[2] Unfortunately in some of the prominent ancient texts, the disease was confused with leprosy and also other skin diseases like psoriasis. This was referred to as *Swethakushtha* (white leprosy) in the *Atharva Veda* (1400 BC).[3] An accurate description also exists in a collection of Japanese Shinto prayers, *Amarakośa*, dating from 1200 BC.[4] In the Old Testament, the white spots were also described in Verse 2 of Chapter 13 of Leviticus under the Hebrew word *Zora at* or *Tzaraat/Tzoraath. Tsoraath* was translated using the Greek word "Lepros", which means a scale or scales. Along with this the phonetic resemblance of the word *Tsoraath* (which in Ashkenazi pronunciation would read *tsoraas*) led to the belief that "leprosy" was psoriasis. In truth, in all likelihood, most cases of biblical "leprosy" were achromic or hypochromic disorders that would include vitiligo, some cases of psoriasis, cases of pityriasis alba, probably albinism, and also leprosy. The word got translated as "lepra" in the Greek and English translations of the Bible. Also the theory of vitiligo as a dirty/polluted/contaminated disease was initiated, as the word *Tzaraat* refers to a group of skin diseases, which according to the Old Testament, renders one ritually unclean.[5] The exact word "vitiligo" may have been derived from the Latin word *vitium* meaning "blemish", or possibly *vitulum* meaning "small blemish".[5] Another theory is that the Latin derivation is from the white, glistening flesh of calves (vitelius). Others believe that the actual word was first used by Celsus in his tome De Medicina in the first century AD.[4,6,7] References to this disease can also be found in the ancient Koran and Buddhist scripts.[7] The treatment has undergone an enormous evolutionary change from the Vedic days of *Vasuchika* to the most modern transplantation techniques. However, the ultimate goal remains the same, which is, replenishment of lost pigment.

With standard medical treatment options many patients respond. But several patients remain recalcitrant or respond only partially. Any attempt of repigmentation of these resistant patches with conventional medicinal modalities is often unsuccessful and sometimes exasperating, indicating the absence of melanocytes reservoir to induce repigmentation. Under these circumstances, melanocytes repopulation of the achromic areas is not possible unless a new source of pigment cells is placed by surgical methods within the depigmented lesion.[8]

Different corrective surgical methods have evolved during the last four decades. Some of these are thin Thiersch's graft,[9] epidermal grafting by suction blister,[10] punch grafting,[11] minipunch grafting,[12,13] cultured melanocytes grafting,[14,15] grafting of cultured epidermis,[16] autografting and psoralen plus ultraviolet A (PUVA),[17,18] transplantation of autologous cultured melanocytes, [19] single hair transplant,[20] ultrathin epidermal sheets and basal cell layer suspension,[21] and minigrafting and narrowband ultraviolet B (NB-UVB).[22]

Among all these minipunch grafting is the easiest, fastest, least aggressive, and minimal expensive method.

THE PUNCH INSTRUMENT

The skin punch or surgical punch is an instrument which is used almost solely by dermatologists. It is interesting to note that originally it was used as a trephine to cut through the skull bone. Its use was documented in abscess removal from tibia as early as in 1852.[23] In 1878, Watson described the use of it in the correction of accidental gunpowder disfigurement.[24] But the importance of cutaneous punch instrument in dermatology was first established by Keyes in 1887.[25]

The Keyes punch **(Fig. 1)** has been used in dermatology since then for diagnostic purpose. Its rounded sharp cutting end and thick handle make it very much appropriate for small skin biopsies. Because of the thick walls with angled sides above the cutting edge, tissue leans to be pushed away as the punch is made, causing less dermis to be cut through (in diameter) than overlying epidermis. This is also a function of the bevel, which is outside the barrel of the Keyes punch.[26]

To overcome these difficulties other punches have been developed.[27]

The walls of the Loo trephine **(Fig. 2)** are thinner and less slanted than those of the Keyes punch, making it advantageous to use on depressed scars or minor autotransplants (where a straight vertical incision is needed). This is difficult to do with Keyes punch.

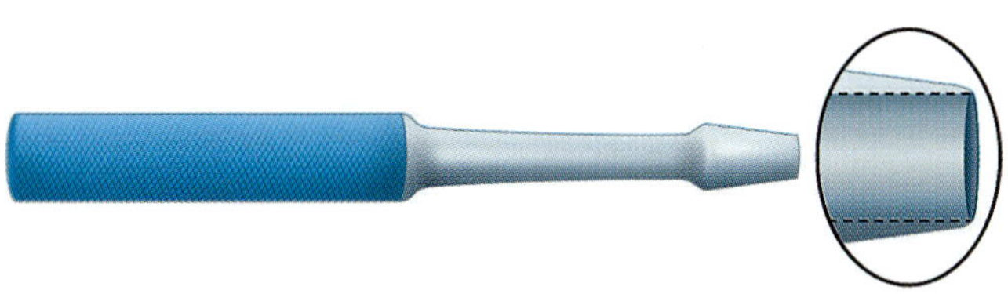

Fig. 1: Keyes punch.

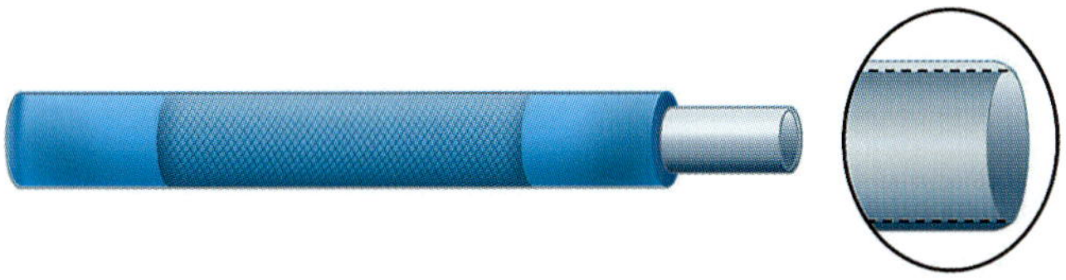

Fig. 2: Loo trephine.

The newer disposable punches **(Fig. 3)** are excellent for punch biopsies or excisional work on cysts. The razor-sharp edge is a great benefit. The punch is made in a number of different dimensions.

EVOLUTION OF MINIPUNCH GRAFTING

In the history of skin grafting, a couple of observations can be mentioned as a preamble to further discussion on punch grafting.

The first documented successful result of experimental skin grafting was described in sheep by Baronio in 1804.[28] But it took another almost one and half century to get the first recorded autograft response of dark-skinned autografts when transplanted to light areas in spotted guinea pigs by Lewin and Peck in 1941.[29]

In 1972, Norman Orentriech first reported autograft repigmentation in human. He treated a black woman with long-standing leukoderma that followed a chemical burn many years back when she was treated with home remedy which included a copper penny dipped in vinegar for presumptive tinea infection on her cheek. Orentriech deployed nine 1 and 2 mm diameter normal skin autografts and observed the "pigment spread phenomenon". He reported a maximum of 1 mm pigment spread from both 1 and 2 mm grafts.[11]

In 1976, Labuono and Shatin made a similar observation after transplanting hair bulbs with hair punch grafting within the leukodermic scars of discoid lupus erythematosus (DLE).[30]

Falabella in 1978 reported a novel method of repigmenting leukoderma. With the help of a power driven dermabrasion unit he used dental burrs to create abrasion 2–3 mm in diameter and <1 mm in depth and 5 mm apart. In the donor area, skin was raised by means of a curved needle, and was snipped off just below it to harvest 1–2 mm size minigrafts. He reported about 3 mm perigraft pigment spread by this technique. Three patients, one with piebaldism, another with chemical leukoderma, and a third with postburn depigmentation were treated by this method.[31] He observed that this superficial split thickness grafts evoked a much better outcome than the full thickness hair punch grafting by Labuono.

In the same article, interestingly, it was concluded that "... true vitiligo is not treatable by transplantation of grafts of normally pigmented, autologous skin".[31]

Miniature punches of 1.5 mm diameter was used by Falabella while repigmenting three cases of segmental vitiligo in 1983.[13]

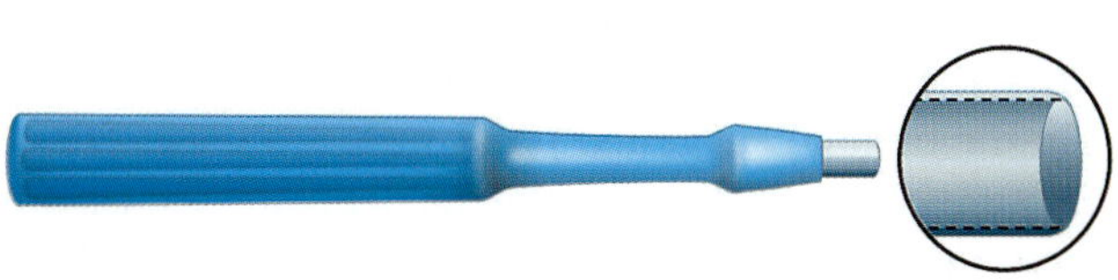

Fig. 3: Disposable punch.

Behl (1985) expressed some reservation while commenting on Falabella's work on minigrafting and claimed better results with thin Thiersch grafting. In a rejoinder Falabella reiterated his faith on miniature punch grafting and countered with his sets of reasons and logics in favor of punch grafting.[32,33]

In the following years Falabella reported success with minipunch grafting in chemical leukoderma, postdermabrasion leukoderma, and focal and segmental vitiligo.[34-36]

While repigmenting stable leukoderma with autologous minigrafting Falabella made an important observation regarding the relationship between the donor graft area and the area of surgical repigmentation and found that a 1 mm donor graft can originate a pigmented spot 25 times larger than its size.[34]

In 1995, it was Falabella again who combined epidermal grafting and minigrafting in treating vitiligo and piebaldism.[37]

Westerhof in 1994 reported success with punch grafting in stable vitiligo and observed a maximum of 5 mm of pigment spread.[38] In the subsequent year (1995), Boersma stressed on the importance of proper selection of cases before minigrafting.[39]

Various studies point toward the high effectiveness of the procedure.[40-43] An assortment of different evaluation parameters of minipunch grafting has also evolved over the years.[44-47]

TEST GRAFTING

Before embarking upon any surgical intervention in vitiligo proper assessment of the stability status is of paramount importance.

Clinically, stability can be judged by three simple indicators:

1. *History:* Lack of progression of old lesions and absence of development of any new lesion within a specified period (6 months to 2 years).
2. *Koebner phenomenon (KP):* Absence of a recent KP either from history (KP-h) or experimentally induced (KP-e).
3. *Test grafting (TG):* On the backdrop of a pervasive incongruity about the minimal period of stability an attempt was made for the first time by Falabella in 1995 to Fathom stability before surgery by introducing minigrafting test.[48]

The objective of this test vowed to serve several purposes:

- Establishing the stability of the depigmenting process
- Determine a means by which patients could be selected
- Identifying patients who may respond to pigment cell transplantation
- To anticipate the response to surgical repair.

In the original suggested procedure, few grafts (1.0–1.2 mm) were placed in the center of the depigmented lesion to be scrutinized. Dressing was done by Micropore® adhesive tape and kept for a couple of weeks. After removal of the tape the area was exposed to sunlight for 15 minutes daily for a period of 3 months. No treatment was permitted during this test period.

All test sites are visualized under Wood's light. The test was considered positive if unequivocal repigmentation takes place beyond 1 mm from the border of the implanted grafts. On the other hand, if <1 mm or no repigmentation was observed the test was considered as negative.

In some of the biggest series, this evaluation has been termed as "TG" and found this to be a more reliable exercise than the unjustified dependence on period of stability alone.[41,42]

Over the years this "test" has been vindicated and acknowledged as a powerful tool for detecting stable vitiligo, which anticipates the repigmentation success in vitiligo when surgery becomes a therapeutic option.

PROCEDURE OF MINIGRAFTING (FIGS. 4 TO 6)[31,40-42]

After proper assessment of the stability status and routine physical examination and investigations an informed consent is taken from the patient. The donor and recipient areas are surgically prepared.

- The instruments required are 1.5 or 1.2 mm punches, small jeweler's or graft holding forceps, and small curved tip scissors **(Fig. 5)**.
- Recipient area is prepared first. 2% lignocaine with or without adrenaline is infiltrated as local anesthetic.
- To minimize the chance of developing any perigraft halo, the initial recipient chambers are made on or very close to the border of the lesion. The punched out chambers are spaced according to the result of TG or at a gap of 5–10 mm from each other.

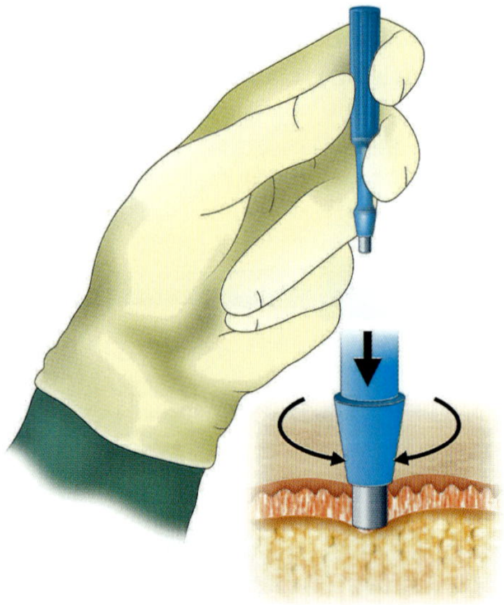

Fig. 4: Correct positioning of the hand while taking grafts with a miniature punch.

- The donor area is either upper lateral portion of thigh or gluteal area. Punch impressions are made very close to each other so that from a small area maximum number of grafts can be taken.
- Same sized punches are used for both donor and recipient area.

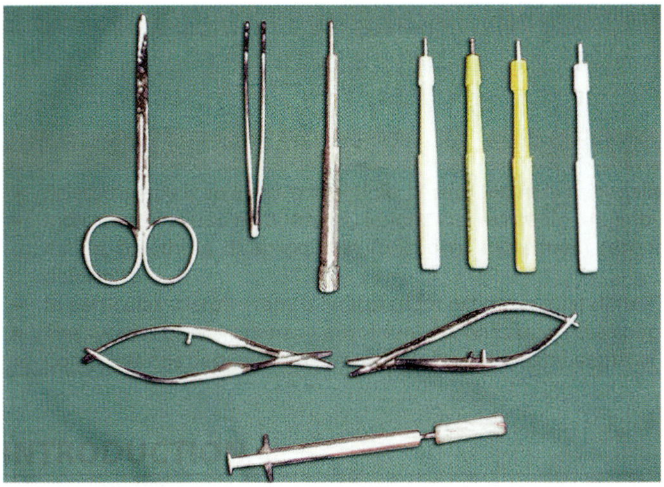

Fig. 5: Instrument needed for minigrafting.

- The grafts were placed directly from donor (buttock/upper thigh) to the recipient areas. This speeds up the procedure and lessens the chance of infection. Care is taken, so that the graft edges are not folded, the tissue is not crushed or placed upside down. The needle of the syringe or the tip of the scissors is used for proper placement of grafts in the recipient chambers.
- Hemostasis is achieved by pressing a saline soaked gauze piece over the area.
- For the recipient area three layers of dressing from inside out were paraffin-embedded nonadherent sterile gauze (Jelonet®), sterile Surgipad®, and bio-occlusive Micropore® **(Figs. 6A to E)**.
- For the donor area only Surgipad® and Micropore® are used.
- The recipient area may be immobilized if necessary. Proper instructions for special areas like lips are necessary. To secure the recipient area these patients are advised to take liquid diet for first 24 hours, preferably with a straw. Patients are allowed normal diet after this period.
- Sometimes dressings are opened after 24 hours to look for any dislodgement of grafts, if found any, they are replaced.
- Finally after 4–7 days the dressings are removed.

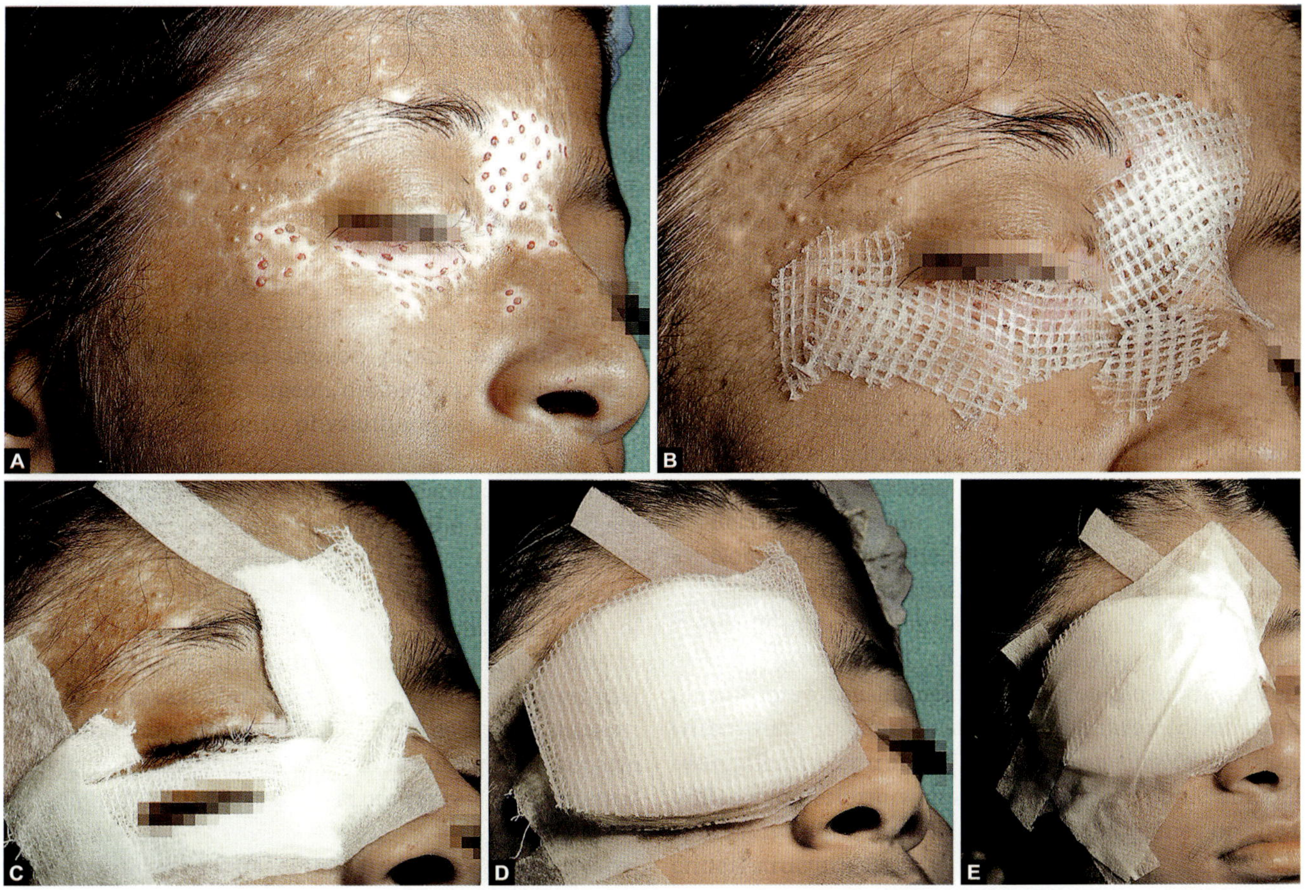

Figs. 6A to E: Three layers of dressing from inside out: Paraffin-embedded nonadherent sterile gauze (Jelonet®), sterile Surgipad®, and bio-occlusive Micropore®.

FOLLOW-UP AND COURSE OF EVENTS

Postsurgically the patients are exposed to PUVA[17,18]/psoralen plus UVA from sunlight (PUVASOL)[41,42] or NB-UVB[22] or even kept as such in some studies.[29] The patients are followed up fortnightly for initial 2 months and then monthly, up to complete repigmentation is achieved.

In the donor site, after healing with secondary intention minimal superficial scarring is expected and acceptable.

Scabs may fall off from the recipient site within 7–14 days. Though in many instances there may not be any scab formation. Perigraft repigmentation is expected to start around 3–4 weeks.[41-43]

The entire depigmented and grafted area is expected to be completely repigmented within 3–6 months, based on the area of grafting and body part involved. Minigrafting can be deployed on any part of the body **(Figs. 7 to 11)**.

COMPLICATIONS[39-41]

Complications are seen in punch grafting frequently and are enumerated in **Table 1**. By proper selection of cases

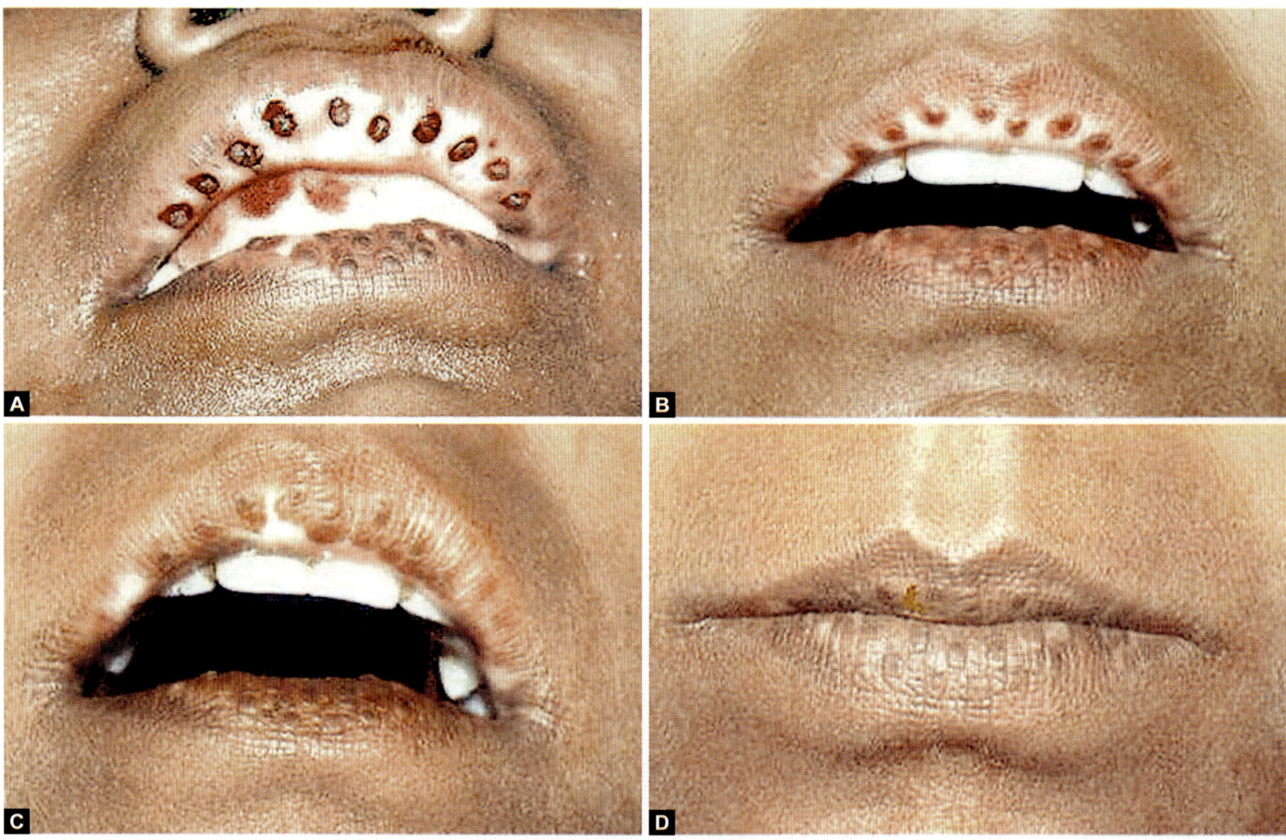

Figs. 7A to D: Minigrafting on lips. Upper lip showing gradual repigmentation. Lower lip showing resolving of cobblestoning.

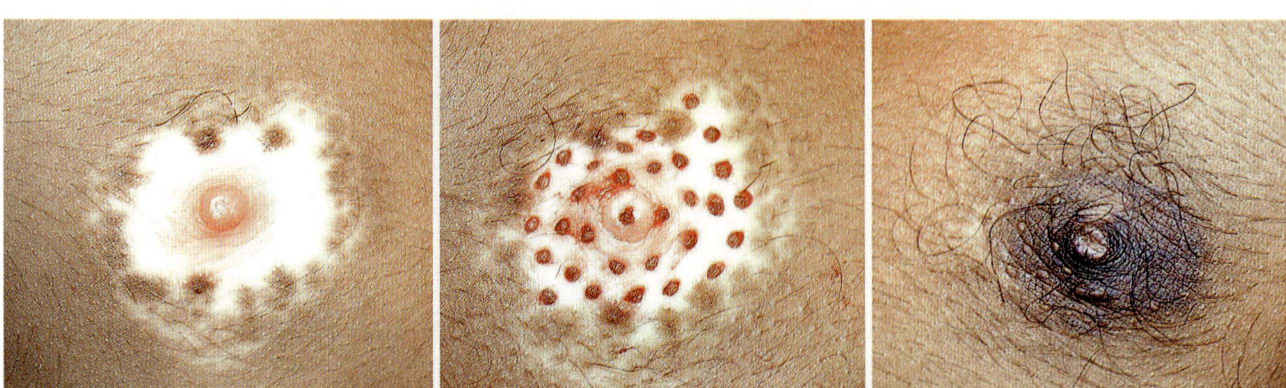

Figs. 8A to C: Minigrafting on male nipple, without any glue or stay suture, showing graft take-up and repigmentation.

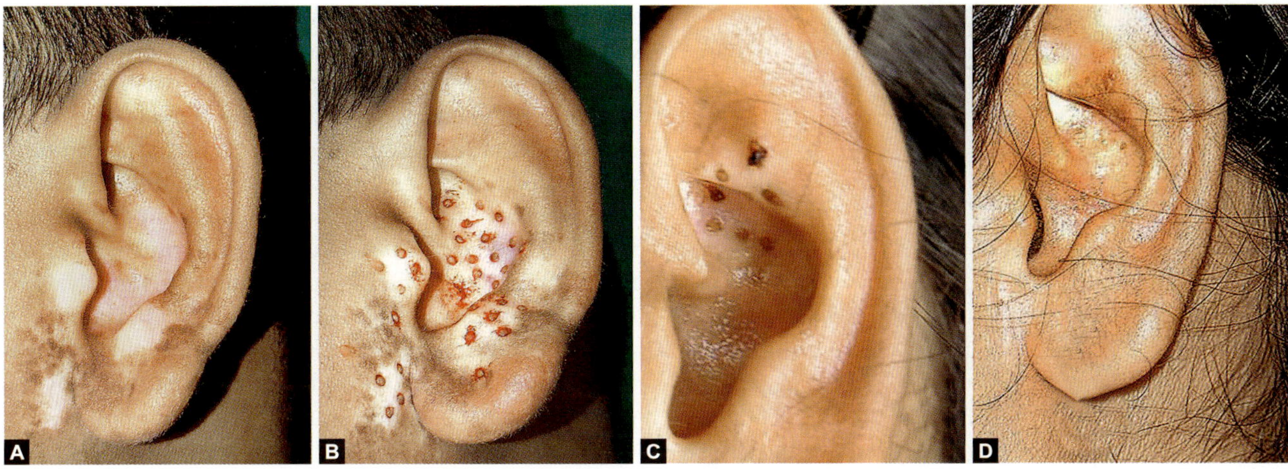

Figs. 9A to D: Minigrafting on inner part of the external ear.

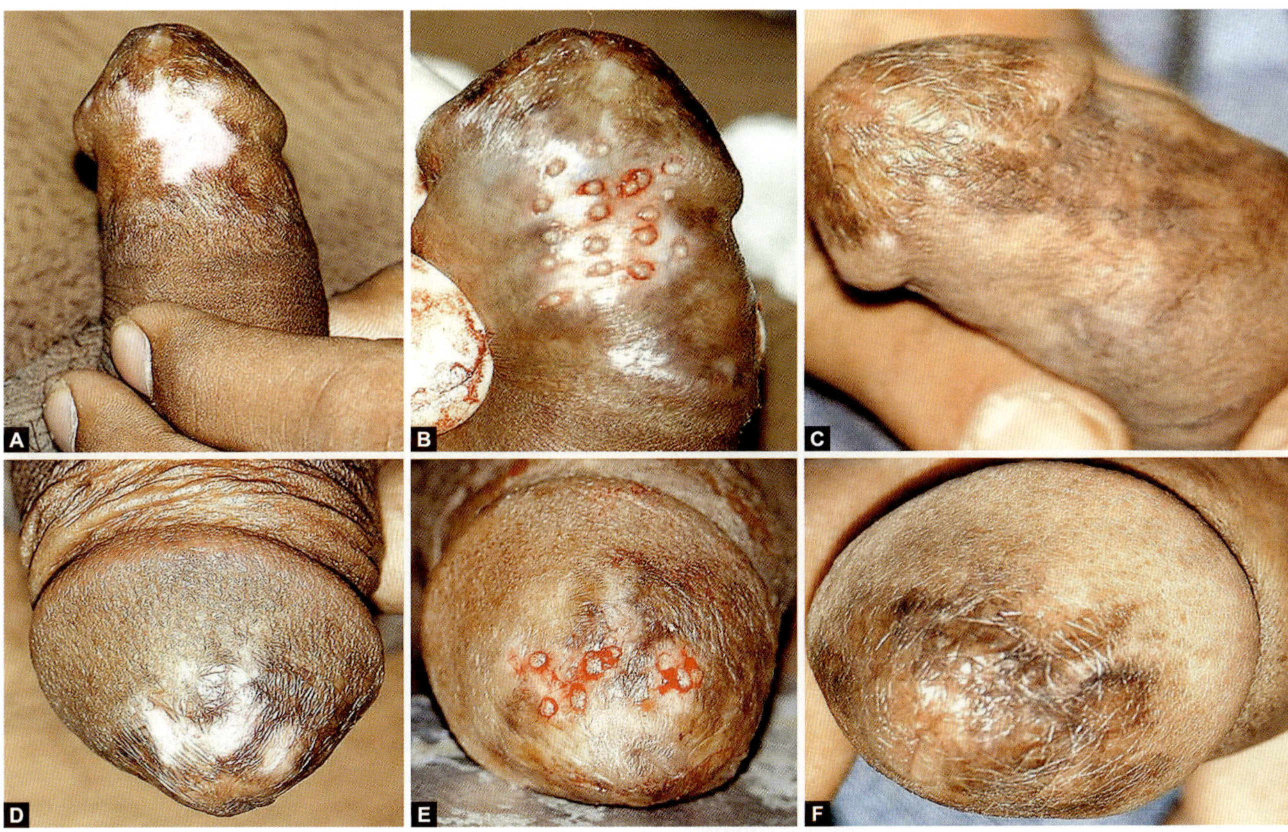

Figs. 10A to F: Minigrafting on ventral and dorsal aspect of glans penis.

and with proper technique, most of these complications are entirely avoidable. Cobblestoning **(Fig. 12)** is regarded as the most common of them all.[40,41,48] It was observed that with time it got corrected in most of the cases.[38] In resistant cases, corrective electrofulguration may be needed.[49] It can be avoided by avoiding punches >1.5 mm in diameter. On face and lips, it should be even smaller (1.2 or 1 mm). Rejection of grafts is another complication, particularly seen in herpes labialis-induced lip leukoderma.[50-53]

By proper selection of cases most of these complications are entirely avoidable. Cobblestoning is regarded as the most common of them all.[41,42,48]

It was observed that with time it got corrected in most of the cases.[41] In resistant cases corrective electrofulguration may be needed.[49]

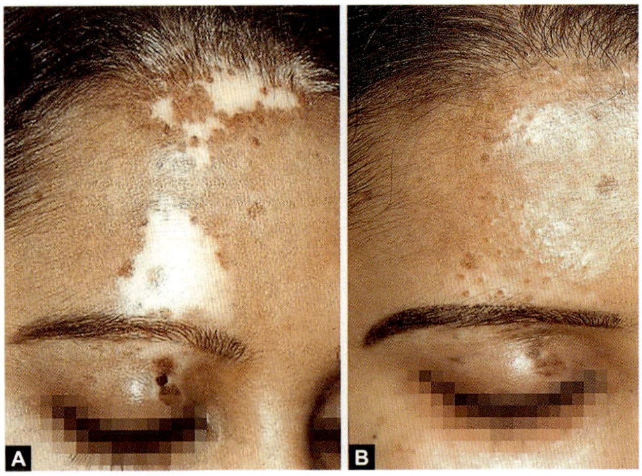

Figs. 11A and B: (A) Segmental vitiligo with leukotrichia; (B) Complete repigmentation with resolving cobblestoning and repigmentation of leukotrichia.

TABLE 1: Complications of minigrafting.

Recipient site	*Donor site*
Cobblestoning **(Fig. 12)**	Keloid
Polka dot	Hypertrophic scar
Variegated appearance and color mismatch	Superficial scar
Static graft (no pigment spread)	Depigmentation/spread of disease
Depigmentation of graft	Contact dermatitis to adhesive tapes
Perigraft halo **(Fig. 12)**	
Graft dislodgement/rejection	
Hypertrophic scar and keloid formation	

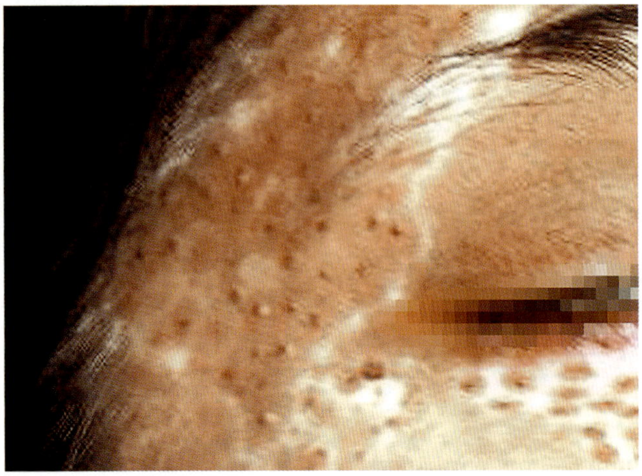

Fig. 12: Cobblestoning and perigraft halo.

DISCUSSION AND ANALYTICAL PERSPECTIVE

Surgical correction of vitiligo and other cutaneous achromia has come a long way in last four decades. But among all other methods, autologous miniature punch grafting has already established its place as the easiest, fastest, least aggressive, and of course one of the most effective means of vitiligo therapy.

When the graft is taken off, the piece of tissue is completely detached from the donor site and then it is placed on the vascular bed in the recipient holes. From this vascular bed it derives its blood supply. Initially the graft adheres to its new bed by fibrin. There is diffusion of nutrients through this fibrinous layer which keep the graft alive initially. Within 2–3 days, capillary linkage occurs with vascularization of the graft. The thinner the graft the denser the capillary network in the superficial dermis and thus earlier is the process of vascularization.[54]

Several Aspects of Punch Grafting Need Special Consideration

- *Mechanism of pigmentation of grafting procedures:* The mechanism of pigmentation of grafting procedures has been studied in several studies. Melanocytes have been shown to spread centrifugally from the infundibulum of hair follicle to the basal cell layer and recolonize the epidermis with active and functional melanocytes.[55,56] But the presence of pilosebaceous apparatus within the minigrafts is not at all necessary for the repigmentation process. Because in suction blister grafts only epithelial cells present in the grafts are enough to induce repigmentation.[57] In 1970, Billingham and Silvers have demonstrated the phenomenon of melanocytes migration from graft's edge within the achromic skin to recolonize and replenish the area with functional and active melanocytes.[58]
- *Relapse after grafting:* The major limitation of all grafting techniques is lack of specific criteria for defining stability.[50,59-63] It is often hard to predict how long the disease will remain stable. Similarly, it is difficult to envisage when it will start to become unstable.[64,65] This fact has made assessment of results difficult. Treatment of relapsed cases is considered difficult. However, repigmentation has been successfully induced in previous graft failure cases under NB-UVB (311 nm) phototherapy.[22] Even after recognizing the significance of stability and after three decades of experience in vitiligo surgery, it is quite ironic to note the little consensus regarding the optimal required period of stability. The complete lack of unanimity can be glaring in some instances **(Table 2)**. In one study the minimal period of stability as a prerequisite for grafting was mentioned to be as little a period as 4 months.[59] While on the other side of the spectrum in another study it was taken as 3 years.[13,14] Other variable figures like 6 months, 1 year, and 2 years can easily be obtained from some other studies as well.[30,31,51]

  Even same author has taken different period of stability into consideration in different articles.[16,32]

TABLE 2: Minimum period of stability in different studies.

Author	*Year*	*Period of stability*
Das SS, Pasricha JS[60]	1992	4 months
Boersma BR, Westerhof W[39]	1995	6 months
Jha AK, Pandey SS, Shukla VK[61]	1992	1 year
Savant SS[40]	1992	2 years
Falabella R[37]	1995	2 years
Falabella R[16]	1992	3 years

TABLE 3: Maximum grafted area in different studies.

Author	*Year*	*Maximum grafted area (cm²)*
Jha AK, Pandey SS, Shukla VK[61]	1992	15
Das S, Pasricha JS[60]	1992	80
Boersma BR, Westerhof W[39]	1995	96
Malakar S, Dhar S[43]	1999	>100
Falabella R[36]	1988	110
Lahiri K, Sengupta SR[42]	1997	144

TABLE 4: Size of graft in different studies.

Author	*Year*	*Size of punch (diameter in mm)*
Das S, Pasricha JS[60]	1992	4
Jha AK, Pandey SS, Shukla VK[61]	1992	3 and 4
Boersma BR, Westerhof W[39]	1995	2
Lahiri K, Sengupta SR[42]	1997	2
Malakar S, Dhar S[43]	1999	2
Malakar S, Lahiri K[49]	2004	1.5
Falabella R[36]	1988	1.2
Orentriech N, Selmanwitz VJ[11]	1972	1 and 2

The curious reverse KP after punch grafting; spontaneous repigmentation of distant nongrafted vitiligo patches after punch grafting have been reported.[66-68] It was attributed to possible release of cytokines from grafts.

Size of the grafted lesion varied between 15 and 144 cm² in different studies **(Table 3)**. Likewise the size of the punch instrument differed in different studies **(Table 4)**. But now the consensus being toward using smaller punches likes 1.2 or 1.5 mm. Falabella even recommends 1 mm grafts for facial region and 1.2 mm for other body parts.[63]

In this way the most common complication of punch grafting can also be avoided. Though the rate of cobblestoning was substantial in most of the study, it was found that with time it got corrected. In resistant cases electrofulguration is helpful.[51]

Repigmentation of leukotrichia with punch grafting and NB-UVB was noticed.[22] The same was also observed and documented before with PUVASOL and punch grafting.[65]

TABLE 5: Appearance of repigmentation (AOR) time in different studies.

Author	*Year*	*Earliest AOR (in days)*
Lahiri K, Malakar S, et al.[22]	2006	14
Lahiri K, Sengupta SR[42]	1997	14
Malakar S, Dhar S[43]	1999	16
Savant SS[40]	1992	30–45

TABLE 6: Maximum pigment spread (MPS) in different studies.

Author	*Year*	*MPS (in mm)*
Orentriech N, Selmanwitz VJ[11]	1972	1
Falabella R[31]	1978	2–3
Falabella R[36]	1988	3–4
Westerhof W, Boersma M[38]	1994	5
Savant SS[40]	1992	5–15
Lahiri K, Sengupta SR[42]	1997	1–10
Malakar S, Dhar S[43]	1999	
Lahiri K, Malakar S, et al.[22]	2006	12

- *Time of appearance of repigmentation (AOR):* Another important parameter is the post-graft AOR time. It was found to be between 2 and 6 weeks in different studies **(Table 5)**.

  After punch grafting and PUVASOL, AOR time in different regions varied between 14 and 39 days, with an overall average being approximately 21.6 days as shown in one study.[41] With the deployment of NB-UVB along with punch grafting AOR time in different regions varied between 14 and 32 days, with an overall average being approximately 20.6 days.[22]
- *Maximum pigment spread:* Orentriech in his original article (1972) observed that whether 1 or 2 mm grafts were employed, the pigment spread was consistently 1 mm.[11]

  Various other results can be found in the literature **(Table 6)**. Falabella while establishing a relationship between donor graft and the area of surgical repigmentation found that a 1 mm donor graft can repigment an area 25 times larger than the graft itself.[33] In a later study with 1.5 mm grafts and NB-UVB in type IV and V skin type subjects, this value was found to be more than double of that (56.21 times).[22] Previously in one study with PUVASOL this relationship was found to be 42 times.[43] Bigger grafts, darker skin types, and deployment of NB phototherapy all may have accounted for this high statistical value.

CONCLUSION

Considering all the indicators and parameters, it can be concluded that minigrafting is an easy, inexpensive, and effective method of treating stable and recalcitrant vitiligo.[69] The advantages and disadvantages are summarized in **Box 1**.

BOX 1: Advantages and disadvantages of minipunch grafting.

Advantages:
- Easiest, fastest, and least expensive method
- Can be performed anywhere on any site (except angle of the mouth)
- Particularly suitable for areola
- It is perhaps the only suitable method for palm, though results may not be fully satisfactory

Disadvantages:
- Side effects are common, particularly cobblestoning
- Phototherapy is always necessary after grafting
- Perfect match may not occur

ACKNOWLEDGMENT

Some Figures and Tables used in this chapter have also been used in the following chapters by me and my coauthors. With the permission of the concerned editors and publisher, I would like to properly acknowledge the original source:

- Lahiri K, Malakar S, Sarma N, Banerjee U. Repigmentation of vitiligo with punch grafting and narrow-band UV-B (311 nm)—a prospective study. Int J Dermatol. 2006;45(6):649-55.
- Malakar S, Lahiri K. Spontaneous repigmentation in vitiligo: why it is important? Int J Dermatol. 2006;45(4):478-9.
- Malakar S, Lahiri K. Minigrafting for vitiligo. In: Gupta S, Olsson MJ, Kanwar AJ, Ortonne JP (Eds). Surgical Management of Vitiligo, 1st edition. Oxford: Blackwell Publishing; 2007. pp. 87-95.
- Lahiri K. Evolution and evaluation of autologous mini punch grafting in vitiligo. Indian J Dermatol. 2009;54(2):159-67.

REFERENCES

1. Millington GW, Levell NJ. Vitiligo: the historical curse of depigmentation. Int J Dermatol. 2007;46(9):900-5.
2. Ebbel B. The Papyrus Ebers: the greatest Egyptian medical document. London: Oxford University Press; 1937.
3. Whitney MD. Atharva-Veda Samhita (Translation and notes). Cambridge: Harvard University Press; 1905.
4. Nair BK. Vitiligo—a retrospect. Int J Dermatol. 1978;17(9):755-7.
5. Freilich AR. Tzaraat—biblical leprosy. J Am Acad Dermatol. 1982;6(1):131-4.
6. Mercurialis H. De morbidis cutaneis et omnibus corporis humani excrementis tractatus. Venezia: Paulus et Antonium Meietos; 1572.
7. Sutton RL. On definition of vitiligo. Arch Dermatol. 1965;91:288.
8. Ortonne JP, Mosher DB, Fitzpatrick TB. Vitiligo and Other Hypomelanoses of Hair and Skin. New York: Plenum Medical; 1983.
9. Behl PN. Homologous thin Thiersch's grafts in treatment of Vitiligo. Curr Med Pract. 1964;8:218-21.
10. Falabella R. Epidermal grafting: an original technique and its application in achromic and granulating areas. Arch Dermatol. 1971;104(6):592-600.
11. Orentriech N, Selmanwitz VJ. Autograft repigmentation of leucoderma. Arch Dermatol. 1972;105(5):734-6.
12. Falabella R. Repigmentation of leukoderma by minigrafts of normally pigmented, autologous skin. J Dermatol Surg Oncol. 1978:4:916-9.
13. Falabella R. Repigmentation of segmental vitiligo by autologous minigrafting. J Am Acad Dermatol. 1983;9:514-21.
14. Lerner AB, Halaban R, Klaus SN, Moellmann GE. Transplantation of human melanocytes. J Invest Dermatol. 1987;89:219-24.
15. Lerner AB. Repopulation of pigmented cells in patients with vitiligo. Arch Dermatol. 1988;124(11):1701-2.
16. Falabella R, Escobar C, Borrero I. Treatment of refractory and stable vitiligo by transplantation of in vitro cultured epidermal autografts bearing melanocytes. J Am Acad Dermatol. 1992;26(2 Pt 1):230-6.
17. Skouge JW, Morison WL, Diwan RV, Rotter S. Autografting and PUVA. A combination therapy for vitiligo. Dermatol Surg Oncol. 1992;18(5):357-60.
18. Hann SK, Im S, Bong HW, Park YK. Treatment of stable vitiligo with autologous epidermal grafting and PUVA. J Am Acad Dermatol. 1995;32(6):943-8.
19. Olsson MJ, Juhlin L. Repigmentation of vitiligo by transplantation of cultured autologous melanocytes. Acta Derm Venereol (Stockh). 1993;73:49-51.
20. Malakar S, Dhar S. Repigmentation of vitiligo patches by transplantation of hair follicles. Int J Dermatol. 1999;38(3):237-8.
21. Olsson MJ, Juhlin L. Long-term follow-up of leucoderma patients treated with transplants of autologous cultured melanocytes, ultrathin epidermal sheets and basal cell layer suspension. Br J Dermatol. 2002;147(5):893-904.
22. Lahiri K, Malakar S, Sarma N, Banerjee U. Repigmentation of vitiligo with punch grafting and narrow-band UV-B (311 nm)—a prospective study. Int J Dermatol. 2006;45(6):649-55.
23. Thompson CJS. The evolution and development of surgical instruments. IV. The trepan. Br J Surg. 1937;25:726.
24. Watson BA. Gunpowder disfigurements. St Luis Med Surg J. 1878;35:145.
25. Keyes EL. The cutaneous punch. J Cutan Geniturin Dis. 1887;5:98.
26. Hagerman D, Wilson H. The skin biopsy punch: evolution and modification. Cutis. 1970;6:1139.
27. Stegman SJ. Commentary: The cutaneous punch. Arch Dermatol. 1982;118:943.
28. Baronio G. Degli innesti animali. Stamperia e Fonderia del genio. Milano; 1804.
29. Lewin ML, Peck SM. Pigment studies in skin grafts on experimental animals. J Invest Dermatol. 1941;4:504.
30. Labuono P, Shatin H. Transplantation of hair bulbs and melanocytes into leucodermic scars. J Dermatol Surg Oncol. 1976;2:53-5.
31. Falabella R. Repigmentation of leucoderma by minigrafts of normally pigmented, autologous skin. J Dermatol Surg Oncol. 1978;4:916-8.
32. Behl PN. Repigmentation of segmental vitiligo by autologous minigrafting. J Am Acad Dermatol. 1985;12:118-9.
33. Falabella R. Reply. J Am Acad Dermatol. 1985;12:119.
34. Falabella R. Repigmentation of stable leucoderma by autologous minigrafting. J Dermatol Surg Oncol. 1986;12:172-9.
35. Falabella R. Post-dermabrasion leucoderma. J Dermatol Surg Oncol. 1987;13:44-8.
36. Falabella R. Treatment of localized vitiligo by autologous minigrafting. Arch Dermatol. 1988;124:1649-55.

37. Falabella R, Barona M, Escobar C, Borrero I, Arrunategui A. Surgical combination therapy for vitiligo and piebaldism. Dermatol Surg. 1995;21(10):852-7.
38. Westerhof W, Boersma B. Grafting Techniques in Leucoderma. Book of Abstract. New Delhi, India: 7th International Congress of Dermatology; 1994.
39. Boersma BR, Westerhof W, Bos JD. Repigmentation in vitiligo vulgaris by autologous minigrafting: Results in nineteen patients. J Am Acad Dermatol. 1995;33(6):990-5.
40. Savant SS. Autologous miniature punch grafting in vitiligo. Ind J Dermatol Venereol Leprol. 1992;58:310-4.
41. Malakar S. Punch grafting. In: Paul A (Ed). An Approach to Dermatosurgery, 1st edition. Calcutta: Palsons Drugs Pvt Ltd.; 1996. pp. 44-6.
42. Lahiri K, Sengupta SR. Treatment of stable and recalcitrant depigmented skin conditions by autologous punch grafting. Ind J Dermatol Venereol Leprol. 1997;63:11-4.
43. Malakar S, Dhar S. Treatment of stable and recalcitrant vitiligo by autologous miniature punch grafting: A prospective study of 1,000 patients. Dermatology. 1999;198:133-9.
44. Lahiri K, Sengupta SR. A regionwise comparative study of post punch graft appearance of repigmentation (AOR) time in cutaneous achromia. Indian J Dermatol. 1998;43(1):13-5.
45. Lahiri K, Sengupta SR. A clinic-microscopic corroboration of surgical repigmentation—a study of 30 cases. Indian J Dermatol. 1998;43(3):99-101.
46. Lahiri K, Sengupta SR. A regionwise comparative study of the extent of post punch graft surgical repigmentation in cutaneous achromia. Ind J Dermatol Venereol Leprol. 1998;64(4):173-5.
47. Lahiri K, Sengupta SR. Relationship between donor graft area and area of surgical repigmentation. Indian J Dermatol. 1999;44(1):11-4.
48. Falabella R, Arrunategui A, Barona MI, Alzate A. The minigrafting test for vitiligo: Detection of stable lesions for melanocyte transplantation. J Am Acad Dermatol. 1995; 32:228-32.
49. Malakar S, Lahiri K. Punch grafting for lip leucoderma. Dermatology. 2004;208(2):125-8.
50. Malakar S, Lahiri K. Electrosurgery in cobblestoning. Indian J Dermatol. 2000;45(1):46-7.
51. Malakar S, Dhar S. Rejection of punch grafts in three cases of herpes labialis induced lip leucoderma, caution and precaution. Dermatology. 1997;195:414.
52. Malakar S, Dhar S. Acyclovir can abort rejection of punch grafts in herpes-simplex-induced lip leucoderma. Dermatology. 1999;199:75.
53. Malakar S, Lahri K. Successful repigmentation of six cases of herpes labialis induced lip leucoderma by micropigmentation. Dermatology. 2001;203:194.
54. Lahiri K, Malakar S. Herpes simplex induced lip leucoderma: revisited. Dermatology. 2004;208:182.
55. Burge S, Rayment R. Free skin grafts. In: Burge S, Rayment R (Eds). Simple Skin Surgery, 1st edition. Bombay. Blackwell Scientific Publications; 1986. pp. 71-84.
56. Parrish JA, Fitzpatrick TB, Shea C, Pathak MA. Photochemotherapy of vitiligo: use of orally administered psoralen and a high-intensity long-wave ultraviolet light system. Arch Dermatol. 1976;112:1531-4.
57. Ortonne JP, Schmnitt D, Thivolet J. PUVA-induced repigmentation of vitiligo, scanning electron microscopy of hair follicles. J Invest Dermatol. 1980;74:40-2.
58. Suvanprakorn P, Dee-Analap S, Pongsomboon C, Klaus SN. Melanocyte autologous grafting for treatment of leukoderma. J Am Acad Dermatol. 1985;13:968-74.
59. Billingham RE, Silvers WK. Studies on the migratory behaviour of melanocytes in guinea pig skin. J Exp Med. 1970;131: 101-17.
60. Das SS, Pasricha JS. Punch grafting as a treatment for residual lesions in vitiligo. Ind J Dermatol Venereol Leprol. 1992;58: 315-9.
61. Jha AK, Pandey SS, Shukla VK. Punch grafting in vitiligo. Ind J Dermatol Venereol Leprol. 1992;58:328-30.
62. Singh KG, Bajaj AK. Autologous miniature skin punch grafting in vitiligo. Ind J Dermatol Venereol Leprol. 1995;61:77-80.
63. Falabella R. Surgical treatment of vitiligo: why, when and how (Editorial). J Eur Acad Dermatol Venereol. 2003;17:518-20.
64. Malakar S, Dhar S. Repigmentation of leukotrichia over vitiligo patches after punch grafting. Indian J Dermatol Venereol Leprol. 1998;64(5):252-3.
65. Malakar S, Lahiri K. How unstable is the concept of stability in surgical repigmentation of vitiligo? Dermatol. 2000;201:182-3.
66. Lahiri K, Malakar S, Banerjee U, Sarma N. Clinico-cellular stability of vitiligo in surgical repigmentation: an unexplored frontier. Dermatology. 2004;209:170-1.
67. Malakar S. Spontaneous repigmentation of vitiligo patches other than the grafted site. Indian J Dermatol. 1997;47(2): 68-70.
68. Malakar S, Dhar S. Spontaneous repigmentation of vitiligo patches distant from the autologous skin graft sites: a remote reverse Koebner's phenomenon? Dermatology. 1998;197(3):274.
69. Malakar S, Lahiri K. Spontaneous repigmentation in vitiligo: why it is important. Int J Dermatol. 2006;45(4):478-9.

CHAPTER 36

Suction Blister Epidermal Grafting

Shyamanta Barua, Seujee Das

KEY MESSAGES

- Suction blister epidermal grafting is a simple, easy, safe, and inexpensive method in surgical management of vitiligo.
- It arguably yields the best cosmetic results among all available methods of tissue grafting employed in vitiligo surgery.
- It is a time-consuming procedure and yields only small grafts that can cover limited area(s) of vitiliginous skin in a single session.
- It is useful to treat small, localized patches of vitiligo, and is best suitable for eyelids, lips, areolae, and face.
- It is not associated with any scarring at either the donor or recipient sites.

INTRODUCTION

Suction blister epidermal grafting (SBEG) is a method of tissue grafting in vitiligo surgery where the pigmented epidermis is harvested from the donor site by prolonged suction at a negative pressure to raise a blister followed by transplantation of the blister roof to the dermabraded or laser ablated vitiliginous recipient site leading to transfer of melanocytes to the underlying dermal surface and resulting in repigmentation of the achromic site.

The suction used in SBEG causes a physiological split at the dermoepidermal junction and results in very thin skin grafts.[1-3] Light and electron microscopic studies have shown that the cleavage in suction blisters takes place between the base of the basal cells and the basal lamina of the basement membrane.[4] These pure epidermal grafts, in the absence of donor dermal tissue, adopt most of the characteristics of the recipient area, thus leading to excellent color match and cosmetic outcome.[2,5,6] Melanocyte transfer from the epidermal grafts to the underlying dermal surface generally occurs within 48–72 hours and complete repigmentation of the achromic recipient site is usually achieved within 3 months.[7]

HISTORICAL ASPECTS

It was Unna[8] in the late 19th century who first observed and documented that dry cupping on intact skin can occasionally produce blisters. In 1950, Blank and Miller[9] achieved the first in vitro separation of epidermis from dermis by the use of suction. The in vivo induction of blister was first reported in 1961 by Slowey and Leider[10] and subsequently by Kiistala and Mustakallio.[11,12] Suction blister technique was first used for transplantation of viable epidermis in achromic lesions by Falabella in 1971.[7] Suvanprakorn et al.[13] reported in 1985 successful repigmentation of lesions of vitiligo by transplantation of epidermis obtained through suction blistering.

Various types of suction apparatus have been used over the years starting from the angiosterrometer,[11] the conventional respiratory or gastrointestinal suction pump,[7] the oil rotatory pump,[14] to the manually operated suction unit.[5] The initial suction blister device consisted of a motor-driven suction pump with cups, vacuum bottle, and a mercury manometer.[15] This heavy, cumbersome, and expensive device underwent several modifications aimed at simplifying the apparatus and the procedure.[16-20]

Mukhtar et al.[16] made a very significant modification by using disposable syringes for production of the blister. This made the device very simple but could not measure the negative pressure inside the syringe. This drawback was overcome by Gupta et al.[17] and they developed a modified suction blister device. This consisted of a disposable syringe of variable capacity (5, 10, or 20 cc) attached to a three-way tap with a latex rubber tube, a 50 cc syringe for aspiration of air to produce the vacuum, and a manometer to measure the negative pressure. Gupta et al., in a subsequent study,[20] made the manometer superfluous by calculating the column of vacuum or the amount of aspirated air that is necessary for the production of a specific pressure gradient. Kaliyadan et al.[21] substituted the 50 cc syringe with a microdermabrasion device having a vacuum pump to generate negative pressure.

Burm et al.[22] developed a suction device consisting of only two units—a portable suction pump (Medi-Pump, Model 1130D, Tomas Ind., Inc., USA) and cylindrical plastic suction cups containing an independent one-way check valve. A negative pressure cutaneous suction chamber system (NPCSCS, Electronic Diversities, MD, USA) that combines high negative pressure (up to –508 mm Hg) and thermal regulation allowing for rapid induction of blisters was designed by Alexis et al.[23]

PATIENT SELECTION

Proper selection of the patient is the most important factor for achieving a good cosmetic result with any grafting procedure in vitiligo. The age of the patient, the site of vitiligo, keloidal tendency, and most importantly, the stability of the disease are the factors that need consideration.[24]

The minimum duration of stability for vitiligo grafting is still a contentious issue with the recommended duration ranging from 6 months to as long as 4 years in different clinical studies.[25-27] The most accepted consensus is to select a patient with no history of progression of lesions, no new lesions, and no history of a Koebner's phenomenon over at least 1 year before the procedure.[28] Another debatable issue is the relative importance of lesional versus disease stability. A recent multicentric study[29] concluded that lesional stability is as relevant as the overall disease stability in selecting patients for surgical intervention in vitiligo.

The indications and contraindications of SBEG are listed in **Box 1**.

PROCEDURE

A written informed consent and preoperative photographic documentation of the vitiliginous areas considered for surgery must be made. Premedication with antibiotics may be necessary only in selected cases, especially if large areas are to be grafted. All instruments and equipment **(Box 2)** required for SBEG must be kept ready in the operating trolley **(Fig. 1)**.

BOX 1: Indications and contraindications of suction blister epidermal grafting (SBEG).[30]

Indications:
- Stable vitiligo
- Secondary leukoderma
- Piebaldism

Contraindications:
- Active unstable vitiligo
- Infection
- Keloidal tendency

BOX 2: Instruments and equipment for suction blister epidermal grafting (SBEG).

- Sterile disposable syringes (5 cc; 10/20 cc; 50 cc)
- Three-way connectors and polyvinyl tubing
- Petroleum jelly (@Vaseline)
- 1% xylocaine vial or topical anesthetic cream
- 0.9% sodium chloride solution
- 10% povidone-iodine and spirit swabs
- Dermabrader—manual or electrical
- Iris scissors
- Jeweler's forceps
- Graft spreading rods and spatula
- Sterile glass slides
- Surgical glue (N-butyl-2-cyanoacrylate)
- Surgical dressing material
- Lasers [CO_2 or erbium: yttrium aluminum garnet (YAG)]—optional

Preparation of Donor Site

Falabella,[7] in his original study, had used the inner aspect of the thigh as the site for raising suction blisters. Other preferred donor sites for SBEG include the medial aspect of forearm and arm, the abdomen, buttocks, and the anterolateral aspect of the thigh or leg.[14,17,30-33] As a rule, covered sites such as the gluteal region or the thigh are preferred since there is always a risk, however minimal, of pigmentary changes occurring at the donor site.[34]

The area is surgically prepared by shaving and local cleaning with 10% povidone iodine and spirit. A topical local anesthetic may be applied as the procedure is painful. Alternatively, especially in patients with lower pain threshold, the donor area is infiltrated with 1% xylocaine as a field block.[30,34]

Suction Application and Blister Induction

Blisters may be raised using syringes[17] or suction pump and suction cups[22] or a NPCSCS.[23] Using syringes to raise blisters is the most commonly employed method.

The plunger of a 20 cc syringe is removed and a three-way connector is attached to its needle end piece through polyvinyl tubing, generally cut from intravenous (IV) infusion set. The basal rim of the syringe is coated with petroleum jelly and then applied to the fully stretched donor site. The needle end piece of the 50 cc syringe is then attached to the other adopter of the three-way connector connected to the 20 cc syringe. The three-way connector is unlocked and air is sucked out from the 20 cc syringe by the 50 cc syringe to create negative pressure. The connector is then locked and the aspirated air from the 50 cc syringe is evacuated. Further unlocking of the connector and aspiration of air can be done to increase the negative pressure within the 20 cc syringe.[2,14,15,33]

Once the desired negative pressure is attained, the three-way connector is locked and the 50 cc syringe is disconnected to maintain constant negative pressure within the 20 cc syringe. This pressure generally sucks in 0.5 cm donor skin

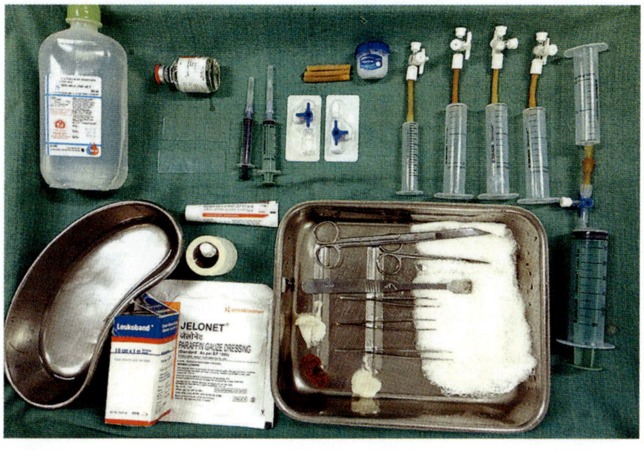

Fig. 1: The suction blister epidermal grafting (SBEG) surgical trolley.

inside the syringe. Multiple such 20 cc syringes can be applied similarly next to each other as per the area of the recipient site required to be grafted **(Fig. 2)**. Instead of 20 cc syringes, 10 cc syringes can be used if the area to be grafted is minimal. It has, however, been noted that syringes larger than 20 cc take a long time to generate a blister, and those smaller than 10 cc provide blisters that are difficult to handle.[31,34]

The use of three-way connector can be avoided by directly connecting the 50 cc syringe to the other end of the IV polyvinyl tube and then can be tied with sutures after achieving the required negative pressure.[35] The 50 cc syringe is withdrawn after securing its attached end of the tube with an artery forceps. Both ends of the IV tube are then tied with Mersilk suture material and artery forceps is withdrawn. There is a very minimal chance of improper blister formation with this method.

Appearance of multiple blisters **(Fig. 3)** can be seen through the 10 cc or 20 cc syringes, as the case may be. These slowly coalesce to form single or one to three unilocular blisters **(Fig. 4)**, large enough to be grafted. This is taken as the end point of suction application when the syringes are disconnected by unlocking the three-way connector.[15]

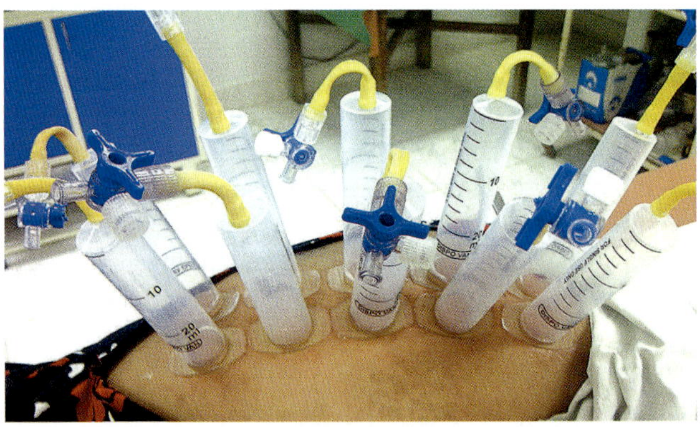

Fig. 2: Multiple 20 cc syringes applied next to each other for suction-induced blistering.

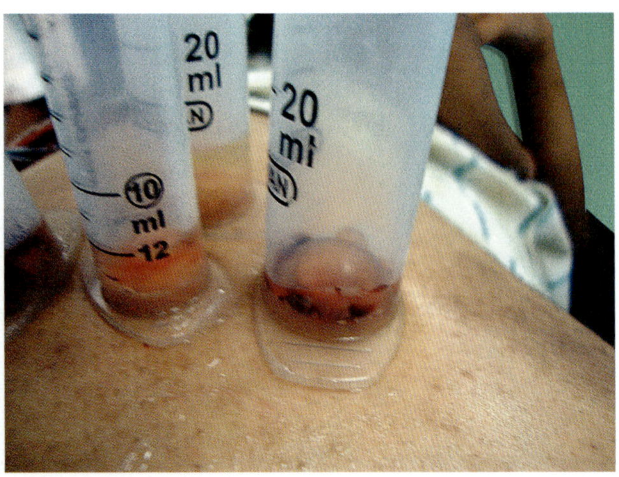

Fig. 3: Appearance of blisters within 20 cc syringes.

Recent literature suggests an easy way of making blister by using "Hijama" therapy cups.[36] "Hijama" or cupping therapy is a form of alternative medicine in which a local suction is created on the skin. The cups are available in varying sizes from 2 to 7 cm in diameter with an attached valve over the upper portion of each cup. After placing an adequate sized cup firmly over the skin, the plunger attached to the valve over the cup is pulled three to five times to create vacuum inside. The plunger is detached from the valve once the skin is visibly lifted inside through the transparent cup. Once a blister of sufficient size is formed the top valve is pulled to release the vacuum, thereby detaching the cup from the skin.

The time reported for suction blistering varies widely in different studies from 45 minutes to >3 hours.[7,14,37,38] Several factors **(Box 3)** can affect suction blister induction time (SBIT).[37] Syringe-induced blister formation in a given patient is mostly dependent on the anatomic site, the pressure gradient generated, and the length of time the gradient is applied.[17] It was observed that the ideal pressure gradient required to produce suction blisters varied according to age and gender of the patient.[20]

Various measures have been devised to reduce the time required for blister formation. The blistering process can be augmented by applying intracavity positive pressure using intradermal normal saline injection passed through normal skin near the imminent bulla formation site.[39] This is also useful if there is a single small blister inadequate for grafting or if there are multiple small blisters separate from each other. Saline infiltration leads to coalescence of these blisters or even enlarges the size of a single blister that is present.[17,34,37] Even

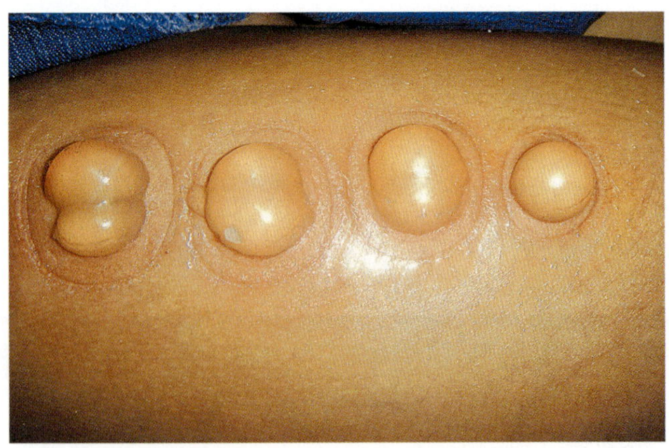

Fig. 4: Formation of unilocular blisters.

BOX 3: Factors that determine suction blister induction time (SBIT).[37]

- Diameter of the suction syringe or cup
- Site of suction blistering
- Age and gender of the patient
- Gradient of negative pressure
- Temperature of suction area
- Pathological variation
- Intradermal injection of saline or anesthetic solution
- Pretreatment with phototherapy or photochemotherapy

ultraviolet A (UVA) exposure[32] and intraepidermal injection of anesthetic solutions[40] have been reported to shorten the time of blister formation. Other measures include application of heat using infrared lamps, Wood's lamp or even hairdryer.[41]

Preparation of Recipient Site

Once the blisters form at the donor site, the recipient site is prepared surgically and infiltrated with 1% lignocaine as field block. It is necessary to de-epithelialize the recipient skin for melanocyte adherence and survival.[42] This can be done with one of the following methods.

Dermabrasion

Controlled mechanical abrasion of the epidermis and a variable segment of the upper dermis can be performed with wire brush, diamond fraise, curette, manual dermabrader, sandpaper, and others.[43] Diamond-impregnated cylindrical fraises are preferred over wire brushes as the latter cause deeper destruction than required for SBEG. Both can be attached to hand-held micromotor controlled by a foot pedal rheostat. The heads are driven at rotational speed between 12,000 and 15,000 rpm to obtain slow and gradual controlled denudation.[44]

Manual dermabraders of appropriate size are more useful for smaller areas or areas with thinner epidermis, such as eyelids. Manual dermabrasion with sterile sandpaper is another alternative. Zaimi et al.[45] recently developed a simple, reliable, and inexpensive manual dermabrasion technique performed with a presterilized scratch pad.

Dermabrasion should be stopped on appearance of uniform pinpoint bleeding points to avoid scarring at recipient site. Dermabrasion is best extended for 1–2 mm beyond the border of vitiliginous area.[24]

Suction Blistering

The recipient vitiliginous patch can be denuded by producing suction blisters. The advantage is that only epidermis is removed and there is no risk of scarring. Moreover, the roof of recipient site blister can be used as an autologous biological dressing. The latter retains the moisture, reduces chances of infection, and helps in faster healing.[46]

Cryoblistering

Liquid nitrogen is applied using a large cotton applicator for 5–10 seconds, usually 2–3 days prior to the date of surgery. Blisters will develop within few hours though grafting is performed 48 hours later when edema and inflammation subside.[47] Just before grafting, the depigmented bullous epidermis is unroofed with scissors and wound bed is cleaned. The main concern with cryoblistering is the risk of postinflammatory hyperpigmentation and hypertrophic scarring.[48]

Laser Ablation

The continuous wave, pulsed, and ultrapulse carbon dioxide laser, and erbium-doped yttrium aluminum garnet (Er:YAG) laser can be used to de-epithelialize the recipient site in SBEG. Laser ablation has several advantages over other methods: it is a faster procedure, there is less thermal damage to the perilesional normal skin, and de-epithelialization can be done precisely on irregular shapes and surfaces. However, it adds significantly to the overall cost of the procedure.[49,50]

Phototoxic Blistering

The lesions are painted with 0.75% 8-methoxypsoralen and then exposed to 15 J/cm^2 of UVA. Care should be taken to protect the surrounding skin with a physical sunscreen. The procedure is repeated after 4 hours. The lesional blisters develop in about 24 hours. The advantages of phototoxic blistering are that it removes only epidermis, there is little or no bleeding and there is easy demarcation of margins as only depigmented skin blisters.[14,51]

Once the recipient bed is created for the epidermal graft, hemostasis is achieved by pressure and area is kept covered with normal saline soaked gauze(s).[52]

Graft Harvesting

The well-formed unilocular blister is cut all along its border with curved iris scissors **(Fig. 5)** parallel to the skin surface. Care should be taken to avoid touching the floor of the blister as it causes pain.[34] One edge of a sterile glass slide, smeared with petroleum jelly or antibiotic cream, is kept near the blister **(Fig. 6)**. A pair of fine tipped or Jeweler's forceps is placed beneath the graft. The graft is lifted gently and is everted on the glass slide with the dermal side facing upward **(Fig. 7)**. This prevents the future chances of graft rejection, due to wrong placement of epidermal side of graft on the dermabraded area.

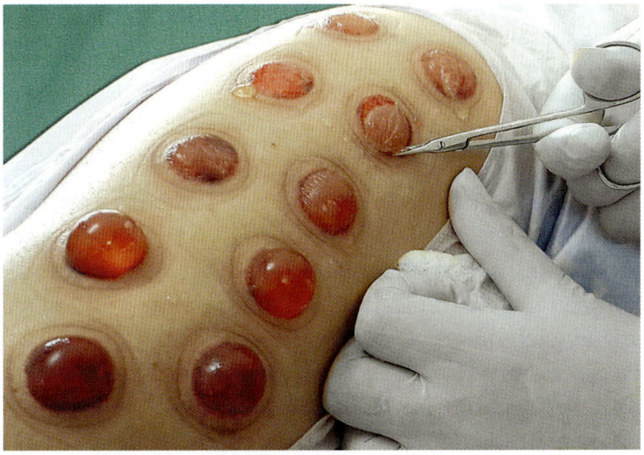

Fig. 5: Curved iris scissors to cut blisters.

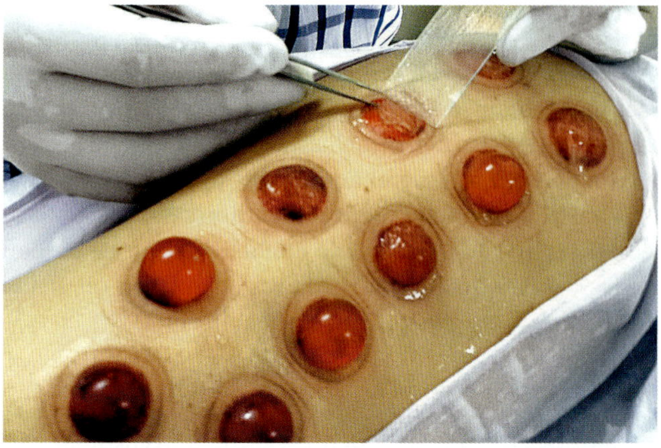

Fig. 6: Vaseline smeared sterile glass slide placed at blister edge to harvest blister graft.

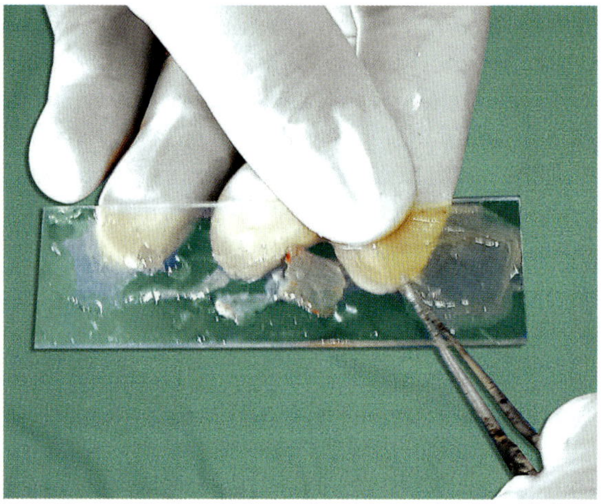

Fig. 7: Blister graft everted on glass slide with dermal side facing upward.

Anchoring filaments attached to the under surface of the graft along with the coagulum of fibrin and blood are delicately scraped away with flat surface of the spatula. The graft is then spread to its maximum size over the glass slide with the help of Jeweler's forceps and kept moist with normal saline. A fine gauze[53] and acetate sheet,[54] latter commonly known as transparency sheet used in overhead projectors, are other alternatives as graft carrier.

Graft Transfer

The glass slide with the spread out graft is then inverted over the denuded recipient area in such a manner that it sticks to the underlying dermabraded or laser ablated raw surface. All the grafts are transferred in similar manner and placed next to each other with overlapping of their borders so as not to leave any raw surface uncovered. Special care is taken to erase the curling tendency of the edges, if any, with the help of graft spreading rods. At the periphery, the graft edges should extend 1–2 mm beyond the dermabraded wound edge, thus crossing over to the rim of normal surrounding skin.[15,30]

A disposable syringe can be made to transfer the graft easily to the recipient site.[55] After separating the graft from its edges at the donor site, a syringe smeared with petrolatum jelly is rolled across the cut graft. The graft gets transferred easily onto the syringe which is than unrolled unto the recipient site. The advantage of this method is that it does not require much skill, there is no rolling in of the graft at the edges, no high-end gadget is required and most importantly it obviates the need to remember the dermal side of the graft.[55]

As blister formation at the donor site is unpredictable, clinicians have to manage with partially formed blisters to cover the recipient area. Moreover, graft placement is difficult in some areas, such as the angle of the mouth. In such circumstances, the paper that sandwiches the sterile petrolatum-soaked gauze can be used to transfer the harvested grafts.[56]

The size of the slide makes it difficult for maneuvering, especially for use in areas like the angle of the mouth. Half the regular size slide can be used for graft placement.[57] The cut slide is as good as the full size and has an additional advantage of easy maneuverability in tricky areas.

GRAFT FIXATION AND DRESSING

The graft is pressed firmly over the recipient site with sterile moist gauze to remove any serous exudate underneath the graft; this also helps the graft to adhere to the under surface. Alternatively, drops of surgical glue (N-butyl-2-cyanoacrylate) are applied along the free and overlapped edges of the grafts, especially in lip vitiligo.[3] Care must be taken to wait for 2 minutes for the glue to dry out so as to ensure firm adhesion. Fibrin glue has also been used as a fixative in SBEG.[58]

Postsurgical dressing significantly impact graft survival and thereby affect repigmentation outcomes.[42] The pressure dressing in the recipient area is done with double layer framycetin tulle, moist gauze, followed by sterile gauze and Elastocrepe bandage **(Figs. 8A to C)**. The donor area is dressed with framycetin tulle and dry sterile gauze(s). The recipient area can be immobilized, if considered necessary. The patient is given a course of antibiotics and anti-inflammatory drugs for 5–7 days.[30]

Dressing Removal

The dressing in the recipient site is removed after 5–7 days. The adhesive plaster is lifted up from one corner and removed slowly with simultaneous downward pressure on the underlying dressing. The dressing pad is then lifted up with forceps and its base is separated from the gauze slowly with artery forceps with simultaneous downward pressure on the underline gauze.[30] The remaining dressing layers, i.e., the gauze, framycetin tulle are then soaked with normal saline

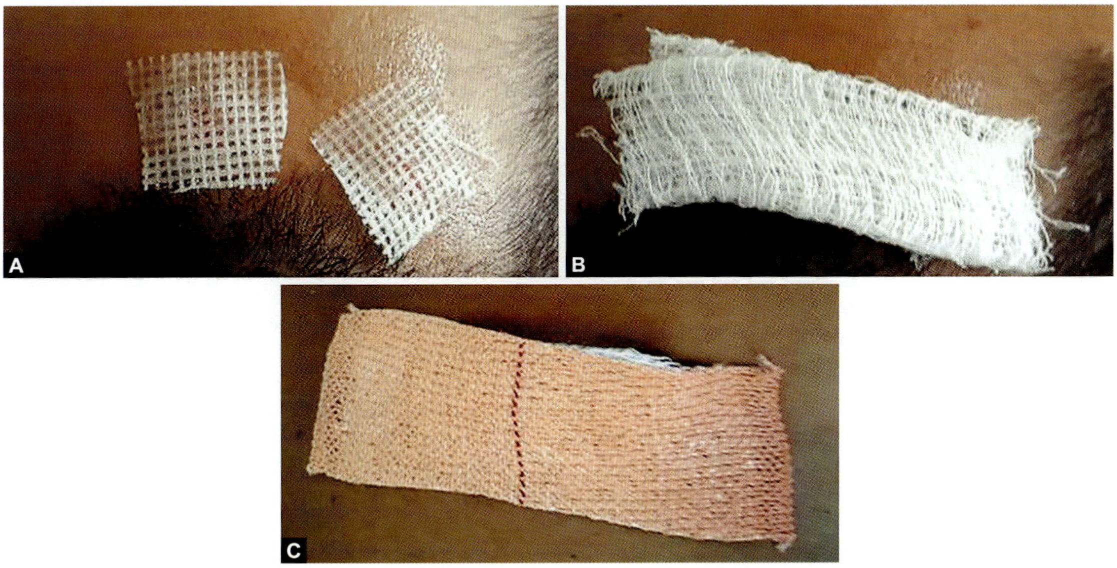

Figs. 8A to C: Layered dressing of recipient site.

and removed in the same manner to avoid tearing of the grafts from its bed. Redressing for another 2–3 days is required. Final dressing is removed on the 10th day and the patient advised to bathe regularly. The dressing over the donor site is removed after 24 hours and cleaned daily.[34]

BOX 4: Advantages and limitations of suction blister epidermal grafting (SBEG).

Advantages:
- It is a simple, safe, and inexpensive procedure
- It offers excellent cosmetic results with no scarring at the donor or recipient sites
- It is useful to treat small and localized patches of vitiligo
- It is the most suitable method for facial vitiligo and for areas such as the lips and areolae

Limitations:
- It is a time-consuming procedure
- It yields only small grafts that can cover limited area(s) of vitiliginous skin in a single session
- It carries the remote risk of failure of blister induction
- It is not suitable for palms and sole

COURSE OF GRAFTS

During the period of contact between grafts and the recipient bed, melanocytes migrate to the depigmented recipient skin resulting in pigmentation.[3] The pigment spreads from the graft to the surrounding area. The melanocyte transfer to the underlying denuded dermal surface takes place within 48–72 hours.[7] The graft either dries off or gets macerated over lips or other mucous membranes by 10–12 days and either comes out or can be peeled off manually leaving behind hyperpigmented and erythematous achromatic areas.

The grafted areas are postoperatively exposed to sunlight directly or treated with psoralen UVA (PUVA) or PUVA solar (PUVASOL) or narrowband ultraviolet B (NB-UVB) phototherapy.[31] Institution of NB-UVB therapy post-transplantation may stimulate melanocyte activity and spreading and thus, accelerate repigmentation of transplanted vitiliginous areas. Moreover, the immunosuppressive action of NB-UVB may provide protection for melanocytes in proliferation and migration.[59] Complete repigmentation with excellent cosmesis due to uniform color match is observed by 2–3 months.[60]

EFFICACY

Suction blister epidermal grafting is one of the most effective methods among all transplantation procedures in vitiligo. A meta-analysis showed that 87% of patients who underwent the procedure achieved >75% repigmentation. This outcome was similar to that of split thickness grafting (87%), but better than minigrafting (68%) and grafting of noncultured epidermal suspensions (31%).[38] The success rate of SBEG was higher in patients younger than 20 years and in segmental and focal vitiligo (91% achieving >75% repigmentation) than generalized vitiligo (53%, $p < .001$).[61] The meta-analyses, however, failed to demonstrate any statistically significant difference in outcomes on different body areas.

COMPLICATIONS

The complications associated with the procedure are perigraft halo of depigmentation, wrinkling and displacement of the graft and graft rejection. Other rare complications include infection, hematoma, and ecchymosis.[24,42]

The advantages and limitations of SBEG are summarized in **Box 4**.

CONCLUSION

Suction blister epidermal grafting is perhaps the simplest, although time-consuming, tissue grafting method for surgical management of medically recalcitrant but stable vitiligo and other secondary leukodermas. It does not require costly equipment or special surgical skills and small-to-medium sized vitiliginous areas can easily be treated by this method. As the split is physiological, the graft obtained is very thin and provides excellent cosmetic results, especially on mucosae-like lips. This method is, however, unsuitable for large areas that require more number of grafts and multiple surgical sessions. It is hoped that future research and innovation will lead to the development of more effective equipment to raise large suction blisters, rapidly and reliably.

REFERENCES

1. Lee DY. The use of suction blisters for recipient site in epidermal grafting: the implications for vitiligo. J Eur Acad Dermatol Venereol. 2009;23:241-2.
2. Gupta S, Jain VK, Saraswat PK. Suction blister epidermal grafting versus punch skin grafting in recalcitrant and stable vitiligo. Dermatol Surg. 1999;25:955-8.
3. Gupta S, Sandhu K, Kanwar A, Kumar B. Melanocyte transfer via epidermal grafts for vitiligo of labial mucosa. Dermatol Surg. 2004;30:45-8.
4. Hunter JAA, McVittie E, Comaish JS. Light and electron microscopic studies of physical injury to the skin. Br J Dermatol. 1974;90:481-90.
5. Kiistala U. Suction blister device for separation of viable epidermis from dermis. J Invest Dermatol. 1968;50: 129-37.
6. Lee AY, Jang JH. Autologous epidermal grafting with PUVA-irradiated donor skin for the treatment of vitiligo. Int J Dermatol. 1998;37:551-4.
7. Falabella R. Epidermal grafting: an original technique and its application in achromic and granulating areas. Arch Dermatol. 1971;104:592-600.
8. Unna P. Zur anatomic der blasenbildung an der man-schlichen haut. Vjschr Derm Syph. 1878;5:1-4.
9. Blank H, Miller OG. A method for separating the epidermis from dermis. J Invest Dermatol. 1950;15:9-12.
10. Slowey C, Leider M. Abstract of a preliminary report: the production of bulla by quantitated suction. Arch Dermatol. 1961;83:1029-30.
11. Kiistala U, Mustakallio KK. In-vivo separation of epidermis by production of suction blisters. Lancet. 1964;1:1444-5.
12. Kiistala U, Mustakallio KK. Dermo-epidermal separation with suction: electron microscopic and histochemical study of initial events of blistering of human skin. J Invest Dermatol. 1967;48:456-77.
13. Suvanprakorn P, Dee-Ananiap SP, Pongsomboon C, Klaus SN. Melanocyte autologous grafting for the treatment of leukoderma. J Am Acad Dermatol. 1985;13:968-74.
14. Koga M. Epidermal grafting using tops of suction blisters in the treatment of vitiligo. Arch Dermatol. 1988;124:1656-8.
15. Gupta S, Goel A. Suction blister epidermal grafting. In: Gupta S, Olsson MJ, Kanwar AJ, Ortonne JP (Eds). Surgical Management of Vitiligo, 1st edition. New Jersey: Blackwell Publishing Ltd; 2007. pp. 96-107.
16. Mukhtar M, Singh S, Shukla VK, Pandey SS. Surgical pearl: suction syringe for epidermal grafting in vitiligo. J Am Acad Dermatol. 1997;37:638-9.
17. Gupta S, Shroff S, Gupta S. Modified technique of suction blistering for epidermal grafting in vitiligo. Int J Dermatol. 1999;38:306-9.
18. Radmanesh M, Ebrahimi A. Double syringe blistering by adding a three-way connector for grafting stable vitiligo patches. J Dermatol Treatment. 2000;11:43-6.
19. Kim HV, Yun SK. Suction device for epidermal grafting in vitiligo: employing a syringe and a manometer to provide an adequate negative pressure. J Dermatol Surg. 2001;26: 702-4.
20. Gupta S, Ajith C, Kanwar AJ, Kumar B. Surgical pearl: standardized suction syringe for epidermal grafting. J Am Acad Dermatol. 2005;52:348-50.
21. Kaliyadan F, Manoj J, Venkatakrishnan S. Using a microdermabrasion machine as a suction blister device. Indian J Dermatol Venereol Leprol. 2008;74:392-3.
22. Burm JS. Simple suction device for autologous epidermal grafting. Plast Reconstr Surg. 2000;106:1225-6.
23. Alexis AF, Wilson DC, Todhunter JA, Stiller MJ. Reassessment of the suction blister model of wound healing: introduction of a new higher pressure device. Int J Dermatol. 1999;38: 613-7.
24. Majid I. Grafting in vitiligo: how to get better results and how to avoid complication. J Cutan Anesthet Surg. 2013;6:83-9.
25. Juhlin L. How unstable is the concept of stability in surgical repigmentation of vitiligo. Dermatology. 2000;201:183.
26. Lahiri K. Stability in vitiligo: what's that? J Cutan Aesthet Surg. 2009;2:38-40.
27. Lahiri K, Malakar S. The concept of stability of vitiligo: a reappraisal. Indian J Dermatol. 2012;57:83-9.
28. Parsad D, Gupta S. IADVL Dermatosurgery Task Force. Standard Guidelines of Care for Vitiligo Surgery. Indian J Dermatol Venereol Leprol. 2008;74:S37-45.
29. Majid I, Mysore V, Salim T, Lahiri K, Chatterji M, Khunger N, et al. Is lesional stability in vitiligo more important than disease stability for performing surgical interventions? Results from a multicentric study. J Cutan Aesthet Surg. 2016;9:13-9.
30. Savant SS. Skin grafting. In: Savant SS (Ed). Textbook of Dermatosurgery and Cosmetology, 2nd edition. Mumbai: ASCAD; 2005. pp. 149-65.
31. Hann SK, Im S, Bong HW, Park YK. Treatment of stable vitiligo with autologous epidermal grafting and PUVA. J Am Acad Dermatol. 1995;32:943-8.
32. Suga Y, Butt KI, Takimoto R, Fujioka N, Yamada H, Ogawa H. Successful treatment of vitiligo with PUVA pigmented autologous epidermal grafting. Int J Dermatol. 1996;35:518-22.
33. Laxmisha C, Thappa DM. Reliable site for suction blister induction and harvesting. Indian J Dermatol Venereol Leprol. 2005;71:321-4.
34. Khunger N, Kathuria SD, Ramesh V. Tissue grafts in vitiligo surgery: past, present, and future. Indian J Dermatol. 2009;54:150-8.
35. Mahapatra S, Sharma RK, James R, Deb KD. Simple but effective blister-forming trick in suction blister technique. Clin Dermatol Rev. 2019;3:151-3.
36. Jain S, Patra S, Choudhary S, Kaur M. An easy way to make blisters in suction blister grafting of vitiligo with Hijama therapy cups. J Am Acad Dermatol. 2022;86(4):e149-50.
37. Gupta S, Kumar B. Suction blister induction time: 15 minutes or 150 minutes? Dermatol Surg. 2000;26:754-6.

38. Njoo MD, Westerhof W, Bos JD, Bossuyt MM. A systematic review of autologous transplantation methods in vitiligo. Arch Dermatol. 1998;134:1543-9.
39. Gupta S, Chandrashekar BS, Reddy R, Jagadish P, Asati D. Rapid induction of suction blisters by intra-cavity positive pressure enhancement. Dermatol Surg. 2011;37:843-5.
40. Hanafusa T, Yamaguchi Y, Nakamura M, Kojima R, Shima R, Furui Y, et al. Establishment of suction blister roof grafting by injection of local anesthesia beneath the epidermis: less painful and more rapid formation of blisters. J Dermatol Sci. 2008;50: 243-7.
41. Arora S, Kar BK. Reduction of blister formation time in suction blister epidermal grafting in vitiligo patients using a household hair dryer. J Cutan Aesthet Surg. 2016;9:232-5.
42. Al-Hadidi N, Griffith JL, Al-Jamal MS, Hamzavi I. Role of recipient-site preparation techniques and post operative wound dressing in the surgical management of vitiligo. J Cutan Aesthet Surg. 2015;8:79-87.
43. Orentreich N, Orentreich DS. Dermabrasion as a complement to dermatology. Clin Plast Surg. 1998;25:63-80.
44. Baker TM. Dermabrasion as a complement to aesthetic surgery. Clin Plast Surg. 1998;25:81-8.
45. Zaimi I, Romanzi A, Gherardini G. Tricks and tips for manual dermabrasion. Dermatol Surg. 2016;42:1393-4.
46. Gupta S, Kumar B. Surgical pearl: autologous biological dressing for epidermal grafting in vitiligo and other achromic disorders. J Am Acad Dermatol. 2003;48:430-1.
47. Falabella R. Repigmentation of leukoderma by autologous epidermal grafting. J Dermatol Surg Oncol. 1984;10: 136-44.
48. Kim HY, Kang KY. Epidermal grafts for treatment of stable and progressive vitiligo. J Am Acad Dermatol. 1999;40:412-7.
49. Lee DY, Park JH, Choi SC, Lee JH. Comparison of recipient site preparations in epidermal grafting for vitiligo: suction blister and CO_2 laser. J Eur Acad Dermatol Venereol. 2009;23: 1448-9.
50. Sachdev M, Krupashankar DS. Suction blister grafting for stable vitiligo using pulsed Er:YAG laser ablation for recipient site. Int J Dermatol. 2000;39:471-3.
51. Albert S, Srinivas CR, Shenoi SD. Phototoxic blister induction in vitiligo surgery. Br J Dermatol. 1999;141:30-1.
52. Savant SS. Suction blister technique. In: Savant SS (Ed). Textbook of Dermatosurgery and Cosmetology, 2nd edition. Mumbai: ASCAD; 2005. pp. 351-8.
53. Tang WY, De Han J, Lu NZ, Chan LY, Lo KK. Surgical pearl: fine gauze is a useful carrier for epidermal graft in the treatment of vitiligo by means of the suction blister method. J Am Acad Dermatol. 1999;40:247-9.
54. Albert S, Shenoi SD. Acetate sheets in the transfer of epidermal grafts in vitiligo. J Am Acad Dermatol. 2001;44:719-20.
55. Singh BSTP, Agrawal I, Kar BR. Use of disposable syringe for transfer of graft in suction blister epidermal grafting. J Am Acad Dermatol. 2022;86(2):e43-4.
56. Ashique KT, Srinivas CR. Resizing blister roof grafts for vitiligo surgery. J Am Acad Dermatol. 2014;71:e39-40.
57. Ashique KT, Kaliyadan F. When half-slide can deliver double efficiency for blister grafting in vitiligo. J Am Acad Dermatol. 2020;83(3):e181-2.
58. Kim H, Kang JN, Hwang SH, Seo JK, Sung HS. Fibrin glue fixation for suction blister epidermal grafting in two patients with stable vitiligo. Ann Dermatol. 2014;26:751-4.
59. Zhang DM, Hong WS, Fu LF, Wei XD, Xu AE. A randomized controlled study of the effects of different modalities of narrow-band ultraviolet B therapy on the outcome of cultured autologous melanocytes transplantation in treating vitiligo. Dermatol Surg. 2014;40:420-6.
60. Falabella R. Surgical repigmentation of leukoderma. In: Wheeland RG (Ed). Cutaneous Surgery, 1st edition, Philadelphia: WB Saunders Company; 1994. pp. 1090-9.
61. Gupta S, Kumar B. Epidermal grafting in vitiligo: influence of age, site of lesion, and type of disease on outcome. J Am Acad Dermatol. 2003;49:99-104.

CHAPTER 37

Thin Split-thickness Skin Grafting for Vitiligo

Niti Khunger, Rajat Kandhari

KEY MESSAGES

- Split-thickness skin grafting (STSG) is a simple and cost-effective technique requiring a fair amount of surgical skill.
- Harvesting uniformly thin split-thickness skin grafts (STSG), dermabrasion, proper graft placement, and Immobilization are the key steps of STSG.
- Among the tissue graft techniques, it covers larger areas with yield coverage of 1:1.

INTRODUCTION

Conventional thin split-thickness skin grafting (STSG) technique is the most successful among all methods of vitiligo surgery.[1] Although, STSG requires a fair amount of surgical skill, it is a relatively simple and cost-effective procedure as compared to melanocyte suspension technique. The ability to cover larger areas in a single sitting, achieving high rates of repigmentation, and producing pigmented skin almost immediately after surgery make this a popular technique for the treatment of stable and recalcitrant vitiligo, when patients require quick results. The technique can be used not only for stable vitiligo, but also for secondary leukoderma (post burns, post herpes infection, contact leukoderma and, post discoid lupus erythematosus) and piebaldism.

HISTORY

Haxthausen first transplanted thin split-thickness skin grafts from normal to vitiliginous skin in three cases to study the pathogenesis of the disease.[2] Behl, in 1964, was the first to report the use of thin Thiersch's skin graft to treat vitiligo.[3] The technique involves the free transfer of epidermis containing melanocytes from one donor site to another recipient vitiliginous site.[4] Kahn et al.[5,6] used a modification of this technique where they used ultrathin epidermal sheets or ultrathin split-thickness grafts (<0.08–0.15 mm) which were obtained with the help of a power dermatome, to successfully repigment large vitiliginous areas. This technique was later employed by Olson and Juhlin[7] to transplant melanocytes to the dermabraded vitiliginous areas.

DEFINITION

Split-thickness skin grafting involves transfer of epidermis and often a thin uppermost part of superficial dermis to achieve transfer of melanocytes and keratinocytes from donor skin to the dermabraded vitiliginous skin.[8] The thickness of the graft ranges from 0.1 to 0.7 mm[9] and different harvesting techniques have been used.[10]

PRINCIPLE OF SPLIT-THICKNESS SKIN GRAFTING

There are three biological changes which are observed following skin grafting.[11]

Graft Uptake and Adherence

The first 72 hours after placement of the graft are the most crucial for graft uptake as fibrin bonding occurs during this time. The graft appears pink at this stage. Bleeding, infection, and mechanical movement due to improper immobilization of the area can lead to graft failure at this stage. The fibrin bonding is followed by onset of vascular anastomosis and fibrovascular growth. The graft imbibes wound exudate by capillary action through the sponge-like structure of the graft dermis and through the dermal blood vessels. This prevents graft desiccation, maintains graft vessel patency, and provides nourishment for the graft.

Graft Revascularization

Revascularization of the graft begins at 2–3 days postgrafting. This stage involves establishment of direct anastomoses between graft and recipient blood vessels, a process known as inosculation. Insufficient vascular proliferation, development of a thick layer of fibrin or hematoma or seroma can lead to failure of graft uptake in this stage. Hence, a compression bandage is useful to prevent this.

Contracture

Graft contracture can occur either immediately after harvesting the graft or after grafting at the recipient site.

This occurs due to contraction of the elastin fibers. Myofibroblasts are said to be responsible for graft contraction. The ability of a graft to resist contraction is related to the thickness of the deep dermal component as it provides inhibition of the myofibroblast function due to unknown mechanisms.[12] The chances of graft contracture in a thin graft are more as compared to a thicker graft since the deep dermal component is lacking. This can lead to achromic fissures and perigraft halo. Overlapping of graft edges at the recipient site can prevent these complications.

PATIENT SELECTION CRITERIA

The most important criteria is stability of the lesion to be grafted. This is dealt with in detail on stability of vitiligo. Briefly the disease should be stable for at least one year before attempting surgery.[13-21] Specific features are as follows:

- *Failure of medical treatment:* STSG can be used to cover large vitiliginous areas, as compared to suction blister technique or miniature punch grafting which are used for relatively smaller areas.
- *Site and extent of lesions:* The success rate of this procedure is low in certain sites. The fingers, elbows or other sites prone to movement show considerably lower success rates than other sites.

REQUIRED EQUIPMENT

Dermabraders

Manual (Dr Manekshaw's hand-held metallic dermabrader) or electrical micromotor with a handpiece and diamond fraises for abrasion (micromotor with a diamond fraise or wire brush attached to the handpiece).

Skin Grafting Equipment

- *For harvesting the graft:* Humby's skin grafting knife, Padget's or Davol's dermatome, straight artery forceps with a razor blade, or Silver's razor blade holding knife are alternatives that can be used. **(Figs. 1A and B)**.
- Graft spreading rods or spatula
- Nontraumatizing ring forceps

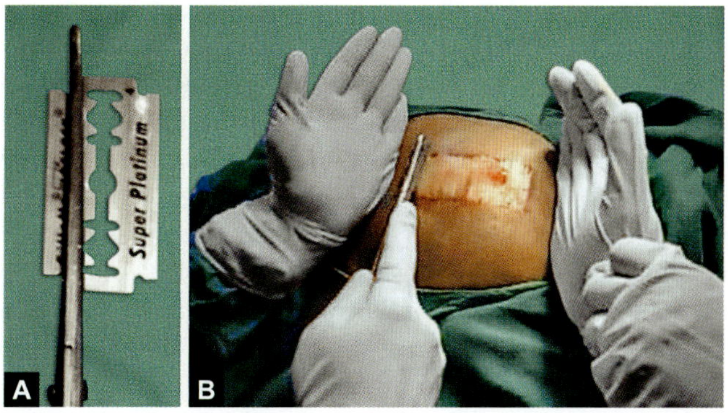

Figs. 1A and B: (A) Stainless steel blade mounted on a straight artery forceps; (B) Harvesting of split skin graft.

- *Surgical glue:* Cyanoacrylate adhesive (N-butyl-2-cyanoacrylate)
- *Other equipment includes:* Iris scissors and sterile Petri dishes

TECHNIQUE

Preoperative Preparation

Shaving of the donor and recipient area is important prior to the procedure. In recipient areas where there is thick terminal hair, as the hair grows, it tends to lift up the graft. Hence, plucking the hair with a forceps after giving anesthesia, instead of shaving is said to delay hair growth, thereby preventing the graft from being lifted up.[21,22] As an alternative, chemical depilation of the hair can be carried out.[21]

Split-thickness skin grafting consists of the following steps which are discussed briefly here.

Harvesting the Graft

Donor Site Preparation and Anesthesia

Harvesting the ideal split-thickness graft with uniform thickness requires special surgical skill. The gluteal area is the most preferred site for obtaining a graft for obvious cosmetic reasons, though it is relatively a difficult area to harvest because of the curvature and needs more skill. Alternatively, the anterolateral aspect of the thigh, the arms,[5] or the abdomen can be used as a donor site. After appropriate surgical cleansing, the required donor area is calculated and marked with a surgical pen. Topical anesthesia with eutectic mixture of local anesthetics (EMLA) may be sufficient, but in certain cases, anesthesia with lignocaine 2% may be needed.[10] A field block with 1% lignocaine at the edges should be given instead of infiltration anesthesia within the donor area to prevent an uneven surface. This can lead to harvesting a graft of uneven thickness.[23]

Graft Harvesting Technique

The procedure is commenced by an assistant stretching the skin firmly at one end, applying downward and outward traction with the help of the flat of his hand and the surgeon providing outward traction at the other end. This is done to flatten the skin as much as possible and thereby decreasing the drag felt while harvesting the graft. A thin split-thickness graft of uniform thickness is harvested using either a sterile razor blade mounted on a Kocher's forceps **(Fig. 1A)** or a blade holding instrument. A straight-tip forceps such as Kelly or Rochester-Pean forceps can also be used to hold the razor blade.[10] Alternatively, a hand dermatome, Silver's knife,[24] Humby's knife,[25] or a motor driven Zimmer dermatome (Zimmer Inc. Warsaw Indiana, USA) can also be used. While harvesting the graft, the cutting blade is held parallel to the skin surface and a sliding to-and-fro motion is then employed to cut tangentially throughout the upper dermis.

The angle at which the blade is applied controls the depth of the graft (usually at 10–15°) and one should aim at obtaining a thin, translucent uniform graft. Pinpoint bleeding at the donor site signifies suitable depth of the graft taken. The harvested graft is then transferred to a sterile Petri dish containing normal saline. Hemostasis is then attained at the donor site with pressure and the area is dressed with a nonadherent dressing.

Donor Area Dressing

Options for dressing the donor site include occlusive dressings (DuoDerm), semiocclusive dressings (Tegaderm),[26] semi-open dressings (Vaseline gauze), and no dressing.[27] The semiocclusive dressings are deemed to be superior as they have the fastest healing rates (average of 9 days to re-epithelialization), lowest subjective pain scores, and lowest infection rates (3%).[26] They also have the advantage of being transparent and allowing ongoing inspection of the site. The rate of healing of the donor site is proportional to the number of epithelial appendages remaining and inversely proportional to the thickness of graft harvested.

Recipient Site: Preparation, Graft Placement, and Immobilization

Preparation of the recipient site is a critical step to achieve successful repigmentation. The objective is to prepare a uniform denudation of the epidermis at the dermoepidermal level to allow for plasmatic imbibition in the first 24–48 hours, and then vascular ingrowth to provide cellular nutrition to the donor graft, which is crucial for graft survival. There are various techniques that have been described, which include mechanical dermabrasion using a motor driven diamond fraise or handheld dermabraders, CO_2, and erbium-doped yttrium-aluminum-garnet (Er:YAG) lasers, blister formation by cryotherapy with liquid nitrogen, suction blisters, and phototoxic blisters induced by psoralen plus ultraviolet A (PUVA).[28] Mechanical dermabrasion using a motor driven diamond fraise is the most commonly used technique.

Preparation

After appropriate surgical cleansing, the vitiliginous area is first marked with a surgical pen. Anesthesia may be administered using 1% lignocaine, infiltrated into four quadrants, deep dermal and subcutaneous, covering the vitiliginous area and the surrounding 4–5 cm of normal perilesional skin. Alternatively, topical anesthetic cream is applied under occlusion 2–3 hours before the procedure is sufficient in most cases.[29] For larger areas, a nerve block or general anesthesia is usually required.

Dermabrasion

The vitiliginous area **(Fig. 2A)** is then abraded with the help of an electric high speed dermabrader with a diamond fraise end piece. Dermabrasion must be done evenly all over the depigmented area and 2–3 mm of the perilesional normal skin, in order to prevent the development of a perigraft halo postoperatively. Dermabrasion is done till punctuate papillary bleeding is seen, which is the level of the dermoepidermal junction at the level of the papillary dermis **(Fig. 2B)**. A manual metallic dermabrader may be used by beginners as it provides better depth control. Alternatively, an Er:YAG laser or an ultrapulse CO_2 laser can be used, particularly for critical anatomical sites. The ultrapulse CO_2 is considered better since it has the ability to achieve an epidermal-dermal split with a single pass and also achieves better hemostasis, as compared to the Er:YAG laser.[30]

Placement of Graft

Once the recipient area is abraded, the graft is transferred onto the dermabraded recipient skin, taking care to place the dermal surface facing down. The graft may be placed over a sterile glass slide with the dermal side up. Two to three punctures with a 24 G needle to make tiny holes in the graft can be made in order to prevent serum accumulation under the graft. The slide is then everted on the recipient area so that the dermal side faces down. Ideally, the graft should be little larger than the recipient site and should extend 3–5 mm beyond the edges of the abraded area. The edges of the graft should be evened out with the help of a spatula. This helps in preventing curling of the graft and thereby preventing a beaded border appearance. Once the graft has been placed one must ensure that no air, blood, serum, or debris from the dermabraded area is trapped underneath the graft.

Immobilization

Proper immobilization of the graft is of utmost importance, and failure to do so may result in wrinkling and beading of the graft resulting in a relative decrease in the size of the graft. Collection of serum under the graft and poor immobilization are the two main factors for failure of graft uptake.

Various methods such as surgical adhesive, octyl-2-cyanoacrylate with a pressure dressing, the composite film and graft unit (FGU),[31] flexible collodion,[3] and sprays such as Opsite spray (Smith and Nephew, United Kingdom)[32] have been tried in order to prevent the earlier mentioned complications. The octyl-2-cyanoacrylate adhesive is excellent to secure the graft and in addition also exhibits antimicrobial properties against staphylococci, *Pseudomonas,* and *Escherichia coli.*[33] It is best applied at the edges of the graft in an interrupted manner **(Fig. 2C)**. In a study of 50 patients of stable, recalcitrant vitiligo, treated with STSG of over 180 lesions, cyanoacrylate adhesive was effective in immobilizing the grafts, especially over the mobile areas.[34] The composite FGU consists of a semipermeable thin film (Tegaderm) and the harvested thin graft, wherein the film is placed over the graft and slightly beyond it. The adhesive nature of the film

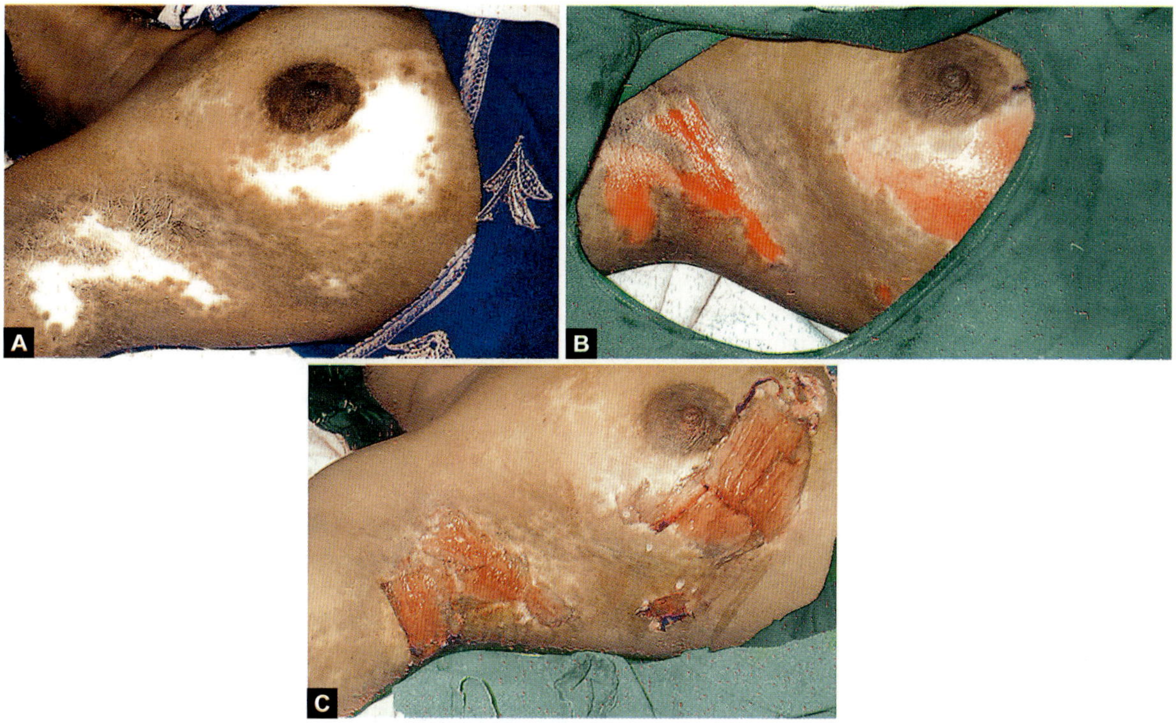

Figs. 2A to C: (A) Lesion before dermabrasion; (B) Dermabraded recipient area; (C) Graft fixed with surgical glue.

prevents beading or curling of the graft. A pressure dressing may be given with an Elastocrepe bandage to avoid hematoma or seroma formation.

POSTOPERATIVE CARE

The patient is counseled regarding strict immobilization of the site where the graft is placed. Antibiotics are administered for a week. The first dressing change is done preferably after 24 hours, to check for formation of any seroma or hematoma underneath the graft. Drainage of the seroma or hematoma is done by making a small incision over the collection and expressing the underlying contents. One should not attempt to express the fluid out from the edge of the graft as this may disrupt the adherence of the whole graft. In case of a flexible collodion dressing windows of 0.5 cm diameter are made with the help of acetone to observe for seroma, blood or air.[16]

Dressing is *subsequently* changed after 1 week by which time the graft is usually taken up and healing is complete. When removing the dressing, one can moisten it with saline to reduce adherence to the graft. The dressing may then be carefully removed to prevent lifting the graft off of the underlying wound bed. Donor site dressing is also changed after 1 week.

EXPECTED OUTCOMES

The systematic reviews by Njoo et al.[35] on autologous transplantation methods show that the highest mean success rates are achieved by STSG, which range from 87 to 91%. Agrawal et al.[36] treated 32 sites in 21 patients with stable refractory vitiligo using this technique. They reported 100% repigmentation in 68% of the patches and 90–95% repigmentation in the remaining patches. It took an average.[6] 3 months to achieve close to a full color match.

Compared to other techniques split-thickness grafting appears to be better than control, suction blister, or combined split-thickness or suction grafts.[37] Compared to blister grafting, the STSG can cover a larger surface area. Ozdemir et al.[24] demonstrated a higher percent of repigmentation with the STSG technique than the suction blister grafting in a single patient. As compared to mini-punch grafting the STSG technique produces far more cosmetically superior results and matching over larger areas. Repigmentation is greater in patients treated with photochemotherapy plus split-thickness skin graft versus punch grafts.[38]

COMPLICATIONS

Complications may occur either at recipient site or donor site.

At the Recipient Site

These include the following:

- Graft rejection
- *Seroma or hematoma formation:* The most common cause of graft rejection is accumulation of air bubbles, serum (seroma), or blood (hematoma) underneath the graft surface. They prevent adherence of the graft to the underlying wound bed, thereby depleting the graft of the required nutrition. Meshing the graft can be considered as an effective way of preventing seroma formation.[39] Movement or shifting of the graft is also a cause of graft

rejection as it results in disrupting the attachment of the graft to the recipient site. One must counsel the patient regarding immobilization, especially if the graft is placed on a joint. Longitudinal strips of grafts arranged parallel to the skin creases can be used at these sites.[8] Another common cause of failure of graft uptake is due to technical error wherein the graft is placed upside down, with the epidermal surface of the graft in contact with the dermal surface of the wound bed. Trauma to the graft or excessive stretching of the graft may also result in partial failure of graft uptake. A recipient site having poor vascularity or surface contamination can also result in graft failure.

- *Textural abnormalities:* Failure to even out the edges of the graft results in "curling" or "branching", resulting in peripheral beading at the graft edge or a "stuck on tire patch" appearance.
- *Hyperpigmentation:* This is a relatively common complication, especially in dark skinned individuals and takes a long time to resolve **(Fig. 3)**.[40] This can be treated with topical retinoids or chemical peeling (personal observation) or with laser resurfacing, or at times, with superficial dermabrasion.
- *Perigraft halo:* Peripheral depigmentation or achromic fissures at the graft edge occurs primarily due to graft contraction **(Fig. 3)**. The graft should ideally extend 3–5 mm beyond the abraded area to avoid this complication. They can be treated with topical or systemic psoralens or narrowband ultraviolet B (NB-UVB).[23] Al-Mutairi et al.[41] have used excimer laser (308 nm) after grafting to minimize the chances of developing perigraft halo or achromic fissures.[26]
- *Hypertrophy:* Thick grafts usually are the cause of hypertrophy. This usually subsides spontaneously in 3–4 months. Topical retinoids or topical midpotent corticosteroids can be used to treat this complication.[23]
- *Milia*: Formation of milia is common on the face and neck, which is due to remnants of epidermis following dermabrasion **(Figs. 4A to C)**. They resolve spontaneously or can be expressed out.

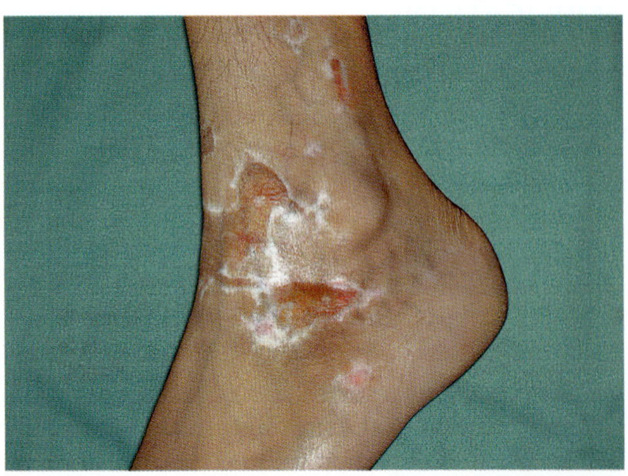

Fig. 3: Split skin graft showing hyperpigmentation and perigraft halo.

- *Secondary infection:* If proper aseptic precautions are maintained, secondary infection is relatively uncommon complication of this procedure.[42]
- *Reactivation of vitiligo:* This may occur at the graft site or the perigraft area.

Complications at the Donor Site

These include the following:

- *Postinflammatory hyperpigmentation:* This is common in darker skins and can persist even up to 1 year.
- *Scarring:* Superficial scarring can occur at the donor site, especially when thick grafts have been harvested.
- *Recurrence or koebnerization:* Occurrence of vitiligo at the donor site.

ADVANTAGES AND DISADVANTAGES OF SPLIT-THICKNESS SKIN GRAFTING

Advantages and disadvantages of STSG are shown in **Box 1**.

TECHNIQUE MODIFICATIONS AT SPECIAL SITES

Certain areas such as eyelids, lips, acral areas, and genital area are difficult areas to graft. Successful results can be attained by managing difficult to treat sites with modifications in the original technique.

Eyelids

The thinnest graft should be selected for the eyelid area. Eye shields may be used by beginners during dermabrasion for protection. Strict immobilization is required for the first 72 hours, and this can be achieved by cyanoacrylate adhesive and pressure bandage **(Figs. 4A to C)**.

Lips

Although, the suction blister technique is considered a good option for small areas on the lip, the split-thickness graft gives optimal results for slightly larger areas. Care should be taken to secure the graft with cyanoacrylate adhesive first along the mucosal side and then straightening out the graft onto the surrounding normal skin.

Alternately, the graft may be secured by 5-0 Prolene® sutures at the edges to prevent graft displacement. It is preferable to admit the patient and give intravenous fluids and nil orally for the first 24 hours. A semisolid or liquid diet through a straw is advised till the dressing is removed. Sutures and dressing are removed in a week.[28]

Acral Areas

The presence of a thicker epidermis, leading to inadequate dermabrasion and inability to prepare a good vascular bed, makes the acral sites one of the toughest sites to treat with

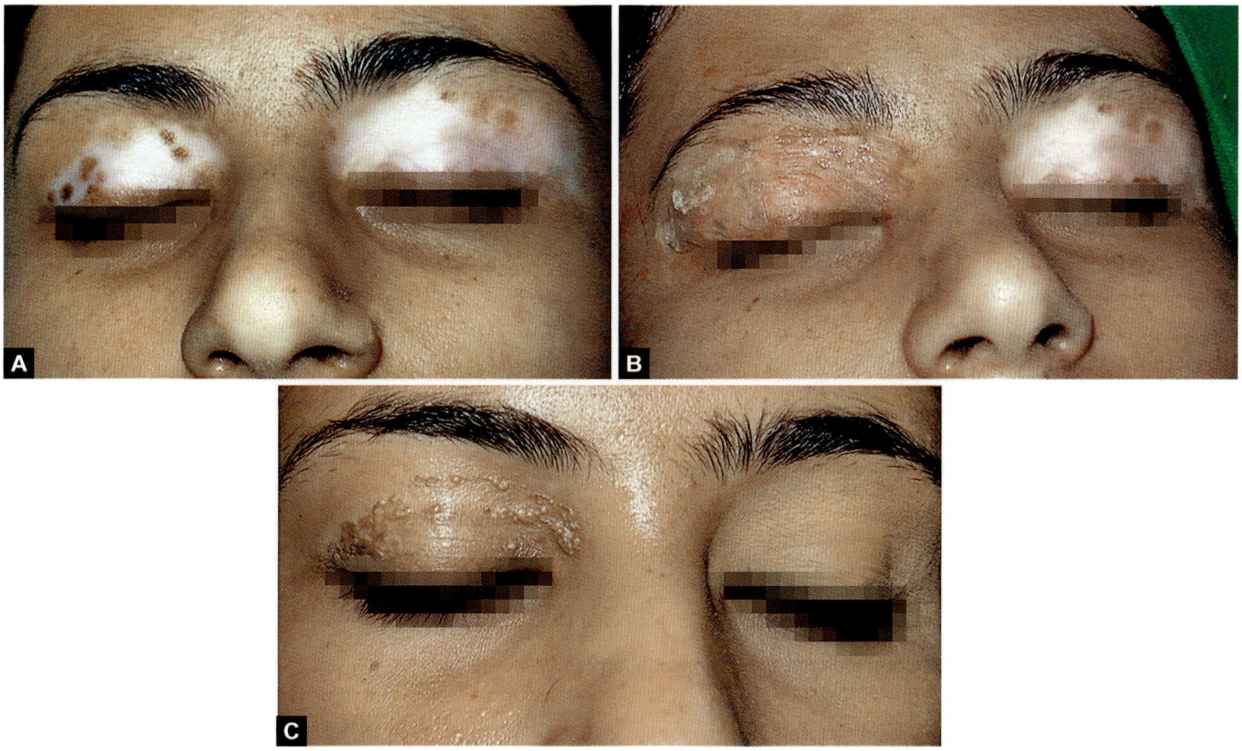

Figs. 4A to C: (A) Vitiligo lesions on eyelids; (B) Vitiligo lesion after grafting on right eyelid; (C) Excellent results, but with milia on right eyelid.

BOX 1: Advantages and disadvantages of split-thickness skin grafting (STSG).

Advantages of thin split-thickness skin grafting:
- Large areas can be covered in a single sitting, resulting in quick results over a short period of time.
- Grafted areas appear skin colored immediately after the operation.
- Excellent cosmetic matching over large areas.
- Uniform pigmentation—no "cobblestoning" as compared to miniature punch grafting.[38]
- Relatively simple and cost-effective procedure. No reagents, laboratory facilities or elaborate equipment is required, as compared to noncultured or cultured melanocyte suspensions.
- Repigmentation of leukotrichia is possible with this technique.[43,44]
- Difficult areas such as eyelids, inner canthus of eyes, areola, and nipples can be treated with relatively successful outcomes.
- Procedure is less time consuming as compared to punch grafting, suction blister grafting and melanocyte suspension methods.

Disadvantages:
- Hyperpigmentation is common, especially in dark skinned individuals and particularly on the exposed areas.
- Superficial scarring may occur at the donor site.
- Multiple sittings may be required when large areas need to be covered.
- Surgical skill is required to take adequate sized, thin grafts. However, the use of electric dermatomes has made it simpler to harvest uniform thin grafts.
- Tips, palms, soles, and mucous membranes are difficult to graft by this method. Inherent differences occur in the histology of the oral mucosa and skin, and any procedure involving partial-thickness grafts from keratinized skin may lead to mismatch in texture and disfigurement.[45] Scarring and contracture at the recipient area in addition to the donor site morbidity is a common phenomenon when split-thickness grafts are applied in the oral mucosa to cover the full-thickness defects.[46,47]
- Furthermore, there is a risk of malignant transformation in such keratinized grafts applied in the oral mucosa.[48]
- The STSG technique provides a yield of 1:1 ratio,[49] although a modification of the technique called the "flip-top" graft may be used; wherein 3–5 mm thinly shaved dermoepidermal fragments are inserted under very thin flaps raised on the recipient site. Repigmentation occurs by coalescence of pigment spread arising from multiple grafts within a few months after grafting.[50]

this technique. These sites are also more prone to friction and trauma, making koebnerization a common phenomenon.[51] Thin split-thickness grafting may be used for dorsal sites, and immobilization is essential, by splinting the fingers. The dorsa of fingers and periungual areas take up mini-punch grafts better than STSGs, wherein graft contracture and rejection are major limitations.

Genital Areas

Conventional surgical therapies such as mini-punch grafts or ultrathin split-thickness grafts from keratinized skin are not suitable for the nonkeratinized mucosa of the glans penis because this may lead to gross mismatch in texture and color.[52] History of genital herpes must be taken before attempting

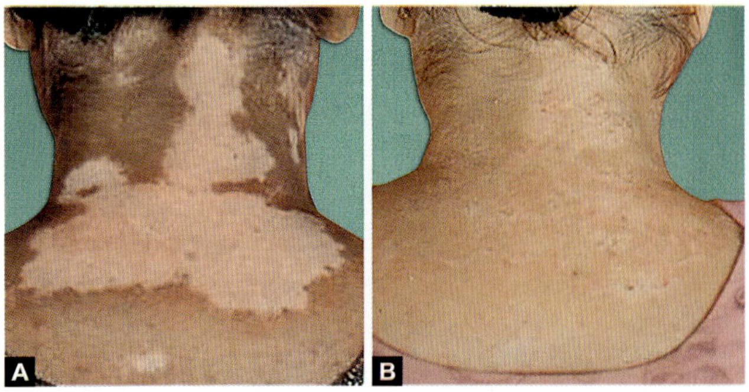

Figs. 5A and B: (A) Vitiligo patch on upper back and neck; (B) Excellent result after split-thickness grafting.

a surgery at these sites, as it can be a potential reason for failure of the surgical procedure. Long-term prophylaxis with acyclovir should be given in proven and doubtful cases and the prognosis is explained.[21] Autologous, noncultured melanocyte-keratinocyte cell transplantation is considered as the preferred and effective surgical option for management of genital vitiligo.[53,54]

The earlier mentioned discussion shows that a surgeon dealing with vitiligo surgery must have adequate expertise of all various methods as often combination treatments give the best results[55] **(Figs. 5A and B)**.

TREATMENT PEARLS

- Acquire training—mastering STSG requires a certain amount of skill, training, and practice—preferably learn the technique, observe, and assist closely before attempting a solo procedure.
- *"Practice makes perfect":* For beginners practice taking small but ultrathin grafts of uniform thickness which is devoid of dermal tissue as this is the key to good cosmesis and an appropriate color match. Slowly graduate to taking larger grafts and attempting larger areas. There are various ways of harvesting the graft, choose one you are most comfortable with.
- Dermabrade the skin 1–2 mm beyond the margins of the vitiligo lesion and place the grafts beyond the dermabraded margins to minimize the chances of perigraft halo formation.
- Proper immobilization is essential after grafting to ensure satisfactory results.
- Use ring blocks at the donor site to ensure a smooth surface for graft placement. Infiltration anesthesia at the donor area may lead to an irregular surface.
- Use NB-UVB, PUVA, or excimer laser if there is a delay in the onset of repigmentation—practice caution as overuse of psoralens may lead to hyperpigmentation.
- Counsel your patient well, regarding the advantages and disadvantages.

CONCLUSION

The thin split-thickness skin graft technique is effective, simple to learn, gives rapid results, provides good cosmesis, and can be used to treat large as well as "difficult to treat" areas. Furthermore, it is a cost-effective procedure which does not require elaborate settings. The mentioned reasons make it one of the most popular surgical modalities used for treating stable vitiligo. However the newer modalities of cellular transplants, which have been simplified and have better textural results are the preferred modalities particularly for larger areas, whereas split-thickness grafting techniques are preferred if immediate results are required.

REFERENCES

1. Mulekar SV, Isedeh P. Surgical interventions for vitiligo: an evidence-based review. Br J Dermatol. 2013;169:57-66.
2. Falabella R. History and chronology of development of surgical therapies for vitiligo. In: Gupta S, Olsson MS, Kanwar AJ, Ortonne JP (Eds). Surgical Management of Vitiligo, 1st edition. Oxford: Blackwell Publishing; 2007. pp. 41-8.
3. Behl PN. Treatment of vitiligo with homologous thin Thiersch's skin grafts. Curr Med Pract. 1964;8:218-21.
4. Skouge JW. Split thickness skin grafting. In: Skouge JW, Gerkin RL (Eds). Skin Grafting, 1st edition. New York: Churchill Livingstone Inc.; 1991. pp. 5-45.
5. Kahn AM, Cohen MJ. Vitiligo: Treatment by dermabrasion and epithelial sheet grafting. J Am Acad Dermatol. 1995;33; 646-8.
6. Kahn AM, Cohen MJ. Repigmentation in vitiligo patients. Melanocyte transfer via ultra-thin grafts. Dermatol Surg. 1998;24(3):365-7.
7. Olsson MJ, Juhlin L. Epidermal sheet grafts for repigmentation of vitiligo and piebaldism, with a review of surgical techniques. Acta Derm Venereol. 1997;77:463-6.
8. Sameem F, Sultan SJ, Ahmad QM. Split thickness skin grafting in patients with stable vitiligo. J Cutan Aesthet Surg. 2011;4:38-40.
9. Khunger N. Vitiligo surgery. In: Robinson JK (Ed). Surgery of the skin: procedural dermatology, 2nd edition. UK: Elsevier Health Sciences; 2010. pp. 683-92.
10. Foroozan M, Pouaha J, Truchetet F. Simple method for harvesting split-thickness skin grafts. Dermatol Surg. 2010;36:1743-5.
11. Khunger N. Thin split-thickness skin grafts for vitiligo. In: Gupta S, Olsson MS, Kanwar AJ, Ortonne JP (Eds). Surgical Management of Vitiligo. Oxford: Blackwell Publishing Ltd; 2007. pp. 108-14.
12. Rudolph R. Inhibition of myofibroblasts by skin grafts. Plast Reconstr Surg. 1979;63(4):473-80.
13. Kim HY, Kang KY. Epidermal grafts for treatment of stable and progressive vitiligo. J Am Acad Dermatol. 1999;41:412-7.
14. Mutalik S, Ginzburg A. Surgical management of stable vitiligo: a review with personal experience. Dermatol Surg. 2000;26:248-54.
15. Boersma BR, Westerhof W, Bos JD. Repigmentation in vitiligo vulgaris by autologous minigrafting: result in nineteen patients. J Am Acad Dermatol. 1995;33:990-5.
16. Kim HU, Yun SK. Suction device for epidermal grafting in vitiligo: employing a syringe and manometer to provide an adequate negative pressure. Dermatol Surg. 2000;26:702-4.

17. Hann SK, Im S, Bong HW, Park YK. Treatment of stable vitiligo with autologous epidermal grafting and PUVA. J Am Acad Dermatol. 1995;32:943-8.
18. Falabella R, Escobar C, Borrero I. Treatment of refractory and stable vitiligo by transplantation of in vitro cultured epidermal autografts bearing melanocytes. J Am Acad Dermatol. 1992;26:230-6.
19. Parsad D, Gupta S. IADVL Dermatosurgery Task Force. Standard guidelines of care for vitiligo surgery. Indian J Dermatol Venereol Leprol. 2008;74:S37-45.
20. Falabella R, Arrunategui A, Barona MI, Alzate A. The minigrafting test for vitiligo: detection of stable lesions for melanocyte transplantation. J Am Acad Dermatol. 1995;32:228-32.
21. Khunger N. Vitiligo surgery. In: Khunger N, Sachdev M (Eds). Practical Manual of Cosmetic Dermatology and Surgery, 1st edition. India: Mehta Publishers; 2010.
22. Van Geel N, Ongenae K, de Mil M, Naeyaert JM. Modified technique of autologous noncultured epidermal cell transplantation for repigmenting vitiligo: a pilot study. Dermatol Surg. 2001;27:873-6.
23. Khunger N, Kathuria SD, Ramesh V. Tissue grafts in vitiligo surgery—past, present and future. Indian J Dermatol. 2009;54(2):150-8.
24. Ozdemir M, Centikale O, Wolf R, Kotoğyan A, Mat C, Tüzün B, et al. Comparison of two surgical approaches for treating vitiligo: a preliminary study. Int J Dermatol. 2002;41(3):1358.
25. McGregor IA, McGregor AD. Fundamental Techniques of Plastic Surgery, 9th edition. Edinburg: Churchill Livingstone; 1995. pp. 35-9.
26. Terrill PJ, Goh RC, Bailey MJ. Split-thickness skin graft donor sites: a comparative study of two absorbent dressings. J Wound Care. 2007;16(10):433-8.
27. Kilinc H, Sensoz O, Ozdemir R, Unlü RE, Baran C. Which dressing for split-thickness skin graft donor sites? Ann Plast Surg. 2001;46(4):409-14.
28. Al-Hadidi N, Griffith JL, Al-Jamal MS, Hamzavi I. Role of Recipient-site Preparation Techniques and Post-operative Wound Dressing in the Surgical Management of Vitiligo. J Cutan Aesthet Surg. 2015;8:79-87.
29. Juhlin L, Olsson MJ. Optimal application times of eutectic mixtures of local anesthetics (EMLA) cream before dermabrasion of vitiliginous skin. Eur J Dermatol. 1995;5:365-70.
30. Oh CK, Cha JH, Lim LY, Jo JH, Kim SJ, Jang HS, et al. Treatment of vitiligo with suction epidermal grafting by the use of an ultrapulse CO2 laser with a computerized pattern generator. Dermatol Surg. 2001;27(6):565-8.
31. Malakar S, Malakar RS. Surgical pearl: composite film and graft unit for the recipient area dressing after split-thickness skin grafting in vitiligo. J Am Acad Dermatol. 2001;44:856-7.
32. Mysore V. Punch grafting in vitiligo. Gulf J Dermatol. 2000;7:27-31.
33. Toriumi DM, O'Grody K, Desai D, Bagal A. Use of octyl-2-cyanoacrylate for skin closure in facial plastic surgery. Plast Reconstr Surg. 1998;102(6):2209-19.
34. Khunger N, Lahiri K, Mysore V. Surgical treatment of vitiligo. In: Robinson JK, Hanke W, Siegel DM, Fratila A (Eds). Surgery of the Skin, 2nd edition. USA: Elsevier Inc.; 2010. pp. 683-93.
35. Njoo MD, Westerhof W, Bos JD, Bossuyt PM. A systematic review of autologous transplantation methods in vitiligo. Arch Dermatol. 1998;134:15439.
36. Agrawal K, Agrawal A. Vitiligo: repigmentation with dermabrasion and thin split-thickness skin graft. Dermatol Surg. 1995;21:295-300.
37. Whitton ME, Ashcroft DM, Gonzalez U. Therapeutic interventions for vitiligo. J Am Acad Dermatol. 2008;59(4):713-7.
38. Khandpur S, Sharma VK, Manchanda Y. Comparison of minipunch grafting versus split-skin grafting in chronic stable vitiligo. Dermatol Surg. 2005;31:436-41.
39. Acikel C, Ulkur E, Celikoz B. Carbon dioxide laser resurfacing and thin skin grafting in the treatment of "stable and recalcitrant" vitiligo. Plast Reconstr Surg. 2003;111:1291-8.
40. Khunger N. Recent advances in the surgical treatment of vitiligo. In: Ghosh S (Ed). Recent Advances in Dermatology, 1st edition. New Delhi: Jaypee Brothers Medical Publishers (P) Ltd.; 2007. pp. 19-40.
41. Al-Mutairi N, Manchanda Y, Al-Doukhi A, Al-Haddad A. Long-term results of split-skin grafting in combination with excimer laser for stable vitiligo. Dermatol Surg. 2010;36(4):499-505.
42. Behl PN, Azad O, Kak R, et al. Autologous thin Thiersch's grafts in vitiligo: experience of 8000 cases 50000 grafts (195998) with modified technique in 198 cases in the year 1997-98. Indian J Derm Venereol Leprol. 1999;65(3):117-21.
43. Agrawal K, Agrawal A. Vitiligo: surgical repigmentation of leukotrichia. Dermatol Surg. 1995;21(8):711-5.
44. Bose SK. Is there any treatment of leukotrichia in stable vitiligo? J Dermatol. 1997;24(9):615-7.
45. Gupta S, Sandhu K, Kanwar A, Kumar B. Melanocyte transfer via epidermal grafts for vitiligo of labial mucosa. Dermatol Surg. 2004;30(1):45-8.
46. Rhee PH, Friedman CD, Ridge JA, Kusiak J. The use of processed allograft dermal matrix for intraoral resurfacing: an alternative to split-thickness skin grafts. Arch Otolaryngol Head Neck Surg. 1998;124(11):1201-4.
47. Mitchell R. The use of collagen in oral surgery. Ann Acad Med Singapore. 1986;15(3):355-60.
48. Sa'do B, Nakamura N, Higuchi Y, Ozeki S, Harada H, Tashiro H. Squamous cell carcinoma of the oral cavity derived from a skin graft: a case report. Head Neck. 1994;16(1):79-82.
49. Falabella R. Surgical approaches for stable vitiligo. Dermatol Surg. 2005;31(10):1277-84.
50. McGovern TW, Bolognia J, Leffell DJ. Flip-top pigment transplantation: a novel transplantation procedure for the treatment of depigmentation. Arch Dermatol. 1999;135(11):1305-7.
51. Mutalik S. Surgical management of acral vitiligo. In: Gupta S, Olsson MS, Kanwar AJ, Ortonne JP (Eds). Surgical Management of Vitiligo. Oxford: Blackwell Publishing Ltd; 2007. pp. 225-8.
52. Gupta S. Commentary on: genital vitiligo treated by autologous, noncultured melanocyte-keratinocyte cell transplant. Derm Surg. 2005;31:1740.
53. Mulekar SV, Al Issa A, Al Eisa A, Asaad M. Genital vitiligo treated by autologous, noncultured melanocyte-keratinocyte cell transplantation. Dermatol Surg. 2005;31:1737-40.
54. Mulekar SV, Al Issa A, Al Eisa A. Treatment of vitiligo on difficult-to-treat sites using autologous noncultured cellular grafting. Dermatol Surg. 2009;35(1):66-71.
55. Pahwa M, Gupta S, Khunger N. Multi modal single step vitiligo surgery (MMSSVS): A novel approach. Dermatol Surg. 2010;36(10):1627-31.

CHAPTER 38

Epidermal Noncultured Cell Suspension in Vitiligo Including Megasessions

Munish Paul

PART A: EPIDERMAL NONCULTURED CELL SUSPENSION IN VITILIGO

KEY MESSAGES

- Tissue grafts have the limitation of smaller area coverage.
- Cellular grafts need a small size of donor, which can then be used to cover a large vitiligo area.
- The vital steps in epidermal noncultured suspension include donor harvesting, trypsinization to separate the cells, centrifugation to make a suspension of cells, preparation of the recipient site by dermabrasion, and transfer of the cells.
- The donor recipient area coverage is in the ratio 1:8–1:10.
- It is suitable for all areas.
- Limitations include higher cost, need for trained staff and a longer learning curve.

INTRODUCTION

As discussed in earlier chapters, medical treatments are not successful in all cases of vitiligo.[1-3] Tissue grafts have the limitations that large amount of donor skin is needed as there is no cell expansion in these methods.[4,5] Hence, transplantation of autologous cultured and noncultured melanocytes which involve cell suspension without culture or keratinocyte/melanocyte co-cultures[6-10] are gaining popularity. Transplantation of noncultured melanocytes/keratinocytes suspension has the advantage that cell culture is not needed and that skin harvesting from the donor area, cell separation, and application of melanocytes can all be undertaken in a single 3-hour procedure.

Indications, contraindications, case selection, preoperative investigations have all been dealt with in earlier chapters. This chapter will deal, therefore, only with specific details of the procedure.

PROCEDURE

- Harvesting a skin graft
- Trypsinization and cell separation
- Dermabrasion of the recipient (vitiligo) site
- Transfer and fixing of melanocyte rich cell suspension

Accompanying **Box 1 and Figures 1 to 8** demonstrate these steps.

Harvesting of Skin Graft

The lateral aspect of the gluteal region is selected as the donor area. Care should be taken to ensure that the donor area has no vitiligo patches. The area of split thickness donor skin taken is one-tenth of the recipient area while dealing with large confluent patches. In cases having multiple scattered small patches, larger donor skin is taken, approximately one-fifth of the recipient area. Under aseptic precautions, a very superficial sample is harvested using a shaving blade held in straight Kocher's forceps or a Silver skin grafting handle or a dermatome as is comfortable with surgeon. The donor area is dressed with liquid paraffin dressing (Fairlee™) and a sterile gauze pad.

Cell Separation Technique (Box 1)

This is the most important step and consists of three steps—trypsinization, removal of excess trypsin by antitrypsin, and centrifugation to obtain a cell suspension.

1. *Trypsinization:* The cell separation is done ideally under aseptic precautions in a laminar flow bench kept in the

BOX 1: Steps in obtaining epidermal noncultured cell suspension (**Figs. 1 to 8**).

- *Step 1:* A split thickness thin graft is harvested under local/topical anesthesia
- *Step 2:* Graft is placed in a Petri dish containing 5 mL of 0.2% trypsin + 0.8% ethylenediaminetetraacetic acid (EDTA) solution
- *Step 3:* Graft is soaked completely in the solution and spread out with epidermal surface facing upward
- *Step 4:* Incubated in an incubator at 37°C for 45 minutes.
- *Step 5:* Trypsin solution is neutralized by 5 mL of 0.5% trypsin inhibitor or phosphate-buffered saline (PBS) or ringer's lactate (RL) solution
- *Step 6:* Dermis is teased out from the epidermis and discarded
- *Step 7:* The cells are separated from the epidermis and transferred to a test tube
- *Step 8:* The test tube with epidermal cells is centrifuged for 7 minutes to obtain a pellet rich in cells
- *Step 9:* The pellet is resuspended in PBS/Ringer's lactate solution/Dulbecco's modified Eagle's medium (DMEM) and transferred to 1 mL tuberculin syringe, ready for application onto the recipient area.

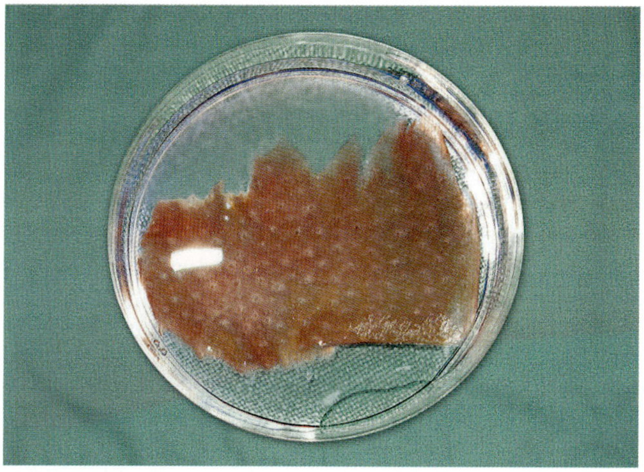

Fig. 1: In the first step a very thin skin graft is taken from the thigh and incubated at 37°centigrade with trypsin enzyme for 45 minutes to induce separation of the various layers of the skin. The size of donor area required is only one-tenth of the vitiligo area to be operated.

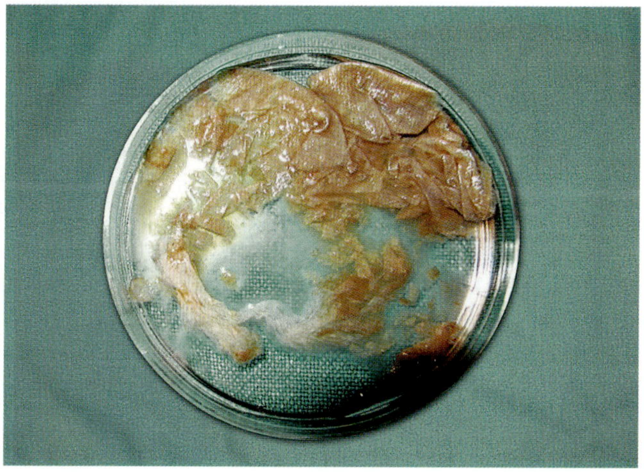

Fig. 2: The trypsin enzyme dissolves the various layers of skin so that the epidermis (upper layer), dermis (middle layer) are separated and skin is now in a liquid state.

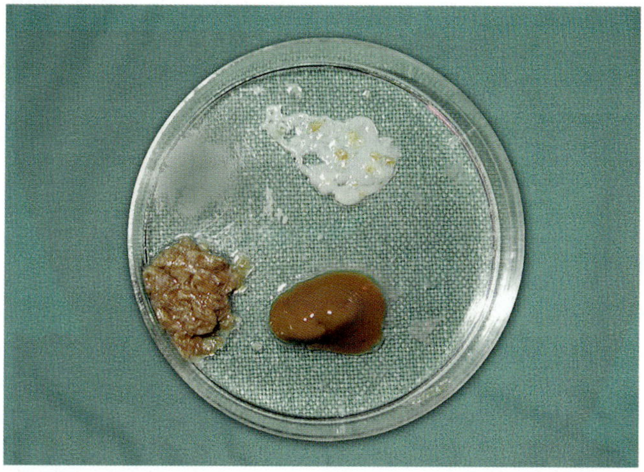

Fig. 3: All the layers of skin have separated: White is dermis, light brown fraction is upper epidermis, and dark brown is melanocyte-rich cell suspension.

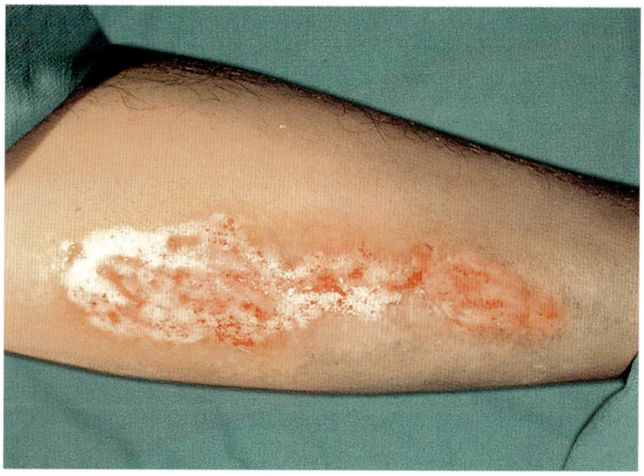

Fig. 4: The skin of the vitiligo area to be treated is removed very superficially with an Er:YAG laser or diamond burs.

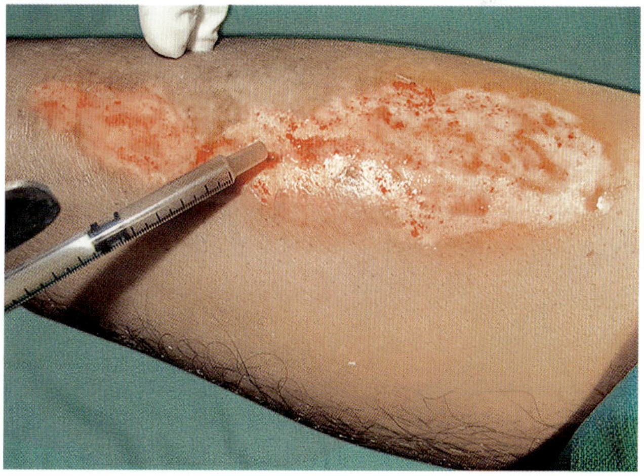

Fig. 5: The melanocyte rich cell suspension (pigment cells) is applied on the laser ablated area uniformly.

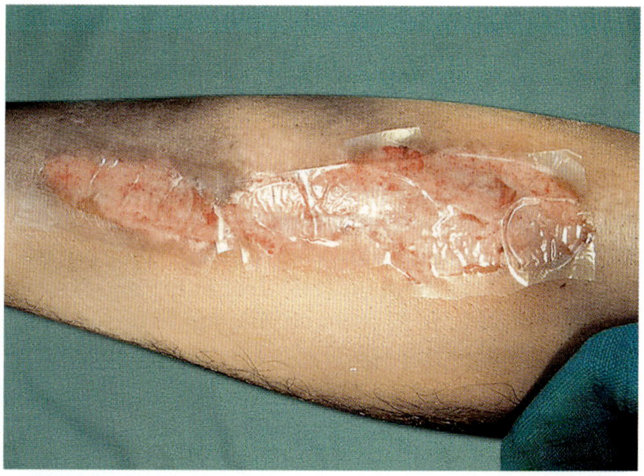

Fig. 6: Collagen dressings are applied on the transplanted cells to ensure that they get fixed completely on the area to be operated.

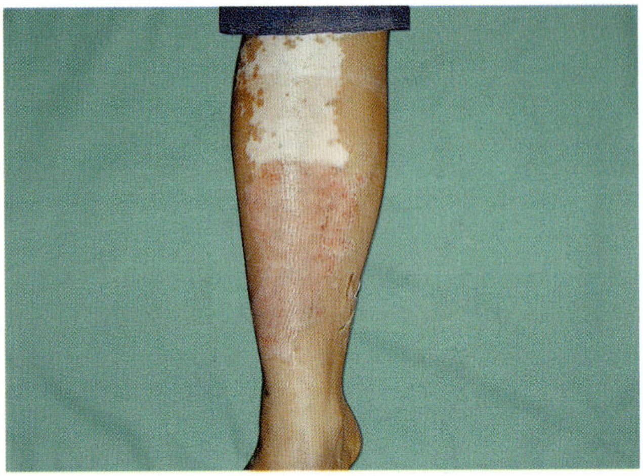

Fig. 7: The operated area heals completely in 7 days and looks pink in color. At this stage, patient can resume normal bath and activity.

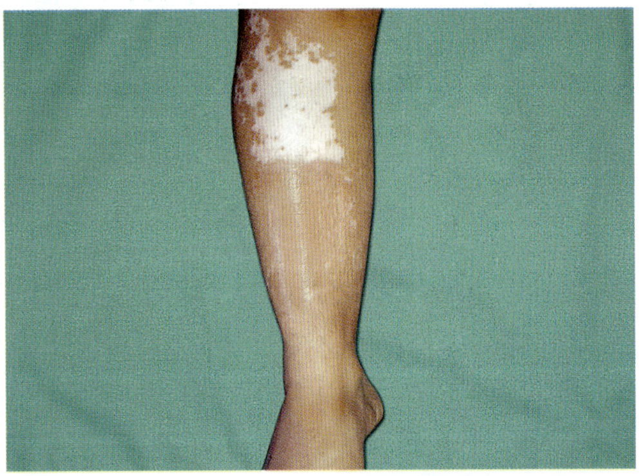

Fig. 8: The operated area has completely achieved pigmentation in 3 months and there is good color and texture matching.

operation theater. If laminar flow bench is not available, the sterile environment of the theater is adequate. The skin sample harvested is transferred to a Petri dish containing 5 mL of the 0.2% w/v trypsin solution, epidermal side facing upward, and incubated for 45 minutes at 37° centigrade.

2. *Removal of excess trypsin:* After incubation for 45 minutes–2 hours, the action of trypsin is neutralized with trypsin inhibitor (Life Technologies, USA). The epidermis is separated from the dermis and transferred to a test tube containing 2 mL of Dulbeccos Modified Eagles Medium (DMEM): Nutrient mixture F-12 (DMEM/F-12) medium (Life Technologies, USA) and vortex-mixed for 15 seconds. The epidermis is further broken into smaller pieces in a Petri dish and washed with the DMEM/F-12 medium and finally transferred to a test tube containing the DMEM/F-12 medium.
3. *Centrifugation:* The test tube is then centrifuged for 6 minutes. The supernatant is discarded and the pellet at the bottom is suspended in a 1-mL insulin syringe. The final volume prepared varies from 0.2 to 0.5 mL depending on the size of the graft taken and the area to be treated.

Dermabrasion of the Recipient Site

The recipient site is abraded with a dermabrader fitted with a diamond fraise wheel (Delasco™). While operating close to the eyelid margins, an erbium:YAG (Er:YAG) laser is used with a fluence of 1,000 mJ, 1–2 passes. The endpoint of ablation is pinpoint bleeding. Hemostasis is achieved and the ablated area is covered with saline-soaked gauze pieces.

Transplantation Technique

The cell suspension is spread evenly on the dermabraded area with 1-mL insulin syringe and covered with collagen dressing (Collomedica Laboratories) to hold the cells applied. This is covered with liquid paraffin dressing and gauze pieces. Patients are instructed to lie still in the same position for at least 1 hour to ensure cell fixation and then shifted to a room and further instructed to avoid excessive movements of the treated area for at least 6 hours.

POSTPROCEDURE INSTRUCTIONS

All patients are instructed to take complete rest and avoid all vigorous physical activities. Patients are prescribed oral antibacterial agents for 5 days and nonsteroidal anti-inflammatory drugs (NSAIDs) for 3 days. The dressings are removed after 1 week in most cases. Patients are asked to follow up at weeks 1 and 3 and then at 3-month intervals. Patients are instructed not to scrub the area. Patients are permitted to use make-up on the treated area 15 days after the removal of dressings.

ONSET OF PIGMENTATION

The onset of pigmentation usually occurs in 3–6 weeks and it can take 3–6 months for the patches to achieve significant pigmentation. Psoralen ultraviolet A (PUVA) with sunlight or phototherapy can be initiated after 3–6 weeks. Vitiligo patches which do not recover even after 6 months will need to be transplanted again. **Figures 9 to 12** show before and after photographs in different areas—hands, neck, and scalp. **Box 2** shows the advantages and disadvantages of non-cultured epidermal cell suspension (NCECS) technique.

Modifications of the Procedure

Noncultured epidermal cell suspension has only four basic steps, i.e., harvesting the graft, cell separation, resurfacing the vitiligo area, and transferring the cell suspension and stabilizing it. Various authors have reported modifications which can be incorporated while performing this procedure:

- *Making the cell suspension more viscous and uniform:*[11] The suspension obtained is often too watery and

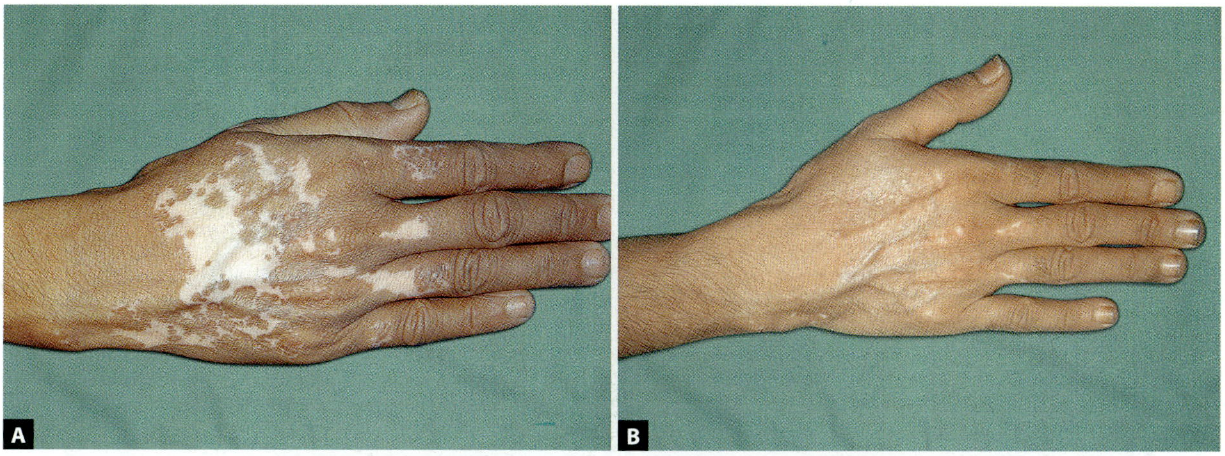

Figs. 9A and B: Vitiligo hand (A) Pretreatment; (B) Postcell transfer.

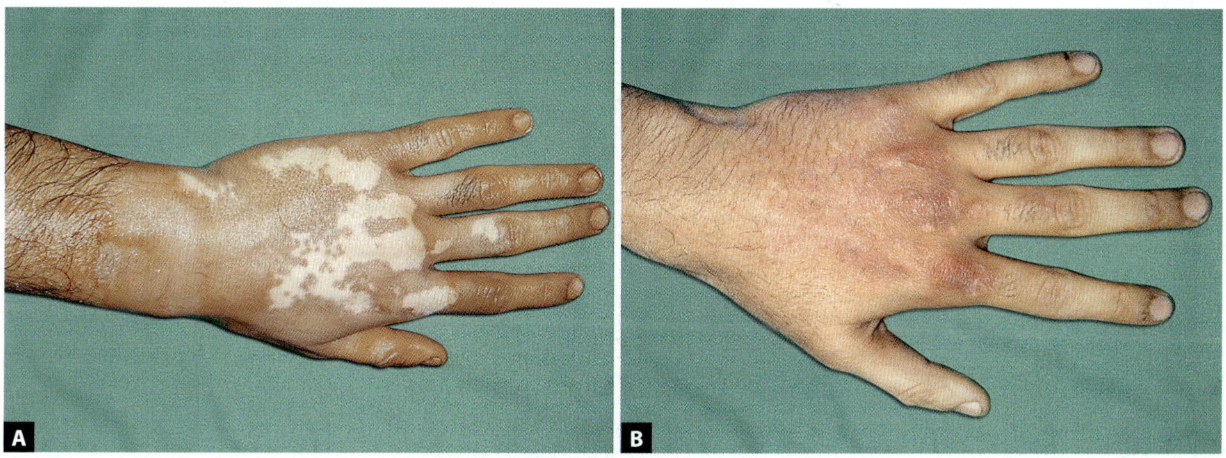

Figs. 10A and B: Vitiligo hand (A) Pretreatment; (B) Postcell transfer.

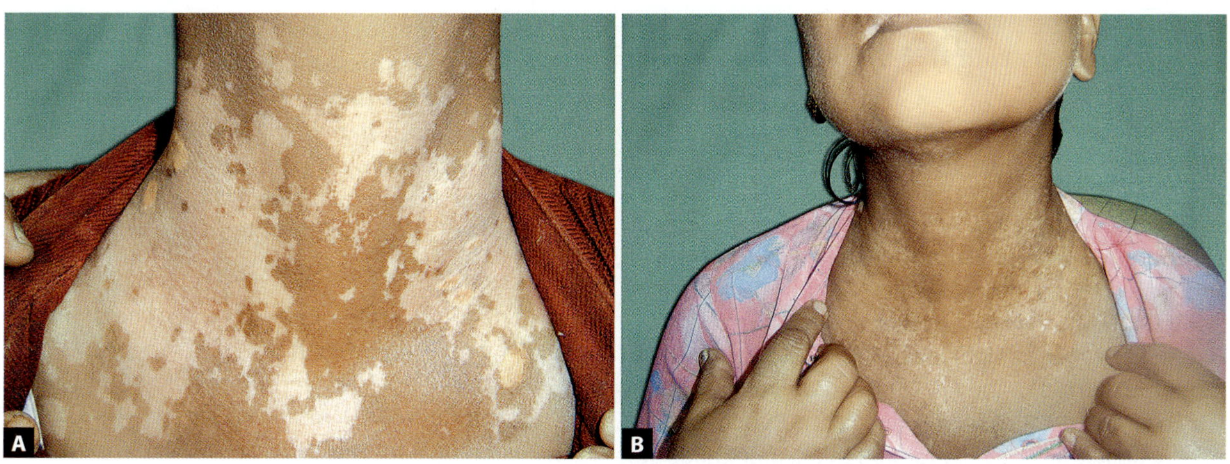

Figs. 11A and B: Vitiligo neck (A) Pretreatment; (B) Postcell transfer.

runs off. Nanny van Geel et al.[11] reported the use of hyaluronic acid to the final pellet, in the ratio reported the use of hyaluronic acid addition to the final pellet in the ratio of 1:1, this increases the viscosity and prevents runaway of the final cell suspension.

- *Cold trypsinization:* Yvon Gauthier et al.[9] described a two-step technique; recipient area is prepared by inducing cryoblisters with liquid nitrogen and then the melanocyte keratinocyte suspension is injected into the blisters. The donor area used is the skin of the scalp which is incubated in 0.25% trypsin for 18 hours at 4°centigrade.

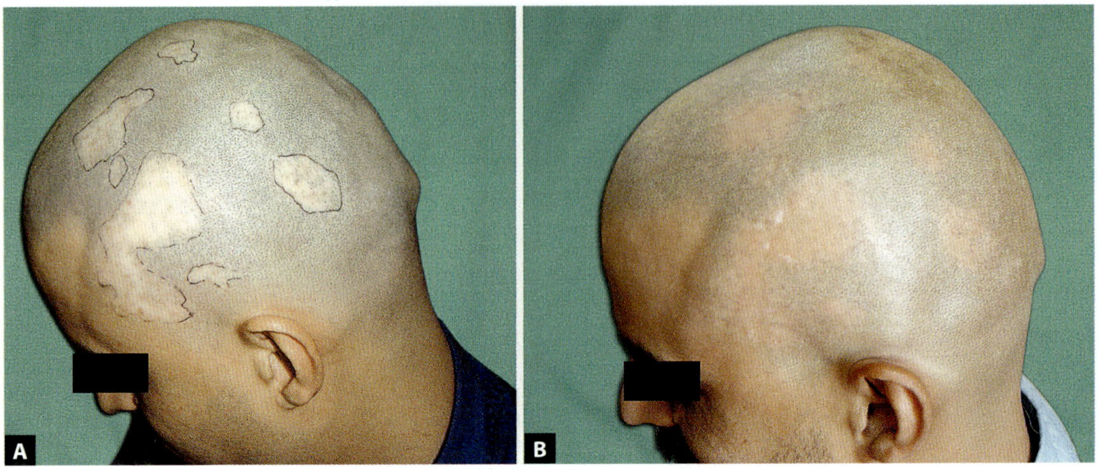

Figs. 12A and B: Vitiligo scalp: (A) Pretreatment; (B) Postcell transfer.

BOX 2: Advantages and disadvantages of the procedure.

Advantages:
- Donor recipient ratio 1:10, i.e., with just 10 cm^2 of donor size a vitiligo patch of 100 cm2 can be treated
- Excellent texture and color matching
- No stuck-on look (as seen in split thickness grafting) or cobblestoning (as with punch grafting)
- Large areas can be treated in a single session
- Patient can use cosmetic camouflage as early as 20 days post-operatively

Disadvantages:
- Complex procedure as compared to simple punch or split thickness grafting
- Longer training and supervision required to perfect the procedure
- Variables such as trypsin strength, media used, temperature and time of incubation, centrifugation can alter results
- More expensive.

This is referred to as cold trypsinization and avoids centrifugation.

- *Cryopreservation of cell suspension*[12]
- *Using suction blister roofs as donor skin*[13]
- *Use of timed surgery for removing epidermis in epidermis.*[14]
- *Four compartment method of NCECS:*[15] Four compartment (FC) method is a simplified and cost-effective method of noncultured epidermal cell suspension for the treatment of vitiligo. A split-thickness graft is taken using a shaving blade held by long straight artery forceps. The skin graft is then transferred to the FC Petri dish in compartment 1 which contains 0.25% trypsin and 0.02% EDTA solution and is incubated at 37°centigrade for 1 hour. After 1 hour, the trypsinized graft is washed sequentially to remove trypsin in phosphate-buffered saline (PBS) in compartments 2 and 3. Then the graft is shifted to compartment 4. In this compartment, the dermis is separated from the epidermis using sterile forceps, and cells are dislodged gently from the basement membrane and suspended in PBS. This suspension of epidermal cells, comprising a mixture of keratinocytes and melanocytes, is used for transplantation over the dermabraded area of the patient **(Figs. 13A to F)**.

  This technique makes the NCECS process cost-effective and simple enough to be performed in the clinic without laboratory equipment. The following items are required in the FC method—a Petri dish with four compartments, forceps, PBS, trypsin solution, and a sterile syringe.

  Advantages of the four compartment method:
  1. *No need for the following items:* Trypsin inhibitor, pipettes, autoclaved tips, centrifuge tube, and centrifuge machine
  2. There is no need for centrifugation; overnight cold trypsinization at 4° centigrade in an ordinary refrigerator is performed.
  3. PBS washing is used to remove trypsin and hence there is no need to use any trypsin inhibitor.
  4. Pipette and tips are replaced by syringes.
- *In vivo preparation of NCECS:*[16] In this process, cell separation and harvesting is performed inside sterile blisters induced by suction on the patient's thigh. This technique is simple, inexpensive, and requires minimal processing and handling of the tissue outside the body.

  Procedure:
  - Suction blisters are raised on the lateral aspect of the patient's upper thigh.
  - With a 24-G hypodermic needle, the blister fluid is aspirated and 1 mL of 0.25% trypsin-0.002% EDTA solution is introduced into the blister cavity, body heat acts as an incubator at a temperature of around 37.8° centigrade
  - Within 45 minutes, epidermal melanocytes and basal keratinocytes, which are in contact with the trypsin-EDTA solution, detach to form a cellular suspension inside the blister cavity. This suspension is aspirated and transferred to a sterile Petri dish following which the dermal side of blisters is scrapped to release basal

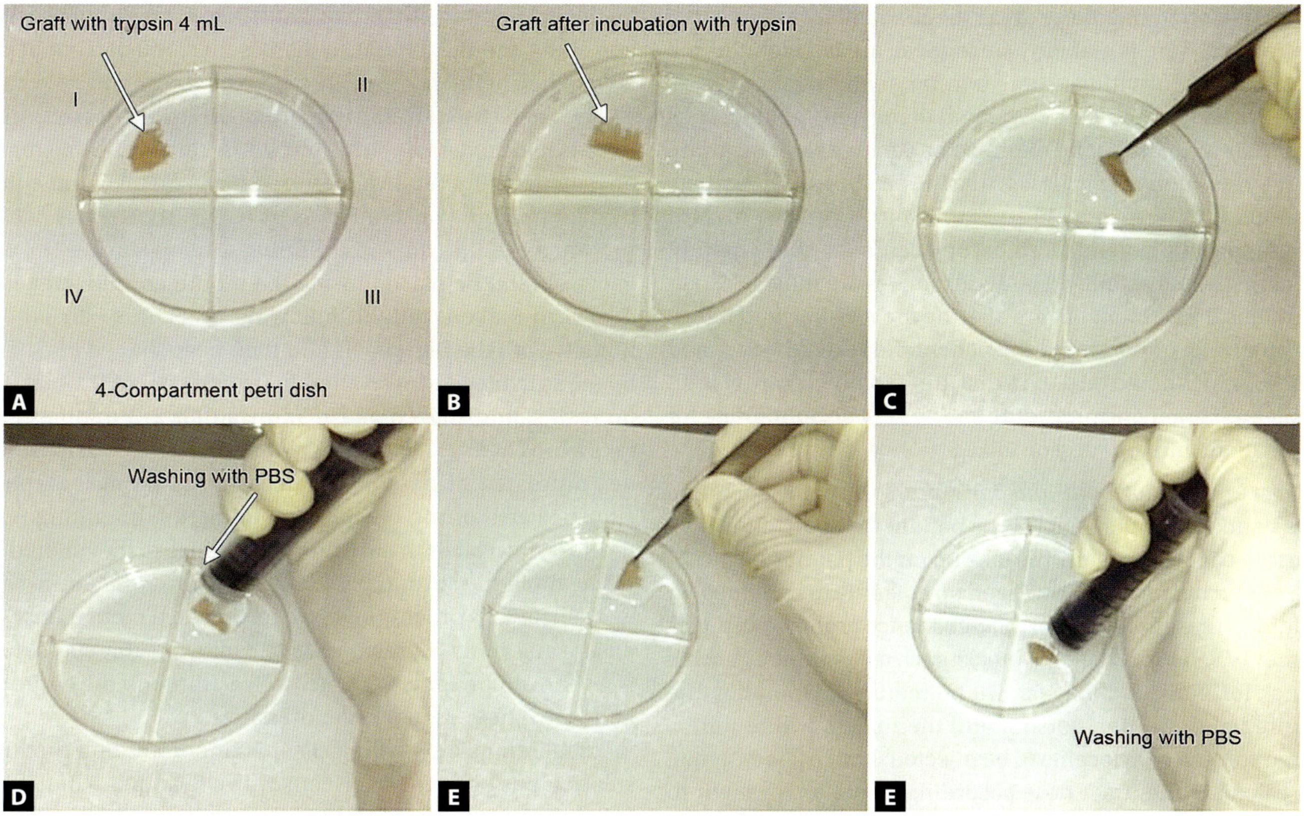

Figs. 13A to F: (A) Trypsin added to skin graft; (B) Skin graft in trypsin after incubation; (C–F) Washing with PBS to remove trypsin in compartments II and III. (PBS: phosphate-buffered saline)

layer cells into the suspension. The suspension is then transplanted onto dermabraded vitiligo patches.

Advantages:
- It does not require specialized training or laboratory equipment.
- There is no lag period between harvesting and transplantation.
- There is minimal handling of tissue outside the body, thus reducing risk of contamination.
- The blister cavity provides a closed system, essentially creating a mini-laboratory in the patient's own skin.
- This procedure is suitable for dermatologists in smaller centers where conventional cellular transplantation cannot be performed because of lack of infrastructure.

- *Using hair as donor:* This is described in detail in the next chapter.

TABLE 1: Modifications of the procedure for specific acral areas.

Site	*Recipient site preparation*	*Retaining the cellular grafts*
Eyes	• Dermabrasion (DA) • Use cylindrical burrs • Stabilize well, use a corneal shield to provide base for dermabrasion	• For small areas, use only collagen and leave it open • *For larger area (full eyelid):* Apply collagen>> paraffin>> gauze>> pad>> close eye for 7 days
Finger tips	Deeper dermabrasion	Dress each finger individually and then the whole hand
Lips	• Use infiltration • Put a gauze inside mouth to make the lips taut • Use CO_2 laser or Er:YAG	Collagen>> paraffin>> suture with 4-0 prolene
Penis/ Scrotum	• Pear-shaped burr for dermabrasion • Pinch skin around to make it taught • Use CO_2 laser or Er:YAG	• Cut collagen in small pieces and sprinkle • Admit patient • Put in urinary catheter • Use drugs to reduce erection

Modifications of NCECS While Operating on the Acral Areas

Acral vitiligo is the most difficult variety of vitiligo to manage. The reason for failure is two fold; firstly the acral areas are difficult to operate; dermabrasion is difficult to perform and secondly the retention of the cell suspension is also difficult. The procedure of NCECS has to be modified to improve the chances of take up of the melanocytes and repigmentation achieved. A few pearls are being described in **Table 1**.

The areas considered to be difficult are the: Fingers, toes, lips, penis, scrotum, and nipple areola complex.

While operating these areas the first and foremost thing to be 100% sure is stability, since these areas belong to the acral variety of vitiligo there can be a very slight spread. Ideally lesions should be compared to previous photographs ascertain stability. Quite often the patient may not be aware or may be withholding the fact that the patches are spreading, so look for signs of stability, i.e., sharp borders, inward migration of pigment. Dermoscopy can offer some help in deciding about stability. The acral patches are most resistant to medical treatment but are also the most visible and hence cosmetically important to the patient. Repeated history and questioning should be done to ensure stability is there else no repigmentation postprocedure can be very disappointing for the patient and the surgeon alike.

Fingers, dorsum of hand, and finger tips/toes: While operating the hand we should counsel the patient that only the dorsal surface can be operated, the take up on the palmar surface is very poor and most cases will end up as failure to repigment in addition these areas are very painful hence proper anesthesia either IV sedation, regional blocks such as wrist block or ring block for individual fingers will be required. Operating the entire hand, i.e., the dorsum and the fingers will require a large volume of Xylocaine to be injected; hence it is essential to calculate the exact dose according to patients weight to avoid overdose or xylocaine toxicity.

After adequate anesthesia is achieved the dermabrasion is carried out using the wheel burs over the dorsum of the hand and pear-shaped burs to be used ear the periungual areas. After DA up to the papillary bleed each finger is wrapped with a saline-soaked gauze to achieve hemostasis.

While transferring the cells it is important that the final solution has been made viscous with the addition of methyl cellulose so it does not run off. Small pieces of dry collagen sheets should be precut and kept ready so that they are applied immediately by the assistant as the cells are being spread uniformly over the DA area. Following this paraffin dressings which are also precut ready according the area are applied; this is followed by applying wet but squeezed gauze pieces which mold with the finger very well. The next layer is dry gauze followed by Micropore tape, finish each finger completely before moving to the next digit else the cells/collagen sheet/paraffin dressing can get dislodged during subsequent cell application.

Once all the fingers have been done then the dorsum of the hand should be dressed in the same fashion after this a gamjee roll dressing or surgical pads need to applied and the whole hand bandaged up to the wrist. We usually do not give a plaster of Paris posterior slab or additional splints but they are used by some dermatosurgeons.

This detailed dressing is essential to maximize the retention of the cells.

Lips: When operating the lips it is important to understand that the lip has a dry and a wet part, and we can implant cells only on the dry lip. Start out by marking the area, take photographs, and show it to the patient so there is no confusion about the area to be operated.

Two percent xylocaine is injected; the lip has been cleaned with betadine, spirit, and draped. After the lip has been anesthetized the removal of the skin can be taken up either by diamond burs or ablative lasers (CO_2/Er:YAG).

Since the lip can keep running around during DA wet gauze should be placed inside the mouth and lip stretched over it to make it taught; following this DA is carried out initially with the big wheels and then pear-shaped burs. The lip tends to bleed a lot so after doing first pass of DA soak the lip with saline-soaked gauze and wait for 2–3 minutes and take a look at the base to ensure that there are no skip zones, i.e., untreated or partially treated areas. Amongst all body sites because of the bleeding clouding the operating field the lip is most likely to have these skip zones so they should be DA again in the second pass and again cover the entire with wet gauze. This process needs to be repeated meticulously to ensure an evenly DA recipient site. Following this stay suture is given with prolene 4-0 which will go through the entire lip and which help us in tie over dressings.

While transferring the cells it is important that the final solution has been made viscous with the addition of methyl cellulose so it does not run off. Small pieces of dry collagen sheets should be precut and kept ready so that they are applied immediately by the assistant as the cells are being spread uniformly over the DA area. Following this paraffin dressings which are also precut ready according the area are applied; this is followed by applying wet but squeezed gauze pieces which mold with the lip very well. The next layer is dry gauze over which the tie over dressing is done. This detailed dressing is essential to maximize the retention of the cells.

Patient should be instructed to have a liquid diet with a wide bore straw or use spoon to eat small bites for the next 5–7 days. Patient counselling about taking care of the dressings should be done in detail and a written instruction sheet should be handed over.

Eyelids: Eyelid vitiligo surgery should ideally be undertaken after the dermatosurgeon has already done many cases over other body parts and he/she is confident about the entire procedure especially the DA.

Eyelid skin is one of the thinnest over the body hence the DA has to be very precise even a slight deep DA can cause scarring and any injury if it occurs to the underlying eyeball can be disastrous.

After disinfecting and draping the area 2% xylocaine is injected to create anesthesia; small size pear shaped/cylindrical burs should be used. While DA the eye the role of the assistant who is stretching the skin is very important because any lack of concentration/distraction leading to lax skin will make the wheel bite/tug/wrap the skin leading to serious injury.

Using an ablative CO_2 or Er:YAG laser is safer on this site, the energy settings will vary according to the device being used but the endpoint is uniform whitening of the skin which when scrapped with a wet saline-soaked gauze will lead to complete deepithelialization.

Following this the cells are applied. While transferring the cells it is important that the final solution has been made viscous with the addition of methyl cellulose so it does not run off. Small pieces of dry collagen sheets should be precut and kept ready so that they are applied immediately by the assistant as the cells are being spread uniformly over the DA area. Following this paraffin dressings which are also precut ready according the area are applied; this is followed by applying dry gauze and finally a pad which is then put across to close the eye. It is desirable to shut the eye for a week so that there is minimum movement and the uptake of the cells is good. Patient is instructed that if they feel excessive pain, they should review early else the dressings are left for 1 week; but obviously only one eye should be operated at one time ideally.

Penis: Vitiligo surgery over the shaft of the penis and the glans should ideally be undertaken after the dermatosurgeon has already done many cases over other body parts and he/she is confident about the entire procedure especially the DA.

Penile skin is one of the thinnest over the body hence the DA has to be very precise even a slight deep DA can cause scarring. After disinfecting and draping the area 2% xylocaine is injected as local anesthesia. Patients having a small areas just topical anaesthesia applied under occlusion can provide a good anaesthesia.

In very apprehensive patients and if the entire shaft and glans needs to be operated a dorsal penile nerve block or IV sedation is preferable. A catheter can also be introduced so that postsurgery micturition will not displace the cells; patient is ideally admitted for 2–3 days.

For dermabrasion small size pear-shaped/cylindrical burs should be used. The skin over the shaft of the penis keeps running around so it needs to be pinched and made taught so that smooth DA can be carried out.

Using an ablative CO_2 or erbium YAG laser is safer on this site the energy settings will vary according to the device being used but the endpoint is uniform whitening of the skin which when scrapped with a wet saline-soaked gauze will lead to complete deepithelialization.

Following this the cells are applied. While transferring the cells it is important that the final solution has been made viscous with the addition of methyl cellulose so it does not run off. Small pieces of dry collagen sheets should be precut and kept ready so that they are applied immediately by the assistant as the cells are being spread uniformly over the DA area. Following this paraffin dressings which are also precut ready according the area are applied; this is followed by applying dry gauze and micropore. Patient should be made to rest for at least an hour immediately following the process on the OT table itself and then transferred to the recovery room on a stretcher. Handling of the operated area should be gentle.

Scrotum: While operating on lesions over the scrotum small lesions can simply be excised and sutured. Larger lesions will require the precautions similar to that described for the penis; special precautions being putting very small bits of collagen so that they can move with expansion and contraction of the skin on this area.

Pearls to Make the NCECS Process More Simple

- Using a simple instrument—*USTRA* to harvest skin grafts.
  - The first and foremost step in NCECS is to harvest an ultrathin graft, because if the graft is thick, i.e., with dermis it cannot be separated by trypsinization **(Figs. 14A to D)**.
  - The ability to cut a split-thickness skin graft free-handedly needs long experience. Several devices have been improvised to simplify this task. However, the size and elaborate arrangements of dermatomes often preclude their use. The various options available are Humby's skin grafting knife, Silver skin grafting knife, and dermatomes: Davol's, Padgett's.
    - Most dermatosurgeons are comfortable using a blade in straight artery forceps.
    - The author has been using *USTRA* which is commonly used shaving handle for harvesting ultrathin grafts. Normal shaving blade can be inserted in this and no complicated adjustments are required.
- Suction blister roofs can be used as donor skin.
- Laminar air flow is not mandatory to conduct cell separation; use of a laminar air flow has been conventionally recommended for carrying out the cell separation procedure, but this adds to the cost of treatment. However, if the cell separation is carried out in a sterile OT, there is no requirement of laminar air flow.
- Incubator is not mandatory; ideally incubation should be done at 37° centigrade in an incubator but even if it is done in the open with room temperature of 25–35° centigrade, cell separation can be achieved.
- *Cutting down the incubation time of the graft in trypsin-EDTA solution:* Recommended incubation time is 45 minutes at 37° centigrade. If the grafts harvested are ultrathin, the incubation time can be cut down to just 30 minutes (instead of 45 minutes) in hot trypsinization method at 37° centigrade.
- *Avoiding trypsin inhibitor:* Antitrypsin solution is the most expensive chemical in the NCECS process. However, DMEM/F-12 media, patients own serum or PBS or Ringer lactate (RL) can be used to neutralize trypsin.

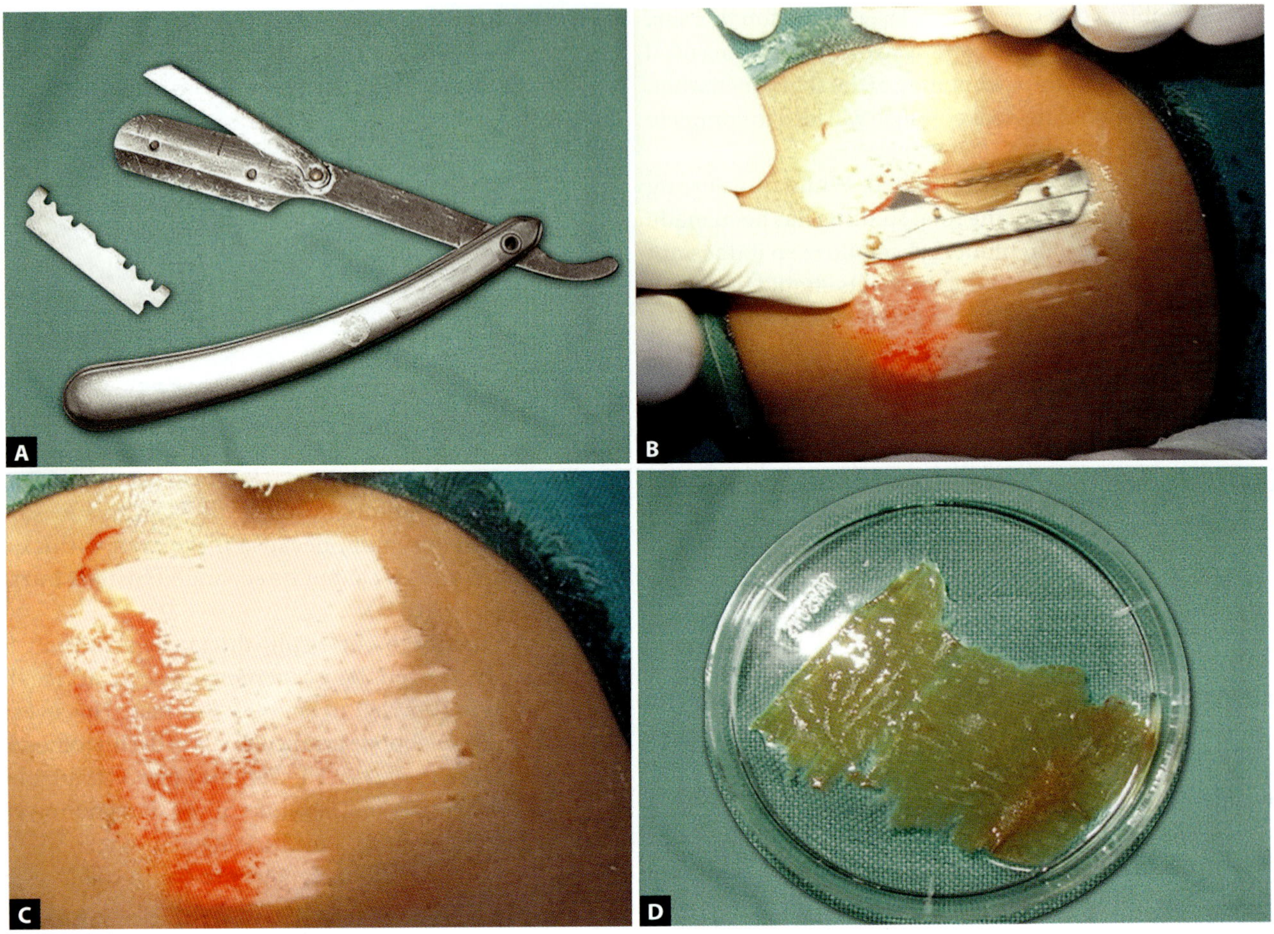

Figs. 14A to D: (A) *Ustra:* A simple device to harvest grafts; (B) Ultrathin graft being harvested with the USTRA; (C) Pinpoint bleed at the donor area shows that the graft harvested is very thin and superficial; (D) Graft harvested with USTRA, graft is floating, not curled up denoting minimum dermis.

- *Using pixel collagen to hold the cells:* Retaining the cell suspension in some areas such as the eyelid, scrotal skin, penile skin, areola, perianal area skin is a challenge because the skin tends to be mobile and expansile. By cutting the collagen sheet into very small pieces, graft take is enhanced, as the multiple small pieces adhere better and are more mobile with the skin stretching. We have coined the term pixel collagen for this step, i.e., cutting the dry collagen sheet in small pixel pieces and applying them.

CONCLUSION

Noncultured epidermal suspension method has established itself as an effective and safe method of treating vitiligo and has replaced split skin grafting in many centers. The several modifications introduced over the last few years have enhanced its utility.

PART B: VITILIGO SURGERY—MEGASESSIONS

KEY MESSAGES

- Local anesthesia permits to operate only small areas in one session, because of issues of pain, apprehension and Xylocaine dosage and toxicity.
- *Extensive areas:* Giga sessions (>400 cm^2), mega sessions (150–400 cm^2) can be performed comfortably and safely under general anesthesia.
- General anesthesia requires OT equipped with anesthesia equipment, cardiac monitors, and trained staff to handle emergencies.
- Nonculture epidermal suspension (NCECS) technique scores over other vitiligo grafting techniques because of the excellent donor recipient ratio, i.e., 1:10.
- Pain para and postoperative, blood loss, are important issues while doing large areas in one session.
- The percentage and extent of repigmentation of the mega and giga session is similar to that of regular sessions.

INTRODUCTION

Surgical management of stable vitiligo[17] has evolved and come a long way. More and more dermatologists are now apt at various vitiligo and other surgeries. Most dermatologists either work from their own clinics or centers or perform various procedures in a minor theater, doing most procedures under local anesthesia. Most vitiligo surgeries are done for small areas, usually of size 50–100 cm^2. This part of the chapter focuses on surgical management of extensive vitiligo and offers tips for performing such surgeries.

A patient of stable vitiligo may have a large area to be operated and may not have time for multiple sessions such as those coming from a foreign country, or those with a marriage in the offing. Currently there are no definite guidelines as to how much maximum area can be operated in a single session. We take up cases with larger areas 150–400 cm^2 for such mega sessions **(Table 2)**.

CASE SELECTION

1. Only patients having disease stability for 1 year are taken up for surgery.
   Stability is taken up on these criteria:
   a. No new patches for 1 year
   b. No extension of existing patches for 1 year
   c. No loss of pigmentation in patches which had achieved repigmentation for 1 year
   d. No vitiligo patches at the site of injury i.e., Koebnerization for 1 year.
2. General anesthesia (GA) should be preferred in these cases:
   a. Extensive area, i.e., 150 cm^2 and above
   b. Young/apprehensive patient having extensive area
   c. Patient is medically fit and does not have major comorbidities which may pose as a contraindication for GA.
3. *Site, area, selection:*
   a. Ideally only one side of the body should be operated, i.e., we should try to avoid doing both hands/both feet/both eyes in one go. Bandaging both hands/feet for a week at a stretch can be quite disabling for the patient.
   b. Since turning or changing a patient's position under GA is difficult and compromises sterility, patches to be operated in extensive cases need to be planned in way that no/minimum change of position is required. Example, areas over the chest and abdomen can be done in one session, lesions over the back need a separate session.
   c. All areas should be photographed, measured, and marked before the GA is induced so that no patches are missed out.
   d. Total recipient area should be calculated so that donor area to be harvested is more precise.

TABLE 2: Terminology used while doing NCECS over large areas.

Terminology	*Area to be operated in cm^2*
Regular NCECS session	Up to 150 cm^2
Mega sessions	150–400 cm^2
Giga sessions	Area >400 cm^2

(NCECS: noncultured epidermal cell suspension)

Anesthesia: Safe upper limit of local anesthetic xylocaine (2%) without adrenaline is 4.5 mg/kg (up to 300 mg) and with epinephrine 7 mg/kg (up to 500 mg). This implies that in safe limits only a small amount of xylocaine can be injected and thus a small area can be operated at one time. Regional blocks can be used but they again require training and expertise to be really effective. Local anesthesia cannot be used in small children and apprehensive adults. The main limitation is pain and its effective management intraoperation and postoperation. Hence transplantation for extensive areas will require general anesthesia and local anesthesia is not suitable while operating on large areas.

The use of GA (general anesthesia) makes the process simpler as the issues of pain relief are taken care of and the surgeon as well as the patient, both are equally comfortable. The setting is thus conducive for taking up extensive cases in single session.

Operation theater setup: It is imperative to have a complete OT setup which is equipped with anesthesia equipment, cardiac monitors, and lifesaving equipment. The staff should be trained to handle emergencies. An anesthetist has to be present throughout the procedure till the patient is completely out of anesthesia; admission facilities are required for short stay to monitor the patient postoperatively for 6–8 hours minimum.

PREOPERATIVE COUNSELING AND INFORMED CONSENT[18]

The surgical process starts with a detailed history of the patient pertaining to vitiligo and general health and associated diseases especially in regard to the use of general anesthesia.

It is important to always remember that general anesthesia requires meticulous planning right from the patient evaluation, OT setup, anesthesia drugs, equipment, gases, emergency drugs, trained staff, and vigilant pre- and postoperative care. Even if the duration of anesthesia is short, the risks and complications can be similar to a long case and if they occur can be very unforgiving.

A detailed consent form elaborating the procedure and possible complications, risks should be signed by the patient and a witness. The consent form should specifically cover the limitations, risks of the noncultured epidermal cell suspension (NCECS) procedure as well as that of the general anesthesia.

Preoperative laboratory studies include complete hemogram including platelet counts, bleeding and clotting time (or prothrombin and activated partial thromboplastin time), thyroid profile, liver function test (LFT), kidney function test (KFT), serum electrolytes, chest X-ray PA view, and electrocardiogram (ECG) in adults. Screening for antibodies for hepatitis B, C, and human immunodeficiency virus (HIV) is recommended. In coronavirus disease (COVID) times a real-time reverse transcriptase-polymerase chain reaction (RT-PCR) for COVID antigen should be done within 48 hours of the surgery.

The type of anesthesia used is to be decided on a case-to-case basis depending on the site, extent of the area, age of the patient, and comorbidities. Most cases can be managed with just IV sedation with drugs combination such as ketamine, midazolam, propofol. Intubation is not required in most of the cases of NCECS and the cocktails of anesthesia drugs used by an experienced anesthetist can make the whole process go smooth.

DURATION OF ANESTHESIA

The duration of anesthesia required is usually short as it is required only for the painful steps of the procedure:

- Analgesia is required at the time of harvesting of skin graft which on an average needs only 2–5 minutes.
- Secondly, analgesia is needed during dermabrasion that varies from 20 to 30 minutes depending on the area to be covered.
- Once the skin grafts are harvested, they are trypsinized immediately while the dermabrasion is being carried out. The cell separation process, dressings, etc., require no further anesthesia and the patient need not be under anesthesia at that point of time.
- Lastly, the application of dry collagen sheets on the dermabraded skin also produces stinging and burning sensation, which warrants a second dose of anesthesia in some patients.

DONOR-RECIPIENT RATIO

This is the second and most important consideration while taking up large vitiligo areas for surgery. Vitiligo is a cosmetic problem and if in the process of repigmenting the vitiligo patch ends up scarring the donor area, the purpose of the procedure is lost.

Noncultured epidermal cell suspension has the advantage that with a small skin graft from the donor area, a large recipient vitiligo area can be treated. The commonest donor recipient ratio being used is 1:10, i.e., if we harvest a skin graft of 3 cm × 3 cm, i.e., 9 cm^2; we can almost treat 90 cm^2 of vitiligo area. A smaller graft implies minimum scar over the donor area.

Other tissue grafting methods are not suitable for large areas for the following reasons:

Punch grafting[19,20] (tissue graft) is the easiest and least expensive method, but it is time consuming, seldom produces even uniform repigmentation. In minipunch grafting, the donor recipient ratio is 1:3, i.e., a punch can only spread the pigment three times its size. Hence it is not suitable for large areas.

In suction blister grafting[21] the donor recipient ratio is 1:1 and although the cosmetic results are good, there is limitation in raising blisters. Hence blister grafting is suitable only in small areas.

In suction blister grafting[21] the donor recipient ratio is 1:1 and although the cosmetic results are good, there is limitation in raising blisters. Hence blister grafting is suitable only in small areas.

Ultrathin epidermal sheet grafting can treat larger areas (up to 200 cm^2) **(Figs. 15 to 17)** but requires skill and experience to take such large grafts. Ultrathin split thickness grafting[22] involves harvesting of large sheets of skin; the donor recipient ratio is 1:1 or at times even 1.5:1, because if the graft harvested is relatively thick it has to be discarded as only the thinnest graft would give a better cosmetic result. Hence a large area is at a risk of donor skin scarring and disfigurement, depigmentation at the donor site. The graft on the recipient site can have a stuck on appearance and in many cases hyperpigmentation, perigraft halo, milia formation are encountered. The overall cosmetic result is not very cosmetically appealing **(Figs. 18 and 19)**.

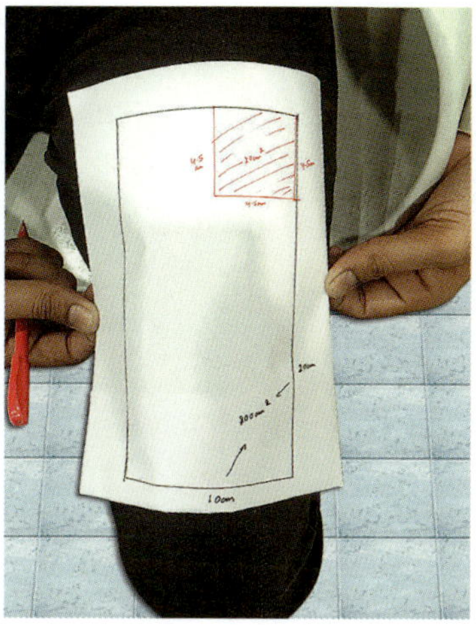

Fig. 15: Donor area calculation to cover 200 cm^2 of vitiligo area. If a split thickness graft is to be harvested 10 × 20 cm^2, i.e., 200 cm^2, if NCECS is planned then 1/10 area, i.e., 4.5 × 4.5 cm, i.e., 20.25 cm^2, if is needed. (NCECS: noncultured epidermal cell suspension)

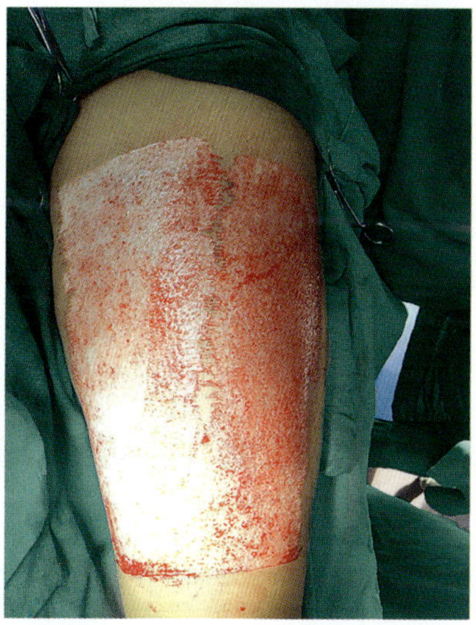

Fig. 16: 200 cm^2 of split thickness graft harvested.

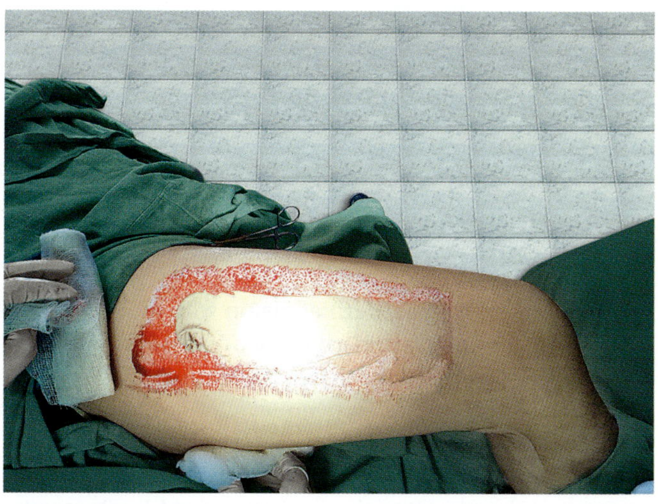

Fig. 17: Large graft harvested, pinpoint to continuous bleed seen on the donor bed suggestive of a level of papillary to reticular dermis.

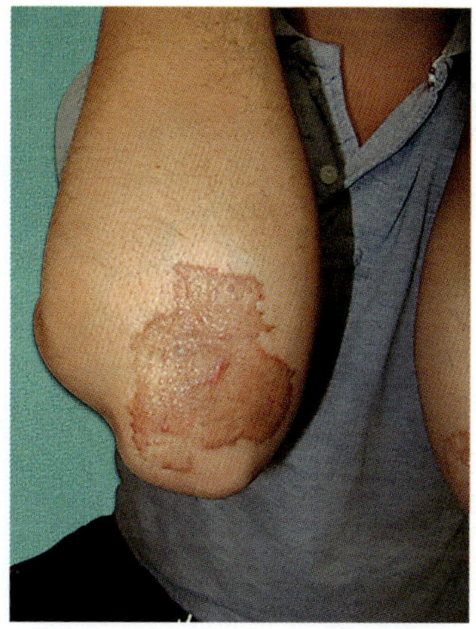

Fig. 18: Limitation of split thickness grafting (STG). Stuck on appearance, milia formation, hypertrophic margins, and perigraft halo.

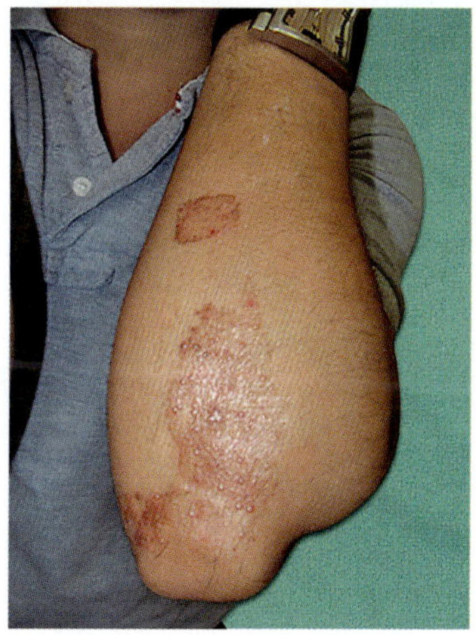

Fig. 19: Limitation of STG: Hyperpigmentation and stuck on appearance.

CULTURED METHODS

Culture methods[7] have a definite edge in that they provide an unlimited number of cells for transplantation, i.e., 100 fold. However, culture methods require extensive laboratories, equipment, and trained personnel and hence the cost of procedure goes up making it unaffordable for most patients. There are also concerns of contamination, bacterial/fungal overgrowths.

Hence the NCECS is the ideally suited for vitiligo surgery of extensive areas. However, punch grafting may be preferred if the dermatosurgeon is not trained for NCECS or split skin grafting. Split skin ultrathin grafts may be preferred by a surgeon who has the expertise for taking large grafts, if facilities do not exist for NCECS.

PROCEDURE DETAILS: SPECIAL ISSUES WHILE DOING LARGE AREA (>200 CM^2)

Preparation of the NCECS[23,24] has already been covered in detail, hence only relevant steps are described here.

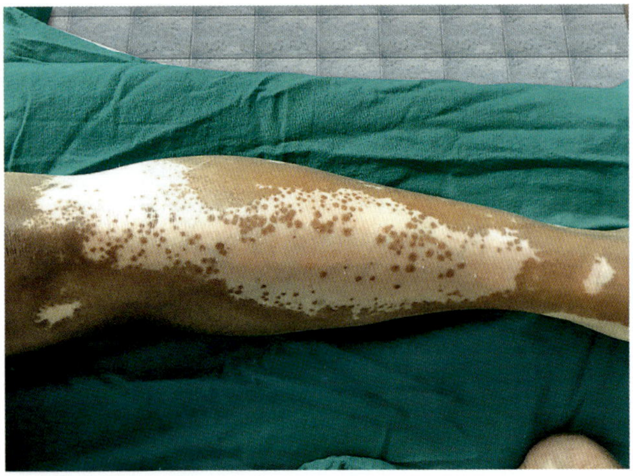

Fig. 20: Extensive vitiligo patches over the shin approximately 250 cm^2.

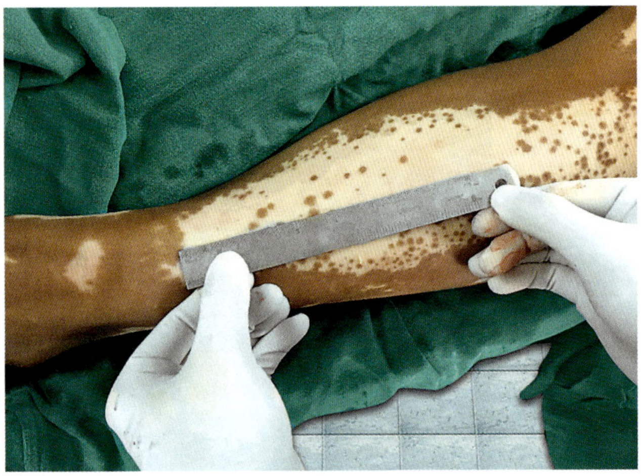

Fig. 21: Area calculation presurgical over the recipient area.

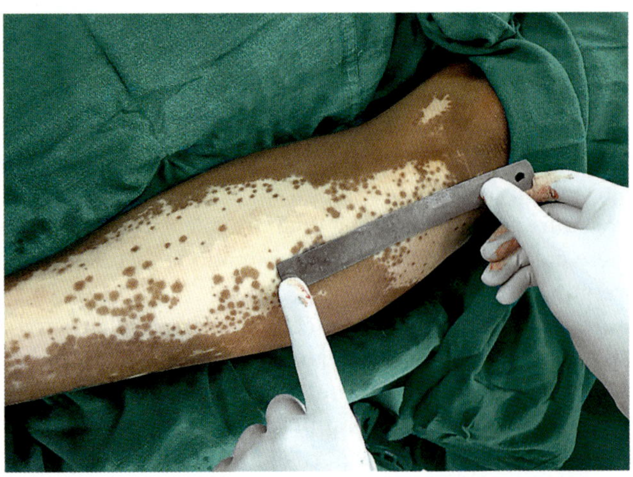

Fig. 22: Area calculation presurgical over the recipient area.

Donor Area Calculation

Preoperatively, all recipient areas are marked and photographed. Calculation of the area that needs to be operated is done **(Fig. 15, Table 3)**. **Figures 16 to 23** show different steps

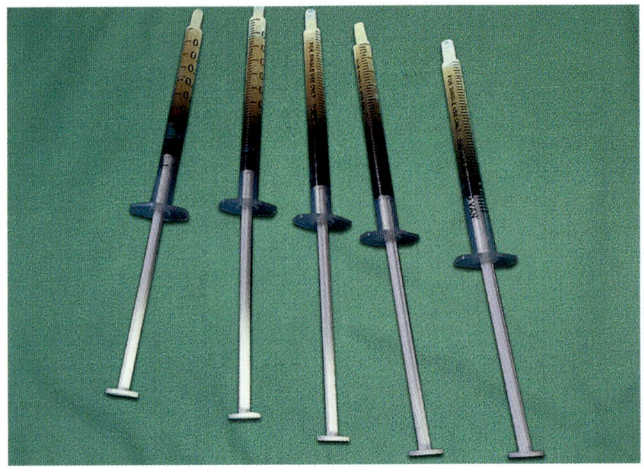

Fig. 23: 4.5 mL of cell suspension for the 250 cm^2 area.

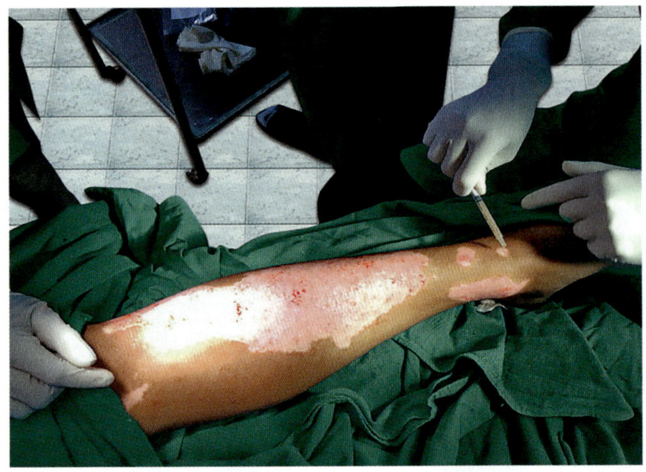

Fig. 24: Uniform spread of the cell suspension over the dermabraded area.

TABLE 3: Rough estimate for deciding the donor-recipient ratio.

Recipient areas	*Donor-recipient ratio*
Single confluent patch	1:10
Few scattered large patches	1:8
Multiple small patches	1:5

of donor harvesting. The process of NCECS is the same as has been described previously.

Recipient Area Preparation in NCECS/STG (Figs. 24 to 29)

While doing large areas, dermabrasion with diamond burrs and with micromotor is preferred since its fast and large areas (200–500 cm^2) can be done in just 20–30 minutes.

While dermabrading an even level of dermabrasion up to the papillary dermis should be achieved–this is evident by fine pinpoint bleeding. At times there can be some skip zones, because of the clouding the operating field by the oozing blood. These are areas of inadequate level of dermabrasion

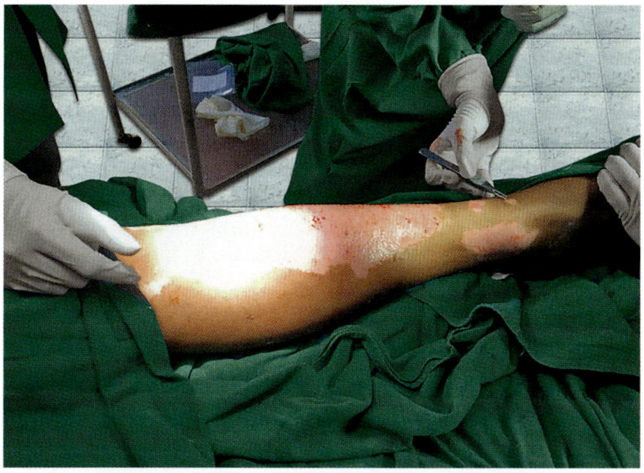

Fig. 25: Collagen dressing to hold the cell suspension in place.

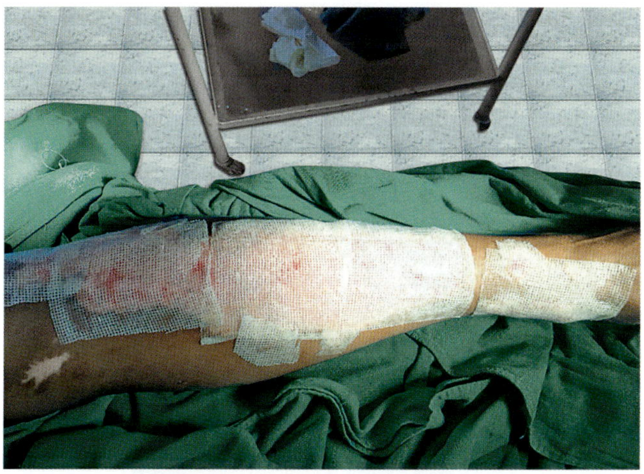

Fig. 26: Single layer of collagen dressing as the second layer of dressing.

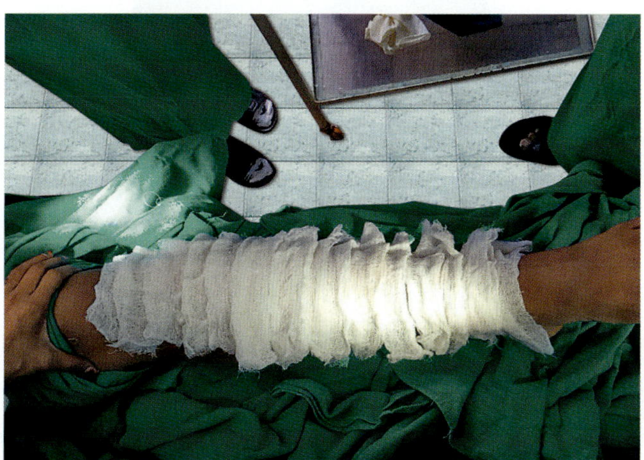

Fig. 27: Dry gauze as the third layer of dressing.

which should be watched for closely. After the entire area has been dermabraded, adequate hemostasis is achieved with saline-soaked gauzes for 10 minutes and a relook is taken. The areas not showing pinpoint bleed are further dermabraded

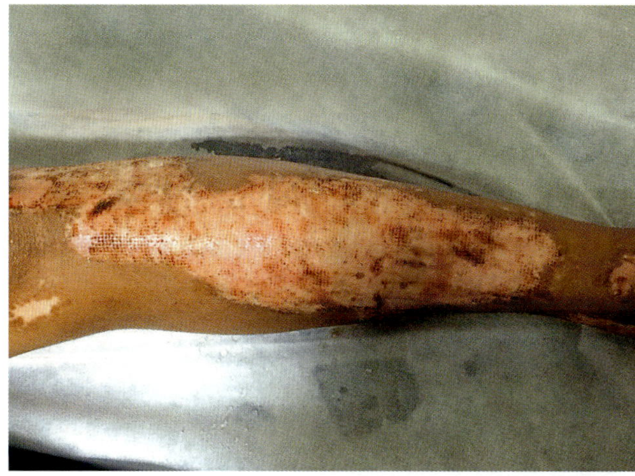

Fig. 28: Complete epithelialization and healing at day 7.

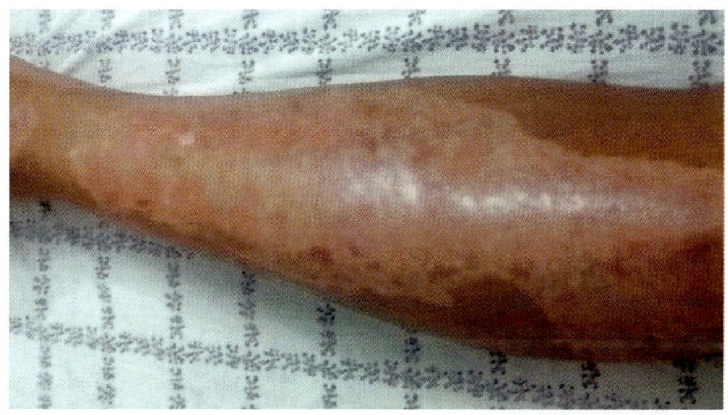

Fig. 29: Early pigmentation at 8 weeks.

to create an even surface. This avoids skip zones in the repigmentation.

While doing margins it is important to go 5 mm into the normal skin, this reduces the incidence of perigraft achromic fissures and perigraft halo.

PAIN MANAGEMENT

Adequate care of the postoperative pain is essential since large amount of skin has been dermabraded. In most of our patients we have found an IM or IV diclofenac 2 mL, i.e., 80 mg injection is adequate to keep the patient comfortable. Few patients would need an additional dose of pentazocine, Phenergan.

FLUID AND ELECTROLYTE MANAGEMENT

Noncultured epidermal cell suspension is a surgery with little blood loss because the level of dermabrasion is only up to the papillary dermis. There is not much bleeding and even in extensive areas, i.e., 400 cm^2 the amount of blood loss is <20 mL. Since a small donor area is required and the grafts are ultrathin there is not much of a blood loss from the donor site as well.

In harvesting extensive sheets of skin as in split thickness grafting there is more blood loss. In punch grafting also there is more blood loss since the punches are up to the mid-dermis there is considerably more bleeding at both the donor and recipient areas.

The patient should be kept well hydrated with IV fluids since most GA patients need to be nil per oral (NPO) for almost 8 hours preoperative and 4–6 hours postoperative and also since a large area is operated there can be oozing postoperative.

RESULTS (FIGS. 30 TO 38)

The percentage and extent of repigmentation of the mega and giga session is similar to that of regular sessions. The onset of pigmentation color and texture matching is not different in these large area surgeries, even the retention of pigmentation and relapse rates were similar to the surgeries of limited

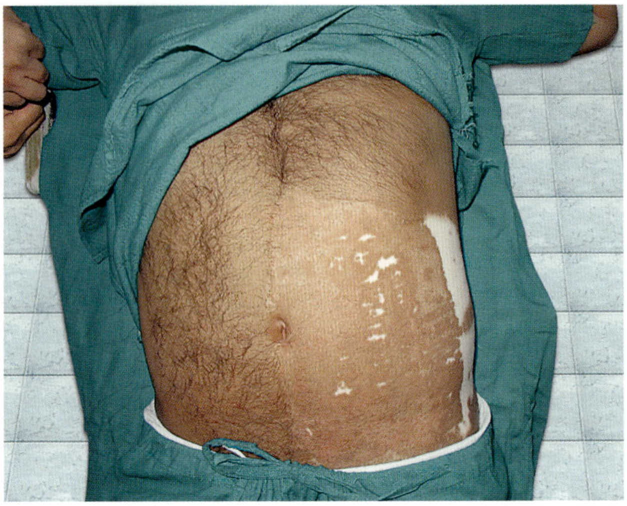

Fig. 32: 6 months postoperation entire area repigmented including the skip zones.

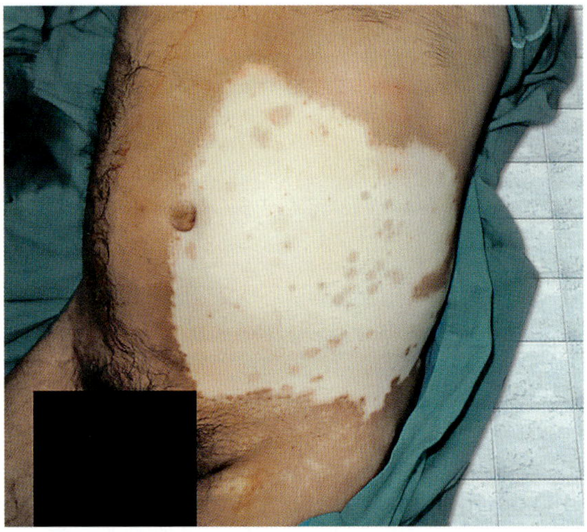

Fig. 30: Extensive vitiligo area (350 cm^2): Segmental variety.

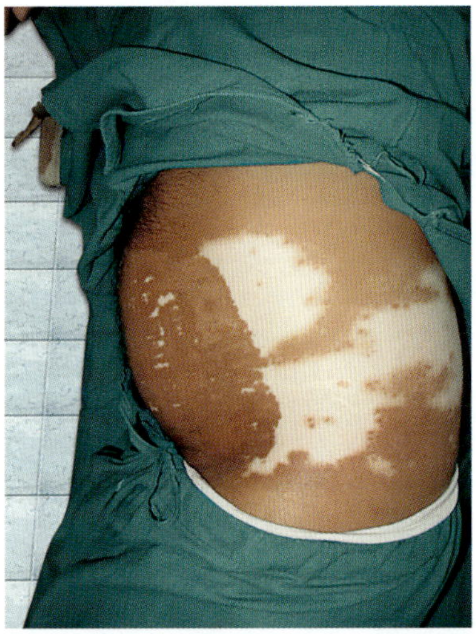

Fig. 33: Second session of cell transplant in the same patient.

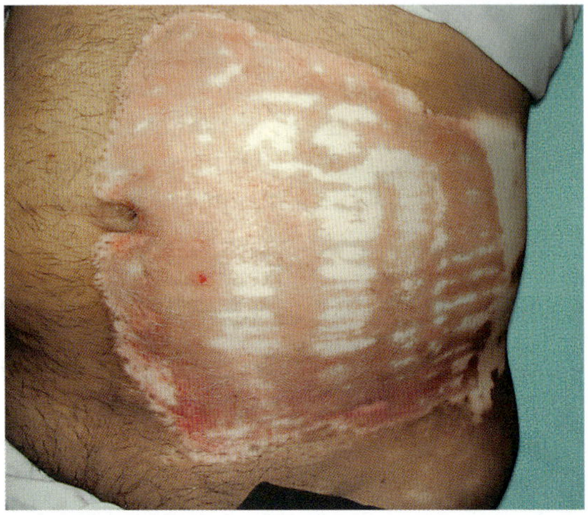

Fig. 31: At 3 weeks' postoperation, entire area epithelized, area appears erythematous, and some skip zones visible indicating a more superficial level of dermabrasion in those areas.

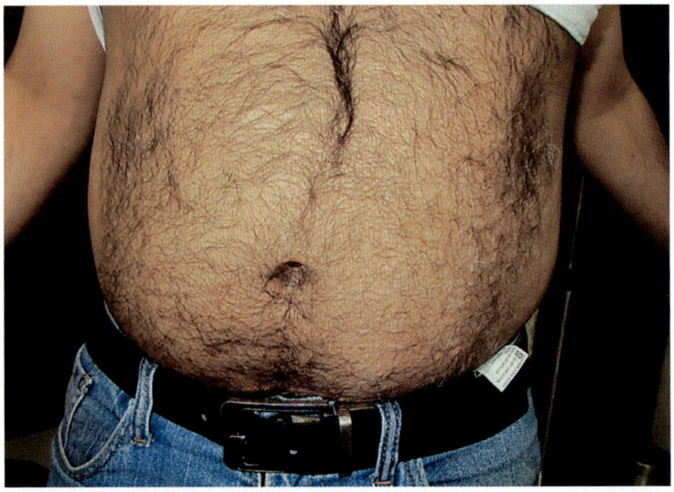

Fig. 34: Entire area repigmented well with leukotrichia also replaced by pigmented hair.

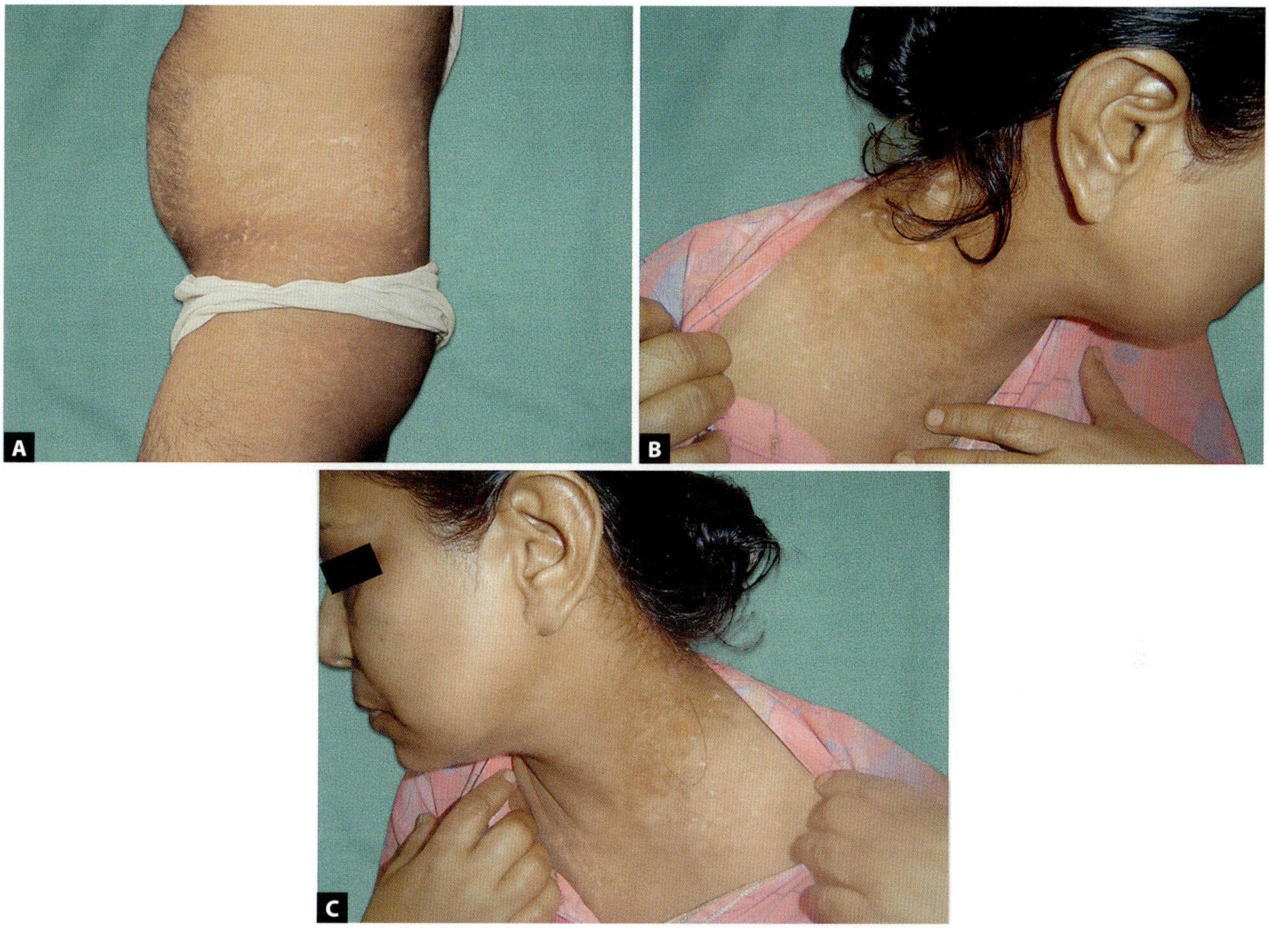

Figs. 35A to C: Good texture and color matching in the entire area.

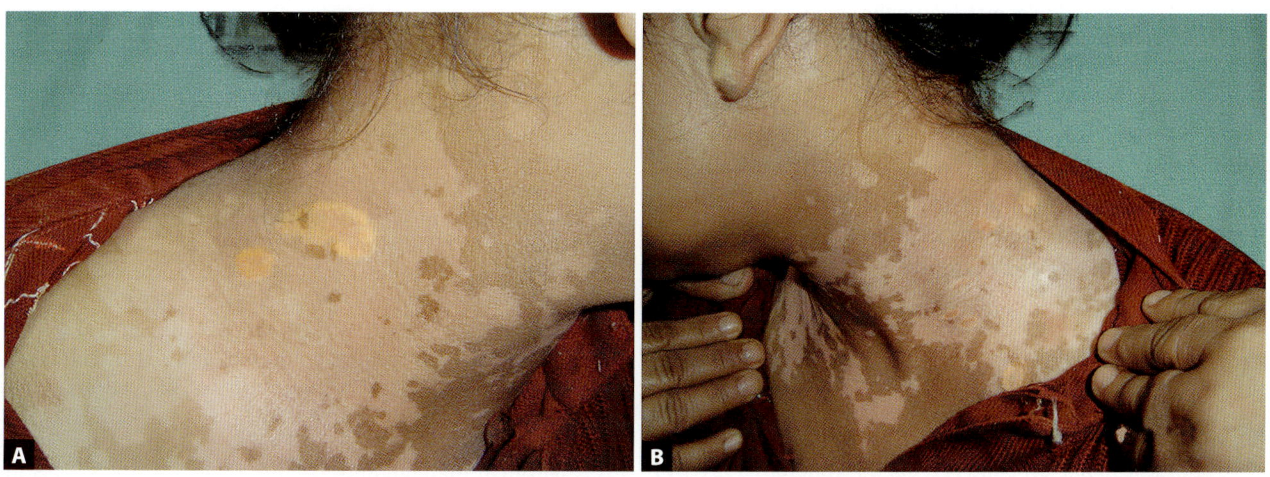

Figs. 36A and B: NCECS over neck, chest, and a previously tattooed area.

area. We did not observe any Koebnerization being induced, i.e., the disease becoming unstable immediately after the procedure. Hence larger areas per session can be taken up to reduce the total number of procedures a patient has to go through to repigment a certain amount of area.

CONCLUSION

Taking up mega or giga sessions of NCECS is safe and effective. Doing large areas in a single session is the best way to manage a patient having extensive vitiligo in minimum

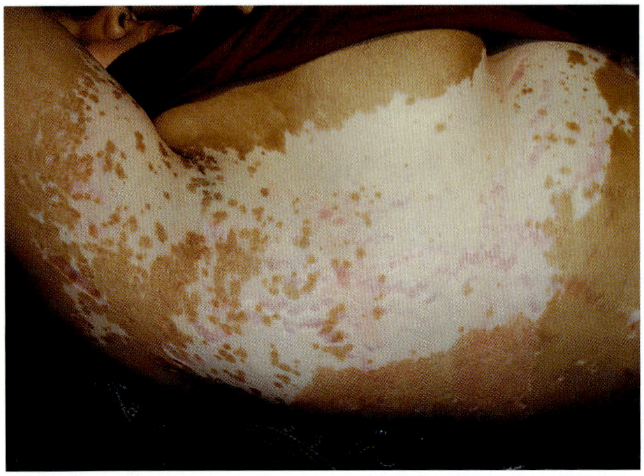

Fig. 37: Extensive vitiligo >400 cm^2 over the trunk, few areas showing stretch marks because of long-term steroid use.

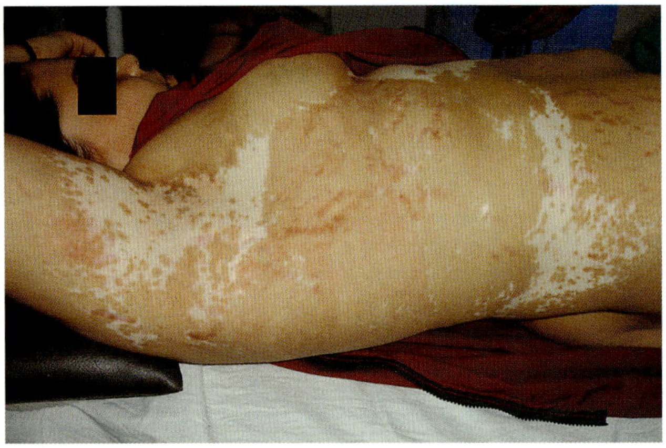

Fig. 38: Good texture and color matching in the entire area, even the stretch marks showing repigmentation.

sessions. However, case selection has to be done carefully and after thorough counseling. The process requires planning and dedicated team of dermatologists, anesthetist, OT nursing staff technicians, and post nursing care to make the procedure safe and comfortable for the patient.

REFERENCES

1. Pasricha JS, Khaitan BK. Oral mini pulse therapy with betamethasone in vitiligo patients having extensive or fast spreading disease. Int J Dermatol. 1993;32:753-7.
2. An appraisal of narrow band (TL-01) UVB phototherapy. Br J Dermatol. 1997;137:327-30.
3. Moshar DB, Pathak MA, Fitzpatrick TB. Photochemotherapy for Vitiligo: An Approach to Diagnosis and Management in Phototherapy in Dermatology. New York: Mosby Yearbook; 1993. pp. 114-6.
4. Falabella R. Treatment of localized vitiligo by autologous minigrafting. Arch Dermatol. 1988;124:1649-55.
5. Savant SS. Autologous miniature punch skin grafting in stable vitiligo. Indian J Dermatol Venereol Leprol. 1992;58:310-4.
6. Lerner AB, Halaban R, Klaus SN, Moellmann GE. Transplantation of human melanocytes. J Invest Dermatol. 1987;89(3): 219-24.
7. Olsson MJ, Juhlin L. Repigmentation of vitiligo by transplantation of cultured autologous melanocytes. Acta Derm Venereol. 1993;73:49-51.
8. Olsson MJ, Juhlin L. Leucoderma treated by transplantation of basal cell layer enriched suspension. BR J Dermatol. 1998;138:644-8.
9. Gauthier Y, Surleve-Bazeille J. Autologous grafting with non-cultured malanocytes: a simplified method for treatment of depigmented lesions. J Am Acad Deramatol. 1992;26:191-4.
10. Mulekar SV. Melanocyte-keratinocyte cell transplantation for stable vitiligo. Int J Dermatol. 2003;42:132-6.
11. Van Geel N, Ongenae K, De Mil M, Naeyaert JM. Modified technique of autologous non cultured epidermal cell transplantation for repigmenting vitiligo: a Pilot study. Dematol Surgery. 2001;27:873-6.
12. Olsson MJ, Moellmann G, Lerner AB, Juhlin L. Vitiligo: repigmentation with cultured melanocytes after cryostorage. Acta Derm Venereol. 1994;74(3):226-8.
13. Chen FY, Chang JS, Yang PY, Hung CM, Huang MH, Hu DN. Transplantation of cultured autologous pure melanocytes after laser abrasion for the treatment of segmental vitiligo. J Dermatol. 2000;27(7):434-9.
14. Guerra L, Capurro S, Melchi F, Primavera G, Bondanza S, Cancedda R, et al. Treatment of "stable" vitiligo by timedsurgery and transplantation of cultured epidermal autografts. Arch Dermatol. 2000;136(11):1380-9.
15. Kumar R, Parsad D, Singh C, Yadav S. Four compartment method: a simplified and cost-effective method of noncultured epidermal cell suspension for the treatment of vitiligo. Br J Dermatol. 2014;170(3):581-5.
16. Gupta S, Sahni K, Tembhre MK, Mathur S, Sharma VK. A novel point-of-care in vivo technique for preparation of epidermal cell suspension for transplantation in vitiligo. J Am Acad Dermatol. 2015;72(2):e65-6.
17. Manchanda K, Bansal M, Pandey SS. Surgical management of vitiligo—an approach to the patient. NJDVL. 2013;11(1): 7-19.
18. Parsad D, Gupta S; IADVL Dermatosurgery Task Force. Standard guidelines of care for vitiligo surgery. Indian J Dermatol Venereol Leprol. 2008;74(Suppl):37-45.
19. Taieb A, Alomar A, Böhm M, Dell'anna ML, De Pase A, Eleftheriadou V, et al. Guidelines for the management of vitiligo. Br J Dermatol. 2013;168(1):5-19.
20. Van Geel N, Ongenae K, Naetert JM. Surgical techniques for vitiligo. Review dermatology. 2001;202:162-6.
21. Oh CK, Cha JH, Lim JY, Jo JH, Kim SJ, Jang HS, et al. Treatment of vitiligo with suction epidermal grafting by the use of an ultrapulse CO_2 laser with a computerised pattern generator. Dermatol Surg. 2001;27(6):565-8.
22. Khunger N. Thin split thickness skin grafts for vitiligo in surgical management of vitiligo. In: Gupta S, Olsson MJ, Kanwar AJ, Ortonne J-P (Eds). Surgical Management of Vitiligo. Blackwell Publishing Ltd. 2007. pp 108-14.
23. Munish Paul. Autologous non-cultured basal cell-enriched epidermal cell suspension transplantation in vitiligo: Indian experience. J Cutan Aesthet Surg. 2011;4(1):23-8.
24. Mulekar SV. Long-term follow-up study of segmental and focal vitiligo treated by autologous non-cultured melanocyte-keratinocyte cell transplantation. Arch Dermatol. 2004:140(10)1211-15.

CHAPTER 39

Noncultured Extracted Hair Follicle Outer Root Sheath Cell Suspension

Rashi Pangti, Savita Yadav, Sanjay Singh, Somesh Gupta

KEY MESSAGES

- Noncultured extracted hair follicle outer root sheath cell suspension also called follicular cell suspension, although relatively recent, is now an established surgical method of repigmentation in vitiligo.
- Procedure is technically minimally demanding and can be completed on the same day.
- Major advantage is the lack of visible scarring at the donor site.
- Large areas can be treated with suspension prepared from a small number of hair follicles.
- Technique of suspension preparation has not undergone much change since its inception.

INTRODUCTION

Autologous noncultured hair follicle outer root sheath cell suspension (NCHF-ORS-CS), also known as hair follicular cell suspension (FCS) is a relatively recent surgical modality for the management of vitiligo. It is a minimally invasive procedure.[1] The technique of FCS preparation has not undergone much change since its inception. The biggest advantage of this method over noncultured epidermal cell suspension (NCECS) is the less scarring at the donor site usually inconspicuous as hidden by the hair on the occipital scalp.[1]

AUTOLOGOUS NONCULTURED HAIR FOLLICLE OUTER ROOT SHEATH CELL SUSPENSION/FOLLICULAR CELL SUSPENSION

Basic Concepts

The maintenance of the melanocytes in the epidermis, and hair follicles, is dependent on melanocyte stem cells (MelSCs). This quiescent cell population is located in the bulge region of the hair follicle and acts as a melanocyte reservoir. These stem cells can migrate into the epidermis and give rise to differentiated pigment-producing melanocytes. Under normal circumstances, these melanocytes remain inactive but become active to produce melanin when stimulated by ultraviolet radiation, wound, or dermabrasion.[1,2]

Repigmentation of vitiligo depends on three possible sources of melanocytes: (1) from the hair follicle where stem cells are found, (2) from the normal skin at margins, and (3) unaffected melanocytes within depigmented areas.[3] This leads to four clinical patterns of repigmentation: (1) follicular, (2) marginal, (3) diffuse, and (4) combined, of which follicular pattern is the most common.[4]

Cui et al. in their study observed dopa-positive melanocytes (active) in the epidermis of normal skin. In contrast, dopa-negative melanocytes (inactive) were seen in the outer root sheath (ORS) of normal hair follicles, which serve as a melanocyte reservoir. In vitiligo patients, the dopa-positive melanocytes in the epidermis were completely absent, whereas the dopa-negative melanocytes present in ORS of hair follicles were unaffected. Treatment leads to stimulation of the inactive melanocytes present in the middle and/or lower parts of the ORS resulting in their proliferation and migration upward along the surface of the ORS to the adjacent epidermis. Continued radial migration of the melanocytes leads to the appearance of perifollicular repigmentation in vitiligo lesions. The melanocytes undergo continuous maturation and become active during their upward migration. In conclusion, these inactive melanocytes in ORS function as reservoirs and are a potential source for repigmentation of vitiligo lesions. These observations signify the crucial role of the hair follicle in the repigmentation of vitiligo lesions.[5]

Meyer et al. studied normal human scalp hair follicles by using immunohistochemistry and quantitative histomorphometry. They found the bulge region, a relatively immune-privileged area of human skin, which leads to the protection of the hair follicle epithelial stem cell reservoir from auto aggressive immune attacks.[6] MelSCs reside in the bulge region that might be responsible for their protection from damage by immune cells, which possibly explains the persistence of pigmented hairs in vitiligo lesions in most cases.

In a recent study, MelSCs were isolated by the "side population" technique, a method frequently employed to isolate hematopoietic stem cells. These hair follicle MelSCs and differentiated melanocytes when fabricated with chitosan/gelatin composite were seen to have the potential to produce pigmentation.[7] Sülflow et al. demonstrated that a copolymer synthesized from pentaerythritol diacrylate monostearate, maleic anhydride, and *N*-isopropylacrylamide or diacetone acrylamide linked with gelatin to form a hydrogel named cGEL, provided a niche for the significant production of melanin as compared with both bovine collagen membrane and polycaprolactone scaffolds.[8]

Theoretical Advantages of Follicular Cell Suspension over Epidermal Cell Suspension

Hair follicle melanocytes differ from epidermal melanocytes in various ways **(Table 1)**. Epidermal and follicular melanin are independent units and this fact is strongly approved by the presence of white hair on highly pigmented skin.[9] The follicular melanin unit consists of one melanocyte to five keratinocytes in the hair bulb and 1:1 in the basal layer of the hair bulb, while in the epidermal melanin unit, there is one melanocyte for every 36 keratinocytes. One of the most striking differences between the two melanocyte subpopulations is that the hair bulb melanocytes are cyclically active during the anagen phase, whereas epidermal melanogenesis is a continuous process.[10] Furthermore, even a small number of hair melanocytes can produce sufficient melanin to pigment up to 1.5 m of the hair shaft. Because of these properties, the hair appears to be a better source of melanocytes than the epidermis for cell suspension techniques. The FCS has many other advantages besides the unique characteristics of hair follicle melanocytes. FCS requires few hair follicles, which means less volume of tissue in comparison with NCECS. There is an intact interfollicular area after follicular extraction by using a 1 mm punch. This leads to earlier and better wound healing at the donor site than the conventional shave biopsy technique in NCECS, where a continuous sheet of the epidermis is taken from the thigh. Follicular unit extraction (FUE) wound heals by minimal scarring. Furthermore, these scars are located over hairy sites and practically invisible leading to cosmetically very acceptable donor sites to the patients, while with the NCECS technique there is a risk (though low) of keloid or hypertrophic scar formation over the donor site with its associated cosmetic disfigurement. The technique of preparation of FCS is relatively simple when compared to NCECS as it does not require the separation of the epidermis from the dermis and manual breaking of epidermal samples into small pieces.

TABLE 1: Comparison of follicular and epidermal melanin units.

	Follicular melanin unit	*Epidermal melanin unit*
Activity	Cyclical activity, tightly coupled to hair growth cycle	Continuously active
Ratio with keratinocytes	1:1–1:5	1:36
Size	Larger, have longer and extensive dendrites	Smaller, less dendritic
Melanosomes	Larger	Smaller (2–4 times smaller)
Melanin granules	Minimally degraded in hair cortex	Completely degraded in the differentiating keratinocytes
Golgi apparatus and rough endoplasmic reticulum	More developed	Less developed
Susceptibility to immune destruction	Relatively less due to their immunologically privileged location (the bulge area)	More
Aging	More influenced by aging (hair graying)	Less influenced by aging

Procedure of Follicular Cell Suspension

Step 1: Follicular Unit Extraction

The occipital scalp is the preferred donor site by most cutaneous surgeons. Few hairs are delineated in this area and trimmed to a length of approximately 2 mm. Anagen hairs are preferred for extraction as they have a more significant number of active melanocytes. Field block anesthesia using 2% lignocaine with adrenaline (1:1,000) is given encircling the delineated donor area. With the help of a 1 mm punch (manual or motorized), intact hair follicles are extracted. This is a very critical step as hair follicles should be taken in toto to avoid the transaction of hair follicles. Then the hair follicle is gently extracted using a hair follicle holding forceps. Depending on the area to be transplanted, approximately 50–100 pigmented follicles are extracted. On average, 15–25 hair follicles are sufficient to repigment approximately 20 cm^2 area.[1] The intact hair follicles are collected in normal saline and transferred immediately to the laboratory. The donor area is dressed using mupirocin ointment and sterile cotton pads.

Step 2: Preparation of Cell Suspension

The extracted hair follicles are washed three times under aseptic conditions with phosphate-buffered saline (PBS) containing various antibiotic and antifungal agents such as penicillin, streptomycin, kanamycin, and amphotericin B. The extracted hair follicles are incubated in test tubes with 0.25% trypsin and 0.05% ethylenediaminetetraacetic acid (EDTA) at 37°C for 30 minutes, to prepare the single-cell suspension.[4] Within 15–20 minutes of first incubation, the cells from the ORS start separating from each other. After 30 minutes of incubation, the hair follicles are gently stroked with forceps to separate the loosened-up cells and hair follicles are then transferred to the second test tube for further incubation for 30 minutes. At this point, we add trypsin inhibitor to the first test tube to arrest continued digestion of the loosened cells, which have remained behind in the first test tube. The same procedure is repeated in the second and third test tubes. Only thin keratinous shafts are left behind at the end of three such cycles. Finally, the contents of all three test tubes are collected in a single test tube and the single-cell suspension is prepared by filtering with a 70 μm cell strainer. The final cell pellet is obtained by centrifuging the combined cell suspension at 1,000 rpm for 5 minutes. The cell pellet thus obtained is resuspended in a small amount (0.25 mL or 0.5 mL, depending on the size of the recipient area) of PBS or Dulbecco's Modified Eagle's Medium (DMEM). The whole laboratory process usually takes around 2–3 hours.

The trypsin used can be either porcine or bovine source derived or recombinant trypsin. Trypsin from a porcine or bovine source has a risk of zoonotic disease transmission such as the transmission of endogenous retroviruses. Manira et al. compared animal-derived trypsin and recombinant trypsin on human skin cell culture expansion. They found similar results in both groups in terms of cell yield and expression of specific cellular markers.[11]

Step 3: Transplantation

Under strict aseptic measures, the recipient site is cleaned and topical lignocaine is applied for anesthesia. Most cutaneous surgeons avoid using adrenaline with lignocaine as it leads to vasoconstriction that might result in poor graft intake or complete failure. Besides, it masks the bleeding, which may result in deeper dermabrasion. The recipient site is abraded with manual or motorized dermabrader until tiny bleeding points appear which suggest the appearance of the dermoepidermal junction, after which dermabrasion should not be carried out as it might lead to scarring. Five millimeter of normal-looking skin beyond the margin of vitiliginous skin is also abraded to avoid the halo phenomenon.

The cell suspension is aspirated using a pipette, and the suspension is evenly spread over the recipient site, followed by five-layered dressing composed of a collagen sheet, antiseptic-containing paraffin gauze, surgical cotton gauze/pad, thin transparent dressing film, and an elastic adhesive bandage from inside out. There are no specific existent guidelines regarding the quantity of the suspension to be used per unit area. The most commonly used collagen sheet is of fish origin. In India, it is marketed by the name of NeuSkin-F (Chennai). It is considered to support epidermal cells and to help in their migration.[12] Chlorhexidine, as an antiseptic, integrated with paraffin gauze is preferred. Transparent dressing film (Tegaderm) and elastic adhesive bandage (Dynaplast) are used to stabilize the graft. The patient should be kept under observation for at least 1–2 hours after the procedure.

Postoperative Care

Restriction of the recipient site's movement, keeping the area clean and dry, and minimizing local manipulation are essential measures to be taken in the postoperative period for at least 7 days. Systemic antibiotics preferentially covering *Staphylococcus aureus* should be prescribed for 5–7 days. The dressing is removed on the 8th day at the follow-up visit. At this time, the recipient site has taken up the graft adequately. Topical tacrolimus 0.1% is then started to induce rapid repigmentation at the recipient site.

Response Following Follicular Cell Suspension Transplantation (Fig. 1, Tables 2 and 3)

There is a scarcity of literature regarding response following FCS transplantation. Only a few studies have assessed the results of this technique to date. Vanscheidt et al. in their study on five patients of stable vitiligo used autologous ORS cell suspension prepared by using trypsin on plucked anagen scalp hair follicles. Erbium-doped yttrium aluminum garnet (Er-YAG) laser was used for dermabrasion at the recipient site. Post-reepithelialization, lesions were treated with narrowband ultraviolet B two to three times weekly. The authors found almost complete (>90%) repigmentation in three out of five patients with vitiligo, around 50% repigmentation in one patient, and <10% repigmentation in the other.[13] Mohanty et al. in their prospective study on 14 patients of stable vitiligo (at least for 3 months) used extracted FCS and found >75% repigmentation in 9 out of 14 patients. Three patients in the study had <1 year of disease stability and none of them had >75% repigmentation, while 11 patients had at least 1 year of stability, 9 of which showed >75% repigmentation. This study further emphasizes the concept of stability of 1 year before undergoing any vitiligo surgery. The authors used 15–25 follicular units, which provided 25,000–50,000 cells that were sufficient to treat up to 25 cm^2 area.[14] Similarly, in their study on 25 patients of stable vitiligo, Shah et al. noticed excellent repigmentation (90–100%) in 60% of cases with the FCS technique.[15] A randomized comparative study on 30 patients with 47 vitiligo lesions has compared FCS with NCECS. There was excellent repigmentation (90–100%) in 83.3% of lesions in the NCECS group and 65.2% of lesions in the FCS group.

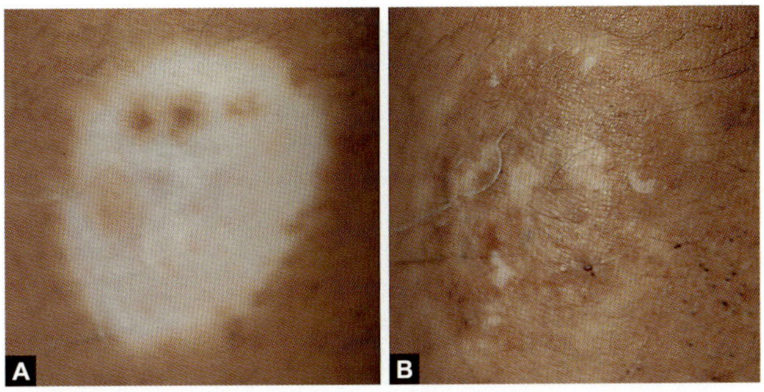

Figs. 1A and B: Vitiligo patch before surgery and 6 months post-hair follicular outer root sheath cell suspension transplantation with around 90% repigmentation.

There was a significant improvement in the dermatology quality-of-life index (DLQI) score in both but patients in the NCECS group were significantly more satisfied than the patients in the FCS group. Both groups showed similar color match and pattern of repigmentation.[16]

A recent study comparing NCECS and FCS with 10 patients in each group found both the methods to be similar in efficacy with comparable results in terms of the extent of repigmentation, color match and patient satisfaction. FCS was not associated with any complications whereas NCECS had mild scarring in 20% and hyperpigmentation in 40% of patients in the donor area.[17] Furthermore, a study on 30 patients with stable vitiligo analyzed factors affecting the repigmentation in patients treated with FCS. Significant repigmentation (>75%) was seen in 21 out of 60 (35%) lesions while 10 out of 21 lesions showed excellent repigmentation (>90%). Authors have concluded that the number of melanocytes and hair follicle stem cells transplanted, and the absence of dermal inflammation were essential determinants of optimal repigmentation.[18] FCS has also shown modest repigmentation in leukotrichia. In the study by Gunaabalaji et al, 10 patients in FCS and 8 patients in NCECS out of the total 19 patients in each group showed repigmentation of leukotrichia. The percentage of hair showing repigmentation was 7.42% in HFCS and 11.42% in NCECS, however, there was no statistical difference found between them.[19]

In a preliminary pilot study on three human subjects, partial loss of stem cell niche was found to be manifested as a low mean percentage of CD200 positive cells during follicular plucking (FP). The average cell yield per follicle was 2,500 and 250 by the FUE and FP method, respectively, which showed a significant statistical difference.[20] Similar result of low cell yield by the FP method as compared with FUE was found in a study by Pangti et al. In this study, the mean repigmentation at 36 weeks was statistically more significant with cell suspension prepared with follicles isolated with the FUE method (74%) than with FP method (18%). NCECS transplantation showed a mean of 79% repigmentation.[21]

In a pilot study, a combination of FCS and NCECS was compared with NCECS alone on a total of 12 patches in five patients. The mean repigmentation was more in the combination arm (94%) than in the NCECS arm (78%).[22] A similar study on 84 patches in 30 patients also saw superior repigmentation with the combination of FCS and NCECS than with NCECS alone (76% vs. 57%).[23]

Vashisht et al., in their pilot study compared FCS prepared using trypsin alone and trypsin combined with collagenase type I. It is recognized that there is a perifollicular dermal sheath comprising of type I collagen around the "bulge region" of the hair follicle. Collagenase type I is hypothesized would digest that sheath thereby leading to a better release of trypsin-treated ORS cells. There was a significant increase in the number of cells obtained in the trypsin plus collagenase group compared to the trypsin-alone group. A higher number of HMB45+ melanocytes and stem cells were also obtained translating to greater repigmentation when collagenase was added, although the difference was not significant.[24]

TABLE 2: Studies on noncultured extracted hair follicle outer root sheath cell suspension.

S. No.	Authors	Year	Number of patients	Percentage repigmentation (Mean ± SD)	Duration of study
1	Mohanty et al.[14]	2011	14	65·7 ± 36.7%	6 months
2	Shah et al.[15]	2016	25	80.15 ± 22.9%	6 months
3	Kumar et al.[25]	2018	25	52 ± 25.1%	6 months

(SD: standard deviation)

TABLE 3: Studies on comparison of noncultured hair follicle cell suspension with other cell-based methods.

S. No.	Authors	Year	Number of patients	Number of patches	Comparison with FCS	Percentage repigmentation (Mean ± SD)	Repigmentation of number of patches	Duration of study	p-value
1	Singh et al.[16]	2013	30	47	FCS versus NCECS	>75%	78% versus 92%		0.425
2	Hamza et al.[17]	2019	20	20	FCS versus NCECS	57.5% versus 50%	-	3 months	0.105
3	Gunaabalaji et al.[19]	2020	19	38	FCS versus NCECS	78.68 ± 30.03 versus 61.58 ± 42.68	-	9 months	0.1618
4	Pangti et al.[21]	2020	10	20	FCS versus PHF FCS versus NCECS	73.6 ± 39.71 versus 87.6 ± 30.83 73.6 ± 39.71 versus 17.5 ± 34.01	-	9 months	0.03 (FCS versus PHF), 0.32 (FCS versus NCECS)
5	Donaparthi et al.[26]	2016	11	60	FCS versus NCECS	>75%	43.34% versus 90%	6 months	Statistically significant
6	Thakur et al.[27]	2020	30	30	FCS versus PHF	>75%	3 versus 0 patients	16 weeks	0.02

(FCS: follicular cell suspension; NCECS: noncultured epidermal cell suspension; PHF: plucking of anagen hair follicles; SD: standard deviation)

CONCLUSION

The FCS is a novel, less invasive, and cosmetically acceptable technique, which requires less expertise. A few studies now establish the efficacy of this procedure and have seen it to be comparable with NCECS. A combination of NCECS with FCS has been found superior to NCECS alone suggesting that the hair follicle cell suspension provides certain cells which add to the overall success. Plucked hair follicles do not work well in repigmenting vitiligo patches, therefore, FUE should be used for donor follicles harvesting. Overall, the FCS technique is an addition to the armamentarium for the surgical management of stable vitiligo.

REFERENCES

1. Kumar A, Mohanty S, Sahni K, Kumar R, Gupta S. Extracted hair follicle outer root sheath cell suspension for pigment cell restoration in vitiligo. J Cutan Aesthetic Surg. 2013;6:121-5.
2. Goldstein NB, Koster MI, Hoaglin LG, Spoelstra NS, Kechris KJ, Robinson SE, et al. Narrow-band ultraviolet B treatment for human vitiligo is associated with proliferation, migration, and differentiation of melanocyte precursors. J Invest Dermatol. 2015;135:2068-76.
3. Falabella R. Vitiligo and the melanocyte reservoir. Indian J Dermatol. 2009;54:313-8.
4. Sawatkar GU, Vinay K, Dogra S. Follicular cell suspension: a new surgical modality for the treatment of vitiligo. Pigment Int. 2015;2:4-8.
5. Cui J, Shen LY, Wang GC. Role of hair follicles in the repigmentation of vitiligo. J Invest Dermatol. 1991;97:410-6.
6. Meyer KC, Klatte JE, Dinh HV, Harries MJ, Reithmayer K, Meyer W, et al. Evidence that the bulge region is a site of relative immune privilege in human hair follicles. Br J Dermatol. 2008;159:1077-85.
7. Zhou X, Ma Y, Liu F, Gu C, Wang X, Xia H, et al. Melanocyte chitosan/gelatin composite fabrication with human outer root sheath-derived cells to produce pigment. Sci Rep. 2019;9:5198.
8. Sülflow K, Schneider M, Loth T, Kascholke C, Schulz-Siegmund M, Hacker MC, et al. Melanocytes from the outer root sheath of human hair and epidermal melanocytes display improved melanotic features in the niche provided by cGEL, oligomer-cross-linked gelatin-based hydrogel. J Biomed Mater Res A. 2016;104:3115-26.
9. D'Mello SA, Finlay GJ, Baguley BC, Askarian-Amiri ME. Signaling pathways in melanogenesis. Int J Mol Sci. 2016;17:1144.
10. Tobin DJ, Slominski A, Botchkarev V, Paus R. The fate of hair follicle melanocytes during the hair growth cycle. J Investig Dermatol Symp Proc. 1999;4:323-32.
11. Manira M, Khairul Anuar K, Seet WT, Irfan AWA, Ng MH, Chua KH, et al. Comparison of the effects between animal-derived trypsin and recombinant trypsin on human skin cells proliferation, gene, and protein expression. Cell Tissue Bank. 2014;15:41-9.
12. Scharffetter-Kochanek K, Klein CE, Heinen G, Mauch C, Schaefer T, Adelmann-Grill BC, et al. Migration of a human keratinocyte cell line (HACAT) to interstitial collagen type I is mediated by the alpha 2 beta 1-integrin receptor. J Invest Dermatol. 1992;98:3-11.
13. Vanscheidt W, Hunziker T. Repigmentation by outer-root-sheath-derived melanocytes: proof of concept in vitiligo and leucoderma. Dermatol Basel Switz. 2009;218:342-3.
14. Mohanty S, Kumar A, Dhawan J, Sreenivas V, Gupta S. Noncultured extracted hair follicle outer root sheath cell suspension for transplantation in vitiligo. Br J Dermatol. 2011;164:1241-6.
15. Shah AN, Marfatia RK, Saikia SS. A study of noncultured extracted hair follicle outer root sheath cell suspension for transplantation in vitiligo. Int J Trichol. 2016;8:67-72.
16. Singh C, Parsad D, Kanwar AJ, Dogra S, Kumar R. Comparison between autologous noncultured extracted hair follicle outer root sheath cell suspension and autologous noncultured epidermal cell suspension in the treatment of stable vitiligo: a randomized study. Br J Dermatol. 2013; 169:287-93.
17. Hamza AM, Hussein TM, Shakshouk HAR. Noncultured extracted hair follicle outer root sheath cell suspension versus noncultured epidermal cell suspension in the treatment of stable vitiligo. J Cutan Aesthet Surg. 2019;12:105-11.
18. Vinay K, Dogra S, Parsad D, Kanwar AJ, Kumar R, Minz RW, et al. Clinical and treatment characteristics determining therapeutic outcome in patients undergoing autologous non-cultured outer root sheath hair follicle cell suspension for treatment of stable vitiligo. J Eur Acad Dermatol Venereol. 2015;29:31-7.
19. Gunaabalaji DR, Pangti R, Challa A, Chauhan S, Sahni K, Arava SK, et al. Comparison of efficacy of noncultured hair follicle cell suspension and noncultured epidermal cell suspension in repigmentation of leukotrichia and skin patch in vitiligo: a randomized trial. Int J Dermatol. 2020;59:1393-400.
20. Kumar A, Gupta S, Mohanty S, Bhargava B, Airan B. Stem cell niche is partially lost during follicular plucking: a preliminary pilot study. Int J Trichol. 2013;5:97-100.
21. Pangti R, Challa A, Chauhan S, Narayanan A, Gupta S. Comparison of cell suspension transplantation prepared from plucked hair shafts, excised hair follicles, and epidermal shave biopsies in vitiligo patients: a randomized study. Dermatol Surg. 2021;47(5):735-8.
22. Razmi TM, Parsad D, Kumaran SM. Combined epidermal and follicular cell suspension as a novel surgical approach for acral vitiligo. J Am Acad Dermatol. 2017;76:564-7.
23. Razmi TM, Kumar R, Rani S, Kumaran SM, Tanwar S, Parsad D. Combination of Follicular and Epidermal Cell Suspension as a Novel Surgical Approach in Difficult-to-Treat Vitiligo: A Randomized Clinical Trial. JAMA Dermatol. 2018;154: 301-8.
24. Vashisht KR, Arava SK, Tembhre MK, Parihar AS, Sharma VK, Das BK, et al. A randomized pilot study to compare hair follicle cell suspensions prepared using trypsin alone versus trypsin in combination with collagenase type I for transplantation in vitiligo. Clin Exp Dermatol. 2020;45:172-9.
25. Kumar P, Bhari N, Tembhre MK, Mohanty S, Arava S, Sharma VK, et al. Study of efficacy and safety of noncultured, extracted follicular outer root sheath cell suspension transplantation in the management of stable vitiligo. Int J Dermatol. 2018;57: 245-9.
26. Donaparthi N, Chopra A. Comparative Study of Efficacy of Epidermal Melanocyte Transfer Versus Hair Follicular Melanocyte Transfer in Stable Vitiligo. Indian J Dermatol. 2016;61:640-4.
27. Thakur DS, Kumar S, Kumaran MS, Srivastava N, Parsad D. Comparison of follicular unit extraction vs. plucking of hair follicles as technique of harvesting hair follicles in non-cultured hair follicular cell suspension in vitiligo. J Eur Acad Dermatol Venereol. 2020;34:e34-6.

CHAPTER 40

Cultured Melanocyte Transplantation

Debdeep Mitra, Davinder Parsad, Krishna Talukdar

KEY MESSAGES

- Cultured melanocyte transplant represents a major advance in vitiligo surgery as it has the big advantage of a donor to recipient area of around 1:100 and hence a very small donor graft is adequate to cover a very large area. The cultured human melanocytes are generally multidendritic, and many mature melanosomes are observed using both L-DOPA staining and S-100 protein immunohistochemical staining.
- Multiple sessions like one limb at a time can be planned by harvesting the donor tissue in just one sitting and reusing the melanocyte cell culture cells.
- The other major advantage of this technique is it contains the possibility to cryopreserve these cells in cell banks and reculture them whenever these are needed for transplantation in future.
- However, the need for expensive laboratory equipment and technical knowledge of cell culture limits the use of this modality to a few centers only at present and the technique still needs to evolve before it can find widespread practical application. There is still lack of complete standardization; relatively inadequate data and no long-term follow-up data on transplantation of cultured melanocytes.

INTRODUCTION

The ideal surgical treatment modality for treating vitiligo should be effective in all cases, rapid, cheap, easy to perform, and safe. None of the currently available modalities have all the mentioned advantages. Tissue grafts possess several limitations such as inability to cover large areas in a single sitting and nonuniform repigmentation and textural change (especially punch grafting and split-thickness skin grafting). Cultured melanocyte (CM) grafting has overcome these problems as they are able to cover large areas with uniform pigmentation, from small grafts in a smaller number of sittings, hence contributing to greater patient comfort, with less textural changes of donor skin. The other major advantage of this technique is the possibility to cryopreserve these cells in cell banks and reculture them whenever these are needed for transplantation in future. Hence, cellular graft represents a major advance in vitiligo surgery. However, the lack of complete standardization, relatively inadequate data, the need for expensive laboratory equipment and technical knowledge of cell culture limit the use of this modality to a few centers only at present and the technique still needs to evolve before it can find widespread practical application.

Cultured melanocyte suspensions are of two types, i.e., pure melanocyte cell suspension and coculture with keratinocytes. The latter are more manageable and make it easier to treat many large achromic patches at the same time. In addition, these cocultures allow melanocytes to grow in more physiologic conditions. The maintenance of an optimal numerical relationship with the keratinocytes provides a more suitable environment for their development, possibly owing to the release of growth factors essential for their functions. The maintenance of a physiological melanocyte keratinocyte unit is the basis of this technique and leads to better results. This epidermal melanin unit is composed of one melanocyte and approximately 36 neighboring keratinocytes, working in synchrony to produce and distribute melanin. Melanin is synthesized in melanosomes, transferred to the dendrite tips, and translocated into keratinocytes, forming caps over the keratinocyte nuclei. The molecular and cellular mechanisms involved in melanosome transfer and the keratinocyte-melanocyte interactions required for this process are not yet completely understood. Suggested mechanisms of melanosome transfer include melanosome release and endocytosis, direct inoculation (injection), keratinocyte-melanocyte membrane fusion, and phagocytosis. Studies of the keratinocyte receptor protease-activated receptor-2 (PAR-2) support the phagocytosis theory. PAR-2 controls melanosome ingestion and phagocytosis by keratinocytes and exerts a regulatory role in skin pigmentation. Modulation of PAR-2 activity can enhance or decrease melanosome transfer and affects pigmentation only when there is keratinocyte-melanocyte contact. Moreover, PAR-2 is induced by ultraviolet (UV) irradiation and hence the role of phototherapy postprocedure leads to better surgical outcomes. Also, there is ongoing research on the role of UV radiation during the keratinocyte-melanocyte coculture for a better and faster yield without increasing the underlying risk of cell atypia.

BACKGROUND AND HISTORY

The first clinical use of cultured epidermis was reported in the 1980s to treat burns,[1] and later extended to the treatment of many other depigmenting disorders including vitiligo. The idea of obtaining a large population of melanocytes from small samples of normally pigmented skin by growing them in the laboratory thus seemed attractive and plausible. However, initial attempts at culturing melanocytes were unsuccessful because of the slow multiplication rate and the overgrowth of other more rapidly multiplying cells like fibroblasts and keratinocytes. The first successful culture of melanocytes was from tissue obtained from metastatic melanoma patients, but at that time, attempts to culture them from normal skin or nonmetastatic melanoma failed. The first break came in 1980 when Eisenger and Marko[2] were able to successfully culture melanocytes from newborn foreskins and adult skin by the addition of phorbol-12-myristate-13-acetate (PMA) and cholera toxin. The technique was further refined by the addition of isobutylmethylxanthine (IBMX) and human placental extract. Cholera toxin and IBMX served to keep intracellular levels of cAMP high. The placental extract was believed to be a source of basic fibroblast growth factor (bFGF) while at a concentration of 10 ng/mL PMA was found to be toxic to human keratinocytes but not melanocytes; and in fact, was found to promote the attachment and proliferation of melanocytes. They observed that PMA at 10 ng/mL had a toxic effect mainly on keratinocytes, whereas 10 nM cholera toxin inhibits growth of fibroblasts. In 1984, Gilchrest et al.[3] reported the selective cultivation and long-term maintenance in culture, of human melanocytes from newborn and adult epidermis, which they were able to serially passage up to six times. The next breakthrough occurred in 1987 with the first report of the use of CMs to pigment leukodermas, when Lerner et al. successfully treated a patient of piebaldism by injecting CMs into suction blisters prepared at the depigmented site. This opened new avenues in the field of the application of tissue cultures for treatment of cutaneous depigmenting disorders. The procedure included obtaining a thin skin graft (from roofs of suction-induced blisters) which was enzymatically dissociated to provide a suspension which was later cultured in vitro in a medium containing 12-O-tetradecanoylphorbol-13-acetate (TPA), newborn calf serum and cholera toxin to yield a growth of melanocytes after 1 month of incubation. Initial cultivation which yielded growth of melanocytes mixed with fibroblasts was later supplemented with 100 μg/mL Geneticin to eliminate fibroblasts and yield pure melanocyte cultures. However, reports on mutagenicity of phorbol esters later led to their exclusion from media and it had to be later replaced by bFGF.[4] In the last few decades, the procedure has undergone several modifications. Donor skin has variously been obtained using biopsy (punch biopsy/split-thickness skin graft/full-thickness skin grafts/CelluTome) or suction/cryo-induced blisters. Several methods have been used to prepare the recipient site including dermabrasion, suction/cryo-induced blisters, or lasers [erbium-doped yttrium aluminum garnet (Er:YAG) or CO_2]. Recently, the use of hyaluronic acid sheets[5] and amniotic membrane (AM)[6] as scaffolds for CMs has been reported to be successful. The reagents and their function of a melanocyte culture medium are summarized in **Table 1**.

PATIENT SELECTION

The technique of cultured autologous melanocytes can be used for repigmentation of skin in all types of vitiligo, postinflammatory depigmentation, and piebaldism. Case selection should be done carefully, as discussed in earlier chapters, as per existing guidelines.[7,8] Apart from the general recommendations for vitiligo surgery, cultured autologous melanocyte transplantation is particularly useful for patients with large achromic patches. However, it must be explained to patients that involvement of large body surface area by vitiligo is in itself a poor prognostic factor for repigmentation by both medical and surgical means. In addition, acrofacial vitiligo, especially involvement of tips of fingers and toes, may have a poorer response to CM grafting compared to lesions on other sites. In a large study of the use of the procedure in

TABLE 1: Components of melanocyte culture medium.

S.No.	*Reagent*	*Remarks*
1.	Phorbol-12-myristate-13-acetate (PMA)	Toxic to human keratinocytes but not melanocytes so help prevent keratinocyte overgrowth. Also enhances the proliferation and attachment of melanocytes to keratinocytes
2.	Human placental extract	Source of basic fibroblast growth factor (bFGF). No mutagenic potential so ideal for melanocyte proliferation
3.	Cholera toxin	*Cyclic AMP (cAMP)-inducer:* Mitogenic effect on melanocytes so promotes melanocyte proliferation
4.	Isobutylmethylxanthine (IBMX)	*Cyclic AMP (cAMP)-inducer:* Mitogenic effect on melanocytes so promotes melanocyte proliferation
5.	4-(2-hydroxyethyl)-1-piperazineethanesulfonic acid (HEPES) buffering agent	HEPES is a zwitterionic sulfonic acid buffering agent. It is widely used in cell culture, largely because it is better at maintaining physiological pH despite changes in carbon dioxide concentration (produced by aerobic respiration) when compared to bicarbonate buffers, which are also commonly used in cell culture

105 achromic lesions, it was reported that generally there were poor results in the treatment of extremity lesions and those in periorificial areas. The average percentages of repigmentation of extremities and periorificial sites were 8% and 35% respectively compared to 88–96% repigmentation of all other body sites.[9]

TECHNIQUE

The ideal donor recipient (DR) ratio is not yet accurately defined. Interestingly, in a study by Hong et al.,[10] found no significant differences in repigmentation after CM transplantation based on donor-recipient ratio. They divided 102 patients undergoing transplantation of cultured pure melanocytes into two groups, (1) a low DR ratio group, with DR ratio ≤1:10 (mean 1:8 in 35 cases) and (2) a high DR ratio group with DR ratio >1:10 (mean 1:27 in 67 cases) and found results to be comparable between the two groups. They concluded that although cultured autologous melanocyte transplantation is an expensive and complicated procedure, it provides the highest DR ratios (>1:10 and up to 1:60).

The following steps are involved in melanocyte culture:

- Technique of culture
- Preparation
- Donor site
- Recipient site
- Dressing and follow-up.

Technique of Culture

Collection of the Samples

The skin biopsies are obtained from the normally pigmented skin for transplantation, and if necessary, additionally from lesional or perilesional skin for experimental purposes. Various methods have been used to obtain skin samples from donor site, including punch grafts, split-thickness skin grafts, full-thickness skin grafts, and roofs of suction blisters. However, for transplantation purposes the ideal graft is a split-thickness skin graft comprising of epidermis and superficial part of dermis. It provides a good yield of melanocytes and does not leave behind any scarring. The CelluTome Epidermal Harvesting System is another technique which consists of a control unit, vacuum head, and a harvester. The system produces autologous epidermal microdomes for use as skin grafts. A 3M Tegaderm™ film is currently used to transfer the microdomes onto the recipient site.

A 4 × 4 cm size graft is usually obtained from the upper thigh or gluteal area under lignocaine infiltration and/or topical eutectic mixture of local anesthetics (EMLA) anesthesia, with proper aseptic precautions. The graft is collected in phosphate-buffered saline (PBS) with antibiotics (50 U/mL penicillin and 0.05 mg/mL streptomycin), in a sterile container (labeled with patient details) and immediately transported to the laboratory on ice. If the lag period is >4 hours, then the graft is placed in complete M2 melanocyte medium (M7167 Sigma-Aldrich or PromoCell, Heidelberg, Cat. No. C-24300) and kept at 8°C. The donor area is dressed with sterile nonadherent chlorhexidine gauze (Bactigras, TJ Smith & Nephew Ltd., Hull, UK or Sofra Tulle Dressing 10 × 10 cm, Sanofi India Limited Pharma) followed by a sterile surgical pad that is kept in place with a sterile transparent occlusive dressing (Tegaderm O, 3M Health Care, St. Paul, MN).

Processing of the Graft

In the laminar air flow chamber, the grafts are trimmed with sharp scissors to remove all fat and the deeper dermis. They are then transferred to a Petri dish with trypsin-ethylenediaminetetraacetic acid (EDTA) (0.25% trypsin and 0.02% EDTA) and the sample is turned back and forth with the help of jeweler's forceps to ensure that it comes in complete contact with the solution. The grafts are placed with the epidermal side facing upward, and then cut into pieces of about 5 × 5 mm. This is followed by incubation at 37°C for 1 hour in an incubator. Dulbecco's Modified Eagle's Medium (DMEM) is added and the epidermis is separated from the dermis using sterile forceps. The tissue is then pipetted well so as to separate cells of the dermoepidermal junction from the tissue and the solid waste of tissue is removed. The DMEM containing cells is then centrifuged at 1,000 rpm for 5 minutes to obtain a pellet. The supernatant and the floating fragments are removed and the pellet is resuspended in 5 mL DMEM medium and transferred to a 75 or 150 cm^2 culture flask containing M2 medium and placed flat to prevent cells from adhering to the sides of flask. The empty centrifuge tube is rinsed twice with M2 medium, which is also transferred to the T-25 tissue culture flask, to ensure that all cells are collected **(Figs. 1 and 2)**. The cell number is adjusted to 2.5 × 104 cells /cm^2 which is counted using a Neubauer chamber **(Fig. 3)**. Care is taken to avoid media containing phorbol esters when the culture is being done for transplantation purposes due to mutagenic potential.

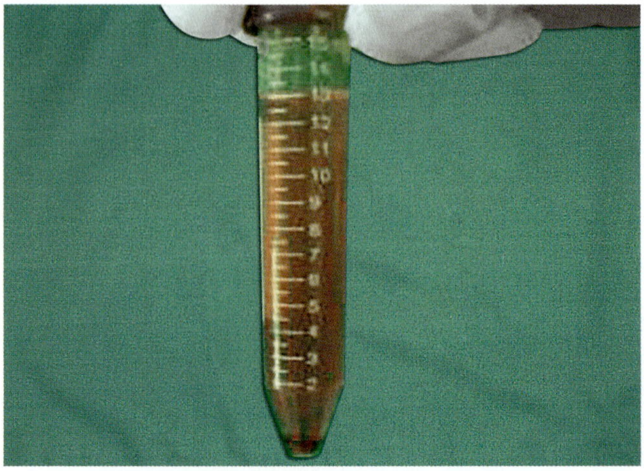

Fig. 1: Cell pellet obtained after centrifugation.

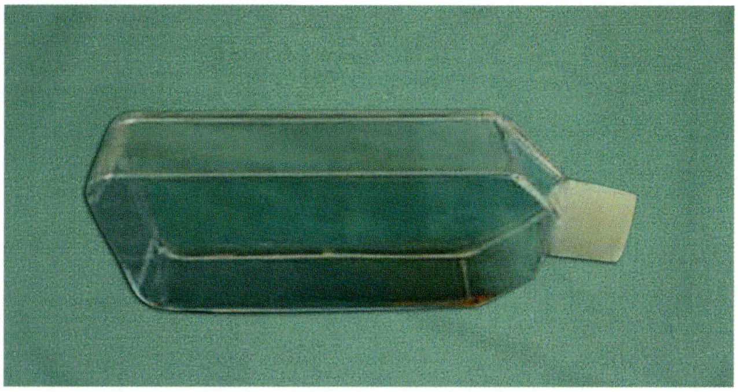

Fig. 2: T-25 tissue culture flask.

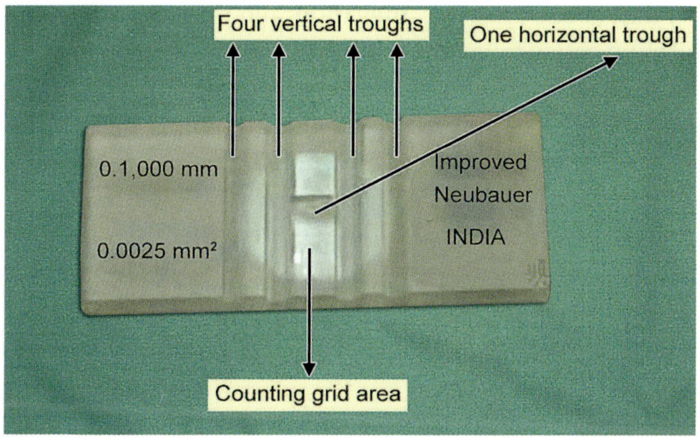

Fig. 3: Neubauer counting chamber.

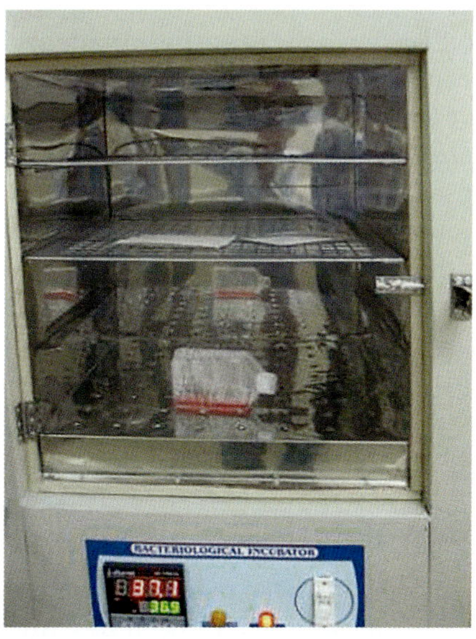

Fig. 4: Melanocyte cell culture inside incubator at 37°C.

The culture is maintained at 37°C **(Fig. 4)** in a humidified, 95% air and 5% CO_2 atmosphere using anaerobic gas chargers. The medium is to be changed at 1–2 days intervals and the cells should be examined daily microscopically to look for contamination or infection and also to look for outgrowth of cells. When confluence occurs, the cells are split by trypsin treatment for 5 minutes at room temperature and subcultured.

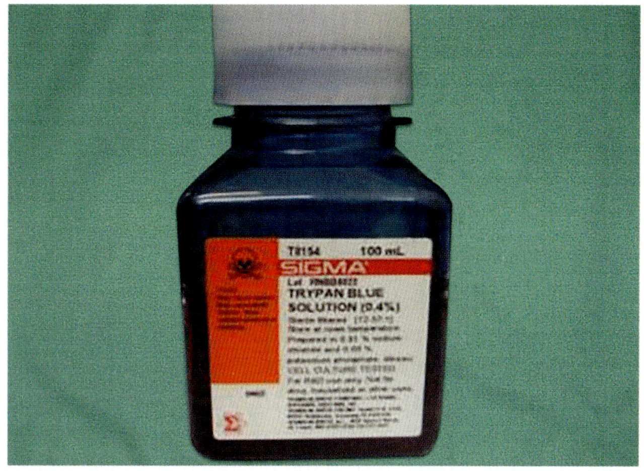

Fig. 5: Trypan blue stain.

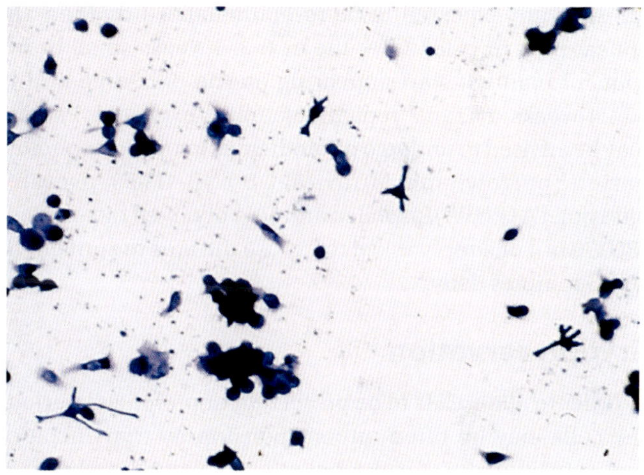

Fig. 6: Trypan blue staining for melanocyte vitality.

Cell viability may be assessed by trypan blue exclusion assay, which is based on uptake of trypan blue dye by nonviable cells as a result of disintegration of the cellular membrane **(Figs. 5 and 6)**. If a 100% pure melanocyte culture is needed for research purpose, 45 µg/mL Geneticin (G418; 45 µg/mL) can be added to the medium for 3 days, starting from the 10th day of the culture. Geneticin selectively suppress the fibroblasts. To eliminate keratinocytes, the level of Ca^{2+} levels may be elevated to 1.6 mM for 2 days, since high Ca levels are toxic to keratinocytes but not melanocytes. However, for therapeutic purposes these interventions are not necessary since they do not interfere with melanocyte growth to a sufficient degree. In fact, few remaining keratinocytes may in fact aid in the growth and differentiation of melanocytes. Usually, between 10×10^6 and 50×10^6 cells are obtained at the end of 3 weeks at which stage, the cells are ready for transplantation. To harvest the cells for transplantation, after removing culture medium from the flask, a small amount of trypsin/EDTA solution is added and the flask is shaken slightly to allow the solution to come in contact with all the cells. The cells are hence incubated for 5 minutes and then the flask is tilted to check whether the cells have detached sufficiently. The suspension is then pipetted out and the solution centrifuged at 1,000 rpm for 5 minutes and the pellet resuspended in M2 medium and transplanted onto the recipient site.

Recipient Site

Patient preparation, donor area and recipient area, and follow-up have been discussed in earlier chapters and are essentially similar to what is followed for tissue grafts. Application of the cultured cell suspension is similar to what has been discussed in noncultured epidermal cell suspension. The patient is asked to give rest to the operated area and to limit mobility at the site. First follow-up visit is at 7 days when the dressing at both donor and recipient sites is removed. Both the sites are expected to be re-epithelialized by then and appear pink in color. Over the next 2–4 weeks small brown spots of pigment start appearing on the pink area and by 16–24 weeks maximal repigmentation is expected. Patients may be advised to undergo phototherapy in the postoperative period [narrowband ultraviolet B (NB-UVB)/psoralen ultraviolet A (PUVA)/psoralen and UVA obtained by solar light (PUVAsol)] or simply asked to expose the area to sunlight for 10–15 minutes daily.

Cryopreservation

In order to allow CMs to be preserved for prolonged periods, the cells may be lifted into suspension by trypsinization and centrifuged to form a pellet as explained earlier. The pellet is to be then resuspended in cryoprotectant, which is a solution consisting of 8% dimethyl sulfoxide (DMSO) in undiluted newborn calf serum (or a commercially available cryoprotectant). Usually, 1 mL of cryoprotectant is to be used for each 10 million cells and the suspension is transferred to cryotube which is kept on ice for 10 minutes and then placed in a freezer and frozen at a temperature of –70°C to –85°C. Whenever needed, these cells can be thawed by placing in a 37°C water bath, after which the suspension is transferred to a test tube containing culture medium. This is centrifuged at 1,000 rpm for 5 minutes and pellet is resuspended in culture medium or PBS for transplantation. About 70% of cells retain viability after 1 year.

MODIFICATIONS AND NEW DEVELOPMENTS

Phorbol 12, 13-dibutyrate for Melanocyte Culture

A study has attempted to compare the efficacy of another phorbol ester, phorbol 12, 13-dibutyrate (PDBu) in melanocyte culture because of its less hydrophobic nature compared to PMA. In PDBu, melanocytes acquired proliferative status and bipolar morphology quicker with less survival of keratinocytes. PDBu has also been found to have a higher proliferative induction capacity than PMA and melanocytes survived longer in PDBu compared to PMA.[11]

Amniotic Membrane as a Scaffold for Melanocyte Transplantation

In a pilot study on four patients, Redondo et al.[6] replated cultured epidermal melanocytes onto the basement membrane (BM) side of AM at a density of 5–25 × 10^3 cell/cm^2 after which they allowed the melanocytes to grow for another 3–4 days. Following this, they mounted these AMs on sterile Vaseline gauze following which the AMs were placed on the dermabraded recipient site with the BM side down. They were able to achieve excellent repigmentation in all patients and observed repigmentation of the marginal area also, which is found to persist as a halo of depigmentation following other surgical procedures in some patients. They hypothesized that AMs are an easily available substrate which offer anti-inflammatory and antimicrobial properties with lack of antigenicity which facilitates the re-epithelialization of skin and reduces scarring.

Hyaluronic Acid Micropore Sheets as Scaffold[5]

Another modification is the use of hyaluronic acid micropore sheet as a scaffold for culture of melanocytes. Andreassi et al. transferred CMs and keratinocytes from suspension onto a 10 × 10 cm sized sheet of hyaluronic acid fixed on the bottom of a dish of same shape and size. The cells were allowed to proliferate and form a keratinizing stratified epithelium that reproduces the structure of epidermis. This sheet was then transferred to dermabraded recipient sites and repopulation of the areas occurred via passage of cells through the micropores. In their experience on 85 patients treated in the course of 7 years, they observed more or less intense repigmentation in most of the treated lesions.

Preparation of Recipient Site

A number of methods have been used for dermabrasion of the recipient site which have been described in earlier chapters. The new ones are use of Er:YAG laser,[12] CO_2 laser, and recently Timedsurgery. Timedsurgery is a programmed diathermosurgery device which allows precise control of all operational parameters (electric power, appropriate shape of the output waveform, emission time, and dimension of the electrode). Guerra et al.[9] used the earlier mentioned device for denudation of epidermis by coagulating it at 1 W using the dull portion of a 0.2 mm electrode bent at an angle, so as to allow the electrode to skim over the skin surface. The coagulated epidermis was then gently removed with the same electrode, but without electric power.

RESULTS

There has been a study by the authors comparing the results of CM transplantation with noncultured epidermal suspension (NCES) transplantation and it was found that excellent response was seen in 62.17% cases with the NCES technique and in 52% with the CM technique. Thus though results were comparable, CM offers the potential for significant expansion of donor-recipient ratio from 1:10 to 1:100.[13] Another similar study found better repigmentation followed CM transplantation as compared to NCES transplantation in vitiligo.[14] Bao et al. compared blister grafting with NCES and CM transplantation and found blister roof grafting (BG) inferior to both CM and NCES while both the cellular techniques were not significantly different.[15] There have been two recent reports that highlighted the repigmentation of leukotrichia after CM transplantation.[16,17]

CONCLUSION

Cultured melanocyte transplantation is a promising technique for the management of resistant stable vitiligo with a special advantage of being able to cover large areas with small grafts. However, it requires technical expertise and expensive laboratory set-up and hence has not gained widespread popularity. In the hands of experienced personnel, it has the potential to give satisfactory and gratifying results.

REFERENCES

1. O'Connor NE, Mulliken JB, Banks-Schlegel S, Kehinde O, Green H. Grafting of burns with cultured epithelium prepared from autologous epidermal cells. Lancet. 1981;1:75-8.
2. Eisinger M, Marko O. Selective proliferation of normal human melanocytes in vitro in the presence of phorbol ester and cholera toxin. Proc Natl Acad Sci U S A. 1982;79:2018-22.
3. Gilchrest BA, Vrabel MA, Flynn E, Szabo G. Selective cultivation of human melanocytes from newborn and adult epidermis. J Invest Dermatol. 1984;83:370-6.
4. Löntz W, Olsson MJ, Moellmann G, Lerner AB. Pigment cell transplantation for treatment of vitiligo: a progress report. J Am Acad Dermatol. 1994;30:591-7.
5. Andreassi L, Pianigiani E, Andreassi A, Taddeucci P, Biagioli M. A new model of epidermal culture for the surgical treatment of vitiligo. Int J Dermatol. 1998;37:595-8.
6. Redondo P, Gimondo de Azcarate A, Marquar L, GarcGa-Guzman M, Andreu E, Prosper F. Amniotic membrane as a scaffold for melanocyte transplantation in patients with stable vitiligo. Dermatol Res Pract. 2011;2011:532139.
7. Prasad D, Gupta S; IDVAL Dermatosurgery Taskforce. Standard guidelines of care for vitiligo surgery. Indian J Dermatol Venereol Leprol. 2008;74 (Suppl):S37-45.
8. Falabella R, Arrunategui A, Barona MI, Alzate A. The minigrafting test for vitiligo: detection of stable lesions for melanocyte transplantation. J Am Acad Dermatol. 1995;32: 228-32.
9. Guerra L, Capurro S, Melchi F, Primavera G, Bondanza S, Cancedda R, et al. Treatment of 'stable vitiligo by Timedsurgery and transplantation of cultured epidermal autografts. Arch Dermatol. 2000;136:1380-9.
10. Hong WS, Hu DN, Qian GP, McCormick SA, Xu AE. Ratio of size of recipient and donor areas in treatment of vitiligo by autologous cultured melanocyte transplantation. Br J Dermatol. 2011;165(3):520-5.
11. Padma D, Bhat KM. A comparison between Phorbol 12 Myristate 13 Acetate and Phorbol 12, 13 Dibutyrate in Human Melanocyte Culture. J Clin Diagn Res. 2016;10(1):GC01-4.
12. Kaufmann R, Greiner D, Kippenberger S, Bernd A. Grafting of in vitro cultured melanocytes onto laser-ablated lesions in vitiligo. Acta Derm Venereol. 1998;78(2):136-8.
13. Verma R, Grewal RS, Chatterjee M, Pragasam V, Vasudevan B, Mitra D. A comparative study of efficacy of cultured versus non cultured melanocyte transfer in the management of stable vitiligo. Med J Armed Forces India. 2014;70(1):26-31.
14. Verma G, Varkhande SR, Kar HK, Rani R. Evaluation of repigmentation with cultured melanocyte transplantation (CMT) compared with non-cultured epidermal cell transplantation in vitiligo at 12th week reveals better repigmentation with CMT. J Invest Dermatol. 2015;135(10):2533-5.
15. Bao H, Hong W, Fu L, Wei X, Qian G, Xu A. Blister roof grafting, cultured melanocytes transplantation and non-cultured epidermal cell suspension transplantation in treating stable vitiligo: a mutual self-control study. J Dermatolog Treat. 2015;26(6):571-4.
16. Yao L, Zhong SX, Hu DN, Guo JW, Li SS, Xie XL, et al. Repigmentation of leukotrichia in vitiligo with transplantation of cultured autologous melanocytes. Int J Dermatol. 2014;53(8):1016-8.
17. Wu XG, Xu AE. Successful treatment of vitiligo on the scalp of a 9-year-old girl using autologous cultured pure melanocyte transplantation. Pediatr Dermatol. 2017;34(1):e22-3.

CHAPTER 41

Vitiligo: Other Modalities of Treatment

Dilip Kachhawa

KEY MESSAGES

- Over the years, many surgical techniques have been introduced in order to overcome the limitations of the conventional techniques.
- Jodhpur technique, introduced in 2008, require minimal surgical expertise and a simple procedure with the advantage of treating multiple large areas mat the same time with very few limitations.
- Follicular unit extraction transplant, is mainly used for leukotrichia over vitiligo patches.
- Micropigmentation or tattooing uses the concept of camouflaging the vitiliginous patches.

INTRODUCTION

Surgical mode of treatment has been an integral part of vitiligo management and is gold standard in resistant areas. This chapter includes few of such surgical techniques.

JODHPUR TECHNIQUE WITH KERATINOCYTES–MELANOCYTES CELL SUSPENSION (FIGS. 1A TO D)

One of the newest and popular techniques in stable vitiligo surgery is Jodhpur technique with many new advancements in the technique, which has high success rates in terms of repigmentation not only in accessible areas but also in difficult areas. In this technique, we take skin graft mostly from the lateral side of the thigh and can also take perilesional graft and transplant in a stable vitiligo patch. These modalities of treatment are discussed below.

The authors have described a revolutionized surgical method in vitiligo in which material consisting of epidermis and dermis is collected by dermabrasion from the donor area and applied directly on the dermabraded recipient area. This is the only method in which split thin grafts are not taken.

They described the Jodhpur technique based on their observations while performing dermabrasion on acne-scarred facial skin. During the procedure, they experienced macroscopic skin particles spatter on their face, which they thought could be used as a grafting material with the presumption of the presence of melanocytes in it.

Indications

- Stable vitiligo
- Secondary leukoderma due to burns
- Chemical trauma, etc.
- Other—Nonhealing ulcer

Contraindications

- Active vitiligo
- Secondary infection
- Keloidal tendency
- Autoimmune disorders
- Inflammatory disorders
- Bleeding disorders.

Procedure

Written informed consent

- Shaving of donor area and recipient area
  - Preparation of recipient site should be done before donor site because:
    - Oozing is reduced and hemostasis is achieved by the time donor graft is collected
    - The obtained graft can be directly transferred to the recipient site

Recipient area:

- Vitiliginous patch should be prepared by cleaning with spirit and povidone iodine, and thereafter mark the area including 2–3 mm of normal perilesional area.
- *Local anesthesia:* 1% lignocaine given as a quadrant infiltration, deep dermal, and subcutaneous.
- Dermabrade the vitiliginous patch with a diamond fraise disk till there is appearance of uniform pinpoint bleeding, which is seen when we reach up to the dermoepidermal junction. This dermabrasion should be done up to the edge of the marked area so as to ensure that perigraft halo does not develop. Cover the denuded area with gauze pieces soaked with normal saline after achieving adequate hemostasis.

Donor area:

- The site of choice is the lateral area of the thigh for collection of graft material, which is approximately one-third of the recipient area.

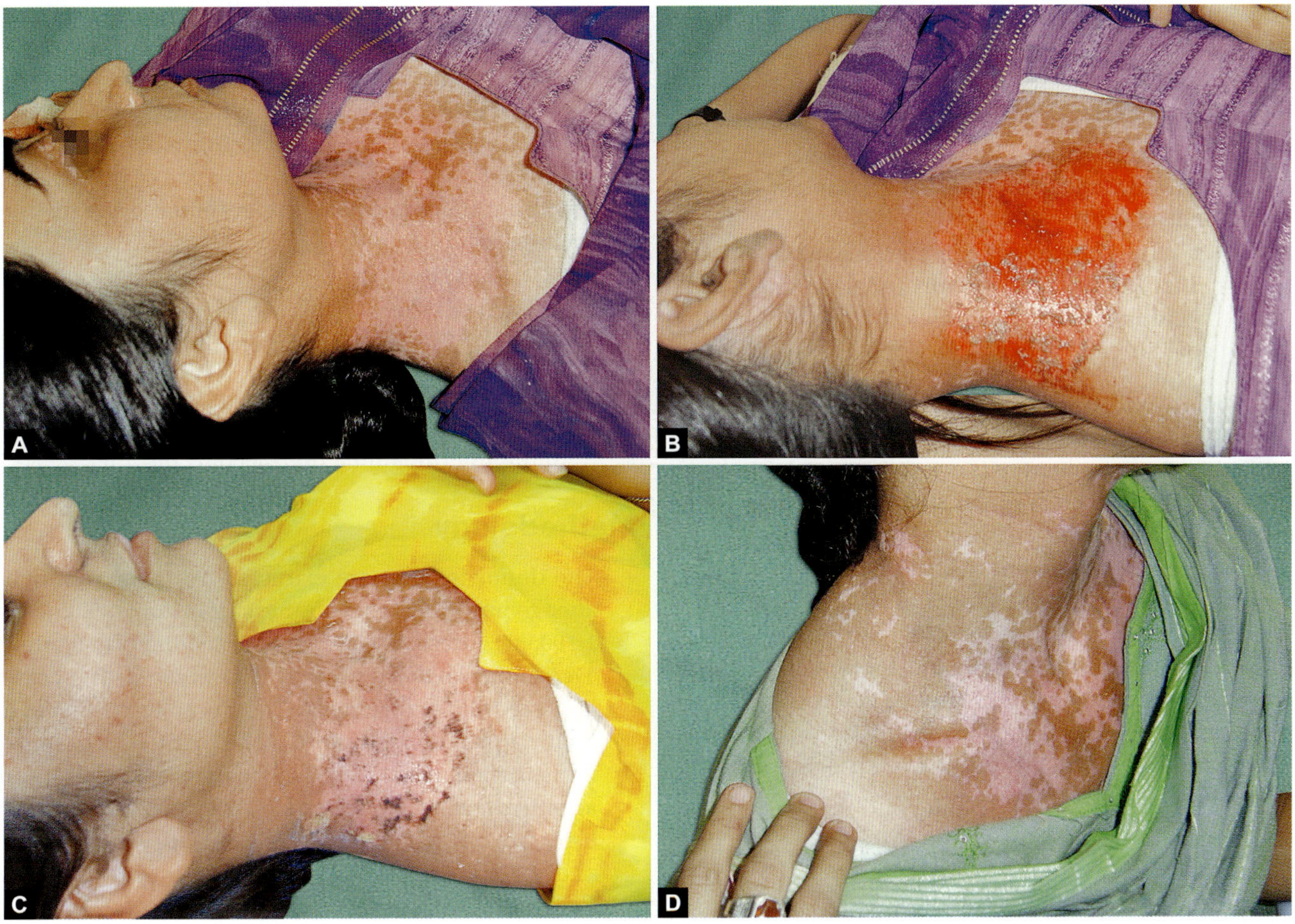

Figs. 1A to D: (A) Before surgery; (B) Just after grafting with paste-like material containing melanocytes; (C) After one week of grafting; grafted material is seen as black eschar; (D) After 20 weeks, pigmentation is seen over grafted sites.

- Marking of the donor area to be dermabraded for collecting the grafting material (approximately one-third of the recipient area).
- Surgical preparation with povidone iodine, spirit, and marking need to be done.
- Local anesthesia with 1% xylocaine is to be given as a four quadrant infiltration deep dermal and subcutaneous to achieve a flat surface.

Preparation of donor area:

- Make the donor area flat and taut by stretching.
- 2% mupirocin ointment is applied over the donor area.
- Hold the handpiece of the electrical dermabrader in a safety razor grip and roll the fraise two to three times all over the donor area gently, initiating from periphery of the donor site.
- Dermabrader is rotated in small circles in clockwise direction so that the abraded epidermal particles, containing melanocytes and keratinocytes, blends with the mupirocin ointment leading to decreased spraying of particles.
- Mixture of keratinocytes and melanocytes blended with mupirocin forms a paste which is collected with the help of spatula and transferred to a glass slide
- A drop of 1% methyl cellulose or NS is added to make it a homogeneous paste.
- Hemostasis is achieved at the donor area by a pressure bandage
- Transfer the graft material obtained from the donor area evenly on the dermabraded recipient area and spread uniformly all over the surface with the spatula.
- Cover the area with collagen dressing followed by ointment soaked gauze pieces and then dry cotton gauze pieces and support it with elastocrape bandage.
- Patient is allowed to go after immobilization for 30 minutes
- *Side effects:*
    - Erythema, edema, transient postinflammatory hyper/hypopigmented lesion at both donor and recipient areas
- *Advantages:*
    - It is a simple, cheap, and less time-consuming surgery for vitiligo.
    - No laboratory setup, enzymes, machines, etc. required.

- It can be performed on an outpatient department (OPD) basis.
- High successful rates of repigmentation and even large areas can also be treated at one time.
- It does not need costly instruments.
- No scarring is seen at donor or recipient site

- *Disadvantages:*
    - It results in terms of complete pigmentation seen after a delay of 3–6 months and not immediately.
    - Achromic and hypochromic skip areas may be left behind.

MODIFIED JODHPUR TECHNIQUE

Modified Jodhpur technique is a modification of Jodhpur technique in which perilesional skin of vitiliginous patch consisting of normal skin can serve as a donor area.

The procedure is the same as that of Jodhpur technique except the chosen site for the donor area. The advantage of this technique over the conventional Jodhpur technique is that the procedure is more time-saving and the patient only needs manipulation of the lesional site, and no new areas will need anesthesia and dermabrasion. This technique can be used for difficult areas to treat such as the head and neck, bony areas, and periorificial and acral parts.

Chronic nonhealing ulcer (CNHU): Researchers attempted repurposing of the Jodhpur technique for chronic NHU involving the leg, refractory to multiple ulcer-treatment modalities.

FOLLICULAR UNIT EXTRACTION TRANSPLANT

Follicular unit grafting is another refined technique that is useful for a stable vitiligo lesion.

Indications

- Stable segmental vitiligo located in hairy areas with or without leukotrichia
- Secondary leukoderma due to burns, chemical, and trauma
- Leukotrichia over facial vitiligo patch eyebrows and eyelashes.

Contraindications

- Active vitiligo
- Secondary infection
- Keloidal tendency
- Autoimmune/inflammatory/bleeding disorder.

Methodology

- The donor follicles are extracted using micropunches after giving tumescent anesthesia, that is, lignocaine with 1:100,000 adrenaline diluted in 1:10 with normal saline.
- Depending on the number of hairs required, the occipital or postauricular region of the scalp can be chosen as the donor area **(Figs. 2A and B)**. The hair follicles are then transplanted intact as follicular units. After infiltrative anesthesia at the recipient site, transplantation is done using an 18G needle to create slits in the recipient area and the hair follicle is gently inserted using a jeweler's forceps.
- Topical corticosteroids, tacrolimus, and topical PUVAsol therapy are given to enhance repigmentation after a few weeks.
- Extraction of individual follicular units from the occipital area, chest, and back can be usefully employed even in a surgically difficult site such as nonglabrous skin, eyelash, or the angle of the mouth **(Figs. 3A and B)**.

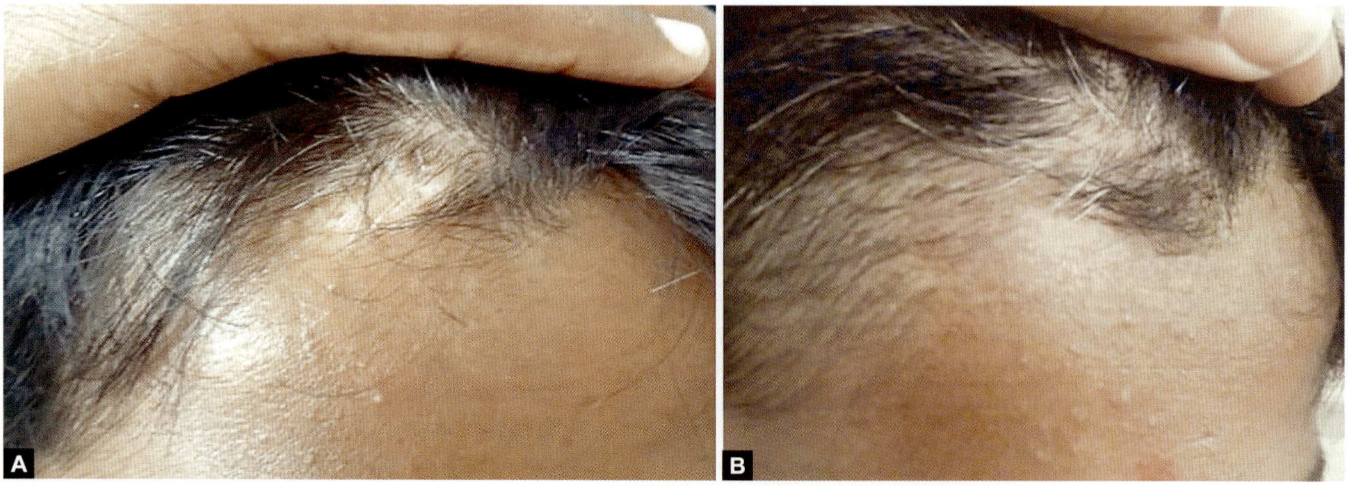

Figs. 2A and B: (A) Vitiligo lesion over scalp before the procedure; (B) 6 months after the procedure; improvement in vitiligo and leukotrichia with excellent color match.

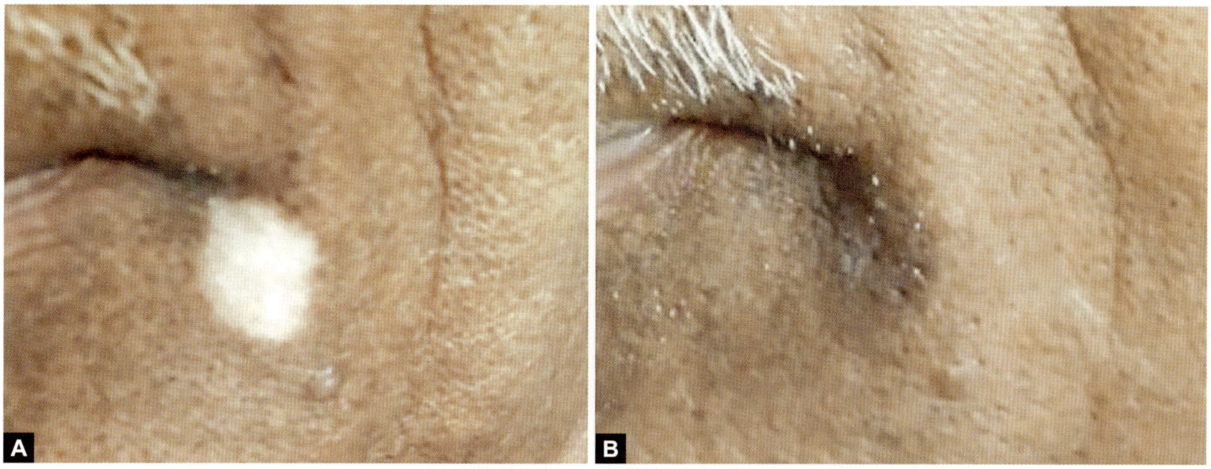

Figs. 3A and B: (A) Vitiligo lesion over the mustache before the procedure; (B) Two months after the procedure.

- This technique avoids scarring and is also devoid of complications such as cobblestoning, hypertrophic scar, and postoperative hyperpigmentation, which may be seen with other grafting procedures.
- However, using this technique, it is difficult to treat medium-to-large lesions and glabrous areas. The grafted melanocyte requires a long time to spread so vitiliginous skin heals slowly with this method.

Complications

Pain, graft rejection, localized hyperpigmentation, pseudo-folliculitis, epidermal cyst, and scarring around the graft can occur.

Limitations

- It is a time-consuming, skilled, and tedious procedure.
- Repigmentation occurs slowly as hair follicle melanocytes spread gradually.
- Unaesthetic results if performed over nonhairy areas.

SMASH GRAFTING

Smash grafting is a modification of split-thickness grafting (STG). In this technique, STG is cut into very small pieces and a paste-like material is prepared and used as a graft on the predermabraded recipient site.

Advantages of this technique are as follows:
- Thick graft can be used
- Uniform pigmentation is seen
- Avoids stuck on appearance of graft.

Surgical Removal of Depigmented Areas

- This method is followed for a small patch of vitiligo over the lip and mucosal areas since the retention of cellular grafts over the mucosal surface is poor.
- In situations of urgency to get rid of the small lesion, surgical removal followed by primary closure of a small depigmented patch of vitiligo can be done and most grafting methods need few weeks for the repigmentation to occur.
- This modality is useful as long as the lesion is amenable for surgical excision, and closure with a good resultant scar is acceptable to the patient.

THERAPEUTIC WOUNDING

- In this method, superficial wounding of the epidermis is done for small and stable patches of vitiligo.
- This technique is suited for hairy areas and in this, dermabrasion is performed by other means without subsequent grafting procedures.
- This methodology works by inducing the repigmentation of the lesion by altering the cytokines milieu, which stimulates active melanocyte present in the outer sheath of the hair.
- The melanocytes which appear after 8–10 days in the epidermis are two to three times larger than normal melanocytes with a hypertrophic cellular body, elongated dendrites, and intense 3,4-dihydroxyphenylalanine (DOPA) oxidase activity.
- The wounding/dermabrasion can be performed by various modalities such as laser ablation by CO_2, cryosurgery, 30–50% trichloroacetic acid, 5-fluorouracil, needling, and motor dermabrasion.
- *Limitations:* The method cannot be used for places such as mucosa, palms, and soles where the hair follicles are absent.

MICROPIGMENTATION/TATTOOING

- Micropigmentation is a therapeutic modality in which inert artificial small particles of various pigments, mostly

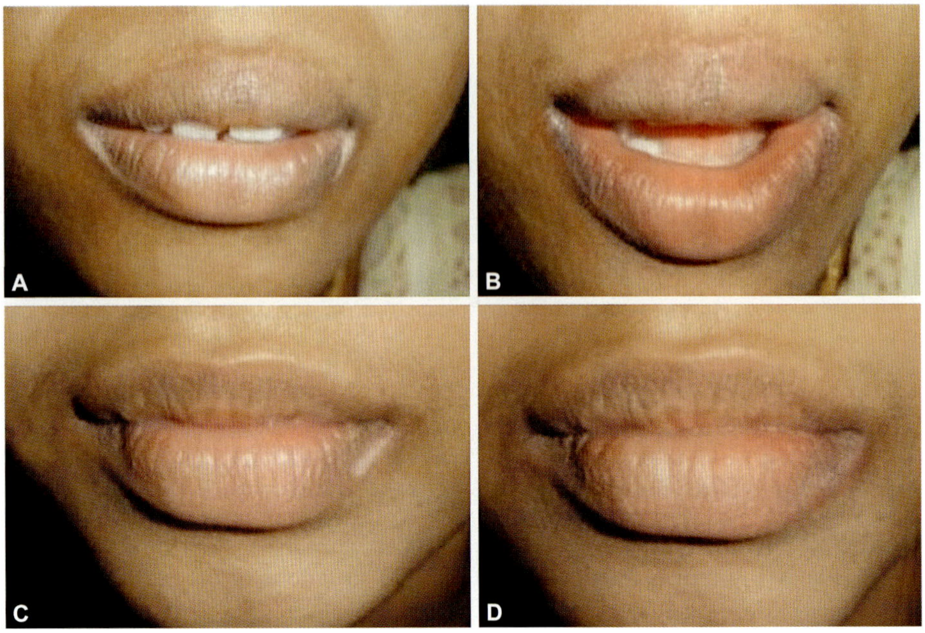

Figs. 4A to D: Vitiligo of lower lateral lip before and after micropigmentation.
Courtesy: Journal of Cutaneous and Aesthetic Surgery (JCAS).

of iron oxide, are implanted into the middle layer of the dermis, similar to a tattoo.

- This modality is used in various combinations of different pigments to match the patient skin color. The procedure is sometimes called permanent cosmetics.
- Micropigmentation is a useful procedure for the cosmetic camouflage of vitiliginous patches, especially involving mucosal and mucocutaneous areas **(Figs. 4A and B)**.
- Tattooing as the treatment of vitiligo is performed for the following indications:
  - In a situation which needs urgent pigment correction of the depigmented patch
  - In special sites such as angles of the mouth where graft retention is poor

Various tattoo pigments include:

- *White:* Titanium dioxide
- *Red:* Cinnabar, mercuric sulfate
- *Black:* Iron oxide
- *Yellow:* Cadmium sulfate
- *Camel yellow:* Iron oxide light
- *Brown:* Iron oxide
- *Dark brown:* Iron oxide.

  All tattoo pigments must be autoclaved before use.

Procedure

- Informed consent is needed.
- Clean the vitiliginous area with normal saline followed by tumescent anesthesia with injection 2% xylocaine.
- Tattoo pigments are mixed in a desired proportion depending on the site and to get an appropriate color match.
- Micropigmentation can be done with a no. 10 pony sewing needle after sterilization in Cidex solution or a motorized tattoo instrument can also be used. This is done until the color matches the surrounding skin.
- Pressure is given with a gauge to stop bleeding if any.
- Clean the area with saline whole procedure.

Side effects of the procedure such as bleeding and hematoma can sometimes be seen.

Advantages of Micropigmentation

- It blends the vitiligo patch to the color of the surrounding skin.
- It breaks up the texture of the vitiligo skin by softening and flattening it.

Disadvantages of Micropigmentation

- Blackening due to oxidation and fading of pigmentation can occur over a period of time.
- Greenish discoloration due to Tyndall effect may also be seen.
- Reaction to tattoos can include allergic hypersensitivity, lichenoid, granulomatous, and pseudolymphomatous types.
- Swelling in the treated area resolves either spontaneously or with ice pack application.

CONCLUSION

To get around the drawbacks of conventional surgical methods, numerous new approaches have been developed over time. Introduced in 2008, the Jodhpur approach is a straightforward operation that requires no surgical experience and has the advantage of treating numerous big areas at once with very few limitations. The primary application of follicular unit extraction transplantation is for leukotrichia over vitiligo patches. The concept of camouflaging the vitiliginous patches is used in micropigmentation, or tattooing.

BIBLIOGRAPHY

1. Kachhawa D, Kalla G. Keratinocytes—Melanocyte graft technique followed by PUVA therapy for stable vitiligo.
2. Indian J Deramatol Venerol Leprol. 2008;74:622-4.
3. Lamoria A, Agrawal A, Rao P, et al. A Comparative Study between Follicular Unit Transplantation and Autologous Non-cultured Nontrypsinized Epidermal Cells Grafting (Jodhpur Technique) in Stable Vitiligo. J Cutan Aesthet Surg. 2020;13(3):204-9.
4. Verma M, Saini S, Rao P, et al. Tertiary Health Care-Based Randomized Controlled Study to Compare Autologous, Non-cultured, Nontrypsinized Epidermal Cell Transplant (Jodhpur Technique) with Split-Thickness Skin Grafting (STSG) in Stable Vitiligo. J Cutan Aesthet Surg. 2022;15(1):33-9.

CHAPTER 42

Surgical Management of Non-Vitiligo Leukoderma

Sanjeev Mulekar, Madhulika Mhatre

KEY MESSAGES

- Non-vitiligo leukodermas form an important spectrum of hypopigmented disorders.
- Conditions include piebaldism, nevus depigmentosus, halo nevus, postburn leukoderma, postdiscoid lupus erythematosus (DLE) depigmentation, postlaser leukoderma, and postdermabrasion leukoderma.
- Piebaldism and postburn leukoderma respond to various surgical transplantation methods consistently.
- Nevus depigmentosus may recur postsurgery.
- Halo nevus shows consistent results.

INTRODUCTION

Leukoderma and hypopigmentation are generic terms used to designate disorders characterized by lightening of the skin due to reduced epidermal melanin. Hypomelanosis is a more specific term that denotes the absence or reduction of melanin in the skin, while amelanosis indicates the total absence of melanin. The term depigmentation refers to the total loss of skin color.[1]

Leukodermas may be genetic or acquired. Among the genetic hypomelanotic disorders, vitiligo is by far the most common leukoderma encountered in clinical practice: Piebaldism and nevus depigmentosus are also commonly seen. Postinflammatory leukodermas may result from many inflammatory dermatoses such as burns, DLE, and treatment with laser and dermabrasion. Halo nevus is a specific type of leukoderma that occurs around a melanocyte nevus. These are not genetically determined but can be considered as experiments of nature that demonstrate that there are mechanisms in humans that can selectively damage pigment cells.[2]

Leukodermas are most striking of all human disease phenotypes due to their characteristic stark patches of white skin, exposing patients to cosmetic embarrassment and social stigma in many societies. However, many of them with absolute stability do not respond to conventional conservative therapies such as psoralen plus ultraviolet A (PUVA) or narrowband ultraviolet B (NB-UVB); therefore, surgical therapies need to be considered. While there are many published reports on surgical treatment for vitiligo, there is a paucity of data on surgical treatment modalities for other hypopigmented disorders.

In this chapter, we review published studies on the surgical management of non-vitiligo leukoderma. PubMed search of all published English literature was conducted by using keywords: Leukoderma, piebaldism, nevus depigmentosus, halo nevus, postdiscoid depigmentation, and postburn leukoderma. The level of evidence was graded on a five-point scale as follows:[3] (I) At least one properly designed randomized controlled trial; (II-1) a well-designed controlled trial without randomization; (II-2) a well-designed cohort or case–control analytic study, preferably more than one center or research group; (II-3) multiple time series with or without intervention or dramatic results from uncontrolled studies; and (III) clinical experience, descriptive studies, or reports of expert committees.

SURGICAL TREATMENT MODALITIES

- *Tissue grafting:*
  - Split-thickness tissue grafting
  - Punch grafting
  - Suction blister roof grafting

  Pieces of pigmented skin are used to transfer melanocytes from normal pigmented parts of a patient's body to hypomelanotic or achromic areas. A dermatome is used to obtain a split-thickness thin graft in the first technique. Punch grafting uses a punch tool to harvest the skin sample. In suction-blister grafting, the roof of an induced blister is the source of melanocytes.
- *Cellular grafting:* Epidermal cells are extracted from a skin sample and transplanted as a suspension. Cellular grafting can be accomplished either by in vitro culture of melanocytes and/or keratinocytes or by noncultured cell suspension.

INDICATIONS

- Piebaldism
- Nevus depigmentosus

- Halo nevus
- Postburn leukoderma
- Post-DLE leukoderma
- Postlaser leukoderma
- Postdermabrasion leukoderma.

Piebaldism (Figs. 1A and B)

Piebaldism is an autosomal dominant genetic skin disease characterized by a white forelock and large vitiligo-like amelanotic macules, generally located on the forehead, ventral and lateral chest and abdomen, mid-upper arms to wrists, and mid-thighs to mid calves.[4] Melanocytes are either absent or greatly reduced in piebald lesions, although islands of hyperpigmentation may occur within leukodermic patches.[5] It does not respond to medical therapy.[4] Several surgical methods, such as minigrafts, epidermal grafts, and split-thickness skin grafts, have been used to treat piebaldism successfully.[6-9] Repigmentation of achromic areas of piebaldism has also been reported with noncultured epidermal cellular grafting[10] and pure melanocyte and epidermal cultured techniques which has the advantage of treating large surface areas with a smaller skin biopsy sample.[11-14] However, the value of this data is limited by the low number of patients and/or by the small size of treated lesions except by Guerra et al. who reported treatment of very large areas without any scarring by epidermal culture **(Table 1)**.

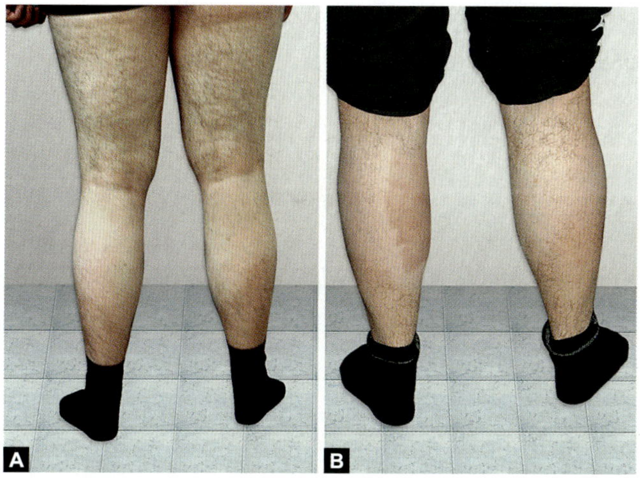

Figs. 1A and B: (A) Piebaldism pretreatment; (B) Piebaldism post-treatment. Please note color mismatch.

Nevus Depigmentosus (Figs. 2A and B)

Nevus depigmentosus is a congenital, nonprogressive cutaneous hypomelanosis, which can present as a circumscribed irregular, oval, or round macule or as a unilateral band or streak with a block-like configuration or arranged along Blaschko's lines.[15] The lesions are hypomelanotic and remain unchanged throughout life although they may enlarge proportionately with the growing child. Different therapeutic attempts have been made to achieve repigmentation of nevus, such as epidermal grafting, noncultured melanocyte-keratinocyte suspension, and cultured epidermis bearing melanocytes.[10,16-21] All authors except Olsson have reported successful repigmentation varying from 80 to 100%. Long-term outcome has been monitored over a period of 2.5 years with sustained repigmentation by Raskovic et al.,[21] but Kim et al. reported recurrence of nevus 8 years after successful repigmentation.[17] Mulekar et al.,[20] in a prospective uncontrolled study, observed 80–100% repigmentation, but uneven repigmentation in two, and 100% good-quality repigmentation in one of six patients treated with noncultured melanocyte transplantation, while two failed to repigment. Based on the available evidence, it can be concluded that though repigmentation of nevus depigmentosus is possible by grafting techniques, the results are inconsistent and recurrence is possible **(Table 2)**.

TABLE 1: Piebaldism.

Method	*Study*	*Patients*	*Repigmentation*	*Type of study*	*Level of evidence*	*Reference*
Cultured autologous	Lerner et al.	1	Excellent	Case report		J Invest Dermatol. 1987[11]
Cultured autologous	Kumagai and Uchikoshi	1	Normal			Ann Plast Surg. 1997[13]
Split-thickness graft	Njoo et al.	12	95–100%			Br J Dermatol. 1998[8]
Cultures autologous	Guerra et al.	6	95%			Br J Dermatol. 2004[14]
Punch grafts	Selmanowitz					Cutis. 1979[6]
Epidermal sheet grafts	Olsson and Juhlin					Acta Derm Venereol. 1997[7]
Cultured and noncultured autologous melanocytes, autologous ultrathin epidermal sheets	Olsson and Juhlin			Retrospective questionnaire study	III	Br J Dermatol. 2002[9]
Noncultured cellular	van Geel et al.	3	Mean 85–90%			Br J Dermatol. 2010[10]
Cultured epidermis+ minigrafting	Falabella et al.	1	100%			Dermatol Surg. 1995[12]

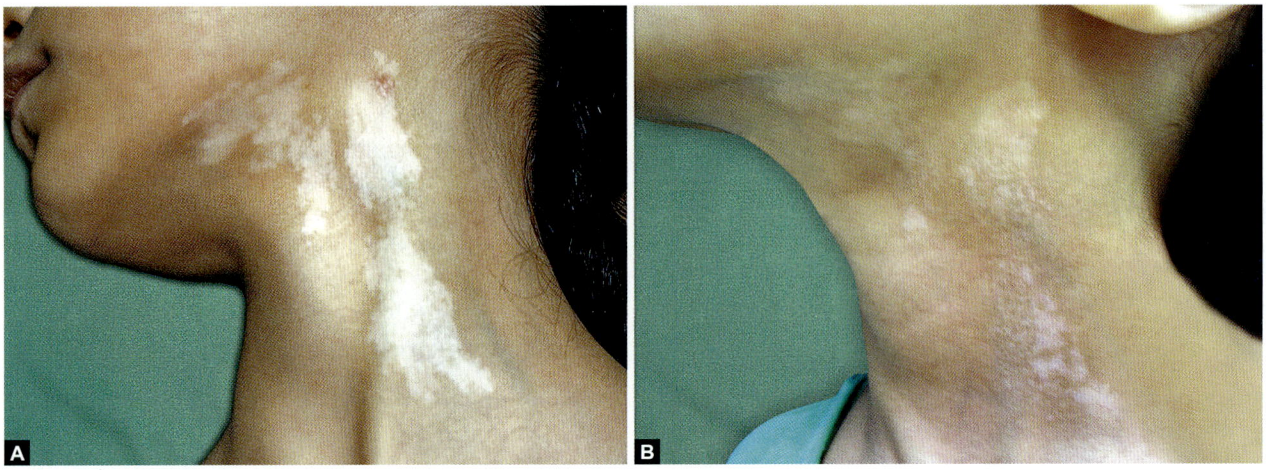

Figs. 2A and B: (A) Nevus depigmentosus pretreatment; (B) Nevus depigmentosus post-treatment. Please note incomplete repigmentation.

TABLE 2: Nevus depigmentosus.

Method	*Study*	*Patients*	*Repigmentation*	*Type of study*	*Level of evidence*	*Reference*
Epidermal graft	Gupta and Goel	1	Good in grafted area	Single case report	III	Dermatol Surg. 2005[16]
Epidermal graft	Kim et al.	1	Good but recurred after 8 years	Single case report	III	J Am Acad Dermatol. 2008[17]
Cultured epidermis	Raskovic et al.	1	Complete	Single case report	III	J Am Acad Dermatol. 2006[21]
Noncultured epidermis	Gauthier et al.	1	80%		III	J Am Acad Dermatol. 1992[18]
Noncultured epidermis	Olsson and Juhlin	1	0%		III	Br J Dermatol. 1998[19]
Noncultured epidermis	Mulekar et al.	5+1	Poor—2 80–100%—3			J Cutan Aesthet Surg. 2011[20]
Noncultured epidermal cellular grafting	van Geel et al	1	78%			Br J Dermatol. 2010[10]

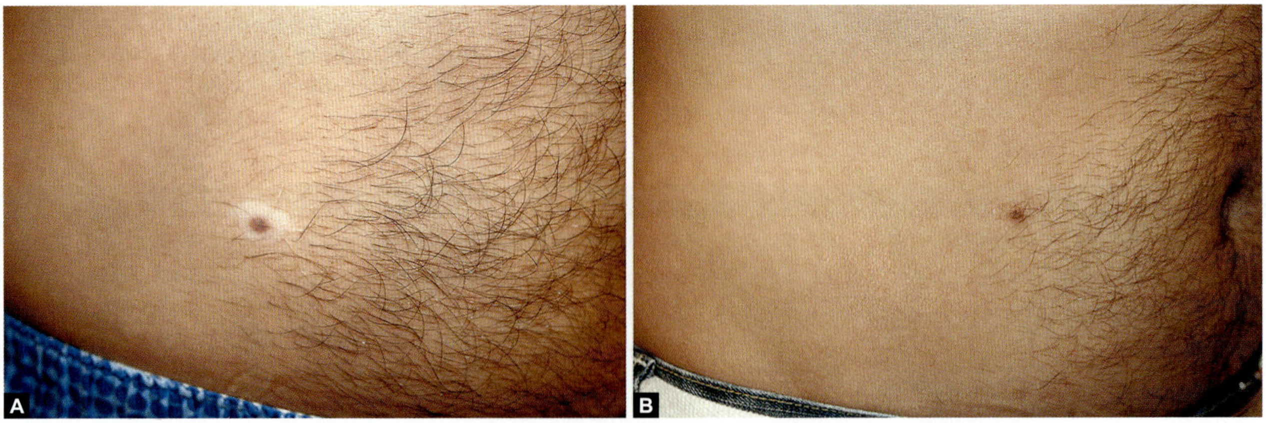

Figs. 3A and B: (A) Halo nevus pretreatment; (B) Halo nevus post-treatment.

Halo Nevus (Figs. 3A and B)

Halo nevus is a pigmented nevus, surrounded by a ring of depigmentation that may progress to spontaneous disappearance of the nevus.[22] The cause of the halo is difficult to explain solely by cellular or humoral mechanism and could be attributed to a product released from damaged nevus cells or a cytokine produced by the inflammatory cells.[2] The treatment of halo nevus is controversial because it is suspected but unproven that it (halo nevus) may result from nevus cells that are atypical or undergoing malignant transformation. Recommendations range from observation requiring no therapy to excision biopsy.[2] PubMed search revealed only two studies which reported long-term results of different surgical therapies. Van Geel et al. reported 11 patients of halo nevi treated with noncultured epidermal cellular grafting with a mean repigmentation of 91 and 90% of patients achieving repigmentation of ≥75%. A diffuse hypopigmented color mismatch was more frequently observed. In some exceptional cases, a peripheral white ring also was present.[10] Olsson and Juhlin reported three cases of halo nevi each treated by transplantation of cultured autologous melanocytes, autologous ultrathin epidermal sheets, and autologous basal cell layer suspension, respectively.[9] Two patients who received cellular grafting showed 65–95% repigmentation and one who was grafted with ultrathin epidermal sheet showed 22–64% repigmentation of the trunk and the neck. We have experienced consistent repigmentation with very good color matching of most halo nevi treated in patients with skin type 3–5[23] **(Table 3)**.

Postburn Leukoderma (Figs. 4A and B)

Postburn leukoderma usually results when deeper burns heal with secondary intention. It is characterized by chalk-white depigmented lesions of variable sizes and shapes with the disappearance of melanocytes which appear at the site of the burn injury and remain unchanged subsequently. The exact mechanism of developing leukoderma following burn injuries is not known. Medical therapies are not known to be effective in the treatment of postburn leukoderma. Tissue grafting methods reported to treat postburn leukoderma are chip skin grafting, epidermal grafting, and thin skin grafting. There are three prospective uncontrolled studies and two case report series. Kahn and Cohen reported excellent graft take in 29 of 30 operative procedures performed on 21 patients with depigmentation following burn injuries. Color match was rated excellent in 34% (n = 10) of the procedures and good in 62% (n = 19). The follow-up period varied from 2 weeks to 94 months with an average of 17 months. Among the adverse effects, most patients developed milia following the procedure.[24] Açikel et al. treated 13 patients with thin split-thickness grafting with a follow-up period of 1–12 months (average 8 months). The surface area of the treated leukoderma sites ranges from 0.5 to 3% of the total body surface area. The skin graft take was 100% in 12 patients while 1 graft was lost due to hematoma. The color match was rated excellent in five of the procedures (38.5), good in six (46%), and fair in two (15%).[25] Three patients of postburn gas leukoderma treated with epidermal grafts showed 100% repigmentation with good color matching. The follow-up period was 6–14 months. The size of the lesions treated is not mentioned.[26] In another series, three patients were treated with minigrafting with adequate repigmentation. Cobblestone appearance was seen in one of them.[27] Falabella described for the first-time epidermal grafting in three patients with postburn leukoderma with 100% take of the grafts.[28] Mulekar et al. reported for the first time good to excellent repigmentation in postburn leukoderma with noncultured melanocyte-keratinocyte transplantation[29] **(Table 4)**.

TABLE 3: Halo nevus.

Method	*Study*	*Patients*	*Repigmentation*	*Type of study*	*Level of evidence*	*Reference*
Noncultured epidermal cellular grafting	van Geel et al.	11	91%		III	Br J Dermatol. 2010[10]
Cultured and noncultured autologous melanocytes, autologous ultrathin epidermal sheets	Olsson and Juhlin	2 1	65–95% 22–64%	Retrospective questionnaire study	III	Br J Dermatol. 2002[9]

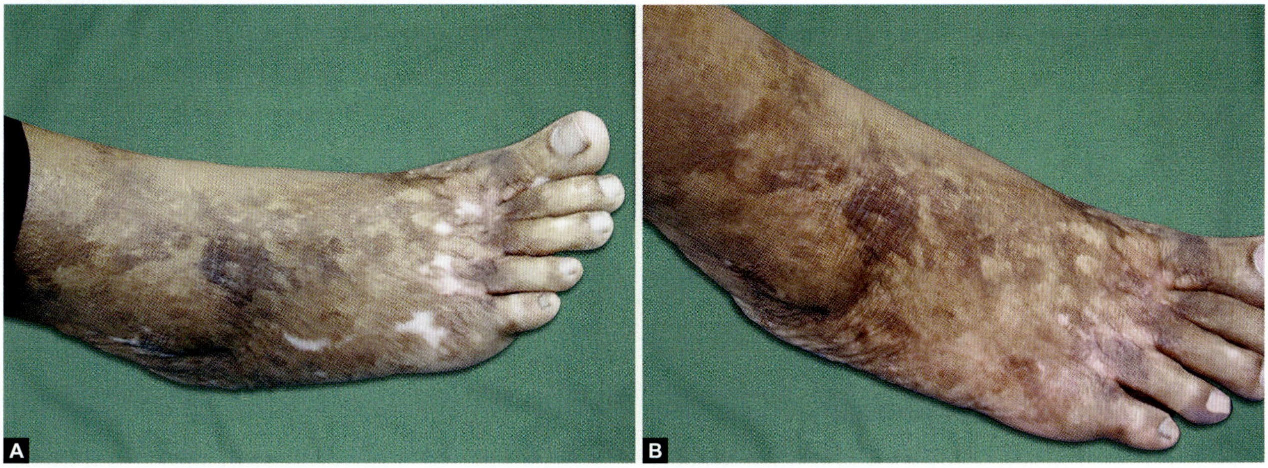

Figs. 4A and B: (A) Postburn leukoderma pretreatment; (B) Postburn leukoderma post-treatment.

TABLE 4: Postburn leukoderma.

Method	Study	Patients	Repigmentation	Type of study	Level of evidence	Reference
Dermabrasion + chip skin graft	Harashina T et al.					Br J Plast Surg. 1985[35]
Dermabrasion + thin skin graft	Onur Erol O et al.					Plast Reconstr Surg. 1990[36]
Thin skin graft	Kahn and Cohen	20	Good, excellent	Prospective uncontrolled		Burns. 1996[24]
Thin minigraft	Fuji et al.	3	Excellent	Case report		Dermatol Surg. 2007[27]
Epidermal graft	Falabella	4		Case report		Arch Dermatol. 1971[28]
Autologous graft	Suvanprakorn et al.	3	Good	Prospective uncontrolled study		J Am Acad Dermatol. 1985[26]
CO_2 laser + dermabrasion + thin skin graft	Açikel et al.	13	Excellent	Prospective uncontrolled		Plast Reconstr Surg. 2000[25]
Noncultured epidermis	Mulekar et al.	7+3	Excellent			Burns. 2011[29]

TABLE 5: Postdiscoid lupus erythematosus (DLE).

Method	Study	Patients	Repigmentation	Type of study	Level of evidence	Reference
Epidermal graft	Gupta	1		Case		Dermatology. 2001[30]
Noncultured melanocyte–keratinocyte transplantation procedure (MKTP)	Mulekar et al.	1	98%	Case		Dermatol Surg. 2008[31]

Postdiscoid Lupus Erythematosus Leukoderma

Long-standing lesions of DLE may heal with depigmented scars and is very difficult to induce repigmentation by conventional methods such as the use of topical steroids and topical or systemic photosensitizers. In addition, histopathologically, DLE lesions destroy areas deep into the hair follicles in the skin, thus destroying the main reservoir for melanocytes. Epidermal grafts by suction blister, which is well known to improve recalcitrant vitiligo, were used to treat four patients of postdiscoid depigmentation with repigmentation of >100% of the grafted area due to the peripheral spread of the pigment.[30] Use of noncultured melanocyte–keratinocyte suspension is another modality to treat post-DLE depigmentation[31] **(Table 5)**.

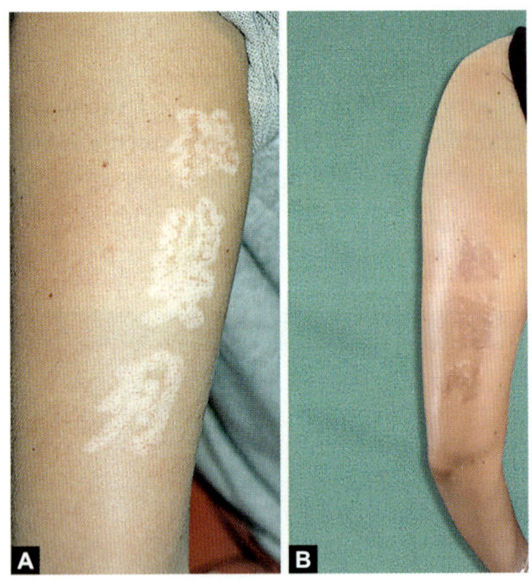

Figs. 5A and B: (A) Postlaser leukoderma pretreatment; (B) Postlaser leukoderma post-treatment. Please note initial hyperpigmentation.

Postlaser Leukoderma (Figs. 5A and B)

Various lasers are used in the treatment of melasma, tattoo removal, telangiectasia, etc. This may result in loss of pigment and is usually restricted to the area of treatment. We treated one patient of depigmented macules on the face that resulted from the treatment of telangiectasia with V beam laser with noncultured melanocyte–keratinocyte transplantation. Olsson reported his experience of treating leukoderma caused by laser. However, these reports are anecdotal and in the form of personal experience.[32]

Postdermabrasion Leukoderma

Mechanical dermabrasion using diamond fraise wheels was commonly practiced by plastic surgeons for facial resurfacing. There is only a single report by Flabella of treatment of postdermabrasion leukoderma which may be a rare complication.[33]

DISCUSSION

Non-vitiligo leukoderma makes an important spectrum of hypopigmented disorders; most of them are responsive to surgical intervention. However, there seems to be unawareness among patients and physicians about the possible ways of intervention. This has led to a lack of sufficient literature supporting the therapeutic options.

Among the conditions discussed, piebaldism and postburn leukoderma respond to various surgical transplantation methods consistently. Therefore, these conditions may be recommended to be treated by surgical transplantation methods. Hypopigmentation observed in halo nevus shows repigmentation when treated with cell suspension transplantation. Patients with halo nevi are psychologically disturbed due to their cosmetic appearance resembling the headlights of a car as described by one, especially after tanning in summer in the European continent, and due to its resemblance to vitiligo in South and Middle East Asia. Initial reports of successful repigmentation should be followed up with long-term observation to assess the potential recurrence and development of atypical melanocytes. No untoward effects have been reported by any of the investigators till date.

Nevus depigmentosus is a matter of concern for both the patient and the physician. Though positive results have been reported by many, the quality of repigmentation remains an area of uncertainty, and recurrence is possible. More studies are indicated to find the mechanism of melanosome distribution in nevoid lesion. We advise caution and in-depth discussion with the patient and his/her parents before exercising the surgical intervention.

Hypothetically, postinflammatory depigmentation should respond well to surgical transplantation unless associated with an underlying autoimmune cause. Laser procedures are on the rise, especially for tattoo removal; treatment of telangiectasia and hypopigmentation due to laser is likely to increase in the near future. Awareness of the potential of surgical transplantation methods will increase the reports of such cases.

Questions may be raised about the lack of controlled studies to prove the efficacy of the surgical methods in these disorders. However, studies by Lerner et al.[11] and van Geel et al.[34] support the efficacy of cellular suspension against a placebo in the case of piebaldism and vitiligo patients, respectively. The efficacy of cellular transplantation seems to be beyond doubt at least in those conditions associated with complete loss or absence of melanocytes.

CONCLUSION

Non-vitiligo leukodermas form an important spectrum of hypopigmented disorders; treatment with surgical modalities should be better studied in the management of these patients.

REFERENCES

1. Ortonne JP. Vitiligo and other disorders of hypo-pigmentation. In: Bolognia J, Jorizzo JL, Rapini RP (Eds). Dermatology. London UK: Mosby; 2003. pp. 947-73.
2. Brochez L, Boone B, Naeyaert JM. Hypomelanoses associated with melanocytic neoplasia. In: Nordlund JJ, Boissy RE, Hearing VJ, King RA, Oetting WS, Ortonne JP (Eds). The Pigmentary System, 2nd edition. Oxford UK: Blackwell Publishing Ltd.; 2006. pp. 705-24.
3. Harris RP, Helfand M, Woolf SH, Lohr KN, Mulrow CD, Teutsch SM, et al. Current methods of the US Preventive Services Task Force: a review of the process. Am J Prev Med. 2001;20(3 Suppl):21-35.
4. Mosher DB, Fitzpatrick TB, Ortonne J-P, Hori Y. Hypomelanoses and hypermelanoses. In: Freedberg IM, Eisen AZ, Wolf K, Austen KF, Goldsmith LA, Katz SI (Eds). Dermatology in General Medicine, 5th edition. New York: McGraw-Hill; 1999. p. 961.
5. Spritz RA. Piebaldism, Waardenburg syndrome, and related disorders of melanocyte development. Semin Cutan Med Surg. 1997;16:15-23.
6. Selmanowitz VJ. Pigmentary correction of piebaldism by autografts. II. Pathomechanism and pigment spread in piebaldism. Cutis. 1979;24:66-73.
7. Olsson MJ, Juhlin L. Epidermal sheet grafts for repigmentation of vitiligo and piebaldism, with a review of surgical techniques. Acta Derm Venereol. 1997;77:463-6.
8. Njoo MD, Nieuweboer-Krobotova L, Westerhof W. Repigmentation of leucodermic defects in piebaldism by dermabrasion and thin split-thickness skin grafting in combination with minigrafting. Br J Dermatol. 1998;139: 829-33.
9. Olsson MJ, Juhlin L. Long-term follow-up of leucoderma patients treated with transplants of autologous cultured melanocytes, ultrathin epidermal sheets and basal cell layer suspension. Br J Dermatol. 2002;147:893-904.
10. van Geel N, Wallaeys E, Goh BK, De Mil M, Lambert J. Long-term results of noncultured epidermal cellular grafting in vitiligo, halo naevi, piebaldism and nevus depigmentosus. Br J Dermatol. 2010;163:1186-93.
11. Lerner AB, Halaban R, Klaus S, Moellmann GE. Transplantation of human melanocytes. J Invest Dermatol. 1987;89:219-24.
12. Falabella R, Barona MI, Escobar C, Borrero I, Arrunategui A. Surgical combination therapy for vitiligo and piebaldism. Dermatol Surg. 1995;21:852-7.
13. Kumagai N, Uchikoshi T. Treatment of extensive hypomelanosis with autologous cultured epithelium. Am Plast Surg. 1997;39:68-73.
14. Guerra L, Primavera G, Raskovic D, Pellegrini G, Golisano O, Bondanza S, et al. Permanent repigmentation of piebaldism by erbium:YAG laser and autologous cultured epidermis. Br J Dermatol. 2004;150:715-21.
15. Di Lernia V. Segmental nevus depigmentosus: analysis of 20 patients. Pediatr Dermatol. 1999;16:349-53.
16. Gupta S, Goel A. Letter to the Editor: nevus depigmentosus needs transplant of epidermal sheets. Dermatol Surg. 2005;31:1746-7.
17. Kim DY, Park YK, Hann SK. Recurrence of nevus depigmentosus after an autologous epidermal graft. J Am Acad Dermatol. 2008;58:527-8.
18. Gauthier Y, Surleve-Bazeille JE. Autologous grafting with noncultured melanocytes: a simplified method for treatment of depigmented lesions. J Am Acad Dermatol. 1992;26:191-4.
19. Olsson MJ, Juhlin L. Leucoderma treated by transplantation of a basal cell layer enriched suspension. Br J Dermatol. 1998;138:644-8.
20. Mulekar SV, Al Issa A, Al Eisa A. Nevus depigmentosus treated by melanocyte-keratinocyte transplantation. J Cutan Aesthet Surg. 2011;4:29-32.
21. Raskovic D, Bondanza S, Gobello T, Luci A, Zambruno G, Happle R, et al. Autologous in vitro reconstituted epidermis in the treatment of a large nevus depigmentosus. J Am Acad Dermatol. 2006;54(5 Suppl.):S238-40.
22. Wayte DM, Helwig EB. Halo nevi. Cancer. 1968;22:69-90.

23. Mulekar SV, Al Issa A. National Center for Vitiligo and Psoriasis, Riyadh, Saudi Arabia. Personal communication.
24. Kahn AM, Cohen MJ. Treatment for depigmentation following burn injuries. Burns. 1996;22(7):552-4.
25. Açikel C, Ulkür E, Güler MM. Treatment of burn scar depigmentation by carbon dioxide laser-assisted dermabrasion and thin skin grafting. Plast Reconstr Surg. 2000;105(6): 1973-78.
26. Suvanprakorn P, Dee-Ananlap S, Pongsomboon C, Klaus S. Melanocyte autologous grafting for treatment of leukoderma. J Am Acad Dermatol. 1985:13;968-74.
27. Fuji M, Terashi H, Hashikawa K, Nomura T, Omori M, Tahara S. Thin minigrafting technique for postburn leukoderma. Dermatol Surg. 2007;33:1368-73.
28. Falabella R. Epidermal grafting. An original technique and its application in achromic and granulating areas. Arch Dermatol. 1971;104:592-600.
29. Mulekar SV, Al Issa A, Al Eisa A. Treatment of post-burn leucoderma with non-cultured melanocyte-keratinocyte transplantation (MKTP). Burns. 2011;37:448-52.
30. Gupta S. Epidermal grafting for depigmentation due to discoid lupus erythematosus. Dermatology. 2001;202:320-3.
31. Mulekar SV, Ghwish B, Al Issa A, Al Eisa A. Melanocyte-Keratinocyte transplantation for postdiscoid lupus erythematosus depigmentation. Dermatol Surg. 2008;34: 261-3.
32. Olsson MJ. Surgical treatments of leukodermas other than vitiligo vulgaris. In: Gupta S, Olsson MJ, Kanwar AJ, Ortonne JP (Eds). Surgical Management of Vitiligo. Oxford UK: Blackwell Publishing; 2007. pp. 238-45.
33. Falabella R. Repigmentation of stable leukoderma. J Dermatol Surg Oncol. 1987;13:44-8.
34. van Geel N, Ongenae K, De Mil M, Haeghen YV, Vervaet C, Naeyaert JM. Double-blind placebo-controlled study of autologous transplanted epidermal cell suspensions for repigmenting vitiligo. Arch Dermatol. 2004;140:1203-8.
35. Harashina T, Iso R. The treatment of leukoderma after burns by a combination of dermabrasion and "chip" skin grafting. Br J Plast Surg . 1985;38(3):301-5.
36. Onur Erol O, Atabay K. The treatment of burn scar hypopigmentation and surface irregularity by dermabrasion and thin skin grafting. Plast Reconstr Surg. 1990;85(5): 754-8. doi: 10.1097/00006534-199005000-00016. PMID: 2326358.

CHAPTER 43

Complications of Vitiligo Surgery

Niti Khunger, Alka Goel

KEY MESSAGES

- Complications in vitiligo surgery include those which are specific to vitiligo surgery and others which are nonspecific and common to any surgery such as infection, scarring, and keloids.
- Specific complications include failure of complete pigmentation due to poor choice of patient (unstable disease), poor choice or execution of technique, partial pigmentation, perigraft halo of depigmentation, and poor cosmetic color matching and texture with surrounding normal skin.
- Punch grafting is associated with the highest number of side effects. Cellular grafts are associated with the least incidence of side effects.
- Since the criteria for case selection (stability) are inadequately defined, relapse is a possibility in all cases and this needs to be emphasized during counseling.

INTRODUCTION

Complications in vitiligo surgery include those which are common to any surgical procedure such as reactions to medications and anesthetic agents, infections, delayed healing, scars and keloid formation, and those that are specific to the technique of vitiligo surgery **(Box 1)**. To minimize the risk of complications, the surgery should be performed in an operation theater setting, with all aseptic precautions. Preoperative evaluation to identify patients at risk, adequate counseling of the patient, explaining all limitations and likely complications, and clear postoperative instructions are the keys to prevent patient dissatisfaction following surgery. A motivated patient who diligently follows instructions and takes all precautions is equally important for a successful surgery.

BOX 1: General complications of vitiligo surgery.

Nonspecific:
- Reaction to anesthetic agents and medications
- Pain
- Bleeding
- Infection
- Delayed healing
- Scarring
- Keloids

Specific to vitiligo surgery:
- Inadequate graft material
- Failure of graft uptake
- Failure of pigmentation
- Partial repigmentation
- Textural mismatch
- Cosmetic mismatch
- Relapse of disease with reversal of pigmentation

GENERAL COMPLICATIONS

General complications can be immediate or delayed. Immediate complications are bleeding, pain, damage to important structures, and adverse reactions to anesthetic. Delayed complications include infection at donor or recipient site, delayed healing, and scarring.

Bleeding

Generally, bleeding is not common in vitiligo surgery as most surgery is superficial and limited to the upper dermis. However, bruising can occur on the forehead, face, and eyelids, and bleeding on the scalp may be seen in patients with bleeding disorders or on medications such as aspirin, warfarin, dipyridamole, clopidogrel, dabigatran, and heparin. A history to rule out the above factors is important as bleeding can also lead to hematoma and graft failure.

Reactions to Anesthetics

Local anesthetics are generally safe. However, adverse reactions may occur if a large volume is injected in large areas or if the anesthetic is inadvertently injected into a blood vessel. Hence, aspiration before injecting is absolutely important. With large volumes, mild reactions can occur such as tingling of mouth, dizziness, and metallic taste. Severe reactions are rare and include slurring of speech, confusion, diplopia, muscle twitching, and even seizures. Coma and cardiovascular toxicity such as arrhythmia and cardiac arrest are potential complications of overdose of lignocaine. Hence, the safe limit should not be crossed and the volume of anesthetic administered must be recorded. Local anesthetics are often given with adrenaline to minimize bleeding and prolong the action. Large volumes of adrenaline can cause headache, tachycardia, chest pain, high blood pressure, and tremors. True allergy to local anesthetics is very uncommon, especially with the amides.

Damage to Important Structures

These are very rare complications in vitiligo surgery as the surgery is not deep enough. However, where nerves are superficial, paresthesia or sensory impairment can occur.

Infection

Infection occurs if aseptic precautions are not followed, such as inadequate sterilization of instruments, improper surgical setting, long duration of surgery, and infection near the surgical site. Patient factors such as immunosuppression, uncontrolled diabetes, malnutrition, poor blood supply to the areas, old age, and sites such as lower legs and flexures are more prone to infection. Proper hand hygiene of the surgical team and optimum operating room environment are essential to reduce the risk of infection.[1] Localized redness, pain, and edema are the first signs of infection and the physician and patient must be alert to these signs so that treatment can be started early.

SPECIFIC COMPLICATIONS

Specific complications can occur in the donor as well as the recipient sites. Some complications occur in relation to improper case selection, poor choice of method, or poor technique, which are common to all vitiligo surgeries. Such complications are shown in **Box 1**. Complications related to a specific technique are enumerated in **Box 2**. In general, cellular grafts appear to have the least incidence of side effects, whereas tissue grafts are reported to be associated with more adverse effects. The maximum number of adverse events is seen when minipunch grafting (MPG) and thin split thickness skin grafting.[2]

BOX 2: Complications observed at the recipient and donor areas in transplantation procedures.

Recipient area:
- Hyperpigmentation
- Perigraft halo- or hypopigmented borders
- Cobblestone appearance
- Contact dermatitis to topical medication
- Milia/inclusion cysts
- Thick margins/stuck-on appearance
- Variegated appearance
- Infection
- Scarring

Donor area:
- Hyperpigmentation
- Hypopigmentation
- Scarring
- Koebner's phenomenon
- Infection
- Hypertrophic scar/keloid formation

Inadequate Graft Material

Inadequate graft material, which is less than that required in the recipient area, is more common with ultrathin grafts that contract after harvesting, such as with suction blister technique and ultrathin split-thickness grafts. To avoid this, the donor area should be at least 5–10% more than the recipient area.

Graft Failure

Failure of graft uptake can occur due to inadequate immobilization over mobile areas such as over joints, lips, eyelids, or collection of serous fluid under the graft. This is more common with thin split-thickness skin grafts (STSGs) and suction blister grafts. Strict immobilization by the use of splints over mobile areas and pressure dressings will minimize this complication. Failure of graft uptake can also occur if there is bleeding or hematoma under the graft. To prevent this, hemostasis must be ensured before the dressing, a pressure dressing should be applied using an adhesive bandage, and the patient must be advised to avoid mobility over the grafted area at least for 24–48 hours till neovascularization takes place. Infection or excessive movement, with shifting of grafts and upside-down placement of graft, can also lead to graft rejection.[3] In very thin grafts, it may be difficult to distinguish the epidermal and dermal sides. There will be a failure of graft uptake if the epidermal side is put face down. To avoid this complication, a sterile slide can be pressed on the donor graft after harvesting and everted so that the dermal side faces upward.[3]

Graft failure can be minimized by:
- Placing the graft on the recipient patches after the bleeding is controlled
- Postoperative immobilization by securing the graft by proper pressure dressings and use of splints over mobile areas
- Prophylactic antibiotics.

Failure of graft uptake is more common in the acral areas, particularly fingers and toes. Adequate immobilization with splints and adequate deep level of dermabrasion may minimize the risk of graft failure. Overall, thin splitthickness graft has the highest success rate compared to other methods.

Failure of Pigmentation and Partial Pigmentation

Only a stable case with no signs of active disease should be taken up for surgery. An unstable case leads to failure to repigment. An unstable vitiligo can also lead to depigmentation at the donor site due to Koebnerization. A multicentric report suggested that lesional stability was more important than disease stability.[4] The details of the stability of the disease are discussed in the previous chapter.

Activity of vitiligo is unpredictable and the disease can recur at any time. This should be clearly explained to the patient before the surgery. Relapse of disease with depigmentation of the graft can occur in spite of correct technique due to reactivation of vitiligo.

Color Mismatch (Hyperpigmentation and Hypopigmentation)

Repigmentation may not occur in the same manner in all patients. A slight degree of hyperpigmentation is frequently observed with all methods, and especially in darker skin types, Fitzpatrick phototype IV–VI.[5] A possible role of arachidonic acid metabolites has been suggested due to higher levels of tyrosinase and immunoreactive blocus protein found when pigment cells were in vitro cultured for 2 days with prostaglandin D2, leukotriene B4, C4, D4, E4, thromboxane B2, and 12hydroxyeicosatetraenoic acid.[6] Prostaglandin E2 has also been thought to have a similar role.[7] Some patients have a tendency for hyperpigmentation, which may be determined by examining areas of recent superficial skin trauma. Such patients should be counseled regarding the risk of hyperpigmentation at the donor and recipient sites. This hyperpigmentation may persist for years **(Figs. 1A and B)**. It is difficult to manage due to the possible risk of reactivation of the disease associated with hypopigmenting agents. Sunscreens should be advocated on the exposed areas once repigmentation has occurred. Topical steroids like fluticasone propionate or mometasone furoate may be used. Topical tretinoin 0.025% and salicylic acid peels have been found to be beneficial in persistent cases (personal observation).

Hypopigmentation is more common with noncultured melanocyte cell suspensions, if the concentration of melanocytes in the suspension is not adequate or the suspension is spread too thin. It may also occur due to reactivation of vitiligo. This can be managed with psoralen plus ultraviolet A (PUVA) therapy, narrowband ultraviolet B (NBUVB),[8] or the excimer lamp or laser,[9] if topical therapy is not successful **(Fig. 2)**. Nowadays, for cosmetically acceptable repigmentation at the recipient site, newer techniques like CO_2 laser and Er:YAG laser are being utilized to prepare the recipient site.[10]

Cosmetic disfigurement and color mismatch of graft are more common with tissue grafts and infrequent with cellular grafts. Hence, cellular grafts are preferred, particularly in cosmetically important areas such as the face.[11]

PERIGRAFT HALO AND ACHROMIC FISSURES

Perigraft halo is a rim of depigmentation that persists at the outer edge of a grafted vitiligo lesion, while achromic fissures are areas of depigmentation between the grafts **(Figs. 3A and B)**. They are caused by the combined effect of initial

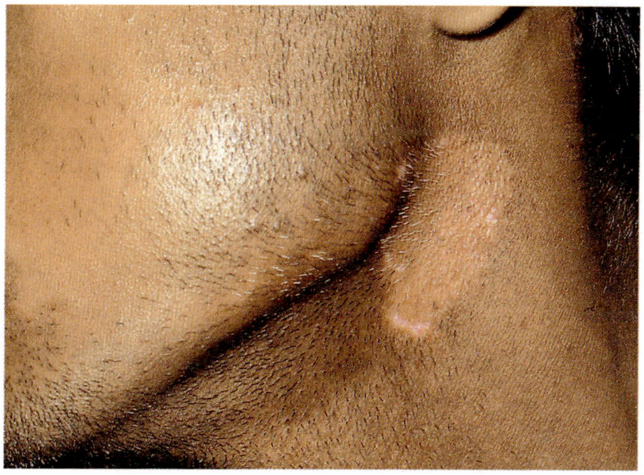

Fig. 2: Hypopigmentation following grafting.

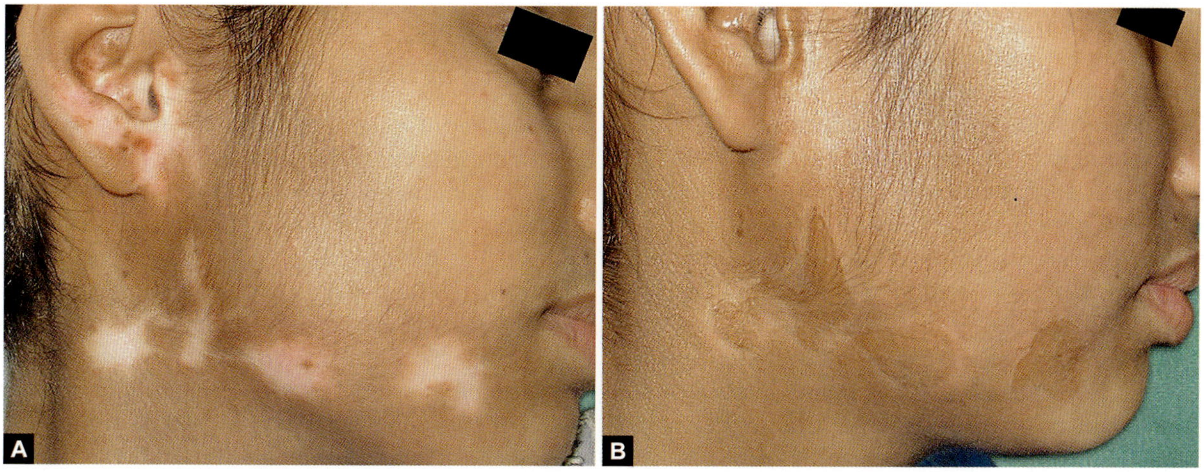

Figs. 1A and B: Persistent hyperpigmentation on the face after split skin grafting.

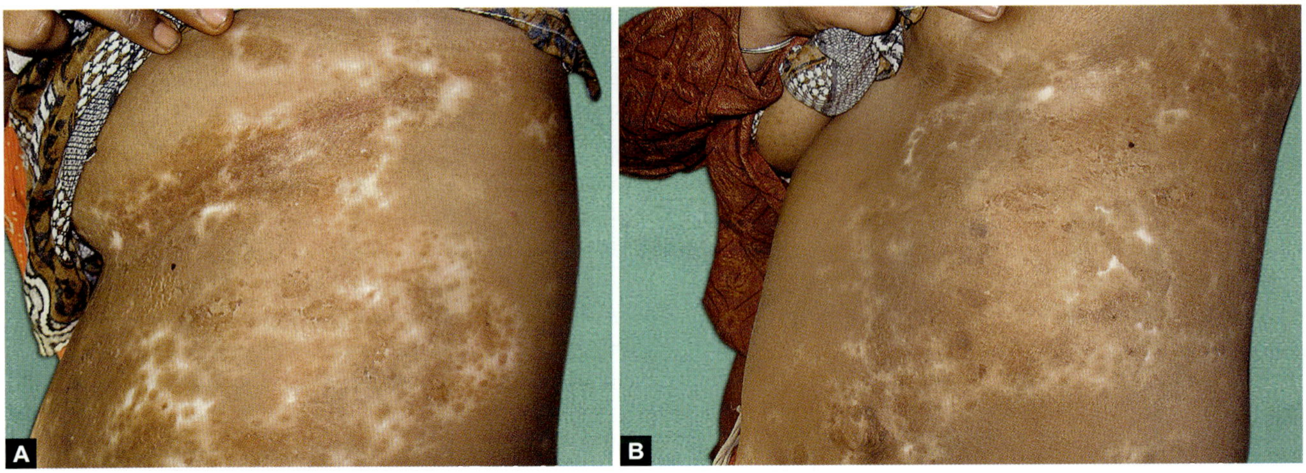

Figs. 3A and B: Perigraft halo with achromic fissures, gradually improving with phototherapy.

contracture of the graft when it is harvested and contraction of the dermal elastin fibers occurring at the recipient site.[11] Immunological reactions at the periphery of the recipient area may also be responsible. Pigment spread may also not be complete, particularly in tissue grafts leading to perigraft halo. This complication may be prevented by overlapping of graft edges at the recipient site and applying the graft 1–2 mm beyond the depigmented area.[12] Proper postoperative dressing and splinting and prolonged application of pressure will also prevent contracture. Postoperative PUVA therapy, NBUVB therapy, or excimer laser is usually corrective.

Cobblestoning (Raised Grafts) and Sunken Pits (Sunken Grafts)

Cobblestone appearance at the recipient site is one of the most common and distressing complications seen with MPG **(Fig. 4)**. Various studies have reported cobblestone appearance in 22–47% of the patients.[13,14] This occurs when large punches are used to obtain donor grafts or when punch recipient sites are not deep enough leading to variable protrusions. Cobblestoning may be prevented by using punches of smaller size (ideally 1–1.5 mm),[12] using thinner grafts, trimming excess dermis if any from the bottom of grafts, and punching the recipient pits 1 mm deeper than the size of the donor grafts. The recommended sizes of biopsy punch to be used for MPG are 1.0 mm for facial areas and 1.2 mm at other sites, particularly in young patients.[12,14] Preventing overcrowding by keeping the grafts at least 5 mm apart from each other also reduces this complication.[15] Silicone gel sheets may be used to prevent or minimize the chances of cobblestoning.[16] It has been observed that with time, cobblestoning gets corrected in most of the cases. In resistant cases, corrective electrofulguration may be needed.[17] Sinking pit or sunken graft is seen when the minigrafts used are smaller than the punched hole sizes. To avoid sunken grafts, appropriate thickness grafts should be chosen.

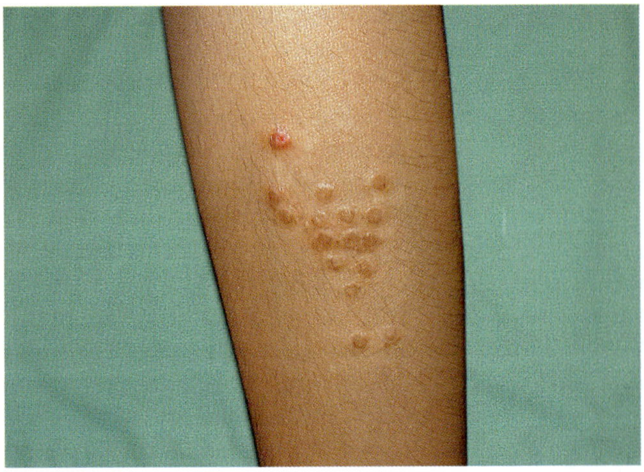

Fig. 4: Persistent cobblestoning in a punch grafting.

Graft Hypertrophy

Graft hypertrophy is seen when the donor grafts are thick **(Fig. 5)**. It usually resolves spontaneously over a period of 3–4 months. Topical steroids and topical retinoids may be used if it is persistent.

Scarring at Donor Site

Some degree of scarring is inevitable while harvesting punch grafts and split-thickness grafts. Scarring at the donor site is not seen with suction blister grafting as the grafts are purely epidermal. Hence, the donor site should be selected with care such as the unexposed area (gluteal region). Scarring on the thigh is more visible and hence should be avoided. To avoid scarring in punch grafting, the donor punches should be very superficial and smaller than 2 mm. Scarring following graft can be prevented by taking very thin dermoepidermal grafts of preferably 0.1–0.3 mm thickness with a suitable dermatome. Plain knives or surgical blades are not preferred for shaving large grafts as they do not provide regular and

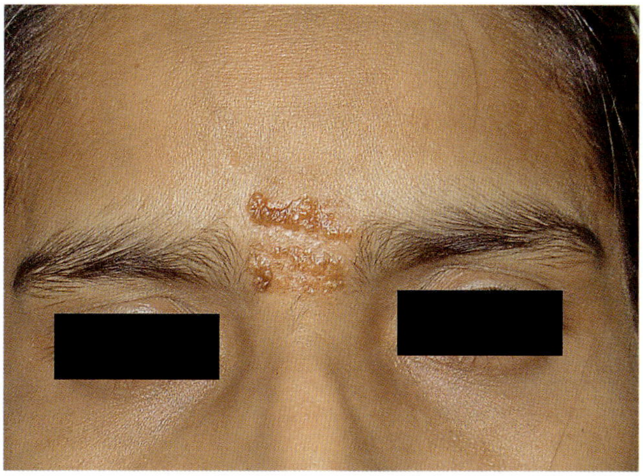

Fig. 5: Graft hypertrophy along with milia formation.

even graft thickness. Surgical skill is acquired with experience and harvesting thin grafts without scarring leads to good cosmetic results, with the added advantage of being able to reuse the same donor site, if required. Dermatomes are ideal for harvesting large thin grafts of even thickness.

Hypertrophic Scars or Keloids

Hypertrophic scars, thick grafts, and grafted areas with uneven surfaces may be seen with all tissue grafts. Hypertrophic scars can also develop at the donor site due to the inability to regulate the depth while attempting to obtain ultrathin grafts or punch grafts. The risk is high in dark-skin individuals with a tendency to keloid formation. Hence, before performing the procedure, old scars should be carefully examined. The motor-driven diamond fraise or wire brush used for dermabrasion at the recipient sites might lead to the formation of hypertrophic scar if dermabrasion is done deeply.[15] Hypertrophic scarring, if it occurs, subsides spontaneously over 3–4 months in most cases. Topical retinoids may be used to hasten the response.[11] Individuals prone to keloids should be evaluated and surgery should preferably be avoided. Suction blister grafting or cellular techniques are better options in such patients, if vitiligo surgery is an absolute necessity. Punch grafting or split-thickness grafting should not be performed in such patients. Appropriate evaluation of old scars, accidental or surgical, should be done and if doubts still persist, a minigrafting test area should be done before the definitive procedure.[18]

Curling of Borders with Beaded Appearance of the Periphery of Grafts

It is usually seen in mesh grafting and fliptop pigment transplantation when grafts with inappropriate thickness are taken. Curling of borders can be prevented by stretching the grafts and smoothening out the edges after placement of the grafts. Postoperative pressure and splinting are also helpful. Once beading has occurred, the "beads" can be snipped off with the scissors or can be lightly dermabraded.

Thick Margins or Stuck-on Tyre Appearance

These occur due to thick grafts. These usually subside spontaneously over a period of 3–4 months as the development of scar tissue below the graft will smooth out the graft but may persist for longer periods.

Inclusion Cyst and Milia Formation

Milia are small epithelial cysts seen commonly in the first 6 months following splitthickness grafting **(Fig. 5)**. They develop due to persistence of remnant of epithelial cells following dermabrasion or due to occlusion of sweat ducts where the outflow is blocked in combination with rapid proliferation of epithelial cells at the end of sweat ducts.[19] It is a temporary phenomenon, commonly seen over the face and neck following split-thickness grafts and not seen with surgical techniques using cellular grafts. Untreated milia resolve spontaneously after some time and do not recur or they can be expressed out with a sterile needle. The incidence of milia formation can be reduced by uniform and even dermabrasion and thorough cleaning of the dermabraded recipient site before application of the graft.[11]

Variegated Appearance

Depending on the technique used, the final results of repigmented areas may vary from patient to patient. The graft may initially appear variegated but later, they lighten up and the border merges so as to match the surrounding skin color in most patients, except a few who may have permanent hyperpigmentation. For successful repigmentation, preparation of the recipient site is important and newer techniques may be helpful in it.[20]

Infection

Infection is a very infrequent complication observed in the available literature. Prevention of infection is important, and appropriate aseptic precautions should be taken while performing transplant procedures.[1,21]

Koebner's Phenomenon

Reactivation of vitiligo at the donor or recipient site or appearance of new lesions may occur in unstable cases or if the disease becomes reactive after a period of stability. This can be minimized with a proper selection of stable vitiligo patients.

INDIVIDUAL TRANSPLANT PROCEDURES AND THEIR COMPLICATIONS

Table 1 summarizes the side effects seen in each type of grafting technique.

TABLE 1: Complications of various surgical procedures for vitiligo.

		PG	SBG	STSG	NCES	HFCS	CM
Donor site	Hyperpigmentation	+	+	++	+	–	+
	Depigmentation	+	+	+	+	–	+
	Scarring	++	–	+	+/–	–	
Receipient site	Hyperpigmentation	++	+	++	+	+	+
	Hypopigmentation	+	+	–	++	–	–
	Perigraft halo	+	+	++	–	+	+
	Cobblestoning	++	–	–	–	–	–
	Stuck on appearance	+	–	++	–	–	–
	Raised edges	–	–	+	–	–	–
	Milia	–	–	+	–	–	+
	Scarring	+	–	+	–	–	–
	Variegated appearance	+++	+	+	+	+	+

Tissue Grafts

Tissue grafts in general have more complications than cellular grafts.

Minipunch Grafts

Minipunch grafting has perhaps the highest complication rate among all grafting methods. Cobblestone appearance, variegated appearance and color mismatch, perigraft halo, graft dislodgment/rejection, static graft (no pigment spread), depigmentation of graft, hypertrophic scar, and keloid formation are the main complications seen at the recipient site.[22] Superficial scarring, Koebner's phenomenon, and hypertrophic scar formation may be seen at the donor site.

Suction Blisters Epidermal Grafts

Suction blister epidermal grafting (SBEG) is generally a safe technique. Perigraft halo of depigmentation, wrinkling and displacement of the graft, and graft rejection are usually the main complications seen. Temporary hyperpigmentation at donor and recipient sites, Koebner's phenomenon, and keloid formation have also been observed in a few studies.[12] Higher suction pressure, if used to raise blisters, may cause rupture of epidermis and hemorrhagic blisters.[23] Liquid nitrogen, if used excessively, can result in severe inflammation causing hypertrophic scarring and postinflammatory hyperpigmentation. It can also cause cryodamage of peripheral melanocytes resulting in a hypopigmented rim around the recipient site. The chance of scarring at the donor site is minimal because the dermis remains intact.[24,25]

Thin Split-thickness Skin Grafts

Complications in this technique are usually operator-dependent. Scarring at the donor site can occur in inexperienced hands. Recipient area may show complications, such as stuckon appearance, perigraft halo, curling of the graft with beaded appearance, displacement of the grafts, cosmetically mismatched pigmentation, and milia formation.[26]

Hair Follicular Grafts

Hair follicle grafting has been performed by a few authors to treat small patches in hairbearing areas and has been found useful in treating lesions with leukotrichia.[24,26] Previously hair follicles were harvested by small strip grafting of hairbearing scalp from the occipital area followed by separation of single hairs, which are then transplanted into vitiligo patches 5–10 mm apart. Currently, follicular unit extraction (FUE) is the method of choice for harvesting hair follicles. Hair follicles are harvested from the occipital area using 0.9- or 0.1-mm metallic punches mounted on a micromotor. Though no major complications were seen in the available studies, this method has several limitations. Hair dissection is a tedious, timeconsuming, and delicate procedure and needs proper training. It is difficult to treat large vitiligo lesions because of the limited number of donor hairs and vitiliginous skin heals slowly because the grafted melanocytes require a long time to spread.[27] Besides, it can only be used in hair-bearing areas.

Cellular Grafts

Cellular grafts generally have a lesser incidence of side effects.

Autologous Noncultured Epidermal Cell Suspension

Reported adverse effects on recipient and donor areas are, in general, minimal as compared to tissue grafts. Mild textural changes at the donor site, cosmetic mismatch at the recipient site, and either hypo or hyperpigmentation at the recipient site are common complaints. Hyperpigmentation or hypopigmentation and hypopigmented halo at the edge of the graft may be seen.[21,28,32] These can be minimized by taking appropriate concentration of melanocytes in the suspension. In a study on 1,060 vitiligo patches in 300 patients where the cell suspension was injected in the recipient area, pain or infection were not observed at therecipient site, but two patients developed keloid at the donor site, 5-6 weeks after cell transplantation. Postinflammatory hyperpigmentation was observed in 32 (10.67%) patients and the Koebner phenomenon (hypopigmentation at the donor site) was observed in six patients at the donor site.[32]

Hair Follicle Melanocyte Cell Suspension

Melanocyte cell suspension obtained from the outer root sheath of the hair follicle is a recently described technique in vitiligo surgery.[33,34] It is based on the principle that the outer root sheath and bulge area of the hair follicle is a reservoir of inactive melanocytes (melanocyte stem cells), which when activated produce melanin pigment and are responsible for perifollicular repigmentation seen clinically in a repigmenting patch of vitiligo. In this technique, hair follicles are extracted by FUE using a 1-mm biopsy punch from the occipital area, trypsinized for 90 minutes in an incubator, and the melanocytes are suspended in Dulbecco's modified Eagle's medium (DMEM) similar to the epidermal cell suspension method.[35] They are then transplanted to the recipient vitiliginous sites prepared after dermabrasion. In the study by Shah et al.,[34] excellent repigmentation (90–100%) was achieved in 60% of patients. No side effects were observed in the donor site. In the recipient site, hyperpigmentation was observed in 75% of patients, which reduced after few months in a few patients. Pruritis (25%), xerosis (10%), and infection were transient side effects. Hyperpigmentation and color mismatch were also observed by Donaparthi and Chopra.[35] In their comparative study, the results were also inferior when compared to epidermal cell suspension. Clearly, there is a need to further standardize this procedure to obtain uniform excellent results.

Transplantation of Cultured Autologous Melanocytes

This procedure treats larger areas successfully without the need for additional phototherapy and is associated with minimal complications at the donor/recipient site.[36,37] However, cultured epidermis is difficult to handle and manipulation affects cell vitality. Mutagenicity and possible risk of cancer have also been cited as potential risks. One of the additives, TPA, also known as 12otetradecanoylphorbol13-acetate, is a selective growth accelerator of the melanocytes. Since this is a tumor promoter, concerns about its long-term safety have been expressed.[38,39] The availability of TPA-free and serumfree media is a possible solution to this problem. A comparative study of the efficacy of cultured versus noncultured melanocyte transfer reported that there was no significant difference between the two groups, but a larger area could be covered with cultured melanocytes (1:100) as compared to noncultured melanocytes (1:10).[40] Complications seen in their study were reactivation and infection in one patient in each group.

REVIEW OF LITERATURE

A systematic review of autologous transplantation methods[41-43] showed the highest rate of success (87%) with suction blister, while the average success rates for other methods varied from 13 to 53%. The maximum incidence of adverse effects was seen with tissue grafts, mainly punch grafting, i.e., cobblestone appearance on the recipient site (27%) and scar formation on the donor sites (40%), followed by split-thickness grafting and SBEG. Cellular grafting was associated with the lowest number of adverse effects. In the recipient site, cobblestone appearance was the predominant complication in punch grafts, whereas hyperpigmentation and thickening of grafts were common in suction blister epidermal grafts and STSGs. In the donor site, superficial scarring and hypopigmentation are the common findings in punch grafts, whereas hyperpigmentation is the main problem in SBEG and to minimize complications and increase chances of success, certain modifications of the technique can be done at different sites.

TIPS TO MINIMIZE COMPLICATIONS

Selection of the proper technique according to the site and size of the recipient sites and stable disease are the key factors to avoid or minimize complications **(Box 3)**. On the face, cellular grafts are preferred. Once healing has occurred, sunscreens should be advocated as hyperpigmentation is common. If it occurs, it can be managed by judicious use of skin-lightening agents. Topical tretinoin is safer. If hyperpigmentation is persistent, light dermabrasion of laser resurfacing may help. In acral areas, strict immobilization by use of splints is advocated. However, in spite of all precautions, acral areas have a high failure rate and the patient should be counseled. A small test area can be done to see the response to surgery.

BOX 3: Tips to achieve good results and avoid complications.[39]

- Avoid
- Procedures in patients with a keloid diathesis
- Patients with unstable, active vitiligo
- Thick dermoepidermal grafts with knife or dermatome
- Punch grafts larger than 1.2 mm (1.0 mm ideal for facial areas)
- Extensive areas without planning full treatment
- Manipulation of recipient sites with excessively invasive methods

CONCLUSION

To conclude, with the advancement in the techniques and horizontal spread of training, surgical therapies are more frequently practiced, especially in Asian countries. Serious postoperative complications arising from dermatologic surgery are uncommon. Not every patient with vitiligo is a good candidate for surgical repigmentation and the key for success is an appropriate selection of patients since there are specific criteria that must be fulfilled for vitiligo surgery. Proper patient counseling about the nature of the disease and the surgery, limitations of the procedure, and whether more procedures will be needed for optimal outcome should be done. The patient should be counseled for all possible therapeutic options and should be given liberty to choose from the available modalities. Many complications may be prevented by preoperative evaluation, sound surgical technique, and careful followup care.

REFERENCES

1. Gaines S, Luo JN, Gilbert J, Zaborina O, Alverdy JC. Optimum operating room environment for the prevention of surgical site infections. Surg Infect (Larchmt). 2017;18(4):503-7.
2. Gupta S, Narang T, Olsson MJ, Ortonne JP. Surgical management of vitiligo and other leukodermas: evidencebased practice guidelines. In: Gupta S, Olson MJ, Kanwar AJ, Ortonne JP (Eds). Surgical Management of Vitiligo. Oxford, UK: Blackwell Publishing Ltd; 2007. pp. 6979.
3. Khunger N, Kathuria SD, Ramesh V. Tissue grafts in vitiligo surgery—past, present, and future. Indian J Dermatol. 2009; 54:150-8.
4. Majid I, Mysore V, Salim T, Lahiri K, Chatterji M, Khunger N, et al. Is lesional stability in vitiligo more important than disease stability for performing surgical interventions? Results from a multicentric study. J Cutan Aesthet Surg. 2016;9(1):13-9.
5. Falabella R. Surgical approaches for stable vitiligo. Dermatol Surg. 2005;31:127784.
6. Falabella R. Treatment of localized vitiligo by autologous minigrafting. Arch Dermatol. 1988;124:164955.
7. Tomita Y, Iwamoto M, Masuda T, Tagami H. Stimulatory effect of prostaglandin E2 on the configuration of normal human melanocytes in vitro. J Invest Dermatol. 1987;89:299301.
8. Lahiri K, Malakar S, Sarma N, Banerjee U. Repigmentation of vitiligo with punch grafting and narrowband UVB (311 nm)—a prospective study. Int J Dermatol. 2005;45:64955.
9. Linthorst Homan MW, Spuls PI, NieuweboerKrobotova L, de Korte J, Sprangers MA, Bos JD, et al. A randomized comparison of excimer laser versus narrowband ultraviolet B phototherapy after punch grafting in stable vitiligo patients. J Eur Acad Dermatol Venereol. 2012;26:6905.
10. Zhang D, Wei X, Hong W, Fu L, Qian G, Xu AE. A retrospective study of long term follow-up of 2283 vitiligo patients treated by autologous, non-cultured melanocyte-keratinocyte transplantation. Aging (Albany NY). 2021;13(4): 5415-25.
11. Khunger N. Thin splitthickness skin grafts for vitiligo. In: Gupta S, Olson MJ, Kanwar AJ, Ortonne JP (Eds). Surgical Management of Vitiligo. Oxford, UK: Blackwell Publishing Ltd; 2007. pp. 10814.
12. Majid I. Grafting in vitiligo: how to get better results and how to avoid complications. J Cutan Aesthet Surg. 2013;6:839.
13. Malakar S, Dhar S. Treatment of stable and recalcitrant vitiligo by autologous miniature punch grafting: a prospective study of 1,000 patients. Dermatology. 1999;198:1339.
14. Falabella R. Surgical therapies for vitiligo and other leukodermas, part 1: minigrafting and suction epidermal grafting. Dermatol Ther. 2001;14:714.
15. Mulekar S. Surgical management of vitiligo. Expert Rev Dermatol. 2010;5:22939.
16. Agarwal US, Jain D, Gulati R, Bhargava P, Mathur NK. Silicone gel sheet dressings for prevention of postminigraft cobblestoning in vitiligo. Dermatol Surg. 1999;25:1024.
17. Malakar S, Lahiri K. Electrosurgery in cobblestoning. Indian J Dermatol. 2000;45:467.
18. Falabella R, Arrunategui A, Barona MI, Alzate A. The minigrafting test for vitiligo: detection of stable lesions for melanocyte transplantation. J Am Acad Dermatol. 1995;32:22832.
19. Olson MJ. Treatment of leukoderma by transplantation of ultra-thin epidermal sheets. In: Gupta S, Olson MJ, Kanwar AJ, Ortonne JP (Eds). Surgical Management of Vitiligo. Oxford, UK: Blackwell Publishing Ltd; 2007. pp. 115-23.
20. Al-Hadidi N, Griffith JL, Al-Jamal MS, Hamzavi I. Role of recipient-site preparation techniques and post-operative wound dressing in the surgical management of vitiligo. J Cutan Aesthet Surg. 2015;8(2):79-87.
21. Mulekar SV. Longterm followup study of 142 patients with vitiligo vulgaris treated by autologous, noncultured melanocytekeratinocyte cell transplantation. Int J Dermatol. 2005;44:8415.
22. Lahiri K. Evolution and evaluation of autologous mini punch grafting in vitiligo. Indian J Dermatol. 2009;54:159-67.
23. Parsad D, Gupta S. Standard guidelines of care for vitiligo surgery. Indian J Dermatol Venereol Leprol. 2008;74: S37-45.
24. Maleki M, Banihashemi M, Sanjari V. Efficacy of suction blister epidermal graft without phototherapy for locally stable and resistant vitiligo. Indian J Dermatol. 2012;57:282-4.
25. Baweja S, Chand S. A prospective observational comparative study of novel autologous negative pressure epidermal harvesting system (ANPEHS or EHS) and suction blister grafting (SBG) in treatment of stable vitiligo. J Cutan Aesthet Surg. 2020;13(4):283-91.
26. Sameem F, Sultan SJ, Ahmad QM. Split thickness skin grafting in patients with stable vitiligo. J Cutan Aesthet Surg. 2011;4:38-40.
27. Thakur P, Sacchidanand S, Nataraj HV, Savitha AS. A study of hair follicular transplantation as a treatment option for vitiligo. J Cutan Aesthet Surg. 2015;8(4):211-7.
28. van Geel N, Wallaeys E, Goh BK, De Mil M, Lambert J. Long-term results of noncultured epidermal cellular grafting in vitiligo, halo naevi, piebaldism and naevus depigmentosus. Br J Dermatol. 2010;163:118693.
29. van Geel N, Goh BK, Wallaeys E, De Keyser S, Lambert J. A review of noncultured epidermal cellular grafting in vitiligo. J Cutan Aesthet Surg. 2011;4:1722.
30. Vakharia PP, Lee DE, Khachemoune A. Efficacy and safety of noncultured melanocyte-keratinocyte transplant procedure for vitiligo and other leukodermas: a critical analysis of the evidence. Int J Dermatol. 2018;57(7):770-5.
31. Gill BS, Brar MS, Chaudhary N, Randhawa A. Non-cultured melanocyte transfer in the management of stable vitiligo. J Family Med Prim Care. 2019;8(9):2912-6.

32. Orouji Z, Bajouri A, Ghasemi M, Mohammadi P, Fallah N, Shahbazi A, et al. A single-arm open-label clinical trial of autologous epidermal cell transplantation for stable vitiligo: a 30-month follow-up. J Dermatol Sci. 2018;89(1):52-9.
33. Kumar A, Mohanty S, Sahni K, Kumar R, Gupta S. Extracted hair follicle outer root sheath cell suspension for pigment cell restoration in vitiligo. J Cutan Aesthet Surg. 2013;6:1215.
34. Shah AN, Marfatia RK, Saikia SS. A study of noncultured extracted hair follicle outer root sheath cell suspension for transplantation in vitiligo. Int J Trichol. 2016;8:6772.
35. Donaparthi N, Chopra A. Comparative study of efficacy of epidermal melanocyte transfer versus hair follicular melanocyte transfer in stable vitiligo. Indian J Dermatol. 2016;6:6404.
36. Chen YF, Yang PY, Hu DN, Kuo FS, Hung CS, Hung CM. Treatment of vitiligo by transplantation of cultured pure melanocyte suspension: analysis of 120 cases. J Am Acad Dermatol. 2004;51:6874.
37. Czajkowski R, Placek W, Drewa T, Kowaliszyn B, Sir J, Weiss W. Autologous cultured melanocytes in vitiligo treatment. Dermatol Surg. 2007;33:102736.
38. Li J, Chen S, Uyama T, Wu W, Xu J. Clinical application of cultured stratified epithelial sheets grown under feeder or feeder-free conditions for stable vitiligo. Dermatol Surg. 2019;45(4):497-505.
39. Khunger N. Commentary on clinical application of cultured stratified epithelial sheets grown under feeder or feeder-free conditions for stable vitiligo. Dermatol Surg. 2019;45(4): 506-7.
40. Verma R, Grewal RS, Chatterjee M, Pragasam V, Vasudevan B, Mitra D. A comparative study of efficacy of cultured versus non cultured melanocyte transfer in the management of stable vitiligo. Med J Armed Forces India. 2014;70(1):26-31.
41. Njoo MD, Westerhof W, Bos JD, Bossuyt PM. A systematic review of autologous transplantation methods in vitiligo. Arch Dermatol. 1998;134:15439.
42. Mulekar SV, Isedeh P. Surgical interventions for vitiligo: an evidence-based review. Br J Dermatol. 2013;169 Suppl. 3:57-66.
43. Bergqvist C, Ezzedine K. Vitiligo: a review. Dermatology. 2020;236:571-92.

CHAPTER 44

Innovations in Vitiligo Surgeries

Somesh Gupta, Sanjeev Gupta, Dilip Kachhawa, Ashique KT, Neha Taneja

KEY MESSAGES

- Innovation involves seeking new and improved methods beyond conventional ones. It is driven by a desire to enhance techniques, embrace subjectivity, brainstorm, and share knowledge, leading to better outcomes, simplified techniques, and cost-efficiency.
- Vitiligo surgeries have advanced from simpler noncultured techniques to complex methods using cultured melanocytes. Dermatosurgeons have significantly contributed to innovating these techniques, making them more effective and economically viable.
- Minigrafting for small depigmented areas has evolved with smaller punches and motorized micropunches. Innovations include using a hypodermic needle for graft transfer and motorized devices for improved precision.
- Suction blister epidermal grafting (SBEG) techniques have undergone innovations in creating epidermal blisters, including using suction syringes, vacuum pumps, and nonelectric alternatives. Heat, household hair dryers, and alternative cups have also been explored to expedite blister formation.
- Various methods for graft transfer have been proposed, such as using microscope glass slides, dressing materials, and household items like hair dryers and eyelid plates for challenging areas.
- Innovations in dermabrasion techniques involve using disposable hypodermic needles, chemical agents, and lasers to optimize de-epithelialization. Dermabrasion alternatives like ultrasonic aspirators and callus removers have been suggested.
- Graft fixation techniques have been refined, including using cyanoacrylate glue, autologous biological dressings, and fibrin glue, leading to improved healing, protection, and graft uptake.
- Thin skin grafting has seen innovations in graft harvesting using disposable razor blades, mesh grafting, and techniques like needling micrografting to enhance graft coverage.
- Innovations in noncultured epidermal cell suspension (NCES) include incubation alternatives like refrigeration and axillary temperature regulation. Modifications in donor area preparation using epidermal brushing and using patient-derived serum or plasma have been proposed.
- Techniques involving hair follicle extraction have been refined, resulting in higher cell yield and improved outcomes for vitiligo repigmentation.

INTRODUCTION

Innovation means trying to find a new and better method, idea, or device to do the work beyond conventional methods. It is a result of wanting to improvise a technique rather than accepting the same, as the final word written or said on the same. It begins by appreciating and recognizing highly subjective insights, frequent brainstorming, and sharing ideas and knowledge with colleagues. It requires oneself to be able to ask the right questions at the right time and to have a firm belief in his ideas, intelligence, hard work, communication skills, and madness about work in small, yet acceptable quantities. The advantages of innovations include better outcomes, simplified techniques, and sometimes easy availability and cost-cutting.

Dermatologic surgery is a well-established segment of dermatology and vitiligo surgeries are evolving continuously for the past half a century with new improvisations and discoveries. In vitiligo surgery, interestingly, cultured melanocytes using complex and advanced culture methods were used first in the late 1980s and simple noncultured cell suspensions were introduced later and this extreme simplification of cell-based therapies without a significant loss of efficacy. Subsequently, with the help of several innovations, the technique has become even simpler.

The last decade has witnessed the birth and/or evolution of a lot of new techniques and instruments in vitiligo surgeries. There have been quite a few dermatologists, including Indian dermatologists, who have made a tremendous contribution in improving outcome, simplifying the different vitiligo surgeries, and made them economically viable. This chapter will focus on describing some of the salient innovations from those.

MINIGRAFTING

This is an easy, simple, and classical procedure used for repigmenting small depigmented areas. As it is not a very popular technique, very few advancements have happened in this technique. The punches used for minigrafting have evolved from Keyes punch to Loo trephine punch and disposable cylindrical punches. Miniaturization itself is an innovation. Earlier, 2.5 mm and 2 mm punches were used, which have been changed to 1.2 mm or even smaller now to improve complications such as cobblestoning.[1] The latest in this is the use of motorized micropunch of 0.7 mm in size.[2]

Laxmisha et al. suggested the use of hypodermic needle to transfer minigrafts to recipient area instead of forceps (cumbersome due to small size of grafts).[3] They used a 23-gauge hypodermic needle to secure the graft by slightly piercing from epidermal side and transfer them from the saline gauze to the recipient area. This modification minimized the trauma, speeded up the procedure, and helped in a smooth transfer of the grafts.

SUCTION BLISTER EPIDERMAL GRAFTING

Suction blister epidermal grafting (SBEG) is one of the established modalities among various vitiligo surgeries. Majority of the innovations and advancements have been made to establish an easy, adequate, and effective method to create suction and form epidermal blisters for grafting. Suction was first used to produce epidermal blisters using angio-sterrometer by Kiistala et al. in 1964.[4] They produced blisters within 2 hours by applying suction at a pressure of -20 mm Hg, to intact healthy human skin, and the roof of which consisted solely of epidermis including the basal layer. This technique of producing epidermal blisters was further modified by using a gastric or respiratory suction machine by Falabella,[5] (who was the first to treat vitiligo with SBEG), foot pedal operated machine and plastic cups,[6] and oil rotary vacuum pump with manometer and suction cups, with pressures of about 200 mm Hg.[7] These techniques required complex instruments, which were expensive, heavy, and cumbersome and may not be easily available. Hence, the technique was further simplified by Indian dermatologists by using suction syringe, where a 20-mL disposable syringe was modified in order to produce the blister.[8] They cut the needle end of syringe and introduced the plunger through this end. To generate negative pressure, they pulled the plunger, which was held in position by a small metal rod. Although this was a cheap and small apparatus that could be assembled in the dermatologist's own office, limitations included inability to measure and control the force and pressure applied and the technique of syringe preparation was a little complex. They also had erroneously concluded that the height of the column of vacuum within the syringe had no effect on the magnitude of the suction generated such that the final height of the piston is arbitrary. Lewis objected to this by applying the Boyle's law.[9] He suggested that the height of the piston within the syringe is directly related to the pressure gradient, thereby, generated. Hence, the magnitude of the gradient will be determined by the height of piston within the syringe. To overcome this limitation, another breakthrough milestone in the history of suction blister grafting was achieved by Gupta et al. who used a cylindrical funnel connected with a three-way tap and suction was given by a 50-mL syringe.[10] The pressure inside the suction cup was retained by changing the position of the lock of the three-way tap. The pressure was measured by connecting the three-way tap to a vacuum gauge. This technique simplified the procedure, had pressure control of 300 mm Hg, and helped to reduce the cost and time required. The glass funnels/cups were replaced by disposable syringes applied upside down on the patient's skin after removal of plunger in further modifications. The authors described another surgical pearl where they used disposable syringe and calculated the column of vacuum or the amount of aspirated air that is necessary to produce a specific pressure gradient in the syringe.[11] They found that the volume of air aspirated by 50 mL syringe through 5 mL, 10 mL, and 20 mL syringe to achieve -300 to -400 mm Hg pressure was 9–13 mL, 14–21 mL, and 25–40 mL, respectively. Generally, 10 mL syringes are the most suitable. Determination of the amount of aspirated air obviated the need to use manometer and, hence, further simplified the technique. The time required for raising suction blisters depends on several factors such as diameter of the suction syringe, site of suction blistering, age of the patient, negative pressure, corticosteroid-induced atrophy, pre-treatment of the site with psoralen plus ultraviolet A (PUVA), and laxity of the skin (especially, pathological variations due to underlying disease states such as cutis laxa and Ehlers–Danlos syndrome). The authors also suggested to use some maneuvers to reduce the blister time formation, e.g., intradermal injection of saline **(Figs. 1A to C)**,[12] intradermal injection of local anesthetics,[13] application of heat, increasing the negative pressure by 100 mm Hg when small vesicles appear in suction area, and choice of skin overlying the greater trochanter of the femur as the donor site. Wood's lamp[14] and infrared lamp[15] have been used for faster induction of suction blister formation (up to 50% reduction in blister formation time), but they may not be readily available in clinics. The use of household hair dryer to reduce the blister formation time in SBEG by increasing the surface temperature to 44°C was suggested by Arora et al.[16] In their study, the mean time taken for the formation of blister reduced from 121 to 70 minutes using hair dryer. Gupta and Kumar used 2, 5, 10, 20, and 50 mL syringes as suction cups and noted the difference in suction blister induction time.[17] They demonstrated that suction blister induction time is directly proportional to the diameter of the suction syringe/cup. They concluded that use of 10 or 20 mL syringes as suction cups and -300 mm Hg pressure are appropriate choices for suction blister induction and produce blisters in about 1-2 hours. Innovating the use of syringe further, it was suggested that a cut syringe can be used as a suction cup, as the entire long syringe attached to skin for 2 hours is cumbersome.[18] Kaliyadan et al. suggested use of a microdermabrasion machine having a vacuum pump (Dermapeel Gold® manufactured by Derma India) along with 20 mL or 50 mL syringes and three-way connectors.[19] The method was similar, except that instead of 50 mL syringe, the vacuum tube of the microdermabrasion machine was used

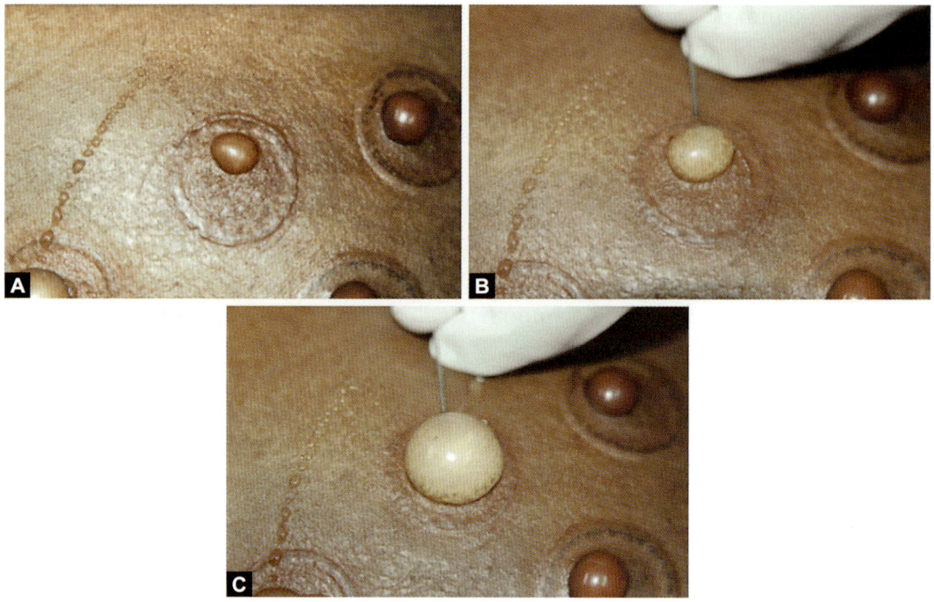

Figs. 1A to C: (A) A small blister; (B) Introducing needle into the blister cavity through the normal skin just outside the suction area and slowly injecting saline to generate intracavity positive pressure; (C) Full-size blister is ready in approximately 1 minute.

to produce suction. Burm developed another suction device consisting of only two units: a portable suction pump and suction cups containing an independent one-way check valve.[20] The suction pump is commercially available (Medi-Pump, Model 1130D, Thomas Industries, Inc., USA) and contains a manometer to permit readings up to 760 mm Hg. The suction cups are cylindrical plastic cups with a one-way check valve. These are available in two sizes: 15 mm and 22 mm in inside diameter. Suction cups are placed on the donor skin, which is moisturized with tap water. These cups are individually connected with every suction pump until the negative pressure within each cup reaches up to 250–300 mm Hg. Small vesicles begin to appear 1–1.5 hours later, which coalesce to form a single bulla 3–4 hours later. The maximum size of a harvested epidermal sheet is approximately 1.7 cm in diameter for small cup and 2.5 cm in diameter for a large one. A negative pressure cutaneous suction chamber system (NPCSCS; Electronic Diversities, MD, USA) has been developed to induce blisters rapidly.[21] The apparatus consists of temperature-controlled suction chambers connected to a control unit incorporating a diaphragm pump, which can generate up to –508 mm Hg of pressure. A slightly higher (40°C) temperature facilitates blister formation. In this device, heat is produced by applying a low AC voltage to incandescent lamps within the chambers. Each of the chambers is attached to an orifice plate that has multiple openings. This plate is applied directly to the subject's skin and secured in place by a belt placed around the limb/trunk. The combination of high negative pressure and thermal regulation allows for rapid blister formation. Awad has reported the successful use of a Chinese cupping device (commercially available with Beijing Kangzhu Baguanqi Medical Appliance Center), which produces larger blisters and does not need electrical instruments and connections.[22] It is composed of multiple transparent plastic cups (1.5–6.5 cm in size) and a pistol for the induction of negative pressure. A randomized split body study to compare Chinese cups with syringes of similar diameter in inducing suction blisters showed no difference in suction blister induction time, diameter of blisters, and the number of complete blister formation.[23] Similarly, "Hijama" therapy cups have been used as an alternative easy methods for creating suction blisters.[24]

Carvalho et al. studied real-time tomographic imaging of epidermal–dermal separation using optical coherence tomography (OCT) during suction blistering of human skin (freshly excised human abdominal skin tissue samples).[25] They observed three phases during suction blistering: (1) skin doming phase, (2) growth phase, and (3) steady-state phase. They also showed that while the blister time is inversely proportional to the applied suction pressure, the relationship between the blister time and the applied temperature is described by an exponential decay.

The next step in SBEG is graft transferring. Because of its flimsiness, the graft easily curls toward the dermal or epidermal surface. Moreover, even the most careful handling of the graft to spread it out on the recipient site with forceps often causes its disruption, making it useless. Many means for safely transferring the graft onto the recipient site have been proposed and used conventionally: an antibiotic-smeared microscope glass slide,[5] moistened plain fine gauze,[26] Tegaderm dressing (Medical Surgical Division, 3M, St. Paul, MN), and acetate sheets.[27] Use of saline-soaked gloved index or middle finger for spreading the graft over recipient site has been suggested by Laxmisha et al.[28] Insulin syringe has been suggested to be used like a sardine tin key to roll up the epidermal graft from the donor blister and safely roll it out on the affected skin.[29] Also, placing the graft on the lip and angle of mouth during SBEG is difficult with a standard-sized microscope glass slide (3 × 1 inch). Using half the regular size, slide (1.5 × 1 inch) for graft placement can be done to overcome this difficulty, as it can have an additional advantage of easy maneuverability **(Fig. 2)**.[30]

The blister roof is so thin that sometimes it becomes difficult to identify the dermal and epidermal sides. Therefore, Kim et al. devised a simple method to differentiate the dermal side from the epidermal side through writing a numeral "4" with a semipermanent marker over the suction blister.[31] The dermal side showed a reverse numeral "4" and was laid on top, while the epidermal side showing a correct figure "4" was well grafted into the recipient area.

Moreover, it is often difficult to place the grafts in few areas such as the angle of the mouth. To overcome this problem, Ashique et al. suggested using the butter papers that sandwich the sterile petrolatum-soaked gauge (Sofra-Tulle Dressing™).[32] The sticky surface of the paper is pressed on the donor graft site to transfer the blister roof to the paper with the dermal side of the blister roof facing the surgeon. The blister roof placed on the paper can easily be cut into desired sizes and shapes and applied on recipient area such as a sticker and the paper is removed **(Figs. 3A to D)**.

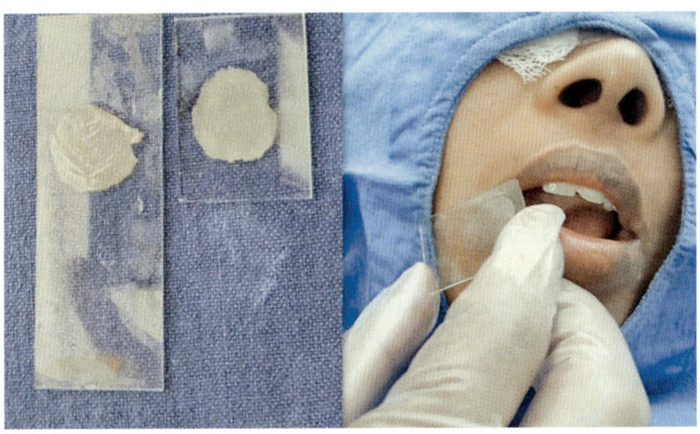

Fig. 2: The conventional slide and the cut slide with the graft ready for placement. The ease of placing the slide (engaging only one hand) on the angle of the mouth at ease.

The next step is the preparation of the recipient site of which dermabrasion remains an important step. The conventional manual dermabraders fail to achieve precision dermabrasion; hence, various modifications, such as the use of diamond-impregnated cylindrical fraises, producing a blister with liquid nitrogen spray, phototoxic reaction (PUVA or PUVASoL) or suction, or carbon dioxide or pulsed erbium-doped yttrium aluminum garnet (Er:YAG) laser, but their availability in limited-resource settings remains a major issue. To overcome this, Gupta et al. suggested the use of disposable hypodermic needle as a dermabrading device. Any size of the needle can be taken depending on the need and is held by the hub with the thumb, index finger, and ring finger at an acute angle to the skin surface keeping the beveled edge in maximum contact with the skin surface. The linear, parallel strokes are given in a crisscross manner on the recipient surface in transverse, longitudinal, and oblique directions until tiny bleeding points are observed.[33] Sometimes, the dermabrasion is difficult to perform on eyelids because of risk of trauma to the eyeball. To overcome this problem, Ashique et al. suggested the use of a long eyelid plate **(Figs. 4A to D)**.[34] The eyelid plate was inserted into the orbit and after which the dermabrasion can be performed without any risk of trauma to the eyeball. Another method described as an adjunct to manual dermabrasion in difficult sites (acral areas and phototherapy-induced thickened skin) is the use of 25% trichloroacetic acid (TCA-25%).[35] TCA-25%

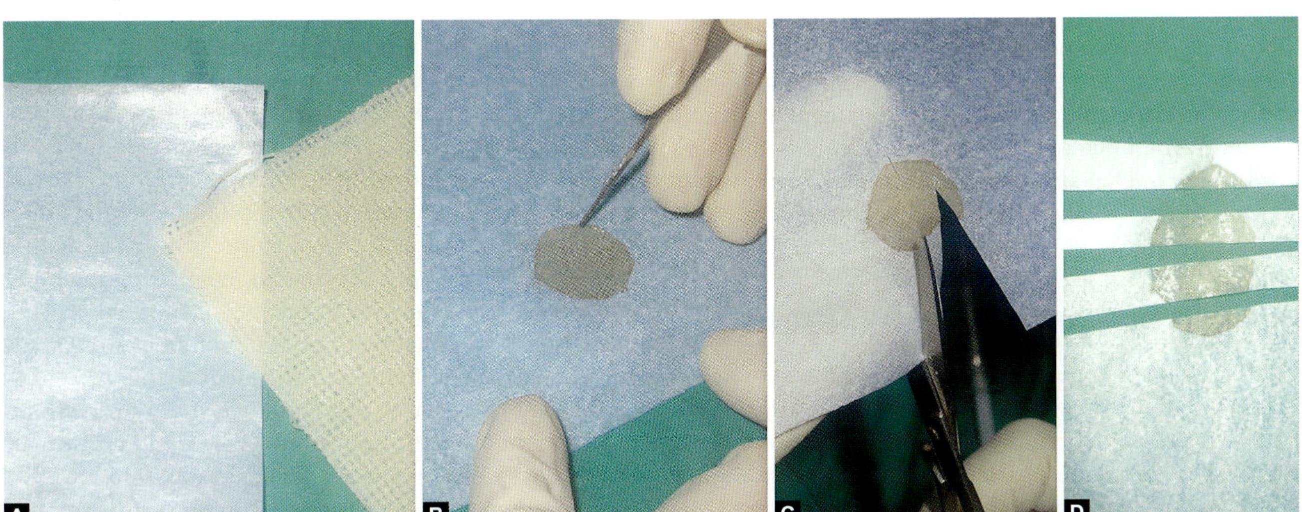

Figs. 3A to D: (A) The oil paper that comes sandwiching the *jelonet* dressing; (B) The blister roof was harvested and placed on the paper; (C) The graft is easily cut with paper; (D) The split grafts are ready for placement at the recipient end.

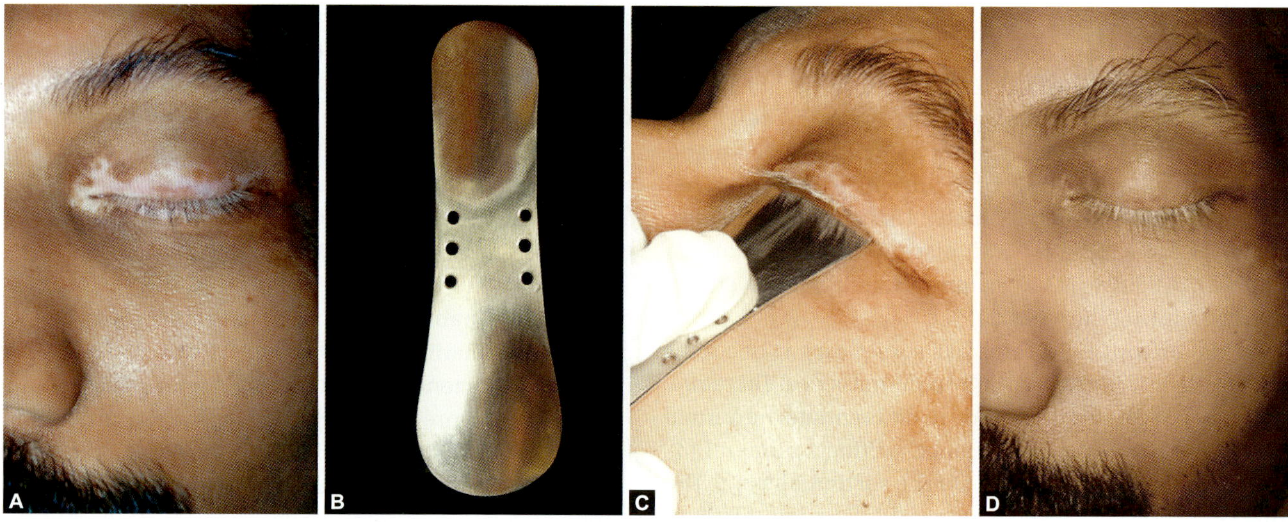

Figs. 4A to D: (A) Vitiliginous area affecting the eyelid margin; (B) The eye plate; (C) The plate used as a physical guard during dermabrasion; (D) Lesion after complete recovery due to the uniform and complete dermabrasion.

is applied using chemical peeling brush to the recipient site followed by air drying for 5 minutes. A sterile, moist cotton pad is placed over the area for further 5 minutes to facilitate controlled maceration. A sterilized manual dermabrader is then used to superficially dermabrade the TCA-25%-treated recipient area.

The final step after grafting the recipient site is dressing the wound. Types, availability, and cost of dressings have always been a matter of debate in the case of blister grafting. To solve this problem, the authors suggested that instead of dermabrading the recipient site, suction or phototoxic blisters may be induced for de-epithelialization and the blister roof can be used as an autologous biological dressing.[36] The roof of the blister is elevated like a flap, the denuded area is covered with grafts, and the flap is then replaced to cover the grafts. The periphery of the flap is sealed with tissue glue (cyanoacrylate), which retains the moisture, reduces chances of infection, and helps in faster healing. Traditionally, while performing SBEG over perioral areas, surgical tapes and stay sutures are put in place to immobilize the graft. Oh et al. have used dressing-free grafting for the treatment of perioral vitiligo.[37] The other means of graft fixation over mobile sites is fibrin glue, which may also improve the "take-up" of graft, confer protection against bacterial infection, and promote hemostasis.[38]

THIN AND ULTRATHIN SKIN GRAFTING

Of all the tissue or cellular grafting techniques, autologous thin and ultrathin skin grafting provide the most rapid onset of repigmentation, but require large grafts from donor area. Traditionally, instruments such as hand dermatome, motor-driven Zimmer dermatome, Humby's knife, or Silvers knife has been used to harvest a graft from the donor area. However, these instruments may not be easily available in resource-poor settings and they require a fair degree of surgical skills in their handling. An easy and cheap alternative is that the graft can be harvested freehand using a halved sterile razor blade mounted on a hemostatic forcep.[39] To increase the surface area of graft to cover large areas, mesh grafting has been undertaken. In this technique, the skin is passed through a machine that makes small slits and stretch it, allowing and cover area larger than itself.[40] Another inexpensive modification of split-thickness grafting is smash grafting, where the donor tissue is harvested in the similar manner as split-thickness skin grafting and then smashed into minute particles using a sterile curved suture cutting scissors, making a thick paste, which is then grafted onto dermabraded recipient site.[41] The smaller the particles, the better the uptake and so is the repigmentation. Another innovative technique in tissue grafting in vitiligo is needling and needling micrografting.[42] In this technique, the recipient area is punctured using an 18-gauge needle at intervals of 1–5 mm. These punctures are then left for a short time, so that the bleeding and oozing halt, following which the area is ready for grafting. For donor graft, split-thickness skin grafts (STSGs) are harvested and cut into small micropieces of size 0.1–0.3 mm with the scalpel. The micropieces are then soaked in normal saline and grasped with either microtweezers or a needle and implanted deeply inside the dermis into the readymade punctures followed by dressing. This seems an easy, inexpensive, and effective tissue grafting method. In another technique of vitiligo grafting, epidermal brushings obtained with dermabrader from donor areas were applied as such on de-epithelialized recipient area by Kachhawa et al. They named this technique as "Jodhpur technique" (autologous noncultured, nontrypsinized keratinocyte–melanocyte cellular graft technique).[43] However, the pigmentation obtained with this technique was cosmetically less satisfactory, as the technique involved transplantation of tiny flakes that included the dermal and epidermal tissue rather than single cells. Also, this technique is associated with morbidity at two sites—donor and recipient. Hence, the authors proposed use of perilesional normally pigmented skin adjacent to the depigmented patch as the donor site for obtaining melanocyte-containing fine epidermal flakes.[44] This eliminates the need for a separate donor site and morbidity is limited to a single site.

NONCULTURED EPIDERMAL CELL SUSPENSION

Noncultured epidermal cell suspension (NCES) transplantation is a well-established technique of vitiligo surgery. Many modifications have been made till date to make this technique easier and economical. Basal layer cells of epidermis can also be separated from the suction blister roof using an in vivo technique.[45] In this technique, the trypsin solution is injected in the cavity of well-formed blisters by introducing the needle from the skin close to the blister into the blister cavity through its floor. The blister fluid is aspirated and the syringe is detached with the needle is still in place. Then, another syringe filled with trypsin-ethylenediaminetetraacetic acid (EDTA) solution is attached to the syringe and the blister cavity is filled with the trypsin solution and the needle is withdrawn. The body heat works as an incubator for about 30–45 minutes and the melanocytes get separated or loosened up from the basal layer. Later, the blister fluid containing these cells is aspirated, blister roofs are removed and gently scrapped, and applied without centrifugation to the de-epithelialized recipient site.

Industrial grade incubators, commonly employed for NCES, occupy a significant volume of space and are expensive. In the absence of an incubator, cold trypsinization can be employed instead.[46] This can be achieved by placing the petri dish containing the donor tissue in 0.25% trypsin-EDTA overnight in a refrigerator at 4°C. Also, the patient's axilla has been used to maintain the temperature in case the incubator is unavailable **(Figs. 5A to I)**.[47] Another indigenous incubator has been designed using a discarded box, a 15-W incandescent light bulb, a dimmable electric fan regulator, and digital temperature sensor, which can maintain temperatures between 36° and 40°C consistently.[48]

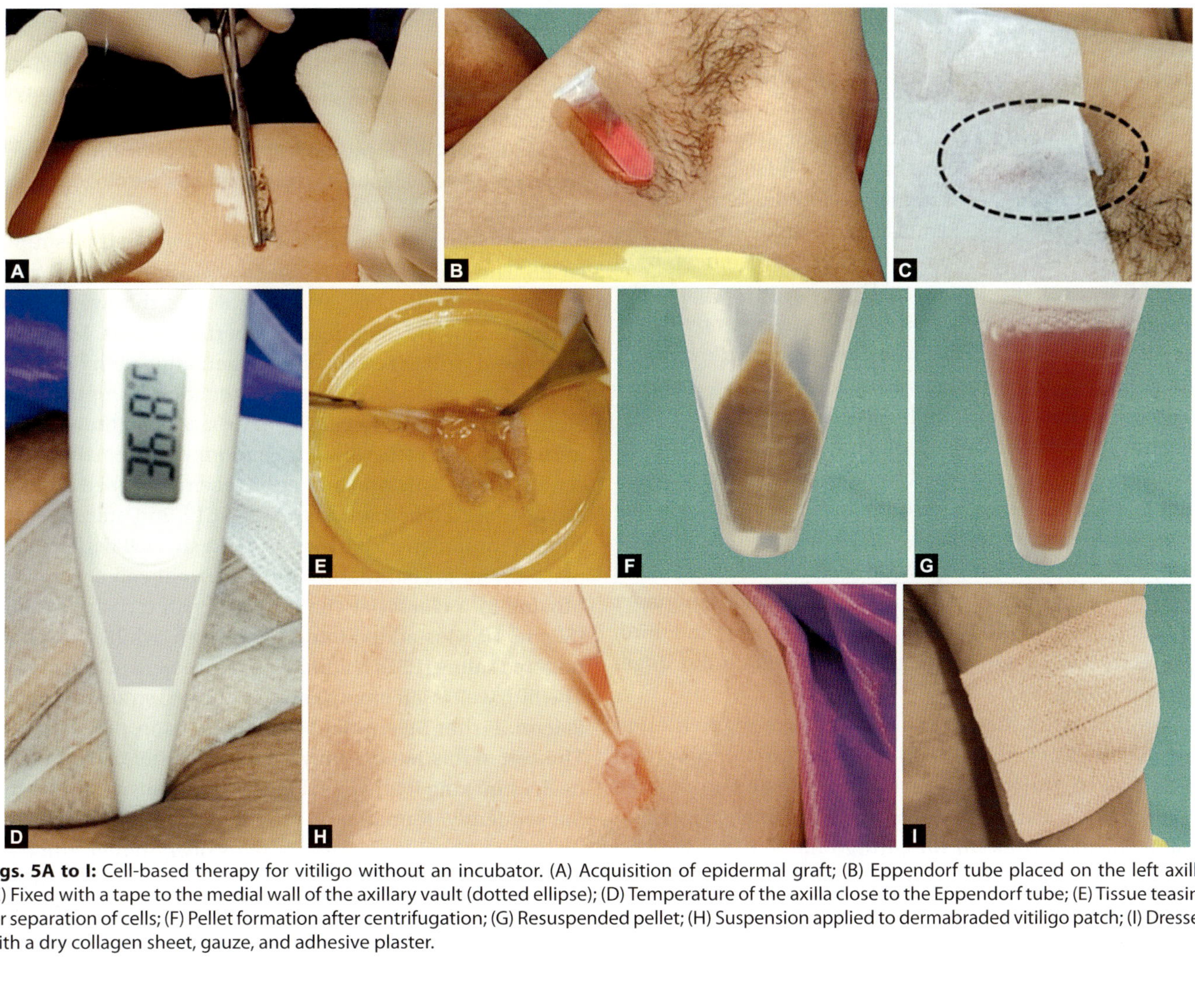

Figs. 5A to I: Cell-based therapy for vitiligo without an incubator. (A) Acquisition of epidermal graft; (B) Eppendorf tube placed on the left axilla; (C) Fixed with a tape to the medial wall of the axillary vault (dotted ellipse); (D) Temperature of the axilla close to the Eppendorf tube; (E) Tissue teasing for separation of cells; (F) Pellet formation after centrifugation; (G) Resuspended pellet; (H) Suspension applied to dermabraded vitiligo patch; (I) Dressed with a dry collagen sheet, gauze, and adhesive plaster.

Another suggested modification is that incubation may be carried out at room temperature. Aljasser et al. showed that it is possible to separate the epidermis from the dermis at room temperature without the need to use an incubator, though the efficacy of such innovation is not tested in vitiligo patients.[49]

Another modification for donor area was introduced by Gupta et al. In the conventional technique of noncultured epidermal melanocytes suspension, a thin Thiersch graft is taken from the donor site for the preparation of epidermal cell suspension. This results in superficial scarring at the donor site and it is difficult to take the graft from the same site in subsequent sessions of surgery. To overcome this problem, Gupta et al. suggested the use of epidermal brushing taken by manual dermabrader instead of a shave biopsy for preparing epidermal cell suspension.[50] Some of superficial epidermal brushings are discarded, as they contain only keratinized horny layer cells and deeper brushings are collected. These brushings are then trypsinized to prepare a single cell suspension. The proposed technique is a much faster and scarless technique for harvesting melanocytes from donor area for the preparation of melanocyte suspension.

Kaufmann et al. and Chen et al. have demonstrated, in their respective studies, that de-epithelialization of the recipient site with the help of Er:YAG or short-pulse carbon dioxide laser in transplantation of melanocytes can produce similar results as with dermabrasion.[51-53] Laser ablations may have advantages over dermabrasion on some delicate sites such as the eyelids. Removal of the epidermis with the help of a device for ultrasonic abrasion has also been used successfully for transplanting melanocytes in vitiligo.[54] The ultrasonic surgical aspirator easily and safely removes only the epidermis, even on spotty lesions or intricate regions, which are difficult to remove using a conventional motor-driven dermabrader or liquid nitrogen. A sterilized ready-to-use device (electric callus remover), which is primarily for pedicures, has been proposed to be used for dermabrasion of recipient vitiligo area in resource-poor settings.[55] Manual dermabrasion using sandpaper has been done in three ways: first, by placing the sandpaper tied to the index finger of the operator with a surgical suture material; second, sandpaper strips affixed onto a disposable tongue depressor; and third, by directly folding and holding it between the index finger and thumb **(Fig. 6)**.[56]

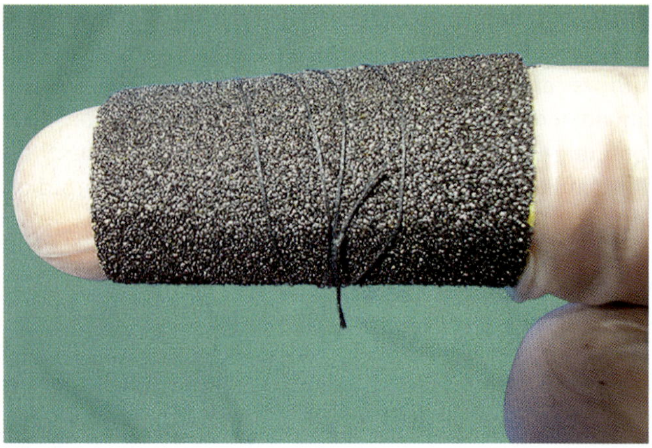

Fig. 6: Sandpaper wound around the index finger of the surgeon and fastened by surgical suture material for dermabrasion of the recipient site.

Another issue that remains is variable pigmentation because the suspension tends to accumulate in certain areas due to gravity and/or surface tension under the collagen sheet. Furthermore, because the final suspension is thin, it often runs off the vitiligo patch often leading to poor repigmentation. van Geel et al. have suggested mixing hyaluronic acid to improve viscosity and retain the suspension on the treatment area.[57] This modification, although effective, has shortcomings because hyaluronic acid dilutes the suspension and adds to the cost of the procedure. Gupta et al. tried a simple technique to overcome this problem. A small piece of monofilament nylon suture (for smaller lesions) or sterilized synthetic nylon mesh such as mosquito net and curtain nets (for larger lesions) was fixed using cyanoacrylate glue around the dermabraded recipient lesion to form a rim.[58] This rim acted as a boundary and prevented the seepage of the suspension beyond the margins of the affected area.

Results of NCES can be improved significantly more by suspending the melanocytes in the patients' autologous serum or platelet-rich plasma than in normal saline.[59,60]

Many other methods have been developed to simplify NCES. The Recell® kit (Avita Medical, Australia) is a portable battery-operated, cell-harvesting device that was initially developed for the treatment of superficial burns. Mulekar et al. showed similar results of repigmentation with Recell® kit as the conventional NCES transplantation in repigmenting vitiligo.[61] Recell® has a certain drawbacks that these devices are expensive and this limits their routine usage in the clinical setting. Six-well plate technique has been developed to obviate the need for a laboratory setup for NCES and utilizes a set of simple equipment.[62] It makes use of a six-well tissue culture plate in the preparation of an epidermal cell suspension. Moving in a clockwise manner, soybean trypsin inhibitor (Sigma, USA) is added into the first well, while phosphate-buffered saline (PBS) is added into the second to fourth wells. The fifth well is left empty and a 40-µm cell strainer (Corning Falcon, Fisher Scientific, USA) is placed in the sixth well. The cost of this setup is only a fraction of that in commercial devices making it an appealing and inexpensive alternative. Subsequently, Kumar et al. modified this technique further by using a four-compartment petri dish, though the basic principles remained the same.[63] Instead of using a separate petri dish, the harvested donor tissue is placed in the first compartment of the petri dish containing 0.25% trypsin-

EDTA and then incubated for 1 hour at 37°C in a portable incubator. The tissue is subsequently rinsed in PBS in the next two compartments to remove residual trypsin. In the fourth compartment, the epidermis of the tissue is separated from the dermis using a pair of fine forceps and the epidermal cells are dislodged. Instead of using a microfilter, the tissue debris is removed using forceps, PBS is added, and the suspension is mixed by aspirating several times using a sterile syringe. The final suspension is then applied to dermabraded vitiliginous recipient sites.

The utility of NCES has also been reported in the treatment of iatrogenic dyspigmentation and textural abnormalities in vitiligo patches, which develop after topical therapies, phototherapy, and various transplantation procedures.[64]

NONCULTURED EXTRACTED FOLLICLE OUTER ROOT SHEATH CELL SUSPENSION TRANSPLANTATION

Transplantation of suspension of outer root sheath (ORS) cells in vitiligo was reported by Vanscheidt et al. in a small case series.[65] But as the suspension was prepared from plucked hair follicles, the procedure suffered from a low cell yield. The method was improvised by obtaining the hair follicle tissue by the follicular unit extraction (FUE) method, which takes out the hair follicle completely along with its stem cell reservoir and a narrow rim of perifollicular dermal sheath, leading to good cell yield and repigmentation.[66] It has been combined with NCES too with significantly better outcomes in terms of repigmentation.[67] Body hair transplantation by FUE has also been developed for treating localized/segmental vitiligo, especially on hairy parts of the skin, including the eyelids and eyebrows and for small areas of vitiligo.[68]

CONCLUSION

These innovative techniques simplify the techniques of vitiligo surgeries, obviating the need of a laboratory setup, and make the procedure more cost-effective and accessible in a clinic setting. Future studies, comparing the simplified versus conventional techniques, will be helpful in determining, if they have similar clinical outcomes.

REFERENCES

1. Kim DS, Ju HJ, Lee HN, Choi IH, Eun SH, Kim J, et al. Skin seeding technique with 0.5-mm micropunch grafting for vitiligo irrespective of the epidermal-dermal orientation: animal and clinical studies. J Dermatol. 2020;47(7):749-54.
2. Bae JM, Lee JH, Kwon HS, Kim J, Kim DS. Motorized 0.8-mm micropunch grafting for refractory vitiligo: a retrospective study of 230 cases. J Am Acad Dermatol. 2018;79(4): 720-7.e1.
3. Laxmisha C, Thappa DM. Surgical pearl: use of hypodermic needle to transfer minigrafts. J Am Acad Dermatol. 2006;54(4):707.
4. Kiistala U, Mustakallio KK. In-vivo separation of epidermis by production of suction blisters. Lancet Lond Engl. 1964;2(7348):1444-5.
5. Falabella R. Epidermal grafting. An original technique and its application in achromic and granulating areas. Arch Dermatol. 1971;104(6):592-600.
6. Mutalik S. Transplantation of melanocytes by epidermal grafting. An Indian experience. J Dermatol Surg Oncol. 1993;19(3):231-4.
7. Koga M. Epidermal grafting using the tops of suction blisters in the treatment of vitiligo. Arch Dermatol. 1988;124(11): 1656-8.
8. Mukhtar M, Singh S, Shukla VK, Pandey SS. Surgical pearl: suction syringe for epidermal grafting. J Am Acad Dermatol. 1997;37(4):638-9.
9. Lewis EJ, Kageyama N. The mechanism of "suction." J Am Acad Dermatol. 1998;39(4 Pt 1):664.
10. Gupta S, Shroff S, Gupta S. Modified technique of suction blistering for epidermal grafting in vitiligo. Int J Dermatol. 1999;38(4):306-9.
11. Gupta S, Ajith C, Kanwar AJ, Kumar B. Surgical pearl: standardized suction syringe for epidermal grafting. J Am Acad Dermatol. 2005;52(2):348-50.
12. Gupta S, Chandrashekar BS, Reddy R, Jagadish P, Asati D. Rapid induction of suction blisters by intra-cavity positive pressure enhancement. Dermatol Surg. 2011;37(6):843-5.
13. Kim T, Roh HJ, Kim JY, Noh S, Oh SH. Rapid formation of suction blister through intradermal injection of local anesthetics in epidermal graft for vitiligo. Dermatol Surg. 2010;36(10):1642-3.
14. Kaliyadan F, Venkitakrishnan S, Manoj J. Use of a wood's lamp as a ultraviolet light source to improve the speed and quality of suction blister harvesting. Indian J Dermatol Venereol Leprol. 2010;76(4):429-31.
15. Laxmisha C, Babu A, Thappa DM. Letter: infrared lamps for faster suction blister induction. Dermatol Surg. 2006;32(8): 1111-2.
16. Arora S, Kar BR. Reduction of blister formation time in suction blister epidermal grafting in vitiligo patients using a household hair dryer. J Cutan Aesthet Surg. 2016;9(4):232-5.
17. Gupta S, Kumar B. Suction blister induction time: 15 minutes or 150 minutes? Dermatol Surg. 2000;26(8):754-6.
18. Mukhtar M. Disposable syringe cup for 3-way cannula-syringe suction. J Am Acad Dermatol. 2020.
19. Kaliyadan F, Manoj J, Venkitakrishnan S. Using a microdermabrasion machine as a suction blister device. Indian J Dermatol Venereol Leprol. 2008;74(4):392-3.
20. Burm JS. Simple suction device for autologous epidermal grafting. Plast Reconstr Surg. 2000;106(5):1225-6.
21. Alexis AF, Wilson DC, Todhunter JA, Stiller MJ. Reassessment of the suction blister model of wound healing: introduction of a new higher pressure device. Int J Dermatol. 1999;38(8): 613-7.
22. Awad SS. Chinese cupping: a simple method to obtain epithelial grafts for the management of resistant localized vitiligo. Dermatol Surg. 2008;34(9):1186-92.
23. Anbar TS, Moftah NH, El-Khayyat MAM, El-Fakahany HM, Abdel-Rahman AT, Saad EK. Syringes versus Chinese cups in harvesting suction-induced blister graft: a randomized split-body study. Int J Dermatol. 2018;57(10):1249-52.
24. Jain S, Patra S, Choudhary S, Kaur M. An easy way to make blisters in suction blister grafting of vitiligo with Hijama therapy cups. J Am Acad Dermatol. 2020.

25. Carvalho JCO, Palero JA, Jurna M. Real-time imaging of suction blistering in human skin using optical coherence tomography. Biomed Opt Express. 2015;6(12):4790-5.
26. Tang WY, De Han J, Lu NZ, Chan LY, Lo KK. Surgical pearl: fine gauze is a useful carrier for epidermal graft in the treatment of vitiligo by means of the suction blister method. J Am Acad Dermatol. 1999;40(2 Pt 1):247-9.
27. Albert S, Shenoi SD. Acetate sheets in the transfer of epidermal grafts in vitiligo. J Am Acad Dermatol. 2001;44(4):719-20.
28. Laxmisha C, Thappa DM. Surgical pearl: gloved finger as a transport platform for epidermal graft of suction blister. J Am Acad Dermatol. 2007;57(5 Suppl):S118-9.
29. Pagliarello C, Calogero P, Paradisi A, Andrea P. An effective way to perform suction-blister grafts: using an insulin syringe as a sardine tin key. Dermatol Surg. 2011;37(4):549-53.
30. Ashique KT, Kaliyadan F. When half-slide can deliver double efficiency for blister grafting in vitiligo. J Am Acad Dermatol. 2020;83(3):e181-2.
31. Kim T, Roh HJ, Kim JY, Noh S, Oh SH. Easy method to distinguish epidermal side through writing figure "4" over a suction blister. Dermatol Surg. 2010;36(9):1457-8.
32. Ashique KT, Srinivas CR. Resizing blister roof grafts for vitiligo surgery. J Am Acad Dermatol. 2014;71(2):e39-40.
33. Gupta S, Gupta S, Kumar A. The hypodermic needle as a dermabrading device for recipient area preparation for skin grafting in vitiligo. J Am Acad Dermatol. 2015;72(4):e105-6.
34. Ashique KT, Kaliyadan F, Iqbal S. Dermabrasion of the eyelids in vitiligo surgery. Dermatol Surg. 2016;42(5):691-2.
35. Razmi TM, Kumaran SM, Parsad D. Trichloroacetic acid 25% peel to facilitate dermabrasion at difficult sites in vitiligo surgery. Dermatol Surg. 2019;45(5):750-2.
36. Gupta S, Kumar B. Surgical pearl: autologous biological dressing for epidermal grafting in vitiligo and other achromic disorders. J Am Acad Dermatol. 2003;48(3):430-1.
37. Oh SH, Shin JY, Kim T, Kim DY, Park SG, Hann SK. Dressing-free epidermal grafting for the treatment of perioral vitiligo. Dermatol Surg. 2011;37(8):1173-5.
38. Kim H, Kang JN, Hwang SH, Seo JK, Sung HS. Fibrin glue fixation for suction blister epidermal grafting in two patients with stable vitiligo. Ann Dermatol. 2014;26(6):751-4.
39. Huang K, Li J, Jiang Z, Fan H, Yu N, Liu D, et al. Razor blade: a simple instrument used in epidermal grafting for vitiligo. J Am Acad Dermatol. 2021;84(1):e17-8.
40. Srinivas CR, Rai R, Kumar PU. Meshed split skin graft for extensive vitiligo. Indian J Dermatol Venereol Leprol. 2004;70(3):165-7.
41. Krishnan A, Kar S. Smashed skin grafting or smash grafting—a novel method of vitiligo surgery. Int J Dermatol. 2012;51(10):1242-7.
42. Sharquie KE, Noaimi AA, Al-Mudaris HA. Melanocytes transplantation in patients with vitiligo using needling micrografting technique. J Drugs Dermatol. 2013;12(5):e74-8.
43. Kachhawa D, Kalla G. Keratinocyte-melanocyte graft technique followed by PUVA therapy for stable vitiligo. Indian J Dermatol Venereol Leprol. 2008;74(6):622-4.
44. Kachhawa D, Kachhawa N, Gupta S. Mechanical harvesting of perilesional normally pigmented tissue to merge donor and recipient sites for transplantation in vitiligo. J Am Acad Dermatol. 2020.
45. Gupta S, Sahni K, Tembhre MK, Mathur S, Sharma VK. A novel point-of-care in vivo technique for preparation of epidermal cell suspension for transplantation in vitiligo. J Am Acad Dermatol. 2015;72(2):e65-6.
46. Gauthier Y, Surleve-Bazeille JE. Autologous grafting with noncultured melanocytes: a simplified method for treatment of depigmented lesions. J Am Acad Dermatol. 1992;26(2 Pt 1):191-4.
47. Bhatia S, Rajput L, Gupta S. Axillary incubator for cell-based therapies in vitiligo. J Am Acad Dermatol. 2020.
48. Agrawal S, Sharma A, Dhurat R. A Do-it-yourself incubator for autologous melanocyte-keratinocyte transplantation surgery—a resource-poor alternative. J Am Acad Dermatol. 2019.
49. Aljasser MI, Mulekar SS, Mulekar SV. Epidermal cell suspension: achieved by incubation at room temperature. J Cutan Aesthet Surg. 2013;6(2):126.
50. Gupta S, Kumar A, Mahendra A, Gupta S. A minimally invasive, scarless technique of donor tissue harvesting for noncultured epidermal cell suspension transplantation in vitiligo. J Am Acad Dermatol. 2015;73(6):e213-5.
51. Kaufmann R, Greiner D, Kippenberger S, Bernd A. Grafting of in vitro cultured melanocytes onto laser-ablated lesions in vitiligo. Acta Derm Venereol. 1998;78(2):136-8.
52. Chen YF, Chang JS, Yang PY, Hung CM, Huang MH, Hu DN. Transplant of cultured autologous pure melanocytes after laser-abrasion for the treatment of segmental vitiligo. J Dermatol. 2000;27(7):434-9.
53. Chen YF, Yang PY, Hu DN, Kuo FS, Hung CS, Hung CM. Treatment of vitiligo by transplantation of cultured pure melanocyte suspension: analysis of 120 cases. J Am Acad Dermatol. 2004;51(1):68-74.
54. Tsukamoto K, Osada A, Kitamura R, Ohkouchi M, Shimada S, Takayama O. Approaches to repigmentation of vitiligo skin: new treatment with ultrasonic abrasion, seed-grafting and psoralen plus ultraviolet A therapy. Pigment Cell Res. 2002;15(5):331-4.
55. Ashique KT, Kaliyadan F, Jayasree P. Ready-to-use device for dermabrasion in vitiligo surgery. J Cutan Aesthet Surg. 2020;13(4):338.
56. Ashique KT, Kaliyadan F, George RR. Dermabrasion of the recipient skin in vitiligo surgery: an easier way out. Indian J Dermatol Venereol Leprol. 2018;84(4):498-9.
57. van Geel N, Ongenae K, De Mil M, Naeyaert JM. Modified technique of autologous noncultured epidermal cell transplantation for repigmenting vitiligo: a pilot study. Dermatol Surg. 2001;27(10):873-6.
58. Gupta S, Jangra RS, Gupta S, Ashique KT. Novel technique for retention of cell suspension in melanocyte-keratinocyte transplantation procedure using glued nylon suture or mesh. Dermatol Surg. 2019;45(1):163-5.
59. Sahni K, Parsad D, Kanwar AJ, Mehta SD. Autologous noncultured melanocyte transplantation for stable vitiligo: can suspending autologous melanocytes in the patients' own serum improve repigmentation and patient satisfaction? Dermatol Surg. 2011;37(2):176-82.
60. Parambath N, Sharma VK, Parihar AS, Sahni K, Gupta S. Use of platelet-rich plasma to suspend noncultured epidermal cell suspension improves repigmentation after autologous transplantation in stable vitiligo: a double-blind randomized controlled trial. Int J Dermatol. 2019;58(4):472-6.
61. Mulekar SV, Ghwish B, Al Issa A, Al Eisa A. Treatment of vitiligo lesions by ReCell vs. conventional melanocyte-keratinocyte

transplantation: a pilot study. Br J Dermatol. 2008;158(1):45-9.
62. Goh BK, Chua XM, Chong KL, de Mil M, van Geel NAC. Simplified cellular grafting for treatment of vitiligo and piebaldism: the "6-well plate" technique. Dermatol Surg. 2010;36(2):203-7.
63. Kumar R, Parsad D, Singh C, Yadav S. Four compartment method: a simplified and cost-effective method of noncultured epidermal cell suspension for the treatment of vitiligo. Br J Dermatol. 2014;170(3):581-5.
64. Taneja N, Sahni K, Gupta S. Autologous noncultured epidermal cell suspension for treatment of iatrogenic variegate repigmentation, textural changes, and color mismatch in vitiligo. Dermatol Ther. 2020;33(6):e14399.
65. Vanscheidt W, Hunziker T. Repigmentation by outer-root-sheath-derived melanocytes: proof of concept in vitiligo and leucoderma. Dermatol Basel Switz. 2009;218(4):342-3.
66. Kumar A, Gupta S, Mohanty S, Bhargava B, Airan B. Stem cell niche is partially lost during follicular plucking: a preliminary pilot study. Int J Trichol. 2013;5(2):97-100.
67. Singh C, Parsad D, Kanwar AJ, Dogra S, Kumar R. Comparison between autologous noncultured extracted hair follicle outer root sheath cell suspension and autologous non-cultured epidermal cell suspension in the treatment of stable vitiligo: a randomized study. Br J Dermatol. 2013;169(2):287-93.
68. Chouhan K, Kumar A, Kanwar AJ. Body hair transplantation in vitiligo. J Cutan Aesthet Surg. 2013;6(2):111-2.

SECTION 6

Procedural Management of Acne Scars

CHAPTER 45

Acne Scars: An Overview

Rajat Kandhari, Jyoti Gupta

KEY MESSAGES

- Early treatment of acne is crucial in order to prevent acne scarring.
- There is no one treatment modality that appears to be a "magic wand" for acne scars.
- The results of treatment vary depending on the depth and morphology of the scar being treated, making it pertinent to classify and make a thorough assessment of the acne scars.

INTRODUCTION

Some degree of cosmetic disfigurement occurs in up to 95% of individuals suffering from active acne. Delayed treatment and acne severity are factors predisposing an individual to a greater extent of scarring, psychological distress, and impairment in the quality of life.[1-3]

In addition, acne scars have also been considered as a risk factor for depression, suicide, low academic performance, and unemployment.[4,5]

Creating awareness and educating the general population regarding the importance of early treatment of acne appear to be essential to prevent the burden of acne sequelae. This chapter aims to provide an overview of acne scars—their formation, grading, and feasible treatment modalities.

EPIDEMIOLOGY

There is limited epidemiologic data available on the prevalence of acne scarring. Scarring has been recorded in 14% of women and 11% of men in patients aged 25 and 58 years.[6] Acne scarring has been demonstrated in 30–95% of patients with acne vulgaris in the Western literature,[7] while Indian data reveals a prevalence of 39.5%.[8]

Most of the acne scars are atrophic in nature and occur on the face. Truncal involvement appears to be more common in males, wherein hypertrophic and keloidal scars may also be noted.[9] There is a lack of robust epidemiologic data on the relative prevalence rates of different types of scarring.[10]

PATHOGENESIS

The pathogenetic factors causing acne lead to a cytokine cascade resulting in an infrainfundibular inflammatory process, follicular rupture, and perifollicular abscess formation, which in turn gives rise to a wound-healing process.[11,12]

Individuals with acne who are prone to scarring appear to demonstrate a slightly different cellular infiltrate and a prolonged inflammatory response at the follicle than those who do not scar. The inflammatory process may result in an aggravated response, forming a raised nodule of fibrotic tissue (hypertrophic scars) or degradation of collagen fibers, resulting in the formation of pitting (atrophic scars). While the textural changes due to alteration in the collagen fibers are permanent, the vascular and pigmentary alterations are transient. Moreover, scars demonstrate a relative absence of skin appendages and elastic fibers histologically.[13]

The wound healing process undergoes through three stages: (1) Inflammation, (2) granulation tissue formation, and (3) matrix remodeling.[14]

Inflammation: Hemostasis during the wound healing process results in vasoconstriction and blanching. Subsequently, the blanching is replaced by vasodilatation and resultant erythema, resulting in post-acne erythema. Moreover, at this stage, melanogenesis may be stimulated, which results clinically as post-acne pigmentation. The severity and duration of the inflammatory component have been shown to have a direct correlation with the extent of scarring.[15]

Granulation tissue formation: The inflammatory mediators set the stage for granulation tissue formation, wherein there are neoangiogenesis and tissue repair. It is in this stage that fibroblast stimulation and proliferation, along with the release of growth factors, result in collagen deposition. Initially, the composition of the new skin is dominated by type III collagen, with type I collagen in very small amount (20%). However, type I collagen dominates in the mature scars (80%).[16]

Matrix remodeling: It is mediated mainly by the extracellular matrix metalloproteinases (MMPs) and tissue inhibitors of MMPs (TIMPs) that are secreted by the fibroblasts and keratinocytes. Activation of NF-κB and activator protein-1 (AP-1) stimulates MMPs such as MMP-1, MMP-8, MMP-9, and

MMP-13, all of which are involved in collagen degradation. MMP upregulation and procollagen synthesis are prolonged in patients prone to acne scarring.[17] Further, the imbalance in the ratio of MMPs to TIMPs results in the formation of atrophic or hypertrophic scars.[18]

CLASSIFICATION

Acne scars are categorized as "atrophic" or "hypertrophic", depending on the net collagen deposition. Majority of the individuals present with atrophic scars (loss of collagen) compared to a minority who show hypertrophic scars and keloids.[14]

Atrophic Scars

Atrophic scars are further subclassified into ice pick, boxcar, and rolling scars according to depth, width, and three-dimensional architecture.[10]

Rolling Scars (15–25%)

Rolling scars are clinically characterized by their wide (up to 5 mm) and undulating nature. They are similar in shape to an "inverted speed breaker". The undulating appearance of rolling scars is a result of the fibrous anchoring of the dermis to the subcutaneous tissue. Correction of this dermal tethering via specific techniques such as subcision and the help of soft-tissue fillers is particularly effective in these scars **(Table 1)**.

Ice Pick Scars (60–70%)

Clinically, ice pick scars are deep, narrow (2 mm), punctiform, cylindrical depressions, akin to an "inverted dagger" that occur at the infundibulum. These scars, though not always, are usually recognized with a wider surface opening than the deep layer (forming a "V" shape). Due to their depth, punch excisions, trichloroacetic acid chemical reconstruction of skin scars (TCA CROSS), and ablative fractional laser (AFL) are useful techniques.[19]

Boxcar Scars

Boxcar scars are round, oval, or ill-defined depressions with defined vertical edges. These scars may be shallow (0.1–0.5 mm) or deep (>0.5 mm) and are usually 1.5–4 mm in diameter. Boxcar scars are wide at the surface and demonstrate a wide base. While shallow boxcar scars are amenable to most treatment modalities, deep boxcar scars are challenging to treat. Surgical modalities of treatment such as punch excision, elevation, and grafting technique help in improving deep boxcar scars,[20] while shallow scars, on the other hand, appear to improve with fractional resurfacing, microneedling, and microneedling radiofrequency.[21]

More often than not, more than one type of scar (cocktail of scars) is clinically seen in an individual presenting with atrophic scars. It is essential that the dermatologist assess each scar well at the initial assessment to form a bespoke treatment plan in order to provide the most optimal outcome.

Hypertrophic and Keloidal Scars

Hypertrophic and keloidal scars are more common in darker-skinned individuals and are seen on the trunk and, at times, around the jawline. These scars are particularly disfiguring for the individual and pose a challenge for the treating physician. While hypertrophic scars are typically confined within the borders of the original injury site, keloidal variants proliferate beyond the original wound borders. These scars are typically reddish-pink in color, raised, papulonodular lesions with firm-to-hard consistency. Histologically, hypertrophic scars demonstrate "excess collagen deposition with thick hyalinized collagen bundles", whereas keloidal scars show "thick bundles of hyalinized acellular collagen arranged in whorls". These scars are typically treated with intralesional steroids (40 mg/mL), fractional lasers, pigment dye laser, and/or cryotherapy.

Other Types of Acne Scarring

Lipoatrophic Acne Scars

Wide areas with loss of tissue lead to the formation of depressed scars, which are seen commonly on the mandibular area and lower cheeks, thereby giving the patients a gaunt and prematurely aged appearance. They are best treated with a filling substance such as a synthetic filler or autologous fat (lipofilling).[22]

Macular Scars

Macular scars can be hyperpigmented, hypopigmented, or erythematous scars localized to the epidermis and superficial dermis. Hyperpigmentation is usually due to the postinflammatory effects of acne that resolve with time, although the resolution may take months to years. Hypopigmented areas, on the other hand, represent true scar healing. Acne-associated erythematous scars may be addressed with topical therapies, chemical peels, fractionated, and pigment or vascular-specific lasers.

ASSESSMENT AND GRADING OF ACNE SCARS

There is no predictive tool to identify patients at risk of scarring from the severity of acne. However, grading of acne scars and assessment of individual scars may give the treating physician a fair direction to create a bespoke treatment plan for the patient.

TABLE 1: Acne scar classification.[21]

Scar type		*Treatment available*
Ice pick	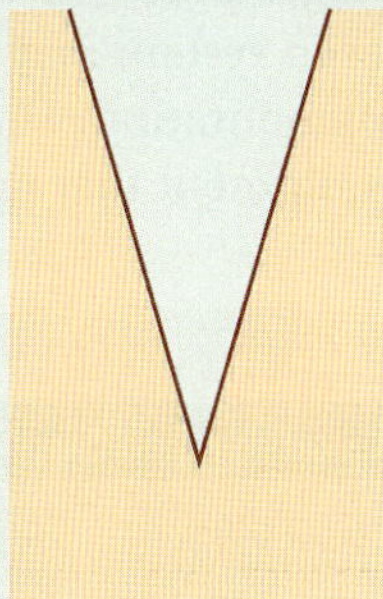	• Punch excision • TCA CROSS • Radiofrequency • Laser skin resurfacing—CO_2 pinpoint irradiation technique
Rolling	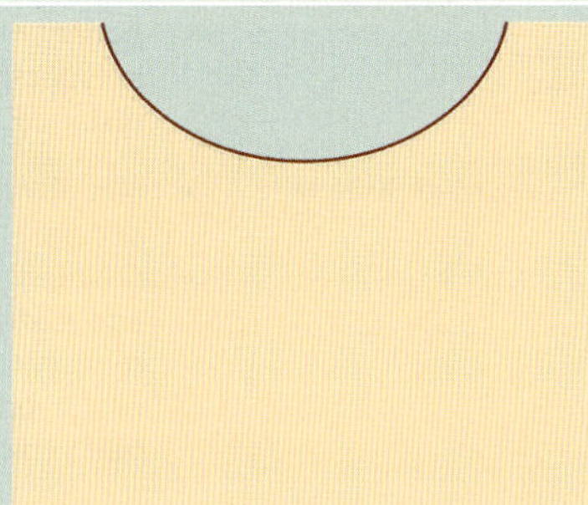	• Subcision • Fillers • Dermabrasion • Microneedling • Radiofrequency • Laser skin resurfacing
Boxcar	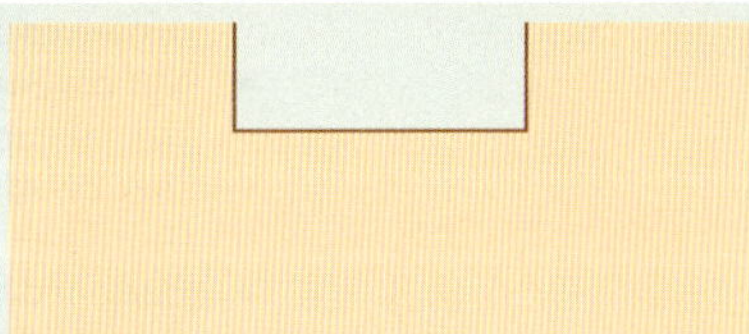	• Shallow boxcar • Laser skin resurfacing • Microneedling • Radiofrequency • Punch elevation
	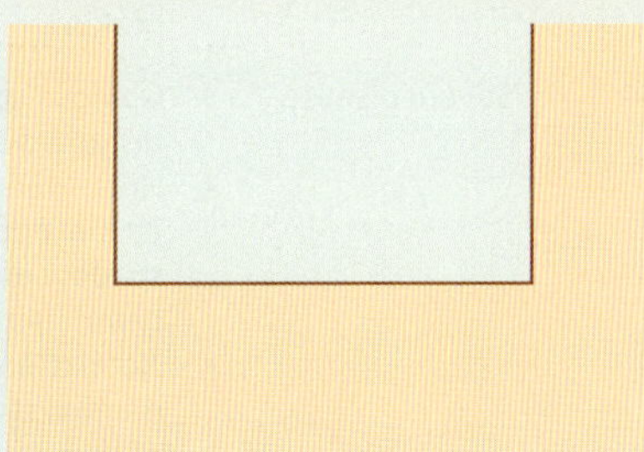	• Deep box scar • Subcision • Punch excision/elevation • Laser skin resurfacing

(CO_2: carbon dioxide; TCA CROSS: trichloroacetic acid chemical reconstruction of skin scars)

An ideal acne scar grading scale should be:

- Reproducible
- Assess the scar color (evaluating hypopigmentation and hyperpigmentation of the lesions)
- Assess the scarring depth and area of involvement
- Should allow for changes to be tracked with time and treatments.

A proper assessment should include a thorough examination, including the depth, width, and color of the scar. The use of directional lighting shined tangentially on the skin may highlight atrophy or textural changes. Palpation of the scars provides help in evaluating underlying tethering or fibrosis, and stretching of the skin provides valuable information regarding whether the scars would be amenable to laser therapy or not.

In grading postacne scars, the most common issues are assessing variation in scarring, three-dimensional assessment, quantification of scars, and quantifying scar changes over time and with treatment modalities.[23]

The current grading scales do not account for depth, color, change over time of the scars, and the appearance in differing lights or tangential lighting. It is recommended that these be introduced to current grading scales to provide more practicality in their usage in real-world clinical settings.

There are four broad approaches to the assessment of acne scarring: (1) Scar subtype counting, (2) subjective self-assessment, (3) global acne scar severity scoring, and (4) multimodal imaging.[2]

Scar subtype or lesion counting involves counting each scar type and allocating a score accordingly. This is not only time-consuming and impractical in a busy clinical practice but also can vary with lighting and visual acuity.[24,25]

The subjective self-assessment scales are useful tools to measure the quality of life of an individual as they are patient-centric methods of assessment. The "Self-assessment of Clinical Acne-related Scars (SCARS)" and "Facial Acne Scar Quality of Life (FASQoL)" are questionnaires providing information about the patient's perspective to the clinician. SCARS is a 5-item patient questionnaire that rates the acne scar severity as seen in a mirror, while FASQoL is a 10-item questionnaire that rates the impact of acne scars on emotions, social functioning, and work/school on a 5-point scale. A subjective self-assessment has been identified as an unreliable measure for the assessment of acne scar severity in comparison to practitioner-rated grading scales.[25,26]

Global scoring allows clinicians and investigators to objectively understand and discuss the efficacy of various interventions or therapies. Goodman and Baron developed the "Qualitative Scarring Grading System" **(Table 2)**. This system subdivides acne scars into four grades based on acne scar severity (macular, mild, moderate, and severe, respectively).[27]

Goodman and Baron also developed the "Quantitative Global Acne Scarring Grading System", which accounts for the number and type of scar based on a point system instead of category. The final score ranges from 0 to 84 **(Table 3)**.

Another quantitative scale is the Echelle d'Evaluation Clinique des Cicatrices d'acné (ECCA) scale, which takes the number and type of scar into consideration. Scores range from 0 to 540. Though it has high inter-investigator reliability, the scale is complex, requiring training, is time-consuming, and is limited to face only.[28]

Further, the Global Scale for Acne Scar Severity (SCAR-S) is independently applied to the face, chest, and back and then summed to provide a composite score. This score ranges from clear to extremely severe and is given a code from 1 to 6.[29]

Imaging techniques can provide an objective measure. A volumetric measurement by three-dimensional photographic images allows tracking of the scars over time, whereas a color-based system may be limited to assessing erythema and dyspigmentation. However, the technologies rely on specific equipment that may be inaccessible to most of the clinicians.[30,31]

TABLE 2: Goodman and Baron Qualitative Scarring Grading Scale.

Grade	*Level of disease*	*Characteristics*	*Example of scars*
1	Macular disease	• Marks visible to patient or observer irrespective of distance	Erythematous, hyper- or hypopigmented flat marks
2	Mild disease	• Not obvious at distances ≥50 cm • Covered adequately by makeup or shadow of shaved beard hair in males	Mild rolling, small soft papular
3	Moderate disease	• Obvious at distances ≥50 cm • Not covered easily by makeup or shadow of shaved beard hair in males • Flattened by manual stretching of skin	More significant rolling, shallow "boxcar", mild-to-moderate hypertrophic or papular scars
4	Severe disease	• Obvious at distances ≥50 cm • Not covered easily by makeup or shadow of shaved beard hair in males • Not flattened by manual stretching of skin	Punched-out atrophic (deep "boxcar"), "ice pick", bridges and tunnels, gross atrophy, dystrophic scars, significant hypertrophy, or keloid

TABLE 3: Goodman and Baron Quantitative Scarring Grading Scale.

			Number of lesions		
Grade	*Type*	*Description*	*1 (1–10)*	*2 (11–20)*	*3 (>20)*
A	Milder scarring (1 point each)	• Macular erythematous or pigmented • Mildly atrophic dish-like	1	2	3
B	Moderate scarring (2 points each)	• Moderately atrophic dish-like • Punched out with shallow bases but small scars (<5 mm) • Shallow but broad atrophic scars	2	4	6
C	Severe scarring (3 points each)	• Punched out with deep but normal bases, small scars (<5 mm) • Punched out with deep abnormal bases, small scars (<5 mm) • Linear or troughed dermal scarring Deep, broad atrophic areas	3	6	9
D	Hyperplastic	• Papular scars	2	4	6
		• Area <5 cm^2	6		
		• Area 5–20 cm^2		12	
		• Area >20 cm^2			18

TREATMENT OF ACNE SCARRING

There is no one treatment modality that appears to be a "magic wand" for acne scars. There are numerous available treatment options; however, their results vary depending on the depth and morphology of the scar being treated. The primary focus of the clinician should be treating the acne and reducing the inflammation, thereby reducing the scarring. The use of topical retinoids in acne scars' prevention is well known, and the use of silicone gel is continually proving its efficacy in this field, especially for hypertrophic scars and keloids.[14] Scar treatment can vary from chemical-based treatment, energy-based treatment, and surgical treatment to cell and filler-based treatment. While the older treatment modalities, including fractional resurfacing, form a foundation for the treatment of acne scars, many novel therapies in the form of platelet-rich plasma, picosecond lasers, radiofrequency subcision, jet volumetric remodeling, autologous noncultured dermal cell suspension, and fibroblast cultures are some of the modalities which show promise. Depending on the depth and predominant type of scars, a tailored treatment plan may be made for the patient, wherein different treatments may be combined either sequentially or in the same session to provide optimal outcomes. An outline of the various treatment modalities available and the type of scar they appear to be beneficial in is given in **Table 4**.[22]

TABLE 4: Treatment modalities of acne scars based on types of lesions.

Type of scar	*Treatment modality/level of evidence*[22]
Superficial pigmented scars	Chemical peel—LA, SA, Jessner's, GA, pyruvic, mandelic, salicylic (LOE 3–4)
Superficial erythematous scars	• Lasers—PDL (LOE 2–3) • IPL (LOE 2–3)
Atrophic scars	• Chemical peel-mandelic + SA peel (LOE 1), GA (LOE 1) • TCA CROSS (LOE 2–3) • Microneedling (LOE 2–3) • MNRF (LOE 3–4) • Lasers—Er:Yag, CO_2, NAFL (LOE 2–3) • Subcision (LOE 1–2) • Punch techniques (LOE 2–4) • PRP plus microneedling or fractional ablative lasers (LOE 2–3) • Dermabrasion (LOE 1–3) • Combination treatments (LOE 1–4)
Lipoatrophic acne scars	• Autologous fat grafting with or without PRP (LOE 1–3) • Synthetic fillers (LOE 1–3) • Dermal cell suspension injection (LOE 1–3) • Cultured fibroblasts (LOE 1–3)
Hypertrophic scars	• Intralesional injections of triamcinolone and 5-FU (LOE 2–3) • Light liquid nitrogen cryotherapy (LOE 2–3) • Fractional cryotherapy (LOE 2–3) • Fractional ablative lasers (LOE 1–3) • Excision and closure (LOE 2–3) • Botulinum toxin (LOE 1–3)
Linear scar	Excision and closure (LOE 2–3)

(5-FU: 5-fluorouracil; CO_2: carbon dioxide; Er:Yag: erbium-doped yttrium aluminum garnet; GA: glycolic acid; IPL: intense pulsed light; LA: lactic acid; LOE: level of evidence; MNRF: microneedle radiofrequency; NAFL: non-ablative fractional laser; PDL: pulsed dye laser; PRP: platelet-rich plasma; SA: salicylic acid; TCA CROSS: trichloroacetic acid chemical reconstruction of skin scars)

CONCLUSION

Acne scarring carries with it considerable psychosocial morbidity, and it is pertinent for the dermatologist to educate the acne patient and address the inflammation associated with acne early on in order to prevent acne scarring. A thorough assessment of the "type" of scar helps the clinician layout a tailored plan for the patient to improve the scarring. Despite an array of modalities available to treat acne scarring, most tend to improve the scar and create a global improvement over a period of time. The treating clinician should spend adequate time counseling and discussing the differing modalities, timeline associated with treatment and the expected outcome of the treatment with the patient.

REFERENCES

1. Agrawal DA, Khunger N. A morphological study of acne scarring and its relationship between severity and treatment of active acne. J Cutan Aesthet Surg. 2020;13(3):210-6.
2. Dréno B. Assessing quality of life in patients with acne vulgaris: implications for treatment. Am J Clin Dermatol. 2006;7(2): 99-106.
3. Clark AK, Saric S, Sivamani RK. Acne scars: how do we grade them? Am J Clin Dermatol. 2018;19(2):139-44.
4. Fife D. Practical evaluation and management of atrophic acne scars: tips for the general dermatologist. J Clin Aesthet Dermatol. 2011;4(8):50-7.
5. Tasoula E, Gregoriou S, Chalikias J, Lazarou D, Danopoulou I, Katsambas A, et al. The impact of acne vulgaris on quality of life and psychic health in young adolescents in Greece. Results of a population survey. An Bras Dermatol. 2012; 87(6):862-9.
6. Cunliffe W. Clinical features of acne. In: Cunliffe WC (Ed). Acne, 1st edition. Chicago: Martin Dunitz-Year Book; 1989. pp. 20-32.
7. Goulden V, Stables GI, Cunliffe WJ. Prevalence of facial acne in adults. J Am Acad Dermatol. 1999;41:577-80.
8. Adityan B, Thappa DM. Profile of acne vulgaris—a hospital-based study from South India. Indian J Dermatol Venereol Leprol. 2009;75:272-8.
9. Layton AM, Henderson CA, Cunliffe WJ. A clinical evaluation of acne scarring and its incidence. Clin Exp Dermatol. 1994;19:303-8.
10. Jacob CI, Dover JS, Kaminer MS. Acne scarring: a classification system and review of treatment options. J Am Acad Dermatol. 2001;45:109-17.
11. Wolfram D, Tzankov A, Pülzl P, Piza-Katzer H. Hypertrophic scars and keloids—a review of their pathophysiology, risk factors, and therapeutic management. Dermatol Surg. 2009;35(2):171-81.

12. Cowin AJ, Brosnan MP, Holmes TM, Ferguson MW. Endogenous inflammatory response to dermal wound healing in the fetal and adult mouse. Dev Dyn. 1998;212(3):385-93.
13. Sobanko JF, Alster TS. Management of acne scarring, part I: a comparative review of laser surgical approaches. Am J Clin Dermatol. 2012;13(5):319-30.
14. Fabbrocini G, Annunziata MC, D'Arco V, De Vita V, Lodi G, Mauriello MC, et al. Acne scars: pathogenesis, classification and treatment. Dermatol Res Pract. 2010;2010:893080.
15. Holland DB, Jeremy AH, Roberts SG, Seukeran DC, Layton AM, Cunliffe WJ. Inflammation in acne scarring: a comparison of the responses in lesions from patients prone and not prone to scar. Br J Dermatol. 2004;150(1):72-81.
16. Baum CL, Arpey CJ. Normal cutaneous wound healing: clinical correlation with cellular and molecular events. Dermatol Surg. 2005;31(6):674-86.
17. Kang S, Cho S, Chung JH, Hammerberg C, Fisher GJ, Voorhees JJ. Inflammation and extracellular matrix degradation mediated by activated transcription factors nuclear factor-kappaB and activator protein-1 in inflammatory acne lesions in vivo. Am J Pathol. 2005;166:1691-9.
18. Chivot M, Pawin H, Beylot C, Chosidow O, Dreno B, Faure M, et al. Acne scars: epidemiology, physiopathology, clinical features and treatment. Ann Dermatol Venereol. 2006;133(10):813-24.
19. Zaleski-Larsen LA, Fabi SG, McGraw T, Taylor M. Acne scar treatment: a multimodality approach tailored to scar type. Dermatol Surg. 2016;42:S139-49.
20. Khunger N, IADVL Task Force. Standard guidelines of care for acne surgery. Indian J Dermatol Venereol Leprol. 2008;74:S28-36.
21. Boen M, Jacob C. A review and update of treatment options using the acne scar classification system. Dermatol Surg. 2019;45(3):411-22.
22. Gupta A, Kaur M, Patra S, Khunger N, Gupta S. Evidence-based surgical management of post-acne scarring in skin of color. J Cutan Aesthet Surg. 2020;13:124-41.
23. Goodman GJ, Baron JA. Postacne scarring: a qualitative global scarring grading system. Dermatol Surg. 2006;32(12):1458-66.
24. Chuah SY, Goh CL. The impact of post-acne scars on the quality of life among young adults in Singapore. J Cutan Aesthet Surg. 2015;8(3):153.
25. Agnew T, Furber G, Leach M, Leach M, Segal L. A comprehensive critique and review of published measures of acne severity. J Clin Aesthet Dermatol. 2016;9(7):40.
26. de Almeida Jr H, Cecconi J, Duquia RP, Souza PR, Breunig J. Sensitivity and specificity of self-reported acne in 18-year-old adolescent males. Int J Dermatol. 2013;52(8):946-8.
27. Goodman GJ, Baron JA. Postacne scarring—a quantitative global scarring grading system. J Cosmet Dermatol. 2006;5(1):48-52.
28. Dreno B, Khammari A, Orain N, Noray C, Mérial-Kieny C, Méry S, et al. ECCA grading scale: an original validated acne scar grading scale for clinical practice in dermatology. Dermatology. 2007;214(1):46-51.
29. Tan JK, Tang J, Fung K, Gupta AK, Richard Thomas D, Sapra S, et al. Development and validation of a scale for acne scar severity (SCAR-S) of the face and trunk. J Cutan Med Surg. 2010;14:156-60.
30. Dey BC, Nirmal B, Galigekere RR. Automatic detection of acne scars: preliminary results. IEEE EMBS Special Topic Conference on Point-of-Care (POC) Healthcare Technologies: Synergy Towards Better Global Healthcare, PHT. 2013.
31. Petukhova TA, Foolad N, Prakash N, Shi VY, Sharon VR, O'Brecht L, et al. Objective volumetric grading of postacne scarring. J Am Acad Dermatol. 2016;75(1):229-31.

CHAPTER 46

Surgical Management of Acne Scars

T Salim, Ragini Ghiya

KEY MESSAGES

- Acne scarring requires a combination approach; each type of scar may need a different treatment.
- A combination of resurfacing techniques, scar revisions, subcision, punch elevation, or excision may be needed.
- Trichloroacetic acid chemical reconstruction of skin scars (TCA CROSS) is a technique advocated for ice pick scars.
- Subcision is recommended for boat-shaped scars.
- Dermal grafts are useful to fill up depressions and are a replacement for fillers.

INTRODUCTION

The previous chapter has dealt with an overview of acne scars, their classification, and pathophysiology. This chapter deals with the surgical management of acne scars.

Numerous invasive, semi-invasive, and noninvasive techniques have been used to remove, replace, or raise acne scars and, in turn, resurface the cutaneous surface and reduce shadows. The currently available treatments for acnescarring include the following:[1,2]

- *Aesthetic approach:* Chemical peels, microdermabrasion, and dermal fillers
- *Surgical approach:* Punch techniques, subcision, dermal grafting, fat transfer, implantation of autologous collagen, cultured and expanded autologous fibroblasts, focal treatment with trichloroacetic acid (TCA), microneedling, dermabrasion, scar revision, and cryoslush
- Laser resurfacing, including ablative, nonablative, and fractional resurfacing.

The treatments vary in severity and efficacy **(Fig. 1)**. Treatment options such as ablative laser resurfacing or mechanical dermabrasion offer significant improvement in facial scars but are invariably associated with considerable morbidity and downtime.[2] On the other hand, treatments such as microdermabrasion, superficial peels, and nonablative laser resurfacing are associated with minimal or no downtime but do not show the same level of therapeutic efficacy.[3,4] This chapter will focus on different surgical techniques for acne scar revision, while laser resurfacing is dealt with in the next chapter. Other techniques, such as scar revisions, chemical peels, and microdermabrasion, have been dealt with in different chapters. This chapter will, therefore, only briefly mention relevant features of these techniques. For details, the reader is referred to individual chapters.

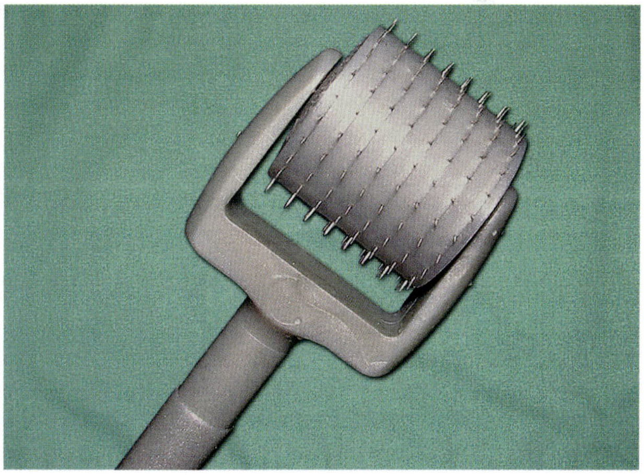

Fig. 1: Microneedling instrument.

The specific surgical techniques for the management of postacne scarring include:

- Microneedling
- Subcision
- Punch techniques
- Trichloroacetic acid chemical reconstruction of skin scars (TCA CROSS)
- Dermal grafting.

MICRONEEDLING

Microneedling[5-12] [skin needling therapy, dermaroller therapy, or collagen induction therapy (CIT)] has been dealt within a separate chapter, and only relevant and specific points are discussed here. It is a relatively new technique with efficacy and safety in the management of atrophic acne scars.

The dermaroller used to treat acne scars is a handheld device with drum-shaped roller studded with 192 fine microneedles of 0.1-mm diameter in eight rows **(Fig. 1)**. The device is available in needle length, ranging from 0.5 to 2 mm. A dermaroller with 1.5-mm needle length is commonly used in acne scar therapy. A deeper atrophic scar may require a 2-mm instrument. There are also motorized dermastamps and homecare dermastamps available for percutaneous collagen induction. Motorized dermastamps are needle cartridges attached to a motor device similar to a mesogun having a to-and-fro movement inducing pricks. The speed and depth of the needling can be adjusted according to the scars.

Indications

- This technique works best on acne scars of grades 3 and 4.
- It is recommended for rolling acne scars and boxcar scars.

Contraindications

- Active herpes labialis
- Keloidal tendency
- Patients on isotretinoin therapy within the preceding 6 months
- Bleeding disorders.

Procedure

The procedure is carried out under topical anesthesia. The patient is prepared in a similar manner to a surgical procedure. The facial skin is disinfected and anesthetized using a thick application of topical anesthetic cream (eutectic mixture of prilocaine and lignocaine). This is left for 30–45 minutes.

The treatment is then carried out by rolling the needling tool over the areas affected by acne scars, four times in four different directions: Horizontally, vertically, and diagonally right and left. This ensured an even pricking pattern, resulting in about 250–300 pricks/cm^2. It has been shown that rolling with a dermaroller (192 needles, 200 μm length, and 70 μm diameter) **(Fig. 1)** over an area for 15 times will result in approximately 250 holes/cm^2.

The microneedles penetrate through the epidermis but do not remove it; the epidermis is only punctured and heals rapidly. As the needles are set in a roller, every needle initially penetrates at an angle and then goes deeper as the roller turns. Finally, the needle is extracted at a converse angle, therefore curving the tracts and reflecting the path of the needle as it rolls into and then out of the skin for about 1.5–2 mm into the dermis **(Fig. 2)**.[8] The epidermis, and particularly the stratum corneum, remains intact except for the minute holes, which are about four cells in diameter.

The endpoint for each treatment is the presence of uniform bleeding points over the scarred area. In patients with deep-seated scarring, the skin is stretched in a perpendicular direction to the dermaroller movement so that the base of the scars could also be reached **(Fig. 3)**.

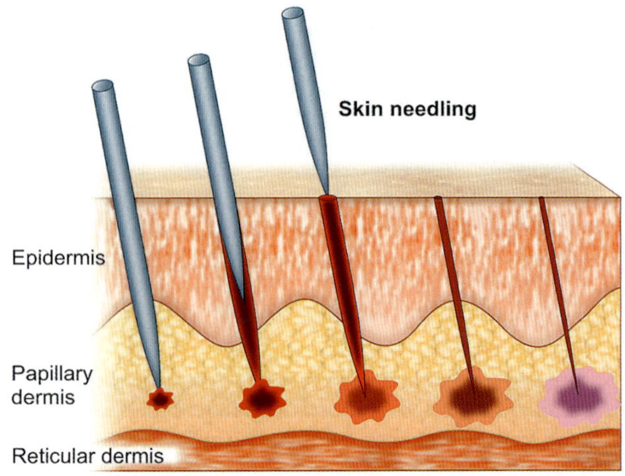

Fig. 2: Microneedling principle.

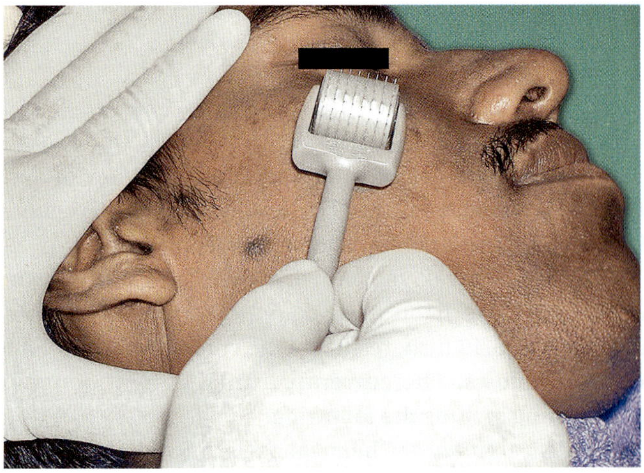

Fig. 3: Microneedling procedure.

Postprocedure Care

Immediately after the procedure, the area is mildly swollen, with superficial bruising. After the initial bleeding stops within a few minutes, there is a serous ooze, which stops within the first few hours after the operation. The treated area is cleaned with sterile saline solution to remove the serous ooze and bleed. The patient may require oral analgesics if the treatment is done with needle size >2 mm. The edema and erythema subside in a few hours. As the epidermis is not abraded, there is no need for photoprotection as postprocedure care.

The total number of treatment sessions required is three to four, repeated at 4–8 weeks' intervals.[8]

Outcome

In accordance with the literature, the full result may take 8–12 months of treatment as the deposition of new collagen takes place slowly **(Figs. 4A and B)**. Improvement in acne scars continues even after 6 months after the last dermaroller therapy. As shown by Fernandes and Signorini,[13]

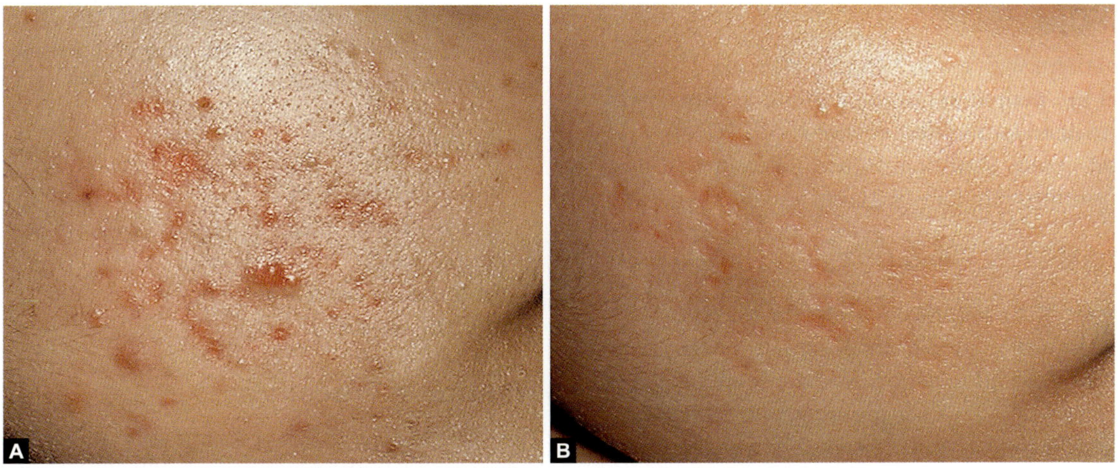

Figs. 4A and B: Dermaroller (A) Before 6 months; and (B) After 6 months.

TABLE 1: Advantages and disadvantages of different surgical modalities of acne scar correction.

Modality	*Advantages*	*Disadvantages*
Chemical peeling	Noninvasive, minimal downtime	Less effective, needs multiple sessions
Microdermabrasion	Noninvasive, minimal downtime	Less effective, needs multiple sessions
TCA CROSS	Noninvasive, minimal downtime Ideal for ice pick scars	Risk of postinflammatory hyper- or hypopigmentation in Indian skin
Microneedling	Easy, safe. Can be combined with topical drug delivery or topical platelet-rich plasma application for better results	Full result may take 8–12 months as collagen deposition occurs slowly
Subcision	Effective for all kinds of depressed scars	Downtime, needs proper training on part of dermatologist
Punch techniques	Effective for box scars, large ice pick scars	Should be combined with laser resurfacing few weeks later, downtime, needs proper training on part of dermatologist
• Fillers • Fat transfer	Effective for all kinds of depressed soft scars	Should be preceded by subcision in most cases, costly (except fat transfer), needs to be followed by laser or chemical peel for skin texture correction
Cryoslush	Noninvasive, minimal downtime	Effective only in superficial scars
Scar revision	Effective for linear scars	Needs proper training for operating dermatologist
Lasers	Noninvasive, minimal downtime	Good for superficial scars only. Has to be preceded by punch techniques or subcision for deep scars

(*TCA CROSS:* trichloroacetic acid chemical reconstruction of skin scars)

microneedling has undisputable advantages compared with conventional methods **(Table 1)**. The most important is that the epidermis remains intact because it is not damaged, eliminating most of the risks and negative side effects of chemical peeling or laser resurfacing.[13]

Many studies have confirmed the effectiveness of microneedling in acne scars. Fabbrocini et al. confirmed that dermaroller therapy was highly effective in the treatment of rolling acne scars.[8] A recent Indian study by Majid found that, in 21 patients with grade 3 scarring treated with microneedling, an excellent response was noted in 16 patients (reduction to grade 1 or less). Overall, 26 out of the total 36 patients (72.2%) showed an excellent response to dermaroller treatment, while six others achieved a good response (16.7%).[14] This technique can be employed in darker skin types without the fear of inducing postinflammatory hyperpigmentation. Relative advantages and disadvantages are mentioned in **Box 1**.

BOX 1: Microneedling in acne scars—advantages and disadvantages.

Advantages:
- Can be done in all types of skin
- Can be done with topical anesthesia
- Skin becomes thicker
- The healing phase is short
- Cost-effective
- Can be done on people who have had laser resurfacing or those with very thin skin
- Reduces telangiectasias along with acne scars
- Simple technique. Easy to master
- Minimal chances for postinflammatory hyper and hypopigmentation

Disadvantages:
- Overaggressive needling may cause scarring
- Mild treatment—it takes a longer time to see the result than with laser resurfacing
- Multiple sessions required
- Unsightly swelling and bruising while using deeper needles (>2 mm)

Practical Tips

- Select patients with grade 2 and 3 acne scars.
- Counsel the patient about the gradual improvement of scars and need for multiple sessions.
- Use good-quality instruments to avoid complications.
- Combine other techniques for faster and improved results.

SUBCISION

Subcision or subcutaneous incision-less surgery is a surgical intervention used to treat a variety of skin depressions, including atrophic acne scars, depressed scars, and wrinkles for years.[6,15] This procedure acts by releasing the subcutaneous fibrotic strands that pull down the overlying tissue in a rolling scar.

History

In 1957, Spangler reported use of Bowmen's iris needle to cut the fibrous strands beneath the deeply depressed facial scar.[16] The same technique was later described by David Orentreinch and Norman Orentreinch under "subcutaneous incisionless surgery" in 1995 with the use of a tri-beveled hypodermic needle.[6]

Principle

The mechanisms of scar improvement in subcision are:

- Releasing fibrotic strands underlying scars
- Organization of blood in the induced dermal pocket
- Connective tissue formation in the area.[6]

Thus, the depressed scar is lifted by the releasing action of the procedure as well as from connective tissue that forms in the course of normal wound healing **(Figs. 5A and B)**.

Indications

- This is the first scar revision technique to be performed in any case of pitted acne scars before taking up other procedures.
- Rolling acne scars—particularly scars that improve with stretching the skin.

Treatment Procedure

The scarred area is marked, and subcutaneous anesthesia (lidocaine 1% with epinephrine 1:100,000) is given. The best needle to perform subcision is an 18 gauge, 1.5 inch Nokor Admix needle. In the absence of Nokor needle, injection needles ranging from 16 to 23 gauge can be used. The needle is inserted with the blade facing upward at the periphery of the scarred area. Afterward, it is turned so that the tip is in a horizontal orientation (parallel to skin surface—side to side) just below the dermal-subcutaneous junction plane and gently swept across the site. A snapping sound is heard as the bands are broken. In addition, a gentle piston-like (to-and-fro) motion has been used to advance needle through fibrous bands to release them. The procedure is done in two directions in each scarred area. For maximal pressure release of the fibrotic strands, it is better to approach larger scars from multiple puncture sites. The needle can be fixed on a 2 cc syringe so that the syringe works as a handle **(Figs. 6A and B)**.

A

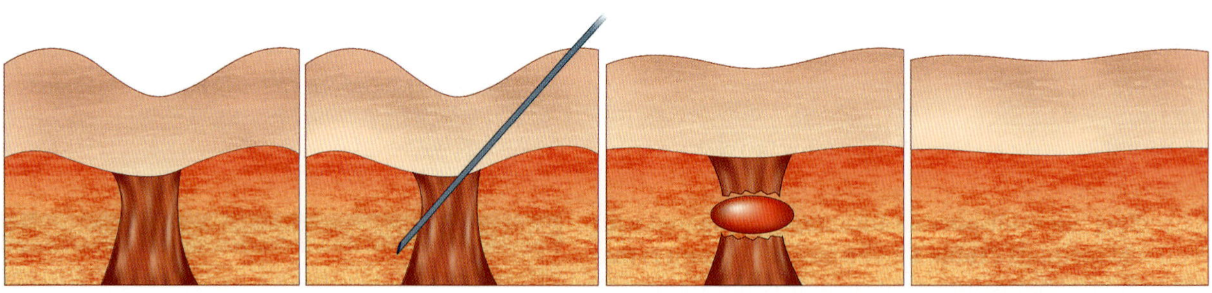

B

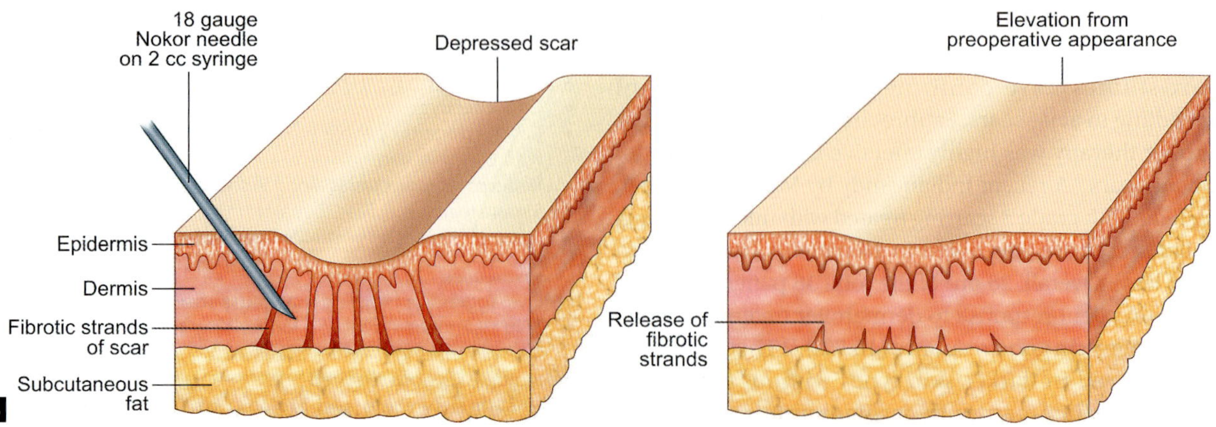

Figs. 5A and B: Subcision principle.

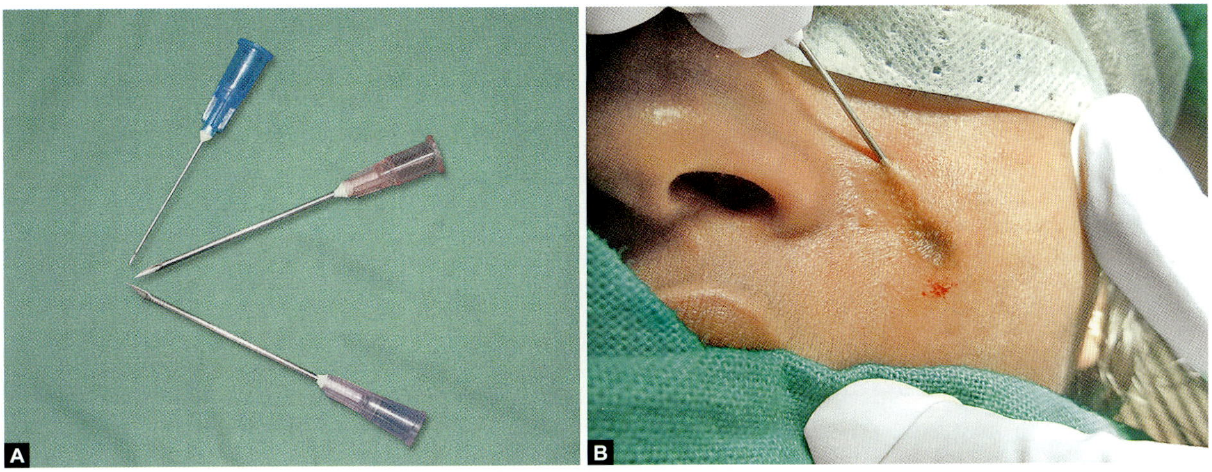

Figs. 6A and B: (A) Nokor needles; and (B) Subcision.

Firm pressure should be applied postoperatively for at least 5 minutes to achieve hemostasis. Treatment can be repeated at an interval of 6 weeks for up to two to three successive treatments.

Complications

Bleeding, hematoma, hypertrophic scarring, and scar recurrence are complications. Some degree of swelling is invariable, and the patient needs to be counseled. Bluish discoloration and swelling persist for 5–7 days.

Practical Tips

- When treating multiple scars with subcision, start with the most dependent area and work upward.
- While mild bleeding is expected and beneficial, a large hematoma may lead to persistent swelling and bruising. Prevent the formation of a large hematoma by allowing blood to flow out, if undue bleeding is noticed.
- Subcision can be combined with suction. Doing repeated suction by microdermabrasion device of the subcised scars may prevent redepression by induction of repeated hemorrhage in dermal pocket, delay in healing, and more new connective tissue formation at the scar area. Aalami Harandi et al. followed a subcision suction method by starting suction sessions on the 3rd day after subcision and continuing every other day for 2 weeks. There was a significant and persistent improvement in a short time, without considerable complication.[17]
- Subcision can be combined with subdermal implants. Balighi et al. treated acne scars with subcision and implantation of absorbable plain catgut pieces passed through the insertion puncture of the needle. However, the subdermal catgut implant led to no significant superior results in the above-mentioned study.[18] Autologous fat or dermal tissue can be used as subdermal implants.[19] The use of these implants may cause an inflammatory response leading to fibrous tissue formation in the subcised area and theoretically improve the result of subcision.
- Subcision can be combined with most other acne scar treatments. Superior results can be achieved by combination therapy.[20]

Bilevel Subcision

The author combined subcision at two different levels in the same session with promising results. Instead of combining two different techniques, a bilevel subcision is done at two different planes so as to break the fibrotic bands of individual scars and induce neocollagenesis at a deeper level. Apart from improvement of scars, this technique also reduces the skin sagging and induces excellent skin tightening. The procedure is done under tumescent anesthesia, thereby protecting all vital structures. Subcision of the individual scars is done at a superficial level as in classical subcision, and further, a deeper full plane subcision is done at the upper subcuticular level. This can be performed, preferably using a blunt cannula or even a Nokor needle. **Figures 7A to D** show the principle of bilevel subcision.

One side of the face can be treated by approaching through three points for deep subcision **(Figs. 8 and 9)**. Each scar can be individually subcised at a superficial level. There is edema and feeling of tightness during the first 1 week. It takes 7–10 days for the swelling to subside. Scars become better over the next few months, and maximum effects are seen at the end of a year along with overall facial tightening and pore reduction.

PUNCH TECHNIQUES

All punch techniques remove a pitted scar with a small rim of normal tissue. There are some scars that are circular, small, punched out in appearance, and have normal or altered texture of skin. Examples of such scars include acne scars with

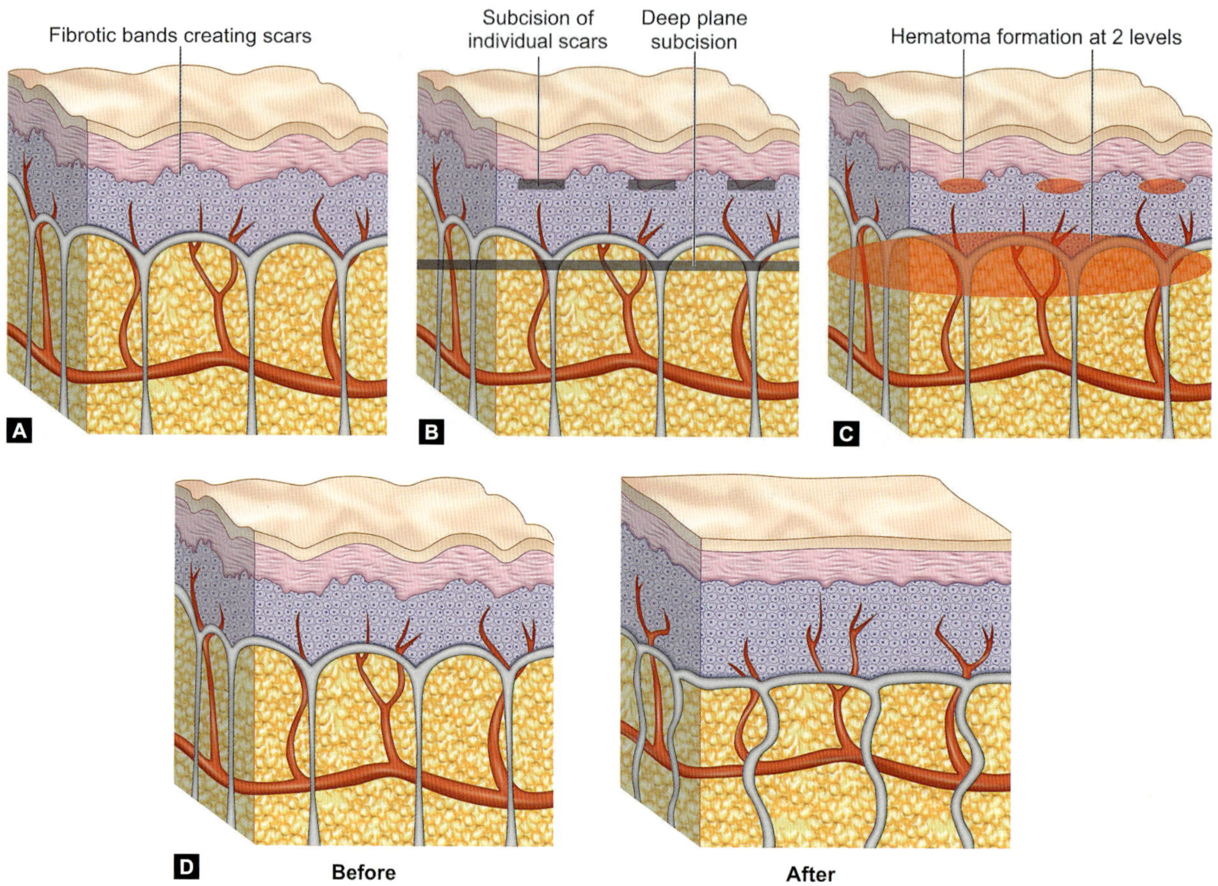

Figs. 7A to D: (A) Schematic representation of scar; (B) Sites of bilevel subcision. Just below individual scars and deeper plane; (C) Hematoma formation; (D) Before and after bilevel subcision.

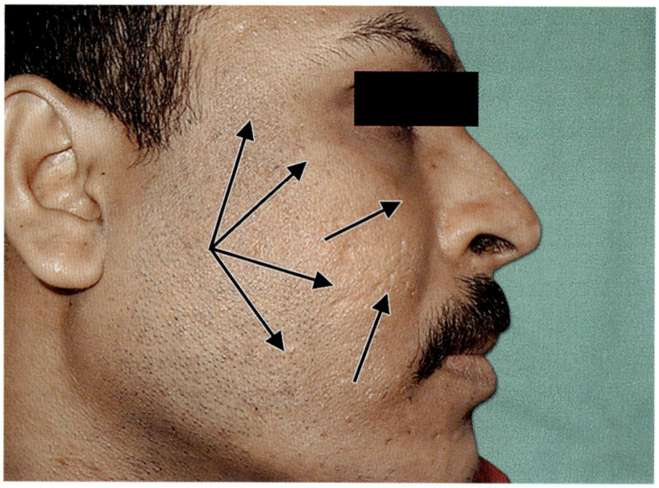

Fig. 8: Three points of entry for deeper subcision. Fanning movement can cover major area over the face.

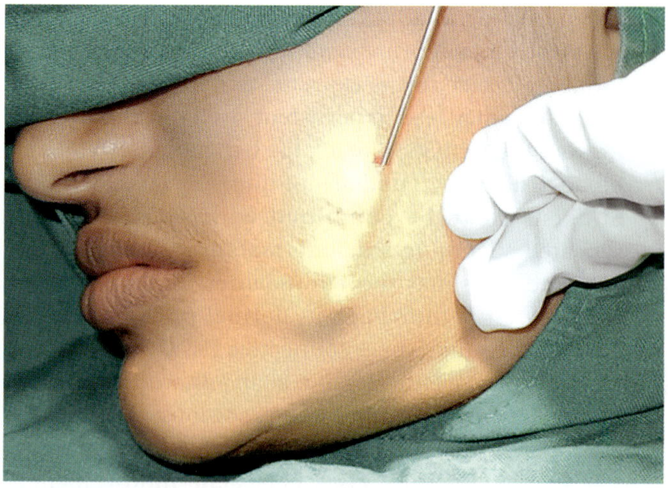

Fig. 9: Deep subcision using a cannula.

white atrophic bases or sharply punched-out "ice pick" scars. Punch techniques can be of use in the management of these scars. The punch techniques include punch excision, punch flotation or punch elevation, and punch replacement grafting.

Punch Excision

Indications

Punch excision is recommended for ice pick scars and deep boxcar scars <3.5 mm diameter **(Fig. 10)**.

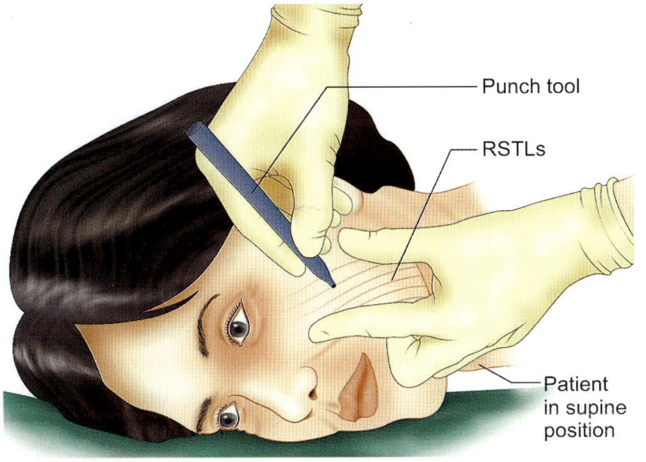

Fig. 10: Punch excision—schematic illustration. Note the use of a nondominant hand to apply outward traction perpendicular to facial relaxed skin tension lines. The punch tool is placed perpendicular to the skin and used with a quick rotating motion to remove the scar. (RSTLs: relaxed skin tension lines)

Procedure

Punch incision is done under local anesthesia. Scars are excised with a 1.5-, 2-, 2.5-, or 3-mm biopsy punch as per the size of the scar **(Figs. 11A and B)**. By placing outward traction on the punch site at the time of excision, the circular wound is changed into an ellipse. To ensure that the ellipse runs parallel to the relaxed skin tension lines, the outward traction should be applied perpendicular to the skin lines. The scar tissue is removed, and the wound is sutured with one to three interrupted sutures using 6-0 nylon or Prolene. If the punch excision is 2.5 mm or greater, a 6-0 vicryl (Ethicon) subcutaneous suture can be placed prior to epidermal closure. This absorbable deep suture helps to promote wound edge eversion and facilitates proper healing **(Figs. 11C and D)**.

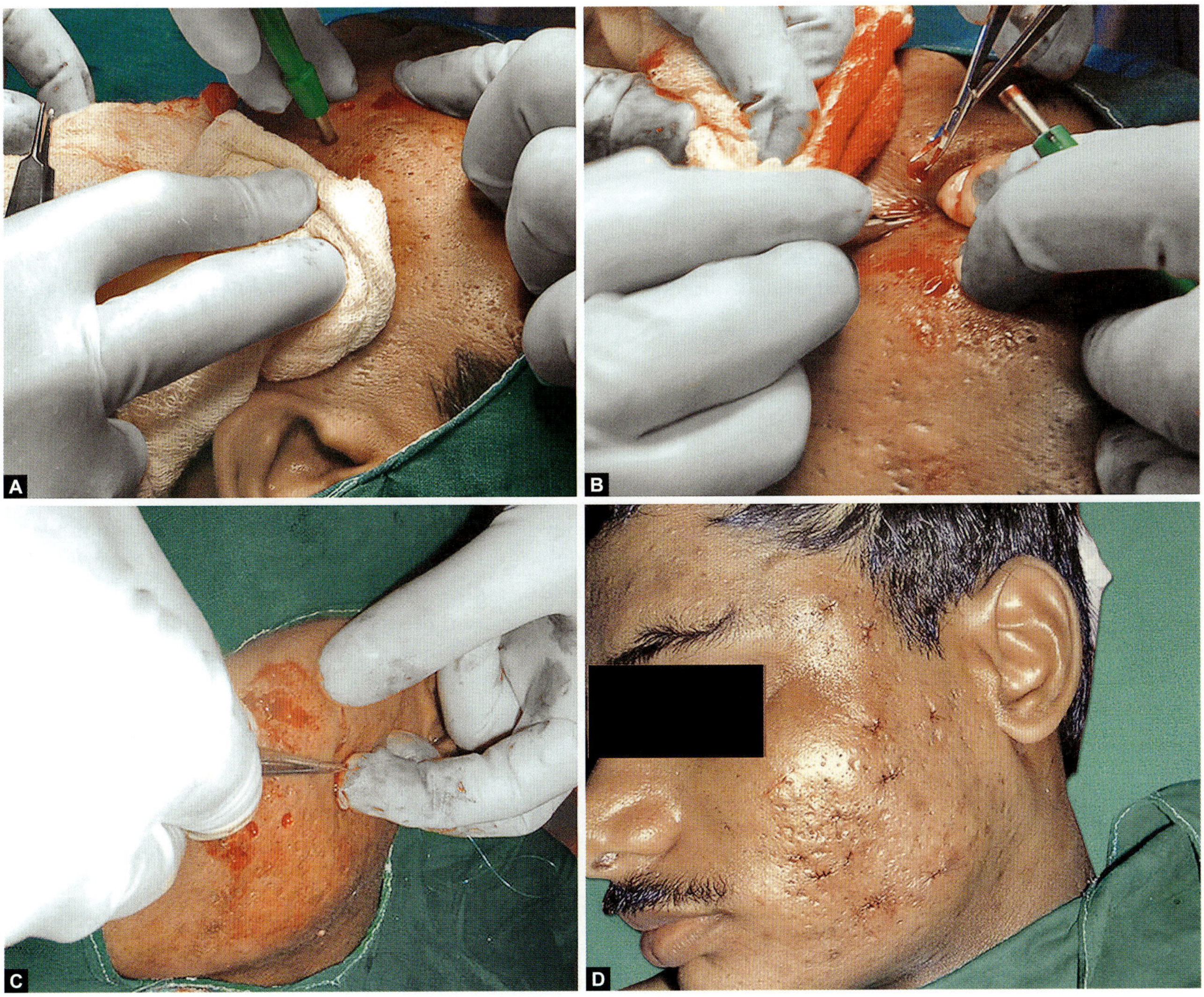

Figs. 11A to D: Punch excision and closure.

Punch Flotation

Indications

Punch flotation works best for wide (>3 mm) boxcar acne scars that do not have significant color or textural irregularities **(Figs. 12A to D)**.

Procedure

A punch that is exactly sized to match the inner diameter of the crateriform scar is selected for treatment. The punch is performed using a quick, rotating motion. This releases the bound-down scar. The plug is elevated with forceps and carefully freed from the underlying tissue. The plug is then elevated and positioned to lie slightly higher than the surrounding skin. The elevated punch can be secured in position by applying cyanoacrylate tissue adhesive and further closing with wound closure tapes like Steri-Strips (3M Corp.).

Punch Replacement Grafting

Indications

This procedure is utilized for deep, irregular pits and tethered boxcar scars with altered skin texture.

Procedure

The technique is similar to that of a punch flotation but replaces the plug with a donor plug instead of elevating the original defect. The scar plug is removed, and a graft plug of tissue obtained from the postauricular area or inner arm is transferred to the plug site. The donor punch graft should be 0.5 mm larger than the punch used to excise the scar. Grafts can be secured into place by cyanoacrylate tissue adhesive and wound closure tapes.

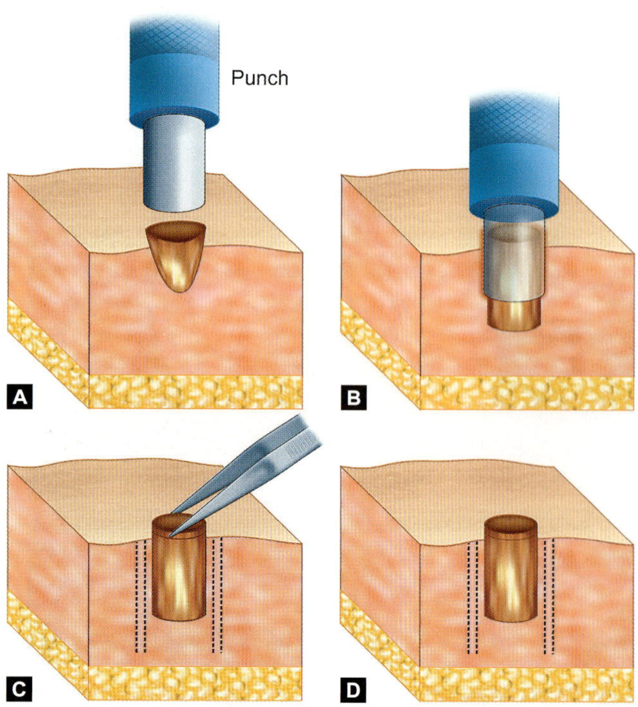

Figs. 12A to D: Punch flotation—schematic.

Limitations of Punch Techniques

Punch replacement and punch flotation techniques are more successful for scars located on less mobile regions of the face, such as the malar area and the forehead, and less successful in perioral sites. Complications that may be observed include poor graft take, graft extrusion, and graft visibility. Poor color and textural mismatch are also frequently observed. Multiple procedures may be needed. Since the advent of lasers, these procedures are performed less frequently.

Practical Tips

- Punch techniques have to be combined with other scar revision modalities for effective management of acne scars.
- Punch techniques followed by resurfacing 4–8 weeks later improve the scar significantly.[20,21] Several studies have suggested that if resurfacing is performed in this postoperative period, the healing takes on almost a fetal type, with distribution of the extracellular matrix glycoprotein, integrin subunits in the epidermis,[22] and dermal collagen fibers becoming unidirectional parallel to the epidermal surface after dermabrasion.
- Dermabrasion after excision, but before closure, improves the subsequent scar appearance.[23]
- Recently, simultaneous resurfacing with a CO_2 laser and punch excision[24] has been advocated.

CHEMICAL RECONSTRUCTION OF SKIN SCARS

Chemical reconstruction of skin scars is a technique using high-strength TCA focally on the atrophic acne scars to induce collagenization and cosmetic improvement. Lee et al. reported the use of high concentration (65 and 100%) TCA applied locally to atrophic acne scars. The authors labeled this technique CROSS.[25]

Trichloroacetic acid is a versatile peeling agent because the peel depth varies according to its concentration.[26] It is also self-neutralizing and not absorbed in the systemic circulation; hence, high concentrations can be safely used without risk of systemic absorption.

Principle

Application of the caustic agent TCA causes precipitation of proteins, coagulative necrosis of cells in the epidermis, and necrosis of collagen in the papillary to upper reticular dermis.[27] There is an increase in dermal volume as a result of an increase in collagen production, glycosaminoglycan, and elastin fragmentation and reorganization of dermal collagen. The dermal remodeling continues for several months. During the remodeling phase, type III collagen is gradually replaced by type I collagen. The fibroblasts are oriented parallel to the epidermis, which leads to improvement of scars.[27,28]

Indications

Trichloroacetic acid chemical reconstruction of skin scars is indicated for ice pick scars. In fact, it is the best treatment for this otherwise difficult-to-treat scar. Since ice pick scars are deep, destruction of the floor and wall of the pits, followed by dermal remodeling, leads to gradual improvement.

Procedure

The scars are marked with a surgical marking pen **(Figs. 13A to D)**. The face is cleaned with spirit and degreased with acetone. The procedure is carried out with the patient sitting comfortably as lying down can cause effacement of appearance of the scars. The skin is stretched, and 100% TCA is focally applied with a wooden toothpick, pressing firmly up to the bottom of the depressed area of atrophic scar, taking care to avoid spillage to the surrounding skin. The skin is monitored carefully and kept stretched until a frosted appearance is seen. Frosting is a result of coagulation of epidermal and dermal proteins and is generally seen in 10–15 seconds. The patient is asked to wash the face after the procedure. Photoprotection is recommended. TCA CROSS can be repeated at 4 week intervals for a total of three treatments.[26,29]

Complications

Transient postinflammatory hyperpigmentation and hypopigmentation are the reported complications of TCA CROSS.[26]

Concentration of TCA ranged from 50 to 100% in various studies.[25,26,29,30] None of the studies have reported any significant side effects even after applying 100% TCA on type V skin.[26] However, the results were better with increased concentration.

In a split-face study comparing TCA CROSS 100% applied twice at 12-week intervals with a 1,550 nm Er:glass fractional laser applied thrice at 6-week intervals, the CROSS technique was reported to be superior for ice pick scars.[30]

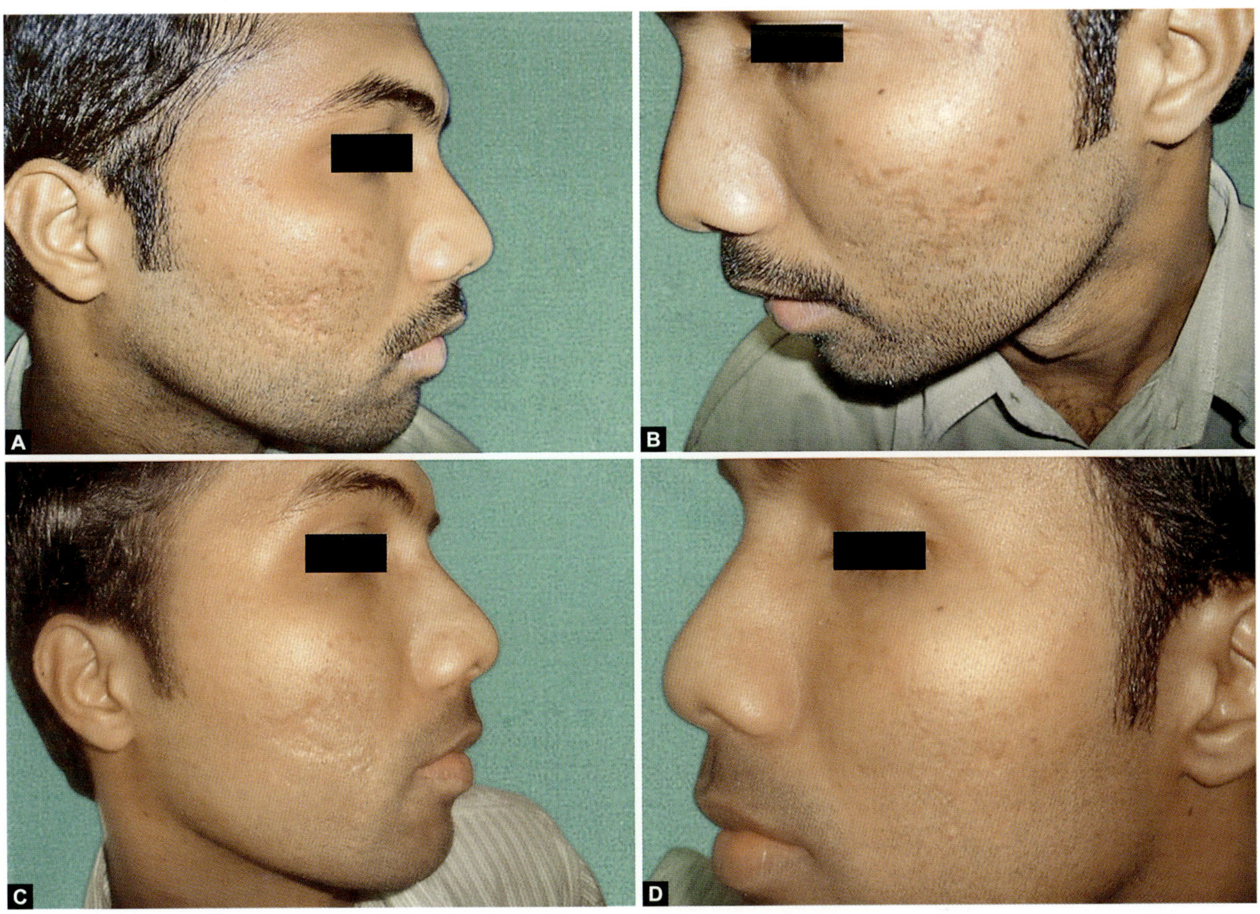

Figs. 13A to D: Trichloroacetic acid chemical reconstruction of skin scars (TCA CROSS): (A and C) Before; (B and D) After.
Courtesy: BS Chandrashekar, Bengaluru.

Practical Tips

- Priming the skin with hydroquinone and tretinoin cream for 2 weeks before the procedure helps in reducing the incidence of postinflammatory hyperpigmentation that is expected after using high concentrations of TCA in dark skins.
- Photoprotection should be strictly followed in all patients on TCA CROSS.
- Care should be taken to avoid spillage of TCA to normal skin.
- Application of TCA should be limited to the ice pick scars, and care should be taken not to apply the agent to the rim of the opening of the pit.

DERMAL GRAFTING[31-33]

Dermal grafts have been reported to be effective as a filler material for treating depressed scars. This technique builds on previous subcision and consists of placing dermal grafts into precise pockets under the skin. A dermal graft is a skin graft from which epidermis and subcutaneous fat have been removed.

Dermis can be used for filling up the defects in a cost-effective way. Dermal grafts have shown long-term survival in various published data and are almost permanent. Survival rates of dermal grafts are much higher than fat transplants.

Advantages of Using Dermal Graft

- Not susceptible to infection
- Can be accurately tailored for a variety of defects
- Creates a permanent spacer between overlying skin and underlying fibrous band of tissue
- Readily available material
- Easy to perform.

Procedure

Two different techniques of dermal grafting using the conventional technique and enzymatic separation are discussed below.

Conventional Technique

The procedure is done under local anesthesia **(Figs. 14 and 15)**.

The scar is subcised using an 18-gauge or Nokor needle 10–14 days before the operation in order to stimulate granulation tissue and achieve some initial correction.

Donor tissue is harvested using any conventional dermatomes or using biopsy punches from the postauricular site down to the fascia level. The epidermal part is trimmed using fine scissors. Alternatively, dermal tissue can also be harvested from a dermabraded area where the whole of the epidermis is completely removed. Excess fat is also trimmed in a similar way. Dermofat graft can be used in larger defects.

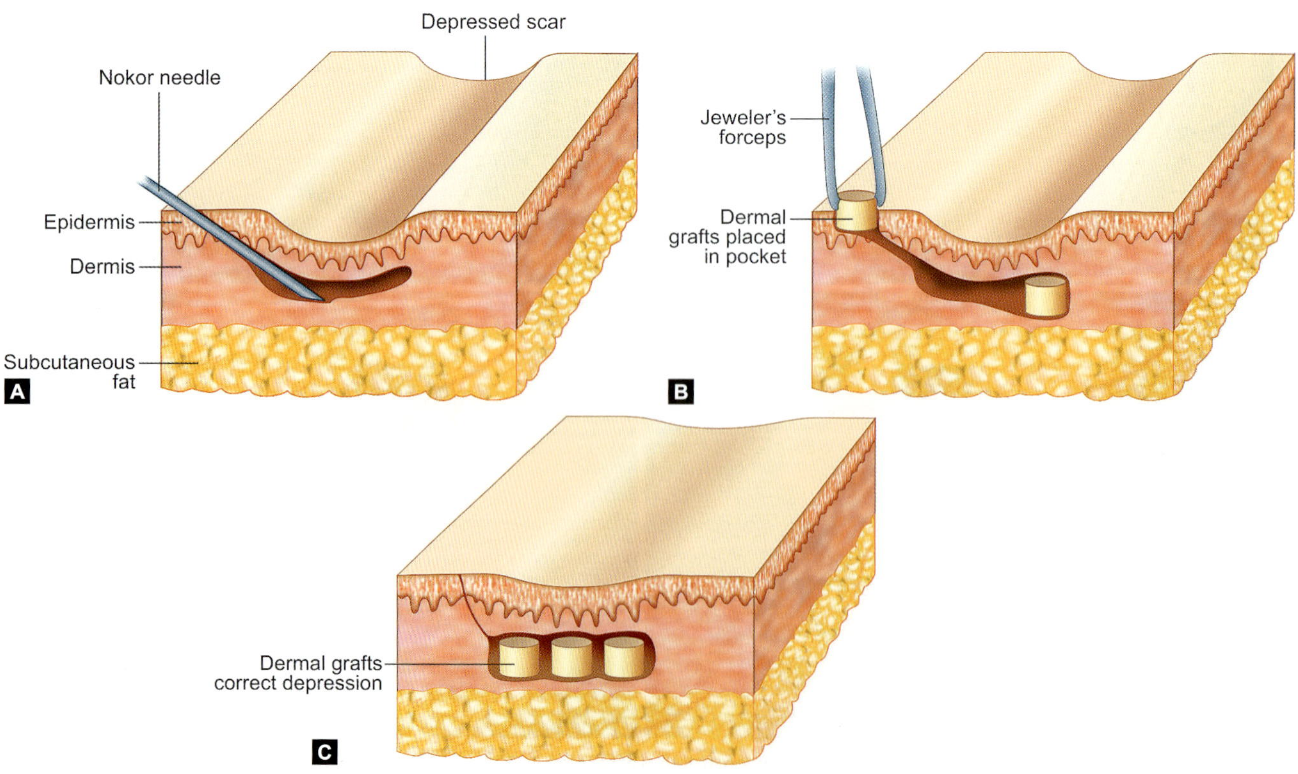

Figs. 14A to C: Dermal grafting conventional technique principle.

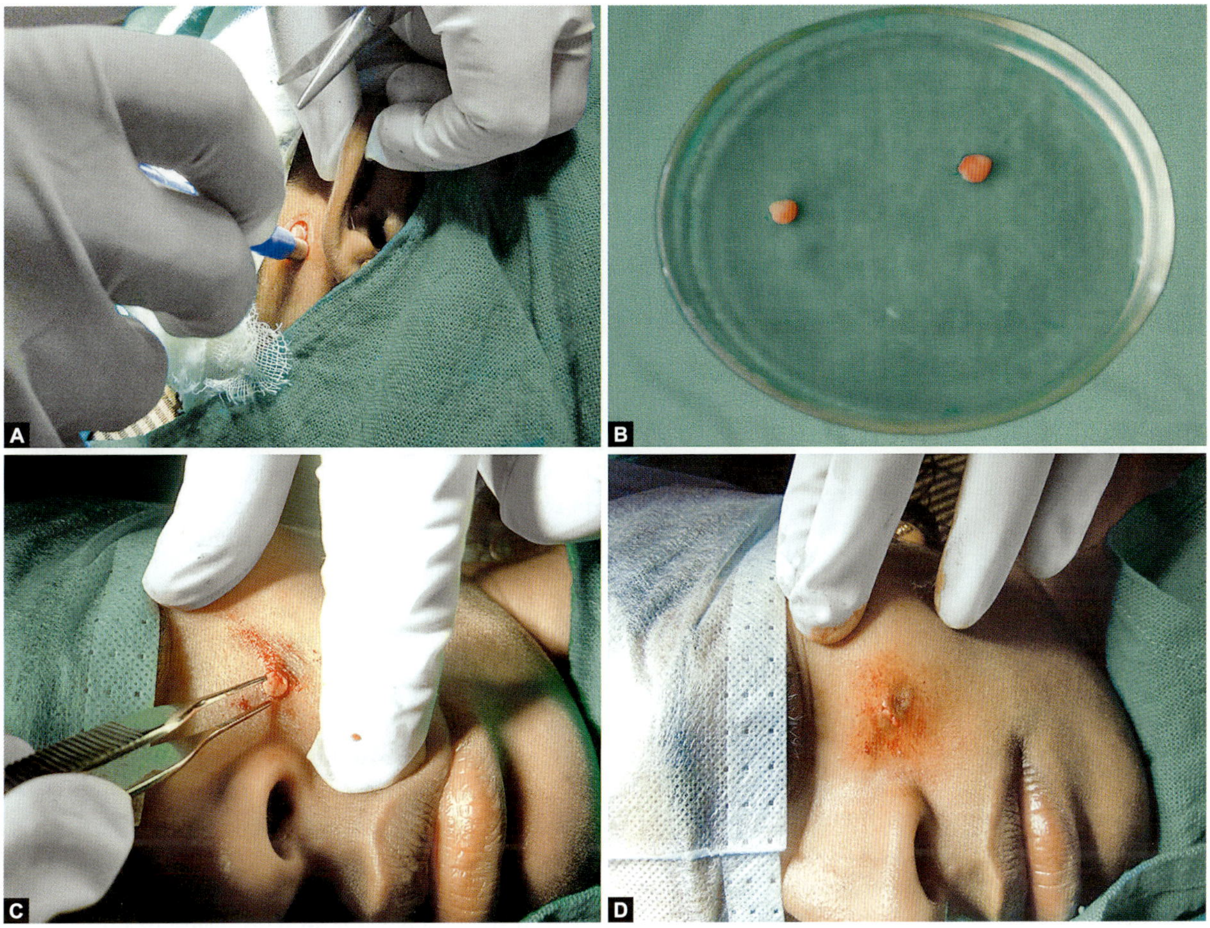

Figs. 15A to D: (A) Dermal grafting—conventional harvesting donor graft; (B) Dermal grafting—conventional donor graft with epidermis removed; (C) Dermal grafting—conventional placement of donor graft in the scar; and (D) Dermal grafting—conventional graft in place after closure.

These punches or long narrow strip of dermis is transferred to saline. The defective area is tunneled to create a space for the graft, as per the size of the defect. A small slit is made to insert the grafts. The grafts are trimmed according to the shape of the defect. The graft is inserted using forceps, and once complete correction has occurred, the slit is sutured with Prolene.

Enzymatic Technique

This is a technique of dermal grafting developed by the author **(Figs. 16A to D)**. The technique uses trypsin to make the firm dermal tissue soft and moldable.

Full-thickness skin graft is harvested as in case of a conventional technique. This is then transferred into a Petri dish containing 0.25% of trypsin in ethylenediaminetetraacetic acid (EDTA) solution. This is incubated at 37°C for 75 minutes. After incubation, the tissue is transferred to phosphate-buffered saline, and the epidermis is manually separated.

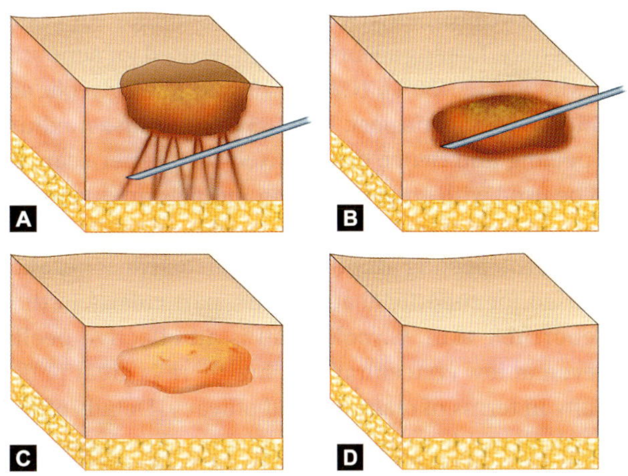

Figs. 16A to D: (A) Initial subcision prior to enzymatic dermal grafting; (B) Creation of a dermal pocket prior to enzymatic dermal grafting; (C) Injection of dermal suspension obtained from enzymatic dermal grafting with a wide-bore needle or directly by syringe; and (D) After injection of suspension.

The dermal tissue separated by enzymatic technique is soft, flexible, and easily moldable in comparison with the firm dermal tissue harvested by the conventional technique. This is filled into the defect as in the case of conventional technique or it can be transferred into a 1-cc syringe and pushed into the defect. The area can be molded by external manipulation. The slit made for inserting the material is then sutured. The result achieved can be gratifying **(Figs. 17A and B)**.

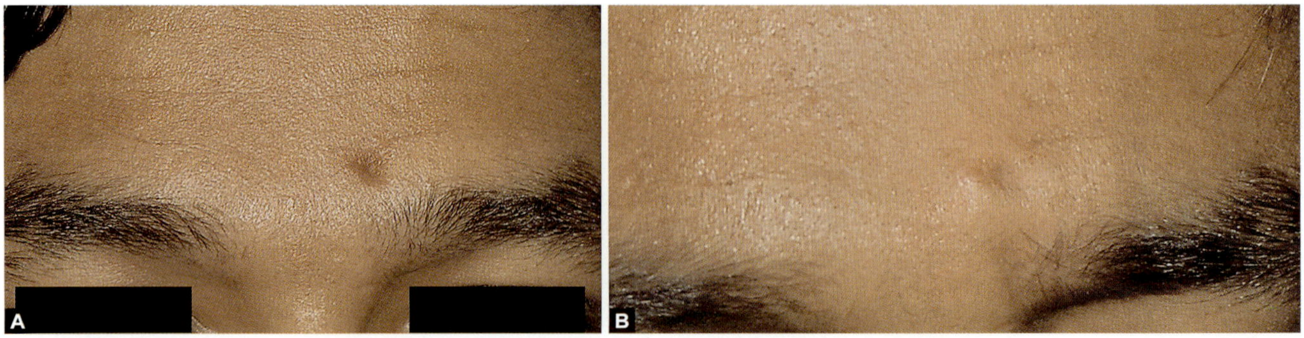

Figs. 17A and B: Dermal grafting—enzymatic separation before and after 3 months.

Practical Tips

- Epidermis should be removed entirely. Any epidermal tissue left along with the dermal graft can induce cyst formation.
- Great care should be taken while handling the dermal tissue. Any contamination can lead to infection and rejection of the graft.

OTHER MODALITIES FOR TREATMENT OF ACNE SCARS

In addition to the above methods, there are a number of other methods which have been described individually in different chapters. Relevant points of these techniques are mentioned here briefly.

Chemical Peeling

As is well known, superficial peels are useful for superficial acne scars only. Peeling agents that can be used for acne scars are salicylic acid (20–30%), TCA (10, 15, and 25%), glycolic acid (25–35%), and Jessner's peel. TCA (35%) can cause medium-depth peeling and hence can be used for deeper scars but should be used with great caution in Indian skin due to high chances of postinflammatory pigmentation. Salicylic acid (20–30%) is the peeling agent of choice in active acne, and it can be used for superficial acne scars, particularly in those with seborrheic skin. Glycolic acid is an effective peeling agent even at low concentrations, but there is great patient variability in terms of reactivity and efficacy. Details of each peel are dealt within a separate chapter on chemical peels.

Microdermabrasion

Microdermabrasion has become popular because of the ease of its technique, safety, and low cost. It is mainly indicated for the treatment of superficial acne scars and is ineffective for deeper scars. The patient must be adequately counseled regarding the limitations of the procedure, the need for multiple sittings, and expected outcome and complications. The key to effective microdermabrasion is stretching the skin under tension for effective abrasion and achieving a vacuum to aspirate the epidermal debris and used crystals. Treatment is repeated weekly until the desired result is obtained. Microdermabrasion is a safe procedure, particularly in darker skin, and requires no downtime.

Soft-tissue Augmentation (Fillers)

The popularity of soft-tissue augmentation with dermal fillers and autologous fat implantation is increasing because of minimal downtime, immediate results, and availability of an array of newer agents. It is mainly indicated for the treatment of soft atrophic acne scars with loss of dermal tissue. Dermal fillers placed under the scars elevate them and bring the surface of the scars in level with the surface of surrounding skin. It may be combined with lasers or other modality to improve skin textural abnormalities. It may be preceded by subcision or microneedling to break the fibrous septa, preventing scars to raise to the surface after filler injection.

Many preparations can be used for this, including hyaluronic acid fillers, autologous fat, etc. Fillers working by fibroplasia, such as poly-L-lactic acid (PLLA, Sculptra) and calcium hydroxyapatite (CaHA, Radiesse), have attracted attention in recent years because of their longer correction duration due to their collagen-stimulating effect. Liquid injectable silicone, one of the permanent fillers, is also being used for correction of acne scars, giving long-term correction.

However, their high cost and temporary duration of result are disadvantages.

Scar Revisions

In selected cases, when scarring is linear and extensive, scar revision techniques such as Z, M, and Y plasty may be useful. These need to be performed by a dermatosurgeon properly trained in performing these procedures. Details of the procedures are given in the section on "Scar Revision."

Cryotherapy

Cryoslush and cryopeel are used for the treatment of nodulocystic acne, inflammatory papule, and pustule.

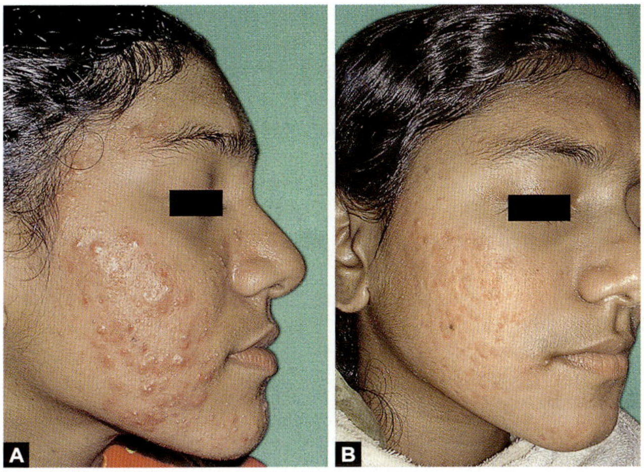

Figs. 18A and B: Cryoslush (A) Before; and (B) After in active acne.
Courtesy: BS Chandrashekar, Bengaluru.

In the cryoslush method **(Figs. 18A and B)**, solid CO_2 is crushed, and a few drops of acetone are added to make a paste. This paste is rapidly applied to the lesions with a gauze ball for 2–10 seconds. Superficial peeling is achieved due to epidermal necrosis, which causes desquamation of comedones and resolution of inflammatory papules, pustules, nodules, and cysts. In the cryopeel method, a spray of liquid nitrogen is used for 2–3 seconds instead of a CO_2 slush. However, pigmentary changes are commonly observed, particularly in darker-skinned patients, so this procedure should be used carefully only after proper counseling of the patient. Persistent erythema and scarring may also occur.

CONCLUSION

The treatment of postacne scars is a multimodality approach, and any single modality usually does not bring satisfactory correction. Each modality has its advantages and disadvantages **(Table 1)**. The main goal of treatment is to achieve maximal improvement rather than perfection in most of the cases. The surgical procedures (punch excision, punch elevation, and subcision) can be combined in one treatment session, if necessary, for different scar types. Most patients who have had punch excision or elevation should undergo laser resurfacing a few months later for further textural refinement. Laser skin resurfacing can be used after subcision but is not always necessary. Laser skin resurfacing alone is not as effective for rolling scars because it does not release the fibrous tethers. Patients must be reminded that collagen remodeling can take several months to occur, and maximum benefit from resurfacing or microneedling may not be evident until that time. Dermal fillers can be combined with any procedure for elevation of scar depressions. Many complications can be prevented by thorough preoperative evaluation, sound surgical technique, and careful follow-up care. Good patient rapport and effective communication with patients are invaluable.

There are multiple surgical options that can be tailored to each individual's needs, tolerance, and goals, along with the physician's assessments, skills, and expectations. The right procedure has to be combined in the right sequence to achieve the best result.

This chapter deals with only some of the surgical methods in acne scar revision. For information on lasers and other adjunctive therapies, please refer to appropriate sections.

TIPS AND PEARLS

- Subcision is an underutilized technique but yields excellent results in trained hands.
- Chemical peeling and microdermabrasion (MDA) give limited improvement and need multiple sessions.
- The main goal of treatment is to achieve maximal improvement rather than perfection in most of the cases.
- Punch excision techniques should be followed by resurfacing to achieve optimum results.
- Dermal fillers can be combined with any other treatment modalities.
- Multiple treatments combined in a rational way can help bring satisfactory improvement rather than any single modality used alone.

REFERENCES

1. Jacob CI, Dover JS, Kaminer MS. Acne scarring: a classification system and review of treatment options. J Am Acad Dermatol. 2001;45:109-17.
2. Alster TS. Cutaneous resurfacing with CO_2 and erbium: YAG lasers: preoperative, intraoperative, and postoperative considerations. Plast Reconstr Surg. 1999;103:619-32.
3. Ang P, Barlow RJ. Nonablative laser resurfacing: a systematic review of the literature. Clin Exp Dermatol. 2002;27:630-5.
4. Shim EK, Barnette D, Hughes K, Greenway HT. Microdermabrasion: a clinical and histopathologic study. Dermatol Surg. 2001;27:524-30.
5. Fernandes D. Minimally invasive percutaneous collagen induction. Oral Maxillofac Surg Clin North Am. 2005;17: 51-63.
6. Orentreich DS, Orentreich N. Subcutaneous incisionless (subcision) surgery for the correction of depressed scars and wrinkles. Dermatol Surg. 1995;21:543-9.
7. Camirand A, Doucet J. Needle dermabrasion. Aesthetic Plast Surg. 1997;21:48-51.
8. Fabbrocini G, Fardella N, Monfrecola A, Proietti I, Innocenzi D. Acne scarring treatment using skin needling. Clin Exp Dermatol. 2009;34:874-9.
9. Rawlins JM, Lam WL, Karoo RO, Naylor IL, Sharpe DT. Quantifying collagen type in mature burn scars: a novel approach using histology and digital image analysis. J Burn Care Res. 2006;27:60-5.
10. Ferguson MW, O'Kane S. Scar-free healing: from embryonic mechanisms to adult therapeutic intervention. Philos Trans R Soc Lond B Biol Sci. 2004;359:839-50.
11. Bandyopadhyay B, Fan J, Guan S, Li Y, Chen M, Woodley DT, et al. A "traffic control" role for TGFbeta3: orchestrating dermal and epidermal cell motility during wound healing. J Cell Biol. 2006;172:1093-105.
12. Aust MC, Fernandes D, Kolokythas P, Kaplan HM, Vogt PM. Percutaneous collagen induction therapy: an alternative treatment for scars, wrinkles, and skin laxity. Plast Reconstr Surg. 2008;121:1421-9.

13. Fernandes D, Signorini M. Combating photoaging with percutaneous collagen induction. Clin Dermatol. 2008;26: 192-9.
14. Majid I. Microneedling therapy in atrophic facial scars: an objective assessment. J Cutan Aesthet Surg. 2009;2: 26-30.
15. Goodman GJ. Therapeutic undermining of scars (subcision). Australas J Dermatol. 2001;42:114-7.
16. Spangler AS. New treatment for pitted scars; preliminary report. AMA Arch Dermatol. 1957;76:708-11.
17. Aalami Harandi S, Balighi K, Lajevardi V, Akbari E. Subcision-suction method: a new successful combination therapy in treatment of atrophic acne scars and other depressed scars. J Eur Acad Dermatol Venereol. 2011;25:92-9.
18. Balighi K, Robati RM, Moslehi H, Robati AM. Subcision in acne scar with and without subdermal implant: a clinical trial. J Eur Acad Dermatol Venereol. 2008;22:707-11.
19. Pinski KS, Coleman 3rd WP. Microlipoinjection and autologous collagen. Dermatol Clin. 1995;13:339-51.
20. Katz BE, Oca AG. A controlled study of the effectiveness of spot dermabrasion ('scarabrasion') on the appearance of surgical scars. J Am Acad Dermatol. 1991;24:462-6.
21. Yarborough Jr JM. Ablation of facial scars by programmed dermabrasion. J Dermatol Surg Oncol. 1988;14:292-4.
22. Harmon CB, Zelickson BD, Roenigk RK, Wayner EA, Hoffstrom B, Pittelkow MR, et al. Dermabrasive scar revision. Immunohistochemical and ultrastructural evaluation. Dermatol Surg. 1995;21:503-8.
23. Caver CV. Versatile dermabrasion. J Dermatol Surg Oncol. 1980;6:665-7.
24. Grevelink JM, White VR. Concurrent use of laser skin resurfacing and punch excision in the treatment of facial acne scarring. Dermatol Surg. 1998;24:527-30.
25. Lee JB, Chung WG, Kwahck H, Lee KH. Focal treatment of acne scars with trichloroacetic acid: chemical reconstruction of skin scars method. Dermatol Surg. 2002;28:1017-21.
26. Khunger N, Bhardwaj D, Khunger M. Evaluation of CROSS technique with 100% TCA in the management of ice pick acne scars in darker skin types. J Cosmet Dermatol. 2011;10:51-7.
27. Yug A, Lane JE, Howard MS, Kent DE. Histologic study of depressed acne scars treated with serial high-concentration (95%) trichloroacetic acid. Dermatol Surg. 2006;32:985-90.
28. Brodland DG, Cullimore KC, Roenigk RK, Gibson LE. Depths of chemexfoliation induced by various concentrations and application techniques of trichloroacetic acid in a porcine model. J Dermatol Surg Oncol. 1989;15:967-71.
29. Fabbrocini G, Cacciapuoti S, Fardella N, Pastore F, Monfrecola G. CROSS technique: chemical reconstruction of skin scars method. Dermatol Ther. 2008;21:S29-32.
30. Kim HJ, Kim TG, Kwon YS, Park JM, Lee JH. Comparison of a 1,550 nm erbium: glass fractional laser and a chemical reconstruction of skin scars (CROSS) method in the treatment of acne scars: a simultaneous split-face trial. Lasers Surg Med. 2009;41:545-9.
31. Arndt KA. Scar revision. Procedures in Cosmetic Dermatology. Amsterdam, Netherlands: Elsevier; 2006. pp. 45-66.
32. Besecker B, Hart CG. A new treatment option for acne scars: allograft dermis. Dermatol Nurs. 1999;11:111-4.
33. Burres SA. Recollagenation of acne scars. Dermatol Surg. 1996;22:364-7.

CHAPTER 47

Acne Scars: Treatment with Lasers

Imran Majid

KEY MESSAGES

- Lasers, particularly fractional lasers, are an integral part of the management of acne scars.
- Both fractional ablative and nonablative lasers are useful.
- Ablative fractional lasers score over nonablative lasers in terms of efficacy of scar amelioration. However, the former are associated with significant downtime.
- Among the different morphological types of acne scars, rolling and superficial boxcar scars respond the best to laser resurfacing treatment.
- In severe types of scarring, lasers have to be combined with other antiscar modalities for optimum results.

INTRODUCTION

Postacne scarring is one of the most feared and long-lasting complications of inflammatory acne.[1] The condition is associated with a lot of psychological trauma as the involved site is most often the face. There is a long list of treatment options available for amelioration of postacne scars, but the outcome from any of these treatment options is still far from being ideal. Lasers are among the most recent additions to this list of therapeutic options. A number of laser and light devices are currently used in managing acne scars, and these devices will be discussed in this chapter. What needs to be remembered, however, is that the majority of patients with acne scars have more than one morphological type and grade of scars, and this warrants the use of multiple treatment options to reach a satisfactory level of improvement.

INDICATIONS OF LASER TREATMENT IN ACNE SCARS

Laser treatment for acne scars can be considered in any patient in whom the scars are causing a significant psychological impact. In general, patients with grade 2 to grade 4 scars by the Goodman and Baron grading system are thought to be the ideal candidates for laser treatment.[2] While patients with grade 1 scars can be managed by simpler scar amelioration techniques such as peels with or without topical retinoids or even microdermabrasion techniques, laser resurfacing can be used in such cases if the psychological impact is really high in an individual patient.[2,3] Patients with the most severe, grade 4 scars are the most difficult to treat and generally do not show a considerable improvement after any single treatment option. These patients have to be treated with a cocktail of multiple treatment options such as surgical techniques, fillers, subcisions, and laser resurfacing.

Lasers are indicated in the treatment of all the different morphological types of acne scars. However, the response to laser resurfacing varies among these morphological variants. Among the different morphological types of acne scars, rolling and superficial boxcar scars respond the best to laser resurfacing treatment.[4,5] Pitted scars and especially deeper boxcar scars usually respond less satisfactorily to laser resurfacing than the abovementioned scar types. In such cases, laser resurfacing needs to be combined with surgical procedures such as punch excision or punch flotation or with trichloroacetic acid (TCA) chemical reconstruction of skin scars (CROSS) technique to improve the therapeutic results.[4-6]

LASERS USED FOR ACNE SCARS

Lasers used in the treatment of postacne scars can be broadly divided into two main groups—ablative and nonablative lasers. This classification is simply done on the basis of whether the laser leads to an ablative injury to the epidermis/dermis or not during the treatment process.

Ablative Lasers

Ablative lasers, as the term denotes, cause an injury or ablation of the epidermis and a part of the dermis with resultant collagen deposition as a part of the healing response. This collagen deposition in the dermis along with a renewal of the epidermal layer is responsible for amelioration of postacne atrophic scars as well as any pigment dyschromias.

The two main ablative lasers used for acne scars are the CO_2 and erbium lasers. The CO_2 laser emits light at the 10,600 nm wavelength and is the more ablative of the two. It causes vaporization of the epidermis and the papillary dermis to a depth of about 50–150 μm.[7] The depth of this vaporization depends largely on the energy level that is used.

In addition to this vaporizing effect, there is an additional thermal injury extending up to another 20–40-µm zone around the vaporization zone.[8] The erbium yttrium aluminum garnet (Er:YAG) laser, on the other hand, emits light in the 2,940 nm wavelength, and the depth of ablation with this laser is less than that achieved with CO_2 laser. In addition, it causes minimal surrounding thermal damage of about 5–15 µm.[8] The depth of ablation can be increased by increasing the number of laser passes (stacking), and similarly, the extent of surrounding thermal damage can be increased by increasing the laser pulse duration (variable pulse). See the chapter on Er:YAG laser for more details.

As a rule, ablative lasers are the most effective in the treatment of postacne scars, but the high incidence of adverse effects limits their use. These adverse effects include a prolonged erythema and exfoliation of the skin, posttreatment hyper- and hypopigmentation, and even the risk of scarring and secondary infections. Another disadvantage of these ablative lasers is the prolonged downtime associated with their use.

Nonablative Lasers

While ablative procedures result in removal of entire epidermis and parts of dermis and cause a dramatic and impressive reduction in scar severity, their side effect profile is equally serious, especially in dark-skinned races.[8,9] This is where the nonablative lasers score as they can also reduce acne scarring without significant downtime. However, the efficacy of these lasers is considered to be less as compared with the ablative lasers. The underlying principle of laser remodeling by nonablative lasers is induction of controlled injury to the dermal collagen without any damage to the epidermis. This controlled injury leads to a healing response with dermal collagen remodeling. This causes a tightening effect on the skin with resultant improvement in the appearance of the scars.[8,9]

The nonablative lasers used for the treatment of acne scars can be divided into two groups:

1. *Infrared lasers:* These include 1,450 nm diode laser, 1,064 nm Q-switched neodymium yttrium aluminum garnet (Nd:YAG) laser, 1,320 nm Nd:YAG laser, and 1,540 nm Er:glass laser.
2. *Visible light lasers:* This list includes the commonly used intense pulsed light (IPL), pulsed dye lasers, light emitting diodes, broadband light sources, etc.

Among the above two groups, infrared lasers are the ones that have been used and studied more commonly than the other group. Treatment with nonablative lasers can provide modest improvement scores in acne scar management. Typically, the treatment comprises multiple sessions at 3–4 week intervals, and the overall score is presumed to improve with more number of sessions. The first nonablative laser that was used for the treatment of acne scars was the 1,450 nm diode laser. This laser provides an additional advantage of treating active acne in addition to the acne scars through its effect on sebaceous glands.[10] Another laser device in the infrared range that has been used in the management of postacne scars is the 1,320 nm Nd:YAG laser.[11] This laser system has been compared with the 1,450 nm diode laser, and the comparison study showed both the lasers to be effective and safe with relatively better efficacy from the latter.[12] A combination of serial TCA peels and 1,450 nm diode laser treatments has also been assessed in a study with a small sample size, and the combination has been shown to be more effective than laser treatment alone.[13]

FRACTIONAL PHOTOTHERMOLYSIS

Fractional photothermolysis is a relatively new concept in laser rejuvenation, wherein the laser system, instead of causing a photoinjury to the whole skin, produces longitudinal arrays of microscopic thermal injury to specific depths in the dermis. These longitudinal thermal wounds are known as microscopic treatment zones (MTZs), and they are separated from each other by normal, noninjured skin. The term "fractional" is in fact derived from this fact that only a fraction of the whole skin is treated rather than the whole skin surface. This "fractionated treatment" minimizes the chances of any serious adverse effects to the skin and also shortens the downtime after treatment. The technology provides a fine balance between the undesirable side effects of ablative lasers and the limited efficacy of nonablative ones. Fractional photothermolysis was initially used for the treatment of photoaging,[14] but the technology is now used in many more indications, especially postacne scarring.

In fractional photothermolysis, the skipped noninjured part of the skin provides the source of keratinocytes that migrate into the laser-treated injured areas.[15] This phenomenon of keratinocyte migration is seen within the first 24 hours after treatment. After migration into the treatment zone, the donated keratinocytes facilitate the removal of necrotic debris from the skin in the form of denatured dermal tissue, melanin, and other constituents.[14,15] This necrotic debris is known by the name of "microscopic epidermal necrotic debris" (MENDs). Elimination of this microscopic debris (MENDs) is followed by laying-down of new collagen in the dermis and a resultant antiscarring and antiaging effect.

Fractional photothermolysis is also divided into the ablative and nonablative platforms depending upon the wavelength of the laser used and the effects of the laser on the skin. In the treatment of acne scars, both the ablative and the nonablative fractional lasers have been used. Fractional photothermolysis is summarized in **Box 1**.

Nonablative Fractional Resurfacing for Acne Scars

Fractional lasers with wavelengths in the range of 1,410–1,550 nm are the ones referred to as nonablative

BOX 1: Summary of fractional lasers.

- Fractional lasers are the most commonly used lasers for acne scars at present
- Fractional lasers treat only a small fraction or part of the skin by causing longitudinal columns of injury known as microscopic treatment zones (MTZs)
- Two main categories of fractional lasers are used: Nonablative and ablative fractional lasers
- Nonablative lasers are associated with minimal downtime and are considered safer than ablative lasers
- Ablative fractional lasers are claimed to be more efficacious than nonablative lasers

TABLE 1: Some studies on nonablative lasers in acne scars.

Laser used	*Study type*	*Results*
1,560 Erbium, Mosaic[6]	Prospective split face study on comparison between laser and CROSS technique in 20 patients	Laser gave better results in rolling scars, while ice pick scars showed similar results with both
1,560 Erbium glass, Fraxel SR[17]	Prospective study in 29 patients	16% patients achieved >75% improvement, while 62% showed 50–75% improvement
1,560 Erbium[16]	Prospective study in 53 cases	50–75% improvement in 90% patients after three sessions
1,540 Erbium, Starlux[21]	Prospective split face study	About 50% patients showed moderate improvement

(CROSS: chemical reconstruction of skin scars)

fractional lasers. These lasers cause columns of coagulative change in the dermis without injuring the epidermis. As the stratum corneum remains intact, the healing is fairly rapid without any sequelae. Among the nonablative fractional lasers, the one that has been the most commonly used till date is the 1,550 nm erbium-doped fiber laser known as Fraxel laser (Reliant Technologies, USA). Most of the studies on this laser device have reported improvements in the scar appearance in the range of 50% or even up to 75% after multiple sessions at monthly intervals.[16-18] The erbium-doped fiber laser has even been used in patients with darker skin with good results.[19,20] The most important advantage of nonablative lasers is that there is no significant downtime after treatment with these devices. This is of significant practical benefit as many patients are not ready to accept downtime over many days after any treatment for acne scars **(Table 1)**.

ABLATIVE FRACTIONAL LASER RESURFACING

Ablative fractional lasers have been designed to deliver the best of both worlds by applying ablative laser technology in a fractionated pattern that provides the efficacy of ablative laser treatment but minimizes the side effect profile to a considerable degree. Fractional ablative lasers cause a direct vaporizing effect on the epidermis and some part of the dermis in a microscopic columnar pattern. In addition, there is a zone of coagulation of variable thickness around these columns. The depth and diameter of these columns depend upon the laser device used as well as the energy and pulse width used during the procedure **(Figs. 1A to C)**.

The use of fractional ablative lasers in acne scars has seen an increasing trend over the last few years. The level of scar improvement achieved with these lasers has been claimed to be more than with nonablative lasers **(Figs. 2 and 3)**. These lasers have been used in almost all races and skin types with good to excellent efficacy and a favorable adverse effect profile.

Two ablative fractional laser devices are reported to be useful in acne scars—fractional CO_2 laser and fractional Er:YAG laser **(Table 2)**.

FRACTIONAL CO_2 LASER IN ACNE SCARS

Among all ablative and nonablative fractional lasers, the one that has been the most commonly used and reported as successful is the fractional CO_2 laser. A number of clinical studies have confirmed the efficacy of this laser system in acne scars.[22,25-27] The range of improvement reported with fractional CO_2 laser has varied from one study to another. This is mainly because of nonuniform means of assessment of treatment response. There is still a lack of reproducible objective means of assessing therapeutic response in acne scars.

STEPS OF FRACTIONAL LASER TREATMENT FOR ACNE SCARS

The procedure is done usually under the effect of topical anesthesia under occlusion. A eutectic mixture of prilocaine/tetracaine and lignocaine is commonly used and kept for 45 minutes to 1 hour.

A smoke evacuator should be available and needs to be used as it removes the viral particles along with the smoke.

Proper fluence and density settings are then selected according to the scar type and severity. Deeper scars need higher fluencies as the depth of penetration of the laser beam is directly proportional to it. It is important to treat the shoulder or margins of scars to achieve a good therapeutic benefit.

A topical noncomedogenic antibiotic cream is advised in the postoperative period. Patients with a history of herpes simplex need to be given antiviral prophylaxis 1 day prior and 5 days after the procedure. Patients are advised to avoid sun exposure after the procedure to minimize the chances of post-inflammatory hyperpigmentation. It is important to counsel the patients about the downtime. Patients do experience erythema and crusting for few days after the procedure, and this may limit their social activities for these days.

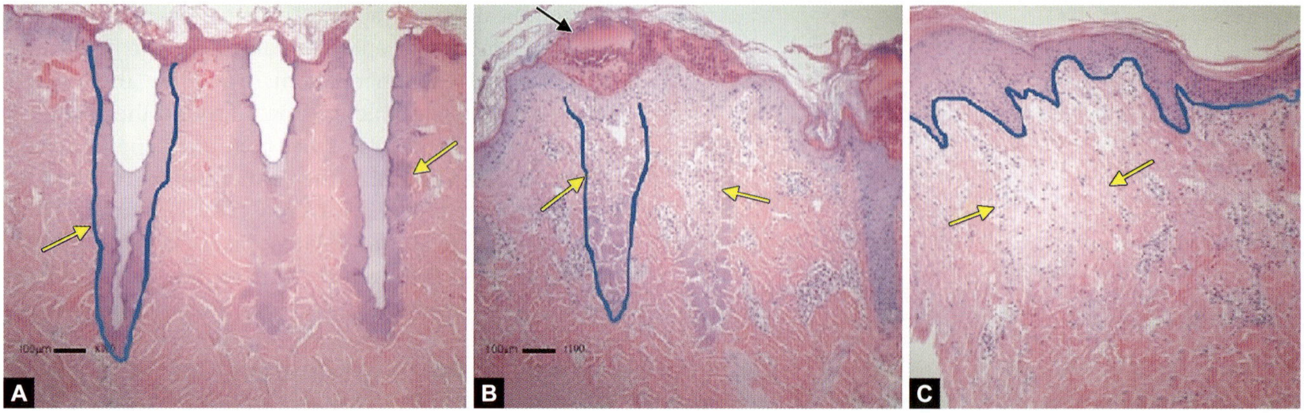

Figs. 1A to C: Histological pictures showing the longitudinal ablation and healing response with fractional CO_2 laser: (A) Immediately after; (B) Post 2 days; (C) Post 14 days.
Courtesy: Lutronics Corp.

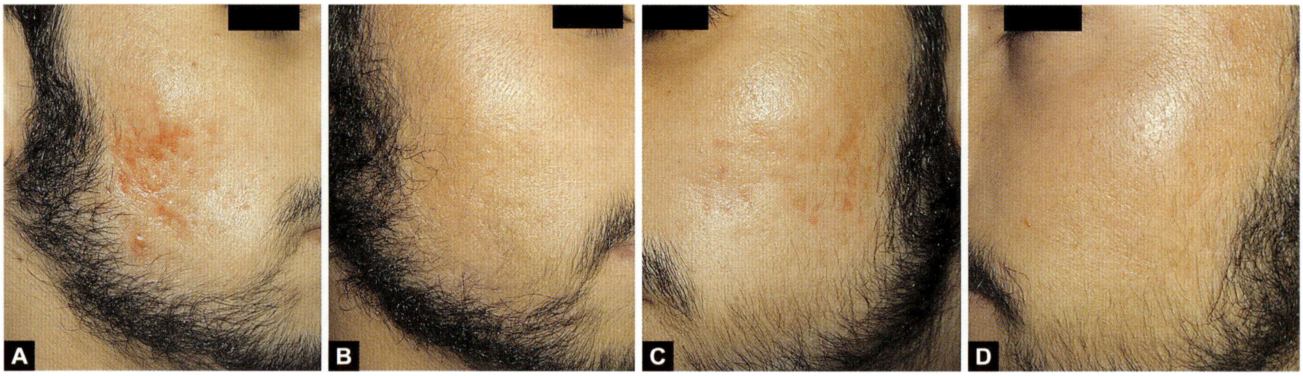

Figs. 2A to D: Predominantly rolling scars showing excellent improvement after fractional CO_2 laser resurfacing.

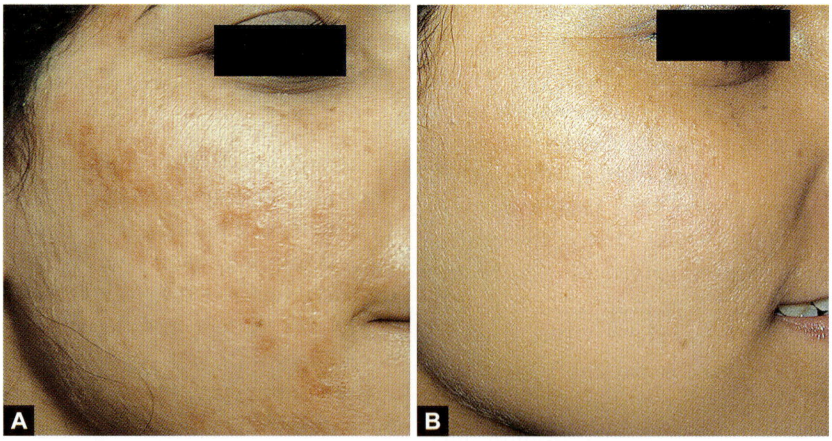

Figs. 3A and B: Early scars show better results after fractional CO_2 laser resurfacing.

COMPLICATIONS OF LASER TREATMENT FOR ACNE SCARS

Adverse effects that are reported most commonly with ablative fractional lasers are erythema and crusting that can remain for 4–7 days after treatment session. In addition, patients may suffer from postinflammatory hyperpigmentation, flaking and dryness of the skin, pruritus, bronzing of skin, and aggravation of active acne.[22,25]

Among all these complications mentioned, the one that is the most important in colored or darker skin is postinflammatory hyperpigmentation and even depigmentation. To avoid this complication, it is important to use lower fluences and lower MTZ densities and to avoid overlapping of laser passes over the skin. It is equally important to avoid any posttreatment sun exposure and to use sunscreens properly in the postprocedure period.

TABLE 2: Some studies on ablative fractional lasers in acne scars.

Laser used	*Study design*	*Results*
Fractional CO_2, Ultrapulse[19]	Prospective study in 20 cases	50% patients showed >50% improvement
Fractional CO_2, Fraxel[22]	Prospective study in 16 cases	43–79.9% improvement on clinician's assessment
Fractional CO_2, Cynosure[23]	Prospective study in 15 cases	Good to excellent improvement reported by 79% patients
Erbium YAG, Pixel[24]	Prospective study in 26 patients	Mean improvement of 79% in all patients treated with 5 treatments 3 weeks apart
Fractional CO_2, Ellipse[25]	Prospective study in 13 cases	85% patients achieved 25–50% improvement
Fractional CO_2, Qray FRX[26]	Prospective study in 60 cases	• Excellent improvement in 43.3% cases and good results in 25% • Rolling and superficial boxcar scars responded better and pits responded the least

BOX 2: Adverse effects of fractional laser resurfacing.

- Erythema and crusting
- Postinflammatory hyperpigmentation
- Acne flare-up
- Pruritus
- Bronzing of skin
- Severe adverse effects include purpura, prolonged erythema, aggravation of scarring, and hypopigmentation

In addition, if the laser is not used cautiously and judiciously, it can also lead to prolonged erythema and edema, purpura especially if the patient is taking nonsteroidal anti-inflammatory drug (NSAID), aggravation of scarring, painful crusting and permanent scarring, and hypopigmentation **(Box 2)**.[28,29]

COMBINATION TREATMENTS WITH LASERS IN ACNE SCARS

Fractional laser resurfacing can be combined with other procedures to cause a synergistic effect in treating acne scars. The most popular combination treatments are TCA CROSS, medium depth peels, and surgical procedures such as subcision, punch elevation, and punch flotation. Combination with TCA CROSS can tackle coexistent pitted scars, which respond less to fractional laser treatment. Similarly, subcision can be used prior to fractional laser resurfacing with significant benefit. Subcision is used to decrease the depth of deep rolling or boxcar scars, and this makes them more amenable to treatment with fractional lasers.

Another popular combination treatment nowadays is platelet-rich plasma. There are few reports of successful combined use of fractional laser resurfacing with autologous platelet-rich plasma. Lastly, fractional laser treatment can be combined with autologous fat grafting or with hyaluronic acid filler injections.[16,30-33]

CONCLUSION

Lasers have found a permanent place in the treatment of facial acne scars. Among the nonsurgical modalities, they are perhaps the most efficacious in causing scar amelioration. Among the different lasers available for this indication, fractional lasers are the ones that are the most favored as of now. However, before using any of these lasers, it is imperative to know the right laser and the right parameters for an individual patient. Using the wrong setting or the incorrect laser can harm and even disfigure the patient.

REFERENCES

1. Orentreich D, Orentreich N. Acne scar revision update. Dermatol Clin. 1987;5:359-68.
2. Goodman GJ, Baron JA. The management of post-acne scarring. Dermatol Surg. 2007;33:1175-88.
3. Goodman GJ. Management of post-acne scarring: what are the options for treatment? Am J Clin Dermatol. 2000;1:3-17.
4. Rivera AE. Acne scarring: a review and current treatment modalities. J Am Acad Dermatol. 2008;59:659-76.
5. Goel A, Krupashankar DS, Aurangabadkar S, Nischal KC, Omprakash HM, Mysore V. Fractional lasers in dermatology—current status and recommendations. Indian J Dermatol Venereol Leprol. 2011;77:369-79.
6. Kim HJ, Kim TG, Kwon YS, Park JM, Lee JH. Comparison of a 1,550 nm erbium: glass fractional laser and a chemical reconstruction of skin scars (CROSS) method in the treatment of acne scars: a simultaneous split-face trial. Lasers Surg Med. 2009;41:545-9.
7. Tanzi EL, Alster TS. Laser treatment of scars. Skin Therapy Lett. 2004;9:4-7.
8. Tanzi EL, Alster TS. Treatment of atrophic facial acne scars with a dual-mode Er:YAG laser. Dermatol Surg. 2002;28:551-5.
9. Alster T, Zaulyanov L. Laser scar revision: a review. Dermatol Surg. 2007;33:131-40.
10. Paithankar DY, Ross EV, Saleh BA, Blair MA, Graham BS. Acne treatment with a 1,450 nm wavelength and cryogen spray cooling. Lasers Surg Med. 2002;31:106-14.
11. Rogachefsky AS, Hussain M, Goldberg DJ. Atrophic and a mixed pattern of acne scars improved with a 1320-nm Nd:YAG laser. Dermatol Surg. 2003;29:904-8.
12. Tanzi EL, Alster TS. Comparison of a 1450-nm diode laser and a 1320-nm Nd:YAG laser in the treatment of atrophic facial scars: a prospective clinical and histologic study. Dermatol Surg. 2004;30:152-7.
13. Carniol PJ, Vynatheya J, Carniol E. Evaluation of acne scar treatment with a 1450-nm midinfrared laser and 30% trichloroacetic acid peels. Arc Facial Plast Surg. 2005;7:251-5.
14. Manstein D, Herron GS, Sink RK, Tanner H, Anderson RR. Fractional photothermolysis: a new concept for cutaneous remodeling using microscopic patterns of thermal injury. Lasers Surg Med. 2004;34:426-38.
15. Khan MH, Sink RK, Manstein D, Eimerl D, Anderson RR. Intradermally focused infrared laser pulses: thermal effects at defined tissue depths. Lasers Surg Med. 2005;36:270-80.

16. Alster TS, Tanzi EL, Lazarus M. The use of fractional laser photothermolysis for the treatment of atrophic scars. Dermatol Surg. 2007;33:295-9.
17. Chrastil B, Glaich AS, Goldberg LH, Friedman PM. Second-generation 1,550-nm fractional photothermolysis for the treatment of acne scars. Dermatol Surg. 2008;34: 1327-32.
18. Rahman Z, Tanner H, Jiang K. Treatment of atrophic scars with the 1,550 nm erbium-fiber fractional laser. Lasers Surg Med. 2006;38:24.
19. Hu S, Chen MC, Lee MC, Yang LC, Keoprasom N. Fractional resurfacing for the treatment of atrophic facial acne scars in Asian skin. Dermatol Surg. 2009;35:826-32.
20. Mahmoud BH, Srivastava D, Janiga JJ, Yang JJ, Lim HW, Ozog DM. Safety and efficacy of erbium-doped yttrium aluminum garnet fractionated laser for treatment of acne scars in type IV to VI skin. Dermatol Surg. 2010;36:602-9.
21. Hedelund L, Moreau KER, Boyer D, Beyer DM, Nymann P, Haedersdal M. Fractional nonablative 1,540-nm laser resurfacing of atrophic acne scars. A randomized controlled trial with blinded response evaluation. Lasers Med Sci. 2010;25:749-54.
22. Chapas AM, Brightman L, Sukal S, Hale E, Daniel D, Bernstein LJ, et al. Successful treatment of acneiform scarring with CO_2 ablative fractional resurfacing. Lasers Surg Med. 2008;40:381-6.
23. Katz B. Efficacy of a new fractional CO_2 laser in the treatment of photodamage and acne scarring. Dermatol Ther. 2010;23: 403-06.
24. Deng H, Yuan D, Yan C, Lin X, Ding X. A 2940 nm fractional photothermolysis laser in the treatment of acne scarring: a pilot study in China. J Drugs Dermatol. 2009;8:978-80.
25. Manuskiatti W, Triwongwaranat D, Varothai S, Eimpunth S, Wanitphakdeedecha R. Efficacy and safety of a carbon-dioxide ablative fractional resurfacing device for treatment of atrophic acne scars in Asians. J Am Acad Dermatol. 2010;63: 247-83.
26. Majid I, Imran S. Fractional CO2 laser resurfacing as monotherapy in the treatment of atrophic facial acne scars. J Cutan Aesthet Surg. 2014;7(2):87.
27. Cho SB, Lee SJ, Kang JM, Kim JK, Chung WS, Oh SH. The efficacy and safety of 10,600-nm carbon dioxide fractional laser for acne scars in Asian patients. Dermatol Surg. 2009; 35:1955-61.
28. Fife DJ, Zachary CB. Delayed pinpoint purpura after fractionated carbon dioxide treatment in a patient taking ibuprofen in the postoperative period. Dermatol Surg. 2009; 35:553.
29. Metelista AI, Alster TS. Fractionated laser skin resurfacing treatment complications: a review. Dermatol Surg. 2010; 36:299-306.
30. Zhu JT, Xuan M, Zhang YN, Liu HW, Cai JH, Wu YH, et al. The efficacy of autologous platelet-rich plasma combined with erbium fractional laser therapy for facial acne scars or acne. Mol Med Rep. 2013;8(1):233-7.
31. Faghihi G, Keyvan S, Asilian A, Nouraei S, Behfar S, Nilforoushzadeh MA. Efficacy of autologous platelet-rich plasma combined with fractional ablative carbon dioxide resurfacing laser in treatment of facial atrophic acne scars: a split-face randomized clinical trial. Indian J Dermatol Venereol Leprol. 2016;82(2):162.
32. Nofal E, Helmy A, Nofal A, Alakad R, Nasr M. Platelet-rich plasma versus CROSS technique with 100% trichloroacetic acid versus combined skin needling and platelet rich plasma in the treatment of atrophic acne scars: a comparative study. Dermatol Surg. 2014;40(8):864-73.
33. Gawdat HI, Hegazy RA, Fawzy MM, Fathy M. Autologous platelet rich plasma: topical versus intradermal after fractional ablative carbon dioxide laser treatment of atrophic acne scars. Dermatol Surg. 2014;40(2):152-61.

CHAPTER 48

Approach to Management of Acne Scars

BS Chandrashekar, Kumudhini S, Mysore Venkataram

KEY MESSAGES

- Adequate counseling regarding possibility to significantly reduce and impossibility to erase acne scars should be done hitherto.
- Multimodality treatment is the right approach to treat acne scars.
- Fractional lasers have become a game-changer in acne scar management.
- Isotretinoin is not a contraindication for laser procedures anymore considering delayed wound healing.
- Scar-associated erythema needs to be addressed before treating acne scars.
- Newer technologies such as microneedling radiofrequency and Tixel® are showing promising results in the management of acne scars.
- In Indian skin tone, dermatologists should be cognizant of the frequent postinflammatory hyperpigmentation (PIH).

INTRODUCTION

There is no single modality which can remove the acne scars completely. Introduction of newer modalities of treatment such as fractional laser, microneedling radiofrequency (MNRF), and Tixel® promises to deliver significant reduction in the visibility of scars from a distance. It is now possible to manage severe scars, with far better results than ever possible before, with minimal side effects and healing time. The previous chapters 45, 46, and 47 have dealt with different aspects of acne scar surgery including classification and pathophysiology, different surgical techniques, and lasers. This chapter deals with a summary of approach to management of acne scars. The reader is also referred to the guidelines of care for acne scars by the taskforce on dermatosurgery, Indian Association of Dermatologists, Venereologists and Leprologists.

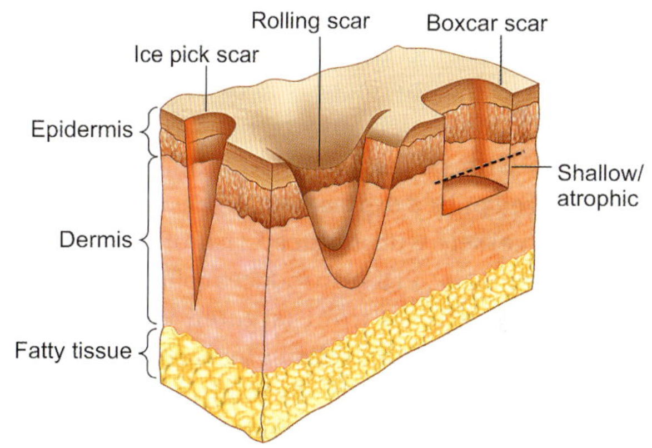

Fig. 1: Types of atrophic (shallow) acne scars include ice pick scar, rolling scar and box car scar.

PRETREATMENT CONSIDERATIONS

Postacne scars are polymorphic and various types of scars can usually coexist in the same individual. Acne scars can be broadly classified as hypertrophic and atrophic acne scars **(Fig. 1)**. It is very important to assess each scar individually and treat accordingly. The method of the intervention depends on the types of the scars, overall appearance of the face, whether erythema is associated with the scar, and the economy of the patient.

A combination of medical and surgical approaches is needed with frequent visits to the clinic over several months. Counseling should include frank and free discussion of all aspects of the treatments such as time taken, number of sessions, outcomes expected, posttreatment course and care, downtime and discomfort, and pre- and post-treatment conditioning regimens. An effort should be made to understand patients' expectations, pain threshold, and work schedules. The pros and cons of each individual procedure need to be addressed clearly. The results and possible complications, if any, from previous patient photographs can be shown beforehand. It is therefore important to establish an open, free communication, and good rapport with patients to gain their trust and confidence.

Informed consent is mandatory and so are pre- and post-treatment photographs. Often the improvement is gradual, and patients may express disappointment at the lack of improvements. Photographs are of great help in such cases. It is important for the patients to have realistic expectations as in all aesthetic treatments, particularly in management of scars. Patients have to be counseled that despite recent advances, severe scarring remains a difficult challenge to manage.

Examination of skin should include an assessment of scars, type, extent, tendency for pigmentation, and keloid formation.

PRETREATMENT ASSESSMENT

Pretreatment assessment of acne scars is shown in **Flowchart 1**.

SCAR-ASSOCIATED ERYTHEMA

The first step is to assess presence of erythema in and around acne scars. In that case, erythematous component has to be addressed first to improve the outlook of the scar.

The treatment options for scar-associated erythema (SAE) are vascular laser such as:

- Pulsed dye laser (PDL)
- Solid-state vascular laser (SSVL)
- Potassium titanyl phosphate (KTP) laser
- Gold toning (595 nm)
- Erbium-doped fractional laser (EDL)
- Intense pulsed light (IPL)

Pulsed Dye Laser

(Level of evidence 1, strength of recommendation A)
Pulsed dye laser is the gold standard treatment for SAE.[1] It works by selective thermolysis of oxyhemoglobin within cutaneous vessels, which absorbs light in the yellow and green range, with peaks at 418, 542, 577, and 589 nm.[2] The long-pulsed pulsed dye laser (PDL) (595–600 nm) slowly heats target vessels with reduced risk of postprocedure purpura. Additionally, PDL also induces collagen remodeling as heat energy diffuses from targeted vessels into the surrounding dermis and results in increased transforming growth factor beta (TGF-β), which ultimately stimulates fibroblasts.[3,4]

Solid-state Vascular Laser

Solid-state vascular laser is a solid-state yellow laser of dual wavelength 1,319 and 589 nm laser. Its solid-state dye is the next-generation alternative to liquid dye that does not require consumable with lesser maintenance and avoids the untoward effects of PDL-like purpura leading to further postinflammatory hyperpigmentation (PIH).[5]

Potassium Titanyl Phosphate Laser

Potassium titanyl phosphate laser (532 nm), also known as frequency-doubled neodymium-doped yttrium aluminum garnet (Nd:YAG), has a target specificity for the first peak of the oxyhemoglobin absorption curve. Here the thermal energy extends only up to the papillary dermis without significant effects on collagen remodeling.[6] The long-pulsed KTP laser is especially successful for SAE with pulse durations of 20–30 ms, fluences of 6–9 J/cm,[2] and spot sizes of 4–5 mm.[7]

Gold Toning (595 nm)

The 595 nm Q-switched Nd:YAG laser applied at low fluences is safe and effective for the treatment of postacne erythema (PAE), early acne scarring, and inflammatory acne. They have some photoinhibitory effect on the endothelial structure and physiology secondary to the primary reaction, such as endothelium dependent relaxing factors; highly selective photocoagulative destruction, as in the extended theory of selective photothermolysis.[8]

The advantages of this new laser treatment compared to others are less pain, greater patient comfort, and almost no downtime.

Flowchart 1: Assessment of acne scars.

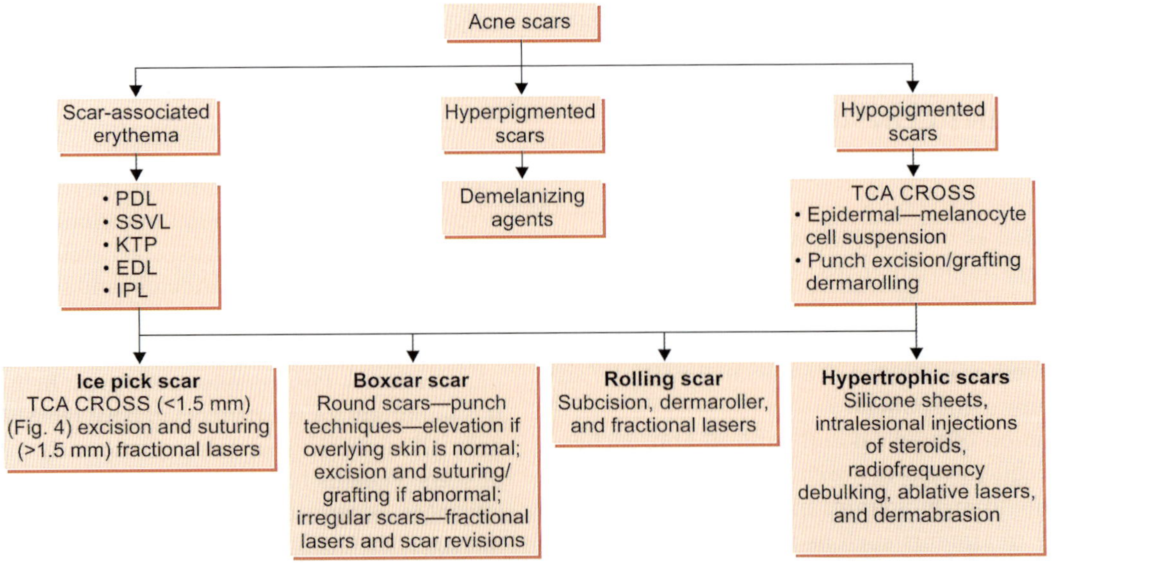

(EDL: Erbium-doped fractional laser; IPL: intense pulsed light; KTP: potassium titanyl phosphate; PDL: pulsed dye laser; SSVL: solid-state vascular laser; TCA CROSS: chemical reconstruction of skin scars using trichloroacetic acid)

Erbium-doped Fractional Laser

Erbium-doped fractional laser (1,550 nm) targets tissue water and penetrates to approximately 1,000 μm into the skin. It produces microvascular destruction of vessels deeper in the dermis.[9]

CLASSIFICATION OF TYPES OF MANAGEMENT FOR ATROPHIC ACNE SCARS WITH LEVEL OF EVIDENCE[10]

Level of evidence and strength of recommendation of each modality of treatments for atrophic acne scars are given in **Table 1**.

TABLE 1: Management of atrophic acne scars with level of evidence.

Topical	• Retinoic acid 0.025–0.5% • Microsphere 0.04% • Glycolic acid 12%[11] • Vitamin C • Niacinamide	LoE III, SoR C
Oral	Isotretinoin 0.5–1 mg/kg weight	LoE III, SoR C
Chemical peels	• Superficial peeling agents (resorcinol, tretinoin, glycolic acid, lactic acid, salicylic acid, and trichloroacetic acid) • Medium-depth peeling agents [phenol, TCA 35–50%, and Jessner solution (resorcinol, lactic acid, and salicylic acid in ethanol)] • Deep peeling agents (Baker-Gordon or Litton phenol formulas) • TCA CROSS • Botulinum toxin	• LoE III, SoR C (for atrophic acne scars) • LoE II, SoR B (for ice pick scars) • LoE III, SoR C (for hypertrophic scar)
Lasers and energy based	• *Ablative fractional*: • Fractional CO_2 (10,600 nm) • Fractional Er:YAG laser (2,940 nm) • Erbium: yttrium scandium gallium garnet (Er:YSGG) (2,790 nm) *Ablative nonfractional*: • Fractional CO_2 (10,600 nm) • Fractional Er:YAG laser (2,940 nm) *Nonablative fractional*: • Erbium-doped laser (1,550 nm) • Erbium glass laser (1,540 nm) • Diode-based laser (1,440 nm) *Nonablative nonfractional*: • Nd:YAG laser (1,320 nm) • Nd:YAG laser (1,064 nm) • Picosecond pulse alexandrite (755 nm) • Diode (1,450 nm) • Radiofrequency microneedling • Tixel® • PRP and lasers	 LoE I, SoR A LoE I, SoR A For papular scar • LoE II, SoR B • LoE II, SoR B • LoE II, SoR B • LoE II, SoR B • LoE III, SoR C • LoE I, SoR A (for mild-to-moderate scars) • Yet to obtain evidence • LoE I, SoR A
Surgical based	• Subcision • Punch techniques • Subcision with MNRF	• LoE II, SoR B • LoE III, SoR C (for moderate-to-severe scars) • LoE I, SoR A
Mechanical trauma based	• Dermabrasion • Microdermabrasion • Microneedling • PRP and microneedling	• LoE II, SoR B (for superficial and small scars) • LoE II, SoR B (for mild-to-moderate scars) • LoE II, SoR B (for mild-to-moderate scars) • LoE I, SoR A
Fat and filler based	• Autologous fat transplant • Hyaluronic acid filler • Calcium hydroxylapatite • Poly-L-lactic acid • Polymethyl methacrylate	• LoE II, SoR B • LoE II, SoR B • LoE II, SoR B • LoE II, SoR B • LoE I, SoR A
Newer therapies	• Autologous noncultured dermal cell suspension • Autologous fibroblast culture • Jet volumetric remodeling • Radiofrequency subcision	• LoE III, SoR C • LoE II, SoR B • LoE III, SoR C • LoE III, SoR C

(Er:YAG: erbium-doped yttrium aluminum garnet; LoE: level of evidence; MNRF: microneedling radiofrequency; Nd:YAG: neodymium-doped yttrium aluminum garnet; PRP: panretinal photocoagulation; SoR: strength of recommendation; TCA: trichloroacetic acid; TCA CROSS: chemical reconstruction of skin scars using trichloroacetic acid)

FRACTIONAL LASER RESURFACING

Scars: Boxcar, rolled-over acne scars, superficial ice pick scars, and also old, quiescent hypertrophic scars and keloid scars

Fractional carbon dioxide laser (10,600 nm) laser and fractional erbium-doped yttrium aluminum garnet (Er:YAG) laser (2,940 nm) are highly efficacious with minimal downtime and side effects and the most comprehensive treatment. The best results with fractional resurfacing depend more on the number of passes per session and the number of sessions than on the fluency and density used on each session. CO_2 fractional laser resurfacing normally requires fewer passes and sessions, and a longer time must be left between the treatments **(Figs. 2A and B)**.

The Er:YAG laser has an absorption coefficient 16 times greater than the carbon dioxide laser. The greater absorption decreases the penetration depth through the epidermis by a factor of ten. The advantage is more precise ablation of skin with even less damage to the surrounding skin and less likely chances of PIH.

The depth of penetration of carbon dioxide ablation is 2 mm and Er:YAG ablation is 1 mm.

MICRONEEDLING RADIOFREQUENCY (FIGS. 3A AND B)

Scars: Ice pick scars, boxcar, and rolling scars

Microneedling radiofrequency system is a novel fractional resurfacing technique for the treatment of acne scars. It creates controlled thermal damage in the dermis and stimulates wound-healing response thus initiating a collagen remodeling process by using thermal production from tissue impedance and subsequent heat diffusion to deeper tissue.

The procedure is repeated four to six times with an interval of 6 weeks between each session, since the time for collagen remodeling lasts around 4–6 weeks. The treatment regimens can be changed depending on the scar type. Needle depths range from 0.5 to 3.5 mm and is modified depending on the anatomical site and pass number. Power levels are adjusted according to the needle depth and site. Exposure times range from 10 to 1,000 ms.

The advantages of fractional radiofrequency include less epidermal disruption by only 5%, compared with 10–70% of that of fractional ablative laser systems, faster healing process, lesser incidence of PIH in darker skin tones, minimal downtime, and control over the depth of treatment.[11]

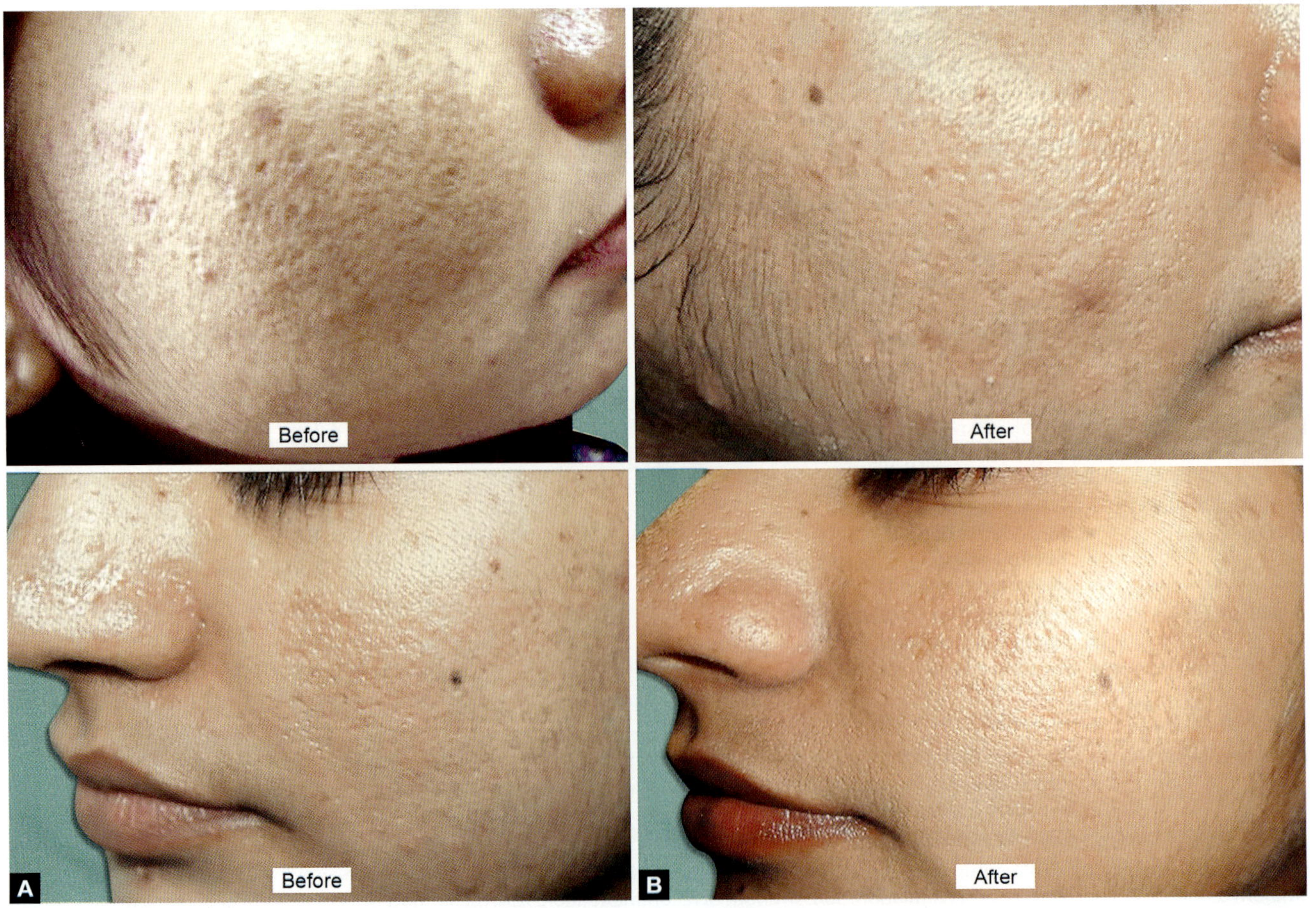

Figs. 2A and B: Before and after three sessions of fractional CO_2 laser.

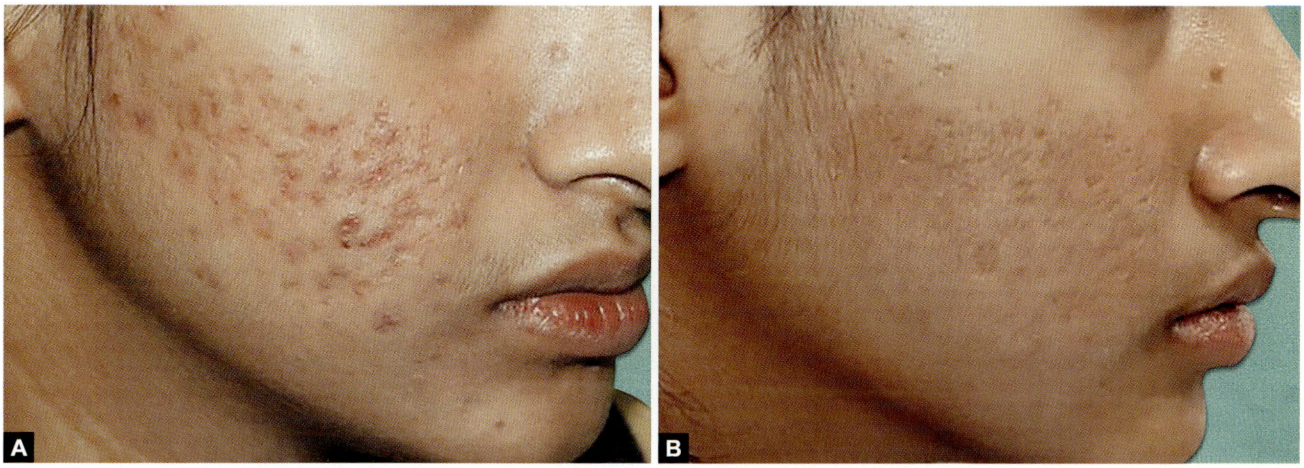

Figs. 3A and B: (A) Before; (B) After four sessions of microneedling radiofrequency (MNRF).

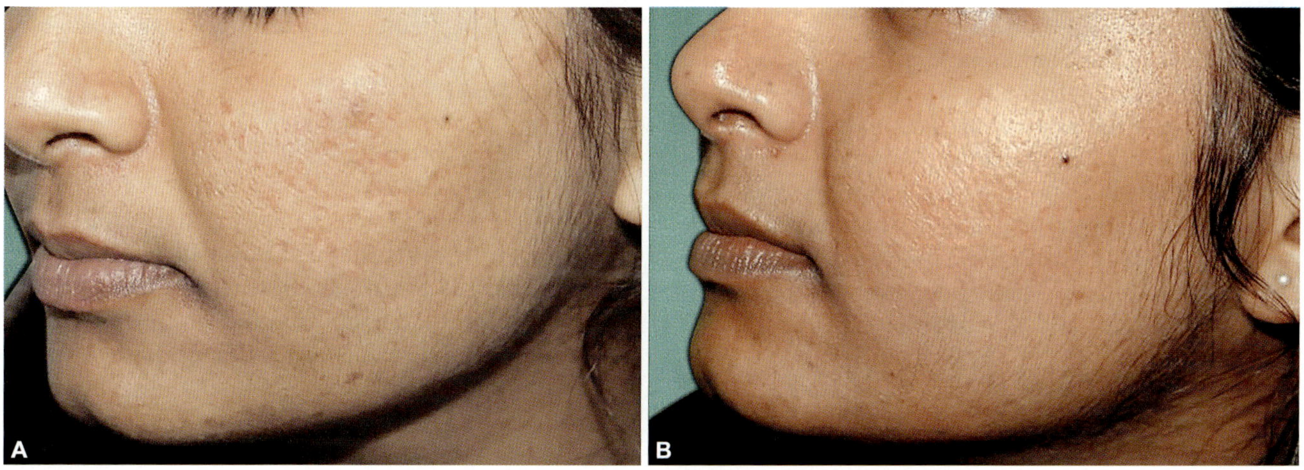

Figs. 4A and B: (A) Before; (B) After four sessions of Tixel®.

Microneedling radiofrequency can reach up to a depth of 3.5 mm and is ideal for all atrophic acne scars.

TIXEL® (FIGS. 4A AND B)

Tixe® is a nonlaser fractional treatment device based on thermomechanical ablation technology similar in effectiveness to fractional CO_2 laser treatment. The energy is emitted through a matrix of 81 tiny pyramid-shaped pins **(Fig. 5)** made of biocompatible materials covering a treatment area of 1 cm^2, heated to a temperature of 400°C. During treatment, the pins are introduced to the surface of the skin at a precisely controlled speed, after which the thermal energy stored in the pins is rapidly transferred upon brief contact with the skin. The ensuing evaporation of water from the skin occurs instantaneously, resulting in the formation of tiny craters in the treatment zone.

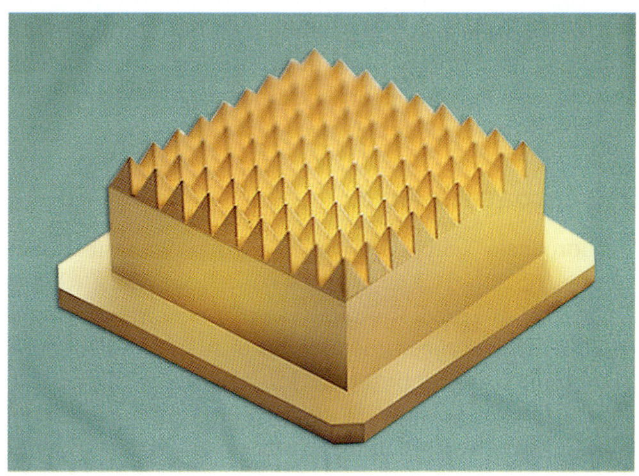

Fig. 5: Tixel® tip.

The parameters for treatment are changed according to the severity of acne scars **(Figs. 6A to D)**. Treatment sessions are spaced 1 month apart and three to five sessions are advised. The extent of thermal damage is closely related to the pulse duration and the type of tip. Longer pulses create a larger crater diameter and deeper thermal damage while shorter pulses create permeable channels for transdermal transfer of drugs. Exposure time (pulse duration) ranges

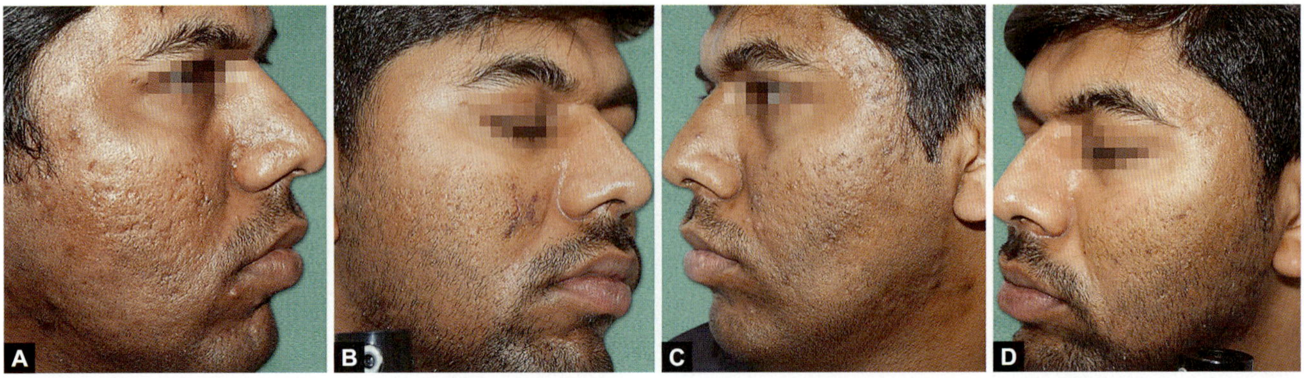

Figs. 6A to D: Acne scars treated with Tixel®.

from 5 to 18 ms. Pulse protrusion is the distance that the pyramid's distal section extends beyond the distance gauge surface and it ranges from 100 to 700 μm with a micropore width of 170 μm.

In contrast to thermal damage created by CO_2 lasers, histopathologic studies have shown that Tixel® has extremely high control over the diameter and depth of craters, which are as deep as CO_2, but narrower. There is less charring and crusting, safe to use with darker skin tones, lesser pain without anesthesia or cooling, absence of fumes during the procedure, and less downtime and postcare.

Grade 4 scars improve poorly with resurfacing procedures, where punch excision and punch elevation can be tried.[12]

CHEMICAL PEELS

Glycolic Acid

Scars: Superficial acne scars

The higher the concentration, the deeper the peel they produce. Glycolic acid acts by thinning the stratum corneum, promoting epidermolysis, and dispersing basal layer melanin. The best results achieved for acne scars include five sequential sessions of 70% glycolic acid every 2 weeks.[13]

Trichloroacetic Acid

Trichloroacetic acid (TCA) can be used in different concentrations; 10–20% TCA is used for superficial peels, whereas 35% is used as a medium-depth peel. Concentrations higher than 35% are not recommended because the results are less predictable and the potential for scarring is higher. TCA application to the skin causes protein denaturation, the so-called keratocoagulation, resulting in a readily observed white frost.

Chemical Reconstruction of Skin Scars Using Trichloroacetic Acid Technique

Scars: Ice pick, narrow boxcar scars, and hypopigmented/depigmented scars

A high-strength TCA solution is placed in the base of these scars to ablate the epithelial wall and to promote dermal remodeling. It can be also applied on the surface of hypopigmented/depigmented scars to induce pigmentation.

Salicylic Peel

Scars: Erythematous scars, pigmented scars, and superficial scar

Salicylic acid is one of the best peeling agents for the treatment of acne scars. It is a beta hydroxy acid agent which removes intercellular lipids that are covalently linked to the cornified envelope surrounding cornified epithelioid cells. The most efficacious concentration for acne scars is 30% in multiple sessions, around three to five times every 3–4 weeks.

Jessner's Peel

Scars: Superficial boxcar and rolling scars

Formulated by Dr Max Jessner, this combination of salicylic acid (14 g), resorcinol (14 g), and 85% lactic acid (14 g) in 95% ethanol is an excellent superficial peeling agent. Resorcinol is structurally and chemically similar to phenol. It disrupts the weak hydrogen bonds of keratin and enhances penetration of other agents. Lactic acid is an alpha-hydroxy acid which causes corneocyte detachment and subsequent desquamation of the stratum corneum.

PYRUVIC ACID

Scars: Moderate acne scars

Pyruvic acid is an alpha-keto acid and an effective peeling agent. It presents keratolytic, antimicrobial and sebostatic properties as well as the ability to stimulate new collagen production and the formation of elastic fibers. The use of 40–70% pyruvic acid has been proposed for the treatment of moderate acne scars. Side effects include desquamation, crusting in areas of thinner skin, intense stinging, and a burning sensation during treatment.[14]

DERMABRASION

Scars: Superficial and moderate depth scars

Under local anesthetic, a high speed brush or fraise used to remove surface skin and alter the contour of scars. Superficial scars may be removed altogether and deeper scars may be reduced in depth.

MICRODERMABRASION

Scars: Only superficial acne scars and pigmentary alterations

It is a superfacial resurfacing technique in which skin surface is abraded with rough aluminum oxide (Al_2O_3) crystals. Microdermabrasion (MDA) unit has two systems namely projection and suction **(Fig. 7)**. Projection system has a compressor generator (power line) responsible for the controlled projection of sterile Al_2O_3 crystals. Suction system rather creates vacuum and aspirates epidermal debris, grime, and used Al_2O_3 crystals. There are two designated independent glass/plastic containers along with their flexible tubings for each of these systems. The connecting tubes of both the systems open into the unit's handpiece near its tip and are the only connection link between the two systems.

When the tip is placed on the surface of the skin and the system is activated, the handpiece gently pulls the skin in. The power line projects the Al_2O_3 crystals on to the skin surface through one opening. These abrade the skin surface and the used crystals along with the epidermal debris and grime are collected by the tubings of the suction system through another opening housed in the tip of same handpiece; thus establishing a close circuit loop of continuous flow and collection simultaneously. The operator can control the pressure (treatment intensity) with the control panel located on the main body and can stop the treatment at any stage by simply lifting the handpiece. Al_2O_3 crystals are preferred as they are inert, nontoxic, and insoluble in water and organic solvents.

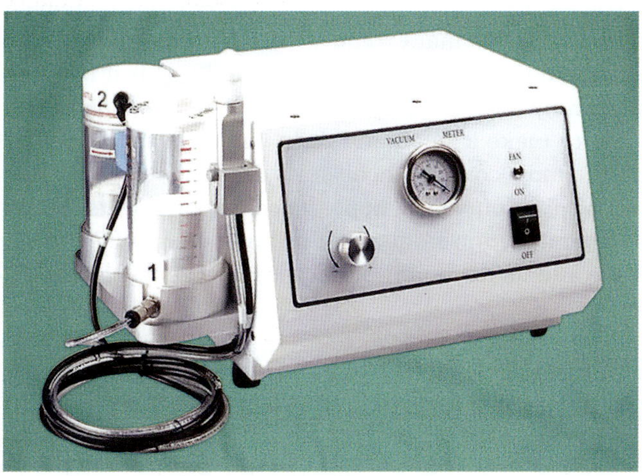

Fig. 7: Microdermabrasion unit.

Crystalline Hydrogen Microderm and Diamond Hydrogen Microderm are the most common ones. As diamond technique is particle free, they have more control and accuracy.

SUBCISION (FIGS. 8A AND B)

Scars: Rolling scars, depressed scar, and ice pick scar

The principle of this procedure is to break the fibrotic strands, which tether the scar to the underlying subcutaneous tissue. Pan subcision is the technique where the entire collagen is focused and not just individual scars. Under tumescent anesthesia, 20% trichloroacetic acid peel, full face CO_2/erbium laser followed by subcision at a dermal-subcutaneous interface using a newly designed tool had proven safe and effective in rolling acne scars.[15]

MICRONEEDLING (FIGS. 9A AND B)

Synonym: Skin needling, collagen induction therapy, needle dermabrasion

Scars: Rolling acne scars, superficial boxcar scars, or erythematous or hypopigmented macular scars

It is the technique of rolling a device composed of a barrel studded with hundreds of needles, which create thousands of micropunctures in the skin to the level of the papillary to mid-dermis.

Dermapen is an electronic microneedling device, which has a detachable head of 33G size consisting of 12 microneedles that can penetrate to variable depths in the skin, depending on preset values.

PUNCH EXCISION TECHNIQUE (FIGS. 10A AND B)

Scars: Deep ice pick acne scars or deep boxcar scars

It is a technique where a disposable punch biopsy instrument is selected that matches the size of the ice pick or narrow boxcar scar, including the walls of the scar. A series of punch excisions can be performed with or without dermal grafting depending on the size of the scar.

DERMAL GRAFTING

Scars: Round/oval acne scar that is soft, prominent, at least 4–5 mm

It is the implantation of appropriately dissected deep dermis (graft) into recipient areas. It is an old procedure that is used to treat atrophic scars.[16]

FILLERS

Scars: Depressed and soft rolling acne scars

Fillers add volume to the skin. Injection of hyaluronic acid filler (HAF) stimulates collagen production by fibroblasts

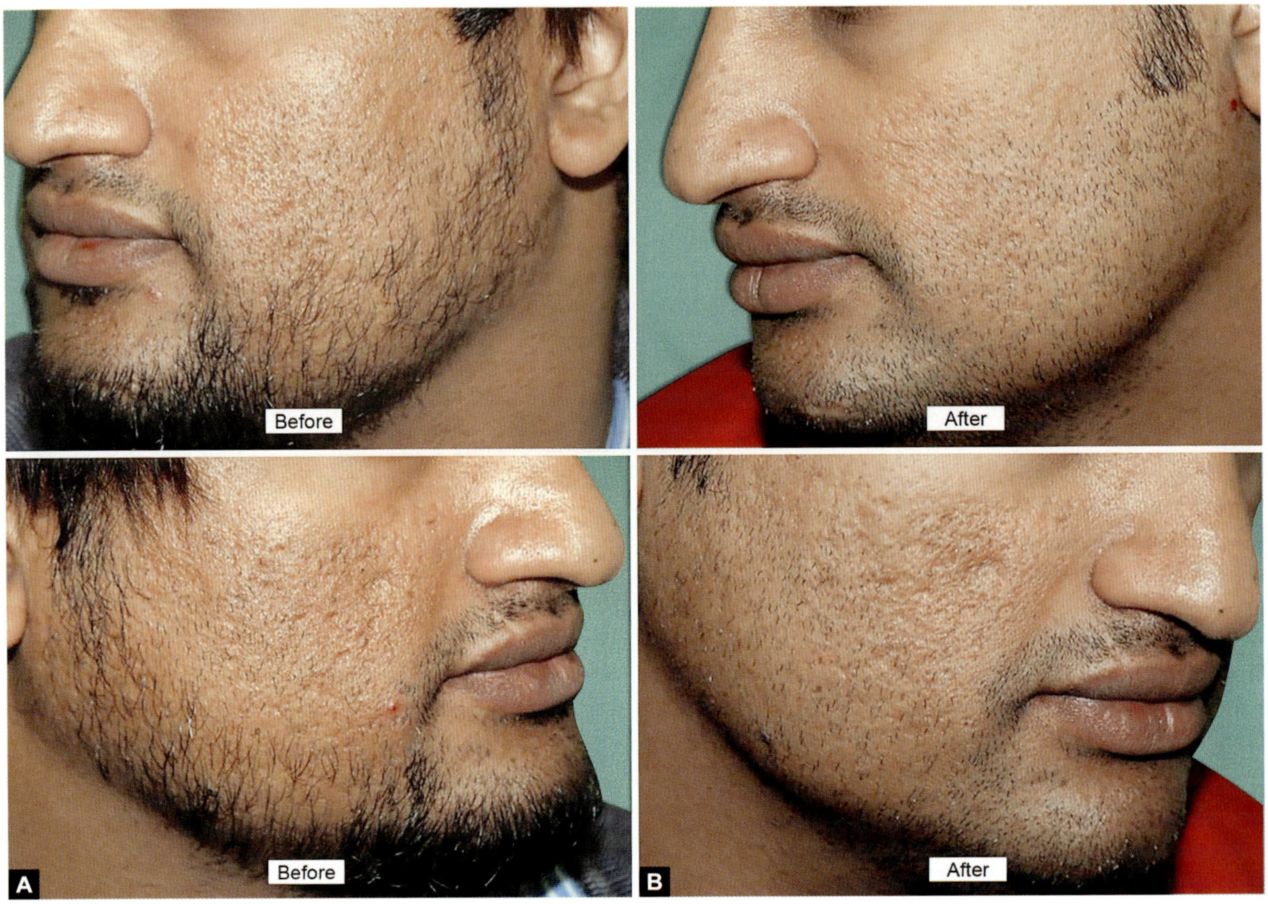

Figs. 8A and B: Before and after two sessions of pan subcision.

contributing to soft-tissue augmentation.[17] They are not useful for ice pick scars. They can be used alone or in combination with other procedures.

Autologous Fat (Figs. 11A and B)

Scars: Depressed and rolling scars

The technique consists of two phases, i.e., procurement of the graft and placement of the graft. The injection phase with small parcels of fat implanted in multiple tunnels allows the fat graft maximal access to its available bloody supply. The fat injected will normalize the contour except where residual scar attachments impede this.

A split-face, prospective clinical trial was conducted in 10 patients comparing intradermal injection of autologous adipose tissue-derived adult stem cells (AT-ASCs), i.e., stromal vascular fraction and fractional carbon dioxide laser resurfacing (FxCR) in patients with postacne scarring. One injection of AT-ASCs was as effective as three sessions of FxCR in the treatment of atrophic acne scars.[24]

HYPERTROPHIC SCARS

The different types of management of hypertrophic scars and their mechanism of action are given in **Table 2**.

STEPWISE APPROACH TO MANAGEMENT OF ATROPHIC SCARS

Among atrophic acne scars, the ice pick type represents 60–70%, boxcar 20–30%, and rolling scars 15–25%.

STEPWISE APPROACH TO MANAGEMENT OF ICE PICK SCARS (FLOWCHART 2)

Ice pick scars are narrow (<2 mm), deep sharply marginated epithelial tracts that extend vertically to the deep dermis or subcutaneous tissue. The skin looks as if it has been pierced by an ice pick or sharp instrument. Ice picks scars seem to make a small and deep “hole” in the skin. They are the most common acne scars that occur on the cheeks and have a “punctate” appearance. Ice pick scars develop after an infection from a cyst or other deep inflamed skin tissue and its way to the surface leaving a long column-like scar.

STEPWISE APPROACH TO MANAGEMENT OF BOXCAR SCARS (FLOWCHART 3)

Boxcar scars are angular scars with sharp vertical edges and resemble the scars left by chickenpox. They may be shallow

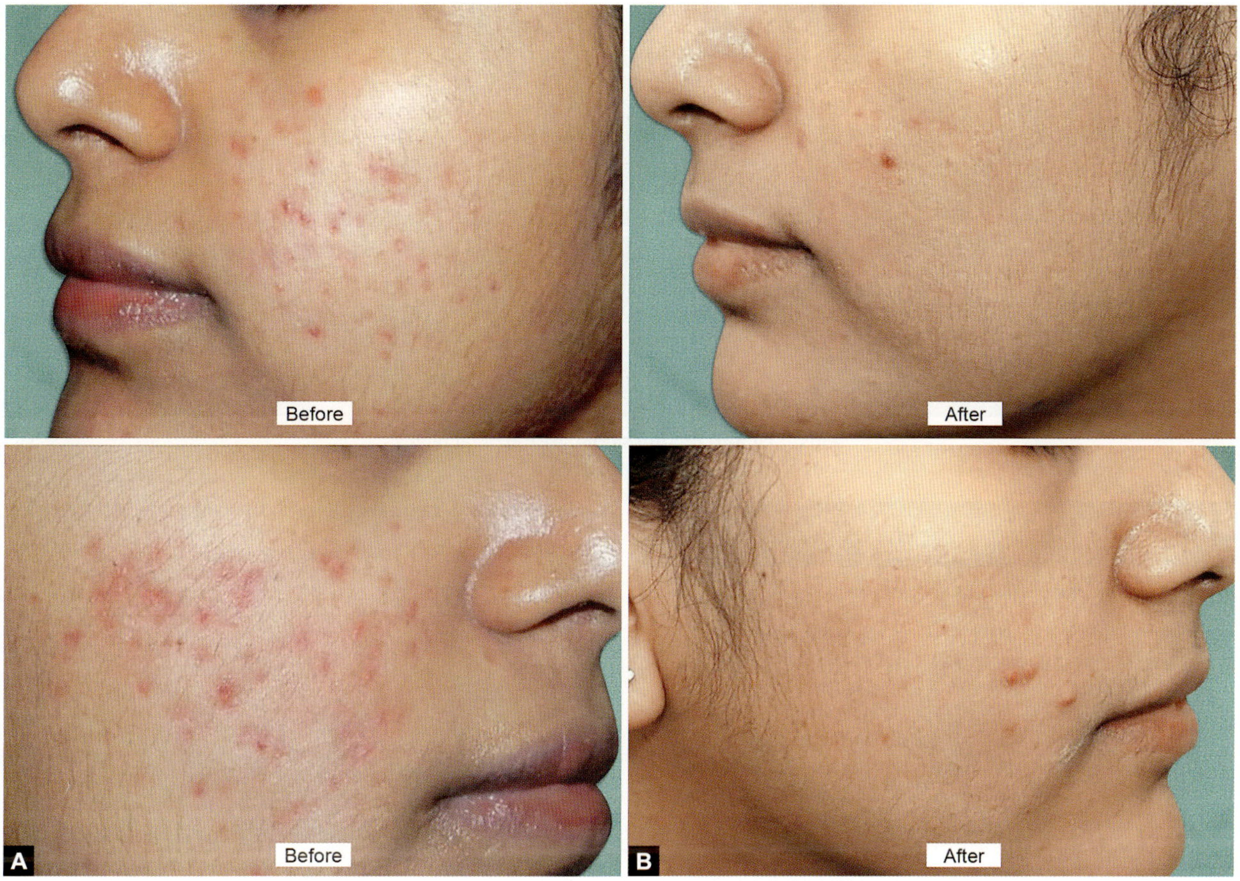

Figs. 9A and B: Before and after four sessions of dermarolling.

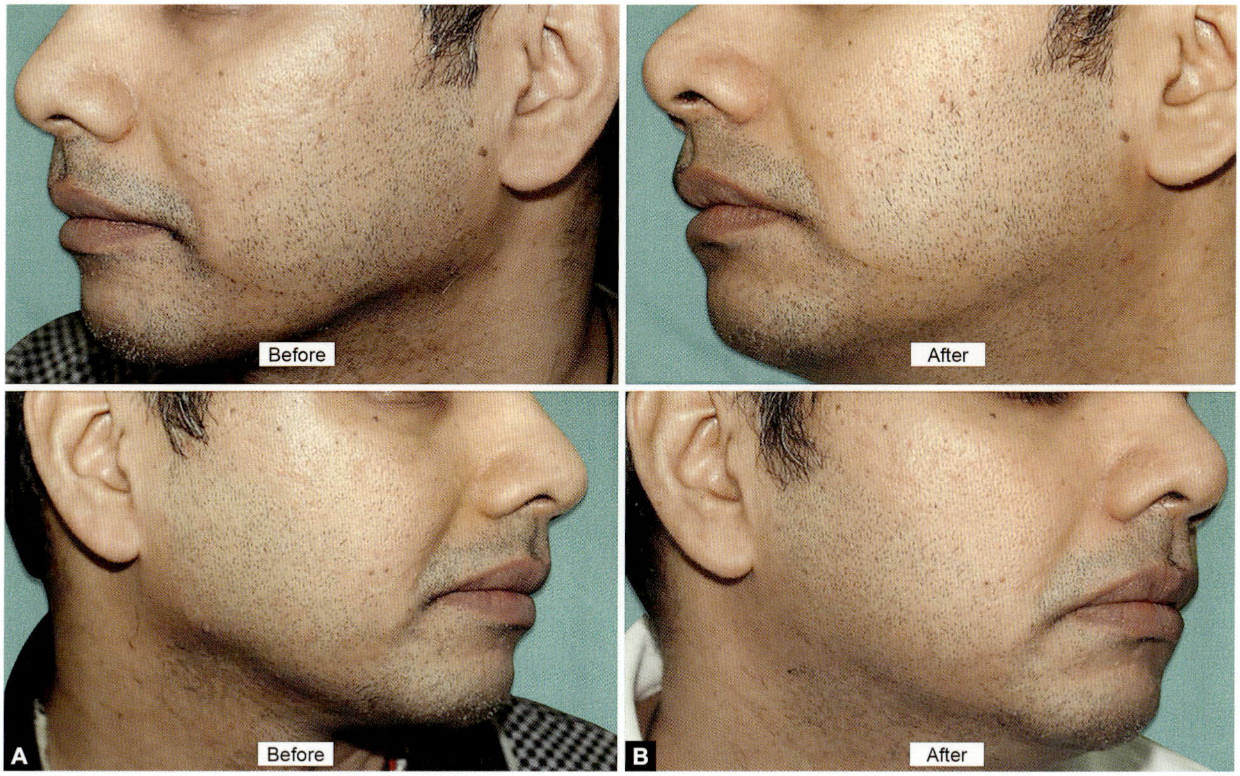

Figs. 10A and B: Before and after single session of punch excision and grafting.

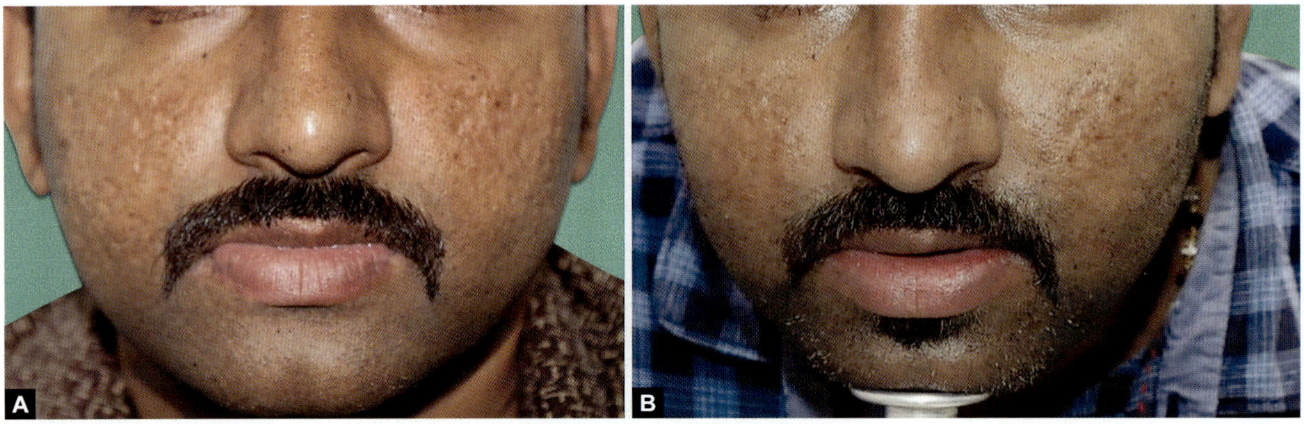

Figs. 11A and B: After single session of fat filler.

TABLE 2: Management of hypertrophic acne scars and their mechanism of action.

Management	*Method*	*Mechanism*
Silicone gel	Applied in small amounts, twice daily for at least 8 weeks	Exact mechanism is not known, proposed mechanisms are: (1) increase in hydration; (2) the increase in temperature; (3) protection of the scar; (4) increased tension of O_2; and (5) action on the immune system[18]
Intralesional triamcinolone	2.5–10 mg/mL	It reduces the volume, thickness, and texture of scars, and they can relieve symptoms such as itching and discomfort in hypertrophic acne scars and keloids
Bleomycin	2 mL/cm^2 at concentration 1.5 IU/mL or multiple puncture technique	It acts by binding to deoxyribonucleic acid (DNA), whether double-stranded and single-stranded, causing strand scissions
Cryotherapy	Two freeze thaw cycles for 15–30 seconds	Younger and smaller scars are most responsive to cryotherapy
Radiofrequency debulking	Once in 3 weeks	Increase in the temperature of the skin, increases the extensibility, and reduces the density of collagen (by a lifting effect due to the radiofrequency)
Botulinum toxin and hyperbaric oxygen	Once in 6 months	Former stimulates collagen formation and latter provides pure oxygen at a pressure slightly higher than atmospheric pressure, leading to decreased growth of atypical fibroblasts and restoration of tissue regeneration

Flowchart 2: A stepwise approach to management of ice pick scars.

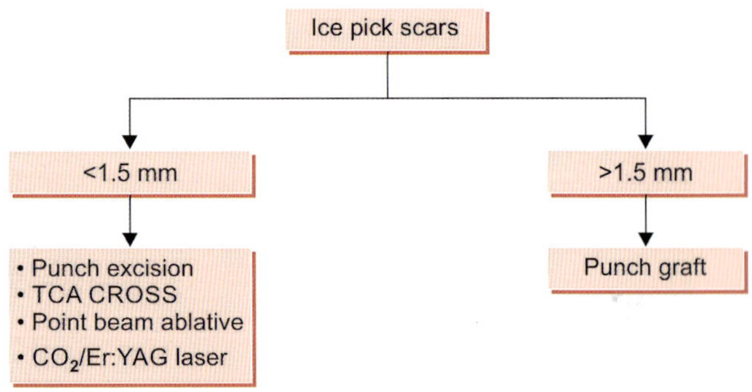

(Er:YAG: erbium-doped yttrium aluminum garnet laser; TCA CROSS: chemical reconstruction of skin scars using trichloroacetic acid)

Flowchart 3: A stepwise approach to management of boxcar scars.

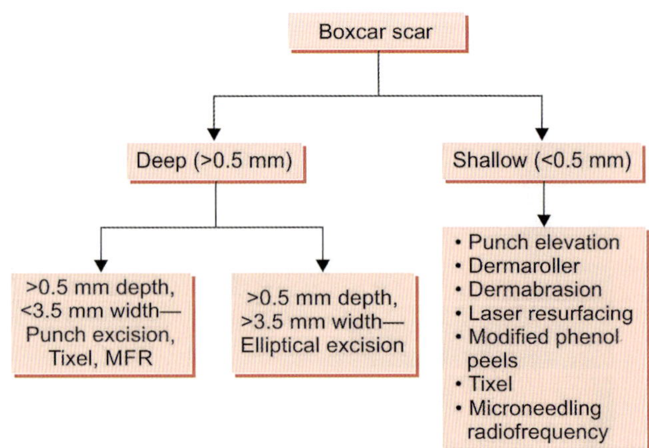

or deep, punched out, and wide at the surface and at the base. They are most often found on the cheeks and temples.

STEPWISE APPROACH TO MANAGEMENT OF SHALLOW/ATROPHIC AND VALLEY SCARS (FLOWCHART 4)

Rolling scars are distensible and depressed scars with gentle sloping edges. Rolling scars are shallow depressions that

Flowchart 4: A stepwise approach to management of shallow/atrophic and valley scars.

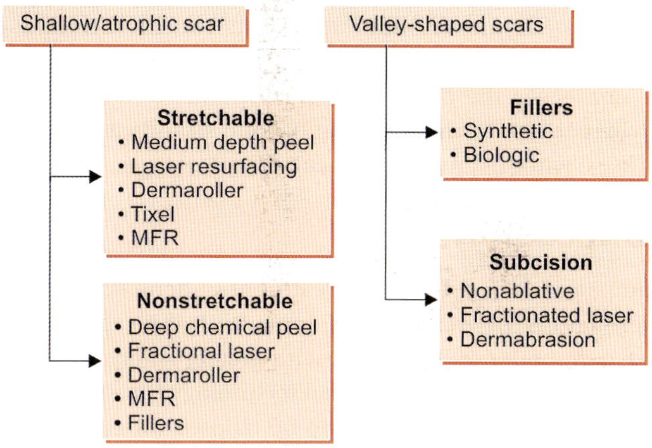

are best appreciated with a change in surface lighting. They can vary in size and often coalesce with neighboring rolling scars. Rolling scars are shallow, wide (>4–5 mm), and have a subdermal fibrous tether. These scars are caused by damage under the surface of the skin. They give the skin a wave-like appearance.

ISOTRETINOIN AND ACNE SCAR MANAGEMENT

It is an established fact that the advent of isotretinoin has greatly enhanced the management of acne vulgaris, even the most severe variants. However, the subject of use of different resurfacing techniques in patients treated with the drug has remained a matter of debate. It is generally agreed that care should be exercised in patients with a history of recent isotretinoin use as the drug may lead to delay in healing and atypical scar formation. A 6–12-month waiting period following discontinuation of isotretinoin has been recommended before performing resurfacing procedures. This recommendation is based on earlier reports of keloid formation and atypical scar formation after use of dermabrasion and argon lasers, which are invasive and ablative procedures. However, several recent publications have documented the safety of different procedures such as laser hair removal and dermabrasion in patients recently treated with isotretinoin.[11]

TIPS AND TRICKS

- Priming with lightening agents and sunscreen should be started at least 3–4 weeks before first treatment. Sunscreen usage is mandatory for any of the earlier mentioned procedure. Enquiry on regular usage of sunscreen should be made during every visit, and in case of recent sun activity, procedure has to be deferred for at least 5–7 days to avoid complications.
- Topical retinoids and benzoyl peroxide has to be stopped 2 days before and 5 days after fractional lasers and strong peels.
- Low-level light therapy (LLLT) can be used to enhance faster recovery post-fractional lasers. It uses the properties of 830 nm light via light-emitting diode (LED) technology.
- While using MNRF and Tixel® for acne scars, bony areas such as the forehead and supraorbital and infraorbital margin should be treated with lesser protrusion and lower contact time to prevent burns.
- Do not use the fluence judiciously in darker skin (Fitzpatrick skin types 3–6) while treating pigmented acne scars with ablative fractional lasers. Parameters to be chosen with caution as chances of postinflammatory pigmentation are very high. Low-fluence and high-density treatments are safer for pigmented acne scars.
- CO_2 laser resurfacing, dermabrasion, and deep chemical peeling used for the treatment of scar ablate the epidermis with subsequent re-epithelialization, and render the skin more sensitive to photodamage and dyschromia. A well-designed postprocedure protocol with oral and topical anti-inflammatories for 3–5 days helps in reducing the dyschromia.
- Infraorbital and mental block is a better option for patients who develop eutectic mixture of local anesthetics (EMLA) patch-associated erythema.
- Patients need to undergo a series of treatment sessions, and the best results are often obtained when laser therapy is combined with another treatment modality (multimodal approach).

NEWER THERAPIES

- Recently, a 577-nm high-power optically pumped semiconductor laser (HOPSL) initially developed for vascular lesions has shown promising results for the treatment of PAE and had demonstrated significant decrease in erythema index.[19]
- Topical brimonidine tartrate 0.33% gel could serve as an effective agent to prevent laser-induced erythema and PIH.
- *Low-level light therapy:* LLLT can be considered for treatment for acne and hypertrophic acne scars. LLLT is a form of treatment (also known as phototherapy or photobiomodulation) that involves the use of light at nonthermal irradiance levels. Coherent (one or more of lasers) or noncoherent light sources (filtered lamps or light-emitting diodes) can be used as a source. Absorption of red or near-infrared frequencies by the mitochondria stimulates a number of biological processes involved in cell proliferation, survival, tissue repair, and regeneration.[20]
- *Autologous smashed dermal graft with epidermal reclosure:* After harvesting epidermal ultra split-thickness graft, dermal tissue was harvested by punches of size 2 mm, excess fat were trimmed, and dermal grafts were transferred to Petri dish containing normal saline. Donor area was closed back with the sheet of epidermis which was spread uniformly and fixed with cyanoacrylate glue which acted as biological dressing. Dermal grafts were held with graft holding forceps and minced with 15 number surgical blade to form smashed dermal grafts which was aspirated into 1 ml tuberculin syringe with 18-gauge needle attached to it. It was injected into the dermal pockets beneath the scars. The advantages of this technique were smashed dermal graft is soft and easily moldable to any shape and can be accurately tailored for all types of acne scars.[21]

- *Autologous bone marrow (BM) stem-cell transplant:*
  - *Scars:* All atrophic facial scars
  - Autologous bone marrow stem cells (BMSCs) seem to be a safe and effective treatment option for the management of all types of atrophic facial acne scars.[22]
  - A pilot study where each patient received 5 mg/kg/day granulocyte colony-stimulating factor (G-CSF) as a single subcutaneous dose for two successive days before BM aspiration. The stem cell containing solution was injected under each scar intradermally. Long-term studies are needed to determine whether these effects are persistent long-term beyond 6 months or if the results are temporary compared to the use of a filler.
- *Jet volumetric remodeling (JVR):* It is a needle-free proprietary technology which accurately delivers kinetic energy and a healing compound at a high speed simultaneously via a tiny entry point in the epidermis. The particles, acting as nano-bullets, disperse in the dermis to create a microtrauma, which promotes neocollagenesis. The JVR device using hyaluronic acid has been used to treat acne scars in two patients in two sessions showing some improvement with minimal downtime.[25]
- *Radiofrequency subcision:* This modification uses radiofrequency energy for subcision. This method decreases the chances of postoperative bleeding and hematoma formation. The fibrotic strands get cut with ease without any mechanical force.[26]

TABLE 3: Summary of treatment modalities for different grades of postacne scarring.

Grades of postacne scarring	*Level of disease*	*Treatment modalities*
1	*Macular:* • Erythematous • Hyperpigmented • Hypopigmented	• IPL, vascular lasers • Hydroquinone, topical retinoids, azelaic, kojic acids, microdermabrasion, salicylic acid and glycolic peels, spot dermabrasion, epidermal—melanocyte cell suspension, Dermaroller, and TCA CROSS
2	Mild	• Microdermabrasion, chemical peels, microneedling, and nonablative lasers
3	Moderate	• Subcision • Scar revisions • Medium depth peels • TCA CROSS • Fractional lasers—Er:YAG, CO_2, and erbium glass • Intralesional steroid/cytotoxic therapy for hypertrophic scars
4	Severe	• Combination of all the earlier mentioned treatments • Fat injections • Dermabrasion • Ablative lasers • Microneedling radiofrequency • Tixel®

Note: The recommendations in the Table are not absolute and variations can exist depending on the preference of the physician and needs of the patient.
(Er:YAG: erbium-doped yttrium aluminum garnet; IPL: intense pulsed light; TCA CROSS: chemical reconstruction of skin scars using trichloroacetic acid)

CONCLUSION

The patient's quest for the treatment of acne scars begins even before the treatment of acne. With the ever evolving research, better technologies with greater safety profile are getting developed. Till the ideal technology for acne scars is perfected, the treatment has to be tailored for each patient according to their type of scars **(Table 3)**.

REFERENCES

1. Alster TS, McMeekin TO. Improvement of facial acne scars by the 585 nm flashlamp-pumped pulsed dye laser. J Am Acad Dermatol. 1996;35:79-81.
2. Anderson RR, Parrish JA. Selective photothermolysis: precise microsurgery by selective absorption of pulsed radiation. Science. 1983;220:524-7.
3. Lee DH, Choi YS, Min SU, Yoon MY, Suh DH. Comparison of a 585-nm pulsed dye laser and a 1064-nm Nd:YAG laser for the treatment of acne scars: a randomized split-face clinical study. J Am Acad Dermatol. 2009;60:801-7.
4. Seaton ED, Mouser PE, Charakida A, Alam S, Seldon PM, Chu AC. Investigation of the mechanism of action of non-ablative pulsed-dye laser therapy in photorejuvenation and inflammatory acne vulgaris. Br J Dermatol. 2006;155:748-55.
5. Gold MH, Wilson A, Mordon SR. Treatment of acne scarring with a novel dual-wavelength laser. J Cosmet Dermatol. 2019;18:1290-3.
6. Cohen BE, Brauer JA, Geronemus RG. Acne scarring: a review of available therapeutic lasers. Lasers Surg Med. 2016;48:95-115.
7. Rao J. Treatment of acne scarring. Facial Plast Surg Clin North Am. 2011;19:275-91.
8. Panchaprateep R, Munavalli G. Low-fluence 585 nm Q-switched Nd:YAG laser: a novel laser treatment for post-acne erythema. Lasers Surg Med. 2015;47(2):148-55.
9. Glaich AS, Goldberg LH, Friedman RH, Friedman PM. Fractional photothermolysis for the treatment of postinflammatory erythema resulting from acne vulgaris. Dermatol Surg. 2007;33:842-6.
10. Gupta A, Kaur M, Patra S, Khunger N, Gupta S. Evidence-based surgical management of post-acne scarring in skin of color. J Cutan Aesthet Surg. 2020;13(2):124-41.
11. Chandrashekar BS, Ashwini KR, Vasanth V, Navale S. Retinoic acid and glycolic acid combination in the treatment of acne scars. Indian Dermatol Online J. 2015;6(2):84-8.
12. Fabbrocini G, Annunziata MC, D'Arco V, et al. Acne scars: pathogenesis, classification and treatment. Dermatol Res Pract. 2010;2010:893080.
13. Van Scott EJ, Yu RJ. Hyperkeratinization, corneocyte cohesion, and alpha hydroxy acids. J Am Acad Dermatol. 1984;11(5):867-79.
14. Berardesca E, Cameli N, Primavera G, Carrera M. Clinical and instrumental evaluation of skin improvement after

treatment with a new 50% pyruvic acid peel. Dermatol Surg. 2006;32(4):526-31.
15. Taylor MB, Zaleski-Larsen L, McGraw TA. Single session treatment of rolling acne scars using tumescent anesthesia, 20% trichloracetic acid extensive subcision, and fractional CO_2 laser. Dermatol Surg. 2017;43 Suppl 1:S70-4.
16. Shilpa K, Sacchidanand S, Leelavathy B, Shilpashree P, Gorur D, Ranjitha R, et al. Outcome of dermal grafting in the management of atrophic facial scars. J Cutan Aesthet Surg. 2016;9:244-8.
17. Wollina U, Goldman A. Fillers for the improvement in acne scars. Clin Cosmet Investig Dermatol. 2015;8:493-9.
18. Berman B, Perez OA, Konda S, Kohut BE, Viera MH, Delgado S, et al. A review of the biologic effects, clinical efficacy, and safety of silicone elastomer sheeting for hypertrophic and keloid scar treatment and management. Dermatol Surg. 2007;33(11):1291-302.
19. Wanitphakdeedecha R, Cembrano KAG, Ungaksornpairote C, Kobwanthanakun W, Phothong W, Eimpunth S, et al. The efficacy and safety of a 577-nm high-power optically pumped semiconductor laser in the treatment of postacne erythema. J Cosmet Dermatol. 2020;19:1642-7.
20. Sánchez Viera M. Management of acne scars: fulfilling our duty of care for patients. Br J Dermatol. 2015;172 Suppl 1: 47-51.
21. Nagaraju U, Chikkaiah MK, Raju BP, Agarwal P. Autologous smashed dermal graft with epidermal re-closure: modified technique for acne scars. J Cutan Aesthet Surg. 2016;9(4): 258-62.
22. Ibrahim ZA, Eltatawy RA, Ghaly NR, Abd El-Naby NM, Abou El Fetouh HM, Abd Elateef AE, et al. Autologous bone marrow stem cells in atrophic acne scars: a pilot study. J Dermatolog Treat. 2015;26(3):260-5.
23. Sahoo AK, Yadav S, Sharma VK, Parihar AS, Vyas S, Gupta S. Safety and efficacy of autologous noncultured dermal cell suspension transplantation in the treatment of localized facial volume loss: A pilot study. Indian J Dermatol Venereol Leprol. 2019;85:44-50.
24. Abou Eitta RS, Ismail AA, Abdelmaksoud RA, Ghezlan NA, Mehanna RA. Evaluation of autologous adipose-derived stem cells vs. fractional carbon dioxide laser in the treatment of post acne scars: a split-face study. Int J Dermatol. 2019; 58(10):1212-22.
25. Munavalli GS, Smith S, Maslowski JM, Weiss RA. Successful treatment of depressed, distensible acne scars using autologous fibroblasts: a multi-site, prospective, double blind, placebo-controlled clinical trial. Dermatol Surg. 2013;39: 1226-36.
26. Yadav S, Gupta S. Radiofrequency-assisted subcision for postacne scars. J Am Acad Dermatol. 2018;78(1):e9-e10.

SECTION 7 Nail Surgery

CHAPTER 49

Basic Surgery of Nails

Sushil Tahiliani, Harsh Tahiliani, Manjit Sandhu Tahiliani

KEY MESSAGES

- Knowledge of nail anatomy is important for successful nail surgeries.
- Conservative surgical approach leads to less downtime and morbidity.
- Nail plate is formed essentially by matrix and hence it should be handled with utmost care.
- Knowledge of clinical conditions leads to planning of nail surgeries in an appropriate manner.
- Most basic nail surgeries can be performed using proximal or distal digital block.

INTRODUCTION

Interest in the field of nail surgery is recent. It has already been introduced in the core curriculum of US dermatology residents, and books devoted to the subject have been published in the Western world more than a decade ago.[1-3] In our country, it still remains a "poor cousin," and a dermatology resident can pass the postgraduate examination without bothering to touch the subject. It is an "orphan" that needs to be adopted by us, and doing so leads to job satisfaction and earns the gratitude of a relieved patient.

Nail surgeries could be classified in one of the following two ways:

1. *Basic/advanced*:
   a. *Basic surgeries* include nail avulsion and nail plate and nail bed biopsy.
   b. *Advanced surgeries* include matricectomy, matrix biopsy, nail fold surgeries, and nail unit tumor surgeries.
2. *Diagnostic (biopsy of nail unit)/therapeutic surgeries*

Basic nail surgery is in the domain of a general dermatologist and can safely be performed as an office procedure under local anesthesia. More advanced nail surgeries require structured training and may require collaboration with an orthopedic or a plastic surgeon, and should be performed in a standard surgical facility.[1]

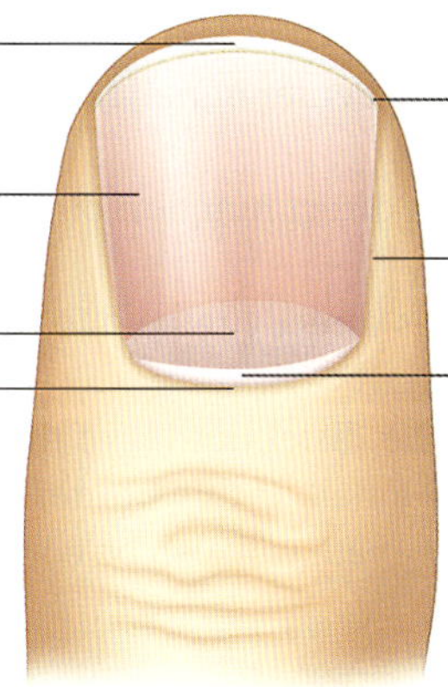

Fig. 1: Nail unit.

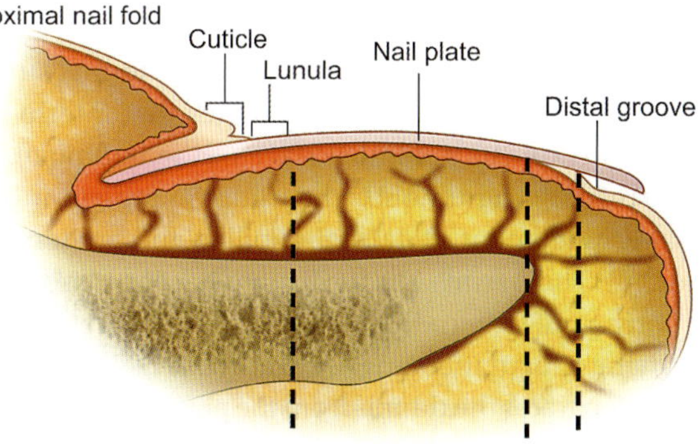

Fig. 2: Sagittal section through nail unit.

RELEVANT AND APPLIED ANATOMY

The nail unit (nail complex) consists of proximal nail fold (PNF), lateral nail fold (LNF), nail matrix, nail bed, nail plate, and hyponychium **(Figs. 1 and 2)**.

Nail Plate

Nail plate is a flat, translucent, rectangular, convex, and hard structure that consists of closely packed adherent, interdigitating cells without nuclei and organelles. It is formed almost exclusively by nail matrix. Proximal matrix forms the dorsal part and distal matrix forms the ventral part of nail plate.[4] There is a small contribution of cells by nail bed to the undersurface of nail plate. Longitudinal brown to black bands seen throughout the length of the nail plate may be a normal finding in Fitzpatrick type IV, V, and VI people.[4-6] The part of nail plate in relation to nail bed is thicker and firmly attached, whereas the part over lunula is thinner and loosely attached.[7,8]

Nail Matrix

The nail matrix is the germinative portion of the nail complex, giving rise to the nail plate.[4,5,7,8] The matrix is at the most proximal point of the nail bed and is seated deep beneath the PNF; it is separated from the distal phalanx by only a few millimeters. The proximal matrix continues proximally and laterally to form the lateral matrix horn. The nail surgeon should be cognizant that the lateral matrix horn may be extensive. The lunula is usually seen through the transparent nail plate, especially on the thumbs and great toes, as the visible distal component of the nail matrix. Several reasons exist why the nail surgeon must attempt to leave the structural and functional boundaries of the nail matrix intact when performing nail surgery;[1,9-11] some of these reasons are mentioned here:

- The matrix is the center of nail formation and the source of the nail plate.
- Nail growth is a direct function of the rate of turnover of matrix cells.
- Nail thickness is directly related to the length or the size of the nail matrix.
- The shape of the distal border of the lunula determines the shape of the nail. If this border is convex, the distal free edge of the plate will also be convex.

Nail Bed

The nail bed extends from the distal lunula to the point of origin of the hyponychium. LNF marks the lateral border of nail bed. The epidermis of the nail bed is relatively thin, with a dimensional thickness of only one to two cells.[7] Like the matrix, it has no granular layer. The epidermal surface of the bed has parallel longitudinal ridges that interlock with similar folds on the ventral surface of the nail plate. There is a corresponding unique, longitudinal, tongue-in-groove spatial arrangement of dermal papillae and epidermal rete ridges.[5,7,12] The dermis has a wealth of glomus bodies and a rich network of longitudinally oriented capillaries. It lacks an underlying subcutaneous layer of adipose tissue. As a result, nothing separates the dermis from the periosteum of the distal phalanx. Melanocytes are not found in the nail beds.

Hyponychium

The hyponychium is the anatomical area that begins at the onychodermal band, where the nail bed ends, and terminates at the distal groove. The distal groove is a transverse demarcation extending across the distal digit that divides the hyponychium from the volar epidermis of the digit. This groove is the first component of the nail unit to be recognized during the embryologic period, and it is the origin point of the volar epidermis.

Proximal Nail Fold

The PNF is a continuation of the dorsal skin of the digit that folds back on itself at the nail root to create two epithelial surfaces: A superficial dorsal layer and a deep ventral layer.[5,7,10,11] The ventral layer travels to the base of the nail plate to create the nail matrix. Where the two epithelial surfaces meet, the cuticle converges onto the distal nail plate. The PNF is contiguous with the LNFs that border the nail plate.

Proximal and Lateral Nail Grooves

These are potential spaces created by overlap of PNF and LNF over the nail plate.

Blood Supply[1,13,14]

Blood supply is derived from lateral digital arteries, which supply the nail unit through the formation of superficial, proximal, and distal arcades **(Figs. 3A and B)**.

Venous drainage follows arterial vasculature, the only difference being that it combines proximally forming two digital veins on either side.

Vascular structure of nail bed is unique in that it must supply a vascular structure between two hard surfaces—the nail plate and distal phalanx.[1]

Large AV anastomoses including glomus bodies are found at the level of the anastomotic arteries and the deep venous circulation in all the areas of nail unit except the PNF.

Nerve Supply[15]

Innervation of the nail unit is through two laterally positioned sensory nerves—dorsal and ventral. Nail unit is richly innervated **(Fig. 4)**.

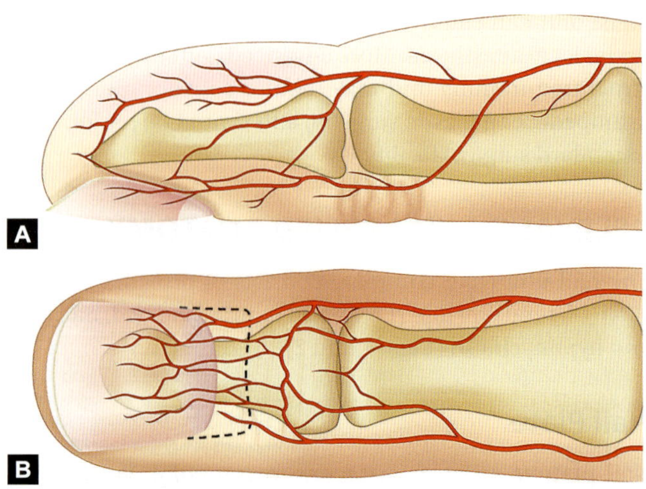

Figs. 3A and B: *Vasculature of nail:* (A) Lateral view; (B) Dorsal view.

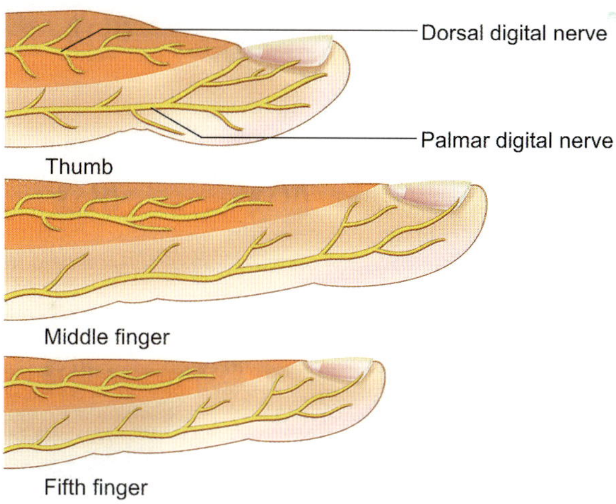

Fig. 4: Nerve supply of nail.

INDICATIONS FOR NAIL SURGERY[1,16,17]

- *Diagnostic dilemmas:* To differentiate between infective and noninfective disorders, accurate diagnosis of "Twenty nail" syndrome, differentiate between subungual hematomas and malignant melanoma are some examples.
- Onychocryptosis
- Acute paronychia and subungual abscess
- *Trauma:* For example, subungual hematoma
- Myxoid cyst
- Benign and malignant growths involving the nail unit: Warts, pyogenic granuloma, glomus tumor, Koenen's tumor, subungual exostosis, malignant melanoma, basal cell carcinoma (BCC), squamous cell carcinoma (SCC), Bowen's disease[18]

CONTRAINDICATIONS[17]

With refinement of technique and availability of better medical care, the contraindications are "relative."

- Established peripheral vascular disease
- Collagen vascular disease
- Uncontrolled diabetes mellitus
- Disorders of hemostasis
- Very acute infections/inflammation of nail unit

Preoperative Evaluation

- To rule out local infection and vasculopathies
- To rule out drug allergies
- To rule out significant systemic disorders and to control existing disorders
- To rule out intake of agents that may interfere with hemostasis
- To evaluate and discuss with the patient the duration of functional impairment and risk of short-term and long-term nail dystrophy
- To take a good clinical photograph
- To take informed consent

Surgical Setting

Nail avulsions, biopsies, and simple excisions can safely be performed in a dermatologist's office under the same conditions as basic skin surgery procedures. Advanced nail surgical procedures should be performed in an operation theater.[1]

Anesthesia

Depending on procedure, indication, and personal preference, we have a choice of various types of digital (local) anesthesia techniques as well as a variety of regional blocks. Surgeries done in a dermatologist's office require only a distal or proximal digital block.

Syringe: Dental syringe/2 mL Luer lock syringe for distal nail blocks

Needle: 27/30-gauge needle.

Anesthetic agent: Plain lidocaine (2% preferred over 1%). Lidocaine with adrenaline is safe for digital anesthesia[19-22] but not very useful as exsanguination is still necessary.[1]

Ropivacaine and bupivacaine are preferred for regional blocks.[23]

- *Digital anesthesia:*
  - *Distal nail blocks*:
    - Distal digital block (wing block)
    - Distal anesthesia through PNF
    - Distal anesthesia through hyponychium
  - Proximal digital block
  - Transthecal digital anesthesia
- *Regional blocks:*
  - Wrist block
  - Median nerve block at wrist
  - Ulnar nerve block
  - Nerve blocks for posterior tibial, deep peroneal, sural nerves[24]

Digital blocks offer total nail unit anesthesia and are hence the preferred methods. These would be discussed in further detail.

Distal Digital Block ***(Figs. 5 and 6)****:* The needle is inserted 2–3 mm proximal to the junction of PNF and LNF. After raising a wheal to minimize pain, the needle is inserted vertically down toward the ventral aspect. While doing so, 0.5–1 mL of anesthetic agent is injected to cover the dorsal and ventral digital nerves. Both sides of digit are injected. The advantages and disadvantages of distal digital block are summarized in **Box 1**.

Proximal Digital Block ***(Fig. 7)****:* The needle is introduced at the base of digit, and a wheal is raised. The needle is then pushed

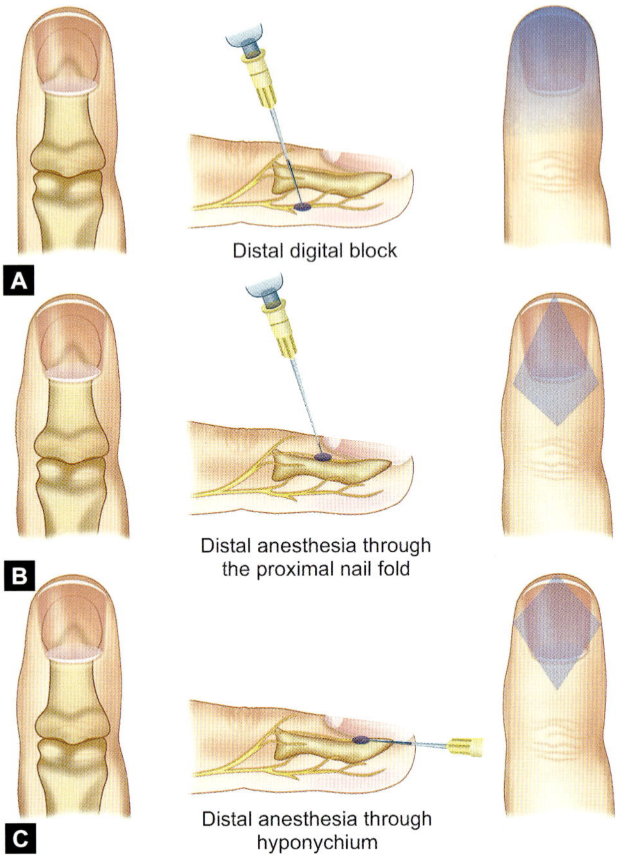

Figs. 5A to C: Three types of distal digital anesthesia with area covered. *Source:* Abimelec and Dumontier (2005).[1]

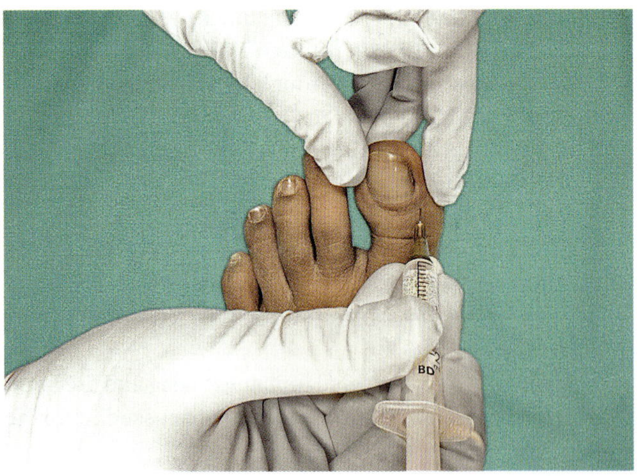

Fig. 6: Distal digital block—given at a point 2–3 mm proximal to the junction of proximal nail fold (PNF) and lateral nail fold (LNF).

gently in a ventral direction, injecting a larger amount near the dorsal and ventral digital nerves (1 mL for each nerve for thumb and 2 mL for toe). It takes 10–15 minutes for full effect to take place. It is not a ring block, which should be avoided.

Transthecal Digital Block: At the level of the palmar flexion crease, 2 mL lidocaine is injected into the potential space of the flexor tendon sheath with a syringe and 26-gauge hypodermic needle. The digit is anesthetized through centrifugal diffusion.[25]

BOX 1: Advantages and disadvantages of distal digital block.

Advantages:
- Immediate effect (in <1 minute)
- Low risk of neurovascular compromise
- Induces compression hemostasis

Disadvantages:
- Injection relatively painful
- Vascular compromise in vasculopathies (e.g., systemic sclerosis)
- May cause inadequate coverage and swelling of surgical field in large surgeries

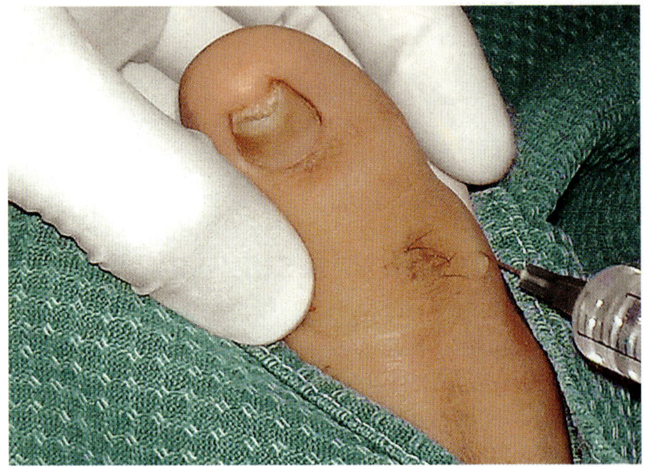

Fig. 7: Proximal digital block.

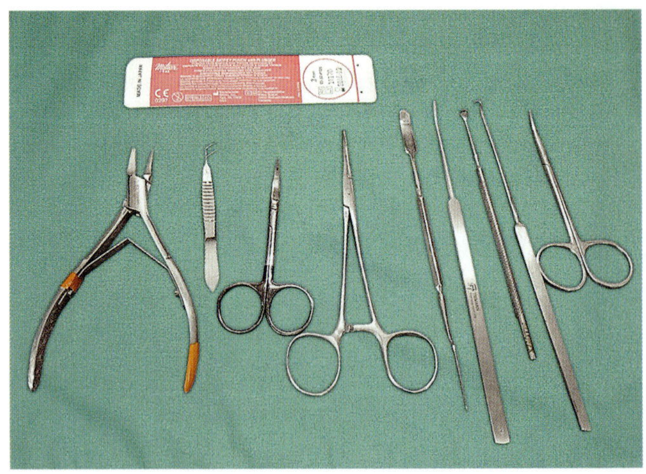

Fig. 8: Nail instruments.

INSTRUMENTS

Most instruments used for nail surgery are not specific.

General Instruments (Fig. 8)

- Binocular magnifying loupe that magnifies 2.5–3.5 times at a distance of 35–45 cm.

- Delicate Adson's forceps with one by two teeth/Castroviejo forceps
- Biopsy punch
- Double-prong Guthrie retractors
- Delicate needle holder
- Stevens/Gradle scissors
- Straight mosquito forceps
- Curette
- Digital tourniquet

Specific Instruments

- *Nail elevator:* Lempert (2–3 mm wide)/Freer septum elevator/dental spatula
- English anvil-action nail splitter
- Nail nipper

SUTURES

- Biopsies and excisions with a diameter ≤3 mm do not require suturing.
- *PNF/LNF:* Absorbable suture (Vicryl Rapide: 4-0 for toes, 5-0 for fingers)
- Nonabsorbable suture such as Ethilon/Prolene can also be used.
- *Nail matrix:* Absorbable suture (Vicryl 6-0)
- *Nail bed:* Absorbable suture (Vicryl 5-0)

HEMOSTASIS

Intraoperative

A bloodless field is mandatory for optimal results.

- Pressure applied to lateral digital arteries—by an assistant—suffices for simple avulsions and biopsies.
- Digital tourniquet at the base of finger is used most commonly. Various agents such as Penrose drain, rubber band, urinary catheter, a gauze strip, and a rolled rubber glove finger whose tip has been removed, have been used. For finger nail surgery, the whole glove (patient's glove size) is a better alternative as it provides adequate (not excessive) and reliable pressure while providing a sterile surgical field.[26] A tourniquet should not be applied for >15 minutes at a stretch.[27]
- *Pneumatic tourniquet:* It is applied to upper arm/forearm after exsanguination. It is used in cases with a digital infection or a distal vascular compromise.

A conscious patient can tolerate a pneumatic tourniquet for about 30 minutes.

Electrocoagulation should be avoided as far as possible to reduce the risk of nail tissue scarring and permanent nail dystrophy.

Postoperative

Bulky dressing, gentle pressure, and overhead limb positioning are sufficient measures in majority of cases.

OPERATIVE PROCEDURES/TECHNIQUES

Nail Plate Avulsion

Nail avulsion is the most common surgical procedure performed on the nail unit. It is the excision of the body of the nail plate from its primary attachments, the nail bed ventrally and the PNF dorsally.

Indications

- To treat recalcitrant onychocryptosis
- To excise tumors of the nail unit
- To allow full examination and exploration of the nail bed, the nail matrix, the PNF and the LNF, and the nail grooves for the presence of pathology
- To use as a preliminary step before performing biopsy on the nail bed and the nail matrix
- Avulsion of the nail plate is frequently used as a therapeutic adjunct in long-standing fungal infections of the nail, such as chronic onychomycosis, and in acute bacterial infections.
- In traumatic nail injuries, avulsion may be used to evaluate the stability of the nail bed or to release a subungual hematoma after failed puncture aspiration.

Nail plate avulsion is done as partial or total. Total avulsion could be chemical (40% urea) or surgical.

Surgical Avulsion[1,28,29]

Steps:

1. *Nail plate, PNF separation* ***(Fig. 9)****:* Dental spatula/Freer septum elevator is pushed back toward the cuticle and gently introduced under the PNF. The instrument is moved laterally in gliding movement to separate the remaining part of PNF from nail plate.
2. *Nail plate and nail bed separation* ***(Fig. 10)****:* The same instrument is introduced under the nail plate at the level of hyponychium and pushed toward lunula. There is

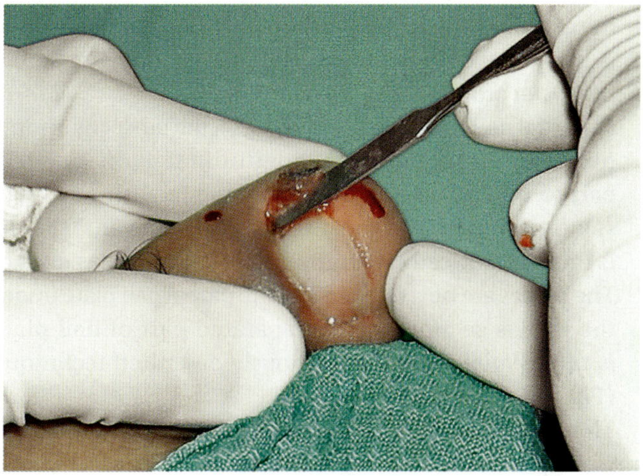

Fig. 9: Separation of nail plate from proximal nail fold (PNF).

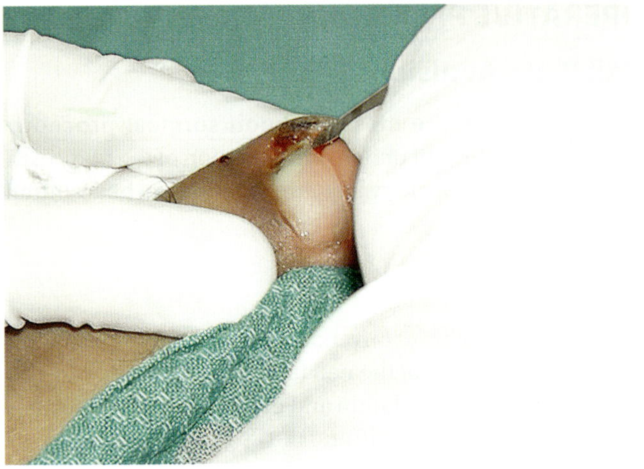

Fig. 10: Separation of nail plate from nail bed.

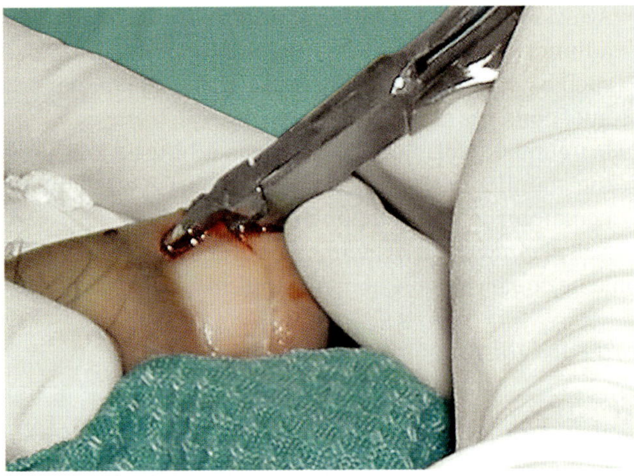

Fig. 11: Sectioning of nail plate with nail splitter.

lesser resistance to the movement of spatula underneath lunula. The instrument is withdrawn and reintroduced in the adjoining region till the entire area to be avulsed is separated. The spatula must not be swept laterally to respect the longitudinal orientation of the ridges and grooves in this region.

3. In case of complete nail avulsion, the separated nail plate is grasped with a hemostat and avulsed by twisting the hemostat around its long axis.
4. In partial nail plate avulsion **(Fig. 11)**, the most commonly performed technique is longitudinal avulsion. The part to be avulsed is sectioned using English anvil nail splitter till the distal-most part of PNF. Stevens' scissor is then introduced under the PNF with its blades closed. The blades are next opened and the part of nail plate under the PNF is sectioned. The separated part of nail plate is then avulsed using a previously described technique **(Fig. 12)**.

The partial nail plate avulsions could also be done as proximal (for nail matrix exposure), distal, or circular in less common indications.

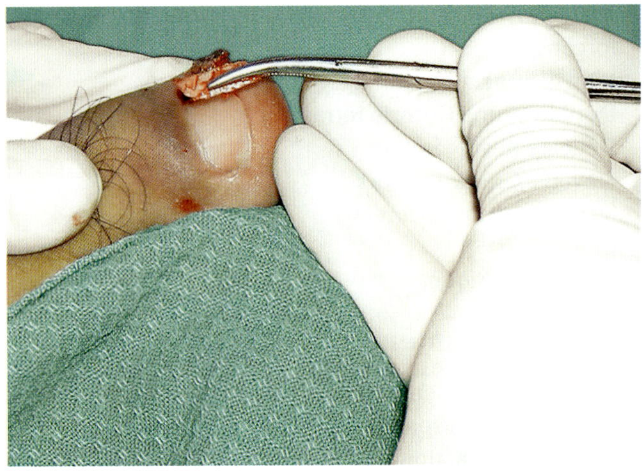

Fig. 12: Avulsion of separated and sectioned parts of nail plate.

In the proximal approach **(Figs. 13A and B)**, the spatula is inserted under the detached PNF and pushed proximally till one feels the proximal edge of the nail plate. It is then flipped and rotated to go under the proximal part of nail plate. The tip of spatula would now be facing the hyponychium. It is gently pushed in that direction to cause separation of nail plate from nail bed.

Complications

- Bleeding
- Pain
- Distorted curvature or hypertrophy of newly grown nail due to trauma to nail matrix and/or nail bed

Nail Plate Repositioning[1]

After some surgeries such as nail matrix biopsy and nail bed tumor removal, the avulsed nail plate is repositioned as this gives a natural and effective protection to the wound, nail matrix, and nail bed for 3–12 postoperative weeks. The repositioned nail also prevents pterygium unguis in event of nail matrix surgeries. It is secured to LNF with one Vicryl Rapide suture on each side.

Proximal Nail Fold Reflection

Proximal nail fold is needed to expose nail matrix and underside of PNF. The procedure is done by taking one/two oblique incisions starting at the junction of PNF and LNF and going proximally toward the DIP crease between dorsal and volar aspects. The separated PNF is reflected with the help of skin hooks or sutures. After the surgery, the PNF is repositioned and the incisions are closed using Vicryl 5-0.

Biopsy (Figs. 14 to 16)

Biopsy is useful for the diagnosis of various skin diseases when careful medical history, clinical examination, and other investigations fail to establish a precise diagnosis.

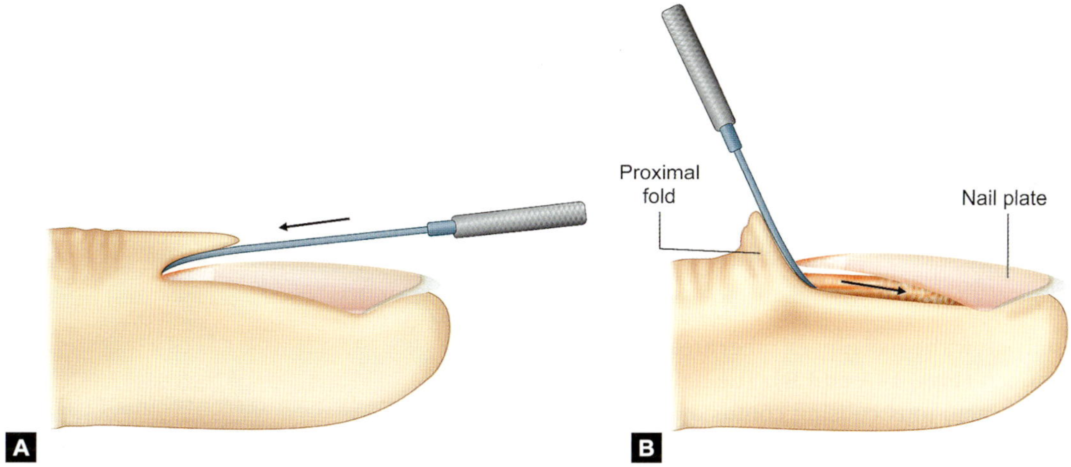

Figs. 13A and B: Proximal approach for nail avulsion.
Source: Salasche (1996).[16]

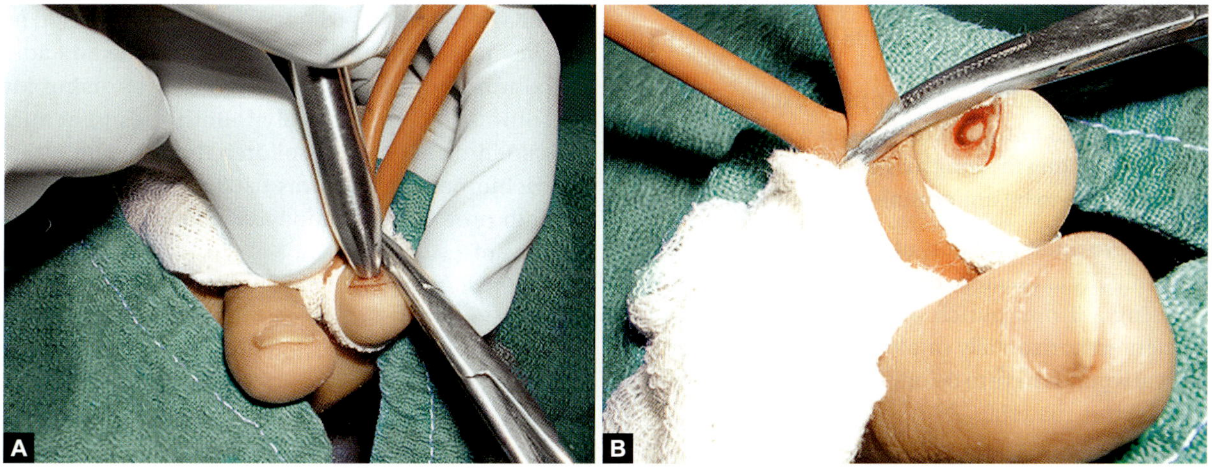

Figs. 14A and B: Nail plate biopsy with subsequent exposure of nail bed.

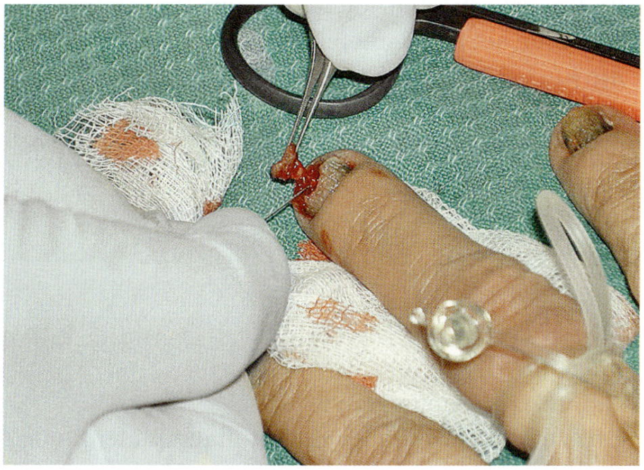

Fig. 15: Nail bed biopsy with a 11 number blade.

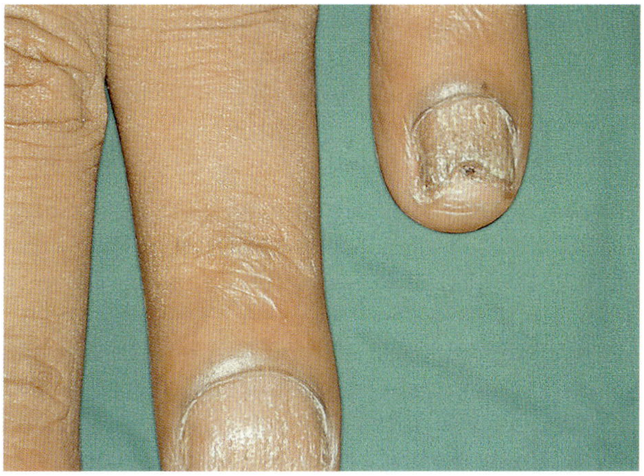

Fig. 16: Healing of the biopsied nail plate, circular defect grows out.

Some Indications[30]

- To differentiate between inflammatory and infective disorders, affecting nail unit, for example, psoriasis *versus* onychomycosis
- To establish the diagnosis in cases with one nail/"twenty nail" dystrophy
- To establish the cause of longitudinal pigmented streaks
- To differentiate between subungual hematoma and malignant melanoma

- To differentiate between benign and malignant tumors
- To identify the cause of pain (e.g., glomus tumor)

Types

Types of biopsy are nail bed, nail plate, nail matrix, nail fold, nail unit (combined biopsy of LNF, lateral nail matrix, and PNF)

Technique[1,30]

Nail plate: Distal part with a nail nipper, other areas with 3- or 4-mm biopsy punch **(Figs. 14A and B)**. The nail plate may get stuck in the punch, thus causing confusion and scare. It should be looked for and removed from there.

Nail bed: Done after partial nail plate avulsion with a 4-mm punch or nail plate lifting. A 3-mm punch is used to take the sample. The punch is moved deeper gently till it touches the periosteum. The base is separated using small iris scissors or 11 number scalpel blade **(Fig. 15)**.

For a larger sample size, elliptical excision with a maximum width of 3 mm should be taken with the long axis of incision being along the long axis of nail. The wound thus created would have to be undermined and sutured.

Nail matrix: Proximal avulsion of the nail plate has to be performed initially to visualize the matrix. The matrix sample is taken using a 3-mm punch or a longitudinal elliptical sample oriented horizontally or along the long axis of digit. The elliptical wounds have to be undermined and closed with absorbable suture material.

Matricectomy[1,16,17]

Matricectomy is destruction of nail matrix to prevent regrowth of nail plate in conditions such as onychogryphosis, pincer nails, onychocryptosis, and permanently split nails. It may involve the entire matrix or part of it (total or partial).

Modalities

- *Chemical* ***(Fig. 17)****:* Done by applying fully saturated (88%) liquefied phenol or 10% NaOH directly to exposed matrix. Phenolization as a method for partial destruction of nail matrix has been in use for >50 years and is the most commonly used method. It is by far the simplest, least traumatic, and most successful of all methods. A recent review in Cochrane Library has endorsed the same and shown that it carries the least rate of recurrence postoperatively at 6 months and above.[31] Phenol has the added advantage of being an antimicrobial agent and of causing damage to nerve endings, thus reducing postoperative pain. It should be applied with the help of cotton-tipped toothpicks, though other methods have been described. Phenol should be kept for 2–3 minutes. The duration of contact for 10% NaOH is 1 minute.[32]

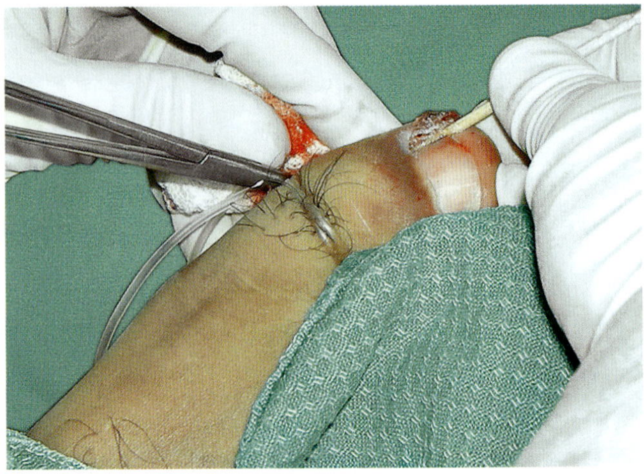

Fig. 17: Application of phenol after securing tourniquet.

  The duration of postoperative drainage is shorter for NaOH (average 9 vs. 17 days). The oozing period has been shown to be reduced by using lidocaine and adrenaline combination for anesthesia[33] and by using Monsel's solution postoperatively.[34] Both these chemicals are safe in diabetics and children. In only one series, 100% trichloroacetic acid was used with results comparable with previously mentioned chemical but with a healing time of 2 weeks.[35]
- *Surgical (removal of matrix, lateral matrix horns, undersurface of PNF):* PNF needs to be reflected. A more extensive surgery (wedge excision) is popular with orthopedic surgeons, but in view of a higher risk of infection, pain, recurrence, and deformity of nail plate, it should not be performed for treating ingrowing nails.
- *CO_2 laser* (ablation with focused mode or vaporization with defocused mode): PNF needs to be reflected.
- Radiosurgery/electrocoagulation (insulated matrix electrode set is commercially available—9 from Ellman Inc.)

Both CO_2 laser and radiosurgery carry a higher risk of postoperative pain as well as periostitis due to overzealous removal of the matrix.

Complications

- Pain
- Bleeding
- Infection
- Failure to prevent regrowth
- Growth of nail spicules due to inadequate damage to matrix
- Nail plate disfigurement

Onychocryptosis (Ingrown Nail)

Management: It is a very painful commonly seen condition due to impacting of the nail plate in periungual soft tissue. The most common variant is seen due to piercing of lateral nail sulcus by the nail plate due to trimming the nail plate too short or wearing shoes with a narrow toe box. Less commonly seen variants are due to increased transverse curvature of nail plate or due to swelling of periungual tissue. In the latter condition, distal embedding of the nail plate happens due to lack of counter-pressure of nail plate on the distal part of pulp.

- *Prophylaxis:*
  - Avoidance of overaggressive trimming of nail plate
  - Cutting the distal edge of nail plate straight and not in a curvilinear shape
  - Avoidance of narrow, closed footwear
- *Conservative management:* Works in cases with tenderness but no granulation tissue/severe discharge. Splinting of nail plate border using a flexible plastic tube,[36] introducing cotton wisp/dental floss between the nail plate and distal part of nail groove,[37] and use of adhesive tape to pull the LNF away from nail plate[38] are some of the methods that have been described as innovative office-based procedures to successfully treat such cases.
- *Surgical management:* Indicated in cases where conservative measures have failed or the condition is extremely painful/recurrent.

Approaches

- Narrowing of the nail plate (partial nail plate avulsion)
- Debulking the soft tissues

Partial nail plate avulsion with matricectomy: For lateral ingrowing nail, vertical avulsion of the involved part of nail plate followed by destruction of the relevant part of matrix chemically is a very successful method to treat more severe cases and cases where the abovementioned methods fail to work.

The procedure has been described under headings of nail avulsion and matricectomy.

Debulking of periungual soft tissue: For distal embedding and very hypertrophic and exuberant LNF, debulking with secondary intention/primary intention healing is the most effective and easy to perform, with great results.[39]

Howard–Dubois procedure, Vandenbos' procedure, Super U technique, Noel's procedure, Tweedle and Ranger's transposition flap are some of the methods described to debulk the soft tissue in PNF and the nail pulp.

A detailed knowledge of anatomy is essential before doing these surgeries. One should also train to acquire commensurate surgical skills. These surgeries need a proper operation theater with facilities matching orthopedic surgery standards.

Surgery for Subungual Hemorrhage

An acute painful reddish hematoma occupying 25% of nail bed needs to be evacuated to cause instant relief from pain and a chance of salvaging the nail. It is done with number

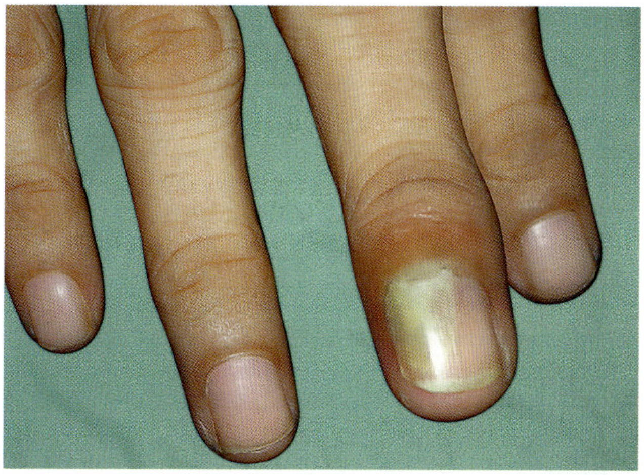

Fig. 18: Subungual abscess.

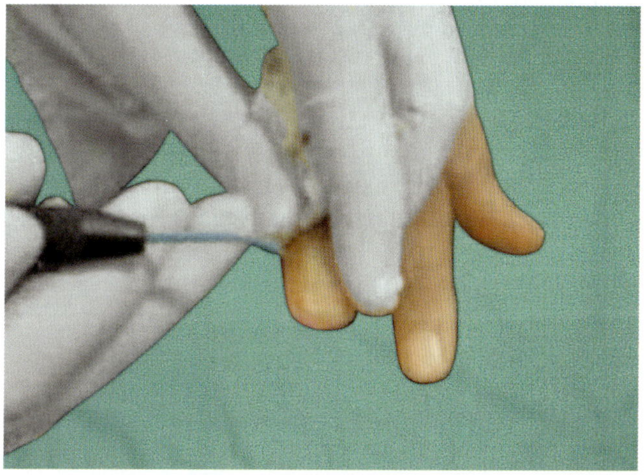

Fig. 19: Ellman RF equipment used to drain a subungual abscess.

18 needle, a pointed scalpel blade, a drill, or electrosurgical apparatus.[40] One should rule out a fracture to distal phalanx and presence of malignant melanoma.[41] Old asymptomatic bluish hematoma should be left untouched.

Nail Unit Infections (Pyogenic)

Acute pyogenic abscesses involving the nail folds should be drained in conjunction with the use of appropriate antibiotics. The incision should be parallel to the nail fold length. Baran and Bureau recommend incising the site of maximum pain rather than the site of maximum soft-tissue induration.[42] Formed septa in the abscess base are destroyed by using the tip of a curved hemostat.[43] In case of nail bed abscess, the methods described for subungual hematoma may be used **(Figs. 18 to 20)**.

POSTOPERATIVE DRESSING AND CARE

A nonadherent gauze coated with petrolatum, or an antibiotic is used to cover the operated area. This is then covered by many layers of absorbent gauze. A roller bandage is next used to secure the gauze and put some pressure. The limb may have to be elevated and immobilized in case of major surgeries. The dressing is changed after 48 hours, and the operated area is examined to look for complications such as infection, hematoma, and dehiscence. Smaller dressing is used in place; the bulky dressing is applied on surgery day. The dressings may be necessary for 10–30 days.[1]

Lasers and the Nail Unit

Multiple laser wavelengths and techniques have shown utility in the treatment of various nail disorders. In particular, CO_2 laser has been used for different purposes:

- Incisional mode for incising nail plate to expose underlying tissue
- Vaporization mode for matricectomy and periungual and subungual verrucae[44]

Advantages

- Hemostasis
- Visualization
- Less traumatic with higher precision
- Sterilization and sealing of tissue leading to noninoculation
- Helps to avoid blotting of surgical site, tourniquet, and bulky dressings
- Improved functional and cosmetic outcomes

Disadvantages

- Cost factor (equipment, training, operational and setup time)
- Lack of robust evidence

Lasers can be used for the management of the following disorders of the nail apparatus:

- Subungual hematoma
- Nail fold and plate dystrophies
- Onychomycosis
- Periungual/subungual verrucae
- Matricectomy
- For making incisions
- Laser-assisted drug delivery

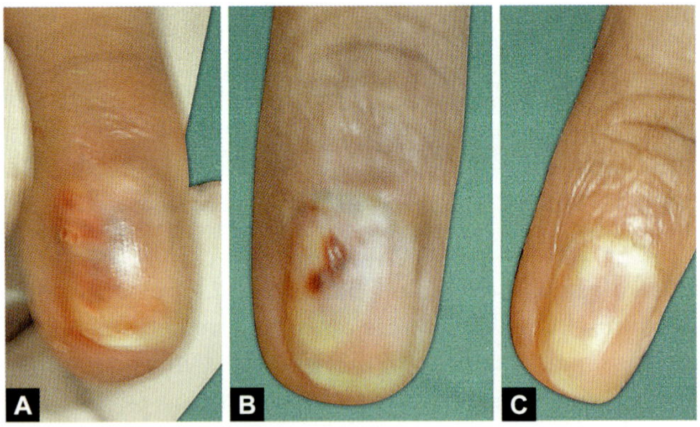

Figs. 20A to C: *Results after drainage of subungual abscess:* (A) Immediately postprocedure; (B) After 3 days; (C) After 9 days.

Onychomycosis

Laser treatment in onychomycosis have been approved by the Food and Drug Administration (FDA); however, doubts still exist over the fungicidal effect of lasers. There is a lack of literature of high methodological quality or evidence through randomized placebo-controlled studies comparing their efficacy with systemic therapy in onychomycosis.

Lasers may be considered due to:

- Poor penetration of topical drugs through the nonporous nail plate
- Long-term systemic therapy
- Pain, discomfort, and prolonged nail regrowth time postoperatively

Fractional CO_2 laser has been used to aid the delivery of topical antifungal agents[45,46] **(Figs. 21A and B)**, and fractional CO_2 laser associated with photodynamic therapy[47] has been used for the management of onychomycosis.

Long pulsed Nd:YAG laser delivers extremely brief microsecond bursts of energy resulting in ablative thermal

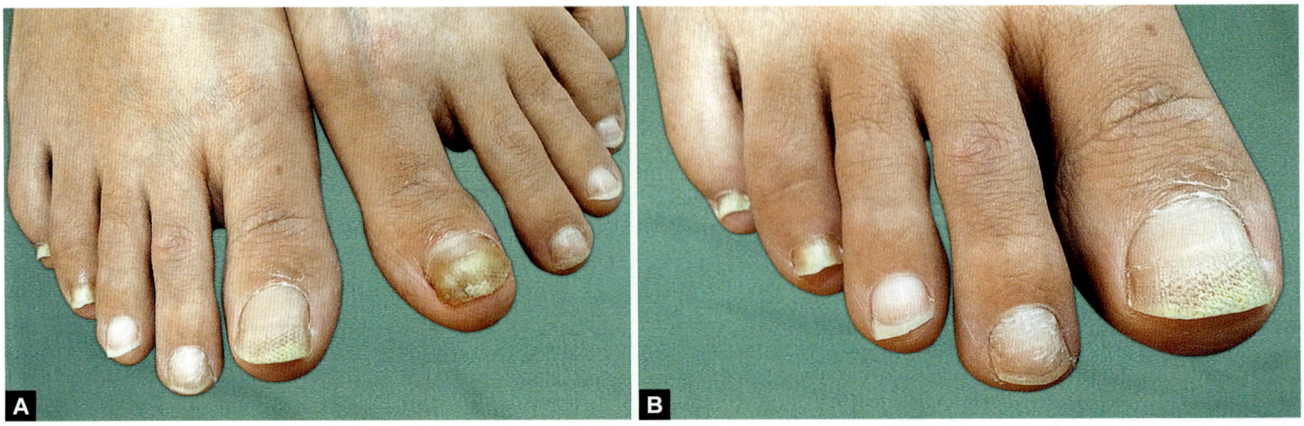

Figs. 21A and B: Fractional CO_2 laser-assisted drug delivery.

destruction of the fungi with minimal damage to the surrounding epidermal tissue.[48] Toenails have a higher cure rate as compared to fingernails with this laser.[49]

Diode laser at 870 and 930 nm has also been used, but questions have been raised over the mechanism of action and effectiveness of this laser.

TIPS AND TRICKS

- Learn your anatomy, be a good clinician
- Nail surgery is not difficult to master, take a plunge
- *Anesthesia:* Distal/proximal digital anesthesia should be used. Ring block must be avoided. Though 1–2% lidocaine is the agent of choice, bupivacaine could be injected postoperatively to prolong pain-free period
- There is no need to routinely exsanguinate the digit
- Tourniquet is not needed in all cases. When required, it should not be put for >15 minutes. Pressure on digital vessels by an assistant is sufficient to get a "bloodless" field
- During a punch biopsy of nail bed through the nail plate, a 4-mm punch should be used for nail plate and a 3-mm punch should be used for nail bed. The nail plate gets separated from nail bed and may get embedded in punch
- One should combine technologies to get optimum results
- One should be innovative and adapt to available facilities
- One should be conservative as reduced operative trauma leads to lesser downtime
- One should accept the limitations and take the help of orthopedic/plastic surgeons wherever needed

CONCLUSIONS

A willingness to embrace onychology would result in more scientific approach while seeing a patient with nail disorders. Office-based procedures done under local anesthesia would result in better and early diagnosis and more complete management. Many nail disorders with no medical management would be successfully treated with simple surgical approach. It would not be inappropriate to mention that onychology is an integral part of dermatology and hence it is imperative that dermatologists should be well trained in the subject. This chapter is a step in that direction.

REFERENCES

1. Abimelec P, Dumontier C. Basic and advanced nail surgery. In: Scher RK, Daniel CR (Eds). Nails: Diagnosis Therapy, Surgery, 3rd edition. Philadelphia: Saunders; 2005. pp. 265-306.
2. Dumontier C. L'Ongle. Paris: Elsevier; 2000.
3. Krull EA, Zook EG, Baran R, Haneke E. Nail Surgery: A Text and Atlas. Philadelphia: Lippincott, Williams and Wilkins; 2001.
4. Zaias N. The Nail in Health and Disease. Norwalk, CT: Appleton & Lange; 1990.
5. Ditre CM, Howe NR. Surgical anatomy of the nail unit. J Dermatol Surg Oncol. 1992;18(8):665-71.
6. Fleegler EJ. A surgical approach to melanonychia striata. J Dermatol Surg Oncol. 1992;18(8):708-14.
7. Dawber RP, Baran R, Berker D. Science of the nail: gross anatomy. In: Baran R, Dawber RP (Eds). Diseases of the Nails and their Management. Oxford, England: Blackwell Science; 1994. pp. 1-34.
8. Gonzalez-Serva A. Structure and function. In: Scher RK, Daniel CR (Eds). Nails: Therapy, Diagnosis, Surgery. Philadelphia, PA: WB Saunders; 2005. pp. 12-31.
9. Scher RK. The nail. In: Roenigk RK, Roenigk HH, Ratz JL (Eds). Dermatologic Surgery: Principles and Practice. New York, NY: Marcel Dekker; 2006. pp. 281-8.
10. Siegle RJ, Swanson NA. Nail surgery: a review. J Dermatol Surg Oncol. 1982;8(8):659-66.
11. Samman PD. Tumors producing nail disorders: benign tumours. The Nails in Disease. Boston, MA: Butterworth-Heinemann; 1994. pp. 169-82.
12. Fleckman P. Basic science of the nail unit. In: Scher RK, Daniel CR (Eds). Nails: Therapy, Diagnosis, Surgery. Philadelphia, PA: WB Saunders; 2005. pp. 37-54.
13. Flint MH. Some observations on the vascular supply of the nail bed and terminal segments of the finger. Br J Plast Surg. 1995;8:186-95.
14. Samman PD. Human toe nail: is genesis and blood supply. Br J Dermatol. 1959;71:296-302.
15. Fleckman P, Allan C. Surgical anatomy of the nail unit. Dermatol Surg. 2001;27:257-60.
16. Salasche SJ. Nail unit surgery. In: Robinson JK, Arndt KA, LeBoit PE, Wintroub BU (Eds). Atlas of Cutaneous Surgery. Philadelphia: Saunders; 1996. pp. 189-200.
17. Scher RK. Biopsy of the matrix of a nail. J Dermatol Surg Oncol. 1980;6(1):19-21.
18. Pardo-Castello V, Pardo O. Diseases of the Nails. Springfield, IL: Charles C Thomas; 1960.
19. Denkler K. A comprehensive review of epinephrine in the finger: to do or not to do. Plast Reconstr Surg. 2001;108(1): 114-24.
20. Krunic AL, Wang LC, Soltani K, Weitzul S, Taylor RS. Digital anesthesia with epinephrine: an old myth revisited. J Am Acad Dermatol. 2004;51(5):755-9.
21. Wilhelmi BJ, Blackwell SJ, Miller J, Mancoll JS, Phillips LG. Epinephrine in digital blocks: revisited. Ann Plast Surg. 1998;41(4):410-4.
22. Sylaidis P, Logan A. Digital blocks with adrenaline. An old dogma refuted. J Hand Surg Br. 1998;23(1):17-9.
23. Salam GA. Regional anesthesia for office procedures: part II. Extremity and inguinal area surgeries. Am Fam Physician. 2004;69(4):896-900.
24. Cohen SJ, Roenigk RK. Nerve blocks for cutaneous surgery on the foot. J Dermatol Surg Oncol. 1991;17(6):527-34.
25. Chiu DTW. Transthecal digital block: flexor tendon sheath used for anesthetic infusion. J Hand Surg. 1990;15A: 471-3.
26. Hixson FP, Shafiroff BB, Werner FW, Palmer AK. Digital tourniquets: a pressure study with clinical relevance. J Hand Surg Am. 1986;11(6):865-68.
27. Richert B. Basic nail surgery. Dermatol Clin. 2006;24(3):313-22.
28. Abimelec P. Nail surgery made easy, can it be true? American Academy of Dermatology, New Orleans; 1999.
29. Abimelec P. Tricks and tips of nail surgery: nail symposium. American Academy of Dermatology Annual Meeting, Orlando, FL; 1998.
30. Rich P. Nail biopsy: indications and methods. Dermatol Surg. 2001;27(3):229-34.
31. Rounding C, Bloomfield S. Surgical treatments for ingrown toenails. Cochrane Database Syst Rev. 2005;2:CD001541.
32. Oxdemir E, Bostanci S, Ekmekci P, Gurgey E. Chemical matricectomy with 10% sodium hydroxide for the treatment of ingrowing toenails. Dermatol Surg. 2004;30(1):26-31.

33. Altinyazar HC, Demirel CB, Koca R, Hosnuter M. Digital block with and without epinephrine during chemical matricectomy with phenol. Dermatol Surg. 2010;36(10):1568-71.
34. Aksakal AB, Atahan C, Oztas P, Oruk S. Minimizing postoperative drainage with 20% ferric chloride after chemical matricectomy with phenol. Dermatol Surg. 2001:27(2):158-60.
35. Kim S-H, Ko H-C, Oh C-K, Kwon K-S, Kim M-B. Trichloroacetic acid matricectomy in the treatment of ingrowing toenails. Dermatol Surg. 2009:35(6):973-9.
36. Schulte KW, Neumann NJ, Ruzicka T. Surgical pearl: nail splinting by flexible tube: a new noninvasive treatment for ingrown toenails. J Am Acad Dermatol. 1998;39(4 Pt 1):629-30.
37. Heidelbaugh JJ, Lee H. Management of the ingrown toenail. Am Fam Physician. 2009;79(4):303-8.
38. Haneke E. Nail surgery. In: Rusciani L, Robins P (Eds). Textbook of Dermatologic Surgery. Padua Piccin Nuova Libraria; 2008. pp. 300-1.
39. Richert B. Surgical management of ingrown toe nails: an update overdue. Dermatol Ther. 2012;25:498-509.
40. Herndon JH, Myers SR, Akelman E. Advanced surgery. In: Scher RK, Daniel CR (Eds). Nails: Therapy, Diagnosis, Surgery. Philadelphia, PA: WB Saunders; 2005. pp. 350-62.
41. Clark RE, Madani S, Bettencourt MS. Nail surgery. Dermatol Clin. 1998;16(1):145-64.
42. Baran R, Bureau H. Surgical treatment of recalcitrant chronic paronychias of the fingers. J Dermatol Surg Oncol. 1981;7(2):106-7.
43. Salasche SJ. Surgery. In: Scher RK, Daniel CR (Eds). Nails: Therapy, Diagnosis, Surgery. Philadelphia, PA: WB Saunders; 2005. pp. 326-49.
44. Lim JT, Goh CL. Carbon dioxide laser treatment of periungual and subungual viral warts. Australas J Dermatol. 1992;33(2):87-91.
45. Bhatta AK, Keyal U, Huang X, Zhao JJ. Fractional carbon-dioxide (CO_2) laser-assisted topical therapy for the treatment of onychomycosis. J Am Acad Dermatol. 2016;74(5):916-23.
46. Lim EH, Kim HR, Park YO, Lee Y, Seo YJ, Kim CD, et al. Toenail onychomycosis treated with a fractional carbon-dioxide laser and topical antifungal cream. J Am Acad Dermatol. 2014;70(5):918-23.
47. de Oliveira GB, Antonio JR, Antonio CR, Tomé FA. The association of fractional CO_2 laser 10.600 nm and photo-dynamic therapy in the treatment of onychomycosis. An Bras Dermatol. 2015;90(4):468-71.
48. Moon SH, Hur H, Oh YJ, Choi KH, Kim JE, Ko JY, et al. Treatment of onychomycosis with a 1,064-nm long-pulsed Nd:YAG laser. J Cosmet Laser Ther. 2014;16(4):165-70.
49. Li Y, Yu S, Xu J, Zhang R, Zhao J. Comparison of the efficacy of long-pulsed Nd:YAG laser intervention for treatment of onychomycosis of toenails or fingernails. J Drugs Dermatol. 2014;13(10):1258-63.

CHAPTER 50

Advanced Nail Surgery

Chander Grover

KEY MESSAGES

- A basic understanding of the nail unit anatomy and nail unit procedures and being conversant with these procedures is essential before proceeding to advanced surgical approaches in the nail unit.
- Advanced nail surgeries involve a higher level of complexity and are based on a combination of basic nail surgical approaches as covered in the chapter on Basic Nail Surgery.
- This chapter will deal with surgical interventions involving the nail matrix, which is the sensitive and germinative portion of the nail unit, hence, requires special care.
- Ingrown toenail is a very common condition involving the nail unit. It can be of various types and depending on that, the surgical approach needs to be planned.
- Nail unit is also the site of origin for many benign and malignant tumors of varied origin. They may be difficult to diagnose, as the presenting features may be different from those arising elsewhere. Imaging studies are necessary before any surgical intervention is considered.

INTRODUCTION

The nail unit is complex anatomical structure composed of the nail bed, nail matrix, nail plate, nail folds, and the underlying supporting phalanx and ligamentous structures. It has a rich neural and vascular supply and is yet prone to ischemic or neuropathic damage, if not carefully handled. Nail surgery is a specialized form of dermatosurgery owing to these peculiarities of the nail unit. Hence, certain surgical principles, techniques, and precautions are a must before surgically venturing into this area. These have been detailed in the chapter on Basic Nail Surgery.

The present chapter deals with advanced techniques of nail surgery, which should be practiced only after being conversant with the basics of nail surgery. Various techniques for managing the ingrown nail and nail unit tumors are detailed in this text.

INGROWN NAIL

Ingrown nail is a commonly encountered dermatologic morbidity responsible for much pain and symptoms. It generally presents in the active age group and limits the mobility of its sufferers. Some cases, especially in initial stages, can be dealt with conservatively; however, for most cases, one requires surgical correction to relieve the symptoms and reverse the deformity.

Predisposing factors for developing an ingrown nail include various intrinsic and extrinsic risk factors.[1] These are important to recognize and correct so as to prevent potential recurrences. These include trauma, incorrect nail trimming,[2] tight toe-box of the footwear, plantar hyperhidrosis, systemic diseases such as diabetes, or congenital/acquired nail plate abnormalities, which alter the nail plate growth.[1] Management strategy for ingrown nail depends on identifying the clinical stage and treating accordingly. Surgical correction is required in cases with pain, functional disability, recurrences, or failure of conservative treatment.[3]

Ingrown nail can be classified clinically based on the location of the ingrowing element and inflammation. Thus, it can be proximal, lateral, or distal ingrown nail. Proximal ingrown nail is better known as retronychia.[4] The severity of ingrowing also needs to be graded, as it is useful in deciding optimal management technique.[5] The commonly used severity grading systems include the Heifetz index[6] and the more recent Mozena grading[7] **(Table 1)**.

These grading systems are based on the degree of erythema, infection, swelling, oozing, and hypertrophy of the lateral nailfold, the severity of which decides the scale of intervention.

The surgical procedure resorted to in most of the cases is lateral partial nail avulsion with matricectomy. It is based on the principle of removal of a narrow strip of the ingrowing nail plate, accompanied by permanent matricectomy of a limited part of the matrix (the lateral horn) to prevent recurrence due to ingrowing of a broad nail plate. The permanent matricectomy can be attempted either chemically (more commonly) or surgically. The procedure is outlined below.

Lateral Ingrown Nail

Lateral ingrown nail is the most common type of ingrown nail. It is commonly encountered in adolescents and adults. The distal lateral corner of an improperly trimmed nail plate

TABLE 1: Mozena severity grading[7] for ingrown nail and corresponding treatment options.

Stage	*Nomenclature*	*Clinical features*	*Optimum treatment approach*
I	Inflammatory stage	• Erythema and mild edema • Pain on pressure in the lateral nailfold • No extension of nailfold over to the nail plate	• General measures including avoidance of predisposing factors, appropriate footwear, avoiding improper cutting of nail plate, and warm soaks with topical antibiotic, if needed • Conservative techniques including taping, packing, use of dental floss, toe spacer, nail braces, etc. • Recurrent cases in adolescents and adults or with type I diabetes mellitus—may require excision of the spicule and partial matricectomy
IIa	Abscess stage	• Increased pain, erythema, edema, and hyperesthesia • Oozing and/or infection • Extension of nailfold over nail plate (<3 mm)	Lateral partial nail avulsion with phenol matricectomy, especially in young patients and controlled diabetics
IIb	Abscess stage	• Similar to above • In addition, an extension of hypertrophic nailfold over the nail plate (>3 mm)	Aesthetic reconstruction with wedge resection of the nail and nailfold
III	Hypertrophic stage	• Chronic hypertrophy of nailfold • Granulation tissue covering a wide part of the lateral nail plate	*Winograd technique*: Wedge resection of the toenail and nailfold
IV	Distal hypertrophic stage	• Chronic deformity of the toenail (lateral and distal nailfold) • Hypertrophic tissue completely covering the nail plate (lateral or distal)	• Lateral nail matrix phenolization • Wedge resection of the toenail and nailfold by Winograd technique • May consider total nail avulsion and matricectomy as a last resort

embeds into the distal-lateral nailfold, inciting a cascade of inflammation, which causes nailfold swelling and further worsening of the impingement. To relieve the pain, the patient tries to trim the impinging edge, which upon regrowth again pierces the overgrowing periungual tissue, thus setting up a vicious cycle.

Details about the Procedure

The most commonly used procedure is lateral nail matrix phenolization, which is a combination of distal-lateral partial nail avulsion with chemical matricectomy.[8-11] The technique is proven to have a faster surgical recovery, very low recurrence rate, and is also technically less demanding.

Preoperative Workup or Preparation

The patient should be evaluated for causes or predisposing factors for ingrown toenail. These should be carefully corrected to prevent any recurrences.[1] These include advice regarding appropriate footwear, keeping the feet dry and clean, and advice regarding proper cutting of nails so that the formation of nail spicule is minimized. Any gait abnormalities or anatomical abnormalities should be taken into consideration. A digital radiograph should be done to rule out underlying bony lesion, which may need correction accordingly.

For cases with excessive granulation tissue or secondary infection, a preoperative course of antibiotics can be considered. However, it has been shown to be not much useful and the definitive procedure needs to be done sooner or later.[12] The patient should be advised to maintain cleanliness to avoid chances of secondary infection. They are asked to start cleaning the digit with antiseptic solution/soap morning and evening at least 48 hours in advance. This helps to reduce bacterial carriage and decrease chances of postoperative infections as well.

For patients undergoing surgery, advice regarding coming to the clinic with appropriate open footwear is also a must. The footwear should be able to accommodate the bulky dressing and also permit the patient to walk. The patient should also be made to understand that they may need help being driven back home.

Procedure Itself Step-by-step (Figs. 1A to E)

- The digit to be operated is cleaned and draped.
- The digit is anesthetized with proximal digital block being used commonly for this.
- Exsanguination of digit followed by a tight tourniquet at the base of the digit is tied **(Fig. 1A)**.
- This is followed by lateral partial nail avulsion, which is done by a distal approach. The nail spatula or Freer's septum elevator is used to separate the proximal nailfold and the lateral nail-fold from the dorsal surface of the embedded nail plate **(Fig 1B)**.
- Thereafter, the nail spatula is used to separate the distal nail plate from the nail bed **(Fig. 1C)**. For this, spatula/elevator is inserted in the gap between the distal nail plate and the most lateral part of the nail bed on the side of ingrown nail to separate the connections by performing longitudinal motions.

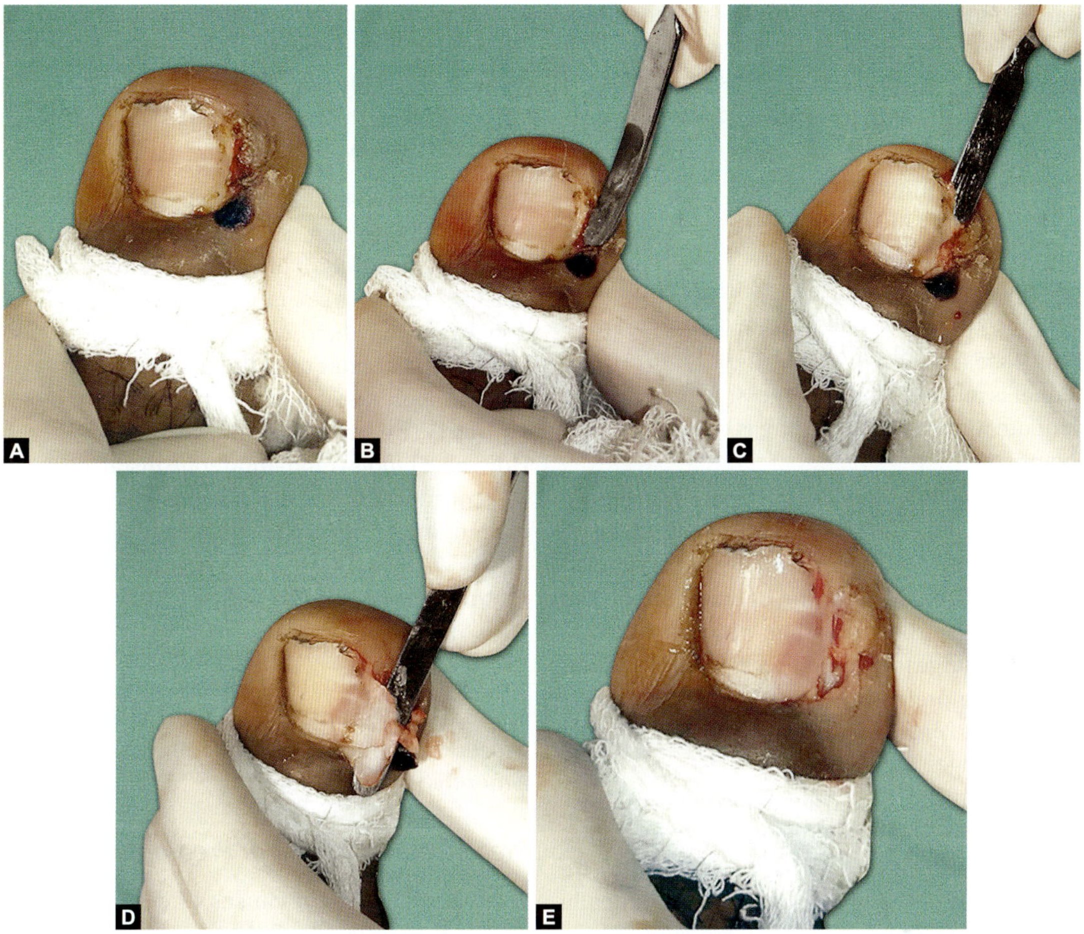

Figs. 1A to E: (A) Lateral ingrown nail with extensive granulation tissue on the lateral nailfold; (B) Distal partial nail avulsion starting by separating the lateral and proximal nailfold from the lateral and proximal nailfolds, respectively; (C) Separation of the nail plate from the distal nail bed with the help of nail spatula; (D) Lateral nail plate lifted up. It shows the extent of embedding. Also, it shows the proximal horn of the nail plate, which reflects complete exposure of the proximal matrix horn; (E) The lateral gutter has been curetted, cleaned, and phenolized.

- The narrow strip of nail plate, which has thus been separated from its proximal and distal attachments, is then lifted up to extract it from embedding **(Fig. 1D)**. The proximal edge of the avulsed nail plate should be carefully examined. It should have a horn-like shape reflecting the shape of the underlying matrix. This helps us to ensure that the nail plate has been removed and the lateral horn of matrix lies exposed in entirety.
- It is then cut with a nail clipper from the distal edge till the PNF. A straight scissors may be used to cut the portion under PNF, if one encounters any difficulty. One should be careful in this final separation. If there are still any attachments of the nail plate perceived, one should not twist and turn the nail plate, rather the nail spatula should be gently reintroduced. This is important to prevent damage to the rest of the nail plate or to the underlying nail bed.
- The separated and split lateral sliver of the nail plate is then lifted out revealing the lateral nail gutter underneath, at the proximal end of which lies the exposed lateral nail matrix.
- Thereafter, a curette with blunt edges is used to remove any tissue remnants or debris from the lateral nail gutter. These should be removed to prevent unnecessary denaturation of phenol solution, which is to be subsequently applied.
- Matricectomy by chemical means is then attempted for the exposed lateral horn of matrix. This is a blind procedure, as the proximal most edge of the nail matrix lies under the PNF, which has not been retracted or opened. Phenol solution is applied using a wooden stick dipped in pure liquefied phenol (BP 80% w/w, USP 89% w/w) in the lateral nail matrix cavity. The author is in favor of using three swabs dipped (but not dripping!) in phenol rubbed vigorously in the cavity for 20 seconds each. This totals to an application time of 1 minute, which has been considered optimum.[9] In case of visible blood or any other debris, the application time may need to be prolonged, as the phenol solution gets quickly denatured.
- The author is *not* in favor of phenolizing the whole lateral nail groove or the whole lateral nailfold to minimize cauterization of healthy tissue. This results in excessive tissue damage with prolonged postoperative oozing

and discharge. This, in turn, predisposes to secondary infection and also prolongs postoperative healing. The more the phenol is applied, the longer is the period of postoperative discharge increasing the need for dressing.

- In case there is formation of pyogenic granuloma or excessively bleeding granulation tissue on the lateral nailfold, phenol can be applied to chemically cauterize the same.
- Postphenol application, neutralization with alcohol swab, and draining the gutter with saline are recommended to remove any excess phenol solution **(Fig. 1E)**.
- The tourniquet is released and firm pressure is applied to secure adequate hemostasis. Dressing is done only after securing hemostasis.
- The digit is cleansed thoroughly with povidone-iodine solution, especially the areas, which turned white. A liberal amount of antibiotic ointment is applied followed by a nonadherent dressing over the operated area. The next layer is of an absorbent dressing, which is aimed at absorbing the discharge to prevent excessive maceration. All these layers are preferably draped in the form of a Y-shaped dressing to ensure grip.[13] The dressing is firmly secured with bandage.
- The patient should be instructed about limb elevation for the first 48 hours (to avoid digital edema). Appropriate postoperative antibiotics and analgesics should be prescribed. The first dressing change should be ideally done in the clinic at 48 hours. Thereafter, dressing change is advised at 1–2-day interval depending on the discharge, for as long as it continues (may vary from 1 to 3 weeks).

Modifications

Although the procedure for lateral nail avulsion remains the same, the technique of lateral horn matricectomy can vary. Various methods used for lateral matricectomy include:

- *Chemical matricectomy*: There are reports of successful matricectomy with 10% sodium hydroxide[11,14] and 100% trichloroacetic acid.[15] Chemical matricectomy being a blind procedure does carry a chance of recurrence, even though minor. Varying durations of application of chemical solutions have been described in literature. A 1-minute application time (by vigorous rubbing) has been found to be optimal.[9,11]
- *Surgical matricectomy*: This involves surgical resection of the matrix horn.[16] It may require incision at the junction of proximal and lateral nailfold to expose the underlying matrix. This is a more traumatic procedure with potentially more scarring. However, the chances of recurrence are the least.
- *Laser matricectomy*: CO_2 laser has been used to selectively destroy the lateral matrix.[17] Recent reports of use of 1,064 nm laser have also reported success.[18]
- *Electrical matricectomy*: Electrocautery and radiofrequency surgery have both been reported to be effective means of destroying the lateral matrix horn.[19]

Distal Ingrown Nail

Distal ingrown nail is less commonly seen. In younger children, it is self-correcting, and hence, it can be conservatively managed. In adults, it often results after total nail avulsion or nail loss. In such a scenario, a massaging of the distal nailfold downward may help to correct less severe cases. However, surgical management of the distal nailfold may be required in cases with distal ingrown nail because of a hypertrophic nailfold. The procedures described in literature include Howard–Dubois (mild–moderate distal ingrown) and "Super U" procedure (severe distal ingrown), which overcome distal embedding by freeing the distal nail plate edge.[3,20,21]

Details about the Procedure

Treatment for distal ingrown nail involves debulking of distal soft tissue so as to free the distal and lateral aspects of the nail unit. As compared to lateral nail matricectomy, these procedures require a much longer downtime (even up to 2 months).[20]

Preoperative Workup or Preparation

One should rule out causes of distal ingrown. A fair trial of distal massaging, pulp taping, and use of emollients and keratolytics should be given, if the condition is not severe. Digital X-ray is needed to rule out underlying bony abnormalities, which may be responsible for the hypertrophic distal nailfold.

For patients requiring this surgery, it should be clarified that postoperative recovery is prolonged. Hence, appropriate footwear modification and need for prolonged dressings should be explained.

Procedure Itself Step-by-Step

- **Howard–Dubois procedure** involves first marking the planned excision margins with a surgical marking pen.[22] This involves a crescentic incision 5 mm below the hypertrophic distal and lateral nail grooves. This continuous incision runs from the medial to the lateral aspect of the distal interphalangeal (DIP) joint, across the distal nailfold.
- The second incision is made in a crescent shape so that it reaches about 5 mm width at the widest portion, which is the distal nailfold. This much is generally enough to remove the excessive soft tissue.
- After marking the crescent, soft tissue is excised between the two incisions with the help of sharp-pointed scissors. This should be done down to the bone. The adequacy can

be checked by evaluating the wound edges to ensure that enough tissue has been removed to free the distal edge of the nail, which can be pulled onward easily and without much traction.

- The margins of the excision are then sutured with simple interrupted technique. Care should be taken that there is no area of excessive traction, which compromises healing of that tissue (avoid necrosis by pulling too much).
- The sutures are removed after a week, depending on the healing.
- ***"Super U" procedure*** is an even more extensive removal of the lateral and distal nailfold soft tissue in cases, which have a complete embedding of the nail plate.[21] This procedure is not commonly resorted in Indian setting and has an even longer surgical downtime.
- The incision in this technique is similar to the one in Howard–Dubois technique, except for the fact that proximal edges of this wedge are not pointed proximally, but are formed by a straight line extending from the nail plate edge to the bulk of the lateral nailfold. Even distally, tissue is removed up to the distal nail edge to practically "unearth" the embedded nail plate.
- The hypertrophic tissue is removed with scissors and toothed Adson forceps. Care should be taken to avoid removing too much fatty tissue to protect the phalanx.
- The wound is closed by a continuous suture.
- Postoperative dressing and advice as detailed above should be ensured.

Proximal Ingrown Nail/Retronychia

Proximal ingrown nail or retronychia refers to an ingrowing of the nail plate into the PNF. It is presumed to be a result of an arrested distal nail growth, because of which there is a heaping up proximally with detachment of the "old" nail, and new nail plate formation under the previous one cyclically.[23,24] The resultant inflammation makes the condition disfiguring and painful with swelling and granulation tissue formation over the PNF in extreme cases. Great toenails in young female patients are most commonly involved. The condition is often the result of repetitive microtrauma.

Retronychia diagnosis is primarily on clinical grounds. However, in doubtful cases, high-resolution ultrasonography can reveal the presence of multiple nail plates clinching the diagnosis.

Early stages may be managed conservatively with topical or intralesional steroids.[25] However, total nail avulsion is the definitive form of therapy, often required in unresponsive cases.

Details about the Procedure

The definitive treatment for retronychia is total nail avulsion which has been detailed in the chapter on Basic Nail Surgery.[22,23] It produces prompt healing, pain relief, and prevention of recurrence. The proximally thickened nail plate shows many underlying nail plates. Care should be taken to remove all of them. Postavulsion regrowth is usually normal, with prompt regression of signs of inflammation.

Preoperative Workup and Preparation

The preoperative preparation remains the same as for previous types of ingrown nail.

Procedure Itself Step-by-step

The procedure and expected complications have been detailed with basic nail surgeries.

NAIL UNIT TUMORS

A tumor refers to a circumscribed swelling. Evidently, these may or may not be of neoplastic origin. Several cellular proliferations, degenerative lesions, reactive lesions, and true neoplasms are referred to as "tumors". This chapter deals with the common nail unit tumors (NUTs) and their management.

The nail unit is the site of involvement with various tumors and clinical manifestations tend to overlap. These are frequently diagnosed late because of covering by the nail plate. Interestingly, they are difficult to diagnose clinically in the nail area and supportive investigations (imaging and histopathology) are routinely recommended and required. Surgical management depends on the tumor type, size, or location within the nail.

Tumors can arise from any of the components of the nail unit. A variety of tumors have been described in the nail unit,[26] including, but not restricted to, as given in **Table 2**.[27] This chapter focuses on surgical management of the most seen nail tumors.

Patient Evaluation: History, Counseling, Photography, and Imaging

Patients with NUT generally present with a *growth* or *swelling* in the subungual or periungual location.[28] Owing to their innocuous and asymptomatic nature, the duration is generally long (many years). Presence of significant pain (or cold sensitivity) points toward a glomus tumor; whereas, significant destruction of the nail plate points toward a possible malignancy. Many lesions commonly present as pressure changes with secondary distortion of nail plate. Any lesion in the subungual or periungual location should be promptly imaged.[29] A routine skiagram may show evidence of bony outgrowth (exostosis) or distortion/depression of bone (due to larger subungual tumors such as the glomus). High-frequency ultrasound can help to delineate the size, location, or type of lesion. However, the investigation of choice is magnetic resonance imaging (MRI), which can pick up even very small lesions.[29]

TABLE 2: Classification of nail unit tumors.

Epithelial tumors	*Onycho-tumors*	*Soft tissue tumors*	*Melanocytic tumors*	*Others*
Benign: • Wart • Syringoma • Eccrine poroma • Distal keratoacanthoma • Keratin cysts	• Onychopapilloma • Onychomatricoma	*Fibrous tumors*: • Koenen's tumors • Acquired digital fibrokeratoma • Infantile digital fibromatosis • Keloid	*Benign*: • Longitudinal melanonychia • Benign melanocytic hyperplasia • Lentigo simplex • Blue nevus	*Pseudotumors*: • Myxoid pseudocyst • Primary osteoma cutis • Subungual calcifications • Foreign body granuloma • Gout
Malignant: • Squamous cell carcinoma • Epithelioma cuniculatum • Sebaceous gland carcinoma		*Vascular tumors*: • Hemangiomas • AV malformation • ALHE • Pyogenic granuloma • Glomus tumor • Lymphangioma circumscriptum	*Atypical:* Melanocytic hyperplasia	Histiocytic and lymphomatous tumors
		Osteocartilaginous tumors: • Exostosis • Osteochondroma • Enchondroma • Osteoid osteoma • Giant cell tumor of bone	Nail melanoma	Metastatic tumors
		• Tumors of peripheral nerves • Synovial tumors • Lipomatous/ myxomatous sarcomas		

(AV: arteriovenous; ALHE: angiolymphoid hyperplasia with eosinophilia)

Surgical Management of Nail Unit Tumor

A thorough knowledge of nail unit anatomy helps to understand the origin of the suspected tumor. It also helps to minimize potential scarring and adverse surgical outcomes associated with nail surgery. Here, we discuss surgical management of commonly observed nail tumors, including warts (periungual or subungual), glomus tumor, acquired fibrokeratomas, and digital myxoid cysts.

Ungual Verrucae (Periungual and Subungual)

Warts arising in the subungual or periungual location are often difficult to treat because of hindrance by overlying nail plate and potential of damage to underlying nail matrix.[30] Routine topical treatments may not be practical requiring removal of nail plate to expose the wart in its totality. The same holds true for destructive options such as electrosurgery, radiofrequency destruction, or lasers. The procedure of choice may be intralesional bleomycin, which is safe as well as effective.

Details about the procedure: Bleomycin is a glycopeptide, which is used as an antimitotic drug.[31,32] It acts by causing DNA strand scission preventing cell replication. The intralesional use of bleomycin is not Food and Drug Administration (FDA) approved but multiple clinical studies have described its use, documenting beneficial response[33] as well as adverse events.[34] Intralesional bleomycin is commonly used for viral warts in difficult-to-treat sites such as subungual, periungual, and palmoplantar mosaic warts. Reported cure rates in ungual warts range from 76 to 94%.[35]

Preoperative workup or preparation: It is imperative to comprehend the extent and number of warts in the subungual and periungual location before treating with intralesional bleomycin. Warts in the PNF area need to be treated carefully to avoid inadvertent damage to underlying matrix. The patient also needs to be assessed for signs of digital ischemia, which may be further worsened by such injections.

Bleomycin is available as a dry powder, which is to be reconstituted to prepare a 5 mL stock solution of 3 U/mL. The stock solution must be stored at 4°C and is stable for 30–60 days.

Procedure itself step-by-step:

- Generally, no digital anesthesia is required. However, a proximal digital block is advisable for very apprehensive patients with multiple warts over a digit.
- The wart to be injected may be debulked prior to injection, by paring with a scalpel blade. This eases penetration into the substance of the wart.
- The stock solution can be injected in strength varying from 1 to 3 U/mL, with the higher strength producing better results. If dilution is required, it may be done with normal saline or 1% lignocaine without adrenaline.

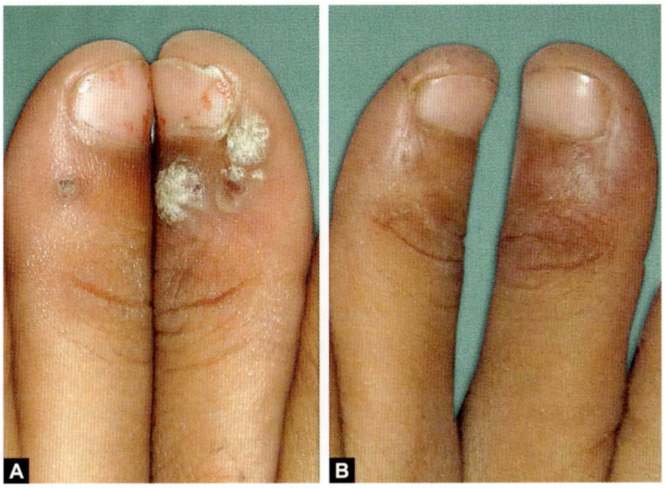

Figs. 2A and B: A 19-year-old girl with multiple periungual and digital warts. The result is seen after three sessions of intralesional bleomycin (3 U/mL) administered at 2-week intervals. There is complete resolution without any scarring or pigmentary changes.

- The solution is injected into the substance of the wart so as to produce blanching. It is preferably given with 1 mL tuberculin syringe with inbuilt 30G needle, which eases penetration into thick warts, minimizes pain, and prevents backsplash.
- Repeated punctures may be needed to infiltrate the substance of the wart depending on its size. Though there are no clear data available, the usual injected volume should generally not exceed 1–2 mL per session.
- For lesions, which are flatter or not possible to inject in, the technique of "bleopuncture" is used. For this, the needle is used to puncture multiple holes into the wart till there is appearance of multiple droplets of blood on the surface. Thereafter, a drop of the bleomycin solution is placed on top of it to allow it to seep into the defects. Continued puncturing can be done with the drop placed. This produces a more superficial necrosis of the wart.
- Following treatment, the patients are advised to use heavy emollients such as petrolatum, which help in softening the lesion and ease the symptoms associated with appearance of necrotic eschar or hemorrhagic bullae. No oral antibiotics or painkillers are required.
- The wart is reassessed in 2–3 weeks by which time most of the eschar would have fallen off revealing any residual lesions. This may be further injected. The average number of injections per wart varies from 1 to 4 **(Figs. 2 and 3)**.

Recent work has demonstrated increased efficacy of bleomycin in conjunction with fractional CO_2 laser and electroporation (electrochemotherapy).[36,37] Ungual warts can also be dealt with nail avulsion (partial or complete depending on the extent of the wart) followed by use of destructive methods such as radiofrequency cautery, electrocautery, or ablative lasers. However, there is a low success rate as well as high risk of recurrence in author's personal experience.

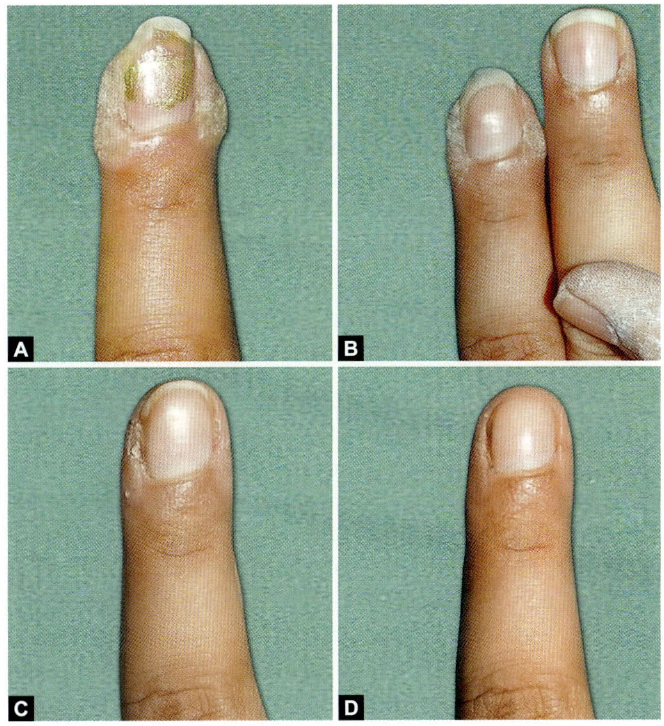

Figs. 3A to D: A 16-year-old girl with extensive periungual and subungual warts treated with intralesional bleomycin. These warts required four sessions (2 weeks apart) to clear. Secondary nail surface irregularities can be seen.

Glomus Tumor

Glomus tumors are vascular tumors common in the subungual location. These are hamartomas of the neuromyoarterial glomus body, which is normally responsible for thermoregulation.[38] Diagnosis is mainly on clinical grounds although imaging may be useful in localizing the lesion and determining its size. Surgical excision is the treatment of choice.

A diagnosis of glomus tumor is suggested by clinical signs and symptoms including spontaneous pain, sensitivity to touch, and cold sensitivity with an area of blue-reddish discoloration.[38] Some cases may have associated nail deformity. Pain may be severe and paroxysmal, often radiating to the shoulder. Love's sign and Hildreth's test are clinical tests and helpful in achieving the diagnosis.[39] Love's sign refers to severe localized tenderness elicited on applying pressure with a pinhead, along with relief of pain when the pressure is removed. Hildreth's test involves reduction or abolition of lesional pain and tenderness on elevating the patient's arm and inflating the blood pressure cuff. Releasing the cuff then causes a sudden return of pain.

Details about the procedure: Treatment of glomus tumors is purely surgical. The major concerns are the postoperative risk of nail deformity and risk of recurrence. Incomplete surgical removal and pre-existing synchronous satellite lesions are associated with a persistent or recurring pain. There are two possible approaches for surgical excision of glomus tumor—(1) transungual[38] and (2) lateral.[40] The former is preferred and routinely resorted to, as it offers a better visualization of the subungual region and easier exploration. If the lesion is believed to be involving the nail matrix, an eponychial flap must be raised to ensure complete removal. Careful handling of tissues during surgery and meticulous repair of the defect created by excision can prevent scarring. Postoperative repositioning of the avulsed nail plate segment helps to prevent adhesions of the eponychium to the matrix, favors repair of nail bed, and reduces pain.

Preoperative workup or preparation: The lesion can mostly be localized on the basis of clinical signs such as Love's test (point of maximal tenderness), the point of visible erythema over the nail plate, or the painful base of a band of erythronychia. Onychoscopic examination also offers useful pointers toward the clinical localization of the tumor. Plain radiographs should be done, although diagnostic yield is low. Changes may be seen only with very large tumors producing a bony depression, erosion, or cortical thinning seen in 30–60% cases. It may be useful for differentiating glomus tumors from subungual exostoses. Ultrasonography can also localize and assess the size of the tumor preoperatively. These are seen as well-circumscribed hypoechoic masses. Doppler ultrasonography can identify low signals within the hypoechoic mass and is preferred over standard ultrasonography.

Magnetic resonance imaging is the investigation of choice, as it can detect lesions as small as 2 mm in size. The classical findings include marked hyperintensity seen on T2-weighted images with a strong enhancement with gadolinium-based contrast.[38] MR angiography also shows a typical appearance of strong arterial enhancement and tumor blush in delayed phase.[41] MRI is also useful for assessment of patients with recurrence or incomplete resolution of symptoms following surgery.

Procedure itself step-by-step ***(Figs. 4A to H)****:*

- The digit to be operated is anesthetized with proximal nerve block using 2% lignocaine hydrochloride solution.
- Digital exsanguination followed by tourniquet at the base helps in achieving a relatively avascular operating field helping in localization of the tumor **(Fig. 4A)**.
- The nail plate overlying the tumor is carefully avulsed either distally or proximally, depending on the location of the tumor **(Fig. 4B)**. Thus, prelocalization of the possible location of the tumor is very useful. As far as possible, only a partial nail plate removal should be attempted. Conservative nail plate avulsion followed by repositioning of the avulsed nail plate after surgery helps to improve postsurgical outcomes in the short term as well as in long term.
- If the glomus tumor is in the nail matrix location, it would require additional retraction of the PNF and raising an eponychial flap (lateral release incisions and stay sutures) to ensure adequate exposure.
- Once the area of nail bed or matrix is exposed, blunt dissection with fine forceps is used to enable separation of the tumor from surrounding tissue **(Fig. 4C)**. This takes a few minutes but helps in removal of the lesion in toto. Punch excision can also be attempted for very small lesions. For larger lesions, there is a risk of incomplete excision with a punch.
- Resultant defect is primarily repaired with 6-0 absorbable sutures, if possible **(Figs. 4D and E)**. For very large tumors (>7–8 mm), this may not be possible.
- The avulsed nail plate can be trimmed and repositioned whenever and wherever possible **(Figs. 4F and G)**.
- If an eponychial flap had been raised, it is allowed to fall back and sutured in place with 4-0 nonabsorbable suture.
- Postoperative dressing is done using antibiotic cream and gauze.
- Patient is prescribed postoperative oral antibiotics and analgesics. They are reviewed at 1 week or are asked to report back earlier, if there is severe pain in the operated digit (suggestive of tight dressing).
- Any nonabsorbable sutures used are removed at the end of the 1st week **(Fig. 4H)**.

Acquired Digital Fibrokeratoma

It is an uncommon and acquired growth, which resembles a cutaneous horn. On the basis of distinctive histopathology, the lesions were named acquired digital fibrokeratoma (ADFK).[42,43] Subsequently, similar lesions were reported on the proximal hand, toes, sole, etc., hence, renamed acral fibrokeratomas. In the ungual or periungual location, they are also known as garlic-clove fibromas **(Fig. 5A)**, owing to their clinical presentation in the form of skin-colored asymptomatic nodule with hyperkeratotic tip. Mostly, it originates from under the PNF, placing itself on top of nail plate. The pressure on the underlying matrix can result in a grooved nail plate surface. Less common sites of origin may be the nail matrix (intraungual fibrokeratoma) or nailbed (subungual fibrokeratoma). Multiple such lesions seen in a patient with tuberous sclerosis are known as Koenen's tumors.

Details about the procedure: The procedure involves removal of the tumor from its most proximal origin in the most proximal part of the ventral surface of PNF.[44] For intraungual fibrokeratomas, the lesion has a matrix origin; and for subungual ones, the nail bed origin is to be delineated. The origin must be removed in toto, without any margin, to prevent recurrences. The attempted removal can be less complete in case of a Koenen's tumor, because there are high chances of recurrence anyways.

Preoperative workup or preparation: Preoperative workup involves routine precautions like those for any nail or digital

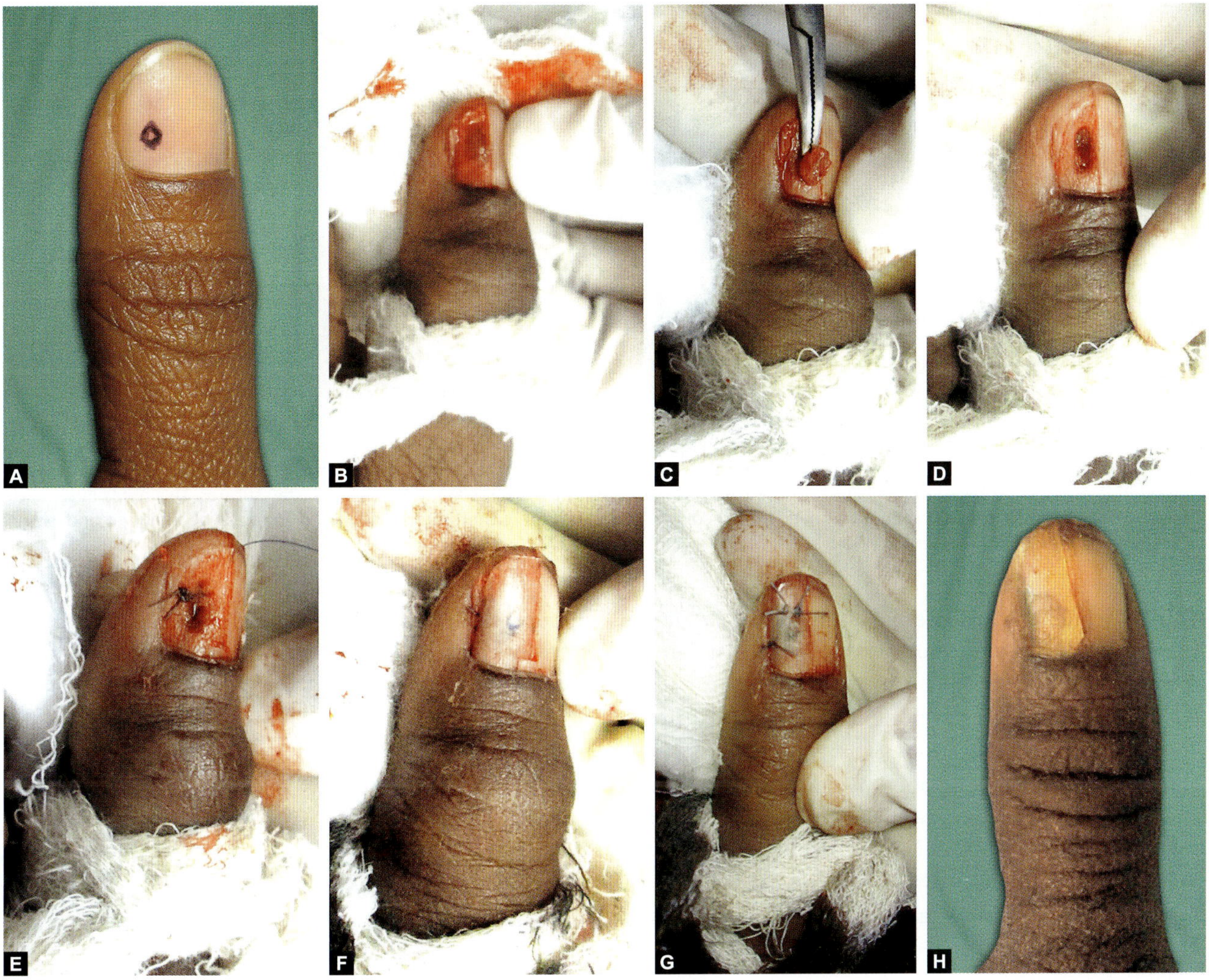

Figs. 4A to H: Surgical management of glomus tumor. (A) An extremely painful area of reddish discoloration in the nail bed of 4 years duration. The point of maximum tenderness is marked before administering anesthesia. This helps in localization of the tumor intraoperatively; (B) After anesthesia, digital exsanguinations, and tourniquet, a lateral partial avulsion of the nail plate has been done using a distal approach. This reveals the longitudinally-oriented bluish swelling in the nail bed; (C) The lesion is gently separated from the surrounding nail bed using blunt dissection. It is advisable to remove the lesion in toto; (D) The resultant linear defect after the glomus tumor has been removed; (E) Primary closure of the defect after mobilizing nail bed tissue by undermining; (F) The nail plate is trimmed (made shorter) and repositioned over the surgical wound; (G) It is held in situ with stay sutures; (H) The stay sutures are removed after a week. The nail plate sheds off subsequently.

surgery. In case of multiple lesions, tuberous sclerosis should be ruled out. Preoperative imaging helps to delineate the extent, if any, of the bone involvement.

Procedure itself step-by-step ***(Figs. 5A to E)****:*

- The digit to be operated is anesthetized with proximal nerve block using 2% lignocaine hydrochloride solution.
- Digital exsanguination followed by tourniquet at the base helps in achieving a relatively avascular operating field helping in localization of the tumor.
- For tumors overlying a thinned nail plate, no nail plate avulsion is needed. Instead, the PNF needs to be retracted fully to visualize the origin of the tumor from the most proximal part of the ventral surface of the PNF **(Fig. 5B)**. For nail bed lesions, partial nail plate avulsion (the part lying above the tumor) is needed.
- For more laterally placed lesions, a lateral release incision at the junction of the PNF and lateral nailfold (LNF) helps to locate the origin of the growth. The separated nailfolds are held back with stay sutures **(Fig. 5C)**.
- For more centrally placed lesions, the PNF is gently separated from the nail plate surface. Thereafter, two lateral incisions are made to fully retract the nailfold.
- The fibrokeratoma is dissected from its ventral aspect down to its base where it is severed from the PNF **(Fig. 5D)**.
- The nailfolds are then allowed to fall back and are sutured in place.
- For nail bed lesions, similar technique is followed after avulsing or laterally curling the nail plate. The resultant nail bed defect can then be primarily repaired with 6-0 absorbable sutures.

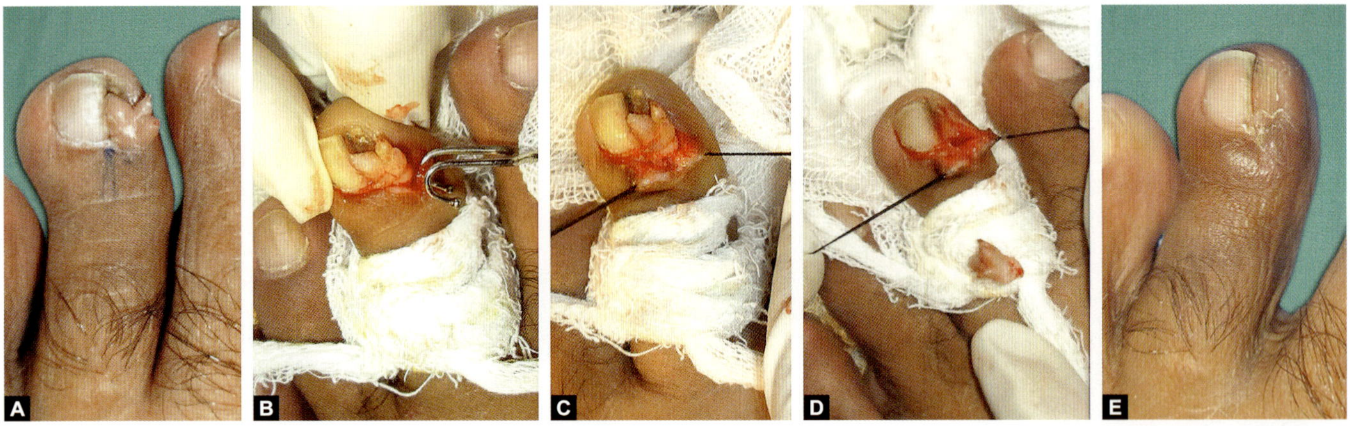

Figs. 5A to E: Surgical management of acquired digital fibrokeratoma. (A) Third toenail of a 40-year-old male showing a fleshy growth for the past 2 years. The lesion has typical "garlic clove" morphology. The underlying nail plate is very much thinned out due to the pressure of the lesion; (B) After administering digital block, exsanguinating, and tying tourniquet, an incision is given at lateral and proximal nailfold junction, overlying the tumor and extended laterally as far back as possible to expose the origin; (C) Both the nailfolds are retracted with stay sutures. This helps in severing the tumor from its base; (D) The tumor has been removed from its origin. The nailfolds are then sutured back preventing any damage to underlying bed or matrix; (E) The surgical wound after 3 weeks.

- The nail plate, if it had been avulsed earlier, should be trimmed and repositioned whenever and wherever possible.
- Postoperative dressing is done using antibiotic cream and gauze.
- Patient is prescribed postoperative oral antibiotics and analgesics. They are reviewed at 1 week or are asked to report back earlier, if there is severe pain in the operated digit (suggestive of tight dressing).
- Any nonabsorbable sutures used are removed at the end of the 1st week **(Fig. 5E)**.

Digital Myxoid Pseudocyst

It is a benign ganglion cyst of the digit, which mostly presents over the DIP joint in PNF. They are more common on the hands. Etiologically, they are a result of mucoid degeneration and are mostly asymptomatic, not requiring treatment. If large, they can produce a cosmetic disfigurement and secondary pressure changes on the nail plate and nail deformity **(Fig. 6A)**.[45] Both injectable therapy and surgical removal of the cyst are worth attempting; the choice of procedure being dependent on the cyst morphology and location. For fluctuant cysts, injections of triamcinolone acetonide as well as of sclerosing agents are described.

Details about the procedure: Pseudomyxoid cysts are a result of mucoid degeneration of connective tissue. They may or may not have a communication with the adjacent DIP joint with or without osteoarthritis.[45] Digital mucous cysts have a good prognosis, though recurrence is common. Radical surgery carries a low recurrence but significant associated morbidity. Several different treatment options exist but recurrence is high. If asymptomatic, the lesion can be left untreated with a possibility of spontaneous resolution. Other treatment options include repeated drainage of cyst fluid, cryotherapy, etc. More destructive modalities to be attempted under local anesthesia include curettage, cauterization, or even isolation of the origin of leakage from joint space by injection of a dye, and subsequent ligation.[46,47] This section describes method of cyst excision.

Preoperative workup or preparation: Digital X-ray is a must to rule out extensive involvement of the joint space or osteoarthritis. Ultrasonography is also very helpful. In cases with an organized cyst with no underlying bony abnormalities, cyst excision can be attempted.

Procedure itself step-by-step ***(Figs. 6A to F)****:*

- The digit to be operated is anesthetized with proximal nerve block using 2% lignocaine hydrochloride solution.
- Digital exsanguination followed by tourniquet at the base helps in achieving a relatively avascular operating field helping in localization of the tumor.
- For cysts in the PNF area, longitudinal incision is oriented over the most prominent part of the cyst **(Fig. 6B)**.
- This is followed by the use of fine artery forceps (mosquito forceps) to carefully separate the organized cyst from the overlying skin and the underlying structures **(Fig. 6C)**.
- The separated cyst is removed in toto **(Fig. 6D)**, followed by primary closure of the PNF incision **(Fig. 6E)**.
- Postoperative dressing is done using antibiotic cream and gauze.
- Patient is prescribed postoperative oral antibiotics and analgesics. They are reviewed at 1 week or are asked to report back earlier, if there is severe pain in the operated digit (suggestive of tight dressing).
- Nonabsorbable sutures used are removed at the end of the 1st week **(Fig. 6F)**.

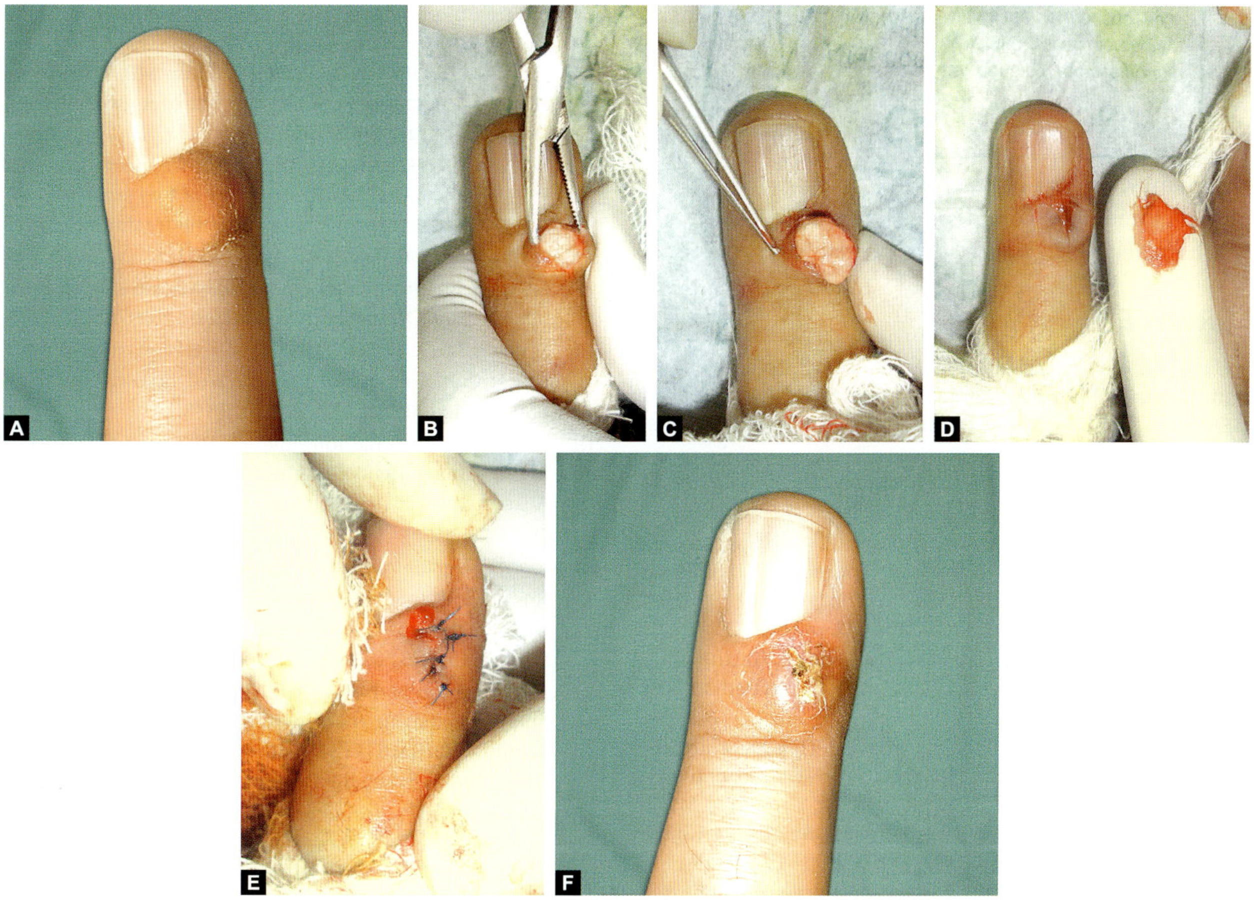

Figs. 6A to F: Surgical management of digital myxoid pseudocyst. (A) A myxoid pseudocyst in the proximal periungual location. Note the pressure effects of the cyst producing a linear depression on nail plate; (B) The cyst is exposed through a longitudinally-oriented incision in the proximal nailfold area; (C) The cyst is dissected from its attachment and extracted. It generally does not have a defined cyst wall; (D) The resultant defect is shown along with the removed organized myxoid cyst; (E) The defect is sutured primarily; (F) Postoperative period. Healing wound at 2 weeks.

Tips for Ensuring Good Results in Advanced Nail Surgical Procedures

- A thorough understanding of the complex nail anatomy and basic principles of operating on the nail unit is a must.
- Preoperative imaging is a must to rule out underlying bone involvement, be it the ingrown nail or a nail tumor.
- Nail plate avulsion should be attempted to the minimum possible extent, depending on the absolute need to expose the underlying nail bed or matrix.
- Chemical cauterization helps in achieving matricectomy blindly, without the need to expose the matrix.
- It is important to preoperatively localize the tumor to plan the approach and extent of nail plate removal.
- Nail bed incisions should be oriented longitudinally, while nail matrix incisions should be oriented horizontally.
- Nail bed or matrix defects can be sutured with fine absorbable suture; whereas, for the nailfold, nonabsorbable sutures are preferred.
- As far as possible, an attempt should be made to reposition the avulsed nail plate after suitably trimming it, wherever possible or not contraindicated.

SUMMARY

- Ingrown nail is a common and painful condition. It is important to recognize the various types of ingrown nails. It can be lateral, distal, or proximal ingrown.
- It is also important to recognize the cases, which are likely to improve conservatively. For others, appropriate surgical avulsion should be attempted promptly.
- Lateral partial nail avulsion with phenol matricectomy is the most commonly used technique for managing ingrown toenail. It gives a high cure rate and fast relief of symptoms.
- Cases with prominent nailfold hypertrophy need nailfold surgery.
- Surgical approaches for distal ingrown and proximal ingrown vary.
- Tumors tend to behave differently in the nail as compared to other sites and presentation depends on the site of origin within the nail unit, rather than on the histological type.
- The surgical approach is also determined by the site of tumor in the nail unit, with an aim to preserve as much structure as possible and to prevent scarring.

- Radiological investigation to assess type and extent of involvement of underlying bone is an absolute must before any surgical intervention.
- Generally, a deformity of nail plate suggests benign disease, whereas, active destruction suggests possible malignancy.
- Glomus tumors are common in subungual location and are characterized by pain and cold sensitivity.

REFERENCES

1. Hassan I, Jeelani S. Ingrown nails: Causes and pathogenesis. In: Grover C, Relhan V, Nanda S, Bansal S (Eds). Textbook of Onychology, 1st edition. Delhi, India: Evangel Publishers; 2021. pp. 451-6.
2. Khunger N, Kandhari R. Ingrown toenails. Indian J Dermatol Venereol Leprol. 2012;78(3):279-89.
3. Richert B, Haneke E, Zook EG, Baran R. Nail Surgery. In: Baran R, de Berker D, Holzberg M, Thomas L (Eds). Baran & Dawber's diseases of the nails and their management, 5th edition. Hoboken: Wiley-Blackwell; 2019. pp. 853-4.
4. Nakouri I, Litaiem N, Jones M, Zeglaoui F. Retronychia (Clinical Features and Surgical Treatment). J Am Podiatr Med Assoc. 2018;108(1):74-6.
5. Richert B, Di Chiacchio N, Caucanas M, Di Chiacchio NG. Definition—Pathogenesis Risk Factors—Classification—Scoring. In: Richert B, Di Chiacchio N, Caucanas M, Di Chiacchio NG (Eds). Management of Ingrowing Nails. Cham, Switzerland: Springer; 2016. pp. 35, 54, 56.
6. Heifetz CJ. Operative management of ingrown toenail. Mo Med. 1945;42:213-6.
7. Mozena JD. The Mozena classification system and treatment algorithm for ingrown hallux nails. J Am Podiatr Med Assoc. 2002;92(3):131-5.
8. Bostanci S, Ekmekçi P, Gürgey E. Chemical matricectomy with phenol for the treatment of ingrowing toenail: A review of the literature and follow-up of 172 treated patients. Acta Derm Venereol. 2001;81(3):181-3.
9. Tatlican S, Yamangöktürk B, Eren C, Eskioðlu F, Adiyaman S. Comparison of phenol applications of different durations for the cauterization of the germinal matrix: An efficacy and safety study. Acta Orthop Traumatol Turc. 2009;43(4):298-302.
10. Andreassi A, Grimaldi L, D'Anello C, Pianigiani E, Bilenchi R. Segmental phenolization for the treatment of ingrowing toenails: A review of 6 years' experience. J Dermatologic Treat. 2004;15(3):179-81.
11. Grover C, Khurana A, Bhattacharya SN, Sharma A. Controlled trial comparing the efficacy of 88% phenol versus 10% sodium hydroxide for chemical matricectomy in the management of ingrown toenail. Indian J Dermatol Venereol Leprol. 2015;81(5):472-7.
12. Reyzelman AM, Trombello KA, Vayser DJ, Armstrong DG, Harkless LB. Are antibiotics necessary in the treatment of locally infected ingrown toenails? Arch Fam Med. 2000;9(9):930-2.
13. Ashique KT, Grover C. The "Y" technique: An attempt to standardize nail dressing. J Am Acad Dermatol. 2018;78(5): e103-4.
14. Tatlican S, Eren C, Yamangokturk B, Eskioglu F, Bostanci S. Chemical matricectomy with 10% sodium hydroxide for the treatment of ingrown toenails in people with diabetes. Dermatol Surg. 2010;36(2):219-22.
15. Kim SH, Ko HC, Oh CK, Kwon KS, Kim MB. Trichloroacetic acid matricectomy in the treatment of ingrowing toenails. Dermatol Surg. 2009;35(6):973-9.
16. Peyvandi H, Robati RM, Yegane RA, Hajinasrollah E, Toossi P, Peyvandi AA, et al. Comparison of two surgical methods (Winograd and sleeve method) in the treatment of ingrown toenail. Dermatol Surg. 2011;37(3):331-5.
17. Serour F. Recurrent ingrown big toenails are efficiently treated by CO_2 laser. Dermatol Surg. 2002;28(6):509-12.
18. Sánchez LC, Zalacaín-Vicuña AJ. Onychoplasty with 1064-nm Laser: Matrixectomy for Treatment of Ingrown Toenails. J Am Podiatr Med Assoc. 2019;109(5):401-6.
19. Singal A, Kaur I. Radiofrequency Ablation for Matricectomy in the Management of Ingrown Toenail: A Pilot Study. J Cutan Aesthet Surg. 2019;12(4):212-4.
20. Di Chiacchio N, Di Chiacchio NG. Best way to treat an ingrown toenail. Dermatol Clin. 2015;33(2):277-82.
21. Rosa IP, Di Chiacchio N, Di Chiacchio NG, Caetano L. "Super U"—a technique for the treatment of ingrown nail. Dermatol Surg. 2015;41(5):652-3.
22. Di Chiacchio N, Borges CD, de Mello F, Di Chiacchio NG. Surgical management of ingrown nails. In: Grover C, Relhan V, Nanda S, Bansal S (Eds). Textbook of Onychology, 1st edition. Delhi, India: Evangel Publishers; 2021. pp. 463-73.
23. Alessandrini A, Piraccini BM. Retronychia. In: Grover C, Relhan V, Nanda S, Bansal S (Eds). Textbook of Onychology, 1st edition. Delhi, India: Evangel Publishers; 2021. pp. 474-9.
24. de Berker DA, Richert B, Duhard E, Piraccini BM, André J, Baran R. Retronychia: proximal ingrowing of the nail plate. J Am Acad Dermatol. 2008;58(6):978-83.
25. Laird ME, Lo Sicco KI, Rich P. Conservative Treatment of Retronychia: A Retrospective Study of 25 Patients. Dermatol Surg. 2019;45(4):614-6.
26. Domínguez-Cherit J, Chanussot-Deprez C, Maria-Sarti H, Fonte-Avalos V, Vega-Memije E, Luis-Montoya P. Nail unit tumors: A study of 234 patients in the dermatology department of the "Dr Manuel Gea González" general hospital in Mexico City. Dermatol Surg. 2008;34(10):1363-71.
27. Tosti A, Richert B, Pazzaglia M. Tumors of the nail apparatus. In: Scher RK, Daniel IIICR (Eds). Nails: Therapy Diagnosis, Surgery, 3rd edition. China: Elsevier Saunders; 2005. pp. 195-204.
28. Grover C, Khurana A. Nail tumors. In: Sacchidanand S, Savitha AS (Eds). Nail and its Disorders, 1st edition. Delhi, India: Jaypee Brothers Medical Publishers (P) Ltd.; 2013. pp. 169-81.
29. Baek HJ, Lee SJ, Cho KH, Choo HJ, Lee SM, Lee YH, et al. Subungual tumors: clinicopathologic correlation with US and MR imaging findings 1. Radiographics. 2010;30(6):1621-36.
30. Tosti A, Piraccini BM. Warts of the nail unit: surgical and nonsurgical approaches. Dermatol Surg. 2001;27(3):235-9.
31. Cordero AA, Guglielmi HA, Woscoff A. The common wart: intralesional treatment with bleomycin sulfate. Cutis. 1980;26(3):319-20.
32. Saitta P, Krishnamurthy K, Brown LH. Bleomycin in dermatology: a review of intralesional applications. Dermatol Surg. 2008;34(10):1299-313.

33. Soni P, Khandelwal K, Aara N, Ghiya BC, Mehta RD, Bumb RA. Efficacy of intralesional bleomycin in palmoplantar and periungual warts. J Cutan Aesthet Surg. 2011;4(3):188-91.
34. Miller RA. Nail dystrophy following intralesional injections of bleomycin for a periungual wart. Arch Dermatol. 1984;120(7):963-4.
35. Shumer SM, O'Keefe EJ. Bleomycin in the treatment of recalcitrant warts. J Am Acad Dermatol.1983;9(1):91-6.
36. Suh JH, Lee SK, Kim MJ, Lee UH. Efficacy of bleomycin application on periungual warts after treatment with ablative carbon dioxide fractional laser: a pilot study. J Dermatol Treat. 2020;31(4):410-4.
37. Di Chiacchio NG, Di Chiacchio N, Criado PR, Brunner CHM, Suaréz MVR, Belda Junior W. Ungual warts: comparison of treatment with intralesional bleomycin and electroporation in terms of efficacy and safety. J Eur Acad Dermatol Venereol. 2019;33(12):2349-54.
38. Grover C, Khurana A, Jain R, Rathi V. Transungual surgical excision of subungual glomus tumour. J Cutan Aesthet Surg. 2013;6(4):196-203.
39. Bhaskaranand K, Navadgi BC. Glomus tumour of the hand. J Hand Surg Br. 2002;27(3):229-31.
40. Vasisht B, Watson HK, Joseph E, Lionelli GT. Digital glomus tumors: a 29-year experience with a lateral subperiosteal approach. Plast Reconstr Surg. 2004;114(6):1486-9.
41. Theumann NH, Goettmann S, Le Viet D, Resnick D, Chung CB, Bittoun J, et al. Recurrent glomus tumors of fingertips: MR imaging evaluation. Radiology. 2002;223(1):143-51.
42. Bart RS, Andrade R, Kopf AW, Leider M. Acquired digital fibrokeratomas. Arch Dermatol. 1968;97(2):120-9.
43. Kint A, Baran R, De Keyser H. Acquired (digital) fibrokeratoma. J Am Acad Dermatol. 1985;12(5):816-21.
44. Haneke E, Richert B, Di Chiacchio N. Surgery of the proximal nail fold. In: Richert B, Chiacchio D, Haneke E (Eds). Nail Surgery, 1st edition. London, UK: Informa Healthcare; 2011. pp. 42-54.
45. Lin YC, Wu YH, Scher RK. Nail changes and association of osteoarthritis in digital myxoid cyst. Dermatol Surg. 2008;34(3):364-9.
46. Salasche SJ. Myxoid cysts of the proximal nail fold: a surgical approach. J Dermatol Surg Oncol. 1984;10(1):35-9.
47. de Berker D, Lawrence C. Ganglion of the distal interphalangeal joint (myxoid cyst): Therapy by identification and repair of the leak of joint fluid. Arch Dermatol. 2001;137(5):607-10.

CHAPTER 51 Innovations in Nail Surgery

Sanjeev Gupta, Deepak Jakhar

KEY MESSAGES

- Simulation models like banana can be used to practice and refine nail surgery techniques.
- Pain during local anesthesia can be minimized by optimizing pH and temperature of anesthetic solution.
- Early stages of ingrown toenails can be managed nonsurgically with methods like cotton nail cast and braces.
- Innovative techniques like syringe method or Y-shaped dressing have made postsurgery dressing of nail unit convenient.
- Innovations pave path for simplifying techniques in various steps of nail surgeries.

INTRODUCTION

In the recent past few years, nail surgery has gained a good popularity and the field of nail surgery is expanding day by day. Many advancements have been made to make nail surgery easy, user friendly, affordable, and interesting. The purpose of this chapter is not to describe the surgical techniques but to highlight the different important innovations in the field of nail surgery so far.

SIMULATION MODELS OF NAIL BED TO LEARN NAIL SURGERY

Most of dermatology residents often learn nail surgery on patients without prior training. Nowadays simulation models having plastic nail finger with nail plate fixed on that are available. Simple nail surgery (e.g., suturing and nail bed fixation) can be very well learnt on these models. In a study conducted to see the effectiveness of such models, the results were encouraging, and the use of such models into the training program of residents was strongly suggested.[1]

USE OF BANANA AS SIMULATION MODEL TO LEARN INGROWN NAIL SURGERIES

Many fruit models have been suggested in the past to learn various surgical techniques. Unfortunately, no animal models are available to learn nail surgeries. To overcome this problem, use of a ripe banana has been suggested owing to its soft peel and core which better simulates periungual soft tissue **(Figs. 1A to D)**. In addition, it also gives a better appreciation

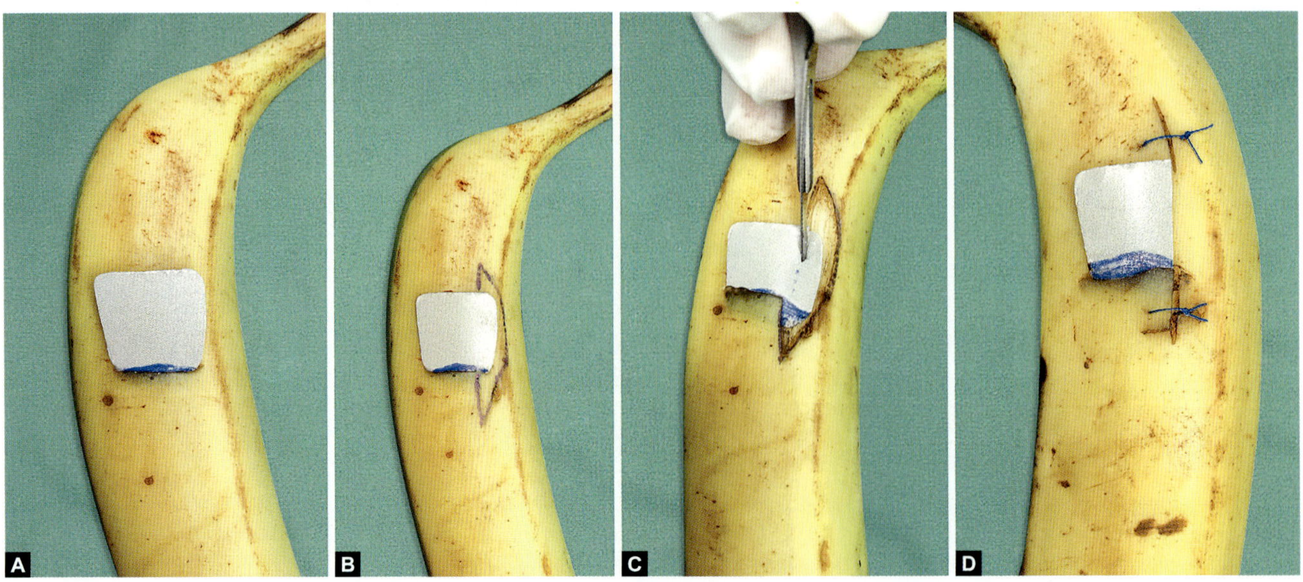

Figs. 1A to D: Use of banana as simulation model to learn nail surgery, different steps of partial nail plate excision are depicted.

of the depth of incision made. A flexible acetate plate was affixed by obliquely inserting it into a banana peel after a single incision. Digital blocks anesthesia, partial nail plate avulsion, and matrixectomy can be very well demonstrated on such models.[2]

USING EMLA CREAM TO REDUCE PAIN OF RING BLOCK

It has been observed that ring block injection for nail surgeries is very painful. To avoid needle prick pain and pain of drug infiltration, the use of EMLA cream has been suggested. The study by Browne J et al.[3] concluded that EMLA significantly reduces the pain associated with digital ring block. However, another study by Serour F et al.[4] showed that there was no clinical benefit in using EMLA during digital nerve block.

USE OF TOPICAL ALKANE VAPOCOOLANT SPRAY TO REDUCE PAIN OF NERVE BLOCK

Needle penetration and local anesthetic infiltration are two painful steps that cause considerable stress and anxiety during digital nerve block, which is the most frequently used regional anesthesia for ingrown nail surgery. In the study conducted by Kose O et al.,[5] alkane vapocoolant spray was applied to patients prior to the digital block. There was significant reduction in visual analog scale (VAS) scores during needle penetration in the intervention group. However, VAS scores during infiltration were similar statistically.

USE OF ICE TO REDUCE NEEDLESTICK PAIN

In a study conducted by Hayward C et al.,[6] it was observed that application of ice significantly reduces the needlestick pain. However, there was subjective variation to this; some patient did not prefer ice application prior to injection. Icing the digit prior to injection may be an effective and inexpensive method to reduce the discomfort of a local anesthesia injection.

REDUCTION OF INJECTION PAIN WITH MASSAGER

Use of a physical stimulus near the injection site through the use of a massager (e.g., head massager) can considerably reduce the injection pain. The physical stimulus decreases pain via the gate theory, thus narrowing or closing the pathway of pain.[7]

BUFFERING THE ANESTHETIC SOLUTION WITH SODIUM BICARBONATE

Local anesthetic agent diffuses into the nerves and works by blocking nerve transduction. The pH of lidocaine 1% with 1:100,000 epinephrine is 4.2 (1,000 times more acidic than physiologic pH). Lidocaine molecules are in unionized state at a physiological pH. Buffering local anesthetic with sodium bicarbonate has the potential to accelerate the passage of more uncharged molecules through lipophilic cell membranes, producing a faster time of onset. When compared to unbuffered lidocaine, a buffered lidocaine with sodium bicarbonate (1:10) can significantly reduce pain during infusion. 1 mL of 8.4% sodium bicarbonate mixed with 10 mL of lidocaine, for a total volume of 11 mL, provides a simple method to achieve the desired 10:1 ratio.[8]

WARMING LOCAL ANESTHETICS CAN REDUCE PAIN DURING INJECTION

Local anesthetics are the main class of analgesics used for pain management during minor surgeries; however, they are administered by injection, which is painful. Warming local anesthetics to body temperature has been proposed as a cost-free intervention that reduces injection pain, and therefore it should be done before administration.[9]

PLATELET-RICH PLASMA FOR REFRACTORY NAIL DISORDERS

Many of the nail disorders are refractory to treatment. Platelet-rich plasma (PRP) is a new modality of treatment which is gaining popularity day by day in aesthetic dermatology because of its regenerative properties. Keeping this in mind, PRP (0.1 mL) was tried as intramatricial injection at 3 weeks interval in two of nail disorders [idiopathic trachyonychia and nail lichen planus (LP)]. A significant improvement was seen within a month without any relapse in follow-up of 16–20 weeks. However, further studies with larger sample size and controls were required to validate the results.[10]

SAFE TECHNIQUE FOR PROXIMAL NAIL FOLD INCISION

Exploration of the nail matrix during nail surgery requires incision and reclination of the proximal nail fold (PNF). Incision with surgical blade at the PNF can sometimes damage the underlying nail matrix, which can lead to nail dystrophy. The damage can be prevented by a simple modification. First, the PNF is separated from the nail plate and the surgical blade is introduced horizontally into the separated space. Then the surgical blade is rotated to place sharp end of blade on the ventral aspect of PNF and incision is performed.[11]

COTTON WISP FOR INGROWN TOENAIL WITH GRANULATION

Ingrown toes nail with granulation tissue (stage 3 ingrown toenail) usually requires surgical intervention. In many cases, patients fear surgery and opt for conservative management. Such patients can be managed with a soaked cotton wisp, which elevates the distal nail plate from the nail bed and lateral nail folds. For this, after soaking the foot in warm water, a cotton wisp soaked with mupirocin can be inserted below the ingrown nail plate. The pain and granulation tissue decreases within 4 weeks.[12]

COTTON NAIL CAST FOR INGROWN NAIL

Conservative treatment of stage 1 or 2 ingrown toenail can be achieved through elevating the nail plate and decreasing the contact with nail bed and lateral nail folds. This can be easily done in an office setting with the help of cotton and cyanoacrylate glue. With the help of forceps, a small piece of cotton can be inserted between the nail plate and periungual tissue. Once the cotton is in place, cyanoacrylate glue can be applied and allowed to dry until a hard cast is formed.[13]

COTTON NAIL CAST FOR ONYCHOCRYPTOSIS

Onychocryptosis is one of the most common painful nail conditions. Conservative treatment may take a long time to obtain effective results. A study used cotton cast to show the effectiveness of a conservative treatment of ingrown nails. Patients with painful stage 1 to 2 onychocryptosis who were not candidates or refused surgery were treated with the cotton cast. The severity and cause of onychocryptosis was clinically evaluated during a 2-month period. A questionnaire was applied to all patients to evaluate pain, final treatment, and possible complications. All patients noticed results in <72 hours. Pain subsided in <24 hours in half of the patients and before 72 hours in 100% of the patients without the need of other treatments. The use of the cast prevented surgery and the accompanying morbidities in most of the patients (80%). The "cotton nail cast" is an effective conservative method for mild nail embedding. It is easy to apply, inexpensive, relieves pain rapidly, and avoids surgery in most patients.[14]

ANGLE CORRECTION TECHNIQUE FOR INGROWN NAIL

In this technique, dome shape (convexity) and thickness of the nail plate is reduced using a nail file, daily. This way, the convexity of the nail is corrected, and the thick nail becomes flatter and smoother. Thus, the curving of the nail plate does not occur in the nail margins.[15]

DEBULKING ONYCHOMYCOTIC NAIL

Fungal nail infections are one of the most common diseases presenting to a dermatologist. Onychomycoses can be really difficult to treat, especially with altered nail plate architecture. It is a chronic and less successfully treated entity due to various factors including slow growth of nail plate, lack of vasculature, poor penetration of drugs, etc. The infected pathological volume of nail plate persists and becomes a constant source of relapses, even during ongoing course of antifungal agents. Since, the diseased nail plate is rough and hyperkeratotic, there are little chances of penetration of topical and oral drugs; hence, debulking the diseased nail plate may increase the chances of drug penetration. Nail plate avulsion is an invasive procedure with poor patient compliance and cosmetic acceptance. Ablative lasers have also been found useful in removing the thick onychomycotic nail plate, but cost, availability, and uncertain efficacy are the limitations. As the nail is avascular, and lacks sensory innervation, it is possible to remove the pathological infected nail plate with the help of micromotor burrs by gradual abrasion done from the dorsal aspect of nail plate toward the nail bed. The routinely used motorized diamond fraises/burrs may not be appropriate for nail plate debulking; hence, the authors started using small-sized burrs with variable shapes. Dental burrs fulfilled this requirement as they are available in wide range of sizes, shapes, and designs. These could be carbide burs **(Figs. 2A and B)** used for cutting and removing the tough part of nail plate; or diamond burrs for fine grinding of nail plate **(Fig. 3)**. These are again attached to the micromotor commonly used in hair transplantation and other procedures.

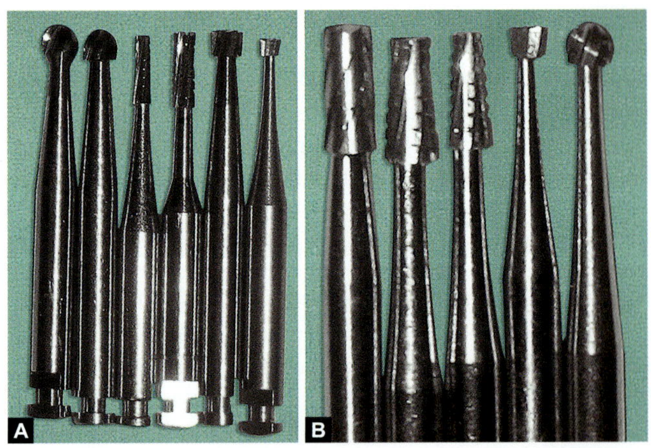

Figs. 2A and B: (A) Carbide burs of contra angle handpiece of micromotor; (B) Carbide burs of straight handpiece of micromotor.

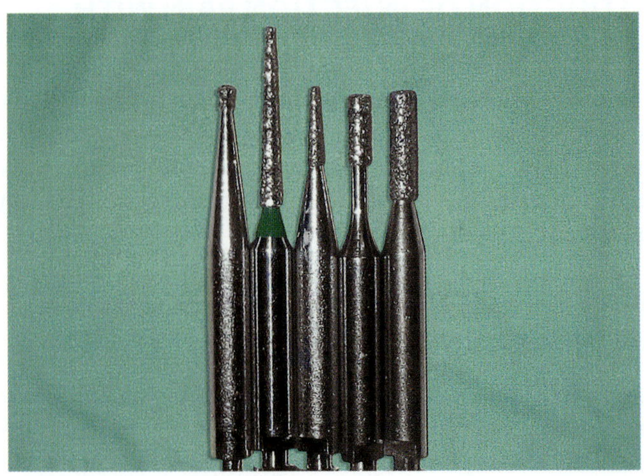

Fig. 3: Diamond burs of contra angle handpiece of micromotor.

The revolution per minute (RPM) is set at approximately 3,000 per minute. A gradual abrasion of nail plate surface is done, starting from the central thick nail part toward the periphery in gradual strokes. As the device is motorized and powerful, the strokes must be gentle to avoid penetration up to the nail bed. A constant normal saline irrigation over the operated area helps keep the field clean and prevents aerosolization of the infected debris. Lastly, the finishing is done by using the diamond burrs for fine grinding of the abraded nail plate **(Fig. 3)**. The procedure requires no anesthesia, is quick and easy, outpatient department (OPD)-based procedure, gives instant aesthetic improvement, ensures good patient compliance, increases the penetration of topical agents, and decreases the fungal load. It does not require any dressing or postoperative care.[16]

KNOT TECHNIQUE FOR INGROWN TOENAIL

Stage 2 or 3 ingrown toenail can be very painful and when untreated becomes a chronic issue. Knot technique is a newly described technique for stage 2 or 3 ingrown toenail. In this technique, the hypertrophied nail fold or granulation tissue is excised in a wedge shape manner. The edges of the wound are approximated with a polypropylene suture. After approximation, 8–10 knots are tied without cutting the stitches. These knots serve the purpose of pushing the soft tissue down and simultaneously raising the nail plate. The ingrown nail plate is raised with a final knot on the nail plate. In a study on 30 patients, Ince et al.[17] found that the knot technique is an efficient technique for treating ingrown toenail. Only one patient reported recurrence in the study in a mean follow-up period of 20 months.

NAIL BRACES FOR INGROWN TOENAIL

Nail braces can be a useful conservative treatment option for ingrown toenail. The principle behind the use of nail braces is that they exert a bending force on the nail through the restoring torque of the wire, which allows for the correction of even severely deformed nail. Most studies do not use local anesthesia before putting nail braces. Prior to application of the nail brace, the ingrown nail is partially removed and cleaned. Any infection or severe inflammation is treated with antibiotics and anti-inflammatory agents. A nail brace consists of two parts; one side is a spring wire and the other is fitted with a plastic pad. The wire is shaped into a hook. The hook is placed under one side of the nail, followed by gluing the pad to the nail plate. Finally, the pad is sealed with gel used for gel nails.

In a study by Liu et al.,[18] out of the 76 affected ingrown toenail sites, 81%, 94%, and 100% showed an excellent or fair outcome at 1, 3, and 6 months, respectively. Recurrence rates were 10.3% and complication rates were 7.7%. While, in the first 3 months, acute inflamed (AI)-type ingrown toenails tended to achieve excellent results more rapidly than chronic dystrophic (CD)-type nails; outcomes were similar at 6 months.

In the study by Wang et al.,[19] out of the 96 affected sites, 80.9%, 94.9%, and 100% achieved an excellent or fair result at 1, 3, and 6 months, respectively. Treatment duration and follow-up period were 179.2 ± 96.8 days and 281.6 ± 120.9, respectively. The recurrence rate was 7.4%. The treatment course and response were different between the two types of ingrown toenails.

USE OF MIXTURE OF ANESTHETICS TO PREVENT POSTSURGERY PAIN

In day-to-day practice, patients are given proximal block anesthesia with lidocaine 2%. Unfortunately, the effect of lignocaine is not long lasting and patients feel pain postprocedure. To overcome this problem, the patients were divided in two groups; the one group received only lignocaine during procedure and another group received antipain solution containing mixture of ropivacaine and triamcinolone (1 mL of the solution containing 0.5 mL of ropivacaine and 0.5 mL of triamcinolone) into the surgical wound after the surgical procedure. Both groups received anti-inflammatory tablets. Follow-up and assessment using the VAS were applied after 48 hours, when the dressing was removed. On the VAS scale, a score of 0 represented no pain and a score of 10 represented the worst pain that the patient ever had. Patients treated with the antipain solution had a VAS of 2 (± 1.07), compared with 7.88 (± 0.84) in the nontreatment group.[20]

INNOVATIVE PROTECTIVE COVERING OVER FINGERNAIL

Local wound dressings of the nail unit post-nail surgery and nail/finger injuries are tricky due to their shape and acral location. The dressing often tends to slip out of the finger. Moreover, as the fingers are constantly in use, minor trauma while working becomes unavoidable. Even a properly cushioned dressing may not provide adequate protection from external injuries while performing daily personal chores. Following a nail surgery or an injury to finger/fingernail, dressing is usually required for approximately 2–3 weeks in majority of cases. To overcome this problem, the authors suggest the use of a section or portion of a disposable syringe as a protective covering in such cases. After nail surgery, first of all hemostasis is achieved with local pressure. The area of surgery is then cleaned and covered with antiseptic, soft paraffin dressing to be wrapped around with a piece of gauge. Approximately two inches section/portion of a 10–20 mL syringe depending upon the size of finger is cut. In this transparent cylinder (cut piece of syringe) **(Figs. 4A to D)**, a vertical slit is then made so that it may

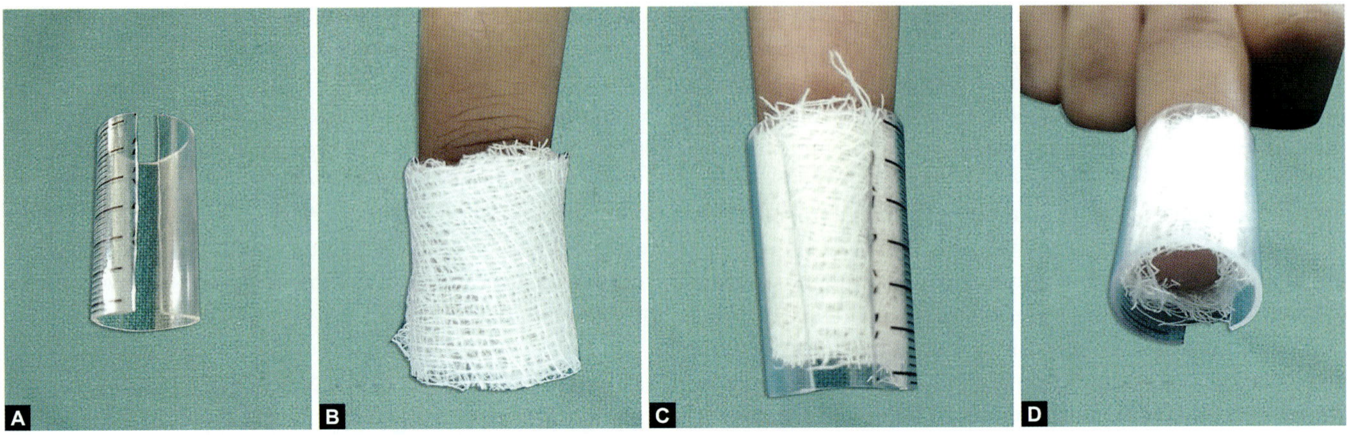

Figs. 4A to D: Use of cut piece of syringe as protective dressing post-nail surgery.

be slipped easily and snugly around the bandaged finger **(Figs. 4A to D)**. As the syringe is transparent, it is easier to visualize any unexpected ooze or bleed. In addition, this adjustable plastic dressing serves two purposes; first it provides reasonable protection to the site of surgery from the external inadvertent trauma and secondly it helps to maintain the pressure over the bandaged finger.[21]

THE "Y" TECHNIQUE FOR POSTOPERATIVE DRESSING

Postoperative dressing can be challenging after nail surgery primarily because with the functional mobility of the digits the dressing can be displaced. To overcome this challenge, a new innovative "Y"-shaped dressing for the nail surgery has been proposed. In this technique, a nonadherent paraffin gauze is cut in the shape of a "Y". The dimensions of the "Y" can be modified depending on the toe or finger. The first step is winding the base layer of this paraffin gauze which provides adequate grip for the dressing and prevents dislodgement. The limbs of the "Y" are crossed in the opposite directions to promote grip. The second layer is the adsorbent gauze (again "Y" shaped) and wound over the first layer in the same fashion. This layer further promotes the grip. The second layer takes care of the reasonably profuse and prolonged discharge **(Figs. 5A to E)**.[22]

SAW-TOOTHED MOTORIZED PUNCH FOR NAIL BIOPSY

Diagnosis of nail disorders is usually on a clinical basis; however, confirmation requires histopathological examination. Because of the cumbersome procedure of nail biopsy, this investigation is often neglected. The routine skin biopsy punch is commonly used but the nail being a rigid structure is not easily penetrated with the main problem of breakage of punch during the procedure. A great amount of pressure needs to be applied to pierce the nail plate. Based on the concept of motorized FUE punches, authors designed a serrated/saw-toothed motorized punches for nail biopsy. Unfortunately, the FUE punches available in market are of small sizes (maximum size of 1.2 mm); whereas, we need punches of sizes varying from 2 to 4 mm. To overcome this problem, the authors devised a motorized nail biopsy punch which is a cylindrical device made of metal (brass or stainless steel) **(Figs. 6A to C)**. The edge of the hollow tube is saw-toothed with various sizes and angulated tips. For a thick, hard, and tough nail plate the angulations of saw-toothed end were kept acute and the numbers of angulated tips were increased.

The size of the hollow tube can vary depending on the diameter of tissue to be taken. Size can vary from 2 to 4 mm in most of the nail pathologies.

A window was also provided on the side so that if the tissue sample gets stuck inside the hollow tube, it can be pushed out by using fine-tipped forceps. The other end is a solid rod which is suitable for fitting into commonly used micromotor **(Figs. 6A to C)**. It is the same micromotor which can be used in hair transplantation procedures. It should be borne in mind that the device is motorized and the tool is rotating at a very high RPM; hence, the tissue penetration must be extremely slow and in vertical axis only. A constant irrigation of the site with normal saline can help reduce friction by draining the powder of the nail plate and keeping the tissue temperature low.

As soon as the nail plate is penetrated, there is a sudden decrease in the resistance offered. This is the indication to switch off motor and withdraw the punch if only nail plate sample is required. In case sampling of nail bed or matrix is to be done, the device is further penetrated for approximately 1 mm and then withdrawn. The tissue can be lifted with the help of fine-tipped forceps and separated from the base with help of small scissor or surgical blade. A firm pressure is given to stop the bleeding, and antiseptic dressing is done. Using motorized punch with saw-toothed edges for nail biopsy makes the procedure easy and quick.[23]

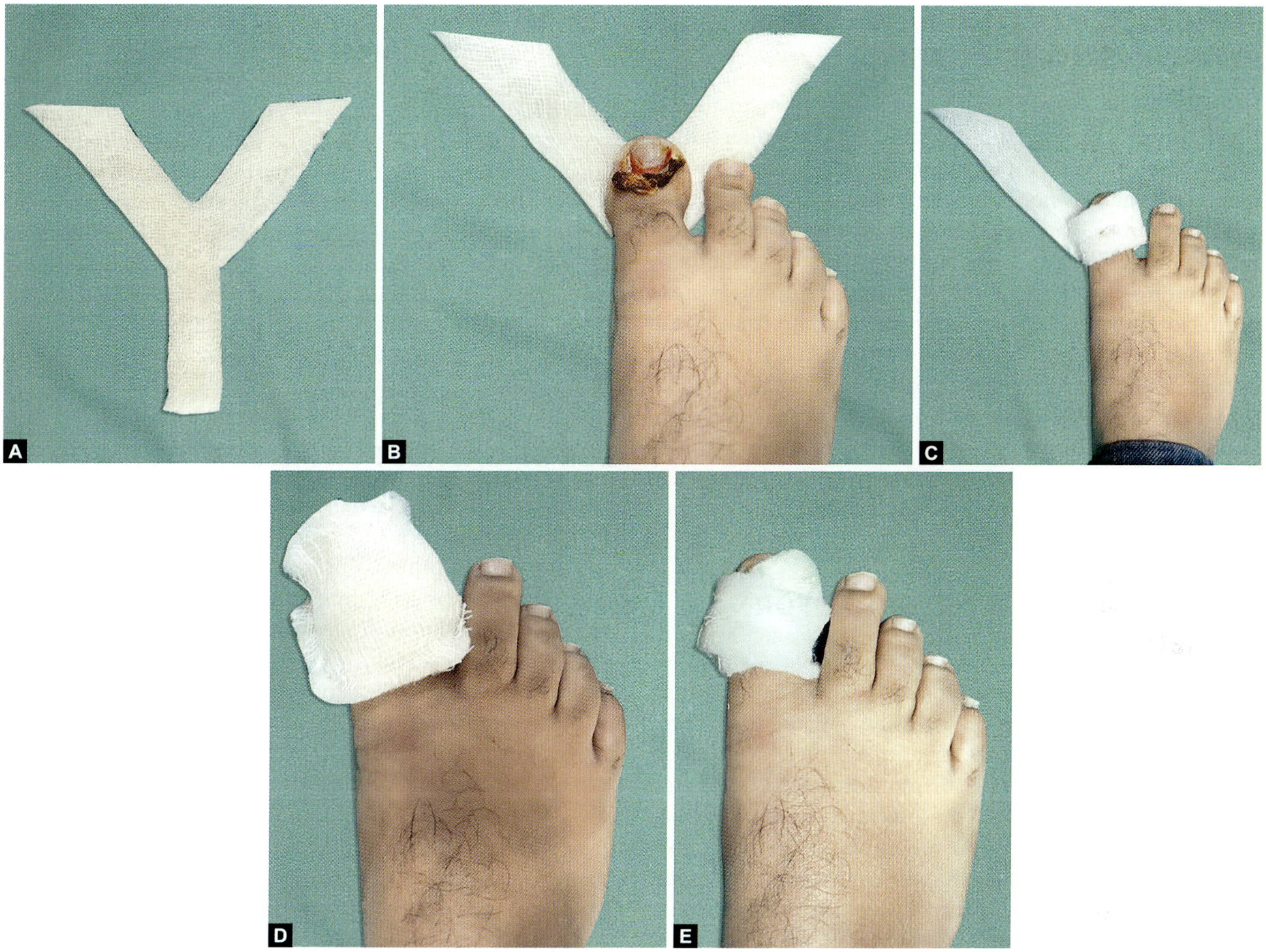

Figs. 5A to E: Different steps of "Y" shape dressing post-nail surgery.

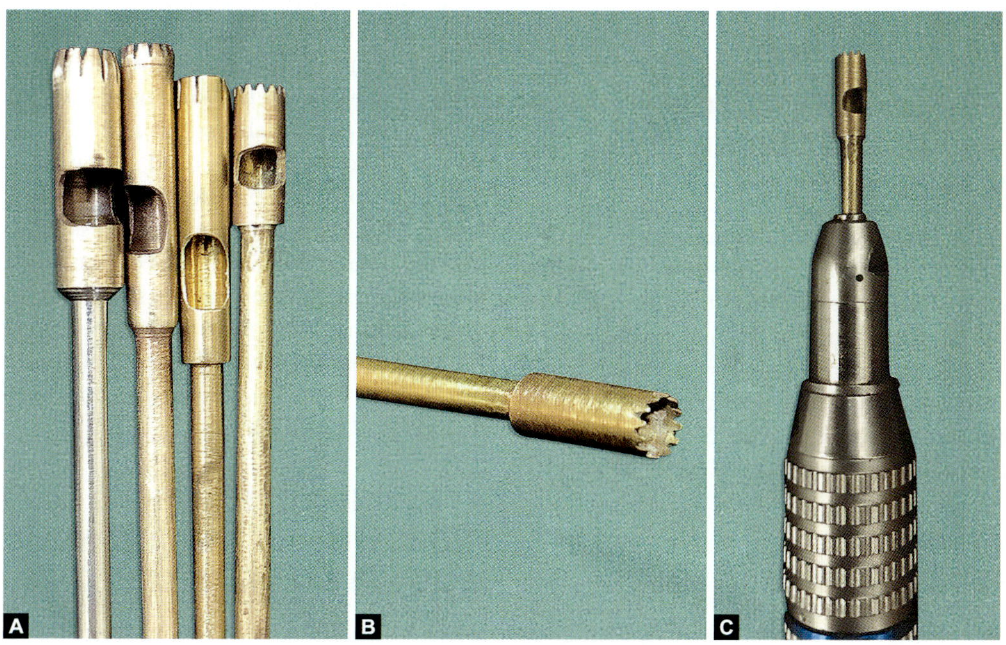

Figs. 6A to C: (A and B) Saw-toothed power punch for nail biopsy; (C) Punch fixed in micromotor.

TOPICAL HEMOCOAGULASE FOR ACHIEVING HOMEOSTASIS

Hemostasis has always been a concern in all dermatosurgical procedures as the bleeding hinders proper visualization of the surgical field. Topical hemocoagulase is a nontoxic fraction of snake venom obtained from the Brazilian snake *Bothrops jararaca* or *atrox*. It is being sold with different brand names all over the world. It promotes coagulation by accelerating the formation of fibrin monomers and hastens fibrin clot formation when used topically, apart from that, it acts on factor X11a and stabilizes the fibrin. It is widely used as topical solution in ear, nose, and throat (ENT) department for treatment of epistaxis and in dental surgeries. It can also be a good alternative to stop bleeding in nail surgeries (especially where use of adrenaline is controversial) and can be cheap, efficacious, easy to use, and without any reported adverse effect.[24]

KAOLIN-IMPREGNATED GAUZE FOR HOMEOSTASIS

Achieving a bloodless field is important during nail surgeries. It can be effectively achieved by using a digital tourniquet, direct pressure with gauze or application of aluminum chloride, ferric subsulfate, brimonidine 0.33% gel, and absorbable gelatine, but with these techniques, there are risks of adverse effects such as postoperative wound infections and delayed wound healing. Kaolin is an aluminum silicate that promotes hemostasis by initiating the extrinsic clotting pathway. After digital tourniquet removal, authors applied kaolin-impregnated gauze to the nail unit with firm pressure for 3 minutes, until hemostasis was achieved. It is absorbent and flexible, and it may be cut and molded to fit the uniquely shaped nail unit.[25]

USING AIR-COOLING DEVICE FOR IMPROVED ANALGESIA DURING LOCAL ANESTHETIC INFILTRATION

The use of an air-cooling device can serve as an alternative to any contact cooling method. It does not cause any physical interference with the anesthetic infiltration and is independent of the topography of the area to be treated. The air-cooling device uses a compressor system to deliver a stream of cold air through a thin tube with a flow of 500–1,000 L/min at a temperature as low as 2308C. This technique minimizes pain in patients.[26]

CRYOTHERAPY FOR ONYCHOGRYPHOTIC NAILS

Onychogryphosis refers to nail plate thickening with gross hyperkeratosis and increased curvature of the nail plate. Definitive cure is achieved with surgical avulsion followed by destruction of the nail matrix. It results in permanent nail loss. Trimming the onychogryphotic nails can be time consuming. Before nail trimming, authors performed cryotherapy on onychogryphotic nails with liquid nitrogen. Liquid nitrogen was emitted toward the targeted nail from a distance of 1–2 cm until an ice ball formed over the target area. The nail became very brittle after cryotherapy, presumably because of the rapid decrease in the water content of the nail plate. Nail trimming with a pair of stainless nail pliers was performed immediately after the freezing cycle. Using cryotherapy on nails before nail trimming is a safe, easy, clean, and efficient modality for patients with onychogryphosis.[27]

USE OF GASKET FOR FINGER TOURNIQUET

The biggest challenge in nail surgery is obtaining a bloodless field. Authors used a simple gasket, usually applied at the junction of two pipes to prevent water leakage in garden watering systems as a digit tourniquet. Varied sizes are available for different finger and toe calibers and can be obtained from local hardware stores and used after proper sterilization. This device can be easily applied, opened, and readjusted during surgery by the operator, without the need for an assistant. The tourniquet time is the same as that for other tourniquet methods and it can easily be removed. The device can be reused after proper disinfection/sterilization, or, as it is cheap, it can be disposed of after each operation.[28]

FINGER-SHAPED DRESSING FOR FINGERS AND TOES POST-NAIL SURGERIES

It remains challenging how to dress fingers or toes post-nail surgeries like onychectomy or tumor excision. Applying an appropriate dressing is critical. Foam dressing has advantage of strong fluid absorbance ability and nonadherent property which make it ideal dressing used after the nail surgeries. However, foam dressing is flat and it is challenging to fix it closely. Here the authors used an innovative finger-shaped technique to ensure the dressing wrapped tightly around the wound. The top half of the foam dressing was cut into strips and the operated digit was put on the uncut foam part right below the first strip and the first strip was folded over the digit. Then the other strips were folded one by one while wrapping the foam dressing around the operated digit. Lastly, a bandage was used as the second layer with appropriate pressure and fix it **(Figs. 7A and B)**.[29]

A NONINVASIVE METHOD FOR TREATING INGROWN NAIL RECURRENCE DUE TO INCOMPLETE MATRICECTOMY

Excision of an ingrown nail and partial matricectomy is a commonly used technique. In some cases, however, the matrix

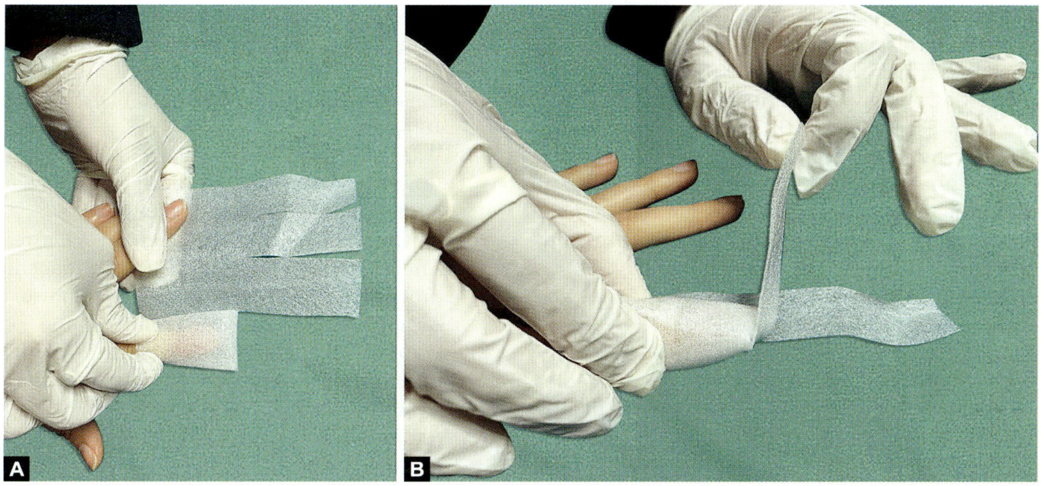

Figs. 7A and B: Different steps of foam dressing.

is not totally destroyed. Though it is a widely used method, it can cause scars and contractures. Authors treated these cases with a cotton splint. An ethanol-soaked 5-mm-diameter cotton pellet is packed between the inflamed periungual tissue and the nail plate by using a plastic filling instrument. Dental adhesive can be applied to the cotton pellet and the adjacent nail plate. This splint is hardened by ultraviolet curing. After that a superelastic wire was applied onto the nail plate to prevent the nail plate from being buried in the nail bed. The device stays on the nail plate for about 3–6 months.[30]

PINCER NAIL TREATMENT USING DENTAL CORRECTION PRINCIPLES

Pincer nail deformity (PND) is characterized by excessive transverse curvature of the nail plate. The authors used dental correction methods to improve PND. Portion of the nail plate buried in periungual tissue was removed. The nail plate was bent with a forceps to check its flexibility. Dental devices such as G-aenial bond and M-flex archwire were used to correct the curvature of nail. The ratio of nail tip height to width (HW ratio) was used to measure the effectiveness of the treatment. The improvement of the HW ratio was statistically significant. Besides successful clinical improvement, this method has three advantages. First, it can be tailored. The elastic force of wire increases proportionally to the thickness and the amount of transformation. Second, it can be performed in nails other than those of the big toe. Third, it is noninvasive and does not restrict patient lifestyle.[31]

SUTURING THE NAIL PLATE DURING MATRICECTOMY

One of the most challenging steps in a matricectomy can be suturing the nail plate to the adjacent skin to facilitate creation of a new lateral fold. If nail plates are thickened because of dystrophy or onychomycosis, manually drilling through a hardened nail plate usually causes alteration of the needle curvature of the nail. By using a carbon dioxide (CO_2) laser to drill the suture holes through the nail plate, nail suturing can be performed quickly and easily. This method helps avoid mechanical trauma and bleeding of the soft tissue underneath and improve the aesthetic outcome.[32]

NAIL SPLINT USING NASOPHARYNGEAL TUBE TO PREVENT PTERYGIUM AFTER NAIL SURGERY

A dorsal pterygium may develop as a complication after nail surgery. It may cause a scar that over which the nail plate grows resulting in a permanent deformity. Surgical correction is possible but difficult. A sterile nasopharyngeal tube can be used as a nail splint. In cases of nail bed or matrix surgery, the risks of dorsal pterygium increase dramatically. When the plate is missing, the nasopharyngeal tube is used to create a nail splint. The tube is inserted under the PNF, over the matrix or bed defect, and secured with absorbable suture, fixing it to the nail fold skin. The nail tissues re-epithelialize quickly and the tube can be removed when the risk of pterygium has passed, usually at 2 weeks postoperatively. Advantages of this technique involve ease of use and cost.[33]

CONCLUSION

Innovative modalities and techniques are essential to solve day-to-day issues faced during nail surgery. It is essential to keep a track about the growing advancements in this field for a safe and up-to-date practice.

REFERENCES

1. Giurin I, Bréaud J, Rampal V, Rosello O, Solla F. A simulation model of nail bed suture and nail fixation: description and preliminary evaluation. J Surg Res. 2018;228:142-6.

2. Abbade LP, Silva F, Guiotoku MM, Miot HA. Banana: a new simulation model to teach surgical techniques for treating ingrown toenails. Dermatol Surg. 2013;39(8):1274-6.
3. Browne J, Fung M, Donnelly M, Cooney C. The use of EMLA reduces the pain associated with digital ring block for ingrowing toenail correction. Eur J Anaesthesiol. 2000;17:182.
4. Serour F, Ben-Yehuda Y, Boaz M. EMLA cream prior to digital nerve block for ingrown nail surgery does not reduce pain at injection of anesthetic solution. Acta Anaesthesiol Scand. 2002;46(2):203-6.
5. Kose O, Saylan S, Ediz N, Yigit S. Effects of topical alkane vapocoolant spray on pain intensity prior to digital nerve block for ingrown nail surgery. Foot Ankle Spec. 2010;3(2):73-5.
6. Hayward SC, Landorf KB, Redmond AC. Ice reduces needle-stick pain associated with a digital nerve block of the hallux. Foot. 2006;16:145-8.
7. Jellinek NJ, Vélez NF. Nail surgery: best way to obtain effective anesthesia. Dermatol Clin. 2015;33(2):265-71.
8. Strazar AR, Leynes PG, Lalonde DH. Minimizing the pain of local anesthesia injection. Plast Reconstr Surg. 2013;132(3):675-84.
9. Hogan ME, vanderVaart S, Perampaladas K, Machado M, Einarson TR, Taddio A. Systematic review and meta-analysis of the effect of warming local anesthetics on injection pain. Ann Emerg Med. 2011;58(1):86-98.e1.
10. Kaur I, Jakhar D. Intramatricial platelet-rich plasma therapy: a novel treatment modality in refractory nail disorders. Dermatol Ther. 2019;32(2):e12831.
11. Di Chiacchio N, Fonseca Noriega L, Borges Figueira de Mello CD, Di Chiacchio NG, Ocampo-Garza J. Do Not Hurt the Nail Matrix: Safe Technique for Proximal Nail Fold Incision. Skin Appendage Disord. 2018;4(4):347-8.
12. Du JF, Xi XY, Liu ZH. Successful conservative treatment with cotton wisp for ingrown toenail with granulation. Dermatol Ther. 2016;29(6):486-7.
13. Gutiérrez-Mendoza D, De Anda Juárez M, Ávalos VF, Martínez GR, Domínguez-Cherit J. "Cotton nail cast": a simple solution for mild and painful lateral and distal nail embedding. Dermatol Surg. 2015;41(3):411-4.
14. d'Almeida LF, Nakamura R. Onychocryptosis Treatment Pearls: The "Rolled Cotton Padding" Maneuver and the "Artificial Resin Nail" Technique. Dermatol Surg. 2016;42(3):434-6.
15. Ozdil B, Eray IC. New method alternative to surgery for ingrown nail: angle correction technique. Dermatol Surg. 2009;35(6):990-2.
16. Gupta S, Jangra RS, Gupta S, Mahendra A, Kumar A. A painless, minimally invasive technique for debulking onychomycotic nails. J Am Acad Dermatol. 2017;76(1):e17-9.
17. Ince B, Dadaci M, Altuntas Z. Knot technique: a new treatment of ingrown nails. Dermatol Surg. 2015;41(2):250-4.
18. Liu CW, Huang YC. Efficacy of a new nail brace for the treatment of ingrown toenails. J Dtsch Dermatol Ges. 2018; 16(4):417-23.
19. Wang HH, Yang TH, Liu CW, Tsai TY, Huang YC. Efficacy of Nail Braces for Acute and Chronic Ingrown Toenails: A Prospective Study. Dermatol Surg. 2020;46(2):258-66.
20. Di Chiacchio N, Ocampo-Garza J, Villarreal-Villarreal CD, Ancer-Arellano J, Noriega LF, Di Chiacchio NG. Post-nail procedure analgesia: A randomized control pilot study. J Am Acad Dermatol. 2019;81(3):860-2.
21. Gupta S, Shankar Jangra R, Singal A, Singla R. Innovative protective covering over finger nail surgery dressing. J Am Acad Dermatol. 2020;82(2):e45-6.
22. Ashique KT, Grover C. The "Y" technique: an attempt to standardize nail dressing. J Am Acad Dermatol. 2018; 78(5): e103-4.
23. Gupta S, Jangra RS, Gupta S, Mahendra A, Singla R. Saw-toothed power punch for effortless nail biopsy. J Am Acad Dermatol. 2016;75(3):e109-11.
24. Gupta S, Jangra RS, Gupta SS, Gakhar A. Topical hemocoagulase: a novel method for achieving hemostasis. J Am Acad Dermatol. 2020;82(3):e81-2.
25. Ricardo JW, Lipner SR. Kaolin-impregnated gauze for hemostasis following nail surgery. J Am Acad Dermatol. 2021;85(1):e13-4.
26. Ricardo JW, Lipner SR. Air cooling for improved analgesia during local anesthetic infiltration for nail surgery. J Am Acad Dermatol. 2021;84(5):e231-2.
27. Yang TH, Tsai HH. Performing cryotherapy on onychogryphotic nails before nail trimming. J Am Acad Dermatol. 2016;75(2): e69-70.
28. Beksaç B, Caliskan E. Use of a gasket for finger tourniquet. J Am Acad Dermatol. 2020;82(3):e75-6.
29. Yang S, Li Z. Finger-shaped dressing for fingers and toes after nail surgeries. J Am Acad Dermatol. 2023;88(2):e83-4.
30. Won JH, Chun JS, Won YH. A noninvasive method for treating ingrown nail recurrence due to incomplete matricectomy. J Am Acad Dermatol. 2019;81(2):e31-2.
31. Won JH, Chun JS, Park YH, Kim SJ, Won YH. Treatment of pincer nail deformity using dental correction principles. J Am Acad Dermatol. 2018;78(5):1002-4.
32. Eirís Salvado N, Rodríguez Prieto MA. Suturing the nail plate during matricectomy. J Am Acad Dermatol. 2016;75(3): e107.
33. Jellinek NJ, Cressey BD. Nail Splint to Prevent Pterygium After Nail Surgery. Dermatol Surg. 2019;45(12):1733-5.

SECTION 8 Regional Dermatosurgery

CHAPTER 52

Eyelid Surgery

Manas Chatterjee, Dipali Rathod, Ruchi Hemdani, Harish Prasad BR

KEY MESSAGES

- Majority of the eyelid surgeries are office procedures and therefore dermatosurgeons need to be fully aware of them and include them in their armamentarium.
- Proper planning and execution of these procedures require good understanding and knowledge of eyelid anatomy and vascular and nerve supply which would aid in preventing serious surgical events.
- Various procedures undertaken for the common correctable eyelid disorders in dermatology such as simple excision and suturing, tarsorrhaphy, blepharoplasty, vitiligo surgeries, ocular leprosy surgeries, and few others would be discussed in detail in this chapter.
- Eyelash transplantation has created a new ray of hope in vitiligo patients with leukotrichia of the eyelashes.
- The eyelid procedures should be meticulously performed as inappropriate techniques may result in scarring and may further cause ectropion.

"I shut my eyes and all the world drops dead; I lift my eyes and all is born again."

—Sylvia Plath

INTRODUCTION

The eyelids consist of a complex structure with multiple subunits; hence, knowledge and understanding of the anatomy and dynamics of eyelids is of vital importance for the treating dermatologist and the aesthetic surgeon in order to avoid any injury to the underlying structures. This chapter is intended to give a comprehensive account of all the common diseases that affect the eyelids, for which a dermatologist needs to be alerted and if need be, advice an urgent referral to an ophthalmologist **(Fig. 1)**.

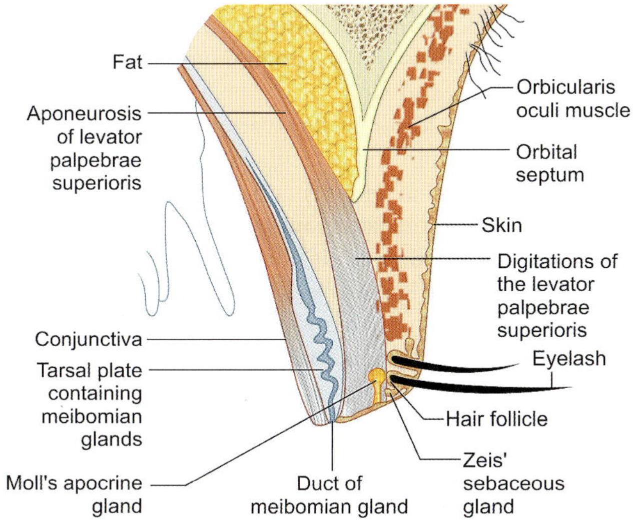

Fig. 1: Eyelid anatomy.

ANATOMY OF EYELID

The contour of the eyelid is highly dependent on the race, gender, and age of the individual. The lateral canthus of a typical eyelid is approximately 2 mm superior to the medial one. In Asians, this vertical elevation may be slightly higher and this is referred to as the "mongoloid slant." The palpebral fissure in the adult measures 10–12 mm vertically and 28–30 mm horizontally. In adults, about 1–2 mm of the superior cornea is covered by the upper eyelid margin and the apex of the upper lid margin is found nasal to a vertical line drawn through the center of the pupil. The vertical palpebral fissure and position of the upper eyelid crease varies among different ethnic groups. This finding has important implications in both ptosis and upper eyelid blepharoplasty surgery.

The upper eyelid crease (formed by attachment of the levator aponeurosis to skin) in Caucasians is situated 7–8 mm above the lid margin in men and 10–12 mm in women. In Asians, the crease is lower and the upper sulcus is more full. This occurs because the orbital septum and levator aponeurosis fuse lower on the lid, below the superior tarsal border. However, a recent study by Kakizaki et al. showed that this fusion occurred above the tarsal border.[1]

In either case, the preaponeurotic fat pad (PFP) descends and prevents a higher insertion of the levator aponeurosis to the upper lid skin.[2] These variations result in an inferiorly positioned or absent upper eyelid crease in Asians.

The skin of the eyelids is the thinnest (0.05 mm) as compared to the other parts of the body. The subcutaneous tissue consists of loose connective tissue. Fat is absent from the pretarsal skin and very sparse in the preseptal and preorbital skin. Also, the medial and lateral palpebral ligaments show absence of subcutaneous tissue and therefore, the skin here adheres directly to the underlying fibrous tissue. Relaxed skin tension lines (RSTLs) around the eyes can be used easily as they follow the lid creases. Upper eyelid can be excised without any deformity as it has more elastic skin.

The most important function of the eyelid is to protect the eyeball. It contains fine hair (cilia) at its outer margin (eyelashes), both apocrine and eccrine sweat glands and sebaceous glands. About 300 eyelashes are arranged in two rows along the lid margin, two thirds of which are in the upper lid. The lids lack the arrector muscles. The tarsal plate of each eyelid gives the palpebral aperture its shape and stability. Additional components of the eyelid include the superior palpebral fold, the palpebral fissure, the medial limbus, and the medial canthus. Just lateral to the bony orbital margins, the thin and smooth eyelid skin transforms into a coarse and thicker skin with numerous sebaceous glands. Significance of this transition is the different manner in which each of them recovers from a surgical incision. The distinct anatomical layers of the eyelids comprise the skin, subcutaneous tissue, tarsal plate, and conjunctiva and striated muscles which affect the movement of the eyelids. The four layers of eyelids are (1) (2) skin, (3) muscle, tarsus, and (4) mucous layers.

Skin of Eyelid

In the eyelid, the dermis lies directly on the orbicularis oculi muscle. It is composed of connective tissue and contains blood vessels, lymphatics, and nerve fibers in addition to fibroblasts, macrophages, and mast cells. Sebaceous, eccrine, meibomian glands, glands of Zies and Moll, all lie deep in the dermis or within the tarsal plates.

Muscle Layer

Muscle layer comprises the following:

- The horizontal concentric fibers of orbicularis oculi, major protractor of eyelids.
- The levator palpebral superioris, which is the major retractor of upper eyelid, ends in an aponeurosis which is inserted into three points—(1) the skin of the upper lid, (2) upper border of the tarsus, and (3) conjunctiva at the fornix. The levator aponeurosis is supplanted by the preaponeurotic fat compartments (pockets) of the eyelids **(Fig. 2)**.
- Müller's muscle, also known as superior tarsal muscle.

The upper lid margin is positioned over the upper cornea at midpoint between the upper edge and the pupillary border. Sometimes in a normal eye, there is visible sclera below the cornea. The lateral and medial angles of the palpebral aperture lie along a single horizontal plane. The superior palpebral sulcus in upper eyelid results from insertion of the levator aponeurosis into the lid skin. This insertion varies considerably in different persons. Measured

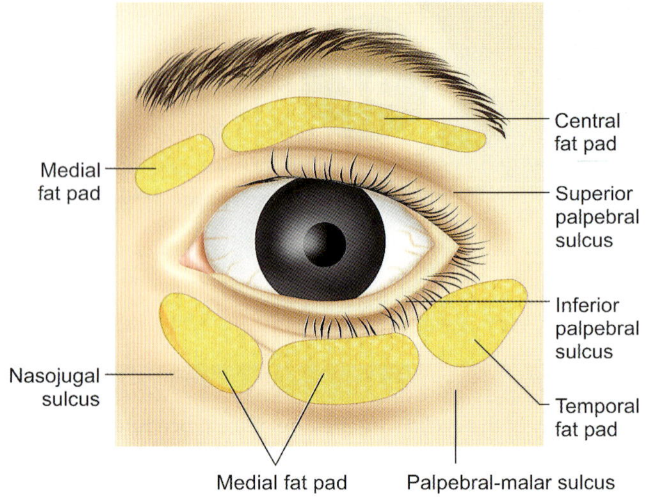

Fig. 2: Fat pockets and sulci.

from the lid margin, the fold or sulcus may be as high as 12 mm in eyes that have a high prominent, supraorbital rim. Conversely, the lid fold may be as low as 5–6 mm above the lid margin in an eyelid that usually appears to be heavy and full. The inferior palpebral sulcus marks the lower margin of the inferior lid tarsus.

Tarsus Layer

Tarsus layer consists of the tarsal plates. The tarsi (tarsal plates) are two comparatively thick, elongated plates of dense connective tissue, about 2.5 cm (1.0 inch) in length; one is found in each eyelid and contributes to its form and support. They are located directly above the lid margins. Embedded in it are enormously developed sebaceous glands—the meibomian glands.

Mucous Layer

Mucous layer is formed by the palpebral conjunctiva. The lid margin consists of the following:

- Eyelashes—arranged in two to three rows anteriorly. The normal eyelashes point forward.
- Opening of the ducts of the meibomian gland posteriorly
- Glands of Zies and Moll

The upper and lower eyelid layers are classically divided into the anterior (skin and orbicularis oculi muscle of upper eyelid), middle (orbital septum), and posterior lamellae (tarsal plate, eyelid retractors, and conjunctiva). The gray line is a darker line in the middle of the lid margin that is between the anterior and middle lamellae of the lid. Any lesion extending beyond the gray line or if there is a possibility of malignancy, a full-thickness lid excision is required.

BLOOD SUPPLY

The eyelid has a rich blood supply, mainly through the medial and lateral palpebral arteries, which are branches of the ophthalmic artery. There is also a rich anastomosis between adjacent arteries arising from the internal and external carotid arteries. The blood drains through a network of veins to the facial and orbital veins and the cavernous sinus.

The rich vascularity enables rapid healing of eyelid wounds with relative lack of infection.

NERVE SUPPLY (TABLE 1)

TABLE 1: Nerve supply of eyelids.

Motor	Sensory
• Facial nerve (VII) supplies orbicularis oculi, frontalis, procerus, and corrugator supercilii muscles, thereby enabling eyelid protraction • Oculomotor nerve (III) supplies levator palpebrae superioris • Sympathetic fibers innervate superior (Müller's) and inferior tarsal muscles, causing respective lid retractions	*Trigeminal nerve (V):* • Ophthalmic division (V1) supply the upper eyelid as the lacrimal, supraorbital, and supratrochlear nerves (lateral to medial) and the medial aspect of both upper and lower lids as the infratrochlear nerve • Terminal branches of the maxillary division supply the lower eyelid as the zygomaticofacial (lateral lower lid) and infraorbital nerves (lower eyelid proper)

LYMPHATIC DRAINAGE

The eyelid consists of superficial and deep lymphatic system with respect to the orbicularis oculi muscle which are interconnected by lymphatic channels and additionally, the conjunctival lymphatic network.[3]

The superficial lymphatic channels travel in the subcutaneous fat within the nasolabial and lateral orbital fat compartments. The lateral deep lymphatic channels travel beneath the orbicularis oculi muscle, then through the superficial orbicularis retaining ligament, travel further into the suborbicularis oculi fat in the roof of the prezygomatic space. Further, these vessels descend to the preperiosteal fat at the level of zygomatico-cutaneous ligaments to reach adjacent to the facial nerve and then into the preauricular nodes. The lymphatic pathways finally drain laterally to the parotid nodes and medially to submandibular nodes.

Incisions and dissections in the infraorbital area make the superficial system vulnerable to damage, while dissection around the orbicularis-retaining ligament and the zygomatico-cutaneous ligaments damages the deep system. Therefore, concurrent damage to both the lymphatic systems, especially laterally, may be responsible for postoperative chemosis and edema.

Common disorders of the eyelids and eyelashes are given in **Table 2**.

GENERAL PRINCIPLES OF THE EYELID SURGERY

One should possess a thorough knowledge regarding the vascular and nerve supply of eyelid in order to prevent serious surgical events during the operation.

TABLE 2: Common disorders of the eyelids and eyelashes.

Disorders of eyelids[4-6]	*Disorders of eyelashes*
Structural abnormalities: Lagophthalmos, entropion, ectropion, epicanthal fold, tear trough, dermatochalasis, lid laxity, ptosis	Trichiasis
Infections: Molluscum contagiosum, verruca, leprosy sequelae	Eyelash ptosis
Autoimmune: Vitiligo, alopecia areata	Trichomegaly
Premalignant: Cutaneous horn, actinic keratoses	Madarosis
Benign tumors: Milia, syringomas, hidrocystomas, nevi, seborrheic keratoses, acrochordons, dermatofibroma, xanthelasma, etc.	Leukotrichia
Malignant tumors: Basal cell carcinoma, squamous cell carcinoma, malignant melanoma, Merkel cell carcinoma, etc.	Poliosis

- Local anesthesia using a mix of lidocaine 2% with epinephrine (1:100,000) is commonly used.
- As blood supply of the eyelid is good, always use adrenaline 1/100,000 along with the local anesthetic agent.
- In case the patient is anxious, sedation is advised and avoid adrenaline in hypertensive patients.
- A newer agent that has been tried is ropivacaine, which produces less intraoperative or postoperative bleeding and swelling with epinephrine 1:100,000.[7]
- During the surgery, if the eyelid is fixed and kept taut, it becomes much easier to perform the procedure. This can be done with a lid guard or a clamp. The exercise of holding the lid steady and secure also helps to protect the cornea from accidental damage anytime during the operation. Because of the pressure, the guard or the clamp lessens the bleeding. However, they should be applied just tight enough to occlude the marginal arteries as too much of pressure may permanently damage the tissues.
- Avoid placing the knots on the inner conjunctival surface which may otherwise irritate the cornea. The suture generally used during eye surgeries is 5-0 polypropylene (prolene), which is a nonabsorbable monofilament suture.
- Always try to approximate the skin and conjunctiva so as to avoid any "bare areas." In case a bare area is left, it may fill up with granulation tissue, which may eventually get converted to fibrous tissue causing lid deformity few months later.
- Ensure good hemostasis from the marginal arteries at the medial and lateral margins of the tarsal plates and try to avoid excessively tight padding of the eye postoperatively.
- As the eyelid skin heals very quickly, sutures may be removed early (4–5 days). However, mattress sutures used to rotate or to alter the position of some tissue should be left in for about 2 weeks to ensure a permanent correction. In case the patient cannot return in 2 weeks, then absorbable mattress sutures should be used. Buried sutures ideally should be absorbable but may be nonabsorbable. However, the buried suture technique in double-eyelid blepharoplasty, which is a popular aesthetic

surgery, is associated with complications related to the suture thread implantation. This complication can be addressed with a suture removal surgery.[8]

Preoperative Evaluation

Preoperative evaluation should include proper history and examination of the patient to rule out any local infection, significant systemic disorders, drug allergies, and intake of agents that may interfere with the hemostasis while operating. Proper clinical photographs and informed consent are mandatory.

INDIVIDUAL PROCEDURES OF COMMON CORRECTABLE EYELID DISORDERS IN DERMATOLOGY

Excisions and Destructive Procedures

Most of the excisions can be done as an outpatient procedure under topical or injectable anesthesia. The skin lesions may be removed using various modalities depending upon the type of lesion.

Indications

- *Benign growths:* Warts, molluscum contagiosum, nevus, acrochordons **(Fig. 3)**, dermatosis papulosa nigra, seborrheic keratosis, actinic keratosis, neurofibroma **(Fig. 4)**, syringoma, pilomatricoma, eccrine hidrocystoma, milia, etc.
- *Malignant growths:* Squamous cell carcinoma, basal cell carcinoma (BCC), melanoma, etc.
- *Other conditions:* Xanthelasma palpebrarum

Procedures

The following procedures can be utilized depending upon the pathology:
- Simple scissor excision
- Shave excision
- *Skin excision and suturing* ***(Figs. 5 and 6)***
- *Cryotherapy:* The disadvantage of using cryotherapy around the eyes is the thin skin reducing safety and possibility of ocular damage by contiguous spread or spillage.
- Electrosurgery

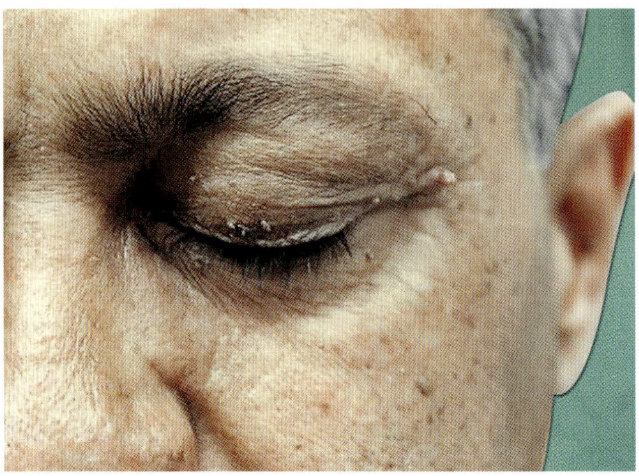

Fig. 3: Acrochordons of upper eyelid.

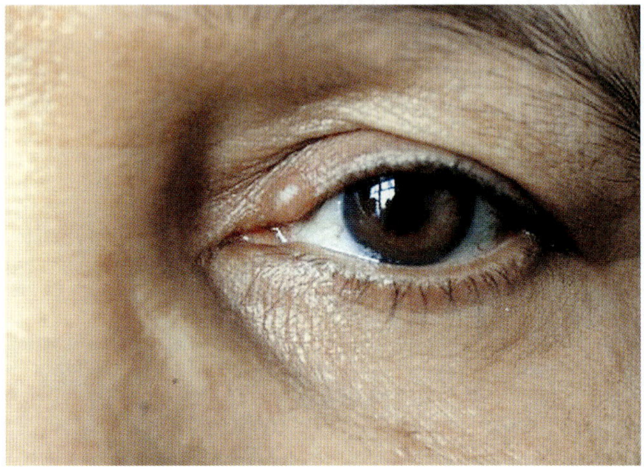

Fig. 4: Neurofibroma (biopsy proven) of upper eyelid margin.

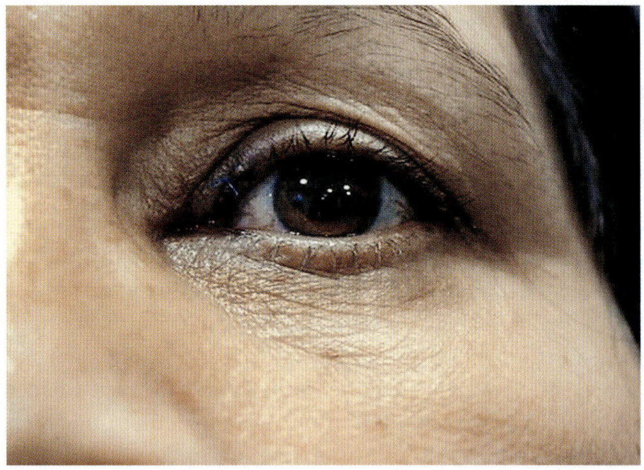

Fig. 5: Immediate postexcision of neurofibroma of upper lid margin.

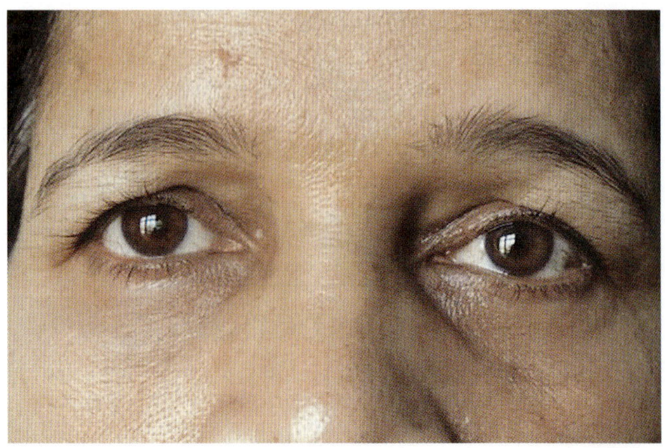

Fig. 6: 10 days postoperative following excision of neurofibroma upper eyelid margin.

- Radiofrequency (RF) excision **(Figs. 7 and 8)**
- Moh's micrographic surgery
- *Laser excision:* Ablative lasers are used, predominantly the carbon dioxide laser.

Tarsorrhaphy[9]

Tarsorrhaphy is the procedure of joining a part or the entire upper and lower eyelids so as to attempt partial or complete closure of the eye **(Figs. 9 and 10)**.

The term tarsorrhaphy is most commonly used in the western countries, whereas in Russia, the term blepharorrhaphy is widely accepted. The latter seems to be a more appropriate term as the sutures are passed through all the palpebral layers and not just the cartilage.

Blepharorrhaphy may be temporary or permanent. Temporary procedure implies use of only sutures to bring the eyelids together and therefore should be called simple blepharorrhaphy. But in the permanent procedure, the goal is to cause ankyloblepharon; hence, ankylosing blepharorrhaphy is recommended instead of permanent.

Indications

- To protect the cornea when there is inadequate closure of the eyelids as in:
  - Facial nerve palsy, ocular leprosy, postburn scarring, proptosis, and infrequent blinking as in intensive care unit (ICU) patients or those with severe brain injuries, protection of the anesthetic cornea from the risk of damage and infection, etc.
- To promote healing of the cornea in patients of corneal ulcer
- Exposure after ocular surgery to retain a conformer or other device, e.g., in children with anophthalmia or adults after evisceration or enucleation.

Procedure

- *Temporary tarsorrhaphy:* It can be performed by using a drawstring, botulinum toxin (the upper lid levator muscle is paralyzed with the toxin), or by using cyanoacrylate glue to appose the lids.

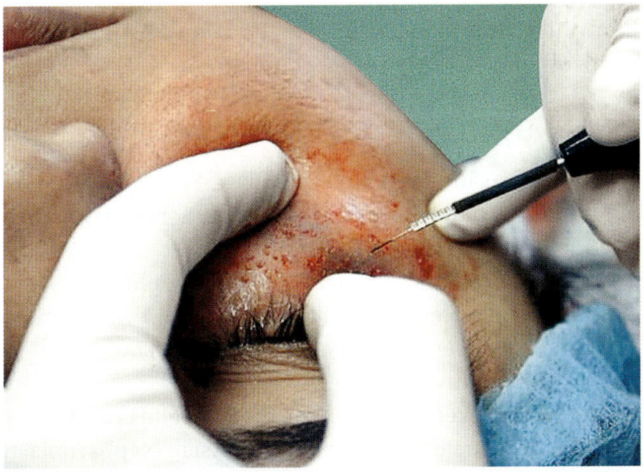

Fig. 7: Extensive milia being treated with radiofrequency needle electrode.

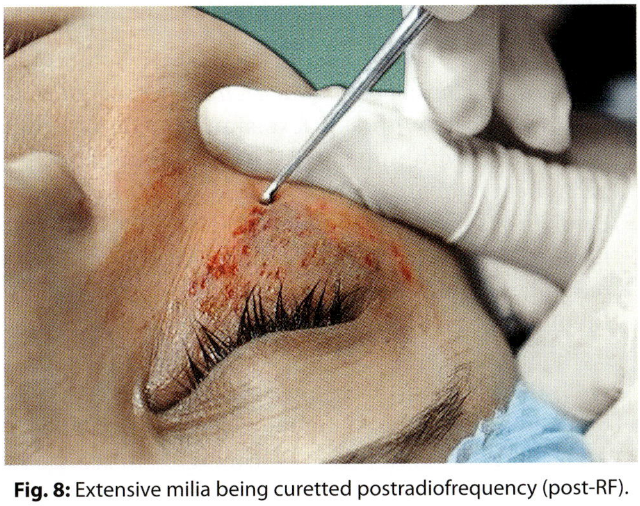

Fig. 8: Extensive milia being curetted postradiofrequency (post-RF).

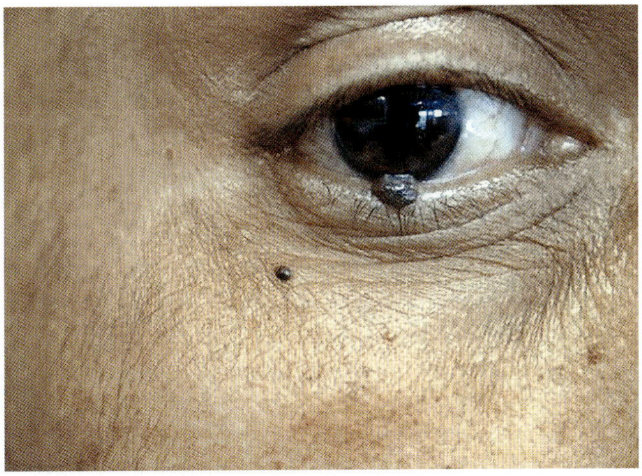

Fig. 9: Melanocytic nevus of lower eyelid.

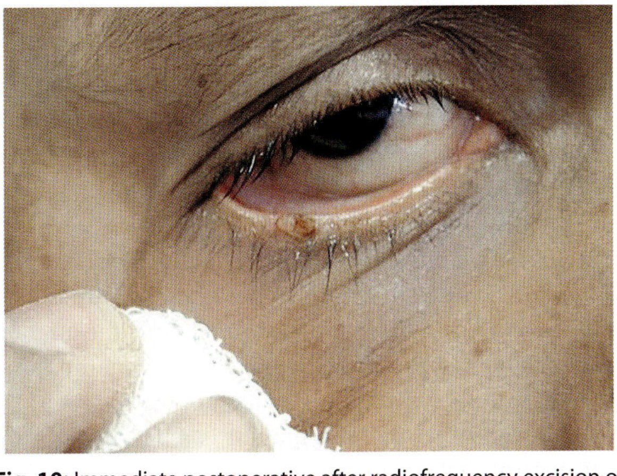

Fig. 10: Immediate postoperative after radiofrequency excision of melanocytic nevus.

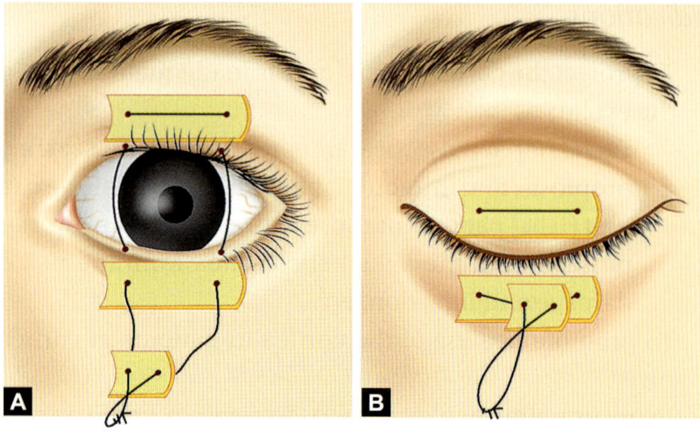

Figs. 11A and B: Temporary tarsorrhaphy procedure: (A) Alignment and threading of bolster; and (B) Using sutures and bolster to close the eye.

- After cleaning and dressing of the operation site, local infiltration is given. The procedure of temporary central tarsorrhaphy using a drawstring is as described **(Figs. 11A and B)**.
- After cleaning the area with 5% povidone iodine, anesthetize central part of both the eyelids with lidocaine and adrenaline. For each eye, prepare three bolsters (e.g., small cotton wool balls or plastic tubing), two with size 2 × 2 cm each and one of 1 × 1 cm size. The sutures are passed and tied over the bolsters to prevent them from cutting the skin. A double-armed nonabsorbable suture (e.g., silk, prolene, or nylon 4-0, 5-0, or 6-0) is passed straight through one of the 2 cm bolsters, 2 mm from the end. After aligning the bolster in the middle of the upper lid, pass the same needle 3–4 mm above the upper eyelid margin, through the tarsal plate and come out of the gray line of the lid margin. Pass the same needle into the gray line of the lower lid, then into the tarsal plate, and out of the skin 2–3 mm below the lower eyelid margin. After aligning the lower lid bolster centrally, pass the needle through it a few millimeters from one end. Similarly, pass the suture through the other end of the upper bolster → upper lid → lower lid → lower bolster in the same fashion as the previous step.
- The needles should be passed through the shorter length of bolster, 2 mm from each bolster end. Slide the two lower lid bolsters upward to close the eye. The smaller bolster "locks" and closes the lid. To separate the lids, the smaller bolster should be pulled down and the lids will open up easily.
- A slight modification of this procedure is also practiced, where instead of the bolster, a sterile button is used.

- *Permanent tarsorrhaphy:* In this procedure, the lid margin is debrided which allows the lids to stick together as they heal. It is almost always restricted only to the lateral part of the eyelids, so that the patient is able to see through the central eyelid opening and therefore, the eye can still be examined. It may last at least 3 months (sometimes lifelong). In this technique, the anterior and posterior lamellae of the lateral third of the upper and lower lids is split along the gray line using a no. 11 blade (preferably over no. 15 blade) up to a depth of 2 mm.
  - The split should be continued over the lid for about 5 mm with the same blade or spring scissors. Care should be taken to keep the split parallel to the tarsal plate so that the eyelid separates into anterior and posterior lamellae neatly. In order to remove the epithelium of the eyelid, excise 1 mm of the posterior lamella which is then closed using 5-0 or 6-0 absorbable suture. This is followed by closure of the anterior lamella (eyelid skin) by 4-0 to 6-0 sized nonabsorbable suture **(Figs. 12A to D)**.
  - These tarsorrhaphies almost often last forever, but if they need to be divided, this can be done by cutting the sutures under the effect of a local anesthetic agent and the lids look perfectly normal.

Blepharoplasty

The term blepharoplasty was coined by Karl Ferdinand von Grafe[10] in 1818, where the technique was used for repairing deformities caused by eyelid cancer. Upper blepharoplasty improves the palpebral fissure **(Figs. 13A and B)**.

Indications

The indications involved are as follows:

- Redundant and lax eyelid skin (dermatochalasis), causing double-eyelid fold creation
- Preaponeurotic fat herniation (steatoblepharon), which may result in either functional visual symptoms or cosmetic concerns in the affected patients
- Periorbital rejuvenation
- *Aesthetic:* Correcting low-lying upper eyelid crease or creating supratarsal fold in Asians (aka Asian blepharoplasty)

The goal of blepharoplasty should be to achieve the eyebrows at an appropriate level, neat-looking eyelids with well-hidden scar, correction of fat bulges without too much excision, or creating a sunken eye.

Situations where it can be combined with other procedures:[11]

- Blepharoplasty with skin excision may be indicated for patients with upper eyelid–skin redundancy and prominent double eyelids.
- Blepharoplasty with skin excision and nonburied suture fixation may be indicated for patients with upper lid–skin redundancy and weak, double eyelids.
- Blepharoplasty with skin excision and buried suture fixation may be indicated for patients with upper lid–skin redundancy but no double-eyelid folds.
- Blepharoplasty with simultaneous ptosis (lid or lacrimal) correction may be indicated for patients with senile or subclinical ptosis requesting upper blepharoplasty.

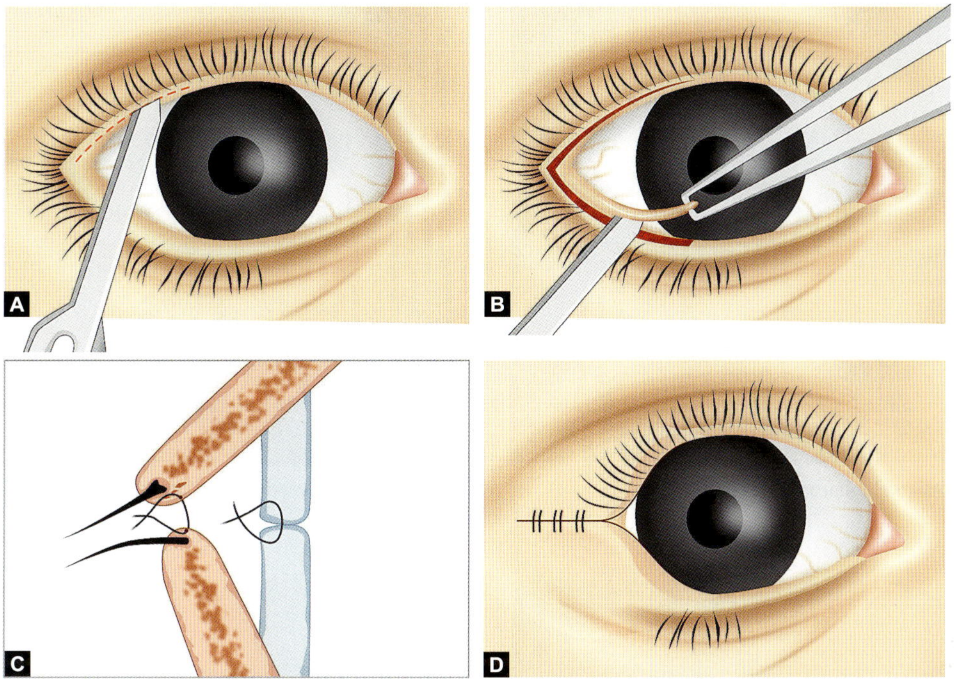

Figs. 12A to D: Permanent tarsorrhaphy: (A) Splitting the anterior and posterior lamella; (B) Excising 1 mm of the posterior lamella; (C) Closing the anterior and posterior lamella; and (D) After the procedure.

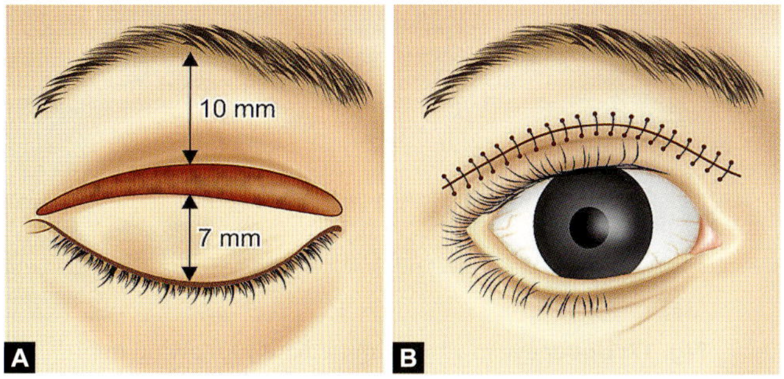

Figs. 13A and B: Upper eyelid blepharoplasty.

Procedure of Asian Blepharoplasty (Figs. 14 and 15)

Infiltration with 2% xylocaine with adrenaline mixed with 0.25% sensorcaine gives a very good anesthesia.[12] The marking of the required skin to be excised should be done preoperatively in a sitting position. A curved line 9–10 mm above the lid margin in the midpupillary line is marked which corresponds to the supratarsal fold. The line should gently curve down to 7 mm above the lid margin at the medial and lateral ends. The excessive skin is thereafter marked by pinching it with a nontoothed forceps or marking the upper line 10 mm below the inferior margin of the eyebrow

A scalpel or RF electrosurgical device may be used to make the incisions after cleaning and local infiltration. After excising the desired amount of eyelid skin, the orbicularis oculi fibers are excised. The preaponeurotic fat is made to protrude by a gentle pressure on the globe and also to help in identifying the septum and incising it. The septum is incised along its entire length to expose the levator aponeurosis lying under it. The fat pads are excised if in excess. Avoid giving traction to the fat pads and to the superior oblique tendon while dissecting the medial fat pad. The excessive skin and muscle are resected with scissors. Correction of the lid ptosis and lacrimal gland ptosis may be carried out. Hemostasis may be achieved with pressure or cautery and the incision is closed with interrupted 5-0 or 6-0 nylon or prolene sutures. The hitching suture should include the aponeurosis, orbicularis muscle, and the skin so that when the patient blinks the eyelid moves with the contraction of the muscle and so that the upper eyelid crease is created. At last, the cutaneous sutures are taken in a simple, interrupted manner. It differs from standard blepharoplasty in the hitching of levator aponeurosis to skin. This step is not undertaken in standard blepharoplasty.

With upper lid blepharoplasty, the degree of lash ptosis was found to be reduced, thereby improving the visual quality.[13] The brow position does not seem to change in patients who undergo upper eyelid blepharoplasty for simple dermatochalasis.[14]

In the Asian population, too high eyelid folds after blepharoplasty may cause an unsatisfactory aesthetic outcome which is difficult and challenging to correct.

It may be attempted to correct with a procedure called "secondary blepharoplasty," wherein the levator is advanced and intervened between the levator aponeurosis and the overlying skin by in situ tissue or fat grafting.[15]

Lower lid blepharoplasty: The aim of lower eyelid blepharoplasty is to remove the pseudoherniated fat via skin incision. The procedural details have been dealt in the

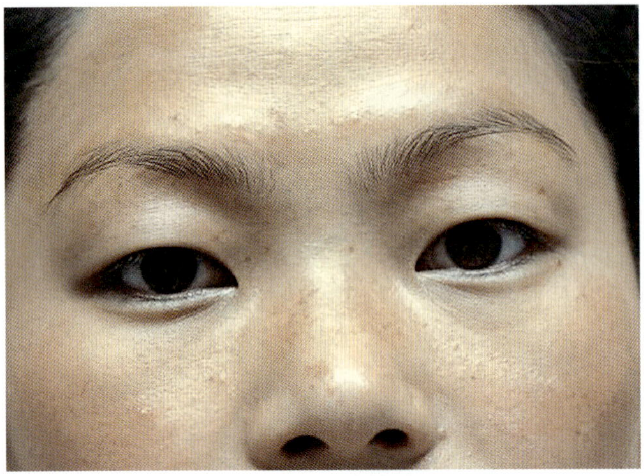

Fig. 14: Asian blepharoplasty preoperative.

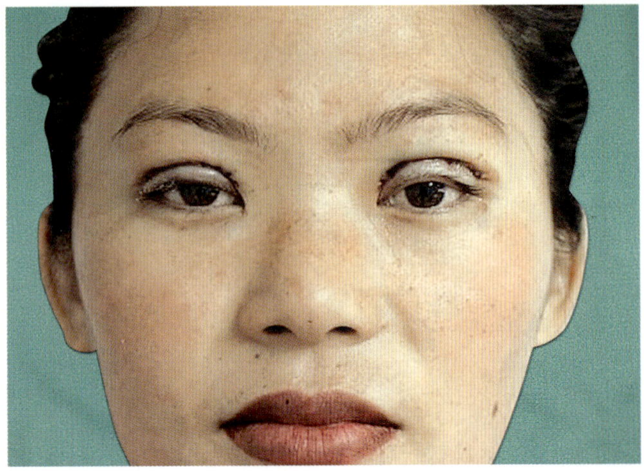

Fig. 15: Asian blepharoplasty immediate postoperative.

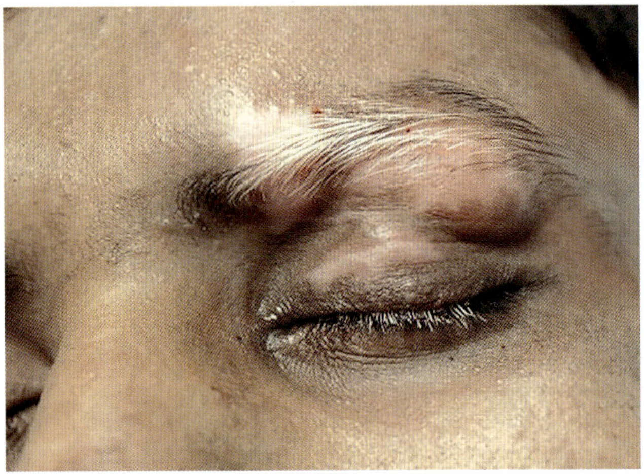

Fig. 16: Upper eyelid vitiligo.

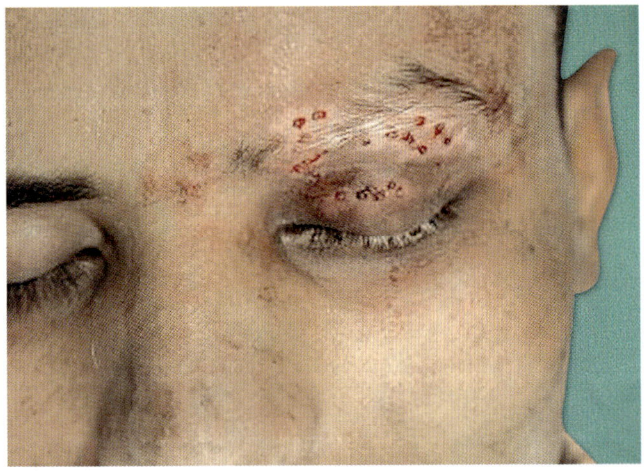

Fig. 17: Upper eyelid vitiligo immediately following mini punch grafting.

TABLE 3: Complications post blepharoplasty.

Complications post blepharoplasty	*Management*
Retrobulbar hemorrhage, bulbar hematoma	Immediate referral to an ophthalmologist
Lagophthalmos	Corrective surgeries
Conjunctival scarring, diplopia, symblepharon	Corrective surgeries
Pyogenic granuloma	Excision with RF/EF

(RF/EF: radiofrequency/electric frequency)

next chapter. Complications post blepharoplasty have been mentioned in **Table 3**.

VITILIGO SURGERIES

Involvement of the head and neck area is associated with leukotrichia of the eyelashes and eyebrows.[16,17] In many cases, the surgical management of vitiligo may cause repigmentation of leukotrichia;[18] however, eyelash leukotrichia involving periocular region is generally resistant to medical or surgical therapy.[19]

Various factors to be kept in mind before conducting the surgeries on the eyelids are:

- Age of the patient
- Type of vitiligo (segmental vitiligo or vitiligo vulgaris)
- Size of the depigmented area
- Assessment of stability of vitiligo
- Patient expectation

Various operations recommended for eyelid vitiligo are:

- Suction blister roof grafting
- Mini punch skin grafting **(Figs. 16 and 17)**
- Hair follicle grafting **(Figs. 18 and 19)**
- Ultrathin (Thiersch) or split-thickness skin grafting **(Figs. 20 and 21)**
- Autologous noncultured melanocyte transplantation **(Figs. 22 to 26)**
- Cultured melanocyte transplantation

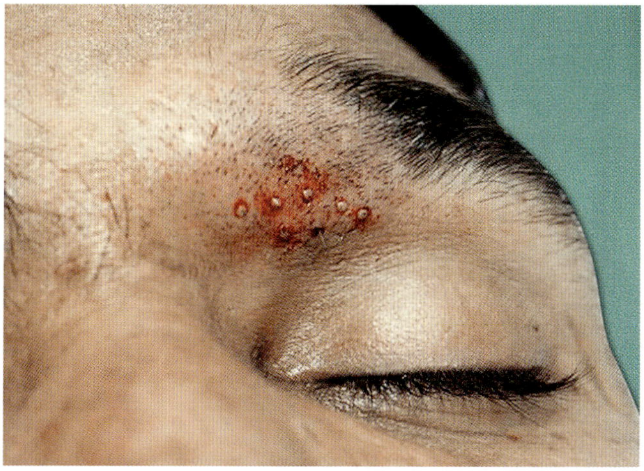

Fig. 18: Immediate postfollicular unit extraction and hair follicle grafting onto vitiliginous macule.

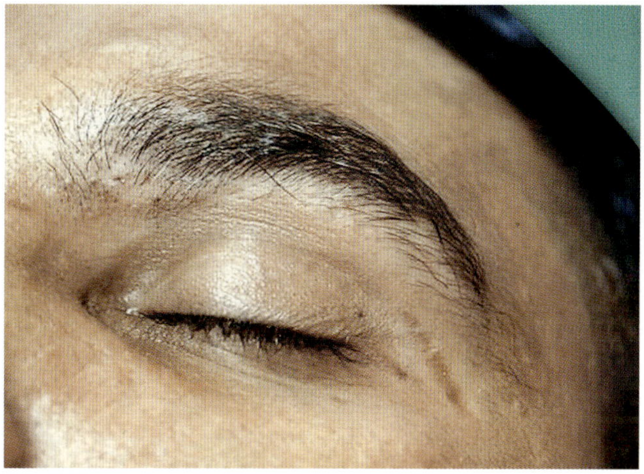

Fig. 19: Hair follicle graft: 1-month postoperative.

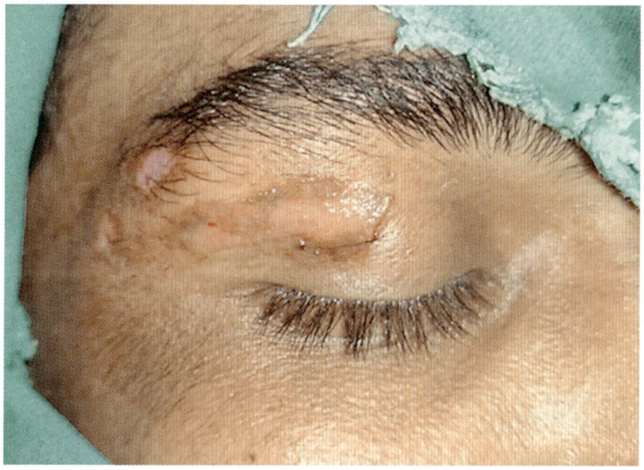

Fig. 20: Thin Thiersch's graft for vitiligo upper eyelid.

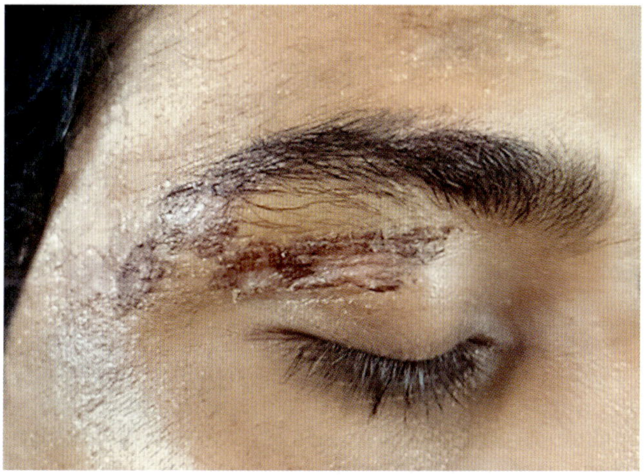

Fig. 21: One week after thin Thiersch's grafting over upper eyelid.

All of these procedures are carried out the same way as on any other site of body.

Contraindications to the above surgeries are:

- Patients with unrealistic expectation
- Unstable vitiligo
- Children
- Keloidal tendency

EYELASH TRANSPLANTATION (FOLLICULAR UNIT TRANSPLANTATION)

Eyelash transplantation is a procedure in which the hair follicles from hair-bearing areas are transplanted in the eyelashes. It has been used as a therapeutic option for:

- The loss of eyelash as a result of the following diverse etiologies (trauma, trichotillomania, and alopecia areata)
- May also be performed for aesthetic purposes for:
  - Patients who demand denser eyelashes
  - Vitiligo-associated leukotrichia **(Figs. 27 and 28)**

Procedure

Half an hour prior to the procedure, mild sedation can be achieved by giving the patient tablet diazepam 10 mg orally. Corneal eye shield should be applied after topical anesthesia with lignocaine eye drops. Local anesthesia is achieved by infiltration of 2% lignocaine with adrenaline in the donor and recipient site.

The donor area is prepared by clipping the hair of the temporal area. Only single hair follicles are harvested using 0.8 mm punch with the help of follicle unit extraction motor. The involved eyelashes of recipient area are removed with 20-gauge needle. The hair obtained are harvested in a similar way as in hair transplant surgery and the single hair follicles are grafted, using fine Jewelers forceps or implanters into the chambers created. Implantation can be carried out in one row in a fan-shaped manner. In a single sitting, 15–20 hair can be transplanted in each eyelid. Thereafter, the donor lashes are trimmed to the size of other eyelashes and the operated eye

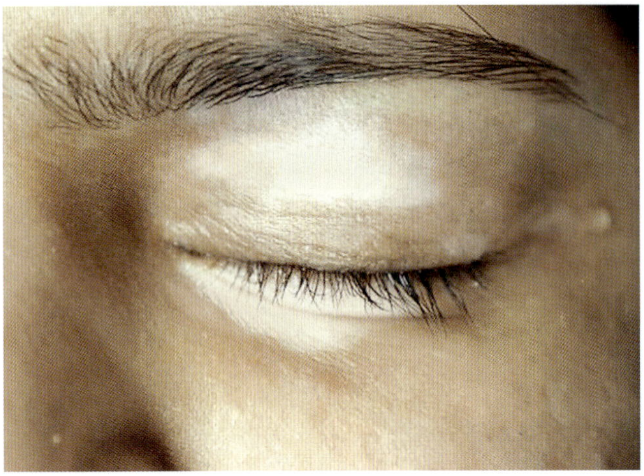

Fig. 22: Upper eyelid vitiligo.

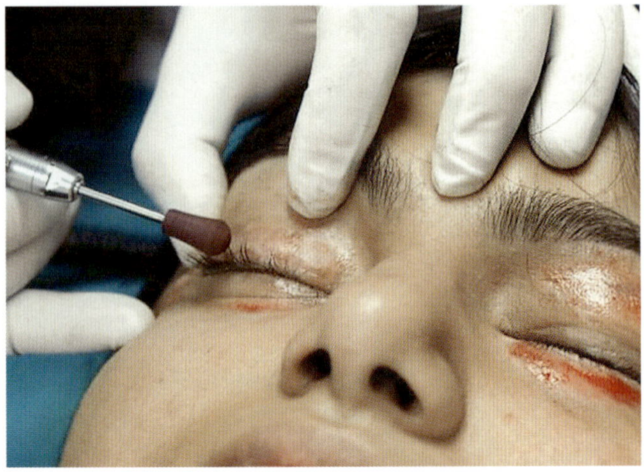

Fig. 23: Dermabrasion of recipient area.

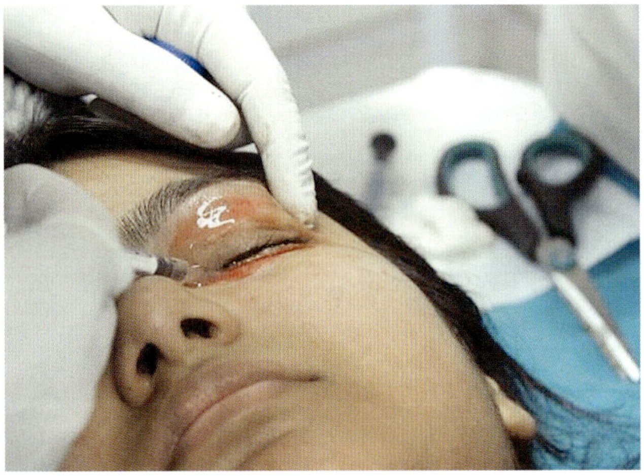

Fig. 24: Application of melanocyte–keratinocyte suspension.

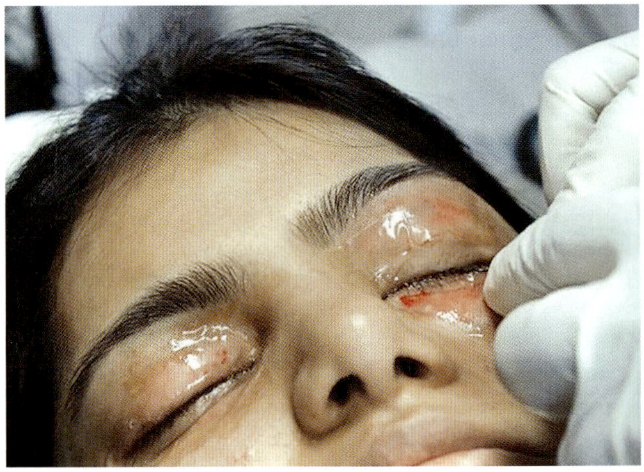

Fig. 25: Application of dry collagen sheet dressing.

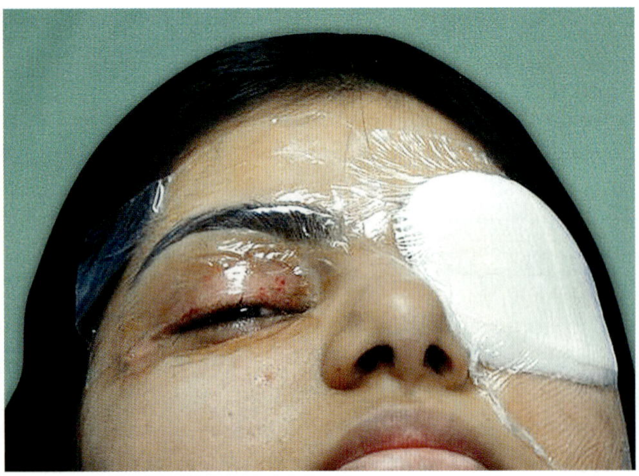

Fig. 26: Application of eye pad dressing with eyes closed.

is padded with a bandage for a week. Few patients may need two to three sittings at the interval of 4 weeks. The surgery takes about 2–3 hours.

The procedure of eyelash transplantation can be performed by various other methods. It can be performed using Choi and Kim hair transplanter,[20] with single-hair grafts or by strip composite eyebrow graft as described by Kasai.[21] It can also be performed using the "pluck and sew technique" as described by Caputy and Flowers.[22]

The present first author has harvested single unit grafts using motorized punches of 0.8 mm similar to hair transplantation and implanted them in the chambers created after removal of leukotrichic eyelash using forceps or implanter with excellent repigmentation of the leukotrichic eyelashes. Use of the implanter makes the procedure simpler and faster as compared to the manual forceps technique.

Postprocedure, the author observed that the transplanted eyelashes matched closely with natural eyelashes and were cosmetically elegant.

Postprocedure Care

Capsule amoxicillin clavulanic acid 625 mg and tablet ibuprofen 400 mg 8 hourly are advised for 5 days. Protective

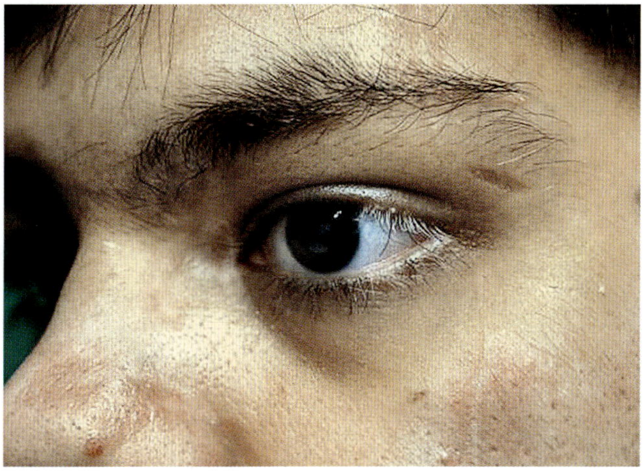

Fig. 27: Residual eyelash leukotrichia following vitiligo treatment.

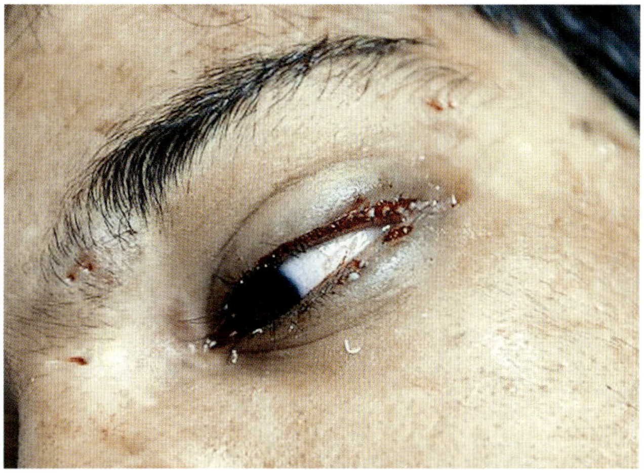

Fig. 28: Immediately following eyelash transplantation.

goggles are advised for 4–6 weeks. The curvature of the eyelashes may be maintained with the regular use of mascara or a curling device.

Postprocedure, there is scab formation around the transplanted follicle and the transplanted hair which falls off by 2–3 weeks and regrowth of the eyelashes are first noticed by 8–10 weeks. The results are assessed at the end of 6 months. Surgery is most of the time free from major complications and most common complications noticed are swelling and bruising of eyelids and blepharitis. As the scalp hair grow faster, the patient should be advised to trim these lashes at regular intervals.

SURGERIES IN LEPROSY

Lagophthalmos

Lagophthalmos is a common complication of leprosy, where there is a visible lid gap due to incomplete closure of the eyelids. This condition puts the eye at risk of exposure and external injuries, further giving rise to sequelae of exposure keratitis, secondary infection, corneal ulcer, and finally vision loss. At times, the infection may involve the deeper tissues causing panophthalmitis. It may be aggravated by anesthesia of the cornea due to fifth nerve involvement. Role of medical management is limited. The patient is observed for 6 months on medical measures; if the lid gap persists for more than 5 mm, then surgery is often required.[23]

Surgical Management[24]

- *Dynamic procedures:* Gillie's and Johnson's temporalis muscle transfer (TMT) procedures are commonly carried out. However in the Indian subcontinent, Johnson's TMT procedure **(Figs. 29A and B)** is considered the surgery of choice. The procedure has few limitations which include prolonged admissions, well-motivated patient, well-trained oculoplastic surgeon, good corneal sensitivity, and postoperative intensive physiotherapy. In this procedure, strips of the temporalis muscle are tunneled through the tarsal plates and anchored to the medial canthal ligaments.
- *Static procedures:* Various procedures have been carried out which include the canthopexies, canthoplasty, slings, springs, gold implants, ear cartilage grafts, etc. Two procedures that are effective in corneal blindness are tarsal strip (Kuhnt-Szymanowski) and tarsorrhaphy (discussed earlier in this chapter).

Trichiasis

The term trichiasis means that some of the eyelashes point backward and hence rub against the cornea. Usually, every patient with entropion will have trichiasis. However, sometimes the misdirected lashes may turn inward without the turning in of the whole eyelid (i.e., trichiasis without entropion). Treatment of this condition is removal of the incriminating eyelashes.

Methods to remove the lashes are as follows:

- *Epilation:* The offending lashes are plucked out with the epilation forceps after which the patient may temporarily heave a sigh of relief. The symptoms usually recur as the lash nearly always grows again. This procedure requires repeated epilation to keep the eyes comfortable and therefore, patients with only slight trichiasis are the ideal candidates.
- *Cutting the lashes:* Scissors are used to cut off the offending lashes which also gives temporary relief. But at times, it may be worse as after cutting, the eyelash end becomes sharper and therefore it may be an irritant.
- *Excision of misdirected lashes:* This procedure is undertaken in patients who present with just one or two small tufts of abnormal eyelashes. It involves excision of the affected lashes along with their roots without affecting the eyelid. This procedure may be an alternative to electrolysis or cryotherapy (described later) in milder cases of trichiasis.

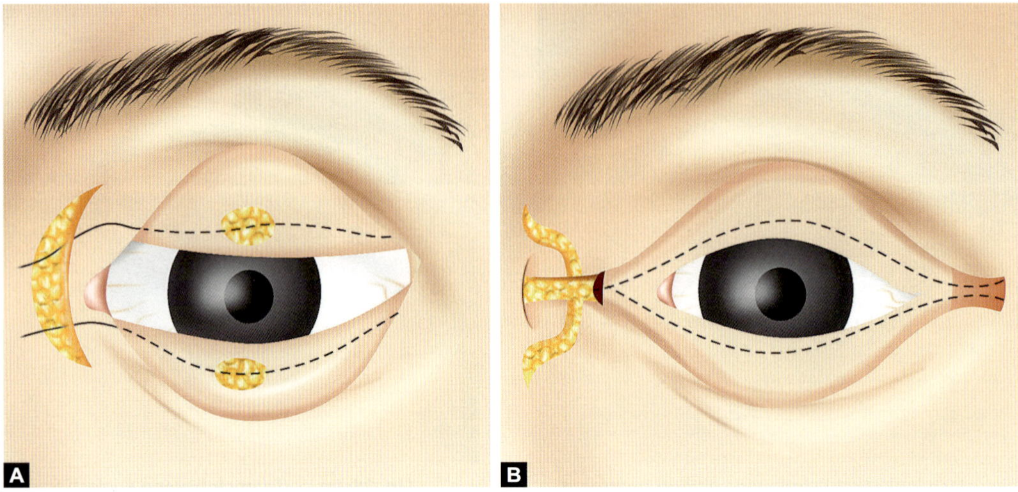

Figs. 29A and B: Temporalis muscle transfer (TMT) through eyelids to medial canthal ligaments and tarsal plates.

- *Electrolysis:* The principle of electrolysis is to pass a low-voltage current through a fine needle inserted along the direction of eyelash up to its root (approximately 3 mm), causing a localized burn enough to destroy the lash root. It is an ideal procedure in patients with few ingrowing eyelashes and commenced under local anesthesia. The current is passed for at least 5 seconds. Tiny bubbles may appear on the surface of the eyelid at the entry point of the needle. Even when the local anesthesia effect is adequate, patient may feel some discomfort with the passage of current. In order to check the adequacy, lift the lash out with an epilation forceps; if it comes out easily, the lash root has been destroyed. However, if there is any resistance, the procedure is continued till each ingrown eyelash root has been destroyed. Repeated treatment may be required.
- *Cryoepilation:* Use of a chalazion clamp is recommended while performing cryoepilation as it facilitates exposure of the surgical field and supports cryodestruction of the follicle by reducing blood flow to the gland, thereby speeding the freeze and slowing the thaw. It is the least risky procedure, where the cryoprobe is applied over base of the affected Meibomian gland on the palpebral conjunctiva (3–4 mm behind the eyelid margin). A double freeze–thaw (–25°C) cycle spares adjacent normal tissue but destroys the affected follicles.
- *Surgery:* Orbicularis oculi fibers' shortening is useful in the management of trichiasis and cicatricial entropion of the upper or lower eyelids.

Ectropion

Ectropion (eversion) is commonly seen in old cases of leprosy in those who have thin tarsal plate and orbicularis oculi. It may be associated with trichiasis.

Ectropion surgery: Lateral tarsorrhaphy, electrosurgery, and suture repair can be done.

The surgical outcome after the tarsal strip procedure for lower eyelid ectropion was similar with both the absorbable and nonabsorbable sutures.[25]

MISCELLANEOUS SURGERIES

Xanthelasma Palpebrarum

Treatment entails removal of the lesion. Before choosing the surgical modality, one should always keep in mind that if the xanthelasma extends deep into the orbicularis muscle, it may not respond to the surface ablation techniques.

Various options available for the removal of xanthelasma palpebrarum are as follows:

- *Chemical cauterization:* Use of chlorinated acetic acids has been found to be effective in the removal of xanthelasma. Monochloroacetic acid, dichloroacetic acid, and trichloroacetic acid (TCA) have been used with good results. They dissolve the lipids and precipitate and coagulate the proteins. Dichloroacetic acid (100%) has been used with excellent results and minimal scarring.
- *Electrodessication/RF and cryotherapy:* Xanthelasma may be destroyed with the above methods when they are superficial but may require repeated treatments. Cryotherapy may cause hypopigmentation and scarring. In comparison to the TCA application, RF ablation required fewer sessions in order to achieve more than 75% clearance of lesions; however, TCA applications were associated with fewer complications.[26]
- *Surgical excision:* Smaller lesions may be removed with incision and dissection (uncapping), followed by replacement and suturing of the flap. In case there are small linear lesions, total excision is recommended as the scarring would blend along with the surrounding eyelid tissue. Sometimes, excision of xanthelasma along with depigmentation caused by previous TCA application may need to be done **(Figs. 30 and 31)**. In case of full-thickness

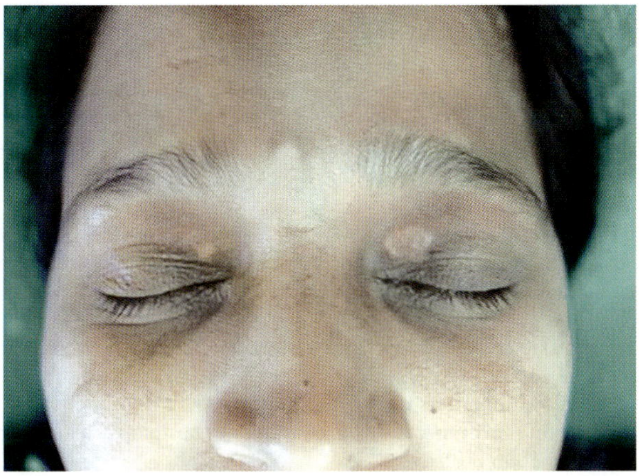

Fig. 30: Xanthelasma with depigmentation post 50% trichloroacetic acid application.

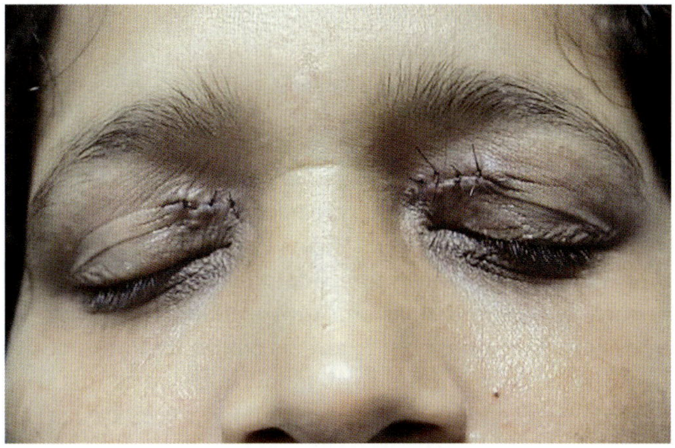

Fig. 31: Postsurgical excision of xanthelasma and depigmented area.

excisions, the lower lid is more prone for development of prominent scarring as the tissue here tends to be thicker. Simple excision of larger lesions increases the risk of eyelid retraction, ectropion, and need for more complicated reconstructive procedures. Incorporation of xanthelasma removal into routine blepharoplasty may increase the risk of ectropion formation by extending the incisional limits.

- *Carbon dioxide and argon laser ablation:* Better visualization, lack of suturing, enhanced hemostasis, and speed have been cited as the reasons to use this technique; however, scarring and pigmentary alterations are inevitable. A couple of case reports have shown conflicting results in the context of using Q-switched Nd:YAG (neodymium-doped yttrium aluminum garnet) in the treatment of xanthelasma.[27,28]

Basal Cell Carcinoma

Various modalities are useful for the treatment of BCC. For the superficial lesions, excision remains the treatment of choice. Other modalities can be used in patient where surgery is contraindicated. Excision by RF, with mild curettage has been done, which has been proved effective and yielded satisfactory therapeutic results.[29,30]

Sometimes, an extensive procedure in the form of eyelid reconstructive surgery is required. This procedure has triple objective of tumor removal, functionality, and an aesthetic outcome. BCC of the eyelids has a high risk of recurrence. Recurrences have a considerably poorer rate of cure than the primary tumors and are more severe, aggressive, infiltrative, and destructive.

Moh's Micrographic Surgery

Moh's micrographic surgery procedure involves complete excision of the tumors with predetermined margins in different sized BCCs. Surgeons need to be trained for this procedure to do this surgery. It is a skin-sparing technique that allows skin cancer to be removed with less damage to the healthy skin around it. Patients who undergo Moh's micrographic excision for the indication of an eyelid cancer may present with a full-thickness defect of the lower lid. Hughes flap (tarsal-conjunctival flap) is commonly undertaken to address this defect. The disadvantages of this procedure are that the edge of the flap is often edematous (eye is closed) and erythematous postoperatively and a second stage is often required. To avoid this, an excellent one-step procedure is undertaken in which lateral stabilization[31] of the posterior lamella with a periosteal strip and myocutaneous advancement flap is carried out.

Grafting

The periorbital region requires different and special care in terms of reconstruction because of its complex anatomy and important structures.

- *Indications:* Soft-tissue defects such as trauma, tumors, burns, radiation, infection, and congenital anomalies
- *Method:* Simple, full-thickness grafting over eyelids is done in a similar manner as over other body sites.

Chalazion Excision

Chalazion is one of the most common eyelid lesion requiring surgical excision. When the lesion presents on the anterior lid, the chalazion clamp is placed encircling the lesion and a horizontal incision is made over the mass. The cyst is evacuated, necrotic debris is curetted, and fibrous tissue is excised. The skin is closed with 5-0 or 6-0 prolene. The horizontal scar blends well with the normal skin crease.

When the lesion presents on the posterior lid surface, a chalazion clamp is applied and the lid is everted. A vertical incision is then made over the mass. The procedure is then repeated as mentioned earlier. Suturing is not necessary here and bleeding can be controlled with a cautery which is usually very minimal. The advantage of using the chalazion clamp is that it provides a bloodless field while operating.

Sclerotherapy

Using sclerotherapy, smaller hemangiomas and small visible periocular veins can be safely treated with sodium tetradecyl sulfate (STD) in 1:4 dilution. However, one should be careful while injecting making sure that adequate protection of cornea is achieved as sclerosant can damage the cornea and cause ulcerations. It is always advisable to direct the injection away from the cornea and midface as much as possible to avoid untoward complications. Recently, a series of 50 adult female patients underwent successful sclerosing of their visible periocular veins without experiencing any ophthalmological or neurological sequelae.[32]

Medial Canthus Reconstruction

At this site, simple defects should be closed in a diamond-shaped manner. To restore the normal canthal angle in all types of medial canthus reconstruction, whether allowing it to heal with secondary intention or by using full-thickness skin graft or glabella flap,[33] the edge of the lid remnants must be attached to the posterior reflection of the medial canthal tendon.

This may be achieved by placing a strong permanent suture such as 5-0 prolene through the tarsal remnant of both upper and lower lids and then attaching it to the posterior reflection of the medial canthal tendon. In most situations, the best result is obtained by allowing defects of the medial canthus that are equal above and below the caruncle to heal by secondary intention.

COMMON COMPLICATIONS AND MISTAKES TO AVOID

Complications are bound to occur even in the hands of an astute and experienced dermatosurgeon, despite most of these being simple and reliable outpatient-based procedures. The risks may be minimized by careful patient selection, performing the surgeries meticulously by a trained personnel, early recognition, treatment of complications, and appropriate keep pre- and postoperative skin care.

CONCLUSION

To conclude, most of the abovementioned procedures are within the reach of an eminent dermatosurgeon, provided they are done meticulously in a setup well equipped with all the required materials and instruments. Thus, the expectations of a digitally savvy patient of today's era of having a perfect outcome, rapid postoperative recovery with no complications can be addressed.

TIPS AND PEARLS

- Local anesthetic infiltration in the sublesional plane lifts the lesion away as a result of "ballooning" effect which protects the tarsal plate during a destructive surgery
- While performing surgeries which necessitate the eyes to be open, use a corneal eye shield after topical anesthesia to prevent damage to the cornea
- A 27-gauge needle and a 26-gauge-filling cannula may be utilized to give anesthesia, which reduces the number of punctures, and thereby decreases the incidence of postoperative hematomas and bruising[34]
- As the skin of the eyelids is extremely thin and at the free margin continues with the conjunctiva, precaution should be taken to maintain the borders of the margin to prevent asymmetry due to contractures postoperatively (e.g., ectropion postbiopsy or excisional surgery around the eyes)
- During grafting, attempt should be made to harvest thin grafts in order to maintain the proper functioning and contour of the eyelids.
- Graft may be rejected in the eyelid area because of the increased folds and rugosity. In order to prevent this and corneal xerosis, a pad dressing must always be given keeping the eye in the closed position with stay sutures or proper taping
- Cyanoacrylate glue has been successfully used in stabilizing the skin grafts and flaps in the immediate postoperative period[35]
- While padding the eye, care should be taken to avoid inward upper eyelid push on the lower eyelid which may otherwise result in an involutional lower eyelid entropion[36]

REFERENCES

1. Kakizaki H, Leibovitch I, Selva D, Asamoto K, Nakano T. Orbital septum attachment on the levator aponeurosis in Asians: in vivo and cadaver study. Ophthalmology. 2009;116(10):2031-5.
2. Chen WP. Asian blepharoplasty: update on anatomy and techniques. Ophthal Plast Reconstr Surg. 1987;3(3):135-40.
3. Shoukath S, Taylor GI, Mendelson BC, Corlett RJ, Shayan R, Tourani SS, et al. The lymphatic anatomy of the lower eyelid and conjunctiva and correlation with postoperative chemosis and edema. Plast Reconstr Surg. 2017;139(3):628e-37e.
4. Jakobiec FA, Zakka FR, Tu Y, Freitag SK. Dermatofibroma of the eyelid: immunohistochemical diagnosis. Ophthal Plast Reconstr Surg. 2017;33(6):e134-8.
5. Betharia SM, Ramakrishna K, Sen S, Kashyap S, Thanikachalam S. Dermatofibroma of the eyelid: a case report. Orbit. 2000; 19(3):161-4.
6. Ovhal A. Pilonidal sinus of eyelids: A rare presentation. Indian J Dermatol Venereol Leprol. 2013;79(1):113-5.
7. Ensat F, Heinrich K, Kholosy HM, Wimbauer J, Hladik M, Wechselberger G. A double-blind randomized prospective study comparing prilocaine versus ropivacaine in upper blepharoplasty. J Plast Reconstr Aesthet Surg. 2017;70(3): 375-9.
8. Mizuno T. Treatment of suture-related complications of buried-suture double-eyelid blepharoplasty in Asians. Plast Reconstr Surg Glob Open. 2016;4(8):839.
9. Boiko EV, Chernysh VF. Medical terminology: Blepharorhaphy. Vestn Oftalmol. 2016;132(5):93-5.
10. Rees TD. Aesthetic Plastic Surgery. Philadelphia: WB Saunders Company; 1980. p. 459.
11. Park KS, Park D. Objective outcome measurement after upper blepharoplasty: an analysis of different operative techniques. Aesthetic Plast Surg. 2017;41(1):64-72.
12. Subramanian N. Blepharoplasty. Indian J Plast Surg. 2008; 41(Suppl):S88-92.

13. An SH, Jin SW, Kwon YH, Ryu WY, Jeong WJ, Ahn HB. Effects of upper lid blepharoplasty on visual quality in patients with lash ptosis and dermatochalasis. Int J Ophthalmol. 2016; 9(9):1320-4.
14. Nakra T, Modjtahedi S, Vrcek I, Mancini R, Saulny S, Goldberg RA. The effect of upper eyelid blepharoplasty on eyelid and brow position. Orbit. 2016;35(6):324-7.
15. Wattanakrai K, Chiemchaisri N, Wattanakrai P. Secondary blepharoplasty: correction of the high fold. Aesthetic Plast Surg. 2016;40(6):914-20.
16. Ezzedine K, Eleftheriadou V, Whitton M, van Geel N. Vitiligo. Lancet. 2015;386(9988):74-84.
17. Lee DY, Park JH, Lee JH, Yang JM, Lee ES. Is segmental vitiligo always associated with leukotrichia? Examination with a digital portable microscope. Int J Dermatol. 2009;48(11):1262.
18. Gan EY, van Geel N, Goh BK. Repigmentation of leucotrichia in vitiligo with noncultured cellular grafting. Br J Dermatol. 2012;166(1):196-9.
19. Lee DY, Kim CR, Park JH, Lee JH. The incidence of leukotrichia in segmental vitiligo: implication of poor response to medical treatment. Int J Dermatol. 2011;50(8):925-7.
20. Choi YC, Kim JC. Single hair transplantation using the Choi hair transplanter. J Dermatol Surg Oncol. 1992;18(11):945-8.
21. Kasai K. Eyelash reconstruction with strip composite eyebrow graft. Ann Plast Surg. 2008;60(6):649-51.
22. Caputy GG, Flowers RS. The "pluck and sew" technique of individual hair follicle placement. Plast Reconstr Surg. 1994;93(3):615-20.
23. Rajan MA. The Eye in Leprosy 1980 to 2005: A Study of 30, 121 patients. Kolkata, India: Proceedings of the First International Symposium on Ocular Leprosy; 2005. pp. 86-9.
24. Joshua J. Surgical Management of Lagophthalmos in Leprosy. Kolkata, India: Proceedings of the First International Symposium on Ocular Leprosy; 2005. pp. 125-35.
25. Sommer F. Surgery of lower eyelid ectropion with the tarsal strip procedure, using absorbable or non-absorbable sutures for periosteal fixation. Klin Monbl Augenheilkd. 2017;234(1):59-63.
26. Reddy PK, Kunneth ST, Lakshminarayana SP, Yallappa SM, Chandrashekara R, Nanjundaswamy SK. Comparative study to evaluate the efficacy of radiofrequency ablation versus trichloroacetic acid in the treatment of xanthelasma palpebrarum. J Cutan Aesthet Surg. 2016;9(4):236-40.
27. Fusade T. Treatment of xanthelasma palpebrarum by 1,064-nm Q-switched Nd:YAG laser: A study of 11 cases. Br J Dermatol. 2008;158:84-7.
28. Karsai S, Schmitt L, Raulin C. Is Q-switched neodymium-doped yttrium aluminium garnet laser an effective approach to treat xanthelasma palpebrarum? Results from a clinical study of 76 cases. Dermatol Surg. 2009;35(12):1962-9.
29. Wolff K, Johnson RA, Suurmond D (Eds). Color Atlas and Synopsis of Clinical Dermatology. London: McGraw-Hill; 2005. pp. 282-9.
30. Savant SS. Radiosurgery. In: Savant SS, Shah RA, Gore D (Eds). Textbook and Atlas of Dermatosurgery and Cosmetology. Mumbai: ASCAD; 2005. pp. 305-14.
31. Perry CB, Allen RC. Repair of 50–75% full-thickness lower eyelid defects: Lateral stabilization as a guiding principle. Indian J Ophthalmol. 2016;64(8):563-7.
32. Green D. Removal of periocular veins by sclerotherapy. Ophthalmology. 2001;108(3):442-8.
33. Meadows AE, Manners RM. A simple modification of the glabellar flap in medial canthal reconstruction. Ophthalmol Plast Reconstr Surg. 2003;19(4):313-5.
34. Trapasso M, Veneroso A. Local anesthesia for surgical procedures of the upper eyelid using filling cannula: our technique. Plast Reconstr Surg Glob Open. 2014;2(5): e143.
35. Jackson CM, Nguyen M, Mancini R. Use of cyanoacrylate glue casting for stabilization of periocular skin grafts and flaps. Ophthal Plast Reconstr Surg. 2017;33(3):218-220.
36. Sun MT, O'Connor AJ, Wood J, Casson R, Selva D. Tissue engineering in ophthalmology: Implications for eyelid reconstruction. Ophthal Plast Reconstr Surg. 2017;33(3): 157-162.

BIBLIOGRAPHY

1. Collin JRO. A Manual of Systematic Eyelid Surgery, 3rd edition. Oxford: Elsevier Butterworth-Heinemann; 2006.
2. Saw V, Leonard J. Dermatoses of the eye, eyelids and eyebrows. In: Griffiths C, Barker J, Bleiker T, Chalmers R, Creamer D (Eds). Rook's Textbook of Dermatology, 9th edition. New Jersey, United States: Wiley Blackwell; 2016. pp. 109.1-109.51.
3. WHO. Trichiasis Surgery for Trachoma—the Bilamellar Tarsal Rotation Procedure. Geneva: WHO; 1993.

CHAPTER 53

Blepharoplasty, Brow Lift, and Ptosis Surgery

Milind N Naik, Ruchi Hemdani

KEY MESSAGES

- Facial aging changes are most prominent in the periorbital region.
- The concern about visual function, clubbed with the need for hidden incisions, makes the periocular region a highly specialized surgical area, which needs to be handled by a properly trained aesthetic surgeon with ophthalmic background.
- Knowledge of anatomy and physiology of the periocular region is vital to ensure satisfactory results.
- The management of periorbital aging changes includes both medical and surgical options. A proper knowledge of limitations of medical treatment and when to suggest a surgical correction is the key to deliver the most accurate aesthetic result.
- Upper and lower eyelid blepharoplasty can be combined with other facial aesthetic procedures such as brow lift, ptosis correction, and facelift.
- Appropriate surgical correction of specialized eye disorders such as blepharoptosis and prominent eyes (proptosis) is also of equal aesthetic importance.

INTRODUCTION

Lambros has summed up periocular aging with "the eyes seem to get smaller as one ages, the entire lid aperture gets smaller because the lower lid rises, the upper lid falls, the lid gets shorter from the side, and the fat pads enlarge."[1,2] Ophthalmic cosmetic surgery therefore primarily deals with disorders of the eyelid, lacrimal apparatus, orbit, and periocular region. This chapter provides an overview of common periocular and facial aesthetic procedures. For the purpose of description, they are divided into upper and midface which represent the periocular region.

UPPER FACE

The upper face lies between the trichion superiorly and the canthi inferiorly. It includes the forehead, eyebrows, upper eyelid, and the mimetic muscles of the forehead and the eyebrows. The most common aesthetic procedures for the upper face include upper eyelid blepharoplasty, brow lift surgery, brow volume augmentation, and cosmetic correction of blepharoptosis.

Upper Eyelid Blepharoplasty

The eyes are an important component of facial aesthetics and blepharoplasty has a vital positive effect on facial harmony and the perception of aging. Blepharoplasty is one of the most commonly performed facial cosmetic procedures. Symptoms such as tired-looking eyes, excess skin, droopy eyelids, or circles around the eyes may benefit from blepharoplasty.[3] Other facial and skin rejuvenation procedures such as brow or midface lift, lasers, or chemical skin resurfacing can often be performed at the same time.[4]

Indications

Upper eyelid blepharoplasty is most commonly performed for "dermatochalasis" which represents excessive, overhanging inelastic upper eyelid skin due to aging **(Figs. 1A to D)**. Blepharochalasis represents excessive papery thin skin in the upper eyelid in young patients and can also benefit by blepharoplasty. Less frequently, a "blepharoplasty-like" excision is required for extensive xanthelasma.

Preoperative Evaluation

Preoperative patient evaluation for blepharoplasty should document medical and ocular evaluation. In addition to a complete eye examination, the evaluation of the periorbital area should take into account skin quality and quantity, underlying three-dimensional soft-tissue contours, and the bony skeletal support. Ophthalmologic history should be obtained including vision, corrective lenses, allergic reactions, excess tearing, and dry eyes.

Anesthesia

Blepharoplasty may be performed under either local or general anesthesia, depending upon the surgical plans, patient and surgeon preference, and need for concomitant operations. A simple upper or lower eyelid blepharoplasty where only skin or fat is excised can be performed under local anesthesia. Other more invasive procedures, such as lower

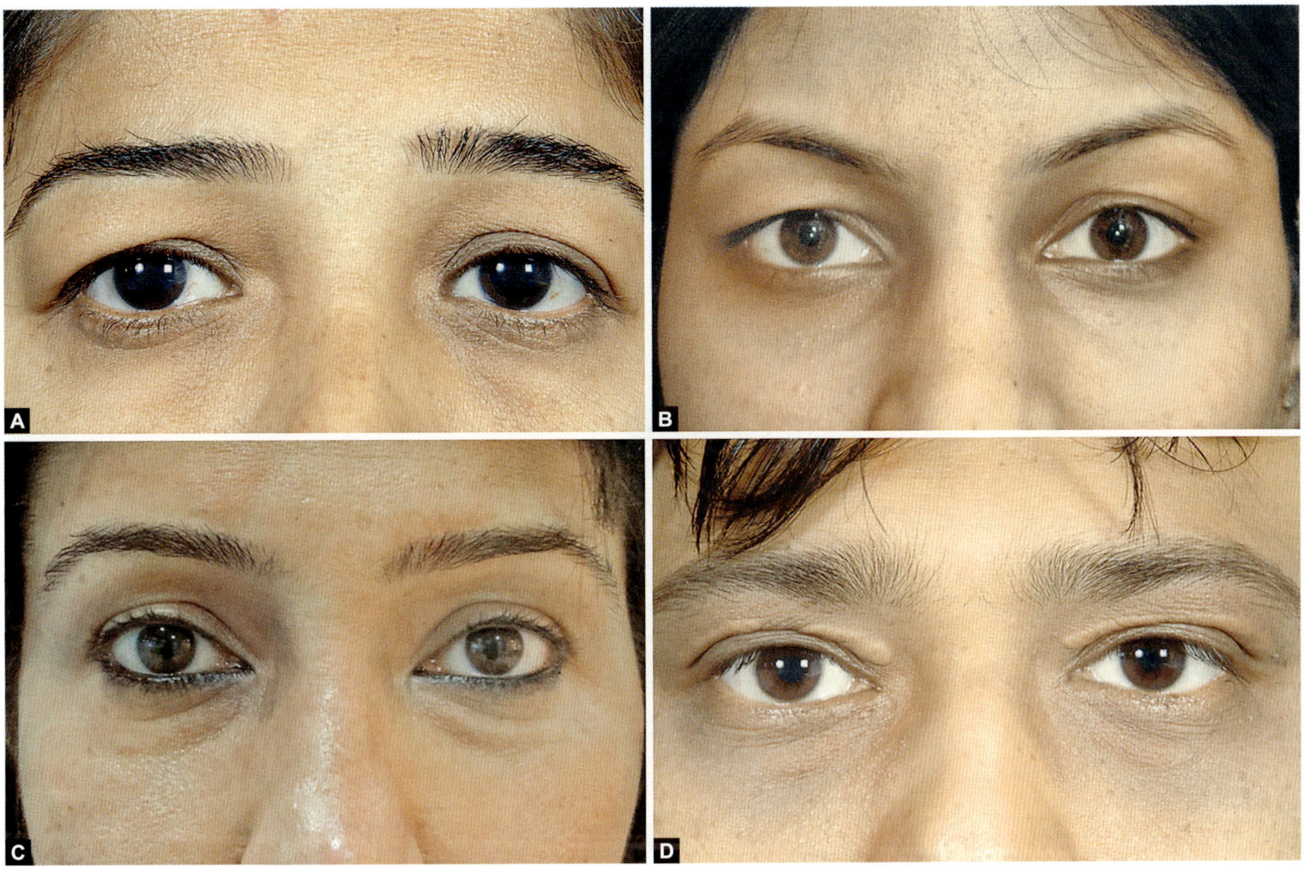

Figs. 1A to D: (A) Typical indications for blepharoplasty include excessive overhanging skin in the aged, termed dermatochalasis; and (B) Excessive papery thin skin in young patients is called blepharochalasis; (C) Loss of brow fat volume can give an appearance of excess upper eyelid skin that needs brow volume augmentation rather than blepharoplasty; (D) Rarely, a blepharoplasty-like incision may be needed for extensive xanthelasma.

blepharoplasty combined with fat repositioning, midface lift, or endoscopic brow lift may need intravenous sedation or general anesthesia.

Surgical Technique

Upper eyelid blepharoplasty is almost always performed via anterior approach (skin excision). Additional steps include fat sculpting, recontouring brow fat pad, and a transbleph browpexy if that is planned. Preoperative markings are made with the patient sitting upright, in straight gaze. The lower limit of excision is along the eyelid crease, which is situated 7–9 mm above the lash line. The lateral extent of the marking is limited by an imaginary line joining the lateral end of the brow to the lateral canthus. The upper extent of excision should be at least 10 mm from the inferior border of the brow, making a pattern of skin excision as shown in **Figures 2A to D**. Minimum 20 mm of vertical lid height should be preserved for normal eye closure. The location of fat should be determined and marked preoperatively.

After the markings, the eyelid should be injected superficially, with 2% lignocaine with 1:100,000 epinephrine using a 30-gauge needle. Skin incision can be made either with the surgical blade, empire tip of radiofrequency monopolar cautery, or CO_2 laser. Either skin alone or skin with orbicularis oculi is excised with meticulous hemostasis. Conservative fat excision can be performed as a part of upper lid blepharoplasty. There are two fat compartments, medial and central, that can be accessed through small incisions in the septum, gently prolapsed out and resected using radiofrequency monopolar tip. The sub-brow fat pad can be repositioned during wound closure with the use of periosteal suspension sutures. This is the most crucial step of an upper eyelid blepharoplasty **(Figs. 3A to D)**.

The skin incision is closed using running or interrupted sutures with either absorbable or permanent materials or cyanoacrylate glue to achieve an aesthetic outcome **(Figs. 4 and 5)**.

Postoperative Care

Postoperatively, ocular pad dressing should be given. Patients should be advised to use ice packs on the surgical site for 3 days to minimize postoperative swelling and topical antibiotic (ciprofloxacin ophthalmic ointment) application two to three times a day over the suture line for 2 weeks. Oral antibiotics and analgesics should be given for 5 days. Pain is usually very minimal which subsides with

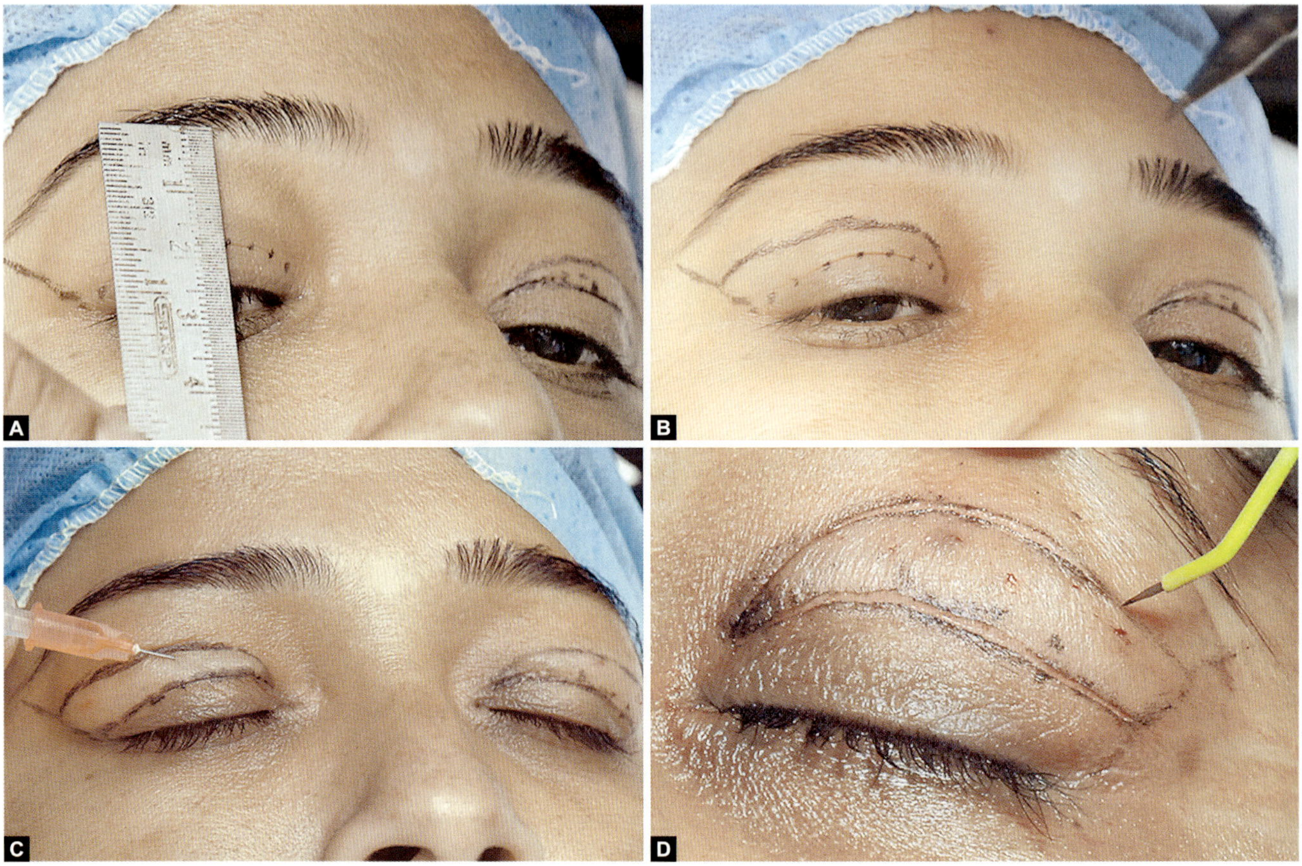

Figs. 2A to D: Upper eyelid blepharoplasty: (A) Skin marking and measurement is performed to leave minimum 20 mm vertical lid height; (B) The medial and lateral extent of skin excision is marked; (C) Subcutaneous injection of local anesthetic agent is slowly given; (D) Skin incision is placed with radiofrequency fine monopolar empire tip.
Source: Adapted from Naik MN, Honavar SG, Das S, Desai S, Dhepe N. Blepharoplasty: an overview. J Cutan Aesthet Surg. 2009;2:6-11.

analgesics. If the pain still continues despite analgesics, rule out retrobulbar hemorrhage which is a dreaded complication. Nonabsorbable sutures, if used, can be removed after 1 week. Artificial tear drops may be prescribed. Patients should be advised to avoid the use of contact lenses and no bending and lifting heavy weights for at least 2 weeks. Patient must be advised to wait for 6 weeks for the swelling to resolve before judging the final results.

Complications

Possible complications include upper eyelid retraction with scleral show from anterior lamellar inadequacy, lagophthalmos, acquired diplopia, and corneal exposure. The most common complication of cosmetic surgery is failure to meet the patient's expectations. This can be avoided by preoperative counseling and identifying reasonable expectations.

Endoscopic Brow Lift and Brow Volume Augmentation

In periocular aesthetic evaluation, the eyebrow receives special attention as it is a functionally integral part of upper eyelid complex. Two classical aging changes noted in the eyebrow include deflation (volume loss) and descent (brow ptosis). The former requires filling (Filler or fat), whereas the latter is best handled by a brow-lift procedure.

Indications

Volume augmentation of the eyebrow is performed to restore the lost brow fat pad to restore its convex contours. Brow lift is indicated for aesthetically or functionally significant brow ptosis.

Assessment of the Eyebrow

Deflation or loss of volume is indicated by loss of the round contour of eyebrow fat pad, leading to skin hooding. It can be best appreciated by comparing the findings with the individual's old photographs. Brow ptosis should be assessed by evaluating the position of the hair-bearing eyebrow in relation to the superior orbital rim. Normally, it is placed at or above the superior orbital rim. Brow deflation as well as brow ptosis leads to an appearance of "excess" upper eyelid skin and a blepharoplasty is erroneously thought of. Eyebrow asymmetry is commonly noted as a part of facial asymmetry but can also be an indicator of subtle eyelid ptosis on the side with a higher brow.

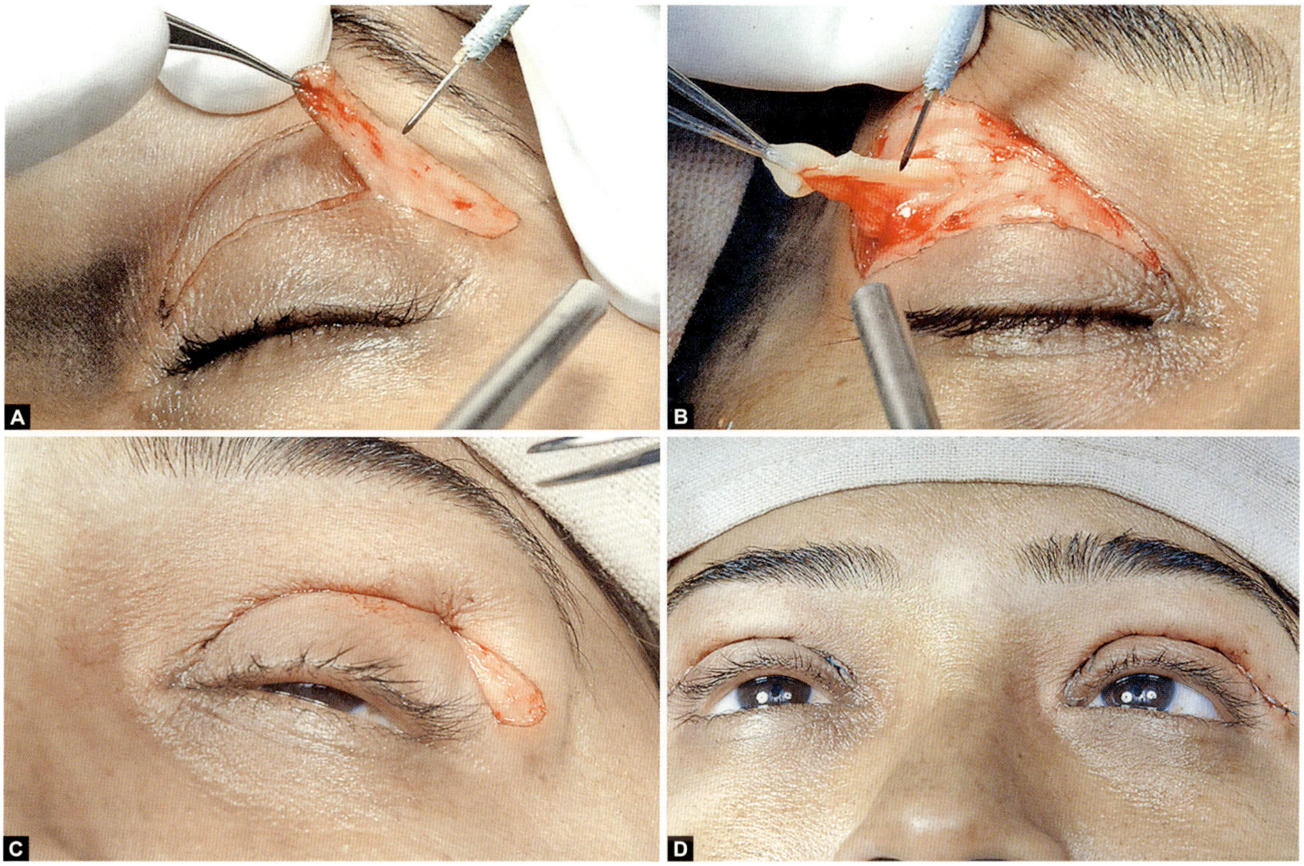

Figs. 3A to D: Upper eyelid blepharoplasty. (A) Either skin alone, or skin with orbicularis (temporal orbicularis excised when temporal elevation of brow is desired) is excised; (B) Conservative fat sculpting is followed by (C) the "brassiere" suture to reform the brow fat pad; (D) Final wound closure can be with continuous or interrupted suture.

Brow Volume Augmentation

Loss of brow volume can lead to an erroneous appearance of excess skin in the upper eyelid (pseudodermatochalasis) and these patients are often advised blepharoplasty. However, a simple brow volume augmentation by hyaluronic acid fillers or autologous fat transfers can improve their appearance.[5] It achieves a fuller brow, eliminates the appearance of "pseudodermatochalasis," and to some extent, also elevates the eyebrow **(Figs. 6A to F)**. It is always prudent to perform hyaluronic acid filler first and then graduate to a fat transfer after the patient is convinced about the appearance.

Brow Lift

Brow lift can be performed by several techniques mentioned in **Table 1**.[6,7]

The goal of forehead rejuvenation is to elevate the brows and to address glabellar frown lines by weakening the corrugator and procerus muscles. It is best suited for brows with mild-to-moderate ptosis of up to 1.5 cm.[6]

Surgical Technique

Preoperative marking is done with the patient in an upright position for placement of temporal and paramedian incisions. Lidocaine 1% and epinephrine 1:100,000 are locally injected at the incision sites and supraorbital and supratrochlear nerve exits. The forehead and upper midface are injected with tumescent solution to facilitate dissection and reduce bleeding.

One central and paracentral and two temporal incisions are made behind the hairline, to the depth of the periosteum centrally, and deep temporalis fascia laterally. The entire forehead soft-tissue complex is then dissected off the skull in a subperiosteal plane and endoscope-assisted dissection is performed to lyse the periosteal attachments along supraorbital region to allow lifting the eyebrow. The corrugator and procerus muscles can be lysed or sharply dissected. The freed forehead complex is then fixated at a higher position by fixing it to temporalis fascia temporally and to the calvarium centrally.

The endoscopic approach to forehead lift has become a popular method due to improved aesthetics, minimal scarring, decreased healing time, and greater patient satisfaction **(Figs. 7 and 8)**. A described limitation of endoscopic brow lift is the inability to predict the long-term results of forehead elevation.

A recently introduced technique is gliding brow lift in which the brow gets elevated without raising the forehead's height.[1,9] The procedure involves only two small 3 mm scalp

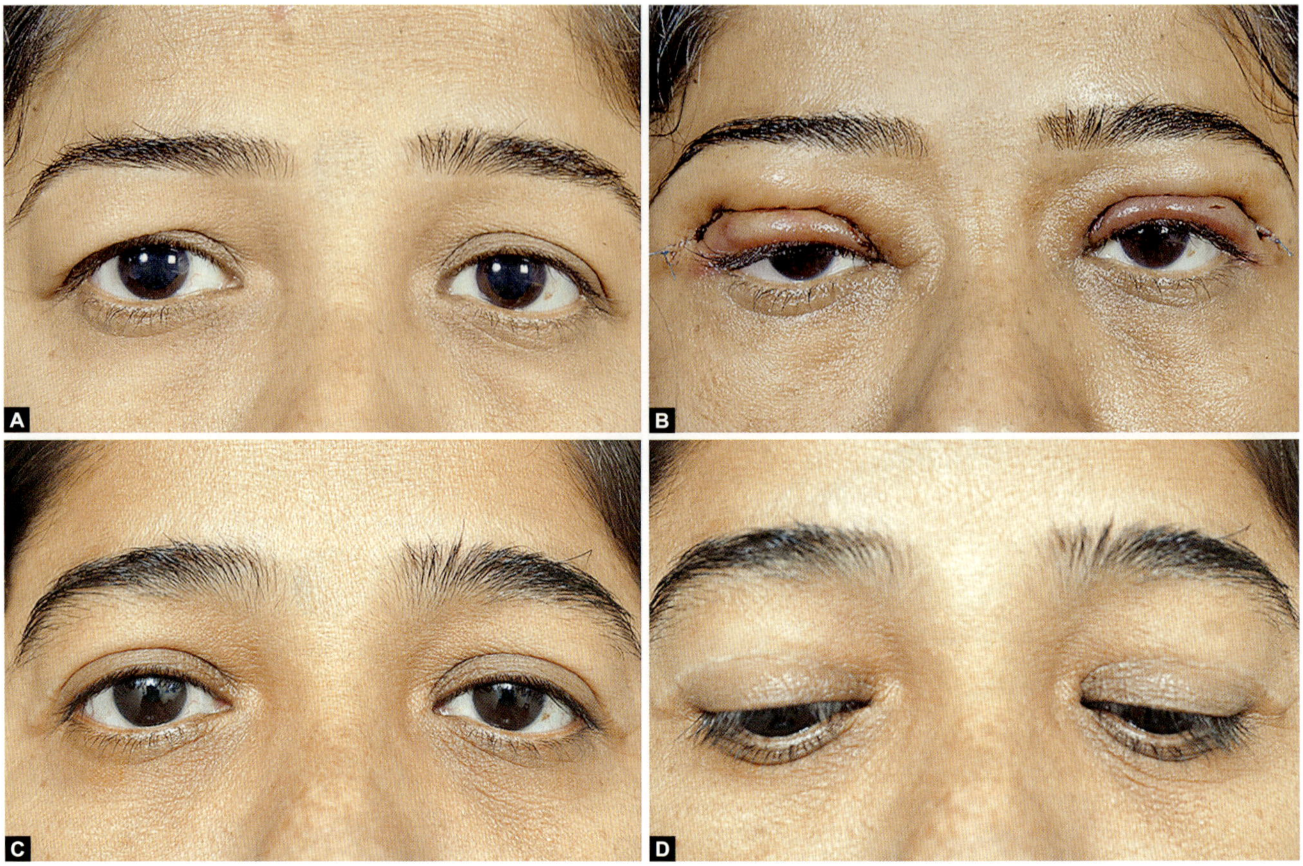

Figs. 4A to D: Upper eyelid blepharoplasty for dermatochalasis. (A) Preoperative appearance; (B) Day-1 postoperative, with upper eyelid edema; (C) Three months postoperative appearance showing symmetrical eyelid crease; (D) A barely visible scar hidden in the eyelid fold.

incisions in the frontotemporal area. Undermining is done directly above the frontalis and galea till 1 cm below the eyebrows followed by lifting a plane of subcutaneous tissue and then suturing to the frontalis and galea via a hemostatic net which maintains brow elevation. Gliding brow lift is gaining superiority as chances of scarring are minimal.[1]

Ptosis Surgery

Blepharoptosis means drooping of the upper eyelid and it can be either congenital or acquired. Both pose a cosmetic blemish to the patient and acquired aponeurotic ptosis is often a common aging change leading to sleepy or droopy eyes.

Indications

Adult ptosis surgery is almost always indicated for cosmetic reasons, though it also adds to the functional value by improving the superior field of vision.

Preoperative Evaluation

Ptosis results from suboptimal functioning of the levator palpebrae superioris muscle. The cause of ptosis can be diagnosed by an accurate history, duration, progress, and clinical evaluation. Assessment of ptosis includes measurement of the amount of ptosis using the margin reflex distance (MRD_1), the levator function, skin crease level from the lid margin, ocular movements, and Bell's phenomenon and the vision. Check for jaw-winking phenomenon and rule out myasthenia gravis when myogenic cause is suspected.

Surgical Technique

The surgical technique of ptosis correction entirely depends upon the residual levator muscle action. Mild ptosis can be corrected by Müllerectomy surgery **(Figs. 9A to D)** that tightens the posterior eyelid lamina (conjunctiva and Müller's muscle) to predictably raise the eyelid. Moderate ptosis requires anterior approach levator resection surgery **(Figs. 9A to D)** performed through an eyelid-crease incision. Severe ptosis requires a sling surgery, where the ptotic eyelid is connected to the frontalis muscle, thereby lifting the eyelid.

MIDFACE

The midface lies between the lateral canthal angle and the top of the nasolabial fold. It includes the medial and lateral canthal tendon, lower eyelids, suborbicularis oculi fat (SOOF), malar fat pad, orbitomalar ligament, orbital septum, and origins of the zygomaticus major and minor muscles and levator labii superioris.

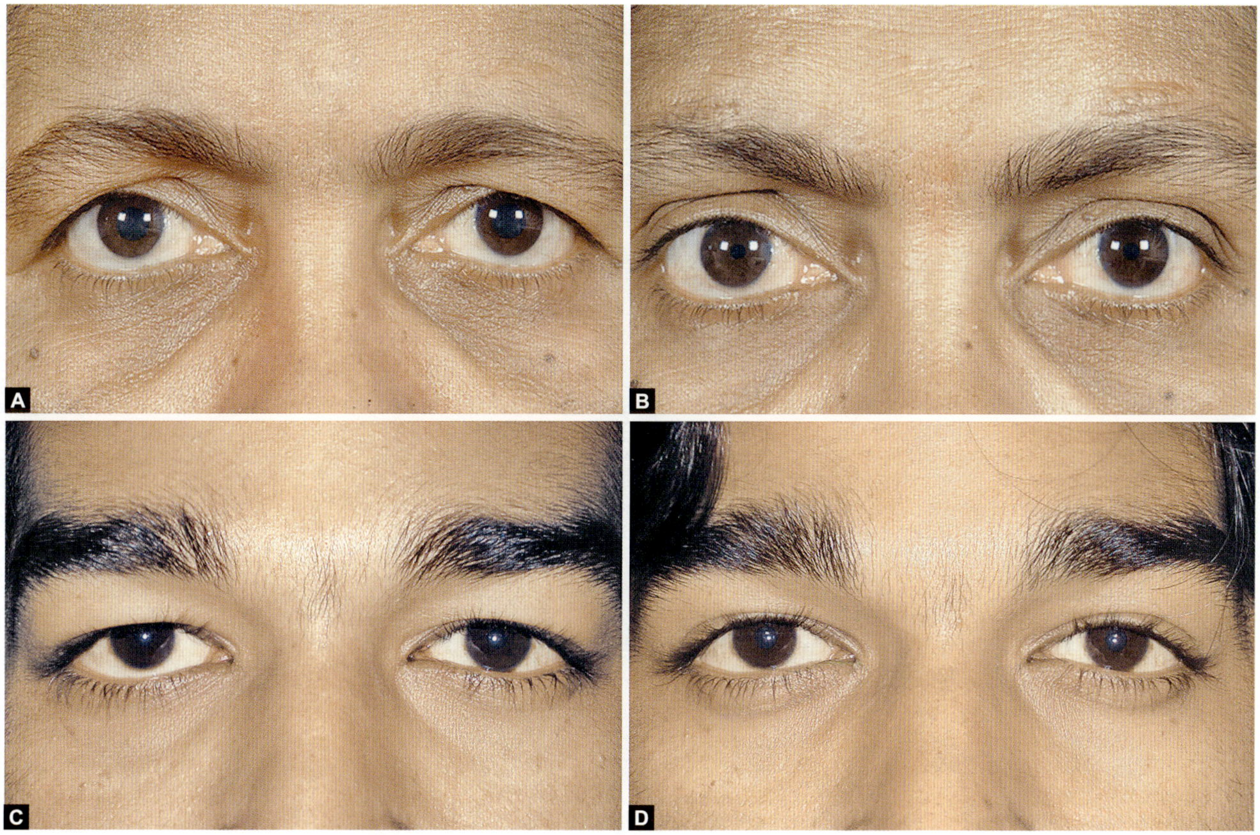

Figs. 5A to D: (A and B) Pre- and postoperative photographs following upper eyelid blepharoplasty combined with external brow lift; (C and D) Upper eyelid blepharoplasty combined with retro-orbicularis oculi fat (ROOF) excision.
Source: Adapted from Naik MN, Honavar SG, Das S, Desai S, Dhepe N. Blepharoplasty: an overview. J Cutan Aesthet Surg. 2009;2:6-11.

Volumetric distribution of the midface soft tissues is an important factor in the youthful appearance of the human face. If these tissues are full relative to the lower face, the individual appears healthy and young.[10]

The most common aesthetic procedures in the midface include lower eyelid blepharoplasty, lower lid fat repositioning, midface lift, and volume augmentation of lower eyelid hollows (fillers/fat).

Assessment of the Lower Eyelid and Midface Region

Lower eyelids should be assessed for skin excess and fat herniation. Fat bags should be differentiated from fluid festoons, since the management is entirely different. Fat prolapse typically presents as medial, central, and lateral fat pads; it is limited inferiorly by the orbital rim and becomes more prominent in upgaze and less prominent in downgaze **(Figs. 10A to D)**. Fluid festoons, on the other hand, are primarily within the skin, not restricted by the orbital margin and are not compartmentalized. Downward displacement of the lateral canthus is an aging change. Orbital rim hollow (tear trough deformity), though an aging sign, can also be found to be significant in young adults **(Figs. 10A to D)**. Another typical aging change in the lower eyelid midface region is the appearance of a double bubble—lower eyelid fat bag (hill), followed by a prominent orbital rim hollow (valley). Prominent or deep-set eyes should be documented with exophthalmometry. Malar anatomy should be evaluated for periorbital hollows **(Figs. 10A to D)**.

Aging can lead to a number of aesthetic changes in the lower eyelid including laxity of the skin, orbicularis or orbital septum, orbital fat prolapse (eyelid bags), canthal laxity, malar festoons, and periocular wrinkles and pigmentation.[6] Lower eyelid rejuvenation is more complex and has several treatment options such as fillers, blepharoplasty, and skin resurfacing. Most cosmetic surgeons today have developed a customized approach to eyelid surgery in which the specific anatomic problems are identified and the operation is individualized to address these problems.

Lower Eyelid Blepharoplasty

The approach to the lower eyelid remains a controversial issue within plastic surgery. The transconjunctival approach is preferred because it leaves no external scar and reduces the chance of eyelid retraction, scleral show, and postoperative ectropion than other methods.[1,11-14]

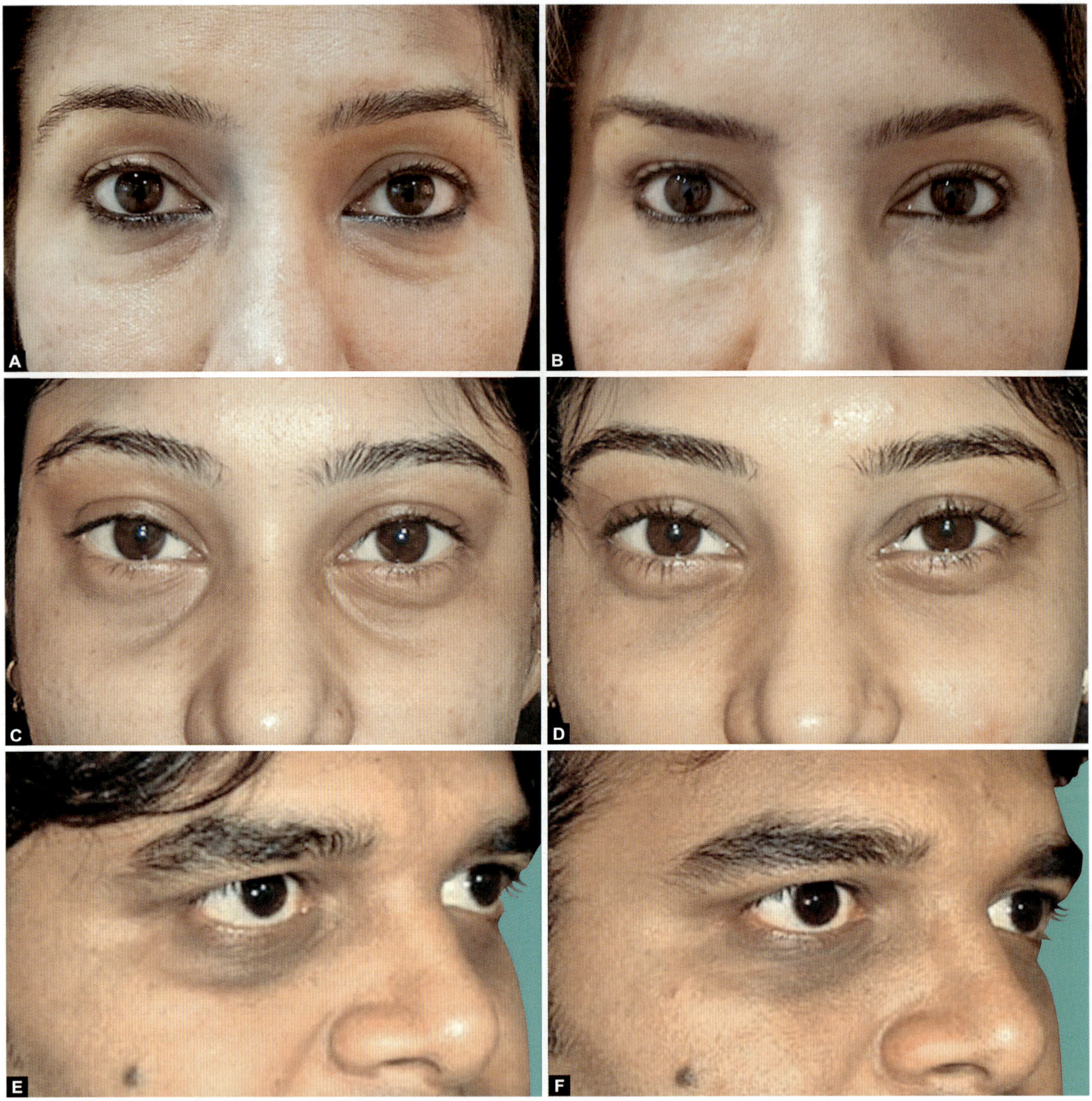

Figs. 6A to F: (A and B) Brow volume augmentation with hyaluronic acid filler. Note the loss of brow volume (A), which when adequately filled, eliminates the overhanging skin and gives a fuller eyebrow with convex contours (B). A tear trough filler was also performed, along with chemodenervation of the forehead to reshape the eyebrow; (C and D) Orbital rim hollow (tear trough deformity) is another common indication for periorbital filling with hyaluronic acid or autologous fat; (E and F) Undereye hollow filled with autologous fat transfer. The under eye pigmentation that is caused by shadowing effect has significantly improved just by filling the tear trough.

TABLE 1: Brow lift techniques.

Procedure	*Surgical principle*
Direct brow lift	Skin above the eyebrow is excised to lift the brow[8]
Pretrichial brow lift	Reduction in vertical height of forehead by excising skin just in front of the forehead hairline
Internal brow pexy	Fixation of the brow to the supraorbital periosteum through a transblepharoplasty incision
Coronal brow lift	Excision of a part of coronal scalp so as to raise the eyebrow and forehead

Transconjunctival approach is also preferred in men undergoing lower lid blepharoplasty as they desire correction in deep palpebromalar groove and tear trough deformity.[15,16] The transcutaneous approach is preferred only if there is excess skin that requires excision.[17]

Surgical Procedure

For transconjunctival lower lid blepharoplasty, the inferior fornix, eyelid skin, and lateral canthus are anesthetized with

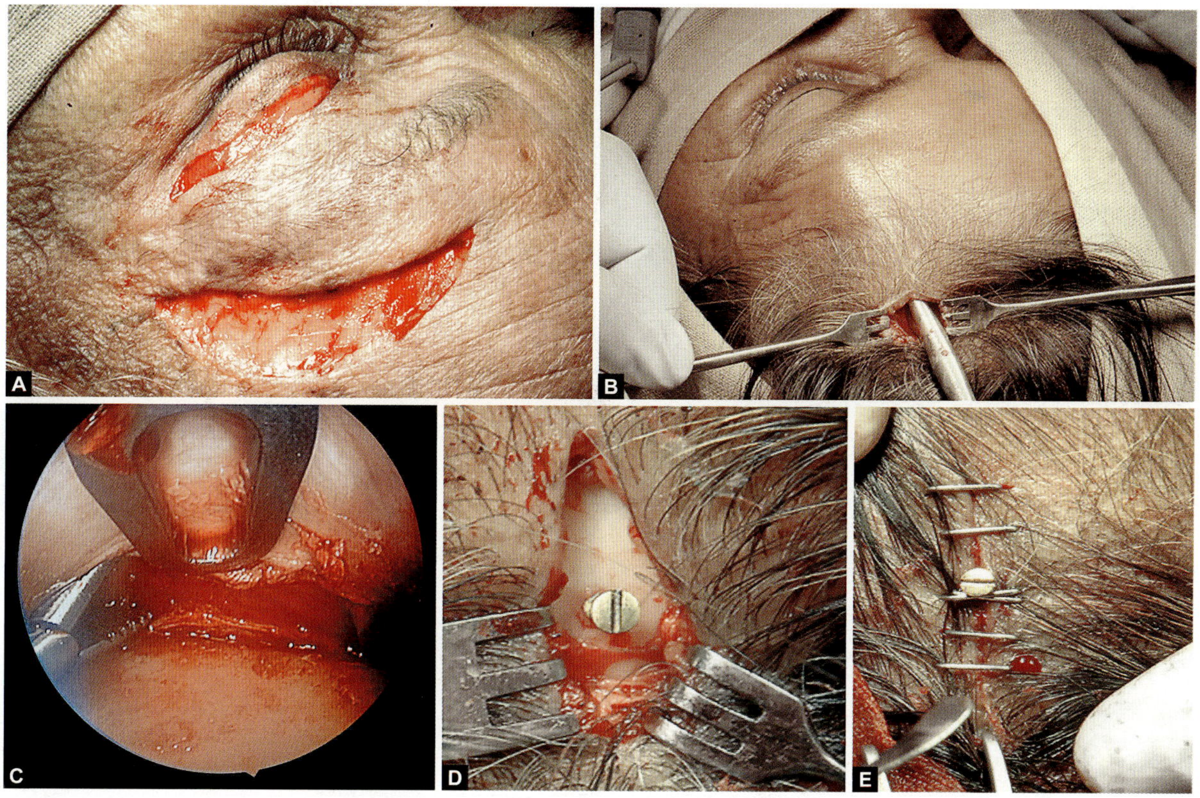

Figs. 7A to E: Techniques of surgical brow lift. External brow lift (surgeon's view) showing: (A) Excision of forehead skin above the temporal half of the eyebrow; (B) Endoscopic brow lift showing the forehead dissection through a stab incision in the scalp; (C) Endoscopic view of the supraorbital periosteum that is released; (D) Calvarial fixation with titanium screws within the parasagittal scalp incisions; and (E) Finally, fixation of the entire forehead–brow complex at a higher position on the skull using staples.

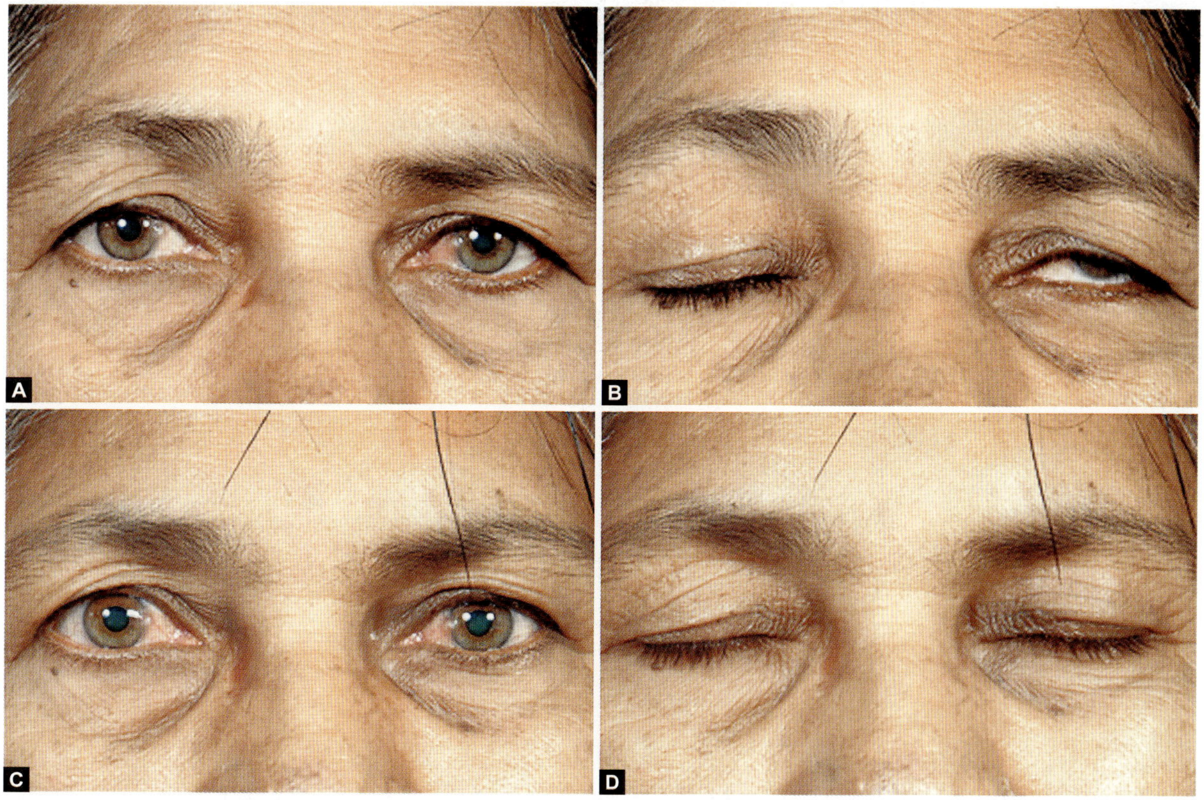

Figs. 8A to D: (A) Patient with left facial palsy showing left brow ptosis; (B) Lagophthalmos; (C) Corrected by endoscopic brow lift; and (D) Eyelid gold weight implant.

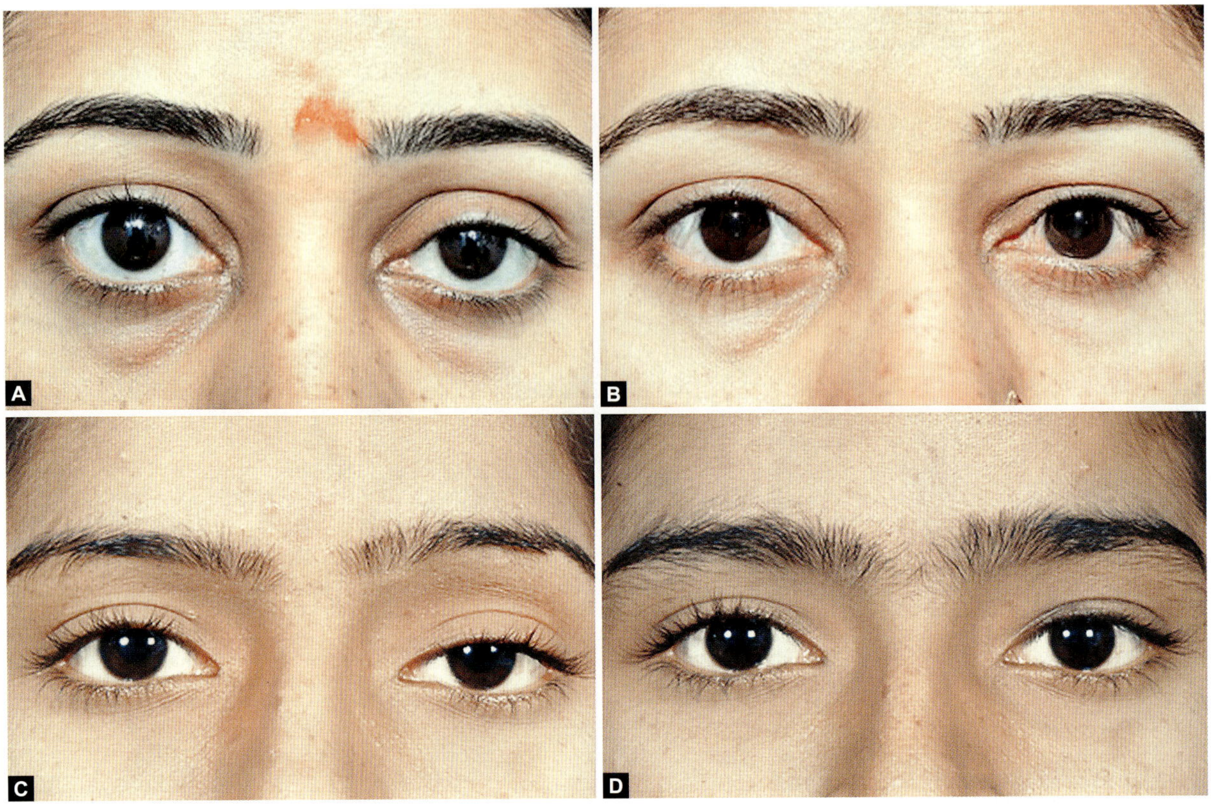

Figs. 9A to D: (A and B) Mild upper eyelid ptosis (aponeurotic) corrected by Müllerectomy surgery that leaves no cutaneous scar; and (C and D) Moderate congenital ptosis corrected by anterior approach levator resection surgery, where the scar is hidden inside the eyelid fold.

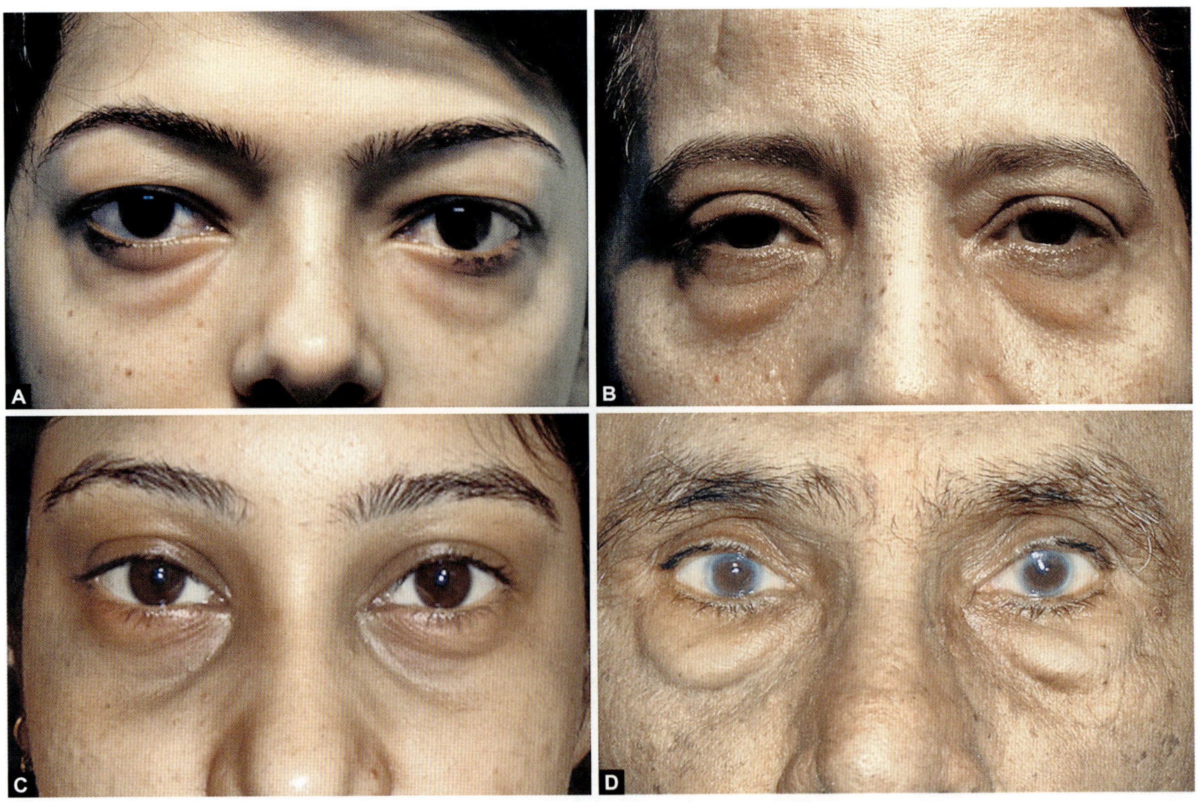

Figs. 10A to D: Typical aging changes in the lower eyelid and midface region. (A) Lower eyelid fat prolapse (fat bags) is compartmentalized into lateral, central, and medial; (B) Fluid festoons look similar to fat bags but need to be differentiated; (C) Lower eyelid tear trough (orbital rim hollow) can also appear in young patients; and (D) A double-bubble appearance needs a fatrepositioning procedure.

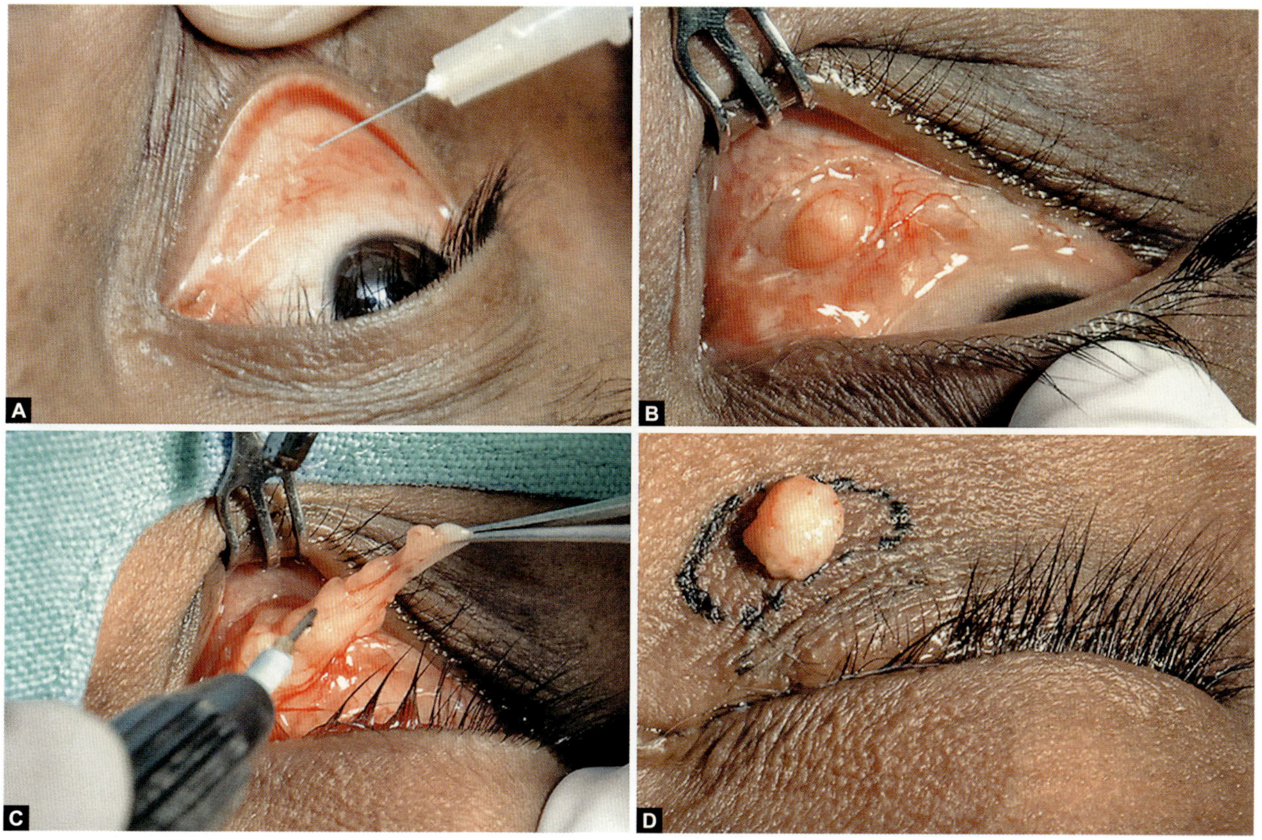

Figs. 11A to D: Transconjunctival blepharoplasty (surgeon's view). (A) Injection of local anesthetic into the inferior conjunctival fornix; (B) Forniceal incision to expose orbital fat; (C) Conservative fat excision with radiofrequency monopolar tip; and (D) Assessment of contours on table.
Source: Adapted from Naik MN, Honavar SG, Das S, Desai S, Dhepe N. Blepharoplasty: an overview. J Cutan Aesthet Surg. 2009;2:6-11.

1% lidocaine containing 1:100,000 epinephrine **(Figs. 11A to D)**. Surgery is performed through an incision made 4–6 mm below the lid margin through the conjunctiva and lower eyelid retractors with a radiofrequency monopolar cautery or CO_2 laser. Gentle pressure on the eyeball prolapses the fat compartments and aids in identification of the medial, central, and lateral fat pads. Conservative fat removal is achieved using radiofrequency monopolar or bipolar cautery. The tarsoconjunctival incision is left to heal by epithelization without any sutures. Excellent aesthetic outcome is achieved in most cases **(Figs. 12A to D)**.

Some surgeons perform lateral canthopexy along with lower eyelid blepharoplasty. It eliminates unnecessary skin resection and is believed to restore tone and youthful contour of the lower eyelid.[6,14,18]

Wrinkles and excess of vertical skin can be dealt with skin resurfacing techniques, such as chemical peeling and fractional laser resurfacing.

Transcutaneous Lower Lid Blepharoplasty

Transcutaneous lower lid blepharoplasty is chosen when excess skin or orbicularis needs to be excised along with the prolapsed fat **(Figs. 13A to D)**. The "skin pinch" technique removes only skin and is ideal for skin laxity alone.[19] The more aggressive "skin-muscle flap" method is also approached through a subciliary incision, undermining the skin and orbicularis. Dissection can be continued along the orbital septum to the level of the orbital rim. Periorbital fat is approached through small incisions in the septum. Orbicularis muscle fibers and skin can be excised at closure; however, damage to the orbicularis may lead to lower lid malposition and orbicularis denervation.

There is an increasing shift in lower blepharoplasty from fat resection to volume redistribution or augmentation through fat transposition or micro- and nanofat grafting.[1]

Lower Eyelid Fat Repositioning

In youth, the eyelid-cheek complex has a single, smooth convex profile. With advancing age, thinning of septum, and receding bony orbital rim, pseudoherniation of intraorbital fat occurs producing a double convex deformity **(Fig. 10D)** of the lower eyelid.[20] Simple removal of orbital fat in this situation can result in a hollow appearance of the lower eyelid.

Preservation of the lower orbital fat is a new concept in facial rejuvenation.[21] Preservation of the fat along with repositioning creates a smooth transition to the malar eminence **(Figs. 14A and B)**, blending nicely into the upper face.[22]

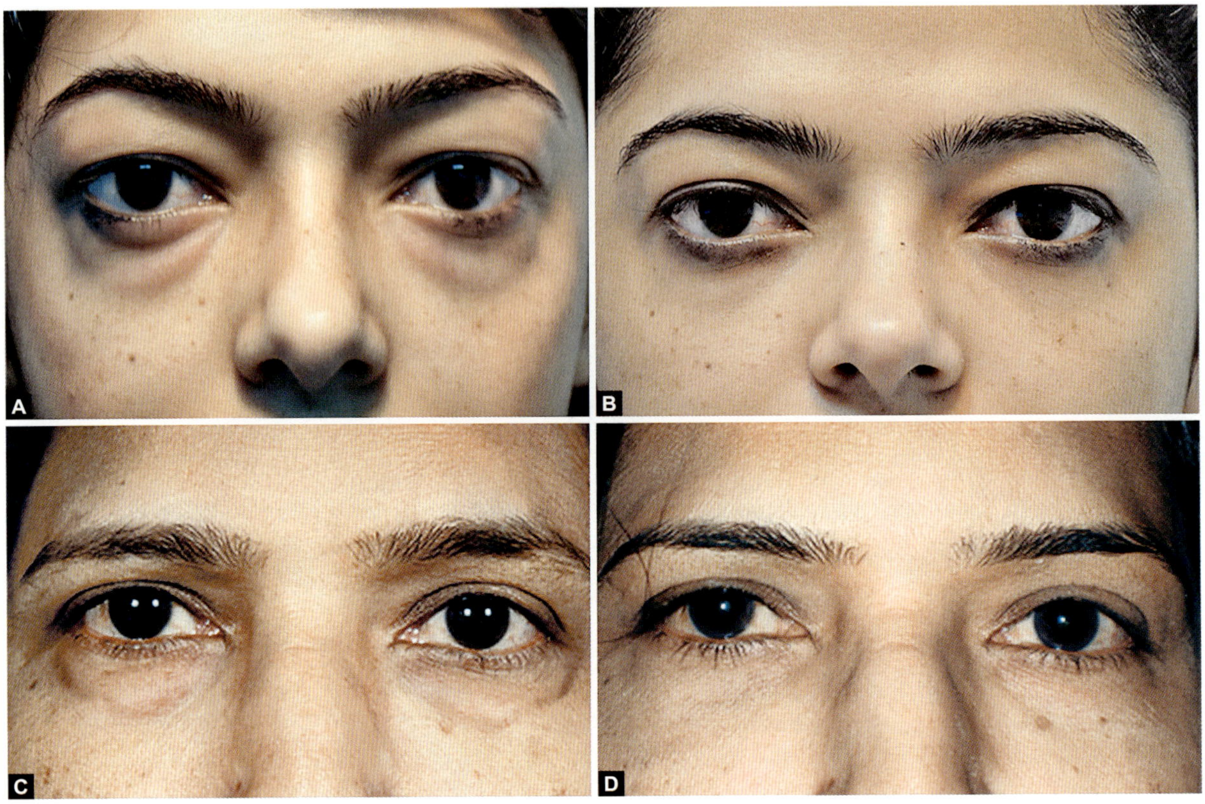

Figs. 12A to D: (A and C) Preoperative; (B and D) Postoperative photographs following transconjunctival lower eyelid blepharoplasty with conservative fat excision. No external scar, no conjunctival sutures, and no scarring of the orbital septum are the advantages of the transconjunctival approach.

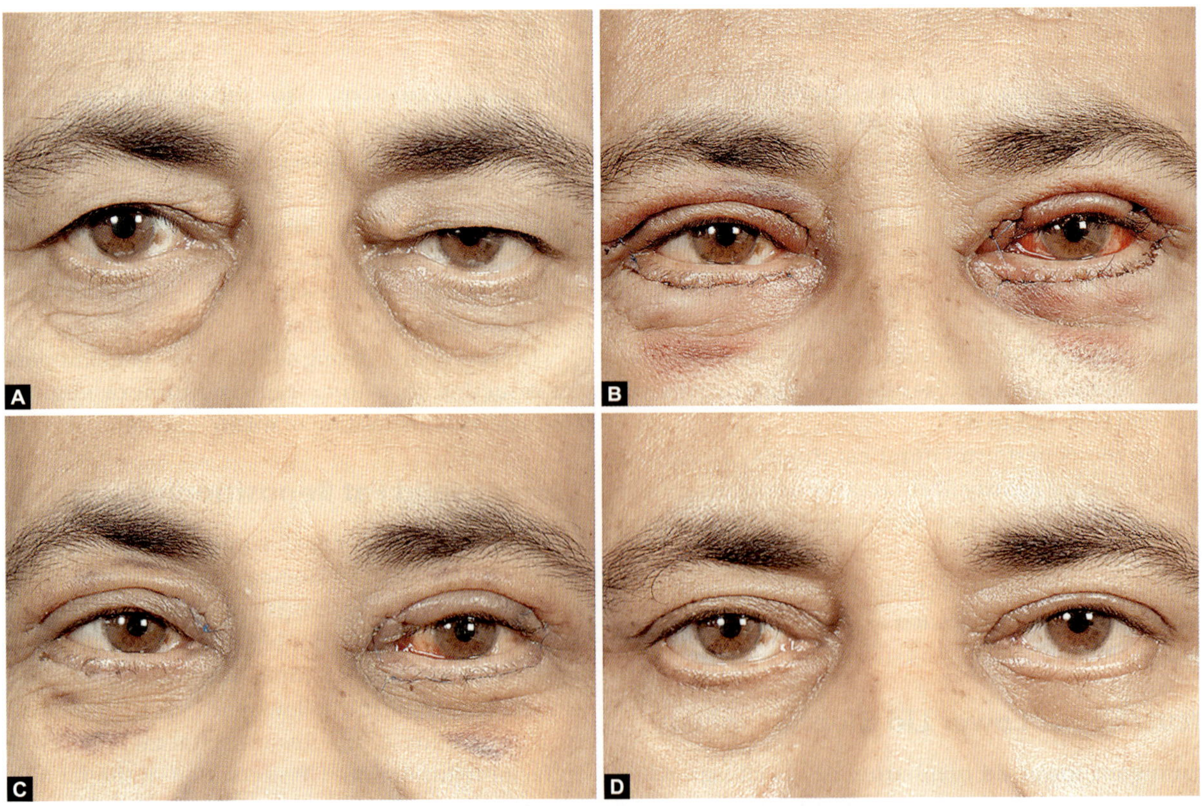

Figs. 13A to D: (A) A middle-aged patient with upper eyelid dermatochalasis, left upper eyelid ptosis, excess lower eyelid skin, and lower lid fat bags. He underwent a transcutaneous blepharoplasty with conservative fat excision and left Müllerectomy for ptosis; (B) Appearance on day 1 postoperative; (C) One week postoperative; and (D) Three months postoperative.

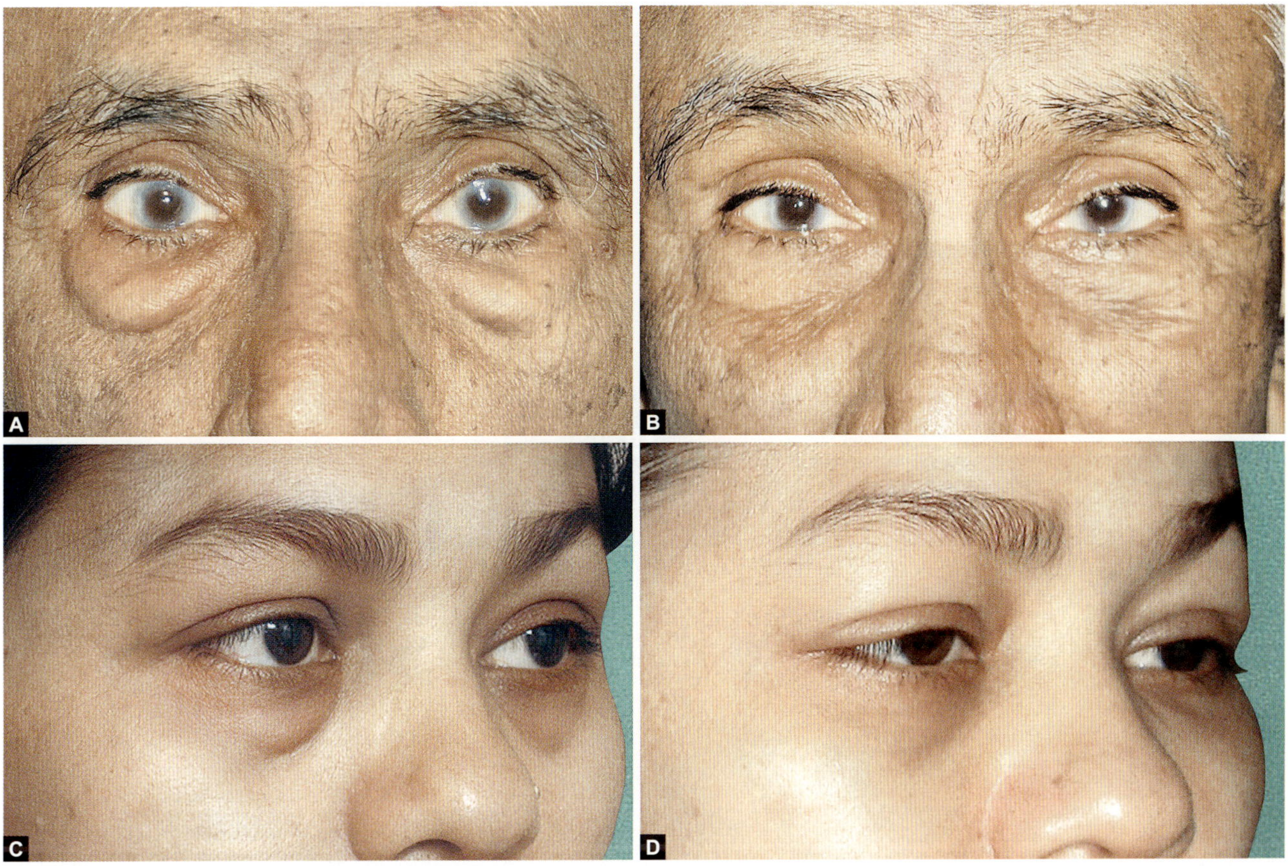

Figs. 14A to D: (A and B) Transconjunctival lower eyelid fat repositioning that eliminates the double-bubble appearance; (C and D) Transconjunctival midface lift that elevates the descended midface soft tissue. Residual tear trough may need hyaluronic acid fillers or an autologous fat transfer.

Surgical Technique

Fat repositioning surgery includes release of the arcus marginalis and advancement of the orbital fat beyond the infraorbital rim underneath the orbicularis muscle with the help of temporary exteriorized sutures. The fat can be placed either in the subperiosteal or supraperiosteal plane, with no apparent effect on aesthetic results. This technique camouflages the lower orbital rim anatomy and provides more youthful rejuvenation of the midface.[20,22,23]

There is risk of injury to blood vessels in supraperiosteal plane of dissection and inefficient release of orbicularis retaining ligament (ORL), tear trough, and lid cheek junction in subperiosteal plane. Therefore, a newer approach of using midcheek spaces for lower eyelid fat repositioning has evolved,[24] which results in an enhanced cosmetic outcome particularly in patients who require lid fat repositioning in combination with midface rejuvenation.[25]

Other methods suggested to correct tear trough deformity include orbital fat removal, fat injections or grafts, and alloplastic cheek implants. In general, transconjunctival fat repositioning results in leveling of the tear trough deformity, a smooth contour of the lower eyelid, and high patient satisfaction.[26]

Midface Lift

Aesthetically, the goal of midface lift is to achieve facial rejuvenation by increasing malar fullness and reduce the "skeletonized" appearance of the inferior orbital rim **(Figs. 14C and D)**. It also reduces the prominence of the nasolabial and nasojugal (tear trough) folds.[27] Functional indications for midface lift include lower eyelid retraction secondary to lower blepharoplasty and cicatricial ectropion.[28]

Surgical Technique

In patients with tear trough deformity, transconjunctival approach is adequate and yields good aesthetic results. For correction of mild midface descent, a preperiosteal dissection is extended along inferior orbital rim, beyond the inferior margin of the tear trough deformity. Anchoring sutures from the SOOF pad to the periosteum of the infraorbital rim are placed along the horizontal extent of the deformity. The conjunctival incision is then closed.

When a more robust midface suspension necessitates freeing of the cheek soft tissue, from the skin anteriorly and the bone posteriorly. Incisions are made at the temporal scalp, inferior conjunctiva, and alveolar oral mucosa. Dissection is aimed at creating a temporal pocket, mobilizing the midface by

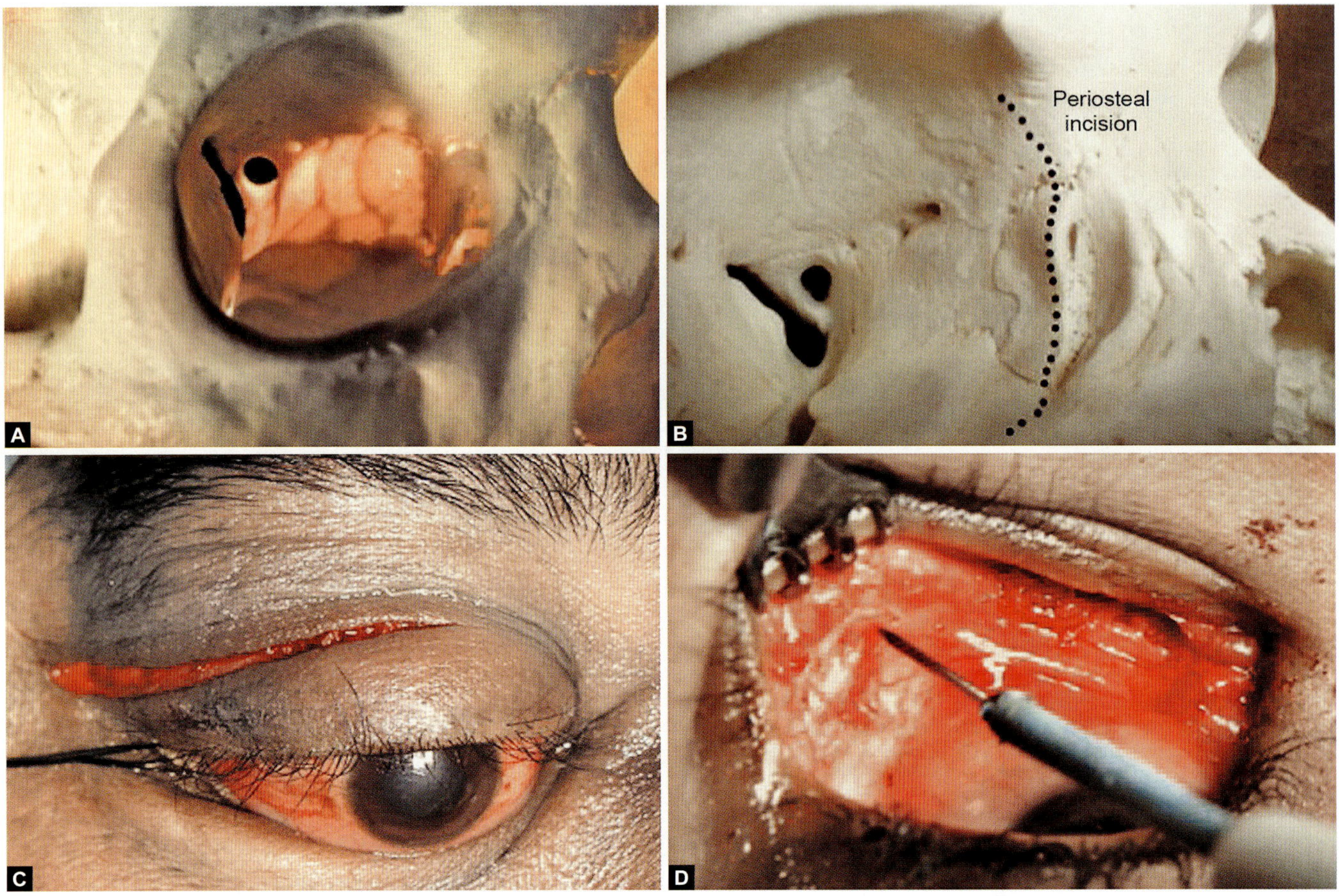

Figs. 15A to D: (A) Minimally invasive techniques of orbital decompression target the ethmoidal air cells medially (B) via transcaruncular incision; (C) The lateral orbital wall is approached through an eyelid–crease incision; and (D) the orbital floor through inferior transconjunctival incision to achieve orbital decompression through hidden incisions.

subperiosteal dissection and lifting the mobilized face toward the deep temporalis fascia while securing the SOOF pad to the inferior orbital rim.[29]

Orbital Decompression for Prominent Eyes

Prominent eyes (proptosis) can be a cosmetic blemish and is seen in high myopias as a familial trait or as a sequel of thyroid eye disease. Decompression surgery involves removal of excessive fat from behind the eye or widening the bony orbit. This allows the prominent eyes to relax back into the socket, giving a more natural look.

Minimally invasive orbital decompression surgery is performed through incisions hidden within the upper eyelid crease, inferior conjunctival fornix, or transcaruncular approach.

Essentially, there are three orbital walls available for decompression—medial, inferior, and lateral wall. Today, all three walls can be reached via orbital approach by an ophthalmic plastic surgeon trained in orbital surgery. The medial wall and the floor can be accessed through hidden conjunctival incisions, including the transcaruncular incision.[30]

The deep lateral wall (sphenoid bone) can be accessed through an orbital approach with substantially less morbidity compared to an open craniotomy.

Removing orbital fat is a major technical change in orbital decompression. For many surgeons, removal of intraconal fat is the "first wall" of orbital decompression. Typically, decompression begins with orbital fat removal and removal of bony wall is added if required as the deep lateral wall, medial wall, and floor in that order **(Figs. 15 and 16)**.

CONCLUSION

The periocular region is the first to reveal aging changes on the face. The upper face and midface can be significantly improved by minimally invasive procedures. In practice, the rejuvenation of this complex anatomical area requires a combination of therapies including fat excision, repositioning or transfer, simultaneous brow or midface lift, and adjunctive treatment for skin resurfacing and periorbital hollows.

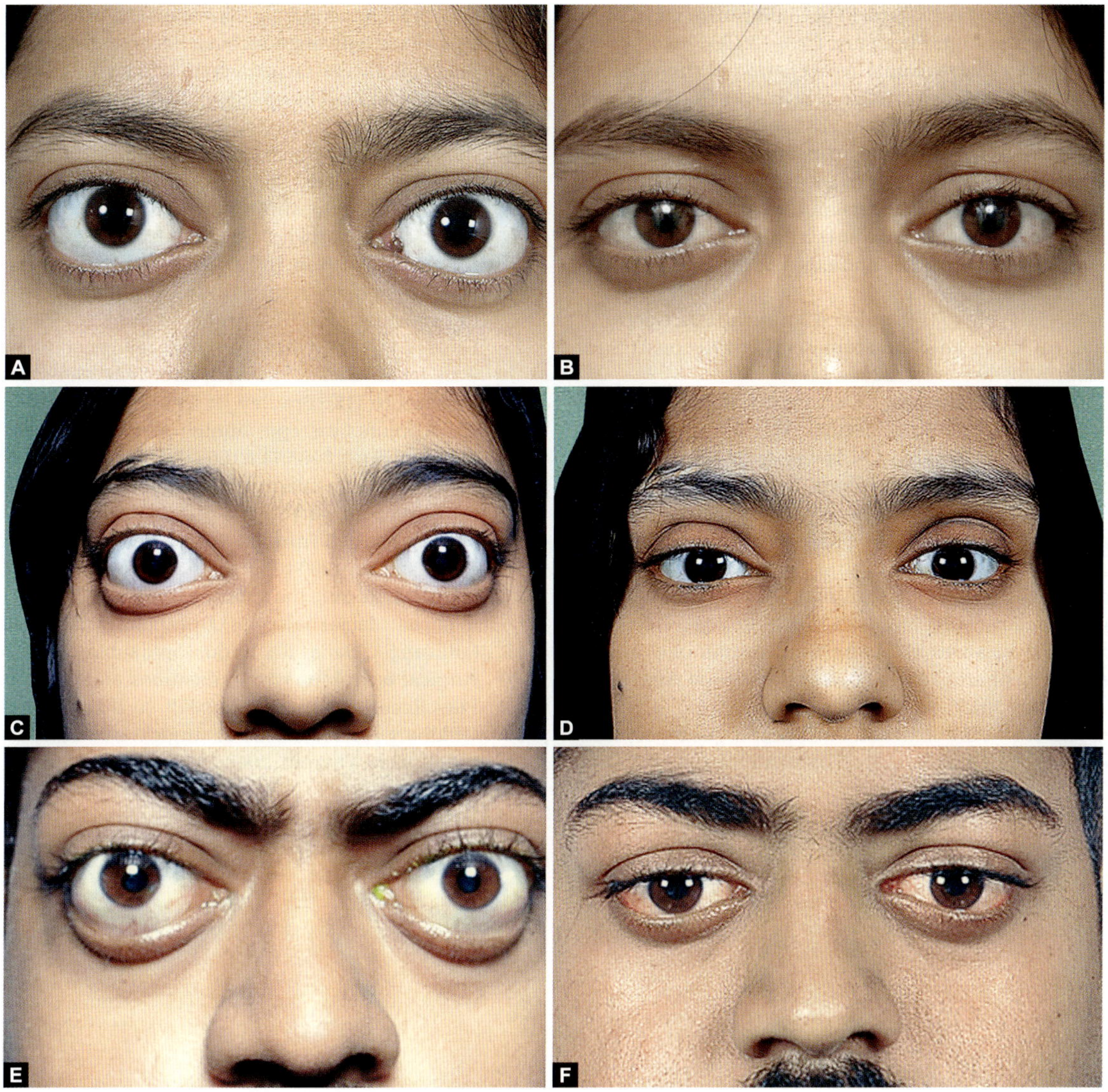

Figs. 16A to F: Pre- and postoperative photographs of orbital decompression for (A and B) Mild; (C and D) Moderate; and (E and F) Severe prominence of the eyes secondary to thyroid eye disease. Extent of decompression (fat and bony walls) depends upon the extent of prominence of the eyeballs and is performed through hidden conjunctival incisions.

TIPS

Tips for periocular injectables and periocular surgery.

Periocular injectables:

- Use pinch technique to avoid bleeders
- Inject away from orbital rim to prevent ptosis
- *Fillers:* Inject slowly and use cannulas

Periocular surgery:

- Use of hyaluronidase with local anesthesia
- Hide incisions within the eyelid crease for better cosmetic results
- Be conservative in removal of fat
- Use deep injections for autologous fat transfer
- In upper eyelid blepharoplasty, use deep periosteal (brassiere) sutures to recreate brow volume

REFERENCES

1. Kuruoglu D, Salinas CA, Kirk DS, Wong C, Sharaf BA. Brow and eyelid rejuvenation: trends from the 100 most cited articles over 30 years. Medicina. 2023;59:230.
2. Asaad M, Kelarji AB, Jawhar CS, Banuelos J, Taslakian E, Wahood W, et al. Eyebrow height changes with aging: a systematic review and meta-analysis. Plast Reconstr Surg Glob Open. 2019;7:e2433.
3. Castro E, Foster JA. Upper lid blepharoplasty. Facial Plast Surg. 1999;15:173-81.
4. Jacono AA, Moskowitz B. Transconjunctival versus transcutaneous approach in upper and lower blepharoplasty. Facial Plast Surg. 2001;17:21-8.
5. Lewis CD, Perry JD. A paradigm shift: volume augmentation or 'inflation' to obtain optimal cosmetic results. Curr Opin Ophthalmol. 2009;20:389-94.
6. Ben Simon GJ, McCann JD. Cosmetic eyelid and facial surgery. Surv Ophthalmol. 2008;53:426-42.
7. Karimi N, Kashkouli MB, Sianati H, Khademi B. Techniques of eyebrow lifting: a narrative review. J Ophthalmic Vis Res. 2020;15:218-35.
8. Perry JD, Hwang CJ. Direct Browlift. Clin Plast Surg. 2022; 49:409-14.

9. Viterbo F, Auersvald A, O'Daniel TG. Gliding brow lift (GBL): a new concept. Aesthetic Plast Surg. 2019;43:1536-46.
10. Little JW. Three-dimensional rejuvenation of the midface: volumetric resculpture by malar imbrication. Plast Reconstr Surg. 2000;105:267-85; discussion 286-9.
11. Rizk SS, Matarasso A. Lower eyelid blepharoplasty: analysis of indications and the treatment of 100 patients. Plast Reconstr Surg. 2003;111:1299-306; discussion 1307-8.
12. Zarem HA, Resnick JI. Minimizing deformity in lower blepharoplasty. The transconjunctival approach. Clin Plast Surg. 1993;20:317-21.
13. Zarem HA, Resnick JI. Expanded applications for transconjunctival lower lid blepharoplasty. Plast Reconstr Surg. 1991;88:215-20; discussion 221.
14. Flowers RS. Canthopexy as a routine blepharoplasty component. Clin Plast Surg. 1993;20:351-65.
15. Rostami S, de la Torre JI, Czyz CN. Lower Eyelid Blepharoplasty. In: StatPearls [Internet]. Treasure Island (FL): StatPearls Publishing; 2024.
16. Rao V, Sullivan PK. Lower lid blepharoplasty in men. Clin Plast Surg. 2022;49:213-20.
17. Adamson PA, Strecker HD. Transcutaneous lower blepharoplasty. Facial Plast Surg. 1996;12:171-83.
18. Honrado CP, Pastorek NJ. Long-term results of lower-lid suspension blepharoplasty: a 30-year experience. Arch Facial Plast Surg. 2004;6:150-4.
19. Parkes M, Fein W, Brennan HG. Pinch technique for repair of cosmetic eyelid deformities. Arch Ophthalmol. 1973;89:324-8.
20. Hamra ST. Arcus marginalis release and orbital fat preservation in midface rejuvenation. Plast Reconstr Surg. 1995;96:354-62.
21. Baker SR. Orbital fat preservation in lower-lid blepharoplasty. Arch Facial Plast Surg. 1999;1:33-7.
22. Goldberg RA. Transconjunctival orbital fat repositioning: transposition of orbital fat pedicles into a subperiosteal pocket. Plast Reconstr Surg. 2000;105:743-8; discussion 749-51.
23. Loeb R. Fat pad sliding and fat grafting for leveling lid depressions. Clin Plast Surg. 1981;8:757-76.
24. Jin Y, Gao W, Teo HMT, Lin X. Transconjunctival lower blepharoplasty using midcheek spaces for orbital fat transposition (S.O.F.T.). Ann Plast Surg. 2021;86:620-6.
25. Liao HT. Lower eyelid and midface rejuvenation: suborbicularis oculi fat lift. Facial Plast Surg Clin. 2021;29:497-509.
26. Kawamoto HK, Bradley JP. The tear "TROUF" procedure: transconjunctival repositioning of orbital unipedicled fat. Plast Reconstr Surg. 2003;112:1903-7; discussion 1908-9.
27. Patipa M. Transblepharoplasty lower eyelid and mid-face rejuvenation: part I. Avoiding complications by utilizing lessons learned from the treatment of complications. Plast Reconstr Surg. 2004;113:1459-68; discussion 1475-7.
28. Olver JM. Raising the suborbicularis oculi fat (SOOF): its role in chronic facial palsy. Br J Ophthalmol. 2000;84:1401-6.
29. Sullivan SA, Dailey RA. Endoscopic subperiosteal midface lift: surgical technique with indications and outcomes. Ophthal Plast Reconstr Surg. 2002;18:319-30; discussion 329-30.
30. Goldberg RA. Advances in surgical rehabilitation in thyroid eye disease. Thyroid. 2008;18:989-95.

CHAPTER 54

Dermatologic Surgery of the Lips

R Raghunatha Reddy, Shashikumar BM, Savitha AS

KEY MESSAGES

- The vermilion border is a very important structure for aesthetic appearance of lips and it should not be distorted during procedures.
- Incisions should be vertical all around except at the commissures.
- Dehiscence and notching of the lip can occur because of the high mobility of the area. If this occurs, conservative management may be all that is necessary; notch formation will require surgical revision.
- Lip contracture with elevation of the vermilion border may require a Z-plasty.

INTRODUCTION

The lips are graceful structures that symmetrically occupy the lower third of the facial profile. Lips represent the anterior border of the mouth. The skin of the lips contains hair, sebaceous glands, and eccrine glands. In the male, the skin of upper lip and central portion of the lower lip are hair bearing. The vermilion border is the mucocutaneous junction between the skin and the dry mucosa of lip; lips are red in color because of lack of keratinization and the proximity of underlying capillary plexus to skin **(Fig. 1)**. In males, the entire keratinized upper lip and central lower lip is hair bearing. Sebaceous glands are found in normal vermilion tissue 50% of the time, although no hair follicles are seen. The dry vermilion becomes a wet mucous membrane proximally in the oral cavity. The bulk of the tissue comprising the lips consists of striated muscle, primarily the orbicularis oris. The vasculature of the lips consists mainly of the inferior and superior labial arteries, which are the main branches of the facial artery **(Fig. 2)**.[1]

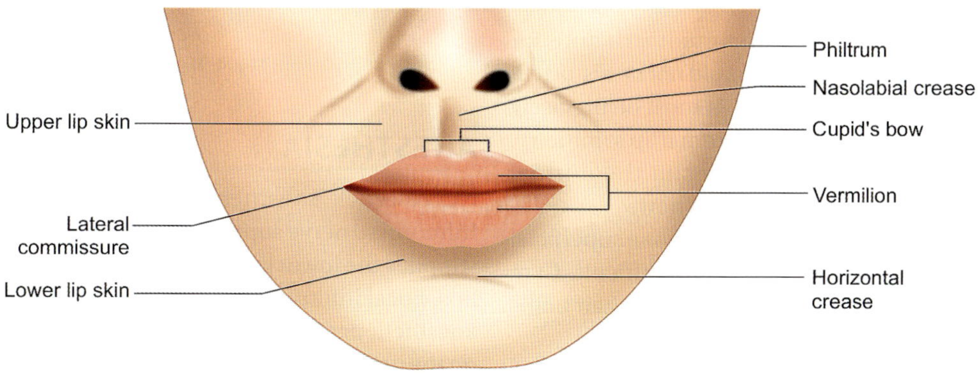

Fig. 1: Lip anatomy.

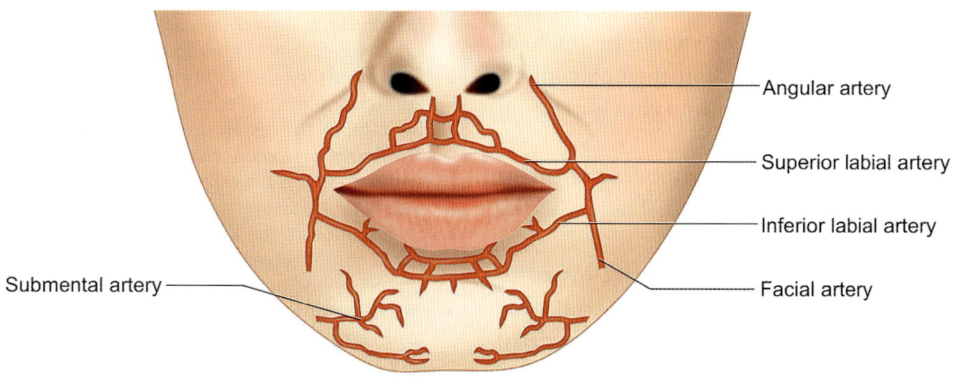

Fig. 2: Blood supply of lip.

TABLE 1: Commonly performed procedures by dermatologists.

Sl. No.	*Conditions*	*Surgical methods*
1.	Lip biopsy	• Diagnostic • Therapeutic
2.	Lip vitiligo	• Mini-punch grafting • Suction blister grafts • Simple excision and closure • Ultrathin split skin graft • Mucosal advancement flap • Noncultured epidermal cell suspension
3.	Mucous cyst	• Simple excision • Radiofrequency • Deroofing and removal • Sclerotherapy
4.	Benign lesions, premalignant and malignant lesions	• Simple excision and closure • Shave excision • Flap surgery
5.	Lip enhancement surgery	• Autologous fat graft • Fillers • Dermal graft • Vermilion advancement • Lip implants • Surgical lip lift
6.	Hair transplantation	• *For scars on upper lip:* Post-traumatic or postsurgery cleft lips

Commonly procedures performed by dermatologists are enumerated in **Table 1**. This chapter deals with surgical procedures performed on lips.

PRINCIPLES OF PROCEDURES

- The vermilion border is a very important structure for aesthetic appearance of lips and it should not be distorted. In an inevitable situation, if violated, it must be precisely reconstructed surgically to preserve normal lip symmetry. Every attempt should be made to retain the normal contours, with the philtrum and Cupid's bow.
- Undermining in the philtral area has to be done superficial to underlying muscle, and may be more difficult. Care should be taken to avoid damage to subdermal hair bulbs in male patients.
- Incisions around lips should follow skin tension lines. Incisions should be vertical all around except at the commissures. **Figure 3** illustrates the relaxed skin tension lines (RSTLs) over the face. Incisions should be made at the junction of natural boundaries to hide their placement (i.e., vermilion border, nasolabial fold, and chin horizontal crease).
- Defects involving up to one-third of the upper or lower lip can be closed primarily in a layered fashion. Larger defects may require local or pedicle flap closure.
- Nonirritating suture materials are preferred over the mucosa. A comparative study of suture material over mucosa showed faster wound healing with polyglactin 910 (Vicryl Rapide®) compared to polyglycolic acid and catgut.[2]

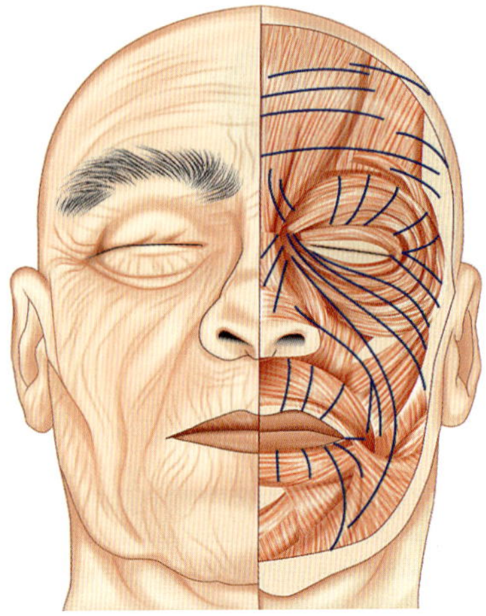

Fig. 3: Relaxed skin tension lines around the lips.

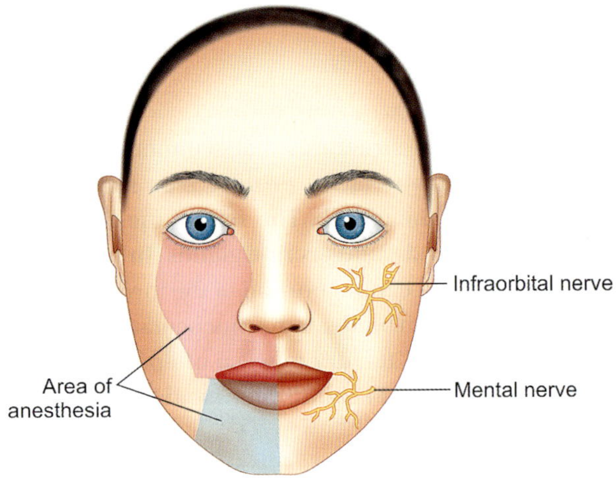

Fig. 4: Nerve supply of lip.

ANESTHESIA

Nerve block anesthesia is better tolerated by patients. Infraorbital nerve supplies the upper lip and the mental nerve supplies the lower lip. **Figure 4** illustrates the nerve supply of lips. Local infiltration of either local anesthetic or tumescent anesthetic agent may then be added for hemostasis. For details on the nerve blocks, please refer to the chapter "Nerve Blocks".

TIPS

- Marking lip margins with marker pen, methylene blue, 7-0 silk suture, or with scalpel nicks prior to administering local anesthesia can help to identify the border during closure.
- For excision of smaller lesions, use of chalazion ring forceps helps to stabilize the lesion on the lip/tongue during biopsy/excision. The ring of the forceps also helps to achieve circumferential pressure and hemostasis providing a bloodless field during surgery. As the instrument is self-retaining, need of the assistant is eliminated.
- Stabilization of the lip may also be achieved with dental rolls (or rolled gauze) between the lip and gums, suture ligatures temporarily placed, or instruments like long artery forceps.
- Airway maintenance is of utmost importance both during and after surgical procedures. Postoperative edema may impair the airway.

COMMON PREOPERATIVE AND POSTOPERATIVE INSTRUCTIONS AND CARE

- Rule out any foci of infection at the site of surgery
- Take an informed consent including for photographs
- Lignocaine test dose to be given prior to procedure
- Surgical preparation with povidone-iodine and spirit.

Postoperative Dressing and Care

Dressing is to be applied in layers, first topical antibiotic followed by sterile Vaseline gauze, cotton gauze, and cotton pad in that order **(Figs. 5A and B)**.

Antibiotics and analgesics are prescribed for 5–7 days. Patient is advised liquid diet on the day of procedure followed by soft food to be taken for few days carefully with a spoon and liquids with a straw to prevent wetting of the dressing. Dressing to be changed once in 2–3 days after surgery and may be left open after 7 days depending on the healing. For small lesions of the lip, no dressing is needed.

Dehiscence and notching of the lip can occur because of the high mobility of the area. If this occurs, conservative management may be all that is necessary; notch formation will require surgical revision. Lip contracture with elevation of the vermilion border may require a Z-plasty. In females, the use of lip color may provide the finishing touch to conceal scars and give a more pleasing appearance.

Lip Biopsy

Lip biopsy is performed to identify the histopathology of a visible oral lesion or to assist in the diagnosis of a systemic disorder like Sjögren syndrome (SS) or sarcoidosis. Like any other skin biopsy either a punch biopsy, incisional or excisional biopsy can be performed on the lip with a scalpel. Using a chalazion forceps helps to stabilize the biopsy site as well as helps to achieve hemostasis.

Indications

- Any oral lesion that persists despite removal of any irritative stimulus
- Findings suggestive of malignancy such as red or white discoloration, induration or fixation to deeper tissues, rapid growth, friability, or ulceration
- Submucosal minor salivary gland biopsy should be done if the diagnosis of SS cannot be made by history and serologic testing.

Anesthesia

Lip biopsy is typically done under local anesthesia, using 1% lidocaine with 1:100,000 adrenaline. Topical anesthetic sprays are not usually sufficient for anesthesia in the case of biopsies. Inject the lip at the desired biopsy location using a 27- or 30-gauge needle and a 1- to 3-mL syringe.

Ensure that adequate lighting is available, either by a head mirror, headlight, or surgical light.

Procedure

After surgical preparation, plan and mark the elliptical incision before infiltration. Orientation of the ellipse should take into account the vascular and neural structures in the area, as well as any functional or cosmetic concerns. The incision should be parallel to the long axis of the lip to most easily allow the recommended 3:1 length:width ratio. In large resections, the vermilion of the lip may be reduced or the white roll at the vermilion junction may be retracted. Incisions perpendicular to the long axis cause less of this distortion but may require extension beyond the vermilion

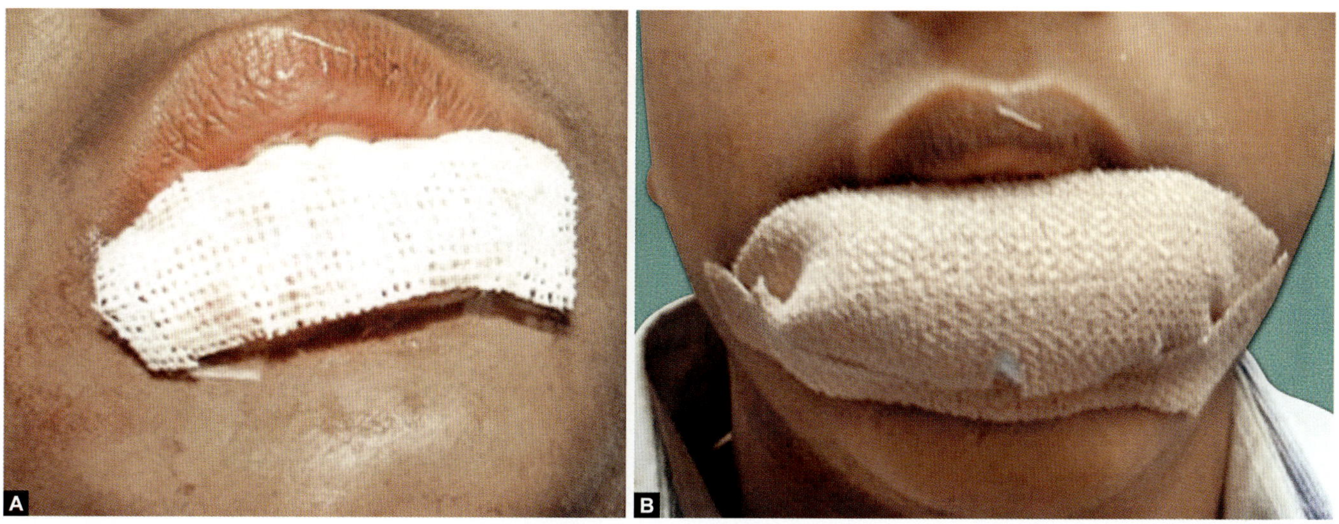

Figs. 5A and B: Postoperative dressing in layers.

border or onto gingival tissue to maintain the 3:1 ratio. After infiltration, the incision is done along the markings. Delicately grasp the edge of the ellipse with fine forceps. Dissect beneath the ellipse with fine sharp scissors. The depth of dissection should be determined by the lesion characteristics. In most mucosal lesions, the plane of dissection is in the layer that contains the minor salivary glands, leaving the orbicularis oris muscle intact. Alternately, a punch of optimum size can be used to take a biopsy. The specimen is sent to the pathology laboratory in the appropriate tissue media. Obtain hemostasis via manual pressure, silver nitrate cautery, or electrocautery. Closure of the wound may be aided by circumferential undermining, depending on the size of the resultant defect. Suture the mucosa to reapproximate the edges. Postoperative dressing is not required usually.

VITILIGO SURGERY OVER LIP MUCOSA

Lip vitiligo has much more impact on the social and psychological well-being of the individual compared to localized vitiligo elsewhere, however, small it may be. Repigmentation of lip is slower with medical lines of management due to the lack of hair follicles, thus surgical treatment becomes essential in most of the cases of lip vitiligo. Basic principles of vitiligo surgery regarding stability should be followed.

Miniature Punch Grafts

Extraction of punch grafts from the donor area is similar to standard procedure. The 1 mm punches are used for both donor and recipient areas. Preferred donor site is retroauricular area. Uniform wells are created using 1 mm punches at an average distance of 0.5–1 mm. Grafts should be placed along the margins to prevent perigraft halo. Application of glue is optional, if needed, should be applied after hemostasis is achieved, to prevent the glue getting entry to the punch thereby causing graft rejection **(Figs. 6A and B)**. Bleeding is controlled by applying pressure with wet gauze. Dressing and postoperative care are as mentioned earlier. Phototherapy is advised once the dressing is removed. This procedure is the easiest, least expensive, and fastest. Cobblestone appearance is the most common complication noticed.

Suction Blister Graft

Induction of blister and removal of graft from donor area are similar to standard procedure of harvesting suction blister. Local anesthesia with saline infiltration to the lip produces tumescence swelling with anesthesia. This swelling everts the lip making the vitiliginous area more accessible as well as gives a firm surface for dermabrasion. Lip as a recipient bed can be prepared either with triangular probe of radiofrequency in cut-coagulation mode with low energy and with a gentle and fast movement of the probe very superficially **(Fig. 7A)**, erbium-doped yttrium aluminum garnet (Er:YAG) or carbon dioxide laser by superficially deepithelializing the tough epidermal layer followed by superficial dermabrasion by either manual or motor dermabrader **(Fig. 7B)**. The dermabrasion should always be superficial and optimal for graft uptake, to prevent possibility of hematoma formation and for faster healing. The graft is then gently placed on the lip with dermal side down **(Figs. 8A and B)**. Ensure that the edges are smoothened out to avoid folds and incurving of borders, otherwise there will be thickening of the graft due to rolling of edges **(Fig. 8C)**. The grafts should be placed to cover the entire depigmented area and also about 2–3 mm from the margins **(Fig. 8D)**.

The grafts can be secured in place by application of glue to the edges or by stay sutures with 5-0 or 4-0 suture material of choice or Steri-Strip. A hypodermic needle can be fixed to the glue for easier and nonmessy application **(Fig. 9)**.

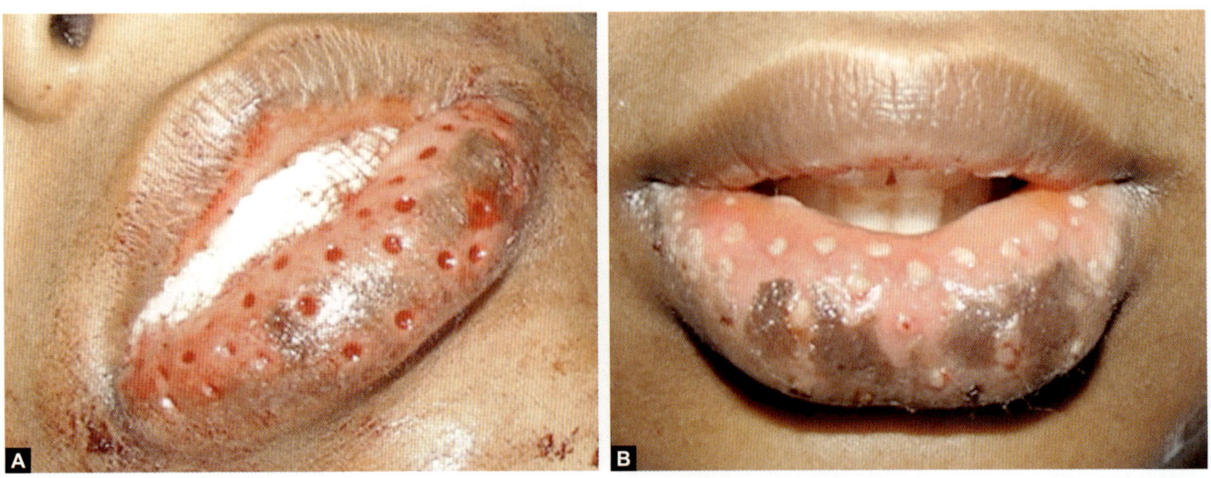

Figs. 6A and B: (A) Uniform wells created using 1 mm punch at the recipient area; (B) Grafts in place and taken up 5 days after grafting without glue.

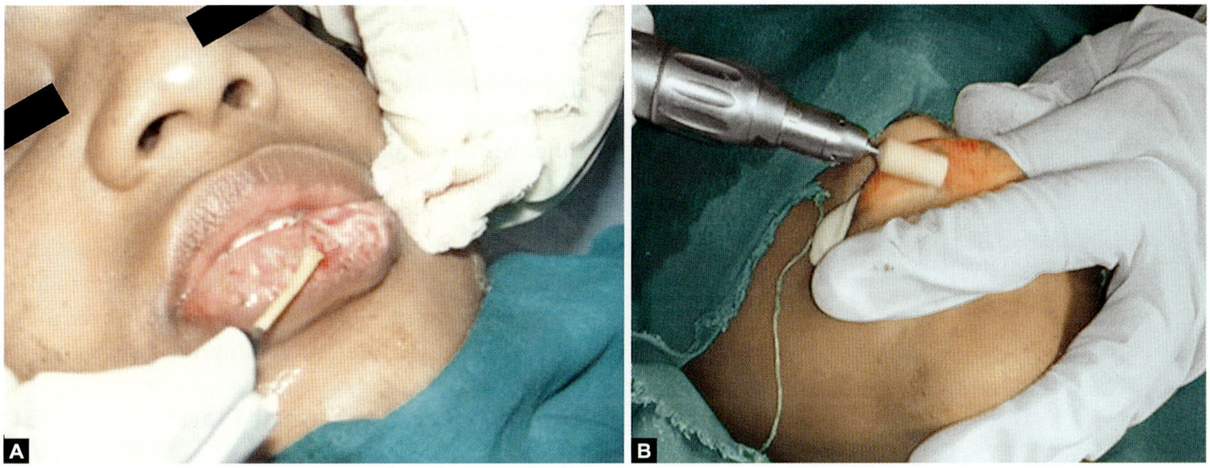

Figs. 7A and B: De-epithelialization of lip. (A) Triangular loop of radiofrequency; (B) Motor dermabrasion.

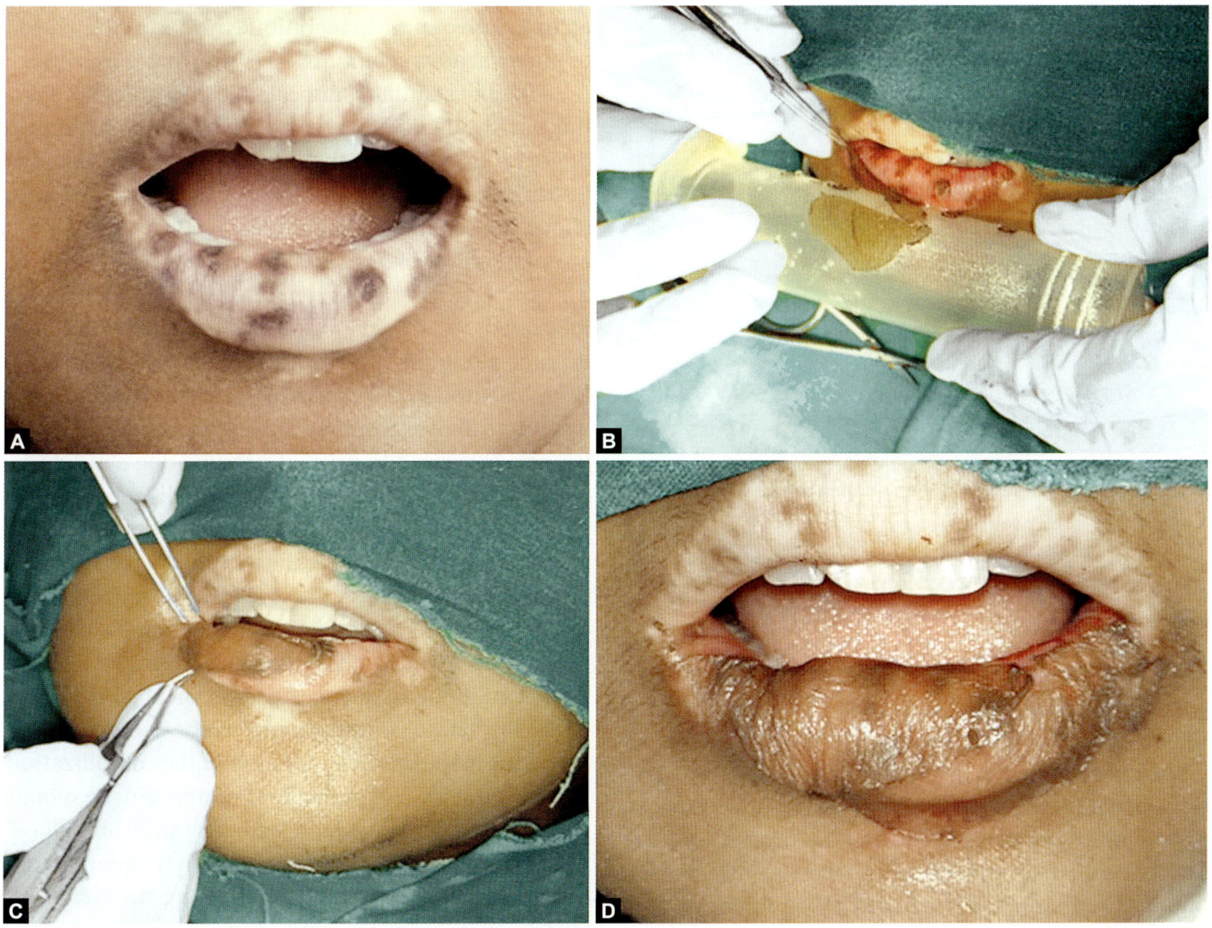

Figs. 8A to D: (A) Preprocedure; (B) Placing graft on prepared lip; (C) Smoothening out the edges; (D) Immediately postprocedure.

Dressing and postoperative care are as discussed earlier.

As the dermoepidermal grafts retain the characteristics of site of origin, there are reports of development of cutaneous diseases which normally do not involve the oral mucosa. A modification to improve the aesthetic outcome of pure epidermal grafts is to remove the graft along with the dressing after 1 week. During this period of contact melanocytes are transferred to the dermabraded area and the chances of change in texture or keratinization is reduced.[3]

Suction blister grafts are as efficacious as noncultured epidermal cell suspension and do not require expensive reagents. However it is a time-consuming procedure and complications are irregular uneven pigmentation and thickening of grafts **(Fig. 10)**.

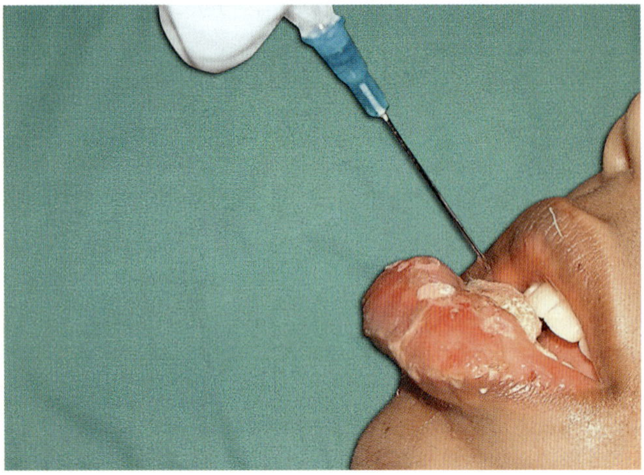

Fig. 9: Securing with glue.

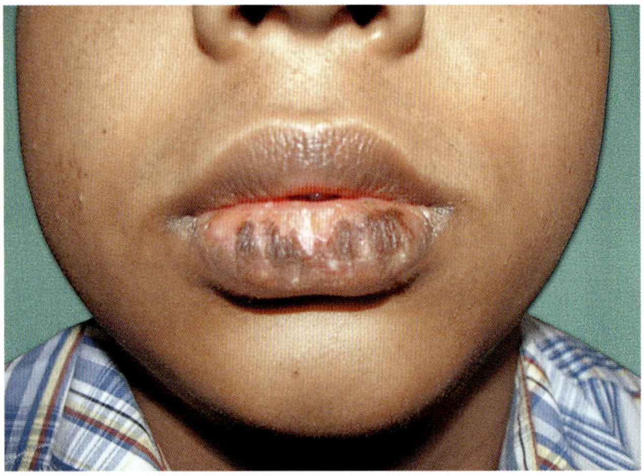

Fig. 10: Irregular and uneven pigmentation in postblister graft.

Excision and Closure for Small Depigmented Areas

The borders of the area to be excised have to be marked before infiltrating the lesion. Nerve blocks are better than local infiltration **(Fig. 11A)**. This procedure is ideal only for smaller or linear lesions which can be excised and sutured without distorting the shape of the lip. A sponge holding forceps can be used to achieve homeostasis during the procedure. Care should be taken not to crush and traumatize the lips. Incision is put along the premarked lines and the vitiliginous area excised **(Figs. 11B and C)**. Wound edges are approximated with running sutures or percutaneous interrupted sutures **(Fig. 11D)**. Undermining to be done where deemed necessary. Caution to be exercised to prevent lip inversion or distortion of the shape by undermining.

Ultrathin Graft

Conventional thin split-thickness skin grafting technique continues to be the most commonly practiced and also the most successful among all methods of vitiligo surgery.[4] With ultrathin grafts without any dermal component present, excellent results can be achieved at both the recipient as well as donor sites **(Fig. 12)**. Ultrathin grafts are harvested either with a dermatome or Silver's knife. It needs a properly trained person to do the procedure. The quality of the grafts can be gauged by means of their translucent nature and by their ability to float on isotonic saline. The edges should not be rolled upon itself.[5] The graft placement and follow-up are similar to that of suction blister grafting, however, the graft has to be fixed with sutures, preferably 5-0 absorbable.

Mucosal Advancement Flap[6]

The mucosal advancement flap is a novel procedure practiced as a therapeutic modality to cover excised lip lesions of varying etiologies. This principle has been applied to treat lip vitiligo as an innovative surgical technique by the author. The principle of mucosal advancement flap is shown in **Figure 13**.

After the standard surgical precautions and preparation of the part, the depigmented patch is marked. Two perpendicular lines are drawn from the lateral edges of the depigmented lesion over the lower lip, extending downward up to 1 cm above the junction of gingivolabial sulcus. Burow's triangles are marked on either side at the lower end of the marking, 2 cm above the anterior sulcus **(Fig. 14)**. The area is infiltrated with 2% xylocaine hydrochloride, and an incision is made along the markings. Depigmented mucosa is excised **(Figs. 15A and B)**. The flap is dissected in the submucosal plane up to 2 cm above the gingivolabial sulcus **(Fig. 15C)**. A Burow's triangle is excised to prevent possible dog ear deformity as a result of mucosal advancement. The dissected mucosal flap with the intact attachment at the lower end is advanced and mobilized forward to cover the excised defect and sutured with preferably absorbable sutures **(Figs. 15C and D)**.

The possible complications of the mucosal advancement flap are lip inversion, flap necrosis, rounded appearance of the vermilion, and decreased anterior-posterior dimensions of the lip. These complications can be avoided by taking the following steps: sufficient length of flap mobilization with a Burow's triangle and proper undermining in the subcutaneous plane to avoid lip inversion, ensuring sufficient blood supply from the base of the flap and the fresh recipient bed, and not disturbing the vermilion and excising the lesion of the lip clearly away from the vermilion. This procedure being an innovative and skilled-surgical procedure, it may be practiced only in special situations where other methods have failed or not suitable **(Table 2)**.

Noncultured and Cultured Melanocyte Grafting

These procedures provide excellent cosmetic coverage and are better suited for larger areas. They are not of any

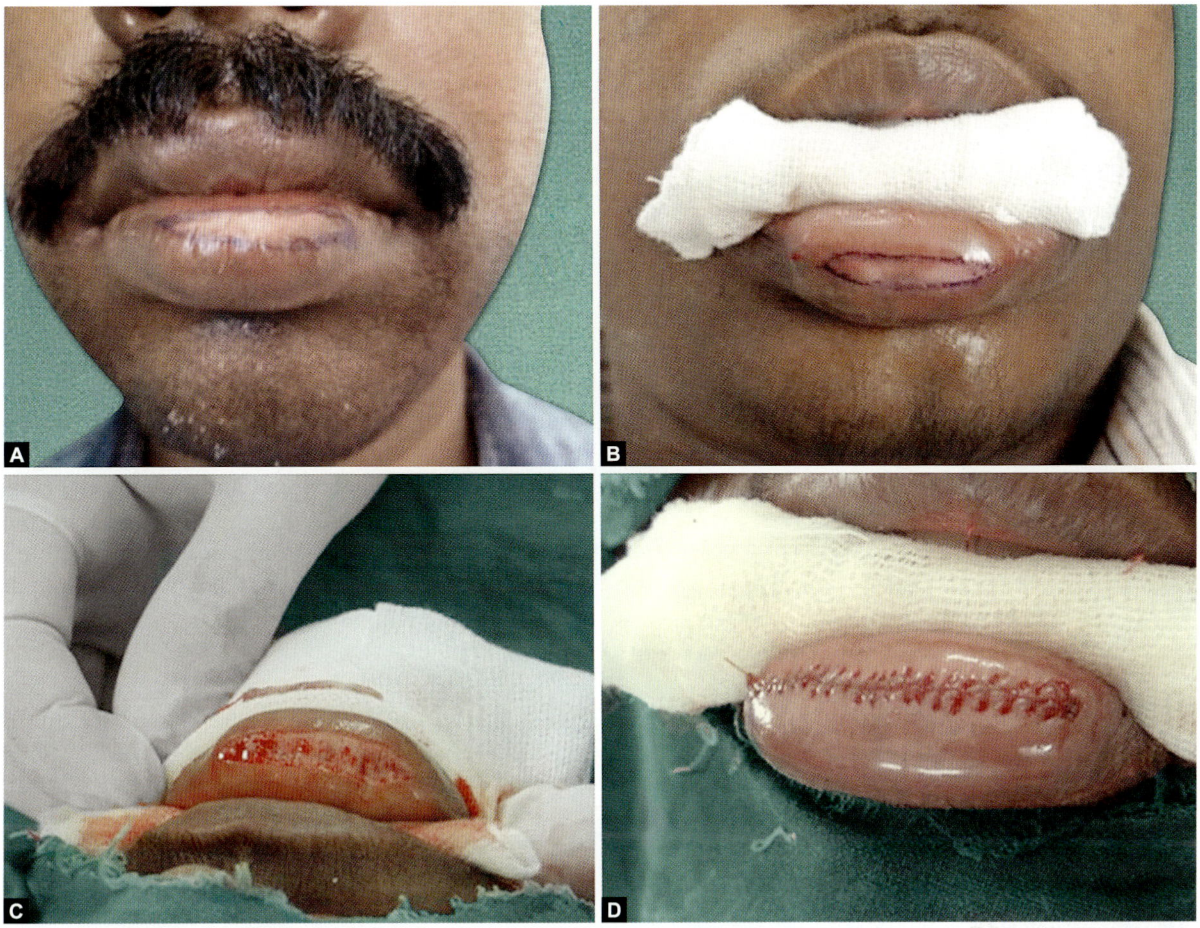

Figs. 11A to D: (A) Marking the area before infiltration; (B) Local infiltration; (C) Vitiliginous area excised; (D) Primary closure with continuous sutures.

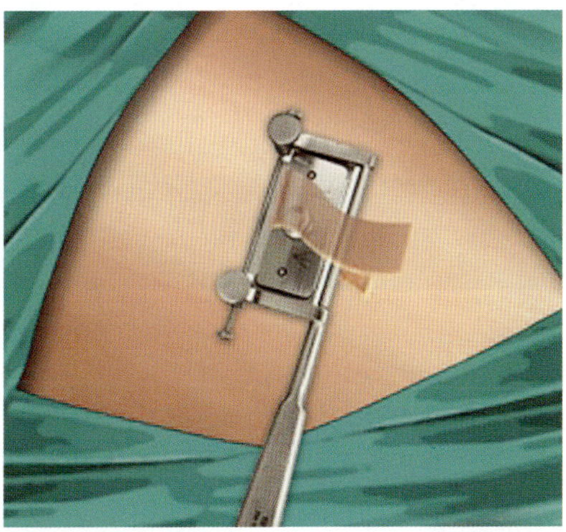

Fig. 12: Ultrathin split-thickness graft obtained from the upper thigh.

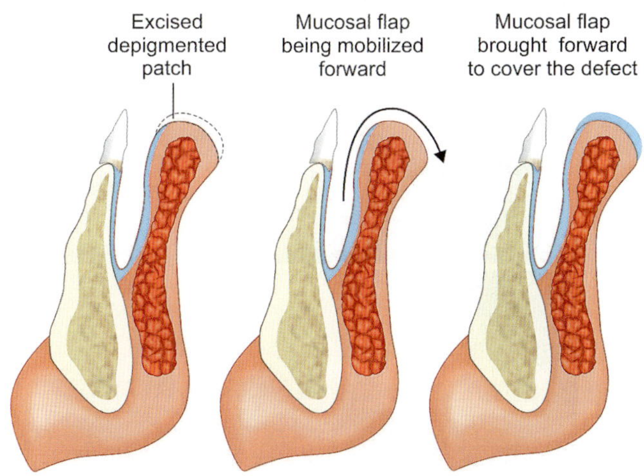

Fig. 13: Principle of mucosal advancement flap.

additional advantage in small areas like lips in comparison to suction blister grafting. It is not recommended by most experts and guidelines for the management of lip vitiligo due to either technical difficulties or poor response rates at this site. Cultured melanocyte grafting is a complex process, expensive, and involves high level of technical expertise.[7]

PROCEDURES FOR MUCOUS CYST

Mucous cyst arises either due to extravasation of mucus from the damaged salivary gland duct or due to obstruction of the duct. Lower lip is the most common site for mucous cyst. High rate of recurrences are common as feeding mucous glands are left behind. Modalities of treatment include the following.

Excision and Closure

There are various modalities of excision of mucous cyst as explained here.

Deroofing the Cyst

It is always better to mark the margins of the cyst before infiltration of anesthesia. After infiltration, the mucocele can be stabilized with chalazion forceps. The cyst roof is deroofed with scissors or scalpel blade and all contents removed. Then the base of the cyst is electrofulgrated. After removal of chalazion forceps, the wound is left open to heal by secondary intention. The risk of recurrence is slightly higher with this method.

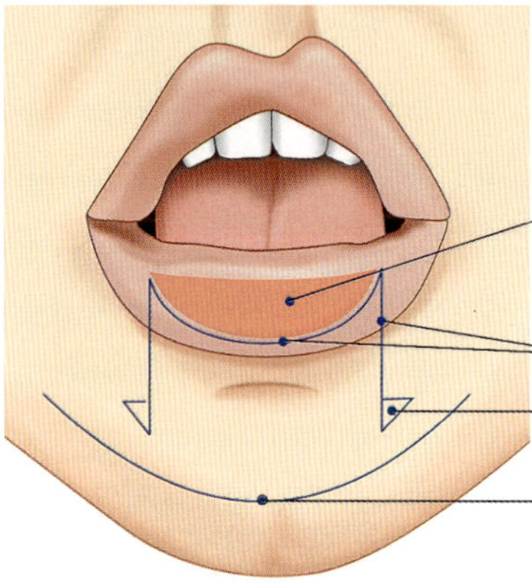

Fig. 14: Surgical markings for mucosal advancement flap inside the oral cavity.

Simple Excision and Closure

After marking the margins of the cyst and infiltrating the surrounding skin with lignocaine 1% with adrenaline **(Fig. 16A)**. A linear or elliptical incision is placed over the cyst superficially taking care not to rupture the cyst preferably. When the mucosa is incised, the cyst pops out **(Fig. 16B)** or dissect it carefully to excise it in total. If the cyst ruptures remove the cyst wall and sack in total **(Fig. 16C)**. The cyst is removed and mucosa sutured with prolene 5-0 with simple interrupted sutures or with absorbable sutures **(Fig. 16D)**. Healing is complete in a week without any scar **(Figs. 17A and B)**.

Complete Excision

Mucous cysts can be completely excised and sutured. The rate of recurrence will be almost nil with this method.

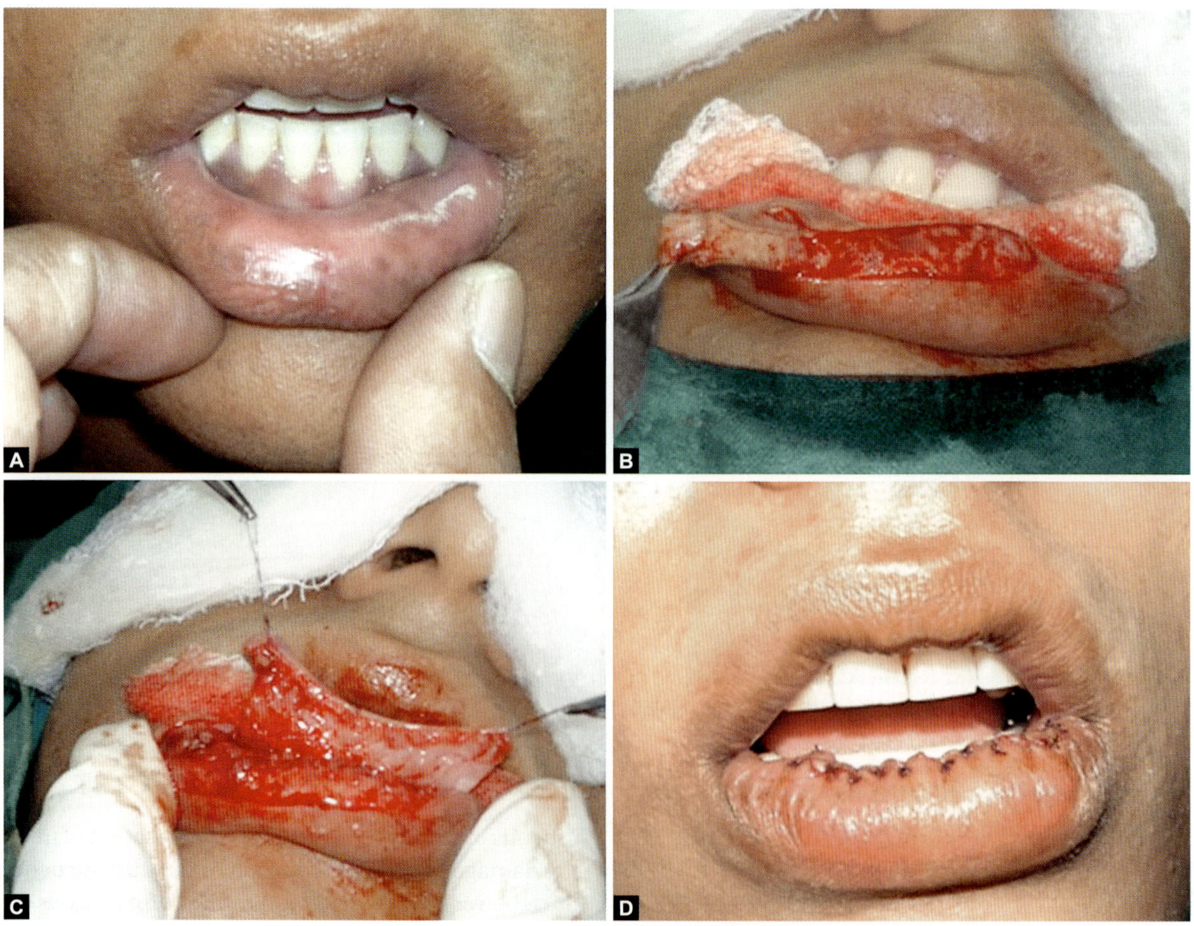

Figs. 15A to D: (A) Vitiligo patch on lower lip mucosa; (B) Excision of depigmented mucosa; (C) Mobilized mucosal flap; (D) The defect is sutured with 5-0 Vicryl interrupted sutures.

TABLE 2: List of transplantation procedures commonly used for lip vitiligo with their advantages, disadvantages, and outcome in various studies.[8]

Type of grafts for lip leukoderma	*Advantages*	*Disadvantages*	*Summary of the outcome of literature analysis for surgical treatment of lip vitiligo [successful/total (%)]*
Thin and ultrathin split-thickness skin grafts (STSGs)	High success rates with immediate results, but not a best choice	Color and texture mismatch, donor area scarring, recipient area contracture, occurrence of dermatological diseases, such as psoriasis, malignant transformation, and expertise skill needed. Lip may look heavy with stuck on appearance	2/2 (100%)
Suction blister grafting (SBG)	The ease of procedure, the high success rate, and the excellent cosmetic results. No scarring at donor site as the graft consists of only epidermis	Time-consuming, hyperpigmentation at the recipient site and donor site, and unsuitable for larger areas. Lip should not be covered partially. Even if the lesion is small grafting should be done for the entire lip to have uniformity in color	40/45 (88.88%)
Miniature punch grafting	Easy to perform and can take care of a relatively larger vitiligo area	Cobblestone appearance, polka-dot appearance, depigmentation of the grafts, perigraft halo, graft rejection, hypertrophic scarring, variegated appearance with color mismatch at the recipient sites, and scarring at the donor site. Usually requires postsurgical medical management	102/132 (77.21%)
Noncultured melanocyte grafting of epidermal suspensions	Larger area can be treated with a smaller size of donor graft. Excellent color match	Time-consuming, need for specialized equipment, such as centrifuge, incubator, and reagents, training and experience to obtain standardized uniform results and hence there is an initial learning curve. The epidermal cell suspension may run away and produce irregular pigmentation. Not a best procedure for the lip compared to other sites	6/14 (42.9%)
Cultured "pure" melanocytes (CM) and epithelial grafts (CE)	Large area can be treated in a single session	Time-consuming and labor intensive technique, requires a sophisticated laboratory setup for cell culture	Not available at all places except in specialized centers
Micropigmentation	Relatively inexpensive, simple office procedure with instant results may be performed for vitiligo of the angle of the mouth where graft placement is difficult	Difficult to adjust or homogenize tone of skin color, pigment migration, and bluish discoloration due to Tyndall effect. It is almost an obsolete procedure	100%. However, the author's experience does not recommend this since the long-term results are poor with undesirable results such as color change of pigmentation. It should be discouraged due to availability of much better procedures
Mucosal advancement flap	Single-case report. Best and suitable graft to replace the excised mucosa due to various causes, since it is a natural replacement of lip mucosa with oral mucosal tissue	If performed in a suitable case where the patch is small, the results are excellent with complete natural appearance and function. Is a skilled procedure and requires surgical expertise	Though a single-case report in published literature, author's experience is good with eight cases performed in a situation where other grafting techniques have failed

After marking the margins of the cyst and infiltrating the surrounding skin with lignocaine 1% with adrenaline. An elliptical incision is placed around the mucous cyst and the cyst is dissected from the surrounding tissue to be removed in total. After achieving hemostasis by compression, sutures are placed **(Figs. 18A to D)**.

Application of Caustic Chemicals

The caustic agents like phenol can be used to treat mucoceles. No local anesthesia is required. Under aseptic precautions, a very small quantity of 88% phenol is injected into the cyst cavity using insulin syringes. No dressing is given afterward. Patients are given analgesics postprocedure for 1 day **(Fig. 19)**.[9]

Sclerotherapy

Sclerosing agents like polidocanol or sodium tetradecyl sulfate can also be injected into the mucous cysts. The minimum concentration required to produce desired results with least complications is 1.5%. In those patients who

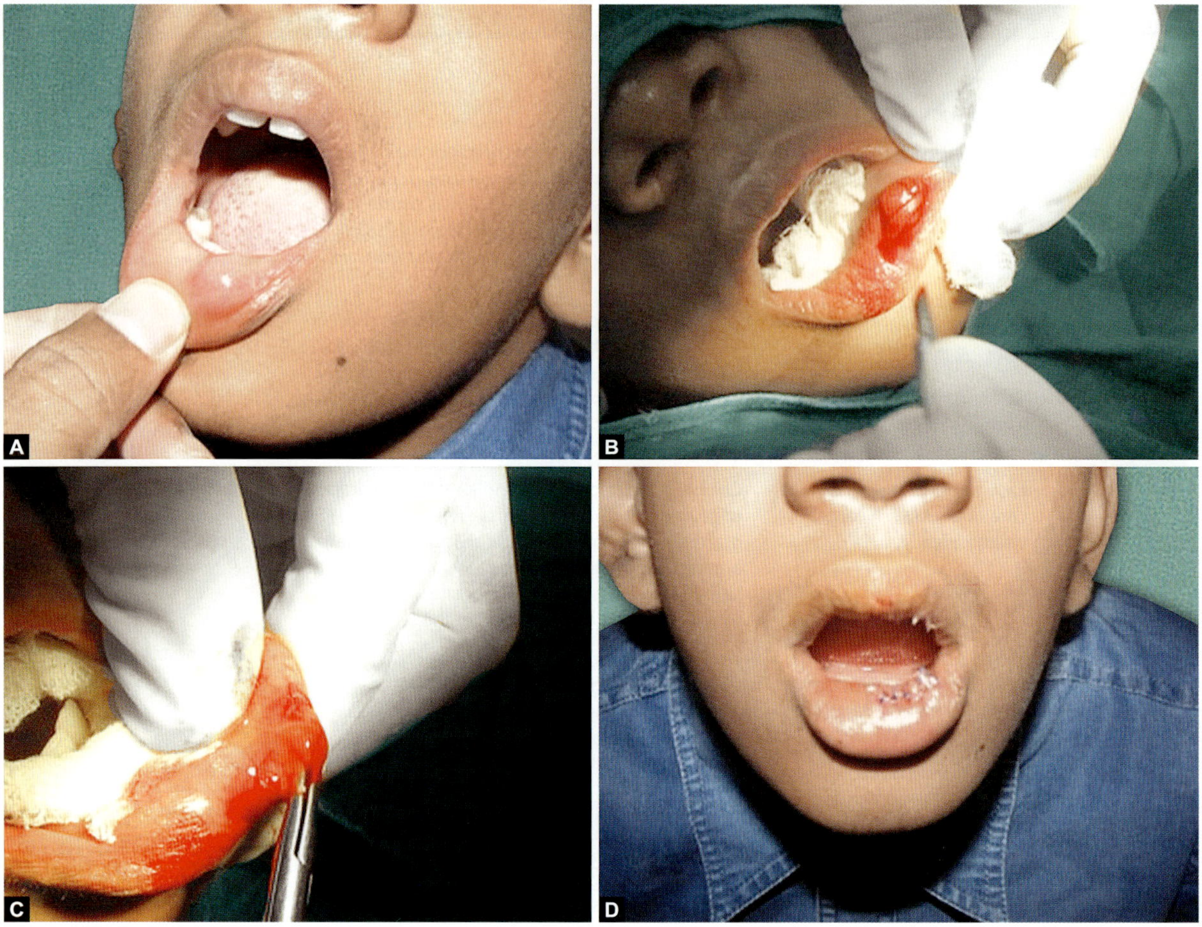

Figs. 16A to D: (A) Mucous cyst over lower lip; (B) The cyst pops out when the mucosa is incised; (C) If the cyst ruptures remove the cyst wall and sack in total; (D) Mucosa sutured with prolene 5-0 with simple interrupted sutures.

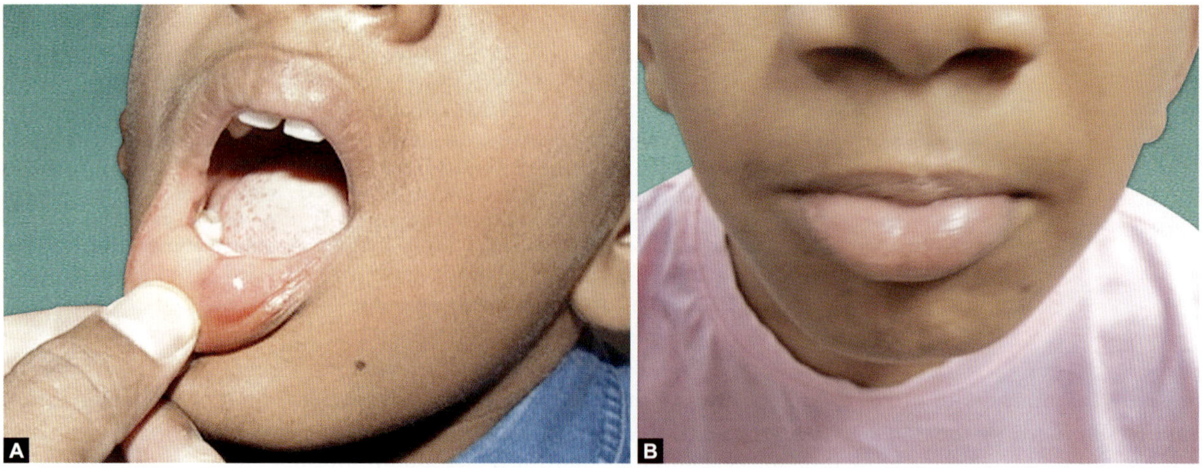

Figs. 17A and B: Healing is complete in a week without any scar.

show partial response in initial sittings, concentration can be increased to 2%. Common complications include pain on injection, erythema, and healing with postinflammatory hyperpigmentation **(Figs. 20A and B)**.

Removal of Superficial Growths

Small superficial lesions around the lip removed by shave excision with a number 15 blade heal well by secondary

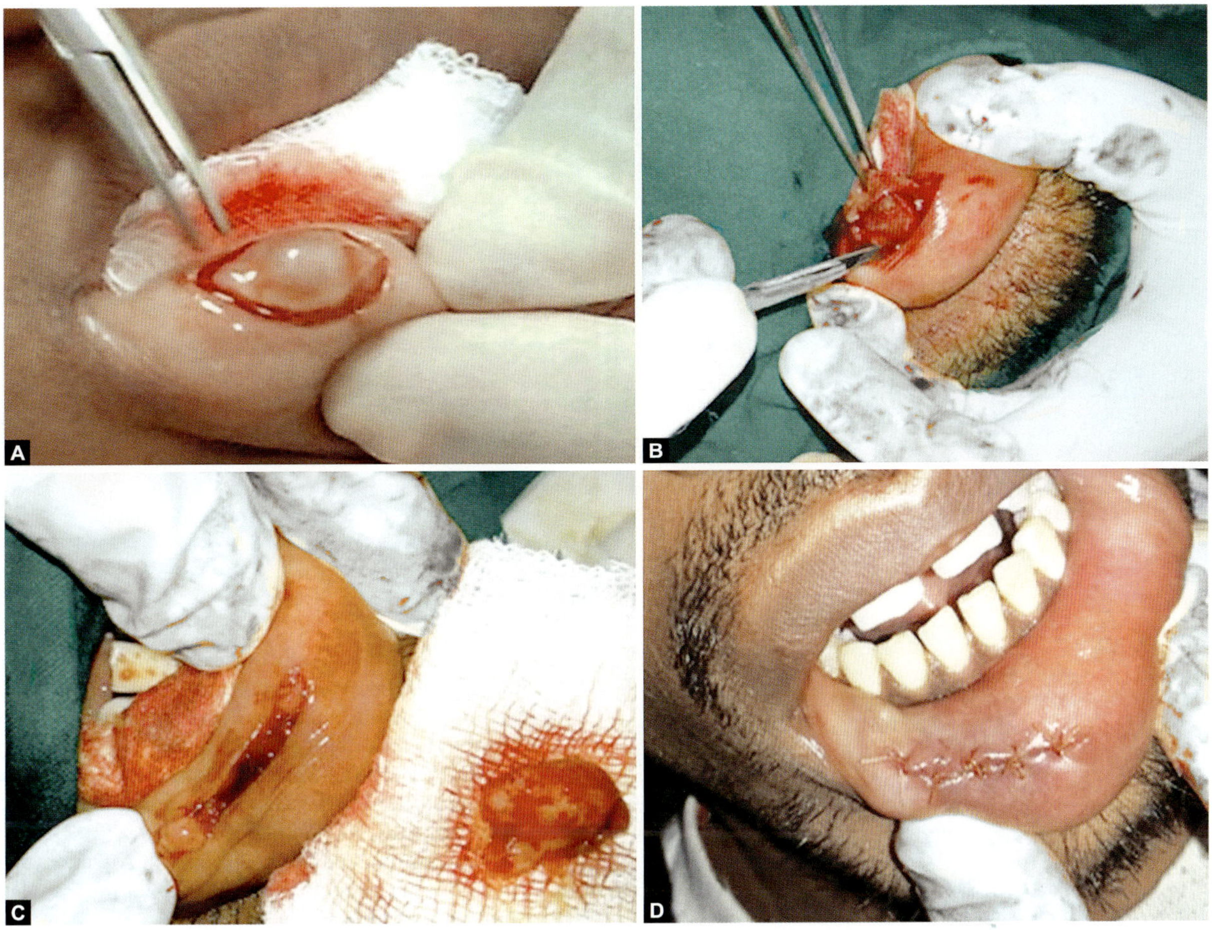

Figs. 18A to D: (A) Elliptical incision is placed around the mucous cyst; (B) The cyst is dissected from the surrounding tissue; (C) The cyst is removed in total; (D) Wound closed with interrupted sutures.

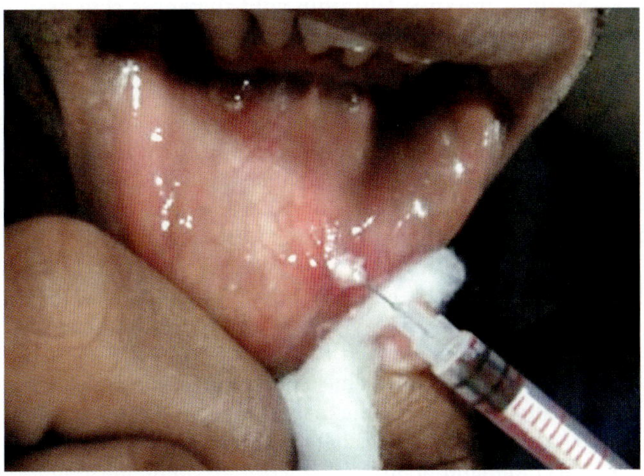

Fig. 19: Injection of phenol into the mucous cyst.

intention with excellent cosmetic results **(Fig. 21)**. Small excision or punch biopsy also will heal satisfactorily by secondary intention but may heal more rapidly by simple primary closure.

HAIR TRANSPLANTATION

Hair transplantation on upper lip is frequently requested by patients for scars: post-traumatic or postsurgical (due to cleft lip surgery). Occasionally, patients seek hair transplantation for moustache enhancement. While a detailed discussion is out of scope of this chapter, the following salient points need to be kept in mind:

- Donor hair can be obtained from scalp or beard since the number of grafts needed is small, extraction method is preferred for harvesting.
- Direction of hairs varies according to location; in the center of the lip, hairs grow vertically down, but grow downward and laterally in the lateral parts of the lip.
- Only single-hair units are preferred.
- Lip is a mobile and vascular area and hence graft placement and stabilization cause challenges.
- Patient should be advised to avoid undue movements of the lips for 5 days till grafts get stabilized.
- Postoperative edema may occur.

Despite these challenges, results are satisfying.

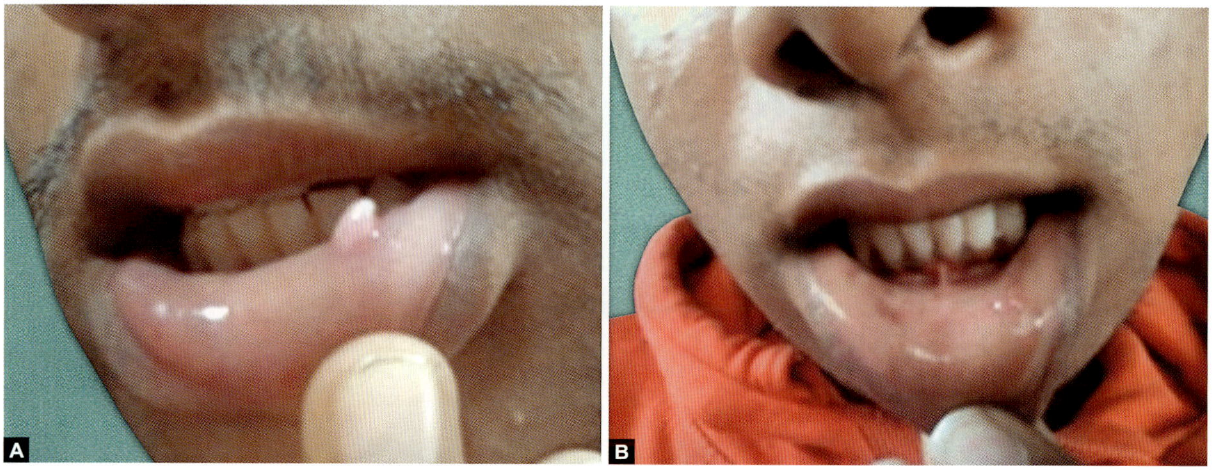

Figs. 20A and B: Before and 1 week after sclerosant injection.
Courtesy: Dr Shruthi C, Department of Dermatology, Bangalore Medical College and Research Institute, Bengaluru.

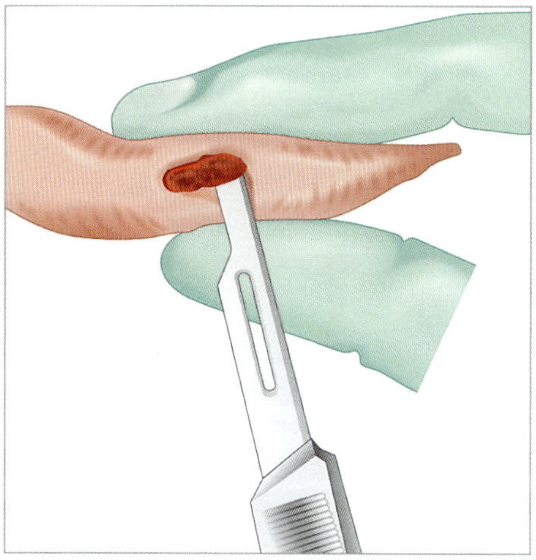

Fig. 21: Schematic diagram of shave excision.

CONCLUSION

- Lips are an important component of facial aesthetics. While performing procedures the shape of the lip and vermilion border should be maintained.
- Nerve blocks are better tolerated by patients.
- Use of chalazion ring forceps helps to stabilize the lesion on the lip/tongue during biopsy/excision and provides adequate hemostasis.
- Airway maintenance is of utmost importance both during and after surgical procedures.
- Marking lip margins with marker pen, methylene blue, 7-0 silk suture, or with scalpel nicks prior to administering local anesthesia can help identify the border during closure.

REFERENCES

1. Greenway HT. The lips and oral cavity. In: Roenigk RK, Ratz JL, Roenigk HH (Eds). Roenigk's Dermatologic Surgery: Current Techniques in Procedural Dermatology, 3rd edition. New York: Informa Healthcare; 2007. pp. 231-8.
2. Mirković S, Durdević-Mirković T, Branislav B, Sarcev I. Choice of surgical suture material used in oral cavity-clinical study. Med Pregl. 2010;63(7-8):497-501.
3. Gupta S, Sandhu K, Kanwar A, Kumar B. Melanocyte transfer via epidermal grafts for vitiligo of labial mucosa. Dermatol Surg. 2004;30(1):45-8.
4. Khunger N. Recent advances in the surgical treatment of vitiligo. In: Ghosh S (Ed). Recent Advances in Dermatology, 1st edition. New Delhi: Jaypee Brothers Medical Publishers (P) Ltd.; 2007. pp. 319-40.
5. Majid I, Imran S. Ultrathin split-thickness skin grafting followed by narrowband UVB therapy for stable vitiligo: an effective and cosmetically satisfying treatment option. Indian J Dermatol Venereol Leprol. 2012;78:159-64.
6. Reddy RR, Basavapura SM, Chandramouli GA. Mucosal advancement flap: an innovative surgical technique for treatment of lip vitiligo. Dermatol Surg. 2013;39(2):334-7.
7. Bhatia R, Gupta S. Surgical Management of Vitiligo of Lips, Eyelids, and Genitals. In: Gupta S, Olsson MJ, Parsad D, Lim HW, Geel NV, Pandya AG [Eds]. Vitiligo: Medical and Surgical Management, 1st edition. Oxford: Wiley-Blackwell; 2018. pp. 371-88.
8. Shilpa K, Sacchidanand S, Savitha S, Ranjitha R, Lakshmi DV, Divya G. A study of the outcome of primary excision and closure technique in the management of lip leukoderma in 30 patients. J Cutan Aesthet Surg. 2016;9(1):20-6.
9. Sacchidanand S, Sujaya SN, Purohit V. Phenolisation as a mode of treatment of mucosal cysts. J Cutan Aesthet Surg. 2012;5(3):210-1.

CHAPTER 55

Surgery on the Ear

R Raghunatha Reddy, Savitha AS, Shashikumar BM

KEY MESSAGES

- Repair of cleft earlobe and keloid surgeries are the commonly performed procedures on the ear.
- Dermatologists with basic surgical skills and regular dermatosurgical practice can safely perform these procedures.
- Nonsurgical closure techniques are better avoided in earlobe repair due to the weak scar, high recurrence rates, and ugly scar following nonsurgical closure.
- It is preferable to avoid simple closure techniques and advisable to practice complex closure techniques such as unilateral Z-plasty and lower border advancement flap repair to prevent recurrences and to avoid lower border notching.
- Recurrence rate of earlobe keloid is much less after surgery and postsurgical preventive measures compared to other sites, making it more amenable for surgical reduction and management by dermatologists.

INTRODUCTION

Surgery on the ear is for keloids and ear lobe repairs are frequently sought by patients. Understanding the anatomy and vascular supply of the ear, helps in better planning of the procedure and avoiding complications.

EAR ANATOMY

The parts of the ear are depicted in **Figure 1**.

Most of the auricle has a cartilaginous framework, with the lobule being the only part not supported by cartilage.

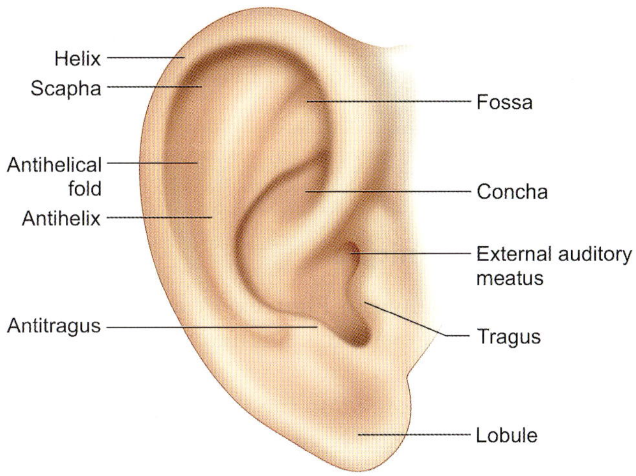

Fig. 1: Anatomy of external ear.

Sensory Innervation of External Ear (Figs. 2 and 3)

The sensory innervation of the external ear is composed of the following:

- The greater auricular nerve supplies the lower two-thirds of the anterior and posterior external ear
- The auriculotemporal nerve supplies anterior superior one-third
- The lesser occipital nerve supplies the posterior surface of the superior one-third
- The auricular branch of vagus nerve innervates the external auditory canal floor and concha.

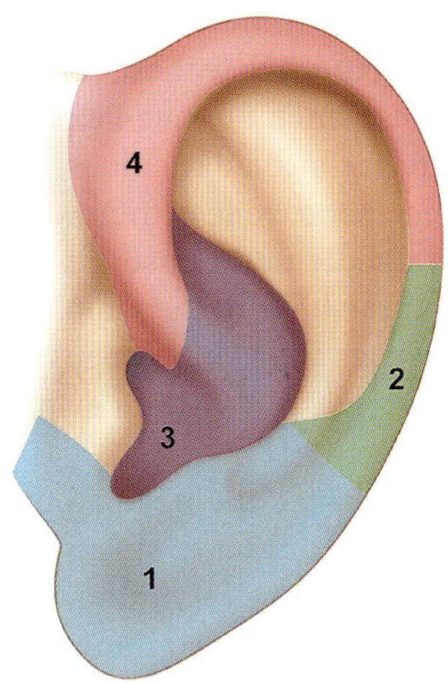

Fig. 2: Sensory supply of external ear: (1) Greater auricular nerve; (2) Lesser occipital nerve; (3) Auricular branch of vagus nerve; (4) Auriculotemporal nerve.

Vascular Supply

The earlobe is supplied by a rich plexus of perforators from both the superficial temporal and posterior auricular arteries, which are the branches of external carotid artery. Venous drainage is from the accompanying vein.[1] Rich vascularity of the earlobe is an advantage for all earlobe surgeries as it

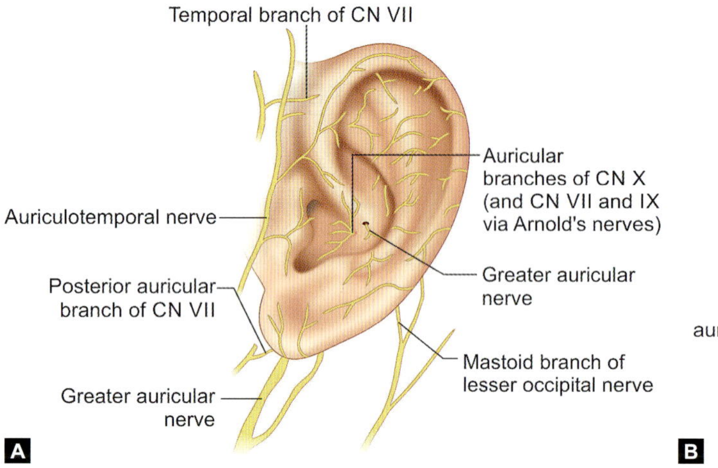

Figs. 3A and B: Innervations of the ear. (CN: cranial nerve)

helps in better and faster healing, due to which flap necrosis following the earlobe repair is uncommon.

The auricle develops from six mesenchymal proliferations located at the dorsal ends of the first and second pharyngeal arches. These swellings are called *auricular hillocks*. Congenital earlobe cleft is probably the result of failure of fusion between the first and sixth hillocks, the tragus and lobule, respectively.[2]

ANESTHESIA

Ring Block Technique

The ring block, shown in **Figures 4A and B**, provides anesthesia to the entire ear, excluding the concha and external auditory canal.

- The needle is inserted into the skin just inferior to the attachment of the earlobe to the head. *Do not insert the needle into the earlobe itself.* Advance the needle just anterior to the tragus. Aspirate and then inject 2–3 mL of anesthetic while withdrawing the needle slowly back toward the puncture site without removing it.
- Redirect and advance the needle posteriorly along the inferior posterior auricular sulcus, aspirate and inject 2–3 mL of anesthetic while withdrawing the needle.
- Remove the needle and reinsert it just superior to the attachment of the helix to the scalp. Direct and advance the needle just anterior to the tragus, aspirate and inject 2–3 mL of anesthetic while withdrawing the needle toward the puncture site.
- Redirect and advance the needle posteriorly along the superior posterior auricular sulcus, aspirate and inject 2–3 mL of anesthetic while withdrawing the needle.
- Be aware that the superficial temporal artery, located medial to the ear, crosses over the zygomatic arch. If the artery is cannulated by accident, maintain firm pressure with gauze for at least 20–30 minutes.

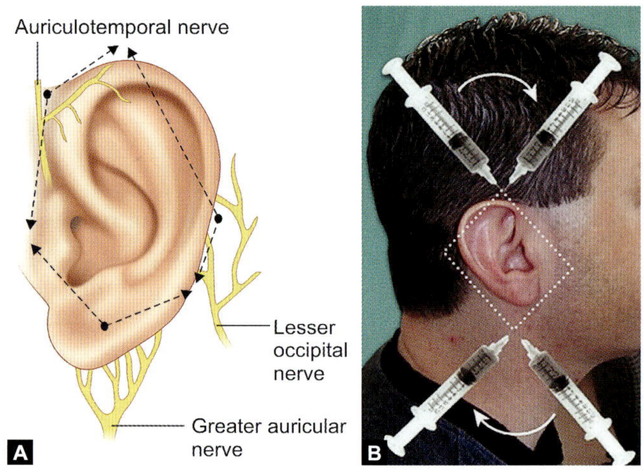

Figs. 4A and B: Ring block.

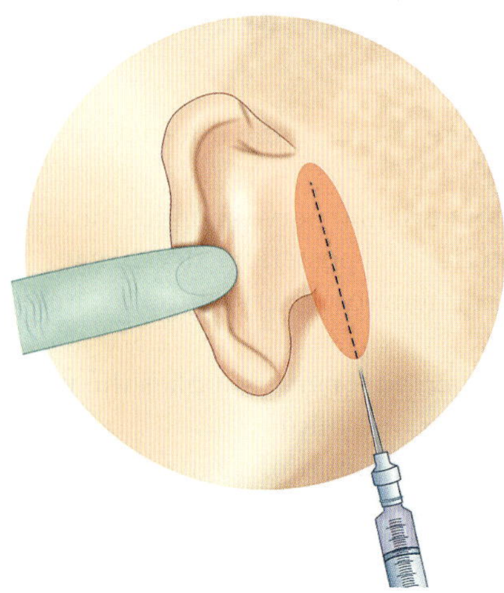

Fig. 5: Field block.

Field Block Technique

The field block, depicted in **Figure 5**, provides anesthesia to the earlobe and lateral helix (greater auricular and lesser

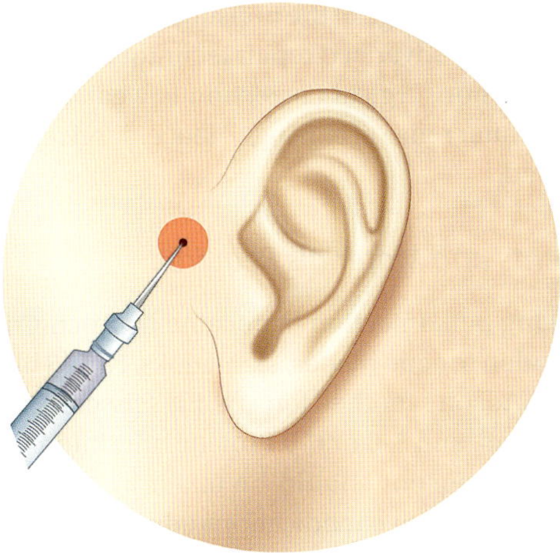

Fig. 6: Auriculotemporal nerve block.

occipital nerve branches). Insert the needle just posterior to the inferior attachment of the auricle (behind the earlobe). Aspirate and inject a total of 3–4 mL of anesthetic while advancing the needle superiorly, following the curvature of the posterior sulcus.

Auriculotemporal Nerve Block (Fig. 6)

Auriculotemporal nerve block provides anesthesia to the helix and tragus. Insert the needle anteriorly and superiorly to the tragus. Aspirate and inject 3–4 mL of anesthetic **(Fig. 6)**. The block is explained earlier in the nerve blocks chapter.

EARLOBE REPAIR

Ear piercing has been practiced across the globe irrespective of race, religion, and region, to adorn the ear with earrings and ornaments. It has also been practiced during religious customs since time immemorial. However, many patients present with complications as a result of wearing heavy earrings or due to sudden or prolonged pull. Partial or complete tears or enlarged ostium are the common complaints. Torn earlobes or cleft earlobes may be classified as either a complete or partial cleft. A complete cleft usually occurs when the earring is pulled suddenly, forming a divided medial and lateral limb. A partial cleft occurs when piercing canal is elongated or deformed, due to the practice of wearing heavy earrings or due to persistent and prolonged pulling habits, but has not severed through the earlobe.[3]

The pathology of the tear concerns around the torn edges of the lobe becoming epithelialized, thus forming a fistula or cleft. The principle in all earlobe tear repair techniques is to de-epithelize the margins and approximation of freshened edges.

Causes for Cleft Earlobe

Congenital earlobe clefts show a wide range of severity from simple notching to extensive tissue deficiency. These variable forms have been subtyped by several authors. Kitayama et al. described four subtypes as longitudinal, transverse, triple lobe, and defective types. Yamada et al. classified them as anterior, posterior, and double lobe types. Usually, a congenital earlobe cleft has soft tissue deficiency and curved cleft margin.

Acquired cleft of the earlobe is usually due to tear through the lobe by a sudden pull on an earring or by prolonged pull of a heavy earring or because of direct trauma. Factors influencing the clefting of the earlobe are congenital alterations, local trauma, facial aging, keloids, earlobe tumors, and as a result of the treatment for the same. Several retrospective studies have reported a 1–2% incidence rate of torn earlobes in patients wearing earrings.[3] Pierced earlobes may encounter trauma due to sudden pull on ear by children, friction from headgear, or entanglement in clothes.

TABLE 1: Classification of split earlobe.

Types of split earlobe	*Subtypes*
Type I: Elongated perforation with length less than that of normal tissue measured from lower end of the cleft to the inferior margin of the earlobe	• *IA:* Inferior contour normal, no ptosis of earlobe • *1B:* Inferior contour abnormal, ptosis of earlobe present
Type II: Elongated perforation with length more than that of normal tissue measured from lower end of the cleft to the inferior margin of the earlobe	• *IIA:* Inferior contour normal, no ptosis of earlobe • *IIB:* Inferior contour abnormal, ptosis of earlobe present
Type III: Total split of earlobe	• *IIIA:* Total split of earlobe with preservation of soft tissue with or without ptosis • *IIIB:* Total split of earlobe with loss of soft tissue or retraction of split ends needing local flaps for repair
Recurrent cleft earlobe: Any of the above suffixed with "r"	

Classification of Earlobe Tears

Sadasivan et al.[4] proposed a classification of earlobe tears taking into account the length of the defect and inferior margin changes **(Table 1)**.

Earlobe Repair Techniques

Torn earlobes can be repaired either by surgical or nonsurgical methods.

Nonsurgical Methods

Epithelium around the cleft is de-epithelialized by various nonsurgical method and the cleft is closed by applying a glue and a tubular bandage, allowing the de-epithelialized edges to be united, thus closing the cleft. But the resultant closure will be a weak scar, and the recurrence is almost invariable following wearing of earrings, postnonsurgical repair.

Incomplete earlobe cleft repair can be done by using various methods to de-epithelialize the tissue by:

- Trichloroacetic acid (TCA) 90%
- 88% phenol solution
- Ablative laser or radiofrequency de-epithelialization
- Dermabrasion by manual or motorized dermabraders followed by applying surgical glue or tubular dressing to unite the de-epithelized edges.

Surgical Methods

Partial cleft repair:

- Excision followed by simple repair
- Punch excision (for defects <4 mm in length) with simple closure
- Parallel opposed flaps
- Purse string repair
- Wedge excision with Z-plasty

Complete cleft repair:

- *Without preservation of piercing site:*
  - Excision and closure
  - Z-plasty
  - L-plasty
  - Interlocking V-incisions
  - Partially incised V-plasty
  - Rotation flap
  - Z-plasty and advancement flap
- *With preservation of piercing site:*
  - Pardue technique
  - Z-plasty

Nonsurgical Techniques for Cleft Earlobe Repair

Various nonsurgical techniques have been described in the literature and are being practiced. Most of the nonsurgical methods for the earlobe repair are practiced by dermatologists since the surgical techniques require proper training and certain degree of surgical skills.

Freshening of the edges for de-epithelialization and application of surgical glue with dressing is the simplest procedure. De-epithelialization of the cleft is done by various chemical agents such as TCA and phenol, dermabrasion, and lasers.

Maria Cristina Cardoso de Mendonça et al.[5] have reported a nonsurgical technique for incomplete earlobe cleft repair. Selected patients were subjected to a noninvasive incomplete earlobe cleft repair consisting of application of TCA 90% inside the cleft with nonsurgical incisions until frosting was achieved. No acid neutralization was needed. The cleft was then occluded with micropore tape until complete cicatricial adhesion of the cleft borders was achieved. The complete coagulation of the cleft borders may require several TCA 90% applications and the patients were advised to return weekly for evaluation of the cicatricial process. The major disadvantage of the nonsurgical technique without suturing or other advanced repair techniques is that, the scar following the nonsurgical correction is weak and prone for recurrences after reuse of earrings. Hence, surgical techniques are preferred.

Instruments and Materials Required

Skin marking pen, injection lignocaine hydrochloride 1–2%, sterile wooden tongue blades, skin hooks, No. 15 blade, No. 3 B.P. handle, Adson's toothed forceps, iris scissors, Castroviejo's needle holders, and 5-0 or 6-0 Prolene or Ethilon.

Informed consent should be taken in all patients and necessary preoperative medications administered.

Preoperative Preparation

The entire area is prepared by standard methods of sterilization. After the anesthesia either a field block or ring block, a small quantity of anesthetic may be injected along the slit with the extension beyond the margins.

Surgical Technique

Various surgical techniques have been advocated for both complete and partial cleft earlobe repair to provide a good, cosmetically acceptable and stronger scar with less possibility of recurrences. If the cleft is partial with more than one-third portion of the earlobe being intact, the deformity may be corrected without cutting through the intact portion to convert into a complete cleft. But it is always preferable to convert a partial cleft into a complete tear-through, if the cleft is large with remaining portion of the intact skin minimal.

Reiter and Alford, in a study involving 68 earlobe clefts, suggested that lobe thickness is also an important factor to be considered before choosing the technique to repair the clefts. Lobes measuring <4 mm at their greatest thickness have the greatest likelihood of developing elongation of the piercing site or complete clefting. Patient should be informed about this before repiercing the repaired earlobe.[6]

Partial cleft repair: Partial cleft repair methods include excision followed by simple repair, punch excision with simple closure, parallel opposed flaps, purse string repair, and wedge excision with Z-plasty.

- *Simple excision and closure (McLaren side-to-side closure):*[7] Excision of the skin margins of the cleft with No. 15 blade on anterior and posterior margins was first described by McLaren. Suture from side-to-side the opposing edges with simple interrupted sutures using 5-0 or 6-0 Prolene and suture similarly on the opposing posterior sides. Using mattress sutures causes wound eversion and gives better cosmetic results. Hemostasis may be achieved by application of pressure and dress with antibiotic ointment **(Figs. 7 and 8)**.

- *Punch excision with simple closure: Tan's technique*[8] punch excision for defects <4 mm in length is done after stabilizing the ear with chalazion forceps **(Fig. 9)** followed by punch excision of the elongated slit and simple closure of the wound. The punch, 1 mm larger than the cleft, is positioned perpendicular to the lobe, and its rotation movement de-epidermises the cleft from its front to the back side, i.e., throughout its length. The skin should be pulled by the tip of the lobe during the punch action, which results in an incision and consequent transverse suture in relation to the lobe **(Figs. 10 and 11)**. Repiercing should be done 3 months after complete healing.

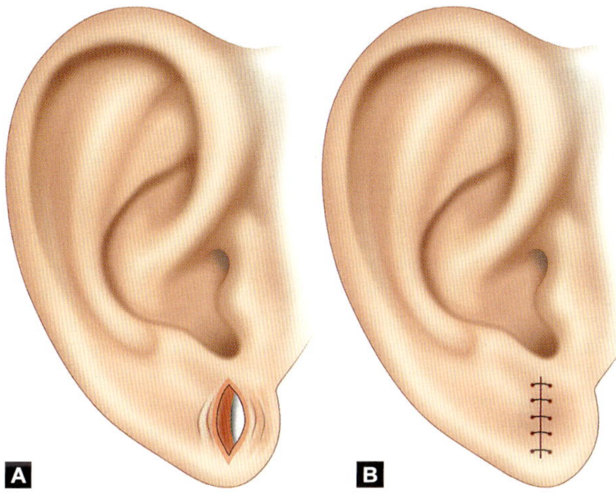

Figs. 7A and B: Schematic of side-to-side repair.

One shortcoming of a side-to-side partial cleft closure is the resultant elongation of the inferior lobule. In the instance of small tears, this may be negligible; however, in a longer partial tear, this resultant elongation may look unsightly. Suturing the slit transversely reduces the risk of elongation **(Fig. 11 D)**.

- *Parallel opposed flaps (Reiter and Alford technique):*[6] Here flaps are created with pedicles along the edge of the slit, one in front at the right side and another in the back at the left side of the lobe. The flaps are rotated as saloon doors (each flap is pulled through the cleft) trimmed at the end, and closed in the form of a "C" on each side of the lobule. Each one will cover the raw area of the other when sutured, making the cleft disappear. While this elegant repair preserves the inferior contour of the lobule, it is time consuming in comparison to a simple side-to-side closure **(Figs. 12A to D)**.
- *Repair of partial earlobe cleft using a "purse-string" repair was described by Justin Vujevich and Suzan Obagi:*[3] Using a No. 15 blade, a full-thickness elliptical incision is made around the partial cleft, hemostasis is obtained, a running 5–0 Prolene or 5–0 Ethilon suture is placed in a purse-string manner through the intradermal tissue. After encircling the defect, the free ends of the suture are pulled together and knotted from the anterior, superior edge of the lobule. Any scar that remains is easily camouflaged when the earlobe is subsequently repierced. The sutures are removed after 7 days **(Figs. 13A to D)**.

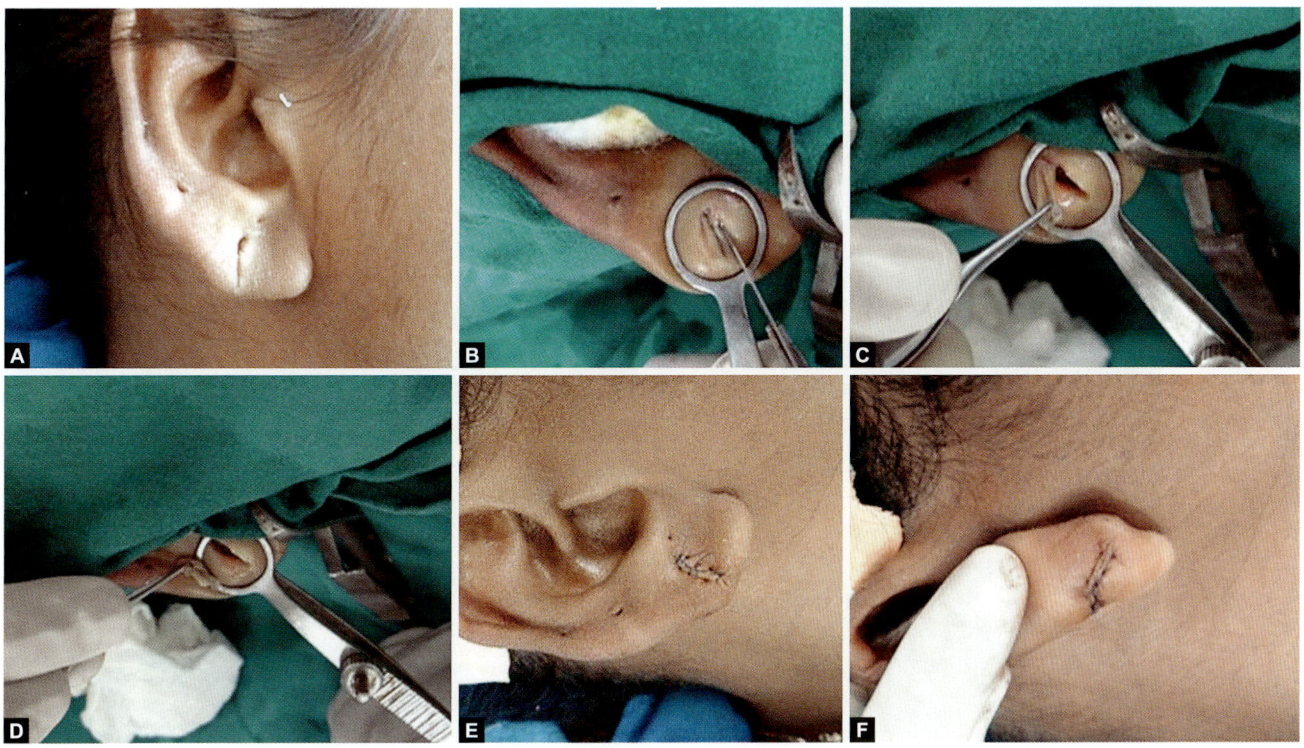

Figs. 8A to F: Side-to-side closure of partial cleft. (A) Partial tear; (B) Chalazion clamp applied for pressure and hemostasis, freshening of edges with scalpel; (C and D) Epithelized portion removed from the cleft; (E and F) edges opposed with simple interrupted sutures.

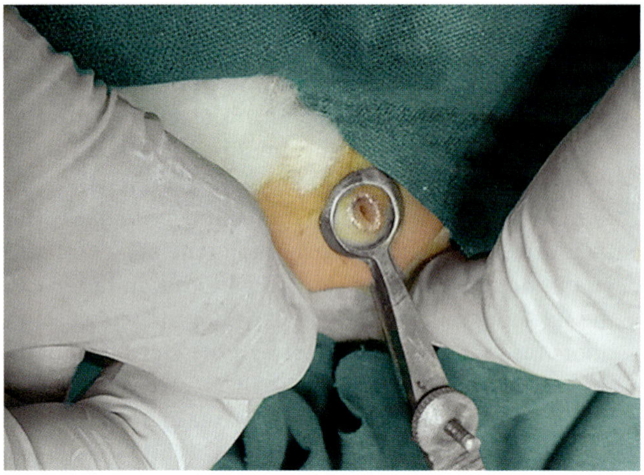

Fig. 9: Using a chalazion clamp to stabilize the earlobe, it also provides hemostasis.

- *Side-to-side closure with half Z-plasty:* Abenavoli described a side-to-side closure incorporating a half Z-plasty **(Figs. 14A to C)**. Once the limbs of the Z-plasty are made, the inferior margins of the cleft are freshened, and the flaps are transposed onto one another. This technique allows preservation of the earring canal and a staggered suture line away from the line of gravity.[9] Unilateral Z-plasty and partial advancement flap can also be done **(Figs. 15A to D)**.

Complete cleft repair methods without preservation of piercing site: Different methods have been employed as follows:

- *Side-to-side closure:* The simplest way to repair a complete cleft earlobe is to incise the cleft with an inverted V-shaped excision as described by Apesos and Kane. Once excised, the anterior and posterior edges of skin are undermined

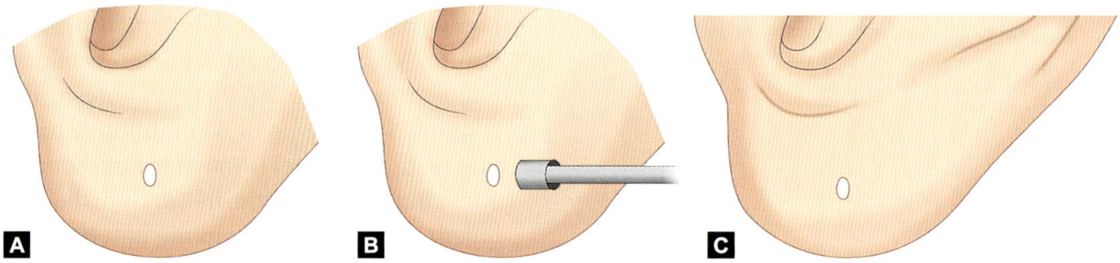

Figs. 10A to C: Schematic of punch excision.

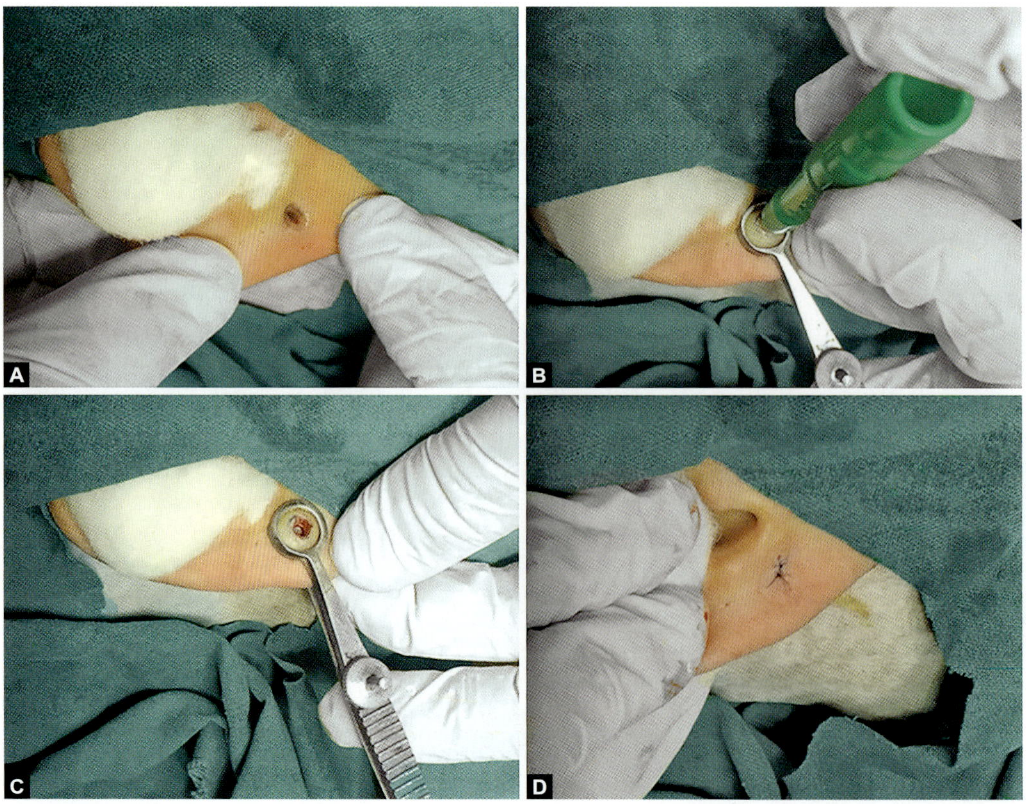

Figs. 11A to D: Punch excision and closure. (A) Stretching the love to make the defect prominent; (B) Placing the tight-sized punch to de-epithelize the margins; (C) Raw surface throughout the defect; (D) Suture is placed transversely to prevent elongation of the lobe.

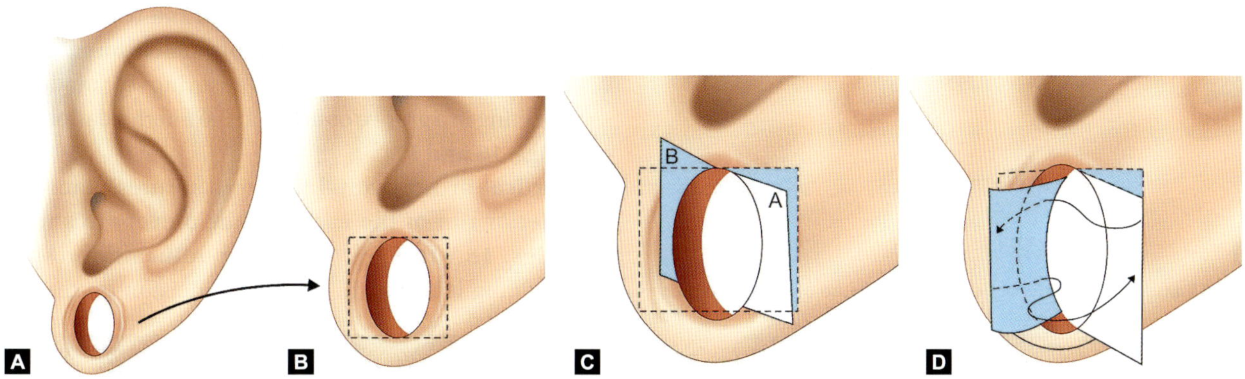

Figs. 12A to D: Reiter and Alford technique (parallel opposing flaps): Frontal flap and dorsal flap.

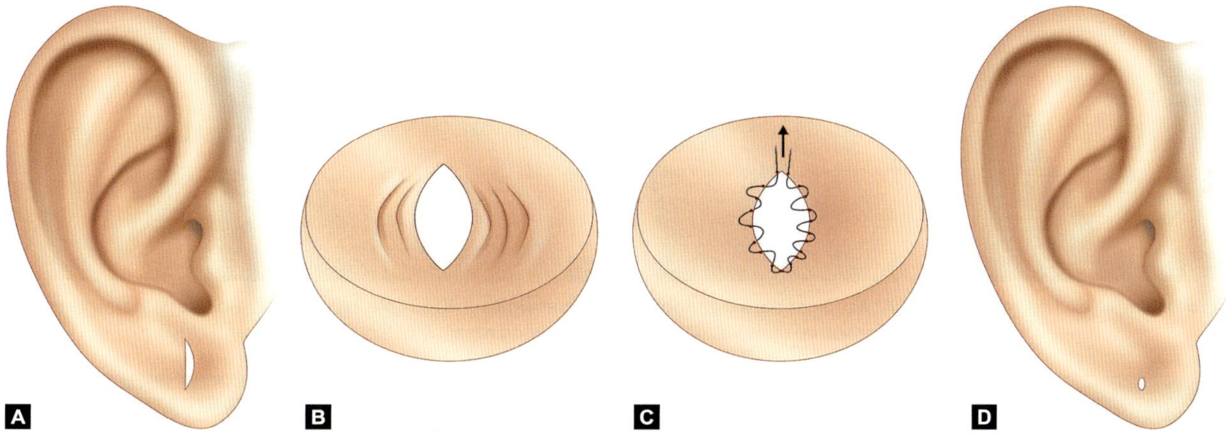

Figs. 13A to D: Illustration of purse string repair.

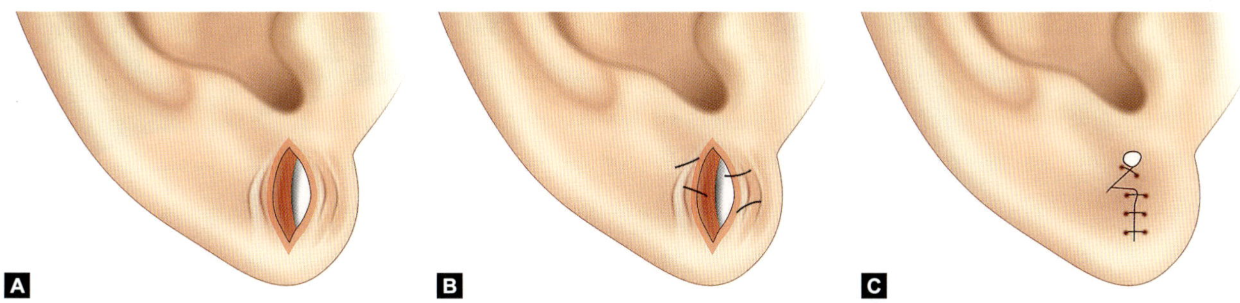

Figs. 14A to C: Illustration of side-to-side closure with half Z-plasty.

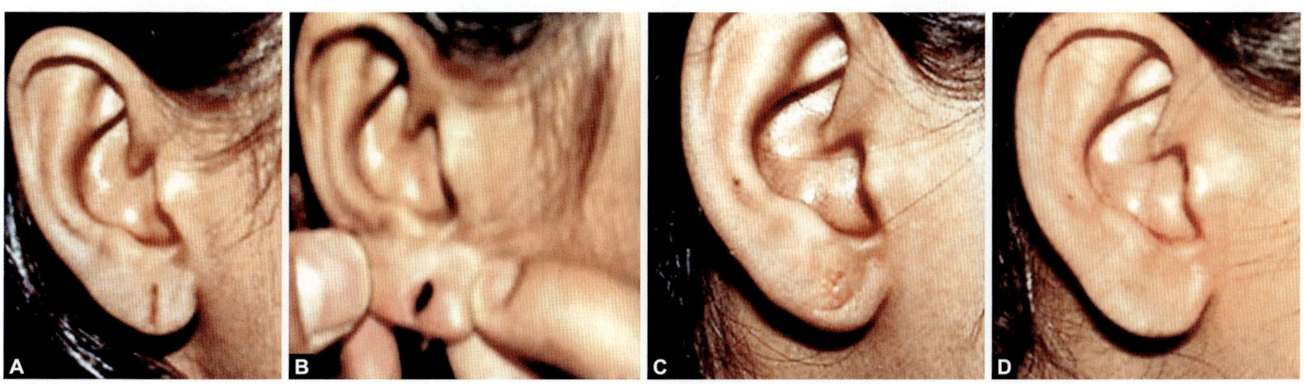

Figs. 15A to D: Unilateral Z-plasty and advancement flap for partial cleft.

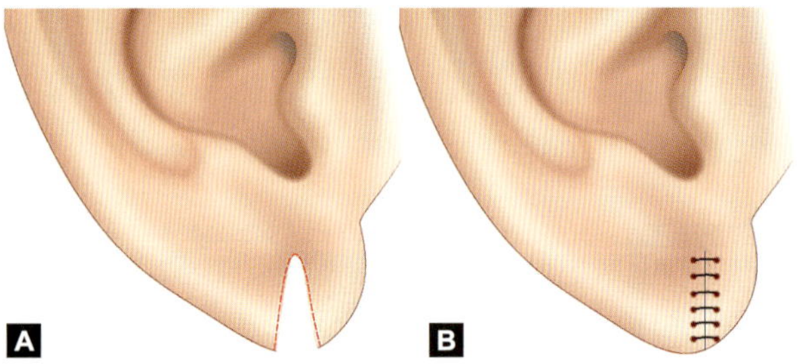

Figs. 16A and B: Schematic of side-to-side closure of complete tear.

to about approximately 1 cm and the wound edges are reapproximated with a straight line closure. While this repair is quick and simple, the ensuring scar may contract, resulting in a groove or notch at the inferior earlobe border **(Figs. 16 and 17)**.

Vertical or horizontal mattress sutures placed in the inferior rim of the earlobe may prevent this notching **(Figs. 18A to F)**.[10] Another modification to prevent notching is to create a Z-plasty incision on the inferior

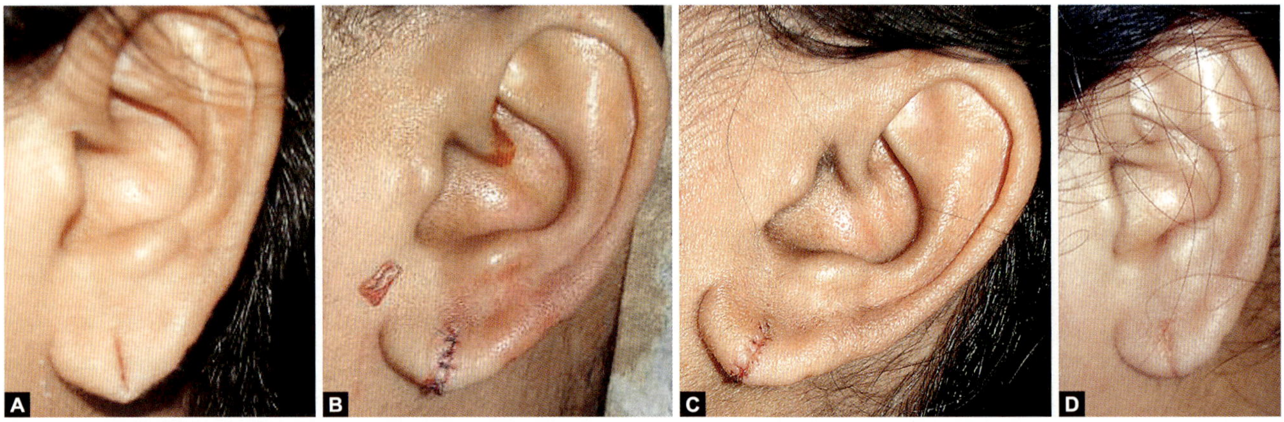

Figs. 17A to D: Simple excision and closure: (A) Acquired partial earlobe defect (presurgical); (B) Simple excision and closure with simple interrupted sutures; (C) Immediately after suture removal; (D) Notching following repair with simple excision and closure.

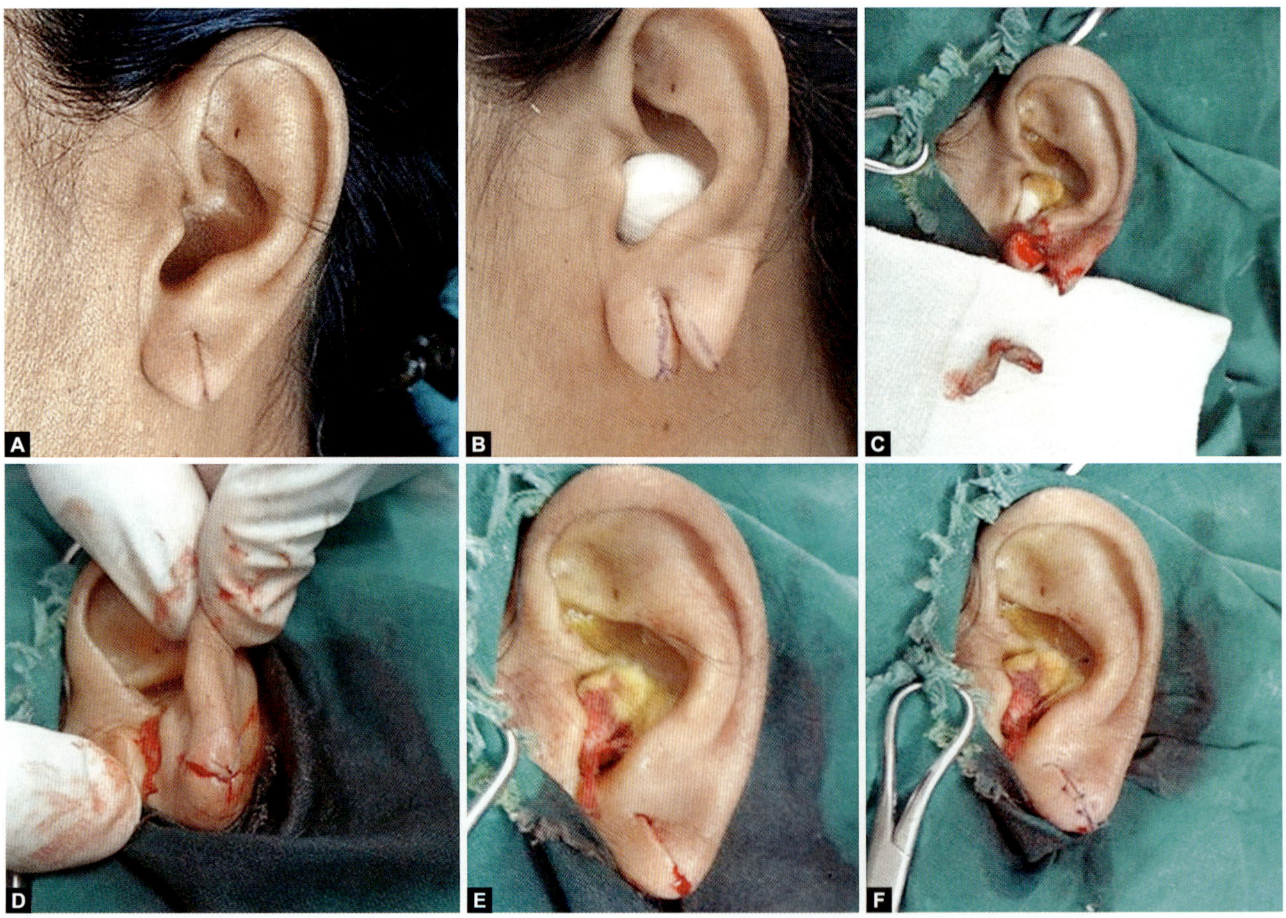

Figs. 18A to F: Simple excision and closure. The mattress suture at the lobule prevents notching.

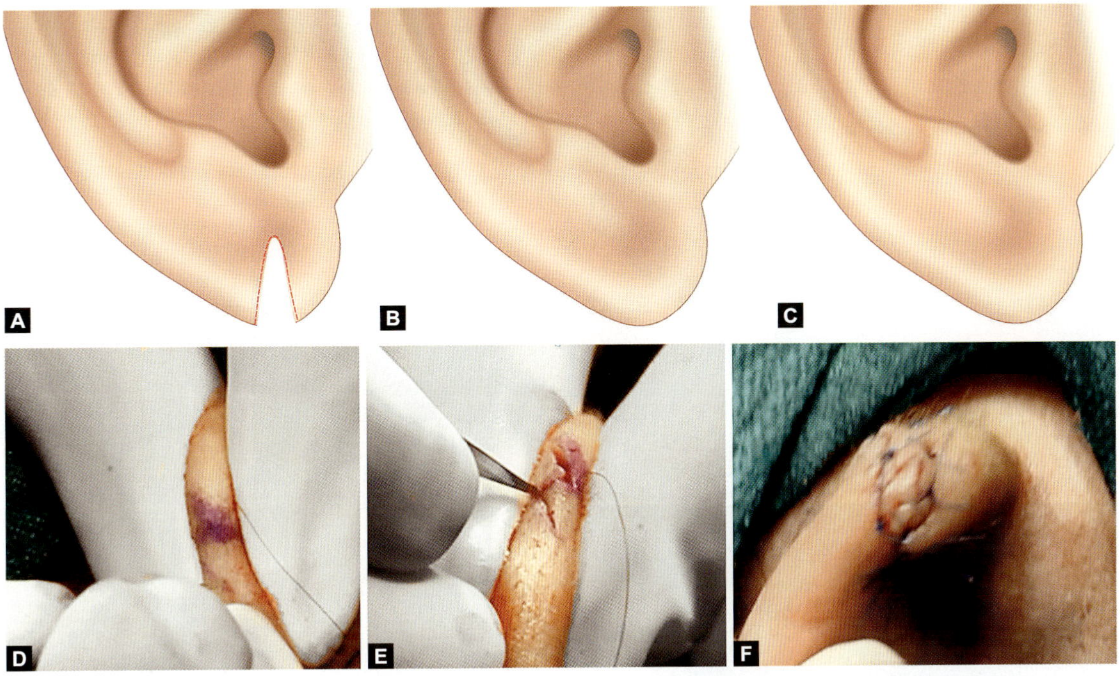

Figs. 19A to F: Z-plasty at the edge of the lobule. (A to C) Schematic diagram; (D) Marking of the Z; (E) incisions along the Z at the tip; (F) Z-plasty sutured.
Courtesy: Dr Madura C, CUTIS Academy of Cutaneous Sciences, Bengaluru.

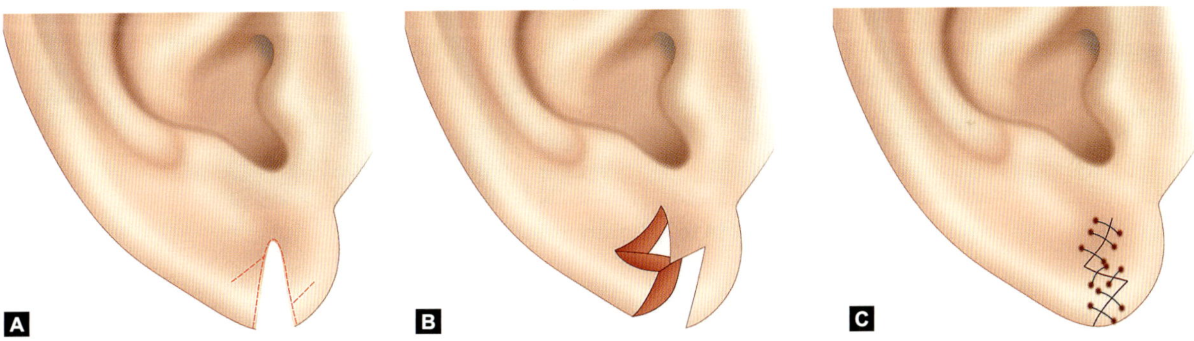

Figs. 20A to C: Schematic for full-thickness Z-plasty.

margin of the lobule and transpose the resultant flaps over each other and closed with interrupted sutures **(Figs. 19A to F)**.[11]

- Reiter and Alford described utilizing a full-thickness Z-plasty for complete cleft earlobes thicker than 4 mm **(Figs. 20 and 21)**. Alternatively for earlobe <4 mm thickness, the same author advocated the use of partial-thickness Z-plasty on the lateral surface of the earlobe, and a linear closure on the medial sides of the lobe **(Figs. 22A to C)**. One disadvantage of utilizing a Z-plasty, however, is the requirement of a precisely angled small incision on a small amount of skin on the lobe.[6]
- *Side-to-side closure with L-plasty:* Fatah MF described the creation of an L-shaped flap on the medial or lateral side of excised cleft and a complementary L-shaped defect on the other side of the earlobe. The lateral flaps are inserted onto one another and sutured together and the medial flaps are inserted onto one another and sutured together **(Figs. 23A to C)**.[12]

  A modification of L-plasty is to create a L-shaped flap on the anterior and posterior sides of the lobule, then a partial incision is made on the anterior and posterior surface lobule, the flaps are inserted with a Z in the lower end **(Figs. 24A to C)**.[13]
- *Side-to-side closure with a V-flap:* Two small 3 mm incisions are made in the shape of a V on the free margin of the inferior lobe. The V-flap is then inserted together and the superior portion is sutured together in a straight-line fashion. The advantages of using this flap are the prevention of notching at the earlobe rim, and the utilization of a simpler flap than the Z-plasty **(Figs. 25A to C)**.[14]
- *Side-to-side closure with a rotational flap:* After the edges of the cleft are split, a short segment of posterior edge

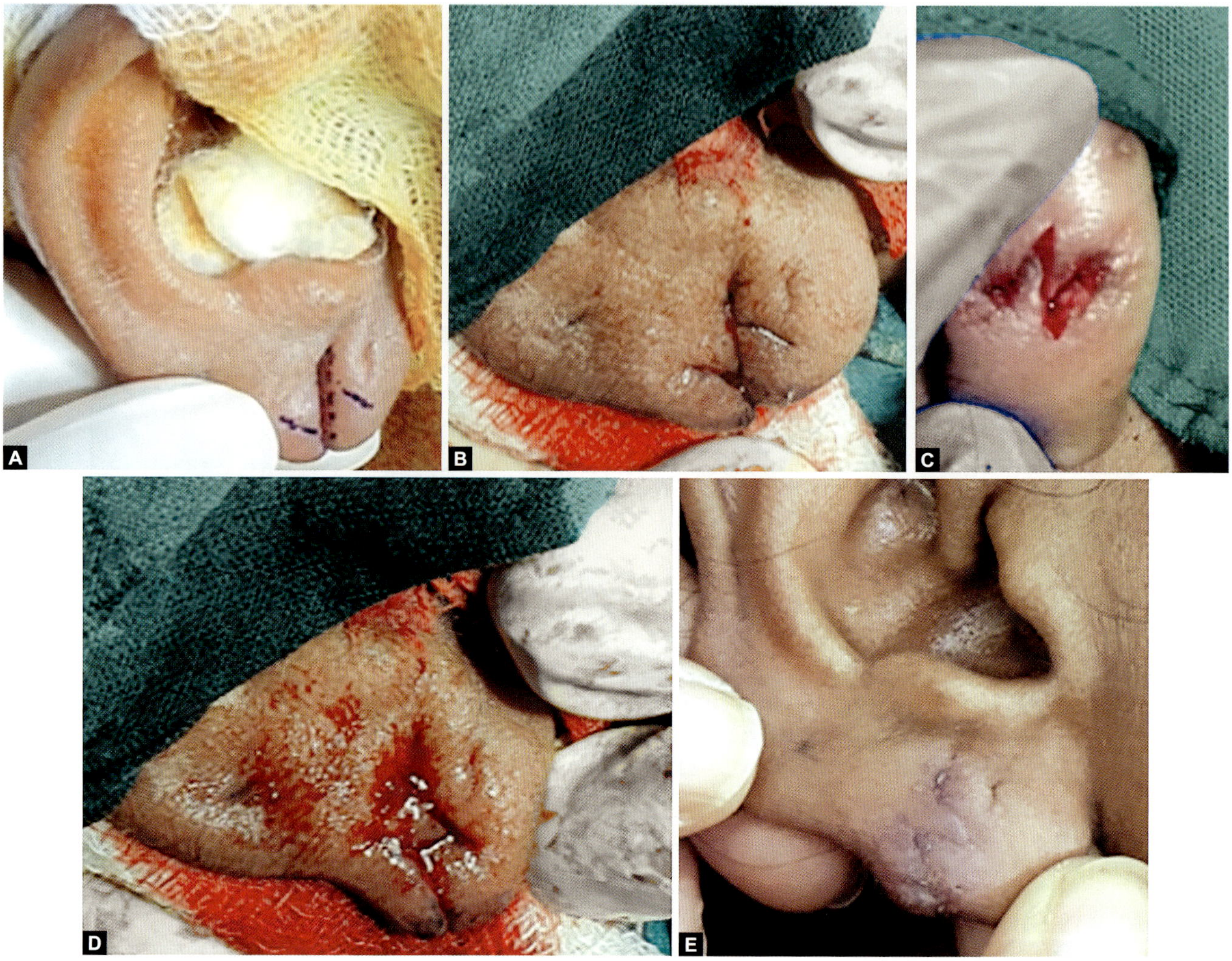

Figs. 21A to E: Z-plasty for earlobe repair.

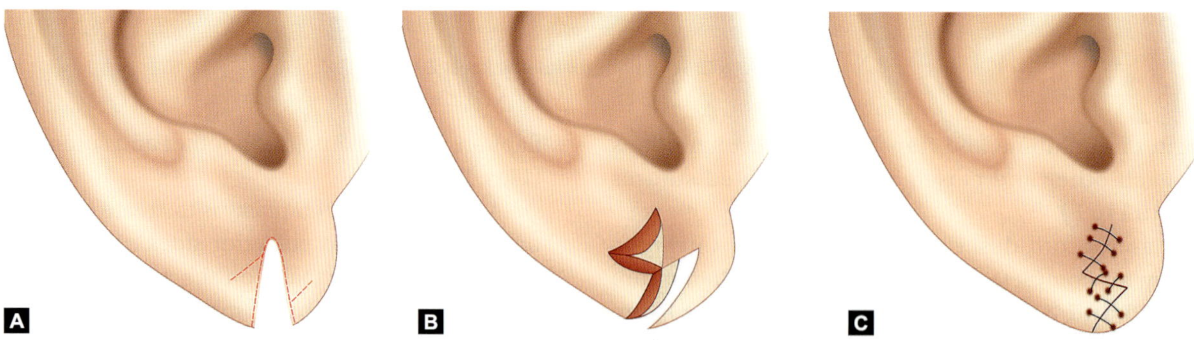

Figs. 22A to C: Schematic of partial-thickness Z-plasty.

of the cleft is de-epithelialized and curled back into the cleft. This technique, however, may produce a "trap door" deformity in the vertical and horizontal planes, resulting in notching of the rim **(Figs. 26A to C)**.[15]

Complete cleft repair with preservation of piercing site:

- *Side-to-side closure with preservation of apical skin*: This is performed by excising 80% of the lining epithelium leaving an intact superior lining edge. The anterior and posterior opposing edges are then sutured side-to-side retaining a small ostium at the superior pole of the sutured linear tract. The ostium is maintained by passing a light gold wire or silk suture at same sitting. While this technique is relatively easy to perform, the resulting earring canal is typically unable to withstand the weight of the earring, leading to cleft recurrence **(Figs. 27A to C)**.

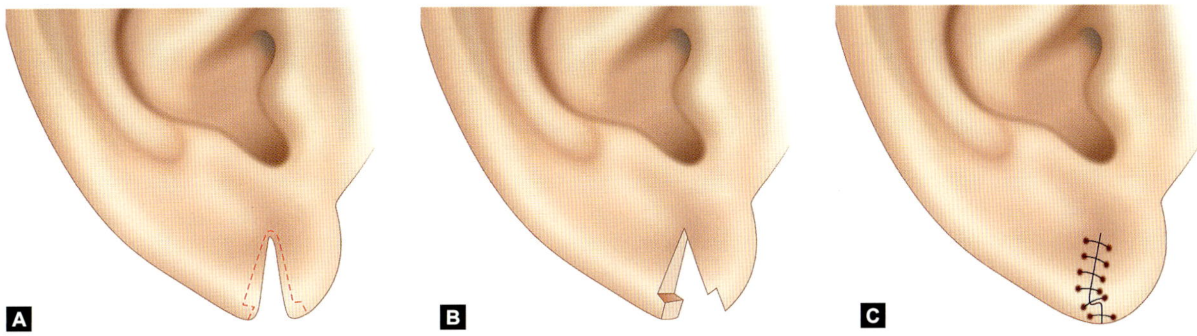

Figs. 23A to C: L-plasty.

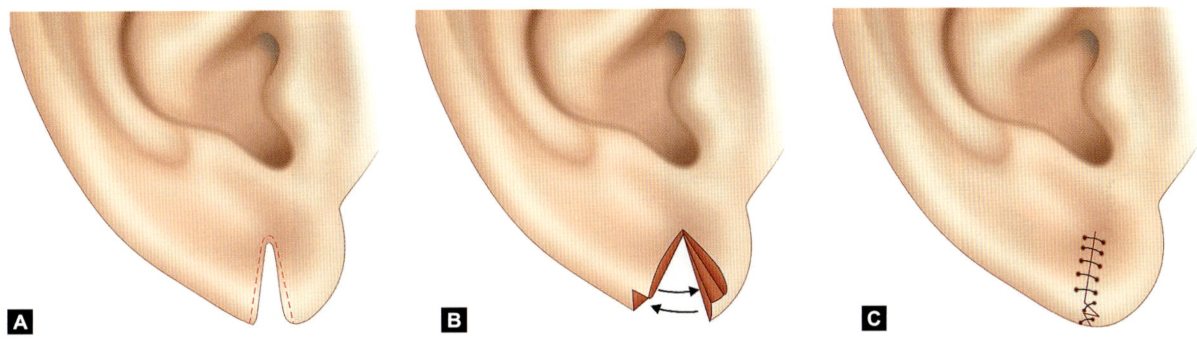

Figs. 24A to C: Modified L-plasty.

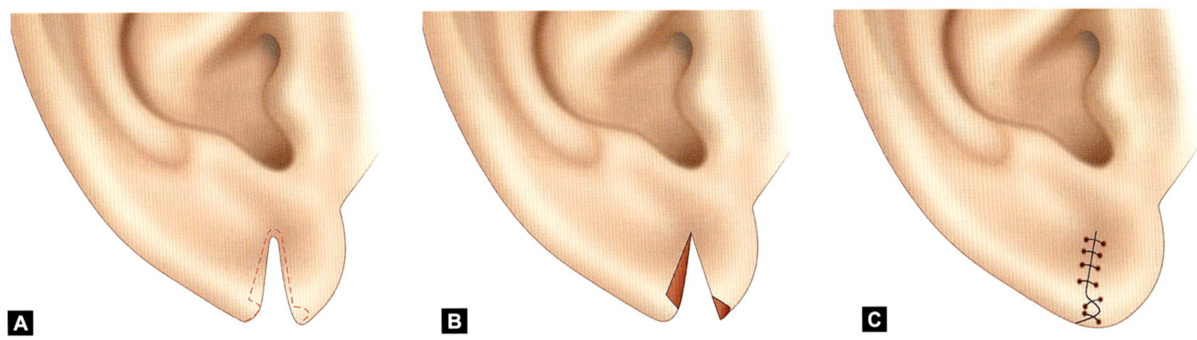

Figs. 25A to C: Side-to-side closure with V flap.

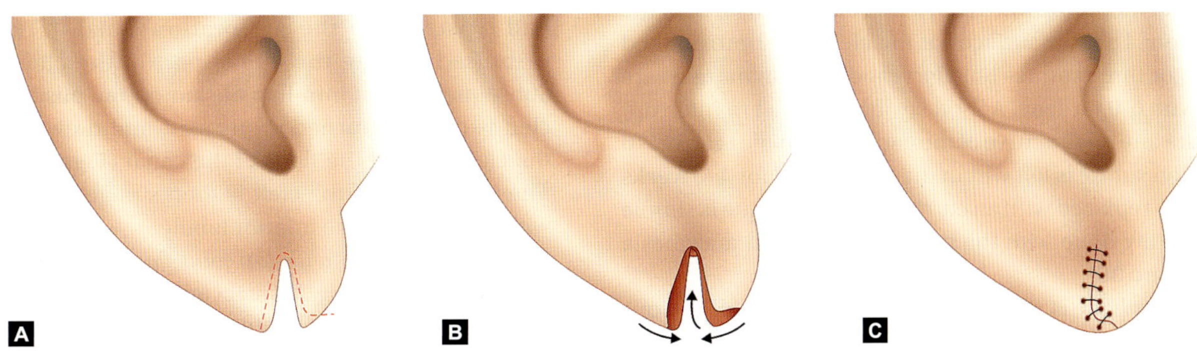

Figs. 26A to C: Rotational flap.

If patients insist on retaining the aperture in spite of counseling, an intravenous (IV) cannula or a small wire can be placed in the aperture during the procedure, and a suture can be passed through it after surgery **(Figs. 28A to D)**.

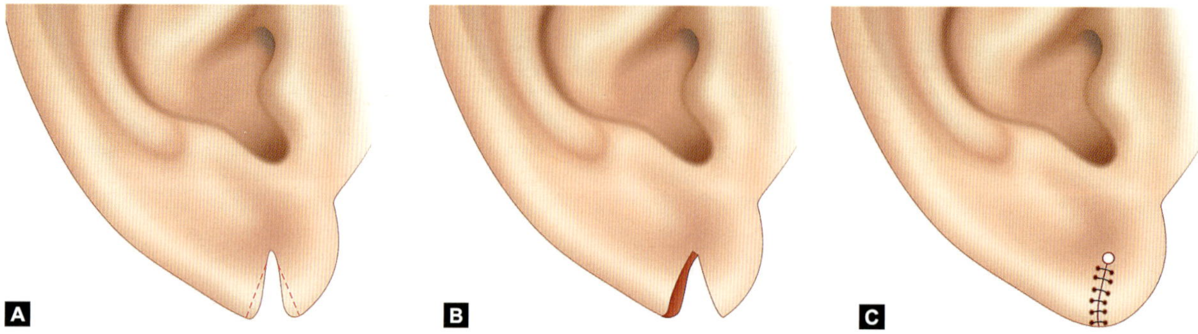

Figs. 27A to C: Side-to-side closure with preservation of apical piercing site.

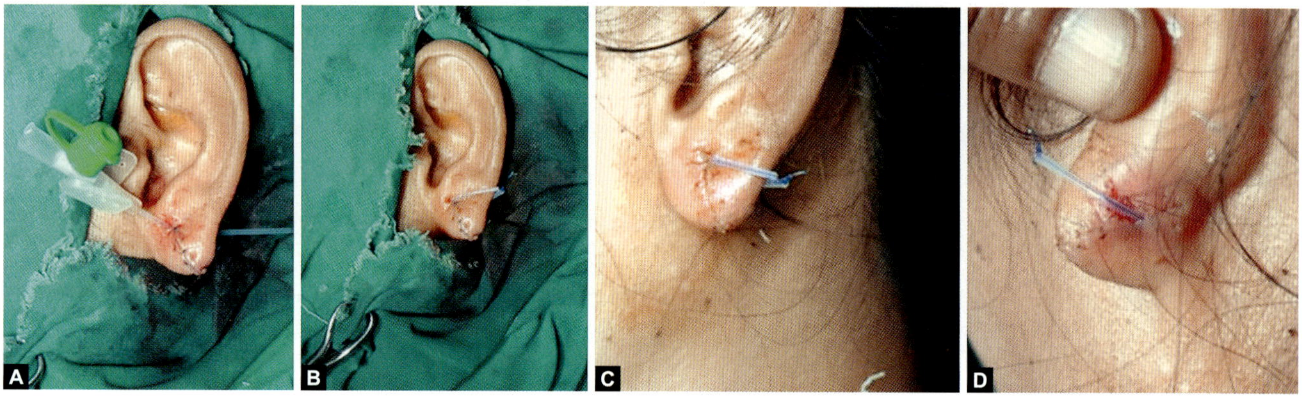

Figs. 28A to D: Maintaining the aperture during procedure.

- *Side-to-side closure with apical-lateral flap:* This technique was described by AM Pardue. The flap is based superiorly to one side of the upper end of the cleft. The width of the flap is the width of the inner surface of the cleft near its superior end. The flap is approximately 3 mm long and 1 mm thick.[1]

Operative technique: The procedure starts with outlining the flap and the area to be excised. The margins of the cleft are excised, and a small flap is raised on one side at the upper end of the cleft. The distal edge of the flap is sutured to the opposite side so that the suture line is not at the dependent area of the perforation. The raw surfaces of the cleft are approximated with two or three sutures 5-0 Vicryl and the skin margins are closed with 6-0 Prolene. A Z-plasty may be used to interrupt the suture line on the curve of the earlobe. A single loop of 2-0 clear nylon suture is left within the perforation for 4–6 weeks and then is replaced with an earring. The technique is simple and is readily done with the patient under local anesthesia **(Figs. 29 and 30)**.

The drawback is that this repair requires small tedious incisions to recreate the flap. In addition, the flap is composed of thin, already scarred skin, which may lead to cleft recurrence.

Clinical results: Results with this technique have been uniformly good for both complete and incomplete clefts. There have been no reports of failures of the flap. The patient should be instructed not to wear heavy earrings again or ones that might be snagged easily, thereby retearing the earlobe.

This technique is further modified by doing a Z-plasty at the inferior rim of the lobule.

The Z-plasty serves to prevent notching and creates a more aesthetic nonlinear scar at the inferior lobule.[11]

- A different technique using a posterior transposition flap has been reported, but the design of this flap requires excising more normal skin from one side of the cleft, with possible distortion of the flap as it is transposed and twisted into the perforation canal.[16] The cleft is excised leaving the apical part of the cleft intact. Subsequently, a 2 mm flap of skin on the posterior side cleft is created, turned on its axis, and drawn through the cleft to form the floor of the canal **(Figs. 31A to E)**. The remainder of the cleft is then straight-line sutured with a Z-plasty at the inferior lobule.
- *Side-to-side closure with lap-joint flap:*[17] The cleft edges are first pared leaving an intact apical portion of the cleft. Then, each half of the lobule is split into two triangular flaps overlapped onto one another and sutured together. This method reconstructs the apical earring canal, avoids the formation of a notch, staggers the scar on the lobule, and allows the surgeon to create a thinner or thicker lobule based on the construction of the flaps **(Figs. 32A to C)**.

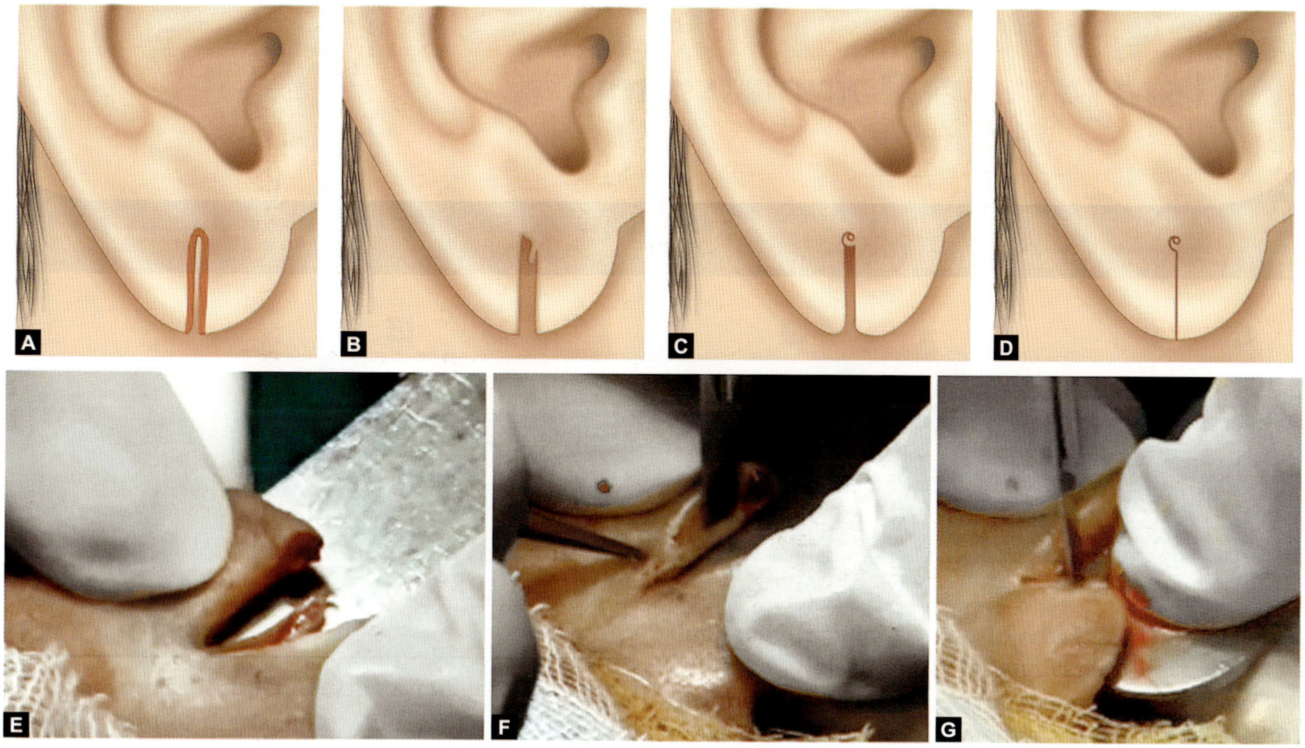

Figs. 29A to G: (A to D) Pardue technique; (E to G) A and B—flaps raised on the torn edges.

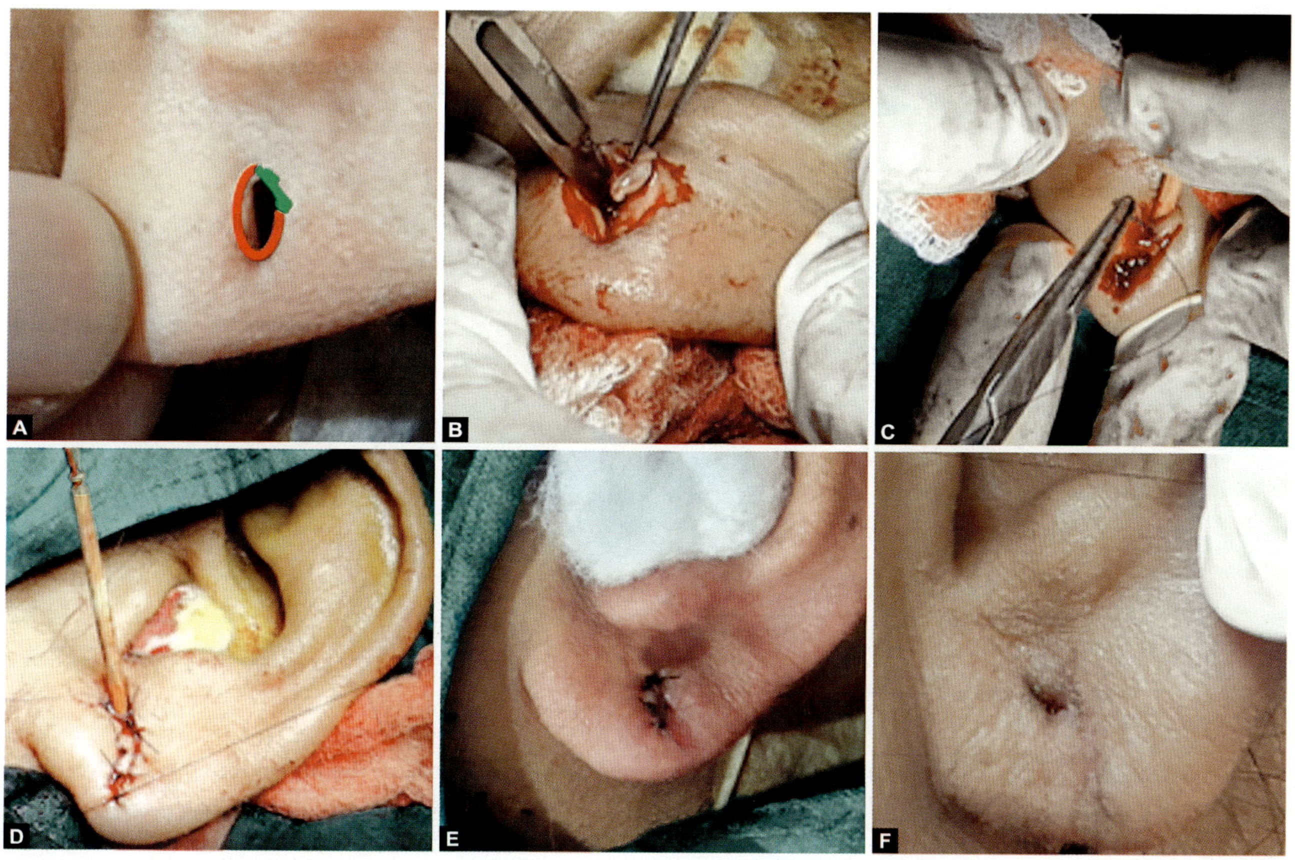

Figs. 30A to F: (A) Red portion is the area which is excised, green portion is the flap at the tip; (B) Flap raised at the apical tip; (C) The flap sutured to maintain the aperture; (D) The remaining defect sutured; (E) Immediately after procedure with stud in place; (F) On 10th postoperative day.

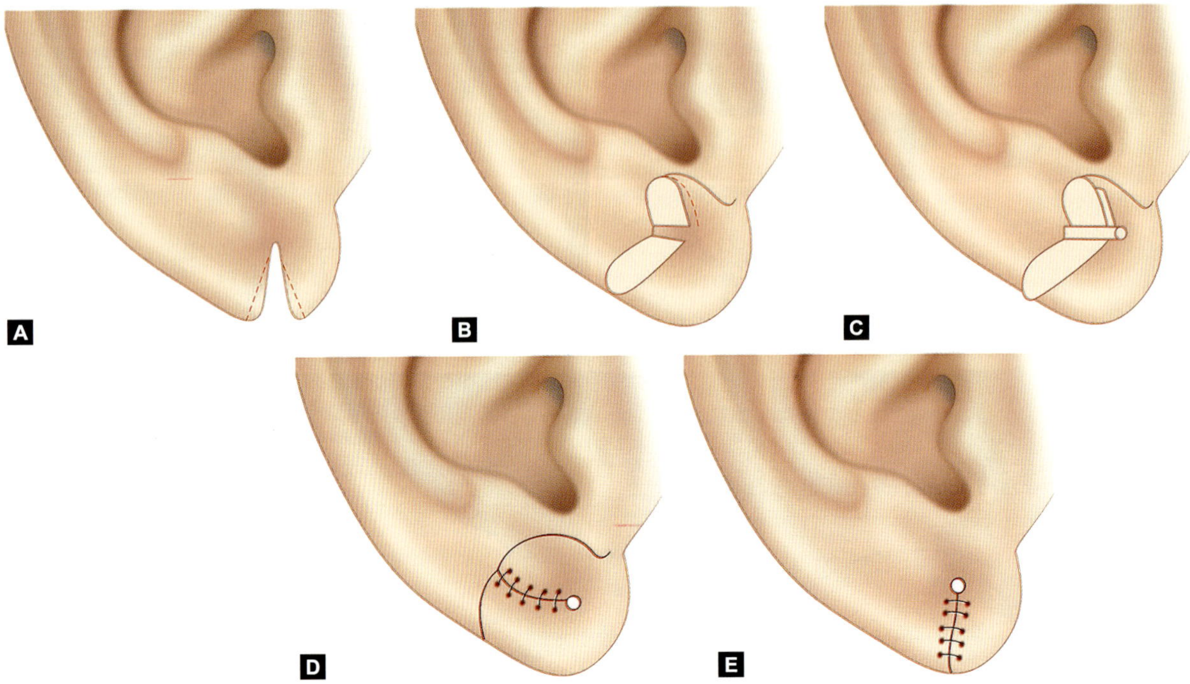

Figs. 31A to E: Posterior transposition flap.

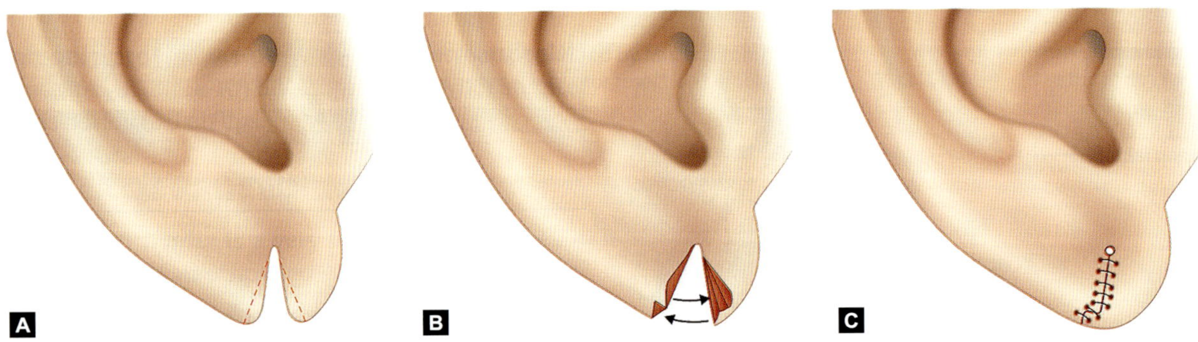

Figs. 32A to C: Schematic representation of lap-joint repair.

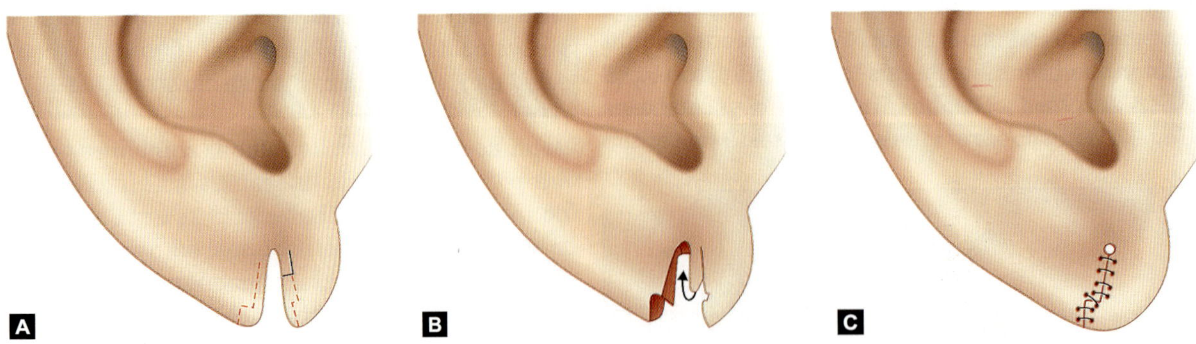

Figs. 33A to C: Lap-joint flap with Pardue's flap.

- *Modification of lap-joint flap with Pardue's flap:* This method combines a small apical-lateral flap, similar to Pardue's flap, with L-flap to repair the split lobe **(Figs. 33A to C)**.
- *Side-to-side closure with rectangular flap:* Once the cleft is excised leaving the apical portion intact, rectangular flaps are created on the anterior and posterior aspects of the cleft. Each flap is half the thickness of the lobule and extends up to the apical earring canal. The flaps are then overlapped onto one another and sutured together **(Figs. 34A to C)**.[18]

- *Side-to-side closure with superior-based flap:* Parallel incisions are placed on both sides of the cleft to create hanging flaps **(Figs. 35A to D)**. The upper ends of the superior-based flaps are sutured together to create an earring tract. A nylon loop is then passed through the canal. The remaining parts of the hanging flaps are excised and the edges of the cleft are sutured together. Alternately the first flap can be sutured to the tip of the split to recreate the earring hole. The second flap is sutured to the raw surface of the first flap. Finally, the remaining inferior portion of the cleft is sutured together. The authors state that the use of two flaps produces a stronger "cradle" of tissue for the new earring to rest. This technique, however, is rather complicated and requires a fair amount of time and suturing of tiny strands of tissue **(Figs. 35E to H)**.
- *Excision followed by unilateral Z-plasty and advancement flap* ***(Figs. 36A to C)****:*[2] The two unequal, unilateral Z-plasties are transposed in a superior direction. An incision on posterior limb of the cleft bisects this limb, using the lower third as the advancement flap and the upper two-thirds becomes the lower unilateral Z-plasty. An incision on the anterior limb of the cleft creates the second unilateral Z-plasty. Inferior border of the anterior limb of the cleft is de-epithelialized to accept the advancement flap.

An advancement flap from the posterior limb of the cleft provides the rounded contour of the lower edge of the lobule. The inferior limb of the cleft is de-epithelialized to accept the advancement flap **(Figs. 37A to F)**. Two unequal, unilateral Z-plasties are transposed in a superior direction.

Postoperative Precautions and Instructions

Appropriate systemic antibiotics for 7–10 days and nonsteroidal anti-inflammatory drugs (NSAIDs) for 2–3 days are prescribed. Suture removal is usually done between 5 and 7 days. Patient is advised to wait for minimum of 3 months

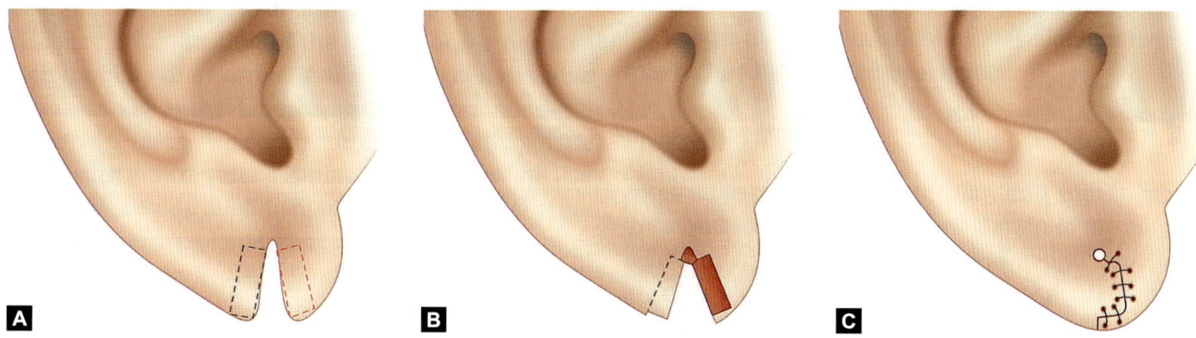

Figs. 34A to C: Side-to-side closure with rectangular flap.

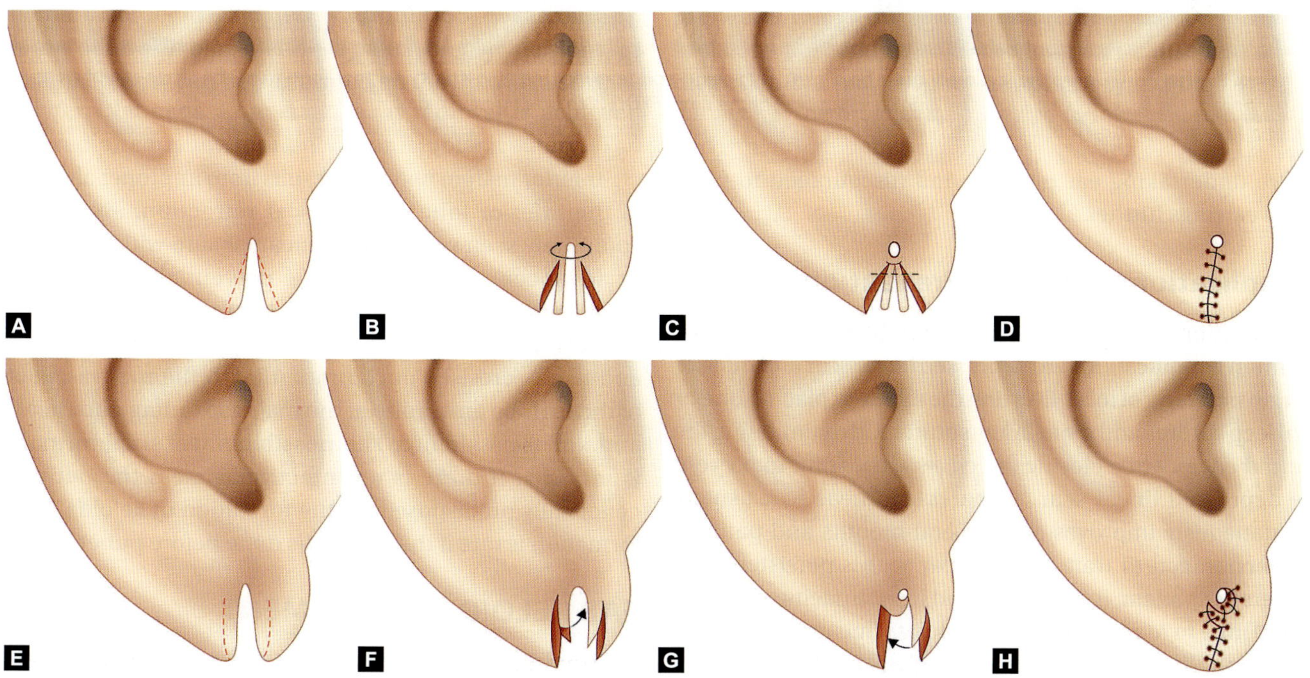

Figs. 35A to H: Superior-based flap side-to-side closure.

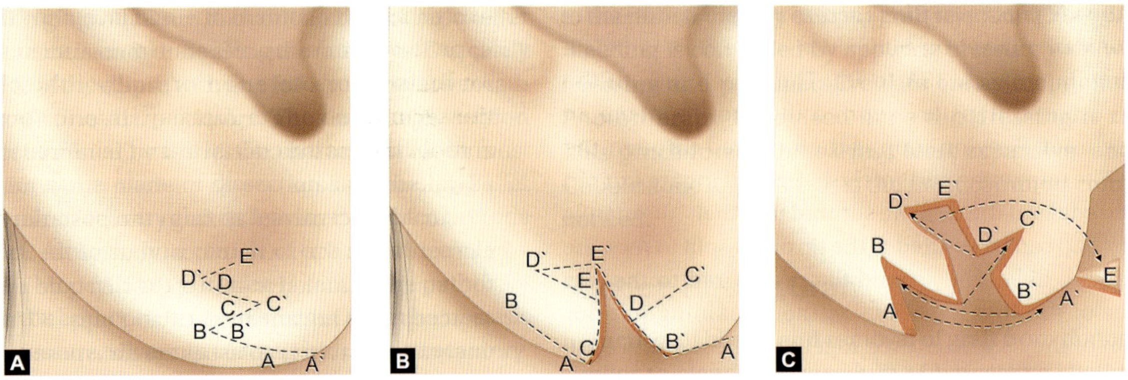

Figs. 36A to C: Excision followed by unilateral Z-plasty and advancement flap—diagrammatic design of the flap.

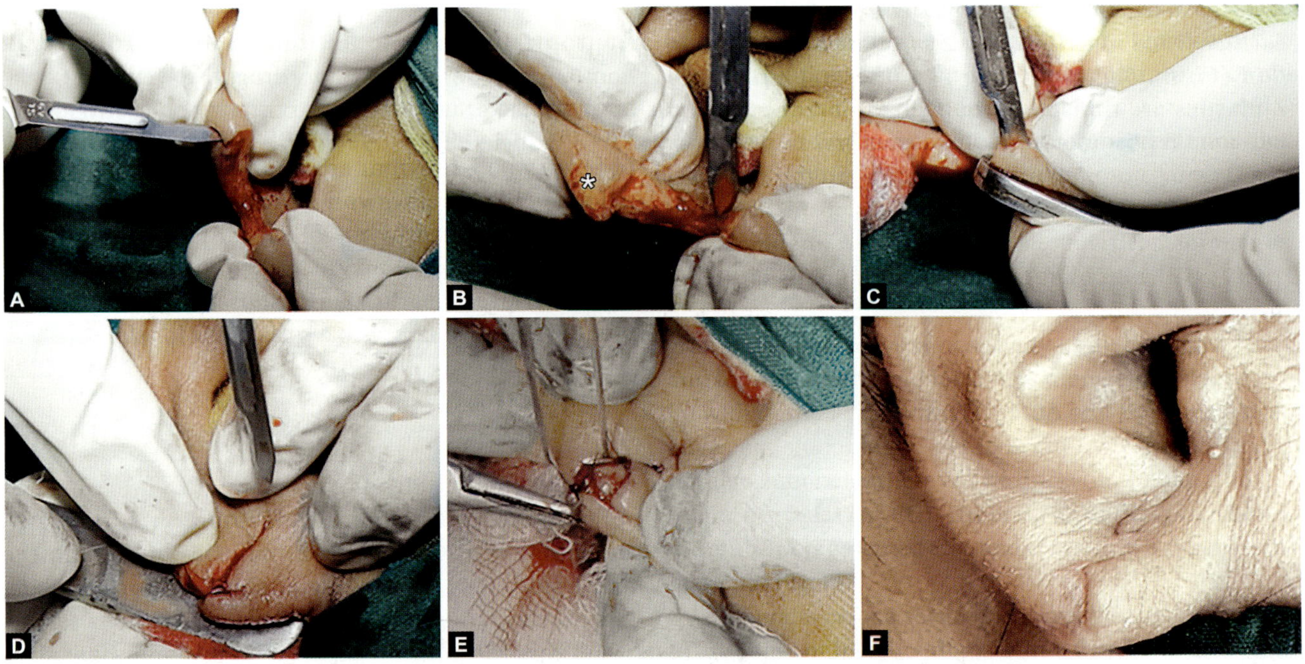

Figs. 37A to F: (A) De-epithelization of one end of cleft; (B) The de-epithelialized area (*); (C and D) Flap raised from the other end of cleft; (E) Transposition of the flap; (F) On 10th postoperative day.

before undertaking ear piercing and discouraged to wear heavy earrings further.

Complications and Their Prevention

Complications are infrequent with earlobe repair. The most common complications are depressed linear scar and inferior margin notching of lobe. Everting the edges by placing one or two deep sutures and a single key suture, and maintaining the everted edges while closing the edges are helpful to prevent the depressed linear scar. A depressed linear scar usually spontaneously improves over several months and patients are encouraged to wait. If the linear scar is persistent and bothers the patient, it may be treated by resurfacing with CO_2 laser. Three to four passes with moderate fluence and energy will gradually ablate the area and gives a good cosmetic acceptance.

Inferior margin notching results from improper alignment of the inferior lobe or from scar retraction, and is more commonly seen with simple linear closure without Z-plasty or advancement flap. It can be prevented by performing advancement flap repair at the lower margin.

Postoperative infection is infrequent, healing is quick and flap necrosis is uncommon due to the rich vascularity of the earlobe and is one of the major advantages for healing and scar remodeling. The possibility of keloid formation is minimal if there is no infection, unless the patient is genetically predisposed for the formation of keloids. Keloid formation is rare if the surgery is done before puberty.

EAR KELOID MANAGEMENT

External ear is one of the most common sites for keloid formation, more common after puberty due to hormonal influences. External ear keloids occur commonly after ear piercing. The incidence is about 2.5% after ear piercing.[19] Due to its location, ear keloids are cosmetically disfiguring and treatment is also challenging. There are various modalities of treatment of keloids, however no single method has been found to be completely successful. Combination of techniques offers better results. Surgical excision of keloids alone has a poor success with a high recurrence rate of 55%.[20] Simple excision is thought to promote additional collagen synthesis, resulting in fast regrowth and frequently an even larger keloid.[21] A study by Aköz et al. found combination of surgery, intralesional injection, and silicone gel sheets to be effective.[22]

If keloid is smaller in size, intralesional injections of various medications such as intralesional triamcinolone acetonide 10–40%, 5-fluorouracil (5-FU), and bleomycin either alone or in combination can be used. However, combination of triamcinolone acetonide and 5-FU is best studied.

Liquid nitrogen cryotherapy is one of the important modalities of treatment either given alone or with various intralesional medications. If the keloid is small and flat, surface cryotherapy with intralesional medication of earlier mentioned agents works in synergy and yield superior results compared to either of them used alone. If keloids are bulky, intralesional cryotherapy is the best option.

Intralesional Cryotherapy

After local anesthesia, depending upon the size of the keloid, an 18 G hypodermic needle or spinal needle is inserted through the summit of the keloid from one side to another. Either single or multiple needles depending upon the size of the keloid can be used. Padding with cotton gauge to be done at the exit point of the needle to protect the surrounding skin. Liquid nitrogen is sprayed from the handheld cryo gun either directly into the hub of the needle or with a modified rubber tubing fitted to the spray tip of handheld cryo gun. Freezing is done till the entire keloid mass is frozen from within the core of the keloid without freezing the surface of the skin. Freeze time may vary depending upon the size of the keloid from 1 to 3 minutes. Complete thawing to be allowed which is usually two to three times that of freezing. Two freeze thaw cycles to be done depending upon the size and bulk of keloid. Patient is advised to take analgesics for 2–3 days. The procedure may be repeated after 2–4 weeks depending on the response. Intralesional cryo has been reported to give good results with lesser complications compared to surface cryo. Intralesional steroid or combination with 5-FU may be given 10–15 minutes after complete thawing.

Surgical Excision

Surgical excision is one of the commonly practiced treatments for earlobe keloids. Excision should be performed gently and atraumatically so that the borders of the wound can be approximated without tension. Intrakeloidal excision without traumatizing the normal skin and excising the keloid with incision within the keloid is ideal.

Fillet Technique

Fillet technique involves strict intramarginal keloid excision in which the keloid scar is sharply dissected from the covering skin and the keloid mass is completely removed. Skin over the keloid is termed a "keloid fillet flap". Subcutaneous sutures are not used, and the keloid fillet flaps are closed with 6-0 nylon sutures after trimming. The keloid mass functions as an endogenous expander of the skin, and removal results in an excess of skin so as to adapt the wound edges without tension. According to Kim et al., the "five As and one B" (asepsis, atraumatic technique, absence of raw surface, avoidance of tension, accurate approximation of wound margin, and complete bleeding control) are important factors in reducing the recurrence rate of earlobe keloids in surgical excision.[23] The flap is marked so that the pedicle is toward the free edge of the earlobe and the line of incision close to the retroauricular crease, if the keloid is on the posterior aspect of earlobe, since it would be more cosmetically acceptable. If the keloid is on the anterior aspect of the earlobe, the flap is marked so that the pedicle is in the posterior position. Marking the incision and flap is very important and it varies depending on the type, size, and location of keloid. Marking should always be done before injecting the local anesthetic agent. A local anesthetic (2% lidocaine with 1:100,000 epinephrine) is infiltrated at the surgical site, after delineation of the line of incision so that borders of the mass are not obscured. Then, the cutaneous compartment is separated from the main keloidal mass using a curved blunt iris scissor until the keloid mass was completely separated, with normal skin all around. A sharp tipped scissor is used to separate the mass from its bed without perforating normal skin on either side. The thickness of the flap should be not too thin to prevent necrosis. If perforation occurred, it is closed using nylon 5-0 interrupted sutures. Bleeding is controlled by pressure.[24] Care should be taken not to overzealously excise the keloid mass. Sufficient tissue should be left attached to the earlobe all around to enable primary closure of the flaps after removing the core keloid tissue at the base. The thickness of the flaps should not be too thin to prevent necrosis considering the less vascularity of keloid tissue **(Figs. 38 and 39)**.

If keloids are involving the undersurface or lower border of earlobe altering the normal anatomy, flaps has to be raised posteriorly and the core of the keloid to be debulked from behind and the flap sutured on posterior aspect maintaining the near normal rounded anatomy of the earlobe. Incision of the skin at lower margin to be avoided **(Figs. 40A to C)**.

Keloids which reach the other skin side, at the site of ear piercing, i.e., dumbbell keloid, can be excised both anteriorly and posteriorly leaving behind a sufficient skin flap for primary closure ensuring the core of the keloid tissue which is connecting both the sides is removed completely. The skin flaps harvested are closed with primary closure using 5-0/6-0 suture similar to core fillet. Before proceeding to wound closure, meticulous palpation of the wound all around and also the bed is done to make sure that there is no residual fibrous tissue. A pressure dressing is applied and sutures are removed 7–10 days later.

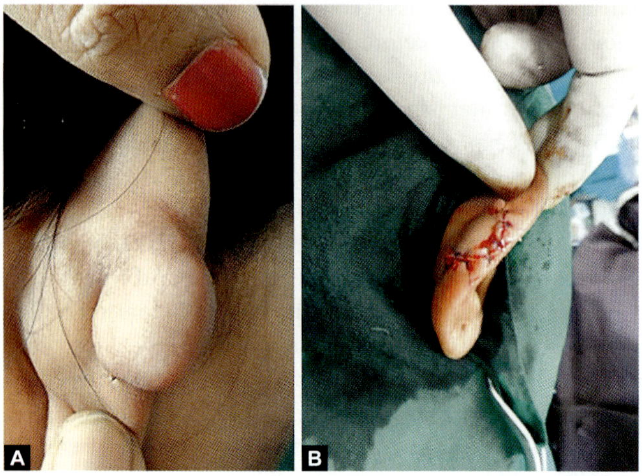

Figs. 38A and B: Excision of intrakeloidal tissue and closure with C flap.

In contrast, extramarginal keloid excision, which is defined as an incision of physiological skin and removal of the entire lesion, produces a linear scar. The disadvantage occurs in maintaining tension in the suture. Particularly after resection of larger keloids, skin grafts or local flaps often are required to perform the primary wound closure.

If the keloid is a pedunculated mass, mark the incision leaving behind a pedicle which will be sufficient for primary closure. Excise the mass leaving behind a pedicle, debulk the keloidal tissue from within the left out base with No. 15 surgical blade carefully without nicking or cutting the flaps, leaving behind bulky flaps on either side at the base, and closure of the flaps with primary closure without dead space. Pressure bandage is applied. Suture removal to be done 7–10 days later **(Figs. 41A to D)**.

Various surgical methods are available for debulking of keloids tissue with primary intention of reducing the size of keloid without cutting the normal tissue; however, surgery alone leads to high rate of recurrences, hence postsurgical preventive strategies are most important for prevention of recurrences of earlobe keloids.

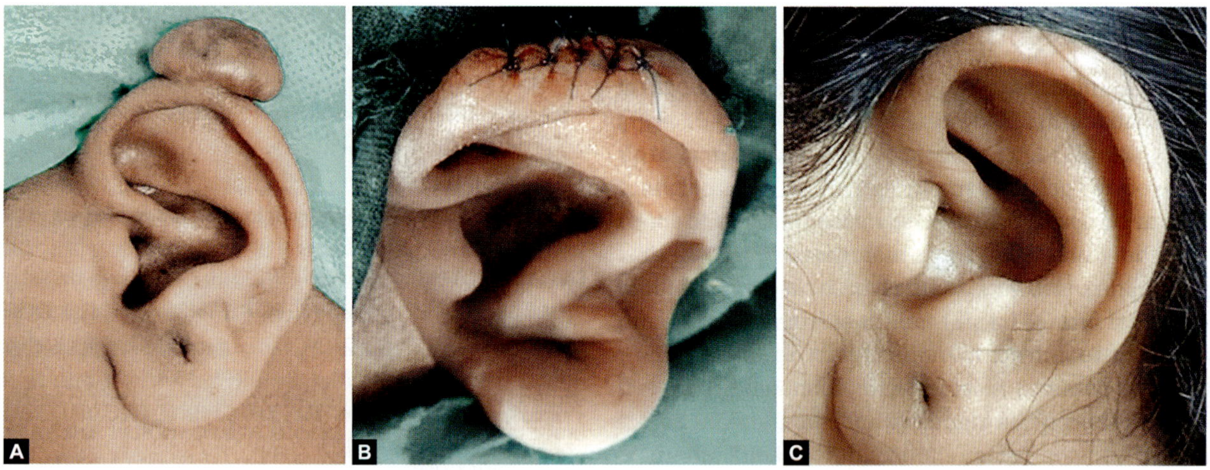

Figs. 39A to C: Keloid excision and closure.

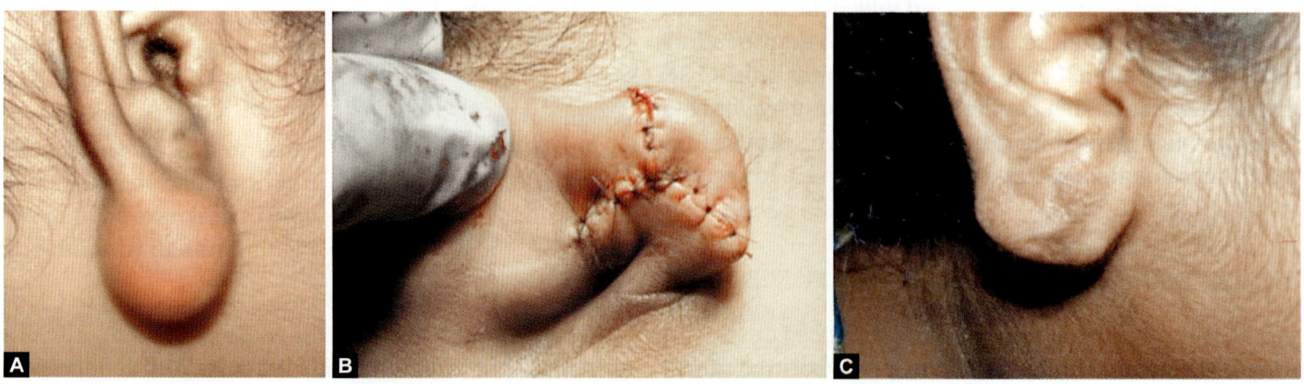

Figs. 40A to C: Excision of keloid over lobule, debulking of keloid with flaps on posterior aspect, and sutures applied posteriorly.

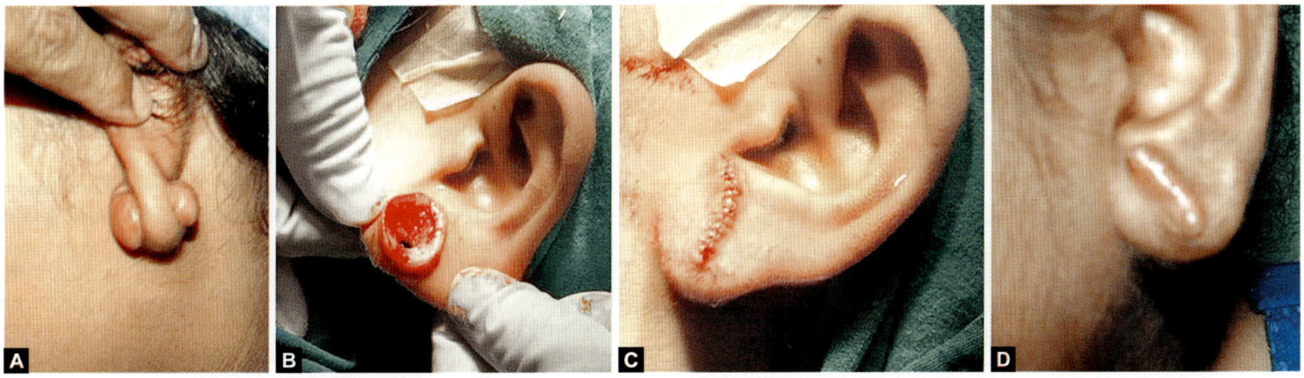

Figs. 41A to D: Intrakeloidal surgical debulking of dumbbell keloid on both anterior and posterior.

LASERS

Roles of lasers have been described in the literature in the management of earlobe keloids. Photothermal effect of lasers produces collagen denaturation. The heat energy ruptures collagen stabilizing intermolecular and molecular cross-links. In addition, the concurrent superheating of collagen fibers could also dissociate disulfide bonds with a subsequent realignment of these fibers.[25] However, lasers have limited role in the authors experience. Flash-lamp pulsed-dye laser (FPDL) has been used for the treatment of keloids with achievement of promising results, however, the treatment by FPDL alone is suitable only for small keloids with a limited volume.[26] Neodymium-doped yttrium aluminum garnet (Nd:YAG), carbon dioxide, and diode laser have been used to treat earlobe keloids.[27,28]

However, the role of lasers in keloids is limited in a large bulky keloids, which are firm and hard with less vascularity.

To reduce recurrence rates, surgery is often combined with adjuvant treatment:

- *Corticosteroid injections.* In addition to their anti-inflammatory effect, corticosteroids reduce collagen and glycosaminoglycan synthesis and the proliferation of fibroblasts. Triamcinolone acetonide, 10–40 mg, is often used as an active ingredient in intralesional injections. Injection at the correct depth in the mid- dermis is important to prevent undesired adverse effects, such as atrophy of the skin, telangiectasia, or pigmentary abnormalities. Steroids can be either first line or adjuvant to surgery. Injections are given perioperatively and then every three weeks.
- *Corticosteroid injection* in association with 5-FU, pulsed dye laser, and cryotherapy has been reported to be more efficient than corticosteroid alone.[29]
- *Verapamil hydrochloride* is a widely used calcium channel antagonist which inhibits the synthesis/secretion of extracellular matrix molecules including collagen, glycosaminoglycans, and fibronectin while increasing collagenase. It can be injected locally, intraoperatively before application of the pressure dressing, then postoperatively every 2 weeks for 1 month, then monthly for 3 months. The injection is given along suture lines and also into the wound bed.[24]
- Topical controlled pressure is reported to reduce the capillary perfusion that causes local hypoxia and leads to a decrease of myofibroblasts and collagen synthesis, acceleration of collagen maturation, and consequent flattening of the keloid.[30] The pressure exerted should be at least 24 mm Hg, in order to exceed the inherent capillary pressure, but must be <30 mm Hg, otherwise it diminishes the peripheral blood circulation. This therapy is performed especially for ear keloids, for which pressure is applied at the front and back to build an abutment.[31] Making an auricle splint is demanding due to complex anatomy of external ears. To overcome this custom-made devices have been tried.

Custom-made methyl methacrylate stent can be used as pressure devices. This is applied 2 weeks postexcision to ensure primary healing. Since, the fabricated pressure device is unique for each ear, the natural folds of the ear are not compromised during application, enhancing its usage as postoperative pressure therapy.[32] Pressure devices should be used up to 20 hours per day during 12 months; and then 12 hours per day for another 6 months. Other modification to this is U-shaped screw-and-pin system which helps to adjust auricle pressure.[33]

- *Cryotherapy:* The freeze induces vascular damage that may lead to anoxia and ultimately tissue necrosis. Fikrle reported good results using cryotherapy alone for ear keloids in young patients.[34]
- *Other adjuvant therapies* are silicone gel sheets, radiation therapy, and imiquimod.

CONCLUSION

Earlobe cleft and keloids present commonly to dermatologists.

A proper knowledge of various techniques for the earlobe repair and keloid surgery followed by proper postsurgical preventive methods is essential. These procedures can be very well-handled by dermatologists with surgical skills. Each procedure has its own advantages which a surgeon can make use of, depending on the type of earlobe deformity and type, site, and size of earlobe keloid.

REFERENCES

1. Pardue AM. Repair of torn earlobe with preservation of the perforation for an earring. Plast Reconstr Surg. 1973;51:472-3.
2. Strauch B, Keyes-Ford M. Repair of the cleft earlobe with an advancement flap and two unilateral Z-plasties. Plastic Reconstr Surg. 1997;99:924-6.
3. Vujevich J, Obagi S. Repair of partial earlobe cleft using "purse string" repair. Dermatol Surg. 2006;32:969-7.
4. Sadasivan K, Kochunarayanan A. A Revised Classification and Treatment Algorithm for Acquired Split Earlobe, With a Description of the Composite Technique and its Outcome. Cureus. 2020;12(9):e10422.
5. de Mendonça MC, de Oliveira AR, Araújo JM, Silva M, Gamonal A. Nonsurgical technique for incomplete earlobe cleft repair. Dermatol Surg. 2009;35:446-50.
6. Reiter D, Alford EL. Torn earlobe: a new approach to management with a review of 68 cases. Ann Otol Rhinol Laryngol. 1994;103:879-84.
7. McLaren LR. Cleft earlobe: a hazard of wearing earrings. Br J Plast Surg. 1954;7:162-5.
8. Tan EC. Punch technique: an alternative approach to the repair of pierced earlobe deformities. J Dermatol Surg Oncol. 1989;15:270-2.
9. Abenavoli FM. Split earlobe: repair using a half Z-plasty technique. Plast Reconstr Surg. 1996:98:372-3.
10. Apesos J, Kane M. Treatment of traumatic earlobe clefts. Aesthetic Plast Surg. 1993;17:253-5.
11. LaRossa D, Hamilton R. Method for repair of cleft earlobes. Plast Reconstr Surg. 1973;51:472-3.
12. Fatah MF. L-plasty technique in the repair of split earlobe. Br J Plast Surg. 1985;38:410-4.
13. Harahap M. Repair of split earlobes. A review and a new technique. J Dermatol Surg Oncol. 1982;8:187-91.
14. Kalimuthu R, Larson BJ, Lewis N. Earlobe repair: a new technique. Plast Reconstr Surg. 1984;74:299-300.
15. Effendi SH. Reconstruction of the middle-aged torn earlobe: a new method. Br J Plast Surg. 1988;41:174-6.
16. Buchan NG. The cleft ear lobe: a method of repair with preservation of the earring canal. Br J Plast Surg. 1975;28:296.
17. Argamaso RV. The lap-joint principle in the repair of the cleft earlobe. Br J Plast Surg. 1978;31:337-8.
18. Zoltie N. Spilt earlobes: a method of repair preserving the hole. Plast Reconstr Surg. 1987;80:619-21.
19. Simplot TC, Hoffman HT. Comparison between cartilage and soft tissue ear piercing complications. Am J Otolaryngol. 1998:19:305-10.
20. Cosman B, Wolff M. Correlation of keloid recurrence with completeness of local excision. A negative report. Plast Reconstr Surg. 1972;50:163.
21. Niessen FB, Spauwen PH, Schalkwijk J, Kon M. On the nature of hypertrophic scars and keloids: a review. Plast Reconstr Surg. 1999:104:1435-58.
22. Aköz T, Gideroqluk, Akan M. Combination of different techniques for the treatment of earlobe keloids. Aesth Plast Surg. 2002;26:184-8.
23. Kim DY, Kim ES, Eo SR, Kim KS, Lee SY, Cho BH. A surgical approach for earlobe keloid: keloid fillet flap. Plast Reconstr Surg. 2004;113(6):1668-74.
24. El-Kamel MF, Selim MK, Alghobary MF. Keloidectomy with core fillet flap and intralesional verapamil injection for recurrent earlobe keloids. Indian J Dermatol Venereol Leprol. 2016;82:659-65.
25. Alster TS. Laser scar revision: comparison study of 585 nm pulsed dye laser with and without intralesional corticosteroids. Dermatol Surg. 2003;29(1):25-9.
26. Dierickx C, Goldmann MP, Fitzpatrick RE. Laser treatment of erythematous/hypertrophic and pigmented scars in 26 patients. Plast Reconstr Surg. 1995;95(1):84-90.
27. Norris JE. The effect of carbon dioxide laser surgery on the recurrence of keloids. Plast Reconstr Surg. 1991;87:44-9.
28. Kassab AN, Kharbotly AEl. Management of ear lobule keloids using 980-nm diode laser. Eur Arch Otorhinolaryngol. 2012;269:419-23.
29. Sobec R, Dobreanu C, Fodor L, Comcutean A, Cichil I, Cosgarea M. Ear keloids: A review and update of treatment options. Clujul Medical. 2013;86(4):313-17.
30. Macintyre L, Baird M. Pressure garments for use in the treatment of hypertrophic scars. Burns. 2006;32(1):10-5.
31. Bran GM, Brom J, Hörmann K, Stuck BA. Auricular keloids: combined therapy with a new pressure device. Arch Facial Plast Surg. 2012;14(1):20-6.
32. Kadouch DJ, van der Veer WM, Delavary BM, Kerkdijk D, Niessen FB. An alternative adjuvant treatment after ear keloid excision using a custom-made methyl methacrylate stent. Dermatol Ther. 2010;23:686-92.
33. Tanaydin V, Colla C, Piatkowski A, Beugels J, Hendrix N, Kerckhove EV, et al. Management of ear keloids using custom-molded pressure clips: a preliminary study. Eur J Plast Surg. 2014;37:259-66.
34. Fikrle T, Pizinger K. Cryosurgery in the treatment of ear lobe keloids: report of seven cases. Dermatol Surg. 2005;1:1728-31.

CHAPTER 56

Hidradenitis Suppurativa

Kumaresan M, Eswari L

KEY MESSAGES

- Hidradenitis suppurativa (HS) is a chronic disorder which can lead to severe morbidity. There is no satisfactory medical or surgical treatment available.
- Medical treatments include antibiotics, dapsone, retinoids, intralesional steroids, and biologics.
- Lasers (CO_2 laser, Nd:YAG laser) have been tried with variable success.
- Surgery is needed in most cases and consists of deroofing, limited local excision, and wide excision.

INTRODUCTION

Hidradenitis suppurativa (HS), derived from the Greek words "hidros" meaning sweat and "aden" meaning glands, is also known as Verneuil's disease, acne inversa, or smoker's boils. HS is a chronic, recurrent, debilitating disease that presents usually after puberty with painful, deep-seated, inflammatory lesions in the apocrine glands of the body. HS is seen usually after puberty during the second and third decade of life and onset after menopause is rare.[1] HS in prepubertal age group is associated with premature adrenarche.[2,3] It is seen more commonly in females than the males.[1] Autosomal dominant type of inheritance has been reported in families.[1,4]

PATHOGENESIS

The pathogenesis of HS is not clearly understood. Initially, it was thought to be a disorder of apocrine origin, but recent evidence states that HS is caused primarily by follicular occlusion with secondary involvement of the apocrine glands.[5] Follicular plugging leads to occlusion and dilation of the pilosebaceous unit, with subsequent rupture.[1] Extrusion of follicular contents, primarily consisting of corneocytes, bacteria, sebum products, and hair into the dermis produce a chemotactic inflammatory response.[1] The resulting influx of neutrophils, lymphocytes, and histiocytes leads to abscess formation.[6] This facilitates infection with further suppuration. With recurrence, sinuous and fistulous tracts evolve.[6,7] The role of hormones in HS is controversial and it is likely that hyperandrogenism does not play a role in the pathogenesis.[1] Some investigators postulate that there may be an underlying immunologic aberration involved in the pathogenesis of HS.[1]

The bacterial species isolated from HS include *Streptococcus viridans*, *Staphylococcus aureus*, *Streptococcus milleri*, anaerobes (*Peptostreptococcus* species, *Bacteroides melaninogenicus*, and *Bacteroides corrodens*), coryneform bacteria, gram-negative rods, gram-negative bacteria such as *Escherichia coli*, *Klebsiella*, and *Proteus*. No single bacterial species predominated in the culture, and this indicates that the bacteria are secondary colonizer rather than a primary agent. The most common bacteria isolated are *Staphylococcus epidermidis* and *S. aureus*.[8] Increased prevalence of smoking has been found among patients with HS, suggesting that tobacco is a potential trigger for HS.[9,10] A significant association with obesity has been reported in HS.[11] Obesity aggravates disease through sweat retention, maceration, and shearing of follicular or ductal outlets.[12]

CLINICAL FEATURES

Hidradenitis suppurativa is insidious in onset and usually seen in postpubertal males and females who are otherwise healthy.[13] Lesions are most frequently seen in the intertriginous apocrine glands as the axillary, inguinal, perianal, perineal, mammary, inframammary, buttock, pubic, chest, scalp, retroauricular, and eyelid areas.[14] This distribution pattern corresponds for the most part with the "milk line" distribution of apocrine-related mammary tissue in mammals.[1] The sites affected in HS correspond not only to the location of apocrine glands in the body but also to that of terminal hair follicles dependent on low androgen concentrations.[7] Lesions begins usually in axillae and anogenital regions, but as the disease progresses, new lesions develop in areas of friction including the submammary region, nape of the neck, waistband area, and in the inner thighs. Perineal HS is associated with higher recurrence and poor prognosis than axillary HS.[15] HS lesions are characterized by tender subcutaneous nodules. With time, nodules rupture spontaneously or coalesce to form painful, deep dermal abscesses. These abscesses are rounded without central necrosis or pus pointing and exude a purulent foul-smelling discharge. Double comedone is a black head with

TABLE 1: Hurley staging system for hidradenitis suppurativa.

Hurley stage	*Extent of disease in tissue*
I	Abscess formation (single or multiple) without sinus tracts and cicatrization
II	One or more widely separated recurrent abscesses with tract formation and scars
III	Multiple interconnected tracts and abscesses throughout an entire area

multiple apertures that communicates below the skin and is typical for HS.[16] Early symptoms include burning, pruritus, local warmth, hyperhidrosis, and pain. HS may be divided into acute and chronic forms. Acute HS presents with a few deep-seated nodules, which may coalesce developing into cord-like red-to-bluish red structures.[1] Chronic HS is characterized by multiple abscesses, internetted working sinus tracts, foul exudate from draining sinuses, inflammation, both atrophic and hypertrophic scars, ulceration, and infection which may extend deep into the fascia.[1] Hurley separated patients into three groups based largely on the presence and extent of cicatrization and sinuses **(Table 1)**. Over time, sinus tracts can coalesce into large regions of subcutaneous honeycombing.[17] They can potentially dissect into deep structures including muscle, fascia, lymph nodes, the urethra, and the bowels.[6,14] They release a serous-to-purulent malodorous discharge, resulting in ulceration,[18] soiling of clothes, and social embarrassment. The ulcers characteristically present with rolled, boggy, ragged edges and clean granulating bases.[18] Patients with anogenital HS may also have disease in the anal canal.[19] The severity of disease varies considerably. The diagnosis of HS is made clinically by the features such as chronicity, recurrence of disease, failure to completely clear with antibiotics, characteristic multifocal lesion distribution, sinus formation, scarring, dermal contracture, presence of double comedones, multiple open comedones, nodules, papules, tenderness of lesions, and malodorous discharge.[1]

PROGNOSIS AND COMPLICATIONS

Contractures, strictures, serious infection, and anemia are also potential sequelae of HS.[1] Risk of squamous cell carcinoma (SCC) is increased in those with HS.[1] The ratio of SCC in HS favors males (4:1).[20] Majority of SCC occurred in perineum or buttocks.[20]

DISEASE ASSOCIATION

Hidradenitis suppurativa has been associated with many disorders. The other disorders of follicular occlusion (acne conglobata, dissecting cellulitis of the scalp, and pilonidal cyst) are well-known associations with HS, and make up the so-called follicular occlusion tetrad.[21] Acne vulgaris and Crohn's disease are the other common associations.[1]

TREATMENT

There is no single effective therapy for HS. Treatment modality depends on the disease severity. Treatment for HS is classified as either medical or surgical **(Flowchart 1)**.

Flowchart 1: Treatment algorithm.[22]

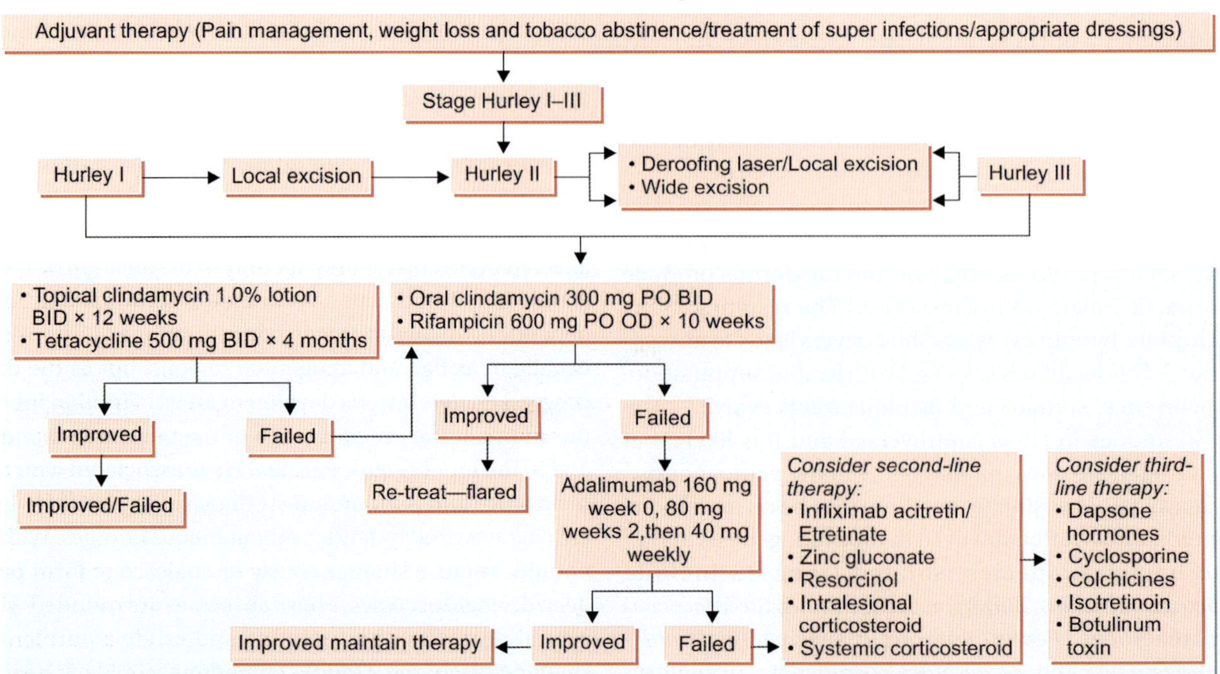

Medical Treatment

Conservative Measures

Conservative measures include warm baths, avoidance of shaving if irritation occurs, avoiding prolonged exposure to heat, humidity, hydrotherapy, weight loss, and use of topical cleansing agents to reduce bacterial load.

Nonsteroidal anti-inflammatory drugs (NSAIDs) can be used to alleviate pain as well as inflammation. Antibiotics either topical or systemic agents are used as the first-line agents or in Hurley's stage I disease. Though antibiotics are used to improve HS, complete remission is rarely achieved with antibiotics. The only topical antibiotic that has been proven effective in a randomized controlled trial is clindamycin. Topical 1% clindamycin phosphate applied twice daily for a period of minimum 3 months has been shown to be effective in Hurley stage I and II disease.[23] Combination of rifampicin (600 mg) and clindamycin (300 mg twice daily) for 10 weeks has been shown to be effective in moderate-to-severe HS.[24,25] Dapsone had been reported to be an effective and safe alternative, therapeutic option for HS at a dose of 25–150 mg/day (4–12 weeks) and may be particularly useful for women in the reproductive age group.[26] The other combination reported to improve refractory HS is rifampicin, moxifloxacin, and metronidazole.[27] Antistaphylococcal agents are best for axillary disease, and more broad-spectrum coverage is preferred for perineal disease.[28] There is no evidence that chronic suppressive antibiotic therapy alters the natural history of HS. Oral retinoids work by inhibiting sebaceous gland function and abnormal keratinization. Pretreatment with isotretinoin at a dosage of 0.5–1.0 mg/kg daily for a few months before surgery has been recommended to reduce the inflammatory components.[28] Acitretin appears to be an effective treatment for refractory HS, leading to reduction of pain from painful nodules and reducing the extent of the disease for a prolonged period.[29] Hormonal therapy should be considered in females presenting with HS.[30] Oral contraceptive agents that contain a high estrogen-to-progesterone ratio and low androgenicity of progesterone, finasteride at a dosage of 5 mg daily, and cyproterone acetate, have been reported to be effective in HS.[28] Immunosuppressive drugs such as cyclosporine, azathioprine, and prednisone are occasionally successful.[31] The use of biologic drugs for the treatment of HS has variable long-term results and is laden with significant adverse effects.[32] Among the biological agents, infliximab, etanercept, and adalimumab have been reported to be effective in HS.[32]

Botulinum Toxin

Botulinum toxin (BTX) has been reported to be effective in HS by decreasing apocrine gland sweat secretion and limiting tendency toward follicular rupture.[33] Prepubertal HS has been successfully treated with BTX.[34] Dose ranges from 50 to 100 units and injected intradermally as in hyperhidrosis. BTX treatment appears to be suppressive with the effect lasting for 6 months. The inhibitory effect of BTX on neurogenic inflammation and nociceptive mast cell innervations has been reported as a possible additional mechanism of action.[35]

Radiotherapy

Radiotherapy has been suggested as efficacious for early lesions of HS but not for sinuses.[36] Hair follicle destruction is the suggested mechanism of action.[36] When more radical and invasive surgical options fail, radiotherapy is a viable option.[37] Doses of 7.5 Gy at 2.5 Gy per fraction have been reported to be beneficial in refractory cases.[37] Caution should be exercised when offering this therapy to younger patients. Brachytherapy has been successfully utilized for treating HS.[38]

Cryotherapy

Cryosurgery has been studied as a potential HS treatment. Complications like pain, ulceration, secondary infection, and prolonged healing limit its routine use in HS.[39]

LASERS AND LIGHT DEVICES

Laser and light devices act in two main ways: selective and ablative. Internal pulsed light (IPL) and lasers such as Nd:YAG (neodymium-doped yttrium aluminum garnet), Alexandrite, and Diode act in a selective manner and are useful in Hurley stage I or II to reduce the number of hair follicles and sebaceous glands and thereby bacterial load in the treated areas, deocclusion of the follicle followed by drainage of the inflammatory lesion and destruction of the follicular unit, while the CO_2 laser debulks the diseased tissue and established sinus tracts, and hence more useful in stage II–III disease. CO_2 laser does not prevent the formation of new lesions. Hair removal lasers do not have a downtime but require repeated session to reduce the symptoms. Laser offers a safe, effective, and alternative treatment for moderate stage HS.[40]

Nd:YAG Laser

Prospective randomized controlled studies have shown that long-pulsed Nd:YAG lasers are effective in controlling the existing lesions and preventing the new lesions of HS.[40,41] As the inflammatory lesions of HS are located in the midreticular dermis and the subcutaneous tissue, a longer wavelength device like Nd:YAG would increase the efficacy of treatment. Treatment with Nd:YAG laser in patients with HS is characterized by rupture of nodules, abscesses, and sinus tracts with relative increase in the discharge in the initial few days, followed by a rapid healing of HS lesions.[3] Areas with dark, coarse terminal hair like the axilla show faster and greater degrees of improvement than areas with fine vellus hair, such as the inframammary region.[3] Improvement in the inframammary areas can be explained by nonspecific thermal damage of the laser on the skin with water being the likely chromophore.[40] Excessive scarring present in chronic stages of the disease leads to decreased penetration of the laser beam and hence results in lesser efficacy in patients with long-standing disease with extensive scarring.[40] The parameters for skin types IV–VI are: fluence: 25–35 J/cm², pulse duration: 35 ms, and spot size of 10 mm.[39]

Carbon Dioxide Laser

CO_2 lasers offer a promising treatment option in HS. The advantages are good hemostasis, excellent operative field visualization, and reduced risk of postoperative scar contractures, infection, and recurrence.[42] CO_2 laser ablation is also termed as carbon dioxide laser stripping (CLS). CLS can also be performed as an office procedure, offering rapid recovery and reduced patient costs.[42]

CO_2 laser treatment aims at focal radical vaporization of all nodules, abscesses, and fistulas, leaving healthy tissues in between the pathological lesions. The lesions are vaporized under local anesthesia from "inside and out" until surrounding healthy tissues are reached, superficially and deep. In this way, the technique can be tissue-sparing and at the same time radical. Usually, the vaporization reaches the deep subcutaneous fat or fascia. In the axillary and inguinal region, major vessels and the nerve plexus must be protected, but this depth is seldom reached in Hurley stage II lesions. The smaller blood vessels are coagulated by the laser, but bleeding from vessels larger than 0.5–1 mm in diameter is usually controlled with electrocoagulation or ligation. CO_2 laser can also be used to excise smaller or larger skin areas en bloc with or without laser coagulation of remnants (marsupialization) in the deep tissues, with less bleeding and better visualization than in standard excisions **(Figs. 1 and 2)**.[43,44]

Wound Healing[45]

The wound is generally left to heal by secondary intention. The wound is immediately covered with dry dressings or ointment-impregnated dressings and a covering bandage attached with surgical adhesive tape or gauze underwear. The dressings are initially left on for 2 or 3 days without changing to prevent early bleeding. Thereafter, the wound is cleaned, and the bandage is changed as often as necessary, sometimes daily, pending complete healing. Healing time ranges from 6 to 8 weeks. CO_2 laser excision followed by split skin grafting has been reported to accelerate wound healing **(Fig. 3)**.[46]

Complications

The common complications encountered are secondary infection, prolonged healing time, scarring, and scar contracture. Fractional CO_2 laser has been reported to reduce the scar contracture and improve the healing of chronic ulcers in cases who had undergone CO_2 laser excision earlier.[47]

Internal Pulsed Light and Diode Laser

Internal pulsed light and diode laser works on the same principle as Nd:YAG. IPL has also been shown to have anti-

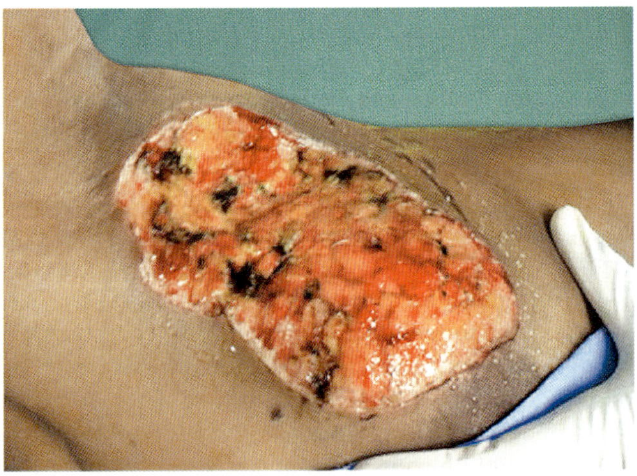

Fig. 2: Post-CO_2 laser excision of the affected tissue.

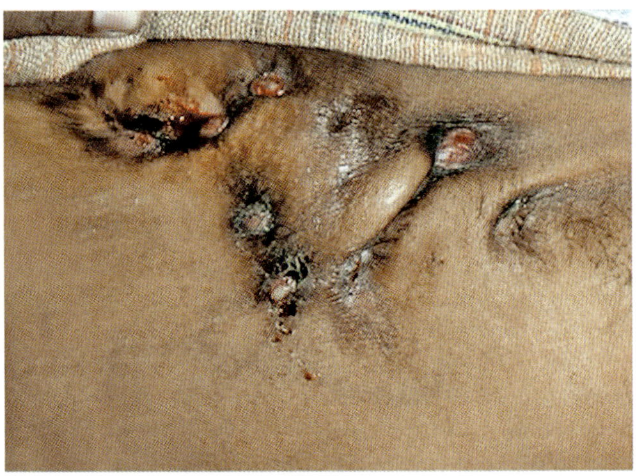

Fig. 1: Hidradenitis suppurativa (HS) before CO_2 laser surgery.

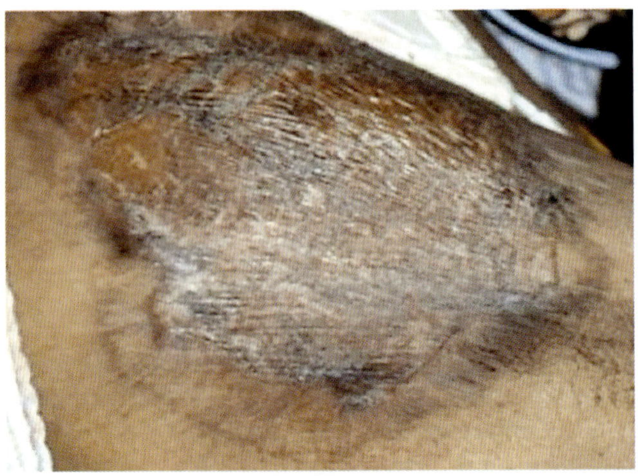

Fig. 3: Postoperative image following skin grafting at the end of 12 months.

inflammatory effect and has the ability to eliminate the chronic inflammation within the diseased tissue.[48]

Combination of two different laser systems has been reported to be beneficial in HS; first stage of Nd:YAG laser for targeting the hair follicles followed by CO_2 laser to deroof the lesions.[49,50]

Photodynamic Therapy

The mechanism of action of photodynamic therapy (PDT) in HS treatment is the cytotoxic effects, which cause selective cell necrosis, immunomodulatory effects, and the ability of aminolevulinic acid (ALA) or its methyl ester [PDT-methyl aminolevulinate (MAL)] to break up the biofilm produced by coagulase-negative *Staphylococcus* (CONS) and other antibacterial effects in patients in whom biofilm plays a pivotal part of their pathogenesis.[51] PDT is not a first-line treatment for HS but in some cases could be added as an adjuvant. More studies are needed to establish the role of PDT treatment in HS.

INTRALESIONAL CORTICOSTEROIDS

The use of intralesional triamcinolone acetonide 5–10 mg/mL has been advocated for the rapid reduction of inflammation associated with acute flares and for management of recalcitrant nodules and sinus tracts.[52] It is utilized as both monotherapy and as adjunct to systemic therapies. When effective, clinical response (flattening, resolution, or spontaneous discharge of nodules) is seen within 48–72 hours. Therapy is contraindicated if clinical suspicion of bacterial infection exists. Local complications include atrophy, infection, pigmentary change, and telangiectasia.[53]

Surgical

Surgery is largely regarded as one of the most effective treatments for intractable HS.[1] Patients should be advised that surgery treats only the disease that is present at the site of the excision and a recurrence at a new site is possible. Incision and drainage of abscesses is not recommended because it is only transiently beneficial and does nothing to halt progression of the disease.[28] On an individual basis, however, incision and drainage might be indicated to relieve excessive lesional pain in large nonrecurrent abscesses.[28] Single nodules may be injected with intralesional triamcinolone (3–5 mg/mL) to decrease inflammation.[54] The efficacy of the surgical treatment depends upon the number of lesions and the disease duration. A better outcome is seen with fewer lesions and shorter duration. Deroofing, limited local excision, and wide excision are the routine surgical modalities practiced in HS.

Deroofing

The deroofing technique was first described by Mullins et al. in 1959.[55] The deroofing technique is an effective, simple, minimally invasive, tissue-saving surgical intervention for the treatment of mild-to-moderate HS lesions at fixed locations and it is suitable as an office procedure.[55] This technique converts, with limited surgery and maximal preservation of the surrounding healthy tissue, painful recurrent lesions into cosmetically acceptable scars.[55] The lesions to be deroofed are marked with an ink. After cleansing the target area, local anesthesia should be infiltrated into the lesion and the surrounding area. The discharging sinus tracts should be explored with the help of a blunt probe introduced into the sinus through the opening, if there are no openings detectable, incisions are done over the sinus tract to introduce the probe. The roof of the tract is surgically removed leaving the floor open. The purulent discharge and other exudates on the floor of the tracts are curetted out and the ulcer is allowed to heal by secondary intention. The defects heal with cosmetically acceptable scars **(Figs. 4 to 8)**.

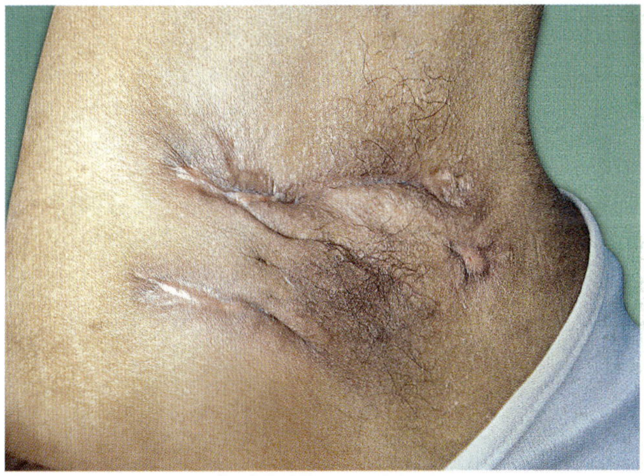

Fig. 4: Axillary hidradenitis suppurativa (HS) with sinus tracts before deroofing.
Courtesy: Dr Venkataram Mysore and Dr Anita.

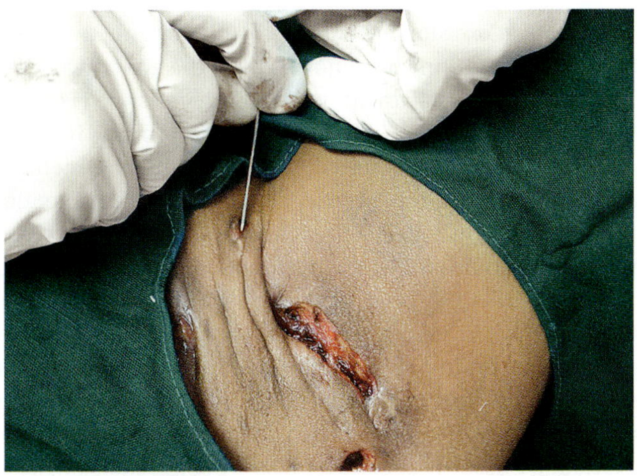

Fig. 5: Blunt probe to visualize the sinus tract.
Courtesy: Dr Venkataram Mysore and Dr Anita.

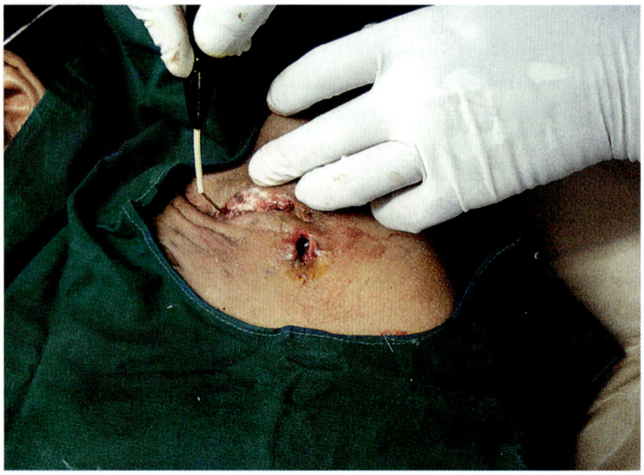

Fig. 6: Deroofing the sinus tract.
Courtesy: Dr Venkataram Mysore and Dr Anita.

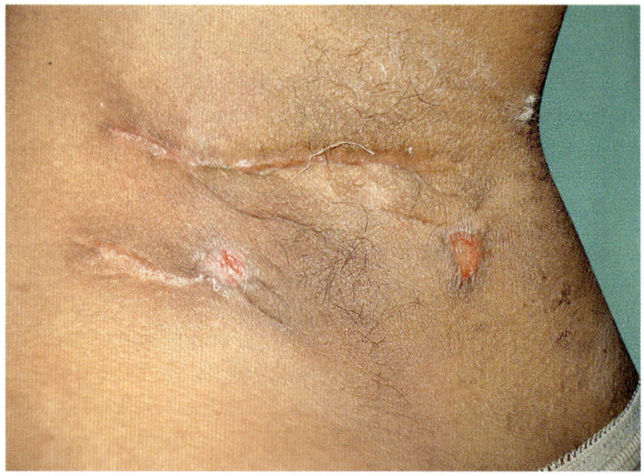

Fig. 8: Complete healing of wound by secondary intention after deroofing.
Courtesy: Dr Venkataram Mysore and Dr Anita.

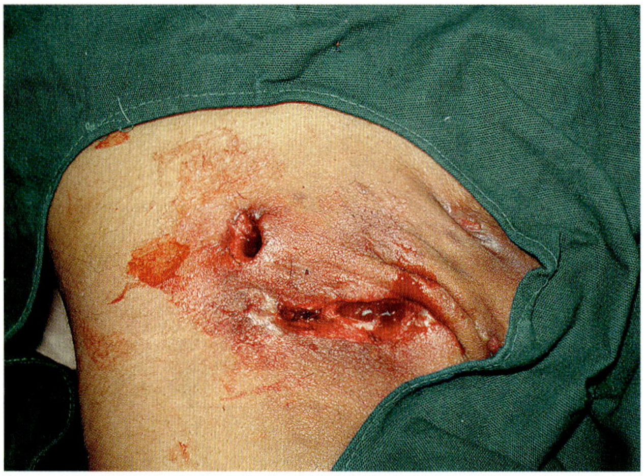

Fig. 7: Wound after deroofing.
Courtesy: Dr Venkataram Mysore and Dr Anita.

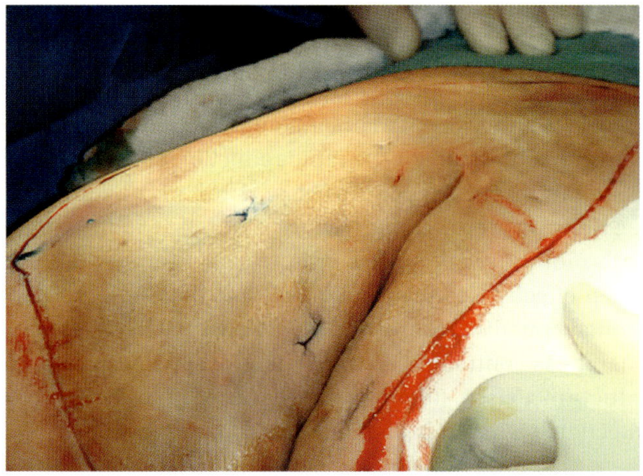

Fig. 9: Perianal hidradenitis suppurativa (HS) before wide surgical excision.
Courtesy: Uwe Wollina, Germany.

EXCISION

Limited local excision is associated with more recurrence.[56] Wide excision is done by removing all of the apocrine glands from hair-bearing skin to the deep underlying fascia **(Fig. 9)**.[57] Reconstruction after wide excision is important in terms of wound healing time and cosmetic results, the methods commonly practiced are primary closure, secondary intention healing, and graft and flap closure.[58] Primary closure is appropriate in minor defects surrounded by lax skin.[56] High recurrence rate has been associated with primary closure, which may be due to inadequate excision.[59] The usual purse-string suture frequently leads to premature suture extrusion and wound dehiscence.[55] Secondary intention healing gives satisfactory results in wounds up to 20 cm **(Figs. 9 to 13)**.[51] New granulation tissue in secondary healing eliminates the risk of recurrence because it does not include apocrine glands.[58]

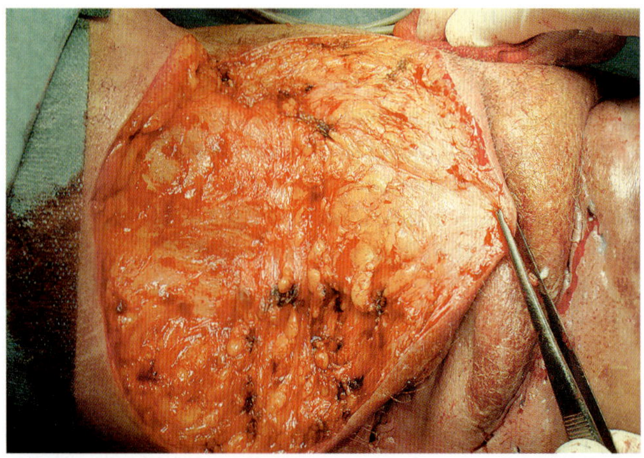

Fig. 10: Surgical removal of the inflamed subcutaneous tissue, sinus tract, and fistula.
Courtesy: Uwe Wollina, Germany.

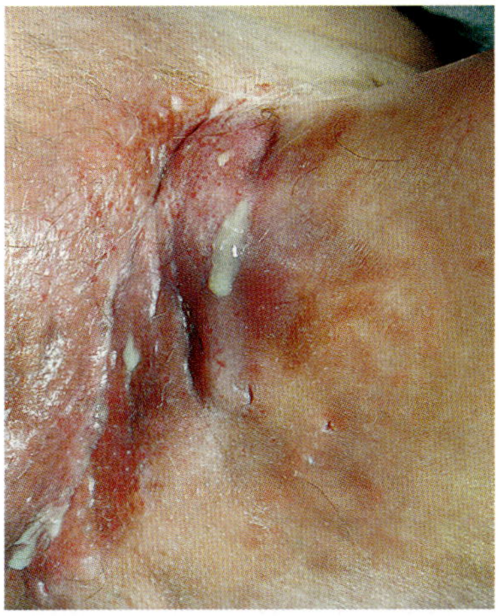

Fig. 11: Hidradenitis suppurativa on the groin before surgical excision.
Courtesy: Uwe Wollina, Germany.

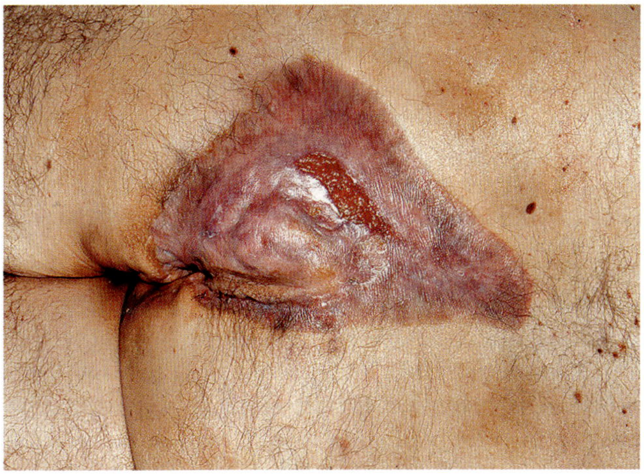

Fig. 13: Healed wound at the end of 3 months.
Courtesy: Uwe Wollina, Germany.

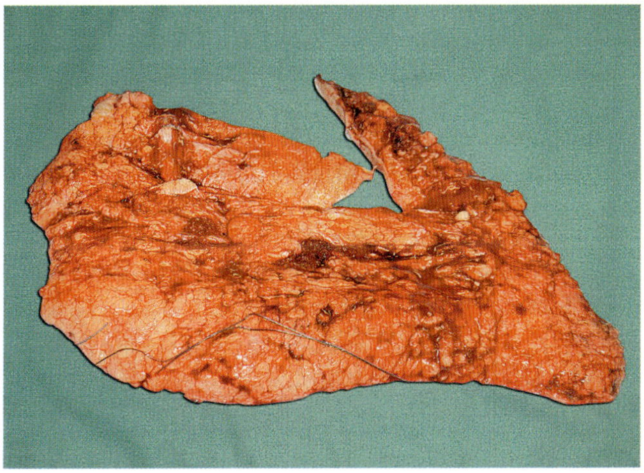

Fig. 12: Excised tissue from the groin.
Courtesy: Uwe Wollina, Germany.

Major drawback in secondary healing is long duration for healing (6–12 weeks) and need for supervision by a physician.[55] Closure of wounds with split-thickness graft is associated with low recurrence rates.[58] Bacterial contamination of skin in the axillary, perineal, and perianal region may lead to graft loss.[58] Other shortcomings of surgery include contracture development and limitation of movement.[58] Flap techniques described for the closure of defects in HS are lipocutaneous, fasciocutaneous, myocutaneous, and free flaps. In axillary, perineal, and perianal regions, repair with fasciocutaneous or musculocutaneous flaps is recommended. Contracture development and limitation of movement are observed less frequently in flap repair methods. The common complications after surgical methods in HS are pain, wound infection, contracture, bleeding, and excessive proliferation of hypertrophic granulation tissue.[55] Recurrence following surgery is more likely related to insufficient excision than closure technique.[58] Great majority of recurrence occurs in perineal, perianal, gluteal, and inguinal sites.[58] The use of magnetic resonance imaging (MRI) and ultrasound will help in preoperative assessment of the extension of the lesions and planning of radical surgery.[55] The lesions at the scrotum, gluteal region, perianal, and perineum should be treated surgically because the lesions in these areas are more painful, cause movement restriction, and carry the risk of urethral fistula. In the perianal, perineal, and gluteal area, colostomy helps in control of postoperative infection and contributes to the success of radical surgical excision.[55]

Surgical intervention is typically reserved for diseases that is uncontrolled by pharmacologic care. Medical therapy for HS should be initiated or continued without interruption, as the risk for surgical complications is likely higher from poorly controlled disease.[59,60]

SURGICAL TREATMENT OF AXILLARY HYPERHIDROSIS

Surgical treatment for axillary hyperhidrosis is generally reserved for those who did not respond to the other modalities of management and to those who have poor quality of life due to hyperhidrosis. The various surgical modalities available can be categorized into the following:

- Minimally invasive surgical treatment
- Radical surgical excision
- Thoracic sympathectomy

Minimally Invasive Surgical Treatment[61]

Type IA: Removal of the subcutaneous cellular tissue (SCCT) without excision of the skin (superficial liposuction)

This procedure involves removal of axillary sweat glands using liposuction with tumescent anesthesia as an outpatient setting. Under tumescent anesthesia, incisions are made over the area of axilla to be treated (demarcated by starch-iodine test) and the liposuction cannula inserted through the incision. Criss-crossed tunnels are created against the undersurface to scrape the underside of the dermis to remove glands rather than adipose tissue. The wound can be sutured or left to heal by secondary incision to facilitate the drainage of fluid. Possible complications of axillary liposuction include recurrence, bleeding, infection, pain, hematoma, and seroma.

Type *IB*: Removal of the SCCT and deep dermis without excision of the skin (curettage/suction)[62,63]

A surgical access is created by two to three small incisions over the area to be treated. Subsequently, a volume of 100–500 mL of tumescent solution is infiltrated, as superficially as possible, into the premarked area of each axilla, creating a "Peau d'orange" effect in the overlaying tissue. Subcutaneous tunnels are created by sharp dissection, in a back-and-forth movement, in order to separate the dermis from the subcutaneous tissue. The subcutaneous sweat glands are thus mobilized. Subsequently, a Cassio cannula (or curette) for suction–curettage is inserted in order to perform the dermal curettage. Suction of the removed tissue can be performed manually or by using a device. Pressure dressing and suturing are performed at the end of the surgery.

The procedure is currently performed in outpatient settings, with tumescent anesthesia.

Possible complications include hematomas, ecchymosis, seromas, superficial erosions of the skin, loss of local sensitivity, skin necrosis, infection, reduction in the number of hairs, fibrosis, formation of subcutaneous adherences, scars, and recurrence of hyperhidrosis.

Type II: En bloc resection of the SCCT and overlying skin

Type III: En bloc excision of a small part of the central axillary region, and removal of the SCCT of the adjacent area[64]

In this procedure, the axillary skin and superficial subcutaneous tissue is removed under local anesthesia through an elliptical incision made at the central portion of the axillary hair-bearing area, with the longer axis perpendicular to the axillary crease. The widest diameter should be kept at no <3 cm, and both tips of the incision located at the highest and lowest points of the axillary hairline.

The adjacent skin should be undermined for about 0.5 cm beyond the hair-bearing area.

The skin flap should be turned over using skin forceps, and the subcutaneous apocrine glands and hair follicles are removed by excision. The incision should be closed in one layer and wound edges should be anchored to the subcutaneous tissue with sutures, so as not to leave dead space. Compression dressings are advised post-surgery. Both axillae can be operated at one sitting. Scarring on the surgical site is the major drawback of this method.

Minimally invasive techniques offer the following advantages, reduction of the infection risk/postoperative pain, shorter recovery time, and reduced scarring, when compared to traditional surgical methods, these methods are associated with high relapse rate.[62,63]

Radical Surgical Excision[65]

The affected tissue is excised with wide margins to eliminate all deeply burrowed glands. The resultant defect, when allowed to heal secondarily, may result in contractures and shoulder stiffening. To avoid this, primary healing using direct closure, split skin grafting, or local flap application is generally recommended. Direct closure is associated with a high incidence of recurrence, presumably because of limited resection, while skin grafting poses problems of graft take, repeated dressings, cosmesis, and scarring. A flap is a good option to facilitate soft tissue coverage while avoiding axillary contractures.

Thoracic Sympathectomy[66-68]

This procedure has evolved from an open surgical procedure to an endoscopic one which involves cutting, cauterization, or clipping sympathetic nerves. Referral for endoscopic thoracic sympathectomy may be indicated when less invasive therapies are ineffective. Although the procedure decreases or eliminates sweating in the original problem area, a common late complication is compensatory sweating in other areas, usually in the abdomen, back, gluteal region, and legs.[66] This treatment has been found to be effective in eliminating axillary hyperhidrosis in 68–100% of cases.

CONCLUSION

Though there are numerous options available for treatment of HS, there is no universally effective single therapy. Therefore,

TABLE 2: Category of evidence/strength of recommendation rating scale.[22]

Treatment modality	*Category of evidence*	*Strength of recommendation*
Excision or curettage of individual lesions	III	C
Total excision of lesions and the surrounding hair-bearing skin	IIb	B
Secondary intention healing	IIb	B
Primary closure	III	C
Reconstruction with skin grafting	III	C
Reconstruction with skin flap plasty	Ia/IIa	A/B
Deroofing	IV	D
CO_2 laser	Ib	A
Nd:YAG laser	Ib	A
IPL	IV	D
Intralesional steroids	IV	D
Botox	IV	D

(Nd:YAG: neodymium-doped yttrium aluminum garnet)

the treating physician must weigh the risks and benefits of each option based on the patient's disease severity and personal circumstances and manage accordingly.

Category of evidence and strength of recommendation rating scale[22] are shown in **Table 2**.

REFERENCES

1. Alikhan A, Lynch PJ, Eisen DB. Hidradenitis suppurativa: a comprehensive review. J Am Acad Dermatol. 2009;60:539-61.
2. Lewis F, Messenger AG, Wales JK. Hidradenitis suppurativa as a presenting feature of premature adrenarche. Br J Dermatol.1993;129:447-8.
3. Mengesha YM, Holcombe TC, Hansen RC. Prepubertal hidradenitis suppurativa: two case reports and review of the literature. Pediatr Dermatol. 1999;16:292-6.
4. Gao M, Wang PG, Cui Y, Yang S, Zhang YH, Lin D, et al. Inversa acne (hidradenitis suppurativa): a case report and identification of the locus at chromosome 1p21.1-1q25.3. J Invest Dermatol. 2006;126:1302-6.
5. Pironi D, Caruso F, Panarese A, Vendettuoli M, Mascagni D, Moraldi L, et al. Chronic hidradenitis suppurativa in the inguinal, perineal and scrotal regions: a case report and review of the literature. Ann Ital Chir. 2010;81:465-70.
6. Mortimer PS, Lunniss PJ. Hidradenitis suppurativa. JR Soc Med. 2000;93:420-2.
7. Yu CC, Cook MG. Hidradenitis suppurativa: a disease of follicular epithelium, rather than apocrine glands. Br J Dermatol. 1990;122:763-9.
8. Jemec GB, Faber M, Gutschik E, Wendelboe P. The bacteriology of hidradenitis suppurativa. Dermatology.1996;193:203-6.
9. Rompel R, Petres J. Long-term results of wide surgical excision in 106 patients with hidradenitis suppurativa. Dermatol Surg. 2000;26:638-43.
10. Freiman A, Bird G, Metelitsa AI, Barankin B, Lauzon GJ. Cutaneous effects of smoking. J Cutan Med Surg. 2004;8: 415-23.
11. Revuz JE, Canoui-Poitrine F, Wolkenstein P, Viallette C, Gabison G, Pouget F, et al. Prevalence and factors associated with hidradenitis suppurativa: results from two case-control studies. J Am Acad Dermatol. 2008;59:596-601.
12. Edlich RF, Silloway KA, Rodeheaver GT, Cooper PH. Epidemiology, pathology, and treatment of axillary hidradenitis suppurativa. J Emerg Med. 1986;4:369-78.
13. Wiseman MC. Hidradenitis suppurativa: a review. Dermatol Ther. 2004;17:50-4.
14. Slade DE, Powell BW, Mortimer PS. Hidradenitis suppurativa: pathogenesis and management. Br J Plast Surg. 2003;56:451-61.
15. Williams ST, Busby RC, De Muth RJ, Nelson H. Perineal hidradenitis suppurativa: presentation of two unusual complications and a review. Ann Plast Surg. 1991;26:456-62.
16. Larralde M, Abad ME, Muñoz AS, Luna P. Childhood flexural comedones: a new entity. Arch Dermatol. 2007;143:909-11.
17. Brown TJ, Rosen T, Orengo IF. Hidradenitis suppurativa. South Med J. 1998;91:1107-14.
18. Anderson MJ, Dockerty MB. Perianal hidradenitis suppurativa: a clinical and pathologic study. Dis Colon Rectum. 1958;1:23-31.
19. Culp CE. Chronic hidradenitis suppurativa of the anal canal: a surgical skin disease. Dis Colon Rectum. 1983;26:669-76.
20. Maclean GM, Coleman DJ. Three fatal cases of squamous cell carcinoma arising in chronic perineal hidradenitis suppurativa. Ann R Coll Surg Engl. 2007;89:709-12.
21. Scheinfeld NS. A case of dissecting cellulitis and a review of the literature. Dermatol Online J. 2003;9:8.
22. Gulliver W, Zouboulis CC, Prens E, Jemec GBE, Tzellos T. Evidence-based approach to the treatment of hidradenitis suppurativa/acne inversa, based on the European guidelines for hidradenitis suppurativa. Rev Endocr Metab Disord. 2016; 17:343-51.
23. Jemec GB, Wendelboe P. Topical clindamycin versus systemic tetracycline in the treatment of hidradenitis suppurativa. J Am Acad Dermatol. 1998;39:971-4.
24. van der Zee HH, Boer J, Prens EP, Jemec GB. The effect of combined treatment with oral clindamycin and oral rifampicin in patients with hidradenitis suppurativa. Dermatology. 2009;219:143-7.
25. Gener G, Canoui-Poitrine F, Revuz JE, Faye O, Poli F, Gabison G, et al. Combination therapy with clindamycin and rifampicin for hidradenitis suppurativa: a series of 116 consecutive patients. Dermatology. 2009;219:148-54.
26. Kaur MR, Lewis HM. Hidradenitis suppurativa treated with dapsone: a case series of five patients. J Dermatolog Treat. 2006;17:211-3.
27. Join-Lambert O, Coignard H, Jais JP, Guet-Revillet H, Poirée S, Fraitag S, et al. Efficacy of rifampin-moxifloxacin-metronidazole combination therapy in hidradenitis suppurativa. Dermatology. 2011;222:49-58.
28. Shah N. Hidradenitis suppurativa: a treatment challenge. Am Fam Physician. 2005;72:1547-52.
29. Boer J, Nazary M. Long-term results of acitretin therapy for hidradenitis suppurativa. Is acne inversa also a misnomer? Br J Dermatol. 2011;164:170-5.
30. Kraft JN, Searles GE. Hidradenitis suppurativa in 64 female patients: retrospective study comparing oral antibiotics and antiandrogen therapy. J Cutan Med Surg. 2007;11:125-31.
31. Mitchell KM, Beck DE. Hidradenitis suppurativa. Surg Clin North Am. 2002;82:1187-97.
32. Shuja F, Chan CS, Rosen T. Biologic drugs for the treatment of hidradenitis suppurativa: an evidence-based review. Dermatol Clin. 2010;28:511-21.
33. O'Reilly DJ, Pleat JM, Richards AM. Treatment of hidradenitis suppurativa with botulinum toxin A. Plast Reconstr Surg. 2005;116:1575-6.
34. Feito-Rodríguez M, Sendagorta-Cudós E, Herranz-Pinto P, de Lucas-Laguna R. Prepubertal hidradenitis suppurativa successfully treated with botulinum toxin A. Dermatol Surg. 2009;35:1300-2.
35. Grimstad Ø, Kvammen BØ, Swartling C. Botulinum toxin type B for hidradenitis suppurativa: a randomised, double-blind, placebo-controlled pilot study. Am J Clin Dermatol. 2020;21:741-8.
36. Zeligman I. Temporary X-ray epilation therapy of chronic axillary hidradenitis suppurativa. Arch Dermatol. 1965;92: 690-4.
37. Trombetta M, Werts ED, Parda D. The role of radiotherapy in the treatment of hidradenitis suppurativa: case report and review of the literature. Dermatol Online J. 2010;15:16.
38. Paul S, Bach D, LeBoeuf NR, Devlin PM, Lipworth AD. Successful use of brachytherapy for a severe hidradenitis suppurativa variant. Dermatol Ther. 2016;29:455-8.
39. Bong JL, Shalders K, Saihan E. Treatment of persistent painful nodules of hidradenitis suppurativa with cryotherapy. Clin Exp Dermatol. 2003;28:241-4.
40. Mahmoud BH, Tierney E, Hexsel CL, Pui J, Ozog DM, Hamzavi IH. Prospective controlled clinical and histopathologic study

of hidradenitis suppurativa treated with the long-pulsed neodymium:yttrium aluminium-garnet laser. J Am Acad Dermatol. 2010;62: 637-45.
41. Tierney E, Mahmoud BH, Hexsel C, Ozog D, Hamzavi I. Randomized control trial for the treatment of hidradenitis suppurativa with a neodymium-doped yttrium aluminium garnet laser. Dermatol Surg. 2009;35:1188-98.
42. Crocco EI, Dalapicola MC, Suzuki NM, Alves RO. Surgical treatment of chronic hidradenitis suppurativa: CO_2 laser stripping—second intention technique. Dermatol Surg. 2016; 42:429-31.
43. Finley EM, Ratz JL. Treatment of hidradenitis suppurativa with carbon dioxide laser excision and second-intention healing. J Am Acad Dermatol.1996;34:465-9.
44. Hazen PG, Hazen BP. Hidradenitis suppurativa: successful treatment using carbon dioxide laser excision and marsupialization. Dermatol Surg. 2010;36:208-13.
45. Zouboulis CC, Desai N, Emtestam L, Hunger RE, Ioannides D, Juhász I, et al. European S1 guideline for the treatment of hidradenitis suppurativa/ acne inversa. J Eur Acad Dermatol Venereol. 2015;29:619-44.
46. Natarajan K, Srinivas CR, Thomas M, Aruchamy M, Kumar SR. Hidradenitis suppurativa treated with carbon dioxide laser followed by split skin thickness graft. Indian J Dermatol Venereol Leprol. 2014;80:376-8.
47. Nicholson CL, Hamzavi I, Ozog DM. Rapid healing of chronic ulcerations and improvement in range of motion after fractional carbon dioxide (CO_2) treatment after CO_2 excision of hidradenitis suppurativa axillary lesions: a case report. JAAD Case Rep. 2016;2:4-6.
48. Jain V, Jain A. Use of lasers for the management of refractory cases of hidradenitis suppurativa and pilonidal sinus. J Cutan Aesthet Surg. 2012;5:190-2.
49. John H, Manoloudakis N, Stephen Sinclair J. A systematic review of the use of lasers for the treatment of hidradenitis suppurativa. J Plast Reconstr Aesthet Surg. 2016;69:1374-81.
50. Saunte DM, Lapins J. Lasers and intense pulsed light hidradenitis suppurativa. Dermatol Clin. 2016;34(1):111-9.
51. Scheinfeld N. The use of photodynamic therapy to treat hidradenitis suppurativa: a review and critical analysis. Dermatol Online J. 2015;15:21.
52. Jemec GBE, Revuz J, Leyden J. Hidradenitis suppurativa. Berlin, Heidelberg: Springer. 2006. pp. 138-40.
53. Alikhan A, Sayed C, Alavi A, Alhusayen R, Brassard A, Burkhart C, et al. North American Clinical Management Guidelines for Hidradenitis Suppurativa: A Publication from the United States and Canadian Hidradenitis Suppurativa Foundations: Part II: Topical, intralesional, and systemic medical management. J Am Acad Dermatol. 2019;81:91-101.
54. Krbec AC. Current understanding and management of hidradenitis suppurativa. J Am Acad Nurse Pract. 2007;19:228-34.
55. van der Zee HH, Prens EP, Boer J. Deroofing: a tissue-saving surgical technique for the treatment of mild-to-moderate hidradenitis suppurativa lesions. J Am Acad Dermatol. 2010; 63:475-80.
56. Büyükaşik O, Hasdemir AO, Kahramansoy N, Çöl C, Erkol H. Surgical approach to extensive hidradenitis suppurativa. Dermatol Surg. 2011;37:835-42.
57. Parks RW, Parks TG. Pathogenesis, clinical features and management of hidradenitis suppurativa. Ann R Coll Surg Engl. 1997;79:83-9.
58. Bieniek A, Matusiak L, Okulewicz-Gojlik D, Szepietowski JC. Surgical treatment of hidradenitis suppurativa: experiences and recommendations. Dermatol Surg. 2010;36:1998-2004.
59. Alikhan A, Sayed C, Alavi A, Alhusayen R, Brassard A, Burkhart C, et al. North American clinical management guidelines for hidradenitis suppurativa: a publication from the United States and Canadian Hidradenitis Suppurativa Foundations: Part I: Diagnosis, evaluation, and the use of complementary and procedural management. J Am Acad Dermatol. 2019;81:76-90
60. Watson JD. Hidradenitis suppurativa: a clinical review. Br J Plast Surg. 1985;38:567-9.
61. Lee MR, Ryman WJ. Liposuction for axillary hyperhidrosis. Australas J Dermatol. 2005;46:76-9.
62. Bechara FG, Sand M, Sand D, Altmeyer P, Hoffmann K. Surgical treatment of axillary hyperhidrosis: a study comparing liposuction cannulas with a suction-curettage cannula. Ann Plast Surg. 2006;56:654-7.
63. Huang YH, Yang CH, Chen YH, Chen CH, Lee SH. Reduction in osmidrosis using a suction-assisted cartilage shaver improves the quality of life. Dermatol Surg. 2010;36:1573-7.
64. Fan YM, Wu ZH, Li SF, Chen QX. Axillary osmidrosis treated by partial removal of the skin and subcutaneous tissue en bloc and apocrine gland subcision. Int J Dermatol. 2001;40:714-6.
65. Teo WL, Ong YS, Tan BK. Radical surgical excision and use of lateral thoracic flap for intractable axillary hidradenitis suppurativa. Arch Plast Surg. 2012;39:663-6.
66. Doolabh N, Horswell S, Williams M, Huber L, Prince S, Meyer DM, et al. Thoracoscopic sympathectomy for hyperhidrosis: indications and results. Ann Thorac Surg. 2004;77:410-4.
67. Cerfolio RJ, De Campos JR, Bryant AS, Connery CP, Miller DL, DeCamp MM, et al. The society of thoracic surgeons Expert Consensus for the Surgical Treatment of Hyperhidrosis. Ann Thorac Surg. 2011;91:1642-8.
68. de Andrade Filho LO, Kuzniec S, Wolosker N, Yazbek G, Kauffman P, Milanez de Campos JR. Technical difficulties and complications of sympathectomy in the treatment of hyperhidrosis: an analysis of 1731 cases. Ann Vasc Surg. 2013; 27:447-53.

CHAPTER 57

Surgery of Male Genitalia: Circumcision

Eswari L

KEY MESSAGES

- *Circumcision:* Removal of foreskin. Benefits include: prevention of UTIs, penile cancer, and STDs.
- *Indications for circumcision:* Phimosis, paraphimosis, balanitis, STD prevention, and lichen sclerosis, while contraindications include anatomical abnormalities and bleeding disorders.
- The surgical principle involves ensuring asepsis, adequate excision of skin layers, hemostasis, and protection of the glans and urethra and to achieve cosmesis.
- *Surgical methods:* Forceps guided, dorsal slit, and sleeve resection methods.
- *Complications of circumcision:* Bleeding, infection, urethrocutaneous fistula, excess or inadequate foreskin removal, and rarely sexual dysfunction.

INTRODUCTION

Circumcision is the removal of some or the entire foreskin (prepuce) from the penis. The word "circumcision" comes from Latin words, circum (meaning "around") and cædere (meaning "to cut"). Circumcision is a popular practice in certain cultural and ethnic groups. Globally, the prevalence of circumcision is thought to be about 30%.[1] Multiple medical organizations have brought out various recommendations and guidelines which have added to the confusion. The American Academy of Pediatrics addresses several areas of potential benefit from neonatal circumcision, including prevention of urinary tract infection (UTI), penile cancer, and sexually transmitted diseases (STDs). Male circumcision is recognized as an additional important step in curbing heterosexually acquired human immunodeficiency virus (HIV) in men.[2]

EMBRYOLOGY

Understanding the development of the male genitalia is key to identifying congenital anomalies—many of which are grounds for deferring newborn circumcision. Sex-determining region Y (SRY) protein initiates differentiation of the male primitive sex cords into Sertoli cells, which is the initial step in testicular development. Subsequent development of the Leydig cells results in production of testosterone, which is converted (by 5-alpha-dehydroxlase) to dihydrotestosterone (DHT), the hormone responsible for the differentiation of genital tubercle and urogenital folds into the male phallus.

The prepuce or foreskin in humans is defined as the fold of skin that covers the glans penis. The prepuce forms in concurrence with urethral development and by 8 weeks' gestation appears as a ring of thickened epidermis at the base of the glans penis/coronal edge. By 16 weeks' gestation, the prepuce extends from the penile shaft skin and folds over itself at the distal glans penis forming a mucocutaneous junction and serving as a physical barrier between the glans penis and the environment.

Almost all newborns exhibit a state of physiologic phimosis or inability to fully retract the prepuce. According to Gairdner, only 4% of newborns will have a retractable prepuce at this stage and 90% will have a fully retractable prepuce at 3 years of age.[3] The prepuce separates naturally from the glans over time by desquamation of underlying cells forming the prepucial space.

APPLIED ANATOMY

A good understanding of "normal anatomy" is the best way to spot an abnormal condition, be it anatomical or procedural. The groove that delineates the glans (head of the penis) from the penile shaft is called the coronal sulcus. The coronal sulcus is discernable through the foreskin and is a valuable landmark for circumcision. First, it is the point to which the foreskin is removed in neonatal circumcision. Second, a good rule of thumb is to defer circumcision where there is <1 cm of dorsal shaft skin (the distance between the dorsal junction and the coronal sulcus) and/or ventral shaft skin.

The nerve supply of the penis is the twin dorsal penile nerves. These nerves are located on the top and sides of the penis, at the 11 and 1 o'clock positions near the base of the penis. They fan out toward the glans.

INDICATIONS

Phimosis

Phimosis represents a condition in which the retractable portion of the foreskin (prepuce) is unable to be reduced over the glans penis. This can result in pain with erection and intercourse. Diabetes is a risk factor.[4]

Paraphimosis

When there is a partially phimotic band and the foreskin does not reposition or reduce itself over the glans, the band acts like a tourniquet. This creates edema of the distal foreskin and as this increases, retraction of the foreskin becomes even more difficult. Furthermore, the glans will subsequently become edematous, causing reduction of the retracted foreskin to become even more difficult. This can become a urologic emergency.

Balanitis

Balanitis refers to inflammation of the glans penis. When there is inflammation of the foreskin also it is termed balanoposthitis. Causes of balanitis include both infectious and noninfectious. Candidal fungal species are a common infectious source. Noninfectious causes include allergic dermatitis, trauma, and Zoon's balanitis.

Sexually Transmitted Disease Prevention

Circumcision is preventive in the spread of HIV and acquired immunodeficiency syndrome (AIDS). The inner prepucial skin is rich in Langerhans cells, which contain CD4 receptors and other coreceptors for the HIV virus. As such, removing the bulk of the Langerhans cells on the penis, via circumcision, was theorized to be efficacious in preventing the spread of HIV.[5] Additionally, the inner prepucial skin contains little to no keratin relative to the outer foreskin, rendering it less mechanically resistant to injury than the keratinized outer layer and more likely to serve as a nidus for HIV transmission.[6] No increase in HIV transmission was seen at 3–6 months for men having sexual contact <42 days after circumcision.[7]

It was also shown that there was decrease in the prevalence of human papillomavirus (HPV) and herpes simplex virus (HSV) infections in the circumcised group.[8]

Lichen Sclerosis

Lichen sclerosis (LS), also known as lichen sclerosis et trophicus and balanitis xerotica obliterans (BXO), affects both pediatric and adult populations. LS has been known by many names, including lichen sclerosis et trophicus and BXO.

CONTRAINDICATIONS

Absolute Contraindications

- *Anatomical abnormalities:* These include congenital abnormalities of the phallus such as hypospadias, epispadias, megalourethra, webbed penis, prematurity, bleeding problems, myelomeningocele, and anorectal anomaly.[9]
- Chronic paraphimosis
- Genital ulcer disease
- Urethral discharge
- Bleeding disorders

Relative Contraindications

- A tight foreskin as a result of scar tissue
- Scar tissue at the frenulum
- Penile warts

INFORMED CONSENT

A well-crafted informed consent document outlining the procedure, goals of surgery, risks, benefits, and expected outcomes of the procedure allows an opportunity to confirm that the patient/parent has understood and retained the information needed to reach a meaningful decision.

PRINCIPLES AND GOALS OF CIRCUMCISION

The principles of circumcision are asepsis, adequate excision of outer and inner prepucial skin layers, hemostasis, protection of the glans and urethra, and cosmesis. The goal of the procedure is to expose the glans sufficient to prevent phimosis or paraphimosis.

PREPARATION

Surgeon should rule out a history of bleeding abnormalities and all medications affecting platelet function should be stopped 7–10 days prior to elective surgical circumcision [nonsteroidal anti-inflammatory drugs (NSAIDS), aspirin, clopidogrel, warfarin, etc.].

INSTRUMENTS REQUIRED

- Instrument tray wrapped with sterile drape
- Dissecting forceps (finely toothed)
- Artery forceps (two straight, two curved)
- Curved Metzenbaum's scissors
- Stitch scissors
- Mayo's needle holder
- Sponge-holding forceps
- Scalpel knife handle and blades
- "O" drape (80 × 80 cm, with ~5 cm hole)

- Gallipot for antiseptic solution (e.g., povidone iodine)
- Povidone iodine (50 mL of 10% solution)
- Plain gauze swabs (10 × 10 cm; 10 for the procedure, 5 for dressing)
- Petroleum jelly-impregnated gauze (5 × 5 cm or 5 × 10 cm; tulle gras) and sticking plaster
- 15 mL of 1% plain lidocaine (without epinephrine) anesthetic solution
- Syringe 10 mL
- Injection needles (18- or 21-gauge)
- Suture material (chromic gut or vicryl 3-0 and 4-0) with 3/8 circle reverse-cutting needle
- Gentian violet (no more than 5 mL) or sterile marker pen

PROCEDURES IN DETAIL

Skin Preparation and Draping

Prepare the skin with povidone iodine antiseptic solution, starting with the glans and the shaft of the penis, and moving out to the periphery. Holding the penis with a swab, retract the foreskin in order to clean the glans. The prepared area should include the penis, the scrotum, the adjacent areas of the thighs, and the lower part of the abdomen (suprapubic area), so that there is no risk of the surgeon touching unprepared skin during the procedure.

Draping

Draping provides a sterile operative field and helps prevent contamination of the wound. Leave uncovered only the operative area and the areas where the anesthetic will be administered.

Anesthesia (Fig. 1)

The local anesthetic most often used is 1% plain lidocaine. The maximum dose that can safely be given is 3 mg/kg of body weight. Lidocaine with epinephrine must not be used because there is a risk of constriction of the blood vessels to the whole penis, which can cause gangrene and loss of the penis. The advantage of lidocaine is that it works rapidly. An alternative is a mixture of 5 mL of lidocaine, 1%, and 5 mL of plain bupivacaine, 0.25%. This provides longer lasting anesthesia (up to 4–5 hours after the operation).

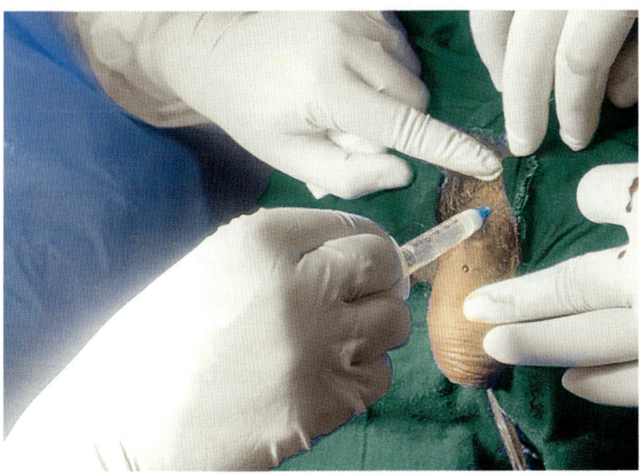

Fig. 1: Infiltration of anesthesia.

Dorsal penile block: This involves local infiltration of the dorsal nerve of the penis with local anesthetic, typically lidocaine or a longer-acting agent such as bupivacaine. As the penis is a terminal extremity without distal collateral blood flow, it is suggested that no sympathomimetic (e.g., epinephrine) is used, in order to prevent the theoretical complication of penile ischemia. The dorsal nerve to the penis originates as one of the branches from the pudendal nerve, which arises from the S2–S4 nerve roots. The dorsal penile nerve runs through the suspensory ligament of the penis and continues distally below Buck's fascia, passing lateral to the penile arteries and terminating on the glans penis. Many practitioners will also do a ring block at the base of the penis in conjunction with the dorsal block. More reliable anesthesia can be achieved by also in filtrating the distal penile tissue near the area of the frenulum.[10]

Ring block technique: Using a fine needle (23-gauge), approximately 0.1 mL of anesthetic is injected subcutaneously at the 11 o'clock position. Then, without withdrawing the needle, the needle is advanced into the subdermal space. At this point, 2–3 mL of anesthetic is injected to block the dorsal penile nerves. Then needle is advanced subcutaneously around the side of the penis and an additional 1 mL of anesthetic is injected. Needle is withdrawn and procedure is repeated, starting at the 1 o'clock position so as to complete a ring of anesthetic. In some cases it may be necessary to make an additional injection on the underside of the penis to fully complete the ring of anesthetic. After injection, the base of the penis is massaged for 10–20 seconds to increase the diffusion of the lidocaine into the surrounding tissues. Surgeon should wait for 3–5 minutes for the anesthesia to act. Sensation should be tested before starting the surgery. This can be done by gently pinching the foreskin with an artery forceps.

EMLA cream can be applied 1 hour prior to circumcision so that dorsal block is less painful.

RETRACTION OF THE FORESKIN AND DEALING WITH ADHESIONS

This step is common to all the methods of circumcision described below. After effective local anesthesia has been achieved, the foreskin should be fully retracted. If the opening of the foreskin is tight, it may be necessary to dilate it with a pair of artery forceps, but this is not usually necessary in adults and adolescents. Care must be taken to stretch just the aperture of the foreskin and not to push the forceps in too far because there is a risk of dilating the urethra and causing injury to the urethra and glans. Once the foreskin has been retracted, adhesions have to be separated by gentle traction or using a blunt probe, such as a pair of closed artery forceps.

MARKING THE LINE OF THE CIRCUMCISION

This step is common to all the methods of circumcision described below. With the foreskin returned to a natural "resting" position, intended line of the incision is indicated with a marker pen. The line should correspond with the corona, just under the head of the penis. Some uncircumcised men have a very lax foreskin, which is partially retracted in the resting position. In such cases it is better to apply artery forceps at the 3 and 9 o'clock positions, to apply a little tension to the foreskin before marking the circumcision line. Gentian violet or pinch marks made by toothed forceps can also be used in place of marking pen.

SURGICAL METHODS

Surgical Methods

Three widely used methods of circumcision are described below. All three methods produce a good long-term result, but require different levels of skill. The sleeve method produces an excellent result, but requires the highest level of surgical skill. The forceps-guided method produces a less tidy result initially, but has the advantage that it is a simple technique with low complication rates. The dorsal slit method is probably the most widely used method.

Forceps-guided Method of Circumcision (Fig. 2)

This is a simple step-by-step procedure, with easy learning curve. A disadvantage of the procedure is that it leaves between 0.5 and 1.0 cm of mucosal skin proximal to the corona.

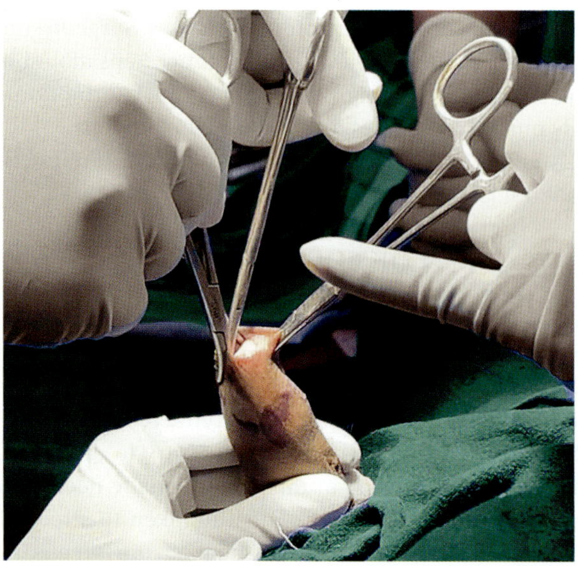

Fig. 2: Forceps-guided method.

Step 1: Skin is prepared, draped, and anesthesia is administered.

Step 2: Foreskin is retracted and adhesions are separated as described above.

Step 3: Intended line of the incision is marked.

Step 4: Foreskin is grasped at the 3 and 9 o'clock positions with two artery forceps. Forceps are placed on the natural apex of the foreskin, in such a way as to put equal tension on the inside and outside surfaces of the foreskin. If this is not done correctly, there is a risk of leaving too much mucosal skin or of removing too much shaft skin.

Step 5: Sufficient tension on the foreskin is applied to pull the previously made mark to just beyond the glans. Taking care not to catch the glans, a long straight forceps is applied across the foreskin, just proximal to the mark, with the long axis of the forceps going from the 6 to the 12 o'clock position (taking the frenulum as the 6 o'clock position). Once the forceps is in position, the glans is felt to check that it has not been accidentally caught in the forceps.

Step 6: Using a scalpel, the foreskin is cut away flush with the outer aspect of the forceps. The forceps protects the glans from injury, but nevertheless, particular care is needed at this stage.

Step 7: Skin is pulled back to expose the raw area. Any bleeding vessels are clipped with artery forceps. Each vessel is tied or underrun with a suture and tied off. Hemostatic stitches should not be too deep. When dealing with bleeding in the frenular area or on the underside of the penis, care must be taken not to injure the urethra.

Step 8: Horizontal mattress suture is placed at the frenulum. When placing the frenulum suture, midline skin raphe is aligned with the line of the frenulum. It is helpful to leave a long end on the horizontal mattress suture at the frenulum (at the 6 o'clock position) and on the vertical mattress suture opposite (at the 12 o'clock position). The long ends of the sutures can be held by an assistant with artery forceps to stabilize the penis during suturing.

Step 9: After placement of the sutures at the 6, 12, 3, and 9 o'clock positions, two or more simple sutures are placed in the gaps between them.

Step 10: Once the procedure is finished, dressing is done.

Dorsal Slit Method of Circumcision (Fig. 3)

The dorsal slit method requires more surgical skill than the forceps-guided method. There is a risk that more skin is cut away from one side than the other, giving an asymmetric result.

Step 1: Skin is prepared, draped, and anesthesia is administered.

Step 2: Foreskin is retracted and adhesions are separated as described above.

Step 3: Intended line of the incision is marked.

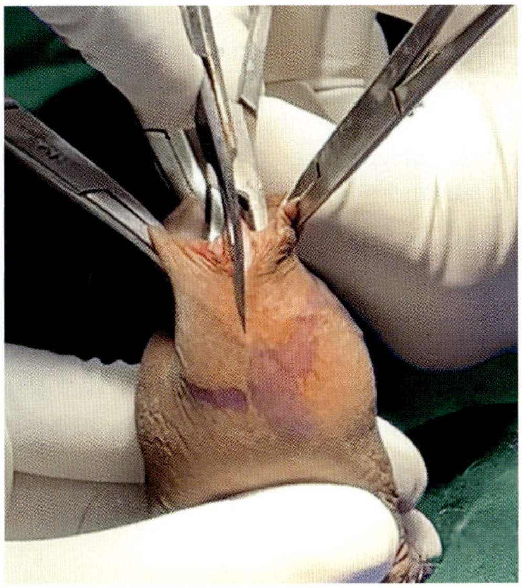

Fig. 3: Dorsal slit method.

Step 4 (optional): Some surgeons prefer to mark the line of incision by making a very shallow incision using a scalpel. This is useful on a deeply pigmented man on whom it is difficult to see the line of the marking pen or dabs of gentian violet. Before making the shallow incision, check carefully that the incision line is in level with the corona and that even amounts of skin are marked for removal from each side of the penis. The incision should be made just through the skin; it is very important not to cut too deeply and divide blood vessels.

Step 5: The foreskin is grasped with artery forceps at the 3 and 9 o'clock positions. The artery forceps is applied so that there is equal tension on the inner and outer aspects of the foreskin.

Step 6: Two artery forceps are placed on the foreskin in the 11 and 1 o'clock positions. Check that the inside blades of the two artery forceps are lying between the glans and foreskin, and have not been inadvertently passed up the urethral meatus.

Step 7: Between the two artery forceps, in the 12 o'clock position, use dissection scissors to make a cut (the dorsal slit) up to but not beyond the previously marked incision line.

Step 8: Using dissection scissors, foreskin is cut free, following the previously marked circumcision line.

Step 9: Any skin tags on the inner edge of the foreskin can be trimmed to leave approximately 5 mm of skin proximal to the corona. Care must be taken to trim only the skin and not to cut deeper tissue.

Step 10: Bleeding should be stopped and sutured.

Step 11: Dressing is applied.

Sleeve Resection Method of Circumcision (Figs. 4 to 8)

The sleeve resection method requires good surgical skill and is better suited to a hospital rather than a clinic setting. If bipolar diathermy is available the procedure can be virtually

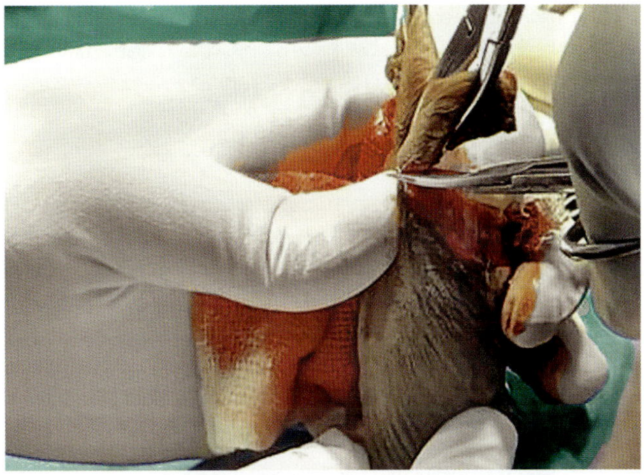

Fig. 4: Sleeve resection method.

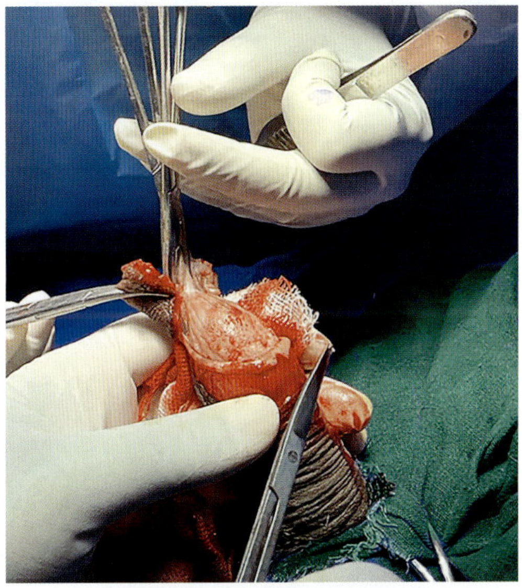

Fig. 5: Postresection of foreskin.

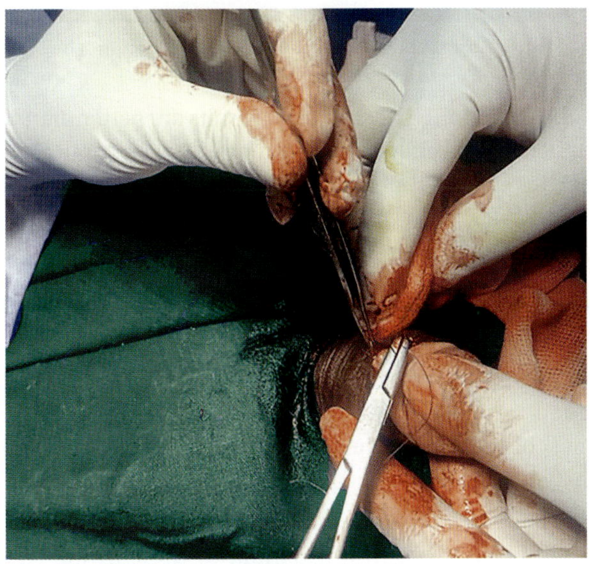

Fig. 6: Suturing.

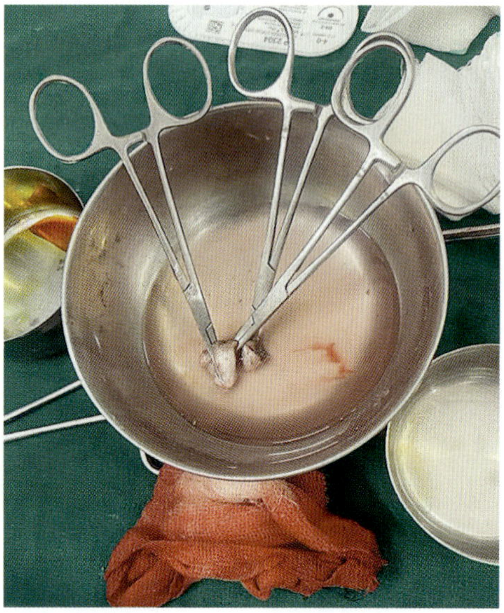

Fig. 7: Resected foreskin.

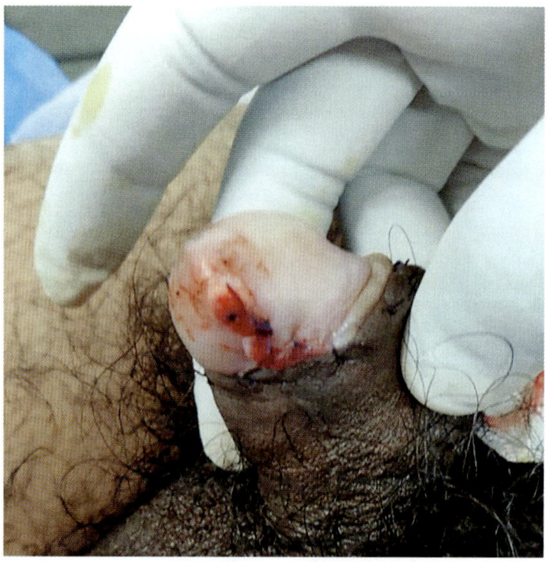

Fig. 8: Absorbable sutures placed following circumcision.

bloodless. Although the cosmetic results are better than with the other two techniques, there is more room for surgical error, either by cutting too deep when making the two circular incisions or cutting too deep when dissecting the skin flap-free.

Step 1: Skin is prepared, draped, and anesthesia is administered.

Step 2: Foreskin is retracted and adhesions are separated as described above.

Step 3: Intended line of the incision is marked with a V shape, pointed toward the frenulum, on the underside (ventral aspect) of the penis. The apex of the V should correspond with the midline raphe.

Step 4: Foreskin is retracted and the inner (mucosal) incision line is marked, 1–2 mm proximal to the corona. At the frenulum, the incision line crosses horizontally.

Step 5: Using a scalpel, incisions are marked along the marked lines, taking care to cut through the skin to the subcutaneous tissue but not deeper. As the incision is made, the assistant should retract the skin with a moist gauze swab. Any significant bleeding vessels should be clipped with an artery forceps and tied or secured with an underrunning suture.

Step 6: Skin between the proximal and distal incisions is cut with scissors.

Step 7: Sleeve of foreskin is held under tension with two artery forceps, and skin is dissected from the shaft of the penis, using dissection scissors. Bleeding vessels are tied with underrunning sutures.

Step 8: Bleeding is stopped and sutured.

Step 9: Dressing is applied.

DRESSING

Irrespective of the method of circumcision, a standard penile dressing technique is used. Check that there is no bleeding. Minor bleeding from a skin edge will often stop after five minutes of pressure with a gauze. Once all bleeding has stopped, petroleum-jelly-impregnated gauze (tulle gras) is placed around the wound. A sterile dry gauze is placed over this, and secured in position with adhesive tape. Dressing should not be applied tightly. The dressing should be left in position no longer than 48 hours. It is important not to disrupt the wound by pulling at a dressing that has dried to the wound.

NEONATAL CIRCUMCISION TECHNIQUES

Besides classical surgical methods, three different circumcision clamps can be used in neonates: Gomco, Plastibell, and Mogen clamps. The more frequently used Gomco clamp provides a superior cosmetic appearance in the neonatal period. However, glans injuries are rarely seen with the Mogen clamp, and although the Plastibell clamp can be easily used, it is not generally preferred due to the longer stay of the device on the neonate penis.

Anesthesia

Different analgesic applications exist for neonatal circumcision, including topically applied lidocaine–prilocaine (EMLA) cream, dorsal penile blockage, subcutaneous ring blockage, sucrose–glucose, and acetaminophen.[11]

Complications of Neonatal Circumcision

Common complications of circumcision include hemorrhage, wound infection, meatitis, and UTI. Opening of the wound, insufficient removal of the foreskin, skin bridges and inclusion cysts, amputation of the glans penis, sepsis, frenulum breve, and buried penis are rarely seen.

COMPLICATIONS

Postoperative bleeding, when present, can be dealt with by gentle manual compression; however, if the bleeding is emanating from the skin edges, placement of a hemostatic stitch under local anesthesia can be performed. If the wound appears slightly prone to bleeding at the completion of the circumcision, a gentle compressive dressing can also be applied. Care should be taken in not making the dressing too occlusive as difficult voiding, wound ischemia, and, rarely, urinary retention can occur.[12]

Infection has been reported to occur in approximately 10% of circumcisions yet, in general, antibiotics are not necessary. Most infections are self-limited, resulting in local inflammation and erythema, but purulence and systemic manifestations can be present. With evidence of a local wound infection, the patient should receive systemic antibiotics with coverage against gram-positive flora, such as a first-generation cephalosporin.

An *urethrocutaneous fistula* is a rare but dreaded complication of circumcision. Such a complication usually occurs during suture ligation of a bleeding vessel located at the frenulum. Concomitant ligation of the underlying urethra inadvertently occurs, increasing the possibility of a fistula. Burn injuries from cautery causing urethral necrosis and localized infection are other sources of fistula formation.

Removal of excess foreskin during circumcision can be a source of frustration among patients undergoing circumcision. This can result in penile–scrotal webbing, chordee, or frank shaft skin loss. Removal of excess foreskin highlights the importance of placing the penis on stretch to aid in the decision of incision lines. Whereas neonatal penile skin loss can often be managed with local wound care, this is not necessarily true with adult patients. Options for penile skin loss management include local skin flaps and full- or split-thickness skin grafts.[13]

Removal of too little foreskin is chiefly a cosmetic problem.

Sexual dysfunction: Alteration in sexual function after circumcision is controversial.

CONCLUSION

Adult circumcision is a safe procedure with infrequent but measurable complications. Unlike neonatal circumcision, where the procedure is largely elective, there are several concrete indications including phimosis, paraphimosis, balanitis, and LS. Recent studies in Africa also indicate that circumcision can be preventive in HIV transmission and some sexually transmitted infections. Several methods of performing an adult circumcision exist, but the sleeve method remains the most common. Although sensation appears to be diminished in circumcised adults relative to their uncircumcised cohorts, studies have not discovered a difference in sexual function when compared to uncircumcised men.

REFERENCES

1. World Health Organization, Joint United Nations Programme on HIV/AIDS. (2007). Male circumcision: global trends and determinants of prevalence, safety, and acceptability. [online] Available from https://apps.who.int/iris/bitstream/handle/10665/43749/9789241596169_eng.pdf?sequence=1&isAllowed=y [Last accessed September, 2023].
2. World Health Organization, Jhpiego Corporation. Manual for early infant male circumcision under local anaesthesia. Geneva: World Health Organization; 2010.
3. Gairdner D. The fate of the foreskin, a study of circumcision. Br Med J. 1949;2:1433-7.
4. Bromage S, Crump A, Pearce I. Phimosis as a presenting feature of diabetes. BJU Int. 200;101:338-40.
5. Patterson BK, Landay A, Siegel JN, Flener Z, Pessis D, Chaviano A, et al. Susceptibility to human immunodeficiency virus-1 infection of human foreskin and cervical tissue grown in explant culture. Am J Pathol. 2002;161:867.
6. McCoombe SG, Short RV. Potential HIV-1 target cells in the human penis. AIDS. 2006;20:1491-5.
7. Mehta SD, Gray RH, Auvert B, Moses S, Kigozi G, Taljaard D, et al. Does sex in the early period after circumcision increase HIV-seroconversion risk? Pooled analysis of adult male circumcision clinical trials. AIDS. 2009;23:1557.
8. Tobian AA, Serwadda D, Quinn TC, Kigozi G, Gravitt PE, Laeyendecker O, et al. Male circumcision for the prevention of HSV-2 and HPV infections and syphilis. N Engl J Med. 2009;360:1298-309.
9. Gerharz EW, Haarmann C. The first cut is the deepest? Medicolegal aspects of male circumcision. BJU Int. 2000;86:332-8.
10. Long RM, McCartan D, Cullen I, Harmon D, Flood HD. A preliminary study of the sensory distribution of the penile dorsal and ventral nerves: implications for effective penile block for circumcision. BJU Int. 2010;105(11):1576-8.
11. Circumcision policy statement. American Academy of Pediatrics. Task Force on Circumcision. Pediatrics. 1999;103:686-93.
12. Williams N, Kapila L. Complications of circumcision. Br J Surg. 1993;80:1231.
13. Black PC, Friedrich JB, Engrav LH, Wessells H. Meshed unexpanded split-thickness skin grafting for reconstruction of penile skin loss. J Urol. 2004;172(3):976.

SECTION 9

Miscellaneous Surgical Procedures

CHAPTER 58

Chemosurgery

Niti Khunger, Ridhima Lakhani, Gulshant Panesar

KEY MESSAGES

- Chemosurgery or chemical cautery is defined as the use of chemical substances to destroy diseased or unwanted tissues.
- Phenol (88%), trichloroacetic acid (TCA) (30–100%), sodium hydroxide (10–20%), potassium hydroxide, urea, salicylic acid (>30%), and glycolic acid (>70%) are popular agents used for chemosurgery.
- Xanthelasma, warts, ingrown toenail are some of the conditions that can be successfully treated with chemosurgery.

INTRODUCTION

Chemosurgery or chemical cautery is defined as the use of chemical substances to destroy diseased or unwanted tissues, by resurfacing, destruction or exfoliation.[1] The chemical reagent is transferred to the skin lesion, by various means, most commonly a wooden stick or swab, producing the desired effect. Various chemicals that are used for cauterization are phenol (88%), trichloroacetic acid (TCA) (30–100%), sodium hydroxide (10–20%), potassium hydroxide, urea, salicylic acid (>30%), and glycolic acid (>70%). The main principle involved in using such chemicals is abrading the superficial layers and subsequent rejuvenation. Based on the pH and concentration of chemical, there may be difference in level of penetration. Generally higher strength of aforementioned chemicals is used for chemosurgery. Some of the commonly used chemosurgical procedures are described in this chapter.

CHEMISTRY OF CHEMICALS USED IN CHEMOSURGERY

Trichloroacetic acid is a common, inexpensive agent widely used for chemical cauterization. It is an analog of acetic acid in which three hydrogen atoms of methyl group have been replaced by chlorine atoms, $C_2HCl_3O_2$ (CCl_3COOH). It exists as white crystalline form in its natural state. It is strongly acidic. Aqueous solution of 0.1 mol of solution has pH of 1.2. TCA with concentration 30% or less is difficult to be stored for a long period of time and gradually gets decomposed to chloroform, HCl, etc. It is stored in colored bottles to prevent decomposition. It acts by precipitating macromolecules like DNA, RNA, and proteins.

Phenol also known as carbolic acid is extracted from coal tar. In its purest form, it resembles needle-like crystals which are pink to colorless, but tarnish to brown on exposure to air or light. It also has a characteristic odor. It is diluted to attain a desired strength; 88% phenol being most commonly used in chemosurgery. Phenol penetrates the superficial reticular dermis to reach deeper layers and cause coagulation of proteins, thus causing tissue destruction. Epidermal regeneration starts after 48 hours but takes around 7–10 days to heal completely.

Sodium hydroxide is a basic salt that is also found as white crystals and dissolved to attain desired concentration generally around 10%. Sodium hydroxide causes basic tissue destruction and produces a liquefaction necrosis rather than the coagulation necrosis produced by phenol; hence healing is faster.

Indications

Some of the common indications of chemosurgery are given in **Table 1**. Xanthelasma palpebrarum (XP), verruca plana,

TABLE 1: Common indications of chemosurgery.

Indication	*Chemical*
Xanthelasma palpebrarum	Trichloroacetic acid (TCA) 25–100%
Cystic acne	Phenol 88%
Ice pick acne scars	TCA 50–100%
Ingrown toe nail	Phenol 88%, sodium hydroxide 10%
Chemical nail avulsion	Urea 40%
Warts—verruca vulgaris, plantar warts	Wart lotion containing 16.5% salicylic acid and 16.5% lactic acid, TCA 50%
Facial planar warts	TCA 15–30%
Genital warts	Podophyllin 25%, TCA 50–100%
Molluscum contagiosum	5–10% potassium hydroxide (KOH)
Freckles and lentigines	TCA 15–25%
Seborrheic keratosis, dermatosis papulosa nigra	TCA 50–100%, ammonium lactate and 70% glycolic acid

ingrown toenail, and chemical nail avulsion are some of the common indications that can be treated with chemosurgery. It is user-friendly in treatment of molluscum contagiosum and warts particularly in children.

Precautions

Sensitive areas such as the face, around the eyes and mucosal surfaces should be done with care. Eye covers can be used, if necessary. Emergency eye irrigation equipment such as a syringe filled with saline should be at hand when carrying out chemosurgery on the face. It should be done cautiously in children as it is difficult to keep them still when applying the chemical. Restless children may be given oral sedation, if necessary. Active herpes simplex, or any infection, and erosions and raw areas at the site of application of chemical should be treated before chemosurgery.

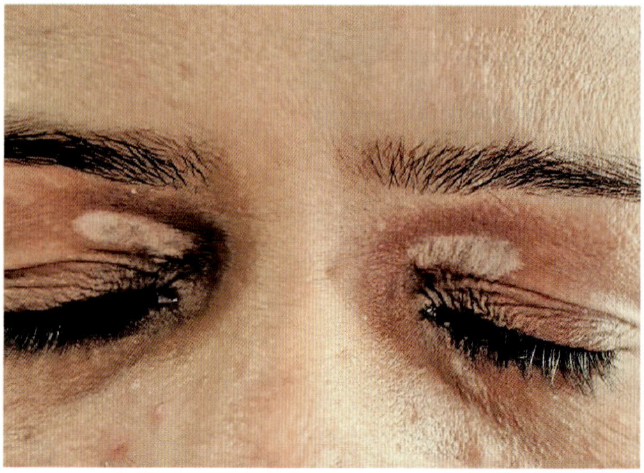

Fig. 1: Dense white frost due to application of 50% TCA for xanthelasma palpebrarum.

Procedures

Xanthelasma

Xanthelasma palpebrarum is most common cutaneous xanthoma, clinically characterized by yellowish plaques over eyelids—most commonly, medially over the inner canthus of the upper lid and lower lid. It is triggered by diabetes, hyperlipidemia, and thyroid dysfunction and may also be seen in normolipemic individuals. So, a systemic workup is important. Lee et al.[2] classified XP into four grades depending on the extent and location of the lesion. Grade I has lesions on the upper eyelids only. Grade II has lesions extended to the medial canthal area. Grade III has lesions on the medial side of both lower and upper eyelids. Grade IV has diffuse involvement on medial and lateral sides of both eyelids. Grade IV generally has deeper muscle involvement and surgical management is the best resort. The other three grades can be appropriately managed with TCA.[3]

Procedure: 70–100% TCA can be used but 100% TCA gives the best results. 50% TCA may be used initially in patients with thin lesions. To prepare 100% solution, 100 g TCA crystals are dissolved in 100 mL of distilled water. There should be utmost precaution to avoid dripping of TCA to ocular areas. The patient is seated comfortably in a semirecumbent position. Toothpick/or swab applicator may be used. The eyelids are degreased with alcohol or acetone. The surrounding normal skin is protected with Vaseline. The technique requires the applicator to be moved in a circular fashion with the greater amount of TCA to be applied at the margin of the lesion. Frosting is observed within a minute. Complete frosting with the presence of uniform densely white color and cessation of burning sensation is the end point of treatment **(Fig. 1)**. The area is cleaned with normal saline and the patients are asked to wash the face. A dark, brownish-black crust forms which should be kept soft by application of petroleum jelly and allowed to come off by itself. This usually takes 10–14 days. If the lesion still persists, TCA is reapplied. The procedure can be repeated every 15 days or till complete healing. The common side effects seen are hypo- or hyperpigmentation, which are usually transient. Transient edema may be seen in older patients with thin lax skin. However, scarring and ectropion formation are uncommon serious side effects especially with higher strengths.

The results of prospective treatment of 24 patients with eyelid xanthelasma with 70% TCA indicated that this was a simple and effective method, achieved a satisfactory cosmetic result, had an acceptable recurrence rate, and high patient satisfaction.[4] Three strengths of TCA were used on 51 patients by Haque et al. randomly after categorizing their xanthelasma into papulonodular, flat plaques and macular lesions. The average number of sittings was calculated in each category and patients were reviewed fortnightly. The study concluded that 100% TCA gives the best results in papulonodular lesions, 100% or 70% TCA gave similar results in flat plaque xanthelasma and in macular lesions 50% was sufficient. Hypopigmentation was the most common side effect, followed by hyperpigmentation. Scarring was a minor problem.[5] In a study by Mourad et al. 70% TCA was found to be more effective as compared to 35 or 50% TCA, with hypopigmentation seen as a side effect with 70% TCA and hyperpigmentation with 50% TCA.[6] In a comparative study by Goel et al.[7] 30% TCA was compared with the ultrapulsed CO_2 laser. It was observed that for clinically mild lesions, both TCA and laser were good options, with comparative effect, but the laser was found to be a better option for severe lesions. However, the TCA concentration used in this study was only 30%. Recurrence was seen in both groups.

Chemoablation of Warts

Most modalities for the treatment of warts focus on destruction of the lesion through electrocautery, chemosurgery by TCA

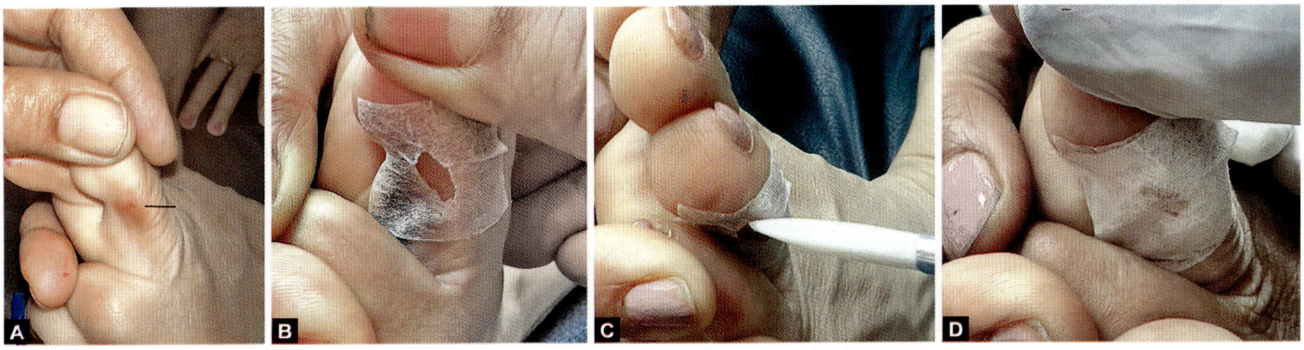

Figs. 2A to D: (A) Wart on the 4th toe; (B) Application of fenestrated micropore taope to prevent damage of surrounding normal skin; (C) Application of 100% TCA; (D) Use of micropore tape for occlusion.

or wart solution (salicylic acid 16.5% and lactic acid 16.5%), cryotherapy, or immune mediators. Radiofrequency ablation is considered gold standard for the treatment of warts. Certain circumstances in which TCA cauterization is preferred are planar warts on face, anogenital warts specially in pregnancy, in verruca vulgaris if patient is hesitant for radiofrequency ablation, and finally in plantar warts where TCA is used after paring. It is a preferred technique in children and in patients with multiple lesions, where ablation with radiofrequency or CO_2 laser is not feasible. It is less painful as compared to cryotherapy. In plantar warts, it is the treatment of choice as it causes least pain and scar formation as compared to ablation with electrosurgery, radiofrequency, or CO_2 laser.

Wart solution containing 16.5% salicylic acid and 16.5% lactic acid is most commonly used. It is self-applied by the patient as a home preparation, with proper instructions. The wart solution is carefully applied to the lesion with a pointed toothpick or cotton bud, depending on the size of the lesion. In case of plantar warts, the surrounding skin is protected with tape or Vaseline **(Figs. 2A to D)**, the wart solution is allowed to dry and then the lesion is occluded with micropore tape.

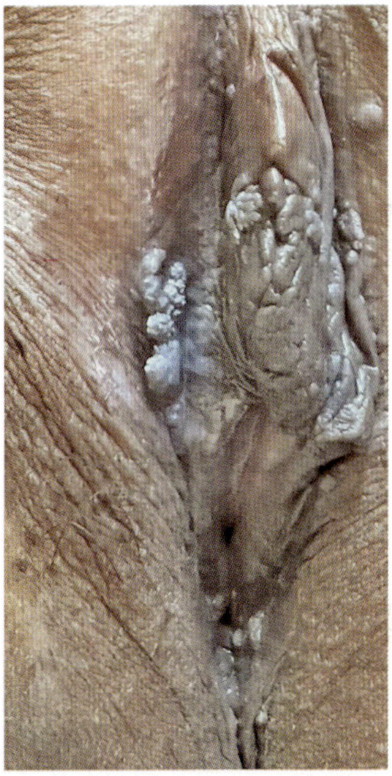

Fig. 3: Frosting with TCA in genital warts.

Procedure: TCA solution has a low viscosity comparable with that of water and can spread rapidly and damage adjacent tissues if applied excessively. A small amount should be applied only to the warts and allowed to dry (i.e., develop white frost on tissue) before the patient sits or stands. If pain is intense or an excess amount of acid is applied, the area can be covered with sodium bicarbonate (i.e., baking soda), washed with liquid soap preparations, or be powdered with talc to neutralize the acid or remove unreacted acid. TCA treatment can be repeated weekly if necessary. In office application of TCA 50–100% is an alternative. For facial verruca plana TCA 15–25% is safer. Podophyllin 25% is the agent of choice for anogenital warts, but in pregnancy, TCA is preferred **(Fig. 3)**.

Trichloroacetic acid leads to 70–100% clearance of anogenital warts. In a study recurrence was observed in 18–36% of patients.[8] Topical 85% TCA is one of the accepted cytotoxic therapies for condyloma and is recommended by Centers for Disease Control and Prevention (CDC) as one of the first-line treatments for condyloma acuminatum. 30% TCA has been used for plane warts with good results.[9] The procedure is to be repeated every week for 4–6 weeks or till complete clearing.

Phenol can be used as a means to chemically cauterization of verruca. It is less painful than TCA, hence more preferred in children.[10]

Potassium and sodium hydroxide have also been used.[11]

Molluscum Contagiosum

It is a common cutaneous viral infection seen especially in children. Phenol, sodium hydroxide, and TCA all have been used successfully but phenol requires lesser number of applications for complete clearance and is also better tolerated by children.[12] Potassium hydroxide 2.5–5% as a self-application by the patient at home is another alternative. But it should be used with precaution as excess application on the surrounding normal skin can lead to crusting.

NAIL SURGERY

Chemical Matricectomy for Ingrown Toenail

Ingrown toenail is a common painful nail condition and a significant number of cases require surgical management in the form of lateral partial nail avulsion of the ingrown edge. A simple avulsion of the nail is associated with high chances of recurrence. Destruction of the lateral horns of the matrix (lateral matricectomy) is an essential component in the management of ingrown toenail. This may be achieved by surgical, or more commonly, by chemical destruction of the lateral matrix (chemical matricectomy). The matrix destruction should be selective to minimize damage to the surrounding normal structures, but at the same time it must be complete and reliable to prevent recurrences. Chemical matricectomy uses various chemical agents to destroy the lateral nail matrix. Among these, phenol is the most common agent used. It is an effective protein denaturant which shows its cauterizing effect by producing a coagulation necrosis in the matrix and the surrounding soft tissue **(Figs. 4A to E)**. Sodium hydroxide has also been used for chemical matricectomy.

Procedure: Phenol crystals dissolved to 88% concentration, toothpick, nail plate elevator, nail spatula, skin hook, and nail splitter/clipper are the reagent and equipment required for chemical matricectomy for ingrown toenail. Patient is laid supine and the feet are properly cleaned and draped. The affected nail is anesthetized with a ring block. Tourniquet is applied for hemostasis and time is noted as the total time should not exceed 20 minutes. The lateral and proximal nail folds are retracted using a nail spatula and skin hook. The nail spatula is inserted beneath the nail plate to separate the nail plate from nail bed and then the entire nail plate is pulled along with the lateral horn. Then toothpick or swab with phenol is applied over the lateralmost part of the nail matrix for 1–2 minutes. Finally pressure dressing is done and tourniquet is removed. After complete or partial nail avulsion, phenol is locally applied on lateralmost part of matrix for 1–2 minutes. The phenol is then neutralized with povidone-iodine lotion. Recurrence rates reported are <5%.[13]

Good results have also been reported with TCA, but postoperative pain is more.[14] Sodium hydroxide has also been used. A 1-2-minutes application has very good efficacy with reduced postoperative morbidity.[15] Sodium hydroxide is a strong basic salt that, in contrast to phenol, causes basic tissue destruction and produces a liquefaction necrosis that is known to heal more rapidly than the coagulation necrosis produced by phenol. It has been shown to have an efficacy similar to phenol, but with a shorter recovery time. It offers a slightly better adverse effect profile.

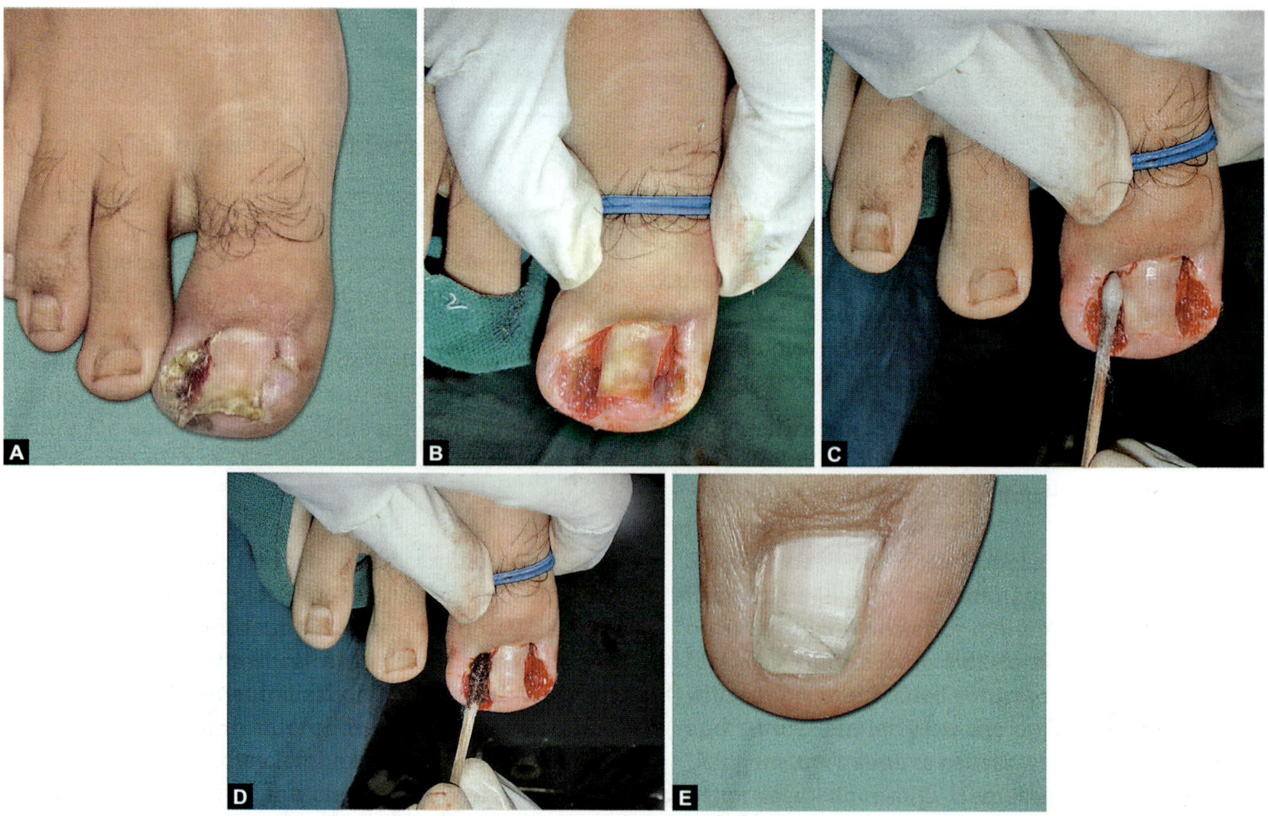

Figs. 4A to E: (A) Ingrown toenail; (B) Avulsion of lateral nail plate; (C) Application of 88% phenol; (D) Application of betadine; (E) No recurrence till final result at 1 year.

Other methods used are surgical matricectomy and ablative methods such as carbon dioxide laser, electrocautery, and radiofrequency. The latter techniques are more technically demanding and more expensive compared with chemical matricectomy.

Chemical Nail Avulsion

Avulsion of the nail can be achieved by surgical or chemical means. Though surgical avulsion is more commonly employed, chemical avulsion is more popular in the elderly population, or when the patient is not fit or unwilling for surgery or when multiple nails are involved.[16]

Urea ointment is used for chemical nail avulsion. It is indicated for the treatment of onychogryphosis, onychomycosis particularly due to mold infections in the elderly, psoriasis, and recalcitrant candidial and bacterial infections. Urea ointment paste is formulated to include 40% urea, 5% white beeswax or paraffin, 20% anhydrous lanolin, and 35% white petrolatum.[17] Urea acts by dissolving the bond between the nail bed and the nail plate, and it also softens the nail plate. The paronychial area is protected with adhesive tape before applying urea paste to prevent chemical irritation of the soft tissues. The ointment is liberally applied to the nail plate, and hypoallergenic tape is used to create a well around the treated thickened nail, to hold the paste. The patient is instructed to keep the nail occluded and to avoid wetting the treated area. After 1 week of occlusion, the dystrophic nail is removed by using a nail elevator and a nail clipper. In onychomycosis, antifungals may be prescribed as an adjunct.

Dystrophic nails may respond better to chemical avulsion, and it is the ideal management for symptomatic dystrophic nails in patients with diabetic neuropathy, vascular disease, or immunosuppression. In addition, chemical avulsion may be used as a palliative, pain-relieving therapy in onychogryphosis. Minimal to absent pain, a low risk of infection, hemorrhage, and lesser downtime are the advantages of chemical over surgical avulsion. Requirement of prolonged application and irritation are some disadvantages of the procedure. Further, patients with gross thickening of the nail without significant nail dystrophy may respond poorly to chemical avulsion due to poor penetration.

ACNE SURGERY

Phenolization for Cystic Acne

This is a simple office procedure to drain the cysts in acne. It achieves quicker healing with minimal scarring.[18]

Procedure: The face is first surgically cleaned with alcohol, povidone-iodine and again alcohol. Local anesthesia is infiltrated around the cyst, taking care not to puncture the cyst. The contents of the cyst are drained by making a fine, small nick with a No. 15 surgical blade. The cyst should be thoroughly evacuated. The walls of the cyst are then destroyed with 88% phenol by introducing a fine cotton swab on a toothpick dipped in phenol. Care should be taken to prevent spillage of excess phenol on the surrounding normal skin. The procedure is repeated with fresh phenol dipped swabs two to four times. The phenol is then neutralized with povidone-iodine dipped fine swabs. Intralesional and perilesional triamcinolone acetonide 5–10 mg/mL is then injected to reduce fibrosis and scarring. The advantages of this procedure are that the cysts heal quickly, inflammation is reduced and deep scars, typical of nodulocystic acne, are avoided or minimized. The disadvantage is that improper technique can lead to complications. It is important that the nick should be small to prevent a large scar. Phenol should be neutralized with povidone-iodine to prevent prolonged inflammation. This can otherwise result in postinflammatory hyperpigmentation (PIH). Complications are however uncommon and it is a safe, simple technique.

TCA–CROSS Technique for Acne Scars

Chemical reconstruction of skin scars (CROSS) is a technique using high concentrations of TCA (50–100%) focally on the atrophic acne scars to induce inflammation and collagenization.[19] The CROSS technique is an excellent treatment strategy for ice pick acne scars in all skin types including Fitzpatrick skin types IV to VI. TCA is a caustic agent that causes precipitation of proteins and coagulative necrosis of cells in the epidermis along with necrosis of collagen in the papillary to upper reticular dermis, when used in high strengths. An increase in dermal volume as a result of an increased collagen production, glycosaminoglycan, and elastin fragmentation and reorganization is also seen. The clinical effects of TCA are due to dermal collagen remodeling and an increase in the content of collagen, glycosaminoglycan, and elastin.[20]

Ice pick scars are most commonly treated with this method, followed by boxcar scars.[21,22]

It can be combined with laser skin resurfacing using 1,550-nm erbium:glass laser or fractional CO_2 laser or percutaneous microneedling to enhance results and improve other types of scars.

Procedure: Priming for 2–4 weeks before the procedure is essential before doing CROSS technique as PIH is common in darker skin.[23] Tretinoin 0.025% cream at night and a sunscreen containing avobenzone, octinoxate, and 2% hydroquinone in morning is most ideal. Informed consent and pretreatment photographs are essential before treatment. It is best to do the procedure with the patient sitting or inclined at 45°. No anesthesia is needed. A sharp, pointed toothpick is dipped in the TCA solution, taking care to see that there is no dripping. The skin is stretched and TCA is focally applied to reach the bottom of the scar by pressing hard and rotating a few times, taking care to avoid spillage to the surrounding skin **(Fig. 5)**. The skin is kept stretched and monitored carefully

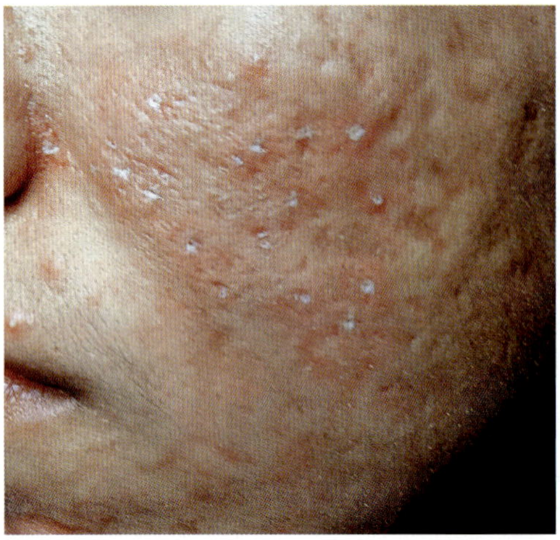

Fig. 5: Pinpoint frosting in icepick scars due to application of 100% TCA with a sharpened toothpick.

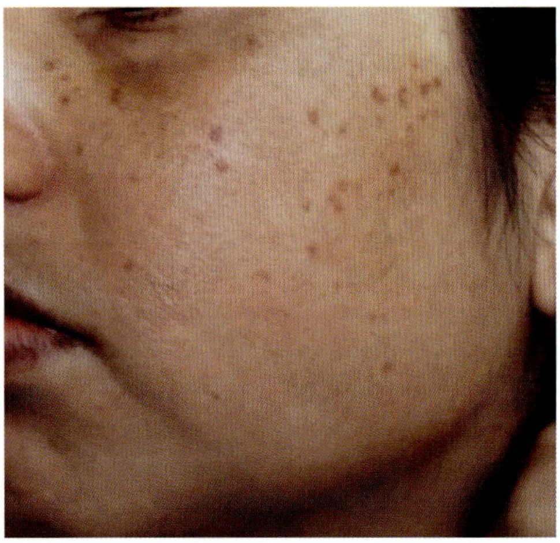

Fig. 6: PIH following TCA CROSS.

until frosting occurs. The face is then washed and the patient is sent from the clinic with application of sunscreen. A black crust forms in 3–4 days and heals in 7–10 days. The procedure can be repeated every 2–4 weeks, till the desired results are obtained. Better results are observed with 100% TCA as compared to 50–65%[23] using CROSS method. The advantage is that it is an efficacious cost-effective technique to treat ice pick scars. Persistent erythema, PIH **(Fig. 6)**, and widening of the scar are complications that can occur, with improper technique. Approximately a third of patients with darker skin type may develop PIH, which may persist in some patients.[24] Caution to be exercised for Fitzpatrick skin types V and VI.

Phenol is another agent which can be used in CROSS technique in a similar methodology. It is a painless technique when compared to TCA but the downtime is higher.[25]

Spot Cauterization for Seborrheic Keratosis, Lentigo, and Freckles

Four to five monthly sessions with TCA or phenol are used for treatment of solar lentigo, seborrheic keratosis, and melanocytic nevi.[26]

Anal Intraepithelial Neoplasia

Trichloroacetic acid has also been used as potentially attractive treatment approach for anal intraepithelial neoplasia (AIN) It is inexpensive, is generally well tolerated by patients, has no systemic side effects, and is safe to use in pregnancy. TCA may be a safe, inexpensive, and effective treatment in patients with two or fewer discrete AIN lesions, particularly for patients under 50 years of age. TCA was applied through the anoscope using a cotton-tipped applicator. It was directed toward the lesion under colposcopic guidance.[27]

NOVEL USES IN OTHER DERMATOLOGICAL DISEASES

Trichloroacetic acid has been recently used in treatment of depigmentation post-Q-switched Nd-YAG (neodymium-doped yttrium aluminum garnet) laser. In a case reported, after 15 sessions of Q-switched Nd-YAG, the patient developed postinflammatory depigmentation. He was initially treated with excimer laser for 10–15 sessions with no repigmentation, all depigmented macules were marked within 1 cm^2 area, and 65% TCA was applied using toothpick. Frosting was seen in 10–15 sessions. It was done in five sessions in divided areas. Complete repigmentation was seen in 2–4 weeks.[28]

Studies have also been done for inducing pigmentation in vitiligo[29] and idiopathic guttate hypomelanosis,[30] and the results are better with higher concentration of TCA and phenol. The procedure is simple but the only disadvantage being that it can be used in cases of limited involvement only.

Phenol has also been tried in alopecia areata (AA). 88% phenol can be considered as a treatment of choice for stable AA due to its ease of application, easy availability, and low cost.[31]

Phenol application can be used to cause fibrosis of the tract of pilonidal sinuses. Inadequate debridement and hair that is stuck in the sinus are responsible for poor healing and recurrence. Phenol application, owing to its sclerosing effects, provides quick recovery and the anesthetic effect of phenol leads to minimal pain in the postoperative period.[32]

Precautions

Avoid sensitive surfaces (eyes, mucosal surfaces), where eye covers can be used, if necessary. Emergency eye irrigation equipment should be at hand. Rule out active herpes labialis or any other infection at the site of application of chemical.

Postprocedure Instructions

Frosting of the surface may last up to 12 hours. Skin on the treated area may be red and sore for few days but if persistent, topical steroids may be prescribed. Scabs will form after 3 days and fall off by 1 week. Postprocedure edema may last for a day or two specially after use of TCA for xanthelasma over eyelids. Antihistaminics, anti-inflammatory, or topical steroids may be prescribed. Emollients should be prescribed to avoid excessive dryness and for procedures on face, broad-spectrum sunscreen with SPF 40 or above is mandatory in follow-up period.

Contraindications

Pregnancy and lactation are an absolute contraindication as exposure to phenol has been linked to birth defects and low birth weight.

Herpes/infection at the site of application should be ruled out.

Adverse Effects

Systemic

Systemic toxicity is feared in cases of larger quantity (>3 mL) use of phenol, which may lead to renal damage and cardiac arrhythmias. Use of endovenous fluids and adequate hydration during and postprocedure may prevent such circumstances.[33]

Cutaneous[34]

Pigment alteration especially permanent hypopigmentation is very specific with phenol. PIH may also occur in darker skin types. Scars and keloids are also common if patient has a tendency. Infections due to *Staphylococcus*, *Streptococcus*, *Pseudomonas* can be prevented by keeping strict asepsis during the procedure and giving antibiotics postprocedure. Adhesions or lower eyelid ectropion may occur if use of phenol is too close to eye. Milia can also be seen rarely in case of use of higher percentage of chemicals. Prolonged erythema may be treated with mild steroid.

CONCLUSION

Chemosurgery with various chemical agents is a simple office procedure that can be an effective tool in selected skin disorders. It needs to be done cautiously to prevent complications.

REFERENCES

1. Matarrasso SL, Hanke CW, Alsters TS. Cutaneous resurfacing. Dermatol Clin. 1997;15(4):569-81.
2. Lee HY, Jin US, Minn KW, Park YO. Outcomes of surgical management of xanthelasma palpebrarum. Arch Plast Surg. 2013;40(4):380-6.
3. Nair PA, Singhal R. Xanthelasma palpebrarum—a brief review. Clin Cosmet Investig Dermatol. 2017;11:1-5.
4. Nahas TR, Marques JC, Nicoletti A, Cunha M, Nishiwaki-Dantas MC, Filho JV. Treatment of eyelid xanthelasma with 70% trichloroacetic acid. Ophthalmic Plast Reconstr Surg. 2009;25(4):280-3.
5. Haque MU, Ramesh V. Evaluation of three different strengths of trichloroacetic acid in xanthelasma palpebrarum. J Dermatolog Treat. 2006;17(1):48-50.
6. Mourad B, Elgarhy LH, Ellakkawy HA, Elmahdy N. Assessment of efficacy and tolerability of different concentrations of trichloroacetic acid vs. carbon dioxide laser in treatment of xanthelasma palpebrarum. J Cosmet Dermatol. 2015;14(3):209-15.
7. Goel K, Sardana K, Garg VK. A prospective study comparing ultrapulse CO_2 laser and trichloroacetic acid in treatment of Xanthelasma palpebrarum. J Cosmet Dermatol. 2015;14(2):130-9.
8. O'Mahony C, Gomberg M, Skerlev M, Alraddadi A, de Las Heras-Alonso ME, Majewski S, et al. Position statement for the diagnosis and management of anogenital warts. J Eur Acad Dermatol Venereol. 2019;33(6):1006-19.
9. Jayaprasad S, Subramanyan R, Devgan S. Comparative evaluation of topical 10% potassium hydroxide and 30% Trichloroacetic acid in the treatment of plane warts. Indian J Dermatol. 2016;61(6):634-9.
10. Banihashemi M, Pezeshkpoor F, Yazdanpanah MJ, Family S. Efficacy of 80% phenol solution in comparison with cryotherapy in the treatment of common warts of hands. Singapore Med J. 2008;49(12):1035.
11. Al-Hamdi KI, Al-Rahmani MA. Evaluation of topical potassium hydroxide solution for treatment of plane warts. Indian J Dermatol. 2012;57(1):38-41.
12. More YE, Chavan D, Gokhale N. A comparative study of treatment of Molluscum Contagiosum with 100% Trichloroacetic Acid and 88% Phenol. Int J Sci Research. 2014;3(1).
13. Muriel-Sánchez JM, Becerro-de-Bengoa-Vallejo R, Montaño-Jiménez P, Coheña-Jiménez M. The Treatment of Ingrown Nail: Chemical Matricectomy With Phenol Versus Aesthetic Reconstruction. A Single Blinded Randomized Clinical Trial. J Clin Med. 2020;9:845.
14. Terzi E, Guvenc U, Türsen B, Kaya Tİ, Erdem T, Türsen Ü. The effectiveness of matrix cauterization with Trichloroacetic acid in the treatment of ingrown toenails. Indian Dermatol Online J. 2015;6:4-8.
15. Ozdemir E, Bostanci S, Ekmekci P, Gurgey E. Chemical matricectomy with 10% sodium hydroxide for the treatment of ingrowing toenails. Dermatol Surg. 2004;30:26-31.
16. Averill RW, Scher RK. Simplified nail taping with urea ointment for nonsurgical nail avulsion. Cutis. 1986;38(4):231-3.
17. Pandhi D, Verma P. Nail avulsion: Indications and methods (surgical nail avulsion). Indian J Dermatol Venereol Leprol. 2012;78:299-308.
18. Khunger N; IADVL Task Force. Standard guidelines of care for acne surgery. Indian J Dermatol Venerol Leprol. 2008;74:28-36.
19. Lee JB, Chung WG, Kwahck H, Lee KH. Focal treatment of acne scars with trichloroacetic acid: chemical reconstruction of skin scars method. Dermatol Surg. 2002;28(11):1017-21.
20. Stegman SJ. A comparative histologic study of the effects of three peeling agents and dermabrasion on normal and sundamaged skin. Aesthetic Plast Surg. 1982;6(3):123-35.
21. Fabbrocini G, Annunziata MC, D'Arco V, De Vita V, Lodi G, Mauriello MC, et al. Acne scars: pathogenesis, classification and treatment. Dermatol Res Pract. 2010;2010:893080.
22. Gupta A, Kaur M, Patra S, Khunger N, Gupta S. Evidence-based Surgical Management of Post-acne Scarring in Skin of Color. J Cutan Aesthet Surg. 2020;13(2):124-41.

23. Khunger N, Bhardwaj D, Khunger M. Evaluation of CROSS technique with 100% TCA in the management of ice pick acne scars in darker skin types. J Cosmet Dermatol. 2011; 10:51-7.
24. Agarwal N, Gupta LK, Khare AK, Kuldeep CM, Mittal A. Therapeutic response of 70% trichloroacetic acid CROSS in atrophic acne scars. Asit Mittal Dermatol Surg. 2015;41(5): 597-604.
25. Dalpizzol M, Weber MB, Mattiazzi AP, Manzoni APD. Comparative Study of the Use of Trichloroacetic Acid and Phenolic Acid in the Treatment of Atrophic-Type Acne Scars. Dermatol Surg. 2016;42(3):377-83.
26. Chun EY, Lee JB, Lee KH. Focal trichloroacetic acid peel method for benign pigmented lesions in dark-skinned patients. Dermatol Surg. 2004;30(4):512-6.
27. Singh JC, Kuohong V, Palefsky JM. Efficacy of trichloroacetic acid in the treatment of anal intraepithelial neoplasia in HIV-positive and HIV-negative men who have sex with men. J Acquir Immune Defic Synd. 2009;52(4):474-9.
28. Chandrashekar BS, Sriram R, Madura C. Novel Method of Treatment of Post-Q-switched Nd-YAG Laser depigmentation with Trichloroacetic acid: A report of two cases. J Cutan Aesthet Surg. 2014;7(1):56-7.
29. Puri N, Puri A. A comparative study on 100% TCA versus 88% phenol for the treatment of vitiligo. Our Dermatol Online. 2012;3(3):184-6.
30. Ravikiran SP, Sacchidanand S, Leelavathy B. Therapeutic wounding—88% phenol in idiopathic guttate hypomelanosis. Indian Dermatol Online J. 2014;5(1):14-8.
31. Chikhalkar S, Jerajani H, Madke B. Evaluation of utility of phenol in alopecia areata. Int J Trichology. 2013;5(4):179-84.
32. Emiroğlu M, Karaali C, Esin H, Akpınar G, Aydın C. Treatment of pilonidal disease by phenol application. Turk J Surg. 2017;33(1):5-9.
33. Stuzin JM. Phenol peeling and the history of phenol peeling. Clin Plast Surg. 1998;25(1):1-8.
34. Conning DM, Hayes MJ. The dermal toxicity of phenol: an investigation of the most effective first-aid measures. Br J Ind Med. 1970;27:155-9.

CHAPTER 59

Leg Ulcers

Reena Rai, R Jayashree, CR Srinivas

KEY MESSAGES

- Leg ulcers may be either acute or chronic.
- They are commonly due to venous, arterial, and neuropathic causes.
- Clinical presentation varies according to whether it is venous, arterial, or neuropathic ulcer.
- Treatment should be aimed at treating the underlying cause.
- For venous ulcers, compression therapy is the mainstay of treatment, along with local wound care and periwound protection.
- For arterial ulcers, treatment is aimed at establishing adequate arterial supply.
- For neuropathic ulcers, treatment is aimed at minimizing pressure with aggressive debridement of dead tissue and callus.

INTRODUCTION

Ulcers of the lower extremities are a common cause for visits to the surgeon, vascular surgeon, or dermatologist. Leg ulcers refer to full-thickness skin loss on the leg or foot due to any cause. They occur in association with a range of disease processes and may be acute or chronic. Acute ulcers are those that follow the normal phases of healing; they are expected to show signs of healing in <4 weeks and include traumatic and postoperative wounds. Chronic ulcers are those that persist for longer than 6 weeks and are often of complex nature.[1] Of the various causes of leg ulcers, 70% are due to venous disease, 20% have mixed arterial and venous disease, and 10% result from other causes such as neuropathy, infections, malignancy, and inflammatory causes.[2]

CAUSES OF LEG ULCERS

The causes of leg ulcers are elaborated in **Box 1**.

CLINICAL FEATURES OF LEG ULCERS

The clinical features of venous, arterial, and neuropathic ulcers according to their characteristics are elaborated in **Table 1**.

VENOUS ULCERS

Pathophysiology of Venous Ulcers

Figure 1 shows the normal anatomy of the venous system of the legs.

The venous system in the lower extremities comprises three systems of veins: Superficial veins, deep veins, and communicating veins **(Fig. 1)**. Blood flows from the superficial

BOX 1: Causes of leg ulcers.

- *Vascular diseases:*
  - Venous
  - Arterial
    - Atherosclerosis
    - Thromboangiitis obliterans
    - Arteriovenous malformation
    - Hypertensive ulcers (Martorell's ulcer)
    - Cholesterol embolism
  - Mixed (arterial and venous)
  - *Vasculitis:*
    - Idiopathic
    - Small-vessel vasculitis
      - Rheumatoid arthritis
      - Lupus erythematosus
      - Hypersensitivity vasculitis
      - Scleroderma
      - Behçet's disease
    - Medium- and large-vessel vasculitis
      - Polyarteritis nodosa
      - Wegener's granulomatosus
      - Nodular vasculitis
  - *Vaso-occlusive states:*
    - Calciphylaxis
    - Cryofibrinogenemia
    - Cryoglobulinemia
  - *Hypercoagulable states:*
    - Antiphospholipid antibody syndrome (APLA)
    - Protein C or S deficiency
  - Lymphatics
    - Lymphedema
- *Neuropathic diseases:*
  - Diabetes mellitus
  - Leprosy
  - Tabes dorsalis
  - Syringomyelia
- *Hematological diseases:*
  - *Disorders of red blood cells*
    - Sickle cell anemia
    - Hereditary spherocytosis

Contd...

Contd...

- ◆ Thrombocytosis
- ◆ Thalassemia
- – *Disorders of white blood cells:*
  - ◆ Leukemia
- – *Dysproteinemias:*
  - ◆ Cryoglobulinemia
- – *Physical causes:*
  - ◆ Trauma
  - ◆ Burns (thermal, chemical)
  - ◆ Cold injury (frostbite)
  - ◆ Radiation dermatitis
  - ◆ Factitial ulcers
- – *Infections:*
  - ◆ *Bacterial*
    - Furuncle, ecthyma, gram-negative infections, anaerobic infections
    - Mycobacterial, spirochetal infections, diphtheria, tropical ulcers
    - Septic emboli
  - ◆ *Fungal*
    - Deep fungal infections, Majocchi's granuloma, Protozoal
    - Infestations and bites
- *Skin diseases:*
  - Pyoderma gangrenosum
  - Epidermolysis bullosa
- *Neoplasm:*
  - Squamous cell carcinoma (SCC)
  - Basal cell carcinoma (BCC)
  - Kaposi's sarcoma
  - Lymphomas
  - Metastatic tumors
- *Metabolic diseases:*
  - Diabetes mellitus
  - Gout
  - Prolidase deficiency
- *Drugs:*
  - Ergotism
  - Hydroxyurea
  - Halogenoderma
- *Genetic:*
  - Klinefelter's syndrome
  - Werner's syndrome

to deep veins through the communicating veins, then up from the foot to the thigh and thence to the abdomen, before venous blood returns to the heart. These veins contain valves which prevent backflow of blood and allow unidirectional flow. During muscular activity, a high pressure develops in the deep venous system allowing blood to flow from deep to the superficial veins. When the calf muscle relaxes, high pressure in the superficial veins allows blood to flow from superficial to deep veins.

This mechanism is called "calf muscle pump". Failure of this pump, which could be due to incompetence of the valves, muscle weakness, and distension of veins, might lead to reflux of blood from deep to superficial veins causing high pressure in the superficial venous system and chronic venous insufficiency (CVI).

Various theories have been postulated to explain the mechanism of cutaneous ulceration.

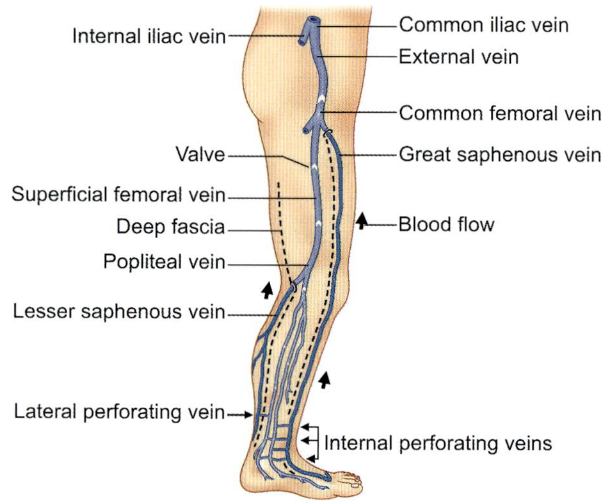

Fig. 1: Normal venous anatomy.

TABLE 1: Clinical features of leg ulcers.

	Venous ulcer	*Arterial ulcer*	*Neuropathic ulcer*
Complaints	Heaviness, pain, and swelling of limbs, which is aggravated on standing and relieved by limb elevation	• Claudication pain in the calves upon walking; relieved by rest • Rest pain in advanced stages	Burning, numbness, itching, pain, or paresthesias of distal extremities
Location	Gaiter area of the leg (medial malleolar region)	Pressure sites such as toe and ankle	Pressure sites such as plantar surface of the first and fifth metatarsal heads, plantar surface of the great toe **(Fig. 4)**
Morphology	Single or multiple ulcers with irregular borders, shallow depth, and sloping edges **(Fig. 2)**	Round with sharp borders with a dry necrotic base **(Fig. 3)**	Punched out with a thick rim of callus around
Surrounding skin	Pigmentation and lipodermatosclerosis	Shiny with loss of hair, cold limbs	Dryness and fissuring of skin with decreased or loss of sweating
Other features	Varicose veins, ankle edema, inverted champagne bottle appearance (stasis dermatitis)	Poor or absent peripheral pulses, pallor on limb elevation with rubor in dependent position	Features of peripheral neuropathy, deformities of the foot

Homan stated that stasis of venous blood could lead to tissue anoxia leading to venous ulcers.[3] Browse and Burnand postulated that venous hypertension could lead to endothelial distension causing leakage of fibrinogen into the interstitial fluid, which forms a pericapillary fibrin "cuff" that acts as a barrier to diffusion of oxygen causing ischemia and ulcer formation.[4] Coleridge Smith et al. thought that white blood cells disappear from the venous blood when the leg is in a dependent position. These leukocytes might get trapped in the capillaries and obstruct the flow causing ulceration.[5] Adhesion molecules, like intercellular adhesion molecule-1 (ICAM-1) and vascular cell adhesion molecule-1 (VCAM-1), also become overexpressed in CVI leading to continuous migration of leukocytes to the dermis.[6,7] Falanga and Eaglestein suggested that in patients with CVI, the pericapillary fibrin cuffs prevent the transfer of growth factors, which leads to delayed wound healing.[8] Another theory suggests that elevated pressure on the venular side of capillaries leads to the widening of interendothelial spaces and disintegration of collagen IV. This is laid down around capillaries leading to decreased availability of various growth factors required for wound healing.[9] Another theory suggests that fibroblasts present in chronic wounds may become senescent leading to impaired wound healing.[10]

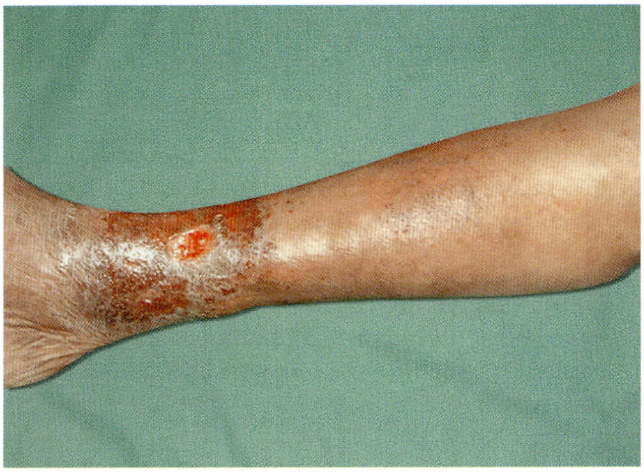

Fig. 2: Venous ulcer over the medial aspect of the leg with varicose veins and surrounding pigmentation.

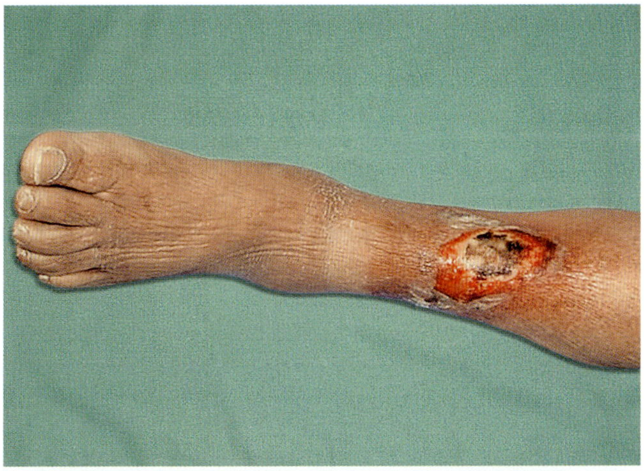

Fig. 3: Arterial ulcer with a necrotic slough at the base.

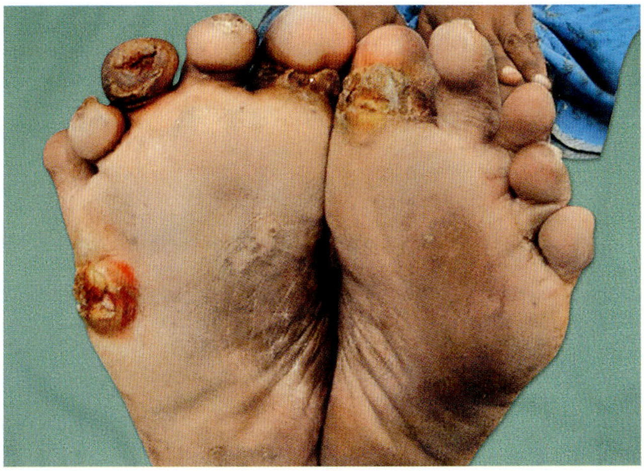

Fig. 4: Trophic ulcer on the plantar aspect of the toes and lateral aspect of the right sole.

Pathogenesis of Arterial Ulcers

Cigarette smoking, diabetes mellitus, hypertension, and high lipid diet are thought to encourage the development of atheroma, which leads to the accumulation of cells, tissue debris, and cholesterol plaques in the vessel intima leading to the narrowing of arterial lumen of vessels of the heart and lower limb.

Inadequate collaterals or occlusion from thrombosis before collaterals develop causes tissue infarction leading to ischemic ulceration of the skin.[11]

Pathogenesis of Neuropathic Ulcer

In neuropathy, there is a loss of pain sensation so repetitive trauma, shearing, and frictional forces lead to ulceration. Moreover, autonomic neuropathy leads to hypohidrosis of the foot causing dry skin and development of fissures and calluses leading to ulcers.[12]

LABORATORY EVALUATION OF LEG ULCERS

Leg ulcers need proper evaluation and often a battery of tests as mentioned below may be needed.

Complete blood count: To rule out infection, anemia, and polycythemia—blood sugars, glycated hemoglobin (HbA1C) for diabetic status.

- Serum albumin, transferrin, ferritin, vitamins A and C, zinc, and iron—to rule out nutritional deficiency
  - Vitamins A and C; iron and zinc are important in wound healing.[11,13]
  - Serum homocysteine levels—increased in vitamins B_6 and B_{12} and folate deficiency

- Screening for lupus anticoagulant, anticardiolipin antibodies
- Antinuclear antibody (ANA), rheumatoid factor, antineutrophil cytoplasmic antibody (ANCA) (P and C), cryoglobulins[14]

Protein C, protein S, and antithrombin III, factor V

- Leiden[14]
- Wound swabs for bacterial culture and sensitivities.[15] Tissue for mycobacterial and fungal cultures.

Deep wedge biopsies including ulcer margin and bed—to rule out malignancy, vasculitides, panniculitis,[15] and venous Doppler (color Doppler duplex ultrasound):

- For information on venous anatomy and reflux.[16,17]

Doppler ultrasound:

- When peripheral pulses are impalpable, Doppler flow meter is used to hear the pulsation over the dorsalis pedis and posterior tibial arteries, and ankle brachial pressure index (ABPI) is calculated as follows:

$$\text{ABPI} = \frac{\text{Systolic pressure in the ankle}}{\text{Higher of the two systolic pressure obtained from brachial arteries in both arms}} = 1.1$$

- ABPI 0.5–0.8 indicates occlusive arterial disease and arteriography should be performed.
- ABPI <0.5 indicates severe arterial obstruction.[18]

Plain radiograph—to rule out osteomyelitis

- Patch testing—to rule out allergic contact dermatitis to medicaments and preservatives, especially when the patient has been applying topical medication for a long time. Common allergens that have been detected include neomycin, lanolin, bacitracin, formaldehyde, and parabens.[15]

TREATMENT

Venous Ulcers

After arterial disease has been excluded, the primary aim of treatment of venous ulcers is to reduce venous hypertension, promote wound healing, prevent recurrences, and make the patient ambulant as early as possible.

Venous hypertension can be reduced by various ways. These include simple leg elevation and compression therapy. Simple leg elevation should be above the level of the heart and various compression devices.

Compression therapy: The aim of compression therapy is to achieve sustained graded compression of 30–40 mm Hg at the ankle, thereby reducing the edema and improving the function of the calf muscle pump and promoting ulcer healing.[19-21]

Various compression devices that can be used are elaborated in **Table 2**.

Wound Care for Leg Ulcers

Wound can be managed by dressings, debridement, topical treatment, systemic treatment, and biophysical treatment modalities.[22]

Dressings

Maintaining a moist environment, which accelerates wound healing, is very important. This can be accomplished by frequent application of saline dressings over the wound, which helps to keep the wound surface moist, debrides the wound, and removes the surface bacteria.

Recent research on wound care has resulted in increased use of interactive and active dressings rather than passive dressings that cover and absorb. Active dressings deliver

TABLE 2: Compression devices.

Types	*Functions*
Unna's boot A preparation consisting of zinc oxide 5 parts, gelatin 5 parts, boric acid 1 part, glycerin 8 parts, and water 6 parts. Ichthyol 1 or 2 parts are incorporated into it. Moist gauze impregnated with this paste is wrapped from behind the first metatarsal up to an inch below the knee, either in a figure-of-8 pattern or adding pleats while wrapping. It can be left in place for 7 days before changing	Protects against trauma and maintains the ambulatory status of the patient but cannot be used in highly exudative wounds. Pressure variation can also occur
Graduated compression stockings Three classes are available depending on the desired degree of ankle pressure in mm Hg *Class-I* (18–21 mm Hg) Indicated in mild varicosis, early varicosis in pregnancy, and heaviness of legs *Class-II* (23–32 mm Hg) Indicated in severe varicose veins, moderate edema, pronounced varicosis in pregnancy, posthealing minor ulcerations, superficial thrombophlebitis, and postsclerotherapy *Class-III* (34–46 mm Hg) For severe chronic venous insufficiency, marked edema and induration of skin	Improves the venous return, raises the hydrostatic pressure, and decreases the superficial venous pressure; therapy reducing the leak of solutes and fluid into the interstitial space also enhances the release of plasminogen activator, which helps in the breakdown of pericapillary fibrin deposits and restores defective fibrinolysis

Contd...

Contd...

Orthotic devices	*Bulky*
Four-layered bandaging (Velfour™) High compression bandage system (sub-bandage pressure of 35–40 mm Hg at the ankle) that incorporates elastic layers to achieve sustained compression **(Figs. 5 and 6)**[23] Layer 1 is orthopedic wool Layer 2 is a cotton crepe bandage Layer 3 is a light-weight elastic compression bandage Layer 4 is a cohesive compression bandage and it retains the bandage in position	Promotes healing of ulcer in patients with superficial, deep venous incompetence and mixed ulcers (arterial and venous). Also used in lymphatic disorders
Intermittent pneumatic compression Used in those who do not respond to stockings or compression bandages[24]	Relieves edema and promotes healing in patients with venous ulcers, also used to treat lymph edema

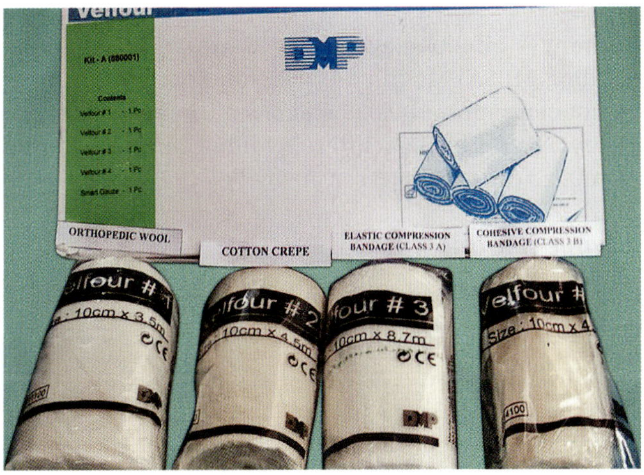

Fig. 5: Four-layered bandage.

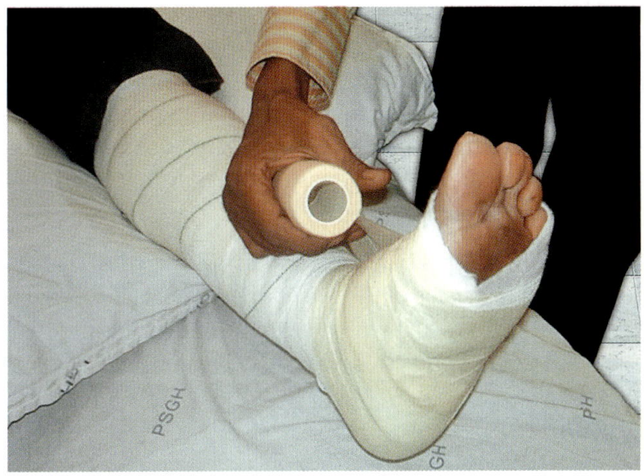

Fig. 6: Application of four-layered bandage.

substances, such as growth factors, which are important in the healing cascade. Interactive dressings are occlusive dressings. They provide a favorable microenvironment for the growth of new tissue. Moist occlusive dressings control the exudates, while epithelial cell migration is encouraged. Eschar is liquefied and fibrin is lysed to allow convenient debridement. Infection is managed through wound fluid rich in leukocytes. These dressings are also believed to provide symptomatic relief such as decreased pain and pruritus.

The various dressings and their advantages and disadvantages[21,24] are elaborated in **Table 3**.

Periwound protection: The skin surrounding the ulcer can be damaged due to excess moisture, wound fluid proteases, and adhesives present in the dressings.[21,25] Barrier creams and ointments are available, which protect the skin around the ulcer. These include the following:

- *Vaseline petroleum jelly:* Protects the periwound skin but interferes with dressing adherence
- *Unna's paste:* It is a preparation containing zinc oxide 5 parts, gelatin 5 parts, boric acid 1 part, glycerin 8 parts and water 6 parts with ichthyol 1 or 2 parts. It protects the skin around the wound, has anti-inflammatory effect, and promotes healing. It can also interfere with dressing adherence.[26,27]

Debridement

Standard wound care consists of debridement, which removes the necrotic debris and helps in the formation of healthy granulation tissue.[21,28] Various methods of debridement include the following:

Surgical debridement: This is done using a curette and scissors where a chronic wound is converted into an acute wound. Neutrophils and macrophages, which are recruited to the area, secrete growth factors and phagocytize the bacteria and nonviable tissue.[21,29]

Autolytic debridement: This is the gentle separation of slough from wound bed that occurs slowly in a moist wound environment. It is accomplished by placing an occlusive dressing on a wound and allowing proteases within the wound space to liquefy the necrotic tissue. It is useful in patients with bleeding tendencies where surgical debridement is not feasible.[21,30]

TABLE 3: Types of dressings.

Types of dressings	*Availability*	*Indications and adverse effects*
Films	Thin transparent adhesives, made of polyurethane to be changed every 12–24 hours, e.g., Tegaderm	Protects the wound from contamination but may strip away the newly forming granulation tissue. Used in wounds with moderate exudates
Hydrogels	Gel-like sheets. Semitransparent and nonadhesive. To be changed every 1–3 days, e.g., restore hydrogel	Helps in desloughing the wound and can also be used as drug vehicles. Causes incarceration of skin around the ulcer
Hydrocolloids	Occlusive dressing composed of hydrocolloid with a polyurethane outer coating. Can be changed once a week, e.g., DuoDERM	Cost-effective. Traps the fluid under the dressing producing an offensive odor. Can be used in wounds with moderate exudates. Early removal strips off the newly formed epidermis
Alginates	Biodegradable. Derived from seaweeds Can be left in place until soaked with exudates, e.g., Sorbsan	Highly absorbent and hemostatic. Dries out the exudating wound making it more painful
Collagen	• Available in particle and sheet form • Obtained from human, porcine, and bovine sources. Forms a biodegradable gel over the wound surface, e.g., Promogran	Promotes wound healing by laying down a matrix that leads to new tissue formation and depletion of free radicals and proteases that hinder the healing process

Enzymatic debridement: It consists of the application of topical protease preparation that targets the fibrin and collagen of necrotic tissue. These include papain urea preparations—papain obtained from papaya contains protease and urea is a protein denaturant.[25] Collagenase, derived from *Clostridium histolyticum,* targets collagen.[30,31]

Biodebridement: This is achieved by using maggots. They are the larvae of a species of fly (*Lucilia sericata*), also known as "green bottle" blow fly, which selectively debride the dead tissue and tissue debris by secreting collagenase.[32]

Topical Treatment

Wound healing is impaired when bacterial colonization exceeds 10^5 organisms per gram of tissue.[33] As systemic antibiotics are reserved only for patients with evidence of cellulitis or systemic infection, topical antiseptics and antibiotics have been used to reduce the wound bioburden. The various preparations used are as follows:

- *Acetic acid:* Acetic acid 0.25% is used in the treatment of wounds infected with *Pseudomonas aeruginosa.*[34]
- Twenty percent benzoyl peroxide has antimicrobial properties when applied under occlusion.[35,36]
- *Silver compounds:* Silver ions have proven efficacy against various gram-negative bacteria. They are incorporated into various wound dressing products, creams, and gels and are used for their bactericidal properties.[37]
- *Iodosorb (cadexomer iodine):* A complex of iodine with cadexomer (starch-based polymer bead) promotes absorption of wound fluid, debris, and bacteria from wound bed by controlled release of iodine.[38]

Other topicals: Metronidazole gel provides good anaerobic coverage. Retapamulin, the first drug in the class of pleuromutilin antibiotics, acts by inhibiting bacterial protein synthesis by interacting at a site on the 50S ribosome subunit of bacterial ribosome. When used as a topical antibiotic, it is effective against gram-positive bacteria including methicillin-resistant *Staphylococcus aureus* (MRSA).[39] Mupirocin ointment is effective against gram-negative organisms including MRSA. Modified Dakin solution (hypochlorite) at a concentration of 0.025% elicits antimicrobial effects. Neomycin and bacitracin are avoided because of their potential to cause contact sensitivity.[39,40]

Systemic Treatment

Antibiotics are recommended only for patients with evidence of cellulitis or systemic infection.[41]

Fibrinolytics: Browse et al. have demonstrated that patients with lipodermatosclerosis have reduced fibrinolytic activity.[42] The commonly used fibrinolytic is stanozolol, an anabolic steroid, in the dose of 2 mg twice daily which reduces the pain and dermal thickness in acute lipodermatosclerosis.[43] Pentoxifylline, a substituted xanthine, in a dose of 400 mg thrice a day also has fibrinolytic properties. It acts by decreasing blood viscosity, increases red blood cell deformability, and inhibits platelet aggregation and production of proinflammatory cytokines.[44,45]

Other drugs which can be used as an adjuvant to compression therapy are oral enteric-coated aspirin (300 mg), micronized purified flavonoid fraction (Daflon 500), etc.

Biophysical Treatment Modalities

Electrical stimulation: It promotes wound healing by inhibiting bacterial growth, attracting fibroblasts toward the wound and expressing transforming growth factor (TGF) on fibroblasts.[46-48]

Low-frequency ultrasound: Continuous wave low-frequency ultrasound of 34 kHz has a temporary stimulatory effect on microcirculation mainly due to improved oxygenation and improved wound healing.[49-51]

Topical negative-pressure devices: They consist of a fenestrated evacuation tube embedded in a foam dressing covered with an airtight dressing. This tube is attached to a vacuum source, and a subatmospheric pressure of 100–125 mm Hg is applied in a continuous or an intermittent manner. This promotes wound healing by absorbing the exudates and promoting healthy granulation tissue formation.[52]

Hyperbaric oxygen therapy: It is based on the theory that tissue hypoxia results in the failure of chronic wounds to heal; 100% oxygen is breathed in at superatmospheric pressure while inside a compression chamber to facilitate wound healing.[53]

Surgical Options for Covering the Wound

Skin grafting is indicated when there is slow epithelialization with nonsurgical measures.

Pinch grafts: They are useful for small nonhealing ulcers, provided the ulcer bed is clean with healthy granulation tissue **(Fig. 7)**.[54]

Procedure: One percent lidocaine is injected into the anterior aspect of the thigh (donor area) to raise a number of wheals. Skin around the wheal is stretched firmly so as to pinch up the wheals and grafts are harvested by shaving off the top of each wheal with a number 11 Parker blade and placed on the ulcer bed with the dermal side down. Multiple grafts are placed on the ulcer bed, spacing them few millimeters apart from one another and then both donor and recipient sites are covered with a dressing for a week.

Advantage: It is a simple technique that can be done on an outpatient basis.

Disadvantage: Cobblestoning of the ulcer site and scarring over the donor site.

Split-thickness skin grafting (SSG): It consists of an epidermis and a portion of the dermis from the selected donor site and grafting onto the recipient site. The thickness of the graft may vary depending on the amount of dermis included in the graft.

Preoperative preparation of recipient site: Ulcer is debrided to remove the necrotic tissue and a healthy granulating base is created before SSG.

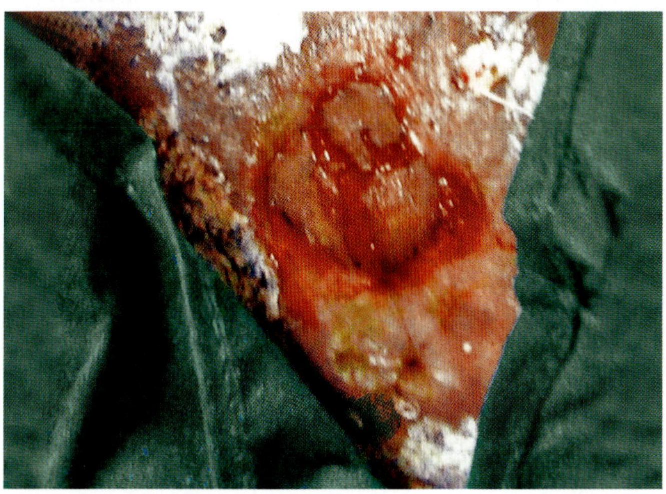

Fig. 7: Pinch graft over the ulcer.

Procedure: It is done under local, spinal, or general anesthesia. After cleansing the donor and recipient sites with povidone-iodine or surgical spirit, the skin over the donor area is stretched and the cutting edge of the knife or a razor blade is held at a 15–30° angle to the skin surface and sunk to the desired depth. The blade is moved back and forth gently by sawing movement to obtain a translucent graft, which is then placed on the recipient site, with the dermal side down, and secured with sutures and covered with a nonadhesive pressure dressing. Sutures can be removed after a week.[55]

Advantage: It covers large defects.

Disadvantage: It is less durable and might undergo contraction.

Skin Substitutes

Cultured epidermal grafts: Another approach in the treatment of leg ulcers secondary to CVI is the use of cultured epidermal cells (keratinocytes) as skin grafts, which can be derived from the patient's own skin (autograft) or from an unrelated donor (allograft). Growth factors released by the skin keratinocytes promote wound healing.[56,57]

Dermal substitutes: They are manufactured from human newborn foreskin fibroblast cells seeded onto a bioabsorbable mesh scaffold, which when implanted onto the wound secrete various growth factors and cytokines, persist in the wound for several months, and are eventually replaced by host tissue.[58]

Composite graft: Apligraf (has both dermal and epidermal components).

Apligraf is a living bilayered skin substitute manufactured using neonatal foreskin keratinocytes and fibroblasts with bovine type-I collagen. As it contains living cells, it should be kept sealed in its nutrient medium and 10% CO_2 or air atmosphere under a controlled temperature of 68–88°F (20–31°C) and used within 15 minutes of opening. It is used in leg ulcer due to venous insufficiency of >1 month duration along with standard compression therapy.[59]

LASER FOR LEG VEINS

Pulsed dye laser (PDL): At a wavelength of 585 nm and a pulse duration of 1–40 ms, PDL is capable of treating leg veins <0.2 mm in diameter. For larger veins up to 1.5 mm, long pulsed (595 mm) PDL can be used.[60,61]

Diode laser (800 mm): Long pulsed Nd:YAG laser (1,064 mm), long pulsed alexandrite laser (755 nm), and intense pulsed light (515–1,200 nm) are also used for treating leg telangiectasias.

Long pulsed Nd:YAG laser (1,064 nm): It has a maximum penetration of 3 mm, making it ideal for the destruction of large vessels of 0.5–3 mm diameter in the mid-dermis.[62]

Long pulsed alexandrite laser: With a wavelength of 755 nm and pulse duration of up to 20 ms or longer, alexandrite lasers penetrate 2–3 mm into the skin. It is ideal for treating medium-sized vessels (0.4–1 mm) and larger vessels (1–3 mm).[63]

Diode lasers: At 800–930 nm, the diode lasers can be used to treat deeper and larger reticular veins. More recently, 940-nm diode lasers have been found to be efficacious in the treatment of leg veins up to 1 mm in diameter.[64]

Intense pulsed light: It is a noncoherent, 515–1,200 nm flash lamp pumped light source with a fluence of 90 J/cm^2 and a pulse duration of 2–100 ms. To increase the selectivity, IPL uses filters that remove lower wavelengths. Filters (550 and 570 nm) are useful for vascular lesions that deliver light of yellow and red wavelengths and some infrared light. Broadband source of 515–1,200 nm helps in treating the smaller superficial vessels and large deeper vessels simultaneously.[65]

Endovenous Laser and Radiofrequency Treatment

Under duplex ultrasound guidance, a needle is inserted into the saphenous vein followed by a guide wire. Finally, either radiofrequency energy or light from 810-nm diode, 940-nm diode, or 1,320-nm Nd:YAG laser is delivered into the incompetent saphenous vein using a fibrotic catheter. Ninety percent of clearance has been reported after a single treatment.[66,67]

INDICATIONS FOR SURGICAL INTERVENTION IN LEG ULCERS SECONDARY TO CHRONIC VENOUS INSUFFICIENCY

- Recurrent episodes of hemorrhage
- Development of lipodermatosclerosis
- Recurrent, hard-to-heal ulcers despite conservative treatment.

Surgical options: They include surgical ligation and endoscopic perforator ligation combined with superficial vein ligation.[68,69]

Ambulatory Phlebectomy

Ambulatory phlebectomy is the removal of diseased venous segments by hook avulsion wherein incisions are made parallel to the diseased venous segments along the long axis. The vein is then exteriorized using a phlebectomy hook and avulsed after clamping both the proximal and the distal aspects. This process is repeated at 3–5-cm intervals along the entire length of the vein until the diseased vein is removed. The patient can be ambulant after the procedure so that normal gait and calf muscle pump function return quickly.[70]

Shave therapy: This is a simple and effective treatment for recalcitrant leg ulcer with deep venous insufficiency (post-thrombotic type). Under general/spinal anesthesia, the ulcer and the surrounding lipodermatosclerosis are removed or shaved off in horizontal layers followed by the application of a meshed split-skin graft from the thigh on the (0.4–0.6 mm thick) wound area.[71]

Treatment of Arterial Ulcers

The aim of the therapy is to establish adequate arterial supply[29] and wound care.

General Measures

The patient is advised to keep the extremities warm, quit smoking, lose weight if obese, maintain low-cholesterol diet, and keep diabetes and hypertension under control.

Lipid-lowering drugs such as statins and antiplatelet drugs such as aspirin, clopidogrel [inhibits adenosine diphosphate (ADP)-induced platelet aggregation], and cilostazol (phosphodiesterase III inhibitor) prevent ischemic events.[29,72]

Referral to a vascular surgeon for assessment and revascularization by angioplasty or arterial bypass surgery may be necessary in selected cases.

Treatment of Neuropathic Ulcers

The patient is advised to inspect the feet daily for any blisters, moisturize the feet adequately but to keep the interdigital spaces dry, and use proper footwear with offloading of pressure. Aggressive debridement of the dead tissue and the surrounding callus is followed by saline gauze dressings which are changed thrice a day.[12] Occlusive dressings like alginates, which absorb the exudates and maintain a moist environment, are also helpful.

Becaplermin gel: A topical recombinant platelet-derived growth factor has been approved by the Food and Drug Administration (FDA) as an adjunctive for the treatment of diabetic neuropathic ulcers.[12,73] Vascular surgery is to be considered if there is severe vascular impairment after confirming by arteriography or magnetic resonance imaging (MRI) of limb vessels.

Biological and Bioengineered Therapies

Biological therapies refer to tissue-based treatments (acellular and cellular), autologous platelet-rich plasma (PRP), as well as recombinant human growth factor, recombinant human platelet-derived growth factor (rhPDGF), recombinant human fibroblast growth factor (rhFGF), and recombinant human epidermal growth factor (rhEGF) therapies. Numerous other growth factors have been isolated and investigated, such as vascular endothelial growth factor (VEGF), keratinocyte growth factor-2, TGF-β, and granulocyte-macrophage colony-stimulating factor, but these currently are not approved for use in wound care.

Recombinant human epidermal growth factor is perhaps the best-studied growth factor for cutaneous ulcers and wounds. Applied as a topical cream or, more commonly, by intralesional injections, EGF has also been found to expedite the healing of a variety of types of cutaneous wounds. Several small trials attest to the healing benefits of EGF compared with controls.[74]

Recombinant human epidermal growth factor is considered a potent angiogenic growth factor and also has an isoform [fibroblast growth factor-10 (FGF-10)] commonly known as keratinocyte growth factor-2 or repifermin, which is reported to accelerate wound healing.[75]

Platelet concentrates are a concentrated suspension of growth factors found in platelets, which act as bioactive surgical additives that are applied locally to induce wound healing. Platelet concentrates can be used as (1) PRP and (2) platelet-rich fibrin (PRF). PRP (also referred to as platelet-enriched plasma, platelet-rich concentrate, autologous platelet gel, and platelet releasate) is a volume of autologous plasma that has a platelet concentration above baseline, five times more than the normal.

The cocktail of growth factors in PRP by virtue of platelets alone (stored as alpha granules in platelets) includes platelet-derived growth factor (αα, αβ, ββ), TGFsβ1 and β2, VEGF, epidermal growth factor, hepatocyte growth factor, and fibroblast growth factor. These growth factors are pivotal in the modulation of tissue repair and regeneration. The plasma proteins in PRP, namely fibrin, fibronectin, and vitronectin, act as a scaffold for the bone, connective tissue, and epithelial migration. Degranulation of the prepackaged growth factors in platelets occurs upon "activation", i.e., on coming in contact with coagulation triggers. The secreted growth factors in turn bind to their respective transmembrane receptors expressed over adult mesenchymal stem cells (MSCs), osteoblasts, fibroblasts, endothelial cells, and epidermal cells. This further induces an internal signal transduction pathway, unlocking the expression of a normal gene sequence of a cell-like cellular proliferation, matrix formation, osteoid production, collagen synthesis, angiogenesis, mesenchymal cell recruitment, proliferation, and extracellular matrix (ECM) synthesis, thereby augmenting the natural wound healing process.[76]

Platelet-rich fibrin is a second-generation platelet concentrate which contains platelets and growth factors in the form of fibrin membranes prepared from the patient's own blood free of any anticoagulant or other artificial biochemical modifications. The PRF clot forms a strong natural fibrin matrix, which concentrates almost all the platelets and growth factors of the blood, harvesting a complex architecture as a healing matrix with unique mechanical properties which make it distinct from other platelet concentrates.[77] PRF is superior to other platelet concentrates like PRP due to its ease and inexpensive method of preparation and also it does not need any addition of exogenous compounds such as bovine thrombin and calcium chloride. Thus, PRF has emerged as one of the promising regenerative materials for wound healing.

Acellular Therapies

The most common types of advanced biological therapies for chronic wounds are acellular therapies—those dermal, amniotic, or collagen-based tissues (human or animal) that have been decellularized during their processing. Often referred to as acellular and/or ECM, these biological products serve as substrates into which cells can migrate and initiate angiogenesis, thereby promoting granulation tissue development and tissue regeneration. ECMs contain not only structural collagen but also glycosaminoglycans (including hyaluronan), proteoglycans, and glycoproteins—all essential components to replace the defective ECM of injured tissues. Human dermal allografts have become increasingly popular in recent years for augmenting tissue regeneration in chronic lower extremity wounds and these are harvested from screened donors, and each is prepared with proprietary processes to decellularize and cryopreserve the dermis while maintaining the natural structure of the collagen and ECM. The dermal matrices serve as scaffolds for cellular repopulation and angiogenesis, with varying degrees of incorporation into the recipient wound.[78]

Amniotic membranes (AMs) and umbilical cord tissues have been used for many years for corneal ulcers and were actually the earliest reported biomaterials used for wound repair. In recent years, they have been tried for chronic wounds, likely due to the wide availability of placental tissues after cesarean deliveries. Due to their rich cellular content, AMs contain a number of cytokines and growth factors bound to the ECM after decellularization and preparation that remain available to augment angiogenesis and tissue repair when implanted into chronic wounds.[79] AMs are available in the cryopreserved state or as dehydrated products for direct implantation.[80] Several products are also available in a micronized formulation that can be applied topically or hydrated for injection into wounds to augment healing.[81,82]

Stem Cell Therapies

The most recent advancements for wound care therapies are those of stem cell therapies, primarily bone marrow-derived and, most recently, placental-derived stem cells. Both sources are considered as adult stem cells, and the cell lineage of interest is MSCs. They are multipotent progenitor cells that can directly differentiate into mesenchymal tissues, such as bone, tendon, and cartilage. Their ability to affect cutaneous repair, however, is through an indirect paracrine function (trophic activity), whereby they synthesize essential growth factors and cytokines that affect cell migration, proliferation, and metabolic activity of host cells and tissues. In this manner, MSCs play an active role in the inflammatory, proliferative, and remodeling phases of wound repair. Stem cells can respond to the host environment by upregulating anti-inflammatory cytokines in the presence of inflammation and respond to hypoxic environments by upregulating the release of VEGF to induce angiogenesis. During the remodeling phase, MSCs produce growth factors, such as TGF-β3, to limit excessive scarring as well as modulate the balance between matrix metalloproteinases and tissue inhibitors of metalloproteinases while regulating collagen deposition. Important for allogeneic implantation, MSCs are characterized as being immune privileged since they lack cell surface antigens that would typically engender a foreign body reaction.[83]

Bone marrow-derived stem cells (BMSCs) have been of interest for some time now and studies have indicated their ability to augment the repair or regeneration of numerous tissues, including cardiac, bone, cartilage, blood vessels, and skin.[84]

Placental tissues—including the umbilical cord, the amnion, and the chorion—are a rich source of MSCs and are readily available without the ethical concerns of embryonic stem cells.[85] Placental-derived MSCs show minimal differences from those obtained from different sites and yet retain all of the metabolic, paracrine, and immunomodulative properties previously described while maintaining their immune-privileged status.[84]

CONCLUSION

Chronic leg ulcer is a difficult-to-treat condition with a 20% chance of recurrence. Hence, a methodical approach to identify and treat the factors influencing underlying wound healing would go a long way in preventing recurrences.

TIPS AND PITFALLS

Tips for better results and pitfalls to avoid.

- Compression is the mainstay of treatment for venous ulcers. High compression is better than low compression.
- Graduated sustained compression reduces pressure in the superficial venous system, aids venous return to the heart, and promotes ulcer healing.
- When peripheral pulses are impalpable, ABPI should be calculated and if ABPI is <0.5, compression is contraindicated.
- Topical medicaments are to be avoided as they may lead to contact sensitization.
- Bilayered skin substitutes promote better wound healing when combined with standard compression therapy.
- Surgery is indicated in ulcers secondary to CVI when there are recurrent episodes of hemorrhage, lipodermatosclerosis and when ulcers fail to heal with conservative treatment

REFERENCES

1. Nelzén O, Bergqvist D, Lindhagen A, Hallböök T. Chronic leg ulcers: an underestimated problem in primary health care among elderly patients. J Epidemiol Community Health. 1991;45:184-7.
2. Abbade LP, Lastória S. Venous ulcer: epidemiology, physiopathology, diagnosis and treatment. Int J Dermatol. 2005;44:449-56.
3. Homan SJ. The etiology and treatment of varicose ulcer of the leg. Surg Gynecol Obstet. 1917;24:300-11.
4. Browse NL, Burnand KG. The cause of venous ulceration. Lancet. 1982;2:243-5.
5. Coleridge Smith PD, Thomas P, Scurr JH, Dormandy JA. Causes of venous ulceration: a new hypothesis. Br Med J (Clin Res Ed). 1988;296:1726-7.
6. Peschen M, Lahaye T, Hennig B, Weyl A, Simon JC, Vanscheidt W. Expression of the adhesion of molecules ICAM-1, VCAM-1, LFA-1 and VLA-4 in the skin is modulated in progressing stages of chronic venous insufficiency with and without atrophie blanche. In: Maessen-Visch MB (Ed). Atrophic Blanche (Thesis). Nijmegen: Drukkerij Hendrix Volharding; 1999. pp. 77-87.
7. Veraart JC, Verhaegh ME, Neumann HA, Hulsmans RF, Arends JW. Adhesion molecule expression in venous leg ulcers. Vasa. 1993;22:213-8.
8. Falanga V, Eaglestein WH. The "trap" hypothesis of venous ulceration. Lancet. 1993;341:1006-8.
9. Neumaan HA, Van den Broek MJ. Increased collagen IV layer in the basal membrane area of the capillaries in severe chronic venous insufficiency. Vasa. 1991;20:26-9.
10. Mendez MV, Raffeto JD, Phillips TJ, Menzoian JO, Park HY. The proliferative capacity of neonatal skin fibroblasts is reduced after exposure to venous ulcer wound fluid: a potential mechanism for senescence in venous ulcers. J Vasc Surg. 1999;30:734-43.
11. Philips TJ, Dover JS. Leg ulcers. J Am Acad Dermatol. 1991;25:965-87.
12. Caputo GM, Cavanagh PR, Ulbrecht JS, Gibbons GW, Karchmer AW. Assessment and management of foot disease in patients with diabetes. N Engl J Med. 1994;331:854-60.
13. Ruberg RL. Role of nutrition in wound healing. Surg Clin North Am. 1984;64:705-14.
14. Bello YM, Philips TJ. Management of venous ulcers. J Cutan Med Surg. 1998;3:6-12.
15. Ouahes N, Philips TJ. Leg ulcers. Curr Probl Dermatol. 1995;7:109-42.
16. Coleridge-Smith P, Labropoulos N, Partsch H, Myers K, Nicolaides A, Cavezzi A. Duplex ultrasound investigation of the veins in chronic venous disease of the lower limbs—UIP consensus document. Part-1. Basic principles. Eur J Vasc Endovasc Surg. 2006;31:83-92.
17. Cavezzi A, Labropoulos N, Partsch H, Ricci S, Caggiati A, Myers K, et al. Duplex ultrasound investigation of the veins in chronic venous disease of the lower limbs—UIP consensus document. Part II. Anatomy. Eur J Vasc Endovasc Surg. 2006;31:288-99.
18. Vowden K, Vowden P. Doppler and the ABPI: how good is our understanding? J Wound Care. 2001;10:197-202.
19. Partsch H. Compression therapy of the legs. A review. J Dermatol Sur Oncol. 1991;17:799-805.
20. Coleridge-Smith PD. Leg ulcer treatment. J Vasc Surg. 2009;49:804-8.
21. Fonder MA, Lazarus GS, Cowan DA, Aronson-Cook B, Kohli AR, Mamelak AJ. Treating the chronic wound: a practical approach to the care of nonhealing wounds and wound care dressings. J Am Acad Dermatol. 2008;58:185-206.

22. Paquette D, Falanga V. Leg ulcers. Clin Geriatr Med. 2002;18:77-88.
23. Blair SD, Wright DD, Backhouse CM, Riddle E, McCollum CN. Sustained compression and healing of chronic venous ulcers. BMJ. 1988;297:1159-61.
24. Philips TJ. Current approaches to venous ulcers and compression. Dermatol Surg. 2001;27:611-21.
25. Bishop SM, Walker M, Roger AA, Chen WYJ. Importance of moisture balance at the wound-dressing interface. J Wound Care. 2003;12:125-8.
26. Agren MS. Studies on zinc in wound healing. Acta Derm Venerol Suppl (Stockh). 1990;154:1-36.
27. Strömberg HE, Agren MS. Topical zinc oxide treatment improves arterial and venous leg ulcers. Br J Dermatol. 1984;111:461-8.
28. Steed DL. Debridement. Am J Surg. 2004;187:71S-4S.
29. Williams D, Enoch S, Miller D, Harris K, Price P, Harding KG. Effect of sharp debridement using curette on recalcitrant nonhealing venous leg ulcers: a concurrently controlled, prospective cohort study. Wound Repair Regen. 2005;13:131-7.
30. König M, Vanscheidt W, Augustin M, Kapp H. Enzymatic versus autolytic debridement of chronic leg ulcers: a prospective randomised trial. J Wound Care. 2005;14:320-3.
31. Alvarez OM, Fernandez-Obregon A, Rogers RS, Bergamo L, Masso J, Black M. A prospective, randomized, comparative study of collagenase and papain-urea for pressure ulcer debridement. Wounds. 2002;14:293-301.
32. Ziffren SE, Heist HE, May SC, Womack NA. The secretion of collagenase by maggots and its implication. Ann Surg. 1953;138:932-4.
33. Robson MC, Stenberg BD, Heggers JP. Wound healing alterations caused by infection. Clin Plast Surg. 1990;17:485-92.
34. Lineweaver W, Howard R, Soucy D, McMorris S, Freeman J, Crain C, et al. Topical antimicrobial toxicity. Arch Surg. 1985;120:267-70.
35. Pace WE. Treatment of cutaneous ulcers with benzoyl peroxide. Can Med Assoc J. 1976;115:1101-6.
36. Alvarez OM, Mertz PM, Eaglstein WH. Benzoyl peroxide and epidermal wound healing. Arch Dermatol. 1983;119:222-5.
37. Ip M, Lvi SL, Poon VK, Lung I, Burd A. Antimicrobial activities of silver: an in vitro comparison. J Med Microbiol. 2006;55: 59-63.
38. Zhou LH, Nahm WK, Badiavas E, Yufit T, Falanga V. Slow release iodine preparation and wound healing: In vitro effects consistent with lack of in vivo toxicity in human chronic wounds. Br J Dermatol. 2002;146:365-74.
39. Jones RN, Fritsche TR, Sader H, Ross JE. Activity of retapamulin (SB-275833), a novel pleuromutilin, against selected resistant gram-positive cocci. Antimicrob Agents Chemother. 2006;50:2583-6.
40. Zaki I, Shall L, Dalziel KL. Bacitracin: a significant sensitizer in leg ulcer patients? Contact Dermatitis. 1994;31:92-4.
41. Valencia IC, Falabella A, Kirsner RS, Eaglstein WH. Chronic venous insufficiency and venous leg ulceration. J Am Acad Dermatol. 2001;44:401-21.
42. Browse NL, Gray L, Jarrett PE, Morland M. Blood and vein-wall fibrinolytic activity in health and vascular disease. Br Med J. 1977;1:478-81.
43. Vesic S, Vukovic J, Mendenica LJ, Pavlović MD. Acute lipodermatosclerosis: an open clinical trial of stanozolol in patients unable to sustain compression therapy. Dermatol Online J. 2008;14:1.
44. Jarret PE, Moreland M, Browse NL. The effect of oxypentifylline ('Trental') on fibrinolytic activity and plasma fibrinogen levels. Curr Med Res Opin. 1977;4:492-5.
45. Phillips TJ, Dover JS. Leg ulcers. J Am Acad Dermatol. 1991;25:965-87.
46. Gault WR, Gatens Jr PF. Use of low intensity direct current in management of ischemic skin ulcers. Phys Ther. 1976;56:265-9.
47. Barran SD, Spardaro JA, Berger TJ, Becker RO. In vitro effect of weak direct current on *Staphylococcus aureus*. Clin Orthop Rel Res. 1974;100:250-5.
48. Erickson CA, Nucitelli R. Embryonic fibroblast motility and orientation can be influenced by physiological electric fields. J Cell Biol. 1984;98:296-307.
49. Ernst E. Ultrasound for cutaneous wound healing. Phlebology. 1995;10:2-4.
50. Johannsen F, Gam AN, Karlsmark T. Ultrasound therapy in chronic leg ulceration: a meta-analysis. Wound Repair Regen. 1998;6:121-6.
51. Wollina U, Heining B, Naumann G, Scheibe A, Schmidt WD, Neugebauer R. Effects of low-frequency ultrasound on microcirculation in venous leg ulcers. Indian J Dermatol. 2011;56:174-9.
52. Shirakawa M, Isseroff RR. Topical negative pressure devices: use for enhancement of healing chronic wounds. Arch Dermatol. 2005;141:1449-53.
53. Kranke P, Bennett M, Roeckl-Wiedmann I, Debus S. Hyperbaric oxygen therapy for chronic wounds. Cochrane Database Syst Rev. 2004;CD004123.
54. Ceilley RI, Rinck MA, Zuchlke RL. Pinch grafting for chronic ulcers on lower extremities. J Dermatol Surg Oncol. 1977;3: 303-9.
55. Skouge JW. Techniques for split-thickness skin grafting. J Dermatol Surg Oncol. 1987;13:841-9.
56. Kirsner RS, Falanga V, Kerdel FA, Katz MH, Eaglstein WH. Skin grafts as pharmacological agents: pre-wounding of the donor site. Br J Dermatol. 1996;135:292-6.
57. Límová M. Active wound coverings: bioengineered skin and dermal substitutes. Surg Clin North Am. 2010;90:1237-55.
58. Harding KG, Moore K, Philips TJ. Wound chronicity and fibroblast senescence—implications for treatment. Int Wound J. 2005;2:364-8.
59. Karr JC. Retrospective comparison of diabetic foot ulcer and venous stasis ulcer healing outcome between a dermal repair scaffold (Primatrix) and a bilayered living cell therapy (Apligraf). Adv Skin Wound Care. 2011;24:119-25.
60. Garden JM, Backus AD. Treatment of leg veins with high energy pulsed dye laser. Lasers Surg Med. 1996;8:34.
61. Bernstein EF, Lee J, Lowery J, Brown DB, Geronemus R, Lask G, et al. Treatment of spider veins with the 595 nm pulsed-dye laser. J Am Acad Dermatol. 1998;39:746-50.
62. Eremia S, Li CY. Treatment of leg and face veins with a cryogen spray variable pulse width 1064-nm Nd:YAG laser—a prospective study of 47 patients. J Cosmet Laser Ther. 2001;3:147-53.
63. Kauvar AN, Lou WW. Pulsed alexandrite laser for the treatment of leg telangiectasia and reticular veins. Arch Dermatol. 2000;136:1371-5.
64. Kaudewitz P, Klovekorn W, Rother W. Treatment of leg vein telangiectasis. 1-year results with a new 940 nm diode laser. Dermatol Surg. 2002;28:1031-4.
65. Goldman MP, Eckhouse S. Photothermal sclerosis of leg veins. ESC Medical Systems, LTD Photoderm VL Cooperative Study Group. Dermatol Surg. 1996;22:323-30.

66. Goldman MP. Intravascular lasers in the treatment of varicose veins. J Cosmet Dermatol. 2004;3:162-6.
67. Weiss RA. Endovenous techniques for elimination of saphenous reflux: a valuable treatment modality. Dermatol Surg. 2001;27:902-5.
68. Padberg Jr FT. Surgical intervention in venous ulceration. Cardiovasc Surg. 1999;7:83-90.
69. Van Gent WB, Hop WC, van Praag, Mackaay AJ, de Boer EM, Wittens CH. Conservative versus surgical treatment of venous leg ulcers: a prospective, randomized, multicenter trial. J Vasc Surg. 2006;44:563-71.
70. Sadick NS. Multifocal pull-through endovascular cannulation technique of ambulatory phlebectomy. Dermatol Surg. 2002;28:32-7.
71. Schmeller W, Gaber Y, Gehl HB. Shave therapy is a simple, effective treatment of persistent venous leg ulcers. J Am Acad Dermatol. 1998;39:232-8.
72. Hiatt WR. Medical treatment of peripheral arterial disease and claudication. N Engl J Med. 2001;344:1608-21.
73. Choucair MM, Philips TJ. What is new in clinical research in wound healing. Dermatol Clin. 1997;15:45-58.
74. Singla S, Garg R, Kumar, Gill C. Efficacy of topical application of beta urogastrone (recombinant human epidermal growth factor) in Wagner's Grade 1 and 2 diabetic foot ulcers: comparative analysis of 50 patients. J Nat Sci Biol Med. 2014;5:273-7.
75. Ohura T, Nakajo T, Moriguchi T, Oka H, Tachi M, Ohura Jr N, et al. Clinical efficacy of basic fibroblast growth factor on pressure ulcers: case-control pairing study using a new evaluation method. Wound Repair Regen. 2011;19: 542-51.
76. Lacci KM, Dardik A. Platelet-rich plasma: support for its use in wound healing. Yale J Biol Med. 2010;83:1-9.
77. Dohan DM, Choukroun J, Diss A, Dohan SL, Dohan AJJ, Mouhyi J, et al. Platelet-rich fibrin (PRF): a second-generation platelet concentrate. Part II: platelet-related biologic features. Oral Surg Oral Med Oral Pathol Oral Radiol Endod. 2006;101:e45-50.
78. Iorio ML, Shuck J, Attinger CE. Wound healing in the upper and lower extremities: a systematic review on the use of acellular dermal matrices. Plast Reconstr Surg. 2012;130:232S-41S.
79. Litwiniuk M, Grzela T. Amniotic membrane: new concepts for an old dressing. Wound Repair Regen. 2014;22:451-56.
80. Koob TJ, Rennert R, Zabek N, Massee M, Lim JJ, Temenoff JS, et al. Biological properties of dehydrated human amnion/chorion composite graft: implications for chronic wound healing. Int Wound J. 2013;10:493-500.
81. Fetterolf DE, Snyder RJ. Scientific and clinical support for the use of dehydrated amniotic membrane in wound management. Wounds. 2012;24:299-307.
82. Zelen CM, Gould L, Serena TE, Carter MJ, Keller J, Li WW. A prospective, randomised, controlled, multi-centre comparative effectiveness study of healing using dehydrated human amnion/chorion membrane allograft, bioengineered skin substitute or standard of care for treatment of chronic lower extremity diabetic ulcers. Int Wound J. 2015;12:724-32.
83. Wu Y, Huang S, Enhe J, Fu X. Insights into bone marrow-derived mesenchymal stem cells safety for cutaneous repair and regeneration. Int Wound J. 2012;9:586-94.
84. Maxson S, Lopez EA, Yoo D, Danilkovitch-Miagkova A, Leroux MA. Concise review: role of mesenchymal stem cells in wound repair. Stem Cells Transl Med. 2012;1:142-9.
85. Gu C, Huang S, Gao D, Wu Y, Li J, Ma K, et al. Angiogenic effect of mesenchymal stem cells as a therapeutic target for enhancing diabetic wound healing. Int J Low Extrem Wounds. 2014;13:88-93.

CHAPTER 60

Nerve Biopsy: Technique and Role in Dermatology

Shekhar Neema, Sunmeet Sandhu

KEY MESSAGES

- Nerve biopsy is a key diagnostic procedure to definitely diagnose pure neuritic leprosy in a situation of diagnostic dilemma either to confirm or to rule out neuritic leprosy.
- It is commonly performed on a pure cutaneous nerve such as sural nerve and radial cutaneous nerve. Biopsy of mixed or motor nerve is done very rarely in special circumstances.
- Complete circumference of the nerve taken for biopsy is better than taking a few fascicles. However, partial-thickness nerve biopsy may be done if the cutaneous nerve trunk is grossly thickened.
- Nerve biopsy can also be done for the diagnosis of vasculitis, inflammatory, congenital, and metabolic disorders.

INTRODUCTION

Nerve biopsy is an invasive procedure where a nerve is sectioned either fully or partially to identify potentially treatable causes of neuropathy. The evaluation of a nerve biopsy is often the final step in the diagnostic workup of a neuropathy of unknown origin.[1] Etiology of a peripheral neuropathy is difficult to ascertain in many cases and nerve biopsy may be essential to confirm diagnosis when all other available diagnostic methods fail to establish the diagnosis.

INDICATIONS

Being an invasive procedure, a nerve biopsy is recommended when:

- The neuropathy is progressive
- It threatens to become debilitating.
- Other examinations and investigations fail to identify a cause.

Common indications for nerve biopsy are enumerated in **Table 1**.[1-3]

TABLE 1: Common indications for nerve biopsy.

Genetic	• Charcot-Marie-Tooth (CMT) diseases • Hereditary motor and sensory neuropathies • Familial amyloid neuropathy • Giant axonal neuropathy • Infantile and juvenile neuroaxonal dystrophy (Seitelberger disease)
Vasculitides	• Polyarteritis nodosa • Microscopic polyangiitis • Eosinophilic granulomatosis with polyangiitis • Rheumatoid arthritis
Infectious neuropathies	• Leprosy • Herpes zoster and simplex • Human immunodeficiency virus (HIV) • Lyme disease or borreliosis neuropathy
Inflammatory and immune alterations	• Sarcoidosis • Ganglionitis • Chronic inflammatory demyelinating polyradiculoneuropathy (CIDP) • Monoclonal gammopathy
Storage disorders	• Amyloidosis • Glycogen storage disorders
Metabolic disorders	• Diabetic uremic and nutritional neuropathies
Toxic neuropathies	• Amiodarone • Chloroquine • Antiretroviral drugs • Industrial agents such as n-hexane, methyl n-butyl ketone, and acrylamide
Tumors	• *Primary and secondary nerve tumors:* Schwannomas and neurofibromas • Malignant peripheral nerve sheath tumors • Paraneoplastic neuropathy
Ischemic injury of nerve	• Chronic nerve compression
Others	

PREPARATION

Before considering nerve biopsy, other less-invasive investigations should be considered to know the cause of pathology. In a situation of thickened nerve with infective etiology like Hansen's disease, it is worthwhile to do fine-needle aspiration cytology (FNAC) of the thickened affected nerve as it might not only offer diagnostic help but also aid in the classification of leprosy for treatment purpose and follow-up.[4] However, negative aspiration findings cannot rule out the diagnosis. Electromyography and nerve conduction studies should be carried out along with other investigations for vasculitis screening, genetics, diabetes, erythrocyte sedimentation rate (ESR), vitamin deficiency, autoimmune disease (e.g., rheumatoid arthritis or systemic lupus erythematosus), renal function tests, liver function tests, and toxin panel if indicated.[5] All patients should have a full blood count with or without clotting studies depending on the hematological history preoperatively.

Informed consent for the surgery should be obtained, clearly indicating the possible clinical diagnoses and the need for the biopsy, the procedure involved, and its possible consequences. All preoperative evaluations, preoperative and postoperative instructions, and medications are similar to other minor surgical procedures.

SELECTION OF BIOPSY SITE

Nerve biopsy is performed most often on a pure cutaneous nerve. Sural nerve at the level just above the ankle, superficial radial and dorsal cutaneous branches of the ulnar nerve at the wrist, and superficial peroneal nerve in the leg are the nerves usually chosen for nerve biopsy.[6] Rarely the biopsy of combined nerve and muscle (in vasculitis) or a nerve supplying to muscle which is either suspected to be affected or located nearer to the affected site on the body can be biopsied. Partial fascicular biopsy of a mixed nerve trunk is practiced very rarely in special and unavoidable situations.

Nerve biopsy should target a cutaneous nerve that is constant in an anatomical location and readily accessible. **Table 2** summarizes the common nerve biopsied along with site and indication. In comparison with full-thickness nerve biopsy, fascicular biopsy causes fewer complications or lesser sensory deficit but provides less tissue for analysis. This is of particular importance in focally located or patchy lesions including inflammatory processes where pathology may vary considerably from one fascicle to the next as well as producing localized changes within a fascicle.[6] Such foci are less likely to be detected if just a portion of the nerve is examined. Therefore, biopsy of the complete cross-section of the nerve is recommended wherever possible.[7] The minimum recommended length of the biopsied nerve segment should be 5 cm.[2] Less than minimum may give unsatisfactory results.

Combined nerve and muscle biopsies can be obtained by the same skin incision but in separate pieces. The possibility of detecting inflammatory changes, in particular vasculitis, is significantly higher in a combined biopsy compared to either nerve or muscle biopsy alone.[6] In addition, other disorders that can affect both nerve and muscle, such as amyloidosis and certain hereditary diseases including neuropathy and myopathies, can benefit from combined biopsy. In a patient with pure motor neuropathy, biopsy of a nerve supplying a muscle with little functional importance (e.g., the nerve to gracilis) is preferred.

TABLE 2: Site of nerve biopsy.[2,3,5]

Nerve	*Site of incision*	*Indication*	*Remarks*
Distal sural nerve	Behind the lateral malleolus	Vasculitis and Hansen's disease	With minimal postoperative problems or complications
Superficial peroneal (fibular nerve)	Junction of the middle and distal thirds of leg on lateral aspects	Vasculitis	Access to the peroneus brevis muscle through the same incision
Medial sural nerve	Junction of the gastrocnemius muscle bellies	Vasculitis	Concomitant gastrocnemius muscle biopsy can be done. Very minimal sensory loss
Distal superficial radial nerve (radial cutaneous nerve)	Anatomical snuff box	Upper limb neuropathy, including Hansen's disease	Visible scar, neuroma common, and no major postprocedure complications
Dorsal cutaneous branch of the ulnar nerve	Wrist	Upper limb neuropathy, including Hansen's disease	
Obturator nerve biopsy	4 inches distal to the pubis bone over medial aspect of thigh	Useful to differentiate motor neuropathies and lower motor neuron diseases such as motor neuron disease, Guillain–Barré syndrome, and mixed neuropathy with prominent motor symptoms	Very rarely done. Concomitant gracilis muscle biopsy is taken
Greater auricular nerve	Sterno-cleidomastoid muscle at the upper and lateral aspect of the neck	Hansen's disease	Considered rarely for biopsy

BIOPSY SAMPLE HANDLING[2]

The biopsy nerve samples are prepared in three different ways to fully assess the tissue for diagnostic purposes **(Table 3)**.

COMPLICATIONS

The rate of complications varies from center and with the expertise of surgeon. Surgery-related complications such as persistent pain, dysesthesia, paresthesia, allodynia, sensory impairment, and neuroma formation have been reported in approximately 10% of the patients **(Table 4)**.[6] In case of pure

TABLE 3: Biopsy sample handling.

Segment	*Length*	*Method of fixation or processing*	*Uses*
1st piece	0.5 cm	Formalin-fixed and paraffin-embedded	Hematoxylin and eosin (H&E) and special stains are useful in diagnosing vasculitis, amyloidosis, sarcoidosis, leprosy, and lymphoma
2nd piece	0.5 cm	Transported in Michel's medium and frozen	Staining of light chains is useful in diagnosis of amyloidosis
3rd piece	2–2.5 cm	Glutaraldehyde fixed for transverse semithin plastic sections	Useful for analysis of myelinated fibers

TABLE 4: Complications of nerve biopsy and its prevention.[2,3,5,6,8-10]

Complication	*Prevention*
Hematoma	Hemostasis, postoperative compression dressing, limb elevation, and stopping anticoagulants at least 1 week prior to surgery
Muscle herniation (only if motor nerves deep to muscles are biopsied)	Proper closer of fascia
Wound dehiscence	Adequate rest and support
Wound infection	Adequate antibiotics
Neuroma	Transected nerve can be sutured into the surrounding muscle
Pain, dysesthesia, and paresthesia	Immobilizing the leg in plaster cast for 7–10 days

cutaneous nerve biopsy, such as sural or radial cutaneous nerves, except for paresthesia or anesthesia over the small area supplied by the respective biopsied nerve, no major side or adverse effects are reported. Many times, it has been reported that the nerve trunks get reunited or form collateral reinnervation and thus may re-establish the sensations.[6]

SURAL NERVE BIOPSY

Nerve biopsy has been a well-established diagnostic procedure for the investigation of peripheral neuropathies including leprosy. Leprosy is one of the most common treatable causes of peripheral neuropathy, but diagnosing leprosy in the absence of typical dermatological features is challenging, especially in patients who present with pure neuritic leprosy without any skin lesions. Despite the availability of multiple noninvasive diagnostic tools, such as nerve conduction studies, electromyography, ultrasound examination, and other imaging techniques, in a situation where both clinical examination and these diagnostic modalities cannot either confirm or rule out Hansen's disease, the nerve biopsy becomes crucial particularly where FNAC of thickened nerve also fails to show features of leprosy. Here, nerve biopsy remains the most conclusive diagnostic test. Thus, the nerve biopsy may give useful information in diagnosing pure neuritic leprosy.

The sural nerve is the most often biopsied nerve because:[6,8]

- Sural nerve is a pure sensory nerve and thus there is no motor loss on biopsy.
- Resulting sensory loss is confined to a small area on the dorsolateral aspect of the foot.
- It is usually readily accessible at the level of the lateral malleolus.
- Its structure has been studied extensively in health and disease.

Anatomy of Sural Nerve[5] (Fig. 1)

Sural nerve is a pure sensory nerve and supplies sensation to the dorsolateral aspect of the foot and ankle region. The distal sural nerve is formed by joining of the medial sural nerve (branch of the tibial nerve that is found approximately 6 cm proximal to the fibular head) and the lateral cutaneous sural nerve (branch of the common peroneal nerve). The two branches meet in the distal third of the leg at approximately 11–20 cm proximal to the lateral malleolus. Distally, it courses subcutaneously in a fascial sling between the deep crural fascia and superficial fascia adjacent to the short saphenous vein and lateral to the Achilles tendon.

Anatomical Variation

Amalgamation of medial and lateral sural nerves may occur in the popliteal fossa in 12% of cases rather distally.[10] Anatomical variations include early union or nonunion of the medial or lateral cutaneous sural nerves or very rarely the sural nerve may be completely absent.[11]

Procedure (Figs. 2 and 3)

After obtaining informed consent, the skin is prepared, draped, and anesthetized with the infiltration of a local anesthetic agent. The leg is flexed at the knee to 30° with a soft bolster and the ankle is slightly everted at 90° to keep the sural nerve under slight tension and to aid localization. Surface marking is done along the course of the nerve. A superficial, vertical incision is made halfway between the Achilles tendon and the lateral border of fibula, commencing at the lateral malleolus and extending 5 cm upward along the course of the nerve following Langer's lines **(Fig. 2)**. With sharp dissection and careful undermining of tissues, proceed through the superficial fascia until the lesser saphenous vein is identified and retracted posteriorly to reveal the sural nerve immediately medial to it.[12] The nerve trunk is identified by its white, glistening appearance crossed with oblique dark and light bands (spiral bands of Nageotte).[6] Care should be taken to preserve the saphenous vein. Prior to the nerve

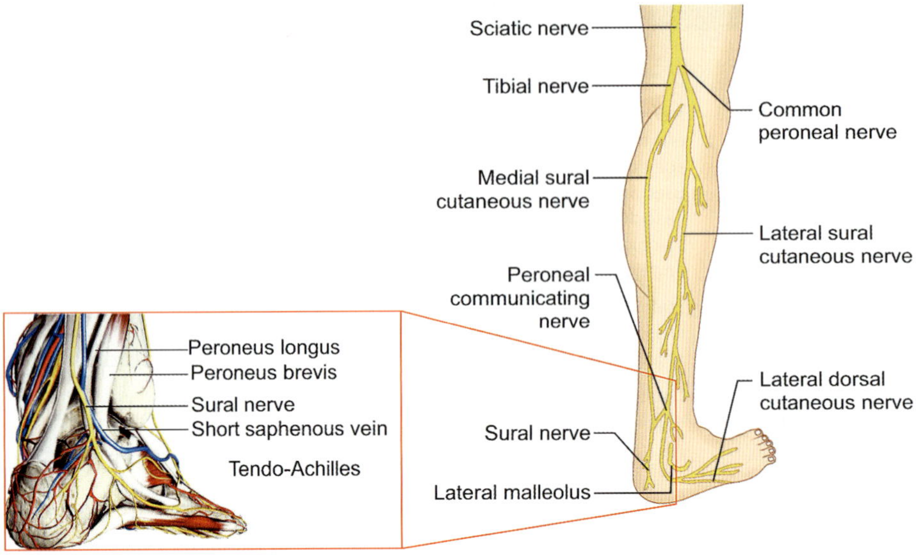

Fig. 1: Anatomy of sural nerve.

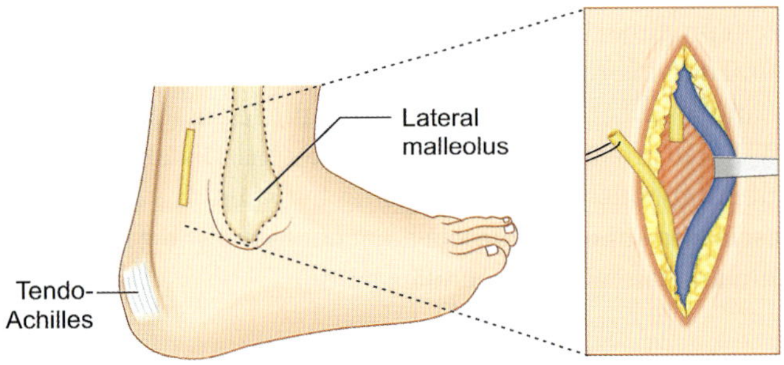

Fig. 2: Distal sural nerve biopsy technique. A superficial, vertical incision is made halfway between the Tendo-Achilles and the lateral border of fibula, commencing at the lateral malleolus and extending 5 cm upward along the course of nerve.

section, a small bolus of local anesthetic can be injected into the proximal nerve as sectioning of nerve is painful (but not necessary always). A single 3.0 nylon suture is placed proximally through the nerve: it is important that the nerve is only minimally manipulated using the proximal suture for moving it **(Figs. 3A to I)**. The nerve is sharply cut with a scalpel (scissors will produce compression trauma artifact) proximally first to prevent pain when the distal end is subsequently sectioned. The nerve is left alone or buried in the adjacent muscle. In case of fascicular biopsy, a few fascicles are separated and sectioned **(Box 1)**. The wound is sutured in layers. The specimen is processed as mentioned in **Table 3**.

Postoperative Care

Immediate postoperatively look for appropriate hemostasis and possibility of hematoma if any. Patients are advised to keep the wound dry for 48 hours and avoid strenuous activity for 2 weeks. Optionally, the leg can be immobilized in a plaster cast for 7–10 days. Skin sutures may be removed after 10 days. Appropriate antibiotics and anti-inflammatory drugs are to be given for a required duration.

DISTAL SUPERFICIAL RADIAL NERVE BIOPSY[5]

Anatomy

The distal superficial radial nerve is a direct continuation of the radial nerve. It travels under the brachioradialis along the anterolateral aspect of the forearm. It pierces the deep fascia in the distal forearm and lies subcutaneously. The nerve can usually be palpated directly over the distal radius or in the anatomical snuff box laterally over the extensor carpi radialis longus, which aids in planning the approach. The boundaries of the anatomical snuff box include posteriorly the extensor pollicis longus tendon, anteriorly the tendons of the extensor pollicis brevis and abductor pollicis longus, and proximally the styloid process of the radius, while the floor consists of both the trapezium and the scaphoid.

Procedure (Figs. 4 and 5)

Preoperative preparations are the same as described earlier. The region around the anatomical snuff box is cleaned and draped. The operating field is then infiltrated with 2% lignocaine. Identify and mark the course of radial artery to avoid injury or inadvertent cutting anterior-laterally; a longitudinal or a transverse incision is placed over the distal radius or anatomical snuff box. The cephalic veins lying medially are retracted to visualize the nerve lying superficial to the extensor retinaculum. The nerve is ligated proximally to 3–5 cm of nerve and is resected mostly in total thickness or partial thickness if it is grossly thickened. After achieving hemostasis, the wound is closed in layers. Postoperative care is done as described earlier.

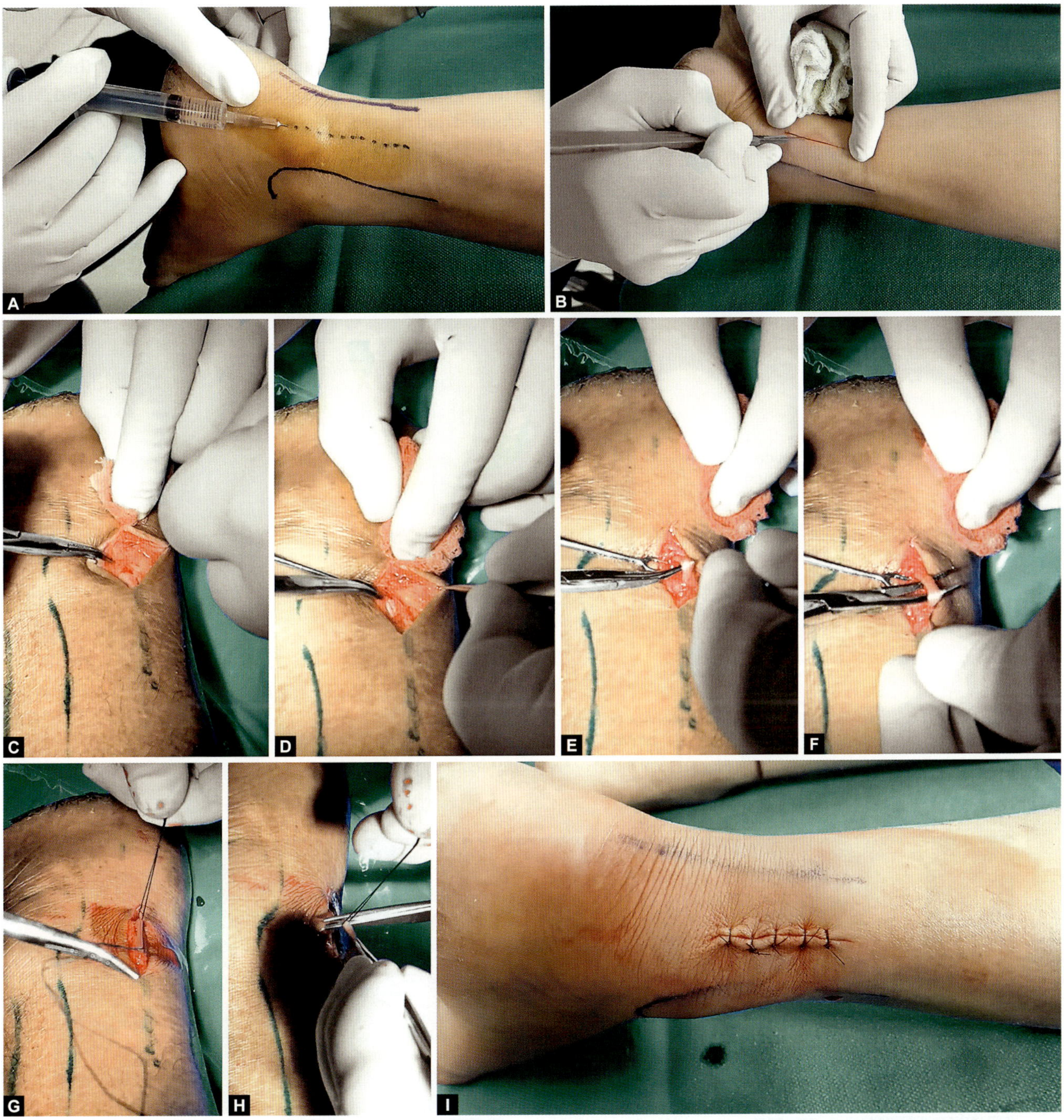

Figs. 3A to I: (A) Sural nerve course is marked and local anesthesia given; (B) Superficial vertical incision given; (C) Sharp dissection and careful undermining of tissues; (D to F) Identify and retract lesser saphenous vein and separate sural nerve; (G) Proximal nerve is ligated; (H) Nerve segment is cut with sharp blade; (I) Hemostasis achieved and wound is sutured.

BIOPSY OF DORSAL CUTANEOUS BRANCH OF THE ULNAR NERVE

Anatomy (Fig. 6)

The dorsal cutaneous branch of the ulnar nerve (DCBUN) is a terminal ramus of the ulnar nerve. It originates from the medial side of the ulnar nerve at the distal third of the forearm, lying between ulna and the *flexor carpi ulnaris* muscle. At the level of its tendon, it is situated posteromedially. It leaves the ulnar nerve, piercing the antebrachial fascia, 4–10 cm above the ulnar styloid process, taking a posterior

BOX 1: Differentiating nerve from vessel.[8]

- Nerve is glistening white and solid in appearance; if examined carefully, fascicles can be visualized.
- Vessels will have true lumen and tributaries.
- Nerve has a pattern of alternating longitudinal lighter and darker bands.

direction. It then courses around the ulnar styloid process medially and dorsally and, at the fifth metacarpal joint (2- or 3 cm distally to the ulnar styloid process), it gives off two or three main branches. It is a purely sensory nerve that supplies sensation to the dorsoulnar aspect of the hand, dorsum of the fifth finger, and dorso-ulnar aspect of the fourth finger.

Procedure (Figs. 7A to D)

Preoperative preparations are the same as described earlier. The region over the dorsal ulnar aspect of hand and wrist is cleaned and draped. Identify and mark the course of thickened DCBUN over the fifth metacarpal joint; a longitudinal incision is placed over the landmark. DCBUN is separated

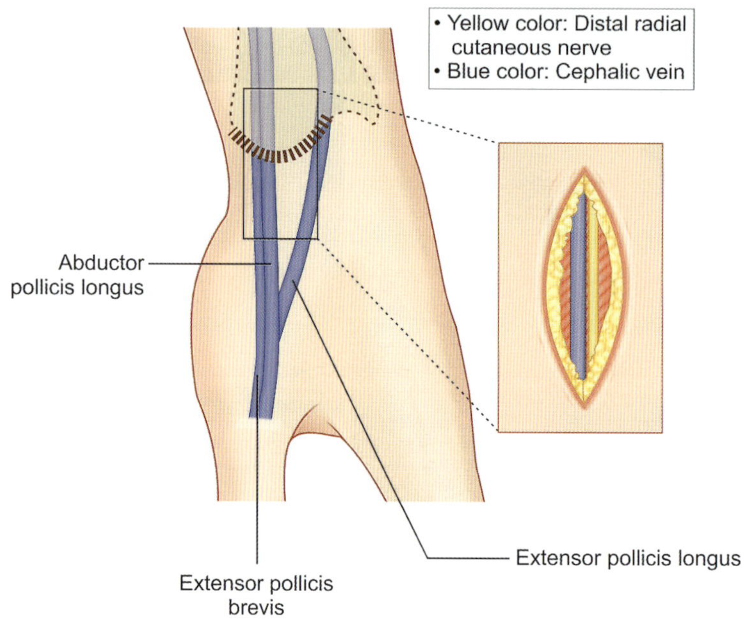

Fig. 4: Distal radial nerve biopsy anatomy technique.

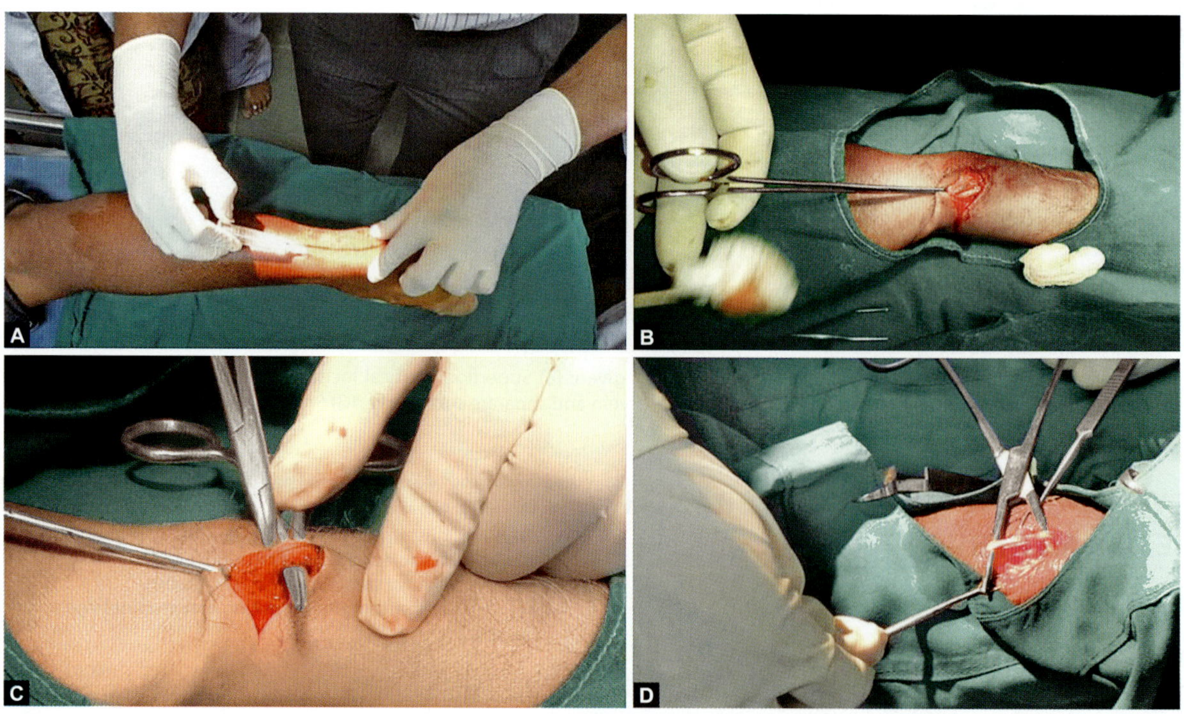

Figs. 5A to D: Distal radial nerve biopsy technique. (A) Local anesthesia infiltration; (B) Incision and blunt dissection; (C) Identification of nerve; (D) Separation and ligation of nerve.

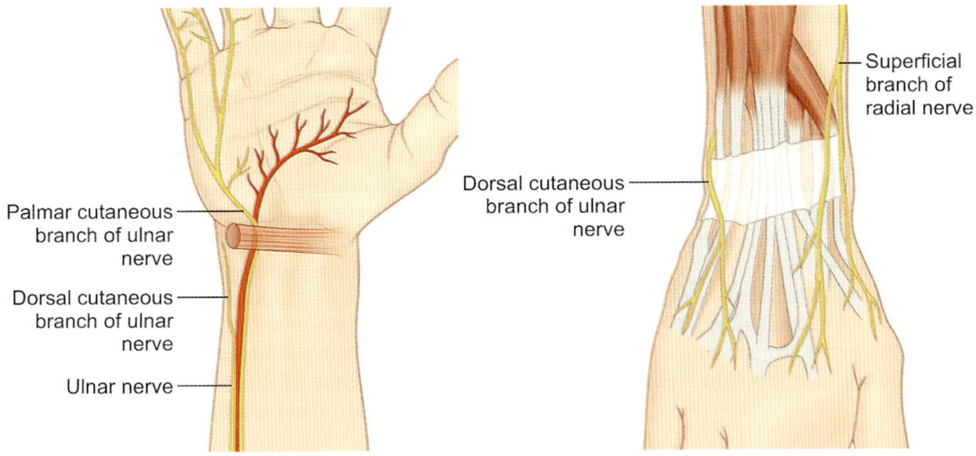

Fig. 6: Dorsal cutaneous branch of ulnar nerve anatomy.

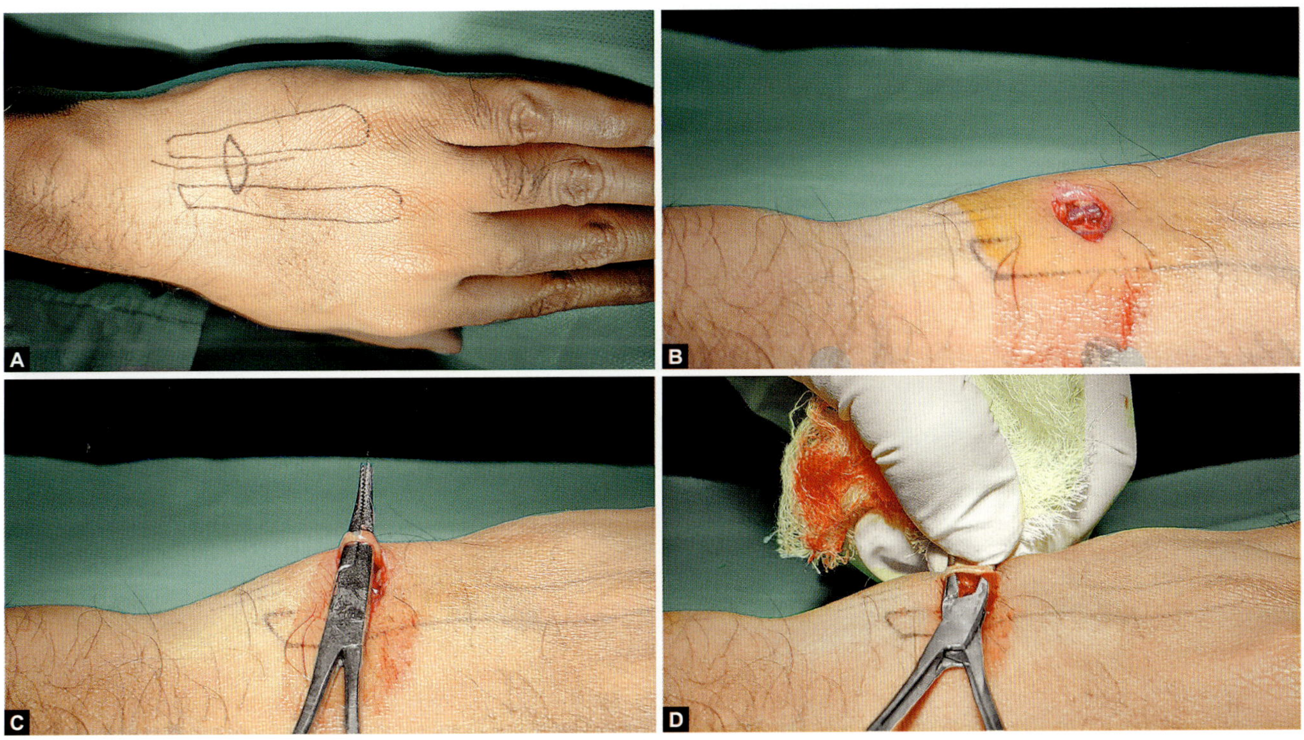

Figs. 7A to D: Dorsal cutaneous branch of ulnar nerve biopsy technique. (A) Surface markings made; (B) After incision and blunt dissection; (C) Identification of nerve; (D) Separation and ligation of nerve.

and gradually retracted from adjoining vessels. The nerve is ligated proximally to 3–5 cm of nerve and is resected mostly in total thickness or partial thickness if it is grossly thickened. After achieving hemostasis, the wound is closed in layers. Postoperative care is done as described earlier.

TIPS

For surgery:
- Sural nerve is the most common nerve biopsied by a dermatologist, mainly to rule out Hansen's disease
- Knowing proper anatomy and variation is crucial before planning surgery
- Gentle handling of nerve with blunt dissection is crucial
- Sharp section of nerve is important

CONCLUSION

Nerve biopsy is the confirmatory test in pure neuritic leprosy. Knowledge of the anatomy of the nerve is important. If performed by an experienced surgeon, it is a safe procedure without any sequela.

REFERENCES

1. Sommer C, Brandner S, Dyck PJ, Magy L, Mellgren SI, Morbin M, et al. 147th ENMC International Workshop: Guideline on Processing and Evaluation of Sural Nerve Biopsies, 15–17 December 2006, Naarden, The Netherlands. Neuromuscul Disord. 2008;18(1):90-6.

2. Weis J, Brandner S, Lammens M, Sommer C, Vallat JM. Processing of nerve biopsies: a practical guide for neuropathologists. Clin Neuropathol. 2012;31(1):7-23.
3. Vallat JM, Funalot B, Magy L. Nerve biopsy: requirements for diagnosis and clinical value. Acta Neuropathol. 2011;121(3):313-26.
4. Sandhu S, Raman DK, Sood A, Sinha P, Singh PY, Dixit PK. Cytomorphological patterns of nerve aspirates in pure neuritic leprosy: A single centre cross-sectional observational study. J Cytol. 2021;38(1):14-20.
5. Hart MG, Santarius T, Trivedi RA. Muscle and nerve biopsy for the neurosurgical trainee. Br J Neurosurg. 2013;27(6):727-34.
6. King R, Ginsberg L. The nerve biopsy: indications, technical aspects, and contribution. Handb Clin Neurol. 2013;115: 155-70.
7. Pollock M, Nukada H, Taylor P, Donaldson I, Carroll G. Comparison between fascicular and whole sural nerve biopsy. Ann Neurol. 1983;13(1):65-8.
8. Ginsberg L, King RH, Orrell RW. Nerve biopsy: how to do it? Pract Neurol. 2003;3:306-13.
9. Mellgren SI, Lindal S. Nerve biopsy: some comments on procedures and indications. Acta Neurol Scand Suppl. 2011;(191):64-70.
10. Ducic I, West J. A modified approach to sural nerve biopsy: minimizing complications. Ann Plast Surg. 2009;62(2):220-2.
11. Devi SK, Sharmila BP, Susan PJ, Gajendra K. Variant formation of sural nerve and its distribution at the dorsum of the foot. Int J Anat Var. 2009;1:33-4.
12. Bevilacqua NJ, Rogers LC, Malik RA, Armstrong DG. Technique of the sural nerve biopsy. J Foot Ankle Surg. 2007;46(2):139-42.

CHAPTER 61

Leprosy Surgery

Sanjay Bhalchandra Sane

KEY MESSAGES

- Diagnosis of nerve involvement and aggressive treatment of neuritis will prevent occurrence of deformity.
- Perineural steroid injection and nerve decompression play an important role in prevention of deformities.
- Patient to be referred for surgery should be medically stabilized/cured by multidrug therapy (MDT).
- Protective footwear plays an important role in management of neuropathic plantar ulcers.
- High plantar pressures, precursors of neuropathic plantar ulceration, can be diagnosed by foot pressure measurement system.

INTRODUCTION

Hansen's disease patients, even after the medical cure with multidrug therapy (MDT), are stigmatized due to the disability and deformity left by the disease. This needs intervention by a leprosy reconstructive surgeon and correction of the deformities, giving the patient the cosmesis and functional hands and feet. Surgeon has an important role in prevention of neural damage, if diagnosed early, and further deformities by timely nerve decompression surgery.

In prevention of deformities, the primary role is of the dermatologists to diagnose and treat neuritis, by medication, adequate rest, and physiotherapy. Surgeon may be called for either giving perineural steroid injection or perform surgical nerve decompression.

In established deformities, primary role is of the surgeon to reconstruct the paralyzed limb by reconstructive surgical procedures. Cosmetic surgery is resorted to correct the loss of eyebrows, depression of nose, and other deformities. The physiotherapist has an important role to prepare the hand or foot for reconstructive surgery by splinting, exercises, etc.

Surgery can be considered only for patients who are medically stabilized or cured. Lepromatous cases should have completed the required MDT and should not have history of reaction for 12–18 months prior to surgical intervention.

INDICATIONS FOR SURGICAL INTERVENTION IN A CASE OF HANSEN'S DISEASE PATIENT

Indications for surgical intervention are shown in **Box 1**. Out of these indications, nerve biopsy has been explained in a separate chapter.

Nerve Decompression Surgery

To understand the role of nerve decompression surgery, it is important to understand the pathophysiology of nerve damage **(Fig. 1)**.

Hansen's neuritis causes nerve damage by two mechanisms. First is *internal nerve compression* caused by the disease inflammatory process progressing in a closed compartment of thickened epineurium, leading to increased intraneural pressure. In situ destruction of nerve tissue leads to

BOX 1: Indications for surgical intervention in a case of Hansen's disease.

- Nerve biopsy, skin biopsy for diagnostic purposes
- Nerve decompression surgery
- Reconstructive surgery for claw fingers and thumb, foot drop
- Cosmetic surgery for facial deformities, viz., depressed nose, loss of eyebrows, lagophthalmos, and gynecomastia
- Surgery for the neuropathic trophic ulcers

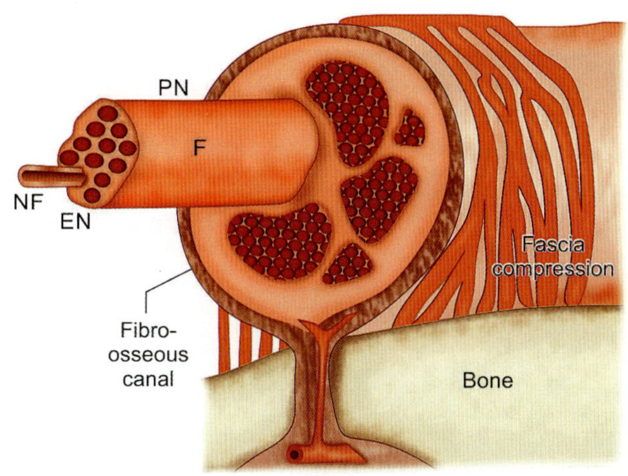

Fig. 1: Pathophysiology of nerve damage in Hansen's disease. (EN: endoneurium; F: fascicle; NF: nerve Fiber, PN: perineurim)

development of intraneural abscess due to caseation necrosis. Second is the external compression on the inflamed nerve because of the nerve and the adjoined morphological structures in the anatomical compartments through which nerves traverse. Thus, the inflamed ulnar nerve traversing through the fibro-osseous canal behind the medial epicondyle is subjected to external compression.

Treatment of neuritis, thus aims at reducing the internal compression by anti-inflammatory medicines systemic steroids, rest and proper splintage of the limb, and managing external compression by surgery.

Management of Internal Compression

Medical management of neuritis: Hansen's neuritis pain is one of the worst pains to suffer and requires rest to the affected limb in form of splint, anti-inflammatory analgesics and judicious use of steroids to control intraneural inflammation. Steroids form an important part of drug regime to combat the neuritis, aid in decompressing the nerve to relieve the intraneural pressures, and save the axons from damage. Giving systemic steroids for a long time either orally or parenterally invites gastrointestinal and systemic side effects. Hence, giving perineural or paraneural steroids by injection is an excellent way to administer maximum steroid dose at the specific site with minimal systemic side effects.

Long-acting steroids like dexamethasone or triamcinolone are administered, diluted with distilled water. One has to be certain that the injection is given by the side of the nerve and not intraneurally. Intraneural injection destroys the already damaged nerve. The whole procedure has to be done with total aseptic precautions preferably in an operation theater. During the treatment, physiotherapy plays an important role in splinting the fingers, electrical stimulation of the weakened muscles, and joint mobilization.

Procedure of perineural injection: The steroid injection is given peri- or paraneurally and never intraneurally. The drug has to be diluted with saline or distilled water and is given along the whole length of clinically thickened nerve. One has to use a long, thin needle, e.g., 23 or 24 spinal needle. The needle has to remain subcutaneous. It is first advanced the whole length and after confirming that it is not in a vessel, withdraw the needle slowly injecting the drug.

Common complications: These include intraneural injection and injury to adjoining vessel.

Splinting of the affected limb: The splinting is done across the joint along which the nerve traverses, e.g., for ulnar nerve, above elbow posterior slab is given. If fingers show early paralysis, splints to prevent clawing are given.

Management of External Compression

Surgical management of neuritis: If there is predominantly external compression, it can only be tackled by surgical decompression and freeing the nerve from the fibro-osseous canal. External compression is surgically treated by external neurolysis and division of fibro-osseous canal, and the internal compression treated by epineurotomy, partial excision of thickened epineurium, and interfascicular nerve decompression under magnification. In practice, both procedures are performed together. Additionally, procedures like medial epicondylectomy and anterior transposition of ulnar nerve may be required to relieve external compressive forces.

Patient with neuritis should be referred to a surgeon in the following instances:

- Occurrence of nerve abscess, absolute indication for surgical intervention
- Neuritis not responding to the medical line of treatment
- Intractable pain and progressive motor loss in the muscles supplied by the nerve

If patient is on steroids, it is advisable to taper oral steroids before surgery.

The nerves that are amenable for surgical decompression are:

- Ulnar nerve, at medial epicondyle of elbow **(Figs. 2A and B)**
- Median nerve, in carpal tunnel

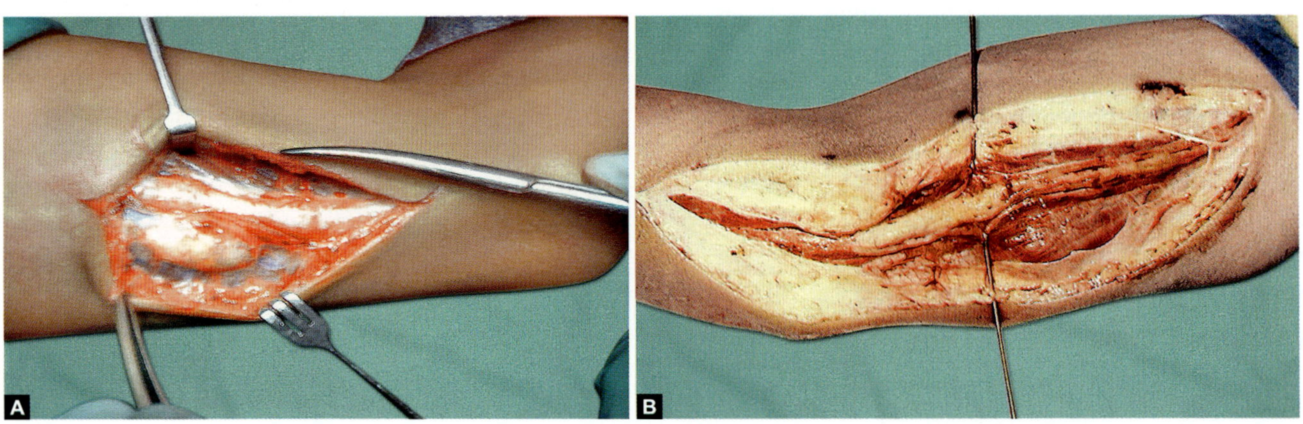

Figs. 2A and B: (A) Ulnar nerve single paraneural abscess and thickened nerve; (B) Ulnar nerve decompression at medial epicondyle of elbow; note inflamed nerve partially decompressed above the medial epicondyle and near normal nerve below the epicondyle.

- Posterior tibial nerve, in the tarsal tunnel
- Lateral popliteal nerve, around neck of fibula

Reconstructive Surgery

Patients may be referred for reconstruction provided:

- There is no active neuritis and disease is stabilized. Patient is medically released from treatment, i.e., cured.
- Deformity is established and at the same time is mobile and surgically correctable.
- Patient must have taken adequate preoperative physiotherapy.

Preoperative physiotherapy involves wax therapy and oil massage to soften the skin and mobilize the joints, plaster and dynamic splints to passively mobilize, and correct the deformities; isolation and strengthening the muscle to be transferred are mandatory for good surgical correction. Physiotherapy time duration may vary from 3 to 10 weeks depending on the duration of the deformity.

Reconstructive Surgery of the Hand

Hand: Hand is involved following the involvement of the ulnar nerve at the elbow and/or median nerve at the wrist, leading to ulnar claw hand and clawed thumb or inability to oppose the thumb against the palm respectively. This is due to the paralysis of intrinsic muscles of fingers and the thumb leading to hyperextension of the metacarpophalangeal (MCP) joints and flexion of interphalangeal (IP) joints. In a normal hand, the fingers function due to the action of long extensors and the finger flexors, and are kept straight in all functional positions by the stabilizing action of the intrinsic muscles. Intrinsics strike a delicate balance between the extensors and flexors, while they act on the triple joint chain of fingers. Once the intrinsics are paralyzed, there is unopposed action of the extensors at the MCP joint and the unopposed action of flexors at the IP joints.

The reconstructive surgery either involves the correction of the deformity by dynamic procedures such as intrinsic muscle power replacement by another muscle, tendon transfers, or by passive procedures such as, mechanical correction of MCP hyperextension, e.g., MCP joint volar capsulorrhaphy.

Ulnar claw hand or the claw fingers can be corrected by using different motor tendons, e.g., flexor digitorum sublimis of one of the fingers, palmaris longus, extensor carpi radialis longus, and distribute the muscle power by four tendon strips to all clawed fingers. There are many variants in the procedures and surgical details are beyond the purview of this chapter.

Thumb correction surgery: Thumb paralysis is a result of loss of action of the thenar muscles and surgery aims at restoring the action by tendon transfer. Muscles of choice are flexor digitorum sublimis from ring finger, extensor indicis or palmaris longus with a fascia extensor graft.

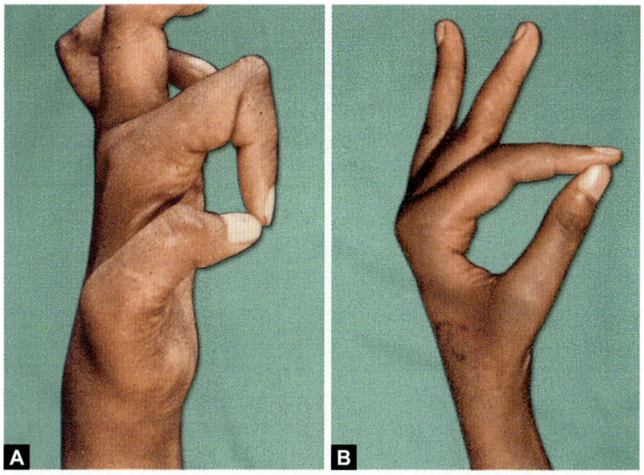

Figs. 3A and B: (A) Preoperative deformity; (B) Postoperative result after opponensplasty.

The aim is to restore the lost abduction and opposition function **(Figs. 3A and B)**.

Surgery for the Foot Drop Correction

Involvement of the lateral popliteal nerve leads to first the paresis, and later total irreversible paralysis of anterolateral group of leg muscles, i.e., the ankle and toe dorsiflexors and the evertors of the foot. Paralysis leads to the foot drop, i.e., loss of foot and toe dorsiflexion and foot eversion. The anesthetic foot is liable to strike on the forefoot and the lateral border at each step, making the foot prone to forefoot high plantar pressure injury and instability. Long-standing foot drop is complicated by the tendo-Achilles contracture, which first has to be addressed by preoperative physiotherapy and at times by surgical tendo-Achilles lengthening.

Reconstruction of the foot drop is done by transferring the tibialis posterior tendon to the dorsum of the foot, either by circumtibial or trans-interosseous membrane approach, and suturing by two slips, one to the insertion of paralyzed tibialis anterior and the extensor hallucis longus and second slip to the toe extensors. The transferred slips have to be balanced delicately, so that the foot is held in dorsiflexion and eversion. Position is maintained with below-knee (BK) plaster for 5–6 weeks. After removal of plaster, graded supervised physiotherapy is necessary for 4 weeks to teach the patient to use the transferred tendon for foot dorsiflexion, to walk again.

Surgery for Correction of Facial Deformities

Following deformities are amenable for correction: depressed nose **(Figs. 4A and B)**, lagophthalmos or inability to close the eyes, loss of eyebrows, partial or total facelift operation to remove the facial wrinkles, and correction of elongated ear lobules.

Eyelid closure is restored by static procedure such as lateral tarsorrhaphy, where the palpebral fissure is permanently reduced from lateral side by suturing the two

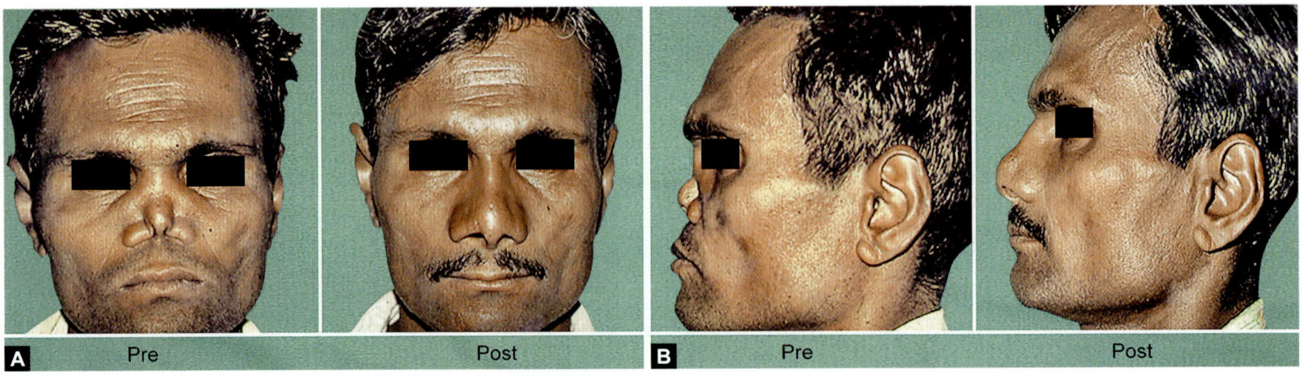

Figs. 4A and B: *Nose reconstruction:* Preoperative and postoperative.

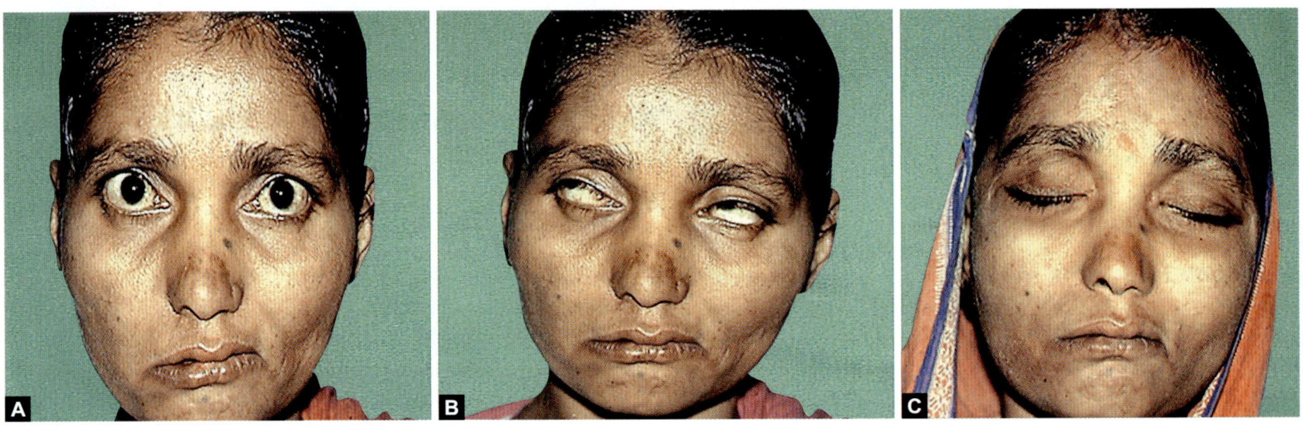

Figs. 5A to C: Lagophthalmos surgical correction. (A) Eyes open before surgery; (B) Eyes closed before surgery; (C) Eyes closed after surgery.

eyelids. Dynamic procedure uses part of temporalis muscle tendon unit, extending it with a fascia graft, and is used to achieve dynamic eyelid closure when person mildly clenches his teeth **(Figs. 5A to C)**.

Neuropathic Foot Ulcers

To understand the mechanism of how foot ulcers are caused, one needs to understand the walking cycle.

Each walking cycle comprises of three phases:

1. *Heel strike:* Foot in dorsiflexion comes in contact with the ground, also called as heel contact phase. Heel structures bear maximum weight-bearing stress **(Fig. 6)**.
2. *Midstance phase:* Whole foot is in contact with the ground.
3. *Push-off phase* **(Fig. 7)**: This is the propulsive phase; forefoot bears maximum body weight and is under tremendous pressure, with almost total body weight from above and the ground reaction from below. These high plantar pressures in neuropathic foot are responsible for tissue injury in neuropathic foot. These ulcers occur on the sole of the foot, on the areas where the metatarsal heads and the heel bone bear the maximum body weight to the ground **(Fig. 8)**.

The ulcers occurring on the sole of the feet in Hansen's disease are due to tissue injury following trauma (such as

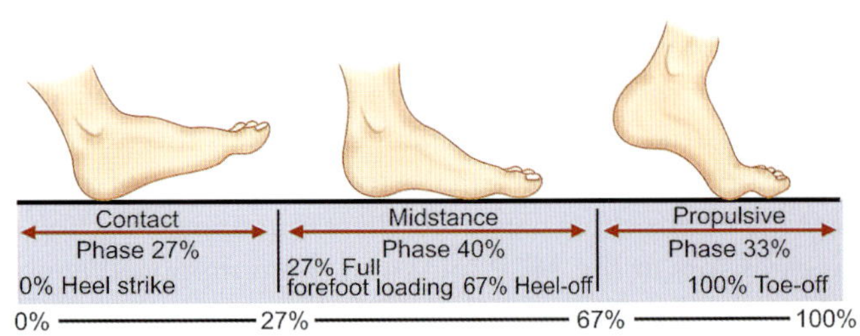

Fig. 6: Phases of walking cycle.

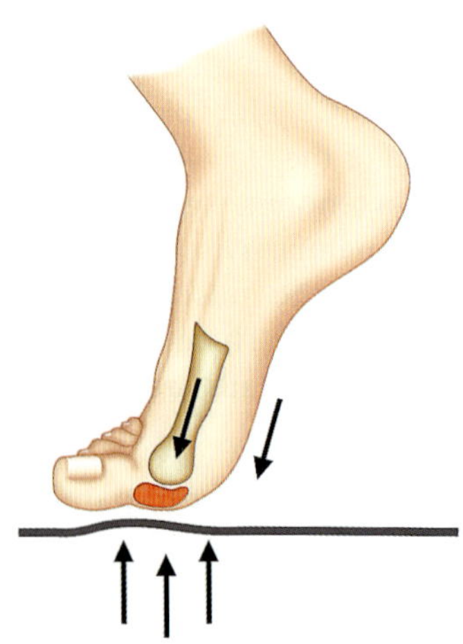

Fig. 7: Propulsive phase.

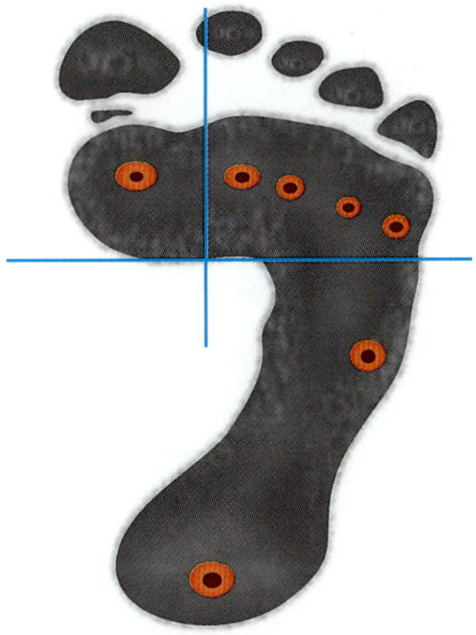

Fig. 8: Location of foot ulcers.

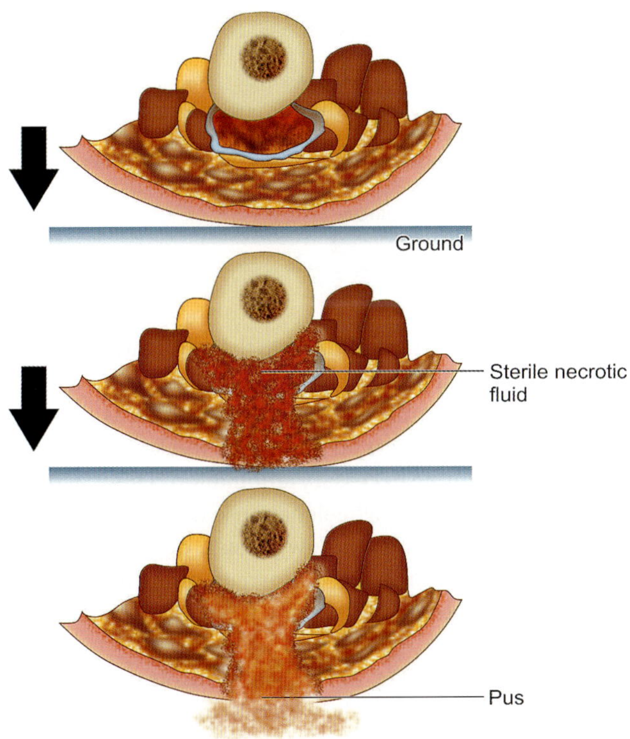

Fig. 9: Ulcers due to high plantar pressures occur from within outside.

cuts, nail prick, footwear injury) on the sole of the foot. Ulcers occurring due to nail prick, shoe bite, etc., occur from skin to the deeper tissues, whereas ulcers due to high plantar pressures occur from within outside **(Fig. 9)**. Weakening of the foot occurs due to loss of sensation, the intrinsic muscle paralysis, and resultant weakening of the foot architecture. This trauma, coupled with the walking stresses and strains, exerted on the weakened neuropathic foot leads to foot ulcers.

Autonomic neuropathy leads to dry plantar skin, excessive fissures and cracks which make sole vulnerable to ulceration. Perceived trauma is the causative factor in about 20% of cases. In 80% of cases, unperceived trauma during normal daily walking on neuropathic weakened foot is responsible for foot ulceration.

The tissue injury starts deepest below the bony points and aseptic tissue necrosis starts. Person unaware of the damage due to neuropathy continues to walk and compounds the damage. As a result, the damage reaches the plantar skin and opens on the plantar skin as ulcer.

Ulcers are frequently preceded and underlie a preexisting corn or callus, frequently indicative of high plantar pressure. Traumas from heat, cold, shoe bite, or penetration by a sharp object are also potential causes. Neuropathy allows the lesions to develop because the normal warning sense of pain has been lost and they go unrecognized. Continued pressure or walking on the injured skin creates even further damage and the ulcer will worsen. The open sore will frequently become infected and may even penetrate to bone.

Ulcer Management

Neuropathic foot with ulceration needs constant expert attention, X-rays to rule out osteomyelitis, antibiotics, and at times, surgical interventions. Proper protective footwear in the form of microcellular rubber (MCR) sandals and use of orthotic supports to aid off-loading are needed.

Ulcers are categorized as acute and chronic.

Acute ulcers: Acute ulcer requires rest to the foot with elevation, at times, admission if infection is severe and use of antibiotics. Once infection is under control, adequate rest and off-loading of the foot will achieve tissue healing. If not cared for, ulcers turn chronic and nonhealing and will need more aggressive treatment. Foot X-ray to rule out osteomyelitis of bones is necessary.

Chronic ulcers: Osteomyelitis is most common cause of nonhealing of ulcers. Such ulcers require in addition, surgical intervention in the form of wound debridement and removal of dead, osteomyelitic bone. Postoperative care involves rest and off-loading till ulcer heals. Constant use of protective footwear for lifetime is always necessary to keep the foot ulcer-free.

Footwear as a therapy: Once we understand that high pressures on the sole of the feet of Hansen's disease patients are responsible for majority of foot problems, it will not be an exaggeration if we say that protective footwear protects the foot, just as a helmet protects the head while driving a two-wheeler. While standing on our feet, footwear is the only interface between the sole of the foot and the ground below which we can suitably alter and use to counteract the bad effects of pressures on the sole of the foot. The footwear should be made according to individual measurements, sewed or glued, without any nails or rivets, and with a hard outer sole for protection. It is used with cotton socks. Most of the neuropathic feet have lost the capacity to hold the *chappal* while walking and can lead to friction between the sole and the

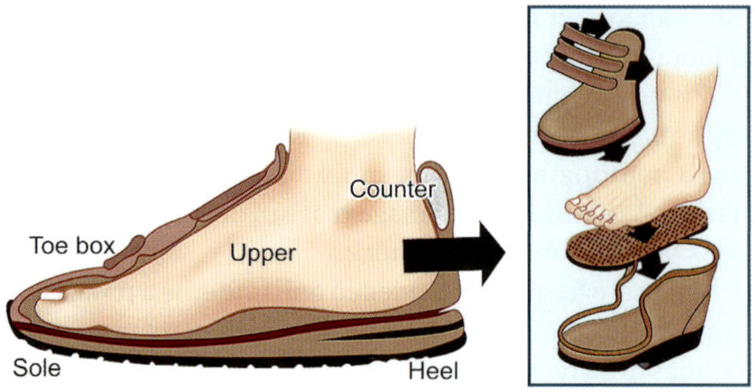

Fig. 10: Insole, the important part in the footwear.

foot, leading to injuries and ulceration. In these cases, a sandal pattern is ideal as it holds the footwear with the back strap.

Microcellular rubber: MCR is the material available in India which is soft, comfortable, gives a good cushioning effect and helps in redistribution of plantar pressures from area of high pressure prone to ulceration to the whole area of foot in contact with the ground. It has 25–30% shore hardness and reduces ground reaction forces acting on the sole of the foot. It has been tested and compared favorably with polyurethane, sorbothane, and other similar materials available abroad. It is used as an insole material and to fabricate orthotic pads.

Shoes when prescribed must always fit comfortably and have adequate width and depth for the toes. Canvas shoes and good-quality leather shoes easily adapt to the shape of your feet and allow them to "breathe". Athletic shoes, jogging shoes, and sneakers are usually excellent choices, if they are well fitted and provide adequate cushioning. "Extra-depth" shoes or custom-molded shoes may be required to adapt to patient's particular needs, or orthoses to provide cushioning and support.

Patient should be given the following instructions:

- Always check your shoes for foreign objects or torn linings before putting them on.
- You should have two or three pairs of shoes each day, so that, one pair is not worn for >4–6 hours. This will minimize the possibility of injury due to footwear.
- New footwear should be worn for only a few hours at a time and you should take care to inspect your feet for any points of irritation.
- Socks should be well fitted without seams or folds. They should not be so tight as to interfere with circulation.
- Well-padded socks can be very protective, if there is an abundance of room in your shoes.
- Avoid wearing open-toed shoes or sandals, until you have discussed this with your surgeon.
- Above all, do not walk with barefoot.

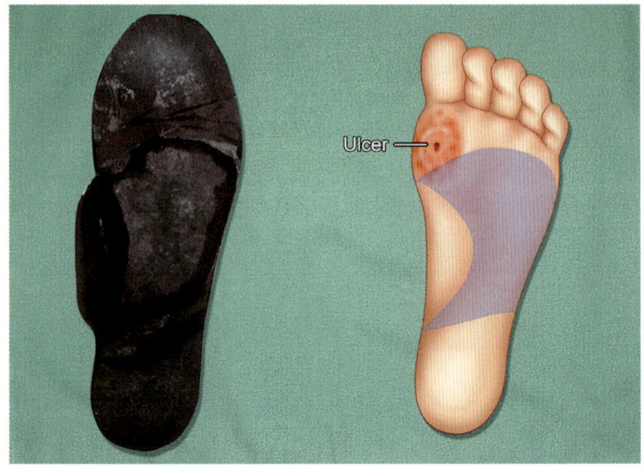

Fig. 11: Orthotic support.

BOX 2: Important aspects of foot care.

- Examine the feet daily.
- Soak both the feet in water daily for 10–15 minutes.
- Mop dry especially between the toes and apply white soft paraffin or petroleum jelly.
- Use well-fitting sandals or canvas shoes with cotton socks.
- Do not walk barefoot.
- Avoid walking long distances.
- Do not treat your foot yourself.
- Report to doctor for the slightest foot complaint.

Insole/orthotic modifications ***(Fig. 10)****:* These are to be worn inside protective footwear. These are the devices which support the weakened foot, help to redistribute the plantar pressures, and help to take off the high plantar pressures from an area of ulceration and give rest to the part, and at the same time allow the patient to carry out the daily routine.

- *Off-loading:* In simple terms, it can be defined as avoidance of all mechanical stress on the injured weakened extremity, while maintaining necessary ambulation. This is achieved by crutches, walker, wheelchair, use of total contact cast (TCC), or a walking window plaster, depending on the severity of the ailment. Footwear modifications like protective shoes or sandals and fixed ankle brace can be used.
- *Orthotic supports* ***(Fig. 11)****:* These are insole modifications, used in shoes or sandals, which help to redistribute the plantar pressures and help to take off the high plantar pressures from an area of ulceration, support the weakened neuropathic foot, give rest to the part, and at the same time allow the patient to carry out the daily routine.

Foot care: Important aspects of foot care are shown in **Box 2**.

NEWER INVESTIGATIONS TO DIAGNOSE HIGH PLANTAR PRESSURES

It is now well known that the normal walking and standing can generate high plantar pressures sufficient to damage the insensitive and weakened foot. These pressures, if diagnosed before their pathological manifestations, can be effectively managed by scientific footwear and external foot supports to be used inside the shoes (orthotic supports).

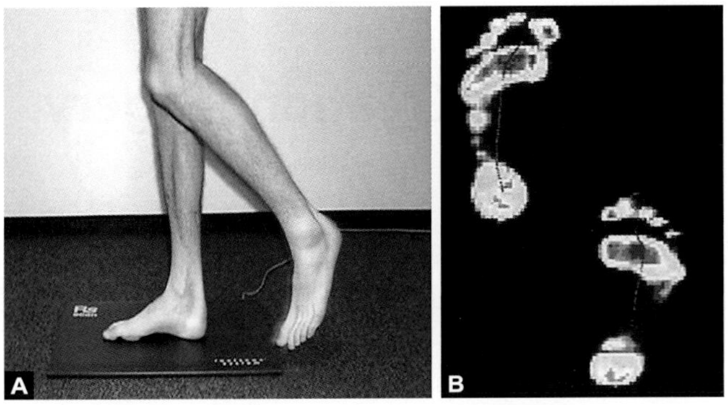

Figs. 12A and B: Footscan plate and scan report.

In footscan plate, patient puts a single step on the platform and pressures below the sole of the foot are recorded instantly, and with the help of unique software information is transformed into a multicolored picture. Each color represents a different pressure; red and pink areas denote highest pressures **(Figs. 12A and B)**.

Based on these foot pressure records, external foot supports, to be used inside the shoes, are prepared with the help of a special MCR. They are called as orthotic supports. They help to correct the foot stance, posture, and support the weakened arch of the foot. They also help in giving rest to the painful foot, keeping the patient ambulatory.

CONCLUSION

It is important for the physician to diagnose and treat the Hansen's disease in early stage, to prevent the occurrence of disability and deformities. Perineural steroid injection and nerve decompression resorted before the onset of deformity can prevent the occurrence of deformities and social stigmatization and segregation. Physicians treating the disease should learn to perform diagnostic nerve biopsy, give perineural steroid injection, and play an important role in prevention of deformities.

Treatment of plantar ulceration needs rest, antibiotic cover, and if complicated by osteomyelitis, good surgical debridement needs to be done. This can be done by any qualified surgeon. Important feature which is lacking is prescription of a protective footwear, which should be done on a priority basis. Foot pressure measurement or footscan is an important investigation to diagnose and prevent plantar ulceration due to high plantar pressures.

RECOMMENDED READING

1. Anderson GA. The surgical management of deformities of the hand in leprosy. J Bone Joint Surg Br. 2006;88:290-4.
2. Dandapat MC, Sahu DM, Mukherjee LM, Panda C, Baliarsing AS. Treatment of leprous neuritis by neurolysis combined with perineural corticosteroid injection. Lepr Rev. 1991;62:27-34.
3. Duerksen F, Schwarz R. Ulnar nerve palsy. In: Schwarz R, Brandsma W (Eds). Surgical Reconstruction and Rehabilitation in Leprosy and other Neuropathies, 1st edition. Kathmandu: Ekta Books Distributors Pvt Ltd; 2004. p. 47-64.
4. Gore D, Atal Shah R. Surgery in leprosy. In: Savant SS (Ed). Textbook of Dermatosurgery and Cosmetology, 2nd edition. Mumbai: ASCAD; 2005. pp. 289-96.
5. Jopling WH, McDougall. Handbook of Leprosy, 5th edition. New Delhi: CBS Publishers and Distributors; 2005.
6. Margery I, Joyce P, Job CK. Role of nerve biopsies in the diagnosis of leprosy in the post multidrug therapy era. Indian J Lepr. 2008;80:279-82.
7. Nilsen R, Mengistu G, Reddy BB. The role of nerve biopsies in the diagnosis and management of leprosy. Lepr Rev. 1989;60:28-32.
8. Parkes AR. Paralytic claw fingers—a graft tenodesis operation. Hand. 1973:5;192.
9. Ramaratnam S. (2023). Leprosy Neuropathy. [online] Available from emedicine.medscape.com/article/1165419 [Last accessed September, 2023].
10. Reddy RR, Singh G, Sacchidanand S, Okade R, Shivakumar V, Uday A, et al. A comparative evaluation of skin and nerve histopathology in single skin lesion leprosy. Indian J Dermatol Venereol Leprol. 2005;71:401-5.
11. Richard B. Surgical management of neuritis. In: Schwarz R, Brandsma W (Eds). Surgical Reconstruction and Rehabilitation in Leprosy and other Neuropathies, 1st edition. Kathmandu: Ekta Books Distributors Pvt Ltd; 2004. pp. 25-32.
12. Ruth A, Schulmeyer FJ, Roesch M. Diagnostic and therapeutic value due to suspected diagnosis, long-term complications, and indication for sural nerve biopsy. Clin Neurol Neurosurg. 2005;107:214-7.
13. Schwarz R. General principles of reconstructive surgery for leprosy and other peripheral neuropathies. In: Schwarz R, Brandsma W (Eds). Surgical Reconstruction and Rehabilitation in Leprosy and other Neuropathies, 1st edition. Kathmandu: Ekta Books Distributors Pvt Ltd; 2004. p. 1-10.
14. Sharma VK, Malhotra AK. Leprosy: Classification and clinical aspects. In: Valia RG, Valia AR, editors. IADVL Textbook of Dermatology. Mumbai: Bhalani Publishing House; 2010. pp. 2046-9.
15. Srinivasan H, Palande DD. (1996). Essential surgery in leprosy: Techniques for district hospitals. [online] Available from https://apps.who.int/iris/bitstream/handle/10665/63357/WHO_LEP_96.2.pdf?sequence=1&isAllowed=y [Last accessed September, 2023].
16. Srinivasan H. Leprosy: Disablement-its prevention and management. In: Valia RG, Valia AR, editors. IADVL Textbook of Dermatology. 3rd ed. Vol. 2. Mumbai: Bhalani Publishing House; 2010. pp. 2119-38
17. Srinivasan H. Prevention of disabilities in patients with leprosy: a practical guide. Geneva: World Health Organization; 1993.
18. Warren G, Schwarz R. Surgery of the nose and other aesthetic surgery. In: Schwarz R, Brandsma W (Eds). Surgical Reconstruction and Rehabilitation in Leprosy and other Neuropathies, 1st edition. Kathmandu: Ekta Books Distributors Pvt Ltd; 2004. pp. 271-301.
19. Warren G. Neuropathic feet. In: Schwarz R, Brandsma W (Eds). Surgical Reconstruction and Rehabilitation in Leprosy and other Neuropathies, 1st edition. Kathmandu: Ekta Books Distributors Pvt Ltd; 2004. pp. 148-74.

CHAPTER 62

Dimple Creation Surgery

T Salim, Laila Arif

KEY MESSAGES

- Dimple creation surgery is aimed to create a scar in the dermis which adheres to the underlying buccinator muscle there by creating a dynamic dimple.
- It is a simple and safe technique done as a daycare procedure with a predictable outcome.
- Positioning of the dimple should be explained well to the patient before the surgery.
- Proper aseptic precautions should be taken in order to prevent postoperative complications.

INTRODUCTION

Cheek dimples are usually considered as an attractive feature of facial beauty. They enhance facial beauty and expression. They occur in both sexes with no particular preponderance and may express unilaterally or bilaterally. Bilateral cheek dimples are more common than unilateral ones. The characteristic inheritance of cheek dimples is in an autosomal dominant fashion on chromosome 16, with variable penetrance.[1,2]

Dimples are considered as a sign of good luck and prosperity in some cultures and they brighten and add character to a beautiful smile. Regardless of the cultural background, there is an increased demand for the creation of facial dimples, and many people seek the expertise of cosmetic and dermatologic surgeons to achieve facial dimple creation.

This chapter will explain the technique of dimple creation, which can be easily performed by a dermatologic surgeon.

ANATOMY OF DIMPLE

Anatomically, dimples are caused by the presence of dermocutaneous insertion of the fibers of double or bifid zygomaticus major muscle. This dermocutaneous insertion causes a dermal tethering effect.[3] Dimple creation surgery involves creating a region of scar tissue through a suture between the buccinator muscle and the dermis.

PRINCIPLE

The surgery is aimed to create a scar in the dermis, which adheres to the underlying buccinator muscle and becomes a natural dynamic dimple. This can be achieved with transcutaneous sutures or by an open technique that is performed through the mouth, which would show no scarring.

POSITIONING OF DIMPLE

Ideally, the position of the dimple is marked by the patient in front of the mirror.

While positioning a dimple, the ideal location would be the area where a less obvious faint dimple is present while smiling, and thus the pre-existing dimple is made more prominent. The patient is asked to create a negative suction and suck the cheeks inside. The site of the maximum depression is the marked site of the dimple.

If one cheek has a dimple, the ideal location for the other dimple would be marked at the corresponding site, which would create symmetry of the face.

If a pre-existing dimple is not present, as per the cosmetic viewpoint, the ideal location would be the intersection between a horizontal line from the angle of the mouth and a vertical line from the lateral canthus of the eye[4] **(Fig. 1)**.

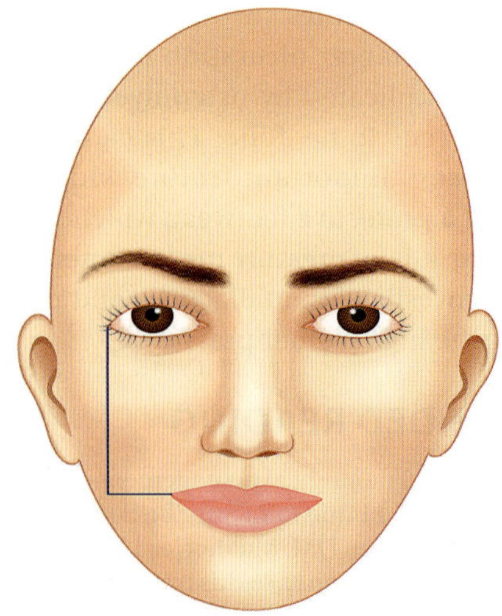

Fig. 1: Positioning of the dimple. Intersection between a horizontal line from the angle of the mouth and a vertical line from the lateral canthus of the eye.

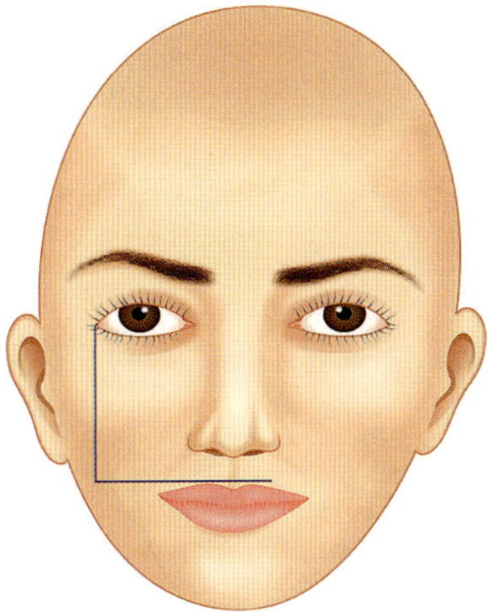

Fig. 2: Positioning of the dimple. Intersection between a horizontal line from the highest point of Cupid's bow laterally and a vertical line from the lateral canthus of the eye.

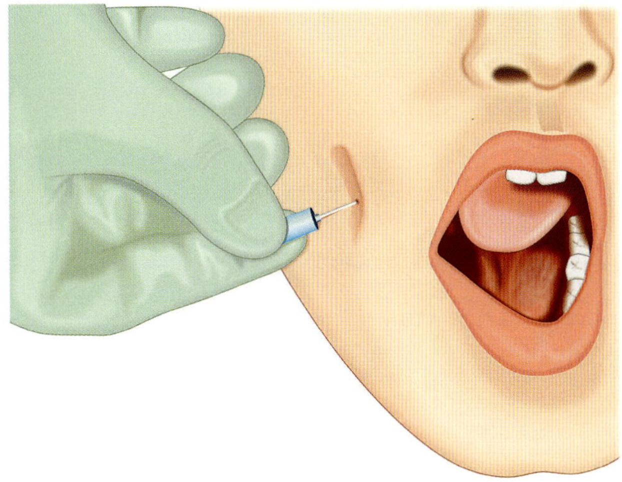

Fig. 3: Needle passed from the skin surface through the point marked for dimple creation.

However, few authors feel that the position of the dimple marked by this method is too low. The point of intersection of the perpendicular line dropped from the external canthus and horizontal line drawn from the highest point of Cupid's bow laterally was suggested as a better landmark for positioning the dimple[5] **(Fig. 2)**.

SURGICAL TECHNIQUE

Dimple surgery can be performed by a skilled dermatologic surgeon under local anesthesia, after obtaining an informed consent. The patient's face and mouth are prepared, and local anesthesia is administered. Around 2–3 mL of 0.5% lignocaine adrenaline solution is injected from the skin side down to the mucosal side at the marked site. A period of 10 minutes is allowed to lapse.

A needle is passed from the skin surface through the point marked on the skin into the buccal cavity so as to act as a guide **(Fig. 3)**. A 6-mm punch inserted from the mucosal side is used to remove the tissue in full depth keeping the needle as a guide. Care should be taken not to injure and cut the skin including the dermal tissue. A soft-tissue cylindrical fragment consisting of the mucosa, a small portion of the buccinator muscle, and a part of the fat pad is removed using scissors, leaving the skin with the dermis intact. The defect is widened by scraping with a no. 15 blade and separating the mucomuscular attachments **(Figs. 4 to 7)**.

Alternatively, a no. 15 blade can be used instead of a punch to make a stab incision followed by separation of the mucomuscular attachments. To create a wider dimple, a wider area is scraped, so that dermal and mucosal raw areas are created. This will adhere to each other and create the dimple. Similarly, if a smaller dimple is to be created, a proportionately smaller area is scraped. A dent is felt if palpated bimanually. If the desired depression is not created, it means that the scraping is inadequate and needs further scraping.

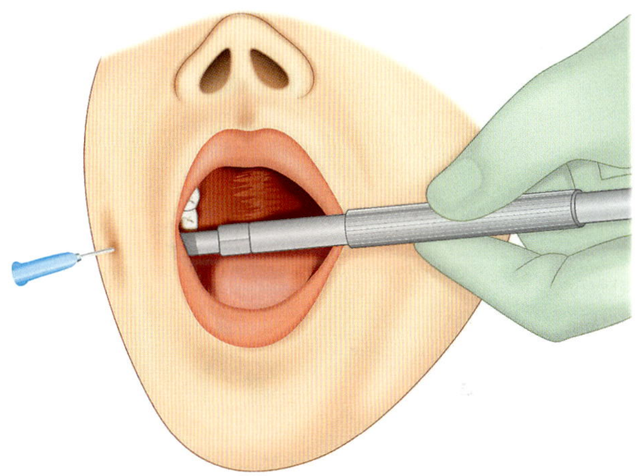

Fig. 4: A 6-mm punch paced at the buccal surface keeping the needle as a guide.

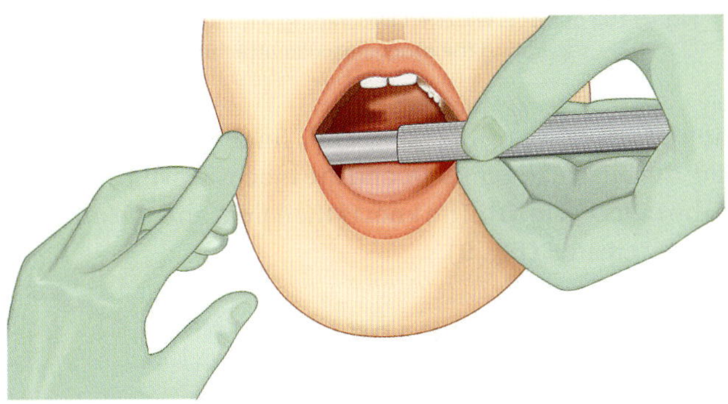

Fig. 5: The needle is removed and the punch is used to remove the tissue in full depth without injuring the skin including the dermal tissue.

The next step is to create and maintain the adhesion. The defect closure is performed by placing an absorbable suture (no. 3-0 Vicryl, Ethicon) through the cheek mucosa, muscle, and fat pad on one side of the defect, then through

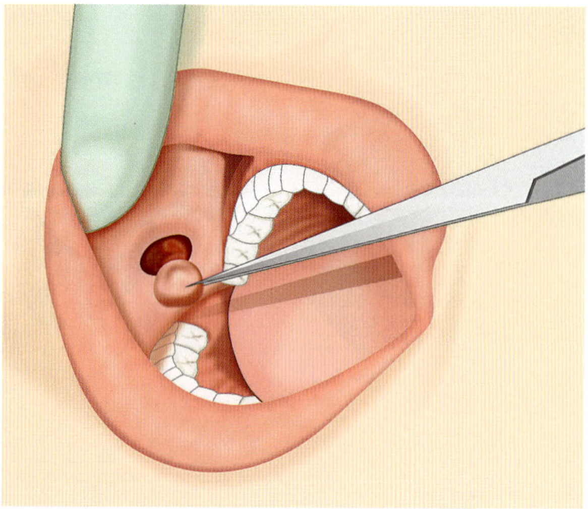

Fig. 6: The soft-tissue cylindrical fragment consisting of the mucosa, a small portion of the buccinator muscle, and a part of the fat pad are removed using scissors.

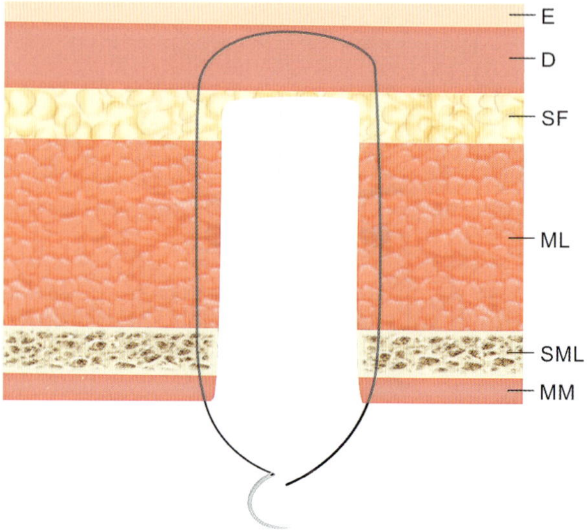

Fig. 8: The suture is passed through the cheek mucosa, muscle, and fat pad on one side of the defect; then through the dermis layer of the skin; and, finally, through the fat pad, the buccinator muscle, and the mucosa on the other side of the defect.

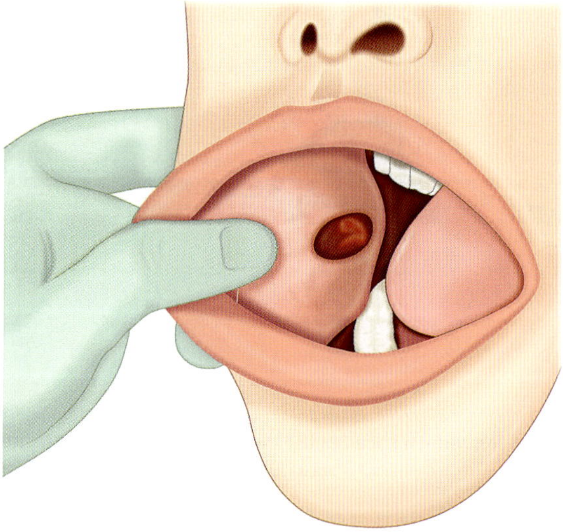

Fig. 7: The defect is widened by scraping with a no. 15 blade and separating the mucomuscular attachments.

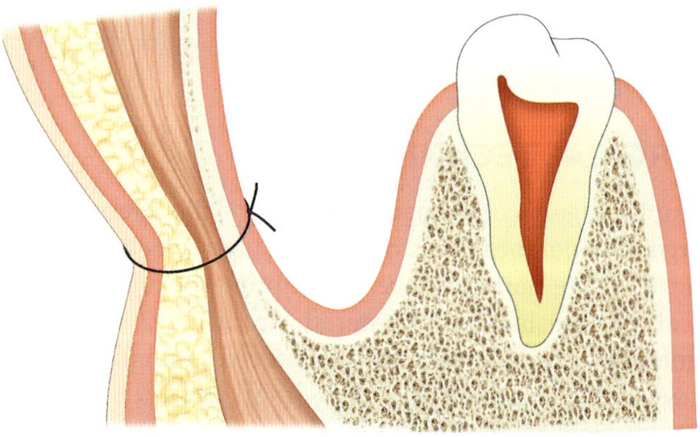

Fig. 9: The knot is tied, and the dimple is created.

the dermis layer of the skin, and, finally, through the fat pad, the buccinator muscle, and the mucosa on the other side of the defect **(Fig. 8)**. The knot is then tied, and the dimple is thereby created **(Fig. 9)**.

POSTOPERATIVE CARE

The patient is discharged immediately with antibiotics and analgesics. The patient is instructed to maintain good oral hygiene with mouthwash and oral rinse in the immediate postoperative period. It is also advised not to smile fully during the first 2 weeks.

Initially, there is a static dimple which deepens on animation, but gradually with time there is only a hint of dimple when static and accentuates on animation. It resembles a natural dimple (appearing only on smiling) within 4–6 weeks **(Figs. 10 to 13)**.

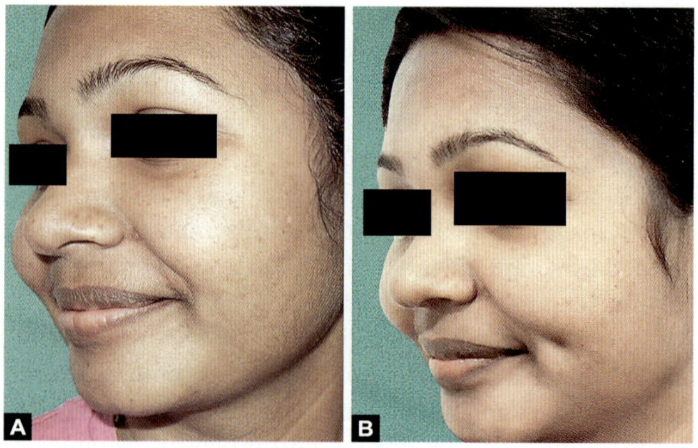

Figs. 10A and B: (A) Before and (B) After 6 months while smiling.

Complications of dimple surgery are given in **Box 1**.

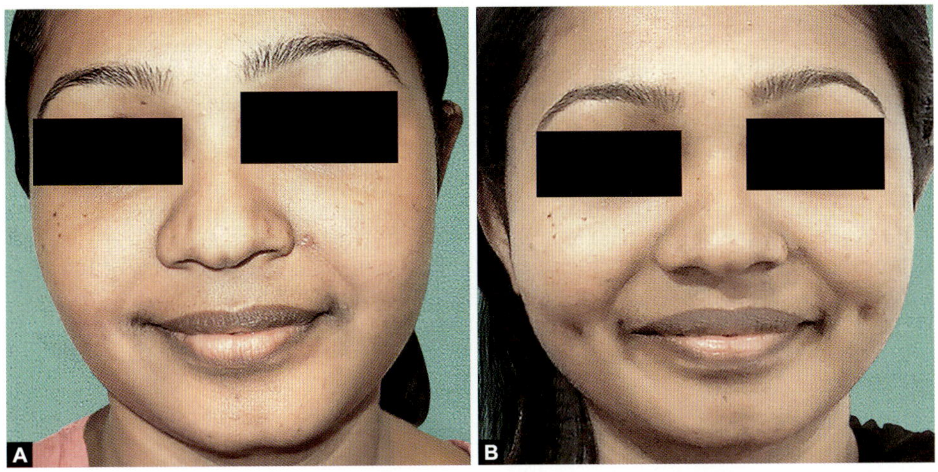

Figs. 11A and B: (A) Before and (B) After 6 months while smiling.

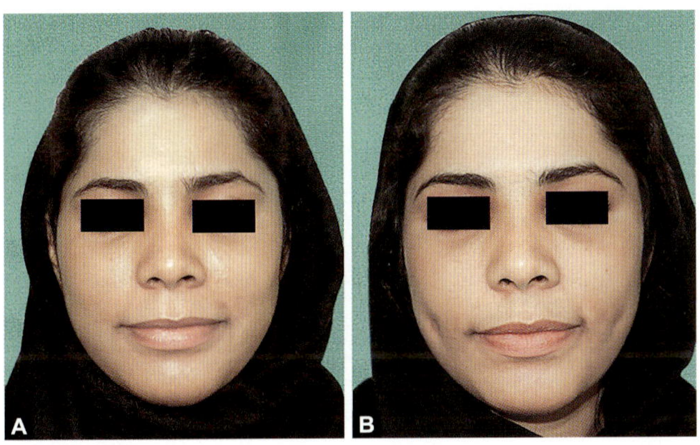

Figs. 12A and B: (A) Before and (B) After 6 months while smiling.

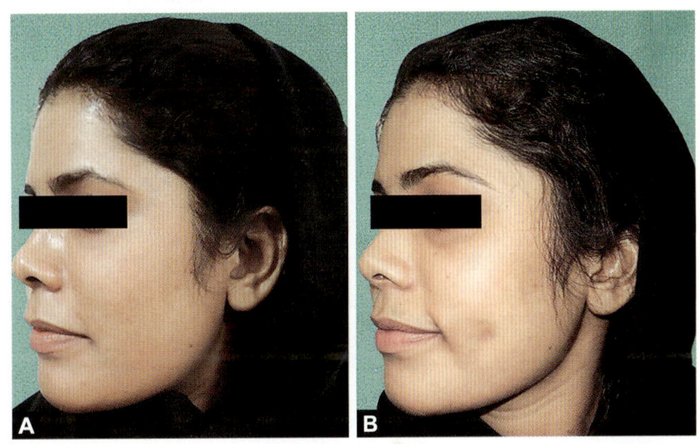

Figs. 13A and B: (A) Before and (B) After 6 months while smiling.

DISCUSSION

Literature reveals various techniques used by different authors for dimple creation.

Boo Chai used a nonabsorbable suture as a sling between skin and buccinator muscle; in effect, this simulated integumentary insertion of the muscle.[4] Bao et al. used a syringe needle to guide a monofilament nylon suture through the dermis and the buccinator muscle. They formed a sling between the skin and buccinator muscle, and a knot was tied and a dimple was created.[5] Saraf and Pillutia used a punch biopsy instrument and an intraoral approach to create a dimple.[6] Thomas et al. have described an open technique that replicates the anatomical basis of a natural dimple without requiring any soft-tissue removal.[7] Lari and Panse used a new and simple technique for dimple creation, passing a transcutaneous bolster stitch after scraping off the dermis of all mucomuscular attachments.[8]

We feel that the method described here is simple and safe and can be done by a dermatologic surgeon as a daycare procedure. This simple and open procedure described in this chapter for placing a facial dimple provides a predictable outcome with minimal morbidity.

BOX 1: Complications of a dimple surgery.

- Sudden disappearance of the dimple (failure of surgery)
- Asymmetry
- Foreign body reaction
- Infection
- Bleeding
- Injury to a nerve (buccal branch of the facial nerve) or salivary gland duct (Stensen duct)

CONCLUSION

Dimples tend to accentuate a smile, thus increasing the perception of attractiveness, sociability, and facial beauty. Unfortunately, not all pretty girls have dimples. But with simple techniques, dimples can be created with much ease. Consideration of vascular anatomy, shape of the face, and smile direction are important aspects for the outcome. Most of the published articles have claimed dimple creation surgery to be a very safe procedure with good results and a very low complication rate.

ACKNOWLEDGMENT

The authors thank Ms Heba J, a final year medical student at VIMS, Wayanad, Kerala, for the drawings.

REFERENCES

1. Argamaso RV. Facial dimple: Its formation by a simple technique. Plast Reconstr Surg. 1971;48(1):40-3.
2. Pentozos Daponte A, Vienna A, Brant L, Hauser G. Cheek dimples in Greek children and adolescents. Int J Anthropol. 2004;19(4):289-95.
3. Pessa JE, Zadoo VP, Garza PA, Adrian EK Jr, Dewitt AI, Garza JR. Double or bifid zygomaticus major muscle: anatomy, incidence, and clinical correlation. Clin Anat. 1998;11(5):310-3.
4. Boo Chai K. The facial dimple: Clinical study and operative technique. Plast Reconstr Surg Transplant Bull. 1962;30:281-8.
5. Bao S, Zhou C, Li S, Zhao M. A new simple technique for making facial dimples. Aesthetic Plast Surg. 2007;31(4):380-3.
6. Saraf S, Pillutia R. Complication of dimple creation. Indian Dermatol Online J. 2010;1(1):42-3.
7. Thomas M, Menon H, D'Silva J. Improved surgical access for facial dimple creation. Aesthet Surg J. 2010;30(6):798-801.
8. Lari AR, Panse N. Anatomical basis of dimple creation–a new technique: our experience of 100 cases. Indian J Plast Surg. 2012;45(1):89-93.

CHAPTER 63

Mohs Micrographic Surgery

Nicholas J Collier, Venura Samarasinghe, Vishal Madan

KEY MESSAGES

- The Mohs micrographic surgery (MMS) procedure allows histological verification of tumor clearance prior to wound closure. This treatment offers unsurpassed cure rates along with maximal conservation of adjacent healthy skin, thus reducing morbidity and mortality.
- MMS is a specialized procedure to treat selected cutaneous tumors.
- It is most commonly used in the treatment of basal cell carcinomas (BCCs) on the face and squamous cell carcinoma (SCC). It is also used to treat squamous cell carcinoma, lentigo maligna, and a number of rare aggressive cutaneous tumor types.
- Limitations of the use of MMS include the time and cost of the surgeon and technician and the cost of specialized equipment such as the cryostat.

INTRODUCTION

Conventional surgery involves excision of a tumor with a preselected wide margin of normal skin and then processing of the pathology specimen in vertical sections at 2–4-mm intervals, akin to a "bread loaf" series of sections through the tumor. Less than 1% of the tumor margin is examined in this method of sampling, and thus there is a possibility of the tumor being present at sites not sectioned during processing. Histopathology reports from this method of sectioning will commonly state that "the tumor *appears* excised from the levels viewed."

Mohs micrographic surgery (MMS) is a specialized method of skin cancer removal allowing unparalleled clearance rates and maximal preservation of healthy skin. The initial stage involves the removal of the tumor with a narrow margin of clinically normal skin. This layer of skin is marked to allow orientation, flattened, frozen, and sectioned horizontally to ensure visualization of the complete peripheral and deep margins. Intraoperative microscopic examination is performed with areas of residual tumor carefully marked and layers of skin adjacent to the involved margins removed. This process continues until complete tumor clearance is assured.

Thus, MMS offers a higher cure rate than standard surgery for skin cancer treatment, reducing the morbidity and mortality from future recurrence and simultaneously allowing maximal conservation of adjacent healthy skin. This is especially important when managing reconstructions in the cosmetically and functionally sensitive sites of the face.

HISTORY

In the mid-1930s, when working as a cancer research assistant during medical school, Frederick Mohs observed that the injection of 20% solution of zinc chloride induced in situ tissue fixation, preserving the cells for microscopic examination. From this finding, Mohs developed a process of fixing tissue using zinc chloride in vivo and excising the tumor in horizontal layers under microscopic control until complete clearance had been achieved.[1]

The new technique, called chemosurgery, was first reported by Mohs in 1941.[2] The main complication of chemosurgery was the use of zinc chloride as the in vivo tumor fixative as it caused significant pain and tissue irritation. From 1953, zinc chloride fixation was replaced by the production of fresh frozen tissue sections for microscopic examination. This allowed multiple stages to be completed in a single day and averted tissue irritation to permit immediate repair of the wound.

In 1969, using his technique, Mohs reported 66 basal cell carcinomas (BCCs) and 4 squamous cell carcinomas (SCCs) with 100% 5-year cure rate.[3] In 1974, Tromovitch and Stegman presented a further series of patients managed to further acclaim.[4,5] Subsequently, the technique was renamed MMS and has become the treatment of choice in high-risk, large, contiguous skin tumors, especially over critical anatomical sites of the head and neck.

INDICATIONS

Mohs micrographic surgery has been widely reported to provide greater cure rates in multiple cutaneous tumors in comparison to all other treatment modalities. In general, large tumors, critical site tumors requiring the greatest tissue conservation, locally aggressive tumors, and recurrent tumors are best treated by MMS.

Table 1 provides a list of some cutaneous malignancies managed by MMS.[6-8] Some of the more common indications for MMS are discussed in further detail.

BASAL CELL CARCINOMA

Basal cell carcinoma is the most common skin cancer worldwide and also the most common indication for MMS. The main subtypes of BCC are nodular, superficial, and infiltrative.[9] Rarer subtypes include cystic, morphoeic, and basosquamous. Subtypes may coexist, forming a mixed pattern and having pigmented variants. The histopathological findings are dependent on the subtype but are characterized by palisading basaloid cells connected to the epidermis with retraction artifact on hematoxylin and eosin staining. High-risk BCCs are optimally treated by MMS. Features compatible with high-risk BCC are listed in **Table 2**.[10] Rowe et al. published a review of all BCC studies published since 1947.[11] The group found a recurrence rate of 10.1% at 5-year follow-up for standard excision compared to 1% for MMS at 5-year follow-up. Results were even more striking for recurrent BCC (rBCC). MMS provides recurrence rates of 5.6% at 5 years for rBCC in comparison to 17.4% at 5 years for SE.[11]

Malhotra et al. performed a retrospective analysis for periocular BCC utilizing data from the Australian Mohs database. Of 1,295 patients treated with MMS, 5-year recurrence rates were found to be 0% for primary tumors and 7.8% for rBCC.[12] Treatment of periorbital BCC is particularly important as recurrences may be associated with orbital invasion, and if extensive, may even require orbital exenteration.

A Dutch randomized clinical trial comparing MMS and surgical excision for the treatment of facial BCCs demonstrated a trend toward lower recurrence rates of SE (4.1%) in comparison to MMS (2.1%) for primary facial BCC at 5-year follow-up ($p = 0.23$).[13] The 10-year-follow-up results were published in 2014.[14] Recurrence rates for primary and rBCC treated by MMS and surgical excision were 4.4 versus 12.2% (p = 0.1) for primary lesions and 3.9 versus 13.5% ($p = 0.02$) for recurrent lesions. It was noted that a substantial number of primary (56%) and recurrent (14%) BCCs were found to recur >5 years after treatment.

TABLE 1: Cutaneous tumors treated with Mohs surgery.

Basal cell carcinoma	*Squamous cell carcinoma*
Dermatofibrosarcoma protuberans	Leiomyosarcoma
Microcystic adnexal carcinoma	Atypical fibroxanthoma
Extramammary Paget's disease	Melanoma
Sebaceous carcinoma	Adenoid cystic carcinoma
Bowen's disease	

TABLE 2: High-risk basal cell carcinomas (BCCs).

Large size >2 cm	*Recurrent BCC*
Morphoeic or micronodular subtype	Perineural/perivascular invasion
H-zone of face	

SQUAMOUS CELL CARCINOMA

Squamous cell carcinoma usually presents as enlarging red or skin-colored keratotic papules, nodules, or plaques, which may be ulcerated, tender, and bleeding. Cutaneous SCC most often develops over chronically, actinically damaged skin on the head, neck, and other photoexposed sites.

The typical histological findings are malignant keratinocytes invading into the dermis and are described in further detail in various dermatopathology books. Mortality from SCC occurs predominantly within a high-risk subgroup of patients. This high-risk subgroup can be identified from factors listed in **Table 3**.[15]

For primary cutaneous SCC, a retrospective review of all studies found that MMS provided an overall cure rate of 97% at 5 years. When the data were further analyzed, the following cure rates of MMS compared to SE were found, respectively: 96.9 versus 89.1% (lip), 94.7 versus 81.3% (ear), 74.8 versus 59.3% (size over 2 cm), 67.4 versus 46.4% (poorly differentiated histologic subtype), and 90 versus 77.7% (recurrent SCC).[16]

Leibovitch et al. undertook a prospective study of 5-year survival rates for 1,263 patients treated with MMS for cutaneous SCC from 1993 to 2002. The 5-year cure rates were 97.4% in patients presenting with primary SCC and 94.1% for patients presenting with recurrent SCC.[17] For organ transplant recipients, subclinical invasion of SCC can occur up to 6 mm wide of the macroscopic tumor margins, and often the SCC is biologically more aggressive.[18] MMS would be indicated in these high-risk patients.

Dermatofibrosarcoma Protuberans

Dermatofibrosarcoma protuberans (DFSP) is a slow-growing cutaneous fibrohistiocytic malignancy. Extensive subclinical invasion often occurs, contributing to the high recurrence rates after standard excision. DFSP usually presents as an asymptomatic purplish-red nodule or plaque. Areas of induration, telangiectasia, or atrophy may be present. Approximately 10% of DFSP transform into a high-grade sarcoma variant. Histological examination shows monomorphic spindle-shaped cells forming a cartwheel arrangement. The deeply invading tumor cells create a honeycomb appearance and stain positive for CD34 and negative for factor XHIa.[19]

Paradisi et al. carried out a retrospective review of all published reports of DFSP treated with MMS versus

TABLE 3: Factors indicating high-risk squamous cell carcinomas (SCCs).

Tumor size >2 cm	*Tumor depth >4 mm*
Moderate, poorly differentiated SCC	Ear, lip, hand, genital anatomic location
Perineural or perivascular invasion	Recurrent SCC
SCC arising from scars or chronic ulcers	SCC arising in immunosuppressed patients

standard excision. The pooled data for MMS revealed that out of 463 patients, 6 tumors recurred [1.3%, confidence interval (CI) 4.4–28.1%] compared with 288 recurrences from 1,394 patients treated with SE (20.7%, 95% CI 18.6–22.9%). DFSP treated with SE were 16 times more likely to recur than those treated with MMS.[20]

A recent large single-center retrospective review of 158 patients with dermatofibrosarcoma treated by MMS (67) and wide local excision (91) demonstrated substantially lower recurrence rates with MMS (30.8 vs. 3.0%, $p < 0.001$). Additionally, the mean defects were smaller with MMS (10.7 vs. 8.8 cm, $p = 0.004$).[21]

Microcystic Adnexal Carcinoma

Microcystic adnexal carcinoma (MAC) is a locally aggressive cutaneous malignancy with follicular and sweat gland differentiation. MAC presents as a smooth, skin-colored, or yellowish slow-growing indurated plaque or cystic nodule usually located on the central face. Clinical differential diagnoses include benign adnexal tumors (e.g., trichoepithelioma, trichoadenoma, syringoma), morphoeic BCC, and SCC. Histological examination reveals the presence of islands of cells forming pilar and gland-like structures, with keratin cysts and a desmoplastic stroma. Perineural and muscular invasion help to differentiate MAC from syringomas histologically. Immunohistochemistry with carcinoembryonic antigen (CEA), epithelial membrane antigen (EMA), and cytokeratin may help with the histological diagnosis.[22]

A retrospective review of 44 patients with MAC was performed using data in the Australian Mohs database over a 9-year period. Perineural invasion occurred in 18% of the cases, and 32% of the cases were recurrences from other treatment modalities. The 5-year cure rates with MMS were found to be 5%.[23] In comparison, SE had a reported recurrence rate of at least 30%. Defects managed by MMS have clinical margins four times larger than predicted, highlighting the invasive nature of the neoplasm and importance of microscopic margin control.[24]

Leiomyosarcoma

Primary leiomyosarcoma (LMS) is a rare mesenchymal malignancy arising from smooth muscle and occurs in cutaneous and subcutaneous forms. The cutaneous type develops from hair follicle arrector pili muscles and the subcutaneous type from the smooth muscles of the blood vessel vasculature. Secondary LMS arises from visceral metastasis. LMSs typically present as red or light brown nodules that may ulcerate. Histology classically shows dermal spindle-shaped cells with blunt-ended nuclei and are actin and vimentin positive.[25]

Standard excision has a reported recurrence rate of 30–45%. Humphreys et al. reviewed 15 cases of LMS treated with MMS in the literature and found the overall recurrence rate to be 13%.[26] Subsequently, Starling and Coldiron reported a further 11 patients treated over a 16-year period by MMS. The average defect size was 15.0 cm^2, and recurrence rates were 0% at 4.5 years.[27]

Atypical Fibroxanthoma

Atypical fibroxanthoma (AFX) is a fibrohistiocytic tumor usually developing over sun-exposed areas in elderly men and presents as a rapidly enlarging pink, red, or brown nodule, often with ulceration. Histological examination reveals atypical spindle cells and epithelioid fibrohistiocytic cells, often with multinucleated giant cells. Immunohistochemistry is positive for actin and vimentin. These features may be indistinct from those of undifferentiated pleomorphic sarcoma (UPS), and some authors believe AFX to be a superficial variant of UPS.[28]

Ang et al. reviewed 88 cases of AFX treated at the Mayo Clinic over a 24-year period. 23 cases were treated with standard excision and 59 cases were treated with MMS. Recurrence rates for SE were 8.7% with median follow-up of 8.7 years in comparison to 0% for MMS at median follow-up of 4.5 years.[29]

Porocarcinoma

Porocarcinomas are malignant tumors that develop from the eccrine duct and acrosyringium. They are estimated to account for between 1 in 10,000 and 1 in 20,000 cutaneous cancers.[30] Porocarcinomas present as firm, erythematous to violaceous nodules, usually <2 cm in diameter. They can develop from an existing poroma or arise de novo. Whilst they can affect a wide age range, they predominately affect patients between 60 and 80 years of age.[31] Lesions occur most commonly on the lower leg but, unlike poromas, are not common on the acral skin.[32]

Wide local excision was historically the treatment of choice; however, recurrence rates affected approximately 20%, with distant metastases in 10% and mortality rates of 5–10%.[33,34] A recent review from the Mayo Clinic included nine cases with a mean follow-up period of 3.3 years, demonstrating no recurrence or disease-related mortality.[35]

Extramammary Paget's Disease

Primary cutaneous extramammary Paget's disease (EMPD) is an adenocarcinoma originating most likely from apocrine glands or epidermal stem cells. Secondary EMPD is associated with an underlying adnexal carcinoma or a regional visceral carcinoma, usually rectum, bladder, urethra, cervix, prostate, or vulva. Clinical presentation is of scaly or macerated plaques with indistinct margins, most commonly over genital skin. Histology shows Paget cells, which are large round cells with big nucleoli. EMPD cells have high mucopolysaccharide levels, staining positive for periodic acid-Schiff and Alcian blue at pH 2.5.[36]

Lee et al. reviewed 35 Korean patients with EMPD over a 10-year period. Recurrence rates at mean 5.3-year follow-up were 36.4% with SE in comparison with 18.2% for MMS.[37]

Hendi et al. performed a literature review for recurrence rates after MMS in comparison to other modalities. Results showed a 5-year cure rate of 80% with MMS for primary EMPD and 56% for recurrent EMPD in comparison to other treatment modalities with a 33–60% 5-year cure rate. The group recommended that if SE is performed, 5-cm wide margins would be required to clear 97% of all tumors.[38]

Lentigo Maligna Melanoma

Melanoma usually presents as a changing pigmented lesion, which, dependent on Breslow thickness, is associated with a substantial risk of local, regional, and distant metastasis. Subtypes include superficial spreading, nodular, lentigo maligna melanoma (LMM), and acral lentiginous melanoma. Histopathology is characterized by invasive melanocytes, and it may pose a significant diagnostic challenge for a pathologist.[39-41] SE involves 5-mm clinical margins of normal skin for LM and 10-mm margins for thin melanoma of <1.0 mm Breslow thickness. The adequacy of 5-mm margins to consistently achieve clearance of in situ melanoma has been questioned.[42]

Zitelli et al. reported on 625 consecutive patients diagnosed with melanoma of the head and neck region. Margins of 9 mm were required to remove 98.5% of in situ lesions, whilst 12-mm margins removed 96.6% of melanomas of Breslow thickness 2.01–4.00. Patients had a mean follow-up of 4.8 years. The 5-year survival results compared favorably with matched results from standard wide local excision. The authors argued for wider than standard margins of 9 mm for in situ disease and melanoma <1 mm Breslow but narrower margins of 12 mm for lesions with a Breslow thickness between 1 and 4 mm.[43]

Thus, in areas where tissue needs to be conserved, such as the head and neck region, MMS may be advantageous for LMM.[43,44] However, the use of MMS for melanoma has been contentious due to both the inferior quality of slides produced with frozen section in comparison to traditional paraffin-embedded sections and the difficulty in differentiating malignant melanocytes from atypical melanocytes in photodamaged skin. With the improvement in immunohistochemistry techniques on frozen sections for melanoma and reduction in turnaround time to produce the sections, MMS may become more widely utilized in melanoma treatment. Further randomized controlled trials are required comparing SE to MMS.

MOHS SUITE (SURGICAL FACILITY)

The Mohs suite is best designed with the surgical theater in close proximity to the Mohs laboratory containing the cryostat machine (used to produce the frozen sections) and the office where the microscope is situated. This will facilitate the transportation of the tissue between the locations and allow optimal communication between the Mohs surgeon and the histotechnician.

Equipment required for the cryostat include surgical blade, specimen button or chuck, antiroll brush, forceps, inking dyes to mark tissue margins, optimal cutting temperature (OCT) medium for embedding, mounting medium, tissue fixing solutions, tissue stains, slides, cover slips, chemical disposal area, wash basin, and eye wash station. The laboratory requires adequate ventilation to remove chemical fumes from the staining process, and most laboratories have a backup cryostat in case of malfunction of the primary machine.

DEVELOPING TECHNIQUES

Mohs micrographic surgery techniques have been in continuous development for many decades, and the excellent outcomes and degree of skill required set a high bar for the introduction of changes in the technique. The technique is, however, both time consuming and associated with high costs compared with standard surgery. Therefore, improvements are constantly being sought and noninvasive methods for in vivo determination of tumor margins developed. The goal of these approaches is to save time and cost while maintaining efficacy; the more important developing ones are discussed below.

Confocal Microscopy

Confocal microscopy is capable of providing images of a quality sufficient to be considered as a potential alternative to the traditional histopathology approaches used in MMS. This has potential advantages as the histological quality of the frozen sections normally used in MMS is inferior than that of traditional histopathology based on formalin fixation and paraffin-embedded sections. This quality sacrifice is being traded off for increased speed, and a similar trade-off might be attainable using confocal microscopy.

The technique enables collection of images at different skin depths (down to the penetration limit), and these images are then manipulated by software to create the desired image output. The confocal microscope uses point illumination and only takes images at one depth level at a time. It is this that gives it an optical resolution much better than with the usual wide-field microscopes, this improved resolution being particularly marked in the depth direction. By focusing on a specific focal plane, the image is freed from interference from adjacent planes, both above and below. This increased optical resolution and contrast are achieved by eliminating all light reflected from other than the focal point. This is accomplished by adding a small pinhole before the detector in the confocal plane, hence the name. As the pinhole produces an ellipsoid of much greater length than width, there is an intrinsically lower axial resolution. Thus, the horizontal images can achieve a resolution of 1.25 μm axially but only 5 μm laterally; however, this is sufficient to observe cellular morphology.

In order to maximize the detection depth in the skin, near-infrared light (830 nm) is used. This is produced by a laser diode, thereby achieving good resolution down to at least 200 μm. In practice, images are produced en face, horizontal and parallel to the skin, and are visually sectioned to resemble the histopathology specimen in MMS.[45]

As only a small point inside the tissue is in focus at any one time, it is necessary to scan the resultant images and recreate composite images using a computer. This allows for the composite images to be manipulated. Two forms of output have proved particularly useful; these are the stack mode and the mosaic mode. In the stack mode, the skin is viewed at consecutive levels from the epidermis down to the papillary dermis, at which point the resolution begins to deteriorate. In the mosaic mode, a composite image is made (stitched together) from the individual images, the resulting mosaics displaying large areas of tissue at the low magnification needed for MMS.[46]

Reflectance Confocal Microscopy

This seems to be the best of the newer techniques for lateral margin detection, allowing the identification of tumor characteristics at the cellular level.[47]

In reflectance confocal microscopy (RCM), no staining is required. The images are grayscale, and the reflectivity of the tissue determines the contrast.

In detecting BCC tumor during MMS, RCM has been shown to have a sensitivity of 96.6% and a specificity of 89.2%, with a positive predictive value of 93.0% and a negative predictive value of 94.7%.[48]

Fluorescence Confocal Microscopy

Fluorescence confocal microscopes (FCM) have been shown to have application to the MMS technique in the examination of ex vivo tissue.[46,48] Ex vivo FCM can be used for real-time imaging of tissue arising directly from MMS excisions. There are differences and similarities between RCM and FCM.

In contrast to RCM, where no staining is used, FCM does use stains as contrast agents. For example, a common technique used in FCM is staining with acridine orange, which by specifically staining the nuclei increases the contrast of nucleated cells, and hence these cells show up clearly in contrast to the weak fluorescence arising from the dermis.[46] This offers an advantage over RCM, as in RCM, the dermis reflects brightly, hindering observation.

As with RCM, FCM produces high-resolution individual images that are manipulated by software to produce mosaics; the images are said to be "stitched together." Again, the images are thin optical sections, but in the case of FCM, the individual images are larger, typically 750 μm × 750 μm, and these are stitched together to give wide field-of-view mosaics, typically 12 mm × 12 mm, which show large areas of tissue at low magnification, which is the desirable output for MMS. In FCM, this image collection and manipulation take <3 minutes, thereby enabling real-time pathology.[46]

Mohs micrographic surgery predominately treats BCCs. Up to 1% of BCCs, termed locally advanced BCCs, are clinically determined as nonamenable to curative surgery or radiotherapy.[49] BCCs develop through inappropriate activation of the hedgehog pathway. Newly approved hedgehog pathway inhibitors (vismodegib and sonidegib) are available, and both have been shown to substantially shrink tumors in 40–50% of patients. Their long-term use is often limited by resistance, and tumors often recur. Adverse effects frequently include muscle cramps, alopecia, and dysgeusia.[50] An area of current research involves their neoadjuvant use to shrink the tumor, thereby enabling surgery and potentially limiting functional or cosmetic impairment from surgery. A crucial question is whether the tumor shrinkage occurs coherently, without residual islands of BCC being left behind. For excision to be effective, clear margins are essential, and for this, shrinkage induced by hedgehog inhibitors would need to occur evenly without leaving BCC cells behind in the vacated areas. It is not yet clear how much of a problem this will prove to be, but this aspect is receiving attention.[51-54]

An investigator-initiated open-label clinical trial of vismodegib as a neoadjuvant to surgery was conducted with 15 patients with high-risk BCC; 11 of these completed the trial and 4 patients could not complete >3 months due to the adverse effects from vismodegib.[52]

This trial showed that 2–6 months of vismodegib treatment produced a 27% reduction in the surgical defect area from baseline.[52] These 11 patients had 13 BCCs selected as targets for excision, mainly of the infiltrative BCC subtype. It was found that vismodegib treatment was needed to last for a minimum of 3 months in order to produce a significant reduction in BCC size.[52]

MOHS MICROGRAPHIC SURGERY TECHNIQUE

Performing successful MMS is dependent on the production and interpretation of high-quality frozen horizontal (en face) sections. The procedure involves different steps as shown in **Box 1**. If a residual tumor is present on microscopic examination, the involved microscopic margins are identified on the defect utilizing the Mohs map, and further Mohs layers are removed precisely from the areas of residual tumor. The process is repeated until the entire tumor has been removed.

BOX 1: Steps of Mohs micrographic surgery.

1. Preoperative screening
2. Removing of the first Mohs layer
3. Accurate paper mapping of the removed tissue in relation to the defect created
4. Inking of margins for orientation
5. Tissue grossing (flattening), embedding, cutting of tissue sections (cryotomy)
6. Fixing of the cut sections, staining
7. Interpretation of the slides produced
8. Repetition of steps 2–7 if residual tumor is present

Step 1: Preoperative Assessment

Mohs micrographic surgery is a lengthy procedure and may not be suitable for all patients, for example, those with dementia. It is important to offer a choice of treatment modalities to patients, with discussion of the benefits and disadvantages of each treatment, and to allow patients to make informed decisions.

A routine preoperative assessment will include a review of current and past medical problems, medications, herbal treatments, smoking and alcohol consumption, and discussion of the risks of surgery. Anticoagulants should not be stopped prior to the operation due to an increased risk of postoperative venous thromboembolism.[55] Patients are requested to stop smoking to aid local tissue perfusion and to stop alcohol consumption and relevant herbal treatments (e.g., garlic, ginger, ginkgo) to reduce hemorrhagic complications. Patients should be provided with written information on the procedure.

Large tumors may require preoperative imaging to assess for muscle or bony invasion. If the defect is likely to be large, preoperative liaison with the relevant plastic, oculoplastic, ear-nose-throat, or maxillofacial surgeon may be necessary to coordinate the complex repair post-MMS.

Step 2: Excision of First Mohs Layer and Mapping of the Tumor

Prior to the infiltration of local anesthesia (LA), the clinical margins of the tumor must be marked in addition to important skin tension lines and anatomic subunits using a skin marker pen. A premixed solution of 1% lignocaine and epinephrine (1 in 200,000) as local anesthetic is typically used for injection. Marcaine may be injected additionally or in combination to provide anesthesia of longer duration.

Prior to excising the first Mohs layer, curettage is used for initial tumor debulking **(Fig. 1)**. In addition to debulking of the tumor, reports have suggested that the curettage can be used to precisely remove subclinical extension of the tumor by palpation of abnormal tissue, thereby reducing the number of Mohs stages required. However, other studies have shown that wider curettage may unnecessarily remove extra normal tissue and result in a larger Mohs defect.[56]

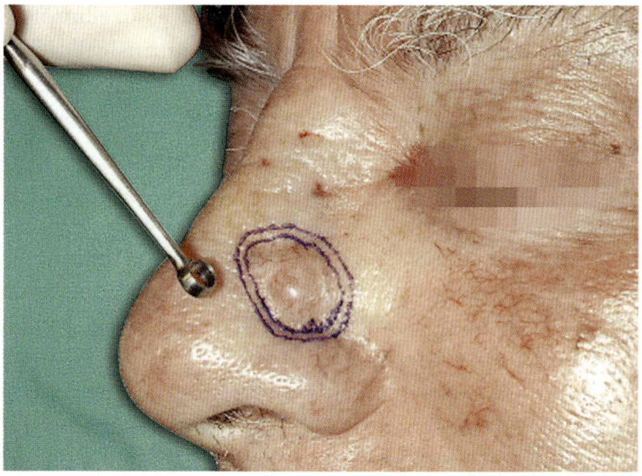

Fig. 1: Curetting or debulking the tumor.

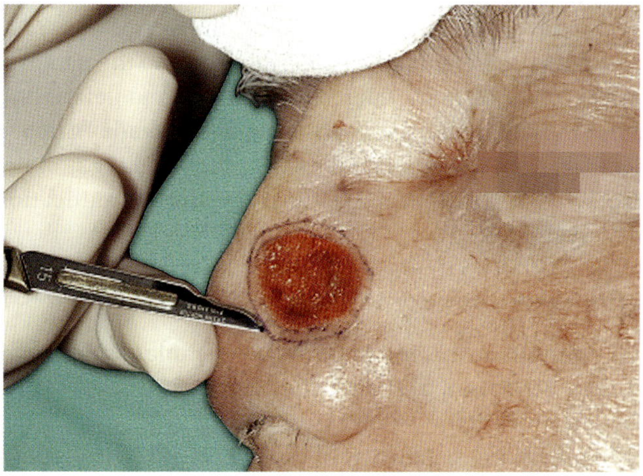

Fig. 2: Incising the Mohs layer at 45° angle.

Following debulking of the tumor, the margin of the first Mohs layer is scored with a 1–2-mm narrow width of epidermis. Perpendicular marking nicks are made through the scored peripheral margin onto the surrounding skin for future orientation. Typically, nicks are made at 12, 6, and 9 o'clock positions. The blade is then classically held at a 45° angle to the skin, incision is made up to the subcutaneous tissue, maintaining the angle, and then the tumor is removed in a horizontal deep plane to provide a "saucer"-shaped layer of tissue **(Fig. 2)**. "Saucerization" facilitates the flattening of the tissue and allows the entire peripheral and deep margin to be examined in one plane. It is important to ensure that the complete margin of epidermis is present and the incision has not incised through the curetted tissue. Radiofrequency ablation or hyfrecator is used to cauterize any bleeding points after the removal of the first layer, and the surgical area is bandaged. The patient is then asked to wait in the waiting hall until the results of the first layer are microscopically interpreted.

The excised tissue is placed on a square of gauze. A hand-drawn Mohs map of the wound is created to represent the in vivo wound with marking nicks **(Fig. 3)**. Large specimens

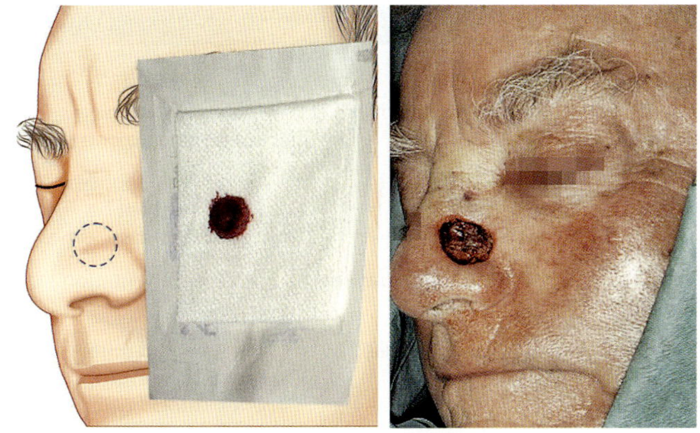

Fig. 3: Mohs template design.

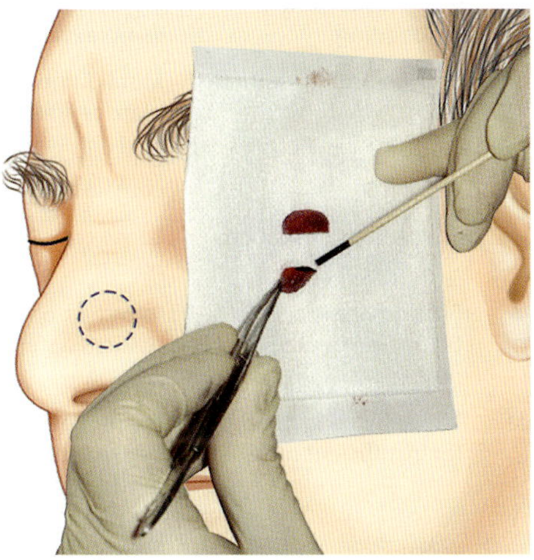

Fig. 4: Color coding the sections.

may require division for placement onto a glass slide. Each subdivision must be numbered and marked on the Mohs map. Digital photographs may be used in place of hand-drawn maps and printed to provide greater accuracy of defect site, size, and orientation.

The tissue margins are marked using ink, and the corresponding site and color are drawn onto the Mohs map. One color is standard on a superior or medial edge while another color at the inferior or lateral edge **(Fig. 4)**. The same color coordination should be used for all Mohs stages and procedures to reduce errors of orientation.

Step 3: Tissue Grossing, Embedding, and Sectioning

The tissue is placed on a slide and carefully checked to ensure that the entire margins are flat and in contact with the slide surface. The edges can be maneuvered flat using cotton tip applicators or forceps. Relaxation incisions may be required through the superficial surface to help gross (flatten) the specimen.

Next, an embedding medium (e.g., OCT compound) is applied around the periphery of the tissue, and the entire

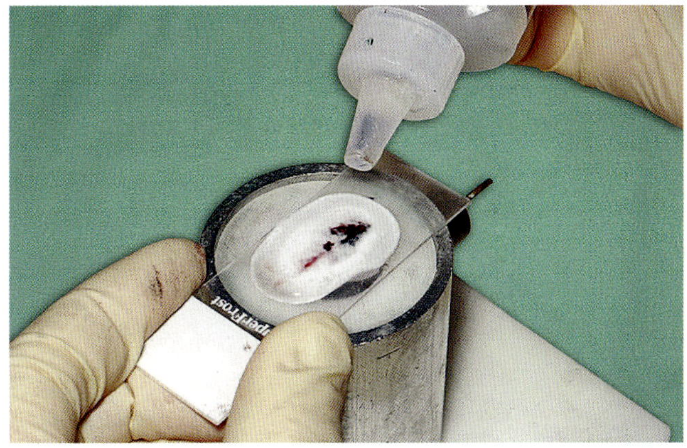

Fig. 5: Embedding medium [e.g., optimal cutting temperature (OCT) compound] is applied around the periphery of the tissue.

block is frozen in the cryostat freeze bar **(Fig. 5)**. The freezing process should occur quickly to avoid the formation of ice crystal and subsequent tissue artifact.

The frozen block is then placed, deep margin face up, on a chuck using further OCT medium for adherence, and the entire button mounted on the cryostat stage ready for sectioning. Alternative techniques of embedding include using a heat extractor, embedding machine, or isopentane histobath.

The frozen tissue block is next sectioned in the microtome. The block should be carefully sectioned until a complete skin edge is obtained, which can be checked for by the histotechnician using a microscope prior to proceeding to fixation. If a complete margin is not present, deeper cuts are required.

Step 4: Tissue Fixation and Staining

The section is placed on a positively charged slide to improve adherence. Two or three sections may be placed simultaneously on one slide. The tissue is then fixed, most commonly using either 10% neutral buffered formalin, alcoholic formalin, alcohol, or acetone. Once the tissue has been fixed, the next step is staining of the tissue.

Hematoxylin and eosin is the most frequently used tissue stain. Toluidine blue may be used in BCC to highlight mucopolysaccharides surrounding islands of tumor. Once the tissue is stained, excess dye is cleared using xylene substitutes.

Increasingly, immunohistochemical staining is also performed on the frozen sections. These include cytokeratin stains for BCC and SCC, Ber-EP4 for BCC, CD34 for DFSP and HMB-45, and Mel-5, S-100, and Melan-A for melanoma.[57]

Cytokeratin staining for BCC in MMS is a useful adjunct in morphologically complex cases where there is a dense inflammatory infiltrate surrounding suspicious cells that can hinder identification of scanty tumor cells, which are difficult to determine with hematoxylin and eosin or toluidine blue staining. A recent study demonstrated pancytokeratins

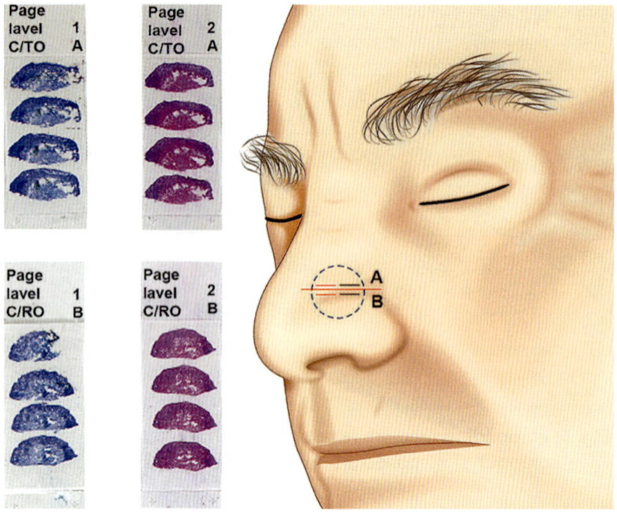

Fig. 6: Sections are ready to be read by the Mohs surgeon.

AE1/AE3 to be a highly effective stain for BCC in MMS and showed consistent staining, both in terms of intensity of staining and sensitivity of >99%.[58] Finally, a coverslip is placed over the section using a coverslip adhesive, and the slide is ready to be reviewed by the Mohs surgeon.

Step 5: Interpreting the Frozen Section

Examination of the Mohs frozen section allows review of the entire peripheral and deep margin for residual tumor **(Fig. 6)**. If a residual tumor is present, further Mohs layers are required. The site of the residual tumor is marked onto the Mohs map and then reflected onto the in vivo defect on the patient. The patient is brought back to the operative room, and utilizing the orientation nicks made onto the skin in step 3, the residual tumor site is marked, and further Mohs layers are taken. A 1–2-mm margin of normal skin is taken from both peripheral and deep involved margins for future orientation, and the entire process is repeated until all of the tumor has been removed. The wound can then be repaired to provide optimum cosmetic and functional result. The choice of wound repair is dependent on the anatomical site, the quality of the adjacent tissue, and individual patient characteristics. The ideal repair for one patient will not necessarily be the best repair for another patient. Commonly used modalities of wound repair include secondary intention healing, skin grafting, and the utilization of local skin flaps, which can be performed on the same or next day.

TABLE 4: List of potential errors in technique.

Step	*Error*	*Adverse consequence*
Step 2: Excision	Incision angle over 45°	Difficulty flattening specimen into one plane
	Incising through curetted area when taking Mohs layer	Complete peripheral margin will not be available for assessment
Step 2: Mapping	Inaccuracy of drawing Mohs map	Incorrect orientation
	Too much ink used	Ink spill onto other margins confusing orientation
Step 3: Grossing	Edges not unrolled during grossing	Tangential sections
Step 3: Embedding	Slow freeze during embedding	Ice formation in tissue sample causing artifact
Step 3: Sectioning	Sections curl on antiroll plate	Misalignment of antiroll plate or cold blade
	Torn sections	Dull blade or blade contains nicks
	Thin and thick sections	Loose chuck or blade holder
	Foreign tissue on blade from a previous procedure	Introduction of foreign tissue (floater) into section
Step 4: Tissue fixation	Tissue in fixing medium for insufficient time	Inadequate dehydration of tissue resulting in reduced quality of staining
Step 4: Tissue staining	Foreign tissue in staining medium from a previous procedure	Introduction of foreign tissue into section (floater)
	Incorrect labeling of slides	Errors of tumor mapping
Step 5: Interpreting frozen section	Misinterpretation of benign histology for malignant and vice versa	Errors of false-negative or false-positive margins
	Inflammation masking underlying tumor cells	Errors of false-negative margins
	Misinterpretation of perineural invasion	Errors of false-negative margins

SLOW MOHS MICROGRAPHIC SURGERY

The classical technique for MMS described above has also been modified to use traditional formalin fixation and paraffin-embedded sections to still ensure 100% margin control. This method is known as slow Mohs, and each stage takes 24–48 hours. The advantage is a higher quality of histological sections than standard Mohs frozen sections, especially useful for melanoma which may be difficult to interpret on frozen sections.

A large series of 750 BCCs treated with slow Mohs found a cure rate of 97.8% for primary tumors and 95.3% for recurrent tumors at 5-year follow-up.[59] Slides were read jointly by the Mohs surgeon and dermatopathologist. The primary disadvantage of slow Mohs is the 1–2 days turnaround time for the production of the paraffin-embedded slides. This necessitates several patient visits but is a viable option when traditional MMS is not feasible. Slow Mohs has also been reported for use with SCC with equivalent cure rates and can be used with any tumor type.[60]

BOX 2: Limitations of Mohs micrographic surgery.

- Time-consuming process
- Quality of frozen sections inferior to standard paraffin-embedded sections for histological interpretation
- Dedicated histotechnician required for preparation of frozen sections
- Tumors that grow in a noncontiguous manner may be associated with falsely negative margins

Cost Effectiveness of Mohs Micrographic Surgery

Mohs micrographic surgery is more expensive than conventional surgery; the main expenses of MMS arise from the labor costs of the Mohs surgeon, nurses, assistants, histotechnicians, and receptionists and increased length of time taken to perform MMS in contrast to standard surgery.

A study by Smeets et al. and Essers et al. found MMS to be significantly more expensive than SE for primary and rBCC, independent of the BCC subtype or anatomical site.[13,61] However, Bialy et al. found MMS to be cost comparable to SE when tumor recurrence rates postprocedure, thus necessitating further procedures, were accounted for.[62] Cook and Zitelli described 400 consecutive tumors and also showed the cost of MMS to be equivalent to SE.[63]

POTENTIAL ERRORS AND LIMITATIONS OF MOHS MICROGRAPHIC SURGERY

Errors can occur at all steps along the process of performing MMS. **Table 4** highlights potential areas of difficulty to be aware of in the procedure and **Box 2** summarizes some of the common limitations of MMS.

CONCLUSION

Surgical treatment of skin tumors can have a significant impact on the quality of life for a patient. MMS provides the highest cure rates, utilizing margin control while sparing the maximum amount of healthy tissue.

This allows for optimum functional and cosmetic repair. MMS should be the treatment of choice for high-risk skin tumors in critical anatomical sites on the head and neck. MMS is a technical procedure requiring specialized training for 1–2 years before independent practice is commenced. A Mohs surgeon in Australia performs on average 200–300 cases per year; while in the USA, the number of cases is on average 1,000.[64] India has a lower incidence of skin cancer, and it should be mandatory that dermatologists in India performing MMS have followed a suitable training program and subsequently completed a minimum number of MMS cases per year to ensure that the highest standards of the MMS technique are maintained.

REFERENCES

1. Wood LD, Ammirati CT. An overview of Mohs micrographic surgery for the treatment of basal cell carcinoma. Dermatol Clin. 2011;29(2):153-60.
2. Mohs F. Chemosurgery: a microscopically controlled method of cancer excision. Arch Surg. 1941;42:279-95.
3. Mohs FE. Cancer of eyelids. Bull Am Coll Chemosurg. 1970;3:10-1.
4. Tromovitch TA, Stegman SJ. Microscopically controlled excision of skin tumors: chemosurgery (Mohs): fresh tissue technique. Arch Dermatol. 1974;110:231-2.
5. Tromovitch TA, Stegman SJ. Microscopie-controlled excision of cutaneous tumors: chemosurgery, fresh tissue technique. Cancer. 1978;41:653-8.
6. Berlin AL, Amin SP, Goldberg DJ. Extraocular sebaceous carcinoma treated with Mohs micrographic surgery: report of a case and review of literature. Dermatol Surg. 2008;34:254-7.
7. Xu YG, Hinshaw M, Longley BJ, Ilyas H, Snow SN. Cutaneous adenoid cystic carcinoma with perineural invasion treated by Mohs micrographic surgery—a case report with literature review. J Oncol. 2010;2010:469049.
8. Leibovitch I, Huilgol SC, Selva D, Richards S, Paver R. Cutaneous squamous carcinoma in situ (Bowen's disease): treatment with Mohs micrographic surgery. J Am Acad Dermatol. 2005;52:997-1002.
9. Arits AH, Mosterd K, Essers BA, Spoorenberg E, Sommer A, De Rooij MJ, et al. Photodynamic therapy versus topical imiquimod versus topical fluorouracil for treatment of superficial basal-cell carcinoma: a single blind, non-inferiority, randomised controlled trial. Lancet Oncol. 2013;14:647-54.
10. Samarasinghe V, Madan V, Lear JT. Focus on basal cell carcinoma. J Skin Cancer. 2011;2011:328615.
11. Rowe DE, Carroll RJ, Day Jr CL. Long-term recurrence rates in previously untreated (primary) basal cell carcinoma: implications for patient follow-up. J Dermatol Surg Oncol. 1989;15:315-28.
12. Malhotra R, Huilgol SC, Huynh NT, Selva D. The Australian Mohs database, part II: periocular basal cell carcinoma outcome at 5-year follow-up. Ophthalmology. 2004;111:631-6.
13. Smeets NW, Krekels GA, Ostertag JU, Essers BA, Dirksen CD, Nieman FH, et al. Surgical excision vs Mohs' micrographic surgery for basal-cell carcinoma of the face: randomised controlled trial. Lancet. 2004;364:1766-72.
14. van Loo E, Mosterd K, Krekels GA, Roozeboom MH, Ostertag JU, Dirksen CD, et al. Surgical excision versus Mohs' micrographic surgery for basal cell carcinoma of the face: a randomised clinical trial with 10 year follow-up. Eur J Cancer. 2014;50:3011-20.
15. Samarasinghe V, Madan V, Lear JT. Management of high-risk squamous cell carcinoma of the skin. Expert Rev Anticancer Ther. 2011;11:763-9.
16. Rowe DE, Carroll RJ, Day Jr CL. Prognostic factors for local recurrence, metastasis, and survival rates in squamous cell carcinoma of the skin, ear, and lip. Implications for treatment modality selection. J Am Acad Dermatol. 1992;26:976-90.
17. Leibovitch I, Huilgol SC, Selva D, Hill D, Richards S, Paver R. Cutaneous squamous cell carcinoma treated with Mohs micrographic surgery in Australia I. Experience over 10 years. J Am Acad Dermatol. 2005;53:253-60.
18. Brodland DG, Zitelli JA. Surgical margins for excision of primary cutaneous squamous cell carcinoma. J Am Acad Dermatol. 1992;27:241-8.

19. Angouridakis N, Kafas P, Jerjes W, Triaridis S, Upile T, Karkavelas G, et al. Dermatofibrosarcoma protuberans with fibrosarcomatous transformation of the head and neck. Head Neck Oncol. 2011;3:5.
20. Paradisi A, Abeni D, Rusciani A, Cigna E, Wolter M, Scuderi N, et al. Dermatofibrosarcoma protuberans: wide local excision vs. Mohs micrographic surgery. Cancer Treat Rev. 2008;34:728-36.
21. Lowe GC, Onajin O, Baum CL, Otley CC, Arpey CJ, Roenigk RK, et al. A comparison of Mohs micrographic surgery and wide local excision for treatment of dermatofibrosarcoma protuberans with long-term follow-up: the Mayo Clinic experience. Dermatol Surg. 2017;43:98-106.
22. Wetter R, Goldstein GD. Microcystic adnexal carcinoma: a diagnostic and therapeutic challenge. Dermatol Ther. 2008;21:452-8.
23. Leibovitch I, Huilgol SC, Selva D, Lun K, Richards S, Paver R. Microcystic adnexal carcinoma: treatment with Mohs micrographic surgery. J Am Acad Dermatol. 2005;52:295-300.
24. Chiller K, Passaro D, Scheuller M, Singer M, McCalmont T, Grekin RC. Microcystic adnexal carcinoma: forty-eight cases, their treatment, and their outcome. Arch Dermatol. 2000;136:1355-9.
25. Annest NM, Grekin SJ, Stone MS, Messingham MJ. Cutaneous leiomyosarcoma: a tumor of the head and neck. Dermatol Surg. 2007;33:628-33.
26. Humphreys TR, Finkelstein DH, Lee JB. Superficial leiomyosarcoma treated with Mohs micrographic surgery. Dermatol Surg. 2004;30:108-12.
27. Starling 3rd J, Coldiron BM. Mohs micrographic surgery for the treatment of cutaneous leiomyosarcoma. J Am Acad Dermatol. 2011;64:1119-22.
28. Iorizzo 3rd LJ, Brown MD. Atypical fibroxanthoma: a review of the literature. Dermatol Surg. 2011;37:146-57.
29. Ang GC, Roenigk RK, Otley CC, Kim Phillips P, Weaver AL. More than 2 decades of treating atypical fibroxanthoma at Mayo Clinic: what have we learned from 91 patients? Dermatol Surg. 2009;35:765-72.
30. Wick MR, Goellner JR, Wolfe 3rd JT, Su WP. Adnexal carcinomas of the skin. I. Eccrine carcinomas. Cancer. 1985;56:1147-62.
31. Robson A, Greene J, Ansari N, Kim B, Seed PT, McKee PH, et al. Eccrine porocarcinoma (malignant eccrine poroma): a clinicopathologic study of 69 cases. Am J Surg Pathol. 2001;25:710-20.
32. Riera-Leal L, Guevara-Gutierrez E, Barrientos-Garcia JG, Madrigal-Kasem R, Briseño-Rodríguez G, Tlacuilo-Parra A. Eccrine porocarcinoma: epidemiologic and histopathologic characteristics. Int J Dermatol. 2015;54:580-6.
33. Song SS, Wu Lee W, Hamman MS, Jiang SI. Mohs micrographic surgery for eccrine porocarcinoma: an update and review of the literature. Dermatol Surg. 2015;41:301-6.
34. Skowron F, Poulhalon N, Balme B, Touzet S, Thomas L. Primary eccrine porocarcinoma: a clinicopathological study of 50 cases. Ann Dermatol Venereol. 2014;141:258-64.
35. Tolkachjov SN, Hocker TL, Camilleri MJ, Baum CL. Treatment of porocarcinoma with Mohs micrographic surgery: the Mayo Clinic experience. Dermatol Surg. 2016;42:745-50.
36. Lam C, Funaro D. Extramammary Paget's disease: summary of current knowledge. Dermatol Clin. 2010;28:807-26.
37. Lee KY, Roh MR, Chung WG, Chung KY. Comparison of Mohs micrographic surgery and wide excision for extramammary Paget's Disease: Korean experience. Dermatol Surg. 2009;35:34-40.
38. Hendi A, Brodland DG, Zitelli JA. Extramammary Paget's disease: surgical treatment with Mohs micrographic surgery. J Am Acad Dermatol. 2004;51:767-73.
39. Higgins 2nd HW, Lee KC, Galan A, Leffell DJ. Melanoma in situ: part II. Histopathology, treatment, and clinical management. J Am Acad Dermatol. 2015;73:193-203; quiz-4.
40. King R. Lentiginous melanoma. Arch Pathol Lab Med. 2011;135:337-41.
41. Kallini JR, Jain SK, Khachemoune A. Lentigo maligna: review of salient characteristics and management. Am J Clin Dermatol. 2013;14:473-80.
42. Felton S, Taylor RS, Srivastava D. Excision margins for melanoma in situ on the head and neck. Dermatol Surg. 2016;42:327-34.
43. Bricca GM, Brodland DG, Ren D, Zitelli JA. Cutaneous head and neck melanoma treated with Mohs micrographic surgery. J Am Acad Dermatol. 2005;52:92-100.
44. Stigall LE, Brodland DG, Zitelli JA. The use of Mohs micrographic surgery (MMS) for melanoma in situ (MIS) of the trunk and proximal extremities. J Am Acad Dermatol. 2016;75:1015-21.
45. Que SK, Fraga-Braghiroli N, Grant-Kels JM, Rabinovitz HS, Oliviero M, Scope A. Through the looking glass: basics and principles of reflectance confocal microscopy. J Am Acad Dermatol. 2015;73:276-84.
46. Bennassar A, Vilata A, Puig S, Malvehy J. Ex vivo fluorescence confocal microscopy for fast evaluation of tumor margins during Mohs surgery. Br J Dermatol. 2014;170:360-5.
47. Venturini M, Gualdi G, Zanca A, Lorenzi L, Pellacani G, Calzavara-Pinton PG, et al. A new approach for presurgical margin assessment by reflectance confocal microscopy of basal cell carcinoma. Br J Dermatol. 2016;174:380-5.
48. Gareau DS, Karen JK, Dusza SW, Lorenzi L, Pellacani G, Calzavara-Pinton PG. Sensitivity and specificity for detecting basal cell carcinomas in Mohs excisions with confocal fluorescence mosaicing microscopy. J Biomed Opt. 2009;14:034012.
49. Dreier J, Dummer R, Felderer L, Nägeli M, Gobbi S, Kunstfeld R. Emerging drugs and combination strategies for basal cell carcinoma. Expert Opin Emerg Drugs. 2014;19:353-65.
50. Sekulic A, Von Hoff D. Hedgehog pathway inhibition. Cell. 2016;164:831.
51. Wolfe CM, Green WH, Cognetta Jr AB, Hatfield HK. Basal cell carcinoma rebound after cessation of vismodegib in a nevoid basal cell carcinoma syndrome patient. Dermatol Surg. 2012;38:1863-6.
52. Ally MS, Aasi S, Wysong A, Teng C, Anderson E, Bailey-Healy I, et al. An investigator-initiated open-label clinical trial of vismodegib as a neoadjuvant to surgery for high-risk basal cell carcinoma. J Am Acad Dermatol. 2014;71(5):904-11.
53. Alcalay J, Tauber G, Fenig E, Hodak E. Vismodegib as a neoadjuvant treatment to Mohs surgery for aggressive basal cell carcinoma. J Drugs Dermatol. 2015;14:219-23.
54. Sofen H, Gross KG, Goldberg LH, Sharata H, Hamilton TK, Egbert B, et al. A phase II, multicenter, open-label, 3-cohort trial evaluating the efficacy and safety of vismodegib in operable basal cell carcinoma. J Am Acad Dermatol. 2015;73:99-105.e1.
55. Stables G, Lawrence CM. Management of patients taking anticoagulant, aspirin, non-steroidal anti-inflammatory and other anti-platelet drugs undergoing dermatological surgery. Clin Exp Dermatol. 2002;27:432-5.

56. Guardiano RA, Grande DJ. A direct comparison of visual inspection, curettage, and epiluminescence microscopy in determining tumor extent before the initial margins are determined for Mohs micrographic surgery. Dermatol Surg. 2010;36:1240-4.
57. El Tal AK, Abrou AE, Stiff MA, Mehregan DA. Immunostaining in Mohs micrographic surgery: a review. Dermatol Surg. 2010;36:275-90.
58. Orchard GE, Wojcik K, Shams F, Georgaki E, Quaye CJ, Fernando P, et al. Pan-cytokeratin markers for rapid frozen section immunocytochemistry from head and facial Mohs cases of basal cell carcinoma: a comparison and evaluation to determine the marker of choice. Br J Biomed Sci. 2015;72:61-6.
59. Lawrence CM, Haniffa M, Dahl MG. Formalin-fixed tissue Mohs surgery (slow Mohs) for basal cell carcinoma: 5-year follow-up data. Br J Dermatol. 2009;160:573-80.
60. Turner RJ, Leonard N, Malcolm AJ, Lawrence CM, Dahl MG. A retrospective study of outcome of Mohs' micrographic surgery for cutaneous squamous cell carcinoma using formalin fixed sections. Br J Dermatol. 2000;142:752-7.
61. Essers BA, Dirksen CD, Nieman FH, Smeets NW, Krekels GA, Prins MH, et al. Cost-effectiveness of Mohs micrographic surgery vs surgical excision for basal cell carcinoma of the face. Arch Dermatol. 2006;142:187-94.
62. Bialy TL, Whalen J, Veledar E, Lafreniere D, Spiro J, Chartier T, et al. Mohs micrographic surgery vs traditional surgical excision: a cost comparison analysis. Arch Dermatol. 2004;140:736-42.
63. Cook J, Zitelli JA. Mohs micrographic surgery: a cost analysis. J Am Acad Dermatol. 1998;39:698-703.
64. Rutherford T, Elliott T, Vinciullo C. Mohs surgery in Australia: a survey of work practices. Australas J Dermatol. 2011;52:98-103.

ACS(I)
Textbook of
Cutaneous and Aesthetic Surgery

Under the Aegis of Association of Cutaneous Surgeons (I)

ACS(I) *Textbook of* Cutaneous and Aesthetic Surgery

Third Edition

Volume 2

Editor-in-Chief

Manas Chatterjee
MD DNB (Dermatology and Venereology)
Brigadier
Armed Forces Medical Services and
Consultant Dermatologist
Base Hospital Delhi Cantt
New Delhi, India

Associate Editor

Biju Vasudevan MD
Professor and Head
Department of Dermatology
Armed Forces Medical College
Pune, Maharashtra, India

Emeritus Editor

Mysore Venkataram
DVD MD DNB DipRCPath (London) FRCP (Glasgow) FISHRS
Consultant Dermatologist and
Hair Transplant Surgeon
Director
Venkat Charmalaya—Centre for
Advanced Dermatology and
Postgraduate Teaching Centre
Bengaluru, Karnataka, India

JAYPEE

JAYPEE BROTHERS MEDICAL PUBLISHERS

The Health Sciences Publisher

New Delhi | London

Editorial Board

Jaypee Brothers Medical Publishers (P) Ltd

Headquarters
Jaypee Brothers Medical Publishers (P) Ltd
EMCA House, 23/23-B
Ansari Road, Daryaganj
New Delhi 110 002, India
Landline: +91-11-23272143, +91-11-23272703
+91-11-23282021, +91-11-23245672
Email: jaypee@jaypeebrothers.com

Corporate Office
Jaypee Brothers Medical Publishers (P) Ltd
4838/24, Ansari Road, Daryaganj
New Delhi 110 002, India
Phone: +91-11-43574357
Fax: +91-11-43574314
Email: jaypee@jaypeebrothers.com

Overseas Office
JP Medical Ltd
83 Victoria Street, London
SW1H 0HW (UK)
Phone: +44 20 3170 8910
Fax: +44 (0)20 3008 6180
Email: info@jpmedpub.com

Website: www.jaypeebrothers.com
Website: www.jaypeedigital.com

ACS(I) Textbook of Cutaneous and Aesthetic Surgery (Volume 2)

First Edition: 2012

Reprint: 2013

Second Edition: 2017

Third Edition: **2024**

ISBN: 978-93-90595-83-9

Printed at: Samrat Offset Pvt. Ltd.

Contributors

Aakash Gupta
MD DNB FRGUHS (Dermatosurgery)
Consultant Dermatologist and Dermatosurgeon
Leelawanti Skin and Laser Institute
New Delhi, India

Aarti Sarda MD FAGE SCE (Dermatology)
Consultant Dermatologist
Wizderm—Specialty Skin and Hair Clinic
Kolkata, West Bengal, India

Abdul Latheef EN
DVD MD MSc (Psychology) FRCP (Glasgow)
Professor
Department of Dermatology and Venereology
Government Medical College
Kozhikode, Kerala, India

Abhishek De
MD FAGE SCE (Dermatology) FRCP (Edinburgh)
Consultant Dermatologist, Aesthetician and Laser Surgeon
Associate Professor
Calcutta National Medical College
Kolkata, West Bengal, India

Adit Mohan Garg MD (DVL)
Consultant Dermatosurgeon
Divya Alok Hospital
Kota, Rajasthan, India

Afreen Ayub MD DNB MRCP (SCE)
Assistant Professor
Department of Dermatology
INHS Kalyani
Visakhapatnam, Andhra Pradesh, India

Alka Goel MD DNB MNAMS
Consultant Dermatologist
Dr Alka Goel's Skin and Laser Clinic
New Delhi, India

Aman Dua MD (Dermatology)
Managing Director
AK Clinics Pvt Ltd
Ludhiana, Punjab, India

Ameet Dandale DNB
Consultant, DNB Teacher Gr-1, and Head
Department of Dermatology
Bharat Ratna Dr Babasaheb Ambedkar General Hospital
Mumbai, Maharashtra, India

Amit Kerure MD (DVL)
Consultant Dermatologist and Hair Transplant Surgeon
Dr Amit Kerure Skin Clinic
Navi Mumbai, Maharashtra, India

Amit Luthra DNB
Consultant Dermatologist
Ishira Skin Clinic
New Delhi, India

Aneesh Kunnath Parambath
MD (DVL)
Specialist Dermatology
Aster DM Healthcare
Dubai, UAE

Aniketh Venkataram
MS (General Surgery) MCH (Plastic Surgery)
Consultant Plastic Surgeon
The Venkat Center for Skin ENT and Plastic Surgery
Bengaluru, Karnataka, India

Anil Ganjoo MD
Founder Director and Consultant Dermatologist
Skinnovation Clinics
New Delhi, India

Anil K Garg
MS MCh MA (Yoga) FISHRS ABHRS
Plastic Surgeon and CEO
Rejuvenate Plastic and Hair Transplant Centre
Indore, Madhya Pradesh, India

Anirudha Gulanikar
MBBS DVD DNB (Skin and VD)
Professor
Department of Dermatology
MGM Medical College
Aurangabad, Maharashtra, India

Anjali Pal
MD (Dermatology, Venereology and Leprology)
Consultant Dermatologist
Navpreet Hospital
Amritsar, Punjab, India

Ankan Gupta MD MNAMS EBDVD
Associate Professor
Christian Medical College
Vellore, Tamil Nadu, India

Ankur Talwar MD
Professor and Head
Department of Dermatology
Hind Institute of Medical Sciences
Lucknow
Consultant Dermatologist
Talwar Skin Centre
Lucknow, Uttar Pradesh, India

Anuj Pall MD PhD FISD (USA)
Chief Director
Escallent Institute of Lasers and Aesthetic Medicine (EILAM)
Gurugram, Haryana, India

Anurag Tiwari DVD DNB
Director and Consultant Dermatologist
Center for Skin Disease and Laser Treatment
Bhopal, Madhya Pradesh, India

Anusha H Pai MD (Dermatology)
Consultant Dermatologist
Derma-Care
Mangaluru, Karnataka, India

AP Balaji MD (DVL)
Consultant Dermatologist and Dermatosurgeon
Bhairavi Skin and Hair Clinic
Chennai, Tamil Nadu, India

Apratim Goel MD DNB FAGE
Medical Director
Cutis Skin Solution
Mumbai, Maharashtra, India

Arpita Arghya MBBS DDVL
Consultant Dermatologist and Cosmetologist
Skinchime—Skin, Hair, and Cosmetic Clinic
Bengaluru, Karnataka, India

Arvind Poswal MBBS
Director
Dr A's Clinic Pvt Ltd
New Delhi, India

(Sqn Ldr) Aseem Sharma
MD DNB MBA FAGE IFAAD
Chief Dermatologist
Skin Saga Centre for Dermatology
Mumbai, Maharashtra, India

Ashique KT
MBBS DDVL PGDHS FRCP (London)
Medical Director and Senior Consultant Dermatologist
Amanza Skin Clinic
Malappuram, Kerala, India

Atul Bothra
MD (Dermatology, Venereology and Leprosy)
Fellow
Department of Dermatosurgery
CUTIS Academy of Cutaneous Sciences
Bengaluru, Karnataka, India

Avitus John Raakesh Prasad DDVL
Managing Director
SP Derma Center
Madurai, Tamil Nadu, India

Ayushi Bothra MD (Dermatology)
Consultant Dermatologist
Skinvest
Mumbai, Maharashtra, India

Banani Choudhury
MD DNB MNAMS
Consultant Dermatologist
Jaslok Hospital and Research Centre
Sir HN Reliance Foundation Hospital and Research Centre
Mumbai, Maharashtra, India

Bhanu Prakash MD DHM PGDMLE
Professor
Department of Dermatology
Vydehi Institute of Medical Sciences and Research Center
Bengaluru, Karnataka, India

Biju Vasudevan MD
Professor and Head
Department of Dermatology
Armed Forces Medical College
Pune, Maharashtra, India

Bipin Deshpande MBBS DVD IFAAD
Dermatologist, Dermatosurgeon
Cosmetic Dermatologist
Chaitanya Clinic
Pune, Maharashtra, India

BS Chandrashekar MD DNB
Chief Dermatologist and Medical Director
CUTIS Academy of Cutaneous Sciences
Bengaluru, Karnataka, India

C Shanmuga Sekar MD
Associate Professor
Department of Dermatology
PSG Hospitals
Coimbatore, Tamil Nadu, India

Chander Grover
MD DNB MNAMS
Professor
Department of Dermatology and STD
University College of Medical Sciences and GTB Hospital
New Delhi, India

Chintan Subhash Gujarathi
MS (General Surgery) MCh (Plastic and Reconstructive Surgery) DNB (Plastic and Reconstructive Surgery)
Consultant Plastic, Cosmetic and Reconstructive Surgeon
Ruby Hall Clinic
Pune, Maharashtra, India

CR Srinivas MD (DVL)
Professor
Department of Dermatology
Kalinga Institute of Medical Sciences
Bhubaneswar, Odisha, India

D Dinesh Kumar
MD FRCP (Glasgow, London)
Consultant Dermatologist and Head
Dr Dinesh's Skin and Hair Clinic
Chennai, Tamil Nadu, India

Davinder Parsad MD
Professor
Department of Dermatology
Postgraduate Institute of Medical Education and Research
Chandigarh, India

Debdeep Mitra
MD DNB (Dermatology)
Professor
Department of Dermatology
Command Hospital Air Force
Bengaluru, Karnataka, India

Deepak Jakhar MD
Consultant Dermatologist
Dermosphere Clinic
New Delhi, India

Dhanashree S Bhide MD DNB
Dermatologist, Venereologist and Leprologist
KEM Hospital
Deenanath Mangeshkar Hospital
Pune, Maharashtra, India

Dilip Kachhawa
MD (Dermatology, STD, and Leprosy)
Principal and Controller
Senior Professor
Dr SN Medical College
Jodhpur, Rajasthan, India

Dinkar Sreekumar
DrNB (Plastic and Reconstructive Surgery)
Associate Consultant
Baby Memorial Hospital
Kozhikode, Kerala, India

Dipali Rathod
DNB DDVL FIDD FIADVL (Dermatopathology) MNAMS
Assistant Professor
Seth GS Medical College and KEM Hospital
Mumbai, Maharashtra, India

Divya Gorur
MD (Dermatology) FRGUHS (Dermatosurgery)
Consultant Dermatology
Cosme Skin and Hair Clinic
Bengaluru, Karnataka, India

Eswari L
MDDVL FRGUHS (Dermatosurgery) FAADV (Dermatopathology)
Associate Professor
Bangalore Medical College and Research Institute
Bengaluru, Karnataka, India

Feroze Kaliyadan
MD DNB MNAMS FRCP (London)
Professor
Sree Narayana Institute of Medical Sciences
Ernakulam, Kerala, India

Ganesh S Pai MD DVD FAAD
Medical Director
Department of Dermatology
Derma-Care
Mangaluru, Karnataka, India

Gautam K Singh MD (Dermatology)
Professor
Base Hospital Delhi Cantt
Army College of Medical Sciences
New Delhi, India

Gillian Roga
MD DNB (Dermatology) Fellowship in Hair Transplantation and Cosmetology
Consultant Dermatology, Cosmetologist and Hair Transplant Surgeon
Dr Gillian's Skin, Hair, Laser and Cosmetology Clinic
Chikmagalur, Karnataka, India

Govind S Mittal
MD DVL FRGUHS (Dermatosurgery)
Consultant Dermatologist and Dermatosurgeon
Therapeia Skin Hair and ENT Centre
Bengaluru, Karnataka, India

Garehatty Rudrappa Kanthraj MD
Professor and Head
Department of Dermatology, Venereology and Leprosy
JSS Medical College and Hospital
JSS Academy of Higher Education (Deemed To Be University)
Mysuru, Karnataka, India

GR Rajput
MD (Dermatology, Venereology, and Leprosy)
Assistant Professor
Institute of Naval Medicine
INHS Asvini
Mumbai, Maharashtra, India

Gulhima Arora DNB MNAMS
Senior Consultant and Dermatologist
Mehektagul Dermaclinic
New Delhi, India

Gulshant Panesar
MD (Dermatology)
Associate Professor
Department of Dermatology
Santosh Medical College and Hospital
Ghaziabad, Uttar Pradesh, India

Gunjan Shah DDV
Director
iBrow Academy
Ahmedabad, Gujarat, India

Harish Prasad BR
MD (Dermatology) FRGUHS (Dermatosurgery)
Consultant Dermatosurgeon
Vitals Skin, Hair, Laser, Vitiligo Klinic
Bengaluru, Karnataka, India

Harsh Tahiliani
MD (Dermatology)
Consultant Dermatologist
Dr Tahiliani's Clinic
Visiting Consultant Dermatologist
Bhartiya Arogya Nidhi Hospital
Mumbai, Maharashtra, India

Harvinder S Marwah
MD DVD DDV MCPS
Consultant Dermatologist and Head
Dr Marwah's Skin, Hair, Laser, and Cosmetic Centre
Mumbai, Maharashtra, India

HM Omprakash MBBS DVD
Consulting Dermatologist
Department of Dermatology
Samastha Skin Clinic
Mysuru, Karnataka, India

Imran Majid
MD FRCP (Edinburgh)
Director
CUTIS Institute of Dermatology
Srinagar, Jammu and Kashmir, India

Indrashis Podder MD DNB MNAMS
Assistant Professor
Department of Dermatology
College of Medicine and Sagore Dutta Hospital
Kolkata, West Bengal, India

Ishmeet Kaur MD (Dermatology)
Assistant Professor
Department of Dermatology
NDMC Medical College and Hindu Rao Hospital
New Delhi, India

Jaishree Sharad MBBS DDV
Dermatologist
Skinfinitii Aesthetic Skin and Laser Clinic
Mumbai, Maharashtra, India

Jayadev B Betkerur MD
Professor
Department of Dermatology Venereology, and Leprosy
JSS Medical College and Hospital
JSS Academy of Higher Education (Deemed to be University)
Mysuru, Karnataka, India

Jayashree Venkataram FRCOG
Director
Venkat Charmalaya—Centre for Advanced Dermatology
Bengaluru, Karnataka, India

Jyoti Gupta MD
Consultant Dermatologist and Hair Transplant Surgeon
Dr Jyoti Gupta Dermatology Clinic
New Delhi, India

Kabir Sardana
MD DNB MNAMS
Director, Professor and Head
Department of Dermatology
Atal Bihari Vajpayee Institute of Medical Sciences and Dr Ram Manohar Lohia Hospital (PGIMER)
New Delhi, India

Kanika Sahni MD
Additional Professor
Department of Dermatology and Venereology
All India Institute of Medical Sciences
New Delhi, India

Kapil Dua
MS (ENT) Dip (ABHRS, USA) Diplomate of American Board of Hair Restoration Surgery
Chairman and Chief Hair Transplant Surgeon
AK Clinics
Ludhiana, Punjab, India
Imm Past President, ISHRS (USA)
Past President, AHRS (India)
Board Member
AAHRS Asia and ABHRS (USA)

Kavish Chouhan
MD (Dermatology)
Director
DermaClinix, KSK Surgicals, Expertified
New Delhi, India
Co-Founder, FUE Asia

KC Nischal
MD (Dermatology)
Chief Dermatologist and Director
Nirmal Skin and Hair Clinic
Bengaluru, Karnataka, India

KH Satyanarayana Rao
MD PGDMLE PGDHHM
Consultant Dermatologist
Central Health Service
Bengaluru, Karnataka, India

Koushik Lahiri
DVD (CAL) FIAD iFAAD FFAADV FRCP (Glasgow, Edinburgh, London)
Professor and Senior Consultant Dermatologist
Apollo Multispecialty Hospital
Honorary Medical Director
Wizderm Speciality Skin and Hair Clinic
Kolkata, West Bengal, India

Krishna Talukdar MD (Dermatology)
Professor and Head
Department of Dermatology
Jorhat Medical College and Hospital
Jorhat, Assam, India

Kshama Talwar MD
Associate Professor
Department of Dermatology
Hind Institute of Medical Sciences
Consultant Dermatologist
Talwar Skin Centre
Lucknow, Uttar Pradesh, India

Kumaresan M
MD FISHRS Diplomate American Board of Hair Restoration Surgery
Consultant Dermatologist
Cutis Skin Clinic and Hair Transplant Center
Coimbatore, Tamil Nadu, India

Kumudhini S
MD FAGE DNB FRGUHS
Chief Dermatologist
Deep Skin Dialogues
Chennai, Tamil Nadu, India

Laila Arif MBBS DVD
Consultant Dermatologist
Cutis Institute of Dermatology and Aesthetic Sciences
Kozhikode, Kerala, India

Lakshyajit D Dhami
MS (Gen Surg) MCh (Plastic Surg)
Consultant Cosmetic, Laser, and Plastic Surgeon
Mumbai, Maharashtra, India

(Late) Sanjeev Mulekar MD
Senior Consultant and Dermatologist
Mulekar Vitiligo Clinic
Mumbai, Maharashtra, India

Madhulika Mhatre MD FRGUHS
Director
Skin Saga Centre for Dermatology
Mumbai, Maharashtra, India

Madhuri Agarwal MD (Skin & VD) DDV
Consultant Dermatologist
Yavana Aesthetics Clinic
Mumbai, Maharashtra, India

Madura C
MD FRGUHS (Dermatosurgery)
Consultant Dermatologist and Dermatosurgeon
CUTIS Academy of Cutaneous Sciences
Bengaluru, Karnataka, India

Malavika Kohli MD DVD DNB
Director and Founder
Skin Secrets
Consultant Dermatologist
Jaslok Hospital and Research Centre
Breach Candy Hospital Trust
Mumbai, Maharashtra, India

Manas Chatterjee
MD DNB (Dermatology and Venereology)
Brigadier
Armed Forces Medical Services
Consultant Dermatologist
Base Hospital Delhi Cantt
New Delhi, India

Manish Gautam DVD DNB (Dermatology)
Chief Dermatologist
Skin Solutions, Vashi
Consultant Dermatologist
Apollo Hospitals
Navi Mumbai, Maharashtra, India

Manjit Sandhu Tahiliani DDVL
Consultant Dermatologist
Dr Tahiliani's Clinic
Mumbai, Maharashtra, India

Manjot Marwah
MD (Dermatology)
Consultant Dermatologist and Director
Dr Manjot's Clinic and LHR Clinic
Jalandhar, Punjab, India

Maya Vedamurthy
MD DD MAMS FRCP (Edinburgh, Glasgow)
Consultant Dermatologist
RSV Skin and Research Centre
Apollo Hospitals
Chennai, Tamil Nadu, India

Milind N Naik
MS (Ophthalmology)
Consultant Ophthalmologist
LV Prasad Eye Institute
Hyderabad, Telangana, India
Adjunct Professor
Department of Ophthalmology
University of Rochester
New York, USA

Milind S Wagh
MS (Gen Surg) MCh (Plastic Surg)
Consultant Plastic and Aesthetic Surgeon
Make A Change—A Centre for Cosmetic Surgery
Mumbai, Maharashtra, India

Mukta Sachdev
MD FAAD DpD(UK) DD (UK) FAAD (USA)
Head
Department of Dermatology
Manipal Hospital, Bengaluru
Medical Director
MS Skin Centre
MS Clinical Research Pvt Ltd
Bengaluru, Karnataka, India

Munish Paul
MD (Dermatology)
Consultant Dermatologist
Skin Laser Centre
Manipal Hospital
New Delhi, India

Murali Chakravarthy MD DA DNB
Director
Department of Anesthesia, Critical Care and Pain Relief
Director
Clinical Affairs
Fortis Hospitals
Bengaluru, Karnataka, India

Mysore Venkataram
DVD MD DNB DipRCPath (London) FRCP (Glasgow) FISHRS
Consultant Dermatologist and Hair Transplant Surgeon
Director
Venkat Charmalaya—Centre for Advanced Dermatology and Postgraduate Teaching Centre
Bengaluru, Karnataka, India

Nagendra Singh Beniwal
DNB (Dermatology)
Associate Professor
Department of Dermatology
Military Hospital
Jalandhar, Punjab, India

Naina Jain MD DVL
Assistant Professor
SGT Medical College
Gurugram, Haryana, India

Narendra Patwardhan
MD DV (London) DVD
Consultant Dermatologist
Joshi Hospital, Deenanath Mangeshkar Hospital
Pune, Maharashtra, India

Nazneen Arsiwala MD DVD
Co-Founder
Renewderm Skin, Hair, Laser and Aesthetics Centre, Mumbai
Consultant Dermatologist
Masina Hospital
Mumbai, Maharashtra, India

Neha Taneja MD DNB MRCP (SCE)
Consultant Dermatologist
DermaClinix—Hair Transplant and Skin Clinic
New Delhi, India

Nicholas J Collier
BM BS MSc MMedSci MD
Consultant Dermatologist and Mohs Surgeon
Mohs Unit
Department of Dermatology
Salford Royal Hospital NHS Foundation Trust
Northern Care Alliance NHS Group
Salford, England
Manchester, UK

Nikhil Mehta MD
Senior Resident
Department of Dermatology and Venereology
All India Institute of Medical Sciences
New Delhi, India

Nilesh N Goyal
MRCP UK DNB (Dermatology and Venereology) DVD SCS Dip IFAAD
Consultant Dermatosurgeon
Juvenis Clinic
Lilavati Hospital and Bombay Hospital
Mumbai, Maharashtra, India

Nirav V Desai DNB (Dermatology)
Dermatologist and Hair Transplant Surgeon
NISH (National Institute of Skin and Hair)
Skin Clinic and Hair Transplant Centre
Surat, Gujarat, India

Niteen V Dhepe
MD FAAD Fellow ASDS ASLMS EADV ISHRS IADVL ACSI
Medical Director
Skin City
The Postgraduate Institute of Dermatology Camp
Pune, Maharashtra, India

Niti Khunger MD DDV DNB
Head, Professor and Consultant Dermatologist
Department of Dermatology and STD
Vardhman Mahavir Medical College and Safdarjung Hospital
New Delhi, India

Nitika Deshmukh MD DNB
Consultant Dermatologist
Deenanath Mangeshkar Hospital
Pune, Maharashtra, India

Nitika Nijhara MD (Dermatology)
Consultant Dermatologist
BLK-Max Multi-Specialty Hospital
New Delhi, India

Pallavi Ailawadi MD DNB
Consultant Dermatologist
Skinacea Clinic
Faridabad, Haryana, India

Pankaj Das MD (Dermatology)
Assistant Professor
Armed Forces Medical College
Pune, Maharashtra, India

Pradeep Kumari MBBS DVD FCPS DNB
Dermatologist
Skin and Surgery International and Asia Institute of Hair Transplant
Pune, Maharashtra, India

Pradeep Sethi MD
Co-Founder
Eugenix Hair Sciences
Mumbai, Maharashtra, India

Pradyumna Vaidya MBBS DVD DNB
Consultant Dermatologist
Deenanath Mangeshkar Hospital and Jehangir Hospital
Pune, Maharashtra, India

R Jayashree DDVL
Consultant Dermatologist
Skin Hair and Nail Laser Clinic
Coimbatore, Tamil Nadu, India

R Raghunatha Reddy
MD DNB FRGUHS (Dermatosurgery)
Professor and Medical Director
Roots Institute of Dermatological Sciences
Bengaluru, Karnataka, India

Rachana Shilpakar MD
Consultant Dermatologist
Rainbow Children's Hospital
Bengaluru, Karnataka, India

Rachita Dhurat MD (Skin)
Professor and Head
Department of Dermatology
LTM Medical College and Hospital
Mumbai, Maharashtra, India

Rachita Talwar MD
Consultant Dermatologist
NMC Specialty Hospital
Al-Ain, UAE

Ragini Ghiya MD
Dermatologist and Hair Transplant Surgeon
Siddharth Hair Transplant Centre
Surat, Gujarat, India

Ragunatha S MD
Associate Professor
Department of Dermatology, Venereology and Leprosy
Sri Siddhartha Medical College
Tumkur, Karnataka, India

Rajat Kandhari MD MSc
Consultant Dermatologist
Dr Kandhari's Skin and Dental Clinic and Veya Aesthetics
New Delhi, India

Rajetha Damisetty MD (Dermatology)
Additional Medical Director
Oliva Hair and Skin Clinic
Hyderabad, Telangana, India

Rashi Pangti MD (Dermatology)
Assistant Professor
Lady Hardinge Medical College
New Delhi, India

Rashmi Sarkar MD FAMS IFAAD
Director Professor
Department of Dermatology
LHMC and Associated KSCH and SSK Hospital
New Delhi, India

Rasya Dixit MD (Dermatology)
Medical Director
Dr Dixit Clinic
Bengaluru, Karnataka, India

Ravina Surve MD (DVL) DNB (DVL)
Senior Resident
Kanachur Institute of Medical Sciences
Mangaluru, Karnataka, India

Reena Rai MD (DVL)
Professor and Head
Department of Dermatology
PSG Institute of Medical Sciences and Research
Coimbatore, Tamil Nadu, India

(Surg Cdr) Reetu Agarwal
DVD MD (Dermatology)
Professor
Base Hospital Delhi Cantt
New Delhi, India

Richa Kumar MD DNB (Dermatology)
Assistant Professor
Military Hospital
Pune, Maharashtra, India

Ridhima Lakhani MD DNB (Dermatology)
Consultant Dermatologist
Fortis Hospital
New Delhi, India

Rohit Batra MD
Consultant Dermatologist
Sir Ganga Ram Hospital
New Delhi, India

Roshni Singh MD
Senior Resident
Assam Medical College and Hospital
Dibrugarh, Assam, India

Ruchi Hemdani MD
Assistant Professor
Himalayan Institute of Medical Sciences
Dehradun, Uttarakhand, India

S Sacchidanand
MD (DVL) DVD DHA FRCP (Glasgow)
Executive Director
Siddaganga Medical College and Research Institute
Bengaluru, Karnataka, India
Vice Chancellor, RGUHS (2018–2021)

Sachin Dhawan MD DVD
Senior Consultant Dermatologist
Fortis Hospital, Gurugram
Director, Skin 'n Smiles
Gurugram, Haryana, India

Sadhana Deshmukh
DNB FCPS DDV (Dermatology and Venereology)
Founder and Medical Director
Dr Sadhana Deshmukh's Forever Young Skin Hair Laser Clinics, Bandra
PD Hinduja Hospital and Medical Research Centre, Khar
Mumbai, Maharashtra, India

Sandeep Arora MD
Professor and Head
Department of Dermatology
Army College of Medical Sciences and Base Hospital Delhi Cantt
New Delhi, India

Sanjay Bhalchandra Sane
MS (General Surgery)
Consulting Foot Surgeon
Joshi Hospital
Pune, Maharashtra, India

Sanjay Singh MD (Dermatology)
Consultant Dermatologist
Gorakhpur, Uttar Pradesh, India

Sanjeev Gupta MD DNB
Professor and Head
Department of Dermatology
MM Institute of Medical Sciences and Research
MMDU, Ambala, Haryana, India

Sanjeev J Aurangabadkar MD
Consultant Dermatologist
Dr Aurangabadkar's Skin and Laser Clinic
Hyderabad, Telangana, India

Satish S Savant MD FAMS FCPS DVD DDV
Director
The Humanitarian Clinic Skin Hair and Laser Center
Dr Savant's Institute of Dermatosurgery Cosmetology, Trichology and Laser Medicine
Mumbai, Maharashtra, India

Savita Yadav MD (Dermatology)
Consultant Dermatologist
Gurugram, Haryana, India

Savitha AS MD DNB FRGUHS
Professor
Sapthagiri Institute of Medical Sciences and Research Centre
Bengaluru, Karnataka, India

Seema Garg MBBS MSc FISHRS ABHRS
CEO, Rejuvenate Plastic and Hair Transplant Centre
Indore, Madhya Pradesh, India

Senkadhir Vendhan MD (Dermatology)
Specialist
Department of Dermatology
Dr Babasaheb Ambedkar Memorial Hospital (Central Railway)
Mumbai, Maharashtra, India

Seujee Das MD
Consultant Dermatologist
Apollo Clinic
Guwahati, Assam, India

Shashikumar BM
MD (DVL) FRGUHS (Dermatosurgery)
Associate Professor
Department of Dermatology
Mandya Institute of Medical Sciences
Mandya, Karnataka, India

Shehnaz Arsiwala MD DDV
Founder, Renewderm Skin, Hair, Laser, and Aesthetics Centre, Mumbai
Consultant Dermatologist
Saifee Hospital, Masina Hospital
Mumbai, Maharashtra, India

Shekhar Neema MD
Associate Professor
Department of Dermatology
Base Hospital
Lucknow, Uttar Pradesh, India

Shilpa K MD (Dermatology) DVL
Professor and Head
Bangalore Medical College and Research Institute
Bengaluru, Karnataka, India

Shital Poojary MD DNB
Professor and Head
Department of Dermatology
KJ Somaiya Medical College
Mumbai, Maharashtra, India

Shrenik Balegar MD (Dermatology)
Director
Cutibless—Skin and Hair Treatment Clinic
Former Consultant and Hair Transplant Surgeon
AK Clinics
Mumbai, Maharashtra, India

Shyamanta Barua MD (Dermatology)
Professor and Head
Department of Dermatology
Assam Medical College and Hospital
Dibrugarh, Assam, India

Siddharth Mani
MD (Dermatology)
Assistant Professor
Department of Dermatology
Indian Naval Hospital Ship (INHS)
Kochi, Kerala, India

Silonie Sachdeva MD FISD (USA)
Senior Consultant Dermatologist
Dr Silonie Skin and Laser Clinic
Amritsar, Punjab, India

Sindhuja T MD MRCP (SCE)
Consultant Dermatologist
Ankura Hospitals
Hyderabad, Telangana, India

Smriti Naswa MD (Skin VD)
Observer (IADVL)—Pediatric Dermatology
Consultant Dermatologist
Fortis Hospital
Mumbai, Maharashtra, India

Somesh Gupta MD
Professor
Department of Dermatology and Venereology
All India Institute of Medical Sciences
New Delhi, India

Somodyuti Chandra
MD (Gold Medalist) DNB MNAMS MRCP-SCE (UK) FRGUHS
Consultant Dermatologist
Medica Superspecialty Hospital
Kolkata, West Bengal, India

Sonal Bansal
MD (Dermatology, Venereology and Leprosy)
Dermatologist, Aesthetic Dermatologist
Dermaspace Skin Clinic
Gurugram, Haryana, India

Sonal Jain
MD DNB (Skin & VD) FRGUHS (Dermatosurgery)
Assistant Professor
Department of Skin and VD
ICARE Institute of Medical Science and Research
and Dr BC Roy Hospital, Haldia
Consultant Dermatologist and Hair Transplant Surgeon
Narayana Hospital
Kolkata, West Bengal, India

Soni Nanda
MD (Dermatology)
Founder and Director
Ojas Skin Care, New Delhi
Consultant
Max Hospitals
New Delhi, India

Shristi Shrestha
MD FRUGHS
Fellowship Student
Venkat Charmalaya—Centre for Advanced Dermatology
Bengaluru, Karnataka, India

Subodh Jane MD FRGUHS
Consultant Dermatologist
Skintotal Clinic
Amravati, Maharashtra, India

Sudarshan R
MD (Dermatology)
Assistant Professor
Department of Dermatology
SSPM Medical College and Lifetime Hospital
Sindhudurg, Maharashtra, India

Sujala S Aradhya MD
Consultant Dermatologist and Dermatosurgeon
Sujala Polyclinic and Laboratory
Bengaluru, Karnataka, India

Sujay Khandpur
MD DNB MNAMS
Professor
Department of Dermatology and Venereology
All India Institute of Medical Sciences
New Delhi, India

Sujit Shanshanwal MD
Consultant
SkinAmour Clinic
Mumbai, Maharashtra, India

Sunmeet Sandhu MD
Assistant Professor
Command Hospital
Bengaluru, Karnataka, India

Suraj Sachidanand MD MSEd
Specialist
Department of Dermatology
Manipal Hospital
Bengaluru, Karnataka, India

Surbhi Rajput
MD DNB (Dermatology and Venereology)
Graded Specialist Dermatology
Military Hospital
Meerut, Uttar Pradesh, India

Suresh Talwar MD
Medical Director and Consultant Dermatologist
Talwar Skin Centre
Lucknow, Uttar Pradesh, India

Sushil S Savant MD (Gold Medalist)
Assistant Director
The Humanitarian Clinic—Skin Hair and Laser Center
Dr Savant's Institute of Dermatosurgery Cosmetology, Trichology, and Laser Medicine, Mumbai, Maharashtra, India

Sushil Tahiliani MD (Dermatology) DVD
Director and Consultant Dermatologist
Dr Tahiliani's Clinic
Visiting Consultant Dermatologist
Hinduja Hospital
Mumbai, Maharashtra, India

Suvarna Samudrala MD
Consultant Dermatologist
Citrine Clinic
Gurugram, Haryana, India

Swapnil Shah MD (Dermatology)
Consultant Dermatologist
Private Clinic
Solapur, Maharashtra, India

T Salim MD DNB
Medical Director and Clinical Head
Cutis Institute of Dermatology and Aesthetic Sciences
Kozhikode, Kerala, India

Tanvi Dev MD DNB MRCP (SCE)
Assistant Professor
Department of Dermatology
Maulana Azad Medical College
New Delhi, India

Trupti Agrawal MD
Associate Dermatologist
Kokilaben Dhirubhai Ambani Hospital
Mumbai, Maharashtra, India

TS Nagesh MD
Professor and Head
Department of Dermatology, STD, and Leprosy
Sapthagiri Institute of Medical Sciences and Research Centre
Bengaluru, Karnataka, India

TS Vidya
MD FRGUHS (Aesthetic Dermatology)
Consultant Dermatologist and Cosmetologist
Sagar Hospitals and Skin and Cosmetic Clinic, Bengaluru, Karnataka, India

Tushar D Kshirsagar DNB (Dermatology)
Dermatologist and Hair Transplant Surgeon
Nuleaf Skin Clinic and Hair Transplant Centre
Pune, Maharashtra, India

Uday Kelkar
DIM MD (Microbiology)
Senior Chief Medical Officer
Senior Administrative Grade
In-Charge, Laboratories
Central Government Health Scheme
Pune, Maharashtra, India
Ministry of Health and Family Welfare
Government of India

Vaishalee Kirane
DVD DNB (Dermatology)
Dermatologist and Trichologist
Dr Vaishalee's Skin and Hair Clinic
Pune, Maharashtra, India

Venura Samarasinghe
MBChB MRCP (Dermatology)
Consultant Dermatologist and Mohs Surgeon
Department of Dermatology
St George's Hospital NHS Foundation Trust
London, UK

(Col) Vikas Pathania MD (Dermatology)
Professor and Head
Base Hospital
Lucknow, Uttar Pradesh, India

Vinay Saraf MD DVD
Senior Consulting Dermatologist
Dr Balabhai Nanavati Hospital and Research Centre
Mumbai, Maharashtra, India

Vishal Madan MD FRCP
Consultant Dermatologist, Laser, and Mohs Surgeon
Northern Care Alliance, Stott Lane
Salford, UK

Vishwanath Jigjinni MS FRCS
Head
Department of Plastic Surgery
Ruby Hall Clinic, Pune
Head
Department of Plastic Surgery
Indrayani Hospital and Cancer Institute
Pune, Maharashtra, India

Yogesh S Marfatia MD (Skin-VD)
Professor (Skin-VD)
SBKS Medical Institute and Research Centre
Vadodara, Gujarat, India

Zeba Chhapra DDVL
Consultant Dermatologist
CUTIS Skin Solution
Mumbai, Maharashtra, India

Message from President ACS(I)

The composite subspecialty of surgical, laser and aesthetic dermatology has grown by leaps and bounds in recent years. It is imperative for all concerned to keep abreast of the exponential expansion in new concepts and keep pace with the innovations in the subspecialty.

The third edition of this textbook is a comprehensive compendium that is well-illustrated with excellent clinical images and extensively covers the latest developments in the specified fields. It is hoped that this treatise will further embellish the composite subspecialty and be a handy reference for both practicing dermatosurgeons and residents in training.

I, on behalf of the Association of Cutaneous Surgeons (I) National Executive, thank all those who were involved in bringing out this edition of the textbook. My deepest appreciation for the hard work and sustained commitment of our Editor-in-Chief, Dr (Brig) Manas Chatterjee and Associate Editor, Dr (Col) Biju Vasudevan. I am grateful to all members of the Editorial Board and each and every author for their valuable contributions. My sincere thanks to M/s Jaypee Brothers Medical Publishers (P) Ltd, New Delhi, India, for their help in bringing out this edition.

Shyamanta Barua
Professor and Head
Department of Dermatology
Assam Medical College and Hospital
Dibrugarh, Assam, India
President, Association of Cutaneous Surgeons (I)

Preface to the Third Edition

The third edition of the *ACS(I) Textbook of Cutaneous and Aesthetic Surgery* was on the table very early after the second edition, since the sale of both the first and the second editions have been unprecedented. The progress made by the ACS(I) Textbook from the first to the second has been attempted to be maintained in the third edition. From 2020 when the project was envisioned and we were asked to chaperone the preparation of the third edition, it has been a roller-coaster journey, not in small measure impacted by the COVID-19 pandemic during which time, editorial assistance suffered due to obvious reasons. As happens during such a time, a large number of authors were impacted in various ways which affected their submission of chapters. Another thing that happened during that time was the slowing down of the reviewing process as reviewers were saddled with other responsibilities. With the loss of continuity, it became an uphill task getting everyone on board once we saw the back of the pandemic's worst phase and getting them to submit their material. However, at last we are ready with the book, which has now been rationalized to 140 chapters in 18 sections of two volumes for ease of navigation. A number of chapters, which were either felt to be superfluous at the current time or could be clubbed to avoid duplication of material, were reorganized to ensure a better experience for the reader. Most of the chapters have been revised by the original authors while some have been rewritten. A few new chapters have been added to keep-up with the recent advances in the field of procedural dermatology. A chapter format was prepared to attempt uniformity of all the chapters, which has been achieved to an extent.

With this textbook coming to its logical conclusion of publication, it has been a pleasure working with Dr (Colonel) Biju Vasudevan as always, for he has been the workhorse of this effort. The Emeritus Editor Dr Mysore Venkataram has always been at our side guiding and directing us in the right path. The Deputy and Assistant Editors have been tireless ensuring that the final product has the desired quality. I would fail in my duty if I do not sincerely appreciate the efforts of Dr (Lt Col) Shekhar Neema, already a star in the field of dermatologic surgery, who has been the backbone of the editorial effort. The members of the editorial board have been ever-ready to pitch in with their contribution.

I would sincerely thank the ACS(I) executive from 2020 till date who has been my pillars of strength and most understanding of the delays that this project has had to suffer due to unforeseen circumstances.

All at M/s Jaypee Publishers Medical Publishers (P) Ltd, New Delhi, India, from Shri Jitendar P Vij (Group Chairman), Mr Ankit Vij (Managing Director), Mr MS Mani (Group President), Ms Chetna Malhotra (Senior Director—Professional Publishing, Marketing, and Business Development), and Ms Nedup Denka Bhutia Pillai (Senior Development Editor), and the production team have been most tolerant of my schedules and have dovetailed their efforts to ensure a quality product.

I wish that this book is of benefit to those for whom it is intended, which is the budding dermatologic surgeons and procedural dermatologists of this country and elsewhere.

Jai Hind!

Manas Chatterjee

Preface to the First Edition

Dermatosurgery has been passing through interesting times, as disease dermatology paves the way for desire dermatology, as illness gets replaced by wellness and patients are replaced by clients—today's interventional dermatology seeks to dominate over armchair dermatology of yesterday. What we now have is a youthful, vibrant, fast-changing subspecialty. Change has been so striking over the last decade that, in some ways, dermatosurgery represents a Theseus' paradox, *"This is my grandfather's axe. My father replaced the shaft, and I put a new head on it. It is my grandfather's axe."*

Despite rapid progress, there have been few books in this field, especially focusing on brown skin, and the need for a comprehensive book, encompassing all the aspects of cutaneous surgery, lasers and aesthetics, has long been felt. Sensing this need, the Association of Cutaneous Surgeons (I) decided to bring out this book.

The rapidly changing profile, range, and scope of the subject, with multitudes of procedures being performed, necessitated a multi-authored book. Fortunately, our association is blessed with the talent that was needed for authoring the chapters—the result is what you see; an exhaustive compilation with 66 chapters, including nearly 33 subchapters, by as many as 105 authors. Every aspect of cutaneous surgery has been comprehensively dealt with, keeping in mind the recent advances.

The brown skin has many peculiarities and variations—in fact, it defies any classification! Pigmentation response, healing and scarring reactions, aging changes are all different in the brown skin. Similarly, the epidemiological situations are also different; vitiligo surgery is more relevant than skin cancer surgery! The textbook aptly seeks to address these challenges and requirements.

Our effort has been to keep the book comprehensive, yet simple; to make the book all-inclusive, yet reader-friendly; exhaustive and yet relevant—to the beginner and the expert, the novice, and the connoisseur. We hope that we have succeeded in achieving this objective.

Writing a book is an experience, exhilarating at times, excruciating at others. And, in a multi-authored book, it is even more so, as deadlines are chased furiously and frenetically. Despite the highs and the lows, I must say the experience has been something to cherish—it has been my privilege to have been the Editor-in-Chief for this effort—and on behalf of the editorial board, I thank each author for his contribution. It truly has been a **great work done by a number of smaller things together!**

I was indeed fortunate to have an experienced editorial board of senior dermatosurgeons, available at all times for counsel and advice. My heartfelt gratitude to each one of them. And I record with a touch of pride and happiness the splendid work done by my young team of Deputy and Assistant editors, who toiled for long hours in correcting proofs, and drafts. The book would not have been possible without their long endeavors.

Lastly, an effort of this size is never possible without the support and understanding from the family—my wife Dr Jayashree, my son Aniketh (both of whom contributed as authors) and daughter Ankitha (who supported silently)—my heartfelt thanks to them.

M/s Jaypee Brothers Medical Publishers (P) Ltd have done an outstanding work in bringing it out on time—in particular, my thanks to Shri Jitendar P Vij (CEO), Ms Sunita Katla (PA to CEO), Ms Shagufta Khan (Executive Assistant to MD), Mr Sumit Kumar and Mr Ram Murti (Graphic Designers), Ms Geeta Srivastava and Laxmidhar Padhiary (Proofreaders) and Mr Venugopal (Branch Manager). My gratitude to them.

I earnestly hope that the book will be appreciated by the readers, and welcome comments and feedback. My earnest hope is that the book will serve as an instrument in furthering progress in the field, and *the grandfather's axe shall improve further!*

Mysore Venkataram

Contents

Volume 1

Section 1: Basic Principles of Cutaneous Surgery

Section 2: Standard Surgical Techniques

Section 3: Heat and Cold Energy-based Procedures

Section 4: Needle-based Basic Procedures

Section 5: Vitiligo Surgery

Section 9: Miscellaneous Surgical Procedures

Volume 2

Section 10: Hair Transplantation Surgery

Section 11: Aesthetic Procedures: Basics

Section 12: Chemical Peels

Section 13: Injectables

Section 14: Liposuction

Section 15: Lasers

SECTION 10

Hair Transplantation Surgery

CHAPTER 64 The History of Hair Transplantation

Aniketh Venkataram, Mysore Venkataram

KEY MESSAGES

History of hair restoration is replete with hits and misses and several discoveries have been ignored only to be rediscovered later:

- Norman Orentreich is heralded as the father of modern hair transplantation.
- Japanese pioneers had done great work in hair transplantation, the famous among is Shoji Okuda.
- The anatomical and histological concept of follicular unit was described by Headington in 1984.
- The concept of follicular unit transplantation (FUT) was introduced by Bernstein and Rassman.
- Technique of trichophytic closure was described by Drs Patrick Prechet, Paul Rose, and Mario Marzola.
- The FOX procedure/follicular unit extraction (FUE) is credited to Bernstein and Rassman.
- Introduction of robot is another important milestone.

Those who forget history are condemned to repeat it.

INTRODUCTION

History of hair transplantation makes for fascinating reading. It is replete with missed opportunities and wrong choices and rediscovery of the old. This chapter outlines the major milestones in the evolution of hair transplantation.

The history of alopecia and hence the search for a treatment is nearly as old as the history of mankind. The earliest mention of treatment options for alopecia can be found in the Ebers Papyrus of ancient Egypt, circa 1500 BC. It has evolved through different eras: era of punch grafting, mini- and micrografting, strip [follicular unit transplantation (FUT)], follicular unit extraction (FUE), and robotics.

ERA OF PUNCH GRAFTS

The origins of hair transplantation as we know it today can be traced back to the early twentieth century **(Figs. 1A to C)**. The New York dermatologist, *Norman Orentreich is heralded as the father of modern hair transplantation* due to his pioneering work in the 1950s. Orentreich was investigating whether common skin conditions showed donor or recipient site dominance when he discovered that grafts transplanted from occipital scalp survived on bald scalp. He coined the term *donor dominance* to explain this basic principle of hair transplantation which is that hair transplanted to a balding area will continue to grow as if it were in its original location. He first performed hair transplant surgery in 1952 by harvesting hair in groups with 4-mm punch. His paper was initially rejected by a skeptical medical community but was eventually published in 1959 in the Annals of the New York Academy of Sciences.[1]

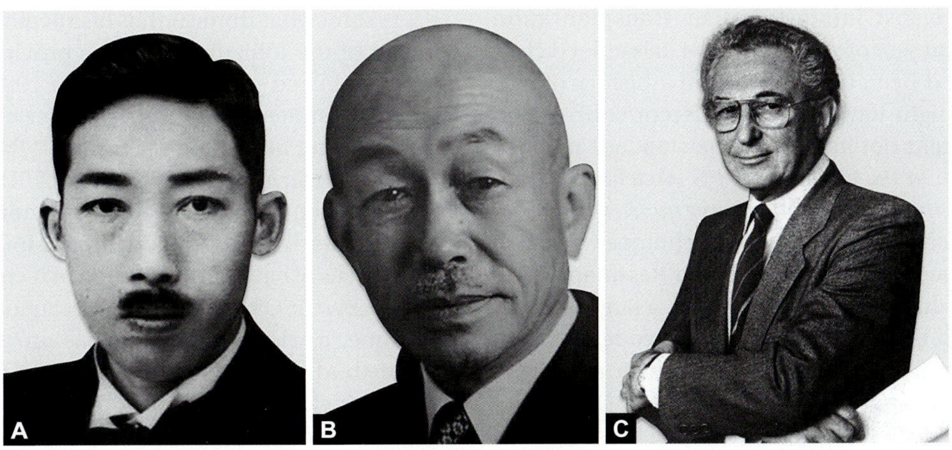

Figs. 1A to C: (A) Dr Shoji Okuda; (B) Dr Hajime Tamura; (C) Dr Norman Orentreich.

As we now know, several Japanese dermatologists were using small autografts for treating alopecia even before Orentreich. *The fallout of World War II prevented these works, originally written in Japanese, from reaching the western world for several years.* These dermatologists included Sasagawa,[2] Okuda, Tamura, and Fujita. Perhaps the most famous of these is *Shoji Okuda*. He published a series of article in the Japanese journal of dermatology entitled "Clinical and Experimental Study of Living Hair Transplantation" in the year 1939 (nearly 20 years before Orentreich).[3] He reported nearly 200 cases and his technique included special round saws which were very similar to Orentreich's punches. Okuda's papers contained most of the principles of modern hair transplantation but he did not mention male pattern hair loss (MPHL) as a treatable condition, which is perhaps why Orentreich is credited with being the first to use this technique for MPHL.

ERA OF MINI- AND MICROGRAFTS

Orentreich's 4-mm punch grafting technique remained the basic procedure till 1975. The benefits of using smaller grafts had occurred to several practitioners, but at the time, there was no satisfactory method to harvest smaller grafts and the dominant influence of Orentreich as a dermatosurgeon was growing. This meant that results were frequently punctuated with an unnatural dolls' hair look. In the 1980s, smaller grafts were prepared by dissecting the punch grafts into halves or quarters. The technique evolved further with Carlos Uebel in Brazil[4] and the Moser Clinic in Vienna,[5] who harvested a donor strip that was then dissected into grafts containing 3–7 hairs. *Mini- or micrografting ultimately signaled the end of punch grafting.*

In hindsight, it is highly regrettable that the work of *Hajime Tamura* of Japan was not known to the western world earlier. He performed many hair transplant procedures in Tokyo. He reported good results starting from 1939.[6] What is most remarkable is how closely his procedure resembled modern hair transplantation. He harvested donor grafts with an elliptical incision, prepared recipient site with a thick needle, stored grafts in saline, and observed postoperative shedding. Most importantly, he advocated that single hair grafts produced better results than larger grafts. Unfortunately, he seems to have lost interest in hair transplantation after becoming professor of urology in 1944. It is indeed clear that if his work had been better known, the history of hair transplantation might have taken a different course, and punch grafting might not have been the standard practice for nearly 30 years. *In the words of Sir PG Wodehouse, "Half the world doesn't know how the other three quarters lives!"*

A major advance occurred when the technique was taken a step further by surgeons such as William Rassman of Los Angeles who introduced mega sessions with a large number of technicians.[7] To hasten dissection, multiblade knives of up to ten blades were developed. Other automatic dissection devices included those of Boudjema in France (1992) and Tony Maugubat in 1996.[8] The problem with all these devices, however, was that they were often difficult to use and more importantly caused injury to follicles (sometimes in the range of 25%). Gradually, multibladed knifes were abandoned.

One of the most important steps in hair transplantation was introduction of *microscope-aided dissection.* This was initially started by Bob Limmer of Texas in 1987,[9] and popularized by others such as Seager in 1996.[10] This stereomicroscopic dissection of grafts became so ubiquitous in hair transplantation that it is now impossible to imagine the technique without a microscope.

ERA OF FOLLICULAR UNIT TRANSPLANTATION

With microscopic dissection, *the concept of "follicular unit transplantation"* was born. This concept recognized the "existence and utility of hairs in naturally occurring groups" and the term FUT was *coined by Bernstein and Rassman* in 1995.[11] Initially, FUT was met with resistance by members of the hair transplant community, as it was perceived as difficult and time-consuming. However, it gained popularity, mainly through increased patient demand, fueled by improved results being posted on the internet. By 2000, it was regarded as the gold standard of surgical hair transplantation. The popularity of FUT ushered in the concept of the hair transplant team, as it was no longer possible for one surgeon to complete the entire procedure by himself.

At the same time, the technique was also developing in Asia. The most significant of these developments was the implanter developed by Choi et al. of South Korea, reported in 1996.[12] This was an ingenious device into which units containing 1–4 hairs could be loaded and implanted into the scalp with a plunger. A similar implanter was developed by Jung Chul Kim, also of South Korea. Choi and Kim also recognized the units as bundles (or units as known in the west). As hair transplantation grew in popularity, it was natural that the procedure was tried in areas of the body other than the scalp, such as eyebrows, chest, and pubic region. This led Hwang to study *the effect of recipient site influence on hair follicles,* and he concluded that the recipient site does affect the characteristics of transplanted hair, including their growth and survival rates.[13]

It is somewhat ironical that histological evidence for the concept of the follicular unit was provided in a landmark paper published earlier, as early as 1984 by Headington, who demonstrated the units in biopsies of scalp which were examined after horizontal sectioning.[14] Rassman, Bernstein, and Kim who developed the concept of FUT were unaware of this paper when they developed their technique. History of hair transplantation is thus replete with such missed opportunities.

The focus of hair transplantation in recent years has shifted to the donor scar. Often, despite all precautions and a meticulous technique, a wide donor scar was an undesirable result. One method to offset this problem was the technique of trichophytic closure, described by Drs Patrick Prechet, Paul Rose, as well as Mario Marzola.[15,16] In this procedure, one of the wound edges is deepithelialized so that hair grows through the scar.

ERA OF FOLLICULAR UNIT EXTRACTION

However, as donor scars were still unacceptable to many, *the technique of removing follicular unit grafts individually by punches instead of using a donor strip, once again became popular—the wheel was reinvented.* Known as the FOX procedure, FUE and FUSE (follicular unit separation extraction), this technique is credited to Bernstein and Rassman for their paper in 2002 **(Figs 2A and B)**.[17] FUE was first attempted by Rassman in the 90s, but he was unsuccessful due to high rate of follicular damage. It was when the work of Masumi Inaba was brought to his attention, that the technique was perfected. Inaba solved the problems that Rassman was encountering by advocating that follicular damage could be reduced by cutting only partially into the dermis. However, here too there was a missed opportunity. Dr Woods from Australia was the first one to harvest single follicular units in 1995, and presented his technique to the Australian Medical Association. However, he failed to produce a paper in a widely read journal, describing his methods.[18]

This technique of FUE shows that the technique of hair transplantation has come full circle in a sense, back to the days of individual graft harvest (albeit follicular unit grafts instead of larger punch grafts).

ERA OF ROBOTICS

More recently, in order to address the main drawback of FUE which is its time-consuming nature, robotic devices have been developed to harvest follicular units. One such device is the ARTAS robotic system by Restoration Robotics Inc, San Jose, CA, which received Food and Drug Administration (FDA) approval in 2011. This system extracts follicular units one at a time, using a 6-axis articulated robotic arm, with stereo cameras and force sensors. This system shows promising results and is improving with new generation of robotics **(Box 1)**.[19]

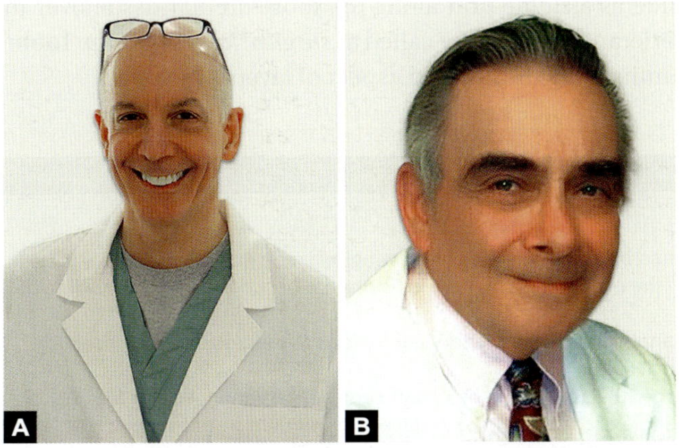

Figs. 2A and B: (A) Dr Robert Bernstein; (B) Dr William Rassman.

BOX 1: Timeline.

- *Pre-World War II:* Sasagawa,[2] Okuda, Tamura, and Fujita's works
- *1950s:* Orentreich's pioneering work, coined term donor dominance
- *1980s:* Mini- or micrografting using donor strips
- *Early 1990s:* Microscope-aided dissection
- *Late 1990s:* Follicular unit transplantation
- *In 1996:* Choi implanters
- *2000s:* Follicular unit extraction
- *2010s:* Robotic surgery

CONCLUSION

This fascinating history of hair transplantation surgery highlights the need to study the techniques used in the past, in order to drive the advances of the future. After all, to paraphrase Sir Isaac Newton, *"If we can see far, it is because we stand on the shoulders of giants".*

REFERENCES

1. Orentreich N. Autografts in alopecias and other selected dermatological conditions. Ann NY Acad Sci. 1959;83:463.
2. Sasagawa M. Hair transplantation (in Japanese). Jpn J Dermatol. 1923;30:493.
3. Okuda S. Clinical and experimental studies on hair transplanting of living hair. Jpn J Dematol Urol. 1939;46: 537-87 (in Japanese)
4. Uebel C. 1000 grafts per session. Hair Transplant Forum. 1992;3:9-12.
5. Hugeneck J, Kokott R. Non-tufted incisional slit grafting. Hair Transplant Forum 1992;3:6-7.
6. Tamura H. Pubic hair transplantation. Jpn J Dermatol. 1943;53:76.
7. Rassman W. Mega-transplants in transition. Hair Transplant Forum. 1993;3:11.
8. Boudjema P, Boolauch SJ. Automated hair transplant system. In: Stough DB, Haber R (Eds). Hair Replacement Surgical and Medical. Philadelphia: Mosby; 1996. pp. 370-4.
9. Limmer R. Bob Limmer does it all one hair at a time. Hair Transplant Forum Int. 1991;2:8-9.
10. Seager D. Binocular stereoscopic dissection microscopes-should we all be using them? Hair Transplant Forum Int. 1996;6:2-5.
11. Bernstein R. Follicular transplantation. Int J Aesth Restor Surg. 1995;3:119-32.
12. Choi JC, Kim JC. The Choi hair transplanter. In: Stough DB, Haber R (Eds). Hair Replacement Surgical and Medical. Philadelphia: Mosby; 1996. pp. 125-7.
13. Hwang S, Kim JC, Ryu HS, Cha YC, Lee SJ, Na GY, et al. Does the recipient site influence the hair growth characteristics in hair transplantation? Dermatol Surg. 2002;28:795-8.
14. Headington JT. Transverse microscopic anatomy of the human scalp. A basis for a morphometric approach to disorders of the hair follicle. Arch Dermatol. 1984;120(4):449-56.
15. Frechet P. Donor harvesting with invisible scars. Hair Transplant Forum Int. 2005;15(4):119-20.
16. Marzola M. Trichophytic closure of the donor area. Hair Transplant Forum Int. 2005;15(4):113-6.
17. Rassman WR, Bernstein RM. Follicular unit extraction. Minimally invasive surgery for hair transplantation. Dermatologic Surgery. 2002;28:720-8.
18. Williams KL Jr. Current practices and controversies in cosmetic hair restoration. Dermatol Surg. 2013;39:797-801.
19. Shin JW, Kwon SH, Kim SA, Kim JY, Na JI, Park KC, et al. Characteristics of robotically harvested hair follicles in Koreans. J Am Acad Dermatol. 2015;72(1):146-50.

CHAPTER 65

Applied Aspects and Approach to a Patient of Androgenetic Alopecia for Hair Transplantation

BS Chandrashekar, Madura C, Atul Bothra

KEY MESSAGES

- Androgenetic alopecia needs a thorough understanding of the needs of the patient and proper understanding of scalp anatomy and physiology are vital for hair restoration surgeries.
- After assessing the patient's global appearance, the hair and scalp are evaluated, aided by a hair-pull test, hair-card test, hair mount, trichoscopy, video dermoscopy and trichogram.
- Counseling the patient with respect to the disease process, possible effects, and adverse effects of the medications along with the probable expected outcome plays a vital role.
- Depending on the type, grade, and severity of hair loss, the management options such as drugs, surgery are decided.

INTRODUCTION

Androgenetic alopecia (AGA) is the most common cause of hair loss, affecting approximately 50% of population. Though medically benign condition it causes significant psychosocial impact on patients. The early recognition and treatment prevent the distress and have better treatment outcome. This chapter will highlight relevant anatomy, applied importance, diagnosis and organized approach to the patient with AGA.

RELEVANT ANATOMY

Thorough understanding of scalp anatomy and its innate characteristics are vital to any successful surgical procedure performed on the scalp and thus crucial for hair restoration surgeons. The scalp anatomy is discussed in detail in chapter regional anatomy, here relevant applied aspects with respect to hair transplantation are discussed.

Layers of the Scalp

The scalp is composed of five distinct layers. These layers are often referred to by the acronym SCALP: *Skin, subcutaneous layer, aponeurotica (galea), loose connective tissue, and pericranium.* The first three layers are bound together and glide as a single unit along the loose areolar tissue over the pericranium, together called as *surgical layers of scalp.* **Table 1** summarizes the applied aspect of layers of scalp.

TABLE 1: Surgical ramifications of scalp anatomy.

Layer	*Applied importance*
Skin: The hair follicle and adnexal structures course through these layers. Its thickness varies from 3 mm at vertex to 8 mm at the occiput	• The incisions on the scalp should be closed vertically following relaxed skin tension lines (RSTLs) **(Figs. 1A and B)**, except for in the occipital area where incisions are best horizontal, paralleling the skin crease lines. • Scalp incisions must be at an angle and parallel to the hair follicles to minimize their transection and to avoid localized scarring alopecia • Angularity of hair follicle and the direction of the hair shaft can change within 2 cm or less. Also it is important to note that the angle of the hair at the surface is usually slightly different at the level of the fat and dermis. This knowledge helps in harvesting follicular unit extraction (FUE) grafts with minimal transactions and also while performing coronal slits
Subcutaneous layer: It consists of a network of fibrous septa which divides it into multiple compartments and binds down the skin to the muscle and aponeurosis. The main arteries, veins, lymphatics, and nerves of the scalp are located at the bottom of this layer just above the galea. The dissection in this plane is difficult and bloody	• The sheets of connective tissue in second layer, bind the blood vessels to the dermis and fibrous septae in such a way that vasoconstriction and vasospasms are prevented when a vessel is cut. Thus, profuse bleeding that can be observed during surgery • Extensive undermining done blindly will traumatize blood vessels and nerves • A good tumescent anesthesia, manual compression and coagulation and ligation are most effective way of controlling bleeding • Anesthetic fluid must be deposited in this layer during scalp block

Contd...

Contd...

Layer	*Applied importance*
Galea aponeurotica: It extends as a fibrous sheet over the vertex area, connects the occipitalis posteriorly to the frontalis anteriorly. Laterally, the aponeurosis blends with the temporal fascia. The tensile strength of this layer makes it useful when suturing various types of scalp reduction, flap procedures, and strip harvesting in donor zone	• Galea is substantially stronger and site to secure retaining sutures • It is the anchoring point during artificial hair implantation • The galea is resistant to stretch and the top of the galea is strongly adherent to the subcutaneous layer, making dissection between these two layers extremely difficult and bloody • In deeper wounds, galea must be reapproximated properly by grabbing a large bite of galea with the suture needle to minimize tension resulting in a good scar. Wounds superficial to the aponeurosis gape less because aponeurosis holds the skin tight
Subgaleal layer: A relatively avascular space, allows for the free movement of the scalp	• Surgical dissection of the subgaleal space does not compromise the blood supply to scalp tissue in any way. The subgaleal layer lends itself to easy avascular dissection during scalp reduction surgeries • The emissary veins connect surface of scalp to the brain, infections in the subgaleal layer might communicate to the intradural venous sinus (thus also known as dangerous layer of scalp) • The space extend beneath the orbicularis oculi and into the eyelids and root of the nose, hematoma may spread and lead to black eye. This gives the answer for developing forehead and periorbital edema post-hair transplant (HT) when there is injection of lot tumescence fluid into this layer in spite of skin and subcutaneous tissue
Pericranium: This is the periosteum that is attached to the skull and is the deepest layer of the scalp	The pericranium is a dense membranous or fibrous sheet loosely fused on its outer aspect to the galea aponeurotica, from which it is readily separable via the subgaleal space

Neurovascular Supply

Scalp receives blood supply through three branches of the external carotid artery: (1) the superficial temporal artery, (2) the posterior auricular artery, and (3) the occipital artery; and two branches from the internal carotid artery—the end branches of the ophthalmic artery: (1) the supratrochlear artery; and (2) the supraorbital artery. Most scalp veins follow the arterial network and drain into the jugular system. Emissary veins perforate the skull and drain into the dural venous sinuses. It is important to understand the sensory pathways of the scalp because procedures such as hair restoration surgeries are often performed under local anesthesia with field or nerve blocks. The sensory innervation is primarily derived from the three divisions of the trigeminal nerve: ophthalmic, maxillary, and mandibular. The motor nerve supply is primarily by branches of the facial nerve. The lymphatic fluid from the scalp drains into the pericervical complex of lymphatics, consisting of the submental, submandibular, mastoid, parotid, and occipital nodes. The drainage from those nodes enters into the deep cervical lymph nodes **(Fig. 2 and Box 1)**

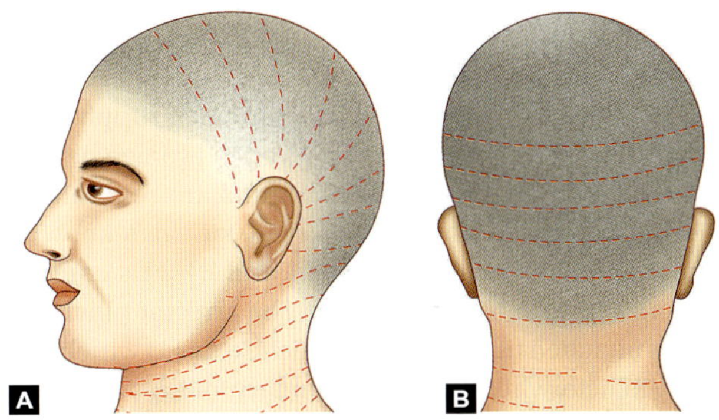

Figs. 1A and B: Relaxed skin tension lines (RSTLs) of scalp.

Scalp Laxity

Careful evaluation of the donor area is crucial when planning hair transplantation. The scalp laxity, elasticity, and glidability are important factors in this assessment. It expedites the choice of a suitable surgical method, preoperative planning, and prediction of surgical outcome.

The extent of surgical scalp excision possible is dependent on the laxity of the scalp. The more lax the tissue, the greater is the surgical excision. It is one of the limiting factors in donor strip harvest and is a function of two components—first, the ability of the scalp to slide or glide on the underlying pericranium. It is known as glidability. This is facilitated by the loose fibroareolar tissue in the subgaleal compartment, which allows the scalp to be moved on the cranium, often for a distance of several centimeters.[1] Second, elasticity of the scalp, i.e., the ability to extend or stretch (stretchability or extensibility). It depends on the viscoelastic properties of the scalp skin and is more relevant to wound closure. Both of these factors are subjected to individual variations either in loose fibroareolar tissue or in content of elastic tissue, this explains why some scalps are tight and some are loose and stretch better. Scalp laxity is defined as the sum of elasticity and glidability. Strip surgery within the range of glidability will result in a complication free surgery. In patients with hyperelastic skin, scar widening can occur, as explained by the laxity paradox.[2]

Follicular Unit

Hair follicles naturally grow in units of one to four hairs known as hair follicular unit (FU). The term was first described by Headington in 1984.[3] A follicular unit consists of 1–4 terminal

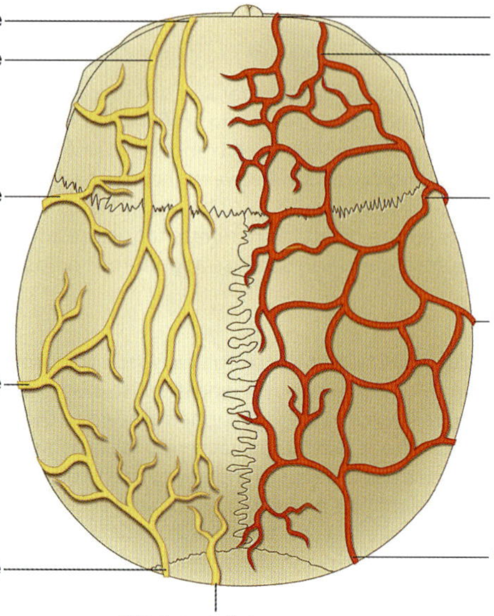

Fig. 2: Neurovascular supply of the scalp.
Source: Reproduced from Wells MD, Skytta C. Scalp and forehead reconstruction. In: Neligan P, Rodriguez ED (Eds). Plastic Surgery, 3rd edition. London: Elsevier Saunders; 2013.

hairs, with their arrector muscle, sebaceous gland, 1–3 vellus hairs, perifollicular collagen, nerves and vessels supplying the unit. FU density on the scalp is believed to average between 75 and 100 FU/cm^2. Two follicular units are separated by 1–1.5 mm of normal non-hair-bearing skin, also known as the interfollicular distance **(Figs. 3A and B)**. FUs comprise of a primary and secondary follicle. The arrector pili muscle (APM) is attached tightest to one follicle in an FU which is the primary follicle, while multiple secondary follicles arise distal to the APM. In contrast, hairs over the beard, trunk, and limbs do not give rise to secondary hairs and exist singly or in groups of 3, known as Meijeres trios.[4] There is a hierarchy of androgen responsiveness within FU, with preferential miniaturization of secondary follicles. The secondary follicles miniaturize first followed by the primary follicle.

Anatomical Divisions of Hair Follicle (Fig. 4)

The hair follicle is anatomically divided into an upper, middle and lower region. These three regions are respectively termed the infundibulum, the isthmus, and the inferior segment. The infundibulum and isthmus comprise the permanent portions of the hair follicle while the inferior segment is transient and undergoes cyclical regeneration.

Infundibulum: The upper region, or infundibulum, of the follicle consists of the area from the opening of the sebaceous duct to the follicular opening on the surface of the skin. It contains the fully formed hair shaft as it exits the epidermis. The epithelium of the epidermis is contiguous with the wall of the infundibulum.

Isthmus: The middle region, or isthmus, begins at the opening of the sebaceous duct and continues down until it reaches the insertion of the AP muscle. At the level of the insertion of the AP muscle is the bulge area. The bulge, considered a part of the outer root sheath (ORS), contains follicular stem cells that are critical for the regeneration of the FU. The bulge area appears to be inundated with nerve endings, as well as Merkel cells. Such a network may be involved in providing signals for hair growth and cycling. APM plays an important role in maintaining follicular integrity by holding together each of the hair follicles in the follicular unit at the isthmus level.

BOX 1: Applied aspects of neurovascular supply.

- All nerves and vessels of the scalp originate below the level of the brow as it is extended circumferentially around the scalp following centripetal distribution from periphery to center and the rich anastomoses between them explains why scalp flaps survive well. Also this anatomical location of the arteries and nerves of the scalp makes central scalp surgeries easy with minimal neurovascular trauma. The incisions in the peripheral scalp can transect nerve trunks and result in large areas of permanent hypoesthesia, a complication that can be avoided or explained to the patient if one is familiar with the anatomical locations of these nerves
- There is relative loss of vascular network and decrease in midline anastomoses with aging, that can affect wound healing. The center of scalp is called watershed area, more prone for necrosis if vascularity is compromised by deeper tissue injury and high density packing of grafts
- Knowledge of anatomy of nerves is important during scalp blocks. Infiltrating local anesthetic around the scalp's periphery (through which all the sensory nerves traverse) can produce total scalp anesthesia
- The arteries travel just superior to the galea in the subcutaneous layer. The subcutaneous layer of the scalp is a particularly poor plane for dissection because of the presence of these large vessels and fibrous septa, which interfere with blood vessel constriction
- This high degree of vascularity also accounts for the extremely low incidence of infection associated with scalp surgery

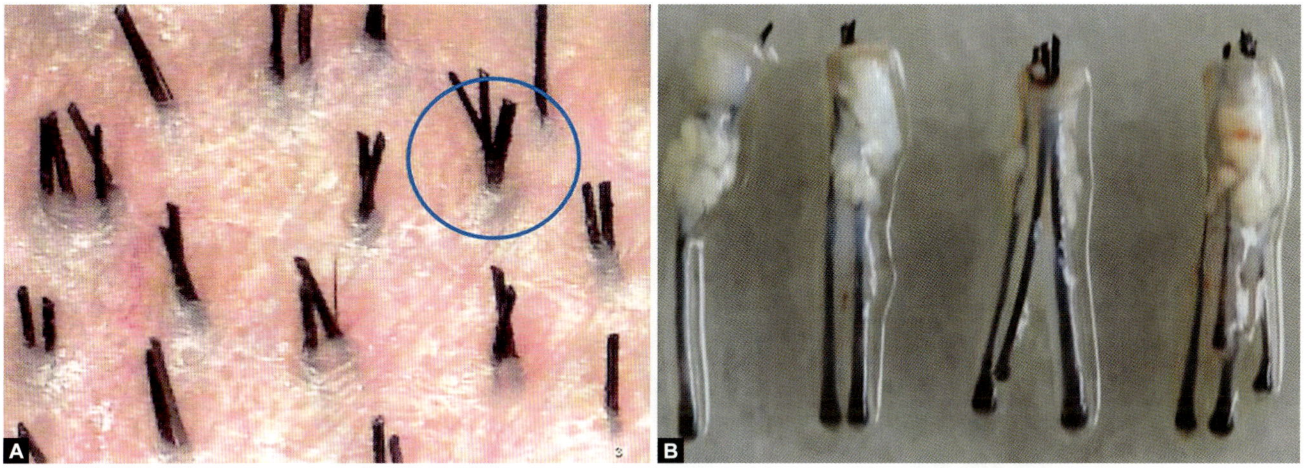

Figs. 3A and B: (A) Follicular units as seen on dermatoscope; (B) Follicular units postextraction.

Inferior segment: This inferior segment of the hair follicle is the area from the base of the follicle to the insertion of the AP muscle. This area is transient and cyclically regenerates itself in a controlled fashion.

The bottom—most portion of the inferior segment is referred to as the hair bulb and contains the rapidly dividing undifferentiated matrix cells and melanocytes which are of epithelial origin. The hair bulb surrounds the dermal papilla. The combination of the hair bulb and the dermal papilla, with its associated nerves and blood vessels, constitutes the hair root.

The dermal papilla is a power house of growth factors and growth factor receptors, which play a role in hair growth. The dermal papilla contains specialized fibroblasts with powerful hair follicle inductive properties needed for initiation of a new hair cycle believed to regulate matrix cell division and the caliber of the hair. It also contains androgen receptors which are the hormonal targets in androgenetic alopecia.

The matrix cells are located directly above the papilla. These cells are undifferentiated, actively dividing, and immunologically "privileged". Melanocytes are present between the basal cells of the matrix. Melanin produced by the melanocytes is incorporated into new hairs by phagocytosis. The matrix cells differentiate into the multiple components of the hair follicle, including the hair shaft, the inner root sheath, and the outer root sheath.

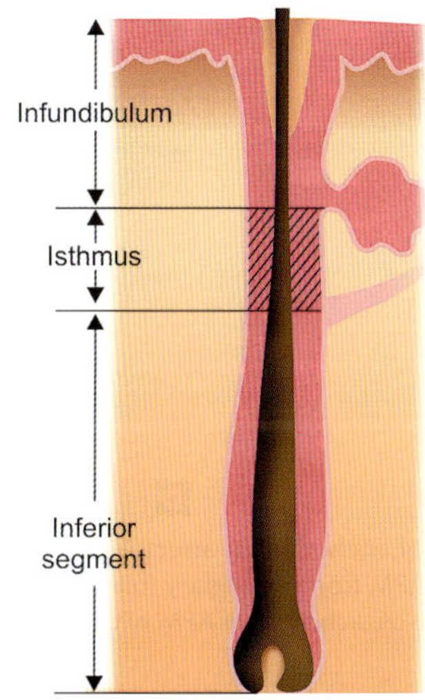

Fig. 4: Anatomical divisions of hair.

Role of Arrector Pili Muscle (Box 2)

The APM comprises of a small band of smooth muscle that connects the hair follicle to the connective tissue of the adjacent upper dermis. It mediates thermoregulation by contracting to elevate hair shafts, thereby increasing air-trapping and hence insulation. It was thought to be vestigial in humans, but recent studies suggest that the human APM plays an important role in maintaining follicular integrity by holding together each of the hair follicles in the follicular unit at the isthmus level. The hair bulge and part of the outer root sheath (ORS) contains follicular stem cells that are critical for

BOX 2: Applied aspects of arrector pili muscle.

- Arrector pili muscle attached to tightest to one follicle in particular—primary HF—least susceptibility to miniaturization. Secondary hairs miniaturize first-those with less intimate contact with the APM. There is a hierarchy of androgen responsiveness within FU, with preferential miniaturization of secondary follicles
- Loss of attachment between the bulge stem cell population and the APM also explains why miniaturization is irreversible in AGA but not alopecia areata. In AGA where follicle miniaturization is either irreversible or only partially reversible—consistent loss of attachment of the APM to vellus hair follicles. In AA, in which the APM maintained contact with the ORS of the miniaturized secondary vellus follicles
- In early stages of hair loss, the APM remains attached to the primary follicle but loses its attachment to some of the regressing secondary follicles in some FUs. Miniaturization of secondary follicles and detachment of the APM from these follicles extend to the rest of the FUs. At this stage, patients may complain of hair thinning and loss of volume in their pony tail without visible baldness
- With further progression, miniaturization continues and the muscle loses attachment to the secondary follicles in affected FUs completely. Primary follicles eventually miniaturize and this leads to visible baldness. When primary follicles lose muscle attachment, the hair loss becomes irreversible[5]

(APM: arrector pili muscle; HF: hair follicle; FU: follicular unit; AGA: androgenetic alopecia; AA: alopecia areata; ORS: outer root sheath)

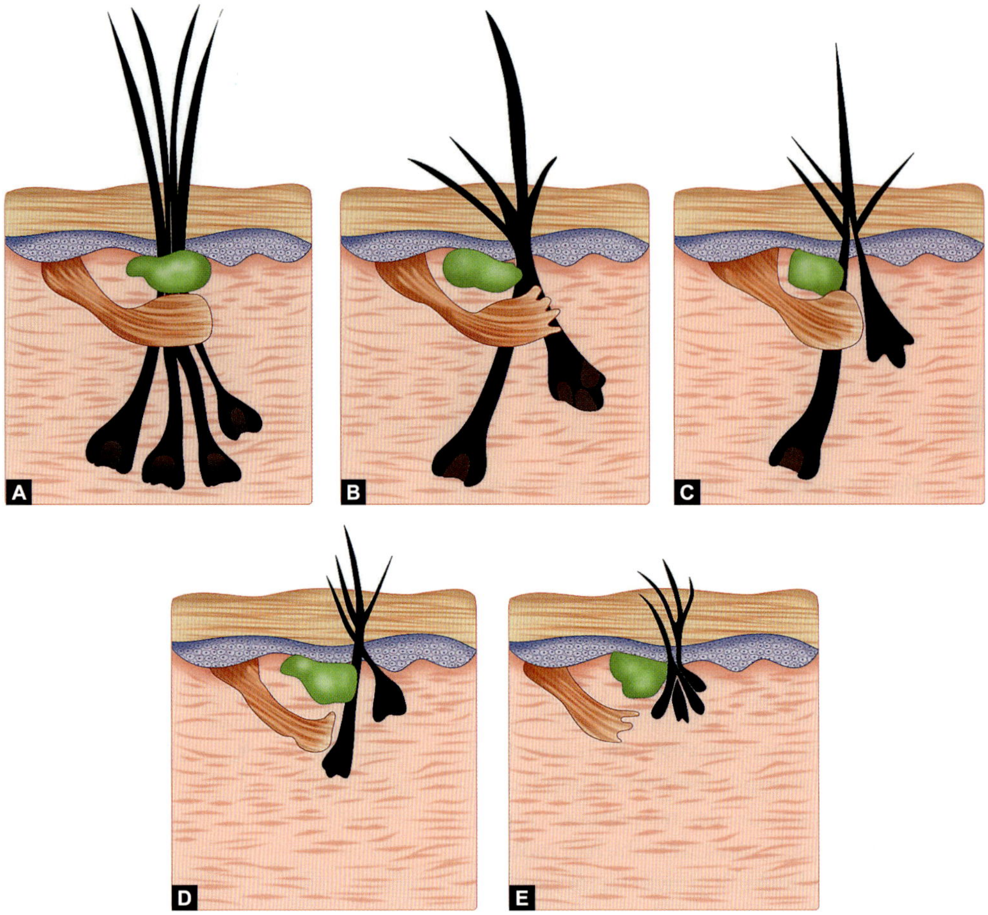

Figs. 5A to E: Loss of anchorage of arrector pili muscle (APM) resulting in progressive follicular miniaturization. (A) Follicles held together by APM; (B) Detachment of APM from secondary follicles; (C) Complete detachment of APM from secondary follicles; (D) Detachment of APM from primary follicle; (E) Complete detachment of APM with complete follicular miniaturization.

the regeneration of the follicular unit. Follicles within the same follicular unit share an APM. The proximal APM attaches via a tendon to the bulge, a known stem cell niche and the bulge cells interact closely with the APM.[5,6]

The APM-bulge connection persists throughout the hair growth cycle and has been suggested to play an important role in morphogenesis and renewal of hair follicles. APM is attached tightly to one follicle in particular within a follicular unit, called the primary hair follicle and has less intimate contact with rest of the follicles known as the secondary hair follicles. The first step of miniaturization involves the loss of anchorage of arrector pili muscle from the hair follicles. There is a hierarchy of androgen sensitivity within FU, with preferential miniaturization of secondary follicles. The secondary hair follicle is the first to miniaturize, where as the primary hair follicle is least susceptible to miniaturization. This process is seen in only few follicular units ("herald units") in the early stages of the disease. This is perceived by the patients as thinning of hairs or decrease in their hair volume. The loss of attachment of the APM with the hair follicle is due to the degeneration of the APM and fat infiltration **(Figs. 5A to E)**. The APM support stimulates stem cell populations in the bulge or dermal sheath, through uncharacterized mechanical or biochemical mechanisms. Hence loss of contact with the APM, disrupts the function of stem cells niche and induces miniaturization

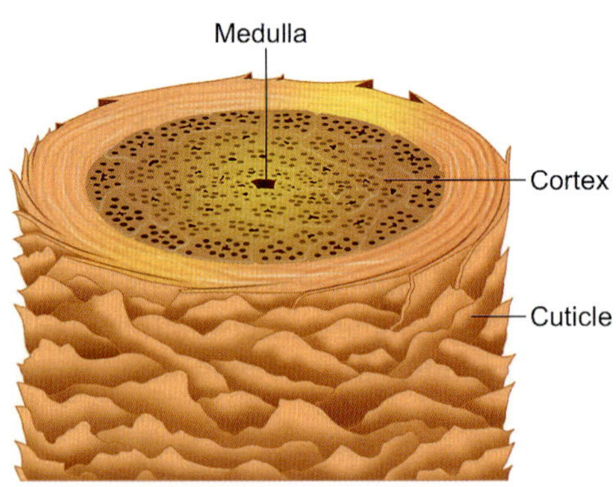

Fig. 6: Parts of the hair shaft.

Hair Shaft

The hair shaft is the only part of the hair follicle to exit the epidermis. It, in itself, is also made up of three layers: the medulla, the cortex, and the hair shaft cuticle **(Fig. 6)**.

HAIR CYCLE

The hair cycle is classically composed of three distinct phases: *anagen* (growth) phase, *catagen* (involution phase), and *telogen* (resting) phase. A fourth *exogen* stage has been described which denotes the shedding of hair during the cycle. Anagen generally lasts from 3 to 10 years, catagen 2–3 weeks, and telogen 3–4 months. In the human scalp, the cycle is asynchronous. At any one time, an average of 13% of the hair is in telogen, although it can range from 4 to 24%. Only 1% is in the catagen phase.

Anagen to Catagen

At the end of the anagen (growth) phase, an unknown signal propels the hair follicle to enter the catagen phase. The matrix cells cease proliferating, and the production of melanin terminates. The dermal papilla contracts and the middle portion of the follicle constricts with the lower portion expanding to become the *club hair.* This lower portion retracts up to the level of the arrector pili muscle leaving behind a thin band (streamer) of undifferentiated epithelial cells.

Catagen

Catagen is the dynamic transition between anagen and telogen. During catagen, the lower "cycling" portion of each hair follicle regresses entirely by apoptosis of epithelial cells in the bulb and outer root sheath (ORS), the outermost epithelial layer.[7] The club hair moves upward till it reaches the permanent, noncycling upper follicle, where it remains anchored during telogen. As the lower follicle recedes, a temporary structure forms—the epithelial strand—which is unique to catagen. This connects the dermal papilla to the upper part of the hair follicle, contains many apoptotic cells.

Telogen

Following catagen, follicles lie dormant in a resting phase (telogen). The transition from telogen to anagen occurs when one or two quiescent stem cells at the base of the telogen follicle, near the dermal papilla, are activated to produce a new hair shaft.[8] These cells now begin to proliferate rapidly, and become the transit-amplifying daughter cells that are fated to form the new hair follicle. The new follicle forms adjacent to the old pocket that harbors the club hair, which will eventually be shed (exogen). Complex molecular signals are involved during progression through each stage.

BODY HAIR CHARACTERISTICS

With limited availability of scalp hair, surgeons sometimes need to opt for body hair as potential donor hair for transplantation. Majority of the body hair remains vellus. In areas such as axilla, pubis, face, chest and back of females it becomes terminal at puberty. Body hair differs from scalp hair in the following ways:

- *Hair cycle:* Hair cycle is significantly shorter in body hair and a large number (close to 60%) of hair are in telogen phase of hair cycle. The hair cycle at different body sites is denoted in **Table 2.**[9]
- *Rate of growth:* Body hair is slower to grow as they have a longer telogen phase and short anagen phase. The rate of growth for scalp hair is 0.37–0.44 mm/day while body hair usually grows at 0.27 mm/day. Moreover, they are thinner in diameter and grow shorter. However, facial hair in men are the thickest hair in the body.
- *Type of units:* Body hair has usually single hair follicular units with very few units of 2–3 hairs.
- *Gray hair:* Body hair is slow to gray as compared to scalp hair.
- *Pattern of hair:* Body hair usually appears curlier compared to scalp hair and the angle of emergence is usually more acute in body hair. Thus, higher transection rates are observed in body hair as compared to scalp. Body hair often grows in variable direction in the same area and occasionally forms whirls.

TABLE 2: Hair cycle at different parts of the body.

Body area	*Anagen hair (%)*	*Telogen duration (months)*	*Density (follicle/cm²)*	*Follicle depth (mm)*	*Anagen duration (months)*
Scalp	85–90	3–4	350	3–5	35–40
Beard (chin)	65–70	1.5–2.5	500	2–4	3–4
Upper lip	65–70	1–2	500	1–2.5	3–4
Axilla	30–60	3	65	3.5–4.5	3-6
Pubic	30	4	70	3.5–4.5	3-6
Legs	20–25	4–6	60	2–4	4–5
Chest	30–40	3	30–60	-	3–4
Eyebrow	10	3	100	2–2.5	2–3
Eyelash	35–40 (upper eyelash) 15 (lower eyelash)	4–9	50–75 (upper) 30–50 (lower)	1.5–2.5	1–2

- *Location:* Body hair lies superficially in the upper dermis as compared to scalp hair which extends down to lower dermis and subcutis.
- *Recipient influence:* Body hair when transplanted into the scalp tends to acquire characteristics of scalp hair and vice versa. This concept is known as recipient influence, first described by Tommy Hwang.[10]

Applied Physiology

- Hair growth on scalp is different from rest of body. Anagen hair is identified by accentuated hue.
- In AGA decreased duration of the anagen stage.
- The terminal hairs are replaced by thin, vellus hairs.
- The ratio of anagen/telogen hairs decreases (from a normal 6 to 8:1 ratio to an abnormal 0.1 to 3:1 ratio.
- Each hair follicle has its own biological clock independent of its neighboring hairs.
- Each hair follicle goes through the hair cycle 10–20 times.
- The cycle varies in beard, chest and other body parts.
- If use of multiple donor areas → knowing where and how source hair will be implanted is important.
- Increase in anagen:telogen ratio of source area by pretreatment with minoxidil.

CLINICAL APPROACH

Androgenetic alopecia is characterized by progressive patterned hair loss.[11] Although, it is not life-threatening, it is associated with negative psychological effects, including low self-esteem, depression, and a general dissatisfaction with body appearance.[12] The first task of physician is to understand the psychology of patient, build good rapport, followed by organized diagnostic approach, and lastly framing a suitable therapeutic regimen.

CLINICAL PRESENTATION (BOX 3)

It begins at puberty, as early as 12 years and most of the cases start between the age of 15 and 25 years.[13] The women with hyperandrogenic state can present as early as 12–15 years. Usually, there is a positive family history; inheritance can be maternal or paternal. First- or second-degree relatives can be affected in the family. The patients present with hair thinning and baldness that follows distinctive pattern. It progresses gradually with acute episodes of increased loss between normal daily shedding. The shedding may be seasonal in few patients. For many individuals, the condition may be stable for years. Most men reach their maximum-stabilized pattern by their forties. This is usually followed by senescent aging (decrease in hair density as they age).

Hair loss affects the androgen-sensitive follicles and clinically progresses from bitemporal to vertex with sparing of occipital scalp. The earliest manifestation of AGA in men is a bitemporal recession of the scalp hairline. Sometimes, there is diffuse hair loss with preservation of the frontal hairline, as in anterior pattern and female pattern hair loss (FPHL), where the prominent presentation is hair thinning or seen through scalp.[14] The hair loss and progression can be rapid in diffuse patterns of AGA, and in such cases, the physician should rule out other history related to diffuse causes of hair loss (hypothyroidism, hyperthyroidism, nutritional deficiency). It can be associated with hyperandrogenic syndrome. Hair loss may be trigged by hormonal changes such as postpartum, peri- or postmenopause state and starting or stopping oral contraceptives (OCPs). These situations may unmask a tendency for AGA.[15] In author's experience, patterned hair loss in women begins as postpartum hair loss, progressing as chronic telogen loss, and ends up with FPHL. Psychological stress is common in AGA both in men and women, and hence complete evaluation is important in patients seeking for surgical option, especially when they have unrealistic expectations. AGA has been linked to anabolic syndrome. A study conducted by Herrera et al.[16] showed extent of baldness was not associated with coronary artery disease (CAD), however rapid progression of baldness was a risk factor of CAD. An age-matched case-control study in men supported the hypothesis that early AGA can be clinical marker of insulin resistance.[17] Hence, men with vertex baldness, rapidly progressing, and early onset AGA must be screened for CAD and insulin resistance.

BOX 3: History—hair loss evaluation questionnaire for androgenetic alopecia.

- Duration
- Pattern of loss (frontotemporal pattern, anterior pattern, vertex, and diffuse pattern)
- Hair fall (it is main complaint in initial and acute phase of AGA)
- Hair thinning (it is more in later stage of disease)
- Associated symptoms (oily and seborrheic scalp)
- Associated systemic disease (CAD and insulin resistance)
- Family history
- Psychological history
- Menstrual history and androgen excess history in women

(AGA: androgenetic alopecia; CAD: coronary artery disease)

CLINICAL EXAMINATION (BOX 4)

During inspection, visible scalp infers reduction in hair density of 50% of normal.[18] On palpation, run your finger around scalp and compare the density all over from frontal hairline to crown and occiput to crown. Decide the pattern and distribution of hair loss. Based on degree of miniaturization the hair may feel rough, soft, or silky. This will also be a guide to assess the treatment response.

Androgenetic alopecia is a patterned, nonscarring alopecia. Based on progression and types of baldness, there are four patterns of AGA. They are typical frontotemporal pattern, anterior pattern, vertex, and diffuse pattern. Women present with frontal or vertex thinning with Ludwig pattern. In men, most of them present with anteroposterior recession

BOX 4: Examination.

- Inspection (type of PHL) **(Boxe 5)**
- Palpation (pattern, elasticity, and surface changes such as seborrhea, oiliness are recorded)
- Hair (color, caliber, and texture of hair)
- *Clinical tests:*
  - Hair pull test
  - Hair card test
  - Hair mount test
- Trichoscopic examination

(PHL: pattern hair loss).

BOX 5: Modified Norwood-Hamilton classification **(Figs. 7A and B).**

This modified Norwood-Hamilton classification divides pattern hair loss in men into seven types according to severity:[19,20]

- *Type I*: Minimal recession of the hairline along the anterior border in the FT region
- *Type II*: The anterior border of the hair in the FT region has triangular areas of recession that tend to be symmetrical. These areas extend no further posterior than approximately 2 cm anterior to a line drawn in a coronal plane between the external auditory meatus on both sides. Hair is either lost or sparse along the midfrontal border of the scalp
- *Type III*: Characterized by deep FT hair recession, usually symmetrical and either bald or sparsely covered with hair. These areas of hair recession extend further posterior than a point that lies approximately 2 cm anterior to a line drawn in a coronal plane between the external auditory meatus on either side
- *Type IIIv (vertex)*: Hair is mainly lost in the vertex. There may be some frontal recession, but it does not exceed than that seen in type III
- *Type IV*: The frontal and FT recession is more severe than type III. There is also sparseness or absence of hair in the vertex area. These bald areas are extensive, but separated from each other by a band of moderately dense hair that joins the fully haired fringe on each side of the head
- *Type V*: The hair loss over the vertex and FT areas is larger than in type IV, and the band of hair between them is narrower and sparser
- *Type VI*: The hair loss over the FT and vertex regions is confluent and the bridge of hair that crosses the crown is absent
- *Type VII*: There is only a narrow horseshoe-shaped band of hair that begins laterally just anterior to the ear and extends posteriorly on the sides and fairly low on the occipital area
- *Variants (Type variants-"a")*: Constitutes 3% of all cases of AGA: (1) The entire anterior border of the hairline progresses posteriorly without the normal island of hair in the midfrontal region; and (2) There is no simultaneous development of a bald area on the vertex. Instead, the anterior recession just advances posterior to the vertex
- *Type IIa*: The entire anterior border of the hairline lies high on the forehead. The usual midfrontal island of hair is represented by only a few sparse hairs. The area of denudation extends no farther than 2 cm from the frontal line
- *Type IIIa*: The area of denudation reaches the mid-coronal line
- *Type IVa*: The area of denudation extends beyond the mid-coronal line and there may be considerable thinning of hair posterior to the actual hairline
- *Type Va:* Most advanced degree of alopecia; however, the bald area does not reach the vertex. This pattern appears to be the most common type in clinical practice

(AGA: androgenetic alopecia; FT: frontotemporal)

of hairline, few may only show vertex thinning. Sometimes, women can present with bitemporal recession and men can present with Ludwig pattern. There are various classifications of AGA in both men and women **(Table 3)**. The modified Norwood-Hamilton classification is the most accepted one. In women, Ludwig and Sinclair scales are frequently employed.[19-21] *Apart from these classifications, there are some variations such as diffuse and reverse patterns, which should never be overlooked during examination* **(Boxes 5 and 6, Figs. 7 to 9)**.

Variations in Androgenetic Alopecia

Diffuse Patterned Alopecia and Diffuse Unpatterned Alopecia[22-24] (Figs. 10A to D)

Diffuse patterned alopecia (DPA) and diffuse unpatterned alopecia (DUPA) are other presentations of AGA, which lack emphasis in literature. In DPA, the pattern of hair loss is same as in the male-pattern hair loss (MPHL). It gradually affects frontotemporal, mid-scalp and vertex, with a stable permanent zone. It differs from MPHL by two points. First, the progression of miniaturization does not pass through the typical Norwood stages. Second, the areas involved do not become totally bald, only the hair density decreases. DUPA is another rare entity that poses challenge for hair transplant surgeon. It is seen in both men and women. It differs from MPHL by lacking the stable permanent zone. It presents early and rapidly progresses to a state resembling the Norwood type VII. However, unlike the Norwood type VII, the stable zone looks sparse due to lower density **(Box 7)**. Hence, differentiating between DPA and DUPA is very important because unlike DUPA, DPA patients often make good candidates for transplantation.

Therefore, DUPA should never be missed, as DUPA patient can never be a candidate for hair transplantation. If transplantation is done, they inevitably suffer extensive hair loss as they do not have safer zone.[25]

Reverse Pattern Androgenetic Alopecia

The usual course of balding is from anterior to posterior, but one can also see ascending hairline, i.e., thinning from nape of neck toward the safe donor area. This is called ascending hairline. The presence of this pattern in AGA signifies shrinkage of safe zone.

CLINICAL TESTS

Hair Card Test

It is a simple technique to differentiate growing hair and also quality of hair shaft. A white paper (for black hair) or black (for white hair) of size 8 × 12 cm paper is placed against hair shafts in affected area **(Fig. 11)**.

Inference

Miniaturized hairs have small caliber, broken hairs have blunt tip and new growing hairs have pointed tips. Thus, differentiates newly grown hair from broken hair.[18,26]

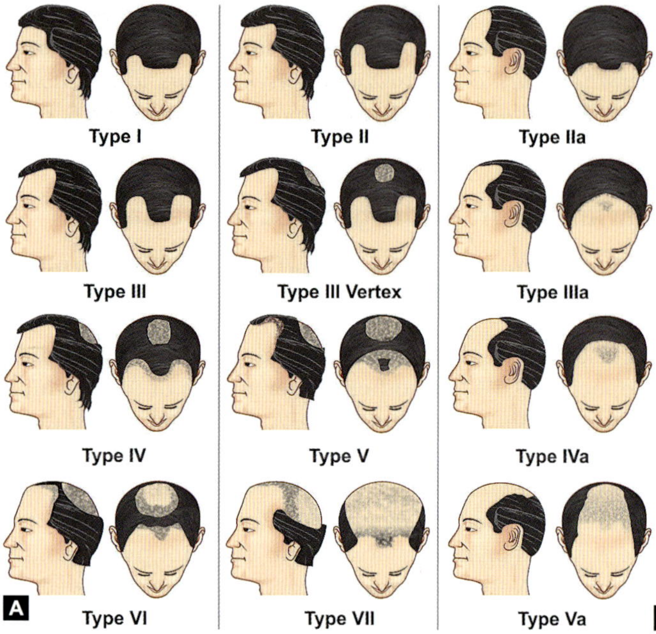

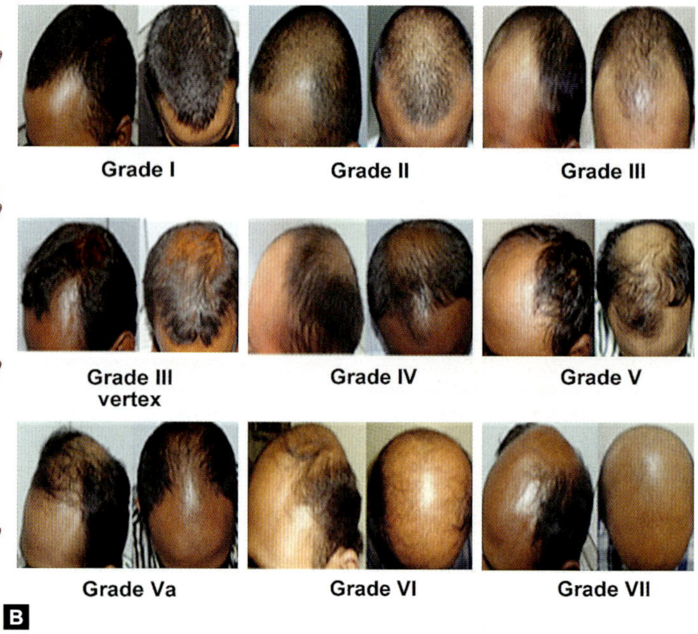

Figs. 7A and B: Norwood-Hamilton classification.

TABLE 3: Various classifications of androgenetic alopecia.

Modified Norwood[19,20]	Types I–VII, anterior pattern, vertex, variants
Ludwig scale[21]	I, II, and III
BASP classification	Types L, M, C, U, F, and V
Variation of AGA	DPA and DUPA[22-24]

(AGA: androgenetic alopecia; BASP: basic and specific; DPA: diffuse patterned alopecia; DUPA: diffuse unpatterned alopecia)

BOX 6: Ludwig's scale (**Figs. 8 and 9**): it is a grading scale for female pattern hair loss. It can also be used in grading men-patterned hair loss.

- *Grade I:* Thinning of hair is seen mainly over the anterior part of the crown with minimal widening of the parting width—indicates 25% loss in hair density
- *Grade II:* Thinning of the crown becomes more evident because of an increase in the number of thin and short hairs—indicates 50% loss in hair density
- *Grade III:* The crown becomes almost total bald. There is significant widening of the parting width, but the frontal hairline is still maintained—indicates 75% loss in hair density

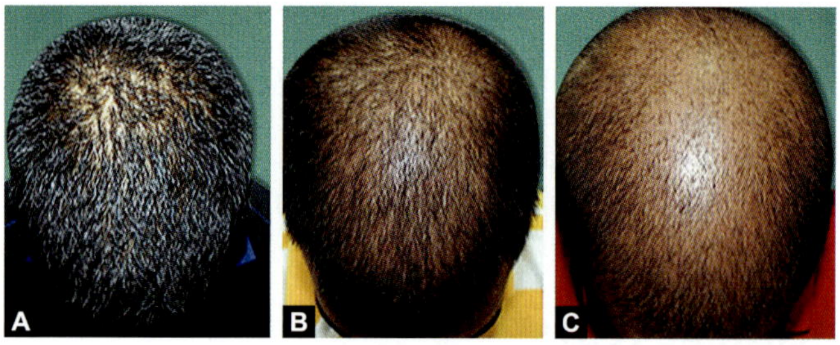

Figs. 8A to C: Ludwig pattern in male-pattern hair loss. (A) Grade I; (B) Grade II; (C) Grade III.

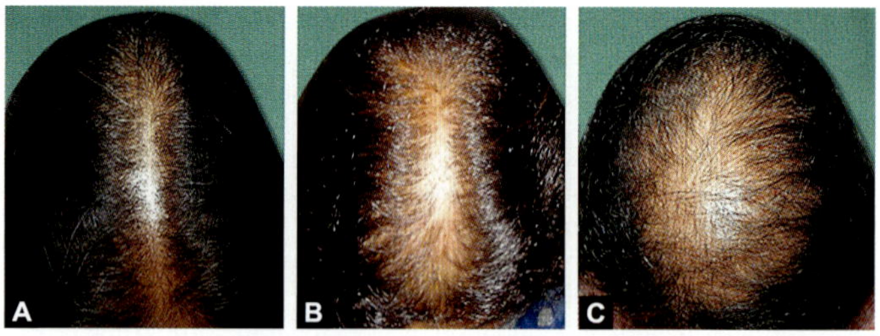

Figs. 9A to C: Ludwig pattern in female-pattern hair loss. (A) Grade I; (B) Grade II; (C) Grade III.

Hair Pull Test

It is a simple test done to determine the severity and the site of hair loss. The patient should not have washed their hair for at least 1 day. The test is performed by grasping 50–60 hairs between thumb and index finger and pulling it firmly with gentle pressure away from scalp and along hair shafts. It is performed in three different sites of scalp (frontal, occipital, and bilateral temporal region). The presence of 5–6 hairs is considered as positive hair pull.[12,15,16] Hair pull test is negative, there is increased telogen hair in affected area only **(Fig. 12)**.

The authors way of doing hair pull test is faster and has advantage of examining large areas at one go and is friendly test. Approximately, 50–100 hairs are grasped between the finger clefts of medial four fingers and hairs are pulled away from scalp. The number of pulled hairs is counted in each cleft. The test is positive, if more than 10% of hairs are shed in each cleft.

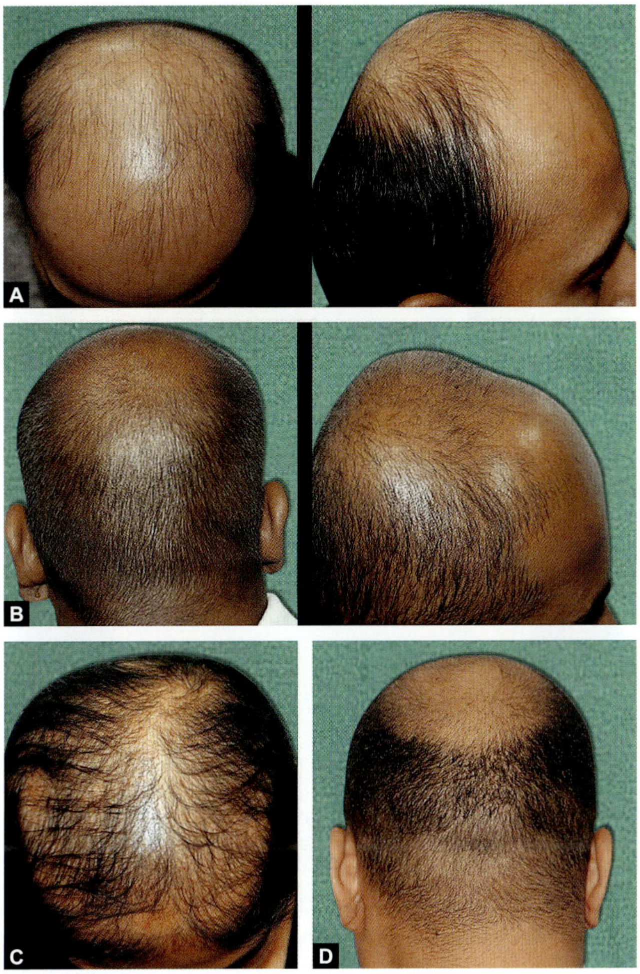

Figs. 10A to D: (A) Diffuse patterned androgenetic alopecia with stable zone; (B) Diffuse unpatterned androgenetic alopecia (DUPA) with transparent safe zone; (C) DUPA in female; (D) Reverse pattern androgenetic alopecia.

BOX 7: Early warning signs of diffuse unpatterned alopecia.

- Rapid decrease in hair volume and a change in hair texture at an early age
- Well-maintained adolescent hair pattern and persistent frontal hairline in spite of volume loss
- A "see-through" safe zone of occipital area
- Significant miniaturization of the donor area (greater than 35%)
- Donor density of less than 1.5 hairs per mm^2

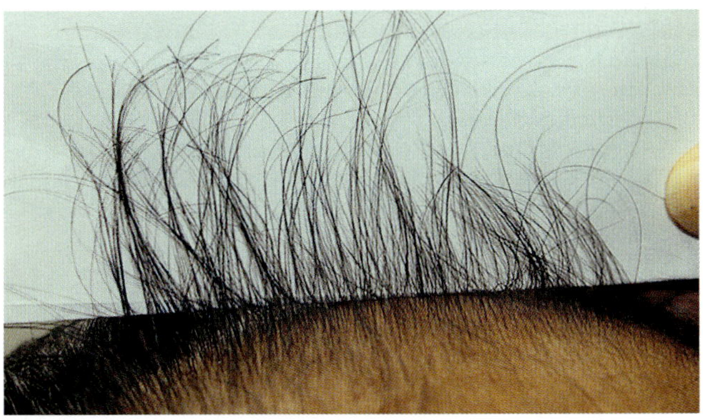

Fig. 11: Hair card test.

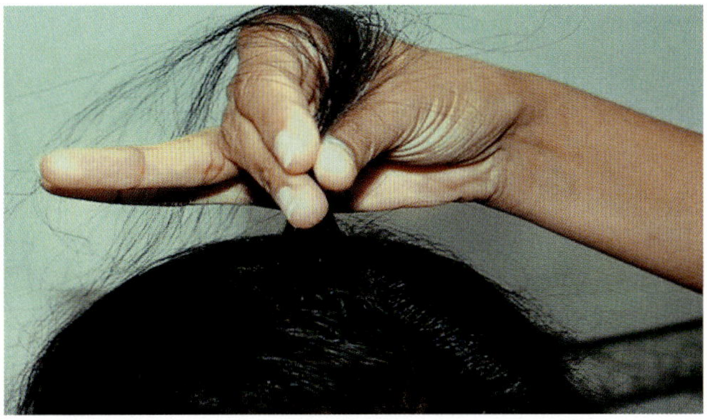

Fig. 12: Hair pull test.

This has advantage of doing it faster and covering large areas at a time **(Figs. 13A to C).**

Hair Mount Test

It is assessment of hair bulbs and shafts using light microscopy. Epilated hair roots are mounted on glass slide to examine the bulbs. Coverslip is placed over roots with mounting medium and examined under microscope for different types of bulbs:[18,26,27]

- Dark-pigmented bulb with preserved inner root sheath is anagen bulb
- Light-pigmented to nonpigmented bulb without inner root sheath and club shaped is telogen bulb
- Dystrophic anagen—"hockey stick" appearance.

DIAGNOSIS

The diagnosis of MPHL is straightforward with typical pattern of hair loss without any evidence of scarring. Diagnosis is supported by the presence of cardinal features as listed in **Box 8**. The diagnostic tests mentioned in literature include hair pull test, phototrichogram (PTG), and trichogram. The relevant bedside investigations that aid diagnosis of AGA are trichoscopy, video dermatoscope, and scalp biopsy.

Trichoscopy (Fig. 14)

It is a simple noninvasive tool to visualize scalp and hair shaft. It is performed by either hand-held dermatoscope (10 times magnified) or digital dermatoscope (10–50 times magnified). The common trichoscopic findings in AGA **(Box 9)** are hair diameter diversity of more than 20%, perifollicular brown scales called peripilar sign (early AGA) and brown dots. The other findings include yellow dots, scattered form of white dots (WD), multihair follicular unit (MHFU), honeycomb pattern pigment (HCPP) and hidden hair. The less severe AGA shows MHFU and peripilar sign, whereas WD, HCPP, and brown dots are seen in severe grades. Though follicular units with single hair are more common in AGA compared to other conditions such as telogen effluvium and anagen hair

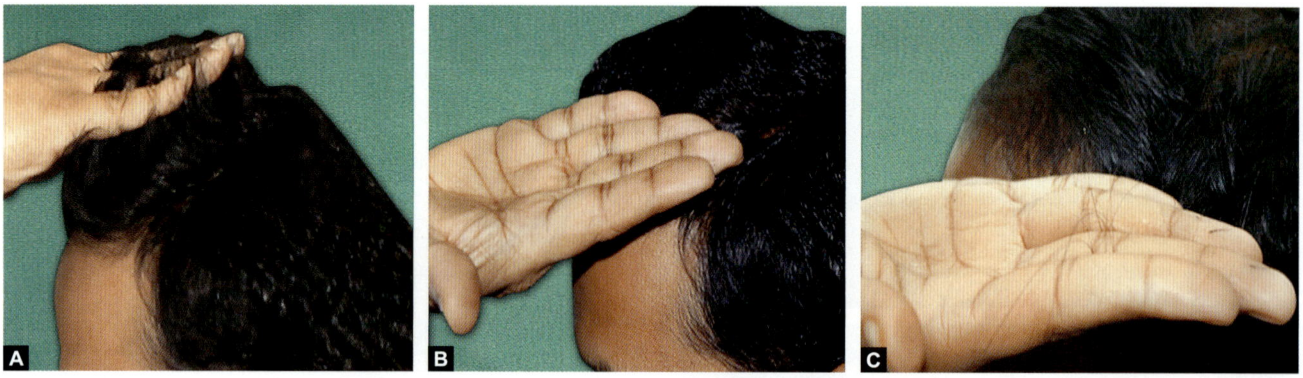

Figs. 13A to C: Hair pull test showing negative and positive results.

BOX 8: Cardinal features of androgenetic alopecia.

- The balding pattern with miniaturized hairs
- Gradual onset with progression
- Onset after puberty
- A history of baldness in the family
- Signs of hyperandrogenism in women
- Thinning with or without gradually developing bare patches
- Negative hair pull test

loss, the MHFU described in early AGA is due to inflammatory release of cytokines and growth factors in combination with anabolic effects of testosterone, which might provoke this augmentation. These trichoscopic findings are more pronounced in frontal than in vertex area.[23,24,28]

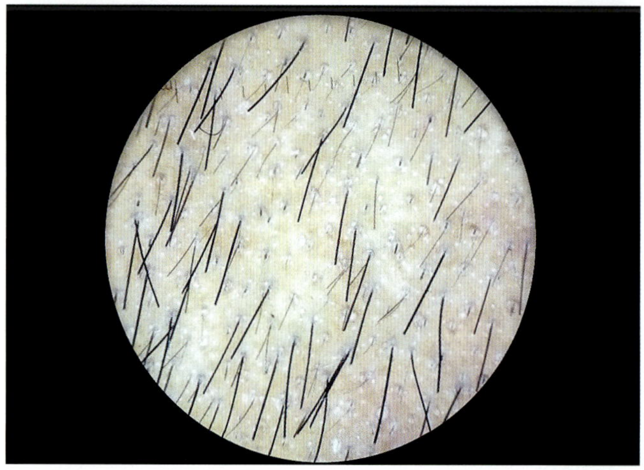

Fig. 14: Trichoscopy showing hair diameter diversity and white dots.

BOX 9: Trichoscopic findings (Fig. 14).

- Hair shaft thickness diversity—presence of thin, intermediate thick hairs
- Increase in vellus hair number
- Follicular units with single hair
- White dots—indicate empty follicular ostia
- Yellow dots—suggest sebaceous gland hypertrophy
- Peripilar sign is perifollicular discoloration—suggests dermal infiltrates in AGA
- Honeycomb pigment pattern
- Multihair follicular unit (MHFU)—seen in early AGA

(AGA: androgenetic alopecia)

Ancillary Laboratory Tests

In men, no laboratory workup is necessary unless there is associated diffuse hair loss. However, as AGA is increasingly associated with cardiovascular risk factors and insulin resistance, it is worthwhile to investigate for lipid profile and do cardiac evaluation in patients with vertex baldness and early onset rapidly progressing AGA.[16,29] Hormonal assay is indicated in hyperandrogenism in women and also to rule out non androgenetic causes of alopecia such as anemia and thyroid abnormality. Scalp biopsy is required to confirm diagnosis when there is diagnostic dilemma such as diffuse alopecia areata (AA) versus diffuse unpatterned AGA **(Box 10)**.

BOX 10: Laboratory workup.

- Blood tests:
  - Hormonal evaluation (to rule out androgen excess and PCOD)
  - Thyroid profile
  - Serum ferritin
  - Extended tests (serum vitamin D, B_{12} serum insulin, lipid profile, etc.)
- Scalp biopsy
- Trichogram
- Phototrichogram

(PCOD: polycystic ovary syndrome)

Scalp Biopsy

It is simple office-based bedside procedure, performed with 4 mm biopsy punch under local anesthesia. The biopsy is taken from the center of the most affected area with 4 mm punch for both transverse and vertical sections, in ambiguous case and also to confirm diagnosis in anxious patients. The main indications of biopsy are to differentiate AGA from diffuse AA, DUPA and also to rule out coexisting pathology. In AGA, the ratio of terminal to vellus hair is less than 3:1 and there is increase in telogen to anagen ratio. The other findings include follicular stellae and minimal perifollicular lymphohistiocytic infiltration with or without fibrosis in upper part of follicle.[30]

Video Dermatoscope or Folliscope

This is used to enhance the images of scalp and hair, and detect the hair shaft in the follicle its length, diameter, and possible anomalies. Author prefers to examine target area about 12 cm from glabella or line joining two tragus on either side to meet on the midscalp in the center. Videodermatoscopy helps to calculate terminal to vellus hair ratio, counts and measures vellus hairs (hairs less than 0.03 mm). Follicular ostea shows predominately single hairs on video dermatoscopy. Perifollicular yellow dots may be seen in some advanced cases of MPHL. The yellow dots correspond to degenerated follicular keratinocytes and sebum contained within the dilated ostium and miniaturized hair follicles.[31]

Trichogram or Pluck Test

The trichogram is a semi-invasive microscopic method for hair-root and hair-cycle evaluation. The hair should not be washed for 5 days before plucking. A rubber-armed forceps is used to pull 60–80 hairs. Location depends on the hair disorder. For example, in pattern hair loss, the first site is 2 cm behind the frontal hairline and 2 cm from the midline, with the second site being 2 cm lateral to the occipital protuberance. The hair is grasped at about 0.5 cm above the scalp and rotated to ensure a firm grip. With perpendicular pull, the hairs are removed and embedded with roots on a glass slide. The hair roots are evaluated under a magnifying lens or a microscope. This test is painful and time consuming, and is reserved for selected cases.[32]

Phototrichogram

The phototrichogram (PTG) is noninvasive and allows in vivo measurement of the total number of hair, anagen hair, hair density, hair thickness, and hair growth rate. Contrast-enhanced PTG has become a valuable tool in the diagnosis of hair loss. It is used in pattern hair loss to detect early changes of decreased hair density and hair miniaturization before the disorder becomes clinically evident **(Fig. 15)**. In pattern hair loss two areas of progression, such as vertex and receding hairline, are chosen and a control area on the occipital scalp is observed. Photographs are taken. At the first visit, all hairs are trimmed 1 mm from the skin surface in all three well-defined areas (1 cm^2). At both visits the hair sites are covered with transient hair dye for contrast enhancement. At the second visit, a photograph is taken using the scalp immersion proxigraphy method, which involves using close-up photography, where by the scalp is viewed under a glass slide with a drop of immersion oil.[31] Exactly, the same area must be seen on both photographs. The individual hairs on both photographs are located pairwise and compared. Substantial hair growth on the second photograph reflects hair growth and indicates anagen. Moderate elongation reflects catagen, and no elongation reflects resting. A missing hair in the second picture suggests hair shedding. This method is again time consuming and is used frequently in clinical and therapeutic trials.

Gene Testing for Androgenetic Alopecia

It is done to determine androgen sensitivity in a patient. The androgen receptor gene is the major determinant of MPHL, which is found on X chromosome. The nucleotide sequence of cytosine-adenine-guanine (CAG) repeats on androgen receptor gene will determine the androgen sensitivity in men and women. The androgen sensitivity is calculated by evaluating CAG repeats on *AR-CAG* gene, which is obtained from a simple cheek swab. The score of less than 24 indicates androgen sensitivity. Lower the number of CAG repeats, higher is the androgen sensitivity and risk of developing AGA. The positive gene indicates 60% chance of going bald by the age of 40. The CAG score can determine the response to finasteride treatment in both sexes. The low CAG score is associated with increase response to finasteride, and score of less than 22 gives good response.

DIFFERENTIAL DIAGNOSIS

The diagnoses that may be difficult to distinguish are both acute and chronic telogen effluvium and alopecia areata (AA) **(Figs. 16A and B)**.[22] Telogen effluvium is acute in onset, generalized with a known trigger factor. Hair shedding is more prominent with positive hair pull test.

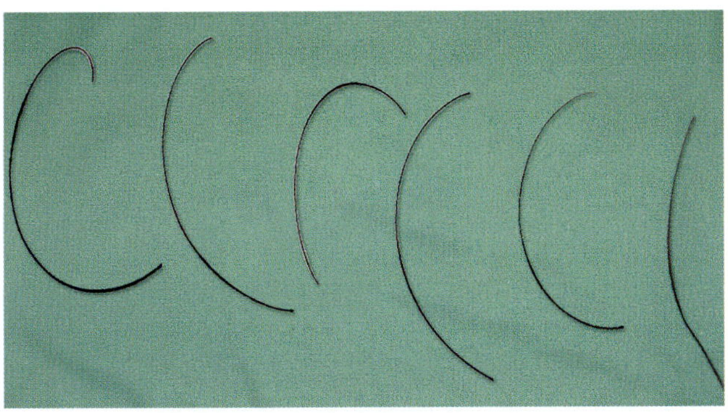

Fig. 15: Miniaturization of hairs.

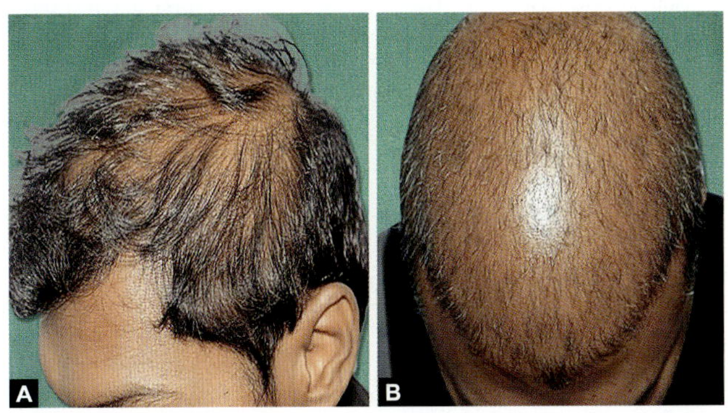

Figs. 16A and B: (A) Diffuse alopecia areata; (B) Androgenetic alopecia with coexistent alopecia areata.

Alopecia areata can present with random patches or generalized/diffuse pattern. Onset is abrupt, generally with remissions and relapses. It can affect any age group. Shedding is prominent, with a positive hair pull test for both dystrophic anagen and telogen hairs. Overlapping of AGA and AA is not an infrequent association in authors' experience, and is important to warn patients undergoing hair transplantation, regarding the possibility of recurrence after surgery. Diffuse AA must be differentiated from DUPA. In DUPA, there is diffuse miniaturization without patchy loss. Dermoscopic examination helps to differentiate both the conditions. Author would prefer to take scalp biopsy for transverse section in such diagnostic dilemmas.[31-33]

MANAGEMENT

In context to the impact of AGA on patient's well-being, psychological stress has to be addressed before implementing medical or surgical treatment. The treatment regimen depends on the grade of AGA, amount of miniaturized hair that can be salvaged, age, and preference of topical or oral or surgical options and cost-effectiveness.

Medical and surgical management are always complementary to each other **(Table 4)**. Medical treatment is effective only if they have sufficient hair to salvage (miniaturized hair capable for terminal conversion). In patient with advanced hair loss with few miniaturized hair, surgical option with topical treatment is the option. In patient undergoing hair transplantation of grades III–VI, finasteride administration should be recommended in all patients.

Hair transplantation can cover rest of bald area in permissible limits. The steps in medical management include—stabilizing the disease, preventing progression and maintenance of growth. Finasteride and minoxidil are the only US Food and Drug Administration (FDA) approved drugs for AGA **(Table 4)**. The combined administration of the two drugs has an additive effect. Most of AGA patients get dissatisfied with treatment because of need for long-term application and compliance and follow-ups, so counseling is very important. Thus, success of managing AGA is simply holding the patient and, it includes good counseling and offering individualized treatment regimens **(Flowcharts 1 and 2; Table 4 and Box 11)**.

How to Hold on Patients?

- The AGA consultations are usually long with long-term follow-ups. The consultant must offer all available options to patients with realistic expectation on treatment outcome
- Pre- and post-treatment photography is mandatory in standard position and need to be reviewed in each visit to appreciate the growth
- Keep the expectation of advanced baldness patients realistic

TABLE 4: Therapeutic options for androgenetic alopecia*.

Options in male	*Options in female*	*Adjuvant therapies in both*[41-43]
• Minoxidil, 5%, topical, twice a day[34,35] • Finasteride, oral, 1 mg/day[36,37] • Dutasteride 0.5 mg/day[38,39] • Topical minoxidil 5% and finasteride 0.1%[40] • Hair transplantation • Hair camouflage	• Minoxidil, 5%, topical, once a day or 2% twice a day[34,35] • Topical minoxidil 5% and finasteride 0.1%[40] • Antiandrogens (finasteride 5 mg/day, cyproterone acetate and spironolactone) • Hair transplantation • Hair piece or camouflage	• Tretinoin, 0.01% (combination with minoxidil) • Aminexil (once a day in combination with minoxidil) • Peptides (Procapil 3% and capixyl 3%) and allium cepa • Saw palmetto, oral, 320 mg/day • Caffeine complex, topical, once a day • Ketoconazole 2% shampoo/2–4 times a week • Hair nutrition (biotin, copper, niacin and amino acids) • Platelet-rich plasma therapy • Low-level laser hair therapy

*These treatments lack high-quality evidence.

Flowchart 1: Treatment algorithm for male pattern hair loss.

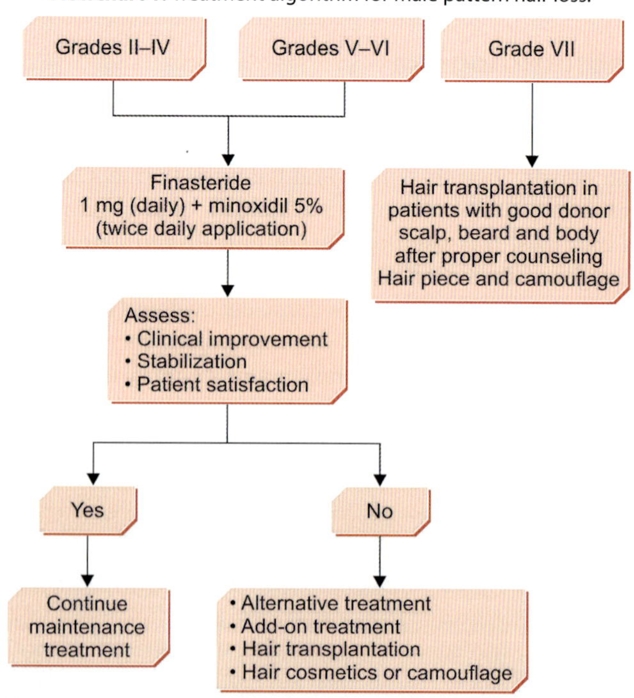

Note:
- In anterior pattern or Ludwig pattern, be conscious while choosing patients for hair transplantation for good recipient density
- In patient undergoing hair transplantation of grade III-VI, it is recommended to take finasteride pre- and post-hair transplantation.

Flowchart 2: Treatment algorithm for female pattern hair loss.

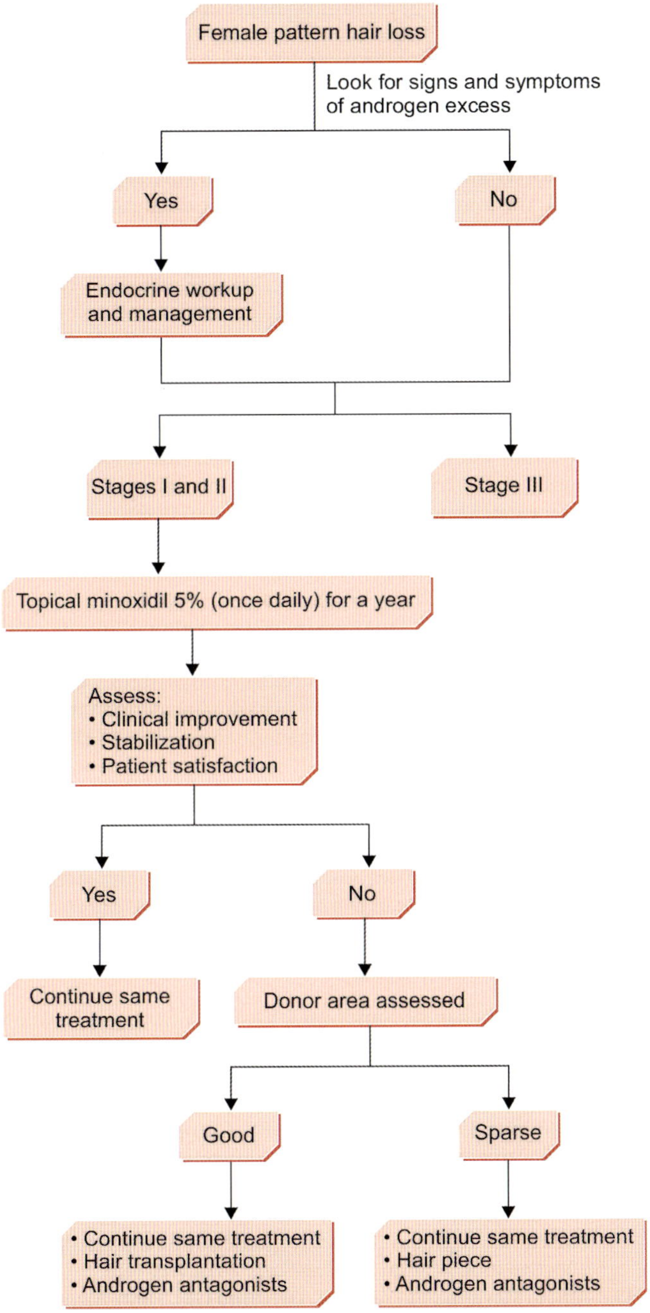

BOX 11: Tips for counseling.

- Counseling the patient with respect to the disease process, possible effects, and adverse effects of the medications along with the probable expected outcome plays a vital role
- Emphasize on prevention of progression of disease and need for maintenance treatment
- Author counsels the treatment of AGA into two phases, phase I (stabilization phase), to grow hair and phase II, to maintain the grown hair for lifelong irrespective of whatever surgical correction they undergo
- Counsel on application methods, to apply adequate quantity, adequate times, and need for shampooing
- Stress on regular follow-ups
- Counsel on realistic expectation. Promise less and deliver more

- In grades II and III, patients must be counseled about disease progression and need for stabilization
- Patients with AGA grades III and IV are the most suitable for management. Emphasis must be made on prevention and maintenance
- In patient with advanced hair loss with few miniaturized hair, surgical management with topical treatment is the option
- Rotational therapy with various formulations (gels, lotions, foams) and add-on therapy at appropriate intervals is the key in developing long-term compliance.

CONCLUSION

The diagnosis of AGA is straightforward. The grading systems help in predicting progression of disease, planning the treatment, and to anticipate future baldness and roughly calculate the required number of grafts to be transplanted in case the patient chooses hair transplantation. DUPA entity is under diagnosed and its poor prognosis to be stressed to patients. The possibility of missing the diagnosis of DUPA and performing hair transplantation at an early age can prove disastrous for both patient and surgeon. It is important to present patients with all therapeutic options, while addressing realistic expectations.

REFERENCES

1. Seery GE. The donor area: a new slant. Hair Transpl Forum. 2001;11:16.
2. Bernstein RM, Rassman WR. The scalp laxity paradox. Hair Transpl Forum Int. 2002;12:9-10.
3. Headington JT. Transverse microscopic anatomy of the human scalp: a basis for a morphometric approach to disorders of the hair follicle. Arch Dermatol. 1984;120(4):449-56.
4. Sinclair R, Torkamani N. Androgenetic alopecia: how it happens. Hair Transpl Forum Int. 2015;25(3):93-101.
5. Sinclair R, Torkamani N, Jones L. Androgenetic alopecia: new insights into the pathogenesis and mechanism of hair loss. F1000Res. 2015;4(F1000 Faculty Rev):585.
6. Yazdabadi A, Whiting D, Rufaut N, Sinclair R. Miniaturized hairs maintain contact with the arrector pili muscle in alopecia areata but not in androgenetic alopecia: a model for reversible miniaturization and potential for hair regrowth. Int J Trichology. 2012;4(3):154-7.
7. Tumbar T, Guasch G, Greco V, Blanpain C, Lowry WE, Rendl M, et al. Defining the epithelial stem cell niche in skin. Science. 2004;303:359-63.
8. Lavker RM, Sun TT, Oshima H, Barrandon Y, Akiyama M, Ferraris C, et al. Hair follicle stem cells. J Investig Dermatol Symp Proc. 2003;8(1):28-38.
9. Lanigan SW. Lasers in Dermatology, 1st edition. London: Springer-Verlag; 2000. pp. 81-9.
10. Hwang ST, Kim HY, Lee SJ, Lee WJ, Do Won Ki, Kim JC. Recipient-site influence in hair transplantation: a confirmative study. Dermatol Surg. 2009;35(6):1011-4.
11. Wang TL, Zhou C, Shen YW, Wang XY, Ding XL, Tian S, et al. Prevalence of androgenetic alopecia in China: a community-based study in six cities. Br J Dermatol. 2010;162:843-7.

12. Wells PA, Willmoth T, Russell RJ. Does fortune favour the bald? Psychological correlates of hair loss in males. Br J Psychol. 1995;86:337-44.
13. Orfanos C. Androgenetic alopecia: clinical aspects and treatment. In: Orfanos C (Ed). Hair and Hair Diseases. Berlin: Springer-Verlag; 1990. pp. 485-527.
14. Oslen EA. Hair disorders. In: Freedberg MI, EissenAZ, Wolff K (Eds). Textbook of Dermatology in General Medicine, 5th edition. New York: McGraw Hill-Inc.; 1999. pp. 729-51.
15. Venning VA, Dawber RP. Patterned androgenic alopecia in women. J Am Acad Dermatol. 1988;18:1073-7.
16. Herrera CR, D'Agostino RB, Gerstman BB, Bosco LA, Belanger AJ. Baldness and coronary heart disease rates in men from the Framingham Study. Am J Epidemiol. 1995;142:828-33.
17. Matilainen V, Koskela P. Early androgenetic alopecia as a marker of insulin resistance. Lancet. 2000;356:1165-6.
18. Ackson AJ, Price VH. How to diagnose hair loss? Dermatol Clin. 2013;31:21-8.
19. Hamilton JB. Patterned loss of hair in man: types and incidence. Ann NY Acad Sci. 1951;53:708-28.
20. Norwood OT. Male pattern baldness. Classification and incidence. South Med J. 1975;68:1359-65.
21. Ludwig E. Classification of the types of androgenetic alopecia (common baldness) occurring in the female sex. Br J Dermatol. 1977;97:247-54.
22. Shapiro J. Hair Loss: Principles of Diagnosis and Management of Alopecia, 1st edition. New York: Taylor & Francis e-Library; 2004. pp. 83-119.
23. De Lacharrière O, Deloche C, Misciali C, Piraccini BM, Vincenzi C, Bastien P, et al. Hair diameter diversity: a clinical sign reflecting the follicle miniaturization. Arch Dermatol. 2001;137:641-6.
24. Deloche C, de Lacharrière O, Misciali C, Piraccini BM, Vincenzi C, Bastien P, et al. Histological features of peripilar signs associated with androgenetic alopecia. Arch Dermatol Res. 2004;295:422-8.
25. Bernstien RM. Follicular unit hair transplantation. In: Robinson JK, Hanke CW, Siegel DM (Eds). Surgery of Skin, 2nd edition. Mosby: Elsevier; 2010. pp. 485-512.
26. Mubki T, Rudnicka L, Olszewska M, Shapiro J. Evaluation and diagnosis of the hair loss patient: part I. History and clinical examination. J Am Acad Dermatol. 2014;71:415.e1-415.e15.
27. Blume-Peytavi U, Hillmann K, Guarrera M. Hair growth assessment techniques. In: Blume-Peytavi U, Tosti A, Whiting DA (Eds). Hair Growth and Disorders. Heidelberg, Germany: Springer; 2008. pp. 125-57.
28. Rudnicka L, Olszewska M, Rakowska A, Kowalska-Oledzka E, Slowinska M. Trichoscopy: a new method for diagnosing hair loss. J Drugs Dermatol. 2008;7:651-4.
29. Sasmaz S, Senol M, Ozcan A, Dogan G, Tuncer C, Akyol O, et al. The risk of coronary heart disease in men with androgenetic alopecia. J Eur Acad Dermatol Venereol. 1999;12:123-5.
30. Kaliyadan F, Nambiar A, Vijayaraghavan S. Androgenetic alopecia: an update. Indian J Dermatol Venereol Leprol. 2013;79:613-25.
31. Tosti A, Whiting D, Iorizzo M, Pazzaglia M, Misciali C, Vincenzi C, et al. The role of scalp dermoscopy in the diagnosis of alopecia areata incognita. J Am Acad Dermatol. 2008;59:64-7.
32. Chartier MB, Hoss DM, Grant-Kels JM. Approach to the adult female patient with diffuse non-scarring alopecia. J Am Acad Dermatol. 2002;47:809-18.
33. Whiting DA. Diagnostic and predictive value of horizontal sections of scalp biopsy specimens in male pattern androgenetic alopecia. J Am Acad Dermatol. 1993;28:755-63.
34. Price VH, Menefee E, Strauss PC. Changes in hair weight and hair count in men with androgenetic alopecia, after application of 5% and 2% topical minoxidil, placebo, or no treatment. J Am Acad Dermatol.1999;41:717-21.
35. Olsen EA. Topical minoxidil in the treatment of androgenetic alopecia in women. Cutis. 1991;48:243-8.
36. Kaufman KD, Olsen EA, Whiting D, Savin R, DeVillez R, Bergfeld W, et al. Finasteride in the treatment of men with androgenetic alopecia. J Am Acad Dermatol. 1998;39:578-89.
37. Finasteride Male Pattern Hair Loss Study Group. Long-term (5-year) multinational experience with finasteride 1 mg in the treatment of men with androgenetic alopecia. Eur J Dermatol. 2002;12:38-49.
38. Olsen EA, Hordinsky M, Whiting D, Stough D, Hobbs S, Ellis ML, et al. The importance of dual 5-alpha reductase inhibition in the treatment of male pattern hair loss: results of a randomized placebo-controlled study of dutasteride vs. finasteride. J Am Acad Dermatol. 2006;55:1014-23.
39. Stough D. Dutasteride improves male pattern hair loss in a randomized study in identical twins. J Cosmet Dermatol. 2007;6:9-13.
40. Chandrashekar BS, Nandhini T, Vasanth V, Sriram R, Navale S. Topical minoxidil fortified with finasteride: an account of maintenance of hair density after replacing oral finasteride. Indian Dermatol Online J. 2015;6:17-20.
41. Khandpur S, Suman M, Reddy BS. Comparative efficacy of various treatment regimens for androgenetic alopecia in men. J Dermatol. 2002;29:489-98.
42. Khatu SS, More YE, Gokhale NR, Chavhan DC, Bendsure N. Platelet-rich plasma in androgenic alopecia: myth or an effective tool. J Cutan Aesthet Surg. 2014;7:107-10.
43. Afifi L, Maranda EL, Zarei M, Delcanto GM, Falto-Aizpurua L, Kluijfhout WP, et al. Low-level laser therapy as a treatment for androgenetic alopecia. Lasers Surg Med. 2017;49(1):27-39.

CHAPTER 66

Basic Principles of Hair Transplantation

Aniketh Venkataram, Mysore Venkataram

KEY MESSAGES

- The concept of follicular unit has made major contributions to several aspects of follicular unit transplantation—both strip dissection and extraction methods.
- It has enabled accurate calculation the number of grafts needed by knowing the density in donor and area of recipient.
- It has allowed dense packing and consistency in results.

INTRODUCTION

There are three basic principles of hair transplantation:

1. The principle of donor dominance—that the occipital area consists of androgen resistant hairs and are therefore permanent—and they retain this property when transplanted to other areas.
2. In addition to donor dominance, there is also the concept of recipient influence enunciated by Tommy Hwang who demonstrated that body hair when transplanted to scalp assumes the property of scalp hair and grows longer (vice versa is also true)—a property used in body hair transplantation.
3. Since, the donor area is smaller than the potential bald area, a small area of donor hair needs to be used to cover a much larger recipient site—hence what is done in any hair transplantation is to create an illusion of hair, to cover the bald area. The logic behind this seemingly imbalanced equation needs to be well understood in order to understand the possibilities and limitations of this procedure. This will enable the surgeon to maximize donor usage, achieve satisfactory recipient cover, as well as plan the overall treatment plan.

The above three principles basically govern the logic of hair transplantation discussed here.

The logic of hair distribution and the follicular unit-donor area:

Logic 1: Follicular unit (FU) transplantation gives natural looking results as the original natural architecture and distribution is preserved.

A follicular unit consists of 1–4 terminal hairs, with their arrectores muscle, sebaceous gland, 1–3 vellus hairs, perifollicular collagen, nerves, and vessels supplying the unit. These are naturally occurring units and each person has a different proportion of these units; 1/2/3/4/5/rarely 6 hairs **(Fig. 1)**. These are transplanted as such and hence give natural results and are the basis of logic 1.

Logic 2: The FUs are smaller, it takes smaller holes to place them in and hence more holes can be made in a given area; more units can be placed in a given area allowing denser packing, leading to better results. The unit is pyramid in shape, the narrowest part being at the junction of arrectors and widest at the bottom where the hairs splay. There is a small amount of dermis in between these units. In contrast, in the minimicrografts, two neighboring follicles or follicular units were clubbed together, with a lot more dermis in between as below. This means the grafts were larger and needed wider holes to place them in **(Figs. 2A and B)**.

Logic 3: Because of limited donor hairs, it is never possible to provide a normal density in any patient nor is it possible to cover entire balding scalp in stage 7 baldness satisfactorily with only units from occipital scalp. What is possible to

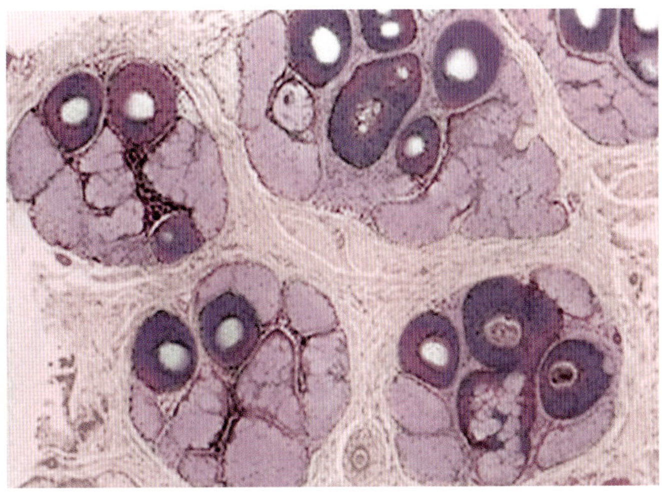

Fig. 1: Follicular units seen by horizontal section at the level of sebaceous gland.

achieve is cosmetic density, to create an impression or an illusion of density.

An average scalp is usually 500 cm^2 (50,000 mm^2) in area, with a follicular unit distribution of 1 per mm^2. Each follicular unit (in an Indian Scalp) has on an average 2–2.3 hairs. This leads to a total hair count of 100,000.[1] Out of the total 50,000 follicular units on the scalp, 75%, i.e., 37,500 are on the frontal region and vertex and hence are at risk of being lost. The permanent donor area has 25%, i.e., 12,500 units. As we need 50% to appear normal, this means that a maximum of 6,250 follicular units are available for transplantation. So, in a worst case scenario, *patient would have 12.5% (6,250) follicles available to cover 75% (37,500) area achieving a density of 1/6 (18%) of normal.*[2,3] Therefore, we have roughly one-fourth the numbers of units to cover the entire scalp.

It must be, however, noted that availability of beard and body hair has expanded the donor available.

Logic 4: A person with greater follicular unit density will have a better result than a person with lesser unit density. A person with more larger units containing 3–4 hairs will have a better result than a person with smaller units containing 1–2 hairs **(Figs. 3A and B)**.[4,5]

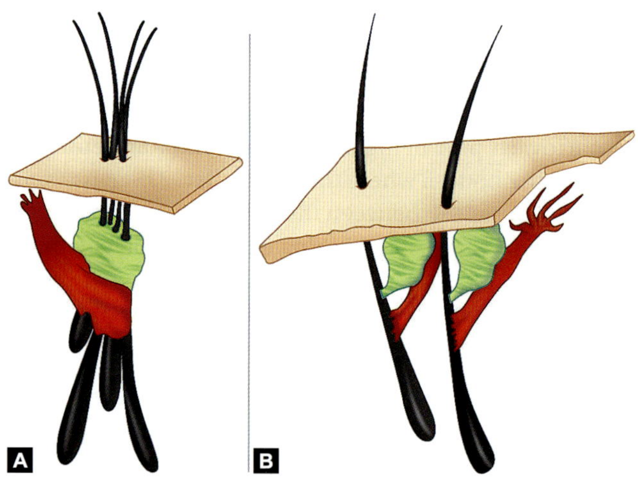

Figs. 2A and B: (A) Schematic diagram of follicular unit; (B) Micrograft—note the larger micrograft even though it contains only two hairs.

It is important to differentiate follicular unit density, which remains relatively constant at $1/mm^2$ from hair density, which varies from 1.5 to $3/mm^2$ (normal = $2/mm^2$). Hence, the hair density is a function of the number of hairs per follicular unit, rather than the total number of follicular units.[2,3] This differentiation is important as it means that a donor area with a lower hair density will need more number of follicular units than a donor with a higher hair density to achieve the same result, as will be elucidated in the following paragraphs.

Logic 5: Along with number, diameter of hair and length of hair play an important role in creating the illusion of thick hairs. A person with thicker hairs gets better results than thinner hairs. Length, curliness and color of hairs are also important factors affecting hair volume and hence appearance.

Hair is a cylinder and the volume is given by the formula $\pi r^2 h$. So, a small increase in radius increases volume geometrically. Likewise, length helps a greater area to be covered. For example:

- Volume of 1,000 hairs with thickness 0.6 μm height 1 cm: $3.14 \times 0.6 \times 0.6 \times 1{,}000 = 1{,}130\ cm^3$
- Volume of 1,000 hairs with thickness 0.7 μm height 1 cm: $3.14 \times 0.7 \times 0.7 \times 1{,}000 = 1{,}538\ cm^3$ which is 36% more, i.e., an 11% increase in radius increases volume by 36% by geometric progression.

  Longer hairs create greater volume and cover greater area.

Importance of length: Length can help cover the gaps - longer the hair more the volume and more area it covers and thicker it appears. For example:

- Volume of 1,000 hairs with thickness 0.6 μm height (length) 1 cm: $3.14 \times 0.6 \times 0.6 \times 1{,}000 \times 1 = 1{,}130\ cm^3$
- Volume of 1,000 hairs with thickness 0.6 μm height 10 cm: $3.14 \times 0.6 \times 0.6 \times 1000 \times 10 = 113{,}000\ cm^3$

  Ten time more length increases total volume ten times.

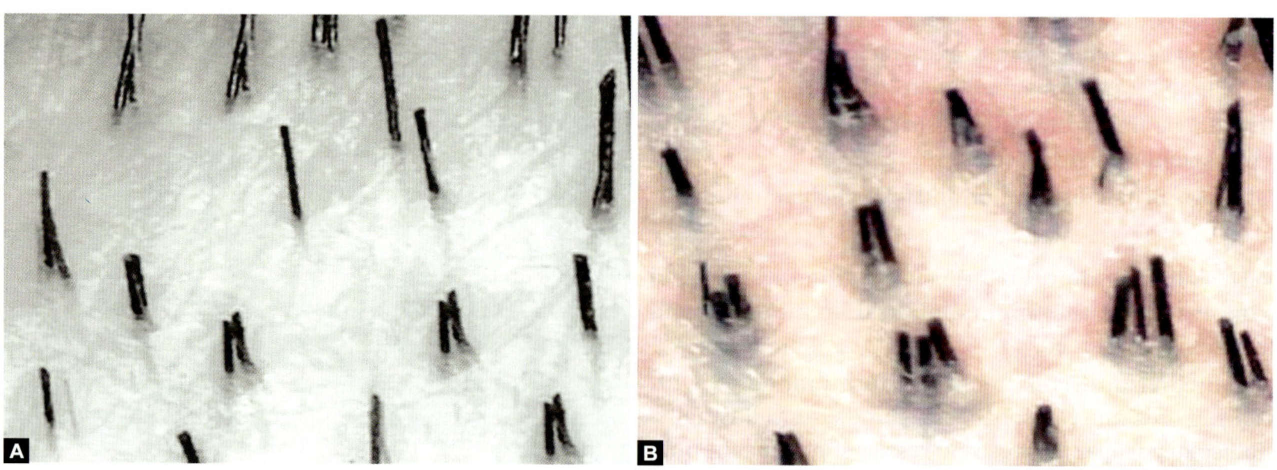

Figs. 3A and B: (A) TrichoScan® with low hair density—most of the units have 1–2 hairs; (B) TrichoScan® with medium hair density—most of the units have 2–3 hairs.

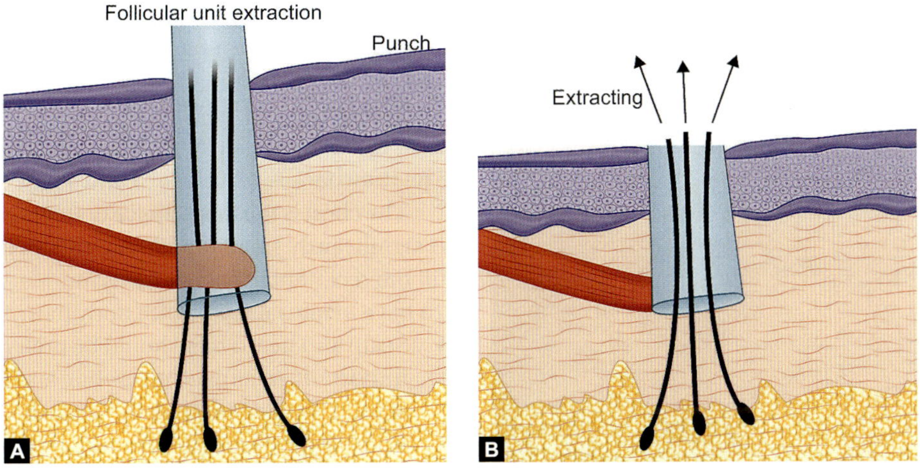

Figs. 4A and B: (A) Introduction of punch; (B) Extraction of unit.

Logic 6: Density needs to be greatest where it matters most; in the front and on the left side when hairs are combed from left to right. *Giving 40–50% of original density is sufficient to create an excellent result. This is called cosmetic density.*

Early on, in the process of balding, the number of follicular units/mm^2 remains constant (though ultimately all hairs in a unit disappear); the thinning appearance is due to the reduction in the number of hairs per follicular unit. The average person can lose up to 50% of his hair, before it is noticeably thin (i.e., a hair density of 1/mm^2).

Hence, while performing transplantation from the unaffected donor area, a follicular unit density of 0.5/mm^2 is required in the frontal hairline to appear normal. In areas behind the hairline, where layering and weighting can add value, less than 50% of the original density may be enough to achieve fullness.

These facts emphasize one premise; we need to use our precious supply of FUs judiciously and long-term planning is necessary as recipient area can increase in future, hence each session should be planned keeping the future possibilities in mind. If the first stage is done at the age of 25, for example, it should be done to achieve the overall density that will be present at the age of 45, else we would end-up having high fullness in one area, low in another.[5] In the donor area, density can vary from area to area; it is greatest in the center of the occipital scalp and least at the lateral edge of the strip.

In the recipient area, density needs to vary depending on the cosmetic significance of the area. Patients expect to look very good in the front—this area therefore needs a higher density and the density can be lower over central scalp. Also if a person combs from left to right, more density needs to be placed on left than right part of the bald area—hence, larger units need to be placed on the left side than the right side, as hairs would flow from left to right, and hence create a visual impression as they flow in to right. This logic also explains why it is difficult to achieve impressive results over vertex—this flow of hairs in one direction does not happen over vortex which is circular in shape and hence hairs spread in all directions like spokes of a wheel.

Logic 7: Follicular unit transplantation (FUT): FUT consists of removing a strip of skin and all its follicles and suturing the wound closed. Hence, the most important thing to remember is that the *density of the donor area does not change noticeably* along with the number of units, the area of skin is also being reduced.

Logic 8: Follicular unit extraction (FUE): The narrowest part of hair unit is at the site of arrectores where the hairs are held by the muscle. So, a small diameter (0.8–1 mm) punch is needed to reach up to this level and loosen the hold of the muscle. Below the muscle is the inferior segment of the hair which is the temporary part of the hair (as it disappears during telogen phase). So, once the muscle is loosened, the entire unit becomes loose and comes out easily. The size of the hole made is small and heals with minimal scarring. This is the basis of FUE **(Figs. 4A and B)**.

The most important thing to remember with FUE is that *the donor density reduces*. This is because while the number of units is reducing, the area stays the same. Hence, as far as possible no two neighboring units should be taken (in either direction) so that the density does not noticeably reduce. This means that total numbers of hairs that can be taken out safely is one in 4 hair units and hence does not exceed 3,000–4,000 in a person who has 12,000–16000 units in safe donor area. If more is taken out, then the ratio 1:4 is breached. If this happens, as in mega sessions (more than 3,000 units are taken out), gaps between neighboring hair units will reach 3 mm, the area looks mottled and hence patient needs longer hairs to cover the gaps—which will defeat one of the premises of FUE that patient can keep trim shorter hairs.

Logic 9: Combining FUT and FUE—this technique combines the maximum advantages of both **(Fig. 5)**.

Follicular unit extraction gives accesses to greater donor area by taking *some hairs* from everywhere—it helps us

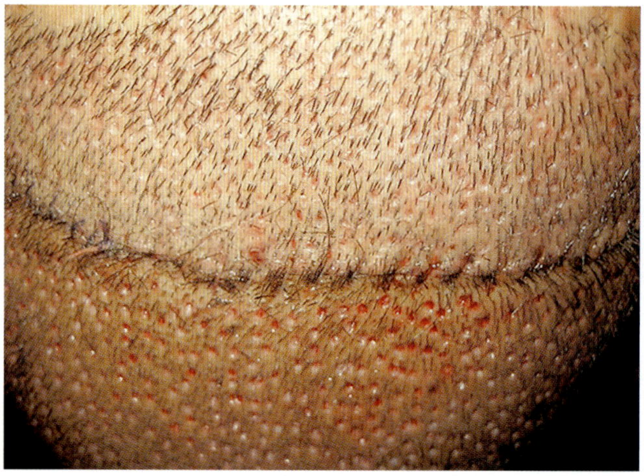

Fig. 5: Strip technique can be combined with FUE to optimize donor harvesting.

to harvest from areas where strip would never have been possible.

Follicular unit transplant or follicle unit strip surgery allows the surgeon to take *all hairs* from one small area and retains the option of taking from the same area by including the previous scar (due to the stretchable property of skin). Hence, combining the two techniques can give larger number of hairs.

A strip can give 2,500 units. An FUE from above and below the strip can give another 1,500 units in the same session. Hence, 4,000 units can be obtained in one session.

Logic 10: Body hair transplantation: The concept of recipient influence was enunciated by Tommy Hwang,[6] who demonstrated that body hair when transplanted to scalp assumes the property of scalp hair and grows longer—a property used in body hair transplantation. This has made it possible to transplant body hair from beard, chest, and other areas when scalp hair is exhausted, and has ensured unlimited number of hairs being available. Hence, almost any area in any extent of bald scalp can now be covered. This area of hair transplantation is now assuming increased importance as patients are insisting on FUE only, and are shying away from FUT.

The beard is the second choice donor area after the scalp as its hair diameter matches scalp hair and the hair grows long. The drawback is the lack of 3 and 4 hair units.

The chest is the third choice donor area as its hair diameter is significantly smaller and hair growth is hampered initially till the recipient influence kicks in.

To have a natural result with body hair:

- Scalp and beard hair should be preferred for cosmetically important areas like the hairline and the vertex. Body hair should be used for the mid-section
- Body hair should be interspersed with scalp hair to camouflage them.

CONCLUSION

Thus, understanding the above mathematical principles with regards to hair loss, enables the surgeon to plan and economize donor graft supple to achieve a balanced, aesthetically pleasing appearance in the long run, and avoids mistakes and short sightedness.

REFERENCES

1. Bernstein RM, Rassman WR. The aesthetics of follicular transplantation. Dermatol Surg. 1997;23(9):785-99.
2. Bernstein RM, Rassman WR. Follicular transplantation. Patient evaluation and surgical planning. Dermatol Surg. 1997;23: 771-84.
3. Bernstein RM, Rassman WR. The logic of follicular unit transplantation. Dermatol Clin. 1999;17(2):277-96.
4. Venkataram M. Changing trends in hair restoration surgery. Indian J Dermatol Venereol Leprol. 2006;72:103-12.
5. Bernstein RM, Rassman WR. Follicular unit hair transplantation. Dermatol Surg. 1997;23:771-84.
6. Hwand ST, Kim HY, Lee SJ, et al. Recipient-site influence in hair transplantation: a confirmative study. Dermatol Surg. 2009;35:1011-4.

CHAPTER 67

Counseling and Case Selection for Hair Restoration Surgery

Vaishalee Kirane

KEY MESSAGES

- A successful outcome of hair restoration surgery also depends, among other factors, on proper counseling and patient selection.
- Counseling is an integral part of a patient's consultation, necessary throughout the hair transplant journey and beyond.
- Counseling done with compassion and genuine interest in the patient will help to develop a good rapport and build a strong patient–physician relationship.
- Counseling is of utmost importance to educate the patient about the nature of hair loss as well as explain the benefits and limitations of hair transplantation.
- Importance of selecting an appropriate patient for hair restoration surgery cannot be understated to achieve good results and requires a detailed consultation and thorough examination.

INTRODUCTION

An individual perceives having a good mane of hair on the head to play a very important role in determining the external beauty, to project a good body image and boost his/her self-confidence.

Suffering from hair-loss, mainly from the scalp, but also from the eyebrows or from moustache or beard area in males, thus causes a lot of anxiety and psychological distress.

This psychological aspect needs as much attention and time, if not more, along with the medical and surgical management of alopecia and thus comes the role of good counseling.

COUNSELING

Physicians have to recognize that any hair issue goes well beyond the simple physical aspect of hair loss and that it is also very important to address its psychosocial and economic impact.[1] Counseling done with a compassionate attitude, taking care not to be judgmental or impatient, goes a long way to gain their trust and goodwill. Many a time, the patient gains therapeutic benefit simply by talking out their concerns with a caring physician. This attitude should be developed and emphasized along with the other important aspects of evaluation, investigations, prescribing medicines or performing hair transplant surgery. Counseling will help to develop a good rapport with the patient and build a strong patient–physician relationship.

The first interaction of the patient starts with either the doctor or more commonly with the receptionist or the front-desk person while taking an appointment for their hair concerns. It is important that they are trained in the soft-skills while dealing with the patients. He/she being warm and knowledgeable will in turn become useful for the subsequent consultation done by the physician.

Providing informational material either via digital platforms such as our website, other social media or giving the patients printed brochures and handouts in the clinic will also be very helpful. Another useful practice is to encourage the presence of the patient's family or close friend in the clinic during the consultation and counseling, especially when hair restorative surgery is being planned.[2-4]

Counseling for hair transplant surgery will also involve explaining the various factors relevant to the patient, elicited during the detailed history, thorough examination and necessary test results. This will range from discussing the patient's lifestyle, nutritional status, hormonal assay and any internal medical issues, as they will also contribute in determining the success of hair transplant surgery.

Continued communication with the patient even after surgery will help them to remain faithful to you and even recommend you to others. It will also help to mitigate the negative impact and decrease the possibility of any litigation if any problem should ever arise from your treatment.[2]

Counseling is thus an integral part of patient care and is required throughout our interaction with the patient, right from when he/she first contacts the doctor or clinic for an appointment, till much beyond the hair restoration surgery (HRS).

Preoperative Counseling for Hair Restoration Surgery

Primary aim of HRS is to carefully tailor an optimal surgical approach to the patient's expressed concerns and particular

BOX 1: Preoperative counseling for hair restoration surgery.

- Eliciting history of medicines
- Previous use of cosmetic hair replacement and camouflage products
- Counseling regarding the use of FDA approved Minoxidil and Finasteride for the male and only Minoxidil for the female patient prior to and post HRS to retard further hair loss as well as to counter the unbearable, albeit temporary, telogen effluvium postoperatively
- Photo documentation of design of the area of hair reconstruction preoperatively
- Explanations regarding the progressive nature of hair fall, and that HRS is not a one-time solution
- Counsel regarding treating a large recipient area in order of priority and addressing it in more than one session

regional hair deficit **(Box 1)**. Goal should also be to determine a surgical plan appropriate for the age and the expected long-term donor-recipient area ratio.

Counseling will involve discussing some points and objectives which can be realistically achieved by the surgery, given further.

a. The nature of the medical problem of hair loss.
b. Benefits and limitations of hair transplantation.
c. Visual or cosmetic density which will help to camouflage the bald scalp area versus the actual density.
d. Fate of the existing hair.
e. Longevity of results.
f. Need of continuation of medical line of treatment before and after transplant.
g. Psychologically unfit patients,[4] especially who exhibit symptoms of major depressive or body dysmorphic syndrome, should be discouraged from undergoing HRS and referred to a trained psychiatrist for further counseling.

Counseling for hair restoration surgery will thus involve a detailed explanation regarding:

- Balance between realistic expectations and therapeutic limitations.
- Multifactorial etiology and associated psychological impact.
- Combining modalities of treatment for better results, e.g., pharmacotherapy, cosmetic aids, procedures or surgical hair restoration if indicated.

Use of camouflage products as an adjuvant therapy can be advised to hide thinning or baldness when the medical and surgical treatments take time to show result, not found effective or not desired by the patient. We can outline the various products available such as pigmented hair fibers, powders, wigs, hair pieces or hair extensions which would be more natural, weigh less and can be customized.

CASE SELECTION FOR HAIR RESTORATION SURGERY

The number of patients coming to dermatology OPDs for problems of hair fall, hair thinning and baldness is showing a rising trend over the years. They also tend to be more aware of various aspects about hair restoration, both surgical and nonsurgical modalities such as hair pieces and wigs. Sometimes they themselves insist on which method of hair restoration they want, having heard about the experience from their friends, colleagues, or media. It thus becomes very much necessary for us to evaluate thoroughly in order to determine whether the patient is a suitable candidate for surgery. This in turn becomes crucial for the final successful outcome of HRS.

Proper case selection requires detailed history, thorough examination, and correct diagnosis of the alopecia. The primary aim should be to tailor an optimal cosmetic coverage of the bald area, taking into consideration the expectations of the patient, the donor hair availability, and particular regional hair deficit. Surgical plan appropriate for his/her age should be decided, keeping in mind the expected long-term donor-recipient area ratio.[5,6]

1. *Case selection according to indications for HRS:* Androgenetic alopecia was and still is, the primary and most common indication for hair restoration surgery (HRS). But now, with the harvesting of smaller follicular units being made possible by method of follicular unit extraction (FUE), improved surgical skills, advanced techniques and specialized instruments, various other causes of alopecia including cicatricial alopecia, smaller areas like eyebrows, can also be selected as well as making it possible to harvest body hairs for HRS, as given in **Table 1**.
2. *According to the pattern and severity.*
   Various aspects for case selection and planning are:
   i. How the patient styles his/her hair is an important aspect in surgical planning. A patient would be a good candidate for HRS if the design and hairstyle which can be adopted after the surgery is acceptable and pleasing.
   ii. Classification of pattern baldness has always been the main key factor in determining the patient selection, with more severe the baldness, more difficult or creative the planning will have to be.
   iii. Norwood emphasizes six major factors and three minor donor hair characteristics to be taken into consideration when selecting patients and planning procedure for hair transplants.[7] The six major factors are classification, color, curl, texture (caliber), density and amount of donor hair. The three minor factors are amount of terminal and vellus hair that remain in the bald area and the color of the skin.
   Along with the classification and extent of the hair loss, the hair characteristics and density also assume importance.
      a. More the contrast between the hair and scalp color, more the difficulty in getting a natural look. Dark hair on a white skin will cause a problem in undetectability. Gray hair gives little contrast between the hair and scalp color, so any plan or

TABLE 1: Indications for hair restoration surgery (HRS).

Male pattern androgenetic alopecia (Receding frontotemporal hair line ± vertex with sparing the parietal and occipital scalp)	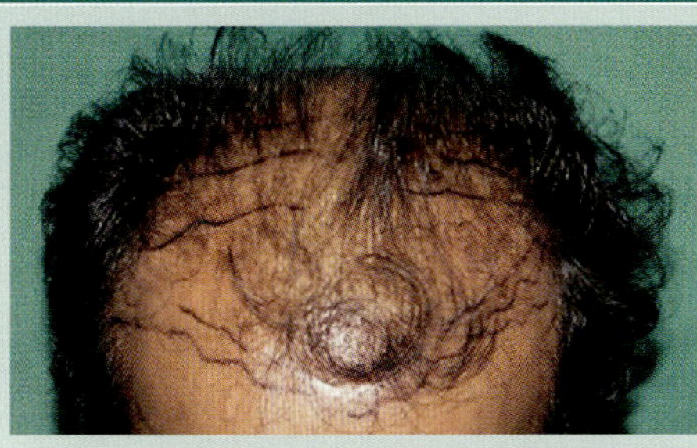 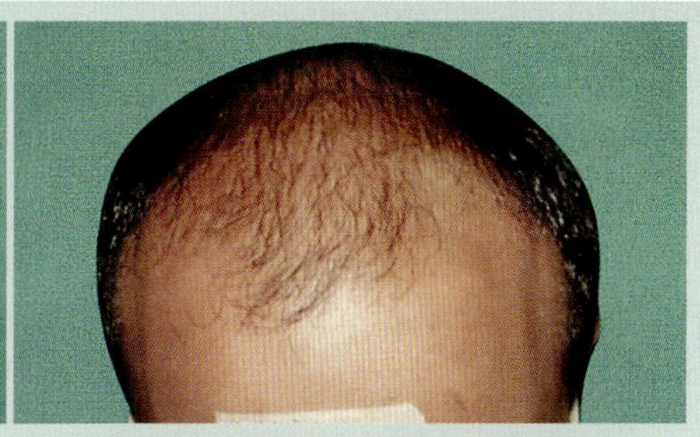
Female pattern hair loss (FPAGA) (Hair partition widening ± hair thinning on top of scalp)	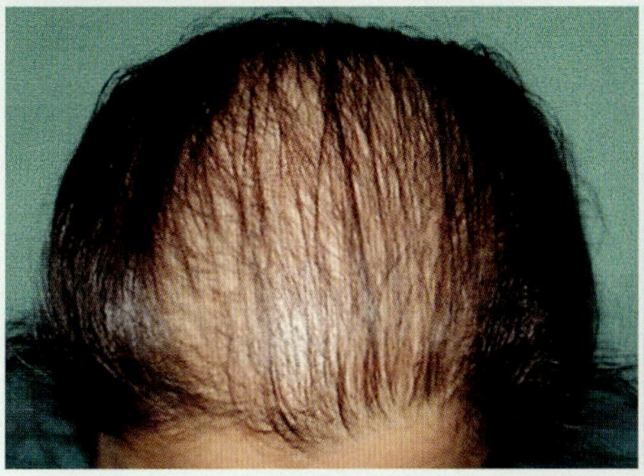 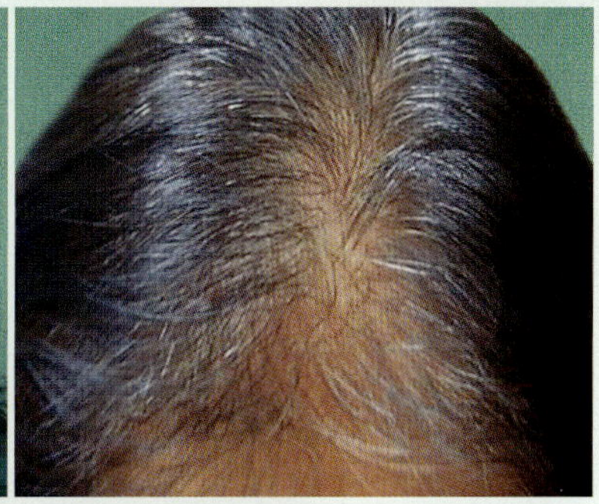
Congenital causes of hair loss: **En coup de sabre**	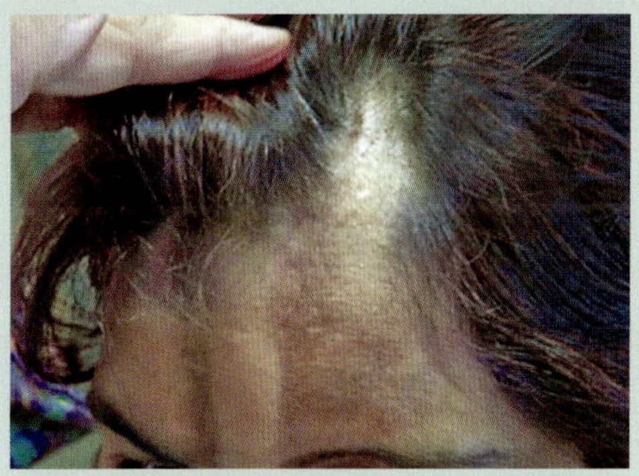
Congenital triangular alopecia (CTA)	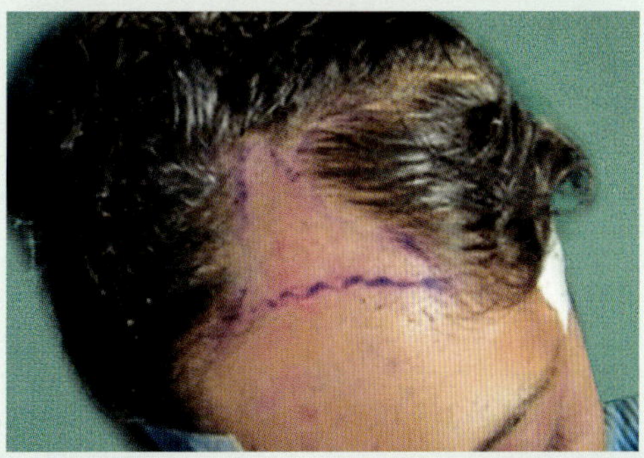
Scarring alopecia patches after injury or burns	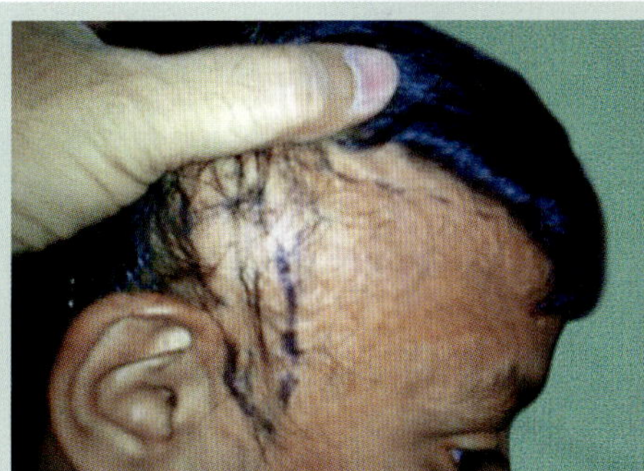 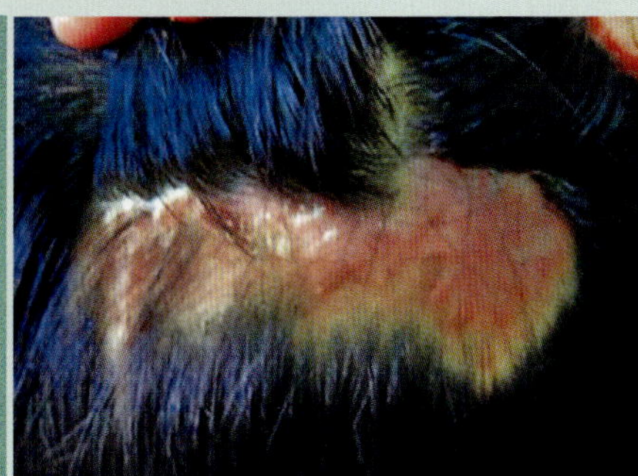

Contd...

Contd...

Burnt-out inflammatory alopecia patches: Frontal fibrosing alopecia (FFA)	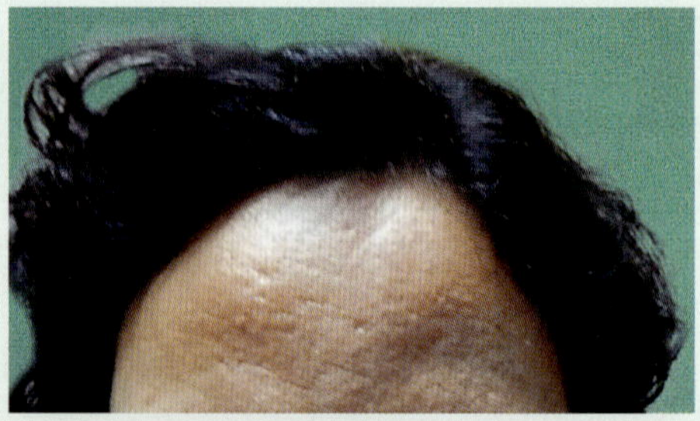
Pseudopelade of Brocq (after careful consideration of disease activity in very selected cases)	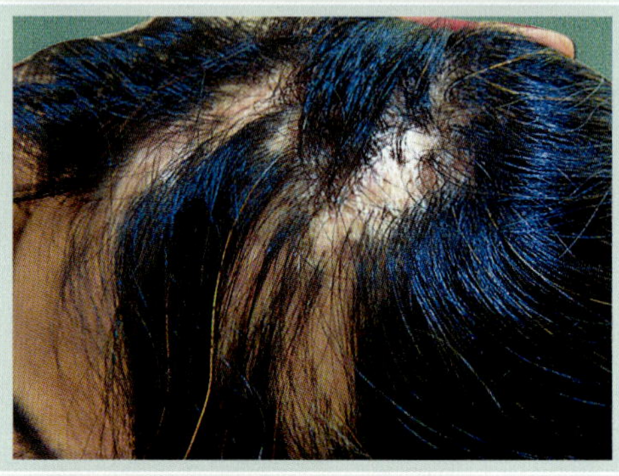
Hair bearing area other than scalp like: Eyebrows	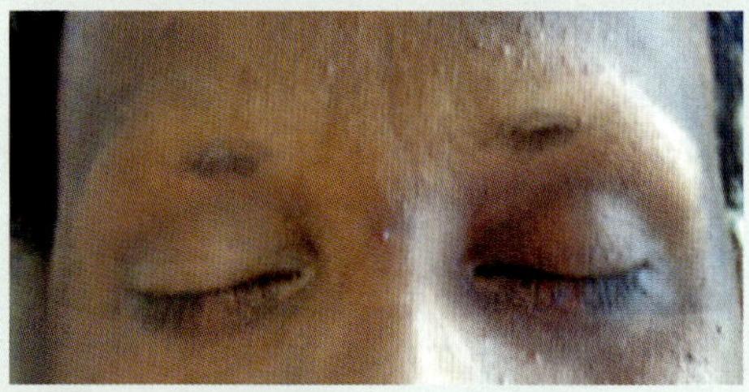
	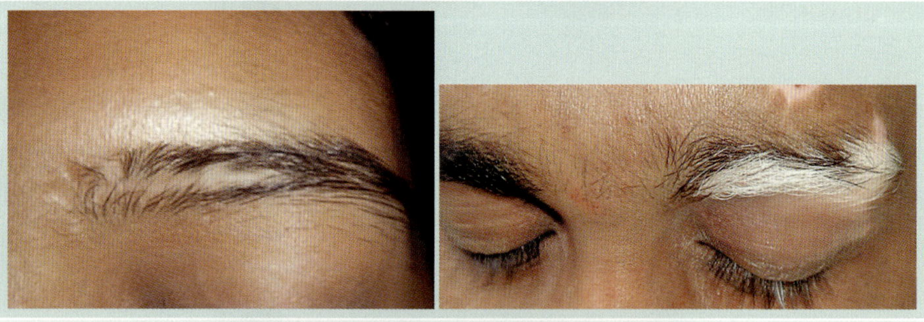
Moustache area	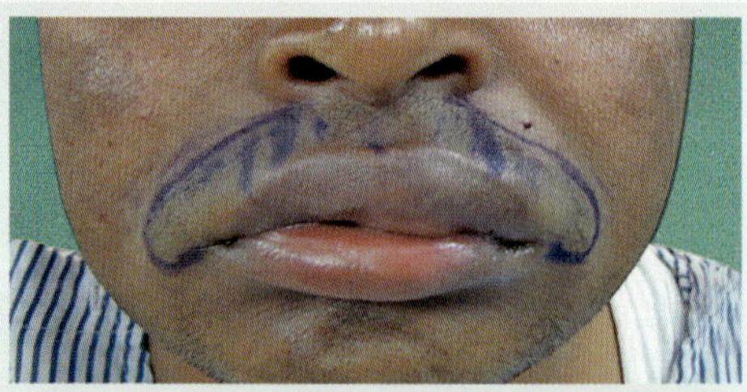
Side locks area	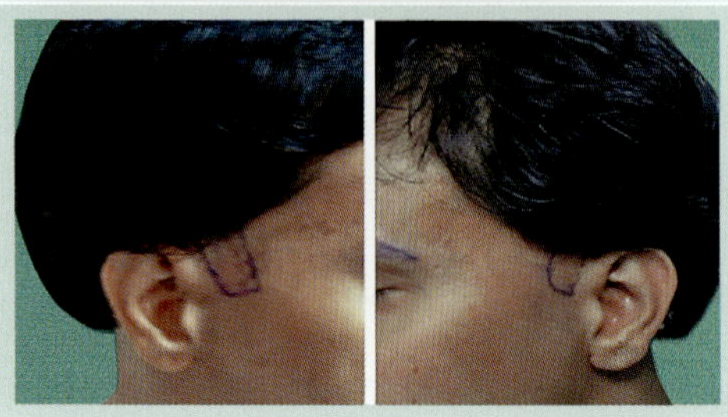

Source: Tricho-transform HT team, Pune.

design will look natural. Fine single hair grafts are useful to construct the front hair line to give a softer look, while two to three hair grafts, which will add volume, are inserted onto the mid-scalp and vertex to give better central density.

b. Hair with thicker caliber and more curl will give an illusion of high visual perceived density.

c. Laxity and elasticity of the donor area of the scalp is also very important as it will determine the availability of number of donor hair and also the risk of a wider donor scar.

d. The temporal hair density supports the frontal hair line to give a more natural look. It should thus be included in planning its position and the density of the frontal region as a whole.

Dr Alejandro Camps Fresneda from Spain added age of the patient as another factor in his article. Depending on the age of the patient, a different approach would be necessary for the same type of alopecia extent.[8] It will be prudent to give a patient above 50 years of age a higher hairline in contrast to a younger patient.

3. *According to examination of the scalp:* Proper examination of the scalp for any problems such as psoriasis, dermatitis or any inflammatory process as well as thorough evaluation of the hair characteristics and its density is essential before selecting any candidate for transplant surgery.
   i. *The recipient area* of the scalp should be examined regarding the nature and extent of thinning or baldness, its classification, and the minor factors as mentioned earlier. These should then be recorded in the preoperative notes. Photo documentation is very much an essential preoperative aspect. Trichoscopy and scalp biopsy should also be done as required. Any pathological findings of the scalp or hair, which may prove to be relative or absolute contraindications for surgery, are also noted. For example, psoriasis, alopecia areata or any inflammatory skin condition of the scalp, infective lesions, any associated scarring or frizzy and easily breakable hair shafts, etc., need to be noted. Evaluation of the recipient site will also include examination of previously transplanted hairs for favorable or poor results.
   ii. *Donor area* evaluation will similarly include examination of the occipital scalp skin for its elasticity, hair density, and hair characteristics. Good elasticity of the donor area of the scalp is important to get more number of available donor hairs and better wound scar. Hair density and characteristics such as caliber, curl and color of donor hairs is also noted. This will be useful to determine the final outcome of coverage with high visual or cosmetic density. Patient may have a hidden alopecia areata patch, scar or a nevus, which may affect outcome of the surgery.

4. *According to the contraindications for HRS and the method used, whether FUE or FUT (Strip technique):*
   Most of the contraindications would be relative rather than absolute, for undertaking a hair transplant surgery. Plus the various advances in all aspects of the procedure have helped to circumvent such reasons.
   They are the following:
   i. Very sparse donor hair on the occipital area of the scalp, especially in the case of retrograde hair loss occurring from the nape of neck upwards.
   ii. Large extensive baldness on the top of scalp like Grade VI-VII of Norwood classification of AGA in males.
   iii. Scarring alopecia affecting the graft uptake and survival.
   iv. Chronic inflammatory scalp problems like lupus, lichen planus, which are still in the active stage of inflammation or infective lesions of folliculitis decalvans.
   v. Young patient in early twenties, as one needs to be mindful of the permanent nature of the transplanted hairs in the face of a progressive nature of alopecia and dwindling supply of donor hairs.
   vi. Medically unfit person as also deemed by the treating physician.

   Further evaluation for any internal medical problems, laboratory workup, and relevant medical intervention would be necessary before selecting the patient for surgery.
   Hair transplantation, thus, can be performed in any person with good donor area hair, in good general health and reasonable expectations.[9] Caution should be exercised in very young patients whose early alopecia is still evolving, patients with Norwood grade VI or VII with poor hair density, patients with unrealistic expectations and patients with significant systemic health problems.

5. *Considerations in special areas/situations:*
   i. *Vertex or crown baldness:* The front hairline and mid-scalp in male pattern hair loss (MPHL) should be considered a priority over the vertex or the crown area, as they form the frame for the face and visualized more by the onlookers than the back of the scalp. Obviously the crown can be transplanted if that is the only area of hair loss and age is beyond mid-thirty. Medical management with Minoxidil and Finasteride used for at least a couple of months before surgery as well as continuing them after transplant will surely help.
   ii. *HRS in females:*[10] Female pattern hair loss (FPHL) is unique in females in that, it does not usually cause complete alopecia other than increasing thinning in affected area of hair partition and top of scalp. This requires the hair transplant surgery to focus on improving density of affected thinned out region. Thorough consultation regarding pertinent medical

history, hormonal and nutritional status or any telogen effluvium along with the genetic pattern hair thinning should be looked for and treated accordingly before taking up the patient for surgery. Surgery should not be performed until regrowth of any recent temporary hair loss has occurred (usually 6 months) with proper medical management. Female pattern hair loss is usually diffuse and complete coverage is rarely possible. Thus, extensive counseling needs to be done with respect to the area to be covered, possible hair style preferences, and the need for concomitant medical treatment.

iii. *Body hair transplant:*[11] In the scenario of limited scalp donor hair, other hair bearing body areas can be used as source, to increase the potential follicle supply. The method of FUE provides the hair restoration surgeon with a useful surgical means for accessing this valuable source of donor hair reserve. Drawbacks of using body hair are that the procedure is more tiring and time consuming, provide mostly single hair which are thinner and smaller in length than the scalp hair, and needs multiple sessions to cover big areas. It is for this reason that harvesting body hair can be useful to restore smaller areas such as eyebrows, eyelashes and moustache where we only need single and smaller length hair.

Counseling and case selection will also include the method of HRS to be chosen and performed, whether FUT or FUE or both together. Thus, few points about FUE[4] are being included in this chapter.

Propaganda of scarless surgery or with minimal scars has increased the popularity and practice of FUE over strip surgery. It has rightfully found a place in the surgical management of hair loss.

However, during counseling and patient selection, patients need to be informed that the surgery is not entirely scarless, has a higher transection rate which becomes less with experience and is a time consuming procedure, thus more than one session may be needed to cover large bald areas. It may be unsuitable for women as the entire donor area hair needs to be trimmed.

Indications for performing FUE would be:

- Patients who want to wear their hair very short (and hence the linear scar is unacceptable).
- When a patient specifically requests an FUE procedure and enough grafts can be harvested to meet his or her needs.
- In patients with limited hair loss or those who require small sessions.
- In the treatment of widened scars resulting from traditional strip excisions.
- Patients having inadequate laxity of donor scalp for a strip excision.
- For scarring alopecia from burnt out dermatologic conditions or trauma where FUT is not possible.
- When previous scars of strip surgeries make further strips impossible.
- In patients, who tend to heal with wide or thickened scars.
- For patients with an inordinate fear of pain or scars.
- When body or beard serves as a donor area.

CONCLUSION

- Counseling is an integral part of management of any trichology problem and hair transplantation surgery and is required throughout our interaction with the patient.
- Counseling should be done with compassion which will help to develop a strong patient–physician relationship.
- It is very important to educate the patient about the nature of the hair loss as well as the benefits and limitations of hair transplantation procedure.
- It also involves making the patient understand and have realistic expectations regarding the result of HRS and need for concomitant medical treatment.
- Selecting the right patient for HRS will go a long way in ensuring a successful outcome.
- Thorough consultation and examination of the patient as regards to donor and recipient areas of the scalp, extent of hair loss, donor hair density and hair characteristics and other internal medical problems are needed to determine suitable candidacy.

TIPS AND PEARLS

- Be thorough in counseling
- Always underpromise and overdeliver
- Rule out body dysmorphophobia
- Emphasize the need for medical treatment to prevent further hair loss
- Keep in mind unusual patterns such as diffuse androgenetic alopecia and reverse pattern AGA
- Choose the right technique for the right patient.

REFERENCES

1. Cash TF. The psychosocial consequences of androgenetic alopecia: a review of the research literature. Br J Dermatol. 1999;141:398-405.
2. Shiell R. The initial interview and evaluation. In: Unger WP, Shapiro R, Unger R, Unger M (EDs). Hair Transplantation, 5th edition. New York: CRC Press; 2011. pp. 63.
3. Teutsch C. Patient-doctor communication. Med Clin North Am. 2003;87:1115-45.
4. Rassman WR, Bernstein RM, McClellan R, Jones R, Worton E, Uyttendaele H. Follicular unit extraction: minimally

invasive surgery for hair transplantation. Dermatol Surg. 2002; 28:720-7.

5. Unger WP. Surgical planning and organization. In: Unger WP, Shapiro R, Unger R, Unger M (EDs). Hair Transplantation, 5th edition. New York: CRC Press; 2011. pp. 113.
6. Konior RJ, Simmons C. Patient selection, candidacy, and treatment planning for hair restoration surgery. Facial Plast Surg Clin North Am. 2013;21(3):343-50.
7. Norwood OT. Patient selection, hair transplant design, and hairstyle. J Dermatol Surg Oncol. 1992;18(5):386-94.
8. Camps-Fresneda A. Age and patient selection in planning hair transplantation procedures. J Dermatol Surg Oncol. 1994;20(3):221.
9. Patwardhan N, Mysore V, IADVL Dermatosurgery Task Force. Hair transplantation: standard guidelines of care. Indian J Dermatol Venereol Leprol. 2008;74(Suppl):S46-53.
10. Unger RH. Female hair restoration. Facial Plast Surg Clin North Am. 2013;21(3):407-17.
11. Umar S. Use of body hair and beard hair in hair restoration. Facial Plast Surg Clin North Am. 2013;21(3):469-77.

CHAPTER 68

Design of Anterior Hairline in Male Pattern Baldness

Pradeep Sethi

KEY MESSAGES

- Design of anterior hairline (AHL) is the most critical step in hair restoration surgery.
- It should be designed in a way that it not only fulfills the present demand, but also matches aesthetically with changes in the facial features and hair loss with advancing age.
- Density, direction, angulation, thickness of hair, and multifollicular units, all need to be kept in mind while creating a hairline and the different zones.

INTRODUCTION

Designing of the anterior hairline (AHL) is perhaps the biggest challenge and most critical step in hair restoration surgery. Hairline should be designed in a way that it not only fulfills present aesthetic demand, but also of the future, keeping in mind the changes in facial features and hair loss with advancing age. It should suit the patients' emotional requirements and also confirm to accepted scientific principles. Another challenge is to give a natural-looking hairline with undetectable grafted look and enough density. In short, it should aesthetically frame the face. Patients are needed to be explained about three points:

1. Reconstructed line will remain the same but facial features will keep on changing as age advances. Most patients demand a hairline which they had in childhood, however doing so may not look natural.
2. Secondly, there will be progressive hair loss and patient will continue to lose hair from remaining frontal and mid scalp regions. Hence, a low level of hairline will look unnatural with the passage of time.
3. To lower the AHL (over vertical part of scalp which is actually the forehead), greater number of grafts are needed as this area needs high density of hair follicles to give a natural look. This would deplete the donor for future sessions.

HAIRLINE CONSTRUCTION

Construction of the hairline is discussed under various headings as given further:

- AHL
- Temporal or lateral fringe
- Parietal fringe
- AHL zone.

LANDMARKS FOR THE HAIRLINE

It is important to know major landmarks **(Figs. 1A and B)**.

- *Mid-frontal point:* It is the most anterior point on the frontal hairline in the sagittal plane.
- *Frontotemporal angle:* The point where frontal hairline meets the temporal hairline.
- *Temporal triangle:* It is the triangular protrusion of the temple beyond the line extending from anterior sideburn border.
- *Temporal points:* Anterior peak point of temporal triangle.
- *Vertex transition point*: It is the anterior-most point of the vertex and is the point where the sagittal plane of the skull transits from being mostly horizontal to vertical.

FACTORS TO BE CONSIDERED WHILE DESIGNING THE ANTERIOR HAIRLINE

Following are the factors that need to be considered while designing the AHL:

- *Age of the patient:* The age of the patient is of prime importance. In patterned hair loss and even in otherwise normal individuals, hairline recedes with advancing age. This factor should be kept in mind while planning the hairline in young patients. Young patients often demand a low hairline without recession and these patients need to be counseled in detailed.
- *Hair characteristics:* Several features such as number of hair follicles per follicular units (FUs), thickness, color, and curvature of hair need to be taken into account while reconstructing AHL. A natural hairline has a softer look with hair matching the local skin color, with gradual transition of hair density from ill-defined zone to well-defined denser zone. This is best matched by single hair units, which are thin, with color matching the scalp color. Coarser and thicker hair implantation will give a hard

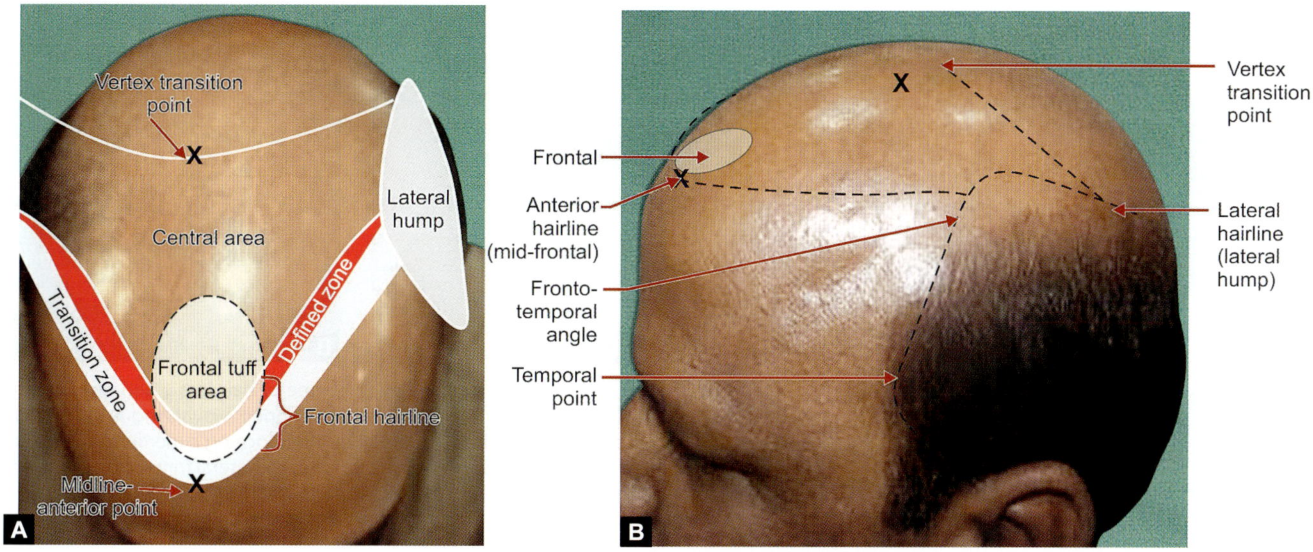

Figs. 1A and B: Scalp zone: (A) Top view; (B) Side view.

look, similarly multiple follicle FUs in AHL will give an unnatural look. More contrast of color of implanted hair with scalp color will show less density and less fullness. Natural curvature or curling enhances visual impact of density.

- *Facial features:* A natural AHL matches with facial aesthetics. The broad, flat forehead will need to have a more flat hairline but a narrow head will need a less flat hairline. So, all facial aesthetics (curvatures) should be considered while reconstructing to give a custom-made hairline.
- *Sex:* Male pattern baldness shows a natural receding hairline while in female pattern hair loss, AHL remains intact. Female face needs a narrowed forehead with more anteriorly placed hairline. But a male has a well-defined frontotemporal angle.
- *Ethnicity:* There is an ethnic variation in AHL. Blacks, Asians, and Hispanics have a broader and flatter hairline, as compared to Caucasians who have an oval AHL.

PLACEMENT OF ANTERIOR BORDER OF THE HAIRLINE

As explained earlier, the rule of thumb "never place AHL too low". A high-placed hairline can be shifted anteriorly but the reverse is not possible.

Few guidelines to place the mid-frontal point include:

- Four finger width above the glabella
- 7–9 cm above the glabella
- A point on forehead where the vertical plane of forehead and horizontal plane of scalp meet **(Figs. 2A and B)**.

Final placement of the AHL is to be individualized depending on size and shape of the head, degree of alopecia, and after understanding patient's expectations.

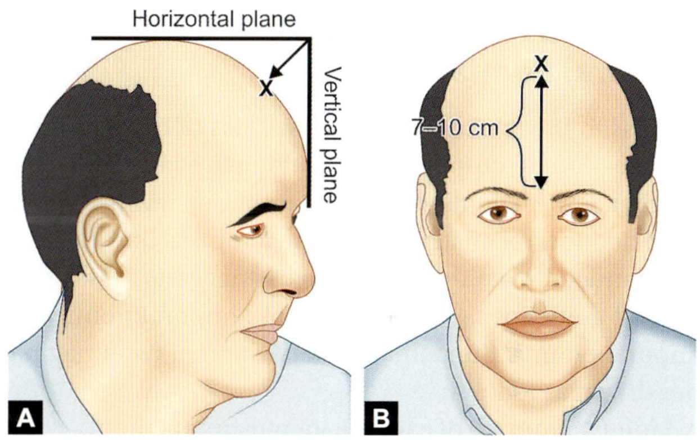

Figs. 2A and B: Placement of midfrontal point. (A) Point at junction of vertical and horizontal plane; (B) A point 7–10 cm from glabella in midline.

FRONTOTEMPORAL ANGLE

Frontotemporal angle is formed by frontal and temporal lines and is a basic characteristic of male pattern hair loss. Proper positioning of this point and recreating a soft frontotemporal angle is one of the most important and also difficult aspects of hairline creation. Blunting this angle or placing it too low will cause an unnatural look.

Guidelines for estimating the frontotemporal points:

- Drawing a line from lateral epicanthus of eye backward to a point where it meets the remaining temporal hair.
- Make sure that the hairline created by this point does not slope downward toward the ear but looks parallel or slopes upward when viewed from the side.
- In mild-to-moderate hair loss, where there is only a little loss of temporal hair, these rules work well. The existing temporal hair becomes the inferior border of the angle while the future AHL becomes the superior border of the

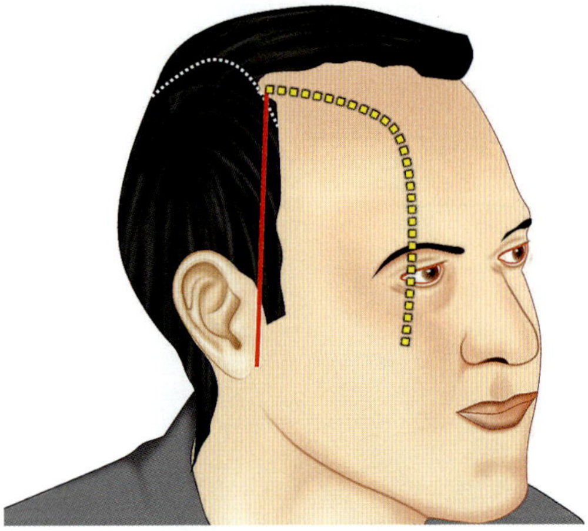

Fig. 3: Placement of frontotemporal angle.

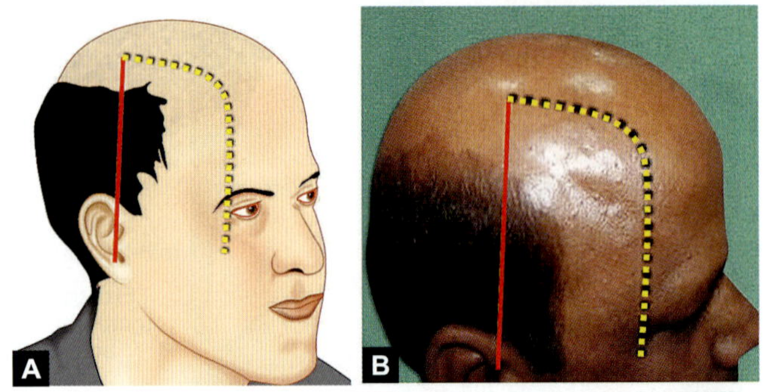

Figs. 4A and B: In more severe degree of hair loss when temporal hair has receded and lateral fringe has dropped, visualizing and recreating "lateral hump" helps. The lateral hump is located superior to the ear and is a semicircular area of hair that bridges the lateral fringe to the mid-scalp region.

angle. The apex of the angle lies on the line that was drawn superiorly from the lateral epicanthus of the eye **(Fig. 3)**.

Recreating the Temporal Fringe and Temporal Points

Hair loss in the temporal area causes loss of temporal point and recession of temporal line resulting in a larger forehead. In earlier days, patients were reluctant about having temporal hump but now reconstruction of the temporal line and point is demanded by patients and hence is necessary. Mayer has outlined guidelines for placement of temporal points. This temporal point is the point of intersection of two imaginary lines drawn as follows:

- Line 1 is from tip of ear lobe to mid-frontal point.
- Line 2 is from base of nose to center of pupil extending to intersect line 1.
- The temporal point is placed lateral and above the lateral end of eyebrow. The angle of hair in this area should be kept as flat as possible. The existing hair help to determine the direction of the hair roots to be implanted, usually pointing downward and backward facing the ear. Single hair units are preferred for the temple area.

PARIETAL HAIRLINE: LATERAL HUMP OR FRINGE

In advanced baldness, the lateral fringe will have dropped to a point where the frontal hairline cannot connect to it. In such cases, there is a need to uplift or restore the lateral fringes. Visualizing and recreating the "lateral hump" helps as the lateral hump is located superior to the ear and is a semicircular area of hair that bridges the lateral fringe to the mid-scalp region. Temporal line and AHL intersects anterior to the hump or approximately 1 cm anterior to a line drawn vertically from the auditory meatus. The temporal line usually becomes the inferior border of the frontotemporal angle **(Figs. 4A and B)**.

Direction of hair should be carefully noted while creating the lateral fringe area. In the upper part, the hair point forward, while in lower part of the fringe, the hair point downward. The anterior portion of the parietal hump blends into the upper temporal line. The existing hair always helps in deciding the angle for implantation of the follicles. The hair in this region are fine in texture and thin in diameter **(Figs. 5 and 6)**.

ANTERIOR HAIRLINE ZONE

Anterior hairline zone consist of three subareas:

1. The anterior-most portion is called the transition zone (TZ).
2. The posterior portion is called the defined zone (DZ).
3. A small oval area in the center of DZ is called frontal tuft area.

Collectively, all the three zones contribute to the overall appearance of the hairline zone.

Transition Zone

Transition zone is the anterior-most zone of the hairline which is approximately 0.5–1.0 cm wide. It is an irregular zone of hair and merges in the DZ. It has some unique features. TZ is composed of micro and macro irregularities.

Micro Irregularity (Figs. 7A and B)

In a normal hairline, there are small intermittent triangular-shaped areas of higher density which contribute a great deal to the appearance of irregularity. This is called micro irregularity. Parsley has called these areas of intermittent density "clusters" and the area between them as "gaps".

Macro Irregularity (Fig. 8)

When we look at the hairline from a distance, the hairline is serpentine or curvaceous than linear. This irregularity is called macro irregularity. Martinine has used the term snail tracking

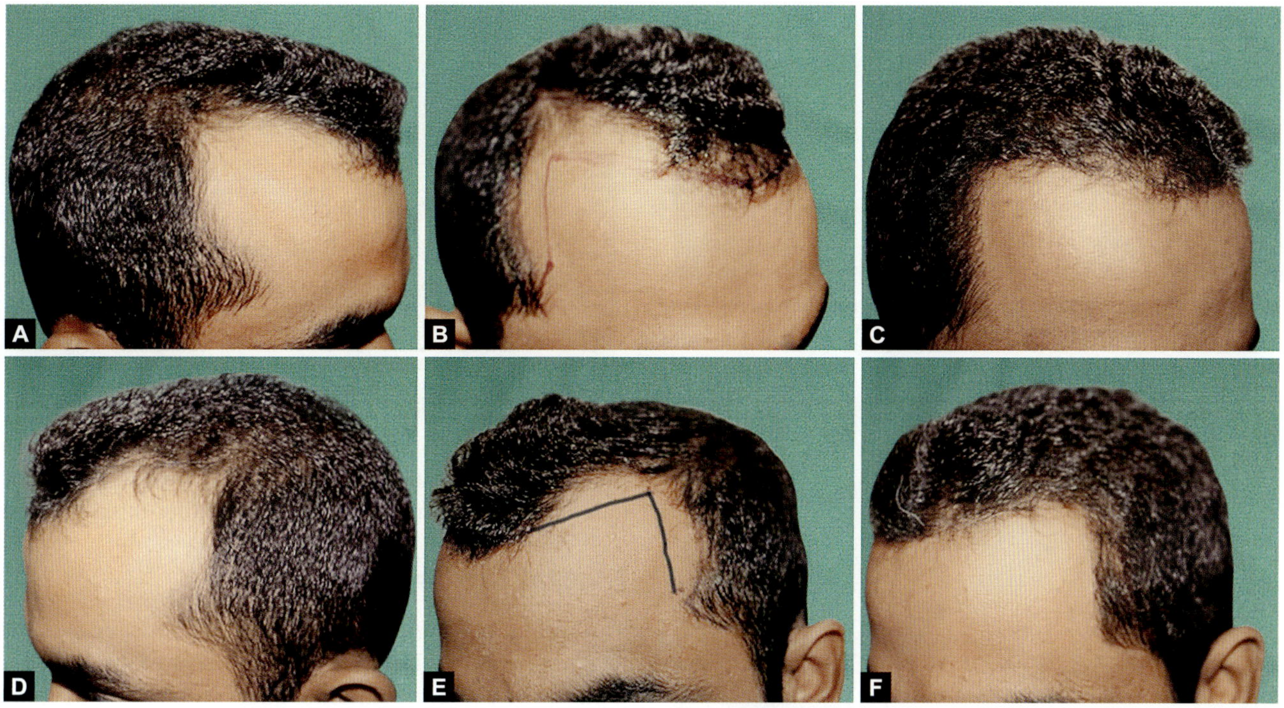

Figs. 5A to F: Creation of frontotemporal angle, temporal fringe, and temporal point.

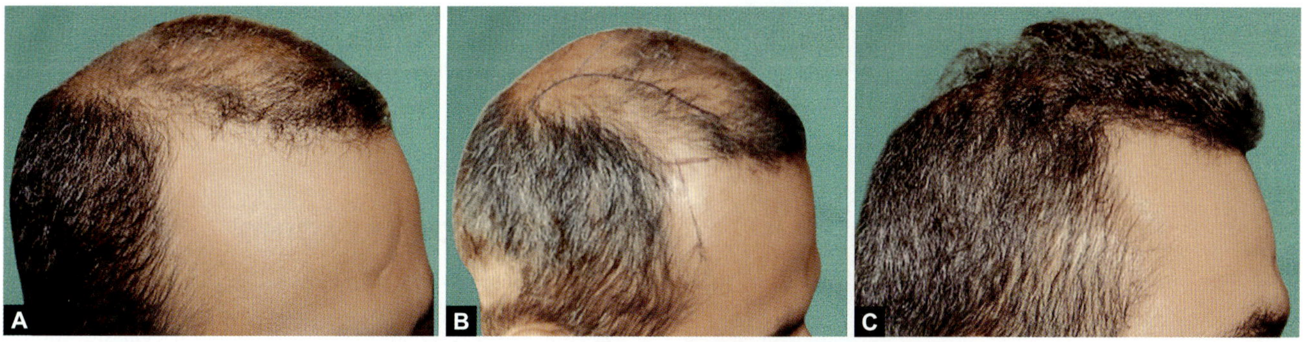

Figs. 6A to C: Restoration of parietal hump with temporal fringe.

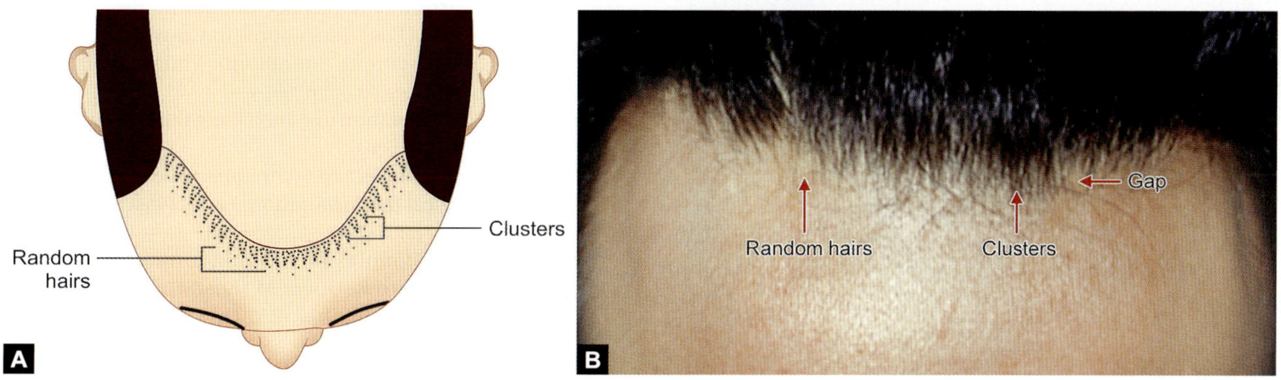

Figs. 7A and B: (A) Cluster and random hair pattern in anterior hairline zone; (B) Clusters of hair and random hair making anterior hairline zone.

to describe it. Parsley has attributed this macro irregularity to existence of one to three mound or protrusions along the path of the hairline. He describes one central mound (the widow's peak) and two lateral mounds in either side of this central mound. Micro irregularity and macro irregularity work together in the TZ to create a natural-looking hairline.

While designing the anterior portion of the TZ, single hair units are preferred, with a shift to two hair FUs toward

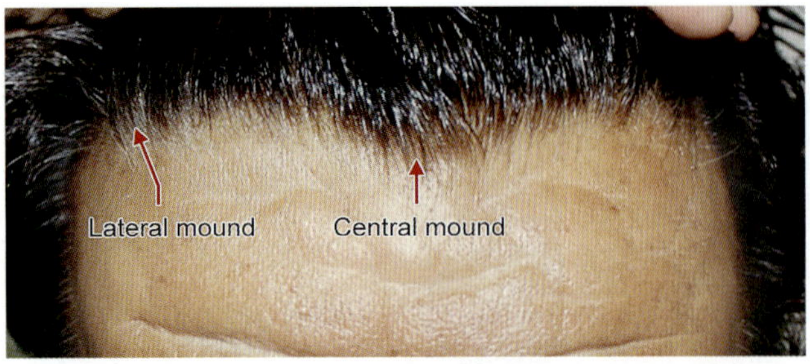

Fig. 8: Central mound (the widow's peak) and two lateral mounds on either side of this central mound.

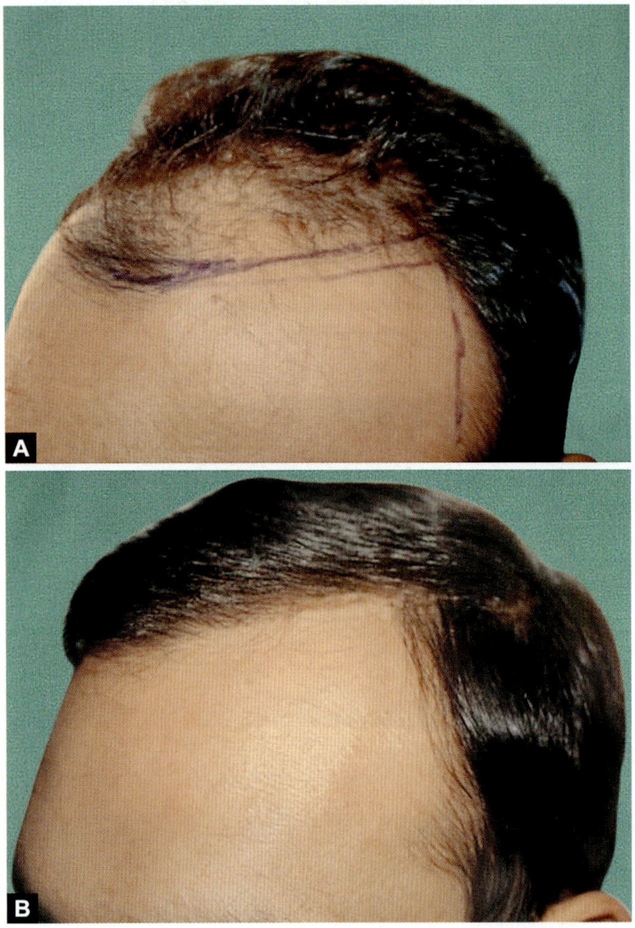

Figs. 9A and B: Restoration of anterior hairline zone and central tuft area.

its posterior. Sometimes, a few isolated, very fine single hairs called sentinel hairs can be transplanted in a scattered manner in front of TZ.

Defined Zone

The DZ is a 2–3 cm wide area that is directly posterior to TZ. In this area, the hairline should develop a higher degree of definition and density. This area is filled with two and three hair FUs. Density in this zone creates a fuller-looking hairline.

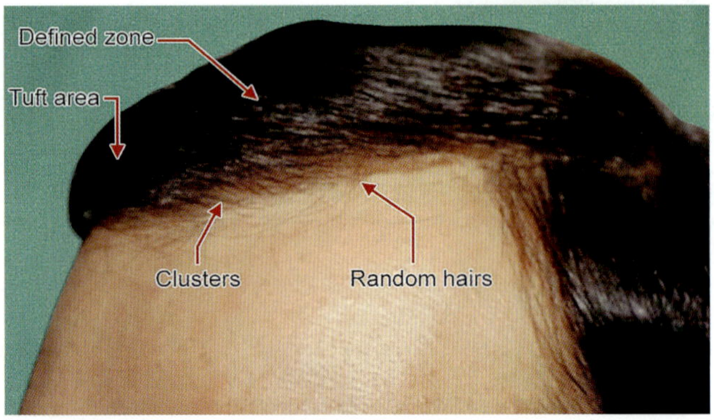

Fig. 10: Arrows showing all zones of anterior hairline zone.

Frontal Tuft Area

The frontal tuft area is a small, but aesthetically significant oval area that overlies the central portion of the DZ directly behind the TZ in the midline. This can be filled by three to five hair FUs or even coupled or multi-FUs **(Figs. 9 and 10)**.

CONCLUSION

Hairline design needs proper training and experience and hence should be learnt systematically by a beginner. The density variation, angulation, direction, thickness of hair, and the levels need close attention.

RECOMMENDED READING

1. Beehner M. Where is thy crown, your Majesty? Hair Transplant Forum Int. 1998;8:18-9.
2. Mayer Ml, Perez-Meza D. Temporal points: classification and surgical techniques for aesthetic results. Hair Transplants Forum Int. 2002;12:147-58.
3. Rose PT, Parsley WM. Science of hairline design. In: Haber RS, Stough DB (Eds). Procedures in Cosmetic Dermatology: Hair Transplantations, 1st edition. Philadelphia, PA, USA: Saunders-Elsevier; 2006. p. 55.
4. Rose PT. Consideration in establishing the hairline. Int J Aesth Rest Surg. 1998;1:24-6.
5. Shapiro R. Principles and techniques used to create a natural hairline surgical hair restoration. Facial Plast Surg Clin North Am. 2004;12(2):201-17.
6. Shapiro R. Principles of creating a natural hairline. In: Unger WP, Shapiro R, Unger M (Eds). Hair Transplantation, 5th edition. Philadelphia, PA, USA: CRC Press (Informa Healthcare); 2011. pp. 374.
7. Simmons C. Five old lines and three new lines that can help when designing a male temporal hairline or when transplanting the frontotemporal apex. Hair Transplant Forum Int. 2004;14(6):201-3.

CHAPTER 69

Donor Area Strip Dissection

Anil K Garg, Seema Garg

KEY MESSAGES

- Preoperative assessment of scalp laxity and elasticity is must before planning of follicular unit transplantation (FUT).
- Safe donor area should be marked before strip excision.
- Calculation of average follicular units (FUs) density in the donor strip helps in determining length and width of strip.
- Use of magnification is recommended, during the process of strip harvesting and FU dissection in order to prevent/reduce follicle transection.
- The goal of donor strip harvesting is to ensure the optimum number of hairs, quick healing, and minimal scarring.
- Proper knowledge of scalp anatomy and basic surgical principles is essential.
- Do not cut deeper to galea while harvesting the strip.
- Avoidance of wound tension, use of double-layer suturing, trichophytic closure, and proper choice of suture materials help in obtaining a minimal scar.

INTRODUCTION

Headington in 1984 described that hair grows in bundles of 1–4 or more individual follicles called FUs.[1] FUT/follicular unit grafting (FUG) implies the transplantation of follicle unit grafts harvested from the donor area to the recipient area as they naturally occur. It maximizes the cosmetic benefit of hair transplant (HT). Limmer described single-strip harvesting and stereomicroscopic dissection, and this led to the term FUT.[2] The term FUT can better be called follicular unit strip surgery (FUSS).

The goal of strip harvesting is to excise the strip from the safe donor area, with minimal injury to the neurovascular bundle and minimal scarring. Indian skin is prone for hypertrophic scar, and hence case selection, considerations of elasticity, prevention of wound tension and proper surgical technique is essential. Careful adherence to standard principles of surgery is necessary to ensure a satisfactory postoperative outcome.

All patients are not for hair transplantation, and also every patient may not be a candidate for FUSS. A young patient whose hair loss is not yet stable is a better candidate for medical treatment.

A patient having baldness wanting hair, with appropriate donor area, otherwise fit for surgery and having reasonable expectations, can undergo a hair transplantation.

Inadequate counseling, improper examination, and wrong technique increase complications. Complications in the donor area are usually technique dependent.

CONTRAINDICATIONS TO FOLLICULAR UNIT STRIP SURGERY (FOLLICULAR UNIT TRANSPLANTATION) SURGERY

Systemic factors: All uncontrolled systemic diseases are making patient unfit for any surgery such as hypertension, cardiac diseases, diabetes, and epilepsy. Psychologically unstable patients having very high expectations in terms of coverage and density and patients having body dysmorphic disorder are also not fit for HT.

Local factors:

- Patients with scarring alopecia or inflammatory scalp diseases affecting hair follicle survival
- Diffuse unpatterned hair loss (DUPA)
- A patient with a keloidal tendency is a relative contraindication.
- Patient with the tight scalp
- Patients who wish to keep short hair, want to resume job early, and who do not like to have a linear scar are not good candidate for strip harvesting.

Steps before harvesting the strip:

1. Planning of the recipient area
2. Detailed counseling with patients and attendants, explaining the importance of medical treatment and limitations of hair transplantation.
3. Assessment of the donor area and its laxity.
4. Calculation of the required number of hair follicles to cover the recipient area.
5. Explanation to the patient of how much density he/she will have after surgery.

DONOR AREA ASSESSMENT

The success of HT depends on the quality of the donor area. The donor area is to be evaluated for skin elasticity and glidability, number of available FUs, and number of hair in FUs. The thickness, curvature, and color of hair are as important as the number of follicles.

Donor Area Evaluation

- Scalp laxity/elasticity and glidability
- Hair/FUs density/number of hairs in FU
- The thickness of hair
- Color of hair
- The curvature of hair
- Anagen–telogen ratio

Scalp Laxity and Elasticity

The concepts of laxity and elasticity are essential for proper strip harvesting. Laxity of the skin is the ability to stretch the skin. Elasticity is the ability of the skin to return to its usual stage after stretching. More the elasticity of skin less will be laxity of skin.

Scalp laxity and elasticity affect the tissue tension during wound closure. Also, the width of skin strip that can be safely removed depends upon laxity of skin.

A wider skin strip in the young individual with limited laxity can lead to excessive tension over suture line, which may result in a wide scar, hypertrophic scar or keloid formation, shock loss, or effluvium near suture line. Tissue necrosis may lead to a gap in the suture line. Repeat surgeries will be difficult in such cases.

Glidability

Mobility of scalp skin not only depends on skin elasticity but also glidability of skin. The scalp can glide over the pericranium, and it is facilitated by a loose layer of fibroareolar tissue below the galea. Most of HT surgeons assess laxity of the skin by merely moving the skin up and down or pinching it between fingers. Depending upon their clinical experience, they decide approximate laxity and determine the width of the skin strip.

Laxity of skin should be assessed at minimum three points in the donor region of the occipital, parietal, and temporal region.

The laxity is maximum in the central occipital area and minimum over the mastoid region. If equal width of skin is taken during the entire length of skin strip, there will be more tension over suture line on both lateral sides of the strip in the mastoid region, so while planning for strip the width on both mastoid areas should be narrower.

Scalp Laxity Exercise

The scalp examination for scalp laxity is important at the time of prior consultation. If the laxity is less than desirable, it is advisable to have the patient to do scalp stretching exercise for at least 4–6 weeks before surgery.

Method: The two hands clasped at the back of the scalp, and donor skin is pressed and stretched up-down and side to side for 4–5 minutes at a time, 8–10 times a day. This will increase the laxity of donor scalp skin, which will help in both being able to take a wider strip and close the wound under low tension. **Figure 1** shows laxity exercise (**1**).

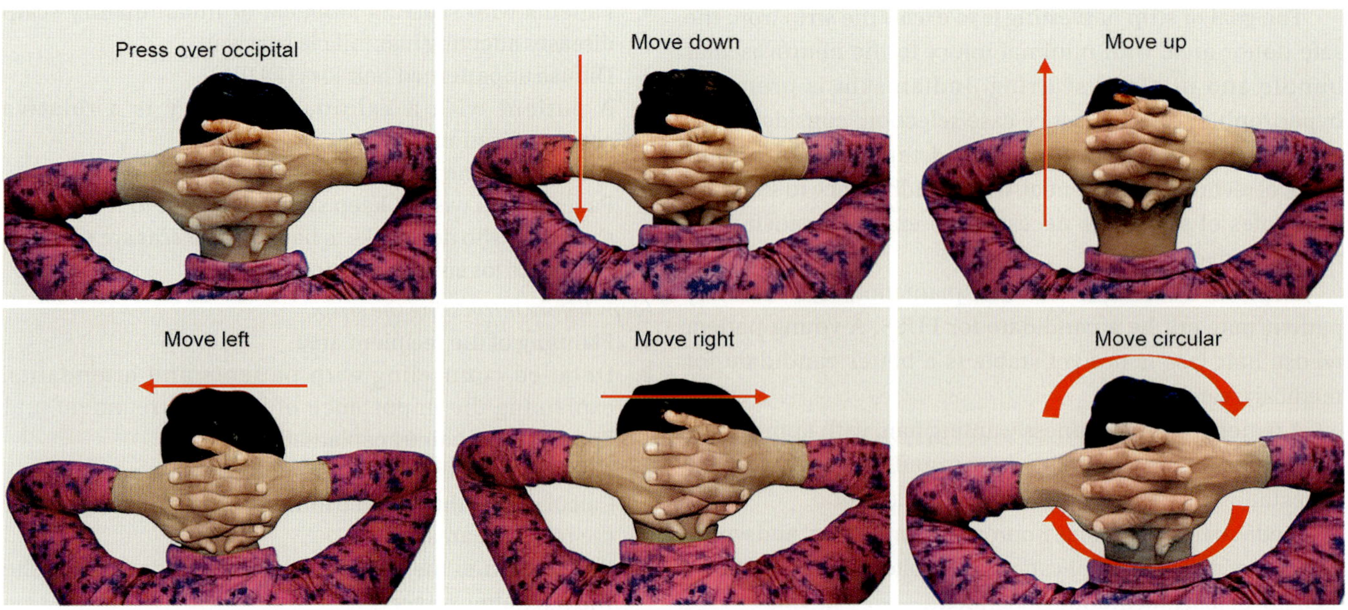

Fig. 1: Scalp laxity exercise (**1**).

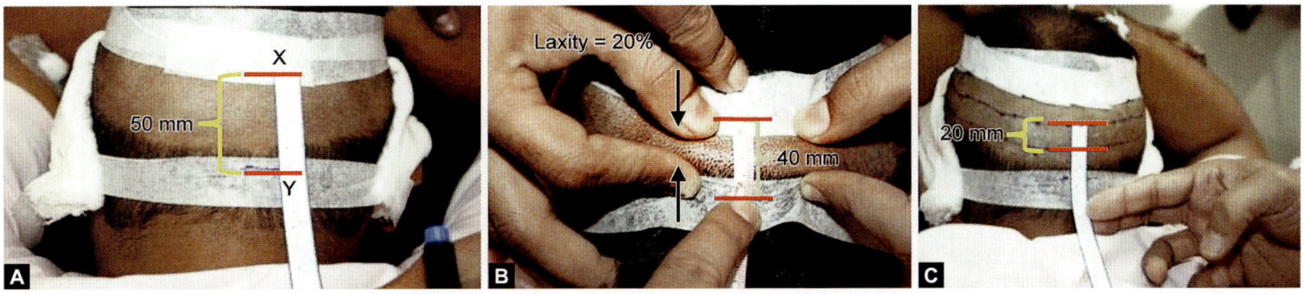

Figs. 2A to C: Method to asses scalp laxity. (A) Two points X and Y are marked at 50 mm apart; (B) Both points are compressed toward each other and distance between both points is measured, which is after 40 mm; (C) Laxity percentage measured as per Mayer's formula, which is 20%. So, a 20-mm wide strip can be taken in center and a 15-mm wide laterally.

Measurement of scalp laxity at three different points before harvesting strip is an important step in order to avoid complications related to tension over the suture line.

1. Bosley in 1980 described a method to measure scalp mobility for scalp reduction.[3]
2. Mohebi proposed the use of a mechanical device called "Laxometer" for measurement of scalp laxity.[4]
3. Mayer and Paul devised a technique to assess the scalp elasticity in an objective and reproducible manner[5] **(Figs. 2A to C)**.

Scalp elasticity = (50 mm – X)/50 mm × 100%

By this calculation, the distance between two points that were 50 mm apart in the horizontal axis when compressed maximally by the examiner's thumbs is measured as X. For example, if the distance between the points measured is 40 mm after compression, X = 40 and then the elasticity is:

50 mm – 40 mm/50 mm × 100% = 20%

Safe donor trip width based on Mayer–Pauls elasticity scale:

- 10% elasticity = 10 mm central occipital and 8 cm lateral region
- 15% elasticity = 15 mm central occipital and 10 mm lateral area
- 20% elasticity = 20 mm central occipital and 15 mm laterally
- 25% elasticity = 22 mm central occipital and 15 mm laterally
- 30% elasticity = 22 mm central occipital and 15 mm laterally

In general, it is preferable to avoid too wide strip. The author believes that strip width in the central occipital region should never exceed 20 mm and in the lateral part 15 mm. Beginners should not exceed 10–12 mm; instead, try to increase length in the safe donor area. Do not stray too far front into the anterior temporal area because of the presence of superficial temporal artery. Damage to this artery will lead to profuse bleeding with chances of decreased circulation in the area, which may cause donor effluvium. In general, Indian skin donor elasticity is limited as compared to western skin. Indian skin is also prone to hypertrophic scar. A wide donor scar is the worst advertisement for strip surgery. Never increase the width of the strip beyond the safe limit just to harvest more grafts.

A straightforward equation for strip width is to add 5 mm to the amount of skin, which can be compressed. For example, if we could compress 7 mm the width which can be taken is 7 + 5 = 12 mm and so on.

Preoperative assessment of scalp laxity saves many complications of strip surgery.

Hair/Follicular Units Density/Number of Hairs in Follicular Unit

Hair density is the measurement of hair per square centimeter of scalp. FUs density is the number of FUs per square cm. Hair/FU density varies from area to area of donor scalp. It is maximum in the center of the occipital area, while lower in the area closer to ear.

For a more accurate assessment, it is advisable to calculate density at a minimum of three locations and then take an average of three. It is important to remember that density varies from patient to patient and from area to area, within each patient **(Figs. 3A and B)**.

Thickness of Hair

The thickness of hair affects the visual impact of hair density. Bernstein has described, "The total volume of hair determines the visual impact. Doubling hair density doubles the hair volume, while doubling the hair diameter quadruples the hair volume."[6] Vellus hairs have a diameter <30 μm. Fine hair is between 60 and 65 μm, medium hair is 65–80 μm, and coarse hair has a diameter >80 μm.

Methods for Assessing Donor Area Hair Density and Diameter of Hair

There are two methods for assessing donor area hair density. One is subjective, which depends on the experience of the physician. Another is the objective in which information is driven through instruments. Several instruments ranging from simple devices to advance options are available.

- *Use of 1 cm² box* **(Fig. 4A)**: An area/box is marked using a rubber stamp of 1 cm² area. The number of hair counted

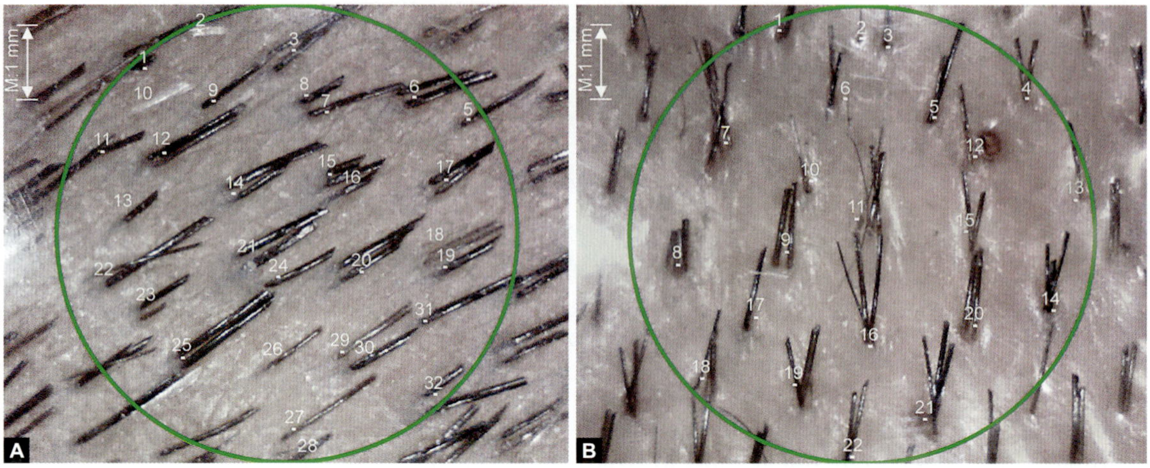

Figs. 3A and B: The trichoscan images show two different FUs density and hair diameter. (A) Density 128 FUs/cm^2. Thickness 0.82 mm; (B) Density 69 FUs/cm^2. Thickness 0.52 mm.

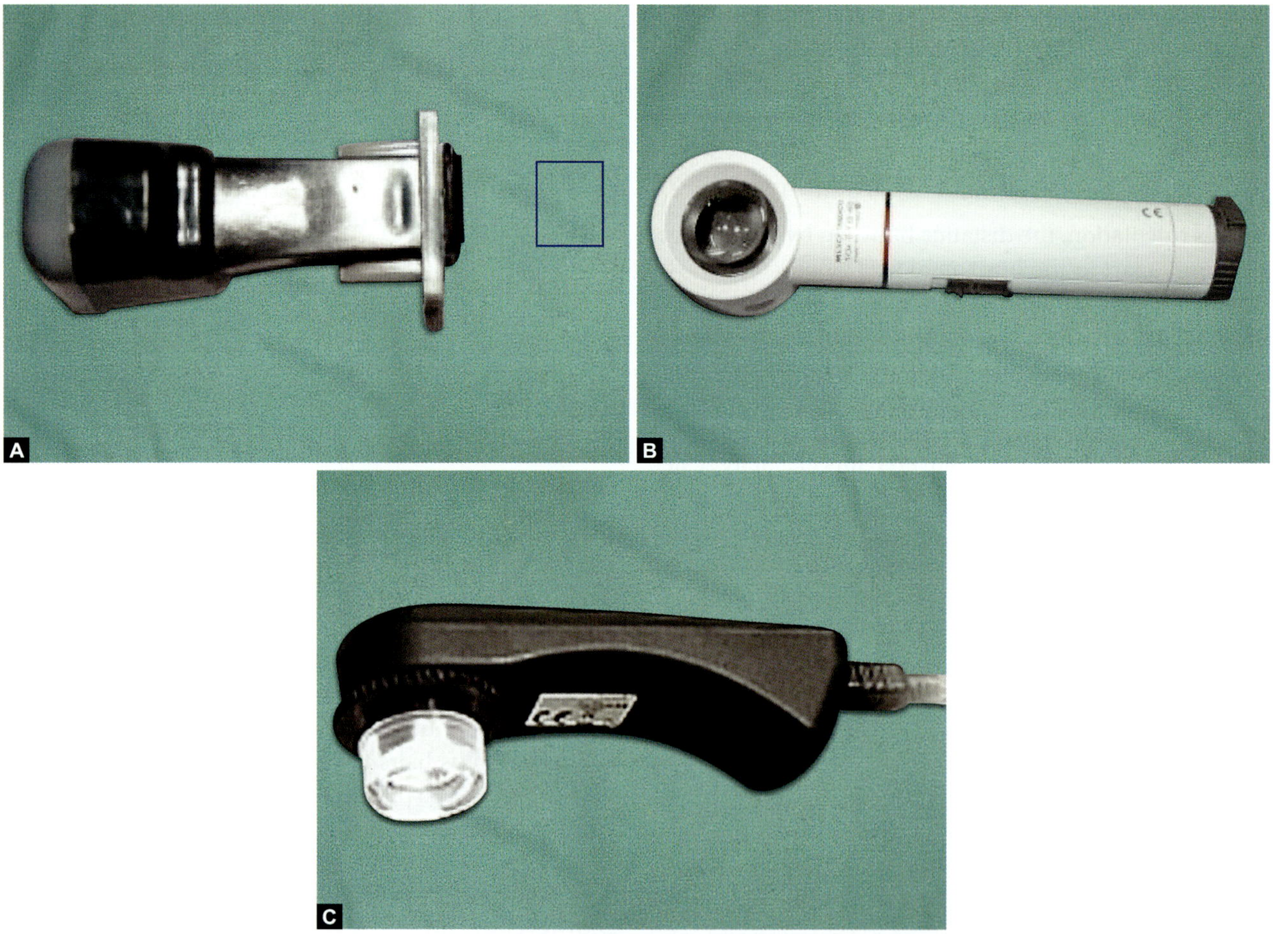

Figs. 4A to C: (A) 1 cm^2 box; (B) Self-illuminated hair densitometer; (C) Tricoscan.

from two sides (length and width) multiply and take density.

- *Hair densitometer* **(Fig. 4B)**: It is a simple device in which magnifying lens with illumination is used to count hairs in 1 cm^2 area.
- *Tricoscan/folliscope* **(Fig. 4C)**: A digital camera is attached to a computer. Picture of the scalp is taken and analyzed by software. By this technique, we can calculate terminal hair count, vellus hair count, FUs count, number of follicle per FUs, and thickness of hair.

Every hair restoration surgeon should have a tricoscope/folliscope or a dermoscope in his clinic and shall examine all cases of hair loss as a routine scalp examination.

- *Color of hair:* The color contrast affects the visual density. More the color contrast between the hair and scalp skin color, more the visual density looks.
- *The curvature of hair:* More the curl of hair, the more visual density is. The straight hair reflects less light as compare to curved or wavy hair.
- *Anagen-telogen ratio:* Normal scalp has 85–90% anagen and 10–15% telogen hair. If the percentage of telogen increases >30%, such donor area is not suitable for hair follicles harvesting. In such cases the underlying cause shall be treated before harvesting hair follicles.

Donor Strip Size Calculation

Based on the average donor hair density, the required length of the donor strip can be calculated as follows:

$$\text{Number of FUs} = \text{length} \times \text{width} \times \text{donor density}$$

Strip length for 1 cm wide donor strip = Number of FUs for transplant/donor density/cm^2. For a person requiring 3,000 FUs with a donor density of 100 FUs/cm^2: Strip length for 1 cm wide donor strip = 3,000/100 = 30 cm^2 or 30 cm long and 1 cm wide strip.

If the maximum possible length of the strip that can be harvested is only 25 cm, then the strip width needs to be increased to 1.5 cm at the central occipital region for a length of 10 cm and a width of 1 cm for the remaining 15 cm length on both lateral ends.

SAFE DONOR AREA

It is generally believed that hairs in the occipital area are androgen resistant, and hence the occipital area is referred to the safe donor area. While harvesting for transplant, if hair beyond safe zone, i.e., the occipital and temporal fringe is taken, there will be a risk of future hair loss of grafted hairs.

To outline safe donor area, three points are marked on the scalp **(Fig. 5)**.

- Midpoint in a sagittal plane over external occipital protuberance (A).
- Lateral point is 1.5 cm behind postauricular hairline and 1.5 cm above the superior aspect of the helix. This point is lateral most limit of a conservative length of strip (B).
- The point (C) is 2 cm above the superior aspect of helix along a line drawn vertically through anterior tragus. This is the lateral/anterior most limit of an extensive strip.

The line joining these three points A, B, and C is a lower limit of safe hair zone. The area below this level is not the scalp but neck region. Hairs harvested from this region are susceptible to fall. Also, strong neck muscles are present in this area, so tension over the suture line is high, and the scar may get widened.

Width of safe donor area at the most anterior (lateral) limit is 6–7 cm wide. In the center of safe zone width is decided by taking a horizontal line drawn from point "C", (i.e., 2 cm above superior helix in a plane anterior to helix), which will intersect midline of occiput. This will be the superior limit of the safe donor area in the midline. 1 cm below and 2 cm above permanent hair-bearing area should be left to camouflage donor scar.

Hair transplant surgeon should carefully examine donor area for a progressive pattern of hair loss in crown, retrograde hair loss, thinning, or miniaturization.

Rassman and Bernstein have suggested that the "safe donor area" consists of approximately 25% of the scalp.[7] Cole advised that the total size of the safe donor area is 203 cm^2 and average FUs in Caucasians are 16,649 FUs, and Asian have 15,718 FUs.[8]

Demand and Supply Gap

The common questions asked by a patient before HT are:

- How many grafts/hairs does he/she need to cover his bald area?

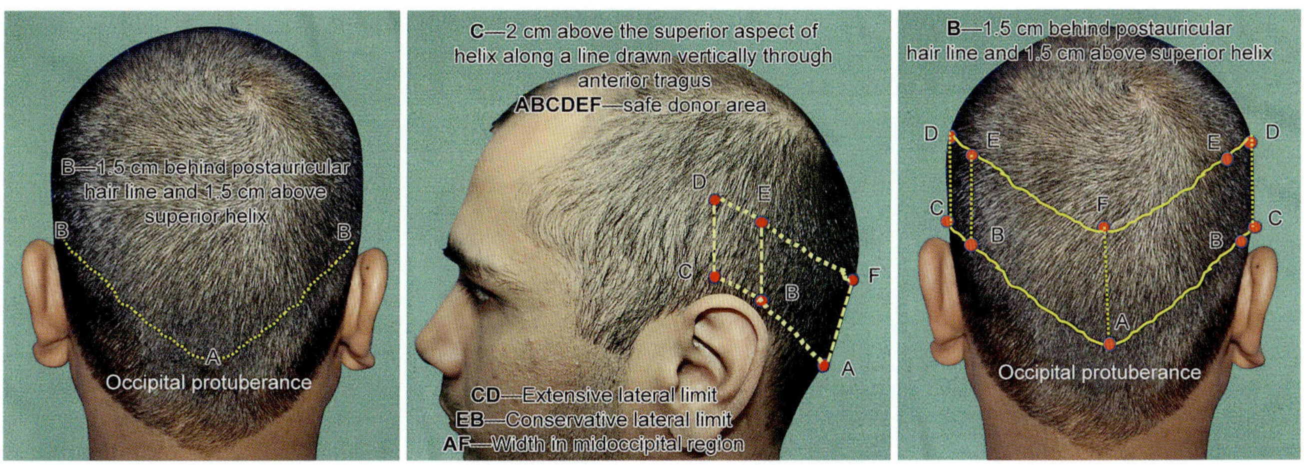

Fig. 5: Safe donor area scalp.

- How much will be hair density after transplantation?
- How many grafts can be harvested?
- How will he/she look?

To answer these questions, a surgeon should know:

- How big is the bald area in cm^2? And what is his Norwood scale of baldness?
- How many numbers of FUs are available from safe donor area?
- List out priorities and discuss with patients. Framing of the face should be preferred.
- Quality of hair in terms of thickness, color, and curl and also scalp of color

Calculation of hair density—sample calculation for a patient:

- Total recipient area = 100 cm^2
- Donor area = 30 cm^2
- Donor density = 80 FUs/cm^2
- Total FUs harvested = 30 × 80 = 2,400 FUs

 Recipient density = No. of FUs transplanted/Area

 Final recipient density = 2,400/100 = 24 FUs/cm^2

With these simple calculations, a surgeon can make a master plan for an individual patient and match the donor density with the recipient area that needs to be covered. Beginners should not give high density. A recipient density ranging from 25 to 40 FU/cm^2 is good enough.

Shaving of donor area and head wash ***(Figs. 6A to C)****:* The occipital protuberance is palpated **(Fig. 6A)**, and donor strip area trimming is done using a motorized trimmer **(Fig. 6B)**.

Generally, hairs are trimmed to keep hair length, 0.5–1 cm, which can give the idea about the direction of the hair and at the same time prevent entanglement of hair during dissection. Trimming of hair 1 cm on either side (above and below) of the strip gives clear field during cutting and suturing. Authors prefer to wash the head after trimming of hairs, using antibiotic scrub (povidone-iodine scrub) **(Fig. 6C)**.

Position of Patient

Key to successful surgery is that both patient and surgeon should be in a comfortable position. Operating table can be a routine surgery table with a horseshoe-shaped head side, which avoids suffocating effect during prone position. One can also use a dental chair or a specially designed table for HT. Use of soft silicone cushion around the face and below chest gives comfort to the patient. Various types of custom-made silicon cushions are available. Position of the patient

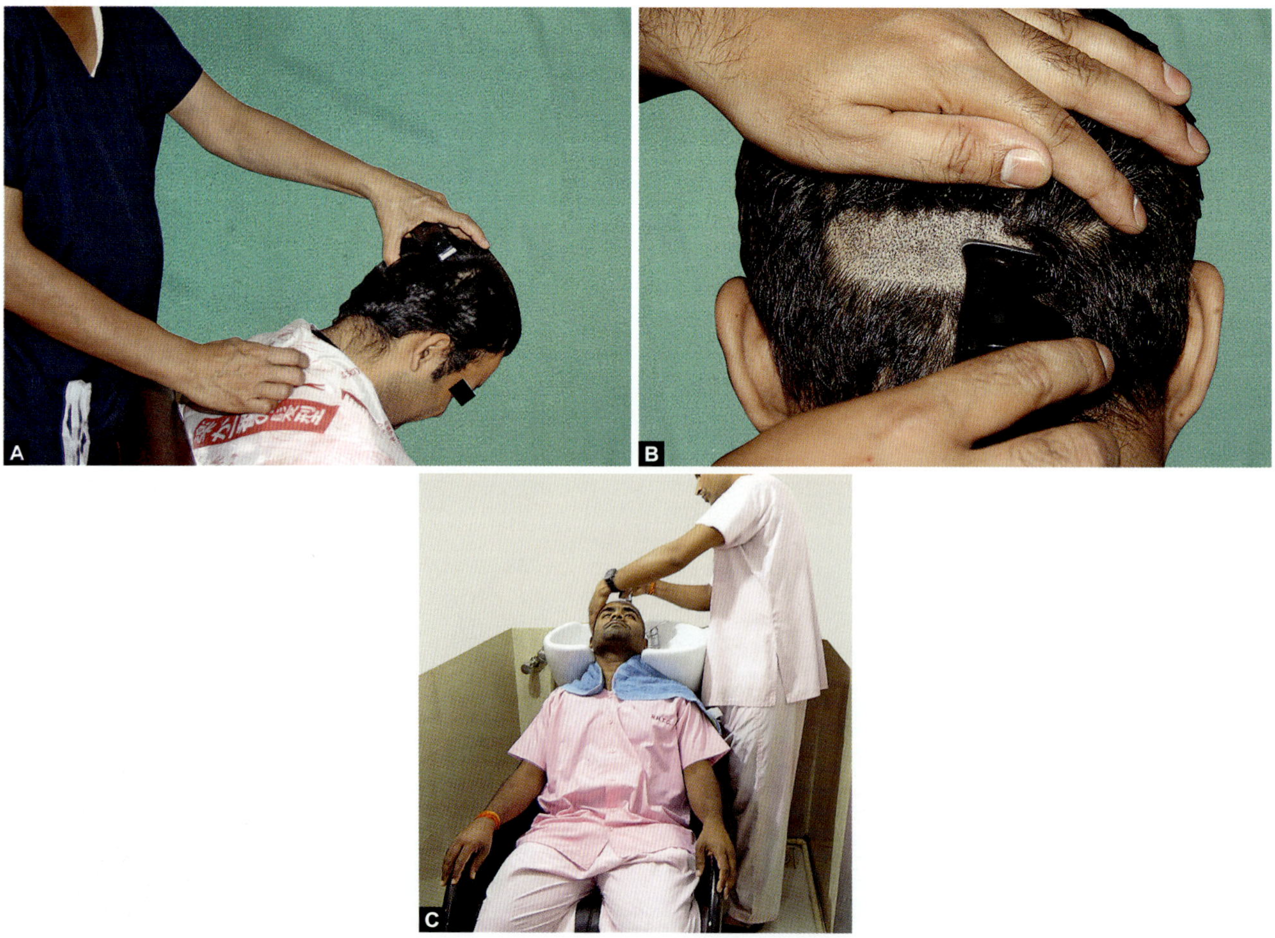

Figs. 6A to C: (A) Palpation of occipital protuberance; (B) Trimming of hair along the donor area; (C) Head wash using povidone-iodine scrub.

is as per the preference of the surgeon. Different positions such as sitting (reclining) position, prone position, and lateral positions have been used.

Vital Parameters Monitoring and Presence of Anesthetist

It is essential to monitor for blood pressure, pulse, and oxygen saturation. Monitoring while in prone position and presence of anesthetist is undoubtedly a great asset to the HT unit. However, most of the HT units do not have anesthetist as a protocol. In such cases, a person who is trained in advance life support should be there, and an anesthetist should be available on call. It is mandatory to take an intravenous line for any emergency. In all high-risk patients, continuous electrocardiogram (ECG) monitoring and presence of anesthetist are advisable.

We should know patients medical history and also of any medicine he is taking. Detailed knowledge of drug interactions, management of emergency like vasovagal syncope, anaphylaxis, hypotension, etc. should be known to HT surgeon **(Table 1)**.

TABLE 1: Possible problems during FUT and their management.

Problem	*Cause*	*Preventive measures*	*Management*
Itching, urticaria, angioedema	Allergic reactions or anaphylaxis to drugs or food	• Preoperative history about allergic reaction to any drug or food • Xylocaine sensitivity test	• Epinephrine subcutaneous • Oxygen • Symptomatic treatment
Syncope/fainting attack	Vasovagal attack, anxiety	Premedication with diazepam or midazolam, keeping the OT environment friendly. Giving local anesthesia in lying down position	• Elevation of limb with head low in supine position • Keep atropine ready if bradycardia persist
Palpitation/anxiety	β1, and α-adrenergic effects of epinephrine	• Premedication with midazolam/ diazepam • Administer adrenaline in diluted form (1:100,000) and slowly	Wait for some time, it will settle by its own (half-life of epinephrine is short). Keep lidocaine ready for arrhythmias
Hypertension with bradycardia	Drug interaction of epinephrine and β-blockers	Switch to selective β1 blocker for hypertension before planning for surgery	Treat it as cardiac emergency, use α-adrenergic blockers
Agitation, confusion, perioral numbness	Lidocaine toxicity	Be very cautious about total dose of anesthetic agent per kg of body weight	Intravenous fluids, IV lipids, oxygen, diazepam
Excessive bleeding	Increased blood pressure	Continue antihypertensive medications as prescribed by the physicians. Stop antiplatelet agents	Antihypertensive must be added if BP is raised. Use of adrenaline in tumescence in diluted form (1:100,000–1:200,000)
Postoperative edema	Nonsteroidal anti-inflammatory agents	Use of kenacort in tumescence, systemic corticosteroid pre- and postoperative. Keep recipient sites small	Lie in supine position, head elevation, postoperative corticosteroid if needed
Sterile folliculitis	Too much tumescence, buffered anesthetic, surgical trauma	Do not burry grafts too much, keep epidermal end with hair shaft above the skin. Size of slits must be appropriate for the graft	Wait and watch, will settle with its own. If persistent, incision and drainage is required
Cyst formation at graft site	Foreign body reaction to imbedded grafts	Avoid inserting one graft over other in the same site (piggy backing)	Topical and systemic antibiotics. Incision and drainage may be needed
Bacterial folliculitis	Secondary to infected sterile folliculitis or cyst, poor hygiene	Keep the area clean, proper head wash as advised by physician, topical corticosteroids for itching	Topical and systemic antibiotics
Infected donor wound	Wound closure is too tight with large suture bites, causes vascular compromise, and postoperative edema	Harvest a narrow donor strip under less tension. Improve suturing technique	Systemic antibiotics; if wound closure is under excess tension leave a portion of it to heal by secondary intension
Hiccups	Stimulation of C2-C4 (phrenic nerves)	Use tumescence anesthesia in donor area to limit donor depth to deep subcutaneous layer	Oral chlorpromazine

(BP: blood pressure; FUT: follicular unit transplantation; IV: intravenous; OT: operation theater)

Donor Area Marking

The marking for donor strip is done in safe scalp donor area only. The dimensions of the strip depend on the number of grafts required, donor area density, and the laxity of skin; the strip shall be narrow in the mastoid region as compare to the mid occipital region, because the skin in the mastoid region has relatively less laxity **(Fig. 7)**.

Isolation of Strip Area

The nearby hair-bearing area is isolated using micropore tape. The author prefers to put a cotton pad in the post-auricular area and the neck area and fix it with micropore. It will prevent the trickling of blood over the face and neck **(Figs. 8A to C)**.

Painting and Draping of Area

Paint scalp donor area by antimicrobial solution (povidone-iodine 10% solution), and the patient is covered with sterile surgical drapes.

Local Anesthetic Infiltration

The author prepares anesthetic solution in the following concentration:

- *Tumescence solution*:
  - 5 mL xylocaine (2%)
  - 5 mL ropivacaine (0.5%)
  - 90 mL of normal saline
  - 0.5 mL of adrenaline (1:100,000)
  - 1 mL of triamcinolone (40 mg/mL)
- *Anesthetic solution for nerve block*:
  - 20 mL of xylocaine
  - 20 mL of 0.5% ropivacaine
  - 40 mL of normal saline
  - 0.5 mL of adrenaline (1:100,000)

Tumescent solution is administered in the subcutaneous plane till the skin becomes firm and swollen. It should not be infiltrated below galea. The author prefers cold pack both to reduce preanesthetic pain and also to induce vasoconstriction **(Figs. 9A and B)**. The use of vibrator near injection site reduces the pain of injection significantly.

STRIP HARVESTING

After checking the anesthesia, the skin scoring incision is given up to dermis level only. The gap between incision margins is increased using two double skin hooks,[9] or using Haber's spreader or using fine mosquito forceps to deepen the incision. Whatever be the method adopted, it is advisable to choose and practice one method so that mastery can be achieved and obtain zero transection during strip harvesting. Depth of incision is significant. The incision should be in upper subcutis and certainly do not cross the galea **(Fig. 10)**. All neurovascular structures run over galea below subcutaneous level. An incision given deeper to galea will injure the neurovascular structures, leading to blood loss. Partial nerve injury may lead to the formation of neuroma, resulting in a painful scar. Complete nerve transection may give neurological deficit, i.e., hypoesthesia or anesthesia in the area of nerve supply. A painful scar and/or neurological deficit in the donor area are the result of faulty technique of strip harvesting and a very stressful complication. See **Box 1** for do's and donot of strip harvesting.

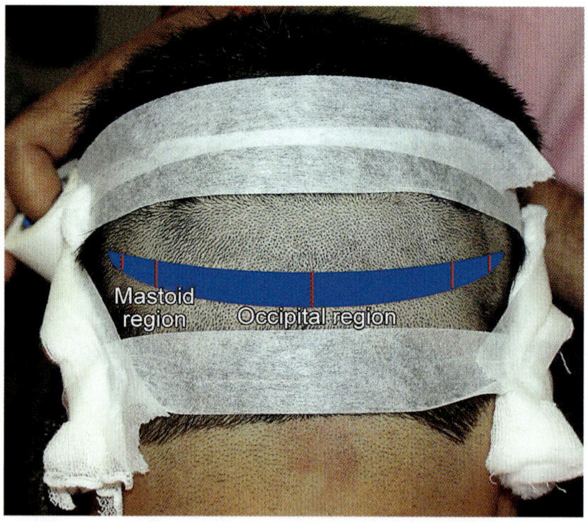

Fig. 7: Strip marking in the scalp donor area. The width in the mastoid region should be narrower than the width in the occipital region.

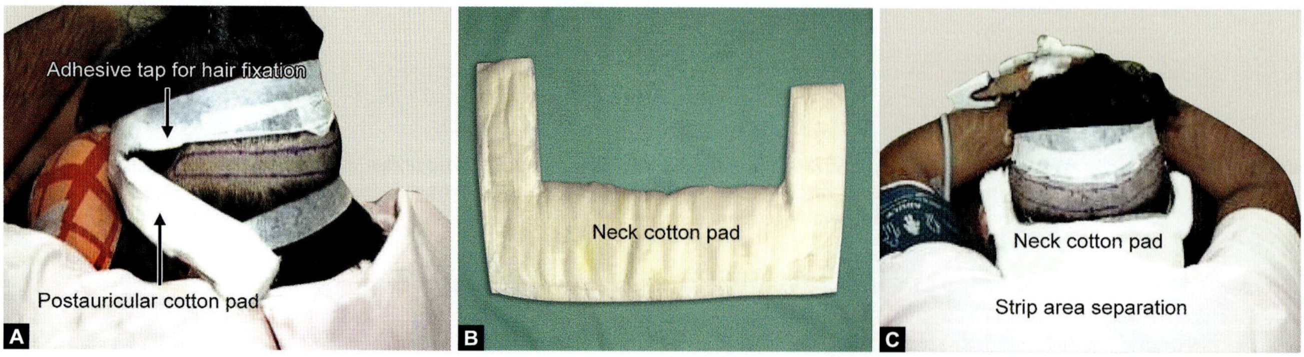

Figs. 8A to C: Isolation of the strip area by dressing material to prevent seepage of blood from the face and neck area.

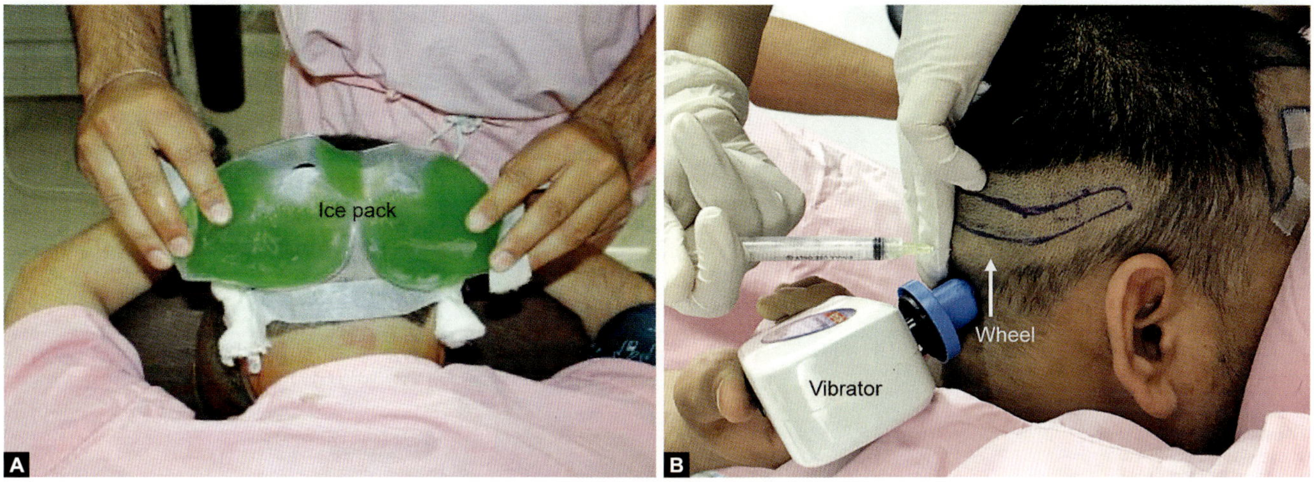

Figs. 9A and B: Local anesthesia infiltration. Use of ice pack and vibrator to reduce the pain of anesthesia injection.

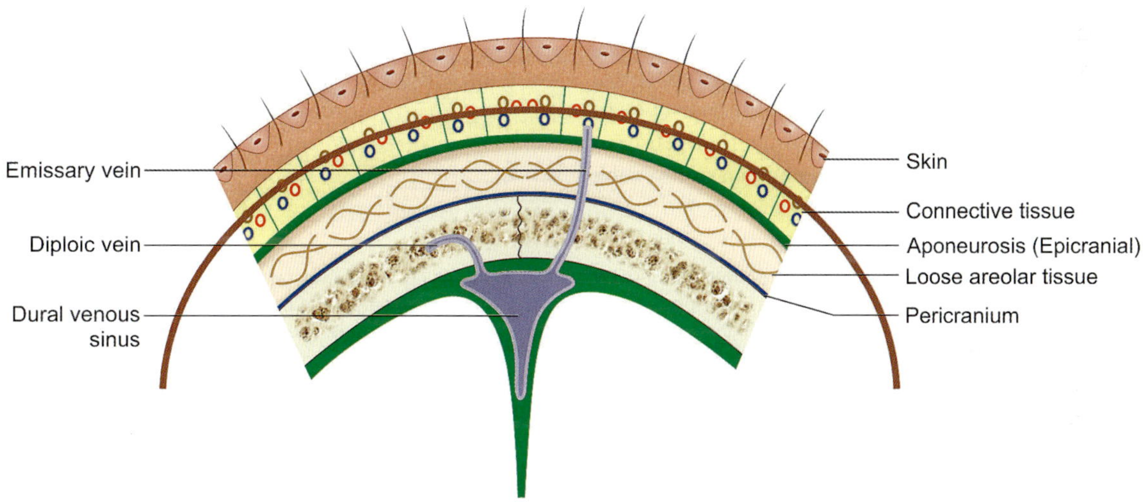

Fig. 10: Strip incision should be limited above the galea. The red line shows the limit of the depth of the incision.

BOX 1: Strip harvesting tips.

Do's:
- Preoperative scalp laxity estimation
- Preoperative scalp laxity exercises
- Detailed counseling
- Prefer to take a narrower and longer strip
- If necessary minimal undermining above galea
- Two-layer closure if skin strip is wider than 1 cm. Deep layer through deep dense connective tissue or galea
- Strip harvesting in safe zone only
- Wider strip in central occipital region and narrower in mastoid region

Don'ts:
- Never cut galea. Strip incision depth should be up to subcutaneous level
- Do not cut/injure nerves and major vessels
- Never undermine below galea

After the incision, the strip is raised and carefully dissects it from galea, avoiding injury to nerve and vessels, which are crossing over it **(Fig. 11)**.

Surgical pearl: For beginners, it is advisable to take strip in two to three parts. This has several advantages:
- It allows judgment of elasticity.
- It allows dissection work to start early.
- It allows a cleaner surgical field as bleeding points can be controlled in each area.

Hemostasis

If a strip is taken out well, hemostasis is rarely a problem, with only a few superficial bleeders. Any arterial bleeder needs to be either cauterized or sutured **(Fig. 11)**. Cautery should be kept to the minimum to prevent postoperative pain and promote healing.

Undermining

Undermining of skin margins is not routinely needed. If the skin is not lax enough for closure, then limited undermining

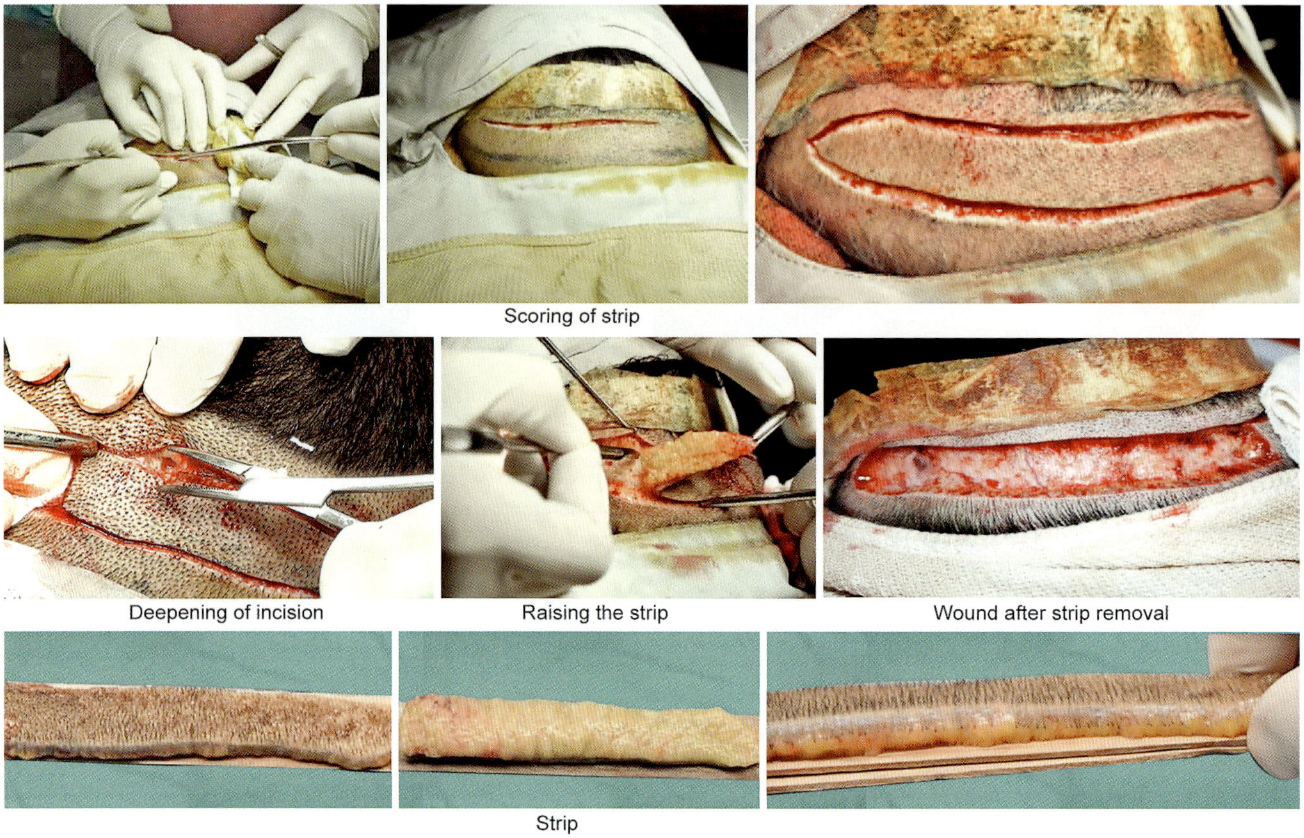

Fig. 11: Strip harvesting. First scoring incision up to dermis. Then widening of incision using fine hemostat forceps. The strip is raised by dissection just above galea aponeurotica. The dissection is done in the plane between the galea and fat below the bulb. Keep the surface of the blade parallel to galea and use the tip of the blade to cut the tissue taking care not to injure the nerves and vessels. The wound is ready for closure after achieving hemostasis. Last three bottom figures show the three different views of the strip.

in the subcutaneous plane is done. It is preferable to avoid undermining in the subgalea plane. It is recommended that beginners limit the width of the strip to about 1 cm, so that undermining is not needed.

Wound Closure

After careful hemostasis, wound closure is started; most surgeons prefer two-layer suturing as it helps to distribute tension into two layers. The usual recommendation is—if the strip width is <1 cm then a single layer of absorbable suture can be used. In case of strip width >1 cm, two-layer closure is advocated. Superficial closure needs to be done, with the careful alignment of hairs above and below the suture. The suture material used is as per individual preference. The author prefers to use Vicryl rapid **(Figs. 12A to E)** (**2**).

The deeper suture is placed in the subcutaneous layer—a deep, dense connective tissue layer is present below the fatty layer, which is a relatively more robust layer. Subcutaneous suture bites are taken through this layer with Vicryl or polydioxanone (PDS) 3-0. However, if this layer is not strong enough to hold suture, then galea suture is taken to bridge the gap. Suture material PDS takes longer time for absorption; it, therefore, holds incision margin together for a longer period and reduces chances of scar widening. Deep suture holds the skin margins and diverts the skin tension in a deeper plane, so the secondary effect of tension over the skin margins is avoided. Deep holding suture works against the elasticity of the skin and helps to promote crepe phenomenon of the skin, which helps in the expansion of the skin.

While suturing, taking a bite through isthmus portion of hair (which harbors the bulge area) needs to be avoided. Care should be taken to see that hairs in the upper edge of the wound and lower edge are aligned for a natural effect. Avoid tight skin margin closure. In cases of tight closure, it is preferable to have 1–2 mm of the gap between skin margin rather than tension closure, which may lead to necrosis of skin, which is a more severe complication than a wide scar.

TRICHOPHYTIC CLOSURE TECHNIQUE

A long linear scar in the donor area is the sequela of the strip technique of HT.

When the scar is wide and hypopigmented, it may show through hair. The risk of a visible scar is the major reason that patients are hesitant to undergo the strip method of hair transplantation.

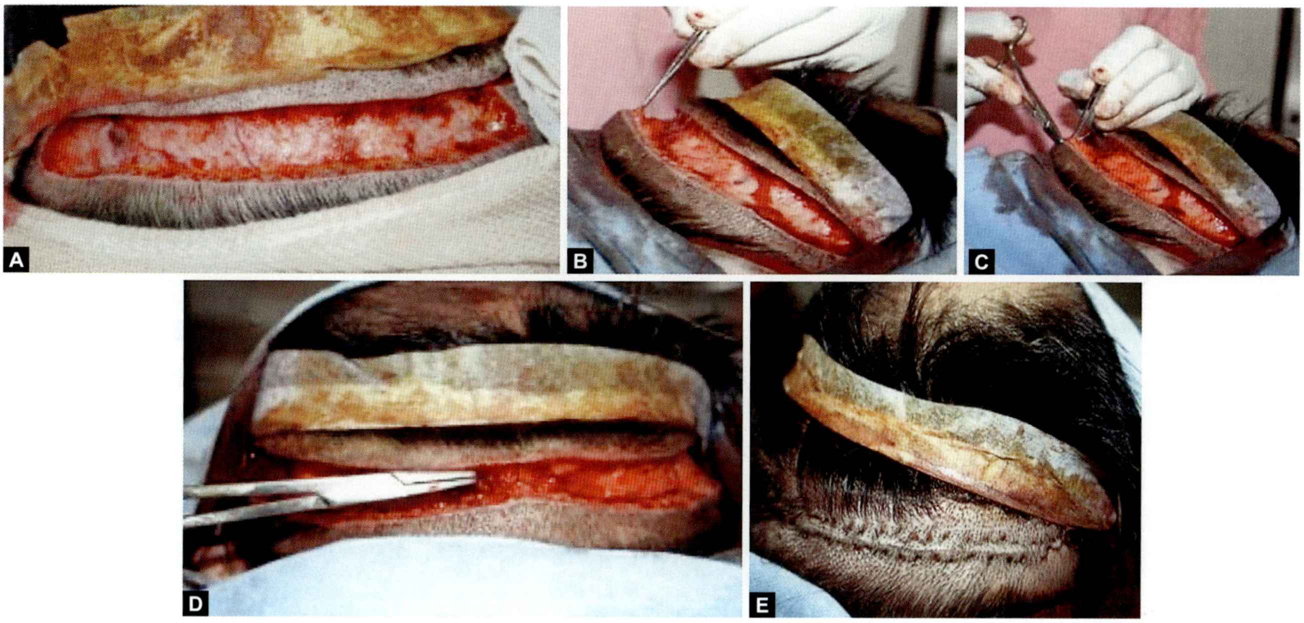

Figs. 12A to E: Wound closure. (A) Wound after strip removal showing no active bleeding; (B) Catch deep, dense connective tissue; (C) Take subcutaneous suture using absorbable Vicryl or polydioxanone (PDS); (D) Both the margins of wound are brought together by suture; (E) Final skin suture using either absorbable (rapid Vicryl) suture or nonabsorbable nylon suture. Author does continuous mattress sutures for perfect closure (**2**).

The trichophytic technique of closure solves the problem of the hairless scar.[10]

The basic principle of trichophytic closure is de-epithelization of one edge of the wound (usually the lower edge) while keeping the underlying hair follicles intact. During the closure of the wound upper edge overlaps the de-epithelized lower edge. After healing, hairs start growing through the scar line. These intermittent hairs growing through the scar can significantly make the scar less visible even with very short hair.

During de-epithelization of the lower edge, avoiding damage to the sebaceous gland and the bulge region is essential, as both are required for follicular regrowth. For this reason the epidermis removed from the lower edge should not exceed 1 mm in depth and width. This shallow depth also reduces cyst formation.

Method of Trichophytic Closure

After harvesting strip, a sharp scissor is used to cut the lower margin of the wound. A skin that shall not be wider than 1 mm and also in-depth <1 mm is cut from one end to another end of the lower margin of the wound. The wound closure is done as a routine (**Figs. 13A to E**).

SLIVERING

After strip harvesting, multiple strips of single FUs thickness are separated from the large skin strip, usually under stereomicroscope—this separation is called slivering. Single FUs thick skin strip is known as a sliver. Slivers can be obtained across the width of the strip or the length of the strip (**Figs. 14 and 15**) (**3**).

FOLLICLE DISSECTION

From sliver, individual FUs are dissected. The follicle dissection should be done preferably under a stereomicroscope, as this provides virtual color, depth perception, and even the white hair follicle dissection is possible under it. The sliver is kept over a wooden spatula or other platforms. One end of sliver is stretched outside by fine-tooth forceps in nondominant hand to increase the gap between the follicles. The scalpel blade in dominant hand cut the tissue between two follicles taking care not to cut any part of the follicle and enough perifollicular tissue is left around each FU. The ideal FU is pear shaped, having intact sebaceous gland, intact follicles, perifollicular tissue, and some fat below the bulb. It is very important to prevent dehydration of graft during follicle dissection, so the rule is the sliver should swim in a pool of saline. The author has innovated a very simple device "dynamic follicle dissection board."[11]

These individual FUs are than transplanted on the recipient area. During the entire process, from strip harvesting to FUs dissection use of magnification is recommended, in order to prevent/reduce follicle transection (**Figs. 16A and B**) (**4**).

TRAINING AND PRACTICE

Novice surgeon should visit a center to see the entire process of strip harvesting to follicle dissection carefully, practice it

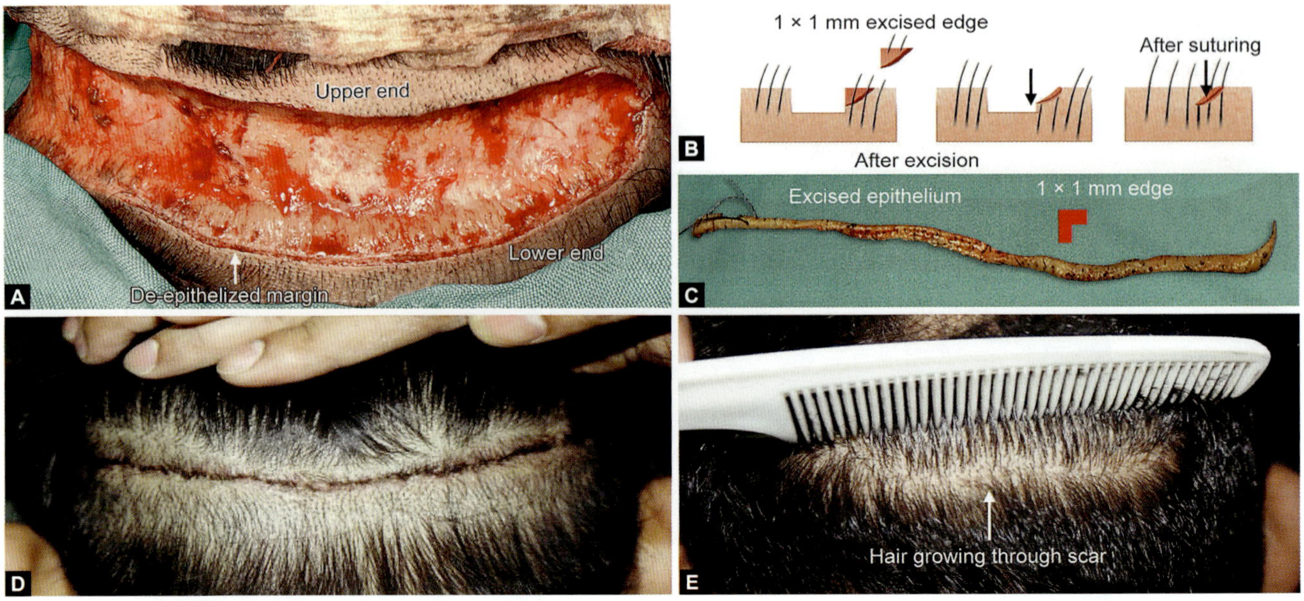

Figs. 13A to E: Trichophytic closure technique. (A) Lower margin of wound is de-epithelized; (B and C) The excised margins dimensions should not be more than 1 × 1 mm; (D) The sutured wound; (E) Hair growing through scar.

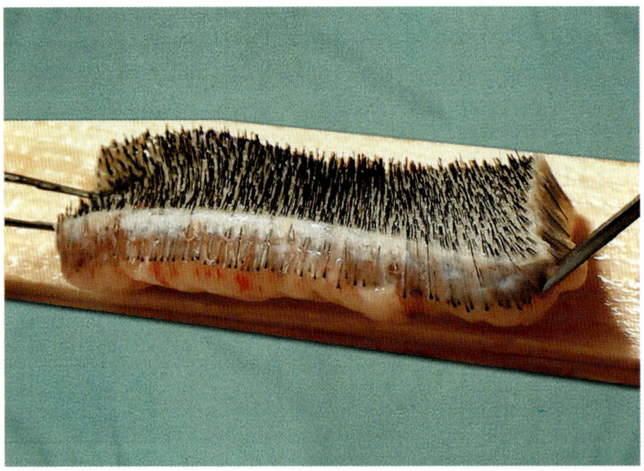

Fig. 14: Slivering. The skin strip is fixed to a wooden spatula, and a saline-soaked gauzed is wrapped around the strip piece to prevent dehydration. A scalpel having surgical blade 20/22 is used by dominant hand to dissect. A fine-tooth forceps is used by another hand. Catch the upper outer end of skin strip at the dermoepidermal junction by tooth forceps and stretch outward and slightly upward to increase the gap between the rows of the follicles. Using the tip of blade dissect in between the two parallel rows of follicles. Keep the tip of the blade in between the rows of the follicle and dissect up to bottom till you separate the one follicle thick skin strip named as a sliver. Keep spraying the saline to prevent dehydration of slivers and skin strip (**3**).

thoroughly and start by taking small cases initially. Author has devised a training module to learn and practice all the steps of HT.[12]

STORAGE OF DISSECTED FOLLICLE UNITS

All the grafts are stored in a graft storage solution, which usually is saline or lactated ringer, or autologous plasma

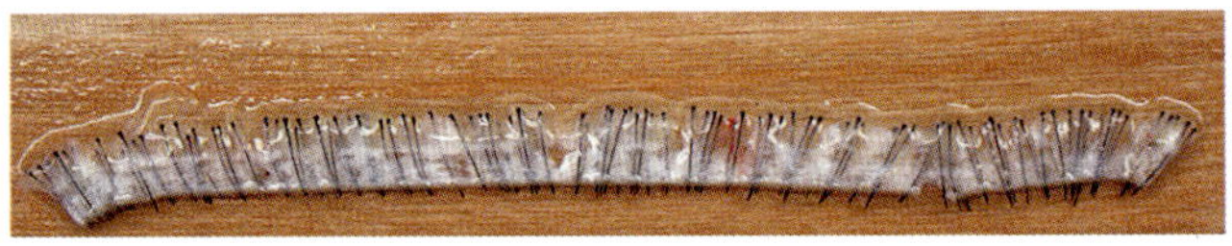

Fig. 15: Longitudinal sliver.

(Fig. 17). If graft out body time is more than 2 hours than intracellular graft holding solution like hypothermosol with or without adenosine triphosphate (ATP) can be used. It is advisable that the grafts are implanted within the 2 hours of ischemia time to get the best result of HT. The author used plasma as a graft-holding solution.[13] Limmer[14] and Kim and Hwang[15] have proved in their studies that grafts kept out of the body in saline for <2 hours have a similar survival rate compared with freshly harvested grafts reimplanted immediately. For this period, the grafts kept in normal saline, or other graft solutions do not have better results. Kim finds normal saline at 4°C does not improve graft health unless >6 hours out of the body.

POSTOPERATIVE CARE

Postoperative Pain

Pain after strip surgery is one of the common fears, which the patient has. The postoperative pain depends on the tension over the suture line. A wider strip excised in a scalp having less laxity is the cause of pain. The author has done a study of the relation of the width of the strip and postoperatively pain. In all cases of strip surgery author give nerve block anesthesia below the suture line, which makes the area numb. This postoperative nerve block not only relieves the pain but also

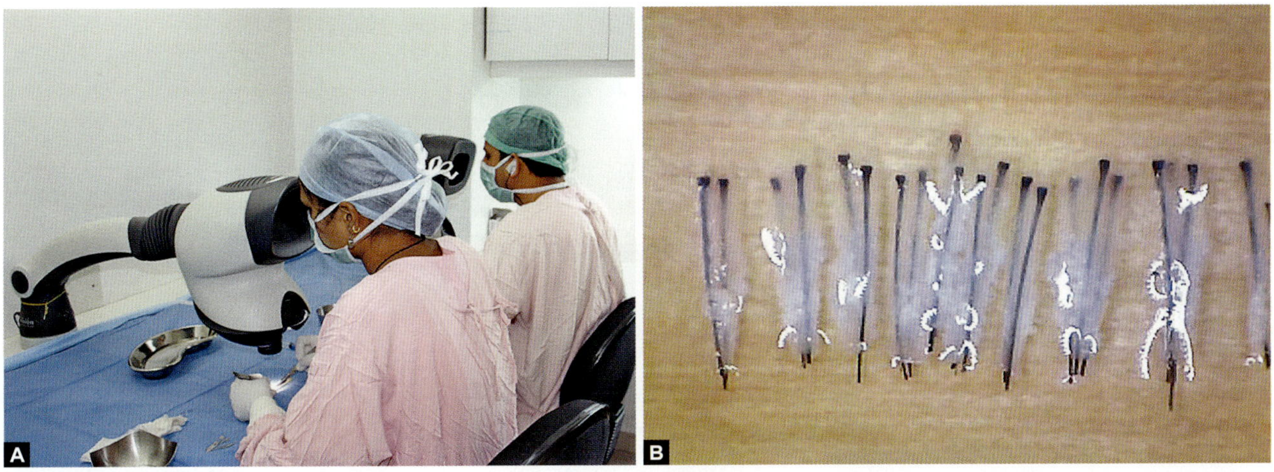

Figs. 16A and B: Follicle unit (graft) dissection under stereo microscope; (B) Dissected follicles immersed in a pool of water to prevent dehydration **(4)**.

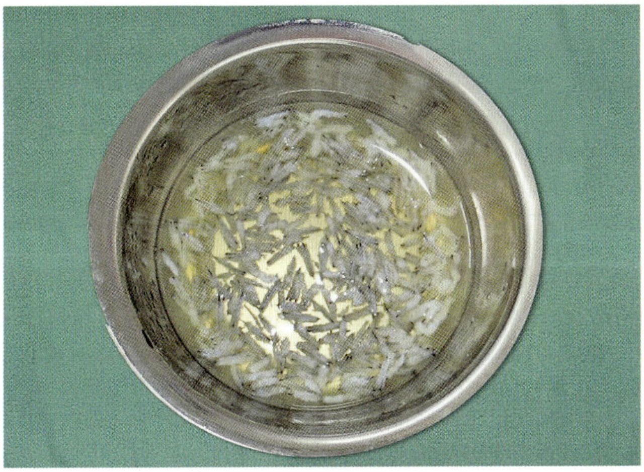

Fig. 17: Grafts in autologous plasma.

reduces fear of pain, which makes the patient comfortable and he sleeps well.[16]

Dressing

After wound closure, proper cleaning of the area is done and antiseptic ointment is applied over suture line and area is dressed with a gauge and cotton pad **(Figs. 18A to C)**.

Recipient area does not require any dressing. A saline solution having antibiotic in it (some preparations are commercially available) can be sprayed over recipient area four to five times a day to prevent drying of recipient area.

Donor area dressing can be removed next day and area is cleaned with antibiotic solution and any topical antimicrobial ointment can be applied over the suture line.

Postoperative antibiotics can be given for 5 days. Some surgeons do not give antibiotic postoperatively. Generous amount of analgesics to reduce postoperative pain is recommended. Some surgeons give oral prednisolone to reduce edema, but the authors do not give.

The authors prefer to give water head wash without soap and shampoo from the third postoperative day, and betadine scrub head wash from 8th to 10th day for 3–5 days.

Use of minoxidil can be started from 3rd to 10th postoperative day.

SECOND STRIP HARVESTING

Subsequent sessions of strip harvesting should be done at an interval of a minimum of 9–12 months. Before planning for second strip harvest one should examine the donor area to see the quality and width of the scar, skin laxity, and the presence of hypertrophic or keloid formation in the scar. If the scar is too wide and the skin laxity is not enough to allow a second strip, it is better to avoid a second strip surgery. If possible, laxity is enough and scar is not hypertrophic or very wide than first, remove the scar of the previous surgery as part of the next strip harvested.

Most patients can undergo two to three strip surgeries if they heal with fine scars and the scars are removed with each surgery.

COMBINATION OF FOLLICULAR UNIT STRIP SURGERY AND FOLLICULAR UNIT EXTRACTION

The combination method of follicle harvesting is the technique in which both strip and follicular unit extraction (FUE) method of follicles harvesting are done on the same patient. The advantage of the combination is that harvesting of a maximum number of the FU without violating the basic principles of each technique. Sometime in an attempt to harvest more graft surgeon may harvest a wider strip, which may give complication in the form of widening of scar or wound dehiscence. If during FUE more grafts are harvested, there is the possibility of harvesting either from the unsafe area or overharvesting. So to avoid these complications,

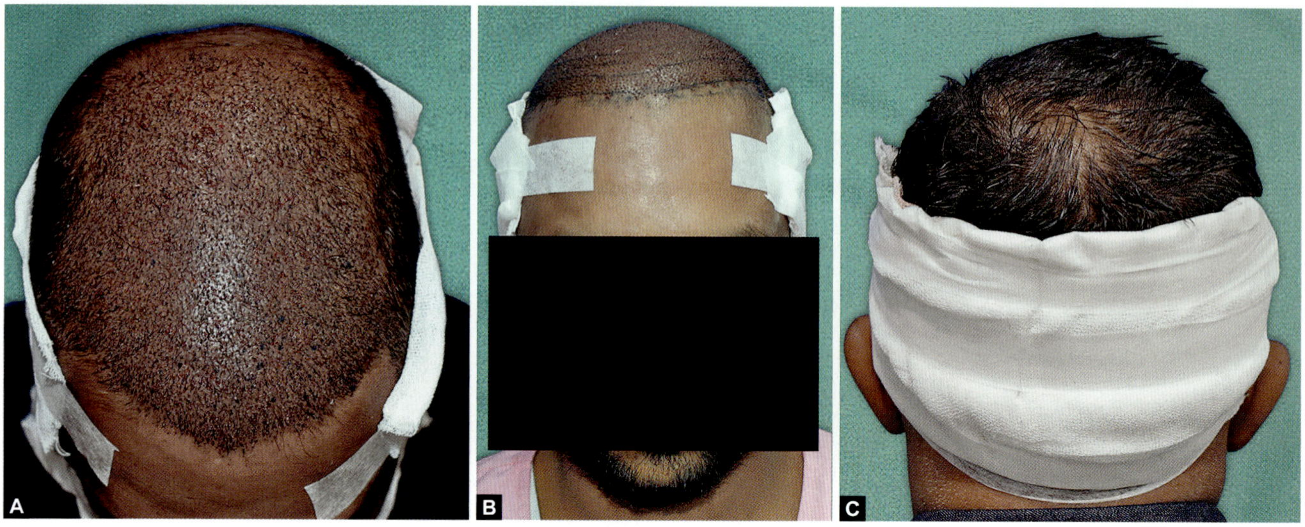

Figs. 18A to C: Postoperative dressing of donor area and no dressing required over recipient area.

both techniques are done together or one after another. By combining FUSS and FUE, a total of more number of grafts can be harvested in comparison of individual method of follicles harvesting.

COMPLICATIONS OF HAIR TRANSPLANT

The problems encountered can be classified as complaints and complications.

- *Nonsurgical complaints:* Patient's dissatisfaction
- *Surgical complaints:* Pain, edema, itching, graft dislodgement, and bleeding
- *Aesthetic complications:* Visible scaring, keloid, hypertrophic scar, and donor hair effluvium
- *Medical complications:* Infection, wound dehiscence, necrosis of skin, neuralgia, painful neuroma, and arteriovenous (AV) fistula.

The most common postoperative complaints are pain, edema, itching, graft dislodgement, and bleeding and sometimes hiccups. Later complaints which are more common and severe are dissatisfaction and poor aesthetic outcome, which can be very well dealt by detail counseling and proper assessment of donor and recipient area and patient's goal.

CONCLUSION

Despite the progress in FUE, strip surgery FUT/FUSS holds its place in HT. Proper planning for the strip surgery includes assessment of safe donor area, estimation of average FUs density, the diameter of the hair, scalp laxity, and elasticity. There are various subjective and objective tools to measure these mentioned parameters. Surgeons can utilize their experience in modifying these tools to suit their practice and better planning of the surgery.

Strip harvesting procedure involves the proper marking of the donor area in the safe zone, a good anesthesia technique and dissection of the strip without the damage to the neurovascular bundle. The donor area can be closed with either a single-layer or two-layer closure. Trichophytic closure prevents the wide hairless scar. Whatever the technique is used the final scar depends on the individual skin characteristics.

Most of the complications of HT surgery are avoidable. History of medical illness, medication, tobacco and smoking, detailed counseling, and discussion before surgery help in proper planning and avoid patient unsatisfaction. It is crucial to estimate the gap between donor supply and recipient requirement. Preoperative scalp massage help in the reduction of donor scar complications. Every patient should be individualized, planned, and operated with aim to zero down complaints and complications.

VIDEOS

Video 1: Laxity Exercise
Video 2: Strip Harvesting
Video 3: Silvering
Video 4: Graft Dissection

Above videos can be accessed by redeeming code given on the front-in of the book cover.

REFERENCES

1. Headington JT. Transverse microscopic anatomy of human scalp. Arch Dermatol. 1984;120:449-56.
2. Bernstein RM. Follicular unit transplantation. In: Robinson JK, Hanke CW, Mark Siegel D, Fratila A (Eds). Surgery of the Skin: Procedural Dermatology, 3rd edition. Elsevier Health Sciences; 2014. p. 480.
3. Bosley LL, Hope CR, Montroy RE, Straub PM. Reduction of male pattern baldness in multiple stages: a retrospective study. J Dermatol Surg Oncol. 1980;6:498-503.

4. Mohebi P, Pak J, Rassman W. How to assess scalp laxity. Hair Transplant Forum Int. 2008;18(5):16.
5. Mayer M, Pauls T. Scalp elasticity scale. Hair Transplant Forum Int. 2005;15(4):9-10.
6. Bernstein RM. Accurate follicular unit transplantation. In: Haber R, Stough D (Eds). Hair replacement: surgical and medical. St. Louis: Mosby; 1996. pp. 138-42.
7. Bernstein R, Rassman W. The logic of follicular unit transplantation. Dermatol Clin. 1990;17:227-92.
8. Cole J, Devroy J. A calculated look at donor area. Hair Transplant Forum Int. 2001;11(5):150-4.
9. Pathomvanich D. Donor harvesting: a new approach to minimizing transection of the hair follicle. Hair Transplant Forum Int. 1998;8(5):4-5.
10. Marzola M. Tricophytic closure of donor area. Hair Transplant Forum International. 2005;15(4):113-6.
11. Garg AK, Garg S. Dynamic hydration follicle dissection board-an innovative device. Hair Transplant Forum International. 2014;24(6):214.
12. Garg AK, Garg S. A learning module in hair restoration: a simple and economical method to learn all the steps of strip method of hair follicle harvesting and implantation. Indian J Plastic Surg. 2017;50:230-5.
13. Garg AK, Garg S. A Histological and Clinical Evaluation of Plasma as a Graft Holding Solution and Its Efficacy in Terms of Hair Growth and Graft Survival. Indian Journal of Plastic Surgery: Official Publication of the Association of Plastic Surgeons of India. 2019;52(2):209-15.
14. Limmer R. Micrograft survival. In: Stough D (Ed). Hair Replacement. St. Louis, Missouri: Mosby Press; 1996. pp. 147-9.
15. Kim JC, Hwang S. The effects of dehydration, preservation temperature and time, and hydrogen peroxide on hair grafts. In: Unger WP, Shapiro R (Eds). Hair Transplantation, 4th edition. New York: Marcel Dekker; 2004. pp. 285-6.
16. Garg S, Garg A. Study of ropivacaine block to reduce post-operative pain after strip harvesting, and the relationship of strip width with post-operative pain. Hair Transplant Forum International. 2009;29(5):186-8.

CHAPTER 70

Donor Area: Follicular Unit Extraction

Aman Dua, Nirav V Desai

KEY MESSAGES

- Follicular unit extraction (FUE) is one of the most important innovations in the field of hair restoration.
- Patients who want to avoid linear scar and patients without adequate laxity of scalp are good candidates for FUE.
- Previously considered as a procedure for small areas or repair surgery, it has now become recognized as a solution for most cases of baldness.
- FUE is the only method for harvesting beard and body hair.
- Power machines and robotics have improved speed of procedure.

INTRODUCTION

Follicular unit extraction (FUE) has proved to be a significant advancement in the field of hair restoration surgeries. Though strip surgical method was successful in providing excellent results, there were several problems:

- Poor donor scar often due to aggressive strip harvesting
- Problematic donor harvesting in subsequent sittings due to wide donor strip scar
- Pain associated with the strip surgery
- Limited access to donor area in strip surgery.

Follicular unit extraction technique has enhanced the armamentarium of the surgeon, expanded the donor area to beard and body and also has removed the fear of surgery from the minds of patients and has led to increasing popularity of the surgery.

Donor area of scalp for FUE is defined as same for any hair transplant surgery, which is the permanent zone where the dihydrotestosterone (DHT) resistant hair follicles are located, i.e., occipital zone. Besides scalp, the advantage with FUE method is that it expands the donor area beyond the scalp and technically any hair-bearing body area can serve as donor. However, since the characteristic of hair in different body parts is different, beard and chest are the preferred nonscalp donors. These alternative donor areas are helpful in cases where the baldness is extensive and donor hair in scalp is limited. In rare case, if patient agrees, pubic hair can also be considered as additional source. Similarly, the hair on the forearms and legs can also be considered as additional source of hair follicles if they are sufficiently thick and large.

PRINCIPLE OF FOLLICULAR UNIT EXTRACTION

Introduction of FOX procedure by Bernstein and Rassman for the hair transplantation without strip harvesting was a breakthrough in the history of modern hair restoration. The basic principle behind FUE is that the hair follicular unit is tightly attached with surrounding dermis up to the level of attachment of arrector pili muscle and below that it is loosely attached in lower dermis and subcutaneous tissue. Once this area above and around the attachment is made loose and separated from the surrounding dermis, the inferior segment can be extracted easily. The follicular unit is narrowest at the surface, thus one can use small micropunches of size 0.7–0.9 mm to dissect the follicular units and therefore the resulting scar is too small to be recognized.

The main anatomical limitation of the technique is that it is not possible to identify the bulge of the hair from outside and hence the procedure is blind. Also, since the hairs within the intact unit splay at the lower end and diverge in different directions, the process of extraction can result in a higher transection rate. The procedure is also slow as each unit has to be pulled out slowly. However, with experience and using appropriate type of punches with motorized device, the speed of the surgery and transection rate can be improved greatly **(Figs. 1A to C)**.

METHODS OF FOLLICULAR UNIT EXTRACTION

The FUE was first published in literature by Rassman and Bernstein[1] in USA in 2002 who described the use of tiny punches to dissect the follicular units followed by extraction of the unit by using a forceps. It was very slow and the transection rate was very high. Later on, the introduction of technically more sophisticated and powered instruments by Jim Harris,[2] John Cole, suction-assisted machines by NeoGraft™, and Robotic FUE device by Restoration Robotics have reduced the time of the procedure as well as the transection rates.

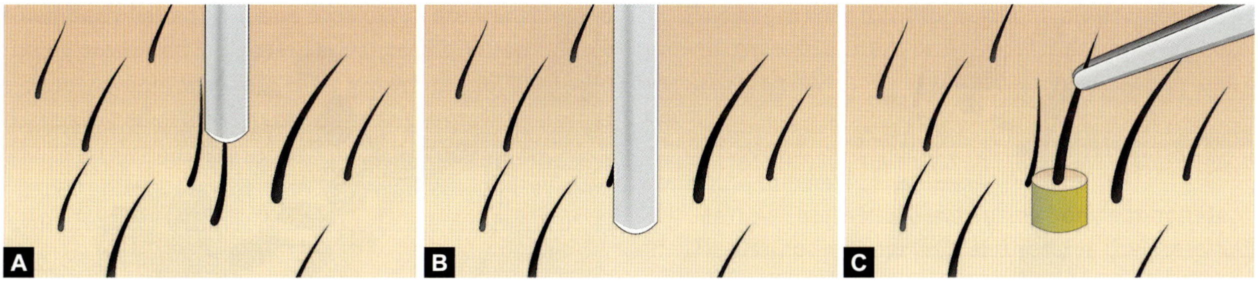

Figs. 1A to C: (A) Follicular unit; (B) Dissection by insertion of the punch; (C) Removal of the follicular unit.

By Manual Punches

Two Steps Method (By Single Forceps and Double Forceps Methods)

In this method, during first step a single punch is used to mark the skin and then rotated in one direction or alternate directions (oscillation) till it suddenly gives way and penetrate deep into the skin. This sudden giving way is due to release of attachment of arrector pili muscle around the follicular unit and below that the attachments are loose and tissue with low resistance. Once the follicular unit is dissected, the punch is removed.

Now in second step, upper part of follicular unit/graft is held by a single forceps and pulled in the direction parallel to the angle of emergence of the hair. At the same time the assistant pushes the skin on the superior aspect of the circular incision down in the direction opposite to that in which hair is being pulled[4] (single forceps method). This gentle traction to the top of the follicular unit is applied until the unit is pulled loose from its deep dermal and subcutaneous connections and comes out. In case, if the graft is not taken out easily by single forceps then one has to hold the graft with fine forceps from top portion just below the epidermis and gentle pull is applied in outward direction so that the bulge potion of graft will come above the skin surface, and another forceps is used to hold the graft is held just below the bulge level and pull is applied in the direction of first forceps to aid it.

Three Steps Dissection Method by Harris

The three steps procedure to extract the follicles was first described by James Harris. In step one, a sharp punch is used to score the epidermis (rather than cut through the full thickness to the dermis) and then in second step a dull punch is used (through a back-and-forth twisting motion) to bluntly dissect the follicular unit graft from the surrounding epidermis and dermis. Harris also invented an instrument for this procedure with a sharp punch on one side and dull punch on the other side.[5] Step three involves the use of forceps to remove the unit and is similar to step two of two steps method described earlier. This variation has several advantages over the original two-step process. Using a dull punch avoids follicle transection and allows intact follicular units to be extracted more easily with an easy-to-learn methodology. One great advantage of this addition is that it opens the technique to the inherent FOX negative population: those with very fine hair and those with African kinky hair types. Some drawbacks of the three steps technique are a possible higher incidence of buried grafts and more time consumption compared to two-step method.[4]

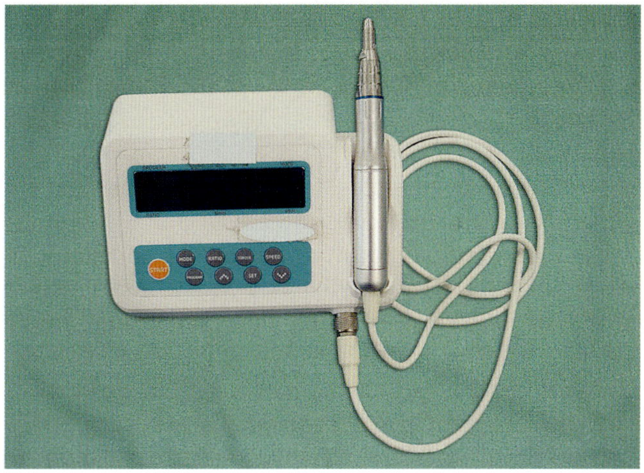

Fig. 2: Motor with handpiece.

By Motorized Device

While using manual punches one has to spin (rotate it in clockwise or anticlockwise direction) or oscillate (alternate movement in both the directions) with application of some axial force to enter into the skin. Such manual rotatory movement is more time consuming and physically tiring, thus limiting the number of grafts per session. By using a motor to rotate the punch one can overcome this problem. With such motor the speed of rotation can also be adjusted as per need so that the required axial force to penetrate the skin can be greatly reduced resulting in faster dissection of the follicular unit thus more number of grafts per session **(Fig. 2)**.

Specialized System

Cole Isolation Technique

It was developed by Dr John Cole. This technique incorporates a variety of highly sharpened, thin wall punches along with a precise depth control mechanism. The goal is to minimize the follicular transection rate and increase the speed of

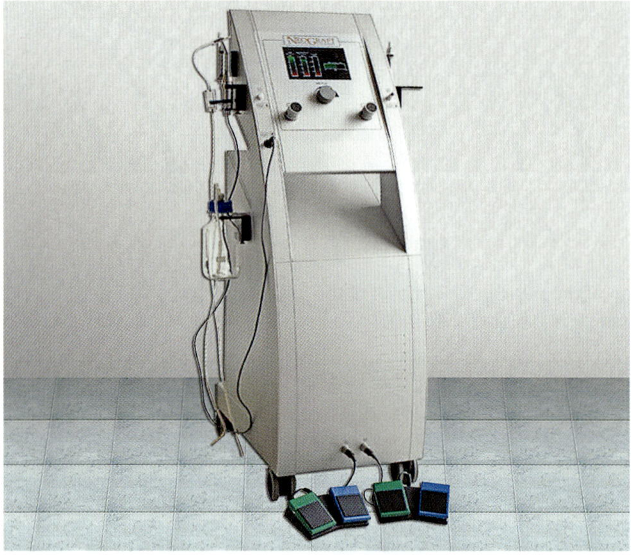

Fig. 3: NeoGraft™ device.

donor harvesting by using punches of different diameter and of varying geometry, precise depth control by using depth controller and altering the tangential forces. The objectives of Cole Isolation Technique (CIT) are to match the donor harvesting methods to the individual physical characteristics of each patient.[6]

Harris Surgically Advanced Follicular Extraction Technique

After introduction of three steps method of grafts harvesting by using sharp and dull punches together in 2004, Dr Harris made some more modifications and attached the dull punch to a rotating drill resulted in introduction of powered surgically advanced follicular extraction (SAFE) system of graft harvesting which works on principle of blunt dissection resulting in low follicular transection rate.[7]

Suction-assisted Automated Devices (NeoGraft™ Device and Smart Graft)

These machines for hair transplant surgery are handheld surgical devices and not a robotic system. They extract follicular units from the donor area and implant them in the recipient area via an air-pressure/suction-based system. The machines are partially automated and do not have the precision of the computer-driven image-guided system that guides and relies on manual control provided by a human operator in order to select and extract follicular unit/grafts **(Fig. 3)**.

Robotic Follicular Unit Extraction: ARTAS Robot for Harvesting

This is computer-assisted and physician control system that combines the numerous features including image-guided robotic arm, dissection punch, and vision mapping as well as tracking technology.[3] The major drawbacks of this system are **(Fig. 4)**:

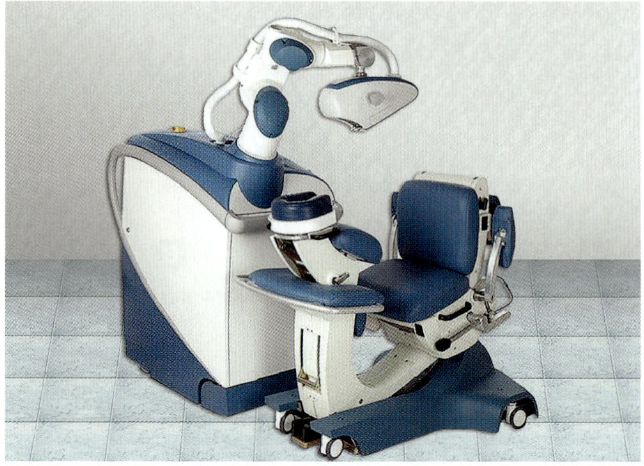

Fig. 4: ARTAS robot of harvesting.

- Very expensive
- Removal after dissection and storage of grafts is still manual.
- Does not perform implantation and still that has to be done manually.

INSTRUMENTS FOR FOLLICULAR UNIT EXTRACTION (FIGS. 5A AND B)

- Motor with handpiece
- Punch
  - Sharp Punch
    - Cutting edge is at outer side/outer cutting edge—inside bevel
    - Cutting edge is in the center—middle bevel
    - Cutting edge is at inner side/inner cutting edge—outside bevel
  - Blunt punch/dull punch
  - Various modifications, e.g., semi-sharp punch, hybrid trumpet punch by Dr Jean Devroye, hex punch by Dr James Harris, contour surface punch, etc.
- Extraction forceps.

STEPS OF EXTRACTION BY MOTORIZED FOLLICULAR UNIT EXTRACTION

Among the various methods of FUE, motorized FUE or the powered FUE is the most commonly performed method of graft harvesting. Following are the various steps involved in this method.

Preparation of Donor Area

Trimming is usually done on the day of the surgery and hair is kept about 1–2 mm of length in the donor area. A typical case, e.g., 2,000 grafts require full trimming of the donor area.

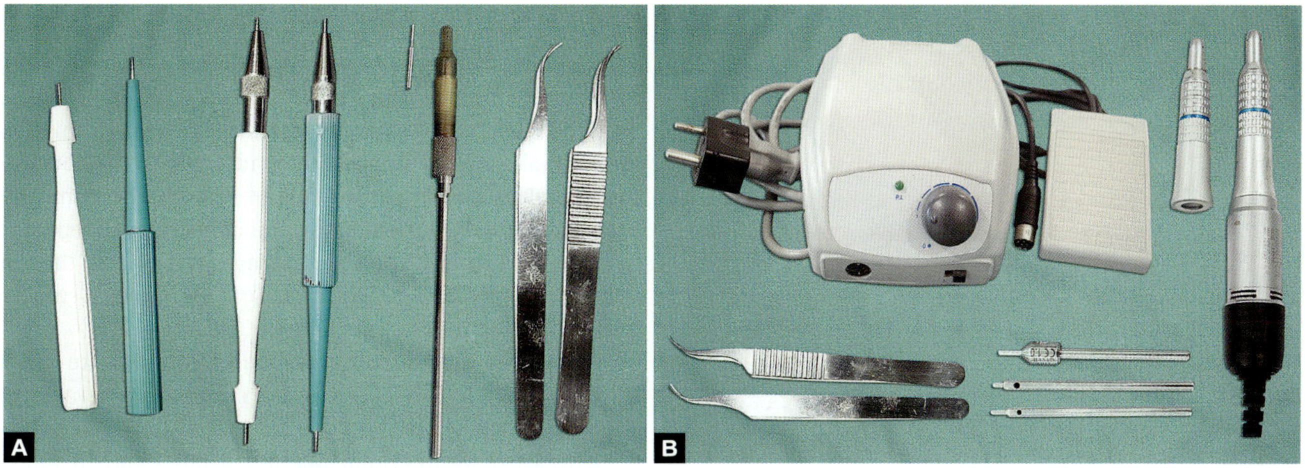

Figs. 5A and B: Instruments for follicular unit extraction: (A) Manual method; (B) Motorized method.

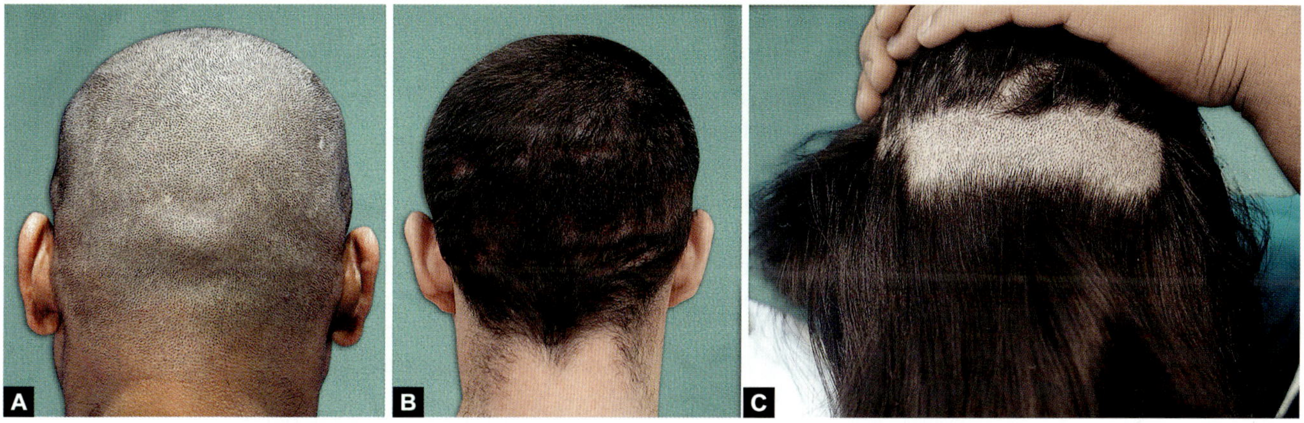

Figs. 6A to C: (A) Full trim donor area; (B) Multiple layered trimming; (C) Partial trim.

If the requirement is less, i.e., around 1,000 grafts, then multiple layered trimming can be done; if the requirement is even less, i.e., around 500 grafts only, then a partial trim can be done. In very rare cases, no-trim technique in which no trimming of hair in the donor area can be used **(Figs. 6A to C)**.

Complete shaving is not recommended as one needs to see the exit angle of hair to judge the angle of follicle within the skin.

Positions of the Patient and Surgeon

Make the patient lie down in the prone position by keeping his face down or turned on one side depending upon the area from where extraction is being done. Some surgeons prefer to use prone chair to make the patient sit during the extraction. Depending upon his/her preference and comfort surgeon may choose a sitting position or standing position. The position of patient as well as surgeon may change during the extraction depending upon the alignment of the grafts and the ease of the extraction **(Fig. 7)**.

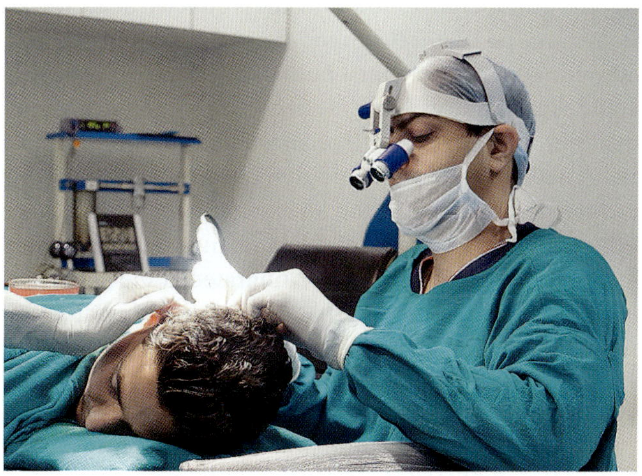

Fig. 7: Positions of the patient and surgeon.

Local Anesthesia

Pain during the surgery is one of the major concerns for any patient undergoing any kind of surgery and when it comes to a surgery done for aesthetic purpose the importance

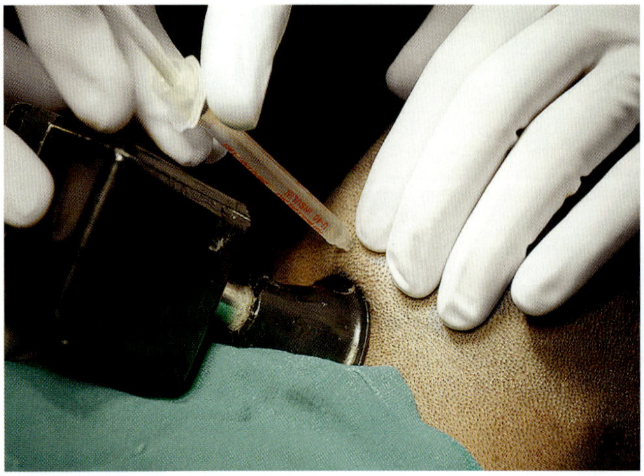

Fig. 8: Anesthesia in donor area—greater occipital nerve block.

increases many fold, so complete pain-free state during the entire surgery is one of the key factor in the overall experience for the patient.

Eutectic mixture applied in form of topical anesthesia approximately 40–60 minutes before the actual local anesthetic is injected can greatly help to reduce the pricking pain associated with needle insertion into the skin while giving the local anesthesia. Along with this vibrator can be used to dampen the discomfort associated during the tissue expansion due to injection of anesthesia. Also the speed of infiltration should be slow to minimize the discomfort.

Greater Occipital Nerve Block

To give this nerve block place three fingers at the level of superior nuchal line with the middle finger on the external occipital protuberance, now a needle is directed at 90° toward the occiput just lateral to the lateral fingers until a bony endpoint is obtained. Once bone is reached withdraw the needle slightly and aspirate to check to prevent intravascular injection. Now inject 1 mL of anesthetic solution on each side. A needle is then inserted dermally through previously anesthetized wheal and the anesthetic is injected slightly to the right and left until solid line of anesthetic is created. Finally, the whole donor area is infiltrated at the superficial dermal level with a mixture of 0.5% lignocaine adrenaline and saline **(Fig. 8)**.

Follicular Dissection

Setting the Speed of the Motor

The speed of the motor should be minimum possible that allows easy penetration in the skin. While working with the blunt punches the speed is more than that required for the sharp punches. For blunt punch, the range of speed is between 1,000 and 2,000 rpm whereas for the sharp punch it is 500–700 rpm.

Infiltration of the Donor Area

After giving local anesthesia in the donor area, one should infiltrate 1 mL of normal saline mixed with adrenaline in around 1 cm × 2 cm of an area (around 0.5 mL/cm) from where one can take out 60–80 grafts depending upon the density of the follicular units. Once the grafts are removed from that area, then again infiltrate them in the adjacent area and repeat the same procedure and keep on moving forward from the right to left side of the patient in the case of right-handed surgeon. The infiltration helps in the following ways:

- It reduces the bleeding on the extraction site due to vasoconstriction effect of adrenaline present in the mixture.
- It increases the interfollicular unit distance and thus allows the easy engagement of the punch.
- It reduces acuteness of angle of follicle by making them straight allowing easy advancement into the skin.
- It helps to decrease the wound surface area by reducing the acuteness of the angle of the follicle as well as by stretching the skin which will shrink later when the infiltrated fluid is drained away.[8]
- It creates high pressure in the lower part of dermis and subcutaneous plane, so once the adhesions around the follicular unit are released by dissection the isolated follicular units/grafts pop up on the skin surface. These popped up grafts are easy to take out by the assistant with single forceps. Thus, making the scoring and extraction simultaneously, reduces the total time of the graft harvesting.

Applying Traction: Counter Traction

Once the infiltration is given, the surgeon should hold the handpiece in their dominant hand and apply traction toward the head end with the nondominant hand. The assistant stands on the other side and applies counter traction toward the opposite end. This helps to reduce the fluidity of the skin, makes it firm and increases the exit angle of the hair which further facilitates the entry of the punch into the skin.

Alignment of the Shaft of the Punch

Alignment of the punch is to place the shaft of the punch parallel to the direction of targeted hair follicle emerging from the scalp. The surgeon has to be careful as the direction of the hair and the exit angle of the hair change every few centimeters, as a result of which, the alignment changes accordingly.[9] The beginner should practice this step by holding the handpiece along the direction of hair shaft in different areas such as the occipital and the temporal to appreciate the difference between different exit angles **(Fig. 9)**.

Engagement of the Punch

The next step is one of the most important steps of the surgery, i.e., engagement. It refers to the part when the tip of

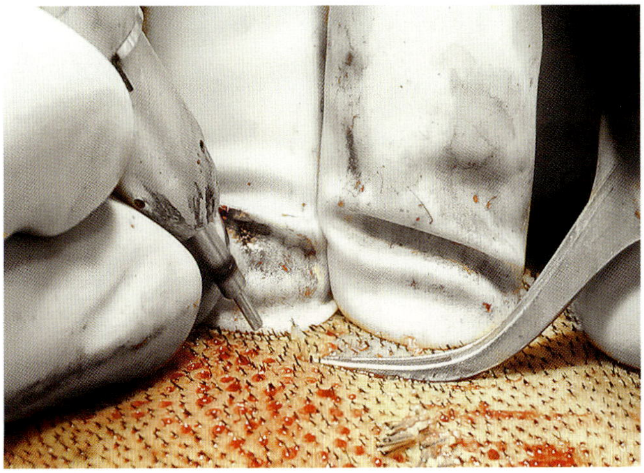

Fig. 9: Alignment.

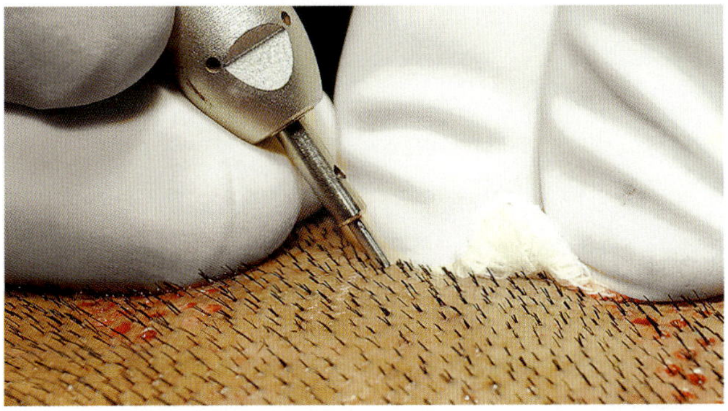

Fig. 10: Engagement.

the punch touches the epithelium around the targeted hairs. The surgeon should make sure that the targeted hair is either in the center of the circular impression of the punch or in the superior part. If the hair is in the inferior part, then the graft is transected (mainly with sharp punch and occasional with blunt punch) or get partially loosened and buried under the skin (mainly with blunt punch) **(Fig. 10)**.

Advancement of the Punch

Advancement is insertion of the punch forward into the skin after successful engagement to loosen the attachment up to the pilosebaceous unit to release the follicular unit. Whenever a surgeon uses a sharp punch, a general dictum is to stay as superficial as possible to loosen the pilosebaceous unit otherwise it can lead to transection of the follicular unit. However, while working with blunt/dull punch, one has liberty of going deeper because of less chance of transection.

When the surgeon passes a blunt punch across the tightest point (attachment of the arrector pili muscle around the follicular unit), there is a "give way" feeling which is an indicator to stop the advancement of the punch. But, even if the surgeon advances deeper, there is hardly any transection of the follicle coming across its path as the edge of the punch

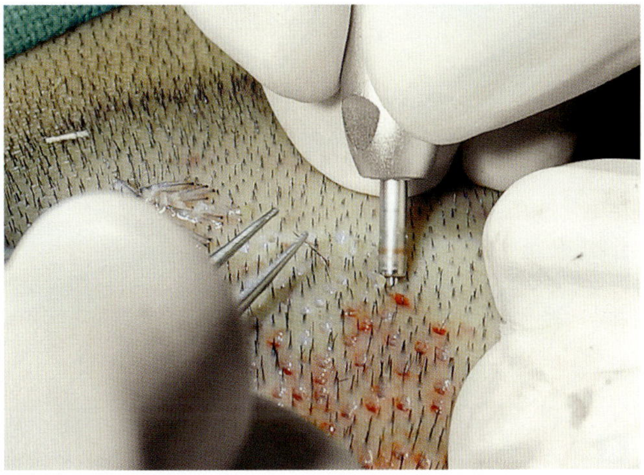

Fig. 11: Advancement of the punch.

is blunt. In fact, introducing the punch deeper not only frees the pilosebaceous unit efficiently, but also makes it easier to remove the graft with minimum force **(Fig. 11)**.

Removal of Grafts

Removal of grafts can be done either separately once the scoring is done or can be done simultaneously. Once the follicular dissection is done the assistant can take out the grafts with the forceps. If the sharp punch was used to score the skin and the incisions are very superficial, one may have to use two forceps to remove the grafts. If grafts are dissected sufficiently, they will slightly pop up 0.5–1 mm above the skin surface and lie loosely. Such grafts can be easily removed simultaneously by the assistant with a forceps in one hand while giving counter traction with the other hand. This leads to increased speed of harvesting of grafts. The assistant can also give a feedback in the real time whether the grafts being removed are fully intact, fully or partially transected and the surgeon can immediately make the necessary adjustments to correct the angle of alignment to harvest the grafts with minimal wastage **(Figs. 12A and B)**.

MEGA SESSIONS AND GIGA SESSIONS

Earlier, FUE was not considered as first-line treatment for the hair restoration of the scalp by many and it was recommended to repair the donor scar after strip surgery or to cover small area.[10] Continuous untiring work and research by many physicians across the globe has led to significant improvements in technique and instrumentation which resulted in faster speed of extraction, lower wastage in terms of transection rates, and ultimately more number of graft extractions per session. So now it is possible to transplant 2,000–2,500 grafts easily from scalp. Some centers with experienced surgeons have shown that one can extract approximately 3,000–3,500 grafts from scalp alone if the donor density is good; however, thinning and overharvesting

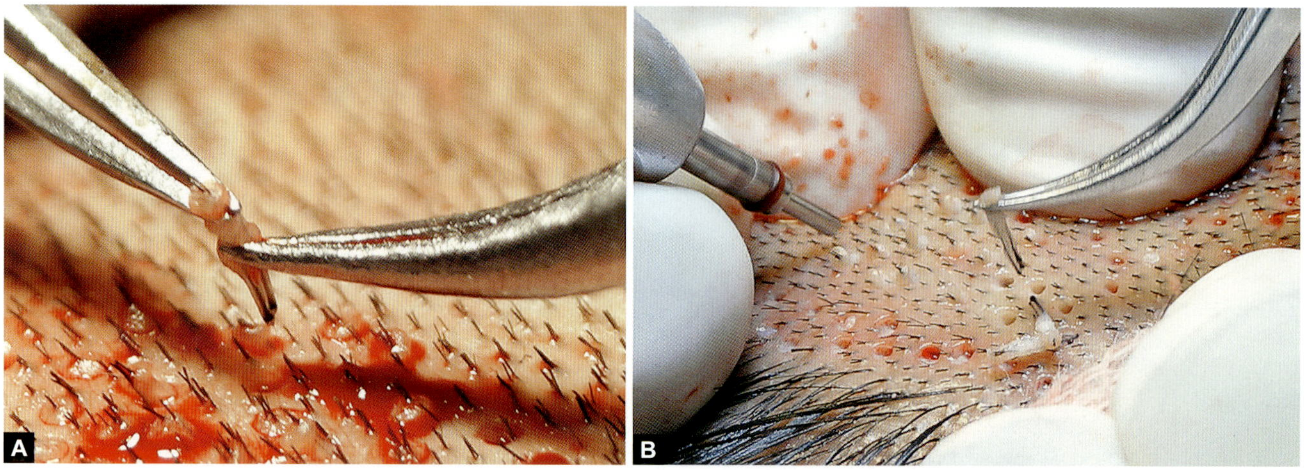

Figs. 12A and B: (A) Graft removal with two forceps after scoring of the skin; (B) Simultaneous graft removal with single forceps.

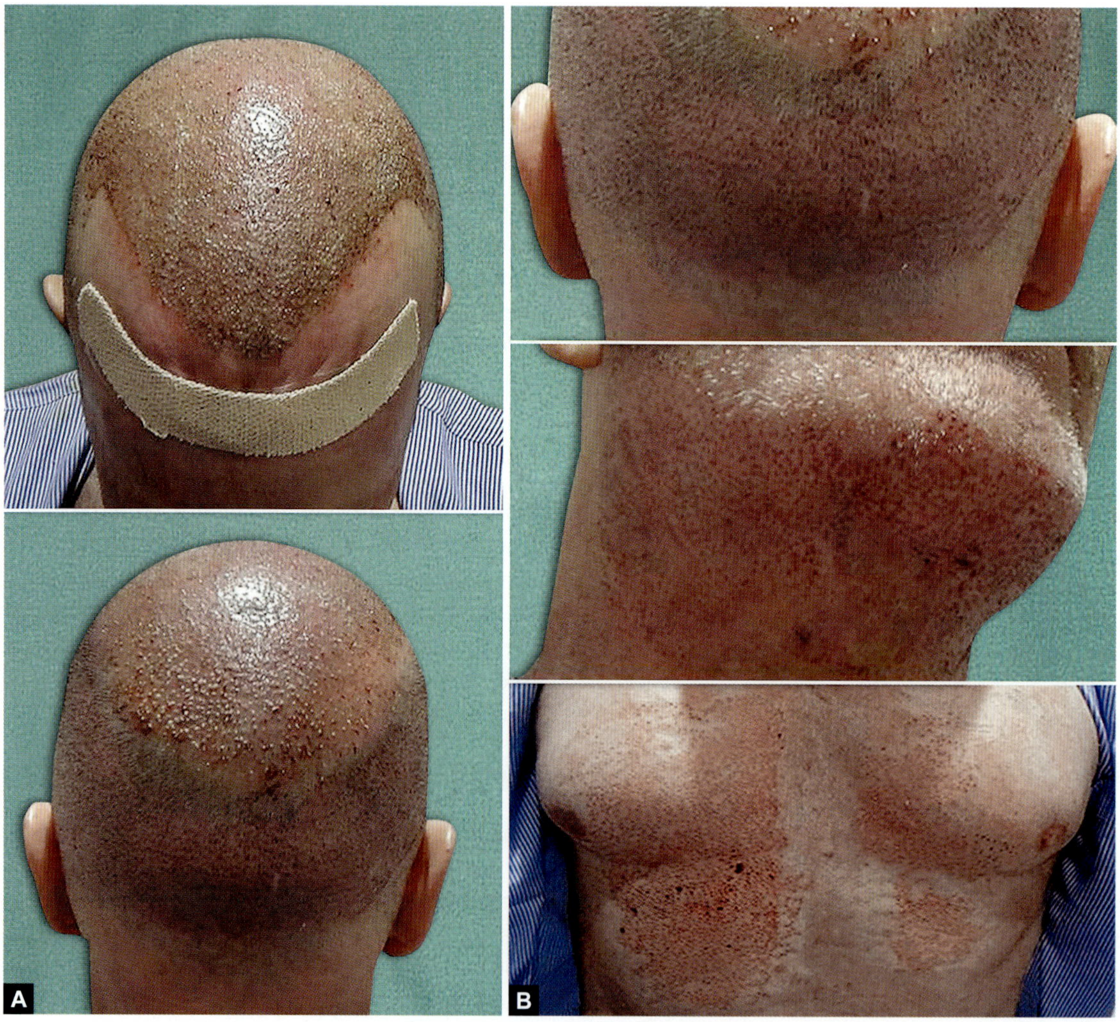

Figs. 13A and B: Giga session. (A) Recipient site after implantation of total 5,000 grafts from scalp and body; (B) Donor sites after extraction—scalp: 2,800 grafts, beard: 1,000 grafts, and chest: 1,200 grafts.

of donor area must be considered before attempting such high number of grafts in single sitting. By combining FUE from scalp with FUE from other body parts such as beard and/or chest, one can transplant around 4,000–5,000 (Giga session) grafts in one surgical sitting over 2–3 days, but this requires high level of experience as extracting grafts from chest and other body parts is difficult in comparison to the scalp extraction **(Figs. 13A and B)**.

COMPLICATIONS RELATED TO HARVESTING

General Postoperative Complaints/ Complications

Follicular unit extraction is relatively less invasive method of graft harvesting still some complications may occur which are as follows:

- *Postoperative pain and discomfort:* The postoperative pain and discomfort is minimal. This may occur on the evening of the surgery and disappears in next couple of days. Analgesics such as paracetamol and nonsteroidal anti-inflammatory drugs (NSAIDs) are given to avoid the pain, especially for first 5–7 days.
- *Oozing and minor bleeding:* Postoperative oozing can occur from the donor site, although it is mild. This occurs more when the patient lies supine on the surface, due to pressure on the donor area. We advise the patient to keep a folded towel on the pillow to avoid spoiling of pillow cover and bed sheet. The patients are also advised to apply firm pressure with gauze piece for few minutes when he/she notices any bleeding from the operated site.
- *Infection:* Infection is rare if proper aseptic measures are taken by surgeon during the surgery followed by proper postoperative care along with the course of prophylactic oral antibiotic prescribed for 5–7 days.
- *Numbness or paresthesia:* There is hardly any numbness or paresthesia in donor area postoperatively after FUE as compared to strip removal in which there is possibility of the transection of the superficial cutaneous nerves.
- *Pruritus:* Some patient may experience mild itching in the donor area once the healing starts and scabs are formed. Most of the time, it gets relieved within couple of days if patient takes proper head bath and clean the area appropriately and applies antibiotic cream regularly. One can apply aloe vera gel or mild steroid cream if the itching is severe.
- *Vasovagal episodes:* Vasovagal episodes or postural hypotension can be seen in some patients due to prolong period of lying down during the surgery.

Complications Specific to FUE in the Donor Area

Early Complications

- *Buried grafts:* This is usually seen with blunt punches. During the follicular dissection when the punch is advanced onto the skin, if the follicle is not in the center of the punch (more commonly when the follicular unit is in inferior part of punch during the advance); the follicular unit is pushed inside the dermis or into the subcutaneous tissue and gets embedded there. Such buried grafts should be taken out as failing to do so can lead to pseudofolliculitis or cyst formation later on.
- *Pseudofolliculitis:* It can occur when the grafts are not taken out completely and parts of them remain buried within the dermis and are left inside the skin. Clinically, this is seen as folliculitis like painful swelling in the donor area, which resolves spontaneously when the growing hair comes out completely on its own. If it does not come out, then one has to take out manually on the surface to stop the inflammatory reaction induced by growing hair within the skin.
- *Necrosis of the donor area:*[11] It is rare to seen with FUE but can occur if the extraction of the grafts are not properly spaced out and too much adrenaline is used.
- *Postoperative effluvium:* Donor hair effluvium can occur after surgery and can be seen as diffuse hair loss from the donor site but in practice it is relatively less visible or appreciable due to complete trimming of the hair during surgery. The reason for such hair fall is not very much clear but possible reasons are numerous trauma to site, interrupted blood supply, overharvesting may lead to some trauma to adjacent follicles, etc. Such hair loss resolves spontaneously and does not require any separate medication besides what is prescribed postoperatively in the form of minoxidil and multivitamins.

Late Complications

- *Pinpoint white scars in the donor area:* Many people have misconception that FUE is "scarless" procedure, however, in truth it is not so. FUE donor site usually heals with contracted circular scars which are difficult to recognize from a distance by naked eye. In some patients, the scarring becomes prominent and seen as depigmented tiny area without hair when hair is kept short or trimmed. It is more prominently seen in dark skin patients, especially in Indians, whereas in Caucasians, it is less visible due to the fair skin color **(Fig. 14)**.
- *Overharvesting leading to scarring and thinning of the donor area:* Sometimes in an attempt to perform large

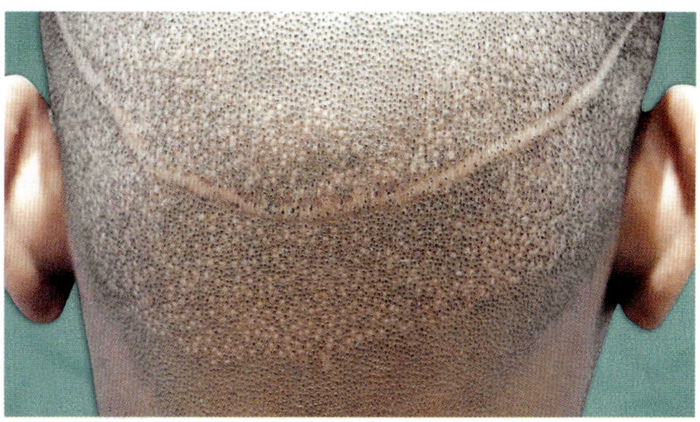

Fig. 14: Prominent hypopigmented scarring in a dark-skinned individual.

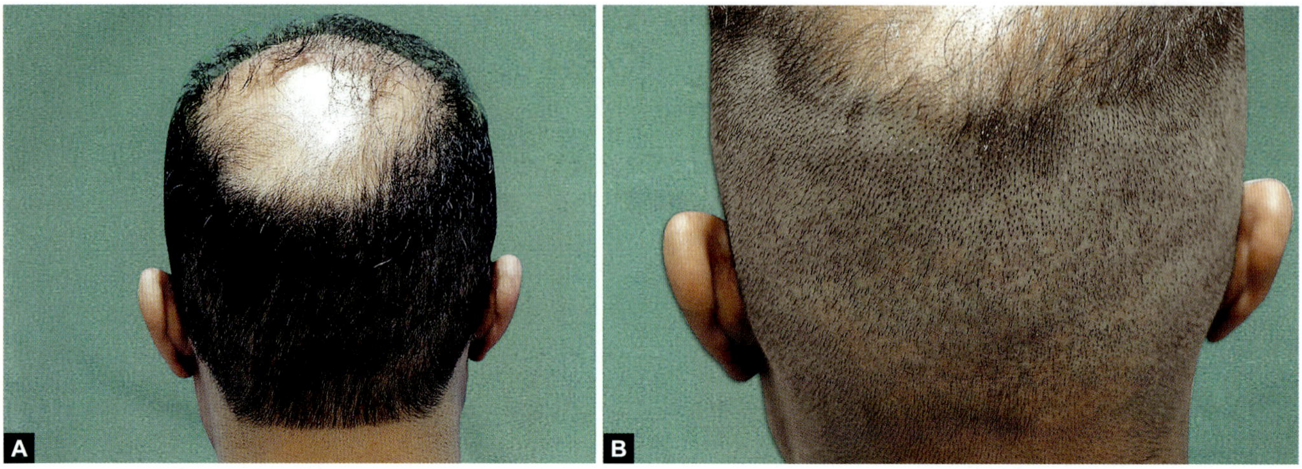

Figs. 15A and B: Donor area thinning due to overharvesting: (A) Before trimming; (B) After trimming.

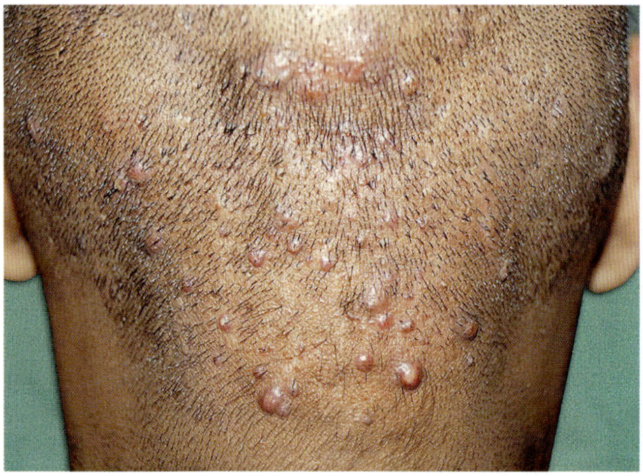

Fig. 16: Epithelial cyst.

session with more number of grafts, the donor area is harvested beyond the safe limits resulting in the permanent damage to the existing hair in that area. This damage can be seen as uneven thinning in various parts of donor area and patchy area of hair loss. Such area with patchy hair loss can be due to the greater area of traumatized skin after harvesting compared to the remaining healthy skin in that particular area, extensive damage at microvascular level, and hidden transections during the follicular dissection **(Figs. 15A and B)**.

- *Moth eaten or pseudosyphilitic appearance:* FUE also has a risk of clinically apparent depletion of hair from the donor region similar to strip cases. This can result in moth eaten or pseudosyphilitic appearance.
- *Epithelial cyst formation:*[12] When the buried grafts subluxate below the surrounding dermis into the subcutaneous tissue and are not taken out, they will grow at that place leading to formation of epithelial cyst which can be found later as multiple painless swellings in the donor area. Later excision is required to remove them **(Fig. 16)**.
- Harvesting of grafts which are at an increased risk of future loss resulting in failure of surgery in later years. When grafts are harvested from outside the safe zone, especially in the younger patients with ongoing process of hair loss, the resulted hair growth from such grafts can fall off later after few years depending upon the progress of hair loss. This usually occurs when higher number of grafts is committed in single sitting which creates the psychological pressure on the surgeon to meet the figures and surgeon may go above and below the "safe zone" to harvest the required number of the grafts.

PEARLS

- Performing FUE requires excellent eye-hand coordination, patience, stamina, and commitment
- Low transection rate during harvesting is essential to deliver the good result to the patient and even planning subsequent sittings of the surgery in future to meet the requirement of balding area
- Proper lightening, correct position of patient and surgeon, and well-maintained instruments are some of the essential things for successful harvesting with minimal transection rate
- Selection of patient having realistic expectation in regards to scarring in the donor area is equally important as opposed to what is claimed in marketing and media; the surgery leaves multiple tiny, hypopigmented, atrophic scars on the donor site which may be visible prominently in patients with dark skin when head is shaved completely

CONCLUSION

Follicular unit extraction is breakthrough advancement in the field of the hair restoration that has given it truly minimally invasive status. The promise of a stitchless surgery without any linear scar on the back of the scalp is attractive to both patient and surgeon. Although the techniques have improved, issues of patient selection, donor area healing by secondary intention after large sessions, and embedded grafts still remain. Training period is extensive and risks of less than desirable results due to inability to harvest intact, undamaged follicular units are high for the beginners.

Follicular unit extraction clearly has a valuable place in a growing number of hair transplant candidates. The reasons for selecting FUE rather than a strip harvest may be the avoidance of a linear scar, the desire for a virtually pain-free recovery period, or simply the idea of having a minimally invasive procedure.

REFERENCES

1. Rassman WR, Bernstein RM, McClellan R, Jones R, Worton E, Uyttendaele H, et al. Follicular unit extraction: minimally invasive surgery for hair transplantation. Dermatol Surg. 2002;28(8):720-8.
2. Harris JA. New methodology and instrumentation for follicular unit extraction: lower follicle transection and expanded patient candidacy. Dermatol Surg. 2006;32(1):56-61.
3. Harris JA. Robotic assisted follicular unit extraction for hair restoration: case reports. Cosmet Dermatol. 2012;25(6):284-7.
4. Haber RS, Stough DB. Hair Transplantation. Maryland, USA: Elsevier Saunders; 2006. pp. 133-7.
5. Bernstein RM, Rassman WR. New instrumentation for three step follicular extraction. Hair Transplant Forum Int. 2006;16:229-37.
6. Cole J. Harvesting the Fallows. San Diego, California: ISHRS Meeting; 2006.
7. Harris JA. Follicular unit extraction: the SAFE system. Hair Transplant Forum Int. 2004;14:163-4.
8. Zontos G, Rose P, Nikiforidis G. A mathematical proof of how the outgrowth angle of hair follicles influences the injury to the donor area in FUE harvesting. Dermatol Surg. 2014;40:1147-50.
9. Dua A, Dua K. Follicular unit extraction hair transplant. J Cutan Aesthet Surg. 2010;3:76-81.
10. Knudsen R. Is FUE a repair technique or small case technique rather than a first option for MPM? Hair Transplant Forum Int. 2011;21(6):192.
11. Karaçal N, Uraloğlu M, Dindar T, Livaoğlu M. Necrosis of the donor site after hair restoration with follicular unit extraction (FUE): a case report. J Plast Reconstr Aesthet Surg. 2012;65:e87-9.
12. Poswal A, Bhutia S, Mehta R. When FUE goes wrong! Indian J Dermatol. 2011;56(5):517-9.

CHAPTER 71

Hair Transplantation: Recipient Area

Mysore Venkataram, Aniketh Venkataram

KEY MESSAGES

- Surgery in recipient site involves different steps such as hairline design, anesthesia, density, methods of implantation and postoperative care.
- Different aspects of transplantation in the recipient site that need consideration include distribution, shape and direction of slits, density, packing and hairline design.
- A surgeon needs to be aware of different methods of implantation.
- Postoperative care is of importance in ensuring optimum results.

INTRODUCTION

Recipient area is the canvas in a hair transplant surgery, where the surgeon can truly display his artistic creativity and to deliver an aesthetic masterpiece—after all hair transplantation is as much about art as science. Understanding the recipient area helps in recreating the most natural results. Studying the progress and pattern of hairline regression, helps in achieving this target. Steps in the recipient area that need important consideration are:

- Hairline design and estimation of the number of grafts
- Anesthesia
- Methods of implantation and site creation
- Density, dense packing and other issues
- Postoperative care.

Ultimately the result of hair transplantation depends on the systematic implementation of these steps along with a timely adequate supply of grafts from the donor area. Hence, each of these steps needs to be understood to get optimum results.

ESTIMATION OF GRAFTS AND HAIRLINE DESIGN

Estimation of Grafts

It can be done by calculation of bald area in sq cm and multiplying it by about 35.[1] 35 grafts/cm^2 is the minimal density required to give an acceptable result in Asian patients. However, this number is relative. If a patient has a donor area where most of the follicular units comprise of 1–2 hair follicles only, then a higher density will be required to give a dense look. Another method to measure the density is using a graph paper, tracing paper and a gel marker pen. The area to be transplanted is marked with the gel pen and then a transparent paper or butter crepe paper is kept on the marking. This duplicates the marking by making an impression on it. This marked trace paper is kept on the sq cm graph paper. This helps in counting how many grafts will be required in each area, frontal, temporal and vertex. Since different densities are needed in different areas, this method helps to get a more accurate measure.

Hairline Design

Designing the anterior hairline is a challenging and demanding step in hair restoration surgery. It should be designed in a way so that it not only fulfils present demand but also adapts to the changing facial architecture of the patient in future as aging advances. Another challenge is to design a natural looking hairline with undetectable pluggy look and just enough density. Extensive discussions are therefore needed during counseling and these have been dealt with in the chapter on counseling and patient selection. The topic of hairline design is complicated and a full discussion on this topic can be found in the "Hairline Design" (Chapter 97).

ANESTHESIA FOR RECIPIENT AREA

This can be done either of the following two methods:

1. *Nerve blocks such as supraorbital and supratrochlear blocks:* The reader is referred to the chapter on Nerve Blocks for details.
2. Ring block along the periphery of the recipient area and infiltration into recipient area, on the lines similar to donor area anesthesia (dealt with earlier in Chapter 98 on Donor Area).

Usually, a combination of both methods is needed; nerve block followed by ring block and infiltration.

Whether entire area is anesthetized in one go or part by part depends on the method of implantation adopted. Author follows preformed slit technique and hence prefers to anesthetize the entire area in one go.

IMPLANTATION

Implantation consists of two steps:
1. Slit creation.
2. Placement of graft within the slit.

Slit Creation

The following aspects need to be considered during slit creation:
- *Type:* Sagittal versus coronal
- *Shape of slits:* Slits versus holes
- Density and packing
- Mega sessions
- Arrangement of units in the recipient area.[2,3]

Type of slits: Slits can be made either sagittally or coronally.

Sagittal slits (from front to back, longitudinal) have the advantage of being easier to perform and at the same time posing less danger to the radially arranged blood supply of the scalp. However, in acute angled slits, one edge of the lower end of the slit may be at a higher level than the other, causing bleeding (deeper penetrating edge) or superficial placement of graft (superficial penetrating edge).

Coronal slits (left to right or horizontal) are said to produce better appearance of density of hair by preventing reflection of light from scalp, and penetrate to the same depth throughout the width of the blade even in acute angled slits but are more time-consuming to make. They are also thought to affect the radially arranged blood supply of the scalp and may cause increased bleeding.

While there are advocates for both methods, most surgeons prefer sagittal slits or use combinations of both.[4]

Slits versus Holes

Earlier, recipient sites were created by coring out tissue using punches. This was used in the era of micrografts. However, they were large and this would remove large amount of tissue, cause trauma, bleeding, and also lead to less density. This technique went out of favor with the advent of the follicular unit concept, where the graft is small with little dermis. So small slits are preferred now. However, it is also true that in selected cases, when multifollicular units are planned, particularly in central part of scalp, larger round or rectangular holes can be used to create additional dense appearance.

Density[3-11]

This has been a matter of great debate as to what density is to be given for good results. The usually accepted density required for optimum results is about 35–40 units per sq cm, which is roughly half of the normal density. There have been claims, by surgeons, that they can pack 50-60-70/cm^2. There has also been an opinion that packing too much would affect dermal vasculature and create an environment of ischemia leading to less graft survival. In any case since there is limited number of units available in the donor area, there is also a limit on the number that can be packed. The recent availability of body hair has made larger number of donor hairs available and removed this limit, at least in some patients.

Hence, the general principle is to give optimum density of 35–40/cm^2. Greater density in specific instances, if required, can be given in a second session, instead of too much packing in the first session. It is also important to take in to account all the factors for optimum results, not just density, that contribute to appearance. These include *the thickness of the hair, number of follicular units of different types, the color, direction, frizziness, etc.*

Innovation in marking slits:
- There are specialized blade holders available now to make slits that can count the number of slits made simultaneously
- The newer version of the ARTAS® robotic hair transplant device can now implant too. And embedded with artificial intelligence, the machine can aid in distribution of different types of grafts in different areas.

Mega Sessions

It is generally agreed, that first sessions yield best results and hence mega sessions to place as many grafts as possible in one session, is widely practiced. This is also convenient to the patient as he would have one surgery and get results at one time. There is no one definition as to what constitutes megasessions, and the definition has varied over time. Hence, one may arbitrarily propose that any session with greater than 2,500 grafts is a megasession. A megasession requires a well-trained surgeon and a well-trained team to complete.

Arrangement of Units in the Recipient Area (Fig. 1)[3,5-7,11]

The hairline and frontal tuft zone is the most visible zone and hence they require more denser placement of hair follicles, about 40 per square centimeter.

A transition zone in front of this needs about 25 units per sq cm, which is made with thinner needle (19 g) in sparsely arranged irregular mounds. Single hairs followed by two hair units are preferred in this area.

The next region of importance is the lateral crease region which is a thin strip extending from the frontotemporal point in front to the vertex transition zone. Most people part their hair along this line and hence the area should have good density to cover the scalp well. Secondly, the hairs growing in this region will overlap the mid-scalp region. In general, since most people comb from left to right, more units are packed on left than right side.

Next zones of importance are the frontal tuft region and the mid-scalp. One can gradually decrease the density of follicles as one progress backwards. 3, and 4 hair units are packed into this area for maximum volume.

Temporal hump is an area which needs particular attention and is packed with single hairs.

Vertex area is circular and hence there is a radial arrangement of units that has to be planned. Whorls also need to be recreated. Cross-hatching helps in getting a more denser look. Vertex transplantation is a complex issue and the reader is referred to advanced text book on hair transplantation for this information.

Placement of Grafts

There are three main methods for implantation:

1. Preformed slits.
2. Stick and place (individual slit creation).
3. Implanters.

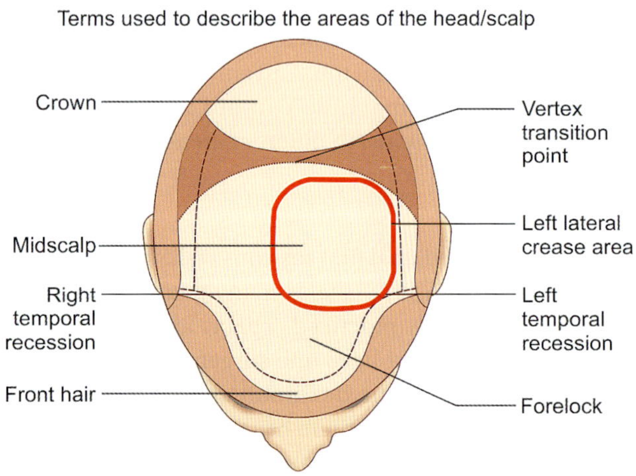

Fig. 1: Different zones for implantation.

Preformed Slit Method

The method basically consists of making all the slits in one go over the entire area to be transplanted, followed by implanting all the grafts together.

Instruments needed for slit creation **(Figs. 2 and 3)**:

- 18, 19, and 20 gauge needles. Nokor needles have been used in earlier days[12,13]
- Designer blades of various sizes.

We prefer to make our own blades from razor blades, with different sizes for 1, 2, and 3 hair grafts. These cut blades are held firm with needle holders. Using the stem of the needle holder, slits can quickly be made. Microsphere blades and Kolkata slits can also be used.

For insertion:

- Angled jewelers forceps in dominant hand
- 18, 19, and 20 gauge needle in nondominant hand
- Angled jewelers forceps can also be in both hands
- A self-made insertor can be created by separating the implantation forceps at its bend and using one of its arms in the nondominant hand.

Technique: Implantation needs magnification of 1.5–2.5X to ensure proper visualization. At the same time very high magnification can prove to be hindrance to viewing the overall design.

The entire region is anesthetized and infiltrated with tumescence:

- The nondominant hand is used to stretch the skin and the instrument of choice is held with a tripod grip in the dominant hand
- The slits are then created in rows as per the overall design plan decided previously. The rows are staggered so that slits do no fall behind each other and are randomly spaced one behind the other
- *Depth control:* It is important to ensure the slit is not too deep in which case the graft is buried or too superficial in which case the graft pops out. Instruments with depth control are available

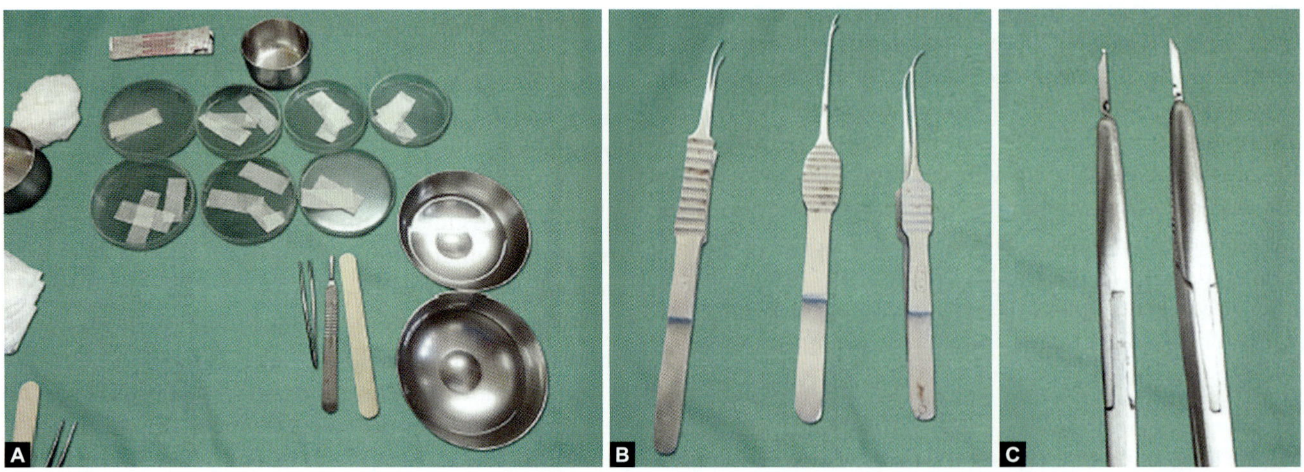

Figs. 2A to C: Instruments needed for slit creation.

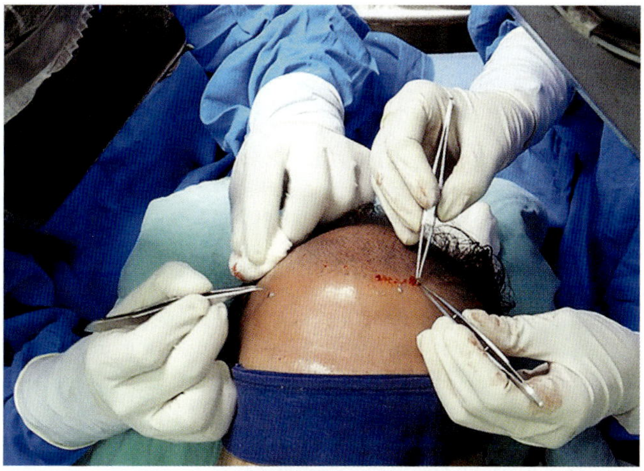

Fig. 3: Two people transplanting together.

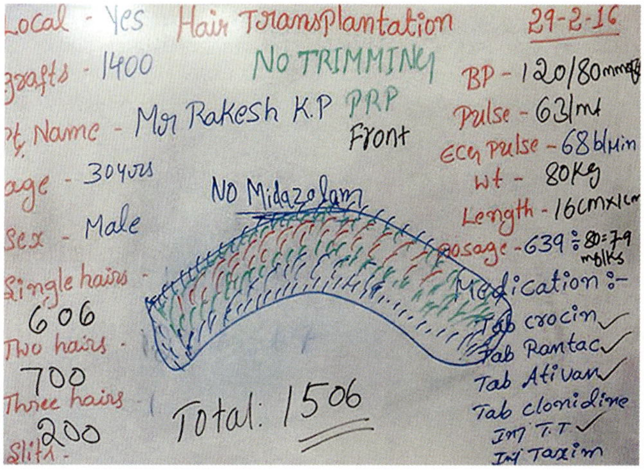

Fig. 4: Counting and marking on a board.

- After creating the slits it is useful to draw a color-coded diagram outlining where each type of grafts go, for easy reference during insertion **(Fig. 4)**. This avoids placing grafts in improper sized slits
- The scalp is then washed to remove any blood clots. Pressure is applied over any sites of bleeding
- The slits are then painted using methylene blue **(Fig. 5)** or gentian violet, and then cleaned with saline. The slits get stained with a few dye particles. This enables easy identification during insertion, particularly in patients with black skin
- *Counting:* It is important to maintain an accurate count of how many slits are made, and that too of each type of graft. As it is easy to lose count, it is helpful for an assistant to mark every 100 slits on a board or paper. Foot operated counters are available too. Automated incision counting devices can help at this stage.

Sources of Error

- *Skip areas:* Sometimes while making slits, some areas might be packed more densely and others more sparsely.

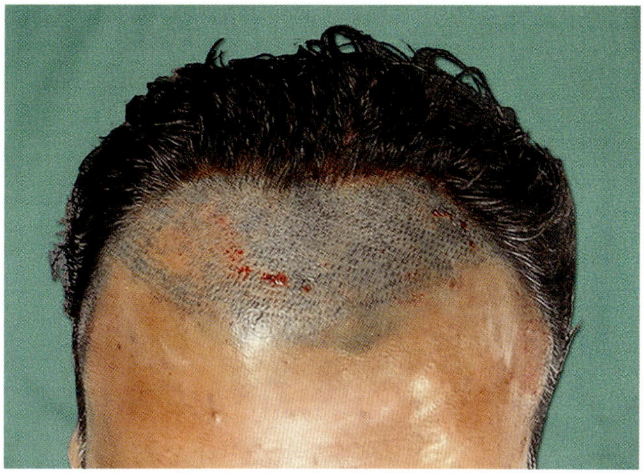

Fig. 5: Staining of slits by using methylene blue.

Hence, it is important to check the entire site once after making all the slits and fill in any gaps
- Depth of slits should be uniform and appropriate. Taking photos with mobile camera and then studying it in magnification can identify skip areas
- Direction of slits should be appropriate and should simulate the direction of vellus hairs or miniaturized hairs
- Identification of slits might be a problem for beginners, in dark-skinned patients especially with continuous irrigation, that may wash out the markings
- Attention should be paid to which grafts are being placed in which slits. The initial plan for the various sized grafts should be adhered to so that the right sized graft should goes in the right sized site.

The process of site creation can be summarized by 4 Ds: depth, density, direction and distribution.

Graft insertion: The technique of graft insertion in the preformed slit method is by nature a tedious process, and hence can be quite frustrating initially while learning. Up to three people can simultaneously implant to speed up the process. It is ideally done under 1.5–2X magnification. While there are variations in methods adopted by different surgeons, the following is the process followed by authors **(Fig. 6)**:

- The grafts are arranged neatly on cloth pieces which are usually placed on the dorsum or index finger of the nondominant hand, or the patient's forehead. The idea is to minimize movement in between successive grafts
- One assistant should constantly provide fresh sets of grafts as well as keep the field clean with continuous irrigation with normal saline
- It is important to keep washing the grafts with saline to prevent drying and desiccation
- The graft is grasped in the dominant hand by subcutaneous tissue below or just above to the side of the bulb. Avoid crushing the bulb or the bulge area
- The slit is identified and gently opened with the non-dominant hand (using needle or forceps). With practice

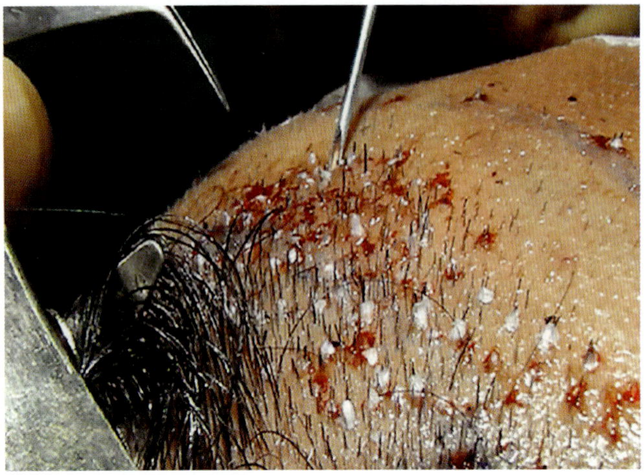

Fig. 6: Graft insertion.

BOX 1: Causes for popping.

- Chubby grafts
- Small slit
- Shallow slits
- Intersecting direction of slits in the hairline
- Excessive bleeding
- Too much density
- Improper technique of insertion
- Increased elasticity of skin

this might be unnecessary and all the work is done by the dominant hand

- The graft is then inserted partially into the slit, following the direction of the slit. A common source of error by beginners is not to remember the direction and follow the angle of the slit, or failure to account for the curvature of the forceps. This will lead to graft curling and damage. Then using both the dominant and nondominant hand in an up-down motion, the graft is eased gently into the slit
- Once one graft is in place the nondominant hand identifies the next slit, while the dominant hand gathers the next graft. This should be a fluid motion to save time and reduce fatigue.

Popping: This is one of the most frustrating problems particularly for a beginner. Causes of popping have been listed in **Box 1**. Excessive maneuvering to place a graft might dislodge an adjacent graft. This can be extremely frustrating and is one of the reasons why preformed slit technique is recommended for surgeons after they have gained some experience with the stick and place technique.

To avoid popping, the following tips may help that are illustrated in **Box 2**.

Table 1 lists different advantages and disadvantages of preformed slit technique.

Note: All disadvantages mentioned earlier are relative. With experience these can easily be overcome and it needs to be recognized that preformed slit technique is the most popular technique amongst surgeons.

BOX 2: Tips to avoid popping.

- One method is to place grafts in every alternate slit initially, and then come back and cover the remaining slits once the grafts are a little more stable due to hemostasis
- Ensure proper hemostasis
- Implanting from back to front
- Slide the graft along the direction of the slit
- Using traction with the nondominant hand. This is usually done only in the frontal direction on the forehead but can be given in the posterior direction by the thumb of the nondominant in case of excessive popping
- Raising the patients head, as close as possible to 90°, helps in decreasing the bleeding and popping eventually. The surgeon may have to stand and implant in such a scenario

TABLE 1: Different advantages and disadvantages of preformed slit method.

Advantages	*Disadvantages*
• Faster • Lesser surgeon involvement: It allows time for the surgeon to do other tasks • Allows for overall planning	• Needs coordination to avoid disparity between number of slits and grafts and is therefore suited for experienced surgeons • Identification of slits might be difficult in dark-skin patients • Skip areas might occur • It is difficult to adopt this technique in between existing hair • Depends on well-trained assistants, otherwise, grafts would be outside the body for a long time and survival is affected • Since surgeon is involved only while making slits, patient often feels neglected

Stick and Place Method

This method consists of creating each slit individually and immediately filling it with a graft. It can be done by one person, where one hand creates the slit and the other hand inserts the graft. Else it can also be done by two people where one person makes the slit, and the other immediately places the graft.

Instrumentation

- *Hypodermic needles:* 19–21 G for creating slits
- Angled jewelers forceps for grasping and placing the graft
- Magnifying loupes.

Technique: The needle is chosen as per the graft size needed from 19–21G. The needle is held in the nondominant hand. The needle is inserted till the bevel and then slightly angled so the slit puts open. The grafts are placed on the dorsum of the nondominant hand so that minimal time is wasted in between grafts. The graft is picked up using the angled forceps in the dominant hand. The graft should be well-trimmed. It is held by the subcutaneous tissue below the bulb or lateral to it. It is important to avoid trauma to the bulb. It is preferred to hold the graft on the concave side of the forceps as this enables better visualization in the next step. The needle is slightly withdrawn. The graft is inserted into the needle bevel using the forceps, following the direction of the slit with the angle of the

TABLE 2: Advantages and disadvantages of stick and place technique.

Advantages	*Disadvantages*
• Less bleeding due to immediate graft placement • Less popping • Can work in between existing hair easily. This is especially important in female patients • Can be adapted to special areas such as eyebrow, and moustache • Can change direction, pattern at any time. You are not committed unlike preformed slits • Can and should be used along with preformed slit method to fill in gaps at the end of the procedure • Allows full control for the surgeon as he is present throughout the surgery	• More time-consuming for the surgeon • Needs good surgical coordination • More effort needed from the surgeon who needs to be present throughout the surgery, cannot be left to assistants • Possibility of difference in angle, density if done by two people

forceps. Once the graft is at least half into the slit, the needle is withdrawn and the graft is pushed in with a simultaneous coordinated movement of both hands. The most common mistake is to not follow the direction of the slit.

The next slit is immediately made, and the graft picked up while the bevel is within the skin. It is important to keep the slit making hand relatively fixed, and minimize time between grafts to avoid fatigue. Multiple passes are needed to achieve density.

Table 2 lists different advantages and disadvantages of slit and place technique.

Implanters

Implanters were designed to automate the process of implantation and make it easier. An ideal implanter should be small, light, durable and easy to use.

Some of the various implanters designed include the Boudjema implanter pen, Rassman implanter, Choi implanter, and the NeoGraft™ implantation device. Of these only the Choi implanter gained popularity and underwent several modifications.

Choi implanter ***(Fig. 7)****:* It consists of a needle with a bevel where the graft is placed, a body, and a plunger which pushes the graft into the slit.

The hair is placed into the bevel using plain forceps, with the bulb toward the bevel of the needle. The implanter is held steady and located on the skin at the appropriate angle. The needle is then inserted to the skin to the desired level or the marked guard. The plunger is then pushed which pushes the graft into the slit. The implanter is then removed.

Four implanters are most commonly used at the same time with an assistant reloading the implanters, so that minimal

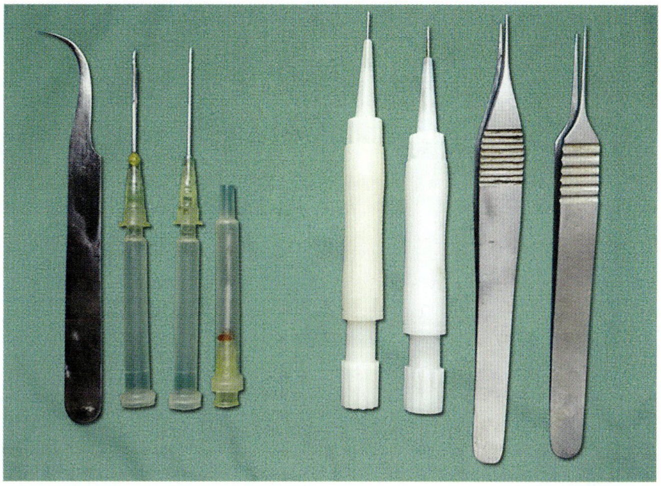

Fig. 7: Sava implanter with placer (yellow) and Choi implanter (white).

time is lost in between grafts. They are available in different sizes, such as 0.8, 0.9, 1 mm, etc., and two different sizes are used during surgery for the different types of grafts.

Other implanters—the SAVA implanter; one of the criticisms of the Choi implanter was the fact that it had many moving parts which could break down and was comparatively more expensive. To address these issues, the SAVA implanter was designed in India as a low cost alternative. In the original Sava implanter it consists of a transplanter and an introducer. The graft is placed in the transplanter which is used to make a hole, the graft is then slide in using the introducer. However, surgeons fatigue was more with the SAVA implanter since both the hands are involved during implantation, hence SAVA plus was introduced. It is an upgraded version which is more similar to the Choi implanter.

The newest implanter introduced is the KEEP implanter **(Figs. 8A to D)** and has several advantages. This implanter has a slit in the needle in to which the grafts can be rolled in to and hence avoids graft handling by forceps. The graft is then slid in to a premade slit.[14] It is therefore particularly suitable for the FUE grafts which are more vulnerable. It does not require separate technicians for loading the grafts as the grafts are kept on the nondominant hand and rolled onto the implanter with the dominant hand. It also saves time for the surgeon.

Table 3 lists different advantages and disadvantages of implanter technique.

Overview (Table 4)

- All the different methods of implantation have their own pros and cons
- Greatest advantage of premade slits is that it reduces the surgeon's involvement. But it can lead to errors between the dissecting time and the implanting time, as it needs proper coordination. Hence, it is a suitable method for an experienced surgeon with a good team

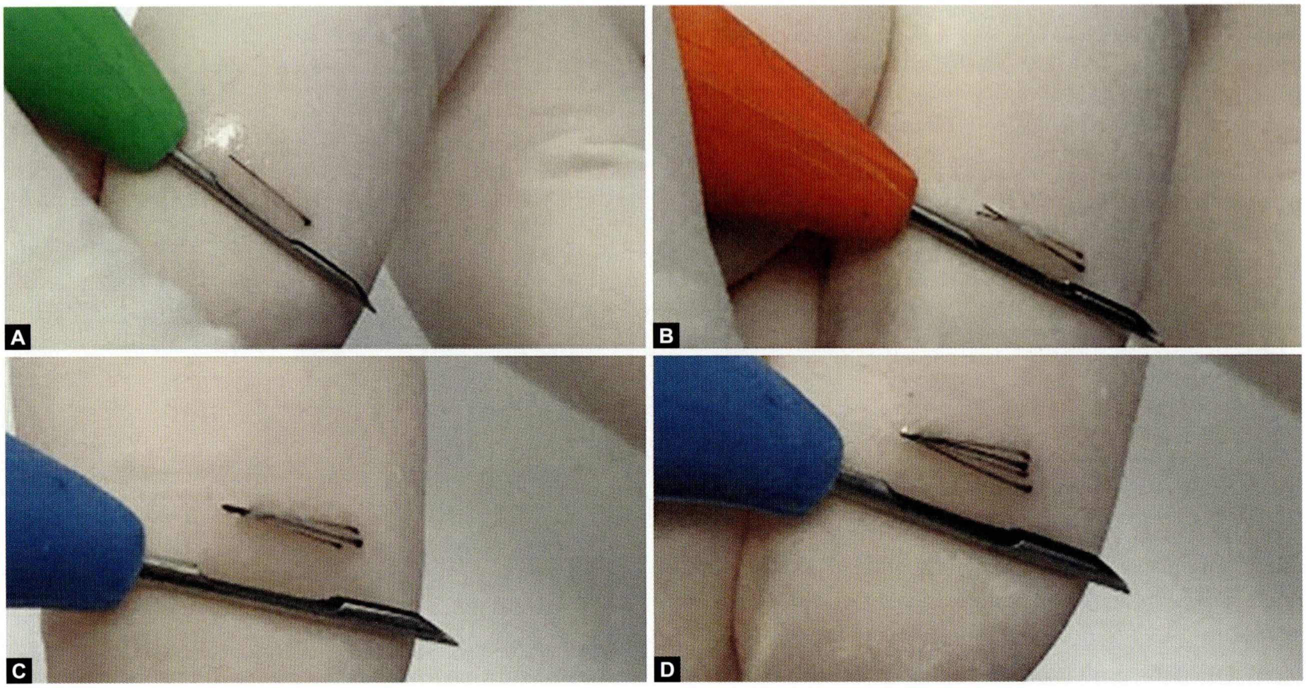

Figs. 8A to D: KEEP implanters which allow grafts to be rolled in to the implanter without handling by forceps.

TABLE 3: Different advantages and disadvantages of implanter technique.

Advantages	*Disadvantages*
• Implanters make handling of the graft minimal • Implantation is quick • It is easy to use in between existing hairs • Implantation in different angles is possible • Depth control is possible • Popping can be avoided by changing the direction of insertion more tangentially to find the avascular plane	• Additional cost as they are disposable • Dissection needs to be precise as graft needs to be loaded into the slit on the needle of the implanter. This is not a problem in follicular unit extraction (FUE) • Loading the implanter with thegraft needs training and additional staff • Popping can occur, in which case graft has to be place by theearlier other method • Only one surgeon can implant at one time hence may be time-consuming till the surgeon gains experience

TABLE 4: Comparison of different recipient methods.

Features	*Preformed slit and graft placement*	*Slit and place*	*Implanters*
Description	All slits are performed in one go and grafts are placed by assistants, one by one after all slits are made	Each slit is performed followed by placement of each graft	Slit and placement in one step using a device
Speed	Quick	Slower	Quick
Staff	2–4 staff can perform at the same time	Usually 1–2 persons	2–4 person
Surgeon's dependency	Surgeon can make the slits and then assistants can place grafts, less surgeon time	Surgeon dependent	Some implanters are Surgeon dependent The newer keep implanters can be used by assistants
Accuracy	Calculations may go wrong in inexperienced hands	Accurate	Accurate; less popping Minimal handling of grafts
Placement	Some slits may be missed, some slits may close	Accurate	Accurate
Bleeding	Bleeding may occur during initial place	Bleeding while making slit making graft placement difficult	Bleeding may push the graft out
Identification of slits	May be difficult with time	Not a problem	Not a problem
Grafting in between existing hairs	Difficult	Easy	Very easy
Angulation, precision of placement	Since done by assistants, may vary	Accurate	Accurate
Cost	Cheap	Cheap	Cost of devices

- The greatest advantage of stick and place is its ease, accuracy and control. However, it is time-consuming. It is a good method for beginners and is also necessary to know for combining with the other methods when needed
- The greatest advantage of the implanters is its ease; however, it can be more expensive.

Ultimately it is necessary to have all the arrows in one's quiver to choose the appropriate one for each scenario.

NATURAL COURSE OF EVENTS AFTER HAIR TRANSPLANTATION

The grafts when transplanted, undergo a shift from anagen phase to telogen phase. Hence, there is a natural loss of hairs in the second week about which patient needs to be forewarned about. The growth then occurs after a lag phase of about 3 months. The hairs then grow 1–1.25 cm a month which is the natural pattern of scalp hair. However, since each hair has its own cycle, it is not necessary that all hair fall. Early use of minoxidil may decrease this hair fall. It is also important to differentiate this hair fall from shock loss which denotes loss of existing hairs after surgery and is particularly common over the donor area adjacent to suture area and also over recipient area, when grafting is done amidst preexisting hairs.

POSTOPERATIVE CARE

Postoperative care after hair transplant surgery is important both from the view of current surgery and also from the view of possible future surgeries. Postoperative pain, edema, healing, etc., all affect patient comfort, particularly in strip technique. Patient education is, therefore, particularly important.

A detailed postoperative instruction sheet needs to be provided so that earlier events do not come as a surprise to the patient. It is in fact preferable to hand over this sheet before surgery, so that patient is prepared to face the issues.

Bandaging

There are many surgeons who prefer not to cover the wound at all—in their view and in the view of some patients, bandaging draws attention to the surgery. However, bandaging is preferred by others as it prevents postoperative bleeding, graft displacement and may also help in providing a moist environment to the grafts. It is also helpful in anxious patients, with anxious relatives who may be intimidated by the appearance immediately after surgery. Others prefer to cover only donor strip wound, but not the recipient area. The author prefers to provide a bandage to both recipient and donor areas. *It is further recommended that a bandage be mandatorily used whenever there has been excessive intraoperative bleeding, patients who have had popping, an agitated patient, patients who have had multifollicular grafts (which are more likely to be displaced) and if in the opinion of surgeon there is a risk of anticipated bleeding.*[15]

Bath and Shampooing

Many surgeons prefer to shampoo the recipient area at the end of surgery. Others prefer to do it on the next day. A third method, followed by author, is a gentle spray of a solution containing saline with hydrogen peroxide on day 1 after surgery. The hydrogen peroxide helps to clean the grafts better and to remove the crusts. The wound is inspected, any displaced graft reinserted, and cleaned.

Several solutions have been promoted for facilitating postoperative wound care.[16,17] These include:

- Platelet-rich plasma
- Solutions containing copper
- Solutions containing growth factor such platelet-derived growth factors.

Evidence is lacking for these and hence it is a matter of individual preference.

Bathing

Use of a mild shampoo (author prefers a baby shampoo) is usually preferred. Tepid water, which is allowed to trickle on to grafts than a forceful shower is advised. Frequent wetting with saline helps to avoid crusts. Most patients are afraid to touch either donor or the recipient area and need adequate counseling. It is not unusual to see patients return a week later with greenish dust settled on the grafts.

Postoperative Edema

This can be a major concern for patients, particularly those who need to travel or return to work early. It is important, therefore, to factor in the possibility of forehead and eyelid edema occurring on 4–5 day and often persisting for 3–5 days. In the author's experience, this edema is more common in elderly patients, perhaps due to the lax skin. Several measures such as use of a head band, injection of steroid triamcinolone into frontal scalp, oral steroid for 3–5 days, mixing steroid in tumescent solution (Abbasi solution) and lying down for prolonged periods to avoid effect of gravity have all been advocated.[18,19] Once it occurs, it persists for 3–5 days and in the authors experience, masterly inactivity, frequent counseling and watchful expectancy are all that is needed. Cold compresses are usually advised, and while their efficacy is doubtful they at least help in keeping the patient engaged and focused.

Minoxidil Use

Early minoxidil is advocated as it may prevent postoperative telogen effluvium and promote growth by enhancing blood supply. However, evidence for such assumption beliefs is debatable.[20] Minoxidil frequently causes itching and hence, may lead to dislodgement of grafts. It is therefore the authors practice to start the application after 7 days.

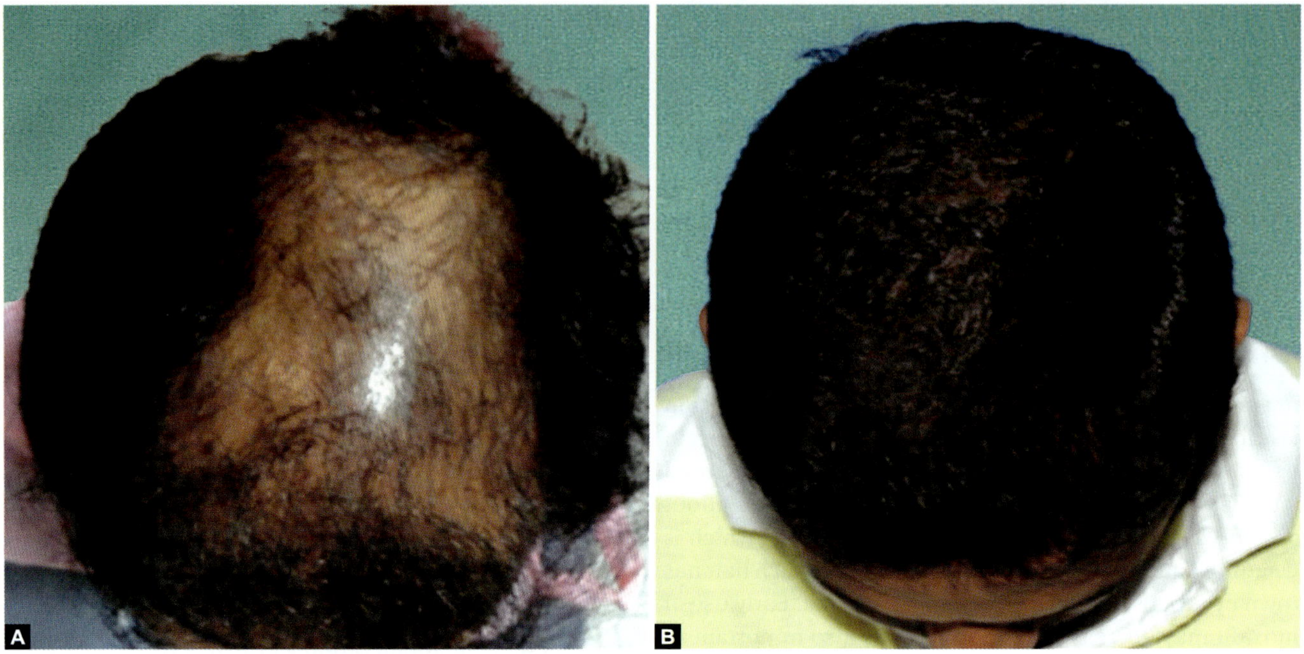

Figs. 9A and B: Result after 10 months 3,000 grafts [follicular unit transplant (FUT)].

Recipient area in female pattern hair loss: Hair transplantation in women presents special difficulties:[21]

- Recession and hence, needs to be carefully planned[22]
- Trimming of hair is not possible for cultural and aesthetic reasons and hence is more time consuming
- Since in female pattern hairloss, complete baldness rarely results and follicular units persist, albeit with miniaturized hairs, implantation will have to be done in between existing hairs. Hence, implanters are very useful
- Hair loss in women is more diffuse and hence, proper planning is essential to ensure grafting in to the most visible area
- Hairline in women is concave downward and descends into temporal area.

CONCLUSION

Recipient area is the area where the artistic skills of the surgeon can truly make a difference in creating an impactful result. The art and science of hair transplantation need to be fully understood.[23] The tendency of some surgeons to leave the entire work to assistants is not acceptable. Hair transplantation is usually associated with an uneventful and predictable recovery period. Detailed counseling will ensure such a smooth recovery.

Excellent results are possible with proper technique **(Figs. 9A and B)**.

ACKNOWLEDGMENT

Thanks to Dr Greeshma Bharathan for assisting in copy editing the draft.

REFERENCES

1. Chang SC. Estimation of number of grafts and donor area. Hair Transplant Forum Int. 2001;11(4):101-3.
2. Nakatsui T, Wong J, Groot D. Survival of densely packed follicular unit grafts using the lateral slit technique. Dermatol Surg. 2008;34(8):1016-22.
3. Alhaddab M, Kohn T, Sidloi M. Effect of graft size, angle, and intergraft distance on dense packing in hair transplant. Dermatol Surg. 2005;31(6):650-3.
4. Ginzburg A, Agrawal S. Alternate coronal and sagittal slits in recipient area of hair transplantation to ensure the correct graft implantation by assisting surgeon. J Am Acad Dermatol. 2020;83(3):e189-e190.
5. Unger WP. Different grafts for different purposes. Am J Cosm Surg. 1997;14:177-83.
6. Brandy DA. The art of mixing follicular units and follicular groupings in hair restoration surgery. Dermatol Surg. 2004;30(6):846-5.
7. Brandy DA. A technique for hair-grafting in between existing follicles in patients with early pattern baldness. Dermatol Surg. 2000;26(8):801-5.
8. Limmer B. The density issue in hair transplantation. Dermatol Surg. 1997;23:747-60.
9. Unger WP. Density issue in hair transplantation. Dermatol Surg. 1998;24(2):297.
10. Marritt E. The death of the density debate. Dermatol Surg. 1999;25(8):654-60.
11. Farjo B, Farjo N. Dense packing: surgical indications and technical considerations. Facial Plast Surg Clin North Am. 2013;21(3):431-6.
12. Brandy DA, Meshkin M. Utilization of No-Kor needles for slit-micrografting. J Dermatol Surg Oncol. 1994;20(5):336-9.
13. Arnold J. Mini-blades and a mini-blade handle for hair transplantation. Am J Cosm Surg. 1997;14(2):195-200.
14. Bansal A, Kumar A, Jain V, Reed G, Puri R, Kalra A, et al. Use of implanters in premade recipient sites for hair transplantation. Cutan Aesthet Surg. 2019;12(4):250-4.

15. Perez-Meza D, Leavitt M, Trachy R. Clinical evaluation of GraftCyte moist dressings on hair graft viability and quality of healing. Int J Cosm Surg. 1998;6:80-4.
16. Hitzig GS. Enhanced healing and growth in hair transplantations using copper peptides. Cosm Dermatol. 2000;13:18-22.
17. Hwang S. Gravity position to prevent facial edema in hair transplantation. Hair Transplant Forum Int. 2009;19(3):80.
18. Gholamali A, Sepideh P, Susan E. Hair transplantation: preventing postoperative oedema. J Cutan Aesthet Surg. 2010;3(2):87-9.
19. Nordstrom RE, Nordstrom RM. The effect of corticosteroids on postoperative edema. In: Unger WP, Nordstrom R (Eds). Hair Transplantation, 2nd edition. New York: Marcel Dekker; 1988. pp. 391-4.
20. Kassimir JJ. Use of topical minoxidil as a possible adjunct to hair transplant surgery. A pilot study. J Am Acad Dermatol. 1987;16(3 Pt 2):685-7.
21. Avram MR. Hair transplantation in women. Semin Cutan Med Surg. 1999;18(2):172-6.
22. Park JH, You SH, Kim N. Frontal hairline lowering with hair transplantation in Asian women with high foreheads. Int J Dermatol. 201;58(3):360-4.
23. Marwah MK, Mysore V. Recipient area. J Cutan Aesthet Surg. 2018;11(4):202-10.

CHAPTER 72

Complications of Hair Restoration Surgery

Narendra Patwardhan, Vaishalee Kirane

KEY MESSAGES

- Complications in hair transplantation can be either due to general causes or those specific for the hair restoration surgery.
- Most complications are infrequent, minor, and can be avoided by proper technique and taking all due prior precautions.
- The most common donor area complication is scarring in the donor area after the strip excision, especially if a wider strip than 1.5 cm is excised in a lesser elastic donor skin.
- The most common recipient area complication is postoperative edema.

INTRODUCTION

Hair restoration surgery (HRS) is usually a safe procedure and associated with very few complications. They too would result more due to not taking the necessary precautions before surgery, improper case selection, or faulty surgical technique.

However, as in all surgeries, complications can occur and which can be classified as follows:

- Complications which are common to all surgeries such as lignocaine reactions, pain, infection, bleeding, and keloids.
- Others which are specific for hair transplantation:[1-5]
  - Complications during anesthesia
  - Complications in donor area—intraoperative and postoperative
  - Complications in recipient area—intraoperative and postoperative
  - Poor results
  - Complications in special areas and situations
  - Complications of special techniques such as follicular unit extraction (FUE).

The factors which may be responsible for these complications include:

- Selection of an unsuitable candidate, improper preoperative counseling, errors in preoperative assessment and inappropriate surgical planning
- Poor technique during donor area harvesting
- Errors during storage of the grafts
- Poor technique during recipient area implantation.

GENERAL COMPLICATIONS

Causes and management of general complications are depicted in **Table 1**.

DONOR SITE COMPLICATIONS IN FOLLICULAR UNIT TRANSPLANTATION (TABLE 2)

Strip technique involves excision of a strip of skin from the donor area from the occipital scalp followed by suturing. This is a step which is associated with most common problems as it is the step which needs proper surgical expertise.

COMPLICATIONS AFTER FOLLICULAR UNIT EXTRACTION

Follicular unit extraction is a less invasive method and hence complications are generally infrequent. However, several complications such as cutaneous necrosis, lichen planopilaris, folliculitis, pitting, and persistent pain have all been reported.

Lichen planopilaris has been reported after FUE possibly due to precipitation of autoimmune reaction of transacted hairs.[17,18] *Alopecia areata* is another rare complication.[19] *Trichorrhexis nodosa* too has been reported.[20]

RECIPIENT AREA COMPLICATIONS

- *Poor hairline:* A proper hairline in HRS is very important to give a natural frame to the face as onlookers' visualize a person mainly from the front. The mid-scalp and the vertex play the next important role. Shapiro felt that proper selection and use of FUs combined with artistry and skill provide surgeons with the tools to follow nature's lead in creating natural-appearing, soft hairlines while establishing the illusion of density.[21]

  Several problems can occur due to improper frontal hairline, which are as follows:
  - *Asymmetry:* Unnatural straight line hairlines with poor temporal angles are very common and reflect poor technique entirely. It is essential to design a natural,

TABLE 1: Causes and management of general complications.

Cause	*Management*
Adverse systemic reactions to local anesthetics fall into four categories: toxic, psychogenic, idiosyncratic, or allergic. They are mainly psychogenic in nature and true immunologic reaction to the molecule is rare	• Prior history should be taken whether any local anesthetic injection given in the past • Otherwise to do prior testing of the local anesthetic
Drug-induced gastritis to analgesics and antibiotics	Administration of prior antacids and H2 blockers
Intraoperative complications: • Tachycardia due to adrenaline in tumescent fluid. Risk is more in a cardiac compromised patient	Do an electrocardiogram (ECG) and physician assessment above 40 years
• Syncope can occur at the end of a surgery, especially if it is many hours long. It is either due to pain, hypoglycemia, postural hypotension, or Xylocaine toxicity	*Avoided by:* • Proper anesthesia and analgesia • Making the patient sit before he gets up • Minimizing Xylocaine usage by completing surgery quickly. • Proper water, electrolytes, and nutrition balance • Preoperative administration of clonidine 0.5 mg helps by its anticholinergic and analgesic activity
• Pain during surgery or postoperative. Factors which can contribute to pain include excision of wide strip, bleeding, wound tension, large sessions with inadequate anesthesia	• Proper surgical technique and use of analgesics • Postoperative administration of prednisolone which reduces wound edema
Postoperative hiccups: Postoperative hiccups are another rare but important complication as it can last up to 2–3 days. The cause is not known but may be due to stimulation of sensory divisions of C2, 3, 4 nerves which also innervate diaphragm through phrenic nerve[6]	

TABLE 2: Donor site complications in follicular unit transplantation.

1. *Bleeding:* • Scalp being highly vascular, bleeding is expected • The possibility is more if the patient is on warfarin or any other antiplatelet drug[7] • After consulting with relevant physician such medicines need to be stopped at least 1 week before surgery	*Bleeding can be prevented by adhering to few simple tips:* • Tumescence to raise hair follicles away from underlying neurovascular plane • Anxiolytics and sedatives are prescribed the night before and morning of surgery to allay anxiety and lower blood pressure, e.g., clonidine • Removing the strip in parts and not in one piece • Monitoring blood pressure • Avoiding deep incision. To first score superficially and then stretch the wound edges by a Haber spreader or skin hooks • Once bleeding occurs, it needs to be controlled by pressure, using an artery forceps or electrocautery used if really necessary
2. *Folliculitis and pits:* • Inflammation of one or more hair follicles can occur in the donor area. While suturing, hair can get stuck in the suture line and lead to folliculitis. Pits can occur due to improper suturing • Folliculitis decalvans like recurring and persistent condition has also been reported, which becomes very chronic and distressing to the patient **(Fig. 1)**[8]	• Proper suturing technique • Prophylactic antibiotics[9] • If infection occurs, appropriate antibiotics after sensitivity testing is necessary[10] • Lower risk of infections has been reported by treating nasal colonization of *Staphylococcus aureus* by the application of mupirocin ointment and preoperative shampooing of scalp hair with use of chlorhexidine gluconate-medicated soap the night before and the morning of surgery[11,12]
3. *Infection:* May occur due to nonadherence to aseptic norms of surgery or lowered patient resistance	
4. *Wound dehiscence or necrosis* of the donor wound site is a very unusual complication and mostly due to excessive tissue removal of width >1.5 cm, wound closure under extreme tension, overzealous use of cautery and malnourished patients[13]	• Restrict width of the strip excised <1.5 cm • Proper wound care, dressings, and antibiotics
5. *Numbness:* Usually transient, can occur because of transection of superficial sensory branches during donor strip excision	
6. *Pain:* Can result especially if donor wound is closed under extreme tension or due to damage to the underlying neurovascular supply	Prevented by injecting sufficient tumescent solution of saline with 0.5% lidocaine/bupivacaine and 1: 50,000 epinephrine to raise the donor tissues and enabling cutting above the plane of the deeper neurovascular structures[14]

Contd...

Contd...

7. *Persistent pain:* Possibly to development of neuropraxia and neuromas	Gabapentin, intralesional steroid injection
8. Suture extrusion	
9. *Keloids* can occur rarely	
10. Donor hair effluvium or shock loss	Temporary, reassure the patient
11. *Donor site scarring:* • Occurs in all techniques used in hair restoration surgery (HRS) with the scars ranging from imperceptible to noticeable and very unsightly and disfiguring **(Figs. 2A and B)** • In strip excision technique of graft harvesting, a wide linear donor scar is the most feared consequence of modern HRS. This mainly results due to an increased tension on the donor wound closure in the occipital scalp area and mainly determined by the laxity of the occipital scalp skin	Various preventive and corrective steps to avoid a wide unsightly donor scar are:[15] • Scalp laxity exercises started 4 weeks prior to the surgery[16] • Not extending the width of the donor strip to >1–1.5 cm, and closing the donor wound using sound surgical principles • Double layer suturing • Trichophytic closure method • Minimizing the use of electrocautery to stop bleeding and instead applying compression for minimum 5–6 minutes • Corticosteroid like 3.33 mg/mL solution of triamcinolone acetonide mixed with bupivacaine 0.5% (prolongs the anesthetic effect) in dose of 5–6 mL is injected intralesional inferior to the closed wound immediately after • Oral steroids have also shown to decrease edema and wound tension

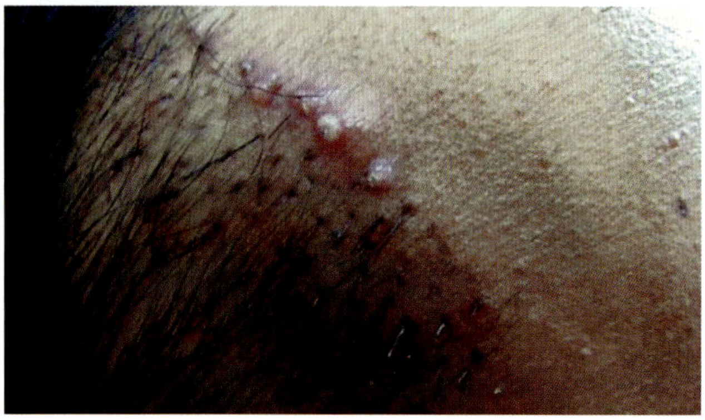

Fig. 1: Folliculitis.
Courtesy: Dr Narendra Patwardhan, Pune.

age-related proper hairline, taking efforts so as to avoid asymmetry. This can be done two-dimensionally with the help of mirror and three-dimensionally when the hairline is examined straight on. Ruler and laser guiding system additionally can be used to help plan an appropriate hairline by the starting surgeon who has not developed an eye for symmetry. Hairlines differ based on gender with female hairlines appear more rounded without the bitemporal recession occurring in males.

- *Cornrow plugs* resulted in the time of the old punch grafting technique and are unaccepted in the modern follicular unit hair transplant method. They especially are exposed as the residual hair recedes and then necessitate correction. It can still occur if larger units are used for hairline.
- *Too low positioned hairline on the forehead and blunting of the temporal angles.* The hairline should never be placed below a point 6 cm from the glabella which can result in dissatisfaction of the patient over time, especially in the case of evolving progressive hair loss behind the transplanted hairline.

- *Low perceived cosmetic density and unnatural coverage* of the bald area reflect errors in surgical and aesthetic judgment, performing procedures on noncandidate patients, surgical distribution of grafts that failed to consider the possibility of progressive hair loss in young patient of genetic pattern hair loss, and failure to communicate successfully with patients about realistic expectations also remain major problems even with latest follicular unit transplant technique. The surgeon needs to consider whether there will be sufficient projected donor hair to cover future hair loss.

Correction and repair of hair transplants require great skill and judgment. The focus is on creative aesthetic solutions to solve the supply/demand limitations inherent in most repairs. Corrective hair transplant procedure involves removal of the plugs partially leaving behind a few hairs which will look soft and natural, combining with scalp reduction surgery, if needed, and camouflage with transplanting additional follicular units using FUE method either from the scalp occiput or body hairs to give further density.[22,23]

- *Recipient area edema:* This is common on third to fifth day of surgery, starting on the forehead and gradually spreading on to eyelids and nose. The precise relevance varies, but may occur in 3–8% of patients. The precise reason is not known, but several factors are thought to be responsible:
  - Large quantity of tumescent anesthetic fluid
  - Gravity which pulls the fluid down
  - Lymphatic drainage of frontal scalp

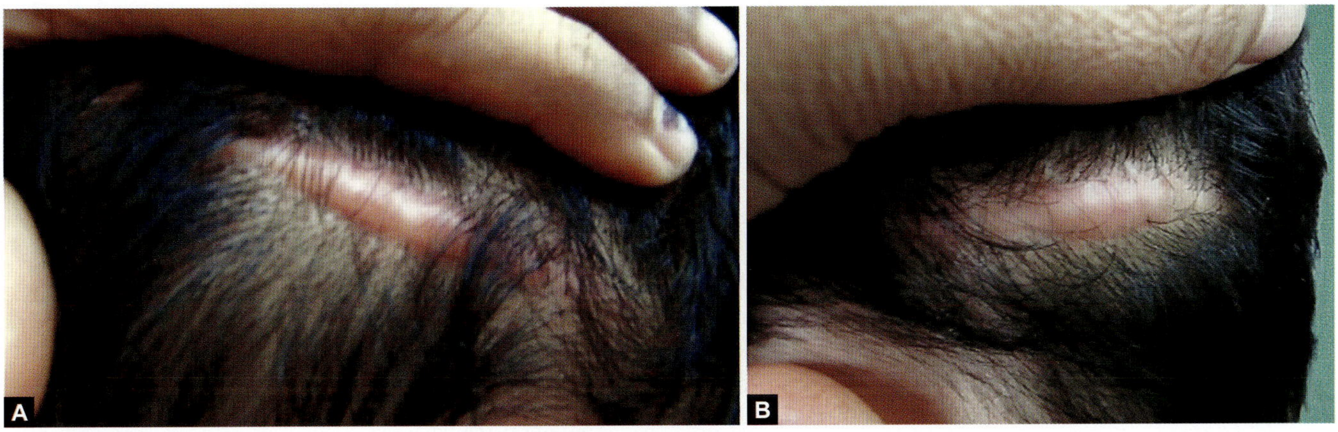

Figs. 2A and B: Hypertrophic scar at donor area.
Courtesy: Dr Narendra Patwardhan, Pune.

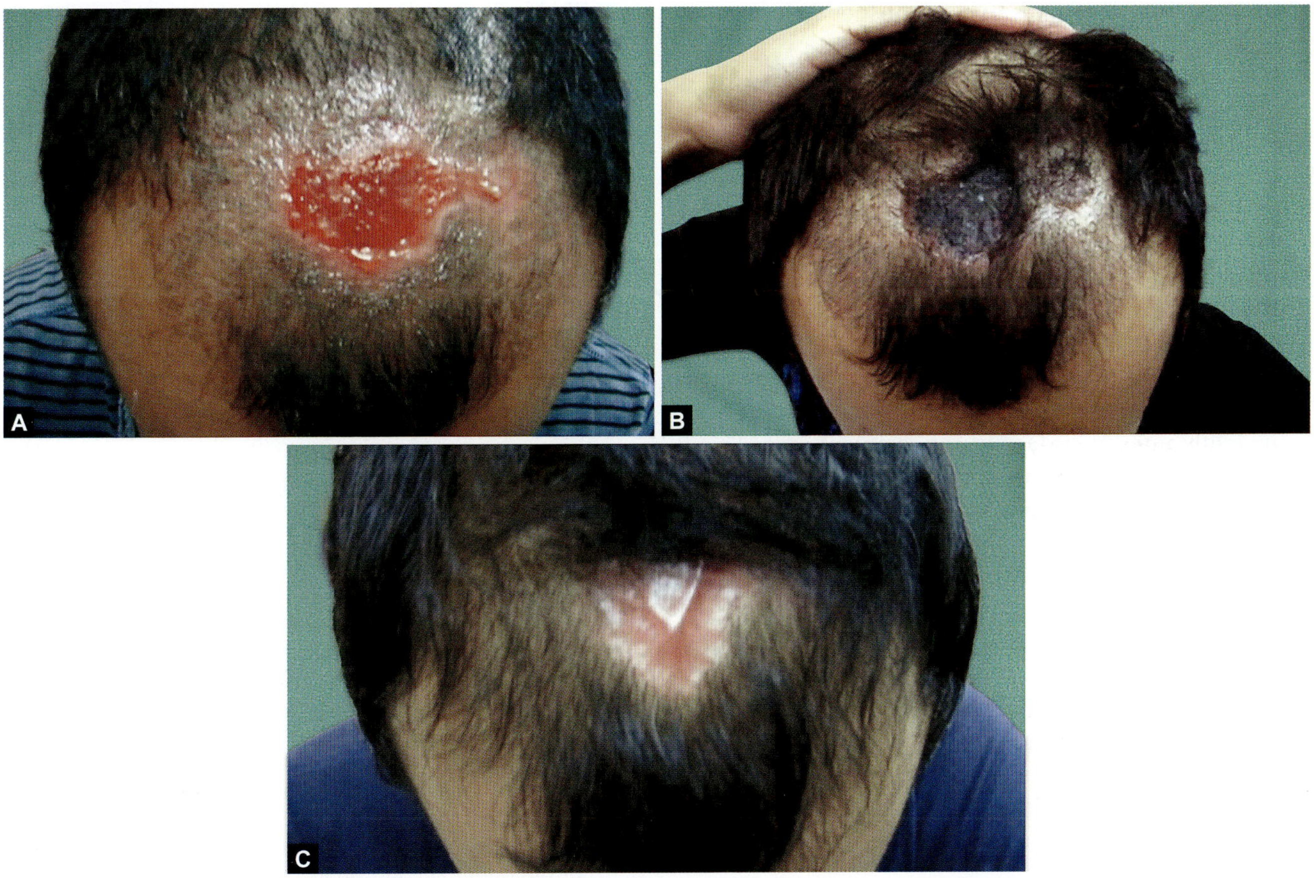

Figs. 3A to C: (A) Necrosis in recipient area; (B) Eschar formed after necrosis; and (C) Scar resulting from necrotic area.
Courtesy: Dr Narendra Patwardhan, Pune.

- Loose donor skin, large sessions, and elderly patients are more likely to experience it
- An Elastoplast band on the forehead at the end of surgery may also help. Abbasi solution was shown to prevent it. Reclining position for 24 hours though impractical may help. Ice packs used frequently once it develops, manual massage to push fluids to the sides are also useful.[24]

- *Postoperative pustules* which occur 1–3 months after surgery is related to presence of poorly dissected grafts and is related to graft dissection technique. It is sterile, usually heals by itself and may need drainage of pus.
- *Central scalp necrosis* **(Figs. 3A to C)** can occur after large sessions in elderly with vascular compromise. It is characterized by a dusky red discoloration of scalp followed by extensive crusting. It heals with central scar. While the

exact cause is not known, it is postulated to the fact that central scalp receives comparatively less blood supply. Smoking, diabetes, and actinic damage may predispose to the condition.[25]

- *Poor hair growth* can occur when there is traumatic dissection of the hair grafts from the harvested strip or traumatic placement or desiccation of the grafts. It can also be a result of poor quality donor hair like vellus hair which should be identified before surgery and thus such patient not selected for surgery. Patient should be counseled regarding the shedding of the transplanted hairs at around 6 weeks and the onset of new growth from 10 to 12 weeks with full growth achieved at 10–12 months. Decreased growth can also be due to factors such as heavy smoking, diabetes is there proof that diabetes can lead to poor result, and excessive sun damage to the scalp skin or sometimes due to nonspecific individual anatomic factors.
- *Temporary hair loss* called as shock loss is a kind of telogen effluvium of the surrounding hairs occurring due to the trauma of the surgery in 10–15% of males and more number in females. The patient can be forewarned about its possibility to alleviate anxiety or alarm. Use of topical minoxidil in males and females and oral finasteride only in males, for at least 4–6 months prior to surgery can help to minimize this hair loss.
- *Arteriovenous fistula* can occur but is extremely rare.[26]
- *Cobblestoning* occurs from elevations and indentations of the scar tissue around the hair graft resulting in an unsightly uneven surface in the recipient area. This is when follicular unit grafts are implanted into too small hole or at incorrect depth. Grafts should be placed only 1–2 mm above the surrounding surface to avoid this. The cobblestoning mostly improves with time or the scars may need to be excised.
- *Cysts* appear as small skin-colored swellings around the transplanted hair follicles which can become erythematous and painful. They result due to small grafts slipping under the skin or from piggybacking one graft on top of the other. Treatment consists of incising the cysts and expressing out the contents, warm compresses, or sometimes topical antibiotics.

TIPS AND PITFALLS

Thorough preoperative counseling regarding the benefits and limitations and also about the risks of HRS and recording of the same in the medical chart goes a long way in preventing complications.

- Selection of a suitable candidate for surgery, proper evaluation, and surgical planning of the recipient area are of paramount importance
- Good design using sound surgical skills and techniques combined with artistry for hairline reconstruction and for high perceived mid-scalp or vertex cosmetic density and to record the same are essential.
- Avoid complications by meticulous preoperative assessment and good postoperative management
- Quality control for every step of the surgery should be on a continuous basis, improving whenever and wherever possible

CONCLUSION

The success of HRS involves not only keeping up-to-date with the technical expertise but also knowledge and learning from experience of avoiding the complications, recognize them in time, and their correction. HRS involves a team of many assistants, thus supervising their quality control is also necessary to avoid complications.

REFERENCES

1. Loganathan E, Sarvajnamurthy S, Gorur D, Suresh DH, Siddaraju MN, Narasimhan RT. Complications of hair restoration surgery: a retrospective analysis. Int J Trichology. 2014;6(4):168-72.
2. Salanitri S, Gonçalves AJ, Helene A Jr, Lopes FH. Surgical complications in hair transplantation: a series of 533 procedures. Aesthet Surg J. 2009;29(1):72-6.
3. Konior RJ. Complications in hair-restoration surgery. Facial Plast Surg Clin North Am. 2013;21(3):505-20.
4. Perez-Meza D, Niedbalski R. Complications in hair restoration surgery. Oral Maxillofac Surg Clin North Am. 2009;21(1):119-48.
5. Lam SM. Complications in hair restoration. Facial Plast Surg Clin North Am. 2013;21(4):675-80.
6. Arnold J. Hiccups following surgery of the scalp. Complications. In: Stough DB, Haber RS (Eds). Hair Replacement. St. Louis: Mosby; 1996.
7. Otley CC, Fewkes JL, Frank W, Olbricht SM. Complications of cutaneous surgery in patients who are taking warfarin, aspirin, or nonsteroidal anti-inflammatory drugs. Arch Dermatol. 1996;132:161-6.
8. Otberg N, Wu WY, Kang H, Martinka M, Alzolibani AA, Restrepo I, et al. Folliculitis decalvans developing 20 years after hair restoration surgery in punch grafts: case report. Dermatol Surg. 2009;35(11):1852-6.
9. Kaiser AB. Antimicrobial prophylaxis in surgery. N Engl J Med. 1986;315(18):1129-38.
10. Zoumalan RA, Rosenberg DB. Methicillin-resistant Staphylococcus aureus—positive surgical site infections in face-lift surgery. Arch Facial Plast Surg. 2008;10(2):116-23.
11. Van Rijn MM, Bode LG, Baak DA, Kluytmans JA, Vos MC. Reduced costs for Staphylococcus aureus carriers treated prophylactically with mupirocin and chlorhexidine in cardiothoracic and orthopaedic surgery. PLoS One. 2012;7(8): e43065.
12. Farjo N. Infection control and policy development in hair restoration. Hair Transplant Forum International. 2008;18(4):141-4.
13. Karaçal N, Uraloğlu M, Dindar T, Livaoğlu M. Necrosis of the donor site after hair restoration with follicular unit extraction (FUE): a case report. J Plast Reconstr Aesthet Surg. 2012;65(4):e87-9.
14. Wesley CK, Unger RH, Rosenberg M, Unger MA, Unger WP. Factors influencing postoperative hyperesthesia in hair restoration surgery. J Cosmet Dermatol. 2011;10(4):301-6.
15. Unger WP. Correction of cosmetic problems secondary to hair transplantation. In: Unger WP, Shapiro R (Eds). Hair Transplantation, 4th edition. New York: Marcel Dekker; 2004. pp. 372-9.
16. Mayer ML, Pauls T. Scalp elasticity scale. Hair Transplant Forum International. 2005;15(4):122-3.
17. Donovan J. Lichen planopilaris after hair transplantation: report of 17 cases. Dermatol Surg. 2012;38(12):1998-2004.

18. Chiang YZ, Tosti A, Chaudhry IH, Lyne L, Farjo B, Farjo N, et al. Lichen planopilaris following hair transplantation and face-lift surgery. Br J Dermatol. 2012;166(3):666-70.
19. Rodrigues Barata AR, Camacho-Martínez F. Alopecia areata as a complication of hair restoration surgery. Eur J Dermatol. 2012;22(6):813-4.
20. Hwang ST, Park BC. Trichorrhexis nodosa after hair transplantation: dermoscopic, pathologic and electron microscopy analyses. Dermatol Surg. 2013;39(11):1721-4.
21. Shapiro R. Principles and techniques used to create a natural hairline in surgical hair restoration. Facial Plast Surg Clin North Am. 2004;12(2):201-17.
22. Bernstein RM, Rassman WR, Rashid N, Shiell RC. The art of repair in surgical hair restoration part I: basic repair strategies. Dermatol Surg. 2002;28(9):783-94.
23. Vogel JE. Correcting problems in hair restoration surgery: an update. Facial Plast Surg Clin North Am. 2004;12(2):263-78.
24. Gholamali A, Sepideh P, Susan E. Hair Transplantation: Preventing Post-operative Oedema. J Cutan Aesthet Surg. 2010;3(2):87-9.
25. Yildiz H, Ercan E, Alhan D, Sezgin M. Recipient Site Necrosis After Tumescent Infiltration with Adrenaline in Hair Transplantation. Acta Dermatovenerol Croat. 2015;23(3):233-4.
26. Unger W. Re: Arteriovenous fistula following hair transplantation. Dermatol Surg. 2011;37(12):1816-7.

CHAPTER 73

Body Hair Transplantation

Arvind Poswal

KEY MESSAGES

- While body hair to scalp transplant offers hope and opportunity for individuals with advanced hair loss, it is crucial to approach the procedure with realistic expectations and a commitment to ongoing collaboration between patients and practitioners.
- Different body hair differ in their characteristics (including curl and A:T ratios). So, the doctor has used his artistic ability to put the best graft/combination suited to each specific recipient area.
- With continued research and advancements, the future holds promise for further refining this technique and improving outcomes, underscoring the importance of innovation, compassion, and partnership in the field of hair restoration.

INTRODUCTION

The BHT stands for body hair to scalp transplants. We propose the more accurate short form as body hair to scalp transplants (BHTs).

Body hair transplants have evoked widespread interest and fascination in the minds of hair loss sufferers as well as hair transplant doctors. However, results vary widely (patient-to-patient as well as doctor-to-doctor).

Here we are going to discuss what to expect from body hair and beard hair-to-scalp transplants, how best to prepare the proposed donor areas, how best to utilize the extracted grafts in terms of aesthetics, management of patient expectations, and how to customize the donor hair usage depending on the individual's body and beard hair growth and depending on the hair growth cycles and various characteristics of the donor hair.

WHY DOES ONE NEED BODY HAIR?

The *idea* is to use the hair growing on the body as an additional donor supply. The *hope* is to get rid of the "donor limitation" that exists with scalp donor. For most patients that are Norwood 5 or more degree of hair loss, scalp donor hair is not sufficient to provide full coverage (i.e., hair growth in all/most of the bald scalp). BHT (or BHTs) aims to rectify the situation in suitable patients.

As per author's knowledge, the first documented case of body hair *only* to scalp hair transplant was documented and published in peer reviewed, indexed medical journal—*Indian Journal of Dermatology* (Volume 52, Issue 2, Year 2007).[1] *(http://www.e-ijd.org/article.asp?issn=0019-5154;year=2007;volume=52;issue=2;spage=104;epage=105;aulast=Poswal)*

As per author's knowledge, the first documented/published study of beard hair to scalp hair transplant was documented and published in *Indian Journal of Plastic Surgery* (Volume 46, Issue 1, January–April 2013).[2]

http://www.ijps.org/article.asp?issn=0970-0358;year=2013;volume=46;issue=1;spage=117;epage=120;aulast=Poswal

OVERVIEW: BODY HAIR TRANSPLANTATION

Hair transplants are all about numbers. The scalp donor area provides a good, but limited resource. Many patients with advanced hair loss must tap additional donor resources to achieve satisfying results. By opening up body hair supply, some patients have access to significant resources of previously untapped donor hair.

Body hair extractions from abdomen, armpits/axillary areas, back, back of hand, beard, chest, forearms, legs/calves, thighs, and pubic provide the additional donor hair supply.[1] This treatment option is *essential for patients with advanced degrees of hair loss and those who may have lost scalp donor supply* due to various reasons.

Follicular unit separation extraction (FUSE) is a proprietary technique of extracting grafts individually invented by the author. It is a form of follicular unit extraction (FUE) used by the author for difficult to extract hair. For the purpose of this text and pictures, FUSE and FUE shall be used interchangeably **(Figs. 1 to 3)**.

BODY HAIR CHARACTERISTICS

Body donor hair differs in characteristics from the scalp donor hair in terms of:

- Length
- Caliber
- Color
- Growth cycles

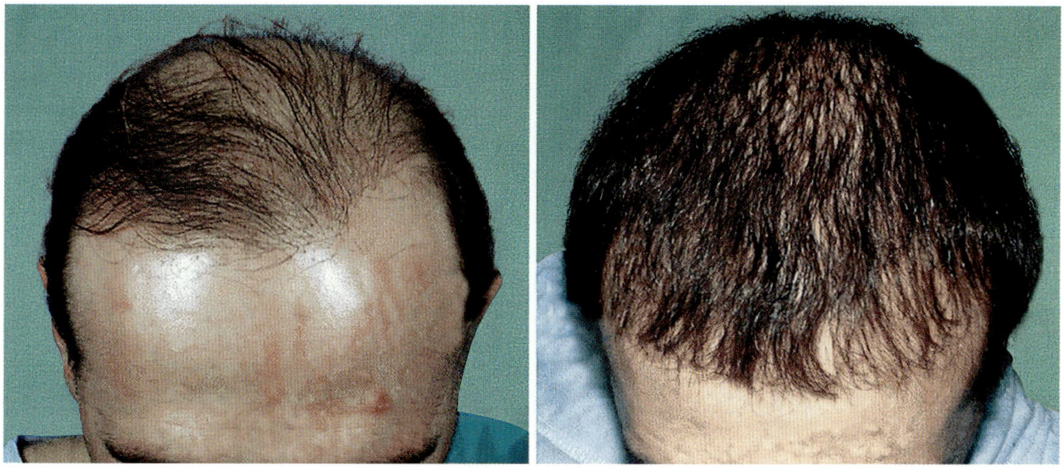

Fig. 1: Comparison picture (11,460 fue grafts).

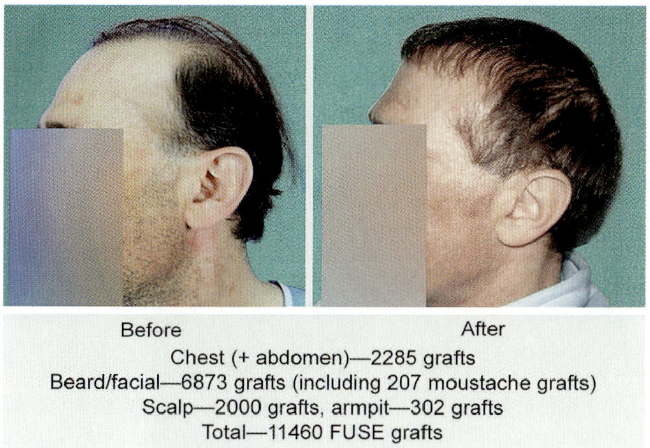

Fig. 2: Comparison picture.

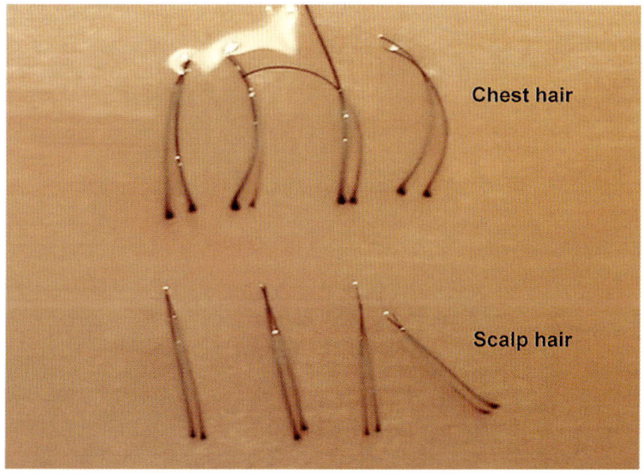

Fig. 4: Distinguishing chest and scalp follicular unit grafts.

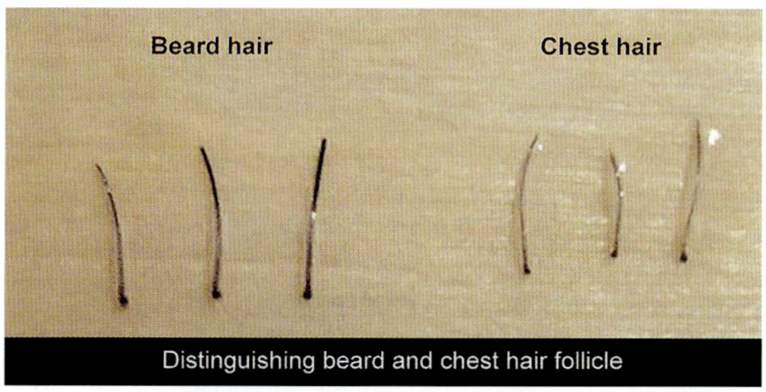

Fig. 3: Body hair varies in caliber, texture, and color. So, mixing of body hair with scalp hair gives a uniform look and feel.

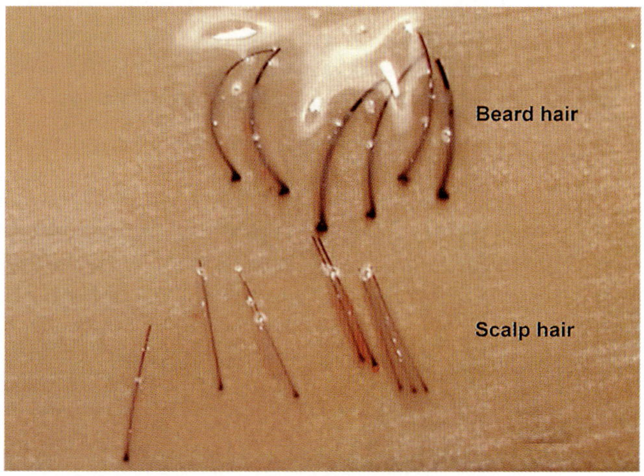

Fig. 5: Distinguishing beard and scalp follicular unit grafts.

- Speed of growth
- Predisposition to greying etc., and
- Texture (wave, curl, feel, etc.)

However, with proper planning it is possible to use robust body donor hair to augment donor hair resources, thus, giving fuller hair restorations.

The transplanted body and beard hair will retain their original characteristics after transplant **(Figs. 4 to 6)**.[2]

GUIDELINES OF BODY HAIR TRANSPLANTS

These guidelines are based on the follow-up observations of the author in patients:

- Preshave the body donor areas 3-5 days before the extraction. It is a simple step and very helpful to pinpoint the actively growing anagen hairs that need to be used. Shave with a razor down to the skin **(Fig. 7)**. The growth of hair over 3-5 days gives a length comparable to that of body donor hair trimmed to the correct length for harvesting on the day of surgery.[3]
- Use only the body donor hair in active growing phase for purpose of transplant. Do not use telogen hair.
- Assume the transplanted body hair will retain their original characteristics (length, caliber, color, predisposition to greying, curl, anagen/telogen ratio, and hair growth cycles).
- Factor in the impact of growth cycles and characteristics of the body donor hair proposed to be transplanted.
- Mix the various body as well as scalp donor hair in any particular area of scalp **(Fig. 8)**.

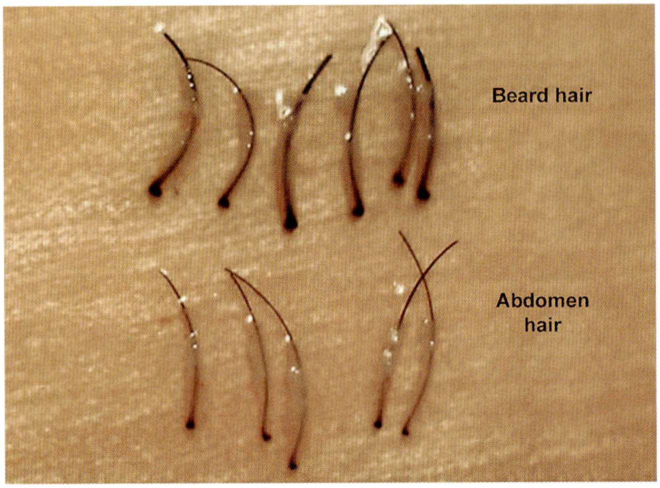

Fig. 6: Distinguishing beard and abdomen follicular unit grafts.

BODY HAIR TO SCALP TRANSPLANTS: THE PRESHAVING PROTOCOL

A larger percentage of hair follicles are in the telogen/resting/nongrowing phase in the body donor areas. It is advisable to use only the actively growing hair for transplant.

Preshaving the body donor areas is a simple, noninvasive method to locate the actively growing hair.[3]

Please note: The body donor areas should be wet shaved with a razor (trimming with a hair trimmer alone will not suffice), 3-5 days before the procedure.

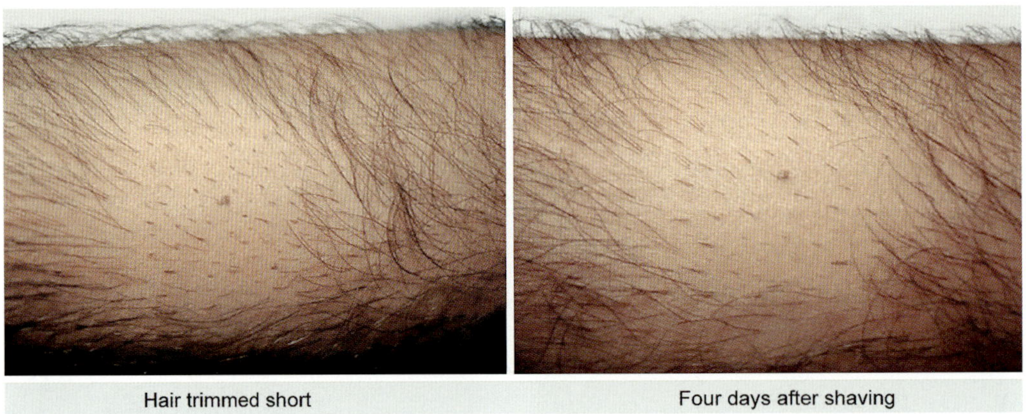

Fig. 7: Guidelines of BHT—preshave the body donor areas. (BHT: body hair to scalp transplants)

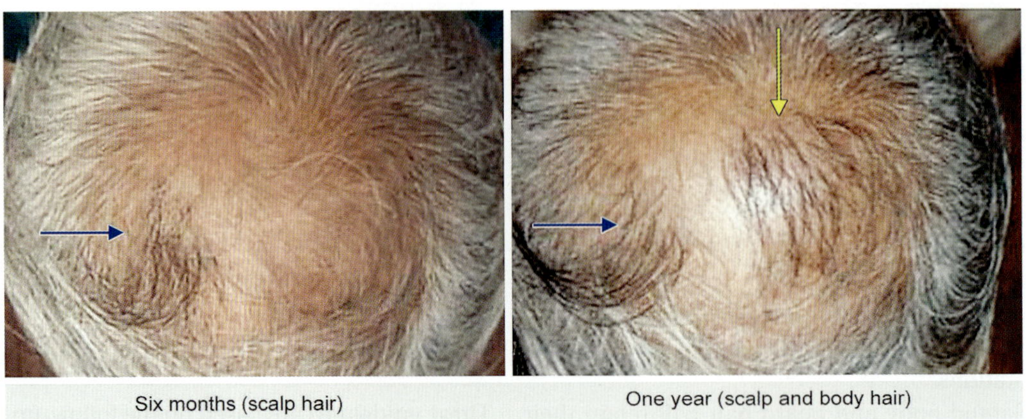

Fig. 8: Distinguishing scalp and body hair growth. (Blue arrows: scalp hair; Yellow arrow: body hair).

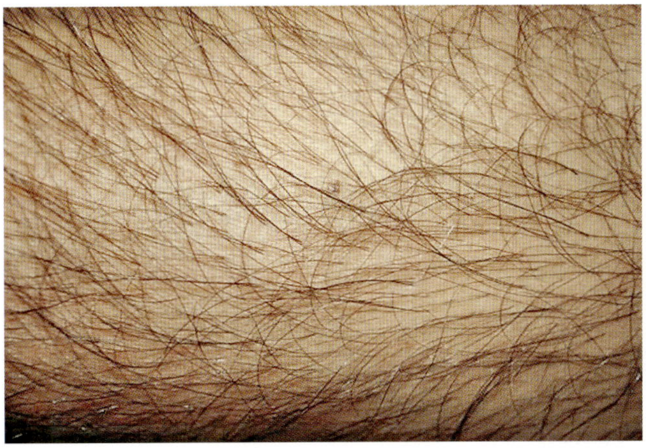

Fig. 9: Before picture.

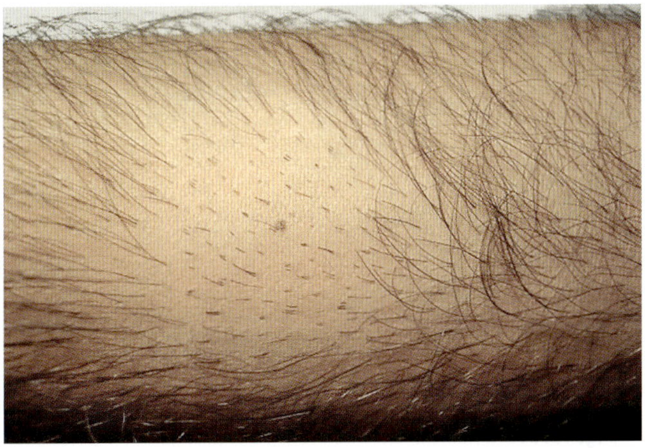

Fig. 10: Hair trimmed—not shaved.

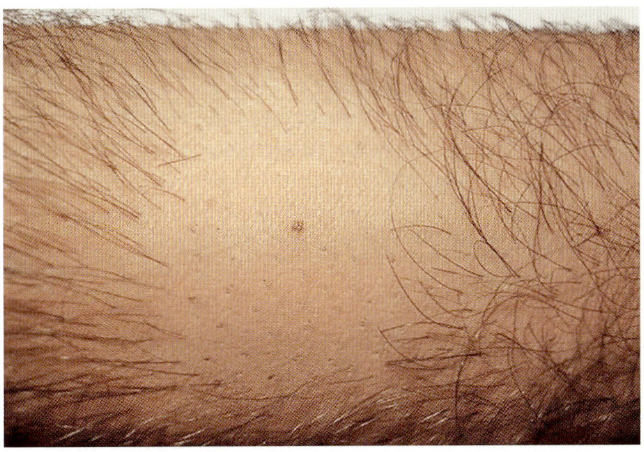

Fig. 11: Hair wet shaved with razor.

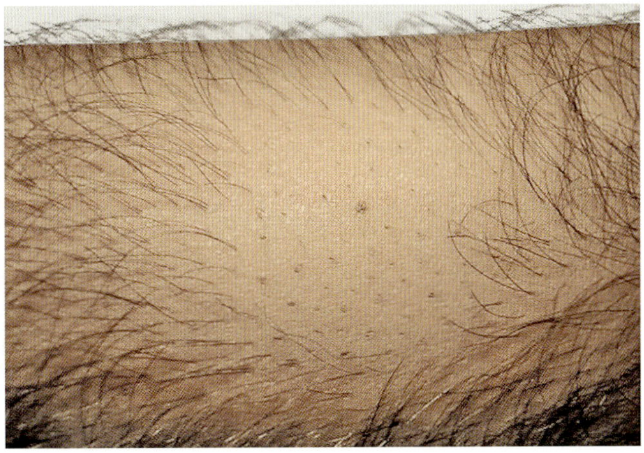

Fig. 12: One day after wet shaving.

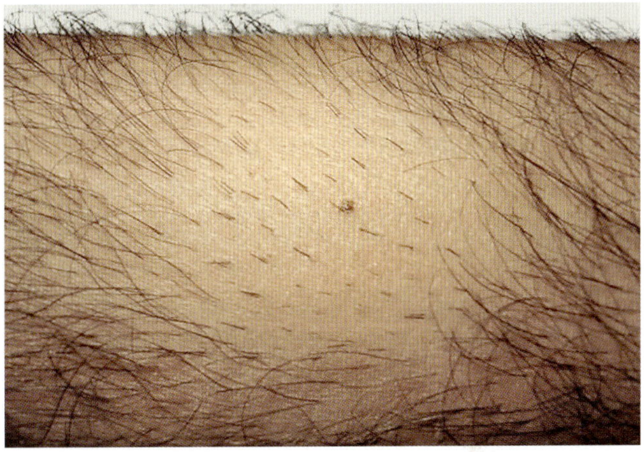

Fig. 13: Four days after wet shaving.

In case of very dense and long hair growth, first buzz cut the hair with a trimmer, followed by shaving the hair flush with the skin using a razor **(Figs. 9 to 14)**.

The duration of the anagen/telogen phases plays an important part overall, while the percentage of hair in telogen gains increasing importance with each passing hair cycle (read disintegration of synchronicity further ahead).

Talking of durations—following is an extract:

Hair Growth Tables (Table 1)

There are many factors that affect individual hair growth. These growth tables should only be used as a very generalized guide.

While the scalp donor hair has a growth phase of an average 3 years, most body hairs have a growth phase lasting approximately 4–5 months.

Therefore, unlike scalp to scalp transplants, BHTs may show a cyclic variation in density and coverage.

Also while 85% of the scalp hairs are in growth phase at any particular time, 40–80% of the body hair may be in telogen (nongrowth phase).

Thus, the significance of the preshaving protocol.

Shaving the proposed body donor area with a razor 3–4 days before extraction is a simple method of identifying actively growing hair.

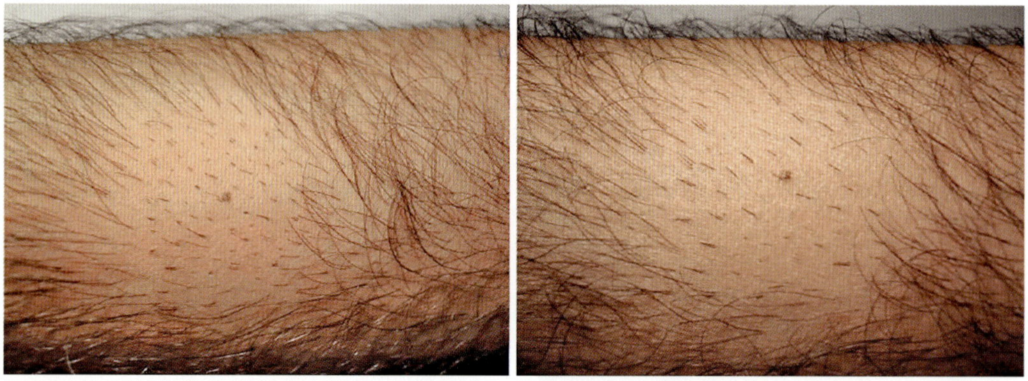

Fig. 14: Comparative pictures.

TABLE 1: Hair growth.			
	Telogen (%)	*Anagen (%)*	*Duration of activity*
Scalp	15	85	2–6 years
Eyebrows	90	10	4–8 weeks
Cheeks	40–50	50–60	50–60 days
Beard (Chin)	40	60	1 year
Moustache	45	55	16 weeks
Armpit	70	30	16 weeks
Pubic area	70	30	4 months
Arms	80	20	13 weeks
Legs and thighs	80	20	16 weeks

Source: Bushong CW, Martin RA, Jr., Westwood KL, et al.

More work and studies need to be done to crosscheck the hair growth cycles in different human races and different ages.

INDICATIONS FOR BODY HAIR TRANSPLANTS

Body hair to scalp transplant is ideal for patients:
- With extensive hair loss (Norwood 5 and above)
- When scalp donor hair is not sufficient to cover all areas of baldness (whether due to donor depletion, previous surgeries, or congenitally thin hair).

When coupled with existing donor supplies, body hair gives patients more graft placement options.

These options include:
- Aggressive hairlines
- Conservation of scalp hair
- Greater density
- An excellent choice to conceal scarring from strip or extraction procedures

Beard hair can substitute for scalp hair, which is ideally suited for the frontal region. In addition, thick beard hair mixed in with thinner scalp hair results in a very natural look. Other options include:
- Beard hair to scalp transplant
- Beard hair to scar transplant
- Using body hair to recreate temple points
- Refining the hairline
- Creating side burn (beard-to-beard hair transplant)
- Eyebrow transplant
- Beard reshaping/eyebrow reshaping/nape reshaping
- Transplant into previous surgical scars unrelated to hair transplants **(Fig. 15)**.

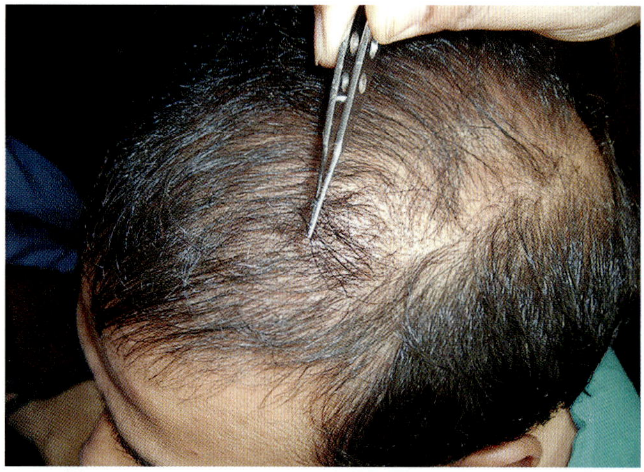

Fig. 15: Beard hair transplanted to the scalp; retain their original characteristics.

OBSERVATIONS WITH BODY HAIR TRANSPLANTS

Hair in different parts of the body including beard, armpits, eyebrows, and other areas has different growth cycles and shows marked variations **(Figs. 16 to 18)**.

In scalp, approximately 85% hairs are in anagen, 12–14% hairs are in telogen, and 2–4% hairs are in catagen. But this is not same for body hair.

Table 2 can be used as a very generalized guide.

PREOPERATIVE ASSESSMENT (FIG. 19)

- As explained previously, a larger proportion of hair follicles are in resting/nongrowing phase in the body donor areas.

- It is advisable to use only the actively growing hair for transplant.
- Preshaving the body donor areas is a simple, noninvasive method to locate the actively growing hair.[3]

Please note: The body donor areas should be wet shaved with a razor (trimming with a hair trimmer alone will not suffice), 3–5 days before the procedure.

Please follow the preshaving protocol discussed above for body hair transplants.

FOLLICULAR UNIT SEPARATION EXTRACTION: THE TECHNIQUE OF FOLLICULAR UNIT EXTRACTION

Follicular unit separation extraction is a method of extracting individual hair follicles with microsurgical precision but without scalpel and stitches. It is a unique variant of FUE technique which is safe, minimally invasive, and a virtually nonscarring technique of extracting single follicular unit (FU).

In patients with extensive hair loss (Norwood 5 and above), scalp donor hair is not sufficient to cover all areas of baldness. FUSE thus makes it possible to extract the individual follicular units from the body and beard donor areas expanding the available donor supply.

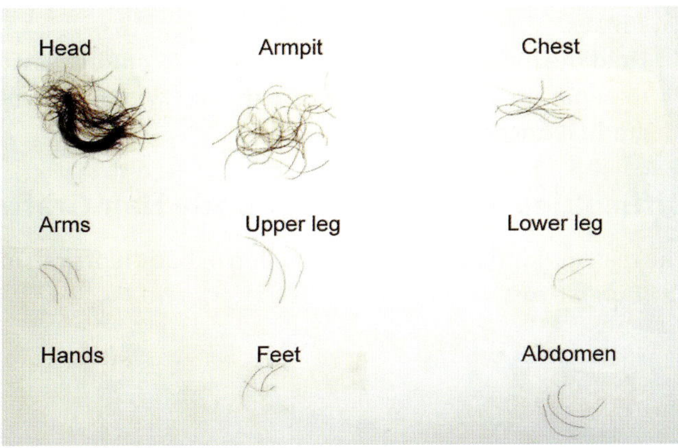

Fig. 16: Hair from different parts of the body.

This method involves separation of the graft bearing skin till the level of mid-dermis with tiny but sharp micro punches (similar to all FUE), followed by separation of the follicular unit by careful microscope/magnifier-aided needle dissection (under direct vision) from its remaining dermal attachments, before gently sliding it out of its location for grafting into the recipient bald area.

The punches are used to score around the follicular unit till the mid-dermis level. Gentle traction is applied to the graft thus scored. The extracted grafts are then trimmed and placed in the recipient slits created in the bald or balding scalp. Since the extraction sites/holes are very small (1 mm or less), no suturing is required. The wounds heal by secondary intention. The follicular units are extracted one by one in a random pattern. The tiny donor sites are left to heal on their own. There is no need of any wound suturing or repeated antiseptic dressing as the donor sites are very small **(Fig. 20)**.

Figure above shows a typical scalp donor area from where the follicular units have been extracted. A 26-gauge needle (needle diameter 0.45 mm) is juxtaposed in the picture above for sake of comparison. As can be seen from the **Figure 20**, the follicular units are extracted in a random pattern, so that no two adjacent units are extracted.

Follicular unit separation extraction technique provides a safe method of extracting follicular units and also provides an additional source of hair from other body parts for fuller and denser hair restoration results and, simultaneously, it gives minimal/no visible scarring on the donor sites.

For patients with robust body hair, BHTs increase the availability of donor hair supply. This treatment option is essential for patients with advanced degrees of hair loss and those who have lost scalp donor supply due to other reasons (burns, head surgery, previous hair restoration surgeries, accidental injuries, etc.).

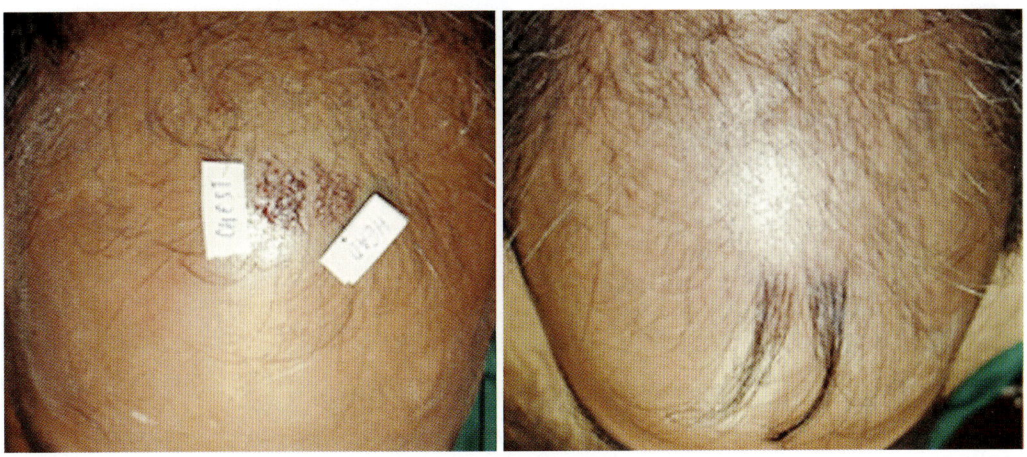

Fig. 17: Scalp and body hair test session.

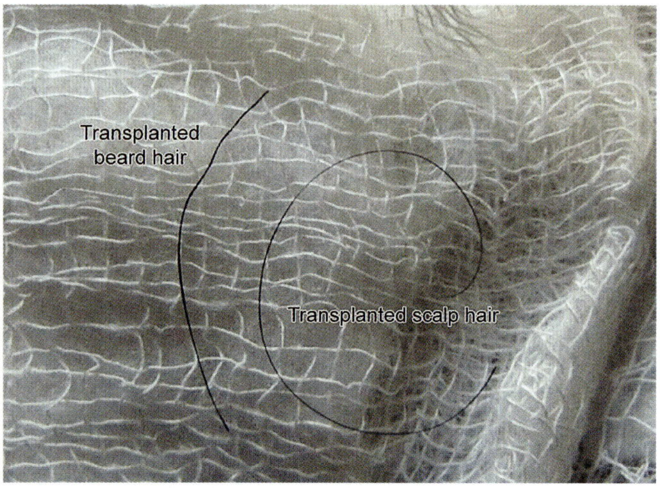

Fig. 18: A comparison of transplanted beard and scalp hair after growth.

TABLE 2: Hair in different parts of the body has different growth cycles.

Parts of body	*Telogen (%)*	*Anagen (%)*	*Duration of activity*
Scalp	15	85	2–6 years
Eyebrows	90	10	4–8 weeks
Cheeks	40	60	50–60 days
Beard (Chin)	40	60	1 year
Moustache	45	55	16 weeks
Armpit	70	30	16 weeks
Pubic area	70	30	4 months
Arms	80	20	13 weeks
Legs and thighs	80	20	16 weeks

Source: Bushong CW, Martin RA, Jr., Westwood KL, et al.

EXTRACTION OF GRAFTS

Traditional punch based FUE extraction of the body hair grafts has following disadvantages:

- Large extraction sites
- Higher transection rates

A non-punch based grafts extraction technique has been, therefore, devised.

EXPANDING NEEDLE CONCEPT

In traditional FUE technique a 0.8–1.4 mm punch is used to cut the dermis to a level of attachment of erector pili muscle so that FU can be extracted. Expanding needle concept (ENC) provides a new method to increase the yield of intact grafts. The use of ENC for extracting body hair grafts is a different extraction methodology in body hair to scalp transplantation.[4] The use of hypodermic needle has overcome the difficulties faced in traditional punch method especially when extracting difficult body hair.

Method of Using Needle (Fig. 21)

- Use the tip of the needle to score around the FU graft scoring the entire circumference requires 3–4 needle strokes.
- Hold the top of graft and use needle tip as cutting device to separate any adhesions/uncut skin while applying gradual traction.

Difficulties in Extraction of Body Hair Grafts

The reasons for difficulties in extraction of body hair graft are attributable to:

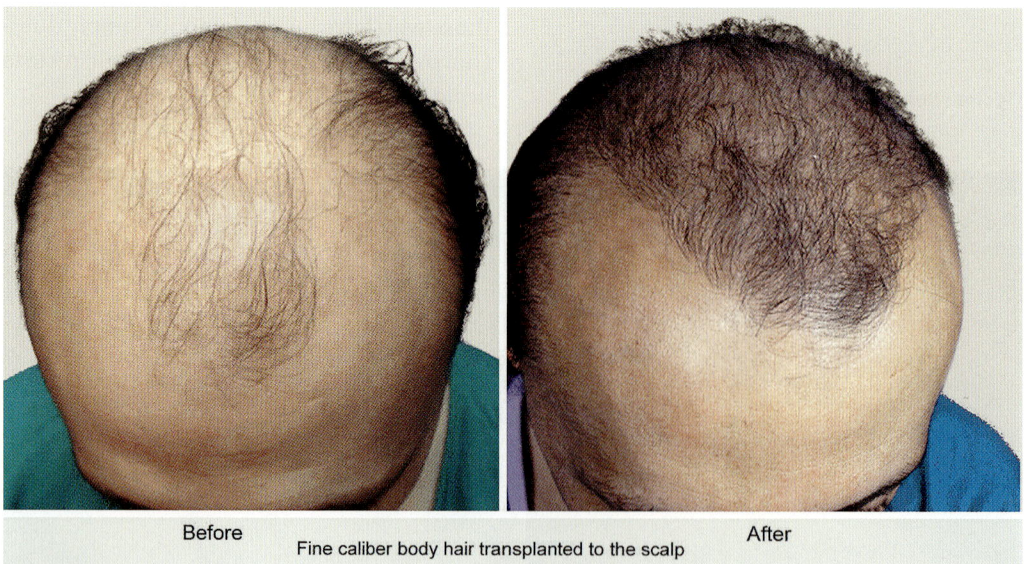

Fig. 19: Body hair from chest, leg, calf, pubic, and armpit donor areas transplanted in the bald scalp recipient. No scalp or beard hair was used as donor source. 7,000 BHT grafts were transplanted. Of the 7,000 body hair grafts, 700 were transplanted into the right temple and 200+ into the left temple. The rest were distributed over the entire scalp.

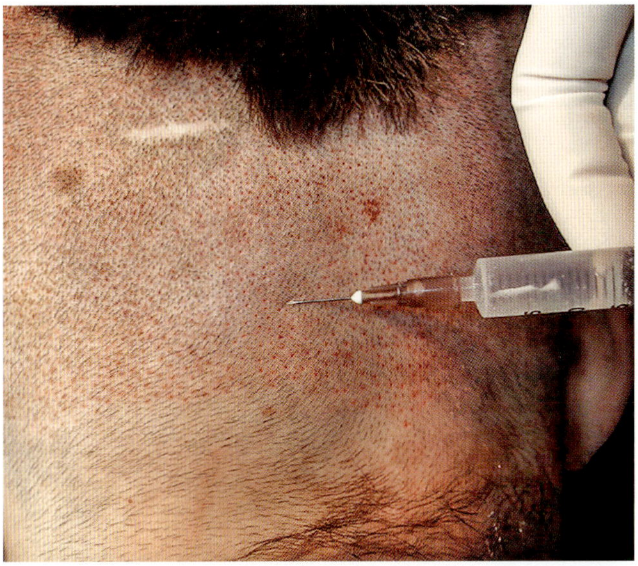

Fig. 20: A 26 gauge needle juxtaposed for comparison of the donor extraction sites.

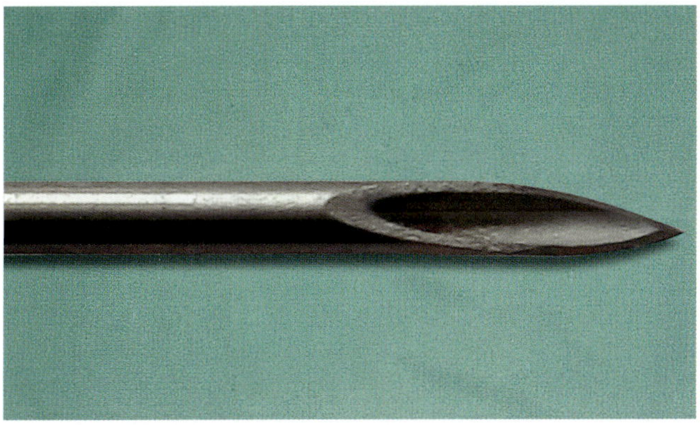

Fig. 21: Needle tip is used to score around the body donor area follicular unit.

- Laxity of skin (skin in most body area is freely mobile over the underlying surface)
- Acute angle of hair shaft (hair follicles in most body donor areas lie at very acute angles)
- Loose arrangement of follicles in the follicular units (in some places the hair follicles of the follicular unit are spread 1.5–2 mm apart)**(Figs. 22 and 23)**

Disadvantages of Traditional Punch

When using the traditional punch for body donor follicular unit graft extraction, the following are some common difficulties encountered:

- Torsion of the follicular units (due to excess skin laxity)
- Downward pressure of the punch.
- Damage to the follicular units due to splaying of the roots (during downward motion of the punch)
- Due to the loosely arranged hair follicle in the body donor area follicular units, larger diameter punches are required giving rise to more visible scarring **(Figs. 24 and 25)**.

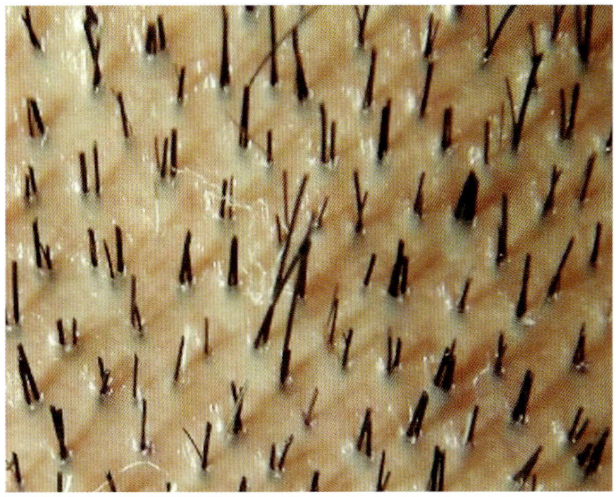

Fig. 22: Scalp donor area.

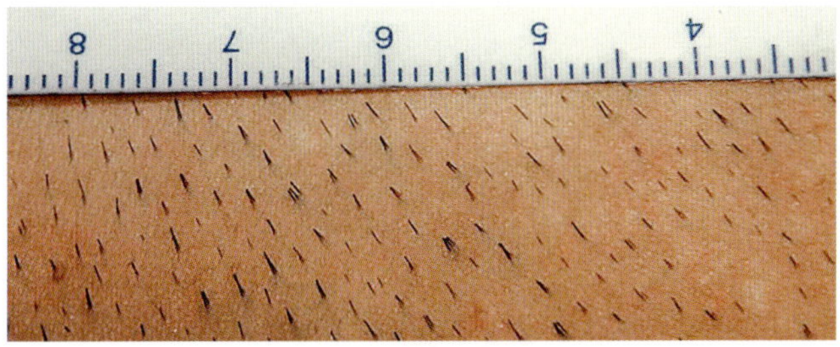

Fig. 23: Chest donor area.

A Different Approach (Expanding Needle Concept)

The extraction occurs as if the needle/punch had expanded as it went inside, adjusting to the shape and diameter of the follicular unit **(Fig. 26)**.[4]

Needle tip is used to score around the follicular unit. A total of 3–4 strokes are used to score around the entire circumference **(Fig. 27)**.

Needle tip is used to score around the body donor area follicular unit. A sharp tip is mandatory. Replace needle as often as required **(Fig. 28)**.

Advantages of Using Needle for Extraction

Using needle tip for scoring and dissecting around the hair follicle of the body donor area hair grafts has certain advantages **(Figs. 29 to 39)**:[4]

- No rotation motion (no torsion)
- No significant downward pressure
- Less damage to follicular units by scoring with needle, as the direction of the needle tip can be customized to the direction of emergence of individual hair follicle of the follicular unit.
- Smaller extraction sites (as the scoring around the body donor area hair graft can be customized as per the shape/lie of the individual hair follicles, and overall smaller extraction wound results).

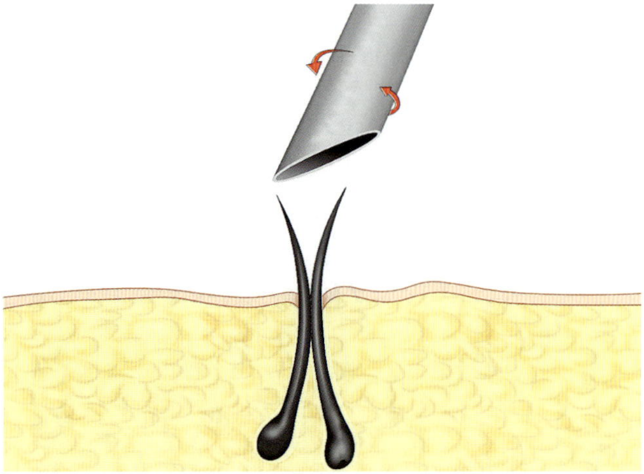

Fig. 24: Downward pressure of the punch.

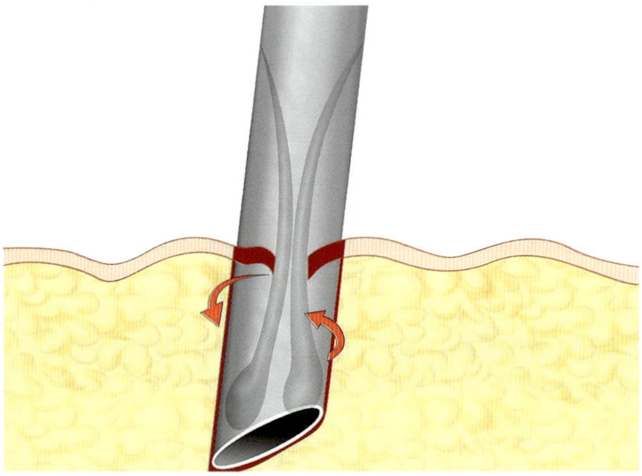

Fig. 25: Large diameter punches.

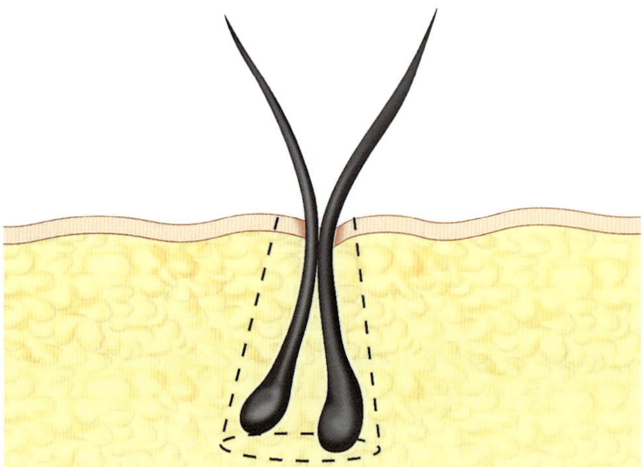

Fig. 26: Adjustment of shape and diameter.

- Part of the extraction/dissection of the deep dermal adhesions is done under direct magnified vision. This improves the yield of the intact grafts from the body donor areas.

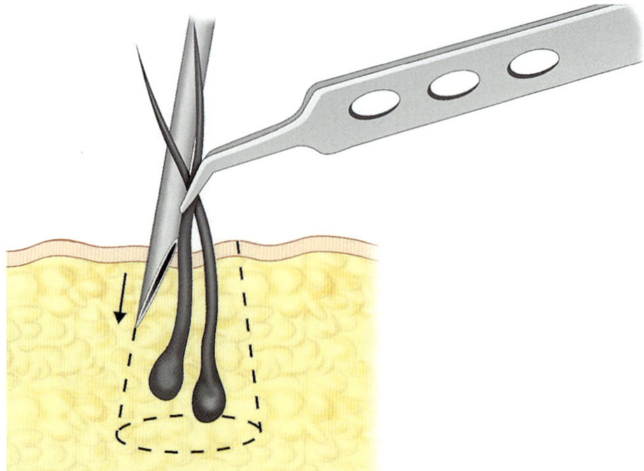

Fig. 27: Needle tip is used to score around the follicular unit.

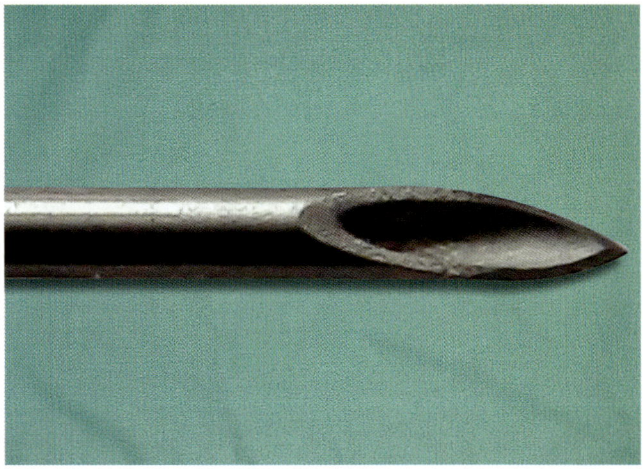

Fig. 28: Needle tip is used to score around the body donor area follicular unit. A sharp tip is mandatory. Replace needle as often as required.

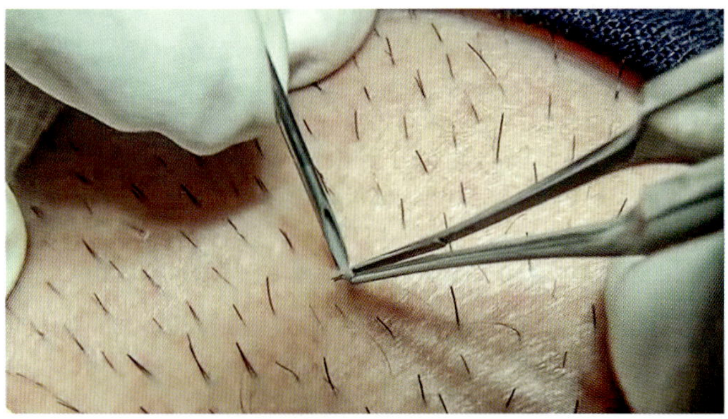

Fig. 29: Step 1.

MY OBSERVATIONS WITH BODY HAIR TRANSPLANTS

- I have monitored the growth and characteristics of the transplanted body and beard hair.[1]

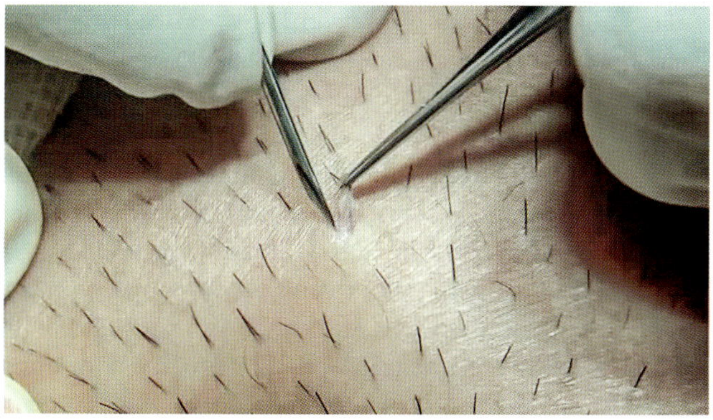

Fig. 30: Step 2.

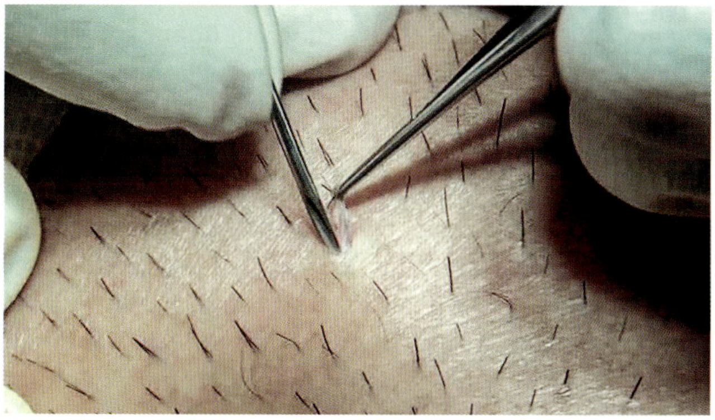

Fig. 31: Step 3.

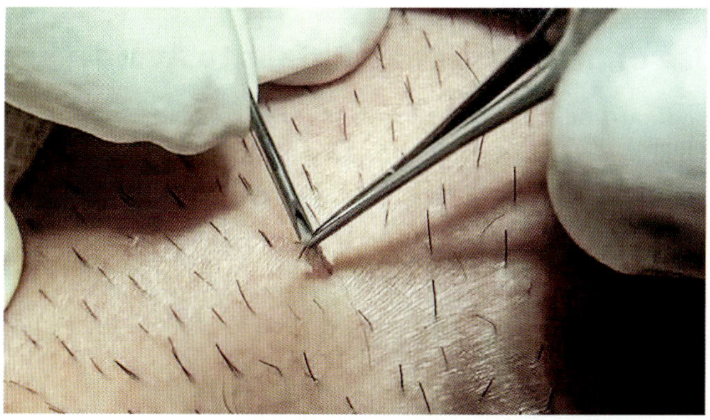

Fig. 32: Step 4.

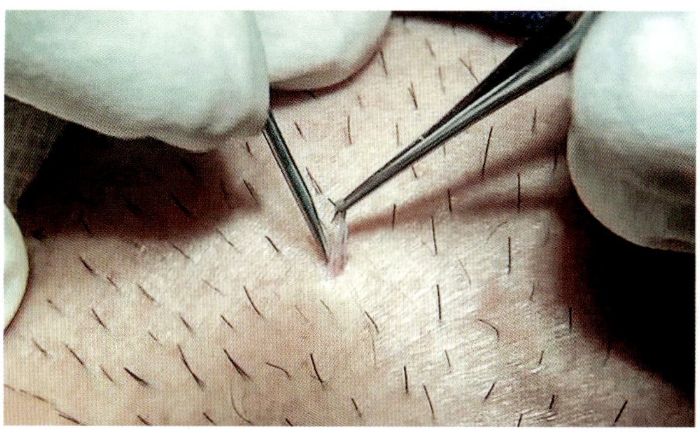

Fig. 33: Step 5.

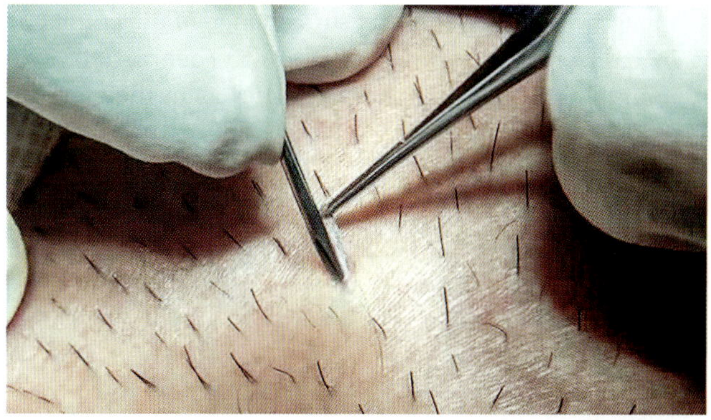

Fig. 34: Step 6.

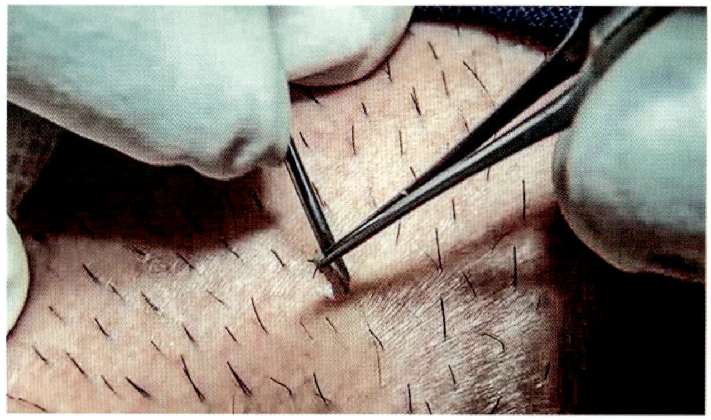

Fig. 35: Step 7.

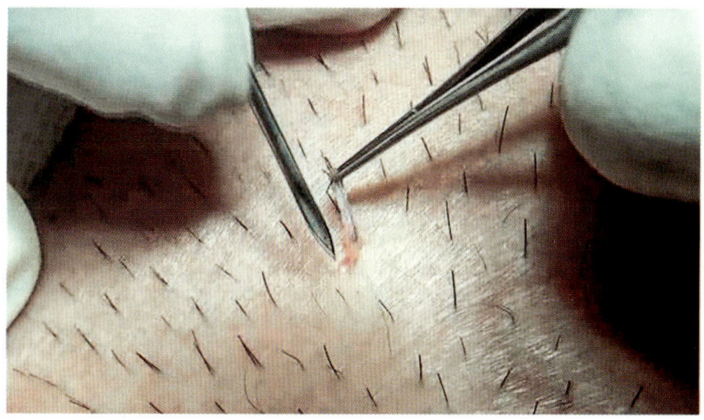

Fig. 36: Step 8.

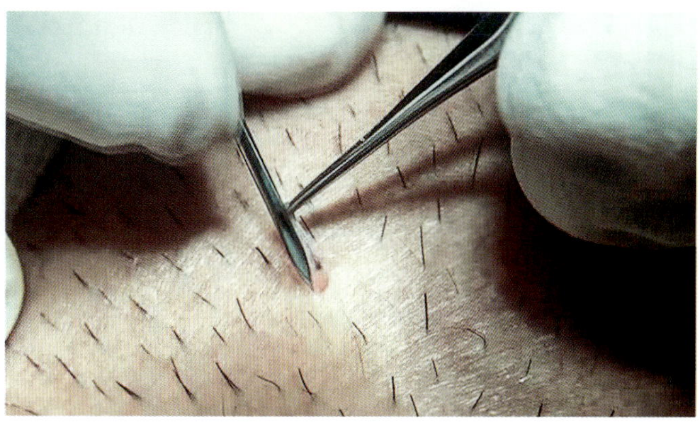

Fig. 37: Step 9.

- In all the patients, there was no change in the color, curl, or caliber of the transplanted body/beard hair. They maintained the same characteristics as in their original location.[1]

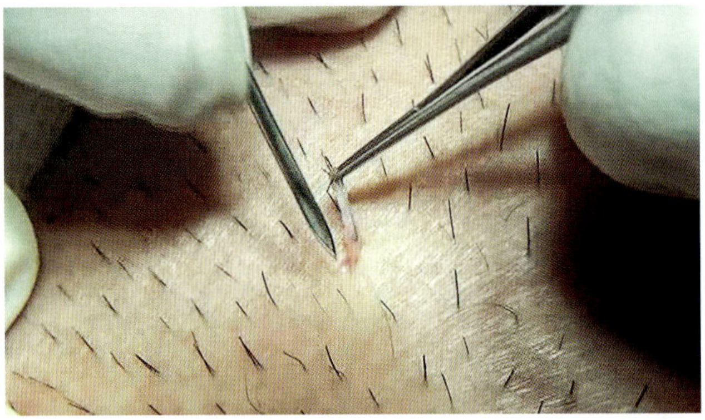

Fig. 38: Step 10.

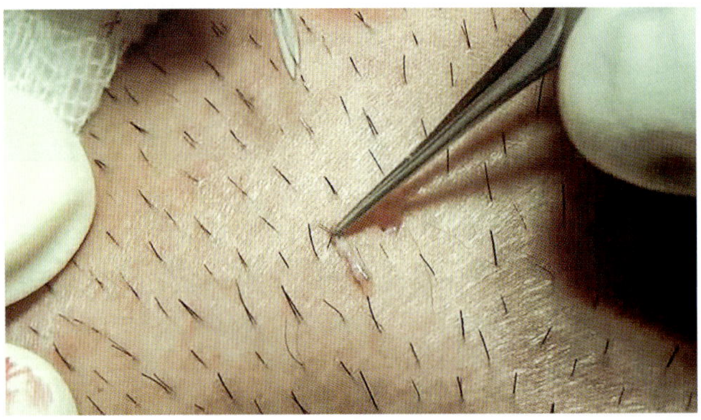

Fig. 39: Step 11.

- The beard hair, due to its thicker caliber provided cosmetically better coverage in the scar tissue, compared to the thin caliber body hair.[2]
- The curl of the hair is a significant factor in patient acceptability of beard/body hair, if the beard/body donor hair is used alone in a slick bald area of the scalp, especially if the patient's own scalp hair is straight.[2]
- The use of the needle tip as a cutting instrument reduced the difficulty posed by larger extraction sites and at the same time lowered the transection rates of the body donor hair.[4]

PATIENT ACCEPTABILITY (FIGS. 40 TO 47)

- The patient acceptability of different donor sources was highest when the beard and/or body donor hair were mixed with scalp donor hair. This held true even in cases where the patient's scalp hair was fine caliber and straight, while the beard donor hair was thick caliber and wavy.
- Transplanted body hair blends in nicely with the scalp hair.
- Body and beard hair can be used as additional donor resource for treating androgenic alopecia. These hairs, however, do not change their color and shaft diameter (caliber). Thus, proper planning is a must when using these different types of donor hair for transplanting.

PITFALLS/MYTHS

Use of Beard Hair and Pitfalls to Avoid

- Beard hair is 2–3 times more bulky/coarse as compared to scalp hair, transplanting beard hair close together en masse is not recommended.

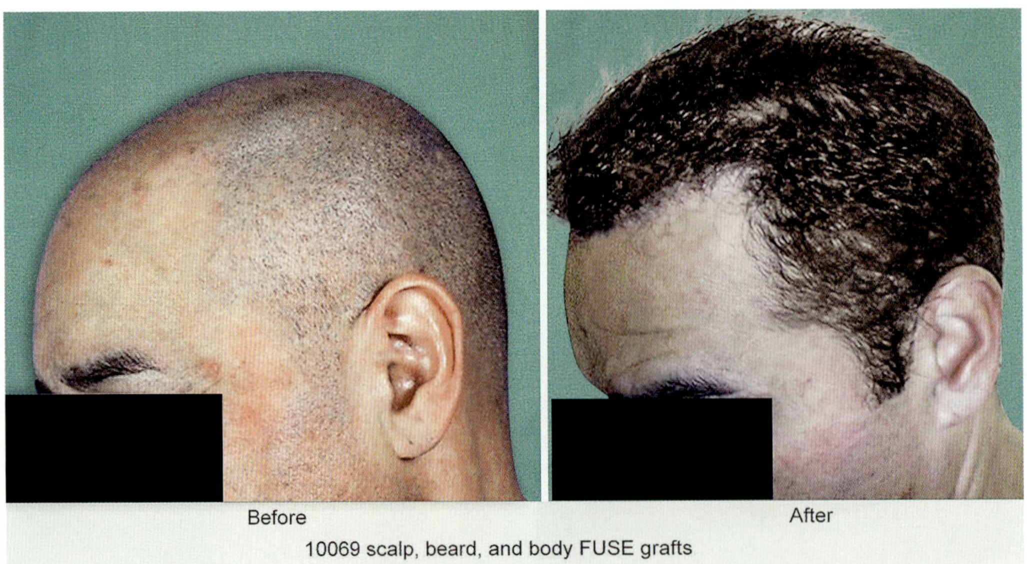

Fig. 40: Comparison picture.
Courtesy: Dr A's Clinic, New Delhi.

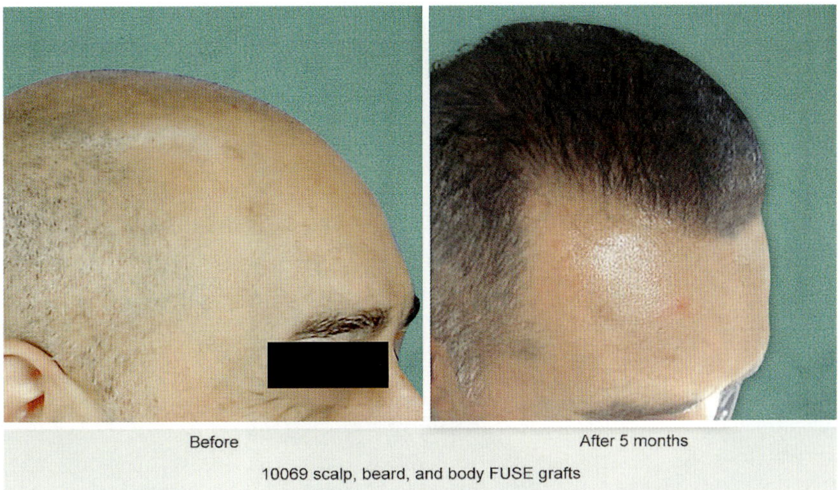

Fig. 41: Comparison picture.
Courtesy: Dr A's Clinic, New Delhi.

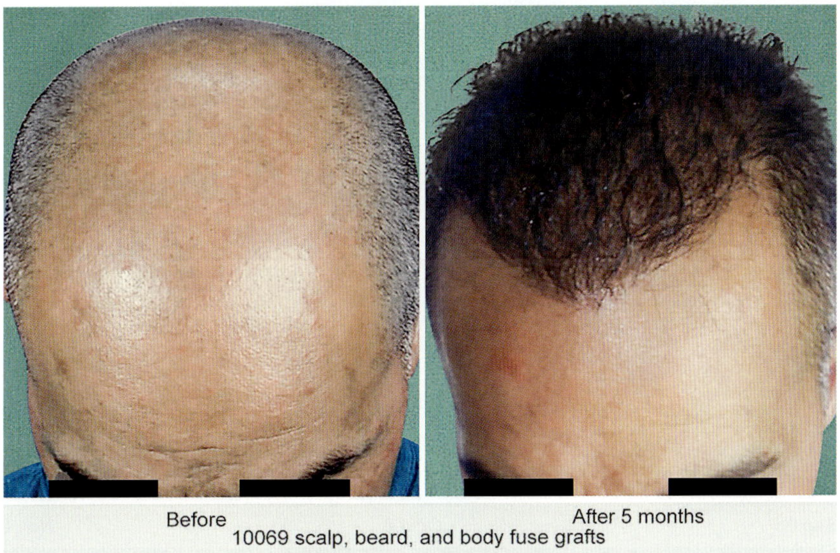

Fig. 42: Comparison picture.
Courtesy: Dr A's Clinic, New Delhi.

- All facial hair is not same. The chin hair, cheek hair, moustache hair, or the hair low down on the neck all differ. They differ in terms of their length, speed of growth, coarseness, etc.

	Telogen (%)	*Anagen (%)*	*Duration of activity*
Cheeks	40–50	50–60	50–60 days
Beard (Chin)	40	60	1 year
Moustache	45	55	16 weeks

- The hair from different parts of the face would be suitable for different purposes.

For example, hairs from the edges of the beard (low down on the neck or high up on the cheek) do not grow very long. They would be better used for areas that do not require long hair length (previous strip scars would be the ideal place for them). Chin hair and hair toward the central parts of the beard grow longer. They would be suitable for adding bulk in the vertex areas.

THE IMPACT OF DISINTEGRATION OF SYNCHRONICITY ON BODY HAIR TRANSPLANTATION

A larger percentage of hair follicles are in resting/nongrowing phase on the body donor areas. It is advisable to use only the actively growing hair for transplant as the extracted telogen hair may not have the entire complement of stem cells to regenerate a full terminal hair.

Preshaving the body donor hair 3–4 days prior to extraction is a simple noninvasive method of isolating the hair in anagen phase that can then be used for transplanting.

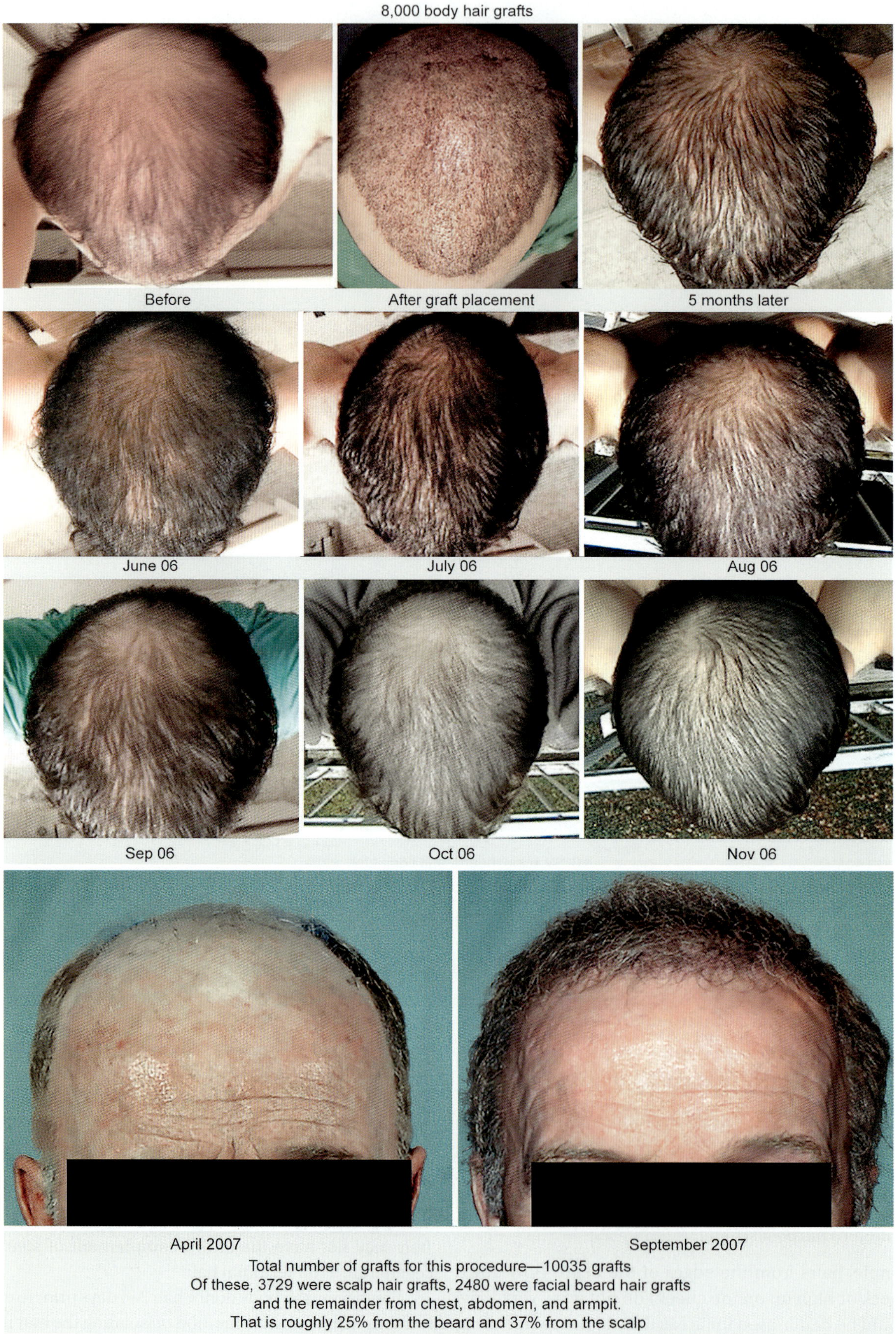

Fig. 43: Comparison picture.

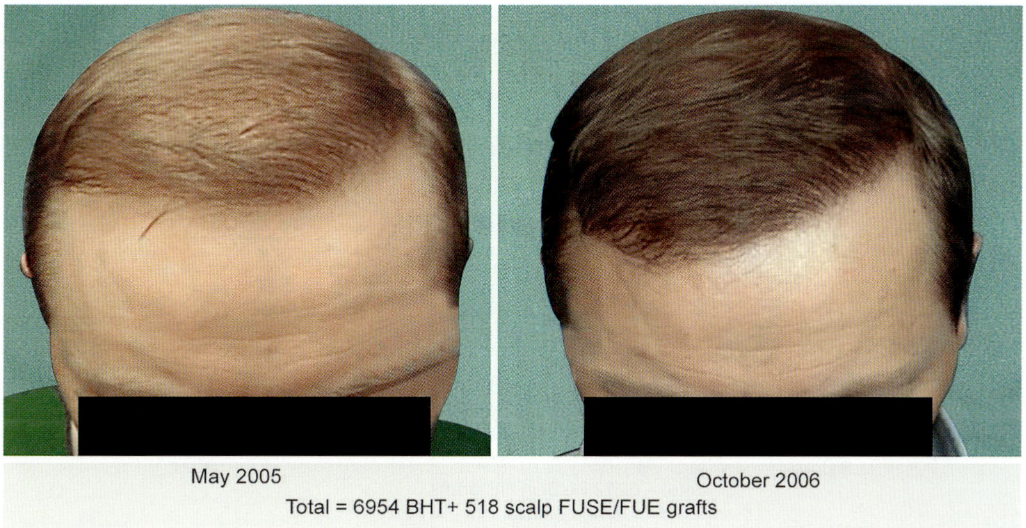

Fig. 44: Comparison picture.

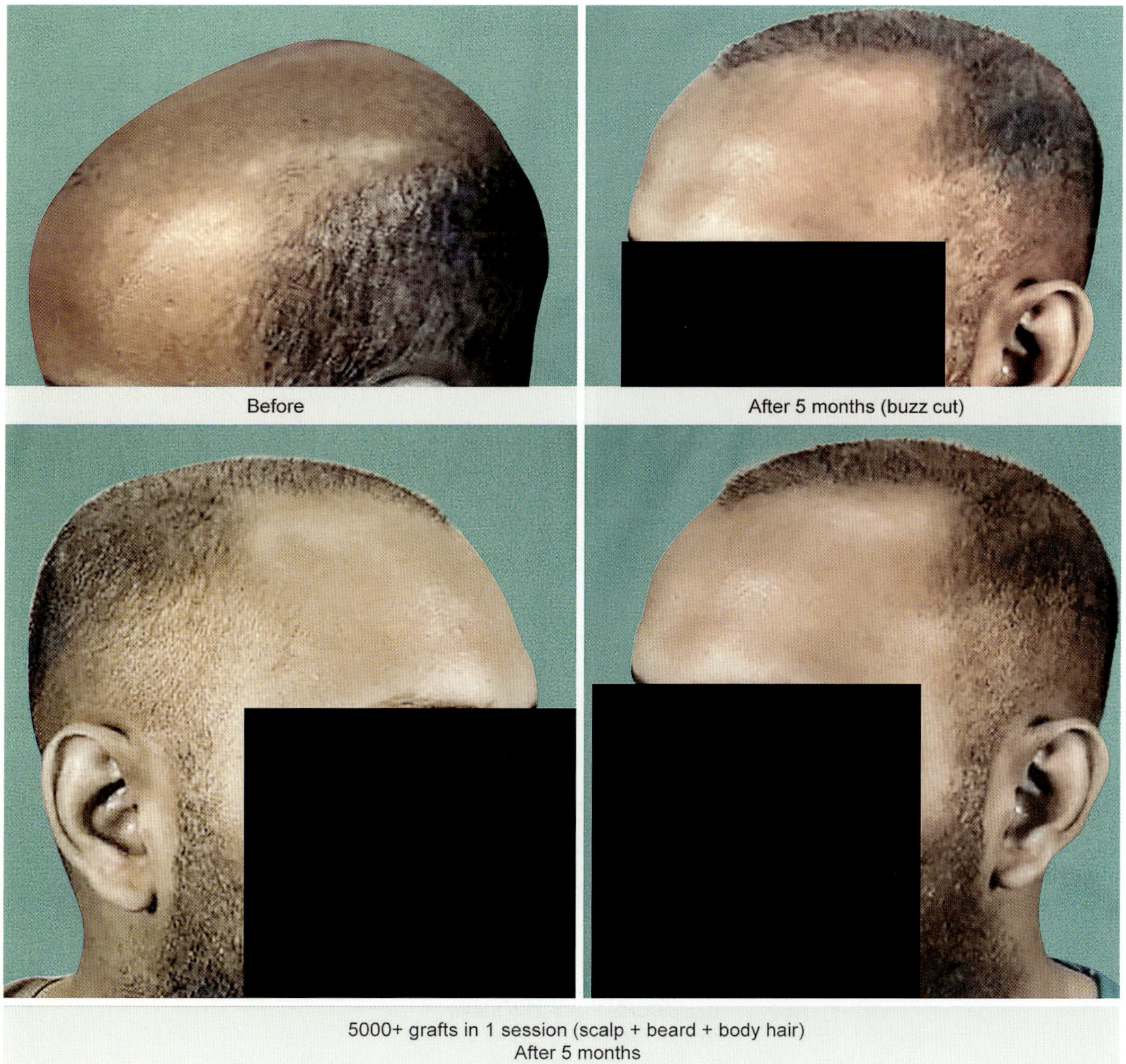

Fig. 45: Comparison picture of hair transplant in an NW 7 patient.

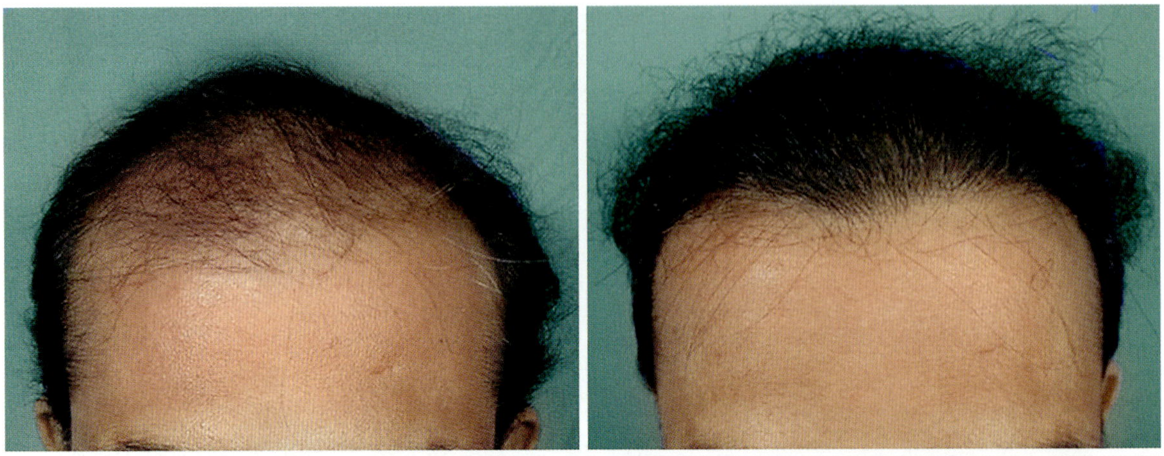

Before After

Total – 6212 FUSE/FUE grafts
Grafts details:
Scalp FUSE/FUE—2338 grafts
Beard/facial—2850 grafts
Chest—1024 grafts

Fig. 46: Comparison picture.

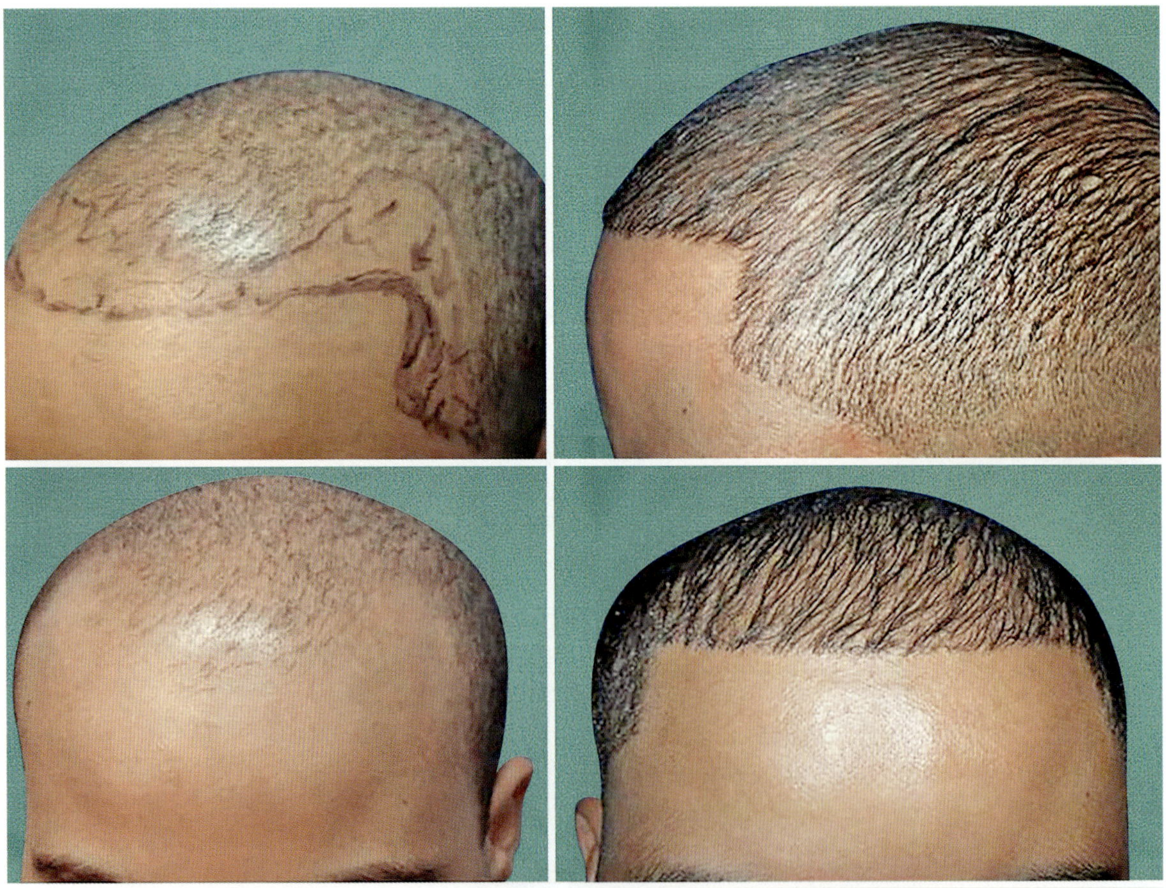

Before After hair removal

Total = 8869 FUSE/FUE grafts
Grafts details:
Scalp FUSE/FUE—869 grafts
Body hair FUSE/FUE—8000 grafts

Fig. 47: Comparison picture.

When body hairs (from one area only), are transplanted after being preshaved 3–5 days in advance, the hairs are likely to be closely synchronized in their growth phase. That is to say, that almost all of those hairs will be in the growth phase at the time of extraction. As a result, for the first couple of cycles, their growth phase may be closely synchronized. However, that synchronicity will not continue. There are two factors that one has to keep in mind:

1. All the hairs will not be in the same part of the growth phase at the time of extraction. Some hairs may have just entered anagen while others may be almost at end of anagen. Still others would be in different stages in between.
2. Even when extracting from the same area, for example, the chest, the hair growth cycles for each hair will not be identical. One tends to categorize these cycles in fixed number of days per area, but nature does not bother to see it the same way. The hair nearer the center of the chest and those to the periphery will have slightly different duration of cycle. If the anagen for 1 hair is 140 days and another 130 and still another 150, then, even if they are harvested on exactly one same day of their growth cycle (say, day 90), their cycles will become asynchronous with time.

The graphic illustration **(Fig. 48)** given shows how the synchronization of the hair cycles disintegrates over time:

The graph above shows how a decrease is seen in the visible growing transplanted hair after sometime. The transplanted body hairs are not rejected, but seem to follow their own hair growth cycles.

Thus, when hair is extracted from any particular donor area, the transplanted hairs will be in different phases of anagen. As extracted hairs are in their active growing phase, their initial growth is more closely synchronized. But with successive growth cycles, the individual hair cycles lose their synchronicity.

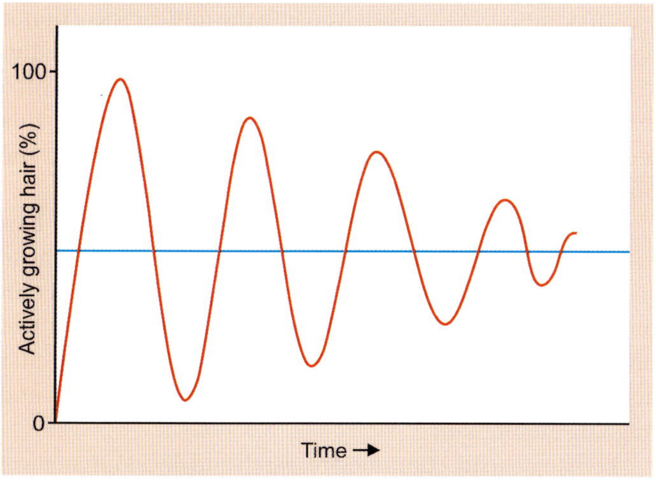

Fig. 48: Disintegration of synchronicity.

One has to keep this disintegration of synchronicity in the growth cycles in mind to understand the temporary observed variations in hair coverage when more body hair has been used.

There are three different options that one can opt for while venturing into hair transplant:

1. Use up all scalp hair before using body donor hair.
2. Use the body donor hair and reserve the scalp hair for touch up work.
3. Use a mix of scalp and robust body donor hair (from various areas), in pre-planned manner from start to finish.

When one uses a mixture of scalp and body donor hair, the scalp donor hair will provide scaffolding and the body donor hair will provide the filler. As we go backward from the hairline toward the vertex and crown-swirl areas, the percentage of scalp hair can be decreased and body donor hair increased.

While using options 1 or 2, there are chances of certain scalp areas having only scalp donor and others having only body donor hair, which may not look aesthetic.

In addition, a higher proportion of body donor hair may be in the resting and shedding phase (as compared to the scalp hair).

Using option 2 and later attempting to fill in the visible gaps at the time with scalp donor hair may lead to damage of the dormant body hair in that part of the scalp.

Therefore, when performing BHT, one should make it a point to mix the robust body hair from different areas with the scalp donor hair in a planned manner. All body donor hairs are not the same. Due consideration needs to be given to the hair diameter, color, curl, etc., at time of planning which hair to relocate in which scalp recipient areas.

Example 1: Temple points—the hair in this area is thinner, slower growing, and length is shorter than scalp hair in vertex or occiput. Axillary/nape area hair and other thin caliber body donor areas are more suitable for these points **(Fig. 49)**.

Example 2: Hairline feathering—using thin/fine caliber hair (from the axilla or nape area) mixed with scalp donor hair gives more natural and aesthetically pleasing outcome **(Fig. 50)**.

Example 3: Scars—whether due to hair restoration surgery or otherwise, it is unadvisable to replace the entire scar with beard hair for example (the smiley scar would be replaced by a smiley moustache—definitely not the desired outcome) **(Fig. 51)**.

HOW PATIENT CAN IMPROVE THE OUTCOME?

Things the patients can do:

- No Yo-Yo haircuts (refer different speed of hair growth). The patient should not repeat/alternate between keeping long hair and shaving/buzz cutting the scalp hair.

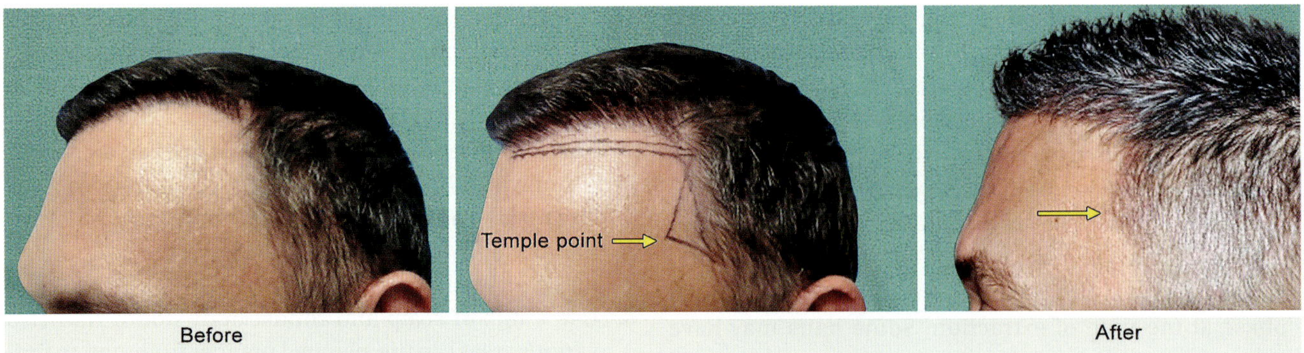

Fig. 49: Temple points recreation with fine caliber hair.

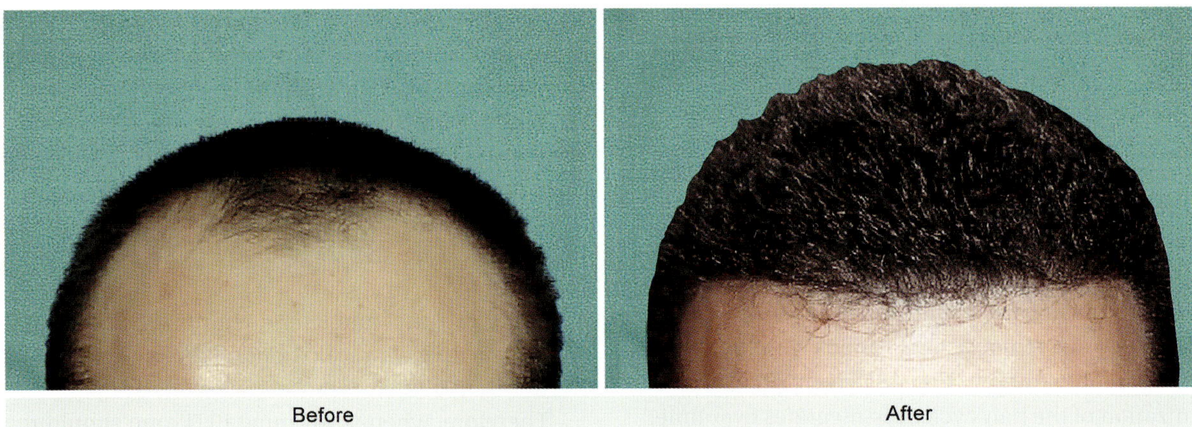

Fig. 50: Hairline feathering.

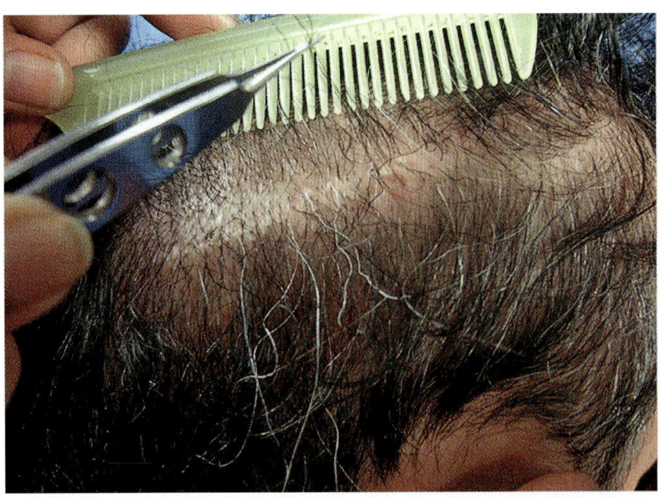

Fig. 51: Beard hair growing in FUT scars.

- Keep buzz cut (between 3 and 5 mm), if possible.
- Handle transplanted body hair gently and try to delay exogen (once the hair is in telogen phase). That includes treating the hair gently (no rough massages) at the same time keeping the scalp thoroughly clean.

RESULTS

Comparison pictures **(Figs. 52 to 66)**.

CONCLUSION

In conclusion, body hair to scalp transplant represents a significant advancement in the field of hair restoration surgery. Through meticulous research, innovative techniques, and the expertise of skilled surgeons, this procedure has emerged as a viable option for individuals with advanced hair loss and limited donor hair on the scalp.

Throughout this chapter, we have explored the principles, methodologies, and outcomes associated with body hair transplantation. We have delved into the intricacies of donor hair characteristics, surgical approaches, patient selection criteria, and postoperative care protocols. We have also examined the challenges and limitations inherent in this technique, as well as the promising advancements on the horizon.

As we conclude our journey, it is evident that body hair to scalp transplant offers hope and opportunity for those seeking to restore their hairline and regain confidence in their appearance. However, it is essential to approach this procedure with realistic expectations, understanding that achieving optimal results may require multiple sessions and ongoing maintenance.

Looking ahead, continued research and development will undoubtedly enhance the efficacy and refinement of body

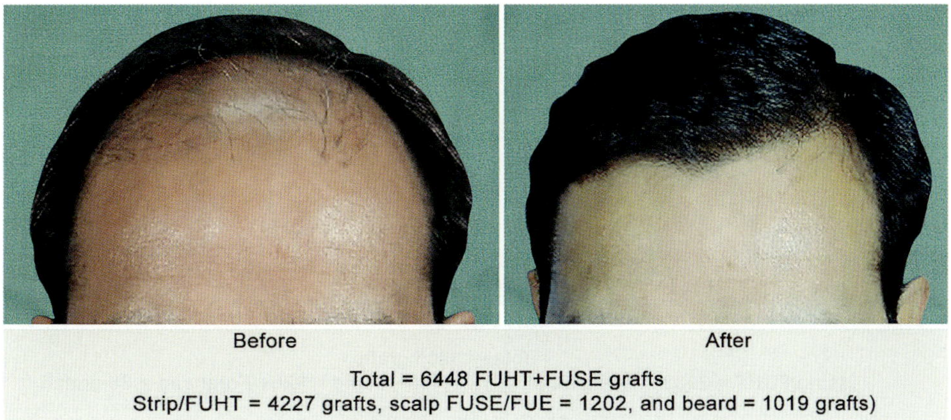

Fig. 52: Comparison picture.

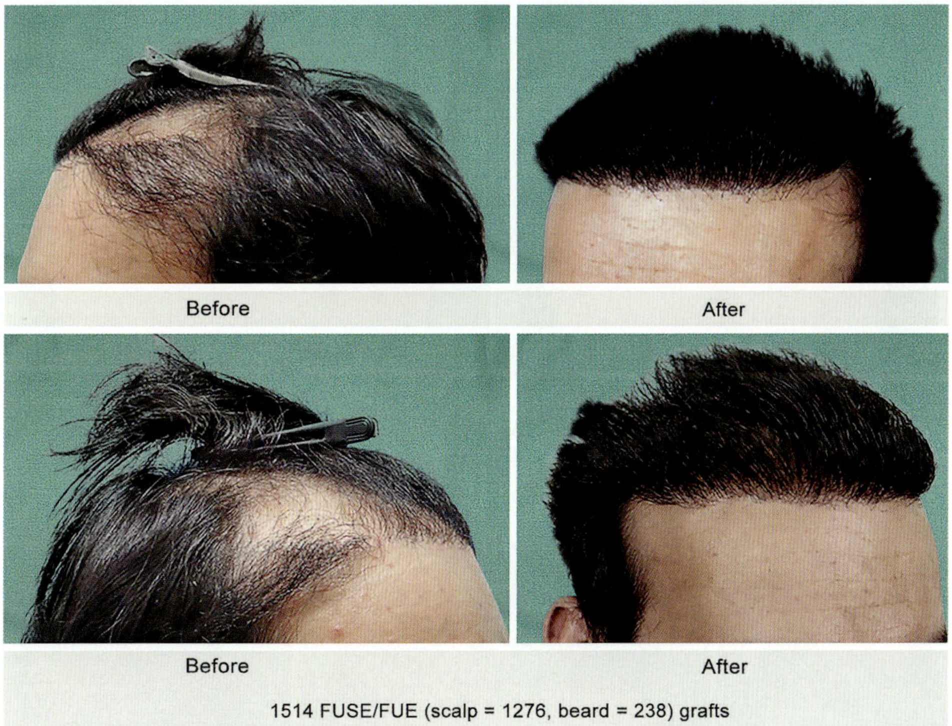

Fig. 53: Comparison picture.

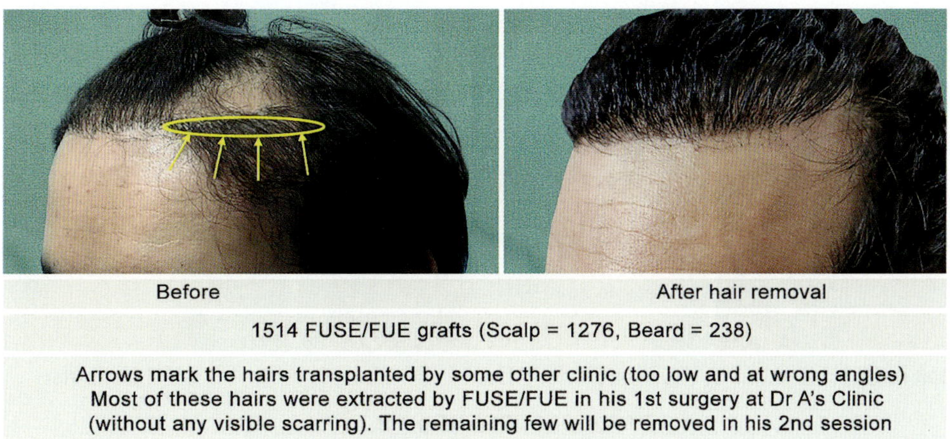

Fig. 54: Comparison picture.
Courtesy: Dr A's Clinic, New Delhi.

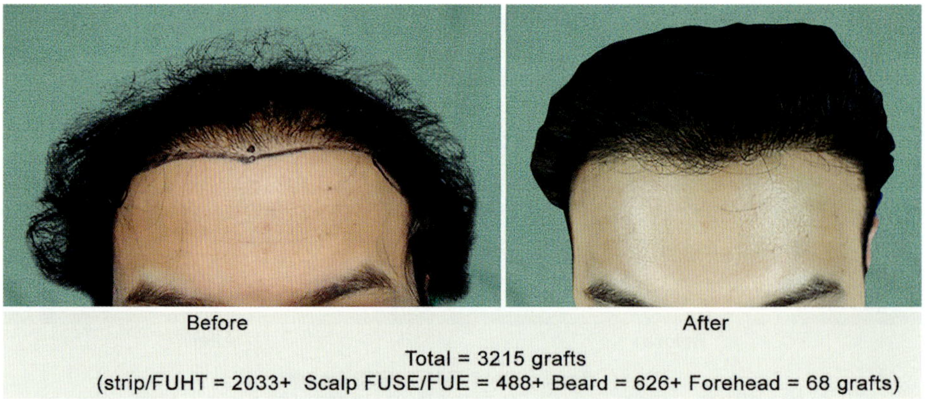

Fig. 55: Comparison picture.

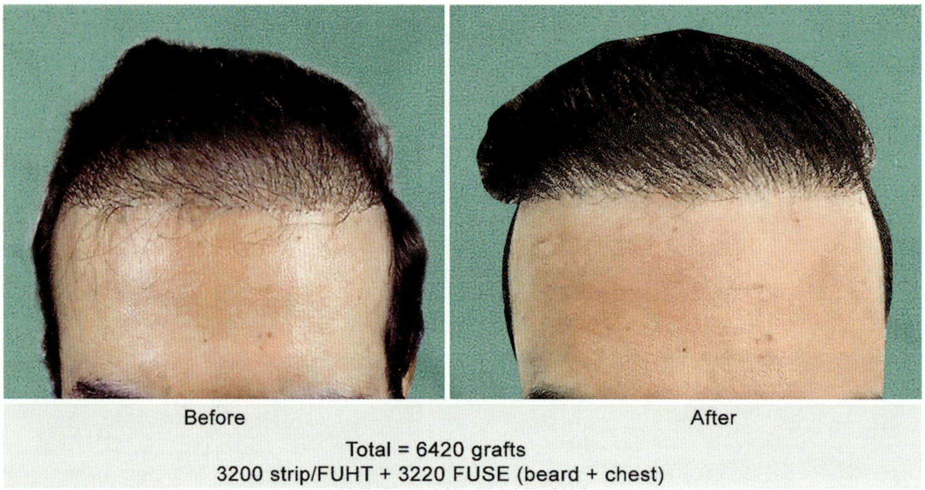

Fig. 56: Comparison picture.

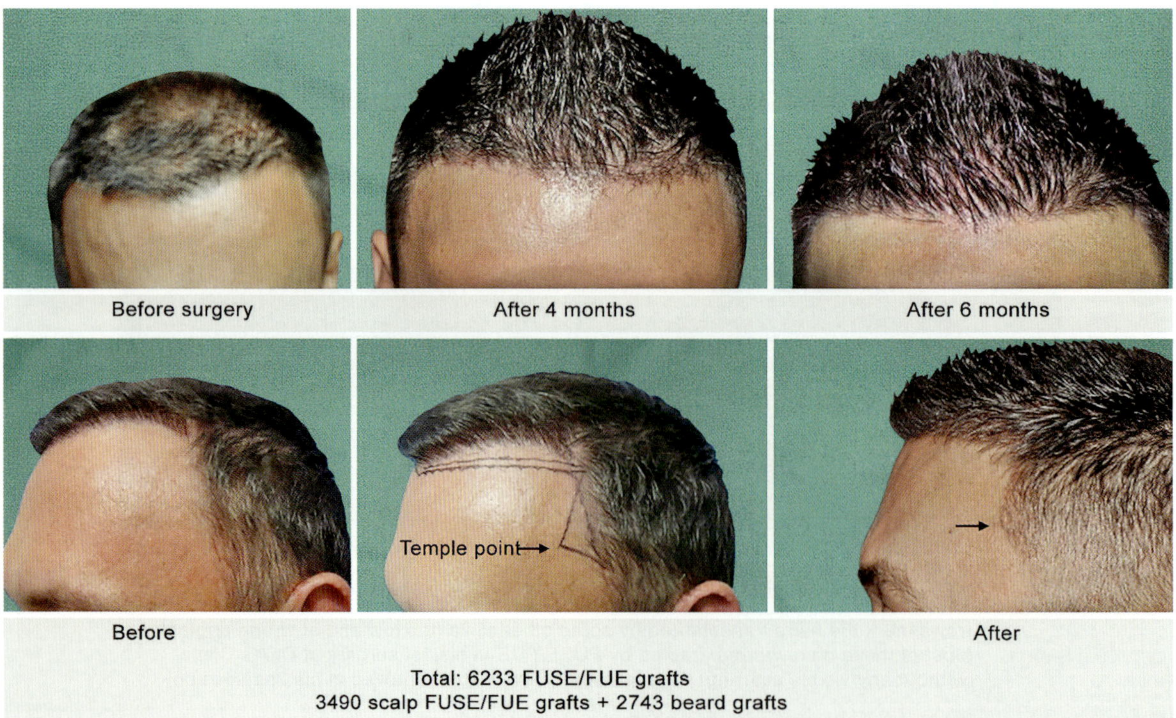

Fig. 57: Comparison picture.

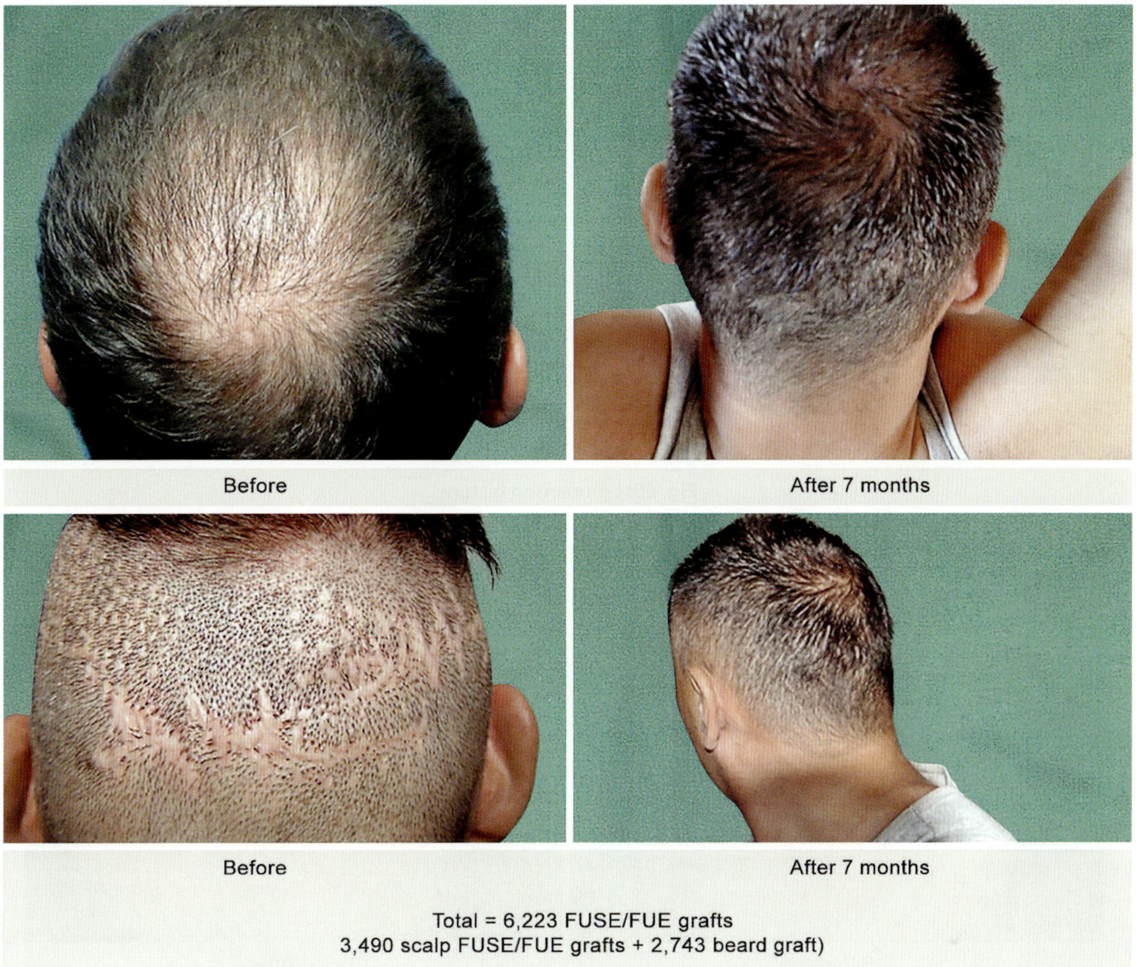

Fig. 58: Comparison picture.

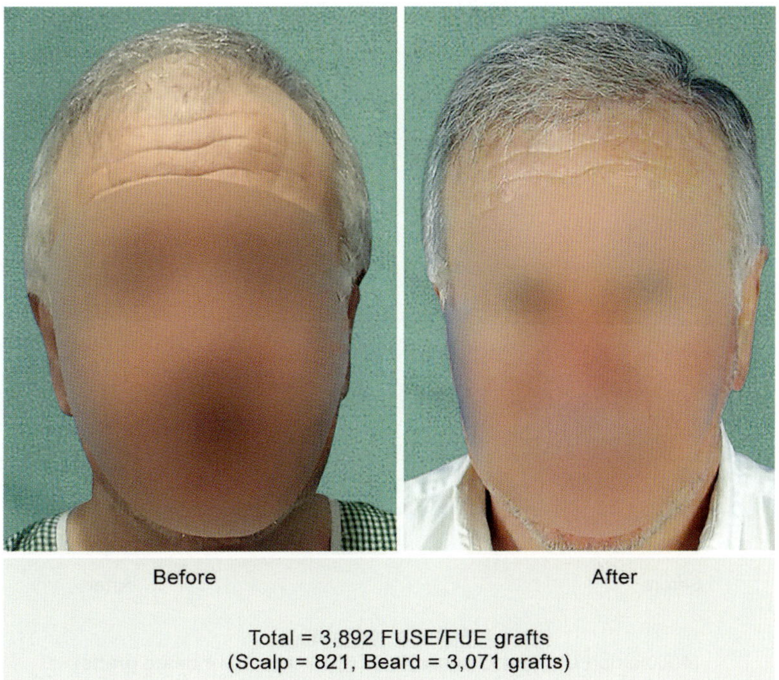

Fig. 59: Comparison picture.

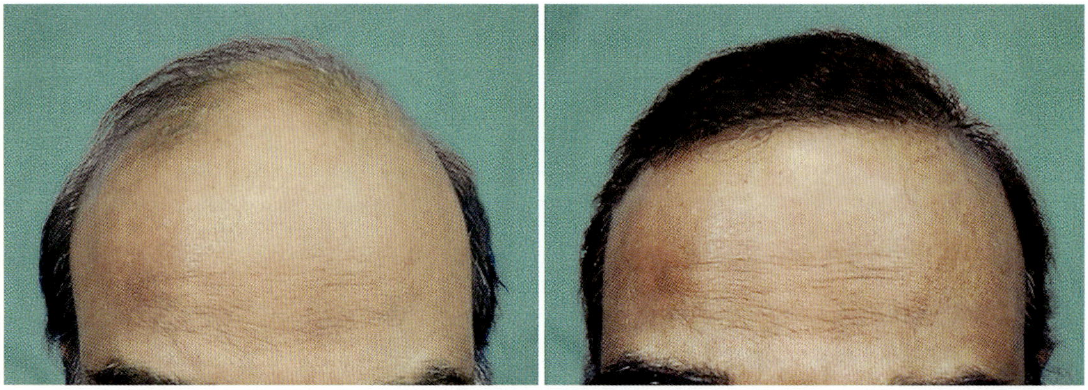

Before After

Total = 3,225 grafts (2,650 strip/FUHT + 575 beard graft)

Fig. 60: Comparison picture.

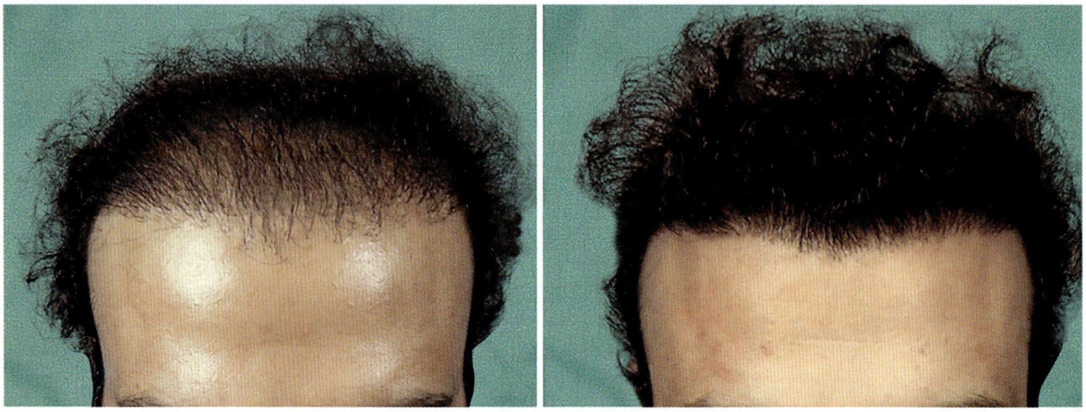

Before After

Total = 2,979 graft (1,907 strip/FUHT + 240 scalp + 832 beard grafts)

Fig. 61: Comparison picture.

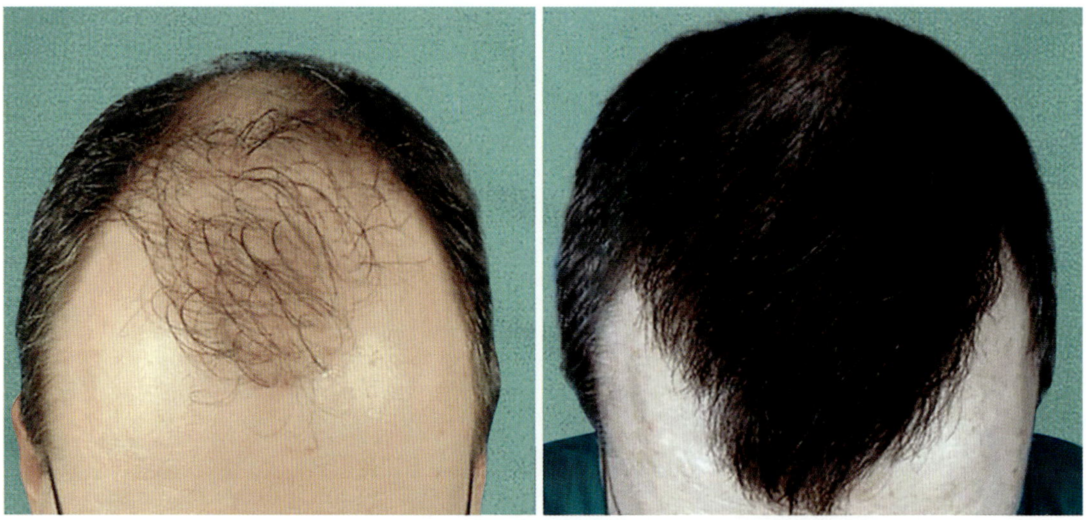

Before After

Total = 6,505 grafts
(4080 strip/FUHT, 1411 scalp FUSE/FUE, and 1014 beard grafts)

Fig. 62: Comparison picture.

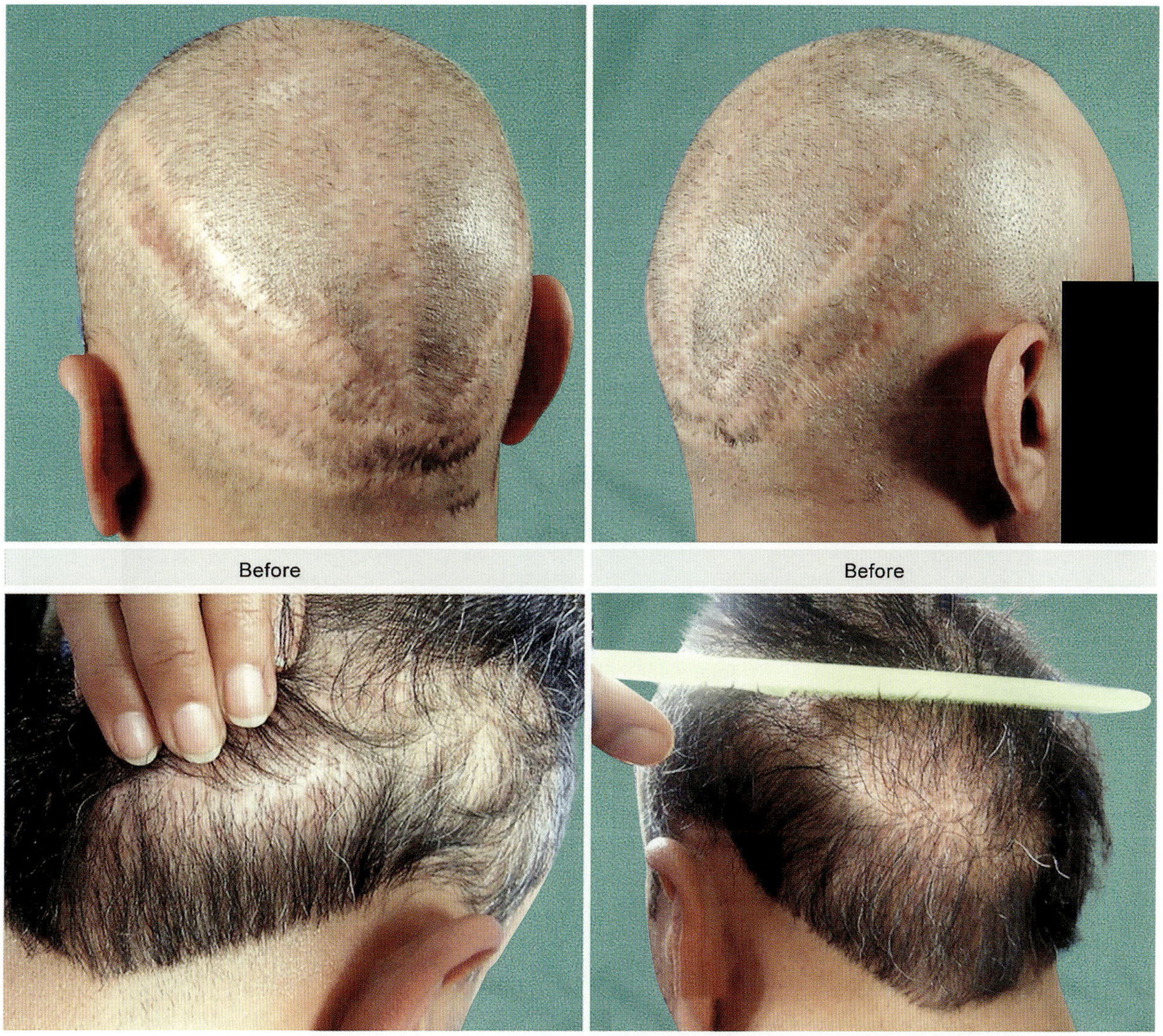

Before Before

After After

Total = 3983 grafts into scar tissues
Beard = 2410, Chest = 1101, Scalp = 312, Pubic = 143, Thigh = 17 grafts

Fig. 63: Comparison picture showing good beard hair growth in scars.

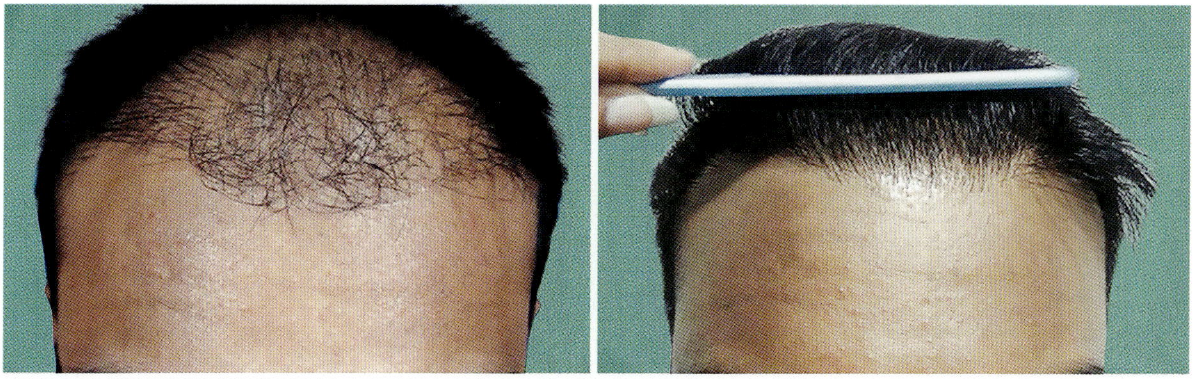

Before After

Total = 3743 strip/FUHT + FUSE/FUE grafts (2615 strip/FUHT + 1128 beard graft)

Fig. 64: Comparison picture.

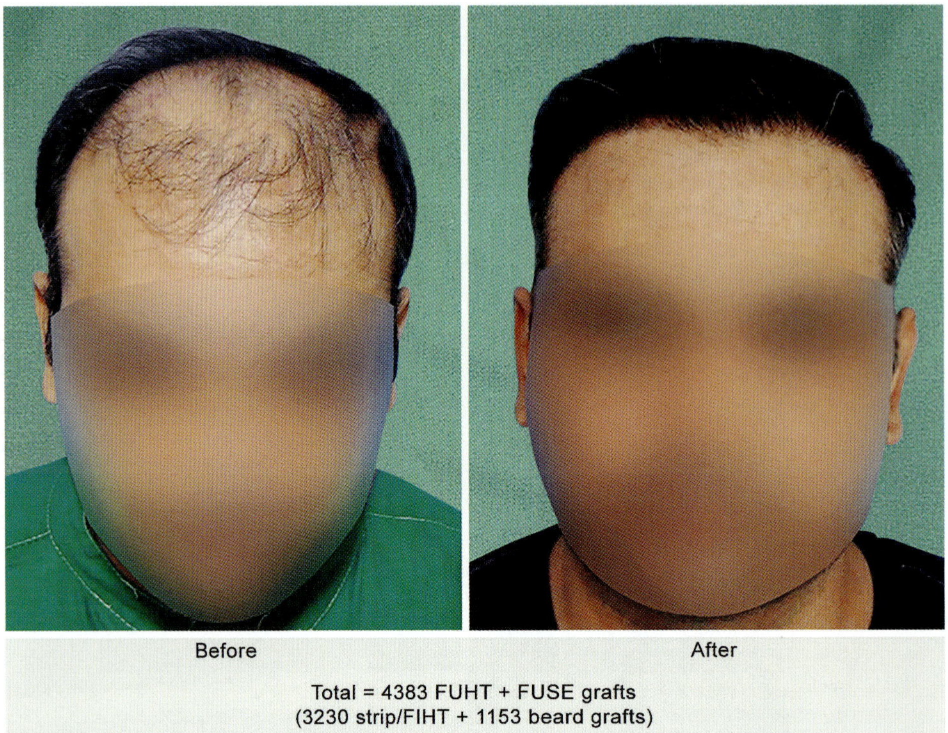

Fig. 65: Comparison picture.

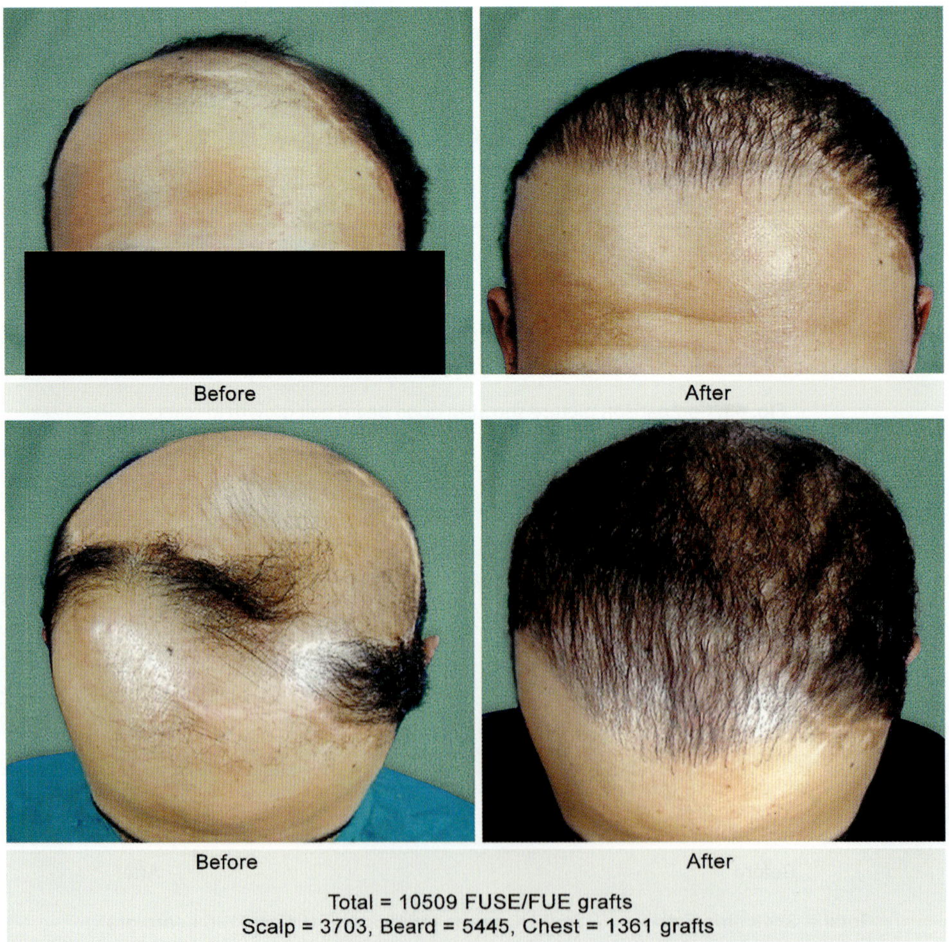

Fig. 66: Comparison pictures showing corrective surgery using beard, body and scalp hair grafts.

hair transplantation. With ongoing advancements in surgical techniques, instrumentation, and biotechnology, we can anticipate even better outcomes and expanded opportunities for patients in the future.

Ultimately, the success of body hair to scalp transplant lies not only in the hands of skilled surgeons but also in the partnership between patients and practitioners. By fostering open communication, mutual understanding, and a commitment to excellence, we can continue to push the boundaries of hair restoration and improve the lives of individuals affected by hair loss.

REFERENCES

1. Poswal A. Body hair transplant: an additional source of donor hair in hair restoration surgery. Indian J Dermatol. 2007;52(2):104-5.
2. Poswal A. Use of body and beard donor hair in surgical treatment of androgenic alopecia. Indian J Plast Surg. 2013;46(1):117-20.
3. Poswal A. The preshaving protocol in body hair to scalp transplant to identify hair in anagen phase. Indian J Dermatol. 2010;55(1):50-2.
4. Poswal A. Expanding needle concept for better extraction of body hair grafts. Indian J Dermatol. 2013;58(3):240.

CHAPTER 74

Scalp Micropigmentation

Rachita Dhurat, Sujit Shanshanwal, Ameet Dandale

KEY MESSAGES

- Scalp micropigmentation decreases the contrast between skin and hair, thereby acting as a concealer to camouflage the loss of hair.
- Scalp micropigmentation is useful in men as well as women suffering from alopecia.
- Scalp micropigmentation is a useful adjunct to medical and surgical interventions for hair loss.
- Scalp micropigmentation requires in depth understanding of its variables to give optimum results.

INTRODUCTION

With increasing hair loss there is decrease in density of hair and as a result the scalp skin can be seen easily due to increase in contrast between skin and hair. Despite medical and/or surgical line of therapy, some patients of androgenetic alopecia (AGA) may not get desirable density. This contrast between the hair and skin can be minimized by providing an illusion using various camouflaging or concealing techniques. Camouflaging techniques such as biofibers, wigs or concealers like hair powder are all temporary methods with their own shortcomings. Compared to these modalities, tattooing is a permanent concealer and thus has a role to play in such patients.

Tattooing is an art of inserting metabolically inert pigments in a desired pattern and at the optimum level into the skin. Scalp micropigmentation (SMP) is a method of placing microdots less than 1 mm in size with the help of one or three pronged needles, creating an illusion of hair by decreasing contrast between hair and skin. The process is performed using manual or electrically driven needles, whereby the pigment that is deposited beyond the epidermis is taken up the dermal macrophages and fibroblasts where it resides permanently, resulting in the desired change in color and pattern on the skin.[1,2] The terms "micropigmentation" and "dermatography", often used interchangeably, reflect the medical application of tattooing.

Scalp micropigmentation is a complex process of math and science, the outcome of which depends on several variables. The size of dots used and pattern of placement varies as per the mutually decided goals between the patient and the surgeon; and depends on the hair density in the affected area.

HISTORICAL ASPECTS

Skin marking with pigments has been used by people for at least the last 4 millennia.[3,4] The initial mentions of tattooing in literature for its use in medical indications in dermatology and ophthalmology appeared by the mid-1800s.[5-7] In 1976, the term "tattoo" was coined by Captain Cook, who mentioned about the Polynesian practice of permanently marking the skin by using black pigments, which in their language was referred to as *Tattow*.[8] In 2001, scalp micropigmentation (SMP) was reported for the first time by Traquina, where the procedure was performed in 62 patients who had scarring on the scalp.[9]

However, this method was crude and the pigmentation was quite detectable. Since then, the procedure of micro-pigmentation has greatly refined over time.

PRINCIPLES OF MICROPIGMENTATION

The purpose of SMP is to act as a permanent concealer in such a way that the targeted artistic effect is similar to the visual effect of a stippled painting as dots are created between the pores of a balding scalp.[2,10]

When performing the procedure, the operator does not need to match the density of stippling with the number of hair follicle openings that would normally be present on the scalp of an average adult. As the dots diffuse over time, overcrowding of dots can result in a patchy appearance. To get the desired effect, there are several variables that influence the deposition of optimum quantity of pigment, at the appropriate level, into the skin. The level of deposition is the papillary dermis so that it can be engulfed by macrophages and retained.

FACTORS AFFECTING SCALP MICROPIGMENTATION

Rassman et al. mentioned numerous variables influencing SMP, having a mathematically proportional "relationship", that can be represented as follows:[11]

Deposition of pigment corresponds to:

$a[(A) \times (D) \times (T) \times (S) \times (N)/(R)] \times C \times V$

A = Needle angle with the skin
D = Needle depth into the skin
T = Contact time of needle with the skin (exposure time)
S = Speed of the rotor
R = Resistance of scalp
C = Color of pigment
V = Viscosity of dye
N = Needle number and thickness
a = Proportionality with the variables

Needle Angle with the Skin and Needle Depth into the Skin

While placing the pigment, needle should be inserted perpendicular to the surface of the skin. If the needle is inserted at an acute angle it does not form round dots. With a highly acute angle of insertion the pigment will be get deposited in a linear fashion which will result in an unnatural look **(Figs. 1A to D)**.

Needle Depth into the Skin

Depth of needle penetration into the skin is a crucial parameter influencing the placement (deposition) of pigment into the dermis. If the depth is too superficial (near epidermis) **(Fig. 2)** then the pigment may not remain in the skin and will be washed off in 3–4 weeks.

If deposition is too deep, down in the dermis **(Fig. 3)**, there is diffusion of pigment into the surrounding skin, leading to enlargement of size of dot giving a patchy appearance over time and also change in color of pigment. Ideal deposition of pigment is in the papillary dermis **(Fig. 4)**.

Contact Time of Needle with the Skin and Speed of the Rotor

There is an inverse relationship between the two parameters. However, if one of these parameters is kept fixed, with an increase in the other parameter, the amount of pigment deposition would proportionately increase. As the speed of the rotor increases, one needs to decrease the contact time of the needle with the skin to compensate for the increased

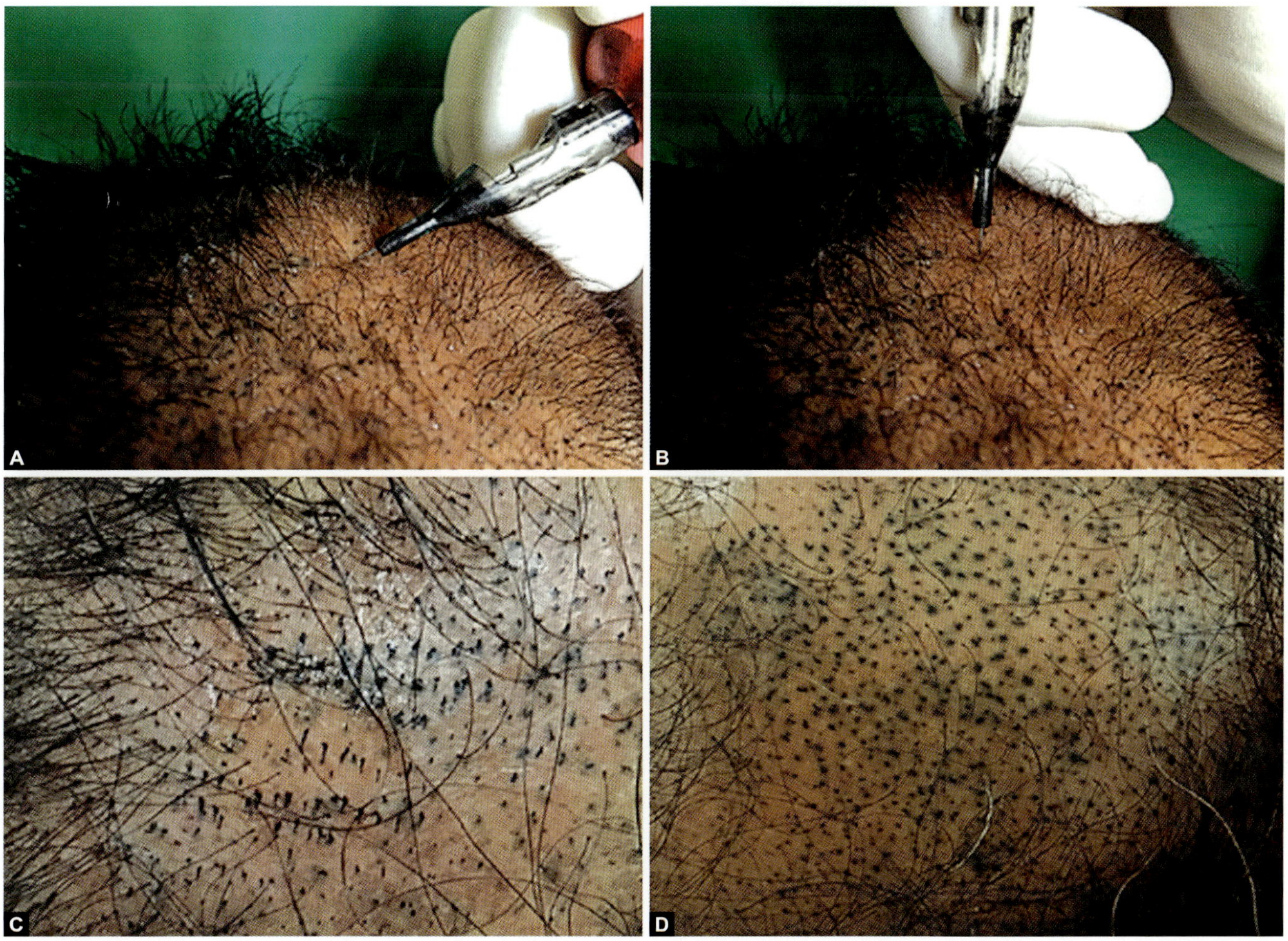

Figs. 1A to D: When the needle is inserted at an angle it results in linear pigment placement compared to the needle being inserted vertically which results in the desired round dot placement. The round dots provide a better illusion of follicular dots.

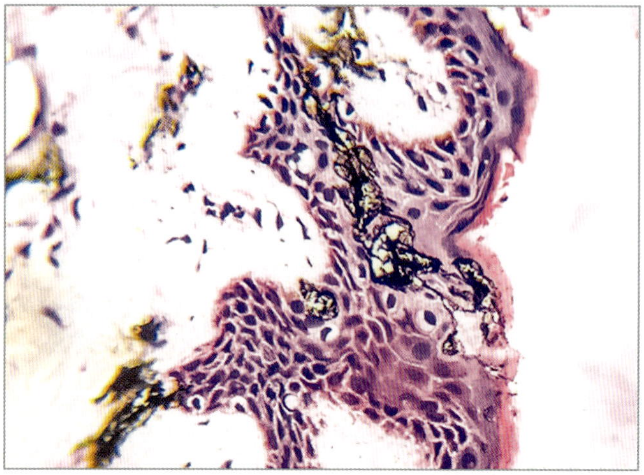

Fig. 2: When the pigment is deposited superficially as shown in this figure, it gets washed off soon and does not give the desired effect.

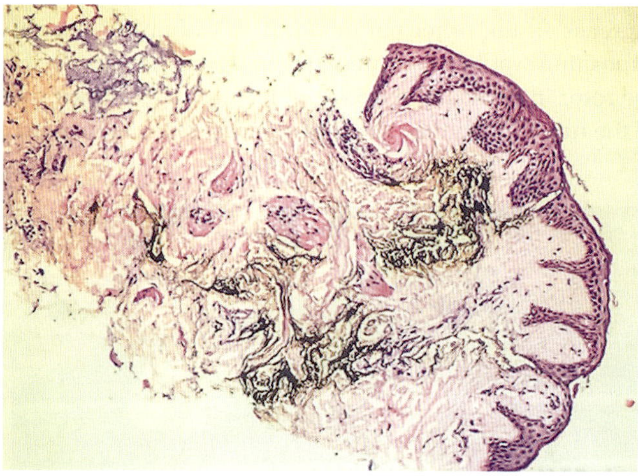

Fig. 3: When the pigment is deposited in deeper dermis as shown in the figure, there is diffusion of pigment and results in a blotchy appearance.

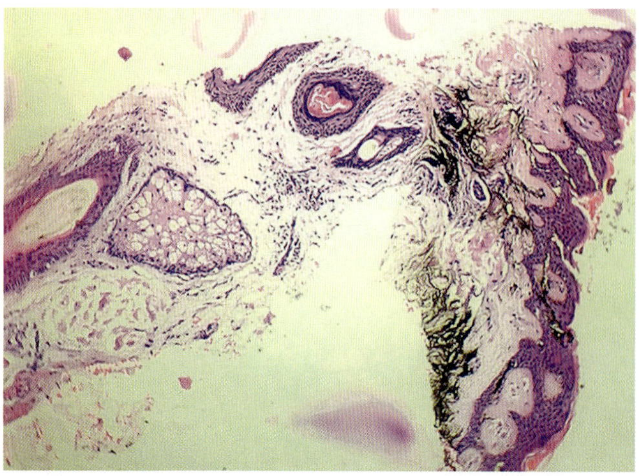

Fig. 4: Pigment should be placed as high in the dermis as possible. Proper deposition of pigment controls the degree of darkness.

number of oscillations of the needle. The speed of the rotor should be adjusted to 5,500–6,500 cycles per minute and the time of needle-to-skin contact should be 0.5–1.0 second. If the speed of the rotor is high, the surgeon would have to decrease the needle contact time to avoid over deposition of pigment. If the rotor speed is kept very slow the needle would not penetrate the skin due to lack of adequate force. Similarly, in certain situations like in cicatricial alopecia where the skin resistance is high, higher speed of rotor is required for penetration into the skin.

Resistance of Scalp

Various disease processes or scalp surgeries lead to changes in the structure of the skin. Epidermis of elderly patients or in individuals who undergo transplant or scalp skin which has developed chronic photodamage in advanced alopecia is not the same as normal skin. Atrophic or scarred skin would not react in the same way to pigment deposition as normal skin. The reduced blood supply and dermal fat in atrophic skin would also affect pigment deposition. In view of these variables, the depth of needle and speed of rotor would need adjustment accordingly. In such cases, it is advisable to start with a test patch to get an estimate on the parameters before proceeding to rest of the scalp.

Color of Pigment

The color of the pigment would influence the final color of the dots deposited.

Authors experimented using black, brown-black, and brown pigment and found that brown ink showed poor retention over time in Indian patients **(Figs. 5A and B)**. Thus, authors prefer to use plain black color for SMP. Sunlight may cause the ink to break down and make it is less visible. NCTR (National Center for Toxicology Research) researchers have found that Pigment Yellow 74 decomposes in sunlight, breaking down into components that are colorless. The pigment components may still be there and they could be potentially toxic. Therefore, yellow color is best avoided for mixing.

Viscosity of Dye

Viscosity of the dye used also influences the proper deposition of dye. If the dye is more watery in consistency its deposition is inadequate due to the dilution of the pigments.

Needle Number and Thickness

The needles that are used for SMP are either single pronged or triple pronged. The choice of needle used varies with the target area. Single pronged needle is used for the area close to the scalp hairline or eyelid tattooing to create fine dots. Triple pronged needle is used when covering the rest of the scalp.

Apart from these earlier mentioned variables, authors believe there are additional factors that would greatly influence the aesthetic appearance of the procedure.

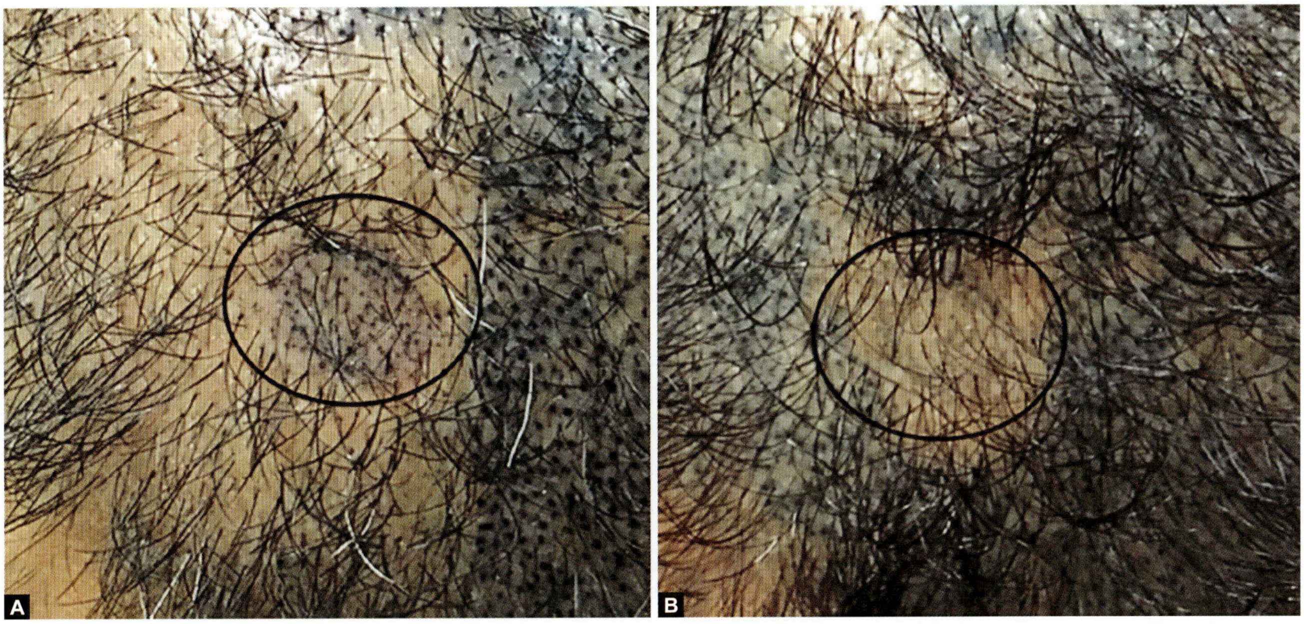

Figs. 5A and B: Experiment of using brown pigment in ratio was done in a patient. In the same patient deposition of pigment with black color was also done to assess influence of depth of deposition. After 3 weeks the brown pigment deposited in the area marked by the circle was washed off compared to the retention of the black pigment in the surrounding area.

Pattern of Dot Placement

The pattern is a very important parameter influencing the outcome of the procedure. Dots should not be placed in a regular grid or a linear fashion. Instead, the dots should be equidistant in an irregular fashion.[11] By placing dots in a random fashion it prevents the pattern from being caught readily to the naked eye thereby augmenting the aesthetic utility of SMP by eliminating the "see-through" effect **(Fig. 6)**.

Expertise of Operator

It requires considerable skill and experience of the operator to gauge the feel of resistance and master depth control while performing SMP. In addition to the earlier variables, only with experience can the operator perform the procedure effectively by considering the anticipated loss of superficially deposited pigment in the epidermis as well as slight diffusion of pigment that occurs over time.

INSTRUMENTS FOR SCALP MICROPIGMENTATION

There are various machines which can be used for SMP ranging from the basic machine that is used by tattoo artists to specialized medical tattoo machines **(Fig. 7)**.

The specialized medical tattooing machine has its advantages over its conventional counterpart by being light in weight and allowing precision for accurate needle depth insertion to the ideal depth of 0.8–1.0 mm and thereby also decreasing the pain and discomfort caused to the patient. In the conventional tattoo machine, the needle length has to be set manually by rough estimation by adjusting the needle chamber and locking it on the handle using a screw. Both the machines have provisions for selecting the desired rotor speed as needed.

The conventional tattoo machine has a power adapter attached to a primary unit which has a digital display and dial to adjust the speed to the rotor. The unit is connected to the handle with a wire which supplies the current for achieving desired speed. The handle has a hollow center through which the needle (single or triple pronged) is inserted, and a disposable transparent plastic chamber is placed over the needle which covers the needle. The cylindrical tube at the tip of the plastic chamber acts as reservoir to hold the dye while performing SMP.

The medical tattooing machine consists of a single handpiece which is attached to a power supply. The handpiece has a button to select one of the desired presets of rotor speed. The tip of the handpiece must be attached to a disposable cartridge which has a prefixed needle inside, which can be used for SMP. The cartridge has a conical tip through which the needle projects and it also acts as a reservoir for the ink during the procedure.

The tattoo inks are available in gel base as well as alcohol base. The alcohol-based dye is the one commonly used but in patients with oily scalp the gel-based dye can be used. There are various inks available in the market in a wide range of quality and cost.

PROCEDURE

1. Appropriate selection of patient as per the indication so that the procedure leads to satisfactory results.

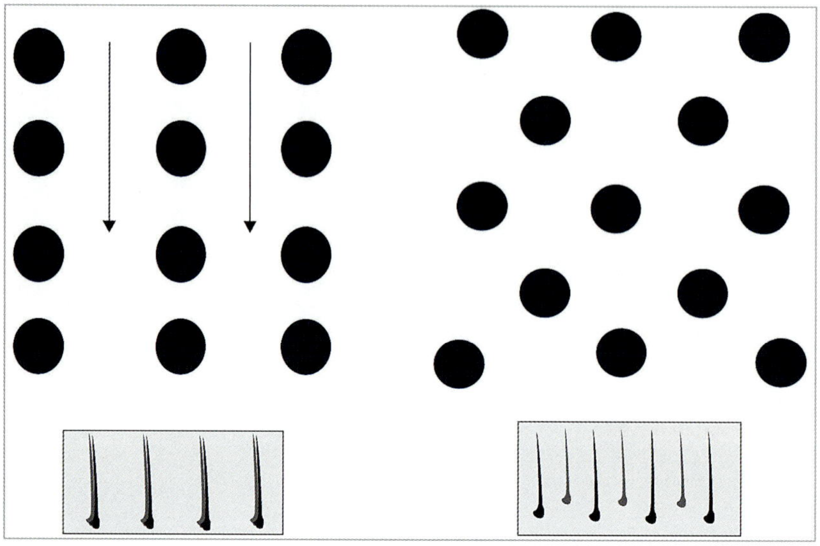

Fig. 6: Placement of dots in a linear grid fashion would result in a "see-through" effect which can be eliminated by placing the dots in a random brick fashion.

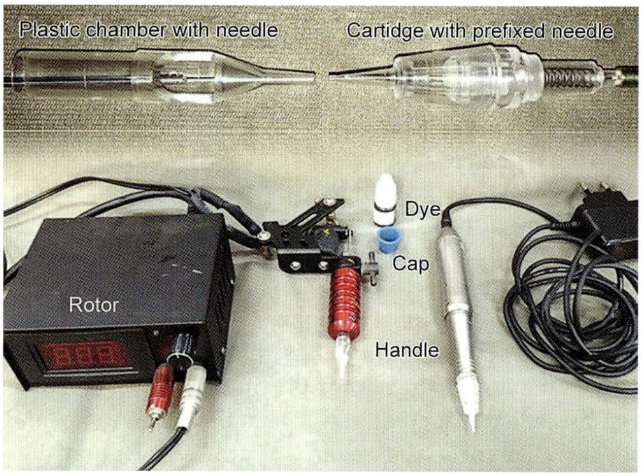

Fig. 7: The conventional tattoo machine with its chamber containing the needle on the left which is commonly used by tattoo artists. The specialized medical tattoo machine with its cartridge containing needle on the right.

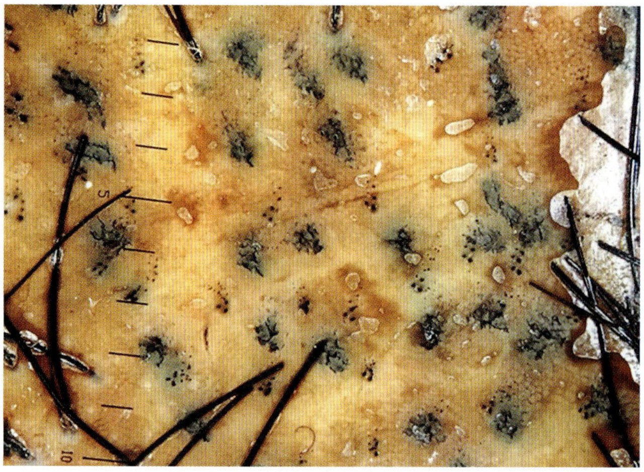

Fig. 8: Trichoscopic evaluation for assessment of adequate pigment deposition.

2. Explaining the procedure to patient and taking consent for the procedure.
3. Certain drugs and herbs which may lead to increased bruising or bleeding and hence should be avoided for 10–14 days prior to the procedure. These include nonsteroidal anti-inflammatory drugs (NSAIDs), aspirin, *Ginkgo*, ginger, vitamin E, Ginseng and *G. biloba*.
4. Local anesthesia is usually not required. However, in uncooperative or apprehensive patients, topical anesthesia may be used.
5. Clean the area with betadine and spirit to prepare the treated area.
6. Set up the machine by selecting appropriate needle number, needle length, and rotor speed
7. The pigment is taken in sterile plastic well and the conical tip of the activated handle is dipped into the ink whereby the ink is sucked into the chamber around the needle by capillary action.
8. The handle of the tattoo machine is held vertically in a pen holding fashion perpendicular to the surface of the skin and the pigment is placed as needed.
9. At regular intervals, the tip must be dipped in the ink to refill the chamber as needed.

Trichoscopy can be used for gauging proper placement of dots. Immediately after the procedure over a small area (test patch), wipe the excess dye and examine with a dermatoscope. If the dots are faint with marking only on the surface they will disappear with the epidermal turnover in a few weeks. For ideal placement, some dye should be visible in the underlying dermis when seen through the dermatoscope **(Fig. 8)**. After the initial test area, entire area is treated.

Postprocedure

- Apply antibiotic ointment over the performed area for 2 days.
- Patient is advised to avoid washing the treated area for 48 hours.
- Retouch can be done after 1 month if required.
- Patient should be explained that it would be necessary to dye the hair black on a continuous basis if there are many gray hairs. For the same reason, SMP would not be recommended for patients who frequently change their hair color.[12]

PIGMENTS

Manufacturers of inks and pigments are not required to reveal the contents. The information is proprietary—a trade secret—so you may or may not get answers to questions **(Table 1)**. Pigments and tattoo inks are not regulated by the US Food and Drug Administration (FDA). However, the FDA is examining tattoo inks to determine the chemical composition of the inks, learn how they react and break down in the body, how light and magnetism react with inks, and whether there are short- and long-term health hazards associated with ink formulations or methods of applying the tattoos.

TABLE 1: Composition of tattoo pigments.[13]

Color	*Materials*	*Comment*
Black	Iron (II III) Oxide (Fe_3O_4) Iron (II) Oxide (FeO) Carbon Logwood	Natural black pigment is made from magnetite crystals, powdered jet, wustite, bone black, and amorphous carbon from combustion (soot) Logwood is a heartwood extract from Haematoxylon campechianum, found in Central America and the West Indies
Brown	Ochre	Ochre is composed of iron (ferric) oxides mixed with clay. Raw ochre is yellowish. When dehydrated through heating, ochre changes to a reddish color
Red	Cinnabar (HgS) Cadmium Red (CdSe) Iron (III) Oxide (Fe_2O_3) Naphthol-AS pigment	Iron (III) oxide is also known as common rust. Cinnabar and cadmium pigments are highly toxic. Naphthol reds are synthesized from Naphtha. Fewer reactions have been reported with naphthol red than the other pigments, but all reds carry risks of allergic or other reactions
Orange	Disazo diarylide and/or Disazo pyrazolone Cadmium selenide sulfide	The organics are formed from the condensation of 2 monoazo pigment molecules. They are large molecules with good thermal stability and color fastness
Yellow	Cadmium Yellow (CdS, CdZnS) Ochres Curcuma Yellow Chrome Yellow ($PbCrO_4$, often mixed with PbS) Disazo diarylide	Curcuma is derived from plants of the ginger family; aka turmeric or curcumin. Reactions are commonly associated with yellow pigments, in part because more pigment is needed to achieve a bright color
Green	Chromium Oxide (Cr_2O_3), called Casalis Green or Anadomis Green Malachite [$Cu_2(CO_3)(OH)_2$] Ferrocyanides and Ferricyanides Lead chromate Monoazo pigment Cu/Al phthalocyanine Cu phthalocyanine	The greens often include admixtures, such as potassium ferrocyanide (yellow or red) and ferric ferrocyanide (Prussian Blue)
Blue	Azure Blue Cobalt Blue Cu-phthalocyanine	Blue pigments from minerals include copper (II) carbonate (azurite), sodium aluminum silicate (lapis lazuli), calcium copper silicate (Egyptian Blue), other cobalt aluminum oxides, and chromium oxides. The safest blues and greens are copper salts, such as copper phthalocyanine. Copper phthalocyanine pigments have FDA approval for use in infant furniture and toys and contact lenses. The copper-based pigments are considerably safer or more stable than cobalt or ultramarine pigments
Violet	Manganese Violet (manganese ammonium pyrophosphate) Various aluminum salts Quinacridone Dioxazine/carbazole	Some of the purples, especially the bright magentas, are photoreactive and lose their color after prolonged exposure to light. Dioxazine and carbazole result in the most stable purple pigments
White	Lead White (Lead Carbonate) Titanium dioxide (TiO_2) Barium sulfate ($BaSO_4$) Zinc oxide	Some white pigments are derived from anatase or rutile. White pigment may be used alone or to dilute the intensity of other pigments. Titanium oxides are one of the least reactive white pigments

Flowchart 1: Components of tattoo ink.

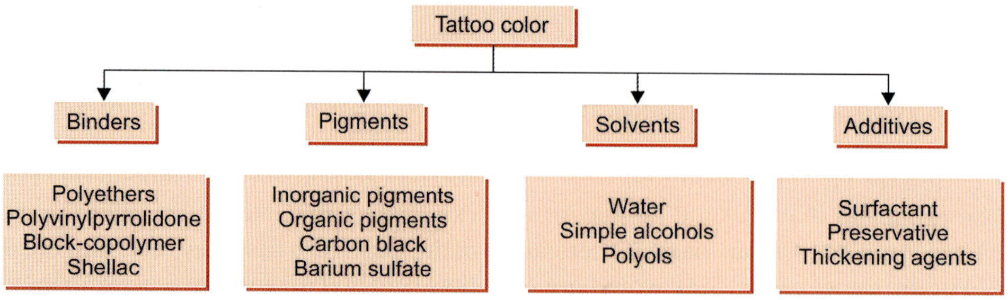

TABLE 2: Average molar masses of binding agents.

Polymer	*Molar mass*
Polyethylene glycol	200–600 g-mol^{-1} (liquid); >4,000 g-mol^{-1} (solid)
Poloxamer 188	7,680–9,510 g-mol^{-1} (solid)
Polyvinylpyrrolidone	2,500–2,500,000 g-mol^{-1} (solid)
Shellac	1,500–2,500 g·mol^{-1} (solid)
Acrylate	10,000–200,000 g·mol^{-1} (solid)

TABLE 3: Purposes of solvents used in tattoo inks.

Solvent	*Purpose*
Water	Solvation of binder
Ethanol	Regulates drying properties, masks smells
Isopropyl alcohol	Regulates drying properties, masks smells
Glycerin	Increasing viscosity, humectant
Propylene glycol	Humectant, increases dispersability

Chemistry of Pigments

The liquid of tattoo ink consists of two components: (1) a binder and (2) a solvent. The fine-dispersed pigment mixture is stabilized by additives **(Flowchart 1)**. Preservatives can be added to prevent microbiological spoilage.[14]

Binding Agents

Binding agents, or binders, are the nonvolatile compounds of tattoo ink, not including pigments and filler but including additives **(Table 2)**. Binder binds the pigment particles to each other and to the tattooing needle for easier injection of the ink into the skin. Because of their high molar mass, the binding agents are limited in their bioavailability and are not seen as an acute hazard.[14]

Solvents

All the above-mentioned binders are soluble in water. Simple and polyvalent alcohols are used to define characteristics such as drying properties, viscosity, and dispersibility **(Table 3)**.[14]

Additives

Additives are auxiliary materials that are added to exclude unwanted characteristics or to enhance wanted characteristics. The concentration of additives used in tattoo inks is not higher than 5%.

Surface active additives: Tensides are used in tattoo inks to better disperse and stabilize the pigments during the production process, leading to a longer shelf life.[14]

Preservatives

As products with a high portion of water, tattoo inks must be protected against microbiological spoilage. To reduce the risk of allergic reaction, it is best practice to waive preservatives. Water rich media provide better reproduction opportunities than water-scarce media. The water activity, as a unit for the availability of water, and not the portion of water in a medium is crucial for the reproduction of microorganisms.[14] To deny microorganisms the opportunity to reproduce in tattoo ink, the water activity value should be <0.6.

Pigment versus Dye

By definition, pigments are insoluble, organic or inorganic colorants in medium, whereas dyes are soluble organic colorants in medium. Dyes are not suitable as tattoo ink because they are soluble and will be biodegraded very fast after application.[14]

Inorganic Pigment used in SMP

Iron oxide pigments: Many variants of iron oxide are used as yellow, red and brownhued pigments. The iron oxides have a dull and nonbrilliant hue compared to inorganic pigments. Iron oxide pigments have a very high opacity. Iron oxide red, which is heat stable to temperatures up to a 1,000°C, yellow and brown iron oxides are not heat stable. In general, tattoos made of iron oxide pigments tend to change to a red hue over time.[14]

Inorganic pigments always have unwanted and quality-diminishing impurities. Nickel, chromium, copper, and cobalt are commonly found in the analyses of iron oxide pigments, but these do not lead to allergic reactions as often as expected. Perhaps the reason is the encasing of these different metals in the spinel structure. Further research is required on this matter. [14]

Carbon black: Soot, also called carbon black, is one of the pigments most suited for tattoo ink. Depending on the manufacturing process and curing, these pigments are very different in size and therefore are different in their dispersibilities. Often, the end product is described to have an aerodynamic diameter of 0.1 µm. Depending on the manufacturing process, carbon black can contain impurities in the form of polycyclic aromatic hydrocarbons.[14]

COLOR CHANGES OF PIGMENT

The excess pigment that is deposited on the surface of the skin is washed away during the first hair wash, at 48 hours after the procedure. Over the course of few weeks, there would be slight softening of the pigment as the epidermal turnover dislodges the keratinocytes with the ink in the epidermal layer. With experience, the operator learns to anticipate some loss of the pigment in the initial few days after the procedure from the superficially deposited pigment in the epidermal layers. Over the course of 1–2 weeks, ink particles start aggregating more focally in the upper dermis. Biopsy samples taken from the pigment deposited areas after 2–3 months or 40 years after procedure have shown the ink to be present mostly in the dermis intracellularly (perivascular dermal fibroblasts) or extracellularly, without any trace of pigment in the epidermis. Dermis may show signs of some fibrosis and on occasion giant cell reactions (foreign body type). The speed of development of pigment-induced foreign body reaction depends on various factors such as subjective variation, quantity, and quality of ink and the physiological or pathological condition of the treated skin.

It has been observed by the authors that using only black pigment leads to a bluish-green tinge. The bluish-green color resulting from the use of black pigment can be compared with the blood vessels carrying red blood that appear green under the surface of the skin. This phenomenon results from absorption of majority of the red spectrum of light which can be explained through the trichromatic theory of color vision.[11] In author's experience, the amount of pigment retention over time varies with each individual and on an average, there is 20–40% reduction in the pigment by 1 year which might warrant a repeat procedure to reinforce the camouflage.

INDICATIONS

- In female pattern hair loss (FPHL), there is reduction in overall hair density without the recession of frontal hairline resulting in a "see-through appearance".[10] SMP can serve as an effective therapeutic option in such patients by camouflaging the hair loss.
- *For donor scarring after hair transplantation:* Micropigmentation can be used to hide the donor area scars seen as hypopigmented dots after follicular unit extraction or linear scars after follicular unit transplantation.
- After hair transplantation if the patients are not satisfied with the results, SMP can be used to further augment the results **(Figs. 9A and B)**.
- Scalp micropigmentation has been effectively used in piebaldism.[15]
- Scalp micropigmentation also works well for camouflaging scalp scars such as[12] cicatricial alopecia on the scalp which can be congenital (aplasia cutis congenita, incontinentia pigmenti), post-traumatic (burns, radiation-induced,

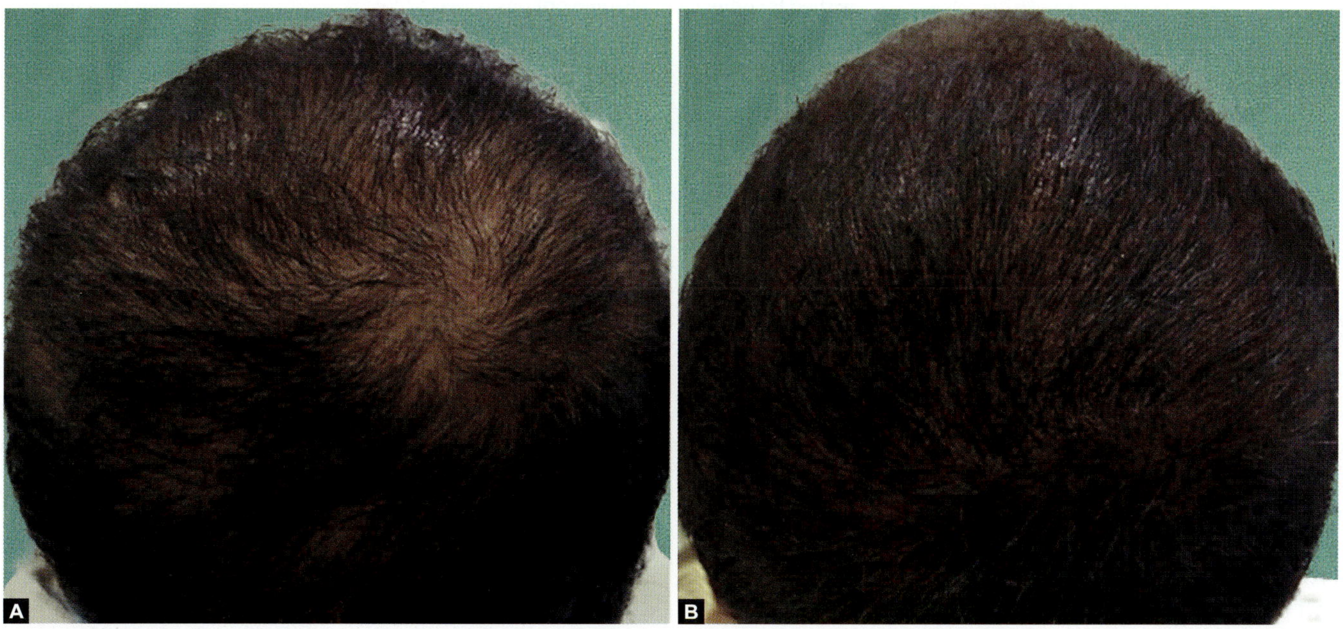

Figs. 9A and B: Pre- and post-SMP in a 28-year-old male patient with androgenetic alopecia who had undergone hair transplantation but was unsatisfied with the results on the recipient site.

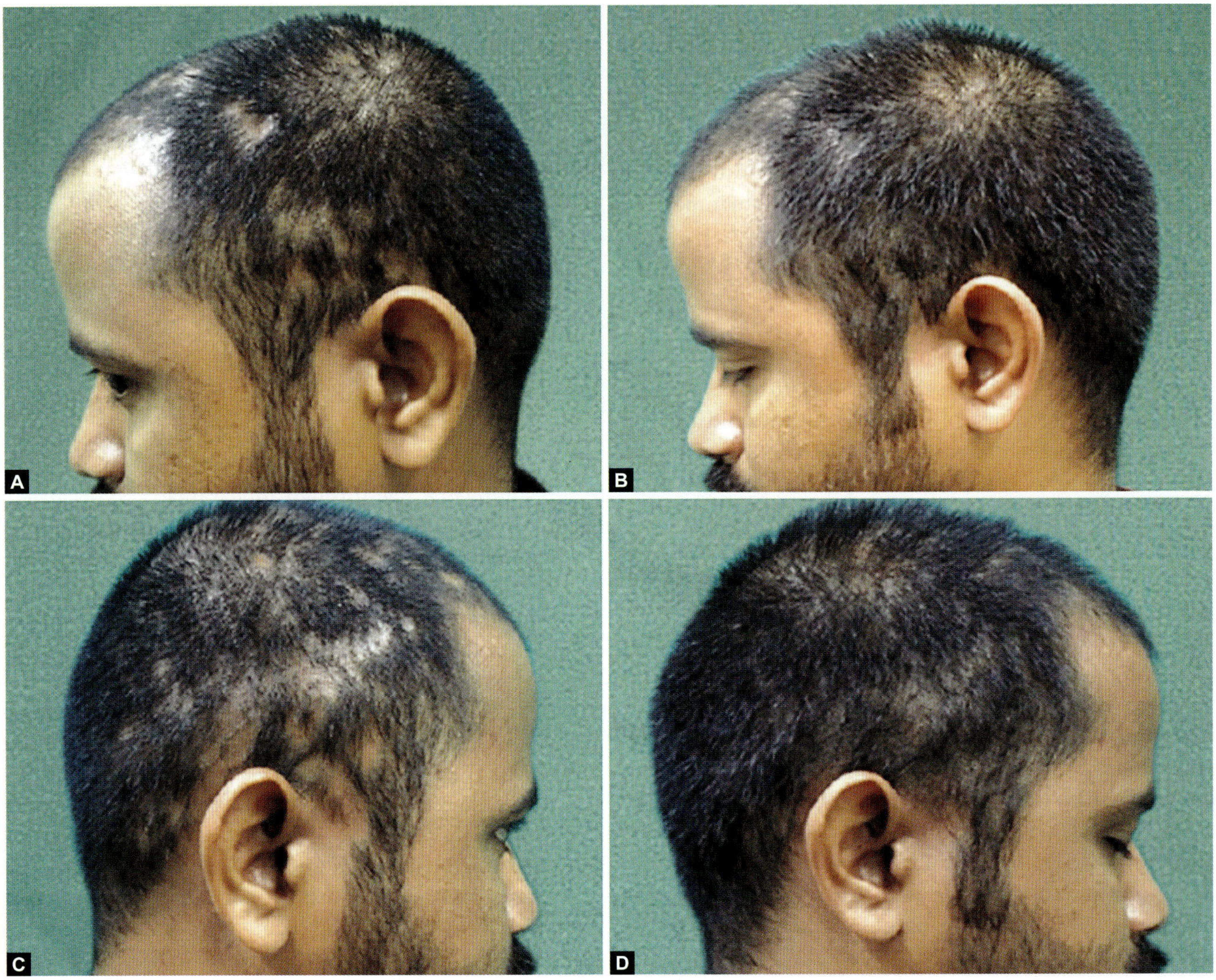

Figs. 10A to D: Pre- and post-SMP in a 32-year-old male patient with inactive lichen planopilaris who was unwilling for hair transplantation and wished for other camouflaging options.

pressure alopecia), iatrogenic (postcraniotomy) or secondary to disease processes such as discoid lupus erythematosus, lichen planopilaris **(Figs. 10A to D)**, folliculitis decalvans, inflammatory tinea capitis, dissecting cellulitis, central centrifugal cicatricial alopecia, acne keloidalis nuchae, keratosis follicularis spinulosa decalvans, etc. If the scar area is too wide the results can be further augmented by combining hair transplantation with SMP.

- Van der Velden et al. have reported excellent response in 30 out of 33 patients with alopecia areata with involvement of the eyebrows.[16]

DESIGNING A DENSER HAIRLINE

Frontal hairline consists of 2–3 cm wide area that connects and bridges the nonhairy forehead to the hairy area of the scalp. Creating a natural hairline is an essential part of hair transplant procedure which greatly influences patient satisfaction. In certain instances, due to inadequate graft availability or lack of patient satisfaction there is need for further augmenting the aesthetic appeal of the hairline; this can be achieved using SMP.

To create an appealing natural looking hairline, simply using a fine paintbrush would not be enough as the operator also needs to know how to paint. The hairline area, for better understanding can be further segregated into three zones: (1) the transition zone which is formed by the anterior portion (0.5–1 cm of frontal area), (2) the defined zone formed by the posterior portion, and (3) a frontal tuft area which is a part of the defined zone in the central portion in the shape of a small oval **(Fig. 11)**. Each of these zones contribute uniquely to give the appearance of a natural hairline.[17] A hairline that stands out and looks abrupt like a harsh wall does not look natural. The severity of hair loss determines the density and width of the transition zone. If the degree of hair loss is great, the transition zone would need to be wider and more diffuse. A natural hairline should start soft to provide transition to increasing density posteriorly over a few millimeters to a centimeter.

Defined zone which lies posteriorly to the transition zone and is 2–3 cm wide, needs to have a higher density and definition, but continue to appear undetectable on close inspection. Frontal tuft which is formed by the central oval part of the defined zone needs to have an even higher density than the rest of the defined zone which helps in further adding to the aesthetic significance of the hairline. Also, the hairline is never a straight uniform line but consists of micro- and macroirregularities. Closer inspection of normal hairlines reveals triangle-shaped, small, "intermittent" areas of density which leads to the appearance of irregularity, which is also an important component of a natural hairline. This irregularity which is noticed on a close examination is termed as *microirregularity*. If a normal hairline is examined from a little distance once can appreciate that it is not along a uniform line but is more curvaceous or serpentine; this irregularity is known as *macroirregularity*. A straight hairline would appear like a harsh wall which would be abnormal and not look natural.[17]

For these reasons, while performing SMP in the transition zone, single pronged needles are preferred whereas when targeting the defined zone, triple pronged needles are preferred to give a more filling effect **(Figs. 12A and B)**.

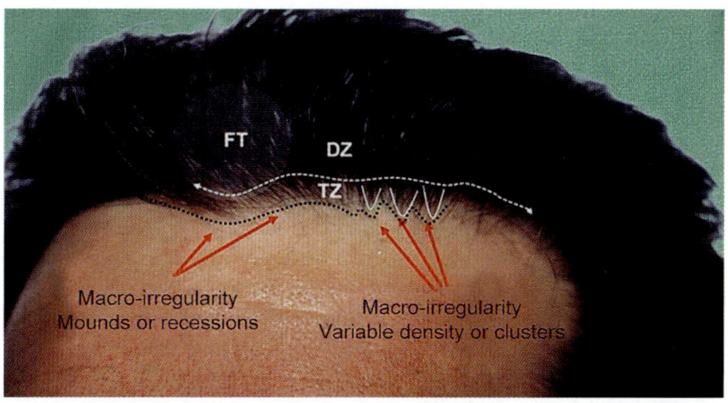

Fig. 11: This picture is an example of a natural hair line. The white dotted line separates the transition zone (TZ) from defined zone (DZ) and frontal tuft (FT). The black dotted line follows the "macroirregular" anterior border of the TZ. Notice the "microirregularity" created by areas of intermittent increased density within the transition zone.
Source: Dr Ronald Shapiro.

CONTRAINDICATIONS

As SMP is a form of tattooing, it is often perceived as a harmless, risk-free procedure. There are certain situations when caution has to be exercised by the physician before recruiting a patient for SMP:[18]

- Chronic skin diseases which may be exaggerated due to Koèbnerization
- Past history of tattoo reaction with a black ink
- Personal or family history of melanoma
- Atypical mole syndrome with lesions over the scalp
- Past history of immunosuppressive conditions [leukemia, human immunodeficiency virus (HIV)] or intake of immunosuppressive treatment(s)
- Inherited or acquired blood disorders (hemophilia, von Willebrand disease)
- *Pregnancy or breast feeding:* For the mother, the complications are the same as for any other individuals getting a tattoo. For the fetus, the risks of transmission of infection and toxic chemicals through the placenta and the milk have never been evaluated
- Complete graying of hair is a relative contraindication.

COMPLICATIONS

In comparison to the magnitude with which SMP is performed in the Western countries the incidence of reported complications is relatively sparse. Majority of the reported complications to tattoos have been seen when procedure was performed in parlors. The complications mainly occur when unsterile pigments are used or if the procedure is performed without sterile precautions. They can present from days to years from the time of procedure depending on the type of reaction developing at the site of tattooing. The following complications are:

- Patient can develop infection at the site of procedure. Bacterial or viral infection can present in days to weeks after the procedure. However, mycobacterial or fungal infections can take months or years to develop.
- Skin diseases such as vitiligo, lichen planus or psoriasis may be exacerbated due to Koèbnerization after tattooing.[19]
- Allergic reactions to the tattoo pigment can be seen but this is more common when mercury salt (red), cadmium (yellow), cobalt (blue) and dichromate (green)-based

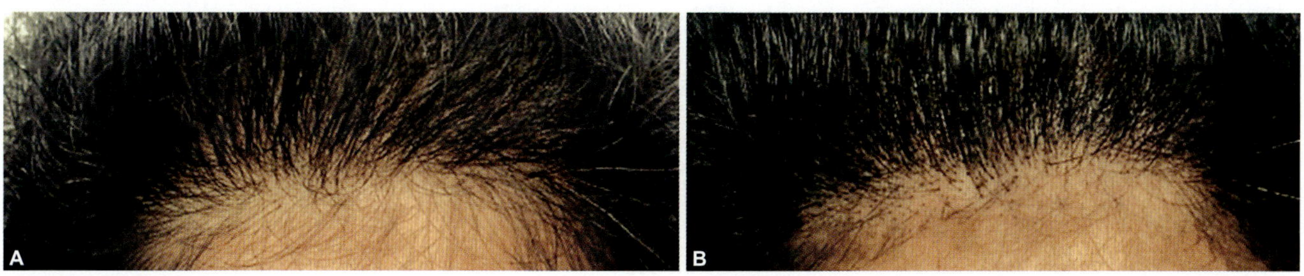

Figs. 12A and B: Note closely placed thicker dots in the dense zone with relative sparsity and use of finer dots in the transition zone.

pigments are used. Also, allergic reactions can occur if the pigment is contaminated by nickel sulfate.[20]

- Occurrence of keloids.
- Tattooing can also lead to granulomatous reactions which can be present either as sarcoidal granulomas or can also present as other granulomatous reactions like foreign body granulomas.[21]
- Tattooing can lead to formation of benign lesions in the form of milia, epidermal cysts and seborrheic keratosis; or in rare instances malignant lesions may be seen as malignant melanoma, basal cell carcinoma, squamous cell carcinoma, keratoacanthoma and dermatofibrosarcoma protuberans.[22] A case of primary non-Hodgkin lymphoma arising in the tattoo has also been reported.[22] In comparison to the large number of people who undergo tattooing the few rare instances of malignant lesions could be just coincidental. However, it is possible that various factors could play a role such as use of black ink containing benzapyrene which is a carcinogenic substance, genetic factors or exposure to ultraviolet (UV) radiation.[20]
- FDA has not approved any tattoo pigments for injection into the skin. This applies to all tattoo pigments, including those used for ultraviolet (UV) and glow-in-the-dark tattoos. Many pigments used in tattoo inks are industrial-grade colors suitable for printers' ink or automobile paint. The use of henna in temporary tattoos has not been approved by FDA. Henna is approved only for use as a hair dye. Do-it-yourself tattoo removal products are non-FDA approved acid-based products and can cause bad skin reactions.[23]

CONCLUSION

Scalp micropigmentation can be a useful mode of managing hair loss, particularly in selected patients, proper technique is essential, and this can only be acquired by proper training.

TIPS AND PEARLS

- Use good quality pigment for optimum results
- Proper designing and use of the right equipment are key to produce satisfactory results
- Proper counseling and education of patient should be undertaken in all patients
- Right depth and design of SMP can be acquired by proper training.

REFERENCES

1. Vassileva S, Hristakieva E. Medical applications of tattooing. Clin Dermatol. 2007;25(4):367-74.
2. Garg G, Thami GP. Micropigmentation: tattooing for medical purposes. Dermatol Surg. 2005;31(8 Pt 1):928-31.
3. Grumet GW. Psychodynamic implications of tattoos. Am J Orthopsychiatry. 1983;53(3):482-92.
4. Van der Velden EM, de Jong BD, van der Walle HB, Stolz E, Naafs B. Tattooing and its medical aspects. Int J Dermatol. 1993;32(5):381-4.
5. Pauli. Ueber das Feuermaal und die einzig sichere Methode, diease ensteullung zu heilen. J Geburttsh. 1835;15:66-72.
6. Turell R, Marino AW. Technic of tattooing with mercury sulfide for pruritus ani. Ann Surg. 1942;115(1):126-30.
7. Von Wecker L. Das Tätowiren der Hornhaut. Arch Augenheilkunde. 1872;2:84-7.
8. Earley MJ. Basal cell carcinoma arising in tattoos: a clinical report of two cases. Br J Plast Surg. 1983;36(2):258-9.
9. Traquina AC. Micropigmentation as an adjuvant in cosmetic surgery of the scalp. Dermatol Surg. 2001;27(2):123-8.
10. Limmer BL. The density issue in hair transplantation. Dermatol Surg. 1997;23(9):747-50.
11. Rassman WR, Pak JP, Kim J, Estrin SF. Scalp micropigmentation: a concealer for hair and scalp deformities. J Clin Aesthet Dermatol. 2015;8(3):35-42.
12. Park JH, Moh JS, Lee SY, You SH. Micropigmentation: camouflaging scalp alopecia and scars in Korean patients. Aesthetic Plast Surg. 2014;38(1):199-204.
13. Helmenstine AM. Tattoo Ink Chemistry. New York: ThoughtCo.; 2020.
14. Serup J, Kluger N, B.umler W. Tattooed skin and health. Curr Probl Dermatol. 2015;48:118-27.
15. Offidani A, Cellini A, Peramezza C, Di Giuseppe A, Di Benedetto G. Tattooing: an alternative treatment for piebaldism. Eur J Dermatol. 1993;3:508.
16. van der Velden EM, Drost BH, Ijsselmuiden OE, Baruchin AM, Hulsebosch HJ. Dermatography as a new treatment for alopecia areata of the eyebrows. Int J Dermatol. 1998;37(8):617-21.
17. Shapiro R. Creating a natural hairline in one session using a systematic approach and modern principles of hairline design. Int J Cosm Surg Anesth Dermatol. 2001;3(2):89-99.
18. Kluger N. Cutaneous and systemic complications associated with tattooing. Presse Med. 2016;45(6 Pt 1):567-76.
19. Khunger N, Molpariya A, Khunger A. Complications of tattoos and tattoo removal: stop and think before you ink. J Cutan Aesthet Surg. 2015;8(1):30-6.
20. Kaatz M, Elsner P, Bauer A. Body-modifying concepts and dermatologic problems: tattooing and piercing. Clin Dermatol. 2008;26(1):35-44.
21. Wenzel SM, Rittmann I, Landthaler M, Bäumler W. Adverse reactions after tattooing: review of the literature and comparison to results of a survey. Dermatology. 2013;226(2):138-47.
22. Armiger WG, Caldwell EH. Primary lesion of a non- Hodgkin's lymphoma occurring in a skin tattoo: case report. Plast Reconstr Surg. 1978;62(1):125-7.
23. Think Before You Ink: Are Tattoos Safe? FDA. [online] Available from: https://www.fda.gov/consumers/consumer-updates/think-you-ink-are-tattoos-safe. [Last Accessed April, 2021].

CHAPTER 75

Hair Transplant Repair

Nirav V Desai, Tushar D Kshirsagar

KEY MESSAGES

- The repair surgeries are not uncommon now a days and the demand will increase in future as there is steep rise in the number of hair transplant surgeries done all over and many of such surgeries are done by freelancing technicians or untrained and unskilled persons leading to unsatisfactory and poor outcomes.
- Broadly the hair transplant repair is classified as repair of the recipient site and repair of the donor site. The recipient site repair is the commonest type of hair transplant repair.
- Repair includes methods to salvage and redistribute viable grafts, scar revision in cases of poor donor area, camouflaging scars, including SMP (Scalp Micropigmentation) or specific hair styling methods.
- We have classified each hair transplant error individually in order to discuss in detail how to correct each one of them. In reality, however, often multiple errors are present together which requires a good assessment of the problem, patient's expectation, available treatment options and detailed counseling for the satisfactory outcome.

INTRODUCTION

There has been a steep rise in demand for hair transplantation during the last decade, making it one of the most common cosmetic surgeries done across the globe. However, at the same time, there has been a rising unsavory trend of untrained and unqualified individuals performing hair transplants at almost every corner. This has resulted in numerous instances of poorly aesthetic and unsatisfactory outcomes. The procedure carried out to correct the errors of previously failed transplants is called a repair hair transplantation. Although most of repair hair transplants are for recipient sites, a good number of patients still require repair of the donor area.

REPAIR OF RECIPIENT SITE

The reasons for having poor outcomes of the hair transplant surgery requiring repair at the recipient site can be as follows:

- Poor designing and improper technique to create recipient sites
- Poor hair growth due to damage to the hair follicles during extraction, storage, and implantation
- Combination of both.

Repair of the recipient site can be divided into the following four sections:

1. Repair of hairline
2. Correction of frontotemporal angels and temples
3. Correction of density (grafts distribution) in various parts
4. Repair of complications due to poor graft placement

Repair of Hairline

Poor and unnatural-looking hair growth after a hair transplant is the prime reason for the need of repair surgery. It can be seen as an isolated problem or in association with poor growth in the central zone of the scalp. In the past, repair methods have been described by Manfred Lucas known as "Lucas Method", and by Vance Elliott known as "PASSO Algorithm".[1]

"LUCAS" Method

"LUCAS method" of hair transplant repair involves extraction of the misplaced grafts by using an electric-powered rotary punch. This method, described by German hair transplant surgeon Manfred Lucas, involves using a 2.25-mm diameter punch for graft extraction. This was mostly used for correcting the old cases of "mini-graft hair transplant", the utility of this method in current era is limited.

"PASSO" Algorithm

Hair transplant repair methods have been described with the help of the "PASSO" algorithm of hair transplant repair. This method involves taking into consideration the following:

- P—Position, i.e., position of the planted hairline relative to the other facial structures.
- A—Angles, i.e., angles of the planted hair in sagittal and coronal planes.
- S—Shape, i.e., the shape of the hairline, whether it appears natural and matches the face.

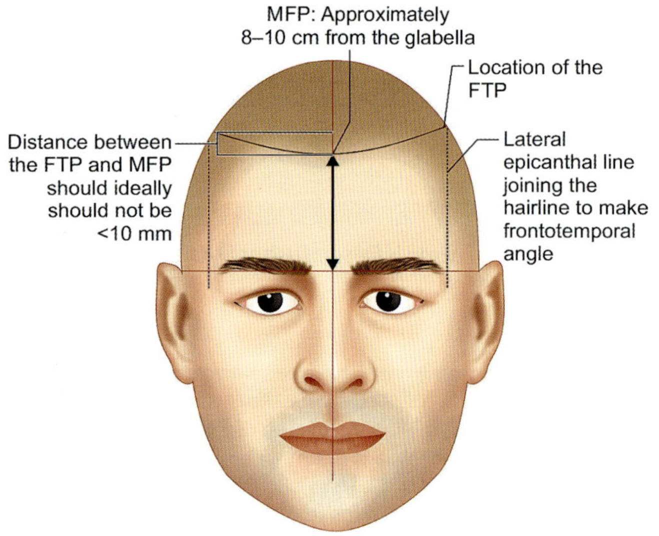

Fig. 1: Midfrontal point (MFP) and frontotemporal point (FTP) for hairline design.

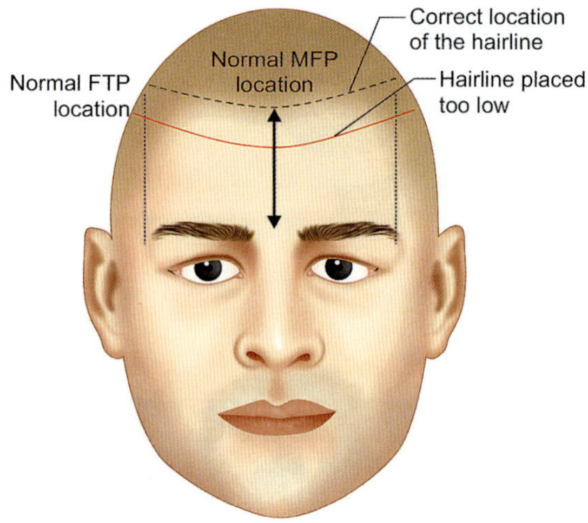

Fig. 2: Schematic of hairline placed too low. (FTP: frontotemporal point; MFP: midfrontal point)

- S—Softness, i.e., whether the hairline begins softly or abruptly, drawing undue attention to the hairline.
- O—Others, i.e., any other errors that do not fit in the categories described earlier.

The PASSO algorithm is mainly focusing on correcting the hairline errors. Apart from hairline, we have tried to include the errors seen at central zone of the scalp and their respective correction.

For the purpose of a repair, we have divided the repair of the hairline into two categories:

1. Repair of hairline to create good facial framing
2. Repair of frontal hairline to give it softness.

Repair of Hairline to Create Good Facial Framing

Correction of the position of frontal hairline: The ideal position of the hairline is not too low, as it may appear unnatural. Also, not too high hairline as it may not give a good cosmetic coverage **(Fig. 1)**. Common methods[1] for locating the anterior border of the hairline include:

- Four fingerbreadths above the glabella
- 8–10 cm above the glabella
- A line is drawn to the curve of the forehead from the point at which the horizontal plane of the scalp meets the vertical plane of the face.

Hairline too low: If hairline is placed too low giving a very unnatural look, the surgeon must consider removing all the implanted hair **(Fig. 2)**. It can be done with either follicular unit extraction (FUE) method or laser hair reduction. In both the methods multiple sessions may be required to achieve a near complete removal. Patient must be counseled about the possibility of scarring and pigmentary changes.

Alternatively, if there are too many grafts to remove, a surgeon can plan to remove anterior portion of the hairline by horizontal strip excision. Forehead skin is then undermined and brought upward to be sutured. After this, a narrow transition zone should be created on stitch line utilizing fine single-hair follicular units (FUs) to hide the scar. The FUs can be prepared by dissecting the removed strip and reutilized in same or the other area. The disadvantage of this approach is a horizontal full-thickness scar at anterior border of scalp, which may affect the vascular supply of the area. If a wide strip is removed, there is possibility of prominent forehead lift with clown-like raised eyebrows.

Hairline too high: This is the easiest situation when sufficient donor area is still available. The new hairline should be created anterior to the old hairline to achieve a good aesthetic appearance. The position of the new hairline should be decided according to the availability of donor hair. The gap between old and new hairlines should be filled by placing multihair FUs in good density. This will hide the errors related to angle and direction of old hairline (if any) without the need of extracting them **(Figs. 3A to E)**. If limited donor hair is available, then one can create a new hairline by creating a wider and more diffuse transition zone by using single hair FUs, then convert the transition zone of previous hairline into a defined zone by adding more two hair FUs. When donor supply of FUs is limited, one should not try to give a high density, rather spread the FUs evenly mimicking the pattern found when more severe hair loss occurs naturally with age.

Correction of errors related to the shape of the frontal hairline: Very straight/flat hairline: Hairline appears flat when midfrontal point (MFP) and frontotemporal point (FTP) are placed at the same level and macroirregularities are absent **(Figs. 4 and 5)**. If the hairline is placed too low as well, extraction of the grafts remains the only option as mentioned earlier.

If the hairline is normally positioned, then 1–3 macro-irregularities should be created in medial hairline. A central peak (widow's peak) and one or two lateral peaks can be

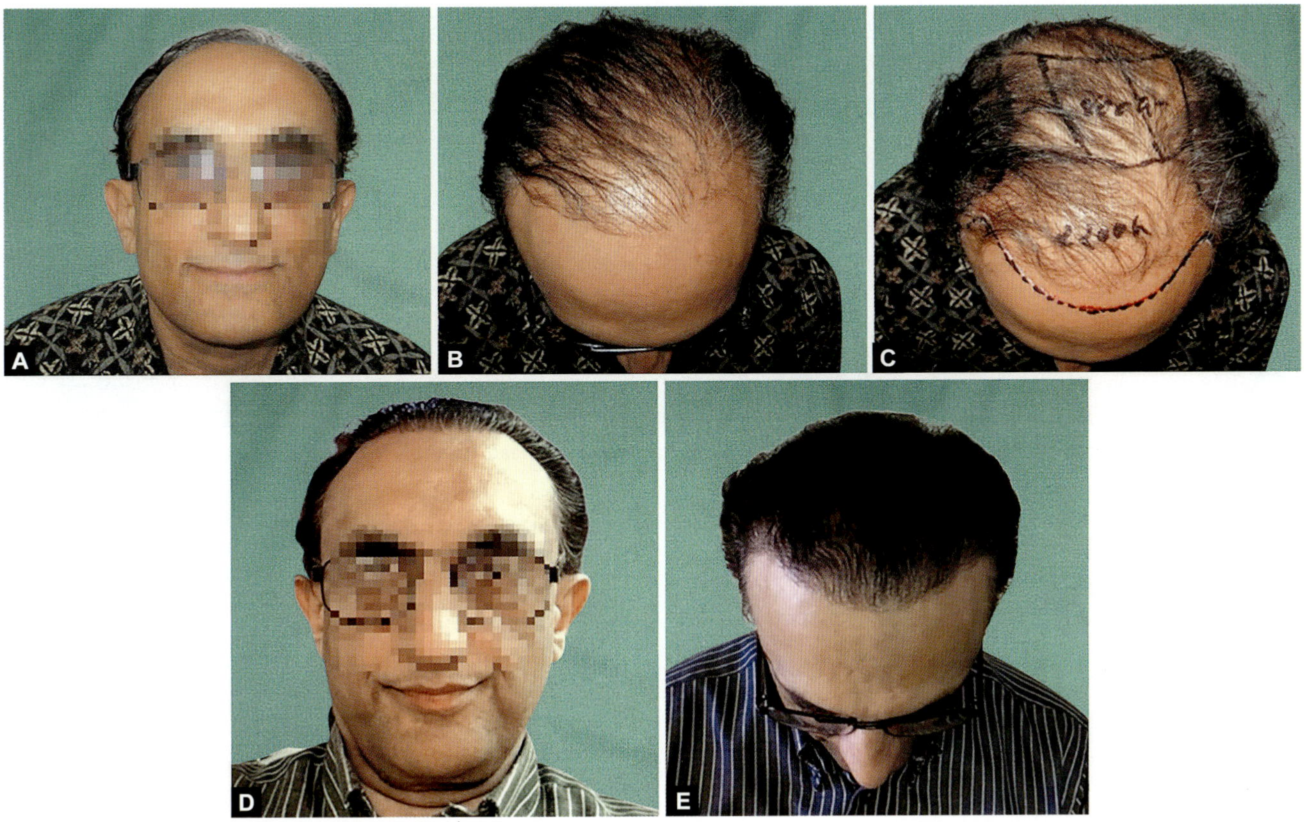

Figs. 3A to E: Correction of very high hairline. (A and B) After first surgery by follicular unit transplantation (FUT) method, the hairline created was very high with poor density; (C) Planning of repair surgery: Lowering of hairline, forelock along with whole frontal area is planted with more density compared to midscalp region where already some hairs are present. Thus, whole frontal and midscalp region looks uniformly covered; (D and E) Results 1 year after repair surgery.

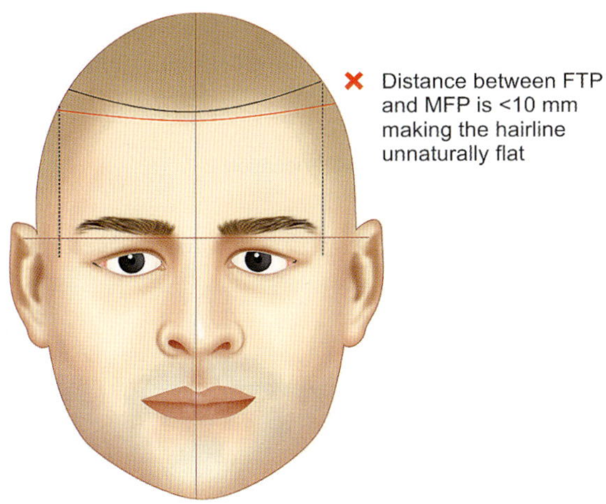

Fig. 4: Schematic of too flat hairline. (FTP: frontotemporal point; MFP: midfrontal point)

created. In addition to this, grafts from the both lateral end of the hairline can be removed, especially having thick hair and poor angulation. This will give an upward curve to the hairline and also reduce the blunting of temporal angle.

If hairline is placed too high, a new hairline below the existing one should be made as we have discussed earlier.

Concave-shaped hairline: This abnormality is opposite of naturally appearing "V"-shaped hairline **(Fig. 6)**. This occurs when MFP is placed at a higher level in comparison to the FTP. This gives a concave shape to the hairline resembling a female hairline. To correct this type of error, the surgeon should lower down the MFP in comparison to the FTP and by adding more FUs **(Figs. 7A and B)**. If required remove some of the grafts from the later ends of hairline near the temples. This will change the shape of hairline from concave to usual "V" or "U" shape, making it appear more natural.

Narrow "V"-shaped hairline: Rarely, excess lowering of the MFP along with a high FTP results in a narrow "V"-shaped hairline **(Fig. 8)**. This might be because of very conservative approach by the surgeon. Patients are often not happy with the result as it gives too big forehead with deep frontotemporal angles. Correction involves reducing the excess concavity of hairline. It is done by removal of FUs from the midportion of hairline to shift the MFP higher. Along with this, FUs should be placed at the lateral part of the anterior hairline and if required bring forward the temporal hairline. This will lower the FTP and also soften the angles.

Asymmetric hairline: Apart from earlier mentioned errors, asymmetric hairline is also commonly observed. Asymmetry can be in the form of shape, position on each side, and density of the hair. Keeping hairline slightly lower and giving more density on parting side is a common practice **(Figs. 9 and 10)**

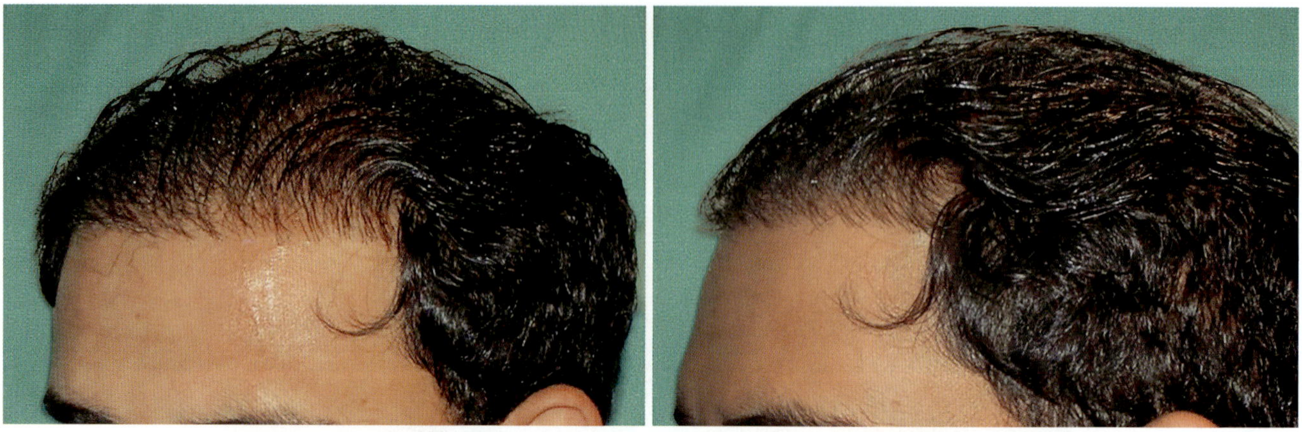

Fig. 5: Multiple errors in the hairline: Low hairline placed on forehead, relatively flat with poor density.

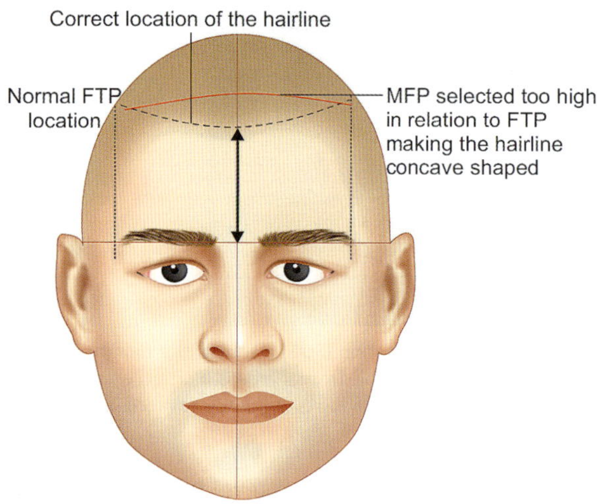

Fig. 6: Schematic of concave-shaped hairline. (FTP: frontotemporal point; MFP: midfrontal point)

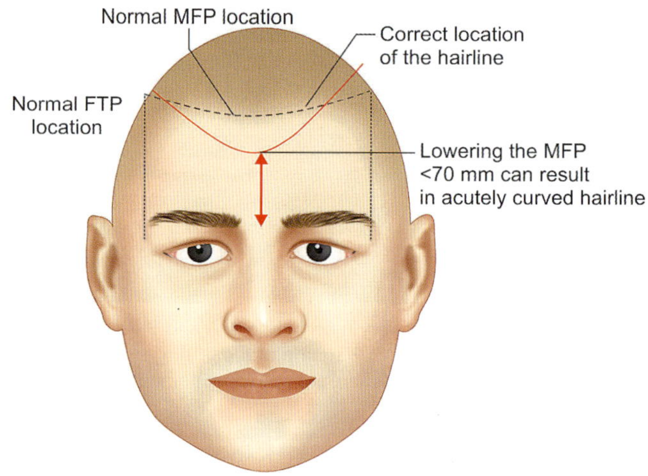

Fig. 8: Schematic of a narrow "V"-shaped hairline. (FTP: frontotemporal point; MFP: midfrontal point)

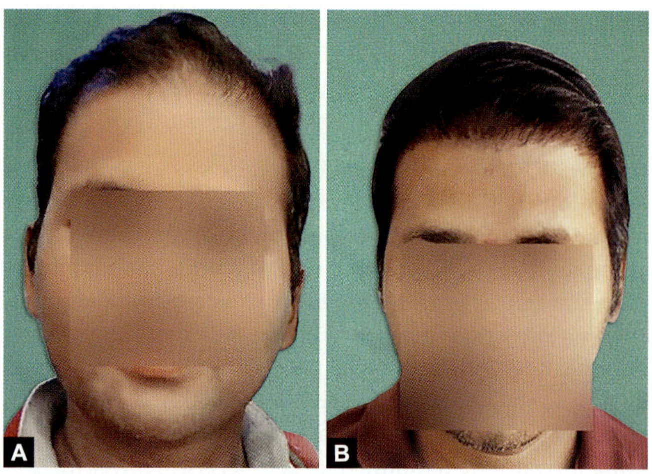

Figs. 7A and B: Repair of concave-shaped hairline (A) Concave hairline created in first hair transplant; (B) Restoring normal shape by lowering the hairline in center with single hair grafts.

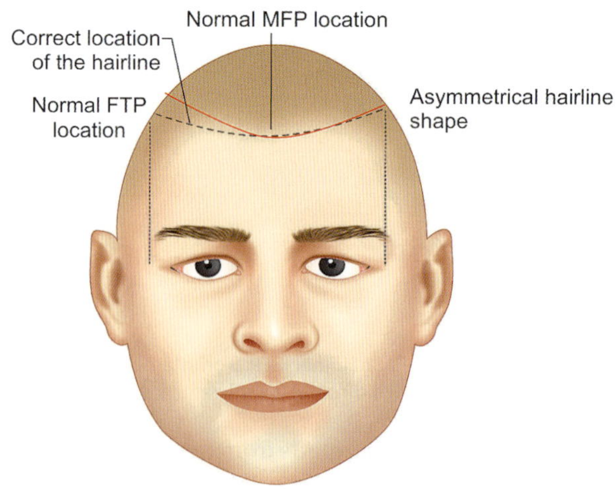

Fig. 9: Schematic of an asymmetric hairline. (FTP: frontotemporal point; MFP: midfrontal point)

among many hair transplant surgeons to effectively create an illusion of larger coverage and denser look. Exaggeration of this practice can result in an obvious asymmetric appearance. Combination of methods mentioned earlier can be used by adding or extracting FUs to rebalance the position, shape, and density of hairline.

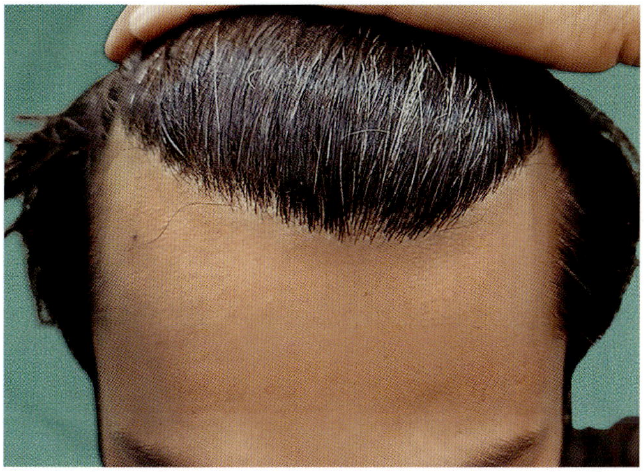

Fig. 10: Asymmetric hairline and lack of other details such as sentinel hairs, macro-, and microirregularities.

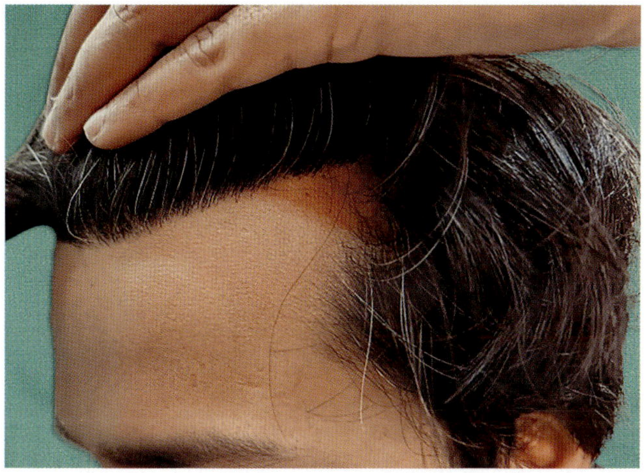

Fig. 12: Abrupt-looking hairline devoid of macro- and microirregularities.

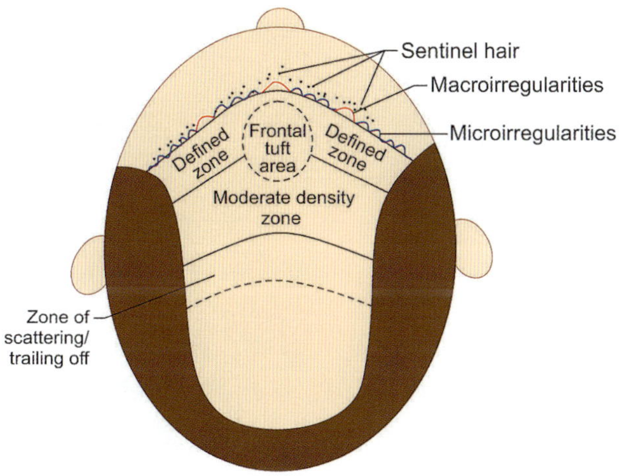

Fig. 11: Characteristics of hairline region.

Repair of Errors Affecting the Softness of Hairline

Softness of hairline is difficult to define in words but according to Vance Elliot[1] "Soft hairline do not unduly draw the attention of your eyes". Surgeons' abilities to create a natural hairline have increased dramatically over the years. Still, errors in hairline designing remain the most common cause of dissatisfaction amongst the patients. Creating a natural-looking hairline is an art. To repair poorly designed hairline, one must have better understanding and recognition of the visual characteristics that make up normal hairlines.

The hairline is not just the first few rows of hairs in frontal area[2], but it is a larger and more extended region, approximately 2–3 cm deep, bridging the bald forehead to the area of central density. This extended hairline region can be divided into three smaller zones **(Fig. 11)**.

1. The anterior portion of hairline know as transition zone.
2. Defined zone
3. A small, oval area in the central portion of the defined zone called frontal tuft area.

Commonly seen errors which affect the softness of hairline are: (1) Absence of micro- and macroirregularities making the hairline appear abrupt and flat, (2) Correction of errors in pattern of recipient site creation, (3) Incorrect angles and direction of hair, (4) Poor grafts placement—use of thick multihair grafts in hairline, especially in transition zone, (5) Incorrect density in transition and defined zone, and (6) Doll's head appearance is not commonly seen nowadays. It was common in the era of mini punch grafting where 4-mm size punches were used to take grafts and are arranged in clusters with large gaps in between giving an unnatural appearance.

Correction of abrupt-looking flat hairline due to absence of micro- and macroirregularities: Absence of macro- and microirregularities will make the hairline appear without any features and hence appears abrupt and flat **(Fig. 12)**. Both irregularities are part of transition zone of the hairline and are made up of single hair FUs. Correcting is relatively easy task. This requires creation of these irregularities specifically with single hair FUs from the scalp. At times, sentinel hairs can be created with finer hair.

Correction of errors in pattern of recipient site creation: Recipient sites should be created in a "brick wall" pattern or an "offset" triangular pattern **(Fig. 13)** to create an illusion of fullness. If the FUs are placed in parallel rows, it not only causes more vascular damage but also leads to a "see-through" effect when the hair grows. The resultant hair growth is going to appear highly unnatural and less dense. Correction is very straightforward and done by placing FUs in between parallel rows, breaking the regular pattern of exiting hair **(Fig. 14)**.

Incorrect angle, direction of hair in the hairline: In most normal scalp hairs, beginning from the hairline, the direction of the hair exiting the skin is either facing forward or facing frontomedially. And the angle of existing hair follicles in the hairline region is acute, ideally <30°. This gradually increases

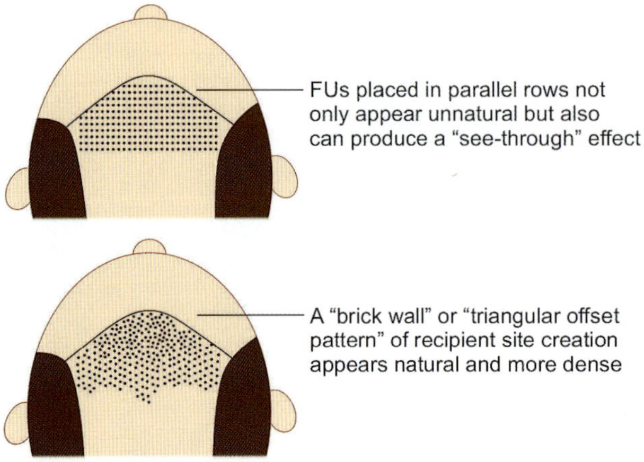

Fig. 13: Schematic showing unnatural recipient site creation versus natural-looking recipient site creation. (FUs: follicular units)

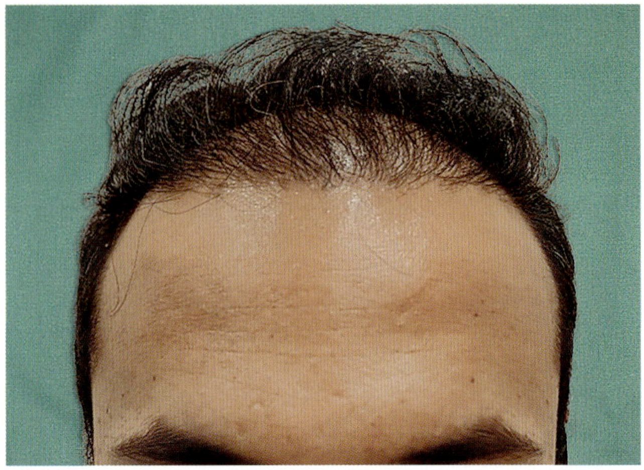

Fig. 15: Hair directed laterally as well as excessively vertical exit angle.

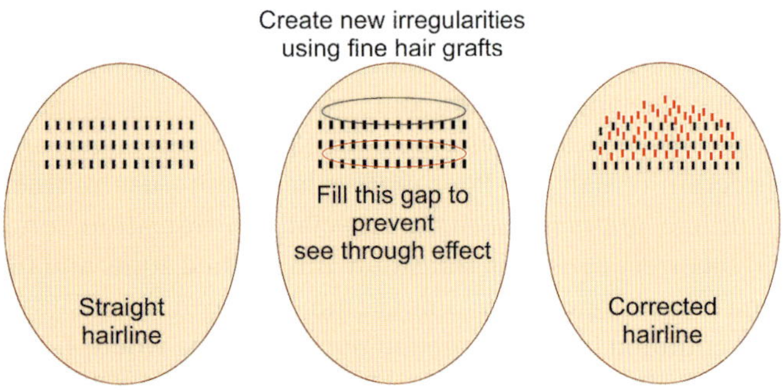

Fig. 14: Schematic representing correction of parallel recipient site creation as well as a straight hairline.

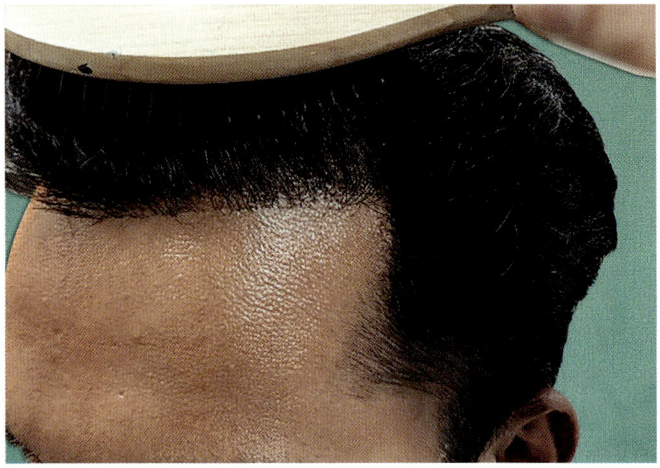

Fig. 16: Placement of multihair follicular units (FUs) in the hairline give a "pluggy" appearance to the hairline.

to 60° going posteriorly till the vertex transition zone. Samuel Lam suggests that in order to make a natural-looking hairline, a general rule to be followed is that all the FUs in the hairline are pointed down and toward the tip of the nose, i.e., in a fronto-inferio-medial direction.

If FUs are placed nearly vertical in the hairline, then it gives a "surprised look" to the hairline. Similarly, strong multihair FUs placed closely, facing laterally give an appearance, which some have described as "Statue of Liberty" appearance **(Fig. 15)**.[2] Both errors also exacerbate the spacing between the implanted hair. This makes the hairline appear much less dense than it actually is due to see through effect. Some patients face an issue while combing and setting hair, as these hairs are difficult to part and do not set down properly. Correcting this is challenging. Since the angle and direction of implanted hair cannot be changed. This problem appears to be exaggerated when multihair grafts are placed in front row. The correction is discussed along with correction of poor graft placement.

Poor placement of multihair grafts in transition zone: This often occurs due to inexperienced technicians not separating and isolating the grafts into single hair, two hair, and multihair grafts before implantation. This leads to incorrect implantation of double and triple FUs in the transition zone. With strong, large multihair grafts, the hairline typically appears "Pluggy" and artificial **(Fig. 16)**. Along with this error, if the FUs are also planted with a low density, it classically gives an appearance of "doll's hairs." This is more common with implanter pen where grafts are usually not identifiable after loading. In preslit method, this can only happen when surgery is done by inexperienced person who has no knowledge about hairline design as grafts are visible at the time of implantation.

Usually, the errors of angle, direction, and poor grafts placement are present altogether, and repair approach is more or less similar. In cases, where grafts are placed at a low density, adding more single hair grafts creates a new transition zone in front of old hairline and merges both the hairline. The newly placed single hair FUs with correct density, angles, and directions will dominate the overall appearance of hairline, and extraction of wrong grafts is not necessary. However, extraction of FUs is almost always needed if the wrongly angled and directed hairs are planted at a high density and in setting of lower positioned hairline. In such cases,

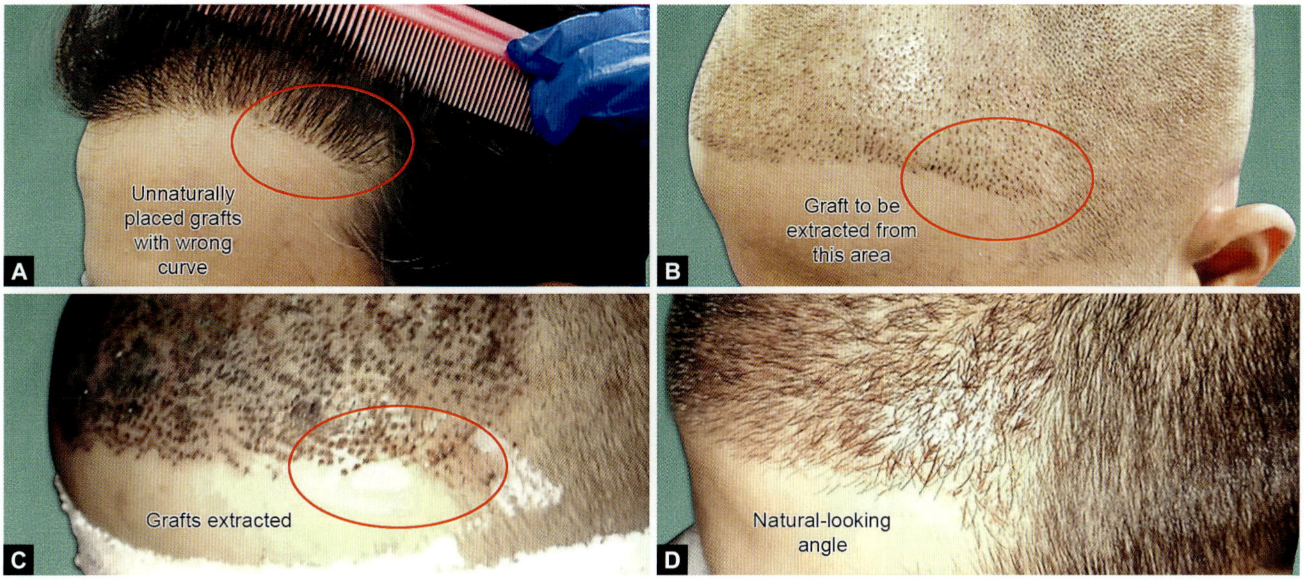

Figs. 17A to D: (A) Misdirected hair multihair grafts at frontotemporal angle; (B) After trimming, frontal hairline shows downward slope and blunt frontotemporal angle; (C) Correction: the grafts in marked area were removed by follicular unit extraction (FUE) to correct the downward slope; the single hair grafts were placed to give softness; (D) Final result: now frontotemporal angles look much softer and natural.

repositioning of hairline can be done as discussed previously with creation of an entirely new hairline.

Correction of Frontotemporal Angles and Temples

Mature male hairlines have a frontotemporal angle, which is formed by the junction of the frontal and temporal hairlines. The superior border of this angle is created by frontal hairline, whereas the temporal hairline forms its inferior border. It has to be noted here that the exit angle of hair in temples is very acute and almost parallel to skin, and direction is slowly turning posteriorly and downward. Proper positioning and recreating a soft frontotemporal angle is one of the most difficult aspects, and so it is one of the most seen errors during a repair hair transplant.

Because of the ongoing hair loss, the apex of the frontotemporal angle moves posteriorly creating deep frontotemporal recession, gradually this angle widens and makes the forehead appear broader. Patients often insist to fill these temporal recessions to make the forehead appear smaller. Usually, due to a poor understanding of hairline among the patients and inexperienced surgeons, the anterior hairline is lowered to fill the gap in frontotemporal angle. By doing this, it not only blunts the frontotemporal angle but also the angle and direction of hair are not matching with that of the temporal hairline. Hair can be seen coming out perpendicular to the temples and gives very ugly and unnatural appearance. Correction of this type of defect always involves removal of all of the misplaced grafts from temporal angles by FUE method **(Figs. 17A to D)**. Additionally, one may bring the temporal hairline forward by placing the grafts in posteroinferior direction at very acute angle to restore the temples and thereby making the forehead appear less broad. This will also soften the frontotemporal angle and give it usual couture. Large multihair grafts should be replaced with fine single hair grafts at temporal hairline and posteriorly one can use fine two hair grafts to mimic natural pattern. Such grafts can be obtained from lower part of occipital scalp near the nap of neck. Alternatively, one can use fine chest hair for the correction purpose.

Another problem, which is commonly seen in this area, is island of hair present in front of temporal hairline. This is due to partial creation of temporal fringe during first hair transplant. With time, temporal hairline slides backward due to hair loss. Thus, a gap is created between implanted hair and temporal hairline, and looks unsightly. Correction is done by removing all the hair present in the island and recreation of temporal fringe according to the grade of baldness and position of frontal hairline **(Figs. 18 and 19)**.

Correction of Density (Grafts Distribution) in Various Parts of Recipient Site

Only one-hair FUs should be used in the anterior portion of the transition zone with a shift toward two-hair FUs to its posterior portion. The defined zone is the 2–3-cm wide area that sits directly posterior to the transition zone. Using two and three hair grafts in this area gives it higher degree of definition and density giving it natural appearance even on close examination. Density in this zone creates a fuller-looking hairline by limiting the distance that can be seen past the transition zone. It creates this effect without placing hair directly in the transition zone, thereby limiting the chance

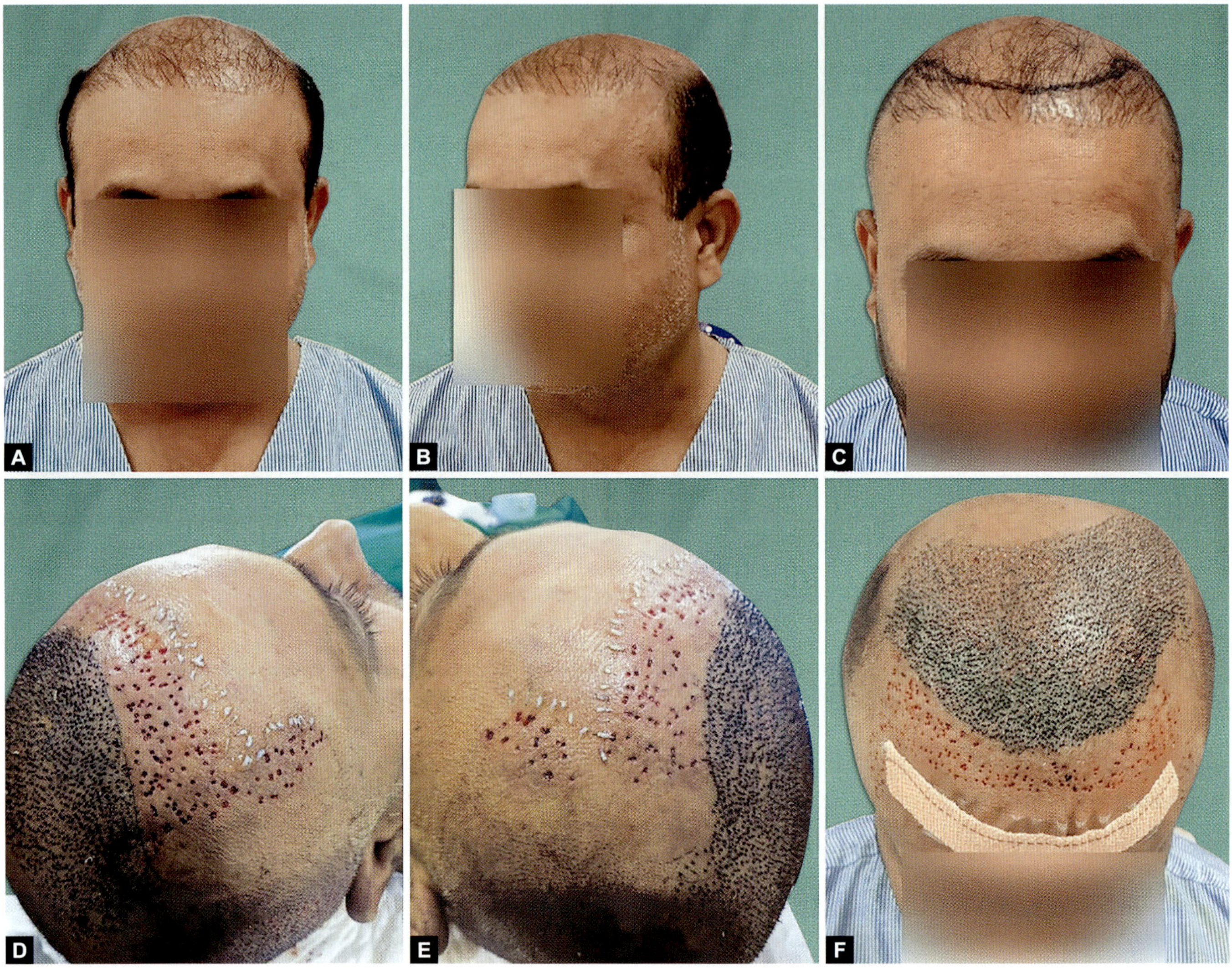

Figs. 18A to F: Correction of the island of hairs remaining in frontal area. (A and B) Remaining hair are low density, multihair follicular units (FUs) with incorrect shape as well as direction; (C) Plan for new hairline; (D and E) Extraction of all remaining FUs done by follicular unit extraction (FUE); (F) Additional FUs planted to make the new frontal are denser.

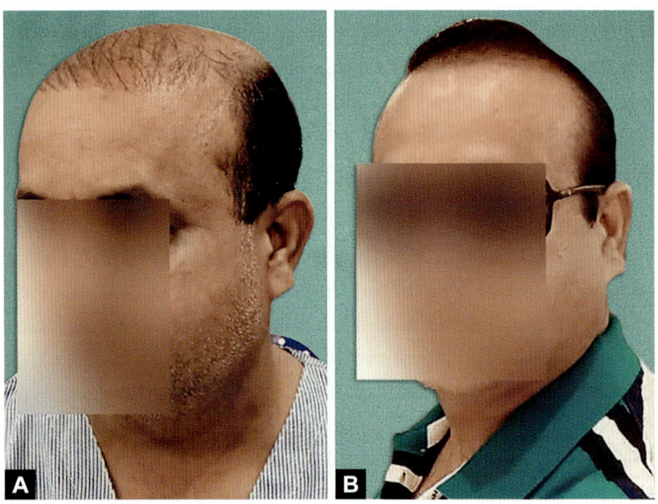

Figs. 19A and B: Results of the correction.

of creating a too straight or solid-appearing hairline. Any deviation from this can lead to density errors and hairline appears unnatural.

Correction of High Density in Transition Zone

In normal hairline, density starts increasing as we move posteriorly to defined zone. When high density is given in transition zone, even with single hair grafts, it lacks the softness and appears more or less flat. It can be corrected by creating microirregularities using single hair grafts. It is almost similar to correction of abrupt-looking flat hairline.

Correction of Low Density in Defined Zone

Defined zone is high density area, and low density typically results in a "see-through" effect. This zone ideally should

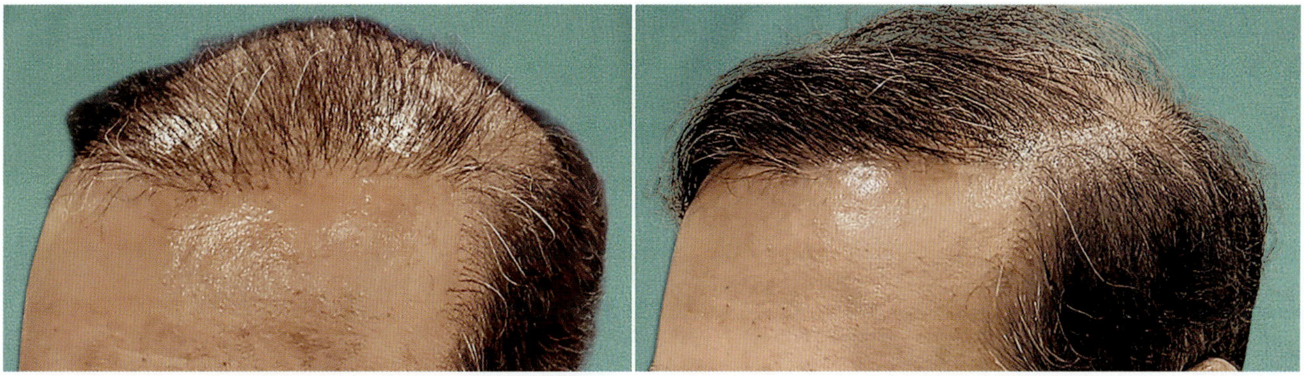

Fig. 20: Correction of low density in the parting line with remaining available follicular units (FUs)

get predominantly double hair grafts placed at high density. To achieve this, new grafts should be placed carefully in space in between existing hair. In absence of multihair grafts, two single-hair grafts are placed in slit to increase the hair volume giving it fuller look.

Correction of Low Density in Forelock

A normal forelock serves the purpose of providing the appearance of a volume. While doing a hair transplant, this should be kept in mind and preferentially given a higher density, ideally with two and three hair grafts. Lack of density in this region makes the overall hair growth appear a flat and lacking volume. Correction involves placement of larger sized grafts (two and three hair grafts in the forelock zone).

Correction of Parting Line Defect

Parting line depends on the individual preference of the patient and can be either left to right or right to left. In any case, even if the patient says the preferential direction of parting, density in the parting lines on either side should be given as high as possible. As hairs in these areas are going to be split and parted, any lack of density will make the scalp skin overly visible and can appear bald. Also, these regions are vulnerable to miniaturization spreading laterally in temporal areas. This miniaturization combined with low density in the parting line will make a lateral defect very obvious. Correction of this region is straightforward with placement of two and three hair grafts in between the existing hairs **(Fig. 20)**.

Correction of Density in Central Zone

Central zone is area which starts at the end of defined zone and extends up to vertex transition zone. The errors in central zone are not seen from the front as they are hidden behind the hairline, but when seen from top they are clearly visible. Usual problem seen in this area is that there is sudden drop in density from hairline to central zone, so patients have to keep their hair long and comb them backward. This can be corrected by adding more grafts into this area. Additional grafts can be taken from beard, chest, and other nonscalp donor areas when scalp donor area is depleted. Grafts should be placed with uniform density in this area, and one may give gradual reduction in density as we move toward vertex transition zone to give smooth merging to crown. If significant scalp visibility through implanted hair is still present, one can use SMP to create an illusion of fuller look.

Correction of Low-density Errors with Scalp Micropigmentation

Scalp micropigmentation provides a quick density correction without going for a repeat hair transplant surgery. SMP works only with the combination of existing hair when there is slightly low density in central zone of crown area. If the density and number of hairs in one particular area are too low, SMP will not improve the density appearance. However, it is a good option to be tried. Alternatively, if patient agrees for completely "shaved head" look then SMP can be a useful tool **(Figs. 21A to D)**.

Repair of Complications due to Poor Graft Placement

Pitting

Pitting in the recipient site happens when FU placement is done below the skin surface. Hair appears to come out of the scalp skin from a small pit such as depression. It is mostly apparent in the hairline or if the scalp is shaved. Correction of this involves extraction and reimplanting the hair grafts at the correct depth. Considering the possibility of graft damage while extraction, this should be done only in places where it is aesthetically a problem, such as the hairline and temporal triangles. Alternatively, it can be hide by correctly placing single hair grafts in front of it.

Cobblestone Appearance

Cobblestone appearance **(Fig. 22)** happens due to the exact opposite reason to that of pitting, i.e., when the hair grafts are planted superficial in the upper dermal level.

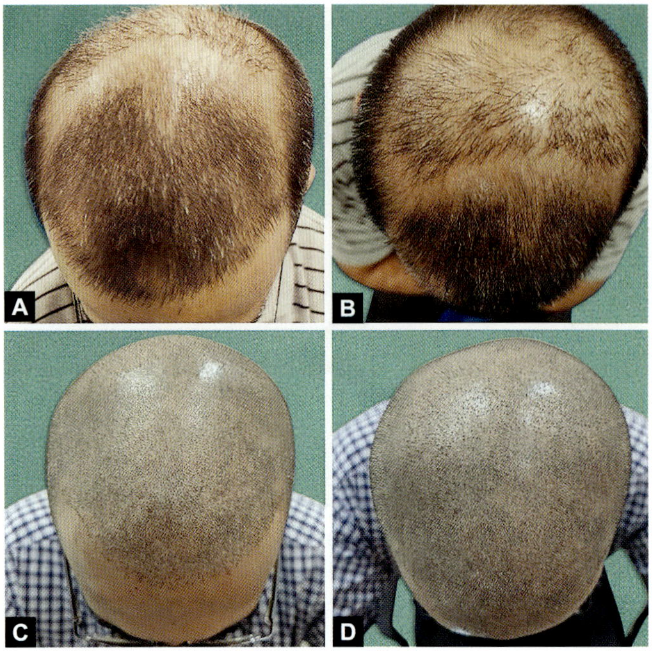

Figs. 21A to D: Recipient site repair by scalp micropigmentation (SMP). Patients who do not want a repair hair transplant and opting for shaving their scalp, a creation of "shaved head appearance" by SMP can be an effective option.

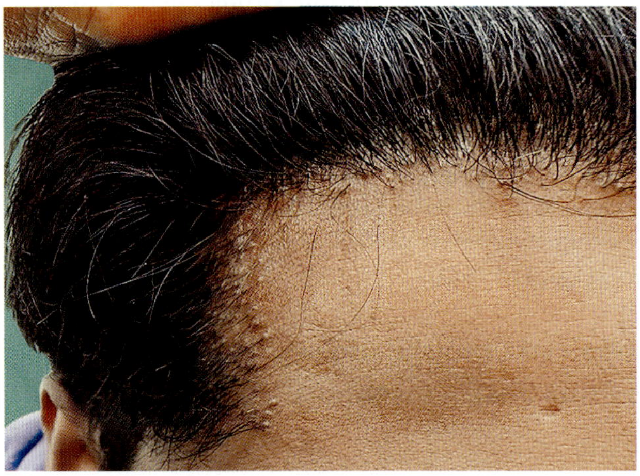

Fig. 22: Cobblestone appearance in the hairline and temporal region.

Another common reason for cobblestone appearance is when large sized. Common reasons for cobblestone appearance are when large-sized multihair grafts are placed at very acute angles close to the skin surface. This is a common occurrence in the temporal angles, moustache, and beard region. It can be seen along the hairline where grafts are not trimmed and are placed above the skin surface and not exactly at the level of skin surface. Correction involves extraction and reimplanting at a correct depth. In the moustache and chin regions, resurfacing with CO_2 laser may offer some benefits.

Excessively Curly Hair

Hair can get some curled appearance during the early stage of hair growth after a hair transplant. However, excessive hair curling of the original straight hair is not normal after hair transplant. Most common cause is tissue damage resulting from poor storage and handling of the grafts. If found in localized area in smaller numbers, the problematic FUs can be removed with FUE.

If larger number of hairs are affected, salon methods, such as chemical straightening, may give some benefits.

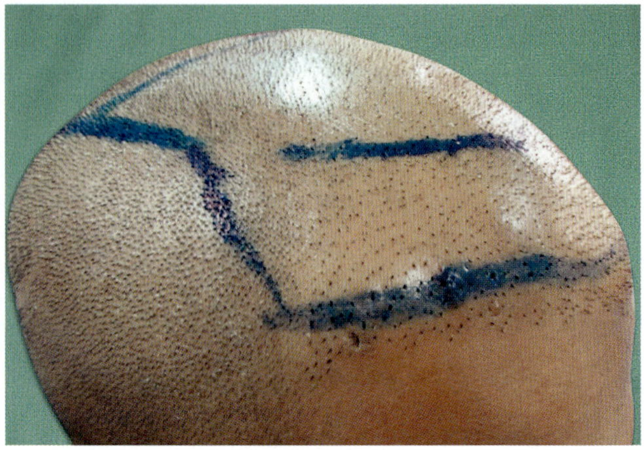

Fig. 23: Cyst formation and severe pitting over the planted area. Another error is regular, parallel rows of implantation, and less density.

Cyst Formation

Cyst formation **(Fig. 23)** occurs at recipient site when grafts are completely buried inside the skin. These cysts are eventually rupture on their own within 2–4 months. They typically involve buried grafts. These result in graft loss and resultant atrophic scarring. Rarely, smaller cysts calcify and result into inert nodules, which remain unchanged for prolonged periods of time. Unless aesthetically problematic, these also do not require a hasty removal. However, when grow larger requires surgical removal.

Scarring Alopecia Resulting from Vascular Damage or Central Scalp Necrosis

The most common location for this is the forelock region. This is a dreaded complication, which can happen due to variety of reasons ranging from advancing age, diabetes, vascular diseases, using long blades, or needle to prepare recipient site, giving very high density in forelock region, etc. However, a basic cause of necrosis is generally a high vascular damage. This results in complete failure of hair growth in the forelock region due to compromised vascularity, leading to atrophic scarring. Since this scarring further compromises the blood supply of the region, a repair hair transplant is challenging. If repair is attempted, care should be taken so as not to pack the area too densely and to avoid making deep slits.

REPAIR OF DONOR AREA

There are patients who undergo multiple sessions of hair transplant surgery to cover the area being bald due to ongoing

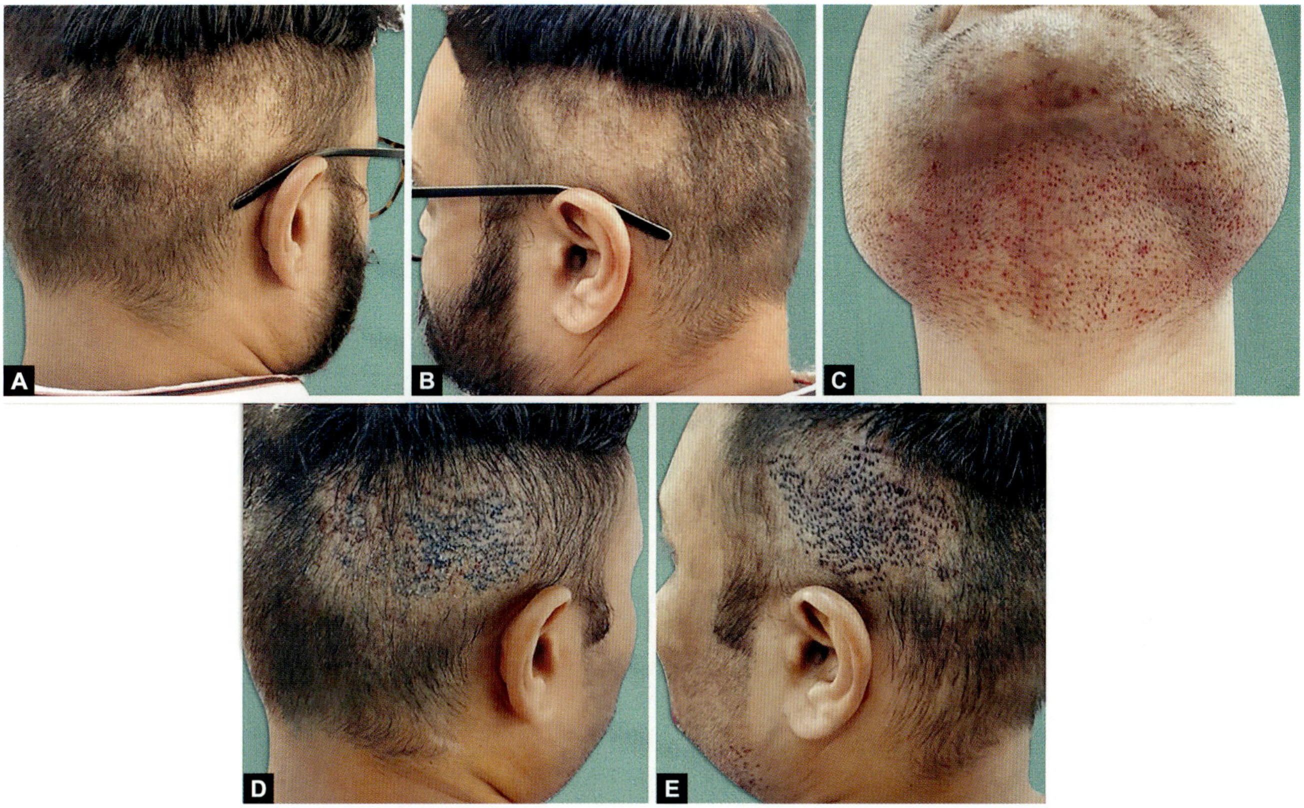

Figs. 24A to E: Repair of the donor area: (A and B) Patchy alopecia was developed in this patient due to multiple sessions of FUE surgeries and subsequent over harvesting; (C) Due to nonavailability of extractable grafts from occipital scalp, beard grafts were taken to covered the alopecia patches in scalp donor area; (D and E) Repair of the scalp donor area using beard grafts—immediate postoperative.

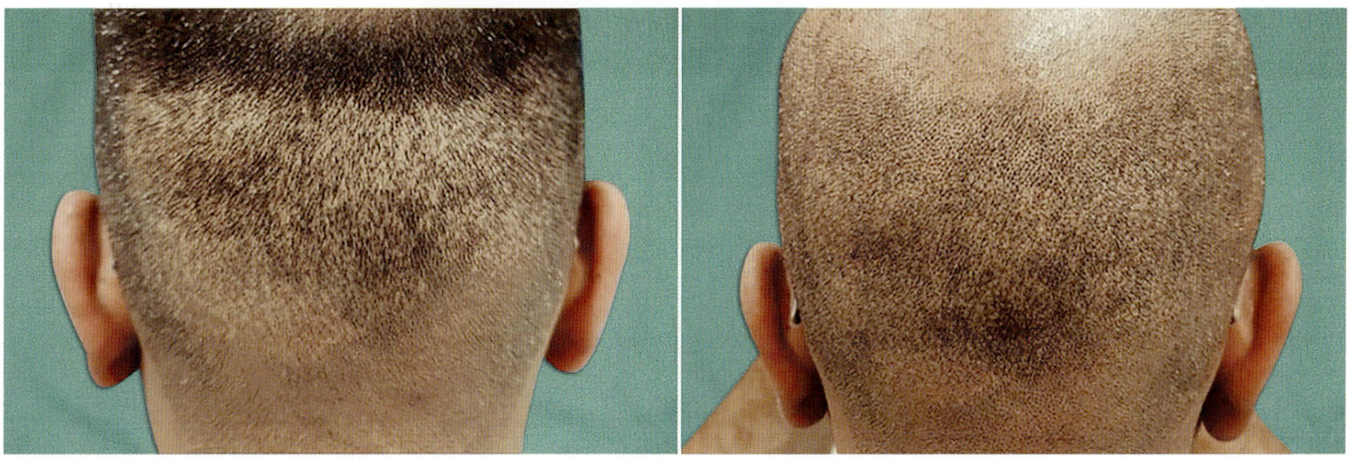

Fig. 25: Repair of donor area by scalp micropigmentation (SMP). SMP done over the follicular unit extraction (FUE) scars to hide hypopigmented and atrophic scars.

hair loss or to achieve the desired density in an already transplanted area. This leads to progressive depletion of hair in the donor area. This is associated with the risk of having low density or uneven density in the donor area. Harvesting a higher number of grafts in one session is another reason where such situations arise. There are cases where more grafts are taken from one particular area of donor scalp, and it can lead to localized baldness, especially in the inexperienced hands. In such cases, patients start worrying about the irregular and uneven growth in the donor area rather than the actual baldness. Such incidence may require to repair the donor area.

The principle here is to make donor area aesthetically acceptable by adding some hair in area where density is too less, or bald patch is present, so that overall the density in donor area looks uniform. This can be achieved either by adding the hair to donor area or by SMP.

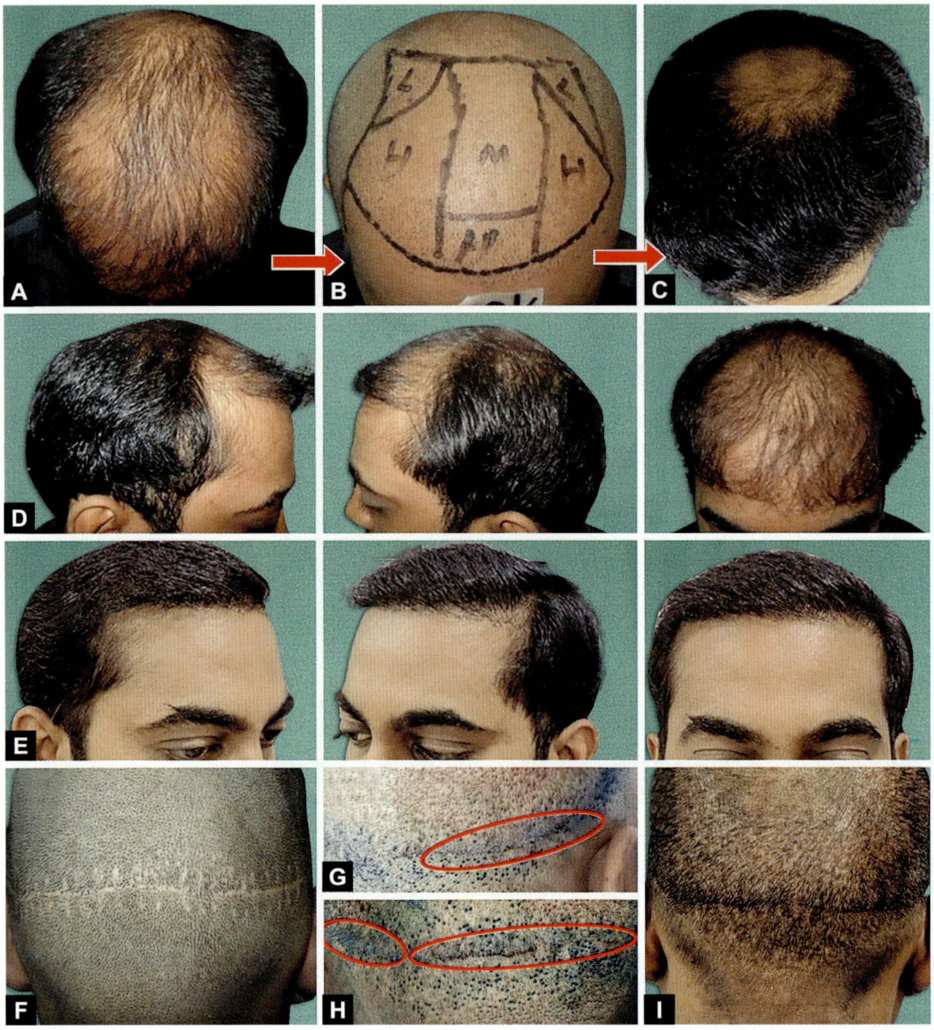

(A) This patient had first surgery by FUT method and had poor hair growth after. The hair near temporal angel were slightly misdirected and very less in number. Patient was not ready for removal of those hair;

(B) For repair surgery grafts were taken from scalp and beard. There are areas, which had low density were given high density and the area where density was slightly more were given medium density as seen in planning

(C) Result after 8 months: Front and mid scalp covered uniformly. Crown baldness is seen, which was not addressed during the repair surgery. (D) Photos from side and front before repair. Side profile shows present of misdirected hair at both the frontotemporal angles (E) After 8 months of repair surgery. As, the errors at frontotemporal angles were minimal, they merge with new hair and barely visible. So every time removal of wrongly placed hair is not necessary.

Correction of FUT scar in same patient later. The grafts were taken carefully from the adjacent area of scar. The idea was to take out the grafts from pockets of high density and use then to fill the pockets of low density. So, whole area appears uniform and graft requirement can be reduced; (F) FUT scar in donor; (G) and (H) implanted grafts in FUT scar-marked with red line, above and below blue dots are seen from where grafts were taken for repair; (I) Result after FUT scar repair.

Figs. 26A to I: Repair surgery. (A to E) Repair of recipient site; (F to I) Repair of follicular unit transplantation (FUT) scar later in same patient.

Role of Hair grafting in donor area repair: Hair grafting in donor area is mainly done to repair either localized area of relatively low density or localized bald area. Such areas are usually developed due to uneven extraction from donor area and harvesting a greater number of grafts from one particular area. To repair this, one can either extract the grafts from area with relatively high density and place them in area with less or no hair, making the density in whole area uniform. Alternatively, one can extract the grafts from beard or other nonscalp donor areas and fill-in the gaps in the affected area **(Figs. 24A to E)**. This will make the density uniform in donor area and reduce the visual contrast. The scar of follicular unit transplantation (FUT) surgery can also be repaired in similar way by adding grafts taken from beard or any other donor area.

Role of scalp micropigmentation in donor area repair: In cases of severe thinning of donor area, SMP can be carried out to reduce the scalp visibility **(Fig. 25)**. SMP only works in those patients with black hair. Patients who developed hypopigmented scarring after extraction can also be benefitted with SMP as part of donor area repair.

In some cases, both of the techniques described earlier can be combined to get optimum results. A wide FUT scar on the donor area can also be treated in the same way either by adding grafts or by SMP or combination of both to make it virtually invisible to those patients who are conscious about their scar and want to hide it.

Excision of donor area: In cases of severe thinning, where getting adequate grafts to cover the damaged donor area by earlier said method is not possible—in such situations, surgeon may plan to excise the donor area horizontally similar to a strip/FUT method, to remove most of the affected area. This can be followed by hair grafting and/or SMP later to cover remaining donor area **(Figs. 26A to I)**.

REPEAT HAIR TRANSPLANT VERSUS REPAIR HAIR TRANSPLANT

A repeat hair transplant is done when the first transplant was successful, but the hair loss progressed to another area and second hair transplant is needed for the same. This is not considered as repair surgery. When the surgery requires the removal of previously planted grafts or addition of grafts to previously operated area or both, it is called repair hair transplant.[3]

CONCLUSION

The goal of repair surgery is to achieve best possible aesthetic outcome by identifying and correcting the errors of the previous hair transplant. When errors are only related to hairline and there is not much of bald area present, usual repair includes removal of undesired FUs, adding more single hair FUs to camouflage misplaced follicles, or combination of both.

If repair is needed due to poor growth, the successful outcome depends upon the availability of adequate donor hair. Surgeon must assess the available donor supply and accordingly plan the repair. When scalp donor area is not adequate, surgeon must look for availability of other nonscalp donor areas like beard, chest, and other hairy areas. If donor supply is adequate, repair surgery can be undertaken. Nonsurgical treatments options like SMP or hair wigs/hair patches can be explained in extreme cases where donor supply is poor and repair seems impossible.

REFERENCES

1. Lam S (Ed). Hair Transplant 360: Advances, Techniques, Business Development, and Global Perspectives, 1st edition, Volume 3, Part 1. New Delhi: Jaypee Brothers Medical Publishers (P) Ltd; 2014.
2. Shapiro R. Principles and techniques used to create a natural hairline in surgical hair restoration. Facial Plast Surg Clin North Am. 2004;12:201-17.
3. Bernstein RM, Rassman WR, Rashid N, Shiell RC. The art of repair in surgical hair restoration part 1: Basic repair strategies. Dermatol Surg. 2002;28(9):783-94.

CHAPTER 76

Hair Transplantation for Other Indications

Kavish Chauhan, Gillian Roga

KEY MESSAGES

- Hair transplantation can be used to successfully treat many other conditions other than androgenetic alopecia, which is the most common known indication.
- Cicatricial alopecia (primary and secondary), alopecia areata, tractional alopecia, facial hair restoration, and vitiligo have shown promising results with follicular unit extraction (FUE), provided certain requisites are satisfied.
- With adept surgical skill and insightfulness, we can restore good density coverage in even a compromised recipient area.

INTRODUCTION

Hair transplant is rapidly becoming one of the most popular aesthetic procedures. Today, follicular unit extraction (FUE) is the most commonly accepted method for hair transplantation. Hair transplantation in today's generation has gone beyond its horizon and is not just indicated in androgenetic alopecia as opposed to common belief but is successfully practiced in correction of cicatricial alopecia, postburn or surgical scars (facelift scars), cleft lip scars, vitiligo, and as an adjuvant to multiple maxillofacial surgical procedures such as reconstruction of eyebrows, eyelashes, beard, and mustache.[1] Hence, in this chapter, we have discussed and reviewed various other conditions where FUE is successfully indicated:[2]

- *Noncicatricial alopecia:*
  - Androgenetic alopecia
  - Stable alopecia areata
  - Tractional alopecia
  - Trichotillomania
  - Facial hair restoration (eyebrow, beard) for cosmetic enhancement of density
- *Cicatricial alopecia:*
  - Primary cicatricial alopecia
  - Secondary cicatricial alopecia
    - Traumatic scars
    - Burn scars
    - Surgical scars
- *Miscellaneous:*
  - Focal stable vitiligo
  - Hirsutism (white hair)
  - FUE in follicular unit transplantation (FUT) scar.

HAIR TRANSPLANTATION IN CICATRICIAL ALOPECIA

In 1885, Brocq first described cicatricial alopecia.[3] Cicatricial (scarring) alopecia is further classified as primary cicatricial alopecia where the hair follicles are directly affected by the disease process and secondary cicatricial alopecia where the hair follicles undergo damage by an external process.[4] Cicatricial alopecia differs from noncicatricial alopecia in the fact that there is inflammation around the bulge area in cicatricial alopecia versus inflammation in the bulb area in noncicatricial alopecia. According to Unger, cicatricial alopecia can also be classified into stable and unstable cicatricial alopecia. In 1939, Dr S Okuda described the first case of hair transplantation in a case of traumatic alopecia. In today's generation of hair transplantation, cicatricial alopecia has become a common indication for FUE.[5-7]

Outcome of Hair Transplantation in Various Types of Cicatricial Alopecia

It is well known that hair transplantation in cicatricial alopecia has lower growth survival rates (50%) in comparison to noncicatricial alopecia (>90%) in view of recipient area dominance.[8] In stable cases of cicatricial alopecia, the result of hair transplant is generally successful. However, in unstable cicatricial alopecia, disease reactivation has led to compromised surgical results. In a study by Ekelem et al.,[9] the outcome of hair transplant in various types of cicatricial alopecia was found to be positive in central centrifugal cicatricial alopecia (60%), morphea (85%), pseudopelade of Brocq (60%), discoid lupus erythematosus (72%), and folliculitis decalvans (40%). However, in certain conditions such as lichen planopilaris and frontal fibrosing alopecia, it has been found to be a mixed outcome of both successful and unsuccessful graft survival. This study corroborated the direct correlation between the stability of information before surgery and graft survival in the successful cases.[9]

Outcome of Surgery in Primary Versus Secondary Cicatricial Alopecia[5]

Hair restoration surgery in cicatricial alopecia depends on multiple factors that are vital to be considered in the preoperative stage.

- *Disease stability:* In primary cicatricial alopecia, if the disease affects the recipient area, transplanted hair may be lost in the due course. On the other hand, if the disease affects the donor area, it may create a donor–recipient area mismatch. Thus, in such cases of primary cicatricial alopecia, due to unfavorable long-term donor–recipient area ratio, surgical excision is a better choice.
- *Donor hair availability:* In primary cicatricial alopecia, there is always a chance of future areas of cicatricial alopecia developing; hence, the donor–recipient area ratio must be kept in mind while planning surgery. If this ratio happens to be unsatisfactory in the current scenario, we need to treat both existing and possibly future areas of new cicatricial alopecia along with areas of noncicatricial alopecia, for example, androgenetic alopecia that may develop in the near future.
- *Vascular perfusion:* If vascular perfusion is compromised, surgical excision is chosen over hair transplant since the transplanted follicular units may undergo ischemic injury and tissue necrosis due to inadequate perfusion, thus resulting in poor graft survival **(Fig. 1)**.
- *Laxity of the scalp:* FUE method of transplantation is more preferable in cases having less scalp laxity.

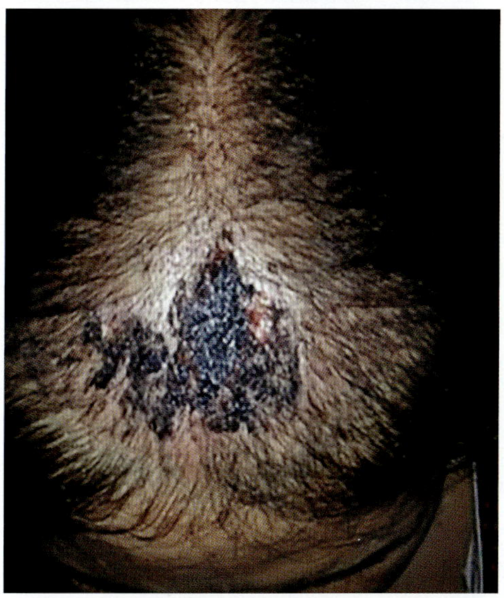

Fig. 1: Necrosis in the recipient area in a case of primary cicatricial alopecia posthair transplantation surgery due to high density.

- *Location of cicatricial alopecia:* Hair transplant surgery is the treatment of choice if the location of cicatricial alopecia is in an easily visible area such as the eyebrow or frontal hairline.
- *Healing characteristics of an individual:* Patients having past history of hypertrophic/keloidal scars, poorly healing scars, less scalp laxity, coagulative/bleeding disorders, and Ehlers–Danlos syndrome are considered poor candidates for surgical intervention.

Hence, hair transplantation is used to treat small, easily visible, areas of stable or secondary cicatricial alopecia in patients with history of good healing characteristics, good vascular supply, and favorable donor–recipient area ratio.

Management of a Case of Cicatricial Alopecia

Preoperative Stage

The best tools for diagnosis of a case of cicatricial alopecia are histopathology and trichoscopy. Prior to hair transplant surgery, trichoscopy is an important tool for assessing the donor and recipient areas for disease activity. The general accepted guidelines available, about when to do hair transplant in cicatricial alopecia, are after 1–2 years of stable disease (inactivity) in cases of primary cicatricial alopecia. Disease activity can be assessed histopathologically, where two biopsies 1 year apart showing disease inactivity are considered sufficient. As far as the method of hair transplantation preferred in cicatricial alopecia is concerned, both FUT/FUE methods have been widely used. However, in cases of secondary cicatricial alopecia, such as traumatic scars and burns scars, since the scalp is tight and atrophic, FUE is the preferred surgical method. The second advantage of FUE over FUT is the ability to "cherry pick" desirable follicular units. Beard and body hair can be used in cases of extensive cicatricial alopecia where the donor area is already compromised. The third advantage of FUE is the absence of suturing and hence negligible scarring.[9-17]

Intraoperative Stage

- *Anesthesia:* Ring block in combination with 2% lidocaine with 1:100,000 adrenaline, along with 0.5% bupivacaine, can be used in both the donor and recipient areas. However, it is important to limit the use of adrenaline, in tumescent anesthesia, due to inadequate vascularity in cicatricial alopecia as it can further lead to vasoconstriction.[13]
- *Recipient area density:* In cases of cicatricial alopecia, it is advisable to keep lower density of <30 grafts/cm^2 as compared to noncicatricial alopecia. The ideal method of determining the appropriate density is by first assessing the vascularity by testing the recipient area with an 18G needle and observing for bleeding points. In case of less vascularity, a lower density of 15–20 grafts/cm^2 is

planned, whereas in cases of better vascularity, a density of 20–30 grafts/cm^2 can be planned. In larger scars, the periphery has higher vascularity as compared to the center. Thus, higher density can be given at the periphery with lower density toward the center. In certain cases where the patient may desire a higher density in cicatricial alopecia cases, it is better to undergo the first session with <30 grafts/cm^2, followed by a second sitting after 9 months to increase the density. Neovascularization around the transplanted hairs is more likely to increase the vascularity in the surrounding areas, thus resulting in better graft survival rate during the second surgery.[10,18-20]

- *Recipient area designing:* This involves two major factors, that is, the size and the depth of the slits. In case of the recipient area being fibrotic and tight, large slits are preferred to avoid more handling of the graft during graft insertion. On the other hand, if the skin has reduced dermal recoil, smaller slits are better in order to reduce popping up of the grafts during insertion. In case of hypertrophic scars, the grafts need to be placed deeper during implantation in order to ensure enough blood supply. In atrophic scars, it is preferable to place the grafts at a more acute angle, hence making it more difficult for the grafts to pop out in the recipient area.[5] A test patch, prior to planning the surgery, can be performed by transplanting a few follicular units to observe the graft uptake and survival rate.[21]
- *Recipient area vascularity:* Since graft survival rates are highly dependent on the vascularity in the recipient area, various different methods have been tried to increase the blood flow prior to surgery in cicatricial alopecia. Minoxidil usage 2–5 weeks before and after the surgery has been recommended according to certain studies. Oral pentoxifylline 400 mg three times a day for 2 weeks can also be given before the surgery. Fractional carbon dioxide laser resurfacing prior to the surgery in the recipient area has also shown good results.[22-24]
- *Donor area:* In cases of cicatricial alopecia, with no scarring in the donor area, usually the occipital, parietal, and posterior parietal regions are preferred in men, whereas occipital and parietal are preferred in women.[25,26]

Postoperative Stage

Liposomal adenosine triphosphate (ATP) can be used as a spray, every 2–4 hours, in order to improve graft survival rate. Painkillers, antibiotics, and oral steroids are given for the initial 3–5 days. After removal of the dressing on the third day, hair wash is started. Similar to hair transplant in cases of noncicatricial alopecia, telogen effluvium post transplant will start within 4–6 weeks, and hair growth begins at 4–6 months. Posttransplant results can be assessed over the next 6–9 months. Repeat second session is done only after 9–12 months. It is advisable to observe for ischemia necrosis infection and promptly manage these complications.[5,27] Results postoperatively can be observed at 6 and 9 months, respectively **(Figs. 2 to 5)**.

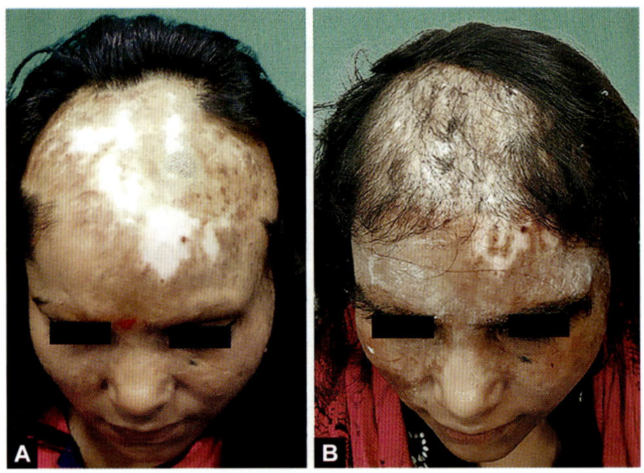

Figs. 2A and B: Postoperative results in an acid burns scar case at 6 months.

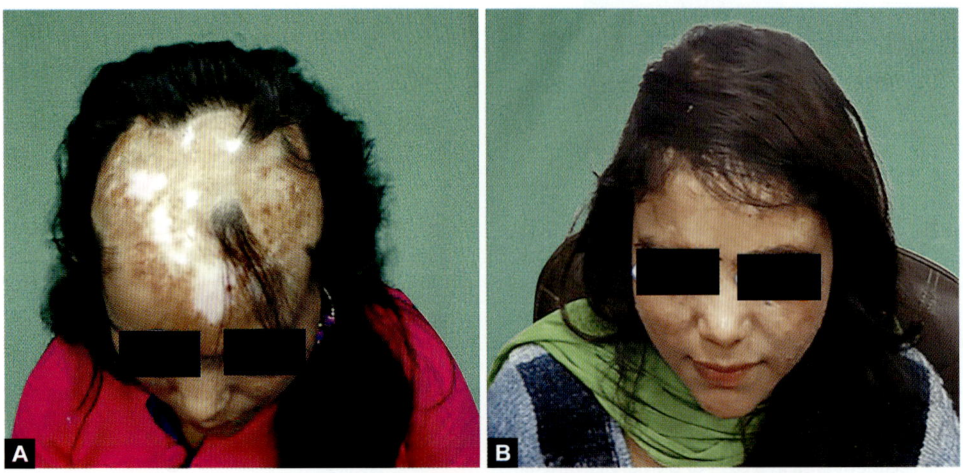

Figs. 3A and B: Postoperative results in an acid burns scar case at 9 months.

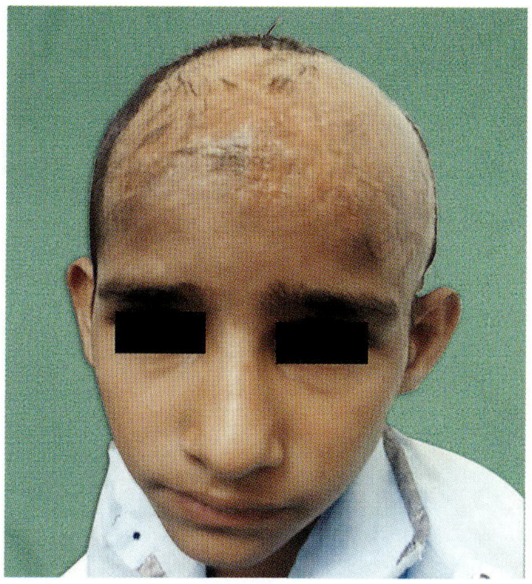

Fig. 4: Preoperative burns scar case recipient area.

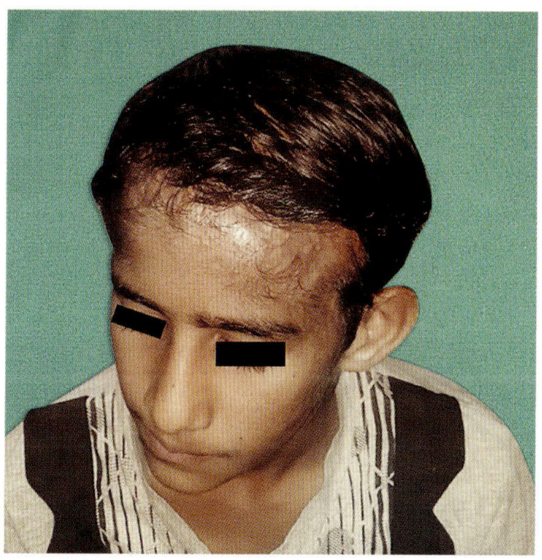

Fig. 5: Postoperative results in a burns scar case at 12 months.

HAIR TRANSPLANTATION IN EYEBROWS, EYELASHES, AND BEARD

Preoperative stage: In facial transplants, especially beard and eyebrow hair restoration, the patient should be counseled that it is ideal to provide cosmetically desired density in a two-staged manner rather than in a single surgical procedure.[28] The most common indications for facial hair transplant are as follows:

- Traumatic scars
- Tractional alopecia in beard
- Congenital hypotrichia/atrichia, ectodermal dysplasia, Netherton's syndrome
- Stable cicatricial alopecia
- Stable alopecia areata
- Repair of cleft lip cases
- Burns injury (chemical, electrical).

Operative stage:

- *Anesthesia:* In cases of facial hair restoration, it is better to give nerve blocks to limit the pain from multiple injections given in field block. The three common nerve blocks that are practiced in facial hair restoration surgery are (1) Auriculotemporal, (2) infraorbital, and (3) mental nerve blocks. After giving nerve blocks, the field block is given into the subcutaneous tissue in a less painful manner. In cases of eyebrow transplant, it is better to give a ring block, and the use of tumescence is restricted to minimum to prevent postprocedure swelling; pressure taping is advised just below the eyebrow on the eyelid.[29,30]
- *Donor area:* Midoccipital region of the scalp provides optimal follicular units for donor graft, matching the caliber and texture of beard and mustache hair. Selecting single and double follicular units from the donor area provides much better yield for a more natural coverage.[28] In case of eyebrow follicular units from the occipital area, preauricular or nape of the neck is preferred.[31]
- *Recipient area designing:* The ideal size of the recipient area slits is between 0.8 and 0.9 mm for the beard and mustache and usually 0.7–0.8 mm for the eyebrow area. Coronal slits are preferred over sagittal slits as they are smaller in size and can therefore offer higher density and better coverage. Tumescent anesthesia is given in the facial area more superficially as compared to other areas, in order to minimize laxity of the skin, which assists in creating the recipient area slits at a very acute angle of 10–20°.[28]
  - *Mustache area designing:* The natural direction of the hair in the mustache area is slightly outward and downward. Coronal slits are preferred over sagittal slits as they are smaller and give better alignment to prevent cobblestoning. Approximately 300–400 grafts on each side are required to give a density of about 35–40 grafts/cm^2. Single follicular units are placed on the outer upper border of the mustache to give a more natural result **(Fig. 6)**.[29]

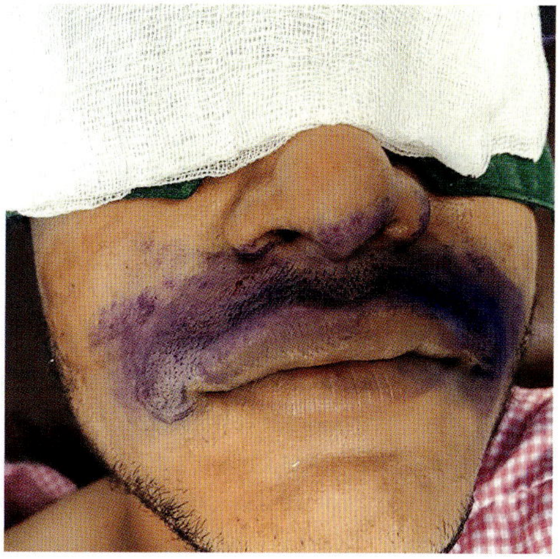

Fig. 6: Recipient area designing in mustache area hair restoration.

  - *Goatee area designing:* The natural direction of the hair in the goatee area is directed downward and is almost parallel to the skin. Approximately 600–700 grafts are required to give a density of 35–40 grafts/cm^2.

- *Sideburns area designing:* The natural direction of the hair in the sideburn area is directed downward and parallel at an acute angle to the skin. Approximately 200 grafts on each side are required.
- *Cheek area designing:* In the cheek area the natural direction of the hair are downwards and laterally, thus the slits are created accordingly and are arranged in a skewed pattern. In the border of the cheek, single hair follicular units are placed to give a soft look; in the body of the beard, double and triple follicular units are placed to give a fuller look to the beard.
- *Jawline area designing:* This area is concealed by the grafts transplanted in the cheek area, which grow longer and give coverage by an overlapping effect.
- *Eyebrow area designing:* The natural direction of the hair in the eyebrow varies in the head, body, and tail. In the head region, the direction of the hair is vertical or superior; in the body, the direction becomes horizontal, creating a "herringbone" pattern; and in the tail, the direction is lateral with crosshatching at the end. Single hair follicles are implanted in the eyebrow. Sagittal slits are preferred over coronal slits for better control of the curling of the eyebrow hair. The angle of the hair in the eyebrow is very acute and as flat as possible at a density of about 30–35 grafts/cm^2.[31]

- *Implantation:* Due to laxity, mobility, and vascularity of the facial skin, implantation is difficult in facial hair transplant. Single hair follicle units are placed using jeweler's forceps at the border of the sideburns, cheek beard, and goatee area to give a softer and fluffier look for a cosmetically aesthetic appearance. In the cheek beard and jawline area, double and triple hair follicular units are implanted to give a dense look. Implanters and "stick-and-place" method can be used to minimize bleeding. Grafts are preferably implanted in groups of fifties to reduce the out-of-body time for the graft. Implantation is done using the "no touch to root" technique with the use of two forceps. De-epithelialization and trimming of the grafts are not required in FUE technique extraction if the appropriate-sized punch of 0.75–0.8 mm is used **(Fig. 7)**.[28,31]

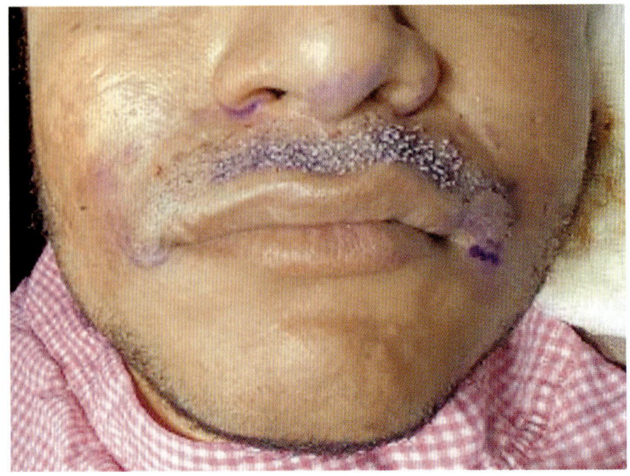

Fig. 7: Recipient area after implantation of follicular units in mustache area.

Eyelash Hair Transplantation[32]

Preoperative stage: Eyelash hair transplant surgery is indicated in patients with thin sparse eyelashes due to alopecia areata, trichotillomania, trauma, blepharitis, eyelid surgery, thyroid disease, ectodermal dysplasia, etc.

Operative stage:

- *Anesthesia:* The cornea is first anesthetized with proparacaine hydrochloride solution (0.5%), after which corneal eye shields are inserted. Local anesthetic infiltration with lidocaine and bupivacaine is injected into the subcutaneous layer of the lower two-thirds of the upper eyelid.
- *Recipient area designing:* A normal upper eyelid and lower eyelid contain about 100 and 60 lashes, respectively. The ideal size of the recipient area slits is between 0.7 and 0.8 mm, along the tarsal border of the eyelid at an angle parallel to the direction of natural hair growth. Single hair follicular units are used for implantation in a retrograde fashion.
- *Donor area:* Donor area for eyelash transplant is from the nape of the neck or area above/behind the ears, due to the fine quality of the hair.

Postoperative stage: To prevent dislodging of grafts, the patient is advised to sleep with glasses. Coat the new eyelashes with lash oil, use an eyelash curler to encourage proper curl, and trim regularly. The transplanted hair in the eyelash must be trimmed every 2–4 weeks.

HAIR TRANSPLANTATION IN VITILIGO[33-35]

Hair transplantation is also being used in the treatment of stable vitiligo not responding to other treatment options. The reason behind this is that when compared to epidermal melanocytes, follicular melanocytes are denser and more melanogenic. Being immunologically privileged, they are also less susceptible to immunological damage after transplantation. The multiple advantages of treating vitiligo by hair transplantation are as follows:

- Donor scars can be minimized by FUE.
- Follicular units in the recipient area do not leave any residual scar as compared to cobblestoning, which occurs in punch grafting.
- Difficult areas such as eyebrow, eyelash, and angle of the mouth are easily possible.
- Touch-up procedure for pigmentation can be achieved by inserting more grafts.

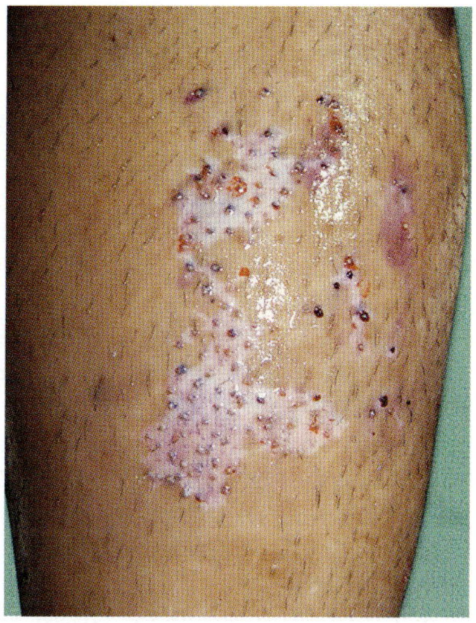

Fig. 8: Postoperative results in a vitiligo case after implantation of grafts using follicular unit extraction method.

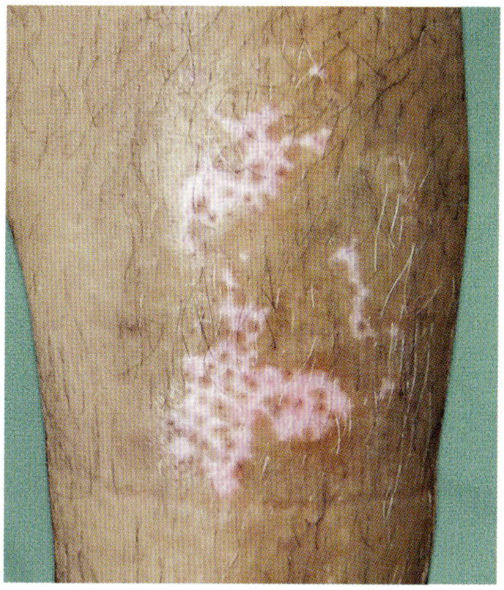

Fig. 9: Postoperative repigmentation results in a vitiligo case, post-PUVA therapy at 4 weeks.

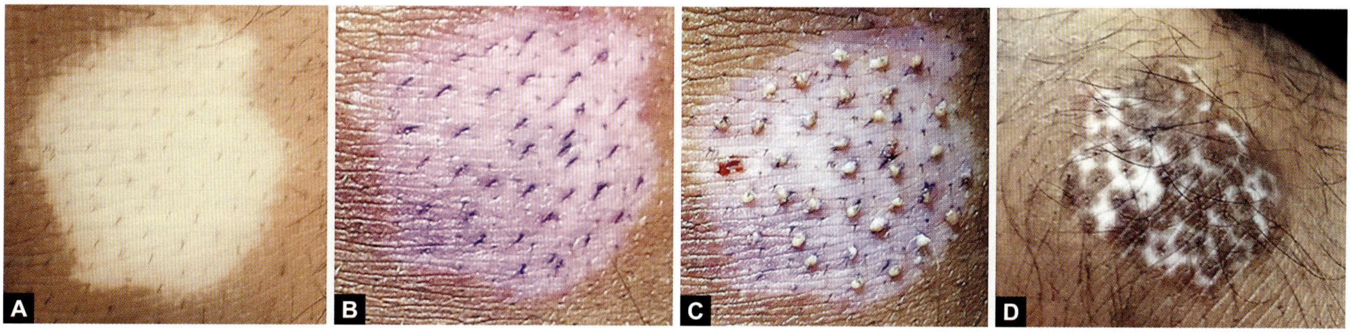

Figs. 10A to D: Steps of recipient area designing, implantation and repigmentation post-PUVA therapy results in a case of vitiligo.

Preoperative stage: The FUE method of hair transplant is recommended in stable cases of focal vitiligo (nonglabrous skin) with leukotrichia, not responding adequately to medical treatment.

Operative stage:

- *Anesthesia:* Recipient area is infiltrated using ring and field block.
- *Donor area:* Follicular units from occipital, postauricular region, or body hair such as the thigh can be used.
- *Recipient area:* Slits are created using an 18G needle, following the natural direction and angle of the hair in the recipient area 3–5 mm apart, at a density of 6–8 grafts/cm^2.
- *Implantation:* Grafts are implanted using a jeweler's forceps into the created slits.

Postoperative stage: Parraffin swab dressing is done under aseptic precautions, followed by which "PUVAsol" therapy and topical tacrolimus are used. Phototherapy post-operatively stimulates melanocytes in their migration from the hair follicle to the epidermis. The perifollicular spread of pigmentation occurs from 5 to 12 mm around the hair follicle. Repigmentation is observed in about 3–6 weeks **(Figs. 8 to 10)**.

FOLLICULAR UNIT EXTRACTION IN HIRSUTISM (WHITE HAIR)[2]

In a patient with hirsutism associated with white hair, laser hair reduction is not a suitable option. Electrolysis is generally recommended; however, it may take multiple sessions and lead to hyperpigmentation. FUE can prove as a great option in these cases, where a 0.7-mm serrated punch is used to minimize scarring and hyperpigmentation. FUE will ensure removal of the hair bulb along with the bulge region and thus minimize the chances of recurrence and repeat sessions.

CONCLUSION

Follicular unit extraction is an adaptable technique in treating various conditions ranging from cicatricial alopecia, non-cicatricial alopecia, and vitiligo. A skilled surgeon with proper clinical assessment, surgical technique, and a well-trained team can achieve excellent results even in rare cases. FUE surgery has a steep learning curve and is a relatively time consuming and meticulous surgery that can yield exceptional results in skilled hands. With hair transplant surgeons around the world, perfecting and modifying the technique, the science of FUE is expected to undergo major advancements in the future years.

TIPS

For hair transplantation in other indications:
- FUE is the preferred method of hair transplantation in other indications such as cicatricial alopecia, vitiligo, and facial hair restoration due to the ability to "cherry pick" the grafts.
- In primary cicatricial alopecia, assessing disease stability and recipient area vascularity are the most vital steps prior to surgery.
- The ideal recipient area density to be followed in cases of cicatricial alopecia is about 30–35 grafts/cm^2.
- The ideal recipient area density to be followed in cases of facial hair restoration in eyebrow, mustache, and beard is about 35–40 grafts/cm^2.
- The ideal recipient area density to be followed in cases of vitiligo in nonglabrous skin is about 6–8 grafts/cm^2.
- Implantation is preferred with implanters or two-forceps method following the "no root touch" technique.

REFERENCES

1. Sharma R, Ranjan A. Follicular unit extraction (FUE) hair transplant: curves ahead. J Maxillofac Oral Surg. 2019;18(4):509-17.
2. Kerure AS, Deshmukh N, Agrawal S, Patwardhan NG. Follicular unit extraction [FUE]—one procedure, many uses. Indian Dermatol Online J. 2021;12(3):381.
3. Brocq L. Alopecia. J Cutan Vener Dis. 1885;3:49-56.
4. Messenger AG, Sinclair RD, Farrant P, de Berker DA. Acquired disorders of hair. Rook's Textbook of Dermatology, 9th Edition. 2016. pp.1-88.
5. Unger W, Unger R, Wesley C. The surgical treatment of cicatricial alopecia. Dermatol Ther. 2008;21(4):295-311.
6. Filbrandt R, Rufaut N, Jones L, Sinclair R. Primary cicatricial alopecia: diagnosis and treatment. CMAJ. 2013;185(18):1579-85.
7. Inui S, Itami S. Dr Shoji Okuda (1886-1962): the great pioneer of punch graft hair transplantation. J Dermatol. 2009;36(10):561-2.
8. Callender VD, Lawson CN, Onwudiwe OC. Hair transplantation in the surgical treatment of central centrifugal cicatricial alopecia. Dermatol Surg. 2014;40:1125-31.
9. Ekelem C, Pham C, Atanaskova Mesinkovska N. A systematic review of the outcome of hair transplantation in primary scarring alopecia. Skin Appendage Disord. 2019;5(2):65-71.
10. Dahdah MJ, Iorizzo M. The role of hair restoration surgery in primary cicatricial alopecia. Skin Appendage Disord. 2016;2(1-2):57-60.
11. Mendes-Bastos P, Camps-Fresneda A. Hair transplantation for frontal fibrosing alopecia: part of the solution? Actas Dermosifiliogr. 2016;107(1):3-4.
12. Farjo B, Farjo N, Williams G. Hair transplantation in burn scar alopecia. Scars Burn Heal. 2015;1:2059513115607764.
13. Roga G, Gupta J, Kumar A, Chouhan K. Management of cicatricial alopecia by hair transplantation using follicular unit extraction. Clin Dermatol Res Ther. 2017;1(1):112.
14. Thakur BK, Verma S, Raphael V. Clinical, trichoscopic, and histopathological features of primary cicatricial alopecias: a retrospective observational study at a tertiary care centre of North East India. Int J Trichol. 2015;7(3):107.
15. Martínez-Velasco MA, Vázquez-Herrera NE, Misciali C, Vincenzi C, Maddy AJ, Asz-Sigall D, et al. Frontal fibrosing alopecia severity index: a trichoscopic visual scale that correlates thickness of peripilar casts with severity of inflammatory changes at pathology. Skin Appendage Disord. 2018;4(4):277-80.
16. Al-Refu K. The role of dermoscopy in assessment of the activity and scarring response in discoid lupus erythematosus. Open Dermatol J. 2018;12(1).
17. Mani S, Manickam N, Gopalan K, Vellaisamy SG. Role of dermoscopy in the diagnosis of alopecia. J Pakistan Assoc Dermatol. 2018;28(3):320-8.
18. Nakatsui T, Wong J, Groot D. Survival of densely packed follicular unit grafts using the lateral slit technique. Dermatol Surg. 2008;34(8):1016-22.
19. Unger WP. Density issue in hair transplantation. Dermatol Surg. 1998;24(2):297.
20. Yoo H, Moh J, Park JU. Treatment of postsurgical scalp scar deformity using follicular unit hair transplantation. Biomed Res Int. 2019;2019:3423657.
21. Loganathan E, Sarvajnamurthy S, Gorur D, Suresh DH, Siddaraju MN, Narasimhan RT. Complications of hair restoration surgery: a retrospective analysis. Int J Trichol. 2014;6:168-72.
22. Avram MR, Cole JP, Gandelman M, Haber R, Knudsen R, Leavitt MT, et al. The potential role of minoxidil in the hair transplantation setting. Dermatol Surg. 2002;28:894-900.
23. Rose P, Shapiro R. Transplanting into scar tissue and areas of cicatricial alopecia. In: Unger WP, Shapiro R (Eds). Hair Transplantation, 4th edition. New York: Marcel Dekker; 2004. pp. 606-9.
24. Madura C, Vinay N, Kusuma MR, Harsha S, Chandrashekar BS. The assessment of hair transplantation outcomes in cicatricial alopecia. Int J Trichol. 2020;12(4):164-7.
25. Moser K, Hugeneck J, Rohrbacher W, Moser C. The pairing technique of the Moser Medical Group. Hair Transplant Forum Int. 2005;15:41-6.
26. Unger W, Solish N, Giguere D, Bertucci V, Coleman W, Loukas M, et al. Delineating the "safe" donor area for hair transplanting. Am J Cosmet Surg. 1994;11:239-43.
27. Kim JC, Hwang SJ, Lee JJ, Oh BM, Lee SJ, Kim DW, et al. The effects of dehydration, preservation temperature and time on the hair grafts. Ann Dermatol. 2002;14:149-52.
28. Dua K, Verma V, Dua A. Beard and moustache reconstruction. Indian J Plast Surg. 2021;54(4):483-8.
29. Dua K, Chahar M. Facial Hair Transplantation. New Delhi, India: Jaypee Brothers Medical Publishers Ltd.; 2016. pp. 313-20.
30. Arndt KA, Burton C, Noe JM. Minimizing the pain of local anesthesia. Plast Reconstr Surg. 1983;72(05):676-9.
31. Gupta J, Kumar A, Chouhan K, Ariganesh C, Nandal V. The science and art of eyebrow transplantation by follicular unit extraction. J Cutan Aesthet Surg. 2017;10(2):66.
32. Gandelman M, Epstein JS. Hair transplantation to the eyebrow, eyelashes, and other parts of the body. Facial Plast Surg Clin. 2004;12(2):253-61.
33. Ng B. The potential role of hair transplant surgeons in treating vitiligo: a case report. Hair Transplant Forum Int. 2010;20(2):37-45.
34. Kumar AV, Parthasaradhi A. Follicular unit extraction technique in treating stable vitiligo with leukotrichia. J Dermatol Dermatol Surg. 2018;22(2):72.
35. Sacchidanand S, Thakur P, Purohit V, Sujaya SN. Follicular unit extraction as a therapeutic option for vitiligo. J Cutan Aesthet Surg. 2013;6(4):229.

CHAPTER 77 Innovations in Hair Restoration

Kapil Dua, Shrenik Balegar

KEY MESSAGES

- Hair transplantation has undergone a lot of advancements in recent times.
- Innovations in the surgical management includes new excision and implanting systems, punches and storage solutions.
- Trivellini's system, Devroye's WAW FUE system, Umar's U punch system, ARTAS 9X, and NeoGraft™ technique are the new excision tools which have eased the process of extraction with least damage to the grafts.
- New punches like Trivellini's edge out punch, Dua's flat punch, hybrid punch, UPunch and many other innovative punches have reduced the rate of transection and increased the graft survivability.
- Innovations in implantation methods include Choi, SAVA, KEEP, Devroye's multigraft Implanter system and INRUT implanters. These have made the process easier with reduced handling and damage of the grafts.

INTRODUCTION

Hair restoration is getting refined with every passing day. From the earlier days of punch grafting, the trend shifted to follicular unit transplantation (FUT). Then came the follicular unit excision (FUE) method, which has become the most popular method in recent times. Subsequently, surgeons all across the globe went on improving the technique of FUE with innovative methods, instruments, and robotics. In the last decade, there have been drastic advances in the field of hair restoration. These advances can be classified as follows:

- *Innovations in surgical management:*
  - Harvesting machines
  - Implantation methods
  - Innovation in storage solutions
- *Innovation in nonsurgical management:*
  - Regenerative medicines—RegeneraActiva, exosomes, etc.

In this chapter, we will be briefly dealing with the innovations in surgical management only as nonsurgical management is beyond the scope of this textbook.

INNOVATIONS IN SURGICAL MANAGEMENT

Harvesting Machines

When FUE was introduced, harvesting was done with sharp manual punches. The speed was slow and the follicular transections were higher. This was overcome by mortised FUE machines, which were introduced by Cole and Harris.

Powered SAFE Scribe Method

Harris first described the SAFE Scribe[1] technique of harvesting grafts with a two-step process. In the first step, a sharp punch scored the skin up to the level of the epidermis and in the second step, a blunt punch would dissect the dermis and separate the follicular unit (FU) from its surrounding. This two-step technique was modified to a single step using a dull punch but with added rotation. This method facilitated harvesting in a single step with less transection (Powered SAFE Scribe) **(Figs. 1A and B)**.

Powered Cole Isolation Device System

Cole, in 2004, introduced the Cole Isolation Technique in which a sharp thin-walled punch with depth control was used.[2] In this punch system, the depth of incision can be adjusted to accommodate for FU variation and scalp characteristics of individual patients. These punches cut just deep to the arrector pili muscle in order to effectively release the FU graft.

These were the first generation of the harvesting machines. But over the passage of time, the surgeons kept on trying to develop newer machines which had more speed and less transection of grafts, which are described below.

Trivellini's System and Technique

Trivellini invented a multiphasic suction-assisted FUE device that removed grafts with more precision, less transection, and greater speed. In normal FUE, the control on the advancement of the punch into the skin varies with the type of skin, punch,

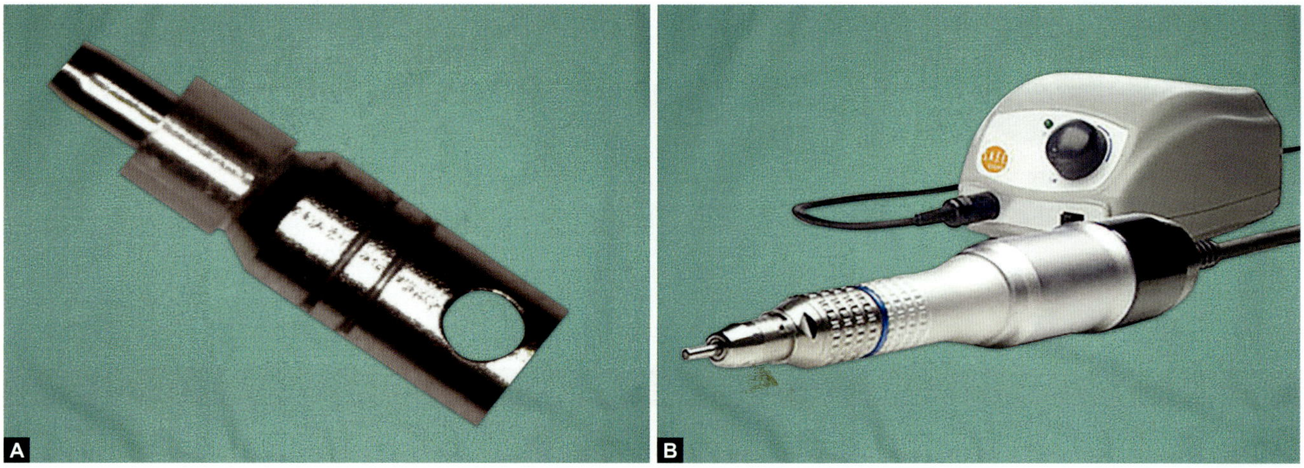

Figs. 1A and B: HARRIS Powered Scribe system with a motor.
Courtesy: https://www.hairsciencescenter.com/s-a-f-e-system/

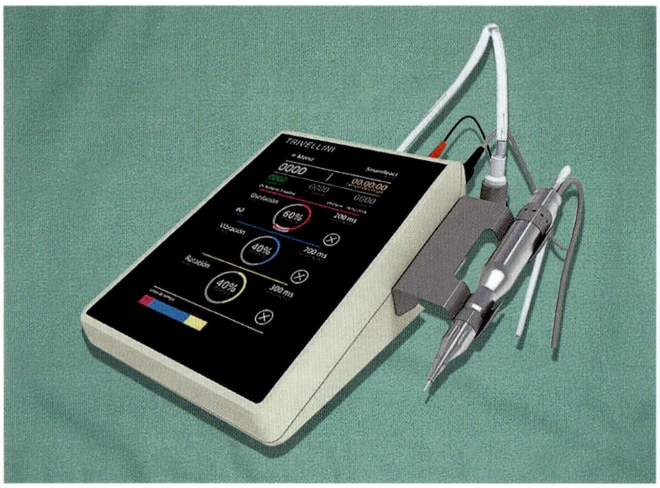

Fig. 2: Trivellini's SmartReact™ system.
Courtesy: https://www.trivellinitech.com/.

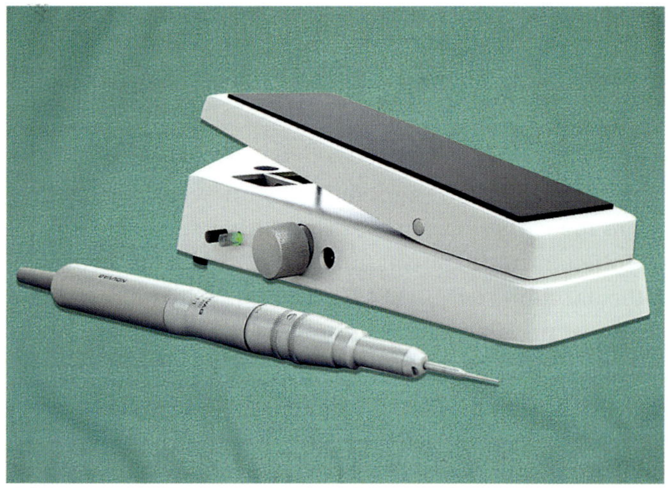

Fig. 3: Devroye's WAW system with smart foot pedal system.
Courtesy: http://www.devroyeinstruments.com/.

and the surgeon's experience.[3] When the advancement into the dermis is more, the chances of damage to the follicles are more, and when the advancement is not adequate, it will result in capping and difficulty in removing the graft.

These variables can be reduced with Trivellini's device. The system allows for repetition of the same sequence of action for every graft, thousands of times a day, and can work on any type of skin and hair. In addition, trauma to the follicles is minimized by directing the graft toward the center of the punch.

It has two essential components, suction and vibration. It provides a multiphasic approach that adjusts the punch mode and speed of motion as it enters different layers of the scalp. The device has various modes such as rotation, oscillation, vibration, and oscillating asynchronous variation modes. All these modes can be combined, and the force and timing can be adjusted as per the type of skin by using touch screen SmartReact™ system[4] **(Fig. 2)**.

SmartReact is an intelligent computerized system that operates automatically when the tip of the punch is positioned over the FU. The operator only needs to focus on following the exit angle of the follicles and placing the tip on the skin.

Devroye's WAW Follicular Unit Excision System[5]

Jean Devroye invented an innovative FUE system which comprised a foot pedal system called WAW pedal and Hybrid Tornado punch which enables the surgeon to do FUE with great precision and less damage to the grafts **(Fig. 3)**. This punch fits into the Nouvag autoclavable handpiece, which provides excellent support. When both are combined with a Nouvag motor, the FUE surgery proceeds with ease. One can adjust the oscillation speed and angulation freely with the support of the motorized handpiece.

The Hybrid Tornado punch has features of both sharp and dull punch **(Fig. 4)**. The tip of the tornado punch has a 90°

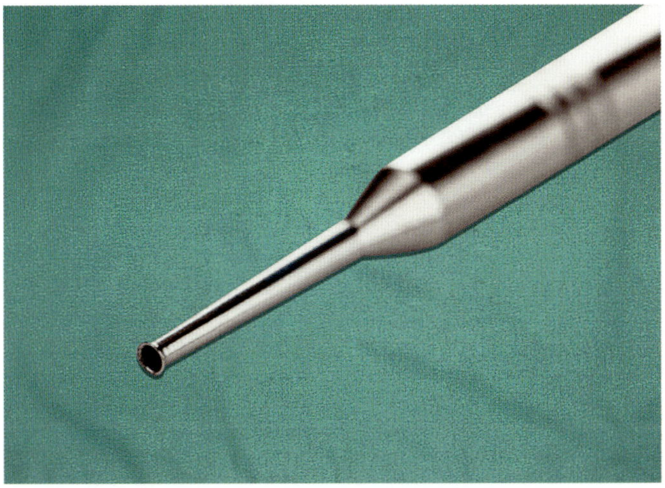

Fig. 4: Hybrid Tornado punch.

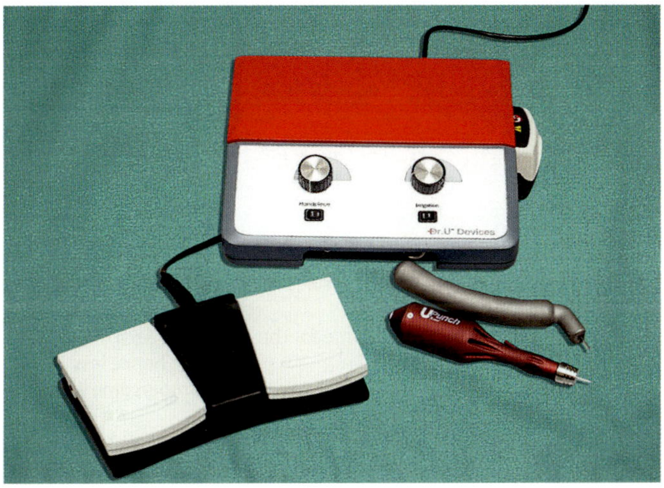

Fig. 5: UPunch system.
Source: Umar (2016).[7]

outer edge and a smooth funnel-shaped inner edge, which makes penetration into the skin gentle and less traumatic.

It works like a dissection tool rather than a cutting one. It has a suction effect also so that the grafts are less transected, chubbier, and richer in hair.

Umar's Machine and Technique

Umar developed nonrotary curved punches (the UPunch Curl),[6] prototyped by Keck Craig, Inc. (Pasadena, CA) **(Figs. 5 and 6)**. These punches have a curved end, which can easily maneuver through the curled Afro-textured hairs.

They have a strategically situated U-shaped cut along the circumference of the tubular edge.[7] The long axis of the punch is first aligned with the direction of the hair as it exits the skin **(Fig. 7)**. The curved tip follows the curl of the hair when plunged into the skin. The punch is pushed to the base of the follicles or even deeper, at which point the follicle is seen to pop out of the skin. Typically, the follicle stays loosely tethered to the extraction hole and is easily pulled out using forceps.

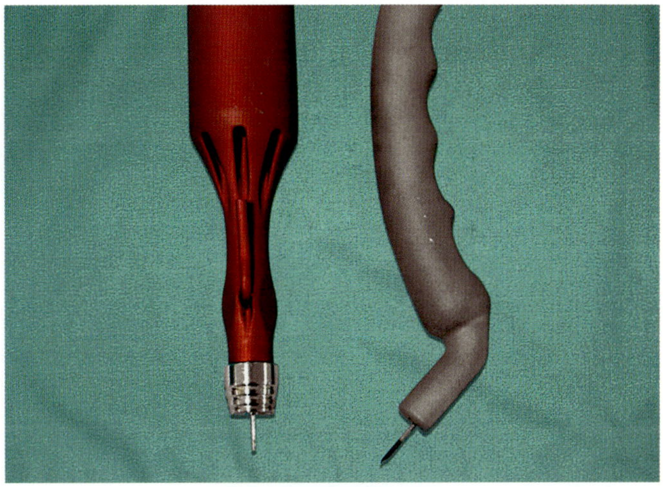

Fig. 6: Umar's handpiece.
Source: Umar (2016).[7]

Alternatively, it can attach to the punch, in which case the fluid mechanism is employed to flush the graft into a Petri dish by the aid of a foot-pedal-activated flushing system that discharges a pulse of physiologic solution to the tip of the punch. As per the inventors of this machine, the UPunch and U graft are best suited for curly hairs, which can be harvested with <10% transection.

Robotic Hair Transplantation

All the above machines have gone a long way in yielding high grafts during harvesting but still the surgeon needs some experience and becomes tired while doing larger sessions. So, this problem has been overcome by the robotic technique.

The robotic technique has been developed by Restoration Robotics (San Jose, CA). The ARTAS system (Restoration Robotics, Sunnyvale, CA)[8] is the first and only robotic device developed specifically for the FUE procedure and is approved for use only in men for the purpose of hair transplantation **(Fig. 8)**. The robotic system was approved by the Food and Drug Administration for hair transplantation in 2011.

The device has a robotic arm with a 1-mm punch which harvests FUs from the donor area, an ergonomic chair for the patient to sit and present the donor area to the surgeon with proper orientation, a video display screen **(Fig. 9)**, multiple cameras, and a computer interface. The device has a sharp inner punch and a blunt outer punch. The former cuts the skin to 1 mm deep and the latter then dissects the FUs from the surrounding tissues. A suction system also helps in retrieving the graft easily. It also has software which identifies the angle of exit of the hairs with precision.

The robot can harvest 1,000–1,200 grafts per hour. The software requires a minimum distance of 1.6 mm between extracted follicular groupings to minimize the risk of overharvesting donor hair. The surgeon can control the machine by a "pendant" that has various buttons controlling the harvesting parameters. The recipient site creation is the

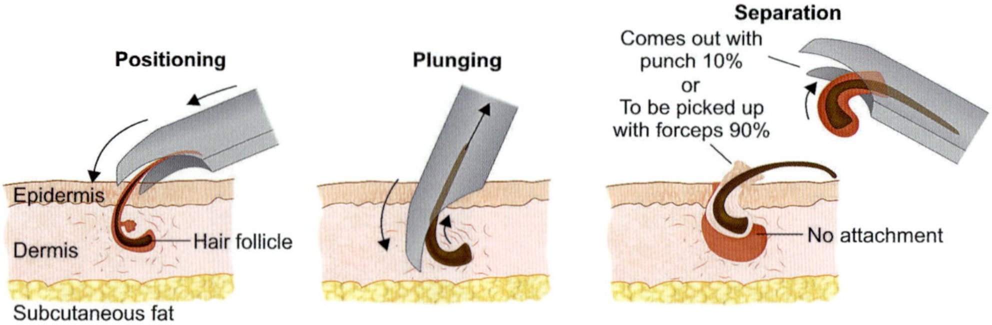

Fig. 7: Mechanism of UPunch system in curly hairs.
Source: Umar (2016).[7]

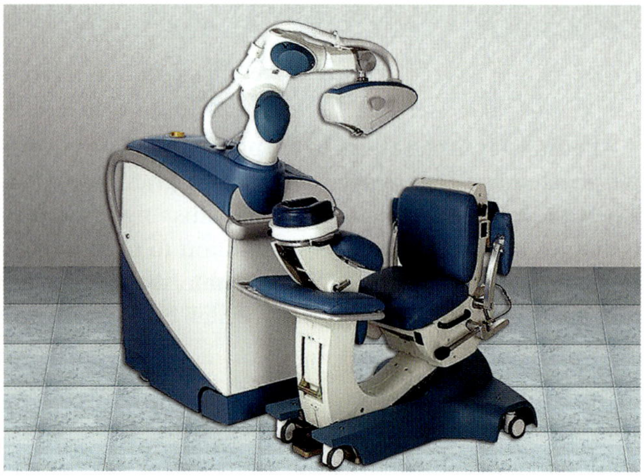

Fig. 8: ARTAS robotic hair transplantation device.
Source: Avram and Shannon (2014).[9]

TABLE 1: Comparison of ARTAS and ARTAS 9X character exercise.

	ARTAS	*ARTAS 9X*
Automation	Automated	Automated
Punch system	18G needle, 1 mm diameter used	20G needle with 1 mm diameter
Scar detection	Low-level detection	High-level scarf detection
Speed of extraction	800–1,000 grafts per hour	1,200–1,400 grafts per hour
Assisted force-drag technology	Absent	Present
Cameras	Monochrome	Color
Ergonomics	Somewhat cumbersome for the patient	Long arm and long reach of the arm, hence less cumbersome

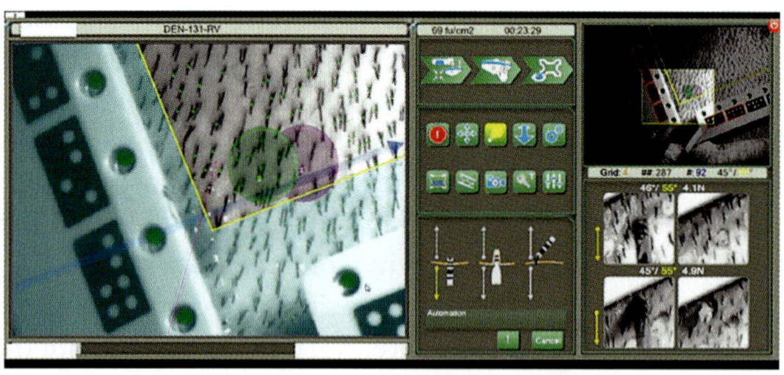

Fig. 9: Video display screen of ARTAS.
Source: Avram and Shannon (2014).[9]

same as in conventional FUE. Cut-to-size (CTS) blades or 18G needles are used to create the openings for the grafts to be placed. Postoperative steps and complications are identical to conventional FUE.[9]

ARTAS 9X

ARTAS 9X is a major upgrade of the hair transplant robot, enabling faster and more precise robotic FUE procedures. It has a lot of improvements in both hardware and software. Few upgrades are white light light-emitting diode (LED), color camera and tensioner, 20G harvesting needle, robotic base extender, new needle mechanism cover, and more comfortable headrest and halo.[9] Software upgrades include better scar detection, faster harvesting, ability to zoom into the main viewing screen, and improved ARTAS Hair Studio software.

The new optical system uses color cameras and white LED lights so surgeons can excise grafts while the system is still harvesting without the risk of eye fatigue. The color cameras also allow the robot to associate colors with shapes increasing the visual sharpness and accuracy of the system.

The ARTAS 9X also has an assisted force-drag technology,[10] which enables the robot to self-align as soon as the indicators are detected by the optical system. This speeds up the procedure and makes it more efficient by minimizing setup time between grids. It has a longer robotic arm with a long reach and minimizes the repositioning of the patient. **Table 1** shows the comparison between the older ARTAS system and the latest ARTAS 9X robotic system.

NeoGraft™ Technique

NeoGraft™ technique is a newer technique introduced by Lee in 2014.[11] It uses a surgical device with a handheld wand

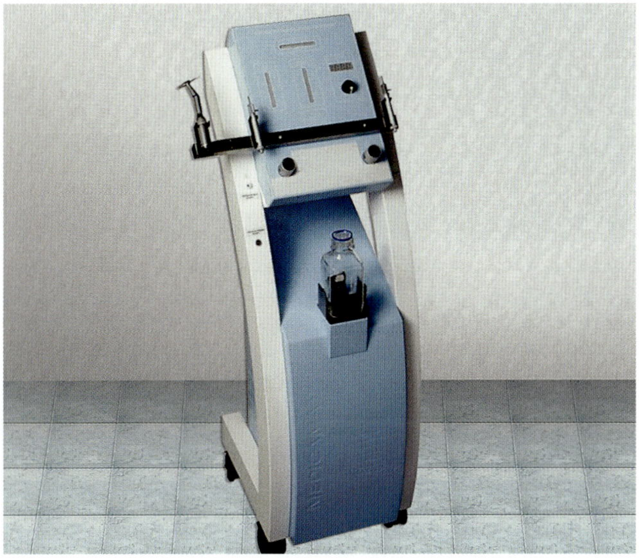

Fig. 10: NeoGraft™ machine.
Source: Lee (2018).[11]

that excises FUs from the donor area and implants them in the recipient area via an air pressure/suction-based system **(Fig. 10)**. The device requires the surgeon to select and harvest the grafts. However, it has vacuum assist technology, which reduces trauma to the grafts during excision.

The vacuum mechanism can be reversed to implant the grafts. This minimizes human intervention and thus achieves better graft survival.

The NeoGraft™ device is used to first separate the graft from the surrounding donor tissue with a rotating sharp punch that is connected to a suction unit.[12] Once the upper part of the graft is dissected by the punch, the suction pulls the graft out, separating it from the remaining tissue. The graft is sucked through a tube into a small holding chamber. This process has the advantage of not requiring a person to manually remove the graft from the scalp, but it can expose the graft to dry air, requiring the regular addition of a preserving solution to the holding chamber.

Once approximately 50 grafts are harvested, the collection chamber is opened and the harvested grafts are placed into a Petri dish that contains a preserving solution. In the placement phase of a hair transplant using NeoGraft™, a small number of extracted grafts are removed from the holding solution, and a second arm of the NeoGraft™ device is used to draw up the grafts one at a time via suction into the needle-tipped device. They are then individually inserted into the recipient sites using the pneumatic implanter or they can be inserted with other implanting devices such as forceps or hand-powered implanter.

The NeoGraft™ device is a semiautomatic device that lessens the burden of follicular excision. But it has a longer learning curve, and many procedures are required to achieve excellent results.

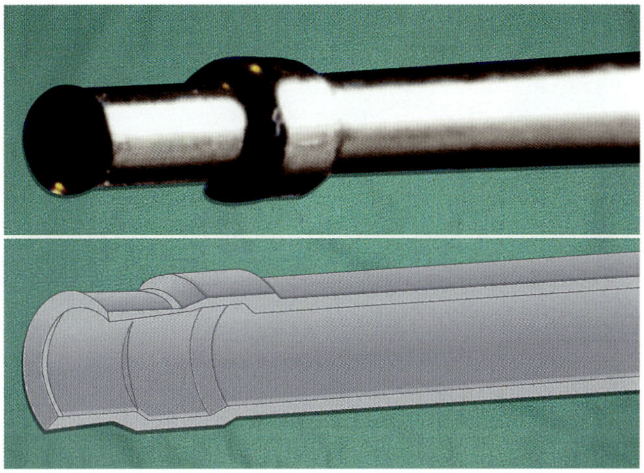

Fig. 11: Trivellini's Edge Out punch.
Source: Trivellini (2018).[4]

Endoscopic Hair Transplantation/Piloscopic Hair Transplantation

Wesley has developed an innovative method of obtaining FUs by FUE/follicular isolation technique (FIT).[12] It is called piloscopic harvesting of FUs. He has developed prototypes of an endoscopic device that can harvest grafts from under the skin. With this device, a small incision is made in the donor area, and the endoscopic device is inserted into the level of the fascia. A camera displays the bulbs of the various FUs, and the device is then manipulated so as to grasp the selected FUs at a level approximately 1 mm below the skin. With this method, the outer surface of the skin is not penetrated, and no evidence of the surgery in terms of a donor scar would be present. This does not cause any visible large scars or hypopigmented scars that result from FUE.

Innovations in Punches

It is not only the machine which is important for harvesting but the punches which penetrate the skin are also equally important. The earlier used punches for FUE had no depth control and hence would cause more transections. To overcome the issue of follicular splay, many newer punches with different shapes and unique features were developed.

These innovative punches are discussed below.

Flare-shaped Punches

Trivellini's Edge Out™ punches ***(Fig. 11)****:* The Edge Out™ punch design by Trivellini has the cutting edge on the outside of a thick-walled punch, with an internal bevel.[13] This shape also keeps the cutting edge away from the follicles when incising through the deeper dermis.

Hybrid punch ***(Fig. 12)****:* A flare was given toward the tip to keep the cutting edge away from splaying follicles.

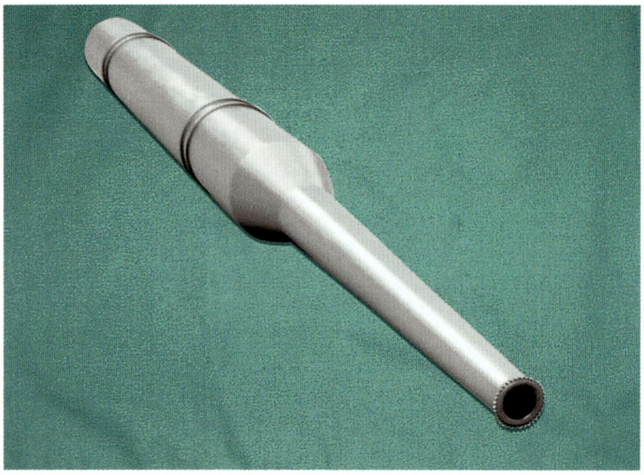

Fig. 12: Hybrid Tornado punch.
Courtesy: https://www.trivellinitech.com.

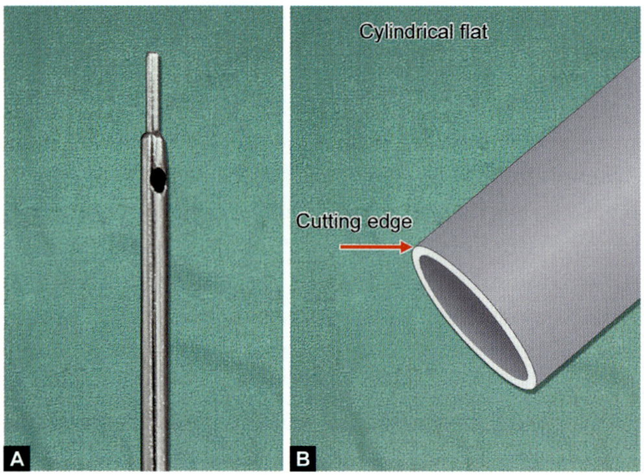

Figs. 13A and B: Dua's Flat punch.

Devroye developed a new Hybrid Tornado punch with a flat-surfaced bevel perpendicular to the axis and a sharp outer edge.[5] This minimized the injury caused due to rotation of the punch within the dermis. The yield with Devroye punches is very good with minimal partial transections of the graft.[12]

UPunchi™: The Dr.UPunchi™ developed by Umar incorporates the curvature of the curly hairs seen in persons with African descent.[14] The flared tip of this punch expands as the punch penetrates the skin, thus resulting in less everted wound profiles with smaller donor scars.

The Window punch: This was introduced by Cole and has an opening above the dissecting edge, where one can see through the punch, resulting in less axial and torsional friction, and providing a better view of the operation of the punch insertion.

Dua's Flat punch ***(Figs. 13A and B):*** The author has developed a Flat punch, which is a modified dull punch made longer in length to accommodate the longer hair follicles of Asian patients.[15] The standard punch length is 4 mm, whereas Dua's

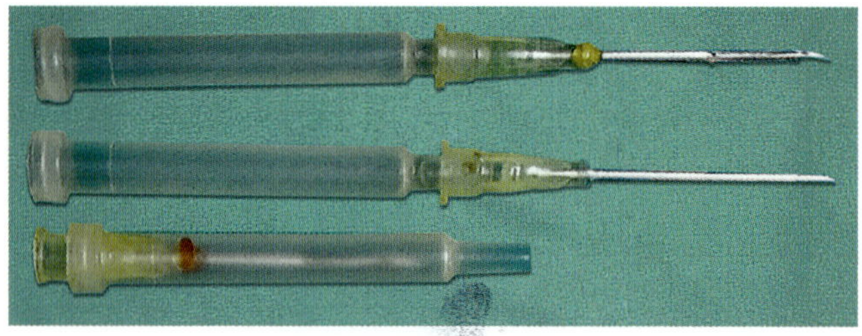

Fig. 14: SAVA implanter.

Flat punch comes in a variety of lengths ranging from 3.75 to 5.5 mm. The advantage of this punch is that the transection of grafts is significantly lesser than the sharp punches, but the force required to insert through the skin is more as compared to the latter.

Innovations in Implantation Methods

The method of implantation is as important as harvesting the grafts. Initial methods of implantation were "stick and place" and "forceps" methods. Then, implanters were introduced which made the process easier and reduced handling and damage of the grafts.

Implanter pens were first invented in the 1990s by Yung Chul Chou of the Kyungpook National University.[16] An implanter pen shortens the out-of-the-body time of grafts, which in turn increases the survivability. Some of the various implanters designed include the Boudjema implanter pen, Lion implanter, Rassman implanter, Choi implanter, SAVA implanter, KEEP implanter, NeoGraft™ implantation device, and Devroye's WAW implanter.

Choi Implanters[17]

A pen-like device with a hollow beveled needle and a plunger is currently popular. The grafts can be loaded by an assistant and then handed over to the surgeon who places the grafts directly on intact skin.

SAVA Implanters[18]

The SAVA implanter was designed in India by Sanjiv Vasa. Similar to other implanters, the assistant loads the graft into the SAVA implanter before handing it to the surgeon. This implanter comes with an additional device called the introducer. After the graft is placed in the implanter, it is inserted into the skin and then the graft is slid in using the introducer **(Fig. 14)**.

KEEP Implanters

Erdogan's "KEEP" implanter (Koray Erdogan's Embedding Placer) **(Fig. 15)** is a newer entry into types of modern implanters. The loading is made on the side of the needle, but more important, the graft is gently slid into a premade incision with angled forceps.[19] However, the KEEP implanter has three disadvantages: It holds only one graft at a time, is very fragile, and is very difficult to manage the orientation of the hair's curve.[20]

Devroye's Multigraft Implanter System (WAW Implanter)

This is another newer implanter invented by Devroye in which the needle edges are blunt and attached to a Luer lock tip.[20] The grafts can be loaded, similar to other implanters, from the tip **(Fig. 16)**. The grafts are gently slid into the lumen of the implanter. They are moved from the tip to the top. Special attention is taken to give good orientation to the hair curve. In contrast to the traditional implanter, the curve has to be directed face down.

The reason is that the implanter is used with the slit placed upward. The number of grafts loaded varies from 5 to 8, and a maximum of 10 grafts can be loaded. Hence, the loading process is faster. The implanter does not move; the grafts placed near the implanter tip, on the finger, get engaged in the lumen very quickly. The beauty of the system is that now, a placer needs only one loader instead of the two required with the classical dull needle implantation (DNI) technique.[20] The placing is also faster. Multiple loaded implanters can be held and soaked in a chilled or room-temperature storage solution.

INRUT implanter: Kim Moon-kyu of Kyungpook National University Hospital, Korea, developed a multihair implanter in which multiple hair follicles (up to 10 follicles) can be loaded at a time and implanted. This implanter comes with a cartridge that can be rotated and loaded with 10 hair follicles quickly, which significantly reduced the loading time **(Fig. 17)**. Hence, the implant time is reduced by more than an hour, and the procedure is less tiring for the patients as well as for assistants. This reduces out-of-the-body time and hence improves graft uptake and survivability.

Mohebi inserter:[21] It is a dull implanter designed by Parsa Mohebi **(Figs. 18A and B)**. This implanter potentially reduces the manipulation of the hair follicles during the placement process into premade sites.[20] With these inserters, the technicians can load their own grafts and can use only one hand for insertion. They can switch hands depending on the angle of slits and maintain distance from the patient's head. It reduces the manpower and space required for implantation.

Dull implanters: Speranzini has developed an implanter with a dull tip.[22] The advantages of this implanter are that there is minimal trauma to the fragile FUE grafts and optimal growth. It also allows smaller incisions which in turn, allows

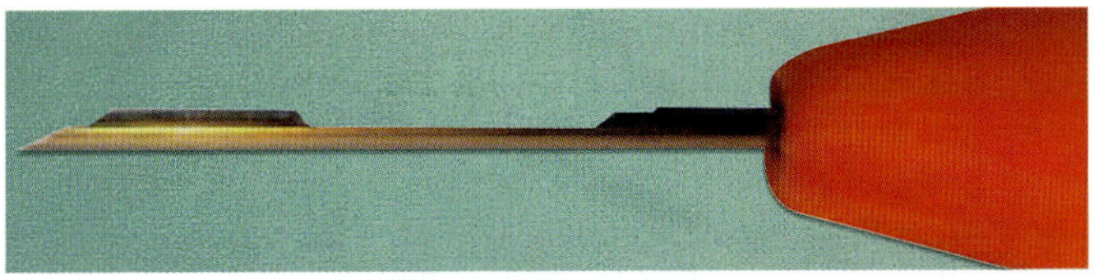

Fig. 15: KEEP implanter.
Source: Erdogan (2016).[19]

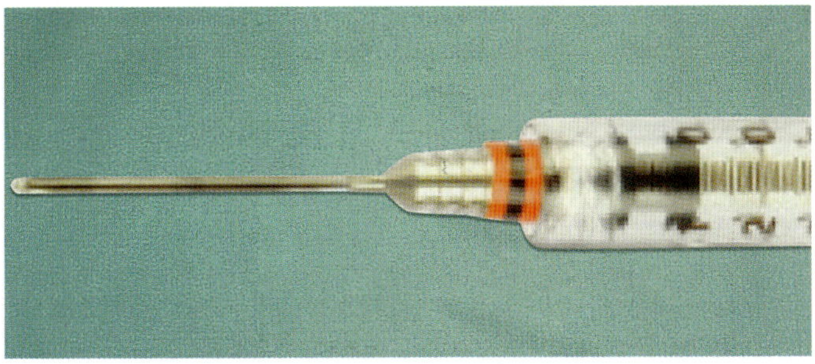

Fig. 16: Devroye's multigraft implanter system (WAW implanter).
Courtesy: http://www.devroyeinstruments.com.

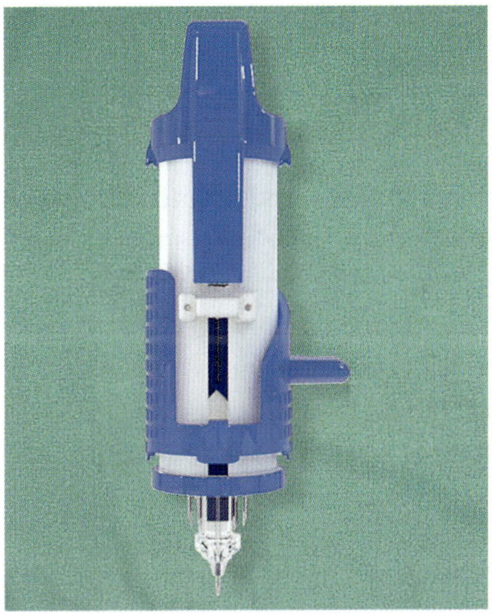

Fig. 17: INRUT multihair implanter.
Courtesy: https://www.inrut.co.kr/.

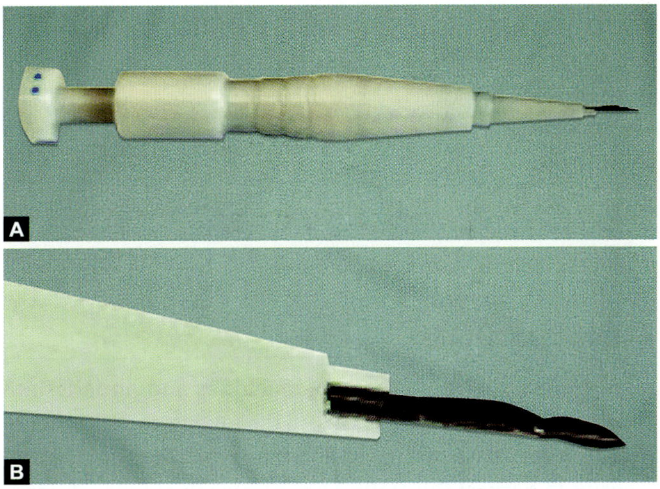

Figs. 18A and B: (A) Mohebi inserter; (B) Close-up of Mohebi inserter.
Courtesy: https://parsamohebi.com/resources/dr-mohebis-innovations/inserter/.

TABLE 2: Storage solutions.[23]

Medium	*pH*	*Osmolality*	*Buffer*	*Comments*
Serum	7.4	289 (280–310)	Bicarbonate	Bicarbonate is a suboptimal pH buffer for cold storage solutions
Saline	5.0		None	Extracellular balance
Ringer's lactate	6.5		Lactate	Extracellular balance
Plasma-Lyte A	7.4		Acetate gluconate	Extracellular balance
HypoThermosol-FRS	7.6		HEPES	Intracellular-like balance
Custodiol-HTK	7.4–40°C 7.25–room temperature (RT)*		Histidine	• Intracellular-like balance • Tryptophan (membrane stabilizer) • Ketoglutarate (energy substrate)

*An indoor temperature around 20 or 22°C (68 to 72°F) according to American Heritage Dictionary of the English Language.

higher densities of the slits and less trauma in the recipient site. Easier learning curve and inexpensiveness are few other advantages.

Innovations in Storage Solutions (Table 2)

In order to increase graft survival and achieve greater results, many storage solutions have been studied. Storage solutions are of two types: One is extracellular balance type and the other is intracellular balance type. In extracellular balance solutions, the Na^+ concentration is high and K^+ concentration is low. In intracellular balance solution, it is the opposite with K^+ being high and Na^+ being low. The commonly used storage solutions having extracellular ion balance are:

- Normal saline
- Ringer's lactate
- Tissue culture media
- Plasma-Lyte A.

These solutions can cause electrolyte imbalance in the grafts when chilled, leading to cell swelling and graft damage. Newer storage solutions have intracellular ion balance.[24] Few of them are:

- HypoThermosol
- Viaspan
- Custodiol[25]
- ACell+PRP[26]

These are expensive and are thought to be more beneficial than extracellular storage solutions.

CONCLUSION

As described above, a variety of machines and punches are available for harvesting in FUE. All the inventors are trying to decrease the transection of grafts while harvesting and making it easier to harvest the grafts. However, each of these devices has a certain learning curve and the surgeon should choose the device with which he/she is the most comfortable.

REFERENCES

1. Harris JA. New methodology and instrumentation for follicular unit extraction: lower follicle transection rates and expanded patient candidacy. Dermatol Surg. 2006;32(1):56-62.
2. Cole JP. Enhanced follicular extraction punch and method. Patent US8753354B2. 2014.
3. Trivellini R. An innovation in suction assisted FUE. Hair Transplant Forum Int. 2016;26(2):58-9.
4. Trivellini R. The Trivellini system and technique. Hair Transplant Forum Int. 2018:28(5):188-90.
5. Devroye J. Powered FU extraction with the short-arc-oscillation flat punch FUE system (SFFS). Hair Transplant Forum Int. 2016;26(4):129-36.
6. Umar S. What is the Dr.UGraft™ FUE Hair Transplant System? [online] Available from: https://ugraft.com/what-is-dr-ugraft-hair-transplant-system/. [Last accessed September, 2023].
7. Umar S. Comparative study of a novel tool for follicular unit extraction for individuals with Afro-textured hair. Plast Reconstr Surg Glob Open. 2016;4(9):e1069.
8. Vandruff CL. ARTAS system: how technology is changing the hair restoration industry. Aesthet Trends. 2011;1-5.
9. Avram MR, Watkins SA. Robotic follicular unit extraction in hair transplantation. Dermatol Surg. 2014;40:1319-27.
10. ARTAS 9x—Bernstein Medical introduces major upgrade to ARTAS Robotic Hair Transplant System. [online] Available from: https://www.bernsteinmedical.com/news/artas-9x-upgrade-robotic-hair-transplant-system/. [Last accessed September, 2023].
11. Lee IJ. NeoGraft™: my experience in Asians. In: Pathomvanich D, Imagawa K (Eds). Practical Aspects of Hair Transplantation in Asians. Tokyo: Springer; 2018.
12. Wesley C. Endoscopic follicular extraction. Presented at: American Academy of Cosmetic Surgery Annual Meeting, January 14–17, 2015, New Orleans, LA. Lecture.
13. Umar S. Dr.UGraft™ solves low hair transplant growth from graft torsion injuries. [online] Available from: https://ugraft.com/solving-low-hair-transplant-growth-from-graft-torsion-injuries/. [Last accessed September, 2023].
14. Tykocinski A. Dealing with a hybrid trumpet punch. Hair Transplant Forum Int. 2017;27(1):14-6.

15. Trivellini RL. Trivellini Flared. [online] Available from: https://www.trivellinitech.com/product/trivellini-flared/. [Last accessed September, 2023].
16. Dua K, Dua A, Desai NV. FUE techniques: motorized with blunt. In: Unger WP, Shapiro R, Unger R, Unger M (Eds). Hair Transplantation, 6th edition. London: Informa Healthcare; 2022.
17. Choi YC, Kim JC. Single hair transplantation using the Choi hair transplanter. J Dermatol Surg Oncol. 1992;18:945-8.
18. Marwah MK, Mysore V. Recipient area. J Cutan Aesthet Surg. 2018;11:202-10.
19. Erdogan K. Keep implanters. [online] Available from: www.youtube.com/watch?v=z9o9S8lrrXA. [Accessed September, 2023].
20. Devroye JM. A new multi-graft implanter system. Hair Transplant Forum Int. 2018;28(3):100-1.
21. Mohebi P. A novel device to insert FU grafts into premade sites. Hair Transplant Forum Int. 2018;28(4):146-8.
22. Speranzini M. FUE graft placement with dull needle implanters into premade sites. Hair Transplant Forum Int. 2016;26(2):49-56.
23. Parsley WM, Perez-Meza D. Review of factors affecting the growth and survival of follicular grafts. J Cutan Aesthet Surg. 2010;3:69-75.
24. Krugluger W, Moser K Hugeneck J, Laciak K, Moser C. New storage buffers for micrografts enhance graft survival and clinical outcome in hair restoration surgery. Hair Transplant Forum Int. 2003;13:333-4.
25. Perez-Meza D, Cooley J, Parsley W. Custodiol vs. hypothermosol. Hair graft survival at 24 and 48 hrs outside the body. ISHRS Annual Meeting, San Diego, CA, 2006.
26. Kim JS, Kaminsky AJ, Summitt JB, Thayer WP. New innovations for deep partial-thickness burn treatment with ACell MatriStem Matrix. Adv Wound Care. 2016;5:546-52.

CHAPTER 78

Ethics of Hair Transplantation

Mysore Venkataram

KEY MESSAGES

- Ethical considerations are the subject of focus in hair restoration practice because of rapid commercialization.
- The areas of focus are physician qualifications, role of technicians, training of doctors and staff, advertisement and promotion, ways of charging patients, and documentation.
- There are no regulatory guidelines for who, when, and where hair restoration surgery can be done.
- Ethical practice is of utmost importance to ensure patient satisfaction and safety.

INTRODUCTION

Medical ethics is a system of moral principles that apply values to the practice of clinical medicine and scientific research. It is based on a set of values that professionals can refer to in the case of any confusion or conflict. These values include respect for autonomy, nonmaleficence, beneficence, and justice **(Box 1)**.[1]

Medical ethics is not just a thought process. It also involves people skills, such as gathering the facts needed to make a decision and presenting your decision in a way that wins over the confidence of all parties. Medical ethics is important to maintain the respect of your patients; to help resolve disputes between family, patients, physicians, or other parties; to maintain respectful relationships with other clinicians; and to maintain efficiency and a safe satisfactory and joyful practice.[2]

THE IMPORTANCE OF QUALITY AND ETHICS IN HAIR TRANSPLANTATION

The field of hair transplant (HT) has grown exponentially in the past decade, especially after the introduction of follicular unit excision (FUE). There is much variation in criteria for case selection, the technique, and pre- and postprocedure protocols by different surgeons. Techniques continue to evolve and evidence in the form of controlled data is not available for all techniques and protocols being used; there is also a debate as to who can do what, what should be the training for staff, and the role of technicians. This has led to a situation wherein medicolegal issues have cropped up as to what is the minimum acceptable.[3]

BOX 1: Values of medical ethics for professionals.

- *Autonomy:* Patients have the right to determine their own healthcare
- *Justice:* Distributing the benefits and burdens of care across society
- *Beneficence:* Doing good for the patient
- *Nonmaleficence:* Making sure you are not harming the patient

What complicates the issue is that hair restoration surgery is a technique practiced by different specialties, both by surgeons and by physicians. Being a cosmetic surgery and not covered by insurance, the field of surgical hair restoration is poorly regulated, both by the medical community and by the government. This implies that, legally speaking, any licensed doctor can claim to be a qualified HT surgeon and undertake HT surgery even without training and/or any license. The advent of FUE, mechanization and automation, the need of assistants, the perception of an easy and safe surgery, minimal need for investment, and the lure of attracting a desperate, eager, sometimes poorly informed young clientele have all led to explosion of clinics performing the surgery often led by nonmedical personnel or poorly qualified personnel. Social media publicity, the potential of exploitation of social media by digitally savvy entrepreneurs, and the possibilities of medical tourism have contributed to the increasing need for ethical practices in the field.[4] Occurrence of two deaths, blindness, and necrotizing fasciitis all are examples of a field being led astray. This chapter deals with several ethical aspects of hair transplantation **(Box 2)**.

Physician Qualifications, Role of Technicians, Training of Doctors and Staff

Hair transplant surgeons: There is no uniform opinion as to which specialties can perform HT. Even medical councils have not categorically resolved this issue and different associations

BOX 2: Ethical aspects of hair transplant.

- Physician qualifications
- Role of technicians
- Training of doctors and staff
- Ethical advertisement and promotion
- Ethical and transparent ways of charging patients
- Honest documentation

have different criteria for membership. The International Society of Hair Restoration Surgery (ISHRS) allows all MBBS doctors to perform HT, while many maxillofacial surgeons also perform the surgery.[5]

The Association of Hair Restoration Surgeons-India (AHRS-I) in October 2015 resolved that the only specialties eligible to become members of AHRS-I and practice HT surgery would be:[6,7]

- The Master of lastic Surgery (MCh)/Diplomate of National Board (DNB) plastic surgery
- Doctor of Medicine (MD) or postgraduate in dermatology
- Master of Surgery (MS) or postgraduate in Ear, Nose, and Throat (ENT) surgery
- General Surgery (MS).

Modern medicine practitioners (MBBS doctors/specialists not included in the above qualifications) who have passed the American Board of Hair Restoration Surgery (ABHRS) exam are also eligible to perform HT surgery. Ayurvedic doctors, homeopathic doctors, and dentists are not qualified to perform HT surgery.

Any procedure that involves tissue removal from the scalp or body, by any means, should be performed by a licensed physician in the field of medicine. The following aspects of hair restoration surgery should only be performed by a qualified HT surgeon and not by technicians:

- Preoperative diagnostic evaluation and consultation
- Surgery planning
- Surgery execution including:
  - Donor hair harvesting
  - Hairline design
  - Recipient site creation
- Management of other patient medical issues and possible adverse reactions
- Postoperative care.

Role of Assistants (Technicians)

Hair transplant practice needs assistants, also called HT technicians. It is both ethical and necessary that such assistants be from a medical background, such as nurses, lab technicians, pharmacists, and MBBS doctors. However, they need to be provided structured systematic proper training in aspects of HT as well as disinfection, sterilization, patient communication, etc. Unrelated nonmedical personnel such as arts graduates and industrial training institute (ITI) technicians should not be used as they have little understanding of sterilization and cannot handle any medical emergency which may arise during the procedure. The concept of nonphysicians removing human tissue and primarily performing HT surgery is improper and not acceptable. It is not consistent with the standard of care in the medical community.

Technicians can be involved only in the following steps of the HT surgery:

1. Picking up the grafts (extraction) after scoring
2. Arranging the grafts
3. Implantation into premade slits
4. Postoperative dressings.

Surgical assistants/technicians should perform only under the supervision of a physician and they are allowed to perform only those steps that do not involve incision of the body. Hence, they should not perform scoring (incision), slit making, and suturing. Assistants shall be offered training on models initially, then placed as observers for the surgical process, and then be deputed for the HT surgery. At least one of the assistants should be a paramedical staff and trained in basic life support/advanced cardiac life support (BLS/ACLS).[5,6]

Training

Hair transplant is not taught as a subject in any of the above courses that were listed as the eligibility criteria for an HT surgeon. While surgical specialties such as MCh/DNB plastic surgery, MS general surgery, and MS ENT provide adequate surgical background, training in trichology is lacking. Likewise, MD/DNB/Diploma in dermatology provides adequate training in trichology, but surgical training is lacking.

Physicians who perform HT surgery must possess the education, training, and current competency in the field of hair restoration surgery. Membership in the National Hair Restoration Society/Global Society and regular attendance in annual conferences and workshops facilitate education and training. Fellowship courses from ISHRS would be an added qualification.

In view of this, the AHRS Task Force on HT recommended the following:[5]

- MCh/DNB plastic surgery, MS general surgery, and MS ENT doctors should undergo further training in trichology in a clinic which provides such training under a dermatologist/HT surgeon, preferably for 3 months, but at least for a period of 1 month.
- Likewise, MD/DNB/Diploma in dermatology should undergo adequate training both hands on and observational under the supervision of an experienced HT surgeon. While no legal guideline exists to define how much observation and supervision is needed, this task force recommends that at least 50 surgeries be observed and 25 surgeries be performed under supervision before starting independent practice. This training should also include training in basic surgical practices, sterilization, disinfection, and emergency resuscitation.

Ethical Issues

Use of trademarks or service marks as commercial names for a hair restoration procedure, without disclosing the scientific basis for the procedure, its complications, and side effects, is not in the public interest nor is it in the public interest to use a commercial name to market a procedure that is described under a commonly accepted name in the medical literature, without revealing the name used in the medical literature. Professional disagreements should be aired in a forum of peers. Denigration that aims to destroy another physician's practice is morally reprehensible. Physicians who market their services have a responsibility for "truth in advertising".

The following advertisements are considered misleading to the public:[5]

- *Inaccurate credentials:* Incorrectly claiming to be certified by the AHRS-I, ABHRS, or claiming to be a member or fellow of the ISHRS, and otherwise stating or suggesting any expertise in hair restoration surgery that is false.
- *Misrepresenting board certification:* Physicians should identify their specific medical specialty certifying board when marketing their board certification in the public domain language; for example, "board-certified hair restoration surgeon" is not acceptable.
- *Misrepresenting photographs:* Publishing photographs of other physicians' patients in any manner that states or suggests they are patients of the publishing practice.
- *Copyright/trademark violations in general:* Republishing or otherwise representing the photographs, publications, trade names, logos, or other trademarks of another practitioner without permission in violation of the owner's copyrights and/or trademarks.
- *Misleading language:* Use of the following terms and phrases in marketing by a hair restoration surgeon may mislead the public:
  - "Scarless surgery"
  - "No incision"
  - "No touch"
  - "No cutting"
  - "Cloning"
  - "Hair multiplication"
  - "Noninvasive"
  - "Eliminates the need for additional procedures"
  - "Pain free or no pain"
  - "Unlimited grafts"
  - "Guaranteed results".

Charges for the Surgery

The surgery cost shall be based on the number of follicular units/follicles/packages for a particular surface area as per the surgeon's routine pricing practice. However, each term unit/graft/follicle should be explained and the patient should be familiar with the terminology. Costs shall be informed prior to the patient and documented in the consent form.

Transparency

Transparency in the HT surgery is needed in the following aspects:[5]

- Physician, who will be performing the surgery, and the role of assistants shall be informed to the patient prior to the surgery.
- Role of the surgeon and the assistants should be documented—who does what.
- Hairline design once accepted by the patient and the surgeon shall be documented with an image.
- Number of grafts/follicles/area to be covered initially planned and actually performed should be disclosed to the patient and documented with images. Discharge slip should document the number of units of each type, 1/2/3/4 hairs total; number of units and total number of hairs separately.
- Provision of counting the grafts can be explained to the patient.
- The need for medical management/chances of inadequate growth/thinning of grafted follicles with time post-HT shall be discussed with the patient and documented.
- Charging for the surgery should be only for viable follicles which are transplanted.

Documentation and Consent

Medical record is admissible as documentary evidence in a legal suit.[8] So it is important to maintain a meticulous record of clinical details of the patient; counseling process; consent taking; detailed preoperative, operative, and postoperative notes and instructions; and follow-up visits.

Photographs taken before, during, and after the procedure provide adequate proof of the outcome of the procedure.[9,10]

Preoperative documentation should include the details about any preexisting health issues, drug allergy, photo ID lignocaine test dose, baseline vital parameters, hairline design planned, planned number of grafts to be harvested, expected results with duration, donor adequacy, continuation of medical management if required, and the possibility of second surgery after a particular period.[11]

Consent in the medical field can be defined as an instrument of mutual communication between doctor and patient with an expression of authorization/permission/choice by the latter for the doctor to act/not act in a particular way.[12-14]

Lack of informed consent is a frequent cause of allegations of medical negligence.

Consent should have the following details:

- Procedure details—in language that the patient understands
- Risks involved
- Complications that can arise
- Outcome expected
- Duration of treatment (average)
- Expenses involved (approximate).

Intraoperative records should include the vital parameters, drugs administered and their dosage, complications if any, the remedial measures that were carried out, number of grafts

BOX 3: The American Board of Hair Restoration Surgery (ABHRS) Code of Ethics.

- Use every opportunity to improve public understanding of the role of the hair restoration surgeon
- Cooperate in every reasonable and proper way with other physicians and work with them in activities contributing to the advancement of quality patient care
- Maintain the confidentiality of privileged information entrusted or known to me by virtue of my role as a hair restoration surgeon within the constraints of the law
- Accept no personal compensation from any party that would influence or require special consideration in the provision of care to any patient
- Provide patient care impartially, provide no special privilege to any individual patient based on the patient's race, color, creed, sex, national origin, or handicap
- Use only legal and ethical means in the provision of care to my patients and strive to expose those physicians deficient in character or competence, or who engage in fraud or deception
- Maintain the highest standard of personal conduct
- Abide by the highest ethical standards in activities designed to attract patients to my practice including recognition of the ABHRS advertising policy which requires membership status should not be embellished, to utilize truthful advertising, and to designate my ABHRS membership as ABHRS diplomate as opposed to board certified by the ABHRS
- Maintain loyalty to the goals and objectives of the ABHRS as stated in the ABHRS by-laws
- Promote and encourage the highest level of medical ethics in providing competent medical service with compassion and respect for human dignity
- Recognize and discharge my responsibility and that of the medical and/or osteopathic profession to uphold the laws and regulations relating to the practice of hair restoration surgery
- Strive for excellence in all aspects of medical practice
- Continue to study, apply, and advance scientific knowledge; make relevant information available to patients, colleagues, and public; obtain consultation; and use the talents of other health professionals when the best interests of a patient so indicate

planted, the area of scalp covered, the details of the surgical team, and the duration of the surgery with the timings of the beginning and the end of each stage of the surgery.

Immediate postoperative records should have the following details: Vital parameters after the surgery, duration of observation post surgery, complications if any at the end of the surgery, remedial measures taken, postoperative prescription and advice, emergency contact number for communication, and the details of the follow-up visit.

Patient's failure to adhere to postprocedure consultations, neglect of precautions, and noncompliance of instructions, if any, should also find a place in the record.

Both manually signed records and computerized data help in standardization, storage, and easy retrieval of records.

Medical records of hair transplantation must be preserved for 5 years, but those pertaining to malpractice suits must be preserved till the final settlement of the case.

Custodial ownership of records vests with the aesthetic surgeon or the hospital. But on request, they should be provided to the patient within 72 hours.

Consumer Protection Act can condone a delay in filing a case of negligence beyond the prescribed limitation of 2 years from the date of occurrence.[15,16]

Counseling for the Medical Management

Hair transplant surgery should not be considered as a single-step permanent solution for androgenetic alopecia (AGA), since hair loss in AGA is a continuous process. Every patient should be educated about the importance of continuing the medical management even after the HT surgery. Topical minoxidil 2–5% and oral finasteride at a dosage of 1 mg/day are the approved medications for AGA. Dosage and duration should be individualized according to the degree of hair loss.[17,18]

American Board of Hair Restoration Surgery Code of Ethics[19]

The ABHRS or International Board of Hair Restoration Surgery (IBHRS) certifies doctors for the safe practice of hair restoration surgery. They require that certified surgeons pledge themselves to the guidelines mentioned in **Box 3**.

CONCLUSION

- Hair restoration is no magic and should not be taken lightly.
- All protocols need to be adhered to strictly.
- Honesty and transparency are of utmost importance.

REFERENCES

1. de Fontaine S. Ethics in aesthetic surgery. Rev Med Brux. 2013;34(4):287-90.
2. Sacchidanand SA, Bhat S. Safe practice of cosmetic dermatology: avoiding legal tangles. J Cutan Aesthet Surg. 2012;5(3):170-5.
3. Rassman WR. Areas of unethical behavior practiced today. Hair Transplant Forum Int. 2009;19(5):149-53.
4. Kumaresan M, Mysore V. Controversies in hair transplantation. J Cutan Aesthet Surg. 2018;11:173-81.
5. ISHRS.orgcapitals pls. Geneva, IL, USA: International Society of Hair Restoration Surgery; 1993. [online] Available from http://www.ishrs.org/. [Last accessed September, 2023].
6. AHRSINDIA.orgcapitals pls. Ludhiana: Association of Hair Restoration Surgeons-India; 2011. [online] Available from http://www.ahrsindia.org/. [Last accessed September, 2023].
7. Standard guidelines of AHRS taskforce on hair transplantation. Accepted for publication. J Cutan Aesthet Surg. 2021;14(3): 265-84.
8. Patwardhan N, Mysore V, IADVL Dermatosurgery Task Force. Hair transplantation: standard guidelines of care. Indian J Dermatol Venereol Leprol. 2008;74:S46-53.

9. Nair AG, Santhanam A. Clinical photography for periorbital and facial aesthetic practice. J Cutan Aesthet Surg. 2016;9: 115-21.
10. Khavkin J, Ellis DA. Standardized photography for skin surface. Facial Plast Surg Clin North Am. 2011;19:241-6.
11. Satish M, Menon R, Rao KV. Professional Accountability and Patients' Rights, 2nd edition. Bengaluru: The Institute of Law and Ethics in Medicine, National Law School of India University; 2002. pp. 57-68.
12. Mousavi SR. The Ethics of Aesthetic Surgery. J Cutan Aesthet Surg. 2010;3:38-40.
13. Bastia BK, Kuruvilla A, Saralaya KM. Validity of consent—a review of statutes. Indian J Med Sci. 2005;59:74-8.
14. Satyanarayan Rao KH. Informed consent: an ethical obligation or legal compulsion? J Cutan Aesthet Surg. 2008; 1:33-5.
15. Trehan SP, Sankhari D. Medical Professional, Patient and the Law: The Institute of Law and Ethics in Medicine, 2nd edition. Bengaluru: National Law School of India University; 2002. pp. 57-68.
16. Mavroforou A, Giannoukas A, Michaldimitrakis E. Medical litigation in cosmetic plastic surgery. Med Law. 2004;23:479-88.
17. Mysore V, Parthasaradhi A, Kharkar RD, Ghoshal AK, Ganjoo A, Ravichandran G, et al. Expert consensus on the management of Androgenetic Alopecia in India. Int J Trichology. 2019;11(3):101-6.
18. Blumeyer A, Tosti A, Messenger A, Reygagne P, Del Marmol V, Spuls PI, et al. Evidence-based (S3) guideline for the treatment of androgenetic alopecia in women and in men. J Dtsch Dermatol Ges. 2011;9(Suppl. 6):S1-57.
19. American Board of Hair Restoration Surgery. [online] Available from https://abhrs.org/. [Last accessed September, 2023].

CHAPTER 79

Setting Up a Hair Clinic

Aseem Sharma, Ravina Surve, Madhulika Mhatre, Amit Kerure

KEY MESSAGES

- *The growing need for specialized hair clinics:* The surge in individuals seeking treatment for hair issues, influenced by social media and greater awareness, underscores the necessity for dedicated hair clinics. These clinics offer comprehensive care for conditions such as alopecia areata, androgenetic alopecia (AGA), and female pattern hair loss (FPHL), which have significant psychosocial impacts.
- *Holistic approach and diverse facilities:* Effective hair clinics must adopt a holistic approach to hair diseases, providing diagnostic facilities, medical and surgical treatments, and support through a competent team. This includes setting up trichology clinics, trichoscopy centers, and hair transplant operating theaters, ensuring a broad spectrum of care for patients.
- *Infrastructure and accessibility:* A successful hair clinic must be easily accessible and designed to be welcoming and informative, with clear signage and an interior that reflects the specialty of hair treatment. Collaboration with nearby hospitals can enhance emergency response capabilities, ensuring patient safety.
- *Comprehensive team and consent protocols:* Building a skilled team, including assistants trained in basic life support and knowledgeable about procedures and equipment, is crucial. Additionally, thorough consent protocols that cover all aspects of treatment, risks, and privacy concerns are essential for ethical practice.
- *Innovative treatments and technologies:* Embracing advanced technologies and treatments, such as platelet-rich plasma (PRP), low-level laser therapy (LLLT), scalp micropigmentation (SMP), and microneedling, can significantly improve treatment outcomes. Detailed attention to the setup of hair transplant facilities and emergency preparedness further ensures the clinic's capability to deliver high-quality care.

INTRODUCTION

Due to the huge influence of social media and increasing awareness among people, there has been a huge surge in the number of people consulting a cosmetologist and a trichologist or a trichiatrist. People from every age group are facing hair problems. The stressful life and shift from a balanced diet to fad diets or increased intake of unhealthy food as well as exposure to different chemical treatments for hair have manifested a lot of hair problems. Hair loss, specifically alopecia areata, androgenetic alopecia (AGA), and female pattern hair loss (FPHL) have a huge psychosocial impact as well. Due to this, a dedicated hair clinic is a need of the hour to diagnose and treat different hair problems. With the growing market of hair treatment and the revolution in hair restoration techniques, patients now prefer a clinic with all the facilities and comfort.

OBJECTIVES

- A holistic approach to hair disease
- Facilities to diagnose hair disease
- Provision of all medical as well as surgical treatments for hair disorders
- Forming a competent team including assistants, technicians, counselors, etc.

A complete trichology clinical unit consists of the following:

- Setting up a trichology clinic
- Setting up a trichoscopy center
- Setting up a hair transplant operating theater (OT).

Setting Up a Trichology Clinic

Exterior and Interior

Clinic should be easily accessible by all kinds of transportation systems. Exterior and interior of the clinic should be attractive and should convey a message regarding the availability of dedicated hair treatments. Clinic's name and doctor's name along with qualifications should be displayed on the board. The Registered Medical Practitioner (RMP) shall display as a suffix to his/her name only National Medical Commission (NMC)-recognized and accredited medical degrees/diplomas as provided in the nomenclature of the regulations and listed on the NMC website. Clinic's name and logo can be attractive and suggestive of the treatments provided. Interiors should be simple with adequate spacing and proper display of video testimonials, display of work, and services provided. A tie-up with a nearby well-equipped hospital is helpful to handle any medical emergency.

Consultation Room

Consultation room should have adequate space to accommodate the doctor himself with his desk, the patient and their

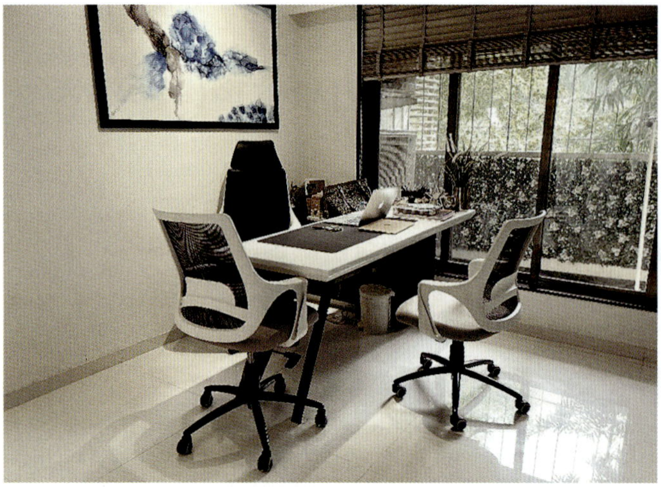

Fig. 1: Consultation room.

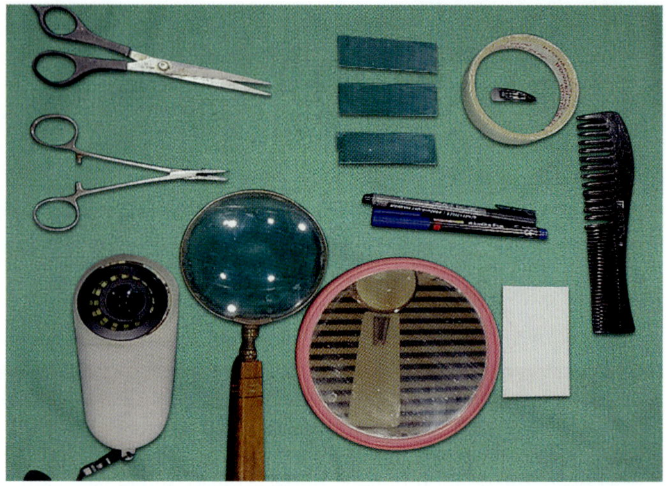

Fig. 2: Necessary things in the hair outpatient department (OPD).

accompanying person, and an examination bed surrounded by a curtain **(Fig. 1)**.

Room should be well illuminated. Top-to-bottom light helps in better visualization of hair thinning on first look. Patient sitting preferably should be such that a complete inspection of the scalp can be done without asking the patient to shift the sitting arrangement. Diagnostic tests like hair pull test, trichoscopy, card test, KOH, hair mount, trichogram,[1] etc. can all be done in the same position. Hair tray consisting of a clean hair comb, glass slide, hand lens, cello tape, dermoscope (handheld or videodermoscope), mirror, marker pen, and card (3 × 5 inch, white on one side and black on the other) should be ready **(Fig. 2)**. Desktop can be used to show pre- and post-treatment photographs to boost the confidence of patients.

A curtained examination bed is a must since other body parts need to be examined for hair growth in conditions like alopecia areata, hirsutism, etc.

Reception Area

Reception comprises the waiting area and front desk.

Front desk is the first point of contact between a patient and a clinic. Hence, the receptionist should be soft-spoken and should handle work smoothly. Waiting area should be comfortable and study materials or brochures regarding normal hair cycle, AGA, and treatments available for these diseases can be kept handy. Videos related to hair treatments can be on display.

Receptionist should be well trained for taking appointments and consents, and should ensure a smooth flow of patients. They should have good communication skills and phone etiquette.

Assistants

Two well-trained assistants are sufficient to help out in most of the procedures like platelet-rich plasma (PRP), scalp micropigmentation (SMP), and microneedling. The assistants should be well trained in basic life support (BLS) course. For hair transplantation OT, usually three assistants are required for a faster and more efficient process. Especially if performing follicular unit transplantation (FUT), then a couple of assistants can help in slivering of graft while the surgeon prepares the recipient area and one technician can help in graft counting. The assistants should be well trained about the various instruments used and aseptic precautions which need to be taken, and should identify various injectables used.

One well-trained laboratory assistant is required for PRP blood collection, preparing KOH mount, etc.

Consent

Proper consent form should be available since consent is a must prior to all procedures and even before taking photographs. Consent form should include complete details of procedures to be performed, information about complications which may be encountered, different treatment options available, and risks related to anesthesia. Consent is even required before starting some drugs, e.g., dutasteride in FPHL. In case the patient is unable to give consent, the consent of the legal guardian or a family member must be taken. We should not publish photographs or case reports of patients without their permission in any medical or another journal in a manner by which their identity could be revealed. Always ensure that the patient's consent is documented before photographing, especially if the shots are taken during a surgical procedure when the patient may not be aware of the same.

Medical Records

According to NMC guidelines, every self-employed RMP shall maintain medical records of patients (outpatients or inpatients) for 3 years from the date of last contact with the patient for treatment in a standard proforma laid down by the NMC. In case of medical emergencies, the medical records should be made available on the same day. Efforts shall be made to computerize patient's medical records for quick retrieval and security. Numerous software are available for patient appointment, appointment cancellations, financial transactions, reminders to patients, etc., for smooth functioning and future references.

Photography

Photography is very important in a hair clinic either for documentation or treatment evaluation in terms of response and improvement. Preoperative photographs assist in surgical planning and comparison of preoperative and postoperative photographs allow surgeons and patients to accurately evaluate the outcome of the procedure.

Photography Equipment

Nowadays, smartphones have developed a lot and inbuilt cameras give great results.[2] Digital single-lens reflex cameras are high-resolution cameras and cameras with 8 megapixels or higher are sufficient for clinical photography. A macro lens with a focal length of 90–105 mm is recommended to capture relevant details of the face and scalp.[3]

Photography Room and Lighting

If possible, a dedicated room should be allotted for photography with dimensions as small as 5 × 8 ft. The best background would be a plain light blue or green nonreflective surface, like a linen cloth.

Photographs of hair disorders often require close-up or macro modes. Inbuilt camera flash units and sharp overhead lamps should be avoided as they tend to whiten out the area of interest and also produce sharp reflections, especially on black hair. For adequate depth perception, two light sources placed at 45° angles to patients are ideal. Additionally, a single backlight mounted centrally above, 1–3 ft from the background, should be used to eliminate shadows in the background. Patients should be positioned at least 2–3 ft from the background. Light diffusers, such as softboxes or umbrellas, should be placed in front of the main lights to provide even, soft lighting to the face.[4]

Photographs should be taken at the same distance to ensure uniform magnification, also the same lighting setup should be used consistently.[5]

Markings on the floor may be placed to indicate the position of the patient's stool and foot placement. A camera can be fixed on a tripod to ensure standardized imaging of hair.

The Canfield technique uses a positioning device on which the patient's chin and forehead are fixed, and on which a given camera and flash device are mounted, assuring that the view, magnification, and lighting are the same at consecutive study visits.[5]

In Indian patients, oiled hair clumps tend to produce more reflections. Hence, it is preferable to take photographs always when the hair is clean and dry or wipe and dry out the oil prior to photography of the scalp. Make it a point to remove accessories like hair bands and clips, which unnecessarily divert focus from the lesion of interest.

Setting a Trichoscopy Center

Trichoscopy helps in better visualization of hair and scalp thereby aiding in the diagnosis of hair disorders. Trichoscopy may be performed with handheld dermoscopes or with advanced digital dermoscopes and handheld ones[6] **(Fig. 3)**. Handheld dermoscopes may be divided into three groups: Contact dermoscopes, polarized light contact dermoscopes, and polarized light noncontact dermoscopes.[7] Hybrid dermoscopes are handheld dermoscopes that work in either contact or noncontact mode. Nonpolarized dermoscopy is better for inspecting structures in the *superficial skin layers*. Polarized dermoscopy is better for evaluating the *deeper skin layers* **(Figs. 4A and B)**.

Handheld dermoscopes provide a magnification of around 10–20× and the image can be viewed by the operator only; cannot simultaneously show to the patient. It can be connected to the smartphone with an adaptor.

Videodermoscopes offer a magnification of 10–100×. It is to be connected to a laptop with a USB port or wireless videodermoscopes are also available, which can be connected to cell phones. With these, the patients can simultaneously be shown the images, which helps in a better understanding of their hair disorder.

Trichoscopy is important in guiding toward the diagnosis of various hair disorders. Trichoscopic features of alopecia areata consist of black dots, exclamation mark hair, broken hair, and yellow dots. In AGA hair diameter diversity (HDD),

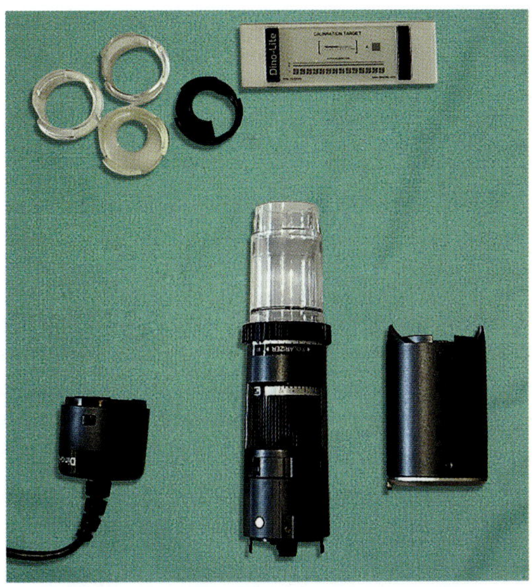

Fig. 3: Wi-Fi dermoscope with an adaptor.

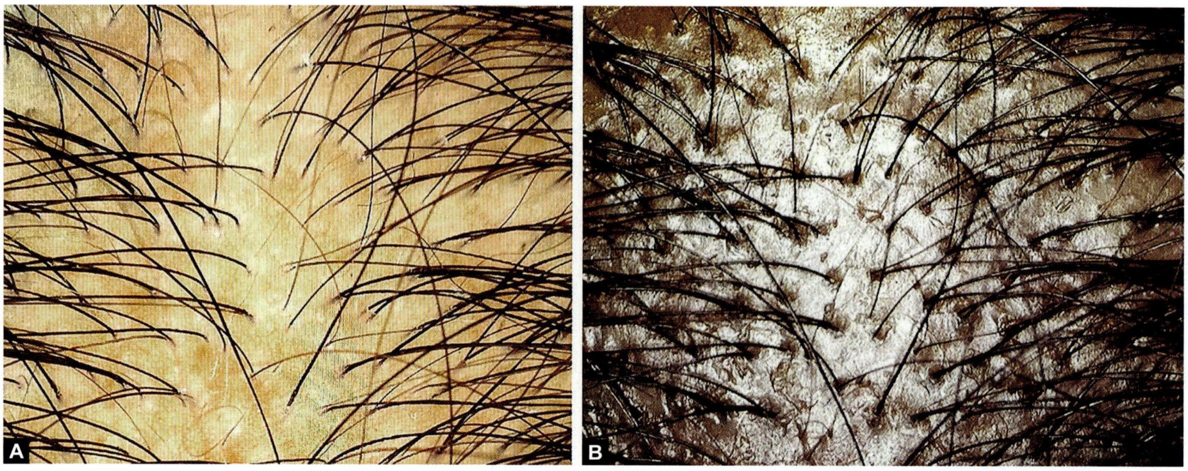

Figs. 4A and B: (A) Polarized mode; (B) Nonpolarized mode.

peripilar sign and yellow dots are observed. Loss of orifices is noted in cicatricial alopecia. Hence, trichoscopy helps in better diagnosis and sometimes the need for biopsy, i.e., invasive procedures, can be avoided.

Apart from these, certain advanced techniques like TrichoScan (measuring hair diameter, density, growth, and anagen–telogen ratio) and cross-sectional trichoscopy can be incorporated into practice.

TrichoScan is a software program based on the statistical growth pattern of hair, it can help in objective post-treatment analysis by comparison.[8]

Hair Transplant Setup[9]

Hair transplantation has undergone a lot of revolution over the years. For a hair transplant setup, proper training, skilled technicians, good infrastructure, and good instruments are a must. Hair transplant is a long-standing procedure, it is time consuming and requires a team effort. Proper advertising should be done in the form of informative videos about the procedure and pretreatment and post-treatment which can be displayed in the waiting room. Hair transplant OT can be setup in an existing clinic or an attachment to a tertiary care hospital OT should be ensured. Hair transplantation, though being an outpatient procedure, should be carried out with proper surgical protocol.

Hair Transplant OT

Well-equipped and well-designed surgical theater improves the outcome of hair transplantation with less complications. There should be a separate hair transplantation theater unit with a sterile and clean environment and backup of advanced life support since it is a time taking procedure and we use large quantities of lignocaine so the patients can suffer from anxiety, vasovagal syncope, anaphylaxis, etc. **(Fig. 5)**.

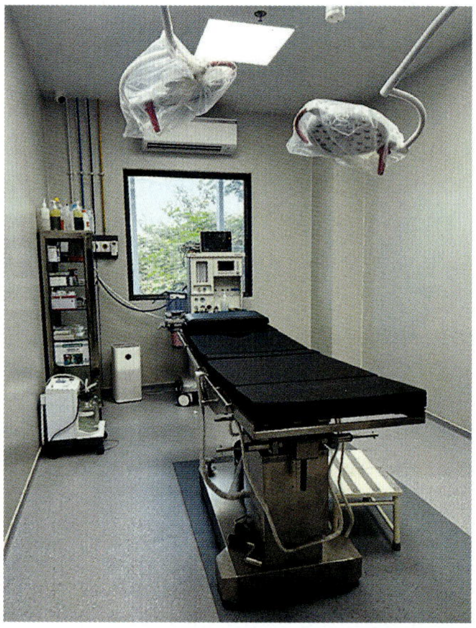

Fig. 5: Operating theater (OT).

There are four well-defined zones depending on the degree of cleanliness:

1. *Protective zone:* Waiting area, preanesthetic examination room, changing rooms, and theater supply rooms
2. *Clean zone:* Theater pack preparation, preoperative room, recovery room
3. *Aseptic or sterile zone:* Sterilization room, OT
4. *Disposal zone or dirty zone:* Soiled instruments and dissected tissues are washed or disposed of here.

Dimension of surgical theater should preferably be 12 × 12 ft or more and height around 10 ft.

The door should be preferably of width >24 inches to facilitate the movement of the trolley and doors should be of opaque material. The door of the complex should be two-leaf type with self-closing hinges.

Floor should be easily washable like marble or concrete floor. The floor and the side of the passage should be tilted to withstand repeated washings. The side walls can be painted with washable paint and light color.

Scrub zone should have elbow-operated or foot-operated taps and elbow-operated hand disinfectant dispenser.

Since water can harbor *Pseudomonas* and other microbes, the water should be ultraviolet (UV) and heat treated.

Careful planning of electrical supply in the theater is a must. Floor or ceiling-mounted sockets are better. A fire extinguisher should be handy. Avoid using extension cords or boards. Sockets should have a capacity of 5 Ampere (on an average of 4 on each wall) and 15 Ampere. Online uninterruptible power supply (UPS) for lasers and OT lights is a mandate. Standby generators will safeguard in terms of electricity problems.

Separate changing and patient preparation room is desirable for shaving, trimming, shampooing, etc.

OT Lights

Factors to be considered are intensity of light, size of the illuminated field, production of heat and shadows, and ease of changing the position of light.

Operating theater can have windows which are sealed but allow natural light inside.

General lighting can be provided by ceiling-mounted fluorescent tube at the rate of 1 W per square foot.

Artificial light in the form of fluorescent tubes, compact fluorescent lamp (CFL), or light-emitting diode (LED) should match the color of the objects as seen in natural sunlight (color rendering index). Lighting should be shadowless and luminaire should produce at least 120,000 lux or 3,000–8,000 foot candles.

Two OT light domes can allow to do various steps of hair transplantation simultaneously (e.g., simultaneous extraction from the chest and implantation in the scalp).

Air conditioning (AC) in the form of an office type system with 10 μm dust filter is required. Temperature should be 21 degree Celsius and humidity 50–55%. National Accreditation Board for Hospitals (NABH) does not recommend split and windows AC for restricted type OT.

Ergonomics is very important in hair transplant OT since hair transplantation is a long and time-consuming procedure. Patient and surgeon both should be in a comfortable position throughout.

Dialysis chair or dental chair can be used as an OT table for hair transplant, which can incline and recline and has easy maneuverability in terms of height adjustment and hand rests. Chair should go completely flat like a bed **(Fig. 6)**.

The OT table should be foldable at the knee end; a knee angle can help in additional support for the patient.

To increase comfort, silicon pillows are also available for head and neck rest.

Surgeons, due to prolonged sitting and standing, experience pain mainly in the lower limb, back, neck, arms, and wrist. Hence, to avoid improper posture, proper positioning of the chair, distance between the chair and OT table, and height of OT table are important. Surgeon's stool with wheels and pneumatic height adjustment controlled by foot and backrest is ideal; an additional armrest will also provide comfort and support.

Instrument Trolley

Mayo stand with four wheels is most preferred.

Autoclavable rubber sheet/Mackintosh should be draped over which sterile pack is placed every time.

Two types of hair transplantation techniques predominate, including FUT and follicular unit extraction (FUE) techniques. Currently, FUE represents the more common approach due to its potential advantages over FUT.[10]

The basic set of instruments required for an OT are as follows:

Forceps: Cheatle's sponge holding forceps, Adson toothed forceps, Adson nontoothed forceps, jeweler's forceps, mosquito artery, Spencer suture removal forceps

Sharp instruments: Bard-Parker handle no. 3, 4, 5 and disposable surgical blade no. 11 and 15, disposable punches.

Lister's scissors (blunt and sharp), iris scissors, and scissors.

Miscellaneous: Skin hooks, graft counters, graft implanters.

Instruments for FUE (Fig. 7)

Manual as well as motorized punches are available. There are multiple types of motors available for the extraction of

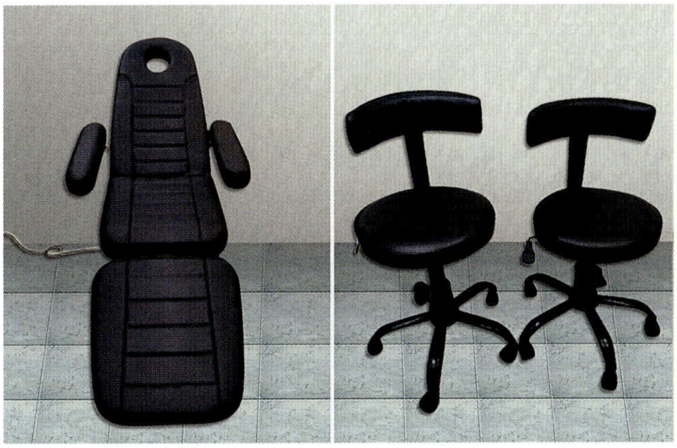

Fig. 6: Operating theater (OT) chair and surgeon's stool.

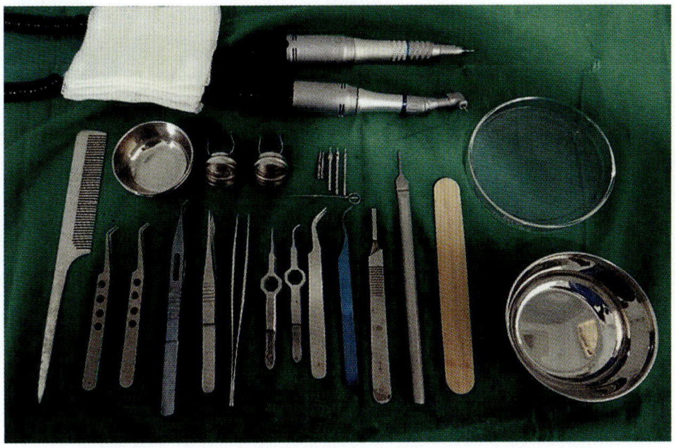

Fig. 7: Instruments for follicular unit extraction (FUE).

hair from simple dental motors to sophisticated Powered Cole Isolation Device (PCID) or surgically advanced follicular extraction (SAFE) system where depth and rotation speed can be controlled. Punches can be blunt or sharp to extract a high number of grafts with speed; sharp punches are more useful but chances of transection of grafts and associated bleeding are higher as compared to blunt punches but with the use of proper technique and training, these problems can be overcome very easily. Shape of punches can be round, hexagonal, or serrated. Different sizes are available, most commonly used are <1 mm for better healing. Magnification loupes (Carl Zeiss, Keeler, Heine) with magnification >2.5× should be used during extraction to lower the transection rate.

Instruments for FUT (Fig. 8)

For strip harvesting, scalpel with blade (no. 21–23), skin hook, and scissors are required. In addition, hemostat, cautery, and suction device should be there to stop bleeding. For blunt dissection at the hair roots, a graft spreader like Haber's spreader can be used to avoid follicular damage. To suture the wound, absorbable as well as nonabsorbable sutures should be there. For graft slivering, self-illuminated stereoscopic microscope or mantis microscope is required for better visualization and to avoid graft transection.[11]

There can be a separate dissection room for slivering of graft where the stereoscopic microscope can be attached to the screen and technicians can be trained to efficiently carry out graft dissection.

Receptor area: Slits can be made with instruments like Nokor needle or 18 gauge sterile needles, or cut to size blades are available. Different implanters are available, which can be used to place grafts without premade slits. Choi, KNU, or SAVA implanters may be used.

Holding medium: Normal saline, Ringer's lactate solution, and PRP can be used to keep grafts hydrated. Chiller trays are required and chilled normal saline is time tested and is the most commonly used holding solution.

For hairline formation, marker pens and hairline design measuring instruments are available.

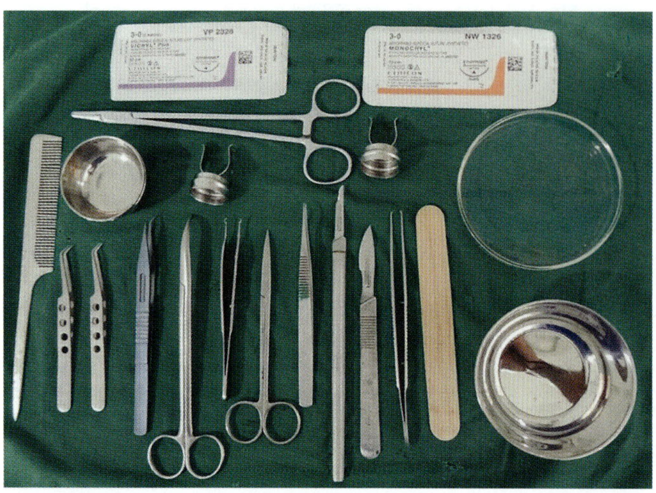

Fig. 8: Instruments for follicular unit transplantation (FUT).

OT Sterilization

Before surgery, the floor should be mopped using 0.5% chlorine solution and using a cloth, operation table and trolleys should be wiped with 0.5% chlorine solution or 500 mL of 40% formalin in 1,000 mL of water for 1,000 cu ft of OT area in a fumigator is the ideal concentration. Nonirritating fumigants like peracetic acid could also be considered.[12]

The theater linen and instruments may be sterilized or chemically disinfected.

Table top autoclave machine can be used for sterilizing instruments to be used on the same day. For sharp instruments like *scissors, curettes, and electrosurgical electrodes*, chemical disinfectant is used.[13]

Cotton, disposable paper, or plastic drapes should be used. Disposable surgical cap, surgical suits and gowns should be used. Cloth instrument packing is a traditional way of securing instrument tray but it has to be laundered every time. Hence, nowadays, disposable paper, crepe type or medical grade paper, reels are available.

Biomedical waste management: Adequate facilities for waste disposal should be ensured with proper segregation of soiled waste, chemical waste, sharps, etc. as per biological waste management rules given by the Government of India **(Box 1)**.

OT Emergency

Emergency resuscitation equipment including drugs, airway resuscitation (Ambu bag, laryngeal airway mask, equipment for intubation, ventilator, and oxygen), defibrillator, and capnograph to deal with any emergency situation because some of the procedures, especially hair transplantation involves local anesthesia use **(Fig. 9)**.

Technicians in the OT should be familiar with BLS and advanced life support. It is always preferable to maintain a liaison with a local hospital with an intensive care unit (ICU) facility.

BOX 1: Biomedical waste management.

- *Black bag*: For cytotoxic waste, expired medications, etc.
- *Red bag*: For used and disposable plastic items like plastic/latex gloves, intravenous (IV) sets, catheters
- *Blue bag*: Infectious waste like glass bottles, glass ampoules, injection vials
- *Green bag*: For office stationery, tissue papers, kitchen waste
- *Yellow bag*: For infectious dressing material, cotton, gauze, disposable gowns, masks, caps

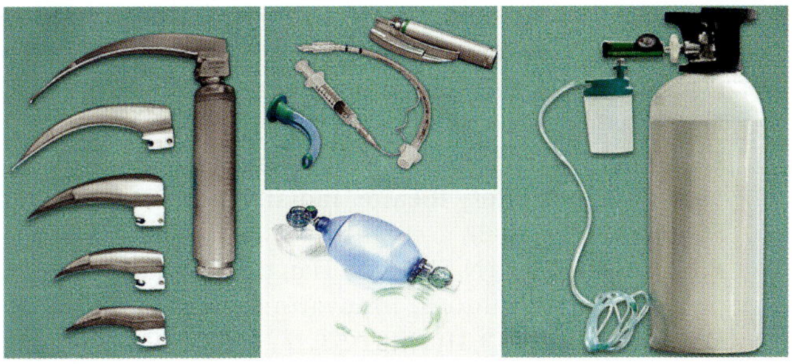

Fig. 9: Emergency equipment.

FACILITY FOR OTHER TREATMENTS LIKE PLATELET-RICH PLASMA PREPARATION, LOW-LEVEL LASER THERAPY, SCALP MICROPIGMENTATION, SCALP BIOPSY, AND MICRONEEDLING

Platelet-rich plasma has a beneficial role in AGA as well as in FPHL and works as an adjuvant along with other treatments like minoxidil. But preparation of PRP needs a good centrifuge machine, preferably in which temperature can be maintained. One such machine is REMI centrifuge, which is like a small refrigerator.

Newer modalities include growth factor concentrate (GFC) treatment which is also derived from the patient's blood, and high concentrations of growth factors are derived from platelet activation. Therefore, there is no platelet loss, and the overall procedure is effortless to perform.

Platelet-rich fibrin (PRF) is a new platelet concentrate concept, which accumulates platelets and released cytokines in a fibrin clot. Advanced-PRF™ (A-PRF™) and injectable-PRF (i-PRF) are different from conventional PRF and are based on the concept that low speed of centrifugation yields maximum results and significantly higher number of leukocytes, platelets, and growth factor concentration. Hair regeneration with i-PRF is relatively new.[14]

For low-level laser therapy (LLLT), there should be a separate comfortable sitting area where patients can take it wearing an LLLT helmet. LLLT appears to improve a variety of nonscarring alopecias—AGA, areata (AA), and chemotherapy-induced alopecia.

Scalp micropigmentation: Instruments required are mainly medical tattooing machines, pigments, and needles. Lightweight pens which are easy to hold, stable, and capable of delivering precise pigment implantation can be used. The SMP process involves inserting a microdroplet of pigment through the skin and into the upper dermis, using a standard tattoo instrument, which supports between one and six needles cycling between 100 and 150 cycles per second. It is a quick and satisfactory procedure.

Microneedling: It can be performed with dermaroller, microneedling and radiofrequency machine, or tattoo machine. This process helps in hair growth by the release of growth factors and stimulating stem cells in the bulge region.[15] It is widely used by many dermatologists as an adjuvant to minoxidil for AGA cases **(Fig. 10)**.

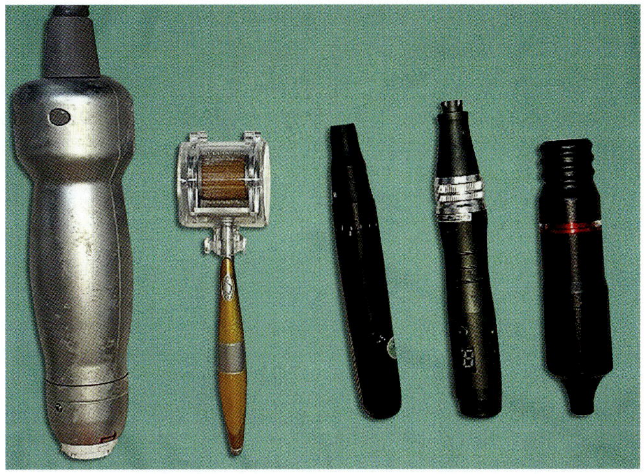

Fig. 10: Microneedling instruments.

Scalp biopsy: It is a diagnostic procedure required to be performed in cases like diffuse alopecia areata, cicatricial alopecia, etc. It is to be performed with aseptic precautions. Punches of sizes 3–5 mm may be used; biopsy site should always be sutured due to high vascularity in that area. A 3-0 nonabsorbable suture can be used.

INSURANCE

Property damage insurance coverage is a must including electronic devices. Electronic insurance plan should be taken for the system that covers all the parts and electronics of the device. Besides that, professional liability insurance, which protects the doctor against financial consequences of an error or omission during the service or professional act, should also be on the list.

Specialized hair clinic is becoming a vital and important branch of medicine. To meet and anticipate patient needs, it is necessary to ensure that the treatments offered and technologies being invested in are tried and true. Maintain a center of excellence in all aspects. One should have an integrated practice of clinical dermatology, dermatosurgery, and cosmetic dermatology to get desirable results and patient's trust as well.

CONCLUSION

In the current landscape where the demand for hair treatment solutions is escalating, establishing a specialized hair clinic represents a pivotal advancement in dermatological care. To meet and exceed patient expectations, such clinics must integrate a holistic approach with cutting-edge treatments and technologies, underpinned by a well-trained team and robust infrastructure. Ensuring patient safety, comfort, and satisfaction through meticulous planning and execution of services is paramount. By adhering to these principles, hair clinics can not only provide effective solutions to a range of hair disorders but also solidify their position as centers of excellence within the field of dermatology.

REFERENCES

1. Dhurat R, Saraogi P. Hair evaluation methods: merits and demerits. Int J Trichology. 2009;1(2):108-19.
2. Ashique KT, Kaliyadan F, Aurangabadkar SJ. Clinical photography in dermatology using smartphones: an overview. Indian Dermatol Online J. 2015;6(3):158-63.
3. Witmer WK, Lebovitz PJ. Clinical photography in the dermatology practice. Semin Cutan Med Surg. 2012;31(3):191-9.
4. Ashique Kt, Kaliyadan F. Clinical photography for trichology practice: tips and tricks. Int J Trichology. 2011;3(1):7-13.
5. Canfield D. Photographic documentation of hair growth in androgenetic alopecia. Dermatol Clin. 1996;14:713-21.
6. Kaliyadan F. The scope of the dermoscope. Indian Dermatol Online J. 2016;7:359-63.
7. Argenziano G, Soyer HP. Dermoscopy of pigmented skin lesions—a valuable tool for early diagnosis of melanoma. Lancet Oncol. 2001;2:443-9.
8. Rudnicka L, Rusek M, Borkowska B. Introduction. In: Rudnicka L, Rusek M, Borkowska B (Eds). Atlas of Trichoscopy Dermoscopy in Hair and Scalp Disease. London: Springer-Verlag; 2012. pp. 1-10.
9. Rajendran SC, Omprakash HM. Standard guidelines for setting up a dermatosurgery theatre. Indian J Dermatol Venereol Leprol. 2009;75:76-82
10. Bunagan MJ, Banka N, Shapiro J. Hair transplantation update: procedural techniques, innovations, and applications. Dermatol Clin. 2013;31(1):141-53.
11. Bernstein RM, Rassman WR. Follicular unit transplantation: 2005. Dermatol Clin. 2005;23(3):393-414.
12. Perez M, Lodha R, Nouri K. Surgical equipment and instrumentation. In: Nouri K, Khouri SL (Eds). Techniques in Dermatologic Surgery. Missouri: Mosby; 2003. pp. 25-6.
13. Post MH. The sterilization of sharp instruments by chemical solutions. Trans Am Ophthalmol Soc. 1940;38:37-53.
14. Arora R, Shukla S. Injectable-platelet-rich fibrin-smart blood with stem cells for the treatment of alopecia: a report of three patients. Int J Trichology. 2019;11(3):128-31.
15. Dhurat R, Sukesh M, Avhad G, Dandale A, Pal A, Pund P. A randomized evaluator blinded study of effect of microneedling in androgenetic alopecia: a pilot study. Int J Trichology. 2013;5(1):6-11.

SECTION 11

Aesthetic Procedures: Basics

CHAPTER 80

Basics of Aging Skin

Manjot Marwah, Shashikumar BM

KEY MESSAGES

- Aging skin, a result of intrinsic and extrinsic factors, undergoes significant structural and functional changes.
- Intrinsic aging progresses naturally over time, influenced by genetics and physiological processes, while extrinsic aging is accelerated by environmental factors such as UV radiation and pollution.
- Reactive oxygen species (ROS) play a crucial role in aging, damaging cellular components and contributing to oxidative stress. UV radiation is a primary source of ROS production, leading to photoaging characterized by wrinkles, sagging skin, and pigmentation changes.
- Mitochondrial dysfunction and altered cellular growth patterns, including cellular senescence and telomere shortening, also contribute to the aging process. Additionally, genetics, hormonal changes, dietary habits, and lifestyle choices like smoking influence the rate of skin aging.
- Clinical features of aging skin include thinning, xerosis, graying of hair, and the development of fine lines and wrinkles, with different skin types exhibiting varying responses to aging and sun exposure.
- Assessing facial aging involves evaluating changes in facial contours, skin texture, and the severity of wrinkles using classification systems like the Glogau score and Fitzpatrick wrinkle score.
- In Asian populations, including Indian skin types, differences in melanosome size and dermal thickness affect susceptibility to pigmentation disorders and the incidence of facial wrinkles.
- Understanding these key factors is essential for effectively addressing the signs and effects of aging skin.

INTRODUCTION

Skin is the exposed part of the body and hence the most vulnerable. As we age, the skin not only changes in structure but also in function. Hence, it is important to understand its anatomy, physiology, and function to maintain its integrity. Research on this topic started way back in the year 1956, wherein Denham Harman stated that reactive oxygen species (ROS) was the main factor behind aging and this theory was confirmed by studying skin aging.[1] Skin is the only organ with the largest amount of ROS resulting from intrinsic (genetic inheritance, cellular functions, hormonal and metabolic dysregulation) and extrinsic (continuous sun exposure, pollutants, and xenobiotics) factors. Cumulative physical and physiological changes are caused due to these factors. They bring about sequential modifications in each skin layer, especially on the sun-exposed areas.

Skin is not the same in all ages. As dermatologists, before we advise a patient an antiaging treatment protocol, or before we start injectables for the same, it is important to know the basics. A patient in their 20s is going to require more of sun protection to prevent premature photoaging, while a patient in their 50s will require more of hydration therapies. Doctors can individualize treatment strategies as per age and personal lifestyle of patients by understanding in detail the pathophysiology of skin aging.

WHAT IS AGING?

Aging is a dynamic, biological, and degenerative process that involves multiple systems including skin and skin support systems such as the bone, cartilage, and subcutaneous tissues. It is a genetically predetermined and environmentally modulated process; hence besides the intrinsic factors, it is the environmental damage on aging skin that will finally determine its ultimate appearance.[2]

TYPES OF AGING

Intrinsic Aging or Chronological Aging

Aging due to the passage of time and our genetic inheritance is called intrinsic aging. Other physiological factors, such as cellular metabolism, hormonal influences, and metabolic processes, are also included in intrinsic aging. The signs of intrinsic aging are typically not visible for decades. It can be well appreciated as thin transparent skin, xerosis in non-sun-exposed areas, loss of underlying pad of fat, graying of hair, unwanted hair due to hormonal disturbances, etc.

Extrinsic Aging

Environmental factors such as sun exposure and lifestyle choices lead to extrinsic aging or photoaging. This type of premature aging or photodamaged skin is seen only in areas exposed to light. In nonexposed areas, elasticity and epidermal regeneration capacity show no change till advanced aging.[3] Physiological factors such as exaggerated expressions and gravity contribute in deepening of wrinkles and sagging of skin with age. Other factors included in extrinsic aging are pollution, chemicals, smoking, and exposure to radiation **(Box 1)**.

BOX 1: Intrinsic and extrinsic causative factors of aging.

Intrinsic factors:
- Genetic or chronological aging
- Hormonal influences
- Cellular metabolism

Extrinsic factors:
- Ultraviolet rays (UV rays)
- Exaggerated expressions
- Gravity
- Smoking
- Pollution
- Exposure to toxins, chemicals, etc.

CAUSES OF SKIN AGING

- *Oxidative stress:* Damage from the free radicals represented by the various ROS causes aging, such as superoxide radicals (O^{-}_2), hydrogen peroxide (H_2O_2), and hydroxyl radical (-OH).[4] ROS gets accumulated due to sun exposure and various internal factors at the cellular level. The stratum corneum has a defensive mechanism against ROS by various protective enzymes; hence, more of the damage by ROS is seen in the dermis.[5]

Effects of Reactive Oxygen Species

Epidermis: As seen in **Figure 1** in the epidermis, there are nonenzymatic [vitamins E and C, coenzyme Q10 (CoQ10), and beta-carotene] and enzymatic (superoxide dismutases, catalases, glutathione peroxidases, ferritin, and peroxiredoxins) antioxidants to combat the ROS. However, with chronic or excessive exposure, oxidative stress and cellular damage may occur. This leads to damage of cellular proteins, deoxyribonucleic acid (DNA), and lipids. This further causes the production of soluble epidermal factors and proteolytic enzymes, resulting in changed composition of stratum corneum.

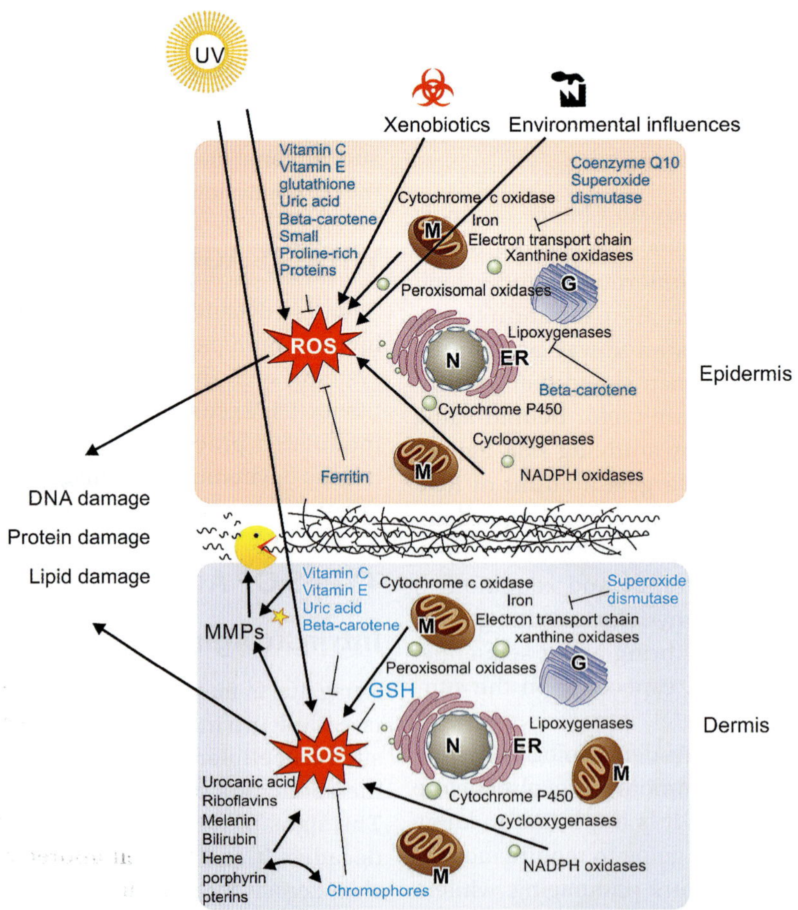

Fig. 1: Reactive oxygen species (ROS) and antioxidants in the skin. Black font shows the extrinsic and intrinsic sources of reactive oxygen species while blue font shows the antioxidants in the epidermis and dermis. (DNA: deoxyribonucleic acid; ER: endoplasmic reticulum; GSH: glutathione; MMP: matrix metalloproteinase; NADPH: nicotinamide adenine dinucleotide phosphate; UV: ultraviolet)

Calcium concentration should be low for renewal and division of cells and high for differentiation of cells. With the change in the composition of the epidermis due to oxidative stress, this gradient is disrupted and the barrier function of epidermis is lost.[6]

Additionally, lipid damage has a significant role not only in skin aging but also in various skin disorders. A mixture of sebum and keratinocyte membrane lipids forms the skin surface lipid (SSL) film protecting the skin from the environment. This film contributes to the defense mechanism of the epidermis against oxidative stress and ultraviolet (UV) rays. When an external or internal factor replenishes the antioxidant defense system of SSL, oxidation of squalene and cholesterol starts. This gives rise to reactive by-products penetrating deeper into skin layers. Qualitative modifications of SSL represent a pathogenetic sign of diagnostic value in dermatological disorders involving altered sebum production, such as pityriasis versicolor, acne, atopic or seborrheic dermatitis, as well as photoaging.[7]

Dermis: ROS in the dermis causes activation of matrix metalloproteinases (MMPs). This in turn causes degradation of collagen and elastin fibers (extracellular matrix components) resulting in wrinkles.[8] The ROS generated in the dermis also contributes to the DNA and protein damage as seen in the epidermis:[9]

- UV radiation causes photoaging by generation of ROS. This extrinsic factor is the main contributor to ROS production. ROS production by sun exposure is mainly driven by UVA, in the range of 320–400 nm.[10] The UVB light does not have the capacity to penetrate into the deeper sections of the epidermis.[10,11] The UVA light induces different changes in the dermis, and these seem to be mainly responsible for the process and progression of photoaging.
- *Mitochondrial theory of aging:* Mitochondria are producers and also targets of oxidative stress and hence play a vital role in aging.[4] Mitochondrial dysfunction and ROS production form a vicious cycle, which is the basis of the mitochondrial free radical theory of aging.[4,12]
- *Cellular senescence and telomers:* The permanent arrest in the growth of individual mitotic cells is known as cellular senescence. As a result, these cells with altered phenotype accumulate and cause tissues to undergo disease progression. The surrounding cells and tissues are affected by these changes, leading to unfavorable effects causing various diseases, cancer, and skin aging.[4] Recent studies have confirmed the role of cellular senescence in skin aging.[13-16]
- *Genetics:* Aging in humans is partly heritable. The role of genetics in aging has always been a debatable issue, but it has been proposed that, though not directly, genes may indirectly influence underlying aging processes.[17]
- *Steroid hormones:* As we age, the human steroid hormone profile changes, especially after menopause in women. Estrogen levels decline in both men and women with age. Estrogen protects the skin from several contributory factors of aging such as ROS, cellular senescence, and shortening of telomeres.[18]
- *Role of diet:* Various researches and studies have been done to find the link between skin aging and nutrition. However, the topic still remains a controversy.[19] Various vitamins, carotenoids, flavonoids, and extracts with antioxidant properties are used either topically or in the form of supplements in the skin care industry to delay aging.[20] These have been aimed at replenishing the natural antioxidants in the epidermis. Hence, nutrition and skin aging may be related; however, the evidence is limited.[21] A balanced diet with a good amount of fruits and vegetables is sufficient to supply a natural source of antioxidants to the skin.
- *Smoking:* Tobacco smoke decreases hydration of the skin. It reduces blood flow to the skin and hence depletes oxygen and vital nutrients in the skin.[22] It also works along the ROS pathway for causing premature skin aging and delayed wound healing and inhibits inflammatory responses. At the cellular level, tobacco smoke extract induces MMPs, which degrade collagen and trigger aryl hydrocarbon receptor, which mediates the toxicity of several environmental contaminants.[23] Vasoconstriction of the blood vessel in the skin causes loss of elastic fibers and collagen.

  Smokers have more wrinkles; they develop hollow cheeks due to repeated drawing of cigarettes resulting in a skeletal appearance. Their skin also shows signs of premature aging.[24]
- *Advanced glycation end products (AGEs) in skin aging:*[4] One of the causes of aging is AGEs.[25] They are a heterogeneous group of molecules that can be ingested or formed inside the cell. A nonenzymatic reaction between a sugar and a protein, or nucleic acid or lipid, results in the formation of AGEs. AGEs cause biological modifications and enzyme activation of MMPs; hence, they cause maximum damage in the dermis. UV radiation also acts on AGEs generating ROS and contributing to the aging process by an extrinsic pathway.[26,27]

CLINICAL FEATURES OF AGING

Clinical Features of Intrinsic Aging

Intrinsic aging, also referred to as natural aging, is a continuous progressive process in which skin changes occur as a consequence of longevity. These changes start to occur as early as in the 20s; however, the actual signs of chronological aging are typically not noticeable for decades **(Fig. 2 and Table 1)**.

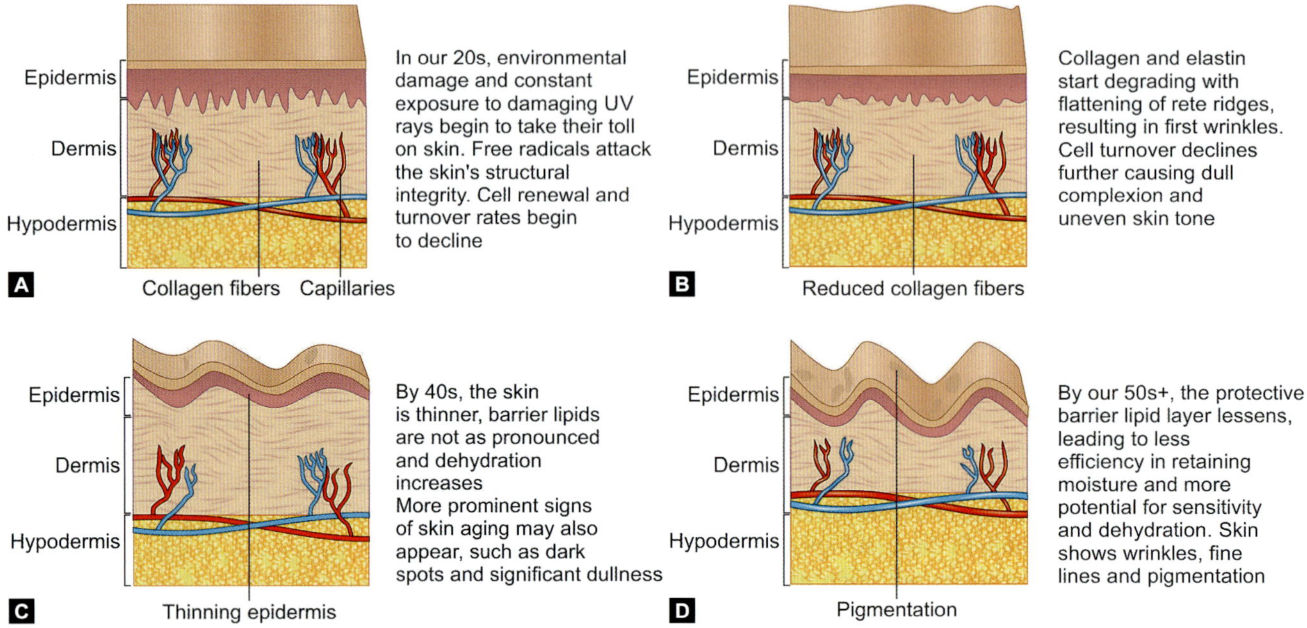

Figs. 2A to D: Changes in epidermis and dermis seen with aging in every decade: (A) 20s; (B) 30s; (C) 40s; (D) 50s+.

TABLE 1: Clinical features of intrinsic aging and pathophysiology behind them.

Signs of intrinsic aging	*Pathophysiology behind it*
Susceptibility to blister formation	Thinning of the dermal–epidermal interface and decreased adherence of epidermis to the underlying dermis because of loss of flattening of stratum basale[28]
Xerosis or roughness	Increase in epidermal turnover time and age-related decrease in intercellular keratinocyte adherence
Irregular pigmentation (solar lentigines)	The melanocyte count reduces by 8–20% every decade after the age of 30 years; still, there is a twofold rise in the melanocyte count in habitually exposed skin in comparison with protected skin[29]
Propensity to tear-type injury	There is a decrease in collagen by 1%/year during adult life.[30] The remaining collagen fibers become thicker, less soluble, and have more tensile strength, thus resulting in tear-type injuries following blunt trauma
Fine wrinkles	In aged skin, elastic fibers in the papillary dermis disappear and are replaced by an abundant quantity of microfibrils resulting in fine wrinkles[31]
Loss of underlying fat	Decrease in fat cell size, fat cell function, and redistribution of fat cells[32]
Prominent nasolabial folds	Volume loss occurs in the tear troughs below the eyes and in the cheek area. As a result of these changes, the nasolabial folds become prominent resulting in midface aging[33]
Sagging skin	Results from shrinkage of bones away from the skin due to bone loss
Inability to sweat sufficiently to cool the skin	Due to a decrease in the number of eccrine glands or glandular dysfunction
Sebaceous gland hyperplasia	Sebaceous gland output is diminished in the elderly causing a paradoxical increase in sebaceous gland size
Graying hair, hair loss, and increased terminal-type hairs	Senescent baldness is characterized by modest reduction in the size of hair follicles; the hair follicle units are not "miniaturized" nor inflammation I present as occurs in androgenic alopecia[34]
Nail fragility	The nail plate thins out, lunula disappears, surface is lusterless, and nail plate is prone to fracture
Osteomalacia	Epidermal photosynthesis of vitamin D is reduced due to a decrease in available 7-dehydrocholesterol, which decreases linearly by 75% in the second decade[35]

Clinical Features of Extrinsic Aging or Photoaging

The normal aging process is influenced by external factors such as repetitive facial movements, sun, gravity, sleeping positions, and smoking, which ultimately lead to premature aging of our skin.

Fine lines and wrinkles are caused by repetitive facial expressions. A groove forms beneath the surface of the skin due to the repetitive use of a facial muscle. This groove becomes permanent as we age because of the loss of elasticity of the skin and failure to spring back to its line-free state leading to fine lines and wrinkles.

Gravity-induced changes become more pronounced in middle age during which the skin elasticity declines. These changes are drooping of the tip of the nose, elongation of the ears, sagging of the eyelids, disappearance of the upper lip, and prominence of the lower lip.

Sleeping in the same direction every night for years eventually leads to sleep wrinkles which no longer disappear.

People who smoke for years develop an unhealthy yellowish hue and deeply wrinkled, leathery skin not seen in nonsmokers.[36]

The primary dermal histologic abnormality in photoaged skin is aggregates of thick, interwoven bands of fibrous material that stain basophilic, present in the papillary dermis and superficial portion of reticular dermis.[37] The abnormal basophilic material is characterized by an increased uptake of elastic tissue stains; hence, it is termed elastosis.[38]

The constellation of skin findings resulting from chronic sun exposure is collectively known as dermatoheliosis. Clinical findings range from elastosis to benign and malignant neoplasms **(Box 2)**.

Solar elastosis is manifested as wrinkled, inelastic skin with a thickened, leathery look. The damaged skin has an underlying yellowish hue due to degenerative changes of the dermal elastic and collagen fibers admixed with overlying epidermal melanocytic dyspigmentation. These findings, which are most typical of chronic sun exposure, are referred to as Milian's citrine skin.[39]

Cutis rhomboidalis nuchae is a clinical manifestation of severe sun damage to the normally redundant skin over the posterior nuchal area. Farmers are usually affected. Solar elastosis in this area results in deep furrows that form a geometric, rhomboidal pattern. In severe cases, cysts and comedones also develop in this area.

BOX 2: Signs of photoaging (dermatoheliosis).[40]

- Solar elastotic syndromes
- Citrine skin (Milian)
- Cutis rhomboidalis nuchae (Jadassohn)
- Nodular elastoidosis with cysts and comedones (Favre–Racouchot)
- Diffuse elastoma (Dubreuilh)
- Elastotic nodule of the ear
- Acrokeratoelastoidosis marginalis
- Striated beaded lines
- Senile purpura **(*see* Fig. 8)**
- Stellate pseudoscars
- Actinic granuloma
- Actinic comedonal plaque
- Venous lake
- Telangiectasia
- Dyspigmentation
- Freckling, lentigines
- Guttate hypomelanosis
- Wrinkling
- Fine surface lines and deep furrows **(*see* Fig. 2)**
- Neoplasms
- Seborrheic and actinic keratosis
- Lentigo maligna and lentigo maligna melanoma
- Basal cell carcinoma and squamous cell carcinoma

Favre–Racouchot syndrome is more prevalent in men and usually affects periorbital and upper lateral aspects of the cheeks, manifested as patulous pilosebaceous orifices filled with keratinous debris similar to acne comedones, but superimposed on the background of sun-damaged skin as seen in **Figure 3**. The pathogenesis is due to weakened dermal support around pilosebaceous units caused by sun damage to the elastic and collagen fibers.

Diffuse elastoma of Dubreuilh is a solitary, asymptomatic, yellowish, thickened papule or plaque that appears on the skin of the nose.

Elastotic nodule of the ear is discrete, semitranslucent, asymptomatic papules measuring 5 mm in size that develop on the anterior crus of the antihelix. They may be confused with basal cell carcinoma.

Acrokeratoelastoidosis marginalis appears as a group of glistening papules in a linear arrangement, often forming plaques along the margins of the fingers.[41]

Striated beaded lines develop in profoundly sun-damaged skin in men overlying the anterior chest. Hyperplastic sebaceous glands, arranged in closely set parallel lines, are seen against the background of atrophic skin.

Stellate pseudoscars are multiangulated hypopigmented lesions that occur predominantly on the extensor aspects of the forearms of elderly patients with severe actinic elastosis featured in **Figure 4**.

The lesions are secondary to trauma and are usually preceded by senile purpura.

Actinic granulomas are annular lesions that develop on habitually sun-exposed skin, especially on the face. Lesions have a smooth, raised border with normal or slightly atrophic skin.

Actinic comedonal plaque is an erythematous to bluish lesion consisting of nodules and plaques, which occurs on the extensor aspect of arms.

Venous lakes are common on the ear and lower lip of men with severe sun damage. They are deep blue in color measuring 5 mm in diameter and disappear with application

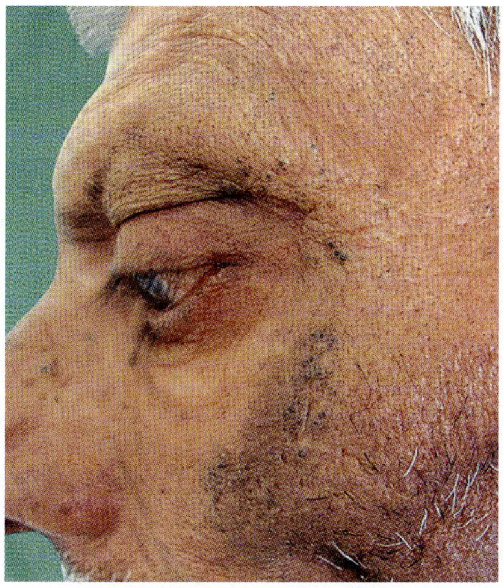

Fig. 3: Favre–Racouchot syndrome.

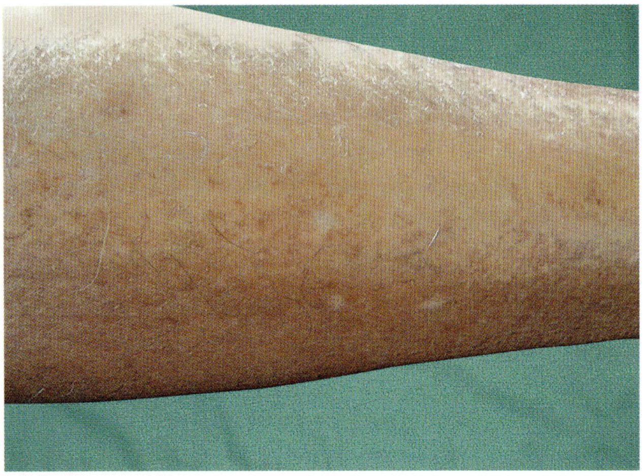

Fig. 4: Stellate pseudoscars over forearm.

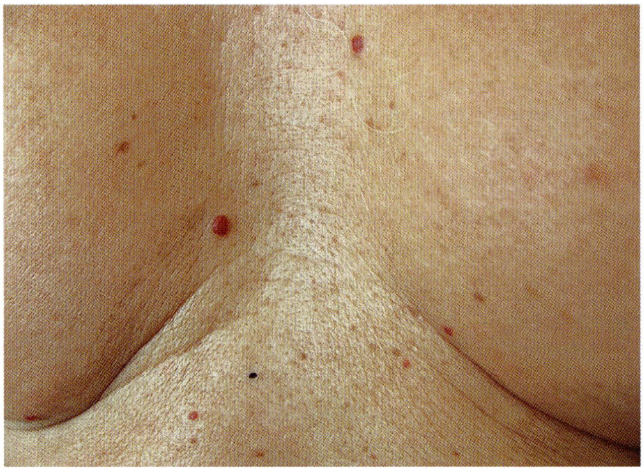

Fig. 6: Cherry angioma.

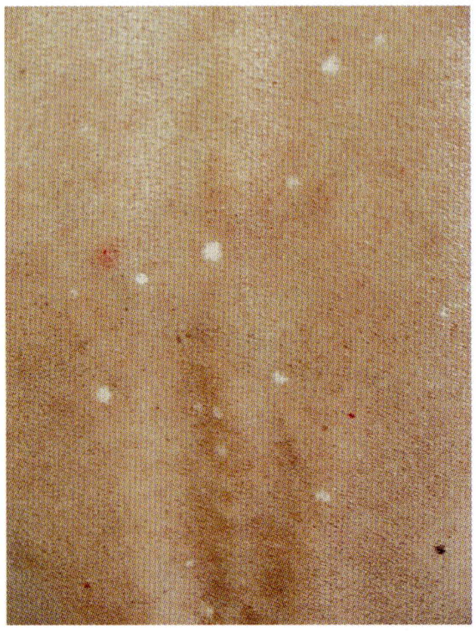

Fig. 5: Idiopathic guttate hypomelanosis.

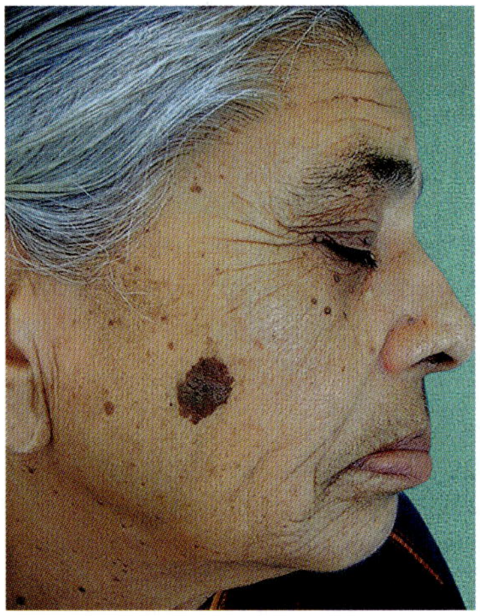

Fig. 7: Seborrheic keratosis.

of pressure (diascopy). They occur due to a lack of stromal support for weakened, bulging blood vessel.

Freckles or ephelides are stellate-shaped, small brown macules of hyperpigmentation seen on sun-exposed skin mainly over the face. The lesions become more prominent during summer months and pigmentation lightens during winter months. They are usually seen in lighter-skinned individuals and genetically predisposed children.

Idiopathic guttate hypomelanosis is an acquired pigmentary disorder characterized by sharply defined, round-to-oval porcelain-white macules of approximately 2–6 mm in size, which increase in number with aging. The lesions are mainly seen on sun-exposed surfaces of the legs and forearms of elderly patients in both sexes as seen in **Figure 5**.

Solar lentigo (also known as actinic lentigo, senile lentigo, sun spots, and liver spots) presents as small (usually <1 cm) circumscribed macular lesions that are associated with an increased number of melanocytes in the dermoepidermal junction. They appear later in adult life in chronically sun-exposed areas. These lesions may enlarge and show minimal darkening or fading with variations in sun exposure.

Cellular heterogeneity within the basal region of the epidermis increases as we age. This explains the plethora of benign neoplastic lesions such as cherry angioma, seborrheic keratosis **(Figs. 6 and 7)**, and skin tags that develop as people age.

PHOTOAGING IN DIFFERENT SKIN TYPES

Sun-induced cutaneous changes vary considerably in Fitzpatrick skin types I and II from that of types III and IV as shown in **Box 3**.

Comparison of intrinsic and extrinsic aging is shown in **Table 2**.[42]

SIGNS OF AGING OF THE FACE

Aging of the face can be described by multiple individual changes that occur in the contour of the face and in the texture of the skin.[43] These are enumerated in **Box 4**.

BOX 3: Sun-induced cutaneous changes in different skin types.

Skin types I and II:
- Proliferative exhaustion
- Epidermal atrophy
- Focal depigmentation
- Pseudoscars
- Mutations and dysplasia
- Freckles
- Nevi
- Lentigo maligna
- Melanoma
- Actinic keratoses
- Basal cell carcinoma
- Squamous cell carcinoma

Skin types III and IV:
- Protective hyperplasia
- Tanning
- Lentigines
- Epidermal thickening

TABLE 2: Comparison of intrinsic aging and photoaging.

Feature	*Intrinsic aging*	*Photoaging*
Clinical appearance	Smooth texture, unblemished surface. Fine wrinkles. Some deepening of skin surface markings. Some loss of elasticity, redundant skin	Nodular, leathery surface. Sallow complexion, yellowish mottled pigmentation. Coarse wrinkles. Severe loss of elasticity
Epidermis	Thin and viable	Marked acanthosis, cellular atypia, skin field carcinogenesis, most skin cancers
Elastic tissue	Increased but almost normal	Tremendous increase, altered as elastotic amorphous mass
Collagen	Thick, disoriented bundles	Marked decrease of bundles and fibers
Glycosaminoglycans	Slightly decreased	Markedly decreased
Reticular dermis	Thinner, fibroblasts decreased, inactive mast cells decreased, no inflammation	Thickened, elastosis. Fibroblasts increased, hyperactive mast cells markedly decreased, mixed inflammatory infiltrate
Papillary dermis	No grenz zone	Solar elastosis with grenz zone
Microvasculature	Moderate loss	Great loss, abnormal and telangiectatic
Subcutaneous fat	Focal shrinkage, focal hypertrophy	Unaffected
Hair	Thinning, graying hair. Hypertrichosis	Discoloration

BOX 4: Age-related changes in the face.

- *Upper face:*
  - Brow arch becomes flattened
  - Sustained contraction of frontalis muscle results in horizontal forehead skin creases
  - Eyelid skin becomes redundant
  - Pseudofat herniation
  - Dynamic rhytides develop at lateral canthus
- *Midface:*
  - Downward migration of the malar soft tissue accentuates skeletonization of the orbital rim
  - Ptosis of central cheek fat results in accentuation of nasolabial folds
- *Lower face:*
  - Platysmal muscle ptosis and cheek fat ptosis along the mandible produce "jowls" overlying the jawline
  - Soft-tissue atrophy anterior to jowls forms "prejowl sulcus" accentuating skeletonized appearance
  - "Turkey neck" deformity results from platysmal ptosis of the upper neck

Age-related textural changes:
- Loss of skin elasticity
- Telangiectasia formation
- Rhytides
- Pigmentary disturbances
- Actinic keratosis

Wrinkles

One of the telltale signs of aging is increased wrinkling of the face, which are configurational changes in skin surface in the form of creases and furrows.[44] There are secondary factors causing these wrinkles of the face, including the constant pull of gravity, frequent and constant positional pressure on the skin of the face (e.g., during sleep), and repeated facial movements caused by contractions of mimetic muscles of facial expression.[45]

Two types of facial wrinkles are as follows:
1. Static wrinkles are the wrinkles which result due to loss of elasticity of the skin as we age. They occur due to the breakdown of the skin's collagen, and as a result of this, the tissues become lax. These changes are further influenced by genetics, sun exposure, poor diet, and smoking. Fine lines around the corners of the mouth, around the cheeks, and neck wrinkles are examples of static wrinkles. They are seen even when the facial muscles are at rest.
2. Dynamic wrinkles are caused due to repetitive muscle contractions as during frowning, smiling, etc. Deep lines become permanent due to these repeated muscle contractions. Examples are frown lines, bunny lines, crow's feet, etc. They are seen only when people express their facial expression.

The combined effects of chronological skin aging and photodamage can lead to the degradation of collagen and accumulation of abnormal elastin in the superficial dermis, causing the skin to lose its thickness and elasticity and develop wrinkles.[46] Hence, skin that has lost its suppleness retains the lines formed by facial expressions such as smiling or frowning. Over a period of time, these "expression lines" deepen into wrinkles.[47]

The commonly used classifications for wrinkles are Glogau score, Fitzpatrick wrinkle score, and Lemperle score.

TABLE 3: Fitzpatrick wrinkle scale and elastosis scale.

Class	*Wrinkling*	*Score*	
I	Fine wrinkles	1–3	Mild fine texture changes with subtly accentuated skin lines
II	• Fine to moderate depth wrinkles • Moderate number of lines	4–6	Moderate-distinct popular elastosis (individual papules with yellow translucency under direct lighting) and dyschromia
III	• Fine to deep wrinkles, numerous lines • With or without redundant skin folds	7–9	*Severe:* Multipapular and confluent elastosis (thickened, yellow, and pallid) approaching or consistent with cutis rhomboidalis

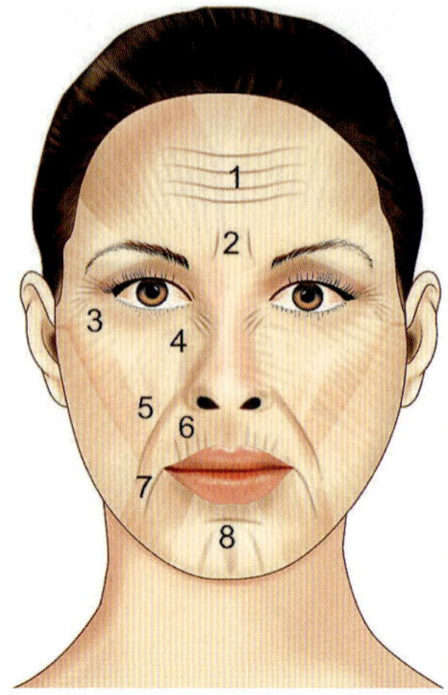

Fig. 8: Different types of wrinkles.

TABLE 4: Classification of facial wrinkle—Lemperle scale.

Class	*Description*
0	No wrinkles
1	Just perceptible wrinkle
2	Shallow wrinkles
3	Moderately deep wrinkle
4	Deep wrinkle, well-defined edges
5	Very deep wrinkle, redundant fold

Note: Locations considered: Horizontal forehead lines, glabellar frown lines, periorbital lines, preauricular lines, cheek lines, nasolabial lines, radial upper lip lines, radial lower lip lines, corner of mouth lines, marionette lines, labiomental crease, horizontal neck folds.

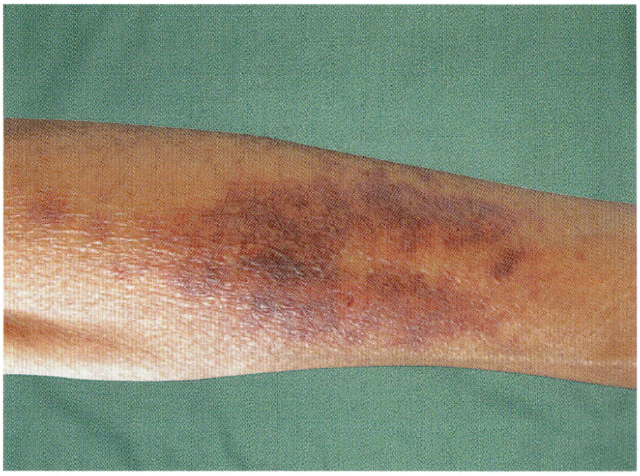

Fig. 9: Senile purpura.

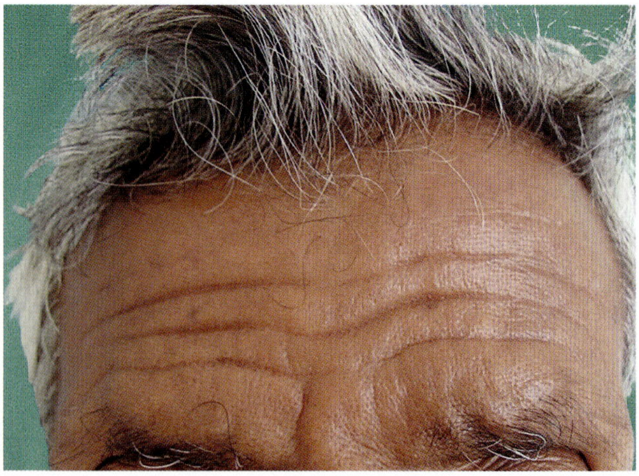

Fig. 10: Horizontal forehead lines.

Glogau score: This classification is confined to generalized wrinkles and does not address specific mimetic wrinkles or folds.

- *Type I:* No wrinkles
- *Type II:* Wrinkles in motion
- *Type III:* Wrinkles at rest
- *Type IV:* Only wrinkles.

Fitzpatrick wrinkle score: This score determines generalized wrinkling and elastosis. Wrinkle depth is not considered in this scoring **(Table 3)**.

Wrinkle assessment scale by Lemperle illustrated in **Table 4**[48] was specifically designed to know the wrinkle depth, which was very important to assess the therapeutic response with injectable fillers.

Specific types of wrinkles may develop on different anatomic sites of the face as shown in **Figure 8.**[49]

Clinical photographs are depicted in **Figures 9 to 13**.

AGING IN INDIAN SKIN

Indian skin usually falls under Fitzpatrick skin types IV–V. This type of skin usually has larger, nonaggregated melanosomes that contain more melanin compared with the smaller, aggregated, less melanin-containing melanosomes that occur in lighter persons. This confers protection from accelerated aging and skin cancers induced by UV radiation in Indian skin.[50] However, it has its own disadvantage, like the Indian skin type is more prone to developing dyspigmentationwhen compared to their Western counterparts.

Indian skin has a thicker and more compact dermis than white skin, with the thickness being proportional to the degree of pigmentation. This likely contributes to the lower incidence of facial rhytides in Asians.[51]

From Lambros's theory of facial aging, it was suggested that skeletal remodeling may be summarized as a clockwise rotation of the maxilla relative to the cranial base.[52] But it is difficult to reinforce Lambros's theory in Indians for aesthetic corrections as the width of the bony framework in Indian men and women is comparably smaller than their North American Caucasian counterparts.[53] Also, Indian faces tend to get fuller and tissues descend downward and medially making it complicated for aesthetic correction.

Sen et al. have developed a 13-item rating scale **(Table 5)** for the evaluation of facial aging in Indian subjects through clinical examination of skin changes. All items were scored on a scale of 0–3 according to an increasing order of severity. The group selected two items from the upper third of the face, four from the middle third, five from the lower third, and one additional item as general attributes of facial aging.[54]

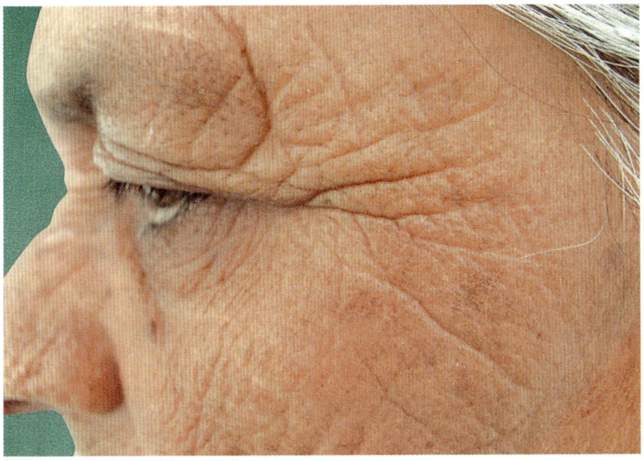

Fig. 11: Crow's feet.

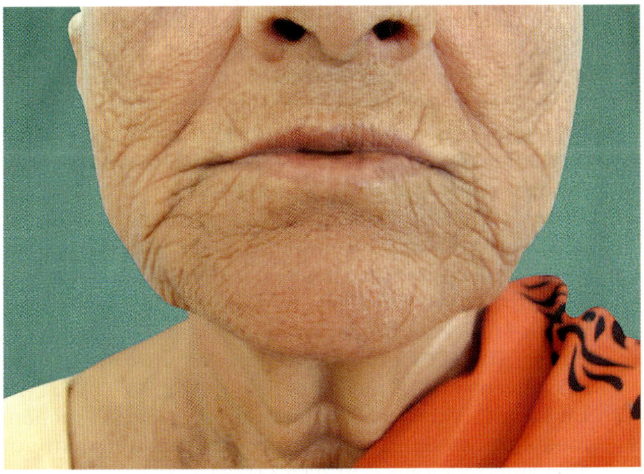

Fig. 12: Nasolabial folds.

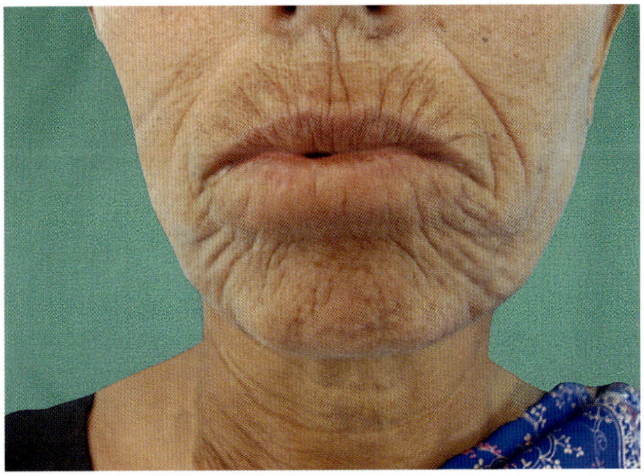

Fig. 13: Radial lip lines and chin lines.

TABLE 5: 13-item rating scale for the evaluation of facial aging in Indian subjects.[31]

Item number	*Item description*	*Score 0*	*Score 1*	*Score 2*
1	Forehead lines at rest	None (no lines)	Mild (1 line)	Moderate (2 lines)
2	Upper eyelid laxity	None	Mild	Moderate
3	Infraorbital laxity	None	Mild	Moderate
4	Visible malar prominence	None	Mild	Moderate
5	Fullness of buccal fat pad	Full	Mildly sunken	Moderately sunken
6	Nasolabial fold at rest	None	Mild	Moderate
7	Cheek skin elasticity	Supple	Toward supple	Toward flaccid
8	Lip wrinkles at rest	None	Mild (a few)	Moderate (some)
9	Descent of corner of mouth	No downturn	Mild downturn	Moderate downturn
10	Perioral wrinkles at rest	None	Mild	Moderate
11	Jawline at rest	No sagging	Mild sagging	Moderate sagging
12	Neck volume at rest	No sagging	Mild sagging	Moderate sagging
13	Pigmented spot	Absent	Few macules	Many macules

CLASSIFICATION OF AGING

- *Glogau classification of photoaging:* This is widely used and is given in **Table 6**.
- *Rubin classification:* It is classified as levels I–III as depicted in **Figure 14**.
- *Numerical score of photoaging:* It has been developed by Dr Monheit and Fulton. The score relates to the recommendation of a rejuvenation program. Each of the 12 features of aging is given a score of 1–4.

CONCLUSION

In conclusion, aging skin represents a multifaceted interplay between intrinsic and extrinsic factors, with cellular mechanisms and environmental influences contributing to its progression. Reactive oxygen species, UV radiation, and lifestyle choices significantly impact the aging process, leading to characteristic clinical features such as wrinkles, sagging, and pigmentation changes. Assessing facial aging through established classification systems provides a framework for understanding individual differences and guiding treatment strategies. Recognizing the unique characteristics of diverse skin types, including variations in melanosome size and dermal thickness, underscores the importance of personalized approaches to skincare. By comprehensively understanding the basics of aging skin, clinicians and skincare professionals can tailor interventions to effectively mitigate the signs of aging and promote skin health across diverse populations.

TABLE 6: Glogau classification.

Types	*Age*	*Features*
Type I—"early wrinkles"	20s–30s	• Early photoaging, mild pigment changes • Minimal wrinkles, no age spots • Requires little or no makeup
Type II—"wrinkle in motion"	30s–40s	• Early to moderate photoaging • Appearance of smile lines • Early brown age spots • Skin pores more prominent • Little makeup
Type III—"wrinkle in rest"	50s or older	• Advanced photoaging • Visible brown age spots • Prominent brown pigmentation • Discoloration with telangiectasia and actinic keratosis • Always wear makeup
Type IV—"only wrinkles"	60s or 70s	• Severe photoaging • Yellow-gray skin color • Multiple actinic keratosis • Wears makeup with poor coverage

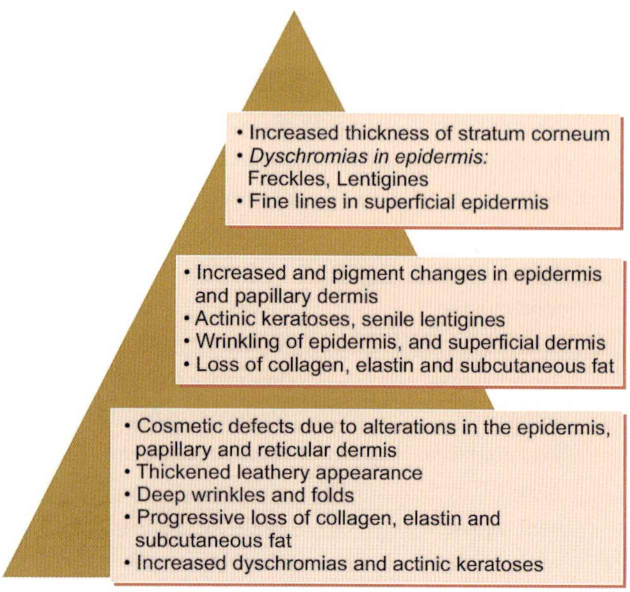

Fig. 14: Levels of Rubin classification.

REFERENCES

1. Harman D. Aging: a theory based on free radical and radiation chemistry. J Gerontol. 1956;11:298-300.
2. Draelos ZD. Concepts in a multiprong approach to photoaging. Skin Therapy Lett. 2006;11:1-3.
3. Yaar M, Gilchrest BA. Aging of skin. In: Freedberg IM, Eisen AZ, Wolff K, Austen KF, Goldsmith LA, Katz SA, Fitzpatrick TB (Eds). Fitzpatrick's Dermatology in General Medicine, 5th edition. New York: McGraw-Hill; 1999. pp. 1697-706.
4. Gragnani A, Cornick S, Chominski V, de Noronha SMR, de Noronha SAAC, Ferreira LM. Review of major theories of skin aging. Adv Aging Res. 2014;3:265-84.
5. Thiele JJ, Dreher F, Packer L. Antioxidant defense systems in skin (reprinted from cosmeceuticals). In: Elsner P, Maibach H (Eds). Drugs vs. Cosmetics: Cosmeceuticals? New York: Dekker; 2000. pp. 145-88.
6. Smyth JT, Hwang SY, Tomita T, DeHaven WI, Mercer JC, Putney JW. Activation and regulation of store-operated calcium entry. J Cell Mol Med. 2010;14(10):2337-49.
7. De Luca C, Valacchi G. Surface lipids as multifunctional mediators of skin responses to environmental stimuli. Mediators Inflamm. 2010;2010:321494.
8. Rattan SI, Ali RE. Hormetic prevention of molecular damage during cellular aging of human skin fibroblasts and keratinocytes. Ann N Y Acad Sci. 2007;1100:424-30.
9. Landau M. Exogenous factors in skin aging. Curr Probl Dermatol. 2007;35:1-13.
10. Rinnerthaler M, Bischof J, Streubel MK, Trost A, Richter K. Oxidative stress in aging human skin. Biomolecules. 2015; 5(2):545-89.
11. Wang CH, Wu SB, Wu YT, Wei YH. Oxidative stress response elicited by mitochondrial dysfunction: implication in the pathophysiology of aging. Exp Biol Med (Maywood). 2013; 238(5):450-60.
12. Kohl E, Steinbauer J, Landthaler M, Szeimies RM. Skin ageing. J Eur Acad Dermatol Venereol. 2011;25:873-84.
13. Burton DGA, Sheerin A, Ostler EL, Smith K, Giles PJ, Lowe J, et al. Cyclin D1 overexpression permits the reproducible detection of senescent human vascular smooth muscle cells. Ann N Y Acad Sci. 2007;1119:20-31.
14. Campisi J. Aging and cancer: the double-edged sword of replicative senescence. J Am Geriatr Soc. 1997;45(2):482-8.
15. Campisi J. The biology of replicative senescence. Eur J Cancer. 1997;33:703-9.

16. Browner WS, Kahn AJ, Ziv E, Reiner AP, Oshima J, Cawthon RM, et al. The genetics of human longevity. Am J Med. 2004;117(11):851-60.
17. Kirkwood T. Ageing: too fast by mistake. Nature. 2006;444: 1015-107.
18. Emmerson E, Hardman MJ. The role of estrogen deficiency in skin ageing and wound healing. Biogerontology. 2012;13(1): 3-20.
19. Draelos ZD. Aging skin: the role of diet: facts and controversies. Clin Dermatol. 2013;31(6):701-6.
20. Higami Y, Barger JL, Page GP, Allison DB, Smith SR, Prolla TA, et al. Energy restriction lowers the expression of genes linked to inflammation, the cytoskeleton, the extracellular matrix, and angiogenesis in mouse adipose tissue. J Nutr. 2006;136: 343-52.
21. Schagen SK, Zampeli VA, Makrantonaki E, Zouboulis CC. Discovering the link between nutrition and skin aging. Dermatoendocrinol. 2012;4(3):298-307.
22. Morita A, Torii K, Maeda A, Yamaguchi Y. Molecular basis of tobacco smoke-induced premature skin aging. J Investig Dermatol Symp Proc. 2009;14(1):53-5.
23. Pageon H. Reaction of glycation and human skin: the effects on the skin and its components, reconstructed skin as a model. Pathol Biol (Paris). 2010;58(3):226-31.
24. Li L, Mac-Mary S, Marsaut D, Sainthillier JM, Nouveau S, Gharbi T, et al. Age-related changes in skin topography and microcirculation. Arch Dermatol Res. 2006;297(9): 412-6.
25. Ahmed N. Advanced glycation endproducts—role in pathology of diabetic complications. Diabetes Res Clin Pract. 2005;67(1):3-21.
26. Goldberg T, Cai WJ, Peppa M, Dardaine V, Baliga BS, Uribarri J, et al. Advanced glycoxidation end products in commonly consumed foods. J Am Diet Assoc. 2004;104:1287-91.
27. Fleming TH, Humpert PM, Nawroth PP, Bierhaus A. Reactive metabolites and AGE/RAGE-mediated cellular dysfunction affect the aging process: a mini-review. Gerontology. 2011; 57:435-43.
28. Montagna W, Kirchner S, Carlisle MS. Histology of sun-damaged human skin. J Am Acad Dermatol. 1989;21: 907-18.
29. Gilchrest BA, Blog FB, Szabo G. Effects of aging and chronic sun exposure on melanocytes in human skin. J Invest Dermatol. 1979;73:141-3.
30. Shuster S, Black MM, McVitie E. The influence of age and sex on skin thickness, skin collagen and density. Br J Dermatol. 1975;93:639-43.
31. Lavker RM. Structural alterations in exposed and unexposed aged skin. J Invest Dermatol. 1979;73:59-66.
32. Johannsson G, Bengtsson BA. Growth hormone and the metabolic syndrome. J Endocrinol Invest. 1999;22(Suppl. 5): 41-6.
33. van Seumeren I. Weight gain and hormone replacement therapy: are women's fears justified? Maturitas. 2000; 34(Suppl. 1):S3-8.
34. Kligman AM. The comparative histopathology of male-pattern baldness and senescent baldness. Clin Dermatol. 1988;6:108-18.
35. Holick MF, MacLaughlin JA. Aging significantly decreases the capacity of human epidermis to produce vitamin D3. Clin Res. 1981;29:408A.
36. Fisher GJ, Kang S, Varani J, Bata-Csorgo Z, Wan Y, Datta S, et al. Mechanisms of photoaging and chronological skin aging. Arch Dermatol. 2002;138:1462-70.
37. Lever WF, Schaumberg-Lever G. Degenerative diseases. In: Lever WF, Schaumberg-Lever G (Eds). Histopathology of the Skin. Philadelphia: JB Lippincott; 1983. pp. 271-89.
38. Banfield WG, Brindley D. Preliminary observations on senile elastosis using the electron microscope. J Invest Dermatol. 1963;41:9-17.
39. Yaar M, Gilchrest BA. Aging of skin. In: Freedberg IM, Eisen AZ, Wolff K, Austen KF, Goldsmith LA, Katz SI (Eds). Fitzpatrick's Dermatology in General Medicine, 6th edition. New York: McGraw Hill; 2003. pp. 1386-98.
40. Cunliffe WJ. Disorders of connective tissue. In: Rook A, Wilkinson DS, Ebling FJG (Eds). Textbook of Dermatology. Oxford: Blackwell Scientific; 1979. pp. 1611-53.
41. Koscard E. Keratoelastoidosis marginalis of the hands. Dermatologica. 1964;131:161-75.
42. Farage MA, Miller KW, Maibach HI. Physiological variations during aging. In: Farage MA, Miller KW, Maibach HI (Eds). Textbook of Aging Skin. Berlin/Heidelberg: Springer-Verlag; 2010. pp. 25-35.
43. Small R. Aesthetic principles and consultation. In: Richard U, Pfenninger J, Stulberg D, Small R (Eds). Dermatologic and Cosmetic Procedure in Office Practise. Philadelphia: Elsevier/Saunders; 2012. pp. 230-40.
44. Aizen E, Gilhar A. Smoking effect on skin wrinkling in the aged population. Int J Dermatol. 2001;40:431-3.
45. Fujimura T, Hotta M. The preliminary study of the relationship between facial movements and wrinkle formation. Skin Res Technol. 2012;18:219-24.
46. El-Domyati MM, Attia SK, Saleh FY, Ahmad HM, Uitto J. Effect of topical tretinoin on photoaged facial skin: a histometric, immunohistochemical and ultrastructural study. J Cosmet Dermatol. 2004;3:191-201.
47. Burton JL. Disorders of connective tissue. In: Champion RH, Burton JL, Ebling FJG (Eds). Textbook of Dermatology, 5th edition. Oxford: Blackwell Science; 1992. pp. 1763-825.
48. Lemperle G, Holmes RE, Cohen SR, Lemperle SM. A classification of facial wrinkles. Plast Reconstr Surg. 2001; 108:1735-50.
49. Small R. Botulinum toxin injection for facial wrinkles. Am Fam Physician. 2014;90(3):168-75.
50. Kaidbey KH, Agin PP, Sayre RM, Kligman AM. Photoprotection by melanin—a comparison of black and Caucasian skin. J Am Acad Dermatol. 1979;1(3):249-60.
51. Montagna W, Prota G, Kenney J. The structure of black skin. In: Montagna W, Prota G, Kenney J (Eds). Black Skin Structure and Function. Oxford: Gulf Professional Publishing; 1993.
52. Pessa JE. An algorithm of facial aging: verification of Lambros's theory by three-dimensional stereolithography, with reference to the pathogenesis of midfacial aging, scleral show, and the lateral suborbital trough deformity. Plast Reconstr Surg. 2000;106:479-88.
53. Jagadish Chandra H, Ravi MS, Sharma SM, Rajendra Prasad B. Standards of facial esthetics: an anthropometric study. J Maxillofac Oral Surg. 2012;11:384-9.
54. Sen S, Choudhury S, Gangopadhyay A, Halder C, Biswas P, Jain A. A clinical rating scale for the assessment of facial aging in Indian population. Indian J Dermatol Venereol Leprol. 2016;82:151-61.

CHAPTER 81

Cosmeceuticals and Systemic Nutraceuticals

Ankur Talwar, Rajetha Damisetty, TS Vidya

PART A: COSMECEUTICALS

KEY MESSAGES

- Cosmeceuticals are cosmetic products that have a drug-like benefit.
- Botanicals are chemicals extracted from leaves, barks, roots, and flowers of plants whose benefits are yet to be established by full research.
- Skin-lightening agents such as phenolic and nonphenolic compounds decrease tyrosinase synthesis, increase tyrosinase degradation, melanocyte toxicity, increase keratinocytes desquamation, or decrease melanosome transfer to keratinocytes.
- Enzymes which are topically applied are now being developed for photodamaged skin.
- Growth factors need further research to define their role as topical skin care preparations.
- Irritant and allergic dermatitis is common with over-the-counter (OTC) skin care products.

INTRODUCTION

Cosmeceutical is defined as a cosmetic that has or claimed to have medicinal properties. Professor Albert Kligman introduced this term in 1984 at the National Scientific Meeting of the Society of Cosmetic Chemists.[1] From the late 20th century, the concept has taken the world of aesthetics by storm and the term has entered common parlance.

DRUGS, COSMETICS, AND COSMECEUTICALS: JUST SEMANTICS?

The United States Federal Drugs and Cosmetics (FD&C) Act defines drugs[2] as those products that cure, treat, mitigate, or prevent disease or that affect the structure or function of the human body. A cosmetic is defined by the US Federal Food, Drug and Cosmetic Act, 1938, as "articles intended to be rubbed, poured, sprinkled, or sprayed on, introduced into, or otherwise applied to the human body or any part thereof for cleansing, beautifying, promoting attractiveness, or altering the appearance," without affecting structure or function. While drugs are subject to a review and approval process by the Food and Drug Administration (FDA), cosmetics are not subjected to this approval process. Cosmeceuticals, as a class part from cosmetics,[3] are not recognized in most countries, including India and the USA. Presently, only Korea and Japan have legislation that distinguishes three categories: (i) cosmetic products, (ii) functional (quasi-drug) cosmetics, and (iii) drugs.

Cosmeceuticals have biologically active ingredients that affect the skin barrier and overall skin health. Ideally, the cosmeceutical should be clinically tested for efficacy to ensure a proven skin benefit and also to substantiate marketing claims. However, proof of improved skin function would remove the cosmeceutical from the cosmetic category and place it in the drug category. Herein lies the challenge of defining the cosmeceutical category. For this reason, good manufacturers limit testing of cosmeceuticals to their ability to improve skin appearance but not function.[3] The most disturbing part of the whole cosmeceutical category debate is the definition of a dermatologic drug as an agent that alters the structure and function of the skin.[3] This was the language used in the original Cosmetics and Toiletries Act of USA. The Act was written in 1938, at a time when the skin was thought to be nothing more than a covering on the outside of the body, with little biologic activity. We now know that the skin is enzymatically and immunologically active, participating in important metabolic functions required to sustain life.

In Kligman's own words, "the distinction between a drug and a cosmetic is somewhat arbitrary." Antiperspirants are over-the-counter (OTC) drugs in the US and cosmetics in Europe. Most antidandruff products are prescription drugs in the US and OTC formulations in Europe. In many cases, the manufacturer's claims decide how the product is categorized. For example, a drug labelled "antiaging" but a cosmetic "improves wrinkles." The concept of cosmeceutical is political depending on the country where the product is marketed.

CURRENT TRENDS IN COSMECEUTICALS

It is anticipated that the global cosmeceuticals market will reach US$ 61 billion by 2020.[4] Major factors that fuel the growth of cosmeceuticals market include increasing consumer consciousness regarding their appearance and increasing number of urban populations. Increase in disposable incomes,[4] along with the attractively packaged and aggressively advertised products are contributors too. Among skincare, antiaging subsegment is expected to contribute maximum revenue during 2017–2021.

Cosmeceuticals can be purchased OTC without a prescription from a healthcare professional. Yet, one of latest trends in the market is rising preference for physician-recommended cosmeceuticals over nonprescription products. Companies operating in the cosmeceuticals market are investing huge amounts in research and development (R&D) activities. Unfortunately, the scope for pseudoscience is huge in this arena.

NEED FOR COSMECEUTICALS

For seekers of youthful and beautiful skin who do not suffer from skin ailments and are not keen on using drugs or "harsh chemicals" in the long run but want more than mere cosmetics, cosmeceuticals offer the perfect via media. OTC availability prevents the necessity of visiting a doctor, except, possibly for an initial consult to get their skin analyzed and a regimen prepared. For patients with acne[5] or pigmentary concerns, cosmeceuticals act as adjuncts to regular prescriptions, improve adherence to treatment and reducing adverse events of irritant drugs.

For the manufacturer, getting a cosmeceutical into the market avoids costs of clinical trials and approvals of FDA, cuts down time, dependence on doctors, and hugely increases scope as these OTC products can be advertised.

COSMECEUTICAL PRODUCT CATEGORIES

Cosmeceuticals are divided into categories based on their active ingredients:

- *Antioxidants:* They reduce the harmful effects of free radicals, which are molecules that injure the skin's cells and cause inflammation, increase sun damage, and contribute to the development of skin cancer.
- *Peptides:* They are small proteins that stimulate the production of collagen and thicken the skin.
- *Growth factors:* They are compounds that act as chemical messengers between cells and play a role in cell division, new cell, and blood vessel growth and in the production and distribution of collagen and elastin.
- *Combination products:* The newer cosmeceuticals contain combination products. These products might contain ingredients, such as multiple antioxidants, retinol plus antioxidants, growth factors plus vitamin C and other unique combinations. Although the individual ingredients, in combination products have been studied, the combinations of their active ingredients are not. Rigorous scientific studies are needed to ensure that biologic activity is maintained when ingredients are formulated together.

Cosmeceuticals can also be classified according to their primary intended action. These include sunscreens, antiaging products, pigmentation lightening products, etc. **(Box 1)**. Amongst these, antiaging cosmeceuticals are the most sought after, followed by hydration, skin lightening, and antiacne preparations.

COSMECEUTICAL INGREDIENTS

There are many constituents **(Table 1)**, including retinoids, peptides, and plant stem cells. A number of agents, otherwise used as drugs, have been used in OTC preparations, often in low concentrations. Delivery systems can be in the form of emulsions, polymeric systems (liposomes), microparticles, nanostructures, and patches.

Retinoids

Topical retinoids (e.g., tretinoin) and retinoid analogous (e.g., adapalene and tazarotene) help normalize hyperkeratinization and have demonstrated significant anti-inflammatory effects. Retinoids promote a reversal of comedogenesis leading to a reduction in microcomedones. Further, it reverses the thickening of the stratum corneum

BOX 1: Cosmeceuticals product categories.

- Sunscreen
- Antioxidant
- Anti-inflammatory
- Pigment lightening, antiaging (collagen repair), and exfoliation
- Moisturizers (hydration/barrier repair)

TABLE 1: Common ingredients of cosmeceuticals.

Retinoids	• Retinol • Retinal • Retinoic acid
Alpha-hydroxy acids	• Glycolic acid • Lactic acid • Tartaric acid • Citric acid
Beta-hydroxy acids	• Salicylic acid • Beta-lipohydroxy acid • Tropic acid
Polyhydroxy acids	• Gluconic acid • Lactobionic acid • Galactose
Antioxidants	• Vitamins A, E, C, and B • Lipoic acid • Coenzyme Q10 • Glutathione • Niacinamide • Polyphenols • Dimethylaminoethanol (DMAE)
Skin-lightening agents	Phenolic, nonphenolic combinations

and the abnormal desquamation of keratinocytes. Topical retinoids also demonstrate anti-inflammatory activity, including the inhibiting the activity of leukocytes, the release of proinflammatory cytokines and other transcription factors and toll receptors involved in immunomodulation.

Several new retinoids have significant all-trans-retinol, which is considered to be a parent form of vitamin A and the addition of this compound in OTC products is not considered to be a drug. Some of the claimed benefits of OTC products containing all-trans-retinol could potentially occur because all-trans-retinol is oxidized to form tretinoin after absorption into skin cells.[6] However, such as all cosmeceuticals, it is difficult to determine the actual amount of the active agent and the efficacy of these unregulated products.

Most of the research concerning cosmeceutical retinoid ingredients is based upon the effects of retinoic acid (RA) on the skin. RA can, however, be irritating to the skin, limiting its use in some patients. Retinol (ROL) and retinaldehyde (RAL) are of interest to the scientific community and cosmetic industry as gentler yet still effective alternatives to RA. Clinical trials concerning retinol and retinaldehyde are scant and lacking in statistical evaluation for significance. However, the other cosmeceutical retinoids, retinyl palmitate, and retinyl acetate, are retinoid esters and are not considered effective against photoaging.

Adapalene is a unique second-generation retinoid and it possesses retinoid properties by reason of a synthetic naphthoic acid derivative. It targets abnormal desquamation of the skin, modulates cellular differentiation, and possesses anti-inflammatory properties. Adapalene is characterized by selectivity for the nuclear retinoic acid receptor (RAR) β/γ, and a potent activity on cell differentiation. This selectivity may contribute to an improved tolerance associated with adapalene.[7] Tazarotene is pharmacologically inactive until metabolic conversion to the active drug transpires (Wolverton, 2001). This prodrug is hydrolyzed rapidly in tissues to the active metabolite, tazarotenic acid. The RAR-β nuclear receptor is the predominant receptor present in the epidermis for which tazarotenic acid has a high affinity. Additionally, tazarotene has the ability to bind with RAR-α and RAR-γ, but not to RXRs. Tazarotene downregulates the abnormal expression of keratinocytes, epidermal growth factor (EGF) receptor, and hyperproliferative keratins.[8]

Antioxidants

Commonly used antioxidants include vitamins B_3, B_5, E, and C, and alpha lipoic acid. The newer antioxidants include omega-3 fatty acids, hyaluronic acid, copper peptide, coenzyme Q10 among others.

- *Alpha-lipoic acid:* Alpha-lipoic acid is both fat- and water-soluble antioxidant. It is a gentle yet powerful antioxidant. It protects the skin from depletion of other antioxidants such as vitamin C and E. Due to this quality, it is believed that alpha-lipoic acid can provide the greatest protection against damaging free radicals when compared with other antioxidants. Alpha-lipoic acid is thought to diminish fine lines, gives skin a healthy glow and boosts levels of other antioxidants, such as vitamin C.
- *Dimethylaminoethanol:* Dimethylaminoethanol (DMAE) helps maintain tone and firmness of face and neck by keeping adequate levels of neurotransmitters and access to vitamin C ester and alpha-lipoic acid for the skin. DMAE is considered to be good for skin tone. It is claimed to prevent and reverse skin sagging. It is present in anchovies, salmon, and sardines. DMAE in skin care products has been marketed for its effects in the reduction of fine lines and wrinkles.[9]
- *Omega-3 fatty acids:* The omega-3 fatty acids have been studied for many years for their beneficial effects. The most commonly consumed omega-3 fatty acid foods are fish, roasted or ground flax seeds, walnuts, hemp, salmon, and spirulina. They are not naturally occurring in the body and thus need to be consumed through diet and supplementation. Sea food and algae are better sources than whole grains, as the body converts the acids consumed in seafood and algae form into usable omega-3s in the body more efficiently. In contrast, only a small percentage of all docosahexaenoic acid (DHA) and eicosapentaenoic acid (EPA) are converted from the whole grain sources.

  The beneficial effects of omega-3 fatty acids in antiaging may be directly linked to their ability to control cell inflammation. Omega-3 fatty acids reduce the inflammation that may occur in the cell due to high levels of omega-6 levels. While all of their antiaging benefits are yet to be discovered, there is little doubt that an increase in omega-3 fatty acids in the body when combined with a decrease in omega-6 fatty acids can help the heart and the lifeline.
- *Hyaluronic acid:* Skin care products containing this substance are often used in conjunction with vitamin C products to assist in effective penetration. Hyaluronic acid [also known as a glycosaminoglycan (GAG)] is often touted for its ability to "reverse" or stop aging. This substance occurs naturally and quite abundantly in humans and animals, and is found in young skin, other tissues, and joint fluid. Hyaluronic acid is a component of the body's connective tissues and is known to cushion and lubricate the tissues. As we age, the content of hyaluronic acid reduces. Diet and smoking can also affect body's level of hyaluronic acid over time. Skin care products with hyaluronic acid are most frequently used to treat wrinkled skin.
- *Copper peptide:* Copper peptide is often referred to as the most effective skin regeneration product, even though it has only been on the market since the year 1997. Copper peptide promotes collagen and elastin production and also acts as an antioxidant. It also promotes

production of GAG. The substance helps to firm, smoothen, and soften skin and is claimed to do it in time less than most other antiaging skin care products.

- *Coenzyme Q10:* Coenzyme Q10, which is a naturally occurring antioxidant in the skin in all organisms helps firm up skin and may retard aging process. Coenzyme Q (ubiquinone, 2-methyl-5,6-dimethoxy-1,4-benzoquinone), a soluble natural fat quinine, is crucial to optimal biological function. The coenzyme Q molecule has biphasic properties due to the hydrophilic benzoquinone ring and the lipophilic polyisoprenoid side chain. It was demonstrated that coenzyme Q in addition to its role in electron transport and proton transfer in mitochondrial and bacterial respiration, acts in its reduced form (ubiquinol) as an antioxidant. Coenzyme Q10 functions as a lipid antioxidant regulating membrane fluidity, recycling radical forms of vitamin C and E, and protecting membrane phospholipids against peroxidation. The antioxidant property, high degree of hydrophobicity, and universal occurrence in biological system suggest an important role for ubiquinone and ubiquinol in cellular defense against oxidative damage.[10]

Alpha-hydroxy Acids

Alpha-hydroxy acids (AHAs) are a group of organic carboxylic compounds, most commonly used in cosmetic applications. They are typically derived from food products including glycolic acid (from sugar cane), lactic acid (from sour milk), malic acid (from apples), citric acid (from citrus fruits), and tartaric acid (from grape wine).

For any topical compound, including AHA, it must penetrate into the skin where it can act on living cells. Bioavailability is one characteristic that is important in determining compound's ability to penetrate the top layer of the skin. Glycolic acid having the smallest molecular size is the AHA with greatest bioavailability and penetrates the skin most easily, this largely accounts for the popularity of this product in cosmetic applications. Glycolic acid has an effect on epidermal remodeling by accelerated desquamation which leads to quick pigment dispersion on pigmented lesions. It also reduces melanin formation in the melanocytes by tyrosinase inhibition.[11]

Alpha-hydroxy acids have a profound effect on keratinization, which is clinically detectable by the formation of a new stratum corneum. It appears that AHAs modulate this formation through diminished cellular cohesion between corneocytes at the lowest levels of the stratum corneum. AHAs with greater bioavailability appear to have deeper dermal effects. Glycolic acid, lactic acid, and citric acid, on topical application to photodamaged skin, have been shown to produce increased amounts of mucopolysaccharides and collagen and increased skin thickness without detectable inflammation, as monitored by skin biopsies.[12]

Over-the-counter skin care products containing AHAs (glycolic, lactic, tartaric, and citric acids) have become increasingly popular over the last 5 years. Creams and lotions with AHAs may help reduce fine lines, irregular pigmentation, age spots, enlarged pores, sun damage, and may help lighten pigment and dark spots. Side effects of AHAs include mild irritation and sun sensitivity which can be avoided by starting with a product with concentrations of AHA of 10–15%.

- *Lactic acid:* It is used for diminishing fine lines and wrinkles, reducing the appearance of age spots, reducing hyperpigmentation, improving skin texture, and stimulating collagen production. It has humectant properties, increases water content of the epidermis, increases natural ceramides (barrier lipids) in the skin, and causes skin whitening. At concentrations over 5% lactic acid inhibits tyrosinase and also stimulates biosynthesis of GAG, thus plumping skin via hydration. Lactic acid has intense hydrating property, helps with photoaging and sun damaged skin, acts as an exfoliant to the skin leaving it softer and rejuvenated, acts as an antibacterial agent and astringent.

This AHA is used in many skin care formulations because it is a good humectant and helps the skin retain water. In the cosmetic industry it is used in shampoos, shower gels, hand creams, facial soaps, moisturizers, and antiwrinkle products.

Beta-hydroxy Acids

The main difference between AHAs and beta-hydroxy acid (salicylic acid) is their lipid solubility. AHAs are water soluble only, while beta-hydroxy acid is lipid soluble. This means that beta-hydroxy acid is able to penetrate into the pore which contains sebum and exfoliate the dead skin cells that are built up inside the pore. Because of this difference in properties, beta-hydroxy acid is better used on oily skin with blackheads and whiteheads. AHAs are better used on thickened, sun-damaged skin where breakouts are not a problem.

Salicylic acid also has been studied for its effect on skin that has aged prematurely due to exposure to ultraviolet (UV) rays from the sun. It exfoliates skin and can improve the texture and color of the skin. It also reduces the oiliness of the skin. There are many skin care products available that contain salicylic acid. Some are available OTC and others require a doctor's prescription. Studies have shown that salicylic acid is less irritating than skin care products containing AHAs, while providing similar improvement in skin texture and color.

Polyhydroxy Acids

Polyhydroxy acids (PHAs) are the new generation hydroxyl acids with less irritation than AHAs. They include lactobionic acid, galactose, and gluconic acid. They are larger, multiple strand molecules with slower skin penetration, slower absorption, and less irritancy. They can be used in patients with sensitive skin.

Botanicals

Botanicals are chemicals extracted from leaves, barks, roots, and flowers of plants. A number of botanicals are used in OTC products, but research and more studies are necessary to know about the benefits, concentrations to be used and side effects. Because of the vigorous processing, most of these extracts lose their beneficial properties. They are excluded from FDA regulations as their efficacy is not based on scientific investigations.

The various botanicals that are used as ingredients of cosmeceuticals are listed in **Table 2**. A few common ones are described here in detail.

- *Soy:* A naturally occurring substance, it increases skin thickness, promotes collagen gene expression and is an antioxidant.
- *Curcumin:* It is derived from turmeric root. It has antioxidant and anti-inflammatory functions. It also inhibits collagenase, elastase, and hyaluronidase.
- *Silymarin:* It is extracted from thistle plant. It is a potent antioxidant.
- *Pycnogenol:* It is derived from French marine bark. It is a free radical scavenger and antioxidant. It augments the antioxidant effect of vitamin A and C. Orally, it prevents cardiovascular disease and topically prevents cutaneous oxidative damage.
- *Kinetin:* It is a type of cytokine in the class of plant hormone that promotes cell division. Kinetin was originally isolated, as a compound from autoclaved herring sperm DNA that had cell division-promoting activity. It was given the name kinetin because of its ability to induce cell division provided that auxin was present in the medium.[13] Since 1994, kinetin has been thoroughly tested for its powerful antiaging effects in human skin cells and other systems. At present, kinetin is a widely used component in numerous skin care cosmetics and cosmeceuticals.
- *Other botanicals: Ginkgo biloba* is an extract from the plant terpenoids. Tea, tea tree oil, grape seed, soothing agents such as aloe vera, allantoin, witch hazel, papaya are all used in topical cosmeceuticals. Tea leaves are a rich source of polyphenols and are strong antioxidants. Tea tree oil has an antimicrobial property. Grape seeds have potent antioxidant, anti-inflammatory and anticarcinogenic properties. N-acetyl glucosamine, alpha acid, gentisic acid, soybean extract, and mulberry extract are also used in several products available in the market.

TABLE 2: Botanicals used as cosmeceuticals.

Flavonoids	• Soy • Silymarin • Hesperidin (lemons and oranges) • Diosmin (lemons and oranges)
Carotenoids	• Astaxanthin (tomatoes) • Lutein (tomatoes) • Lycopene (tomatoes)
Polyphenols	• Rosmarinic acid (rosemary) • Hypericin (St John's wort) • Ellagic acid (pomegranate) • Curcumin (turmeric root) • Pycnogenol (marine pine bark) • Terpenoids (*Ginkgo biloba*) • Procyanidin (grape seed) • Epigallocatechin (green tea)

Skin-lightening Agents

Skin-lightening agents have been classified under phenolic and nonphenolic compounds.

Phenolic Agents

- *Hydroquinone:* Skin care products containing hydroquinone are popularly referred to as bleaching creams or lightening agents. These skin care products are used to lighten hyperpigmentation, such as age spots and melasma. Some OTC skin care products contain hydroquinone, but the dermatologist can also prescribe a cream with a higher concentration of hydroquinone if the skin does not respond to OTC treatments. Its mechanism of action depends on its ability to inhibit tyrosinase synthesis. It also has the ability to inhibit deoxyribonucleic acid (DNA) and ribonucleic acid (RNA) synthesis and to degrade melanosomes.

  Hydroquinone has received a lot of scrutiny because of the exogenous ochronosis, which is seen mainly in long-term usage in concentrations higher than the OTC topical preparations. It is usually used at 2% concentration in topical cosmeceutical preparations, and the benefits are seen after 4–6 weeks of use and increases at 4 months of use beyond which it is generally not recommended. All patients should be warned against the long-term use and the side effects.[14]
- *N-acetyl-4-S-cysteaminylphenol:* It inhibits the activity of tyrosinase. It is supposed to be more stable and cause less irritation than hydroquinone. It is a phenolic agent and acts as an alternative substrate for tyrosinase.
- *Arbutin:* It inhibits tyrosinase activity but does not inhibit the synthesis of tyrosinase.[15]

Nonphenolic Agents

- *Kojic acid:* Kojic acid (5-hydroxy-2-hydroxymethyl-4-pyrone) is a more recent remedy for the treatment of pigment problems and age spots. Discovered in 1989, kojic acid has a similar effect as hydroquinone. Kojic acid is derived from a fungus and studies have shown that it is effective as a lightening agent, inhibiting production of melanin. It acts by inhibiting the production of free tyrosinase. It is used in a concentration of 1–4%, it is a potent antioxidant. It is usually combined with hydroquinone or with glycolic acid.

- *Liquorice derivative:* It is obtained from the root of the perennial herb *Glycyrrhiza glabra*. Glabridin is oil soluble derivative of liquorice extract, which has both tyrosinase inhibitory and anti-inflammatory properties.[16]
- *Niacinamide:* The biologically active amide of vitamin B3 can reversibly prevent the transfer of melanosomes from melanocytes to the keratinocytes. It has no effect on tyrosinase activity. Clinical studies show that it significantly reduces hyperpigmentation.[17]
- *Azelaic acid:* It is a naturally occurring dicarboxylic acid isolated from Pityrosporum ovale. It inhibits thioredoxin reductase, an enzyme needed for DNA synthesis and therefore has antiproliferative and cytotoxic effect on melanocytes. It is used as a 10–20% cream for the treatment of acne, rosacea, lentigines, and hyperpigmentation.[18]
- *Aloe:* Aloe vera is a noncompetitive inhibitor of tyrosinase and a competitive inhibitor of dihydroxyphenylalanine (DOPA) oxidation.
- *L-ascorbic acid:* Ascorbic acid has antioxidant properties. It also affects melanogenesis by reducing dopaquinone to DOPA. It prevents free radical production and promotes absorption of ultraviolet (UV) radiation. Vitamin C is the only antioxidant that is proven to stimulate the synthesis of collagen which is essential since our body's natural collagen production decreases as we age. Sun exposure will also accelerate the decrease in collagen.

There are many skin care products in the market today that claim to have vitamin C derivatives as an ingredient (magnesium ascorbyl phosphate or ascorbyl palmitate, for example), but L-ascorbic acid is the only useful form of vitamin C in skin care products. Ascorbic acid is the natural form of vitamin C and is water soluble. However, it can be irritating to the skin. It is very unstable. In contrast, vitamin C ester is nonirritating and nonstinging. It is fat soluble and absorbed by the skin. However, the efficacy of the esterified derivative has not been properly evaluated.

Although many cosmeceutical formulations contain vitamin C and/or vitamin E, very few are actually effective in topical application. First because the concentration is too low, second because the stability is compromised as soon as the product is opened and exposed to air and light and third because the form of the molecule (an ester or a mixture of isomers) is not absorbed or metabolized effectively by the skin.[19] However, when a stable formulation delivers a high concentration of the non-esterified, optical isomer of the antioxidant, vitamins C and E inhibit the acute UV damage of erythema, sunburn and tanning as well as chronic UV photoaging and skin cancer. Both are highly effective depigmenting agents. Vitamin C also reduces fine lines and wrinkles. Topical vitamin C also increases collagen synthesis in both young and old fibroblasts. Because vitamin C regenerates oxidized vitamin E, the combination in a cosmeceutical formulation is synergistic particularly in UV protection.[20]

Enzymes

Papain, which is derived from papaya fruit is an enzyme that digests intracellular protein bonds. It can improve epidermal exfoliation when used topically.

Growth Factors

Growth factors such as EGF, transforming growth factor (TGF), and platelet-derived growth factor (PDGF) are included in skin care products. They regulate intercellular signaling, cell growth, cell development, and tissue repair. New techniques such as liposomal transdermal delivery, microporation, phonophoresis, and iontophoresis are under study to evaluate the delivery system of growth factors with higher molecular weight.

EVALUATING COSMECEUTICAL SAFETY

The cosmeceutical market is unregulated; however, the cosmetics industry does an excellent job of self-policing the safety of products introduced into the marketplace. No cosmetic manufacturer worth the name wants to introduce formulations that might tarnish the hard-earned company reputation.

Botanical extracts are considered to be safe and meet the US Food and Drug Administration criteria for substances that can be put in OTC formulations. It is generally believed that substances that are safe for oral consumption can be assumed safe when applied topically, e.g., topical lycopene from tomatoes or topical avocadin from avocados. Alternatively, extensive animal testing may be undertaken by the raw material supplier to determine that the new ingredient is appropriate for human use.[3]

EVALUATING COSMECEUTICAL EFFICACY

According to Dr Albert Kligman, it is important to ask three questions to ascertain whether a new cosmeceutical product has a beneficial physiological effect **(Table 3)**.[21]

The stratum corneum is an effective barrier to the penetration of exogenous substances. Typically, the substances that cannot penetrate the SC easily include highly charged molecules, proteins, sugars, peptides, and nucleic

TABLE 3: Three major questions used to evaluate cosmeceutical ingredients.

Question 1	Can the active ingredient penetrate the stratum corneum and be delivered in sufficient concentrations to its intended target in the skin?
Question 2	Does the active ingredient have a known specific biochemical mechanism of action in the target cell or tissue in human skin?
Question 3	Are there published, peer-reviewed, double-blind, placebo-controlled, statistically significant, and clinical trials to substantiate the efficacy claims?

acids with molecular weights greater than approximately 1,000 kDa. In addition, it is important to determine whether threshold concentration (the minimum concentration of ingredient required to produce the desired effect) is achieved.

BIOENGINEERING TESTS FOR COSMECEUTICAL TESTING

Clinical trials are not mandatory for approval by regulatory authorities; most clinical trials of cosmeceuticals are not controlled, involve small number of subjects and rely only on subjective assessment of users by investigators, thus grossly limiting their reliability. Clinical trials should not rely on photographic improvement. There are major pitfalls in standardized clinical photography. In addition, it is difficult to measure appearance clinically because it is highly subjective, and endpoints are difficult to establish.

It is important to ensure that cosmeceuticals are compared with the vehicle and not with a placebo as the vehicle itself may have tangible effects.

Histopathology/biopsy studies or other invasive evaluations are not conducted because this would indicate that the cosmeceutical demonstrated drug effects rather than cosmetic benefits. This need has led to the development of noninvasive assessment techniques classified as skin bioengineering. Measurements of transepidermal water loss (TEWL), water content of skin, colorimetry, skin elasticity, colorimetry, surface replica analysis, etc. A few methods are described in **Table 4**.[22-28]

The human eye is still the best measure of cosmeceutical efficacy, in the absence of the abovementioned technologies.[3] Most cosmeceutical claims are based on the evaluations of the study participant and the investigator, which are accurate if the study is a well-designed, double-blind, and vehicle-controlled trial.

TABLE 4: Bioengineering tests for cosmeceutical testing.

Assessment technique	*Principle of assessment*
Evaporimetry	Measures transepidermal water loss (TEWL), barrier improvement and time to recovery after cosmeceutical application[22]
Corneometry	Evaluates skin water content by measuring conductivity of skin to low current electricity
Profilometry	Polymerizing silicone is placed onto the skin surface to obtain a silicone replica of the skin topography. This is then analyzed with a laser scanner. Used to evaluate skin texture and improvement in skin fine lines and wrinkles[23]
Chromametry	Used to evaluate brown and red skin tones[24,25]
Laser Doppler flowmetry	Uses Doppler effect to measure the speed of blood flow in the skin.[26,27] Used to evaluate any redness of skin
A-scan ultrasound imaging	Uses ultrasound waves to measure alterations in skin thickness.[28] Used to substantiate claims that a cosmeceutical increases skin thickness

COSMECEUTICAL MYTHS

The plant kingdom is a rich source of raw materials for cosmeceuticals. Herbal, organic, and natural have become catchwords that fascinate consumers. Phrases such as hypoallergenic, paraben free and preservative free are used to charge unduly high prices. It is imperative that dermatologists understand the nitty-gritties of cosmeceutical labels.

- *Myth 1:* Hypoallergenic cosmeceuticals do not produce allergic reactions.

  The term hypoallergenic is a marketing term.[29] There is nothing in this world that is not "non-allergenic." There are no regulatory guidelines that apply to the hypoallergenic concept. One cannot assume that companies making the hypoallergenic claim have conducted repeat insult patch testing, especially in those with poor epidermal barrier, such as rosacea or atopic dermatitis, as part of their product safety assessment. In general, hypoallergenic cosmeceuticals do not contain added fragrances or any of the ingredients on the standard patch test series. "Unscented" is a more appropriate term.[30] Dermatologists and consumers should view the hypoallergenic claim only as a marketing claim.
- *Myth 2:* Preservative-free cosmeceuticals produce fewer skin reactions.

  "Preservative-free" is a term devoid of meaning, since all products must contain preservatives to stay free of microbial contamination, except for pure petrolatum. Products that contain vitamin-derived antioxidants may be called preservative free because they do not contain "synthetic" preservatives.[29]
- *Myth 3:* Botanical cosmeceuticals are natural.

  Most botanical extracts are modified and chemically synthesized to obtain a form that can be easily incorporated into a skin preparation. It is far too expensive, in most cases, to use plant extracts for commercial formulations.[29] An example is allantoin, botanically obtained from the root of the comfrey plant. However, most allantoin used cosmeceuticals is obtained from uric acid. It is similar to plant-derived allantoin, but synthesized in a chemical plant, not grown by "mother nature."
- *Myth 4:* All natural ingredients are safer in skin care products.

  All plant derived ingredients are not necessarily safer in skin care products. Even poison ivy[14] which causes an intense allergic contact dermatitis is "natural"!
- *Myth 5:* Numerous botanicals in cosmeceuticals are better.

  Botanical and other cocktails are extremely problematic for the dermatologist who has to identify the culprit ingredient causing a patient's allergic contact dermatitis.[29]
- *Myth 6:* Topical botanical cosmeceuticals minimize postmenopausal skin changes.

  Postmenopausal skin changes are typically due to a low estrogen state leading to an increase in facial folds and rhytides. A number of topical botanical preparations containing genistein, an extract of fermented soy, which is structurally similar to human estrogen and can, thus, bind to some of the same receptors have been introduced to minimize postmenopausal wrinkling. Sadly, these effects are seen only with orally consumed fermented soy.[29]

CONCLUSION

Cosmeceuticals are currently defined by the claims that are made about their intended use. A product that "eliminates wrinkles" is a drug, whereas a product that "minimizes the appearance of wrinkles" is a cosmetic, even though they may both contain the same ingredients. It seems rather unscientific to define product functioning on the basis of package labeling and advertising; yet this is our current level of sophistication. Cosmeceuticals that function too well would alter the structure and function of the skin and become drugs. The current state of the cosmeceutical marketplace is not due to the industry's lack of desire to perform thoughtful research and develop quality products, but rather due to limitations imposed by the present regulatory climate regarding product claims. This is the reason for this category of products hitting the glass ceiling. It cannot be breached unless principles of the scientific method are applied to the clinical study of cosmeceuticals.

The best cosmeceutical research is being performed in industry. They have extremely rigid research standards and evaluate cosmeceuticals in the same manner as drugs. None of the research work on cosmeceuticals is being done in academic dermatology. Unless that changes, dermatologists have to look to partner with the industry to learn.[1]

In the words of the queen of cosmeceuticals Zoe Diana Draelos, "dermatology will move the cosmeceutical category forward, and the cosmeceutical category will move dermatology forward."

PART B: SYSTEMIC NUTRACEUTICALS

KEY MESSAGES

- The cosmeceutical label applies only to products applied topically.
- Products which are similar but ingested orally are known as nutraceuticals.
- Agents which are otherwise used as drugs are used in OTC products in lower concentrations.
- Many antioxidants work synergistically to regenerate and enhance the power of each other.

INTRODUCTION

Consumers are willing to pay a premium for skin and hair care products that they perceive as high-performance.[31]

The term "cosmeceutical" is often used in cosmetic advertising and may be misleading to the consumer.

If the consumer interprets a cosmeceutical to be similar to a pharmaceutical product, he or she may conclude that cosmeceuticals are required to undergo the same testing for efficacy and quality control as required for medication. This may allow the retailer to charge the consumer more for a product which may actually be less effective and/or of poorer quality than perceived.[32]

However, according to the United States FDA, the Food, Drug, and Cosmetic Act "does not recognize any such category as "cosmeceuticals." A product can be a drug, a cosmetic, or a combination of both, but the term "cosmeceutical" has no meaning under the law."[33]

Additionally, the FDA states that: "Food, Drug and Cosmetic Act defines drugs as those products that cure, treat, mitigate, or prevent disease or that affect the structure or function of the human body. While drugs are subject to an intensive review and approval process by FDA, cosmetics are not approved by FDA prior to sale. If a product has drug properties, it must be approved as a drug."[34]

To avoid inquiry and punitive action by the United States Federal Trade Commission, cosmeceuticals which do not intend to be regulated as drugs by the FDA are carefully labeled to avoid making statements which would indicate that the product has drug properties. Any such claims made regarding the product must be substantiated by scientific evidence as being truthful.

Generally speaking, it is to the financial benefit of the cosmeceutical manufacturer that their products are not regulated by the FDA as drugs, because the FDA review process for drugs can be very costly and may not yield a legally marketable product if the FDA denies approval of the product. However, as mentioned above, the reputation of the product may be falsely enhanced if the consumer incorrectly believes that a "cosmeceutical" is held to the same FDA standards as a drug.

DEFINITION

Cosmeceuticals are the combination of cosmetics and pharmaceuticals. Cosmeceuticals are cosmetic products with bioactive ingredients purported to have medical or drug-like benefits.

Dermatological research suggests that the bioactive ingredients used in cosmeceuticals have benefits beyond the traditional moisturizer.

However, despite reports of benefits from some cosmeceutical products, there are no legal requirements to prove that these products live up to their claims.

The "cosmeceutical" label applies only to products applied topically, such as creams, lotions, and ointments. Products which are similar in perceived benefits but ingested orally are known as nutricosmetics.

CLASSIFICATION OF COSMECEUTICALS

The term cosmeceuticals can be used with different terms. For all the terms the definition remains the same, i.e., cosmeceuticals formulations which are neither pure cosmetics, like lipsticks, nor pure drug, like corticosteroids. It is a hybrid category of products lying on the spectrum between drugs and cosmetics. The various terms by which Cosmeceuticals can be substituted are:

- Active cosmetics
- Nutricosmetics
- Performance cosmetics
- Functional cosmetics, and
- Dermaceuticals

A new concept, such nutricosmetics are also known as "beauty pills," "beauty from within," and even "oral cosmetics."[35]

CATEGORIES OF COSMECEUTICALS

Further cosmeceuticals are divided into different categories based on their active ingredients **(Table 5)**.

However, the perceived notion that the natural or organic ingredients are safer than the synthetic ones is a misconception, and there is no scientific data to support this fact. The topical cosmoceuticals have been dealt with in detail in the previous chapter. This chapter deals with systemic agents (nutraceuticals).

Systemic Agents

The free radical theory of aging proposed in 1956[36] is one of the most widely accepted theories to explain the cause of aging. Although antioxidants are present in food sources, many believe that higher levels can be achieved by supplementation.

TABLE 5: Classification of cosmeceuticals.

Antioxidants	Reduce the harmful effects of free radicals
Peptides	Small proteins that stimulate the production of collagen
Growth factors	Compounds that act as chemical messengers between cells and play a role in cell division, blood vessel proliferation, and in production and distribution of collagen and elastin
Combination products	Contain ingredients, such as multiple antioxidants

Therefore, the use of antioxidants as protective agents in oral supplements is extremely popular. Many antioxidants work synergistically to regenerate and enhance the power of each other.[37] These include vitamins C and E, glutathione, alpha lipoic acid, coenzyme Q 10, green tea (polyphenols), melatonin, and selenium.

Vitamin A, C, beta-carotene, selenium, coenzyme Q10, estrogen, testosterone, silymarin, pycnogenol, procyanidins are the major players in antiaging therapies.[38,39] Antioxidants, all of which display various distinguishing characteristics and activities, are believed to be an important focus in prevention of aging, as these free radical scavengers protect the skin via several mechanisms.

Vitamins

L-ascorbic Acid (Vitamin C)

Vitamin C, also named L-ascorbic acid, is water soluble, photosensitive and is the most important antioxidant in the hydrophilic phase. Vitamin C is not naturally synthesized by the human body and therefore adequate dietary intake of vitamin C is required.

The richest natural sources are fresh fruits and vegetables, such as citrus fruits, blackcurrant, rose hip, guava, chili pepper, or parsley. Stability of the vitamin C molecule depends on aggregate condition and formulation. L-ascorbic acid can be used orally and topically for skin benefits. Vitamin C is a cofactor for lysyl and prolyl hydroxylase, which stabilize the triple helical structure of collagen.[40] It also plays a role in cholesterol synthesis, iron absorption, and increases the bioavailability of selenium. The most commonly described cutaneous manifestations accompanying vitamin C deficiency are attributed to the impaired collagen synthesis. Enlargement and keratosis of hair follicles mainly of the upper arms and curled hairs, the so-called "corkscrew hairs," are usually described. The follicles become hemorrhagic with time and they sometimes mimic the palpable purpura of leukocytoclastic vasculitis.[41]

Nutricosmetic products with L-ascorbic acid work as free radical scavengers and repair the membrane-bound oxidized vitamin E.[42] A long-term study observed the effects of a combination of ascorbic acid and d-α-tocopherol (vitamin E) administered orally to human volunteers on UVB-induced epidermal damage. The treatment was well-tolerated and could be used prophylactically against the hazardous effects of solar UV irradiation and skin cancer.[43]

There are many preparations of vitamin C-based products available in the market, but these are predominantly based on more stable esters and other derivatives of vitamin C which more readily penetrate the skin but are not necessarily converted to the only active vitamin C, L-ascorbic acid.[44] These topical or oral products do not have the effects provided by L-ascorbic acid.

Tocopherols (Vitamin E)

The vitamin E complex is a group of eight compounds called tocopherols. Tocopherol is a fat-soluble membrane-bound antioxidant and consequently a free-radical scavenger especially of highly reactive singlet oxygen. Tocopherol is like vitamin C, a naturally occurring endogenous non-enzymatic antioxidant.

Vitamin C and vitamin E act synergistically. When UV-activated molecules oxidize cellular components, a chain reaction of lipid peroxidation in membranes rich in polyunsaturated fatty acids is induced. The antioxidant d-α-tocopherol is oxidized to the tocopheroxyl radical in this process, and it is regenerated by ascorbic acid to d-α-tocopherol.[45,46] Beside ascorbic acid, glutathione, and coenzyme Q10 can also recycle tocopherol.

Higher amounts of tocopherol are available in vegetables, vegetable oils such as wheat germ oil, sunflower oil, safflower oil and seeds, corn, soy, and some sorts of meat. The intake of natural vitamin E products helps against collagen cross linking and lipid peroxidation, which are both linked to aging of the skin.

D-α-tocopherol is involved in stabilizing the cell membrane by inhibiting oxidation of polyunsaturated fatty acids, such as arachidonic acid of membrane phospholipids. Topically applied vitamin E is described to reduce erythema, sunburned cells, chronic UVB-induced skin damage and photo carcinogenesis in the majority of the published studies. Vitamin E deficiency has been associated with a syndrome of edema with papular erythema or seborrheic changes, dryness, and depigmentation in premature infants.[47,48]

There are many clinical studies, which have tested the effects of tocopherol.

Oral combination treatments of vitamins C and E, partly with other photoprotective compounds, did increase the photoprotective effects dramatically compared with monotherapies. This synergetic interplay of several anti-oxidants should be considered in research on cutaneous photoprotection.[49]

Carotenoids (Vitamin A, β-carotene, Astaxanthin, and Retinol)

Carotenoids are vitamin A derivatives such as β-carotene, astaxanthin, lycopene, and retinol, which are all highly effective antioxidants and have been documented to possess photoprotective properties.

β-carotene is the most prominent member of the group of carotenoids, natural colorants that can be found in the human diet.[50]

Compared with other carotenoids, the primary role of β-carotene is its provitamin-A activity. β-carotene can be cleaved by BCMO1 enzyme into two molecules of all-*trans*-retinal. There is no difference between naturally occurring and chemically synthesized β-carotene. Furthermore, β-carotene can also act as a lipid radical scavenger and as a singlet oxygen quencher, as demonstrated in vitro. Based on the distribution of BCMO1 in human tissues, it seems that β-carotene metabolism takes place in a wide variety of organs, including the skin.[51]

Carrots, pumpkin, sweet potatoes, mangoes, and papaya are some examples of β-carotene containing fruits and vegetables. Upon dietary supplementation, β-carotene can be further enriched in skin, in which it is already a major carotenoid. β-carotene is an endogenous photoprotector, and its efficacy to prevent UV-induced erythema formation has been demonstrated in various studies.[52,53]

The systemic photoprotecting effect of β-carotene depends both on dose and duration of treatment. In studies documenting protection against UV-induced erythema, supplementation with carotenoids lasted for at least 7 weeks, with doses >12 mg/day of carotenoids.[54-56] With treatment periods of only 3–4 weeks, studies reported no protective effects. Furthermore, β-carotene supplementation can significantly reduce the rate of mitochondrial mutation in human dermal fibroblasts after UV irradiation.

Astaxanthin is found in microalgae, yeast, salmon, trout, krill, shrimp, crayfish, and crustacea. Astaxanthin is biosynthesized by microalgae or phytoplankton, which are consumed by zooplankton or crustacea. They accumulate astaxanthin and, in turn, are ingested by fish which then accrue astaxanthin in the food chain.

Astaxanthin shows a significant photoprotective effect and counteracts UVA-induced alterations to a great extent. A recent study of Suganuma et al. showed that astaxanthin could interfere with UVA-induced matrix- metalloproteinase-1 and skin fibroblast elastase/neutral endopeptidase expression. Both studies suggest that effects of UVA radiation, such as skin sagging or wrinkling can be prevented or at least minimized by topical or oral administration of astaxanthin.[57-59]

Lycopene is a bright red carotene and carotenoid pigment and phytochemical found in tomatoes and other red fruits and vegetables, such as red carrots, watermelons, and papayas. Although lycopene is chemically a carotene, it has no vitamin A activity.

β-carotene and lycopene are usually the dominating carotenoids in human blood and tissues and are known to modulate skin properties when ingested as supplements or as dietary products. While they cannot be compared with sunscreen, there is evidence that they protect the skin against sunburn, by increasing the basal defense against UV light-mediated damage.

A study confirmed that the amounts of lycopene in plasma and skin are comparable to or even greater than those of β-carotene. When skin is exposed to UV light stress, more skin lycopene is destroyed compared with β-carotene, suggesting a role of lycopene in mitigating oxidative damage in tissues. Lycopene and tomato products are also mentioned for preventing cancer.[60,61]

Retinol is important for the human body; however, the body itself cannot synthesize it. Retinol, a fat-soluble unsaturated isoprenoid such as its two important metabolites retinaldehyde and retinoic acid, is essential for growth, differentiation and maintenance of epithelial tissues and influences reproduction. In human skin two retinoid receptors are expressed, which can be activated by retinol and its metabolites.[62]

Retinaldehyde, additionally being important for vision, is created by in vivo oxidation of retinol in a reversible process. The normal plasma concentration of vitamin A in humans is 0.35–0.75 μg/mL.

Retinol must be derived from diet.

Natural retinol and retinol ester are contained in liver, milk, egg yolk, cheese, and fatty fish etc. Naturally occurring and synthetic vitamin A show similar biological activities. Different retinol products, both for cosmetic (topical) and pharmaceutical (topical, systemic) use can be found in the market.

Also, the effects of UV protection by using sunscreens and topical antioxidants are reviewed. The topical retinoid treatments inhibit the UV-induced, matrix metalloproteinase (MMP)-mediated breakdown of collagen and protect against UV-induced decreases in procollagen expression.

Endogenous retinoids cannot be linked to the pathogenesis of common skin diseases such as acne and psoriasis. Oral treatment with retinol or retinal derivatives has not been proposed as a possible antiaging treatment. Humans require 0.8–1 mg or 2,400–3,000 IU vitamin A per day (1 IU = 0.3 μg).[63,64]

Unfortunately, the large CARET trial mentioned lung cancer-promoting effects of 25,000 IU retinyl palmitate combined with 30 mg β-carotene intake in smokers.[65] Thus, the belief that chemical quenching of free radicals by natural compounds such as retinyl palmitate and β-carotene exerts always beneficial effects has been challenged. Omenn's data showed that an artificial systemic increase of antioxidants by dietary supplementation intended to modify UV erythema thresholds may have severe internal adverse effects which even may not only increase risk of cell aging but of tumor promotion. However, experts still recommend dietary intake of fruits and vegetables.

Vitamin D

In humans, vitamin D serves two functions, it acts as a prohormone and the human body can synthesize it itself through sun exposure. Skin is the major site for UV-B mediated vitamin D_3, and 1,25-dihydroxy vitamin D_3 synthesis.

Smaller amounts of vitamin D_2 and D_3 come from the dietary intake of animal-based foods such as fatty fish or egg yolk. Some products such as milk, cereals, and margarine can be enriched with vitamin D.

Excess of vitamin D is stored in fat of the body and can result in toxic effects. This toxicity presents with nausea, vomiting, poor appetite, weakness, weight loss, and constipation. Food-intake of vitamin D high enough to cause toxicity is very unlikely.

With increasing age, the capacity of the skin to produce vitamin D_3 declines and consequently the protective effects of the vitamin. There are several factors contributing to this deficiency state among them behavioral factors, for example limited sun exposure or malnutrition, which can be partially altered by behavior modification and various intrinsic factors such as reduced synthetic capacity. In skin, the concentration of 7-dehydrocholesterol—a vitamin D_3 precursor—showed an approximately 50% decline from age 20 years to age 80 years[66] and the total amount of pre-vitamin D_3 in the skin of young subjects was at least two times greater than when compared with that of the elderly subjects. Vitamin D and calcium supplementation is therefore of great importance in the elderly population.[67]

Niacin and Niacinamide

These are forms of vitamin B_3. Vitamin B_3 is found in many foods including yeast, meat, fish, milk, eggs, green vegetables, beans, and cereal grains. Niacin and niacinamide are also found in many vitamin B complex supplements with other B vitamins.

Niacinamide can be made from niacin in the body. Niacin is converted to niacinamide when it is taken in amounts greater than what is needed by the body. Niacin and niacinamide are easily dissolved in water and are well-absorbed when taken by mouth.

Niacinamide suppresses melanin from reaching the surface of the skin and protects the skin from further UV damage. Too much melanin (which is a naturally occurring substance in the body that is responsible for both its color the skin's absorption of UV rays) can result in age spots, freckles, and hyperpigmentation.

Oral and topical niacinamide have been shown to reduce UV-induced immunosuppression. Oral niacinamide reduces the onset of actinic keratosis, indicating that this vitamin may be helpful in reducing more terminal forms of photo aging including skin cancer formation.[68]

Topical niacinamide is a potent cell-communicating ingredient that offers a variety of antiaging benefits, and there is also growing evidence that it can mitigate acne and its marks. But according to the National Institutes of Health, there is not enough evidence to recommend taking vitamin B_3 supplements orally to treat acne. Vitamin B_3 works better when applied topically than when taken orally as a supplement, as it is water-soluble, and our body does not use right away, and it is quickly excreted, so taking extra amounts, that is, more than provided by a healthy, balanced diet via supplements does not make much sense. In fact, very few people are ever deficient in vitamin B_3 because it is so prevalent in the foods many of us routinely eat.

Pantothenic Acid

Vitamin B_5, also known as pantothenic acid, is a water-soluble vitamin that is found in all living cells within the body. It helps fight acne and to maintain the health of skin and hair. Vitamin B_5 can reduce the appearance of premature aging such as wrinkles, dark spots, and discolorations. Studies have also shown that it plays an important role in the pigmentation and growth of hair follicles. Vitamin B_5 can help prevent hair from losing its color during the aging process.

According to recent studies, people who were given supplements containing vitamin B_5 were shown to have a reduction in acne outbreaks compared to those who did not take the vitamin. Study results show that pantothenic acid-based dietary supplements in healthy adults with acne facial lesions, are effective, safe, well tolerated and reduced total facial lesion counts.

The results indicated that taking vitamin B_5 can help clear area-specific and inflammatory skin acne blemishes while not causing any known side effects. This may be due partially to the role that vitamin B5 plays in immunity and lowering the general inflammation.[69]

Polyphenols

Polyphenols have drawn the attention of the antiaging research community over the last decade, mainly because of their antioxidant properties, their great intake amount in our diet and the increasing studies showing their probable role in the prevention of various diseases associated with oxidative stress, such as cancer and cardiovascular and neurodegenerative diseases. Their total dietary intake could be as high as 1 g/day, which is much higher than that of all other classes of phytochemicals and known dietary antioxidants.

They are mostly found in fruits and plant-derived beverages, such as fruit juices, tea, coffee, and red wine. Vegetables, cereals, chocolate, and dry legumes are also sources for the total polyphenol intake.[70,71]

Several thousand molecules having a polyphenol structure have been identified in plants being generally involved in defense against UV radiation or aggression by pathogens. Depending on the number of phenol rings and the way that these rings bind to one another, polyphenols can be divided into many different functional groups, such as the phenolic acids, flavonoids, stilbenes, and lignans.[70] Flavonoids are also further divided into flavones, flavonols, isoflavones, and flavanones, each with a slightly different chemical structure.

It has been reported that the polyphenolic content of foods can be easily affected or seriously reduced by methods of meal preparation and culinary traditions. For example, onions, which are a major source of phenolic acids and flavonoids, and tomatoes lose between 75 and 80% of their initial content when boiled over 15 minutes, 65% when cooked in a microwave oven and 30% when fried.[72]

Laboratory studies of different polyphenols, such as green tea polyphenols, grape seed proanthocyanidins, resveratrol, silymarin and genistein, conducted in animal models on UV-induced skin inflammation, oxidative stress and DNA damage, suggested that these polyphenols, combined with sunscreen protection, have the ability to protect the skin from the adverse effects of UV radiation, including the risk of skin cancers.[73]

Flavonoids

Phlorizin

Phlorizin belongs to the group of dihydrochalcones, a type of flavonoid and it is naturally occurring in some plants.

It is be found in the bark of pear, apple, cherry, and other fruit trees.

- Its antiaging effects have only been reported in the last few years.
- Further investigations on humans are needed.
- Many other botanical extracts, such as silymarin, apigenin, and genistein have been demonstrated to have beneficial effects on skin aging parameters.[74]

Resveratrol

Resveratrol is an antioxidant, natural polyphenol, abundant in the skin of grapes. It has been the subject of intense interest in recent years due to a range of unique antiaging properties. High concentrations of natural resveratrol and resveratrol oligomers are found in grape shoots from Vitis Vinifera. Resveratrol works both as a chelating agent and as a radical scavenger and in addition it takes part in inflammation by inhibiting the production of IL-8 by LPS-induced MAPK phosphorylation and a block of NFKB activation.[75]

As far as skin is concerned, resveratrol has been recently shown to possess a protective action in vitro against cell death after exposure of human epidermal keratinocytes (HaCaT) cells to the nitric oxide free radical donor sodium nitroprusside. Furthermore, Giardina et al. reported in 2010 that in experiments in vitro with skin fibroblasts treated with resveratrol there was a dose-related increase in the rate of cell proliferation and in inhibition of collagenase activity.[76]

Curcumin

Curcumin is the principal curcuminoid of the popular Indian spice turmeric, which is a member of the ginger family (Zingiberaceae) and is frequently found in rice dishes to add yellow color to the otherwise white rice. Curcumin has been shown to protect against the deleterious effects of injury by attenuating oxidative stress and suppressing inflammation. In human fibroblasts curcumin-induced cellular stress responses through phosphatidylinositol 3-kinase/Akt pathway and redox signaling, thus providing evidence that curcumin-induced hormetic stimulation of cellular antioxidant defenses can be a useful approach toward antiaging intervention.[77,78]

Green Tea Polyphenols

Green tea polyphenols (GTPs) derivating from the leaves of the *Camellia sinensis* have been postulated to protect human skin from the cutaneous signs of photo aging. Studies have shown that green tea extract also possesses anti-inflammatory activity. These anti-inflammatory and anti-carcinogenic properties of green tea are due to their polyphenolic constituents present therein. The major and most chemopreventive constituent in green tea responsible for these biochemical or pharmacological effects is (–)-epigallocatechin-3-gallate (EGCG). EGCG can directly inhibit the expression of metalloproteinases such as MMP-2, MMP-9, and MMP-12, and is a potent inhibitor of leukocyte elastase, which is instrumental in tumor invasion and metastasis.[79-81]

Ubiquinol (Coenzyme Q10)

Coenzyme Q10 is a fat-soluble, endogenous vitamin-like substance that is mainly stored in the fat tissues of our body. It is present in most eukaryotic cells, primarily in the mitochondria and plays an important role as a component of the electron transport chain in the aerobic cellular respiration, generating energy. Ubiquinol is also a well-known powerful antioxidant compound. In the skin, CoQ10 is mainly to be found in the epidermis where it acts in combination with other enzymic and non-enzymic substances as the initial barrier to oxidant assault.[82]

Primary dietary sources of CoQ10 include oily fish (such as salmon and tuna), organ meats (such as liver), and whole grains.

The amount of CoQ10 needed in human organism can be gained through a balanced diet; however, in the market, CoQ10 is available in several forms as a supplement, including soft gel capsules, oral spray, hard shell capsules, and tablets. As a fat-soluble substance it is better absorbed when taken with fat rich meals. CoQ10 is also added to various cosmetics. In cases of primary CoQ10 deficiency in vitro experiments have shown that they should be treated with CoQ10 supplementation and that complementary administration of antioxidants with high bioavailability should be considered if oxidative stress is present.[83]

Essential Fatty Acids (Vitamin F)

Essential fatty acids (EFAs) are long-chain polyunsaturated fatty acids derived from linolenic, linoleic, and oleic acids. They cannot be produced in the human body, and they have to be consumed through our daily dietary intake. EFAs have also been known as vitamin F. Arachidonic acid is a semi-EFA, as it can be synthesized in the body from linoleic acid. The two families of EFAs are ω-3, derived from linolenic acid, and ω-6, derived from linoleic acid, with the number indicating the position of the first double bond continuing from the terminal methyl group on the molecule.[84]

They are present in multiple food sources such as fish and shellfish, flaxseed, hemp oil, soya oil, canola oil, chia seeds, pumpkin seeds, sunflower seeds, leafy vegetables, walnuts, sesame seeds, avocados, salmon, and albacore tuna.

Essential fatty acids are essential for the synthesis of tissue lipids, play an important role in the regulation of cholesterol levels and are precursors of prostaglandins.[85]

Oral administration of an antioxidant mixture containing vitamin C, vitamin E, pycnogenol and evening primrose oil significantly inhibited wrinkle formation caused by chronic UVB irradiation through significant inhibition of UVB-induced MMP activity accompanied by enhancement of collagen synthesis on hairless mouse skin.[86]

Essential fatty acids can also be found as artificial supplements in the market. Fish oil supplements are usually made from mackerel, herring, tuna, halibut, salmon, cod liver, whale blubber, or seal blubber, are rich in omega-3 fatty acids and often contain small amounts of vitamin E.

They might also be combined with calcium, iron, or vitamins A, B_1, B_2, B_3, C, or D.

SKIN-LIGHTENING AGENTS

Glutathione

The most commonly used systemic skin whitening agent is glutathione (GSH) used alone or in various combinations, both as oral, and intravenous formulations. GSH is an antioxidant synthesized in all mammalian cells from three amino acids-glutamate, cysteine, and glycine.

It is also available naturally in watermelon, avocado, broccoli, spinach, and tomatoes.

Glutathione exists in cells mostly in the reduced form which is constantly oxidized forming oxidized GSH and its supply is replenished by the action of GSH reductase. GSH is involved in various biochemical processes especially those involving scavenging of free radicals and detoxification of toxic compounds. It acts as coenzyme and helps in the transport of amino acids across the cell membranes. Lower GSH levels are implicated in many diseases and GSH has been tried in the management of Alzheimer's disease, Parkinson's disease, multiple sclerosis, alcoholic hepatitis, atherosclerosis, acquired immunodeficiency syndrome, and chronic fatigue syndrome. It has been commonly used to combat the neuro- and nephrotoxicity-associated with cisplatin chemotherapy and this is the only Food and Drug Administration approved indication for the intravenous form of GSH.

The role of GSH as a skin whitening agent was an accidental discovery when skin whitening was noticed

BOX 2: Proposed mechanism of action of glutathione in disorders of pigmentation.

- Interference with cellular transport of tyrosinase
- Direct inactivation of the enzyme tyrosinase by binding with the copper-containing active site of the enzyme
- Mediating the switch mechanism from eumelanin to pheomelanin production as GSH is the major physiologic reservoir of cysteine and increase in cysteine levels results in switching of eumelanogenesis to pheomelanogenesis
- Quenching of free radicals and peroxides that contribute to tyrosinase activation and melanin formation
- Modulation of depigmenting abilities of melanocytotoxic agents

as a side effect of large doses of GSH. This led to studies establishing its role in melanogenesis and the recent controversial use of GSH as systemic skin whitening agent.

Glutathione exerts its action as skin whitening agent at various levels of melanogenesis **(Box 2)**.[87]

Glutathione for skin whitening is available in both tablet and injectable form. When taken orally, GSH is hydrolyzed by intestinal and hepatic gamma-glutamyl transferase resulting in reduced bioavailability. Even when large oral doses were administered, it was found that most of the absorbed GSH remains within the gut luminal cells and only small and transient increases of GSH could be detected in the general circulation.[74] Thus, the effectiveness of exogenously administered GSH is hindered by its instability when crossing cell membranes and its rapid hydrolysis in the circulation by gamma-glutamyl transpeptidase found on the extracellular surfaces of cells.[88,89]

On the contrary, intravenous GSH delivers very high doses directly into the systemic circulation, overloading the renal circulation.

Oral GSH is in the "generally regarded as safe" category of FDA and is usually marketed as a food or dietary supplement and hence it does not certainly need to be FDA or Bureau of Food and Drug (BFAD) approved. There are no provisions in the law for FDA to approve dietary supplements for effectiveness before they reach the consumer. However, Department of Health, Philippines has recently issued a statement stating, "The use of glutathione IV as a skin whitener is not approved by the FDA. The public is strongly warned to refrain from using glutathione for this purpose in light of potential harm associated with such use."[90]

The promoters of GSH promote it at a dose of 20 and 40 mg/kg/body weight/day which is divided into two doses with a maintenance dose of 500 mg/day. They claim that gradual systemic effect will be seen in 1–3 months in medium brown skin, in 3–6 months in dark brown skin, in 6–12 months in very dark skin and in 2 years are more in black skin. Injectable GSH is given at a dose of 900 mg weekly by intravenous or intramuscular method and the sessions can be repeated 2–3 times a week. They claim skin whitening to occur as early as 2–3 weeks.

Glutathione is also combined with many other agents such as vitamin C to increase its absorption, N-acetyl cysteine to boost its level, alpha lipoic acid, and other antioxidants such as vitamin E and grape seed extract. Some oral preparations have dangerous combinations such as monobenzone which causes irreversible depigmentation and hydroquinone which is banned by FDA as a carcinogen.[91]

L-cysteine Peptide

Another agent promoted for skin whitening is L-cysteine peptide, which is claimed to be 3–5 times more potent than GSH and is BFAD approved. Natural sources of L-cysteine include poultry, yogurt, egg yolks, red peppers, garlic, onions, broccoli, Brussel sprouts, oats, and wheat germ.

L-cysteine along with L-glutamic acid and glycine is the rate-limiting precursor in the synthesis of GSH peroxidase and has been found that high concentrations of L-cysteine reduced the tyrosinase activity and produced more pheomelanin by way of cysteinyl dihydroxyphenylalanine (DOPA), the building block of pheomelanin. The cysteinyl DOPAs can be formed in two ways-directly by nucleophilic addition of cysteine to DOPA quinone or indirectly from GSH DOPA by action of gamma-glutamyl transferase and peptidase. Hence L-cysteine peptide is promoted as skin-whitening agent but without much scientific evidence to support its use for this indication.[92,93]

Tranexamic Acid

Tranexamic acid (trans-4-aminomethyl cyclohexane carboxylic acid), a plasmin inhibitor, commonly used as a hemostatic agent owing to its antifibrinolytic action is also promoted as a systemic skin-whitening agent especially as oral or intradermal injections for melasma. The skin-whitening effects of tranexamic acid were incidentally found when it was used in the treatment of aneurysmal subarachnoid hemorrhage. It is a synthetic derivative of lysine and its therapeutic role in melasma was first studied by Nijor as early as in 1979, but only limited data exist in the literature regarding its use in melasma. Plasmin is a protease that enhances the intracellular release of arachidonic acid, a precursor of prostanoid, and also elevates alpha-melanocyte stimulating hormone (α-MSH) processed from proopiomelanocortin. Both arachidonic acid and α-MSH can activate melanin synthesis by melanocytes. Tranexamic acid by way of its antiplasmin activity depletes the keratinocyte pool of arachidonic acid involved in ultraviolet (UV) induced melanogenesis.[94-97]

It has been used at a low dose of 250 mg twice a day for at least 3 months for the treatment of melasma and found to be effective.[96] But, it is not safe to use it for a long duration in view of its antihemorrhagic property resulting in side effects such as venous thromboembolism, myocardial infarction, cerebrovascular accidents, and pulmonary embolism. It is contraindicated in patients with acquired defective color vision, an active intravascular clotting condition, and hypersensitivity to tranexamic acid.[96] However, there is no scientific data available demonstrating the role of tranexamic acid as an overall skin-whitening/lightening agent. It is even being promoted as intravenous injection for skin whitening at a dose of 500 mg every week for 1 or 2 months and 500 mg every month for maintenance. Tranexamic acid has been found to produce good synergistic effect when combined with ascorbic acid or its derivatives and L-cysteine.

Pycnogenol

Pycnogenol obtained from the bark of French maritime pine, is standardized to 65–75% procyanidin compounds by weight and is evolving for its use in hyperpigmentation. Its main constituents are procyanidins, polyphenolic monomers, phenolic, or cinnamic acids. It has antioxidant and anti-inflammatory properties and hence scavenges free radicals. Pine extract has been used in various market preparations. Oral Pycnogenol has been found to reduce melasma severity although, studies on topical use are lacking.[98]

Silymarin

The active ingredient in milk thistle is an antioxidant that can protect against depletion of glutathione, which is a "master antioxidant" that is extremely useful at helping prevent disease formation. Glutathione is found naturally in the human body, as well as in some plants, mushrooms, fungus, and algae.

Its biggest role is to help fight oxidative stress that leads to such diseases as cancer, diabetes, heart disease, and neurodegenerative diseases. It can help prevent damage to important cellular components caused by reactive oxygen species, such as free radicals.

One of the biggest milk thistle benefits is that it preserves glutathione. The modern American diet, pollution, toxins, medications, stress, trauma, aging, infections, and radiation all work to deplete liver capabilities and also glutathione in the body. Milk thistle helps increase glutathione levels by improving liver detox functions. Milk thistle strengthens the liver cell walls, buffering them from invading toxins, and supports liver regeneration and glutathione formation.

Alpha Lipoic Acid

Also known as lipoic acid is a powerful antioxidant and is fat and water-soluble. It also has anti-inflammatory properties that enable it to be the best skin tightening and whitening remedy. Lipoic acid contains sulfur and helps in restoration of other antioxidants, such as vitamins C and E. Lipoic acid is synthesized by the body and produces energy through breaking down carbohydrates. The more the energy is produced by Lipoic Acid, the much younger the skin looks, hence eliminating wrinkles and keeping the skintight and beautiful. It is found in tomatoes, spinach, broccoli, peas and Brussel sprouts, yams, potatoes, carrots, etc. Other foods that have lipoic acid include yeast, fish, chicken, red meat, and specific meat organ such as heart, kidney, and liver.

Problems with Systemic Skin-whitening Agents

These agents are not FDA approved for skin whitening and no scientific evidence exists for their use.

Collagen peptides are natural bioactive ingredients used in many nutricosmetic products, orally taken nutritional supplements which provide skin health and beauty benefits. Collagen peptides present as a mix of specific peptides of different lengths with high abundance of the amino acids hydroxyproline, glycine, and proline, which are produced by enzymatic hydrolysis of native collagen extracted from animal connective tissues. Investigations using radio-actively labeled collagen peptides have demonstrated that the absorbed peptides reach the skin and are retained in the tissue for up to 2 weeks.

A growing body of evidence demonstrates the efficacy of collagen peptides to improve parameters of skin physiology in preclinical studies. Collagen peptides were shown to increase hyaluronic acid production in dermal fibroblasts and to improve skin barrier function by increasing the water content of the stratum corneum. Further, collagen peptides induce the synthesis of collagen on the mRNA and protein level as well as the production of stronger collagen fibrils, promote growth of skin fibroblasts, and induce fibroblast migration.[99]

Metformin

Metformin is a drug, approved to treat diabetes but appears to target a number of aging-related mechanisms. Specifically for aging, metformin leads to decreased insulin levels, decreased IGF-1 signaling,[100] inhibition of mTOR, inhibition of mitochondrial complex 1 in the electron transport chain[101] and reduction in DNA damage.[102]

Metformin favorably influences metabolic and cellular processes closely associated with the development of age-related conditions, such as inflammation and cellular senescence. More specifically, there is evidence that metformin can delay aging and increase healthy lifespan in vivo in several rodent strains.[103] It increases mean lifespan in female outbred mice by 40%.[103] Further, metformin delays the onset of carcinoma and extends lifespan by a mean of 8% in a breast cancer model.[104]

Targeting Ageing with Metformin (TAME) is a novel clinical trial that will test whether the drug metformin, a widely-used treatment for type 2 diabetes, can delay the onset of age-related diseases and conditions including cancer, cardiovascular disease, and Alzheimer 's disease.

Miscellaneous Agents

Apart from these, large doses of vitamin C, hyaluronic acid, epidermal growth factor and combinations of multiple natural extracts natural collagen extracts, bearberry extract, glycyrrhiza glabra extract, lycopene, kelp, olive leaf extract, hawthorn, jujube, sea buckthorn, starch, pearl extracts, etc., are also promoted for skin whitening in the form of food or dietary supplements with no scientific evidence.

CONCLUSION

Cosmeceuticals are used to maintain and improve the appearance of the skin.

The strong demand from the consumers to constantly look youthful and flawless has driven the research and development as well as sale volumes of cosmeceuticals.

This promises noninvasive antiaging procedures, however well designed, randomized, placebo-controlled studies are necessary and important.

REFERENCES

1. Kligman A. The future of cosmeceuticals: an interview with Albert Kligman, MD, PhD. Interview by Zoe Diana Draelos. Dermatol Surg. 2005;31:890-1.
2. Cornell University Law School. Federal Food, Drug and Cosmetic act sec (21 USC 301-392). [online] Available from https://www.law.cornell.edu/uscode/text/21/chapter-9 [Accessed March, 2024].
3. Draelos ZD. Cosmeceuticals: undefined, unclassified, and unregulated. Clin Dermatol. 2009;27:431-4.
4. PR Newswire. (2016). Global Cosmeceuticals Market Outlook 2020. [online] Available from https://www.prnewswire.com/news-releases/global-cosmeceuticals-market-outlook-2020-300239151.html [Last accessed March, 2024].
5. Goh CL, Noppakun N, Micali G, Azizan NZ, Boonchai W, Chan Y, et al. Meeting the challenges of acne treatment in Asian patients: a review of the role of dermocosmetics as adjunctive therapy. J Cutan Aesthet Surg. 2016;9:85-92.
6. Prystowsky JH. Topical retinoids. In: Wolverton SE (Ed). Comprehensive Dermatologic Drug Therapy. Philadelphia: WB Saunders; 2001. pp. 578-91.
7. Michel L, Jomard A, Démarchez M. Pharmacology of adapalene. Br J Dermatol. 1998;139:3-7.
8. Phillips TJ, Gottlieb AB, Leyden JJ, Lowe NJ, Lew-Kaya DA, Sefton J, et al. Efficacy of 0.1% tazarotene cream for the treatment of photodamage: a 12-month multicenter, randomized trial. Arch Dermatol. 2002;138:1486-93.
9. Grossman R. The role of dimethylaminoethanol in cosmetic dermatology. Am J Clin Dermatol. 2005;6:39-47.
10. Hoppe U, Bergemann J, Diembeck W, Ennen J, Gohla S, Harris I, et al. Coenzyme Q10, a cutaneous antioxidant and energizer. Biofactors. 1999;9:371-8.
11. Usuki A, Ohashi A, Sato H, Ochiai Y, Ichihashi M, Funasaka Y. The inhibitory effect of glycolic acid and lactic acid on melanin synthesis in melanoma cells. Exp Dermatol. 2003;12: 43-50.
12. Ditre CM, Griffin TD, Murphy GF, Sueki H, Telegan B, Johnson WC, et al. Effects of alphahydroxy acids on photoaged skin: a pilot clinical, histologic, and ultrastructural study. J Am Acad Dermatol. 1996;34:187-95.
13. Reszko AE, Berson D, Lupo M. Cosmeceuticals: practical applications. Dermatol Clin. 2009;27:401-16.
14. Zawar VP, Mhaskar ST. Exogenous ochronosis following hydroquinone for melasma. J Cosmet Dermatol. 2004;3: 234-6.
15. Chakraborthy AK, Funasaka Y, Komoto M, Ichihashi M. Effect of arbutin on melanogenic proteins in human melanocytes. Pigment Cell Res. 1998;11:206-12.
16. Yokoto T, Nishio H, Kuboto Y, Mizoguchi M. The inhibitory effect of glabridin from liquorice extracts on melanogenesis and inflammation. Pigment Cell Res. 1998;11:355-61.
17. Greatens A, Hakozaki T, Koshoffer A, Epstein H, Schwemberger S, Babcock G, et al. Effective inhibition of melanosome transfer to keratinocytes by lectins and niacinamide is reversible. Exp Dermatol. 2005;14:498-508.
18. Del Rosso JQ, Baum EW, Draelos ZD, Elewski BE, Fleischer AB Jr, Kakita LS,, et al. Azelaic acid gel 15% clinical versatility in the treatment of rosacea. Cutis. 2006;78:6-19.
19. Kobayashi S, Takehana M, Itoh S, Ogata E. Protective effect of magnesium—L-ascorbyl-2 phosphate against skin damage induced by UVB irradiation. Photochem Photobiol. 1996;64:224-8.
20. Alam M, Gladstone HB, Tung RC. Cosmetic Dermatology. New York: Saunders/Elsevier; 2009;27-8.
21. Levin J, Momin SB. How much do we really know about our favorite cosmeceutical ingredients? J Clin Aesthet Dermatol. 2010;3:22-41.
22. Idson B. In vivo measurement of transepidermal water loss. J Soc Cosmet Chem. 1976;29:573-80.
23. Grove GL, Grove MJ. Objective methods for assessing skin surface topography noninvasively. In: Leveque JL (Ed). Cutaneous Investigation in Health and Disease. New York: Marcel Dekker; 1988. pp. 1-32.
24. Babulak SW, Rhein LD, Scala DD, Simion FA. Quantification of erythema in a soap chamber test using the Minolta Chroma (Reflectance) Meter: Comparison of Instrumental Results with Visual Assessments. J Soc Cosmet Chem. 1986;37:475-9.
25. Pierard GE, Nikkels AF. Rating sensitive skin by colorimetry of the skin and of D-squame collections. International Symposium on Irritant Contact Dermatitis. Groningen: Holland; 1991.
26. Nilsson GE, Otto U, Wahlbert JE. Assessment of skin irritancy in many by laser Doppler flowmetry. Contact Dermatitis. 1982;8:401-6.
27. Willis CM, Stephens CJM, Wilkinson JD. Assessment of erythema in irritant contact dermatitis. Contact Dermatitis. 1988;18:138-42.
28. Agner T, Serup J. Skin reactions to irritants assessed by non-invasive bioengineering methods. Contact Dermatitis. 1989;20:352-9.
29. Draelos ZD. Botanical cosmecutical myths. In: Draelos. Z (Ed). Cosmeceuticals, 3rd edition. Philadelphia: Elsevier; 2015.
30. Newburger AE. Cosmeceuticals: myths and misconceptions. Clin Dermatol. 2009:27;446-52.
31. Epstein H. Cosmeceutical vehicles. Clin. Dermatol. 2009; 27(5):453-60.
32. Nutraingredients. (2005). Cosmeceutical makers can charge a premium. [online] Available from http://www.nutraingredients.com/news-by-product/news.asp?id=62920&k=cosmeceutical-makers-can [Last accessed March, 2024].

33. U.S. Food and Drug Administration. (2012). Is It a Cosmetic, a Drug, or Both? (Or Is It Soap?). [online] Available from https://www.fda.gov/cosmetics/cosmetics-laws-regulations/it-cosmetic-drug-or-both-or-it-soap [Last accessed March, 2024].
34. Cfsan.fda.gov. (2006). What are cosmeceuticals? [online] Available from http://www.cfsan.fda.gov/~dms/qa-cos5.html. [Last accessed March, 2024].
35. Ramos-e-Silva M, Ribeiro Celem L, Stella Ramose-Silva S, Fucci-da-Costa A. Anti-aging cosmetics: facts and controversies. Clin Dermatol. 2013;31:750-8.
36. Harman D. Ageing: a theory based on free radical and radiation chemistry. J Gerontol. 1956;11:298-300.
37. Packer L, Colman C. The Antioxidant Miracle. John Wiley and Sons: New York; 1999.
38. Varghese D, Patni P, Palekar N, Jain DK. Anti-aging therapy: a boon in sustaining human quest for youth. IJPS;2007.
39. Callaghan TM, Wilhelm KP. A review of aging and an examination of clinical methods in the assessment of aging skin Part 2: Clinical perspectives and clinical methods in the evaluation of aging skin. Int J Cosmet Sci. 2008;30:323-6.
40. Draelos ZD. Nutrition and enhancing youthful-appearing skin. Clin Dermatol. 2010;28:400-8.
41. Ryan AS, Goldsmith LA. Nutrition and the skin. Clin Dermatol. 1996;14:389-406.
42. Chan AC. Partners in defense, vitamin E and vitamin C. Can J Physiol Pharmacol. 1993;71:725-31.
43. Placzek M, Gaube S, Kerkmann U, Gilbertz KP, Herzinger T, Haen E, et al. Ultraviolet B-induced DNA damage in human epidermis is modified by the antioxidants ascorbic acid and D-alpha-tocopherol. J Invest Dermatol. 2005;124(2):304-7.
44. Kockaert M, Neumann M. Systemic and topical drugs for aging skin. J Drugs Dermatol. 2003;2:435-41.
45. Fryer MJ. Evidence for the photoprotective effects of vitamin E. Photochem Photobiol. 1993;58:304-12.
46. Chan AC, Tran K, Raynor T, Ganz PR, Chow CK,. Regeneration of vitamin E in human platelets. J Biol Chem. 1991;266:17290-5.
47. McVean M, Liebler DC. Prevention of DNA photodamage by vitamin E compounds and sunscreens: roles of ultraviolet absorbance and cellular uptake. Mol Carcinog. 1999;24:169-76.
48. Passi S, Morrone A, De Luca C, Picardo M, Ippolito F. Blood levels of vitamin E, polyunsaturated fatty acids of phospholipids, lipoperoxides and glutathione peroxidase in patients affected with seborrheic dermatitis. J Dermatol Sci. 1991;2(3):171-8.
49. Eknayake-Mudiyanselage S, Thiele J. Sebaceous glands as transporters of vitamin E. Hautarzt. 2006;57:291-6.
50. Britton G, Liaaen-Jensen S, Pfander H. Carotenoids. Basel: Birkhäuser; 2008.
51. Lindqvist A, Andersson S. Cell type-specific expression of beta-carotene 15,15'-mono-oxygenase in human tissues. J Histochem Cytochem. 2004;52:491-9.
52. Köpcke W, Krutmann J. Protection from sunburn with beta-Carotene—a meta-analysis. Photochem Photobiol. 2008;84:284-8.
53. Sies H, Stahl W. Nutritional protection against skin damage from sunlight. Annu Rev Nutr. 2004;24:173-200.
54. Mathews-Roth MM, Pathak MA, Parrish J, Fitzpatrick TB, Kass EH, Toda K, et al. A clinical trial of the effects of oral beta-carotene on the responses of human skin to solar radiation. J Invest Dermatol. 1972;59:349-53.
55. Lee J, Jiang S, Levine N, Watson RR. Carotenoid supplementation reduces erythema in human skin after simulated solar radiation exposure. Proc Soc Exp Biol Med. 2000;223:170-4.
56. Heinrich U, Gärtner C, Wiebusch M, Eichler O, Sies H, Tronnier H, et al. Supplementation with beta-carotene or a similar amount of mixed carotenoids protects humans from UV-induced erythema. J Nutr. 2003;133:98-101.
57. Lyons NM, O'Brien NM. Modulatory effects of an algal extract containing astaxanthin on UVA-irradiated cells in culture. J Dermatol Sci. 2002;30:73-84.
58. Camera E, Mastrofrancesco A, Fabbri C, Daubrawa F, Picardo M, Sies H, et al. Astaxanthin, canthaxanthin and beta-carotene differently affect UVA-induced oxidative damage and expression of oxidative stress-responsive enzymes. Exp Dermatol. 2009;18:222-31.
59. Suganuma K, Nakajima H, Ohtsuki M, Imokawa G. Astaxanthin attenuates the UVA-induced up-regulation of matrix-metalloproteinase-1 and skin fibroblast elastase in human dermal fibroblasts. J Dermatol Sci. 2010;58:136-42.
60. Etminan M, Takkouche B, Caamaño-Isorna F. The role of tomato products and lycopene in the prevention of prostate cancer: a meta-analysis of observational studies. Cancer Epidemiol Biomarkers Prev. 2004;13:340-5.
61. Pohar KS, Gong MC, Bahnson R, Miller EC, Clinton SK. Tomatoes, lycopene and prostate cancer: a clinician's guide for counseling those at risk for prostate cancer. World J Urol. 2003;21:9-14.
62. Zouboulis CC, Schagen S, Alestas T. The sebocyte culture: a model to study the pathophysiology of the sebaceous gland in sebostasis, seborrhoea and acne. Arch Dermatol Res. 2008;300:397-413.
63. Safavi K. Serum vitamin A levels in psoriasis: Results from the first national health and nutrition examination survey. Arch Dermatol. 1992;128:1130-1.
64. Reichrath J, Lehmann B, Carlberg C, Varani J, Zouboulis CC. Vitamins as hormones. Horm Metab Res. 2007;39:71-84.
65. Bayerl C. Topical treatment of skin aging. Hautarzt. 2005;56:328,330-4, 336-9.
66. MacLaughlin J, Holick MF. Aging decreases the capacity of human skin to produce vitamin D3. J Clin Invest. 1985;76:1536-8.
67. Makrantonaki E, Zouboulis C. Skin alterations and diseases in advanced age. Drug Discov Today Dis Mech. 2008;5:e153-62.
68. Surjana D, Halliday GM, Maartin AJ, Moloney FJ, Damian DL. Oral nicotinamide reduces actinic keratosis in phase II double-blinded randomized controlled trials. J Inves Dermatol. 2012;132:1497-1500.
69. Yang M, Moclair B, Hatcher V, Kaminetsky J, Mekas M, Chapas A, et al. A randomized, double-blind, placebo-controlled study of a novel pantothenic acid-based dietary supplement in subjects with mild to moderate facial acne. Dermatol Therapy. 2014;4(1):93-101.
70. Manach C, Scalbert A, Morand C, Rémésy C, Jiménez L. Polyphenols: food sources and bioavailability. Am J Clin Nutr. 2004;79(5):727-47.
71. Scalbert A, Williamson G. Dietary intake and bioavailability of polyphenols. J Nutr. 2000;130(Suppl):2073S-85S.
72. Crozier A, Lean M, McDonald M, Black C. Quantitative analysis of the flavonoid content of commercial tomatoes, onions, lettuce, and celery. J Agric Food Chem. 1997;45:590-5.
73. Nichols JA, Katiyar SK. Skin photoprotection by natural polyphenols: anti-inflammatory, antioxidant and DNA repair mechanisms. Arch Dermatol Res. 2010;302:71-83.

74. Katiyar SK. Treatment of silymarin, a plant flavonoid, prevents ultraviolet light-induced immune suppression and oxidative stress in mouse skin. Int J Oncol. 2002;21:1213-22.
75. Di Franco R, Calvanese M, Murino P, Manzo R, Guida C, Di Gennaro D, et al. Skin toxicity from external beam radiation therapy in breast cancer patients: protective effects of Resveratrol, Lycopene, Vitamin C and anthocianin (Ixor®) Radiat Oncol. 2012;7:12.
76. Giardina S, Michelotti A, Zavattini G, Finzi S, Ghisalberti C, Marzatico F, et al. Efficacy study in vitro: assessment of the properties of resveratrol and resveratrol + *N*-acetyl-cysteine on proliferation and inhibition of collagen activity. Minerva Ginecol. 2010;62:195-201.
77. Heng MC. Curcumin targeted signaling pathways: basis for anti-photoaging and anti-carcinogenic therapy. Int J Dermatol. 2010;49:608-22.
78. Lima CF, Pereira-Wilson C, Rattan SI. Curcumin induces heme oxygenase-1 in normal human skin fibroblasts through redox signaling: relevance for anti-aging intervention. Mol Nutr Food Res. 2011;55:430-42.
79. Katiyar SK, Elmets CA. Green tea polyphenolic antioxidants and skin photoprotection (Review). Int J Oncol. 2001;18:1307-13.
80. Demeule M, Brossard M, Pagé M, Gingras D, Béliveau R. Matrix metalloproteinase inhibition by green tea catechins. Biochim Biophys Acta. 2000;1478(1):51-60.
81. Sartor L, Pezzato E, Garbisa S. Epigallocatechin-3-gallate inhibits leukocyte elastase: potential of the phyto-factor in hindering inflammation, emphysema, and invasion. J Leukoc Biol. 2002;71:73-9.
82. Shindo Y, Witt E, Han D, Epstein W, Packer L. Enzymic and non-enzymic antioxidants in epidermis and dermis of human skin. J Invest Dermatol. 1994;102(1):122-4.
83. López LC, Quinzii CM, Area E, Naini A, Rahman S, Schuelke M, et al. Treatment of CoQ (10) deficient fibroblasts with ubiquinone, CoQ analogs, and vitamin C: time- and compound-dependent effects. PLoS One. 2010;5:e11897.
84. Horrobin DF. Essential fatty acids in clinical dermatology. J Am Acad Dermatol. 1989;20:1045-53.
85. Simopoulos AP. Omega-3 fatty acids in inflammation and autoimmune diseases. J Am Coll Nutr. 2002;21:495-505.
86. Cho HS, Lee MH, Lee JW, No KO, Park SK, Lee HS, et al. Anti-wrinkling effects of the mixture of vitamin C, vitamin E, pycnogenol and evening primrose oil, and molecular mechanisms on hairless mouse skin caused by chronic ultraviolet B irradiation. Photodermatol Photoimmunol Photomed. 2007;23:155-62.
87. Villarama CD, Maibach HI. Glutathione as a depigmenting agent: an overview. Int J Cosmet Sci. 2005;27:147-53.
88. Arjinpathana N, Asawanonda P. Glutathione as an oral whitening agent: a randomized, double-blind, placebo-controlled study. J Dermatolog Treat. 2012;23:97-102.
89. Hong SY, Gil HW, Yang JO, Lee EY, Kim HK, Kim SH, et al. Pharmacokinetics of glutathione and its metabolites in normal subjects. J Korean Med Sci. 2005;20(5):721-6.
90. FDA. (2011). [online] Available from http://www.fda.gov.ph/advisories/cosmetic/38960-doh-fda-advisory-no-2011-004. [Last accessed March, 2024].
91. Levitt J. The safety of hydroquinone: a dermatologist's response to the 2006 Federal Register. J Am Acad Dermatol. 2007;57:854-72.
92. Smit NP, Van der Meulen H, Koerten HK, Kolb RM, Mommaas AM, Lentjes EG, et al. Melanogenesis in cultured melanocytes can be substantially influenced by L-tyrosine and L-cysteine. J Invest Dermatol. 1997;109:796-800.
93. del Marmol V, Ito S, Bouchard B, Libert A, Wakamatsu K, Ghanem G, et al. Cysteine deprivation promotes eumelanogenesis in human melanoma cells. J Invest Dermatol. 1996;107(5):698-702.
94. Ando H, Matsui MS, Ichihashi M. Quasi-drugs developed in Japan for the prevention or treatment of hyperpigmentary disorders. Int J Mol Sci. 2010;11:2566-75.
95. Tse TW, Hui E. Tranexamic acid: an important adjuvant in the treatment of melasma. J Cosmet Dermatol. 2013;12:57-66.
96. Karn D, S KC, Amatya A, Razouria EA, Timalsina M. Oral tranexamic acid for the treatment of melasma. Kathmandu Univ Med J (KUMJ). 2012;10:40-3.
97. Wu S, Shi H, Wu H, Yan S, Guo J, Sun Y, et al. Treatment of melasma with oral administration of tranexamic acid. Aesthetic Plast Surg. 2012;36(4):964-70.
98. Ni Z, Mu Y, Gulati O. Treatment of melasma with pycnogenol. Phytother Res. 2002;16:567-71.
99. Asserin J, Lati E, Shioya T, Prawitt J. The effect of oral collagen peptide supplementation on skin moisture and the dermal collagen network: evidence from an ex vivo model and randomized, placebo-controlled clinical trials. J Cosmet Dermatol. 2015;14:291-301.
100. Liu B, Fan Z, Edgerton SM, Yang X, Lind SE, Thor AD. Potent anti-proliferative effects of metformin on trastuzumab-resistant breast cancer cells via inhibition of erbB2/IGF-1 receptor interactions. Cell Cycle. 2011;10:2959-66.
101. Bridges HR, Jones AJ, Pollak MN, Hirst J. Effects of metformin and other biguanides on oxidative phosphorylation in mitochondria. Biochem J. 2014;462:475-87.
102. Algire C, Moiseeva O, Deschênes-Simard X, Amrein L, Petruccelli L, Birman E, et al. Metformin reduces endogenous reactive oxygen species and associated DNA damage. Cancer Prev Res. 2012;5:536-43.
103. Anisimov VN, Bartke A. The key role of growth hormone-insulin-IGF-1 signaling in aging and cancer. Crit Rev Oncol Hematol. 2013;87:201-23.
104. Anisimov VN, Egormin PA, Piskunova TS, Popovich IG, Tyndyk ML, Yurova MN, et al. Metformin extends life span of HER-2/neu transgenic mice and in combination with melatonin inhibits growth of transplantable tumors in vivo. Cell Cycle. 2010;9:188-97.

CHAPTER 82

Approach to Management of Aging Skin

Shital Poojary, Madhuri Agarwal

KEY MESSAGES

- Management of aging skin has to be a multipronged approach targeting the various pathogenic factors and changes in layers of the skin.
- Therapies have to be individually tailored depending on the needs of the patients and their ethnic, social, and psychological profiles.
- Preventive care, medical therapies, and interventional therapies are the cornerstones of antiaging management.

INTRODUCTION

Aging occurs as a result of complex synthesis of two overlapping processes: Intrinsic and extrinsic.[1,2] Intrinsic aging is primarily due to genetic factors and changes in the endocrine environment and is seen on both sun-exposed and non-sun-exposed areas; extrinsic aging occurs primarily due to sun exposure as well as other harmful events and habits, such as smoking, dietary habits, alcohol consumption, inadequate sleep, stress, and exposure to atmospheric pollution. Due to the primary role of sun exposure, extrinsic aging is seen on the photo-exposed areas. Morphologically, extrinsically aged skin tends to be dull with a leathery texture, deep coarse wrinkles, and pigmentary changes. Intrinsically aged skin tends to be thin, dry with fine wrinkles. Apart from these changes in the skin, the aging face also involves loss of volume, reduction and redistribution of fat, facial muscle action, and resorption in underlying facial bone architecture. Aging skin in Asians tends to have pigmentary problems as typical initial characteristics, while fine wrinkling heralds aging of skin in Caucasian population.[3]

EVALUATION OF PATIENT

History Taking

Age of patient: Preventive care, including moisturization and sunscreen use, should start by age 20 years. With advancing age, cosmeceuticals, antioxidants and later procedural intervention are required.

Sex of the patient: Facial skin tends to be thicker in men. In females, it is important to look for associated polycystic ovary disease (PCOD).

Attitudes and Needs of the Patient

Understanding patient needs and psychological profile: It is important to understand patient needs as it helps to decide which aspect of the aging face needs intervention in a particular patient. The patients' needs can differ according to social background and occupation.

Associated Conditions

Medical conditions such as diabetes and hypothyroidism should be noted. History of drug intake, especially those affecting coagulation, is important. Patients with atopic dermatitis tend to have sensitive skin and also tend to pigment easily. Choice of topical products and interventional procedures needs to be made carefully in these patients.

Habits and Lifestyle

History of smoking: Smoking especially affects the elastin component of the dermis and causes a typical smoker's face with prominent perioral lines and crow's feet.

Excessive sun exposure and dietary habits are contributory factors for aging of skin.

CLINICAL EXAMINATION OF THE AGING FACE

Clinical examination of the aging face includes the following.

Individual skin type, racial, and ethnic background: Skin types IV and V tend to have pigmentary changes as a significant and early manifestation of photoaging much more than wrinkles and rhytides, which are less prominent and are seen after the fifth decade of life.

Type and degree of aging: It is important to assess whether extrinsic or intrinsic type of aging is predominant in a particular patient as it helps tailor treatment accordingly; e.g., in photoaged skin, pigmentary changes are prominent and will require appropriate therapy.

The face is divided into three aesthetic units for evaluation, and changes in color, texture, and shape should be noted in each.

Examination of the neck area as well as forearms and hands should be done for an overall assessment. Examination of specific areas such as periorbital and perioral areas is important.

All clinical signs of aging, including wrinkling, alteration in pigmentation, change in texture, skin sagging, and volume loss, are to be carefully documented in writing and maintaining photographic records. Special features of aging skin such as dermatoporosis are to be noted.[4,5]

Glogau's classification of photoaging is useful for assessing the degree of photoaging.

Other useful methods of assessment include:
- Fitzpatrick nine-point classification system (photodamage and wrinkles)
- Lemperle's score (0–5) for wrinkles
- Ptosis scale (I–V)
- Leal's skin laxity score
- Confocal microscopy.[6,7]

MANAGEMENT

The cornerstone of antiaging management is to achieve healthy, smooth, and blemish-free skin. This requires complete or at least partial reversal of intrinsically as well as extrinsically induced changes in the epidermis and dermis. In the dermis, three primary components—collagen, elastin, and glycosaminoglycans—are the primary targets of antiaging therapies. In addition, structural changes such as loss/redistribution of fat pads, bone, and muscle changes also require intervention. Management of aging skin requires a multistep approach, including a focus on general health, lifestyle changes, photoprotection, and rejuvenation of each skin layer.[8]

It is also important to remember that as a person ages, the epidermal turnover rate is much reduced, and the cell cycle is much longer, thus affecting wound healing and affecting outcome in antiaging aesthetic procedures.

Management of aging skin can be done at three levels:
- *Level I: Primary intervention:* Primary intervention starts with prevention or slowing down of skin aging.
  Photoprotection: Sun protection using sunscreens to block or reduce skin exposure to ultraviolet (UV) radiation. A broad-spectrum sunscreen with sun protection factor (SPF) of at least 30, as well as avoidance of excess sun exposure, especially in peak hours, is recommended. Avoidance of exposure to artificial light is also important.
  - *Lifestyle changes*:
    - Dietary changes:
      - Avoidance of foods which give rise to advanced glycation end products (AGE; e.g., highly processed foods)
      - Inclusion of fresh fruits and vegetables
      - Avoidance of crash dieting
    - Regular exercise and adequate sleep
    - Avoidance of smoking and alcohol
    - Protection from environmental pollutants
- *Level II: Secondary intervention:* Detection and treatment of early signs of skin aging. This primarily includes topical and systemic medical management and superficial interventional procedures.
- *Level III: Tertiary intervention:* Treatment of established aging skin. This requires a combination of topical and systemic medical therapy and surgical modes of therapy.

  Box 1 depicts the broad components of antiaging regimens.

BOX 1: Components of antiaging regimens.

Skincare:
- Daily skin care: With appropriate moisturizer
- Appropriate sun protection: Broad-spectrum sunscreen and physical protection

Avoidance of exogenous factors of aging:
- Smoking
- Environmental pollution
- Sun exposure and artificial UV sources
- Stress
- Correct diet, avoidance of high glycemic foods
- Nutritional supplementation

Topical medical agents:
- Antioxidants
- Cell regulators

Systemic agents:
- Antioxidants
- Hormone replacement therapy

Interventional therapies:
- Chemical peeling
- Visible light devices
- Ablative and nonablative laser photorejuvenation
- Radiofrequency
- Injectable skin fillers for biostimulation and rejuvenation
- Prevention of dynamic wrinkles with BTX-A
- Restoration (redistribution) of fat: HIFU

(BTX-A: botulinum toxin A; HIFU: high-intensity focused ultrasound; UV: ultraviolet)

Medical Management of Aging Skin

Medical management of aging skin including topical and systemic therapy is summarized in **Table 1**.

Procedural Management of Aging Skin

Procedural interventions in management of skin aging can be classified into noninvasive, minimally invasive, and invasive types:
- *Noninvasive:*
  - Medifacials
  - Low energy nonablative lasers

TABLE 1: Medical management of aging skin.

Drug	*Functions*	*Comments*
Topical		
Topical retinoids	• Increases type I, III, and VII collagens • Decreases MMPs • Reorganizes elastic fiber • Normalizes GAG deposition. Decreases fine wrinkles, loss of skin elasticity • Decreases pigmentary dyschromia • Smoothens skin	• *Adverse effects:* Retinoid dermatitis (erythema, peeling and burning sensation, photosensitivity) • Tretinoin 0.025–0.05% to be applied at night • Newer microsphere retinoid formulations have lesser side effects and can be used in higher concentrations[9]
AHAs β-hydroxy acids Polyhydroxy acids	• Exfoliates skin causing skin to become smoother with reduction of dyschromia • Increases collagen, elastin, and glycosaminoglycan synthesis in dermis leading to increased dermal hydration	• Include glycolic, lactic, pyruvic and malic acid, citric acid, gluconolactone • Lower concentrations of AHAs are used in topical preparations • Higher concentrations are used in chemical peels • Most common side effect is irritation
Moisturizer	• Maintains hydration of skin • Decreases fine wrinkles	It is usually combined with sunscreens and AHAs
Vitamins C, B_3, E[10,11]	• Antioxidant effect • *Vitamin C:* Induces production of collagen • *Vitamin B_3:* Cell regeneration • *Vitamin E:* Maintains moisture of the skin, increases epithelialization, photoprotectant	• Vitamin C: Used in concentrations 5–15% • Vitamin B_3: 5% • Combination of both has higher antioxidant effect • *Vitamin E:* 2–20% • Topical vitamin C can be unstable; its ester derivative is nonirritant and stable
Polyphenols: • Green tea polyphenols • α-lipoic acid • Isoflavones	• Antioxidant effect • *Epigallocatechin gallate:* Photoprotective effect[12] • *α-lipoic acid:* Promotes collagen synthesis	α-lipoic acid is useful for stabilization of epigallocatechin gallate
Idebenone[13]	• Antioxidant • Increases collagen synthesis • Decreases collagen breakdown	• It is an analog of coenzyme Q10 • Concentration: 0.5, 1% • *Adverse effects:* Allergic contact dermatitis
Peptides: • Signal peptides: Palmitoyl pentapeptide-3 • Neurotransmitter-affecting peptides: Acetyl hexapeptide-3 • Carrier peptides; glycyl-l-histidyl-l-lysine (GHK:Cu)	• Increased collagen synthesis • Improve periorbital and perioral wrinkles, roughness, and mottled pigmentation • Repair of photodamaged skin	More clinical or in vivo studies required
Plant extracts: • Milk thistle (silymarin) • Turmeric (curcuminoids) • Pine bark extract (pycnogenol) • Grape seed extract (proanthocyanidin) • Licorice extract	• Anti-inflammatory • Antioxidant • Photoprotective effect • Inhibition of tyrosinase (licorice extract)	More clinical studies required
Hormones: • 17-β-estradiol 0.01% • Progesterone 2% • Dehydroepiandrosterone	• Increased epidermal thickness • Induces collagen production • Improves skin elasticity • Increases collagen; reduces wrinkle counts • Differentiation of keratinocytes • Increased collagen	Long-term studies on the efficacy and toxicity of topical hormonal preparations are necessary
Oral		
• Antioxidants[14] • Vitamins A, C, E • Carotenoids • Coenzyme Q10[15] (ubiquinone)	• Neutralize free radicals • Absorb iron to decrease reactive oxygen species production • Reduces collagenase expression, DNA oxidative stress	Reduces wrinkle formation

Contd...

Contd...

Drug	*Functions*	*Comments*
Oral isotretinoin	• Improves wrinkles, thickness and color of skin • Decreases pigmented lesions • Decreases size of pores • Improves skin elasticity and tone	10–20-mg isotretinoin can be given in combination with rejuvenation treatment procedures[15]
Hormones[16,17] HRT	• Decreases wrinkling due to increase in skin collagen content • Increases skin elasticity	• Cannot be used as primary treatment for aging • *Possible adverse effects:* Thromboembolism
Oral tranexamic acid[18]	• Anti-inflammatory • Skin-lightening agent • Decreases proliferation of mast cells and increases the proliferation of fibroblasts	Improves pigmentation
Polypodium leucotomos[19,20]	• Anti-inflammatory • Decreases DNA mutagenesis • Reduces UV-induced immunosuppression	Protective effects against photoaging and PUVA-induced phototoxicity
Oral glutathione[21]	• Antioxidant • Reduces wrinkles by improving skin elasticity	Antiaging and antimelanogenic

(AHAs: alpha-hydroxy acids; DNA: deoxyribonucleic acid; GAG: glycosaminoglycan; HRT: hormone replacement therapy; MMPs: matrix metalloproteinases; PUVA: psoralen plus ultraviolet A; UV: ultraviolet)

  - Nd:YAG (neodymium-doped yttrium aluminum garnet) laser
  - Infrared laser therapy
  - Radiofrequency (RF) (unipolar, monopolar, bipolar, multipolar RF, plasma fractional RF, transcutaneous temperature-controlled RF)
  - Intense pulsed light (IPL) treatment
  - High-intensity focused ultrasound (HIFU)
- *Minimally invasive:*
  - Chemical peels
  - Microdermabrasion
  - Hydroporation
  - Platelet-rich plasma (PRP)
  - Adipose-derived stem cells
  - Microneedling
  - Botulinum toxin injection
  - Filler treatment
  - Skin boosters (low cross-linked, low cohesive rheology hyaluronic acid skin conditioning fillers)
  - Thread lifts
  - Plasma lift
  - Fractional photothermolysis
- *Invasive:*
  - Dermabrasion
  - CO_2 and erbium:YAG laser resurfacing
  - Surgical excision
  - Liposuction
  - Lipolysis

All these treatment modalities have been discussed in detail in respective chapters and are briefly summarized in **Table 2**.

Choice of Treatment Modalities for Skin Aging

- Choice of treatments can be made depending on the type of skin aging concern according to patient needs and clinical evaluation.
  Table 3 is a ready reckoner for choice of nonsurgical treatments according to skin aging concern.
- Selection of treatment can also be done depending on which structural component of the skin and deeper tissues is affected and needs to be treated.
  Table 4 depicts various treatments for facial rejuvenation with a layered approach.
  Table 5 elaborates on all treatment options for wrinkles.
- *Combination of treatments:* Every patient will have multiple signs of aging. Hence, no single treatment can generally achieve desired results in an aging face, and combination therapy is the mainstay of management. The treatment modalities can be used simultaneously or sequentially.

  Few examples:
  - A combination of botulinum toxin A (BTX-A) for forehead wrinkles and crow's feet and chemical peels for pigmentation
  - A combination of fillers for midface and fractional resurfacing *LASER* for improvement of texture.

Chronological Aging Management

An algorithm for chronological aging management, useful in clinical practice, is described below.

Face antiaging protocols in late 20s–early 30s:

- A broad-spectrum sunscreen is essential.
- Regular use of gel-based and oil-free moisturizers

TABLE 2: Procedural interventions for the aging skin.

Treatment	*Mechanism of action*	*Indications*
Noninvasive photorejuvenation method (IPL, long pulsed Nd:YAG laser, infrared light)[22]	Stimulates collagen synthesis	Improves fine to moderate wrinkles, facelift, periorbital tissue tightening
Chemical peels[23]	• Epidermal exfoliation • Epidermal and dermal rejuvenation • Decreases pigmentation	Improves fine wrinkles, photoaging, melasma, freckles, lentigines, superficial scars
Microdermabrasion[24]	• Mild exfoliation • Epidermal regeneration • Collagen formation	Improves fine wrinkles, superficial scars
Medifacial[25]	• Epidermal exfoliation • Epidermal and dermal rejuvenation • Decreases pigmentation	Improves fine lines, texture improvement, increased skin homogeneity
Hydroporation[26]	Increased collagen and procollagen levels	Improves photodamaged skin, fine wrinkles, melasma, freckles
Radiofrequency[27]	Stimulates collagen synthesis	Improves skin laxity and reduces wrinkles
High-intensity focused ultrasound[28]	Neocollagenesis and SMAS tightening	Tightening and lifting of sagging facial and neck skin and improvement in the appearance of wrinkles
Microneedling and microneedling RF[29-31]	Collagen remodeling	Skin tightening, facelift, wrinkles, scars
Botulinum toxin[32]	Inhibits neuromuscular transmission and weakens the injected muscle	Forehead horizontal lines, glabellar frown lines, crow's feet, *Marionette* lines
Fillers[33]	• Corrects volume loss • Tissue augmentation • Correction of wrinkles	Nasolabial folds, deep forehead lines, deep perioral wrinkles, lip augmentation
Skin booster (low cross-linked, low cohesive rheology hyaluronic acid skin conditioning fillers)[34,35]	Hydration, improves collagen and elasticity of skin	Can be used all over the face and neck, hands
Thread lifts[36]	Pulls up and tightens skin	Sagging cheeks, brow lift, chin lift
Fractional photothermolysis	Stimulates collagen synthesis	Fine wrinkles, dyschromia
Plasma lift[37]	Promotes collagen production, reduction of elastosis, and progressive skin rejuvenation	Droopy eyelids, brow lifts, all facial wrinkles and lines
Platelet-rich plasma[38,39]	Skin regeneration through their effects on fibroblast proliferation, collagen production, and the growth of keratinocytes	Fine, moderate, deep wrinkles, texture improvement, increased skin homogeneity
Adipose-derived stem cells[40,41]	• Antioxidant • Skin lightening • Wound healing effects • Increases growth factors	Mild-to-moderate wrinkles, skin lightening
Dermabrasion	• Epidermal and dermal resurfacing • New collagen synthesis	Fine wrinkles, vertical perioral wrinkles
CO_2 and erbium:YAG laser resurfacing[42]	Wounds the skin to the level of dermis and during wound healing organized ultrastructural remodeling of dermis produces smoother, firmer, and rejuvenated skin	• Deep wrinkles • Fine wrinkles
Surgical excision (blepharoplasty, rhytidectomy)	Removal of excess fat pads and skin, tightening of muscle	Droopy eyelids, brow lifts, all facial wrinkles and lines
Autologous fat transfer	Correction of volume loss	Facial recontouring, correction of scars, hand rejuvenation

(IPL: intense pulsed light; Nd:YAG: neodymium-doped yttrium aluminum garnet; RF: radiofrequency; SMAS: superficial musculoaponeurotic system)

- Retinol-based topical creams twice weekly
- Medifacials, chemical peels, and nonablative laser rejuvenation for surface texture
- BTX-A for upper face motor wrinkles
- Correction of midface deficit with filler
- BTX-A and fillers for desired facial contouring.

TABLE 3: Choice of antiaging nonsurgical treatment depending on skin aging concern.

Recommendation in descending order	*Skin textural benefits*	*Skin tightening*	*Volume loss correction*	*Dynamic wrinkles*
1	Resurfacing lasers	HIFU	Dermal fillers	Botox
2	Chemical peels	Radiofrequency	Threads	Threads
3	MNRF	Resurfacing lasers	HIFU	HIFU
4	Radiofrequency	Threads		Resurfacing lasers
5	Skin boosters	Plasma lift		Plasma lift
6	GFC[43]	MNRF		

(GFC: growth factor concentrate; HIFU: high-intensity focused ultrasound; MNRF: microneedling radiofrequency)

TABLE 4: Facial rejuvenation treatments.

Objective	*Treatment options*
Superficial rejuvenation	Superficial peels, microdermabrasion, hydroporation, intense pulsed light treatment, skin boosters, medifacials
Dermal remodeling	Nonablative facial rejuvenation laser, fractional laser resurfacing, PRP, microneedling, radiofrequency, HIFU, plasma lift
Muscle relaxation	Botulinum toxin type A injection
Soft-tissue augmentation/volume replacement	Fillers, fat transfer
Deeper rejuvenation	CO_2 laser, erbium:YAG laser, medium-depth peels, deeper peels, HIFU and RF, threads, plasma lift

(HIFU: high-intensity focused ultrasound; PRP: platelet-rich plasma; RF: radiofrequency; YAG: yttrium aluminum garnet)

TABLE 5: Treatment of wrinkles.

Type of wrinkle	*Treatment options*
Fine wrinkles	Topical tretinoin, alpha-hydroxy acids, chemical peel, microdermabrasion, hydroporation, low-energy nonablative lasers, PRP, microneedling, radiofrequency, skin boosters, threads, medifacials
Moderate wrinkles	Fillers, botulinum toxin injection, HIFU, facelift, threads
Deep wrinkles (difficult to treat)	Dermabrasion, ablative lasers, fillers, plasma lift, HIFU, threads, facelift

(HIFU: high-intensity focused ultrasound; PRP: platelet-rich plasma)

Face antiaging protocols in late 30s:
- Usage of broad-spectrum sunscreen
- Moisturizers can be changed to a formulation that is light but does have some oil for maturing skin needs.
- A topical antioxidant such as vitamin C with ferulic acid can be added before sunscreen application.
- Increase use of retinol products to three to four times a week.
- Textural changes can be treated with chemical peel.
- Lasers and light therapy for visible blood vessels on the face
- Botulinum toxin for dynamic wrinkles on upper and lower face
- Correction of midface and lower face deficit with fillers
- Tear trough improvement with fillers.

Face antiaging protocols in 40s:
- Usage of broad-spectrum sunscreen
- Moisturizers need to be richer and thicker.
- Topical antioxidant containing skin care product
- Retinol-based cream to be used daily
- Stem cells and peptides can be added to the regime.
- Microneedling RF with growth factor concentrate (GFC)
- IPL (vascular filter) for erythema and texture
- Fillers for midface, nasolabial folds, lips and chin aging
- Nose contouring to correct the nose elongation and droop
- HIFU for superficial musculoaponeurotic system (SMAS) and sagging skin
- Monopolar RF for skin tightening
- Threads for additional contouring
- Plasma lift for eyelid droop and neck lines.

Face antiaging protocols in above 50s:
- Continue using daily skincare regimen of sunscreen, peptides, and retinol products
- BTX-A for dynamic wrinkles and lower face muscles hypertrophy
- HIFU for SMAS and sagging skin
- Monopolar RF for skin tightening
- Midface and lower face fillers
- Nose and lip fillers to contour and shape the nose and lips respectively
- Qswitch Nd-YAG LASER and GFC for pigmentation
- Threads for additional lift
- Plasma lift for eye and lower face/neck lines.

FUTURE PROSPECTS

Future prospects in antiaging treatments:
- *Newer therapeutic targets for antiaging treatment:*[44,45]
  - Wnt/β-catenin signaling pathway that is involved in epidermal renewal
  - *Calcium channel Orai-1:* Involved in epidermal proliferation
  - *p16 INK4a pathway:* Involved in human epidermal stem cell self-renewal

- *Drugs targeting senescence:* Senolytics (drugs inducing apoptosis of senescent cells) and senostatics (drugs aborting senescence). Some known drugs and nutraceuticals target senescence, for example, catechins, resveratrol. Fisetin (a polyphenol) found in fruits and vegetables and quercetin (Q), a natural flavonol and micronutrient, have senolytic properties.[46]
- *microRNA (microribonucleic acid):* miR-29 and miR-155 have been shown to have a role in skin aging, especially collagen generation. AntagomiR of miR-29 has been tried for skin aging. Ultra-flexible liposomes and skin-penetrating peptides complexed with microRNA are possible transepidermal topical delivery systems.[47]
- *Nutraceuticals:* Nutraceuticals catering to the fast-paced lifestyle coupled with poor nutrition are growing in demand. Multiple new formulations containing specific nutritional elements addressing specific skin needs of aging will be in demand.[48] Newer formulations such as nanocarriers for enhanced skin permeation are also being researched.[49]
- Artificial mitochondria transfer/transplant (AMT/T) has been proposed to treat skin aging by transferring healthy mitochondria to senescent cells.[50]

CONCLUSION

Skin aging is multifactorial in origin and requires a combined and tailored approach to management.

REFERENCES

1. Zouboulis CC, Ganceviciene R, Liakou AI, Theodoridis A, Elewa R, Makrantonaki E. Aesthetic aspects of skin aging, prevention, and local treatment. Clin Dermatol. 2019;37(4):365-72.
2. Chaudhary M, Khan A, Gupta M. Skin ageing: pathophysiology and current market treatment approaches. Curr Aging Sci. 2020;13(1):22-30.
3. Venkatesh S, Maymone MBC, Vashi NA. Aging in skin of color. Clin Dermatol. 2019;37(4):351-7.
4. Kaya G, Kaya A, Sorg O, Saurat JH. Dermatoporosis, a prevalent skin condition affecting the elderly: current situation and potential treatments. Clin Dermatol. 2019;37(4):346-50.
5. Wollina U, Lotti T, Vojvotic A, Nowak A. Dermatoporosis—the chronic cutaneous fragility syndrome. Open Access Maced J Med Sci. 2019;7(18):3046-9.
6. Robic J, Nkengne A, Perret B, Couprie M, Talbot H, Pellacani G, et al. Clinical validation of a computer-based approach for the quantification of the skin ageing process of women using in vivo confocal microscopy. J Eur Acad Dermatol Venereol. 2021;35(1):e68-70.
7. Wurm EM, Longo C, Curchin C, Soyer HP, Prow TW, Pellacani G. In vivo assessment of chronological ageing and photoageing in forearm skin using reflectance confocal microscopy. Br J Dermatol. 2012;167(2):270-9.
8. Ganceviciene R, Liakou AI, Theodoridis A, Makrantonaki E, Zouboulis CC. Skin anti-aging strategies. Dermato-endocrinology. 2012;4(3):308-19.
9. Weiss JS, Shavin JS, Nighland M, Grossman R. Tretinoin microsphere gel 0.1% for photodamaged facial skin: a placebo-controlled trial. Cutis. 2006;78:426-32.
10. Humbert PG, Haftek M, Creidi P, Lapière C, Nusgens B, Richard A, et al. Topical ascorbic acid on photoaged skin. Clinical, topographical and ultrastructural evaluation: double-blind study vs. placebo. Exp Dermatol. 2003;12:237-44.
11. Yap WN. Tocotrienol-rich fraction attenuates UV-induced inflammaging: a bench to bedside study. J Cosmet Dermatol. 2018;17(3):555-65.
12. Jeon HY, Kim JK, Kim WG, Lee SJ. Effects of oral epigallocatechin gallate supplementation on the minimal erythema dose and UV-induced skin damage. Skin Pharmacol Physiol. 2009;22:137-41.
13. Farris P. Idebenone, green tea, and coffeeberry extract: new and innovative antioxidants. Dermatol Ther. 2007;20:322-9.
14. Oresajo C, Pillai S, Manco M, Yatskayer M, McDaniel D. Antioxidants and the skin: understanding formulation and efficacy. Dermatol Ther. 2012;25(3):252-9.
15. Inui M, Ooe M, Fujii K, Matsunaka H, Yoshida M, Ichihashi M. Mechanisms of inhibitory effects of CoQ10 on UVB-induced wrinkle formation in vitro and in vivo. Biofactors. 2008;32:237-43.
16. Rosenthal A, Jacoby T, Israilevich R, Moy R. The role of bioidentical hormone replacement therapy in anti-aging medicine: a review of the literature. Int J Dermatol. 2020;59(1):23-9.
17. Borda LJ, Wong LL, Tosti A. Bioidentical hormone therapy in menopause: relevance in dermatology. Dermatol Online J. 2019;25(1):13030.
18. Hiramoto K, Sugiyama D, Takahashi Y, Mafune E. The amelioration effect of tranexamic acid in wrinkles induced by skin dryness. Biomed Pharmacother. 2016;80:16-22.
19. Villa A, Viera MH, Amini S, Huo R, Perez O, Ruiz P, et al. Decrease of ultraviolet A light-induced "common deletion" in healthy volunteers after oral Polypodium leucotomos extract supplement in a randomized clinical trial. J Am Acad Dermatol. 2010;62:511-3.
20. Middelkamp-Hup MA, Pathak MA, Parrado C, Goukassian D, Rius-Díaz F, Mihm MC, et al. Oral Polypodium leucotomos extract decreases ultraviolet-induced damage of human skin. J Am Acad Dermatol. 2004;51:910-8.
21. Weschawalit S, Thongthip S, Phutrakool P, Asawanonda P. Glutathione and its antiaging and antimelanogenic effects. Clin Cosmet Investig Dermatol. 2017;10:147-53.
22. Houreld NN. The use of lasers and light sources in skin rejuvenation. Clin Dermatol. 2019;37(4):358-64.
23. Kadhim KA, Al-Waiz M. Treatment of periorbital wrinkles by repeated medium-depth chemical peels in dark-skinned individuals. J Cosmet Dermatol. 2005;4:18-22.
24. Savardekar P. Microdermabrasion. Indian J Dermatol Venereol Leprol. 2007;73:277-9.
25. Diaz D, Boonsiri M, Okawa J, Dekranes D, Ditre CM. Oxygeneo®—a unique three-in-one treatment of exfoliation, infusion, and oxygenation via the Bohr effect and TriPollar™ radiofrequency for skin rejuvenation. J Clin Aesthet Dermatol. 2017;10(11):22-5.
26. Chae JB, Yang SH, Byun SY, Choi HR, Shin JW, Park KC. The effects of hydroporation on melasma with anti-aging cocktail. J Cosmet Dermatol. 2016;15:399-406.
27. Krueger N, Sadick NS. New-generation radiofrequency technology. Cutis. 2013;91(1):39-46.
28. Fabi SG. Noninvasive skin tightening: focus on new ultrasound techniques. Clin Cosmet Investig Dermatol. 2015;8:47-52.

29. Ablon G. Safety and effectiveness of an automated microneedling device in improving the signs of aging skin. J Clin Aesthet Dermatol. 2018;11(8):29-34.
30. Tanaka Y. Long-term three-dimensional volumetric assessment of skin tightening using sharply tapered non-insulated microneedle radiofrequency applicator with novel fractionated pulse mode in Asians. Lasers Surg Med. 2015;47:626-33.
31. Gold M, Taylor M, Rothaus K, Tanaka Y. Non-insulated smooth motion, micro-needles RF fractional treatment for wrinkle reduction and lifting of the lower face: International study. Lasers Surg Med. 2016;48:727-33.
32. Dover JS, Monheit G, Greener M, Pickett A. Botulinum toxin in aesthetic medicine: myths and realities. Dermatol Surg. 2018;44(2):249-60.
33. Cabral LRB, Teixeira LN, Gimenez RP, Demasi APD, de Brito Junior RB, de Araújo VC, et al. Effect of hyaluronic acid and poly-l-lactic acid dermal fillers on collagen synthesis: an in vitro and in vivo study. Clin Cosmet Investig Dermatol. 2020;13:701-10.
34. Niforos F, Ogilvie P, Cavallini M, Leys C, Chantrey J, Safa M, et al. VYC-12 injectable gel is safe and effective for improvement of facial skin topography: a prospective study. Clin Cosmet Investig Dermatol. 2019;12:791-8.
35. Nikolis A, Enright KM. Evaluating the role of small particle hyaluronic acid fillers using micro-droplet technique in the face, neck and hands: a retrospective chart review. Clin Cosmet Investig Dermatol. 2018;11:467-75.
36. Cobo R. Use of polydioxanone threads as an alternative in nonsurgical procedures in facial rejuvenation. Facial Plast Surg. 2020;36(4):447-52.
37. Foster KW, Moy RL, Fincher EF. Advances in plasma skin regeneration. J Cosmet Dermatol. 2008;7(3):169-79.
38. Yuksel EP, Sahin G, Aydin F, Senturk N, Turanli AY. Evaluation of effects of platelet-rich plasma on human facial skin. J Cosmet Laser Ther. 2014;16:206-8.
39. Alam M, Hughart R, Champlain A, Geisler A, Paghdal K, Whiting D, et al. Effect of platelet-rich plasma injection for rejuvenation of photoaged facial skin: a randomized clinical trial. JAMA Dermatol. 2018;154(12):1447-52.
40. Kim JH, Jung M, Kim HS, Kim YM, Choi EH. Adipose-derived stem cells as a new therapeutic modality for ageing skin. Exp Dermatol. 2011;20:383-7.
41. Godic A. The role of stem cells in anti-aging medicine. Clin Dermatol. 2019;37(4):320-5.
42. Worley B, Cohen JL. Combination ablative approach to laser therapy in advanced aging of the face. J Drugs Dermatol. 2018;17(7):796-9.
43. Díaz-Ley B, Cuevast J, Alonso-Castro L, Calvo MI, Ríos-Buceta L, Orive G, et al. Benefits of plasma rich in growth factors (PRGF) in skin photodamage: clinical response and histological assessment. Dermatol Ther. 2015; 28(4):258-63.
44. Barnes L, Saurat JH, Kaya G. Senescent atrophic epidermis retains Lrig1+ stem cells and loses wnt signaling, a phenotype shared with CD44KO mice. PLoS One. 2017;12:e0169452.
45. Darbellay B, Barnes L, Boehncke WH, Saurat JH, Kaya G. Reversal of murine epidermal atrophy by topical modulation of calcium signaling. J Invest Dermatol. 2014;134:1599-608.
46. Kang C. Senolytics and senostatics: a two-pronged approach to target cellular senescence for delaying aging and age-related diseases. Mol Cells. 2019;42(12):821-7.
47. Lawrence P, Ceccoli J. Advances in the application and impact of microRNAs as therapies for skin disease. BioDrugs. 2017;31(5):423-38.
48. Dhanjal DS, Bhardwaj S, Sharma R, Bhardwaj K, Kumar D, Chopra C, et al. Plant fortification of the diet for anti-ageing effects: a review. Nutrients. 2020;12(10):3008.
49. Maione-Silva L, de Castro EG, Nascimento TL, Cintra ER, Moreira LC, Cintra BAS, et al. Ascorbic acid encapsulated into negatively charged liposomes exhibits increased skin permeation, retention and enhances collagen synthesis by fibroblasts. Sci Rep. 2019;9(1):522.
50. Balcázar M, Cañizares S, Borja T, Pontón P, Bisiou S, Carabasse E, et al. Bases for treating skin aging with artificial mitochondrial transfer/transplant (AMT/T). Front Bioeng Biotechnol. 2020;8:919.

SECTION 12 Chemical Peels

CHAPTER 83

Basics of Chemical Peels and Glycolic Acid Peels

Niti Khunger, Jyoti Gupta

KEY MESSAGES

- Chemical peels are versatile procedures and remain among the top five minimally aesthetic procedures worldwide.
- The basic procedure involves three steps of priming, application of the appropriate chemical agent, and postpeel care.
- Glycolic acid is an alpha hydroxy acid, with a dual mode of action. The depth of penetration increases with the concentration and duration. It requires neutralization to stop the action.

CHEMICAL PEELING

Introduction

Chemical peels remain a popular method of rejuvenating aging and sun-damaged skin and improving pigmentary disorders, despite the advent of many technologies. Since they offer many advantages, there has been a resurgence in the use of chemical peels. According to statistics from the International Society of Aesthetic Plastic Surgery (ISAPS), in 2022 chemical peels were among the top 5 minimally invasive aesthetic procedures world wide, with a 57% increase since 2021.[1] In this technique, an exfoliating chemical agent or combination of agents is applied to the skin, which leads to a controlled destruction of the layers, depending on the type of peel. This is followed by regeneration, leading to an improved appearance in texture and tone.[2] Based on the level of exfoliation, chemical peels can be very superficial (up to stratum corneum only), superficial (entire epidermis up to basal layer), medium depth (epidermis and papillary dermis), and deep peels (epidermis and dermis up to mid-reticular dermis). They are versatile and can be used singly or in combination and simultaneously or sequentially with other procedures to enhance results.

History of Chemical Peels and Resurfacing[3]

Skin resurfacing for beauty is an ancient procedure when rocks, shells, and pumice stone were used in ancient Babylonia and India to abrade the surface of their skin. The concept of skin rejuvenation by chemicals was also popular. The Egyptians, Greeks, and Romans are documented to have used acids and balms, and Gypsies were reportedly the first group to use phenol for deep chemical peels, passing secret chemical peel recipes between generations. The rejuvenating properties of alpha-hydroxy acids (AHAs) were well known. Cleopatra used sour milk, which contains lactic acid, as a beauty bath, and French women used old wine-containing tartaric acid. In 1871, Tilbury Fox described the use of 20% phenol to lighten the skin. In 1882, Unna reported the properties of salicylic acid, resorcinol, phenol, and trichloroacetic acid (TCA). The modern era of peeling began in the 1960s with the development of modified phenol solutions (addition of croton oil, Septisol, and water) by Baker and Gordon. The scientific properties of AHAs were first recognized by Van Scott and Yu in 1974.[4] They identified AHAs as a special category of substances with special benefits in the treatment of disorders associated with or caused by abnormal keratinization. In the ensuing years, clinical and laboratory investigations on an expanded array of hydroxy acids have revealed that the presence of additional hydroxyl groups on the molecule, which thereupon becomes a polyhydroxy acid (PHA), adds additional desirable properties to an AHA. Glycolic acid (GA), the smallest of the AHAs, is the most well studied and considered the gold standard. During the mid-1800s, a Viennese dermatologist, Ferdinand Hebra, heralded the use of chemical peels for professional treatment. The AHAs called fruit acids were scientifically studied by Van Scott and Yu and became popular. During the 1970s, the use of phenol and TCA peels became more common among dermatologists and plastic surgeons, and chemical peels evolved into what they are today. The field is evolving with newer agents being added day by day.

Mechanism of Action[3,5]

Chemical peels act by causing injury to the skin that is followed by remodeling and regeneration, through mechanisms of wound healing. The results depend on the depth of wounding, with very superficial peels exfoliating the stratum corneum only and superficial peels exfoliating the entire epidermis from the stratum corneum down to the papillary dermis at a depth

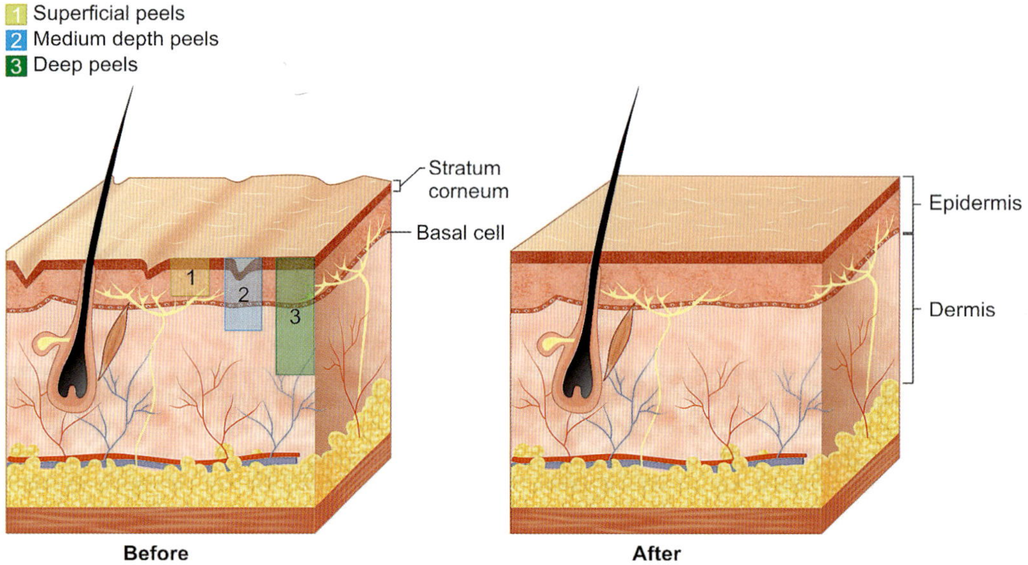

Fig. 1: Depth of chemical peels.

of about 60 μm. There is thinning of the stratum corneum due to decreased corneocyte adhesion, increase in epidermal thickness, and uniform distribution of melanin, which leads to improvement in skin texture and skin tone, with increased collagen deposition in the dermis. Medium-depth peels cause exfoliation of the epidermis and papillary dermis and reach the upper reticular dermis at a depth of 450 μm, causing coagulative necrosis of cells by precipitation of proteins. Deep peels reach up to the mid-reticular dermis, leading to extensive cell necrosis up to a depth of about 600 μm **(Fig. 1)**. Regeneration of epidermis occurs by reepithelialization and repair, and neocollagenesis takes place following mechanisms of wound repair.

In superficial peels, epithelial cells migrate from the intact basement membrane, and normal epidermis is restored in 2–3 days. In deeper peels, keratinocytes migrate from appendages and surrounding normal skin. The appendages, particularly the stem cells in the bulge area of the pilosebaceous follicles, contribute to the regeneration; hence, reepithelialization of the facial skin is faster as compared to nonfacial skin because of a greater number of pilosebaceous follicles on the face. During medium depth and deep peels, the mechanisms of dermal wound healing are stimulated with collagen remodeling, leading to rejuvenation. New collagen formation can continue to improve texture and rhytides for a period up to 4–6 months, particularly with deeper peels.

Indications

Chemical peels are basically cutaneous resurfacing procedures and can be used for a wide variety of conditions such as pigmentation, photodamage, acne, mild facial scarring, dilated pores, and skin rejuvenation **(Box 1)**. Though deep peels with phenol–croton oil give dramatic results in a single sitting, they are rarely used nowadays and have been supplanted by lasers, due to delayed healing and increased risk of complications.

BOX 1: Indications of chemical peels.

- *Pigmentary disorders:*
  - Melasma
  - Lentigines
  - Ephelides
  - Postinflammatory hyperpigmentation
  - Lichen planus pigmentosus
  - Macular amyloidosis
  - Frictional melanosis
- *Inflammatory disorders:*
  - Acne
  - Rosacea
- *Photoaging:*
  - Senile lentigines
  - Superficial wrinkles
  - Uneven texture
  - Dilated pores
  - Rough sallow skin
  - Senile comedones
- *Scarring:*
  - Acne scars
  - Traumatic scars
  - Surgical scars
- *Precancerous lesions:*
  - Actinic keratosis
- *Miscellaneous:*
  - Keratosis pilaris
  - Skin glow
  - *Acanthosis nigricans*

Contraindications

Chemical peels are contraindicated in the presence of open wounds, active infections such as folliculitis, warts, herpes simplex, and recently tanned skin. These should first be treated before beginning chemical peels to prevent exacerbation and complications. Prophylactic acyclovir a week before and till complete healing following a peel should be given to patients with a history of herpes simplex. Peels should be done cautiously in patients with history of photosensitivity, on medications causing photosensitivity, and in patients with unrealistic expectations. Deep peels are relatively contraindicated in dark skins as they can cause permanent depigmentation and scarring.

Principles of Chemical Peels

The basic principles and steps of chemical peels include patient assessment, prepeel counseling, documentation, photographs, selection of the appropriate peeling agent, priming of the skin before the peel, performing a standardized peel procedure, aftercare, and managing complications if they arise.

Patient assessment begins by taking a detailed history, diagnosis of the skin condition, and assessment of risk factors. The focus should be not only on the physical factors but also on the mental makeup and motivation of the patient. A professional psychological assessment may be sought in patients suspected of body dysmorphic disorder. Prepeel counseling should include discussion of patient expectations, alignment, downtime involved, number of sessions required, probable adverse effects, and costs. Documentation involves informed consent and standardized pretreatment photographs. Selection of the appropriate peeling agent and peeling depth is the most important part of the procedure. The selection depends on the pathology of the target condition and patient skin type[6] **(Table 1)**.

Priming is an essential step and the foundation to perform safe peeling. It should be started at least 2–4 weeks before the first peel. It prepares the skin for a uniform peel, reduces the chances of postinflammatory hyperpigmentation (PIH), and can help to detect intolerance to products. A typical priming should include a sunscreen, a skin lightening agent, and preferably a retinoid for reducing the risk of PIH and faster healing. A standardized peel technique should be followed to give optimum results. Postpeel care and a maintenance regimen are important to maintain results as peels are not one-time procedures, and treating conditions such as aging are dynamic and can recur.

TABLE 1: Selection of common peeling agents according to the skin condition.[7]

Condition	*Depth*	*Peeling depth required*	*Peeling agent*
Pigmentary disorders			
Melasma epidermal	Up to basal layer	Superficial	• GA 50–70% • TCA 10–30% • SA 30–50% • MA 40%
Melasma mixed (epidermal and dermal)	Up to dermis	Medium-depth peel	• GA 50–70% + TCA 10–30% • Jessner's + TCA
Freckles	Up to basal layer	Superficial	• GA 50–70% • TCA 10–30% • SA 30–50%
Lentigo	Up to papillary dermis	Superficial to medium	• GA 70% • TCA 35–50% • Jessner's + TCA 35%
PIH	Variable	Superficial to medium	• GA 50–70% • TCA 10–30% • SA 30–50%
Lichen planus pigmentosus	Mid to deep dermis	Medium-depth peel	• GA 50–70% + TCA 10–30% • Jessner's solution + TCA
Inflammatory conditions			
Acne comedonal	Stratum corneum	Very superficial	• SA 20–30% • GA 30–50% (applied for 1–2 minutes) • TCA 10%
Acne active	Up to basal layer	Superficial	• MA 40% • SA 30–50% • GA 50–70% • TCA 10–30%
Acne scars superficial	Up to papillary dermis	Superficial to medium	• GA 70% • TCA 35–50% • Jessner's + TCA 25–35% combinations
Photoaging			
Skin rejuvenation	Up to basal layer	Superficial	• GA 50–70% • TCA 10–30% • SA 30–50%
Wrinkles—mild	Up to basal layer	Superficial	• GA 50–70% • TCA 10–30% • SA 30–50%
Wrinkles—moderate	Up to mid-dermis	Medium-deep	• GA 50–70% • TCA 10–30% • SA 30–50% combinations

(GA: glycolic acid, MA: mandelic acid; SA: salicylic acid; TCA: trichloroacetic acid)

Techniques of Chemical Peels[7]

Basic Procedure

Anesthesia is not required for superficial peels as mild burning that can occur is tolerable and for short duration. Medium-depth peels may require pain control in anxious patients. A cooling fan or ice pack is usually sufficient. Deep phenol peels require an operating theater (OT) setup and sedation, regional or general anesthesia.

Prior to peeling, the face is cleaned with alcohol or prepeel cleanser, and all makeup is removed. Oily skin is degreased with acetone. The hair is kept away with a band or cap, and the patient should be upright or reclining at least 45°. The neutralizing agent and timer must be kept ready. The sensitive areas such as medial and inner canthi, and nasal and oral commissures may be protected with petrolatum. The desired peeling agent is poured into a small glass cup and applied with firm even strokes using a brush or cotton bud. Application should be along cosmetic units of the face, beginning with the forehead, followed by cheeks, nose, chin, and lastly perioral and periocular areas **(Fig. 2)**. The peel should be feathered at the edges. The skin should be stretched before applying the peel in areas of wrinkled skin to prevent pooling of the peeling agent. The peel should be neutralized with cold saline or neutralizing agent once the endpoint is reached. The endpoint of GA peel is erythema, whereas the endpoint of TCA peel is frosting, which occurs due to coagulation of proteins. The degree of frosting depends on the concentration of TCA **(Fig. 3)**. A sunscreen should be applied before the patient leaves the clinic. Some peels such as gel peels are leave-on peels, and the patient is sent home, advising photoprotection.

Combination Peels

Standard peels are single-agent formulations, whereas combination peels combine two or more different agents in a single formulation. This increases the range of action, depth, and efficacy and improves safety as lower concentrations of individual agents are used. Jessner's solution is the most widely used combination peel; however, many other combination peels are proprietary.

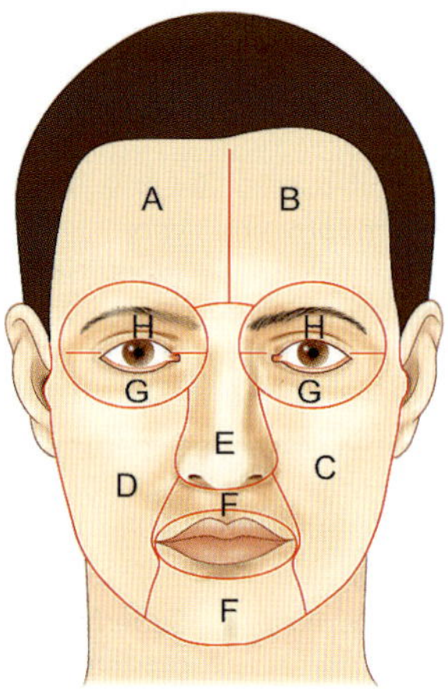

Fig. 2: Application of the peeling agent according to facial cosmetic units.

Enhanced Peels

Enhanced chemical peels are basic peels that are customized by adding an enhancer to match individual skin requirements, for example, adding a skin-lightening agent in darker skins to prevent PIH.

Sequential Peels

Sequential peels are those when more than one peel is applied at a time in a sequential manner as they may not be compatible in a single formulation. The peel that is applied first exfoliates the skin and enhances penetration of the second peel, increasing the depth of the peel. Since these are mostly medium-depth peels, they should be carefully used. Priming with sunscreens and skin-lightening agents should be done at least 2–4 weeks prior to sequential peels.

Segmental Peels

Segmental peels are the technique of using different peels in different cosmetic units at the same session. For example, a patient with sensitive skin, with an oily T-zone, can be treated with a gel peel on the cheeks and an alcoholic peel on the nose and forehead.

Switch Peels

In switch peels, peels are switched to a different peel in serial peeling sessions. This gives a greater flexibility in choosing a peeling agent according to the patient's condition and increasing customization.

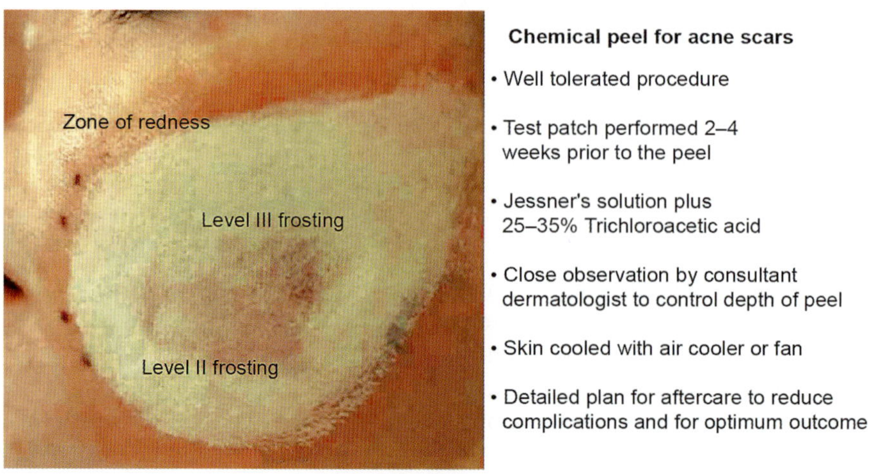

Fig. 3: Levels of TCA frost. Level I—faint frost with patchy erythema, superficial peel, depth epidermal. Level II—white frost, medium depth peel. Level III—solid white frost, deep peel.

TABLE 2: Activity of glycolic acid according to pH of the solution.

pH	1.5	2	2.7	3	3.5	4	4.5	5	5.5	6	6.5	7
% active	99.53	98.54	95.53	87.11	68.13	40.34	17.61	6.33	2.09	0.67	0.21	0.07

Postpeel Care

Postprocedure care is essential to enhance outcomes, reduce complications, and maintain results. Written clear instructions regarding sun protection and topical applications must be provided. Mild peeling or flaking of the skin can occur, and patients should be instructed not to forcibly peel off the skin as it can delay healing. A noncomedogenic moisturizer can be applied if it is severe and uncomfortable. In a superficial peel, the skin returns to normal in 3–5 days, whereas reepithelialization may take 5–7 days in a medium-depth peel.

Complications

Chemical peels are relatively safe procedures, and serious complications are rare provided they are performed under supervision following the basic principles. Choosing the right peel for the right indication and skin type reduces the incidence of complications. The risk increases with increasing depth, darker skin types prone to PIH, sensitive skin, outdoor occupations, and poorly compliant patients.[8] Complications with superficial peels are rare, and unmet expectations are the most common complication. Prolonged erythema, sensitive skin, and PIH are common complications that can occur with overzealous peeling.

GLYCOLIC ACID PEELS

Introduction

Alpha-hydroxy acids, also called "fruit acids" because they are present in certain fruits, are one of the most commonly used peeling agents. They include GA, lactic acid, mandelic acid, citric acid, tartaric acid, etc. GA is present in sugarcane, citric acid in citrus fruits, malic acid in apples, and tartaric acid in grape wine. GA is considered the gold standard as it is the most well studied.

Basic Biochemistry

Alpha-hydroxy acids are organic carboxylic acids with one hydroxyl group attached to the α-position of the carboxyl group. The hydroxyl and carboxyl groups are both directly attached to an aliphatic or alicyclic carbon atom. The hydroxyl group in the AHA is neutral, and only the carboxyl group provides an acidic property. AHAs are weak acids with dissociation constant (pKa) ranging from 3 to 4, which means that at pH 3–4, the level of free acid is the same as salt of substance, that is, 50% free acid concentration. They do not have self-neutralizing properties, and the duration of the peel affects their penetration levels. GA (aliphatic: Alpha-hydroxy acetic acid) is the shortest AHA, which was originally extracted from sugarcane. However, the acid used in treatment today is synthesized chemically by passing carbon monoxide through formaldehyde solution. It is available as crystals, and a solution is prepared by dissolving the crystals in water with or without the addition of alcohol and propylene glycol. GA is extremely hydrophilic. Activity of GA is determined by the pH of the solution **(Table 2)**. A pure aqueous solution of GA, at a saturated concentration of about 80%, has a pH of 0.5. This pH, considerably lower than its pKa of 3.83, shows that the solution consists mostly of pure acid. The pH as well as pKa of a GA solution determines its acidifying power on the skin; a 3% GA solution at pH 3 can acidify the first five layers of corneocytes, whereas at 10% and pH 3, it causes a deeper and more rapid acidification of the entire epidermis.[9] The contact times for partially buffered AHAs at pH >2.5 are far longer than for pure unbuffered AHA solutions at pH 0.5, which are 100 times more acidic. The natural pH of an aqueous solution of 60% GA is 0.5. The gradual addition of a base slowly raises the pH of this solution. When the pH reaches a value of 3.83 as a result of the gradual addition of the base, we know that this solution contains exactly 50% of active free acid and 50% of salt produced by the reaction of the GA with the base (e.g., sodium glycolate or ammonium glycolate). GA is available as synthetic crystals dissolved in a vehicle. It may be dissolved in water or a combination of water, alcohol, and propylene glycol.

Mechanism of Action

Glycolic acid has a dual mode of action.[10-12] In the epidermis, at low concentrations and acidic pH, GA has a lytic action on corneodesmosomes. Acidification of the skin causes an increase in the epidermal activity of lipases, phosphatases, and transforming growth factor beta (TGF-β). By its metabolic action, it interferes with the working of these enzymes along with kinases, sulfotransferases, and phosphotransferases that are responsible for the adhesion of the corneocytes. Hence, corneocytes are shed more easily, causing an exfoliating action, and the thickness of the stratum corneum is reduced. The disruption of the barrier function of the epidermis leads to a cascade of secondary events stimulating growth in the basal layer of the epidermis, which accelerates the conversion of keratinocytes into corneocytes to restore optimum barrier function as soon as possible. Unfortunately, this can also potentially cause melanocyte stimulation, resulting in PIH. It has been reported that partially neutralized GA formulations retain skin rejuvenating properties without causing irritation and inflammation, at varying concentrations from 8 to 25%; thus, topical creams can be effective without irritation.[11]

In the dermis, there is stimulation of fibroblast proliferation and synthesis of collagen, elastin, and glycosaminoglycans.[12] At a higher pH, it acts as a moisturizer due to its hydrophilic nature. It does not cause coagulation of proteins; hence, there is no frosting seen. The grayish discoloration seen with higher concentrations is due to epidermolysis and a sign of overpeeling. Since they do not bind with proteins, they are not self-neutralizing like TCA and must be neutralized to stop their action. The contact time of the acid with the skin is important as greater the contact time, deeper is the peel. The ultimate effect of the above processes is controlled chemical burns of the skin, which results in the thinning of stratum corneum, regulation of epidermal thickness, and laying down of new collagen and ground substance in the dermis, causing an antiaging effect. Regeneration of the epidermis is histologically visible after 2–7 days. The epidermis is completely replaced by 2 weeks after a single light AHA peel. There is a depigmenting effect which occurs due to increased cell turnover inhibiting excess melanin production and also due to direct tyrosinase inhibition. The summary of actions of GA are in **Boxes 2 and 3**. GA also has antibacterial properties, making it useful in acne. It has been demonstrated that 30–35% GA exhibits antibacterial activity against *Propionibacterium acnes* and can decrease *its* concentrations on the cheeks of acne vulgaris patients.[13]

Formulations

The peel formulation should be chosen with care as the vehicle has a key role in the concentration of free acid and efficacy of the peel. It is used as a peeling agent in a concentration of 35–70%. Various formulations are available.

Free acid: This formulation is an aqueous non-neutralized acidic solution with greater bioavailability of free acid and hence increased reactivity. It causes greater burning and stinging and can easily lead to epidermolysis on sensitive skins with impaired barrier function. However, it is more effective than other formulations. But it is recommended to use buffered or partially neutralized GA, which is safer than free GA.[14]

Partially neutralized: It is a partially neutralized form with addition of a base, ammonium hydroxide. This raises the pH of the solution and is said to be less irritant.

Buffered: It is a partially neutralized stable form and has no advantage over other formulations.

Esterified: It is a solution forming glycol citrate, which is said to be less irritant.

Glycolic acid, purified water, and strontium nitrate: The addition of strontium nitrate is said to reduce irritation by inhibiting type C neurons. On the face, a 50% concentration for 1–3 minutes is effective, whereas for the back a 70% concentration for 4–8 minutes is required to show results.

Gel based: These are formulated in a gel base where less free acid is available and is released slowly. It is said to be less irritant and easy to control though less efficacious and more suitable for sensitive skins.[15]

BOX 2: Summary of actions of glycolic acid.

- At low concentrations, it decreases keratinocyte cohesion by interfering with ionic binding
- At higher concentrations, keratinocytes get totally detached (epidermolysis)
- Stimulation of basal keratinocytes
- Decreased melanin production by direct inhibition of tyrosinase
- Fibroblast modulation
- Antioxidant action
- Moisturizing action

BOX 3: Penetration depth of different concentrations of glycolic acid.

- *Very superficial (upper epidermis):* 25–50% partially buffered, for 1–2 minutes
- *Superficial (papillary dermis):* 50–70% partially buffered, for 2–10 minutes
- *Medium depth (mid-deep dermis):* 70% unbuffered, for 5–10 minutes. Not recommended in colored skin

Indications[2,16,17]

- *Acne:* Comedonal acne, postacne hyperpigmentation, superficial scarring following acne, acne excoriee[18-21]
- *Dyschromias:* Melasma,[22-26] fixed-drug eruptions, facial melanosis, lentigines, freckles, PIH, macular amyloidosis, periorbital melanosis,[27] frictional melanosis.[28]
- *Aesthetic indications:* Dilated pores,[29] fine wrinkling, moderate actinic damage, superficial scars, and photoaging[30]
- *Others*: Facial verrucae[31]

Contraindications

- Active viral, bacterial, or fungal infection, particularly oral herpes simplex
- Inflammatory dermatoses on the face such as seborrheic dermatitis, atopic dermatitis, or contact dermatitis should be treated first.
- Patients on photosensitizing drugs
- Patients who have undergone a deep resurfacing procedure such as dermabrasion, laser resurfacing, deep peels, or any surgeries in the last 6–12 months
- Uncooperative patients or patients with unrealistic expectations

Procedure

Alpha-hydroxy acid peels produce the best results if they are preceded by careful preparation and daily cosmetic care called priming. The products usually used to prepare the skin before

GA peeling are sunscreens, low concentrations of AHAs, and tyrosinase inhibitors. Priming should be started at least 2–4 weeks before the peel.

Two days prior to the peel, the patient should stop:

- Use of tretinoin, tazarotene, adapalene, and any other retinoids
- Glycolic and salicylic acid-based face washes
- Waxing, depilatories, electrolysis, bleaching
- Masques, loofahs, and other sponges
- Hair dyeing, permanent wave, or straightening treatments
- Other resurfacing or exfoliating treatments

On the day of the peel, shaving and threading should be avoided before and after the procedure to avoid discomfort and burning.

Peeling Technique

The technique is similar to a standard peel procedure.

Patients are asked to wash their skin with soap and water to remove dirt, makeup, and grease. The skin is disinfected with alcohol and degreased with acetone, a prepeel cleanser, or ether. These degreasing products allow the peel solutions, which are usually hydrophilic and have difficulty penetrating the skin's protective oils, to penetrate more deeply and evenly. They also break down some of the proteins and phospholipids in the cell membranes, which enhances the action of the peels applied afterward. A GA peel can be applied in an aqueous solution or in a gel, with a gauze pad, a brush, presoaked cotton swabs or pads, or gloved fingers. Compact and opaque AHA masks have been used, but monitoring the skin while the mask is on is neither easy nor certain. The peel is performed with the patient sitting up or lying at 45° angle and hair pulled back with a hairband. The sensitive areas such as the inner and outer canthi of the eye and nasal crease are protected with Vaseline®. The GA solution is applied quickly (15–20 seconds maximum), so that the contact time is the same for the whole face. The peeling agent is applied with a cotton-tipped applicator or a brush. Sequential strokes are given starting from the forehead, right cheek, chin, left cheek, nose, and finally the perioral and periorbital areas. Feathering is done at the edges to prevent demarcation lines. It is important to always use the same system, both for applying and for neutralizing the peel. Massaging the skin lightly with a gloved finger allows more even penetration or deeper local penetration as necessary. The timer should be set, and the patient should not be left unsupervised. The AHA solution can be neutralized by closely monitoring changes in skin color, before any frosting occurs. A faint erythema is the endpoint. This may be difficult to appreciate in darker skins; hence, GA peels can lead to PIH **(Fig. 4)** if the endpoint is exceeded and epidermolysis occurs. This is seen as whitening or blistering. Therefore, in darker skins, monitoring the time is an important criterion. To a certain degree, the contact time is more important than the total quantity of AHAs applied to the skin. If any GA comes into contact with the eyes, it should be rinsed immediately with plenty of water, and drops of artificial tears or physiological solution should be applied. Since GA is not a protein coagulant like TCA or phenol, the risk of damage to the eye after contact is not very high, and dilution from artificial tears appears to be enough to avert danger.

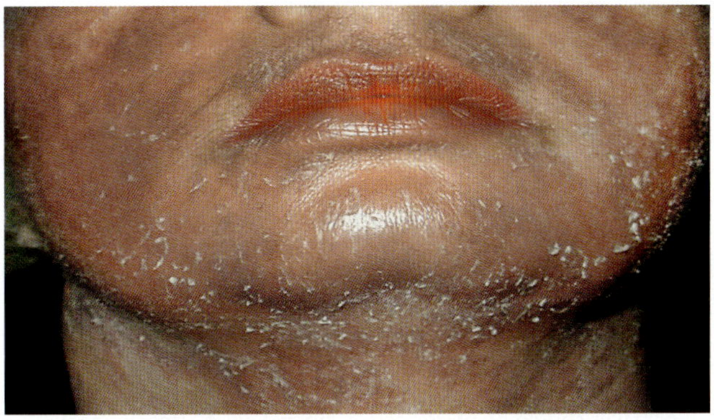

Fig. 4: PIH following a medium depth peel.

Correlation between Skin Appearance and Depth of AHA Peel

- *No erythema:* Hardly any peeling effect
- *Spots of erythema:* Very, very superficial
- *Patches of erythema:* Very superficial
- *Widespread erythema:* Superficial peel, suitable depth for AHAs
- *Small superficial blisters:* Deeper peel causes epidermolysis.
- *Frosting:* Too deep for an AHA peel

Contact Time for a Glycolic Acid Peel

Each patient has a particular level of sensitivity and contact time, which may also vary from one peel to the next peel. Hence, there is tremendous variability in the depth of peeling with GA. A cautious contact time of 2 minutes with 35–50% GA, pH 0.5, on a patient with healthy skin of normal thickness is advised for a first peel. It can gradually be prolonged by 30–60 seconds in subsequent peels if the skin can tolerate it.

Neutralization

An AHA peel should be neutralized as soon as erythema appears and before the first pinpoints of protein coagulation (frosting) appear. GA does not combine with proteins and is not self-neutralizing like TCA. It remains aggressive until it is neutralized, diluted, or picked up by the skin's buffer systems. The peel can be neutralized with a solution saturated with sodium bicarbonate. After neutralization, the patient may continue to feel the acid burning in places. The patient can be given a cotton pad soaked in bicarbonate solution and

BOX 4: Guidelines for postpeel care.

- Patients should be informed that after a peel, erythema and desquamation will occur; this may last for 1–3 days
- A nonsoap cleanser should be used to wash face
- Irritant cleansers such as Dettol, scrubs, and loofahs should be strictly avoided for a week
- If there is crusting, a topical antibacterial ointment should be used to prevent infection
- A moisturizer should be used when the skin is peeling, and it should not be picked
- Broad-spectrum sunscreens should be liberally used and must be applied every 3 hourly for at least a week
- No facial procedures such as steaming, scrubbing, waxing, bleaching, or facials should be performed in the first week after the peel
- The patient should also be advised against getting into chlorinated water for at least 72 hours to prevent postinflammatory hyperpigmentation

BOX 5: Complications.

- Scab formation **(Fig. 5)**
- Delayed healing
- Persistent erythema
- Postinflammatory hyperpigmentation
- Postinflammatory hypopigmentation
- Lines of demarcation
- Acneiform eruptions
- Allergic reactions
- Infections
- Milia
- Scarring

asked to neutralize the more sensitive areas. It can also be neutralized with cold saline or ice-cold water.

Postprocedure Care

A good postprocedure care system is essential to reduce the risk of potential complications and ensure early recovery of normal skin. The postprocedure care depends on the condition being treated. The barrier function of the skin is impaired after a GA peel. Sunscreens are essential to prevent erythema and PIH, particularly in darker skins. If there is excessive desquamation, a nonocclusive water-based moisturizer should be applied to reduce discomfort and excessive picking of the skin, which can delay healing. The peels can be repeated every 2 weeks initially till a satisfactory response is obtained. Thereafter, maintenance peels may be required, particularly for photoaging and melasma. It has been shown that GA peels enhance the efficacy of topical regimens such as the triple-combination creams in melasma.[32] There is a more rapid initial response and overall lightening of skin as compared to topical regimen alone. In a comparative study of GA versus TCA chemical peels in melasma, both were found to be equally effective, though GA was associated with fewer side effects.[33] In another study in melasma, GA peel and 1% tretinoin peel were equally effective, though tretinoin peel was better tolerated.[34] The guidelines of postprocedure care are discussed in **Box 4**.

Complications

Complications, usually minor and preventable with proper priming and postpeel care, are listed in **Box 5**. The best way to avoid complications is to identify patients at risk and use lower concentrations of GA.[35] The deeper the peel, the greater the risk of complications, particularly in darker skins. If epidermolysis occurs during the peel, scab formation **(Fig. 5)** can take place and healing will be delayed. A case report of hyperpigmentation and scarring following 70% GA peel in a patient taking low-dose isotretinoin 10 mg three times per week has been reported.[36] In a 5-year retrospective study of chemical peels in darker skin types, the complication rate was 3.8% in 473 peel treatments. Crusting (2.3%), PIH (1.9%), and erythema (1.9%) were the most frequent complications, and all were located on the face.[37]

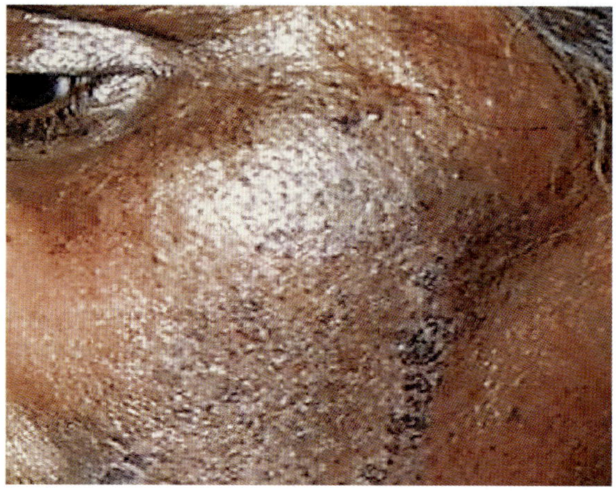

Fig. 5: Scab formation following epidermolysis.

Topical moisturizers and 1% hydrocortisone are usually sufficient to manage it. If there is severe edema, particularly around the eyelids, a short course of systemic prednisolone 30–40 mg as a single morning dose can be administered for 3–5 days. PIH can be treated with broad-spectrum sunscreens, topical corticosteroids, tretinoin, hydroquinone, or AHAs as appropriate.

Combination with Other Aesthetic Treatments

Chemical peels can be combined with other cosmetic procedures such as botulinum toxin, fillers, lasers, and microneedling. Microdermabrasion alone provides the benefits of exfoliation but may provide faster results and increased patient satisfaction when combined with superficial GA (e.g., AHA) peels because of the significant antiaging effects of GA peels. GA peels and microdermabrasion may be done at an interval of 2 weeks. A different approach is to perform both in the same session as microdermabrasion, when used prior to the superficial GA peel, increases the exfoliation and antiaging effects of both treatments. GA 35–70% have been used alternatively with microneedling for superficial acne scarring with better aesthetic outcome.[38,39]

After any peel session, it is important to allow the inflammation to settle down and wound healing to occur before any further resurfacing procedure is done. This will prevent scarring and PIH.[40-44]

TIPS

For ensuring good results

- Combine glycolic acid peels with a good home care program to optimize results.
- Start with the lowest percentage formulation and slowly advance to the higher concentrations.
- Use lower concentrations or combination peels to decrease side effects in darker skin prone to postinflammatory hyperpigmentation.
- Follow all priming and postpeel procedures to avoid complications.
- Contact duration and neutralization are vital to obtain proper results.

CONCLUSION

Chemical peels are time-tested procedures and are here to stay, in spite of the advent of light-based therapies. They are cost effective, evidence-based, safe in all skin types, and versatile. They can be customized and applied in a wide variety of conditions. GA peels are considered the gold standard in chemical peeling because they have undergone more scientific studies than any other peeling agent. They have epidermal as well as dermal effects and have demonstrated clinical and histological value in photoaging, hyperpigmentation, acne, and also photoprotective, anti-inflammatory, and collagen stimulant effects. In darker skins, it is safer to initiate treatment with lower concentrations and gradually titrate to higher concentrations or use them in combination peels, in order to reduce the incidence of PIH.

REFERENCES

1. The International Society of Aesthetic Plastic Surgery (ISAPS) https://www.isaps.org/discover/about-isaps/global-statistics/reports-and-press-releases/global-survey-2022-full-report-and-press-releases/ accessed on 14 March 2024.
2. Khunger N, IADVL Task Force. Standard guidelines of care for chemical peels. Indian J Dermatol Venereol Leprol. 2008;74(Suppl):S5-12.
3. Brody HJ, Monheit GD, Resnik SS, Alt TH. A history of chemical peeling. Dermatol Surg. 2000;26:405-9.
4. Van Scott EJ, Yu RJ. Control of keratinization with alpha-hydroxy acids and related compounds. I. Topical treatment of ichthyotic disorders. Arch Dermatol. 1974;110:586-90.
5. Soleymani T, Lanoue J, Rahman Z. A practical approach to chemical peels: a review of fundamentals and step-by-step algorithmic protocol for treatment. J Clin Aesthet Dermatol. 2018;11:21-8.
6. Lee KC, Wambier CG, Soon SL, Sterling JB, Landau M, Rullan P, et al. Basic chemical peeling: superficial and medium-depth peels. J Am Acad Dermatol. 2019;81(2):313-24.
7. Khunger N. Office-based peels and peel selection. Step by Step Chemical Peels, 3rd edition. New Delhi, India: Jaypee Brothers Medical Publishers; 2021. pp. 40-5.
8. Nikalji N, Godse K, Sakhiya J, Patil S, Nadkarni N. Complications of medium depth and deep chemical peels. J Cutan Aesthet Surg. 2012;5:254-60.
9. Deprez P. Alpha-hydroxy acids: chemistry, pH and pKa, and mechanism of action. In: Deprez P (Ed). Textbook of Chemical Peels. Superficial, Medium, and Deep Peels in Cosmetic Practice. London: Informa Healthcare; 2007. pp. 47-52.
10. Fartasch M, Teal J, Menon GK. Mode of action of glycolic acid on human stratum corneum: ultrastructural and functional evaluation of the epidermal barrier. Arch Dermatol Res. 1997;289(7):404-9.
11. Narda M, Trullas C, Brown A, Piquero-Casals J, Granger C, Fabbrocini G. Glycolic acid adjusted to pH 4 stimulates collagen production and epidermal renewal without affecting levels of proinflammatory TNF-alpha in human skin explants. J Cosmet Dermatol. 2021;20(2):513-21.
12. Okano Y, Abe Y, Masaki H, Santhanam U, Ichihashi M, Funasaka Y. Biological effects of glycolic acid on dermal matrix metabolism mediated by dermal fibroblasts and epidermal keratinocytes. Exp Dermatol. 2003;12:57-63.
13. Takenaka Y, Hayashi N, Takeda M, Ashikaga S, Kawashima M. Glycolic acid chemical peeling improves inflammatory acne eruptions through its inhibitory and bactericidal effects on *Propionibacterium acnes*. J Dermatol. 2012;39:350-4.
14. Becker FF, Langford FP, Rubin MG, Speelman P. A histological comparison of 50% and 70% glycolic acid peels using solutions with various pHs. Dermatol Surg. 1996;22:463-5.
15. Fabbrocini G, Padova MP, Tosti A. Chemical peels: what's new and what isn't new but still works well. Facial Plast Surg. 2009;25:329-36.
16. Grover C, Reddu BS. The therapeutic value of glycolic acid peels in dermatology. Indian J Dermatol Venereol Leprol. 2003;69:148-50.
17. Sharad J. Glycolic acid peel therapy—a current review. Clin Cosmet Investig Dermatol. 2013;6:281-8.
18. Garg VK, Sinha S, Sarkar R. Glycolic acid peels versus salicylic-mandelic acid peels in active acne vulgaris and post-acne scarring and hyperpigmentation: a comparative study. Dermatol Surg. 2009;35:59-65.
19. Kim SW, Moon SE, Kim JA, Eun HC. Glycolic acid versus Jessner's solution: which is better for facial acne patients? A randomized prospective clinical trial of split-face model therapy. Dermatol Surg. 1999;25:270-3.
20. Dréno B, Fischer TC, Perosino E, Poli F, Viera MS, Rendon MI, et al. Expert opinion: efficacy of superficial chemical peels in active acne management—what can we learn from the literature today? Evidence-based recommendations. J Eur Acad Dermatol Venereol. 2011;25:695-704.
21. Handog EB, Datuin MS, Singzon IA. Chemical peels for acne and acne scars in Asians: evidence based review. J Cutan Aesthet Surg. 2012;5:239-46.
22. Sarkar R, Kaur C, Bhalla M, Kanwar AJ. The combination of glycolic acid peels with a topical regimen in the treatment of melasma in dark-skinned patients: a comparative study. Dermatol Surg. 2002;28:828-32.
23. Erbil H, Sezer E, Tastan B, Arca E, Kurumlu Z. Efficacy and safety of serial glycolic acid peels and a topical regimen in the treatment of recalcitrant melasma. J Dermatol. 2007;34:25-30.
24. Puri N. A study on fractional erbium glass laser therapy versus chemical peeling for the treatment of melasma in female patients. J Cutan Aesthet Surg. 2013;6:148-51.
25. Sarkar R, Bansal S, Garg VK. Chemical peels for melasma in dark-skinned patients. J Cutan Aesthet Surg. 2012;5:247-53.

26. Sarkar R, Garg V, Bansal S, Sethi S, Gupta C. Comparative evaluation of efficacy and tolerability of glycolic acid, salicylic mandelic acid, and phytic acid combination peels in melasma. Dermatol Surg. 2016;42:384-91.
27. Dayal S, Sahu P, Jain VK, Khetri S. Clinical efficacy and safety of 20% glycolic peel, 15% lactic peel, and topical 20% vitamin C in constitutional type of periorbital melanosis: a comparative study. J Cosmet Dermatol. 2016;15:367-73.
28. Sacchidanand S, Shetty AB, Leelavathy B. Efficacy of 15% trichloroacetic acid and 50% glycolic acid peel in the treatment of frictional melanosis: a comparative study. J Cutan Aesthet Surg. 2015;8:37-41.
29. Kakudo N, Kushida S, Tanaka N, Minakata T, Suzuki K, Kusumoto K. A novel method to measure conspicuous facial pores using computer analysis of digital-camera-captured images: the effect of glycolic acid chemical peeling. Skin Res Technol. 2011;17:427-33.
30. Yamamoto Y, Uede K, Yonei N, Kishioka A, Ohtani T, Furukawa F. Effects of alpha-hydroxy acids on the human skin of Japanese subjects: the rationale for chemical peeling. J Dermatol. 2006;1:16-22.
31. Rani S, Sharma P. Glycolic acid peel in disseminated facial verrucae. J Cosmet Laser Ther. 2017;19(8):475-8.
32. Godse K, Sakhia J. Triple combination and glycolic peels in post-acne hyperpigmentation. J Cutan Aesthet Surg. 2012;5:60-1.
33. Kumari R, Thappa DM. Comparative study of trichloroacetic acid versus glycolic acid chemical peels in the treatment of melasma. Indian J Dermatol Venereol Leprol. 2010;76:447.
34. Khunger N, Sarkar R, Jain RK. Tretinoin peels versus glycolic acid peels in the treatment of melasma in dark-skinned patients. Dermatol Surg. 2004;30:756-60.
35. Anitha B. Prevention of complications in chemical peeling. J Cutan Aesthet Surg. 2010;3:186-8.
36. Gerber PA, Kukova G, Bölke E, Homey B, Diedrichson E. Severe hyperpigmentation and scarring following glycolic acid peel treatment in combination with low-dose isotretinoin. Eur J Med Res. 2014;19(1):60.
37. Vemula S, Maymone MBC, Secemsky EA, Widjajahakim R, Patzelt NM, Saade D, et al. Assessing the safety of superficial chemical peels in darker skin: a retrospective study. J Am Acad Dermatol. 2018;79(3):508-13.e2.
38. Saadawi AN, Esawy AM, Kandeel AH, El-Sayed W. Microneedling by dermapen and glycolic acid peel for the treatment of acne scars: comparative study. J Cosmet Dermatol. 2019;18(1):107-14.
39. Rana S, Mendiratta V, Chander R. Efficacy of microneedling with 70% glycolic acid peel vs microneedling alone in treatment of atrophic acne scars—a randomized controlled trial. J Cosmet Dermatol. 2017;16(4):454-9.
40. Fulton Jr JE. Dermabrasion, chemabrasion, and laserabrasion. Historical perspectives, modern dermabrasion techniques, and future trends. Dermatol Surg. 1996;22:619-28.
41. Effron C, Briden ME, Green BA. Enhancing cosmetic outcomes by combining superficial glycolic acid (alpha-hydroxy acid) peels with nonablative lasers, intense pulsed light, and trichloroacetic acid peels. Cutis. 2007;79:4-8.
42. Rendon MI, Effron C, Edison BL. The use of fillers and botulinum toxin type A in combination with superficial glycolic acid (alpha-hydroxy acid) peels: optimizing injection therapy with the skin-smoothing properties of peels. Cutis. 2007;79:9-12.
43. Briden E, Jacobsen E, Johnson C. Combining superficial glycolic acid (alpha-hydroxy acid) peels with microdermabrasion to maximize treatment results and patient satisfaction. Cutis. 2007;79:13-6.
44. Kempiak SJ, Uebelhoer N. Superficial chemical peels and microdermabrasion for acne vulgaris. Semin Cutan Med Surg. 2008;27:212-20.

CHAPTER 84

Salicylic Acid and Trichloroacetic Acid Peel

Abhishek De, Aarti Sarda

KEY MESSAGES

- Salicylic acid is a lipophilic slow penetrating acid, useful in acne vulgaris.
- Trichloroacetic acid (TCA) is a versatile peel which can reach all depths depending on the concentration and number of coats. It is used for superficial as well as medium-depth peels.
- Jessner's solution is another type of superficial peel used to treat acne as well as hyperkeratotic skin disorders.

INTRODUCTION

Chemical peeling is a skin resurfacing procedure that utilizes topical agents to remove the outermost layers of the skin.[1,2] This controlled method of wounding stimulates a reparative healing response with regeneration of a healthier epidermis and dermis.[1] Chemical peels are commonly used for skin rejuvenation to improve hyperpigmentation and acne and to smooth rough skin texture and superficial scarring.[3]

Chemical peels address many skin changes. They decrease corneocyte cohesion, promoting a more rapid rate of cell turnover, which normalizes epidermal keratinization. Chemical peels also promote dispersion of melanin accumulated in the basal epidermal layer and transportation of the pigment to the cell surface for exfoliation. Histologic changes in the skin evident after a chemical peel are a compacted stratum corneum, smoother epidermis, and increased dermal thickness with fibroblast production of new collagen, elastin, and glycosaminoglycans.[4]

TYPES OF CHEMICAL PEELS

Chemical peels are categorized based on the depth of the procedure into superficial, medium, or deep.[4] Superficial peels induce necrosis of all or parts of the epidermis. Medium-depth peels penetrate up to the papillary dermis, whereas deep peels reach the reticular dermis.

Therefore, the depth achieved with light chemical peels ranges from very superficial resurfacing with removal of the stratum corneum to superficial resurfacing with penetration up to the upper papillary dermis. Although the type and concentration of chemical peel agent are the main determinants of the depth of penetration in the skin, other factors also influence the depth of penetration **(Box 1)**.

BOX 1: Factors influencing the depth of penetration.[1,5]

- Chemical peel agent
- Concentration
- pH
- Application time
- Application technique
- Number of coats
- Skin preparation
- Skin type
- Area of the body treated

Significance of pKa and pH and Buffered Solutions

In order to use peels properly, one must understand the pKa and how the pH of a peel affects its efficacy. The pKa of a substance measures its capacity to donate protons. The pKa is the pH at which the level of free acid is the same as the level of salt form of the acid. When the pH is less than the pKa, the free acid form which is responsible for the exfoliation of skin predominates. When the pKa is higher than the pH, the salt form predominates. It is important to have a proper balance of the salt and acid forms to have an efficacious peel with minimal irritation.[4] The pKa for salicylic acid (SA) and trichloroacetic acid (TCA) are 2.97 and 0.26, respectively.

As far as pH is concerned, the lower the pH, the more acidic the peel will be. Lower pH equates to increased irritation as well as efficacy.

Buffered solutions contain bases such as sodium bicarbonate or sodium hydroxide. This produces an increased amount of the salt form, which results in less free acid and a higher pH. This increases the tolerability of the peels; however, the efficacy is also reduced.

Although a wide variety of agents have been shown to be effective for superficial peeling, alpha hydroxy acids (AHAs), beta hydroxy acid (BHA), Jessner's solution, modified Jessner's solution, resorcinol, and TCA are the most commonly used peels. Many newer peels have come to the market such as mandelic, lactic, phytic, polyhydroxy, pyruvic, citric, malic, and tartaric acid peels. The newer peels are gentler with lower concentration and may be available singly or in combination. This chapter will focus on SA peel and TCA peel. The newer peels will be discussed in subsequent chapters.

SALICYLIC ACID

Introduction

Salicylic acid (also known as ortho-hydroxybenzoic acid) is a naturally occurring BHA, derived from willow bark, wintergreen leaves, and sweet birch **(Fig. 1)**. It can also be synthesized chemically. SA has been used topically to treat various skin disorders for more than 2,000 years.[4] In the first century AD, Pliny used willow bark (as a source of SA) to treat calluses and corns.

The ability of SA to soften and exfoliate the stratum corneum was discovered in the 1860s which makes it a good agent for peeling. In particular, the comedolytic property of SA makes it a useful peeling agent for patients with acne. The properties and use of SA were first described by Unna, a German dermatologist. Kligman described SA as a BHA, but Yu and Van Scott have classified it as a phenolic aromatic acid.[6,7] Yu and Van Scott have classified it as a phenolic aromatic acid because SA has carboxyl (–COOH) and hydroxyl (–OH) groups directly attached to an aromatic benzene ring, unlike a true BHA, which contains an aliphatic carbon atom chain.[8]

Also, it should be noted that though SA is classified under BHA in the purest chemical terms, the hydroxyl group of BHAs is neutral, and in SA, it is acidic. Also, the carbons of aromatic compounds are traditionally given Arabic numerals rather than the Greek letter designations typical for the nonaromatic structures.[9] **Figure 1** shows the structure of SA.

It was Kligman and Kligman who ushered SA into the current arena of superficial peeling agent.[9] SA is a lipophilic slow penetrating acid which removes the intercellular lipids that are covalently linked to the cornified epithelial cells, thus reducing sebum. This adds to its therapeutic effect in patients with acne.

Owing to its antihyperplastic effect, it is used as a peeling agent. SA should now be regarded as a desmolytic agent because it works by disrupting cellular junctions rather than breaking or lysing intercellular keratin filaments.[10] SA affects the arachidonic cascade and thus exhibits anti-inflammatory capabilities.[11]

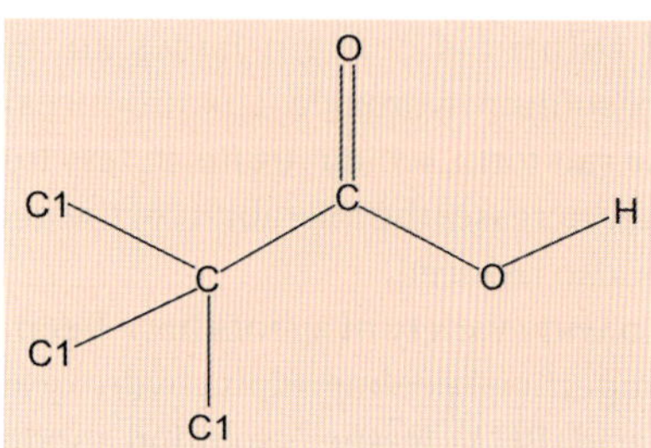

Fig. 1: Structure of salicylic acid.

Salicylates and their derivatives have been used in sunscreen formulations. The aromatic benzene ring in the salicylate converts ultraviolet rays into longer wave radiation, explaining the mechanism of action in sunscreen preparations.[12] SA also has antimicrobial and antifungal properties and is used in Whitfield's ointment.[13]

Salicyclic acid also has an anesthetic effect, which is seen during the peeling procedure and increases the patient's ability to tolerate the procedure.[6]

Formulations[11]

Salicylic acid preparation differs with the indication being treated and the regimen differs for different indications:

- 50% SA ointment paste (croton oil buffered with methyl salicylate)
- 20–30% ethanol formulation/gel
- Combination with mandelic acid and lactic acid.

Indications[8,9,14]

The most important indications for SA peel are acne vulgaris, rosacea, acne-induced postinflammatory hyperpigmentation, and acne-induced superficial scars. It can also be used for various other pigmentary disorders including melasma, postinflammatory hyperpigmentation, freckles, and lentigines **(Box 2)**.

The efficacy and safety of SA peeling in Fitzpatrick skin types I–III as well as in skin types V and VI have been well documented in the literature.

Contraindications[8,9]

Salicylic acid is generally considered a very safe peel. However, it is relatively contraindicated in the presence of active infection and eczema. In patients with known sensitivity to SA, the peel should not be used. Also, the safety of SA is not established in pregnancy and lactation **(Box 3)**.

Prepeel Procedure [8,9,14]

Detailed history and cutaneous examination are to be performed on all patients prior to chemical peeling. Note the patient's Fitzpatrick skin type, Glogau score, skin thickness, dryness, acne, scars, pigmentation, and vascular and pigmented lesions. Assessment of patients' expectations at the time of consultation and commitment to a series of treatments are essential to ensure success with this treatment. The potential risks of the procedure as well as the limitations must be discussed. Obtain an informed consent. Patch testing is recommended for all chemical peels. Standardized photography should be taken of all areas to be peeled,

BOX 2: Indications of salicylic acid peels.

- Acne vulgaris
- Rosacea
- Melasma
- Postinflammatory hyperpigmentation
- Freckles/lentigines
- Mild-to-moderate photodamage
- Texturally rough skin and enlarged pores
- Dull sallow skin/fine lines
- Superficial acne scars
- Keratosis pilaris
- Enhanced penetration of topical products

BOX 3: Contraindications of salicylic acid.[14]

- Active infection/open wound/dermatitis
- Pregnancy/lactation
- Hypersensitivity/allergy to salicylates (for salicylic peels)
- Sunburn or recent suntan
- Impaired healing
- Excessively dry skin
- Patient on isotretinoin
- Unrealistic patient expectations
- Body dysmorphic disorder

preferably full face and frontal and lateral areas. In patients with a history of recurrent herpes infection, antivirals should be started around 2 days before the peel and treated for a duration of 7–10 days.

Priming with topical retinoids or AHAs, hydroquinone, and kojic acid should be started 2–6 weeks prior to the peel. This thins the stratum corneum, increasing the uniform penetration and depth of peel, and enhances epidermal turnover. It also decreases the content of epidermal melanin and expedites the healing. For acne vulgaris, topical retinoids are the priming agent of choice; for pigmentation, depigmenting creams are preferred for priming. Priming agents should be stopped 2 days prior to peeling.

Equipment Required for Salicylic Peel[8,9,14]

Salicylic acid peel is a relatively simple office procedure. It can be done in a properly illuminated procedure room equipped with a derma chair or operating table (OT). The procedure requires very little instrumentation and consumables **(Box 4)**.

Salicylic Acid Chemical Peel Technique

The patient should be comfortably placed in a supine position. Apply a headband to pull hair away from the face and drape a towel on the neck. Set all the products required, most importantly, neutralizer for peels which need to be neutralized. Clean face with prepeel cleanser and degreasing lotion. Apply petroleum jelly to the areas of potential pooling, including the lateral canthi, nasolabial fold, nasal ala, and oral commissures. Eye pads may be applied to protect the eyes. It is wise to perform the initial peel with a 20% SA formulation in order to assess the sensitivity and reactivity of the patient's skin to the peeling agent. Start the peel application with the help of sponge/cotton-tipped applicators/brushes. Begin on a timer, observe the treatment areas at all times, and communicate with the patient regarding any discomfort. Application of peel may be started from the forehead followed by cheeks, chin, nose, and upper lip. Feathering strokes are applied at the edges of the treated area in order to avoid a possible line of demarcation between treated and untreated skin. Inform the patient that he/she will experience mild stinging/burning sensation. Observe the skin for a clinical endpoint. The endpoint for salicylic peel is a white pseudofrost formed as the hydroethanolic vapor evaporates leaving behind a precipitation of SA crystals on the surface of the skin. The penetration of the agent stops once the vehicle has volatilized. At this point, there is no burning or stinging as the agent causes superficial anesthesia to light touch.[11,15] Once pseudofrost appears, apply cool compresses followed by a soothing moisturizer and sunscreen. The desired endpoint of SA peel is pseudofrost and mild erythema. Since SA peels are self-neutralizing, they do not require application of a neutralizing agent.

BOX 4: Equipment required for salicylic peel.

- Prepeel cleanser
- Headband or surgical cap
- Degreasing lotion
- Applicators—cotton-tipped, brushes, and gauze sponges
- Petroleum jelly
- Gloves
- Saline eyewash
- Timer
- Face towels
- Cotton
- Chemical peel
- Dispensing cups
- Neutralizer
- Moisturizer/sunscreen
- Cold compresses

During the procedure, most patients complain of mild burning and a stinging sensation. After 1–3 minutes, some patients may experience anesthesia of the face due to the anesthetic properties of the SA peel. The sensation of burning and stinging can be reduced using a portable handheld fan or ice packs.

Postpeel Care

For the first 48 hours postpeel, bland moisturizers and cleansers are continued or until all postpeel irritation has ceased. Postpeel, the patient is advised to take proper sun protection and apply sunscreen regularly.

Patients can then resume their topical skin care formulations, which may include topical demelanizing agents, topical anti-acne medications, and/or retinoids. Excessive desquamation and irritation in the postpeel period can be treated with low-to-high potency topical steroids.[9] The peels are performed at an interval of 2–4 weeks. Maximal results are achieved with four to six sessions.

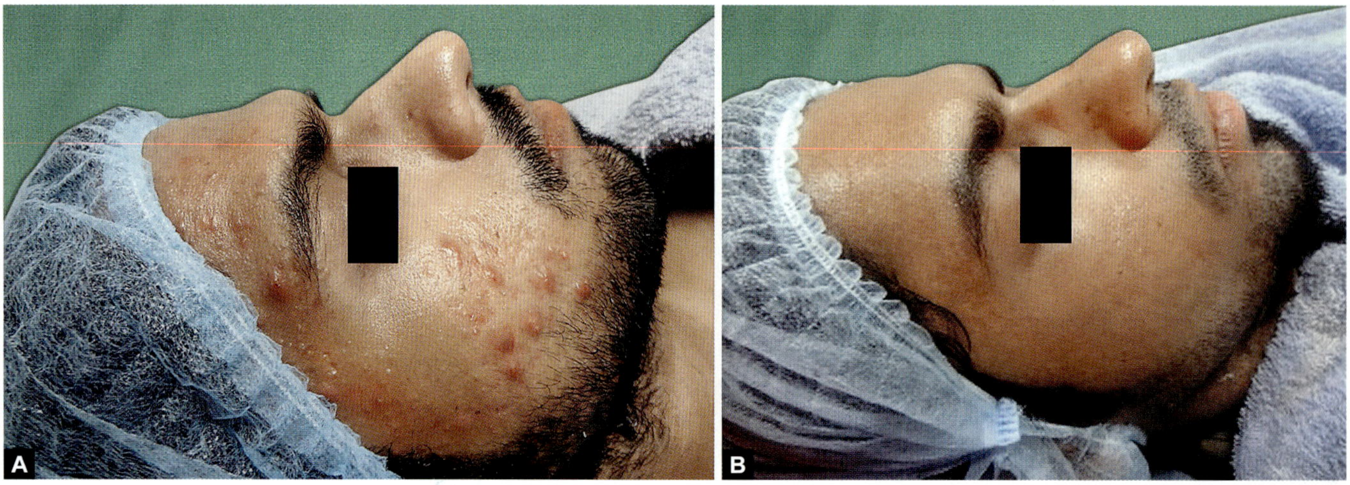

Figs. 2A and B: (A) Before and (B) after four sessions of salicylic peel (30% Sali DS by Sesderma™).

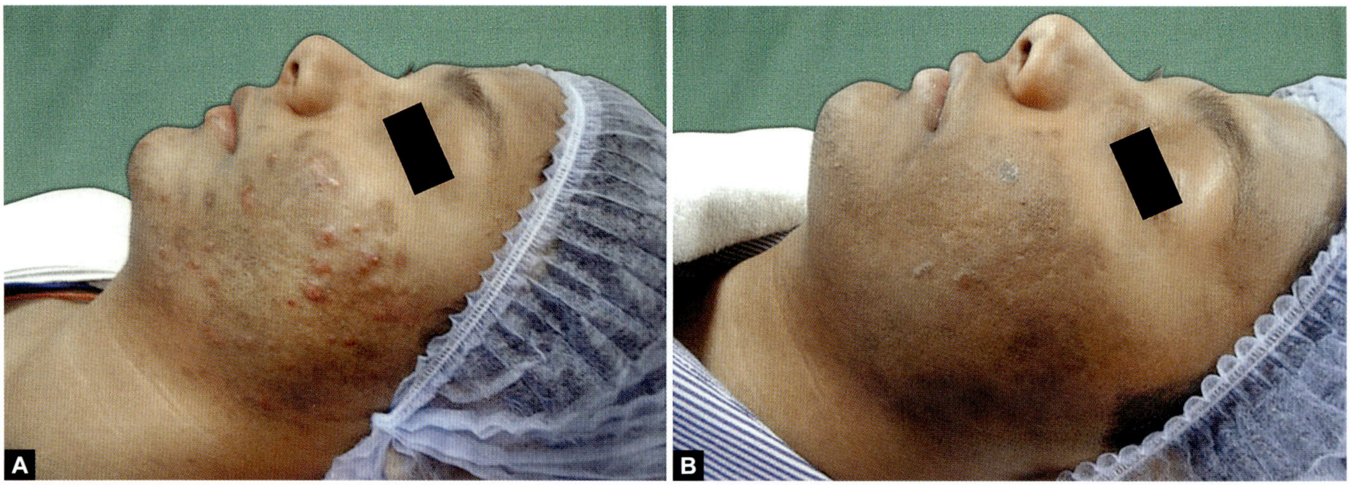

Figs. 3A and B: (A) Before and (B) after five sessions of salicylic peel (30% Sali DS by Sesderma™).

Figures 2 and 3 show before and after images after four and five sessions of salicylic peel, respectively.

Complications[14-18]

Salicylic acid peel is generally a very safe procedure. But inexperience of a dermatosurgeon or the presence of local factors such as active infection or eczema may give rise to complications **(Box 5)**.

The peel solution/soaked applicator should never be passed across the patient's face. If the peel accidentally enters the eyes, the eyes should be copiously flushed with normal saline or water.

Systemic toxicity due to cutaneous absorption is a very rare phenomenon but is a serious concern. In high concentrations, SA is toxic to the central nervous system. SA toxicity may present with nausea, vomiting, dizziness, tinnitus, psychosis, stupor, and consequently coma and death.[19,20,44] Increased labyrinthine pressure can be the cause for tinnitus. Stimulation of the respiratory center in the medulla can occur, leading to hyperventilation and respiratory alkalosis. Systemic absorption of salicylates can affect glucose metabolism and its utilization in cells leading to hypoglycemia, which is mostly seen in patients with uremia.

The advantages and disadvantages of SA peel are shown in **Box 6**.

BOX 5: Complications of salicylic acid peel.

- Pain/discomfort
- Blistering/crusting/desquamation
- Prolonged irritation/erythema
- Hyperpigmentation
- Hypopigmentation
- Excessive dryness
- Milia
- Infections
- Exacerbation of acne/dermatitis
- Allergic reaction
- Scarring
- Contact sensitization
- Salicylism

BOX 6: Advantages and disadvantages of salicylic acid peel.

Advantages:
- Less stinging because salicylic acid (SA) has a mild anesthetic effect
- Visible clinical endpoint (pseudofrost) which ensures even application
- Risk of overpeeling is remote because once the vehicle becomes volatile, which occurs in approximately 2 minutes, there is very little penetration of the active agent
- No requirement of neutralization
- Less downtime
- Can be done on all skin types

Disadvantages:
- More obvious postinflammatory desquamation
- Series of treatments required for best results
- Limited depth of peeling
- Minimal effect in patients with significant photodamage

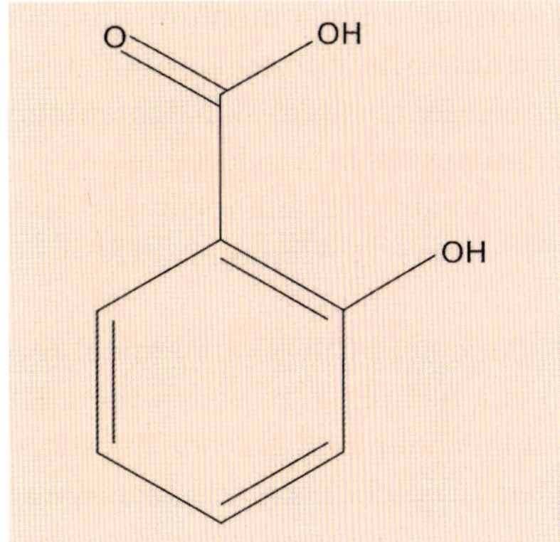

Fig. 4: Structure of trichloroacetic acid.

TRICHLOROACETIC ACID

Introduction

Trichloroacetic acid became popular in the 1960s through the work of Ayres.[20] In 1976, Resnik et al. described the use of TCA in various skin conditions. TCA is a versatile peel which can reach all depths depending on the concentration and number of coats. It is used for superficial as well as medium-depth peels. Lower strength of TCA (10–15%) is used to treat fine lines and dyschromia. Higher strength TCA is used to ameliorate wrinkles. However, it should be used with caution as there is a risk of postinflammatory hyperpigmentation and scarring.[21]

Selection of the appropriate strength of TCA is critical when performing a peel. 10–20% TCA results in a very light superficial peel not penetrating below the stratum granulosum, a strength of 25–35% penetrates full thickness of the epidermis resulting in a light superficial peel, 40–50% results in medium-depth peel injury to the papillary dermis, and >50% results in injury extending to the reticular dermis. The use of TCA above 30% is discouraged except for icepick scars where intentional controlled scarring is desired.

For superficial chemical peels, 10–30% TCA can be used alone or in combination with 10% lactic acid or 15% SA. TCA >40% is known to impart a much greater risk of scarring, pigment dyschromia, and undesired textural change. Also, Fitzpatrick types IV, V, and VI are most prone to developing postinflammatory hyperpigmentation.[22]

After application, TCA causes skin erythema and a whitish discoloration called frosting, which occurs 30 seconds to 2 minutes after application. Histologically, frosting corresponds to coagulation of epidermal proteins and keratinocytes. The intensity of frosting correlates directly with the depth of penetration. The desired endpoint for superficial-depth peels with TCA is level 1 frosting, visible as patchy erythema with faint white discoloration. Coagulation is followed by inflammation and activation of mechanisms of wound repair. This leads to re-epithelialization with replacement of smoother skin with an even skin tone.[23] Medium-depth peels cause collagen modeling, with the production of new collagen in the dermis.

The technique for the application of TCA is very important because the depth of penetration is dependent on the number of coats and the pressure applied. It is usually applied in layers, with a period of 2–3 minutes of observation of clinical endpoints between layers. Neutralization is not required for TCA peels as it is neutralized by serum in superficial dermal blood vessels, but water may be used at the end of treatment to remove the white precipitate. Frosting usually disappears within 1–2 hours and erythema becomes more evident. Erythema may not be seen in dark skin.

Trichloroacetic acid can be applied alone or after use with Jessner's or glycolic peel. Healing time is usually 5–7 days and between 7 and 10 days for patients treated with TCA with Jessner's solution or glycolic acid (GA).

Formulation

Trichloroacetic acid is available as anhydrous, hygroscopic white crystals which are dissolved in distilled water to make a solution. TCA solutions are compounded in a weight-to-volume preparation, and various strengths can be prepared. TCA is stable at room temperature or refrigerated and is not light sensitive and may be stored accordingly. It is hygroscopic so the crystals should be stored in a closed container to limit its absorption of water. Aqueous TCA solution has a shelf-life of 6 months. The structure of TCA is shown in **Figure 4**.

Combination peels with TCA include:
- Brody combination—35% TCA with solid CO_2 ice
- Monheit combination—35% TCA with Jessner's solution
- Coleman combination—35% TCA with 70% GA.

A well-known TCA peel is the Obagi Blue Peel which has TCA 20% peel formulated with a blue-colored base containing glycerin and saponins which slow the penetration and release of TCA in the skin by reducing the surface tension of TCA, water, and glycerin. This results in a homogenous TCA–oil–water solution and provides a gauge to the depth of the peel. A light blue endpoint signifies exfoliation of the papillary dermis, while a medium/dark blue endpoint denotes coagulation to the immediate upper reticular dermis. The lighter procedure results in skin lightening, whereas the deeper procedure results in skin leveling.

Easy TCA is a stabilized, homogenous, and adjuvanted solution with a final TCA concentration of 15% m/m, combined with AHAs , antioxidants, vitamins, and saponins.[25]

Trichloroacetic acid CROSS (chemical reconstruction of skin scars) is a technique in which there is precise and focused spot application of high concentration of TCA into each "pitted" or "icepick" acne scar, avoiding the nonscar areas of normal skin. The resurfacing response that occurs inside the depression stimulates collagen production and increases dermal volume, thereby restructuring the dermal elements within the skin, and this eventually causes the scar to rise up (effacement) and close. TCA CROSS treatments are used alone or in combination with other acne treatments (e.g., fractional laser resurfacing, dermal fillers for rolling atrophic scars, subcision, peels) depending on the severity and type of acne scars they have.

Trichloroacetic acid CROSS technique is a safe, efficacious, cost-effective, and minimally invasive technique for the management of icepick acne scars that are otherwise generally difficult to treat.[19,26]

Indications

The most important indication of TCA peels is photodamaged skin; however, it may be used for a variety of other indications **(Box 7)**.[20]

Contraindications[20]

Trichloroacetic acid peel should not be used in the presence of active infection or eczema. A patient with immediate-type tanning or a recent history of sunburn can develop undesired complications with TCA. The safety of TCA peel in pregnancy and lactation is not established **(Box 8)**.

Prepeel Procedure/Chemical Peel Technique

Trichloroacetic acid peel is performed like other peels. The prepeel preparation is a critical part of the peeling process.

BOX 7: Indications of trichloroacetic acid (TCA) peel.[12,13,24]

- Photoaging
- Textural changes/uneven skin tone
- Seborrheic keratosis/actinic keratosis
- Melasma
- Postinflammatory hyperpigmentation
- Freckles/lentigines
- Frictional melanosis
- Superficial scars
- Keratosis pilaris
- Warts
- Xanthelasma palpebrarum

The endpoint of a TCA peel is frosting **(Table 1)**. Depth of penetration is indicated by the level of frosting. For most indications in darker skin type, TCA should not be used beyond pinpoint or patchy frosting. Once the desired frosting is achieved, it is gently wiped with saline gauze to remove excess acid. The patient is asked to wash his/her face with cold water, followed by the application of moisturizer and sunscreen. The postpeel care is the same as for other peels. **Figures 5A and B** show before and after images after four sessions of TCA peel.

Complications

Complications of TCA peel are the same as for other peels. Medium-depth peel should be done with caution and avoided in patients with keloidal tendency and delayed healing. Pigmentation is a common complication in dark skin types. Deep peels can also cause scarring **(Box 9)**.

A comparative study of 15% TCA peel versus 35% GA peel for the treatment of melasma showed a statistically insignificant difference in the efficacy between the two groups for the treatment of melasma. Another study showed that GA peel is associated with fewer side effects than TCA and has the added advantage of facial rejuvenation.[27,28]

In a study on TCA versus SA in the treatment of acne vulgaris in dark-skinned patients, it was seen that TCA is more superior in treating comedonal lesions, whereas SA is more superior in treating inflammatory lesions without significant difference between their results.[29]

A study showed that superficial peels, such as 70% GA and 15% TCA, proved to be an effective treatment modality for photodamaged facial skin.[30] Microneedling and 10% TCA have been tried for infraorbital dark circles with encouraging results and minor side effects.[31,32]

BOX 8: Contraindications of trichloroacetic acid (TCA) peel.

- Active infection/open wound/dermatitis
- Pregnancy/lactation
- Sunburn or recent suntan
- History of keloid/hypertrophic scar formation
- Impaired healing
- Unrealistic patient expectations
- Body dysmorphic disorder
- Patient on isotretinoin

TABLE 1: Intensity of frosting.[24]

Frosting	*Depth of penetration*	*Clinical findings*
Level I	Superficial	Patchy erythema with patchy white color
Level II	Medium	Even white color with some erythema visible through the white
Level III	Deep	Opaque confluent white

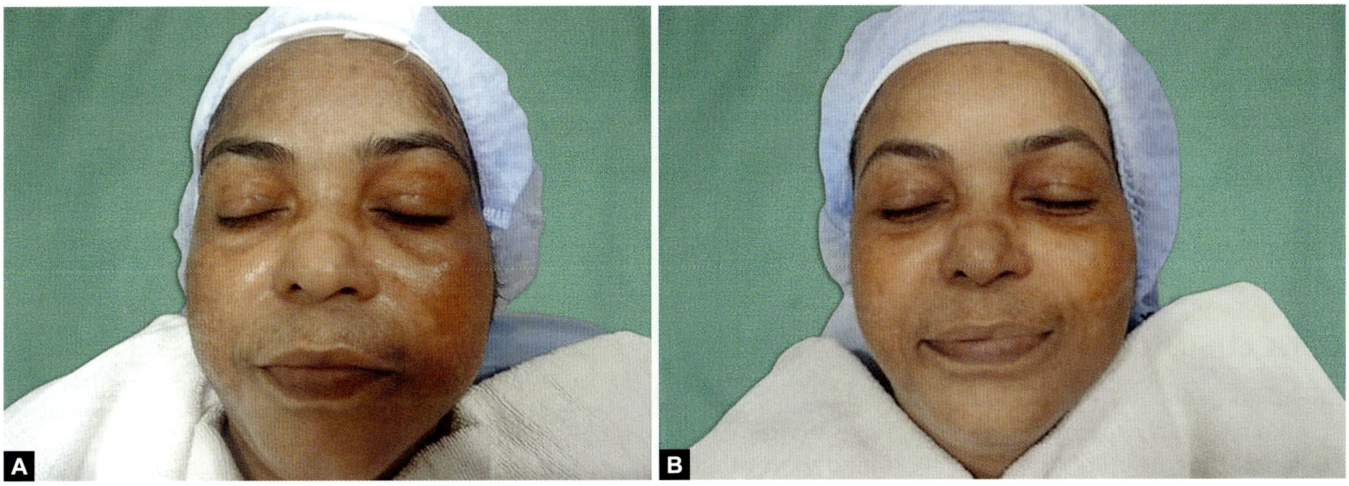

Figs. 5A and B: (A) Before and (B) after four sessions of TCA peel (Easy TCA Basic Protocol by Skintech™). (TCA: trichloroacetic acid)

BOX 9: Complications of trichloroacetic acid (TCA) peel.

- Pain/discomfort
- Crusting/desquamation
- Prolonged irritation/erythema
- Hyperpigmentation
- Hypopigmentation
- Excessive dryness
- Milia
- Blistering/crusting
- Infections
- Exacerbation of acne/dermatitis
- Allergic reaction
- Scarring
- Contact sensitization

JESSNER'S PEEL

Introduction

Jessner's peel is named after Max Jessner, a dermatologist from New York who popularized this peel. The peel became popular in the US army as "Combes peel" after F.C. Combes and was used for the treatment of sun-damaged skin and early actinic keratosis in older field officers. Margaret Ancira is credited with the development of modified Jessner's peel.

Jessner's solution is a superficial peel wherein three keratolytic agents—resorcinol (14 g), SA (14 g), and lactic acid (14 g)—are compounded in ethanol 95% (up to 100 mL).[3] It is a clear, amber-colored solution that needs to be kept in a brown bottle to prevent photooxidation.[2] **Table 2** shows the components of Jessner's peel.

Each constituent of Jessner's solution has specific effects. SA is a lipophilic compound which removes intercellular lipids that are covalently linked to the cornified envelope. Resorcinol is structurally and chemically similar to phenol and disrupts the weak hydrogen bonds of keratin. Lactic acid, an AHA, causes corneocyte detachment and subsequent desquamation of stratum corneum.

TABLE 2: Components of Jessner's peel.

Jessner's peel (Combe's peel)	*Modified Jessner's peel*
Lactic acid (85%)—14 g	Lactic acid—14%
Salicylic acid—14 g	Salicylic acid—17%
Resorcinol—14 g	Citric acid—8%
Ethanol—to make 100 mL	Ethanol—to make 100 mL

Indications

- Acne vulgaris
- Dyschromia
- Photoaging
- Superficial scars
- Benign epidermal growths.

Contraindication

Allergy to resorcinol and salicylates may develop.

Procedure

Following skin preparation, Jessner's solution is applied thinly, with one to three coats depending on the desired depth of penetration. No neutralizing agent is needed. Cool compresses are to be given after washing the face with cold water. The depth of penetration depends on the number of coats and also on the force of application. Instead of a frost, the endpoint is fine, white speckles on an erythematous background. Desquamation occurs over 2–3 days.[33]

Complications

- Allergic reactions
- Systemic toxicity if used over large areas.

Jessner's peel is a relatively safe peel, but it is contraindicated in phototypes IV to VI because of the risk of pigmentary changes. Jessner's solution must be kept in a glass, light-protected sealed bottle. When the solution oxidizes, it turns pink. Contact with the fingernails can turn them orange-yellow.

Modified Jessner's solution (lactic acid 17%, SA 17%, and citric acid 8% in ethanol 95%) without resorcinol, instead of the classic Jessner's solution, can be used to avoid possible allergic reactions and hyperpigmentation problems, which may be created by resorcinol, especially in skin types V and VI.[34]

CONCLUSION

Chemical peels are one of the most common aesthetic procedures which pose minimal risk when performed by educated practitioners. It can be combined with other minimally invasive aesthetic procedures to enhance skin rejuvenation results.[19]

REFERENCES

1. Small R, O'Hanlon K. Chemical Peels in Dermatologic and Cosmetic Procedures in Office Practice. Philadelphia: Saunders; 2012. pp. 259-73.
2. Small R. Aesthetic procedures in office practice. Am Fam Physician. 2009;80(11):1231-7.
3. Kuwahara R, Rsaberry R. (2007). Chemical peels. Emedicine. [online] Available from: https://emedicine.medscape.com/article/1829120-overview [Last accessed September, 2023].
4. Baumann L, Saghari S. Chemical peels. In: Baumann L (Ed). Cosmetic Dermatology: Principles and Practice, 2nd edition. New York: McGraw Hill; 2009. pp. 148-62.
5. Briden ME. Alpha-hydroxy acid chemical peeling agents: case studies and rationale for safe and effective use. Cutis. 2004; 73(2 Suppl):18-24.
6. Kligman AM. Salicylic acid: an alternative to alpha-hydroxy acids. J Geriatr Dermatol. 1997;5:128-31.
7. Yu RJ, Van Scott EJ. Salicylic acid: not a beta-hydroxy acid. Cosmet Derm. 1997;10:27.
8. Arif T. Salicylic acid as a peeling agent: a comprehensive review. Clin Cosmet Investig Dermatol. 2015;8:455-61.
9. Grimes P. Salicylic acid peels. In: Rubin M (Ed). Chemical Peels. Philadelphia: Elsevier; 2006. pp. 47-56.
10. Del Rosso J. Pharmacotherapy update: current therapies and research for common dermatologic conditions. The many roles of topical salicylic acid. Skin Aging. 2005;13:38-42.
11. Vedamurthy M. Salicylic acid peels. Indian J Dermatol Venereol Leprol. 2004;70:136-8.
12. Sacchidanand S, Shetty AB, Leelavathi B. Efficacy of 15% trichloroacetic acid and 50% glycolic acid peel in the treatment of frictional melanosis: a comparative study. J Cutan Aesthet Surg. 2015;8(1):37-41.
13. Monheit GD, Chastian MA. Chemical and mechanical skin resurfacing. In: Bolognia JL, Jorizzo JL, Rapini RP (Eds). Dermatology. Philadelphia: Mosby; 2003.
14. Khunger N. Standard guidelines of care for chemical peels. Indian J Dermatol Venereol Leprol. 2008;74(Suppl):S5-12.
15. Grimes Pearl E. Salicylic acid. In: Antonella T, Grimes Pearl E, Padova D, Pia M (Eds). Color Atlas of Chemical Peels, 2nd edition. New York: Springer; 2012. pp. 49-57.
16. Brackett W. The chemistry of salicylic acid. Cosmet Derm. 1997;10(Suppl 4):5-6.
17. Kinsley M, Metelitsa AI, Somani AK. Chemical peels. In: Wolverton SE (Ed). Comprehensive Dermatologic Drug Therapy, 3rd edition. New York: Elsevier Saunders; 2013.
18. Lee HS, Kim IH. Salicylic acid peels for the treatment of acne vulgaris in Asian patients. Dermatol Surg. 2003;29(12):1196-9.
19. Khunger N, Bhardawaj D, Khunger M. Evaluation of CROSS technique with 100% TCA in the management of Ice Pick Acne scars in darker skin types. J Cosmet Dermatol. 2011;10(1):51-7.
20. Hadly M, Harmon B. Trichloroacetic acid. In: Antonella T, Grimes Pearl E, Padova D, Pia M (Eds). Color Atlas of Chemical Peels, 2nd edition. Springer; 2012. pp.59-67.
21. Paula E, Angela J. Chemexfoliation and superficial skin resurfacing. In: Cheryl M (Ed). Burgress Cosmetic Dermatology. New York: Springer; 2005. pp. 63-82.
22. Leonhardt JM, Lawrence N. Trichloroacetic acid. In: Rubin M (Ed). Chemical Peels. Philadelphia: Elsevier; 2006. pp. 73-86.
23. Deprez P. Trichloroacetic acid: general information, toxicity and formulations. In: Deprez P (Ed). Textbook of Chemical Peels. Florida: CRC Press; 2007. pp. 69-78.
24. Holzer G, Pinkowicz A, Radakovic S, Schmidt JB, Tanew A. Randomized controlled trial comparing 35% trichloroacetic acid peel and 5-aminolevulinic acid photodynamic therapy for the treatment of multiple actinic keratosis. Br J Dermatol. 2017;176(5);1155-61.
25. Deprez P. Easy TCA: basic protocol and skin aging. In: Deprez P (Ed). Textbook of Chemical Peels. Florida: CRC Press; 2007. pp. 109-20.
26. Bhardawaj D, Khunger N. Assessment of the Efficacy and safety of CROSS technique with 100% TCA in the management of ice pick acne scars. J Cutan Aesthet Surg. 2010;3(2):93-6.
27. Puri N. Comparative study of 15% TCA peel versus 35% glycolic acid peel for the treatment of melasma. Indian Dermatol Online J. 2012;3(2):109-13.
28. Kumari R, Thappa DM. Comparative study of trichloroacetic acid versus glycolic acid chemical peels in the treatment of melasma. Indian J Dermatol Venereol Leprol. 2010;76(4):447.
29. Abdel M, Elaziz A, Omar H. Trichloroacetic acid versus salicylic acid in the treatment of acne vulgaris in Dark- Skinned Patients. Dermatol Surg. 2015;41(12):1398-404.
30. Kubiak M, Mucha P, Debowska R, Rotszejn H. Evaluation of 70% glycolic peels versus 15% trichloroacetic peels for the treatment of photodamaged facial skin in aging women. Dermatol Surg. 2014;40(8):883-91.
31. Kontochristopoulos G, Kouris A, Platsidaki E, Markantoni V, Gerodimou M, Antoniou C. Combination of microneedling and 10% trichloroacetic acid peels in the management of infraorbital dark circles. J Cosmet Laser Ther. 2016;18(5): 289-92.
32. Lawrence N, Leonhardt JM. Trichloroacetic acid (TCA) peels. In: Rubin MG, Dover JS, Alam M (Eds). Chemical Peels, 9th edition. Amsterdam: Elsevier Inc; 2006. pp. 77-8.
33. Ekmekçy P, Bostanci S, Gurgey E. The efficacy of chemical peeling performed with Jessner's solution and 35% TCA in the treatment of melasma. Klin J Dermatol. 2001;11:211-6.
34. Safoury OS, Zaki NM, El Nabarawy EA, Farag EA. A study comparing chemical peeling using modified Jessner's solution and 15% trichloroacetic Acid versus 15% trichloroacetic acid in the treatment of melasma. Indian J Dermatol. 2009; 54(1):41-5.

CHAPTER 85

Newer Superficial Peels

Rashmi Sarkar, Pallavi Ailawadi

BOX 1: Newer agents used for superficial chemical peeling.

- Lactic acid
- Mandelic acid
- Azelaic acid
- Pyruvic acid
- Ferulic acid
- Phytic acid
- Arginine
- Retinoic acid
- Obagi blue peel
- Enzyme peels
- Black peels

TABLE 1: Lactic acid (LA) peel.

Indications	*Procedure*	*Remarks*
• Dry or dehydrated skin • Mild acne • Seborrhea • Fine lines and superficial wrinkles • Local peeling for area around the eyes • Striae atrophy of skin	• *Concentration:* 30–90% LA • *Number of coats:* Two coats, applied one over another • *Duration:* 2–10 minutes depending on individual skin features • *End point:* Mild erythema or frosting • *Neutralizer:* Used and is washed off with large amount of cold water	• Gentle peel • Good for sensitive skin • Suitable for both dry and oily skin • Does not cause a strong skin flaking • Does not cause photosensitivity
The first procedure should be performed with low-concentration LA peel and shortest exposure time Some manufacturers offer LA as combination peel with other agents that tend to make it a medium-depth peels rather than superficial. Check the other active ingredients of LA peel solution		

TABLE 2: Azelaic acid (AA) peel.

Indications	*Procedure*	*Remarks*
• Acne and pitted acne scars • Rosacea • Postinflammatory pigmentation • Melasma	• *Concentration:* 15–30% AA with a pH varying from 1.8 to 3 • *Number of coats:* Up to 2 coats • *Duration:* 8–10 minutes • *End point:* Mild erythema • *Neutralization:* Not needed, washed with cold water • Post-peel a sealing cream containing retinol, *Glycyrrhiza* extract, concentrated vitamin E, lactic acid, and other components may be applied for better results	AA does not cause flaking of skin
Commercially available peeling solutions offer AA as a combination peel with include salicylic acid and mandelic acid or other ingredients and can be used effectively for acne		

TABLE 3: Pyruvic acid (PA) peel.

Indications	*Procedure*	*Remarks*
• Mild to moderate acne • Seborrhea • Melasma • Fine lines and wrinkles	• *Concentration:* Starting strength 40% solution, maybe increased to 50% in subsequent sessions • *Number of coats:* Single coat • *Duration:* Short contact time of 2–4 minutes • *End point:* Frosting, erythema and/or severe stinging sensation • *Neutralization:* Used and then washed off with cold water	• Very limited post-peel discomfort • Do not show evident erythema and/or white frost, desquamation
PA is a potent peeling agent and penetrates into the deeper layers. One has to be cautious in using higher concentrations to prevent post-inflammatory hyperpigmentation (PIH) or scarring		

TABLE 4: Ferulic acid peel.

Indications	*Procedure*	*Remarks*
• Fine lines and wrinkles • Mild pigmentary anomalies • Facial rejuvenation	• *Method:* Apply the peel solution and massage it well, leave it for 3–5 minutes and then reapply second coat and massage • *Duration:* Leave on peel, 4–8 hours • *Neutralization:* Not required, washed off with water • Alternatively, the peeling solution can be sealed with a retinol-based cream and washed off after 6–8 hours	• Gentle peel • Does not cause any skin irritation or erythema/frosting or skin flaking • Little/no risk of PIH • Can be used in patients with skin types 5–6 • Can be used as a starting peel before deeper peels are done
It is a useful agent for facial rejuvenation		

TABLE 5: Arginine peel.

Indications	*Procedure*	*Remarks*
• Aging and photoaging • Mild pigmentary anomalies	• *Concentration:* 20% arginine gel peel • *Duration:* 10–20 minutes • *Neutralization:* Removed with water • The peel can be repeated weekly	• Can be used for the area around eyes • Good for patients with sensitive skin intolerant to other peeling agents • Can be performed for the initial preparation of skin for deeper peeling
Arginine is excellently combined with 15–20% lactic acid. This combination enhances the efficiency of the procedure: the stimulation of cellular regeneration increases; removal of skin micro-relief is speeded up; the results of hyperpigmentation control are improved		

TABLE 6: Phytic acid peel.

Indications	*Procedure*	*Remarks*
• Hyperpigmentation • Skin rejuvenation • Fine lines and superficial wrinkles	• Neutralization is not required during the procedure • The peeling solution can be washed off after 1–2 hours in the first few sessions • In subsequent sessions, the peel can be left overnight • In sensitive patients, the peel may be washed off in 10–15 minutes with cold water without neutralization	Post-peel period is characterized by significant flaking and xerosis
Besides phytic acid, special peel solutions often contain a high percentage of glycolic or tartaric acids. These may require neutralization		

TABLE 7: Retinoic acid peel.

Indications	*Procedure*	*Remarks*
• Fine lines and wrinkles • Mild to moderate aging • Comedonal acne • Hyperpigmentation	• *Concentration:* 1–4% • *Number of coats:* 2–3 coats • *End point:* A uniform yellow frost • *Neutralization:* Not required • *Duration:* 7–12 hours, washed off at home • Retinoid-based creams may be applied in post-peel period (after 2 weeks) to increase treatment efficiency • The peel can repeated every fortnight	• Moderate to intense exfoliation may occur after peel • Retinoic acid has photosensitizing potential. Hence, strict sun protection is mandatory • Contraindicated in pregnancy and breastfeeding
Retinoic acid peel is often used in combination with topical vitamin C to enhance the rejuvenating effect and correction of pigmentary anomalies. Topical vitamin C solution is applied first and then the retinoic acid is applied		

TABLE 8: Comparison of different peeling agents at a glance.

Peeling agent	*Salient properties*	*Primary indication*	*Advantages*	*Drawbacks*
Lactic acid	• Powerful moisturizing action • Sebostatic and comedolytic effect	• Dehydrated skin • Mild acne • Seborrhea • Dull uneven skin tone	• Gentle peel • Little or no downtime • Does not cause skin dehydration • Improves deep moisture	Very superficial action hence requires multiple sessions

Contd...

Contd...

Peeling agent	*Salient properties*	*Primary indication*	*Advantages*	*Drawbacks*
Mandelic acid	• Mild comedolytic effect • Bacteriostatic • Anti-inflammatory effect	• Acne and rosacea • Postacne and oily seborrhea	• Good for those with glycolic and retinoic acid intolerance • Useful in combination with salicylic acid	• Require multiple sessions • Used in combination with stronger agents
Azelaic acid	• Antimicrobial effect against *P. acnes* • Reduces hyperpigmentation • Sebostatic action	• Acne and rosacea • Melasma and postacne pigmentation	• Little or no downtime • Potent antimicrobial action • Inhibits tyrosinase activity	Often insufficient as solo peeling agent over repeated sessions
Pyruvic acid	• Strong comedolytic effect • Antimicrobial properties • Stimulates production of production of collagen, elastic fibers	• Acne • Photoaging • Melasma and pigmentary disorders	Medium depth agent which has been found to be effective in acne and photoaging	• Downtime of 2–4 days may be seen • Risk of postinflammatory hyperpigmentation
Ferulic acid	• Strong antioxidant properties • Mild depigmenting effects	• Uneven skin tone • Mild photoaging	Reduces signs of photoaging such as fine wrinkles and promotes even skin tone by reducing hyperpigmentation	• Superficial peel • Multiple sessions are required
Phytic acid	• Significant rejuvenating and lifting effect • Inhibits tyrosinase	• Mild to moderate photoaging • Pigmentary disturbances	• Does not cause any damage to deep epidermal layers • Neutralization is not required	Often combined with other peeling agents, which increase the depth of penetration
Arginine	• Acts on superficial layers alone • Does not penetrate deep	• Early photoaging • Uneven skin tone	• Can be used for the area around eyes • Arginine is excellently combined with lactic acid	Usually used in combination with other peeling agents
Retinoic acid	Regulates the processes of differentiation, proliferation, and intercellular communication	• Skin aging and photoaging • Loss of skin elasticity and strength	Slows down the aging process, improves skin texture with a pronounced rejuvenating and whitening effect	• Prohibited for pregnant and breastfeeding women • Flaking of skin

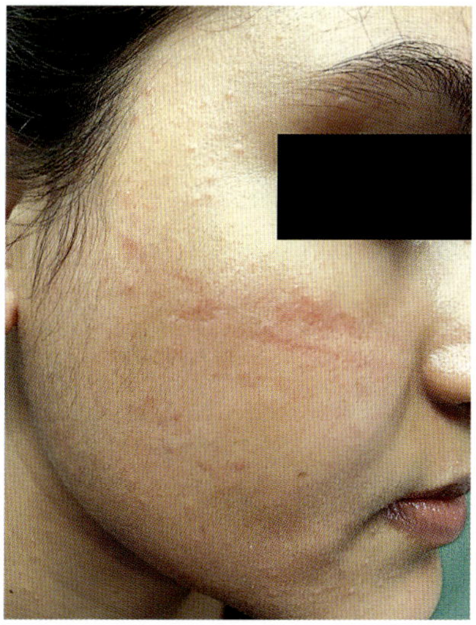

BIBLIOGRAPHY

1. Abdel Hay R, Hegazy R, Abdel Hady M, Saleh N. Clinical and dermoscopic evaluation of combined (salicylic acid 20% and azelaic acid 20%) versus trichloroacetic acid 25% chemical peel in acne: an RCT. J Dermatolog Treat. 2019;30(6):572-7.
2. Chauhan A, Singh S. Comparative Analysis of Efficacy of Lactic Acid with Ferulic Peel (Combination Peel) vs. Ferulic Peel Alone as a Monotherapy for Photoaging. Aesthetic Plast Surg. 2021;45(1):281-8.
3. Chilicka K, Rogowska AM, Szyguła R, Dzieńdziora-Urbińska I, Taradaj J. A comparison of the effectiveness of azelaic and pyruvic acid peels in the treatment of female adult acne: a randomized controlled trial. Sci Rep. 2020;10(1):12612.
4. Cotellessa C, Manunta T, Ghersetich I, Brazzini B, Peris K. The use of pyruvic acid in the treatment of acne. J. Eur. Acad. Dermatol. Venereol. 2004;18(3):275-8.
5. Dayal, S, Kalra, KD, Sahu P. Comparative study of efficacy and safety of 45% mandelic acid versus 30% salicylic acid peels in mild-to-moderate acne vulgaris. J Cosmet Dermatol. 2019;19:393-9.
6. Dayal S, Sangal B, Sahu P. Ferulic acid 12% peel: An innovative peel for constitutional type of periorbital melanosis-Comparing clinical efficacy and safety with 20% glycolic peel and 15% lactic peel. J Cosmet Dermatol. 2020;19(9): 2342-8.
7. Faghihi G, Fatemi-Tabaei S, Abtahi-Naeini B, Siadat AH, Sadeghian G, Ali Nilforoushzadeh M, et al. The Effectiveness of a 5% Retinoic Acid Peel Combined with Microdermabrasion for Facial Photoaging: A Randomized, Double-Blind, Placebo-Controlled Clinical Trial. Dermatol Res Pract. 2017;2017:8516527.
8. Faghihi G, Taheri A, Shahmoradi Z, Nilforoushzadeh MA. Solution of Azelaic Acid (20%), Resorcinol (10%) and Phytic Acid (6%) Versus Glycolic Acid (50%) Peeling Agent in the

Treatment of Female Patients with Facial Melasma. Adv Biomed Res. 2017;6:9.

9. Garg VK, Sinha S, Sarkar R. Glycolic acid peels versus salicylic-mandelic acid peels in active acne vulgaris and post-acne scarring and hyperpigmentation: A comparative study. Dermatol Surg. 2009;35:59-65.
10. Ghersetich I, Brazzini B, Perist K, Cotellessa C, Manunta T, Lotti T. Pyruvic acid peels for the treatment of photoaging. Dermatol Surg. 2004;30(1):32-6.
11. Holland KT, Bojar RA. The effect of azelaic acid on cutaneous bacteria. J Dermatol Treat. 1989;1:17-9.
12. Hong SP, Han SS, Choi SJ, Kim MS, Won CH, Lee MW, et al. Split-face comparative study of 1550 nm fractional photothermolysis and trichloroacetic acid 15% chemical peeling for facial melasma in Asian skin. J Cosmet Laser Ther. 2012;14:81-6.
13. Jaffary F, Faghihi G, Saraeian S, Hosseini SM. Comparison the effectiveness of pyruvic acid 50% and salicylic acid 30% in the treatment of acne. J Res Med Sci. 2016;21:31.
14. Kamila MZ, Helena R. The effectiveness of ferulic acid and microneedling in reducing signs of photoaging: a split-face comparative study. Dermatol Ther. 2020;33(6):e14000.
15. Khunger N, Sarkar R, Jain RK. Tretinoin peels versus glycolic acid peels in the treatment of Melasma in dark-skinned patients. Dermatol Surg. 2004;30:756-60.
16. lknur T, Bicak MU, Demirtasoglu M, Ozkan S. Glycolic acid peels versus amino fruit acid peels in the treatment of melasma. Dermatol Surg. 2010;36(4):490-5.
17. Mokadem S, Al-Aasser O, Nassar A, Al-Sharkawy E. Easy phytic peel as a therapeutic agent in acne vulgaris and melasma. Egypt J Dermatol Venereol. 2013;33:6-11.
18. Nagashima M, Saito K. Antioxidant activity of the new black vinegar "IZUMI". J Nutr Health Aging. 2010;14(10): 845-9.
19. Obagi ZE, Obagi S, Alaiti S, Stevens MB. TCA-based bluepeel: A standardized procedure with depth control. Dermatol Surg. 1999;25(10):773-80.
20. Roberts WE. Chemical peeling in ethnic/dark skin. Dermatol Ther. 2004;17:196-205.
21. Sarkar R, Ghunawat S, Garg VK. Comparative Study of 35% Glycolic Acid, 20% Salicylic-10% Mandelic Acid, and Phytic Acid Combination Peels in the Treatment of Active Acne and Postacne Pigmentation. J Cutan Aesthet Surg. 2019;12(3): 158-63.
22. Sharquie KE, Tikreety MM, Masshadani SA. Lactic acid as a new therapeutic peeling agent in melasma. Dermatol Surg. 2005;31:149-54.
23. Sharquie KE, Tikreety MM, Masshadani SA. Lactic acid chemical peels as a new therapeutic modality in melasma in comparison to Jessner's solution chemical peels. Dermatol Surg. 2006;32:1429-36.
24. Singh R, Goyal S, Ahmed QR, Gupta N, Singh S. Effect of 82% Lactic Acid in Treatment of Melasma. Int Sch Res Notices. 2014;2014:407142.
25. Sumita JM, Leonardi GR, Bagatin E. Tretinoin peel: a critical view. An Bras Dermatol. 2017;92(3):363-6.
26. Szymańska A, Budzisz E, Erkiert-Polguj A. Efficacy of 30% azelaic acid peel in the nonpharmacological treatment of facial acne. J Dermatolog Treat. 2019:1-6.
27. Taylor MB. Summary of mandelic acid for the improvement of skin conditions. Cosmet Dermatol. 1999;12:26-8.
28. Tosson Z, Attwa E, Al-Mokadem S. Pyruvic acid as a new therapeutic peeling agent in acne, melasma and warts. Egyptian Dermatol Online J. 2006;2(2):7.
29. Yildirim S, Gurel MS, Gungor S, Tekeli O, Canat D. Comparison of efficacy of chemical peeling with 25% trichloroacetic acid and 0.1% retinoic acid for facial rejuvenation. Postepy Dermatol Alergol. 2016;33(3):199-205.

SECTION 13 Injectables

CHAPTER 86

Botulinum Toxin: Pharmacology

Rasya Dixit

KEY MESSAGES

- Botulinum toxin remains one of the most popular nonsurgical antiaging therapies in the world.
- Many commercial preparations of botulinum toxin are available. All of them contain toxin type A or B. The different preparations doses are not equivalent and diffusion and effect may vary from preparation to preparation.
- Botulinum toxin is a simple procedure that can be administered in the dermatologists' office. The improvement is gratifying to the performing physician and the patient.

INTRODUCTION

Botulinum toxin is an exotoxin produced by *Clostridium botulinum*, a gram-positive anaerobic bacterium.[1] Botulinum acts as a neurotoxin by inhibiting release of acetylcholine.[2] This is one of the few serendipitous journeys of a drug which was discovered from an agent that was being developed as a bioterror weapon. Today, botulinum toxin remains one of the most popular nonsurgical antiaging therapies in the world.

HISTORY

The recorded history of botulinum toxin started in the 10th century, where deaths were traced due to food poisoning because of the consumption of sausages.[3] These dietary laws possibly indicate the knowledge of life-threatening diseases which were foodborne. It was only in the cases of "sausage poisoning" that systematic research into the disease and the search for the toxin began.

The Napoleonic wars (1795–1813) disrupted the sanitary measures in rural Europe's food production industry.[4] This triggered massive food poisoning-related deaths in Stuttgart, Germany. The source of the food poisoning was traced to smoked blood sausages and the health authorities attributed it to "prussic acid" in the sausages.[3] The term botulism came from the word botulus (Latin for sausages) to describe this disease.[5] Emilie van Ermengem (1851–1922), a microbiologist who trained under Robert Koch, related botulism with a bacterium found in the postmortem tissue of the victims with a bacterium seen in raw pork.[6,7] The bacteria was isolated and named *Bacillus botulinus*,[7] and rechristened *Clostridium botulinum* in later years.

The second world war made the research for the toxin take a macabre turn. At the bequest of the US Government looking for a bioterror weapon, the research was led by Dr Schantz and his colleagues and it was here that the purified crystalline form of the botulinum toxin A was isolated.[8,9]

In 1960s, research on experimental animals showed the effects of botulinum toxin A was at the neuromuscular junctions. Dr Scott, an ophthalmologist who was looking for a treatment of strabismus, tried this toxin to produce a temporary denervation.[10]

Dr Schantz then developed a batch of botulinum toxin A from the Hall strain of *Clostridium botulinum*. This batch was approved by the United States Food and Drug Administration (USFDA) in 1989 for the treatment of facial dystonias. Canadian ophthalmologist Jean Carruthers, in 1987, made an observation in her patients treated for blepharospasm with botulinum toxin type A (BoNTA). The frown lines had markedly disappeared. Together with her dermatologist husband Alistair Carruthers, she had discovered a treatment that would revolutionize the world of medical aesthetics and antiaging treatments.[11] In 1996, and later 1998, the first publications regarding the use of botulinum toxin in medical aesthetic practice came out.[12,13] In 2002, the USFDA approved botulinum toxin for the temporary improvement of glabellar lines associated with procerus or corrugator activity.

PHARMACOLOGY

Synthesis

Clostridium botulinum produces botulinum neurotoxin as a protein complex containing toxin and hemagglutinin and nonhemagglutinin proteins called the neurotoxin-associated proteins (NAPs).[14] Different strains of bacteria produce different types of neurotoxins and associated proteins. There are seven antigenically different serotypes described (A, B, C1, D, E, F, and G). Serotype A is the most potent and only A and B are commercially available.

The active neurotoxin is a relatively inactive molecule of about 150 kDa (a heavy chain of about 100 kDa linked to a light chain of 50 kDa linked by a disulfide bond). This molecule needs to be cleaved by proteases to gain activity. This unique molecule has a metalloprotease enzyme in the light chain, which helps to cleave the protein. The disulfide bond and the NAPs hold the heavy and light chain together. These together make the molecular weight of the injected product, which may determine the distance of diffusion of the toxin from the point of injection.

During the manufacture of neurotoxin for clinical use, the neurotoxin products are manufacturing isolated and purified. This process also removes part of the NAPs. The NAPs may serve critical roles in protecting the neurotoxin against proteolytic enzymes, environmental stress, or pH changes; however, their role in the intramuscular injection is not known. They may protect the neurotoxin core from muscle proteases. Antibodies to the NAPs are described; however, they are non-neutralizing antibodies and do not have an effect on efficacy.[15]

Preparations

Many commercial preparations of botulinum toxin are available. All of them contain toxin type A or B. The different preparations doses are not equivalent and diffusion and effect may vary from preparation to preparation. The physicians are advised to refer to dose recommendation for individual preparations appropriately **(Table 1)**.

Mechanism of Action

Following intramuscular injection, botulinum toxin blocks the release of acetylcholine from the presynaptic nerve terminal. This causes a chemical denervation of the muscle. Muscle function returns after 12 weeks when the new nerve terminals sprout and establish reconnection with the muscle endplate, ending the clinical effect of the toxin. This is why the effect of botulinum toxin is not permanent.

Blocking the acetylcholine release is a multistep process which includes binding to the nerve terminals, internalization, translocation and cleavage, the toxin exerts its inhibition on neuromuscular junction of smooth and striated muscle, and the autonomic nerve terminals that innervate glands.

The 150 kDa neurotoxin is in association with the NAPs, as both are simultaneously produced by the bacteria. During injection, when the saline is added to the lyophilized toxin in the vial, a dissociation of the neurotoxin and NAPs occurs almost instantaneously, as a function of pH and ionic strength **(Flowchart 1)**.[16,17]

Recovery of the neurotransmitter release at the neuromuscular junction occurs over a period of 4–6 months. The inactive muscles send growth factors signal to the nerve. Neuronal sprouts appear at the motor nerve terminals and have been noted as early as 48 hours after botulinum toxin injection. They elongate and establish a rudimentary synapse with the affected muscle. Over time, complete activity returns to the neuromuscular junction. This return in function signals the end of clinical result.[22]

Immunology

Botulinum toxin is now used in treatment of various conditions, and the need for long-term results, calls for the use of repeated treatments. The toxin is a protein and on repeated exposure, it stimulates antibody response. This is a limitation to repeat botulinum toxin. However, the incidence of antibody formation is low.

Two types of antibodies have been described to botulinum toxin, neutralizing antibodies (which affect the efficacy of the repeat treatment) and non-neutralizing antibodies.

TABLE 1: Commercial preparations of botulinum toxin.

	Botox®	*Botox® cosmetic*	*Dysport®*	*Neuronox®*	*Xeomin®*	*PurTox®*	*MyoBloc®*
Company	Allergan	Allergan	Ipsen Inc	Medytox Inc	Merz	Mentor Corp	Elan/Solstice
Type	Type A	Type A	Type A	Type A	Type A	Type A	Type B
Neurotoxin product	Onabotulinum-toxinA	Onabotulinum-toxinA	Abobotuli-numtoxinA	OnabotulinumtoxinA	Incobotuli-numtoxinA		Rimabotuli-numtoxinB
Approvals	In over 75 countries, including US and Canada	In over 16 countries, including US, Canada, Italy, and France	Germany, other European countries	In over 50 countries, including Korea and India and Southeast Asian and European countries	Germany and other European countries	None (phase III trials for glabellar lines, phase I for spasmodic torticollis)	US and Canada
Strength of action	1:1	1:1	1:2–1:4	1:1	1:1	1:1.5	1:52
Units/vial	100	100/50	300/500	100	100	–	2,500, 5,000, 10,000
Reconstitution	0.9% NaCl	0.9% NaCl	0.9% NaCl	0.9% NaCl	0.9% NaCl	0.9% NaCl	Liquid formulation
Storage	2°–8° C or <5°C	2°–8°C or <5°C	2°–8°C	2–8°C	25°C	–	

Flowchart 1: Mechanism of action.

Binding to the nerve terminals

The heavy chain of the toxin binds irreversibly to the dual receptors [ganglioside receptor and secretory vesicle protein 2 (SV2)] on the cholinergic neurons.[18] The ganglioside receptor binds the heavy chain of the botulinum toxin, and during exocytosis, the intravesicular portion of SV2 offers a exposed surface for binding of botulinum toxin type A. Synaptotagmins I and III have been identified as the coreceptors for botulinum toxin B and C[19]

↓

Internalization and translocation

The toxin-receptor complex is translocated into the neuronal cytosol by endocytosis. Inside the endocytotic vesicles, the neurotoxin structure undergoes a conformational change in the presence of a low pH by the presence of proton pumps in the endocytosomal wall.[20] The disulfide bond between the two chains is cleaved and the toxin escapes into the cytoplasm of the neuron through the lipid bilayer of the endosome

↓

Cleavage

The light chain then cleaves one or more of the SNARE (Soluble NSF attachment protein receptor) proteins. The SNARE proteins are responsible for neurotransmitter (acetylcholine) release. Different botulinum toxin serotypes have distinct SNARE protein targets. For example, BoNTA cleaves synaptosomal-associated protein (SNAP 25), BoNTB cleaves synaptobrevin or vesicle-associated membrane-protein (VAMP)[21]

(BoNTA: botulinum toxin type A; BoNTB: botulinum toxin type B)

The formation of the neutralizing antibodies have been found to depend on the following factors:

- *Genetic tendency:* The pattern of neutralizing antibody formation varies between patients and targets the regions binding to the receptors on the nerves. This causes a blocking of the binding of the toxin to the neuron. Patients develop antibodies to the different portions of the toxin molecule, underscoring a genetic role in antibody development.[23]
- *Manufacturing methods and formulation:* The 150 kDa part of botulinum toxin which is produced by the bacteria, though inactive is immunogenic. This inactive antigen needs to be kept as a minimum during the manufacturing process to keep the antigenicity low.[24] To become activated, botulinum toxins are cleaved by the use of a protease, which produces the two peptides. Botulinum toxin A is approximately 95% nicked endogenously before it is released from the cell; however, botulinum B proteins are not nicked endogenously. Botulinum B goes through more exposure to proteases during the manufacturing process. Despite this, 20–25% of product may stay inactive. This may explain the higher immunogenicity with botulinum toxin B.[25]
- *Cosmetic versus noncosmetic treatments:* The need for lower doses in cosmetic treatments possibly lowers the risk of formation of neutralizing antibodies.[26]
- *Difference in the formulations:* Studies in cervical dystonia and spasticity show development of antibodies using abobotulinum toxin showed neutralizing antibody formation up to 3–4% in a long-term dystonia study with three to four treatments.[27] Antibody formation to rimabotulinumtoxinB for the treatment of cervical dystonia was reported at 10% after 1 year and 18% after 2 years.[28] Antibody formation to incobotulinum toxin has not yet been reported.
- *Frequency and dose of toxin:* Greene et al. postulated that large doses of BoNTA (>250 U) and repeated "booster" injections could lead to development of antibodies. This is understandable because resistance is more common in patients receiving larger doses of toxin for the treatment of cervical dytonias than those being treated for blepharospasms.[29] Lange et al. reported that in secondary nonresponders with a frequency between injections <2 months showed higher levels of neutralizing antibodies than those with an injection frequency between 4 and 13 months.[30]

After the development of neutralizing antibodies, a sustained benefit to that serotype is rarely experienced by the patient.[31] The evaluation of the nonresponders should be differentiated into primary clinical nonresponders (who do not respond from the first treatment) and secondary nonresponders. The causes of secondary nonresponse should be carefully evaluated. Some patients may feel the results of the second session were not as dramatic as the first. Errors in toxin preparation, storage, reconstitution and transport, injection into the wrong muscle, and inadequate dosing could also be the cause of secondary nonresponse and should be carefully evaluated as they may be experiencing less dramatic effects than the first session. After all these have been carefully considered, the presence of neutralizing antibodies should be considered. Clinical response to incobotulinumtoxinA, after demonstrating loss of clinical response to onabotulinumtoxinA and rimabotulinumtoxinB has been reported.[32] So, a change in the toxin molecule can be considered in secondary nonresponders.

Dilution and Storage

Here, the dilution and storage of the most commonly used molecule are discussed. Other toxins have to be used and stored as the manufacturer indicates. BOTOX® is available as in 50 U and 100 U and packaged as lyophilized sterile vials. It has to be stored in a freezer at or below –5°C.

Different specialists use a 1–4 mL dilution per 100 units of BOTOX® with sterile saline. More dilute concentration increases the area of spread of toxin effects, whereas lower volumes of dilution are recommended in areas where migration into neighboring areas causes undesirable side effects.[33,34]

The efficacy of BOTOX® is dependent on how it is reconstituted. Bubbling or agitation during the injection of diluent into the vial may denature the product; gently introduce the diluent onto the inside wall of the vial. The diluent is drawn into the vial gently by the vacuum inside the vial.

Once reconstituted, BOTOX® is stored at 2–8°C in a refrigerator and used within 4 hours. Studies showing no loss of activity after 6 hours at room temperature are available; however, most practitioners discard unused reconstituted BOTOX® after 1–7 days.[16]

Therapeutic Uses

The following cosmetic conditions have been treated with botulinum toxin. Newer and noncosmetic indications are listed in **Tables 2 to 4**.

TABLE 2: Cosmetic indications of botulinum toxin.

Dynamic forehead lines	Gummy smile
Glabellar lines	Masseter hypertrophy
Crow's feet	Nefertiti lift
Bunny lines	Nasal flare
Perioral wrinkles	Popley chin
Platysmal bands	Brow lift

TABLE 3: Noncosmetic indications of botulinum toxin.

Axillary, palmoplantar hyperhidrosis	Strabismus, nystagmus
Focal dystonia: Cervical, blepharospasm, laryngeal dystonia	*Chronic pain and disorders of muscle spasms*: Tension headache, chronic migraine
Spasticity: Cerebral palsy, stroke	*Smooth muscle hyperactive disorders*: Neurogenic bladder, achalasia cardia, Raynaud's phenomenon
Nondystonic disorders: Tremors, tics, hemifacial spasm, bruxism, trismus	Frey's syndrome

TABLE 4: Contraindications of botulinum toxin.

Absolute contraindications	*Relative contraindications*
Prior allergic reactions to toxin	*Neuromuscular disorders*: Myasthenia gravis, Eaton–Lambert syndrome
Infection over injection site	Coagulation defects
Pregnancy: Category C	Patient on aminoglycosides, penicillamine, quinine (interfere with neuromuscular transmission and potentiate the effect of toxin)
Lactation	
Unrealistic expectations	

CONCLUSION

Botulinum toxin is a simple procedure that can be administered in the dermatologists' office. The improvement is gratifying to the performing physician and the doctor. A good understanding of the anatomy and the pharmacology forms the basis for great results.

REFERENCES

1. Simpson LL. The origin, structure, and pharmacological activity of botulinum toxin. Pharmacol Rev. 1981;33(3):155-88.
2. Abbruzzese G, Berardelli A. Neurophysiological effects of botulinum toxin type A. Neurotox Res. 2006;9(2-3):109-14.
3. Erbguth FJ. Historical notes on botulism, *Clostridium botulinum*, botulinum toxin, and the idea of the therapeutic use of the toxin. Mov Disord. 2004;19(Suppl 8):S2-6.
4. Erbguth FJ, Naumann M. Historical aspects of botulinum toxin: Justinus Kerner (1786-1862) and the 'sausage poison.' Neurology. 1999;53(8):1850-3.
5. Torrens JK. *Clostridium botulinum* was named because of association with 'sausage poisoning.' BMJ. 1998;316(7125):151.
6. Gunn RA. Botulism: from van Ermengem to the present. A comment. Rev Infect Dis. 1979;1(4):720-1.
7. van Ermengem E. Classics in infectious diseases. A new anaerobic bacillus and its relation to botulism. (Originally published as 'Ueber einen neuen anaeroben Bacillus und seine Beziehungen zum Botulismus' in Zeitschrift fur Hygiene und Infektionskrankheiten 26:1-56;1897). Rev Infect Dis. 1979;1(4):701-19.
8. Sotos JG. Botulinum toxin in biowarfare. JAMA. 2001; 285(21):2716.
9. Lamb A. Biological weapons: the facts not the fiction. Clin Med. 2001;1(6):502-4.
10. Scott AB, Rosenbaum A, Collins CC. Pharmacologic weakening of extraocular muscles. Invest Ophthalmol. 1973;12(12):924-7.
11. Carruthers A, Kiene K, Carruthers J. Botulinum A exotoxin use in clinical dermatology. J Am Acad Dermatol. 1996;34(5 Pt 1):788-97.
12. Carruthers A, Carruthers J. History of the cosmetic use of Botulinum A exotoxin. Dermatol Surg. 1998;24(11):1168-70.
13. Jankovic J, Brin MF. Botulinum toxin: historical perspective and potential new indications. Muscle Nerve Suppl. 1997;6:S129-45.
14. Brin MF. Botulinum toxin: chemistry, pharmacology, toxicity, and immunology. Muscle Nerve Suppl. 1997;6:S146-68.
15. Kukreja RV, Singh BR. Comparative role of neurotoxin-associated proteins in the structural stability and endopeptidase activity of botulinum neurotoxin complex types A and E. Biochemistry. 2007;46(49):14316-24.
16. Huang W, Foster JA, Rogachefsky AS. Pharmacology of botulinum toxin. J Am Acad Dermatol. 2000;43(2 Part 1):249-59.
17. Eisele KH, Fink K, Vey M, Taylor HV. Studies on dissociation of botulinum neurotoxin Type A complexes. Toxicon. 2011;57(4):555-65.
18. Rummel A. Double receptor anchorage of botulinum neurotoxins accounts for their exquisite neurospecificity. Curr Top Microbiol Immunol. 2013;364:61-90.
19. Peng L, Tepp WH, Johnson EA, Dong M. Botulinum neurotoxin D uses synaptic vesicle protein SV2 and gangliosides as receptors. PLoS Pathog. 2011;7(3):e1002008.

20. Yamashiro DJ, Fluss SR, Maxfield FR. Acidification of endocytic vesicles by an ATP-dependent proton pump. J Cell Biol. 1983;97(3):929-34.
21. Sikorra S, Henke T, Galli T, Binz T. Substrate recognition mechanism of VAMP/Synaptobrevin-cleaving neurotoxins. J Biol Chem. 2008;283(30):21145-52.
22. de Paiva A, Meunier FA, Molgó J, Aoki KR, Dolly JO. Functional repair of motor endplates after botulinum neurotoxin type A poisoning: biphasic switch of synaptic activity between nerve sprouts and their parent terminals. Proc Natl Acad Sci USA. 1999;96(6):3200-5.
23. Dolimbek BZ, Steward LE, Aoki KR, Atassi MZ. Regions of recognition by blocking antibodies on the light chain of botulinum neurotoxin A: antigenic structure of the entire toxin. Immunobiology. 2011;216(6):698-706.
24. Jankovic J, Vuong KD, Ahsan J. Comparison of efficacy and immunogenicity of original versus current botulinum toxin in cervical dystonia. Neurology. 2003;60(7):1186-8.
25. Jankovic J, Hunter C, Dolimbek BZ, Dolimbek GS, Adler CH, Brashear A, et al. Clinico-immunologic aspects of botulinum toxin type B treatment of cervical dystonia. Neurology. 2006;67(12):2233-5.
26. Carruthers A, Carruthers J, Lowe N, Menter A, Gibson J, Nordquist M, et al.; for the BOTOX glabellar lines I & II study groups. One-year, randomised, multicenter, two-period study of the safety and efficacy of repeated treatments with botulinum toxin type a in patients with glabellar lines. J Clin Res. 2004;7:1-20.
27. Zuber M, Sebald M, Bathien N, de Recondo J, Rondot P. Botulinum antibodies in dystonic patients treated with type A botulinum toxin: frequency and significance. Neurology. 1993;43(9):1715-8.
28. Myobloc®. Prescribing information. South San Francisco: CA: Solstice Neurosciences, Inc.; 2004.
29. Greene P, Fahn S, Diamond B. Development of resistance to botulinum toxin A in patients with torticollis. Mov Disord. 1994;9(2):213-7.
30. Lange O, Bigalke H, Dengler R, Wegner F, deGroot M, Wohlfarth K. Neutralizing antibodies and secondary therapy failure after treatment with botulinum toxin type A: much ado about nothing? Clin Neuropharmacol. 2009;32(4):213-8.
31. Dressler D, Munchau A, Bhatia KP, Quinn NP, Bigalke H. Antibody-induced botulinum toxin therapy failure: can it be overcome by increased botulinum toxin doses? Eur Neurol. 2002;47(2):118-21.
32. Ramos VF, Karp BI, Lungu C, Alter K, Hallett M. Clinical response to incobotulinumtoxinA, after demonstrated loss of clinical response to onabotulinumtoxinA and rimabotulininumtoxinB in a patient with musician's dystonia. Mov Disord Clin Pract. 2014;1(4):383-5.
33. Carruthers JD, Carruthers JA. Treatment of glabellar frown lines with C. botulinum-A exotoxin. J Dermatol Surg Oncol. 1992;18(1):17-21.
34. Hsu TS, Dover JS, Arndt KA. Effect of volume and concentration on the diffusion of botulinum exotoxin A. Arch Dermatol. 2004;140(11):1351-4.

CHAPTER 87

Botulinum Toxin for the Upper Face

Pradeep Kumari

KEY MESSAGES

- Upper face is the most commonly treated area and usually the first treatment for a patient.
- Safety in this area is good by following basic simple principles of asepsis so often, this is the first injectable treatment for the practitioner too.
- Focus on assessing the patient fully before deciding on dosage and target a softer natural look instead of going overboard. Treatment outcome is centered around creating a softer and natural look.
- There are various formulations available of botulinum neurotoxins type A (BoNT-A), and a number of units mentioned here in this chapter correspond to onabotulinum toxin A (ONA)/incobotulinum toxin A (INCO), using standard reconstitution volume of 2.5 mL preserved/nonpreserved normal saline. The units for abobotulinum toxin A (ABO) are different and a conversion ratio of 1 ONA:2.5 ABO or 1 ONA:3 ABO is used in upper face BoNT-A indications.

INTRODUCTION

The role of BoNT-A in the field of aesthetic as well as various nonaesthetic minimally invasive procedures first started with a report in 1989, where facial asymmetry was corrected using BoNT-A.[1]

This was followed by a study on the safety and efficacy of BoNT-A in 18 patients to treat glabellar frown lines by Carruthers and Carruthers.[2] Over the last 30 years, the use of BoNT-A injection has increased consistently and it has remained the most common cosmetic procedure done globally in injectables and surgeries. Currently, there is a rapidly growing huge list of BoNT-A indications in dermatology as well as other clinical medicine fields. BoNT exerts a specific inhibitory action on cholinergic synapses, and thus can be used for disorders of glandular hyperactivity as well as any hyperkinetic movement disorder. Today, these indications are also supported by a broad literature base.[3]

The first approval for aesthetic indications of BoNT was in 2002 for glabellar rhytids by the US Food and Drug Administration (FDA) and post that multiple indications have been approved in addition to continued usage in multiple off-label indications.[4]

The U S FDA also has mandated, 2009 onward, to mention nonproprietary names for each type of BoNT-A for approved products.[5] This helps clarify that these are different products and have unique chemical and pharmacological properties, and thus their doses are not interchangeable and have different dose–response curves.

Some of the current popular formulations available and in use are as follows:

- *Onabotulinum toxin A (ONA):* Botox Cosmetic, Vistabel, Vistabex, and Botox Vista
- *Abobotulinum toxin A (ABO):* Dysport and Azzalure
- *Incobotulinum toxin A (INCO):* Xeomin, Xeomeen, and Bocouture
- *Prabotulinum toxin A:* Nabota

These products have a similar mechanism of action, but there are chemical differences and their production and method of purification are specific to each manufacturer. Thus, they have different potency units and are not interchangeable.[6]

The potency unit is defined as mouse LD50 by the intraperitoneal route and determined by each company in their own proprietary assay. Another difference in these formulations is the amount of neurotoxin in each individually packed vial and the amount of human albumin in the product. For example, Botox has 0.73 ng neurotoxin per 100-unit vial, Dysport has 3.24 ng per 500-unit vial, and Xeomin has 0.44 ng per 100-unit vial.[7]

There are multiple studies that state conversion factors between various products, and a conversion ratio for ONA:ABO of 1:2 is considered appropriate.[8] In a further study by the same investigator, a change in the conversion ratio of 1:2.5 for ONA:ABO showed significantly different fields of effect, making it clear that a change in dose would change diffusion effect.[9] Incobotulinum toxin A has been shown to have comparable efficacy and a 1:1 conversion ratio with ONA.

A clear understanding of these product differences along with a thorough knowledge of muscle physiology and anatomy can take the process of BoNT-A injections to a satisfying and rewarding procedure for both the injector and the patient. To achieve the desired clinical outcome and avoid complications, the first focus is a good consultation and preprocedure assessment.

PREPROCEDURE ASSESSMENT AND COUNSELING

A comprehensive examination happens at three stages—history taking, formal examination, and final preprocedural assessment. A good examination should include both static and examination as the target tissue, which here is muscle. The most accurate dynamic assessment is when the patient and physician are talking and the panfacial muscle movement shows and this helps seeing the additional muscles being recruited by patient for their emotions in addition to the main muscles. Animation on command during formal examination may not always show the entirety of muscle action and recruitment. Thus, it is crucial to establish good patient–physician rapport.

The dialog during the consultation should include a discussion on patient expectations, beginning and duration of effect postinjections, mention of any specific preferences regarding the nature of results, and possible adverse effects. Verbal education should be supplemented with visual aids, pre–post pictures showing full efficacy, and decreased dosage.

The next step of formal examination should include preoperative photography both at rest and in animation of the target muscle. Validated wrinkle classification and rating scales[10,11] and software programs that depict age-related changes can be used to improve the assessment and explanation[12] further.

In a panfacial context, individual muscle mass, anatomy, and contraction patterns can guide appropriate toxin dosing and avoid adverse events, and palpation of muscles in contraction helps notice these patterns as well as assess muscle mass.[13-15]

During the preassessment or consultation, a brief overview of timeline of procedure should also be offered to the patient. In general, the effect starts as early as 6 hours, maximizes at 7–14 days, and lasts for 2.5–6 months in upper face. This time of onset of response as well as duration of activity are also important markers of efficacy of BoNT-A and also may be related to individual patient genetics, muscle mass, absolute units injected, and injection technique.[16]

Some patients may be aware of improvement in wrinkles within 1 day of procedure, and muscle function generally returns for most patients at 3–6 months.[17]

Younger patients are likely to achieve complete amelioration of any visible rhytids and also prevent rhytids. In older age group, loss of skin elasticity may require a multimodality approach and sometimes lower doses are chosen in older patients in spite of greater visible rhytids because of changing muscle mass/function with age. It is important to discuss the original objective as complete paralysis (frozen look) with a general trend nowadays to modulate activity (natural look) leading to a more natural appearance with decreased dosage as well as increased injection interval.[18]

Patients can be divided into three different groups based on muscle activity level—kinetic, hyperkinetic, and hypertonic:[19]

1. *Kinetic patients:* Regular muscle contraction and wrinkles during active expression but not at rest
2. *Hyperkinetic patients:* They have excessive muscle contractions. These patients are likely to require higher doses and more frequent treatment.
3. *Hypertonic patients:* Some muscles do not relax at all and thus show wrinkles at rest.

Patients should also be made aware of possible adverse effects including unexpected muscle weakness, injection site reactions, or bleeding or bruising. It is advisable to explain the increased risk of a bleed or bruise to patients on anticoagulants and blood thinners instead of stopping/pausing essential life-saving medication.[20]

STANDARD GUIDELINES FOR THE USE OF BOTULINUM NEUROTOXINS TYPE A

Dilution/Storage/Trolley Preparation

The current popular preparations come as freeze-dried powder formulations in vials and need reconstitution before the procedure. For a 100-unit vial, reconstitution is done with 2.5 mL normal saline for ONA/INCO; 2.5 mL dilution makes it very easy to calculate the number of units while withdrawing and injecting as each marking of a 40 unit/mL insulin syringe will contain 1 unit of BoNT.

Usually, manufacturer's guidelines recommend unpreserved saline because of the risk of denaturation of protein with preservatives leading to reduced potency.

Ideally, reconstitution of vial and filling of injection syringes should be done on a sterile surface. After removing the upper cover, exposed rubber should be cleaned with 70% alcohol. Allow this alcohol to evaporate before puncturing the vial. The saline gets drawn in the vial because of negative pressure automatically.

The vial can be gently swirled to dissolve the entire toxin into solution. Once full dissolution has happened, it can be withdrawn into a 31G insulin syringe for injection. Insulin syringes should only be filled with a precalculated amount of units sufficient for two to three punctures or injections. This takes care of keeping the needle sharp and thus making the injection comfortable for the patient. Care should also be taken to pass the needle only through the central thin part of stopper and not touch the vial wall or thick portion of the rubber stopper to avoid needle tip damage as it can make injection painful.

Once withdrawn for injection, under no circumstances should the unused BoNT be pushed into vial to maintain sterility. Recent recommendations allow storage in refrigerator for up to 4 weeks postreconstitution without significant contamination or loss of potency, provided appropriate handling is done, thus allowing usage in multiple patients.[21]

Some injectors may prefer a higher reconstitution amount and hence more injection volume per unit for greater spread. It may, however, make the injection more painful and the injection site may be more visible to others for a longer duration when compared to standard reconstitution.

Injection/Marking

Any procedure involving a breach of the skin surface should always be done with full sterile precautions.

It is a good practice to set up the sterile tray with necessary items such as cleansing agents, antiseptics, sterile gloves, sterile gauze, expected number of syringes, and any other expected items such as reconstitution normal saline **(Fig. 1)**.

From a preparation perspective on patient skin, it is important to remove all makeup and dirt. A headband should be applied to avoid hair coming in the area of injection, once it is sterilized.

Meticulous sterile preparation of skin before injection should be done, and sterile injection technique of not touching any nonsterile items in a sterilized area should be followed to minimize chances of contamination.

In general, two steps of cleansing with a cleansing lotion to help remove dirt, dust, topical anesthetic, etc., and then antisepsis with alcohol swab are followed by most injectors. While using alcohol, exert caution that it is not splashed/sprayed/goes inside eye as alcohol is extremely irritant to cornea. Chlorhexidine has been reported to cause chemical burns on cornea leading to keratitis.

Marking of injection sites is an individual choice, and if being done, things to remember are marking before antisepsis and ensuring that injection should never go through the marks. Marking is traditionally done with a white marker. Another way of marking poststerilizing the area is to do marking with antibacterial cream. Marking helps keep the track of sequence and dose of injections if the process gets interrupted.

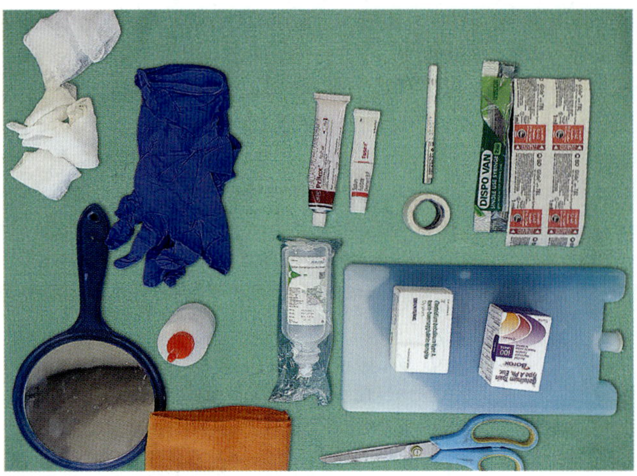

Fig. 1: Trolley preparation.

Injection Techniques

Various techniques described in the literature for injection of BoNT-A are as follows:
- Direct injection
- Two-level injection
- Intradermal wheal technique
- Directed injection
- Electromyograph (EMG)-guided injection

Out of these, only first three are relevant to face injections, and most time, direct injection in muscle belly and intradermal wheal technique get employed. Two-level injections can be used in case of thick muscles such as masseter.

Injector can choose to inject either while standing or while sitting. It is a good practice to keep the needle always away from vital structures such as eyes. The syringe should be held between index and middle fingers with the thumb kept free for placement on plunger for actual injection. The noninjecting hand can be used to directly place on patient skin to either stretch skin for a smoother injection or to provide support to injecting hand.

Steps in Summary

- Do a thorough consultation and assess facial expressions at rest, in dialog, and during animation.
- Evaluate the range of motion for target muscles.
- Evaluate any asymmetries, share with patient, and document these. Also, share the plan to keep asymmetry at the current level or improve symmetry.
- Conduct a final history to look for contraindications and additional precautions to be exerted.
- Take preprocedure photographs of the area to be treated and an informed consent.

Beginners should initially start with the recommended dosage and should make special efforts to follow safety guidelines for the area to be treated. The aim should be to provide a more natural look, and additional injection sites can be done at 10–14-day follow-up if needed.

Patients may resume activities after 4 hours. There is no need to move or avoid moving the muscle that are injected. General strategies to prevent complications mainly come from following sterile precautions and assessing actual muscle movement.[22]

With this baseline, now, we will take up a detailed description of individual face areas.

GLABELLAR REGION/COMPLEX

Glabellar complex is a medial brow depressor and includes the following muscles **(Fig. 2)**:
- *Procerus:* This originates from fascia of the lower nasal bone and inserts into the skin between eyebrows. Procerus is the depressor of the medial aspect of eyebrows and produces a transverse line across the nasal bridge.

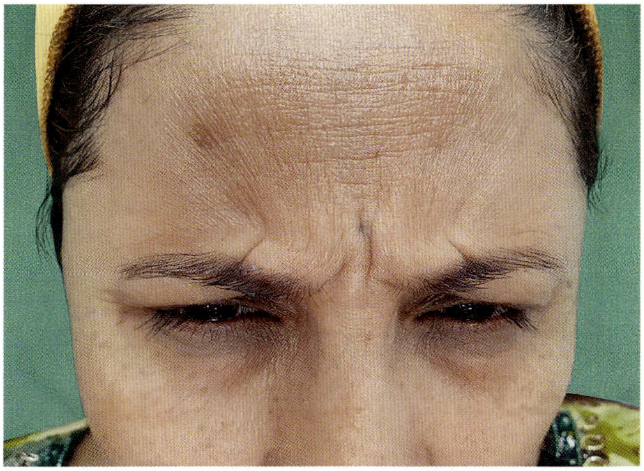

Fig. 2: Glabellar complex muscle.

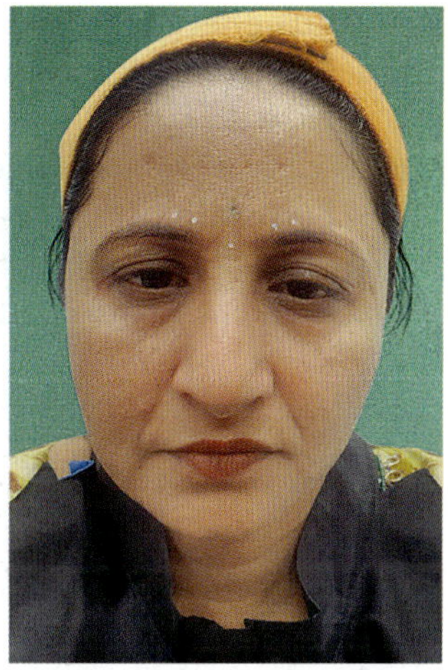

Fig. 3: Glabellar injection point.

- *Corrugators supercilii:* This originates from the medial superciliary arch of the frontal bone and inserts in the skin in the region of the midbrow. This has gradual interdigitations with frontalis. This muscle adducts slight medial brow depression. The plane of this muscle is deep medially and becomes superficial as it extends laterally.
- *Depressor supercilii:* It originates from the nasal portion of the frontal bone approximately 1 cm above the medial canthal ligament. It is a very small thick muscle only recruited in some patients on the lower edge of eyebrow. This needs to be injected only in a more complex treatment of the glabellar region.

Contraction of muscles of these regions forms three distinct creases—Midline crease, corrugators crease, and supraorbital crease.

Glabellar lines play an important role in self-perception as well as perception by others and play a significant role in the emergence of noticeable lines and folds of aging face.[23]

Various studies have been done on BoNT-A injection into the glabellar lines and literature is widely available. It is also a US FDA-approved indication for multiple BoNT formulations in the market.

A combined treatment of lateral canthal lines and glabellar lines when compared with lateral canthal lines alone was assessed to be better by both investigator and patient in a study of 917 subjects.[24]

A meta-analysis of four trials with 621 patients found that a 20-unit treatment of glabellar lines resulted in sustained clinical benefit for 4 months in more than half of responders.[25]

Injection Points (Fig. 3)

The procerus may require one to two injection sites based on the length of the muscle. Corrugators require one to two injections on each side. A more complex treatment may require multiple injections in the procerus if it is long and has intermingled fibers with frontalis. Corrugators may require a deeper medial injection to take care of depressor supercilii and may require more superficial injections and multiple points laterally if multiple insertion points are seen in the skin, as the muscle goes laterally.

So, overall 5-points (1 procerus, 2 each side for corrugators) injections and 12–20 units are required in the majority of patients. These injection points can vary from 3 to 7. Dosage can go up to 40 units. A lower dose in the glabella reduces the risk of medial brow ptosis and splayed eyebrows.

TREATMENT PEARLS

- Nondominant hand grasping the procerus helps in better placement and provides support to the injecting hand.
- As a general rule, in the glabellar area, medial injections are deeper and become superficial as we advance laterally. Needle inside the skin can be used as a guide to depth. So, in procerus, approximately 75% of the needle can be in of 31G 6 mm needle insulin syringe, 50% needle in for medial corrugators' injection, and 25% needle in for lateral corrugators.
- Putting the nondominant hand on the brow rim may prevent unwanted injection/diffusion on orbicularis oculi/orbital septum and thus prevent brow ptosis. Injection direction should be kept upward to avoid undue diffusion.
- Do not inject lateral to midpupillary line as it may cause eyebrow and lid ptosis.
- Brow position, especially in men, may lie below the orbital margin. So, palpate the rim to avoid unwarranted placement in orbit.
- Slight bleeding if any can be controlled by immediate compression with a gauze in nondominant hand or a Q-tip (cotton bud).
- Ptosis, sometimes asymmetric, can occur after uncareful injection into the orbicularis oculi muscle due to unwanted diffusion of the toxin behind the orbital septum. If this happens, limited stimulation of Müller's muscle can be produced by local administration of a sympathomimetic agent such as phenylephrine (e.g., Vasocon eye drops).
- Even if sufficient relaxation of the relevant muscles has been achieved, some individuals can produce frown lines voluntarily by recruiting the medial parts of the orbicularis oculi muscle. If this is the case, small superficial doses can be given into the palpable areas of activity of the orbicularis oculi muscle.

Adverse Effects

A possibility of paralysis of the superior tarsal muscle (Müller's muscle)/levator palpebrae superioris leading to ptosis is the main side effect from upper face BoNT-A injections, and it is necessary to inject above orbital rim to prevent diffusion.[26]

Ptosis can occur as early as 48 hours and up to 2 weeks after injection. It can persist up to 2–4 weeks. An alpha-2 adrenergic agonist apraclonidine 0.5% (Lopidine) eye drops can help the superior tarsal muscle to contract and elevate the upper eyelid.[27]

This is to be treated symptomatic and helps with 1–2 mm elevation of the eyelid. Drops can be put one to three times a day till the ptosis resolves.

FOREHEAD LINES

Forehead lines are caused by a single large muscle frontalis.

Frontalis: Its origin is galea aponeurotica along the coronal suture. Insertion of frontalis is at the level of eyebrows in dermis. Frontalis is intertwined with fibers of procerus, corrugators, depressor supercilii, and orbicularis oculi near its insertion. Laterally, frontalis terminates at the temporal fusion line. The function of the frontalis is to lift/elevate the eyebrows, and this action is more prominent medially. The muscle fibers which are vertical result in horizontal lines across the forehead (wrinkles form perpendicular to the direction of muscle action).

Frontalis is the only elevator in this region and it should not be treated alone without treating depressors (glabella) of the area. Concomitant injection of glabella and forehead is an approved indication since 2017.

Variations/Shapes of Frontalis and Forehead

Uniform band versus V-shaped frontalis: Some patients have a V-shaped frontalis with a relative absence of fibers medially. This is because of two frontalis showing divergence in the middle. This point of divergence is lower in men compared to women.[28]

Uniform band-shape full frontalis muscle leads to more straight parallel lines on forehead attributed to a more acute muscle fascicle angle, and "V" distribution leads to wavy horizontal forehead lines and has more obtuse muscle fascicle angle in frontalis. Thus, based on this, assessing forehead line during consultation can also give ideas about the shape and distribution of frontalis.[29]

Four distinct shapes of frontalis by Abramo et al.[30] **(Fig. 4)**:

- *Type I:* It is full shape and covers the entire forehead, including the central part, giving rise to parallel wrinkles that extend continuously throughout the forehead.
- *Type II:* It is "V-shape" and is formed by two bands separated by aponeurotic tissue in the center.
- *Type III:* It is the central form. Muscle is at the center, aponeurosis is located laterally, and a column of line is seen centrally with lateral part of the eyebrow dropped.
- *Type IV:* It is the lateral form and has characteristic two bands splayed laterally in the forehead with a large portion of aponeurotic tissue at the center.

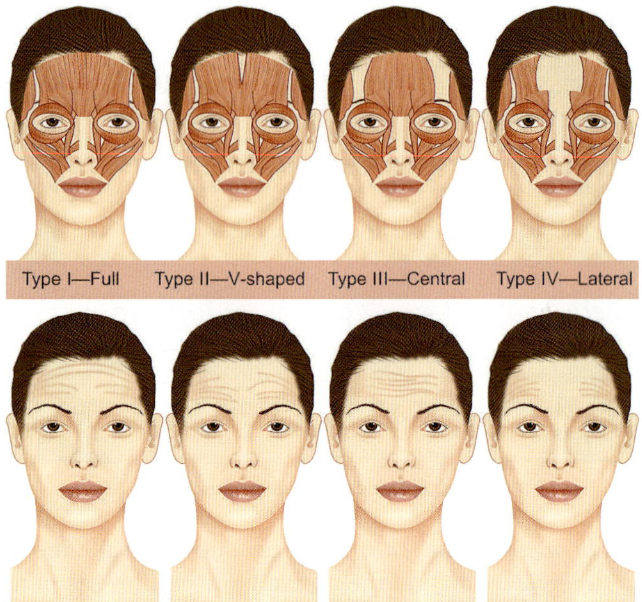

Fig. 4: Various frontalis shapes.

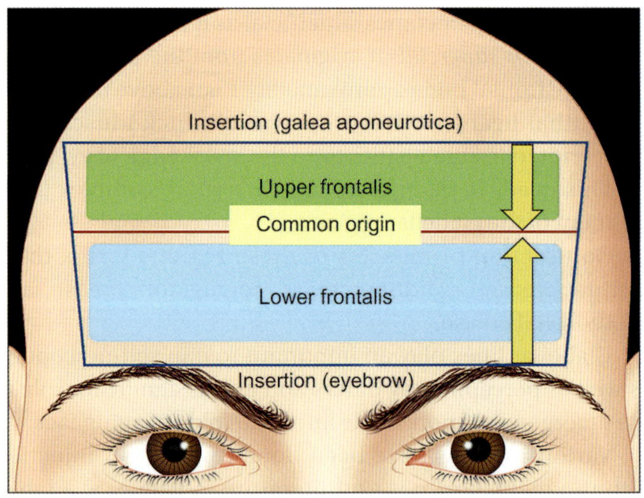

Fig. 5: Frontalis line of convergence.

Frontalis shows bidirectional movement. Eyebrow elevation leads to upward movement of lower forehead skin and lowering of hairline leads to downward movement of upper forehead skin. These two directionally opposite movements converge at a nonmobile horizontal forehead line at approximate 60% height relative to total forehead height. This line of convergence is called C-line and is common across all patient types **(Fig. 5)**. Reduction of BoNT units below C-line helps mitigate the risk of brow ptosis.[31]

Variations to consider while treating forehead:

- Average sized forehead
- High forehead
- *Tendency to Mephisto sign:* The so-called Mephisto sign occurs in some patients when the lateral movement of the frontalis remains after treatment and produces visible wrinkles. It is more common when treatment of the forehead is restricted to the area between the midpupillary lines.
- *Palpebral weakness:* Upper eyelid ptosis may occur when treatment of the frontalis muscle unmasks subtle preexisting weakness of the levator palpebrae superioris muscle, especially in patients with a history of glabellar trauma or surgery for the presence of levator palpebrae muscle separation or weakness.
- *V-shaped frontalis:* The frontalis may either form a uniform band across the forehead or be V-shaped with a relative absence of fibers medially.
- Short forehead
- *Lateral superciliary wrinkles:* It is more common in males. Prominent lateral superciliary wrinkles will require additional injection in the lateral frontalis.

Injection Points/Units (Fig. 6)

The forehead should be treated with a relatively lower dose and in combination with glabella. In general, 4–10 points of injection and 1–2 units per point are sufficient to cover the forehead. Sometimes, in men with larger muscle mass and high forehead, the units can be higher than 20 units. Two points that are consistently covered are anti-Spock points in each side; 1–2 units are required to neutralize the excess action of lateral frontalis to avoid the Mephisto sign. Excessive relaxation can lead to brow ptosis and should be avoided. The injections in the frontalis are intracutaneous to avoid hitting the periosteum and to achieve superficial delivery of depth to avoid ptosis.

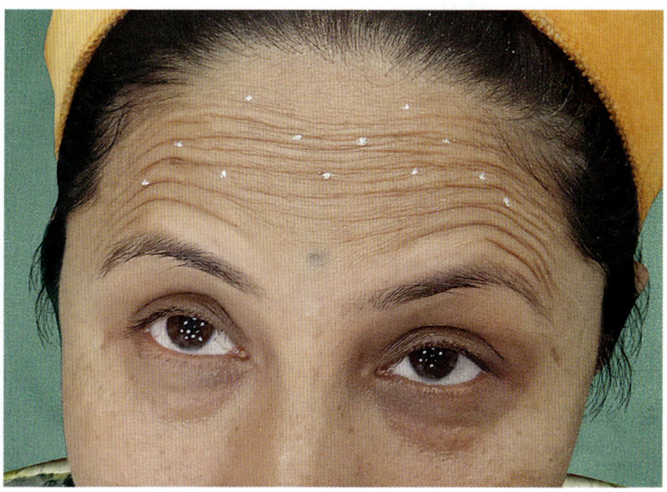

Fig. 6: Frontalis injection point.

TREATMENT PEARLS

- One should stay at least 2 cm above the eyebrow or the first horizontal line seen on contraction.
- Assess for asymmetries in the brow position before starting injections and show it to the patient. An attempt to correct asymmetry by giving 1–2 units extra on overactive frontalis side can be made.
- Start with a low dose in frontalis.
- If not doing together in the same session, brow depressors should be treated first and the forehead later.
- Frontalis shows high interindividual variation, and therefore always follow observed animation of patient rather than predecided points.
- Centrally focused injection can allow lateral brows to elevate; therefore anti-Spock point injection should be given. Antispock point injection should be at least 1.5–2 cm above the bony orbital margin to avoid causing eyebrow ptosis.
- Always assess a functional frontalis where frontalis is helping patients keep the eyes open and not droopy. Treating this may result in heaviness of brow or brow ptosis. Such patients sometimes do better by only treating glabellar complex as that relaxes some of the fibers of the frontalis intertwined with corrugators and procerus.

Adverse Effects

Brow ptosis: This often happens from overtreatment of frontalis and sometimes from injection being placed too low.

Mephisto sign: This is a quizzical eyebrow shape happening because of the left-out untreated lateral fibers. It is easily correctable by giving 1–2 units in the still working part of frontalis to reduce the constant elevating action of working fibers.

LATERAL CANTHAL LINES (CROW'S FEET)

The lateral canthal area has one main muscle that is orbicularis oculi. This is responsible for closure of eye and depression of eyebrow. Orbicularis oculi has three parts: Orbital, preseptal, and pretarsal parts. Extension of orbicularis oculi beyond the lateral orbital margin is responsible for orbital rhytids.

Treatment/Injection Points

Lateral rhytids are a very easy-to-treat area and very beginner friendly. One to three injection points can be marked on each side. In a two-center study, no significant difference was seen between efficacy and adverse events of one injection per side versus three injections per side.[32]

One to four units per injection point at one to three injection sites are usually given. The dosage required is 4–20 units on each side of lateral canthal line, and majority of people do well with 2–3 injection sites and 6–12 units on each side **(Fig. 7)**.

It is important to stay at least 1 cm away from the lateral canthal margin to avoid the complications of diplopia and strabismus by diffusion into extraocular muscles. When giving three injections per side, middle injection is in line with

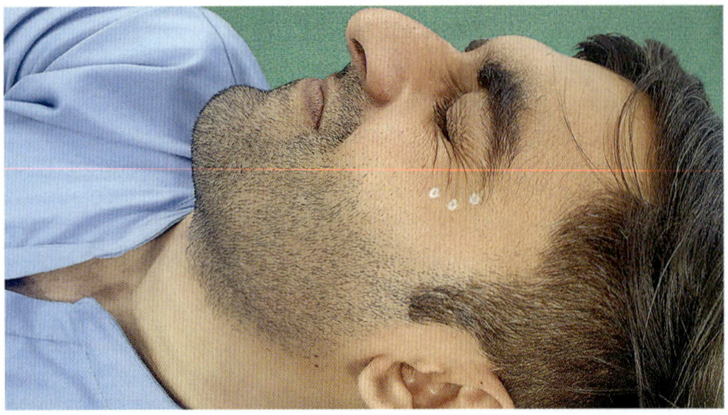

Fig. 7: Crow's feet injection point.

the lateral canthal fold and the remaining in a C shape above or below it, always staying lateral to orbital margins.

A second row of injections can be given in patients having prominent muscle action further laterally, patients with extensive sun damage, and patients who show rhytids in that area as a result of face-lift surgery. The second lateral row of injections should deliberately be avoided in patients having volume loss in the area.

In patients having lines encroaching inferiorly on the cheek, a lowering of dose in the lowermost point in the first row also should be considered to avoid injection in zycomaticus major leading to a lopsided smile.

TREATMENT PEARLS

- A preoperative snap test to evaluate lid laxity should be performed in patients showing severe skin laxity and then the dose adjusted accordingly.
- Stay away from orbital margins to avoid causing ectropion, impaired eye closure, excessive eye tears, and lateral rectus paresis.
- Patients with prominent eye bags may show accentuation of eye bags, so withhold/reduce dose in the lowermost injection point.
- Avoid injecting in the area below zygomatic arch in all patients as it can lead to cheek ptosis or lip ptosis.
- Exercise caution in patients with a history of dry eyes.

Adverse Events

Bruising, diplopia, ectropion or a drooping lateral lower eyelid, and asymmetric smile because of the injection in the zygomaticus major are the rarely encountered complications.[33] Cheek and lid ptosis are other uncommon adverse events.

CHEMICAL BROW LIFT (FIG. 8)

Eyebrow shape is a complex interplay of brow elevator frontalis and medial brow and lateral eyebrow depressors.

- *Medial brow depressors:* Procerus, corrugator supercilii, depressor supercilii, portions of orbicularis oculi
- *Lateral brow depressor:* Lateral orbicularis oculi

Simple lateral brow lift is very easily achieved and can provide 1–3 mm brow elevation leading to a desired shape change.

Medial brow lift is less successful and may require multiple area treatments.

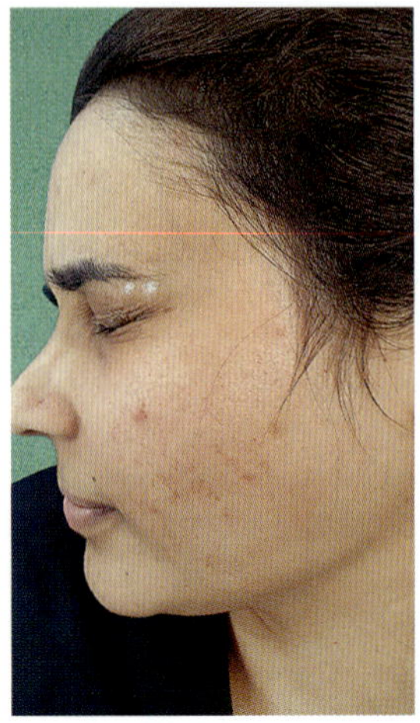

Fig. 8: Brow lift marking.

One to two units are injected in the lateral fibers of orbicularis oculi just below the proper margin in the most prominent visible muscle mass area always staying lateral to the midpupillary line. 1–3 units per side is the total dose needed **(Table 1)**.

Wide Open Eyes/Widening Palpebral Fissures

Jelly roll lines/jelly roll appearance is caused by contraction or hypertrophy of the pretarsal portion of orbicularis oculi on the lower eyelid. In animation/smile, this diminishes the size of palpebral aperture. It can be corrected by giving 1–2 BoNT-A to counteract the contraction leading to opened palpebral aperture.[34]

Skin snap and stretch tests should be performed for this indication to keep treatment safe and to modify treatment accordingly for elderly, repeat treatments, and early proactive preventive treatment of young patients.

Excess injection in this area can lead to sclera show and should be avoided.

Correction of Brow Asymmetry

Pre-existing brow ptosis or as a result of unwanted effect of BoNT-A can be corrected with BoNT-A. Relaxing/neutralizing medial corrugators further by giving 2–4 units and raising the lateral brow by 1–2 units in below brow orbicularis oculi can help level the brow.[35]

Alternatively, the opposite eyebrow can be brought lower for the sake of achieving symmetry. This should only be used if elevating the affected brow has failed.[36]

No Treatment Zones (Fig. 9)

- Lateral corrugator injections should be at least 1 cm away from brow.
- Frontalis should not be injected in an area 1–1.5 cm adjacent to the lateral brow.

TABLE 1: Summary of individual upper face botulinum toxin indications.

Indication	*Target muscle*	*Injection level*	*Injection point*	*Dose per point*	*Average total dose*
Glabellar	Procerus, corrugators supercilii, and depressor supercilii	Intramuscular	3–7	2–4	12–40
Horizontal forehead	Frontalis	Intramuscular/intradermal	4–8	1–2	8–25
Lateral canthal line	Orbicularis oculi	Intradermal	1–5	1–4	6–15 per side
Brow elevation	Orbicularis oculi	Intradermal	1–2	.5–1	1–6

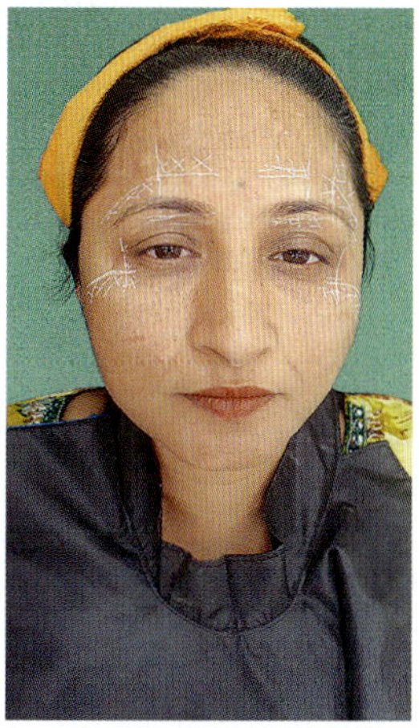

Fig. 9: No treatment zone.

- Lateral canthal fold injections should be always out of the bony margin.
- No injection should be given medial to midpupillary line for brow lift or widening palpebral aperture.

Adverse Effects

Adverse effects that are site-specific have been discussed with each indication. This section is for complications that can arise out of any injection site.

- *Local common complications:* Pain, erythema, ecchymosis, or hematoma at the site of injection can commonly occur and self-resolve without any intervention needed. Topical anesthesia, slower injection rate, and avoiding visible veins are simple preventive steps for these.
- *Local uncommon complications:* Mild and self-resolving headache with facial injections, paresthesia in the area of the injection site, and vasovagal episodes associated with anxiety during the injection procedure.[37]
- *General rare complications:* Antibody formation and immediate allergic reaction to toxin are rare and have severe complications.
- Patients suspected of tolerance or unresponsiveness to BoNT-A should be tested for antibodies, and ideally, they should be stopped being injected for a duration of 6–12 months to stop the development of high titer antibodies.[38]
- A possible immediate allergic reaction to the toxin can start with itching and swelling and may precipitate possible anaphylaxis.[39]

Standard allergic protocols should be used to treat these.

A recent systematic review of 31 randomized or open-label clinical studies of BoNT-A in aesthetic treatments quantified the incidence of treatment-related blepharoptosis (2.5%), brow ptosis (3.1%), eye sensory disorders (3%), and lip asymmetries and imbalances of the lower face (6.9%).[40]

60% of studies in this metanalysis were on ONA, 37% on ABO, and 2.8% on INCO.

CONCLUSION

In summary, BoNT is a safe and efficacious treatment for upper face rhytids with an extremely high patient satisfaction rate. The injector needs to be aware of huge interindividual variations in the muscle anatomy of this area. In addition, it is important to understand each patient's aesthetic preference, particularly with regard to brow aesthetic.[41]

Following a tailored approach is the key to good aesthetic outcomes in this area.

REFERENCES

1. Clark RP, Berris CE. Botulinum toxin: A treatment for facial asymmetry caused by facial nerve paralysis. Plast Reconstr Surg. 1989;84(2):353-5.
2. Carruthers JD, Carruthers JA. Treatment of glabellar frown lines with C. Botulinum-A exotoxin. J Dermatol Surg Oncol. 1992;18(1):17-21.
3. Jankovic J. Botulinum toxin: State of the Art. Mov Disord. 2017;32(8):1131-8.
4. Ong AA, Sherris DA. Neurotoxins. Facial Plast Surg. 2019; 35(3):230-8.
5. U.S. Food and Drug Administration. (2014): Information for healthcare professionals: Onabotulinum toxin A (marketed as Botox/Botox cosmetic), abobotulinum toxin A (marketed as Dysport), and rimabotulinum toxin b (marketed as Myobloc). [online] Available at: https://www.fda.gov/drugs/postmarket-drug-safety-information-patients-and-providers/onabotulinumtoxina-marketed-botoxbotox-cosmetic-abobotulinumtoxina-marketed-dysport-and [last accessed February, 2024].
6. Brin MF, James C, Maltman J. Botulinum toxin type A products are not interchangeable: A review of the evidence. Biologics. 2014;8:227-41.
7. Frevert J. Content of botulinum neurotoxin in Botox®/Vistabel®, Dysport®/Azzalure®, and Xeomin®/Bocouture®. Drugs R D. 2010;10(2):67-3.

8. Hexsel D, Brum C, do Prado DZ, Soirefmann M, Rotta FT, Dal'Forno T, et al. Field effect of two commercial preparations of botulinum toxin type A: A prospective, double-blind, randomized clinical trial. J Am Acad Dermatol. 2012;67(2): 226-32.
9. Hexsel D, Soirefmann M, Porto MD, Siega C, Schilling-Souza J, Rodrigues TC. Fields of muscular and anhidrotic effects of 2 botulinum toxin-A commercial preparations: A prospective, double-blind, randomized, multicenter study. Dermatol Surg. 2015;41(Suppl 1):S110-8.
10. Shoshani D, Markovitz E, Monstrey SJ, Narins DJ. The modified Fitzpatrick wrinkle scale: A clinical validated measurement tool for nasolabial wrinkle severity assessment. DermatolSurg. 2008;34(Suppl 1):S85-91; discussion S91.
11. Carruthers A, Carruthers J, Hardas B, Kaur M, Goertelmeyer R, Jones D, et al. A validated grading scale for crow's feet. Dermatol Surg. 2008;34(Suppl 2):S173-8.
12. Goodman GJ, Halstead MB, Rogers JD, Borzillo D, Ryan E, Riley N, et al. A software program designed to educate patients on age-related skin changes of facial and exposed extrafacial regions: The results of a validation study. Clin Cosmet Investig Dermatol. 2012;5:23-31.
13. Braz AV, Sakuma TH. Patterns of contraction of the frontalis muscle: A pilot study. Surg Cosmet Dermatol. 2010;2(3):191-4.
14. Benedetto AV, Lahti JG. Measurement of the anatomic position of the corrugator supercilii. Dermatol Surg. 2005;31:923-7.
15. de Almeida AR, da Costa Marques ER, Banegas R, Kadunc BV. Glabellar contraction patterns: A tool to optimize botulinum toxin treatment. Dermatol Surg. 2012;38(9):1506-15.
16. Bonaparte JP, Ellis D, Quinn JG, Ansari MT, Rabski J, Kilty SJ. A comparative assessment of three formulations of botulinum toxin A for facial rhytides: A systematic review and meta-analyses. Syst Rev. 2013;2:40.
17. Yu KC, Nettar KD, Bapna S, Boscardin WJ, Maas CS. Split face double-blind study comparing the onset of action of onabotulinumtoxinA and abobotulinumtoxinA. Arch Facial Plast Surg. 2012;14(3):198-204.
18. Erickson BP, Lee WW, Cohen J, Grunebaum LD. The role of neurotoxins in the periorbital and midfacial areas. Facial Plast Surg Clin North Am. 2015;23(2):243-55.
19. De Maio M, Rzany B. Patient selection. In: De Maio M, Rzany B (Eds). Botulinum Toxin in Aesthetic Medicine. Berlin: Springer; 2007. pp. 11-9.
20. Cohn JE, Greco TM. Advanced techniques for the use of Neurotoxins in non-surgical facial rejuvenation. Aesthetic Plast Surg. 2020;44(5):1788-99.
21. Alam M, Bolotin D, Carruthers J, Hexsel D, Lawrence N, Minkis K, et al. Consensus statement regarding storage and reuse of previously reconstituted neuromodulators. Dermatol Surg. 2015;41(3):321-6.
22. Carruthers J, Fournier N, Kerscher M, Ruiz-Avila J, Trindade de Almeida AR, Kaeuper G. The convergence of medicine and neurotoxins: A focus on botulinum toxin type A and its application in aesthetic medicine–a global, evidence-based botulinum toxin consensus education initiative: Part II: Incorporating botulinum toxin into aesthetic clinical practice. Dermatol Surg. 2013;39:510-25.
23. Dessy LA, Fallico N, Mazzocchi M, Scuderi N. Botulinum toxin for glabellar lines: A review of the efficacy and safety of currently available products. Am J Clin Dermatol. 2011;12(6):377-88.
24. Moers-Carpi M, Carruthers J, Fagien S, Lupo M, Delmar H, Jones D, et al. Efficacy and safety of onabotulinumtoxin A for treating crow's feet lines alone or in combination with glabellar lines: A multicenter, randomized, controlled trial. Dermatol Surg. 2015;41(1):102-12.
25. Glogau R, Kane M, Beddingfield F, Somogyi C, Lei X, Caulkins C, Gallagher C. Onabotulinumtoxin A: A meta-analysis of duration of effect in the treatment of glabellar lines. Dermatol Surg. 2012;38(11):1794-1803.
26. Beer JI, Sieber DA, Scheuer JF 3rd, Greco TM. Three-dimensional facial anatomy: Structure and function as it relates to injectable neuromodulators and soft tissue fillers. Plast Reconstr Surg Glob Open. 2016;4:e1175.
27. Scheinfeld N. The use of apraclonidine eyedrops to treat ptosis after the administration of botulinum toxin to the upper face. Dermatol Online J. 2005;11(1):9.
28. Spiegel JH, Goerig RC, Lufler RS, Hoagland TM. Frontalis midline dehiscence: An anatomical study and discussion of clinical relevance. J Plast Reconstr Aesthet Surg. 2009; 62(7):950-4.
29. Moqadam M, Frank K, Handayan C, Hakami M, Benslimane F, Gotkin RH, et al. Understanding the shape of forehead lines. J Drugs Dermatol. 2017;16(5):471-7.
30. Abramo AC, Do Amaral TP, Lessio BP, De Lima GA. Anatomy of forehead, glabellar, nasal and orbital muscles, and their correlation with distinctive patterns of skin lines on the upper third of the face: Reviewing concepts. Aesthetic Plast Surg. 2016;40(6):962-71.
31. Cotofana S, Freytag DL, Frank K, Sattler S, Landau M, Pavicic T, et al. The bidirectional movement of the frontalis muscle: Introducing the line of convergence and its potential clinical relevance. Plast Reconstr Surg. 2020;145(5):1155-62.
32. Fabi SG, Sundaram H, Guiha I, Goldman MP. A two-center, open-label, randomized, split-face study to assess the efficacy and safety of one versus three intradermal injection sites of abobotulinumtoxin A in the treatment of lateral periocular rhytides. J Drugs Dermatol. 2013;12(8):932-7.
33. Klein AW. Contraindications and complications with the use of botulinum toxin. Clin Dermatol. 2004;22(1):66-75.
34. Carruthers J, Carruthers A. Aesthetic botulinum A toxin in the mid and lower face and neck. Dermatol Surg. 2003;29(5): 468-76.
35. King M. Management of Ptosis. J Clin Aesthet Dermatol. 2016;9(12):E1-4.
36. Olson JJ. Balanced botox chemodenervation of the upper face: Symmetry in motion. Semin Plast Surg. 2007;21(1):47-53.
37. Small R. Botulinum toxin injection for facial wrinkles. Am Fam Physician. 2014;90(3):168-75.
38. Wanitphakdeedecha R, Kantaviro W, Suphatsathienkul P, Tantrapornpong P, Yan C, Apinumtham C, et al. Association Between Secondary Botulinum ToxinA Treatment Failure in Cosmetic Indication and Anti-Complexing Protein Antibody Production. Dermatol Ther (Heidelb). 2020;10(4):707-20.
39. Naumann M, Carruthers A, Carruthers J, Aurora SK, Zafonte R, Abu-Shakra S, et al. Meta-analysis of neutralizing antibody conversion with onabotulinumtoxin A (BOTOX®) across multiple indications. Mov Disord. 2010;25(13): 2211-8.
40. Brin MF, Boodhoo TI, Pogoda JM, James LM, Demos G, Terashima Y, et al. Safety and tolerability of onabotulinum toxin A in the treatment of facial lines: A meta-analysis of individual patient data from global clinical registration studies in 1678 participants. J Am Acad Dermatol. 2009;61(6):961. e1-970.
41. Griffin GR, Kim JC. Ideal female brow aesthetics. Clin Plast Surg. 2013;40(1):147-55.

CHAPTER 88

Botulinum Toxin for the Midface, Lower Face, and Neck

Shehnaz Arsiwala, Rajat Kandhari, Nazneen Arsiwala

KEY MESSAGES

- Botulinum toxin treatment of midface, lower face, and neck is used less compared to upper face.
- Intricacies of muscle attachments and innervations need to be understood to obtain precise results in the dynamic rejuvenation of lower face and neck.

INTRODUCTION

The only US Food and Drug Administration (FDA) approved aesthetic indications of botulinum neurotoxin type A (BoNTA) are glabellar lines and more recently lateral canthal lines.[1,2] Other than these indications with the ever-increasing demand for facial rejuvenation the off label uses of BoNTA have immensely widened their horizons. Today, BoNTA, which was essentially used for the upper face and lateral canthal lines, is being increasingly used for wrinkles produced due to contractions of facial mimetic muscles in the midface, platysmal bands, and fine lines on the neck, masseteric hypertrophy or a boxy jaw for a more chiseled jawline, and for a neck lift amongst other advanced indications. Although use of this agent has progressed to other areas of the face, use of BoNTA in the mid and lower face is more challenging, and better cosmetic outcomes may be obtained from the use of soft-tissue fillers, resurfacing techniques or invasive procedures such as rhytidectomy and implants combined with supplementary BoNTA injections.[3]

There are various factors which make injecting the mid and lower face with BoNTA more challenging than the upper face **(Box 1)**.[4]

- The facial musculature of the mid and lower face has a compact spatial arrangement which makes the borders of these muscles indistinct as compared to the muscles of the upper face. Understanding of the facial anatomy is absolutely essential before attempting injections, particularly in the mid and lower face, as diffusion to nearby muscles is not uncommon.
- Muscles of the mid and lower face allow for fine motor movements, and are responsible for laughing, chewing, swallowing, and other complex voluntary and involuntary movements which are characteristic of an individual's mannerisms, as a result of which inadvertent injections or diffusion beyond the intended target may result in unwanted adverse effects.
- Static wrinkles are more common in the midface, and these are enhanced by volume loss and soft tissue—these are more important for aging changes in mid and lower face and need treatment with other modalities such as fillers and lasers. Full effacement of these wrinkles or furrows is not feasible. Persistent treatments with increasing doses only lead to functional imbalance.[5]

BOX 1: Factors important for botulinum toxin type A in mid and lower face.

- Muscles have dynamic functional activity
- Spatial arrangements of fibers
- Functional activity of muscles to be considered
- Volume loss predominates and contributes to static lines

BOTULINUM TOXIN FOR THE MIDFACE

Nasoglabellar Lines (Bunny Lines)

"Bunny lines" or "nasal scrunch" in some individuals wrinkles on the lateral part of the nose, whereas in others these wrinkles may exist on the dorsal part of the nose, and/or extend to the lower eyelids and cheeks. The depth and pattern of these lines may vary on either side of the midline. Tamura et al. noted that after treatment of the nasalis there were certain accompanying persistent or recalcitrant bunny lines, requiring additional treatment. They termed these as follows:[6]

- *Nasociliary rhytides:* Persistent wrinkling at the root on the nose extending superiorly toward the medial margin of the eyebrow and glabella. Contraction of the orbital part of the orbicularis oculi muscle is responsible for these lines.
- *Nasoorbicular rhytides:* Persistent wrinkling at the root of the nose due to contraction of the nasal portion of the orbital orbicularis oculi.
- *Nasoalar rhytides:* This pattern accompanied both the aforementioned patterns, and is a result of the contraction of the alar portion of the levator labii superioris alaeque nasi (LLSAN).

Nasoglabellar lines are produced by asking the patient to squint forcibly, as there is light shining into their eyes.[7]

Bunny lines are usually dynamic wrinkles and appear when patients laugh or frown. They can also be the result of BoNTA treatment on the upper face, when the nasal muscles overcontract to compensate for the paralyzed muscles in the glabellar, forehead, and orbital regions. If bunny lines appear in addition to glabellar lines when patients frown, they should be treated together.

Relevant Anatomy

The nasalis is a horseshoe-shaped muscle, the transverse fibers of which form an aponeurosis interdigitating with the fibers of the procerus over the nasal dorsum and the two lower parts of the muscle are vertical and run down each side of the nose onto the maxillary bone, superior, and lateral to the incisive fossa. The function of the nasalis is sphincter-like, which helps compress the nasal cartilage and is responsible for "flaring" of the nostrils. The nasalis along with the procerus and the depressor septi nasi form the three predominant muscles in the nasal region **(Fig. 1)**. Contraction of the transverse portion of the nasalis usually results in "bunny lines", represented by dynamic horizontal rhytides appearing lateral to bridge of the nose and radiating down along the sides of the nose. Individuals who regularly contract their nose during facial expression develop these lines. Further, in certain individual's treatment of the glabellar complex alone results in recruitment of these muscles, and presence of bunny lines in the absence of glabellar frown lines is a telltale sign of previous neurotoxin treatment and is also known as the "Botox sign" **(Figs. 1 and 2A)**. Subtle treatment of the nasalis while treating the glabellar complex will prevent this occurrence.

Often the medial fibers of the LLSAN, an elevator of the lip and the nose whose fibers at times interdigitate with the fibers of the nasalis and, also contribute to the formation of these lines. The procerus is a pyramid-shaped muscle with its origin at the fascia covering the lower part of the nasal bone and the nasal cartilage, whereas the depressor septi nasi determines the position of the nasal tip. Its fibers originate at the base of the nasal septum and blend with the orbicularis oris.[8]

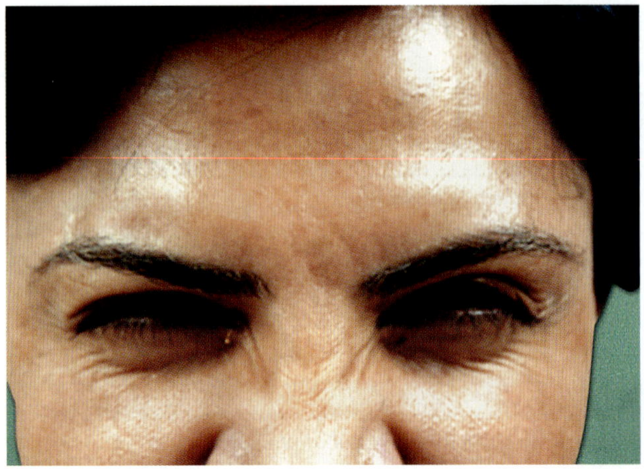

Fig. 1: The Botox sign—post-treatment of the glabellar complex, recruitment of the nasalis muscle.
Courtesy: Dr Rajat Kandhari, New Delhi.

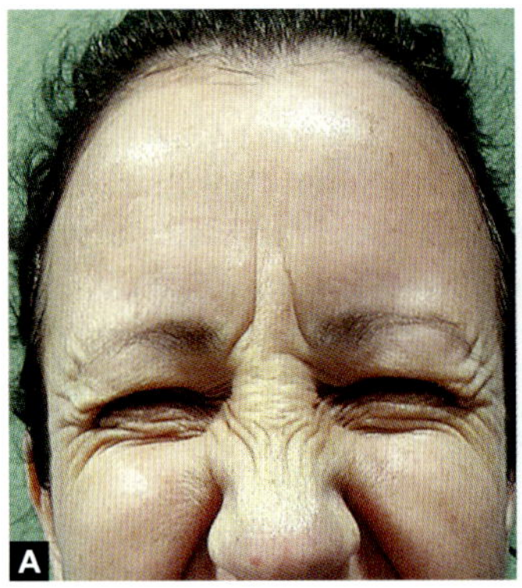

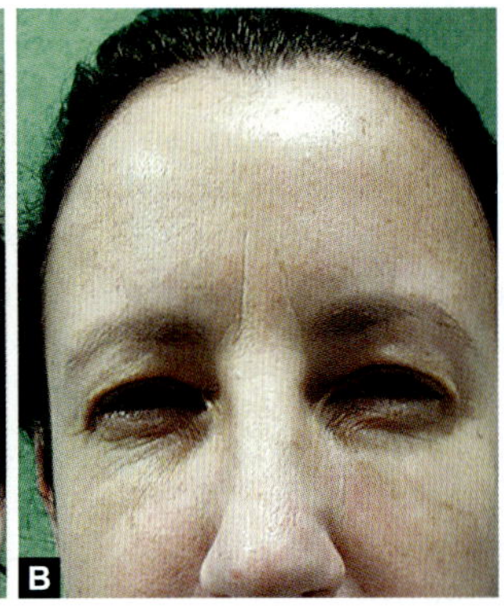

Figs. 2A and B: (A) Bunny lines—nasalis muscle action; (B) After injection botulinum toxin type A for nasalis glabellar complex treated simultaneously.
Courtesy: Dr Shehnaz Arsiwala, Mumbai.

BOX 2: Nasalis.

- 2–4 units of neurotoxin
- Inject superficially
- Avoid nasofacial groove
- Gentle massage
- Avoid vascular injections

Injection Point, Dose, and Technique

Denervation of the nasalis requires 2–4 units of neurotoxin given superficially, so as to raise a visible bleb into the belly of the superficial fibers of the upper nasalis as it runs across the nasal bone. One should exercise caution while treating this region and injections should be high on the lateral nasal wall, away from the nasofacial groove to avoid injecting into the medial fibers of the LLSAN and avoid lid ptosis. Further one must practice caution and avoid the traversing angular vessels in the region. Gentle massage should follow the injection to diffuse the toxin **(Box 2)**.

Some authors have recommended a three-point injection technique which entails one point in the middle and one on each side of the nose into the nasalis superficially **(Fig. 2B)**. The recommended total dose is 6 U (2 U per injection point).[9]

Further, the Asian Facial Aesthetics Expert Consensus Group recommends the use of 2–10 U (94% use ranges that include 4–6 U) into the nasalis.[10]

At times repeated contraction of the lower nasalis may lead to an undesirable flare of the nostrils. The sides of the columella or septum become visible when the nostrils are prominently flared. 5–10 U of BoNTA bilaterally into the lower nasalis fibers draped over the lateral nasal ala, at the most active area of muscle contraction, leads to decrease in this involuntary flare.[11,12]

The latest recommendations by the Global Aesthetic Consensus Group states that 4–8 U may be administered for the nasalis muscle and doses as high as 10 U may be appropriate for some patients.[13]

Complications[14]

- *Lip asymmetry or ptosis:* Injection of the neurotoxin too low along the nasal sidewall may lead to diffusion of the toxin into the medial fibers of the LLSAN or the levator labii superioris (LLS) leading to not only lip ptosis but also functional difficulties such as with speaking, eating, and drinking.
- *Ophthalmic side effects:* Inadvertent diffusion of the toxin into the fibers of the medial palpebral orbicularis oculi results in decreased action of the lacrimal pump leading to epiphora. Rarely, diplopia may occur due to weakening of the medial rectus.
- *Ecchymosis or hematoma:* Since the angular vessels traverse this region intravascular injection of BoNTA into the vessels may result in an ecchymosis or a hematoma.

GUMMY SMILE

The smile is the main facial expression which reflects happiness, pleasure, and good mood[15] and most importantly a smile represents an important aspect of socialization. A beautiful smile makes an individual more desirable. A smile may be voluntary[16] or involuntary, with differing degrees of gingival show caused by singular contraction of involved muscles.[17-20]

Excessive gingival exposure during smiling or laughing is not only considered unsightly but also embarrassing. Many of these individuals are women, seen commonly covering their teeth with their hands while smiling or laughing.

Relevant Anatomy

The aesthetics of ideal tooth exposure while smiling is considered to be three quarters of the dental crown height of the upper incisor and no >1–2 mm of the upper gum mucosa.[21,22]

A gummy smile is defined as a gingival exposure >2 mm above the dental line when smiling.[23] The gum line, upper incisors, and canines are fully revealed. The upper lip length, the distance between the commissure plane and occlusal plane should also be considered when assessing a smile, although a detailed discussion of this is out of the scope of this chapter. Various factors may contribute to the development of a gummy smile which include but are not limited to, a vertical maxillary excess leading to an elongated face, a genetically short upper lip, an increased interlabial space combined with an exacerbated contraction of the upper lip elevators (particularly the LLSAN), and a short crown length with or without malpositioning of the incisors could alone or in combination result in the excessive gum show while smiling or laughing.

The LLSAN muscle retracts the upper lip and produces the upper gum exposure. Weakening of the muscle with botulinum toxin results in a moderate drop in the upper lip sufficient to cover the upper gum.

Three different smile patterns have been described in the literature:[20]

1. *The Mona Lisa smile or commissure smile:* This is the most common pattern seen in close to 67% of individuals. The corners of the mouth are first pulled up and outward, followed by the levators of the upper lip contracting to show the upper teeth. This pattern is produced by the pull of the zygomaticus major muscle.
2. *The cuspid or canine smile:* This smile pattern is represented by the dominance of the LLS. They contract first, exposing the cuspid teeth, then the corners of the mouth contract to pull the lips upward and outward. Seen in close to 31% of the population.
3. *Complex smile:* The elevators of the upper lip, the elevators of the corners of the mouth, and the depressors of the lower lip contract simultaneously, showing all the upper and lower teeth concurrently. This pattern is relatively uncommon and is seen in approximately 2% of the population **(Figs. 3A to C)**.

Injection Technique and Dosing

Injections should be given after careful assessment of the patient who has a definite gummy smile. With your index

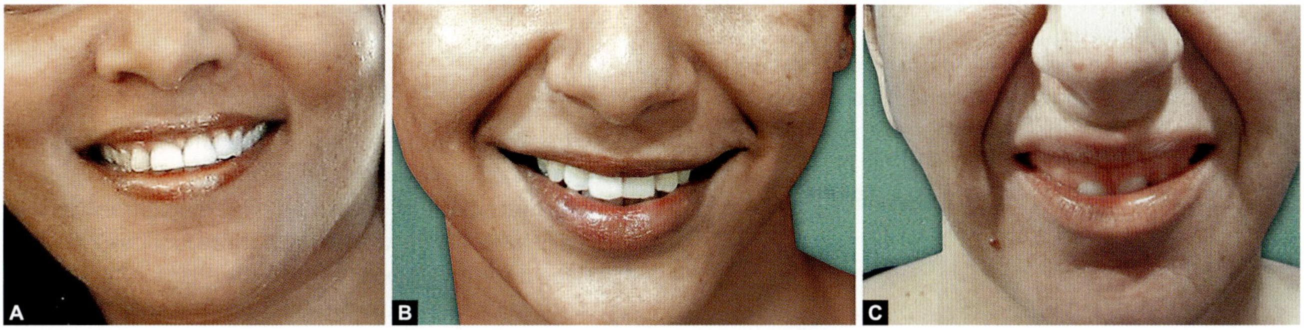

Figs. 3A to C: (A) Commissure smile; (B) Canine smile; (C) Gummy smile.
Courtesy: Dr Shehnaz Arsiwala, Mumbai.

BOX 3: Gummy smile.

- Feel contraction of LLSAN
- 1–2 units, deep IM injection
- 1 in 100 units dilution
- Best combined with DAO injection

(DAO: depressor anguli oris; IM: intramuscular; LLSAN: levator labii superioris alaeque nasi)

finger of nondominant hand identify the nasomaxillary groove and ask the patient to smile, the contraction of the LLSAN will be felt here. Insert your needle deep, perpendicularly where the maximum thickness of the muscle is felt and inject 1–2 U of botulinum toxin into the muscle. Certain authors recommend dilution of 100 units of neurotoxin in 1 mL of saline to prevent unnecessary diffusion of toxin to neighboring muscles in this area. The procedure may be combined with injection into the depressor anguli oris (DAO) to remove antagonistic action against the lateral lip elevators, so that they may have uninhibited action. In a study conducted by Polo, 5 units of neurotoxin per side was best for patients who had at least 5.0 mm of gingival display and for those with <5.0 mm of gingival display lower number of units were considered optimum **(Box 3)**.[24]

Complications

- *Lip asymmetry and upper lip ptosis:* Diffusion of neurotoxin into decussating fibers of the lateral lip elevators such as the LLS, zygomaticus major or minor and the risorius may result in a ptotic lip. This may be accompanied by buccal sphincter incompetence.
- *Sphincter incompetence:* Inaccurate injections or injecting high volumes in this area may result in inadvertent diffusion into the orbicularis oris leading to a buccal sphincter incompetence which in turn results in functional compromise such as difficulty in articulating some words or pucker.
- Relative upper lip lengthening and reduction or flattening of the nasolabial fold.

Note: Even minimal diffusion of the neurotoxin in the earlier mentioned muscles is enough to cause complications. Accurate placement of the injection, appropriate patient selection, and dilution of 100 units of toxin with 1 mL of saline can provide the most optimal results.

Other more advanced indications for the midface include correction of nasal tip ptosis and treatment of the nasolabial folds both of which may be better dealt with soft tissue fillers.

BOTULINUM TOXIN FOR LOWER FACE

Melomental Folds

Also known as "marionette lines" or "labiomandibular creases", these lines extending downward from the corners of the mouth give a negative impression of sadness, disapproval, or melancholy. These lines may vary in severity and have been graded by a five-point scale from no visible folds as grade 0 and extremely long deep folds as grade 5 by Carruthers et al.[22] These lines are treated best by a combination of modalities such as soft-tissue fillers, rhytidectomies, or skin resurfacing along with BoNTA injections as an adjunct, for optimum but temporary results.

Relevant Anatomy

Formation of marionette lines is the result of hyperkinetic activity of the DAO muscle, which pulls on the lateral commissures. The DAO is a triangular muscle which has a wide base originating from the oblique line of the body of the mandible, from where on its fibers converge to be inserted into the angle of the mouth. At its insertion, some of the fibers insert directly onto the undersurface of the skin while others insert into the modiolus interdigitating with fibers of the risorius, orbicularis oris, zygomaticus major, levator anguli oris, and buccinators. At its origin, the muscles lower posterior fibers interdigitate with the platysmal muscle fibers, which also converge toward the oral commissures. The DAO lies superficial to the larger depressor labii inferioris (DLI) and occasionally its fibers cross the midline to interdigitate with its fibers from the opposite side forming a muscular sling.

The modiolus seems to be an important topographic landmark of the lower face. This mobile muscular mass located at the lateral border of the mouth corner is formed by a convergence of the muscle fibers from the DAO and the zygomaticus major, orbicularis oris, risorius, buccinators, and levator anguli oris muscles.[25,26]

The DAO has the potential to alter the position of the modiolus by pulling it down due to its hyperkinetic depressor action, leading to drooping of the mouth corner, while the other muscles inserted at the modiolus are elevators of the mouth corner. Careful inactivation of the DAO by BoNTA will therefore lead to elevation of the oral commissures due to the action of the levator anguli oris and zygomaticus major muscles.

The DAO depresses the labial commissures bilaterally while opening the mouth, giving rise to the marionette lines. These lines also contribute to the formation of the prejowl sulcus.

Injection Technique and Dosing

Injecting the DAO is considered challenging, due to the compact spatial arrangement of the nearby muscles. The medial border of the DAO overlaps with the DLI, and its lateral border is adjacent to the risorius, zygomaticus major, and platysma muscles **(Box 4)**.

Studies have attempted to demonstrate the most appropriate position for injecting the DAO. Hur et al.[24] used the mental foramen as the topographic landmark to delineate

BOX 4: Melomental folds.

- 6–10 units, two points
- 8–10 mm lateral and inferior to the oral commissure
- Avoid injecting high dilution neurotoxin

the safest and most effective site for BoNTA injection into the DAO, while Kim et al. used the modiolus to provide information regarding the most appropriate site for injecting the DAO. They demonstrated that the safest area for injecting the DAO is a fan-shaped area lying between two oblique lines originating from the modiolus down to the mandible, one line lying medially 30° from the modiolus and one line lying laterally 45° from the modiolus. Injection any medial to this fan-shaped region may result in inadvertent injection into the DLI resulting in area more medially to this oblique line which will result in asymmetry of the lip.[27,28]

The point of injection may be identified as a point in the body of the mandible at a point that is most inferior to an imaginary vertical line that passes through the nasolabial sulcus. This point should be approximately 8–10 mm lateral to the oral commissure and 8–15 mm inferior to this point.

Assessment of the patient holds much importance while injecting the DAO, patients who actively contract the muscle and are in the habit of pulling the corners of the mouth down are ideal candidates for this injection. One will be able to visualize the muscle contraction and palpate the muscle in these individuals while they pronounce the letter "e" in an exaggerated manner. Alternatively, a hyperkinetic DAO may also be identified just anterior to the anterior border of the masseter which may be demonstrated by asking the patient to bite down or clench their teeth or just above the lateral platysmal neck band, where the fibers of the platysma and the DAO decussate.

A two-point injection into the DAO (1 point per side) is recommended, with a total dose of 6–10 U (3–5 U per point).[9]

The injection should be intramuscular and perpendicular, although not too deep as that would lead to diffusion of the neurotoxin into the DLI, which lies below the DAO. Further, injections should be closer to the base of the muscle or near its origin where it is wide rather than toward its insertion where the muscle converges into a narrow fasciculus. Injectors should avoid injecting high dilutions of the neurotoxin in this region in order to decrease the chances of adverse events **(Figs. 4A and B)**.[29]

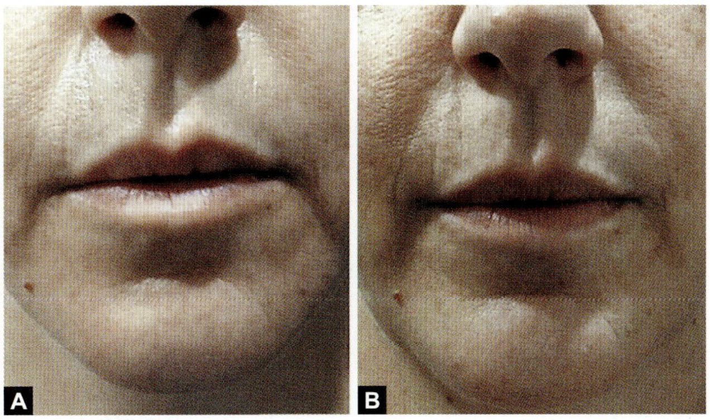

Figs. 4A and B: (A) Melomental lines; (B) After injection of depressor anguli oris: 4 units.
Courtesy: Dr Shehnaz Arsiwala, Mumbai.

Complications

- *Sphincteric dysfunction*: Diffusion of neurotoxin into the fibers of the orbicularis oris may result in inadequate closure of the oral cavity, which leads to a host of difficulties, such as drooling, dribbling, and difficulty in speech and is embarrassing for the patient. Further the patient may feel difficulty in puckering the lips. This may occur when the injections are given high up, in the vicinity of the oral commissure rather than closer to the base of the muscle and/or high volumes are used for dilution of the injected neurotoxin.
- *Asymmetry of the lip*: Injections medial into the DLI may result in flattening of the contour of the lip and an asymmetric smile.

CHIN PUCKERING

Puckering of the chin or hyperactivity of the mentalis is more often noticed by others than the patient themselves. A hyperkinetic mentalis may present itself as a localized "dimpling" or ridges and corrugations involving the whole chin. In some cases, the hyperkinetic mentalis may produce a prominent, deep, and transverse mental crease.

Eversion of the lower lip or pronouncing the letter "F" will accentuate puckering of the chin.

Relevant Anatomy

The mentalis is a short, conical, and paired muscle originating deep to the DLI on the anterior aspect of the mandible on either side of the midline at the level of the incisive fossa and root of the lower lateral incisors.[30] The muscle travels down and converges its two bellies and inserts into the skin of the apex of the chin. Superiorly the fibers of the mentalis mingle with some of the fibers of the orbicularis oris, whereas laterally it interdigitates with the fibers of the DLI. Contraction of the mentalis muscle leads to the upward-inward movement of the soft-tissue complex of the chin, which raises the central portion of the lips in wards against the gums. Further, the mentalis assists other movements such as to protrude, depress, and evert the lower lip.

Injection Technique and Dosing

The 4–8 units of BoNTA may be injected into the muscle in order to relax it. The injection technique employed may vary **(Figs. 5A to C)**:

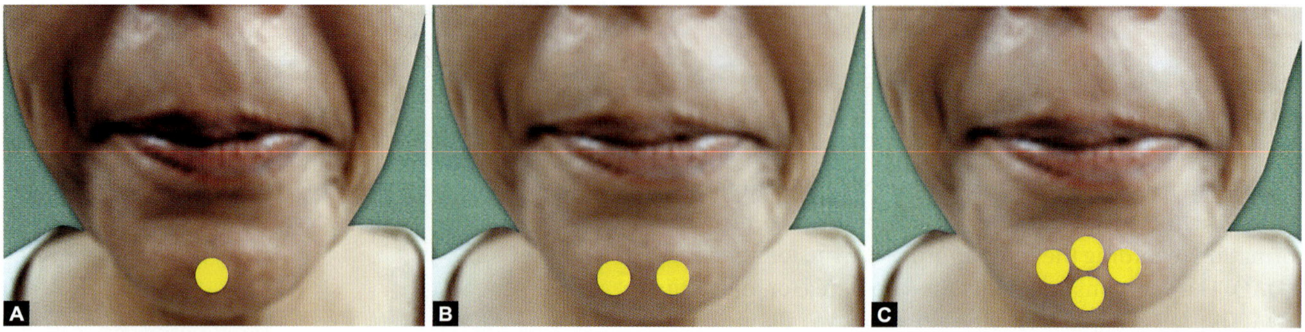

Figs. 5A to C: *Techniques of treating the mentalis muscle:* (A) Single-point technique; (B) Two-point technique; (C) Diamond-shaped technique.
Courtesy: Dr Rajat Kandhari, New Delhi.

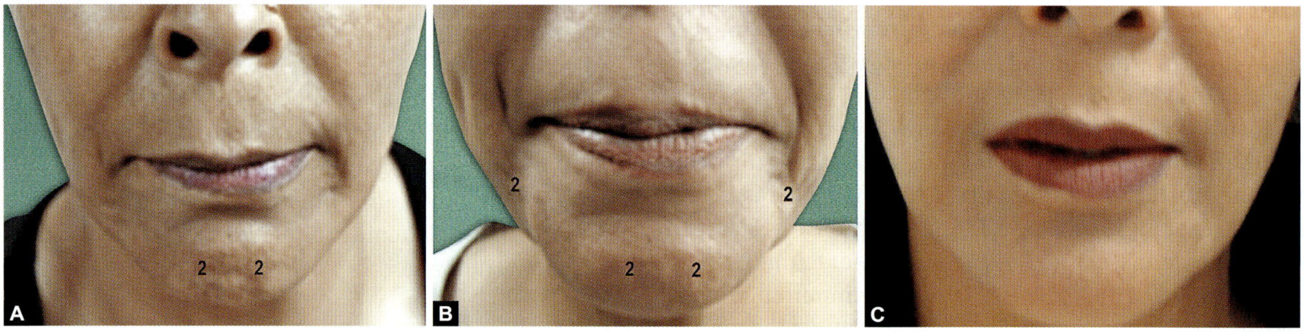

Figs. 6A to C: (A) Treatment of the mentalis with the two-point technique; (B) Treatment of the depressor anguli oris along with the mentalis with 2 units on either side; (C) After treatment of the mentalis and depressor anguli oris.
Courtesy: Dr Rajat Kandhari, New Delhi.

BOX 5: Popley chin.

- 4–8 units directly in mentalis as single or two or four points
- Best results when used with filler

- *Two-point technique:* The 4 units on either side of the midline may be administered directly into the mentalis—appropriate for people with a "squarish" chin or a vertical mental cleft **(Figs. 6A to C)**.
- *Single-point technique*: The 4–6 units into the mentalis at the apex of the mental protuberance—appropriate for those with a pointed or narrow chin.
- *Diamond technique:* Four injection points in the shape of a diamond for equal distribution with 2 units administered at each of these points for a uniform distribution (personal observation).

The global aesthetics consensus on BoNTA recommends the use of 1–4 injection points on either side of the midline with 2–3 units at each injection point.[13]

A deeply placed filler for support along with the use of BoNTA helps in rejuvenation of the chin and is a rewarding indication in aesthetic practice. Moreover, use of soft-tissue fillers with BoNTA, will result in a sustained corrective effect **(Box 5)**.

Complications

- *Sphincter incompetence:* Excessive massage post-injection or injections high up, above, or just below the mental crease can cause diffusion of the neurotoxin to the neighboring orbicularis oris muscle resulting in relaxation of the muscle fibers and an incompetent sphincteric action of the same.
- *Lip incompetence*: Diffusion of the neurotoxin to the adjacent fibers of the DLI will result in lip incompetence. The above two adverse effects can result in difficulty in speech or articulating certain letters or words.
- Over enthusiastic treatment of the mentalis with high doses may freeze the muscle resulting in difficulty in approximation of the lower lip against the gums or teeth and difficulty in approximating a glass or cup to the mouth.

MASSETERIC HYPERTROPHY, "BOXY FACE"

A "boxy face" or squarish, wide lower face is considered undesirable by most individuals, and is perceived as being too "masculine" in women. A wide lower face is commonly seen in India and Asia. A hypertrophic masseter muscle, an enlarged parotid and submandibular gland, and a prominent mandibular angle all contribute to this appearance. Clinically, masseteric muscle hypertrophy is characterized by a symmetrical or asymmetrical increase in the masseter muscle, occurring more frequently between 20 and 40 years age group and is not gender-specific.[31]

The common causes of masseter hypertrophy include masticatory hyperactivity and stomatognathic system dysfunctions, although this may not be the case in all individuals.[32]

Botulinum toxin type A has the potential to decrease lower facial width by inducing atrophy of the masseter muscle and decreasing its volume or size. This results in a narrower face, sharper jawline, and adds a crisp definition to the zygomatic arch and malar eminence.[33]

The use of BoNTA for masseteric hypertrophy has been elaborated upon and proven in the past by ultrasound, electromyography, three-dimensional scanning, as well as by photographic assessment and satisfaction.[34-38]

Relevant Anatomy

The masseter is a thick and rectangular muscle of mastication that extends from the zygomatic arch and the zygomatic bone to the mandible (ramus, mandibular angle, and coronoid process).

The muscle has three overlapping heads:[33]

1. *Deep head*: Originates from the inferoposterior aspect of the zygomatic arch and is inserted into the posterior half of the ascending ramus down to the angle of the mandible.
2. *Intermediate head*: Arises from the middle third of the zygomatic arch and fans downward inserting into the anterior half of the ascending ramus, the condyle, and the angle of the mandible.
3. *Superficial head*: Originates from the anterior half of the zygomatic arch and some aspect of the malar eminence. The superficial head fans downward to insert into the angle of the mandible.

Knowledge of the anatomy of the three heads is critical as the injection of the neurotoxin should be deep so as to affect the motor endplates of the masseter muscle, which are located in the center of the lower half of this muscle.[39,40] In case, injections are not deep, suboptimal outcomes may result.

Injection Technique and Dosing

Prior to injection into the masseter, the muscle is identified by asking the patient to bite down or clench their teeth. The anterior edge of the masseter is easily felt and the other borders comprise the zygomatic arch, the posterior edge of the ramus, and the lower border of the mandible **(Box 6)**. The technique of injecting may vary, while some authors suggest a three-point injection technique in the shape of a triangle, wherein two points are spaced out 1.5 cm apart forming an imaginary line above the body of the mandible and the apex of the triangle is 2 cm above this imaginary line.[41]

Other authors may suggest 5–8 spaced out injections deep into the masseter in the lower half, posteriorly where the three heads overlap, and the muscle is the thickest.[33]

The dosing and the exact site of injection have been a matter of debate while injecting the masseter.

Botulinum toxin type A injections into the masseter not only help decrease muscle volume or the hypertrophic appearance of the muscle but also helps in bony remodeling of the mandible over time. A decrease in the mandibular width over several months has been demonstrated in the past. Further, it helps reduce bruxism, headaches, and teeth grinding in those in whom it is a problem.[42]

BOX 6: Masseter hypertrophy.

- 25–40 units each side
- 2–3 points
- Lower muscle belly points preferred

TABLE 1: Classification of the masseter based on the bulging pattern.

Type	*Pattern*	*Description*
I	Minimal	Even masseter contraction, no obvious bulging palpable
II	Mono	Local single longitudinal bulge
III	Double	Two separate longitudinal bulges of equal or differing height
IV	Triple	Three longitudinal bulges
V	Excessive	Massive single bulge

Xie et al.[39] suggested that the most prominent points of bulging appear to be the appropriate sites for injecting the masseter. They have classified the masseter based on the bulging pattern of the contracted muscle, in order to tailor treatment on the basis of the individual's bulging **(Table 1)**.

The site of most prominent bulging would also be the site of the motor end plates, and an injection near the nerve endings directly at the site of the neuromuscular junction would allow for a reduction in dosage and volume of the neurotoxin and limited dispersion in the region.[43-45] However, injections should be restricted to the posterior, lower quadrant of the masseter muscle in order to avoid injecting into the pterygoid muscles, and other side effects discussed subsequently.

Further, regarding the dosing of the masseter, a minimal dose of 20–25 units per masseter should be administered.[46,47] Although certain authors recommend higher doses (30–50 units per masseter) for increased muscle width in order to achieve optimum results.[38,48] It has been suggested that dosing should be restricted to 60 units per masseter or 1.5 cc in order to avoid inadvertent diffusion of the neurotoxin.[33]

Complications

- *Difficulty in chewing or weakening of the pterygoid muscles:* Care should be taken not to inject into the pterygoid fossa (through the coronoid notch) as this may result in weakening of the pterygoid muscles and difficulty in chewing. Injections should be higher up into the muscle.
- *Asymmetric smile*: Diffusion of the neurotoxin into the neighboring muscles such as the risorius and the levator anguli oris can occur, if the injection is given close to the anterior border of the masseter muscle. High volume injections may also predispose the patient to this side effect.

- *Dull ache on chewing*: The patient might face some difficulty in wide mouth opening, e.g., taking a bite of a burger. This typically settles after repeated treatments.
- *Jowling of the overlying skin envelope*: This complication may arise due to overcorrection or excessive doses of the toxin leading to a fast atrophy of the masseter and sagging of the overlying skin. A thorough assessment of the patient before the injection is important to avoid such adverse effects. Usually, the overlying skin acclimatizes to the shrinking muscles and drapes on it accordingly, but in such cases it may take up to 2–3 months for the skin to acclimatize to the shrunken muscle.
- *Scalloping of the lateral side of the face*: Injecting high up into the masseter especially with larger doses may result in an accentuated scalloping of the lateral side of the face.
- Bruising and hematoma may occur in this region after injection.
- Infrazygomatic hollowing
- Fasciculations in the muscle may occur in the first 2–3 weeks: This represents insufficient dosing.
- Superficial injections may target superficial parts of the muscle, with prolapse of deeper part leading to chipmunk appearance.

PLATYSMA

The neck although frequently neglected is possibly a fairly accurate indicator of a person's age. With age and neck movements, there is loss of elasticity of the skin which becomes lax and redundant, vertical platysmal bands, and horizontal neck lines or creases become apparent and in some individuals, the unsightly "turkey neck" deformity may appear due to the anterior bulging of the vertical platysmal fibers due to loss of tone. Further the hyperkinetic fibers of the upper platysma blunt the jawline along with muscles of the lower face particularly the DAO. BoNTA may be a good treatment option for those patients, who possess some amount of cutaneous elasticity and have platysmal neck bands or horizontal neck lines and are not willing to undergo surgical procedures such as cervicoplasty or rhytidectomy. BoNTA may be used alone or with laser resurfacing, other energy-based devices, threads and/or hyaluronic acid fillers.

Relevant Anatomy

The platysma is a broad, thin, and superficial muscle with two separate bands which originate from the superior portions of the pectoralis major and deltoid muscles, run up the front and lateral aspects of the neck and insert on the inferior mandible at the symphysis, blend with the superficial musculoaponeurotic system (SMAS) in the lower face and with muscle fibers at and around the oral commissure, and few platysmal fibers may extend as high as the zygoma. The platysmal fibers decussate with the fibers of the orbicularis oris and the posterior fibers of the DAO, and together these fibers pull the buccal commissures laterally downward. Relaxation of these decussating fibers with BoNTA injections can give a mini-necklift.[45]

The upper fibers of the platysma comprise three portions contributing to and forming the orbicularis oris complex:[29]

1. *Platysma pars mandibularis*: Insert into the lower border of the body of the mandible below the oblique line and into the skin and subcutaneous tissue of the lower face.
2. *Platysma pars labialis*: These fibers decussate with the muscles around the mouth (orbicularis oris, risorius, mentalis, DAO, and DLI). They act as direct labial tractors and insert within the tissue of the lateral half of the lower lip.
3. *Platysma pars modiolaris*: Fibers posterior to the platysma pars labialis and posterolateral to the DAO make up the platysma pars modiolaris. These fibers pass deep to the risorius and attach into the apical and subapical modiolar attachments.

The structure of the platysma has certain variations as described in a cadaveric demonstration by de Castro:[46]

- *Type I*: In approximately 75% individuals, there is limited decussation of the medial fibers of the platysma. The fibers interdigitate with the opposite counterpart across the midline approximately 1–2 cm below the chin.
- *Type II*: Some part of the platysma appears as a uniform sheet and the unison of the fibers from either side of the midline occurs at the level of the thyroid cartilage. Seen in approximately 15% of individuals.
- *Type III*: In 10% of individuals, the platysma appears as two separate straps of platysma that run parallel to each other and ascend to attach to the mandible without any decussation of fibers from either side.

Other than the muscle itself there are two fat depots in the neck region, namely the submental or submandibular fat which is more superficial and lies anterior to the fibers of the platysma in the subcutaneous plane, and the subplatysmal fat which lies posterior to the platysma. Herniation of the subplatysmal fat depot leads to the so-called turkey neck deformity.

The platysma has the potential to depress the corners of the mouth and mandible and is active during rapid and deep inspiration.

Injection Technique and Dosing

Blunted Jawline (The Nefertiti Lift)

The upper platysmal fibers are responsible for blunting the jawline along with muscles of the lower face. The horizontal wrinkles in the vicinity of the modiolus and adjacent to the oral commissures appear due to contraction of these fibers.

These wrinkles are visible and palpable in individuals when they compress the corners of the mouth. Some individuals have a habit of doing this and may have coexistent Marionette lines and a hypertrophic DAO and mentalis.

The injections are given approximately 2 cm below the mandible, below the region where the wrinkling is visible. The injections are usually 2 units each in spaced out injections at 1–3 points, approximately 1–2 cm apart. Concomitant treatment of the DAO and mentalis will enhance the results and gives a sharper contour to the lower face. The injections should be posterior to the lateral border of the DAO and anterior to the belly of the sternocleidomastoid. Injections in this manner along with treatment of a lateral platysmal band if present comprises the popular "Nefertiti lift". The injection pattern appears like an inverted triangle.[47]

Horizontal Lines and Vertical Neck Bands

Identification of the vertical platysmal bands is simple and is done by asking the patient to clench their teeth or say "e". The platysmal bands can then be grasped between the thumb and index finger of the nondominant hand and 2–3 units of BoNTA is given by raising a wheal intradermally, in spaced out injection 1.5–2 cm apart starting in the submental region about 2 cm below the inferior mandibular border.[49] The Global Aesthetics Consensus Group recommends 1–3 units at each injection site or 6–12 units per band up to a maximum dose of 60 units per session.[13] Other authors recommend a relatively conservative approach of three to four injections per band, with a total dose of 24–32 units.[9]

Patient selection is crucial while treating the platysmal bands and treatment of individuals with extensive skin laxity and flaccid cords can make matter worse.

For treating the horizontal lines on the neck, approximately 1–2 units of BoNTA above and below the lines on the neck at intervals of up to 3 cm may be given in the deep dermis. Further this is one region where a higher dilution of BoNTA may be preferred. Not >25–35 units should be administered per treatment session **(Box 7 and Fig. 7)**.[29]

Complications

Precise injections are the key to optimal outcomes while injecting the platysma, particularly the platysma pars mandibularis (upper platysmal fibers).

- *Distortion of the lower face and/or oral sphincter incompetence*: Inappropriate diffusion of the neurotoxin into the DLI or the deep fibers of the orbicularis oris will result in the malfunctioning of the mouth, an asymmetric smile, and a distortion of the lower face.
- *Difficulty in lateral movement of the neck*: This may occur due to inadvertent diffusion or direct injection into the sternocleidomastoid muscle. This may also lead to difficulty in raising from a supine position.
- Overzealous injections while treating the vertical bands or horizontal lines may lead to xerostomia, dysphagia, dysarthria, and/or neck weakness. This occurs due to the cholinergic nature of the underlying muscles associated with deglutition, phonation, and neck flexion.
- Ecchymosis, transient edema, and erythema are common adverse events and resolve within a few days.

Mesobotulinum for Midface Lower Face and Neck with Dose Variations

Meso- or microbotulinum toxin method employs microdroplets of diluted toxin delivered to the intradermal site of treatment zone to decrease function of sweat and sebaceous glands and achieve superficial muscle relaxation without complete functional inactivity and specifically done in areas where retaining muscle function is important like midface, perioral, jawline, and neck consequently leading to a smooth skin texture and luminosity. The depth of injection in microdroplet technique is more superficial **(Figs. 8A and B)**.

BOX 7: Nefertiti lift.

- *Blunted jawline—upper platysmal fibers*: 2–6 units, mandibular line
- Treat mentalis and depressor anguli oris concomitantly
- *Platysmal bands*: 6–12 units each side
- Horizontal lines on the neck approximately 1–2 units of botulinum toxin type A above and below the lines on the neck

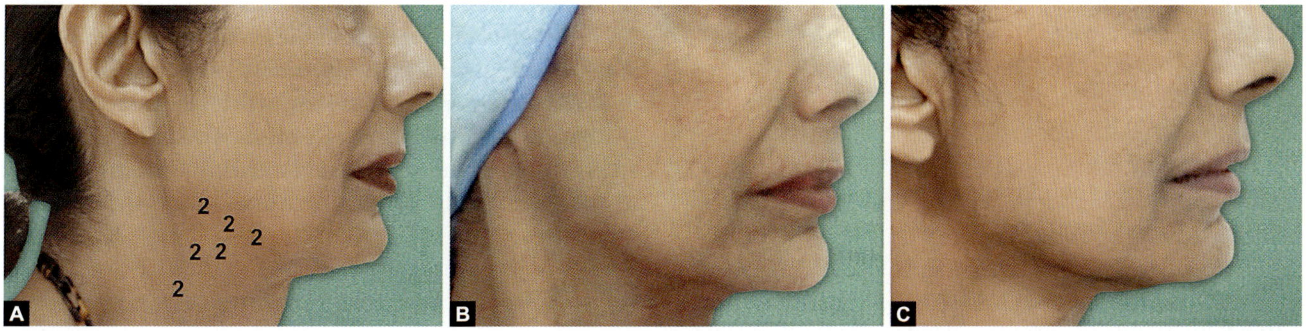

Figs. 7A to C: (A) Injection of the botulinum toxin in the pars mandibularis part of the platysma fibers. The depressor anguli oris was also treated bilaterally with 4 units; (B) After one session of treatment; (C) After two sessions giving the jaw a contoured appearance.
Courtesy: Dr Rajat Kandhari, New Delhi.

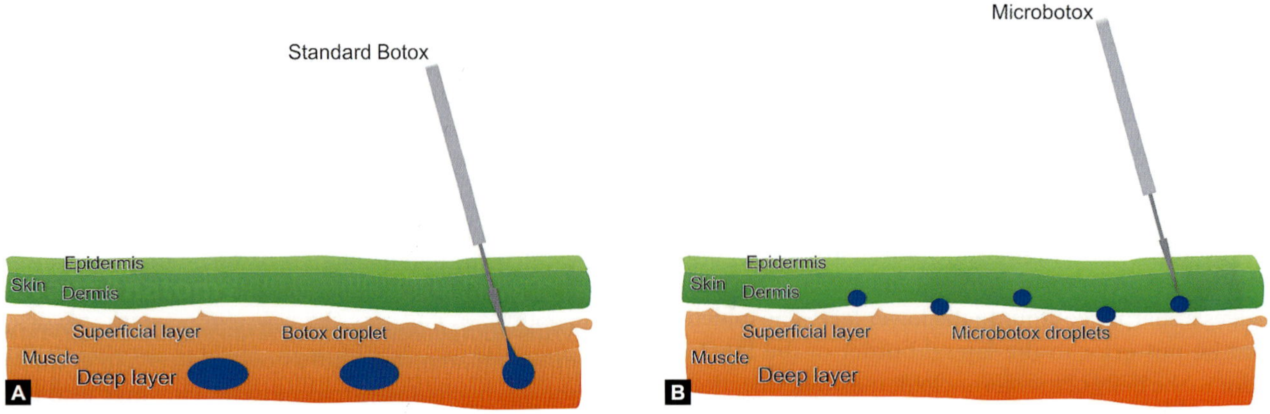

Figs. 8A and B: Difference of depth of injection for standard Bont-A and microbotulinum.

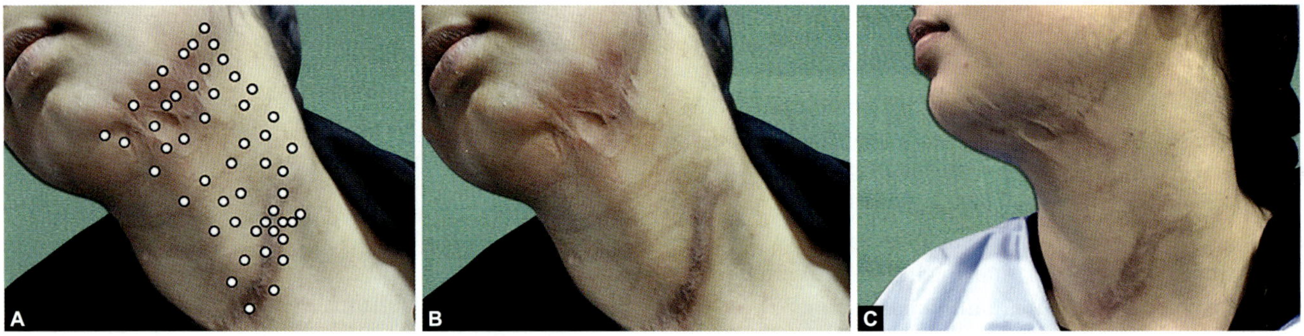

Figs. 9A to C: Mesobotulinum for jawline and neck with dose variation to relax scar tension.

Multiple microdroplets of diluted reconstituted botulinum are injected using 30–32 gauge needle and diluents used can be normal saline and some experts suggest lidocaine for better anesthetic effect and generally lower face and neck require up to 1 mL per site.

Advantages of microdroplet BoNTA are:
- Smoothen the skin texture
- Achieve luminosity
- Smoothen fine lines
- Decrease superficial horizontal and vertical rhytides

Dilution for Midface Lowerface and Neck[50-52]

Dilution depends upon the area to be treated. Standard dilution is achieved to reconstitute botulinum toxin type A (BoNTA) and then double (1:2) or triple (1:3) dilution method with normal saline is employed to prepare microbotulinum doses. This enables the physician to treat areas with standard method like masseter or platysma or DAO and then further dilution to treat neck lines **(Figs. 9A to C)**.

Box 8 highlights the protocol used by Dr Woffles Wu for microbotulinum dilutions pertaining to various areas using 1:10 ratio for open pores and skin luminosity.[52]

BOX 8: Variations from standard doses.[52]

- MB 20–20 U + 0.5 lidocaine for
- Infraorbital, cheeks, T zone, and rosacea acne

- MB 24–24 units +0.5 lidocaine
- Forehead, glabella, and crows' feet

- MB 28–28 units + 0.5 lidocaine
- Jawline, jowls, neck, and scars, keloids

- 1 CC = 100–150 microdroplets
- 1 drop = 0.2 units

(MB: microbotulinum)

Since there is no standardized global technique for microbotulinum microdroplet technique a large variation in dilutions is used by various physicians as per their discretion.

Another technique recently described delivers the solution is delivered intradermally, using an electrical needling pen, and setting the depth penetration of the needles at 3–3.5 mm.[53]

The undesired effects of meso and microbotulinum technique include puncture marks, bruising, uneven distribution, unintended muscle relaxation, and asymmetric smile.[54,55]

TIPS

- Stay intradermal and create a bleb
- Change needle at every 5–6 punctures to prevent bleeding
- Understand anatomy and plan meticulously

CONCLUSION

Botulinum toxin therapy for dynamic rejuvenation of mid and lower face necessitates mandatory knowledge of various muscle attachments and actions. Though units needed are low risk of complications, are high as specific and perfect injection points are necessary. An injecting physician must embark on mid and lower face treatment only after acquiring requisite expertise.

PITFALLS

- Nasalis should be treated with glabellar complex.
- Concomitant treatment of the DAO and mentalis will enhance the results and gives a sharper contour to the lower face.
- Keep the injection point at least 1 cm from the anterior border of the masseter muscle.
- Rejuvenation is dynamic and volumetric when a puckered chin is treated with BoNTA and fillers.
- Consider microbotulinum along with standard injection points to improve skin texture and luminosity.

REFERENCES

1. FDA. (1989). BOTOX Cosmetic (onabotulinum toxin A) for injection, for intramuscular use. [online] Available from http://www.accessdata.fda.gov/drugsatfda_docs/label/2015/103000s5292lbl.pdf [Last accessed March, 2024].
2. US FDA. (2013). FDA approves Botox Cosmetic to improve the appearance of crow's feet lines. [online] Available from http://www.fda.gov/NewsEvents/Newsroom/PressAnnouncements/ucm367662.htm [Last accessed March, 2024].
3. Fagien S. Botox for the treatment of dynamic and hyperkinetic facial lines and furrows: adjunctive use in facial aesthetic surgery. Plast Reconstr Surg. 1999;103(2):701-13.
4. Benedetto AV. Cosmetic uses of Botulinum toxin A in the mid face. In: Botulinum Toxins in Clinical Aesthetic Practice, 2nd edition. Boca Raton: CRC Press; 2011. pp. 101-39.
5. Rohrich RJ, Janis JE, Fagien S, Stuzin JM. The cosmetic use of botulinum toxin. Plast Reconstr Surg. 2003;112(5):177S-88S.
6. Tamura BM, OdoMY, Chang B, Cucé LC, Flynn TC. Treatment of nasal wrinkles with botulinum toxin. Dermatol Surg. 2005;31(3):271-5.
7. Ahn BK, Kim YS, Kim HJ, Rho NK, Kim HS. Consensus recommendations on the aesthetic usage of botulinum toxin type A in Asians. Dermatol Surg. 2013;39(12):1843-60.
8. Wu WT, Liew S, Chan HH, et al. Consensus on current injectable treatment strategies in the Asian face. Aesthetic Plast Surg. 2016;40(2):202-14.
9. Carruthers J, Carruthers A. Aesthetic botulinum A toxin in the mid and lower face and neck. Dermatol Surg. 2003;29(5):468-76.
10. Carruthers A, Carruthers J. Clinical indications and injection technique for the cosmetic use of botulinum A exotoxin. Dermatol Surg. 1998;24(11):1189-94.
11. Sundaram H, Signorini M, Liew S, Trindade de Almeida AR, Wu Y, Vieira Braz A, et al. Global aesthetics consensus: botulinum toxin type A: evidence-based review, emerging concepts, and consensus recommendations for aesthetic use, including updates on complications. Plast Reconstr Surg. 2016;137(3):518e-29e.
12. Peck S, Peck L, Kataja M. The gingival smile line. Angle Orthod.1992;62(2):91-100.
13. Ackerman JL, Ackerman MB, Brensinger CM, Landis JR. A morphometric analysis of the posed smile. Clin Orthod Res. 1998;1(1):2-11.
14. Ackerman MB, Ackerman JL. Smile analysis and design in the digital era. J Clin Orthod. 2002;36(4):221-36.
15. Khanna B. Lip stabilization with botulinum toxin. Aesthetic Dentistry Today. 2007;3:54-9.
16. Tamura BM. Facial anatomy and the application of fillers and botulinum toxin–Part I. Surg Cosmet Dermatol. 2010;2:195-204.
17. Philips E. The classification of smile patterns. J Can Dent Assoc. 1999;65:252-4.
18. Kokich VO, Kiyak HA, Shapiro PA. Comparing the perception of dentists and lay people to altered dental esthetics. J Esthet Dent.1999;11(6):311-24.
19. Sarver DM. The importance of incisor positioning in the esthetic smile: the smile arc. Am J Orthod Dentofacial Orthop. 2001;120(2):98-111.
20. Hexsel D, Trindade de Almeida A. UsoCosméticodaToxinaBotúnica. Porto Alegre, Brazil: Age; 2002. pp. 198-200.
21. Polo M. Botulinum toxin type A in the treatment of excessive gingival display. Am J Orthod Dentofacial. 2005;127(2):214-8.
22. Carruthers A, Carruthers J, Hardas B, Kaur M, Goertelmeyer R, Jones D, et al. A validated grading scale for marionette lines. Dermatol Surg. 2008;34(s2):S167-72.
23. Yu SK, Lee MH, Kim HS, Park JT, Kim HJ, Kim HJ. Histomorphologic approach for the modiolus with reference to reconstructive and aesthetic surgery. J Craniofac Surg. 2013;24(4):1414-7.
24. Hur MS, Hu KS, Cho JY, Kwak HH, Song WC, Koh KS, et al. Topography and location of the depressor anguli oris muscle with a reference to the mental foramen. Surg Radiol Anat.2008;30(5):403-7.
25. Choi YJ, Kim JS, Gil YC, Phetudom T, Kim HJ, Tansatit T, et al. Anatomical considerations regarding the location and boundary of the depressor anguli oris muscle with reference to botulinum toxin injection. Plast Reconstr Surg. 2014;134(5):917-21.
26. Benedetto AV. Cosmetic uses of botulinum toxin A in the lower face, neck and upper chest. Botulinum Toxins in Clinical Aesthetic Practice, 2nd edition. Boca Raton: CRC Press; 2011. pp. 140-89.
27. von LindernJ J, Niederhagen B, Appel T, et al. Type A botulinum toxin for the treatment of hypertrophy of the masseter and temporal muscles: an alternative treatment. Plast Reconstr Surg. 2001;107(2):327-32.
28. Ahn KY, Kim ST. The change of maximum bite force after botulinum toxin type A injection for treating masseteric hypertrophy. Plast Reconstr Surg. 2007;120(6):1662-6.
29. Wu WT. Facial and lower limb contouring. Botulinum Toxins in Clinical Aesthetic Practice, 2nd edition. United Kingdom: Informa Health Care; 2011. pp. 206-22.
30. Wu WT. Botox facial slimming/facial sculpting: the role of botulinum toxin A in the treatment of hypertrophic masseteric muscle and parotid enlargement to narrow the lower facial width. Facial Plast Surg Clin North Am. 2010;18(1):133-40.
31. To EW, Ahuja AT, Ho WS, King WW, Wong WK, Pang PC, et al. A prospective study of the effect of botulinum toxin A on masseteric muscle hypertrophy with ultrasonographic and electromyographic measurement. Br J Plast Surg. 2001;54(3):197-200.
32. Kim HJ, Yum KW, Lee SS, Heo MS, Seo K. Effects of botulinum toxin type A on bilateral masseteric hypertrophy evaluated

with computed tomographic measurement. Dermatol Surg. 2003;29(5):484-9.

33. Lee CJ, Kim SG, Kim YJ, Han JY, Choi SH, Lee SI. Electrophysiologic change and facial contour following botulinum toxin A injection in square faces. Plast Reconstr Surg. 2007;120(3):769-78.
34. Gaofeng L, Jun T, Bo P, Bosheng Z, Qian Z, Dongping L. Evaluation and selecting indications for the treatment of improving facial morphology by masseteric injection of botulinum toxin type A. J Plast Reconstr Aesthet Surg. 2010;63(12):2026-31.
35. Iwasaki S, Tokunaga T, Baba S, Tanaka M, Kawazoe T. Noninvasive estimation of the location of the end plate in the human masseter muscle using surface electromyograms with an electrode array. J Osaka Dent Univ. 1990;24(2):135-40.
36. Mito K, Sakamoto K. Distribution of muscle fiber conduction velocity of m. masseter during voluntary isometric contraction. Electromyogr Clin Neurophysiol. 2000;40:275-85.
37. Trévidic P, Sykes J, Criollo-Lamilla G. Anatomy of the lower face and botulinum toxin injections. Plast Reconstr Surg. 2015;136(5S):84S-91S.
38. Panfilov DE. Nonsurgical facial rejuvenation with the 4r principle: innovative uses of botox and facelifting with the woffles lift, a barbed suture sling. Aesthetic Surgery of the Facial Mosaic. Germany: Springer Science & Business Media; 2007. pp. 636-49.
39. Xie Y, Zhou J, Li H, Cheng C, Herrler T, Li Q. Classification of masseter hypertrophy for tailored botulinum toxin type A treatment. Plast Reconstr Surg. 2014;134(2):209e-18e.
40. Carruthers A, Carruthers J. Botulinum toxin type A. J Am Acad Dermatol. 2005;53(2):284-90.
41. Kim DH, Hong HS, Won SY, Kim HJ, Hu KS, Choi JH, et al. Intramuscular nerve distribution of the masseter muscle as a basis for botulinum toxin injection. J Craniofac Surg. 2010;21(2):588-91.
42. Choe SW, Cho WI, Lee CK, Seo SJ. Effects of botulinum toxin type A on contouring of the lower face. Dermatol Surg. 2005;31(5):502-8.
43. Kwon JS, Kim ST, Jeon YM, Choi JH. Effect of botulinum toxin type A injection into human masseter muscle on stimulated parotid saliva flow rate. Int J Oral Maxillofac Surg. 2009;38(4):316-20.
44. Jaspers GW, Pijpe J, Jansma J. The use of botulinum toxin type A in cosmetic facial procedures. Int J Oral Maxillofac Surg. 2011;40(2):127-33.
45. Prendergast PM. Anatomy of the face and neck. In: Cosmetic Surgery. New York, NY: Springer Verlag Berlin Heidelberg; 2012. pp. 29-45.
46. de Castro CC. The anatomy of the platysma muscle. Plast Reconstr Surg. 1980;66(5):680-3.
47. Levy PM. The 'Nefertiti lift': A new technique for specific re-contouring of the jawline. J Cosmet Laser Ther. 2007;9(4):249-52.
48. de Castro CC. The changing role of platysma in face lifting. Plast Reconstr Surg. 2000;105(2):764-75.
49. Cardoso de Castro C. The changing role of platysma in face lifting. Plast Reconstr Surg. 2000;105(2):764-75; discussion 776-7.
50. Chang S, Hisou HT, Wei-Yu-Chen, Woan-R L, Ping Ling C, Tsung- Hsien T. The wrinkles soothing effect on the middle and lower face by intradermal injection of botulinum toxin type A. Int J Dermatol. 2008;47:1287-94.
51. Cyril J, Samer F, Youssef A, Joseph S, Elio G, Marwan W. Evaluation of the Microbotox Technique: An algorithmic approach for lower face and neck rejuvenation and a crossover clinical trial. Plast Reconstr Surg. 2018;142:640-9.
52. Wu WTL. Microbotox of the lower face and neck: evolution of a personal technique and its clinical effects. Plast Reconstr Surg. 2015;136(5 Suppl):92S-100S.
53. Calvani F, Santini S, Bartoletti E, Alhadeff A. Personal technique of microinfiltration with botulin toxin: the SINB technique (Superficial Injection Needling Botulinum). Plast Surg (Oakv). 2019;27(2):156-61.
54. Joel S, Erin G, Joel L, Cohen, Joel K. New uses of Abotulinum toxin A in Aesthetics. Aesthet Surg J. 2017;37(1 Suppl):S45-S58.
55. Chariya P. Midface lifting with Botulinum toxin: intradermal technique. J Cosmet Dermatol. 2009;8(4):312-6.

CHAPTER 89

Non-cosmetic Indications of Botulinum Toxin

Mukta Sachdev, Rachana Shilpakar

KEY MESSAGES

- Botulinum toxin has been found useful in several non-cosmetic indications.
- These include hyperhidrosis, scars, keloids, rosacea, occipital neuralgia after hair transplant, depression, and rare dermatological conditions such as pachyonychia congenita, pachydermoperiostosis, epidermolysis simplex, etc.
- Dosage regulations need to be followed properly.

"All things are poisons, and there is nothing that is harmless; the dose alone decides that something is a poison."

— **Paracelsus (1493–1541)**.[1]

INTRODUCTION[1-3]

Cosmetic indications for botulinum toxin (BTX) are widely known and are extremely popular. However, the toxin is useful for several non-cosmetic indications in dermatology. While the cosmetic indications have been dealt with in detail in the previous chapter, this chapter deals with non-cosmetic indications. As stated earlier, a fascinating aspect of BTX research in recent years has been development of the most potent toxin into a molecule of significant utility. It is the first biological toxin which is licensed for treatment of human disease. The United States Food and Drug Administration (US FDA) approved BTXA in the management of strabismus, blepharospasm, and related facial spasms in 1989 and cervical dystonias in 2000. Structure, biochemistry, mechanisms of action, and properties have all been dealt in previous chapter and in several publications[3-6] and will not be discussed here.

Dermatological and medical indications of BTX[1,7] are shown in **Table 1**.

NONAESTHETIC DERMATOLOGICAL INDICATIONS OF BOTULINUM TOXIN

Dermatological non-cosmetic indications include hyperhidrosis, hypertrophic scars or keloids, postherpetic neuralgia (PHN), acne scars, painful scars, multiple eccrine hidrocystomas, rosacea, occipital neuralgia post-hair transplant, etc. These will be discussed in detail.

Contraindications have been discussed in earlier chapter and in other reviews.[5,8]

Patients at risk for side effects include:

- Patients with high tendency of bruise formation
- Patients on blood thinning drugs such as aspirin, warfarin, etc.
- Patients with history of herpes simplex infections such as recurrent herpes labialis
- Patients with history of recurrent cutaneous infections, eczema
- Patients needing lots of facial expression by profession, e.g., dancers, actors
- Patients with unrealistic expectations, body dysmorphic disorder.

HYPERHIDROSIS

Hyperhidrosis is defined as the production of excessive sweat beyond the amount required to return elevated body temperature to normal. It is a physically, emotionally, and socially embarrassing condition with considerable difficulties in social situations and in personal relationships due to malodor, wetness, and staining of clothes.

Hyperhidrosis can be divided into primary and secondary forms. Secondary hyperhidrosis, which again may be localized or generalized, may be due to various underlying causes such as neurological disorders, metabolic disorders, elevated catecholamines, febrile illness, etc. Thus, treating the underlying illness will improve such excessive sweating.

Primary or essential hyperhidrosis is the most common cause of excessive sweating associated with comorbidity of psychiatric disorders like anxiety, neurosis, and depression. The management options for primary hyperhidrosis include topical aluminum salts solution, tap water iontophoresis, axillary sweat glands excision, endoscopic thoracic sympathectomy, laser therapy[9-11] with various wavelengths, radio frequency and Mira Dry device and BTX injections.

TABLE 1: Nonaesthetic dermatological and medical indications of botulinum toxins.

Indication	*Examples*
Exocrine gland hyperactivity	Focal hyperhidrosis (axillary, palmar, plantar, forehead) relative sialorrhea, crocodile tears syndrome, Frey's syndrome, stump hyperhidrosis, and eccrine nevus
Dermatology	*Scars:* Hypertrophic scars/keloids, painful scars, facial scar management, acne scars; *Neuralgia:* Postherpetic neuralgia (PHN), occipital neuralgia post-hair transplant; *Inflammatory dermatoses:* Hidradenitis suppurativa, flexural psoriasis, folliculitis decalvans; *Rosacea; Raynaud's phenomenon; pruritic dermatoses:* Pompholyx, lichen simplex, Fox–Fordyce disease, aquagenic keratoderma, nostalgia paresthetica, idiopathic pruritus; *Genodermatoses:* Hailey–Hailey disease, Darier's disease, epidermolysis bullosa simplex, pachyonychia congenita; *Depression; others:* Multiple eccrine hidrocystomas, leiomyoma related pain
Dystonias	Cervical dystonia, oromandibular dystonia, pharyngolaryngeal dystonias, jaw closure/opening dystonias, occupational cramps, limb, and axial dystonias
Spasticity	Cerebral palsy, brain injury, spinal cord injury, post-stroke, multiple sclerosis
Eyelid spasm	Blepharospasm, hemifacial spasm, eyelid twitch
Movement disorders	Tremors, bruxism, tic
Pain syndromes	Migraine, back spasm, fibromyalgia, piriformis syndrome, radiculopathy, myofascial pain, Raynaud's phenomenon
Psychiatry	Depression
Urinary bladder dysfunctions	Sphincter-detrusor dyssynergia, detrusor hyperreflexia
Ophthalmology	Strabismus, entropion, protective ptosis, nystagmus, chronic VI nerve palsy
Gastroenterology	Achalasia, anal fissures, anismus, cricopharyngeal spasm
Gynecology	Vaginismus
Urology	Sterile prostatitis
Dentistry	Muscle spasm associated with temporomandibular joint pathology
Miscellaneous	Stuttering, VII nerve disorders, freezing of gait
Veterinary	Barking dogs

Mechanism of Action of Botulinum Toxin in Hyperhidrosis

Botulinum toxin inhibits cholinergic transmission in post sympathetic fibers to sweat glands leading to temporary chemo denervation of sweat glands with the loss or reduction of activity of the target organ.[12]

Indications and Contraindications of Botulinum Toxin in Hyperhidrosis

- Patients not responding to other modalities of treatment such as aluminum salt solutions, tap water iontophoresis in palmoplantar hyperhidrosis.
- Patients with hyperhidrosis associated with a psychosomatic disorder or with a secondary psychiatric reaction arising from the chronic skin disease such as sociophobia, depression, anxiety who fail to show satisfactory response with the topical treatment.
- Contraindicated in subjects with secondary hyperhidrosis due to underlying diseases.

Preparations Before Procedure[3,13]

- Detailed medical history to rule out any underlying causes of secondary hyperhidrosis as well as the diseases which are contraindicated for BTX injections:
  - *Iodine starch test*: This simple procedure is carried out to document the extent of excessive sweating and also to determine the number of injection sites and the quantity of toxin needed. First the hyperhidrotic area is completely dried. The iodine solution is then applied to the affected area using a swab **(Fig. 1)**. The powdered starch (potato starch or cornflower starch) is sprinkled over the iodine solution. The patient is made to sweat by an external source. The sweat turns the starch black delineating the affected area **(Fig. 2)**. For iodine-sensitive patients, ponceau red tincture is an alternative.
- The affected area is outlined with a marker pen. Photographs are taken for future references.
- The area should be cleansed of all iodine and starch.
- Final cleansing with the isopropyl alcohol should be done before the injection.

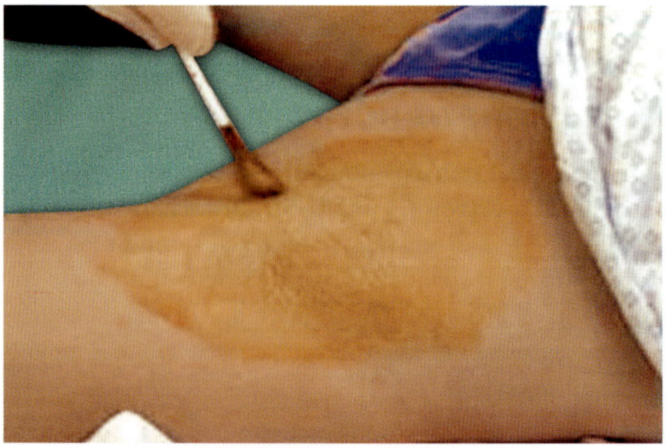

Fig. 1: Application of iodine.

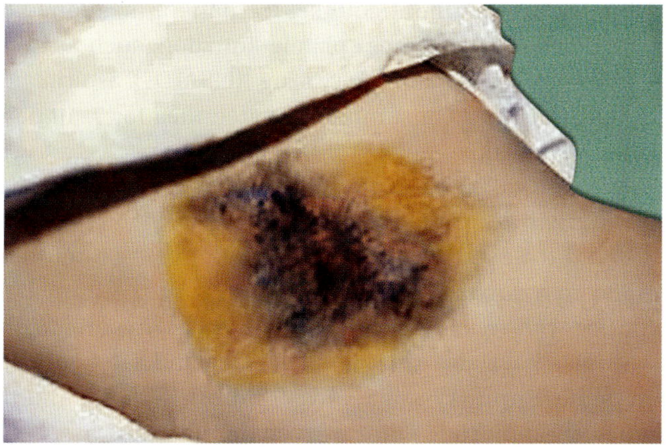

Fig. 2: Dark purple area of hyperhidrosis.

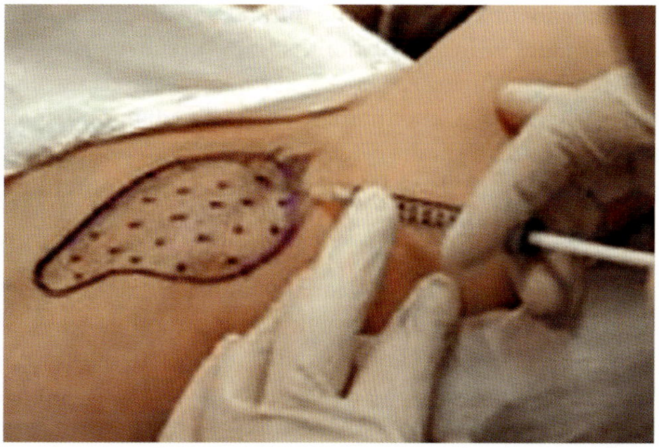

Fig. 3: Injection of botulinum toxin (BTX).

TABLE 2: Suggested dilutions for axillary hyperhidrosis.

Dilution	*Botox® 10 mL*	*Dysport® 10 mL*
U/vial	100	500
U/mL	10	50
U/0.1 mL	1	5
mL/injection site	0.2	0.2

Dose

The dilution and dosage are still the subjects of discussion. The dosage should be defined by the dose per injection point (2 U) and not by the total dose per area, because depending on the extent of the affected hyperhidrotic area the total dose can vary considerably, whereas the dose per injection site always remains constant.[13]

The dose-effect relationship is different for each of these target tissues. The lowest dose needed to gain anhidrotic effect is 2 U of BTX (Botox®) per site.[14]

AXILLARY HYPERHIDROSIS

Anesthesia

It is generally not necessary as BTX injection in this region is almost painless.

Dilution and Dosage

The BTX (Botox®) is diluted with 5.0 cc of preservative free saline yielding 2 U per 0.1 cc.[3] Kreyden OP[13] suggests reconstitution of 100 U of Botox® with 10 mL of normal saline yielding 2 U of BTX A per 0.2 mL. Kreyden's suggestion is influenced by Bigalke et al.[15] a study which showed the enhancement of biologic availability of Dysport® by lowering the concentration of BTX A, increasing the dilution volume, and supplementing reconstituted Dysport® with additional albumin **(Table 2)**. This low dose, high volume technique has several advantages such as:

- Fewer injections

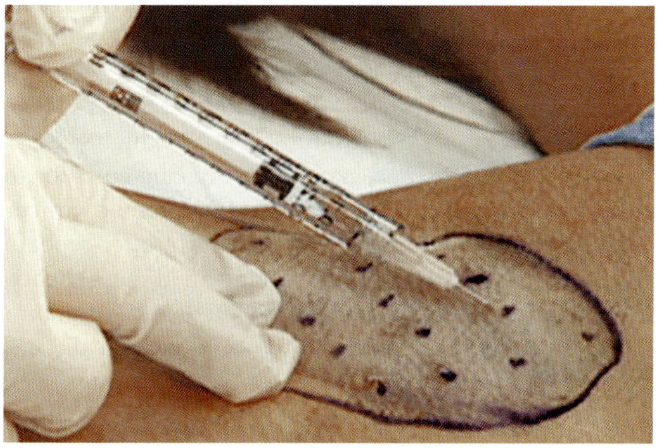

Fig. 4: Raised wheal at injection site.

- Less painful treatment sessions
- Reduced incidence of neutralizing antibody production
- Reduced risk of immunoresistance
- Lower cost.

A study published in 2012 by Güleç AT[16] has concluded that BTX A diluted in 2% of lidocaine with normal saline causes significantly less pain than BTX A diluted in saline alone with equal efficacy and safety.

Procedure[13,17]

The injection sites are marked with a skin marker pen at a distance of about 1.5 cm apart as the diffusion capacity of BTX is about 1.0–1.5 cm in diameter. An antibiotic cream can also be used instead of the skin marker pen to mark the injection site. The diluted BTX A is loaded in insulin syringes. BTX A (0.2 mL) is injected intradermally in each marked area with all aseptic precautions **(Fig. 3)**. In general, 10–20 sites per axilla are injected with approximately 50 units of BTX A.[17] Tiny intradermal wheals are raised **(Fig. 4)** beginning at the periphery of the hair-bearing skin and circling into the center of the axillary vault.[17] The reduction of sweating starts at 2–4 days after injection[18] with complete anhidrosis of the axillary skin after about 1 week.[19-21] The duration of anhidrosis in the axillae ranges from 4 to 10 months.[17-20]

A study conducted by Jain A et al.[18] administered injections only at five sites, at the four corners of the diamond shape hairy area and one at the center with 2.5 U of BTX A (Botox®) of concentration of 10 units/mL and reported the duration of anhidrosis lasting between 4 and 7 months. Similarly, Galadari I et al.[20] also conducted a study in which only five to six points were injected over an elliptical area on each axilla with the result lasting for periods between 1 and 6 months.

However, Wollina U et al.[21] concluded that high-dose of BTX A treatment (200 U in each axilla) is capable of prolonging the antihidrotic effect for >19 months with the percentage of relapses after 12 months of <12% without any clinical evidence of the induction of neutralizing antibodies.

Similarly, Marcella S et al.[22] have concluded in their audit that 35 units of BTX A is a reasonable starting dose and could significantly improve patients' quality of life and reduce the cost of treatment. Dressler D et al.[23] data suggests that the therapeutic effect of BTX A saturates at B50; higher BTX A doses seem not to be necessary thus reducing costs for the treatment substantially. Unlike the documented concept of development of antibodies against toxin after repeated injections, Brehmer F et al.[24] have concluded that repetitive BTX treatments led to a significantly increased duration of efficacy in axillary hyperhidrosis. While the average duration of efficacy continued to increase with each treatment, there were considerable interindividual differences. Similar increase in duration of efficacy was reported in 2019 with repeated use of BTX by Berthin C et al.[25]

In addition, Wu CJ et al.[26] have demonstrated significant reduction in malodor and sweat production at 3 months after BTX A injection with atrophic changes and hypoplasia in apocrine sweat glands in histology.

Side Effects

Common, short-term complications after BTX injections include:

- Pain
- Edema
- Ecchymosis
- Bruise
- Purpura
- Short-term hyperesthesia

Pain, bruising, and ecchymosis can be minimized by:

- Using smaller gauze needles[27]
- Reconstituting the toxin in preserved rather than preservative-frees saline[28]
- Using the single needle for each single prick, that is, changing the needle or syringe for each injection.[29] Repetitive use of the same needle may result in some dulling of the tip.
- Cooling the skin before and after the injection using the ice.[30]
- Proper pretreatment counsel for patient avoidance of medications that hinder platelet function, such as non-steroidal anti-inflammatory drugs (NSAIDs), aspirin and vitamin E, and consumption of green tea for 7–10 days before injection.
- Pain can be significantly lessened by applying topical anesthetics.

Vadoud-Seyedi J et al.[31] in a study have concluded significant reduction in pain on using BTX A reconstituted in lidocaine with equal efficacy in treating axillary hyperhidrosis.

Studies have also shown the efficacy and safety of BTX B in treating primary axillary hyperhidrosis.[32,33] In addition, studies on anhidrotic efficacy of onabotulinumtoxin A and rimabotulinumtoxin B[34] injections, and abobotulinumtoxin A administered by iontophoresis[35] have been documented.

PALMAR AND PLANTAR HYPERHIDROSIS

Palmar hyperhidrosis interferes with nearly all tasks of manual dexterity. Avoidance of handshake can lead to professional embarrassment, and avoidance of touch can lead to social or interpersonal seclusion. These symptoms put patients at risk for higher levels of disability, fear, avoidance, and other physiological symptoms that may encompass social anxiety disorder. Palmar hyperhidrosis usually is accompanied by plantar hyperhidrosis which is easier to conceal but when extreme may cause bromhidrosis, infection, and skin maceration.[36]

Botulinum toxin injection has been a promising alternative to local antiperspirants, tap water iontophoresis, and oral medication such as glycopyrrolate. BTX injections are considered fourth-line treatment for palmoplantar hyperhidrosis.[37]

Anesthesia

The skin overlying palms and soles are thicker and tougher. Thus, a BTX injection at multiple sites at regular intervals is usually a painful procedure. Hence, various modalities of anesthetic methods have been devised to minimize pain during the procedure and provide better comfort to the patient.

Topical Anesthesia

Topical anesthetic creams such as lignocaine gel under occlusion are applied for about 45 minutes to an hour before the procedure. However, this can provide only limited skin surface anesthesia wherein complete painless procedure is not at all possible, probably due to the presence of a thick horny layer which prevents the cream penetration. This method may provide excellent anesthetic effect for the stinging of the needle, but only minimal relief from the burning experienced during the injection of fluid.[13]

Vibration Anesthesia

This technique does not eliminate pain completely. However, it can serve to make the injections much more tolerable.[38]

Jet Injection

Pressurized, needle-free jet injector devices have been used to inject BTX A directly into the dermis in plantar hyperhidrosis without prior anesthesia.[39] The possibility of nerve injury, cost of equipment and cleaning, inability to properly inject the web spaces and digits, and lack of clinical efficacy makes this method unreliable.[38]

Nerve Block[38,39]

Median and radial nerve blocks are used for the hand, and posterior tibial and sural nerve blocks are used for foot. This type of regional anesthesia is an excellent way to provide anesthesia in experienced hands, as it gives a full motor and sensory block. The potential drawbacks of nerve blocks are nerve injury, vascular puncture, and impaired hand dexterity for hours after the anesthesia, and reactive hyperemia which increases the tendency to bleed from the injection sites. The reader is referred to the chapter on local anesthesia for details.

Bier's Block

This intravenous regional anesthesia (IRA) is considered more reliable and an excellent way to provide anesthesia in an experienced hand. The technique consists of exsanguinations, which forces blood out of the extremity, followed by the application of pneumatic tourniquets to safely stop blood flow. The anesthetic agent lidocaine is introduced into the limb and allowed to set in while tourniquets retain the agent within the desired area. After some time, the tourniquet is depressurized to restore circulation. However, systemic effects can result from the sudden release of anesthetic into systemic circulation.[39] A modified Bier block technique has been described which claims to use smaller volume of anesthetic giving patient sensory block and not a major motor block so that the patients can be ambulatory with full use of their hands and feet.[38]

Other Anesthetic Procedures

Cryoanalgesia: Cryoanalgesia with dichlorotetrafluoroethane has shown to lessen the pain of BTX injections for treating palmar hyperhidrosis.[40]

Iontophoresis with 2% lidocaine:[13] Before palmoplantar BTX injection, iontophoresis with 2% lidocaine for 30 minutes (15 minutes for each side) has shown to provide better topical dermal analgesia with only slight stinging and burning, similar to what is felt during injection of BTX for axillary hyperhidrosis. However, this technique does not abolish the burning and stinging completely as it is a very superficial nature of anesthesia.

Lidocaine iontophoresis with cryotherapy:[13] In this novel method, lidocaine iontophoresis is first performed, followed by spraying the marked points on the skin by liquid nitrogen until frozen, leaving a white spot. The BTX then is injected directly into this focus of partially frozen anesthetized skin. A pain-free vertical injection can be achieved with this technique even on the fingertips with overall satisfaction rate of 93.3% in one of the studies. The side effect may be mild blistering at the site of liquid nitrogen spray which can be addressed by using a small hole cone which can give precise anesthesia. To minimize the blister further, a special 10-hole nozzle can be used which produces a defocused iced spray that produces complete anesthesia without any blistering. Although this combined technique requires some training and an assistant to perform, this technique is highly recommended owing to increased patient satisfaction.

Procedure

Dilutions of BTX are shown in **Table 3**.

The dilution of BTX A for the treatment of hyperhidrosis of palms and soles can be the same as that for the treatment of hyperhidrosis of the axilla. However, to avoid attendant muscle weakness after BTX A injections, especially in the hands, the reconstitution volume can be reduced from 10 to 5 mL.

After performing the minor starch test and delineating the area of hyperhidrosis **(Fig. 5)**, the sites are marked with the marker pen around 1.0–1.5 cm interval. Approximately

TABLE 3: Suggested dilutions for palmar and plantar hyperhidrosis.

Dilution	*Botox® 5 mL*	*Dysport® 5 mL*
U/vial	100	500
U/mL	20	100
U/0.1 mL	2	50
mL/injection site	0.1	0.1

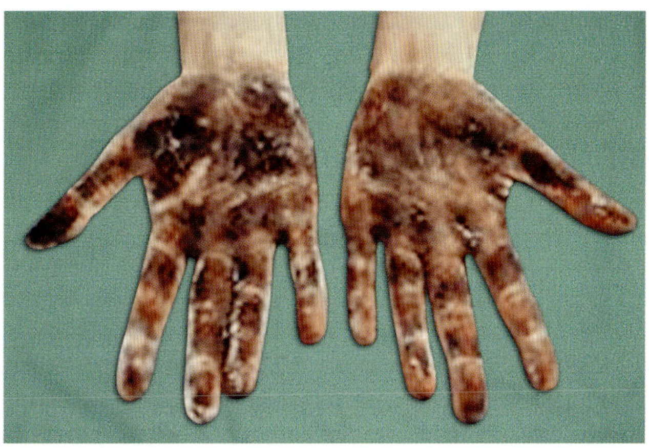

Fig. 5: Positive iodine starch test on palms.

35–40 injection points are planned for each palm and 60–80 injection points for each sole depending upon the site of hyperhidrosis.[13] The BTX A is injected intradermally in each marked site after providing anesthesia. A small zone of visible blanching attests to the deep dermal placement.[17] Subcutaneous injections should be avoided to prevent diffusion into intrinsic muscles of palms and soles. Total doses of approximately 50–165 U of Botox® may be required per palm depending on the area of hyperhidrosis.[13,39,41] Doses for the soles usually exceed that for the palm.

The duration of effect varies from 3 to 12 months.[17] The maximum improvement may persist up to 3 months; from there on, the effects slowly diminish.[42,43] In another study, the remission on average was reported as approximately 7 months for palmar hyperhidrosis and 4 months for plantar hyperhidrosis.[39] The duration of the anhidrotic effects in the plantar zone does not seem to last as long as in any other treated areas (axillae, palms), but the real reason for this difference is not clear.[43]

A study conducted by Marti N et al.[44] has suggested marking at 30 points on each palm, sparing the thenar eminence, and 20 points on the palmar surface of the fingers (one in each proximal and medial phalanx and two in the distal phalanges). 0.1 mL of BTX A of concentration of 25 U/mL was injected at each point resulting in significant reduction in hyperhidrosis.

Similarly, a study conducted by Jain S et al.[18] has described administrating only five sites at each palm and sole, at four corners and one at the center. Each site was then injected with approximately 2.5 U of BTX A of concentration 10 U/mL, and the effect lasted around 7 months.

Complications of Botulinum Toxin Injection at Palms and Soles[41,42,44]

- Pain during injection
- Vasovagal attacks due to pain
- Wrist pain
- Cramps
- Hematomas
- Transitory weakness of small muscles, especially hands, which may affect pinching between the thumb and index finger and can last for 2–8 weeks.

FRONTAL HYPERHIDROSIS

Frontal hyperhidrosis is a social embarrassment which can be triggered by stress, excitement, physical activity, and heat.

Dilution

The dilution should be much less than that used for axillary hyperhidrosis to prevent any diffusion beyond the target area. Low doses and low-volume dilutions (2.5–5.0 mL) of BTX A should be used.[13]

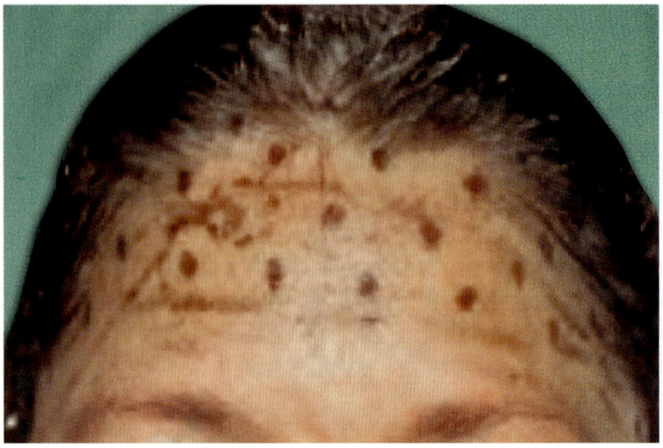

Fig. 6: Marking of injection sites on brow after iodine test.[13]

Procedure

The area of sweating on the forehead is visualized by Minor's iodine-starch test and documented. The injection sites are marked ranging from 1 to 1.5 cm **(Fig. 6)**. About 2–3 U[13,45] of toxin is injected intracutaneously in each site. The toxin should not be injected within 1.5–2.0 cm of the eyebrows to prevent the occurrence of brow ptosis and blepharoptosis. The reduction of sweating is found to be highly significant lasting for approximately 5 months.[45]

Side Effects

The possible common side effects include:

- Pain of injections
- Partial disability in frowning of forehead
- Brow ptosis
- Blepharoptosis
- Hematoma, bruise
- Infection.

GUSTATORY HYPERHIDROSIS (FREY'S SYNDROME)

Gustatory sweating is a common complication following parotid gland surgery, infection, or trauma. This is the pathological sweating of the preauricular area due to an aberrant regeneration of postganglionic parasympathetic fibers feeding the parotid gland that are severed during parotidectomy, which then anastomose with postganglionic sympathetic fibers that supply vessel and sweat gland of the skin. BTX A is an effective therapeutic option for the treatment of gustatory sweating, and it can be considered as a first-line treatment.[13]

Procedure

The Minor iodine starch test is carried out and delineates the area **(Fig. 7)**. The BTX A is injected intracutaneously in

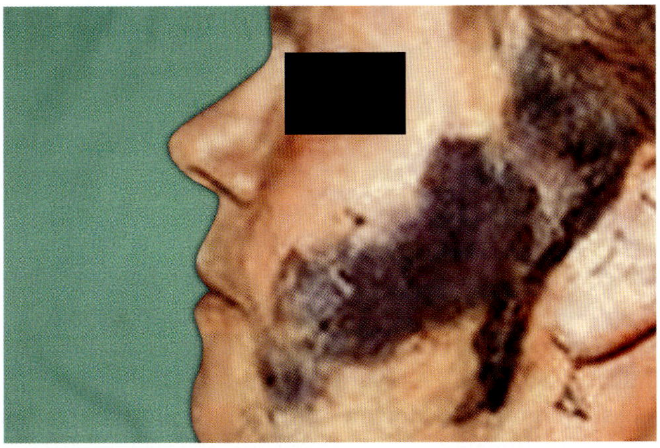

Fig. 7: Positive iodine-starch test for gustatory hyperhidrosis.

arrange of 2–32 units in the affected area.[44] The visible signs of improvement are noticed after 4–7 days.[46,47] The result lasts for the variable periods ranging from 7–10 months[37] to 15–18 months.[47]

Pomprasit M et al.[46] in their study have injected intradermal BTX A 2 U in every 1 cm^2 of involved skin with the mean total dose of 10.6 U. Diaz PM et al.[47] have diluted 100 U of Botox® in 4 cm^3 of saline solution and an average of 38 U of toxin was injected per person in an average area of 26 cm^2. However, Ng S et al.[48] have mentioned the dilution of 100 U of Botox® with 1 mL of isotonic saline to achieve a concentration of 10 U/0.1 mL and 30 U (0.3 mL) was injected in the delineated area.

Cantarella G et al.[49] have concluded in their study about the symptomatic relief from Frey's syndrome with injection of BTX B and considered a potential alternative to BTX A.

Side Effects[47,48]

- Temporary weakness of facial muscles
- Dry mouth
- Difficulty in chewing
- Drooping of the eyelids
- Facial paresis
- Pain
- Edema
- Erythema
- Ecchymosis
- Hyperesthesia
- Allergy reactions.

HYPERTROPHIC SCARS AND KELOIDS

Keloids and hypertrophic scars are benign fibrous overgrowths of scar tissues, which results from an abnormal response to trauma. A scar results from the physiological process of wound healing. Scarring is considered abnormal when it is symptomatic; affects normal function; the fibrous tissues are excessive or suboptimal; and they are aesthetically disfiguring and distressing to the patients. Several treatment options are currently available; however, they do not seem to provide the desired therapeutic outcomes. Currently, BTX injections seem to be a promising treatment option for the hypertrophic scars and keloids.

Mechanism of Action

Botulinum toxin A immobilizes the local muscles, reduces skin tension caused by muscle pull, and, therefore, decreases microtrauma and subsequent inflammation.[50] Reduction of the tensile force during the course of cicatrization and effective regulation of the balance between fibroblast proliferation and cellular apoptosis may represent a novel therapeutic target for treating keloids.[50] It is also suggested that BTX A effectively inhibits the growth of fibroblasts derived from hypertrophic scar and in turn causes a decrease in transforming growth factor-beta 1 protein.[51]

Anesthesia

Topical anesthetic creams are generally not necessary but can be used in a very sensitive patient.

Procedure

A study has presented the use of a concentration of 35 units/mL intralesionally into the keloid with the total dose of 70–140 units per session.[48] The treatment was given at 3-month intervals for a maximum of 9 months, without the signs of recurrence or failure of therapy. Another study conducted by Xiao Z et al.[52] has reported the use of BTX A 2.5 U/cm^3 of lesion intralesionally at 1 month interval for a total of 3 months; wherein the result after 6 months follow-up showed acceptable improvement and high rate of therapeutic satisfaction.

BOTULINUM TOXIN IN MANAGEMENT OF PAINFUL SCARS

Keloids are associated with small-fiber neuropathy and typically present with itching, pain, and allodynia. BTX A injections can be used to treat the painful scars.

Anesthesia

Topical anesthesia is usually not necessary prior to injection but can be used in very sensitive patients.

Dose and Dilution[53]

Botulinum toxin A is reconstituted with normal saline and preservatives. The reconstitution volume does not seem to affect the efficacy. However, to minimize injection discomfort into hypertrophic or keloid scars the smallest possible volume is preferred. Thus, Smith KC et al.[53] have used reconstitution of 1 mL in 100 units of Botox.® In case of very tight tissue and unacceptable discomfort, the author recommends dilution with 0.5 mL of normal saline. The total amount in each treatment may range from 10 to 50 units/mL of scar tissues. The total number of one to four treatments may be required.

Procedure[53]

Prior to the procedure, objective quantification of the patient's pain is of great importance in the management of painful scars. Thus, the followings should be done:

- Visual analog scale for pain perception and global assessment
- Physician global assessment
- Marking the boundaries of the area with pain and then photographing at each visit.

Injections are placed intralesionally using 30-gauge 1-inch needle. The reassessment and retreatment are done every 3–4 weeks as the antinociceptive effect of BTX A seems to reach a maximum at around 3 weeks and is continued till the patient is pain free. The patient typically remains pain free long-term once they have been rendered pain free by BTX A injection. In addition to relief from pain, the scar may become much softer.

BOTULINUM TOXIN IN FACIAL SCAR MANAGEMENT[54]

One of the most important factors determining the final cosmetic appearance of a cutaneous scar is the tension on the wound edges during healing **(Fig. 8)**. In general, relaxed skin tension lines (RSTL) lie perpendicular to the tension vector of the underlying muscular contraction. Scars aligned with RSTL are subject to reduced tension and heal well, whereas scars oriented against RSTL are subject to repetitive tension and result in scar hypertrophy. Mahboub T et al.[54] have strongly recommended the preoperative injection of BTX in muscles underlying the scar before scar revision which will immobilize the muscles pulling on the scar during the critical period of scar healing. This may bring much improvement to the final outcome of scar revision.

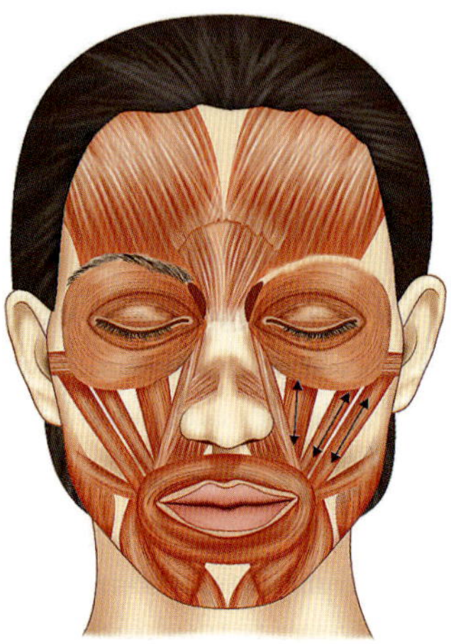

Fig. 8: Diagram of facial muscles to evaluate which facial muscles may have effect on scar.[54]

Procedure

The facial muscles are examined regarding their symmetry and the possible influence of trauma on their activity.

The dose ranging from 5 to 50 U (dilution 5.0 U/0.1 mL) is injected in one or two sessions with 2 weeks intervals. A second dose of BTX A is injected 2 weeks later if there is a degree of persistent hypertonicity on EMG evaluation. The clinical effect of BTX A begins around 1–2 days, peaking 1–4 weeks and gradually declines 6–12 months after injection. BTX can be injected either at the time of scar formation (if anticipated) or at suture removal.[55]

The common side effects may be transient paralysis of the adjacent muscle groups with a resultant temporary functional deficit.

BOTULINUM TOXIN AND POST-ACNE SCARS[55]

The presence of scars, particularly atrophic or mildly hypertrophic, normal muscle movement may have an exaggerated effect on normal aging skin. This seems to be particularly true of rolling scarring or grade 3 atrophic scarring. The movement related to facial expression continues unabated throughout life, but as we age the resistance of dermal tissues that have suffered the twin destructive movements, results in a more prominent visibility of scars.

In the upper face, the forehead and glabellar areas, the marionette lines and the chin and surrounding areas in the lower face seem to cope badly with acne in particular and also appear to age badly once affected. Sometimes mildly hypertrophic scars in these areas may be exaggerated by movement. In the lower face, scars may occasionally be influenced by other movements such as pursing of the lips. Thus, in these areas BTX can be used to the cosmetic advantage of the patient either alone or more usually in concert with other techniques such as fillers, resurfacing, and surgery.

In areas such as cheeks, the role of BTX may be limited due to potential side effects.

POSTHERPETIC NEURALGIA[53]

Botulinum toxin can be used as a treatment option in the neuropathic pain which is refractory to the usual therapies.

Mechanism of Action[53]

Botulinum toxin A has been shown to block release of pain-mediating neurotransmitter substance P (SP), calcitonin gene-related peptide (CGRP), and glutamate from motor and sensory neurons. It may act both by blocking peripheral sensitization and by indirectly reducing central sensitization; and also may reduce various substances that sensitize nociceptors.

Anesthesia

Topical anesthesia is not usually necessary prior to treatment but can be used in patients with intolerable injection discomfort.

Dilution

Botulinum toxin A is reconstituted using normal saline alone or normal saline with benzyl alcohol preservative which has local anesthetic properties and reduces injection discomfort. A reconstitution volume of 2.5 mL/100 units of Botox® are generally used. The reconstitution volume does not seem to influence efficacy.

Procedure[53,56]

Prior to the injection, the patient identifies the area or areas of involvement, the boundaries of which to be marked with a washable pink, fluorescent marker pen and photographed. This needs to be done on all the visits. It is usually better to use a very fine 31-gauge SteriJect needles to reduce discomfort as there is commonly hyperalgesia in the involved areas.

The toxin is injected intradermally or subdermally in the range of 1–2 units/cm^2. The injections are spaced at 2–3 cm apart. The doses range from 2.5 to 5 units per injection. The antinociceptive effect of BTX A seems to peak at around 3–4 weeks. Thus, patients are followed-up for reassessment and possible retreatment every 3–4 weeks until they are pain free. The usual number of treatments required to induce long-term remission of PHN ranges from 1 to 4 and there is frequently a long-term drug-free remission of pain. The explanation may be the gate theory of pain control. The studies have shown the significant effects on average pain intensity from 2 weeks after injections to 14 weeks;[57] and thereby pain relief lasted around 52 days[58] after multiple injections.

The side effects are usually the pain and discomfort during injections and transient weakness of the particular muscles.

OCCIPITAL NEURALGIA AFTER HAIR TRANSPLANT[59]

Occipital neuralgia is defined by the International Headache Society as a neuralgiform headache characterized by paroxysmal shooting or lancinating pain in the greater, lesser, or third occipital nerve dermatomes. Posterior scalp graft harvest for hair transplantation may result in injury to the occipital nerves leading to chronic neuropathic pain. Siefferman J et al.[59] have reported modest additional relief for 3 months after injecting BTX A 100 units in grid-like fashion over the most painful area, the right occiput.

ANDROGENETIC ALOPECIA TREATMENT[60,61]

The pathophysiology of androgenetic alopecia (AGA) is the miniaturization of terminal hairs by dihydrotestosterone (DHT) produced from testosterone by 5-alfa reductase enzyme in genetically prone individuals. DHT is prone for activation under hypoxic condition also leading to hair loss.[60] Several studies suggested that there were hemodynamic abnormalities including microvascular dysfunction and reduced blood flow in the alopecia region of AGA patients. Therefore, improving the scalp blood supply may stimulate hair growth. Possibly, BTX may relax the muscles around the head, increase blood flow and oxygen concentration in the alopecia area, and further inhibit the activation of DHT, ultimately leading to a reduced occurrence of hair loss. Moreover, a high concentration of oxygen can stimulate the hair follicle into the growth phase, resulting in hair regeneration.

Zhou Y et al.[60] in their study injected 30 sites with 100 U of BTX A and patients received BTX A after every 3 months for a total of four times. They demonstrated significant augmentation of hair growth and density, and the area of hair loss was attenuated after each treatment.

Singh S et al.[61] also reported in the pilot study that BTX is an effective therapy in AGA management.

INFLAMMATORY DERMATOSES

Hidradenitis Suppurativa

Studies[62,63] have described the treatment of hidradenitis suppurativa successfully with BTX A. It has been suggested that BTX acts by reducing the production of apocrine sweat and limiting the tendency of follicular rupture, thus not allowing local inflammation and abscess formation.[63,64] O'Reilly DJ et al.[63] have reported successful use of 250 U of Dysport® on bilateral axillae with remission for 10 months. Feito-Rodriguez M et al. in their study have reported the successful treatment of hidradenitis suppurativa with 40 units of Botox® at 10–12 points over the elliptical area on each side with remission for about 6 months.[62] Grimstad O et al.[65] have further pointed out that the anhidrotic effect of BTX B in intertriginous areas may have an impact on the microbiome and bacterial growth, and subsequently inhibit an important factor in the pathogenesis. In addition, the inhibitory effect of BTX on neurogenic inflammation and nociceptive mast cell innervation is a plausible explanation of the results of their study wherein BTX B was injected and followed up at 3 and 6 months.

Flexural Psoriasis

A pilot study of 15 patients with flexural psoriasis showed that 50–100 U of BTX A improved subjective symptoms and objective photographic evidence of disease in 87% of patients at 2, 4, and 12 weeks.[66] Furthermore, patients with psoriasis are known to have a higher concentration of substance P receptors in their skin, meaning BTX should theoretically reduce pruritus by inhibiting substance P and hence prevent binding to the multiple receptors.

Folliculitis Decalvans[67]

Tamura BM et al.[67] found favorable effects on hair regrowth post-injection of 60–150 U of BTX A. They hypothesized that BTX A inhibition of immune factors and cytokines reduced follicular inflammation.

ROSACEA[68-72]

Anecdotal results of reduced erythema and acne with the use of onabotulinumtoxin A for cosmetic purposes led Dayan et al.[69] to experiment further in 13 patients with rosacea. Over the course of 2 years, patients received intralesional micro droplet injections (0.05 mL) of onabotulinumtoxin A in a dilution of 7 mL of saline solution per 100 units. The results indicated a significant reduction in erythema and flushing of the affected area 2–4 weeks after treatment. The mechanism of action through a likely neurogenic component to vascular dysfunction, inflammation, and hyper sebaceous activity is reviewed.[69] Scala J et al.[70] in their discussion on possible mechanism of BTX on rosacea and flushing have mentioned that BTX blocks acetylcholine release from peripheral autonomic nerves of the cutaneous vasodilatory system, and also inhibits the release of inflammatory mediators such as substance P and CGRP that have a relevant effect in vasodilation. The reduction of all those mediators can lead to a reduction of local skin inflammation and allow erythema to fade out relieving at the same time from pain.

Park KY et al.[71] have reported two cases of refractory erythema and rosacea flushing treated with BTX injections. 50 U of BTX A was reconstituted with 2.5 mL of sterile saline to achieve a concentration of 2 U/0.1 mL. A lidocaine-based topical anesthetic cream was applied 1 hour before treatment. A 30-gauge insulin syringe was used for injection. The injection points were staggered 1 cm apart to cover the entire erythematous lesions of the face. The toxin was injected vertically at a 90° angle intradermally. Both patients received two treatments at 1-week interval and around 40–50 U of total BTX A was injected. There was a mild pain during the treatment and one patient had localized bruising afterward, which spontaneously disappeared after 1 week. Both patients voluntarily returned for repeat treatment after 4 months.

No single optimal treatment has been indicated for rosacea, therefore small quantities of intradermal BTX injection may be considered areas on reasonable addition to the therapeutic options for dramatic post-treatment appearance, and the high patient satisfaction with the cosmetic outcome,[72] especially when other established therapies have failed.

RAYNAUD'S PHENOMENON

Raynaud's phenomenon (RP) is an exaggerated vasospastic response in which there is a transient digital ischemia occurring upon exposure to cold temperature or emotional stress leading to pallor and cyanosis. Studies have shown the use of BTX A and a dual mechanism of action has been suggested—inhibition of vasospasm by blocking cold-induced vasoconstriction and by preventing recruitment of alpha-2 receptors to vascular smooth muscle in cold conditions.[73] Neumeister MW[74] and Neumeister MW et al.[75] in their studies have mentioned using 50–100 units of BTX into the palm around each involved neurovascular bundle. Similarly, Iorio ML et al.[76] have injected 10–100 units of BTX in fingers and hands. The result showed pain reduction at rest, a marked improvement in blood flow on laser Doppler scan with tissue perfusion, healed chronic finger ulcers.[75] The pain-free period lasted for 13–59 months.[75]

Segreto F et al.[77] have reported after detailed overview of the use of BTX A in Raynaud's Phenomenon that 75–100% of patients had pain reduction and healing of ulcers after treatment. The most common complication was temporary hand weakness. However, Zebryk P et al.[78] in their systemic review on BTX A in treatment of Raynaud's phenomenon concluded that the results of the majority of studies of BTX A efficacy in RP conducted so far were favorable, current evidence is not strong enough to either prove or disprove its efficacy. Therefore, new randomized clinical trials (RCTs) are needed in order to confidently assess this form of treatment. Meanwhile, Dhaliwal K et al.[79] have reported improvement of cold intolerance, color change and frequency and severity of Raynaud's attacks in cases of RP in scleroderma in feet after injecting 2 U of BTX A in each toe and the result lasted up to 5 months.

Pompholyx[80,81]

An intraindividual study conducted by Swartling C et al.[80] for pompholyx using the untreated side as control (mean dose of BTX A of 162 U) found after 5–6 weeks that 70% of patients subjectively reported an improvement with a 39% decrease in pruritus in the treated side versus a 52% increase in the untreated side. The authors hypothesized that the increase in symptomatic pruritus could be due to compensatory hyperhidrosis. A further study involving six patients corroborated these findings with 100 U of BTX A suggesting that anhidrosis induced by BTX A can improve symptoms of pompholyx and reduce the number of relapses.[81] Thus, BTX A can be a valuable alternative for patients with treatment-refractory hand eczema of the vesicular type, especially with hyperhidrosis or worsening during the summer.

Lichen Simplex-associated Pruritus[82]

Recalcitrant pruritus is a hallmark of lichen simplex and acetylcholine appears to be a dominant pruritic mediator in this condition. Heckmann M et al.[82] have reported injecting intradermally BTX A into five circumscribed lichenoid lesions wherein pruritus subsided within 3–7 days, lesions cleared completely within 2–4 weeks and no recurrence noted over a 4-month follow-up. Wollina U[14] has mentioned that inhibition of SP and CGRP might be involved in mechanism of BTX action on pruritus.

Fox–Fordyce Disease[83]

It is a rare pruritic disorder most evident on skin with high density of apocrine glands. Symptomatic pruritic papules have been shown to be responsive to 100 U of BTX when injected into axillae, with an associated reduction in papules.

Aquagenic Keratoderma

It was suggested that treatment of aquagenic keratoderma with BTX A resolves symptoms of pruritus and pain triggered by immersion in water. Houle MC et al.[84] have reported significant improvement of lesion in case after injecting BTX within 2 weeks and lasted 6 months.

GENODERMATOSES

Hailey–Hailey Disease and Darier's Disease[85]

Hailey–Hailey disease, an autosomal dominant acantholytic disorder, clinically manifesting as a macerated flexural erythema, is aggravated by heat and sweat and results in worsening of discomfort and pruritus. Several case reports have evidenced improvement of Hailey–Hailey with the use of BTX A (50–125 U). Darier's disease is another autosomal dominant acantholytic disorder presenting as greasy warty papules in flexures and heavily eccrine populated areas, which contribute to malodor. Evidence for BTX use is limited with only a letter exampling a case of improvement in one patient who received a 100 U of BTX A.

Pachyonychia Congenita and Epidermolysis Bullosa Simplex with Sweat-Worsened Foot Problem[86,87]

Pachyonychia congenital is a rare genodermatosis which may be associated with painful, focal hyperkeratosis on the soles which can convert into blisters with plantar hyperhidrosis at high ambient temperatures. Similarly, the patients with epidermolysis bullosa simplex may have painful foot blistering. Intracutaneous injections of BTX A or B have been shown as an efficient, long-lasting, and safe treatment of painful blistering and callosities with remarkable relief from of pain on plantar pressure sites.

DEPRESSION

Major depression is a common and serious disease that may be resistant to routine pharmacologic and psychotherapeutic treatment approaches. Positive effects on mood have been observed in subjects who underwent treatment of glabellar frown lines with BTX for the aesthetic reason. Finzi E et al.[88] concluded in their claimed first reported cases that nine of 10 patients were no longer depressed after 2 months of treatment with BTX A at glabellar frown lines, while 10th patient had improvement in mood.

Wollmer MA et al.[89] reported in their randomized double-blind placebo-controlled study that single treatment of the glabellar region with BTX may shortly accomplish a strong and sustained alleviation of depression in patients, who did not improve sufficiently on previous medication. It supports the concept that the facial musculature not only expresses, but also regulates mood states.

Hawlik AE et al.[90] in their reviewed articles identified three studies that evaluated the antidepressant effects of BTX in the treatment of major depression; wherein there have been an improvement in mood and reduction of depressive symptoms after treatment of the glabellar frown lines with BTX injections.

Kruger TH and Wollmer MA[91] have quoted that a series of studies have shown the modulatory effects on mood and affectivity after treating the patients with depression with BTX at glabellar frown lines. Predominantly, female patients suffering from partly chronic, and treatment resistant unipolar depression experienced a quick, strong, and sustained improvement in depressive symptoms after a single glabellar treatment with BTX as a sole or adjunctive therapy. The authors hypothesized that the superficial paralysis of facial muscles may, probably via proprioceptive feedback mechanisms, have profound effects on the emotional brain.

However, we as clinicians should be very vigilant in diagnosing patients with body dysmorphic disorder with prominent depressive symptoms and refer for psychotherapy rather than any aesthetic procedures including BTX injection for meeting their unrealistic expectations, because botulinophilie is not an indication for BTX injection therapy but a psychotherapy.[92]

BREAST LIFT[53]

The position of the shoulders is determined largely by the balance of forces between the pectoralis minor and pectoralis major muscles which tend to rotate the shoulders medially and depress the shoulders.

The ideal candidates are non-obese women with slightly rounded shoulders or who are slightly stooped forward with small to moderate-sized breasts.

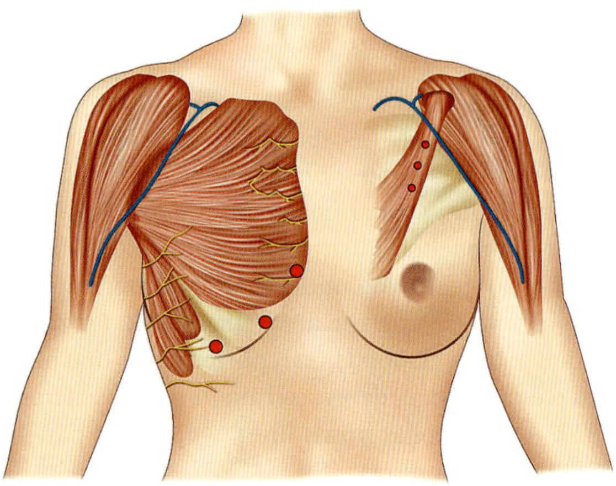

Fig. 9: Injection sites for pectoralis major and minor muscles[53] for breast lift.

Dilution

It is usually recommended to dilute 100 units of Botox® with 2.5 mL of normal saline with benzyl alcohol preservative.

Procedure

The pectoralis major muscle lies medial and inferior to the pectoralis minor muscle. The relaxation of the inferior medial portion of the pectoralis muscle allows the superior portion to lift the ptotic breast. The dose recommended per breast is three injections ranging from 15 U of Botox® at each injection site **(Fig. 9)**; the total dose in one application is around 90 U for both breasts.

The other method is injecting the pectoralis minor muscle which arises on the third, fourth, and fifth ribs and runs under the clavicle to inset on the coracoid process of the scapula. The women with slightly rounded shoulders can attain more erect posture with shoulders back thereby can achieve a more aesthetically pleasing presentation of the breasts. Three injection sites are marked generally about 2.5, 5, and 7.5 cm inferior to the lateral third of the clavicle. The 10 U each of BTX A is injected at a depth of <2 cm at each point.

It has been suggested not to correct naturally occurring breast asymmetry by giving higher doses on the one side.

Side Effects

- Pain at the injected sites which may last for a week.
- Muscle or fascial tenderness for several days.
- Stimulation of nipples which may remain erect for a month.

OTHERS

Multiple Eccrine Hidrocystomas[93,94]

Hidrocystomas are benign cystic tumors of the eccrine or apocrine sweat glands. Multiple eccrine hidrocystomas are benign cystic multiple shining small translucent skin-colored dome-shaped papules with a predilection for the mid face region. The condition runs a chronic course with seasonal variability, exacerbated during heat exposure. Liu TJ et al.[94] have suggested periodic intradermal injection of BTX A (total 40–60 U annually) at a dose of 1–2 U/cm^2. They have noted significant lesional fading 7 days after injection and showed no recurrence 6 months after treatment.[94] The possible side effect can be facial asymmetry which can be avoided by superficial injections.

Leiomyoma-related Pain[95,96]

Cutaneous leiomyomas are benign painful neoplasms with smooth muscle differentiation. Piloleiomyomas are painful benign tumors originating from the arrector pilorum muscle of hair follicle. The results of the local injections of BTX A showed the relief of pain in leiomyomas and also a decrease in the amount of analgesic use.

Chronic Anal Fissure[97]

Chronic fissures are characterized by a sentinel tag, hypertrophic anal papillae, anal spasm, and/or fibrosis of inner sphincter muscle. Pain is less intense during defecation compared to acute anal fissures, but pain increases after defecation. There is increased intra-anal pressure at rest that might contribute to an ischemic state of the anal sphincter muscles. BTX therapy of chronic anal fissures has been performed for >10 years. BTX action on hyperactive smooth muscles such as anal sphincter is mediated by its action on the autonomic nervous system. BTX injection lowers resting intra-anal pressure as demonstrated by sphincter manometry.

Doses of 20–40 U Botox® or 50–100 U Dysport® are useful as long as the patients do not suffer from anal fold hyperhidrosis, in which case, higher doses may be necessary. Injections are given along both sides of a chronic fissure at a distance of 1–2 cm or along the anterior midline. Injections into external sphincter are easier and less painful than into internal sphincter. The earliest effect is the antipruritic effect and the long-lasting outcomes (>12 months) show complete healing rates of about 50%.[97]

Complications include fecal incontinence, flatus incontinence, and perianal thrombosis.

Vulvodynia and Vestibulodynia

Vulvodynia is a multifactorial chronic pain disorder that is distressing to the patient and challenging to the physician.[97] Provoked vestibulodynia is difficult to treat. The beneficial effects of BTX A are being considered because of the muscular anomalies observed in this pathology.[98] A dose of 100 U BTX A injected bilaterally in the bulbospongiosus muscle under electromyographic monitoring significantly reduces pain

3–6 months after injections without side effects. The treatment also improves quality of life and sexual function of patients.[98]

Oily Skin

Rose and Goldberg evaluated the safety and efficacy of BTX on the oily skin of 25 subjects. A 10-point injection was made with BTX (abo-BTX, total amount of 30–45 IU) on the forehead to find significantly lower sebum production and high patient satisfaction.[99] The mechanism by which intradermal BTX results in decreased sebum production is not entirely clear because the role of the nervous system and acetylcholine on sebaceous glands is not well defined.[100]

CONCLUSION

Non-cosmetic and off label indications are constantly being evaluated and explored for varied conditions in medical practice.

Several of these indications have limited evidence or insufficient evidence currently for them to be included in approved treatment indications.

Further clinical trials and proof of efficacy along with official approvals are required prior to these indications becoming officially approved in clinical practice.

REFERENCES

1. Panicker JN, Muthane UB. Botulinum toxins: pharmacology and its current therapeutic evidence for use. Neurol India. 2003;51:455-560.
2. Aoki KR. Pharmacology, immunology and current developments. In: Baumann L, Saghari S, Weisberg E (Eds). Cosmetic Dermatology: Principles and Practice, 2nd edition. McGraw-Hill Companies; 2002. pp. 16-34.
3. Baumann L, Elsaie ML, Grunebaum L. Botulinumtoxin. In: Baumann L, Saghari S, Weisberg E (Eds). Cosmetic Dermatology: Principles and Practice, 2nd edition. McGraw-Hill Companies; 2002; pp. 169-90.
4. Brin MF. Botulinum toxin: chemistry, pharmacology, toxicity and immunology. Muscle Nerve Suppl.1997;6:S146-68.
5. Nigam PK, Nigam A. Botulinum toxin. Indian J Dermatol. 2010;55:8-14.
6. Lipham WJ. What is botulinum toxin and how does it work? In: Lipham WJ (Ed). Cosmetic and Clinical Applications of Botox and Dermal Fillers, 2nd edition. SLACK Incorporated; 2008;5-9.
7. Dhaked RK, Singh MK, Singh P, Gupta P. Botulinum toxin: bioweapon and magic drug. Indian J Med Res. 2010; 132(5):489-503.
8. Coté TR, Mohan AK, Polder JA, Walton MK, Braun MM. Botulinum toxin type A injections: adverse events reported to the US Food and Drug Administration in therapeutic and cosmetic cases. J Am Acad Dermatol. 2005;53:407-15.
9. Leclère FM, Moreno-Moraga J, Alcolea JM, Vogt PM, Royo J, Cornejo P, et al. Efficacy and safety of laser therapy on axillary hyperhidrosis after one year follow-up: a randomized blinded controlled trial. Lasers Surg Med. 2015;47(2):173-9.
10. Caplin D, Austin J. Clinical evaluation and quantitative analysis of axillary hyperhidrosis treated with a unique targeted laser energy delivery method with 1-year follow up. J Drugs Dermatol. 2014;13(4):449-56.
11. Letada PR, Landers JT, Uebelhoer NS, Shumaker PR. Treatment of focal axillary hyperhidrosis using a long-pulsed Nd:YAG1064 nm laser at hair reduction settings. J Drugs Dermatol. 2012;11(1):59-63.
12. Kreyden OP, Scheidegger EP. Anatomy of sweat glands, pharmacology of botulinum toxin, and distinctive syndromes associated with hyperhidrosis. Clin Dermatol. 2004;22:40-4.
13. Kreyden OP. Botulinum toxin in the management of focal hyperhidrosis. Botulinum Toxin in Clinical Dermatology, 1st edition. Taylor and Francis Group, UK; 2006; pp. 321-62.
14. Wollina U. Botulinum toxin: Non-cosmetic indications and possible mechanisms of action. J Cutan Aesthet Surg. 2008;1:3-6.
15. Bigalke H, Wohlfarth K, Irmer A, Dengler R. Botulinum A toxin: Dysport® improvement of biological availability. Exp Neurol. 2001;168(1):162-70.
16. Güleç AT. Dilution of botulinum toxin A in lidocaine vs. in normal saline for the treatment of primary axillary hyperhidrosis: a double-blind, randomized, comparative preliminary study. J Eur Acad Dermatol Venereol. 2012; 26(3):314-8.
17. Shetty MK, IADVL Dermatosurgery Task Force. Guidelines on the use of botulinum toxin type A. Indian J Dermatol Venereol Leprol. 2008;74:S13-S22.
18. Jain S, Tamer SK, Hiran S, Dwivedi MD. Cosmetic effect of botulinum toxin in focal hyperhidrosis. Ann Acad Neurol. 2005;8(1):45-7.
19. Salmanpoor R, Rahmanian MJ. Treatment of axillary hyperhidrosis with botulinum-a toxin. Int J Dermatol. 2002;41:428-30.
20. Galadari I, Alkaabi J. Botulinum toxin in the treatment of axillary hyperhidrosis. Skinmed. 2003;2:209-11.
21. Wollina U, Karamfilov T, Konrad H. High-dose botulinum toxin type A therapy for axillary hyperhidrosis markedly prolongs the relapse-free interval. J Am Acad Dermatol. 2002;46:536-40.
22. Marcella S, Goodman G, Cumming S, Foley P, Morgan V. Thirty-five units of botulinum toxin type A for treatment of axillary hyperhidrosis in female patients. Australas J Dermatol. 2011;52(2):123-6.
23. Dressler D, Adib SF. Towards a dose optimization of botulinum toxin therapy for axillary hyperhidrosis: comparison of different Botox (®) doses. J Neural Transm (Vienna). 2013;120(11):1565-7.
24. Brehmer F, Lockmann A, Gronemeyer LL, Kretschmer F, Schon MP, Thoms KM. Repetitive injections of botulinum toxin A continuously increase the duration of efficacy in primary axillary hyperhidrosis: a retrospective analysis in 101patients. J Dtsch Dermatol Ges. 2015;13(8):799-805.
25. Berthin C, Maillard H. Duration of efficacy increases with the repetition of botulinum toxin a injections in primary axillary hyperhidrosis: a 15-year study in 117 patients. Acta Derm Venereol. 2019;99(13):1237-40.
26. Wu CJ, Chang CK, Wang CY, Liao YS, Chen SG. Efficacy and safety of botulinum toxin A in axillary bromhidrosis and associated histological changes in sweat glands: a prospective randomized double-blind side-by-side comparison clinical study. Dermatol Surg. 2019;45(12):1605-9.

27. Price KM, Williams ZY, Woodward JA. Needle preference in patients receiving cosmetic botulinum toxin type A. Dermatol Surg. 2010;36:109-12.
28. Klein AW. Complications with the use of botulinum toxin. Dermatol Clin. 2004;22:197-205.
29. Lewis T, Jacobsen G, Ozog D. Intrafollicular orifice injection technique for botulinum toxin type A. Arch Dermatol. 2008;144:1657-8.
30. Wollina U, Konrad H. Managing adverse events associated with botulinum toxin type A: a focus on cosmetic procedures. Am J Clin Dermatol. 2005;6:141-50.
31. Vadoud-Seyedi J, Simonart T. Treatment of axillary hyperhidrosis with botulinum toxin type A reconstituted in lidocaine or in normal saline: a randomized, side-by-side, double-blind study. Br J Dermatol. 2007;156:986-9.
32. Nelson L, Bachoo P, Holmes J. Botulinum toxin type B: a new therapy for axillary hyperhidrosis. Br J Plast Surg. 2005; 58:228-32.
33. Baumann L, Slezinger A, Halem M, Vujevich J, Martin LK, Black L, et al. Pilot study of the safety and efficacy of Myobloc (botulinum toxin type B) for treatment of axillary hyperhidrosis. Int J Dermatol. 2005;44(5):418-24.
34. An JS, Hyun Won C, Si Han J, Park HS, Seo KK. Comparison of onabotulinum toxin A and rimabotulinumtoxin B for the treatment of axillary hyperhidrosis. Dermatol Surg. 2015;41(8):960-7.
35. Montaser-Kouhsari L, Zartab H, Fanian F, Noorian N, Sadr B, Nassiri-Kashani M, et al. Comparison of intradermal injection with iontophoresis of abobotulinumtoxin A for the treatment of primary axillary hyperhidrosis: a randomized, controlled trial. J Dermatol Treat. 2014;25(4):337-41.
36. Eisenach JH, Atkinson JLD, Fealey RD. Hyperhidrosis: evolving therapies for a well-established phenomenon. Mayo Clin Proc. 2005;80:657-66.
37. Walling HW, Swick BL. Treatment options for hyperhidrosis. Am J Clin Dermatol. 2011;12:285-95.
38. Solomon P. Modified Bier block anesthetic technique is safe for office use for botulinum a toxin treatment of palmar and plantar hyperhidrosis. Dermatol Online J. 2007;13:6.
39. Benohanian A. What stands in the way of treating palmar hyperhidrosis as effectively as axillary hyperhidrosis with Botulinum Toxin Type A. Dermatol Online J. 2009;15:12.
40. Baumann L, Frankel S, Welsh E, Halem M. Cryoanalgesia with dichlorotetrafluoroethane lessens the pain of botulinumtoxin injections for the treatment of palmar hyperhidrosis. Dermatol Surg. 2003;29:1057-9.
41. Togel B, Greve B, Raulin C. Current therapeutic strategies for hyperhidrosis: a review. Eur J Dermatol. 2002;12:219-23.
42. Perez-Bernal AM, Avalos-Peralta P, Moreno-Ramirez D, Camacho F. Treatment of palmar hyperhidrosis with botulinum toxin type A: 44 months of experience. J Cosmet Dermatol. 2005;4:163-6.
43. Campanati A, Bernardini ML, Gesuita R, Offidani A. Plantar focal idiopathic hyperhidrosis and botulinum toxin: a pilot study. Eur J Dermatol. 2007;17:52-4.
44. Marti N, Ramon D, Gamez L, Reig I, García-Pérez MA, Alonso V, et al. Botulinum toxin type A for the treatment of primary hyperhidrosis: a prospective study of 52 patients. Actas Dermosifiliogr. 2010;101:614-21.
45. Kinkelin I, Hund M, Naumann M, Hamm H. Effective treatment of frontal hyperhidrosis with botulinum toxin A. Br J Dermatol. 2000;143:824-7.
46. Pomprasit M, Chintrakarn C. Treatment of Frey's syndrome with botulinum toxin. J Med Assoc Thai. 2007;90:2397-2402.
47. Díaz PM, Bances del Castillo R, Mancha de la Plata M, Naval Gías L, Martínez Nieto C, Lee GY, et al. Clinical results in the management of Frey's syndrome with injections of Botulinum Toxin. Med Oral Patol Oral Cir Bucal. 2008;13:E248-52.
48. Ng S, Torjek C, Hovan A. Management of Frey Syndrome using Botulinum neurotoxin: A case report. J Can Dent Assoc. 2009;75:651-4.
49. Cantarella G, Berlusconi A, Mele V, Cogiamanian F, Barbieri S. Treatment of Frey's syndrome with botulinum toxin type B. Otolaryngol Head Neck Surg. 2010;143:214-8.
50. Viera MH, Amini S, Valins W, Berman B. Innovative therapies in the treatment of keloids and hypertrophic scars. J Clin Aesthet Dermatol. 2010;3:20-6.
51. Xiao Z, Zhang F, Lin W, Zhang M, Liu Y. Effect of botulinum toxin type A on transforming growth factor beta1 in fibroblasts derived from hypertrophic scar: a preliminary report. Aesthetic Plast Surg. 2010;34:424-7.
52. Xiao Z, Zhang F, Cui Z. Treatment of hypertrophic scars with intralesional botulinum toxin type A injections: a preliminary report. Aesthetic Plast Surg. 2009;33:409-12.
53. Smith KC, Perez-Atamoros F. Other dermatological uses of botulinum toxin. Botulinum Toxin in Clinical Dermatology, 1st edition. Taylor and Francis Group, UK; 2006; pp. 270-90.
54. Mahboub T, Sobhi A, Habashi H. Optomization of presurgical treatment with botulinum toxin in facial scar management. Egypt J Plast Reconstr Surg. 2006;30:81-6.
55. Goodman GJ. The use of botulinum toxin as primary or adjunctive treatment for post acne and traumatic scarring. J Cutan Aesthet Surg. 2010;3:90-2.
56. Smith KC, Alam M. Botulinum toxin for pain relief and treatment of headache. In: Carruthers A, Carruthers J, Dover JS, Alam M (Eds). Procedures in Cosmetic Dermatology: Botulinum toxin; Elsevier Saunders; 2005; pp. 101-11.
57. Ranoux D. Botulinum toxin and painful peripheral neuropathies: what should be expected? Rev Neurol (Paris). 2011;167:46-50.
58. Liu HT, Tsai SK, Kao MC, Hu JS. Botulinum toxin A relieved neuropathic pain in a case of post herpetic neuralgia. Pain Med. 2006;7:89-91.
59. Siefferman J, Khelemsky Y. Occipital neuralgia after hair transplantation and its treatment. Case Rep Neurol Med. 2015;2015:428413.
60. Zhou Y, Yu S, Zhao J, Feng X, Zhang M, Zhao Z. Effectiveness and Safety of Botulinum Toxin Type A in the Treatment of Androgenetic Alopecia. Biomed Res Int. 2020;2020:1501893.
61. Singh S, Neema S, Vasudevan B. A pilot study to evaluate effectiveness of Botulinum toxin in treatment of androgenetic alopecia in males. J Cutan Aesthet Surg. 2018;10:163-7.
62. Feito-Rodriguez M, Sendagorta-Cudos E, Herranz-Pinto P, de Lucas-Laguna R. Prepubertal hidradenitis suppurativa successfully treated with botulinum toxin A. Dermatol Surg. 2009;35:1300-2.
63. O'Reilly DJ, Pleat JM, Richards AM. Treatment of hidradenitis suppurativa with botulinum toxin A. Plast Reconstr Surg. 2005;116:1575-6.
64. Khoo ABS, Burova EP. Hidradenitis suppurativa treated with Clostridium botulinum toxin A. Clin Exp Dermatol. 2014;39:749-50.
65. Grimstad O, Kvammen B, Swartling C. Botulinum Toxin Type B for Hidradenitis Suppurativa: A Randomised, Double-

Blind, Placebo-Controlled Pilot Study. Am J Clin Dermatol. 2020;21(5):741-8.
66. Zanchi M, Favot F, Bizzarini M, Piai M, Donini M, Sedona P. Botulinum toxin type-A for the treatment of inverse psoriasis. J Eur Acad Dermatol Venereol. 2008;22:431-6.
67. Tamura BM, Sortino-Rachou AM, Cuce LC. Letter: folliculitis responds to botulinum toxin: is it possible? Dermatol Surg. 2007;33:1398-400.
68. Weinkle AP, Doktor V, Emer J. Update on the management of rosacea. Clin Cosmet Investig Dermatol. 2015;8:159-77.
69. Dayan SH, Pritzker RN, Arkins JP. A new treatment regimen for rosacea: onabotulinumtoxin A. J Drugs Dermatol. 2012;11(12):e76-9.
70. Scala J, Vojvodic A, Vojvodic P, Vlaskovic-Jovicevic T, Peric-Hajzler Z, Matovic D, et al. Botulin Toxin Use in Rosacea and Facial Flushing Treatment. Open Access Maced J Med Sci. 2019;7(18):2985-7.
71. Park KY, Hyun MY, Jeong SY, Kim BJ, Kim MN, Hong CK. Botulinum toxin for the treatment of refractory erythema and flushing of rosacea. Dermatology. 2015;230(4):299-301.
72. Yuraitis M, Jacob CI. Botulinum toxin for the treatment of facial flushing. Dermatol Surg. 2004;30(1):102-4.
73. Levien TL. Advances in the treatment of Raynaud's phenomenon. Vascular Health and Risk Management. 2010;6:167-77.
74. Neumeister MW. Botulinum toxin type A in the treatment of Raynaud's phenomenon. J Hand Surg Am. 2010;35:2085- 92.
75. Neumeister MW, Chambers CB, Herron MS, Webb K, Wietfeldt J, Gillespie JN, et al. Botox therapy for ischemic digits. Plast Reconstr Surg. 2009;124(1):191-201.
76. Iorio ML, Masden DL, Hggins JP. Botulinum toxin A treatment of Raynaud's phenomenon: A Review. Semin Arthritis Rheum.2012;41:599-603.
77. Segreto F, Marangi GF, Cerbone V, Persichetti P. The Role of Botulinum toxin A in the treatment of Raynaud Phenomenon. Ann Plast Surg. 2016;77(3):318-23.
78. Zebryk P, Puszczewicz MJ. Botulinum toxin A in the treatment of Raynaud's phenomenon: a systematic review. Arch Med Sci. 2016;12(4):864-70.
79. Dhaliwal K, Griffin M, Denton CP, Butler PEM. The novel use of botulinum toxin A for the treatment of Raynaud's phenomenon in the toes. BMJ Case Rep. 2018;2018:bcr 2017219348.
80. Swartling C, Naver H, Lindberg M, Anveden I. Treatment of dyshidrotic hand dermatitis with intradermal botulinumtoxin. J Am Acad Dermatol. 2002;47(5):667-71.
81. Wollina U, Karamfilov T. Adjuvant botulinum toxin A in dyshidrotic hand eczema: a controlled prospective pilot study with left-right comparison. J Eur Acad Dermatol Venereol. 2002;16:40-42.
82. Heckmann M, Heyer G, Brunner B, Plewig G. Botulinum toxin type A injection in the treatment of lichen simplex: an open pilot study. J Am Acad Dermatol. 2002;46:617-9.
83. Gonzalez-Ramos J, Alonso-Pacheco ML, Goiburu-Chenu B, Mayor-Ibarguren A, Heranz-Pinto P. Successful treatment of refractory pruritic Fox-Fordyce disease with botulinum toxintype A. Br J Dermatol. 2016;174:458-9.
84. Houle MC, Dhaybi RA, Benohanian A. Unilateral aquagenic keratoderma treated with botulinum toxin A. J Dermatol Case Rep. 2020;4(1):1-5.
85. Forbat E, Ali FR, Al-Niaimi F. Non-cosmetic dermatological uses of botulinum neurotoxin. J Eur Acad Dermatol Venereol. 2016;30(12):2023-29.
86. Swartling C, Karlqvist M, Hymnelius K, Weis J, Vahlquist A. Botulinum toxin in the treatment of sweat-worsened foot problems in patients with epidermolysis bullosa simplex and pachyonychia congenita. Br J Dermatol. 2010;163:1072-6.
87. Swartling C, Vahlquist A. Treatment of pachyonychia congenital with plantar injections of botulinum toxin. Br J Dermatol. 2006;154:763-5.
88. Finzi E, Wasserman E. Treatment of depression with botulinumtoxin A: a case series. Dermatol Surg. 2006;32(5): 645-9.
89. Wollmer MA, de Boer C, Kalak N, Beck J, Götz T, Schmidt T, et al. Facing depression with botulinum toxin: a randomized controlled trial. J Psychiatr Res. 2012;46(5):574-81.
90. Hawlik AE, Freudenmann RW, Pinkhardt EH, Schonfeldt-Lecuona CJ, Gahr M. Botulinum toxin for the treatment of major depressive disorder. Fortschr Neurol Psychiatr. 2014;82(2):93-9.
91. Kruger TH, Wollmer MA. Depression—an emerging indication for botulinum toxin treatment. Toxicon. 2015;1:107(Pt A): 154-7.
92. Harth W1, Linse R. [Botulinophilia. The new life style venenophilia]. Hautarzt. 2001;52(4):312-5.
93. Blugerman G, Schavelzon D, D'Angelo S. Multiple eccrine hidrocystomas: a new therapeutic option with botulinum toxin. Dermatol Surg. 2003:29:557-9.
94. Liu TJ, Ho JC. Two cases of multiple eccrine hidrocystomas with good response to botulinum toxin. Dermatol Sinica. 2009;27:186-91.
95. Onder M, Adisen E. A new indication of botulinum toxin: leiomyoma-related pain. J Am Acad Dermatol. 2009;60:3258.
96. Sifaki MK, Krueger-Krasangakis S, Koutsopoulos A, Evangelou GI, Tosca AD. Botulinum toxin type A—treatment of a patient with multiple cutaneous piloleiomyomas. Dermatology. 2009;218:44-7.
97. Groysman V. Vulvodynia: new concepts and review of the literature. Dermatol Clin. 2010;28:681-96.
98. Pelletier F, Parratte B, Penz S, Moreno JP, Aubin F, Humbert P. Efficacy of high doses of botulinum toxin A for treating provoked vestibulodynia. Br J Dermatol. 2011;164:617-22.
99. Rose AE, Goldberg DJ, Safety and efficacy of intradermal injection of botulinum toxin for the treatment of oily skin. Dermatol Surg 2013;39:443-8.
100. Campanati A, Martina E, Giuliodori K, Consales V, Bobyr I, Offidani A. Botulinum Toxin Off-Label Use in Dermatology: A Review. Appendage Disord. 2017;3(1):39-56.

CHAPTER 90

General Principles of Soft-tissue Augmentation

Shehnaz Arsiwala, Sadhana Deshmukh, Nazneen Arsiwala

KEY MESSAGES

- Anatomical considerations regarding vascularity and fat compartments are essential for optimal rejuvenation.
- Facial assessment forms the foundation for planning volumetric rejuvenation.
- Focus on global rejuvenation rather than focal wrinkle filling.
- Knowledge of filler particle size, cross-linking, viscoelasticity, and lifting capacity is important for optimum outcome.

INTRODUCTION

Volumetric rejuvenation of the face using fillers has exponentially increased in the last decade. From the days of collagen injections to alleviate lines on the face to the current days of fillers, the dynamics of volumetric rejuvenation have shifted in paradigm from local corrections to global corrections to address volume fat depletion on the face. Advances in the degree of cross-linkage and viscoelasticity have brought in new-generation agents which offer longevity, safety, lifting capacity, gel hardness, and ease of injections.

Progress in anatomical cadaveric studies, vasculature knowledge, and manifestations of aging face have been key to a successful volume replacement sans adverse effect. Fillers along with botulinum toxin are the most gratifying noninvasive procedures for antiaging across the globe. While details are dealt with in other chapters, this chapter presents an overview of general principles of fillers.

VOLUMETRIC CHANGES IN AGING SKIN

Despite tremendous variability over such large geographic area, the diverse population of the Indian subcontinent shares similar anatomical traits on the skull and face. Indian faces have a small, bony framework. The width of malar prominences and mandibular angles along with heights are smaller. Buccal fat gives the cheeks a rounded contour and their lips are typically fuller. Cheekbones are high and hence a support for the aging face. Indian faces tend to get fuller and tissue descends downward and medially. In Indians, the lower one-third of the face is much shorter in comparison to the upper third and middle third. Additionally, the Indian periorbital zone also features a very prominent tear trough.[1]

Commonly published facial proportions that usually represent Greco-Roman standards[2,3] may not be necessarily applicable to Indian faces. Strict adherence to these norms is, therefore, not necessary to obtain satisfying results.

Replacing lost fat pads with filler or fat is one approach to restore the beauty of the aging face.[4] Soft-tissue fillers are commonly categorized by durability.

However, because the face continues to age, temporary or semipermanent products may be preferred. It also gives the ease to the physician and patients to periodically augment the ongoing morphological changes. Aging changes the three-dimensional (3D) view of the underlying facial structures, resulting in deflation, descent deterioration, and disproportion of the face skin and soft tissues. The facial triangle of youth turns upside down with aging **(Fig. 1)**.[5,6]

Injectable Fillers

Injectable fillers are a group of artificial filler substances used for soft-tissue augmentation. Fillers can be classified based on different criteria.

Based on the Site of Placement

- Dermal
- Subdermal
- Supraperiosteal

Based on the Origin of Filler Material

- Heterograft
- Allograft
- Autograft
- Synthetic material

Based on Mechanism of Action

- Replacement dermal fillers
- Stimulatory dermal fillers

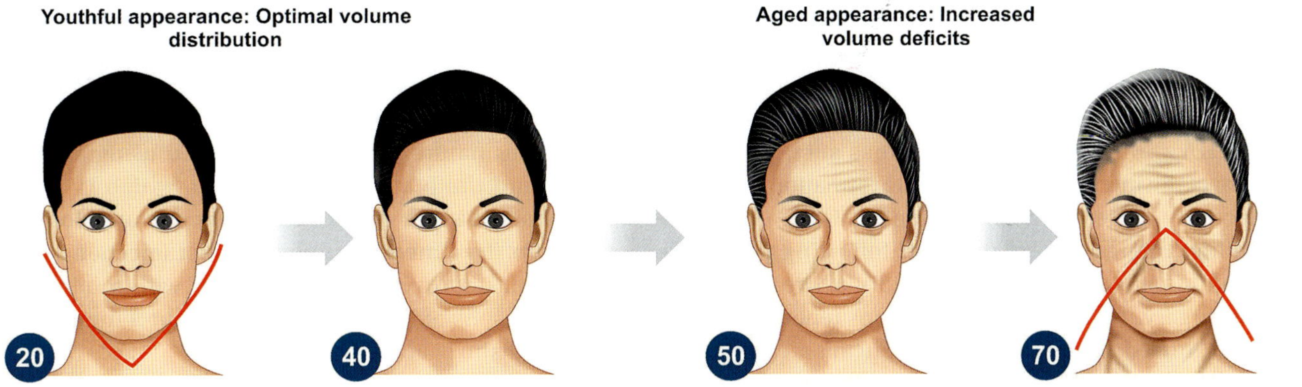

Fig. 1: Volumetric aging changes on the face.

Based on Longevity

- Temporary
- Semipermanent
- Permanent

Soft-tissue fillers are categorized by the material as described in **Box 1**.

Properties of the ideal dermal filler are listed in **Box 2**.

Table 1 shows dermal fillers approved by the US Food and Drug Administration (FDA).

Table 2 shows classification of fillers as per longevity.

The FDA-approved permanent injectable filler contains a suspension of polymethylmethacrylate beads (PMMA) beads in bovine collagen (earlier Artefill later available as Bellafill). They induce fibroplasia and become encapsulated by endogenous collagen. However, due to alarming reports of granuloma formulations, its use is limited and not advocated for lip injections.[7-13] It is now approved by FDA for acne scars.

The nonpermanent dermal fillers are listed in **Box 2 and Table 1**. Collagen dermal fillers are approved for correction of scars and facial filling for volumetric restoration. Although collagen injections made of highly purified cow or human collagen were the first FDA-approved dermal fillers, due to immunogenicity they were withdrawn from the US market by the end of 2010.[12,13]

Poly-L-lactic acid (PLLA) (not available in India) stimulates fibroblast production and is considered a deep tissue regenerator, providing soft-tissue augmentation. It was FDA-approved for lipoatrophy in human immunodeficiency virus (HIV) patients and facial wrinkles in immune-competent individuals. It stimulates collagen synthesis through a foreign body reaction similar to nonabsorbable suture materials. Associated risks include the delayed effect of nonvisible palpable nodules and visible papules.[12,13]

Calcium hydroxylapatite (CaHA) containing carboxymethylcellulose, water, and glycerin is a synthetic inorganic compound of nonanimal origin. Its chemical structure is identical to nonimmunogenic components found in bone and teeth, and it has a minimum risk of an allergic reaction which warrants no pretesting before injecting. The CaHA microspheres are degraded by the body over a period into calcium and phosphate and are excreted by the body. CaHA got FDA approval in 2006 to restore and/or correct lipoatrophy in people with HIV as well as for subdermal placement for

BOX 1: Soft-tissue fillers.

Natural implants:
- *Autologous materials:*
  - Fat transfer
  - Fat autograft muscle injection
  - Cultured human fibroblasts
- *Cadaver-derived materials:*
  - Dermis and extracellular matrix
  - Acellular allogeneic dermis
  - Injectable microparticulate acellular allogeneic dermis
  - Lyophilized human particulate fascia lata
- *Collagen:*
  - Bovine-derived collagen
  - Human-derived collagen from tissue culture
- *Hyaluronic acid (HA):*
  - HA derived from rooster combs
  - Nonanimal stabilized HA from bacterial fermentation
  - Viscoelastic nonanimal HA derived from bacterial fermentation

Synthetic or pseudosynthetic implants:
- Silicone oil
- Expanded polytetrafluoroethylene
- Dual-porosity expanded polytetrafluoroethylene
- Polymethylmethacrylate microspheres in denatured bovine collagen
- Poly-L-lactic acid
- Synthetic calcium hydroxylapatite (CaHA) microspheres suspended in aqueous polysaccharide gel
- Alkylamine gel polymer

BOX 2: Properties of an ideal dermal filler.

The perfect dermal filler should be:
- Safe and effective
- Inexpensive
- Hypoallergenic and requires no pretesting
- Malleable
- Biocompatible
- Easy to distribute, easy to store
- Easy to inject
- Exert no or minimal downtime on the patient
- Have no or minimal risk of complications
- Adequate lifting, long-lasting, consistent, predictable, and easy to remove if necessary
- Nontoxic, noncarcinogenic, no teratogenicity

correction of moderate-to-severe folds, such as the nasolabial fold (NLF). CaHA is best injected deeply.[14]

Studies have shown that the result persists for up to 12 months after the product is injected. It is currently agreed that CaHA should be avoided in areas such as the lips because of the increased risk of nodule formation.

Recently, anterior displacement of CaHA filler due to product migration was reported following periocular injection in patients with a prior history of orbital or periorbital surgery.[15-18] However, publications report that CaHA filler can be used for volume restoration in this area with good safety, tolerability, efficacy, and high patient satisfaction.[19,20]

A biocompatible polysaccharide called *levan* with an elastic modulus higher than hyaluronic acid (HA) has great promise as a novel filler. Levan hydrogel has an interconnected porous structure, similar to the HA hydrogel. The levan hydrogel exhibits a greater collagen induction and augmented anti-wrinkle efficacy when compared with HA hydrogen. Thus, the levan hydrogel is a lucrative alternative to the current commercially available dermal fillers.[21]

TABLE 1: Dermal fillers approved by the US Food and Drug Administration (FDA).

Filler	*Brand name*
Temporary collagen	Numerous
HA gel	Numerous
CaHA	Radiesse
PLLA	Sculptra aesthetic
Permanent	
PMMA beads	Bellafill

(CaHA: calcium hydroxylapatite; HA: hyaluronic acid; PLLA: poly-L-lactic acid; PMMA: polymethylmethacrylate).

TABLE 2: Fillers based on longevity.

Temporary (biodegradable) <1 year	*Semipermanent (biodegradable) 1–2 years*	*Permanent (nonbiodegradable) >2 years*
Collagen	Calcium hydroxylapatite (CaHA)	Polymethylmethacrylate (PMMA)
Collagen—human	DEAE-Sephadex (Dextran)	DEAE-Sephadex (Dextran)
Collagen—Porcine	Poly-L-lactic acid (PLLA)	Polyalkylimide
Hyaluronic acid—avian	Polyvinyl alcohol (PVA)	LIS-Silicon (poly-dimethyl siloxane oil)
Hyaluronic acid—bacterial	Chitosan, hydroxyethyl methacrylate (HEMA), cultured human fibroblasts	

Biofillers using autologous *plasma* filler has been recently introduced into the world of soft-tissue augmentation. This procedure could be done in day care basis relatively economically, without fear of any reactions due to its autologous nature. Biofiller is prepared using autologous serum and the platelet-poor plasma, which is a protein precipitate of a soft, gel-like consistency, is used for wrinkle reduction. Treatment with plasma filler injection results in significant improvement of skin folds with minimal risks, and the results are short-lasting for about 3 months Gupta et al. Doghaim et al.[22-25]

HYALURONIC ACID

Hyaluronic acid is, presently, the most widely used dermal filler across the globe[2] and is dealt with in more detail in a separate chapter.

Though HA fillers have similar origins, they differ from one another in particle size, amount of free HA present, HA concentration, and degree and methods of cross-linkage. These factors are important in determining gel hardness and longevity, which in turn can influence which filler the physician chooses for a particular indication or patient **(Box 3)**.[4,25-29]

At present, the dermal fillers most widely chosen by injectors in India are HA dermal fillers.[1,30-32] Their safety (allergy pretesting is not necessary, the lowest incidence of nodule formation), reversibility (with hyaluronidase), and versatility (usually one treatment is sufficient, and the majority have lidocaine preincorporated) account for their popularity. The main concern about HA fillers is longevity, which seems to be increasing with newer technologies **(Fig. 2)**.[32-36]

Three factors to determine the product choice are: (1) the anatomical area to be injected, (2) the depth of product placement, and (3) the skin thickness.

Regarding the appropriate depth of placement, this is dependent on the products selected and strongly influences the end result.

BOX 3: Characteristics of the hyaluronic acid (HA) dermal fillers approved by the US Food and Drug Administration (FDA).

Restylane:
- Biphasic
- 20 mg/mL particle
- 125 µm 100,000/mL
- BDDE

Perlane:
- Biphasic
- 20 mg/particle
- 325 µm 10,000/mL
- BDDE cross-linked

Juvéderm Ultra Plus:
- Monophasic
- 24 mg/mL homogeneous
- BDDE—8% cross-linked

Juvéderm Ultra:
- Monophasic monodensified
- 24 mg/mL homogeneous
- BDDE—6% cross-linked

Juvéderm Voluma:
- Monophasic monodensified
- 20 mg/mL homogeneous
- BDDE

(BDDE: 1,4-butanediol diglycidyl ether; HA: hyaluronic acid)

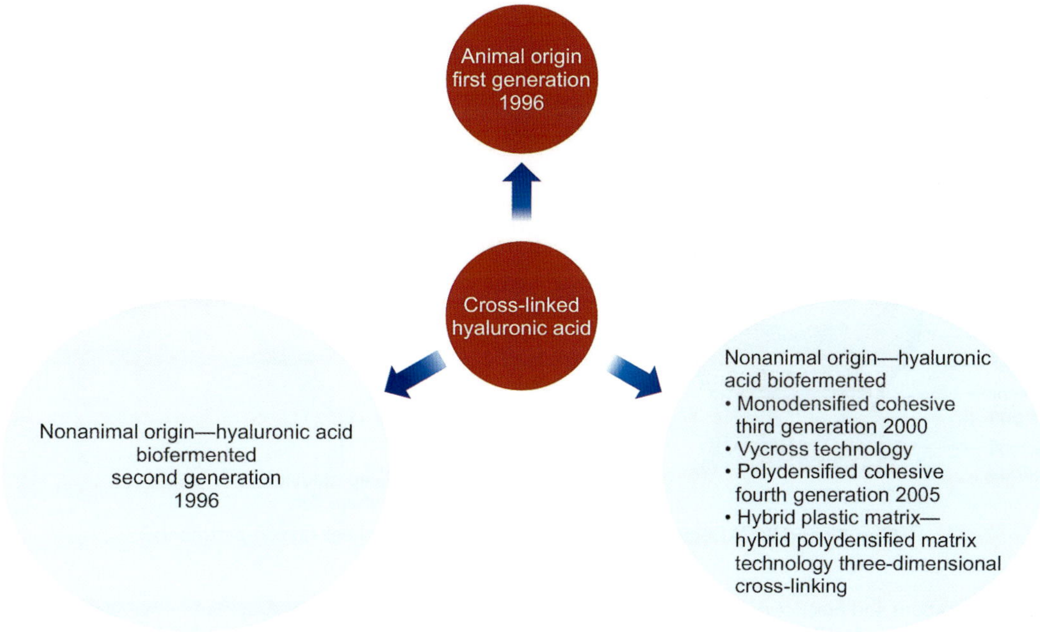

Fig. 2: Generation of cross-linked hyaluronic acid fillers.

The dense/robust filler material are implanted deeper on the supraperiosteum, i.e., on the underlying bone. Therefore, dense fillers are beneficial for filling deeper wrinkles, and softer gels are suitable for more superficial use. In order of depth, medium HA products (Restylane, Juvéderm, and Perlane) should be injected into the mid-to-deep dermis, CaHA (Radiesse) at the dermal-subcutaneous border, and PLLA (Sculptra) into the fat below the dermis. An injection of a dense filler placed too superficially can produce nodules and an uneven surface; therefore, it is usually preferable to err on the deeper side.

Among the HA dermal fillers, more robust/dense HA fillers have a bigger particle size, higher cross-linkage, higher G prime values, and higher concentrations (more particles per milliliter). The G prime value indicates the technical "hardness" of the gel, or how much force it takes to displace the product.[28] The higher G prime products are better at lifting and are frequently used for lifting up the cheeks and oral commissures. The lower-G–G prime products are softer, diffuse into the skin more evenly, and are commonly used for more superficial rhytides or for diffuse filling.[29-32]

Also, in difficult anatomical areas, such as the lips, perioral region, and the periocular region, where nodule formation or product migration can be very detrimental, it is recommended that HA be used rather than any other dermal fillers. Although nodule formation or product migration may occur with any HA fillers, this can be completely removed, if needed, via enzymatic digestion with hyaluronidase.[29-31]

Pain and discomfort would significantly reduce by the incorporation of lidocaine into dermal fillers.[36-38]

FAT COMPARTMENTS IN AGING FACE

Face is divided into superficial and deep fat compartments **(Figs. 3A and B)**.

It is important to know the relation between the ligaments, muscle and fat compartment, and gravity **(Flowchart 1)**. Fat compartment knowledge may help the physician to achieve better aesthetic result **(Figs. 3A and B)**.

Ligaments confine fat areas, and grooves and folds on the skin surface reflect the volume depletion of fat in the area along with ligament fixation. The tear trough is a reflection of the fixation of tear trough and orbital retaining ligament. Mid-cheek groove is by retention of zygomatic cutaneous ligament, NLF of nasolabial ligament, buccal fat groove by parotidomasseteric ligaments, and marionette line by labiomandibular ligament. All the ligaments tend to keep their strength in the central area of the face where a strong fixation exists and become loose laterally **(Flowchart 1)**.[39-41]

INDICATIONS OF DERMAL FILLERS

- Wrinkles and folds
- Forehead contour
- Supraorbital ridge, supraorbital hollow
- Temple
- Tear trough
- Infraorbital hollow
- Malar prominence
- Anteromedial cheek
- Submalar cheek
- Pyriform fossa, NLF
- Lip augmentation

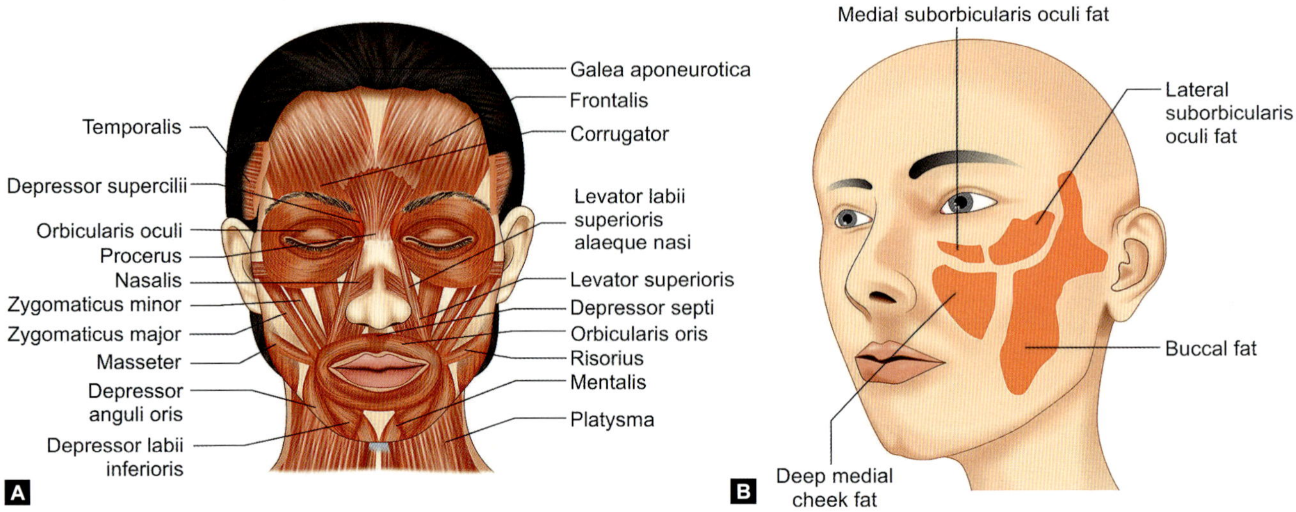

Figs. 3A and B: (A) Depicts muscle attachments; (B) Deep cheek fat compartments.

Flowchart 1: Implications and practice points of facial fat compartments and ligaments.

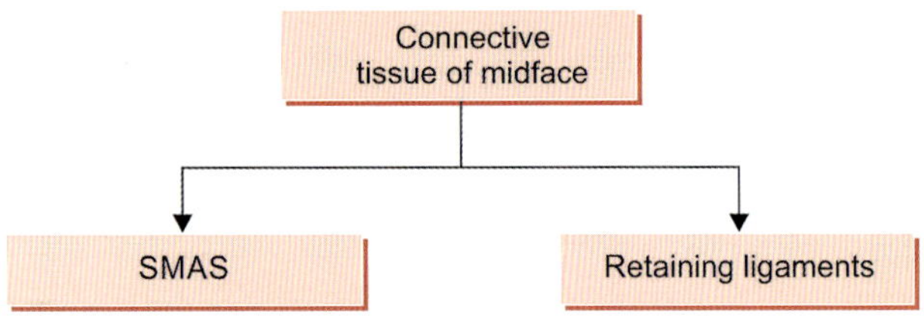

(SMAS: superficial musculoaponeurotic system)

- Commissure turn down
- Hand rejuvenation
- Decollete
- Marionette fold
- Postjowl sulcus
- Prejowl sulcus
- Chin
- Depressed scars—postsurgical, traumatic, postacne, chickenpox, and other diseases
- Dermatological diseases—angular cheilitis, dermal atrophy, acquired immunodeficiency syndrome (AIDS), lipodystrophy
- Earring ptosis, atrophic earlobes

CONTRAINDICATIONS OF DERMAL FILLERS

Contraindications of dermal fillers are shown in **Box 4**.

FACIAL ASSESSMENT

For optimal outcomes, it is necessary for clinicians to have a thorough understanding of facial anatomy as well as an appreciation of the ideal aesthetics.

Full face assessment is a three-step approach.

Consider structural changes, volume loss, and superficial lines and wrinkles.

BOX 4: Contraindications of dermal fillers.

- Pregnancy and breastfeeding
- Recent treatment with other fillers within 6 months to 1 year
- Permanent fillers or implants of any kind
- Skin cancer
- Herpes simplex without prophylaxis
- Known allergy to fillers
- History of anaphylactic shock, fainting, low blood pressure (BP)
- Keloid or hypertrophic scars
- Autoimmune diseases, angina, epilepsy, diabetes
- On drugs like aspirin/warfarin/steroids
- Depression and stress

Design a treatment plan that is:

- Optimally effective
- Natural-looking
- Educate the patient about the aging change in their skin/bone/muscle and the need to plan a long-term antiaging treatment.
- Patient should be educated that facial beauty is a combination of[37] symmetry, balance, and harmony.[42-45]

The left and right sides of the face resemble more as siblings than as twins. But the two sides of the lips are more as twins, with balanced upper and lower vermilion.

Facial photographic view should include frontal [anteroposterior (AP)], right and left lateral, and profile view at rest and animation view.

Facial rejuvenation is not just a two-dimensional (2D) approach (focus on correcting dynamic facial lines), but a 3D approach including loss of facial volume.[46,47]

Recently, focus has shifted on 3D photographic assessment of face using face analytic systems which have inbuilt measurement systems which can not only analyze and assess volume loss with measurements but also are invaluable to establish volumetric rejuvenation consistently after treatment **(Figs. 4 to 10)**.

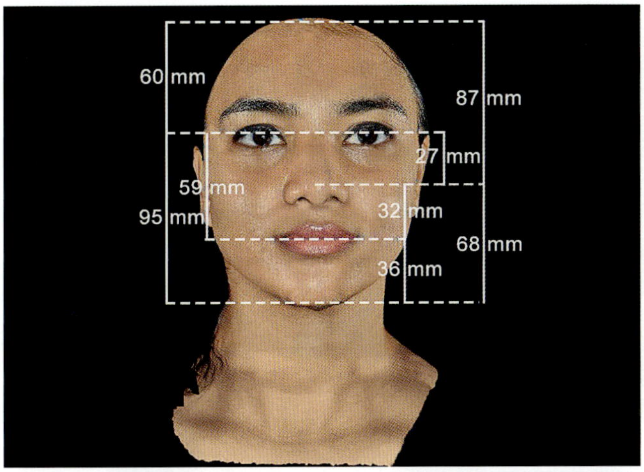

Fig. 4: Horizontal grids for facial measurements using 3D imaging.

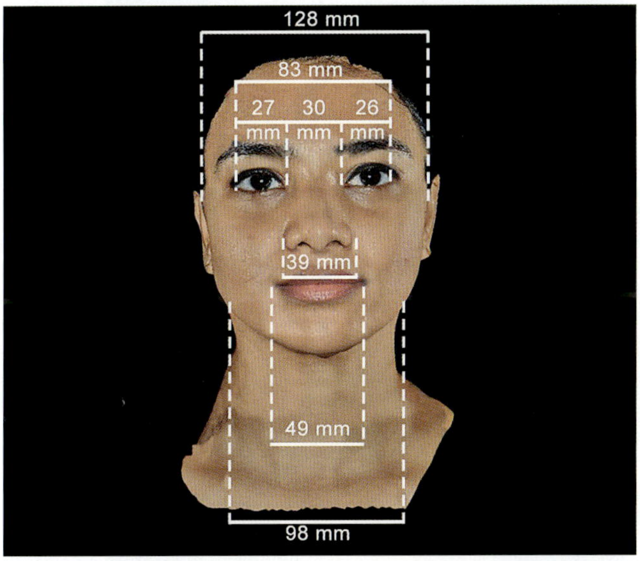

Fig. 5: Vertical grids for facial measurements using 3D analysis.

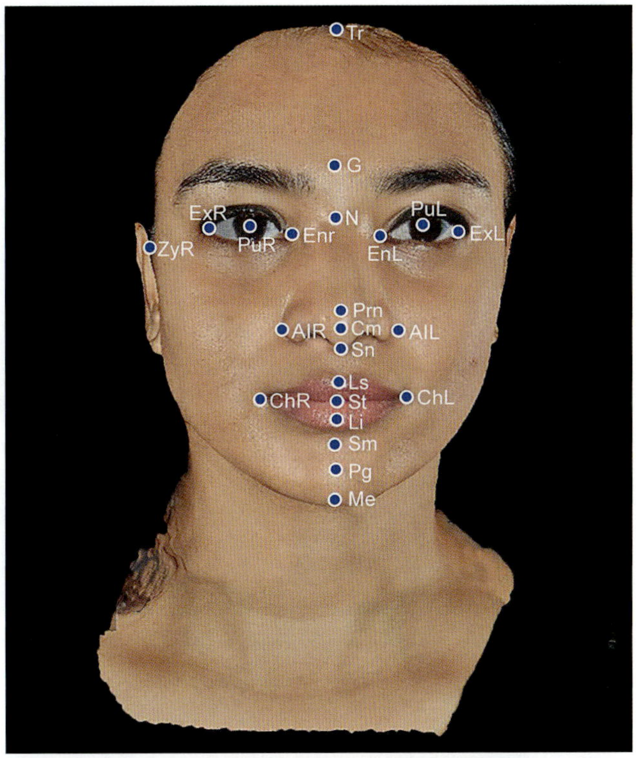

Fig. 6: Landmarks on face.

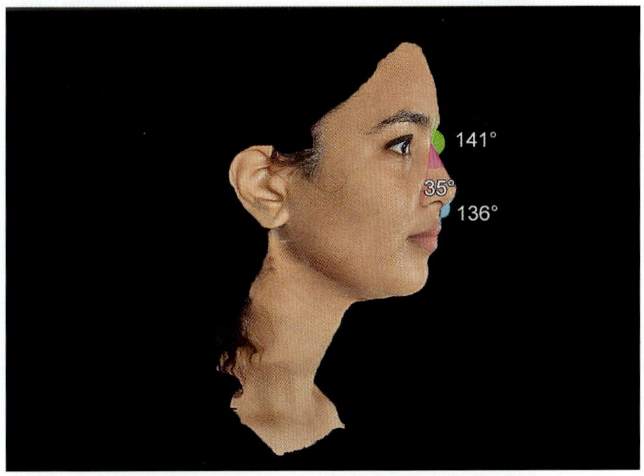

Fig. 7: Measurements of angles using 3D analysis.

PATIENT EDUCATION AND ASSESSMENT

Counseling of the patients should be done about the nature of the filler, expectations from the filler, longevity, possible side effects, and the cost.[48,49] Written informed consent should be taken. Pre- and postphotographs are important. It will help the clinician to critically analyze the results and also, to prepare for medicolegal records.

Patient Education Critical to Avoiding Perceived Adverse Events

Education of patients regarding the rejuvenation process, i.e., the necessity to restore volume rather than filling the individual lines. Explain and demonstrate that facial aesthetic practices have changed from 2D approach to a global, 3D approach with volume restoration and contouring. For example, more emphasis is on medial injection approach than filling up the NLFs itself. It is sometimes reassuring to the patient to show before and after photographs of other patients (who have consented), thus reinforcing that individual treatments and results vary.

PROCEDURE OF FILLER INJECTION

For the patient with temporary fillers, the anesthesia benefit can be 90% technique and 10% filler substance, whereas with permanent fillers, it is usually 99% the technique.[45]

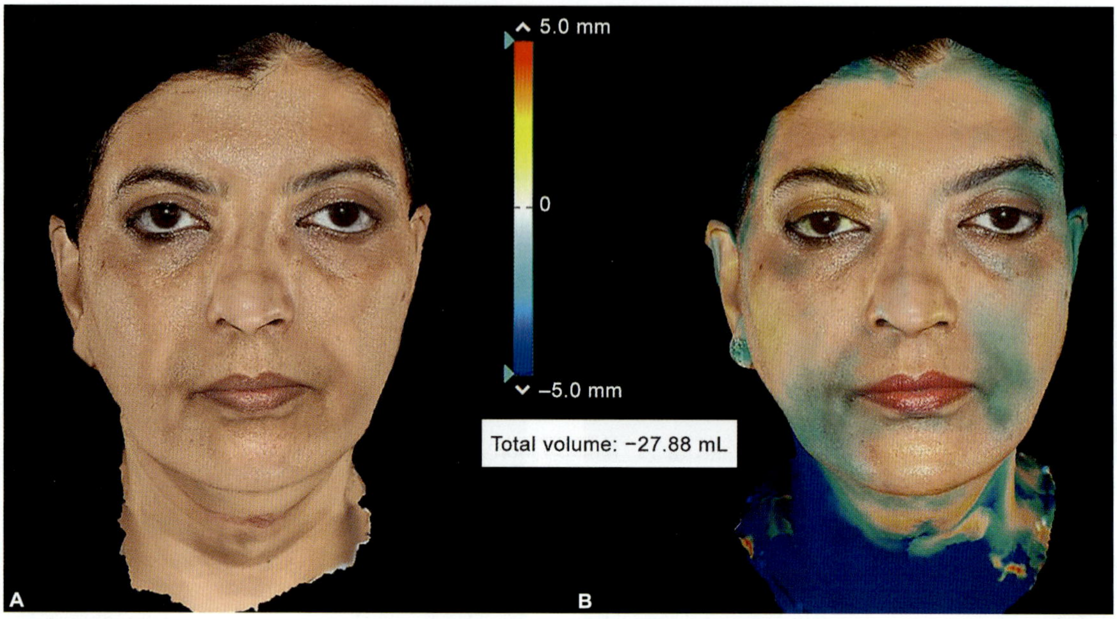

Figs. 8A and B: Post-fillers volumetric assessment using 3D analysis.

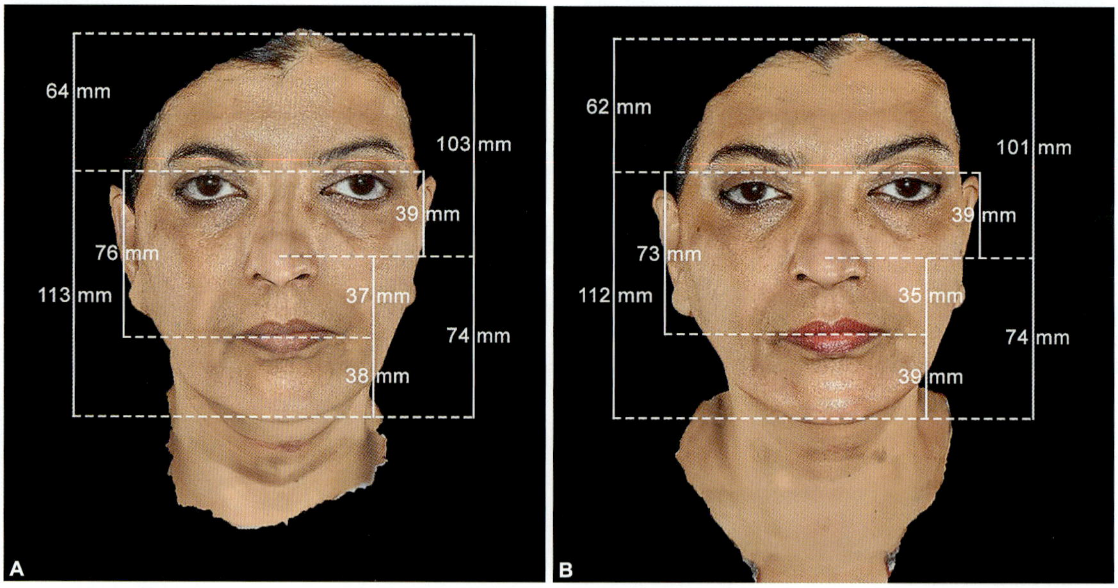

Figs. 9A and B: Before and post-fillers respectively, indicates measurements using 3D face analysis software.

Preparation and Anesthesia

Clean the treatment area and the surrounding skin properly with antiseptics. Topical anesthesia is achieved with following:

- Ice application
- Topical eutectic mixture of local anesthetic (EMLA) cream
- Regional nerve blocks
- *Talkesthesia:* Comforting the patient on a vibration anesthesia by talking in a soothing and comforting manner.

Injection Technique

The choice of injection technique depends on the indication, its location, the filler substance, and the experience of the injector. The techniques are given in **Figures 11A to D and Box 5**.[50]

Before injecting the physician should do the important markings. Infraorbital foramen marking is the most important step to avoid adverse effects **(Figs. 12A and B)**.[47]

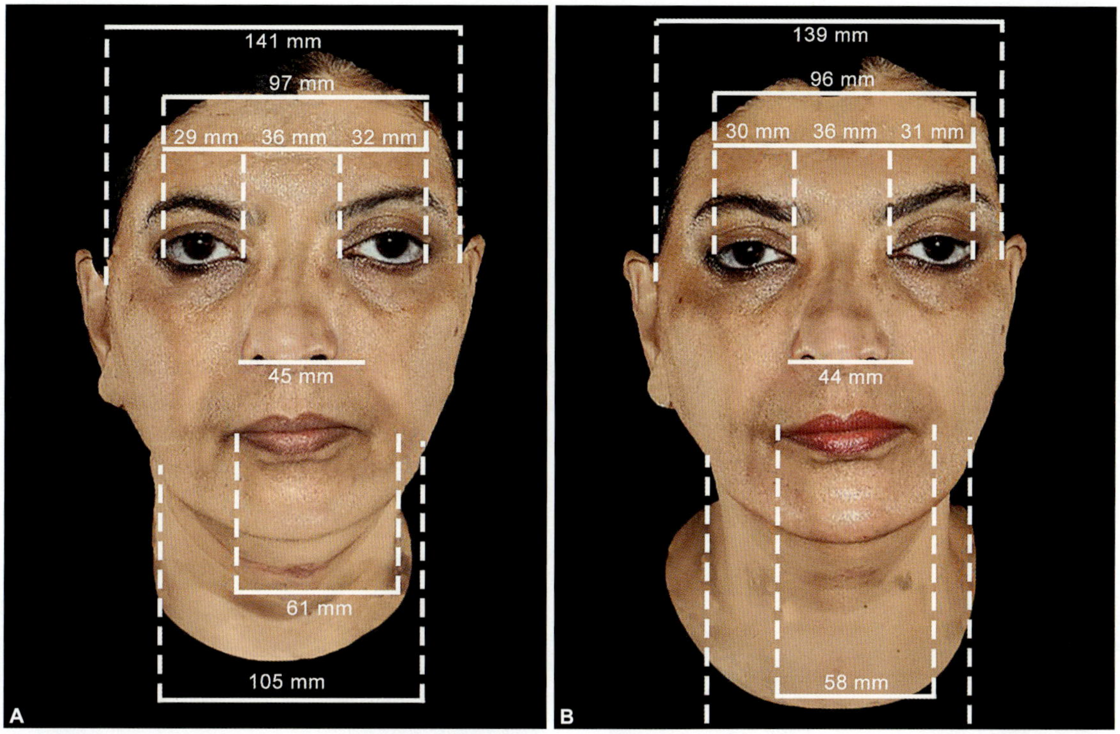

Figs. 10A and B: Before and post-fillers respectively indicates measurements using 3D face analysis software.

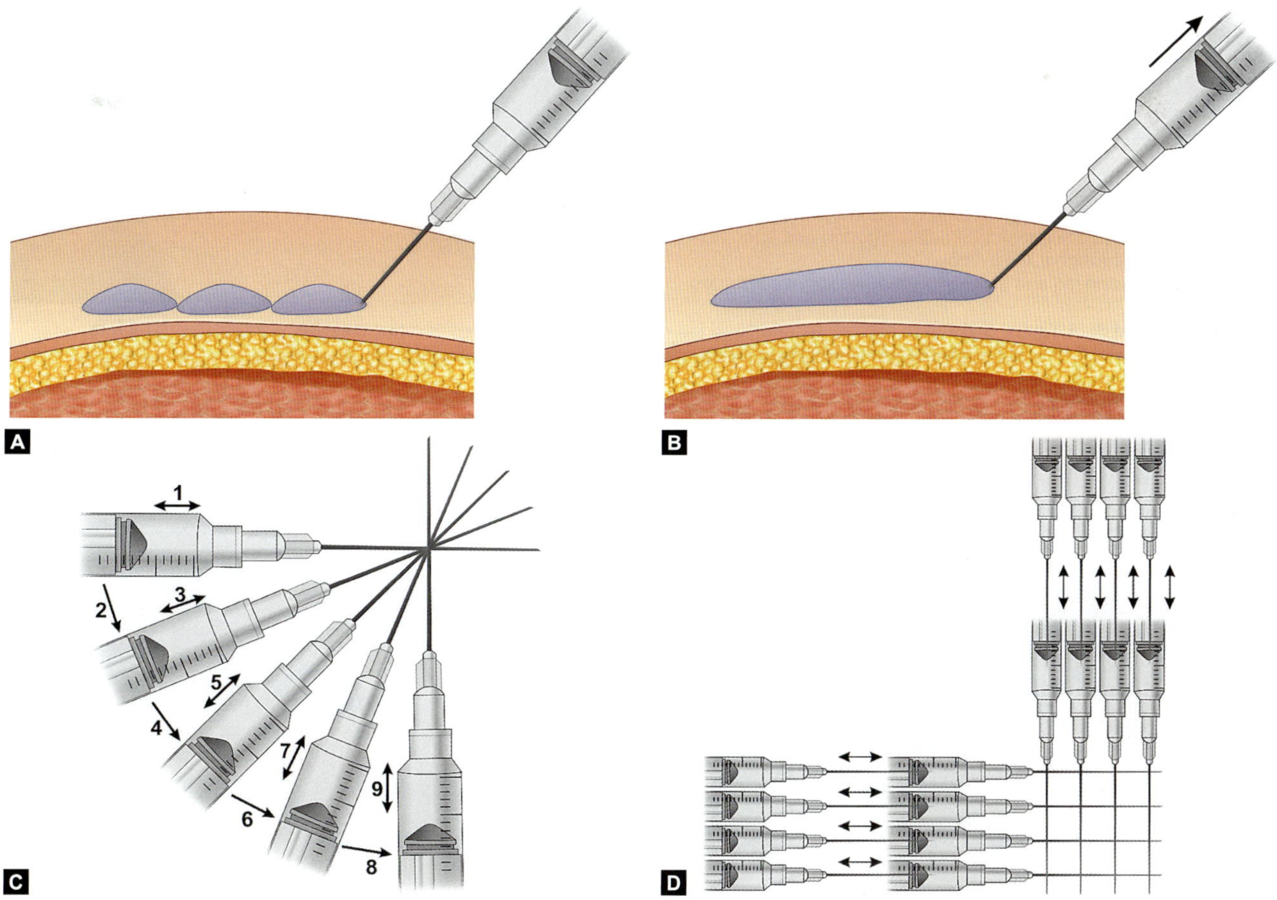

Figs. 11A to D: (A) Serial puncture technique; (B) Linear threading technique; (C) Fanning technique; (D) Cross-hatching technique.

The Hinderer Line

The Hinderer line is a vertical line from the lateral canthus to the oral commissure. An intersecting line is marked from the tragus to the upper alar lobule. Fillers can be put in the outer and lateral quadrant. The Hinderer line helps in establishing the anterior extent of the malar prominence to inject the filler.

BOX 5: Injection techniques.

- Linear threading technique
- Serial puncture
- Fanning
- Cross-hatching
- Depot
- Fern
- Cone

First line is drawn from the lateral commissure to the lateral canthus of the ipsilateral eye (Hinderer line), which is the demarcation for the anterior extent of the malar eminence **(Fig. 13A)**.

A second line is drawn from the lateral commissure to the inferior tragus of the ipsilateral ear (base of the triangle), which demarcates the lateral and inferior extent of the malar prominence eminence. At the level of the limbus of the lower eyelid a horizontal line is marked which is the high point of the cheek (about one-third of the way) from the lateral canthus along the line **(Figs. 13A and B)**.

The injection can be done restoring the ogee curve. The ogee curve is S-shaped consisting of a concave arc flowing into a convex arc. Cheek mound should be restored by injecting on the highest point **(Fig. 13A)**.

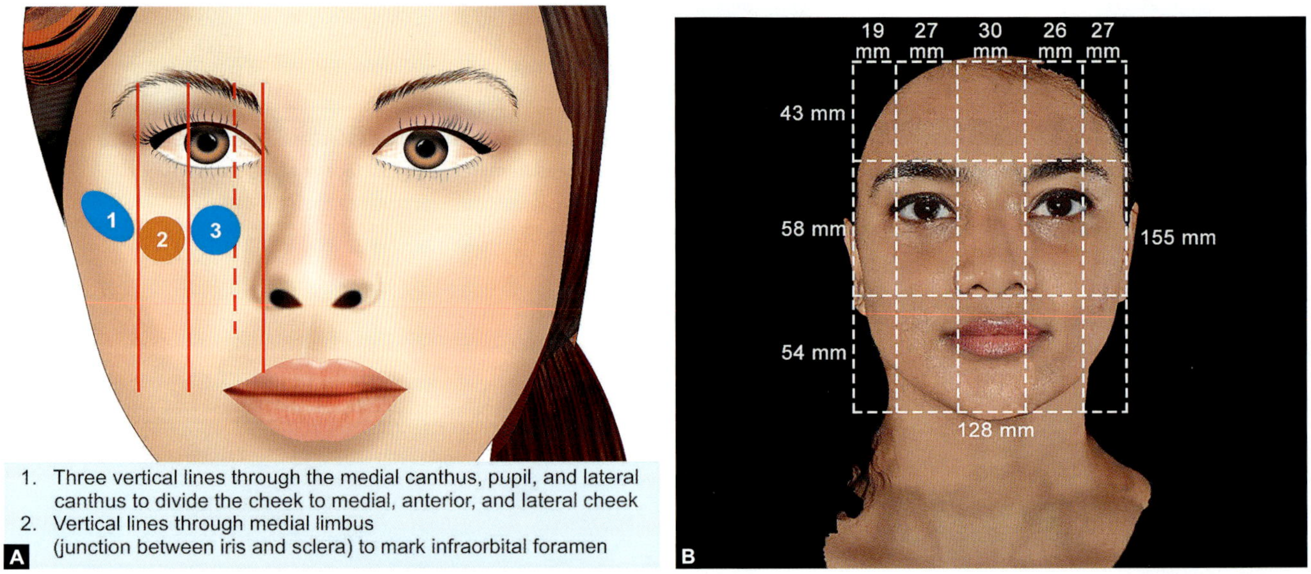

Figs. 12A and B: (A) Cheek division to medial, anterior, and lateral through vertical lines and line marking along infraorbital foramen; (B) Cheek division vertical grid measurements applied practically through 3D analysis.

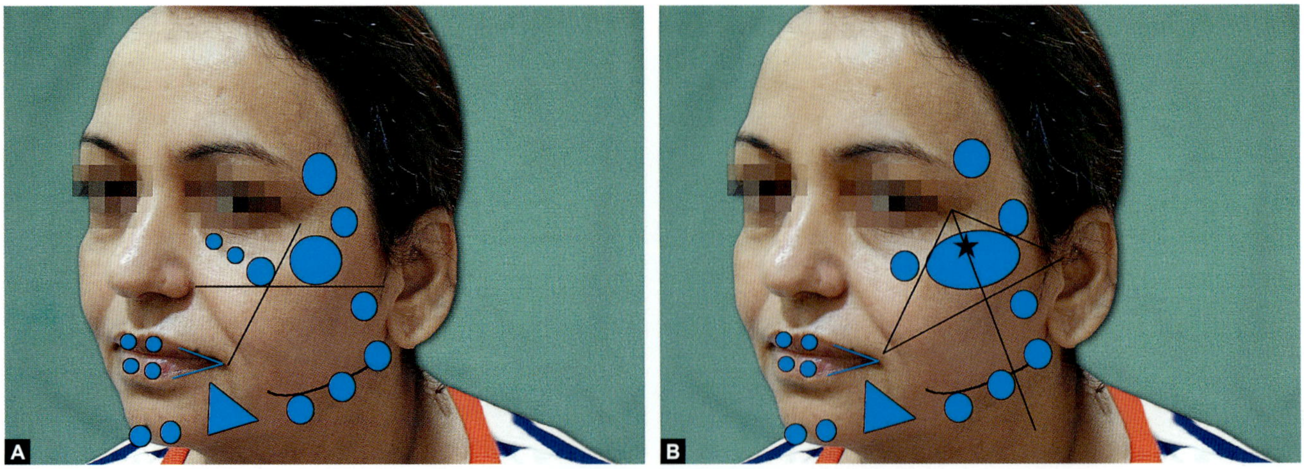

Figs. 13A and B: Hinderers lines, swift point, ogee curve, and key areas of injection on face and lips.

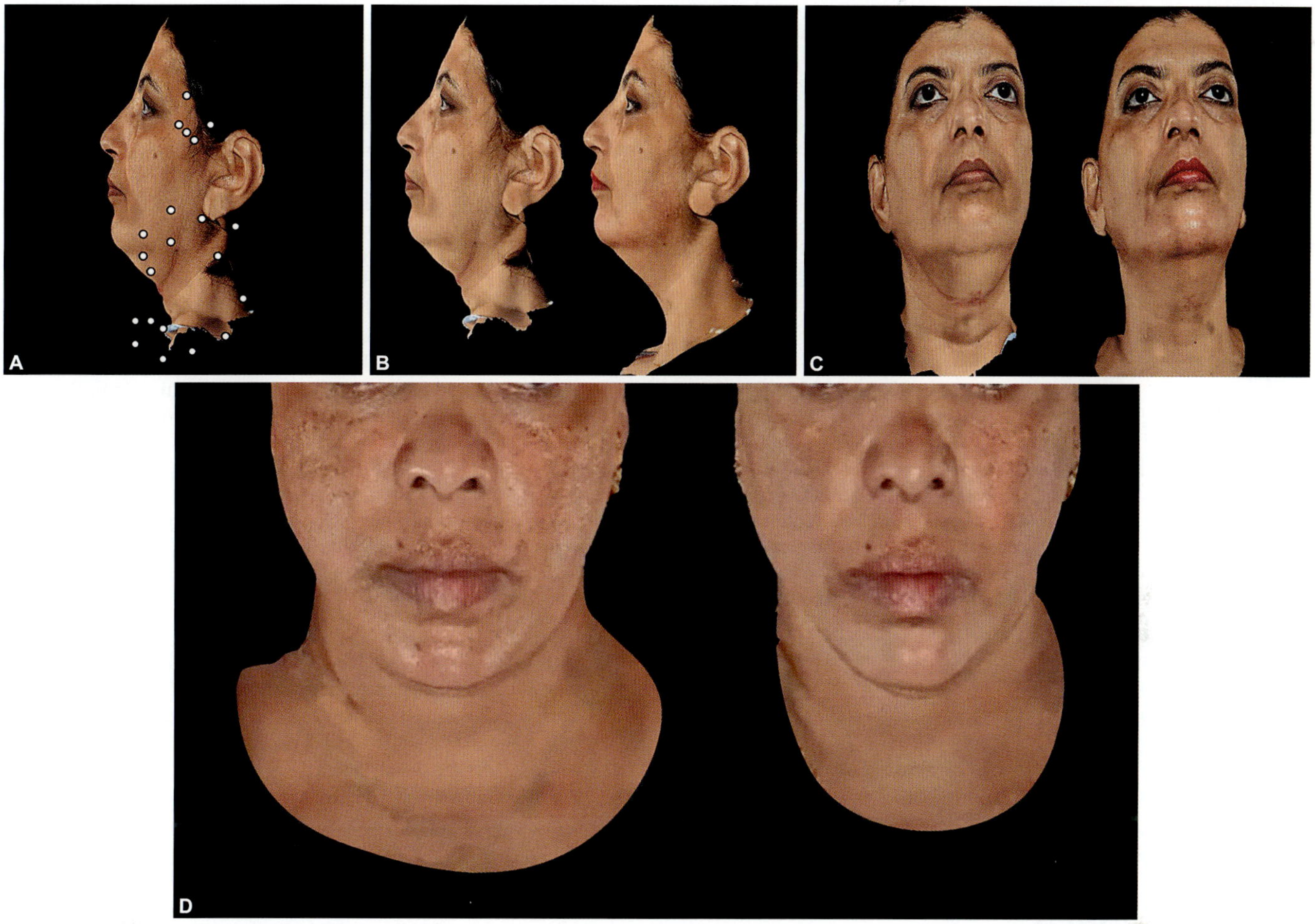

Figs. 14A to D: (A) Injection points for MD codes; (B) Profile view of volumetric rejuvenation pan facial fillers using MD codes; (C) Front view of volumetric rejuvenation pan facial fillers using MD codes; (D) Volumetric rejuvenation after bio filler to achieve slim face.

Thereafter, filler is placed vertically to create two to three pillars on the underlying bone (supraperiosteal plane) with the help of fine needle or microcannula. Injections are placed over the body of the maxilla supraperiosteally as well as subcutaneously. Injections overlying the parotid (preauricular) region, submalar region, and lower anterior cheek are performed in the subcutaneous plane. This technique will soften the NLF and jowl. Often, less product is required for direct correction of whatever deformity may remain along the upper NLF triangle and prejowl sulcus. After treatment mold and massage the product well **(Figs. 13A and B)**.[51]

MD Codes

MD codes™ are originated after point lift techniques in 2010 by Dr de Maio and involves a calculated structured approach to volumetrically rejuvenate the aesthetic subunits of face with desired tool, depth, volume, and type of injection and techniques is identified to give a predictable rejuvenation **(Figs. 14A to D)**.

WARNINGS AND PRECAUTIONS[52]

In general, the following warnings and precautions are applicable to all dermal fillers:

- Do not inject into blood vessels as occlusion of vessel can cause possible subsequent tissue necrosis.
- Before injecting, always make it a practice of aspirating the needle. But negative aspiration does not mean that the vessel has been spared always.
- Blanching in the injected or surrounding area is an alarming sign suggesting vascular compromise. Inject hyaluronidase immediately on visible blanching and pallor.
- Avoid the procedure if any evidence of active infection or inflammation in treatment area.
- In patients with a history of previous herpetic eruption, start prophylactic oral acyclovir as filler procedure causes reactivation of the infection.
- Follow-up should be done after 48 hours to ensure safety, also to see any early signs of vascular compromise if occurred.

TABLE 3: Complications of fillers.

Early onset (occurring up to several days post-treatment)	*Delayed events (occurring from weeks to years post-treatment)*
Injection site reaction: • Erythema • Edema • Pain or tenderness • Bruising • Itching	*Infection (atypical, e.g., mycobacterial)*: • Erythema • Edema • Pain or tenderness • Nodule or abscess • Systemic response to infection • Biofilm
Infection: • Erythema • Edema • Pain or tenderness • Acne papule formation • Nodule or abscess formation	• Foreign body granuloma • Varying from subclinical histological changes to disfiguring nodules
Hypersensitivity: • Erythema • Edema • Pain or tenderness • Non-fluctuant nodules	Migration of material
Lumps, asymmetries, contour irregularities caused by error in technique or placement	• Immune reaction • Local and injection site and generalized
• Skin discoloration • Redness • Whitening • Hyperpigmentation	Persistent discoloration
Local tissue necrosis caused by vascular occlusion	• Persistent scarring • Malar edema

COMPLICATIONS[13]

Complications of fillers are shown in **Table 3**.

CONCLUSION

Facial aesthetics and rejuvenation are evolving rapidly due to changes in products, procedures, and patient demographics. Clinicians can benefit from ongoing guidance on products, tailoring treatments, treating multiple facial areas, using combinations of products, and ways to optimize outcomes. An appreciation that rejuvenation is 3D process involving muscle control, volume restoration, and recontouring helps. Considerable advances in technology have given dermatologists and cosmetic surgeons an array of filler options for soft-tissue augmentation. Fillers with lidocaine give treatment comfort, while maintaining a similar safety and effectiveness. It is our responsibility as injectors to provide patients with safe and effective filler options. Product selection is the result of physicians' experience and comfort with each dermal filler. Selection depends on the appropriate depth of the product placement, the necessity for not performing an allergy test before the treatment, the number of treatments usually necessary to achieve the desired result, whether the product is manufactured with lidocaine or not, the most frequent adverse effects, whether the product is reversible or not, and the longevity of the product.

REFERENCES

1. Lc P, S B, As D, H M, Rh T, Ks S. Facial indices of north and South Indian adults: reliability in stature estimation and sexual dimorphism. J Clin Diagn Res. 2013;7(8):1540-2.
2. Ortman JM, Velkoff VA, Hogan H; United States (US) Census Bureau. (2014). An Aging Nation: The Older Population in the United States. [online] Available from https://www.census.gov/content/dam/Census/library/publications/2014/demo/p25-1140.pdf [Last accessed September, 2023].
3. Fitzgerald R, Graivier MH, Kane M, Lorenc ZP, Vleggaar D, Werschler WP, et al. Update on facial aging. Aesthet Surg J. 2010;30 Suppl:11S-24S.
4. Brandt FS, Kaufman J, Green JB, Ballin AC, Cazzaniga A. Hyaluronic acid fillers. In: Nouri K (Ed). Dermatologic Surgery: Step by Step, 1st edition. Oxford: Wiley-Blackwell; 2012. pp. 259-85.
5. Vleggaar D, Fitzgerald R. Dermatological implications of skeletal aging: a focus on supraperiosteal volumization for perioral rejuvenation. J Drugs Dermatol. 2008;7(3):209-20.
6. Rohrich RJ, Pessa JE. The fat compartments of the face: anatomy and clinical implications for cosmetic surgery. Plastic Reconstr Surg. 2007;119(7):2219-27.
7. Lemperle G, Romano JJ, Busso M. Soft tissue augmentation with artecoll: 10-year history, indications, techniques, and complications. Dermatol Surg. 2003;29(6):573-87.
8. Kontis TC. Contemporary review of injectable facial fillers. JAMA Facial Plast Surg. 2013;15(1):58-64.
9. Conejo-Mir JS, Sanz Guirado S, Angel Muñoz M. Adverse granulomatous reaction to Artecoll treated by intralesional 5-fluorouracil and triamcinolone injections. Dermatol Surg. 2006;32(8):1079-81.
10. Lemperle G, Gauthier-Hazan N, Wolters M, Eisemann-Klein M, Zimmermann U, Duffy DM. Foreign body granulomas after all injectable dermal fillers: part 1. Possible causes. Plast Reconstr Surg. 2009;123(6):1842-63.
11. Lemperle G, Knapp TR, Sadick NS, Lemperle SM. ArteFill permanent injectable for soft tissue augmentation: I. Mechanism of action and injection techniques. Aesthetic Plast Surg. 2010;34(3):264-72.
12. Sclafani AP, Fagien S. Treatment of injectable soft tissue filler complications. Dermatol Surg. 2009;35(Suppl 2):1672-80.
13. Funt D, Pavicic T. Dermal fillers in aesthetics: an overview of adverse events and treatment approaches. Clin Cosmet Investig Dermatol. 2013;6:295-316.
14. Suneva Medical, Inc. (2019). Protocol for the post-approval study of ArteFill for correction of nasolabial folds. [online] Available from https://www.clinicaltrials.gov/study/NCT03299712?term=Protocol%20for%20the%20post-%20approval%20study%20of%20ArteFill%C2%AE%20for%20correction%20of%20nasolabial%20folds&rank=1 [Last accessed September, 2023].
15. Graivier MH, Bass LS, Busso M, Jasin ME, Narins RS, Tzikas TL. Calcium hydroxylapatite (Radiesse) for correction of the mid- and lower face: consensus recommendations. Plast Reconstr Surg. 2007;120(6 Suppl):55S-66S.
16. Daley T, Damm DD, Haden JA, Kolodychak MT. Oral lesions associated with injected hydroxyapatite cosmetic filler. Oral Surg Oral Med Oral Pathol Oral Radiol. 2012;114(1):107-11.
17. Tzikas TL. A 52-month summary of results using calcium hydroxylapatite for facial soft tissue augmentation. Dermatol Surg. 2008;34(Suppl 1):S9-15.
18. Emer J, Sundaram H. Aesthetic applications of calcium hydroxylapatite volumizing filler: an evidence-based review

and discussion of current concepts (part 1 of 2). J Drugs Dermatol. 2013;12(12):1345-54.
19. Sadick NS. A 52-week study of safety and efficacy of calcium hydroxylapatite for rejuvenation of the aging hand. J Drugs Dermatol. 2011;10(1):47-51.
20. Marmur ES, Al Quran H, De Sa Earp AP, Yoo JY. A five-patient satisfaction pilot study of calcium hydroxylapatite injection for treatment of aging hands. Dermatol Surg. 2009;35(12):1978-84.
21. Choi WI, Hwang Y, Sahu A, Min K, Sung D, Tae G, et al. An injectable and physical levan-based hydrogel as a dermal filler for soft tissue augmentation. Biomater Sci. 2018;6(10):2627-38.
22. Abdelfattah NS, Elhusseiny RM, Mahmoud AA. Autologous Plasma Filler in Treatment of Nasolabial Folds. QJM: An Int J Med. 2020;113,Supplement 1.
23. Gupta S, Borde Bisht P, Kannan C. Bio-filler: an effective facial rejuvenation tool—easy on pocket. J Cutan Aesthet Surg. 2020;13:243-6.
24. Doghaim NN, El-Tatawy RA, Neinaa YM. Assessment of the efficacy and safety of platelet poor plasma gel as autologous dermal filler for facial rejuvenation. J Cosmet Dermatol. 2019;18:1271-9.
25. Kablik J, Monheit GD, Yu L, Chang G, Gershkovich J. Comparative physical properties of hyaluronic acid dermal fillers. Dermatol Surg. 2009;35(Suppl 1):302-12.
26. Sundaram H, Voigts B, Beer K, Meland M. Comparison of the rheological properties of viscosity and elasticity in two categories of soft tissue fillers: calcium hydroxylapatite and hyaluronic acid. Dermatol Surg. 2010;36(Suppl 3):1859-65.
27. Edsman K, Nord LI, Ohrlund A, Lärkner H, Kenne AH. Gel properties of hyaluronic acid dermal fillers. Dermatol Surg. 2012;38(7 Pt 2):1170-9.
28. Flynn TC, Sarazin D, Bezzola A, Terrani C, Micheels P. Comparative histology of intradermal implantation of mono and biphasic hyaluronic acid fillers. Dermatol Surg. 2011;37(5):637-43.
29. Lorenc ZP, Fagien S, Flynn TC, Waldorf HA. Review of key Belotero Balance safety and efficacy trials. Plast Reconstr Surg. 2013;132(4 Suppl 2):33S-40S.
30. Sundaram H, Cassuto D. Biophysical characteristics of hyaluronicacid soft-tissue fillers and their relevance to aesthetic applications. Plast Reconstr Surg. 2013;132(4 Suppl 2):5S-21S.
31. Kühne U, Imhof M, Kirchmeir M, Howell DJ. Five-year retrospective review of safety, injected volumes, and longevity of the hyaluronic acid Belotero Basic for facial treatments in 317 patients. J Drugs Dermatol. 2012;11(9):1032-5.
32. Prager W, Wissmueller E, Havermann I, Bee EK, Howell DJ, Zschocke I, et al. A prospective, split-face, randomized, comparative study of safety and 12-month longevity of three formulations of hyaluronic acid dermal filler for treatment of nasolabial folds. Dermatol Surg. 2012;38(7 Pt 2):1143-50.
33. Jones D, Murphy DK. Volumizing hyaluronic acid filler for midface volume deficit: 2-year results from a pivotal single-blind randomized controlled study. Dermatol Surg. 2013;39(11):1602-12.
34. Carruthers J, Carruthers A, Tezel A, Kraemer J, Craik L. Volumizing with a 20-mg/mL smooth, highly cohesive, viscous hyaluronic acid filler and its role in facial rejuvenation therapy. Dermatol Surg. 2010;36(Suppl 3):1886-92.
35. Raspaldo H. Volumizing effect of a new hyaluronic acid subdermal facial filler: a retrospective analysis based on 102 cases. J Cosmet Laser Ther. 2008;10(3):134-42.
36. Levy PM, DeBoulle K, Raspaldo H. Comparison of injection comfort of a new category of cohesive hyaluronic acid filler with preincorporated lidocaine and a hyaluronic acid filler alone. Dermatol Surg. 2009;35(Suppl 1):332-6.
37. Weinkle SH, Bank DE, Boyd CM, Gold MH, Thomas JA, Murphy DK. A multi-center, double-blind, randomized controlled study of the safety and effectiveness of Juvéderm injectable gel with and without lidocaine. J Cosmet Dermatol. 2009;8(3):205-10.
38. Marmur E, Green L, Busso M. Controlled, randomized study of pain levels in subjects treated with calcium hydroxylapatite premixed with lidocaine for correction of nasolabial folds. Dermatol Surg. 2010;36(3):309-15.
39. Ballin AC, Cazzaniga A, Brandt FS. Long-term efficacy, safety and durability of Juvéderm® XC. Clin Cosmet Investig Dermatol. 2013;6:183-9.
40. Tetzlaff JE. The pharmacology of local anesthetics. Anesthesiol Clin North Am. 2000;18(2):217-33.
41. Rhodes G, Proffitt F, Grady JM, Sumich A. Facial symmetry and the perception of beauty. Psychon Bull Rev. 1998;5(4):659-69.
42. Brooks M, Pomiankowski A. Symmetry is in the eye of the beholder. Trends Ecol Evol. 1994;9(6):201-2.
43. Concar D. Sex and the symmetrical body. New Sci. 1995;146:40-4.
44. Enquist M, Arak A. Symmetry, beauty and evolution. Nature. 1994;372(6502):169-72.
45. Grammer K, Thornhill R. Human (Homo sapiens) facial attractiveness and sexual selection: the role of symmetry and averageness. J Comp Psychol. 1994;108(3):233-42.
46. Swaddle JP, Cuthill IC. Asymmetry and human facial attractiveness: symmetry may not always be beautiful. Proc Biol Sci. 1995;261(1360):111-6.
47. Carruthers J, Glogau RG, Blitzer A; Facial Aesthetics Consensus Group Faculty. Advances in facial rejuvenation: botulinum toxin type a, hyaluronic acid dermal fillers, and combination therapies—consensus recommendations. Plast Reconstr Surg. 2008;121(5 Suppl):5S-30S.
48. Vedamurty M. Soft tissue augmentation–use of hyaluronic acid as dermal filler. Indian J Dermatol Venereol Leprol. 2004;70(6):383-7.
49. Lemperle G, Rullan PP, Gauthier-Hazan N. Avoiding and treating dermal filler complications. Plast Reconstr Surg. 2006;118(3 Suppl):92S-107S.
50. Klein AW. Temporary fillers. In: Nouri K, Leal Khouri S (Eds). Techniques in Dermatologic Surgery, 1st edition. Edinburgh: Mosby; 2003. pp. 281-92.
51. Swift A, Remington K. BeautiPHIcationTM: a global approach to facial beauty. Clin Plast Surg. 2011;38(3):347-77.
52. US Food and Drug Administration. (2013). General and Plastic Surgery Devices Panel of the Medical Devices Meeting. [online] Available from https://www.federalregister.gov/documents/2013/05/23/2013-12230/general-and-plastic-surgery-devices-panel-of-the-medical-devices-advisory-committee-notice-of [Last accessed September, 2023].

CHAPTER 91

Soft-tissue Augmentation: Hyaluronic Acid Dermal Fillers

Maya Vedamurthy

KEY MESSAGES

- Soft-tissue augmentation is a useful procedure in both prejuvenation and rejuvenation.
- Dermal fillers are essential tools in soft-tissue augmentation.
- A wide range of dermal fillers is available for use in aesthetic dermatology.
- The future holds great promise and expectations for fillers in cosmetic and noncosmetic indications.
- Thorough knowledge of anatomy and dermal fillers is essential to use them safely and effectively.

INTRODUCTION

Soft-tissue augmentation with fillers has revolutionized the field of aesthetic dermatology as more and more millennials and baby boomers seek antiaging treatment to restore lost shape and volume and hence their youthfulness. With the advent of botulinum toxin, it has been possible to eliminate dynamic wrinkles, while static wrinkles can be addressed only using dermal fillers. Besides, dermal fillers offer a three-dimensional (3D) facelift concept so much that filling not only augments but also replaces pulling.[1]

HISTORY

The history of soft-tissue augmentation dates back to more than 100 years when Neuber, in 1893, used the autologous fat soft-tissue augmentation.[2] Injectable paraffin became popular in the early 1900s but fell into disrepute because of the resultant foreign body granulomas. Lexer in 1901 and Bruning in 1911 modified Neuber's technique to restore lost volume in subcutaneous space.

Later, collagen was widely introduced by dermatologists as the only Food and Drug Administration (FDA)-approved filler to treat facial furrows and rhytids. However, the need for a safer option led to the introduction of hyaluronic acid (HA) fillers, coupled with renewed interest in silicone, poly L-lactic acid, and many more to meet the demands in filler practice.[3] Soft-tissue augmentation is undergoing a Renaissance period as there is an increasing demand for aesthetic procedures with minimal or no downtime and as new fillers seem to flood the market.[4]

AGING SKIN

Skin, in general, undergoes two types of aging processes. The first is intrinsic aging, which occurs with the passage of time and is also referred to as chronologic aging. The second is photoaging, where the degenerative changes occur in overexposed parts of the body, mainly the face. With aging, the skin loses collagen, elastin, and HA in the dermis, along with a decrease in fat and bony structural support.[5] However, HA is a key molecule in skin aging.

The 5 Ds that occur with aging and can be corrected using fillers are:

1. Deterioration of skin architecture
2. Disproportion
3. Descent
4. Dynamic discord
5. Deflation

The clinical result of photoaging is the formation of facial furrows and rhytids. Their terminology varies with the relative change of collagen, elastin, and subcutaneous tissue to the skin, i.e., folds, wrinkles, and lines **(Fig. 1)**. Other causes include trauma and scarring due to diseases that alter collagen and elastin quality in the dermis. All the above changes can be addressed using dermal fillers. Soft-tissue augmentation is a procedure where substances are placed in the skin or under the skin at various levels to restore the 5 Ds of aging.

- *Autologous fat:* Lipoinjection and nanofat (see the chapter on Fat transfer)
- Injectable fillers
- *Surgical implant:* Soft form

Of the above, injectable fillers mainly comprised of HA are the most preferred because of their relative safety, the ease with which they can be injected, and their availability. Dermal fillers have shifted from two-dimensional (2D) to 3D restoration of age-related changes, such as lines, wrinkles and volume loss or pathological changes like scars. Details of classification and general principles[6,7] are discussed in this chapter. This chapter focuses on HA fillers.

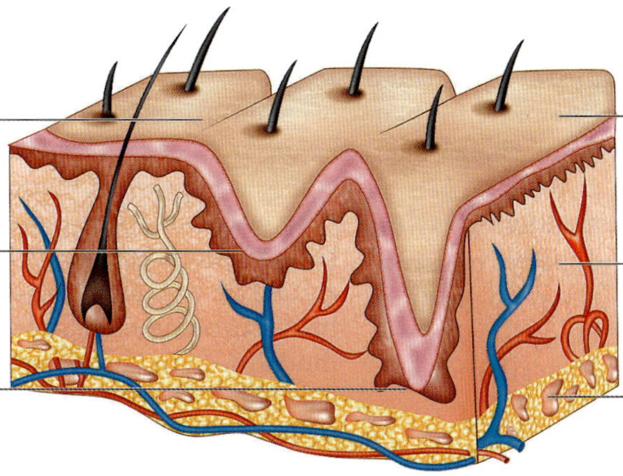

Fig. 1: Physiology of facial wrinkles.

HYALURONIC ACID FILLERS

Hyaluronic acid is a popular and well-accepted material of choice for cosmetic indications. HA is a naturally occurring linear polysaccharide found in all living organisms and is identical in all species and tissue types.

Hyaluronic Acid Dermal Filler Properties

Traditionally, HA has been extracted from rooster combs. The commercial HA sources are bacterial and are termed non-animal stabilized hyaluronic acid (NASHA), as these are biosynthetically produced by bacterial fermentation. HA is a glycosaminoglycan disaccharide composed of alternately repeating units of D-glucuronic acid and *N*-acetyl-D glucosamine[8] **(Fig. 2)**. Multiple changes have been introduced to HA to increase its longevity in the tissues with the least immunogenicity. Several properties contribute to the unique qualities and clinical characteristics of HA **(Fig. 3)**:

- Gel hardness
- Particle size
- Concentration per milliliter
- Cross-linked versus free HA
- Soluble versus insoluble HA
- Swelling/gel's ability to resist dilution
- Presence/absence of xylocaine[9]

The physical characteristics of HA-based fillers[10] **(Table 1)** determine the behavior of the gel placed in tissue and contribute significantly to one of the following features:

- Flexibility during animation
- Lift capacity
- Plasticity
- Elasticity
- Viscosity

History of Hyaluronic Acid

Hyaluronic acid was first isolated from the vitreous jelly of cow's eyes by Karl Meyer and his colleague John Palmer in 1934. They proposed the name HA from hyaloid (vitreous) and uronic acid as the substance contained two sugar molecules, one of which was uronic acid. Hyalos (Greek for glassy) is known for its space-filling and viscoelastic properties. The life of natural HA in tissue is only 1–2 days before it gets degraded in the liver to carbon dioxide and water. Functions of HA in the skin include hydration, a space-filling capacity, and the framework through which cells migrate.[11]

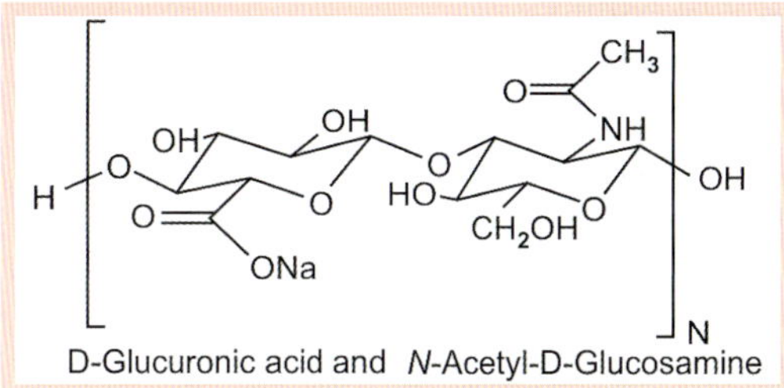

Fig. 2: Molecular structure of hyaluronic acid.

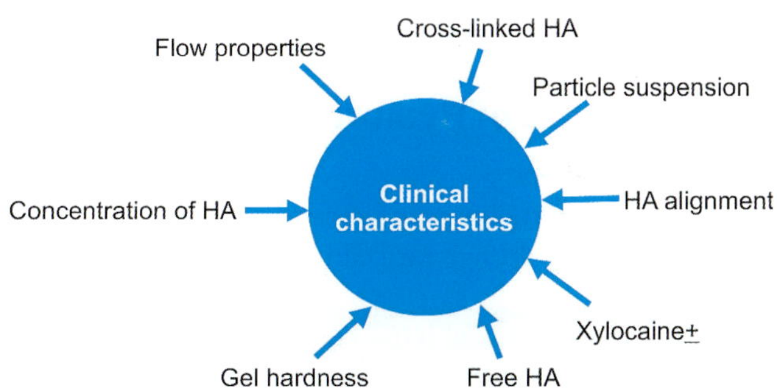

Fig. 3: Variables in hyaluronic acid (HA) product.

TABLE 1: Physical characteristics of HA-based fillers.

Characteristics	*Clinical importance*
G prime	Tissue projection
Particle size	Degree of volume replacement
Cohesivity	Tissue expansion
HA concentration	Durability and stability
Swelling	Degree of inflammation and induration

(HA: hyaluronic acid)

Hyaluronic Acid Products

Hyaluronic acid products are the mainstay of dermal fillers in tissue augmentation. However, they vary in their concentration, gel particle size, cross-linking, and hence their indications. HA products are marketed as biphasic gels in which particles are of varied sizes or as monophasic gels with HA as a homogenous solution. HA has no species or tissue-specific antigenic properties and therefore has no potential for allergic or immunogenic response in humans regardless of its source. Different HA products available are shown in **Table 2 and Box 1**.

Advantages of Hyaluronic Acid

- Convenient procedure/easy to administer
- No pretest required
- Minimal pain/no pain with xylocaine added
- No/minimal downtime
- Looks/feels natural
- Cost-effective
- The versatility of indications from hydration to correction of fine lines to volumization
- Lack of migration
- Minimal side effects
- Compatibility with other cosmetic procedures
- Reversibility with hyaluronidase

Disadvantages of Hyaluronic Acid

- Temporary effect
- Edema and erythema post procedure
- Adverse effects though rare can occur.

TABLE 2: Different filler products and their properties.

Products	*Description*	*Technology*
Restylane	20 mg/mL	NASHA
Restylane Lyft	20 mg/mL	NASHA
Resylane Refyne	20 mg/mL	XpresHAn
Restylane Defyne	20 mg/mL	XpressHAn
Restylane Kysse	20 mg	Optimal balance technology (OBT)
Restylane Volyme	20 mg	OBT
Restylane Vital	20 mg	NASHA
Juvéderm Ultra	24 mg	Hylacross
Juvéderm Ultra Plus	24 mg	Hylacross
Juvéderm Volume	20 mg	Vycross
Juvéderm Volbella	15 mg/mL	Vycross
Juvéderm Volift	17.5 mg/mL	Vycross
Juvéderm Volite	12 mg/mL	Vycross
BELOTERO BALANCE	22.5 mg	Cohesive polydensified matrix (CPM)
Teosyal	23 mg	

(NASHA: non-animal stabilized hyaluronic acid)

CASE SELECTION AND ASSESSMENT

Preprocedure: An insightful patient assessment in the context of patient expectations and overall treatment outcome should be the first step in soft-tissue augmentation. One should also consider age, gender, ethnicity, and need based on the above criteria. Patients with unrealistic expectations and those with body dysmorphic disorder or obsessive–compulsive disorder should be excluded. Expected outcomes with fillers must be discussed in comparison with other available treatment modalities, and appropriate referrals need to be made if warranted. A detailed discussion with the patient should include patient-related factors, product-related factors, and procedure-related factors that form part of an effective strategy of a 10-point plan[13] **(Box 2)**.

Patient-related risk factors include poor periodontal hygiene, the existence of an immunocompromised state, chronic or recurrent skin conditions, or uncontrolled diabetes mellitus.[14]

Product-related factors should include the possibility of reversibility, choice of product, and the number of syringes required to obtain optimum results.

Procedure-related factors to be considered are the pre- and post-photographs, the technique to be used, and injection anatomy in the proposed treatment area.

BOX 1: Desirable characteristics of dermal fillers.[12]

Safety:
- Biocompatible
- Lack of hypersensitivity
- Lack of clinical inflammatory response
- Nonmigratory and nonclumping
- Negligible pain

Efficacy:
- FDA-approved
- Reproducible technique/result
- Ease of use (room temperature storage, requires minimal to no preparation, effortless to inject)
- Results (long-duration, good contouring ability, collagen-stimulating)
- Cost-effective

(FDA: food and drug administration)

BOX 2: Patient, product and procedure-related factors.

Patient-related factors:
- Skin conditions
- Systemic diseases
- Medications
- History of dental procedures
- Dysmorphophobia
- Gender
- Wants versus needs

Product-related factors:
- Reversibility
- Product placement
- Product layering

Procedure-related factors:
- Photographs
- Aseptic technique
- Technical and anatomy knowledge

THEORY OF MYOMODULATION WITH HYALURONIC ACID FILLERS[15]

It is conceived that filler treatment with HA can alter interactions between facial structure and muscle movement and balance action within muscle groups to modify appearance on animation and at rest. This is referred to as mechanical myomodulation in contrast to chemical myomodulation achieved with neurotoxin. The placement of HA filler and the angle with which its injected can either increase or decrease the muscle action based on its relation to the muscle and the angle with which the filler is injected. This controls facial mimetic muscles to improve facial appearance in rejuvenation.

INDICATIONS

The indications may be broadly divided into:

- Facial areas
- Extra-facial areas

Indications in Facial Areas

- Nasolabial folds **(Figs. 4A and B)**
- Fine lines, rhytids—perioral and periocular
- Glabellar complex **(Figs. 5A and B)**
- Brow elevation
- Lip augmentation and contouring **(Figs. 6A and B)**
- Chin, cheek, and temporal fossa augmentation
- Nose reshaping
- Tear trough **(Figs. 7A and B)**
- Sears, traumatic, postacne, and skin diseases **(Figs. 8A and B)**
- Marionette lines
- Oral commissure
- Prejowl sulcus
- Periocular melanoses
- Postacne scars

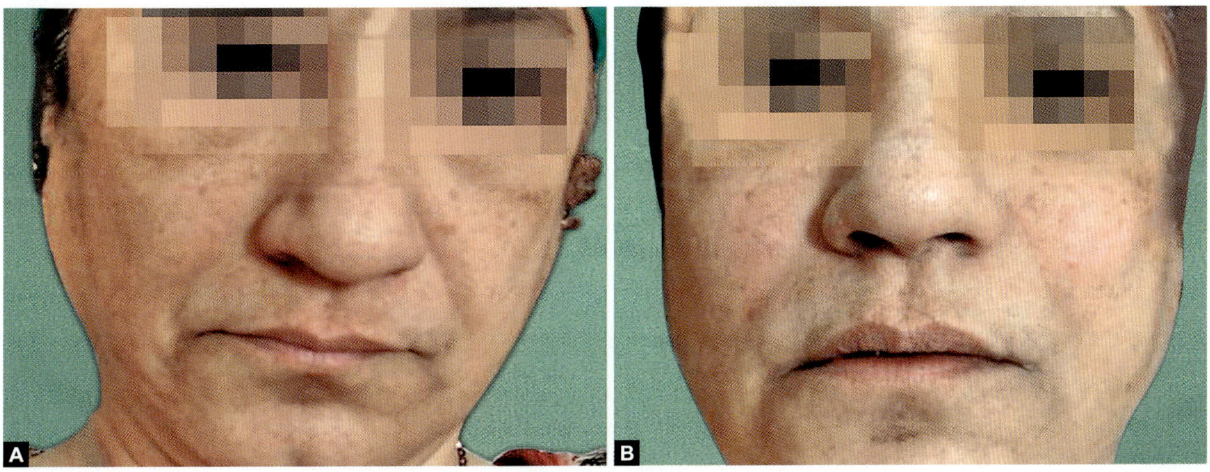

Figs. 4A and B: Nasolabial fold: (A) Pretreatment; (B) Post-treatment.

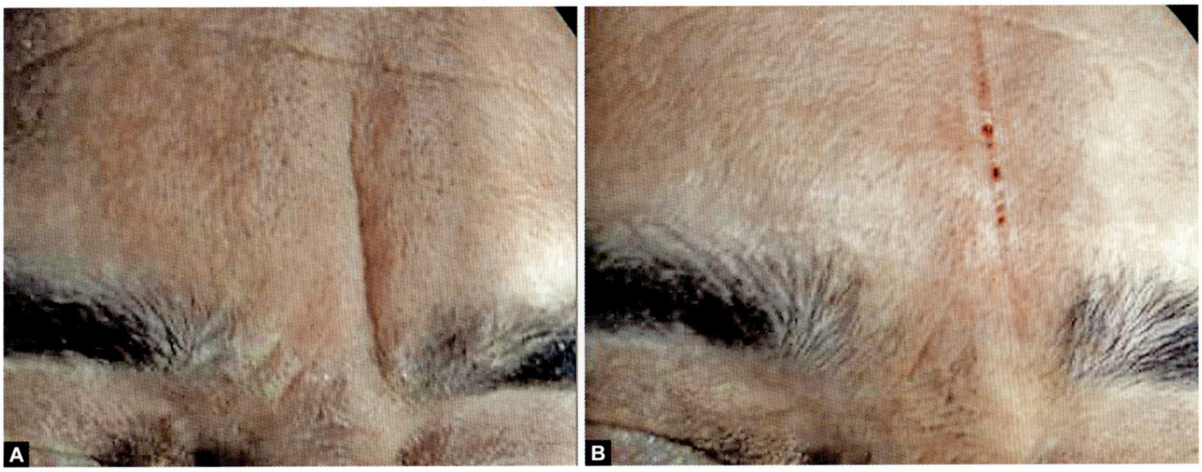

Figs. 5A and B: Glabella—frown line: (A) Pretreatment; (B) Post-treatment.

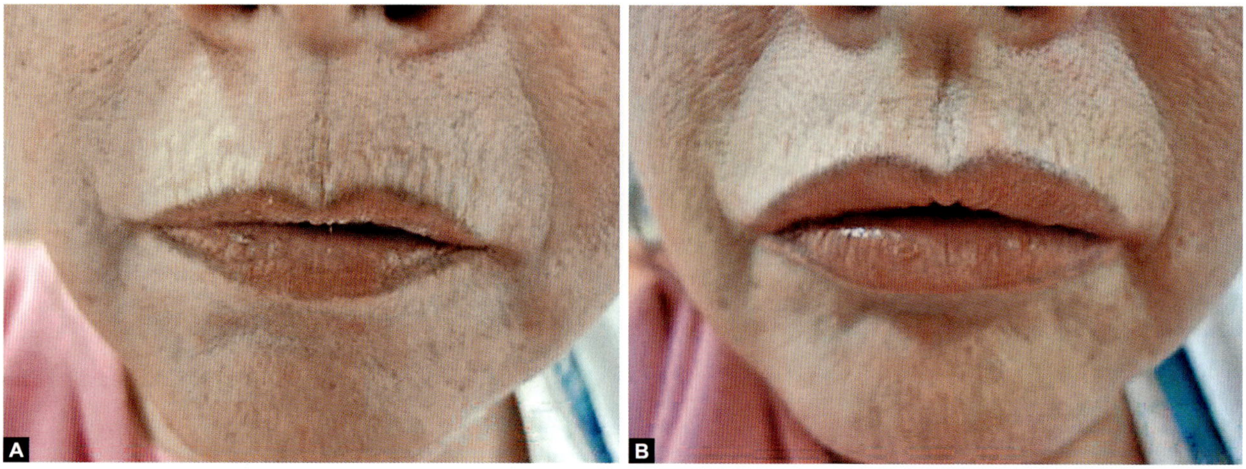

Figs. 6A and B: Lip augmentation: (A) Pretreatment; (B) Post-treatment.

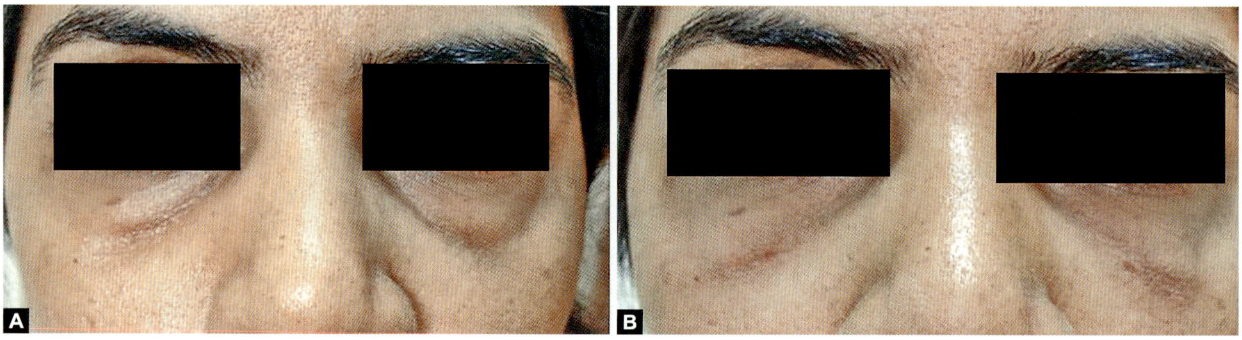

Figs. 7A and B: Tear trough: (A) Pretreatment; (B) Post-treatment.

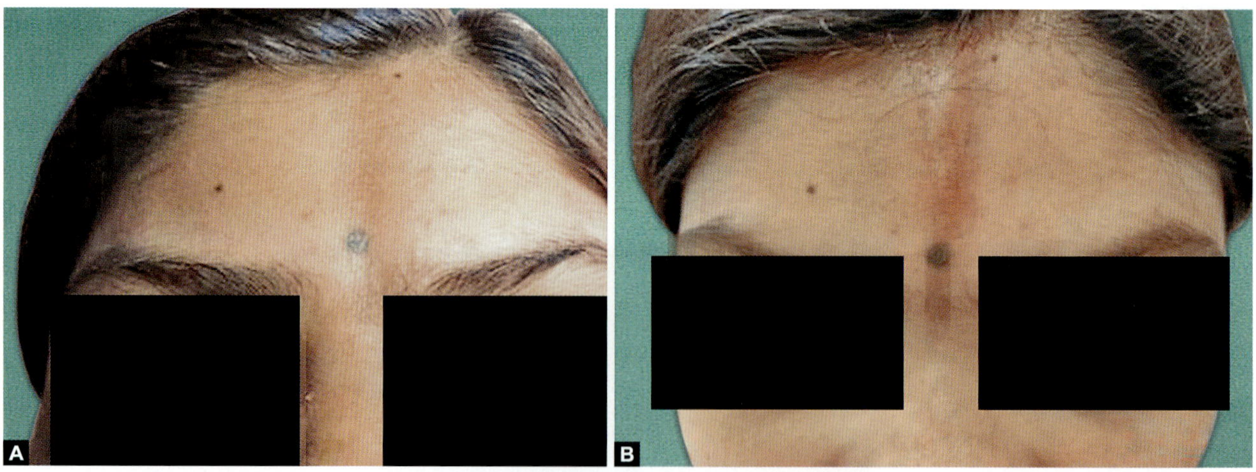

Figs. 8A and B: Morphea: (A) Pretreatment; (B) Post-treatment.

Indications in Extrafacial Areas

- Breast and buttock augmentation
- Hand, neck, and décolleté rejuvenation
- External genital rejuvenation
- Arms
- Traumatic scars
- *Dermatological diseases:* Scleroderma and human immunodeficiency virus (HIV)-associated lipoatrophy
- Earlobe plumping and ear lobe ptosis
- *Feet:* Cushioning effect under corns and calluses[16]

CONTRAINDICATIONS

Contraindications are as follows:

- Unrealistic expectations
- History of allergy/anaphylaxis to one of its components/source
- At sites of inflammation, for example, infections and eczema
- Pregnancy
- Dysmorphophobia

COUNSELING

Counseling sessions must cover both aesthetic and physical considerations from the viewpoint of both the patient and the physician. Physicians should discuss the amount of filler required, the patient's cost, comfort zones like anesthesia, expected outcome, and downtime. Patients need to be counseled about their wants versus needs as well as on their expectation goals versus the physician's expected performance.

PHOTOGRAPHY (BOX 3)

Clinical photography is a powerful tool to record treatment outcomes. 3D imaging is a prerequisite now. The tips for good clinical imaging for filler procedures are given in **Box 3**.

PREOPERATIVE PREPARATION

History should include covering recent use of medications and foods that can cause bleeding and allergies to local anesthetics. A history of herpes simplex is essential to consider antiviral prophylaxis. History of prior use of fillers, especially types of fillers used, and untoward events or reactions, if any has occurred, has to be obtained.

- Instructions to avoid anti-inflammatory drugs, gingko biloba, vitamin E >400 IU/day, green tea, and fish for 7–10 days before treatment
- Antiviral prophylaxis, if needed
- Examine the treatment area for any inflammatory disease.

Equipment Needed

- Alcohol pads/antiseptic solution
- Sterile gloves and gauze
- Marking pencil
- Good lighting and good camera
- Needles/cannulae
- Local anesthetic cream/injections
- Filler material

Informed Consent

Written informed consent is required to ensure compliance with regulatory and legal requirements and satisfy patient's expectations.

Anesthesia

Anesthesia may be recommended to increase the patient's comfort and retention. The products premixed with lidocaine are usually preferred to decrease pain during the procedure. Regular anesthesia involves the use of topical anesthetic agents. Topical anesthesia is applied preferably under occlusion at least 1 hour prior to the procedure. Nerve block anesthesia is rarely preferred nowadays.

Alternative comfort techniques:

- Ice anesthesia[18]
- Vibration Anesthesia **(Fig. 9)**
- Talkaesthesia

PROCEDURES

The procedure steps are given in **Box 4**.

POSTPROCEDURE INSTRUCTIONS

The patient is usually seated comfortably in an upright or semi-reclined position so that gravity helps the wrinkles

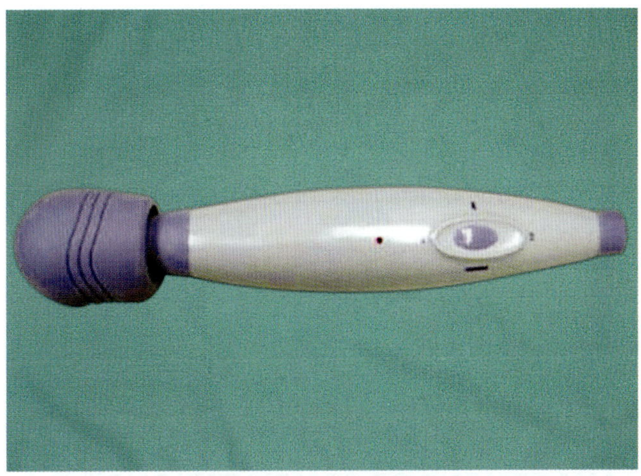

Fig. 9: Vibration anesthesia.

BOX 3: Tips for photography in filler procedures.[17]

- Use a consistent background. For fair-skinned patients, a black background is helpful. For dark-skinned patients, a lighter color like shades of gray or blue can be used
- Use consistent lighting
- Use consistent distance and positioning. Five views recommended are a front view, two oblique views, and two lateral views

BOX 4: Procedure steps.

- Patient assessment
- Medical history
- Consent
- *Photographs:* Pretreatment
- Filler choice
- Injection
- Postprocedure photographs

TABLE 3: Indications and depth of placement.

Indications	*Depth*	*Angle*
Hydration	Deep dermis	<45°
Fine lines and rhytids	Superficial dermis	10–30°
Moderate to deep folds	Mild dermis	30–40°
Deeper folds	Deep dermis and supraperiosteal	45–90°

and folds to be at their maximum. The treatment area is cleaned and disinfected with a suitable antiseptic agent. The appropriate filler is chosen, and usually, the needle prepacked along with the syringe is assembled correctly as per the manufacturer's instructions.

In the anatomical danger zones, a blunt-tipped cannula may be used to inject the product into the subcutaneous plane.

Table 3 gives a quick guide on the indications and depths of placement of fillers. The injection technique is explained in detail in the chapter on general principles of tissue augmentation.

The postoperative instructions are as follows:

- Avoid touching the area for 6 hours.
- Avoid strenuous activity for 6 hours.
- Do not expose to sun/heat/cold till erythema/swelling disappears.
- Sleep with head elevated for one-night following fillers on the face.
- Reduce exaggerated facial movement as much as possible for 3 days.
- Skincare routine to be followed after 24 hours.
- Touch-up treatment can be given after 2–4 weeks, if needed.
- Avoid dental procedures for 3–4 weeks following filler treatment.

The tips for ensuring good results are given in **Box 5**.

TIPS AND TRICKS

Advise patients to avoid nonprescribed anticoagulant agents for about 1 week before treatment.

MANAGEMENT OF COMPLICATIONS[19,20]

Complications of fillers **(Box 6)**, their cause, and management are described in **Table 4**.

ENHANCING PATIENT COMFORT

Products premixed with lidocaine are preferred to deliver filler substances without pain, especially in the lips tear trough, perioral and nasolabial regions.

BOX 5: Tips for good results.[22,23]

- The aim of any cosmetic procedure should be to achieve a successful and satisfactory outcome for both the patient and physician alike
- A good training and experience in the art and science of dermal fillers is necessary to achieve good results. Judicious use of injectable fillers needs knowledge of normal facial anatomy and age-related changes
- A thorough understanding of the filler materials and knowledge of the management of complications is necessary at all times. One must choose the right filler for the correct indication in any given individual. Choosing the right tool for the right job gives a satisfactory outcome[19]
- A proper selection, counseling, assessment, and photographic documentation are necessary to avoid dissatisfied patients. Adopt techniques as appropriate to improve the patient's comfort levels during the procedure. Proper placement of the filler in the correct plane would give the best cosmetic results. Avoid overcorrection at all times, and undercorrection is always a safer and better option. Treat overcorrection judiciously to provide an aesthetically pleasing outcome. Touch-up treatments should usually be offered at 2 or more weeks after the procedure
- Retreatment should usually be encouraged before full aesthetic correction has greatly diminished

BOX 6: Common filler complications and time of onset.[21]

Early (<14 days):

- Ecchymosis
- Edema
- Erythema
- Infection
- Allergic reaction
- Nodules
- Skin necrosis
- Embolism

Late (14 days to 1 year):

- Angioedema
- Hyperpigmentation
- Infection
- Granulomas

Delayed (>1 year):

- Infection
- Biofilm

VASCULAR COMPROMISE

Vascular adverse events, such as necrosis and blindness, should be treated as a medical emergency. All safety protocols to avoid inadvertent injection into the arteries have to be followed strictly.

Avoiding Necrosis

Dermal filler injections can cause necrosis in areas such as the glabella, lips, and nasolabial folds. This occurs due to the inadvertent intravascular injection that causes impediment to the blood flow. Thus, the necrosis is prevented by staying in the safe anatomical plane for that area, injecting in small boluses, and stopping to inject once pallor sets in with the treatment field or adjacent skin.[24]

TABLE 4: Common complications—cause and management.

Complication	*Cause*	*Management*
Anxiety	Anxious personality	• Reassurance • Offer full explanation • Answer all questions and allay anxiety
Pain	Nil anesthesia used	• Use suitable anesthesia
Infection	• Unsterile technique • Pre-existing herpes	• Proper sterile precautions • Antiviral prophylaxis
Biofilms	Dormant infection	• Long-term antibiotics • Excision
Hypersensitivity reactions	Antibody production	• Antihistamines • Intralesional steroids
Immunologic reaction/granuloma **(Figs. 10A and B)**	Allergy to filler substances	• Steroids • Allergy testing preprocedure
Erythema **(Figs. 11A and B)**	Vasodilation	• Photoprotection • Topical tacrolimus • Topical steroids
Acneiform eruption	Occlusion of sweat and sebaceous gland openings	• Firm massaging • Topical astringent lotions
Beading, clumping, and overcorrection **(Fig. 12)**	Too much product deposited	• Firm massaging • Hyaluronidase injection
Necrosis	Intravascular injection	• Firm massaging, nitroglycerine paste, and low molecular heparin
Bluebump **(Figs. 13A and B)**	• Tyndall effect • Superficial placement of filler	• Aspiration of gel • Hyaluronidase injection
Blindness	Embolization of filler into the ophthalmic artery	Early identification and referral to an ophthalmologist

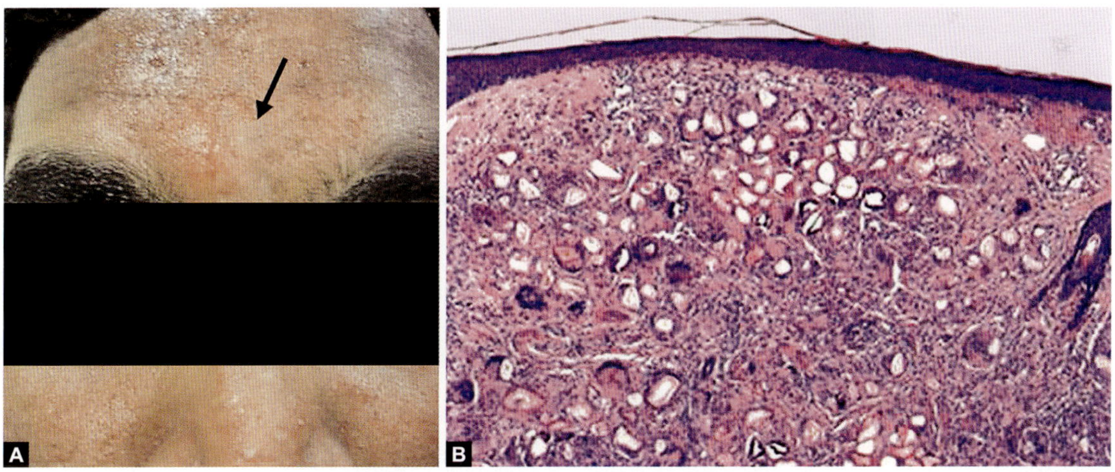

Figs. 10A and B: Immunologic reaction/granuloma.

A new choke vessel spasm concept determines the location and extent of tissue necrosis following inadvertent HA intra-arterial injection.[25]

Blindness

A literature review to identify vision loss for soft-tissue augmentation concluded that autologous fat (47.9%) followed by HA were the most common causes of blindness. The injection sites identified were glabella (38.8%), nasal (25.5%), nasolabial fold (13.3%), and forehead (12.2%). Prevention protocols include an excellent knowledge of anatomy, slow injections in small aliquots under low pressure, and moving the needle tip while injecting. It is recommended to use blunt-tipped cannulae to deposit material in the proper plane of

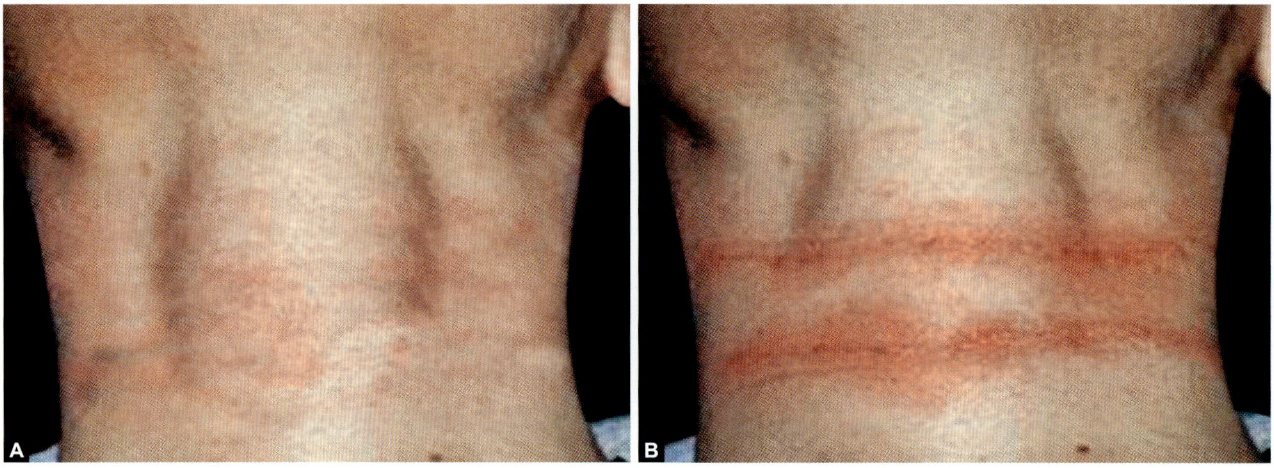

Figs. 11A and B: Erythema: (A) Before; (B) After injection.

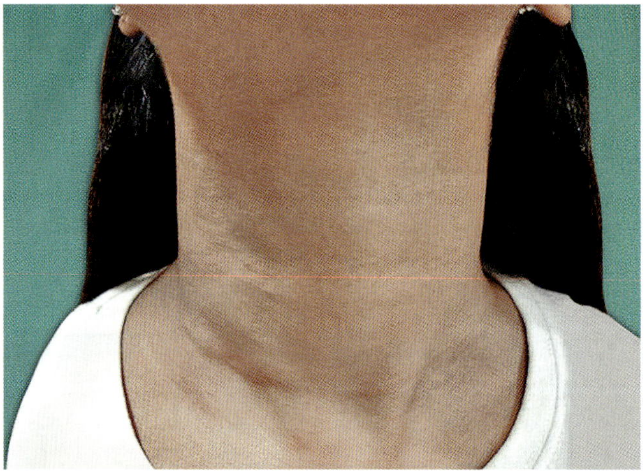

Fig. 12: Beading and clumping.

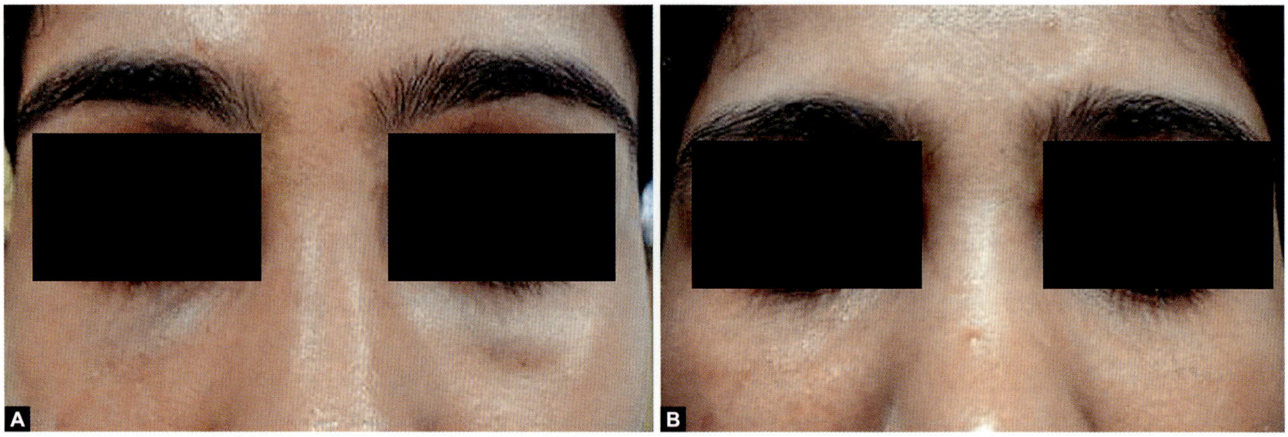

Figs. 13A and B: Tyndall effect: (A) Before treatment; (B) After hyaluronidase injection.

injection. Once blindness sets in, there are fewer chances of reversing the effects. Prompt use of hyaluronidase injections, both extraocular and retrobulbar, is employed or emergency referral to an ophthalmologist is advocated.[26]

LAYERING OF MULTIPLE INJECTANTS

Hyaluronic acid fillers can be used in conjunction with other injectable fillers. Fillers for superficial correction or deeper correction may be layered appropriately in the same session to achieve good results.[27]

TIPS AND TRICKS

Hyaluronic acid fillers may be layered on top of each other or on top of another semipermanent filler.

Current Concepts in the Use of Hyaluronic Acid Fillers in Combination with Lasers, Intense Pulsed Light , and Radiofrequency Devices

Combination therapies are a winning paradigm. The recent trend is to use a multiple-modality approach combining neurotoxins, fillers, threads, and energy-based devices.

A lot of interest is generated regarding the interaction between HA fillers and laser/light treatments in the same individual when treating the same area.

Although the depth of penetration of nonablative laser or superficial ablative laser does not penetrate deep enough to affect any filler material, it is advisable to use the energy-based device first.[28] Similarly, intradermal radiofrequency treatment before HA filler injection may provide synergistic and long-lasting effects. Hence, if a combination approach is performed simultaneously on the same day, it is recommended to start with light/laser treatment or radiofrequency to avoid skin manipulation after HA injection.

The process of cross-linking and other technology platforms in the HA fillers enhances the resistance of HA to heat, mechanical stresses, and enzymatic degradation, thus contributing to its longevity in tissue.

Platelet-rich Plasma and Hyaluronic Acid[29]

Combining platelet-rich plasma and HA injections serves as efficient biostimulation in skin rejuvenation. Both procedures can be combined in the same session or performed sequentially for the best results.

CONCLUSION

There is a surge of interest in soft-tissue augmentation as millennials seek prejuvenation while baby boomers seek rejuvenation. The available treatment options, awareness through social media, and the availability of products and providers have increased over time. The flooding of new HA fillers in the market and new techniques emerging to improve outcomes are a boon to dermatologists practicing aesthetic medicine. The dermatologist's challenge is to have a thorough knowledge of injection anatomy, knowledge of the product, and a proper selection of the right product to suit each patient's requirement.

REFERENCES

1. Klein AW. Skin filling. Dermatol Clin. 2001;19(3):491-508.
2. Klein AW, Elson ML. The history of substances for soft tissue augmentation. Dermatol Surg. 2000;26(12):1096-105.
3. Coleman WP 3rd. Introduction. Dermatol Surg. 2017;43 (Suppl 1):S95.
4. Hanke CW. Filler materials. In: Thiers B, Lang Jr G (Eds). Year Book of Dermatology and Dermatology Surgery. Philadelphia: Mosby; 2004. pp. 1-15.
5. Roenigk HH Jr. Treatment of the aging face. Dermatol Clin. 1995:13(2):245-61.
6. Vedamurthy M; IADVL Dematosurgery Task Force. Standard guidelines for dermal fillers. Indian J Dermatol Venereol Leprol. 2008;74:S23-7.
7. Hamilton TK. Skin augmentation and correction: The new generation of dermal fillers—A dermatologist's experience. Clin Dermatol. 2009;27(3):S13-22.
8. Kablik J, Monheit GD, Yu L, Chang G, Gershkovich J. Comparative physical properties of hyaluronic acid dermal fillers. Dermatol Surg. 2009;35(Suppl 1):1302-129.
9. Monheit GD, Prather CL. Juvéderm: A hyaluronic acid dermal filler. J Drugs Dermatol. 2007;6(11):1091-5.
10. Monheit GD, Coleman KM. Hyaluronic acid fillers. Dermatol Ther. 2006;19(3):141-50.
11. Papakonstantinou E, Roth M, Karakiulakis G. Hyaluronic acid: a key molecule in skin aging. Dermatoendocrinol. 2012;4(3):253-8.
12. Heydenrych I, Kapoor KM, De Boulle K, Goodman G, Swift A, Kumar N, et al. A 10 point plan for avoiding hyaluronic acid dermal filler-related complications during facial aesthetic procedures and algorithm for management. Clin Cosmet Investig Dermatol. 2018;11:603-11.
13. Ferneini EM, Beauvis D, Aronin SI. An overview of infections associated with soft tissue facial fillers: Identification, prevention, and treatment. J Oral Maxillofac Surg. 2017; 75(1):160-66.
14. Matarasso SL, Carruthers JD, Jewell ML. Restylane Consensus Group. Consensus recommendation for soft tissue augmentation with nonanimal stabilised hyaluronic acid (Restylane). Plast Reconst Surg. 2006;117:3S-34S; discussion 35S-43S.
15. Bhatia AC. The clinical image: archiving clinical processes and an entire specialty. Arch Dermatol. 2006;142(1):96-8.
16. Smith KC. Ice anaesthesia for injection of dermal fillers. Dermatol Surg. 2010;36(1):812-4.
17. Van Eijk T, Braun M. A novel method to inject hyaluronic acid: the fern pattern technique. J Drugs Dermatol. 2007;6(8):805-8.
18. De Boulle K. Management of complications after implantation of fillers. J Cosmet Dermatol. 2004;3(1):2-15.
19. Hirsch RJ, Cohen JL, Carruthers JD. Successful management of an unusual presentation of impending necrosis following a

hyaluronic acid injection embolus and a proposed algorithm for management with hyaluronidase. Dermatol Surg. 2007;33(3):357-60.

20. Ashton MW, Taylor GI, Corlett RJ. The role of anastomotic vessels in controlling tissue viability and defining tissue necrosis with special reference to complications following injection of hyaluronic acid fillers. Plast Reconstr Surg. 2018;141(6):818e-30e.
21. Walker L, King M. This month's guideline: visual loss secondary to cosmetic filler injection. Journal Clin Aesthet Dermatol. 2018;11(5):E53-5.
22. Alam M, Gladstone H, Kramer EM, Murphy JP Jr, Nouri K, Neuhaus IM, et al. American Society for Dermatologic Surgery. ASDS guidelines of care: Injectable fillers. Dermatol Surg. 2008;34:S115-48.
23. Urdiales-Gálvez F, Martín-Sánchez S, Maíz-Jiménez M, Castellano-Miralla A, Lionetti-Leone L. Concomitant use of hyaluronic acid and laser in facial rejuvenation. Aesthetic Plast Surg. 2019;43(4):1061-70.
24. Ulusal BG. Platelet-rich plasma and hyaluronic acid—an efficient biostimulation method for face rejuvenation. J Cosmet Dermatol. 2017;16(1):112-9.
25. de Maio M. Myomodulatin with injectable fillers: an update. Aesthetic Plast Surg. 2020:44(4):1317-9.
26. Pinski KS. Soft tissue augmentation for the new millennium. Dermatol Therapy. 2000;13:192-7.
27. Goldman MP. Optimizing the use of fillers for facial rejuvenation. Cosmet Dermatol. 2007;20:14-26.
28. Rohrich RJ, Bartlett EL, Dayan E. Practical approach and safety of hyaluronic acid fillers. Plast Reconstr Surg Glob Open. 2019;7(6):e2172.
29. Carruthers J, Cohen SR, Joseph JH, Narins RS, Rubin M. The science and art of dermal fillers for soft tissue augmentation. J Drugs Dermatol. 2009;8(4):335-50.

CHAPTER 92

Nonhyaluronic Acid Fillers

Jaishree Sharad

KEY MESSAGES

- Nonhyaluronic acid fillers can be biodegradable (calcium hydroxyapatite and polylactic acid) which are semipermanent and nonbiodegradable fillers such as polymethylmethacrylate and polyacrylamide gel which are permanent.
- The safety of permanent fillers is yet to be established.
- Calcium hydroxylapatite is an excellent filler for cheek, chin augmentation, and rhinoplasty as it achieves good volume effect.
- Poly-L-lactic (PLA) acid is useful for human immunodeficiency virus (HIV) lipodystrophy.

INTRODUCTION

Soft-tissue augmentation is an ancient science and dates back to more than 100 years in time, when autologous fat grafts were used to restore facial volume defects.[1] Paraffin was also used for some time, but it caused foreign body reactions frequently, hence was stopped. Liquid silicone as filler was used since 1950 until 1982, when the Food and Drug Administration (FDA) temporarily banned its use. Injectable bovine collagen became available after the 1980. Subsequently, the market was flooded with fillers such as the semipermanent hyaluronic acid (HA) derivatives, calcium hydroxylapatite (CaHA), and poly-L-lactic acid (PLA). Some longer lasting, called "permanent fillers" such as polymethylmethacrylate (PMMA) microspheres which were highly purified forms of liquid silicone and hydrogel polymers were also launched.[2]

While the search for an ideal filler continues, a number of new materials have been introduced, each with its own advantages and disadvantages.[3-7] The HA fillers have been dealt with in earlier chapter and this chapter deals with non-HA fillers.

CLASSIFICATION

The non-HA fillers can be semipermanent (with longevity between 1 and 2 years) and permanent (longevity more than 2 years).

They can also be classified as:

- *Biodegradable fillers:*
  - Polylactic acid (New-fill—Sculptra)
  - CaHA gel (Radiesse®)
- *Nonbiodegradable fillers:*
  - PMMA (Artecoll, ArteFill, Bellafill)
  - Polyacrylamide gel [PAAG (Aquamid, Amazingel)]

SEMIPERMANENT FILLERS

Calcium Hydroxylapatite

Introduction

Calcium hydroxylapatite, represented by the formula $Ca_5(PO4)_3(OH)$, is a compound naturally found in human bone and teeth and has been used as implant or coating material in dentistry and other therapeutic areas for more than 20 years.[2] Available as Radiesse®, its off-label use in facial aesthetics has been reported since 2002, though it got the United States (US) FDA approval in 2006.

Mechanism of Action

Radiesse® is composed of a suspension of 30% CaHA microspheres (size 25–45 microns) in a 70% gel consisting of 1.3% sodium carboxy methylcellulose, 6.4% glycerin, and 36.6% sterile water for injection. CaHA promotes neocollagenesis. Preclinical studies demonstrate that the gel is phagocytosed over a period of 4 weeks, leaving only the microspheres. These CaHA microspheres are substituted with natural collagen from attracted histiocytes and fibroblasts which act as a scaffold that promotes tissue ingrowth. Fibroblasts lay down a collagenous extracellular matrix and as the matrix is deposited, the implant becomes integrated into the surrounding soft tissue.[8] The spherical CaHA particles are gradually broken down and degraded by way of normal metabolic processes and eliminated as calcium and phosphate ions through the kidney. The proliferation of collagen along with the slow breakdown of the CaHA is understood to account for the long-lasting effect of the filler.[9,10]

Safety and Efficacy

Synthetic CaHA has the same biocompatibility profile as of the natural compound and is immunologically inert; hence, skin testing is not required. It is biodegradable. When CaHA is injected directly into bone, osteogenesis may occur. However, when deposited in the deep dermis or subcutaneous border, no osteoblastic activity occurs. It shows no evidence of migration, calcification, or ossification. Though it is visible on computed tomography (CT), its appearance is distinct from the surrounding bony structures, does not obscure underlying structures, and does not interfere with normal analysis.[11]

Indications[2]

- *US FDA-approved indications*:
  - Nasolabial folds (NLFs) **(Figs. 1 and 2)**
  - Correction of human immunodeficiency virus (HIV)-associated facial lipoatrophy
- *Off-label facial uses also include*:
  - Correction of marionette lines and oral commissures
  - Prejowl sulcus[12]
  - Cheek-volume loss[13]
  - Dorsal nasal deformities[14]
  - Soft-tissue augmentation of aging hands[15,16]
  - Acne scars
  - Wrinkling of the décolletage
  - Injecting in the infraorbital hollows is usually not recommended due to the visibility of the product. However, there have been reports of CaHA injected in this area deep on the periosteum with no side effects.[17]

Contraindications

Calcium hydroxylapatite is not appropriate for injecting in the lips and for the nasojugal groove. The carrier methylcellulose dissipates soon after injection and leaves the microspheres clumped, appearing as white, hard calcium nodules.[18] Other contraindications as discussed in chapter on HA fillers are also applicable.

Storage

Calcium hydroxylapatite is available in 1.3 and 0.3 mL prefilled syringes. It requires no special handling and it can be stored at room temperature (15–32°C) for up to 2 years.

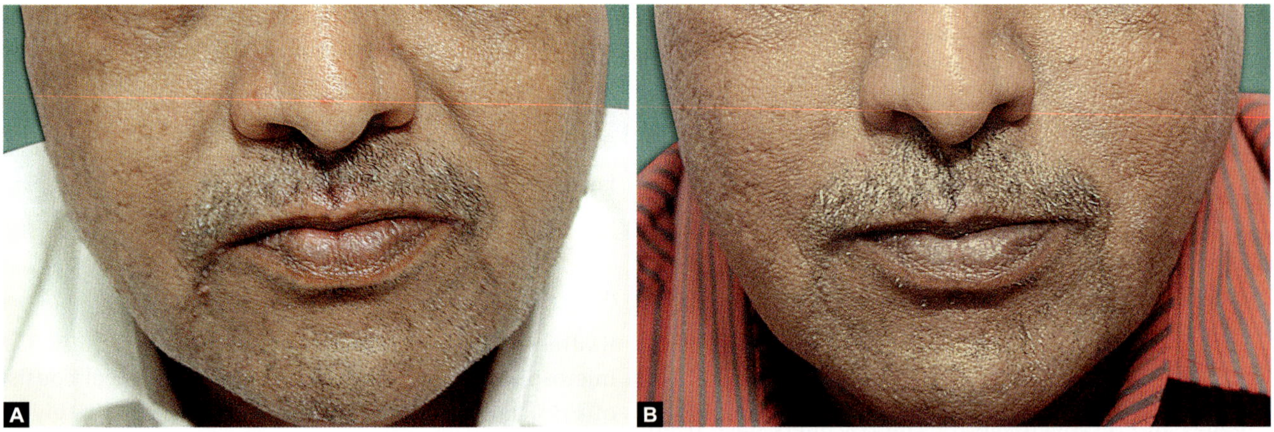

Figs. 1A and B: (A) Nasolabial fold before Radiesse® (calcium hydroxylapatite); (B) Nasolabial fold after Radiesse® (calcium hydroxylapatite).

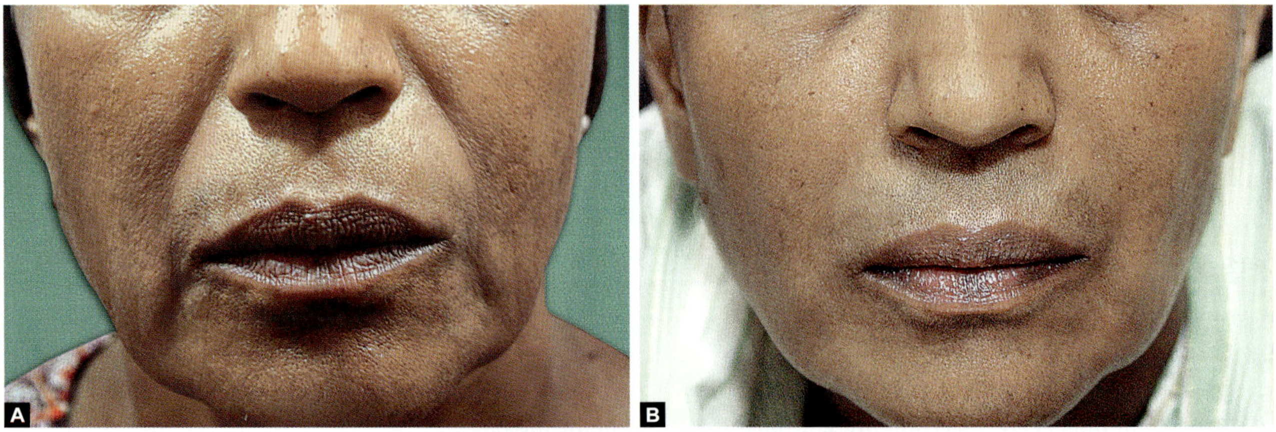

Figs. 2A and B: (A) Nasolabial and Marionette before Radiesse® filler (calcium hydroxylapatite); (B) Nasolabial and Marionette after Radiesse® filler (calcium hydroxylapatite).

Anesthesia

2% xylocaine can be added to CaHA syringes safely without harmful changes in the physical properties of the original soft-tissue filler.[19] Usually, 0.2–0.3 cc of lidocaine is added to 1.3 cc of CaHA using a "Luer lock" connector. A minimum of 10 mixing passes are required to get a uniform mixture.

Technique

The material is provided in sterile syringes and is a milky white suspension. Because it is viscous, CaHA should be injected with a 25- or 26-gauge needle to obtain a regular flow with low resistance.[2,20] CaHA should be injected in small amounts in a retrograde fashion into the immediate subcutaneous plane or supraperiosteal plane using a linear retrograde tunneling technique. Cross-hatched linear threading technique may also be employed. Overcorrection should be avoided. The nondominant index finger should be used to guide the needle and the thumb and forefinger used to mold the product and to remove any contour irregularities. CaHA should be injected very slowly in long, linear microthreads of approximately 0.05 mL per pass. It is important to massage the product immediately after injection to ensure adequate dispersion and to prevent clumping of the CaHA. In case of clumping, the nodule needs to be punctured with #11 blade or 16-gauge needle and contents extruded out. Alternatively, a 2 or 3 mm punch may be used to remove the product. The use of intralesional saline injection followed by massage to mechanically break up the product has been described.[21]

In a randomized study of 205 patients receiving either CaHA or HA fillers for correction of NLFs, CaHA was more effective and longer lasting and had higher patient satisfaction scores.[22] Other studies have confirmed the durability and safety of CaHA as compared with other injectable fillers for correction of the NLFs.[22,23] A 47-month study of 113 patients injected with CaHA filler confirmed a favorable safety profile with low incidence of adverse events and high patient satisfaction. 90% of patients reported very good or excellent results following treatment of multiple facial areas including NLFs, perioral lines, cheeks, acne scars, tear trough depressions, and prejowl sulci.[24]

Post-treatment Care

Apply ice over the injection site to reduce and limit edema and bruising. Patient should follow-up in 8 weeks for a touch-up.

Side Effects

Side effects are transient in the form of erythema, edema, temporary pain, and ecchymoses.[25] A nongranulomatous nodule of lip was reported in one study.[26] Exercise extreme caution when injecting into the subdermal plane around the superior NLF, where the angular artery and its branches are present. Occlusion of this vessel can occur by way of external compression from CaHA or by injection of CaHA directly into the lumen of the vessel; hence, causing embolic ischemia and tissue necrosis of the nasal alar region, i.e., along the distribution of the angular arteries or its branches.

Advantages

- CaHA has high viscosity and elasticity (G prime or G') due to which large areas can be augmented or lifted with a small amount of product.
- It is easy to administer.
- It is biocompatible.
- It is immunologically inert.
- It is long lasting (lasts between 1–3 years)[27]
- It gives a smooth and natural look.[10,28]
- It is easy to store and does not need refrigeration.
- It has a shelf life of 2 years.
- It is available as a ready-to-use, prefilled syringe which does not need reconstitution.

Disadvantages

- Fine wrinkle correction or very superficial injection can result in visible nodules.
- The material may be palpable for up to 2 weeks and should not be confused with nodule formation.

Poly-L-lactic Acid

Introduction

Poly-L-lactic acid is a synthetic polymer from the alpha-hydroxy acid family that is similar to absorbable suture material.[29] It is biodegradable, biocompatible, and resorbable. PLA was approved by the FDA in 2004 for the treatment of HIV-related facial lipoatrophy. PLA (Sculptra) is available as a carton containing two clear glass vials of a sterile freeze-dried preparation composed of 24.5% sodium carboxymethylcellulose (an emulsifying agent), 34.7% nonpyrogenic mannitol (provides osmosity), and 40.8% PLA microparticles.[30]

Mechanism of Action

Immediately and temporarily upon injection, there may be an augmentation response due to tissue edema and fluid from reconstitution. In the long run, PLA stimulates foreign body reaction. PLLA particles are 40–60 μm and impede phagocytosis and diffusion. The microparticles of PLA are surrounded in a capsule of connective tissue, consisting of connective tissue cells and inflammatory cells, such as macrophages, lymphocytes, mast cells, and foreign body giant cells. Volume restoration is a result of a granulomatous inflammation that stimulates neocollagenesis in the deep dermis or subcutaneous tissue.[31]

Histologically, a capsule of mast cells, macrophages, lymphocytes, foreign-body giant cells, and vascular structures are seen surrounding the PLLA particles a month after implantation. The particles are degraded into naturally occurring lactic acid, carbon dioxide, and water, with subsequent deposition of type I collagen. By 18 months, there is no evidence of granulomatous inflammation but evidence of new collagen deposition that is sustained.[21].

Safety and Efficacy

The efficacy of injectable PLA is well established. Although it is well tolerated and no long-term side effects have been reported, its safety beyond 2 years has not been investigated. No skin test is required.

Indications[20,32]

- HIV-related facial lipoatrophy[33]
- Correction of deep NLFs[34]
- Cheek augmentation
- Mid- and lower-facial volume loss
- Jawline laxity[35]
- Temples
- Volume loss in inframalar region
- Chin augmentation
- Prejowl sulcus
- Marionette lines
- Facial asymmetry
- Atrophic scars[36,37]
- Chest wall deformity after breast reconstruction[38]
- Volumization of dorsum of the hands[39,40]

Contraindications

Specific contraindication includes lips, planes of orbicularis oris, and oculi.

Pretreatment Patient Education

Poly-L-lactic acid is usually administered in three or more sessions spread over a period of 3 months or more. Because of the substantial amount of the water in the suspension, patients will leave the office looking well filled; however, they should be made aware that the immediate improvement seen will subside in 2–4 days and then the collagen growth will start, the effect of which will be seen at 6–8 weeks. Best results will be visible only after 4–6 months. Once volumization has been achieved, results can be expected to last for 2–3 years or sometimes longer.[34,41,42]

Storage

The material is stored at room temperature prior to and following reconstitution. The freeze-dried product has a shelf life of 2 years.

Reconstitution[43]

Each vial containing 350 μg of PLA is diluted in 3–5 mL of sterile water. The suspension is allowed to stand undisturbed for 2 hours at room temperature to facilitate reconstitution. Just prior to injection, an additional 1–2 mL plain lignocaine 2% is added to the bottle. The suspension is drawn into a 3 mL syringe with an 18-gauge needle which is then changed to a 25-gauge, 1.5 inch needle for injection.

New treatment protocols involve using higher dilution volumes (8–12 mL total; 5–10 mL of sterile water plus 1–2 mL of 1% lidocaine with or without epinephrine) and earlier reconstitution (a minimum of 24–72 hours before injection). This improves product hydration and reduces the chances of nodule formation. The addition of lidocaine in the injection mixture limits pain after a small amount has been delivered to the treatment area.[21]

Pretreatment Preparation[30]

The area is cleansed and then the areas of concavity are outlined with a wax-based marking pencil (a white eyeliner pencil also can be used). While treating the cheeks, the outlined area should not extend above the infraorbital margin. The area of injection should not extend too far inferiorly in order to avoid accentuation of jowl region in some patients. Additional dots, typically six to eight per side, are marked within the confines of the outline to denote injection sites for both anesthesia and PLA.

Anesthesia[44]

One percent xylocaine with 1:100,000 epinephrine is injected in the area marked; 0.5 mL is injected into the dermis and 0.5 mL into the subcutis. This injection is repeated into each dot for a total of 6 mL. This will result in vasoconstriction and reduce bruising and also prolong the effect of anesthesia. There may be a little swelling and distortion of facial topography; however, since the area to be treated has been marked and placement of filler is not affected.

Injection Technique[45]

Just before injecting, the material is shaken vigorously to obtain a uniform translucent suspension. The needle is inserted repeatedly into the points marked and advanced in the supraperiosteal plane in areas such as temples, piriform aperture, zygoma, and mandible. In the midface/cheek, preauricular, NLFs, marionette lines, mental crease, the product is placed evenly with fan-like sweeps in the subcutaneous region. The material is injected evenly while the needle is withdrawn. Each thread should be equally dispersed and limited to small aliquots.

Fanning helps to reduce discomfort and bleeding as there are fewer puncture sites.

After the injection, it is important for the injector to deeply palpate and massage the treated areas to ensure an even distribution of product and prevent formation of nodules. Injecting into the mid-to-superficial dermis can result in dermal nodules. Focal blanching and outpouching of skin may be a marker that the injection is too superficial. In such a case, firm focal massage should be given at least for 10 minutes until the out pouching disappears.[44] It is essential not to overcorrect because the injection is followed by a delayed fibroblastic reaction. Moreover, overcorrection increases the risk of a delayed formation of bumps.

Use a 25-gauge sharp needle (1–1.5 inches) or a 22- or 25-gauge, blunt-tipped cannula (1.5–2 inches) on a 3 mL syringe to inject PLLA. The product should be adequately mixed 24–72 hours before usage. Once drawn into syringes, it should be shaken consistently to prevent clogging and ensure homogenous dispersion of product. Clogging occurs due to product settling while keeping the syringe on a stand for a long time. It could be a good practice to leave 0.5 cc of air in each syringe to allow mixing of the product. It is best to avoid product settling as it can lead to uneven application and contributes to nodule formation, so some advocate warming the solution or drawing from the vial and injecting one syringe at a time. If particulate separation is seen, pull the plunger back and rock the syringe back and forth to allow easier mixing and then force the material back out through the needle or cannula to ensure it is clear before injecting. It is better to have multiple sessions with lower injection volumes than higher volumes in fewer sessions. No more than two vials are used per visit every 4–8 weeks until a desired effect is seen.[21]

Deep product placement in the subcutaneous and periosteal planes and vigilant avoidance of intramuscular injections (i.e., lip, perioral, and periocular) has reduced the development of visible papules and nodules as well. Other helpful techniques include limiting volume injected per session, aggressive massage by the patient after treatment (the "5/5/5" rule: 5 minutes, 5 times a day, for 5 days), and waiting 4–8 weeks between injections sessions.[46-48]

Post-treatment Instructions

Applying ice packs to the injection sites every 30 minutes over the next 24 hours will greatly reduce the risk of bruising. The area should also be massaged for a week postinjection. Patients should be told that the immediate filling effect is due to tissue edema and mechanical volume and will disappear within 3–4 days. The actual result is seen only 12–15 weeks later.

Side Effects

Swelling, erythema, bruising, and hematoma may occur at the site of injection. If injected too superficially, there may be papules seen weeks after the injection. If the dilution is not proper or if the area is overcorrected, there may be reactionary subcutaneous nodule formation.[49] Injection of sterile water or subcision may be used for early onset lesions. These usually disappear in a few weeks with daily massage. Resistant nodules can be treated with intralesional steroid injections. Hypersensitivity reaction my occur at the site of injection. Thorough removal of makeup and proper prepping of skin should be ensured to reduce the chances of introduction of foreign particles. Prepping also reduces the risk of postprocedural infections. Necrosis is the most concerning complication. It results due to inadvertent product introduction into a vessel, or vascular compression. A thorough knowledge of facial anatomy is essential on the injector's part. Aspiration must always be done before injecting the product to avoid this complication.[50]

Advantages

- Ideal for volume loss
- Does not need skin testing
- Long lasting (18–24 months)

Disadvantages

- Results are not seen immediately and may take up to 8 weeks to become evident.
- Multiple treatment sessions may be required to achieve optimum results.
- The injection has to be reconstituted and allowed to stand for a minimum of 2 hours before injecting.
- Clogging of the needle is a common problem. Needle needs to be changed frequently.

PERMANENT FILLERS

Polymethylmethacrylate

Polymethylmethacrylate is a polymeric microsphere-based permanent soft-tissue filler.

Available as Bellafill, (previously known as Artefill), it is the only FDA-approved permanent filling agent and the only one that contains bovine collagen. It represents a third-generation product that contains fewer nanoparticles (<20 microns), which were thought to be associated with granulomatous reactions observed with previous generations of PMMA fillers (such as Arteplast and Artecoll).[2] Artefill® was approved by the FDA in 2006 for the correction of NLFs.

This dermal filler is a "mixed implant" made of PMMA microspheres measuring from 30 to 42 μm of diameter, suspended in a 3.5% partially denatured bovine collagen solution.[20]

The exact composition is 20% implant volume of nonbiodegradable PMMA microspheres, 80% implant volume of purified bovine collagen gel (3.5%), lidocaine hydrochloride (0.3%), and water for injection (92.6%).[21]

Mechanism of Action[51]

Polymethylmethacrylate appears to stimulate the patient's own collagen production, which then permanently envelopes the PMMA microspheres.[52] A key advantage of the collagen carrier appears to be its viscosity which keeps the microspheres evenly distributed and facilitates tissue ingrowth into the interstices. The residual, inert PMMA acts as a scaffold to engender permanent autologous collagen replacement of the injected bovine collagen carrier.[45] A sustained tissue augmentation effect is achieved only with a nonabsorbable synthetic component in the filler.[53,54] The 30–50 μm diameter of PMMA microspheres seem to be the ideal size for dermal injections as they are large enough to escape phagocytosis yet small enough to be smoothly delivered through a fine 26- or 30-gauge needle.[3] Two key features which prevent dissipation of PMMA into the surrounding network of collagen fibers of the deep dermal and subdermal layers following the injection are:

1. The bovine collagen carrier acts as a glue which embeds the microspheres and prevents clumping. It allows new tissue ingrowth. Thus, the implant becomes part of the patient's own soft tissue, maintaining its integrity over years and decades.
2. The 30–50 μm size of the microsphere prevents phagocytosis and also limits the PMMA particles from entering the interstices of deep dermal fibers, which have a diameter of 10–15 μm where muscle action might disperse them.[55]

The collagen carrier is absorbed within 1 month after injection and is completely replaced by the patient's own connective tissue over a period of 3 months. Each mL of Bellafill contains approximately six million microspheres and histological studies have shown that over a long term, the wrinkle-corrected tissue is composed of 80% of the patient's own connective tissue and 20% microspheres.

Storage

Polymethylmethacrylate should be stored in the refrigerator. However, it should not be frozen.

Indications

- NLFs[56]
- Glabellar frown lines
- Perioral lines
- Marionette lines
- Atrophic acne scars[57]

Contraindications

- Patients who have a positive result to the PMMA skin test
- Patients with history of anaphylaxis or multiple allergies or allergies to bovine products
- PMMA should not be used for lip augmentation.

Technique[2]

Injectable PMMA is supplied as 0.8 mL syringes with 26-gauge, 5/8 inch needles. It should be placed into the dermal-subcutaneous junction using the tunneling or linear threading technique with a 26-gauge needle. Multiple treatment sessions with small aliquots (0.1–0.5 mL per site) of material injected with a 26- or 27-gauge needle into the desired treatment areas using a microdroplet technique will help to optimize volume and prevent nodule formation.

Patients should be evaluated 4–6 weeks after the injection to assess the need for further treatments. Optimal correction usually requires two to three treatments. This is done about 2–3 months after the first implant.

Overcorrection is not recommended. It is preferable to inject deeper than be superficial as the risk of wasted material is less problematic than superficial injection, which can cause permanent skin surface texture or color impairment. Bovine collagen allergy testing is required to minimize the risk of hypersensitivity reactions, especially in patients who are being treated with a bovine collagen product for the first time. An intradermal collagen test injection in the volar aspect of forearm 4 weeks prior to the planned Bellafill implantation should be performed as standard procedure.

It is best to avoid the use of PMMA in areas which are highly mobile such as the lips/perioral or ocular areas, as product clumping can lead to irregularities and nodule formation.[58,59]

Longevity

Polymethylmethacrylate is a permanent filler as established by a large study conducted by the FDA at 8 centers in the US.[51]

Side Effects

Bruising and edema are transient which disappear in 48 hours. Granulomas are rare and treated with intralesional steroid injections or excision.[57]

Nodules may occur if injected into areas such as lips or in case of inadequate massage.

Superficial placement is associated with long-lasting pruritus, redness, and hypertrophic scarring in association with delayed-onset inflammatory nodules or hypersensitivity reactions. Hypertrophic scarring can sometimes be softened by topical or injectable corticosteroids, topical silicone, topical or injectable 5-FU, topical imiquimod, cryotherapy, or various laser technologies such as pulsed dye, potassium titanyl phosphate (KTP), and/or fractional ablative or nonablative laser or fractional radiofrequency; however, results can be permanent and emotionally devastating to both the physician and patient.[21]

Advantages

Bellafill has a dual action of immediate wrinkle correction from collagen lasting about 1–3 months and permanent deep fold ablation from PMMA lasting for more than 5 years.[60]

Disadvantages[60]

- Bellafill contains bovine collagen. Hence, skin testing is necessary.
- Due to its high viscosity, the material is difficult to inject and more pressure is required to inject.
- It should not be given for lip augmentation or superficial wrinkle correction as it may lead to lumps and nodules.
- It is difficult to foretell the long-term appearance of the patient since the skin changes with age and the permanent filler may look displaced.

Polyacrylamide Gel

Polyacrylamide gel represents a newer generation of soft-tissue fillers and is available as Aquamid® gel. It contains 2.5% PAAG and a very high concentration of water (97.5%). It is homogenous, perfectly stable, and nonbiodegradable. It has optimal viscosity and elasticity. It is a biocompatible, non-reabsorbable hydrogel.[20] It had been used in the former Soviet Union for more than 15 years and was authorized for commercial use in Europe only since March 2001 as a new medical product (CE mark 0543) with no guarantee that the product does not have side effects. It is not yet approved by the US FDA.

Indications

- Lip augmentation
- NLFs[61]
- Facial lipoatrophy[62]
- Nonsurgical rhinoplasty[63]

Injection Technique

Because infections have been reported as a side effect with this filler, antisepsis must be scrupulous and on a 5 cm radius around the injection site. Aquamid is available in a 1 mL syringe. It should be injected subcutaneously, with a 27-gauge needle. Injection is done using the fine multiline retrograde technique. The plasticity of PAAG is similar to that of silicon, but PAAG is hydrophilic and has a tendency to absorb water from the surrounding tissue.[6]

Adverse Effects

- Transient bruises, swelling, redness, pain, or itching[64]
- Infection
- Granulomas may be seen even after a year.[65,66]
- Rarely, bony erosion and facial ulcer[67-69]

Advantages

Polyacrylamide gel is biocompatible, nonabsorbable, and long lasting.[70]

Disadvantages[70]

- Local or regional anesthesia is necessary.
- Chances of prolonged swelling, edema, granulomas, and hematomas are not uncommon.
- There is not much data on its safety profile.

CONCLUSION

The use of dermal fillers has advanced significantly from its beginning when fat graft was used in the early 20th century till now when the full array of semipermanent and permanent fillers are available. The clinical persistence of an injectable material and its effect on skin atrophy and wrinkles depends partly on the amount, depth, and shape of the implant. The carrier substance, whether fast or slowly resorbable, may play an important role in persistence as well. Host defense mechanisms react differently to the various filler materials. One should understand the basic property of each filler substance before deciding on the injection. Temporary fillers may be used as a trial or prelude to a permanent or semipermanent filler. This will give the patient an idea of what can be accomplished and whether it is up to their expectations. The side effects and disadvantages of permanent fillers must be explained to the patient and written consent should be taken as excision may be the only way to remove a permanent filler if required later.

The tips for nonhyaluronic acid fillers are mentioned below.

TIPS

Calcium hydroxylapatite:
- It is an excellent filler for cheek, chin augmentation, and rhinoplasty as it achieves good volume effect
- Overcorrection should be avoided
- At the end of a session, feel for nodules and gently massage till they are no longer palpable

Poly-L-lactic acid:
- Shake vigorously before injecting to form a uniform suspension and prevent needle blockage
- Inject into subcutaneous tissue and avoid being superficial in order to prevent lumps from forming
- Massage for 5–10 minutes posttreatment

Polymethylmethacrylate (PMMA):
- Avoid overcorrection or superficial injection. PMMA microspheres are nonabsorbable. Hence, the implantation is permanent and cannot be reversed without excision

Polyacrylamide gel (PAAG):
- Do not inject PAAG if you are a first timer

REFERENCES

1. Klein AW, Elson ML. The history of substances for soft tissue augmentation. Dermatol Surg. 2000;26:1096-105.
2. Jones DH. Semipermanent and Permanent Injectable fillers. Dermatol Clin. 2009;4:433-44.
3. Lemperle G, Morhenn V, Charrier U. Human histology and persistence of various injectable filler substances for soft tissue augmentation. Aesthetic Plast Surg. 2003;27:354.

4. Kablik J, Monheit GD, Yu L, Chang G, Gershkovich J. Comparative physical properties of hyaluronic acid dermal fillers. Dermatol Surg. 2009;35(Suppl 1):302-12.
5. Gold MH. Soft Tissue Augmentation in Dermatology-2009 Update. J Cutan Aesthet Surg. 2010;3:2-10.
6. Von Buelow S, von Heimburg D, Pallua N. Efficacy and safety of polyacrylamide hydrogel for facial soft-tissue augmentation. Plast Reconstr Surg. 2005;116:1137-46.
7. Alster TS, West TB. Human-derived and new synthetic injectable materials for soft-tissue augmentation: Current status and role in cosmetic surgery. Plast Reconstr Surg. 2000;105:2515-25.
8. Coleman KM, Voigts R, DeVore DP, Termin P, Coleman WP 3rd. Neocollagenesis after injection of calcium hydroxylapatite composition in a canine model. Dermatol Surg. 2008;34:S53-5.
9. Berlin AL, Hussain M, Goldberg DJ. Calcium hydroxylapatite filler for facial rejuvenation: a histologic and immunohistochemical analysis. Dermatol Surg. 2008;34:S64-7.
10. Marmur ES, Phelps R, Goldberg DJ. Clinical, histologic and electron microscopic findings after injection of a calcium hydroxylapatite filler. J Cosmet Laser Ther. 2004;6:223-6.
11. Carruthers A, Liebeskind M, Carruthers J, Forster BB. Radiographic and computed tomographic studies of calcium hydroxylapatite for treatment of HIV-associated facial lipoatrophy and correction of nasolabial folds. Dermatol Surg. 2008;34:S78-84.
12. Felderman L. Radiesse for facial rejuvenation. Cosmet Dermatol. 2005;18:823-6.
13. Busso M. Cheek augmentation and rejuvenation using injectable calcium hydroxylapatite (Radiesses). Cosmet Dermatol. 2006;19:583-91.
14. Stupak HD, Moulthrop TH, Wheatley P, Tauman AV, Johnson CM Jr. Calcium hydroxylapatite gel (Radiesse) injection for the correction of postrhinoplasty contour deficiencies and asymmetries. Arch Facial Plast Surg. 2007;9:130-6.
15. Bank DE. A novel approach to treatment of the aging hand with Radiesse. J Drugs Dermatol. 2009;8:1122-6.
16. Marmur ES, Al Quran H, De Sa Earp AP, Yoo JY. A Five-Patient Satisfaction Pilot Study of Calcium Hydroxylapatite Injection for Treatment of Aging Hands. Dermatol Surg. 2009;35:1978-84.
17. Hevia O. Retrospective Review of Calcium Hydroxylapatite for Correction of Volume Loss in the Infraorbital Region. Dermatol Surg. 2009;35:1487-94.
18. Zide BM. Radiance: Short-term experience. Aesthet Surg J. 2003;23:495-9.
19. Busso M, Voigts R. An investigation of changes in physical properties of injectable calcium hydroxylapatite in a carrier gel when mixed with lidocaine and with lidocaine/epinephrine. Dermatol Surg. 2008;34:S16-23.
20. Thioly-Bensoussan D. Non-hyaluronic acid fillers. Clin Dermatol. 2008;26:160-76.
21. Emer JJ, Waldorf H. Nonhyaluronic Acid Fillers. In: Sharad J, Vedamurthy M (Eds). Aesthetic Dermatology: Current Perspectives. New Delhi: Jaypee Brothers Medical Publishers (P) Ltd.; 2018. pp. 240-55.
22. Moers-Carpi M, Vogt S, Santos BM, Planas J, Vallve SR, Howell DJ. A multicenter, randomized trial comparing calcium hydroxylapatite to two hyaluronic acids for treatment of nasolabial folds. Dermatol Surg. 2007;33 (Suppl 2):S144-51.
23. Bass LS, Smith S, Busso M, McClaren M. Calcium hydroxylapatite (Radiesse) for treatment of nasolabial folds: long-term safety and efficacy results. Aesthet Surg J. 2010;30(2):235-8.
24. Sadick NS, Katz BE, Roy D. A multicenter, 47-month study of safety and efficacy of calcium hydroxylapatite for soft tissue augmentation of nasolabial folds and other areas of the face. Dermatol Surg. 2007;33(Suppl 2):S122-6; discussion S126-7.
25. Busso M, Applebaum D. Hand augmentation with Radiesse (calcium hydroxylapatite). Dermatol Ther. 2007;20:385-7.
26. Smith S, Busso M, McClaren M, Bass LS. A randomized, bilateral, prospective comparison of calcium hydroxylapatite microspheres versus human-based collagen for the correction of nasolabial folds. Dermatol Surg. 2007;33:S112-21.
27. Carruthers A, Carruthers J. Evaluation of injectable calcium hydroxylapatite for the treatment of facial lipoatrophy associated with human immunodeficiency virus. Dermatol Surg. 2008;34(11):1486-99.
28. Godin MS, Majmundar MV, Chrzanowski DS, Dodson KM. Use of Radiesse in combination with restylane for facial augmentation. Arch Facial Plast Surg. 2006;8:92-7.
29. Kates LC, Fitzgerald R. Poly-L-lactic acid injection for HIV-associated facial lipoatrophy: treatment principals, case-studies and literature review. Aesthet Surg J. 2008;28:397-403.
30. Leonard AL, Hanke CW. A protocol for facial volume restoration with poly-L-lactic acid. J Drugs Dermatol. 2006;5:872-7.
31. Alam M, Gladstone H, Kramer EM, Murphy JP Jr, Nouri K, Neuhaus IM, et al. ASDS guidelines of care: injectable fillers. Dermatol Surg. 2008;34:S115-48.
32. Rotunda AM, Narins RS. Poly-L-lactic acid: a new dimension in soft tissue augmentation. Dermatol Ther. 2006;19:151-8.
33. Levy RM, Redbord KP, Hanke CW. Treatment of HIV lipoatrophy and lipoatrophy of aging with poly-L-lactic acid: a prospective 3-year follow-up study. J Am Acad Dermatol. 2008;59:923-33.
34. Salles AG, Lotierzo PH, Gimenez R, Camargo CP, Ferreira MC. Evaluation of the poly-L-lactic acid implant for treatment of the nasolabial fold: 3-year follow-up evaluation. Aesthetic Plast Surg. 2008;32:753-6.
35. Vleggaar D. Facial volumetric correction with injectable poly-L-lactic acid. Dermatol Surg. 2005;31:1511-7.
36. Beer K. A single-center open label study on the use of poly-L-lactic acid for the treatment of moderate-to-severe scarring from acne or varicella. Dermatol Surg. 2007;33:S159-67.
37. Sadove R. Injectable poly-L-lactic acid: a novel sculpting agent for the treatment of dermal fat atrophy after severe acne. Aesthetic Plast Surg. 2009;33:113-6.
38. Schulman MR, Lipper J, Skolnik RA. Correction of chest wall deformity after implant based breast reconstruction using poly-L-lactic acid (Sculptra). Breast J. 2008;14:92-6.
39. Burgess CM. Treatment of facial asymmetry with poly-L lactic acid: a case study. Aesthetic Plast Surg. 2008;32:552-4.
40. Engelhard P, Humble G, Mest D. Safety of Sculptra: a review of clinical trial data. J Cosmet Laser Ther. 2005;7:201-5.
41. Mest DR, Humble GM. Duration of correction for human immunodeficiency virus-associated lipoatrophy after retreatment with injectable poly-L-lactic acid. Aesthetic Plast Surg. 2009;33:654-6.
42. Keni SP. Sculptra (injectable poly-L-lactic acid). Facial Plast Surg Clin North Am. 2007;15:91-7.
43. Butterwick K, Lowe NJ. Injectable poly-L-lactic acid for cosmetic enhancement: learning from the European experience. J Am Acad Dermatol. 2009;61:281-93.

44. Lacombe V. Sculptra: a stimulatory filler. Facial Plast Surg. 2009;25:95-9.
45. Cohen SR, Holmes RE. Artecoll: a long-lasting injectable wrinkle filler material: report of a controlled, randomized, multicenter clinical trial of 251 subjects. Plast Reconstr Surg. 2004;114:964-76.
46. Lam SM, Azizzadeh B, Graivier M. Injectable poly-L-lactic acid (Sculptra): technical considerations in soft-tissue contouring. Plast Reconstr Surg. 2006;118(3 Suppl):55S-63S.
47. Woerle B, Hanke CW, Sattler G. Poly-L-lactic acid: a temporary filler for soft tissue augmentation. J Drugs Dermatol. 2004;3(4):385-9.
48. Narins RS. Minimizing adverse events associated with poly-L-lactic acid injection. Dermatol Surg. 2008;34(Suppl 1):S100-4.
49. Hilinski JM, Cohen SR. Soft tissue augmentation with Arte Fill. Facial Plast Surg. 2009;25:114-9.
50. Sickles CK, Nassereddin A, Gross GP (2022) 'Poly-L-Lactic Acid', in StatPearls. Treasure Island (FL): StatPearls. Available at: https://www.ncbi.nlm.nih.gov/books/NKB507871/ (Accessed: 19 March 2024)
51. Nicolau PJ. Long lasting and permanent fillers: biomaterial influence over host tissue response. Plast Reconstr Surg. 2007;119:2271-86.
52. Smith KC, Melnychuk M. Five percent lidocain cream applied simultaneously to the skin and mucosa of the lips creates excellent anesthesia for filler injections. Dermatol Surg. 2005;31:1635-7.
53. Cohen SR, Berner CF, Busso M, Gleason MC, Hamilton D, Holmes RE, et al. ArteFill: a longlasting injectable wrinkle filler material—summary of the US Food and Drug Administration trials and a progress report on 4 to 5-year outcomes. Plast Reconstr Surg. 2006;118:S64-76.
54. Lemperle G, Morhenn VB, Pestonjamasp V, Gallo RL. Migration studies and histology of injectable microspheres of different size in mice. Plast Reconstr Surg. 2004;113:1380-90.
55. Lemperle G, Sadick NS, Knapp TR, Lemperle SM. ArteFill permanent injectable for soft tissue augmentation: II. Indications and applications. Aesthetic Plast Surg. 2010;34: 273-86.
56. Epstein RE, Spencer JM. Correction of atrophic scars with Artefill: an open-label pilot study. J Drugs Dermatol. 2010;9:1062-4.
57. Sachdev M, Anantheswar YN, Ashok BC, Hameed S, Pai SA. Facial granulomas secondary to injection of semi-permanent cosmetic dermal filler containing acrylic hydrogel particles. J Cutan Aesthet Surg. 2010;3:162-6.
58. Al-Qattan MM. Complications related to Artecoll injections for soft tissue augmentation of the hand: 3 case reports. J Hand Surg Am. 2011;36(6):994-7.
59. Baumann L, Blyuminn M, Saghari S. Dermal Fillers. In: Baumann L (Eds). Cosmetic Dermatology Priciples and Practice, 2nd edition. New York: Mc Graw Hill Medical; 2009. p. 203.
60. Pallua N, Wolter TP. A 5-year assessment of safety and aesthetic results after facial soft-tissue augmentation with polyacrylamide hydrogel (Aquamid): a prospective multicenter study of 251 patients. Plast Reconstr Surg. 2010;125:1797-804.
61. Mansor S, Breiting VB, Dahlstrøm K, Andersen AB, Andersen O, Christensen LH. Polyacrylamide Gel Treatment of Antiretroviral Therapy-induced Facial Lipoatrophy in HIV Patients. Aesthetic Plast Surg. 2011;35:709-16.
62. Yagi Y, Kato K, Murakami D, Misaki K, Ota M. Utilization of Aquamid as a filler for rhinoplasty in Orientals. Plast Reconstr Surg. 2009;123:26e-8e.
63. de Cássia Novaes W, Berg A. Experiences with a new nonbiodegradable hydrogel (Aquamid): a pilot study. Aesthetic Plast Surg. 2003;27:376-80.
64. Manafi A, Emami AH, Pooli AH, Habibi M, Saidian L. Unacceptable results with an accepted soft tissue filler: polyacrylamide hydrogel. Aesthetic Plastic Surg. 2010;34: 413-22.
65. Amin SP, Marmur ES, Goldberg DJ. Complications from injectable polyacrylamide gel, a new nonbiodegradable soft tissue filler. Dermatol Surg. 2004;30:1507-9.
66. Liu HL, Cheung WY. Complications of polyacrylamide hydrogel (PAAG) injection in facial augmentation. J Plast Reconstr Aesthet Surg. 2010;63:e9-12.
67. Abenavoli FM, Servili A, Corelli R. Aquamid: where is the reality? Plast Reconstr Surg. 2008;122:32e-3e.
68. Niedzielska I, Pajak J, Drugacz J. Late complications after polyacrylamide hydrogel injection into facial soft tissues. Aesthetic Plast Surg. 2006;30:377-8.
69. de Bree R, Middelweerd MJ, van der Waal I. Severe granulomatous inflammatory response induced by injection of polyacrylamide gel into the facial tissue. Arch Facial Plast Surg. 2004;6:204-6.
70. Baumann L (Ed). Cosmetic Dermatology. New York: The McGraw-Hill Companies; 2009. p. 206.

CHAPTER 93 Tear Trough Correction with Fillers

Amit Luthra

KEY MESSAGES

- Tear trough is an important aesthetic problem.
- Proper knowledge of anatomy and vasculature is essential for management.
- Fillers are a simple and effective mode of managing tear trough.

INTRODUCTION

The deep groove that commonly occurs near the junction of the eyelid and the cheek is called tear trough.[1]

It extends downward and lateral from the inner canthus of the eye.[2]

Tear trough deformity is a common issue in those looking for improvement in the periorbital area.[3] The tear trough deformity does not necessarily only occur in older individuals. A mild trough is seen in youth in many instances.[4]

Sunken appearance of the eyes with a dark shadow-like effect **(Fig. 1)** on the lower eyelid is characteristic of a tear trough deformity. This adds a tired and exhausted look to the patient in spite of adequate rest. This deformity is very difficult to hide with concealers and other cosmetic methods.[3]

The correction of the tear trough can be done both surgically and nonsurgically. Dermal fillers are a noninvasive and nonsurgical option, which in comparison to surgical correction by fat reposition, may have lesser downtime and longevity.

DEFINITION

The term tear trough deformity is the medial periorbital hollow extending obliquely from the medial canthus to the midpupillary line.[3] The indentation that defines the tear trough deformity is at the junction of thin eyelid skin above and the thicker and different nasal and cheek skin below with attenuated subcutaneous tissue overlying the maxillary bone.[4]

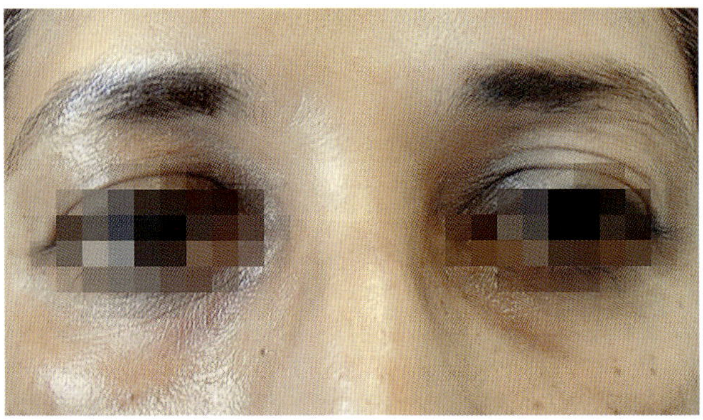

Fig. 1: Shadow effect.

ANATOMY OF TEAR TROUGH

Knowing the anatomy of the periorbital area is important to understand the dynamics of changes with age and to treat and prevent the problem **(Fig. 2)**. The tear trough deformity is a natural consequence of the anatomic attachments of the periorbital tissues.[3]

The tear trough is at the inferior orbital rim most medially with the maximal distance from the rim occurring centrally. Volume loss can be present laterally in more advanced aging, at/or just below the orbital rim, where the retaining ligaments are thicker and less distensible.[4]

The location of the indentation is along the fibers of the orbicularis oculi in the medial third at the orbital rim. The orbicularis oculi muscle has a direct attachment to the inferior orbital rim from the anterior lacrimal crest to the medial limbus or approximately 30% of the orbital rim length.[4]

Lateral to this, the attachment to the bone is by means of the orbicularis-retaining ligaments, which have variable length at different points along the inferior orbital rim. The length increases to a maximum centrally and then decreases laterally until the orbicularis-retaining ligaments merge with the lateral orbital thickening in the lateral canthal region. The levator labii superioris originates just below the orbicularis oculi muscle attachment to the medial orbital rim.[5-8]

In the medial area where the orbicularis oculi muscles attaches to the orbital rim, the tear trough deformity appears for the first time and becomes deeper as time progresses.[4]

A true osteocutaneous ligament called the tear trough ligament is consistently found on the maxilla, between the palpebral and orbital parts of the orbicularis oculi.[3]

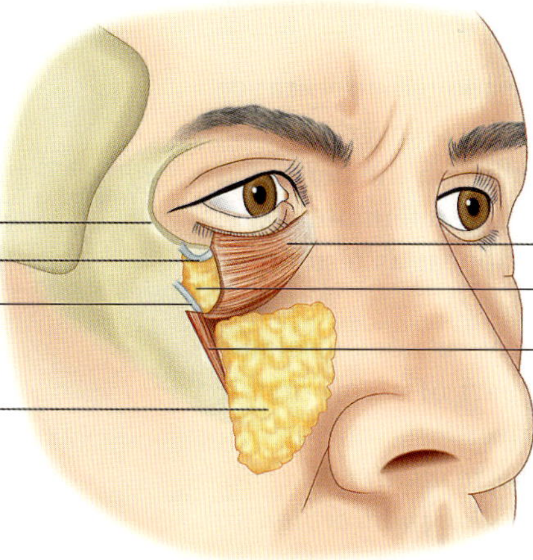

Fig. 2: Periorbital anatomy.

It commences medially, at the level of insertion of the medial canthal tendon, just inferior to the anterior lacrimal crest, to approximately the medial pupillary line, where it continues laterally as the bilayered orbicularis retaining ligament.[3]

The skin of the tear trough area is thin as there is very little subcutaneous tissue between the skin and the orbicularis muscle that is attached to the orbital rim.[4]

Given the fixed attachment of the muscle to the rim and contraction of muscles, notably the orbicularis oculi that the tear trough would show the consequences of volume loss earlier and more dramatically than the rest of the face.[9] The depression of the tear trough is also sometimes associated without pouching of the orbital fat superiorly in the lower lid fat compartments **(Fig. 3)**.

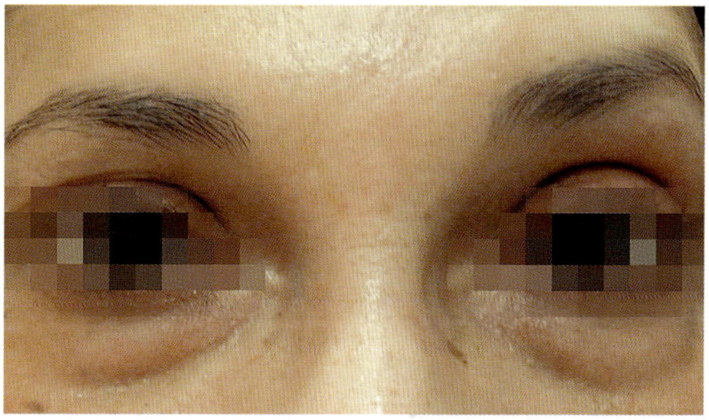

Fig. 3: Orbital fat herniation due to aging.

This herniation, although it takes attention away from the tear trough deformity itself, on its own holds an independent problem.[4]

Volume loss in the periorbital area is variable in depth and morphology from person to person.[4]

As the patient ages, the globe descends within the orbit and the infraorbital fat is displaced anteriorly. This anterior bulge causes the tear trough to deepen. This anteriorly displaced fat causes a shadow to form below it, and it makes the tear trough deformity appear deeper depending on the conditions of lighting. The inferior border of the tear trough is formed by the thick skin of the upper cheek with its abundant subcutaneous fat, suborbicularis oculi fat (SOOF), and portions of the malar fat pad **(Fig. 4)**.[3]

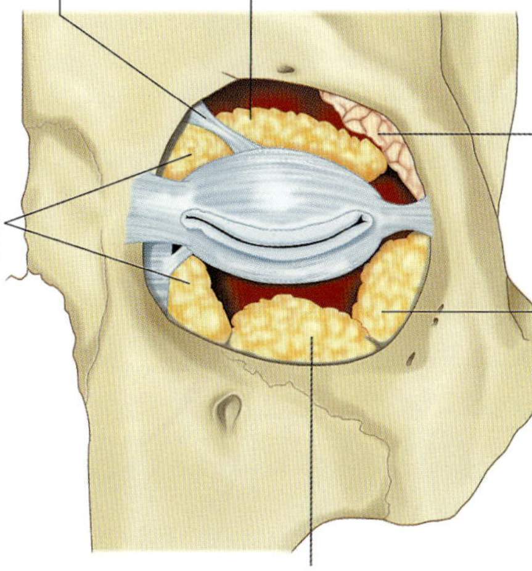

Fig. 4: Periorbital fat pads.

The medial most part of the trough is the deepest, while it starts getting shallow as we move laterally. The skin of the groove is extremely thin with barely any fat under it and this makes the depression worse. With age, loss of osseous support and soft tissue causes the tear trough to deepen further.[3,10]

Suborbicularis oculi fat provides volume and shape to the face and acts as a gliding plane within which muscles of expression can move freely.[2]

Suborbicularis oculi fat herniation occurs when there is compromise to the ligamentous support provided by the orbicularis-retaining ligament and the zygomaticocutaneous ligament. It herniates from under the orbicularis oculi muscle and forms a gentle mound just in the inferolateral portion of the tear trough.

The malar bags **(Fig. 5)** create a festooned appearance over the medial portion of the zygoma just below the lateral portion of the inferior orbital rim. Along with the herniated SOOF, there may be a component of fluid retention, laxity, and descent of malar fat pads, which appear as festooning **(Figs. 6A and B)**.

Volume loss at the orbital rim is of course not an isolated aging event **(Fig. 7)**. In truth, it is part of a volumetric involution that occurs globally in the face.[4,11]

Tear trough deformity takes place due to multiple reasons. Volume loss being one of the main causes along with orbital fat herniation and skin laxity.[4] *Secondary to volumetric changes, ptosis of tissues below could play a role.*

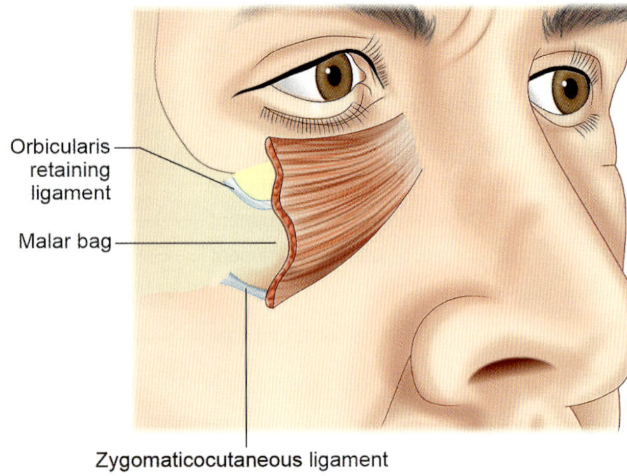

Fig. 5: Zygomaticocutaneous ligament.

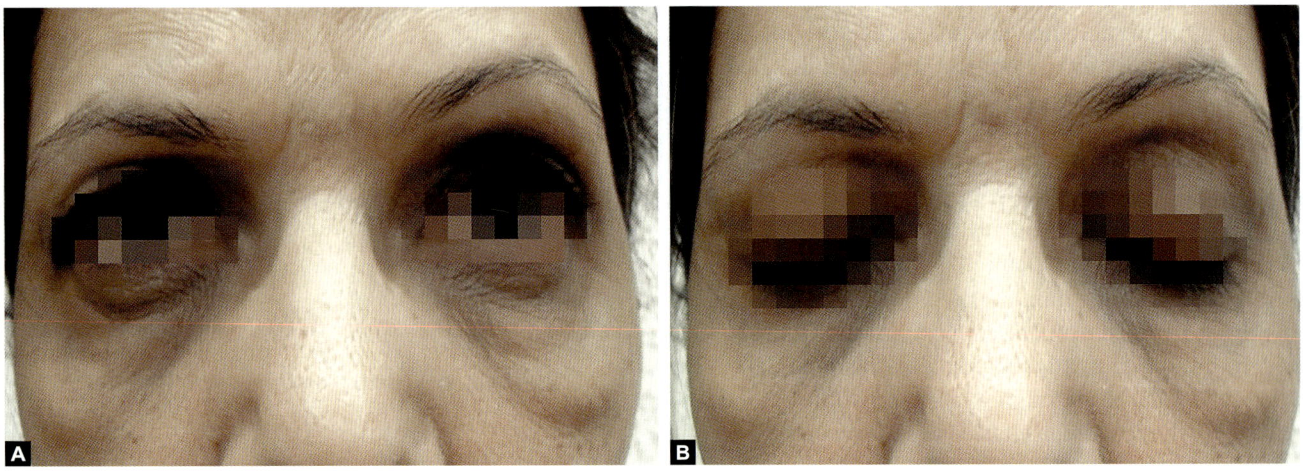

Figs. 6A and B: Suborbicularis oculi fat herniation with malar bags: (A) Eyes open; (B) Eyes closed.

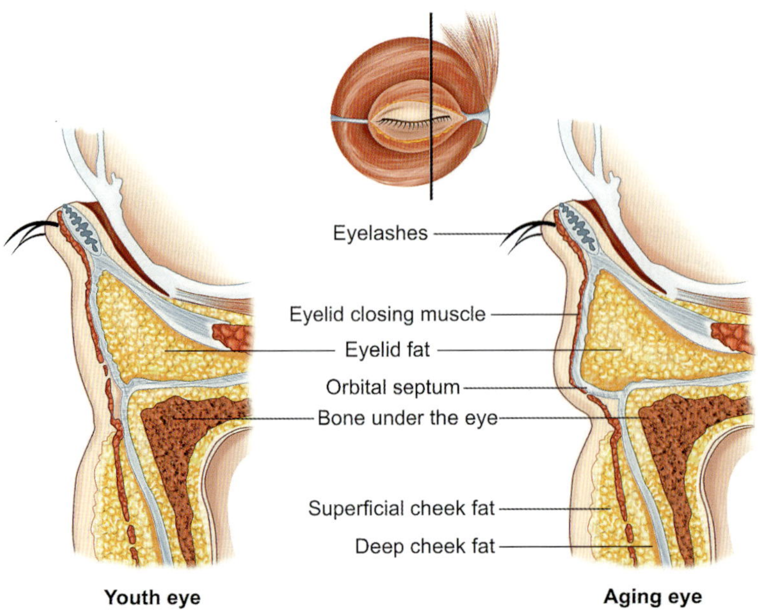

Fig. 7: Periocular changes with aging.

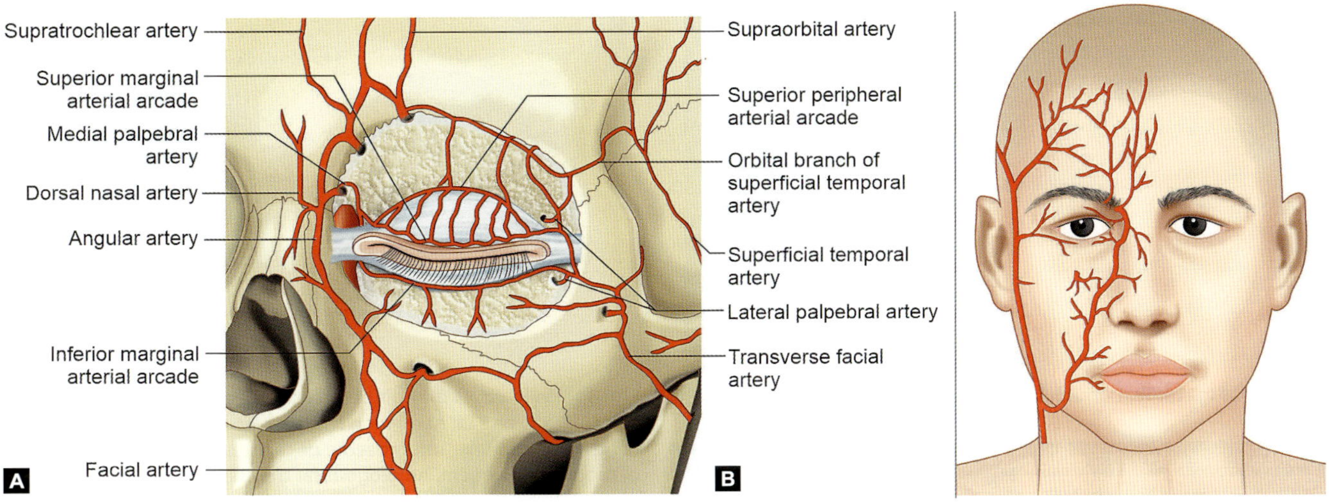

Figs. 8A and B: Supratrochlear and supraorbital arteries.

Periorbital Vascular Anatomy (Figs. 8A and B)

Branches of the external carotid artery (ECA) provide the blood supply to the face excluding the central forehead, upper eyelids, and upper nose, which are supplied by the internal carotid system (ICA) by the ophthalmic artery. Vascular anastomosis between the ECA and ICA is danger zone as intravascular injections here can lead to vascular compromise and permanent blindness.[10]

The vascular watershed areas are:

- *The infraorbital foramen:* The infraorbital vessels arise from maxillary branch of ECA, which anastomose with branches of ophthalmic artery.
- *The supraorbital notch and glabella:* Supraorbital and supratrochlear, infratrochlear, and external nasal branches of ophthalmic artery anastomose with branches of ECA.
- *The temple area:* Superficial temporal artery crosses the zygomatic arch and 2 cm above the arch divides into anterior (which anastomose with branches of ophthalmic artery) and posterior branches.[10]

TYPES OF TEAR TROUGH

Tear trough patients are categorized into two basic groups and corrected accordingly.

Group 1: Structural Tear Trough Deformity

- Can be seen in young patients, where inferior orbital rim deficiency is hereditary.
- In other cases, the periorbital skin is very thin with minimal natural padding of underlying tissue, which highlights the bony trough.
- As early as in the third decade, some individuals may present with complaints of tired look, which is actually due to an early volume loss of infraorbital fat pads **(Fig. 9)**.

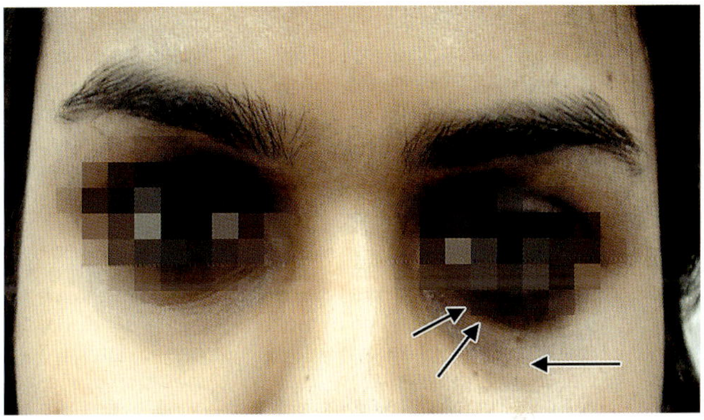

Fig. 9: All three signs can be seen. The left side is worse than the right.

Group 2: Older Individuals with Accentuation of Tear Trough due to Loss of Midfacial Volume

These individuals may or may not have had a preexisting tear trough deformity. In either case, midface volume loss from malar fat pad descent (in early cases), and the middle cheek fat pad loss (in extreme cases) will aggravate tear trough deficiency **(Fig. 10)**. This is of prime importance in choice of product and its placement.

Associated changes of skin laxity of the periorbital and surrounding skin, presence of malar bags, and temporal hollowing need to be assessed before treating the tear trough.

The midface is corrected first with a high concentration of hyaluronic acid (HA) (22–25 mg/mL) deep into fat pads. Midface correction itself offers support that is enough to correct the tear trough in many cases. If the trough persists, then correction of it can be done directly. Correction of lateral cheeks can give some improvement in lateral tear trough, which can be further corrected as described above. If there is herniation of SOOF and presence of malar bags, then less

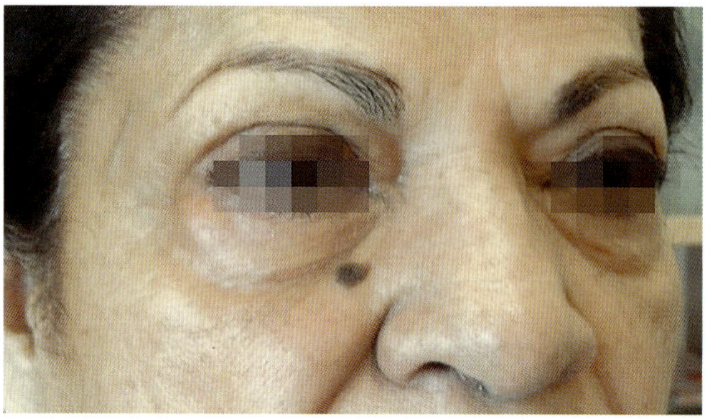

Fig. 10: Tear trough due to loss of midface volume.

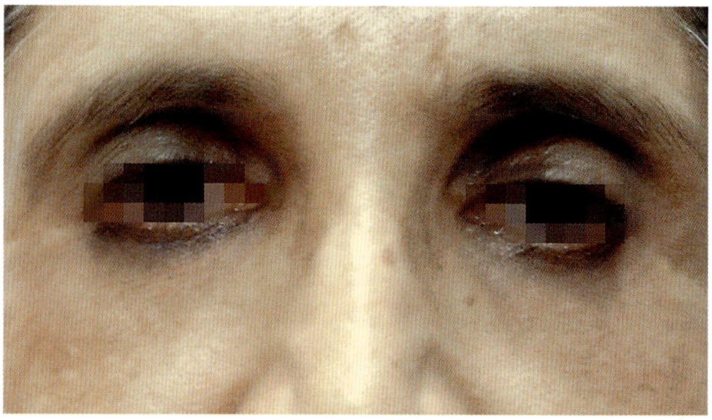

Fig. 11: Hollowness of orbit has occurred as a postsurgical event done for skin laxity and fat herniation with residual scar ring and fibrosis. Here, correction with filler using needle or cannula may result in unevenness of product placement. Autologous fat transfer may be a better choice.

TABLE 1: The periorbital pattern of volume loss.

Classes	*Hirmand's clinical classification*	*Grades*	*Barton's anatomic classification*
I	• Volume loss limited medially to the tear trough • These patients can also have mild flattening extending to the central cheek	0	Absence of medial or lateral lines demarcating the arcus marginal is or the orbital rim, and a smooth, youthful contour without a transition zone at the orbit-cheek junction
II	Volume loss in the lateral orbital area in addition to the medial orbit. They may have moderate volume deficiency in the medial cheek and flattening of the central upper cheek.	I	Mild, subtle presence of a medial line, or shadow; smooth lateral transition of the lid-cheek junction
III	• Full depression circumferentially along the orbital rim medially to laterally • This pattern is often associated with more advanced volume deficiency in the medial cheek, central cheek, and malar eminence	II	Moderate prominence of a visible demarcation of the lid-cheek junction, extending from medial to lateral
		III	Severe demarcation of the orbit-cheek junction with an obvious step between the orbit and the cheek

material needs to be placed and one must be cautious of its placement. The material here plays a more supportive role to the lax tissues and is not injected into the malar bag. Caution should be taken to not injure the true and false ligaments in this area, which are already compromised.

CLASSIFICATION OF VOLUME LOSS

The periorbital pattern of volume loss can be categorized clinically as well as anatomically **(Table 1)**.

Patients of any class may present with excess orbital fat or significant skin laxity. The presence of either of these variables identifies a patient who would benefit from surgery or surgery followed by filling of the tear trough for optimal results. These patients are not good candidates for nonsurgical correction alone **(Fig. 11)**.[4]

PATIENT SELECTION

Assessment for patient selection depends on the following:

- *Skin quality and laxity:* This can be determined by the snap test.
  - A small portion of infraorbital skin is pinched.
  - If it recoils immediately, then the elasticity is good.
  - If it takes time to recoil, then the elasticity is moderate.
  - If it stays pinched, then the laxity is severe.
- *Assessing the skin discoloration in the periorbital area*:
  - Causes of discoloration are:
    - Vascular
    - Hemosiderin
    - Melanin

  Vascular discoloration is due to congestive etiology where vitamin K, decongestants, lymphatic drainage will help in improving the appearance. Correcting the tear trough with fillers, here will not show a significant improvement.

  Melanin contributes to the dark-brown discoloration of the periorbital skin. Lightening and exfoliating agents are of limited value here. HA filler helps in reducing the shadow effect; thus, improving the light reflex but never eliminates the pigment.
- *Periorbital fat pads:* These can only be camouflaged by injecting the tear trough, which decreases the sausage roll. In early cases of fat pad prominence, it can almost correct it but in later cases, the results may be variable.
- *Preexisting periorbital edema:* This can be seen as eye bags in the infraorbital region.

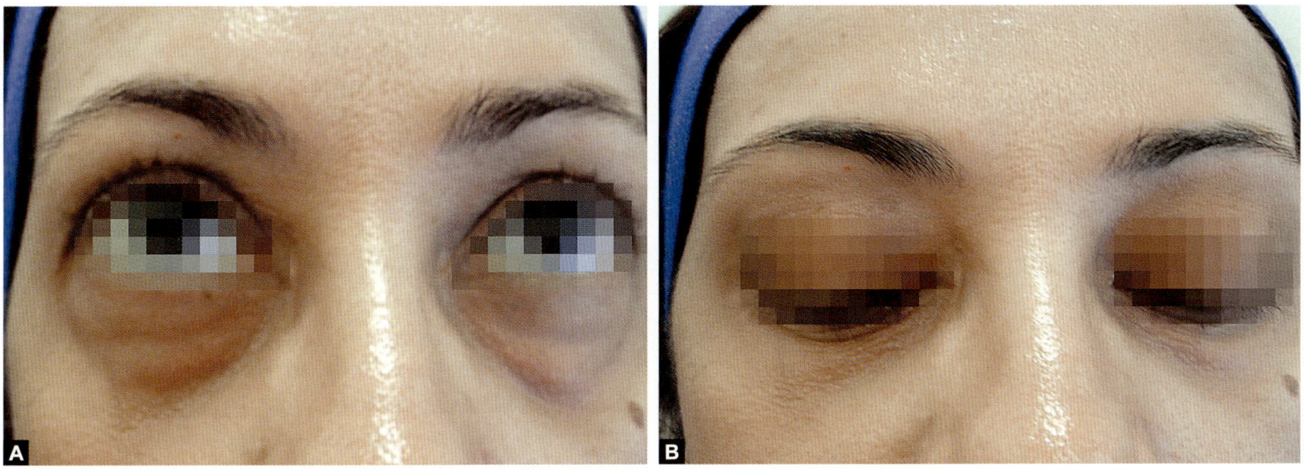

Figs. 12A and B: Differentiate between lower lid fat pad and edema.

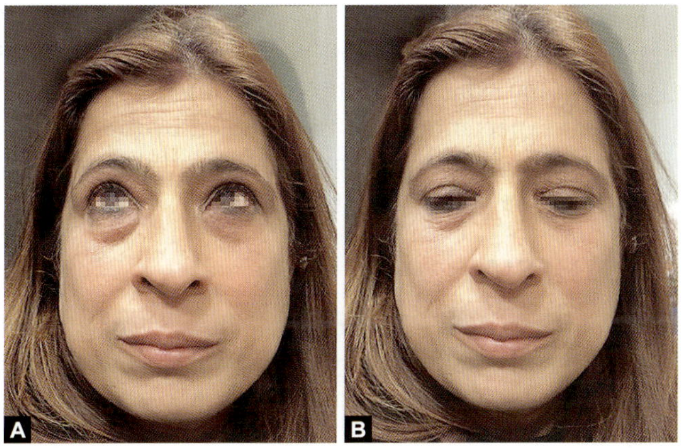

Figs. 13A and B: (A) Patient looking up, the bulge becomes prominent on both the sides (more on the right); (B) Patient looking down, the bulge remains prominent on the right side because of edema but disappears on the left.

Clinical test to differentiate between lower lid fat pad and edema:

- The patient is seated and head is kept steady.
- Ask the patient to roll eyeballs up and down
- True fat pad becomes prominent on rolling up and disappears on rolling down **(Figs. 12A and B)**.
- In edema, the bulge under the eye becomes prominent on rolling down or looking down as shown on the right side in the patient in **Figures 13A and B**.
- This is due to the movement of the orbicularis oculi muscle up and down in its tensed and relaxed form.

By doing this test, the most contributing factor for the periorbital changes can be gauged, according to which the product specific, amount of material and degree of correction achieved without aggravating the preexisting deformity can be outlined.

It is helpful to simulate the effect of filling, in the less than ideal candidate, by pushing on the soft tissues just under the tear trough with the patient observing in the mirror while their reaction is assessed.[4]

COUNSELING

Choosing the right kind of patient is imperative for a good and satisfactory result with fillers, the ideal candidates being those with very less skin laxity, good skin tone, and mild-to-moderately deep-tear troughs.[4]

Patients with severely deep-tear troughs or those with a lot of skin laxity and thin skin are poor candidates. They may obtain improvement in the appearance of the tear trough, but they must be counseled as to the higher risk of visibility, irregularity, and overall suboptimal results.[4]

Many of these, patients still elect to proceed and rarely seek reversal even if the results are not perfect.

Patients with orbital fat herniation and severe skin laxity will benefit from surgery. These patients are unlikely to obtain good results from injecting the tear trough alone and should be advised of this.[4] This procedure has excellent utility in postsurgical patients, who have uncorrected troughs or over-resected orbital fat.

CONTRAINDICATIONS

- Unrealistic expectations[3]
- Infection near the site of injection[3]
- Known allergy or hypersensitivity to the material or to the lidocaine mixed in the syringe of the filler **(Fig. 14)**[3]
- Patients with septal fat herniation[3]
- Severe elastosis[3]
- Scarring or fibrosis in the periorbital area, which may have been a result of past surgeries or trauma.

PRECAUTIONS

- Vitamin E, ginkgo biloba, aspirin, and nonsteroidal anti-inflammatory drugs (NSAIDs) should be avoided at least 5 days before the treatment to prevent bruising.[3]
- Care should be taken in patients with a history of lower eyelid blepharoplasty without lateral retinacular suspension.[3]

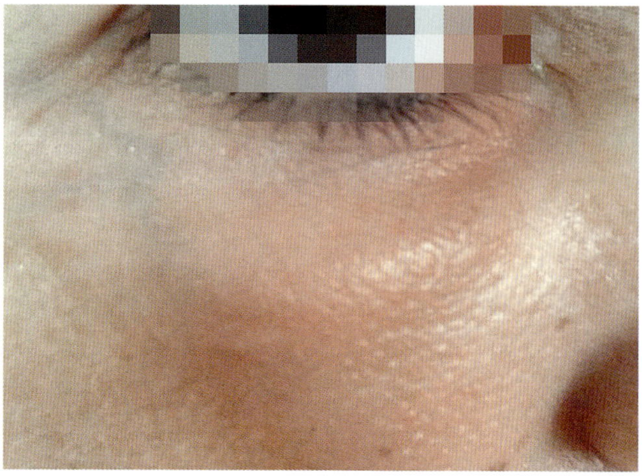

Fig. 14: Local hypersensitivity reaction to hyaluronic acid 6 months after the procedure was done and subsided in 4 days with only anti-inflammatory medications and serratiopeptidase. No oral or topical corticosteroids were used.

- One should be cautious while injecting around the infraorbital foramen to avoid injury to the neurovascular bundle.[3]
- Careful and gentle molding of the product for a more homogeneous distribution of the material after injection to obtain an even distribution of the filler in the lateral part of the hollow may be required.[3]

TYPES OF FILLER

Hyaluronic acid fillers are the most commonly used fillers worldwide.[1,12-15] The material is particularly appealing because it is perceived to be a simple, safe, and reversible nonsurgical procedure. HA is well adapted for tear trough treatment with a high-satisfaction rate,[12] given its limitations.

Lower eyelid hyperpigmentation (dark circles) will improve in its appearance due to the hydration benefits of HA and change in light reflex, which reduces the shadow effect. However, one cannot promise elimination.

Light molecular weight HA is most preferred in the tear trough area but is placed directly, deep in the supraperiosteal plane. Medium weight HA can be placed similarly by an experienced injector but in very small quantities.

Heavy weight HA is ideal to restore volume loss in the midface, which helps to reposition the subluxated tear trough, but is not preferred in the tear trough.

Advantages

With adequate training and reasonable expertise, the injection is relatively easy to perform.[1] The very medial and superior tear trough is where one starts injecting where it is extremely effective in obliterating the trough; there is a high degree of patient satisfaction.[1] This procedure performed with finesse has a minimum downtime. The material is long-lasting (1 year or more) in the tear trough. Most complications are self-limiting and can be treated by massage. In the event of an unsatisfactory effect, the material can be dissolved away.[1]

With this method, a young patient can avoid surgery completely.[1]

Limitations

- It is not permanent.
- The superficial method can easily produce skin irregularities. In patients with large fat pads, only moderate improvement is possible with filler treatment, hence they are not ideal candidates.
- There are no associated improvements in the lower lid as can be obtained with surgery.
- There is a distinct group of patients who will have more improvement by direct fat pad modification than by filling below them.[1]
- Injection of the trough with filler, unlike surgery, does not address any of the deformity's root causes.
- Patient expectations can be matched by the injecting physician, if better communication on the anatomic complexities of tear trough is described with outcome.

ANESTHESIA

Use of local anesthesia depends upon the mode of injection. Topical (cream) anesthesia may be used with needles whereas an entry point infiltration with 2% lignocaine is useful when using a cannula.

PERSONAL TECHNIQUE

Authors do tear trough correction only with HA filler. They use both cannula as well as needle according to preference and both methods are described below. We use lower concentration of HA (20 mg/mL) and 0.2–0.3 mL is put along the inferior orbital rim supraperiosteally and massaged medially and laterally.

Needle

Needle is useful for site specific injections supraperiosteally. As the needle touches the bone, it will scrunch and the patient will wince, which confirms the supraperiosteal position. The authors prefer to tilt the needle by 15° upward to glide it smoothly along the natural curvature of the periosteal plane. This is one indication where the bevel should be facing downward.

The first entry point is to cover the central portion of the tear trough lateral to the midpupillary line. Injection is supraperiosteal with aspiration before injecting. At all times, during the entire duration, injection should be extremely slow, smooth, and controlled; light but firm pressure should be placed on the rim to protect the globe of the eye. Once the needle is withdrawn, the supporting finger is lifted to assess the product placement. It should be smooth and not visible, and slight under correction is usually the rule. We can either place a tiny bolus of 0.05 mL or less or thread and fan as per the desired correction. It is important to stay lateral to the midpupillary area with a needle to avoid any injury to the infraorbital structures.

The next point of entry is lateral to the midpupillary line. Usually, the tissue quality of the skin in this area is superior and the injection is deep below the orbicularis oculi muscle. This may allow a larger bolus of 0.1–0.2 mL to be placed in two points.

The third point is to cover the medial most portion of the tear trough. This can be tricky and is prone to vascular compromises if done incorrectly. It is best to thread in this area as the skin is thinnest and most adherent. If a larger deficit is present, one or two threads can be fanned in the same area. Since, it is impossible to quantify the amount of product used here, it is important to judge the feel of the area rather than the amount injected.

Superficial product placement is evident immediately. Firm pressure along the bone may help in some amount of correction. However, avoid vigorous molding or massaging as this lends to more trauma and edema, worsening the situation. One may need to observe this over the next 15 days and either correct it or redo it. If it is very evident, it may be better to dissolve the product.

The total amount of 0.2 mL can be placed safely, and more can be added in the touch-up. Up to 0.5 mL can be safely put in this area if more volume replacement is required.

Hydrating fillers can be used for improving the hydration of the skin in cases of dry skin and fine lines. Tiny amounts of HA can be used more superficially in drops or threads, more medially in the skin. This can be repeated once every 6 months with the newer products.

Cannula

When using a cannula is your preferred choice, a 25-gauge cannula is the safest as it is thin enough to traverse this delicate area but is blunt enough to avoid trauma and there is less risk of vascular complications including a bruise. One should be extremely gentle and cautious and not be in a very deep plane, especially with a harper cannula like the 27 gauge.

The insertion point of the cannula lies at the intersection of the Hinderer's lines. This I is the safest point of entry as there is no risk of damaging any surrounding structures. If one is trying to correct the midface along with the tear trough, then this is the ideal point. The cannula can be inserted in a deeper and subdermal plane. Gently glide the cannula up, to first correct the midface volume loss both in its medial and lateral aspects. Once adequate product is placed, which may be HA with a higher viscosity placed deep; one can remove the cannula and fix the HA with lower viscosity. Reinsert the

TABLE 2: Merits and demerits of needle and cannula.

Needle	*Cannula*
Short length	Long length
Sharp	Blunt
Multiple entry points required	Single entry point
More traumatic	Less traumatic
More bruising	Less bruising
Placement of material uneven	Uniform placement of product
More specific	More diffuse placement
Less material used	More material used up

cannula, provided it is long enough (measuring externally along the surface of the skin) but the insertion will now follow a more superficial plane. As you approach the tear trough follow caution along the midpupillary area. Avoid going in too deep as you may inadvertently damage the infraorbital structures. Pass the cannula along the infraorbital rim in a supraperiosteal fashion.

Initially, stay under the orbicularis oculi, but as you move medially toward the inner can thus, you will be on the bone as there are hardly any muscle fibers here. You should not be able to see the outline of the cannula, although its shadow must be visible. Bevel down, slowly inject in tiny droplets, with your finger kept above to prevent the material from floating up along the rim or the infraorbital area. Drawback the cannula and change the direction to address the lateral portion of the tear trough. Here, the plane is below the orbicularis oculi, so that the product sits nicely to give a good molding. Injecting above the muscle may result in the Tyndall phenomena and look lumpy.

If both midface and tear trough correction have to be done for the same patient, address the midface primarily and then go ahead with the tear trough correction.

At all times, the amount of product extruded is in tiny droplets with no force or pressure. The flow should be with ease; if resistance is felt then the cannula must be withdrawn and renegotiated smoothly to avoid any trauma to the tissue, vessels, and retaining ligaments, especially in the lateral portion of the tear trough **(Table 2 and Figs. 15 to 17)**.

OTHER METHODS

Several techniques are done for tear trough correction. Each has its own merits and demerits.

Eventually, irrespective of the technique, gaining experience by repetition gives the best results. Some of the techniques are mentioned here.

Kane's Technique

This technique is more medial, injecting small amounts of HA filler at each pass in a parallel threading fashion. In a deep-tear trough, the filler is laid down in a crosshatching fashion.[16]

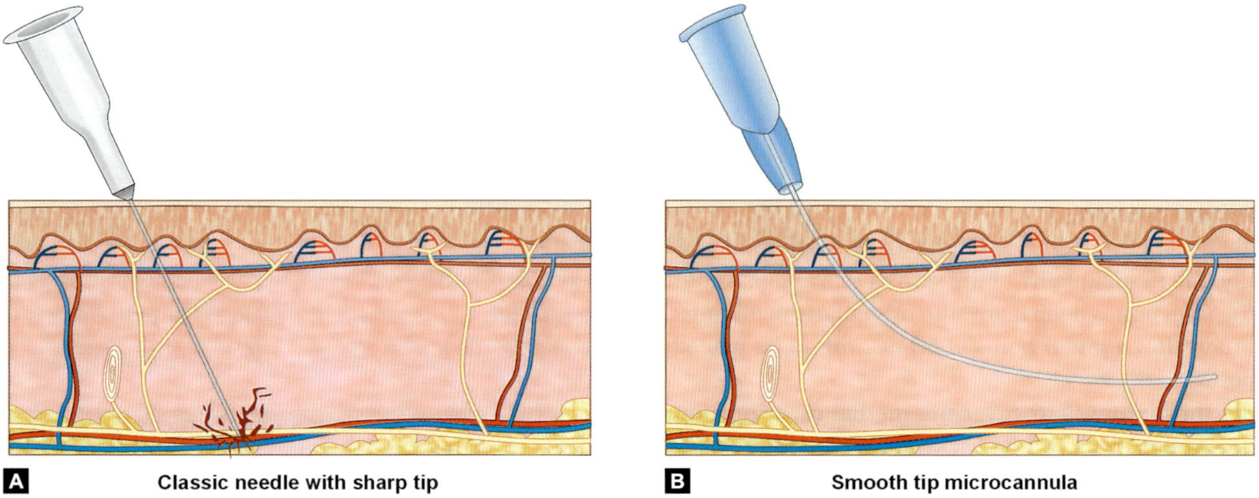

Figs. 15A and B: Merits and demerits of needle and cannula.

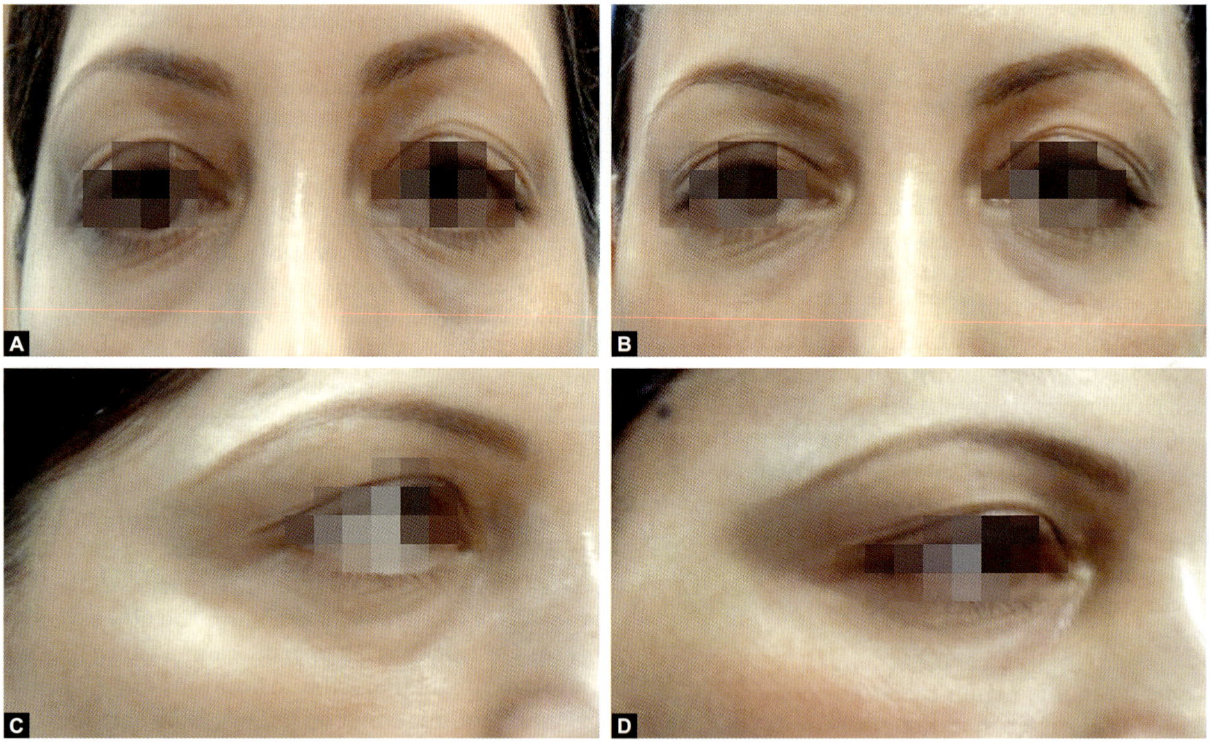

Figs. 16A to D: Pre- and posthyaluronic acid filler done only for tear trough correction by using cannula. The patient desired a natural and subtle look. Midface was not addressed. (A and C) Prefiller; (B and D) Postfiller.

Lambro's Technique

This technique uses a lateral approach where the filler is injected deep into the dermis as the needle is withdrawn and the same process is repeated above and below. Avoid forcefully compressing the product during massage, as this can displace it into the cheek and exaggerate the tear trough.[3,1]

Technique of Stutman and Codner

The filler is injected deep in a crosshatching and linear fashion into the periosteal plane, laterally inferior to the orbicularis-retaining ligament. The product is then lightly massaged.[3,17]

Technique of Kenneth and Samantha Steinsapir

Aliquots of filler are placed in the preperiosteal tissue just inferior to the orbital rim in a serial puncture technique.

The orbital rim is digitally palpated and the needle rotated, so that the bevel is parallel to the skin and advanced to be flush on the periosteum.[3,18]

Technique of Patel and Glaser

Hyaluronic acid filler is injected by using a serial point injection or linear threading technique. Small aliquots of filler just inferior to the orbital rim at a plane between the periosteum and the orbicularis oculi muscle to correct loss of volume in the lower eyelid are a due to pseudoherniation, orbital septal laxity, and atrophy of the midface.[3,19]

COMPLICATIONS AND THEIR TREATMENT

- Uneven filling of the product,[3] which may resolve by light molding 3–7 days later.
- If the unevenness does not resolve by 15 days, then it must be dissolved by using hyaluronidase.
- *Small superficial bruises:* These will resolve within 3–5 days spontaneously and more rapidly if a topical vitamin K and decongestant cream is applied immediately and over the next few days.
- Swelling is inevitable and temporary. It will settle within 3–7 days. Any persistence will need to be addressed.
- Deep bruising may cause hemosiderin deposition, which may persist as a brown stain for months **(Figs. 18A to C)**.[3]

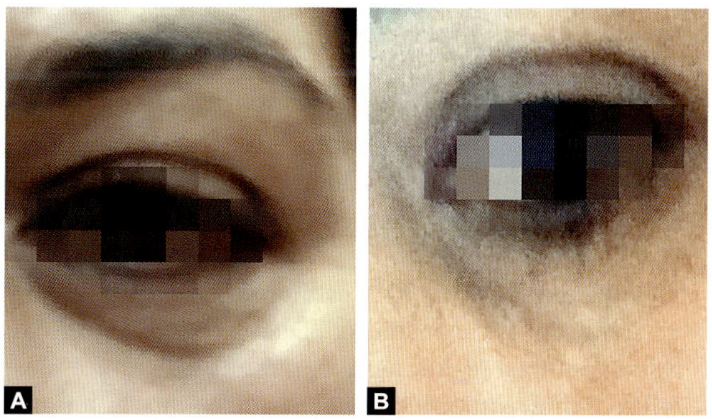

Figs. 17A and B: Needle was used for only tear trough correction as described above: (A) Prefiller; (B) Postfiller (few hours later).

- If an interprocedural bruise is seen or suspected or the patient presents with a delayed bruise, then low levels of intense-pulsed light of 570 nm, pulsed dye laser, neodymium-doped yttrium aluminum garnet (Nd:YAG) laser can be used twice a week to resolve it.
- *The Tyndall effect:* HA when injected too superficially can lead to a bluish discoloration under the skin, which is due to the Tyndall effect where the blue light spectrum is scattered by the colloid particles more strongly.[3] This is highly undesirable and any extra product, which is placed superficially, must always be dissolved. It is not necessary to dissolve all of the filler. Small amounts of hyaluronidase can be injected and the rest of the filler can be molded along the infraorbital rim.
- *Postfiller puffiness may be multifactorial:*
  - Inadequate correction of preexisting bulging fat pads—after an appropriate gap of 2–4 weeks of previous filling, more HA can be injected to further camouflage the puffiness as much as permissible. This may or may not always be successful, especially in those who are surgical candidates but have made an informed choice to do this procedure.
  - Where HA with a higher viscosity has been used, especially in large amounts with: the options can be to either dissolve it immediately or to wait for 2 weeks for complete integration of the product and dissolve if needed.
  - Worsening of preexisting puffiness due to the hydroscopic property of HA. This may or may not resolve over time. If not, this has to be addressed with hyaluronidase.
- *Infection in the form of:*
  - *Persistent edema and erythema:* This will have to be addressed with oral antibiotics like ciprofloxacin 750 mg twice a day for 10–15 days along with NSAIDs and serratiopeptidase. It is advisable to minimize

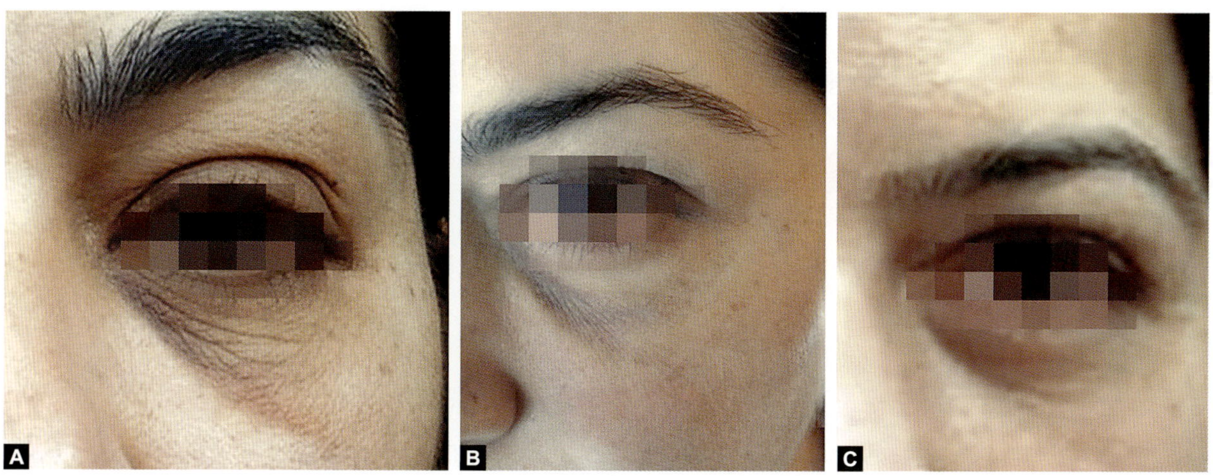

Figs. 18A to C: *Bruising:* (A) Immediate bruising; (B) After 2 months; (C) After 6 months.

handling of the affected area. If still persistent, consider hyaluronidase to dissolve the possibly infected material. This is an advantage of using HA. Semipermanent materials require surgical removal.

- Fluctuant nodules[1] are rare and have been reported. Antibiotics and anti-inflammatories are advised.

If the patient comes with a filler injected from someone else and is confirmed to be HA, it is still worth dissolving the filler. If no improvement is seen, then a non-HA filler or a biofilm may be suspected, which can become very resistant and may require excision.

If the filler is HA, and the nodular inflammation occurs within the first few weeks, it may be due to a hypersensitivity to the product or due to an infection. It is treated with antibiotics and anti-inflammatories and dissolved, if necessary. But, if it occurs after months to years, it is due to biofilm.

Always rule out atypical mycobacteria (biopsy) for persistent stubborn nodules.

But at all times, the general consensus is to avoid intralesional or oral steroids to save the risk of potential biofilm. However, in some individuals despite all efforts and all forms of treatment including supportive as well as dissolution and lasers, the granulomatous reaction just persists.

The authors suggest that thorough asepsis of the area minimal handling of tissue pre-, intra-, and postprocedure greatly help to reduce the risk of infection.

- Vascular accidents
- *Blindness after facial injections:* To prevent blindness via migration of an embolus of filler retrograde through an arteriole into central retinal artery, it is important to know vasculature and anatomical variations, which may throw up a surprise; the emboli may either be intra-arterial or due to pressure occlusion **(Fig. 19)**.

It is important to limit the amount of material or bolus injected in one site.

The possibility of blindness also can be minimized by using blunt cannulas instead of needles. Avoid going too close to the medial canthus; inject slowly in a controlled manner with minimal pressure and minute quantities of filler of lighter weight material at a time.[16]

Rarely, if one is not careful in staying inferior to the orbital rim, one might injure the conjunctival vessels causing a subconjunctival hemorrhage.[20]

DISSOLVING THE FILLER

Hyaluronidase is used to reverse the presence of excess or inappropriately placed filler in the area. There are a variety of hyaluronidase preparations available and hence the reconstitution is product specific. The authors use the brand Hynidase and it is reconstituted as follows:

- One vial of hyaluronidase containing 1,500 units is reconstituted with 1 mL of normal saline and 0.5 mL of 2% lignocaine. This final product is used as filler dissolve and injected deep into the filler.
- The number of units of hyaluronidase required depends on the amount of unwanted filler present. It can range from 25 units for a lump to 500 units for a vascular occlusion. In cases of vascular accidents, it is prudent to overinject the hyaluronidase than underinject, one can even go up to 1,500 units depending on the area of involvement. Prior intradermal sensitivity testing is advised in a nonemergency situation. In case of a vascular compromise, it is advisable to go ahead without testing but with necessary back up for anaphylaxis reaction.
- Hyaluronidase must be freshly prepared and injected as soon as it is reconstituted. Deep, dermal, and robust fillers require a higher number of units of hyaluronidase, while lighter superficial ones require a lesser amount. Care must be taken to not inject more than necessary. Higher concentrations of hyaluronidase may cause hypersensitivity reactions in prone individuals **(Fig. 20)**.

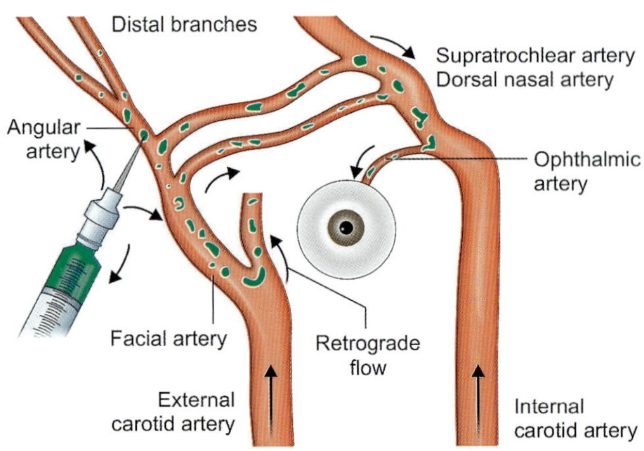

Fig. 19: Embolus formation.

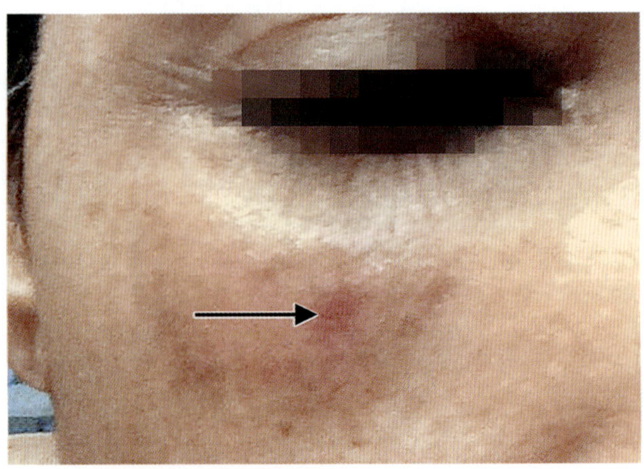

Fig. 20: Hypersensitivity reaction to hyaluronidase.

PEARLS

- Injections are usually supraperiosteal. The mode of injection can be needle or cannula, with the latter preferred because of relative safety and lesser bruisability.
- Fillers for older patients need to be given first in the cheeks followed by the tear troughs.
- The insertion point of the cannula lies at the intersection of the Hinderer's lines. As you approach the tear trough follow caution along the midpupillary area to avoid damage the infraorbital structures.
- If there is herniation of SOOF and presence of malar bags, then less material needs to be placed and one must be cautious of its placement. The material here plays a more supportive role to the lax tissues and is not injected into the malar bag.
- If an interprocedural bruise is seen or suspected or the patient presents with a delayed bruise, then low levels of intense-pulsed light of 570 nm can be used twice a week to resolve it.
- The authors suggest that completed is infection of the area, minimal handling of tissue pre-, intra-, and postprocedure with frequent changing of needles, gentle maneuvering of the cannula, and extreme patient care can greatly minimize the risk of infection.

REFERENCES

1. Lambros VS. Hyaluronic acid injections for correction of the tear trough deformity. Plast Reconstr Surg. 2007;120:74S-80S.
2. Erian A, Shiffman MA. Advanced Surgical Facial Rejuvenation. New York City: Springer; 2012.
3. Sharad J. Dermal fillers for the treatment of tear trough deformity: a review of anatomy, treatment techniques, and their outcomes. J Cutan Aesthet Surg. 2012;5:229-38.
4. Hirmand H. Anatomy and nonsurgical correction of the tear trough deformity. Plast Reconstr Surg. 2010;125:699-708.
5. Muzaffar AR, Mendelson BC, Adams WP Jr. Surgical anatomy of the ligamentous attachments of the lower lid and lateral canthus. Plast Reconstr Surg. 2002;110:873-84; discussion 897-911.
6. Lucarelli MJ, Khwarg SI, Lemke BN, Kozel JS, Dortzbach RK. The anatomy of midfacial ptosis. Ophthalmic Plast Reconstr Surg. 2000;16(1):7-22.
7. Sullivan PK. The anatomic basis for the tear trough and crescent deformity at the lower eyelid-cheek junction. SanDiego, Calif: American Society of Plastic Surgeons, Annual Meeting; 2003.
8. Zide BM. Surgical anatomy around the orbit: the system of zones. Philadelphia: Lippincott Williams and Wilkins; 2006.
9. Guo-Wu Wang, Jin-YeWang. Native polymer-based 3D substitutes in plastic surgery. In: Wang Jin-Ye (Eds). Native Macromolecule-Based 3D Tissues Repair. Singapore: World Scientific Publishing Co. 2014.
10. Aesthetics Journal. Aesthetics March 2015. United Kingdom: 2015.
11. Lambros VS. The dynamics of facial aging. Las Vegas: American Society for Aesthetic Plastic Surgery, 2002.
12. Jiang J, Wang X, Chen R, Xia X, Sun S, Hu K. Tear trough deformity: different types of anatomy and treatment options. Postepy Dermatol Alergol. 2016;33(4):303-8.
13. Goldberg RA, Lee S, Jayasundera T, Tsirbas A, Douglas RS, McCann JD. Treatment of lower eyelid retraction by expansion of the lower eyelid with hyaluronic acid gel. Ophthalmic Plast Reconstr Surg. 2007;23(5):343-8.
14. Morley AM, Malhotra R. Use of hyaluronic acid filler for tear-trough rejuvenation as an alternative to lower eyelid surgery. Ophthalmic Plast Reconstr Surg. 2011;27:69-73.
15. Peckinpaugh JL, Reddy HS, Tower RN. Large particle hyaluronic acid gel for the treatment of lower eyelid retraction associated with radiation-induced lipoatrophy. Ophthalmic Plast Reconstr Surg. 2010;26:377-9.
16. Michael AC, Kane MA. Treatment of tear trough deformity and lower lid bowing with injectable hyaluronic acid. Aesthetic Plast Surg. 2005;29:363-7.
17. Stutman RL, Codner MA. Tear trough deformity: review of anatomy and treatment options. Aesthet Surg J. 2012;32: 426-40.
18. Steinsapir KD, Steinsapir SM. Deep-fill hyaluronic acid for the temporary treatment of the nasojugal groove: a report of 303 consecutive treatments. Ophthalmic Plast Reconstr Surg. 2006;22:344-8.
19. Glaser DA, Patel U. Enhancing the eyes: use of minimally invasive techniques for periorbital rejuvenation. J Drugs Dermatol. 2010;(8 Suppl ODAC Conf Pt 2):s118-28.9:S118-283.
20. Luthra Amit. Subconjunctival hemorrhage post-hyaluronic acid filler for cheeks and tear trough deformity. Dermatol Ther. 2020;33(6):e13902.

CHAPTER 94

Lip Augmentation

Malavika Kohli, Banani Choudhury

KEY MESSAGES

- Lips are the most defining feature of the face; lip augmentation is a commonly done procedure in aesthetic clinics.
- Aesthetic treatment of the lips has changed from localized structural approach to more of a regional treatment approach.
- Assessment is an essential part of treatment. It also helps in the choice, placement, and quantity of product to create natural (naturally looking) beautiful lips.
- Biodegradable hyaluronic acid (HA)-based fillers are most commonly used because of their safety and widespread acceptance.

INTRODUCTION

Lips are one of the most visible of all human organs and perhaps the most emotionally expressive part of the human body, so it is hardly surprising that lip enhancement has become so popular. Soft and pliable, they are also multifunctional, providing an opening for food and beverage consumption, an instrument of both verbal and nonverbal communication, a tactile sensory organ, and an erogenous zone.

DEFINITION

Lips are the upper or the lower fleshy margin of the mouth, consisting of two muscular folds, each with an outer mucosa with a stratified squamous epithelial surface layer.

BASIC FEATURES OF LIPS (FIG. 1)

- *Vermilion border:* The red margin of the upper and lower lip, which commences at the exterior edge of the intraoral labial mucosa (moist line) and extends outward, terminating at the extraoral labial cutaneous junction; a thinly keratinized type of stratified squamous epithelium deeply penetrated by well-vascularized dermal papillae that show through the translucent epidermis to impart the typical red appearance of the lips
- *Vermilion:* Red or pink surface of upper and lower lip
- *Labial or oral commissure:* It is the junction of upper and lower lips lateral to mouth angle
- *Cupid's bow:* The contour of the superior margin of the upper lip
- *Philtrum:* The *vertical* groove in the midline of the upper lip, extending downward from the nasal septum to the tubercle of the upper lip
- *Philtral column:* These are the margins that surround the philtrum
- *Labiomental crease:* The horizontal depression between the lower lip and the chin.

HISTORICAL BACKGROUND

Women of all ethnic and social backgrounds have applied cosmetics to their lips to define or alter their appearance since the Stone Age. Tribal ceremonies involving the introduction

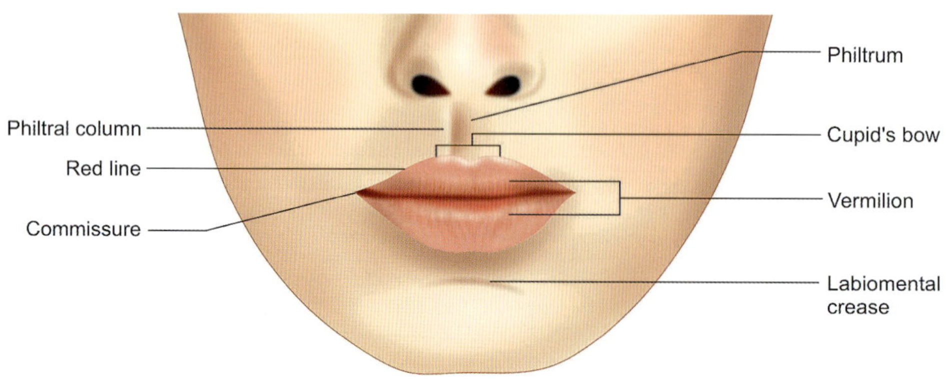

Fig. 1: Basic features of lips: Diagrammatic presentation.

of various materials in the upper and lower lip to alter their shape, usually with the intent to enlarge them, have been practiced in African tribes for centuries.

Rosy lips were desirable, and botanically derived stains such as crushed rose petals were used for their pink color. History of Indian lips is given in **Table 1**.

ANATOMY

Lips are soft pliable anatomical structures that form the oral margin of most vertebrates. They are composed of a surface epidermis (skin), connective tissue, muscle layer, and inner mucosa (from outward in).

Blood supply (through arteries and veins) to the lips has been shown in **Figures 2 and 3**. **Flowchart 1** also describes blood supply of the lips.

Besides supplying the nutrients, blood supply also affects the lip color. For example, in fair skin, which contains no melanocyte, the underlying blood vessels appear through the skin on the lips. Hence, the lips look pink or red.

TABLE 1: Indian lips history.

Era	*Lip trend*
Ancient India, 900 AD	Trend was luscious rosebud lips
Radiant beauty of 1960s and 1970s	Lips were not a separate entity but were seen holistically with face
Glorious smile of 1980s and 1990s	At this time, smile was the attractive part, with beautiful lips being the nonseparable entity
India and worldwide, 2000s: Still big	The ideal of beauty in the 2000s: In last one and half decade, fuller luscious lips became a singular feature of beauty, especially, upper lip is the current preference and most frequently asked for. Indian women avoid over enhanced lips; instead, they express the desire for natural looking refreshed hydrated lips

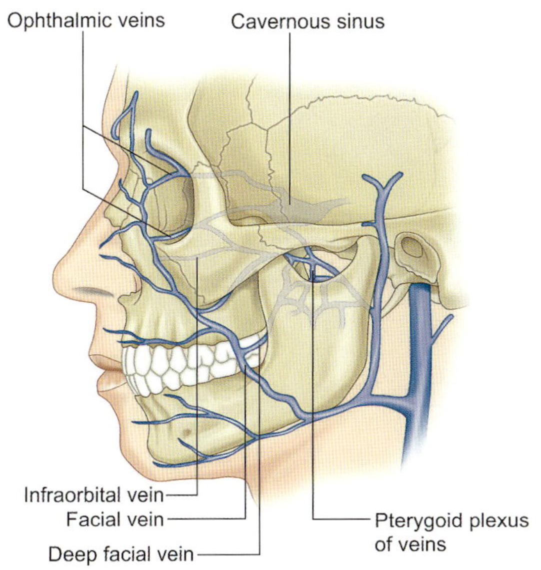

Fig. 2: Veins of the face: Course of facial vein and its anastomosis.

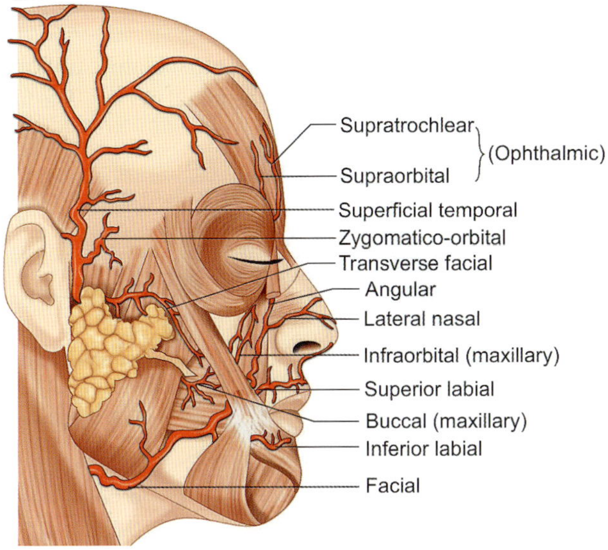

Fig. 3: Arteries of face: Facial artery and its branches supplying the perioral area.

Flowchart 1: Blood supply.

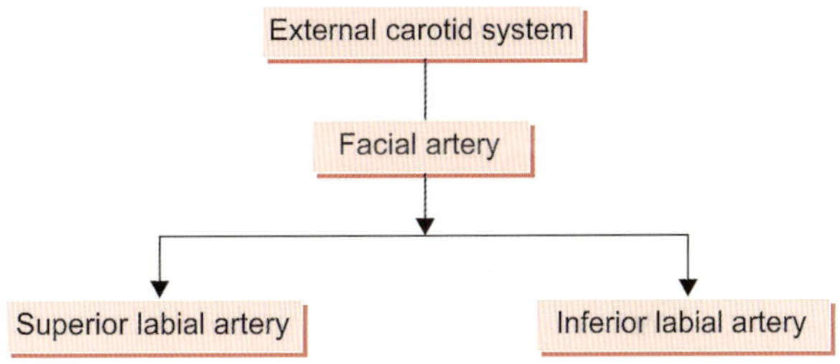

In the case of darker skin, which contains more melanin and is visually thicker, the effect is less prominent.

Lymphatic Drainage (Lips and Perioral Region)[1,2]

Lymphatic drainage from the upper lip is unilateral except for the midline. The lymphatics coalesce to form five primary trunks that mainly lead to the ipsilateral submandibular nodes, with some drainage also going to the periparotid lymph nodes. Occasionally, some drainage may occur to the ipsilateral submental lymph nodes. The lower lip lymphatics also coalesce to form five primary trunks that lead to bilateral submental nodes from the central lip and unilateral submandibular lymph nodes from the lateral lip **(Figs. 4 and 5)**.

Nerve Supply

Lips are packed with nerve endings. Besides making them a highly erogenous zone, it is also extremely sensitive when treating them with injectables.

Motor Nerve

The motor innervation to the perioral musculature uniformly is from the seventh cranial nerve (the facial nerve). The facial nerve has temporal, zygomatic, buccal, marginal mandibular, and cervical branches. The buccal and marginal branches primarily supply innervation to the perioral musculature.

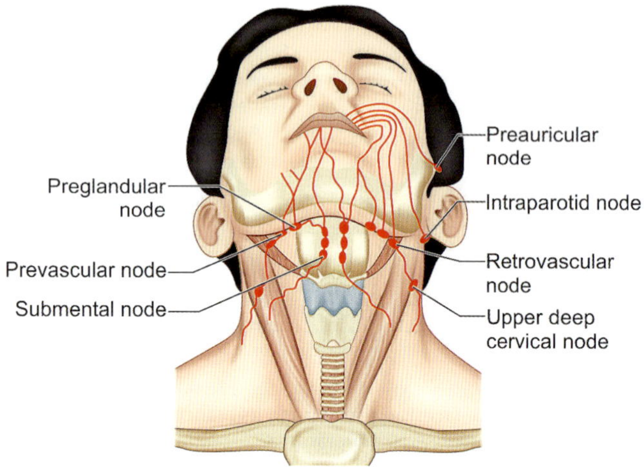

Fig. 4: Lymph nodes draining the perioral area.

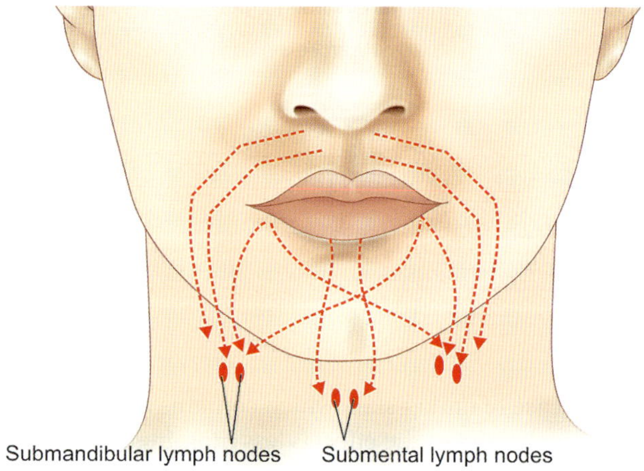

Fig. 5: Lymph drainage from lower and upper lips: Diagrammatic.

Muscle Insertion of Lip

A structure called the modiolus is essential to understand the insertions of the lip musculature. The modiolus is a tendinous thickening at each commissure that serves as an attachment site for several of the upper and lower lip muscles **(Fig. 6)**.[3]

The perioral muscles can be classified into three groups based on function: (1) Lip elevators, (2) lip depressors, and (3) accessory muscles **(Table 2)**.

LIP AUGMENTATION

Ideal Lips

The ideal lips have the following properties **(Fig. 7)**:[4]

- Well-defined philtral columns
- A beautifully shaped Cupid's bow
- Distinct lip edges
- Oral commissures or corners that are neutral or slightly turned up
- Fullness in certain key areas, as indicated by the "+" in **Figure 7**
- Areas of fullness in the lower lip balanced by deficiencies in the upper lip and vice versa

Types of Lips

- *Young lips:* Lips are at a relatively short distance from the base of the nose to the upper vermillion with a distinct vermilion border or "white roll". Good amount of upper tooth shows (4–5 mm) when the upper and lower lips are parted in repose. In young lips, thickness of the lower lip in its central half is 2–3 times the thickness of its upper

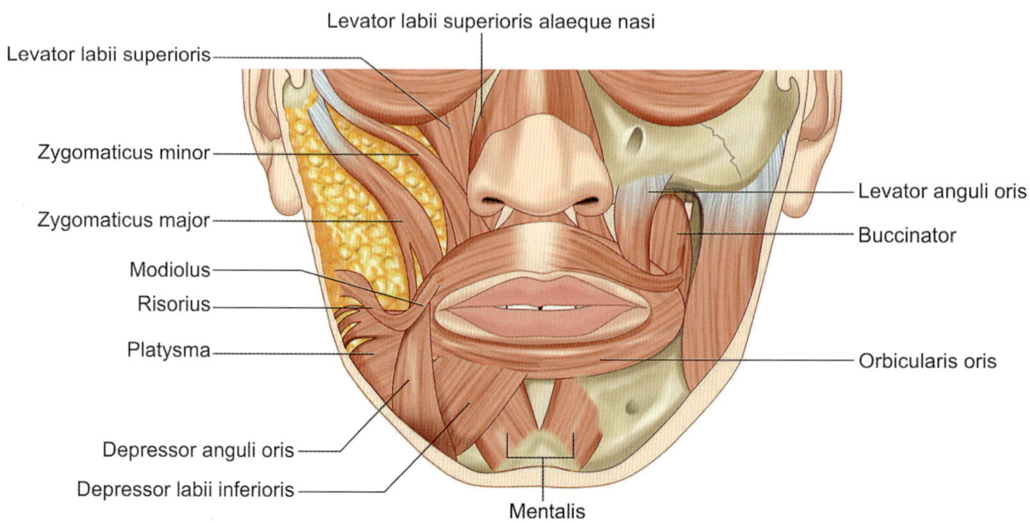

Fig. 6: Muscles around the mouth.

counterpart. The width of the mouth, as measured from corner to corner, is no more than twice the width of the nostril span **(Figs. 8 and 9)**.

TABLE 2: Perioral muscles.

Lip elevators	*Lip depressors*	*Accessory muscles*
• Levator labii superioris alaeque nasi • Levator labii superioris • Zygomaticus major and minor • Levator anguli oris	• Depressor labii inferioris • Orbicularis oris • Mentalis • Depressor anguli oris	• Platysma • Risorius • Masseter

- *Dehydrated lips:* Dryness appears along with flaking and chapping. Scales are also there on lips, in extreme cases, there may also be soreness **(Fig. 10)**.
- *Deflated lips:* Deflated lips have thin vermilion, ill-defined border and/or perioral wrinkles **(Fig. 11)**.
- *Aging lips:* As the lips age, the upper lip flattens and lengthens, philtrum flattens and lengthens, Cupid's bow effaces, and the vermilion thins, leaving a flat, thin profile. The vertical rhytides deepen and appear, the corners of the mouth droops with gravity and volume loss, and the nasolabial folds deepen. All of these changes result in a sad, tired look **(Fig. 12)**.

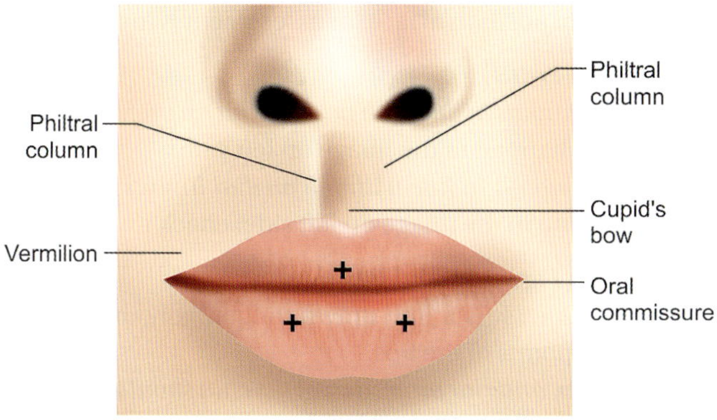

Fig. 7: Ideal lips.

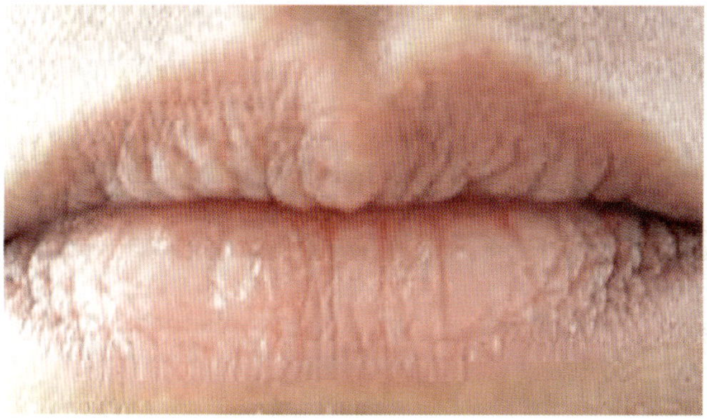

Fig. 10: Dehydrated lips.

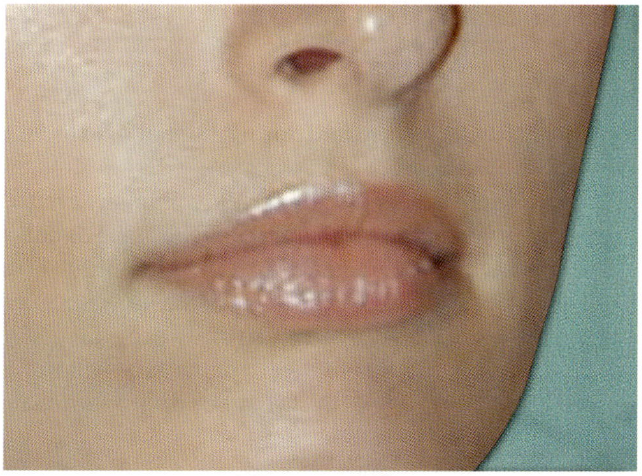

Fig. 8: Caucasian lips.

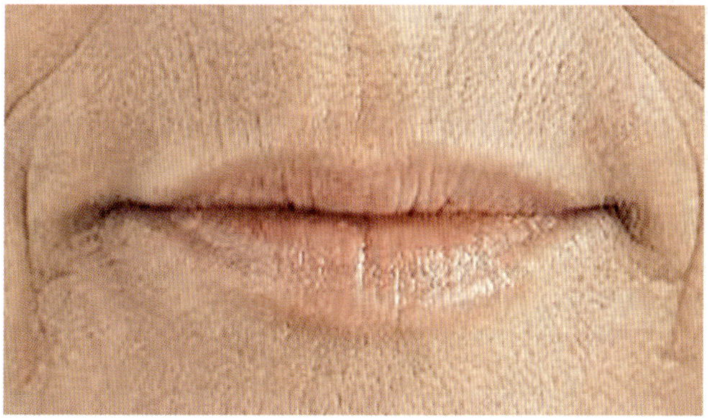

Fig. 11: Deflated lips.

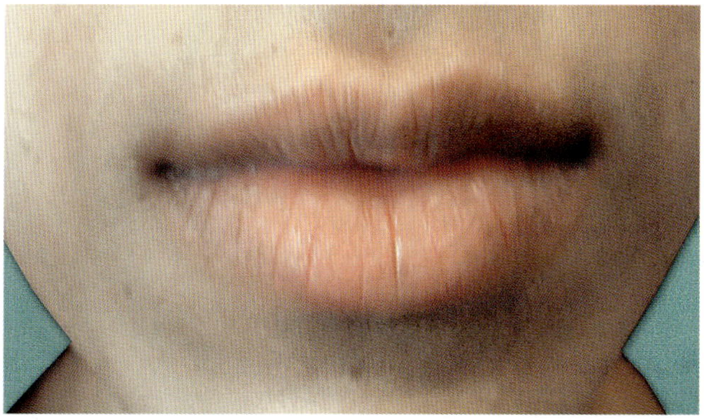

Fig. 9: Indian lips.

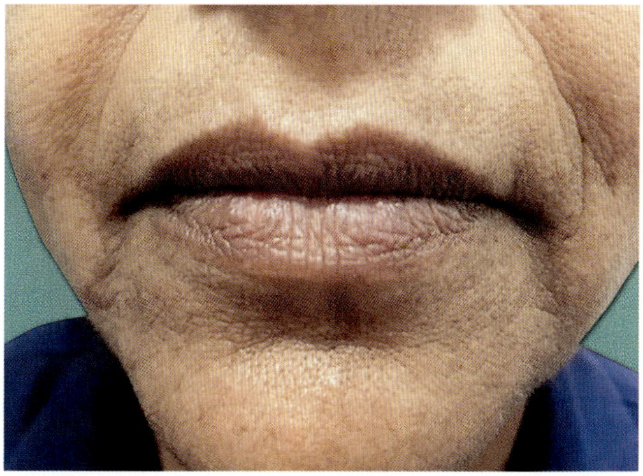

Fig. 12: Aging lips.

Current Trends in Lip Augmentation

In recent years, there is an increasing trend both in young and older women to opt for lip augmentation.

Subtle enhancement of the lip contours and body and lip hydration are trending the most these days. Dark lips are a newer concern and lighter HA fillers or boosters can be injected to get the natural pinkish color of the lips as well as soften and smoothen the dry and dehydrated appearance of younger and older lips.

Pouty lips are no more trending. What is more desired is a natural enhancement of lip borders and shape.

Upper lip volumizing is often asked for by the youth and millennial age groups.

Older people, ask for overall, gentle volumizing as with age the lips tend to get flatter and thinner.

Overall current trends suggest that an injector should be well versed with all the lip augmentation products available that can satisfy their patient needs. A healthy discussion on product choices and longevity will lead to more satisfying and gratifying results.

A well-chosen product and well-planned placement keeping all variables in mind can give well-defined, natural looking lips and not an over filled one.

Relative Contraindications

Contraindications of lip augmentation are given in **Box 1**.

Patient Selection: Assessment of a Patient for Lip Augmentation

After ruling out the contraindications, patient selection is done according to:

- Patient's desire
- Physician assessment

Patient's Desire

It usually depends on the age of the patient—young or old.

- Young patients are usually sure of what they want. Their areas of concern are as follows:
  - Upper lip enhancement
  - Lip border eversion
  - Cupid's bow enhancement
- Old patients want to get rid of sad or tired look but desire natural or fresh look. Their areas of concern are as follows:
  - Vermilion border and vermilion
  - Angle of mouth
  - Marionette lines
  - Perioral aging.

BOX 1: Relative contraindications.

To be handled with caution:

- Patient with history of allergies
- Patient with history of uncontrolled diabetes
- History of connective tissue disorder or poor scarring
- Patient having lupus erythematosus, some products may cause flare ups of lupus
- Patient with blood clotting disorders
- Patient with poor dental health, especially dental abscess/excessive plaque
- History of oral herpes or active herpes
- Person suffering from nerve disorders of the face
- Person with any active diseases that can affect the outcome or increase the risks of lip augmentation including heart disease or asthma

Physicians' Assessment

Patient should be assessed in natural sitting position in a well-lit room. Ideal position of face for assessment is further given.

Front view ***(Fig. 13)****:*

- *Medial canthus in line with nostrils and lip projection:* This does not happen in the image on left side.
- *Angle of mouth in line with the medial limbus:* This does not happen in the image on left side; check image again.

Profile view ***(Figs. 14A and B)****:*[5,6]

- *Riedel plane:* It is a line drawn tangentially through the anterior points of the lips.
- In *women, anterior projection of the chin should be slightly behind or just at the Riedel plane.*

Line in photo is behind chin projection not the same as schematic diagram **(Figs. 14A and B)**.

Lips Examination

Examine lips while relaxed and during animation in order to assess the following:

- *Border* should be clearly defined and minimally everted.
- *Projection:* Maximal projection should be in the middle of the lip, which gently graduates to the medial portion of the lip and slopes laterally to the angle of the mouth.
- *Volume:* Should be in proportion to the face size, e.g., enlarged, full lips in a very petite face will not be aesthetically pleasing as this would be disproportionate.

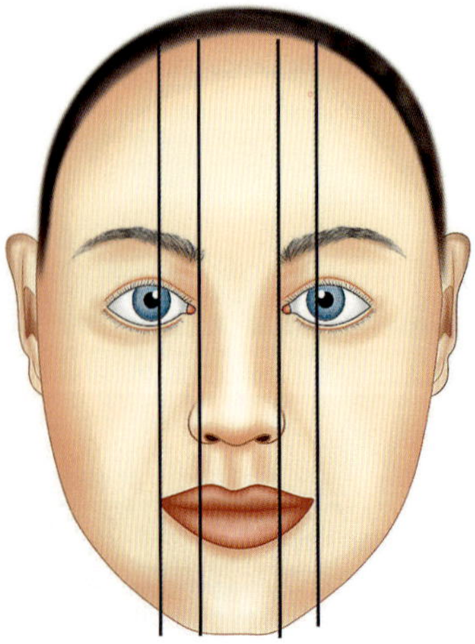

Fig. 13: Front view.

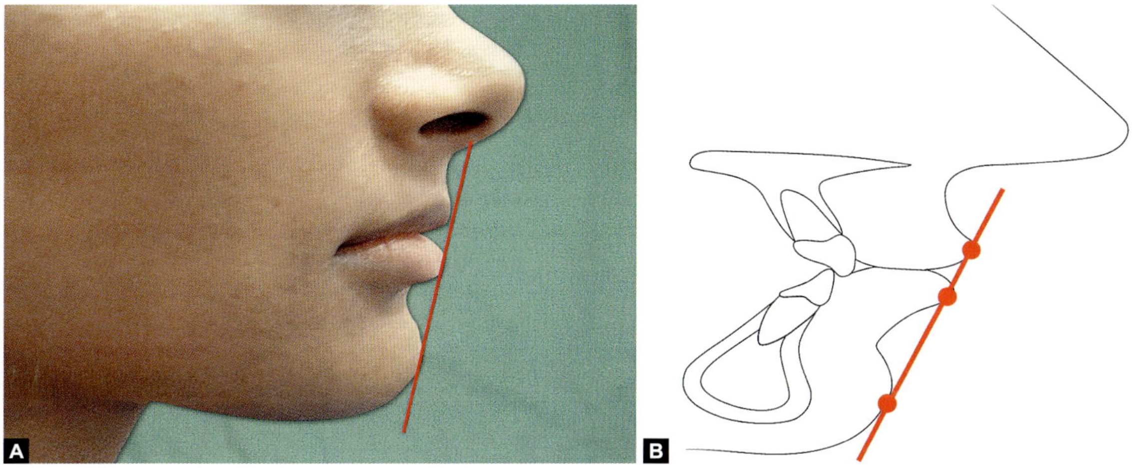

Figs. 14A and B: Profile view.

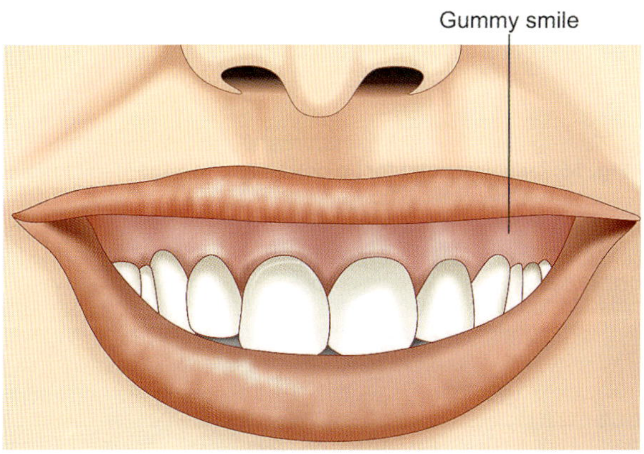

Fig. 15: Gummy smile.

- *Proportions or ratio:* Upper lip (UL): lower lip (LL) (1:1.6).
- *Symmetry:* Look for any deviation from midline or prognathic or retrognathic maxilla, muscle hypo- or hyperactivity.
- Perioral aging.
- *Dental evaluation:* Do a detailed dental evaluation and a dental reference, if necessary, in cases like malalignment or gingival show, etc.
- *Muscle assessment:* Assess muscle activity around the lips as it can contribute to asymmetry and assessment for with botulinum toxin A, if required, in case of hyperactive muscles.
- *Smile evaluation*: *Gummy smile* ***(Fig. 15)****:* The appearance of a person's mouth when smiling in which their teeth appear abnormally small, due to either a high lip line (hypermobile lip), hyperplasia of the gums, which can occur in response to certain medications, e.g., phenytoin, or smaller than normal teeth due to developmental events, tooth eruption abnormalities, orthodontic treatments, and even congenital defects.

Product Selection

Lip Fillers in the Market and their Placement

Name	*Hyaluronic acid (mg/mL)*	*Technology*	*Gel swelling*	*Indication*
1.	12 mg/mL	Patented Vycross	60%	• Used for hydration in case of dry lips • Does not help in shape or size of lips
2.	17.5 mg/mL	Patented Vycross	210%	• Used for plumping and reshaping • Good for younger patients who want visible enhancement
3.	15 mg/mL	Patented Vycross	150%	Used for subtle change and slight enhancement of lips
4.	24 mg/mL	Patented Hylacross	475%	Ideal for patients who want visible pout and volume in lips
5.	20 mg/mL	OBT (Optimal Balance Technology)	-	Used to enhance texture and color of lips, it also helps to smoothen upper lip lines

Procedure

Preparation

- *Tray setting:* Keep emergency tray ready with atropine, adrenaline, and reconstituted hylase in case of vascular occlusion, and nitroglycerin ointment.
- *Procedure room setting:* The room should be well-lit and preferable patients placed facing the light source.
- *Patient preparation:* Patient should be sitting in semireclined position with head supported. Patient is cleansed using betadine solution and spirit gauze.

- *Preoperative photographs:* Photographs to be taken in front and profile view (45° and 90°).
- *Patient consent:* Written informed consent with all the procedural details to be signed by the patient.

INJECTION TECHNIQUES FOR THE LIP REGION[7-9]

For injection purpose, lip can be divided into the following areas:

- Lip border
- Vermilion
- Oral commissures
- Cupid's bow or philtrum.

Lip Border

- Inject in a linear pattern using 1–2 injection sites per quadrant with 0.1–0.2 mL HA filler per quadrant **(Figs. 16 to 18)**.[10]
- Medium-to-heavy-weight product to be injected using 27 G ½" needle.
- Lightweight to be injected using 30 G ½" needle **(Figs. 19A to C)**.

Technical Tips

- Avoid the labial artery and vein in the intraoral submucosal plane.
- When needle is placed in the correct plane, the product flow should be retrograde.

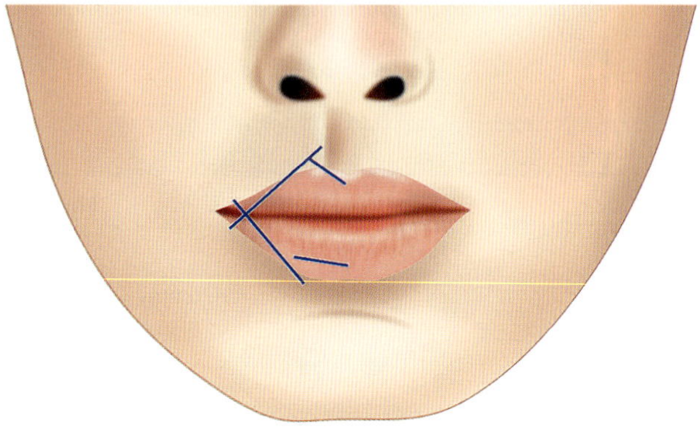

Fig. 16: Injection point for lip border enhancement (pictorial).

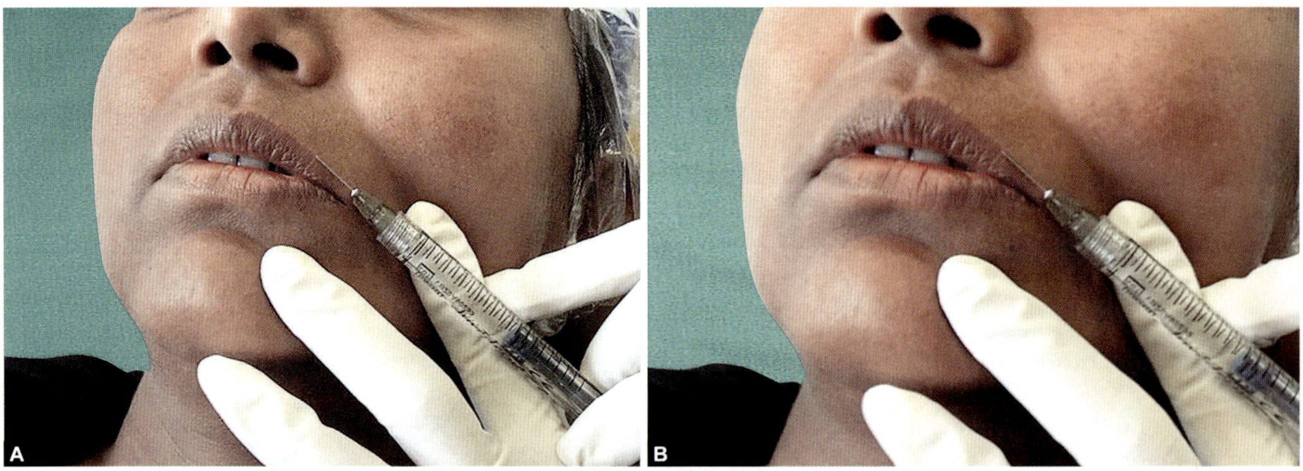

Figs. 17A and B: Upper lip border: Injection points.

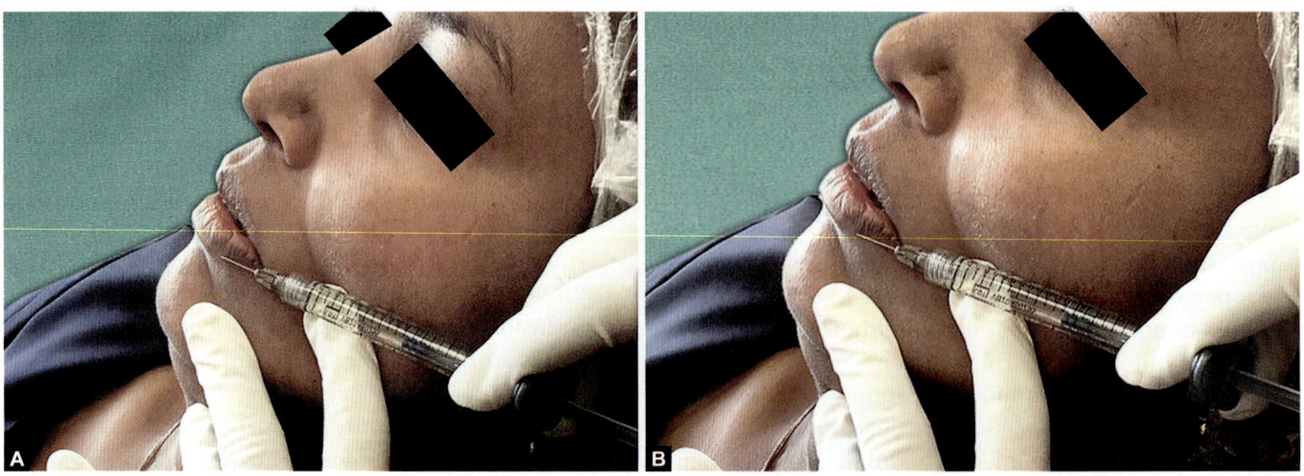

Figs. 18A and B: Lower lip border: Injection points.

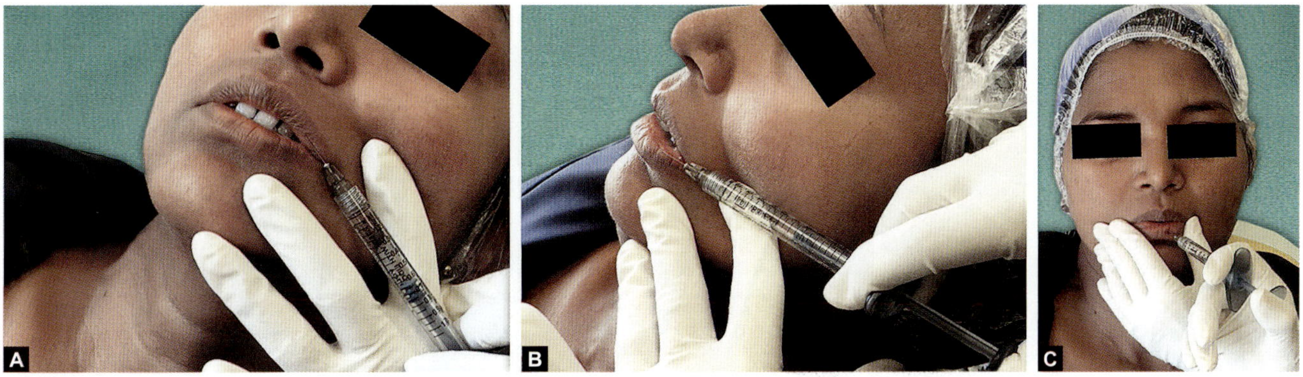

Figs. 19A to C: Injection points: (A) Entry point near the angle of mouth at the junction of wet and dry portion of upper lip; (B and C) Entry point for the lower lip vermilion at the junction of wet and dry.

- Remain superficial.
- When border definition is poor, in case of older patients, product should be placed into the border.
- When border enhancement is desired, in case of young patients, product to be placed just medial to the border which will help in eversion of border and avoid accentuation of white roll.

TIPS

- Inject at the junction of wet and dry portion of the lip, stay in the submucosal plane, neither the needle nor the needle outline should be visible.
- Avoid the labial artery and vein in the intraoral submucosal plane.
- Inject very slowly specially if using a heavier HA product, to avoid lumpiness.
- This is a sensitive area; potential for bruising is high.
- Avoid the labial artery and vein in the intraoral submucosal plane.
- In the upper lip, it is just above the wet and dry junction, in the body of the lip.
- In the lower lip, it is just below the wet and dry junction, in the body of lip.
- To prevent lateral displacement of the bolus, gently stabilize the injected area. between your thumb and forefinger and then inject.
- Assess any asymmetry prior to injection.
- Respect proportion between upper and lower lip.
- Avoid overcorrection.
- Avoid excessive anterior projection of the upper lip.
- Area prone to bruising and edema (suggest use of icepacks).
- Inject very slowly and smoothly.
- Avoid inadvertent displacement of the product which may then appear irregular, bumpy, or beaded.

Vermilion

- *Linear:* Inject in a linear fashion either anterograde or retrograde; choose one site per quadrant using total 0.5–1.0 mL HA filler for both lips.
- Medium-to-high molecular weight (MW) to be injected using 27 G ½" needle.
- Low MW to be injected using 30 G ½" needle.

Bolus Technique 2

Choose three injection sites per quadrant and put a small bolus (<0.05 mL/Bolus), with a total of 0.5–1.0 mL of HA for both lips **(Fig. 20)**.

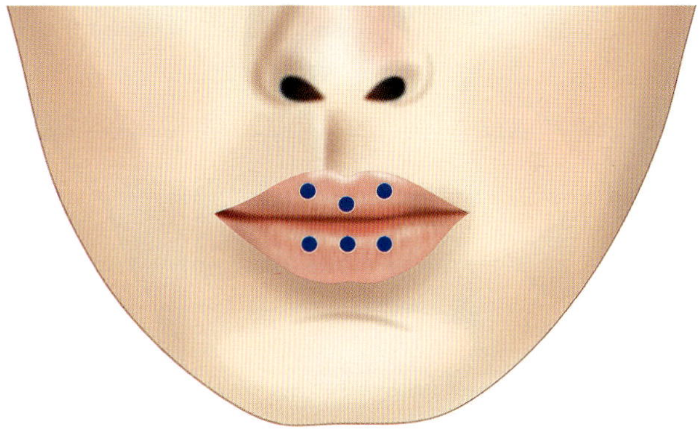

Fig. 20: Injection points for vermilion: Bolus points are three points per quadrant 0.25–0.5 cm apart starting from the bulk of the vermilion (medial to lateral).

Oral Commissures (Figs. 21A to C)

- Inject slowly and observe volume guidelines.
- Give 0.05–0.1 mL bolus, into the oral commissure. Additionally, threading along the upper and lower borders may be required for perioral support of the commissure.

Warning: Stay within 1 cm of the oral commissure to avoid inadvertent placement of product or puncturing of labial artery to avoid a bad bruise or vascular accident.

Cupid's Bow/Kissing Tubercles/Philtrum (Figs. 22A to C)

A very gentle accentuation of the Cupid's bow is desirable without over projection. This can be achieved by placing miniscule amounts in a linear fashion just at the border.

Philtrum column: To be enhanced only if absolutely necessary. In case of ill-defined preexisting column, accentuation can be achieved by injecting few drops of the filler at exact high point of Cupid's bow where philtrum column descends and ends.

Hyaluronic Acid Filler with Lidocaine 0.03%

This product is used to maximize the anesthetic benefit provided by newer HA which has lidocaine 0.03% incorporated. With the linear method, as you enter, a few

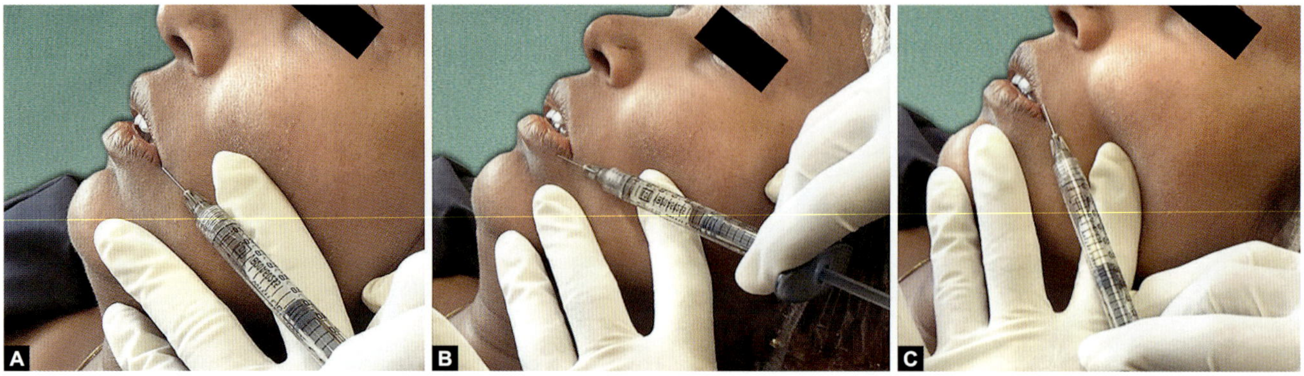

Figs. 21A to C: Needle entry points for oral commissure.

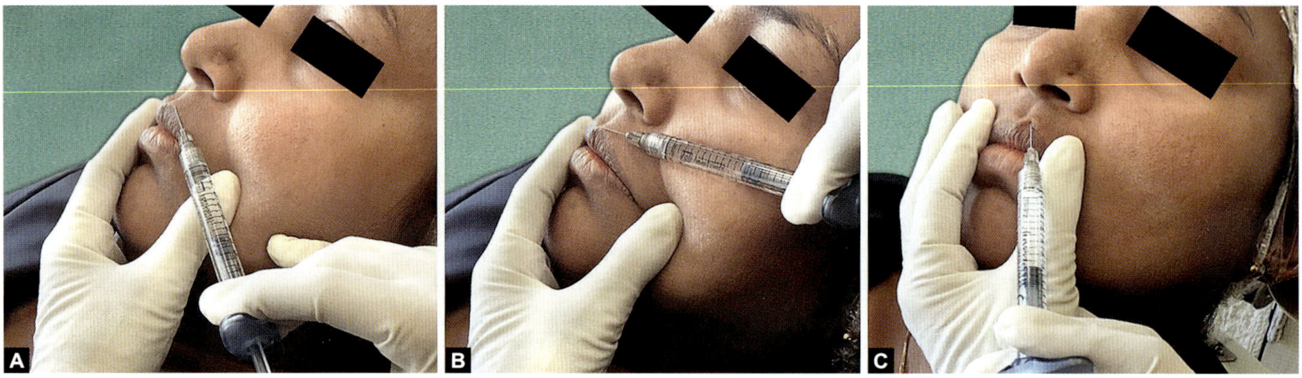

Figs. 22A to C: Injection entry point for Cupid's bow and philtrum.

drops of the product are introduced to immediately initiate the anesthetic effect of lidocaine and reduce the patients discomfort and as the needle is passed upward, small amount of product is injected in antegrade fashion. This is followed by the retrograde threading with the desired amount of product deposition. It reduces pain and discomfort by 80%.[9,10] Necessity of a dental block has been greatly reduced with these filler. For those who are very pain sensitive, a topical lidocaine/prilocaine anesthetic cream can be applied 30 minutes prior.

LIP AUGMENTATION AND MEN

One should always keep in mind following points when performing lip augmentation procedure in males:

- Do not upturn the corners of lips.
- Do not inject complete lips.
- Keep the balance of upper lip and lower lip.
- Use less product. Avoid projection of lips.
- Do not touch the Cupid's bow or philtrum.

Postinjection

- Adequate icing of the injected area
- Antibiotic cream application
- Vitamin K cream
- Gentle massage, only if required.

Instruction to the Patient

Instructions for the patients are given in **Box 2**.

Options Available

Different options are available for lip regeneration and augmentation, which include the following:

- *Fillers:*
  - *Temporary*: HA-based (6–9 months) and autologous stem cell fat transfer (average 5 years)
  - *Permanent*: Polyacrylamide, polymethylmethacrylate (PMMA), collagen, Artecoll,® silicon
- *Machine based*: Lasers like 1064, Q switched Nd: YAG, ablative including fractionated laser
- Platelet-rich plasma (PRP) therapy.

Surgical implants: Artecoll®[11] (Canderm Pharma Inc., Canada), and Gore-Tex™

Out of these options available, HA-based fillers are most commonly used and preferred for lip augmentation because of the following reasons:[12]

- They are safe and have less chances of complications and *least* hypersensitivity reactions.
- HA-based fillers are reversible with hyaluronidase.
- HA-fillers can be used for all parts of the lip allowing for very controlled and predictable results.
- They ease the use.
- They have widespread acceptance.

Strategic positioning helps in aesthetically pleasing results, recreating the same results next time. Many brands are available in the market with different proportions of HA. The methodology used to cross-link light and heavy chain of HA determine the G-prime of the product, its viscosity, gel hardness, and lifting capacity which further determine the depth of the product placement. Hence, the choice of proper product and its correct placement will ensure the best aesthetic results as well as its longevity.

COMPLICATIONS

Hyaluronic acid filler-related or procedure-related immediate and long-term complications may occur as mentioned in the following text.[13]

Short-term/Immediate

- *Swelling:* Multiple injections and handling usually resolves in 2–3 days.
- *Bruise:* Unpredictable, fairly common. Chances of bruising can be reduced by taking detailed history and refining injection technique.
- *Infection:* Aseptic precautions and local antibiotic postinjection can reduce the chance. If occurs, then oral antibiotic may be needed.
- *Asymmetry:* Can be due to swelling, counsel the patient to give 7–15 days for inflammation to settle.
- *Vascular occlusion:* Blanching.

BOX 2: Instructions for the patients.

- Plenty of fluids or water
- No kissing for 48 hours
- No pressing or massaging of lips
- Avoid too much of lip movement
- Postinjection meal preferable with a straw
- Follow-up in 2–3 weeks for a touch up, if required
- Swelling postinjection is fairly common, and may take an anti-inflammatory, if required
- Avoid lip gloss or lip stick for 12 hours
- Avoid soaps or facial cleansers for first 2 days
- Minimize contact between the lips and water for a day

Late

- *Lump/nodule:* Lumps and nodules may occur, which may not be visible but patient may feel it. Mostly lumps resolve in few weeks but, if not, they may have to be dissolved with hyaluronidase.[14]
- Long-term lumps/nodules (delayed inflammatory reaction) with both HA and non-HA filler can occur and may require dissolution through repeated hyaluronidase or extraction through laser or surgery.[15-17]
- *Asymmetry:* It can be corrected by adding or dissolving the filler.

AUTHORS' EXPERIENCE/TECHNIQUE/TIPS

Case 1 (Figs. 23A and B)

Patient wanted natural fresh look, did not want to enhance volume. Also, patient refused to do botulinum toxin (because she is a singer) in depressor anguli oris (DAO) which would have enhanced the effect of filler into the oral commissure.

- *Our opinion:* On assessing, lips have good volume, patient needs *hydration* of lips, angles of mouth, and border correction.
- 1 cc of low molecular weight (LMW) filler was used to correct the border, angles, and vermilion, in older individuals, better to keep angles of mouth in neutral position rather than upturned which may look unnatural.

Case 2: Perioral/Lip Rejuvenation (Cannula) (Figs. 24A and B)

A 60-year-old patient, dehydrated with marked perioral aging (barcode lines):

- *Assessment:* UL:LL ratio is adequate
- *Upper lip:* Border inadequate and volume is less
- Asymmetry
- *Projection:* Incorrect.

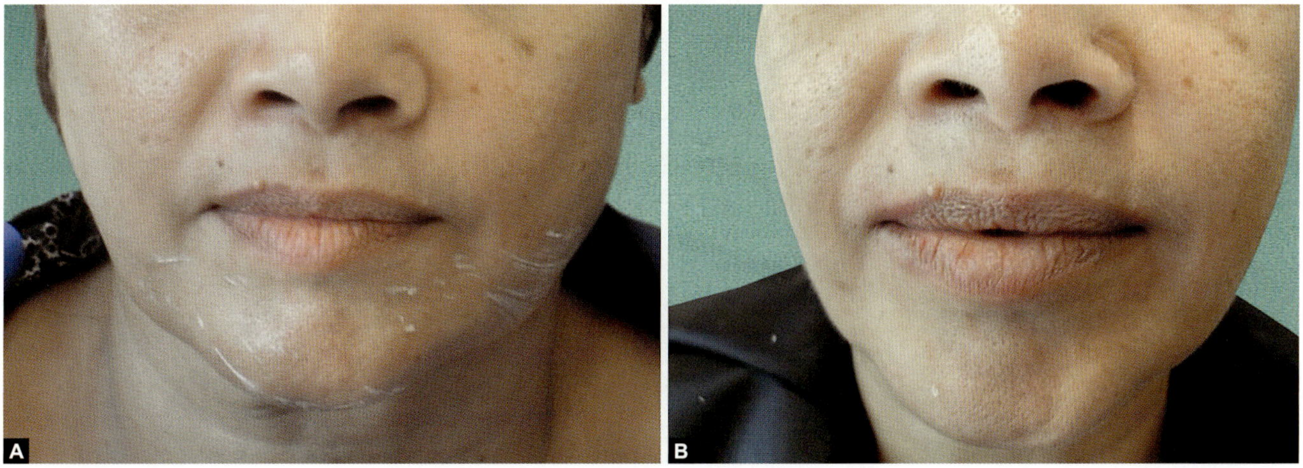

Figs. 23A and B: (A) Before and (B) after immediate postfiller, see the improvement in angle of mouth, no botulinum toxin was used.

Correction: Upper lip was enhanced to complement lower lip which was adequate. A lightweight HA filler with cannula (30 G) was used. To define the vermilion border and vermilion, 0.4 cc of product was used to define the vermilion border, and vermilion. Hydration can be achieved by putting tiny droplets with cannula with no bruising and minimal downtime. Cannula was used for this patient as she could not afford any downtime.

Case 3: Angle of Mouth (Advanced Case) (Figs. 25A and B)

A 55-year-old female with voluminous lips, patient wants angle correction:

- *Assessment:* Very deep nasolabial folds resulting from mid face volume loss, deep marionette lines resulting from lower face volume loss.
- *Correction:* Lips were not touched.

Replaced the volume loss which supported perioral tissue by injecting total 8 cc sequentially in mid-face, nasolabials, and marionette in three sessions over 9 months, improved the angle of mouth and overall lip enhancement.

Case 4: Asymmetry

Right-sided muscle hyperactivity over a period of time.

Plan of action: First treat with botulinum toxin in levator labii superioris and depressor anguli oris, once muscle relaxes, over subsequent sessions, reassess; filler may be considered for remaining asymmetry **(Fig. 26)**.

Case 5: Upper Lip Augmentation (Needle)

Young patient for lip augmentation.

Correction: 0.8-cc lightweight filler was used for the following:

- Eversion of upper lip border
- Projection of vermilion
- Enhancement of Cupid's bow/philtrum/kissing tubercles **(Figs. 27A and B)**.

Case 6: Creating Ideal Lip Proportions

Patient wanted a glamorous/sensuous look: (UL:LL = 1:1) and upper lip should project 1–2 mm beyond lower lip:

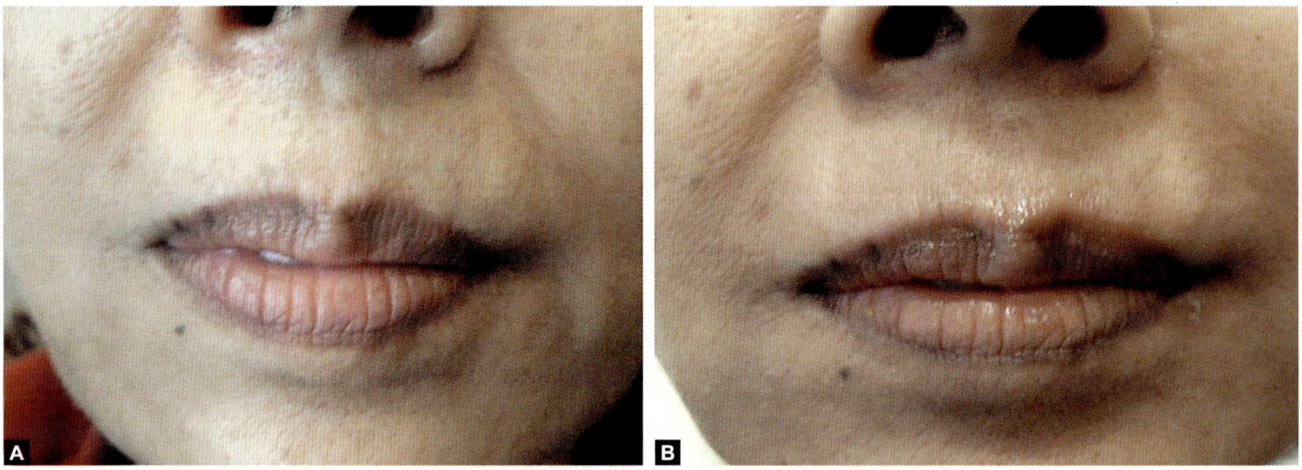

Figs. 24A and B: Change is vermilion border and vermilion post-hyaluronic acid filler: (A) Before; (B) After (immediate).

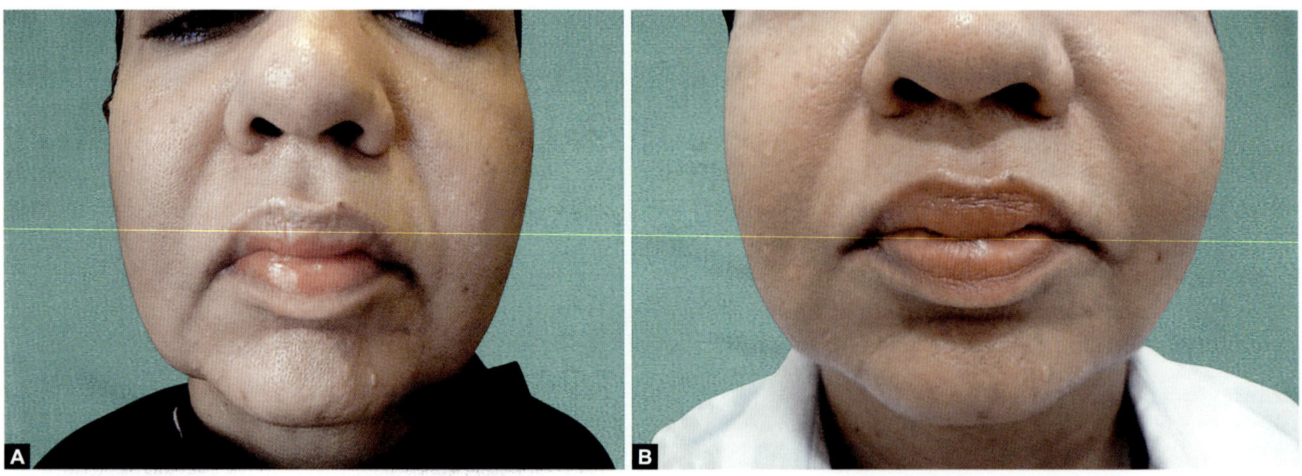

Figs. 25A and B: (A) Before and (B) after (9 months) injecting 8 cc of hyaluronic acid filler in midface which resulted in improvement of angles.

- *Plan of action:* Lower lip was not touched.
- *Upper lip:* Vermilion 1 cc in first session and 1 cc in second session (3 months later).
- *Angle of mouth:* 0.1 mL on each side bolus **(Figs. 28A and B)**.

Case 7: Over the Top

- Patient desired over inflated lips.
- 1.5 cc of medium-weight filler was used in this patient **(Figs. 29A and B)**.

Case 8: Young Lips Filling with Cannula

Light hydrating filler was used for lip rejuvenation and hydration.

Why was a cannula used? To deliver controlled small amount in the lip body, as lips are already full and the patient did not want any downtime. It helped to improve the color of lips **(Figs. 30A and B)**.

Case 9: Hyaluronic Acid Nodule

These appear as cystic, sclerotic, or edematous well-defined palpable lesions which occur either from infections in areas of this soft-tissue coverage or superficial injections **(Figs. 31A to F)**.

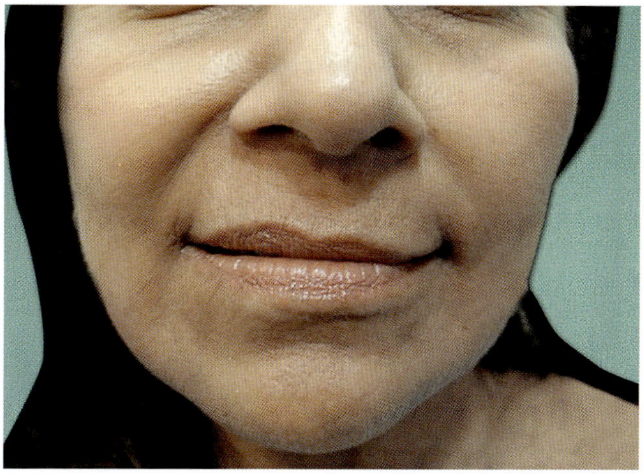

Fig. 26: Pre-existing asymmetry.

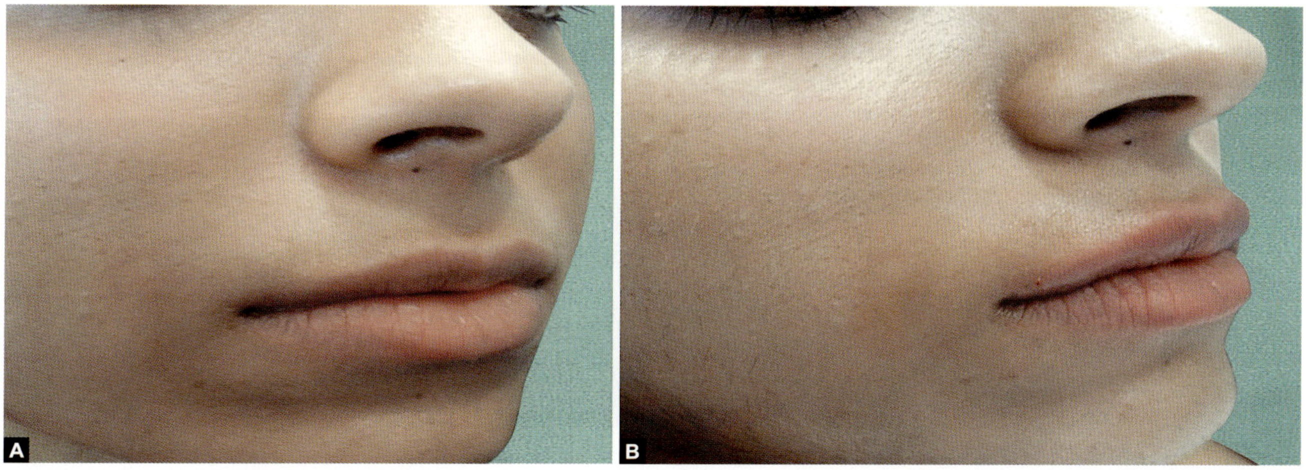

Figs. 27A and B: Young patient desiring luscious lips: (A) Before; (B) After (Immediate post: no bruise).

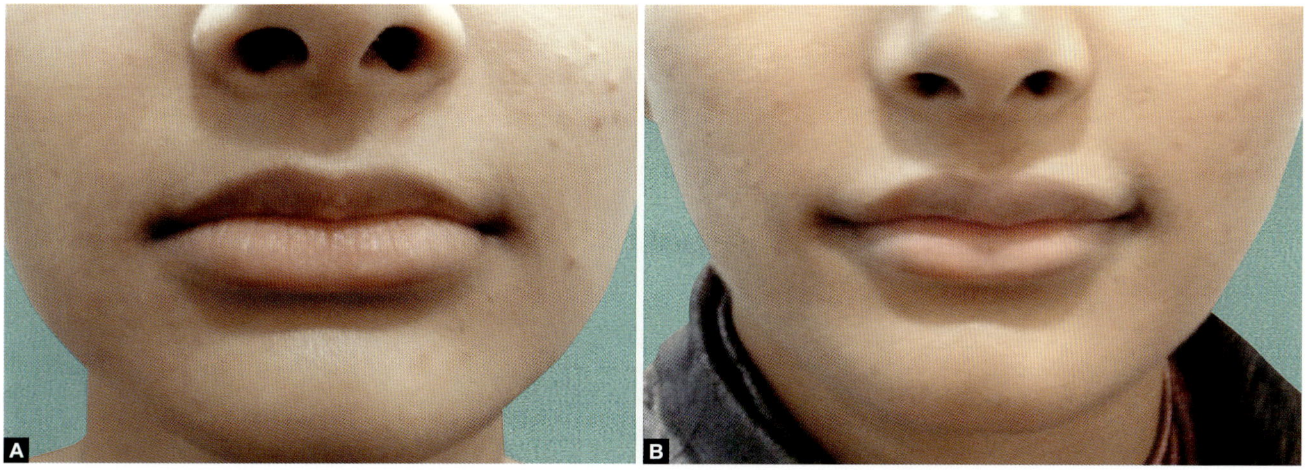

Figs. 28A and B: Young patient desiring glamorous lips: (A) Before; (B) After.

PEARLS

- Indian lips are prone to be darker. Causes are as follows:
  - Lip smacking
  - Nutritional
  - Actinic
  - Smoking
  - Dry/dehydration.
- Patients, especially Indians, seek options for improving color:
  - Change of habits
  - Ultraviolet protection
  - Lightening agents
  - HA fillers provide excellent and instant option in giving pinker/fresher/hydrated lips. In case of fullness, a light HA product can be used.
- HA filler with lidocaine is the preferred choice. Technique has been discussed earlier. It reduces pain and discomfort by 80%. Necessity of a dental block has been greatly reduced with these filler. For those who are very pain sensitive, a topical lidocaine/prilocaine anesthetic cream can be applied 30 minutes prior.
- Sterile ice packs application pre- and postinjection helps to alleviate pain and swelling and reduce chance of bruising.
- Topical anesthesia: Authors have found too thick or prolonged application of topical cream does not give additional anesthetic benefit. So, we prefer to apply a thin layer with a cling film and reapply in 15 minutes. Extra cream may give pseudohydration effect.
- Mapping the amount of product in specific area gives good result.

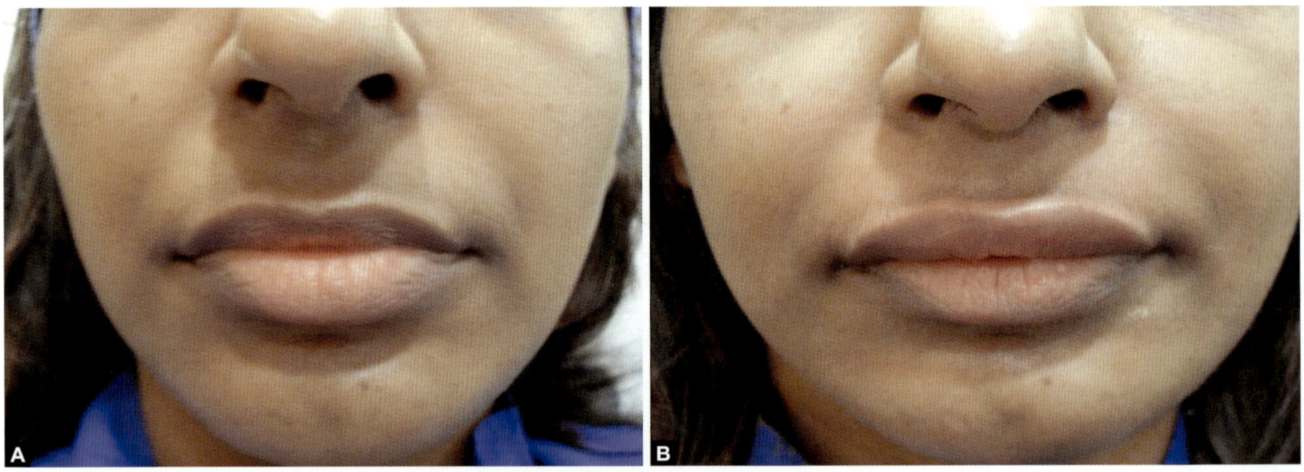

Figs. 29A and B: Over the top lips: (A) Before; (B) After.

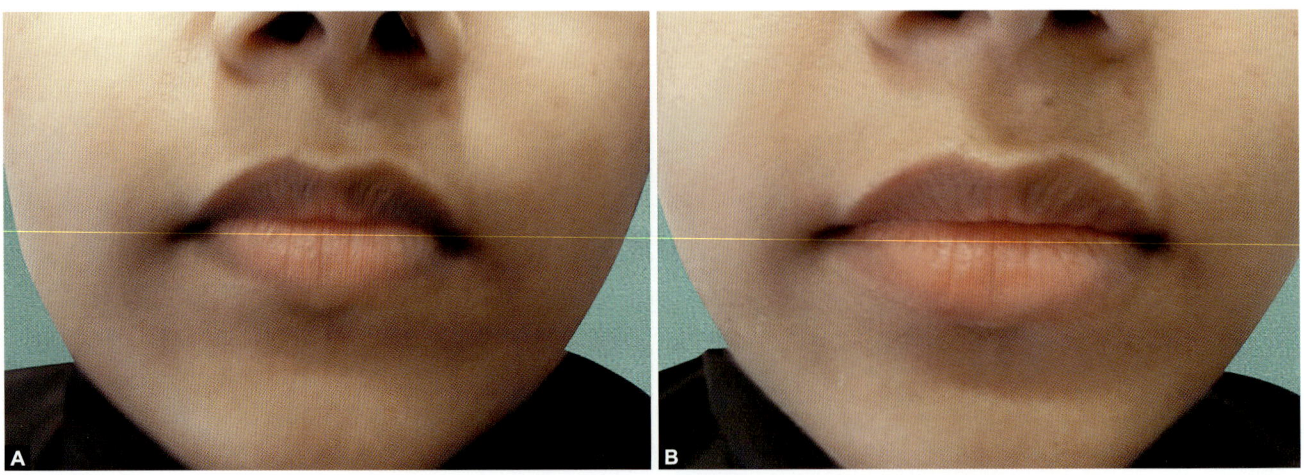

Figs. 30A and B: Lip rejuvenation with a hydrating filler: (A) Before; (B) After.

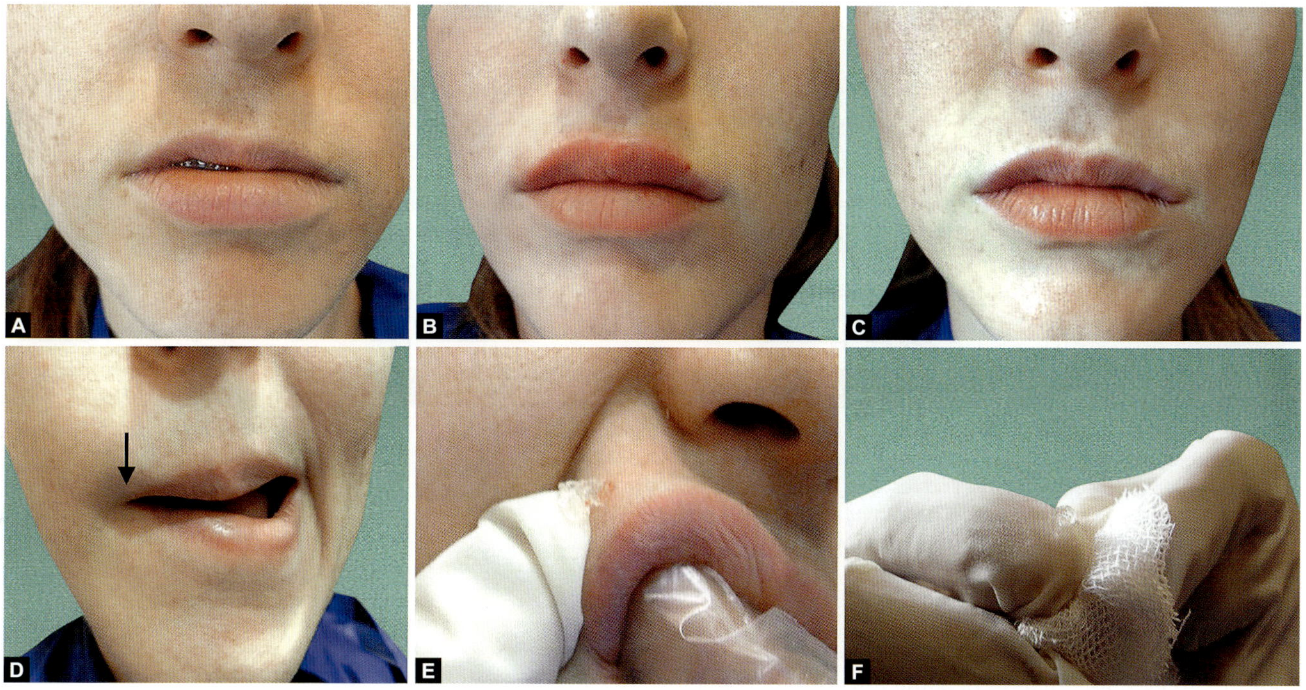

Figs. 31A to F: Hyaluronic acid nodule: (A) Before; (B) Immediately after; (C) After 6 months; (D) Indicating the nodule; (E and F) Extraction of hyaluronic acid lump.

Management: In this case, a simple puncture (incision and drainage) was done to extract the filler.

REFERENCES

1. Parwar BJ. (2013). Lips and perioral region anatomy. [online] Available from: www.emedicine.medscape.com/article/835209. [Last accessed July, 2022].
2. AM-Medicine. (2014). Lymphatic system-Lymphatic drainage of oral cavity. [online] Available from: www.am-medicine.com/2014/10/lymphatic-system-lymphatic-drainage-of- oral-cavity.html. [Last accessed July, 2022].
3. Alfen NV, Gilhuis HJ, Keijzers JP, Pillen S, Van Dijk JP. Quantitative facial muscle ultrasound: feasibility and reproducibility. Muscle Nerve. 2013;48(3):375-80.
4. Reid D, Gordon A. Ideal lips. [online] Available from: www.restoraaustin.com/face/lip-augmentation-austin-tx/ [Last accessed July, 202].
5. Guyuron B, Kinne BM. Aesthetic Plastic Surgery Video Atlas. New York: Elsevier Health; 2011.
6. Carruthers A, Carruthers J, Hardas B. A validated lip fullness grading scale. Dermatol Surg. 2008;34:S161-6.
7. Luthra A. Shaping lips with fillers. J Cutan Aesthet Surg. 2015;8(3):139-42.
8. Chiu A, Fabi S, Dayan S, Nogueira A. Lip injection techniques using small-particle hyaluronic acid dermal filler. J Drugs Dermatol. 2016;15(9):1076-82.
9. Fischer TC, Sattler G, Gauglitz GG. Hyaluron filler containing lidocaine on a CPM basis for lip augmentation: reports from practical experience. Facial Plast Surg. 2016;32(3): 283-8.
10. Fischer T, Sattler G, Gauglitz G. Lidocaine-containing hyaluronic acid filler on a CPM® basis for lip augmentation: Experience from clinical practice. [Article in German]. Hautarzt. 2016;67(6):472-8.
11. Hilinski JM, Cohen SR. Soft tissue augmentation with ArteFill. Facial Plast Surg. 2009;25(2):114-9.
12. Smith SR, Vander Ploeg HM, Sanstead M, Albright CD, Theisen MJ, Lin X. Functional safety assessments used in a randomized controlled study of small gel particle hyaluronic acid for lip augmentation. Dermatol Surg. 2015;41 (Suppl 1):S137-42.
13. Rodrigues-Barata AR, Camacho-Martínez FM. Undesirable effects after treatment with dermal fillers. J Drugs Dermatol. 2013;12(4):e59-62.
14. Shahrabi Farahani S, Sexton J, Stone JD, Quinn K, Woo SB. Lip nodules caused by hyaluronic acid filler injection: report of three cases. Head Neck Pathol. 2012;6(1):16-20.
15. Artzi O, Loizides C, Verner I, Landau M. Resistant and recurrent late reaction to hyaluronic acid-based gel. Dermatol Surg. 2016;42(1):31-7.
16. Curi MM, Cardoso CL, Curra C, Koga D, Benini MB. Late-onset adverse reactions related to hyaluronic acid dermal filler for aesthetic soft tissue augmentation. J Craniofac Surg. 2015;26(3);782-4.
17. Beleznay K, Carruthers JD, Carruthers A, Mummert ME, Humphrey S. Delayed-onset nodules secondary to a smooth cohesive 20 mg/mL hyaluronic acid filler: cause and management. Dermatol Surg. 2015;41(8):929-39.

CHAPTER 95

Hand Rejuvenation

Maya Vedamurthy

KEY MESSAGES

- Hands age at the same rate as the face.
- Hands are one of the first areas in the body to show visible signs of aging.
- Hand rejuvenation complements and restores an overall perceived youthful look.
- Cosmetic hand rejuvenation is now becoming increasingly popular.
- There are several options for hand rejuvenation.

INTRODUCTION

Hands are an essential marker of aging next to the face and have become a popular part of the human body in terms of rejuvenation. Hands are more important not only in utility but also for interpersonal relationships and contact.[1]

Both intrinsic and extrinsic factors contribute to the aging of hands and involve all three layers: Skin, muscle, and bones. Rejuvenation of aging hands, therefore, needs a multimodal approach to restore its youthfulness.[2]

HAND AESTHETICS

Hands age at the same rate as the face and chest and form the most visible parts of the human body. They are also said to reveal the actual age of an individual. An anatomically and functionally healthy hand with less visible veins is a prerequisite to an aesthetically pleasing hand.

Types of hands have been classified by Kretschmer and are based on body habitus as follows:[3]

- *Leptosome (aesthenic) type:* Ectomorph with long slender hands and fingers
- *Athletic type:* Mesomorph characterized by rough wider hands
- *Pyknic type:* Endomorph characterized by short wide dorsum and short conical fingers

An aesthetically pleasing hand should have Phi (φ) proportions, and all rejuvenation procedures should conform to maintain this golden ratio.[4] When a golden Phi caliper is applied to the hand, it will be noticed that each of the phalanges of each finger is golden to the next in all five fingers.

BASIC ANATOMY RELEVANT TO VOLUMETRIC REJUVENATION

The dorsum of the hand has three fatty laminae separated by three thin fascial layers. The dorsal superficial lamina (DSL) is the uppermost and has no apparent structures within it. Beneath this is the dorsal superficial fascia, and below this is the dorsal intermediate lamina (DIL) with large veins and sensory nerves of the dorsum of the hand. The deepest is the dorsal deep lamina (DDL), which contains the extensor tendons of the hand. Beneath the DDL are the dorsal interosseous muscles and metacarpal bones. Generally, dermal fillers are placed into the deep lamina above the metacarpal plane.

Aging of the hand is due to both intrinsic and extrinsic factors and can be distinguished clinically **(Box 1)**.

BOX 1: Signs of extrinsic and intrinsic aging.

Extrinsic	*Intrinsic*
• Solar lentigines	• Wrinkles
• Actinic keratoses	• Fat atrophy
• Solar purpura	• Dermal thinning
• Punctate hyperpigmentation	• Visible veins and tendons
	• Visible skeletal architecture

PATHOPHYSIOLOGY OF AGING HAND

The aged hand is characterized by thinning of the epidermal and dermal layers giving rise to wrinkled and translucent lax skin. Volume loss occurs due to decreased subcutaneous fat, muscle atrophy, and decreased bone density of the metacarpal and carpal bones. The combination of thinning skin and volume loss gives rise to skeletonized look with the prominence of bones, joints, tendons, and veins. There is also a decreased density of adnexal structures such as hair follicles and sebaceous glands with aging.

Photoaging of hands leads to textural and pigmentary changes along with the appearance of solar lentigines, actinic keratosis, and seborrheic keratosis.

TABLE 1: Busso hand volume severity scale.[5]

Rating	*Definition*
0	No tendons are exposed
1	One or two tendons are slightly exposed
2	All three central tendons are partially exposed
3	All three central tendons are partially exposed, with one or two tendons fully exposed
4	All three central tendons are fully exposed

TABLE 2: Merz hand grading scale.[6]

Grade	*Definition*
0	No loss of fatty tissue
1	Mild loss of fatty tissue and slight visibility of veins
2	Moderate loss of fatty tissue and mild visibility of veins and tendons
3	Severe loss of fatty tissue and moderate visibility of veins and tendons
4	Very severe loss of fatty tissue marked by visibility of veins and tendons

There are two grading scales for assessing the severity of volume loss in the hands.

1. Busso hand volume severity scale (BHVSS) based on tendon exposure and visibility **(Table 1)**
2. Merz hand grading scale (MHGS) based on loss of fatty tissue and visibility of veins **(Table 2)**

HAND REJUVENATION MODALITIES

Approach to Management

A routine medical history should be carried out to ascertain the individual's fitness to undergo the chosen hand rejuvenation procedure. History of any local injury, surgery, or previous filler injection is to be obtained.

Counseling should be done regarding different procedures for hand rejuvenation with a focus on downtime and postoperative care. Baseline photographs of the dorsum of the hand should be taken for comparison after the procedure.

Hand rejuvenation procedures aim at both epidermal and dermal changes along with volume loss of subcutaneous tissue.

Epidermal rejuvenation improves cell turnover, corrects pigmentary abnormalities, and stimulates collagen and elastin production in the dermis.

Dermal rejuvenation aims at neocollagenesis to improve the rhytides and wrinkles in the skin and to decrease the skin laxity and visibility of veins.

Restoring volume loss by replacing lost subcutaneous fat helps to plump up the dorsa of hands, thereby reducing vascular and bony prominences **(Box 2)**.

This chapter will focus on the revolumization of hands with fillers.

BOX 2: Options for hand rejuvenation.

Epidermal rejuvenation
- Superficial chemical peels
- Lasers:
  - Q-switched lasers
  - Nonablative resurfacing lasers
  - Ablative fractionated lasers
- Lights and energy devices:
  - Intense pulsed light (IPL)
  - Photodynamic therapy (PDT)
  - Radiofrequency

Dorsal hand vein treatment
- Sclerotherapy
- Endovenous vascular ablation
- Phlebectomy

Volume replacement
- Fat transfer
- Injectables

REVOLUMIZATION WITH DERMAL FILLERS

Fat

Fat was one of the first fillers to be used in soft-tissue augmentation of the hand. Fournier was the first to describe fat transfer for dorsa of hands and fingers. He injected a bolus of fat, which was then massaged all over the hand, including dorsa of fingers.[7] Adipose tissue has several advantages, like it is easy to obtain, is cost-effective, is autologous, and has good tissue integration. However, fat transfer was not favored because of the unpredictable longevity, which ranged from 4 months to 3 years.[8]

The introduction of microautologous fat transplantation (MAFT) can be used in hand rejuvenation. It augments the dorsum of the hand and rejuvenates the skin via adipocyte stem cells.[9]

Hyaluronic Acid

With aging, there is a gradual decrease in hyaluronic acid (HA), leading to dehydration and wrinkling of the skin as well as volume loss. Noncross-linked HA, when injected intradermally, stimulates neocollagenesis leading to an increase in dermal thickness and elasticity.

In contrast, cross-linked HA which is not degraded quickly acts as a volume filler in addition to biostimulation. Therefore, in hand rejuvenation, HA can be used either to increase hydration or due to its benefits as a volume filler. The technique of injecting HA for hand rejuvenation depends on the choice of filler and the indication for which it is used.

Hydrating HA fillers are indicated for injection in the superficial dermis and dermoepidermal junction and are intended to rehydrate the skin to restore the skin's quality and texture.

Volumizing HA fillers are indicated for injection in the deep plane along the tendons and are intended to restore volume loss similar to autologous fat.

The longevity of HA filler depends on the gel particle size and degree of cross-linking and varies from 3 to 18 months.

Calcium Hydroxylapatite

Calcium hydroxylapatite (CaHA) is the first Food and Drug Administration (FDA) approved injectable filler for hand rejuvenation. CaHA filler is made of CaHA microspheres suspended in an aqueous gel, which can be stored at room temperature for up to 2 years. The microspheres in the filler stimulate collagenesis in and around CaHA particles resulting in volume restoration.[10] CaHA filler is mixed with a local anesthetic agent before treatment and administered subcutaneously. Recently, CaHA is injected with concomitant visualization by ultrasound at 15 MHz to ensure safety in the correct plane.[11]

The results obtained with CaHA last up to 1 year approximately.[12]

POLY-L-LACTIC ACID

Poly-L-lactic acid (PLLA) was first used by Redaelli for the rejuvenation of the hand in 2006.[13] It is a semipermanent filler which lasts up to 2 years. It has the property of stimulating neocollagenesis by fibroblasts. PLLA filler (367.5 mg/vial) as a lyophilized powder is to be mixed the day before treatment with 1 mL of 1% lidocaine with or without epinephrine and 5 mL of sterile water. However, larger dilutions and more extended reconstitution periods are preferred for safety. The final product is injected into the reticular dermis and subcutaneous tissue planes and massaged well. Following the procedure, patients are instructed to follow the rule of "5-5-5", i.e., massage the treated area for 5 minutes, 5 times a day for 5 days to prevent nodule formation.[14]

Polycaprolactone

Another biostimulating dermal filler is polycaprolactone (PCL). The PCL microsphere is suspended in carboxymethyl cellulose gel and has the property of stimulating neocollagenesis. The product is injected in the subcutaneous plane and massaged well. The advantage of PCL filler is that it shows immediate results and provides a choice of longevity based on the type of product used.[15] There are four versions of this filler, and the PCL-2 version has been studied in hand rejuvenation. PCL is a medical polymer that has entered the filler market **(Table 3)**.

PREOPERATIVE EVALUATION

A general assessment of the hand, including normal function and anatomy, is essential. One should look for muscle movement, strength, and deformity, if any. A good collateral arterial blood flow has to be ascertained using Allen's test.[16] The dorsal hand's degree of aging has to be graded based on one of the validated systems.

TABLE 3: Injectable fillers for hand rejuvenation.

Fillers	*Products*	*Depth of injections*	*Longevity*
Fat	Autologous	Subdermal or intramuscular	4 months to 3 years
Hyaluronic acid (HA)	Restylane JUVÉDERM VOLUMA	Dermo-epidermal junction, superficial dermis, deep-dermis subcutaneous	6–18 months
Calcium hydroxylapatite (CaHA)	RADIESSE	Subcutaneous	12–15 months
Poly-L-lactic acid (PLLA)	Sculptra	Deep dermis subdermal	18–24 months
Polycaprolactone (PCL)	Ellansé	Subcutaneous	*Tunable longevity:* 3–5 years

CONTRAINDICATIONS

- History of allergy to filler material, lidocaine, and gram-positive bacterial proteins
- Previous hand surgery/trauma
- Advanced photoaged/photodamaged skin
- A poor collateral arterial blood flow
- Indwelling orthopedic hardware
- Raynaud's syndrome
- Carpal tunnel syndrome
- Rheumatoid arthritis
- *History of bruising tendency:* Arnica and bromelain supplements have been advocated 1–2 days before and after treatment to minimize bruising.

PROCEDURE

Counseling includes explaining the procedure in detail and fulfilling all the criteria for a cosmetic treatment. Written informed consent is obtained. A photograph of both hands lying prone on a flat surface, with fingers extended, is taken.

The patient is instructed to remove all ornaments such as finger rings and wash hands thoroughly with chlorhexidine. The treatment area is cleaned with an antiseptic solution. In situations where numbing cream is chosen for the procedure, the cream is applied 45 minutes before the procedure.

The technique is to place the patient in the Trendelenburg position to reduce vein pressure, thus avoiding accidental venepuncture and bleeding. The hand is placed on a flat surface and draped with sterile materials. The injector holds the hands loosely in a semiflexed resting position to allow easy movement of the syringe.

Treatment Protocol

Multiple techniques are available, and their choices depend on the indication and comfort of the injector. The dermal

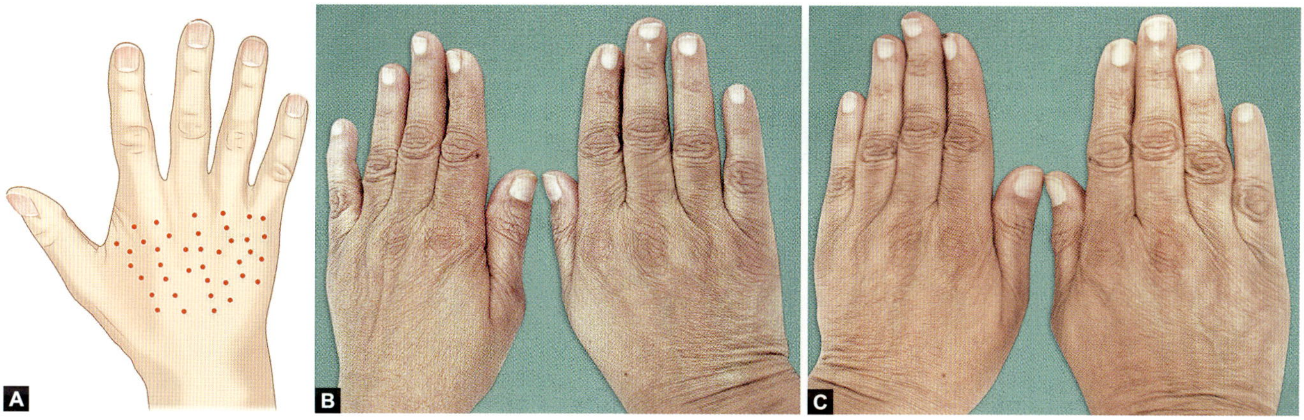

Figs. 1A to C: Technique 1: (A) Microdroplet technique showing injection points; (B) Before; (C) After microdroplet injection technique using hyaluronic acid (HA).

fillers are injected using either a needle or a cannula based on the physician's discretion and choice of the product.

Technique 1: Skin Boosters for Hydration—Microdroplets Technique

Small particle HA (SP-HA) with a low degree of cross-linking rejuvenates the skin by increasing the hydration. This SP-HA is injected as intradermal microdroplets that deposit small quantities (10 μL) of the product throughout the dorsa of hands.

Several techniques like threading, fanning, and puncture may be used, but micro depot injections are preferred for precise delivery into the deep dermis **(Figs. 1A to C)**.

Using a 32G ½ inch needle provided with the product, micro depot injections are carried out, placing the product into the deep dermis at an angle <45° from the skin surface. The injections are spaced approximately 0.5–1 cm apart. Some SP-HAs are delivered using specialized injection devices such as the smart click syringe that comes with the product. A total of 1 mL per hand is injected. The area is massaged using an ultrasound gel to disperse the filler uniformly.

The procedure is usually repeated once a month or once a year based on the product chosen for the purpose.

Technique 2: Bolus Injections—Tenting Technique

This technique is used for dermal augmentation using CaHA or volumizing HA filler. Local anesthesia is administered either in conjunction with or preceding the use of dermal filler. Here, the hand's dorsal skin is lifted between the physician's thumb and index finger to separate the underlying tissues and create a potential space for injection of the dermal filler. A needle is used for this technique and inserted at 45° angle to the skin. The material is then injected slowly into the subdermal space till a sufficient bolus is delivered. After injection, a soapy cleanser or ultrasound gel is applied to the hand to make massage easier and uniform.[17] Firm massage is done to distribute the product evenly into the entire hand **(Fig. 2)**.

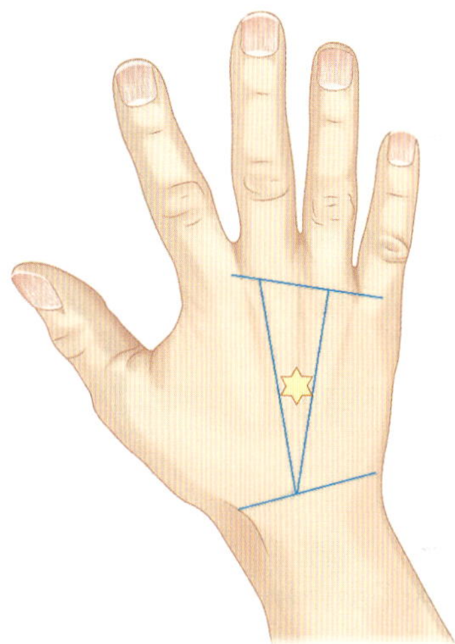

Fig. 2: Technique 2—bolus injection technique showing entry point.

Technique 3: Tunneling or Linear Retrograde Threading

A cannula is used to deliver the material along the tendons. The web spaces between the fingers is anesthetized using lidocaine. An entry point is made in each interdigital web using a 23G needle to allow the cannula to pass through easily. The first cannula is pushed between the fifth and fourth finger interdigital space and injected in a retrograded fashion, next between fourth and third fingers, then between third and second, and then first and second in a total of four lines of the product. The product is delivered as linear threads along the tendons. The products are then massaged for even distribution **(Figs. 3A to C)**.

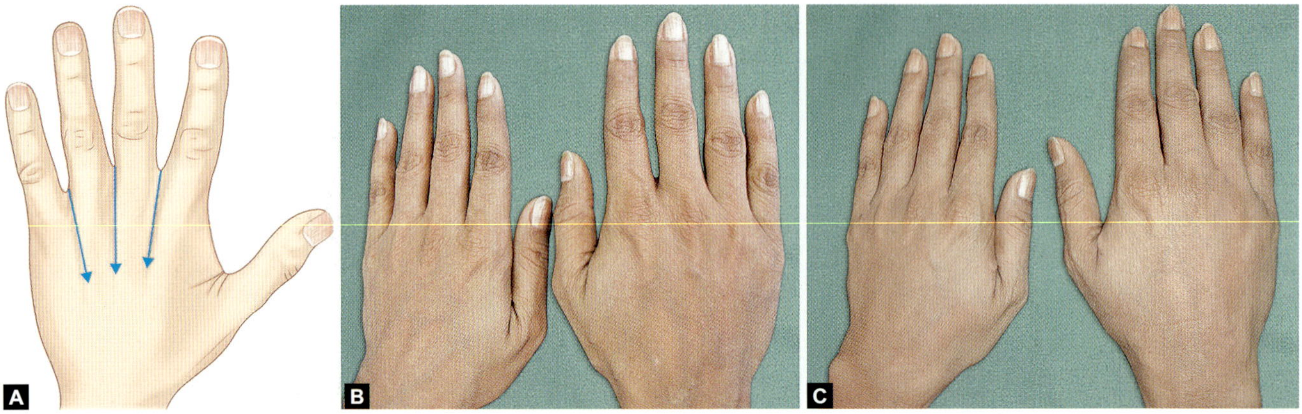

Figs. 3A to C: Technique 3: (A) Tunneling or linear threading technique; (B) Before; (C) After injection by linear threading technique using hyaluronic acid (HA).

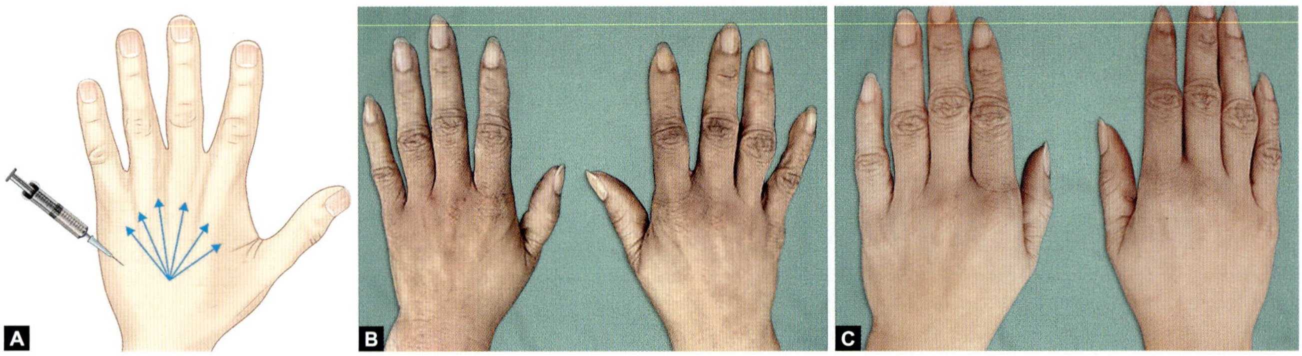

Figs. 4A to C: Technique 4: (A) Fanning technique; (B) Before; (C) After injection by fanning technique using hyaluronic acid (HA).

Technique 4: Fanning Technique

The entry point is below the wrist. An entry point is made on the proximal portion of the hand near the wrist. A cannula is introduced, and threads of filler are injected distally and radially without withdrawing the needle[18] **(Figs. 4A to C)**.

Technique 5: Scrape Skin Threading Technique[19]

This is an optimal technique for the perfect placement of product precisely in the dorsal superficial lamina. To find this plane, the undersurface of the dermis must be scraped with a soft-tipped cannula. The cannula's tip is introduced with the lateral hole pointing toward the dermis to scrape the undersurface of the dermis. The injection is done strictly subdermally as fine threading in a retrograde direction and in a fan-shaped configuration to cover the entire treatment area. It is a safer technique as the cannula is kept away from veins and tendons. For this technique, dilute CaHA is preferred, as it allows easy flow of the product restricted to the fascial layer.

Injection tips:
- Needles are used to inject boluses of HA.
- Cannulas are preferred to inject CaHA.

TIPS AND TRICKS

- The needle should be advanced slowly, and injection is done in a retrograde fashion for safety.
- Small volumes should be introduced with each injection.
- Icing before injection decreases pain and shrinks blood vessels making them less likely to be punctured.
- Knowledge of the anatomy of dorsal arteries of the hand will help minimize complications **(Fig. 5)**.[16] The venous system that runs parallel with the arteries can be easily visualized and act as a guide.

POSTPROCEDURE

After injection, the patient is asked to make a tight fist, and a firm massage is done to distribute the material uniformly. Then, the patient is asked to sit on the dorsum of their hand for 10 minutes. The warmth and pressure of the body flatten the boluses and help to even out the products. The post filler instructions are given in **Box 3**.

Complications following hand rejuvenation are not expected if planned and executed well. However, complications that may arise may be classified as minor and major adverse reactions.

Minor adverse reactions:
- Mild tenderness
- Erythema

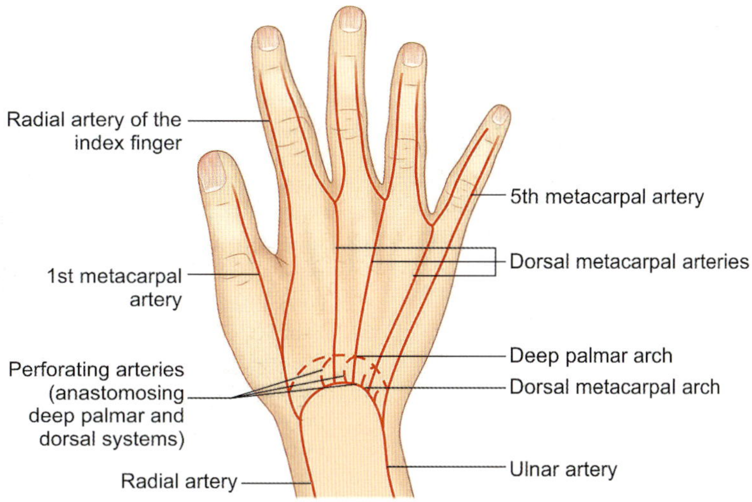

Fig. 5: Anatomy of dorsal arteries—hand.

BOX 3: Postprocedure tips.

- Avoid extreme cold or heat.
- Ice packs can be applied periodically to reduce swelling.
- To alleviate bruising, topical application of arnica is helpful.
- Avoid excessive movement of treated hands.

- Bruising
- Edema
- Temporary numbness
- Mild pruritus

These reactions occur within a few hours after the procedure and resolve without medical intervention within 4–6 weeks.

Major adverse reactions: Significant adverse reactions are more common with semipermanent fillers and less with temporary fillers.

- Infections
- Nodule formation
- Granuloma

MANAGEMENT

Flowchart 1 and Box 4 show the management of complications of fillers in hands.

CONCLUSION

Hand rejuvenation with dermal fillers is a good option as an antiaging therapy. Sound knowledge of injection anatomy and filler properties and proper training for a safe technique are essential for a good outcome.

A three-step combination therapy that includes sclerotherapy for veins, dermal fillers for volume restoration, and laser resurfacing to improve skin texture would be a holistic approach to improve the appearance of aged hands.

Flowchart 1: Algorithm for management of hand rejuvenation complications with fillers.

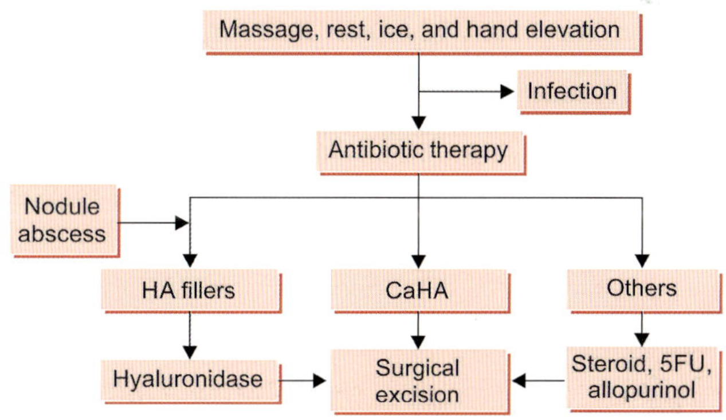

(5FU: 5-fluorouracil; CaHA: calcium hydroxylapatite; HA: hyaluronic acid)

BOX 4: Postfiller instructions for the first 48 hours.[2]

- Elevate hands as much as possible when not in use.
- Apply ice or triamcinolone lotion two to three times per day to minimize edema.
- Avoid strenuous hand movement or manual tabs.
- Wear arthritis gloves at night for the first few days.
- Remove rings for at least 24 hours to avoid entrapment due to swelling.

PEARLS

- A good medical history and clinical assessment is essential.
- Careful patient and product selection is important.
- Temporary fillers are to be chosen when injecting hands for the first time.
- Overcorrection is to be avoided.
- The injection should not infringe upon metacarpophalangeal joints.
- Combination hand rejuvenation procedures like chemical peels, lasers, and fillers give the best results.
- Complications must be recognized and treated immediately.

REFERENCES

1. Inglefield C. Nonsurgical hand rejuvenation with Dermicol-P35 30G. Aesthet Surg J. 2009;29(3 suppl):S19-21.
2. Butterwick K, Sadick N. Hand Rejuvenation using a combination approach. Dermatol Surg. 2016;42(Suppl 2):S108-18.
3. Jakubietz RG, Jakubietz MG, Kloss D, Gruenert JG. Defining the basic aesthetics of the hand. Aesthetic Plast Surg. 2005;29(6):546-51.
4. Ricketts RM. The biologic significance of the divine proportion and Fibonacci series. Am J Orthod. 1982;81(5);351-70.
5. Riyaz FR, Ozog D. Hand Rejuvenation. Semin Cutan Med Surg. 2015;34(3):147-52.
6. Cohen JL, Carruthers A, Jones DH, Narurkar VA, Wong M, Cheskin LN, et al. A randomized blinded study to validate the Merz Hand Grading Scale for use in live assessment. Dermatol Surg. 2015;41(Suppl 1):S384-8.
7. Fournier PF. Fat grafting: My technique. Dermatol Surg. 2000;26(12):117-28.
8. Butterwick KJ. Lipoaugmentation for aging hands: A comparison of the longevity and aesthetic results of centrifuged versus noncentrifuged fat. Dermatol Surg. 2002;28(11):987-91.
9. Villanueva NL, Hill SM, Small KH, Rohrich RJ. Technical retirement in autologous hand rejuvenation. Plast Reconstr Surg. 2015;136(6):1175-9.
10. Haq S, Storck R, Baspeyras M, Thio A, Campion C, Essayagh E, et al. Multinational, multipatient study of calcium hydroxylapatite for treatment of the aging hand: European cosmetic Physician Group on Hand Augmentation. Dermatol Surg. 2010;36(1):782-9.
11. Poggi B. Hand rejuvenation with CaHA guided by ultrasound. J Dermat Cosmetol. 2020;4(2):39-40.
12. Moers-Carp M, Vogt S, Santos BM, Planas J, Vallve SR, Howell DJ. A multicentre, randomized trial comparing calcium hydroxylapatite to two hyaluronic acids for treatment of nasolabial folds. Dermatol Surg. 2007;33(Suppl 2):S144-51.
13. Redaelli A. Cosmetic use of polylactic acid for hand rejuvenation: Report on 27 patients. J Cosmet Dermatol. 2006;5(3):233-8.
14. Fabi SG, Goldman MP. Hand rejuvenation. A review and our experience. Dermatol Surg. 2012;38(7 pt 2):1112-27.
15. Figueiredo VM. A five-patient prospective pilot study of a polycaprolactone based dermal filler for hand rejuvenation. J Cosmet Dermatol. 2013;12(1):73-7.
16. Melton K. Techniques for hand rejuvenation with fillers in aesthetic practice. Journal of Aesthetic Nursing. 2020;9(3): 108-13.
17. Kühne U, Imhof M. Treatment of the ageing hand with dermal fillers. J Cutan Aesthet Surg. 2012;5(3):163-9.
18. Lefebvre-Vilardebo M, Trevidic P, Moradi A, Busso M, Sutton AB, Bucay VW. Hand: Clinical anatomy and regional approaches with injectable fillers. Plast Reconstr Surg. 2015;136(5):258S-75S.
19. Park TH, Yeo KK, Seo SW, Kim JK, Lee JH, Park JH, et al. Clinical experience with complications of hand rejuvenation. J Plas Reconstr Aesthetic Surg. 2012;65(12):1627-31.

CHAPTER 96

Complications of Botulinum Toxin and Fillers

Madhuri Agarwal

KEY MESSAGES

- A detailed understanding of facial anatomy and knowledge about the variety of products available is essential for avoiding complications of botulinum toxin and fillers.
- A well-planned methodical approach and awareness of the algorithms for complication management are a good enabler.
- Understanding of true and perceived adverse effects along with preventing and treating them promptly is crucial for successful outcomes.

INTRODUCTION

The aspiration to look young has led to trending statistics of people undergoing botulinum toxin A (BTX-A) and hyaluronic acid (HA) fillers in recent years. A broad array of toxins and dermal fillers offered in medical aesthetics though safe are potentially adept at causing complications.

Inadequate experience is a contributing factor in the development of complications.

We are aware that most adverse events can be avoided with correct planning and technique. In the event that adverse events do occur, the physician should be equipped with tools for prompt treatment and close follow-up.

The chapter elaborates on factors affecting the occurrence of adverse reactions and practical tips to avoid and mitigate associated unfavorable complications.

PATIENT, PHYSICIAN, AND PRODUCT FACTORS THAT AFFECT THE INCIDENCE OF COMPLICATIONS

Patients often envisage an unrealistic outcome that needs to be managed by the treating physician. Patients must be made aware of the limitations and hazards of botulinum toxin and dermal fillers.[1] Physicians should have a comprehensive knowledge of facial anatomy as well as the probable hazard areas, and distribution of facial arteries and nerves. Textbook anatomy though typical of the overall population, subtle individual disparities are common. Hence, cognizance of the possibility of perforation, laceration, or compromising vessels should be there.

Physicians should be aware of high-risk areas like the glabella, nasal region, and nasolabial folds (NLF) and the muscles adjacent to the treating BTX-A muscles. In addition, the location of the injection is associated with local trauma. For example, implantation immediately above or beneath a muscle, such as in the lip or tear trough sulcus has a higher propensity for swelling and bruising simply due to the highly vascular nature of these regions. The physician should have control over the injection procedure, precisely the injection depth, volume, velocity, and accuracy. Depending on the nature of the filler, outcomes of distinct severity are seen. Product-related considerations include the filler's concentration, rheological properties, and production processes.[1]

COMPLICATIONS OF BOTULINUM TOXIN

Botulinum toxin A injections have a long history of safety and efficacy. The common complications with BTX-A are mentioned in **Box 1**. With the small amounts of BTX-A used for cosmetic applications, serious adverse events are rare and occur far less often than with the larger doses often necessary for therapeutic applications. Adverse events with BTX-A are generally transient and mild to moderate in severity.[2-8] More serious adverse events can result from inappropriate doses or injection sites, and rare incidents of hypersensitivity have been reported.

Complications for BTX-A can be classified into three groups based on their type and are explained in detail as follows:

1. Self-limiting complications
2. Common complications
3. Serious complications

BOX 1: Common complications of botulinum toxin-A (BTX-A).

- Bruising
- Asymmetric result
- Upper eyelid ptosis
- Dysphagia
- Neck weakness
- Perioral droop
- Lagophthalmos
- Diplopia
- Globe perforation
- Exposure keratopathy
- Intravascular injection
- Psychosomatic problems

TABLE 1: Self-limiting complications.

Indications	*Target muscle*	*Erroneous muscle involvement*	*Adverse effect seen*
Frown/forehead lines	Corrugator/procerus/ frontalis	Levator palpebrae superioris/ orbicularis oculi	Lid/brow ptosis
Crow's feet	Orbicularis oculi	Lateral rectus and other extraocular muscles	Ectropion, diplopia, xerophthalmia, and lagophthalmos
Oral commissures	Depressor anguli oris	Depressor labii inferioris	Asymmetric smile due to relaxation
Pebbly chin and ptosis of chin	Mentalis	Depressor labii inferioris	Asymmetric smile due to relaxation
Contour and reshape/square and broad lower face due to hypertrophy	Masseter	Risorius and zygomaticus major	Loss of full smile/asymmetric smile
Prominent neck bands/sagging of the neck	Medial platysmal bands	Mylohyoid and stylohyoid	Dysphagia

PREVENTION AND MANAGEMENT OF BOTULINUM TOXIN A COMPLICATIONS

Self-limiting Complications

Self-limiting complications are usually due to erroneous muscle involvement **(Table 1)** and recover once the effect of BTX-A fades out in 4–6 months. The treatment for this kind of complication is constant reassurance and managing the patient's anxiety till the adverse effect wears out.

Lid and Brow Ptosis

Brow ptosis occurs while treating frontalis muscle for treating horizontal forehead lines with BTX-A **(Fig. 1)**. To evade this complication, the physician should stay at least 2–3 cm above the supraorbital margin or 1.5–2 cm above the eyebrow while injecting into the frontalis, thus sparing the function of inferior frontalis muscle fibers in the area and thereby preventing ptosis.[9,10] In case of patients presenting with glabellar frown lines along with horizontal forehead lines, it is imperative to treat the glabellar area (corrugators and procerus) as well alongside forehead, so as to prevent brow ptosis because of the unopposed depressor action of the glabellar muscles.[10,11] While injecting the toxin in and around the glabella, migration of injected toxin through the orbital septum can cause weakening of the levator palpebrae superioris leading to ptosis of upper eyelid **(Fig. 2)**. This is frequent when the toxin is injected in close proximity to bony supraorbital margin at the mid-pupillary line and when significant volumes of diluted toxin are injected in the area.[11,12]

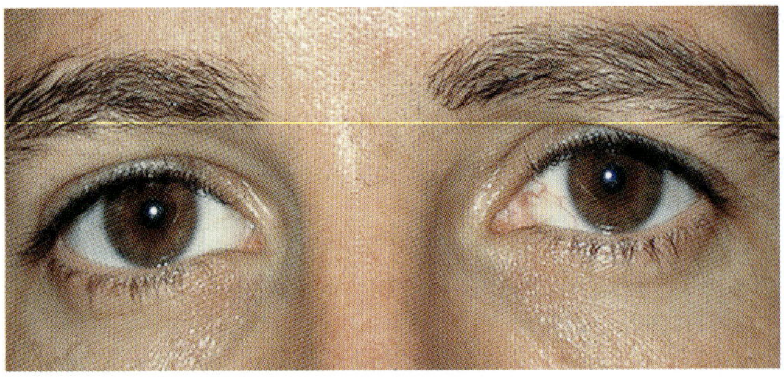

Fig. 1: Brow ptosis after botulinum toxin A (BTX-A).

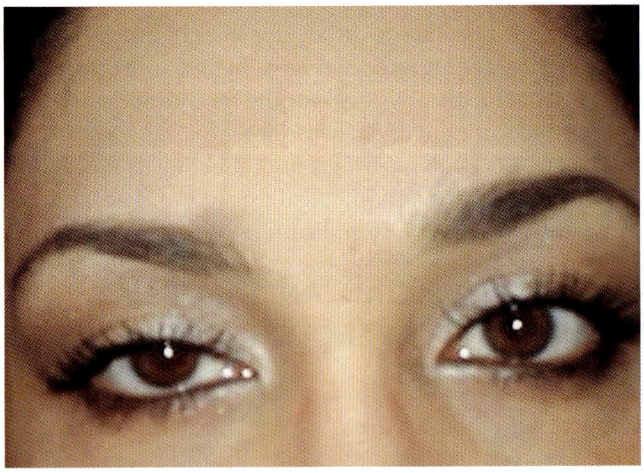

Fig. 2: Lid ptosis after incorrect placement of botulinum toxin A (BTX-A). *Courtesy:* Realself.

Brow and lid ptosis can occur more readily in older patients where senile descent of the brow line is not taken into consideration while treating the forehead; hence, a proper technique is crucial in this case.

Botulinum toxin A needs a thorough pretreatment review of periorbital rhytides in the elderly. Excessive lower eyelid laxity can lead to ectropion or lid lag, detected by a large scleral display or an irregular snap examination. If this complication occurs, application of eye drops containing alpha-adrenergic agonists, such as apraclonidine or phenylephrine 2.5%/ naphazoline 0.025%/pheniramine 0.3% or apraclonidine 0.5%, may be used to elevate the upper eyelid via contraction of the müller muscle.[13]

Ectropion, Diplopia, Xerophthalmia, and Lagophthalmos

Complications such as ectropion, diplopia, xerophthalmia, and lagophthalmos can be caused by injection of high doses of BTX-A into the lateral canthus region. Ectropion occurs due to the inadvertent weakening of the lateral orbicularis muscular sling due to toxin diffusion. Diplopia may occur due to the spread of the toxin through the orbital septum, resulting in the lateral rectus and other extraocular muscles being compromised. If the toxin is injected too deeply into the upper lateral part of the periocular region, xerophthalmia can occur, thereby affecting the secretion of the lacrimal glands. Another unusual complication that results from the loss of the normal sphincteric feature of the orbicularis oculi and the excessive closing of the eyelids is lagophthalmos. When the toxin diffuses into the palpebral portion of the orbicularis oculi, leading to lagophthalmos, loss of sphincteric functions of the orbicularis oculi and eyelid weakness can occur. By injecting the toxin subdermally and laterally through a hypothetical vertical line passing through the lateral canthus, these complications can be decreased.[9,10,14]

Lip Ptosis and Asymmetry

This very rare complication is seen when the toxin is injected below the superior margin of the zygomatic arch or too low along the nasal sidewalls, thereby diffusing into the upper lip elevators, i.e., levator labii superioris alaeque nasi and levator labii superioris, leading to asymmetry and ptosis of the upper lip and even difficulties in speaking and eating.[15-17]

Botulinum toxin A should be injected high on the lateral nasal wall, above the nasofacial groove to prevent this. Injections into the orbicularis oris should be placed superficially and in small doses to avoid significant and asymmetric weakening of the lip sphincter.

Overdosing of the toxin over the upper lip can cause various adverse functional variations such as inability to form certain letters, articulate different sounds, and pronounce various words. Failure to approximate the lips tightly may lead to fluid or even food incontinence and drooling.[18]

Asymmetric Smile

While treating depressor anguli oris (DAO) for oral commissures or mentalis for chin ptosis, one must be extremely cautious while injecting BTX-A because of the danger of producing an incompetent mouth or an asymmetric smile **(Fig. 3)** due to erroneous involvement of depressor labii inferioris.[10] Likewise, while treating masseter to reshape or contour the lower face, erroneous involvement of risorius or zygomaticus major may give rise to an asymmetric smile or loss of a full smile. A reduction in mastication strength is commonly seen while treating masseter.[19]

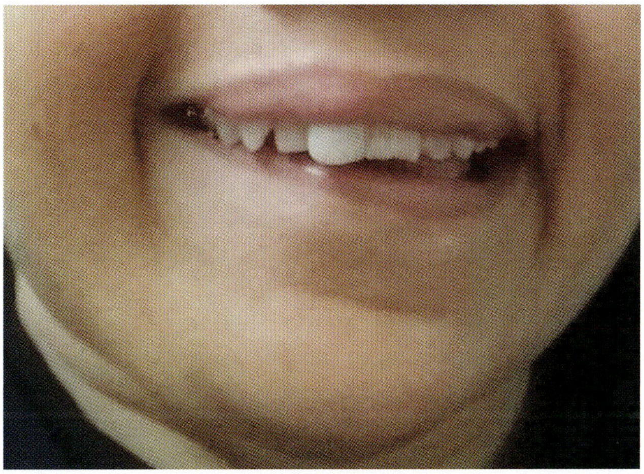

Fig. 3: Asymmetric smile due to inadvertent injection of depressor labii inferioris after botulinum toxin A (BTX-A).

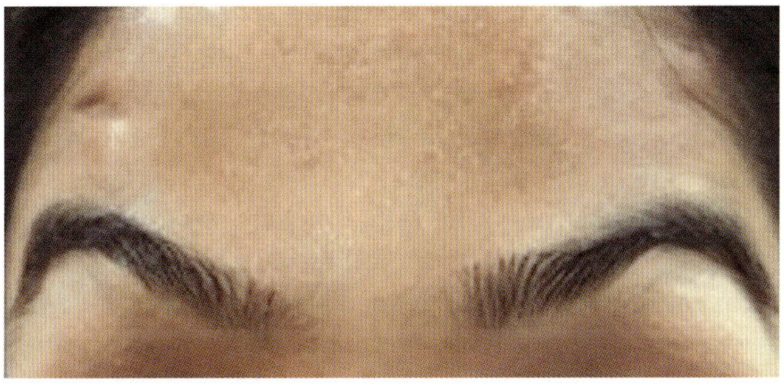

Fig. 4: Spock eyebrow after botulinum toxin A (BTX-A).

Dysphagia, Hoarseness, and Neck Weakness

Botulinum toxin treatment for treating horizontal rhytides and vertical bands in the neck though safe can give rise to complications due to improper technique. As the underlying muscles of deglutition, phonation, and neck flexion are also cholinergic, higher doses or deeper injections of BTX-A can result in xerostomia, dysphagia, dysarthria, and neck weakness.[20,21] The maximum recommended dose in this region ranges from 30 to 100 units of BTX-A per session.[22] It is recommended to use not more than 50 units per session with possible touch-up 2 weeks later. Few patients may complain of either difficulty or rarely an inability to lift the head and to keep it still and erect.

Asymmetry

Asymmetry is a common complication and is usually due to improper placement or a patient's anatomic variation. "Spock" eyebrow **(Fig. 4)** is a common asymmetry presenting as curvature of the lateral brow occurring due to imbalance arising from the deactivation of the central frontalis and the activity of the lateral frontalis that lifts the brow tail, which can be corrected by placing some additional toxin at the active area of the muscle.[10,12]

Common Complications

The most common adverse events associated with BTX-A are related to injection site reactions, such as bruising, edema, pain at the injection and adjacent sites, headache, and general body malaise after the injection.[18,20]

- Bruising can be minimized by advising patients to refrain from taking medications that inhibit clotting, such as vitamin E, aspirin (or medications containing aspirin), and nonsteroidal anti-inflammatory drugs, for up to 2 weeks before and after injection.
- Using a small gauge needle and stretching the skin to visualize the superficial vessels can limit bruising, especially around the lateral canthus region where the skin is thin and veins are superficial.
- Usage of icing or cooling tools like frozen gel packs is recommended to mitigate pain and cause vasoconstriction to minimize bruising. Since ice is not sterile, place it in a sterile glove or in a nonsterile glove after wiping it with alcohol or chlorhexidine to sterilize it.
- Slow injection technique with a gentle and slow extrusion rate, using smaller gauge needles, applying topical anesthetic 10–15 minutes prior to injection, and reconstituting the BTX-A with preservative-containing saline may all help to alleviate the pain considerably. Vibration anesthesia and distraction therapy, such as guided breathing, music, or engaging conversation, can be helpful in reducing pain.
- Headache is due to the initial muscle spasm caused by BTX-A in the first 12 hours, followed by muscle weakness for months thereafter. Headaches can be classified into two types: Minor and severe. Minor headaches can be controlled with standard over-the-counter analgesics, whereas severe headaches can be managed with stronger analgesics and systemic corticosteroids when necessary.

Serious Complications

Serious reactions like anaphylaxis, urticaria, soft-tissue edema, and dyspnea are rare.[23]

COMPLICATIONS OF FILLERS

Adverse reactions of fillers range from minor and self-limited to severe complications. Generally, HA fillers and collagen can cause reversible side effects; calcium hydroxylapatite (CaHA), alginate, dextranomer beads in HA, and polylactic acid can cause longer-lasting side effects and vaseline, paraffin, silicone oil, hydroxyethyl methacrylate fragments, polymethyl methacrylate beads, polyacrylamide, and polyalkylimide gels can cause delayed and permanent side effects. Temporary fillers can cause less serious side effects of shorter duration compared to permanent fillers which can cause long-lasting and more serious side effects.[24,25] These demand timely intervention, close follow-up, and management. Ideal complication management of fillers is an unmet need in the aesthetic domain. Fortunately, a better understanding of anatomy, new techniques, and expert handling can help physicians to achieve reasonably safe filler injections.

Classification of Filler Complications Based on Onset[1]

Complications of fillers can be classified based on the average time to onset:

- *Early onset (up to 4 weeks)*
  - Placement, injection-related (bruising and swellings), vascular, and inflammatory
- *Delayed onset (after 4 weeks)*
  - Inflammatory, nodules, dyspigmentation, and displacement.

The complications due to fillers can also be classified as:

- Allergic/hypersensitivity reactions
- Vascular events
- Infections
- Late-onset nodules or inflammation.

CAUSES AND MANAGEMENT OF FILLER COMPLICATIONS

Early Onset

Edema, erythema, pain, bruising **(Fig. 5)**, and tenderness are due to the effect of filler injected in the treatment region and often resolve in a day or two. The application of local anesthetic cream and slow injection delivery reduces pain. Ice compresses help to alleviate pain and edema and increase the comfort level of the patient while injecting. Bruising can be minimized by ice compresses and adequate pressure. The use of blunt cannula also decreases the bruising risk substantially.[26] Patients should be advised to discontinue anti-inflammatory and blood-thinner medications like aspirin or clopidogrel. They should also be recommended to stop the intake of common nutritional blood thinners like salmon oil, vitamin E, ginkgo biloba, red wine, dark chocolate, and grapefruit for a week prior to treatment to minimize bruising.[27]

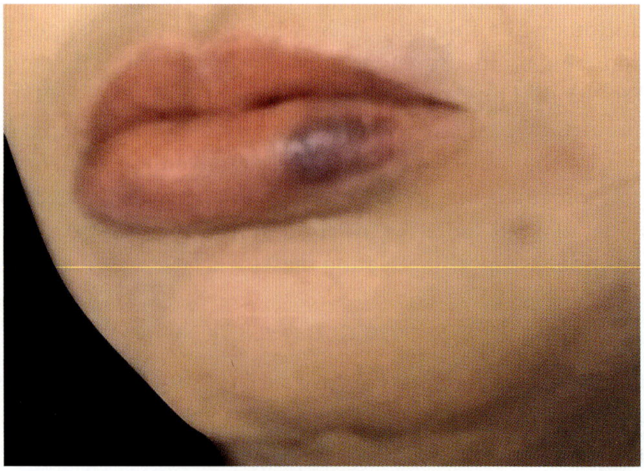

Fig. 5: Bruising is a transient complication after filler injections, more common in lip areas.

Allergic/Hypersensitivity Reactions

Hypersensitivity or allergic reactions may occur when an immune response is activated by the injected filler. This may be a type I hypersensitivity reaction that typically has an early onset (within minutes to hours of injection) or a type IV reaction that has a delayed onset, i.e.,1–3 days to several weeks after injection.[28] Although it does not require the urgent attention that vascular occlusion requires, it may be a problem that causes considerable patient distress. Delayed-onset localized angioedema can be managed with cold compresses and H1-receptor antagonist for histamine-induced hypotension and pruritus reduction. The management of hypersensitivity reactions to fillers is elaborated in **Table 2**.[29,30]

TABLE 2: Management of hypersensitivity reactions to fillers.

Early	*Delayed*
Check vital signs	Cold compresses
• Resuscitation measures • Adrenaline • Intravenous access • Fluids	H1-receptor antagonists
	H2-receptor antagonists
	Leukotriene synthesis inhibitors
	Oral corticosteroids
	Propranolol
	Ibuprofen

Vascular Events

The most severe complication of fillers is vascular compromise, which may be inadvertent but can be attributed to various risk factors like injecting fast under pressure, using wide gauge needles, not aspirating before injecting, and the use of lignocaine **(Table 3)**.[31-33] Vision loss occurs due to central retinal artery occlusion through the external–internal carotid vessels post filler injection. The filler lodges in the retinal tissues, potentially leading to irreversible and severe vision loss.[31,34,35]

The vascular compromise risk is higher in certain areas of the face as mentioned in **Table 4**.[36] The knowledge of these areas can help to subvert the risk of vascular compromise.

Physicians should be able to recognize the early signs of an impending vascular event and need to distinguish it clearly from a bruise **(Box 2)**. The early identification and management of vascular compromise can save the patient from catastrophic outcomes **(Figs. 6A to C)**. Any vascular pattern that looks like fishnet stockings is an intravascular event.

Nowadays, the pain due to impending vascular compromise may be masked due to the common addition of local anesthetics to filler formulations. Careful attention for skin color change that may be located away from the injection point is necessary. Stop injecting the filler on any

TABLE 3: Risk factors for accidental intra-arterial injection of hyaluronic acid (HA) fillers.[33]

Risk factors	*Description*	*Clinical considerations*
Site	Deep injection of filler products at or near the site of named vessels. Needle aspiration may or may not show any flashback of blood	Exercise increased caution near the facial artery, angular artery, along the nasolabial fold, the nose, and glabellar areas. Intimate knowledge of the location named facial vessels is mandatory for injectors
Volume	The volume of product injected into any one area is a risk factor since larger amounts of product can cause a proportionally greater degree of arterial obstruction. Safer practice is to inject no more than 0.1 mL into any one location and change the position for further injections	Attempts to clear a needle obstruction by increasing the syringe pressure is a risk factor since accidental discharge of a large volume of material can result in disastrous consequences if the needle tips in the lumen of an artery. Purposeful large-volume injection (Lake Technique) is also a risk factor for the same reason
Small sharp needles	Small-gauge sharp needles are more likely to penetrate the lumen of an artery than larger needles. Aspiration of arterial blood through a narrow-gauge long needle is an unreliable indicator	Larger caliber needles are more likely to have a "back flash" of blood following aspiration. Although aspiration prior to injection is good practice, the viscous filler material may not allow arterial blood to flash back into the syringe
Previous scarring	Deep tissue scars may stabilize and fix arteries in place, making them easier to penetrate with small sharp needles. This may also occur when injecting sites where arteries pass through bony foramina or deep fascial structures	In fatty tissues, thicker-walled arteries may roll out of the way when prodded by larger needles, as attested to by those experienced in microvascular surgery. Fixation by scarring holds the vessel in place, making it easier to penetrate
Blunt cannulae	Blunt cannulae may reduce—but not eliminate—the risk of accidental intra-arterial injection, especially in the presence of previous scarring (e.g., following years of filler treatments in the same area). There have been several reports of accidental intra-arterial injection with blunt cannulae	Some cannulae possess a bullet tip, and although they have a side port, these fine cannulae (e.g., smaller than 27 gauge) can penetrate arterial walls. Larger diameter cannulae with a rounded tip are less likely to penetrate. There are no LOE 1 or 2 clinical reports that support treatment via cannulae at present, and the author knows of accidental arterial injections that have occurred despite cannulae application
Composition of filler material used	Permanent fillers have no means of dissolving the material. Some fillers promote immediate clotting	HA products have the advantage of being hydrolyzed by hyaluronidase

(HA: hyaluronic acid; LOE: level of evidence)

sign of skin blanching or mottled discoloration. Then, massage the affected area and immediately start hyaluronidase injections. High-dose hyaluronidase (500–1,000 IU) with lidocaine administered every hour for 3 hours is the latest recommended guideline **(Table 5)**. The new protocol of high-dose hyaluronidase helps to resolve the secondary signs of the vascular event within 3 days with few bruises vis-à-vis the 6 weeks or longer of healing by secondary intention.[37] Additionally, aspirin (650 mg) must be given to the patient at the same time.

Hyaluronidase for correction of HA filler complications is an off-label use of its Food and Drug Administration (FDA)-approved indications. The hyaluronidase dosage is related to multiple factors when used for HA filler correction such as the concentration of HA, the amount of cross-linking, the cohesivity, etc. Various HA fillers have varying physiochemical properties and these influence the dose of hyaluronidase. A study by Kim et al. reported that Belotero was the quickest to dissolve followed by JUVÉDERM VOLUMA and Restylane Lyft. The study showed that high cross-linkage and concentration of HA along with large particle size increase the sustainability of HA filler.[38]

TABLE 4: Facial areas with risk of blindness and visual complications.

Risk	*Regions*
Low	Jawline and marionette, lateral cheek (lateral to a vertical line through lateral canthus), submalar, preauricular, and chin augmentation
Moderate	Lips, perioral region, and anterior cheek (between a vertical line through lateral canthus and mid-pupillary line)
High	Temples, nasolabial folds, tear troughs, periorbital, and medial cheek (between mid-pupillary line and side of the nose)
Very high	Glabella, nose, and forehead

BOX 2: Timeline of tissue reaction affected by intravascular embolism.

- Immediate evanescent blanching after filler injection
- Livedo lasting a few days with slow capillary refill time
- Scabbing, pustulation, and blisters starting on 2nd or 3rd day
- Necrosis is seen by about 6th or 7th day
- Secondary healing is slow and occurs over some weeks

A skin sensitivity intradermal patch test is mandatory an hour before injecting hyaluronidase except in critical cases such as impeding vascular compromise. Hyaluronidase is a rapidly acting drug that shows effect in 12–24 hours. It is available as a dried powder vial and needs to be reconstituted for use. Insulin 1 mL syringe of 40 units marking is used to inject in the compromised tissue. Hyaluronidase 1,500 units vial is reconstituted with 1 mL normal saline. Thus, the calculation is:

- 1,500 units in 1 mL of normal saline = 1,500 units per mL
- 1,500 divided by 40 units of insulin syringe = 37.5 units per marking.

For ophthalmic events, the following is suggested:[30]

- Contact the ophthalmologist of choice directly and accompany the patient to his office.
- Respect the absolute 90-minute time frame for saving the loss of vision.
- Have multiple vials of hyaluronidase at hand and be knowledgeable regarding reconstitution and dosage.
- Carry your own hyaluronidase to the ophthalmologist.
- If possible, annotate the time of the vascular event and the visual acuity if lack of light perception (LP) or loss of vision occurs.
- To facilitate accurate ophthalmological follow-up, immediate recording of vision should be annotated as no light perception (NLP), LP, hand motion (HM), and count fingers (CF), followed by a Snellen chart if available. An afferent pupillary defect should be noted if present.
- Attempt rapid ocular pulsed massage. Having the patient hyperventilate in a paper bag may promote retinal vessel dilation.

Late Onset

Infections

Fillers are minimally invasive treatment and have the potential of infecting the skin. The infections due to filler procedure are

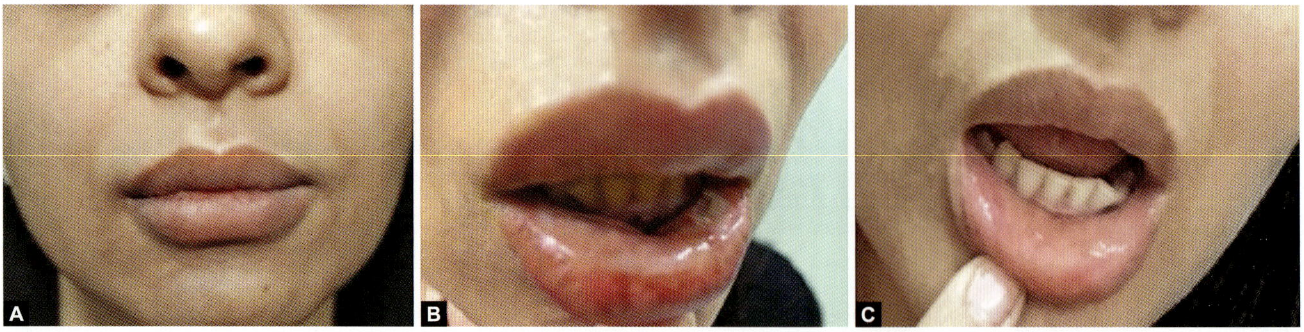

Figs. 6A to C: (A) Normal appearance of lips immediately after filler injection; (B) 3rd day after injection, patient presented with signs of vascular event, and institution of impending necrosis treatments as per protocol **(see Table 5)** were immediately done; (C) 13 days later, extensive necrosis was averted and the skin is normal without any signs of injury.

TABLE 5: Delorenzi's high-dose pulse hyaluronidase protocols.[37]

Dosage	Standard dosage	500 IU per area
	Lip, nose, and forehead	Act as multipliers
	Two areas	1,000 IU per hour
	Three areas	1,500 IU per area
Inject at least every 60–90 minutes until skin color has normalized and capillary refill time has normalized		
Massage to increase embolus contact with the hyaluronidase by propelling the HA distally into thinner-walled arterioles		
Aim to complete treatment within 72 hours of onset for complete resolution		
• Keep the patient in clinic for observation and treatment until the capillary refill has improved (usually three sessions over 3 hours) • Do not apply nitroglycerin paste until the offending HA has been dissolved (day 2 or 3 of treatment) as dilation of adjacent nonobstructed vascular pathways can lead to the propagation of the embolus toward the orbit		

(HA: hyaluronic acid)

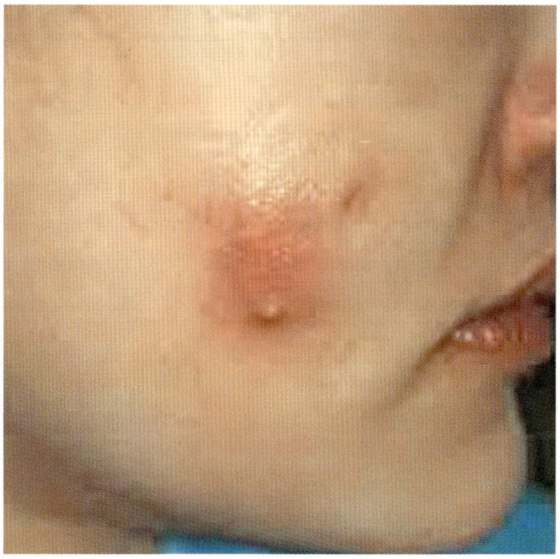

Fig. 7: Biofilm formation after fillers.
Courtesy: med.mahidol.ac.th.

usually categorized as acute and delayed chronic infections. Acute infections appear as acute inflammation or abscesses at the injection site, whereas chronic infection is seen after 2 weeks or more after the filler procedure at times comprising atypical mycobacteria. Biofilm can occur in certain cases, and this is challenging to diagnose as well as treat.[28]

It is vital to distinguish between hypersensitivity and infection as steroid use has to be strictly avoided in infection. The distinguishing features of infection are fever, pain, absence of pruritis, and evidence of abscess **(Fig. 7)**. Any region adjacent to the injection site displaying signs of infection needs to be immediately examined and treated. Investigation such as C-reactive protein (CRP), erythrocyte sedimentation rate (ESR), and other infective markers can contribute to diagnosis. Oral antibiotics that have anti-inflammatory and immunomodulatory properties can be administered to treat the infection. Additional treatments include hyaluronidase, intralesional 5-fluorouracil, and surgical drainage of abscess.

Biofilm presents as a delayed-onset skin reaction. It may appear at any time after treatment, regardless of the duration of effect. Presentation varies from a nonfluctuant red, indurated area to granulomatous inflammation, abscesses, nodules, or full-blown recurrent infection. Management includes:[1,28]

- Broad-spectrum antibiotic
- At least long-term high-dose or two-drug therapy
- Do not use intralesional steroids before antibiotics and until all acute inflammatory reaction is settled
- Hyaluronidase and intralesional high-dose steroids
- If fluctuant, needle-drain and culture
- 5-fluorouracil ± steroids 1
- Laser
- Excision as a last resort.

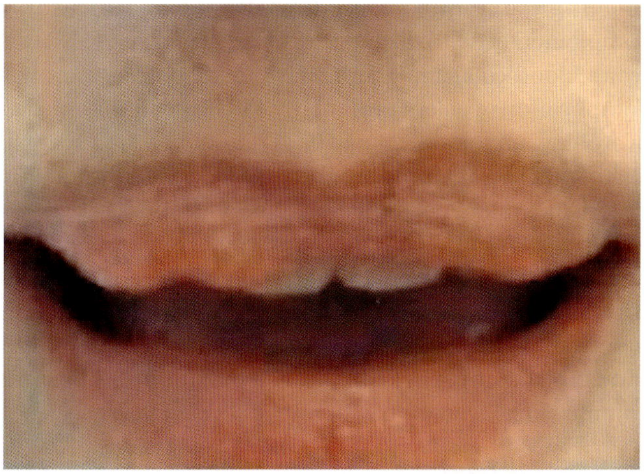

Fig. 8: Delayed-onset nodules after fillers.

Nodules or Inflammation

Delayed-onset nodules are generally infection related including biofilm or inflammatory, i.e., immune response to filler **(Fig. 8)**. They are seen after 4 weeks up to a year and at times may persist as noninflammatory nodules.[39] The nodules can be due to hematogenous implantation of innocuous bacteria from a distant region, for example, dental procedures or persistent mechanical irritation. An immune response mediated by toll-like receptor (TLRs) can occur due to the attachment of nonvirulent infectious agents at the time of filler treatment. The treatment of late-onset nodules is hyaluronidase, oral antibiotics, topical tacrolimus (0.1%), or pimecrolimus (1%). Agents such as cyclosporine, methotrexate, and hydroxychloroquine can be added after evaluating the etiology of nodules.[30,39,40] The protocol for managing late-onset nodules is highlighted in **Table 6**.

TABLE 6: Management of late-onset nodules secondary to fillers.

Single nodule			*Multiple nodules*
Inflammatory		Noninflammatory	Consider systemic diseases
Fluctuant	Nonfluctuant	Encapsulated hematoma	If biofilm or granuloma
Abscess	Biofilm or granuloma	Wait	Topical immunosuppressants
Puncture + drain	Hyaluronidase + antibiotics	Puncture + drain	
Antibiotics	Intralesional steroids	Antibiotics	Antibiotics for example:
		Hyaluronidase	Ciprofloxacin 500–700 mg bd (2–4 weeks)
			Clarithromycin 500 mg bd + Moxifloxacin 400 mg bd (10 days)
			Minocycline 100 mg/day (6 months)
			Levofloxacin (3 weeks) followed by additional clarithromycin (3 weeks)
			Hyaluronidase + antibiotics
			Colchicine

Imaging Techniques

Imaging techniques using high-frequency ultrasound complemented with magnetic resonance imaging (MRI) and white blood cell scintigraphy have made detection of filler complications easier, particularly for suspected abscesses, overfilling, migration, foreign body granuloma, and scarring. Distinguishing features are described between infections, fibrosis, granulomatous inflammation, and product migration. Using conventional X-ray films, computed tomography (CT), and MRI techniques, and a distinction of different materials is often possible. Ultrasound-guided filler placements and detection of specific areas of fat depletion by high-resolution ultrasonic skin probes and scans constitute the future of volumetric rejuvenation with minimal side-effects.

CONCLUSION

Injectable BTX-A and soft-tissue fillers have well-established safety profiles. Most adverse reactions are transient, self-resolving, and mild to moderate in severity. With growing popularity of these minimally invasive facial treatments, physicians are likely to confront a greater rate of occurrence of complications. It is, therefore, important for physicians to be fully mindful of all potential complications, to adhere to known prevention strategies, and to be able to undertake appropriate corrective treatment. Thorough understanding of anatomy and meticulous injection techniques are vital in achieving optimal outcomes. Comprehensive patient counseling and education are also essential elements to enable them.

- Know the injection anatomy. Beware of high-risk areas
- Carefully consider the patient's medical history
- Usually, majority of adverse events related to botulinum toxin A can be attributed to improper injection technique rather than the neurotoxin itself. These adverse events can be prevented with thorough knowledge of muscle anatomy and adequate training in technique
- The remaining adverse events are due to local diffusion of injected botulinum toxin A, leading to weakness of adjacent functionally important muscles. The radius of diffusion of botulinum toxin A ranges from 1 to 3 cm from the injection site. The use of concentrations according to the product information in small volumes (i.e., 0.1–0.2 mL per injection site) will ensure that the toxin does not diffuse to unwanted sites. The spread of toxin can also be affected by muscle contraction in the injected area
- Aspirate before injecting. Slowly inject with the least amount of pressure possible. Move tip with delivery of product
- Incrementally inject 0.1–0.2 mL of product. Use a small syringe to deliver precise aliquots
- Use a small needle to slow injection speed. When indicated, use blunt microcannulae
- Cannula can be a safer substitute to needles in areas such as the brow or lateral and anterior cheek. However, it is not a safe substitute for nasal injection because smaller-gauge cannula (<25 gauge) can act as needles and pierce the blood vessels
- While injecting fillers, reduce the risk of vascular compromise by positioning the needle/cannula perpendicular to primary axial vessels in the anatomical region
- Always ensure that the filler injection is directed away from the eye in high-risk areas like nose, glabella, and nasolabial fold
- Stop injecting when resistance is encountered or the patient experiences pain/discomfort

REFERENCES

1. Signorini M, Liew S, Sundaram H, De Boulle KL, Goodman GJ, Monheit G, et al.; Global Aesthetics Consensus Group. Global Aesthetics Consensus: Avoidance and Management of Complications from Hyaluronic Acid Fillers-Evidence-and Opinion-Based Review and Consensus Recommendations. Plast Reconstr Surg. 2016;137(6):961e-71e.
2. Brin MF, Boodhoo TI, Pogoda JM, James LM, Demos G, Terashima Y, et al. Safety and tolerability of onabotulinum toxin A in the treatment of facial lines: a metanalysis of individual patient data from global clinical registration studies in 1678 participants. J Am Acad Dermatol. 2009;61(6):961-70.
3. Cavallini M, Cirillo P, Fundarò SP, Quartucci S, Sciuto C, Sito G, et al. Safety of botulinum toxin A in aesthetic treatments: a systematic review of clinical studies. Dermatol Surg. 2014;40(5):525-36.
4. Botox [AU package insert]. Gordon, NSW, Australia: Allergan Australia; 2017.

5. Dysport Australia [package insert]. Glen Waverley, Victoria, Australia: Ipsen Pty Ltd.; 2018.
6. Gadhia K, Walmsley AD. Facial aesthetics: Is botulinum toxin treatment effective and safe? A systematic review of randomised controlled trials. Br Dent J. 2009;207(5):E9; discussion 216-7.
7. Giordano CN, Matarasso SL, Ozog DM. Injectable and topical neurotoxins in dermatology: indications, adverse events, and controversies. J Am Acad Dermatol. 2017;76(6):1027-42.
8. Hexsel D, Cartier H, Hedén P, Delmar H, Bergentz P, Camozzato F, et al. Efficacy, safety, and subject satisfaction after abobotulinum toxin A treatment of upper facial lines. Dermatol Surg. 2018;44(12):1555-64.
9. Carruthers A, Carruthers J. Clinical indications and injection technique for the cosmetic use of botulinum A exotoxin. Dermatol Surg. 1998;24(11):1189-94.
10. Klein AW. Complications and adverse reactions with the use of botulinum toxin. Dis Mon. 2002;48(5):336-56.
11. Klein AW. Dilution and storage of botulinum toxin. Dermatol Surg. 1998;24:1179-80.
12. Carruthers A, Carruthers J. Botulinum toxin type A: history and current cosmetic use in the upper face. Semin Cutan Med Surg. 2001;20(2):71-84.
13. Small R. Botulinum toxin injection for facial wrinkles. Am Fam Physician. 2014;90(3):168-75.
14. Carruthers JD, Carruthers JA. Treatment of glabellar frown lines with C. Botulinum-A exotoxin. J Dermatol Surg Oncol. 1992;18(1):17-21.
15. Matarasso A. Discussion: New indications for botulinum toxin type A in cosmetics: mouth and neck. Plast Reconstr Surg. 2003;110:86S-7S.
16. Goldwyn R, Rohrich R. Consensus recommendations on the use of botulinum toxin type A in facial aesthetics. Supplement to Plast Reconstr Surg. 2004;114:1S-22S.
17. Matarasso SL, Matarasso A. Treatment guidelines for botulinum toxin type A for the periocular region and a report on partial upper lip ptosis following injections to the lateral canthal rhytides. Plast Reconstr Surg. 2001;108(1):208-14.
18. Kassir M, Gupta M, Galadari H, Kroumpouzos G, Katsambas A, Lotti T, et al. Complications of botulinum toxin and fillers: A narrative review. J Cosmet Dermatol. 2020;19(3):570-3.
19. Park MY, Ahn KY, Jung DS. Botulinum toxin type A treatment for contouring of the lower face. Dermatol Surg. 2003;29(5): 477-83.
20. Klein AW. Complications and adverse reactions with the use of botulinum toxin. Semin Cutan Med Surg. 2001;20(2): 109-20.
21. Blitzer A, Binder WJ, Aviv JE, Keen MS, Brin MF. The management of hyperfunctional facial lines with botulinum toxin: a collaborative study of 210 injection sites in 162 patients. Arch Otolaryngol Head Neck Surg. 1997;123(4): 389-92.
22. Krishtul A, Waldorf HA, Blitzer A. Complications of cosmetic botulinum toxin therapy. In: Carruthers A (Ed). Botulinum Toxin. Philadelphia, PA: W.B. Sanders; 2007. pp. 111-21.
23. Dayan SH. Complications from toxins and fillers in the dermatology clinic: recognition, prevention, and treatment. Facial Plast Surg Clin North Am. 2013;21(4):663-73.
24. Haneke E. Adverse effects of fillers and their histopathology. Facial Plast Surg. 2014;30(6):599-614.
25. Apikian M, Roberts S, Goodman GJ. Adverse reactions to polylactic acid injections in the periorbital area. J Cosmet Dermatol. 2007;6(2):95-101.
26. Colbert SD, Southorn BJ, Brennan PA, Ilankovan V. Perils of dermal fillers. Br Dent J. 2013;214(7):339-40.
27. Di Minno A, Frigerio B, Spadarella G, Ravani A, Sansaro D, Amato M, et al. Old and new oral anticoagulants: Food, herbal medicines and drug interactions. Blood Rev. 2017;31(4): 193-203.
28. De Boulle K, Heydenrych I. Patient factors influencing dermal filler complications: prevention, assessment, and treatment. Clin Cosmet Investig Dermatol. 2015;8:205-14.
29. De Boulle K. Management of complications after implantation of fillers. J Cosmet Dermatol. 2004;3(1):2-15.
30. Heydenrych I, Kapoor KM, De Boulle K, Goodman G, Swift A, Kumar N, et al. A 10-point plan for avoiding hyaluronic acid dermal filler-related complications during facial aesthetic procedures and algorithms for management. Clin Cosmet Investig Dermatol. 2018;11:603-11.
31. Glashofer MD, Flynn TC. Complications of temporary fillers. In: Carruthers J, Carruthers A (Eds). Soft Tissue Augmentation. Toronto: Elsevier Saunders; 2013. pp. 179-87.
32. Lazzeri D, Agostini T, Figus M, Nardi M, Pantaloni M, Lazzeri S. Blindness following cosmetic injections of the face. Plast Reconstr Surg. 2012;129(4):995-1012.
33. DeLorenzi C. Complications of injectable fillers, part 2: Vascular complications. Aesthet Surg J. 2014;34(4):584-600.
34. Park SW, Woo SJ, Park KH, Huh JW, Jung C, Kwon OK. Iatrogenic retinal artery occlusion caused by cosmetic facial filler injections. Am J Ophthalmol. 2012;154(4):653-62.
35. Carle MV, Roe R, Novack R, Boyer DS. Cosmetic facial fillers and severe vision loss. JAMA Ophthalmol. 2014;132(5):637-9.
36. Goodman GJ, Magnusson MR, Callan P, Roberts S, Hart S, McDonald CB, et al. A Consensus on Minimizing the Risk of Hyaluronic Acid Embolic Visual Loss and Suggestions for Immediate Bedside Management. Aesthet Surg J. 2020;40(9):1009-21.
37. DeLorenzi C. New high dose pulsed hyaluronidase protocol for hyaluronic acid filler vascular adverse events. Aesthet Surg J. 2017;37(7):814-25.
38. Kim DW, Yoon ES, Ji YH, Park SH, Lee BI, Dhong ES. Vascular complications of HA fillers and the role of hyaluronidase in management. J Plast Reconstr Aesthet Surg. 2011;64(12): 1590-5.
39. King M, Bassett S, Davies E, King S. Management of Delayed Onset Nodules. J Clin Aesthet Dermatol. 2016;9(11):E1-5.
40. Urdiales-Gálvez F, Delgado NE, Figueiredo V, Lajo-Plaza JV, Mira M, Moreno A, et al. Treatment of soft tissue filler complications: expert consensus recommendations. Aesthetic Plast Surg. 2018;42(2):498-510.

CHAPTER 97

Skin Boosters

Malavika Kohli, Ayushi Bothra

KEY MESSAGES

Skin boosters are preferred as a final step in treating acne scars as they are a great finisher.

INTRODUCTION

Collagen is an essential scaffold protein that gives smoothness and elasticity to the skin, but its production declines with age. This age-related decrease in collagen synthesis can be reversed by skin boosters.

HYALURONIC ACID

Hyaluronic acid (HA) is a natural moisturizing factor present in skin, muscle, and joints, with an ability to draw 1,000 times its own weight of water and retain the water molecules within itself. This ensures deep and natural hydration of the skin.

Skin boosters are microinjections of HA injected into the skin as aliquots. They not only help in improving skin hydration but also:

- Aid in collagen production
- Improve skin elasticity
- Keep skin firm, soft, and supple
- Give a radiant sheen to the skin by improving its hydration quotient
- Accelerate wound healing
- Provide antioxidative benefits
- Reduce pigmentation and give an even-toned complexion.

Thus, skin booster is a complete rejuvenating treatment that reduces fine lines, hydrates the skin, and makes it fresh and glowing.

Skin boosters are suitable for all age groups and can be placed even in perioral and periorbital areas safely.

TYPES OF SKIN BOOSTERS

Cross-linked

Cross-linked skin booster is the new kid on the block in skin boosters. It contains 12 mg/mL of cross-linked HA per syringe. A single treatment of this type of skin booster is sufficient to boost skin hydration and elasticity for up to 9 months. Intended for intradermal injections, it fills in the superficial cutaneous depressions such as fine lines and superficial acne scars and improves the skin quality, hydration, and elasticity. It utilizes the VYCROSS technology, which is a patented blend of lower and higher molecular weight HA that has undergone a unique cross-linking process to produce an efficiently bound matrix.[1]

Partially Cross-linked

Partially cross-linked HA chains contain up to 20 mg/mL of HA per syringe.[2] The protocol is three treatments spaced 4 weeks apart initially and then maintenance sessions every 6–12 months. They come with the Smart Click technology to ensure precise dispensing of metered dose, which generates an acoustic signal for every 10 μL injected. The clicking sound is produced by a small metal plate that is pressed over the grooved surface of the plastic piston. There are insufficient and nonsustainable results in few studies because it gets neutralized much faster by hyaluronidase due to a lack of cross-links.[3]

Biostimulatory Injectables

Biostimulatory injectable is a stabilized HA-based product designed to remodel multilayered skin tissue. It is usually preferred to treat mature and aging skin with signs of photodamage and where the acne scars are scattered, superficial, and are not the primary concern. The benefit of such kinds of skin boosters is that they have the highest HA concentration of 32 mg/mL. They are also clinically tested. Biostimulatory skin boosters are slowly injected with 10 injection sites, and there is little-to-no risk of bruising or hematomas. Five injection sites are specially planned for each side of the face to support different anatomical regions **(Fig. 1)**. Patients primarily report lifting and skin texture improvements across the cheeks, lip area, and chin.[4]

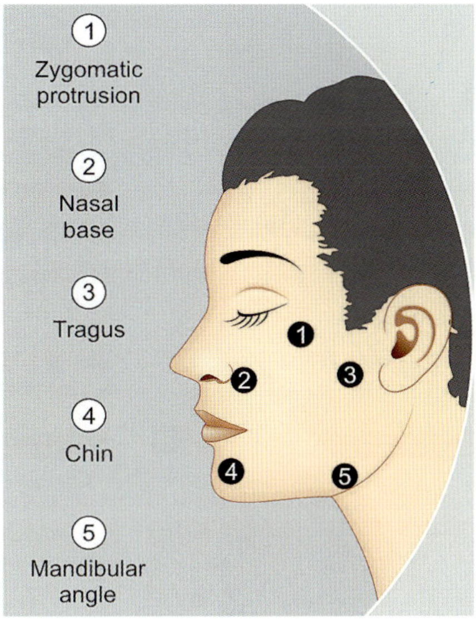

Fig. 1: Five injection sites for biostimulatory injectables.

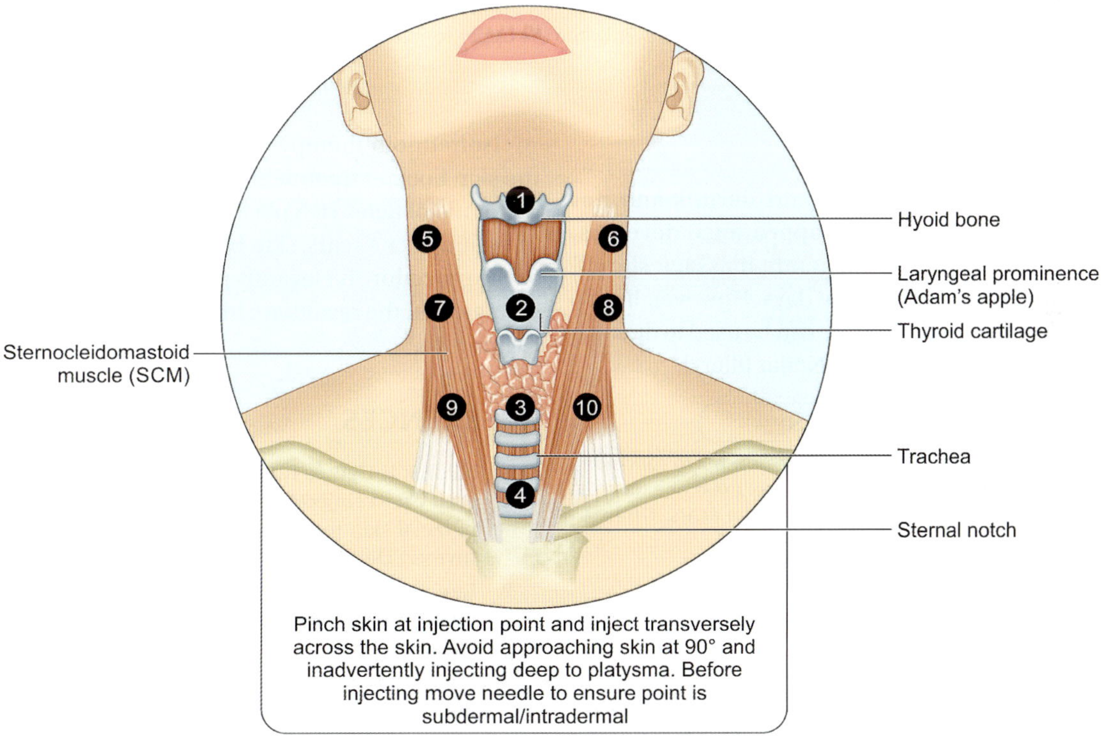

Fig. 2: Injection technique.

PROCEDURE (FIG. 2)

Prior to the procedure, a topical numbing cream is applied, which makes the treatment a comfortable experience. For a full-face treatment, the face is divided into three sections: Upper, mid, and lower. Skin boosters are injected evenly into the upper-to-mid dermis to a depth of 1.5–2 mm **(Figs. 3A and B)**. Each side of the face can receive 1–2 mL of skin booster depending on the requirement.

SIDE EFFECTS[5]

Side effects of skin boosters are as follows:

- Swelling
- Bruising
- Bumpiness or cobblestone appearance, if injected too superficially
- Tenderness
- Itching in the treatment areas.

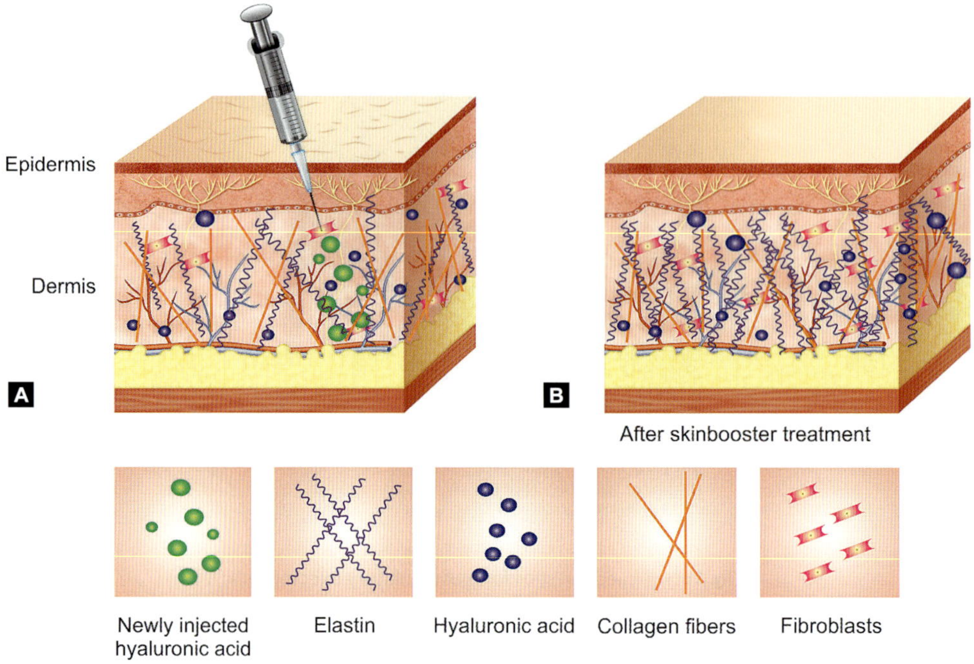

Figs. 3A and B: Skin booster injections evenly into the upper-to-mid dermis: (A) Before and (B) After.

AUTHOR'S EXPERIENCE

Skin boosters are best injected in mid-dermis and not too superficially. In case a beaded appearance develops, especially in areas with thin skin, gentle massage should be done immediately or within a few days. However, if they remain persistent, then hyaluronidase can be used to dissolve them (in the same concentration as regular fillers).

> **SURGICAL PEARLS**
>
> While injecting the skin booster into the acne scars, a micro subcision can be done with the same needle to release and break the fibrotic strands, which would also help smoothening the scars. Often a 27-number needle may suffice for thicker scars.

CONCLUSION

Skin boosters are preferred as a final step in treating acne scars as they are a great finisher. An interval of 4–6 weeks should be kept between using a heat or energy-based device and the final session of the skin booster.

If the patient has a social or personal emergency and wants quick results, a skin booster is the first and the best option for grade 1 and 2 scars with minimal downtime and almost immediate results.

Skin boosters are of minimal value in ice pick scars and longstanding untreated scars. They do not work as monotherapy for boxcar scars. The results are very variable for pitted scars, mainly when used as a sole option.

Isotretinoin therapy can be safely continued along with the skin booster treatment.

While platelet-rich plasma (PRP) therapy is also effective in treating acne scars, skin boosters may score a point over it as the procedure is elegantly performed with a sterile prefilled syringe, and the results are immediately visible and continue to improve.[6]

REFERENCES

1. Niforos F, Ogilvie P, Cavallini M, Leys C, Chantrey J, Safa M, et al. VYC-12 injectable gel is safe and effective for improvement of facial skin topography: A Prospective Study. Clin Cosmet Investig Dermatol. 2019;12:791-8.
2. Lee BM, Han DG, Choi WS. Rejuvenating effects of facial hydrofilling using restylane vital. Arch Plast Surg. 2015;42(3):282-7.
3. Wohlrab J, Wohlrab D, Neubert RH. Comparison of noncross-linked and cross-linked hyaluronic acid with regard to efficacy of the proliferative activity of cutaneous fibroblasts and keratinocytes in vitro. J Cosmet Dermatol. 2013;12(1):36-40.
4. Cassuto D, Delledonne M, Zaccaria G, Illiano I, Giori A M, et al. Safety assessment of high- and low-molecular-weight hyaluronans (Profhilo®) as derived from worldwide postmarketing data. Biomed Res Int. 2020;2020:8159047.
5. Lafaille P, Benedetto A. Fillers: Contraindications, side effects, and precautions. J Cutan Aesthet Surg. 2010;3(1):16-9.
6. Hesseler MJ, Shyam N. 'Platelet-rich plasma and its utility in the treatment of acne scars - A systematic review.' J Am Acad Dermatol. 2019;80(6):1730-45.

SECTION 14

Liposuction

CHAPTER 98

Dermatologic Liposuction Surgery

Nilesh N Goyal

KEY MESSAGES

- Liposuction and fat grafting are an extension of cosmetic procedures offered by a dermatosurgeon to the cosmetically inclined patients.
- Liposuction is an easy to adapt, safe and economically rewarding surgical procedure that can be performed under local anesthesia at a dermatosurgeon's facility offering sterile surgical theater.
- Microcannular tumescent liposuction has been proven to be the gold standard method for safe and effective liposuction.

INTRODUCTION

Liposuction (aka *suction lipectomy, lipoplasty*) is defined as the method of removal of fat from the desired areas under tumescent local anesthesia using vacuum suction and micro cannulas.

Liposuction done traditionally using cannulas with vacuum assistance is said to be the manual way of performing liposuction. The vacuum can be created using syringe or a suction pump.

HISTORY

Dr Arpad Fischer of Roma, Italy first described liposuction when he developed a method of removal of fat using a hollow metal tube.[1] This procedure underwent modifications over the next decade with advent of use of blunt cannulas (Illouz YZ, Paris), syringe liposculpture (Fournier PS, Paris), and tumescent anesthesia (Klein JA, USA).[2-4] Many dermatosurgeons have adopted the procedure across the globe. It has become a part of core training in dermatologic procedures in many countries including the USA and Indonesia.

INDICATIONS

An ideal patient for this procedure is the one who is medically fit not having any systemic disease and has a body weight very close to the ideal body weight for that person with respect to age, gender and height.[5] Patients who have recently gained fat respond better to liposuction.

The procedure aims to redefine the body curves by getting rid of the fat lobules. It does help to a certain extent in reducing the overall fat load in a high body mass index (BMI) individual but the reduction in weight is not the primary objective of the surgery.

Liposuction is a useful method of treating patients with large lipomas on body and extremities. The procedure helps in achieving a cosmetically accepted removal of the grotesque lumps without the need for large incisions and postoperative hospital stay.[6,7] Another condition that presents very commonly to dermatology clinics and can be treated successfully with liposuction is axillary hyperhidrosis. This is a very simple procedure wherein the incriminating sweat glands are curetted under tumescent local anesthesia giving long-lasting results.[8]

CONTRAINDICATIONS

A person with BMI >35 would be thought to be the one benefitting most from this procedure; however, almost all studies show that the best results with liposuction are obtained in those with BMI between 25 and 30.[9] The patient needs to be informed about this prior to procedure. There is a significant increase in complications when liposuction is performed in patients with BMI >30.[10]

It is done under local anesthesia with lidocaine. Hence, it is very important that a detailed history regarding medications is taken. There is a long list of drugs that interfere with the cytochrome P-450 system thereby having an impact on the metabolism of lidocaine and its overall efficacy to provide anesthesia[11] **(Table 1)**.

Patients with hepatic and renal impairment should be excluded.

There is a risk of poor healing and infections in diabetic patients due to development of microvascular channels. Patients with hypertension need to have their blood pressures controlled very well prior to taking up for the procedure.

This procedure is to be avoided in those taking blood thinners and in those with bleeding disorders.

It is advisable to avoid this procedure in those with communicable viral illnesses such as human immunodeficiency virus (HIV), hepatitis B, and hepatitis C. This keeps the risk of transmission to minimum, especially when using nondisposable cannulas.

TABLE 1: Common drugs that affect lidocaine metabolism via cytochrome P-450 enzyme inhibition or stimulation.

Antifungal: • Fluconazole • Itraconazole • Ketoconazole • Miconazole *Benzodiazepines:* • Alprazolam • Diazepam • Flurazepam • Midazolam *Calcium channel blockers:* • Amiodarone • Diltiazem • Felodipine • Nicardipine • Nifedipine • Verapamil	*Macrolide antibiotics:* • Erythromycin • Clarithromycin *Protease inhibitors:* • Indinavir • Nelfinavir • Ritonavir • Saquinavir *Selective serotonin reuptake inhibitors (SSRI):* • Fluoxetine • Paroxetine • Sertraline • Nefazodone • Fluvoxamine	*Miscellaneous:* • Anastrozole • Caffeine • Cimetidine • Ciprofloxacin • Isoniazid • Norfloxacin • Omeprazole • Acetazolamide • Cyclosporine • Danazol • Metronidazole • Grapefruit juice • Quinidine • Troglitazone • Zafirlukast

Source: Adapted from Klein JA. Tumescent Anesthesia.

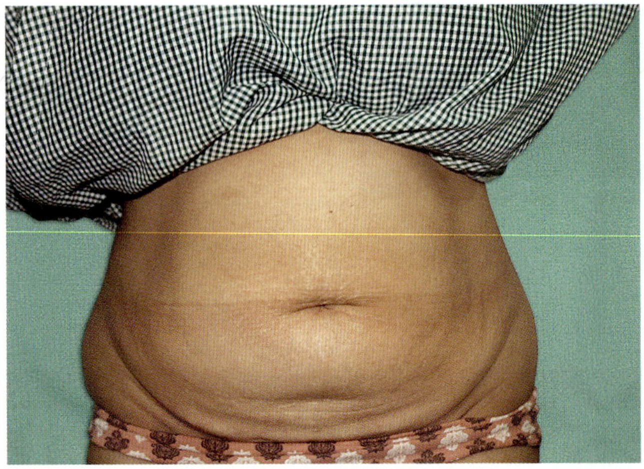

Fig. 1: Front view of abdomen of a 31-year-old lady on the day of liposuction to upper and lower abdomen.

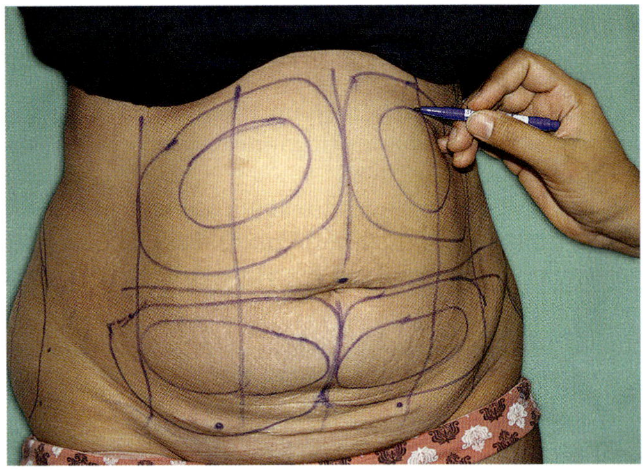

Fig. 2: Marking of upper and lower abdomen showing delineation of mounds of fat and division of the area into smaller quadrants.

Patients who have lost a lot of body weight by diet and exercise tend to have less fat and more fibrous tissue in the subcutaneous area. A liposuction done in such a person does not remove much fat. In such an individual postprocedure skin contraction is limited. This leads to less than desired change in body shape that can result in an unhappy patient.

Smoking can often be a cause of worry for poor healing of the fat compartment. The risk of venous thromboembolism following liposuction is higher in chronic smokers.[12] It can also lead to less than expected retraction of skin following the procedure which results in loose skin postoperatively.

PROCEDURE

Preparation

Counseling

It is advisable to discuss the areas to be treated with patient at the clinic visit. At the same visit, the patient is informed regarding the benefits and risks involved. The patient signs a copy of the consent form with all information at this visit.

Clinical photographs are to be taken in proper lighting with due consideration to patient modesty[13] **(Fig. 1)**.

A record of patient's maximum and current body weight in kilograms is a must. This will help in calculating the maximum dose of lidocaine that can be given on the day of surgery.

For very anxious patients, a prescription for lorazepam 2 mg preoperatively can be given. In addition in some, clonidine 0.1 mg can be given as preoperative sedative. These have least interaction with lidocaine.

On the Day of Surgery

Patient is asked to have a light meal preprocedure.

Patient's vital parameters are recorded by a trained staff nurse. These are repeated every 30 minutes for the entire length of procedure. Any aberration from the normal in the readings is immediately informed to the operating dermatosurgeon.

An intravenous line access with a 21 G cannula is advisable. It can be used to administer antibiotics and, in some cases, painkillers and/or antiemetics.

The area to be worked upon has to be marked with a semipermanent skin marker pen. The fat mounds are delineated in a circular fashion and the entire region is divided into grids with vertical and horizontal lines **(Fig. 2)**. This helps in deciding the amount of tumescent fluid to be infiltrated and for removing fat during aspiration from each grid area.

Marking is done with the patient in standing position and the surgeon at the same level as that of the area being marked.

Cleaning of the surgical area is done using povidone iodine solution followed by surgical spirit. This is easier with the patient standing.

A sterile drape is laid on the operating table. The patient is made to lie on this.

Tumescent Anesthesia

While the patient is being cleansed and prepped, a trained staff is given instructions to prepare the tumescent solution. This is made by adding lidocaine, adrenaline and sodium bicarbonate to 1 L bags of normal saline or Ringer's lactate (Klein's formula) **(Fig. 3)**. The total dose of lidocaine is calculated as per the body weight of patient. It has been proven that up to 55 mg/kg bodyweight of lidocaine can be administered on a day in an obese female patient. Doses up to 45 mg/kg can be safely used for obese male patients.[14] The area of body that is to be anesthetized determines the amount of lidocaine in each bag. For example, around 1,500 mg of lidocaine in 1 L of normal saline is required while working on a female breast but only 800 mg of lidocaine in 1 L of normal saline is adequate for abdomen and waist areas.

The amount of lidocaine is calculated in mg/mL of a 1 or 2% ready available solution. So, a 1% lidocaine solution contains around 10 mg/mL of the drug while a 2% solution contains around 20 mg/mL of the drug. It is essential to stick to the same method of calculating dose of lidocaine so as to prevent confusion among staff and possible overdosing.

The usual amount of adrenaline in each bag varies from 0.5 to 1 mL of a 1:100,000 solution. This works by causing vasoconstriction that helps in reducing the blood loss significantly. The entire mixture with lidocaine tends to have an acidic pH, which results in stinging sensation during administration. To raise the pH sodium bicarbonate is added up to 10 mL of an 8.4 mEq/L solution in each 1 L bag. Raising the pH reduces stinging during infiltration.

Tumescent anesthesia using lidocaine is the most essential feature of microcannular liposuction. Use of multiple drugs for anesthesia, i.e., general anesthetics and local anesthetic can lead to drug interactions within the patient resulting in complications. General anesthesia is associated with accelerated coagulability which is thought to increase the risk of venous thromboembolism.[15,16] It is preferable to avoid multidrug anesthesia. The metabolism of lidocaine when given in high doses has a bearing on drugs concomitantly administered during the procedure. Deaths have been reported when patients have been given sedatives or anxiolytics along with lidocaine.[17]

Infiltration

Once the patient has got on the operating table, a local anesthesia is given at the sites of adits. This is done using up to 2 mL of a ready mixture of lidocaine and adrenaline (1:200,000) at each site under the skin. A 2 mm round skin punch is used to make entry points at the anesthetized sites **(Fig. 4)**. A round hole is preferable as it causes lesser friction during cannula movement and does not seal during the time duration of procedure. Further a round hole can close well postoperatively under pressure dressing resulting in a better scar.

Anesthesia is begun using either a 23 G spinal needle or a 2 mm diameter infiltration cannula with multiple holes distributed circumferentially extending up to 2 inches from the tip. The tumescent solution in 500 mL or 1 L bags is pushed using a pressure bag or a specially designed infiltration pump with a peristaltic infusion system **(Figs. 5 and 6)**. The cannula or the needle is moved forward and backward in each direction from all the adits so as to have a uniform infiltration. To begin with lifting the skin along with superficial fat with the nondominant hand infiltrates the deeper fat **(Fig. 7)**. Once this is achieved then the superficial fat is infiltrated. A record is kept of the time of finishing infiltration and the amount of solution infiltrated.

A waiting/settling time of 45–60 minutes is required for the detumescence to happen (**Figs. 8 and 9**). During this time, the adrenaline works upon the blood vessels causing vasoconstriction. This reduces the systemic absorption of lidocaine preventing a rise in blood lidocaine levels and its consequent metabolism. Monitoring of the patients vital parameters is continued during this phase.

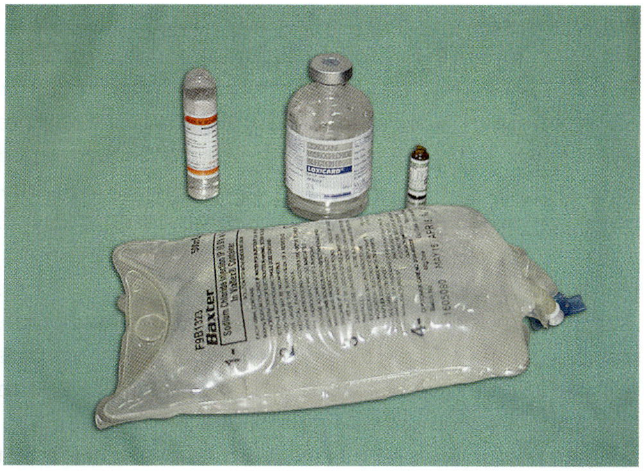

Fig. 3: Ingredients for making of Klein's tumescent anesthesia solution.

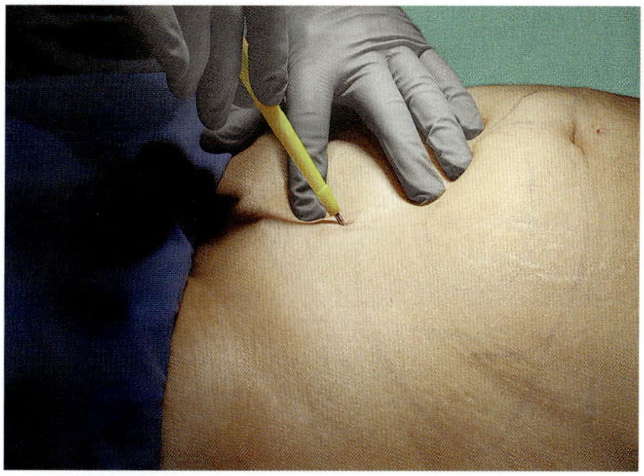

Fig. 4: Making of adits with 2 mm skin punch.

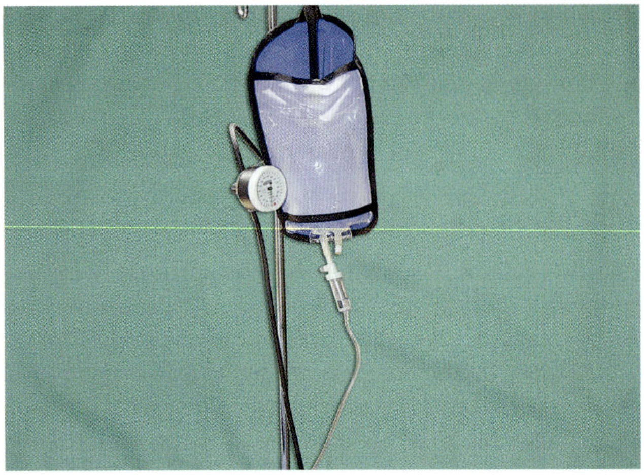

Fig. 5: Pressure infusion bag.

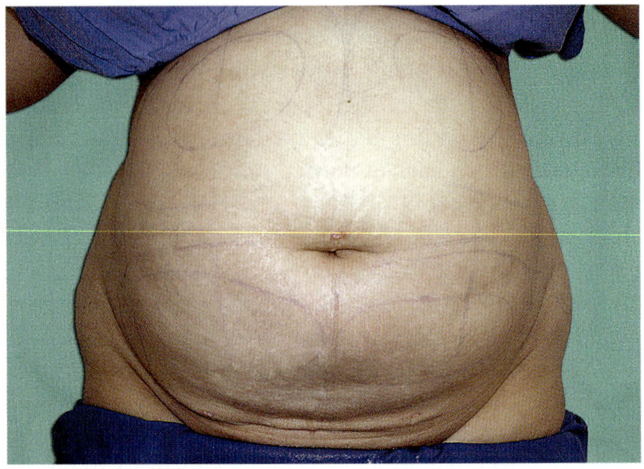

Fig. 8: Area to be treated (upper and lower abdomen) immediately after infiltration of tumescent anesthesia solution.

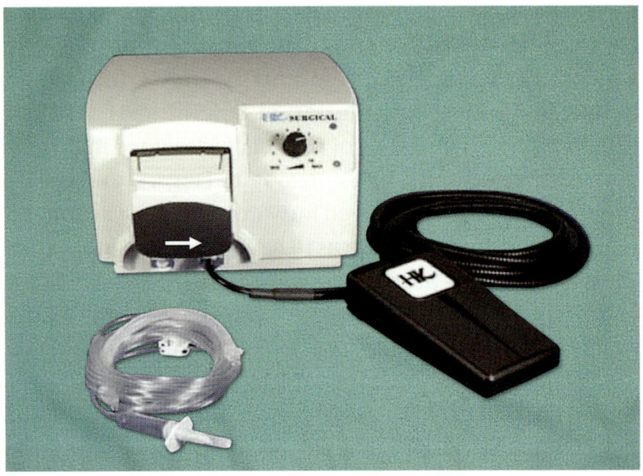

Fig. 6: Infiltration pump with foot *pedal* and specialized rubber tubing.

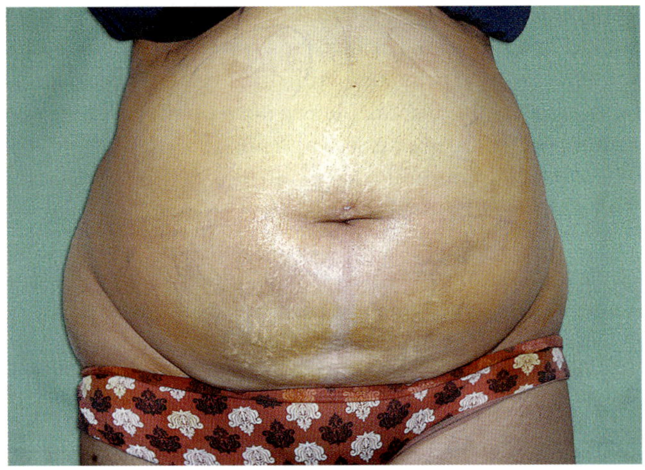

Fig. 9: Area (upper and lower abdomen) infiltrated showing detumescence after settling time.

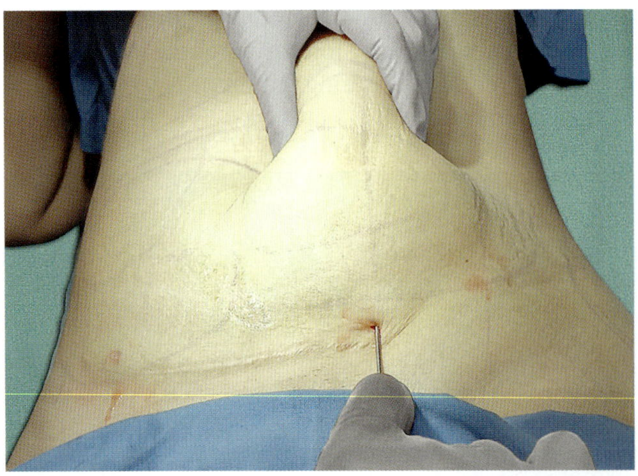

Fig. 7: Infiltration of tumescent anesthesia solution beginning in the deeper plane.

Aspiration

Before starting aspiration of fat, the areas to be treated are once again cleansed using povidone iodine solution and surgical spirit. The patient is made to lie on the operating table and the procedure started by using a 16 G cannula attached to a suction pump or syringe. Strict asepsis is maintained throughout the procedure to prevent infection through the adits. Suction is usually started with the smallest diameter cannula through all the adits. This is followed with higher diameter cannulas (i.e., 14 G, 12 G, and 10 G) till the desired amount of fat has been removed from all the areas **(Fig. 10)**. At frequent intervals during suctioning, the area worked upon is checked for fat remaining under the skin. The author follows the rule of three—after every three strokes, the cannula is withdrawn partially and the direction with the area of suctioning is changed. This prevents unequal fat aspiration that could result in liponots or lipotrops.

At all times, the nondominant hand helps in guiding the aspiration cannula tip into the desired fat plane by pinching the skin and superficial fat along with it **(Fig. 11)**. Suctioning of fat from the superficial plane should be avoided to prevent damage to neurovascular plexus that runs through it. Injury to this plexus can result in skin necrosis and resultant

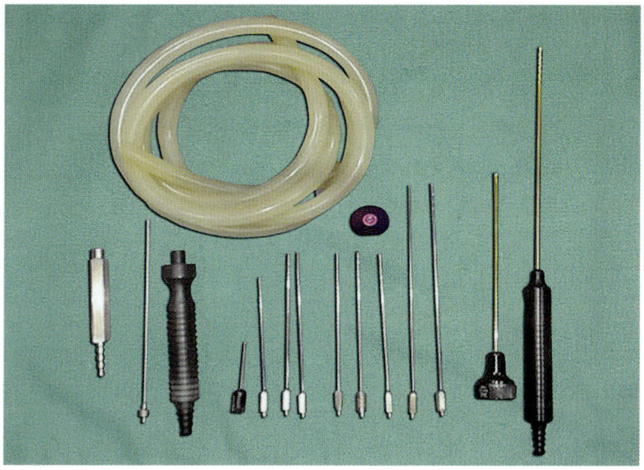

Fig. 10: Lipobodysculpting and fat transfer kit showing cannulas of varying diameters and lengths, silicon tubing, and decant stand.

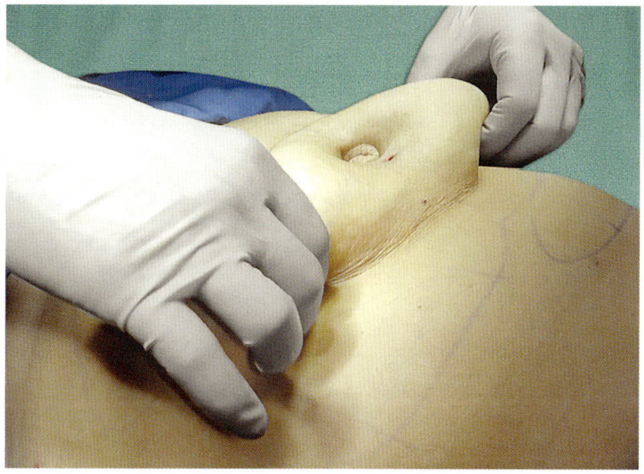

Fig. 12: Pinch test to ascertain adequacy of aspiration of fat; it is advisable to compare the two sides to avoid uneven appearance.

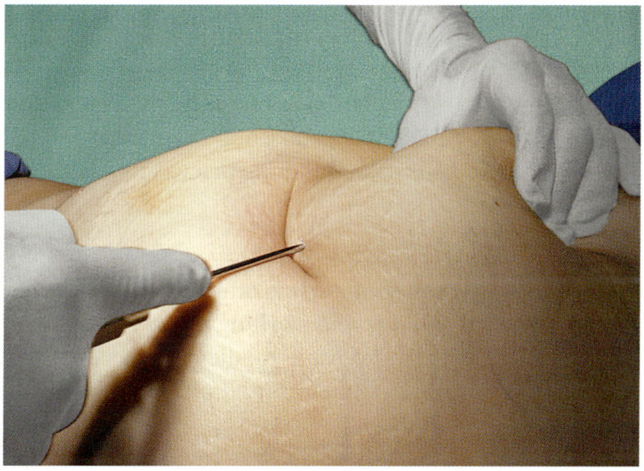

Fig. 11: Fat aspiration—note placement of thumb on the handle hole controlling suction, index finger on upper end of hub of cannula and left hand grasping the skin and superficial fat in a firm grip.

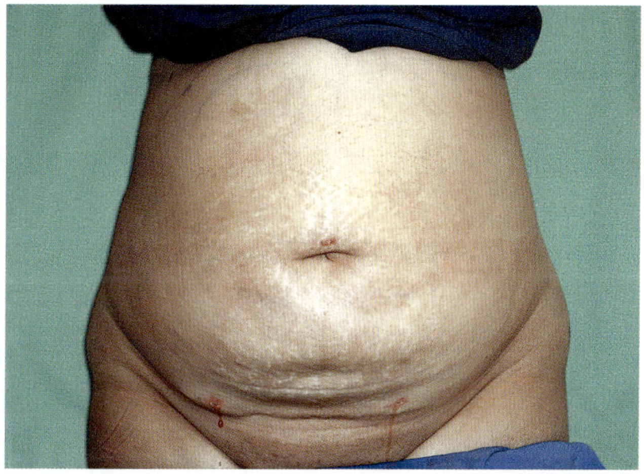

Fig. 13: Immediate intraoperative photograph showing treated area (upper and lower abdomen).

scarring. It can also lead to prolonged numbness after the procedure.[18]

Dressing

Once it is decided on table that adequate fat has been removed and the desired shape has been achieved, the patient is made to stand **(Fig. 12)**. Immediate postoperative photographs are taken of the areas treated **(Figs. 13 and 14)**. Often these show immediate change of body shape. All the adits or wounds are covered with an antiseptic ointment and gauze swab. The entire treated area, in particular, the adits are covered with a thick Gamjee roll dressing **(Fig. 15)**. This soaks all the blood stained discharge coming out of the adits postoperatively. This is further compressed and held in place with a Coban dressing (3M, USA) which helps in squeezing out all the fluid collected inside the treated areas **(Fig. 16)**. This is a variation of the bimodal compression dressing described by Jeffrey Klein.[19]

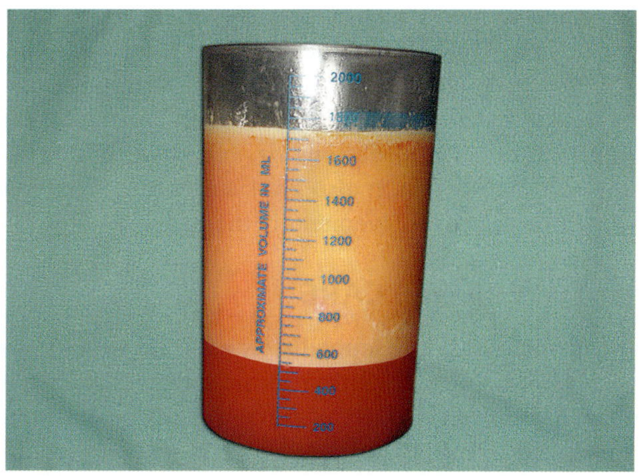

Fig. 14: Suction machine canister showing aspirated material with fat in the upper part separated from the blood-tinged solution at the bottom.

The patient is informed about this discharge that continues for up to 24 hours postoperatively. On top of the above dressing, the patient is made to wear a compression

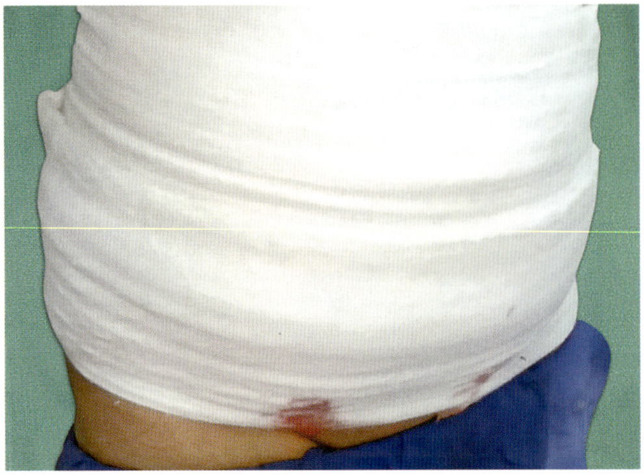

Fig. 15: Gamjee roll dressing to cover treated area over the gauze swabs.

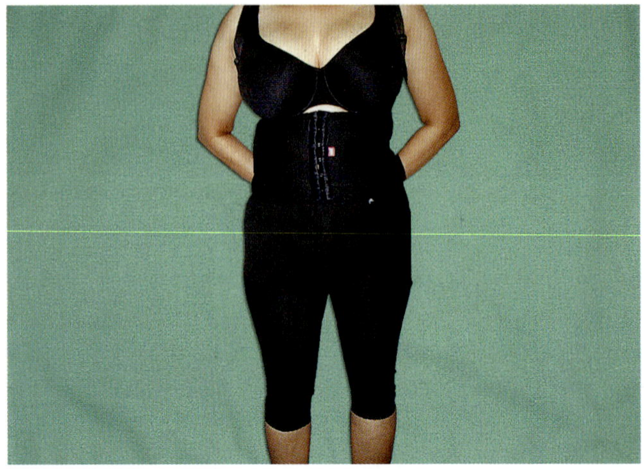

Fig. 17: Final layer of bimodal compression dressing with compression garment.

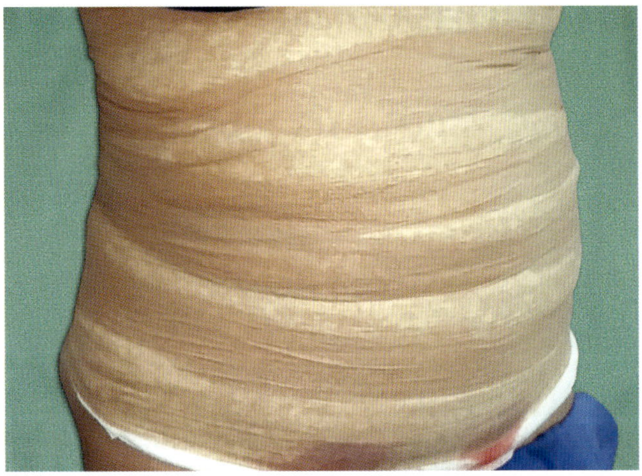

Fig. 16: Coban dressing over Gamjee roll dressing to exert maximal pressure onto the treated area.

garment **(Fig. 17)**. This is made to measure garment specific for liposuction patients that have to be worn daily for up to 2 weeks after the procedure. It helps in preventing early complications of liposuction, viz. bleeding, hematoma, seroma, and infection. It also gives support to the treated tissues allowing easy movements of the body.

POSTOPERATIVE CARE

Patients are sent home immediately after the surgery once their vital parameters are within normal limits. They are given emergency contact numbers of the clinic and doctor who can be contacted in case of any problems. It is generally followed at the author's clinic that all patients are given a call by the clinic staff on the second day to check upon them. This call also helps to find out if patients have encountered any delayed side effects of lidocaine.

The patients are instructed to remove all dressing on the following day and wash all treated areas thoroughly with soap and water. From the second day, no dressing is required. The patient is to apply an antibacterial ointment daily to the adits till they heal. The compression garment is worn daily as instructed. The patient is to take oral antibiotics and pain killers as advised by the doctor for up to a week.

FOLLOW-UP

The patients are seen in the clinic after 7–10 days to check upon the healing of adits and swelling of the treated areas. Pain is treated with appropriate medications at this stage. Gradual start of exercise is permitted after 2 weeks of the procedure.

At this stage when patients are very keen to see the effects of the procedure it is very important to explain that the fat compartment will now take on an indurated feel. This will settle within 4–6 weeks after the procedure and then the overlying skin will contract. The final result will be evident 2–3 months postprocedure.

Safety of Tumescent Liposuction

Liposuction under tumescent local anesthesia without the use of any other form of anesthesia has been found to be safe compared with liposuction done under tumescent anesthesia with regional or sedation anesthesia.[20,21] The doses of lidocaine used for tumescent anesthesia have been extensively studied and found to be safe in the range of 35–55 mg/kg. Aspiration of fat admixed with the anesthetic solution prevents at any time for the maximum serum concentration of lidocaine to cross 6 μg/kg.[22,23] This level is thought to be associated with onset of lidocaine toxicity effects. Studies done by Jeffrey Klein have shown that serum lidocaine levels range between 1.5 and 4.5 μg/kg during the course of a liposuction under tumescent local anesthesia and for up to 48 hours postoperatively. It has been found that most of the serious complications associated with liposuction have occurred when the patient is exposed to more than one form of anesthesia.[24] A survey done among dermatologic surgeons across USA highlighted that the rate of complications was much lower when the procedure was conducted in dermatologic offices than at hospitals.[21] The risk of complications was least when the rules of liposuction under tumescent anesthesia were strictly followed by the operating doctor.[20,25] Guidelines for care of liposuction recommend that a board certified dermatologist with adequate training in liposuction at recognized courses and at surgical table under the tutelage of an experienced dermatologic surgeon specializing in liposuction can very well perform liposuction in his/her practice.[26]

COMPLICATIONS

Immediate

- *Pain:* In the initial phase it can be of sharp nature but soon after it becomes a dull aching pain, which occurs on movement of the treated area of body. This pain is reduced a lot by wearing the compression garment and regular painkillers.
- *Bleeding and bruising:* Immediately after the procedure, there can be some blood-stained discharge from the adits. Frank bleeding is seen when the surgeon employs large bore cannulas. Bruising is often seen when adequate compression of the treated area is not employed. This occurs due to collection of the blood within the superficial tissues of the treated area. Again this is prevented by wearing compression garment regularly **(Fig. 18)**.
- *Hematoma and seroma formation:* These occur due to collection of blood and serous fluid within the treated fat compartment. Wearing compression garment can prevent these **(Figs. 19 and 20)**.
- *Infection:* The risk of infection in an open adit is high, but this can be reduced by following strict asepsis during infiltration and aspiration. The cannula tip should not be touched at any time during surgery. The bimodal compression and open drainage helps in getting rid of the excess fluid collections in the treated fat compartment. All the cannula tracks get apposed due to the tight compression postoperatively. This significantly reduces the chances of infection setting in.[27] To be on safe side, every patient is started on a prophylactic 5-day course of oral antibiotics starting from the day of surgery.
- *Morning after liposuction syncope:*[28] This is the transient episode of dizziness that can be experienced by some patients when they get up the morning after liposuction. It occurs due to postural hypotension secondary to liposuction of the limbs. It could also occur after seeing blood-soaked dressing while changing.
- *Postliposuction edema:*[29] This occurs due to collection of excess fluid in the extracellular space post operatively. It is brought upon by two factors:

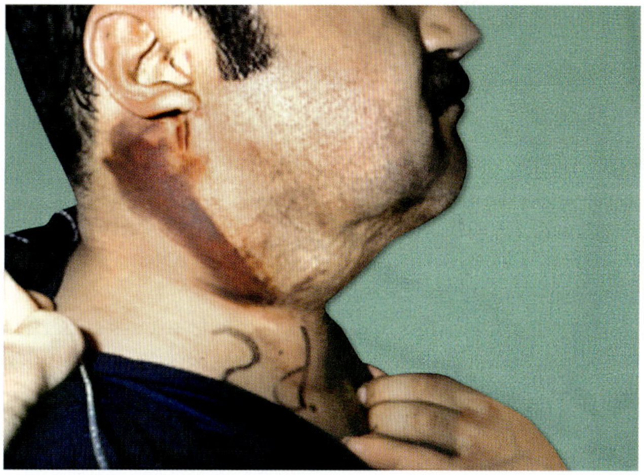

Fig. 19: Hematoma formation after liposuction of neck tracking into the posterior triangle.
Courtesy: Prof Lawrence M Field, USA.

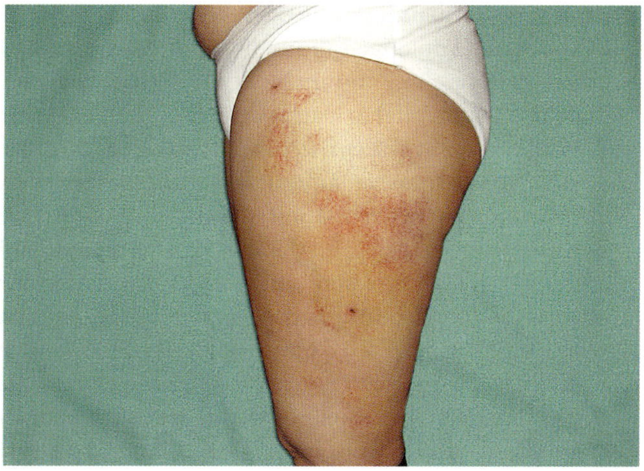

Fig. 18: Significant bruising seen 2nd day after lipobodysculpting done to saddle bags in a young lady.

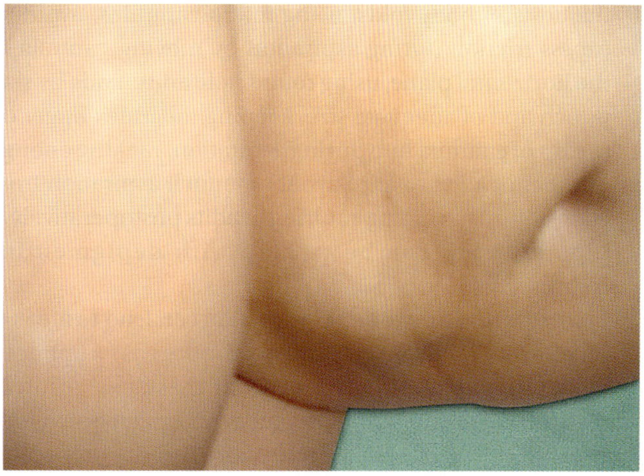

Fig. 20: Seroma formation on lower abdomen.
Courtesy: Dr Ioannis Peros, Greece.

(a) Impaired lymphatic drainage and (b) Excessive capillary filtration. It is seen usually in the areas distal to the treated fat compartments on limbs particularly. Prolonged suctioning can damage lymphatic channels and also capillaries which together result in edema postoperatively. Further, closing the adits after the procedure can prevent the escape of fluid from the treated fat compartments. Open drainage and bimodal compression dressing can greatly help in reducing the swelling. It can last for 3–5 days after the procedure. It usually responds to limb elevation and gentle massage of the area.

- *Irregularity of menstrual cycles:* It has been reported in some patients especially when liposuction is done in the lower abdomen and upper thigh areas.
- *Fascial and muscular injury:* This is more common after excess deep suctioning of fat using large bore cannulas. It can result in frank blood colored aspirate and also tends to be painful in an awake patient. The tissue heals within 7–10 days but can cause restriction of movements of the affected area till it heals.

Delayed Complications

- *Prolonged numbness of skin:* This is more of an issue in patients in whom superficial liposuction has been performed that results in damage to the neurovascular plexus in this compartment. The cutaneous nerves regenerate within 3–6 months with return of normal sensations.
- *Irregularity of skin:* Again this is due to excess superficial compartment liposuction that results in unequal fat removal. The skin overlying the treated area feels granular and lumpy at places and also wrinkled at times. This gets better as the skin contracts over the 3 months postprocedure.
- *Scars:* There is risk of hyperpigmented and prominent scars at sites of adits. This is more so in dark-skinned patients **(Fig. 21)**. This risk can be minimized by placing the adits in body folds, using micro cannulas, avoiding excess friction during aspiration by moving cannula in the horizontal plane, using round hole adits made by skin punch and of adequate size, keeping the index finger on the tip of cannula hub during aspiration, making enough number of adits so as to avoid too much aspiration from each adit and avoiding suturing of adits postoperatively.[28] Pigmentation can be tackled with depigmenting creams.
- *Lipotrops and liponots:*[28] Liposuction can lead to areas of unequal fat removal resulting in raised areas (= liponots) or depressions (= lipotrops). Both these can result in disfigurement and unhappy patient. They can be avoided by regularly doing skin pinch tests during the procedure. Often they need redoing the liposuction to remove the lumps or fat filling in case of depressions **(Fig. 22)**.

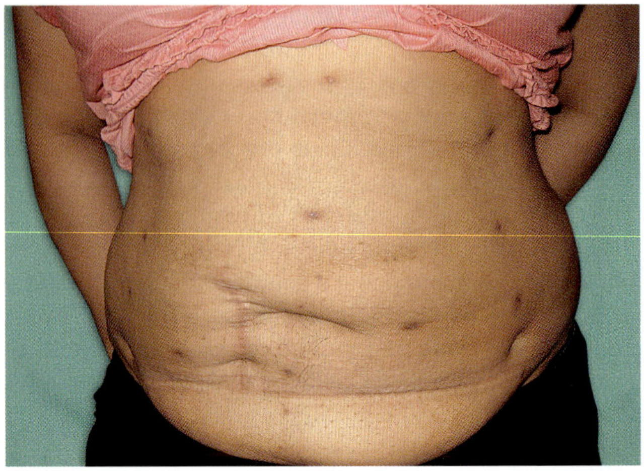

Fig. 21: Hyperpigmented scars seen at sites of adits 1 month post-liposuction to abdomen of this young Indian lady.

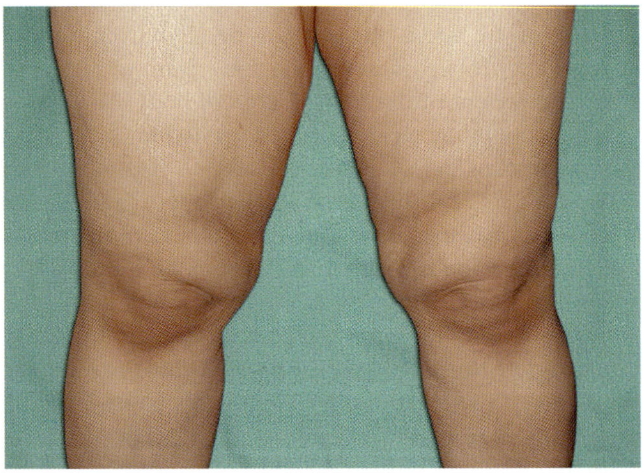

Fig. 22: Excessive lipobodysculpting above knees showing areas of depression.
Courtesy: Prof Lawrence M Field, USA.

- *Necrosis of overlying skin:* This is a serious complication occurring in a shape-changing procedure. It is the result of excessive superficial fat suctioning that damages the subcutaneous neurovascular plexus causing necrosis. The outcome is a prolonged morbidity with daily dressings, possible skin grafting and antibiotics and an unsightly scar that has the potential to lead to legal proceedings.
- *Erythema ab lipoaspiration:*[28] Another problem arising from excessive superficial lipoaspiration is the development of erythematous streaks on the overlying skin akin to those seen in erythema ab igne. It is commonly seen after use of large bore cannulas for aspiration. This again is thought to be due to damage to the subcutaneous vascular plexus. The appearance tends to be permanent.
- *Postliposuction panniculitis:*[28] This is seen occurring in cases where the adits are sutured postliposuction resulting in collection of blood-tinged fluid and serous discharge within the treated fat compartment. It results in formation of microseromas that can present with

increased redness, tenderness, swelling, and warmth of overlying skin. A bacterial culture is to be sent to rule out an infection. The patient is treated with oral antibiotics initially till the results of culture are confirmed and then a short course of oral steroids to settle the inflammation.

- *Increased risk of thromboembolic events:*[30] The risk is enhanced when the procedure is conducted using systemic and local anesthesia. Quite often surgeons employ both methods of anesthesia so as to make the patient comfortable. However, the risk of thromboembolic complications such as deep vein thrombosis and pulmonary embolism increase due to prolonged periods of immobilization and pain postoperatively. Also with use of systemic anesthesia, the patient is often administered excess of IV fluids and gets exposed to hypothermia during long surgeries that further increases the risk of hypercoagulability.[21,24]

  Other risk factors include smoking, oral contraceptive use, and immobility.

- *Necrotizing fasciitis:*[31,32] This is the most dreaded complication following liposuction. It occurs due to spread of infection from the subcutaneous plane to dermis. Perforation of abdominal viscus or poor sterilization techniques or even direct contamination of entry points after surgery can result in this complication. It requires urgent diagnosis and treatment within a tertiary hospital setup.
- *Injury to internal organs:*[33] This is a very rare occurrence with liposuction under tumescent anesthesia as an awake patient can warn the surgeon of severe pain immediately. However, this has often been reported when performing liposuction under systemic anesthesia. Often the surgeons in their zeal to remove excess fat tend to transgress the fat plane and injure an underlying organ. They do not get warned as the patient is under anesthesia. This can lead to serious complications postoperatively and has led to death in many cases.

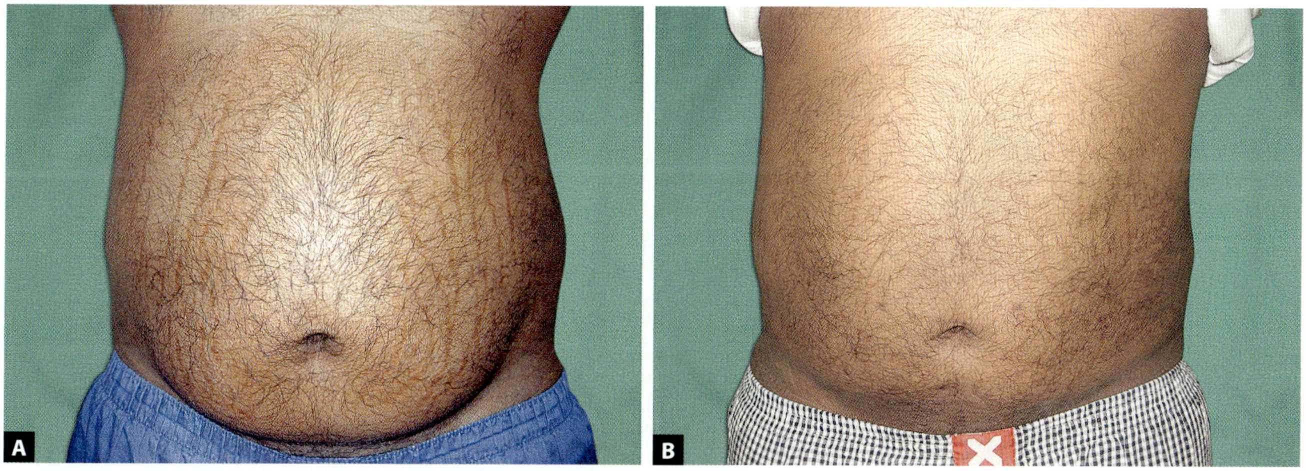

Figs. 23A and B: A 30-year-old male before and 3 months after lipobodysculpting to lower abdomen. Note the significant contraction of skin postprocedure.

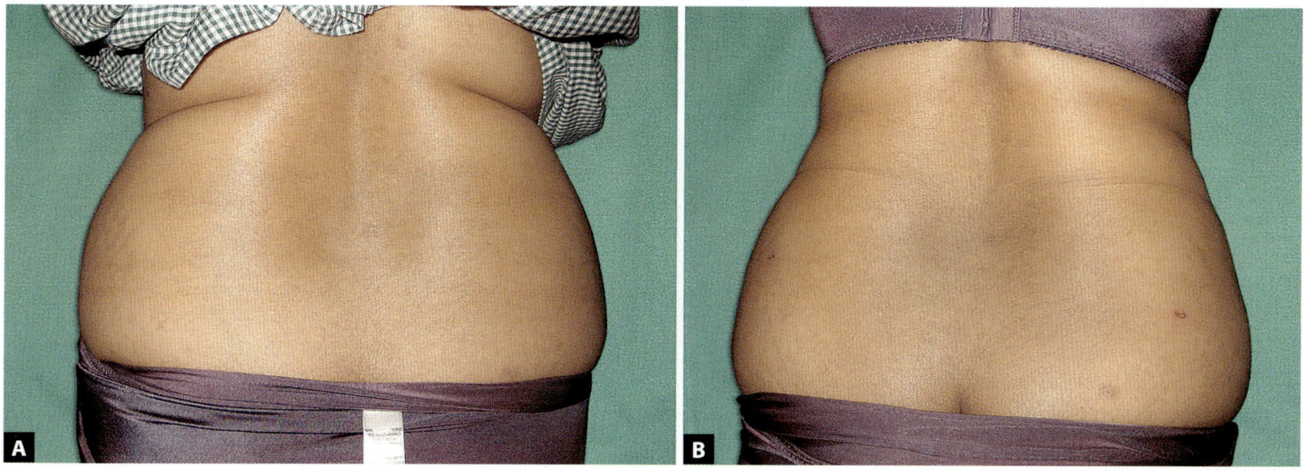

Figs. 24A and B: A 39-year-old female who underwent *lipobodysculpting* to waist and flanks. Note the absence of fold on flank in the 1 week after photograph.

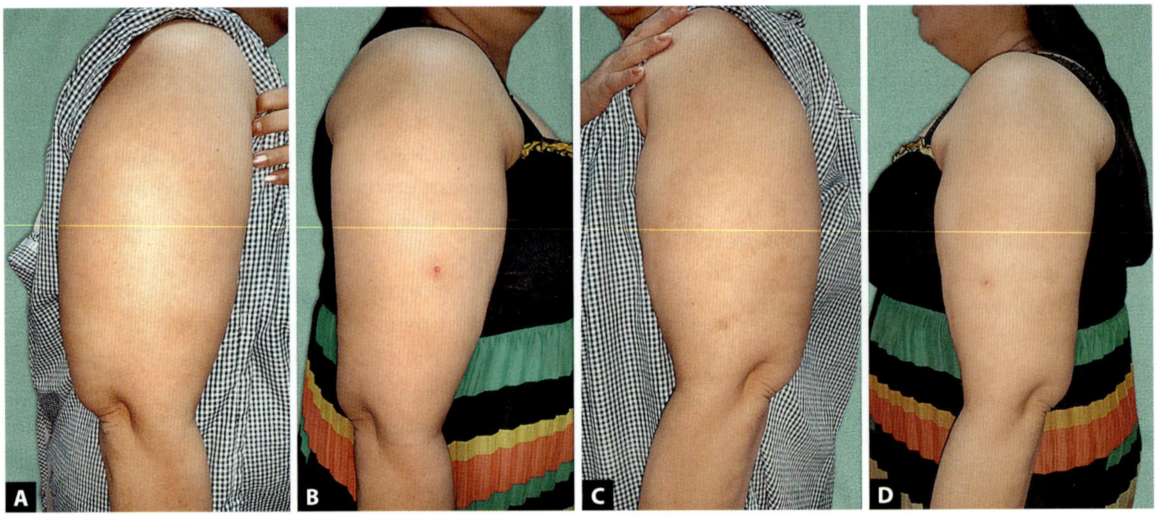

Figs. 25A to D: Views of arms before and 1 month after liposuction in a 48-year-old lady.

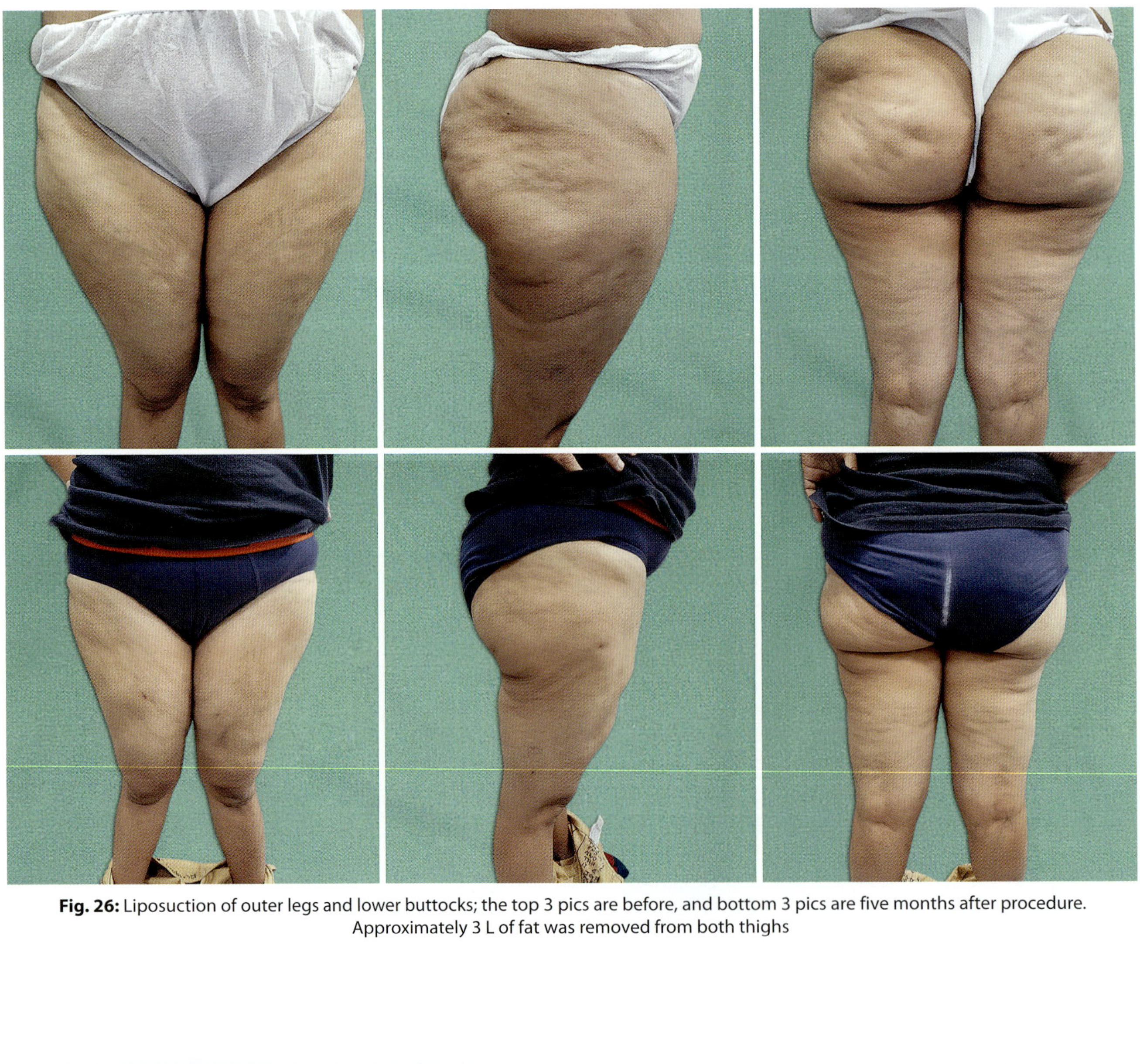

Fig. 26: Liposuction of outer legs and lower buttocks; the top 3 pics are before, and bottom 3 pics are five months after procedure. Approximately 3 L of fat was removed from both thighs

CONCLUSION

Liposuction under tumescent anesthesia is a "practice changing" procedure. The procedure is very safe and effective when performed as per the abovementioned principles. Till date no deaths have been reported across the globe when liposuction has been performed using only tumescent local anesthesia. This procedure can be easily adopted in a busy cosmetic practice as it adds to the armamentarium of procedures that can be offered to the cosmetic patient.

Figures 23 to 25 are showing before and after photographs of patients who underwent liposuction at the author's clinic.

The author also extends his gratitude toward Prof Lawrence M Field from USA and Dr Ioannis Peros from Greece for their help with photos of complications of liposuction.

REFERENCES

1. Fischer A, Fischer G. First surgical treatment for molding body's cellulite with three 5 mm incisions. Bull Int Acad Cosmet Surg. 1976;3:35.
2. Illouz YG. Body contouring by lipolysis: a 5-year experience with over 3000 cases. Plast Reconstr Surg. 1983;72(5):591-7.
3. Fournier PF. Reduction syringe liposculpturing. Dermatol Clin. 1990;8(3):539-51.
4. Klein JA. Tumescent technique for liposuction surgery. Am J Cosm Surg. 1987;4:263-7.
5. Augustin M, Zschocke I, Sommer B, Sattler G. Sociodemographic profile and satisfaction with treatment of patients undergoing Liposuction in Tumescent Local Anesthesia. Dermatol Surg. 1999;25(6):475-9.
6. Girling VRGW, Salisbury M, Ersek RA. Sequential (Serial) Suction. In Clin Plastic Surg. 2006;33(1):75-7.
7. Pinski KS, Roenigk HH Jr. Liposuction of lipomas. Dermatol Clin. 1990;8(3):483-92.
8. Lillis P, Coleman WP III. Liposuction for treatment of axillary hyperhidrosis. Dermatol Clin. 1990;8(3):479-83.
9. Seretis K, Goulis DG, Koliakos G, Demiri E. Short and long term effects of abdominal lipectomy on weight and fat mass in females: a systematic review. Obes Surg. 2015;25:1950-8.
10. Gupta V, Winocour J, Rodriguez-Feo C, Bamba R, Shack RB, Grotting JC, et al. Safety of aesthetic surgery in the overweight patient: analysis of 127,961 patients. Aesthet Surg J. 2016;36(6): 718-29.
11. Klein JA (Ed). Cytochrome P450 3A4 and lidocaine metabolism. In: Tumescent Technique. St. Louis: Mosby Inc. 2000. Chapter 18. pp. 131-40.
12. Valente DS, Carvalho LA, Zanella RK, Valente S. Venous thromboembolism following elective aesthetic plastic surgery: a longitudinal prospective study in 1254 patients. Plast Surg Int. 2014;2014:565793.
13. Toledo LS, Mauad R. Complications of body sculpture: prevention and treatment. Clin Plast Surg. 2006;33(1):1-11.
14. Klein JA (Ed). Pharmacokinetics of tumescent lidocaine. In: Tumescent Technique. St. Louis: Mosby Inc. 2000. Chapter 19. pp. 141-61.
15. Kohro S, Yamakage M, Arakawa J, Kotaki M, Omote T, Namiki A. Surgical/tourniquet pain accelerates blood coagulability but not fibrinolysis. Br J Anaesth. 1998;80:460-3.
16. Jennings S, Cass AJ, Heather BP, Greenhalgh RM. Coagulation changes during major surgery and relationship to postoperative deep vein thrombosis. J Cardiovasc Surg. 1981; 22:327-54.
17. Rao RB, Ely SF, Hoffman RS. Deaths related to liposuction. N Engl J Med. 1999;340:1471-5.
18. Klein JA (Ed). Surgical technique: microcannular tumescent liposuction. In: Tumescent Technique. St Louis: Mosby Inc. 2000. Chapter 28. pp. 248-70.
19. Klein JA (Ed). Postliposuction care: open drainage and bimodal compression. In: Tumescent Technique. St Louis: Mosby Inc. 2000. Chapter 30. pp. 281-93.
20. Habbema L. Safety of liposuction using exclusively tumescent local anaesthesia in 3,240 consecutive cases. Dermatol Surg. 2009;35(11):1728-35.
21. Housman TS, Lawrence N, Mellen BG, George MN, Filippo JS, Cerveny KA, et al. The safety of liposuction: results of a national survey. Dermatol Surg. 2002;28(11):971-8.
22. Klein JA, Jeske DR. Estimated maximal safe dosages of tumescent lidocaine. Anesth Analg. 2016;122(5):1350-9.
23. Ostad A, Kageyama N, Moy RL. Tumescent anaesthesia with a lidocaine dose of 55 mg/kg is safe for liposuction. Dermatol Surg. 1996;22:921-7.
24. Tierney EP, Kouba DJ, Hanke CW. Safety of tumescent and laser-assisted liposuction: review of the literature. J Drugs Dermatol. 2011;10(12):1363-9.
25. Boeni R. Safety of tumescent liposuction under local anaesthesia in a series of 4,380 patients. Dermatology. 2011;222(3):278-81.
26. Coldiron B, Coleman WP III, Cox SE, Jacob C, Lawrence N, Kaminer M, et al. Education/Training. ASDS Guidelines of Care for Tumescent Liposuction. Dermatol Surg. 2006;32(5):710-1.
27. Klein JA (Ed). Miscellaneous complications. In: Tumescent Technique. St Louis: Mosby Inc. 2000. Chapter 8. pp. 43-60.
28. Klein JA (Ed). Postliposuction edema. In: Tumescent Technique. St Louis: Mosby Inc. 2000. Chapter 11. pp. 79-87.
29. Klein JA (Ed). Thrombosis and embolism. Tumescent Technique. St Louis: Mosby Inc. 2000. Chapter 10. pp. 67-78.
30. Sharma D, Dalencourt G, Bitterly T, Benotti PN. Small intestinal perforation and necrotizing fasciitis after abdominal liposuction. Aesthetic Plast Surg. 2006;30(6):712-6.
31. Klein JA (Ed). Infections. In: Tumescent Technique. St Louis: Mosby Inc. 2000. Chapter 12. pp. 88-101.
32. Delliere V, Bertheuil N, Harnois Y, Thiénot S, Gérard M, Robert M, et al. Multiple bowel perforation and necrotizing fasciitis secondary to abdominal liposuction in a patient with bilateral lumbar hernia. Indian J Plast Surg. 2014;47(3):436-40.
33. Talmor M. Hoffman LA, Lieberman M. Intestinal perforation after suction lipoplasty: a case report and review of literature. Ann Plast Surg. 1997;38:169-72.

CHAPTER 99

Powered Liposuction and Specific Aspects of Liposuction

Jayashree Venkataram, Aniketh Venkataram, Mysore Venkataram

KEY MESSAGES

- Powered liposuction reduces extraction time and fatigue.
- Careful choice of machine is necessary.
- Aggressive liposuction can lead to complications and hence adherence to basic principles of safety is necessary.

INTRODUCTION

Manual liposuction has the disadvantages of causing physician fatigue and prolonger surgical duration. Powered liposuction was introduced to overcome these advantages.[1,2] Machines have also been introduced to increase the rate of infiltration and thereby decrease duration of infiltration.[3] This chapter deals with powered liposuction and other specific aspects such as safety of liposuction.

POWER-ASSISTED LIPOSUCTION

Powered liposuction consists of using machines for aspiration of fat. Several advantages have been claimed for power-assisted liposuction (PAL):

- In PAL, the reciprocating motion of the machines mimics the to-and-fro action of the surgeon's hand movement, decreasing the work of the procedure and is therefore, less tiring to the physician.
- In addition, it allows the surgeon to remove fat more completely in "tight" areas, where forceful cannula movements are difficult because of physical space constraints (e.g., periumbilical and waist areas).
- It has also been claimed that these machines help to remove larger amounts of fat.

  However, it should be emphasized that the primary objective of powered liposuction is not larger volume of liposuction, as the size of the cannula used is still the same as in manual liposuction and the use of larger cannula would enhance the risks of bleeding, vascular adverse reactions, and irregularities. The major advantage of powered liposuction is thus the reduced work for the surgeon, with some reduction in time and mild increase in rate of extraction as additional benefits. Reduced surgeon fatigue and reduced time of extraction could result in enhanced efficiency and lowered rate of side effects.
- New instruments for powered liposuction have emerged in the last few years, with each instrument having distinct advantages and disadvantages.[4,5] These machines move the cannula forward and backward 2–12 mm with rapidity. The machines may operate with either compressed air or electric-driven cannulas. Power cannulas may also decrease postoperative pain, ecchymoses, and edema, as well as resulting in higher patient satisfaction scores.[3] A study showed the complication rate to be 0.3%, with three cases of seroma, which compared favorably with manual liposuction.[5] The study also showed that because there is some radial movement of powered cannulas, the resulting tunnels are larger than those formed after manual liposuction. Consequently, a 3 mm powered cannula may produce tunnels of the size expected from a 4 mm manual cannula. A study in 2002 showed the increased rate of fat extraction varying from 20 to 45% between different machines.[4] The overall increased extraction in powered versus non-powered mode was reported to be 30%.[5] PAL has been used in specific indications such as breast,[6] and multiple symmetric lipomatosis.[7]

Disadvantages of Power-assisted Liposuction

Most of these are operator depended and include:

- Too rapid fat extraction, resulting in irregularities particularly in thighs, buttocks, arms.
- Vibration can lead to discomfort for hands.
- Some patients are uncomfortable with vibration.
- Cost of machine.

Which Machine to Buy?

Several factors need to be considered while buying a powered-assisted liposuction machine.

- *Weight of the handle:* The handle should be light and not cause strain on the hands.
- Vibration should be minimal and not cause vibration fatigue on the palms.
- Size of the handle should suit the operator's hand.

- Heat generated should be minimal.
- Ease of operation
- Autoclavable/disposable parts. (Disposable parts enhance the cost.)
- *Cost:* The machines add to the cost.

The machines used by the author are shown in **Figures 1 and 2**. **Figures 3 and 4** show the results obtained in abdomen and for gynecomastia.

Summary of Power-assisted Liposuction

- Main advantage is enhanced physician comfort.
- Helps in infiltration—reduces time.
- Difficult areas become accessible.
- Damage to skin of adits is less and hence less postoperatively pigmentation.
- Decrease in time and enhanced fat extraction—about 25%.
- Useful in large areas, repeat liposuctions, and areas of fibrosis.

ULTRASOUND-ASSISTED LIPOSUCTION

Ultrasound-assisted liposuction (UAL) was introduced to damage the fat cells and thereby facilitate the removal of fat. However the technique has had a chequered course.[8] The earlier machines had significant side effects such as burns of the skin, small cysts containing fluid called seromas, bruising, and prolonged postoperative swelling. Most importantly the ultrasound machines are expensive, increasing the cost of the procedure. Newer machines have been introduced with claims of safety, but still have not gained uniform acceptance. Studies suggesting its efficacy though limited, have been published.[9,10] In a recent study nearly 80% of the patients were completely or mostly satisfied with UAL. A total of 75% reported that they had or would recommend UAL to others.[9] Fibrosis after ultrasound liposuction has been reported.[11] Since fat transfer is commonly performed after liposuction, use of ultrasound would be a disadvantage in such cases.

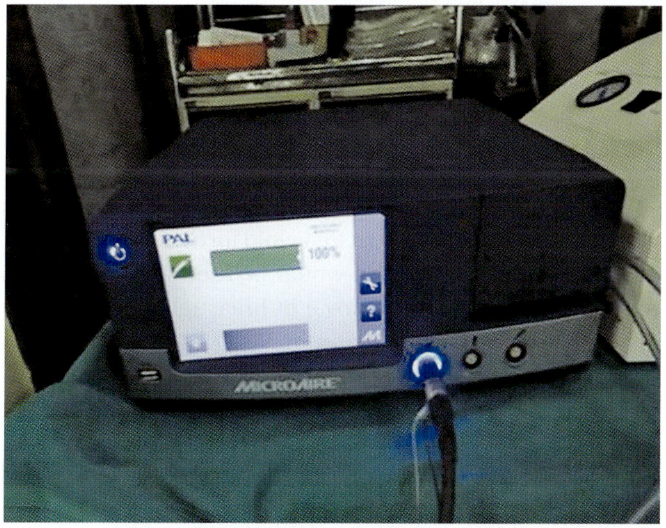

Fig. 1: Powered-assisted liposuction machine.

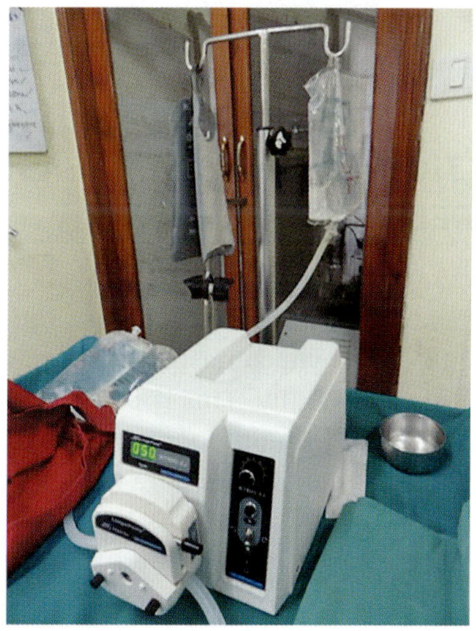

Fig. 2: Infiltration machine.

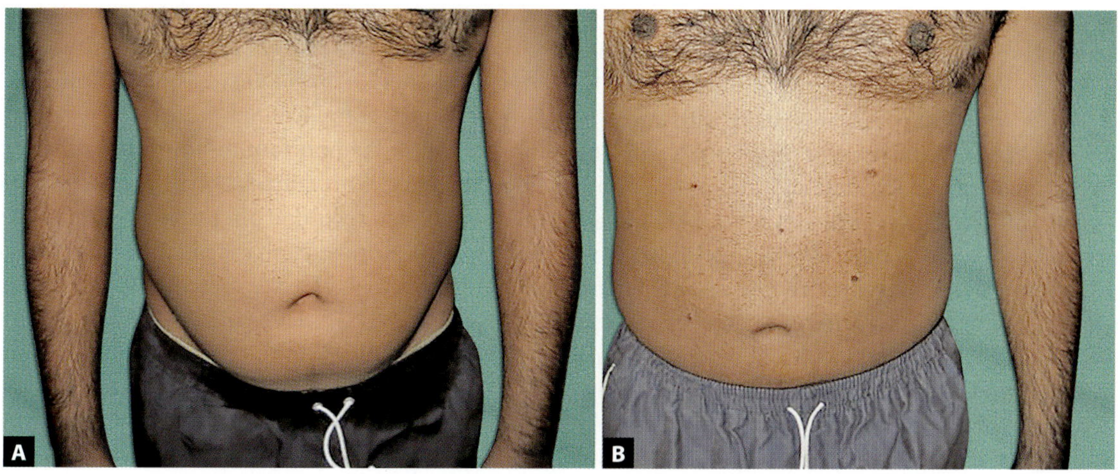

Figs. 3A and B: Abdomen (A) before and (B) after PAL. (PAL: power-assisted liposuction)

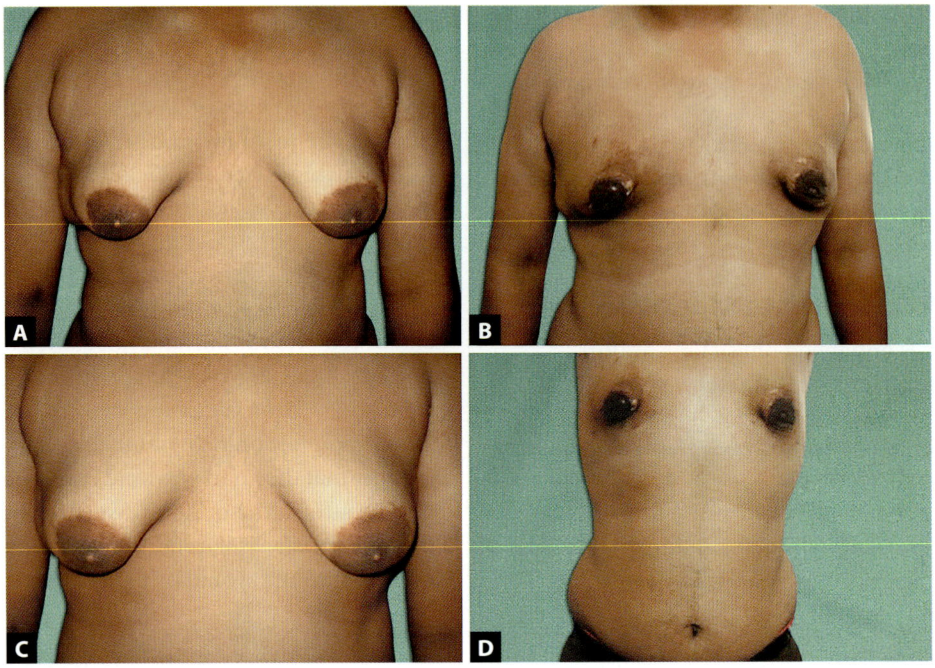

Figs. 4A to D: Gynecomastia (A and C) before and (B and D) after PAL. (PAL: power-assisted liposuction)

LIPOSUCTION OF SPECIFIC AREAS: BREAST REDUCTION

Breast reduction in both men [gynecomastia **(Fig. 4)**] and women with large breasts are excellent indications for liposuction.[8] In men, gynecomastia causes much aesthetic and psychological disability. This is particularly so in men who wish to participate in outdoor activities and in Indian patients, religious ceremonies require the upper torso to be exposed.

Gynecomastia has been classified as mild, moderate, and severe. Mild gynecomastia refers to enlargement of breast around areola. Moderate gynecomastia extends to involvement of infra-axillary area, while in severe gynecomastia, there are large pendulous breasts resembling female breasts.

Gynecomastia presents certain challenges for liposuction. The tissue in gynecomastia consists of fat, breast glands, and fibrous tissue. While fat comes out easily with suction, fibrous tissue and breast tissue presents challenges. For this reason, many surgeons have felt that subtotal mastectomy should be performed in all severe gynecomastia cases. However, several publications have shown that liposuction can yield satisfactory results even in severe cases,[12,13] and author's experience supports this finding. Manual extraction of fibrous tissue through an adit placed just beneath areola is helpful in such cases. Another challenge is the tightness of the area for the suction. Powered liposuction is very helpful in such tight areas. Another important fact to be kept in mind is that the dosage of lignocaine needed is higher up to 1.5 mg/L. Location of adits is an important cosmetic consideration.

Too high a location on the medial aspect would increase visibility, an area also known for keloid formation. In women, an important consideration would be breastfeeding, which may be affected by the removal of breast glands. However, a study revealed that lactation may not be affected by the procedure.[14]

SAFETY OF TUMESCENT LIPOSUCTION

Several serious complications have been reported with conventional liposuction, particularly when liposuction is combined with other procedures such as abdominoplasty, more than one area are treated and in megaliposuctions when large amounts of fat (>5 L) are aspirated. These serious side effects include pulmonary embolism, excessive blood loss, hemorrhagic necrosis of fat and even death.[15,16] However, these complications are extremely rare in tumescent liposuction. It is important to note that while mortality has been reported with conventional liposuction, not a single death had been recorded after tumescent liposuction.[17] In a survey of 9,478 liposuction cases, performed by dermatologic surgeons, the risk of systemic complications was found to be as low as 0.07%.[17] Five patients had "excessive" intra- or postoperative blood loss, and two patients had infection. There were no reported cases of disseminated intravascular coagulation, fat emboli, perforated viscus, thrombophlebitis or death. The risk of local complications was also small. Of these, the most common were postoperative contour irregularities (2.1%), hematoma (0.47%), and persistent postoperative edema (46%). A more extensive survey of data on 15,336 patients undergoing tumescent liposuction also did not find any serious complications.[18]

In 1999, a study by Coleman determined whether the specialty of the physician had an effect on the incidence of malpractice claims.[19] The study showed that <1% of the defendants were dermatologic surgeons, even though dermatologic surgeons performed about 33% of liposuctions in the US. In 2002, in a national survey of over 66,000 liposuction cases performed using the tumescent anesthesia technique, no deaths were reported and the rate of serious adverse events was 0.68/1,000 cases.[20] A review of the State of Florida adverse event data revealed that there were no tumescent anesthesia-related liposuction deaths.[21] In contrast, there were two deaths related to liposuction under general anesthesia. Safety of office-based liposuction as opposed to hospital-based liposuction too has been well documented. It was found that hospital-based liposuction had three times the rate of malpractice settlements when compared with office-based liposuction surgery.[21,22]

Superficial liposuction, which has found its application for maximizing and creating a lifting effect to achieve a better aesthetic result, has been reported to have potential risks for higher complications compared with conventional suction techniques.[23] A recent study revealed that the side effects by this technique could be minimized by proper case selection.[24]

A study by Boeni[25] conducted between 2003 and 2010, in 4,380 consecutive patients who underwent tumescent liposuction revealed no serious complications requiring hospitalization. A survey in 2001 collected data from 267 members of the American Society for Dermatologic Surgery (ASDS) who performed 66,750 liposuction procedures, on the complications that occurred during the 7-year period from 1994 to 2000. No deaths were reported. The overall serious adverse event rate (SAE) was 0.68/1,000 cases and were higher for tumescent liposuction combined with intravenous or intramuscular sedation than without sedation.[19] A study was conducted by the Accreditation Association for Ambulatory Health Care Institute between February 2001 and August 2002. A total of 688 patients who had tumescent liposuction from 39 centers were studied. The overall clinical complication rate found to be 0.7% (five of 702) with major complication in only 0.14% patients, with only one patient requiring hospitalization. A total of 75% of the patients reported no discomfort during their procedures and 91% were happy about their decision to have and 84% had high levels (4 or 5 on a scale of 1–5) of overall satisfaction with the procedure.[26]

However it is important to note that, like in all surgeries, in liposuction too, complications can occur. A retrospective analysis of severe or lethal complications in liposuction in Germany[26] showed 72 cases of severe complications, including 23 deaths following cosmetic liposuction in a 5-year period from 1998 to 2002. The most frequent complications were bacterial infections such as necrotizing fasciitis, gas gangrene, and different forms of sepsis. Insufficient standards of hygiene were responsible for these infections. Further causes of lethal outcome were hemorrhages, perforation of abdominal viscera, and pulmonary embolism which were related to poor technique. Fifty-seven of 72 complications were clinically evident within the first 24 postoperative hours; 41 of these 72 liposuction procedures were performed using tumescent anesthesia and 17 of 72 were performed using true tumescent anesthesia, with four deaths. The study concluded that major risk factors for the development of severe complications are, the infiltration of very large volume of wetting solution, poor technique, liberal postoperative discharge, and poor selection of patients.

Thus, these data have conclusively established the safety of this procedure, particularly when performed by dermatologic surgeons and as an office-based surgery. Hence, tumescent liposuction is now regarded as the gold standard method for liposuction.

SATISFACTION AFTER LIPOSUCTION

Due to its safety profile and mildness of the procedure, tumescent liposuction has achieved a high degree of satisfaction.[27]

In a study, satisfaction with the liposuction was high (about 85% mostly or completely satisfied). The procedure was regarded by most patients as a nonstressful event (>80%). About 40% reported positive effects on social life, about 91% on body feeling, 57% on attractiveness, and 20% on their profession.[28] In another study,[29] a large proportion of patients experienced positive lifestyle outcomes from the procedure: 80.5% were more confident, 74.8% noted an increase in self-esteem, and 87% were more comfortable in clothes.[28]

The time since surgery did not influence results.

It has been suggested[30] that the key to satisfactory outcome after liposuction depends on five physician factors: *(1) Proper case selection, (2) ensuring proper thorough uniform anesthesia, (3) proper experience and training to perform a three-dimensional layered circumferential aspiration, (4) proper knowledge of anatomy to avoid irregularities, and (5) adequate bimodal compression.* In addition, there is one important patient factor—continued exercise, a proper diet, and positive lifestyle changes.[31]

Some special aspects of liposuction: Some tools and modifications have been used to ensure safety and to enhance outcomes.[32] Pigmentation and scarring at the site of adits are frequent complications in brown skin. The barrel flange of an insulin syringe (28G), from which the plunger is removed, can be used as a port for the cannulas. Four-millimeter cannulas can easily pass through this port of entry, and this minimizes the friction with the skin and consequently reduces pigmentation and possible ugly scarring at the site of adits. A topical eye ointment or sterile gel can be applied for lubrication and minimizing friction. Continuous irrigation with saline applied on the adit sites can also help to friction. Placement of adits should be done keeping in mind cultural and racial preferences. In Indian women, the saree worn by women exposes the midriff and hence adit sites can look unaesthetic.[33] Tranexamic acid has been used to reduce bleeding and enhance safety.[34]

CONCLUSION

Tumescent liposuction, as a surgical procedure, requires a combination of:

- Appreciation of beauty, shape, and proportions
- Thorough surgical skill attained through proper training and clinical experience
- Proper knowledge about pharmacology of lignocaine and epinephrine, and fluid balance, and
- Adherence to safety principles and protocols.[35]

In tumescent liposuction, speed and size of aspirate are not the criteria for excellence. The criteria are safety, patient comfort, finesse, and quality of outcome.

TIPS AND PEARLS

- Liposuction is a surgical procedure and needs strict aseptic conditions.
- Adequate documentation of the medical history, proper counseling, and a thorough physical examination of the patient is necessary
- Patients with underlying medical condition such as uncontrolled hypertension, diabetes mellitus should be avoided
- Patients with umbilical and incisional hernia should be avoided
- Tumescent anesthesia is an adequate and safe form of anesthesia in liposuction. However, the total dosage of lignocaine should not exceed 45 mg/kg
- Avoid excessive extraction of fat—avoid too superficial liposuction
- Treat coexisting cutaneous infections prior to surgery
- Liposuction patients should be reexamined within 24 hours after discharge
- Proper training is essential to avoid morbidity and mortality
- Powered liposuction enhances extraction and reduces fatigue but needs careful use of the machine

REFERENCES

1. Coleman WP 3rd. Powered liposuction. Dermatol Surger. 2000;26:315-8.
2. Coleman WP 3rd, Katz B, Bruck M, Narins R, Lawrence N, Flynn TC, et al. The efficacy of powered liposuction. Dermatol Surg. 2001;27(8):735-8.
3. Katz BE, Bruck MC, Coleman WP 3rd. The benefits of powered liposuction versus traditional liposuction: a paired comparison analysis. Dermatol Surg. 2001;27(10):863-7.
4. Flynn TC. Powered liposuction: an evaluation of currently available instrumentation. Dermatol Surg. 2002;28: 376-82.
5. Katz BE, Bruck MC, Felsenfeld L, Frew KE. Power liposuction: a report on complications. Dermatol Surg. 2003;29:925-7.
6. Habbema L. Breast reduction using liposuction with tumescent local anesthesia and powered cannulas. Dermatol Surg. 2009;35(1):41-50.
7. Tremp M, Wettstein R, Tchang LA, Schaefer DJ, Rieger UM, Kalbermatten DF. Power-assisted liposuction (PAL) of multiple symmetric lipomatosis (MSL)—a longitudinal study. Surg Obes Relat Dis. 2015;11(1):155-60.
8. Narins R, Coleman WP III, Brody H, Goldman M, Hanke CW, Lillis PJ, et al. Statement on ultrasonic liposuction. Task Force on Ultrasonic Liposuction of the American Society for Dermatologic Surgery. Dermatol Surg. 1998;24:1035.
9. Masoumi Lari SJ, Roustaei N, Roshan SK, Chalian M, Chalian H, Honarbakhsh Y. Determinants of patient satisfaction with ultrasound-assisted liposuction. Aesthet Surg J. 2010;30(5): 714-9.
10. Omranifard M. Ultrasonic liposuction versus surgical lipectomy. Aesthetic Plast Surg. 2003;27:143-5.
11. Greenhaw BN, Cook J. Painful subcutaneous fibrosis: a complication after high-intensity focused ultrasound for lipolysis. Dermatol Surg. 2015;41(6):744-6.
12. Voigt M, Walgenbach KJ, Andree C, Bannasch H, Looden Z, Stark GB. Minimally invasive surgical therapy of gynecomastia: liposuction and exercises technique. Chirurg. 2001;72(10): 1190-5.
13. Samdal F, Kleppe G, Amland PF, Abyholm F. Surgical treatment of gynaecomastia. Five years' experience with liposuction. Scand J Plast Reconstr Surg Hand Surg. 1994;28(2):123-30.
14. Habbema L, Alons JJ. Liposuction of the female breast: a histologic study of the aspirate. Dermatol Surg. 2010;36: 1406-11.
15. Rao RB, Ely SF, Hoffman RS. Deaths related to liposuction. N Engl J Med. 1999;340:1471-5.
16. Yoho RA, Romaine J, O'Neil D. Review of liposuction, abdominoplasty, and facelift mortality and morbidity risk literature. Dermatol Surg. 2005;31(9 Pt 1);733-43.
17. Bernstein G, Hanke CW. Safety of liposuction: a review of 9,478 cases performed by dermatologists. J Dermatol Surg Oncol. 1988;14:1112-4.
18. Hanke CW, Bernstein G, Bullock S. Safety of tumescent liposuction in 15,336 patients: National survey results. Dermatol Surg. 1995;21:459-62.
19. Coleman WP 3rd, Hanke CW, Lillis P, Bernstein G, Narins R. Does the location of the surgery or the specialty of the physician affect malpractice claims in liposuction? Dermatol Surg. 1999;25(5):343-7.
20. Housman TS, Lawrence N, Mellen BG, George MN, Filippo JS, Cerveny KA, et al. The safety of liposuction: results of a national survey. Dermatol Surg. 2002;28(11):971-8.
21. Coldiron B. Office surgical incidents: 19 months of Florida data. Dermatol Surg. 2002;28:710-3.
22. Hancox JG, Venkat AP, Hill A, Graham GF, Williford PM, Coldiron B, et al. Why are there differences in the perceived safety of office-based surgery? Dermatol Surg. 2004;30(11):1377-9.
23. Kim YH, Cha SM, Naidu S, Hwang WJ. Analysis of postoperative complications for superficial liposuction: a review of 2398 cases. Plast Reconstr Surg. 2011;127(2):863-71.
24. Matarasso A. Discussion. Analysis of postoperative complications for superficial liposuction: a review of 2398 cases. Plast Reconstr Surg. 2011;127(2):872-3.
25. Boeni R. Safety of tumescent liposuction under local anesthesia in a series of 4,380 patients. Dermatology. 2011;222(3): 278-81.

26. Lehnhardt M, Homann HH, Daigeler A, Hauser J, Palka P, Steinau HU. Major and lethal complications of liposuction: a review of 72 cases in Germany between 1998 and 2002. Patricia Plast Reconstr Surg. 2008;121(6):396e-403e.
27. Hanke W1, Cox SE, Kuznets N, Coleman WP 3rd. Tumescent liposuction report performance measurement initiative: national survey results. Dermatol Surg. 2004;30(7):967-77; discussion 978.
28. Augustin M, Zschocke I, Sommer B, Sattler G. Sociodemographic profile and satisfaction with treatment of patients undergoing liposuction in tumescent local anesthesia. Dermatol Surg. 1999;25(6):480-3.
29. Goyen MR. Lifestyle outcomes of tumescent liposuction surgery. Dermatol Surg. 2002;28:459-62.
30. Rohrich RJ, Smith PD, Marcantonio DR, Kenkel JM. The zones of adherence: role in minimizing and preventing contour deformities in liposuction. Plast Reconstr Surg. 2001;107(6):1562-9.
31. Rohrich RJ, Broughton G 2nd, Horton B, Lipschitz A, Kenkel JM, Brown SA. The key to long-term success in liposuction: a guide for plastic surgeons and patients. Plast Reconstr Surg. 2004;114(7):1945-52.
32. Taha A, Tahseen H, Kadry H. Liposuction—gadgets and widgets. Plast Reconstr Surg Glob Open. 2020;8(4): e2759.
33. Field LM, Venkataram J. Ethnic and cultural factors in liposuction scars. J Drugs and Treatment. 2007;6(1):56-8.
34. Cansancao AZ, Condé-Green A, David JA, Cansancao B, Vidigal RA. Use of tranexamic acid to reduce blood loss in liposuction. Plast Reconstr Surg. 2018;141(5):1132-5.
35. Taha AA, Tahseen H. Liposuction: keeping it safe! Plast Reconstr Surg Glob Open. 2020;8(4):e2783.

CHAPTER 100

Laser Lipolysis

Jayashree Venkataram, Mysore Venkataram

KEY MESSAGES

- Laser lipolysis can be used either with liposuction or for lipolysis.
- Using the right wavelength is necessary to ensure efficacy and safety.
- Laser lipolysis has been claimed to reduce bleeding and induce tightening.

INTRODUCTION

Suction lipoplasty or liposuction has been the gold standard for removing fat over the last four decades.[1] Several efforts have been made with technology of different energy sources such as laser, and ultrasound to enhance the efficacy of this procedure. Recent devices have shown gradually increasing efficacy but a perfect device is not yet available. Hence, while tumescent liposuction continues to be the gold standard, these alternatives are being accepted as additional procedures, if not as replacement.[2] This chapter reviews laser-assisted lipolysis (LAL), which is also known as laser lipoplasty or laser-assisted liposuction.

HISTORY

The technology has had a chequered history. The first documented use of LAL was done by Dressel in 1990.[3] Apfelberg et al. later reported efficacy of a 1,064 nm light source.[4] These initial efforts did not show much promise and the field lagged behind as tumescent liposuction (both manual and powered) established its dominance. Recent advances in laser technology such as introduction of a laser beam via a liposuction cannula[5] have piqued interest again in this field and laser lipolysis is beginning to find its place in the sun.

Laser is currently being used in two ways:

1. Laser-assisted liposuction which means destruction of fat by laser followed by suction aspiration as in any liposuction for.
2. Laser lipolysis which means only destruction without aspiration, useful for small fat deposits.

INDICATIONS FOR LASER LIPOLYSIS

In the current scenario, laser lipolysis is useful for the following scenarios:

- Like liposculpture, the main indication for LAL is for body contouring.[6]
- Fibrous tight areas such as upper chest, male breast, and flanks in abdomen which do not allow sufficient tumescent fluid infiltration and where larger aspiration cannulae cause pain; laser cannulae are smaller and hence more easily maneuverable.[7]
- Small areas such as double chin, neck, arms, and periumbilical areas, i.e., liposuction regions where destroyed fat can be left behind without aspiration; here also smaller laser cannulae lead to smaller adits and hence more acceptable scars.[8]
- As an additional technique in large areas wherein limitations of upper limit of tumescent anesthesia does not allow adequate anesthesia and aspiration areas.[9]
- Areas with loose skin where the purported benefits of laser inducing some collagenogenesis and remodeling can lead to skin tightening, e.g., neck and abdomen
- Additional revision or touch up lipolysis for small areas after an initial liposuction.[9,10]

Advantages of Laser-assisted Lipolysis

Several advantages have been purported by laser manufacturers. These include:

- *Lesser downtime:* The most commonly mentioned advantages of LAL relate to the ease of patient recovery.[6,7,11,12] Compared to traditional liposuction, LAL may diminish postoperative pain, and decrease the extent of edema and bruising following the procedure.[6,7,9,12-14] Laser-operated liposculpture reduces trauma to the tissue during fat removal, resulting in improved wound healing.[15] As a result, patients may have a more rapid return to daily activities.[5,15]
- *Lesser bleeding:* Laser-induced thrombosis of blood vessels and closure of lymphatic channels may explain the reduction in severity of bruising and swelling after laser lipolysis.[11] Operator as well as patient safety is increased with the procedure.

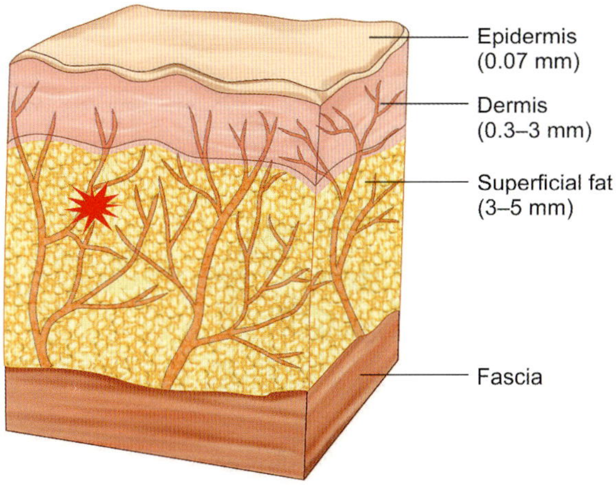

Fig. 1: Superficial lipolysis for skin tightening.

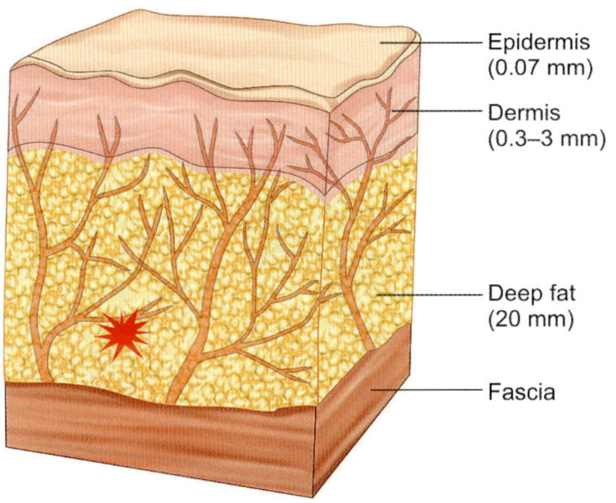

Fig. 2: Deep laser lipolysis.

- *Ease of procedure:* The process of laser-induced fat emulsification allows more efficient fat extraction with less surgeon fatigue.[4,10,11] The need for repeat procedures may also be decreased by use of laser.[8]
- *Skin tightening:* Laser-induced photobiological changes can induce some skin tightening when treating areas of skin laxity by inducing collagen production and subsequent skin contraction.[6,10-12]

  Laser-assisted lipolysis is illustrated in **Figures 1 and 2**.

Disadvantages of Laser-assisted Lipolysis

Several disadvantages exist that are as follows:

- As explained earlier, in most situations it is an adjuvant procedure and not a replacement for traditional liposuction.[9]
- Cost of laser machine is high.
- Efficacy of laser lipolysis as a solo procedure is yet to be established and some studies have not demonstrated any definitive benefit of using the laser.[11,12]
- Since aspiration is essential even after using laser, duration of surgery is increased in an already lengthy procedure.

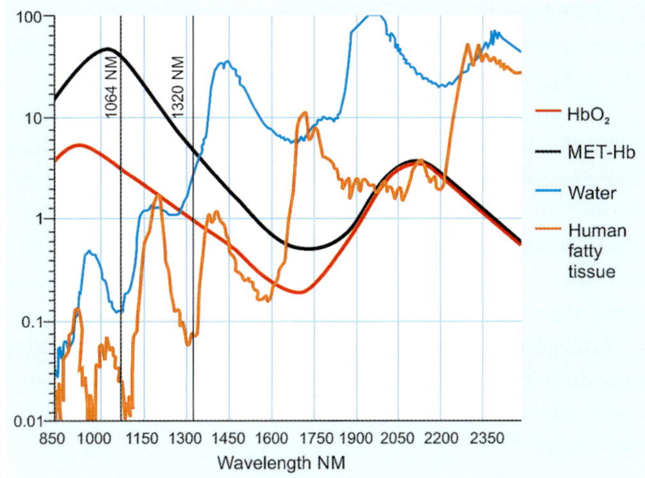

Fig. 3: Absorption coefficients of water and fatty tissue. (MET-Hb: methemoglobin)

  Simultaneous aspiration with laser using dual functioning cannulae allowing laser delivery and aspiration has been attempted in recent machines[16] but are yet to find uniform acceptance.
- As with any laser, burns are a possibility.
- There is a learning curve with the machine.[9]

LASER PHYSICS AND MECHANISM OF ACTION

The basic principle of laser lipolysis, as in all laser indications, is the principle of selective photothermolysis with fat and water, and possibly hemoglobin as chromophores **(Fig. 3)**. According to the theory of selective photothermolysis, these chromophores will preferentially absorb laser energy on the basis of their absorption coefficients at specific wavelengths.[6] Several wavelengths have been found to be absorbed by fat such as 924, 968, 980, 1,064, 1,319, 1,320, and 1,344 nm. Some wavelengths have unique advantages: The 924 nm wavelength has the highest selectivity for fat melting,[12] while 1,064 nm targets oxyhemoglobin leading to coagulation of blood vessels and therefore causes lesser bleeding.[14] 1,320 nm penetrates deeper and hence causes lesser tissue damage in dermis.[12]

Mechanism of Action

Different mechanisms such as photoacoustic,[10] photo-mechanical, photostimulatory, and photothermal effects have been proposed for destruction of fat.[6,17] But the most important mechanism is perhaps a pure thermal effect, referred to as photohyperthermia.[10] Heat produces coagulation of collagen, vessel thrombosis and damage to fat cells by degradation of cell membrane and protein denaturation.[10,15] It is also proposed that the tumescent fluid acts as a heat sink and aids in dissipation of fat to the lower dermis where it leads to neocollagenogenesis as it happens in any laser rejuvenation. This effect is thought to explain the skin tightening benefit of laser lipolysis.[18]

It is said that temperatures of 48–50°C must be reached within the dermis to induce collagen contraction and resultant skin tightening.[12,18,19] Depending on the study, a dermal temperature between approximately 50°C and 70°C translates to a skin surface temperature of approximately 40–41°C.[12,18] Amount of damage depends on total energy delivered and hence determination of optimum levels is important.[2,14]

Collagen damage from thermal damage promotes collagen remodeling, leading to increase in skin tone and texture. These effects continue to improve for 3–6 months after the procedure.[9,16]

LASER LIPOLYSIS TECHNOLOGY

Devices of three wavelengths have been Food and Drug Administration (FDA)-approved for use in the United States (US) for laser lipolysis—diode 924–980 nm (continuous wave), neodymium-doped yttrium aluminum garnet (Nd:YAG) 1,064 nm, and 1,320 nm.[6]

- *Diode laser:* 924 nm wavelength has a high specificity for fat, while the 970 nm targets collagen to promote tissue tightening. A 980-mm device is also available.[12] Dual technology devices are available but have not demonstrated any additional benefit.
- *Neodymium-doped yttrium aluminum garnet laser devices:* Nd:YAG laser at 1,064 nm is one of the earliest lasers to be used to destroy fat. It is absorbed by collagen and fat bound water, though less efficiently than 1,320 nm diode, but it has the advantage of being absorbed by oxyhemoglobin (thus producing hemostasis).
- *1,320 nm:* 1,320 nm is one of the longest wavelengths available and targets water in adipocytes and stimulates to collagen, and hence is thought to produce greater skin tightening.
- Multiplex devices using different wavelengths (1,064 and 1,320 nm) have been introduced. The scientific premise for combining the 1,064 and 1,320 nm wavelengths is to exploit their individual properties and allow them to act synergistically, particularly with regards to hemostasis. The 1,320 nm wavelength converts hemoglobin to methemoglobin. The 1,064 nm not only targets oxygenated hemoglobin, but has a great affinity to methemoglobin, thereby enhancing the effects of the 1,320 nm firing.[12]

  The authors use FOTONA (Slovenia) machine which uses a quasi-continuous pulse Nd:YAG device with maximum power of 35W, pulse energy of 50W, and repetition rate of 100 Hz **(Figs. 4 and 5)**. The machine has been used by us for nearly 4 years since 2013 in 252 patients. The machine is bulky, but easy to use. Our experience shows that the machine is useful in the following ways:

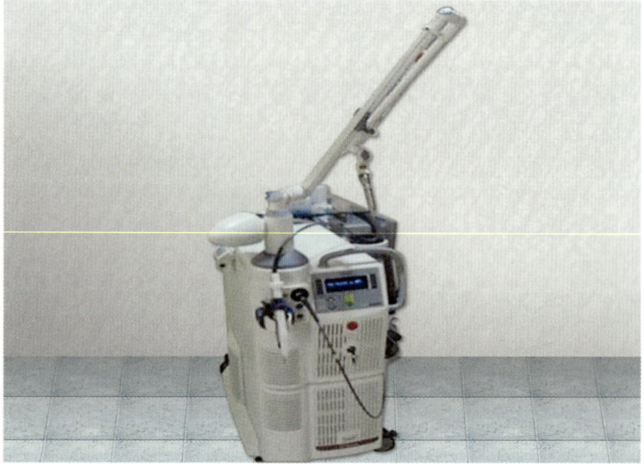

Fig. 4: Neodymium-doped yttrium aluminum garnet (Nd:YAG) laser machine®.

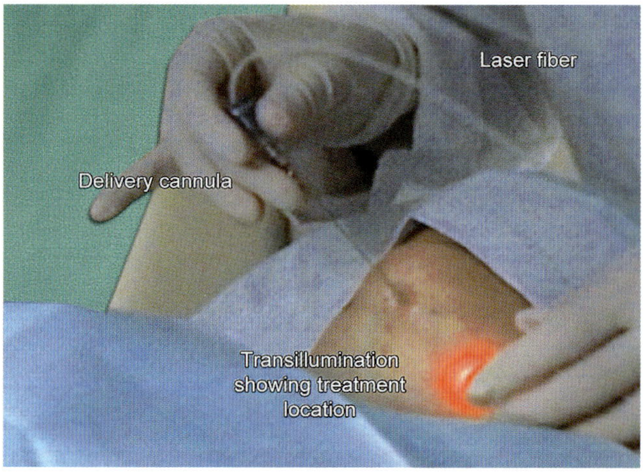

Fig. 5: Laser beam.

- *Initial laser damage to fat to facilitate aspiration:* This is done at 25W fluence of 3000–5000 J over 100 cm^2.
- The laser cannulae are 1.5 mm in size while aspiration cannulae are 3–4 mm in size. This facilitates its use in tight areas such as upper chest, around umbilicus, and flanks.
- At the end of the liposuction, laser is done to create a heat sink in residual tumescent fluid for diffusion into lower dermis, and possible skin tightening.
- While performing large areas, it is difficult to give adequate anesthesia as upper safety limits are approached. In such areas, we use laser as a lipolytic device without aspiration.

A practical advantage of having the machine that the authors have noticed is that it can impress a patient who might be seeking a "high-tech" device, as compared to regular liposuction. However, the machine is expensive if bought for use in liposuction only. This machine, however, is a platform with several applications such as skin tightening, acne, postacne scarring, hair removal, pigmented lesions, etc. This fact is of use in a dermatological setup for other indications.

TECHNIQUE OF LASER LIPOLYSIS

- *Patient counseling:* Patient counseling is in general similar to those undergoing liposuction. Patients often have a high expectation from a high-tech device and it should be properly explained as to what can be reasonably expected.
- *Preparation:* Preparation is similar to the preparation of a liposuction patient. Procedure is performed under tumescent anesthesia. The authors do not advocate the use of intramuscular, spinal or general anesthesia.

Initial phase of infiltration is also entirely similar to that in liposuction and the reader is referred to appropriate books on liposuction for this purpose. If only laser lipolysis is planned as in cases of small areas such as chin, small adits of 2 mm are adequate. If suction is needed after lipolysis as is the case with most procedures, adits of size 3–3.5 mm are needed as in any case of liposuction.

The laser is applied in two ways:

1. Initial lipolysis soon after tumescence at fluence levels 25W and 5000 J over 100 cm^2. The laser movement can be visualized/assessed by the red beam guide. The movements have to be smooth and from below upward in layers. The same area should not be targeted more than once for fear of burning and a fan-shaped movement is advocated. Protective eye glasses should be used by all the staff in the theater. Adequacy of lipolysis is judged by crackling sound (popcorn effect) and the feeling of heat felt by the nonoperating hand. While fluence levels needed may vary depending on the machine, 3,000–5,000 J is what we usually use for 100 cm^2 area. Once adequate soft feeling is felt, aspiration by conventional cannulae is performed.
2. A second use of the laser is at the end of the surgery; at reduced fluences to produce skin tightening. Since the amount of fat left is small, laser has to be used carefully to avoid burning.

After laser lipolysis is complete, the emulsified fat may be removed by aspiration with traditional liposuction. This part is again similar to that done in liposuction and hence will not be elaborated. Adit sites are left open for drainage and wound dressings applied in a manner similar to traditional tumescent liposuction. Patients wear compression bandages or garments for 2–3 weeks. Patients may resume daily activities as tolerated, usually within 24 hours. Pain management usually requires only acetaminophen, and occasionally a codeine-containing medication. Patients can usually resume vigorous physical activity within days. Postoperative physiotherapeutic treatments or lymphatic drainage massage are used by some to accelerate patient recovery and enhance the clinical result **(Figs. 6A to D)**.

COMPLICATIONS/ADVERSE EFFECTS/ PRECAUTIONS

The complication rate after LAL is extremely low in well-trained hands, estimated at 0.93% according to a prospective trial in 537 patients.[8] The following complications/adverse effects/precautions are:

- Ecchymoses, edema, and pain are common but minor and self-limiting, similar to those expected after liposuction.[10,17,20]
- *Laser burns are rare:*[17,20] We have not witnessed this complication in any patient so far.
- Paresthesias and hyperpigmentation have also been reported.[6,20]
- Rare side effects similar to liposuction-related complications are also possible, including seroma, infection, neuropathy, and minor contour irregularities. The presence of tumescent fluid may provide some epidermal protection. According to Mordon et al.,[18] cooled tumescent fluid infiltration decreases skin surface temperature greatly.
- A theoretic concern of laser lipolysis is its effects on serum lipid levels. Laser-induced adipocyte rupture causes the release of intracellular lipid contents, and how this is metabolized by the body is unclear. Studies on lipid levels after laser lipolysis indicate no change in serum lipid levels after the procedure.[18,20]

Mordon et al.[18] followed serial lipid panels in four patients for 30 days after LAL and found no deviation from baseline levels. Goldman et al.[21] conducted LAL with a 1,064 nm and

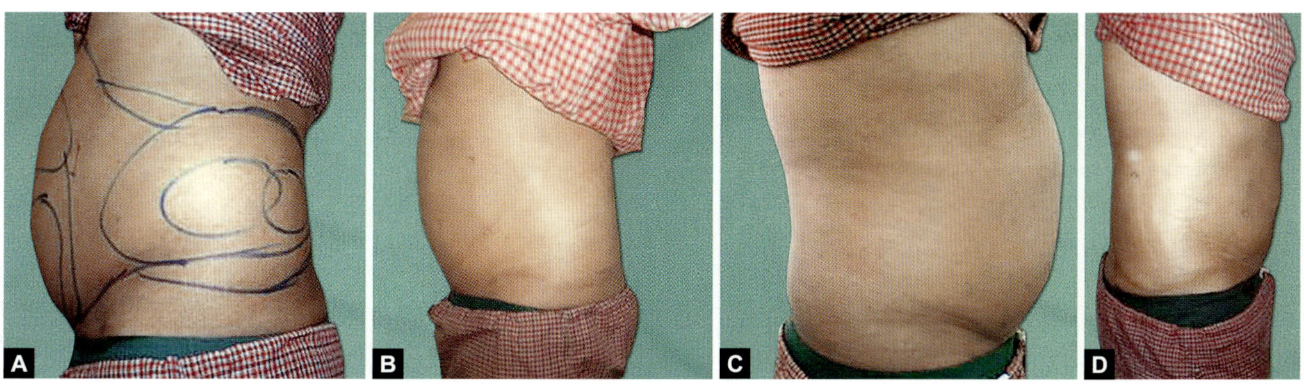

Figs. 6A to D: Results after combination of liposuction and lipolysis.

observed no increase in cholesterol or triglyceride levels after the procedure. Woodhall et al.[16] also found no change in triglycerides in 39 patients undergoing LAL with the 1,064, 1,320 nm, or multiplex (1,064–1,320 nm) device. Given the lack of serum lipid level elevation, there seems to be no lipid-related renal or hepatotoxicity risk. Lipid metabolism after LAL has not been specifically studied although mechanisms of action have been postulated. Lipid metabolism may occur slowly, avoiding changes in serum lipid levels or alternatively, lipids may be cleared through a phagocytic route via macrophage digestion.[18]

CONCLUSION

Despite laser technology being available for a number of years, laser lipolysis is yet to find a pivotal place in routine liposuction. This reflects both the outstanding efficacy and safety of tumescent liposuction and also the evolving phase of laser. While recent machines have shown skin tightening,[22] lesser blood loss[23] and established safety profile,[24,25] further advances are needed to make it a replacement for tumescent liposuction.

PEARLS

- Laser lipolysis is an additional option to conventional liposuction
- Neodymium-doped yttrium aluminum garnet 1,064 nm and diode 980 nm are different effective wavelengths
- Deep laser lipolysis eases suction
- Superficial lipolysis helps in skin tightening

REFERENCES

1. Venkataram J. Tumescent liposuction: a review. J Cutan Aesthet Surg. 2008;1(2):49-57.
2. Mordon S, Eymard-Maurin AF, Wassmer B, Ringot J. Histologic evaluation of laser lipolysis: pulsed 1064-nm Nd:YAG laser versus cw 980-nm diode laser. Aesthet Surg J. 2007;27(3): 263-8.
3. Apfelberg DB. Results of multicenter study of laser-assisted liposuction. Clin Plast Surg. 1996;23(4):713-9.
4. Apfelberg DB, Rosenthal S, Hunstad JP, Achauer B, Fodor PB. Progress report on multicenter study of laser-assisted liposuction. Aesthetic Plast Surg. 1994;18(3):259-64.
5. Uebelhoer NS, Ross EV. Introduction. Update on lasers. Semin Cutan Med Surg. 2008;27(4):221-6.
6. Goldman A, Gotkin RH. Laser-assisted liposuction. Clin Plast Surg. 2009;36(2):241-53.
7. Katz B, McBean J, Cheung JS. The new laser liposuction for men. Dermatol Ther. 2007;20(6):448-51.
8. Katz B, McBean J. Laser-assisted lipolysis: a report on complications. J Cosmet Laser Ther. 2008;10(4):231-3.
9. Badin AZ, Moraes LM, Gondek L, Chiaratti MG, Canta L. Laser lipolysis: flaccidity under control. Aesthet Plast Surg. 2002;26(5):335-9.
10. Goldman A. Submental Nd:YAG laser-assisted liposuction. Lasers Surg Med. 2006;38(3):181-4.
11. Reynaud JP, Skibinski M, Wassmer B, Rochon P, Mordon S. Lipolysis using a 980-nm diode laser: a retrospective analysis of 534 procedures. Aesthetic Plast Surg. 2009;33(1):28-36.
12. Parlette EC, Kaminer ME. Laser-assisted liposuction: here's the skinny. Semin Cutan Med Surg. 2008;27(4):259-63.
13. Mordon SR, Wassmer B, Reynaud JP, Zemmouri J. Mathematical modeling of laser lipolysis. Biomed Eng Online. 2008;7:10.
14. Sun Y, Wu SF, Yan S, Shi HY, Chen D, Chen Y. Laser lipolysis used to treat localized adiposis: a preliminary report on experience with Asian patients. Aesthetic Plast Surg. 2009;33(5):701-5.
15. Badin AZ, Gondek LB, Garcia MJ, Valle LC, Flizikowski FB, de Noronha L. Analysis of laser lipolysis effects on human tissue samples obtained from liposuction. Aesthetic Plast Surg. 2005;29(4):281-6.
16. Woodhall KE, Saluja R, Khoury J, Goldman MP. A comparison of three separate clinical studies evaluating the safety and efficacy of laser-assisted lipolysis using 1,064, 1,320 nm, and a combined 1,064/1,320 nm multiplex device. Lasers Surg Med. 2009;41(10):774-8.
17. Goldman A, Gotkin RH, Sarnoff DS, Prati C, Rossato F. Cellulite: a new treatment approach combining subdermal Nd: YAG laser lipolysis and autologous fat transplantation. Aesthet Surg J. 2008;28(6):656-62.
18. Mordon S, Wassmer B, Rochon P, Desmyttere J, Grard C, Stalnikiewicz G, et al. Serum lipid changes following laser lipolysis. J Cosmet Laser Ther. 2009;11(2):74-7.
19. DiBernardo BE, Reyes J, Chen B. Evaluation of tissue thermal effects from 1064/1320-nm laser-assisted lipolysis and its clinical implications. J Cosmet Laser Ther. 2009;11(2):62-9.
20. Kim KH, Geronemus RG. Laser lipolysis using a novel 1,064 nm Nd:YAG laser. Dermatol Surg. 2006;32(2):241-8.
21. Goldman A, Schavelzon DE, Blugerman GS. Laser lipolysis: liposuction using Nd:YAG laser. Rev Soc Bras Cir Plast. 2002;17:17-26.
22. Min KH, Kim JH, Park HJ, Chung HS, Heo CY. The skin-tightening effects of 1,444-nm Nd:YAG laser on human skin: an in vivo study. Aesthetic Plast Surg. 2014;38(3):585-91.
23. Abdelaal MM, Aboelatta YA. Comparison of blood loss in laser lipolysis vs traditional liposuction. Aesthet Surg J. 2014;34(6):907-12.
24. Przylipiak AF, Galicka E, Donejko M, Niczyporuk M, Przylipiak J. A comparative study of internal laser-assisted and conventional liposuction: a look at the influence of drugs and major surgery on laboratory postoperative values. Drug Des Devel Ther. 2013;7:1195-200.
25. Chia CT, Theodorou SJ. 1,000 consecutive cases of laser-assisted liposuction and suction-assisted lipectomy managed with local anesthesia. Aesthetic Plast Surg. 2012;36(4): 795-802.

CHAPTER 101

Injection Lipolysis and Cryolipolysis

Anjali Pal, Harvinder S Marwah

KEY MESSAGES

- Injection lipolysis and cryolipolysis are targeted fat reduction techniques with minimum downtime and negligible postprocedure complications.
- Injection lipolysis is suitable for small, localized fat deposits, e.g., submental fat.
- Cryolipolysis is based on selective freezing and apoptosis of adipocytes. It can be used for treating larger areas of subcutaneous fat.
- These techniques require around 8–12 weeks for visible results, and multiple treatment sessions may be required.
- They are best used in conjunction with dietary modification, exercise and at times, liposuction.

INTRODUCTION

Aesthetic treatments, both surgical and nonsurgical, have increased in popularity worldwide, in the last few years. Body contouring is one of the most common aesthetic surgical procedures in the USA and UK,[1] and is now a trend that is catching on in India and Asia.

With patients becoming more aware of body contouring procedures, they are expressing increased interest in nonsurgical treatments.[2] The fear of surgery, potential for complications, and morbidity associated with surgical lipoplasty has led dermatologists and plastic surgeons to seek out new ways to refine existing fat reduction techniques.[3]

INJECTION LIPOLYSIS

Injection lipolysis gained attention in recent decades as a nonsurgical alternative to liposuction, for reducing small areas of subcutaneous fat deposits.[3] With recent studies describing physician experience and its excellent safety profile, injection lipolysis is now an established technique, being practiced regularly across the world.[4]

Evolution of Injection Lipolysis

Intravenous phosphatidylcholine (PC) (Lipostabil) was first used in 1966 by Kroupa to prevent posttraumatic fat embolism.[5]

The aesthetic applications of PC evolved from the intravenous uses, and in 1988, Maggiori first reported its use in treating xanthelasma. From then on, its use expanded to include treatment of subcutaneous fat deposits.[3] In 2001, Rittes from Brazil reported subcutaneous injection of PC to reduce infraorbital fat pads.[3]

Sodium deoxycholate (DC) is a bile salt, which is added to solubilize the PC by forming micelles of PC and DC, making it suitable for injection. It is also known to cause reduction of subcutaneous fat when used alone.[3] Both PC and DC have independently been United States Food and Drug Administration (USFDA) approved for treating submental fat (2015)[6] and have been used widely throughout Europe, UK, Asia, and South America for the past 15–18 years, with good results, and minimal side effects.[4]

Lipolytic Solutions in Use[3]

- Phosphatidylcholine **(Fig. 1)**
- Deoxycholate [Kybella (United States)]
- Isoproterenol
- Methylxanthines—caffeine, aminophylline
- Lidocaine
- Buflomedil
- Yohimbine
- Estrogen, thyroid hormone.

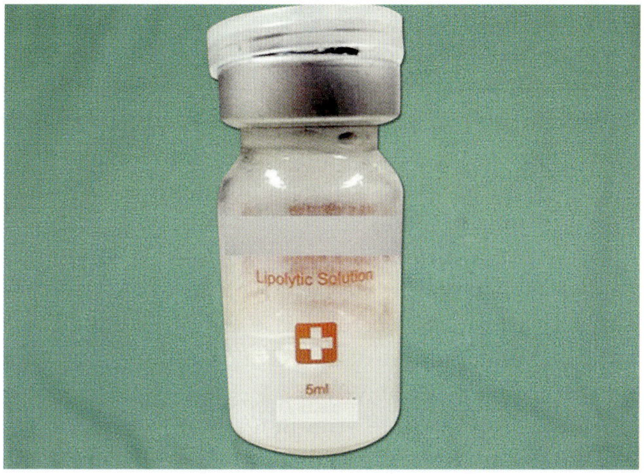

Fig. 1: Lipolytic solution of phosphatidylcholine.

Phosphatidylcholine[3]

It is a naturally occurring glycerophospholipid of glycerol with two fatty acids and choline attached. It has three functions:

1. *Role in digestion:* It is present in bile, and emulsifies dietary fat.
2. *Role as a part of cholesterol metabolism:* It is a component of apolipoprotein.
3. *Role as an essential component of cell membranes:* It is a surfactant in lung alveoli, and plays a part in neuron conduction (precursor to acetylcholine).

Source

In normal diet, as lecithin (in egg yolk, soya beans, whole grains, milk, liver, and kidney) and as oral supplements.

Uses[3]

- *Fat metabolism:* It has a beneficial effect on cholesterol levels.
- *Nervous system:* It is used to guard against low blood choline levels in patients with brain disorders, Alzheimer's disease.
- *Liver conditions:* It is used in drug, alcohol, and toxin-induced liver damage, liver fibrosis, and cirrhosis as a protective agent.

Routes

- Oral and intravenous for earlier mentioned uses.
- Subcutaneous for localized fat reduction.

Injection lipolysis for fat reduction is used in conjunction with dietary modifications, supplements, exercise, correcting hormonal imbalances, liposuction where indicated and not as a stand-alone treatment modality.

Mechanism of Lipolysis

Both PC and DC play a role in the process of lipolysis:[3]

- *Destruction of the lipocyte cell wall:*[3] The PC molecule has a polar head (water soluble), which reduces the interfacial tension of fat globules, enabling their break up into minute particles. Macrophages remove these destroyed fat cells, and apoptotic cascades are stimulated.[7] DC has been found to cause cell lysis directly in a nonspecific fashion by its detergent action.[8]
- *Lipolysis of intracellular fats and triglycerides to fatty acids:* PC activates lipases, which emulsifies triglycerides to fatty acids and glycerol. These are then solubilized in the hydrophobic core of the PC micelle, and transported to the liver and metabolized.
- Phosphatidylcholine stimulates beta-receptors and inhibits alpha-receptors, on adipocyte cell surface, to increase lipolysis.[3]

TABLE 1: Indications and contraindications for injection lipolysis.

Indications (target areas)[9]	*Contraindications*[7]
Double chin	Pregnancy, breastfeeding
Abdomen*	Below age 18 years
Flanks*	Systemic illness (heart or kidney disease, uncontrolled diabetes, hypothyroidism)
Hips*	Active infection
Thighs*	Bleeding tendency, patient on anticoagulants, aspirin, nonsteroidal anti-inflammatory drugs (NSAIDs)
Upper arms	Active or past history of autoimmune condition (lupus, systemic sclerosis)
Areas of lipodystrophy (buffalo hump)	• Microangiopathy, vascular insufficiency[4] • Soy allergy

*Injection lipolysis is not suitable for large areas which need to be treated by liposuction.

- Inflammation and new collagen deposition leads to skin tightening as well.[3]

Indications and contraindications for injection lipolysis are given in **Table 1**.

Procedure[9]

Protocol

Usually 2–3 treatment sessions at least with an interval of 8 weeks.

Materials

- We used a solution of 25–50 mg/mL PC, with 2.5–4.7% sodium DC
- About 27–30 gauge needle or mesogun.

Method[7]

- Written informed consent is taken.
- Weight, height, and body mass index (BMI) are recorded.[4]
- Pretreatment photographs of target areas are taken on a backdrop with fixed vertical lines, with 5 cm spacing, in anterior, posterior, right, and left-lateral positions.[10]
- Circumferential measurement of treatment area is taken, with respect to a fixed bony prominence.[10]
- The treatment areas are palpated and the exact outlines are marked. A grid is drawn on the treatment area, marked into 1.5 cm squares.[11] The distance from the inferior border of the grid to the floor is measured, for duplication in the next treatment session.[11]
- Ice can be applied for 5 minutes prior to injection to reduce stinging and pain.
- Injections of 0.15–0.2 mL are given at a depth of 1 cm (to target the mid-subcutaneous tissue) and are spaced 1–2 cm apart, so as to inject into each square.[9]
- Volume

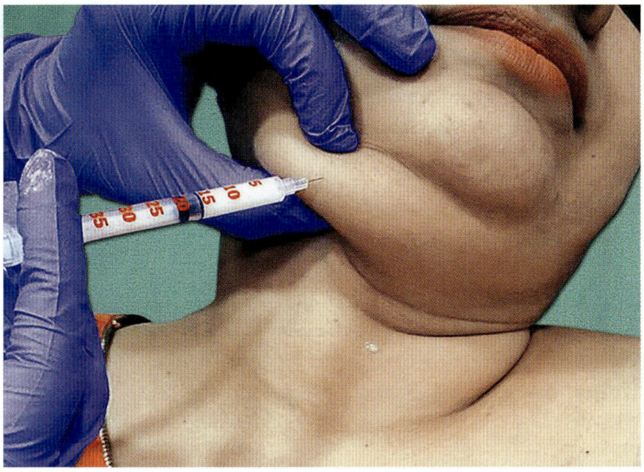

Fig. 2: Injecting lipolytic solution into the submental fat.

TABLE 2: Expected sequelae with injection lipolysis.[9]	
Pain	• Minimal pain or discomfort occurs during injection • Ice the area or use pinch technique • Burning, stinging may occur 30 minutes after injection, then subsides
Swelling	• Appears after 30 minutes • Peaks by 1–3 days, lasts 5–7 days • Gelatinous feel after day 1 • Compression garments reduce swelling
Subcutaneous itching sensation	Lasts for 10 minutes after injection
Immediate erythema	• Transient, up to 24 hours • Occurs 30 minutes after injection
Bruising	• Peaks at week 1 then subsides • Less severe, and resolves quicker than in lipoplasty
Hematoma	Between 1 hour and 1 week, usually small

  - 20–30 mL per flank or outer thigh (saddle bag)
  - 40–60 mL per abdomen area (upper/lower/periumbilical)
  - 3–6 mL for double chin **(Fig. 2)**
- The dosage should be limited to 2,500 mg (100 mL) per treatment session, to limit cholinergic systemic side effects **(Table 2)**.[3]

Postprocedure

- Avoid rubbing postprocedure[7]
- Photographs are taken at 8 weeks, along with measurements of circumference and skinfold thickness.[4] **Table 2** enumerates expected sequelae with injection lipolysis.

Safety Profile and Side Effects

Side effects at the injection site:[3]

- Burning, erythema, edema
- Ecchymosis
- *Urticaria:* It may occur due to allergy to preservative in solution.[4]
- *Hyperpigmentation:* If occurs, is transient, and resolves within 3 months.
- Persistent pain lasting over 2 weeks (<0.015% incidence) occurs more in larger treatment areas, and is associated with DC use.[4]
- Persistent nodules occur when only DC solution is used.
- Superficial injection can cause ulceration.
- Irregular nodularity can occur when given over large areas.

No reports of bacterial or atypical mycobacterial infection at injection site have been reported, when used by a physician.

Systemic side effects with subcutaneous injection are due to cholinergic effects:[3]

- Nausea, dizziness
- Increased salivation
- Abdominal pain
- Diarrhea.

There have been no reports suggesting mutagenicity, teratogenicity.[7]

Studies have shown no significant alterations in blood lipid values, or liver function tests following the procedure.[7,12]

Treatment Pearls[9]

- Soft-fat deposits respond better than fibrous areas.
- Effects of injection are best appreciated over the submental area and arms.[13]
- Areas of excessive skin laxity with minimal underlying fat are not ideal for injection lipolysis.[7]
- *In lipomas:* Mature lipid-filled adipocytes are rather resistant to cytolytic effects which is why multiple treatment sessions are needed.[14]
- Treatment of the lower eyelid fat pad is not endorsed because of chances of retro-orbital bleeding and infection.
- Avoid injecting in the breast or axillary tail of breast (as prolonged inflammation may lead to increased chances of malignancy).
- Avoid injecting too close to ligaments, and below the knee (areas prone to skin breakdown).
- Immediate pain on injection can be reduced by mixing the lipolytic solution with lidocaine.
- High-intensity focused ultrasound performed immediately before or after the procedure may help fat cell lysis.
- About 6–8 weeks are required for the full effect to be seen, before the next injection.
- Results are cumulative and require multiple sessions. Pretreatment patient education is important, for realistic expectations.[4]

CRYOLIPOLYSIS

Liposuction is the most popular method for subcutaneous adipose tissue reduction. However, the procedure is not suitable for all patients, due to its surgical nature and risks involved. Noninvasive procedures for fat reduction have now become increasingly popular in the past decade.

Cryolipolysis has been cleared by the FDA in 2010 as a safe treatment option to reduce subcutaneous fat noninvasively for areas such as abdomen, flanks, thighs, in 2015 for the submental area[15] and in 2016 for the medial axilla bulge, back and underneath the buttock.[16]

Cryolipolysis has been labeled a "lunch time procedure" because it is completed in <2 hours, and with minimal downtime. There is no anesthesia required, no surgical incision, and none of the side effects that may be associated with surgery.[17]

Other noninvasive methods have yet to demonstrate long-term viability and consistency in their results.[18]

History of Cryolipolysis

Cryolipolysis is the controlled application of cooling to reduce subcutaneous fat noninvasively.[19] The phenomenon of cold-induced adipocyte necrosis was originally described by Epstein in 1970, who reported the occurrence of a "red indurated nodule" followed by transient fat necrosis in the cheek of an infant who had been sucking on a popsicle. This became known as popsicle panniculitis.[19] This was also observed in adult patients, and it led to the idea that lipid-rich tissues are more susceptible to cold injury than the surrounding water-rich tissues. Thus, investigators began to explore selective cooling for fat removal, and in 2007, Manstein et al. introduced noninvasive fat reduction by freezing, and coined the term cryolipolysis.[1]

Mechanism of Action

The principle of cryolipolysis is based on the fact that adipocytes are more susceptible to cooling than other cells (skin and nerve).[17] Precise application of cold temperature triggers death of adipocytes, which are subsequently engulfed and digested by macrophages.[17]

- Although its mechanism is not fully understood, it is believed that *vacuum suction with regulated heat extraction* impedes blood flow and induces crystallization of the targeted adipose tissue when cryolipolysis is performed.[20]
- This *cold ischemic injury* may promote cellular injury in the adipose tissue via cellular edema, reduced Na-K-ATPase activity, reduced ATP, elevated lactic acid levels, and mitochondrial free radical release.[20] The temperatures induced have no permanent effect on the overlying dermis and epidermis.[20]
- *Ischemia-reperfusion injury* is thought to compound this effect, causing generation of reactive oxygen species, elevation of cytosolic calcium levels, and *activation of apoptotic pathways*, with a pronounced *inflammatory response*.[20] This leads to the eventual removal of targeted adipocyte cells from the treatment site. Within 3 months, macrophages clear the damaged cells and debris.[20]
- Investigators have suggested that skin tightening also occurs as a somewhat unexpected benefit of cryolipolysis.[2] Pathophysiology of cryolipolysis is given in **Table 3**.

TABLE 3: Pathophysiology of cryolipolysis.[17]

Day 1–3	Influx of inflammatory cells around adipocytes
Day 3–14	Inflammation reaches the peak
Day 14–30	Phagocytes engulf and digest adipocytes
Day 30–60	Adipocyte volume decreases
Day 60–90	Adipocyte volume decreased, interlobular septae thickened

TABLE 4: Indications and contraindications for cryolipolysis.

Ideal candidate for cryolipolysis	*Contraindications for cryolipolysis*
Within ideal weight range:[1] Small amounts of fat in chin, upper arms	*Cold-induced conditions:* Cryoglobulinemia, cold urticaria, and paroxysmal cold hemoglobinuria[20]
Pinchable fat in the target area[1]	Pregnancy, breastfeeding (may alter adipose tissue metabolism, possibly reducing milk production)
Maintain a healthy diet, exercise regularly	*Local factors:* Dermatitis, varicose veins, active infection[20]
Have realistic expectations[17]	Obesity
Alternative for patients unfit for anesthesia for liposuction[18]	High volume removal of fat in a single sitting (it is not a replacement for liposuction)

Indications (Table 4)

Common Treatment Areas[1]

- *Abdomen:* Upper, mid, and lower
- Flanks
- Inner thighs
- Outer thighs
- Infragluteal folds
- Upper arms
- Submental fat
- Medial axilla
- Medial knee.

The procedure described below is in accordance with the CoolSculpting device (ZELTIQ Aesthetics, Inc.) and protocol.[1]

Procedure

- The patient meets the physician for initial consultation, in which areas of concern are discussed, and realistic expectations for fat reduction are established. It is explained to the patient that about 25% reduction of fat in the target area can be expected with a single treatment.

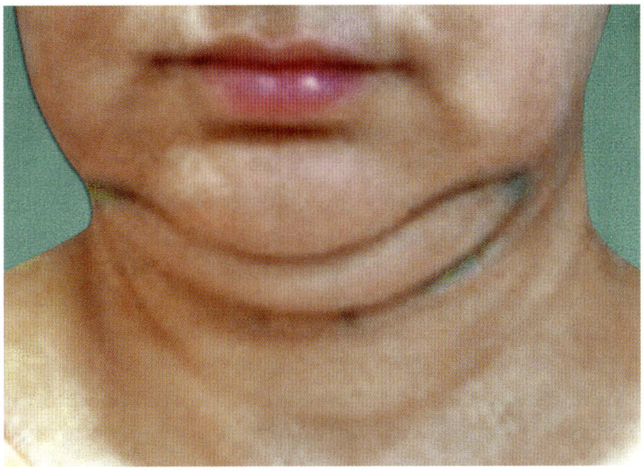

Fig. 3: Marking the submental area where the applicator will be placed.

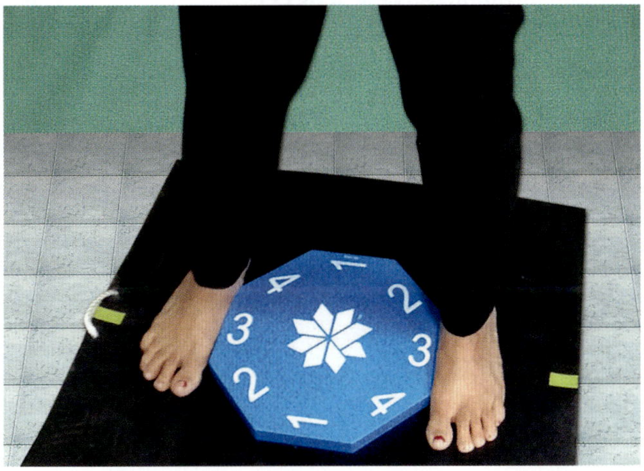

Fig. 4: Floor mat for standardized photography before and after cryolipolysis.

The sites for applicator placement and number of cycles are planned, based on whole body assessment **(Fig. 3)**.[21]

- On the day of treatment, baseline photographs are taken (with the help of a foot mat with fixed markings for capturing front, lateral and oblique views of treatment areas), and weight is recorded **(Fig. 4)**.
- The patient sits comfortably in the treatment chair for the duration of the procedure. A gel sheet is applied over the treatment area, preventing direct contact between the cooling plates and the skin, thus protecting the skin and enabling monitoring of tissue temperature throughout the cycle.
- The treatment device **(Fig. 5A)** utilizes a cup-shaped vacuum applicator with two cooling panels **(Fig. 5B)**. There are a range of applicators, each suited for different target areas. A roll of tissue is drawn into the applicator under moderate vacuum and the selected temperature is modulated by thermoelectric elements, and controlled by sensors that monitor the heat flux out of the tissue **(Figs. 6 and 7)**.[1]

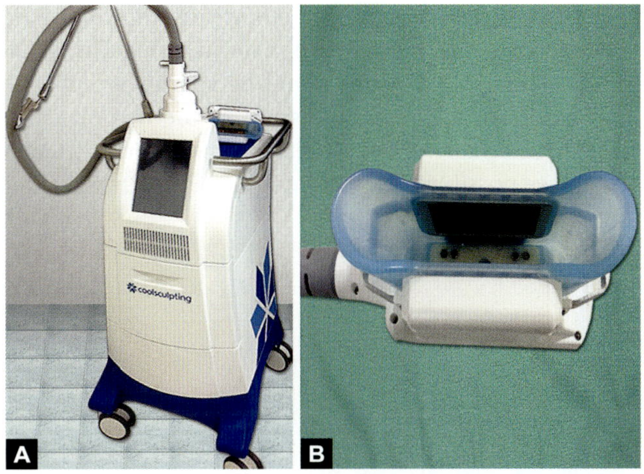

Figs. 5A and B: A cryolipolysis machine (CoolSculpting® by Zeltiq Aesthetics) with applicator used for both abdominal and flank fat.

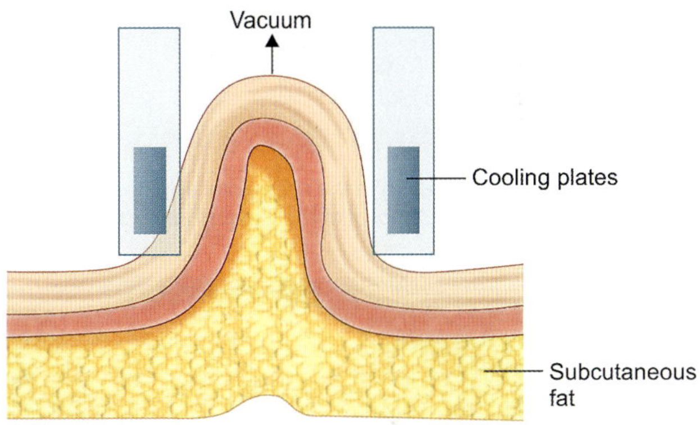

Fig. 6: Diagrammatic representation of a tissue roll in contact with cooling plates of the applicator during the procedure.

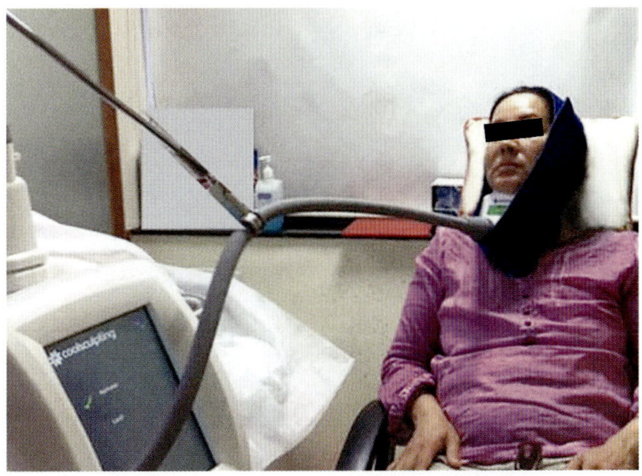

Fig. 7: Cryolipolysis for double chin in progress.

- Typical treatment time is 45 minutes, during which the temperature of the tissue roll decreases to –5°C.[22] At the conclusion of the treatment, the applicator is removed, to reveal firm, frozen tissue.[2] The treatment area is then massaged manually, allowing the tissue to rewarm and obtain its original shape **(Fig. 8)**.[2]

- *Immediate post-treatment 2 minutes manual massage:* This consists of 1 minute of vigorous kneading of the treated tissue between the thumb and the fingers followed by 1 minute of circular massage of the treated tissue against the patient's body (mechanism of action—manual massage possibly adds to tissue-reperfusion injury).[20]

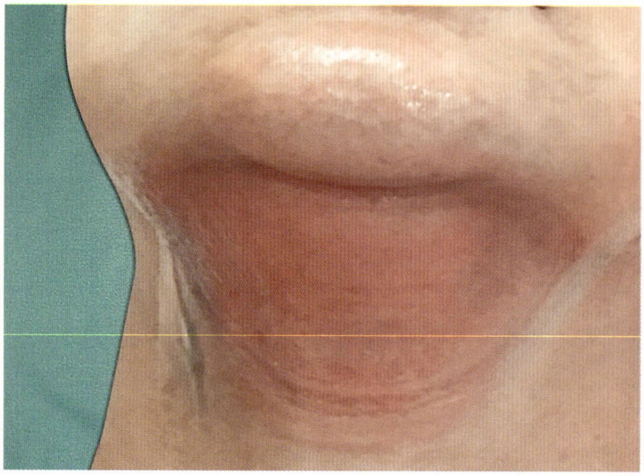

Fig. 8: Erythema and swelling in the submental area immediately postprocedure on removal of the vacuum applicator.

Postprocedure[21]

The patient typically resumes normal activities immediately posttreatment.

Patients should be instructed about expected posttreatment sequelae:

- *Erythema:* Immediately after the treatment, and subsides within a week. It occurs due to the strength of the vacuum and the cold temperature.
- Edema, bruising, and pain due to the same reason.
- *Numbness:* Hypersensitivity and hyposensitivity have both been reported, but normal sensation returns in about 3.6 weeks.[17,18,20] Nerve biopsies taken at 3 months posttreatment have shown no long-term changes to nerve fibers.

Follow-up visits are done at the 8th and 12th week, for weight measurement, photography and discussion of further treatment as required **(Figs. 9 to 11)**.

Modifications in Procedure

- Multiple treatment sessions in the same anatomic area,[20] typically two treatments 8 weeks apart, will maximize the effect of fat reduction.

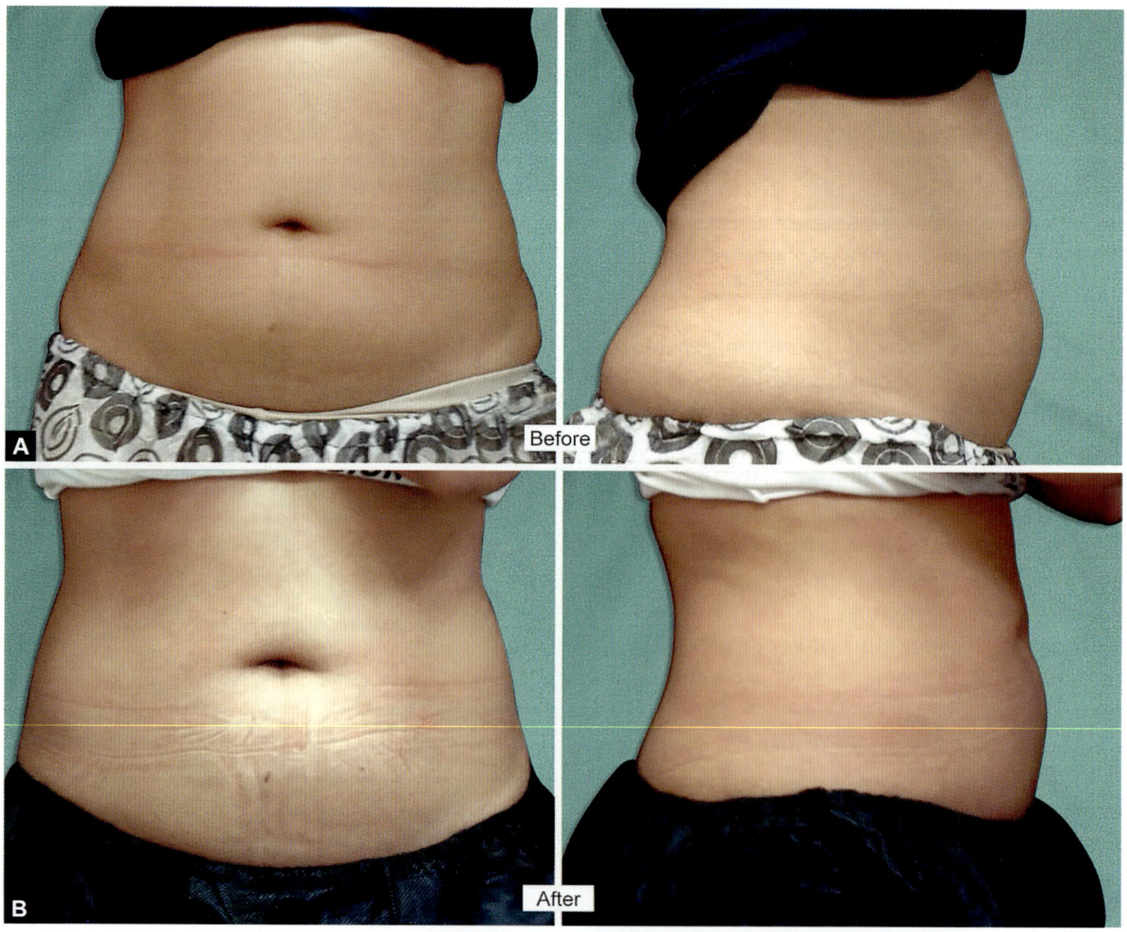

Figs. 9A and B: Lower abdomen front and lateral view: Before and after 8 weeks of one session.
Courtesy: Dr Gurjot Marwah, Mumbai.

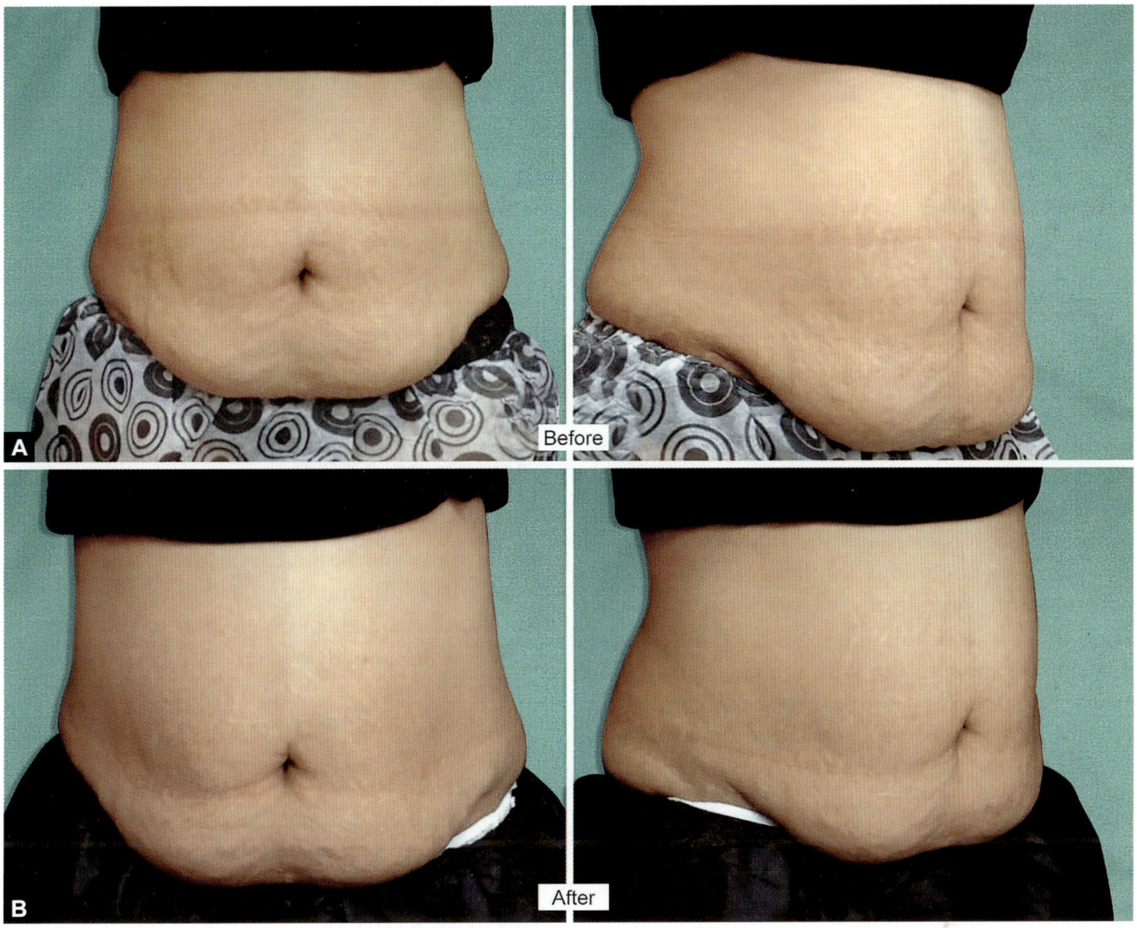

Figs. 10A and B: Lower abdomen front and lateral view: Before and after 8 weeks of one session.
Courtesy: Dr Gurjot Marwah, Mumbai.

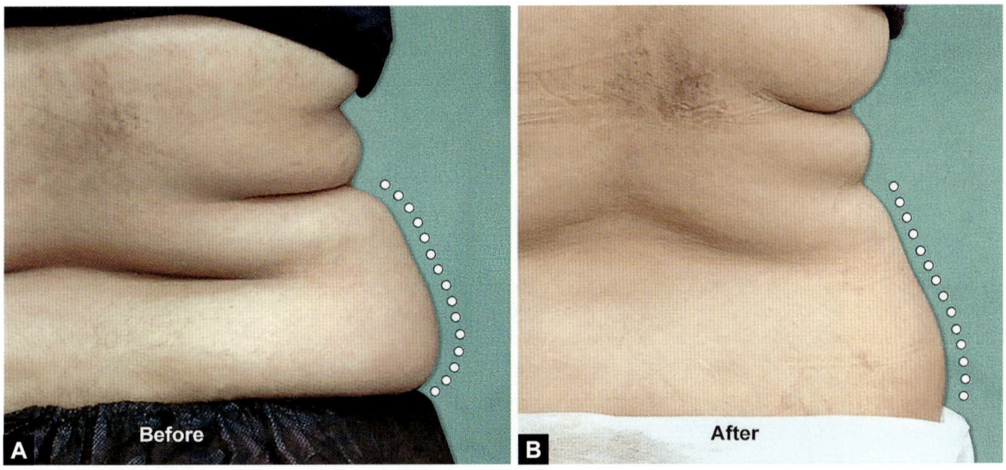

Figs. 11A and B: Flank, posterior view: Before and 12 weeks after one session.
Courtesy: Dr Gurjot Marwah, Mumbai.

- Stacking, or overlapping two cryolipolysis treatments over one area, in one session will also maximize fat reduction.[15]
- Colder cryolipolysis—temperatures lower than -11°C (-12 to -15°C) when applied to the flanks have shown to be effective, resulting in shorter duration of the cycle (30–45 minutes) safely.[15]
- Contrast cryolipolysis—the procedure involves initial heat application (40°C for 10 minutes) followed by a low temperature cooling (at -8°C for 60 minutes) and then another heat application (40°C for 10 minutes). It has been performed on the flanks and abdominal fat successfully. It results in a loss of subcutaneous fat comparable to that

of conventional cryolipolysis.[23] However, there is limited literature on this method, so it has to be studied on more volunteers and over more sessions.[24]

SPECIAL INDICATIONS

Pseudogynecomastia

Pseudogynecomastia refers to benign male breast enlargement due to subareolar fat.[25] It differs from true gynecomastia in that it is a predominantly fat component. There is no proliferation of glandular tissue.[25]

- Clinical assessment is done to rule out true gynecomastia (history taking, physical examination). Manual palpation is done to ensure that breast enlargement is due to idiopathic pseudogynecomastia, i.e., there must be diffuse breast enlargement, without a subareolar palpable nodule.[25]
- Two treatments are ideally required, with 50% overlap of treatment area, in a horizontal fashion.[25]
- It is a more comfortable noninvasive technique with minimal pain, compared to high-frequency ultrasound. Numbing the areolar complex with topical lidocaine for 45 minutes can minimize intra-procedure discomfort.[25]

Ideal candidate: Grade I and II pseudogynecomastia with mild-to-moderate excess of subcutaneous fat (**Figs. 12A and B**).

Double Chin[2]

Increase in fat in the submental compartment plays a crucial role in the perception of aging in the face.[2]

Lower face lift, neck lift, and liposuction are current procedures to invasively treated unwanted submental fat. Here again, cryolipolysis provides great subject comfort and convenience as a noninvasive fat reduction method.

- A protective gel is applied to the skin, and the cup-shaped vacuum applicator is positioned in the center of the treatment area. The patient is seated comfortably, and Velcro straps provide additional support to the applicator (**Fig. 7**).
- The tissue attains a temperature of –10°C, and the cooling cycle is of 45 minutes. Two cycles are usually recommended, ideally 6 weeks apart (**Figs. 13 and 14**).
- An added advantage of cryolipolysis done in the submental area is the "skin-tightening" effect.
  Two cryolipolysis treatments can be overlapped in the same session, to cover the entire central and lateral submental region more efficiently.
- The same applicator can be used for areas such as the knees and axilla.[2,26]
- For patients with excessive skin laxity and platysmal banding, botulinum toxin, fillers or surgical procedures will still be necessary to improve the neckline contour.[2]

SAFETY PROFILE

The FDA cleared a cryolipolytic device in 2010, for the reduction of flank fat. Since then, it has cleared the device for treatment of subcutaneous fat in the abdomen, thighs, double chin, bra-line bulge, back, and infragluteal areas.[17]

No significant adverse effects have occurred—systematic literature reviews[17] have found no reports of scarring, ulceration, disfigurement or nodule formation at the treatment sites.

Studies have shown that cholesterol, triglycerides, liver function tests, and glucose levels remain within normal limits during and after cryolipolysis (3 months posttreatment).[20]

Adverse Effects

A low profile of adverse effects is one of the main advantages with cryolipolysis.[20]

- Expected side effects such as temporary erythema, bruising, transient numbness, resolve within 14 days.[17]
- Late-onset pain (occurring 14 days postprocedure) occurs in 0.1% cases,[27] and it resolves without intervention.
- Persistent tingling.
- Persistent hyperpigmentation that may resolve without intervention within 6 months.[15] This does not depend on

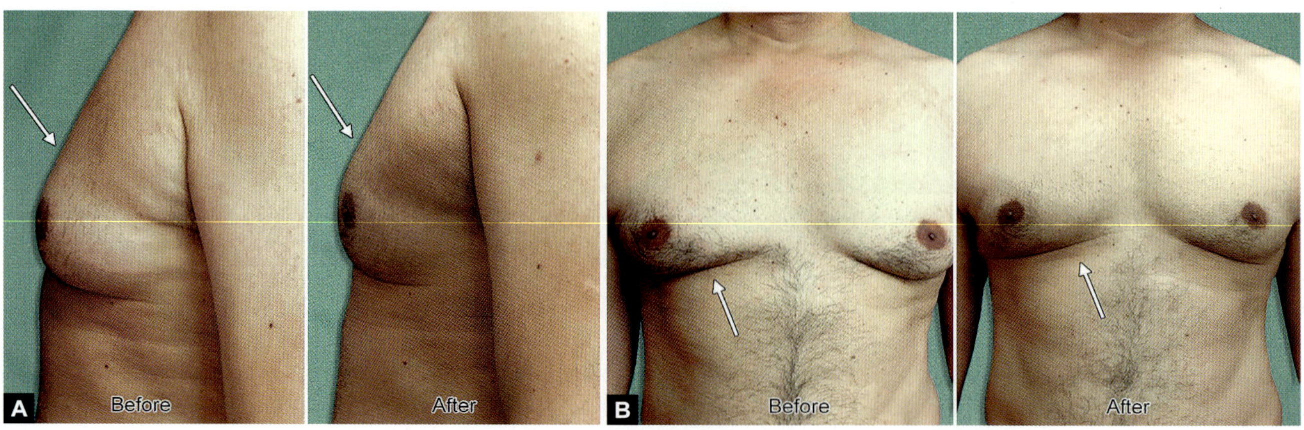

Figs. 12A and B: Male pseudogynecomastia front and lateral view: Before and 12 weeks after one session.
Courtesy: Dr Gurjot Marwah, Mumbai.

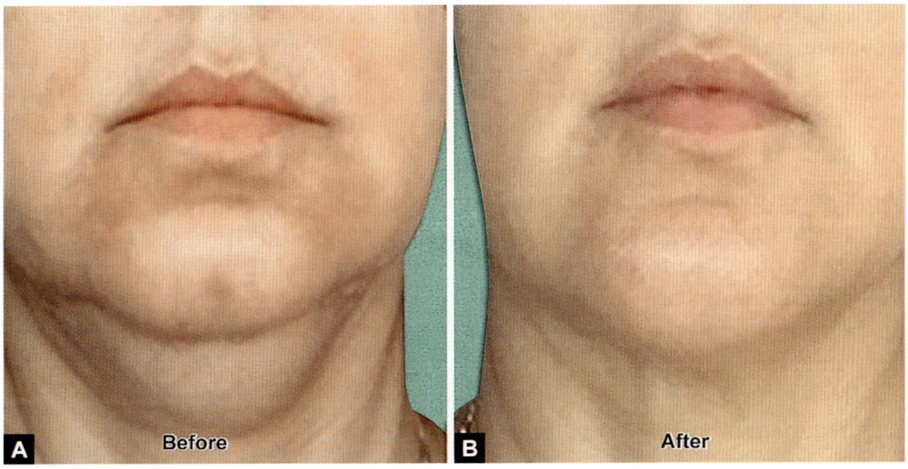

Figs. 13A and B: Double chin anterior view: Before and 12 weeks after one session.

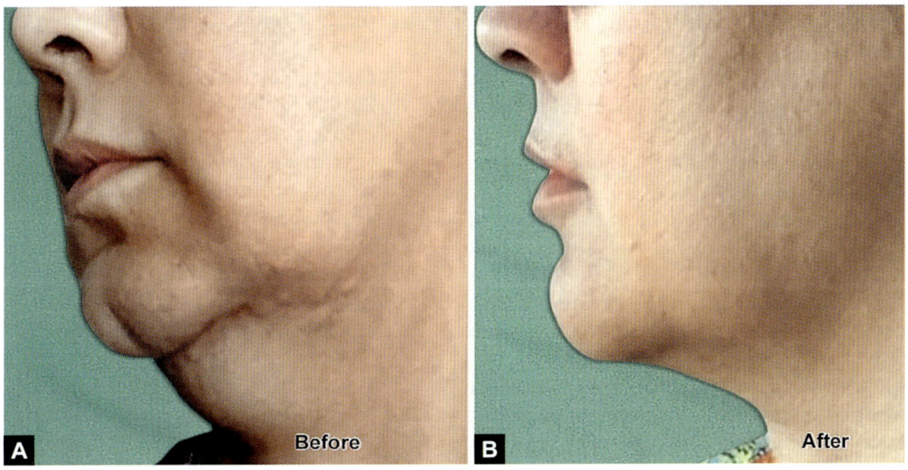

Figs. 14A and B: Double chin lateral view: Before and 12 weeks after one session.

the skin type of the patient, however. It has been shown that cryolipolysis in darker Asian skin types has the same safety profile as in Caucasian skin.[28]

Rare Side Effects

- Vasovagal reaction[20]
- Paradoxical adipose hyperplasia (PAH).[20]

Paradoxical adipocyte hyperplasia: A rare side effect, in which additional fat grows at the treatment site, has been reported in 33 cases.[17]

The estimated incidence of PAH is about 0.021%, or about 2 in 10,000 treatment cycles.[22,25] Certain risk factors have been identified as—male sex, cryolipolysis in the subumbilical region, and use of large size probe.[29] It is noticed to occur usually between 2 and 4 months after the cryolipolysis session.

It has been reported in the flanks, abdomen, and even in the male breast.[22] An initial reduction of subcutaneous fat occurs in the treatment area, followed by the development of a sharply demarcated subcutaneous soft-tissue mass, corresponding to the treatment area, after 2–3 months of treatment.[22] There is no overlying skin change noted.

Pathogenesis: Histopathology of specimen tissue reveals septal thickening, with increased vascularity. It is suggested that the septal thickening could lead to hypoxic injury to the adipose tissue, which in turn increases capillary proliferation and fat hypertrophy.[22]

There is no evidence of spontaneous resolution of PAH. Treatment has relied on liposuction or abdominoplasty.[22]

- The development of morphea in a single case after cryolipolysis, over the sites corresponding to the probe application, was reported in 2018.[27] It could be hypothesized that the local apoptosis of adipocytes triggered an inflammatory response, leading to morphea.

CRYOLIPOLYSIS: LONGEVITY OF RESULTS

While this is not precisely established, a long-term follow-up of two patients (6 and 9 years posttreatment) in which unilateral flank was treated, showed that despite weight changes, the treated area maintained a persistent reduction in size and change in contour, indicating that results may be very durable.[19]

CONCLUSION

For decades, liposuction has been the only accepted procedure for body contouring.[1] In recent times, however, noninvasive modalities for fat reduction have been developed, and are being improved upon. Their results are not immediate, and are less dramatic, but they are useful in the subset of patients who have fear of surgery.[1]

Further clinical studies of these treatment techniques will help in establishing treatment protocols in the future to maximize efficacy and patient benefit.

REFERENCES

1. Demosthenous N. Cryolipolysis: a review of published clinical data. Pmfa news. 2016;3:30-1.
2. Kilmer SL, Burns AJ, Zelickson BD. Safety and efficacy of cryolipolysis for non-invasive reduction of submental fat. Lasers Surg Med. 2016;48(1):3-13.
3. Matarasso A, Pfeifer TM. Mesotherapy and injection lipolysis. Clin Plast Surg. 2009;36(2):181-92.
4. Duncan DI, Chubaty R. Clinical safety data and standards of practice for injection lipolysis: a retrospective study. Aesthet Surg J. 2006;26(5):575-85.
5. Kroupa J. The role of pharmacology in the comprehensive prophylaxis of post-traumatic fat embolism. Acta Chir Orthop Traumatol Cech. 1993;60(2):114-22.
6. Fischer A. (2015). FDA News Release - FDA approves treatment for fat below the chin. [online] Available from: http://www.fda.gov/NewsEvents/Newsroom/PressAnnouncements/ucm444978.htm. [Last accessed August,2023].
7. Mahmud K, Crutchfield CE. Lipodissolve for body sculpting: safety, effectiveness, and patient satisfaction. J Clin Aesthet Dermatol. 2012;5(10):16-9.
8. El Kamshoushy A, Abel Maksoud R, El Mahdy N. Evaluation of the efficacy of injection lipolysis using phosphatidylcholine/deoxycholate versus deoxycholate alone in treatment of localized fat deposits. J Clin Exp Dermatol Res. 2012;3:146.
9. Mann MW, Palm MD, Sengelmann RD. New advances in liposuction technology. Semin Cutan Med Surg. 2008;27(1):72-82.
10. Salti G, Ghersetich I, Tantussi F, Bovani B, Lotti T. Phosphatidylcholine and sodium deoxycholate in the treatment of localized fat: a double-blind, randomized study. Dermatol Surg. 2008;34(1):60-6.
11. Reeds DN, Mohammed BS, Klein S, Boswell CB, Young VL. Metabolic and structural effects of phosphatidylcholine and deoxycholate injections on subcutaneous fat: a randomized, controlled trial. Aesthet Surg J. 2013;33(3):400-8.
12. Hasengschwandtner F. Phosphatidylcholine treatment to induce lipolysis. J Cosmet Dermatol. 2005;4(4):308-13.
13. Thomas M, D'Silva JA, Borole AJ. Injection lipolysis with a cocktail of phosphatidylcholine and deoxycholate: an Indian experience. Plast Reconstr Surg Glob Open. 2016; 4(9):e861.
14. Janke J, Engeli S, Gorzelniak K, Luft FC, Jordan J. Compounds used for 'injection lipolysis' destroy adipocytes and other cells found in adipose tissue. Obes Facts. 2009;2(1):36-9.
15. Leal Silva H, Carmona Hernandez E, Grijalva Vazquez M, Leal Delgado S, Perez Blanco A. Noninvasive submental fat reduction using colder cryolipolysis. J Cosmet Dermatol. 2017;16(4):460-5.
16. Suh DH, Park JH, Jung HK, Lee SJ, Kim HJ, Ryu HJ. Cryolipolysis for submental fat reduction in Asians. J Cosmet Laser Ther. 2018;20(1):24-7.
17. Krueger N, Mai SV, Luebberding S, Sadick NS. Cryolipolysis for noninvasive body contouring: clinical efficacy and patient satisfaction. Clin Cosmet Investig Dermatol. 2014;7:201-5.
18. Chopra K, Tadisina KK, Stevens WG. Cryolipolysis in aesthetic plastic surgery. Eplasty. 2014;14:ic29.
19. Bernstein EF. Long-term efficacy follow-up on two cryolipolysis case studies: 6 and 9 years post-treatment. J Cosmet Dermatol. 2016;15(4):561-4.
20. Ingargiola MJ, Motakef S, Chung MT, Vasconez HC, Sasaki GH. Cryolipolysis for fat reduction and body contouring: safety and efficacy of current treatment paradigms. Plast Reconstr Surg. 2015;135(6):1581-90.
21. Stevens WG, Pietrzak LK, Spring MA. Broad overview of a clinical and commercial experience with CoolSculpting. Aesthet Surg J. 2013;33(6):835-46.
22. Jalian HR, Avram MM, Garibyan L, Mihm MC, Anderson RR. Paradoxical adipose hyperplasia after cryolipolysis. JAMA Dermatol. 2014;150(3):317-9.
23. Meyer PF, Consulin MCD, Rodrigues T, Pereira AM, Lopes PCM, da Silva RMV, et al. Effects of contrast cryolipolysis on flank region adiposity: Case study. J Cosmet Dermatol. 2018;17(6):1059-62.
24. Savacini MB, Bueno DT, Molina ACS, Lopes ACA, Silva CN, Moreira RG, et al. Effectiveness and safety of contrast cryolipolysis for subcutaneous-fat reduction. Dermatol Res Pract. 2018;2018:5276528.
25. Munavalli GS, Panchaprateep R. Cryolipolysis for targeted fat reduction and improved appearance of the enlarged male breast. Dermatol Surg. 2015;41(9):1043-51.
26. Lipner SR. Cryolipolysis for the treatment of submental fat: review of the literature. J Cosmet Dermatol. 2018;17(2):145-51.
27. Ladha M, Poelman S. Cryolipolysis-induced morphea. JAAD Case Rep. 2019;5(4):300-2.
28. Putra IB, Jusuf NK, Dewi NK. Utilisation of cryolipolysis among Asians: a review on efficacy and safety. Open Access Maced J Med Sci. 2019; 7(9):1548-54.
29. Stroumza N, Gauthier N, Senet P, Moguelet P, Nail Barthelemy R, Atlan M. Paradoxical adipose hypertrophy (PAH) after cryolipolysis. Aesthet Surg J. 2018;38(4):411-7.

CHAPTER 102

Autologous Fat Transplantation

Milind S Wagh, Lakshyajit D Dhami

KEY MESSAGES

- Autologous fat transplantation is today one of the most frequently done procedures in aesthetic as well as reconstructive surgery. It entails the utilization of the patient's own fat harvested from one site of the body and injected into a recipient site elsewhere for the desired results.
- Our own body fat has significant advantages over synthetic fillers for soft tissue augmentation in most areas of the body. It is abundant, readily available, inexpensive, and completely biocompatible.
- Fat transplantation is a simple, safe, and relatively noninvasive procedure as long as the treating doctor has proper training and adequate surgical skills.
- Fat transplantation can be combined with liposuction for body contouring.
- Fat is now known as a rich source of stem cells and has clearly shown tremendous regenerative and rejuvenation potential.
- The procedure has rapidly grown in popularity since the 1990s with the increasing demand as tissue fillers and with new discoveries concerning the regenerative capabilities of transplanted fat.
- With much better understanding of the science in the last few years, there have been quantum improvements in the techniques of harvesting as well as transfer, which has helped to improve fat survival and long-term reliability of the procedure.

INTRODUCTION

With the increasing demand for injectable tissue fillers for various indications, autologous fat transplantation (grafting) is a technique, which has been growing in popularity during the last two and a half decades. Synthetic filler substances are expensive, mostly temporary, and have risk of potential allergic and other adverse reactions. In contrast, autologous fat has several advantages; fat not only acts as a filler but also has regenerative capabilities. A properly performed fat transfer has enhanced longevity and stability. Since it is autologous, it also integrates the transferred fatty tissue into the host tissue so that it is hardly detectable. Large amounts can be transplanted, and the surgery can be done in the same session as a liposuction procedure so that patient gets the dual advantage of fat suction from undesired areas for contouring as well as reshaping and augmentation with fat transplantation into the desired areas. The recent discovery of fat as a source of stem cells has further enhanced its role as a rejuvenating procedure. Fat transplantation is also an effective means of changing not only facial and body contours but can also be used for augmentation of other body parts such as breasts, buttocks, calf, penis, and labia; for rejuvenating the dorsum of hands, face, and neck and for revising post-traumatic or burns scars.

Thus, autologous fat has very broad and exponentially increasing applications in aesthetic surgery and dermatosurgery.

HISTORY

Surgeons all over the globe have been experimenting with injections of various substances to alter surface contour of the body, in particular the face, since the 19th century.

The earliest attempts to use adipose tissue can be traced to 1889 when Van der Meulen first attempted to do a fat autotransplantation. He performed a free omentum and autologous fat graft between the liver and the diaphragm to treat a case of diaphragmatic hernia.[1]

Then in 1893, Gustav Neuber transferred fat from the arm to the orbital region to correct adherent depressed scars. He was the first to note that large size grafts were more likely to be unsuccessful, whereas small grafts produced lasting aesthetic results.[2] In 1897, Victor Czerny excised a lipoma and grafted it into the breast of a woman who had had some nodules removed.[3]

In 1908, Eugene Hollander in Berlin first published experiences with injecting fat into the face. In 1912, he published its use for correction of facial atrophy and breast scarring. He published photographic documentation of natural appearing changes after infiltration of fat into two patients with lipoatrophy of the face.[4]

In 1910, Lexer described for the first time the use of adipose tissue in aesthetic surgery to correct aging defects, using fat as a filler for the malar infraorbital area.[5] The donor was a 12 × 12 cm autogenous fat graft from abdomen. In 1919, he published a monogram titled *"Die freien transplantationen"* (free transplantation) in which he described the technique of fat harvesting and grafting in detail **(Fig. 1)** for a wide variety of problems in the face (congenital and post-traumatic), breasts, and hands. In 1925, he published a study on the survival of adipose grafts, emphasizing the need for delicate handling of the harvested tissue to obtain a good result.[6]

In 1911, Brunning was the first to introduce the use of a syringe as an instrument for fat grafting. He was also the first to inject autologous fat into the subcutaneous plane when he used small fragments of adipose tissue to fine-tune the aesthetic outcomes of rhinoplasty. It is he who first noted that the initial good results obtained tended to be lost with time and that this appeared to be due to the reabsorption of the grafted fat.[7]

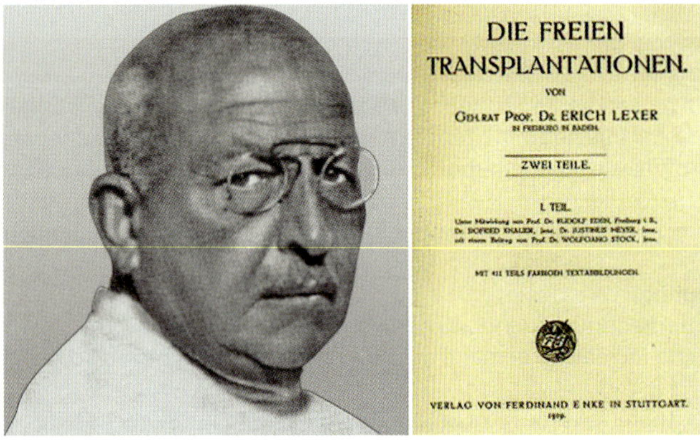

DIE FREIEN TRANSPLANTATIONEN.

VON

GEH.RAT PROF. DR. ERICH LEXER

ZWEI TEILE.

I. TEIL.

VERLAG VON FERDINAND ENKE IN STUTTGART.

Fig. 1: Dr Erich Lexer.

In 1926, Charles Conrad Miller (USA) published an article on the use of cannulae for correction of scar contraction on the face and neck.[8]

In 1941, May described the use of a large free fat graft on one side and a free fascia-fat autograft on the other, taken from the posterolateral surface of the thigh for a bilateral breast reconstruction.[1] He believed that the addition of the fascia to the graft could preserve adipose tissue, reducing its absorption **(Figs. 2A to D)**.

It is absolutely fascinating to note that the use of autologous adipose grafts is also reported during World War II. Salvat made changes to the faces of Allied spies by injecting them with fatty tissue. He has described how he would use autologous fat for permanent results and homologous fat for temporary effects.[9]

Peer studied fat transplantation extensively in the 1950s and he was the first to hypothesize that there was usually a 50% weight loss and volume loss of the fat graft by the end of 1 year.[10,11]

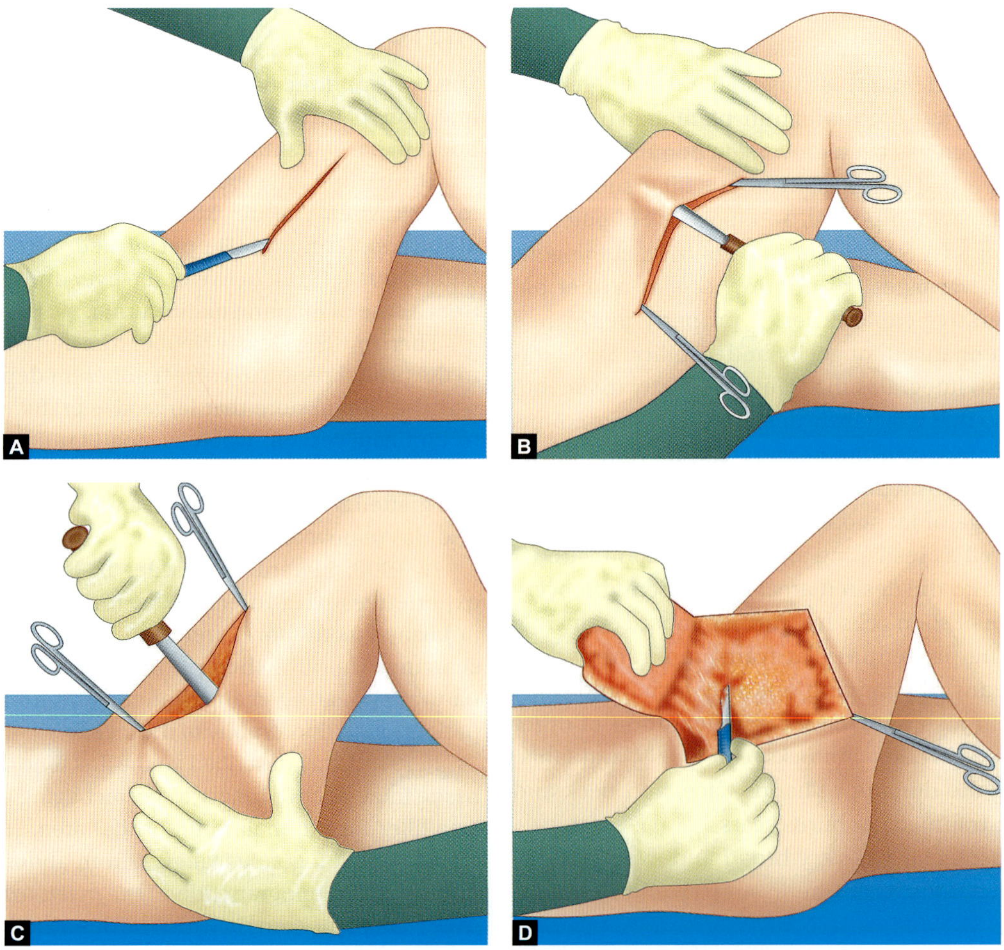

Figs. 2A to D: May's technique to harvest large fat grafts with fascia.

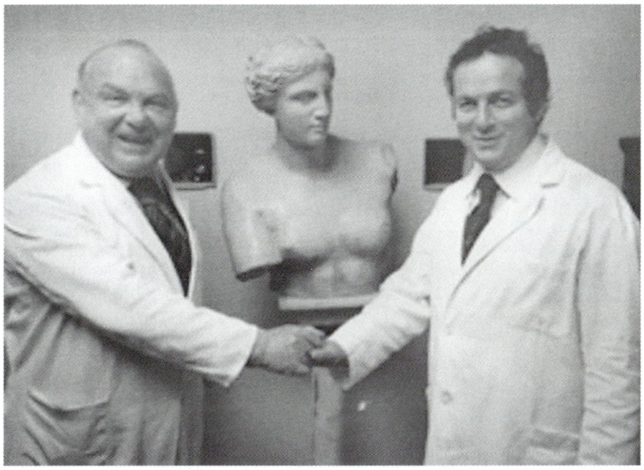

Fig. 3: Arpad and Giorgio Fischer.

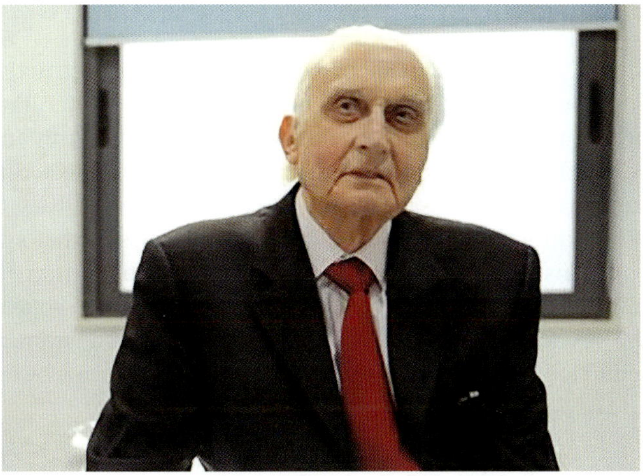

Fig. 5: Dr Pierre Fournier.

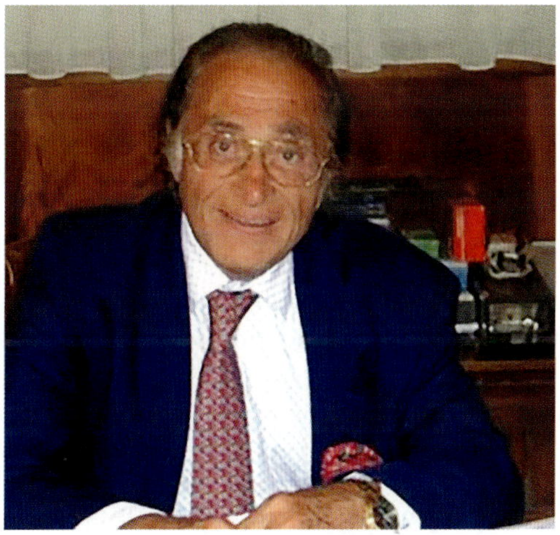

Fig. 4: Prof Yves Gerard Illouz.

As a result of equivocal and unpredictable long-term results, the technique slowly fell into disrepute and disuse. So much so that it was totally forgotten for a period of >25 years. It was the introduction of liposuction in the 1970s, which helped to resurrect the idea of autologous fat injections.[12]

In 1975, father and son duo, Arpad and Giorgio Fischer, developed the modern technique of liposuction **(Fig. 3)**. They were the first to introduce a blunt hollow cannula attached to a suction source and the fan-shaped/criss-cross suctioning technique through multiple incision sites.[13]

In 1977, Yves Gerard Illouz **(Fig. 4)**, also one of the pioneers of liposuction, modified the cannulae for performing liposuction making the technique much less traumatic and reducing bleeding. He was the first to use the semi-liquid lipoaspirated tissue as a filler injection so that fat could be transplanted without donor or recipient incisions. A byproduct of liposuction, the readily available semiliquid fat could be easily reinjected through cannulae and blunt needles.[14,15] In 1978, Pierre Fournier, another pioneer, proposed a new technique for infiltrating adipose tissue, calling it *lipofilling* **(Fig. 5)**. Fournier emphasized a need for overcorrection and also recognized the inconsistency in the results he was getting.[16-19]

In 1984–1985, Mel Bircoll described his experiences of injecting fat obtained by liposuction for enhancement of breasts. In 1987, he reported the advantages of the procedure, namely simplicity, absence of a scar, rapid recovery, and no necessity of implant.[20-24]

In 1986, Ellenbogen reported the use of free pearl fat autografts in a variety of atrophic and post-traumatic facial deficits.[25]

In 1988, Luiz Toledo, in Brazil, developed disposable syringes of different gauges and sizes for aspiration of adipose tissue. The main advantage of syringe liposuction was the precision and accuracy in measurement of the harvested volumes, as well as ability to inject fat less traumatically.[26,27]

From 1986 onward, one man, Sydney Coleman, was largely responsible for completely changing the thinking with regard to this procedure. He made revolutionary changes in the techniques and proposed a strictly atraumatic protocol for the treatment of all adipose tissue. He first used fat for grafting into iatrogenic liposuction contour deformities, then elaborated and refined the technique in the face for aesthetic reasons.[28-30]

He repeatedly showed that the key to successful fat grafting lays in the technique of harvest and refinement of small intact parcels of pure fat. The transfer of these fat parcels into the recipient site needed to be uniform and in multiple planes so that they survive predictably and become integrated into the host tissues to accomplish a desired structural change. He called it *structural fat grafting* and emphasized that the key to attaining these goals is the placement of tiny aliquots of fat droplets with each withdrawal of the infiltrating cannula using small syringes and cannulae.[31,32]

In the year 2001, Zuk made a critical discovery that adipose-derived stem cells (ADSCs) present in the stromal vascular fractions (SVFs) of lipoaspirates are capable of differentiating into many types of tissue and the term "stem cells" finally entered the field of fat grafting.

FAT SURVIVAL

In 1987, the American Society of Plastic and Reconstructive Surgeons reported the problems and difficulties that have been encountered with autologous fat transplantation and concluded that only 30% of injected fat can be expected to survive for 1-year.[33]

In clinical practice, therefore, the main issue that still concerns us as surgeons as well as the patients after fat transfer is the question of fat absorption over time. In spite of the best techniques, several studies have reported an average reduction from 25 to 70% of the total implanted volume by the end of 1 year.[34-36]

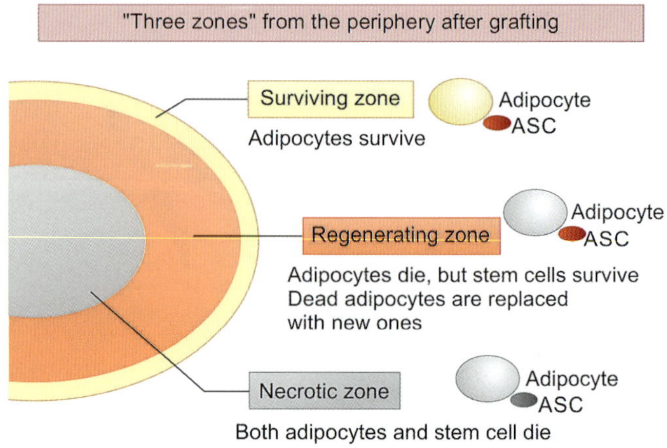

Fig. 6: Zones of ischemia in fat grafts.

Theories of Fat Survival

Host Replacement Theory (Neuhof and Hirschfield 1923)[37]

Fat grafting is followed by degenerative changes in the first few months, which stimulates inflow of histiocytes. As these phagocytize the cellular debris, some of them undergo changes into embryonal fat cells, which eventually transform to adult fat tissue by the end of 5 months or so. They concluded that the originally transplanted fat completely died and was replaced by fibrous tissue and newly formed metaplastic fat.

Cell Survival Theory (Peer)[38]

This states that following a fat transfer, survival depends on the number of vital adipocytes present at the time of transplantation. On day 1, the grafted adipocytes pass through an ischemic phase with macrophages, histiocytes, and polynucleated cells flowing in for phagocytosis to remove all nonviable fat cells. By day 4, revascularization of the graft takes place by neoangiogenesis from the host tissues around the fat cells. This mechanism starts from the periphery and moves inward toward the center. The central core of adipose tissue undergoes a longer period of ischemia and can vascularize only when the size of the droplet is small.

Stem Cells/Preadipocytes-related Theory (Billings and May 1989)[1]

Mature fat cells are very fragile and have a low level of resistance to trauma and ischemia. They return to a primitive cellular state of progenitor immature cells called preadipocytes, which are more resistant to hypoxic and traumatic insults because they have minimal metabolic activity and can survive without nutrition much longer and have a much lower oxygen consumption rate. These preadipocytes and ADSCs in the stromal cell fraction are the only tissues that survive transplantation. Over time, they regenerate into adult fat cells.

Zones of Ischemia

A freshly placed fat graft is now understood to have three zones **(Fig. 6)**:

1. An outermost, "surviving" zone
2. An intermediate, "regenerating" zone
3. A central, "necrotic" zone

It appears that the overall result depends on the degree of survival in the regenerating zone, which contains adipose-derived stromal cells (ASCs) since these have the potential for differentiation and replacement of the adult fat cells destroyed in the necrotic zone.

Adipose-derived Stem Cells

They were first discovered as mesenchymal stem cells in adipose tissue by Zuk et al.[39,40] in 2001, ADSCs are present in the SVF of the lipoaspirate and can differentiate into many types of tissues. ADSCs have also been shown to be critical in encouraging fat graft revascularization.

Fat was already known to be a high-energy reservoir, insulating agent, and thermoregulator but with this discovery, it also appeared to be a *reparative organ* providing a basis for soft tissue regeneration.

Adipose-derived stem cells are believed to facilitate fat survival by the following mechanisms:

- Differentiation into adipocytes and regeneration of adipose tissue
- Differentiation into endothelial cells and thereby promoting angiogenesis and neovascularization
- Release of angiogenic factors such as vascular endothelial growth factor (VEGF), which also aids angiogenesis
- Immunoregulatory effect.

Some ADSCs also survive and then replace the transplanted adipocytes.

TYPES OF FAT TRANSPLANTS

Autologous fat transplant can be of various types:

- *Autologous free fat graft:* A mass of fatty tissue harvested from any inconspicuous subcutaneous area and transplanted *en masse* at a recipient site.
- *Dermo-fat graft:* A piece of skin (dermis only with epidermis removed) along with a thin layer of underlying subcutaneous fat harvested from an area, from where the defect can be closed primarily. A dermo-fat graft can be used as a filler or to act as a spacer between gliding tissues **(Figs. 7A to C)**.
- *Vascularized fat flaps:* Free fat flaps, i.e., omental flaps can be transferred by microvascular means, as a soft tissue filler for conditions such as hemifacial atrophy or to resurface any large defect with an overlying skin graft.
- *Free fat injection:* Fat harvested, processed, and transplanted in a liquid injectable form for various indications.

This chapter focuses on the technique of transfer and transplantation of autologous fat graft in an injectable form. The primary indication for fat injections is its use as an ideal filler to replace "Like with Like." It is also widely used as a spacer, for contour restoration, and for soft tissue augmentation of not only the face, but various body parts. As an advanced indication, it focuses on the regeneration and rejuvenation capabilities of transplanted adipose tissues.

INDICATIONS FOR AUTOLOGOUS FAT TRANSFER

- *For correction of facial volume loss*: Due to aging, infection [e.g., lipoatrophy due to human immunodeficiency virus (HIV)], trauma, Parry–Romberg syndrome, scleroderma, hemifacial microsomia, etc.[29]
- *For augmentation of soft tissue on face*: Correction of post-acne scars, augmentation of lips, nasolabial folds, cheeks, malar region, temporal region, etc.[41-43]
- In aesthetic and reconstructive breast surgery for:
  - Cosmetic breast augmentation[44]
  - Correction of breast lumpectomy defects
  - Correction of breast asymmetry
  - Breast reconstruction after cancer ablation[45,46]
  - Treatment of radiation damage
  - Treatment of breast capsular contracture.
- For augmentation of postliposuction defects on the chest, abdomen, thighs, buttocks, arms, face, etc.
- For restoration of volume and rejuvenation of skin on dorsum of hands[32,47-51] **(Fig. 8)**.
- For buttock augmentation (Brazilian Butt-lift) **(Figs. 9A and B)**.
- For penile girth augmentation[52,53] **(Fig. 10)**.

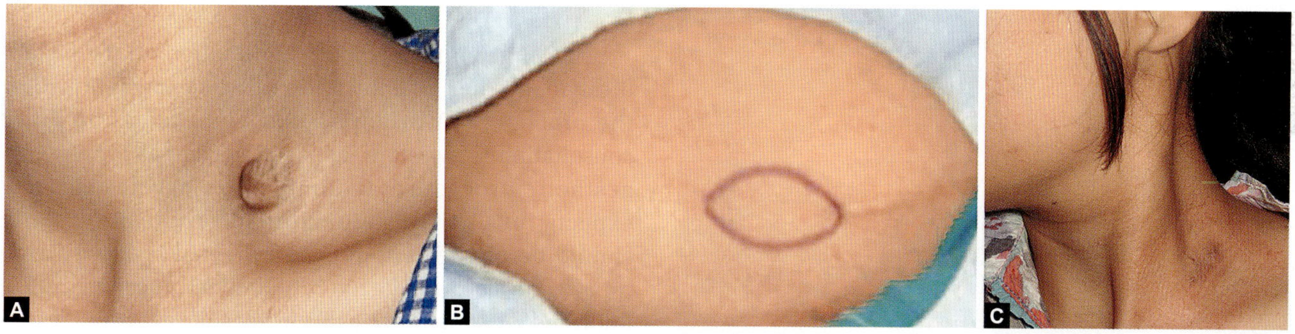

Figs. 7A to C: (A) Defect in left lower neck with a circular depressed scar and loss of tissue volume; (B) Obtaining dermo-fat graft; (C) Result after correction of defect by filling with dermo-fat graft covered by skin advancement and closure.

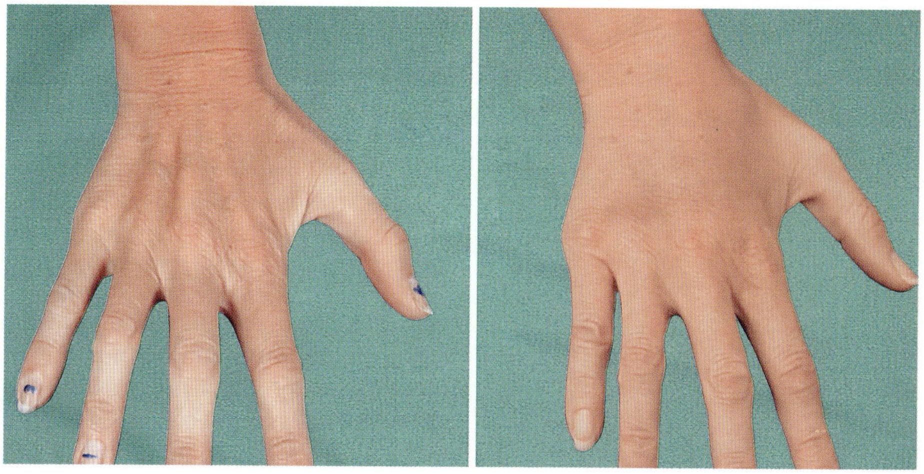

Fig. 8: Rejuvenation of hands by fat injection.

- For augmentation of labia majora as a part of female genital beautification.[54,55]
- For augmentation of calves—acquired or congenital hypoplasia[56-59] **(Fig. 11)**.
- For rejuvenation and improvement in burn scars.[60,61]
- For treatment of sphincteric incontinence by perianal lipoinjection.

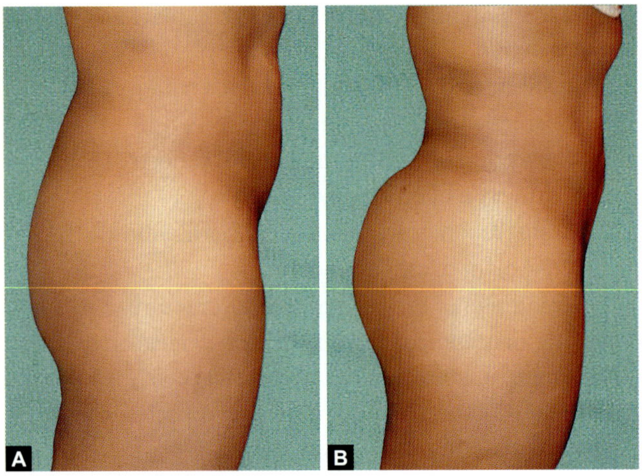

Figs. 9A and B: Buttock Augmentation by fat transfer (Brazilian butt lift). (A) Before; (B) After.

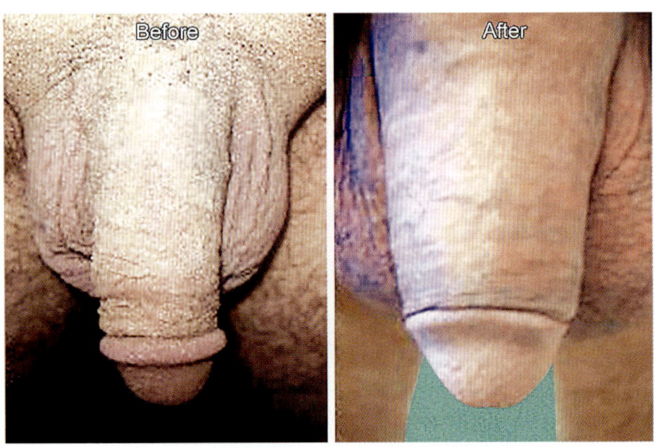

Fig. 10: Penile girth augmentation by fat transfer.

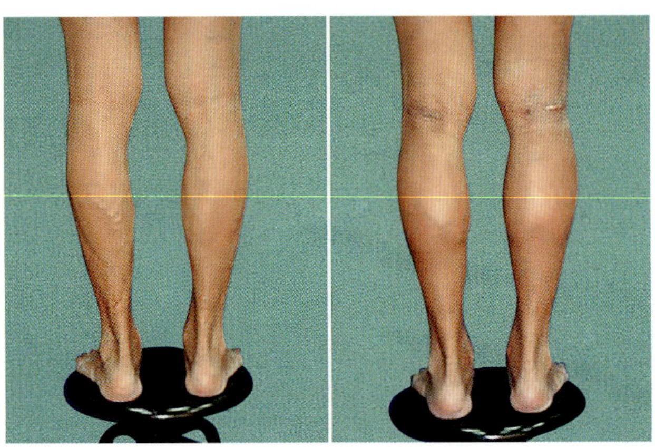

Fig. 11: Calf augmentation by fat transfer.

- For augmentation of paralyzed vocal cords **(Fig. 12)**.
- For treatment of palate-pharyngeal and velopharyngeal incompetence **(Fig. 13)**.

PATIENT SELECTION, PREOPERATIVE ASSESSMENT, COUNSELING, AND PLANNING

In the procedure of autologous fat grafting, precise and detailed preoperative planning as well as collective, informed decision-making between the patient and the surgeon is extremely crucial for the desired outcome and a satisfied patient.

Preoperative assessment must include:

- A thorough history and clinical examination
- History of past aesthetic procedures such as injections of silicone, collagen, other fillers, previous fat injections, or previous implants
- History of unusual or prolonged bleeding, bruising, and unusual swelling after prior procedures
- Indication of any psychiatric problems.

Before any kind of surgical/procedural plan can be made, at the time of consultation itself, the surgeon must also carefully evaluate the patient's present appearance and compare it with photographs of him/her at a younger age to assess past contours, areas of fat atrophy/dystrophy or weight loss.

The surgeon must acquire information on the patient's lifestyle, his/her desires, and realistic expectations from the procedure. A brief psychosocial evaluation during consultation is therefore just as important as for any other aesthetic procedure. Patients often have exaggerated expectations and sustainability of results. Information should be provided about the expected longevity of the transplanted fat, need for future additional procedures, and an informed consent must be taken. Sensible goals and realistic expectations usually result in a satisfied patient.

Patients need to clearly understand all the details of the planned procedure, the areas of treatment (donor and recipient sites), and the postoperative recovery phase including swelling, bruising, and timeline for healing. They should be made aware of their responsibilities during the recovery and healing period, the expected outcome, and are informed of possible sequelae and common complications. *They must be aware that it is NOT "Abracadabra".*

PATIENT EXAMINATION AND EVALUATION

Detailed photographic documentation is essential for successful fat transplantation and it serves as a basis for three-dimensional analysis. All scars, contour irregularities, skin dimpling, and cellulite present before surgery must be documented in detail and pointed out to the patient in advance. Any probability of improvement in these

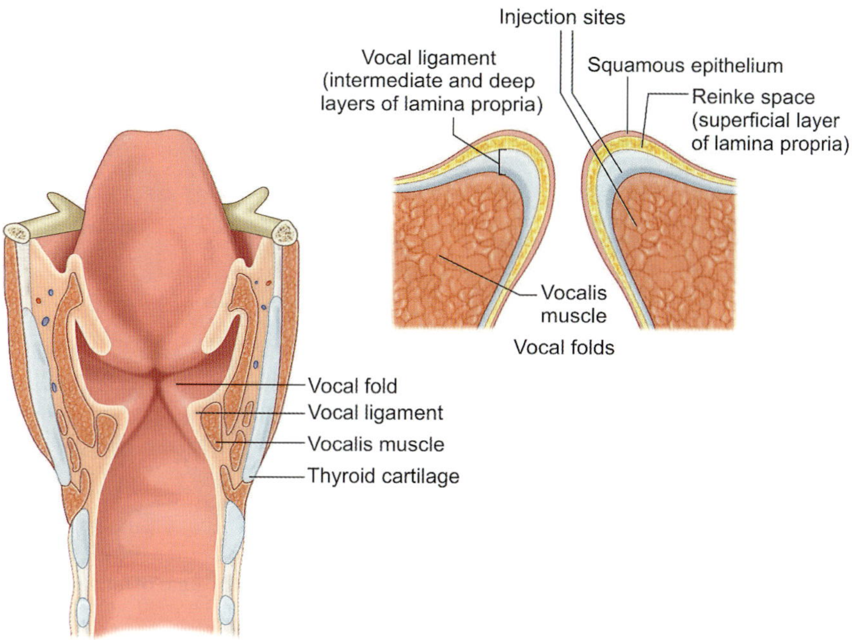

Fig. 12: Augmentation of paralyzed vocal cords.

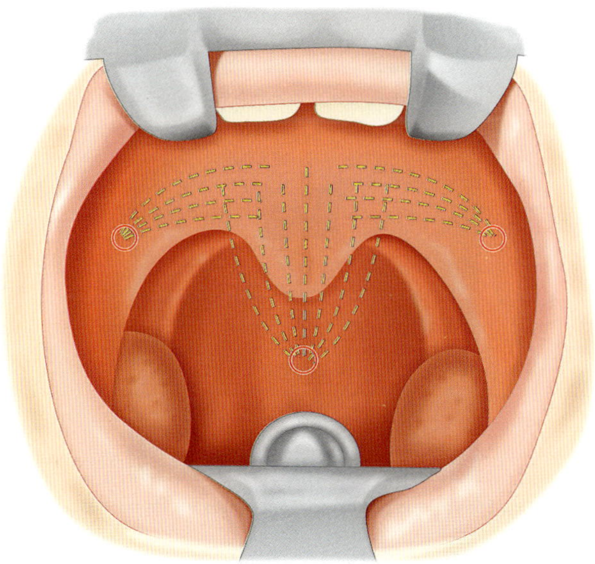

Fig. 13: For treatment of velopharyngeal incompetence.

difficult areas must be clearly informed to the patient. Physical examination of the face and the body is essential to supplement photographic documentation because photographs cannot capture the relationships of underlying structures and the skin. Skeletal landmarks and overlying key soft tissue points and areas must be marked in detail **(Fig. 14)**. Clinical examination should include determination of:

- Loss of facial fullness resulting in hollowing, wrinkling, and/or mild skin laxity
- Unnatural or unaesthetic facial proportions
- Facial asymmetry secondary to congenital abnormalities, trauma, and/or previous surgery
- Sufficient donor area availability for fat harvesting.

Surgical planning then involves determining the specific quantity of fat required, the tissue levels of its injection, and the structural support necessary. A photographic tracing is very useful to document the planned details of areas for fatty tissue placement and the amount to be injected in each subunit of a region **(Fig. 15)**. This also serves as a reference for postoperative evaluation and also acts as a guide to any secondary procedures needed.

SURGICAL TECHNIQUES: HARVESTING, REFINEMENT, AND TRANSPLANT

Over the past two decades, fat transplantation has been a constantly evolving procedure and hence new techniques and methods to maximize results and long-term goals continue to be discovered. Even today, there is no clear consensus on several aspects of fat transplantation such as the best donor sites; degree of negative suction to be applied during harvest; ideal diameter of liposuction cannula and size of its suction holes; exposure of fat to air; effect of concentration of adrenaline and lidocaine in the lipo-infiltrate; role of centrifugation versus decantation versus rinsing to process the harvested fat; diameter of the injecting cannula; amount, depth, and anatomical plane of fat injection; postoperative care and even the timing for a second stage fat transplant if necessary.

The technique discussed here tries to encompass the present state of the knowledge and current concepts accepted by surgeons around the world. It emphasizes on tissue respect and a basic sound knowledge of surgical techniques. Fatty tissues are extremely delicate and can be injured very easily outside the body by both mechanical and chemical insults.

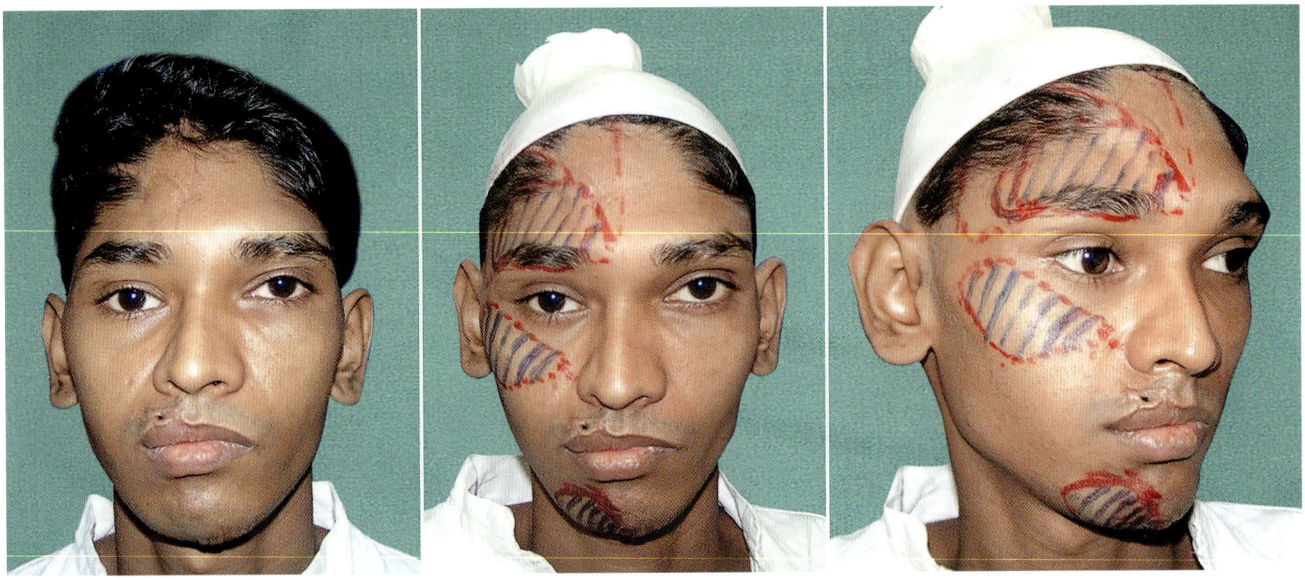

Fig. 14: Contour deformities on right side of face, clearly marked for areas of fat transfer.

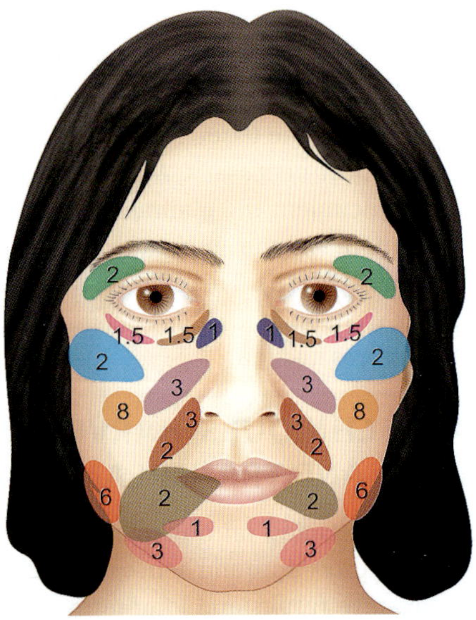

Fig. 15: Rejuvenation with fat transplantation, average volume of fat in milliliters desired and distribution in subunits in different regions of the face (in mL).

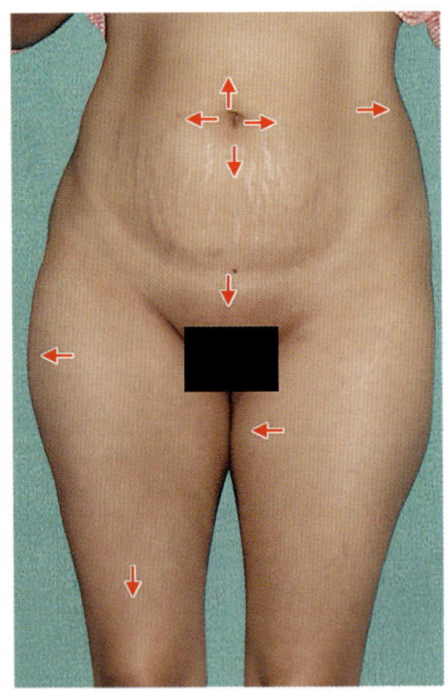

Fig. 16: Various common donor sites for fat harvest.

It must be remembered that for a successful transplantation, fat must survive harvesting, processing, transportation, and implantation as an intact and complete parcel of viable tissue, composed of connective tissues as well as adipose cells.

PRINCIPLES OF FAT GRAFTING

- Infiltration of the donor area with wetting solution
- Harvesting with a blunt cannula and syringe under low suction pressure (up to 200 mm Hg)
- Use of a 2–3 mm aspiration cannula with multiple 1 mm holes
- Refinement of the fat with decantation and/or centrifugation to remove nonliving components
- Meticulous planned placement/transfer into the recipient tissues in multiple planes in small droplet aliquots
- Maintenance of sterility/aseptic precautions throughout the procedure.

HARVESTING

Choice of Donor Site (Fig. 16)

Selected harvesting sites should be those which are convenient to access (usually those easily accessible to the surgeon with the patient in a supine position), usually hidden or covered by clothing and those that may contribute to simultaneous enhancement of the patient's body contour. The lower abdomen, periumbilical area, and upper inner thighs are the most preferred donor sites.

When abdominal or medial thigh fat is in short supply because of prior liposuction or scarcity of body fat, other potential sites which may be considered as donor area are the flanks, suprapubic mound, the anterior, lateral, or posterior thighs, the knee rolls, the lower back, the buttocks, or the upper back region. It is important to lipoaspirate bilaterally from these areas to maintain symmetry.

A higher concentration of ADSCs were found in the lower abdomen and inner thigh in one study.[62] In addition, in a younger age group (<45 years of age), fat grafts harvested from both the lower abdomen and inner thigh have higher viability based on single assay test.[63] The palm and pinch test should be performed in the donor area to determine if there is adequate fat reserve and to quickly estimate the amount of fat that can be harvested. A palm size is roughly measured as 200 cm^2. Whereas pinch test predicts the layer of thickness of the fat graft that can be harvested, e.g., even a thin patient with 0.25 cm of fat layer thickness in surface area of palm size would yield 50 mL of fat graft ($200\ cm^2 \times 0.25\ cm = 50\ mL$) by using super wet infiltration.

Whenever possible, harvesting sites are accessed through incisions placed in natural creases, previous scars, stretch marks, or hair-bearing areas. Meticulous sterile technique is observed with preoperative preparation using antimicrobial scrubs and prep solutions.

Anesthesia

When done for smaller areas such as the face, it is *often* done under local anesthesia on the donor area and using nerve blocks, anesthetic skin creams (EMLA/Prilox cream), and icepacks in the face (preferably with an anesthesiologist as standby). For local anesthesia, a blunt infiltrator attached to a 5 or 10 mL syringe is used to infiltrate 0.04% lidocaine with 1:1,000,000 adrenaline into the desired sites. Lidocaine when used in such super dilution has no adverse effect on fat viability and is still effective.[64]

Intravenous (IV) sedation is also given in cases where deeper plane transfers are planned in the face. For larger areas such as the breasts, buttocks, and hips where larger quantities need to be harvested and transferred or harvest is needed to be done from multiple sites, it is done under spinal/epidural or general anesthesia (GA). In such cases, lactated Ringer solution with 1:1,000,000 adrenaline (1 ampoule of 1:1000 adrenaline per 1 L) is infiltrated to ensure adequate hemostasis. In almost all clinical situations, approximately 1 mL of solution is infiltrated for every 1 mL of fat to be harvested. Tumescent techniques to harvest fat tissue, where a 2:1 ratio of quantity of infiltration solution to quantity of fat aspirated is used, can disrupt the parcels of fatty tissue and may decrease survival, so they are usually avoided.

Syringe Fat Suction

A 15 or 23 cm long harvesting cannula, with a blunt tip and noncutting distal opening with multiple small 1 mm holes

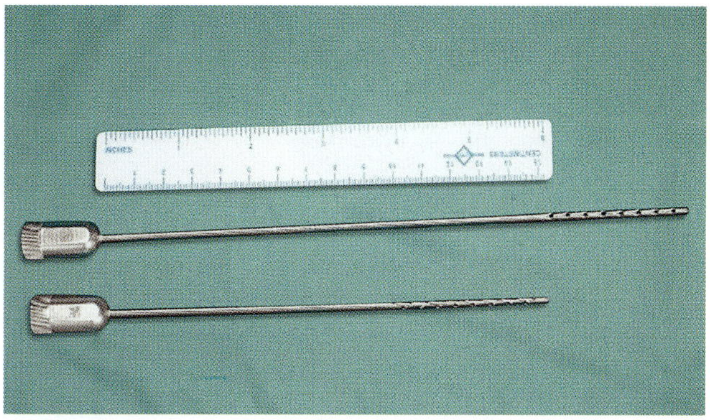

Fig. 17: Blunt noncutting lipo-aspiration syringe cannula with multiple 1 mm sharp holes.

placed on the sides close to the end of the cannula **(Fig. 17)**, is mounted onto a 5 or 10 mL Luer-Lok syringe. The openings of the harvesting cannula being 1 mm, this will allow for an appropriate size and shape of intact fatty tissue parcels that can readily pass through the lumen of a Luer-Lok syringe. If the fatty tissue parcels can pass through the lumen of the Luer-Lok syringe, it will easily, without damage, pass through the much smaller (17-gauge) lumen of the injection cannula.

After inserting the cannula tip into the donor site, the surgeon pulls back on the syringe plunger to create a small amount of negative pressure within the barrel of the syringe. A 10 mL syringe is small enough to be manipulated manually without locking devices to minimize negative pressure. The surgeon pulls back on the plunger of the syringe to create about 1 or 2 mL (not >2–3 mL) of space in the barrel of the syringe while the attached cannula is pushed through the harvest site. Too much negative suction pressure should be avoided to avoid damage to fat cells during suction.[65] Chajchir et al. recommended negative pressures as low as 200–250 mm Hg only (10 inches Hg).[66]

The combination of adequate negative pressure and the curetting action of the cannula's to-and-fro motion through the tissues allows parcels of fatty tissue to move through the cannula and through the Luer-Lok aperture, into the barrel of the syringe with minimal mechanical damage **(Figs. 18A and B)**.

When filled adequately, the syringe is then disconnected from the cannula and replaced with a dual function Luer-Lok plug for capping. After the syringe is sealed at the Luer-Lok end, the plunger is removed from the proximal end of the syringe and the barrel filled up to 10 mL of harvested material and kept aside **(Fig. 19)** before they are either placed into a centrifuge or is allowed for gravity sedimentation (decantation).

PROCESSING OF HARVESTED FAT AND PREPARATION FOR TRANSFER

The aim of processing the harvested fat is to remove contaminants such as excess fluid, cellular debris, oil, and

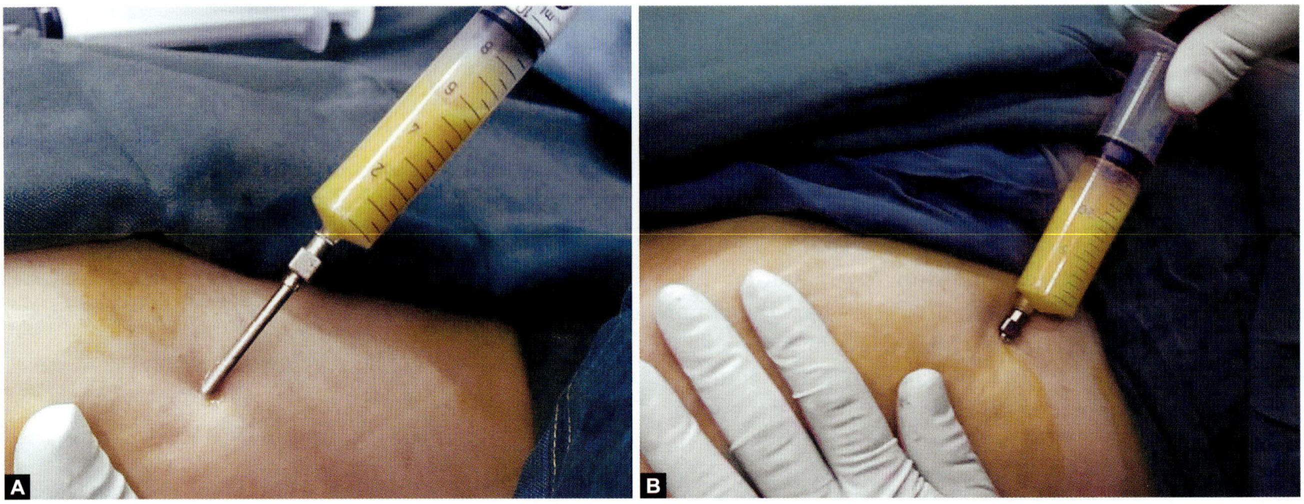

Figs. 18A and B: Donor area on medial thigh for small volume fat harvest using a 10 mL syringe.

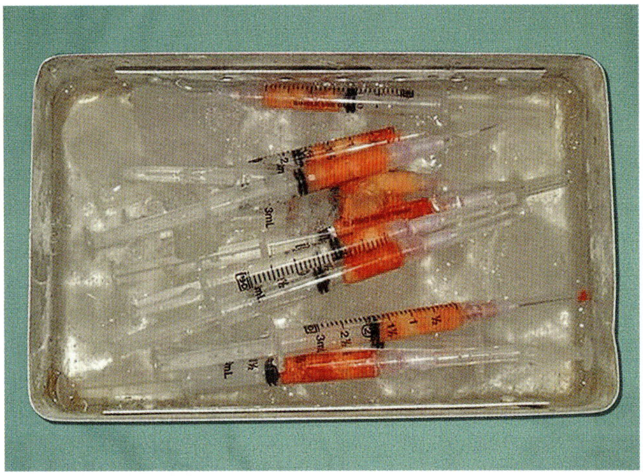

Fig. 19: Syringes filled with harvested fat before processing.

blood cells. Carpaneda and Robeiro[67] have conclusively shown that:

- Blood in the graft accelerates degradation of grafted fat cells
- Free fat, hemoglobin, and clots induce greater cellular damage and thereby stimulate greater inflammatory response
- Maximizing the number of adipose-derived mesenchymal stem cells in the grafted material will obviously improve graft viability.

Also the injection of all this debris gives a wrong estimation of the volume of correction placed in, because all the fluid and debris will be absorbed in a few hours.[68]

Several methods are being used by surgeons to effectively remove the infiltrated solution, oil, and the cell debris within the lipoaspirates and also to concentrate the fat graft. The step of processing and refining is the most controversial and disagreeable issue, in the procedure of fat transplantation, even among seniors and experts in the field. Harvested tissue can have as little as 10% to as much as 90% viable fat even with liposuction from the same site during the same operative procedure.

Common methods among those include gravity sedimentation or decantation, filtration with saline wash, and centrifugation.[69-73]

Decantation

Sedimentation or decantation for 20 minutes is a simple atraumatic method to obtain a good quantity of intact fat cells **(Figs. 20A and B)**. Many surgeons prefer to avoid centrifugation by keeping the test tubes upright for 20 minutes to allow the separation of supernatant oily fraction and infranatant bloody fluid which need to be drained.

The concentration of stem cells is however limited, and the supernatant may still contain a significant amount of fluid, blood cells, and oil which cause an inflammatory effect and are harmful to graft survival. Some publications confirm this, demonstrating lower rates of decanted graft viability relative to centrifuged and washed specimens, whereas others claim equally good results.

Filtration and Washing

Simple filtration through a cotton gauze cloth, nylon cloth, or a stainless-steel sieve mesh while washing with Ringer's lactate also seems to efficiently remove contaminants while maintaining viable adipocytes and a large portion of adipose-derived mesenchymal stem cells **(Fig. 21)**. This processing technique may be more efficient in producing viable graft material for large-volume fat transfers. Washing the lipoaspirate has the goal of removing superfluous tumescent fluid, free lipids, and debris. This technique has previously been demonstrated to preserve both a large number of mesenchymal stem cells and a large number of adipocytes, thus satisfying both current theories for graft survival.[74-77]

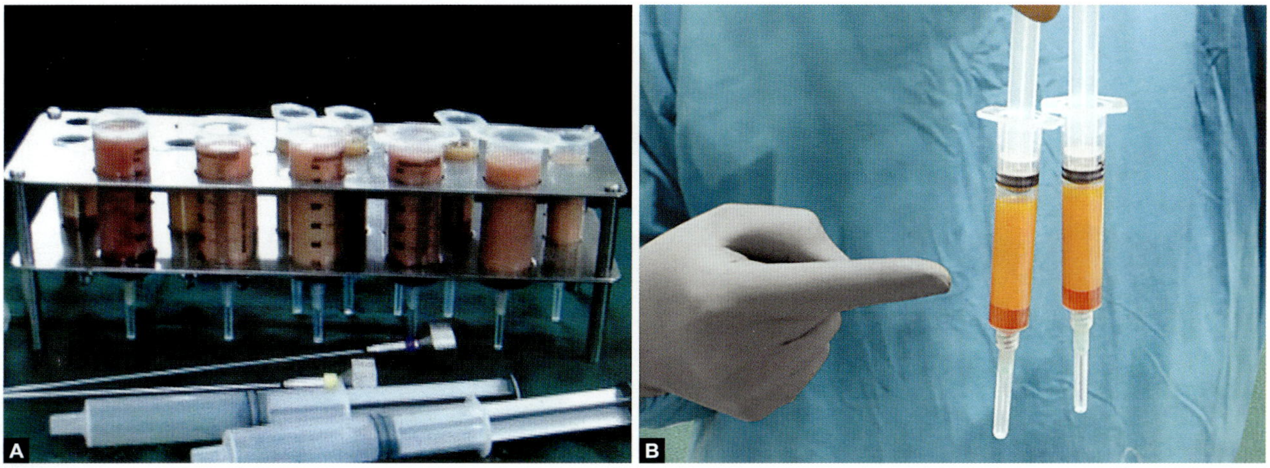

Figs. 20A and B: (A) Harvested fat in syringes kept upright for decantation for 20 minutes; (B) Decanted syringes with infranatant fluid and good quality fat above, after 20 minutes.

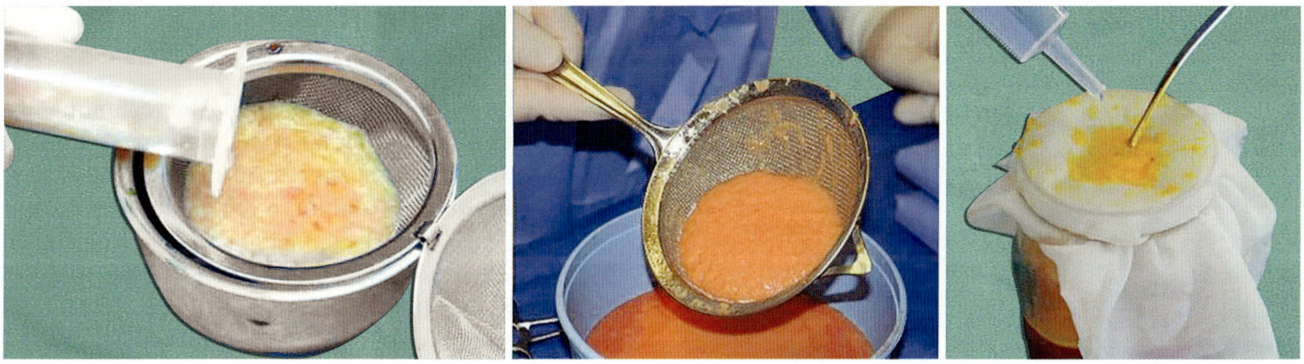

Fig. 21: Processing using the filtration method passing the harvested fat through a stainless-steel sieve or gauze cloth.

This fat can then be filled up in 5/10 mL syringes with spoon, which is then transferred to 1 mL acrylic insulin syringe with bivalve ready to be used for injection. Several surgeons advocate the filtration technique or even just gravity segmentation to process a large or mega-volume of lipoaspirate, especially in cases of breast and gluteal augmentation.

A new technology called the pure-graft filtration system is available which consists of a proprietary closed-membrane filtration system originally designed to prepare fat for isolation of SVF. This is less traumatic than centrifugation and able to clear free lipid, white blood cell (WBC), and red blood cell (RBC) content from the fat graft.

Centrifugation

Centrifugation has been the most common technique for fat processing and was previously considered the ideal method. This method not only makes manipulation of the fat graft easier but also provides reliable viability and results. Recent studies have shown that proper centrifugation can concentrate not only adipocytes and ADSCs but also several angiogenic growth factors within the processed fat grafts.[78-80]

To promote sterility, a centrifuge with a sterilizable central rotor and sleeves that can hold a 5 or 10 mL syringe should be used **(Fig. 22A)**. Manual centrifuges which can be used with the hand are also available **(Fig. 22B)**. Coleman recommended centrifugation speeds of 3,000 rpm for 3 minutes, although excessive centrifugal force may damage intact adipocytes.

Centrifugation separates the denser components from the less dense components to create multiple clearly discernible layers **(Fig. 23)**. The upper level is the least dense and consists primarily of oil. The middle portion is primarily fatty tissue. The lowest layer is blood, water, and any aqueous element. The amount of nonliving components harvested will depend on the quantity of infiltration by the surgeon, the amount of blood in the harvested specimen, and the damage to fatty cells that releases lipids.

Centrifugation obtains the highest possible concentration of stem cells within the lipoaspirate. It has also an increased content of angiogenic growth factors such as fibroblast growth factor (FGF) and VEGF. A higher concentration of stem cells or angiogenic growth factors positively correlates with better fat graft survival both in experimental and clinical studies.

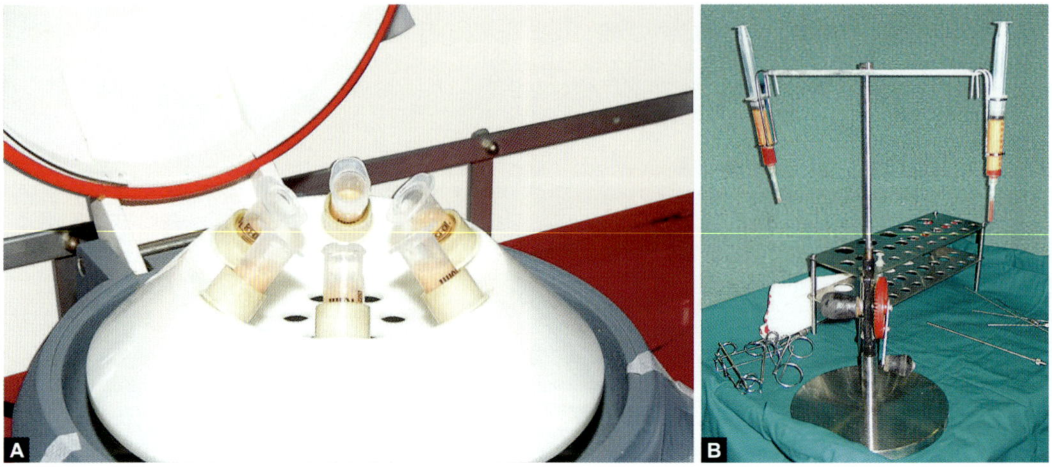

Figs. 22A and B: (A) Electrical centrifuge holding 5 or 10 mL syringes; (B) Manual centrifuge apparatus.

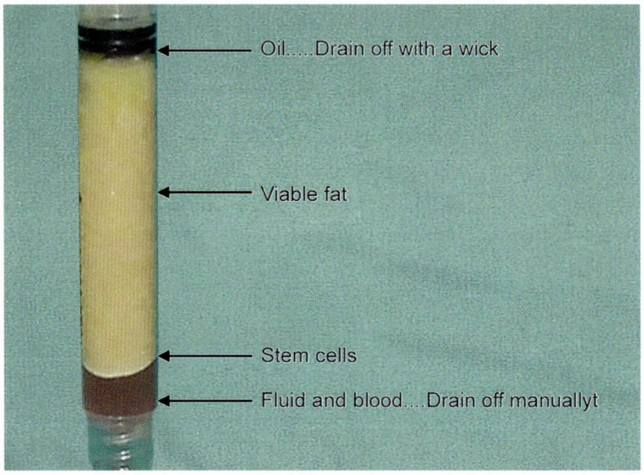

Fig. 23: Separated components after centrifugation showing oil on top, then the viable fat and fluid and blood at the bottom.

The oil layer is decanted from the syringe before the Luer-Lock plug is removed. After the oil is decanted, the Luer-Lock plug is removed to drain the fluid out at the bottom. Blotting paper or other highly absorbent materials can be used to wick off the remaining oil from the exposed end of the harvested fat by capillary action. Care should be taken not to allow the material from the wicks to shred off into the refined tissue. After 4 minutes, the wick can be replaced again if any oil remains. After changing the wick two or three times, the plunger is replaced into the barrel of the 10 mL syringe. This is done by allowing the fat to slide down to the edge of the syringe barrel and then advancing the plunger to obliterate the dead space. The fat is then transferred into 1 mL Luer-Lok insulin syringes ready for transplant **(Figs. 24A and B)**. It is preferable to use acrylic syringe for infiltration as the piston moves smoothly for even distribution of fat transplant.

A summary of the procedure of harvest, processing, and refining prior to transfer is shown in **Figure 25**.

RECIPIENT AREA, INJECTION, AND PLACEMENT

Obviously, one of the crucial steps in the technique of fat transplantation is how the fat grafts are placed (injected/infiltrated). The key to a successful fat transplantation is to achieve an even distribution of fat graft in the recipient area. By doing so, the injected fat graft will have a maximal amount of contact with the host tissue which results in better fat graft survival, stability, and integration through plasmatic imbibition and neovascularization. The fatty tissue parcels must be positioned such that they are separated from each other as much as possible by intervening host tissues. Not only does the grafting with small parcels of fat in each pass gives better surgical outcome but it reduces the complications such as oil cyst formation, calcification, fibrosis, or even potential risk of infection with large boluses fat grafting. *"Fat grafts should be placed via multiple passes within multiple tissue planes and tunnels in multiple directions."*

A small volume (no >0.1 mL) of fat grafts should be injected in each pass. Slow injection of 0.5–1.0 mL per second should be infiltrated during the withdrawal phase in each pass to minimize trauma to the fat graft **(Figs. 26A and B)**. The injection should be as gentle as possible to avoid possibility of injury to blood vessels or nerves. The injecting cannula size usually range from 16 to 20 G for microfat grafting. The cannula size of 22–24 G for nanofat grafting is most appropriate in areas such as in the lower eyelids, nasolabial groove, and under the scars.

The cannulas are blunt with the distal aperture on the side wall just proximal to the tip **(Fig. 27)**. The cannula shape and length vary depending on the area to be grafted. In the face, 7–9 cm long cannulas are the most useful; longer cannulas, up to 15 cm, can be useful in the trunk and extremities **(Figs. 28 and 29)**. A cannula with pointed or sharp end may be used to free up the adhesions or inject into scars and fibrous areas, but

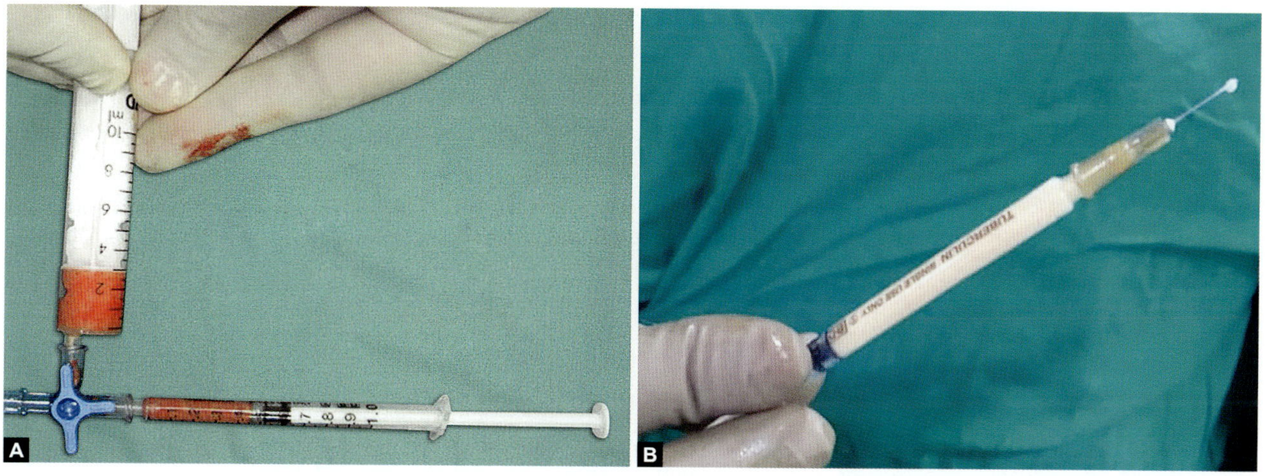

Figs. 24A and B: Transfer to smaller 1 mL acrylic syringes before injection.

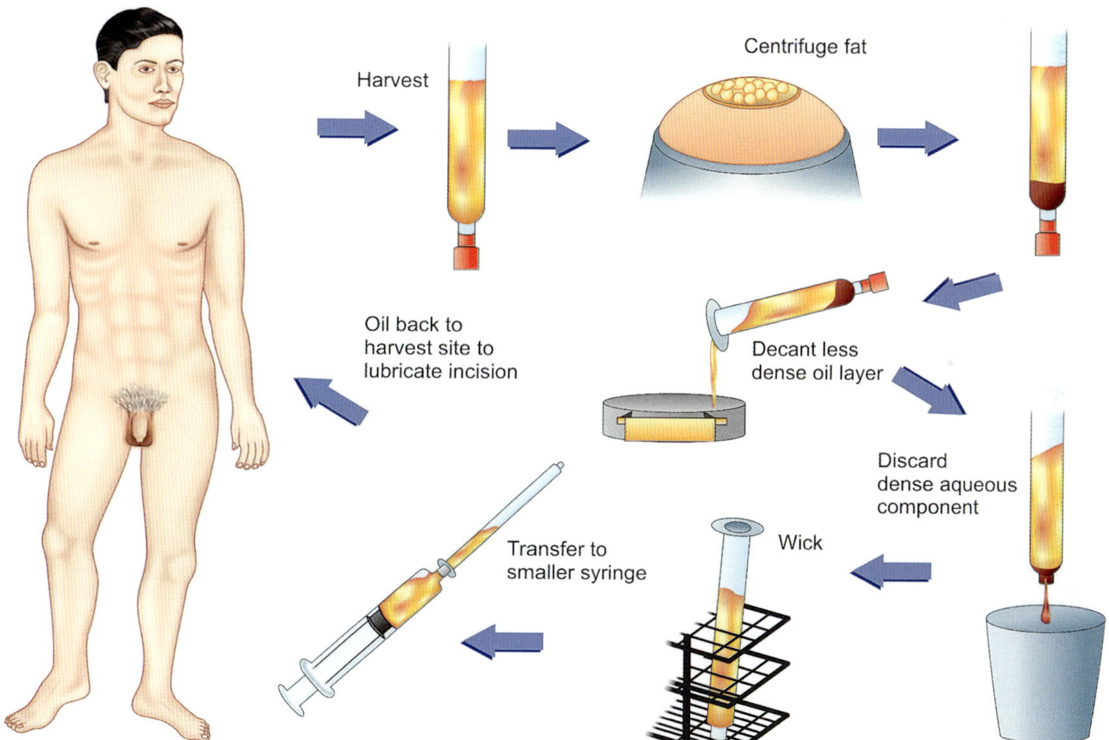

Fig. 25: A summary of fat refinement and preparation techniques prior to transfer.

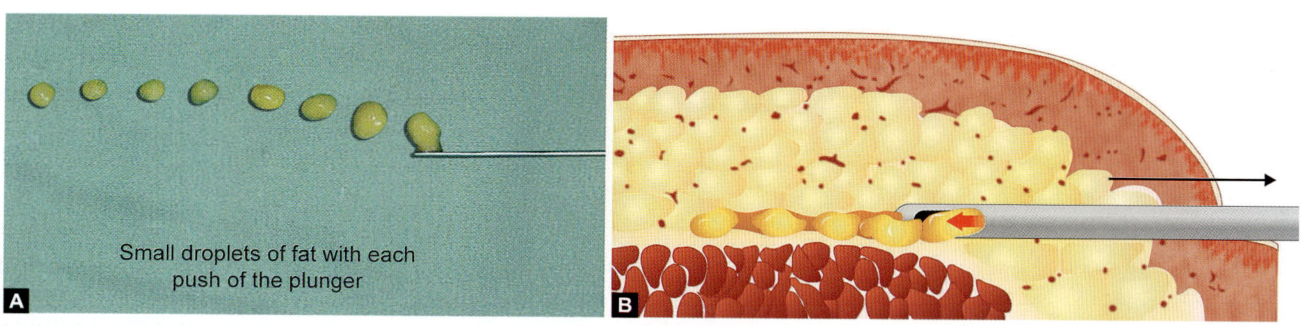

Figs. 26A and B: (A) Demonstration of size of fat graft push with each of the syringe plunger; (B) Way to inject fat graft in beads while withdrawing the cannula in the tissue plane.

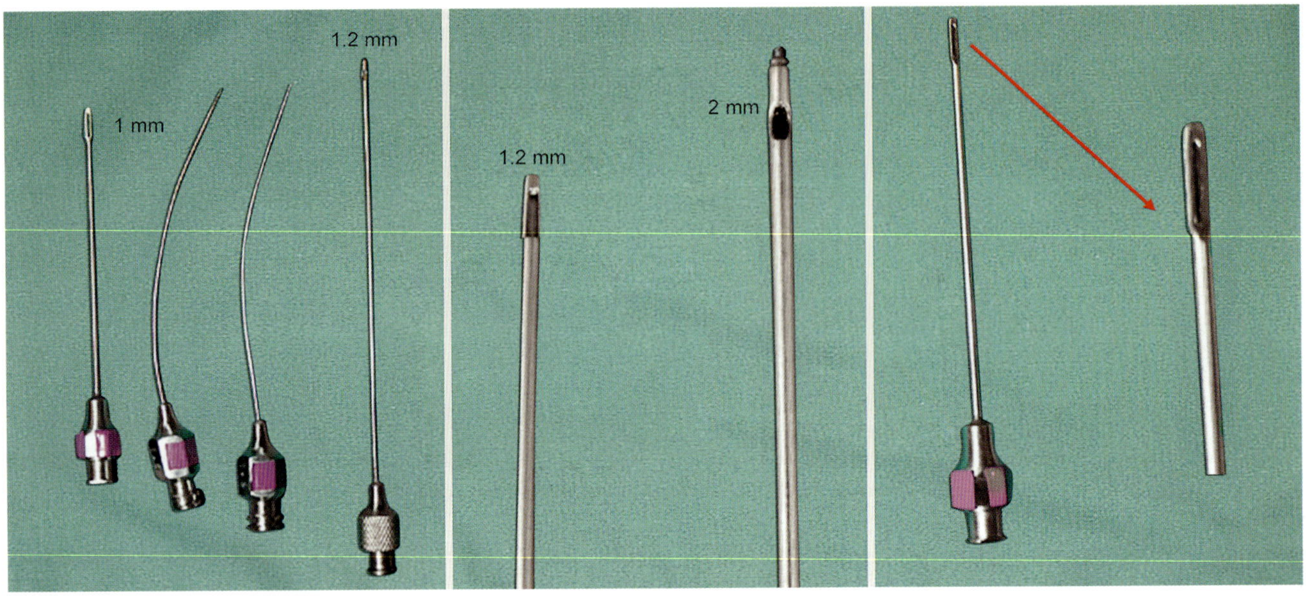

Fig. 27: Various cannulae for fat injection, single hole on the side just proximal to the tip shown.

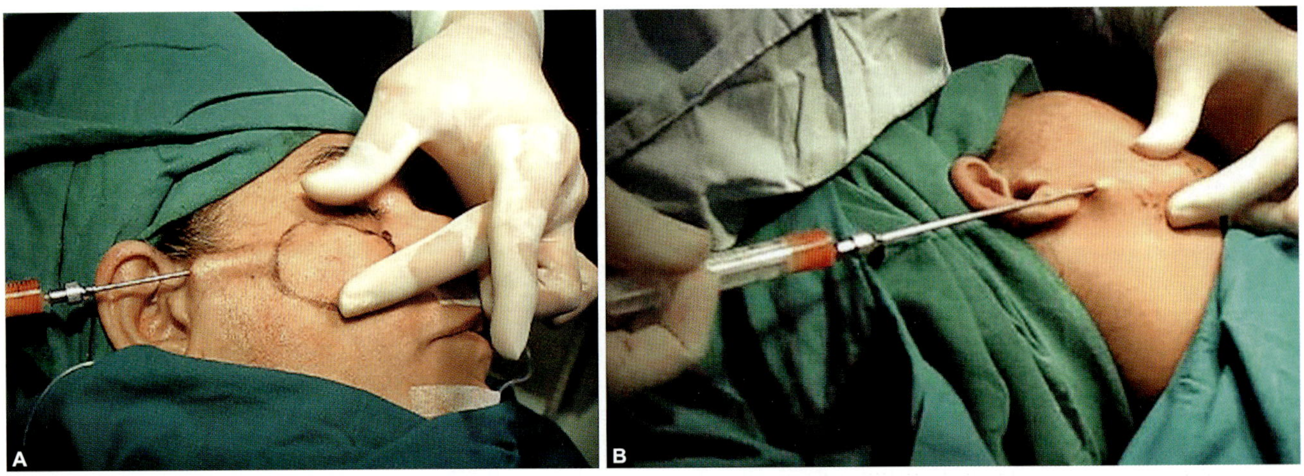

Figs. 28A and B: Fat transplant on the malar and mandibular region by blunt tip cannula.

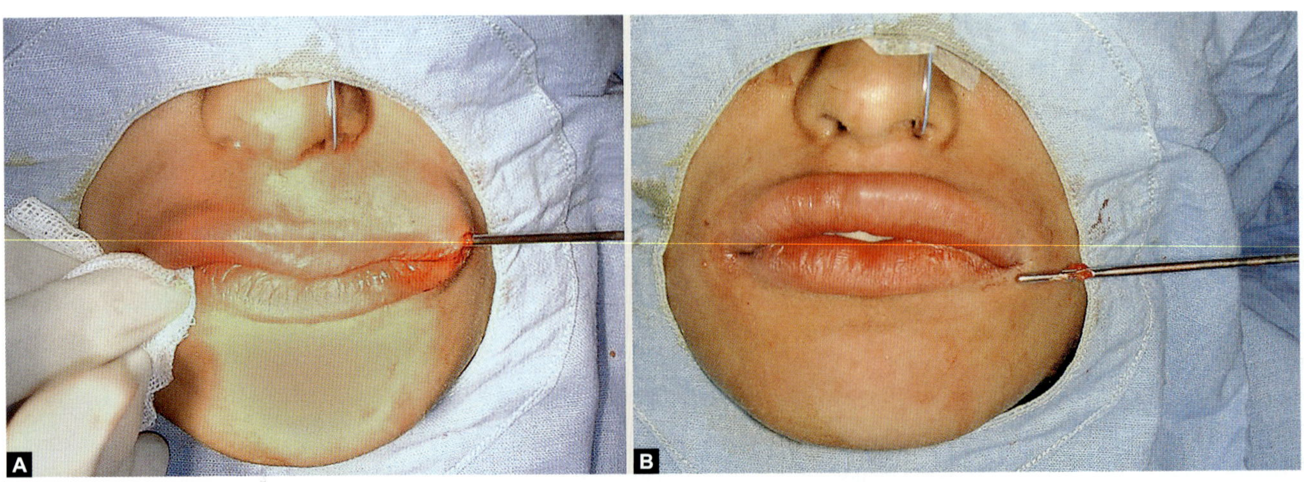

Figs. 29A and B: (A) Fat transplantation for upper lip augmentation; (B) Lips augmentation immediately after fat transplant.

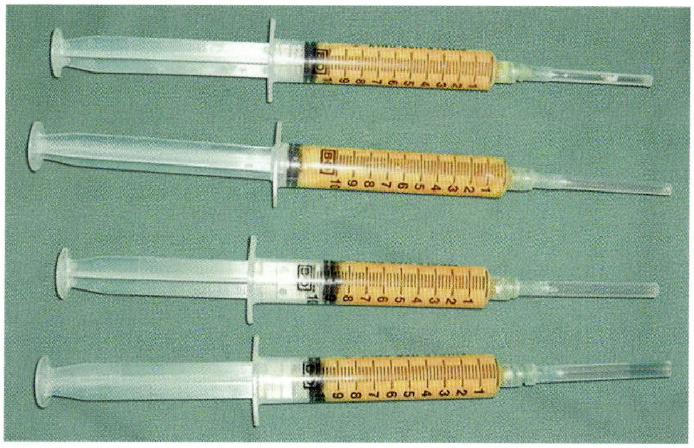

Fig. 30: 10 mL syringes filled with processed fat ready for large volume transfer.

extreme care must be taken to avoid damage to nerves, blood vessels, and other underlying structures and an inadvertent intravascular injection.

Though the use of 1 mL insulin syringes are ideal for fat transplantation in the face and hand, one can use a larger 5–10 mL Luer-Lock syringe for large volume fat transplantation of other body areas such as breast and gluteal region **(Fig. 30)**.

Anesthesia for fat transfer can be local anesthesia, regional blocks, and/or GA. The use of a blunt infiltration cannula minimizes the potential for accidental cannulation of arteries or veins as well as avoids damage to blood vessels and prevents resulting ecchymosis or hematomas.

PROCEDURE

Punctures are made with a no. 20/21 needle through the skin first. Then the blunt injection cannula is inserted through this puncture and slowly advanced through the recipient tissues into an appropriate plane. If resistance is felt at any particular place, it is withdrawn and rethreaded into an adjacent area. No fatty tissue should be injected during the advancement of the cannula. Once the tip of the cannula is placed into the target location, the plunger of the 1 mL syringe is pressed gently while the cannula is being withdrawn. This deposits fatty tissue as small beads or droplets in the pathway of the retreating blunt cannula.

Unlike the sharp tip of a needle, the blunt tip does not cut a defined channel through the recipient tissues. While the blunt cannula is being advanced, the natural tissue planes separate in a somewhat physiologic fashion. As the cannula is withdrawn, the deposited fatty tissue parcels fall into the natural tissue planes as the host tissues collapse around them.

The fatty tissue parcels should be deposited in the desired location with each pass of the infiltrating cannula so that the surgeon places the fat serially creating the desired shape with optimum volume. Accuracy of this initial placement is very important because the infiltrated fatty tissue cannot easily be remodeled or retrieved afterward. If a bolus or a clump forms accidentally, digital manipulation can help to flatten minor irregularities. However, fat parcels should never be placed with the primary idea that digital pressure can later change the shape after placement.

Separating the parcels of fat from each other not only increases the chance of their survival by placing the newly transplanted fat parcels in greater contact with a source of nutrition and respiration, but also encourages better fat adherence and stability in the new recipient sites. Finally, placing the fat in small parcels and separating every parcel with the recipient site tissues in between integrates the grafted fat into the tissues. The newly grafted fat thus feels like the tissue into which it is placed.

Placement of miniscule linear increments is critical to maximizing the surface area of contact and minimizing the potential for irregularities or clumps of tissue **(Figs. 31A to C)**. In the face, the largest amount of tissue that should be placed with each withdrawal is 0.1 mL, but in some areas such as the eyelids, the maximum placed should be closer to 0.03 mL or even 0.02 mL per withdrawal of the cannula. The surgeon should make sure where the cannula tip is during the entire injection process. If there is any doubt about the tip location, tent the cannula tip toward the skin and then see blanching of the skin overlying the advanced cannula to reveal its exact location. If the fat grafts are placed in a correct location, the augmented effect in the grafted area can be easily identified. If the volume does not seem to increase even though grafting is in the right place, other factors that may restrict volume enlargement should be taken into consideration, such as fibrotic adhesions, retaining ligaments, or tight skin envelop.

The end point of placement varies widely between anatomic areas. In the lateral malar cheek and mandibular border, the appearance at the conclusion of infiltration of fat will be similar in shape and size to the final outcome. Conversely, such areas as the lips, eyelids, or hands will be grossly distorted due to edema and not resemble the desired outcome for weeks after placement.

Fibrosis or adhesions can be dissected carefully with a sharp 18/20 G needle or with a forked tip cannula. A tight skin envelope may actually require pre-expansion before the fat grafting. For large or mega volume fat transplantation, the basic principles for the placement of fat graft are the same as small volume fat grafting.

OVERCORRECTION

A modicum of overcorrection by 15–20% was earlier considered acceptable since resorption of at least that much of the injected fat was expected. The present line of thought does not encourage any overcorrection. It is presently believed that precise amounts of fat injection in discrete parcels in multiple planes allow for the best results and avoidance of complications such as fat necrosis and oil cysts. The viable fat grafts are typically observed in the peripheral zone of approximately 1.5 mL from the edge of the graft and the

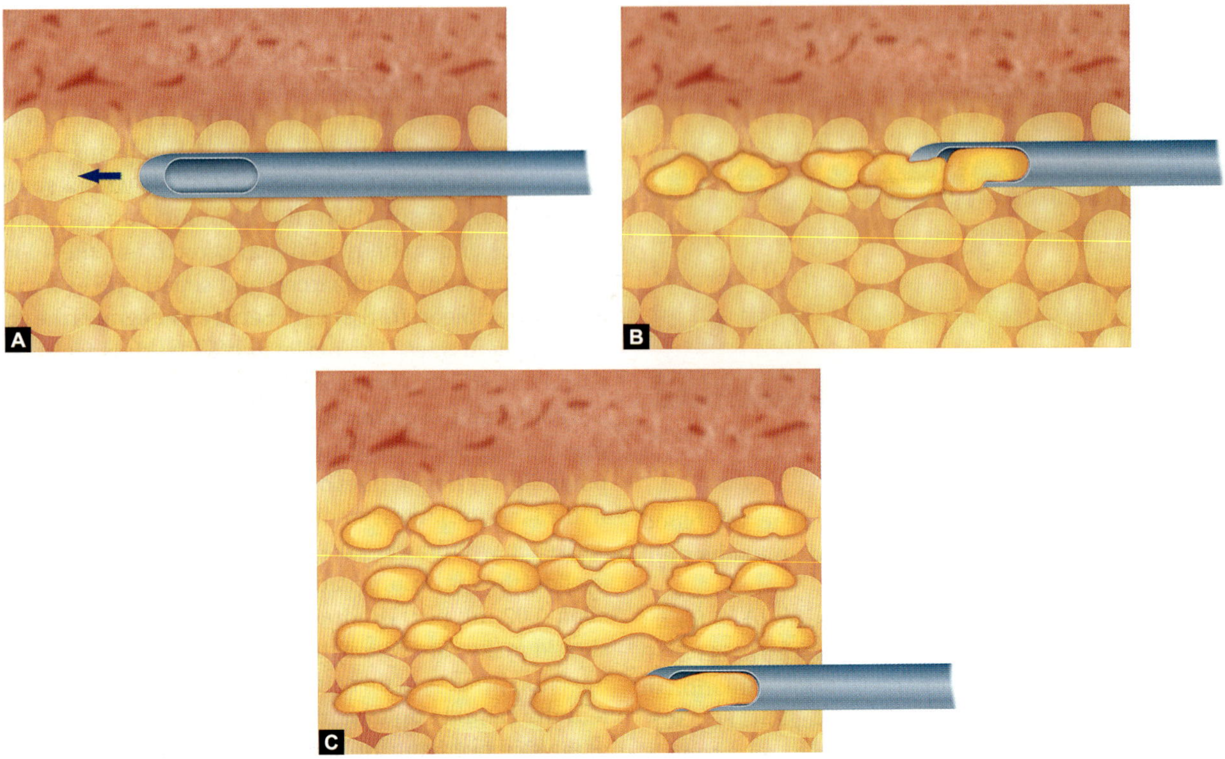

Figs. 31A to C: Levels and planes of placement.

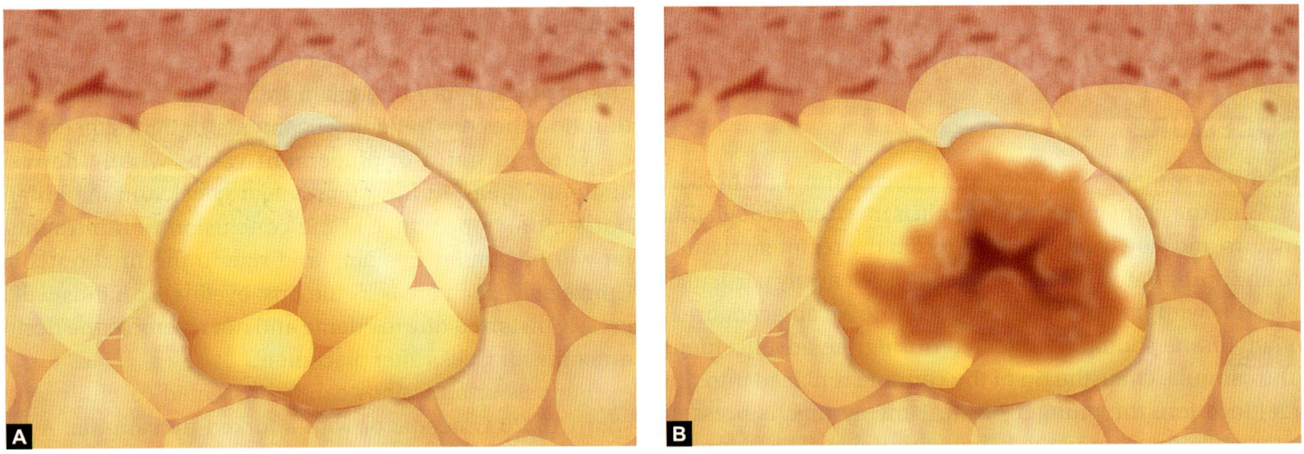

Figs. 32A and B: Fat necrosis following large bolus of fat injection at single spot.

percentage of the graft viability depends on its thickness and geometric shape.

STABILITY OF TRANSPLANTED FAT

After the edema resolves, the texture of the grafted tissue largely resembles the recipient tissue. Unequal access to nutrition and respiration of transplanted fat can cause unequal survival of fat cells and can even cause fat necrosis **(Figs. 32A and B)**. This will result in surface irregularity. As mentioned before, if a small lump or clump forms, digital manipulation may flatten some minor irregularity **(Figs. 33A and B)**.

POSTOPERATIVE CARE

Placement of fatty tissue as described earlier will create noticeable swelling in the recipient tissues. The patient should be prewarned of a recovery period of 4–6 weeks. Even though most patients are socially presentable at 1–2 weeks, they should be prepared for some minimal swelling lasting up to 6 weeks.

Care after fat transplantation should be aimed at minimizing swelling and stabilizing the grafted area to avoid any migration. Elevation, ice fomentation, and external pressure with elastic tape will help prevent excessive swelling **(Fig. 34)**. Local massaging should be avoided to prevent any absorption and migration of the injected fat graft.

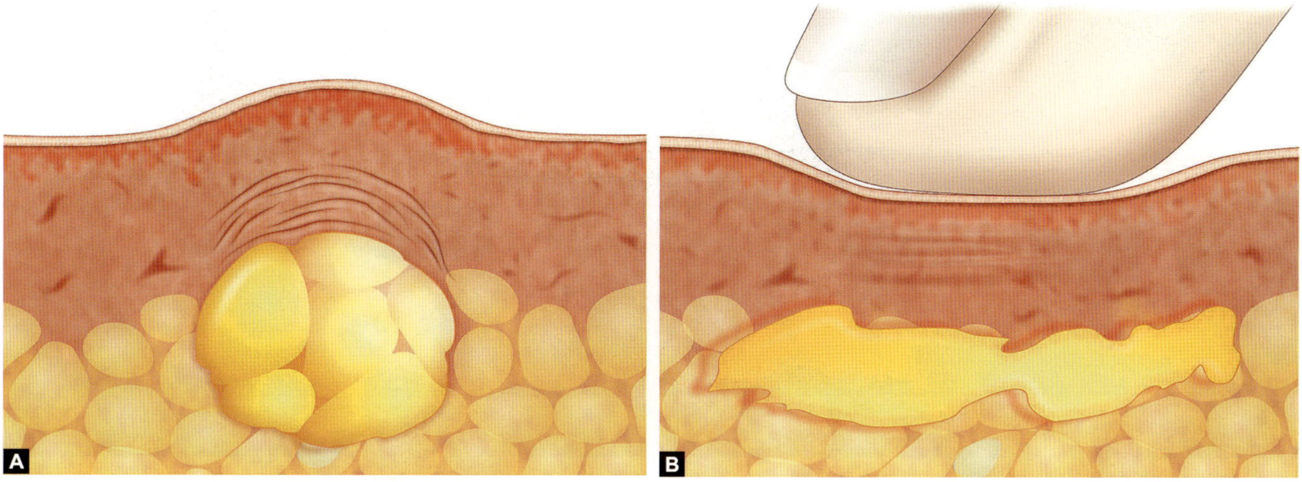

Figs. 33A and B: Massage to flatten any irregularity after accidental extra bolus of fat injection at any site.

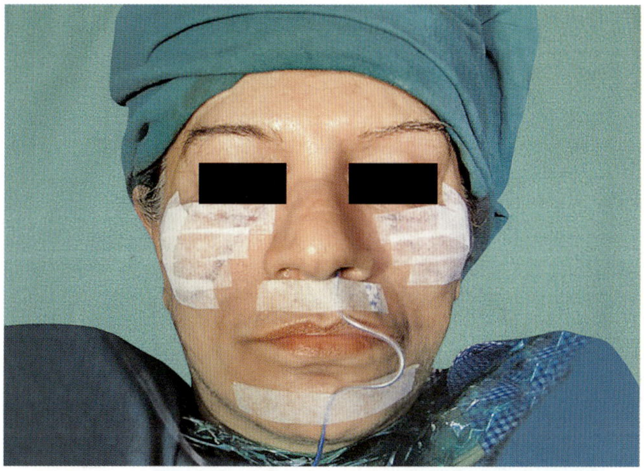

Fig. 34: Postoperative splintage immediately after fat transplant.

COMPLICATIONS

- *Under-correction:* It happens if either insufficient graft was placed or excessive resorption occurred. This can be corrected by subsequent sessions of fat transfer, which should be performed after a minimum interval of 3 months, preferably 6–9 months.
- *Prolonged edema/induration:* In most cases, the postoperative swelling recedes within 4–6 weeks. Rarely, it can last as long as 6 months to 1 year postoperatively **(Fig. 35)**.
- *Migration of fat:* From areas of fibrous attachments, e.g., scars or retaining ligaments. High pressure built up in these relatively unyielding areas can push the fat to lower pressure areas.
- *Lumpiness or palpable ridges:* Due to inadequate feathering or irregular resorption. Gentle massages can generally prevent this problem, if done in the first few weeks after the procedure.
- *Irregular resorption of fat:* This can result in distortion of the anatomy and can be seen especially in case of penile augmentation resulting in deformities and curvatures **(Fig. 36)**.
- *Cellulitis and infection:* Cellulitis can rarely occur due to inadequate aseptic procedure or contamination from intraoral or mucosal surface. Infection is rare but can result from bacterial invasion into poorly vascularized areas, following hematomas or areas of fat necrosis **(Fig. 37)**. It may subside with antibiotics or require surgical drainage.
- *Fat hypertrophy in transplanted autologous fat:* Rarely there can be significant hypertrophy of the fat in the recipient area as the patient gains weight over time **(Figs. 38A to C)**. This can cause abnormal contours. The excess fat then needs to be recontoured by liposuction.
- *Rare and serious complications such as vascular occlusion and fat embolism:* Rare and serious complications have been reported in literature which may include fat emboli to cerebral and retinal arteries leading to aphasia, hemiplegia, and blindness **(Fig. 39)**. These may be as a result of cannulation of arteries or veins and intravascular emboli.[81]

LONGEVITY

Longevity of the result following fat transfer is a hotly debated issue and the duration of survival has varied from 9 months to 3 years to nearly lifetime as reported in different clinical studies. There are cases reported where transplanted fat has grown out of proportion in the recipient site causing asymmetry and clear contour exaggeration. Results not only depend on the technique used but also on recipient site factors. There is in general, a poor survival of transplanted fat under scars, fibrous areas as well as in mobile areas. Additional touch up procedures may be necessary in such cases.

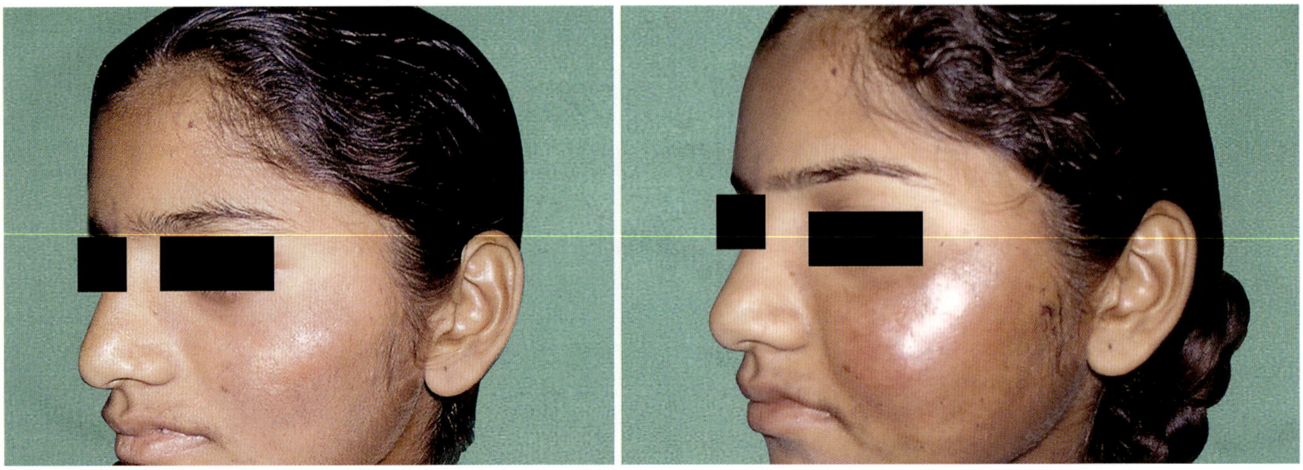

Fig. 35: Fat grafting done over the left cheek in a case of morphea showing persistent edema at 3 months postoperatively.

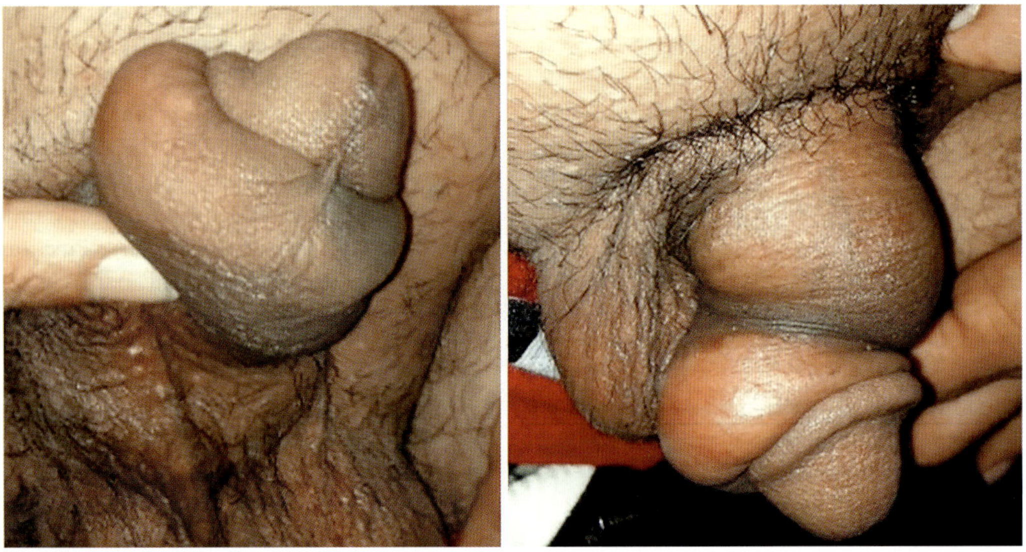

Fig. 36: Subglandular fat accumulation and irregular absorption resulting in deformity in the penis.

TIMING FOR SUBSEQUENT/SECOND STAGE FAT TRANSPLANTATION

As the overall fat graft resorption, even when carried out by an experienced surgeon, ranges anywhere between 15 and 50% in the first 3–6 months, additional fat transplant procedures are frequently necessary to achieve an optimum result. There are no scientific study data available to address the best timing for subsequent fat transplant. Experts suggest that additional fat grafting be deferred till after 6 months of the first procedure to diminish the "inflammatory response" in the grafted area. It is also observed that the transplanted fat gradually loses its volume with time and usually becomes stabilized at 3 months postoperatively. Hence, no secondary procedure should be undertaken during the first 3 months of recovery. Once the transplanted fat is stabilized in 3–6 months, it becomes part of the recipient tissue and will also help in better vascularization and take of the fat graft at a subsequent session.

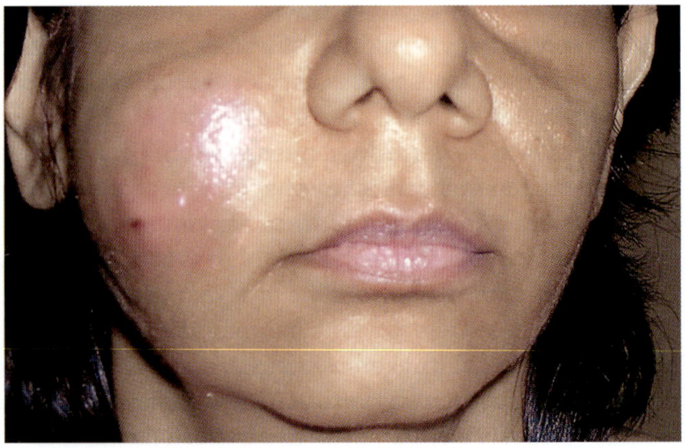

Fig. 37: Fat necrosis and infection in the recipient area on the right cheek.

Results of fat transfer for varied indications on the face and different parts of the body are shown in **Figures 40 to 53**.

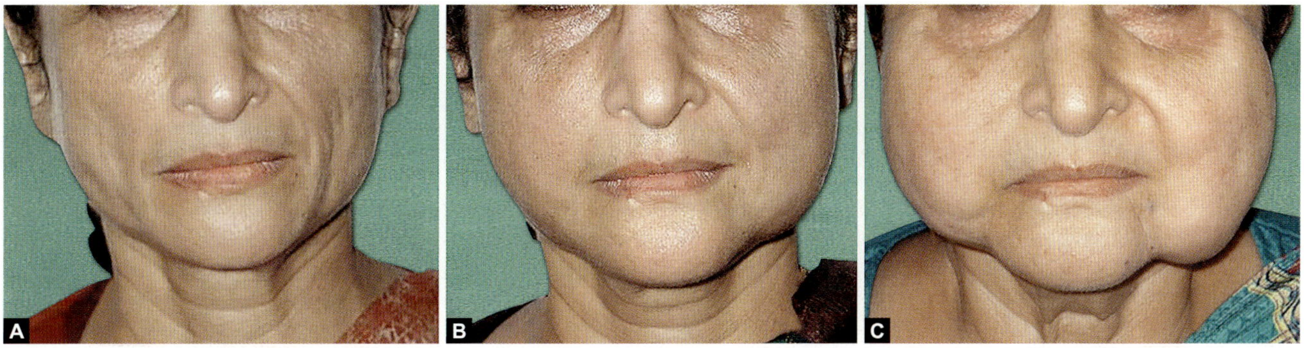

Figs. 38A to C: Fat hypertrophy over time: (A) Preoperative; (B) 3 months postoperative; (C) after a gap of 4 years.

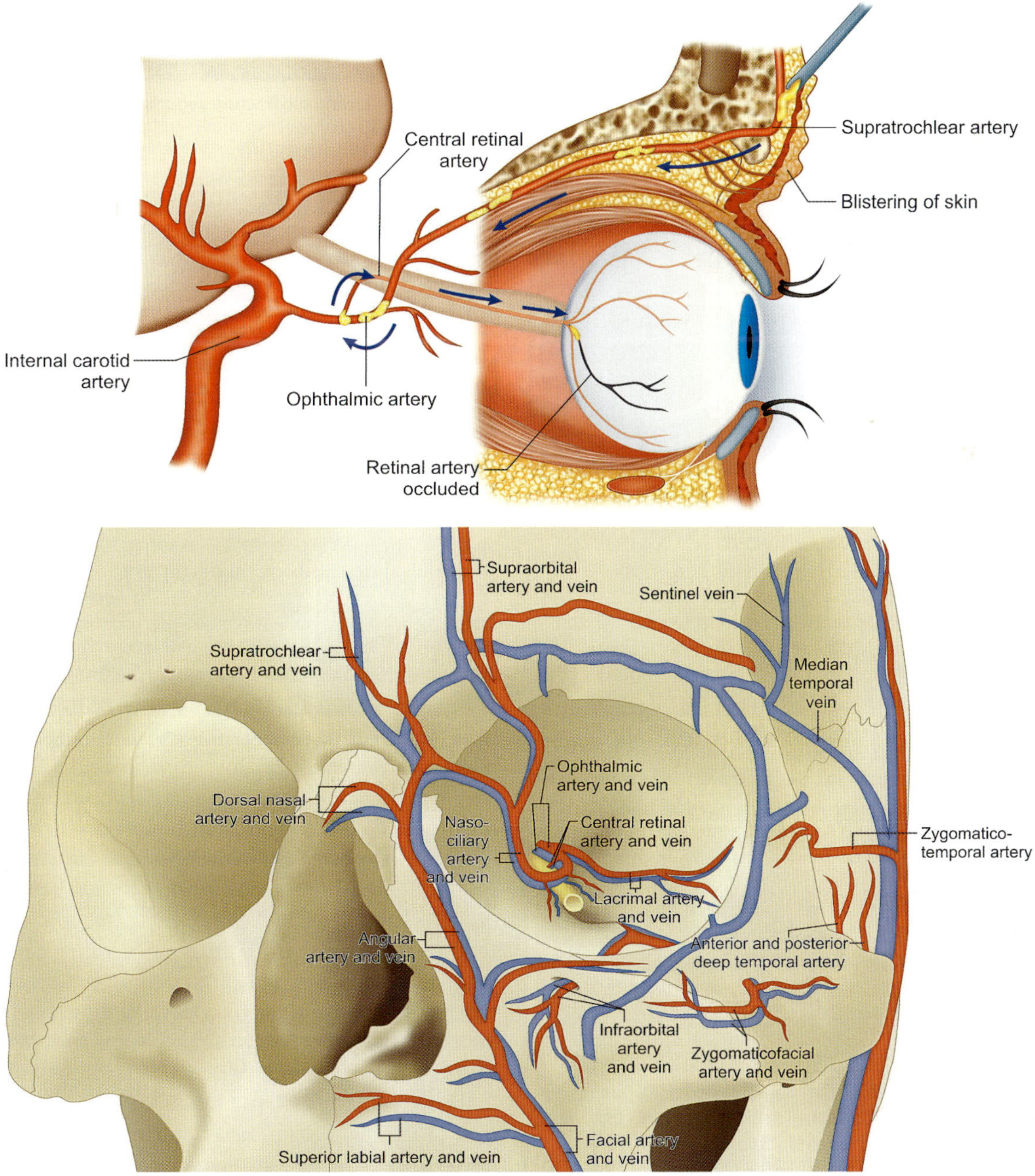

Fig. 39: Fat emboli mechanism leading to blindness.

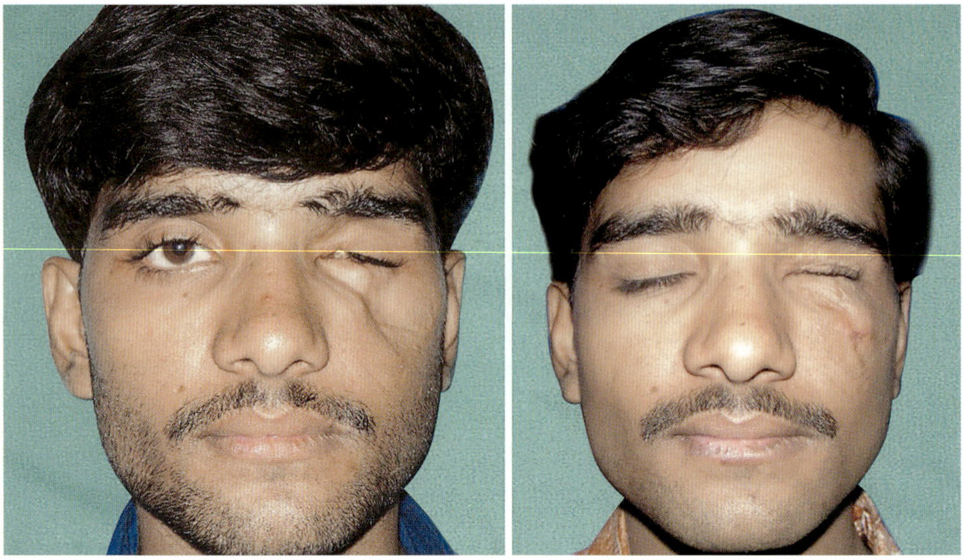

Fig. 40: Fat transfer for contour depression. Left malar area following old fracture zygoma.

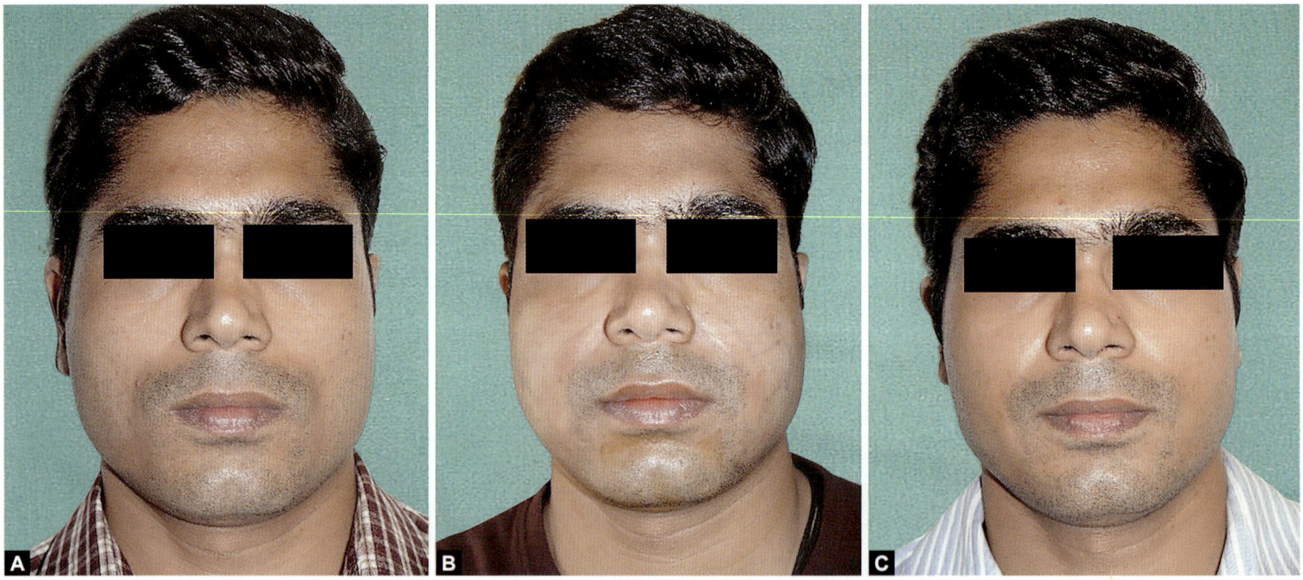

Figs. 41A to C: (A) Cheek augmentation with fat transfer, preoperative; (B) At 2 months postoperative; (C) 1 year postoperative.

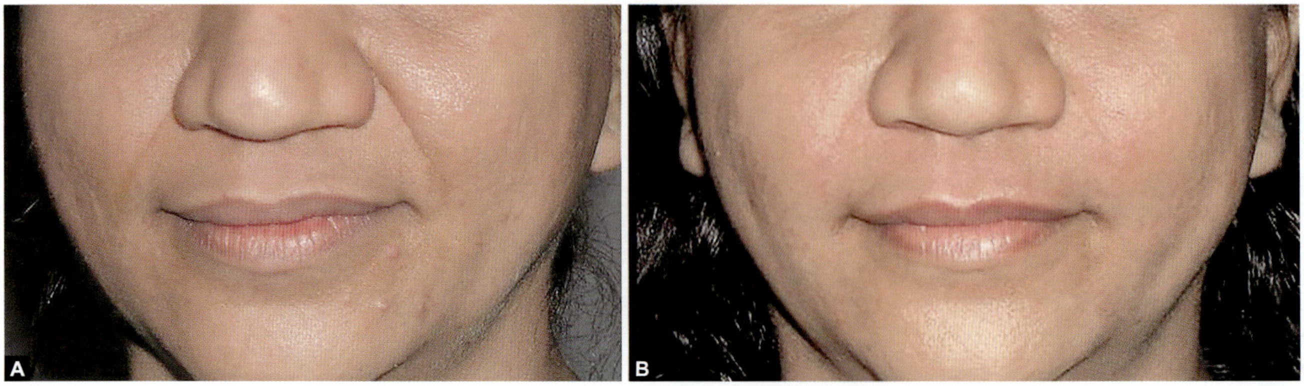

Figs. 42A and B: Fat transfer to nasolabial folds and marionette lines: (A) Preoperative; (B) 8 months postoperative.

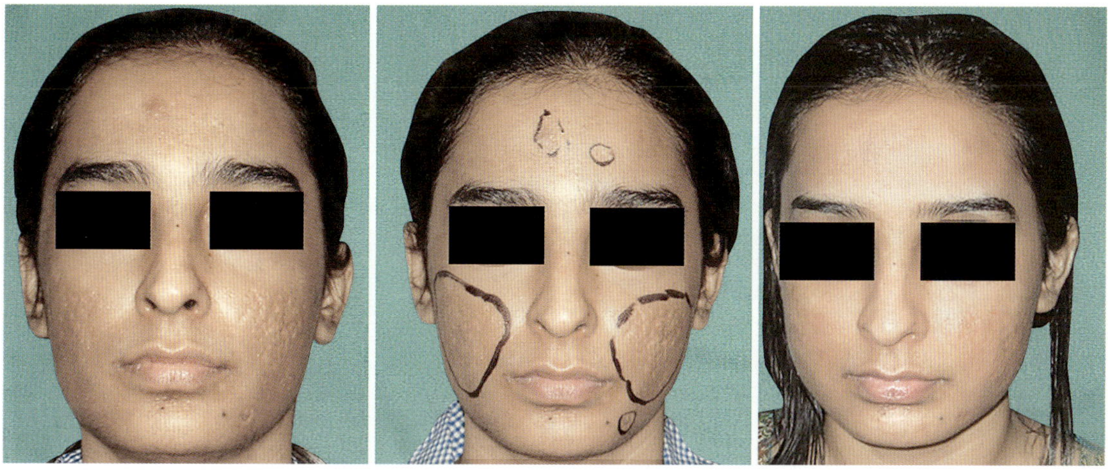

Fig. 43: Acne scars improved following micro-fat grafting.

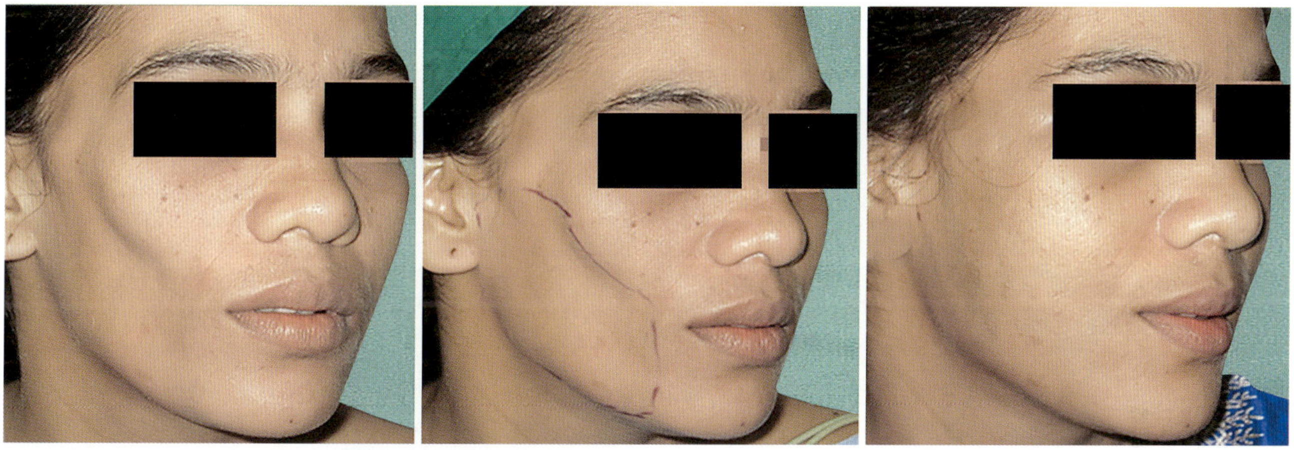

Fig. 44: Right hemifacial atrophy corrected with fat transplantation.

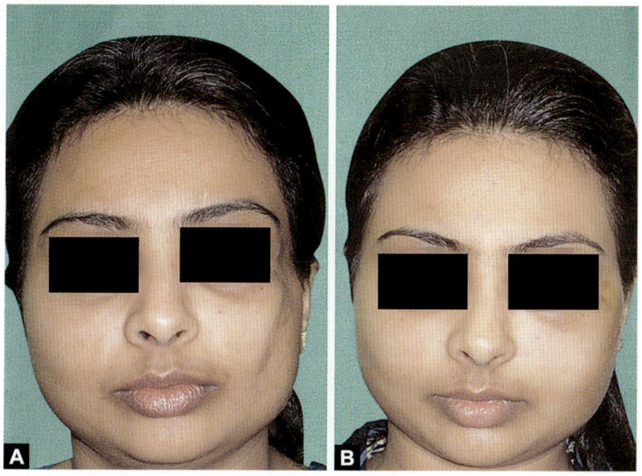

Figs. 45A and B: Morphea left cheek before (A) and after (B) fat transplant.

USE OF ADIPOSE-DERIVED STEM CELLS

Adipose tissue represents an abundant source of autologous cells for tissue engineering and regenerative medicine applications. Fat tissue cells consist of mature adipocytes, pre-adipocytes, and mesenchymal stem cells. Preadipocyte cells can spontaneously differentiate into adipocytes by processing technique. ADSCs have been demonstrated to differentiate into any mesenchymal tissue. Fat is thus not only a high energy reservoir, insulating agent, and thermoregulator, but is also a repair organ providing basis for soft tissue regeneration. Fat transplant, therefore, has enormous potential for solving aesthetic and reconstructive problems **(Fig. 54)**.

Cell-assisted lipo-transfer as proposed, using SVF which contains a heterogeneous group of cells including ADSCs, blood-derived cells (CD45+), endothelial (progenitor) cells, and pericytes, is now practically available **(Fig. 55)**. It is hypothesized that augmentation of the fat graft with SVF can improve fat graft retention by increasing angiogenesis and regeneration of adipocytes in the graft.[82]

FAT GRAFTING FOR BREAST AUGMENTATION AND CONTOUR CORRECTIONS (FIG. 56)

Indications for Fat Grafting to the Breast

- In aesthetic breast surgery:
  - Primary breast augmentation

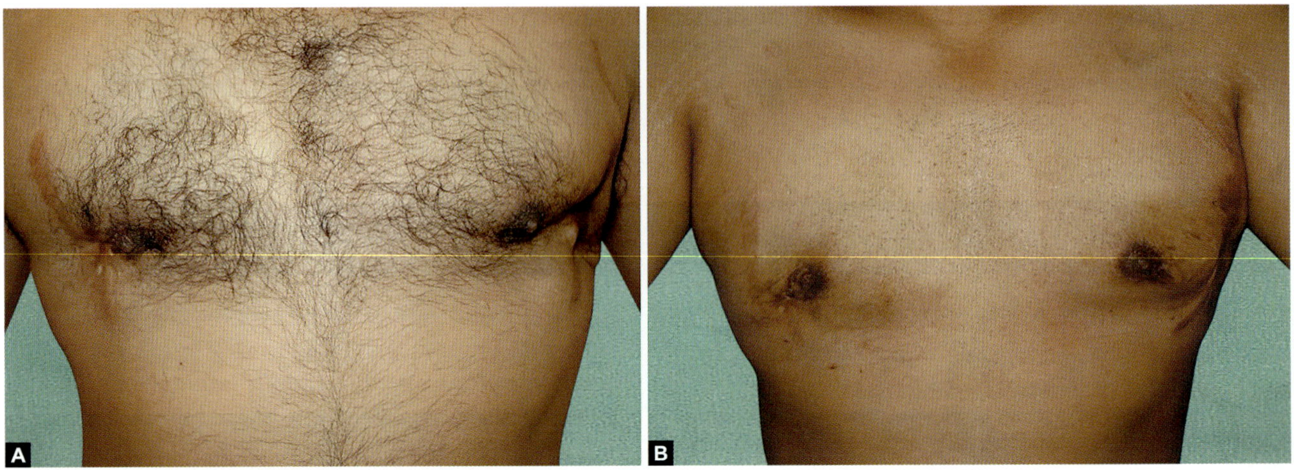

Figs. 46A and B: Contour defect following surgical excision of gynecomastia—corrected by fat transplant.

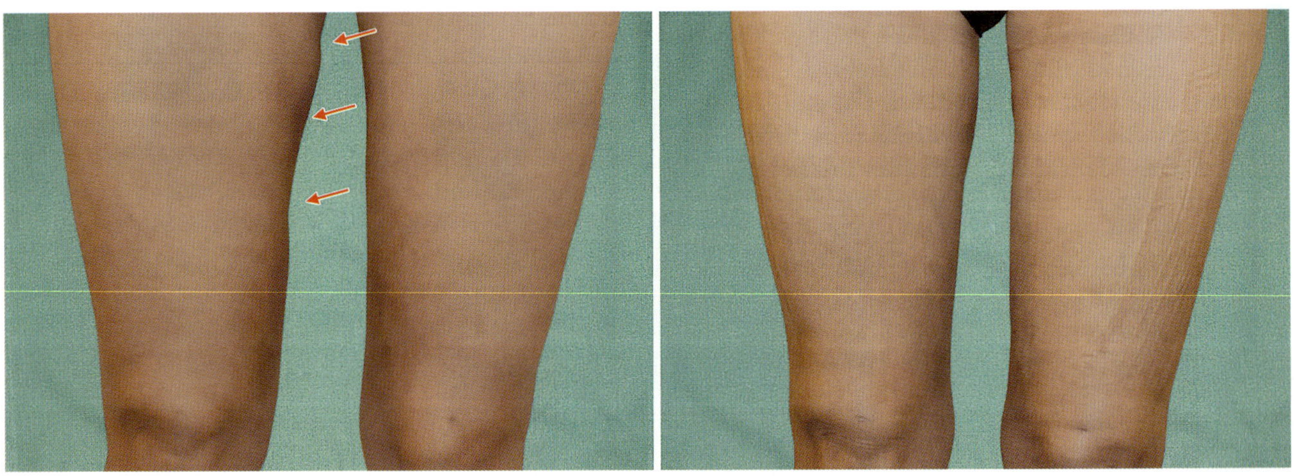

Fig. 47: Contour irregularities after liposuction of thighs corrected by fat transfer.

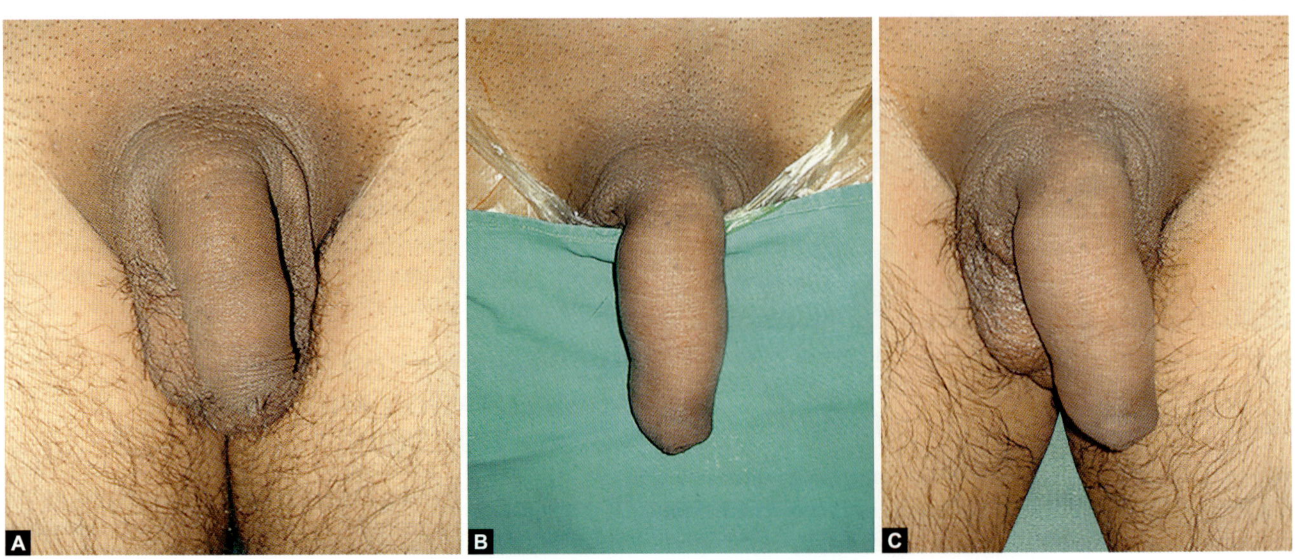

Figs. 48A to C: Penile augmentation with nanofat transplantation to increase the girth and the length.

- Correct the residual contour defects after implant augmentation
- Composite breast augmentation
- Treatment of breast capsular contracture
- Replacement of implants (SIEF.....Del Vecchio)

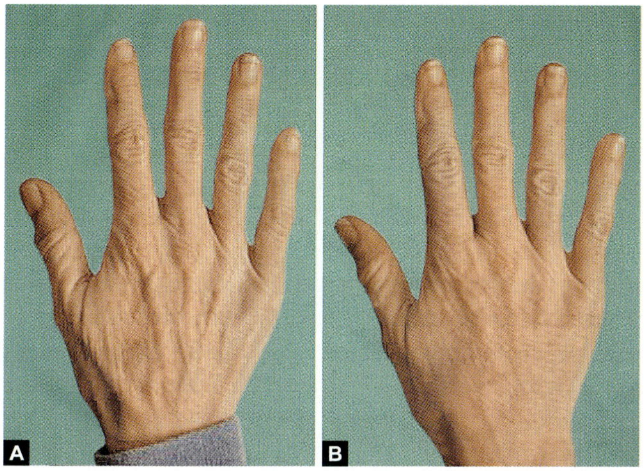

Figs. 49A and B: Hand rejuvenation with fat transplantation.

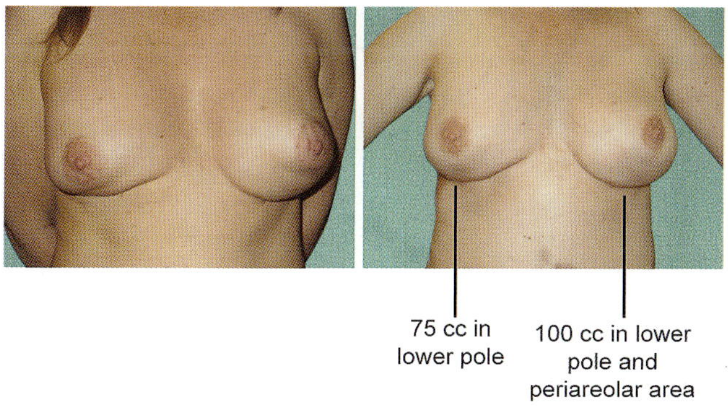

Fig. 50: Fat grafting to lower pole both breasts and left periareolar area to correct contour deformity.

- Tuberous breasts, especially unilateral but also bilateral
- Asymmetrical breasts
- Managing residual sequelae of breast reduction/ mastopexy.

Approximately 100–250 cc per breast is the range of augmentation safely possible in one session. Approximately 300–700 cc of lipoaspirate is therefore necessary to obtain adequate good quality fat after processing.

The abdomen and flanks, medial thighs, trochanteric areas, and arms are potential donor sites without changing the patient's position. Fat is harvested with syringe liposuction using 60 cc Toomey syringes and 3 mm Byron cannula.

After harvesting the fat and processing it by any of the methods mentioned earlier, the fat is transferred to 10 cc syringes and injected in a fan-shaped manner into multiple planes under the breast tissue and in the subcutaneous plane **(Fig. 57)**.

PREPARATION OF THE RECIPIENT SITE WITH EXTERNAL VOLUME EXPANSION FOR FAT GRAFTING TO THE BREAST (BRAVA)

Preparation of the recipient site to be a better environment for the fat graft to survive is another important factor for increasing graft retention. An innovative way of achieving this was first proposed by Roger Khouri and colleagues in the form of pre-expansion of the recipient site using an external device to apply a continued negative pressure on the recipient site skin.[83] Because high graft retention is most critical and difficult to achieve in mega volume fat transplantation such as in cases of breast augmentation or reconstruction, a specially designed external pre-expansion device (BRAVA®) **(Figs. 58A and B)** was first used in fat grafting to the breast. This device has been proved to be successful in increasing long-term fat retention in the breast based on multiple scientific studies. The device increases the overall three-dimensional volume

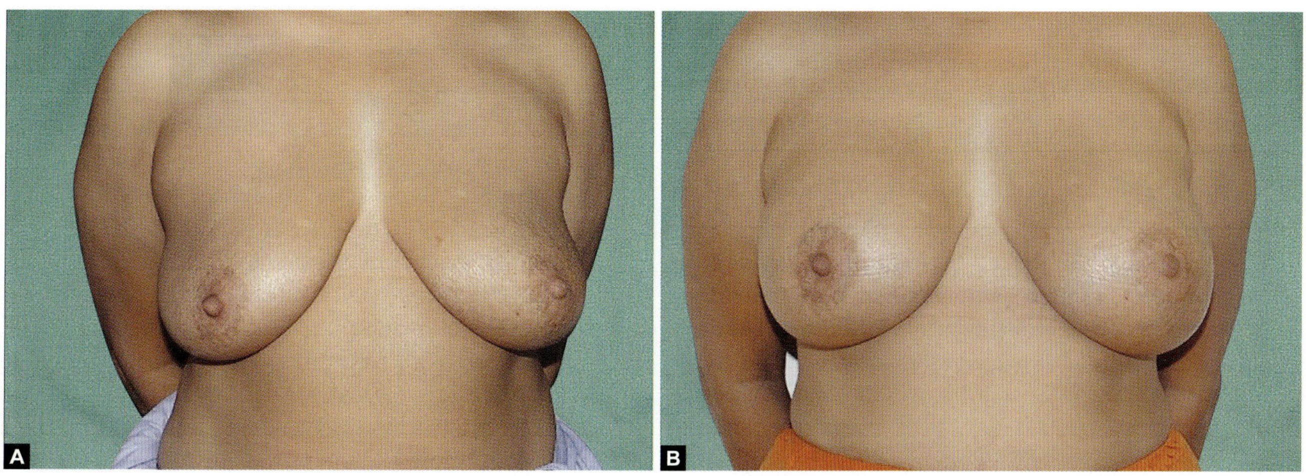

Figs. 51A and B: Breast augmentation with large volume (260 cc) of fat transplant.

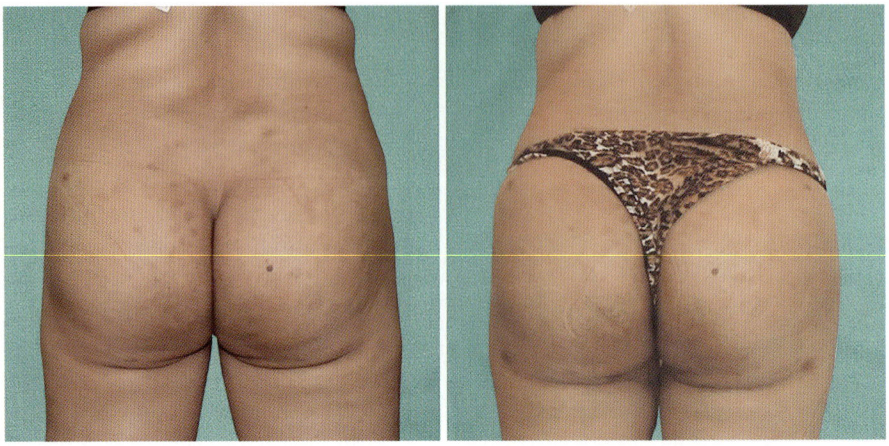

Fig. 52: Gluteal augmentation with fat (400 cc) of fat transfer.

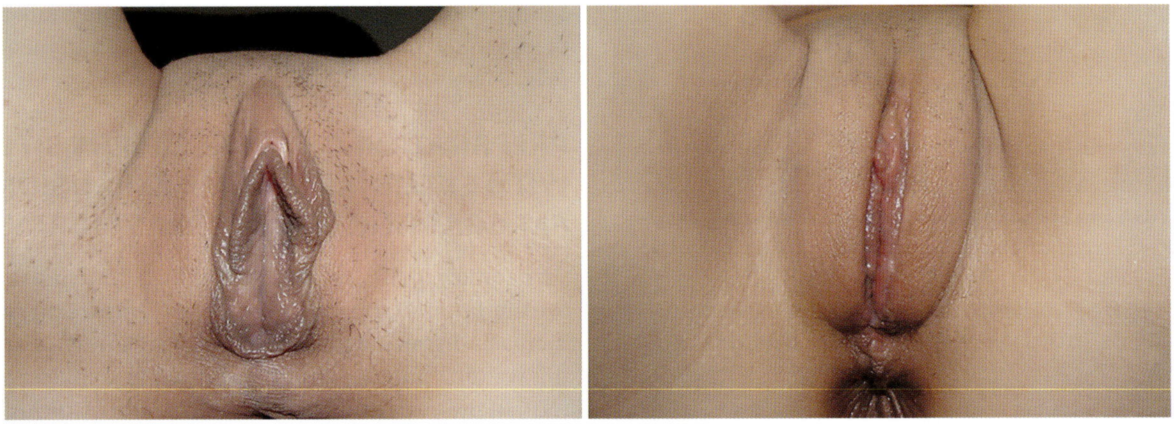

Fig. 53: Labia majora augmentation with fat grafting.
Courtesy: Dr Rakesh Kalra.

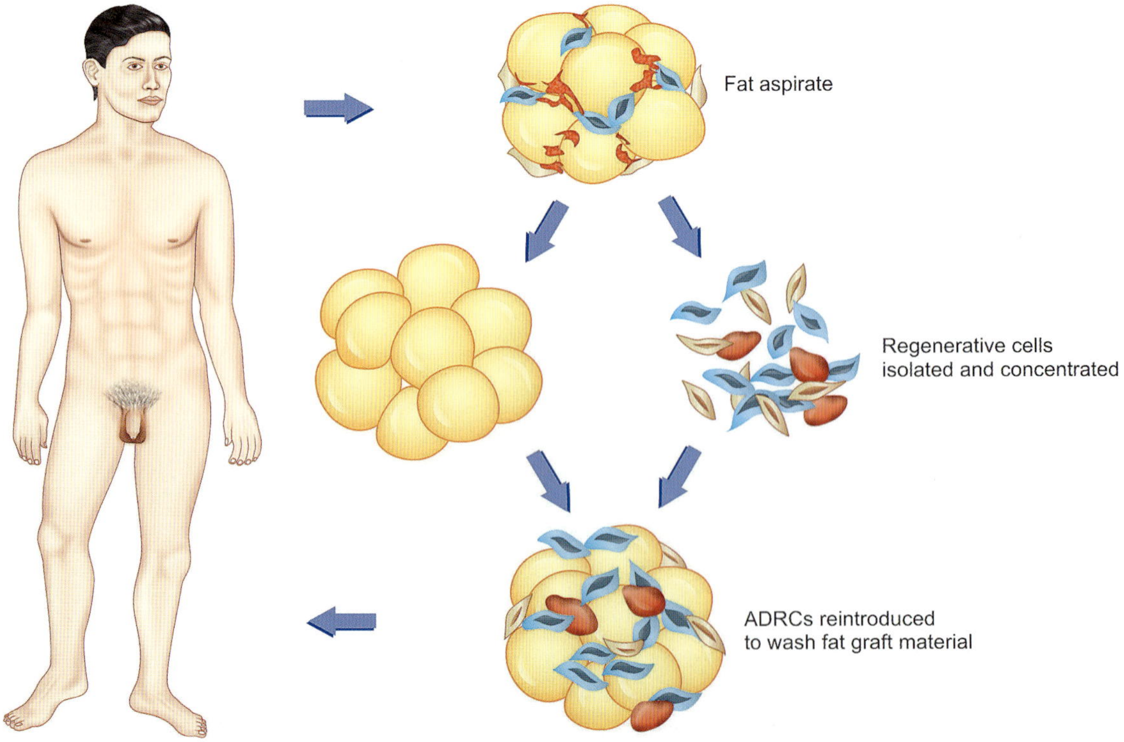

Fig. 54: Adipose-derived stem cells (ADSCs) for rejuvenation. (ADRC: adipose-derived regenerative cell)

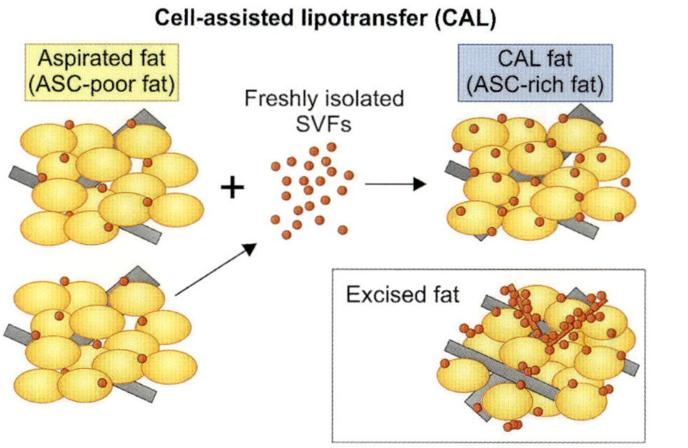

Fig. 55: Addition of stromal vascular fraction to aspirated fat to obtain adipose-derived stem cell (ADSC) rich fat. (ASC: adipose-derived stem cell; CAL: cell-assisted lipotransfer; SVF: stromal vascular fraction)

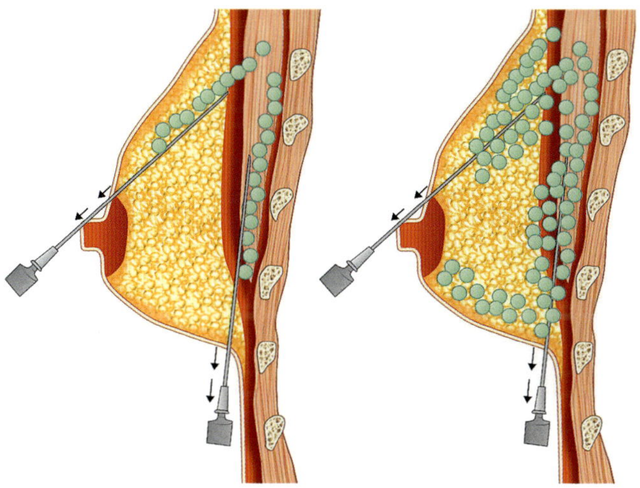

Fig. 56: Fat grafting to the breast in different planes.

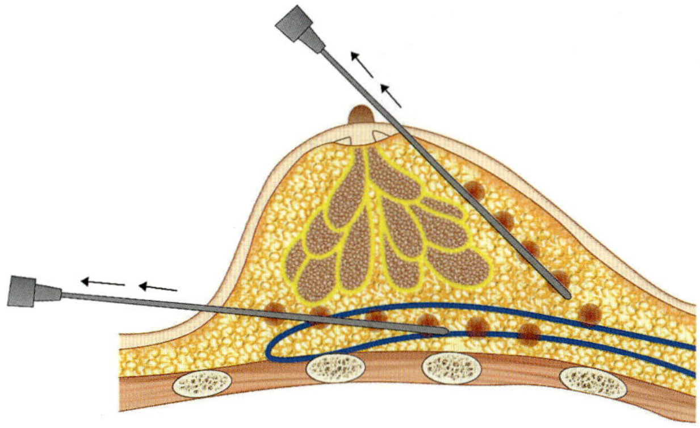

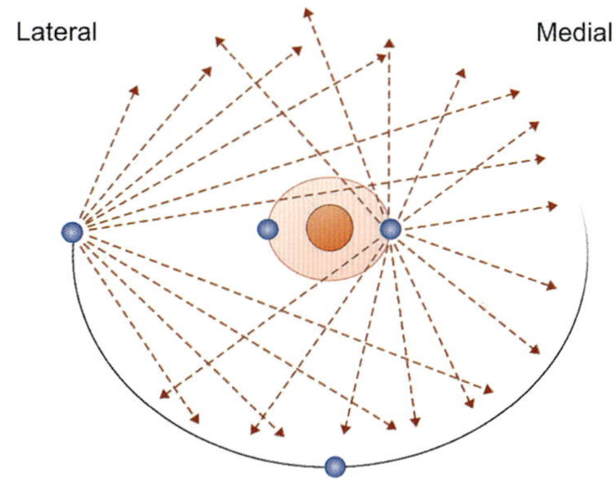

Fig. 57: Injection of fat in a fan shaped criss-cross manner to cover the entire breast.

of the tissue and improves angiogenesis in the recipient site. It also induces adipose tissue enlargement by activating resident progenitor cells combined with controlled release of basic fibroblast growth factors as well as with vascular remodeling.[84,85] Disadvantages of the use of this device include patient commitment and compliance to its continued and uninterrupted use over several months.

FAT GRAFTS TO BUTTOCKS (BRAZILIAN BUTT LIFT): HIGH RISKS IN GLUTEAL FAT GRAFTING

An unusually high mortality rate has been noticed from this cosmetic procedure in many parts of the world, estimated to be as high as *1:3,000*, which is greater than any other cosmetic surgery. In all the cases of mortality reported, the cause was uniformly fatal *fat embolism* due to fat entering the venous circulation associated with injury to the gluteal veins. In every patient who has died, at autopsy, fat was seen within the gluteal muscle. In no case of death has fat been found only in the subcutaneous plane.

A multisociety task force issued an advisory and warning to all surgeons performing this procedure. It concluded that:

- Fat should never be placed in the muscle.
- Fat should only be placed in the subcutaneous tissue. The subcutaneous plane has not been linked to pulmonary fat embolism. Until and unless data emerges that intramuscular injections can be done safely, the subcutaneous plane should remain the standard.
- If the desired outcome might require another procedure, then manage the patient's expectations and discuss the possibility of staging.
- It is easy to unintentionally enter the muscle during subcutaneous injection.
- It is vital to be mentally focused, alert, and aware of the cannula tip at every moment in a gluteal fat grafting procedure.
- The surgeon needs to be vigilant about following the intended trajectory with each stroke and feel the cannula tip through the skin.
- The risk of death should ideally be discussed in the informed consent process, along with alternative procedures (such as gluteal implants or autologous flap augmentation).
- No published series of Brazilian butt lifts (BBLs) done with intramuscular injections is large enough to demonstrate it can be done without the risk of fat embolism.

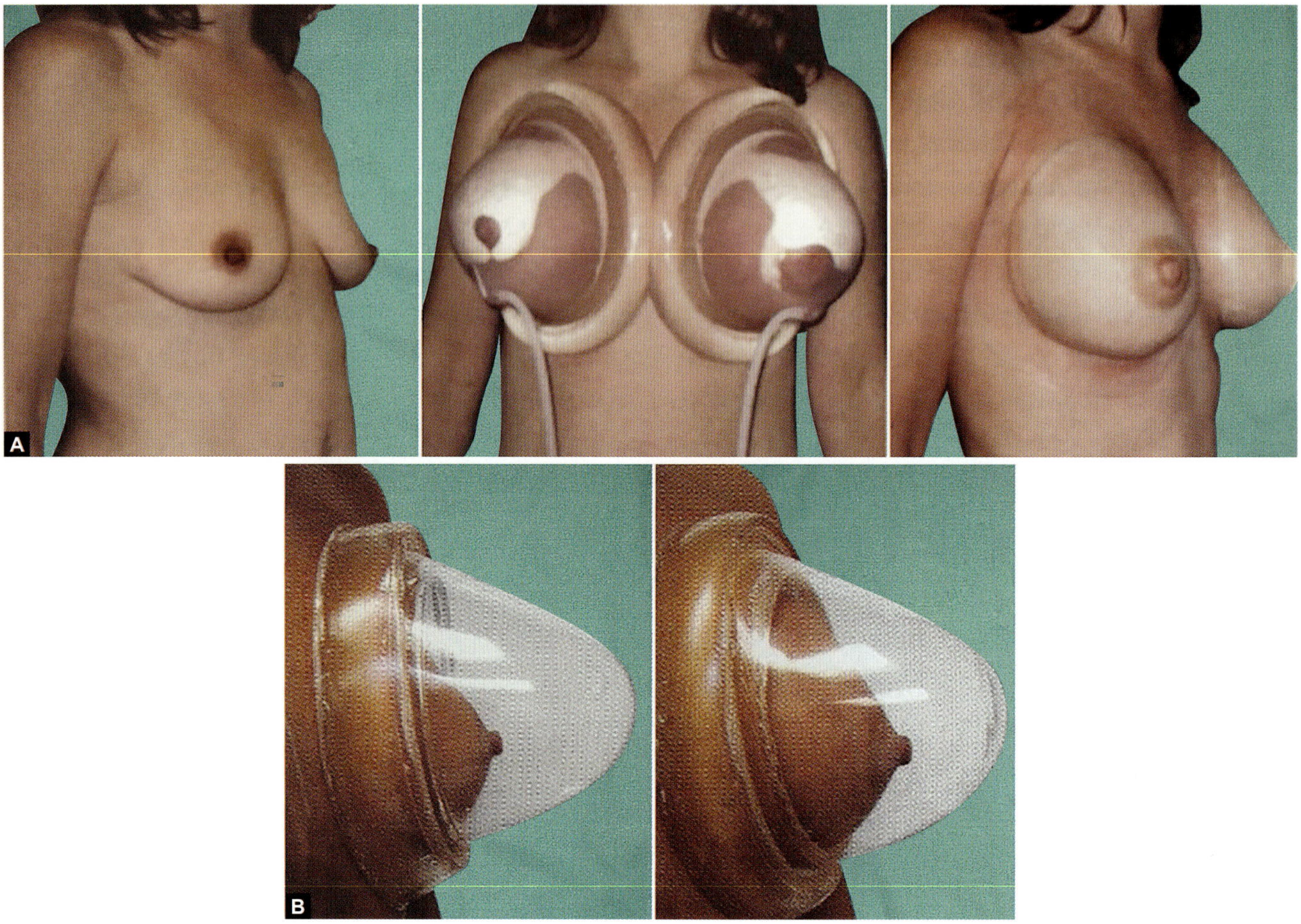

Figs. 58A and B: Breast expansion by using the BRAVA system®.

PEARLS

- Harvest fat gently with a 10 mL syringe to maintain intact tissue parcels.
- Refine the fat using centrifugation and decanting to increase predictability of results.
- Place very small (0.02–0.1 mL) aliquots of fat with each withdrawal of the cannula.
- Do not attempt to mold the grafted fat, but do ensure that it is smooth.
- Start slowly with more forgiving areas of the face and/or the hands.

PITFALLS

- Overcorrection is treatable but is difficult.
- Fat grafting cannot address significant skin laxity.
- Structural fat grafting results in significant bruising and tissue edema.
- The volume of grafted fat can change with significant changes in body weight.
- Fat hypertrophy of transplanted autologous fat is a known entity and can lead to unpredictable results.
- Fat grafting remains somewhat unpredictable and is dependent on the operating surgeon, technique used to harvest, refinement and placement of the fat, the recipient site injected, and an individual patient tissue characteristics.

- Fat injected into the subcutaneous space cannot cross the superficial gluteal fascia and migrate into the muscle; therefore, any intramuscular fat found at autopsy can be concluded to be the result of direct injection into the muscle.
- Surgeons wishing to continue performing this procedure should strictly adhere to these guidelines. The Task Force is actively performing anatomic studies, and more specific technical guidelines will be forthcoming.

CONCLUSION

The authors firmly believe in the potential for long-term fat survival given an atraumatic technique of harvest, centrifugation, and careful, deliberate small injections targeted at maintaining the integrity and preserving the nutrients. However, the technique for large and mega volume fat transplantation has not yet been standardized. This technique of structural fat grafting has achieved successful long-term results in innumerable patients. Improvements in skin quality and evidence of tissue repair have been observed in some patients and fat transfer may have more dynamic benefits than volume restoration alone. It is critical to inform the patient that a subsequent fat transplant procedure may be necessary after the first fat transplantation if the expected results have not been achieved.

REFERENCES

1. Billings E Jr, May JW Jr. Historical review and present status of free fat graft auto transplantation in plastic and reconstructive surgery. Plast Reconstr Surg. 1989;83:368-81
2. Neuber GA. Fett transplantation. Verl Dtsch Ges Chir. 1893;22:66.
3. Czerny M. Reconstruction of the breast with a lipoma. Chir Kongr Verh. 1895;2:216.
4. Hollander E, Joseph M. Cosmetic surgery. Handbuch der Kosmetik. Leipzig, Germany: Veriag von Velt; 1912. pp. 690-1.
5. Lexer E. Freie fett transplantation. Dtsch Med Wochenschr. 1910;36:640.
6. Lexer E. Zwanzig jahre transplantatiosforshung in der chirurgie. Arch Klein Chir. 1925;138:294.
7. Brunning P. Contribution à l'étude des greffes adipeuses. Bull Mem Acad R Med Belg. 1919;28:440.
8. Miller CC. Cannula Implants and Review of Implantation Techniques in Aesthetic Surgery. Chicago: The Oak Press; 1926.
9. Mojallal A, Foyatier JL. Historique de l'utilisation du tissu adipeux comme produit de comblement en chirurgie plastique. Ann Chir Plast Esthet. 2004;49:419-25.
10. Peer LA. Loss of weight and volume in human fat graft, with postulation of a cell survival theory. Plast Reconstr. Surg. 1950;5:217.
11. Peer LA. The neglected free fat graft. Plast Reconstr Surg. 1956;18(4):233-50.
12. Illouz YG. The fat cell "graft": a new technique to fill depressions. Plast Reconstr Surg. 1986;78:122-3.
13. Fischer A, Fischer G. First surgical treatment for molding body's cellulite with three 5 mm incisions. Bull Int Acad Cosmet Surg. 1976;3:35.
14. Illouz Y. Body contouring by lipolysis: a 5 year experience with over 3000 cases. Plast Reconstr Surg. 1983;72:511.
15. Illouz YG. L'avenir de la reutilization de la graisse apres liposuccion. Rev Chir Esthet Lang Franc. 1984;9:36.
16. Fournier PF, Otteni FM. Lipodissection in body sculpturing: The dry procedure. Plast Reconstr Surg. 1983;72(5):598-609.
17. Fournier P. Microlipoextraction et microlipoinjection. Rev. Chir Esthet. 1985;10:40.
18. Fournier P. Facial recontouring with fat grafting. Dermatol Clin. 1989;8:523.
19. Fournier PF. Liposculpture: the Syringe Technique. Paris: Arnette Blackwell; 1991. p. 412.
20. Bircoll MJ. New frontiers in suction lipectomy. Second Asian Congress of Plastic Surgery, Pattyia, Thailand, February, 1984.
21. Bircoll MJ. Autologous fat transplantation with liposuction techniques. California Society of Plastic Surgery, Monterey, California, March, 1985.
22. Bircoll MJ. Autologous fat breast augmentation. Plast Reconstr Surg. 1987;79(2):267-71.
23. Bircoll MJ, Novak, B. Autologous fat transplantation employing liposuction techniques. Ann Plast Surg. 1987;18(4):327-9.
24. Bircoll M. Autologous fat tissue augmentation. Am J Cosmetic Surg. 1987;4(2):141.
25. Ellenbogen R. Free autogenous pearl fat grafts in the face--a preliminary report of a rediscovered technique. Ann Plast Surg. 1986;16(3):179-94.
26. Toledo LS. Syringe liposculpture for face and body. Annals of the International Symposium "Recent Advances in Plastic Surgery". Estadao; Sao Paulo, Brazil: 1989. p. 177.
27. Toledo LS. Syringe liposculpture. Clin Plast Surg. 1996;23: 683-93.
28. Coleman SR. Long-term survival of fat transplants: controlled demonstrations. Aesthet Plast Surg. 1995;19:421.
29. Coleman SR. Facial recontouring with lipostructure. Clin Plast Surg. 1997;24:347.
30. Coleman SR. Structural fat grafts: the ideal filler? Clin Plast Surg. 2001;28:111.
31. Coleman SR. Structural fat grafting: more than a permanent filler. Plast Reconstr Surg. 2006;118:108S–120S.
32. Coleman SR. Hand rejuvenation with structural fat grafting. Plast Reconstr Surg. 2002;110:1731. discussion 1745.
33. Report on autologous fat transplantation. ASPRS Ad-Hoc committee on new procedures. Plast Surg Nurs. 1987;7(4):140-1.
34. Pu LL, Cui X, Fink BF, Cibull ML, Gao D. The viability of fatty tissue within adipose aspirates after conventional liposuction: a comprehensive study. Ann Plast Surg. 2005;54:288-92.
35. Tremolada C, Palmieri G, Ricordi C. Adipocyte transplantation and stem cells: plastic surgery meets regenerative medicine. Cell Transplant. 2010;19:1217-23.
36. Choi M, Small K, Levovitz C, Lee C, Fadl A, Karp NS. The volumetric analysis of fat graft survival in breast reconstruction. Plast Reconstr Surg. 2013;131:185-91.
37. Neuhof H, Hirshfeld S. The Transplantation of Tissues. New York: D Appleton; 1923. pp. 1-297.
38. Peer LA. Cell survival theory versus replacement theory. Plast Reconstr Surg. 1955;16:161-8.
39. Zuk PA, Zhu M, Mizuno H, Huang J, Futrell JW, Katz AJ, et al. Multilineage cells from human adipose tissue: Implications for cell-based therapies. Tissue Eng. 2001;7:211-28.
40. Zuk PA, Zhu M, Ashjian P, De Ugarte DA, Huang JI, Mizuno H, et al. Human adipose tissue is a source of multipotent stem cells. Mol Biol Cell. 2002;13:4279-95.
41. Kaufman MR, Miller TA, Huang C, Roostaien J, Wasson KL, Ashley RK, et al. Autologous fat transfer for facial recontouring: Is there science behind the art? Plast Reconstr Surg. 2007; 119(7):2287-96.
42. Wetterau M, Szpalski C, Hazen A, Warren SM. Autologous fat grafting and facial reconstruction. J Craniofac Surg. 2012;23:315-8.
43. Charles-de-Sá L, Gontijo-de-Amorim NF, Maeda Takiya C, Borojevic R, Benati D, Bernardi P, et al. Antiaging treatment of the facial skin by fat graft and appose-derived stem cells. Plast Reconstr Surg. 2015;135(4):999-1009.
44. Bircoll M. Cosmetic breast augmentation utilizing autologous fat and liposuction technique. Plast Reconstr Surg. 1987;79(2): 267-71.
45. Hang-Fu L, Marmolya G, Feiglin DH. Liposuction fat-fillant implant for breast augmentation and reconstruction. Aesthet Plast Surg. 1995;19:427.
46. Haik J, Talisman R, Tamir J, Frand J, Gazit E, Schibi J. Breast augmentation with fresh-frozen homologous fat grafts. Aesthet Plast Surg. 2001;25:292.
47. Butterwick KJ. Rejuvenation of the aging hand. Dermatol Clin. 2005;23:515-27.
48. Fournier PF. Fat transfer to the hand for rejuvenation. In Shiffman M (ed.). Autologous Fat Transfer. Heidelberg: Springer; 2009. pp. 273-80.
49. Giunta RE, Eder M, Machens HG, Müller DF, Kovacs L. Structural fat grafting for rejuvenation of the dorsum of the hand. Handchir Mikrochir Plast Chir. 2010;42(2):143-7.
50. Villanueva NL, Hill SM, Small KH, Rohich RJ. Technical refinements in autologous hand rejuvenation. Plast Reconstr Surg. 2015;136:1175-9.
51. Fantozzi F. Hand rejuvenation with fat grafting: a 12-year single-surgeon experience. Eur J Plast Surg. 2017;40(5):457-64.

52. Monreal J. Composite augmentation phalloplasty: personal experience after 275 patients Plast Aesthet Res. 2015;2:27-33.
53. Littara A, Melone R, Morales-Medina JC, et al. Cosmetic penile enhancement surgery: a 3-year single-centre retrospective clinical evaluation of 355 cases. Sci Rep. 2019;9(1):6323.
54. Vogt PM, Herold C, Rennekampff HO. Autologous fat transplantation for labia majora reconstruction. Aesthetic Plast Surg. 2011;35(5):913-5.
55. Jabbour S, Kechichian E, Hersant B, Levan P, El Hachem L, Noel W, et al. Labia majora augmentation: a systematic review of the literature. Aesthet Surg J. 2017;37(10):1157-64.
56. Erol OO, Gürlek A, Agaoglu G. Calf augmentation with autologous tissue injection. Plast Reconstr Surg. 2008;121(6):2127-33.
57. Niechajev I. Calf augmentation with autologous tissue injection. Plast Reconstr Surg. 2009;123(6):1891-3.
58. Veber M Jr, Mojallal A. Calf augmentation with autologous tissue injection. Plast Reconstr Surg. 2010;125(1):423-5.
59. Hoppmann R, Meruane M, González D, Wisnia P, Hasbún A, Villalobos B. Calf lipo-reshaping. J Plast Reconstr Aesthet Surg. 2013;66(7):956-61.
60. Bruno A, Delli Santi G, Fasciani L, Cempanari M, Palombo M, Palombo P. Burn scar lipofilling: Immunohistochemical and clinical outcomes. J Craniofac Surg. 2013;24:1806-14.
61. Ranganathan K, Wong VC, Krebsbach PH, Wang SC, Cederna PS, Levi B. Fat grafting for thermal injury: current state and future directions. J Burn Care Res. 2013;34:219-26.
62. Padoin AV, Braga-Silva J, Martins P, Rezende K, Rezende ARDR, Grechi B, et al. Sources of processed lipoaspirate cells: influence of donor site oncell concentration. Plast Reconstr Surg. 2008;122(2):614-8.
63. Geissler PJ, Davis K, Roostaeian J, Unger J, Huang J, Rohrich RJ. Improving fat transfer viability the role of aging, body mass index and harvest site. Plast Reconstr Surg. 2014;134(2):227-32.
64. Keck M, Zeyda M, Gollinger K, Burjak S, Kamolz LP, Frey M, et al. Local anaesthesia have a major impact on viability of preadipocytes and their differentiation to adipocytes. Plast Reconstr Surg. 2010;126(5):1500-5.
65. Lewis CM. Comparison of the syringe and pump aspiration methods of lipoplasty. Aesthet. Plast. Surg. 1991;15(3):203-8.
66. Chajchir A, Benzaquen I, Moretti E. Comparative experimental study of autologous adipose tissue processed by different techniques. Aesthetic Plast Surg. 1993;17(2):113-5.
67. Carpaneda CA, Ribeiro MT. Study of the histologic alterations and viability of the adipose graft in humans. Aesthetic Plast Surg. 1993;17:43-7.
68. Carpaneda CA, Ribeiro MT. Percentage of graft viability versus injected volume in adipose autotransplants. Aesthetic Plast Surg. 1994;18:17-9.
69. Rose JG, Lucarelli MJ, Lemke BN, Dortzbach RK, Boxrud CA, Obagi S, et al. Histologic comparison of autologous fat processing methods. Ophthal Plast Reconstr Surg. 2006;22(3):195-200.
70. Condé-Green A, de Amorim NF, Pitanguy I. Influence of decantation, washing and centrifugation on adipocyte and mesenchymal stem cell content of aspirated adipose tissue: a comparative study. J Plast Reconstr Aesthet Surg. 2010;63:1375-81.
71. Minn KW, Min KH, Chang H, Kim S, Heo EJ. Effects of fat preparation methods on the viabilities of autologous fat grafts. Aesthetic Plast Surg. 2010;34:626-31.
72. Pfaff M, Wu W, Zellner E, Steinbacher DM. Processing technique for lipofilling influences adipose-derived stem cell concentration and cell viability in lipoaspirate. Aesthetic Plast Surg. 2014;38:224-9.
73. Cleveland EC, Albano NJ, Hazen A. Roll, spin, wash, or filter? Processing of lipoaspirate for autologous fat grafting: an updated, evidence-based review of the literature. Plastic Reconstr Surg. 2015;136:706-13.
74. Kuran I, Tumerdem B. A new simple method used to prepare fat for injection. Aesthetic Plast Surg. 2005;29(1):18-22; discussion 23.
75. Ramon Y, Shoshani O, Peled IJ, Gilhar A, Carmi N, Fodor L, et al. Enhancing the take of injected adipose tissue by a simple method for concentrating fat cells. Plast Reconstr Surg. 2005;115:197-201.
76. Botti G, Pascali M, Botti C, Bodog F, Cervelli V. A clinical trial in facial fat grafting: filtered and washed versus centrifuged fat. Plast Reconstr Surg. 2011;127:2464-73.
77. Gerth DJ, King B, Rabach L, Glasgold RA, Glasgold MJ. Long-term volumetric retention of autologous fat grafting processed with closed-membrane filtration. Aesthet Surg J. 2014;34:985-94.
78. Pu LL, Coleman SR, Cui X. Autologous fat grafts harvested and refined by the Coleman technique: a comparative study. Plast Reconstr Surg. 2008;122:932-7.
79. Ferraro GA, De Francesco F, Tirino V, Cataldo C, Rossano F, Nicoletti G, et al. Effects of a new centrifugation method on adipose cell viability for autologous fat grafting. Aesthetic Plast Surg. 2011;35(3):341-8.
80. Kurita M, Matsumoto D, Shigeura T, Sato K, Gonda K, Harii K, et al. Influences of centrifugation on cells and tissues in liposuction aspirates: Optimized centrifugation for lipotransfer and cell isolation. Plast Reconstr Surg. 2008;121:1033-41.
81. Coleman SR. Avoidance of arterial occlusion from injection of soft tissue fillers. Aesth Surg. 2002;22:555-7.
82. Noriyuki A, Yoshimura K, Katsujiro S, Kurita M, Hirohi T, Harii K. Cell assisted lipotransfer for cosmetic breast augmentation: supportive use of adipose-derived stem stromal cells. Aesthet Plast Surg. 2008;32:48-55.
83. Khouri RK, Eisenmann KM, Cardoso E, Cooley BC, Kacher D, Gombos E, et al. Brava and autologous fat transfer is a safe and effective breast augmentation alternative: results of a 6-year 81 patient, prospective multicenter study. Plast Reconstr Surg. 2012;129(5):1173-87.
84. Kato H, Suga H, Eto H, Araki J, Aoi N, Doi K, et al. Reversible adipose tissue enlargement induced by external tissue suspension: possible contribution of basic fibroblast growth factor in the preservation of enlarged tissue. Tissue Eng Part A. 2010;16(6):2029-40.
85. Heit Yl, Lancerotto L, Mesteri I, Ackermann M, Navarrete MF, Nguyen CT, et al. External volume expansion increases subcutaneous thickness, cell proliferation, and vascular remodelling in a murine model. Plast Reconstr Surg. 2012;130(3):541-7.

CHAPTER 103

Stromal Vascular Fat and Nanofat Grafting

Aniketh Venkataram

KEY MESSAGES

- Stromal vascular fraction refers to all components of adipose tissue except adipocytes. It has exciting applications in the field of regenerative medicine due to its high concentration of ADSCs.
- Nanofat is a mechanical method of creating stromal vascular fraction without the need for cell culture or enzymatic techniques.
- Treatment protocols are still being devised, with further research the need of the hour.

INTRODUCTION

One of the holy grails of modern aesthetic surgery is the search for a treatment that is simple, powerful, preventative, therapeutic, and regenerative at the same time. This has led to the growth of regenerative medicine, in particular fat grafting.[1]

There has always been an interest in the use of stem cells for regeneration and rejuvenation, but this interest shifted toward the role of fat when it was noticed that fat grafting often improved the texture of overlying skin along with volume gain. It is found that this was attributable to the stromal vascular fraction and in particular adipose derived stem cells.[2]

STROMAL VASCULAR FRACTION

The stromal vascular fraction refers to all the cellular elements of the adipose tissue, excluding adipocytes. It includes smooth muscle cells, endothelial cells, blood cells, stem cells, and extracellular matrix. Although adipocytes represent 80–90% of the volume of the harvested fat, they only represent 25% of the cell count. The remaining 75% is called the stromal vascular fraction (SVF).[3]

The most important component of the SVF is adipose-derived stem cells or ADSCs.

MECHANISM OF ACTION OF ADIPOSE-DERIVED STEM CELLS[4,5]

- Adipose-derived stem cells are though to stimulate the recruitment of endogenous stem cells and promote their differentiation into cells that are needed.
- They have antioxidant capabilities that mitigate inflammation.
- They are thought to have properties that increase vascularization, the secretion of growth factors, vascular endothelial growth factor (VEGF), hepatocyte growth factor, and insulin-like growth factor.
- Cultured adipose stem cells (ASCs) have also been found to reduce wrinkles through collagen and elastic fiber production and other antiaging effects in the skin through glycation suppression, antioxidation, and trophic effects.

Initially, techniques were focused on culturing and isolating only the ADSCs from the SVF. These involved culture techniques that were complicated, expensive and had regulatory concerns.

However later focus shifted on using all the cellular elements of SVF as it was felt that intercellular cross talking and signaling between cells enhanced activity.[6]

ISOLATION OF STROMAL VASCULAR FRACTION

Stromal vascular fraction was traditionally isolated with chemical or enzymatic methods which broke down the adipose tissue, followed by filtration to separate the cellular components. Chemical methods give a higher cellular yield but are more time consuming.[7]

Tonnard et al. described nanofat in 2013 which was a mechanical way to obtain SVF by emulsification. It gives a lower cellular yield but is simple and can be done in one sitting.[8]

INDICATIONS[9-11]

Aesthetic

- Sun-damaged skin—neck
- Fine lines—perioral, periocular, etc.
- Pigmented skin—dark circles

Clinical

- Scars
- Radiodermatitis
- Pigmentary conditions

Experimental

- Ulcers
- Alopecia

PROCEDURE

The technique is usually done as a day care procedure under local anesthesia. For squeamish patients, intravenous sedation or general anesthesia can be used. There are three parts to the procedure:[12]

1. Harvest
2. Nanofat preparation
3. Injection

Harvest

The harvest is usually done from lower abdomen, flanks or inner thighs. As it requires very little fat tissue, almost everyone has enough for this procedure.

Infiltration is done with Klein's solution. Usually 200–300 cc is adequate. Harvest is done with multihole cannula with 1 mm holes (Tulip Corp, USA). We prefer using a Luer lock 20 cc syringe for harvest as this maintains a closed system for the entire procedure. Around 50–100 cc of aspirate is collected as required. After harvest the donor area is dressed with a simple dressing that is opened by the patient himself/herself the next day (**Fig. 1**).

Nanofat Preparation

The fat is first sedimented allowing the fat to settle by gravity to separate the aqueous and fatty layers. The aqueous layer is discarded. The fatty layer is then prepared by emulsification using the Tulip Nanofat System.

- The fat is transferred to 5-mL syringe with Luer lock.

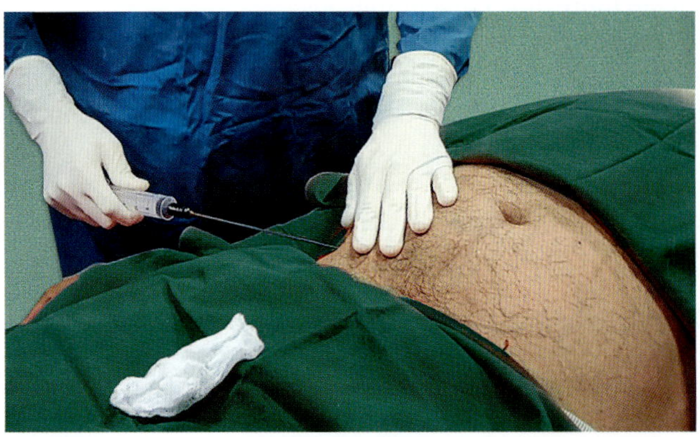

Fig. 1: Fat harvest.

- One full syringe and one empty syringe are used to pass through the connector.
- This aspirate is passed through a 2-, 4-mm connector 20 times.
- Then through a 1.2-mm connector 20 times.

Finally the emulsified material is filtered by passing through a nanofat filter. This filter captures large collagen particles (**Fig. 2**).

Injection

For the face, local anesthesia in the form of nerve blocks is adequate (supraorbital, supratrochlear, infraorbital, and mental). For the neck topical anesthesia in the form of eutectic mixture of local anesthetics (EMLA) is adequate.

Injection is done through 27G needles using 1-mL syringes, into the dermis till a yellow blanching is seen. The entire area is covered as required. Typically 1 mL can cover 1 cm^2 (**Fig. 3**).

After the procedure, the patient can go home immediately. Antibiotics and painkillers are given as needed.

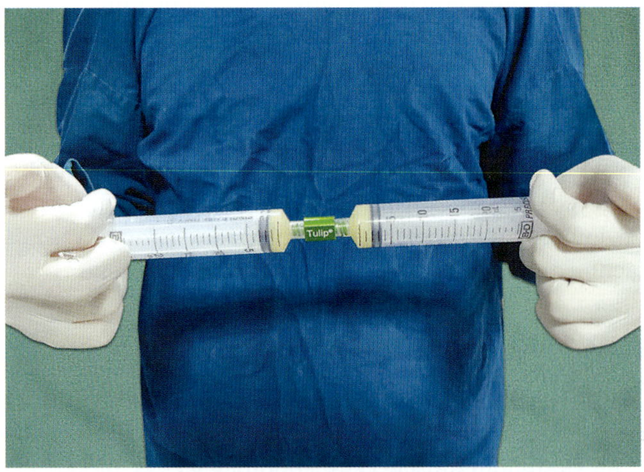

Fig. 2: Nanofat preparation.

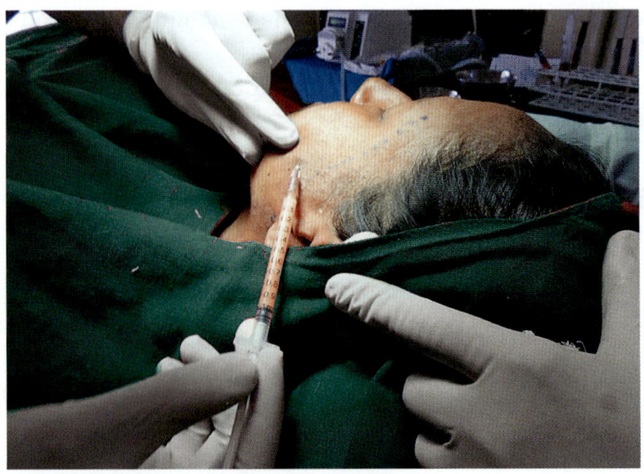

Fig. 3: Nanofat injection.

COMPLICATIONS

- Swelling—5 days
- Bruising—14 days
- Initial yellowish discoloration after injection, last a few hours
- Possible complications of harvest—Deep organ perforation
- Temporary erythema seen when injecting large areas—Can persist for weeks in case of lower eyelids
- Boggy swelling, if injected subdermal instead of intradermal, especially in under eye.

DISCUSSION

Nanofat is not really fat at all, as adipocytes are destroyed. It is a suspension of mesenchymal stem cells which are viable and retain their ability to differentiate. Dr Tonnard et al. have developed what appears to be a very simple method for formulating injectable solutions of stem cells without the use of expensive laboratory equipment or complex isolation procedures.

Limitations of this treatment include:

- Unlike other energy-based treatments such as lasers, this is surgical and more invasive.
- There is some downtime compared to noninvasive techniques.
- There is a lack of standardization in terms of instruments and volumes used.
- There is a lack of consensus on need for repeat treatments.

Future directions for this technique include optimization to achieve as high ADCS population as possible, and standardization of techniques and protocols. Other advances look at combining this technique with other modalities including lasers, microneedling, and microbotox.

PRECAUTIONS

- Unlike platelet-rich plasma (PRP), the emulsified adipocytes may have complications when injected intravascularly.
- Harvest to be done by trained surgeon—Complications of liposuction possible such as deep perforation
- So should not view Nanofat as a new replacement for PRP which can be used with abandon.

CONCLUSION

- Nanofat is an exciting new adipose tissue derivative.
- Might solve the problem of obtaining clinically usable ADSCs with a simple procedure.
- Exciting possible applications for skin rejuvenation and regeneration.
- Technique still in early days, to be used with rationale and caution.

REFERENCES

1. Aafprs.org. (2019). AAFPRS 2018 Annual survey reveals key trends in facial plastic surgery. [online] Available from https://www.aafprs.org/media/stats_polls/m_stats.html. [Last accessed August, 2023].
2. Nowacki M, Kloskowski T, Pietkun K, Zegarski M, Pokrywczyńska M, Habib SL, et al. The use of stem cells in aesthetic dermatology and plastic surgery procedures: a compact review of experimental and clinical applications. Postepy Dermatol Alergol. 2017;34(6):526-34.
3. Alexander RW. Understanding adipose-derived stromal vascular fraction (SVF) cell biology in reconstructive and regenerative applications on the basis of mononucleated cell components. J Prolotherapy. 2013;10: 15-29.
4. Cao Y, Sun Z, Liao L, Meng Y, Han Q, Zhao RC. Human adipose tissue-derived stem cells differentiate into endothelial cells in vitro and improve postnatal neovascularization in vivo. Biochem Biophys Res Commun. 2005;332(2): 370-9.
5. Kapur SK, Dos-Anjos Vilaboa S, Llull R, Katz AJ. Adipose tissue and stem/progenitor cells: discovery and development. Clin Plast Surg. 2015;42(2):155-67.
6. Banyard DA, Sarantopoulos CN, Borovikova AA, Qiu X, Wirth GA, Paydar KZ, et al. Phenotypic analysis of stromal vascular fraction after mechanical shear reveals stress-induced progenitor populations. Plast Reconstr Surg. 2016; 138(2):237e-47e.
7. Oberbauer E, Steffenhagen C, Wurzer C, Gabriel C, Redl H, Wolbank S. Enzymatic and nonenzymatic isolation systems for adipose tissue-derived cells: current state-of-the-art. Cell Regen. 2015;4:7.
8. Tonnard P, Verpaele A, Peeters G, Hamdi M, Cornelissen M, Declercq H. Nanofat grafting: basic research and clinical applications. Plast Reconstr Surg. 2013;132(4): 1017-26.
9. Uyulmaz S, Sanchez Macedo N, Rezaeian F, Hamdi M, Cornelissen M, Declercq H. Nanofat grafting for scar treatment and skin quality improvement. Aesthet Surg J. 2018;38(4): 421-8.
10. Yoshimura K, Sato K, Aoi N, Kurita M, Inoue K, Suga H, et al. Cell-assisted lipotransfer for facial lipoatrophy: efficacy of clinical use of adipose-derived stem cells. Dermatol Surg. 2008;34(9):1178-85.
11. Youn S, Shin JI, Kim JD, Kim JT, Kim YH. Correction of infraorbital dark circles using collagenase-digested fat cell grafts. Dermatol Surg. 2013;39(5):766-72.
12. Tonnard P, Verpaele A, Carvas M. Fat grafting for facial rejuvenation with nanofat grafts. Clin Plast Surg. 2020;47(1): 53-62.

SECTION 15 Lasers

CHAPTER 104

History and Evolution of Energy-based Dermatosurgical Devices, Laser–Tissue Interactions, and their Clinical Relevance

Kabir Sardana, Afreen Ayub

KEY MESSAGES

- 1903—Dr Niels Ryberg Finsen, a Danish physicist, won noble prize for treating lupus vulgaris using carbon arc lamp.
- Dr William Bovie in 1926 built the first electrosurgery device which could cut and coagulate.
- Dr Erving Ellman, in 1970, built the 3.8 MHz radiofrequency device.
- The term LASER was coined by Gordon Gould on November 13, 1957.
- Theodore Maiman created the first working laser on May 16, 1960.
- Ali Javan invented the first gas laser, helium–neon (He–Ne; 633 nm) laser in 1961.
- Neodymium-doped yttrium–aluminum–garnet (Nd:YAG; 1,064 nm) laser was also invented in 1961.
- The Argon (488 nm or 514 nm) laser was developed in 1962.
- Carbone dioxide gas laser (CO_2; 10,600 nm) was invented by C Kumar N Patel in 1,964 nm.
- Rox Anderson proposed the theory of selective photothermolysis in 1983.
- Dr Shimon Eckhouse invented intense pulsed light 1992.
- 1993 saw the white light-emitting diode (LED) invention and later National Aeronautics and Space Administration (NASA) used the same to heal wound in space.
- 1997—intense pulsed light was used for hair reduction.
- 2001—Rox Anderson proposed the concept of fractional photothermolysis.
- Radiofrequency device, in 2002, was approved for treating wrinkles and cellulite.
- 2009 saw the approval of ultrasound for rejuvenating face and neck.
- Most laser interactions are based on laser physics that treat the skin as an optical window.
- The three parameters that are crucial are—the absorption spectrum of chromophores, the pulse duration of lasers, and their depth of penetration.
- In Indian skin, the abundant melanin makes the results complicated.
- Laser tissue interactions can determine most working principles for common dermatological indications.

INTRODUCTION

A century ago, dermatotherapeutics involved sulfur, salicylic acid, steroids, electrosurgery, and cold steel surgery. But in the 21st century, both patients and dermatologists are spoilt for choice; for any cosmetic or dermatosurgical intervention, we have more than one device. For a beginner, the science behind these interventions and terminologies can be intimidating. But if one understands the humble beginning of these devices, one can know the indications and limitations of these energy-based devices. Discovery of different parts of electromagnetic spectrum **(Fig. 1)** by physicists, accelerated the launch of many tools and technologies. But with time, it was clear which technology was worth upgrading out of these and the rest went into oblivion.

UBIQUITOUS ELECTROSURGICAL DEVICE OR RADIOSURGERY DEVICE

Electrosurgery is "safe passage of current or electrons" into human tissue at the speed of light with special attributes to achieve coagulation, desiccation, or tissue cutting with least collateral skin damage. What are these special attributes? The current is high voltage and high frequency with low power. This is best understood by comparing the household current with that delivered to human tissue **(Table 1)**.

The raw household current is taken by the electrosurgery device which has a transformer which increases the voltage and oscillator which increases the frequency **(Fig. 2)**.

The early electrosurgery equipment was built by Thompson in 1889.[1] But to prevent muscular tetanic contraction, the frequency of current was to be above 0.1 MHz. This important discovery was done in 1891 by Jacques Arsène d'Arsonval. Using this device, different clinical applications were discovered—1907 saw fulguration, 1909 saw coagulation, and 1911 saw electrodessication. Another major discovery was the tip of electrosurgery kept small to concentrate current, to pinpoint delivery (compared later in this chapter, to larger electrodes used in dense tissue heating, and used in tissue remodeling—skin tightening and lipolysis, without destroying the epidermis).

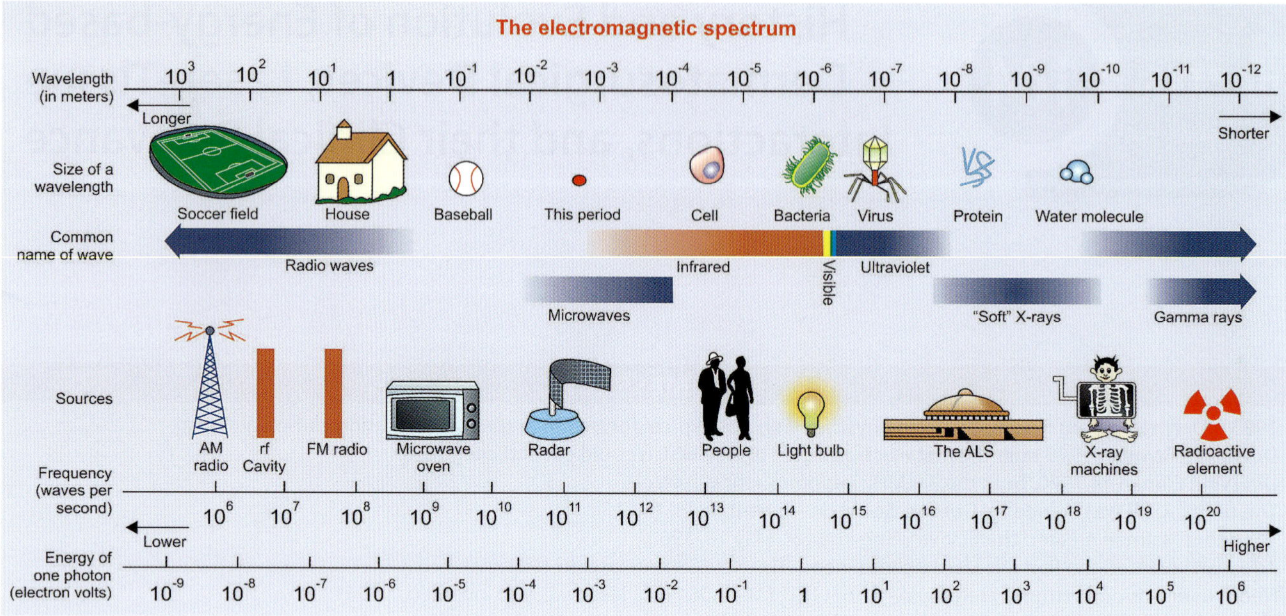

Fig. 1: Electromagnetic spectrum.

- Electromagnetic output is given by atoms. Tungsten in bulb gives light and our body atoms give infrared rays, all a part of electromagnetic spectrum. Both travel at 300,000 km/s.
- Longer the wavelength, lower the frequency, lower the energy. Relatively safe; nonionizing.
- Shorter the wavelength, higher the frequency, higher the energy. Unsafe; ionizing.

Source: Adapted from Advanced Light Source, Lawrence Berkeley National Laboratory.

TABLE 1: Comparison between household power and the power delivered to human tissue.

	Household power (India)	*Electrodessication/fulguration/desiccation*
Voltage (V)	220	2,000
Current (A)	5	0.50–0.75
Frequency (Hz)	50	0.5–4,000,000
Power (W)	1,100	20–35

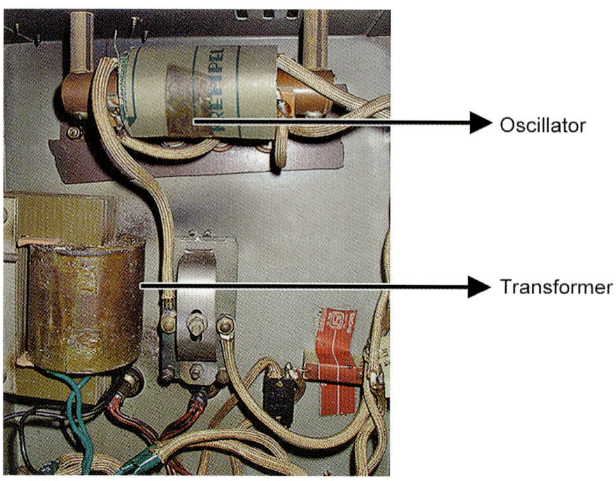

Fig. 2: Early electrosurgery unit.

Probably, the greatest impact on electrosurgery was by a Harvard physicist, William Bovie. He built a hybrid device which could cut and coagulate. Using this device in 1926, Dr Harvey Cushing from Peter Bent Brigham Hospital, Boston, Massachusetts successfully cut and coagulated a brain tumor on October 1st. Thus for some time, electrosurgery unit became synonym as the "Bovie." Ironically, Dr Bovie sold this important patent for just $1.

The modern radiosurgery units are all clones of the 1970s' radiosurgery unit manufactured by Dr Erving Ellman, which works with a frequency of 3.8 MHz. The question of why 3.8 MHz was answered in 1978 by Maness who showed that at this frequency, there is least lateral heat conduction on cutting the skin.

Since MHz frequency is used for frequency modulation (FM) radio transmission, these newer electrosurgery units, which also work in this frequency, are called radiosurgery units.

The current generated are delivered to the skin by either a single electrode—monopolar or two electrode—bipolar **(Figs. 3A to C)**. This is the active electrode. The current transmitted by the active electrode are collected by the antenna plate, which could be called passive electrode. Whether the passive electrode has to be in contact with the patient skin or not has to be ascertained according to the manufacturers recommendation.

Electrocautery equipment is different from electrosurgery/radiofrequency (RF) equipment. In this device, a tungsten filament is heated by direct current and the heat is transmitted to tissue and not the current. This device is useful in patient having cardiac pacemakers. Many dermatologists wrongly

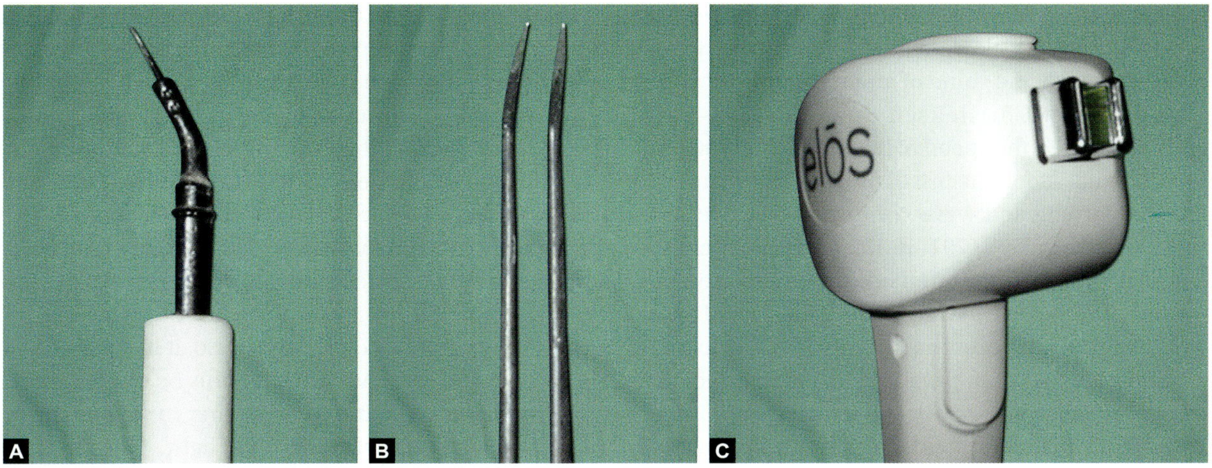

Figs. 3A to C: Different types of electrodes: (A) Monopolar; (B and C) Bipolar.

use the term electrocautery for electrosurgery/radiosurgery. This should be desisted.

The electrode tips could be stainless steel, tungsten, or copper. Larger the size of electrode, more the energy required to work and more the damage to skin. Hence, it is better to work with a thin electrode, except while coagulating where a ball-copper electrode is required.

The next major discovery in dermatosurgery was lasers.

LASERS

"Lasers are to other sources of light, as music is to noise"[2] aptly describes the uniqueness of lasers. The very word, LASER (an acronym; light amplification by stimulated emission of radiation) gives an insight to its creation. Laser is emission of a radiation which is stimulated and light amplifies it further.

The term LASER was coined by Gordon Gould on November 13, 1957, back then in his late 40s.[3] Gould, a graduate student at Columbia University working for his PhD dissertation, during his spare time thought of creating LASER. He had the idea but not the financial backing to realize his dreams. He jotted his concepts in a laboratory notebook and as to its uses he wrote, "it could be used as a spectrometer. The beam could travel long distances essentially unweakened. Applications like communications and radar are obvious." Nearly 3 years later, on May 16, 1960, Theodore Maiman, a young 32-year-old physicist working for Hughes Research Laboratories in California created the first working laser.[4] Maiman, as to its uses noted five uses: Fiberoptic communication, laser spectroscopy, space communication, industry (laser cutting, welding, etc.), and medicine. But in the present day scenario, lasers are ubiquitous. People speed through the supermarket checkout lines, use computers with virtually unlimited storage, communicate via cables that carry their voices across thousands of miles along the beams of light, listen to music, and watch movies in different ways because of lasers. Measurements are easier to make and more precise. Manufacturers weld and drill holes with lasers.

Presidents and Generals dream of them as both swords and shields. Doctors dream of using lasers as a cure for all diseases.

So what is this magic wand? The key principles here are atoms spontaneously emit radiation and this radiation could be augmented by light and sounds like simple, high-school science. But to enjoy the laser creation and its application, one has to travel back along the time machine. Let us begin.

PROLOGUE

To understand how LASER was discovered, it is important to trace how physics evolved in 17th century, from classical physics of Newton to quantum physics in 20th century. In 1666, *Annus mirabilis* (meaning the miracle year of modern physics), Issac Newton (1642–1727) from Woolsthorpe Manor in England, barely 24 years old, laid the foundation for modern physics. He was a farmer's son and a mostly self-taught mathematician. He, during his study days at Cambridge University, was sent home because of plague which was taking a toll of nearly 1,000 people per day. Hence continuing his study at home, sitting in his garden, he wrote the fundamentals of physics—gravity, optics, and calculus. Seeing the apple drop down from the tree, he not only proposed the laws of gravity but also extended the same to the moon that gravity of earth kept the moon in orbit. But if apple falls on the earth, why not then on moon? For this, he proposed the laws of motion which were applicable on earth and in the entire universe. These laws were universal.[5]

More important and relevant from this chapter's point of view, he demonstrated that light is made of seven colors and proposed that light particles are shot out of shining bodies like tiny bullets. But Christiaan Huygens (1629–1695) from Holland thought that light is an undulating wave like ocean wave. Since it was a wave, the different colors bend in the prism at a specific angle, which would not be possible if light was a particle. The particle versus wave controversy raged and almost took away the shine of an important calculation of Danish physicist Christensen Roemer (1644–1710). He roughly calculated the speed of light to be 300,000 km/s, a finding which has stood the test of time for 300 years!

While the particle and wave controversy was yet to be settled, Michael Faraday (1791–1867), an English chemist and physicist studying magnetism, observed iron files arrange from pole-to-pole of magnet in a field-like fashion. These fields were always present, but iron files made it only visibly obvious. Faraday then proposed that light is radiation, electromagnetic radiation (EMR), and it travels as vibrations in fields just like magnetic field. But he did not have the mathematics to prove it.

Then entered James Clerk Maxwell (1831–1879) from Scotland. He learnt that moving magnets create electric current and that moving electrical charges create magnetic fields. He realized that electricity and magnetism are different faces of the same force and that electromagnetic waves travel at the same speed as light, immediately inferring that light is electromagnetic. In fact, the waves of light have electrical and magnetic waves sandwiched at right angles **(Fig. 4)**.

Maxwell also proposed that visible light is a small spectrum of EMR and soon other invisible radiations would be discovered. Radio waves were the first to be discovered, followed by microwaves, X-rays, infrared rays, gamma rays, TV rays, and more. So we have electrical, magnetic, light, and heat energy—all part of a unified EMR **(Fig. 2)** which brought down mankind's dependency on slavery for doing manual work—moving objects, lighting house, cooking, etc. Also, for the first time, mankind had a means of extending their daytime by using light at night.[6]

Just as wave versus particle controversy raged, there arose another intellectual problem; Newton had proposed in his second law of motion: Greater the force on an object, greater is the acceleration. But light could not be pushed beyond 300,000 km/s. His law did not work at particle level so well!

When this controversy was doing rounds, JJ Thomson (1856–1940), an absent-minded Cambridge University professor, discovered that a negatively charged particle exists and its mass is less than that of hydrogen atom. This was an electron particle. Thomson's critics joked that electron will never be of use to anyone. Paradoxically, Thomson's seemingly innocuous discovery shook two fundamental scientific concepts to the core. Nobody had seen atom, the building block of all elements. But everybody believed that it existed. Also, it was accepted that it was uncuttable.[7] (In Greek, *a* means "not" and *tom* means "cut"). This was proved wrong by the existence of electrons, a subatomic particle, according to Thomson. Electron was a particle but traveled like waves in wires to create electric current. So, it had a dual existence, a particle and also a wave. Could this be the same with light? So, Thomson's electrons were nearer to solving the problem of wave versus particle theories of light.

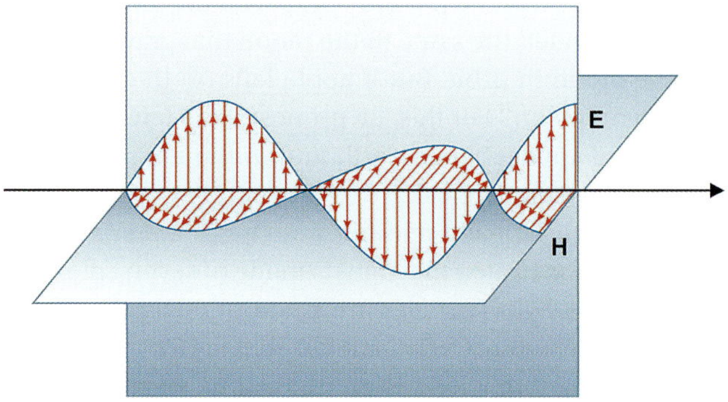

Fig. 4: Electromagnetic wave.

With Newton's laws of motion and Maxwell's equations on electromagnetism, most scientists believed in 1900s that science had all the explanations for the actions in the universe. But there was one question—why does light change color with heat? For this, Max Planck (1858–1947) from Germany came with an equation which associated a particular frequency with particular energy or heat, $E = hf$. His equation also tied the particle with waves. Also, frequency of electromagnetic spectrum is proportional to its energy. It means that violet light of visible spectrum has more energy than red light **(Fig. 1)**. No one in Germany realized the importance of Planck's equation, but Albert Einstein, a German who was at that time in Zurich, Switzerland, did.

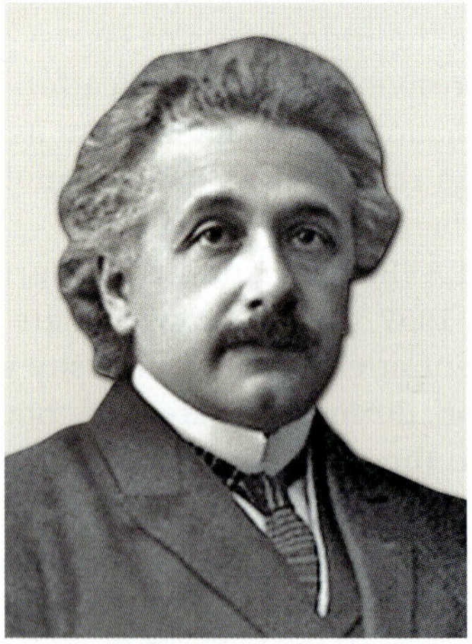

Albert Einstein

Albert Einstein's (1879–1955) initial life had been a wanderer's life. He was born in Germany but had moved out of Germany because his teachers thought that he had a disruptive influence on other students. He did some of his schooling in Italy and later studied physics and mathematics in Switzerland to become a teacher. Einstein was 21 years old when he graduated from Swiss polytechnic. His university record was not very good and he had angered most of his teachers. In fact, he was called "lazy dog" by his professor, for he rarely completed his assignment. But what was the fact? The curriculum at polytechnic only taught Newton's theory.

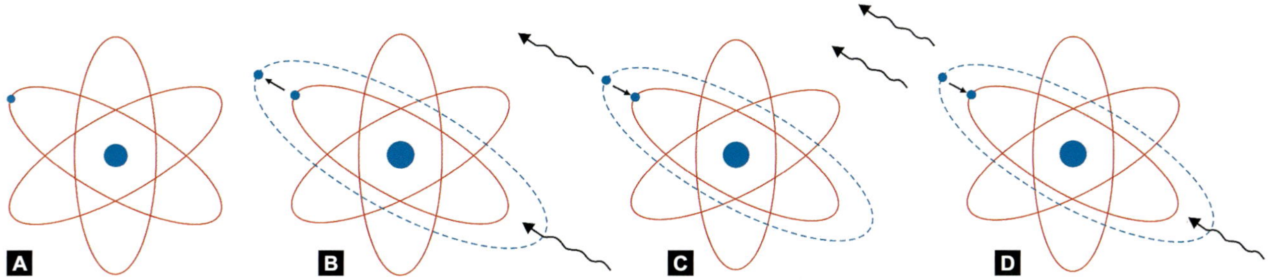

Figs. 5A to D: (A) Electron at rest; (B) Electron shift to inner orbital on photon absorption; (C) Release of energy in the form of photon on returning to resting stage (spontaneous emission); and (D) Stimulated emission.

But Einstein on his own studied Maxwell's electromagnetism, JJ Thomson's electron theory, and his concept of atoms.

Since he had a wife and daughter to support, Einstein settled for a patent office clerical job in Switzerland. The job offered him plenty of free time to think, "What would the world look like if I could sit on a beam of light?" And in the second annus mirabilis of physics, 1905, when he was barely 26 years old, he wrote three epoch-making papers, one of them on "photoelectric effect" for which he was later awarded the Nobel Prize for Physics (the others were on Brownian movement and special theory of relativity). In this paper, he managed to merge, by mathematical equation, the concept that light travels as waves through space and when it meets matter, it behaves like a particle. So from the miracle year of 1666 when Newton said light was made of particle to the second miracle year 1905, it took nearly 250 years to prove the dual existence of light as both particle and waves.[8]

An Einstein contemporary, Niels Bohr (1885–1962), from Copenhagen, then did something remarkable. According to classical physics, the orbiting electrons which have energy should radiate it and come to resting state, hitting the nucleus and ultimately destroying the atom. In other words, the atom would collapse. But this does not take place; the atom does not collapse. So what kept the orbits going and what made atoms stable? Bohr proposed that the nucleus was at the center and electrons, like the planets in the solar system, orbited around the nucleus. The only difference was, unlike planets, which have fixed orbit, the electrons could change orbits. When left alone, the electron stays in the lowest energy orbit. When disturbed, it can jump to a higher energy orbit. Just as a car requiring fuel, an electron needs to absorb energy in order to jump to an orbit where the energy is greater. When it drops to a lower orbit, it gets rid of its extra energy in the form of photon's spontaneous emission. This was the quantum theory. Thus, Bohr, a dyslexic with poor knowledge of English, managed to elucidate the rules of microscopic world of atoms, just as Newton had done with macroscopic world.

In 1917, Einstein, using Bohr's quantum theory, published a series of papers; one of them being on the quantum theory of radiation. He proposed that when matter meets radiation, three things can happen: (1) Absorption, (2) spontaneous emission, and lastly (3) stimulated emission (till then, only the first two concepts were known). The significance of the later concept was that the incident radiation and emitted radiation were identical **(Figs. 5A to D)**. This laid the basis for the concept of LASER physics.[9,10] "A brilliant idea dawned on me about radiation, absorption, and emission" wrote Einstein about this concept.

BUILDING OF THE FIRST LASER

Even though stimulated emission was predicted, nobody took the idea forward because of lack of applications then. Few isolated attempts took place in Germany and the Union of Soviet Socialist Republics (USSR). But the stimulated gain of radiation in laboratory was very weak. Political instability loomed large on Europe and Germany went to war. The United States of America was dragged into this war. It was using 1930s radars to detect enemy planes. The planes appeared like dots on screen and the details were missing. Military planners wanted better radars, so that they could see the details of the aircraft. Previously, radio waves having wavelength equal to that of football field **(Fig. 1)** were being used. Narrow wavelength microwaves **(Fig. 1)**, having wavelength equal to centimeter to millimeter, were required to create these smart radars.

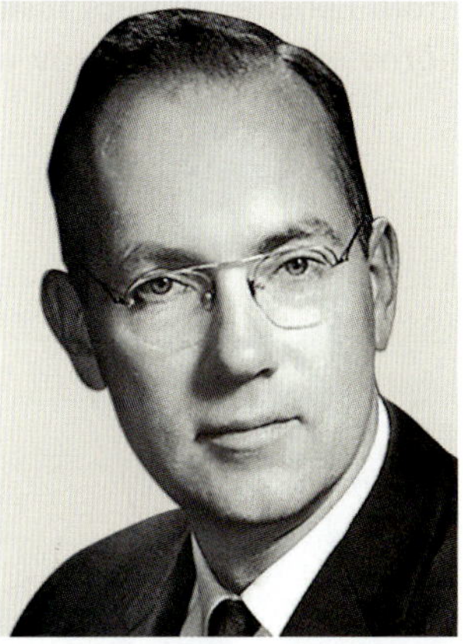

Charles Townes

Charles Townes (1915–2015), a physicist from California Institute of Technology, after obtaining his doctorate in 1939, was looking for academic placement. But he landed in Bell laboratories which had the military radar project. Townes successfully built shorter wavelength radars as per requirement. But military planners wanted even shorter, 1.25 cm (24 GHz) microwave radar. Townes predicted the failure of this technology by his calculations but still managed to build it. This increased his reputation.

After the war, all the scientists were back in their academic tenures. Columbia University was recruiting new minds. One such prized recruit was Charles Townes into the radiation laboratory in 1949 as professor. In this department, Pentagon had put in their money to create microwave communications for military purpose but with loose strings, basic research would not be disturbed. Townes headed this because he could pursue his basic research in spectroscopy.

Each atom in nature gives out its signature EMR. But studying this output, scientist could predict the element present. They could read the radiation from stars and predict the elements present there. For this basic research, spectroscope was required. For creation of this spectroscope, microwaves generators were crucial. At the same time, pentagon also wanted these devices for communication. To create these microwave generators, Einstein's concept of stimulated emission was crucial.

In 1954, using ammonia gas, Townes created stimulated emission. He along with his two graduate students heated ammonia gas. This excited gas was fed into a chamber. In this chamber, microwave would be fired. Gradually, the chamber would be filled with enough microwaves and a powerful beam of microwave emitted. He named this process, Microwave Amplification by the Stimulated Emission of Radiation (MASER). This was what Einstein had predicted, the only difference was, he considered augmenting visible light than microwave. But one should realize microwave and visible light are part of the same electromagnetic spectrum traveling at 300,000 km/s. Later, MASER was used as atomic clock and astronomy.[11] There were sketchy reports in 1954 that even Soviet scientists from Lebedev Physics Institute in Moscow, Alexander Prokhorov and Nikolai Basov were working on MASER.

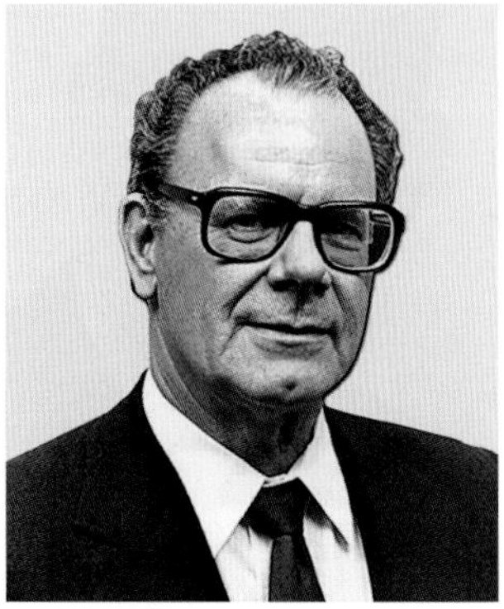

Gordon Gould

At the same time, Gordon Gould (1920–2005), a graduate student, at the same Columbia University physics department also took interest into stimulated emission. Gould had analyzed diamond and graphite. Both were basically made of carbon. The only difference was lattice of carbon. He had the idea of heating graphite in vacuum and creating ultimately diamond. This experiment failed miserably and he decided to study more of physics and enrolled in Columbia University. He chose for his PhD work, to study molecular beam experiment and was assigned to work on thallium element.

Gould, a few years younger to Charles Townes, never liked academic positions. He just wanted to learn physics and settle for patenting a few devices and reap the financial gains. Gould thought that Edison invented things that people needed. His inventions transformed society and individual lives. As much as anyone, he had ushered in the modern age. But what Gould also found compelling about Edison was that he had mastered the business of invention. He had gotten his inventions into the marketplace and reaped their benefits. That meant he had conquered not only the mysteries of the science of his day, but an even greater mystery, the US patent system. Edison had 1,093 patents to his credit.[11]

After joining Columbia University in 1949, Gould passed in PhD exam in February, 1957. Only his dissertation was pending. During this period, he seriously started thinking of optical pumping and creating stimulated emission. He had already mastered this during PhD and was the only person in the country to have done it.

Townes was still using microwaves for creating stimulated emission of microwaves, while Gould was thinking of producing visible light. Townes noted his plans in his laboratory notebook on September, 1957. But there were missing links, for which he approached Gould. Gould for one shared his experience about optical pumping. Townes acknowledged the help from Gould in his October, 1957 notes.

But Gordon Gould sensed trouble and started writing his own notes on November 13, 1957. It was in these notes he coined the term LASER. He also got these notes notarized. But he did not patent his idea because he thought that one has to have a working model before one gets a patent. In March 1958, Gould quit his PhD, just short of dissertation after nearly working 9 years. He with his friends approached Pentagon with his laser idea for funds to realize his dreams.

But by then, Charles Townes shifted his idea of optical maser from Columbia University to Bell Laboratories, where his brother-in-law Arthur L Schawlow (1921–1999) was working. They in 1958 not only patented optical maser (Laser) through Bell Laboratories but also published a paper in Physical Review Letters.

This lead to a patent war between two inventors, one academic Charles Townes and the other entrepreneur, Gordon Gould, for many years. After nearly 30 years, Gordon Gould got his patents from Charles Townes.

Synthetic ruby is made by adding chromium to aluminum oxide. Chromium present in this could absorb visible light and emit red light in range of 692–694 nm. For creating laser, gases were considered but were messy. Solids were considered and ruby was one. But ruby could only emit 10% of incident light and was given up because of the loss.

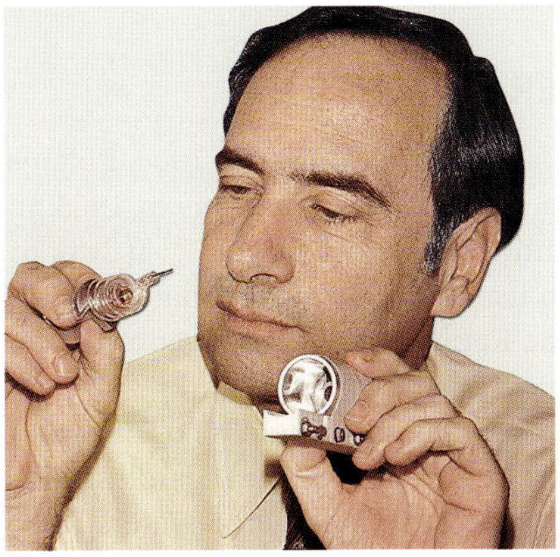

Theodore Maiman

When everybody had given up ruby, Theodore Maiman of Hughes Laboratory from California created the first working laser on May 16, 1960. The physics establishment, till then, had tried bulky tube filled with rare gases or exotic metal vapors to create laser. But Maiman used ruby and succeeded. The dark horse Maiman had crossed the finish line, ahead of thoroughbreds like Charles Townes and Arthur L Schawlow working at Bell Laboratories, Gordon Gould at Pentagon, and four other groups working at Bell Laboratories.[4]

RAINBOW OF LASERS

The birth of ruby lasers ushered in a plethora of new wavelength lasers and newer medium for creating lasers. After ruby, a solid crystal, physicists created lasers using gases and liquid dyes. In 1961, Ali Javan from Tehran, a son of middle-class lawyer, working at Bell Laboratories invented the first gas laser, helium–neon laser (He:Ne; 633 nm). Although this laser was not powerful, its red color was soon used as aiming beam for invisible lasers such as the carbon dioxide (CO_2) laser. Currently, this laser is used in Europe and Asia as a biostimulator to relieve pain and accelerate wound healing.[12]

The same year saw the invention of neodymium-doped yttrium–aluminum–garnet (Nd:YAG; 1,064 nm) laser. This laser emitted energy in the near-infrared (NIR) spectrum, invisible to eye. Early researches found its high emission to be useful to coagulate large blood vessel.

In 1962, the argon (488 or 514 nm) laser was developed. This laser emitted blue-green light, which nonselectively targeted both melanin and oxyhemoglobin (HbO_2).[12] This was the first lesson in skin optics for the dermatologist, for when used to treat vascular lesion, it also targeted melanin and caused hypopigmentation and scarring. In 1981, this argon laser was passed through organic dyes and converted to higher wavelength, yellow light (577 or 585 nm). This increased the HbO_2 targeting with minimal melanin damage.

In 1964, carbon dioxide gas laser (CO_2; 10,600 nm) was invented by C Kumar N Patel (1938–till date).[13] CKN Patel born in Baramati, India, received his Bachelor of Engineering (BE) from the University of Pune, India and the MS and PhD in electrical engineering from Stanford University in 1959 and 1961, respectively. Later, he joined Bell Laboratories and in 1964, invented the CO_2 laser. Initially, CO_2 laser was used for industrial purpose. But by 1970, it turned out be the only laser, highly manipulated to be used in otorhinolaryngology, gynecology, and in the end in dermatology. Early laser applications of CO_2 laser started with congenital vascular malformation. Later, resurfacing of aged skin and ablation of benign and malignant skin lesions found application.[14]

Laser fundamentals

Rule 1: Longer the wavelength, deeper the penetration.

For example, when epidermal freckle is targeted, 532 nm laser is used. To treat dermal Nevus of Ota or hair follicle, 1,064 nm laser is used. To treat the solar elastosis, 1,540 nm laser is used.[15] The ultraviolet, visible, near-infrared, and midinfrared rays penetrate progressively deeper from stratum corneum to deep reticular dermis. But the far-infrared rays—2,940 nm [erbium-doped YAG (Er:YAG) laser] and 10,600 nm (CO_2 laser) would not cross beyond epidermis, despite the above law. This is because of water absorption coefficient of these lasers is very high.

CLINICAL APPLICATION OF LASERS IN DERMATOLOGY (1960–1980): THE DARK AGES

The first use of lasers in medicine was in the field of ophthalmology to spot weld the retinal detachment.[16] However, there was no great progress made in clinical applications during these years. But dermatologists who pioneered and helped in perfecting hair transplantation, liposuction, and sclerotherapy for varicose veins now again provided the leadership in perfecting laser surgery.

Dr Leon Goldman: Father of Laser Surgery and Medicine

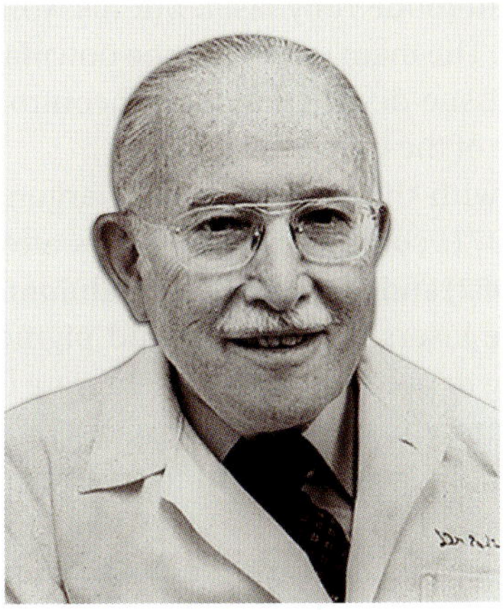

Leon Goldman

In 1961, Dr Leon Goldman,[14,17] a dermatologist, then Chairman of the Department of Dermatology at the University of Cincinnati, started a medical research center at the same university. Ruby laser was just then invented and he wanted to explore the medical uses. At the same time, the National Institute for Occupational Safety and Health wanted to study the safety of ruby laser and Goldman was given the task. Later, with the support of John A Hartford Foundation, he formed a team of biologists, engineers, and physicians of different specialty to work on lasers. He guided this team from 1961 to 1976. Being a true leader, he experimented laser on his own skin and laboratory animals. In 1965, he published his findings on using 500 μs ruby laser for tattoo reduction. He later worked with 50 ns ruby laser and noted more precise tattoo reduction.

This observation is significant because microsecond pulse laser was no better than electro- or chemical cautery for tattoo removal. But with 50 ns pulse ruby laser, there was selective destruction of tattoo with sparing of surrounding tissue. This laid the seeds for selective damage of targets by lasers.

Later, Goldman used Argon laser to treat vascular laser and switched to study CO_2 laser for vascular lesion. In 1981 along with cardiologist Dr Ellet Drake, Goldman formed American Society for Laser Medicine and Surgery (ASLMS). This was a heterogeneous group with dermatologist, surgeons, and physicists as members to foster research and education in lasers.

The Early Decades of "Disease" Laser Dermatology

From 1960s to 1980s, vascular lesions and pigmentary problems were the main targets for dermatologist. In the 1960s, the main lasers to be experimented were ruby laser (694 nm) delivering 500 μs pulse duration and later 50 ns pulse duration and Q-switched Nd:YAG laser (1,064 nm). The first case in dermatology to be treated was malignant melanoma with ruby and neodymium-pulsed laser prior to excision by Dr Goldman.[18] Later, he worked on tattoo's using normal mode and Q-switched mode ruby laser. But his work went largely unrecognized. The main reason for the downfall of ruby laser was that the tissue destruction was uncontrollable and the laser used was of the industrial version.

However, with the introduction of argon laser (488 or 514 nm) in 1971, commercially (9 years after it had been launched in 1962) and CO_2 laser, the pendulum swung toward usage of these lasers for vascular and pigmented lesions. It is interesting to note that these lasers were used as a form of thermal cautery to destroy the target. For a while, argon laser remained the gold standard to treat vascular lesion in children above 12 years.[14]

The argon laser had a 1 mm spot size and it could reach only the papillary dermal blood vessel, leaving behind the deep dermal vessels, leading to incomplete removal or recurrence of vascular lesion. Also, to cover a skin surface area of two square inches, it took nearly one hour making many surgeons handing over the lasers to their incompetent assistants. The two outcomes were scarring and textural changes. This raised the question, should nonphysicians handle lasers?

CO_2 LASER EVOLUTION

After the invention of CO_2 laser in 1964, Polanyi and others developed a medical version of this in 1965 and was used in larynx and middle ear surgery.[19] It was in 1970s that Dr Goldman used this laser in dermatology for skin cancer. In 1972, Issac Kaplan, a plastic surgeon developed the first mass-produced Sharplan CO_2 laser.

The early CO_2 lasers emitted a continuous beam which was absorbed by biologic tissues regardless of pigmentation or vascularity because it targeted water. This was unique compared to ruby, argon, and Nd:YAG laser. Also, it could seal small nerve endings, not leaving frayed ending as occurs with scalpel. It also sealed small lymphatics, causing less postoperative edema. Blood vessels up to 0.5 mm were also coagulated, leading to bloodless surgery. This device could be used in focused and defocused mode. The focused spot size of 0.1–0.2 mm could be used for cutting and defocused beam of up to 5 mm could be used for vaporization of tissues.

"If you don't need the laser, you don't use it"
—Dr Leon Goldman

There were issues with this laser. CO_2 laser being infrared light was invisible. So to help the operator, it was mounted on operating microscope so that the aiming beam of the microscope could guide the surgeon in focusing this invisible beam. This laser was manipulated using joystick. Later with development of tubes with mirrors, the articulate arm, the laser was delivered along with aiming beam. But shortly thereafter, the CO_2 laser was abandoned because the continuous beam caused uncontrolled thermal damage.

Manufacturers later responded to the situation by shuttering mechanically the beam so that the output would be either 1 s or 100 ms. Even this was not good enough. Remember, the thermal relaxation time (TRT) of skin is around 1 ms.[20] Later, super pulsed lasers were developed with pulse duration of 10–100 ms with more power. But even this had drawbacks, leading to development of ultrapulse lasers with pulse duration of 1 ms and peak pulse power of over 500 W.

The thermal relaxation time of skin is approximately 1 ms.

During this decade, CO_2 laser was used only as an expensive electrocautery. The sour part of this evolution was that some doctors charged patients exorbitantly for nail avulsion and some claimed cure for keloids.

This forced Dr Goldman to decry the practice and he displayed these words in his chamber "If you do not need the laser, you do not use it."

THEORY OF SELECTIVE PHOTOTHERMOLYSIS (1983): THE EVOLUTION OF ART OF LASER TO SCIENCE

In 1972, after obtaining his bachelor's degree in physics from Massachusetts Institute of Technology, Rox Anderson joined Harvard Medical School as a technician helping Dr John A Parrish. Dr Parrish, who was part of the team which explored psoralen and ultraviolet A (PUVA) for psoriasis, wanted to try laser and light sources to stimulate psoralen. Together, they published a paper of skin optics, making recommendations like: (1) Melanin in epidermis absorbs EMR from 250–1,200 nm. This absorption is greater in the higher end of the spectrum. Also, beyond 1,200 nm, melanin cannot act like a filter and will allow transmission of radiation to dermis. (2) In dermis, the shorter wavelengths are scattered, but longer wavelength is transmitted with respect to NIR rays.[21]

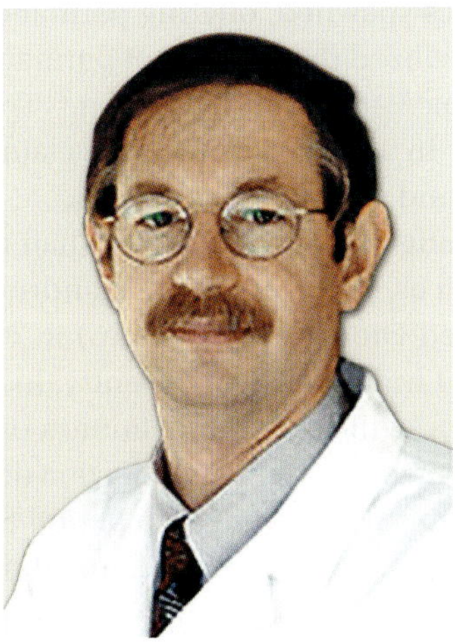

Rox Anderson

Rox Anderson, who was planning on a PhD in physics, had a change of mind after working with Dr Parrish and joined the same medical school and completed his MD in dermatology in 1984 to become both a physicist and a medical doctor. Dr Anderson who had seen Argon laser replacing a vascular anomaly with scar pondered on the same and in 1983 proposed the theory of selective photothermolysis.[21] In this landmark paper, it was proposed that "in targeting pigmented particle or organelles, precise aiming of optical radiation is not necessary because the inherent optical and thermal properties provide target selectivity." Sounds complicated, but the core concept was for a specific target, there is a specific wavelength and to confine the injury by EMR, energy less than TRT of the target should be used.

This theory led to modification of existing lasers and safer lasers for vascular, pigment, and hair reduction were created. The first laser was pulse dye laser (PDL) (577–585 nm) for vascular lesion. It has longer pulse duration of 450 μs and larger spot size. This eliminated the hypertrophic scar of argon laser and even infants could now be treated (previously only children above 12 years could be treated).

DAWN OF LASER CUTANEOUS RESURFACING

The selective photothermolysis also ushered in safer, cutaneous resurfacing lasers. In the 1980s, using the continuous wave (Cw) CO_2 laser, actinic cheilitis, small zone of acne scars, and rhytides were being done. This was more of artistry and required experience. Traditional dermabrasion healed within 2 weeks, but laser took more time and in many cases led to scarring. It was the traditional wisdom that any wound taking more than 2 weeks to epithelize would lead to scarring.

In 1993, Fitzpatrick using modified CO_2 laser with pulse duration of 1 ms and high power of 500 mJ produced less dermal, thermal coagulation zone of 50–100 μm. Previously, it used to be 1000 μm (1 mm). Perhaps, the most significant outcome was reepithelization within 10 days.[20]

If Cw CO_2 laser resurfacing was artistry, so was chemical peel and dermabrasion for resurfacing. Also, dermabrasion led to blood splatter and nonuniform depth of abrasion. This ushered in the era of laser cutaneous resurfacing. Very soon, CO_2 laser became the gold standard for skin resurfacing. But there were issues of prolonged erythema and delayed depigmentation with CO_2 laser. Lastly, the outcome of resurfacing was extremely operator dependent.

If CO_2 laser was getting all the attention in the USA and Germany, Kaufmann[22,23] and colleagues were working on another resurfacing laser, erbium-doped YAG (Er:YAG) laser (2,940 nm), with pulse duration of 250 μs, since 1988. Water is the chromophore for both CO_2 and Er:YAG laser. But the Er:YAG absorption coefficient for water was 10 times greater than CO_2 laser, leading to more precise ablation of epidermis and very little dermal coagulation. The crucial difference between this short-pulsed Er:YAG and pulsed CO_2 laser was the dermal thermal injury. If it was 5 μm for Er:YAG laser, it was nearly 30 μm for CO_2 laser. This precision leads to its introduction in the USA by Goldberg in 1997.[24]

Soon, the pendulum for skin resurfacing swung toward short-pulsed Er:YAG laser. However, it was realized shortly that the results of Er:YAG laser fell short of pulsed CO_2 laser. This led to the introduction of variable pulse Er:YAG laser having pulses from 250 μs to 10 ms. This programmable Er:YAG laser could be used either in short pulse for pure superficial ablation or in long pulse mode of 10 ms for deep ablation and deeper dermal coagulation equivalent to 60 μm, similar to that of CO_2 laser. The clinician now had the choice of safety versus efficacy in resurfacing.[25]

REBIRTH OF Q-SWITCHED LASER FOR PIGMENTARY DISORDERS

Q-Switched laser have output in nanosecond range with high peak power. "Q" stands for quality factor of a resonant circuit. Switching "Q" means varying the circuit quality to store the energy or let it out.

Here, mechanical or optical shutter (pockel cell) is put in the path of photons before laser emission occurs in very high peak power. Dr Leon Goldman had used ruby laser in 50 ns Q-switched mode and shown tattoo reduction in 1967. But the first USFDA approval was given for tattoo removal only in 1989.

Soon there was Q-switched Alexandrite laser (755 nm) and Q-switched Nd:YAG (1,064 nm) laser for pigment reduction. The Nd:YAG light was passed through a crystal (potassium titanyl phosphate, KTP) to frequency double and we had 532 nm. The Q-switched Nd:YAG laser got USFDA approval for tattoo reduction in 1991.

All the above lasers worked by the principle of selective photothermolysis with laser output less than the TRT of melanosome—1 µs. Even the tattoo particles had the TRT of 1–10 ns, equal to or less than the emission time of laser.

Each laser system had its limitation. The Q-switched ruby did cause hypopigmentation even in fairer skin types, the Q-switched Nd:YAG laser could not remove yellow tattoo, and due to oxidation of iron salts in black tattoo, darkening was also noted.

Probably the next greatest step in the evolution of pigment reduction by laser was management of dermal Nevus of Ota. The first report of Q-switched ruby application in Nevus of Ota appeared in 1994.[26] The same year saw early case reports of using Q-switched Nd:YAG laser in treating Nevus of Ota.[27]

Even though epidermal pigmentary disorders such as freckles, lentigines, and dermal lesions like Nevus of Ota and tattoos were manageable, melasma remained an enigma. Also, congenital melanocytic nevi management remained controversial.

Progress in lasers with regard to pigmentation was slow. Few reports of trying femtosecond instead of nanosecond appeared. Perhaps, the significant evolution was change of laser beam profile. Initially, the beam of laser was like a mountain, with more laser output in center and less in the periphery leading to nonuniform skin irradiation. Manufacturers perfected this to top hat profile **(Figs. 6A and B)** with no hot spots or burns on skin.

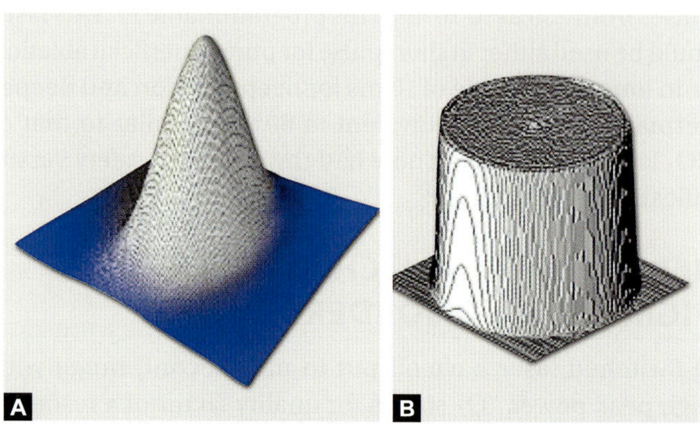

Figs. 6A and B: (A) Gaussian beam profile of laser emission and (B) top hat profile of laser emission.

BIRTH OF DESIRE DERMATOLOGY: HAIR REDUCTION BY LASER

Laser hair reduction was an accidental discovery. It was observed that on tattoo removal by Q-switched ruby laser, the hair shaft in the site was vaporized and the root was bleached with some reduction in number after some days. This observation was documented by Dover et al. in 1989,[27] in guinea pigs. The first human trials were conducted by Grossman et al. using 270 µs ruby laser on 13 patients. A long-term follow-up of 2 years showed nearly four patients had significant hair loss. Next laser to undergo trial was Q-switched Nd:YAG with carbon-based solution application, prior to laser, by Goldberg in 1995.[28] But there was only 25% reduction of hair by 3 months follow-up. But the media went agog and it was widely publicized as permanent hair removal even before reading the small print. Soon, a chain of clinics spawned, offering permanent hair removal. Consumers realized that it was not permanent and in 1997, a paper by Tina Alster nailed the coffin.[29] The chain of clinics faced lawsuit in 1998 for using false claims of permanent hair removal and ultimately wound up.

Things changed for good and laser hair reduction in 1997 saw new devices. Long-pulsed Alexandrite laser (755 nm) in 1997, Pulsed Diode laser (800 nm) in 1998, long-pulsed Nd:YAG (1,064 nm) in 1999 made entry. In 1999, the USFDA made a U-turn with regard to definition of permanent hair reduction. Permanent laser hair reduction does not mean hair will never regrow forever, but for a period equal to or longer than the anagen–telogen phase of growth for the given site. This changed the onus of explaining the laser outcome from the manufacturer to the treating physician.

Laser technology evolved with larger spot size and better skin cooling to prevent burns.[30,31] All lasers required multiple sessions for hair reduction and on an average achieved about 50% reduction.

In 1997, the hair reduction saw the entry of intense pulsed light (IPL) technology. These broadband light devices were more economical and had a larger spot size.

The next major advance in laser hair reduction was in 2004, when laser and RF energy were combined to target the hair [electrical and optical energy synergy (ELOS) technology].[32] Here, first the hair was heated by laser from inside out—hair

Laser fundamentals

Rule 2: Larger the spot size, deeper the penetration of laser beam.
For example, a 3 mm Nd:YAG laser spot size will penetrate 3 mm into dermis, while 10 mm spot size can penetrate up to 10 mm into dermis. So, moustache at the depth of 1–2 mm would require smaller spot size compared to 4 mm depth of bikini hair.

Rule 3: Smaller the spot size of laser, lesser the pain.
For example, when removing a seborrheic keratosis, if one uses 1 mm spot of Er:YAG laser, patient is comfortable compared to using 5 mm spot size.

shaft to external root sheath to destroy the stem cells. This was followed by bipolar RF current delivered to the hair, to heat the hair from the root sheath inward to shaft. This synergy had theoretical advantages such as use of less laser energy, probability of targeting gray hairs, and thin hairs because the RF energy, unlike light, is color blind.

Hair removal in motion: Laser-assisted hair reduction involved using high fluence and single pass. For example, 20 J/cm^2 of diode. But this causes pain and occasional burn. This fluence would have destroyed the stem cell in bulge or dermal papilla in a single pass. But the next novel thinking is using 5 J/cm^2 of fluence and giving four passes on the given area to ultimately achieve 20 J/cm^2. This gradual heating of the stem cells to above 60°C will destroy, without causing epidermal burn or much pain. This is hair removal in motion.

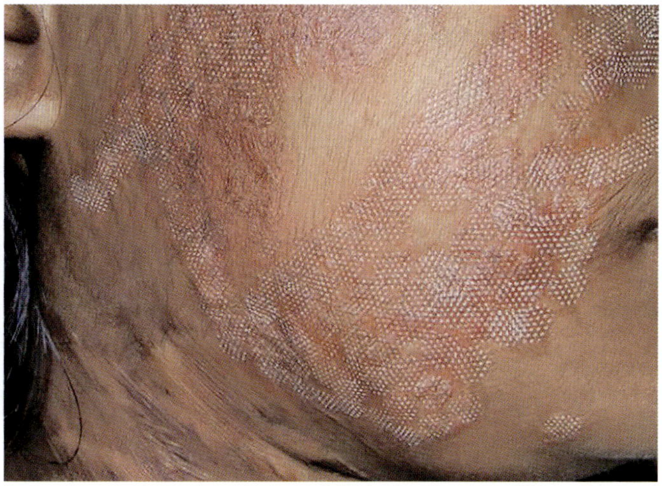

Fig. 7: Fractional ablative resurfacing.

NONABLATIVE DERMAL REMODELING: FOUNTAIN OF YOUTH OR HIGH-TECH SNAKE OIL

Even though CO_2 laser and Er:YAG laser showed promise of reversing the signs of photoaging and acne scars; the downtime was not acceptable for patients. This lead to development of nonablative dermal remodeling, wherein the epidermis is left intact and dermal collagen is heated up to 55°C to stimulate fibroblast to lay new collagen. This is also known as subsurfacing, noninvasive resurfacing, skin toning, or photorejuvenation. For this, laser wavelength in the mid-infrared (MIR) range was used. The first such device was 1,320 nm Nd:YAG laser in 1999. In 2000, the Er:Glass laser (1,540 nm) and in 2002, the 1,450 nm diode laser was introduced. These wavelengths ignore the epidermis and target only the water in the dermis.

In 2002, the technology was in infancy, and in the same year, in the American Society for Laser Medicine and Surgery conference, a plethora of papers were presented. But for the presenters, the audience could hardly differentiate the before from after photos. This elicited puzzled expression from the audience and they wondered whether these interventions were high-tech snake oils.[33]

It was soon realized that dyschromia and telangiectasia component of photoaging responded well with a series of therapies but rhytids and scars not so.[15]

> Permanent laser hair reduction does not mean hair will never regrow forever, but for a period equal to or longer than the anagen–telogen phase of growth for the given site.
>
> —**USFDA**

FRACTIONAL RESURFACING: NONABLATIVE AND ABLATIVE

In 2001, Rox Anderson developed the concept of fractional photothermolysis. In 2003, Huzaira et al. tested this hypothesis using 1,500 nm.[33] In 2004, Manstein further developed this technique and the commercial device was available.[34]

It was during this period that fractional lasers came in to bridge the gap between ablative and nonablative lasers. In this middle path resurfacing, microscopic channels of laser energy are passed into the skin. And here, about 5–90% of the skin surface is treated. The remaining skin is untouched. The best analogy would be water running from a shower head and a tap. In the former, the water output is in small streams and in the later, it comes gushing in toto.[35]

Based on whether the skin is vaporized, ablative or skin is just heated and left in situ, or nonablative, there are two classes of fractional laser: (1) Ablative fractional lasers **(Fig. 7)** and (2) nonablative fractional lasers. The microscopic channel of laser energy path is called microscopic thermal zones (MTZs). In nonablative fractional lasers, the necrotic dermal debris is eliminated transepidermally through channels called microscopic epidermal necrotic debris (MEND) over a short period of time postoperatively. Since 1,400–1,600 nm is absorbed by water in dermis and can penetrate deep into dermis, we have at present 1,440 nm, 1,540 nm, and 1,550 nm wavelengths in the market. As to ablative wavelengths, the old CO_2 laser (10,600 nm) and Er:YAG laser (2,940 nm) have been modified to vaporize and create ablative fractional devices. The laser can be delivered by scanner or stamping devices.

The spot size, density of spot per square centimeter, energy per spot, and depth of penetration varies from device to device. Initially, these devices were tried for rhytides periorbitally and now they are being used to face and off-face sites such as limbs and trunk for pigmentation and antiaging purposes broadly. Compared to conventional ablative technology **(Fig. 8A)**, the fractional modality **(Fig. 8B)** requires many visits. But the complications and downtime has come down dramatically.[36]

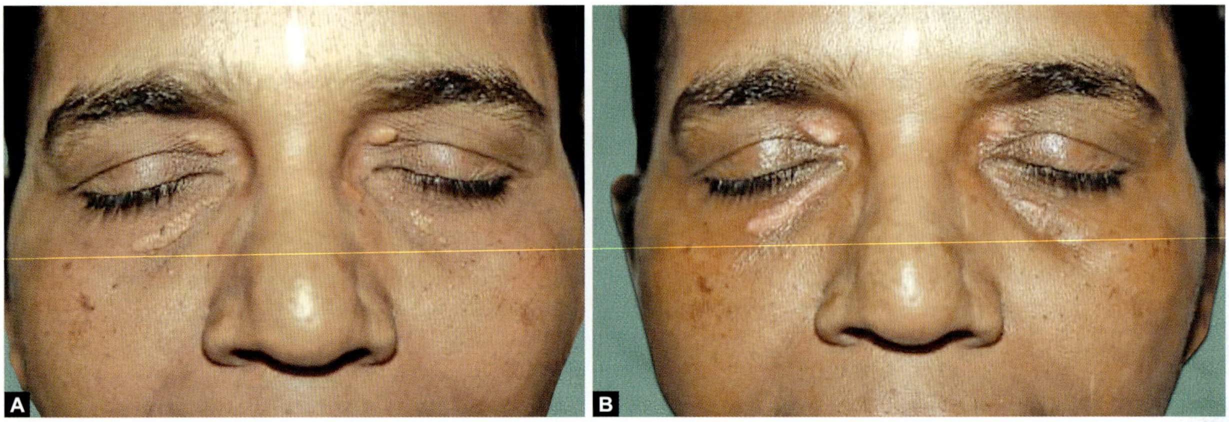

Figs. 8A and B: Ablative resurfacing.

LASERS: A SOLUTION LOOKING FOR A PROBLEM

Lasers in the past five decades have traveled from epidermis to dermis. It has managed pigmentation, vascular pathology, unwanted hairs, and aging issues wherein medical management failed. Probably in the years to come, it would be focused deeper into fat to start a new chapter. The initial emphasis of laser therapy was to destroy, but in the future, it could be used more commonly to conserve. Low-level laser may come in a big way in treating acne, aging, hair loss, and treating pain. Lasers diagnostics, "laser confocal microscopy," may change the way we deal with histopathology. The traditional eosin and hematoxylin stained in vitro technique may be replaced for good by gray scale in vivo laser microscopy.

When laser was created, Irenee D'Haenes, the assistant of Maiman jokingly quipped "a solution looking for a problem." So fire your imagination tempered by Dr Leon Goldman caution—"If you do not need the laser, you do not use it."

Laser fundamentals

Rule 1: Longer the wavelength, deeper the penetration.

Rule 2: Larger the spot size, deeper the penetration of laser beam.

Rule 3: Smaller the spot size of laser, lesser the pain.

INTENSE PULSED LIGHT

Intense pulsed light was introduced in 1992 for aesthetic application. It was invented by Dr Shimon Eckhouse, a PhD in physics from University of California. When this device was first introduced, it was met with lot of skepticism.

Intense pulsed light[37] is produced when electric current is passed through xenon gas. Thus, electric energy is converted to optical energy. This light is polychromatic **(Fig. 9)**, unlike laser which is monochromatic. Another feature is that the light is in millisecond pulse duration. It cannot go down to nanosecond pulse duration like Q-switched laser. Next using various filters, the light, which is emitted from ultraviolet (UV) to infrared spectrum, is modulated depending upon the target chromophore in the skin. Cooling of skin is added for epidermal safety.

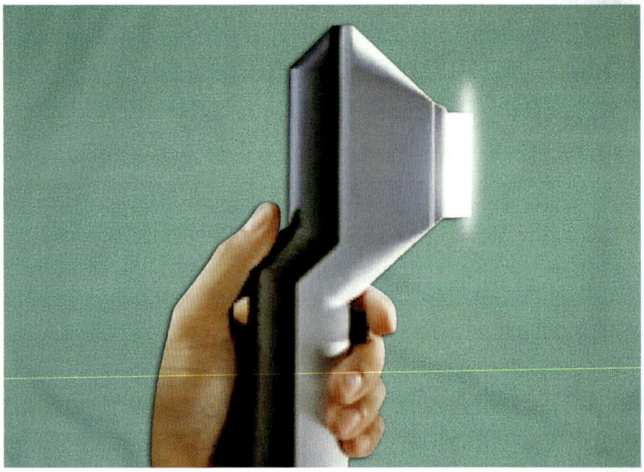

Fig. 9: Intense pulsed light.

The indications of IPL are hair reduction and vascular lesion reduction like rosacea, telangiectasia, and port-wine stain (PWS). Also, acne, photodynamic therapy, photoaging, and cellulite are other indications. IPL is often considered to be the poor man laser, which is jack of all, master of none. Unlike laser, mastering IPL takes time.

The Resurgence of Radiofrequency in Dermatology: Radiofrequency and Aesthetic Applications

Between 1990 and 2000, the laser technology had already peaked. It could handle pigmentation, vascular pathology, and rhytides up to few millimeters in the dermis. However, all this came with a downtime. The reticular dermal aging changes, subcutaneous fat-cellulite problem could not be reached by laser. This required technology which could reach deep down. RF waves which hitherto were used for electrosurgery,

BOX 1: Cosmetic indications for radiofrequency.[38]

- Rhytides
- Skin laxity
- Cellulite
- Noninvasive lipolysis
- Active acne vulgaris

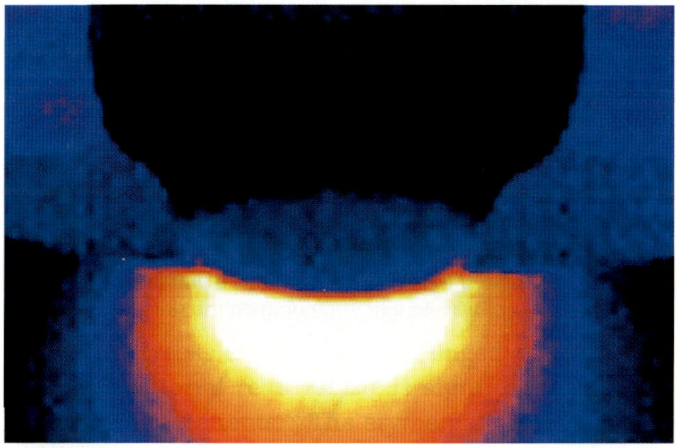

Fig. 10: Thermal image: Monopolar radiofrequency (RF)—deeper penetration.

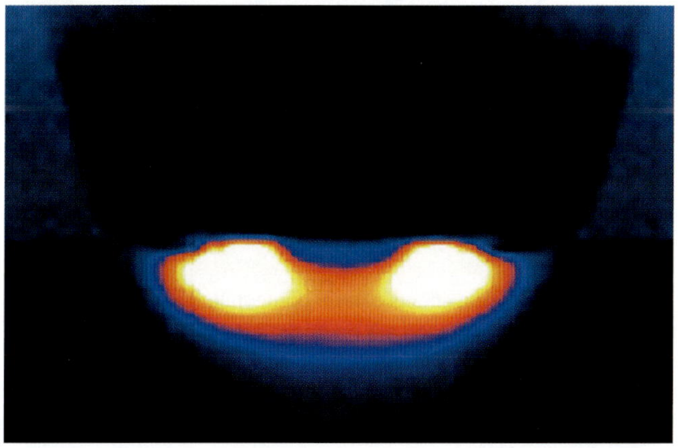

Fig. 11: Thermal image: Bipolar radiofrequency (RF)—superficial penetration.

around 0.5–5 MHz was tuned up to 6 MHz to reach deeper into subcutaneous zone to treat wrinkles and cellulite. The best part of this innovation was less downtime for patient. The first RF device was approved in 2002.

Longer wavelength of lasers like 1,064 nm–Nd:YAG laser or 10,600 nm of CO_2 laser should have penetrated deep into subcutaneous tissue. But the tissue chromophore-water prevents this. However, when you use electrosurgery, you might have noted burns at the distant site of earthing plate applied over the buttock or thigh zone away from face or other operated zone. So, RF waves are chromophore independent—they are color blind **(Box 1)**.[38]

The waves are delivered in various active poles form—monopolar **(Fig. 10)**, bipolar **(Fig. 11)**, tripolar, or multipolar.

These poles deliver radio waves and heat the dermis nonspecifically. The blood in the dermis is warmer and

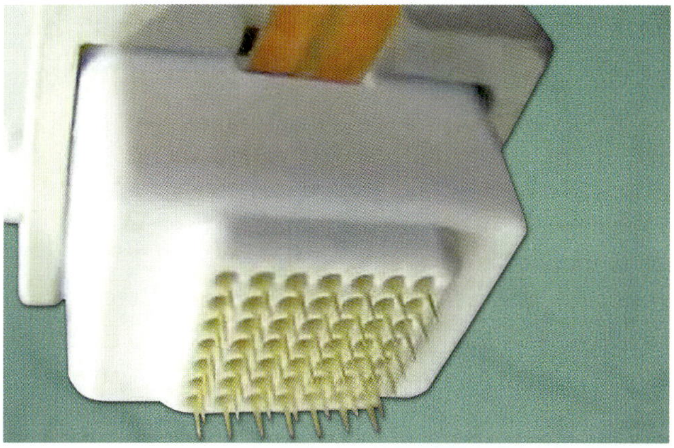

Fig. 12: Fractional radiofrequency (RF) hand piece.

the resistance for current (impedance) is lower and hence, the radio waves are conducted to this zone. This results in increase in collagen, elastic fibers, and mucopolysaccharides. Collagen shrinkage has been noted at temperature around 60°–80°C. However, epidermis at this temperature will burn. Hence, cooling is used to spare the epidermis. When the epidermis is cooled, the radio wave conduction to this zone is reduced. To enhance the safety and deliver the radio waves only to dermis, a needle which penetrates epidermis and localizes heat only to dermis, i.e., microneedle (fractional) RF **(Fig. 12)**, has been introduced.[38] The hybrid technology like RF and IPL also has come to the market.

COSMETIC USES OF ULTRASOUND IN DERMATOLOGY

In 2009, ultrasound in the frequency range of 4–7 MHz was approved for rejuvenating face and neck. Here, low dose of ultrasound is delivered to epidermis and dermis, but incremental energy is delivered to subcutaneous fat. This ablades the adipocytes and noninvasively contours the body to achieve liporeduction.[39] This is a noninvasive way of body sculpting in nonobese individuals.

Another use of ultrasound in the frequency of 5 MHz is drug penetration of ascorbic acid and niacinamide—a process termed phonophoresis.

Microwave technology: Recently, noninvasive microwave technology has been introduced for treatment of axillary hyperhidrosis. Microwaves lead to localized thermolysis of the sweat glands and cause targeted sweat reduction.

LIGHT-EMITTING DIODE-INDUCED PHOTOBIOMODULATION

Light-emitting diode (LED) are solid state semiconductors,[40] which take in electrical energy and deliver incoherent light. In 1960, we had only three colored LEDs—red, green, and yellow. White LED was nonexistent. However in 1993, white

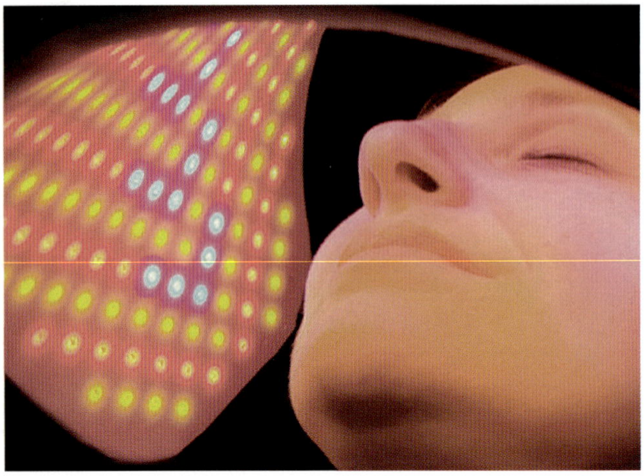

Fig. 13: Light-emitting diode (LED) array used in photorejuvenation.

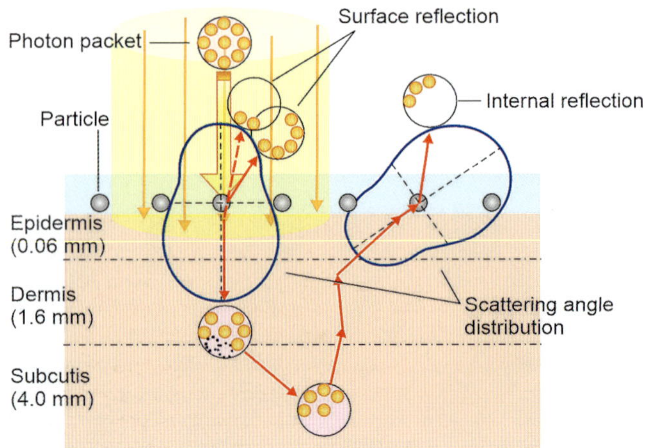

Fig. 14: Schematic diagram of the skin for the simulation model of laser wavelength impinging on the skin.

LED was invented, giving us UV to NIR (247–1,300 nm) spectrum of energy/light.

These LED deliver light to body cells in milliwatt quantity, unlike laser which delivers in watts. Also, LED does not damage eye **(Fig. 13)**.

At cellular level, the mitochondria and nucleus have complex signaling, which decide proinflammatory/healing pathways. LED plays on proinflammatory pathway at the mitochondrial level, which in turn act on nucleus to promote fibroblast proliferation, angiogenesis, and prevention of apoptosis.

This was proven by National Aeronautics and Space Administration (NASA) which documented faster wound healing with LED in space.

Light-emitting diode (LED) application in dermatology
- Reduction of rosacea redness/postlaser erythema
- Wound healing
- Photorejuvenation
- Postinflammatory hyperpigmentation prevention
- Scar prevention postsurgery
- Phototherapy
- Hair growth promotion

BASICS OF LASER–TISSUE INTERACTIONS

Light can be divided into UV (200–400 nm), visual (VIS; 400–760 nm), NIR (760–1,400 nm), MIR (1.4–3 microns), and far-infrared (FIR; 3 microns and beyond) and these also constitute the important wavelength ranges in laser dermatology.[41]

Light behavior conforms to some basic elements which are modified in the skin.[41] Normally, the percentage of incident light reflected from the skin surface is determined by the index of refraction mismatch between the skin surface (stratum corneum $n = 1.55$) and air ($n = 1$).[42,43] The *Fresnel equations* can be used to describe how much light will be reflected from the skin. Depending on the angle between the light beam and the skin surface, this value varies considerably. More light is reflected at "grazing" angles of incidence, while if light impinges at a 90° angle, there is minimum scatter at the epidermis.[42,43]

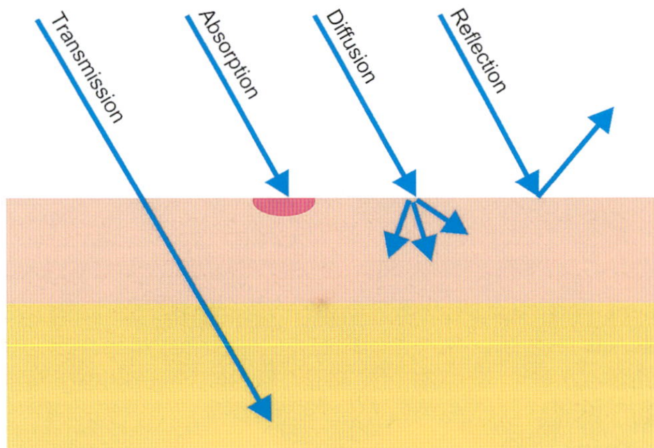

Fig. 15: The varied effects of laser light while impacting on the epidermis and dermis.

It is therefore necessary to deliver light approximately perpendicular to the skin to minimize reflective losses. This regular reflectance is about 4–7% for light incident at right angles to the skin **(Fig. 14)**. One can reduce interface losses by applying an alcohol solution ($n = 1.4$) or even water ($n = 1.33$). This allows for optical coupling. Light not reflected at the skin surface penetrates into the epidermis.[44]

At this point, further light propagation in skin is determined by wavelength-dependent localized absorption and scattering **(Fig. 15)**. Overall, because of scattering, much incident light is remitted **(Fig. 14)** (remittance refers to the total light returned to the environment due to multiple scattering in the epidermis and dermis, as well as the regular reflection from the surface). From a therapeutic point of view, light reflected from the surface is "wasted" energy. The amount of light wasted because of *remittance* varies from 15% to as much as 70%, depending on wavelength and skin type.[21,43] For example, for 1,064 nm, 60% of an incident laser beam may be remitted.

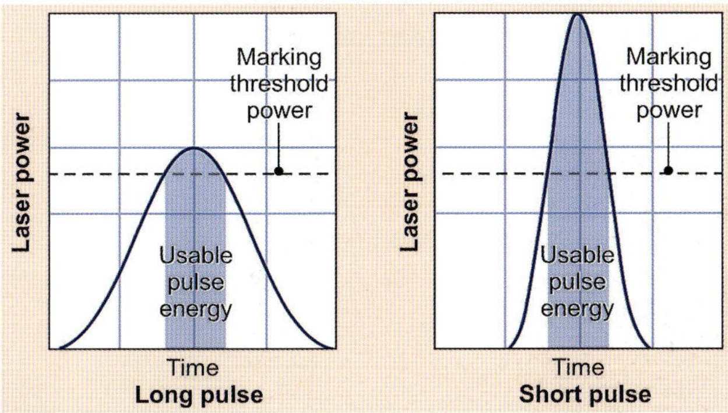

Fig. 16: With longer pulses, much of the usable pulse energy is delivered below the marking threshold and contributes only to unwanted peripheral thermal effects. With shorter pulses, a higher proportion of the pulse energy is delivered above the threshold power level, maximizing marking while minimizing peripheral heating.

One can easily verify this by holding a finger just adjacent to the beam near the skin surface. Considerable warmth will be felt with higher fluence, all of which is due to a remitted portion of the beam.[44]

LASER PARAMETERS AND THEIR IMPORTANCE

Basic *parameters* for any laser depend on the mode. For Cw lasers, power, time, and spot size are important; for pulsed lasers, the important parameters are the energy per pulse, pulse duration, spot size, fluence, repetition rate, and the total number of pulses.[45-47]

- *Energy* is measured in joules (J).
- The amount of energy delivered per unit area is the fluence, sometimes called the dose or radiant exposure, given usually in J/cm^2.
- The rate of energy delivery is called *power*, measured in watts (W). One watt is one joule per second (W = J/s).
- The power delivered per unit area is called the *irradiance or power density (PD)*, usually given in W/cm^2.
- *Laser exposure duration* (called pulse width for pulsed lasers) is the time over which energy is delivered. Dermatology uses EMR exposures ranging from many seconds to nanoseconds.

Fluence (mentioned earlier) is equal to the irradiance times the exposure duration.

This is a very crucial parameter and is useful in pulsed lasers. *Shorter* the pulse duration, lesser is the wastage of energy and if it is less than the TRT of the target organelles, lesser is the thermal damage. Thus, an ultrapulse laser is better than a Cw laser in terms of thermal damage.[45]

For a given pulse energy, a shorter pulse delivers more of its total energy above the threshold power needed to perform material removal and/or transformation **(Fig. 16)**. In contrast, most of the energy of a longer pulse simply goes into heating the material.

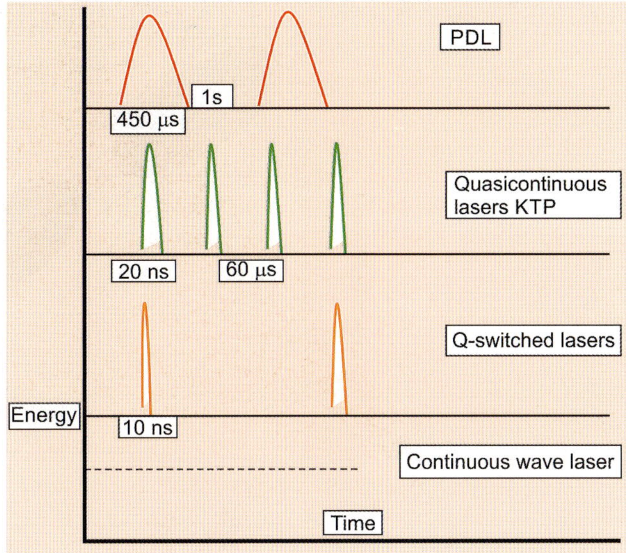

Fig. 17: A figurative depiction of the energy and duration of lasers based on the pulse width. (KTP: potassium titanyl phosphate; PDL: pulsed dye laser)

Clinical implications:[45] Based on pulse width (pw), lasers may be continuous, pulsed, quasicontinuous, and Q-switched **(Fig. 17)**.

The older lasers had pulse durations that varied from seconds to milliseconds (0.01 s/10^{-3}). The CO_2 laser is a classic example of a continuous mode laser.

Here, it must be understood that based on the principles of TRT, if the epidermis is the target, the laser should have a pulse duration < 1 ms, which is the TRT of skin (1,000 µs = 1 ms). Thus, to ensure minimum thermal damage, the laser should have a PD < 1 ms. Microsecond lasers (0.000001 s/10^{-6}) are the ideal lasers (ultrapulse mode) and have a setting of 90 to 900 µs. Most Er:YAG lasers are also microsecond lasers. There is a method which can be used to effectively treat disorders using the superpulse mode, which is based on tissue in vivo or ex vivo effects of the laser by varying the pulse duration while keeping the interval more than TRT of skin.

In the PDLs, a single or a train of pulses is emitted. Pseudocontinuous lasers [potassium titanyl phosphate (KTP)] have very short pulses of light repeated at very high repetition rates. Extremely short pulses are achieved by Q-switching. These nanosecond lasers (0.000000001 s/10^{-9}) are used in pigmented lesions (Q-switched lasers). Recently, picoseconds (0.000000000001 s/10^{-12}) have been used in tattoos.

Operational modes:[45] The operational modes of lasers are Cw, pulsed as interrupted radiation (in ms), pulsed-free running (in hundreds of ms), Q-switched (in ns), or mode locked (in fs).

Continuous wave laser may be differentiated from a pulsed laser, which provides bursts of energy. In the Cw mode, the laser delivers a continuous beam of light with little or no variation in power output over time **(Fig. 17)**. In Cw operation, laser output is controlled by the physician, typically by pressing a foot pedal.

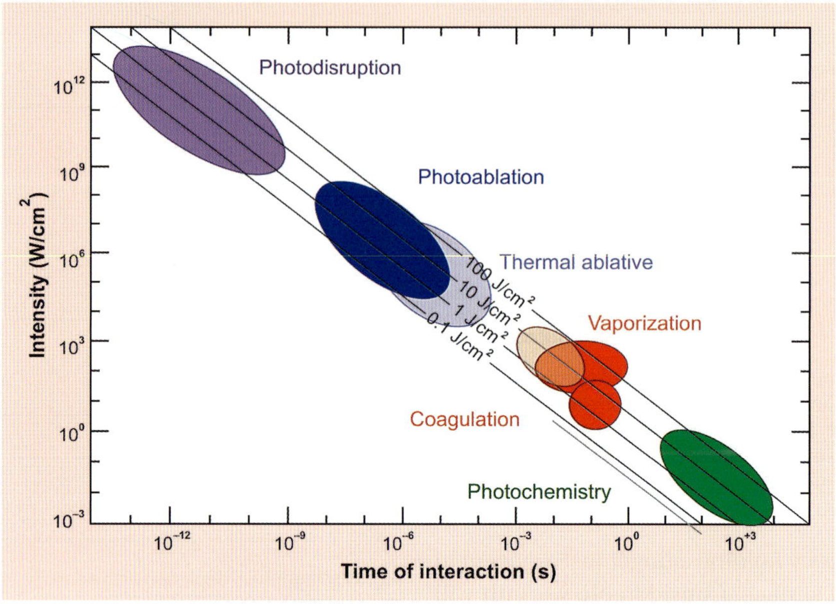

Fig. 18: The tissue effects of laser as a function of power density ranges.

Interrupted radiation of a Cw laser is done by mechanical or electronic switching with modification of the pulse length. The pulse frequency is low-to-moderate, up to 100 Hz. Flashlamp-pumped solid-state lasers in the free-running mode have pulse lengths of 50 ms up to several hundred microseconds. Pulses of medical dye laser systems can vary from microseconds to 50 ms.

Superpulse is a term specific to some CO_2 lasers that have been modified to produce very short pulses with high peak powers in a repetitive fashion, commonly several hundred pulses per second.

Q-switching: Shorter pulses with very high intensities in the nanosecond range are produced by Q-switching (the Q-factor stands for "quality factor," used in electronics theory terminology) of the laser. A single, intense pulse with a duration in the order of nanoseconds is produced. With Q-switching, a fast electromagnetic switch (Pockels cell) in the laser cavity causes excitation of the active medium to buildup far in excess of the level of the medium when the shutter is open. In operation, the flashlamp is turned on and the population inversion gradually grows. Lasing is prevented by the shutter. When the population inversion is at a maximum, the shutter is opened so that lasing occurs and a large burst of energy is emitted as the cavity rapidly depletes the population inversion. The net result is an extremely high peak power ($>10^6$ W) nanosecond duration pulse or series of pulses.

Ultrashort laser pulses are generated by mode coupling due to the coherent properties of the laser. Laser mode coupling is produced by oscillatory motion of a cavity mirror and satisfies the time-dependent boundary conditions. Compared to Q-switching, where the shortest pulse durations are in the range of the resonator period, mode coupling can generate even shorter laser pulses.

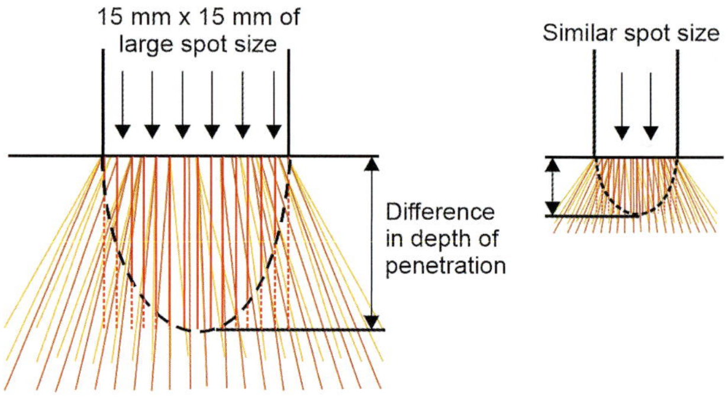

Fig. 19: The effect of the spot size on the depth of penetration of lasers.

- *PD* is one of the most important parameters for it often determines the action mechanism in cutaneous applications **(Fig. 18)**.[45,46] For example, a very low irradiance (typical range of 2–10 mW/cm^2) does not markedly increase tissue temperature and is associated with diagnostic applications, photochemical processes, and biostimulation. On the other extreme, a very short nanosecond pulse can generate high-peak power densities associated with photomechanical effects and even plasma formation. Plasma is a "spark" due to ionization of matter.
- Other important factors are the *laser spot size* (which greatly affects intensity inside the skin), whether the incident light is convergent, divergent, or diffuse and the uniformity of irradiance over the exposure area (spatial beam profile) **(Fig. 19)**.
- The *pulse profile*, i.e., the character of the pulse shape in time (instantaneous power versus time), is another feature that can impact the tissue response.
- *Beam profile*: Top Hat Versus Gaussian[21,44,47]

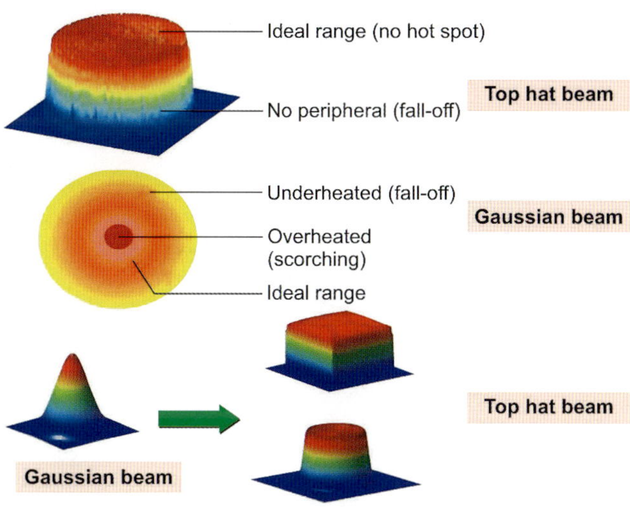

Fig. 20: Comparison of the beam tubes of lasers. In most indications, the top hat profile is preferred. The lower half of the figure demonstrates the conversion of a Gaussian beam into a top hat beam, which can be achieved in certain lasers.

Laser beam profiles can be of various shapes: The Gaussian profile is common. This has the shape of a bell curve and is the fundamental mode of most lasers **(Fig. 20)**. One often sees this shape when the beam has been delivered through an articulated arm (with mirrors at the knuckles). For some wavelengths, this is still the most effective way to deliver energy (CO_2 and erbium).

The Gaussian profile is often disparaged as an inferior profile for lasers. In many applications, the criticism is well-founded. For example, in treating a lentigo with a typical Q-switched ruby laser, one will often observe complete ablation of the epidermis at the center of the "spot" but only whitening at the periphery. On the other hand, sometimes a bell-shaped profile is desirable, for example, when applying a small spot FIR beam with a scanner. In this scenario, the wings of the beam allow for some overlap without delivering "too much" energy at points of overlap.

In most applications, a flat top profile is desirable and with many fiber delivery systems, this is the case as the beam is mixed by the multiple internal reflections within the fiber.

Thermal damage time: In some applications, the immediate chromophore and the final target are not collocated (i.e., hair shaft/bulb contains the chromophore and hair bulge which hosts the stem cells that lie at a distance). In this case, thermal damage time is defined as the time required for irreversible target damage with sparing of the surrounding tissue. For a nonuniformly absorbing target structure, the thermal damage time is the time when the outermost part of the target reaches the target damage temperature through heat diffusion from the heater. In this case, the eventual target (bulge) and the heater (for example, hair shaft) are different and at a considerable distance from each other. Using this model, the thermal damage time can be many times longer than the TRT. This logic also applies to hemoglobin (Hb) and vessel wall.

Thermal kinetic selectivity: Along the same lines is the concept of thermal kinetic selectivity. In this model, one selects larger or smaller targets based on pulse duration. For example, if one wants to heat larger targets while sparing relatively smaller ones, the pulse duration is extended beyond the TRT of the smaller target. In this manner, for example, a melanosome will be heated to a lower temperature than the subjacent vessel.

- *Spot diameter*: In general the spot size should be 3–4× more than *d* (penetration depth), as larger spots make it more likely that photons will be scattered back into the incident collimated beam.[48,49] Photons that are scattered out of the beam are essentially wasted. Traveling "alone," they carry insufficient energy to cause microscopic thermal responses in tissue. The consequences of spot size are explained as follows. Basically, for small beams (narrow), scattered photons are carried out of the beam path after only a few scattering events. A good analogy is a highway with exits. With a narrow highway, any movement obliges the car to "take" the exit and the car does not return to the road. On the other hand, on a superhighway with many lanes, cars can move about and stay within the original boundary of the thoroughfare. Only cars on the extreme left and right are likely to "get" off the road.

Large spots increase the dermal or epidermal damage ratio as well as the relative penetration depth. However, absolute epidermal damage will be greater with the larger spot with the same fluence as the smaller spot. It follows that it is prudent to reduce the fluence by 20%, for example, if one increases the spot size between treatment sessions in care of a PWS. Also, one should note that for any turbid medium, even if the spot is "top hat", there will be an accumulation of photons near the center of the beam such that a greater clinical effect will often be noted at the center of the spot.

For shallow penetrating lasers, such as CO_2 and erbium where the $d <<$ spot size, the diameter of the beam does not intrinsically affect the tissue response. That is why equivalent results can be obtained for skin resurfacing, using pulsed CO_2 lasers versus scanned, tightly focused Cw CO_2 lasers.[50]

ABSORPTION SPECTRUM AND PRINCIPLE OF SELECTIVE PHOTOTHERMOLYSIS

What makes a light source a good choice for a given application is the ability of its emitted light to interact with the tissue so as to achieve the desired effect. This is known as selective photothermolysis.[22] Although Dr Leon Goldman argued for color as a means to selectively damage dermal targets as early as 1963, selective photothermolysis offered an elegant and mathematically rigorous rationale for developing different tissue-selective lasers. As described by Dr Anderson, extreme localized heating achieved with selective photothermolysis relies on: (1) A *wavelength* that reaches and is preferentially absorbed by the desired target structures; (2) an exposure *duration* less than or equal to the time necessary for cooling of the target structures; and (3) sufficient *energy* to damage the target. The heterogeneity of the skin allows for very selective injury in thousands of microscopic targets.

Selectivity is accomplished by matching a specific wavelength of light to a chromophore, i.e., the light-absorbent part of a molecule in the tissue. The energy directed into the target area produces sufficient heat to damage or alter the target while allowing the surrounding area to remain relatively untouched.

The crucial parameters for achieving ideal selective photothermolysis are *wavelength*, *pulse duration*, and *energy level*.[21,42,43,45]

- The wavelength chosen should be such that it achieves selective absorption of light by the target versus the surrounding tissue.
- The pulse duration should be significantly shorter than the target's TRT to avoid interaction with the area outside of the target and the light energy selected should be higher than the damage threshold of the target. Proper selection of these critical parameters ensures the desired results.

Absorption Spectrum[21,43,45-48]

The absorption spectra of major skin chromophores dominate laser transfer implantation (LTI) in dermatology. The *absorption coefficient* is the probability per unit path length that a photon at a particular wavelength will be absorbed.[21,43] It is therefore measured in units of 1/distance and is typically designated μ_a, given as cm^{-1}. The absorption coefficient depends on the concentration of chromophores present. Skin contains pigments and distinct microscopic structures that have different absorption spectra. Common tissue chromophores targeted in dermatology applications are water (which makes up 70% of tissue), Hb (blood), melanin (in the epidermis, pigmented lesions, and hair), lipids (subcutaneous fat and sebaceous glands), and protein (specifically, collagen).[21,43] Each of these has a specific absorption spectra that corresponds to a semiconductor laser material able to produce the matching wavelength **(Fig. 21)**. Because penetration depth depends highly on the wavelength of light, it must be considered when determining the energy needed for a particular application **(Fig. 21)**.

If tissues were clear, then only absorption would be required to characterize light propagation in skin.[21,43,45] However, the dermis is white because of light scatter. Scattering is responsible for much of the light's behavior in the skin (beam dispersion, spot size effects, etc.). The main scattering wavelengths are between 400 and 1,200 nm, where the average distance a photon travels between two scattering events is between 0.05 and 0.2 mm **(Fig. 14)**.

Hemoglobin

There is a large HbO_2 peak at 415 nm, followed by smaller peaks at 540 and 577 nm. An even smaller peak is found at

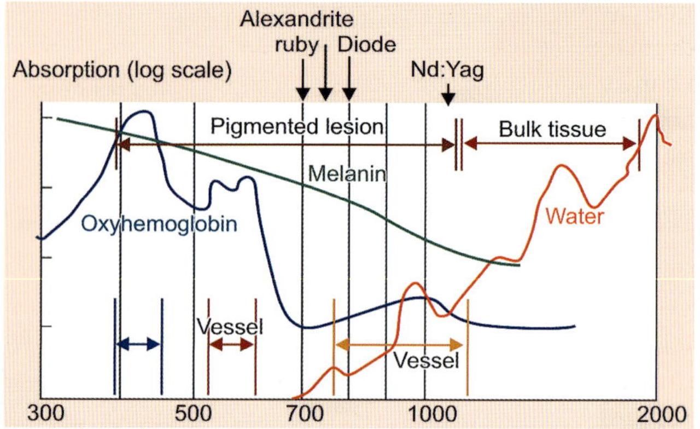

Fig. 21: Each of the major biological chromophores has an absorption spectra. The wavelength of light needed to activate each of these correlates with a semiconductor laser material. Above are shown typical solid-state lasers used for these wavelengths. Penetration depth of light is strongly dependent on wavelength and must be considered when determining the energy for a particular application.

940 nm. For deoxyHb, the peaks are at 430 and 555 nm. Because of the discrete peaks of Hb absorption, the laser physician can optimize heating of the vessel with excellent protection of the surrounding structures.[21,43-45]

Melanin

Most pigmented lesions result from "too" much melanin in the epidermis. By choosing almost any wavelength (<800 nm), one can preferentially heat epidermal melanin **(Fig. 21)**. Shorter wavelengths will tend to create very high superficial epidermal temperatures, whereas longer wavelengths tend to bypass epidermal melanin (i.e., 1,064 nm).

This is why for deeper pigmented disorders such as nevus of Ota, 1,064 nm is used, but in Indian skin, the poor response is because the epidermis is not an optical window and scattering of light occurs. Also, there are variations of color of the nevus of Ota and thus, possibly multiple laser wavelengths may be needed to help in an adequate result.[51]

Water makes up about 65% of the dermis and lower epidermis. Between 400 and 800 nm, water absorption is quite small (which is consistent with our real-world experience that light propagates quite readily through a glass of water). Beyond 800 nm, there is a small peak at 980 nm, followed by larger peaks at 1,480 nm and 1,060 nm. The water maximum is 2,940 nm (Er:YAG). Thus, the Er:YAG is ideally suited for ablation but as it has lesser coagulation than CO_2 laser, it is not preferred for deeper ablation.

Carbon

Carbon is not per se a chromophore but rather a product of prolonged skin heating. Once carbon is formed at the skin surface, the skin become "opaque" to most laser wavelengths (i.e., most energy will be absorbed very superficially). It follows that the dynamics of surface heating changes immediately once carbon is formed. This can be used creatively as an advantage. For example, one could use a layer of carbon paper to convert a deeply penetrating laser to one that would only affect the surface. If the pulse were short enough, a 694 nm laser, for example, could optically act as a CO_2 laser!

Collagen

Dry collagen shows absorption peaks near 6 and 7 μm. With a free electron laser, these peaks can be exploited for selective molecular targeting. In this manner, collagen is directly heated rather than relying on heat conduction due to its close bonds to tissue water (where Er:YAG and CO_2 lasers work). Ellis et al. found that this approach provided more efficient resurfacing and might allow for less tissue irradiation and less thermal damage than CO_2 laser.[52] The *clinical application* of this is immense. The practice of treating pigmented lesions with synergistic lasers is a classic example of lack of science as if an ablative laser even in a fractional mode is used followed by a pigment-specific laser, the former will create a tissue reaction that may obviate the effects of the pigment-specific laser as the chromophores involved may have a change in their absorption spectrum, their size, and depth.

In Indian skin, especially for pigmented lesions, the implications are obvious. A longer wavelength is better as it minimizes damage to the epidermis and there is less scatter; hence, the popularity of the 1,064 nm Nd:YAG.

Thermal Relaxation Time

For effective treatment and to prevent interaction with the surrounding area, the pw should be sufficiently shorter than the TRT of the targeted chromophore.[21,22,43-45] While there is no substitute for testing and experimentation, **Figure 22**, which provides guidance for determining approximate pw, can serve as a starting point. The single limiting factor for using semiconductor lasers is high peak power. Improvements in this area make their use quite compelling since semiconductor lasers also offer performance in the other parameters.

Clinical Application

The TRT explains the futility of using lasers in melasma and postinflammatory pigmentation where the size of the target is variably the melanosome, melanocytes, and clumps of melanocytes, and that too at variable levels; thus, what is needed is a laser that has variable pulse duration, variable depths, and also minimum thermal damage, a combination that is impossible to achieve by any single laser. Hence, it is obvious that monotherapy lasers are of little use in melasma.[53]

HEAT GENERATION AND COOLING

All laser–tissue interactions are guided by the same energy balance rules that guide all of physics. Heat generation can occur in one of two ways. Firstly, it can occur at the site

- **Pulsewidth ≤ TRT**
- **Thermal relaxation time (TRT)**

$$TRT = \frac{d^2}{K^{+\alpha}} \text{ (sec)}$$

where:

$$\alpha = 0.1\left(\frac{cm^2}{sec}\right) \text{(Thermal diffusivity of tissue)}$$

$$8 \leq K \leq 24 \text{ (Geometric factor)}$$

Typical TRT ranges:

- 0.005 mm melanosome ≈ 0.001 ms
- 0.01 mm vessels ≈ 0.010 ms
- 0.1 mm vessels ≈ 1 ms
- Hair follicle ≈ 10–200 ms
- 5 mm of subcutaneous fat ≈ 1 minute

Fig. 22: For effective treatment, the pulse duration should be sufficiently shorter than the thermal relaxation time (TRT) of the targeted chromophore to allow selectivity from surrounding tissue. Typical optical fluence needed for effective treatment targeting is between 1 cm^2 and 100 J/cm^2; the corresponding spot size ranges from 0.1 to 10 cm^2. Typical durations for common treatments include 0.001 ms for a melanosome (the organelle responsible for melanin in animal cells) to 1 minute for 5 mm of subcutaneous fat.

of the chromophore.[48] In this case, there is very precise localized heating consistent with the theory of selective photothermolysis.[48] These hotspots under the skin allow specific damage to the target chromophore while the normal skin is spared, so long as the ratio of absorption coefficients (i.e., blood versus bloodless dermis) is high enough (optimally >10).

When treating by heating tissue water, the injury is typically from "top to bottom," the exception being deeper-penetrating NIR and MIR wavelengths coupled with surface cooling. In this scenario, one can coordinate heating and cooling to damage specific slices of subsurface skin. Spatially selective temperature elevation is possible when: (1) The absorption coefficient of the target exceeds that of collateral tissue (selective photothermolysis) or (2) when the "innocent bystander" tissues are cooled so their peak temperatures do not exceed some damage threshold.

Cooling

Before the availability of surface cooling, fluence thresholds for efficacy, and epidermal damage were often close. There are two purposes of cooling:

1. The first goal of surface cooling is the preservation of the epidermis. Unintentional heating of the basal cell layer can lead to vesiculation, crusting, and at times, scarring.
2. The second and related goal of surface cooling is to allow for delivery of higher fluences to the intended target (i.e., the hair bulb and/or bulge or a subsurface blood vessel). Often, the highest fluence that can be used in targeting hair and/or subsurface vessels is limited by heating of the epidermis.[54] By cooling the epidermis, higher fluences and therefore higher temperature elevations are possible in the targeted structures in the dermis.

Another benefit of surface cooling is analgesia, as almost all cooling strategies will provide some pain relief.[55-58]

Besides protection of the dermal-epidermal (DE) junction from pigment "unfriendly" wavelengths, bulk cooling is sometimes required because the volume heated is large and there is a risk for large volume overheating and catastrophic scarring (i.e., with 1,064 nm).

Overall, shorter wavelengths pose a greater risk to the skin surface because the ratio of epidermal to dermal heating is higher. This ratio derives from (1) a higher absorption of melanin by shorter wavelengths and (2) a tendency for photon scatter to limit penetration of shorter wavelengths. This leads to an accumulation of energy near the DE junction.[59-61]

The *timing* of the cooling relative to the laser pulse is important. Cooling can be pre, during (parallel), or after the pulse (post).[61] All three cooling periods are important. For example, postcooling may prevent retrograde heating (i.e., from the vessel back to the epidermis) from damaging the skin surface.

Clinical Applications

Visible light technologies (especially green-yellow (GY) light sources such as IPL, KTP laser, and PDL) are popular in cutaneous laser surgery, especially in vascular disorders. They are also the wavelength ranges where epidermal damage is most likely. The epidermis is an innocent bystander in cutaneous laser applications where the intended targets, such as hair follicles or blood vessels, are located in the dermis. Specifically, absorption of light by epidermal melanin causes epidermal heating. Melanin is distributed throughout the epidermis but is especially concentrated in the basal cell layer. Melanin absorption of visible light causes heating of melanosomes and through thermal diffusion, subsequent damage to the entire epidermis. This is especially true for GY light, but the risk of selective DE junction-derived epidermal injury extends to wavelengths as long as 1,064 nm.

This also a reason why the results of PDL in Indian skin are poor as the abundant melanin competes with the laser wavelength.

Beyond visible light sources (green, yellow, and red), surface cooling also has been employed in *NIR* and *MIR* lasers. With NIR lasers, surface cooling is important, both to prevent DE junction-derived epidermal heating and to prevent bulk heating caused by deep beam penetration. With MIR lasers (1.32, 1.45, and 1.54 mm), the chromophore is water. It follows that with even very low fluences, surface cooling is imperative. Without cooling, the ubiquitous nature of water in the skin causes laser-induced top to bottom injury. There is no discrete heating. All of the techniques are susceptible to operator error and device failure. It follows that as physicians rely more heavily on cooling devices, any lack of their proper deployment unveils the dark side of cooling.

There are some scenarios where cooling is *unlikely* to prove beneficial: (1) When the absorption of the wavelength is very strong by water (i.e., Er:YAG and CO_2); here, the cooling and heating zone are collocated so that preservation of epidermal viability is unfeasible and also, (2) when using Q-switched lasers in the range from 532 to 1,064 nm, cooling achieves pain reduction but will only modestly reduce the high peak temperatures generated by these ultrashort pulses in melanin and exogenous inks (tattoos).

LASER SKIN OPTICS RELEVANT TO DERMATOLOGIST

The optical properties of human skin determine the penetration, absorption, and internal dosimetry of laser light in skin. The dermatologist can divide the skin into two main components: (1) The epidermis (primarily an absorber of visible light due to melanin) and (2) the dermis **(Fig. 23)**.

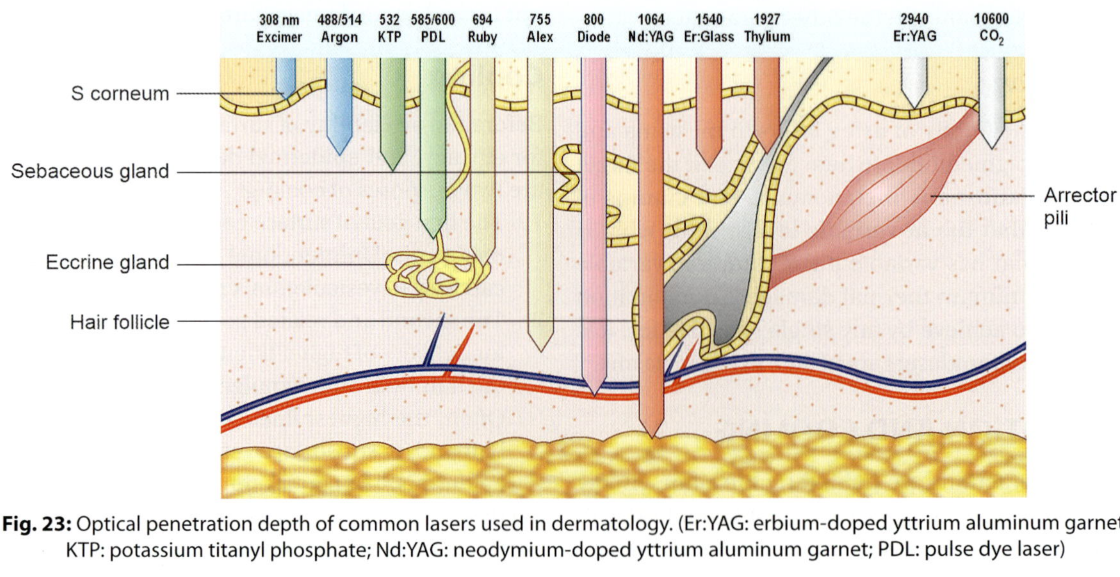

Fig. 23: Optical penetration depth of common lasers used in dermatology. (Er:YAG: erbium-doped yttrium aluminum garnet; KTP: potassium titanyl phosphate; Nd:YAG: neodymium-doped yttrium aluminum garnet; PDL: pulse dye laser)

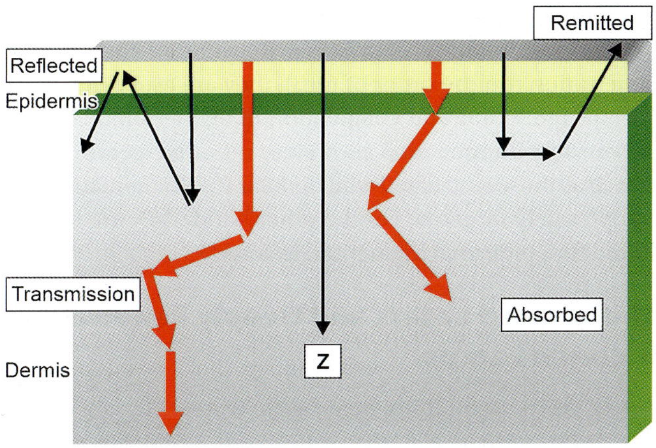

Fig. 24: Laser tissue interaction. Ideal laser penetration is a straight line (z) which is not normally seen as the skin is not an optical window.

One of the most important preconditions to using lasers is to memorize the absorption spectra of the main chromophores in planning the procedure, but it is also crucial to remember that the optical properties of the skin are not static.

Light–tissue interactions can be broken down into (1) transport of light in tissue; (2) absorption of light and heat generation in tissue; (3) localized temperature elevation in the target tissue (and denaturation of proteins), and (4) heat diffusion away from the target.[43-45,48]

In any light–tissue interaction, the thermal or photochemical effects depend on the local energy density at the target. Surface fluence represents the energy per unit area incident on the skin. Once the light penetrates the surface, it undergoes a complex series of *absorbing* and *scattering* events **(Figs. 14, 15, and 24)**. Characterization of the light pathways is best understood by thinking of the incident beam in terms of its constituent photons, where the photons statistically are either scattered or absorbed in a wavelength-dependent fashion.[62] The probabilities of absorption or scattering (designated μ_a and μ_s, respectively) have been determined by experiment. For most visible light, there are typically 100 scattering events before a photon is absorbed. As it turns out, the photon scatters roughly 10 times before it loses its orientation with respect to the initial direction as it migrates in a random walk. With scattering, there is backscattered light that augments the delivered irradiance to yield a higher *effective* fluence beneath the tissue than at the tissue surface (see further).[63]

While the absorption spectrum is detailed earlier, we will focus on scattering in this section. The scattering behavior of biological tissue is important because it determines the volume distribution of light intensity in the tissue. This is the primary step for tissue interaction, which is followed by absorption and heat generation. Scattering of a photon is accompanied by a change in the propagation direction without loss of energy **(Fig. 24)**. Scattering leads to an increase in the light intensity directly below the tissue surface, by a factor of 2–4 as compared with the intensity of the incident beam. The increased fluence rate is caused by scattered photons overlapping with the incident photons.

Clinical Implication[46]

As mentioned earlier, it has been shown that the light intensity directly below the tissue surface is enhanced by a factor of 2–4 as compared with the intensity of the incident beam. The increased fluence is caused by scattered photons overlapping with the incident photons. Because of the scattering effect, the penetration depth depends on the irradiated area. Thus, the penetration depth will double if for the same irradiance, the beam diameter increases from 1 to 5 mm. Thus, for treating PWS or for hair removal, 10–15 mm spot diameters of the laser are recommended as it increases the depth of the laser beam. In tattoos and nevus of Ota, in case there is inadequate response, it is wise to increase the diameter of the probe to increase the depth.

An often-used term is "*penetration depth*" (*d*), which describes the path length that causes light to be reduced to 37% of its surface irradiance. For a clear solution, *d* accurately conveys the depth-dependent fluence attenuation. However, for turbid tissue like the dermis where backscattering can be considerable, the "real" penetration depth can be more than d. This value may be 2–3 × *d*, for example, with 1,064 nm.[61,62]

Jacques notes that a typical bloodless tissue value for μ_a in the visible range is 1 cm^{-1} and the mean free path of a photon is therefore 1 cm.[25] But in real-life scenario, the scattering leads to a augmented energy and depth.

One should consider the choice of laser within the context of the application and the respective absorption and scattering coefficients. If the absorption coefficient is more than 200 cm^{-1}, one typically is looking at a "what you see is what you get" laser (examples are Er:YAG and CO_2). Between 1 and 200 cm^{-1} are the GY lasers (i.e., PDL, KTP, and alexandrite). Finally, when one considers $\mu_a < 1$ cm, we are typically dealing with deeply penetrating light sources where you can injure the skin without obvious surface changes (a "what you do not see can hurt you" laser (an example is Nd:YAG).

Beyond 600 nm, the increase in penetration and a brisk cutoff in Hb absorption make for a therapeutic window between 600 and 1,200 nm. In this range, radiation penetrates biological tissues at a lower loss, thus enabling treatment of deeper tissue structures.

WAVELENGTHS AND ENERGY DEVICES AND CLINICAL APPLICATION

An overview of the absorption spectrum and depth of various lasers is depicted next **(Fig. 23)**. Based on this, we will dwell on the clinical utility of various lasers used in clinical practice.[45]

Green Yellow

These wavelengths are highly absorbed by Hb and melanin and are especially useful in treating epidermal pigmented lesions and superficial vessels.[64-68]

There are two issues concerning these lasers, one is their poor penetration in skin (and the even poorer penetration in blood), which makes them poor choices for treatment of deeper pigmented lesions or deeper larger vessels. Similarly, they are not useful for permanent hair reduction (with the possible exception of very large spots (i.e., IPL) that enhance light depth. The effective portions of many IPL spectra include the green/yellow range.

By the proper manipulation of a laser delivery device, one can optimize parameters for selective heating of pigmented versus vascular lesions as given next.[45]

- Applying a compression handpiece without cooling with 595 nm, blood is depleted as a target and pigment is preferentially heated.
- If the pulse duration is reduced to the nanosecond range, melanosomes are preferentially heated over vessels. For example, extremely short Q-switched 532 nm pulses will cause fine vessels to rupture, but inadequate heat diffusion to the vessel wall precludes long-term vessel destruction. On the other hand, melanosomes are sufficiently heated for single-session lentigo destruction. By choosing specific wavelengths with respect to Hb and melanin, one can achieve some degree of selective melanin or Hb heating.

Red and Near-infrared (I) (630, 694, 755, and 810 nm)[21,43-45]

Deeply penetrating red light (630 nm) Cw wave devices are efficient activators of protoporphyrin after topical application of 5-aminolevulinic acid (ALA). The 694 nm (ruby) laser is optimized for pigment reduction and hair reduction in lighter skin types. The 810 nm diode and 755 nm alexandrite laser, depending on spot size, cooling, pulse duration, and fluence can be configured to optimize outcomes for hair reduction, lentigines, or blood vessels. They are positioned in the absorption spectrum for blood and melanin between the GY wavelengths and 1,064 nm **(Fig. 23)**. They will penetrate deeply enough in blood to coagulate vessels up to 2 mm; also, they are reasonably tolerant of epidermal pigment in hair reduction (with surface cooling) as long as very dark skin is not treated. By decreasing the pw into the nanosecond range, the alexandrite laser is a first-line treatment for many tattoo colors.

Near-infrared (II) 940 nm and Nd:YAG (1,064 nm)

These two wavelengths have been used for a broad range of vessel sizes on the leg and face.[69-71] They occupy a unique place in the absorption spectrum of the "3" chromophores, i.e., blood, melanin, and water. Because of the depth of penetration (on the order of mm), they are especially useful for hair reduction and coagulation of deeper blood vessels. By varying fluence and spot size, reticular ectatic veins, as well as those associated with nodular PWS or hemangiomas, can be safely targeted. On the other hand, they are not well suited for epidermal pigmented lesions.

Midinfrared Lasers and Deeply Penetrating Halogen Lamps

These lasers and lamps heat tissue water. The absorption coefficients for the 1,320, 1,450, and 1,540 nm systems are 3, 20, and 8 cm^{-1}, respectively, and the corresponding penetration depths are 1,500, 300, and 700 μm.[72,73] It follows that for equal surface cooling and equal fluences, the most superficial heating will occur with the 1,450 nm laser, followed by the 1,540 and 1,320 nm lasers. The MIR spectral subset has become the mainstay for fractional nonablative technologies.

Far-infrared Systems

The major lasers are the CO_2 and Er:YAG lasers. Using models, as well as experiments, one can determine relative rates of ablation and heating. Overall, the ratio of ablation to heating is much higher with the Er:YAG laser. However, one can extend the thermal field of the Er:YAG laser by extending the pulse or increasing the repetition rate, and likewise one can decrease the thermal field of CO_2 laser by decreasing pw or increasing fluence.[74,75]

It follows that for applications where precision is required in ablation, Er:YAG is preferred. On the other hand, depending on settings, the CO_2 laser combines an enviable blend of ablation and heating. The depth of residual thermal damage (RTD) is typically more uniform with CO_2 than the depth of ablation with Er:YAG, such that the CO_2 laser is more useful for global skin improvement (fine or moderate wrinkle without severe contour defects) on the face. The thresholds for ablation for CO_2 and erbium lasers vary inversely with their optical penetration depths in tissue (20 and 1 μm, respectively). This assumes thermal confinement. It follows that less surface fluence is required for ablation with the erbium laser. With the CO_2 laser, we are operating at ablation threshold in typical resurfacing applications, so a large fraction of energy is invested in tissue heating. This results in low ablation efficiency and only a small mass of dermal tissue is ablated. In contrast, the erbium laser operates well above threshold (approximately 8–10× at a fluence of 5 J/cm^2), resulting in greater ablation and less thermal denaturation. The CO_2 laser at typical operating parameters performs self-limited controlled heating of the skin, whereas the erbium laser operates in an almost purely ablative regime.

Fractional Technology[76]

Pixilated Injury (Aka Fractional Photothermolysis)

One can create a "pixilated" injury with water as a chromophore in what is called fractional photothermolysis. Thus, the MIR and FIR lasers are commonly used in this technology.

Roughly 100 μm spots have been used with 250–500 μm spacing. The tissue can recover from this fractional injury without the widespread epidermal loss observed after traditional resurfacing applications. Depending on the technology used, two forms are described and though initial enthusiasm was favored toward the ablative fractional lasers, this has been replaced with the fractional RF. But it must be remembered that even with these technologies, the deeper ice pick scars do not completely respond.

Radiofrequency Technology

Radiofrequency skin interactions are fundamentally different than optical ones. Rather than "optical" fluence and absorption coefficients, local heat generation depends on the local resistance and the local current density. With most RF systems, there is a rapidly alternating current that, given the impedance of the skin, generates heat. The distribution of the current density is determined by the configuration of the electrodes relative to the skin anatomy **(Fig. 25)**. Depending on the type of surface cooling, one can create various zones of heating under the skin. There are two types of electrode deployment with variations therein:[77,78]

1. In one scenario, *bipolar electrodes* are combined with either a diode laser or IPL device. In this configuration, there is so-called synergy between the two applications. With the bipolar electrode configuration, electrical field density is intrinsically confined fairly superficially (the field intensity reaches about as deep as one half the distance between the electrodes).

   If both positive and negative electrodes are placed in the contact tip (bipolar electrode), current density tends to flow superficially (path of least resistance from electrode to electrode and therefore, temperature elevation is confined to superficial skin). By placing the electrodes further apart, the current density depth will increase. The control of the tissue heating is determined by variations in electrode type, power, and cooling times.
2. In *monopolar configurations*, the dispersive electrode is located at a distant point on the body. Monopolar skin rejuvenation systems tend to create large volumes of heating. They disperse the electrical energy over the breadth of the electrode through a concept known as capacitive coupling. This type of coupling helps to prevent the natural accumulation of electrical energy at the electrode edge.

Fractional Treatment

Fractional skin treatment was introduced in aesthetic medicine about a decade ago and has become one of the most popular modalities for the improvement of skin quality.[76] This procedure is based on heating or ablation of multiple small foci with a spot size of 100–400 μm. This allows the procedure to be very tolerable and with relatively short downtime.

In contrast to lasers where the thermal effect is limited to the periphery of the ablation crater, RF energy flows through the whole dermis, adding volumetric heating to fractional treatment. This volumetric heating adds a skin-tightening effect. RF fractional technologies can be administered from the surface, using a grid of electrodes, or intradermally, using a grid of microneedles which deliver the RF energy within the dermis.[79] The surface electrodes provide a more superficial effect improving texture and fine lines,[80] while longer needles penetrate deeper, providing deeper dermal remodeling.[81]

The adjustable microneedles allow the depth of delivery of the RF energy to be set depending on the desired result, which allows for the energy to be targeted directly at the tissue being treated with minimal impact on the surrounding tissue and skin. The varying depth of delivery allows the procedure

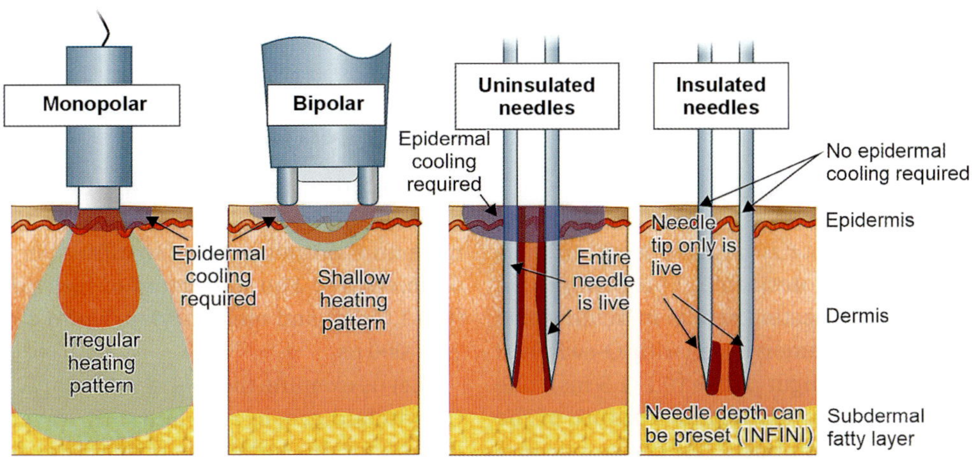

Fig. 25: An overview of the varied radiofrequency (RF) technologies in use in dermatology.

to be precisely customized to address specific problem areas with minimal downtime. The treatment depth can also be varied to allow for resurfacing of the skin, leading to improvement in fine lines, wrinkles, and acne scars.

Minimally Invasive RF Treatment

Minimally invasive RF treatment recently has gained popularity based on the patient's desire to obtain a more dramatic treatment result after a single treatment. Microneedle RF treats the skin in a minimally invasive manner. Dielectric coated needles have become popular in delivering aggressive heating to the reticular dermis without thermal damage to the skin's surface.[82] By heating deep dermal collagen at a higher temperature than could be safely used at the epidermal level, a much stronger collagen contraction effect can be achieved in order to improve deep wrinkles and enhance skin tightening. The combination of deep dermal treatment with superficial fractional treatment has a high potential for complete skin improvement while avoiding skin excision. By introducing larger needle electrodes into the deep dermis, for example, in RF-assisted liposuction, RF can be used to address tightening of the fibroseptal network of the adipose layer with subsequent accommodation of the overlying skin during local fat removal. When energy is applied under the skin, the dermis and epidermis are relatively protected. More aggressive heating up to 60–70°C can be applied during treatment, creating immediate and more pronounced collagen contraction. In some clinical studies,[83,84] up to 42% area skin contraction was achieved after RF-assisted lipolysis.

PRACTICAL APPLICATIONS OF LASER TRANSFER IMPLANTATION

Though there are various applications of LTI, a few examples relevant to common situations are mentioned here. The author would like to emphasize that the use of two or more lasers in one sitting may *not* have a proportionate effect as the LTI of a single laser can be reliably predicted, but the tissue changes that ensue can change the tissue dynamics of the second laser. Thus, concomitant "cocktail" lasers that form part of sundry presentations in conferences have little scientific basis.

Pulse Duration of Lasers[45,48]

With a very short pw, lasers vaporize targets but can produce side effects that may not be desirable. For example, in treating blood vessels, rapid heating results in acute vessel wall damage and petechial hemorrhage (with Q-switched 532 nm). With intermediate length pulses (0.1–1.5 ms), one can gently heat targets without immediate rupture of the vessels. But intravascular thrombosis can create purpura and delayed hemorrhage. With longer pulses (6–100 ms), the ratio of contraction to thrombosis increases and side effects are less likely.

Too long pulses with very small targets can create two problems. With highly absorbing targets, (i.e., tattoo inks), the heat generation is so great and long-lived that significant diffusion occurs to the surrounding dermis. On the other hand, using a long-pulse Nd:YAG for a nevus of Ota results in an insufficient temperature rise as the pigmented nevus cells cool off fast during the delivery of the pulses (also melanin absorption is much weaker than black ink).

Selective Photothermolysis of Tattoos[42,43,45,48]

Amorphous carbon, graphite, India ink, and organometallic dyes, typically found in dark blue–black amateur and professional tattoos, have a broad absorption in the visible and NIR portions of the spectrum. At visible wavelengths longer than 600 nm, Hb and melanin light absorption is minimized and tattoo dyes can be targeted selectively.

The pigment granules characteristically found in tattoos have diameters of 0.5–100 mm, which correspond to TRT of 20 ns to 3 ms. With the development of the Q-switched ruby (694 nm), alexandrite (755 nm), and Nd:YAG (1.06 mm) lasers, tattoo removal without scarring can be achieved. The frequency-doubled, Q-switched Nd:YAG laser (KTP laser) emits at a wavelength of 532 nm, which provides improved removal of red dye. Recently picosecond lasers have been used for tattoos which have been claimed to be superior to conventional Q-switched lasers, but the various parameters that determine tattoo removal, mean that just tweaking the pulse duration may not be a sufficiently good reason to fall for this technology!

But there is an issue of competing pigment in the Indian skin and also the problem of slow results, as the ultimate results are based on the capacity of the macrophages to digest the tattoo pigment. Hence, various modified methods, which include the RTR method, which involves selective ablation of the epidermis, can help to achieve faster results and can be applied to difficult tattoos.[85,86]

Selective Photothermolysis of Pigmented Lesions[45,48]

Pigmented lesions can be divided into epidermal and dermal. Although highest in the UV portion of the spectrum, melanin absorption is also significant in the visible and NIR wavelengths. The diameters of individual melanosomes (0.5–1.0 μm) and melanocytes (7 μm) correspond to TRT of 20–1,000 ns.

Let us examine the role of lasers for lentigines and moles. Q-switched green, red, and NIR wavelengths have been utilized for this indication primarily as their pulse duration corresponds to the target organelle. Though Q-switched lasers are used most commonly, the gentle heating by the millisecond laser can also treat epidermal disorders. With longer pulses (ms), the dermal melanocyte does not become hot enough to achieve pigment reduction, thus ensuring selective epidermal damage.

The geometry (and therefore the microscopic characteristics) of pigmented lesions is important. So in the treatment for a nevus versus a lentigo, the nevus is composed of melanocytes in aggregates (as collectively of a size of 100 μm in diameter), whereas the lentigo is a mere sheet of melanocytes some 10 μm thick. So, the TRT of the nevus cell is about 10 ms, while that of the lentigo is about 0.1 ms. Thus, in treating nevus with a long-pulsed alexandrite laser with a high fluence, the TRT will approach a second. More importantly, the thick slab of melanocytes will take long to cool, such that there will be considerable heat diffusion away from the target. On the other hand, the lentigo represents a slab only tens of microns thick; there will be heat diffusion during the long pulse and rapid cooling after the pulse.

Thus, with millisecond-domain fluences, the nevus might result in scarring and a lighter lentigo might not become hot enough for clearance. If one applies ns pulses to the two lesion types, the lentigo shows a good response with possibly complete clearing, whereas the nevus will require multiple sessions, as each laser application will result in heat confined to the most superficial part of the lesion. Conversely, a microsecond laser might work for nevi.

Thus, the known laser principles of pigment-specific lasers do not apply to all pigmented lesions, especially melanocytic nevi, where ablative lasers are more effective.[87,88]

Selective Photothermolysis and Laser-assisted Hair Removal[49]

The human hair follicle is a complex structure derived from both epidermal and dermal components. The target chromophores, primarily melanin-rich hair shafts, are located deep in human skin (bulge around 1.5 mm and bulb at 2–7 mm). At this depth, only red and NIR wavelengths are useful (690–900 nm). The follicular structure responsible for regeneration has not been conclusively identified and therefore, current systems target the entire follicle. As a result, long pw on the order of milliseconds and high fluences capable of heating large volumes of tissue are required.

Millisecond-domain ruby, alexandrite, diode, and Nd:YAG lasers using high light doses can produce selective injury to human hair follicles, resulting in prolonged growth delay and in some cases, permanent hair loss after a single treatment.

Selective Photothermolysis of Cutaneous Blood Vessels

The pulsed dye lasers at 577–595 nm wavelengths well absorbed by the targeted Hb molecule relative to other optically absorbing structures cause selective thermal damage to dermal blood vessels while minimizing epidermal melanin absorption. Furthermore, because the TRT for cutaneous blood vessels varies between 10 and 300 ms, a variable pulse duration is required for optimal results.

By varying the pulse duration, treatments can be performed purpurically (with bruising) by rupturing the blood vessel or subpurpurically by slowly heating the vessel, causing coagulation of the blood vessel. The V beam PDL lasers have 0.45, 1.5, 3, 6, 10, 20, 30, and 40 ms pulsed durations. The shorter the pulse duration, the more destructive the energy becomes, while with the longer pulse durations, the energy is more gentle, thus causing coagulation of the target without harming structures around the treated area.

For coagulation and treatments without purpura, the laser pulse duration should be shorter than the TRT of the target absorbing the laser radiation in order to confine the thermal damage and spare surrounding tissue. The relaxation time of a target is determined by the target's size (milliseconds or greater for vascular lesions).

But there are numerous variations in pulse duration and absorption of various chromophores (bloodless dermis, HbO_2, and deoxyHb) that can complicate this simplistic interpretation. Moreover, remember that shorter wavelength are absorbed in the epidermis and the epidermal pigment in Indian skin can complicate the laser physics and thus in Indian skin, the results are far from satisfactory.

HOW TO USE THE KNOWLEDGE PRACTICALLY?

The vast amount of data is of little meaning if not used correctly. Thus in practice, *three principles* have to be remembered:

1. *Absorption spectra of various chromophores*: It is important to understand the wavelength that is absorbed by the target chromophore. This is especially relevant in tattoos, thus accounting for the use of 532 nm (green) for a red tattoo and 1,064 nm (blue) for a black pigment. This also accounts for the use of Er:YAG as an ablative tool for dermal tumors, where the target chromophore is water.
2. *Pulse duration of the lasers*: This is directly dependent on the size of the target. This explains why a Q-switched laser is used for a nanosized tattoo and this also explains the logic of using a microsecond laser (Er:YAG) which is used for epidermal ablation (TRT 10 ms).
3. *Penetration depth of laser*: The optical penetration depth is an important consideration especially in pigmented skin. As melanin has a wide range of absorption spectrum, most lasers can be used for pigment disorders. The reason most of us in India use the Q-switched Nd:YAG 1,064 nm is as it penetrates deeper and thus would not interact with the competing epidermal pigment, which is a competing factor in pigmented skin.

Another important aspect is the postinflammatory hyperpigmentation (PIH) that Indian skin is prone for and thus high impact lasers with increased thermal damage should be avoided as they may cause more harm than good. The use of lasers, especially Nd:YAG in melasma,[53] is an example where the patients can have a worsening of the disorder—a fact seen more in practice than talked of in scientific conferences! Minus the use of topical agents,[89] the lasers achieve little to justify their costs.

CONCLUSION

The electromagnetic spectrum has served well dermatology more than any other branch in medicine. The early humble beginning was with electrosurgery in 1891. Later in 1903, a Danish physician Niels Ryberg Finsen won noble prize for treating lupus vulgaris with carbon arc lamp. Next came the big wave of LASER. With helium-neon laser in 1961 started the usage of plethora of lasers, which lasted till 1990s. Following this was IPL, RF, ultrasound, and LED.

The discovery and science behind these energy-based devices should lead us—"From untruth to truth, Darkness to light, and from Death to immortality," an immortal quote which is 5,000 years old.

The above-mentioned concepts may seem extensive and tedious, but they have two important clinical implications. Firstly, the concept of simultaneous combination or sequential use of lasers defies lasers physics as most of the concepts laid earlier are based on a single laser. Hence, the combination of various lasers achieves little, except to add a sense of novelty in conferences discourses. The second problem that has been borne out by numerous practitioners is that excessive and inordinate laser use without understanding the skin type can lead to PIH that tends to spoil results. This is especially true in melasma and cases of PIH treated by lasers.

Hence, it is better to stick to conventional monotherapy use of lasers. It is also useful if laser users also publicize what can go wrong with lasers, especially in Indian skin, instead of highlighting the results in fairer skin types, where the laser optics can be predicted as the epidermis is largely an optical window. I conclude by the famous adage that it is more sensible to be "wiser by learning from others' mistakes than be foolish by learning by one's own mistakes." A working knowledge of LTI would be the first step in following this principle.

REFERENCES

1. Goldman MP, Fitzpatrick RE (Eds). Cutaneous Laser Surgery: The Art and Science of Selective Photothermolysis, 11th edition. Missouri: Mosby Yearbook; 1994.
2. Taylor N (Ed). Laser. New York: Citadel Press Books; 2000. pp. 66-70.
3. Hecht J (Ed). Beam: The Race to Make the Laser. New York: Oxford University Press; 2005. pp. 2-6.
4. Hakim J (Ed). Newton sees the light. The Story of Science: Newton at the Center. USA: Smithsonian Books; 2005. pp. 164-7.
5. Hakim J (Ed). Maxwell's charges. The Story of Science: Newton at the Center. USA: Smithsonian Books; 2005. pp. 356-65.
6. Hakim J (Ed). Getting atom. The Story of Science: Aristotle Leads the Way. USA: Smithsonian Books; 2004. pp. 86-7.
7. Hakim J (Ed). A boy with something on his mind. The Story of Science. Einstein Adds a New Dimension. USA: Smithsonian Books; 2007. pp. 1-9.
8. Einstein A. Zur Quantentheorie Der Strahlung. Physiol Z. 1917;18:121-8.
9. Isaacson W. Einstein, His Life and Universe. New York: Simon and Schuster Paperbacks; 2008. pp. 322-3.
10. Taylor N (Ed). Laser. New York: Citadel Press Books; 2000. pp. 39-165.
11. Lee S. (2010). General Principles and Physics of Lasers. [online] Available from emedicine.medscape.com/article/838099-overview. [Last accessed March, 2024].
12. Marmur ES, Golderg DJ. Nonablative skin resurfacing. In: Goldberg DJ (Ed). Lasers and Lights, Volume-2. Philadelphia: Elsevier Saunders; 2005. pp. 27-41.
13. Patel CKN. (2011). C. Kumar N. Patel. [online] Available from https://en.wikipedia.org/wiki/C._Kumar_N._Patel [Last accessed February, 2024].
14. Brauner GJ. Cutaneous laser surgery: Historical perspectives. In: Kauvar ANB, Hruza GJ (Eds). Principles and Practices in Cutaneous Laser Surgery. New York: Taylor and Francis; 2005. pp. 3-57.
15. Maiman TH. Biomedical lasers evolve towards clinical applications. Hosp Manage. 1966;101:39-41.
16. Wheeland RG, McBurney E, Geronemus RG. The role of dermatologists in the evolution of laser surgery. Dermatol Surg. 2000;26:815-22.
17. Goldman L, Igelman J, Richfield D. Impact of the laser on nevi and melanomas. Arch Dermatol. 1964;90:71-5.
18. Fitzpatrick RE, Goldman MP. CO_2 Laser Surgery. In: Goldman MP, Fitzpatrick RE (Eds). Cutaneous Laser Surgery: The Art and Science of Selective Photothermolysis. St. Louis, MO: Mosby Yearbook; 1994. pp. 198-258.
19. Fitzpatrick RE. The ultrapulse CO_2 laser: selective photothermolysis of epidermal tumors. Lasers Surg Med Suppl. 1993;5:56.
20. Anderson RR, Parrish JA. The optics of human skin. J Invest Dermatol. 1981;77:13-9.
21. Anderson RR, Parrish JA. Selective photothermolysis: precise microsurgery by selective absorption of pulsed radiation. Science. 1983;220:524-7.
22. Kaufmann R, Hibst R. Pulsed erbium: YAG laser ablation in cutaneous surgery. Lasers Surg Med. 1996;19:324-30.
23. Teikemeier G, Goldberg D. Skin resurfacing with the erbium: YAG laser. Dermatol Surg. 1997:23:685-7.
24. Adrain RM. Pulsed carbon dioxide and long pulse 10-ms erbium: YAG laser resurfacing: a comparative clinical and histologic study. J Cutan Laser Ther. 1999;1:197-202.
25. Watanabe S, Takahashi H. Treatment of nevus of Ota with the Q-switched ruby laser. N Engl J Med. 1994;331: 1745-50.
26. Suzuki H. Clinical Use of the Q-Switched Nd:YAG Laser for Treatment of Dermal and Epidermal Pigmented Lesions. Japan: The 8th Congress of International YAG Laser Symposium; 1994.

27. Dover JS, Margolis RJ, Polla LL, Watanabe S, Hruza GJ, Parrish JA, et al. Pigmented guinea pig skin irradiated with Q-switched ruby laser pulses: Morphologic and histologic findings. Arch Dermatol. 1989;125:43-9.
28. Goldberg DJ, Littler C. Topical solution assisted laser hair removal. Lasers Surg Med. 1995;15:47.
29. Nanni C, Alster T. Optimizing treatment parameters for hair removal using a topical carbon-based solution and 1064-nm Q-switched neodymium: YAG laser energy. Arch Dermatol. 1997;133:1546-9.
30. Lepselter J, Elman M. Biological and clinical aspects in laser hair removal. J Dermatol Treat. 2004;15:72-83.
31. Sadick NS, Shaoul J. Hair removal using a combination of conducted radiofrequency and optical energies—an 18-month follow-up. J Cosmet Laser Ther. 2004;6:21-6.
32. Lipper GM. (2002). Shedding light: Nonablative lasers—fountain of youth or high-tech snake oil? [online] Available from https://www.thegeorgiacenter.net/content/uploads/2017/03/Shedding-Light.pdf [Last accessed February, 2024].
33. Huzaira M, Anderson RR, Sink RK, Manstein D. Intradermal focusing of near-infrared optical pulses: a new approach for non-ablative laser therapy. Lasers Surg Med. 2003;15:66.
34. Manstein D, Herron GS, Sink RK, Tanner H, Anderson RR. Fractional photothermolysis: a new concept for cutaneous remodeling using microscopic patterns of thermal injury. Lasers Surg Med. 2004;34:426-38.
35. Gold HM. Update on fractional laser technology. J Clin Aesthet Dermatol. 2010;3:42-50.
36. Pollack SV, Carruthers A, Grekin RC. The history of electrosurgery. Dermatol Surg. 2000;26:904-8.
37. Kunzi-Rapp K, Stiener R. Intense pulsed light technology. In: Raulin C, Karsai C (Eds). Laser and IPL Technology in Dermatology and Aesthectic Medicine. Heidelburg: Springer-Verlag; 2011. pp. 37-40.
38. Lapidoth M, Halachmi S. Radiofrequency in cosmetic dermatology. Karger. 2015;1-108.
39. Kleinerman R, Whang BT, Bard RI, Marmur ES. Ultrasound in dermatology: Principles and application. J Am Acad Dermatol. 2012;67(3):478-87.
40. Barolet D. Light emitting diodes (LEDs) in dermatology. Semin Cutan Med Surg. 2008;27:227-38.
41. Grossweiner L (Ed). The Science of Phototherapy, illustrated edition. Boca Raton: CRC Press; 1994. pp. 217.
42. Hillenkamp F. Interaction between laser radiation and biological systems. In: Hillenkamp FRP, Sacchi C (Eds). Lasers in Medicine and Biology. Series A. New York: Plenum; 1980. pp. 37-68.
43. Neimz M. Laser–tissue interactions, 2nd edition. Berlin: Springer; 2002. pp. 303.
44. Welch A, van Gemert MJ, Starr JC, Star WM, Wilson BC. Definitions and overview of tissue optics. In: Welch AJ, van Gemert MJ (Eds). Optical–thermal response of laser-irradiated tissue. New York: Plenum; 1995. pp. 15-46.
45. Sardana K, Garg VK, Bansal S, Sandhu J, Daulaguphu T. Laser tissue interactions. In: Sardana K, Garg VK (Eds). Lasers in Dermatological Practice, 1st edition. New Delhi: Jaypee Brothers Medical Publishers (P) Ltd.; 2014. pp. 3-24.
46. Boulnois JL. Photophysical processes in recent medical developments. Laser Med Sci. 1986;1(1):47-66.
47. Welch AJ, van Gemert MJ. Overview of optical and thermal interaction and nomenclature. In: Welch AJ, van Gemert MJ (Eds). Optical–Thermal Response of Laser-Irradiated Tissue. New York: Plenum; 1995. pp. 1-14.
48. Anderson R, Ross E. Laser-tissue interactions. In: Fitzpatrick R, Goldman M (Eds). Cosmetic Laser Surgery. St Louis: Mosby; 2000. pp. 1-30.
49. Ross EV, Ladin Z, Kreindel M, Dierickx C. Theoretical considerations in laser hair removal. Dermatol Clin. 1999; 17:333-55, viii.
50. Ross EV, Grossman MC, Duke D, Grevelink JM. Long-term results after CO_2 laser skin resurfacing: a comparison of scanned and pulsed systems. J Am Acad Dermatol. 1997; 37:709-18.
51. Sardana K, Chugh S, Garg V. Are Q-switched lasers for Nevus of Ota really effective in pigmented skin? Indian J Dermatol Venereol Leprol. 2012;78(2):187-9.
52. Ellis DL, Weisberg NK, Chen JS, Stricklin GP, Reinisch L. Free electron laser infrared wavelength specificity for cutaneous contraction. Lasers Surg Med. 1999;25:1-7.
53. Sardana K, Garg VK. Lasers are not effective for melasma in darkly pigmented skin. J Cutan Aesthet Surg. 2014;7(1):57-60.
54. Paithankar D, Ross E. Comparison of cryogen spray and surface contact cooling through heat transfer modeling: Laser Express. 2000;1(2):1-14.
55. Hohenleutner U, Walther T, Wenig M, Bäumler W, Landthaler M. Leg telangiectasia treatment with a 1.5 ms pulsed dye laser, ice cube cooling of the skin and 595 vs 600 nm: preliminary results. Lasers Surg Med. 1998;23:72-8.
56. Greve B, Hammes S, Raulin C. The effect of cold air cooling on 585 nm pulsed dye laser treatment of port-wine stains. Dermatol Surg. 2001;27:633-6.
57. Chan HH, Lam LK, Wong DS, Wei WI. Role of skin cooling in improving patient tolerability of Q-switched alexandrite (QS Alex) laser in nevus of Ota treatment. Lasers Surg Med. 2003;32:148-51.
58. Raulin C, Greve B, Hammes S. Cold air in laser therapy: first experiences with a new cooling system. Lasers Surg Med. 2000;27:404-10.
59. Aguilar G, Majaron B, Karapetian E, Lavernia EJ, Nelson JS. Experimental study of cryogen spray properties for application in dermatologic laser surgery. IEEE Trans Biomed Eng. 2003;50:863-9.
60. Choi B, Pearce JA, Welch AJ. Modelling infrared temperature measurements: implications for laser irradiation and cryogen cooling studies. Phys Med Biol. 2000;45:541-57.
61. Zenzie HH, Altshuler GB, Smirnov MZ, Anderson RR. Evaluation of cooling methods for laser dermatology. Lasers Surg Med. 2000;26:130-44.
62. Jacques SL. Laser-tissue interactions. Photochemical, photothermal, and photomechanical. Surg Clin N Am. 1992; 72:531-58.
63. Jacques S. Simple optical theory for light dosimetry during PDT. In: Tuchin V (Ed). Selected papers on tissue optics. MS 102 vol. Bellingham: International Society for Optical Engineering (SPIE); 1992. pp. 655.
64. Angermeier MC. Treatment of facial vascular lesions with intense pulsed light. J Cut Laser Ther. 1999;1:95-100.
65. West TB, Alster TS. Comparison of the long-pulse dye (590–595 nm) and KTP (532 nm) lasers in the treatment of facial and leg telangiectasias. Dermatol Surg. 1998;24:221-6.
66. Chan H. The use of lasers and intense pulsed light sources for the treatment of acquired pigmentary lesions in Asians. J Cosmetic Laser Ther. 2003;5:198-200.
67. Kauvar AN, Frew KE, Friedman PM, Geronemus RG. Cooling gel improves pulsed KTP laser treatment of facial telangiectasia. Lasers Surg Med. 2002;30:149-53.

68. Lee MW. Combination 532-nm and 1064-nm lasers for non-invasive skin rejuvenation and toning. Arch Dermatol. 2003;139:1265-76.
69. Passeron T, Olivier V, Duteil L, Desruelles F, Fontas E, Ortonne JP. The new 940-nanometer diode laser: an effective treatment for leg venulectasia. J Am Acad Dermatol. 2003;48:768-74.
70. Kaudewitz P, Klovekorn W, Rother W. Effective treatment of leg vein telangiectasia with a new 940 nm diode laser. Dermatol Surg. 2001;27:101-6.
71. Major A, Brazzini B, Campolmi P, Bonan P, Mavilia L, Ghersetich I, et al. Nd:YAG 1064 nm laser in the treatment of facial and leg telangiectasias. J Eur Acad Dermatol Venereol. 2001;15:559-65.
72. Trelles MA, Allones I, Levy JL, Calderhead RG, Moreno-Arias GA. Combined nonablative skin rejuvenation with the 595- and 1450-nm lasers. Dermatol Surg. 2004;30:1292-8.
73. Paithankar DY, Clifford JM, Saleh BA, Ross EV, Hardaway CA, Barnette D. Subsurface skin renewal by treatment with a 1450-nm laser in combination with dynamic cooling. J Biomed Optics. 2003;8:545-51.
74. Smith KJ, Skelton HG, Graham JS, Hamilton TA, Hackley BE Jr, Hurst CG. Depth of morphologic skin damage and viability after one, two, and three passes of a high-energy, short-pulse CO2 laser (Tru-Pulse) in pig skin. J Am Acad Dermatol. 1997;37:204-10.
75. Majaron B, Verkruysse W, Kelly KM, Nelson JS. Er:YAG laser skin resurfacing using repetitive long-pulse exposure and cryogen spray cooling: II. Theoretical analysis. Lasers Surg Med. 2001;28:131-38.
76. Sardana K, Garg VK, Arora P, Khurana N. Histological validity and clinical evidence for use of fractional lasers for acne scars. J Cutan Aesthet Surg. 2012;5(2):75-90.
77. Koch RJ. Radiofrequency nonablative tissue tightening. Facial Plastic Surg Clin N Am. 2004;12:339-46.
78. Sadick NS, Makino Y. Selective electrothermolysis in aesthetic medicine: a review. Lasers Surg Med. 2004;34:91-7.
79. Lapidoth M, Halachmi S. Radiofrequency in Cosmetic Dermatology. Aesthet Dermatol. 2015;2:1-22.
80. Man J, Goldberg DJ. Safety and efficacy of fractional bipolar radiofrequency treatment in Fitzpatrick skin types V–VI. J Cosmet Laser Ther. 2012;14:179-83.
81. Mulholland RS, Ahn DH, Kreindel M, Paul M. Fractional ablative radio-frequency resurfacing in Asian and Caucasian skin: a novel method for deep radiofrequency fractional skin rejuvenation. J Cosmet Dermatol Sci Appl. 2012;2:144-50.
82. Willey A, Kilmer S, Newman J, Renton B, Hantash BM, Krishna S, et al. Elastometry and clinical results after bipolar radiofrequency treatment of skin. Dermatol Surg. 2010; 36:877-84.
83. Paul M, Blugerman G, Kreindel M, Mulholland RS. Three-dimensional radiofrequency tissue tightening: a proposed mechanism and applications for body contouring. Aesthetic Plast Surg. 2011;35:87-95.
84. Duncan D. Improving outcomes in upper arm liposuction: adding radiofrequency-assisted liposuction to induce skin contraction. Aesthet Surg J. 2012;32:84-95.
85. Sardana K, Garg VK, Bansal S, Goel K. A promising split-lesion technique for rapid tattoo removal using a novel sequential approach of a single sitting of pulsed CO(2) followed by Q-switched Nd: YAG laser (1064 nm). J Cosmet Dermatol. 2013;12(4):296-305.
86. Sardana K, Ranjan R, Kochhar AM, Mahajan KG, Garg VK. A rapid tattoo removal technique using a combination of pulsed Er:YAG and Q-Switched Nd:YAG in a split lesion protocol. J Cosmet Laser Ther. 2015;17(4):177-83.
87. Sardana K. The science, reality, and ethics of treating common acquired melanocytic nevi (moles) with lasers. J Cutan Aesthet Surg. 2013;6(1):27-9.
88. Sardana K, Chakravarty P, Goel K. Optimal management of common acquired melanocytic nevi (moles): current perspectives. Clin Cosmet Investig Dermatol. 2014;7: 89-103.
89. Sardana K, Chugh S, Garg VK. Which therapy works for melasma in pigmented skin: lasers, peels, or triple combination creams? Indian J Dermatol Venereol Leprol. 2013;79(3):420-2.

CHAPTER 105

Establishing a Laser Theater

Niteen V Dhepe, Debdeep Mitra

KEY MESSAGES

Location, size, fire suppression systems, laser-opaque and nonreflective surfaces, lighting, electrical needs, air conditioning, ventilation, smoke evacuation, uninterrupted power supply, operation table or chair, operator's chair, eye-protection equipment, prelaser and postlaser kits, surgical instruments, sterilization of devices, asepsis, and emergency management system should all be considered when planning a laser theater.

INTRODUCTION

Light amplification through stimulated emission of radiation is referred to as LASER. It is an electromagnetic radiation source that has the power to cut, coagulate, obliterate, or regenerate tissues.[1] Due to the quest for more precise and minimally invasive treatments, lasers have found a wide and widespread application in dermatology. Indeed, they have a wide range of effective indications. However, using them carries some dangers: Harm to the eyes, fire, burns, and infection.[2] The American National Standards Institute (ANSI), the American Society for Lasers in Medicine and Surgery (ASLMS), the Laser Institute of America (LIA), the National Fire Protection Association (NFPA), the National Institutes of Health (NIH), the National Institute for Occupational Safety and Health (NIOSH), the Occupational Safety and Health Administration (OSHA), and the Canadian Centre for Laser Safety have all established standard norms for laser management and safety.[3]

Globally, lasers are now a standard component of both dermatology practice and academic curricula. The majority of dermatology clinics and educational facilities have laser equipment. In order to prevent emergencies and deliver better patient care, it is crucial to adhere to the accepted rules and safety protocols as a result of the introduction of additional indications and improved lasers. When utilized cautiously by adequately trained personnel in a setting that has been carefully planned, lasers can deliver a variety of beneficial aesthetic treatments. The laser theater facility, which is often referred to as a controlled area, requires careful planning while taking into account the safety of the patient and the operator, as well as the operator's convenience and the best possible handling of expensive equipment. Location, size, nonreflective and laser-opaque surfaces, lighting, electrical requirements, ventilation, smoke evacuation, uninterrupted power supply (UPS), an operating table or chair, an operator's chair, eye-protection gear, pre- and postlaser kits, surgical instruments, sterilization of devices, asepsis, and an emergency management system are all things to take into account.[4]

FACILITY

Since laser treatment is an office outpatient procedure, a full hospital setup is not necessary. However, it is necessary to have backup emergency facilities in place to deal with unfortunate events. Generally speaking, there are two types of laser procedures: Surgical and nonsurgical. Local anesthesia or no anesthesia is used to perform laser operations that produce little to no surface damage. It is extremely possible to turn a procedure room in a dermatologist's office into a laser theater to carry out these nonsurgical laser procedures. However, dermatosurgical theater facilities are required for surgical laser operations needing substantial nerve block or general anesthesia, with anticipated bleeding or predicted bigger raw skin surface injuries.[5,6] The classification of lasers according to the risks engaged is represented in **Table 1**.

Treatment physicians should have a fundamental understanding of laser physics and laser–tissue interaction to ensure successful cosmetic outcomes. A dermatologist or plastic surgeon with experience in executing the treatment, or the medical professionals who work for the equipment provider, should be consulted for proper hands-on instruction. The doctor should be knowledgeable with postlaser (postprocedure) issues such hyper- or hypopigmentation, scars, burns, etc., and how to identify them early, avoid them, and treat them.[7-9]

Many lasers are easy to use, and after receiving the necessary training, a nurse or another nonphysician operator may be permitted to perform the laser. Nonsurgical, nonablative, and semiablative lasers are among them. However, the nonphysician operator should only work with the treating physician's approval; it is not advised for them to work independently.[9] It should also be understood that the

TABLE 1: Classification of lasers according to the NF EN 60825-1/A2 standard of January 2006 (standard applicable for devices put on the market since this date).

Class	*Risks engaged*
Class 1	Lasers considered safe under all reasonably foreseeable conditions of use
Class 1M	Lasers whose direct vision in the beam, especially with optical instruments, can be dangerous
Class 2	• Lasers that emit visible radiation in the wavelength range from 400– 700 nm • The protection of the eye is normally ensured by the palpebral reflex
Class 2M	Lasers that emit visible radiation in the wavelength range from 400 – 700 nm and whose direct vision in the beam, especially with optical instruments, can be dangerous
Class 3R	Lasers where the direct view of the beam is potentially dangerous, but the level of risk remains lower than that of class 3B lasers
Class 3B	Lasers whose direct vision of the laser beam is always dangerous The vision of diffuse reflections is normally safe
Class 4	Lasers that are dangerous when viewed directly but are also capable of producing dangerous diffuse reflections They can cause skin lesions and constitute a fire hazard. Their use requires extreme precautions

primary legal responsibility for results and complications of treatment performed by operator (though trained) lies with the treating physician only.

Laser Procedure Room (Fig. 1)

The room and building design should comply with any existing state and local fire, safety, sanitation, and building regulations.[8,10]

- *Location:* The room in which the laser is used is called a "controlled area". It is recommended that only one patient be treated at any given time in the laser theater. At no time, more than one patient or procedure at the same time in the same room is allowed. A sign must be fitted to the door of the room with the wording: "CONTROLLED AREALASER".
- A notice must be fixed to the laser machine itself as follows: "This device must be used by an authorized operator only".
- A signboard on the entrance similar to as depicted in **Figures 2A to C** should be put up.
- *Dimension:* Laser theater has to accommodate a patient chair (length 6 feet and width 2.5 feet), a trolley carrying the laser machine (about 3 feet × 3 feet), a cart carrying a cooling device (about 2.5 feet × 2.5 feet), a laser operator, and at least one assistant. The ideal dimension should be 12 feet by 12 feet. The room should allow free movement of the operator for proper positioning of laser probes.
- *Laser theater door:* Door should be of 3 feet width for easy movements of laser machines with its trolley. The door should be made of opaque material. This is to prevent the transmission of laser light. The lock should always have preferential access from inside to have an uninterrupted exit in case of emergency. Laser warning signs are to be fixed outside the treatment room.
- *Floor and walls, flooring, cleansing, disinfection:* The flooring should be easily washable and kept clean at all times. Cleaning of the laser theater must always be supervised by an authorized laser operator and care must be taken to protect laser devices and electrical sockets

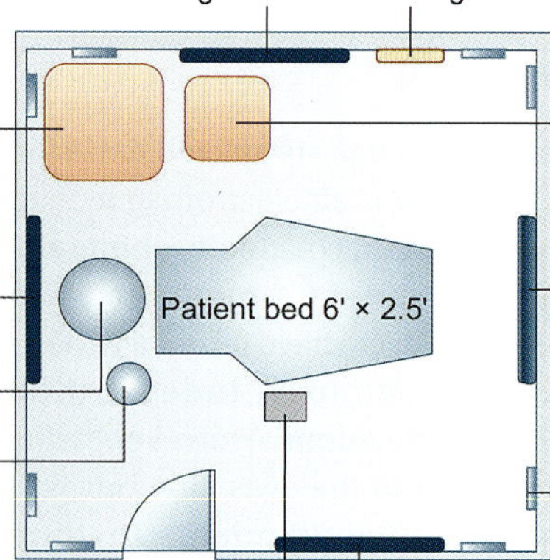

Fig. 1: Laser theater layout (12′ × 12′).

from water. The washing area may be attached to the laser theater but should not be located within it. There should be an adequate hand wash basin (hot and cold water) with long wing taps having long handles, and adjacent soap and paper towel dispenser. Main drainage must be in place. Reflective surfaces should be avoided (walls, ceilings, and worktops.).
- *Windows and ventilation:* The following instructions are given below:
  - All outside air openings to the surgical area are secured against the entrance of insects or other animals.
  - Windows are screened or closed.
- *Electrification and uninterrupted power supply:* A three-phase electric connection is preferable if multiple lasers and/or cooling devices are used.[8] Higher capacity meter is fed with thicker and stable cables and is preferred. Electrical load is calculated on starting load of the equipment which is usually double the labeled working load. The starting load may be calculated by using an ampere meter (ammeter) device. Avoid lower capacity meters fed by thin cables, which in case of overload or

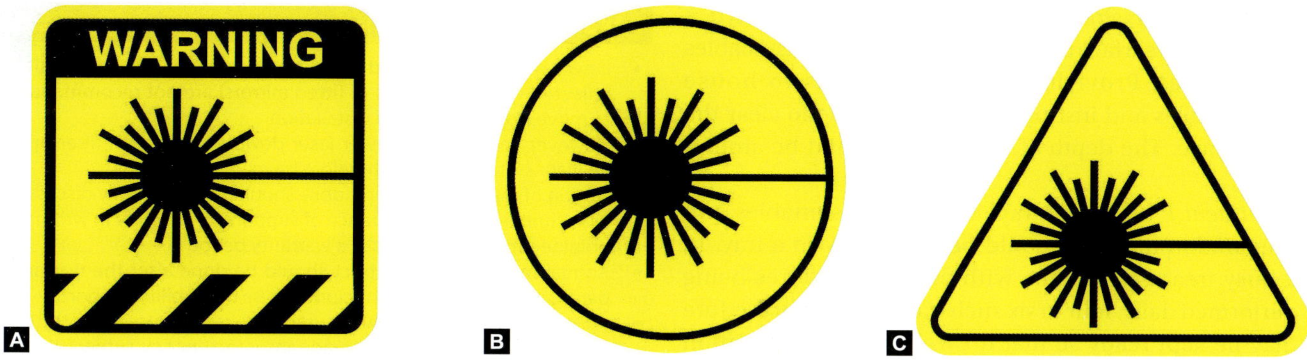

Figs. 2A to C: Laser room entrance board.

BOX 1: Guidelines.

Electrical requirements:
- Each socket board needs to be properly grounded or earthed. Machine productivity is decreased by grounded connections. It can also put the operator at risk of receiving an electric shock
- Imported machine cables may not be supplied with a grounding pin, and this may need to be provided separately
- Three cables from each power plug 15A/5A should run uninterruptedly to the circuit breaker on a control panel. Individual circuiting of plugs protects other machines in case of short-circuit accident in one plug
- Each wall of laser theater should have two panels with two plugs: One 5A and one 15A each. Plug panel should be fitted in each corner one foot off the ground and 2 feet away from the corner. At least five plug panels need to be fitted in a laser theater
- It is possible that the same patient may need to be treated with more than one machine in the same session. During such procedures, crossing of equipment probes or cables over the patient is not advised
- No extension cords should be used in the laser theater as they do not have grounding most of the time. If at all one needs an extension, it must be custom made with grounding and all cable connections tightly fitted. Continuity of grounding cable from the machine to underground attachment must be confirmed periodically. A poorly grounded circuit is a silent killer of a machine's capacity
- Always use a servo stabilizer for lasers. A laser machine should not be plugged directly on without a stabilizer and/or UPS
- A backup lighting system must be of sufficient intensity to permit the completion of any procedure underway at the time of general power failure. The backup system is periodically checked; battery packs (high-intensity flashlights) or backup generators may be used

underload may melt and cause damage to equipment. Some guidelines for ensuring proper and UPS are shown in **Box 1**.

- *Uninterrupted power supply:*[11] UPS online as well as offline is recommended in Indian power supply conditions. UPS should be of 3 kVA or more (minimum 2.5 kVA) with 16 batteries of minimum 60 Amp capacity each. Voltage kVA determines what load UPS can take and battery capacity determines the length of power support when mains are off. UPS and batteries should be installed in a cool and ventilated space. High ambient temperature deteriorates battery life and quality of UPS support. In a laser theater, points fed by UPS and those fed by stabilizer only or directly from mains should be labeled separately. Plugging high-voltage devices like Zimmer, cryo cooling device, or devices with compressor accidentally into UPS points may trip UPS, affecting the function of the laser machine already on UPS.
- *Air conditioning:* Most laser machines require an ambience temperature of 18–22°C for normal functioning, and hence the need for air conditioning in the laser theater. Dust-free and cool environment with well-grounded connections and UPS are necessary for machines' longer working life. Air conditioner (AC) requires a three-phase electric meter connection. Phase feeding AC and laser equipment should be separate so that turning on and off AC will not cause fluctuation in the input of laser. The phase that has less power cut in the load shedding period (reliable phase) may be connected to laser circuit and other unreliable phase to be spared for AC.
- *Treatment chair and operator chair:* It is preferable to have a treatment chair with movable sections. Recommended dimensions include 6 feet length and 22–24 inches breadth to allow the patient to be positioned properly, so the operating team can maintain the airway, quickly alter the position of the patient in an emergency, and provide a firm platform for the management of cardiopulmonary resuscitation (CPR).[12] A dental chair/cosmetic chair/ophthalmic chair with manual or electric manipulation may all be used. The facility of Trendelenburg position is preferable in the treatment chair as it helps in immediate resuscitation in case of a vasovagal attack. A foldable cosmetic chair used in beauty parlors can be a cheaper option for most of laser procedures except for certain procedures on neck. The surgeon's chairs should have adequate back and foot support and should be movable with wheels.
- *Light and illumination:* An adjustable task light, either fitted on the dental/cosmetic chair or situated separately, is preferred. Four 40 watt fluorescent tubelights can be a good alternative fitted preferably on roof or on the wall near treatment end. Switches for each tube should be separate so that the required level of illumination can be selected. A headlight may be used for fine procedures.

- *Laser theater-shelf planning:* A cupboard with a nonreflective surface to store equipment and consumables is essential. Provision for wall cabinets to house consumables and instruments can be made to clear the floor space. The depth of the cabinets could be around 1 foot.
- *Treatment kits:* Plastic trays with all consumables and preparation material should be kept ready in a tray. In a busy treatment center, with many procedures being performed daily, four to six such trays for each procedure may be kept ready so that it saves time of preparation before starting a procedure. A sample treatment kit for laser hair removal may include: Razor, hypoallergic (micropore) tape, marking pen, antiseptic soothing ointment, frozen ice packs, patient's external eye shield, a printed posttreatment instruction sheet, eutectic mixture of local anesthetics (EMLA) cream tube, etc.
- *Waste bin:* Metallic/washable with lid and polythene disposable bag inside should be preferred.

Equipment

- *Maintenance:* Three important prerequisites for longer life of laser machines are: Dustfree environment, low ambient temperature, and well-grounded connections and UPS without voltage fluctuation.[13,14] Machines must be covered during the cleaning of laser theater and when not in use. Regular service visits of a service engineer should be scheduled as per the manufacturer's recommendation. The annual maintenance contract (AMC) from supplier is essential after the warranty period is over. AMC is also essential for insurance. A proper log book should be maintained regarding the date of purchase, service engineer visits, breakdown days, and parts changed during the tenure.
- *Insurance:* Fire insurance is a minimum essential for all costly devices. Breakdown insurance is costly (it has a very high premium), and hence needs to be done. Machines if handled by multiple operators or operated in multiple rooms should always be insured. In mobile laser units, insurance for mobility from one clinic to another or one city to another should be specifically obtained, though this has a high premium. While taking insurance, it is essential that it is clearly specified which parts are covered, e.g., fiberoptics, laser modules, etc. It is important that these terms are included in the cover note and the final policy.
- *Cooling devices:* Cooling is a mainstay in patient safety and getting better results. External cooling devices like Zimmer contain compressors; hence, they require separate electric circuits. Provision should be made for ice cubes or ice packs. Cooling gel packs are a better alternative to ice cooling.
- *Measuring devices:* Measuring tape, measuring scale, Vernier caliper, various molds for measurement of venous diameter, and infrared thermometer are some of the pretreatment measuring devices that help to document results objectively.
- *Molds:* Variously sized molds of laser-opaque and nonreflective material are kept ready when the spot size of the laser is larger than the size of the lesion.

BOX 2: Guidelines for mobile laser unit.

- Lasers with an articulated arm delivery system (whose output is reflected through a series of fitted mirrors) are not recommended to move from the place of installation
- However, most of the newer laser devices come with fiber-optic delivery system and can therefore be made mobile
- Option of making the laser mobile should be thoroughly discussed with supplier and an assurance of support for mobility in writing is obtained if the machine is in a warranty period
- Annual maintenance contract should be done after the warranty period is over, and should include clause of mobility support
- *Insurance:* Usual and routine insurance policies do not cover the risk of mobility. A special tailor-made insurance policy subject to the locations and modes of transport may be designed after discussion with the insurance companies, though this may attract a higher premium rate (also called special contingency insurance)
- The machine should be transported in original manufacturer's packing case designed for shipping
- If a special case is to be designed, polyurethane (PU) foam instead of regular polyethylene (PE) foam with adequate thickness at bottom (minimum 6 inches) is recommended
- Authorized laser operator should always accompany the machine all the time
- Servo stabilizer and/or UPS should be available at other facilities where the mobile laser is to be used. The other clinic also should have class 1 facility
- *Local regulation:* Octroi and entry tax are prevalent in municipal corporation areas in some states. Copies of Octroi payment at original location and prior permission of transport from both the municipal corporations are to be obtained every time

Mobile Laser Unit

In India, a laser machine is often shared between different clinics. So, the machine needs to be shifted from one clinic to another clinic and one city to another city. In the economics of the Indian situation, this is both essential and unavoidable. The task force, therefore, recommends that mobile laser units are acceptable. However, the following guidelines **(Box 2)** are recommended for establishing a mobile laser unit.

CLEANING OF LASER AND OTHER DEVICES

The laser machine is to be cleaned periodically as per the instruction in its user manual by an authorized operator only. No other staff should touch the machine for cleaning purposes. No water is to be used near machine. The outer surface of the device is to be cleaned with spirit swab or acetone swab. Cables of machines are to be checked for snug fitting after cleaning. Laser tips touching patients' skin should be cleaned before using on others patient. Intense pulse light (IPL) tips and covers are to be cleaned off gel with spirit swab. Unclean IPL glass filters can catch fungus and turn opaque, thus blocking output.

Sterilization[15-19]

Adequate procedures that ensure appropriate sterilization or disinfection of instruments and equipment should be in place. Steam, dry heat, or gas sterilization is recommended for critical instruments. Instruments and surgical sets are stored in dry, sterile, and dated packs.

Minimum emergency equipment needed in a laser theater have been discussed in several publications[20-23] and these would be discussed in the chapter on operation theater and on resuscitation.

RECORDS

A clinical history is noted in the patient's record to identify significant medical problems, allergies, bleeding disorders, and current medications. Recording of data in computers is preferred, if feasible. Use of specialized dermatological software is a recent trend but remains optional at this time. There should be a laser treatment register for recording of parameters and relevant findings on a tabular form for subsequent visits. A common procedure register used for other dermatosurgical procedures can be used, if enough space or columns to record laser-specific parameters are provided. A consent form with a questionnaire is covered in a patient's information sheet filled by the patient or a family member. Any contraindications or sensitivity should be brought to notice of the treating dermatologist. A separate day book with records of the date, name of patient, diagnosis, treatment given, and charges may be maintained. It may be useful for income tax audits.

Consent forms and photography are other requirements that are discussed in other relevant chapters.

SAFE LASER PRACTICES

The physician and appropriate staff should be familiar with basic CPR and be able to administer it properly. The staff should be instructed about potential hazards associated with their duties and know how to minimize risks. This includes applicable Occupational Safety and Health Administration (OSHA) standard regulations [e.g., hepatitis B virus and human immunodeficiency virus (HIV) exposure, bacterial contamination, sharps hazards, and hazardous chemical or drug exposures]. The staff should be trained about the proper disposal of medical waste and other biohazardous material. All applicable central government, state, and local regulations should be followed.

Etiquettes

Proper etiquette is very important. A female staff or attendant should always be present while examining or treating a female patient. Patients' privacy, modesty, and dignity should be respected by all staff at all times. The patient must be explained, in detail, about the diagnosis, anesthesia planned, pain involved, and instrument being used—laser or electrosurgery, postoperative care including the necessity of dressing, sunscreens or antibiotics, and complications expected and their remedy. The next follow-up should be informed prior. If the patient is receiving oral sedation, the necessity of an attendant after surgery should be prior informed. The cost of the therapy should be explained. Use of mobile and/telephones in the laser theater should be restricted.

BOX 3: Safe operation practices and emergency protocols.

- *Before administering local anesthetic agents:* Obtain history of xylocaine hypersensitivity and usage of beta-blockers, aspirin, vitamin E, or Ginkgo biloba or any other antiplatelet drug.[16,19-23]
- Never pass electrical cables over the patient
- Avoid using spirit immediately before laser
- Before laser surgery, wear a surgical mask. The pore of the mask should be <1.0 μm. The mask should be covering the nose and mouth. Never put the used mask in apron's pocket
- Smoke evacuator is necessary to suck out laser fumes, which can contain human papillomavirus (HPV) and other viruses, or potent carcinogens, and lung irritants. Plumes of viral infection can cause laryngeal papilloma. Surgical plumes have contents similar to other smoke plumes, including carbon monoxide, polyaromatic hydrocarbons, and a variety of toxic gases. As such, they can produce upper respiratory irritation and have in vitro mutagenic potential. Smoke evacuator contains a filter to adsorb these particulate matters
- Smoke evacuator should have specific attributes, such as suction unit or pump, filter, hose, and inlet nozzle. The capture velocity should be about 100–150 feet per minute at the inlet nozzle. The filter should be high-efficiency particulate air filter (HEPA). The inlet nozzle should be held about 2 inches above the operation site

Safe Operation Practices and Emergency Protocols

These have been discussed in several publications and should include the tips mentioned in **Box 3**.

Fire Precautions

- The CO_2 laser presents a higher risk for ignition of dry and inflammable materials, and appropriate precautions should be taken when necessary, such as the use of moistened towels or sponges to drape the perimeter of laser treatment areas, and avoiding or protecting hair lines that might have hair spray or inflammable prep solutions dried in the hair line. Staff should be aware of the location of office fire extinguishers.
- A fire extinguisher with Indian Standards Institution (ISI) mark should be available. The dry chemical type is most common for general office use. For surgical areas, consider a nonresidue-type fire extinguisher such as Halon or carbon dioxide.

TIPS FOR SAFE LASER PRACTICE[24-26]

The tips mentioned in **Box 4** should be followed for safe laser practice.

BOX 4: Tips for safe laser practice.

- Reflective jewelry worn by the operator and the patient should be removed before the treatment is commenced
- Other dermatological procedures and activities must not take place in the laser theater while the laser is in use
- When the laser is used, the number of persons in the room shall be kept to a minimum
- The operator should be careful to avoid reflections of the beam from reflecting objects close to the beam path and pay particular attention to the possibility of exposure of their own skin to the laser
- Whenever the laser is not under use, it must be switched off and the key withdrawn and placed in safe custody by the authorized operator
- Lasers should be checked for proper operation and test fired prior to each procedure
- The laser should be placed in the standby mode whenever it is not being fired, to prevent accidental firing into the field, prevent accidental fires, and preclude accidents that could occur if the laser and other foot pedals are confused and fired during a procedure
- Except the operator, the person applying the laser to the skin, no other person should control the laser foot pedal or hand switch.
- The laser foot pedal should be situated separately from other foot pedals such as electrosurgery or microscope controls
- If oxygen is to be administered within laser theater, in an emergency, minimum concentration of oxygen, preferably below 40%, should be used to oxygenate the patient with a laser-resistant oxygen chamber.

LASER EYE-PROTECTION EVIDENCE LEVEL B

Lasers have been classified by wavelength and output power into four classes from class 1 (no hazard during normal use) to class 4 (severe hazard for eyes and skin). Medical lasers belong to class 3B and 4, lasers requiring eye protection.[18,27-32] Appropriate protective eyewear is required for all persons within the laser procedure room, during laser use. The IPL (though not a laser) will also require appropriate safety glasses to be worn by personnel within the room.[24] Safety glasses or filters cannot offer eye protection against a direct, close-range impact through the safety material into the eyes. Laser operator will, therefore, not point the laser or fiber directly at any person's face. The laser fiber will always be handled as a "loaded gun" and pointed in a safe direction in the event of an accidental firing. Specific guidelines for the use of eye protection are shown in **Box 5**.

ACCIDENT PROCEDURE

Proper guidelines must be in place in case of accidents, which are outlined in **Box 6**.

DERMATOSURGICAL OPERATION THEATER GUIDELINES

Surgical laser procedures like CO_2 laser or erbium-doped yttrium-aluminum-garnet (Er:YAG) laser, and full face resurfacing where relatively more raw area is expected, should preferably done in dermatosurgical minor theater. Indian Association of Dermatologists, Venereologists and Leprologists (IADVL) guidelines on dermatosurgery theater provide details on this subject and may be referred.[33]

BOX 5: Specific guidelines for the use of eye protection.

- The safety glasses must be specific to the wavelength of the laser being used
- Protective eyewear should be labeled according to the optical density and wavelengths filtered **(Table 2)**
- Safety glasses for the IPL unit should be the generic IPL safety eyewear or the more specific "light-speed" eyewear
- Eyewear and filters should be without defects. Frames should not be broken and separated from the lenses. Side shields, if optionally used, should be in place, and no scratches should be on the front lenses.
- A wet gauze should be wrapped on and around the eyes when laser is used near the eyes
- Goggles should be adequately cleaned between treatments
- *Internal eye shield:* In the event that the laser must be used directly on the eyelid or within the bony orbit of the eye, appropriate laser safety eye shields will be placed between the lid and eye to provide protection. Internal eye shields are metallic and laser opaque. Xylocaine drops are essential for anesthesia
- If an actual or suspected incident of eye exposure to laser happens, an eye examination should be carried out within 24 hours by an ophthalmologist

(IPL: intense pulse light)

TABLE 2: Selecting laser safety glass.

Common lasers used	*OD goggles for treating physician*	*OD goggles for patients*
Excimer	7	7
IPL/Leo 320	3	5
IPL/Leo 420	3	5
IPL/Leo 540	3	5
IPL/Leo 570	3	5
IPL/Leo 650	3	5
ST (infrared laser)	3	5
LP 1064: Nd:YAG	>7	>7
QS Nd:YAG	>7	>7
Erbium:YAG	6	6
Pixel Erbium:YAG	6	6
Light sheer diode	6	6
Soprano	6	6

(IPL: intense pulse light; OD: optical density; LP: long pulsed; Nd: neodymium; QS: Q-switched; ST: surgical tool; YAG: yttrium–aluminum–garnet)

BOX 6: Guidelines for accident procedure.

There should be periodic review training of staff with respect to:
- Power failure protocol
- Fire protocol
- Employees should know the location of fire extinguishers, evacuation procedures, and whom to call
- Adequacy of sterilization
- Periodic checking of autoclave function
- Availability and currency of medical supplies
- Proper functioning of all monitoring equipment
- Items are periodically turned on and tested

ACKNOWLEDGMENT

The author sincerely thanks Dr Niteen Vishwanath Dhepe, MD Dermatology, of Pune for his help with the journal article[4] and the chapter in the previous edition.

REFERENCES

1. Husain Z, Alster TS. The role of lasers and intense pulsed light technology in dermatology. Clin Cosmet Investig Dermatol. 2016;9:29-40.
2. Smalley PJ. Keys to building a safe and effective healthcare laser program. Laser Ther. 2018;27(1):11-20.
3. El Arabi Y, Hali F, Chiheb S. Laser Management and Safety in Dermatology. Cureus. 2022;14(6):e25991.
4. Dhepe N. Minimum standard guidelines of care on requirements for setting up a laser room. Indian J Dermatol Venereol Leprol. 2009;75:10110.
5. Alster TS (Ed). Getting started: Setting up a laser practice. Manual of Cutaneous Laser Techniques, 2nd edition. Philadelphia: Lippincott, Williams and Wilkins; 2000. pp. 24.
6. Dover JS, Arndt KA, Dinehart SM, Fitzpatrick RE, Gonzalez E. Guidelines of care for laser surgery. American Academy of Dermatology. Guidelines/Outcomes Committee. J Am Acad Dermatol. 1999;41:48495.
7. Drake LA, Ceilley RI, Cornelison RL, Dinehart SM, Dorner W, Goltz RW, et al. Guidelines of care for office surgical facilities. Part II. Self-Assessment checklist. American Academy of Dermatology. J Am Acad Dermatol. 1995;33:26570.
8. Hayman MR. Accreditation of the officebased surgical facility. Bull Am Coll Surg. 1995;80(8):811.
9. Alam M. Who is qualified to perform laser surgery and in what setting? Semin Plast Surg. 2007;21(3):193200.
10. Lomando K, Faulconer DR. A workable plan for OR quality assurance. AORN J. 1982;35(7):12915.
11. Olson R. Continuous power to the OR and other critical care areas. Dimens Health Serv. 1975;52(2):2930.
12. Beck WC. Lighting the surgical suite. Contemp Surg. 1978; 12:913.
13. Kerr DR, Malhotra IV. Electrical design and safety in the operating room and intensive care unit. Int Anesthesiol Clin. 1981;19(2):2748.
14. Klebanoff G. Operating room design. Bull Am Coll Surg. 1979;64:610.
15. Bennett RG (Ed). Fundamentals of Cutaneous Surgery. St Louis, Missouri: Mosby; 1988. pp. 18193.
16. Garner JS, Favero MS. Hospital Infections Program Center for Infectious Diseases, Centers for Disease Control and Prevention. (1985). Antiseptics, handwashing, and handwashing facilities. [online] Available from wonder.cdc.gov/wonder/prevguid/p0000412/p0000412.asp [Last accessed__].
17. Centers for Disease Control. Morbidity Mortality Weekly Report. (1987). Recommendations for prevention of HIV transmission in healthcare settings. [online] Available from https://www.cdc.gov/mmwr/preview/mmwrhtml/00023587.htm [Last accessed February, 2024].
18. Simmons BP. CDC guidelines for the prevention and control of nosocomial infections. Guideline for hospital environmental control. Am J Infect Control. 1983;11 (3):97-120.
19. Stegman SJ, Tromovitch TA, Glogau RG. Basics of Dermatologic Surgery. Chicago: Year Book Medical Publishers; 1982. pp. 122.
20. Yakel ME, Cummins RO (Eds). Illustrated Textbook of Advanced Cardiac Life Support, 2nd edition. Dallas: American Heart Association; 1994. p. 267.
21. Gilbert DA, Adamson JE. Procedure manuals in office surgery. Clin Plast Surg. 1983;10(2):269-72.
22. Holzman RS, Cullen DJ, Eichhorn JH, Philip JH. Guidelines for sedation by nonanesthesiologists during diagnostic and therapeutic procedures. J Clin Anesth. 1994;6(4):26576.
23. American Medical Association. Standards and guidelines for cardiopulmonary resuscitation (CPR) and emergency cardiac care (ECC). JAMA. 1986;255(21):290584.
24. United States Department of Labor. Occupational Safety and Health Administration. OSHA Technical Manual. [online] Available from https://sites.ecse.rpi.edu/Courses/CStudio/ham_radio_docs/OSHA%20Technical%20Manual%20(OTM)%20_%20Section%20III_%20Chapter%206%20-%20Laser%20Hazards.pdf [Last accessed February, 2024].
25. Sebben JE. Survey of sterile technique used by dermatologic surgeons. J Am Acad Dermatol. 1988;18:110713.
26. Sebben JE. Surgical antiseptics. J Am Acad Dermatol. 1983;9(5):75965.
27. Chuang LH, Lai CC, Yang KJ, Chen TL, Ku WC. A traumatic macular hole secondary to a highenergy Nd:YAG laser. Ophthalmic Surg Lasers. 2001;32(1):73-6.
28. Elias B. (2005). CRS Report for Congress. Lasers aimed at aircraft cockpits: Background and possible options to address the threat to aviation safety and security. [online] Available from www.fas.org/sgp/crs/RS22033.pdf [Last accessed February, 2024].
29. Breitenbach RA, Swisher PK, Kim MK, Patel BS. The photic sneeze reflex as a risk factor to combat pilots. Mil Med. 1993;158(12):806-9.
30. van Norren D, Keunen JE, Vos JJ. [The laser pointer: no demonstrated danger to the eyes.] Ned Tijdschr Geneeskd. 1998;142(36):197982.
31. Mainster MA, Stuck BE, Brown J Jr. Assessment of alleged retinal laser injuries. Arch Ophthalmol. 2004;122(8):12107.
32. Tobin HA, Lee DR, Stewart G (Eds). Designing the facility. Ambulatory surgery and office procedures in head and neck surgery. Orlando, FL: Grune and Stratton; 1986. pp. 30314.
33. Rajendran SC, Omprakash HM. Standard guidelines for setting up a dermatosurgery theatre. Indian J Dermatol Venereol Leprol. 2009;75:7682.

CHAPTER 106 Laser Hair Reduction: Basic Principles Including Principles of Diode Laser

Sandeep Arora, Gulhima Arora, Pankaj Das

KEY MESSAGES

- Laser light works on the basic principle of "selective photothermolysis."
- Melanin in the hair follicle acts as the chromophore or the selective target for laser hair removal.
- Laser destroys hair by different mechanisms such as photothermal, photomechanical, and photochemical destruction.
- Wavelength, fluence, and pulse duration are the key determining factors for laser efficacy.
- Ideal laser for hair removal would be one with longer wavelength and with sufficient fluence to specifically damage the deep placed hair follicle target but causing lesser collateral tissue and epidermal melanin damage, especially required for Fitzpatrick skin type III–V.
- Extended theory of selective photothermolysis infers that non-uniformly pigmented targets (other than chromophores) can be treated by using pulse width significantly longer than the thermal relaxation time of that tissue. The laser light, by heat diffusion from the target absorber, which is the melanin containing hair matrix cells, thus will also damage the stem cells in the non-pigmented bulge of the pilosebaceous unit.
- Patients must be counseled regarding the scope and realistic outcome of laser hair reduction.
- The ideal patient has thick dark terminal hair, white skin, and a normal hormonal status.
- Photothermal destruction of hair follicles constitutes the fundamental concept of hair removal with red and near-infrared wavelengths suitable for targeting follicular and hair shaft melanin.

INTRODUCTION

Laser- and light-assisted epilation is now established as the standard of care for removal of "unwanted hair."[1,2] Just as any other laser device the principle of "selective photothermolysis," initially introduced by Anderson and Parish in 1983, here, utilizes melanin as its chromophore for hair removal by employing laser light of specific wavelength and sufficient fluence with pulse duration shorter than the thermal relaxation time of the melanocyte.[3,4]

HISTORY OF LASERS FOR HAIR REMOVAL

Traditional physical methods of hair removal such as waxing, epilation, shaving, and tweezing have been in use for a long time. Ancient Egyptians used sugaring techniques and Persians popularized "Bande Abru" or threading for removal of unwanted hair.[5,6] Hair growth retardants and removal methods in history also describe used of walnut oil, vinegar, arsenic sulfide, quicklime, starch, and dried feline feces.[7] Radiograph machines known as the Tricho machines were also used but went out of vogue due to malignancies they induced.[8,9] Electrolysis as a treatment modality was the main method of hair removal before introduction of lase hair removal and is still being used because of its utility in doing away with gray hair, however, it has largely been replaced with optical devices. Laser hair reduction was an accidental discovery when Dover et al. in 1989 observed in guinea pigs that, during tattoo removal by Q-switched ruby laser, the hair shaft in the site vaporized and the root bleached with some reduction in number in a few days **(Fig. 1)**.[10]

Almost all dermatology lasers have been used for taking care of excess hair.[1] Optical devices used in hair removal include Ruby laser, long-pulsed Alexandrite laser (755 nm), pulsed diode laser (800 nm), and long-pulsed neodymium-doped yttrium aluminum garnet (Nd:YAG) (1,064 nm) as well as Intense Pulse Light sources (IPL). Goldberg used Q-switched Nd:YAG with prior application of carbon-based solution by in 1995.[11] Laser technologies have evolved with larger spot size, and better skin cooling to prevent burns.[12] All lasers required multiple sessions for hair reduction and

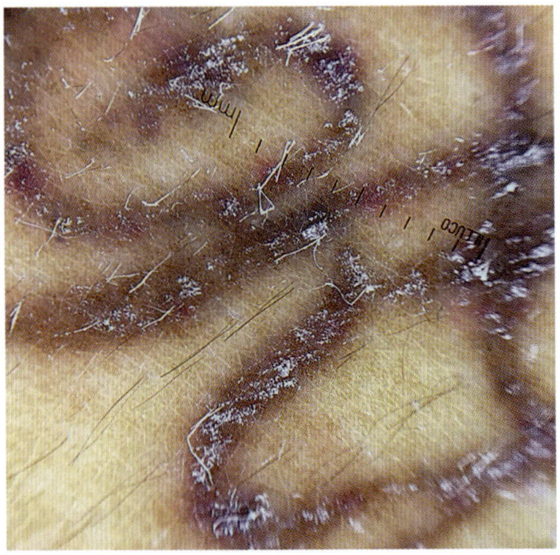

Fig. 1: Q-switched Nd:YAG-induced leukotrichia of hair overlying tattoo.

on an average achieve about 50% reduction in hair growth.[13] In 1997, the hair reduction saw the entry of intense pulsed light (IPL) technology, broadband light devices which were more economical and had a larger spot size. The next major advance in laser hair reduction was in 2004, when laser and radiofrequency energy were combined to target the hair [electro-optical synergy (ELOS) technology].[14] Here, first the hair was heated by laser from inside out—hair shaft to external root sheath—to destroy the stem cells. This was followed by bipolar radiofrequency current delivered to the hair, to heat the hair from the root sheath inward to shaft. This synergy has theoretical advantages such as use of less laser energy and probability of targeting gray and thin hair because the radiofrequency energy, unlike light is color blind. Sadick and Shoul demonstrated a mean 75% reduction in hair count at the end of one year and 40% reduction in white hair count.[15]

DEFINITION OF LASER HAIR REMOVAL

Temporary hair reduction was earlier defined as a delay in hair growth with a 30% decrease lasting 1–3 months.[16] However, this does not translate to permanent hair reduction as it is only consistent with induction of the telogen phase. Temporary hair removal methods such as manual plucking, shaving, waxing, and use of chemical depilatories are only partially effective and in addition cause irritation and pain.[17,18] Permanent hair reduction refers to a significant reduction in the number of terminal hairs after a given treatment, which is stable for a period of time longer than the complete growth cycle of hair follicles at the given body site. It has recently been suggested to add another 6 months to this post-treatment observation time (i.e. the time necessary for a damaged follicle to recover from the laser injury and re-enter a normal growth cycle).[19]

A distinction needs to be made between permanent and complete hair loss. Complete hair loss refers to a lack of regrowing hairs (i.e., a significant reduction in the number of regrowing hairs to zero), which may be either temporary or permanent. Laser treatment usually produces complete but temporary hair loss for 1–3 months, followed by partial but permanent hair loss. Histologically, hair follicles with large, pigmented shafts are damaged more than the hair follicles with small (<25 mm) hypopigmented shafts. Electrolysis is one method for long-lasting hair removal, but is tedious, painful, can result in epidermal side effects and associated with as much as 50% hair regrowth.[20,21]

> Permanent laser hair reduction does not mean—hair will never regrow forever, but for a period equal to or longer than the anagen-telogen phase of growth for the given site.[22]

PHYSICS OF LASER REMOVAL

Relevant Hair Anatomy

With the exceptions of the palms and soles, hair follicles are found over almost the entire body surface area and are approximately 5 million in number for any given person. Factors such as density of hair and variations in color and texture need to be considered when deciding for laser hair removal procedures.

Adult hair is primarily of two types—vellus and terminal. They differ in the amount of pigment, diameter, and depth. Terminal hair is the more darkly pigmented, coarser, with bulb depths at 2–7 mm and longer, found on the scalp, axilla, and groin as also on the moustache, beard and chest area in males while vellus hair are very lightly pigmented, fine and short hair with bulb depths within 1 mm in the skin, found over almost the entire body, except areas such as palms and soles which are devoid of hair. Eyebrows and eyelash hair have characteristics in between terminal and vellus. An individual follicle may shift production from vellus to terminal or otherwise as at puberty or androgenetic alopecia and the bulge maintains a constant depth into the skin.[23]

The hair follicle has traditionally been described in terms of three distinct anatomic units—the infundibulum, the isthmus, and the inferior segment that includes the hair bulb. Located in close proximity and largely enveloped by the hair bulb is the dermal or follicular papilla[24] **(Fig. 2)**. The hair bulb consists of matricial cells with melanocytes.

Trichogenic Stem Cells and Follicular Growth Centers

Hair follicle stem cell niche (HFSC) consists of the traditionally described hair bulb region containing the dividing matrix cells which give rise to the hair shaft and inner root sheath as well as numerous other components which play a part in its activation and rest **(Fig. 3)**.[25-27]

Melanocytes are present in the bulb region as well as the outer root sheath which gives the hair shaft its color. The area of the bulge at the lower end of isthmus at the attachment of the arrector pilorum muscle contains the pluripotent stem cells in the outer root sheath which give rise to the hair bulb and thus a new hair follicle. Although the bulge cells are the main contributors of these stem cells additional stem cells along the hair follicle play a part in the hair cycle **(Fig. 4)**.[28] These cells are not pigmented and reside at some distance from the pigmented hair shaft. Destruction of these stem cell components is essential for laser hair removal.[29] However, targeting the entire hair follicle growth apparatus to effect permanent hair removal is hence a complex issue as is evidenced by the HFSC.

Hair Color

Terminal hair, their hair shaft and bulb matrix in the anagen phase of hair cycle contain melanin.

Melanin is the light-absorbing target chromophore for laser treatment with an absorption spectrum of 250–1,200 nm.[27] Eumelanin (brown black) and phaeomelanin (red) differ in

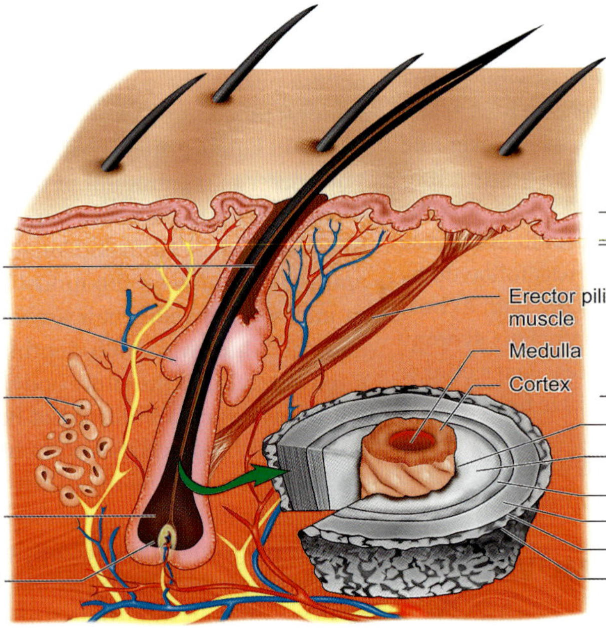

Fig. 2: Anatomy of the hair follicle—longitudinal and cross-section.

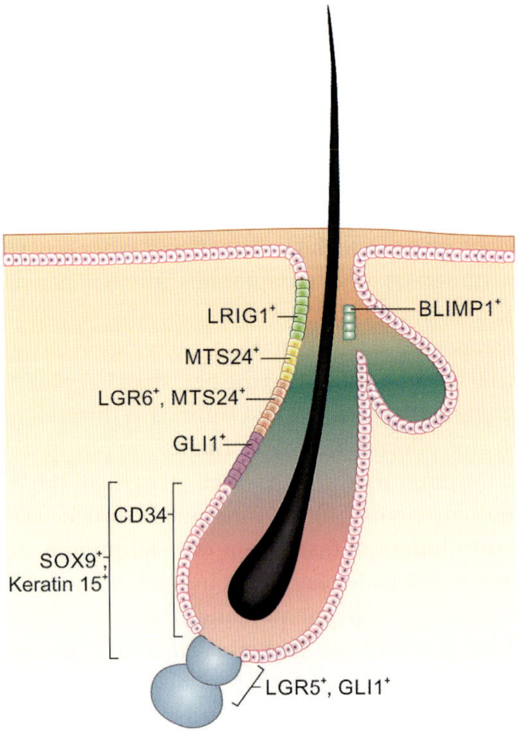

Fig. 3: Follicular stem cells.

their optical properties, pheomelanin absorbing 30 times lesser laser energy at 694 nm.[30] Hair color varies with the type and content of its melanin—highly melanized eumelanosomes produce black or dark brown hair, incomplete melanization of melanosomes results in blond hair, fewer number of melanocytes and poor melanization is seen in gray hair while white hair contain vacuolized areas.[31]

Laser light pulse is absorbed by the melanin present in the hair bulb matrix, thus destroying it by the generated heat. The surrounding nonpigmented tissue is spared from direct thermal injury. However, the higher levels of epidermal melanin in persons with darker skin compete with the hair root melanin for the laser light and can cause side effects such as burns, blistering, or pigmentary changes.

As the non-pigmented bulge of the hair follicle which also contains the stem cells does not absorb this laser light pulse, heat diffusion from the light absorbing melanin to the bulge area will be required to destroy it and result in effective permanent hair follicle destruction. Thus, lasers need to use optimal wavelength, pulse duration, and fluence for effective hair removal with least side effects.

Hair Growth Cycle: Phases

Adult hair has three distinct phases of development: (1) Anagen, (2) Catagen, and (3) Telogen **(Fig. 5)**.

Anagen

Active hair growth takes place in this phase, whereby follicular matrix cells actively divide to produce the hair follicle. Hair in only this anagen phase contains the melanin pigment. The growing anagen hair consists of all histologic divisions and the sequence of events is quite similar to those of fetal development.

Proanagen

Stage 1: Secondary germ cells at base of epithelial sac show mitosis.

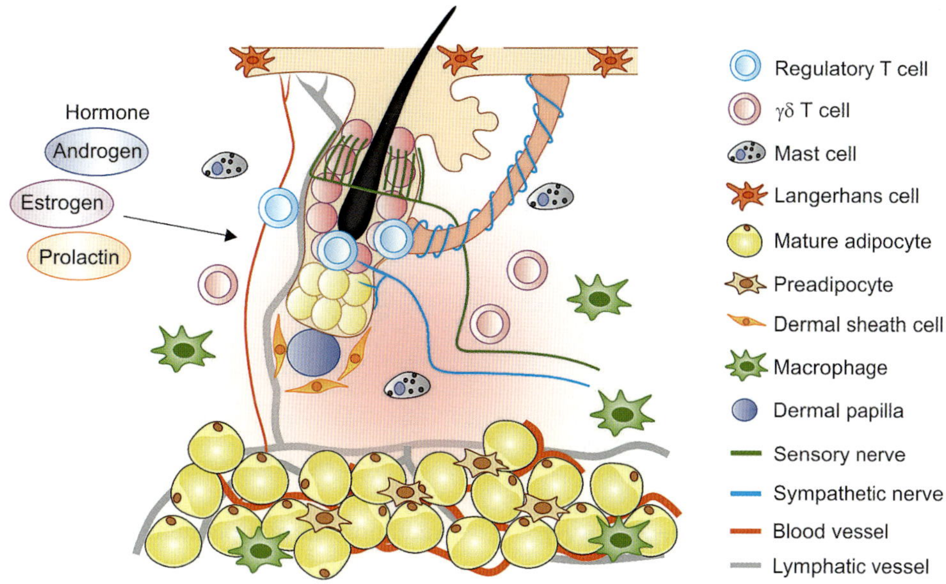

Fig. 4: Hair follicle stem cell niche.

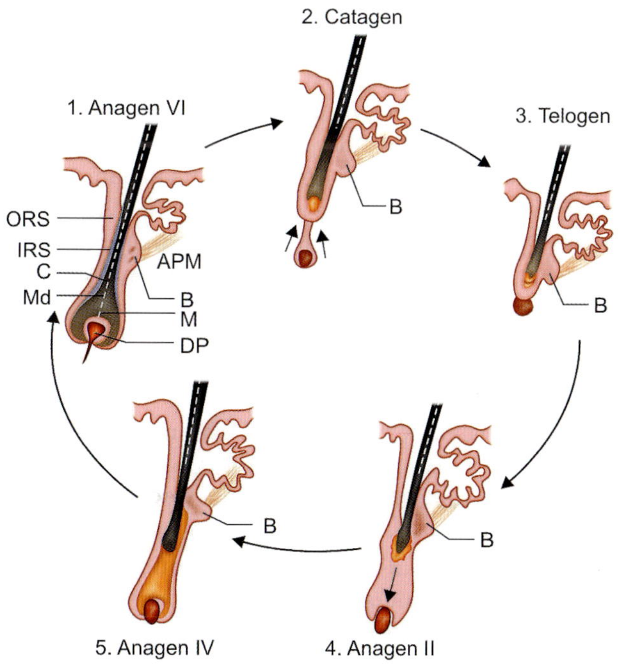

Fig. 5: Hair growth cycle—anagen, catagen, and telogen phases.

Stage 2: Grow down to enclose dermal papilla.

Stage 3: Differentiation into layers of hair shaft and inner root sheath.

Stage 4: Melanocytes form melanin.

Metanagen

Stage 5: Hair emerges from the cone of the outer root sheath to reach surface, extruding earlier telogen club hair.

Stage 6: Till onset of catagen.

Catagen

Catagen is the regression phase, where the matrix cells degenerate and the bulb begins to atrophy, causing the hair follicle to shrink.

Telogen

Telogen is the final resting phase of the hair follicle. Growth of the hair stops, and the follicle contains only the superficial components, the infundibulum, and the isthmus. The hair follicle in the telogen phase does not contain the target melanin pigment.

Exogen

Exogen is the phase which follows telogen where the hair is released from its attachment within the follicle and is extruded out.

Anagen phase of the next hair cycle thereafter begins again to form a new hair.

The length of time spent in each phase depends upon the location of the hair on the body. On the scalp, hair follicles spend up to 10 years in anagen, but on the trunk, brow, and limbs, anagen lasts no longer than 6 months. Catagen lasts only for 2–3 weeks, and telogen lasts for 3–4 months **(Table 1)**.

Approximately 85–90% of hair is in the anagen phase at any given time and as the hair contain melanin only in the anagen phase of development, only these are susceptible to injury during a session of laser-assisted hair removal.

Thus, multiple treatments are necessary to treat all hair follicles on a given body surface area.

Duration of the anagen and telogen phases varies considerably from one anatomic site to another[32] **(Table 1)**.

TABLE 1: Duration of human hair cycles.

Body area	*Anagen*	*Telogen (months)*	*% Telogen*
Scalp	2–6 years	3–4	10–15
Eyelashes	1–1.5 months	–	–
Eyebrows	1–2 months	3–4	85–94
Moustache	2–5 months	1.5	34
Beard	1 year	2.5	–
Chest	–	2.5	–
Axillae	–	–	31–79
Arms	1–3 months	2–4	72–86
Thighs	1–2 months	2–3	64–83
Legs	4–6 months	3–6	62–88
Pubic hair	–	–	65–81

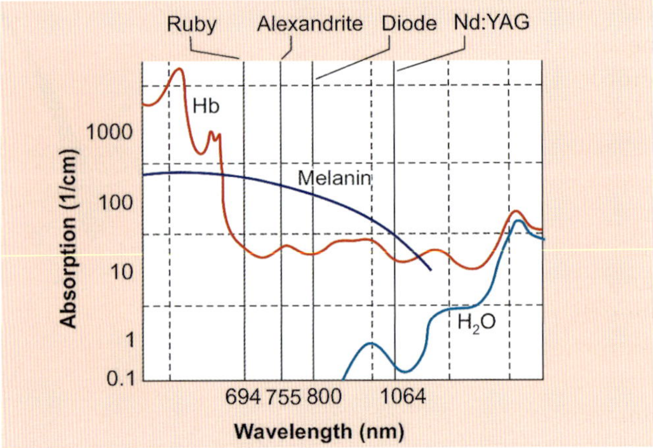

Fig. 6: Wavelength of different laser medium.

Laser-tissue Interactions and Principle of Laser Hair Removal

The interaction of laser energy with tissue depends upon many factors:[33,34]

Energy: Ability of laser to do its work [joules (J)].

Fluence (energy density): Amount of energy applied to unit area of target tissue (joules/cm^2).

Power: Time rate at which energy is emitted by laser. Watts (joules/second).

Power density or irradiance: Power applied per unit area (watts/cm^2).

Laser energy is emitted in continuous wave manner (CW) or in pulse mode.

Laser-hair interactions occur by different mechanisms—photothermal, photomechanical, and photochemical destruction.

Photothermal Destruction

Photothermal destruction is based on the principle of selective photothermolysis.[35] According to this principle, selective damage of a target will take place if enough energy is directed at a wavelength well absorbed by the target in a time frame less than or equal to the Thermal Relaxation Time (TRT) of the target. This TRT is the time taken by the target for to cool to half of its baseline temperature and transfer the heat to its neighboring tissue.[36] This principle is used to selectively damage the target (e.g., hair follicle) while sparing the adjacent tissues. In context of laser hair reduction, the chromophore which absorbs the laser is melanin. The selective targets identified thus far for hair, are either melanin or an exogenous substance,[37] topically applied and absorbed down the follicle. Melanin is found in the anagen hair bulb, the hair shaft, and parts of the outer root sheath. The limiting factors in selecting melanin in laser hair removal are absorptive interference by epidermal melanin and variable hair pigmentation. In addition, the non-pigmented bulge area which contains the stem cells and is located at a distance away from the melanotic target of hair follicle also needs to be targeted for permanent hair removal. To overcome this the concept of thermal damage time (TDT) was proposed wherein the hair follicle were treated for longer than TRT for 200–1,000 ms at fluences up to 115 J/cm^2, ensuring enough time for thermal denaturation of the target proteins.[38,39]

Proper selection of certain laser parameters such as wavelength, fluence, and pulse duration needs to be adhered to in order to cause thermal damage to the melanin of hair follicle root and also the bulge area and at the same time to decrease the competition from the epidermal melanin in absorbing the laser light or causing epidermal adverse effects, especially in darker skin.

Wavelength

Wavelengths ranging between 600 and 1,000 nm of the electromagnetic spectrum can penetrate to the appropriate depth of the dermis (up to 2–4 mm) and cause selective photothermolysis of the target chromophore, it being the melanin pigment of hair follicle **(Fig. 6)**. This is within the "optical window" in which selective absorption by melanin is coupled with deep penetration of laser energy.[40]

Pulse Duration

It is the time of exposure of the tissue to laser or light energy.

Thermal Relaxation Time

Thermal relaxation time is the time required for the tissue to cool to half the temperature achieved after laser exposure.[36] TRT of terminal hair is estimated to be between 10 and 100 ms and that of the epidermis is between 3 and 10 ms. Thus, when we choose the pulse duration of the laser beam to be shorter or equal to the TRT of hair and longer than the TRT of epidermis, hair follicle will remain heated while the epidermis cools down, protecting the epidermal melanocytes. A further corollary of the principle of selective photothermolysis is the principle of "thermokinetic selectivity."[40] This proposes that for a particular chromophore, a longer pulse duration allows swifter intra-pulse cooling of smaller targets than the larger targets. In simple words, larger targets such as hair follicles can be selectively battered more with the help of lasers than the smaller targets of the same chromophore, i.e., epidermis. Theory of "selective photothermolysis" is applicable when the treated target for destruction and the chromophore occupies the same area. However, this becomes inapplicable when the target is a non-uniformly pigmented structure, such as the hair follicle and when the highly pigmented "absorber," and the weakly absorbing "target" are located at a distance. The hair follicle consists of the highly absorbing melanin present in the hair shaft and matrix cells (absorber) and the non-pigmented bulge area of isthmus containing the stem cells (target) which exhibits weak or no absorption and which is located at a distance. The distant target is destroyed by heat diffusion from the absorber and not by direct heating. This will destroy the entire target and thus help to achieve not just hair growth delay but also permanent hair follicle damage. Thus, another theory (Extended Theory of Selective Photothermolysis) was formulated which provided new rationale.[41]

Thermal damage time is the time required for irreversible damage to the outermost part of the target by heat diffusion from the primary absorber with sparing of the surrounding tissue and is significantly longer than the TRT of the target.[39] Thus, the optimal pulse width needs to be shorter or equal to TDT and significantly longer than the target TRT (>100 ms), in contrast to earlier theory of selective photothermolysis.

The wavelength should be chosen to maximize the contrast between the absorption coefficient of the pigmented area and that of the tissue surrounding the target in order to decrease the collateral damage, similar to the earlier theory.

Importance of Shape and Geometry in Heat Diffusion[42]

Heat diffusion from the absorber to the target is strongly dependent on the shape and geometry of the whole target structure. When the three basic geometries: planar, cylindrical, and spherical were studied, TDT/TRT ratio differed greatly, with TDT being several times higher than TRT for a plane dimension, less for a cylindrically shaped and least for a spherical-shaped target. For the same TDT/TRT, the size of the damaged zone and thus the risk of unselective damage are maximal for a plane target and smallest and localized for a spherical shape. Hair bulb is spherical, shaft is cylindrical and epidermis plane. Sphere absorbs maximum heat and also retains it for maximum time, followed by cylinder and then plane; thus, establishing a gradient of heat from the sphere (the bulb) toward epidermis (which is the plane) through the cylinder (the shaft). This gradient is further enhanced by epidermal cooling. This gradient helps diffusion of heat

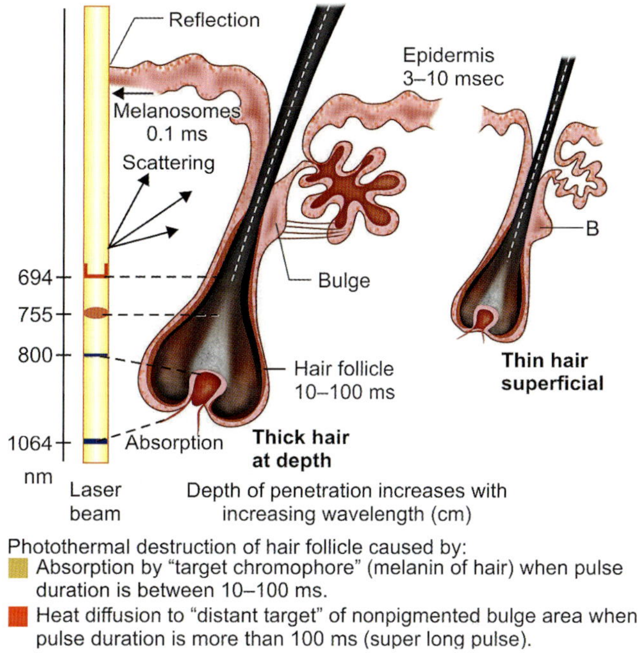

Fig. 7: Laser-tissue interaction depending on wavelength and pulse duration.

from bulb (which houses maximum chromophore) to the bulge which has least chromophore but has the target to be destroyed **(Fig. 7)**.

Fluence

Highest tolerable fluence will give better results by causing effective thermal destruction of hair follicle melanin in the dermis but heat damage to the epidermal melanin, which acts as an innocent bystander, may result in adverse effects of burns, blistering, dyspigmentation, and scarring, particularly in dark-skinned individuals. To reduce this risk, deeper penetrating wavelength and optimal fluence need to be used. The ideal fluence is one which produces perifollicular erythema and edema. However, this end point may be fallacious and difficult to appreciate in darker skin.[43] Lower fluences lead to temporary hair reduction by effecting a shift to telogen from anagen. The use of long pulses and cooling of the epidermis before, during, and after the procedure further enhances safety.

Spot Size

Larger the spot size of the laser beam, deeper is the penetration and lesser is the scattering **(Fig. 8)**. The spot size should be larger than the desired depth of penetration, ideally between 5 and 10 mm. Hence it is useful to increase the spot size rather than fluence in case of ineffective treatment. Dermal collagen causes light to scatter as it traverses the deeper layers into the dermis. A larger spot size ensures photons shall scatter back into the incident beam with the resultant beam delivering greater energy at any given depth.[44,45]

Cooling/Minimizing Epidermal Thermal Damage

When treating dark-skinned patients with lasers, the risk of epidermal damage limits their use as the fluence thresholds for efficacy and epidermal damage were close even in fairer skin. With the advent of cooling, it is possible to decrease this risk of epidermal thermal damage, while delivering energy to the hair follicle placed deeper in the dermis.[46]

Various cooling methods are adopted such as application of ice-pack, cold jelly, cold air by the Zimmer, short bursts of cryogen-spray, or "in built cooling device" such as chilled sapphire window integrated in the laser hand-piece.[42] This chilled sapphire lens gives the advantage of parallel cooling plus the hand-piece can be pressed against the skin. This brings the hair roots closer to the skin surface and thus increases the energy density at the hair bulb. The lens pressure also blanches the underlying blood vessels, minimizing absorption of laser energy by hemoglobin. Pneumatic skin flattening (PSF) uses vacuum-assisted probe with a sapphire window to avoid pain associated with hair removal using diode and lasers. PSF decreases intra-procedure pain as well as post-treatment edema and erythema by employing vacuum-assisted skin flattening against the tip of the hand piece. It is believed that PSF activates the pressure receptors of the skin right before the laser beam blocking the transmission of pain from the laser. Skin flattening also helps bring the hair follicles closer to the laser beam for better efficacy and blanch the dermal vessels so that hemoglobin as a chromophore absorbs minimal energy.[47,48]

Photomechanical Destruction

This occurs due to small local "explosions" from Q-switched laser pulses which are in nanoseconds.[13] These ultra-short laser pulses cause extremely rapid heat confinement at the level of melanosomes of hair follicles, generating photo-acoustic shock waves that cause photomechanical disruption of the melanocytes in the bulb but no complete follicular destruction. This principle has been used in the "Softlight" technique which uses a proprietary suspension of carbon particles applied to the skin followed by Q-switched Nd:YAG laser light (1,064 nm) treatment, with relatively low energy, higher frequency, and larger spot size.

Photochemical Destruction[49]

A photosensitizer is used prior to the use of light to produce a targeted photochemical reaction and therapeutic effect. Aminolevulinic acid, carbon particles, or lipid encapsulated melanin,[37,50] have been used as exogenous chromophores with the aim to target non-pigmented hair. However, at best they cause short term hair reduction and are not very effective.[51] They have been used primarily for white hair or fine hair.[52]

INDICATIONS FOR LASER HAIR REMOVAL[53]

What defines excessive hair growth is at best reductio ad absurdum! The dermatologist must determine if the hair growth is constitutional to the individual hence not needing any additional investigations or has an organic cause which must be addressed before laser hair removal is undertaken, lest it results in ineffective or failure of treatment. The indications where in a patient may report for hair removal are:

- Removal of unwanted hair because of cosmetic disfigurement.
- Facial or body hair in excess of the cultural norm can be distressing to some people, women as well as men **(Figs. 9 and 10)**.
- Hypertrichosis is an increase in hair growth that is not androgen dependent **(Figs. 11A and B)**.
- Hirsutism is characterized by growth of terminal hair in women on androgen-dependent areas of the body such as upper lip, chin, or chest. It may be accompanied by seborrhea, acne, androgenetic alopecia, and acanthosis nigricans due to androgen excess **(Figs. 12A and B)**. Evaluation of hirsutism needs ruling out hyperandrogenism, and polycystic ovarian disease or presence of an androgen secreting neoplasm amongst other causes **(Table 2)**.[54] It must also be distinguished from hypertrichosis **(Table 3)**.

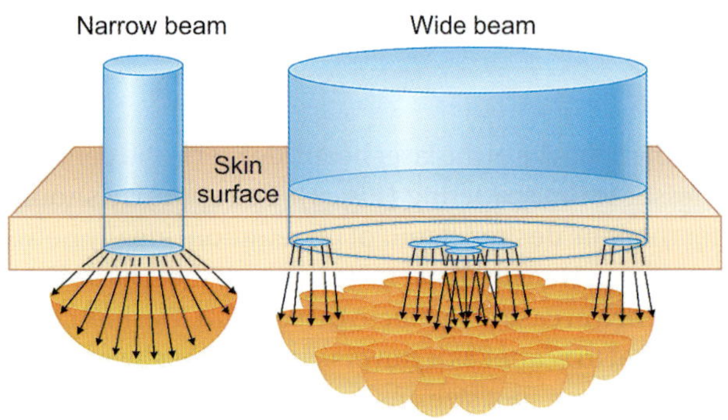

Fig. 8: Effect of spot size on the delivery of laser energy.

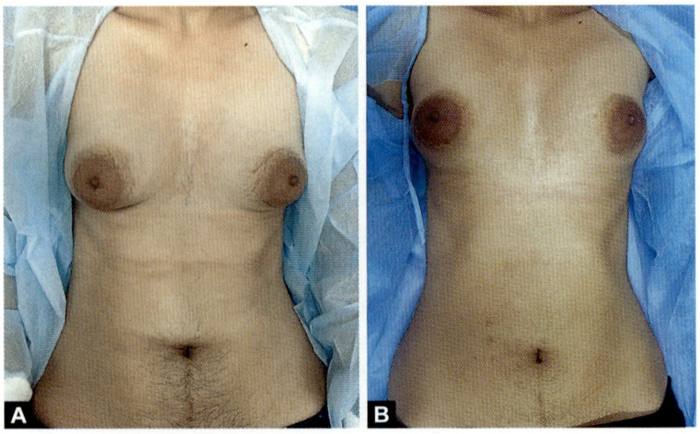

Figs. 9A and B: Excess hair treated with diode laser after three sessions (right).

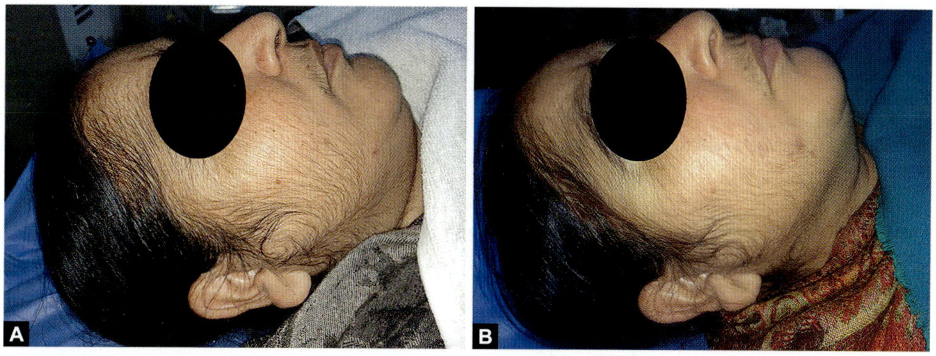

Figs. 10A and B: Hairline reshaping in a young male with intense pulse light, after four sessions (right) using 755–1,200 nm filter.

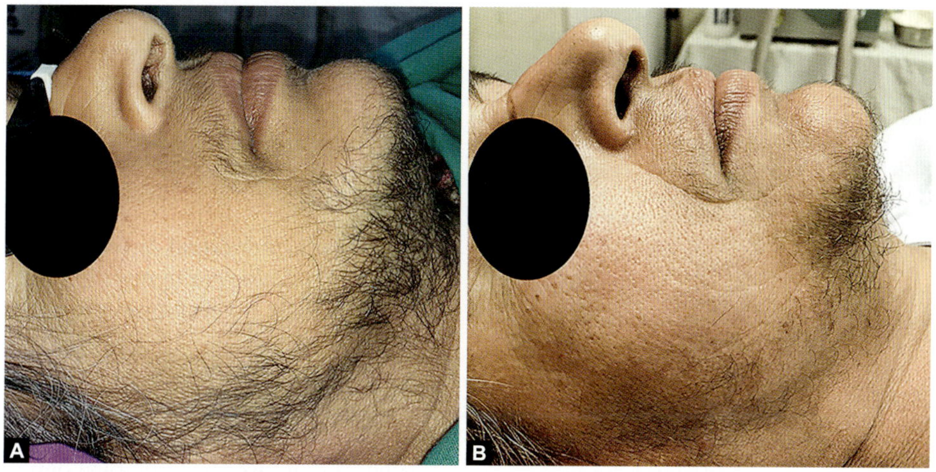

Figs. 11A and B: Persistent cyclosporine-induced hypertrichosis treated with intense pulse light two sessions (right) using 755–1,200 nm filter.

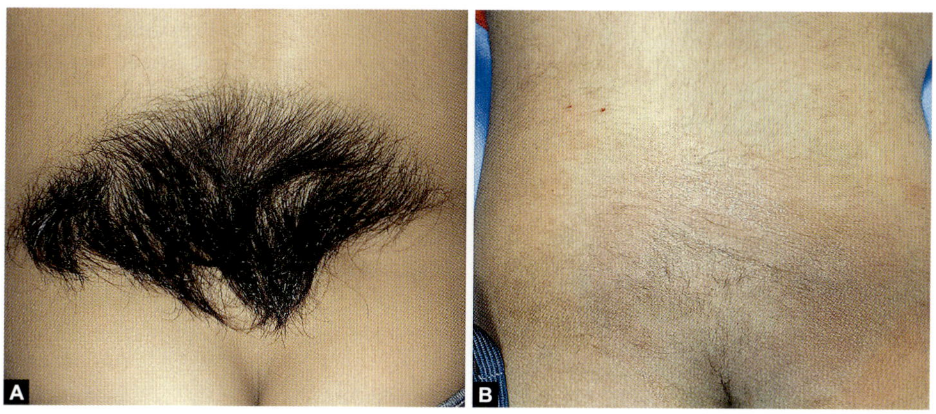

Figs. 12A and B: Idiopathic hirsutism treated with diode laser after four sessions (right).

- Removal of hair for medical treatment purpose, e.g., pseudofolliculitis barbae, pilonidal sinus, hidradenitis suppurativa, acne keloidalis nuchae, or faun tail nevi **(Figs. 13A and B)**.[55-60]
- *Hair from grafted donor site:* Hair-bearing flaps used for reconstruction of any kind may contain unwanted hair that interfere with proper function and thus need to be epilated before surgery.[61] For example, myocutaneous flaps used in urethral reconstruction may cause urinary obstruction, calcification, or infection.

CONTRAINDICATIONS

Contraindications are few.[53] There are no absolute contraindications, hence those patients with the relative contraindications below need evaluation on a case-to-case basis.

- Hair removal for aesthetic reasons is best deferred till the patient is beyond 15 years of age, to allow hormonal changes of pubertal age to settle, although there is no definite consensus of age. However, for therapeutic indications younger children have been treated and it is considered safe.[60]

- Associated photo-aggravated skin diseases and medical illness, e.g., SLE.

TABLE 2: Etiology of hirsutism and hypertrichosis.

Hirsutism[1]	*Hypertrichosis*[2]
• Adrenal • Androgen excess • Cushing syndrome • Ectopic adrenocorticotropic hormone (rare) • Congenital adrenal hyperplasia • Childhood onset adrenal hyperplasia • Delayed (adult onset) adrenal hyperplasia • Androgen secreting tumors • Adenoma • Adenocarcinoma (rare) • Adrenal nest tumors • Adrenal enzyme deficiencies • Early onset 21-hydroxylase deficiency • Late onset 21-hydroxylase deficiency • 11β hydroxylase deficiency • 3β hydroxylase deficiency • Ovarian • Polycystic ovarian disease • Theca/granulosa cell tumor • Hilar/lipoid cell tumor • Arrhenoblastoma • Gynandroblastoma • Krukenberg tumor (metastasis) • Gonadal dysgenesis • Pituitary • Cushing's disease • Hyperprolactinemia • Acromegaly • Other causes • Idiopathic hirsutism • Stress • Drugs • Anabolic steroids • Testosterone • Glucocorticoids • Cyclosporine • Minoxidil • Danazol • Phenytoin • Penicillamine	• Hypertrichosis with lanugo hair • Congenital • Acquired (paraneoplastic syndrome) • Hypertrichosis with vellus hair • *Congenital:* Ambras syndrome • *Acquired:* Drug-induced (bimatoprost) • *Hypertrichosis with terminal hair:* Congenital/localized • Congenital melanocytic nevus • Posterior cervical hypertrichosis • Faun tail • Becker's nevus • Generalized • Fetal alcohol syndrome • Fetal hydantoin syndrome • *Acquired:* – Porphyrias – Hypothyroidism – Anorexia nervosa – Malnutrition – Mucopolysaccharidoses • *Drugs:* – Acitretin – Azelaic acid – Cetirizine – Topical corticosteroids – Cyclosporine – Phenytoin

- Treatment area having active cutaneous infections or wounds, e.g., herpes labialis, staphylococci infections, etc.
- Patient having keloids and keloidal tendencies. It is recommended that these patients should be treated less aggressively. However, the treatment area should not have any keloid.
- Patient having unrealistic expectations
- Psoriasis and vitiligo patients (because of risk of koebnerization of treated area)
- Laser hair removal should be performed cautiously in patients on isotretinoin therapy.

TREATMENT APPROACH[64]

The ideal patient for laser hair removal is one who has realistic expectations, fairer skin, coarse, thick, and dark hair, and normal endocrine status.

Preprocedure

Detailed History

- Underlying endocrinal disorder
- Keloidal tendency or hypertrophic scarring
- Tendency for postinflammatory hyperpigmentation or easy bruising
- Herpes simplex infection, particularly recurrent infections
- Psoriasis or other disorders with koebnerizing potential
- *Pregnancy:* Although no scientific evidence exists to suggest that laser hair removal penetration damages the fetus treatment in pregnancy is best avoided to prevent unnecessary litigation.
- Recent sun-tan or exposure to tanning unit
- Past-treatment for hair removal; sessions, modality, or equipment used if possible.
- Drug intake

TABLE 3: Clinical differentiation hypertrichosis from hirsutism.[62,63]

Hypertrichosis	*Hirsutism*
Male and female	Only female
Independent of age	Onset at puberty or later
Terminal or vellus hairs	Terminal hair in male pattern distribution
Nonandrogen dependent	Androgen-dependent body sites

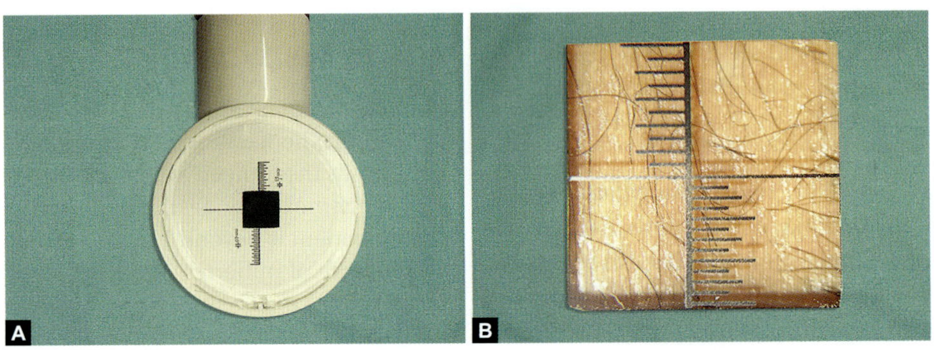

Figs. 13A and B: Faun tail nevus in a 5-year-old girl treated with intense pulse light 755–1,200 nm filter, after eight sessions (right).

Physical Examination

- Evaluation of skin and hair color, hair diameter, density, and anatomic location.
- Evaluate for tan.
- Assess hirsutism using appropriate scales.
- Assess skin response to earlier laser removal procedures particularly—post inflammatory hyperpigmentation and scarring if any.

Evaluation

- Hormonal factors should be evaluated and if necessary, a gynecologist/endocrinologist opinion should be sought.
- Graft site evaluation for healing and reconstructive surgeon review if necessary.
  - *Counseling* must include explanation of hair anatomy and growth cycle and actual method of procedure (if possible, with actual video or power point slides), likely side-effects, number of approximate sittings required, interval between two sittings, per sitting cost, results expected, need for avoiding sun exposure, etc. This counseling would have a very important role to play in making the patient more compliant, cooperative, and in having realistic expectations.
  - *Informed consent* is mandatory.

Instructions

- Patient should be instructed to avoid bleaching, plucking, electrolysis, or waxing in the treatment areas once he/she decides to start with laser hair reduction treatment.
- Sun avoidance must be practiced if laser hair removal is planned on sun-exposed sites and use of sunscreen is recommended.
  - Preprocedure photographs of treatment area should be taken, mentioning name of patient and date of photograph. They should be of good resolution and stored on both hard and soft media. This practice will make the task of practicing doctor easier at a later date in case of dissatisfied patient. For academic purposes either trichoscopic examination with manual hair counts **(Figs. 14A and B)** or use of software may be done.[65]

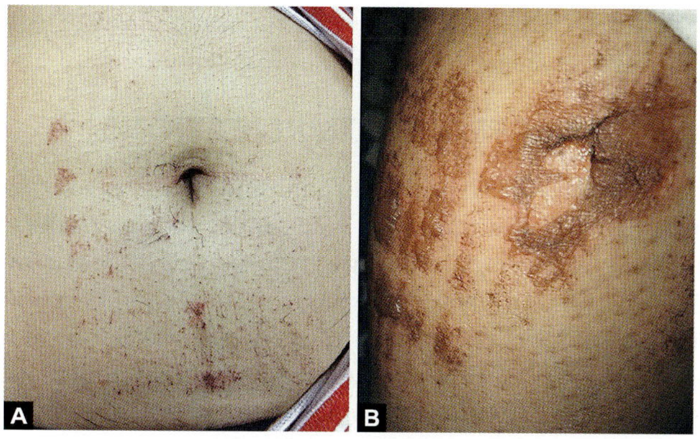

Figs. 14A and B: Trichoscope for measuring hair counts may be used in academic studies.

  - Record tattoos and treat areas overlying tattoos with specific patient consent.
  - If the patient gives a history of recurrent herpes simplex infection, appropriate prophylactic antiviral treatment should be administered.
  - Test patch may be performed before the actual first sitting. Though not mandatory for experienced treating doctors, it is recommended for beginners. It helps to give:
    - Ideal treatment parameters for individual cases
    - Pain threshold of patient
  - Examine the patient for any delayed adverse effects after 72 hours such as erythema, pain, blisters, and pigmentation. If there is no erythema, then the regular sittings for hair reduction procedure can be started.
  - Highest tolerable fluence and the largest spot size are used to obtain the best results. This would be better achieved by three patch tests with three different settings. In general, the treatment fluence should be at 75% of the Nikolsky threshold fluence[66] or that which causes perifollicular erythema. The fluence should be reduced if signs of epidermal damage develop. This will give better and uneventful procedures, decreasing the probability of adverse effects. Authors recommend and practice this in only cases with known photosensitive dermatoses.[67] Details required to be included in the record keeping of test patch are given in **Box 1**.
  - Hair in the area to be treated should be trimmed with an electrical trimmer or shaved before the procedure so as to be not >1–3 mm long.
  - Ensure adequate aseptic precautions.
  - Anesthesia may be required in some cases, especially if the patient was uncomfortable during the time of test patch. Use of topical anesthetic cream of 2.5% lidocaine and prilocaine with a cover of plastic wrap is recommended 45–60 minutes before the actual procedure. Authors recommend use of topical anesthesia in pseudofolliculitis barbae, acne keloidalis nuchae as dense terminal hair growth needs higher effective fluences which can be painful. Similarly in children it ensures better compliance and reduces their anxiety especially in the earlier sessions.[60]
  - Sufficient lights should be there to illuminate the area to be treated, preferably cool white light.
  - Depending upon the system in use—cooling should be used—ice cubes, chilled jelly, short bursts of cryogen

BOX 1: Details which should be included in the record keeping of test patch.

- Details of the patient such as name, age, sex, etc.
- Record of photograph
- Details of the laser parameters such as date and time of test patch, area of test patch, power, fluence, pulse width, cooling used, or not, etc.
- Record of any immediate adverse effects such as blisters, persistent erythema, etc.

spray, etc. However, almost all equipment has "in-built chill sapphire tips."[68]
  - The eyes of patient must be covered with eye protective goggles.
  - Treating doctor and assistant should use manufacturer provided specific goggles.
  - Treatment area should not have any metallic objects such as necklace, bracelets, rings, watches, etc.
  - Use of cosmetic chairs with washable material is encouraged without visible metallic surface which may reflect light-laser beams accidentally leading to adverse effects.
  - Emergency hazard switch should be used (provided in all systems for immediate shut off of the system in case of accidental events).
  - Always see your test patch parameters and use the best result as the starting parameter. Latest fully computerized equipment has the facilities to keep individual patient data, which can be used as and when the patient comes for the next sitting or maintenance touch-ups.
  - Each patient needs individualized parameters. Do not treat all patients with the same parameters. Follow-up with records of earlier session is vital. Special attention to patients who are reporting for follow-up sessions despite being treated elsewhere. Equipment variability and patient response must be accounted for.
  - Handpiece of system should be placed perpendicular to the skin surface and press it gently, but sufficiently to displace blood from capillaries and to bring the hair follicles nearer to the aiming source.
  - Always inform your patient when you are starting with the actual barrage of laser light as the bursts of the laser beam may be associated with slight discomfort.

Procedure

Of paramount importance is the general safety of both the patient and the operating room personnel during laser irradiation. Key laser safety issues include flammability, ocular safety, electric hazards, laser plume, infectious agents, and controlled access to the laser suite.

- Accidental fires are a potential complication of laser use, particularly in the presence of circulating oxygen which should be minimized. Saline-soaked drapes or clothes should be used intraoperatively; exposed hair-bearing areas should be kept moist and alcohol-based skin preparations should be strictly avoided. In addition, lasers should be kept in the standby mode when not in use to avoid inadvertent firing.
- Eye protection is necessary for both patients and operating personnel whenever a laser treatment is performed. Permanent visual loss can result from even minor direct retinal exposure to laser light. All operating room personnel must wear appropriate goggles that filter out the specific wavelength of light. The patient's eyes must also be protected using goggles for non-facial and/or noninvasive procedures or sand-blasted metal contact lenses for complete corneal protection when periorbital laser treatment is performed.
- Electrical hazards can largely be eliminated by dedicating a specific electric outlet for each laser and by avoiding the use of extension cords.
- A smoke evacuator with clean filters and tubing are also essential to contain aerosolized particles and fumes during treatment which has been considered as a health hazard.[69]
- Treat all areas in one sitting simultaneously. Avoid tattoos unless so desired by the patient. Be cautious in skin with moles. Although debatable it is best to avoid lasing over them.[70]
- Watch for any blisters or pain in the treated areas. If observed, either reduce fluence or abandon the procedure (rarely needed if proper selection of patient and test patch is performed).
- After the entire procedure is complete make use of ice packs to reduce postoperative pain and minimize edema.
- Sunblock lotion should be applied at the end of the session.

Postprocedure

- Avoidance of sun exposure and use of sunscreen lotion with proper instructions of its usage during the 1st week after the procedure.
- Prophylactic antivirals, if started, their course must be completed.
- Topical antibiotic cream is prescribed in case of any epidermal injury and mild topical steroid cream to reduce edema and erythema.
- Patient is explained about possibility of any blisters or crusts and to report to the doctor, if any, for proper management. He/she should also be reassured that the damaged hair is often shed in the first few days of treatment and is not a sign of hair growth.
- The patient is explained about the timing of next treatment, which is when regrowth occurs, on an average, after 6–8 weeks, based on the anatomic location.

ADVERSE EFFECTS/COMPLICATIONS

Complications of laser-assisted hair removal using lasers are usually minor and transient.[71] The most common adverse reactions include pain during treatment, erythema, and peri-follicular edema. However, in dark-skinned persons, blister formation, pigmentary alteration, and scarring have also been reported. To reduce side effects, treatment can be performed with concurrent epidermal cooling or selection of the appropriate wavelength, i.e., longer wavelengths [e.g., (Nd:YAG) laser] for darker skin types.

- Pain and discomfort during and after procedure. Cooling and analgesics can be prescribed.
- *Perifollicular erythema and edema:* Topical mild steroid cream can be used.
- Epidermal damage such as blistering, crusting, and secondary infection, if treated aggressively **(Figs. 15A and B)**. Topical antibiotic cream is prescribed.
- Folliculitis if excessive sweating, swimming, or use of hot tub.
- Dyspigmentation is seen in dark-skinned patients or ones with excessive sun exposure. Avoidance of sun exposure and use of sunscreen lotions is advised.
- Patient should be informed of the possibility of Koebner phenomenon occurring in case of vitiligo or psoriasis, though clinically this is rarely seen.
- Ocular retinal injuries may occur if proper eye protection is not taken or treatment is done near the eye. This is due to the presence of melanin which will absorb the laser light used for hair removal.[72]
- The "plume" generated during the procedure can have infective particles and has typical sulfuric smell which can be irritating. Also, the smoke is considered to have many long-term adverse effects. A smoke evacuator is hence recommended.[69,73]
- *Paradoxical hypertrichosis:* Hair growth has been reported when treated by laser or light hair removal especially in face and neck area of young female patients with dark skin types. Other risk factors are—use of hormone supplements, systemic steroids, and underlying hormonal disease such as PCOS. It may be seen in patients treated with suboptimal fluence—too low for therapeutic effect, yet enough to stimulate hair growth. The underlying mechanism is postulated to be due to, either conversion of vellus hair to terminal hair at the site of treatment or induction of hair growth in the immediate vicinity.[67,74] Laser hair removal may also synchronize the hair cycle by converting reversibly injured follicles to anagen, which may falsely give the appearance of hypertrichosis by increasing the hair density.
- *Leukotrichia:* It is said to potentially develop after laser hair removal but is not well documented. It may reflect removal of all dark hairs leaving behind only the white hairs, in an area of mixed hair color. Alternately, destruction of melanocytes leading to gray hairs without damage to stem cells may lead to leukotrichia.[75]

AVAILABLE HAIR REDUCTION SYSTEMS[76]

Currently most devices target melanin in the hair follicle with millisecond-long pulse durations to produce, to some degree, selective photo-thermolysis of hair follicles. These lasers are the ruby, alexandrite, diode, and Nd:YAG. The ruby laser with a wavelength of 694 nm has the shortest penetration depth and the most selective absorption by melanin. The Nd:YAG laser, emitting in the infrared at 1,064 nm, has the deepest depth of penetration but the least selective absorption. The alexandrite (755 nm) and diode (810 nm) lasers sit between these extremes. There is also no consensus on the most preferred and beneficial laser or intense pulse light (IPL) broadband light devices. Each system has its own advantages and disadvantages. Total Reflection Amplification of Spontaneous Emission of Radiation (TRASER) is a simpler optical device which uses a flash lamp to induce the spontaneous emission of photons from a fluorescent dye in solution, or ions impregnated in a crystal structure. Wavelength emission can be varied from UVA to near infra-red.[77,78] It still needs widespread acceptance.

Proper patient selection depending on Fitzpatrick skin type classification **(Table 4)** and tailoring of the fluence remain the most important factors in efficacious and well tolerated laser treatment. The Fitzpatrick scale [Fitzpatrick skin typing test or Fitzpatrick phototyping scale **(Table 4)**] is a numerical classification scheme for the color of skin. It was developed in 1975 by TB Fitzpatrick as a way to classify the response of different types of skin to UV light.[79] It measures several components—genetic disposition, reaction to sun exposure, and tanning habits. Various home-use devices (HUDs) consisting of diode lasers and IPL systems are available which have been manufactured keeping "human factors" in mind reducing the risk of accidental injury to skin and eyes, however safety concerns persist especially in patients with skin of darker color as well as eyes. While the outcome of these devices is significant reduction of hair, the long-term data on efficacy as well as safety are lacking.

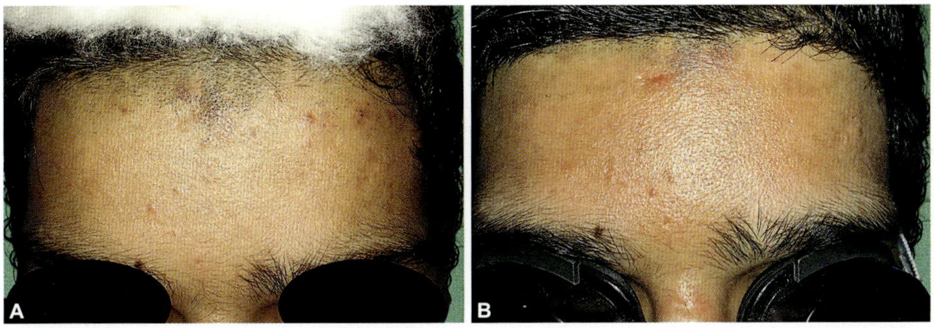

Figs. 15A and B: Superficial epidermal burns with intense pulse light (A) and deeper burns with unsupervised diode laser (B).

TABLE 4: The Fitzpatrick scale.

Skin type	*Skin color*	*Characteristics*
I	White; very fair; red or blonde hair; blue eyes; freckles	Always burns, never tans
II	White; fair; red or blonde hair; blue, hazel, or green eyes	Usually burns, tans with difficulty
III	Cream white; fair with any eye or hair color; very common	Sometimes mild burn, gradually tans
IV	Brown; typical Mediterranean Caucasian skin	Rarely burns, tans with ease
V	Dark brown; mid-eastern skin types	Very rarely burns, tans very easily
VI	Black	Never burns, tans very easily

TABLE 5: Differences between conventional high-fluence single pass diode lasers and newer low-fluence multiple pass diode lasers with "in-motion" technology.

Conventional high-fluence single pass diode laser devices	*Newer low-fluence multiple pass diode laser devices with "in-motion" technology*
Single pass over the areas to be treated in a grid-like fashion	Multiple passes over the areas to be treated
An overlap of 10% is to be given in treating adjacent grids to cover for the area under the margins of the tip of the probe	There are two methods for laser delivery- paint brush method and circular motion method
More discomfort as compared to in-motion technology devices even when using similar fluence	Less discomfort as compared to single pass conventional lasers
The procedure is quicker, but when used under topical anesthesia—may take more time considering the time needed for the topical anesthesia to take effect	The procedure is longer, but topical anesthesia may not be needed, hence no waiting time
Laser hand piece is light and handy	Laser hand piece is bulky
Relatively difficult to operate	Learning curve is gentle, easy to operate

Diode Lasers[80,81]

Semiconductor diode lasers emit energy in the 800–810 nm portion of the electromagnetic spectrum. This longer wavelength is sufficiently absorbed by melanin to make it effective for hair removal, yet less avidly absorbed than that of the ruby or alexandrite, thus, making it potentially safer for individuals with darker skin phototypes. Thus, diode lasers are considered to be the gold standard amongst the various hair removal laser devices. The available diode laser devices can be broadly divided into two groups—conventional high-fluence single pass devices and newer low-fluence multiple pass devices with "in-motion" technology.[81] The single-pass devices may be further classified on the basis of additional option of pneumatic skin flattening (PSF) in some newer devices.[49] Both kinds of devices are available with integrated cooling mechanisms and treatment endpoints being perifollicular erythema. While there are no statistical differences in the outcome of the two, there are a few differentiating points between the two **(Table 5)**.

Fluences in the darker skin are used in the range of 20–24 J/cm^2. Hair reduction at 8 months has been reported at 75% in 91% of individuals after 3–4 treatments at 40 J/cm^2.[82] Lower fluences in darker skin may be countered with longer pulse duration.[83]

Multiplex diode laser with multiple wavelengths in one hand piece helps target superficial and deep, fine, and thick terminal hair. The 755 nm wavelength targets the follicular bulge of and hence found effective for superficially embedded hair in areas such as the eyebrows and upper lip. The 810 nm wavelength penetrates deeper to target the bulge as well as follicular bulb. It is hence suitable for moderate depth penetration as is needed for the arms, legs, beard, and cheeks. Deepest penetration is achieved by 1,064 nm wavelength targeting the bulb and papilla for the deep embedded hair in areas of the scalp, axillae, and pubic areas.[82] Devices with larger spot size of 18 mm help treat larger areas in shorter duration.[84]

Tips are discussed below.

TIPS

- Laser test patch helps to determine the ideal parameters individualized for each patient. It is recommended that the highest tolerable fluence and the largest spot size are used to obtain the best results. This would be better achieved by three patch tests with three different settings. In general, the treatment fluence should be, which causes perifollicular erythema, but if signs of epidermal damage develop, it should be reduced
- For fair skinned individuals long-pulsed Ruby or Alexandrite lasers are preferred whereas long-pulsed Nd:YAG or diode lasers are preferred for dark-skinned patients. Diode lasers may be suitable for both light and dark-skinned patients
- Longer pulse duration and longer wavelength with less fluence would be better for dark skin patients, in order to decrease epidermal adverse effects
- Increase pulse duration instead of fluence to overcome poor response
- Smaller spot size would be better for thin superficially placed hair and larger spot size for thick hair located at more depth. Thus, after few laser sessions when terminal hair starts transforming into vellus hair, type of laser, or its parameters may need to be modified
- Concurrent multiple laser wavelength treatments that have combination effects and dual actions need consideration in poor response cases
- In order to avoid double pulsing or skip areas, a grid may be used. Dark-/metallic-colored marker colors are to be avoided as they interfere with the device optics. A headlamp with a magnifying loupe can be worn to improve visibility
- Cooling the skin between pulses in blister prone skin is beneficial
- Skin-lightening creams for tanned skin should be used prior to laser sessions. This will decrease the risk of laser energy getting absorbed by the epidermal melanin and subsequent epidermal damage. 4% hydroquinone 2–4 weeks before laser sessions especially in darker skin helps prevent complications.[85] However, be cautious in its use over large body surfaces
- Plastic cling film enables aseptic environment and prevents handpiece contamination[86]
- Stacking of pulses may improve outcome in subsequent sessions
- Address the cause of hirsutism before initiating laser hair removal. A lead time of 4–8 weeks of medical management is good enough to start laser sessions

CONCLUSION

Laser hair reduction requires a thorough understanding of the basic principles and physics of laser light and the laser tissue interactions with the hair follicle target chromophore melanin and the bulge area stem cells.

Excellent results in a patient can be achieved if laser hair removal is performed by a trained dermatologist using the optimal parameters in an individualized manner. The first laser system specifically designed to accomplish the long-term hair removal based on the principles of selective photothermolysis received US Food and Drug Administration (FDA) approval in 1995. Subsequently several additional systems have received clearance and come into widespread use. While the advances of the past years have been highly gratifying, the rapidity of development has also brought along a certain level of confusion even among the more experienced laser surgeons. In India IPL, Alexandrite, Ruby, Diode, or Nd:YAG is used for many years now. None of the currently approved systems can yet be said to induce permanent hair loss, nor can physicians expect any system to produce consistent, absolutely predictable results. Most of the available lasers and other light-based systems can achieve a significant delay in regrowth of unwanted hairs lasting 3–9 months, although longer durations have also been observed.

Careful patient selection and evaluation, proper preoperative and postoperative care—all are essential parts to give excellent cosmetic results. The importance of counseling the patient cannot be understated in increasing compliance and ultimately a more satisfied patient at the end of the day.

REFERENCES

1. Haedersdal M, Wulf H. Evidence-based review of hair removal using lasers and light sources. J Eur Acad Dermatol Venereol. 2006;20:9-20.
2. Liew SH. Laser hair removal: guidelines for management. Am J Clin Dermatol. 2002;3:107-15.
3. Barlow RJ, Hruza GJ. Lasers and Light tissue Interactions. In: Lasers and Light, Volume I. Saunders: Elsevier India Pvt. Limited; 2005. p. 1.
4. Anderson RR, Parrish JA. Selective photothermolysis: precise microsurgery by selective absorption of pulsed radiation. Science. 1983;220(4596):524-7.
5. Lin L-Y, Chiou S-C, Wang S-H, Chi C-C. Effects of facial threading on female skin texture: a prospective trial with physiological parameters and sense assessment. Evid Based Complement Alternat Med. 2019;2019:1-8.
6. Lim V, Simmons BJ, Maranda EL, Afifi L, Kallis PJ, Jimenez J. Sugaring—modern revival of an ancient Egyptian technique for hair removal. JAMA Dermatol. 2016;152:660.
7. The Washington Post. (1989). Hair removal in history. [online] Available from https://www.washingtonpost.com/archive/lifestyle/1989/05/26/hair-removal-in-history/85eb869b-29e4-42e4-97ee-eaf85b90adb2/ [Last accessed March, 2024].
8. FitzGerald S. (2013). Tricho System. [online] Available from http://www.museumofquackery.com/ephemera/tricho.htm [Last accessed March, 2024].
9. Lapidus SM. The tricho system: hypertrichosis, radiation, and cancer. J Surg Oncol. 1976;8:267-74.
10. Dover JS, Margolis RJ, Polla LL, Watanabe S, Hruza GJ, Parrish JA, et al. Pigmented guinea pig skin irradiated with Q-switched ruby laser pulses. Morphologic and histologic findings. Arch Dermatol. 1989;125:43-9.
11. Goldberg DJ, Littler CM, Wheeland RG. Topical Suspension-assisted Q-switched Nd:YAG Laser Hair Removal. Dermatol Surg. 1997;23:741-5.
12. Lepselter J, Elman M. Biological and clinical aspects in laser hair removal. J Dermatol Treat. 2004;15:72-83.
13. Dierickx CC, Grossman MC. Laser hair removal. In: Goldberg DJ (Ed). Lasers and Lights, Volume 2. 2005. pp. 74-5.
14. Hammes S, Greve B, Raulin C. Electro-optical synergy (ELOS?) technology for nonablative skin rejuvenation: a preliminary prospective study. J Eur Acad Dermatol Venereol. 2006;20:1070-5.
15. Sadick NS, Shaoul J. Hair removal using a combination of conducted radiofrequency and optical energies-an 18-month follow-up. J Cosmet Laser. 2004;6:21-6.
16. Tope WD, Hordinsky MK. A Hair's Breadth Closer? Arch Dermatol. 1998;134(7):867-9.
17. Marchell NL, Alster TS. Evaluation of temporary and permanent hair removal methods. J Aesth Cosmet Dermatol Surg. 1999;1:3-12.
18. Olsen EA. Methods of hair removal. J Am Acad Dermatol. 1999;40:143-55.
19. Blume-Peytavi U, Tosti A. Hair Growth and Disorders. 1st edition. Springer-Verlag Berlin and Heidelberg GmbH & Co; 2008. p. 440.
20. Richards RN, Meharg GA. Electrolysis: observations from 13 years and 140,000 hours of experience. J Am Acad Dermatol. 1995;33:662-6.
21. Wagner RF. Physical methods for the management of hirsutism. Cutis. 1990;45:199-202.
22. Vaidya T, Hohman MH, Kumar DD. Laser hair removal. In: StatPearls. Treasure Island (FL): StatPearls Publishing; 2024.
23. de Viragh PA, Meuli M. Human scalp hair follicle development from birth to adulthood: Statistical study with special regard to putative stem cells in the bulge and proliferating cells in the matrix. Arch Dermatol Res. 1995;287:279-84.
24. Panteleyev AA. Functional anatomy of the hair follicle: The Secondary Hair Germ. Exp Dermatol. 2018;27:701-20.
25. Chen C-L, Huang W-Y, Wang EHC, Tai K-Y, Lin S-J. Functional complexity of hair follicle stem cell niche and therapeutic targeting of niche dysfunction for hair regeneration. J Biomed Sci. 2020;27:43.
26. Amoh Y, Hoffman RM. Hair follicle-associated-pluripotent (HAP) stem cells. Cell Cycle. 2017;16:2169-75.
27. Ohyama M. Hair follicle bulge: a fascinating reservoir of epithelial stem cells. J Dermatol Sci. 2007;46:81-9.
28. Meilana A, Dewi NM, Wijaya A. Heterogeneous stem cells in skin homeostatis and wound repair. Indones Biomed J. 2015;7:87.
29. Anderson RR. Lasers in dermatology-a critical update. J Dermatol. 2000;27:700-5.
30. Menon IA, Persad S, Haberman HF, Kurian CJ. A comparative study of the physical and chemical properties of melanins isolated from human black and red hair. J Invest Dermatol. 1983;80:202-6.
31. Tsao SS, Hruza GJ. Laser hair removal. In: Robinson JK, Hanke CW, Sengelmann RD, Siegel DM (Eds). Surgery of the Skin. Philadelphia, PA: Elsevier Mosby; 2005. pp. 575-88.

32. Alonso L, Fuchs E. The hair cycle. J Cell Sci. 2006;119 (Pt 3):391-3.
33. Carroll L, Humphreys TR. LASER-tissue interactions. Clin Dermatol. 2006;24:2-7.
34. Nelson S. An introduction to laser and laser-tissue interactions in dermatology. In: Kauvar A, Hruza G (Eds). Principles and Practices in Cutaneous Laser Surgery. 2005. pp. 59-77.
35. Wanner M. Laser hair removal. Dermatologic Therapy. 2005;18:209-16.
36. Choi B, Welch AJ. Analysis of thermal relaxation during laser irradiation of tissue. Lasers Surg Med. 2001;29(4):351-9.
37. Dierickx CC. Photoepilation. In: Blume-Peytavi U, Tosti A, Trüeb RM, (Eds). Hair Growth and Disorders. Berlin, Heidelberg: Springer Berlin Heidelberg; 2008. pp. 427-45.
38. Murphy MJ, Torstensson PA. Thermal relaxation times: an outdated concept in photothermal treatments. Lasers Med Sci. 2014;29:973-8.
39. Rogachefsky AS, Silapunt S, Goldberg DJ. Evaluation of a new super-long-pulsed 810 nm diode laser for the removal of unwanted hair: the concept of thermal damage time. Dermatol Surg. 2002;28:410-4.
40. Fuchs M. Thermokinetic selectivity—a new highly effective method for permanent hair removal: experience with the LPIR Alexandrite laser. Derm Prakt Dermatologie. 1997;5:1.
41. Altshuler GB, Anderson RR, Manstein D, Zenzie HH, Smirnov MZ. Extended theory of selective photothermolysis. Lasers Surg Med. 2001;29:416-32.
42. Ross EV, Ladin Z, Kreindel M, Dierickx C. Theoretical considerations in laser hair removal. Dermatol Clin. 1999;17:333-55.
43. Barolet D. Low fluence-high repetition rate diode laser hair removal 12-month evaluation: reducing pain and risks while keeping clinical efficacy. Lasers Surg Med. 2012;44:277-81.
44. Sardana K, Garg V. Basics of laser-tissue interactions. In: Sardana K, Garg V (Eds). Lasers In Dermatological Practice. 1st edition. New Delhi: Jaypee Brothers Medical Publishers (P) Ltd.; 2014. pp. 3-24.
45. Royo J, Urdiales F, Moreno J, Al-Zarouni M, Cornejo P, Trelles MA. Six-month follow-up multicenter prospective study of 368 patients, phototypes III to V, on epilation efficacy using an 810-nm diode laser at low fluence. Lasers Med Sci. 2011;26:247-55.
46. Bailin PL, Ratz JL, Wheeland RG. Laser therapy of the skin. A review of principles and applications. Derm Clin. 1987;5: 259-85.
47. Lask G, Friedman D, Elman M, Fournier N, Shavit R, Slatkine M. Pneumatic skin flattening (PSF): a novel technology for marked pain reduction in hair removal with high energy density lasers and IPLs. J Cosmet Laser Ther. 2006;8:76-81.
48. Fournier N. Hair removal on dark-skinned patients with pneumatic skin flattening (PSF) and a high-energy Nd:YAG laser. J Cosmet Laser Ther. 2008;10:210-2.
49. Dierickx CC, Grossman MC. Laser hair removal. In: Goldberg DJ (Ed). Lasers and Lights, Volume 2. 2005. p. 64.
50. Trelles MA, Almudever P, Alcolea JM, Cortijo J, Serrano G, Expósito I, et al. Cuttlefish ink melanin encapsulated in nanolipid bubbles and applied through a micro-needling procedure easily stains white hair facilitating photoepilation. J Drugs Dermatol. 2016;15:615-25.
51. Sand M, Bechara FG, Sand D, Altmeyer P, Hoffmann K. A randomized, controlled, double-blind study evaluating melanin-encapsulated liposomes as a chromophore for laser hair removal of blond, white, and gray hair. Ann Plast Surg. 2007;58:551-4.
52. Tierney EP, Goldberg DJ. Laser hair removal pearls. J Cosmet Laser Ther. 2008;10:17-23.
53. Koch D, Pratsou P, Szczecinska W, Lanigan S, Abdullah A. The diverse application of laser hair removal therapy: a tertiary laser unit's experience with less common indications and a literature overview. Lasers Med Sci. 2015;30:453-67.
54. Sachdeva S. Hirsutism: Evaluation and treatment. Indian J Dermatol. 2010;55:3.
55. Minneci PC, Halleran DR, Lawrence AE, Fischer BA, Cooper JN, Deans KJ. Laser hair depilation for the prevention of disease recurrence in adolescents and young adults with pilonidal disease: study protocol for a randomized controlled trial. Trials. 2018;19:599.
56. Ganjoo A. Laser hair reduction for pilonidal sinus—my experience. J Cutan Aesthetic Surg. 2011;4:196.
57. Esmat SM, Abdel Hay RM, Abu Zeid OM, Hosni HN. The efficacy of laser-assisted hair removal in the treatment of acne keloidalis nuchae; a pilot study. Eur J Dermatol. 2012;22: 645-50.
58. Jain A, Jain V. Use of lasers for the management of refractory cases of hidradenitis suppurativa and pilonidal sinus. J Cutan Aesthetic Surg. 2012;5:190.
59. Ogunbiyi A. Pseudofolliculitis barbae; current treatment options. Clin Cosmet Investig Dermatol. 2019;12:241-7.
60. Arora S, Arora G, Totlani S, Chandra M. Faun tail nevus: A series of 15 cases and their management with intense pulse light. Med J Armed Forces India. 2019;75:389-94.
61. García-Zamora E, Naz-Villalba E, Pampín-Franco A, Vicente-Martín FJ, López-Estebaranz J. Laser therapy for hair removal on grafts and flaps. Dermatol Ther. 2019;32(3):e12880.
62. Yilmaz B, Yildiz BO. Endocrinology of hirsutism: from androgens to androgen excess disorders. Front Horm Res. 2019;53:108-19.
63. Blume-Peytavi U. An overview of unwanted female hair. Br J Dermatol. 2011;165(Suppl 3):19-23.
64. Buddhadev RM, IADVL Dermatosurgery Task Force. Standard guidelines of care: laser and IPL hair reduction. Indian J Dermatol Venereol Leprol. 2008;74(Suppl):S68-74.
65. Kuck M. Analysis of the efficiency of hair removal by different optical methods: comparison of Trichoscan, reflectance confocal microscopy, and optical coherence tomography. J Biomed Opt. 2012;17:101504.
66. Dierickx C, Alora MB, Dover JS. A clinical overview of hair removal using lasers and light sources. Dermatol Clin. 1999;17:357-66, ix.
67. Arora S, Gulhima Arora. Laser Hair Removal: Overview and Review of Complications; 2015.
68. Das A, Sarda A, De A. Cooling devices in laser therapy. J Cutan Aesthetic Surg. 2016;9:215.
69. Arora G, Arora S, Talathi A, Kandhari R, Joshi V, Langar S, et al. Safer practice of aesthetic dermatology during the COVID-19 pandemic: recommendations by SIG aesthetics (IADVL academy). Indian Dermatol Online J. 2020;11(4):534-9.
70. Suzuki H, Anderson RR. Treatment of melanocytic nevi. Dermatol Ther. 2005;18:217-26.
71. Lim SP, Lanigan SW. A review of the adverse effects of laser hair removal. Lasers Med Sci. 2006;21:121-5.
72. Huang A, Phillips A, Adar T, Hui A. Ocular injury in cosmetic laser treatments of the face. J Clin Aesthetic Dermatol. 2018;11:15-8.
73. Brownstone ND, Thibodeaux QG, Reddy VD, Myers BA, Chan SY, Bhutani T, et al. Novel Coronavirus Disease (COVID-19) and Biologic Therapy for Psoriasis: Successful Recovery in Two Patients After Infection with Severe Acute Respiratory

Syndrome Coronavirus 2 (SARS-CoV-2). Dermatol Ther. 2020;10(4):881-5.
74. Desai S, Mahmoud BH, Bhatia AC, Hamzavi IH. Paradoxical hypertrichosis after laser therapy: a review. Dermatol Surg. 2010;36:291-8.
75. Radmanesh M, Mostaghimi M, Yousefi I, Mousavi ZB, Rasai S, Esmaili HR, et al. Leukotrichia developed following application of intense pulsed light for hair removal. Dermatol Surg. 2002;28:572-4.
76. Lee CM. Laser-assisted hair removal for facial hirsutism in women: a review of evidence. J Cosmet Laser Ther. 2018;20:140-4.
77. Zachary CB, Gustavsson M. TRASER—total reflection amplification of spontaneous emission of radiation. PLoS One. 2012;7:e35899.
78. Ball K, Gustavsson M, Harris R, Berganza L, Zachary CB. TRASER: acute phase vascular and follicular changes. Lasers Surg Med. 2014;46(5):385-8.
79. Fitzpatrick TB. The validity and practicality of sun-reactive skin types I through VI. Arch Dermatol. 1988;124:869-71.
80. Bouzari N, Tabatabai H, Abbasi Z, Firooz A, Dowlati Y. Laser hair removal: comparison of long-pulsed Nd:YAG, long-pulsed alexandrite, and long-pulsed diode lasers. Dermatol Surg. 2004;30(4 Pt 1):498-502.
81. Koo B, Ball K, Tremaine AM, Zachary CB. A comparison of two 810 diode lasers for hair removal: low fluence, multiple pass versus a high fluence, single pass technique. Lasers Surg Med. 2014;46:270-4.
82. Bhat YJ, Bashir S, Nabi N, Hassan I. Laser Treatment in hirsutism: an update. Dermatol Pract Concept. 2020; e2020048.
83. Roosen GF, Westgate GE, Philpott M, Berretty PJ, Nuijs TAM, Bjerring P. Temporary hair removal by low fluence photoepilation. Lasers Surg Med. 2008;40:520-8.
84. Youssef NJ, Rizk AG, Ibrahimi OA, Tannous ZS. Long-term comparison of a large spot vacuum assisted handpiece vs the small spot size traditional handpiece of the 800 nm diode laser. J Drugs Dermatol. 2017;16:893-8.
85. Alexis AF. Lasers and light-based therapies in ethnic skin: treatment options and recommendations for Fitzpatrick skin types V and VI. Br J Dermatol. 2013;169(Suppl 3):91-97.
86. Arsiwala S, Majid I. Methods to overcome poor responses and challenges of laser hair removal in dark skin. Indian J Dermatol Venereol Leprol. 2019;85(1):3-9.

CHAPTER 107

Different Wavelengths for Hair Removal

Anurag Tiwari, GR Rajput

KEY MESSAGES

- Many technologies are available in the market for laser hair reduction.
- Choice for laser depends on the hair thickness and skin color.
- Laser technologies available in India are Alexandrite (755 nm), diode (810 nm), long pulse neodymium-doped yttrium aluminum garnet (Nd:YAG) (1,064 nm), and intense pulse light (550–1,200 nm).
- Newer machines have two to three wavelengths in a single pulse.
- Different wavelength can be used in same sitting.

INTRODUCTION

Laser hair removal (LHR) was among top six nonsurgical procedure performed in 2020 constituting staggering 735,996 procedures according to the American Society for Aesthetic Plastic Surgery statistic report of 2020.[1] Permanent hair reduction is appropriate term to be used instead of permanent hair removal as maintenance sessions are frequently required to keep the hair growth at bay once the results are achieved.

The standard wavelength for hair removal is between 600 and 1,100 nm.[2,3] The main players are Alexandrite (755 nm), diode (810 nm), and neodymium-doped yttrium aluminum garnet (Nd:YAG) (1,064 nm). These lasers are approved for Fitzpatrick skin types 1-6 for laser hair reduction **(Box 1)**.

Shorter wavelength has a potential to cause more epidermal damage as epidermal melanin absorbs the energy from these wavelengths, especially in Fitzpatrick skin type IV–VI. Longer wavelength bypasses the epidermal melanin and penetrates deeply, so gives more safety and efficacy necessary to treat the darker skin type.

NEWER TRENDS

The need for better hair reduction has led to technological advancements, which have made it possible to get different wavelengths in the same machine and same shot. Many such combinations are available and are listed here.

However, their efficacy and results over conventional laser systems have to be evaluated by a bigger number of practitioners and institutes.

- Combination of Alexandrite and Nd:YAG
- Combination of diode and Nd:YAG
- Combination of triple wavelength Alexandrite, diode, and Nd:YAG
- Combination of laser and radiofrequency (RF)—electro-optical synergy system (ELOS)

BOX 1: Hair reduction wavelengths.

- Ruby laser—694 nm
- Alexandrite laser—755 nm
- Diode laser—810 nm
- Neodymium-doped yttrium aluminum garnet laser—1,064 nm
- Intense pulse light (IPL)—550–1,200 nm

LASER PARAMETERS AND TEST SPOTS

Test spot should be done in an area with similar skin color and hair density as the area to be treated. Generally, two to four different fluences with at least four overlapping shots should be given for each fluence and pulse duration. Begin with safest parameters (longer pulse duration and lower fluences) and progress to shorter pulse duration and higher fluence. The fluence should be lower at areas with high hair density and dark color. Endpoint includes mild redness and perifollicular edema.

In case of blistering, crusting, and prolonged erythema, fluences should be decreased by at least 20% in subsequent sessions postsubsidence of these symptoms.

PRETREATMENT PREPARATIONS

History, Clinical Examination, and Endocrinological Workup

- Thorough history along with clinical examination with relevant investigation is mandatory before venturing into LHR. Clinician should rule out any underlying cause for excessive hair growth and should adequately address the issue before advising the LHR. The outcome of procedure is heavily depended upon treatment of underlying cause and this will help in counseling of patient and setting the appropriate expectation of patient.

- History of keloidal tendencies, parlor procedure, tanning, excessive sun exposure prior to procedure, photosensitizing drug intake, or herpes simplex infection in treatment area is to be recorded. Examination of whole body part with particular attention toward photo-koebnerization-induced disease is to be endorsed. History application of hair dye particularly in beard region is to be asked as this will result in laser burn during procedure.
- History of topical retinoid is to be recorded. Patient is advised to stop topical retinoid for at least 4 days prior to procedure. All topical depigmenting and exfoliating cream to be discontinued at least 3 days prior to procedure. Patient can continue emollient/moisturizer application, if desired.
- Presence of gray and brown hair is to be marked as these are less responsive areas to LHR.

Patient Counseling, Consent, and Photographs

Adequate counseling with information about number of sessions, time interval between sessions, requirement of maintenance sittings, side effect possibilities, possibility of recurrence, and nonresponsive result probability is to be explained before procedure. Cost incurred is to be also conveyed beforehand. The expectation about procedure is to be gauged and if required need to be corrected in unrealistic expectants. Body dysmorphic patients are contraindication for such procedures. Specific consent forms are to be made for different laser machines. Photography before start of procedure, during the sessions and after completing the procedure are must as this will help in judging the response to treatment.

General Instructions

- Tanning of the treatment areas result in laser burns hence patient is advised to avoid intense sunlight exposure prior to treatment. If already tanned then the procedure needs to be deferred till tanning subsides.
- Waxing, parlor procedure, and bleaching procedure to be avoided at least 3 weeks prior to procedure and in between sessions. Bleaching is advised during maintenance phase. The hair removal creams are to be avoided in view if their irritant potential. Patient can shave off hairs in between procedure taking care not to result in cut marks.

LASER SAFETY

The general safety of both the patient and the operating room personnel during laser irradiation is of paramount importance **(Box 2)**.

Alcohol-based skin preparations should be strictly avoided. Lasers should be kept in standby mode when not in use to avoid inadvertent firing. Eye protection is necessary for both patients and operating personnel whenever a laser treatment is performed. Permanent visual loss can result from even minor direct retinal exposure to laser light. All operating room personnel must wear appropriate goggles that filter out the specific wavelength of light. The patient's eyes must also be protected using goggles for nonfacial laser treatments. Electrical hazards can largely be eliminated by dedicating a specific electric outlet for each laser and by avoiding the use of extension cords. A smoke evacuator with clean filters and tubing is also essential to contain aerosolized particles and fumes during treatment.

BOX 2: Laser safety issues.

Key laser safety issues include:
- Flammability
- Ocular safety
- Electric hazards
- Laser plume and infectious agents
- Controlled access to the laser suite

INTRAOPERATIVE PROCEDURE PROTOCOL

Topical Anesthesia

It is not a mandatory requirement. Some patients develop irritant reaction to these creams, and it increases the treatment cost. In case of sensitive patients, the combination of EMLA is to be applied to treatment area at least 45 minutes prior to procedure. Care is to be exercised for large area of treatment and possibility of lignocaine toxicity should always be kept in mind before application over large body surface area.

Test Spot

Test spot at treatment area is good practice point before proceeding for entire area. The parameters are used as per endpoints mentioned earlier. As the thumb rule lower fluences with large spot size and high repetition rate is preferred for Indian skin type.

Site Preparation and Procedure

- Cleanse the area to remove any residual makeup or anesthetic cream.
- Shave off the area before procedure. Always shave in the direction of hair growth and never in opposite direction to avoid any microtrauma.
- It is better to mark the treatment area with white skin marker. For beginners, it is better to divide the area in grids. This will help to avoid skip area or repetition in same area.
- Apply the thin layer of chilled ultrasound gel over treatment area.
- Always complete lasering one area and then move to the other side. Do not move in haphazard directions. This prevents skip areas.
- Use 10–20% overlap depending on the laser used.

- If patient has teeth enamel or braces, protect by overlaying the teeth with moistened gauze.
- Avoid pointing the laser beam toward eyes. The contact tip should be held firmly against skin in perpendicular direction. The movement should be swift and gliding.
- Firmly press the handpiece against skin while firing the beam. This will help in clearing the blood from that area because of compression and will bring the follicle closer to hand piece which will result in better delivery of energy at targeted spot.
- In this era, most of the machines come with inbuilt cooling system. Nevertheless, the surrounding area is to be covered with cold sponge. This will help in preventing heat energy dissipation in nontargeted area. This is particularly important in beard-shaping procedures.
- The handpiece should be checked intermittently to detect any singed hair.
- Distance of at least 1 cm is to be maintained from tattoo borders.
- Melanocytic nevi in treatment area are to be covered with moistened gauge.
- Parameter as well as response is to be noted down in patient records every time.

POST-TREATMENT PROTOCOL

- Cooling pads can be used to decrease discomfort, erythema, and edema.
- Apply mild corticosteroid, if prolonged erythema, edema, and irritation happen.
- Sunscreen applied before the patient steps out of clinic and to be continued for at least week after procedure.
- Avoid topical retinoids, depigmenting, and exfoliating cream till 3 days postprocedure.
- Advised to apply moisturizer/emollient frequently till 1 week postprocedure.
- Shaving to be avoided for at least a week postprocedure.
- In case of burning, crusting oral steroids can be prescribed for 5 days along with steroid antibiotic cream for a week.
- Use of eflornithine cream is to be avoided in between active session. It is more effective as an adjuvant during maintenance phase.

INTERVAL BETWEEN SESSIONS

It is advisable to follow-up after 2–3-weeks post first session to assess the side effects. On an average, laser hair reduction is performed every 3–6 weeks on the face and every 6–10 weeks for body hair. But intervals are individualized it is best to wait for a near complete regrowth of hair and then perform the laser. Spacing is to be gradually increased in next sessions to target the anagen hair. To frequent session without adequate time in between will result in suppression only.

ALEXANDRITE LASER (755 NM)

Conventional Alexandrite lasers used synthetic crystal to emit energy of 755-nm wavelength. It was not used in the darker skin type due to increased chances of complications like blistering and postinflammatory hyperpigmentation, etc.[4-8] Also the high cost and maintenance, lack of safety data, and lack of inbuilt cooling did not make them a popular choice in our country. However, the new age machines have started using diode crystal to emit the 755-nm wavelength. This makes the lasers more durable and less expensive. These new machines have both stamping and in motion technology and contact cooling, thereby gaining popularity.

Parameters most commonly used in stamping mode are:

- 20–40 ms pulse duration
- 13–20 J fluence
- 10% overlap
- 12.5–15 mm spot size.

Alexandrite lasers are said to be more effective in treating light color and thin hair. Indian skin needs to be treated carefully with this wavelength as chances of burns are high. Always use optimal cooling with external devices (Zimmer) and use low fluence. The main use is in treating finer hair, which are present either from the start or are left after treatments with diode or Nd:YAG.

DIODE LASER (800–810 NM)

Diode laser works in the middle of melanin absorption spectrum. They have been proven as safe,[9] relatively cheap, and effective machines having very low maintenance cost. Diode laser is available as machines with stamping mode, in motion technology with scanner, and vacuum-assisted handpieces. They come with chill tip, so there is no need for external cooling device.

Parameters most commonly used in stamping mode are:

- Pulse duration 30–100 ms with fluence 18–22 J and overlap of 10% in stamping mode.

  The in-motion technology uses repeated and fast emission of low energy that progressively heats the chromophore without burning the epidermis. Larger areas can be covered in shorter time and is less painful than the stamping mode.

  Parameters most commonly used for in-motion laser are:

- 8–12 KJ, 10 Hz with movement of handpiece at 10 cm/s. Diode laser is considered the workhorse and gold standard, as they have a balance between efficacy and safety. The technology is stable, and the maintenance of these machines is very low as compared to other wavelengths.

A comparative study about laser transmission ratio to the dermis between diode and Alexandrite laser showed 4% more transmission for diode, thereby reporting diode as a better laser due to better depth of penetration.[10] Another study compared the efficacy, tolerability, and subject satisfaction for axillary hair removal by diode in stamping mode and super hair removal (SHR) mode with conventional scanned Alexandrite laser. Higher efficacy was reported in the stamping mode.[11]

After one treatment of diode laser, a 32–34% reduction has been reported,[12,13] and after multiple treatments, one study described an 84% reduction in hair.[14] Lou et al. studied 50 patients with skin prototypes II and III and found hair regrowth of 47–66% at 6 months after two treatments.[12] In this study, fluencies ranged from 10 to 40 J/cm^2, and pulse duration was 5–30 ms. Bouzari et al. compared different treatment intervals with the diode laser and found the mean hair reduction to be 78.1%, 45.8%, and 28.7%, respectively, in the 45-,60-, and 90-day interval groups.[15]

LONG-PULSED NEODYMIUM-DOPED YTTRIUM ALUMINUM GARNET LASER (1,064 NM)

The longer wavelength of this laser allows for deepest penetration and weakest absorption by epidermal melanin compared to all other wavelengths. This happens as longer wavelength (1,064 nm) leads to less scatter thereby protecting the epidermal melanin the competing chromophore and penetrating deep. It targets the hair structure approximately 5–7 mm below and results in less collateral damage to skin. This safety makes it a laser of choice in the darker skin type.[16-18]

Mittal et al. demonstrated the safety and efficacy of Nd:YAG. Long-pulse Nd:YAG is a good laser to be used in ethnic skin, but requires more sittings to give comparable results.[19]

Parameters most commonly user are 8–10 mm spot sizes with 30–50 ms pulse duration and a fluence of 35–45 J. Long-pulsed Nd:YAG laser is effective, but associated with discomfort and occasional burns and hyperpigmentation in some patients. Recently, submillisecond 1,064 Nd:YAG laser has been introduced and found to be more suitable for skin type IV and V.[20,21]

INTENSE PULSED LIGHT (515–1,200 NM)

These do not qualify technically as lasers, but work on the principle of selective photothermolysis. Unlike laser, intense pulsed light (IPL) uses flash lamps (xenon) to emit incoherent light from 515 to 1,200 nm. Cut-off filters that limit the range of wavelengths are used to exclude the shorter wavelengths.

Intense pulsed light devices have been used to treat hair of all skin types with good results. The main advantage is the large spot size, which makes it easy to treat large areas as back, chest, legs, etc. They are less expensive and one machine can treat multiple conditions. The side effects of these machines are same as lasers, but due to bigger spot size the scars are more unsightly and therefore difficult to hide as compared to lasers.

Intense pulsed light has been reported to have 84% effectiveness after four sessions.[22] Split face comparison with Alexandrite 755-nm laser proved that Alexandrite was more effective.[23] When compared to Nd:YAG (1,064 nm), IPL was shown to be less effective in skin type IV, V, and VI with slightly more risk of postinflammatory hyperpigmentation.[24]

SUPER HAIR REMOVAL IN MOTION™ TECHNIQUE

This is the new technique currently being incorporated specifically in triple wavelength machine. Instead of single pulse the repetitive low fluence pulse is delivered at targeted site in motion. High repetition of this low energy pulses results in uniform dissipation of heat at site resulting in gradual increase in temperature and higher average power in the treatment field with subsequent heating and destruction of hair follicles and sparing of surrounding tissue with good clinical outcome and lesser pain.

RADIOFREQUENCY DEVICES

Diode in IPL has been combined with RF for hair removal.[25] The combination have been studied by several authors and found to be an effective treatment option for hair reduction in all skin types.[26-28]

Radiofrequency causes heat to be focused on hair follicle and bulge whereas laser heats the hair shaft. This leads to uniform distribution of temperature across the hair shaft and follicle. There are reports that the patient gets more discomfort when RF energy is used in therapeutic range.

SIDE EFFECTS AND COMPLICATIONS[29]

- Pain and prolonged erythema
- Crusting
- Postinflammatory hyperpigmentation, usually temporary, can be treated with mild steroid or with depigmenting agents subsides in few days to weeks.[30]
- Postinflammatory hypopigmentation is difficult to manage and requires long-term treatment. Reports of using tacrolimus, topical PUVAsol, and targeted phototherapy are available.
- Rosacea such as lesions, acne aggravation, and follicular depigmentation are some of rare side effects of LHR.
- Paradoxical hypertrichosis is reported with all laser systems.[31] This usually happens due to usage of suboptimal energy thereby leading to paradoxical stimulation of adjacent hair.[32] Using better parameters, cooling the adjacent area while lasering, and switching to a different wavelength can be used to prevent this side effect. This side effect is most frequently seen over chin and in

skin type III and above. Paradoxical hypertrichosis can be treated with increasing the fluences in subsequent sittings.

Complications arising from laser devices are mostly operator dependent; they can happen with all wavelengths to even the most experienced. The idea is to use an optimum fluence and do the treatment as per the protocol explained earlier in the chapter.

TACKLING THE NONRESPONDERS

With the rampant use of laser hair reduction by nondermatologists, beauticians, and untrained individual, there is a subset of dissatisfied patients. Apart from this even after using appropriate parameters few patients get recurrence or are nonresponders.

Despite the best of machine and technique, some patients either do not respond or the improvement becomes stagnant. Here, some tips to handle such patients **(Box 3)**.

BOX 3: Tackling nonresponders.

- *Repeat pass technique:* After finishing the laser session, wait for 20–30 minutes till the erythema and edema disappear, this can be hastened by cooling the area with ice. Once the skin comes back to original, examine carefully to look for persistent erythema, places with impending burn (which can be appreciated as gray/brown color) or any dead hair. If any of these are appreciable then do not do the second session. However, once the skin is back to its original form then laser the entire area again with 20–30% lower fluences and careful monitoring of hot spots
- *Switching of technology:* If one has the luxury of having multiple laser technologies in the setup, then some of these patients can be shifted to another laser. Here, treatments can be switched between diode and Nd:YAG/Alex/IPL
- *Combining of lasers:* One can use a different wavelength for repeat pass technique discussed earlier. Sometime, the patient has both thick and thin hair in one area. One can use diode/Nd:YAG for the thick hair and Alexandrite for the thin hair in the same session
- A submillisecond pulse width can be combined with long-pulse Nd:YAG laser in a second session
- A patient can be called after a shorter interval, after 2 weeks for a repeat session in a resistant area

(Nd:YAG: neodymium-doped yttrium aluminum garnet; IPL: intense pulsed light)

REMOVAL OF GRAY HAIRS

Despite many advances in this field, light-based hair removal is still largely limited to dark hairs. No uniformly effective treatment is available for patients with blonde, white, or gray hair. Research is ongoing to develop efficacious modalities for the removal of light-colored hair. Using RF in addition to laser is one option. Hair loss in blonde, red, or gray-haired patients can be maintained by retreating at approximately 3 months interval. Delivering the chromophore by liposome

BOX 4: Tips for getting better results in laser hair removal.

- Start skin bleaching creams and sunscreen at least 15 days prior to lasering, this helps to lighten the skin thereby reducing the chance of burns. These should be continued in between the sessions as well
- Shave the hair gently. If the shaving is very harsh, it may lead to abrasion which will look unsightly later and is painful. If the hair is not completely shaved, it increases the chances of burn in that area. This can also happen, if the shaved hair is not removed from the skin. A simple micropore tape can be used to lift up the hair by sticking and removing the micropore over the entire area these hair stick on the undersurface of the tape
- It is always better to mark the areas to be lasered with white pencil and shows beforehand to the patient. This is useful when doing isolated areas such as chin, side locks, and eyebrows
- Beginners should make a grid with white pencil to avoid skip areas and retreating the same area
- Always be careful and slow. Do not try to finish the laser quickly and create a personal best time. Remember most of the burns are operator dependent
- Always concentrate on the area treated previously for any hot spots, persistent erythema, etc. These will a give you warning to decrease the fluence and prevent burns in other areas
- If you see any areas, which will potentially lead to complications, it is best to tell the patient while lasing itself. Do it gently but firmly most of the patients accept it. Start on a steroid antibiotic combination immediately for a few days, and at the same time counsel them regarding usage of camouflage for postinflammatory hyper-/hypopigmentation
- If the patient has a mixture of dark- and light-colored hair, change the fluence depending on the requirement in the same sitting (higher fluence for light hair). If one has the luxury of having multiple wavelengths then one can use Alexandrite for thin hair and diode/Nd:YAG for thick hair

(Nd:YAG: neodymium-doped yttrium aluminum garnet)

TABLE 1: Different wavelength lasers used in laser hair removal.

Wavelength (nm)	*Alexandrite (755)*	*Diode (810)*	*Nd:YAG (1,064)*
• Penetration • Absorption coefficient • Source delivery	• Lowest penetration up to 2.5 mm • Absorption 2.5 times than diode • Semiconductor/crystal • Direct/fiber	• Medium penetration up to 4 mm • Absorption three times >1,064 Nd:YAG • Semiconductor • Direct	• Deepest penetration up to 5 mm • Lowest absorption coefficient • Semiconductor/solid state • Direct/fiber
Ideal skin type	III/IV	IV/V	V/VI
Hair	Fine	Fine/coarse	Coarse
Chromophore indication	• Melanin • Hair reduction	Melanin Hair reduction	• Melanin/oxyhemoglobin • Hair reduction/vascular
Maintenance cost	++	+	++
Cooling	Have to use external chiller	Inbuilt	Have to use external chiller

(Nd:YAG: neodymium-doped yttrium aluminum garnet)

encapsulated melanin, then subsequently using laser energy is new approach to tackle these colorless hairs. >50% gray hair in treatment area is relative contraindication for LHR.

CONCLUSION

Laser hair reduction has stood the test of time. We are getting better, safer, and effective lasers for hair reduction. The choice of laser system depends on the expertise and the area of practice. No two machines can perform the same. Learning the parameters of your machine and playing with them gives best results. The search for an ideal hair removal laser goes on. **Table 1** shows a comparison of different wavelengths. **Box 4** describes tips for getting good results in LHR.

REFERENCES

1. American Society for Aesthetic Plastic Surgery. (2020). Cosmetic Surgery National Data Bank Statistics. [online] Available from https://www.surgery.org/sites/default/files/.
2. Van Gemert MJ, Welch AJ. Time constants in thermal laser medicine. Lasers Surg Med. 1989;9:405-21.
3. Commo S, Gaillardo O, Bernard BA. The human hair follicle contains two distinct K19 positive compartments in the outer root sheath: A unifying hypothesis for stem cell reservoir? Differentiation. 2000;66:157-64.
4. Garcia C, Alamoudi H, Nakib M, Zimmo S. Alexandrite laser hair removal is safe for Fitzpatrick skin types IV-VI. Dermatol Surg. 2000;26:130-4.
5. Aldraibi MS, Touma DJ, Khachemoune A. Hair removal with the 3-msec alexandrite laser in patients with skin types IV-VI: efficacy, safety, and the role of topical corticosteroids in preventing side effects. J Drugs Dermatol. 2007;6:60-6.
6. Hussain M, Polnikorn N, Goldberg DJ. Laser-assisted hair removal in Asian skin: efficacy, complications, and the effect of single versus multiple treatments. Dermatol Surg. 2003;29:249-54.
7. Eremia S, Li CY, Umar SH, Newman N. Laser hair removal: long-term results with a 755 nm alexandrite laser. Dermatol Surg. 2001;27:920-4.
8. Lu SY, Lee CC, Wu YY. Hair removal by long-pulse alexandrite laser in oriental patients. Ann Plast Surg. 2001;47:404-11.
9. Shirkavand A, Ataie-Fashtami L, Sarkar S, Alinaghizadeh MR, Fateh M, Zand N, et al. Thermal damage patterns of Diode hair-removal lasers according to various skin types and hair densities and colors: a simulation study. Photomed Laser Surg. 2012;30:374-80.
10. Mustafa FH, Jaafar MS, Ismail AH, Mutter KN. Comparison of alexandrite and diode lasers for hair removal in dark and medium skin: which is better? J Lasers Med Sci. 2014;5:188-93.
11. Paasch U, Wagner JA, Paasch HW. Novel 755-nm diode laser vs. conventional 755-nm scanned Alexandrite laser: Side-by-side comparison pilot study for thorax and axillary hair removal. J Cosmet Laser Ther. 2015;17:189-93.
12. Lou WW, Quintana AT, Geronemus RG, Grossman MC. Prospective study of hair reduction by diode laser (800 nm) with long-term follow-up. Dermatol Surg. 2000:26:428-32.
13. Baugh WP, Trafeli JP, Barnette DJ Jr, Ross EV. Hair reduction using a scanning 800 nm diode laser. Dermatol Surg. 2001;27:358-64.
14. Eremia S, Li C, Newman N. Laser hair removal with alexandrite versus diode laser using four treatment sessions: 1-year results. Dermatol Surg. 2001;27:925-9.
15. Bouzari N, Tabatabai H, Abbasi Z, Firooz A, Dowlati Y. Hair removal using an 800-nm diode laser: Comparison at different treatment intervals of 4,560 and 90 days. Int J dermatol. 2005; 44:50-3.
16. Battle EF Jr. Advances in laser hair removal in skin of color. J Drugs Dermatol. 2011;10:1235-9.
17. Battle EF Jr, Hobbs LM. Laser-assisted hair removal for darker skin types. Dermatol Ther. 2004;17:177-83.
18. Battle EF Jr. Cosmetic laser treatments for skin of color: a focus on safety and efficacy. J Drugs Dermatol. 2011;10:35-8.
19. Mittal R, Sriram S, Sandhu K. Evaluation of long-pulsed 1064 nm Nd:YAG Laser-assisted hair removal vs multiple treatment session and different hair types in Indian patients. J Cutan Aesthet Surg. 2008;1:75-9.
20. Lukac M, Gorjan M, Zabkar J, Grad L, Vizintin Z. Beyond customary paradigm: FRAC3® Nd:YAG laser hair removal. J Laser Health Acad. 2010;1:35-46.
21. Eltarky A, Marko Kazic ML. Avalanche FRAX3® Nd:YAG laser hair removal. J Laser Health Acad. 2013;1:23-31.
22. Feng Y, Zhao J, Gold MH. Skin rejuvenation in Asian skin: the analysis of clinical effects and basic mechanisms of intense pulsed light. J Drugs Dermatol. 2008;7:273-9.
23. McGill DJ, Hutchison C, Mckenzie E, McSherry E, Mackay IR. A randomized, split-face comparison of facial hair removal with the alexandrite laser and intense pulsed light system. Lasers Surg Med. 2007;39:767-72.
24. Goh CL. Comparative study on a single treatment response to long pulse Nd:YAG lasers and intense pulse light therapy for hair removal on skin type IV to VI is longer wavelengths lasers preferred over shorter wavelengths lights for assisted hair removal. J Dermatol Treat. 2003;14:243-7.
25. Yaghmai D, Garden JM, Bakus AD, Spenceri EA, Hruza GJ, Kilmer SL. Hair removal using a combination radiofrequency and intense pulsed light source. J Cosmet Laser Ther. 2004; 6:201-7.
26. Karsai S, Schmitt L, Raulin C, Hammes S. Combination of short- and long-pulsed mode of electro-optical synergy technology for photoepilation: a retrospective study with short- and long-term follow-up. J Eur Acad Dermatol Venereol. 2009;23:46-51.
27. Waldman A, Kreindle M. New technology in aesthetic medicine: ELOS electro-optical energy. J Cosmet Laser Ther. 2003;5:204-6.
28. Sadick NS, Shaoul J. Hair removal using a combination of conducted radiofrequency and optical energies: an 18-month follow-up. J Cosmet Laser Ther. 2004;6:21-6.
29. Wanner M. Laser hair removal. Dermatol Ther. 2005;18:209-16.
30. Lanigan SW. Incidence of side effects after laser hair removal. J Am Acad Dermatol. 2003;49:882-6.
31. Alajlan A, Shapiro J, Rivers JK, MacDonald N, Wiggin J, Lui H, et al. Paradoxical hypertrichosis after laser epilation. J Am Acad Dermatol. 2005;53:85-8.
32. Bouzari N, Firooz AR. Laser may induce terminal hair growth. Dermatol Surg. 2006;32:460.

CHAPTER 108

Nd:YAG Laser: Basic Laser Principles and Indications

Anuj Pall, Richa Kumar

KEY MESSAGES

- Neodymium-doped yttrium aluminum garnet (Nd:YAG) laser is the most versatile and useful available to the dermatologist today.
- It works by targeting the melanosomes/Tattoo particles to give the desired clinical result.
- It can be used to treat various pigmentary conditions; epidermal, dermal or mixed with good response.
- Athena triple spot treatment for effective management of dermal melanosis.
- Athena genesis laser technique for pigmentation, acne, open pores and facial rejuvenation.

INTRODUCTION

The origin of laser dates back to May 16, 1960, when Theodore H Maiman, a physicist at Hughes Research Laboratories in Malibu, constructed the first laser, using a cylinder of synthetic ruby, with silver-coated reflective ends.[1] However in 1963, Leon Goldman, also known as the "father of lasers in medicine", was the first to use the laser in dermatology where he demonstrated the use of lasers for treatment of pigmented lesions, tattoo removal, and also treatment of vascular lesions.[2]

In 1980, the domain of laser therapy was deeply revolutionized by the selective photothermolysis theory, postulated by Rox Anderson and John Parrish which highlighted the use of specific wavelength for destruction of specific molecules (or chromophores), allowing better localization of thermal energy and minimization of damage to the surrounding tissue.[3]

The Nd:YAG laser was invented by Joseph E Geusic and Richard G Smith at Bell Labs in 1964.[4] It has proved to be the most versatile laser with a wide range of indications in clinical dermatology dealing with pigmentary disorders, tattoos, vascular lesions, and facial rejuvenation.

LASER BASICS AND SYSTEMS

The unique characteristic of the laser light is that it is monochromatic, unidirectional, and coherent. The type of laser to be used for a particular skin condition is decided by the target chromophore and its absorption spectrum. For adequate tissue damage a wavelength should be preferentially absorbed by the chromophore in the target tissue and not absorbed by the surrounding tissue, thereby ensuring minimum adverse effects **(Fig. 1)**. For example, in treatment of pigmentary disorders, the chromophore of interest is melanin and light of wavelength from 290 nm up to the range of 1,200 nm is absorbed by melanin. Therefore, the treating dermatologist needs to select an appropriate laser keeping in mind this wavelength.

Wavelength has a dual impact attributable to its absorption coefficient in different chromophores as well as the depth of penetration from the skin surface, which roughly increases as the wavelength increases in the visible and near infrared spectrum.[6] Therefore at longer wavelengths, absorption is lower and the penetration is deeper as compared to the shorter wavelengths in cases of melanin being the chromophore **(Fig. 2)**.

A wavelength that penetrates 2–3 mm into the dermis is suitable for targeting deeper dermal pigmentation, such as found in nevus of Ota. Q-switched Nd:YAG (QS Nd:YAG) laser with a wavelength of 1,064 nm meets this requirement adequately.

By passing the beam in 1,064-nm Nd:YAG laser through the potassium titanyl phosphate (KTP) crystal, the frequency

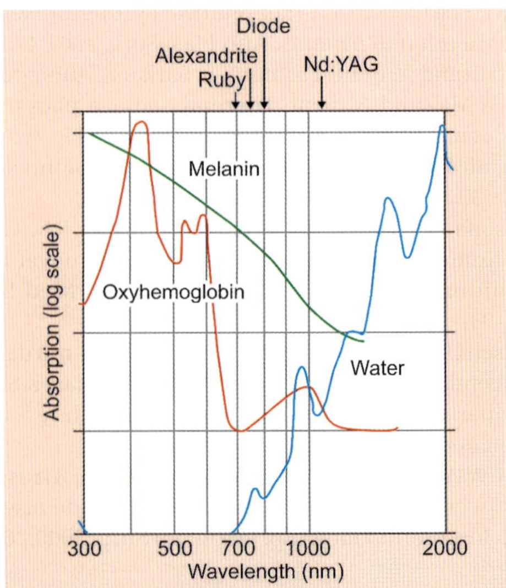

Fig. 1: The absorption of various chromophores as a function of wavelength.[5] (Nd:YAG: neodymium-doped yttrium aluminum garnet)

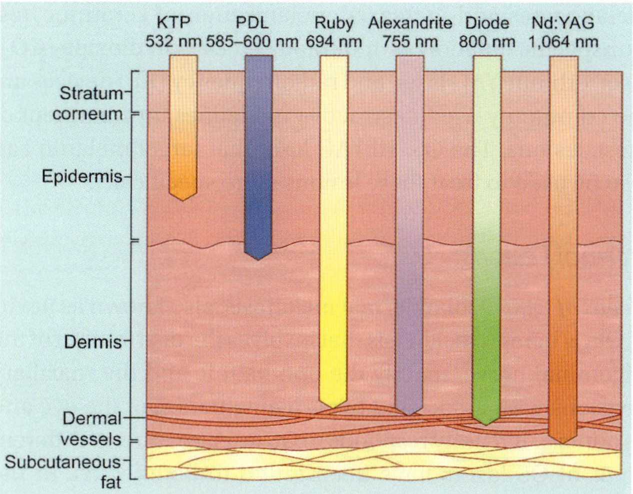

Fig. 2: Depth of penetration by various lasers. (KTP: potassium titanyl phosphate; Nd:YAG: neodymium-doped yttrium aluminum garnet; PDL: pulsed dye laser)
Source: Bolognia JL, Jorizzo JL, Rapini RP. Dermatology, 1st edition. Amsterdam, Netherlands: Mosby Elsevier; 2003. pp. 2148.

is doubled and the wavelength is halved (532 nm). A shorter wavelength will penetrate less deeply and therefore is more useful for removal of epidermal pigment, such as in ephelides.

To be selective, the pulse duration of the laser should be equal or lower than the thermal relaxation time (TRT) of the target. The estimated TRT of epidermis is 1–10 ms and the TRT of tattoo ink particles is 0.1–10 ns, although some newer estimates are in the range of 10–100 picoseconds. TRT of melanosomes is 250–1,000 ns, therefore melanosomes require submicrosecond laser pulses (<1 μs) for their selective destruction when pigmentary conditions are being treated.[7]

The size of the tattoo ink particles is about 10–100 nm and is generally placed at a depth of 1.1–2.9 mm. Laser tissue interaction produces intracellular steam and vacuole formation, which leads to immediate whitening. An audible popping sound is heard during the procedure due to the photoacoustic effect.[8]

The QS Nd:YAG laser matches all the requisite parameters for the same and got the United States Food and Drug Administration (US FDA) approval for tattoo reduction in 1991.

Picosecond lasers have also been recently added as a treatment modality of tattoos and have been found more effective than nanosecond lasers.[9]

PRINCIPLE OF Q-SWITCHING[10]

Q-switched (QS) laser have output in nanosecond range with high peak power. "Q" stands for quality factor of a resonant circuit. Q-switching is a technique for obtaining energetic short pulses from a laser by modulating the intracavity losses which is achieved by putting variable attenuator inside the laser's optical resonator. QS lasers produce nanosecond pulses of high energy and peak power with solid-state bulk lasers. These giant pulses are responsible for the unique laser-tissue interaction that is seen with QS lasers.

The shock produced due to the high energy pulses delivered over short period of time (5–11 ns) leads to rapid thermal expansion leading to rupture of the targets, such as melanosomes and ink particles.[11] The ruptured fragments are cleared by tissue macrophages either to the lymphatic channels or to the regional lymph nodes.

TABLE 1: Pigmented lesions amenable to treatment by lasers.

	Location in the skin	*Examples*
1.	Epidermal lesions	CALM, lentigines, ephelides, solar lentigo, nevus spilus, pigmented seborrheic keratosis, and DPN
2.	Dermal lesions	Nevus of Ota, blue nevus, Hori's nevus (acquired bilateral nevus of Ota-like macules), acquired dermal melanosis, i.e., LPP
3.	Epidermal-dermal lesions	Postinflammatory hyperpigmentation, nevus spilus, periorbital pigmentation, perioral pigmentation, acquired melanocytic nevi (moles), melasma, Becker's nevus, and Riehl's melanosis

(CALM: café-au-lait macule; DPN: dermatosis papulosa nigra; LPP: lichen planus pigmentosus)

INDICATIONS

Pigmented Lesions

Epidermal, dermal, and mixed lesions are amenable to treatment with Nd:YAG laser **(Table 1)**.

Epidermal Lesions

The frequency-doubled QS Nd:YAG laser (532 nm) safely and effectively treats benign epidermal pigmented lesions.[12]

Q-switched ruby (694 nm) and QS Alexandrite laser (755 nm) lasers can also can be used; however, caution has to be exercised in Indian skin type. Epidermal lesions require one to three sessions for clearing. Epidermal lesions can show recurrence few months to years after treatment, therefore, patients should be advised on continued sun protection even after the treatment. If required repeat laser treatments can be offered in cases of recurrence.

Café-au-lait macule (CALM): CALMs are brown to black colored epidermal pigmented lesions of unknown etiology.[13] CALMs are difficult to treat and usually require multiple treatments over months to years. Laser treatment may result in partial or incomplete clearance and recurrences are common, occurring in up to 50% of patients within a year of clearance. Adverse effects such as poor response to laser and pigmentary alteration such as speckled pattern of hyperpigmentation can be noted after laser sessions.

Ephelides and lentigines: Frequency-doubled QS Nd:YAG laser (532 nm) can be used to treat benign epidermal pigmented lesions such as ephelides with good clinical outcome. However, in darker patients even 1,064-nm Nd:YAG can be used. It requires one to two sessions for successful removal, although recurrences are common **(Figs. 3A and B)**. Patient needs to be kept on sun protection and maintenance sessions to prevent recurrence. Todd MM found QS Nd:YAG laser 532 nm to be the most effective laser for epidermal lesions.[14,15]

Nevus spilus: Nevus spilus presents as circumscribed tan colored macule with darkly pigmented macules or small papules. It has both epidermal and dermal components. Nevus spilus can be treated effectively with the QS laser such as ruby, Alexandrite, and Nd:YAG laser. Average number of treatments required may be three to six.[16-18] In such cases, the treating dermatologist needs to modify the spot sizes between various sessions to tackle the pigmentary component at different levels **(Figs. 4A and B)**.

Dermatosis papulosa nigra (DPN) and pigmented seborrheic keratoses: These lesions have significant epidermal proliferation with normal to slightly increased number of melanocytes and increased melanization of keratinocytes. Nonspecific ablation with ultrapulsed carbon dioxide (CO_2) laser, erbium:YAG laser, and radiofrequency (RF) devices are the commonly used destructive modalities for treatment of these lesions. The QS Nd:YAG laser that target melanin can also be used to treat these lesions more specifically.[19-21]

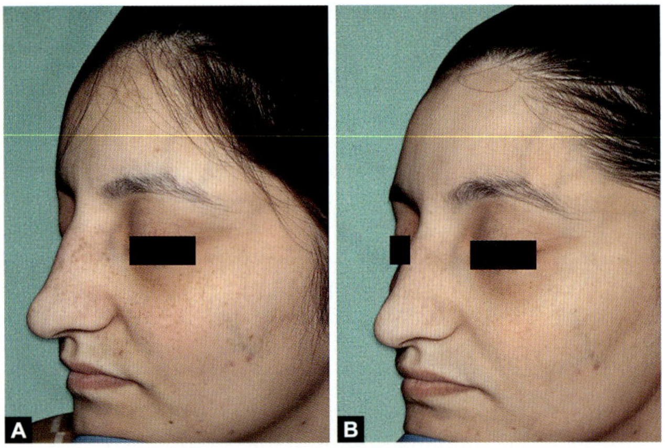

Figs. 3A and B: Freckles before and after two sessions with 1064 nm Nd:YAG laser in a 38-year-old female (polarized view).

Dermal Lesions

Nevus of Ota: Ocular dermal melanosis, also known as nevus of Ota is benign melanosis that involves the distribution of the trigeminal nerve, mainly the ophthalmic and the maxillary divisions with associated hyperpigmentation of the eye and its adnexa. It readily responds to QS laser treatment. Different types of QS lasers have been found to be effective in the treatment of nevus of Ota. The longer wavelength 1,064-nm QS Nd:YAG laser is the most widely used laser to treat, especially in darker skin types **(Figs. 5A and B)**. The longer wavelength along with a large spot size allows deep penetration of photons and is ideally suited to treat this dermal condition. Multiple treatments are necessary (typically more than 10 sessions) with an interval of at least 4–6 weeks between treatments. Kar HK and Gupta L found that QS Nd:YAG is an easy-to-perform and effective treatment in cases of nevus of Ota in Indian patients with fewer side effects.[22]

Q-switched ruby laser can also be effectively used in the treatment of nevus of Ota. Recurrence is rare, but hypopigmentation is common and can be permanent.[23]

Chan HH did a study in Chinese patients and concluded that patients tolerate QS Alexandrite better than QS Nd:YAG based on the pain scores and minimal side effects such as scarring.[24-26]

Nevus of Ito: It is a grayish blue macular hyperpigmentation seen in the distribution of posterior supraclavicular and lateral brachial cutaneous nerves, present over the shoulder or upper arm. The lesion responds well to 1,064-nm QS Nd:YAG laser and requires multiple sessions.

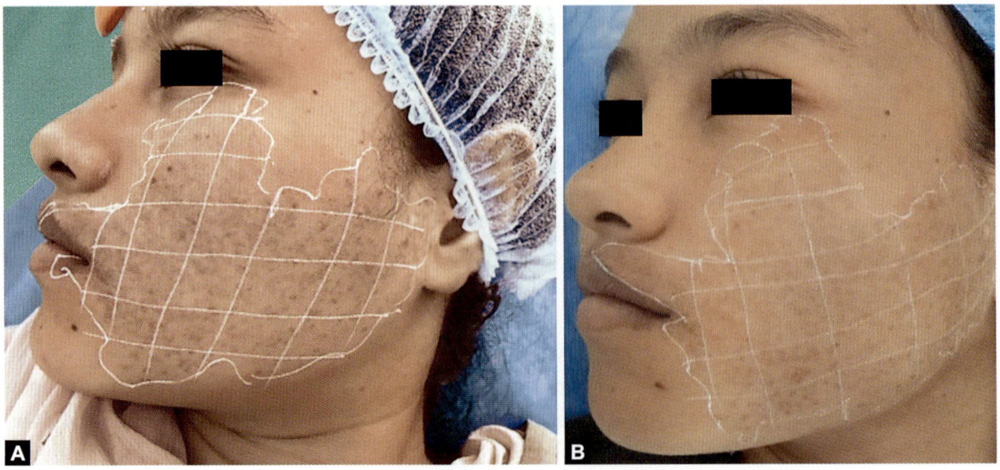

Figs 4A and B: Significant improvement in nevus spilus before and after six sessions.

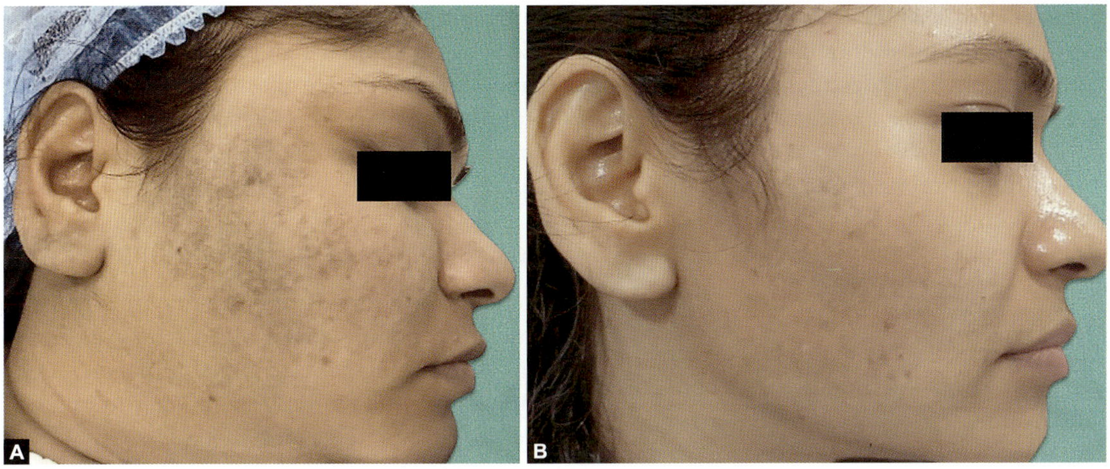

Figs. 5A and B: Nevus of Ota: Before and after seven sessions of treatment with 1,064-nm Q-switched neodymium-doped yttrium aluminum garnet (QS Nd:YAG laser).

Hori's nevus (acquired bilateral nevus of Ota-like macules): In acquired bilateral nevus of Ota-like macules or Hori's nevus, patient presents with late onset and symmetrical blue-brown facial pigmentation similar to nevus of Ota. The mucosal involvement seen in nevus of Ota is absent in Hori's nevus. 1,064-nm QS Nd:YAG laser is a good modality for treatment of such conditions. An average of five to six sessions is needed for good response with an interval of 4–6 weeks. However, the results are not as good as seen in nevus of Ota.[27]

Acquired dermal melanoses:

Riehl's melanosis: Riehl's melanosis (pigmented contact dermatitis) is a hyperpigmentary condition that typically occurs on the face and neck and is characterized by the rapid onset of gray-brown reticular pigmentation.

Kwon et al. in a pilot study using a triple combination approach (low-fluence QS Nd:YAG laser, hydroquinone cream and oral tranexamic acid) for the treatment of Riehl's melanosis in eight patients found significant improvement after 10–18 sessions.

Low-fluence Nd:YAG laser has been found to be an effective and safe treatment modality for Riehl's melanosis. Choi CW studied 10 Korean patients with Riehl's melanosis. The patients received 10–28 treatment sessions at 3-week intervals with low-fluence Nd:YAG laser along with topical hydroquinone and showed good results.[28]

Lichen planus pigmentosus (LPP): It is an acquired dermal pigmentation which presents as bluish gray discoloration over the face, neck, and forearms. It is characterized histopathologically by interface dermatitis and pigmentary incontinence. The pigment is usually stubborn making it a difficult condition to treat. Shah et al. treated 13 patients with quiescent LPP with QS Nd:YAG laser along with topical tacrolimus and found satisfactory results in all patients.

Neodymium-doped yttrium aluminum garnet laser should be used in cases of LPP where active signs of disease activity such as progression of lesions clinically and basal cell vacuolization and perivascular infiltrate are not seen on histopathology. 1,064-nm Nd:YAG can work as an useful tool to tackle the resistant dermal pigment (dermal melanophages) **(Figs. 6A and B)**.[29]

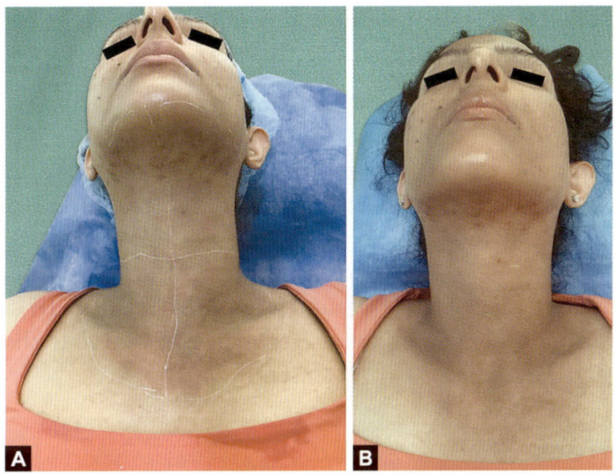

Figs. 6A and B: Remarkable improvement in a lichen planus pigmentosus (LPP) after eight sessions. (Athena Triple Spot Treatment)

Epidermal-dermal Lesions

Melasma: Melasma is an acquired pigmentary condition, presenting as dark brown to black pigmentation over face. It can be epidermal, dermal, or mixed, depending upon the localization of the excessive pigment. Various treatment modalities have been postulated for treatment of this condition. Lasers as a therapeutic option in melasma are considered only in cases of dermal melasma, resistant to conventional treatment options.

Laser toning or low-fluence QS Nd:YAG laser monotherapy also has been found to have good results in melasma in multiple studies.[30] It involves a low fluence, multipass technique, and multiple sessions at weekly intervals and is based on the theory of subcellular selective photothermolysis proposed by Mun et al. in 2011. In this technique, by using a high peak power, ultrashort pulse duration (5 ns), low fluence, and a flat-top beam results in the destruction of only melanin in target cells, keeping the cell alive, thereby minimizing the inflammation.[31]

However in authors experience in Indian skin type, 2 weekly treatments with similar parameters have been found to be more useful.

The results of low-fluence QS Nd:YAG laser (1,064 nm) were found to be better when combined with intense pulsed light (IPL).[32] Low-fluence laser can also be combined with triple combination and it has been found to give better results than individual treatment.[33]

However, it can lead to many side effects such as mottled pigmentation and high rates of recurrence. Chan et al. reported a series of facial depigmentation with the use of low-fluence QS Nd:YAG laser. Hence, caution needs to be exercised while performing this procedure and the risks need to be explained to patients.[34]

Postinflammatory hyperpigmentation (PIH):[35] PIH can result from various dermatological conditions or secondary to topical applications or treatment. It may have epidermal and dermal components. 1064-nm QS Nd:YAG laser has been found an effective modality for the treatment of PIH caused by acne. Zawar VP et al. treated 78 patients with PIH due to acne with 1,064-nm Nd:YAG laser and found good results. PIH due to various other conditions also have been reported to show good response to QS Nd:YAG laser.[36]

Tattoos

Tattoo removal aims on removal of deposited tattoo pigment effectively with minimum adverse effects such as pigmentary changes or keloidal scarring. QS ruby and QS Alexandrite lasers have been earliest lasers for tattoo removal. Since the wavelength of 694 nm is well absorbed by melanin, the most common adverse effect reported is hypopigmentation.[37]

Q-switched Nd:YAG 1,064-nm laser is especially useful in darker patients with Fitzpatrick types V and VI skin due to its longer wavelength. It is most effective for treating black tattoos, especially in more pigmented skin with rare textural changes and almost no hypopigmentation.[38]

A frequency-doubling crystal converts 1,064 nm light to 532 nm green light, which is absorbed well by red ink, as well as by melanin and hemoglobin. >75% removal of red ink within four treatment sessions has been reported. Orange and some purple colors respond almost as well.[39]

Prior to the advent of laser technology, most tattoos were removed by surgical excision, abrasive techniques, cryosurgery, or chemical peels which lead to scarring.

On implantation into the dermis, the tattoo ink particles are engulfed by residing macrophages and they become a "permanent" part of the cell. QS laser pulses fracture the ink into smaller sized particles. Some of the resulting smaller fragments are eliminated transepidermally and the majority are either removed by scavenger cells to the local lymph nodes, or picked up again by resident macrophage cells.[40]

General Principles for Treating Tattoos

Professional tattoos done with tattoo guns, densely pigmented tattoos, decorative tattoos with a variety of colors, and tattoos with metallic pigments (e.g., cadmium, mercury, cobalt, and copper) may be particularly difficult to remove and might require 15–20 sittings for removal.

Amateur tattoos, on the other hand, are typically less dense and are made up of carbon-based India ink that responds more readily to QS laser treatment and may respond in 6–10 sittings.

Adverse Effects[39]

Pigmentary changes: The most common adverse effects following laser tattoo treatment is pigmentary alteration. It may or may not be associated with textural change or scarring. Hypopigmentation is most noticeable when using wavelengths well absorbed by melanin, thereby injuring the melanocytes. The 510- and 532-nm wavelengths invariably leave a temporary hypopigmentation that resolves readily.[41]

Ink darkening: Development of immediate pigment darkening after laser treatment of tattoos is possible if iron oxide and titanium dioxide particles are present due to the reduction reactions. Therefore, a test patch is required before the complete patch is done.

Allergic reaction: Most commonly local allergic responses in the form of erythema and pruritus have been reported after laser treatment. However, systemic allergic reaction is also not uncommon.[42]

Hypertrophic scar and keloid: In certain cases, repeated sessions of laser for deep seated tattoos can result in development of hypertrophic scars and keloid.

Laser Hair Reduction

The long-pulsed 1,064-nm Nd:YAG laser is a safe and effective method of long-term hair reduction in patients with darkly pigmented skin. Alexandrite, diode, and IPL devices are the other options for long-term hair removal. However because of its longer wavelength, the Nd:YAG is the better laser system to use for pigmented skin as the adverse effects of pigmentary changes are minimum.[43,44] It can be used to target the deeper hair follicles without significant damage to the surrounding skin.

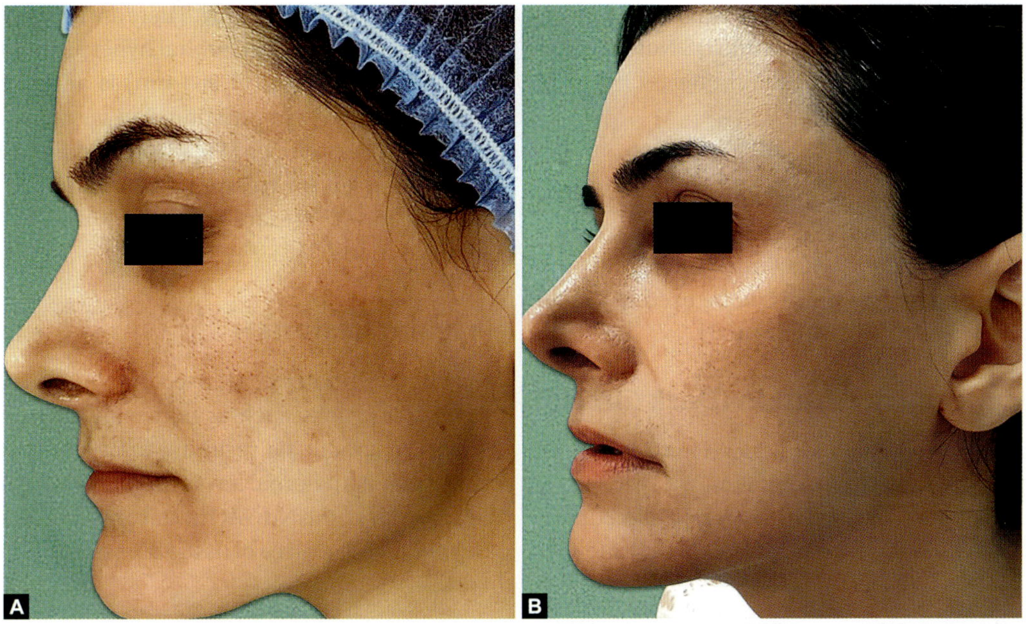

Figs. 7A and B: A 36-year-old patient before and after six sessions of treatment with both TH mode and quasi long-pulsed mode of Q-switched neodymium-doped yttrium aluminum garnet (QS Nd:YAG) laser (Athena Genesis laser treatment).

Quasi Long-pulsed 1,064-nm Nd:YAG (Micropulsed) Technology

In this mode, 1,064-nm Nd:YAG laser is used in the micropulsed mode, pulse fluence of 2–3 J/cm^2 and pulse width of 300 μs. It has been found useful in various skin conditions such as nonablative laser skin resurfacing, treatment of photoaging (wrinkles), treatment of enlarged facial pores, and management of active acne (moderate-to-severe). It can be used alone or in combination with QS Nd:YAG laser. It has been reported by many authors that 1,064-nm Nd:YAG laser-induced thermal damage increases the homogenization of collagen by penetrating into the deep dermal tissue, thereby improving skin texture, wrinkles, and open pores **(Figs. 7A and B)**.

Nonablative Laser Skin Resurfacing

Goldberg D et al. used 1064-nm Nd:YAG laser for photo rejuvenation in comparison to CO_2 lasers. Although the results were less effective than char-free CO_2 lasers in most patients, it was found to be an effective option for skin rejuvenation.[45,46] Multiple studies have demonstrated beneficial role of long-pulsed 1,064 Nd:YAG laser in treatment of photoaging (wrinkles).[47,48] Long-pulsed Nd:YAG laser has been also found useful in treatment of *open pores* with good results.

Treatment of Atrophic Facial Acne Scar and Active Acne

Ablative lasers have been used since long in treatment of acne scars; however, there is always concern over longer down time and chances of pigmentary changes. Nonablative treatment with the 1,064-nm QS Nd:YAG laser offers significant advantages to patients in terms of its minimal recovery period and minimal risk of infectious and pigmentary complications. Friedman PM et al. treated 11 patients with mild-to-moderate atrophic acne scars with 1,064-nm QS Nd:YAG laser and found satisfactory response after 3 months of follow-up in the form of improved texture of the skin.[49]

Artzi O et al. treated moderate-to-severe 19 subjects with 1,064-nm Nd:YAG quasi long-pulsed laser at 8 J/cm^2 fluence at 2 weeks intervals. Significant reduction in Acne Global Severity Scale (AGSS) scores was recorded after two treatments and maintained a statistically significant reduction rate throughout the treatment.[50]

Treatment of Rosacea

Vascular component of rosacea has been tackled by Nd:YAG laser long with other lasers such as KTP laser, pulsed dye laser (PDL), and also IPL devices. The described therapeutic effects include the reduction of vascular abnormalities and even improvement of papulopustular changes. Say EM treated 66 patients with erythemotelangiectatic and papulopustular rosacea were treated using long-pulsed Nd:YAG laser with 15–20 μs pulse width and 2–3 mm spot size. The patient showed good response to therapy.[51]

Carbon Peeling

The Nd:YAG has been used for treatment of dilated pores, aging, and acne along with the carbon lotion with good results. In this procedure, a carbon lotion is applied before the laser treatment (10–20 minutes) after the topical anesthesia **(Figs. 8A and B)**. Carbon peeling has shown good results in inflammatory and noninflammatory acne, done at monthly intervals. Both modes quasi long-pulsed and QS Nd:YAG laser can be used in sequence when using a carbon peel.[52,53]

Dark Lips

Dark lips are a common cosmetic concern in India. Somyas et al. found two to four sessions of QS 532 nm are an effective treatment for lip lightening.[54] In authors experience, 1,064-nm QS Nd:YAG laser with 4 mm spot size can be used in Indian patients with good response **(Figs. 9A and B)**.

Periorbital Hyperpigmentation (Dark Circles)

It is caused by various exogenous and endogenous factors such as genetic or heredity, excessive pigmentation, PIH secondary to atopic and allergic contact dermatitis, periorbital edema, excessive vascularity, shadowing due to skin laxity, and tear trough associated with aging. There are a number of treatment options available for periorbital hyperpigmentation.

The Nd:YAG laser (1,064 nm) is an effective modality in reducing the pigmentation and vascular component of infraorbital dark circles **(Figs. 10A and B)**. Other lasers that have been used for treating dark circles are QS ruby laser (694 nm) and QS Alexandrite laser along with various topical therapy options.[55]

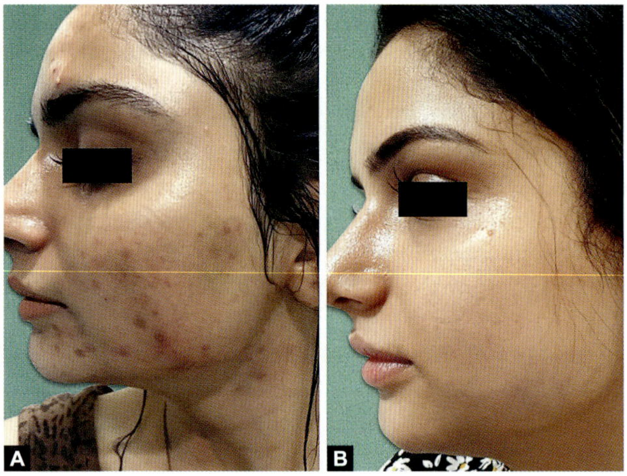

Figs. 8A and B: Before and after five sessions of treatment for active acne with carbon peel followed by quasi long-pulsed and Q-switched neodymium-doped yttrium aluminum garnet (QS Nd:YAG) laser in sequence.

Vascular Lesions

Michael Landthaler et al. used Nd:YAG laser for treatment of vascular lesions such as port-wine stains with a nodular surface, macrocheilia resulting from a port-wine stain, and capillary hemangioma. It was found that in comparison with the argon laser, the Nd:YAG laser coagulates at a much deeper level but higher degree of tissue fibrosis leading more scarring of tissue.[56]

Transcutaneous Laser Treatment of Leg Veins

Leg telangiectasias and reticular veins are a common complaint affecting >80% of the population to variable extent. Sclerotherapy is the gold standard of treatment for most of the patients. However, in conditions where sclerotherapy is contraindicated such as needle phobia, allergy to certain sclerosing agents and the presence of vessels smaller than the diameter of a 30-gauge needle (including telangiectatic matting), transcutaneous laser therapy is a valuable alternative. The 532-nm KTP laser, the 585–600-nm PDL, the 755-nm Alexandrite laser, various 800–983-nm diode lasers, and the 1,064-nm (Nd:YAG) laser and various IPL sources have been evaluated for use in this condition.[57]

The Nd:YAG laser with the wavelength of 1,064 nm, with a high-peak power, and pulse duration ranging from 0.25 to 300 ms is used for treatment of vascular conditions.

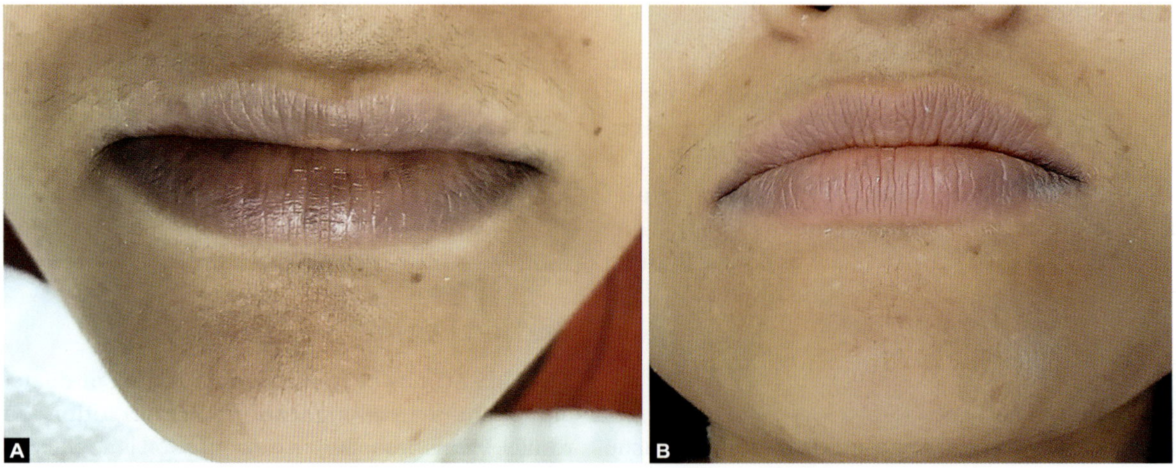

Figs. 9A and B: Dark lips before and after eight sessions of treatment with 1,064-nm Q-switched neodymium-doped yttrium aluminum garnet (QS Nd:YAG) laser with 4-mm spot size.

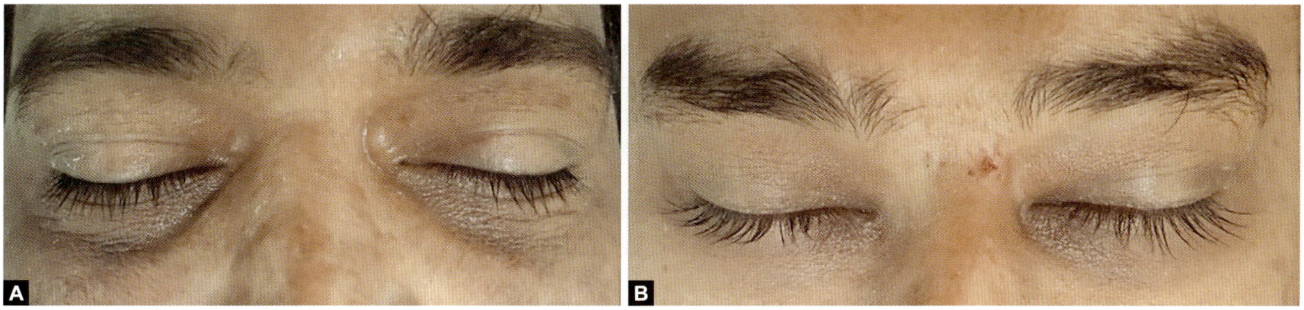

Figs. 10A and B: Improvement in periorbital melanosis and wrinkles after five sessions.

1,064-nm (Nd:YAG) laser has been especially found effective in treatment of deep seated and larger veins due to its deeper absorption. The results and the recurrence rates have been found comparable to sclerotherapy which is considered as the gold standard of treatment. Side effects such as hyperpigmentation or telangiectatic matting may be seen after both sclerotherapy and Nd:YAG laser, although pain scores are higher with the laser.[58,59]

CONTRAINDICATIONS

Absolute contraindications:[8,60]

- Associated photoaggravated skin diseases and medical illness, e.g., systemic lupus erythematosus (SLE)
- Treatment area with active cutaneous infections, e.g., herpes labialis and staphylococcal infections
- Unstable vitiligo and psoriasis for risk of koebnerization of treated area
- Tattoo granuloma
- Localized allergic reactions can occur with almost any color ink and result in urticaria and granulomatous reactions.

Relative contraindications:

- Keloid and keloidal tendencies
- *History of herpes simplex/history of herpes for increased risk of reactivation*: This risk should be seriously considered prior to performing the procedure. If the treating physician decides to perform the procedure, the risk and benefit should be explained to the patient and the procedure should be performed after proper informed consent and only after a course of acyclovir.
- Patient who is not cooperative or has unrealistic expectation.

LASER PROCEDURE

Patient Selection and Counseling[8,60,61]

Proper patient selection is the most important step in a laser treatment. A general medical history, current medical conditions and drug history allergies, past surgeries including bleeding tendencies and wound healing (with or without keloidal tendencies) along with history of previous laser sessions, if any taken, should be taken.

Complete method of laser treatment including the number of procedures, short outline of the events on the procedure day, response to be expected, and the total duration of treatment expected should be explained to the patient in the language understood.

An informed written consent is taken.

Good and representative pretreatment photographs are mandatory. Serial photographs should therefore be taken at successive visits. Various advancement in the form of different imaging systems are available to carry out facial analysis prior to and after the treatment. Reveal imager uses standard white light and cross-polarized flash photography to evaluate surface and subsurface skin conditions. RBX® Technology from Canfield provides extraordinary visualization of melanin and hemoglobin within the epidermis and papillary dermis.

Preoperative Preparation[8,60,61]

Sun Protection

History and examination for tanning is required before starting the laser treatment. If a patient is tanned, epidermal melanin produced by ultraviolet (UV) light exposure may interfere with laser treatment and increase the risks for pigmentary changes. Ideally, treatment should be delayed until the tan has faded as much as possible in the treatment area. Use of broad-spectrum sun protection creams with UVA coverage is crucial.

Oral Retinoids

Recent multicenter studies have documented the safety of oral retinoids while undergoing laser therapy. As per the guidelines there is no requirement to stop oral retinoids before the treatment.[62]

Priming of Skin

Proper priming of the skin with skin-lightening agents such as hydroquinone, kojic acid, and/or other nonhydroquinone skin lightening agents at least 2–3 weeks prior to the initiation of laser therapy for treatment of pigmentary conditions such as melasma is ideal.

Test Patch

It is ideal to do a test patch to confirm the laser parameters. Assessment should be done 4–8 weeks after the test patch to ascertain the effects and then the complete lesion can be treated.

Anesthesia

Topical eutectic mixture of local anesthetic (EMLA) should be applied under occlusion 30–60 minutes before the procedure.

Eye Protection

Q-switched lasers produce ultrashort pulse durations of high energy that produce significant tissue splatter. QS laser light can cause permanent retinal damage and vision loss. Eye protection in the form of optically coated glasses or goggles for the specific laser being used is necessary.

Laser Parameters

Fluence

It is always preferable to begin with the lowest energy fluence that produces a visible frosting. Higher fluence can lead to pinpoint bleeding and erosions which should be avoided.

Spot Size

It is the single most important parameter in a QS laser. Larger spot sizes allow deeper penetration and produce less tissue splatter which can be used for treating dermal lesions. Epidermal lesions would need a smaller spot size.

Frequency

Based on the type of the lesion, location, and the comfort of the dermatologist it can be modified.

Note: Use of a laser with a "top-hat" beam profile, large spot size, and lower fluences in darker skin types is preferable.

Laser Procedure[8,61]

After choosing the correct spot size and the energy fluence (J/cm^2), laser treatment is performed. The handpiece is always held perpendicular to the lesion and the entire area is covered with minimal overlap (up to 10%). QS laser treatment will produce an immediate frosting of the lesion along with a popping sound in cases of tattoos. In pigmentary lesions and laser toning, mild erythema is the targeted endpoint. The entire lesion is covered in one pass. The area is cooled with ice packs/air cooling after laser pulses. A mild topical steroid can be applied for 3–5 days after the session.

Number of Sessions

Epidermal lesions respond in lesser number of sessions (1-2); however, the dermal lesions need larger number of sessions (4–6 or more). Tattoos may need 5–20 sessions depending upon the type of tattoo. Professional tattoos require more treatment sessions for removal. Amateur tattoos are less dense and are often made up of carbon-based ink that responds more readily to QS laser treatment in lesser number of sessions.

The Kirby-Desai scale has been proposed to be used to estimate the approximate number of sessions needed for a given tattoo based on the following factors:

1. Fitzpatrick skin type
2. Location
3. Color
4. Amount of ink used
5. Scarring and tissue damage
6. Ink layering

Each of these six factors are given numerical score and the total of these will give an estimate of the approximate number of sessions required for tattoo removal.[63]

Interval between Sessions

Treatment should be done at least 6–8 weeks apart. Treatment intervals can be longer when treating nevus of Ota (up to 6 months interval has been suggested). While treating tattoos also longer intervals are advisable. Continued clearance of the lesion occurs due to removal of pigment by macrophages and lymphatics between treatments.

Laser Procedure (Newer Methods)

Athena Triple Spot Treatment

It is a well-accepted fact that wavelength and spot size can each impact the depth of penetration of the laser. Depth of penetration is determined by light absorption and scattering in the tissue. In general, longer wavelengths and larger spot sizes have less scattering in the tissue and thus penetrate deeper **(Figs. 11A and B)**. Hence, deeper pigment can be treated at different depths by choosing longer wavelength (1,064 nm) and altering the spot sizes.

Authors recommend a novel scientific approach of treating dermal melanosis by 1,064 QS Nd:YAG laser using three different spot sizes with variable fluence in the same session. Treatment should be carried out by implementing top-hat beam profile and quickly-pulse-to-pulse (Q-PTP) mode, especially at higher fluence. In this technique, patient is treated with three different spot sizes starting with 9 mm, followed by 6 mm and finally at 4 mm using a low fluence for the effective treatment of deep dermal pigmentary dyschromia. The end point would be mild erythema without frosting and petechiae (Athena triple spot treatment). It is then followed by treatment with 300 μs Quasi long-pulsed mode using spot sizes 10 mm and 5 mm **(Fig. 12)** for the improvement of skin texture, wrinkles, and open pores **(Figs. 13 and 14)**. This new innovative technique is known as Athena Genesis laser technique **(Table 2)**.

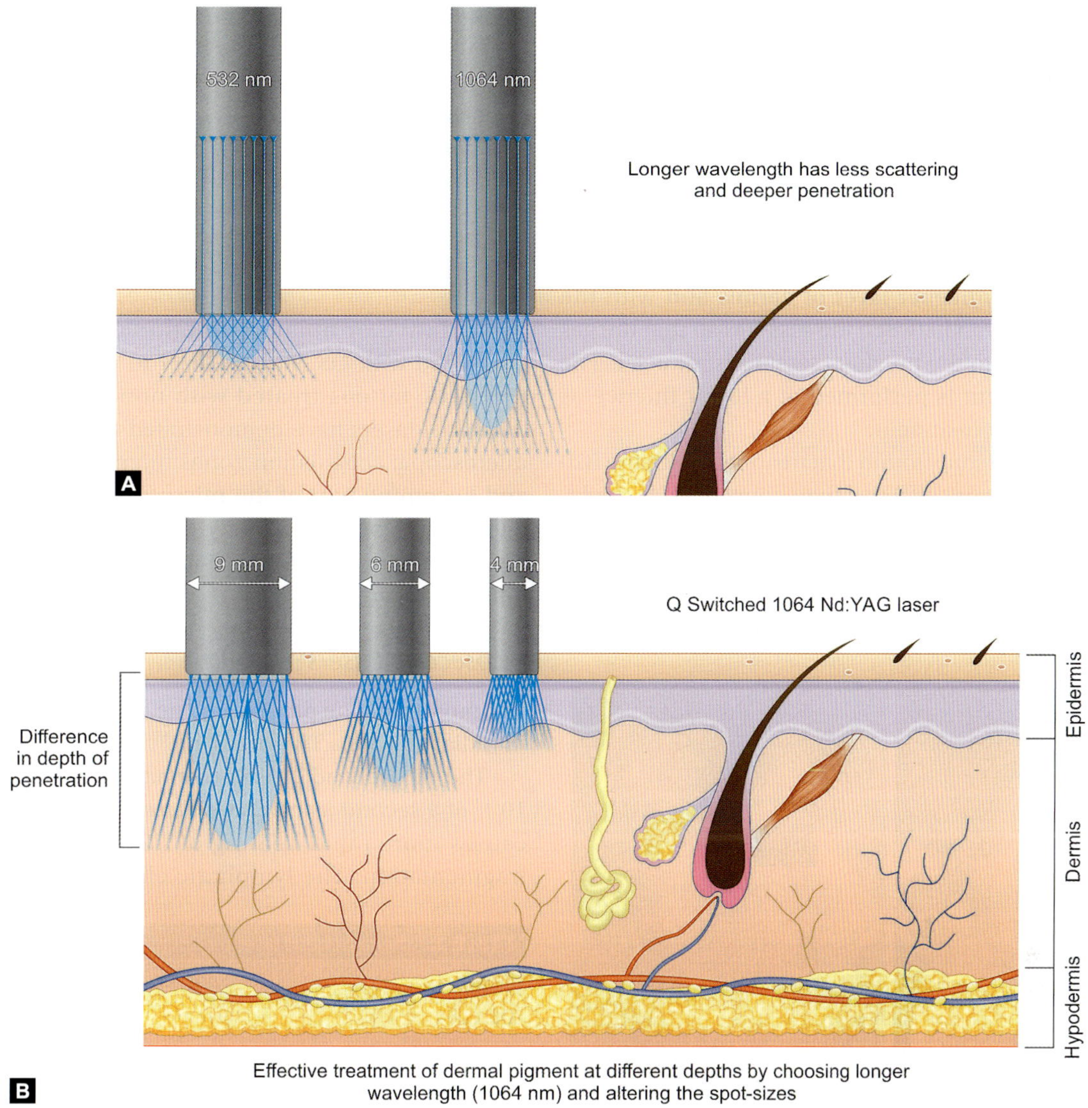

Figs. 11A and B: (A) Effect of wavelength on scattering and penetration of laser; (B) Effect of spot size on penetration depth.

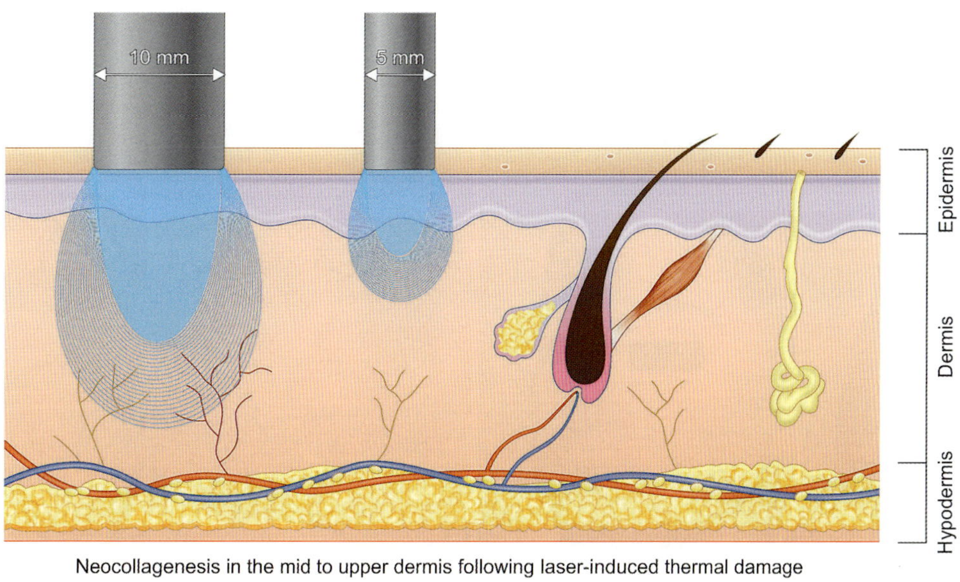

Fig. 12: Quasi long-pulsed mode of 1064 Nd:YAG laser for neocollagenesis.

Newer techniques for laser tattoo removal are:

- R20 technique
- R0 technique
- Combining fractional lasers with QS lasers
- Picosecond lasers

R20 method: Multiple treatments are done with an interval of 20 minutes between the subsequent treatments. It is based on the hypothesis that each pass in the R20 method treats a successively deeper layer of dermis and with the gap of 20 minutes given between the sessions so that the gas bubble formed due to the previous session is reduced. The subsequent treatment is performed at a lower fluence as compared to the first treatment.

Kossida et al. in a study found that treatment with the R20 method was much more effective than conventional single-pass laser treatment without any added adverse effects.[64]

R0 method: Repeated exposure on same day without waiting period can be performed by applying perfluorodecalin (a perfluorocarbon compound, commercially available as "Zero-W") immediately after lasing.

The compound dissolves the gas bubbles formed upon initial laser exposure thereby opening the optical window by reducing scatter. This allows an immediate next pass to be performed without the waiting time of 20 minutes as in the R20 technique.[65]

Combining Lasers

Nonablative or ablative fractional resurfacing can be combined with QS Nd:YAG laser to improve the outcome. Cosmetic tattoos treated with nonablative and ablative fractional lasers have demonstrated tattoo pigments in the microscopic coagulation zones migrating to the epidermis and becoming part of the microscopic exudative necrotic debris that can be exfoliated after 5 days. Such fractional resurfacing when combined with the traditional QS lasers offers a synergistic effect.[66]

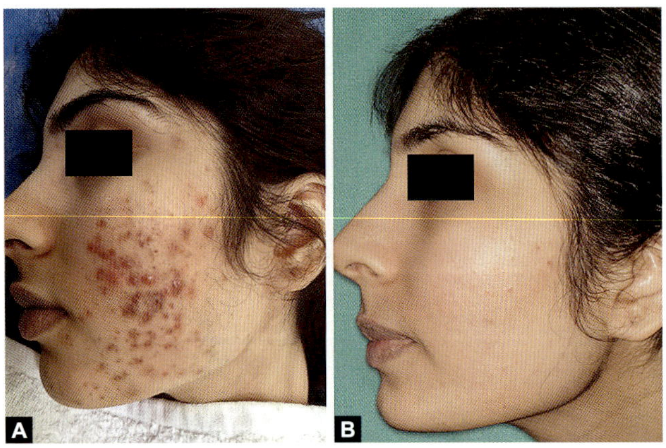

Figs. 13A and B: Athena Genesis laser treatment before and after six sessions. Improvement in acne, postinflammatory hyperpigmentation (PIH), and open pores.

Picosecond Lasers

The most common particle in black tattoo is the carbon black in India ink with a TRT of <10 ns.[67]

The picosecond lasers have narrower pulse duration of 10^{-12} of a second as compared to nanosecond lasers, which causes more rapid heating of the tattoos and thus finer fragmentation. The lymphatic elimination of these finer

TABLE 2: Athena Genesis laser technique.

Mode	*Spot size*	*Fluence*
QS 1,064	9 mm	1.3–1.5
QS 1,064	6 mm	1.8–2.0
QS 1,064	4 mm	1.6–1.8
Quasi long pulse	10 mm	1.5–2.0
Quasi long pulse	5 mm	8–10

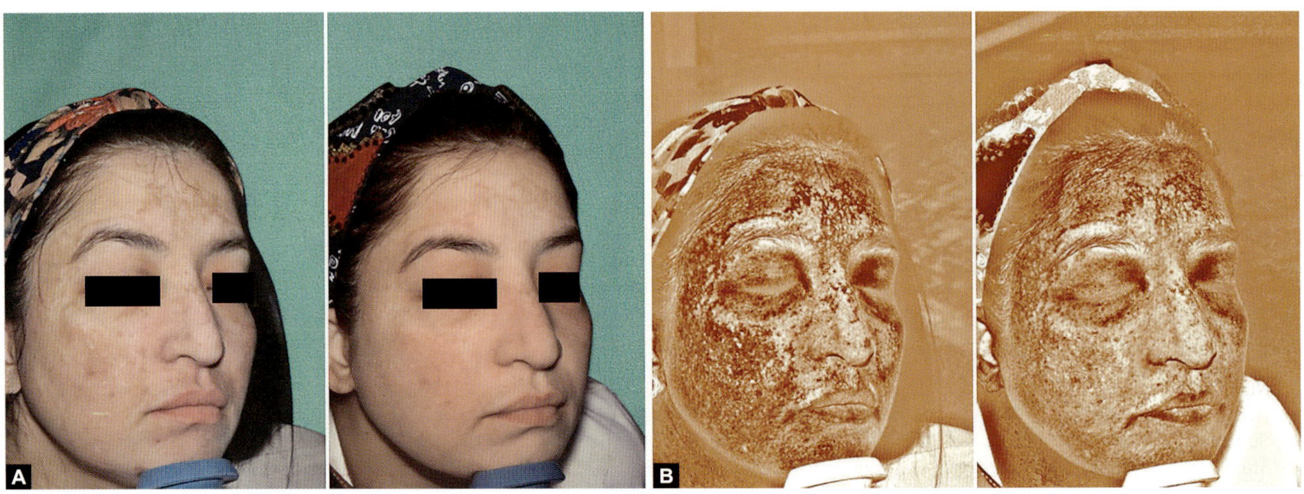

Figs 14A and B: Significant improvement in melasma and skin rejuvenation after Athena Genesis laser treatment. (A) Polarized view; (B) Pigment view.

TABLE 3: Summary of the pigmented conditions treated by Nd:YAG laser.

Level of pigmentation	*Condition*	*Wavelength used*	*Laser parameters*	*Number of sittings*	*Remarks*
Epidermal	Freckles and lentigines	QS, 1,064 nm	Fluence: 3–3.5 J/cm^2 Spot size: 4 mm	One to three	Sun protection to avoid recurrence
	CALM	QS 532 nm (in lighter skin types), 1,064 nm in darker skin tones		Multiple	50% recurrence within a year
	Nevus spilus	1,064 nm	6 mm and 4 mm 3–3.5	Multiple	
	DPN and seborrheic keratosis	532 nm		One to three	
Dermal	Nevus of Ota	QS 1,064 nm	5–6 mm spot size Fluence: 3.5–4	Multiple at intervals of 6–8 weeks	Recurrence uncommon though reported
	Hori's nevus	QS 1,064 nm		Multiple	
	Lichen planus pigmentosus	QS 1,064 nm	9 mm: 1.2–1.5 6 mm: 1.7–2.0 4 mm: 1.6–1.8		Triple spot technique
	Riehl's melanosis	QS 1,064 nm	9 mm: 1.2–1.5 6 mm: 1.7–2.0 4 mm: 1.6–1.8	Five to six sessions	Interval of 4–6 weeks
Mixed epidermal and dermal lesions	Melasma	1,064 nm	9 mm: 1.2–1.4 6 mm: 1.8–2.0 4 mm: 1.5–1.8	Multiple at fortnight intervals	Avoid high energy to avoid rebound pigmentation Response to laser unpredictable, medical management preferred initially
	Postinflammatory hyperpigmentation	1,064 nm	6 mm and 4 mm 1.8–2.0	Multiple	Response to laser unpredictable

(CALM: café-au-lait macule; DPN: dermatosis papulosa nigra; QS: Q-switched; Nd:YAG: neodymium-doped yttrium aluminum garnet)

particles is easier resulting in faster clearing of the tattoos.[9] Picosecond lasers have come up to use in tattoo removal including the colored tattoos such as blue and green tattoos. Beyond tattoo removal its role is also being established for indications such as nevus of Ota, minocycline-induced pigmentation, acne scarring, and rhytides.[68]

Lorgeou A did a split comparative study on 49 patients with all types of tattoos between picosecond lasers to a nanosecond laser and found picosecond lasers showed a statistically significant superiority compared to the nanosecond laser for tattoo clearance. However, they do not show better efficacy for polychromic tattoos and the difference in terms of side effects were also minimal with a tendency of picosecond lasers to be less painful.[69]

However, picosecond lasers are very expensive as compared to its older counterparts, which is why its application for routine use in dermatology is yet to be established.

TIPS AND TRICKS

- Spot size is the most important parameter to be selected in a QS ND:YAG laser treatment.
- Avoid tanned patients.
- Sun protection of the treated part, if sun exposed.
- Start with lower fluence in the beginning, enough to cause a mild frost over the lesion.
- Reassess the response and laser parameters used at each visit.

Pigmented conditions treated by Nd:YAG laser are summarized in **Table 3**.

CONCLUSION

Nd:YAG laser is an excellent modality of treatment for pigmented lesions in almost all skin types. Proper selection of cases, good pretreatment and posttreatment care as mentioned is mandatory for optimum results. Along with treatment of pigmentary conditions, additional use of QS Nd:YAG laser for open pores and skin rejuvenation is an added advantage making it even more versatile.

REFERENCES

1. Maiman TH. Stimulated optical radiation in ruby. Nature. 1960;187:493.
2. Goldman L, Blaney Dj, Kindel Dj Jr, Franke Ek. Effect of the laser beam on the skin. Preliminary report. J Invest Dermatol. 1963;40:121-2.
3. Anderson RR, Parrish JA. Selective photothermolysis: precise microsurgery by selective absorption of pulsed radiation. Science. 1983;220:524-7.
4. Gianfaldoni S, Tchernev G, Wollina U. An Overview of Laser in Dermatology: The Past, the Present and ... the Future (?). Open Access Maced J Med Sci. 2017;5:526-30.

5. Boulnois JL. Photophysical processes in recent medical laser developments: A review. Lasers Med Sci. 1986;1:47-66.
6. Patil UA, Dhami LD. Overview of lasers. Indian J Plast Surg. 2008;41:S101-13.
7. Stratigos AJ, Dover JS, Arndt KA. Laser treatment of pigmented lesions—2000: how far have we gone? Arch Dermatol. 2000;136:915-21.
8. Goldberg DJ. Pigmented lesions, tattoos, and disorders of hypopigmentation. In: Goldberg DJ (Ed). Laser Dermatology Pearls and Problems, 1st edition. Massachusetts: Blackwell Publishing; 2008. pp. 71-114.
9. Ross V, Naseef G, Lin G, Kelly M, Michaud N, Flotte TJ, et al. Comparison of responses of tattoos to picosecond and nanosecond Q-switched neodymium: YAG lasers. Arch Dermatol. 1998;134:167-71.
10. McClung FJ, Hellwarth RW. Giant Optical Pulsations from Ruby. Appl Opt. 1962;1:103-5.
11. Polla LL, Margolis RJ, Dover JS, Whitaker D, Murphy GF, Jacques SL, et al. Melanosomes are a primary target of Q-switched ruby laser irradiation in guinea pig skin. J Invest Dermatol. 1987;89:281-6.
12. Kilmer SL, Wheeland RJ, Goldberg DJ, Anderson RR. Treatment of epidermal pigmented lesions with the frequency-doubled Q-switched Nd:YAG laser. A controlled, single-impact, dose-response, multicenter trial. Arch Dermatol. 1994;130:1515-9.
13. Levy JL, Mordon S, Pizzi-Anselme M. Treatment of individual café au lait macules with the Q-switched Nd:YAG: a clinicopathologic correlation. J Cutan Laser Ther. 1999;1:217-23.
14. Rashid T, Hussain I, Haider M, Haroon TS. Laser therapy of freckles and lentigines with quasi-continuous, frequency-doubled, Nd:YAG (532 nm) laser in Fitzpatrick skin type IV: a 24-month follow-up. J Cosmet Laser Ther. 2002;4(3-4):81-5.
15. Todd MM, Rallis TM, Gerwels JW, Hata TR. A comparison of 3 lasers and liquid nitrogen in the treatment of solar lentigines: a randomized, controlled, comparative trial. Arch Dermatol. 2000;136:841-6.
16. Grevelink JM, Gonzalez S, Bonoan R, Vibhagool C, Gonzalez E. Treatment of nevus spilus with the Q-switched Ruby laser. Dermatol Surg. 1997;23:365-9.
17. Gold MH, Foster TD, Bell MW. Nevus spilus successfully treated with an IPL source. Dermatol Surg. 1999;25:254-5.
18. Moreno-Arias GA, Bulla F, Vilata-Corell JJ, Camps-Fresneda A. Treatment of widespread segmental nevus spilus by Q-switched alexandrite laser (755 nm, 100 nsec). Dermatol Surg. 2001;27:841-3.
19. Fitzpatrick RE, Goldman MP, Ruiz-Esparza J. Clinical advantage of the CO2 laser superpulsed mode. Treatment of verruca vulgaris, seborrheic keratoses, lentigines, and actinic cheilitis. J Dermatol Surg Oncol. 1994;20:449-56.
20. Khatri KA. Ablation of cutaneous lesions using an erbum:YAG laser. J Cosmet Laser Ther. 2003;5:150-3.
21. Mehrabi D, Brodell RT. Use of the alexandrite laser for the treatment of seborrheic keratoses. Dermatol Surg. 2002;28:437-9.
22. Kar HK, Gupta L. 1064 nm Q switched Nd: YAG laser treatment of nevus of Ota: an Indian open label prospective study of 50 patients. Indian J Dermatol Venereol Leprol. 2011;77:565-70.
23. Kono T, Nozaki M, Chan HH, Mikashima Y. A retrospective study looking at the long-term complications of Q-switched ruby laser in the treatment of nevus of Ota. Lasers Surg Med. 2001;29:156-9.
24. Chan HH, King WW, Chan ES, Mok CO, Ho WS, Van Krevel C, et al. In vivo trial comparing patients' tolerance of Q-switched Alexandrite (QS Alex) and Q-switched neodymium:yttrium-aluminum-garnet (QS Nd:YAG) lasers in the treatment of nevus of Ota. Lasers Surg Med. 1999;24:24-8.
25. Alster TS, Williams CM. Treatment of nevus of Ota by the Q-switched alexandrite laser. Dermatol Surg. 1995;21:592-6.
26. Yu P, Yu N, Diao W, Yang X, Feng Y, Qi Z. Comparison of clinical efficacy and complications between Q-switched alexandrite laser and Q-switched Nd:YAG laser on nevus of Ota: a systematic review and meta-analysis. Lasers Med Sci. 2016;31:581-91.
27. Polnikorn N, Tanrattanakorn S, Goldberg DJ. Treatment of Hori's nevus with the Q-switched Nd:YAG laser. Dermatol Surg. 2000;26(5):477-80.
28. Choi CW, Jo G, Lee DH, Jo SJ, Lee C, Mun JH. Analysis of Clinical Features and Treatment Outcomes Using 1,064-nm Nd-YAG Laser with Topical Hydroquinone in Patients with Riehl's Melanosis: A Retrospective Study in 10 Patients. Ann Dermatol. 2019;31:127-32.
29. Shah DSD, Aurangabadkar DS, Nikam DB. An open-label non-randomized prospective pilot study of the efficacy of Q-switched Nd-YAG laser in management of facial lichen planus pigmentosus. J Cosmet Laser Ther. 2019;21:108-15.
30. Sarkar R, Aurangabadkar S, Salim T, Das A, Shah S, Majid I, et al. Lasers in Melasma: A Review with Consensus Recommendations by Indian Pigmentary Expert Group. Indian J Dermatol. 2017;62:585-90.
31. Mun JY, Jeong SY, Kim JH, Han SS, Kim IH. A low fluence Q-switched Nd:YAG laser modifies the 3D structure of melanocyte and ultrastructure of melanosome by subcellular-selective photothermolysis. J Electron Microsc (Tokyo). 2011;60:11-8.
32. Yun WJ, Moon HR, Lee MW, Choi JH, Chang SE. Combination treatment of low-fluence 1,064-nm Q-switched Nd: YAG laser with novel intense pulse light in Korean melasma patients: a prospective, randomized, controlled trial. Dermatol Surg. 2014;40:842-50.
33. Jeong SY, Shin JB, Yeo UC, Kim WS, Kim IH. Low-fluence Q-switched neodymium-doped yttrium aluminum garnet laser for melasma with pre- or post-treatment triple combination cream. Dermatol Surg. 2010;36:909-18.
34. Chan NP, Ho SG, Shek SY, Yeung CK, Chan HH. A case series of facial depigmentation associated with low fluence Q-switched 1,064 nm Nd:YAG laser for skin rejuvenation and melasma. Lasers Surg Med. 2010;42:712-9.
35. Zawar VP, Agarwal M, Vasudevan B. Treatment of Postinflammatory Pigmentation Due to Acne with Q-Switched Neodymium-Doped Yttrium Aluminum Garnet in 78 Indian Cases. J Cutan Aesthet Surg. 2015;8:222-6.
36. Cho SB, Park SJ, Kim JS, Kim MJ, Bu TS. Treatment of post-inflammatory hyperpigmentation using 1064-nm Q-switched Nd:YAG laser with low fluence: report of three cases. J Eur Acad Dermatol Venereol. 2009;23:1206-7.
37. Kupermanbeade M, Levine VJ, Ashinoff R. Laser Removal of Tattoos. Am J Clin Dermatol. 2001;2:21-25.
38. Grevelink JM, Duke D, van Leeuwen RL, Gonzalez E, DeCoste SD, Anderson RR. Laser treatment of tattoos in darkly pigmented patients: efficacy and side effects. J Am Acad Dermatol. 1996;34:653-6.
39. Kilmer SL, Garden JM. Laser treatment of pigmented lesions and tattoos. Semin Cutan Med Surg. 2000;19:232-44.
40. Kilmer SL, Lee MS, Grevelink JM, Flotte TJ, Anderson RR. The QS Nd:YAG laser (1064 nm) effectively treats tattoos: A controlled, dose-response study. Arch Dermatol. 1993;129:971-8.

41. Grekin RC, Shelton RM, Geisse JK, Frieden I. 510-nm pigmented lesion dye laser. Its characteristics and clinical uses. J Dermatol Surg Oncol. 1993;19:380-7.
42. Bailin PL, Ratz JR, Levine HL. Removal of tattoos by CO_2 laser. J Dermatol Surg Oncol. 1980;6:997-1001.
43. Alster TS, Bryan H, Williams CM. Long-pulsed Nd:YAG laser-assisted hair removal in pigmented skin: a clinical and histological evaluation. Arch Dermatol. 2001;137:885-9.
44. Gan SD, Graber EM. Laser hair removal: a review. Dermatol Surg. 2013;39:823-38.
45. Alexiades-Armenakas MR, Dover JS, Arndt KA. The spectrum of laser skin resurfacing: nonablative, fractional, and ablative laser resurfacing. J Am Acad Dermatol. 2008;58:719-37.
46. Dayan SH, Vartanian AJ, Menaker G, Mobley SR, Dayan AN. Nonablative laser resurfacing using the long-pulse (1064-nm) Nd:YAG laser. Arch Facial Plast Surg. 2003;5:310-5.
47. Trelles MA, Alvarez X, Martín-Vázquez MJ, Trelles O, Velez M, Levy JL, et al. Assessment of the efficacy of nonablative long-pulsed 1064-nm Nd:YAG laser treatment of wrinkles compared at 2, 4, and 6 months. Facial Plast Surg. 2005;21: 145-53.
48. Goldberg DJ, Silapunt S. Histologic evaluation of a Q-switched Nd:YAG laser in the nonablative treatment of wrinkles. Dermatol Surg. 2001;27744-6.
49. Friedman PM, Jih MH, Skover GR, Payonk GS, Kimyai-Asadi A, Geronemus RG. Treatment of Atrophic Facial Acne Scars With the 1064-nm Q-Switched Nd:YAG Laser: Six-Month Follow-up Study. Arch Dermatol. 2004;140(11):1337-41.
50. Artzi O, Koren A, Shehadeh W, Friedman O. Quasi long-pulsed 1064nm Nd:YAG (micro pulsed) technology for the treatment of active acne: A case series. J Cosmet Dermatol. 2021;20:2102-7.
51. Say EM, Okan G, Gökdemir G. Treatment Outcomes of Long-Pulsed Nd:YAG Laser for Two Different Subtypes of Rosacea. J Clin Aesthet Dermatol. 2015;8:16-20.
52. Chung H, Goo B, Lee H, Roh M, Chung K. Enlarged pores treated with a combination of Q-switched and micropulsed 1064 nm Nd:YAG laser with and without topical carbon suspension: A simultaneous split-face trial. Laser Ther. 2011;20:181-8.
53. Guida S, Fulgione E, D'Ambra I, Babino G, Pellacani G, Farnetani F. Carbon Peel Laser Technique to Improve Skin Quality: Back to Science!. Dermatol Pract Concept. 2020;10:e2020113.
54. Somyas K, Suntharee K, Pannadda L, Sansanee W. An effective treatment of dark lip by Frequency doubled Q switched Nd:YAG laser. Dermatol Surg. 2001;27:37-40.
55. Sarkar R, Ranjan R, Garg S, Garg VK, Sonthalia S, Bansal S. Periorbital Hyperpigmentation: A Comprehensive Review. J Clin Aesthet Dermatol. 2016;9:49-55.
56. Landthaler M, Haina D, Brunner R, Waidelich W, Braun-Falco O. Neodymium-YAG laser therapy for vascular lesions. J Am Acad Dermatol. 1986;14:107-17.
57. Meesters AA, Pitassi LH, Campos V, Wolkerstorfer A, Dierickx CC. Transcutaneous laser treatment of leg veins. Lasers Med Sci. 2014;29:481-92.
58. Munia MA, Wolosker N, Munia CG. Comparison of laser versus sclerotherapy in the treatment of lower extremity telangiectases: a prospective study. Dermatol Surg. 2012;38:635-9.
59. Coles CM, Werner RS, Zelickson BD. Comparative pilot study evaluating the treatment of leg veins with a long pulse ND:YAG laser and sclerotherapy. Lasers Surg Med. 2002;30:154-9.
60. Kilmer SL, Anderson RR. Clinical use of the Q-switched ruby and the Q-switched Nd:YAG (1064 nm and 532 nm) lasers for treatment of tattoos. J Dermatol Surg Oncol. 1993:19:330-8.
61. Aurangabadkar S, Mysore V. Standard guidelines of care: lasers for tattoos and pigmented lesions. Indian J Dermatol Venereol Leprol. 2009;75:111-26.
62. Mahadevappa OH, Mysore V, Viswanath V, Viswanath V, Thurakkal S, Majid I, et al. Surgical Outcome in Patients Taking Concomitant or Recent Intake of Oral Isotretinoin: A Multicentric Study-ISO-AIMS Study. J Cutan Aesthet Surg. 2016;9:106-14.
63. Kirby W, Desai A, Desai T, Kartono F, Geeta P. The Kirby-Desai scale: A proposed scale to assess tattoo-removal treatments. J Clin Aesthet Dermatol. 2009;2:32-7.
64. Kossida T, Rigopoulos D, Katsambas A, Anderson RR. Optimal tattoo removal in a single laser session based on the method of repeated exposures. J Am Acad Dermatol. 2012;66:271-7.
65. Reddy KK, Brauer JA, Anolik R, Bernstein L, Brightman L, Hale E, et al. Topical perfluorodecalin resolves immediate whitening reactions and allows rapid effective multiple pass treatment of tattoos. Lasers Surg Med. 2013;45:76-80.
66. Ho SG, Goh CL. Laser tattoo removal: a clinical update. J Cutan Aesthet Surg. 2015;8:9-15.
67. Chen H, Diebold G. Chemical generation of acoustic waves: a giant photo- acoustic effect. Science. 1995;270:963-66.
68. Forbat E, Al-Niaimi F. The use of picosecond lasers beyond tattoos. J Cosmet Laser Ther. 2016;18(6):345-7.
69. Lorgeou A, Perrillat Y, Gral N, Lagrange S, Lacour JP, Passeron T. Comparison of two picosecond lasers to a nanosecond laser for treating tattoos: a prospective randomized study on 49 patients. J Eur Acad Dermatol Venereol. 2018;32:265-70.

CHAPTER 109 Lasers for Pigmented Lesions

Sanjeev J Aurangabadkar

KEY MESSAGES

- Laser treatment of pigmented lesions can be extremely rewarding, even in darker skin individuals when appropriate lesions are treated with the right laser.
- Proper patient selection, priming, and adequate sun protection go a long way in clearing the lesions and maintenance of clearance.
- Accurate diagnosis of pigmented lesions is essential prior to initiating laser therapy. A skin biopsy must be performed in case of a diagnostic dilemma.
- Certain controversies exist in the treatment of pigmented lesions, for example, treating melanocytic nevi and treating patients on isotretinoin. Further studies and consensus are needed to resolve these issues:
  - Epidermal lesions need fewer sessions to clear, but recurrences are a problem.
  - Dermal lesions need more number of sessions and recurrences are unlikely upon improvement.
  - Laser therapy is not the first choice for melasma and should only be done in selected resistant cases who fail other treatments or due to intolerance to topical medication.
  - Treatments have to be individualized according to patient skin types and lesion.
  - Choice of parameters depends on the individual laser and manufacturer recommendations are only a starting point which needs to be tailored to the case scenario.

INTRODUCTION

Pigmented lesions are common in Indian skin and pose a challenge to the treating dermatologist. While some of the hyperpigmented lesions, such as postinflammatory hyperpigmentation (PIH), melasma, etc., can be managed medically, their results are variable but not always satisfactory; other lesions such as nevus of Ota do not respond to medical management at all.

The skin of color ages differently than Caucasian skin and shows more pigmentary alterations, such as development of lentigines, solar lentigo, benign skin growths, such as seborrheic keratoses, dermatosis papulosa nigra (DPN). Many of these conditions require dermatosurgical intervention to clear the lesions.

Lasers for pigmented lesions have lagged behind other lasers for resurfacing and hair removal. However, the last decade has seen technological advancements, with new systems being developed that are more effective and yet safe even in darker skin types. Q-switched (QS) lasers (Q-switched = Quality switched or Quantum switched), which produce very high peak powers in ultrashort durations of time (5–100 nanoseconds), have revolutionized the therapy of many pigmented lesions. Picosecond lasers (mode-locking lasers) are the new entrants in the field that show a great deal of potential in the management of pigmentary disorders.

HISTORY

Ruby laser 694 nm was the first laser used to treat pigmented lesions and tattoos in humans by Goldman between the years 1963 and 1967. The first QS laser developed was the Ruby, followed by the neodymium: yttrium-aluminum-garnet (Nd:YAG) and the alexandrite lasers. Polla et al, Dover et al., and Hruza et al. between the years 1987 and 1991 demonstrated the highly selective cellular damage occurring in melanin-containing cells following QS laser therapy.[1-4]

LASER BASICS AND SYSTEMS

Light of wavelength from 290 nm up to the range of 1,200 nm is absorbed by melanin. At longer wavelengths, absorption is lower and the penetration is deeper as compared to the shorter wavelengths. QS lasers produce ultrashort bursts of light in the nanosecond range and target melanin (and ink particles) in the dermis allowing removal or lightening of benign pigmented lesions and tattoos respectively.[1-4]

A wavelength that penetrates 2–3 mm into the dermis is suitable for targeting deeper dermal pigmentation, such as found in nevus of Ota. QS Nd:YAG laser with a wavelength of 1,064 nm meets this requirement adequately. By passing the beam through the potassium titanyl phosphate (KTP) crystal, the frequency is doubled and the wavelength is halved (532 nm). A shorter wavelength penetrates less deeply and therefore is more useful for removal of epidermal pigment, such as in ephelides. The Ruby laser (694 nm) penetrates <1 mm into skin and is used for treating superficial lesions such as freckles or café-au-lait macules (CALM). However, because of its high affinity for melanin and the possible risk of hypopigmentation, the QS Ruby laser is not recommended for use in patients of darker skin types such as the Indian skin. The QS alexandrite laser (755 nm) penetrates deeper than the Ruby laser due to its longer wavelength and hence can be used for removal of both epidermal and dermal pigmented lesions and tattoos.

Besides the QS lasers, long-pulsed (millisecond) lasers, such as the diode 810 nm, long-pulsed alexandrite laser 755 nm, etc., can also be used for treatment of certain pigmented lesions. The intense pulsed light (IPL) systems are polychromatic light sources that use cutoff filters to block shorter wavelengths, thus producing a broad band of IPL. These systems use wavelengths from 530 nm and above, and can be used to treat superficial pigmented lesions such as freckles, lentigines, but are not recommended for dermal lesions or tattoo removal.[1-4]

Fractional photothermolysis, both ablative and nonablative have been used to treat pigmented lesions. They primarily act by elimination of pigment transepidermally through the microablative columns (MAC) or the micro-epidermal necrotic debris (MEND). These lasers are nonselective meaning they do not specifically target melanin but work by producing vaporization or coagulation of tissue followed by remodeling in the dermis.[5]

Newer lasers, such as the copper bromide laser that targets the vascular component of melasma has been used as well.[6]

MECHANISM OF ACTION OF Q-SWITCHED LASERS

Definition of Q-switch or Quality Switch

Q-switching is a method for obtaining energetic pulses from lasers by modulating the intracavity losses. It is a technique for obtaining energetic short (but not ultrashort) pulses from a laser by modulating the intracavity losses, the so-called the *Q* factor of the laser resonator. The technique is mainly applied for the generation of nanosecond pulses of high energy and peak power with solid-state bulk lasers. These giant pulses are responsible for the unique laser-tissue interaction that is seen with QS lasers.[7]

Q-switched lasers work on the principle of selective photothermolysis and also produce an additional photoacoustic effect producing shock waves that cause explosion of target.[3] Very high energy, to the tune of 300 MW, is delivered in a very short period of time (5–100 ns) which leads to rapid thermal expansion. This produces shock waves that rupture the targets, such as melanosomes and ink particles.[4] The ruptured fragments are cleared by tissue macrophages either to the lymphatic channels or to the regional lymph nodes. Some fragments may be eliminated transepidermally. To be selective, the pulse duration of the laser should match the thermal relaxation time (TRT) of the target. The estimated TRT of epidermis is 1–10 ms and the TRT of tattoo ink particles is 0.1–10 ns, although some newer estimates are in the range of 10–100 picoseconds. The size of the tattoo ink particles is about 10–100 nm and is generally placed at a depth of 1.1–2.9 mm. Laser tissue interaction produces intracellular steam and vacuole formation, which leads to immediate whitening. An audible popping sound is heard during the procedure due to the photoacoustic effect.

Though Q switched lasers are considered "gold standard" for pigmented lesions, subnanosecond lasers, such as picosecond lasers are now available. The picoseconds pulse width is in the range of 10-12 of a second. This >10 fold reduction of pulse width may allow better targeting of the tiny melanosomes and tattoo ink particles whose TRT is in nanosecond domain.[8]

Both nanosecond and subnanosecond lasers are available in various wavelengths including 1,064 nm, 532 nm, 755 nm, 585 nm, 660 nm, etc. All these wavelengths (WLs) may not be available in the same system but most newer Q-switched lasers (QSL) and picoseconds lasers have option of having multiple wavelengths. Some newer laser systems have both nano and subnanosecond options in the same device making them very flexible.

Indications

Choosing the right patient for the laser therapy of pigmented lesions especially in skin of color is important. When diagnosis is in doubt, biopsy should be performed. Pigmented dermatological conditions which can be treated by lasers are listed in **Box 1**.[1-3]

Some pigmented lesions amenable to laser therapy are shown in **Figures 1 to 7**.

Contraindications[9-11]

The contraindications for performing the lasers on a particular patient should be borne in mind by the clinician all the time. The contraindications can be relative or absolute are listed hereunder.

BOX 1: Pigmented lesions amenable to treatment by lasers.[12]

- *Epidermal lesions:* CALM, lentigines, freckles, solar lentigo, nevus spilus, pigmented seborrheic keratosis, DPN
- *Dermal lesions:* Nevus of Ota, blue nevus, Hori's nevus (acquired bilateral nevus of Ota-like macules), acquired dermal melanosis, e.g.: Lichen planus pigmentosus (LPP)
- *Epidermal-dermal lesions:* Postinflammatory hyperpigmentation, nevus spilus, periorbital pigmentation, perioral pigmentation, acquired melanocytic nevi (moles), melasma and Becker's nevus, Riehl's melanosis

(CALM: café-au-lait macules; DPN: dermatosis papulosa nigra)

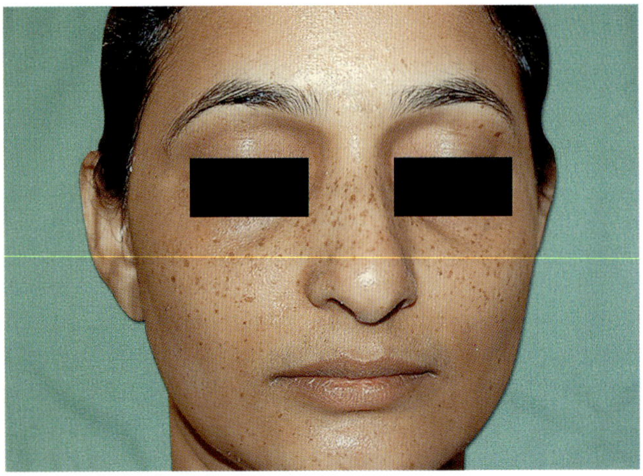

Fig. 1: Lentigines—centrofacial type.

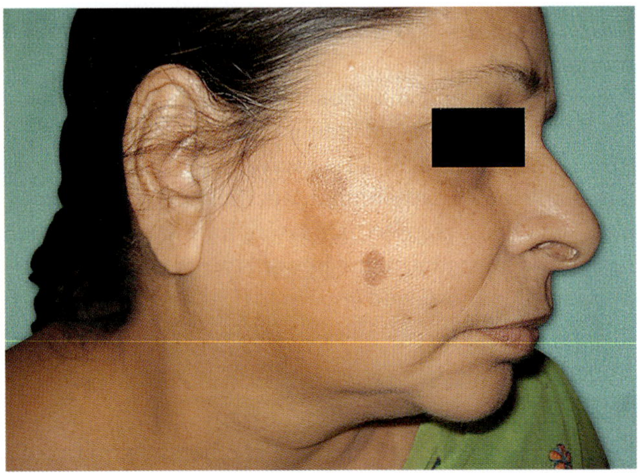

Fig. 2: Solar lentigos on the face.

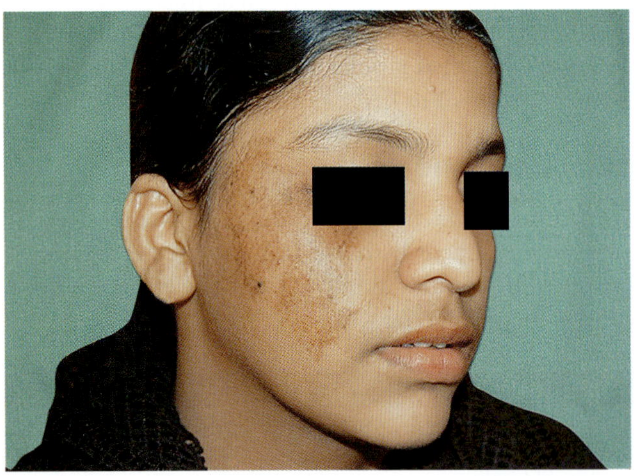

Fig. 3: Nevus spilus.

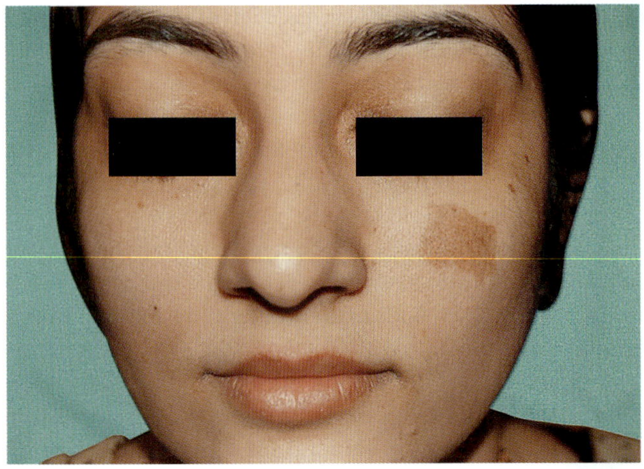

Fig. 4: Café-au-lait macule.

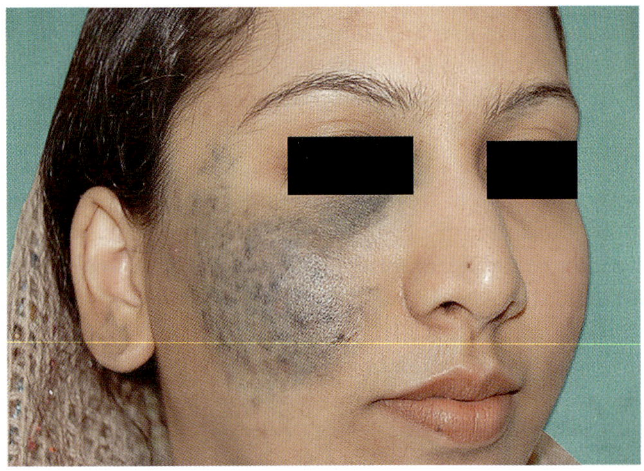

Fig. 5: Nevus of Ota.

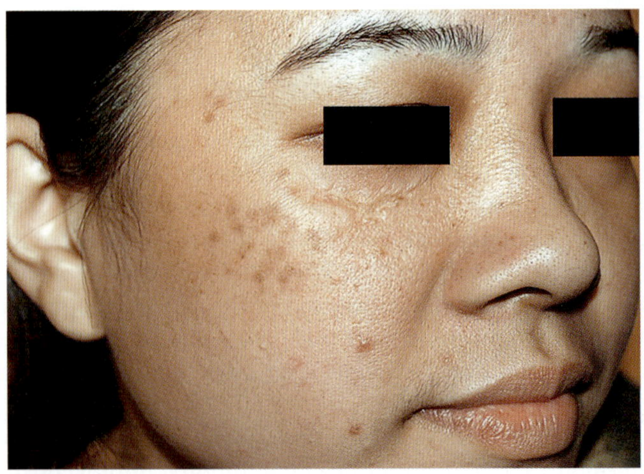

Fig. 6: Hori's nevus; acquired bilateral nevus of Ota-like macules.

Absolute Contraindications

- Associated photoaggravated skin diseases and medical illness, for example, systemic lupus erythematosus (SLE).
- Treatment area with active cutaneous infections, for example, herpes labialis and staphylococcal infections.
- Unstable vitiligo and psoriasis for risk of koebnerization of treated area.

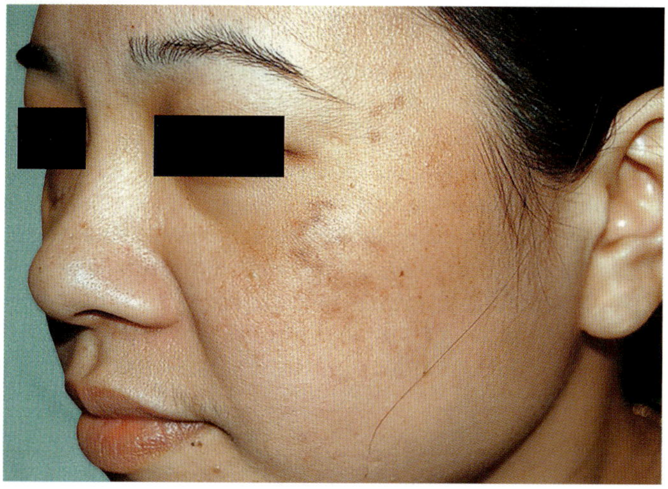

Fig. 7: Hori's nevus.

- Tattoo granuloma.
- Localized allergic reactions can occur with almost any color ink and result in urticaria and granulomatous reactions. If a patient exhibits a cutaneous reaction within a tattoo, QS laser treatment should be used with caution. After QS laser treatment, the ink particles are mobilized, potentially triggering an allergic response. Rarely systemic allergic reactions may occur, particularly common in patients exhibiting a localized allergic response.

Relative Contraindications

In the following situations, laser has to be used cautiously and after proper counseling of the patient; use of laser in these situations depends on individual situation and on treating physician's judgment.

- Keloid and keloidal tendencies.
- Patient on isotretinoin.
- *History of herpes simplex/history of herpes for increased risk of reactivation:* This risk should be seriously considered prior to performing the procedure. If the treating physician decides to perform the procedure, the risk and benefit should be explained to the patient and the procedure should be performed after proper informed consent and only after a course of acyclovir.
- Patient who is not cooperative or has unrealistic expectation.

PATIENT SELECTION AND COUNSELING[10-13]

Patient selection needs utmost care on the part of the clinician. A general medical history, current medical conditions and medications, allergies, past surgeries, including bleeding tendencies and wound healing (response of previous skin injuries whether they heal with hyperpigmentation or hypopigmentation, response to previous laser sessions if any taken) should be obtained.

Thorough counseling of the patient and an informed written consent completes the baseline step required for initiating therapy. Good pretreatment photographs are mandatory, as in any aesthetic procedure. Scarring often occurs during tattoo placement and may be unmasked and become more noticeable once the ink is removed. Serial photographs should, therefore, be taken at successive visits.

PREOPERATIVE PREPARATION

Sun Protection

It is very important to ensure that the patient is not tanned. Epidermal melanin produced by ultraviolet (UV) light exposure may interfere with laser treatment and increase the risks for scarring, hypopigmentation or hyperpigmentation[10,12-16] To check for tanning, it is wise to compare the color of the potential treatment site to that of an unexposed skin site, similar to the buttock or axilla. If a tan is present, treatment should be delayed until the tan has faded as much as possible in the treatment area. Use of broad spectrum sun protection creams with ultraviolet A (UVA) coverage is crucial. Protective clothing and bleaching creams can be useful in treating the tan. Patients with darker skin types and tanned patients are advised to apply hydroquinone-containing compounds (2–4%) or other lightening agents preoperatively to minimize the risk of PIH.

Oral Retinoids

It has been recommended that patients on oral retinoid therapy should not undergo laser treatment of pigmented lesions and tattoos for 6–12 months following discontinuation of the medication, as they have an increased risk of keloidal scar formation.[10-15] Proper evidence to support such a recommendation in Indian patients, particularly for epidermal lesions is lacking. However, caution is advised while treating all patients with history of recent administration of isotretinoin.

Test Patch

A test patch helps determine the treatment parameters for an individual. It is also helpful in medicolegal situations. In particular, it is advisable for all beginners to perform laser test spots in all patients prior to treating an entire lesion, since skin type and color do not always perfectly predict the response to treatment. Even seasoned experts may need to perform small test spots, particularly where response to treatment cannot be judged properly. Always evaluate the patient 4–8 weeks after the test spots.[10,12-16]

Eye Protection

Q-switched lasers produce ultrashort pulse durations that produce significant tissue splatter. QS laser light can cause permanent retinal damage and vision loss.[1,2] Precautions include protective clothing, goggles, masks, and laser cone containment devices which should be used with every patient. Eye protection in the form of optically coated glasses or goggles for the specific laser being used is necessary. All persons present in the room during laser treatment must also wear appropriate eye protection. The eye wear should block the wavelength being used and the lens should provide an optical density (OD) for at least four. Laser protective eye shields (anodized external metal eyecup) must be used when treating periorbital lesions. When treating eyelids, a metal corneal eye shield should be placed on the eye using topical anesthesia to protect the globe (**Box 2**).

Anesthesia

Q-switched laser treatment usually does not require anesthesia. However, if a large area needs to be treated, topical eutectic mixture of local anesthetic (EMLA) should be applied under occlusion 1–2 hours before the procedure.[17,18]

LASER PROCEDURE

Selecting the appropriate laser parameters is of paramount importance while executing the treatment.

Fluence

It is always preferable to begin with the lowest energy fluence that produces a visible response. Fluence may be increased if response is suboptimal. If epidermal debris are significant, the fluence should be lowered.[10-12,16,19-22] Fluence used is device specific (not comparable across different devices) and manufacturers' recommendations need to be kept in mind. This can be further tailored based on the individual situation.

Spot Size

The spot size which is just large enough to accommodate the treated lesion should be selected for epidermal lesions. While treating epidermal lesions, especially in darker individuals, it is important to avoid treating surrounding unaffected area to minimize pigmentary alterations. For dermal lesions, the spot size that elicits immediate brisk whitening on laser irradiation should be selected. Larger spot sizes allow deeper penetration and produce less tissue splatter.[10-12]

BOX 2: Checklist before laser therapy.

- Right indication
- Counseling
- Rule out contraindication
- Test patch
- Sun protection and priming
- Pretreatment photograph
- Informed valid consent
- Eye protection

Endpoint of Treatment

Appropriate endpoints are essential to ensure optimum outcome. With the QS laser, the endpoint of treatment is immediate whitening of the lesion. With an IPL, the endpoint is only erythema. Higher fluences may produce pinpoint bleeding and blistering.

- *Repetition rate*: Choose higher frequency, i.e., 5–10 Hz while doing large area. For smaller discrete lesions a frequency of 2–3 Hz gives better control.[12]

Figures 8 to 11 show immediate whitening and erythema/edema following Q-switched Nd:YAG (QSNY) laser treatment.

LASER TECHNIQUE

After choosing the correct spot size and the energy fluence (J/cm^2), laser treatment is performed with the handpiece held perpendicular to the lesion and the entire area is covered with minimal overlap (up to 10%). QS laser treatment will produce

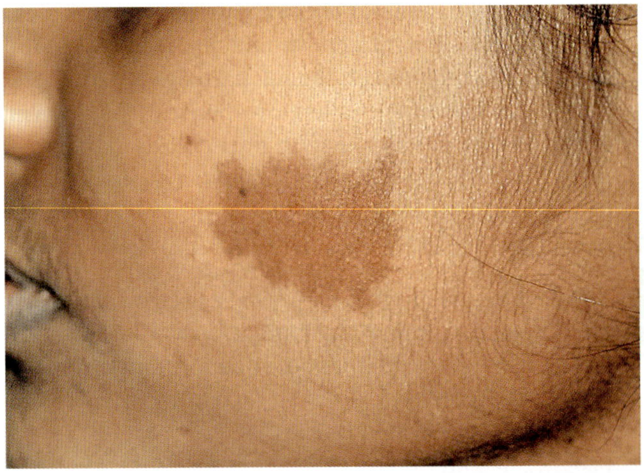

Fig. 8: A café-au-lait macule on the left cheek.

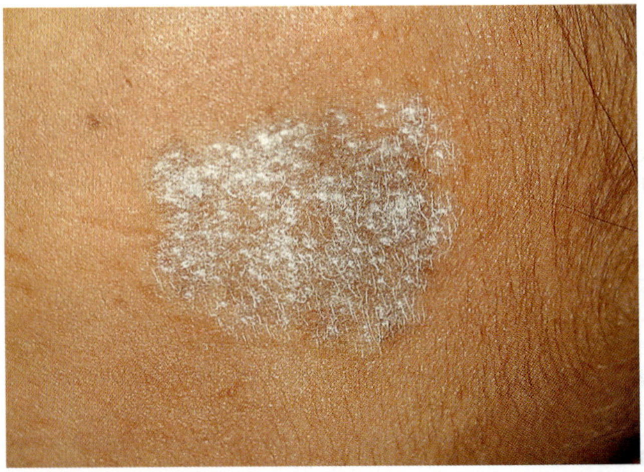

Fig. 9: Café-au-lait macule immediately following 532 nm QSNY laser showing the immediate whitening of the lesion. (QSNY: Q-switched Nd:YAG)

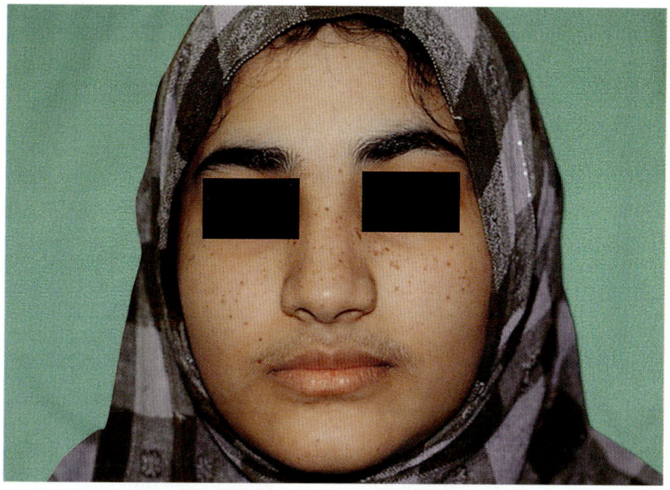

Fig. 10: Centrofacial lentiginosis before laser.

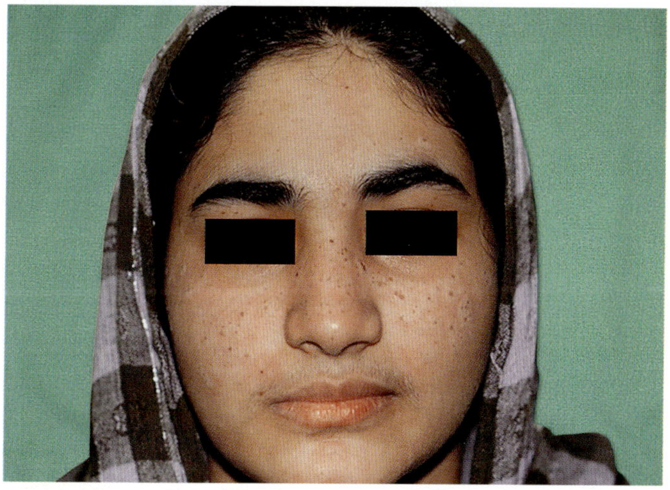

Fig. 11: Lentigines immediately after QSNY laser with 532 nm wavelength showing erythema and edema. (QSNY: Q-switched Nd:YAG)

an immediate whitening of the lesion. Pinpoint bleeding may occur if very high fluences are used. The entire lesion is covered in one pass. A popping sound is heard with each laser shot as the cells containing melanin or ink particles explode. Laser pulses are placed close to each other with minimum overlap. The area is cooled with ice packs/air cooling (e.g., Zimmer) just before and after laser pulses to avoid a buildup of heat and to prevent collateral tissue damage.

Number of Sessions

Epidermal lesions require one to two treatments, dermal lesions may need anywhere between 6 and 10 or even more sessions.

Interval Between Sessions

Treatment should be done at least 6–8 weeks apart. Treatment intervals can be longer when treating nevus of Ota (average of 3 months interval has been suggested). Continued clearance of the lesion occurs due to removal of pigment by macrophages and lymphatics between treatments. Optimal interval between treatments therefore needs to be determined on an individual basis.[10-12,16,19-22]

TREATMENT OF INDIVIDUAL LESIONS

Treatment depends on the type of lesion; epidermal lesions, dermal lesions, tattoos and mixed epidermal and dermal lesions. **Table 1** summarizes the different indications and their treatment parameters.

Epidermal Lesions

Epidermal lesions respond readily to QS laser treatment. The wavelengths used include frequency doubled 532 nm QS Nd:YAG, 755 nm QS alexandrite, 1,064 nm QS Nd:YAG. An average of 1–6 sessions is needed to clear most lesions. Recurrence is common after a few months to years, and patient needs to be advised regarding continued sun protection. The lesions can be retreated with QS laser without any additional risk. A spot size that is contained within the epidermal lesion should be used and the lesion treated with a single pass with minimal overlap. The 532 nm WL is to be used with caution in dark skin types and test spots are recommended. It is best to avoid a tanned patient.

Café-au-Lait Macules

Café-au-lait macules (CALM) are light to tan brown hypermelanotic flat lesions. The size varies 2–20 cm and is sharply demarcated from the surrounding normal skin. CALM are difficult to treat and usually require multiple treatments over months to years. Laser treatment may result in partial or incomplete clearance and recurrences are common, occurring in up to 50% of patients within a year of clearance. The preferred wavelength used is 532 nm particularly in light-skinned individuals. Risk of pigmentary alteration is higher in darker individuals, particularly a speckled pattern of hyperpigmentation.[23-25]

In the author's experience, a combination of 1,064 nm and 532 nm wavelength in the same session gives good results in CALM. First pass of 1,064 nm is made with energy that elicits subtle whitening; this is followed by a pass of 532 nm with energy that produces very light frosting. This is repeated once a month for 5–8 sessions until clearing. Fluence depends on skin type and lesion darkness. Strict sun avoidance and protection is necessary for good results throughout the course of treatment.

Figure 12 shows a CALM on the left cheek before treatment, while **Figure 13** shows CALM post two 532 nm QS Nd:YAG laser sessions showing lightening of the lesion with partial clearance.

TABLE 1: Summary of different indications and their treatment with lasers.

Level of pigmentation	*Condition*	*Wavelength used*	*Number of sittings*	*Remarks*	*Recommendations*
Epidermal	• Freckles and lentigines	• QS 532 nm, 1,064 nm, 755 nm, 660 nm QS • IPL	• 1–3	• Sun protection to avoid recurrence	• QS lasers treatment of choice
	• CALM	• QS 532 nm (in lighter skin types)	• Multiple	• 50% recurrence within a year	• Use with caution as partial or incomplete clearance common
	• Nevus spilus	• 532 nm	• Multiple	• Junctional and compound nevus components clear well, but CALM remains	• Use with caution as partial or incomplete clearance common
	• DPNs and seborrheic keratosis	• Ablative lasers, QS lasers, long pulse lasers	• 1–3		
Dermal	• Nevus of Ota	• QS 1,064 nm, 755 nm	• Multiple	• Recurrence uncommon though reported	• QS 1,064 nm is the preferred wavelength in darker skin types
	• Hori's nevus	• QS 1064 nm, 755 nm	• Multiple		• QS laser is treatment of choice
	• Blue nevus	• QS 1064 nm, 755 nm	• Multiple		• QS laser is treatment of choice
	• Acquired dermal melanosis	• QS 1,064 nm	• Multiple (average of 5–6 sessions)	• Interval of 4–6 weeks	• Initiate laser only after ensuring stability of the condition and withdraw any inciting factors
Mixed epidermal and dermal lesions	• Becker's nevus	• Long pulsed lasers and QS laser • IPL, ablative lasers	• Multiple	• Though many lasers have been tried, response is not satisfactory	• Treat with caution, test patch recommended.
	• Melasma	• Fractional photo-thermolysis, IPL, QS lasers (low fluence QS laser), LED • QS 585 nm if vascular component suspected	• Multiple	• Response to laser unpredictable, medical management preferred	• Use in selected resistant cases, test spots mandatory
	• Nevocellular nevi	• QS 532 nm, 755 nm, 1,064 nm QS	• 1–3		• QS lasers useful but treatment remains controversial
	• Postinflammatory hyperpigmentation	• 532 nm, 1,064 nm	• Multiple	• Response to laser unpredictable	• Lasers of limited value, test spots recommended

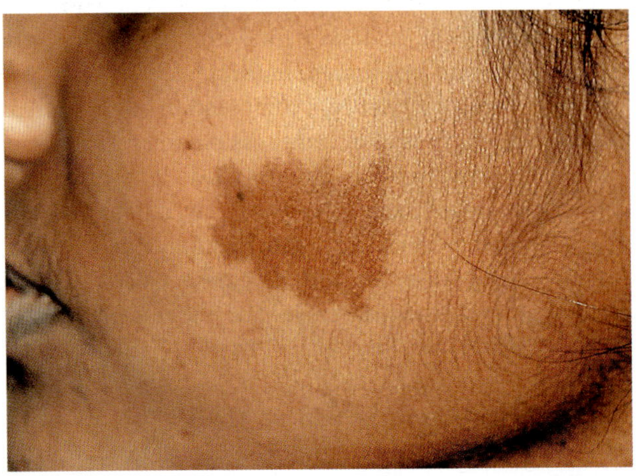

Fig. 12: CALM on the left cheek before treatment with 532 nm QS Nd:YAG laser. (CALM: café-au-lait macules)

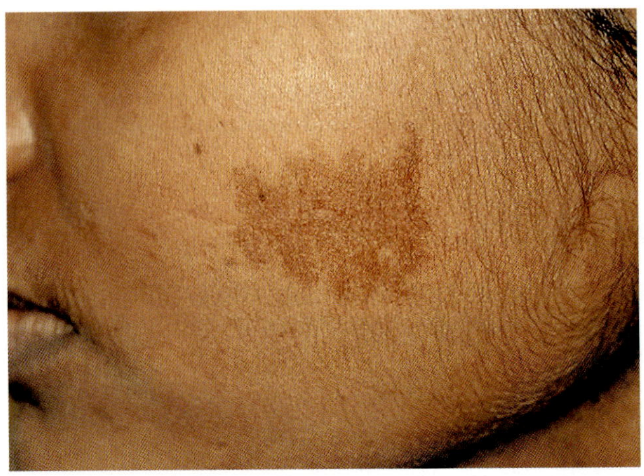

Fig. 13: CALM after two QS laser sessions showing partial clearing and lightening. (CALM: café-au-lait macules)

Lentigines/Solar Lentigo

Lentigines are small, round to oval dark macules that may occur on any cutaneous surface including mucous membranes. They usually measure a few millimeters in diameter. Lentigines can usually be removed completely in 1–3 treatments with the 532 nm QS Nd:YAG laser. In darker patients, the 1,064 nm QS Nd:YAG laser can also be used. The treatment of the lentigines found on the mucosal surface in Peutz–Jeghers syndrome may produce equally good results as those found on the skin surface. Treatment with Q-switched lasers is more effective than with other modalities such as liquid nitrogen, 35% trichloroacetic acid and glycolic acid peels.[23,26-32]

Figures 14 and 15 show a solar lentigo on the nose of an elderly woman, before and after 1,532 nm QS Nd:YAG laser treatment. **Figures 16 and 17** show a case of segmental lentiginosis before and after five sessions with a 1,064 nm QS Nd:YAG laser.

Nam et al. treated 12 patients with low fluence QSNY laser at a fluence of 1.6 J/cm^2 once a month for eight sessions and found excellent clearing of solar lentigo. They concluded that repetitive low fluence QSNY laser could be a safe and effective modality for senile lentigo.[33]

Freckles

Freckles are small brown macules that occur on sun-exposed skin and darken in color on exposure to sunlight. Histology shows normal epidermis without elongation or branching of rete ridges. The number of melanocytes is normal with hypermelanization confined to the basal layers. Melanosomes are larger with more active and larger melanocytes. They respond very well to 532 nm QS lasers with most lesions clearing in 1–2 sessions.[23,27,34] In spite of adequate clearance, freckles are known to recur after treatment, thus maintenance treatments may be necessary and the need for adequate sun protection should be emphasized during counseling.

Nevus Spilus

Darker speckles of flat or raised hyperpigmentation on a background of café-au-lait macule are seen in nevus spilus.

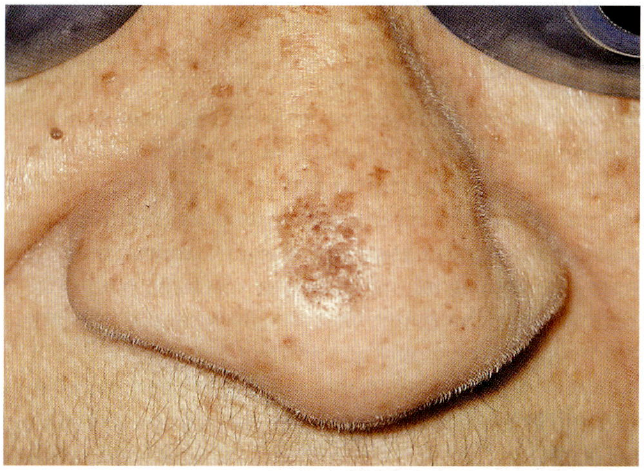

Fig. 14: Solar lentigo on the nose.

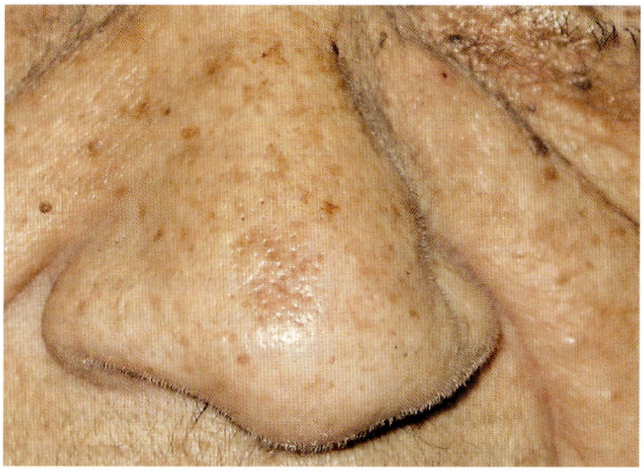

Fig. 15: Solar lentigo on the nose showing good clearing post one 532 nm QS Nd:YAG laser treatment.

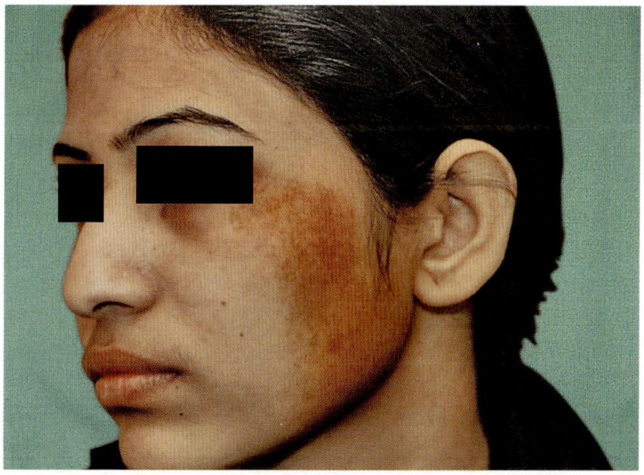

Fig. 16: Segmental lentiginosis.

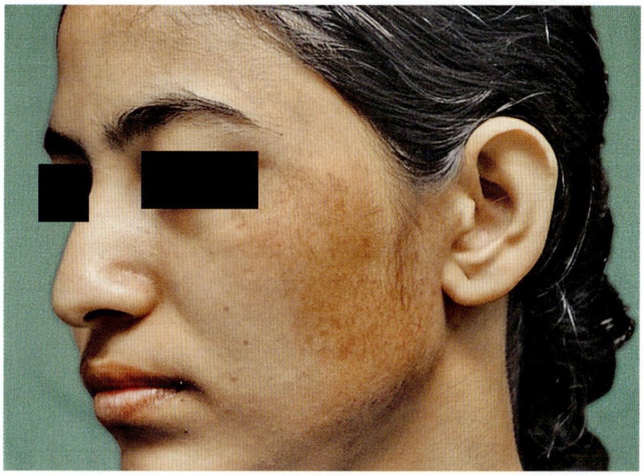

Fig. 17: Segmental lentiginosis post five sessions with QS Nd:YAG 532 nm laser.

Histology shows lentiginous elongation and hyperpigmentation of the rete with increase in melanocytes. There may be nesting of nevus cells within the lesions. The darker speckles are either junctional or compound nevi. Since nevus spilus has a dual component of pigmentation, the entire lesion may not respond uniformly to the laser treatment. The darker macular lesions (junctional or compound melanocytic nevus component) tend to respond better than the lighter component café-au-lait macule (CALM) to the 532 nm QS Nd:YAG laser treatment. Partial or complete clearance has been reported with the use of Q-switched lasers, long-pulsed lasers, and IPLs. Rarely, melanoma has been reported in cases of nevus spilus which has to be kept in mind.[35-38]

Figures 18 and 19 show a nevus spilus before and after 532 nm QS Nd:YAG laser treatment.

Dermatosis Papulosa Nigra and Pigmented Seborrheic Keratoses

These lesions have significant epidermal proliferation with normal to slightly increased number of melanocytes and increased melanization of keratinocytes. These lesions can be readily treated by nonspecific ablation with ultra-pulsed carbon dioxide laser, erbium:YAG laser, radiofrequency (RF) devices and electrofulguration. The QS lasers and long-pulsed lasers that target melanin can also be used to treat these lesions more specifically. Laser spot size should be limited to just below the size of the lesion. The nonspecific ablative methods are preferred means of treatment due to the cost-effectiveness and good results obtained with them.[39-41]

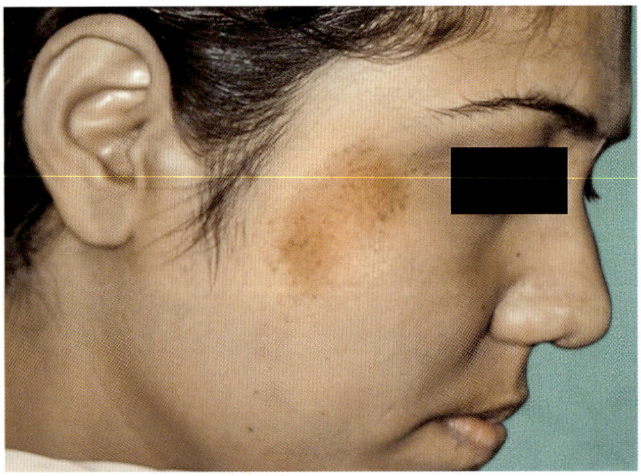

Fig. 18: Nevus spilus before treatment.

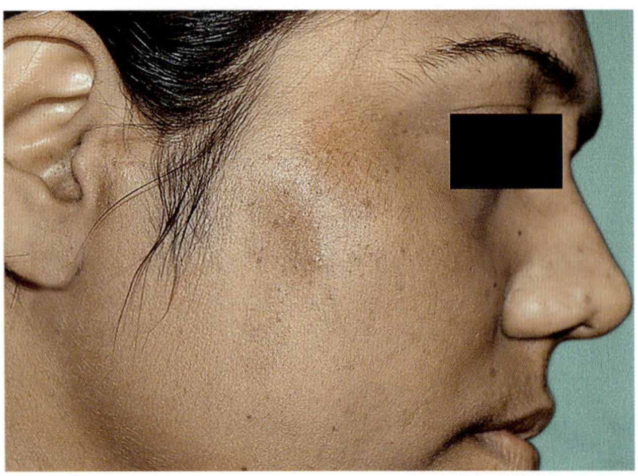

Fig. 19: Nevus spilus after three sessions with QS Nd:YAG laser at 532 nm.

Dermal Lesions

The chromophore for the laser treatment of dermal lesions includes melanin in melanosomes and ink particles, and other pigments that are located in the extracellular matrix or in melanophages. The longer wavelengths, such as 1,064 nm Nd:YAG, allow deeper penetration to target these pigments with minimal damage to the overlying epidermis. Multiple sessions are required to clear the dermal lesions optimally, with an interval of at least 6–8 weeks between sessions. Recurrences are uncommon after complete clearing.

Nevus of Ota

Nevus of Ota, also known as oculodermal nevus, is an acquired bluish gray persistent macular lesion that occurs on the face in the area innervated by the first and second division of the trigeminal nerve.[6,17,18,38-52] It is often associated with ipsilateral ocular pigmentation. Histological examination shows bipolar long, slender dermal melanocytes scattered largely in the upper dermis. The epidermis is usually normal, but focal basal hyperpigmentation may be seen.

Nevus of Ota is extremely satisfying to treat, and it readily responds to QS laser treatment. The longer wavelength 1,064 nm QS Nd:YAG laser is the most widely used laser to treat, especially in darker skin types. The longer 1,064 nm wavelength along with a large spot size allows deep penetration of photons and is ideally suited to treat this dermal condition. Multiple treatments are necessary (typically 6–8 sessions) with an interval of at least 2 months between treatments. In selected cases, one may even do a treatment once in 6 months as lesions continue to clear between sessions. Purpura and pinpoint bleeding may occur if very high fluences are used or if smaller spot sizes are employed. Postinflammatory hyperpigmentation (PIH) and hypopigmentation are common problems in Indian skin and good preoperative and postoperative care is necessary to minimize side effects. The PIH usually clears within a few weeks, without scarring.[42-56]

Figures 20 and 21 show a nevus of Ota on the right cheek before and after ten 1,064 nm QS Nd:YAG laser treatments.

Figures 22 and 23 show a case of bilateral nevus of Ota before and after QSNY laser treatment.

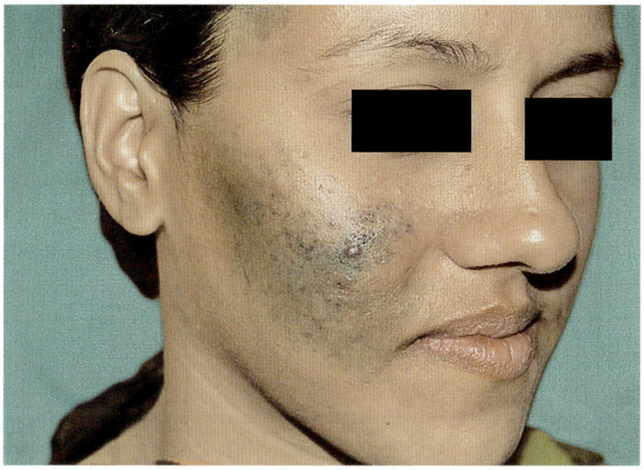

Fig. 20: Nevus of Ota on the right cheek.

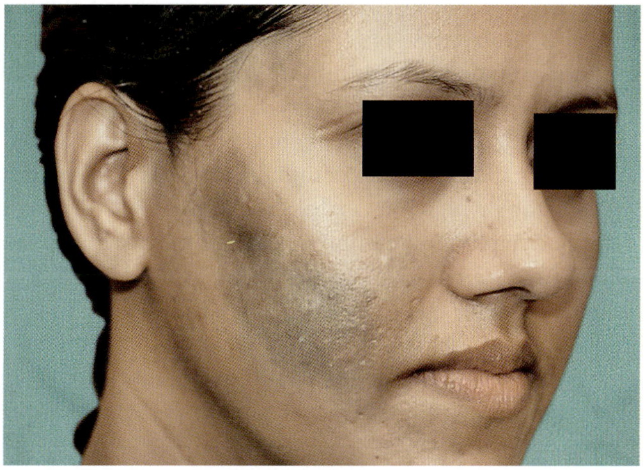

Fig. 21: Nevus of Ota after ten 1,064 nm QS laser sessions.

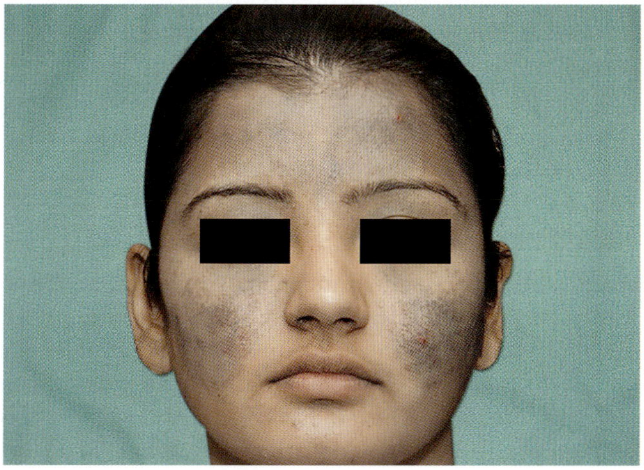

Fig. 22: Bilateral nevus of Ota.

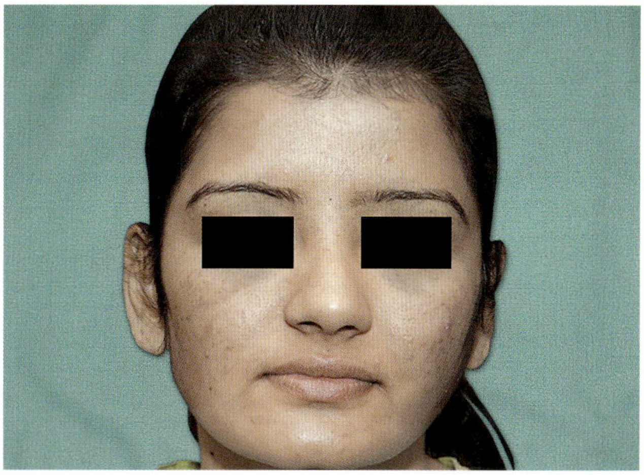

Fig. 23: Bilateral nevus of Ota after eight 1,064 nm QSNY laser sessions. (QSNY: Q-switched Nd:YAG)

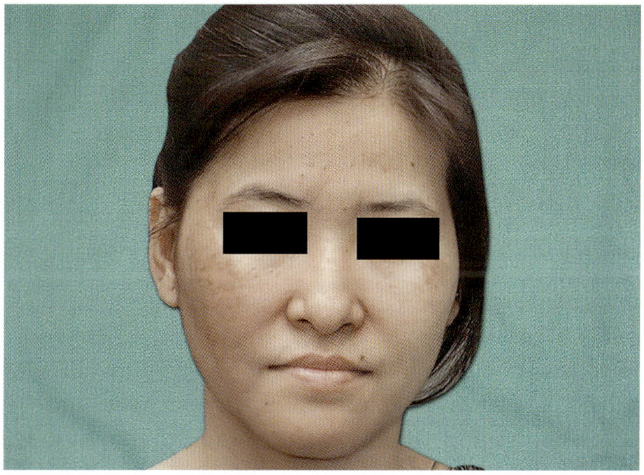

Fig. 24: Hori's nevus.

Nevus of Ito

Nevus of Ito is a grayish blue macular hyperpigmentation seen on the shoulder or upper arm in the area innervated by the posterior supraclavicular and lateral brachial cutaneous nerves. The lesion responds well to 1,064 nm QS Nd:YAG laser.[12]

Hori's Nevus (Acquired Bilateral Nevus of Ota-like Macules)

Acquired bilateral nevus of Ota-like macules or Hori's macules can mimic nevus of Ota. Late age of onset, bilateral nature of lesions, symmetry, and absence of mucosal involvement are features that differentiate Hori's nevus from bilateral nevus of Ota. It is amenable to treatment by longer wavelength QS lasers.[57-60] An average of 5–6 sessions are needed for good response with an interval of 4–6 weeks.

Figures 24 and 25 show a case of Hori's nevus before and after QSNY laser treatment.

Blue Nevus

The blue nevi are characterized by presence of melanocytes deep within the dermis and their blue-black color is a tyndall

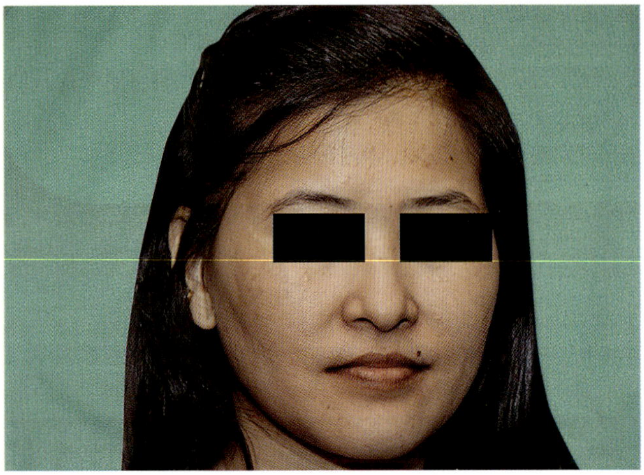

Fig. 25: After five sessions of QSNY laser at 1064 nm. (QSNY: Q-switched Nd:YAG)

effect reflected from the overlying tissues. Like the nevus of Ota and Ito, the blue nevi respond readily to 1,064 nm QS Nd:YAG laser treatment. Lesions that extend into the subcutaneous fat are more difficult to treat.[61]

Other Causes of Epidermal and Dermal Pigmentation

Melasma

Melasma is an acquired, usually symmetrical and bilateral facial hypermelanosis. Histologically, melasma can be classified as epidermal, dermal, or mixed types. Wood's light is useful in clinical assessment of the type of melasma.

Epidermal melasma is enhanced on examination with Wood's light whereas dermal melasma does not show enhancement of pigmentation.[62]

In epidermal melasma, the melanin deposition is seen in the basal and suprabasal layers and the melanocytes are found to contain highly melanized melanosomes. In dermal melasma, melanophages are seen in the superficial and deep dermis along with epidermal hyperpigmentation.[63]

Melasma is best treated medically. Sun protection, short course fixed triple combination creams, hydroquinone (HQ), and non-HQ compounds being the mainstay of therapy. Lasers have a limited role in the treatment of melasma.[6] Lasers can be used to cause thermal destruction of melanosomes as well as elimination of epidermal pigment by resurfacing. Although successful use of QS lasers, fractional lasers, IPL, and combination lasers have all been reported, response to treatment is unpredictable, and pigmentation frequently recurs. Postinflammatory hyperpigmentation is commonly seen in Indian patients. For these reasons, lasers are not routinely recommended as the treatment of choice for treating melasma in Indian patients. It may be used in selected resistant cases, at the discretion of the treating physician, after proper counseling. A test patch may be performed prior to treating the lesion.[64-69]

Recently, the concept of subcellular selective photothermolysis has emerged. By using lower fluences with the QS lasers, only the organelles, such as melanosomes, are targeted thereby destroying the intracellular organelles and preventing destruction of the melanocytes. This also helps reduce the risk of complications, such as postinflammatory hyperpigmentation and hypopigmentation.[70] Weekly sessions of low fluence QS Nd:YAG laser, up to 10 sessions have been used to successfully treat melasma.[71-76]

The traditional QSNY laser treatment is based upon principle of selective photothermolysis which results in destruction and death of pigment containing cell.[3] As a response to this, inflammation ensues and can result in repigmentation and recurrence. The high peak power, ultrashort pulse duration (5 nanoseconds), and flat top beam results in destruction of only melanin in target cell but leaving the cell alive which could be explained by the concept of *Subcellular Selective Photothermolysis* discussed above.[70]

Since fluence used is very less and there is no cell death and inflammation and heating is kept to minimum which could lead to less recurrence.

A number of studies have reported the use of low-fluence QSNY laser treatment (laser toning) at weekly intervals for 8–10 sessions with some success. Though effective, the risk of mottled hypopigmentation following multiple QSNY laser sessions at frequent intervals has been reported in literature. Hence caution needs to be exercised while performing this procedure and the risks need to be explained to patients. In our experience, modified laser toning with low fluence and large spot size of 8–10 mm with treatments performed once in 2 weeks instead of weekly treatments for 6–8 sessions is better as it decreases the risk of hypopigmentation. The chances of recurrence are very high after discontinuing the procedure with some studies noting figures as high as 81%.[71]

Table 2 highlights the current literature evidence for lasers in melasma.[77-85]

Figures 26 and 27 show melasma before and after 10 weekly low fluence 1,064 nm QS Nd:YAG laser sessions demonstrating good improvement.

Becker's Nevus

Becker's nevus is a hamartomatous pigmented hairy lesion that occurs in adolescence and young adulthood. The condition is difficult to treat and uniform results are difficult to obtain. These lesions require multiple lasers for management; long-pulsed lasers for the removal of hairs, QS laser treatment for pigment reduction, and fractional lasers for lesions associated with thickened skin. However, pigment reduction is variable and use of test spots with different pigment-specific lasers is recommended to determine the laser (or combination of lasers) best suited to treat an individual lesion. However, it should be emphasized that the outcome of laser treatment in these conditions may be suboptimal and unpredictable.[86-89]

TABLE 2: Summary of recent studies on lasers in melasma.[77-85]

Journal	*Title and authors*	*Conclusion*	*Remarks*
Lasers Med Sci. 2016 July 23	• Efficacy and safety of fractional Q-switched 1064-nm neodymium-doped yttrium aluminum garnet laser in the treatment of melasma in Chinese patients • Yue B, Yang Q, Xu J, Lu Z	The fractional mode (Pixel) QS Nd:YAG 1064-nm laser is an effective and safe treatment for melasma. The recurrence rate was relatively lower than that reported in studies treating with large-spot low-fluence QS Nd:YAG laser	The lower recurrence could be due to lesser thermal effect due to use of fractionated beam
J Cosmet Dermatol. 2016 June 28	• Long-term results in low-fluence 1064-nm Q-Switched Nd:YAG laser for melasma: Is it effective? • Gokalp H, Akkaya AD, Oram Y	The recurrence of low-fluence 1064-nm QS-Nd:YAG laser rates in melasma was high when the long-term results were considered	This result may be attributed to certain patient and treatment-related factors
Ann Dermatol. 2016 May 25	• Treatment of melasma with the photoacoustic twin pulse mode of low-fluence 1,064 nm Q-switched Nd:YAG laser • Kim JY, Choi M, Nam CH, Kim JS, Kim MH, Park BC, et al	After five sessions of laser therapy alone, about 60% of the subjects showed significant improvement. Few sessions of repeated laser toning treatment using the PTP mode is a safe and effective way to treat facial melasma	PTP involves splitting of the laser pulse into two with an interval of 100 microseconds between the two pulses. The energy is divided into half rather than a single high peak energy pulse
Skin Therapy Lett. 2016 January	• Melasma and postinflammatory hyperpigmentation: management update and expert opinion. • Sofen B, Prado G, Emer J	Combining topical therapy with procedures, such as chemical peels, intense pulsed light (IPL), fractional nonablative lasers or radiofrequency, pigment lasers (microsecond, picosecond, Q-switched), and microneedling, enhances results. With proper treatment, melasma can be controlled, improved, and maintained	Combining medical therapy with procedures enhances results in melasma
Dermatol Surg. 2016 April	• Clinical and histopathologic assessment of facial melasma after low-fluence Q-switched neodymium-doped yttrium aluminium garnet laser • Hofbauer Parra CA, Careta MF, Valente NY, de Sanches Osório NE, Torezan LA	The results confirm the safety and effectiveness of low-fluence QS Nd:YAG laser for treating melasma; however, the high recurrence suggests poor long-term results when the laser is used as a monotherapy	High rate of recurrence precludes use of laser toning as first-line therapy
Ann Dermatol. 2015 May 29	• Changes in melanin and melanocytes in mottled hypopigmentation after low-fluence 1,064-nm Q-switched Nd:YAG laser treatment for melasma • Jang YH, Park JY, Park YJ, Kang HY	In conclusion, laser toning-induced hypopigmentation is characterized by almost destroyed melanosome pigments and a preserved number of melanocytes, which seem to be functionally downregulated not to produce fully matured melanosomes. Thus, early intervention aiming to restore melanocyte function would be required	This study endorses the subcellular selective photothermolysis theory and shows that after laser toning the melanocytes are downregulated rather than destroyed
Lasers Surg Med. 2014 June 4	• A randomized, split-face clinical trial of low-fluence Q-switched neodymium-doped yttrium aluminum garnet (1,064 nm) laser versus low-fluence Q-switched alexandrite laser (755 nm) for the treatment of facial melasma • Fabi SG, Friedmann DP, Niwa Massaki AB, Goldman MP	Both low-fluence Q-switched Nd:YAG and low-fluence QSAL were equally effective at improving moderate to severe mixed-type facial melasma	Both low-fluence QSNY and QSAL seem effective but long-term follow-up is needed with QSAL

Contd...

Contd...

Journal	*Title and authors*	*Conclusion*	*Remarks*
Am J Clin Dermatol. 2014 August	• Low-power fractional CO_2 laser versus low-fluence Q-switch 1,064 nm Nd:YAG laser for treatment of melasma: a randomized, controlled, split-face study • Jalaly NY, Valizadeh N, Barikbin B, Yousefi M	The present study shows that low-power fractional CO_2 laser is safe and effective and can be considered as a valuable approach in the treatment of melasma	The results seem encouraging in this randomized split-face study. Though caution needs to be exercised in darker skin types
Indian J Dermatol. 2017 November–December	• *Lasers in melasma:* A review with consensus recommendations by Indian pigmentary expert group. Indian J Dermatol. 2017;62:477-82 • Sarkar R, Aurangabadkar S, Salim T, Das A, Shah S, Majid I, et al	The authors suggest lasers as third-line therapy for melisma	
Indian J Dermatol Venereol Leprol. 2019 January–February	• Optimizing Q-switched lasers for melasma and acquired dermal melanoses. Indian J Dermatol Venereol Leprol. 2019;85:10-7 • Aurangabadkar SJ	The author suggested modified laser toning with sessions performed once every fortnight for 8–10 sessions for melasma and use of large spot size of 10 mm at 1,064 nm	The study was on skin phototypes IV to V

(PTP: photoacoustic twin pulse; QSNY: Q-switched Nd:YAG; QSAL: Q-switched alexandrite laser)

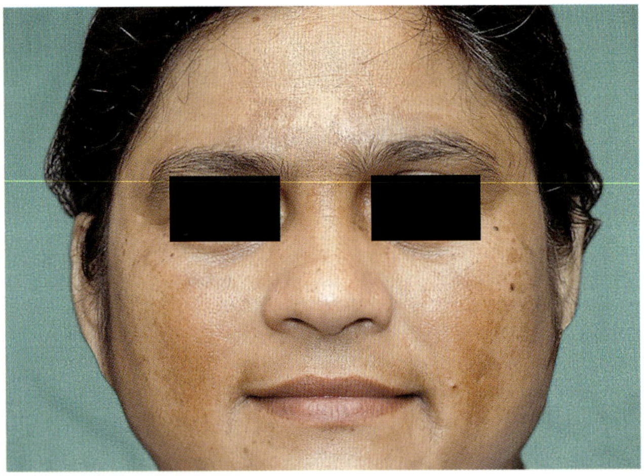

Fig. 26: Melasma before 1,064 nm QS Nd:YAG laser treatment.

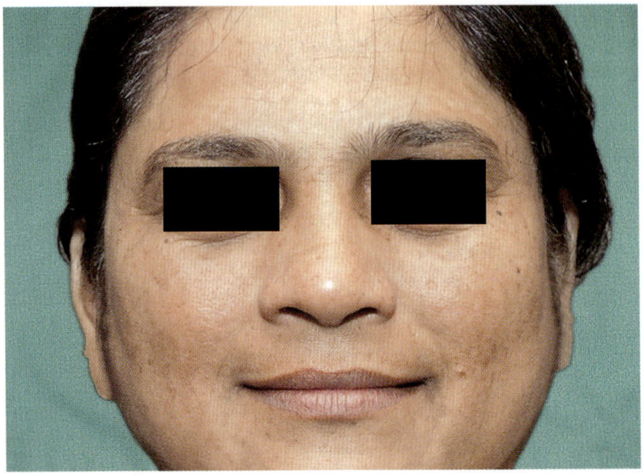

Fig. 27: Melasma after 10 weekly low-fluence 1,064 nm QS Nd:YAG laser sessions.

Zhong et al. in their paper on lasers for Becker's nevus observed that the clinical outcomes were mixed although combination of lasers with different wavelengths appeared to achieve a better efficacy. They concluded that lasers were relatively safe, their efficacy for Becker's nevus was moderate and combination therapy could improve the outcome.[88]

Nevocellular Nevi

Nevocellular nevi may be congenital or acquired. Acquired nevi are further subdivided into junctional, compound, and intradermal types. Any of the currently available QS lasers can be used to treat nevi. Frequency-doubled Nd:YAG at 532 nm are considered suitable for superficial junctional nevi; however, longer-pulsed pigment specific lasers, with pulse duration of up to 3 ms, may also be used for the treatment of nevi. Compound and intradermal nevi are best treated by radiofrequency surgery or surgical excision. While treating junctional nevi, the response is variable. The superficial lesions may lighten or clear only partially and lesions may recur. The QS lasers at 532 nm and 755 nm are more effective than the 1,064 nm wavelength due to better melanin absorption of these wavelengths, though the latter is safer in darker skin types. On an average, 1–3 sessions are required for clearing. The risk of dyschromia and atrophic scarring is high in darker individuals. For these reasons laser treatment should be used with caution and test treatments are recommended.[90-98]

Congenital melanocytic nevi, which are generally very dark and bulky, with a deep dermal component are difficult to treat and need a combination of different approaches, such as excision, grafting, and lasers. Among lasers, high powered pulsed carbon dioxide 10,600 nm laser, Er:YAG 2,940 nm laser, normal mode Ruby and Q-switched ruby 694 nm laser, Q-switched alexandrite 755 nm lasers have all been tried for congenital melanocytic nevi (CMN).[97] Combinations of QS and subsequent longer-pulsed lasers have been reported to be effective, but the lesion may clear only partially and the response is unpredictable. Three to five treatments are usually needed. Patients should be followed up regularly to check for recurrences. Nonpigmented deep nests of nevus cells may persist leading to recurrence.

Laser treatment of large CMN is controversial due to remnant deep nevus cells that can recur or undergo malignant transformation which can either be deep seated or masked. Curettage of CMN has been suggested in neonates and infants but again has risk of recurrence. For giant congenital melanocytic nevi, the risk of developing melanoma has been reported to be as high as 5–7% by age 60 years.[98]

Figures 28 and 29 show a congenital melanocytic nevus before and after QS Nd:YAG laser treatment.

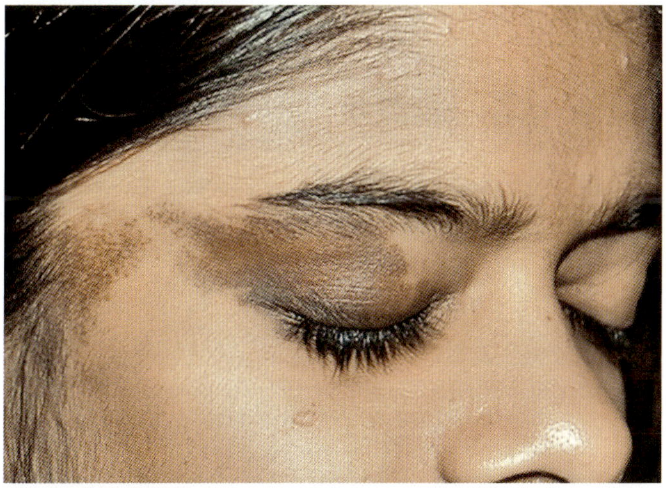

Fig. 28: Congenital melanocytic nevus on the upper eyelid and temple area.

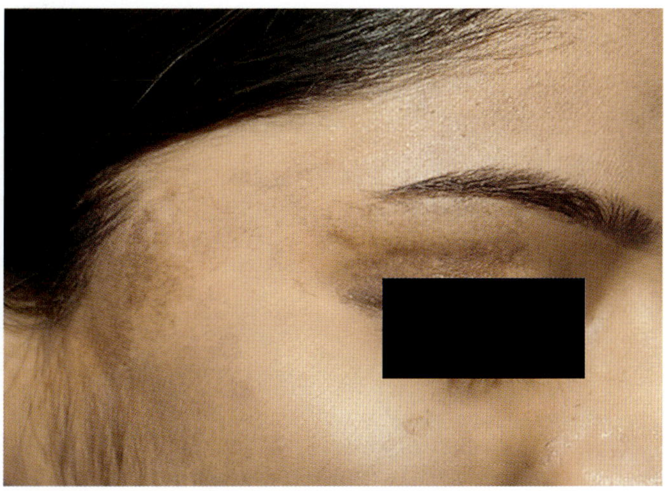

Fig. 29: Congenital melanocytic nevus after six QS laser treatments using a blend of 532 nm and 1,064 nm.

Postinflammatory Hyperpigmentation

Most commonly encountered in skin of color, PIH may have epidermal and dermal components. Although the epidermal component can be targeted with QS lasers and IPL systems, the dermal components are refractory to treatment and the pigmentation may even worsen. Hence, lasers are of limited value.[99]

Riehl's melanosis characterized by diffuse gray to black hyperpigmentation around the face is a challenge to treat. Kwon et al. in a pilot study using a triple combination approach (low-fluence QSNY, hydroquinone cream, and oral tranexamic acid) for the treatment of Riehl's melanosis in eight patients found significant improvement after 10–18 sessions.[100]

Lichen planus pigmentosus is characterized by bluish-gray macular hyperpigmentation that is often distributed on the face, neck, upper trunk, and arms. It is characterized histologically by an interface dermatitis, pigment incontinence, and dermal melanophages. The pigmentation can be persistent and recalcitrant to medical therapy. Once the disease activity ceases, the residual pigmentation can be tackled by a QSNY laser. In the author's experience, multiple sessions (average five) of QSNY at 4–6 week intervals using a large spot size and moderate fluences (which vary with the laser used) yield excellent results. In a series of patients, very good clearing was observed using this protocol as shown in **Figures 30 to 33.**[101]

Table 3 provides an algorithm for laser treatment of pigmented lesions and tattoos.

Box 3 summarizes the approach to pigmented lesions laser treatment.

Box 4 classifies the various pigmented lesions according to their response to QS laser therapy.

POSTOPERATIVE INSTRUCTIONS

- Broad spectrum sunscreens with good UVA/UVB coverage are recommended before and throughout the treatment period.
- Immediately after laser treatment, the treated area appears abraded and inflamed. Apply ice packs till burning sensation subsides, then apply a layer of antibiotic such as mupirocin and cover with gauze. Patient is instructed to clean the area with copious amount of water and apply the ointment twice daily till lesions heal. Healing can take around 5–10 days.
- Oral antibiotics may be used, if considered essential, but are not mandatory. Anti-inflammatory agents may be needed while treating large lesions. Patient should be instructed to avoid sun exposure and cosmetics on the treated area. Treatments are scheduled at an interval of 6–8 weeks.

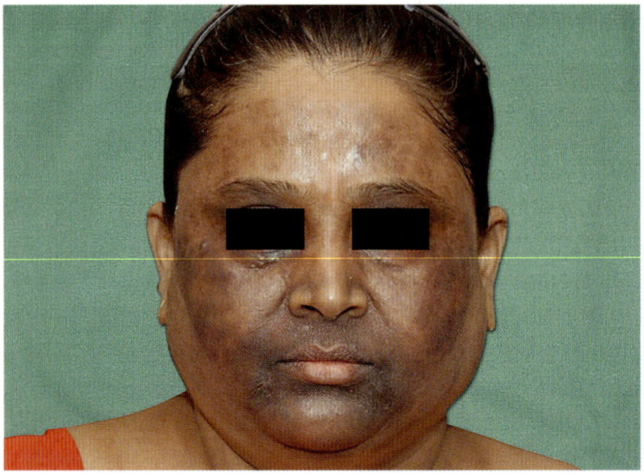

Fig. 30: Lichen planus pigmentosus (LPP) before laser therapy.

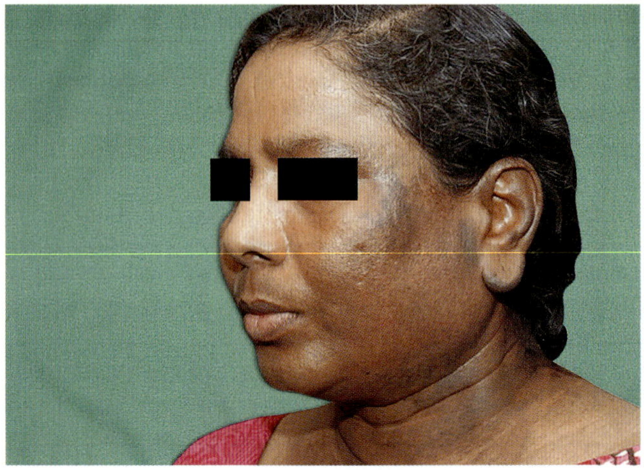

Fig. 32: Lichen planus pigmentosus (LPP) before laser.

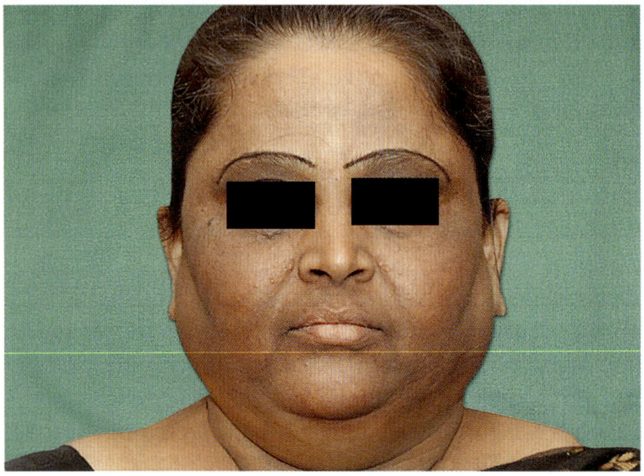

Fig. 31: Lichen planus pigmentosus (LPP) after five sessions of QSNY laser at 1,064 nm. (QSNY: Q-switched Nd:YAG)

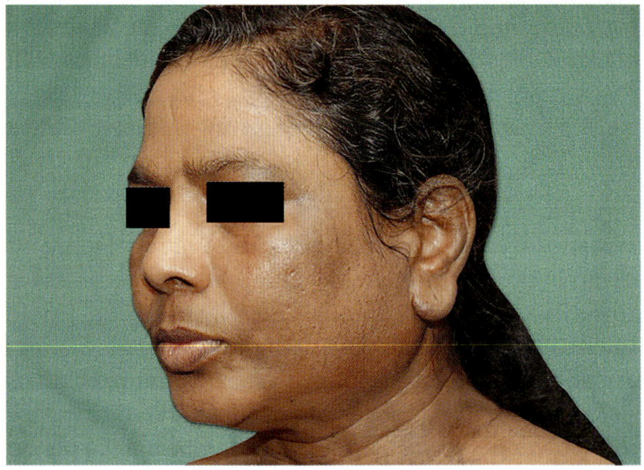

Fig. 33: Lichen planus pigmentosus (LPP) after six sessions of QSNY laser at 1,064 nm. (QSNY: Q-switched Nd:YAG)

TABLE 3: Algorithm for laser treatment of pigmented lesions and tattoos.

Ephelides, lentigines and solar lentigo 532 nm QS Nd:YAG/IPL (in light skin only) ↓	CALM and nevus spilus	Nevus of Ota and Ito/ Hori's nevus ↓	Melasma ↓	Tattoos ↓
	532 QS Nd:YAG (in light skin only)	1,064 nm QS Nd:YAG laser (all skin types)	1,064 nm QS Nd:YAG	Blue-black tattoo ↓
1,064 nm QS Nd:YAG (in all skin types) ↓	1,064 QS Nd:YAG (in all skin types)		Low fluence-laser toning (all skin types) Or	1,064 nm QS Nd:YAG
Ablative lasers like CO_2 and Er:YAG may also be used for lentigines if QS laser not available			• Fractional lasers (nonablative—1,540 and 1,550 nm Er:Glass)/ (ablative 2,940 nm Er:YAG) • Sequential lasers (ablative super pulsed CO_2 10,600 nm followed by QS Alexandrite 755 nm)	Red tattoo ↓ 532 QS Nd:YAG ↓ Green tattoo ↓ 694 QS Ruby laser ↓ Purple or teal color ↓ 755 QS Alexandrite laser

BOX 3: Approach to laser treatment of pigmented lesions in dark skin.

- Strict sun-protective clothing and use of broad spectrum sunscreens of at least 30 SPF and PA +++ prior to starting laser treatment and throughout the course of therapy
- Proper priming with skin-lightening agents, such as hydroquinone, kojic acid, etc., at least 2–3 weeks prior to initiation of laser therapy
- Performing test treatments/test spots to choose the right fluence
- Individualizing the treatment parameters tailored to the patient and indication
- Use of a laser with "top-hat" beam profile, large spot size, etc.
- Avoiding stacking and too much overlap while treating
- Cooling the treated area with continuous air cooling (Zimmer)
- Postoperative ice pack application for a few minutes, application of emollients, steroid-antibiotic ointment for 3–5 days (if blistering or crusting is anticipated)

(SPF: sun protection factor)

BOX 4: Classification of pigmented lesions and tattoos according to response to QS laser therapy.

- *Excellent:* 532 nm/IPL—ephelides, lentigines, and labial melanotic macules
- *Very good:* 1,064 nm—nevus of Ota, Hori's nevus, and junctional nevus
- *Variable:* CALM, nevus spilus, Mongolian spots, segmental lentigines, and PIH
- *Poor:* Melasma, Becker's nevus

(CALM: café-au-lait macules; IPL: intense pulsed light; PIH: postinflammatory hyperpigmentation)

- Patients are instructed to apply an antibiotic ointment or petrolatum ointment for about a week after procedure. Strict sun protection is advised for darker patients. Ice packs may be used after the procedure to minimize discomfort.
- Postprocedure bleaching agents may be used but only after the crust subsides.

COMPLICATIONS AND THEIR MANAGEMENT

Complications may be encountered, especially in darker skin types.[60] These may be minor and transient or major and persistent. The risk of complications increases with more aggressive treatments, poor priming, multiple treatments, choosing inappropriate laser systems, and in unrealistic patients. Some of the complications which demand considerations are:

- Postinflammatory hyperpigmentation resolves with time; some patients may need bleaching agents such as hydroquinone along with sunscreens.
- Postinflammatory hypopigmentation may persist for several weeks to months and may be difficult to treat. Phototherapy may be used to treat the hypopigmentation. **Figures 34 and 35** show guttate/mottled hypopigmentation following multiple QSNY laser sessions using a smaller spot size.
- Textural changes and scarring
- Thermal injury and burns.

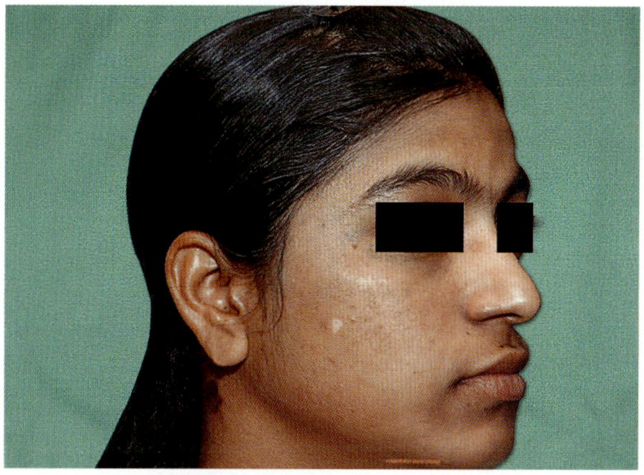

Fig. 34: Hypopigmentation following multiple >10 sessions of 1,064 nm QSNY at 4 mm. (QSNY: Q-switched Nd:YAG)

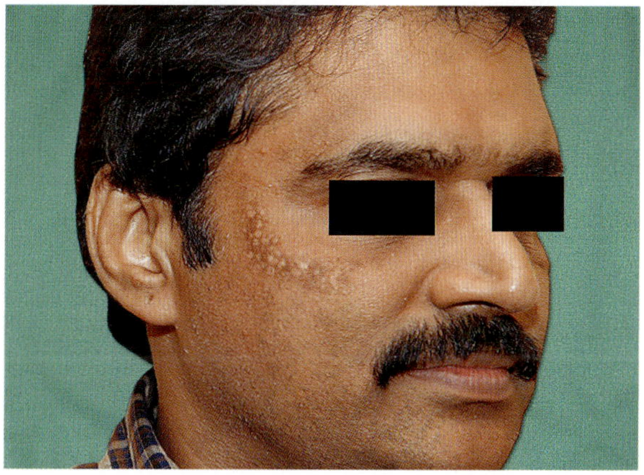

Fig. 35: Mottled hypopigmentation following laser toning in melasma using 4-mm spot, 1,064 nm.

- Scarring may occur if very high fluence is used. A high fluence may result in burns which, if secondarily infected, may lead to scar formation.
- Infection, though uncommon, may occur. An antibiotic ointment and a nonadherent dressing should be applied upon completion of treatment. Patients should be instructed regarding the proper local wound care.

Table 4 summarizes the features of some of the available QS laser machines in India.

CONCLUSION

The current gold standard for pigmented lesion removal remains the QSNY laser, the versatility of the system with the availability of multiple wavelengths, quasi-long pulse mode and large spot size makes this the laser of choice particularly in dark skin. Though the picosecond laser are available in various WLs and spot sizes, the early results show they may not yet replace the QSNY laser. They are very expensive when compared to the QSLs hence are not yet widely available. The newer techniques of laser toning and its modifications hold some promise and fine tuning of the protocols will ensure better outcomes. Low fluence QSNY has been used in a wider

TABLE 4: Some of the currently available Q-switched and picoseconds lasers and their specifications.

Laser	*Manufacturer*	*Spot size*	*Fluence*	*Repetition rate*	*Additional features*
Spectra XT Q-switched Nd:YAG laser	Lutronic	Up to 10 mm variable	2 J @ 1,064 nm	Up to 10 Hz	Extended platform with four wavelengths 1,064 nm, 532 nm, 660 nm, and 585 nm
Tri-beam	Jeisys	2–10 mm	1.6 J @ 1,064	Up to 20 Hz	• 5–10 nanoseconds pulse duration • Dye HP • Zoom HP • Collimated HP • Fractional HP
Helios	Laseroptek	1–7 mm Zoom, 8 mm collimated, 4 × 4 and 5 × 5 fractional	• 1.3 J @ 1,064 nm • 0.5 J @ 532 nm	Up to 10 Hz	10 nanoseconds pulse duration
Alma-Q	Alma	1–8 mm	• 1,064–1,200 mJ • 532–450 mJ	10 Hz	Triple mode Q-switched, quasi long pulse and long pulse mode Nd:YAG laser
RevLite and MedLite	Hoya CONBIO-Cynosure	1.2–8.5	Up to 12 J/cm^2	10 Hz	Pulse duration 5–20 nanoseconds 1,064, 532, 585, and 650 nm wavelengths
Discovery Pico	Quanta	2 × 2; 3 × 3; 4 × 4; 5 × 5; 9 × 9 mm^2; ø 3; 4.5; 6; 7.5; 9; 10.5 mm round; 8 mm fractional round	• Pico 800 mJ @ 1,064 nm • Pico 300 mJ @ 532 nm	Up to 10 Hz	• Q-switched mode pulse duration 6 nanoseconds • Photothermal mode 300 microseconds 2 J
PICOPLUS	Lutronic	1–10 mm, Focused dots handpiece	Up to 2 J	Up to 10 Hz	• Pico and nanosecond range • Pico toning four wavelengths 532, 1064, 660, and 585 nm
PicoSure	Cynosure	2–6 mm Zoom HP, Fixed HP 6, 8 and 10 mm	Up to 200 mJ	10 Hz	• 755 nm Alex Pico • 750 PS pulse duration
PicoWay	Syneron Candela	2–10 mm	• 400 mJ @ 1064 nm • 200 mJ @ 532 nm	Up to 10 Hz	375–450 PS Pulse duration

variety of indications beyond melasma, such as segmental lentigines, solar lentigo, nevus of Ota, etc., and has been effective with the additional benefit of lower side effects.

Overall the QSNY laser is highly effective and safe in darker skin types. It still remains the "Gold Standard" for pigment removal.

TIPS

For laser treatment of pigmented lesions:
- Confirm the diagnosis (perform biopsy if diagnosis is uncertain)
- Avoid a tanned patient
- Choose appropriate QS laser and do a test area if necessary. Epidermal lesions, for example, lentigines use 532 nm QS Nd:YAG
- Dermal lesions, for example, nevus of Ota use 1,064 nm QS Nd:YAG
- Evaluate test spots after 4–8 weeks
- If lesion clears well proceed for rest of area
- If marginal improvement with laser, test the area again at 8 weekly intervals and only after significant pigment dilution is produced, proceed for rest of the area. If any worsening/scarring, stop further treatments.

For approach to laser treatment of tattoos:
- Avoid treating a tanned patient
- Choose appropriate QS laser and do a test area
- *Red tattoo:* Use 532 nm QS Nd:YAG
- *Dark blue and black tattoo:* Use 1,064 nm QS Nd:YAG
- *Green tattoo:* Use 694 nm QS Ruby
- Evaluate test spots after 4–8 weeks
- If the test patch lesion clears well, treat the remaining area
- If any worsening or scarring occurs, stop further treatments

REFERENCES

1. Barlow RJ, Hruza GJ. Lasers and light tissue interactions. In: Goldberg DJ, Dover JS, Alam M (Eds). Procedures in Cosmetic Dermatology: Laser and Lights, 1st edition. Philadelphia: Elsevier; 2005. pp 1-11.
2. OíShea DC, Callen WR, Rhodes WT. Introduction to lasers and their applications. Menlo Park, CA: Addison-Wesley Publishing Co; 1978.
3. Anderson RR, Parrish JA. Selective photothermolysis: precise microsurgery by selective absorption of pulsed radiation. Science. 1983;220:524-7.
4. Polla LL, Margolis RJ, Dover JS, Whitaker D, Murphy GF, Jacques SL, et al. Melanosomes are a primary target of Q-switches ruby laser irradiation in guinea pig skin. J Invest Dermatol. 1987;89(3):281-6.
5. Goel A, Krupashankar DS, Aurangabadkar S, Nischal KC, Omprakash HM, Mysore V. Fractional lasers in dermatology. Current status and recommendations. Indian J Dermatol Venereol Leprol. 2011;77:369-79.
6. Lee HI, Lim YY, Kim BJ, Kim MN, Min HJ, Hwang JH, et al. Clinicopathologic efficacy of copper bromide plus/yellow laser (578 nm with 511 nm) for treatment of melasma in Asian patients. Dermatol Surg. 2010;36:885-93.
7. McClung FJ, Hellwarth RW. Giant optical pulsations from ruby. J Appl Phys. 1962;33:828.
8. Ross V, Naseef G, Lin G, Kelly M, Michaud N, Flotte TJ, et al. Comparison of responses of tattoos to picosecond and nanosecond Q-switched neodymium: YAG lasers. Arch Dermatol. 1998;134(2):167-71.

9. Kilmer SL. Laser eradication of pigmented lesions and tattoos. Dermatol Clin. 2002;20:37-53.
10. Goldberg DJ. Pigmented lesions, tattoos, and disorders of hypopigmentation. In: Goldberg DJ (Ed). Laser Dermatology Pearls and Problems, 1st edition. Massachusetts: Blackwell Publishing; 2008;71-114.
11. Kilmer SL, Garden JM. Laser treatment of pigmented lesions and tattoos. Semin Cutan Med Surg. 2000;19:232-44.
12. Aurangabadkar S, Mysore V. Standard guidelines of care: lasers for tattoos and pigmented lesions. Indian J Dermatol Venereol Leprol. 2009;75:111-26.
13. Schmults CD, Wheeland RG. Pigmented lesions and tattoos. In: Goldberg DJ, Dover JS, Alam M (Eds). Procedures in Cosmetic Dermatology: Laser and Lights, 1st edition. Philadelphia: Elsevier; 2005. pp. 41-66.
14. Kilmer SL. Laser treatment of tattoos. Dermatol Clin. 1997;15:409-17.
15. Grevelink JM, Duke D, van Leeuwen RL, Gonzalez E, DeCoste SD, Anderson RR. Laser treatment of tattoos in darkly pigmented patients: efficacy and side effects. J Am Acad Dermatol. 1996;34(4):653-6.
16. Adrian RM, Griffin L. Laser tattoo removal. Clin Plast Surg. 2000;27:181-92.
17. Koay J, Orengo I. Application of local anesthetics in dermatologic surgery. Dermatol Surg. 2002;28:143-8.
18. Drake LA, Dinehart SM, Goltz RW, Graham GF, Hordinsky MK, Lewis CW, et al. Guidelines of care for local and regional anesthesia in cutaneous surgery. J Am Acad Dermatol. Guidelines/Outcomes Committee: American Academy of Dermatology. J Am Acad Dermatol. 1995;33(3):504-9.
19. Kilmer SL, Farinelli WF, Tearney G. Use of a larger spot size for the treatment of tattoos increases clinical efficacy and decreases potential side effects. Lasers Surg Med Suppl. 1994;6:S51.
20. Chan HH, Lam LK, Wong DS, Leung RS, Ying SY, Lai CF, et al. Nevus of Ota: new classification based on the response to laser treatment. Lasers Surg Med. 2001;28(3):267-72.
21. Ueda S, Isoda M, Imayama S. Response of naevus of Ota to Q-switched ruby laser treatment according to lesion color. Br J Dermatol. 2000;142:77-83.
22. Kilmer SL, Lee MS, Grevelink JM, Flotte TJ, Anderson RR. The Q-switched Nd:YAG laser (1064 nm) effectively treats tattoos. A controlled, dose-response study. Arch Dermatol. 1993;129:971-8.
23. Kilmer SL, Wheeland RJ, Goldberg DJ, Anderson RR. Treatment of epidermal pigmented lesions with the frequency-doubled Q-switched Nd:YAG laser. A controlled, single-impact, dose- response, multicenter trial. Arch Dermatol. 1994;130(12):1515-9.
24. Levy JL, Mordon S, Pizzi-Anselme M. Treatment of individual cafe au lait macules with the Q-switched Nd:YAG: a clinicopathologic correlation. J Cutan Laser Ther. 1999;1:21723.
25. Grossman MC, Anderson RR, Farinelli W, Flotte TJ, Grevelink JM. Treatment of cafe au lait macules with lasers. A clinicopathologic correlation. Arch Dermatol. 1995;131(12):1416-20.
26. Jiang SB, Levine V, Ashinoff R. The treatment of solar lentigines with the Diode (Diolite 532 nm) and the Q-switched ruby laser: a comparative study. Laser Surg Med Suppl. 2000; 12:55.
27. Wang CC, Sue YM, Yang CH, Chen CK. A comparison of Q-switched alexandrite laser and intense pulse light for the treatment of freckles and lentigines in Asian persons: a randomized, physician-blinded, split-face comparative trial. J Am Acad Dermatol. 2006;54(5):804-10.
28. Todd MM, Rallis TM, Gerwels JW, Hata TR. A comparison of 3 lasers and liquid nitrogen in the treatment of solar lentigines: a randomized, controlled, comparative trial. Arch Dermatol. 2000;136(7):841-6.
29. Li YT, Yang KC. Comparison of frequency-doubled Q-switched Nd:YAG laser and 35% trichloroacetic acid for the treatment of face lentigines. Dermatol Surg. 1999;25:202-4.
30. Bjerring P, Christiansen K. Intense pulsed light source for treatment of small melanocytic nevi and solar lentigines. J Cutan Laser Ther. 2000;2:177-81.
31. Kono T, Manstein D, Chan HH, Nozaki M, Anderson RR. Q-switched ruby versus long-pulsed dye laser delivered with compression for treatment of facial lentigines in Asians. Lasers Surg Med. 2006;38(2):94-7.
32. Chan HH, Fung WK, Ying SY, Kono T. An in vivo trial comparing the use of different types of 532 nm Nd:YAG lasers in the treatment of facial lentigines in oriental patients. Dermatol Surg. 2000;26(8):743-9.
33. Nam JH, Kim HS, Lee GY, Kim WS. Beneficial effect of low fluence 1,064 nm Q-switched Nd:YAG laser in the treatment of Senile Lentigo. Ann Dermatol. 2017;29(4): 427-32.
34. Jang KA, Chung EC, Choi JH. Successful removal of freckles in Asian skin with a Q-switched alexandrite laser. Dermatol Surg. 2000;26:231-4.
35. Grevelink JM, Gonzalez S, Bonoan R, Vibhagool C, Gonzalez E. Treatment of nevus spilus with the Q-switched Ruby laser. Dermatol Surg. 1997;23(5):365-9.
36. Gold MH, Foster TD, Bell MW. Nevus spilus successfully treated with an intense pulsed light source. Dermatol Surg. 1999;25:254-5.
37. Moreno-Arias GA, Bulla F, Vilata-Corell JJ, Camps-Fresneda A. Treatment of widespread segmental nevus spilus by Q-switched alexandrite laser (755 nm, 100 nsec). Dermatol Surg. 2001;27(9):841-3.
38. Abecassis S, Spatz A, Cazeneuve C, Martin-Villepou A, Clerici T, Lacour JP, et al. Melanoma within naevus spilus: 5 cases. Ann Dermatol Venereol. 2006;133: 323-8.
39. Fitzpatrick RE, Goldman MP, Ruiz-Esparza J. Clinical advantage of the CO_2 laser superpulsed mode. Treatment of verruca vulgaris, seborrheic keratoses, lentigines, and actinic chelitis. J Dermatol Surg Oncol. 1994;20(7):449-56.
40. Khatri KA. Ablation of cutaneous lesions using erbium:YAG laser. J Cosmet Laser Ther. 2003;5:150-3.
41. Mehrabi D, Brodell RT. Use of the alexandrite laser for the treatment of seborrheic keratoses. Dermatol Surg. 2002; 28:437-9.
42. Chan HH, Leung RS, Ying SY, Lai CF, Kono T, Chua JK, et al. A retrospective analysis of complications in the treatment of nevus of Ota with the Q-switched Alexandrite and Q-switched Nd:YAG lasers. Dermatol Surg. 2000;26(11): 1000-6.
43. Chan HH, King WW, Chan ES, Mok CO, Ho WS, Van Krevel C, et al. In vivo trial comparing patients' tolerance of Q-switched Alexandrite (QS Alex) and Q-switched neodymium:yttrium-aluminum-garnet (QS Nd:YAG) lasers in the treatment of nevus of Ota. Lasers Surg Med. 1999;24(1):24-8.
44. Chan HH, Ying SY, Ho WS, Kono T, King WW. An in vivo trial comparing the clinical efficacy and complications of Q-switched 755 nm alexandrite and Q-switched 1064 nm Nd:YAG lasers in the treatment of nevus of Ota. Dermatol Surg. 2000;26(10):919-22.

45. Kono T, Nozaki M, Chan HH, Mikashima Y. A retrospective study looking at the long-term complications of Q-switched ruby laser in the treatment of nevus of Ota. Lasers Surg Med. 2001;29(2):156-9.
46. Kilmer SL, Anderson RR. Clinical uses of Q-switched ruby and Q-switched Nd:YAG (1064 nm and 532 nm) lasers for treatment of tattoos. J Dermatol Surg Oncol. 1993;19:330-8.
47. Goldberg DJ, Nychay SG. Q-switched ruby laser treatment of nevus of Ota. J Dermatol Surg Oncol. 1992;18:817-21.
48. Watanabe S, Takahashi H. Treatment of nevus of Ota with the Q-switched ruby laser. N Engl J Med. 1994;331:1745-50.
49. Geronemus RG. Q-switched ruby laser therapy of nevus of Ota. Arch Dermatol. 1992;128:1618-22.
50. Alster TS, Williams CM. Treatment of nevus of Ota by the Q-switched Alexandrite laser. Dermatol Surg. 1995;21:5926.
51. Turnbull JR, Assaf Ch, Zouboulis C, Tebbe B. Bilateral naevus of Ota: a rare manifestation in a Caucasian. J Eur Acad Dermtol Venereol. 2004;18(3):353-5.
52. Kopf AW, Bart RS. Malignant blue (Ota's?) nevus. J Dermatol Surg Oncol. 1982;8:442-5.
53. Patel BC, Egan CA, Lucius RW, Gerwels JW, Mamalis N, Anderson RL. Cutaneous malignant melanoma and oculodermal melanocytosis (nevus of Ota): report of a case and review of the literature. J Am Acad Dermatol. 1998; 38(5 Pt 2):862-5.
54. Lowe NJ, Wieder JM, Sawcer D, Burrows P, Chalet M. Nevus of Ota: treatment with high energy fluences of the Q-switched ruby laser. J Am Acad Dermatol. 1993;29(6): 997-1001.
55. Chan HH, Lam LK, Wong DS, Wei WI. Role of skin cooling in improving patient tolerability of Q-switched alexandrite (QS Alex) laser in nevus of Ota treatment. Lasers Surg Med. 2003;32(2):148-51.
56. Aurangabadkar S. QYAG5 Q-switched Nd:YAG laser treatment of nevus of Ota: an Indian study of 50 patients. J Cutan Aesthet Surg. 2008;1:80-4.
57. Kunachak S, Leelaudomlipi P. Q-switched Nd:YAG laser treatment for acquired bilateral nevus of Ota-like maculae: a long-term follow-up. Lasers Surg Med. 2000;26:376-9.
58. Polnikorn N, Tanrattanakorn S, Goldberg DJ. Treatment of Hori's nevus with the Q-switched Nd:YAG laser. Dermatol Surg. 2000;26:477-80.
59. Lee B, Kim YC, Kang WH, Lee ES. Comparison of characteristics of acquired bilateral nevus of Ota-like macules and nevus of Ota according to therapeutic outcome. J Korean Med Sci. 2004;19(4):554-9.
60. Lam AY, Wong DS, Lam LK, Ho WS, Chan HH. A retrospective study on the efficacy and complications of Q-switched alexandrite laser in the treatment of acquired bilateral nevus of Ota-like macules. Dermatol Surg. 2001;27(11): 937-41.
61. Milgraum SS, Cohen ME, Auletta MJ. Treatment of blue nevi with the Q-switched ruby laser. J Am Acad Dermatol. 1995;32:307-10.
62. Katsambas A, Antoniou C. Melasma. Classification and treatment. J Eur Acad Dermatol Venereol. 1995;4:217-23.
63. Kang WH, Yoon KH, Lee ES, Kim J, Lee KB, Yim H, et al. Melasma: Histopathological characteristics in 56 Korean patients. Br J Dermatol. 2002;146:228-37.
64. Nouri K, Bowes L, Chartier T, Romagosa R, Spencer J. Combination treatment of melasma with pulsed CO_2 laser followed by Q-switched alexandrite laser: a pilot study. Dermatol Surg. 1999;25(6):4947.
65. Wang CC, Hui CY, Sue YM, Wong WR, Hong HS. Intense pulse light for the treatment of refractory melasma in Asian persons. Dermatol Surg. 2004;30(9):1196-200.
66. Manaloto RM, Alster T. Erbium:YAG laser resurfacing for refractory melasma. Dermatol Surg. 1999;25:121-3.
67. Rokhsar CK, Fitzpatrick RE. The treatment of melasma with fractional photothermolysis: a pilot study. Dermatol Surg. 2005;31:1645-50.
68. Polnikorn N. Treatment of refractory dermal melasma with the MedLite C6 Q-switched Nd:YAG laser: two case reports. J Cosmet Laser Ther. 2008;10:167-73.
69. Jeong SY, Chang SE, Bak H, Choi JH, KIM IH. New melasma treatment by collimated low fluence Q-switched Nd:YAG laser. Korean J Dermatol. 2008;46:1163-70.
70. Mun JY, Jeong SY, Kim JH, Han SS, Kim IH. A low fluence Q-switched Nd:YAG laser modifies the 3D structure of melanocyte and ultrastructure of melanosome by subcellular-selective photothermolysis. J Electron Microsc (Tokyo). 2011;60(1):11-8.
71. Hofbauer Parra CA, Careta MF, Valente NY, de Sanches Osório NE, Torezan LA. Clinical and histopathologic assessment of facial melasma after low-fluence Q-switched neodymium-doped yttrium aluminium garnet laser. Dermatol Surg. 2016;42(4):507-12.
72. Chan NP, Ho SG, Shek SY, Yeung CK, Chan HH. A case series of facial depigmentation associated with low fluence Q-switched 1,064 nm Nd:YAG laser for skin rejuvenation and melasma. Lasers Surg Med. 2010;42(8):712-9.
73. Jeong SY, Shin JB, Yeo UC, Kim WS, Kim IH. Low-fluence Q-switched neodymium-doped yttrium aluminum garnet laser for melasma with pre- or post-treatment triple combination cream Dermatol Surg. 2010;36(6): 909-18.
74. Na SY, Cho S, Lee JH. Combinational treatment using intense pulsed light and low fluence Q-switched Nd:YAG laser over laser treatment alone. Lasers Surg Med. 2010;42(8): 712-9.
75. Zhou HL, Hu B, Zhang C. Efficacy of 694-nm fractional Q-switched ruby laser (QSRL) combined with sonophoresis on levorotatory vitamin C for treatment of melasma in Chinese patients. Lasers Med Sci. 2016;31(5):991-5.
76. Tian WC. Novel technique to treat melasma in Chinese: The combination of 2940-nm fractional Er:YAG and 1064-nm Q-switched Nd:YAG laser. J Cosmet Laser Ther. 2016;18(2): 72-4.
77. Yue B, Yang Q, Xu J, Lu Z. Efficacy and safety of fractional Q-switched 1064-nm neodymium-doped yttrium aluminum garnet laser in the treatment of melasma in Chinese patients. Lasers Med Sci. 2016;31(8):1657-1663.
78. Gokalp H, Akkaya AD, Oram Y. Long-term results in low-fluence 1064-nm Q-Switched Nd:YAG laser for melasma: Is it effective? J Cosmet Dermatol. 2016;15(4):420-6.
79. Kim JY, Choi M, Nam CH, Kim JS, Kim MH, Park BC, et al. Treatment of melasma with the photoacoustic twin pulse mode of low-fluence 1,064 nm Q-switched Nd:YAG Laser. Ann Dermatol. 2016;28(3):290-6.
80. Sofen B, Prado G, Emer J. Melasma and post inflammatory hyperpigmentation: management update and expert opinion. Skin Therapy Lett. 2016;21(1):1-7.
81. Jang YH, Park JY, Park YJ, Kang HY. Changes in melanin and melanocytes in mottled hypopigmentation after low-fluence 1,064-nm Q-switched Nd:YAG laser treatment for melasma. Ann Dermatol. 2015;27(3):340-2.

82. Fabi SG, Friedmann DP, Niwa Massaki AB, Goldman MP. A randomized, split-face clinical trial of low-fluence Q-switched neodymium-doped yttrium aluminum garnet (1,064 nm) laser versus low-fluence Q-switched alexandrite laser (755 nm) for the treatment of facial melasma. Lasers Surg Med. 2014;46(7):531-7.
83. Jalaly NY, Valizadeh N, Barikbin B, Yousefi M. Low-power fractional CO_2 laser versus low-fluence Q-switch 1,064 nm Nd:YAG laser for treatment of melasma: a randomized, controlled, split-face study. Am J Clin Dermatol. 2014;15(4):357-63.
84. Sarkar R, Gokhale N, Godse K, Ailawadi P, Arya L, Sarma N, et al. Medical management of melasma: a review with consensus recommendations by Indian Pigmentary Expert Group. Indian J Dermatol. 2017;62(6):558-77.
85. Aurangabadkar SJ. Optimizing Q-switched lasers for melasma and acquired dermal melanoses. Indian J Dermatol Venereol Leprol. 2019;85:10-17
86. Nanni CA, Alster T. Treatment of a Becker's nevus using 694-nm long-pulsed ruby laser. Dermatol Surg. 1998;24: 1032-4.
87. Trelles MA, Allones I, Moreno-Arias GA, Vélez M. Becker's nevus: a comparative study between erbium: YAG and Q-switched neodimiyum: YAG; clinical and histopathological findings. Br J Dermatol. 2005;152(2):308-13.
88. Zhong Y, Yang B, Huang L, Elias PM, Man MQ. Lasers for Becker's nevus. Lasers Med Sci. 2019;34(6):1071-9.
89. Kopera D, Hohenleutner U, Landthaler M. Quality-switched ruby laser treatment of solar lentigines and Becker's nevus: a histopathological and immunohistochemical study. Dermatology. 1997;194:338-43.
90. Goldberg DJ, Stampien T. Q-switched ruby laser treatment of congenital nevi. Arch Dermatol. 1995;131:621-3.
91. Grevelink JM, van Leeuwen RL, Anderson RR, Byers HR. Clinical and histological responses of congenital melanocytic nevi after single treatment with Q-switched lasers. Arch Dermatol. 1997;133(3):349-53.
92. Rosenbach A, Williams CM, Alster TS. Comparison of the Q-switched alexandrite (755 nm) and Q-switched Nd:YAG (1064 nm) lasers in the treatment of benign melanocytic nevi. Dermatol Surg. 1997;23:239-44.
93. Waldorf HA, Kauvar AN, Geronemus RG. Treatment of small and medium congenital nevi with Q-switched ruby laser. Arch Dermatol. 1996;132:301-4.
94. Ueda S, Imayama S. Normal-mode ruby laser for treating congenital nevi. Arch Dermatol. 1997;133:355-9.
95. Kono T, Ercocen AR, Chan HH, Kikuchi Y, Nozaki M. Effectiveness of the normal-mode ruby laser and the combined (normal-mode plus Q-switched) ruby laser in the treatment of congenital melanocytic nevi: a comparative study. Ann Plast Surg. 2002;49(5):476-85.
96. Kono T, Ercocen AR, Nozaki M. Treatment of congenital melanocytic nevi using the combined (normal-mode plus Q-switched) ruby laser in Asians: clinical response in relation to histological type. Ann Plast Surg. 2005;54;494-501.
97. Michel JL. Laser therapy of giant congenital melanocytic nevi. Eur J Dermatol. 2003;13(1):57-64.
98. Bett BJ. Large or multiple congenital melanocytic nevi: occurrence of cutaneous melanoma in 1008 persons. J Am Acad Dermatol. 2005;52(5):793-7.
99. Taylor CR, Anderson RR. Ineffective treatment of refractory melasma and postinflammatory hyperpigmentation by Q-switched ruby laser. J Dermatol Surg Oncol. 1994;20: 592-7.
100. Kwon HH, Ohn J, Suh DH, Park HY, Choi SC, Jung JY, et al. A pilot study for triple combination therapy with a low-fluence 1064 nm Q-switched Nd:YAG laser, hydroquinone cream and oral tranexamic acid for recalcitrant Riehl's Melanosis. J Dermatol Treat. 2016;27:1-5.
101. Shah DSD, Aurangabadkar DS, Nikam DB. An open-label non-randomized prospective pilot study of the efficacy of Q-switched Nd-YAG laser in management of facial lichen planus pigmentosus. J Cosmet Laser Ther. 2019;21(2): 108-115.

CHAPTER 110

Lasers for Tattoo Removal

Sanjeev J Aurangabadkar

KEY MESSAGES

- Tattoo removal with lasers requires thorough understanding of the Q-switched laser and the relevant laser-tissue interaction.
- The choice of the laser or wavelength depends on the tattoo type, color, and its location. Sometimes multiple wavelengths may be necessary to clear a professional tattoo. Newer techniques such as R0 and R20 have cut down the treatment duration significantly.
- Combination methods such as ablative fractional lasers together with the Q-switched Nd:YAG lasers have shown a synergistic effect by speeding up the rate of clearance of the tattoo and minimizing adverse effects.

INTRODUCTION

A tattoo is a form of body modification done by inserting ink (either indelible or temporary) into the dermal layer of the skin. The word tattoo or tattow is derived from a Polynesian word "tatau" as was first described in the 18th century.[1] Tattooing has been in vogue since the ancient times for various reasons such as cultural, religious, and decorative. There has been a dramatic rise in the trend in the past few decades with more and more people getting themselves tattooed. Single color amateur tattoos are being superseded by complex multicolored decorative tattoos with the current trend being 3D tattoos, optical illusion tattoos, head mandala tattoos, and foot tattoos to name a few. Present statistics show that nearly 25% of Australians <30 years sport at least one tattoo![2] While tattooing has gained popularity, a fair subset of people with tattoos seek its removal. In the past, before lasers became widely available, limited options existed for tattoo removal. These included dermabrasion, surgical excision, cryotherapy, salabrasion, etc.[3] These methods often led to poor cosmetic results and also scarring in many instances as shown in **Figures 1 and 2**. The advent of lasers, particularly Q-switched lasers (and more recently picosecond lasers) has transformed the tattoo removal scenario and lasers have now become the primary treatment modality for tattoo removal.[4]

Mechanism of Action of Q-Switched Lasers

Q-switching is a method for obtaining energetic pulses from lasers by modulating the intracavity losses—the so-called the *Q* factor of the laser resonator. The technique is mainly applied for the generation of nanosecond pulses of high energy and peak power with solid-state bulk lasers. These giant pulses are responsible for the unique laser-tissue interaction that is seen with Q-switched lasers.[5]

Q-switched lasers (QSL) work on the principle of selective photothermolysis and also produce an additional

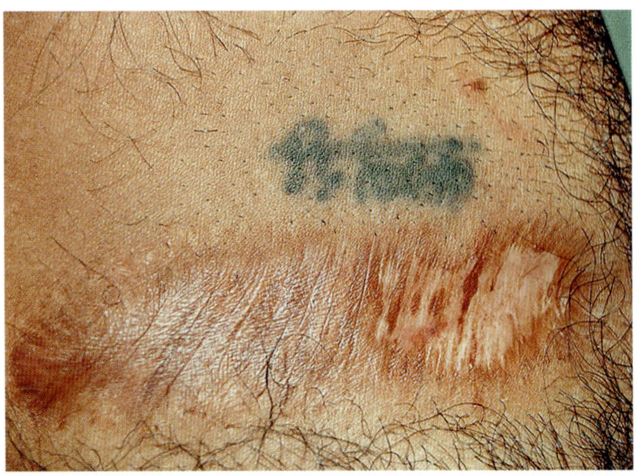

Fig. 1: Dermabrasion done for tattoo removal leading to scarring.

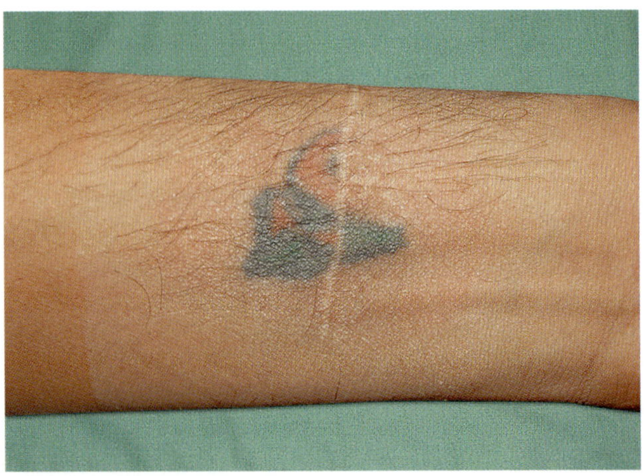

Fig. 2: Partial surgical excision of tattoo with ineffective removal and linear scar.

photoacoustic effect producing shock waves that cause explosion of target.[6] Very high energy, to the tune of 300 MW, is delivered in a very short period of time [5–100 ns (nanoseconds)] which leads to rapid thermal expansion. This produces shock waves that rupture the targets such as melanosomes and ink particles.[7] The ruptured fragments are cleared by tissue macrophages either to the lymphatic channels or to the regional lymph nodes. Some fragments may be eliminated transepidermally. To be selective, the pulse duration of the laser should match the thermal relaxation time (TRT) of the target. The estimated TRT of epidermis is 1–10 ms and the TRT of tattoo ink particles is 0.1–10 ns, although some newer estimates are in the range of 10–100 ps (picoseconds). The size of the tattoo ink particles is about 10–100 nm and is generally placed at a depth of 1.1–2.9 mm **(Figs. 3 and 4)**. Laser tissue interaction produces intracellular steam and vacuole formation, which leads to immediate whitening. An audible popping sound is heard during the procedure due to the photoacoustic effect.[3]

- Size of pigment particles 10–100 nm
- Depth 1.1–2.9 mm from granular layer

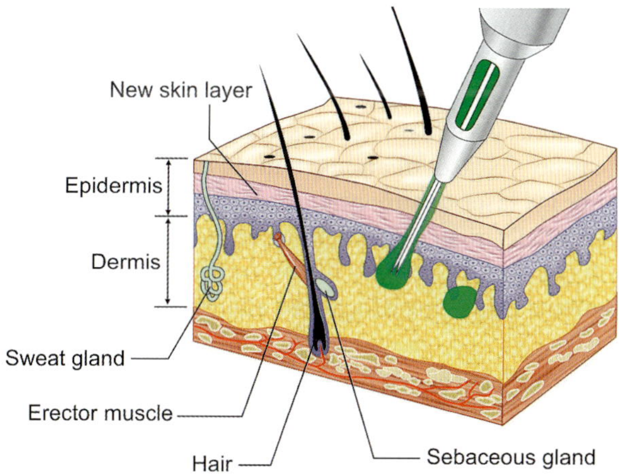

Fig. 3: Depth of placement of tattoo with a tattoo gun.

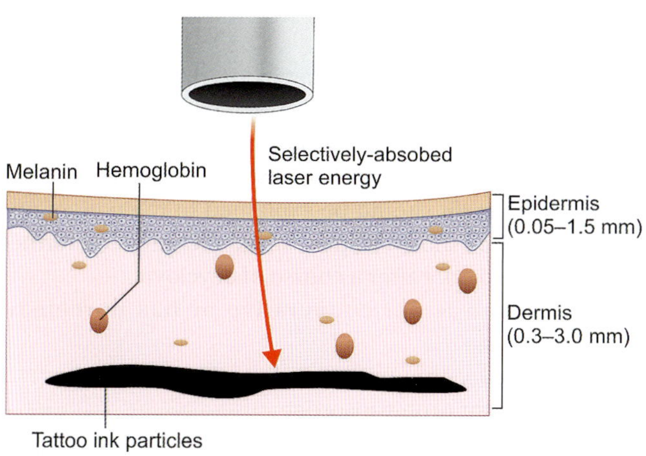

Fig. 4: Selective absorption of laser pulse by tattoo ink in the dermis.

- TRT of particles 0.1–10 ns
- New estimates 10–100 ps.

Basic Principles of Q-Switched Lasing

Tattoos consist of thousands of large particles of pigment suspended in the skin.

Q-switched laser delivers energy in an ultrashort duration, typically in nanosecond range with very high peak power. This energy is then selectively absorbed by tattoo ink because of its preferential wavelength and thermal relaxation time.

The surface temperature of the ink particles can rise to thousands of degrees but this energy profile rapidly collapses into a shock wave.[8] This shock wave then propagates throughout the local tissue (the dermis) causing brittle structures (tattoo pigment) to fragment and leads to vibrational damage to cellular structures and rupture of cell membranes.[8]

The rapid heating of melanosomes converts cytoplasmic water into steam, which results in intracytoplasmic vacuole formation. Due to this, there is sudden change in light scarring properties of skin, which is evident clinically as whitening or frosting. Frosting prevents further penetration of laser into the skin.[9]

The current trends and techniques in laser tattoo removal have attempted to reduce the total number of sessions needed, to shorten the total duration of time required to achieve clearing of tattoos, and also to minimize adverse effects. The choice of laser depends on the skin type, tattoo ink, and type of the tattoo to be treated. The characteristics of the laser, i.e., spot size, pulse width, and fluence are key to successful treatments. Type of the ink used (organic or inorganic, heavy metals, etc.), amount of ink placed, and the depth of ink placement also affect the outcomes. Until now, multiple sessions spaced over a period of time have been the protocol for tattoo removal. The limitations included incomplete clearance, long total treatment duration, and ineffective removal of some colors. Other problems faced in laser tattoo removal include allergic reactions to certain ink, darkening of cosmetic tattoos, tattoo resistance, etc.

INDICATIONS AND TYPES OF TATTOOS (BOX 1)

Amateur Tattoos

They are made of carbon-based ink. They tend to be less dense than professional tattoos. These types of tattoos

BOX 1: Types of tattoos commonly found.[3]

- Amateur (decorative)
- Professional (decorative)
- Cosmetic
- Traumatic, gun powder, and firearm tattoos
- Medical

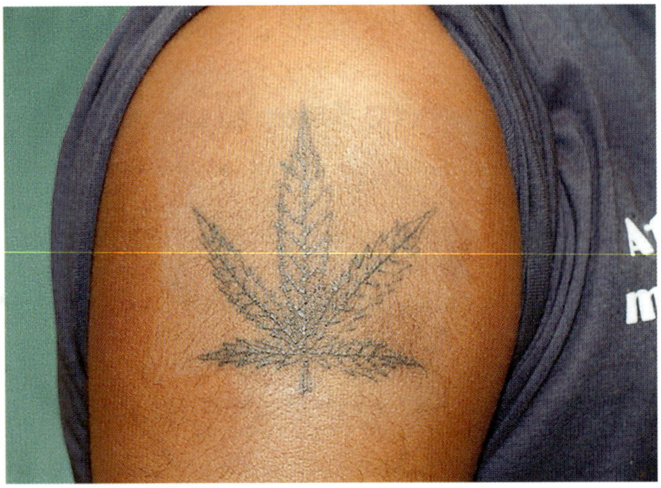

Fig. 5: Amateur tattoo on the right arm of a male.

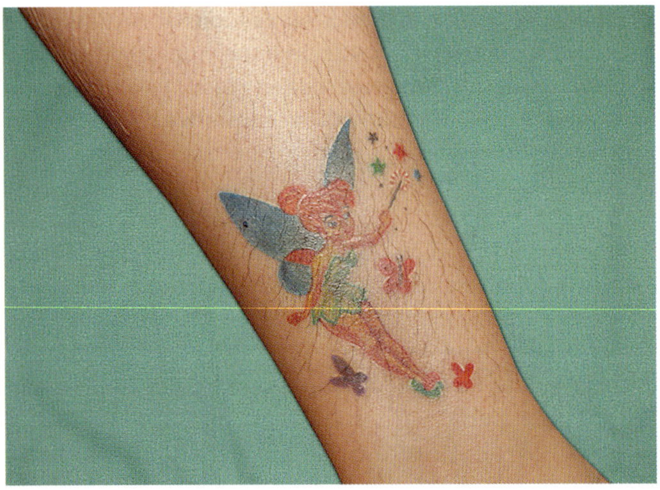

Fig. 6: A multicolored professional tattoo.

respond readily to Q-switched laser treatment. Wavelength of 1,064 nm is the preferred wavelength as it targets black ink in the dermis and also can penetrate deep. Generally, less number of sessions is needed for removal as compared to professional tattoos. **Figure 5** shows a typical black amateur tattoo.

Professional Tattoos

They are more complex and can be multicolored. Inks used include organic (azo dyes) or inorganic compounds (cadmium, mercury, cobalt, copper, cinnabar, ferric oxide, TiO, carbon ink, etc.).[3] Professional tattoos are more dense and intricate than amateur tattoos. These generally need multiple treatments and yet may not clear fully. **Figure 6** showcases a typical multicolored professional tattoo on the leg of a female.

The available wavelengths for tattoo removal are shown in **Box 2**.

BOX 2: Wavelengths used for tattoo removal.

- Q-switched Nd:YAG 1,064 nm—blue black tattoos
- Q-switched Nd:YAG 532 nm—red tattoo ink
- Q-switched 755 nm alex—purple and teal colors
- Q-switched ruby 694 nm—green color
- Picosecond 755 nm alex—blue and green color tattoos
- Q-switched 660 nm—green
- Q-switched 585 nm—sky blue color

CONTRAINDICATIONS OF TATTOOS[10]

The contraindications for performing the lasers on a particular patient should be borne in mind by the clinician all the time. The contraindications can be relative or absolute are listed hereunder.

Absolute Contraindications

- Associated photoaggravated skin diseases and medical illness, for example, systemic lupus erythematosus (SLE).
- Treatment area with active cutaneous infections, for example, herpes labialis, *Staphylococcal* infections.
- Unstable vitiligo and psoriasis for risk of Koebnerization of treated area.
- Tattoo granuloma.
- Localized allergic reactions can occur with almost any color ink and result in urticaria and granulomatous reactions. If a patient exhibits a cutaneous reaction within a tattoo, QS laser treatment should be used with caution. After QS laser treatment, the ink particles are mobilized, potentially triggering an allergic response. Rarely systemic allergic reactions may occur, particularly common in patients exhibiting a localized allergic response.

Relative Contraindications

In the following situations, laser has to be used cautiously, and after proper counseling of the patient; use of laser in these situations depends on individual situation and on treating physician's judgment.

- Keloid and keloidal tendencies.
- Patient on isotretinoin.
- *History of herpes simplex/history of herpes for increased risk of reactivation:* This risk should be seriously considered prior to performing the procedure. If the treating physician decides to perform the procedure, the risk and benefit should be explained to the patient and the procedure should be performed after proper informed consent and only after a course of acyclovir.
- Patient who is not cooperative or has unrealistic expectations.
  - Pregnancy or nursing
  - Body dysmorphic disorder
  - Photosensitizing medication such as tetracyclines, thiazides

- Gold therapy (used for the treatment of arthritis)
- Livedo reticularis (can be exacerbated with heat exposure by laser)
- Erythema ab igne
- Seizure disorder
- Melanoma or suspected melanoma in the treatment area.

BOX 3: Checklist before laser therapy.

- Right indication
- Counseling
- Rule out contraindication
- Test patch
- Sun protection and priming
- Pretreatment photograph
- Informed valid consent
- Eye protection

PATIENT SELECTION AND COUNSELING[11,12]

Patient selection needs utmost care on the part of the clinician. A general medical history, current medical conditions and medications, allergies, past surgeries, including bleeding tendencies, and wound healing (response of previous skin injuries whether they heal with hyperpigmentation or hypopigmentation, response to previous laser sessions if any taken) should be obtained.

Thorough counseling of the patient and an informed written consent complete the baseline step required for initiating therapy. Good pretreatment photographs are mandatory, as in any aesthetic procedure. Scarring often occurs during tattoo placement and may be unmasked and become more noticeable once the ink is removed. Serial photographs should therefore be taken at successive visits. Ideally the photographs should be taken with same or similar camera equipment and settings, distance, uniform light, and background.

PREOPERATIVE PREPARATION

Sun Protection

It is very important to ensure that the patient is not tanned. Epidermal melanin produced by ultraviolet (UV) light exposure may interfere with laser treatment and increase the risks for scarring, hypopigmentation or hyperpigmentation.[13-15] To check for tanning, it is wise to compare the color of the potential treatment site to that of an unexposed skin site, similar to the buttock or axilla. If a tan is present, treatment should be delayed until the tan has faded as much as possible in the treatment area. Use of broad-spectrum sun protection creams with UVA coverage is crucial. Protective clothing and bleaching creams can be useful in treating the tan. Patients with darker skin types and tanned patients are advised to apply hydroquinone-containing compounds (2–4%) or other lightening agents preoperatively to minimize the risk of PIH.

Oral Retinoids

It has been recommended that patients on oral retinoid therapy should not undergo laser treatment of pigmented lesions and tattoos for 6–12 months following discontinuation of the medication, as they have an increased risk of keloidal scar formation.[3] Proper evidence to support such a recommendation in Indian patients is lacking. However, caution is advised while treating all patients with history of recent administration of isotretinoin.

Test Patch

A test patch helps to determine the treatment parameters for an individual. It is also helpful in medicolegal situations. In particular, it is advisable for all beginning practitioners to perform laser test spots in all patients prior to treating an entire lesion, since skin type and color do not always perfectly predict the response to treatment. Even seasoned experts may need to perform small test spots, particularly where response to treatment cannot be judged properly. Always evaluate the patient 4–8 weeks after the test spots.[3,12,14]

Eye Protection

Q-switched laser light can cause permanent retinal damage and vision loss.[16] Precautions include protective clothing, goggles, masks, and laser cone containment devices which should be used with every patient. Eye protection in the form of optically coated glasses or goggles for the specific laser being used is necessary. All persons present in the room during laser treatment must also wear appropriate eye protection. The eye wear should block the wavelength being used and the lens should provide an optical density (OD) for at least four. Laser protective eye shields (anodized external metal eyecup) must be used when treating periorbital lesions. When treating eyelids, a metal corneal eye shield should be placed on the eye using topical anesthesia to protect the globe. **Box 3** shows the checklist before performing laser surgery.

Anesthesia

Q-switched laser treatment usually does not require anesthesia. However, if a large area needs to be treated, topical eutectic mixture of local anesthetic (EMLA) should be applied under occlusion 1–2 hours before the procedure.[17,18]

LASER PROCEDURE

Selecting the appropriate laser parameters is of paramount importance while executing the treatment.

Fluence

It is always preferable to begin with the lowest energy fluence that produces a visible response. Fluence may be increased if response is suboptimal. If epidermal debris are significant, the fluence should be lowered.[19]

Spot Size

For dermal lesions and tattoos, the spot size that elicits immediate brisk whitening on laser irradiation should be selected. Larger spot sizes allow deeper penetration and produce less tissue splatter.[20] The exact spot size selection will depend on the laser system being used, the type and size of the tattoo and the wavelength being used.

Endpoint of Treatment

Appropriate endpoints are essential to ensure optimum outcome. With the QS laser, the endpoint of treatment is immediate whitening of the lesion. Higher fluences may produce pinpoint bleeding and blistering.

Repetition rate: Choose higher frequency, i.e., 5–10 Hz while doing large area. For smaller discrete lesions a frequency of 2–3 Hz gives better control.

Figures 7 and 8 show an amateur tattoo before treatment. **Figures 9 and 10** show immediate whitening of the treated area.

LASER TECHNIQUE

After choosing the correct spot size and the energy fluence (J/cm^2), laser treatment is performed with the handpiece held perpendicular to the lesion and the entire area is covered with minimal overlap (up to 10%). QS laser treatment will produce an immediate whitening of the lesion. Pinpoint bleeding may occur if very high fluences are used. The entire lesion is covered in one pass. A popping sound is heard with each laser shot as the cells containing melanin or ink particles explode. Laser pulses are placed close to each other with minimum overlap. The area is cooled with ice packs/air cooling (e.g., Zimmer) just before and after laser pulses to avoid a build-up of heat and to prevent collateral tissue damage.

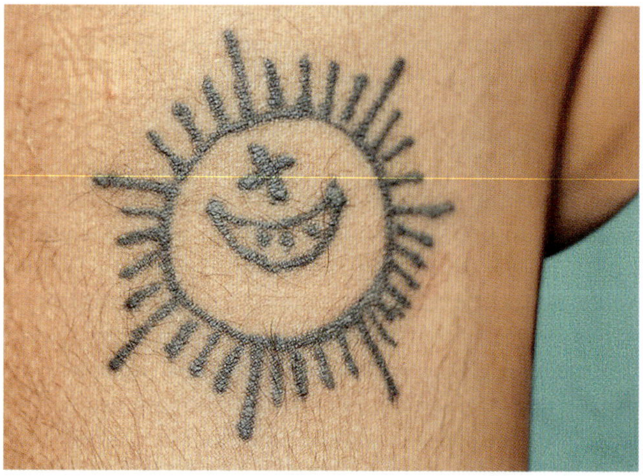

Fig. 7: Amateur tattoo before treatment.

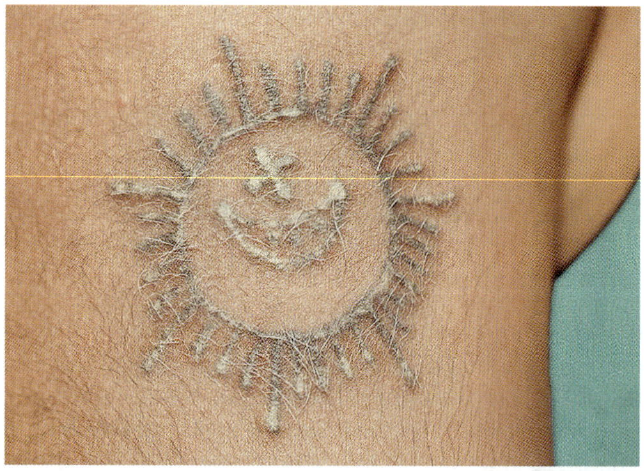

Fig. 9: Immediate post-treatment view showing whitening of the lesion.

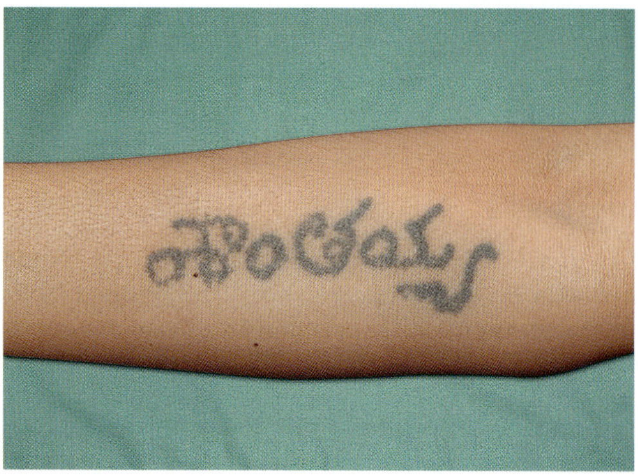

Fig. 8: Amateur tattoo on the forearm.

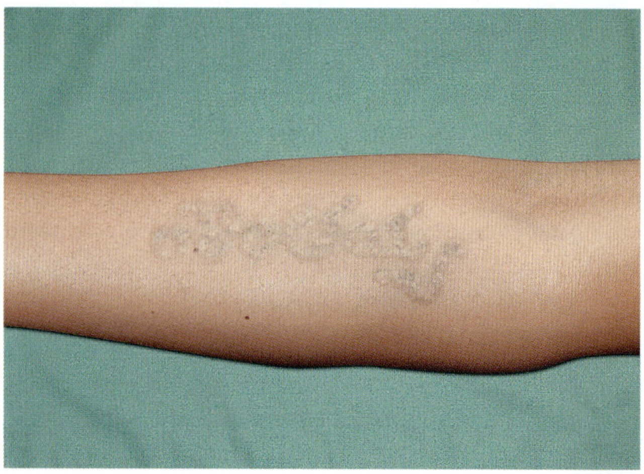

Fig. 10: Amateur tattoo on the forearm immediately after QSNY showing brisk whitening. (QSNY: QS Nd:YAG)

Number of Sessions

Tattoos may need 2–20 sessions for successful lightening. Professional tattoos require more treatment sessions for eradication. Amateur tattoos are less dense and are often made up of carbon-based ink that responds more readily to QS laser treatment. Traumatic tattoos are more superficial with minimal pigment and clear with one or two treatments. Gunpowder and firework tattoos need more care while treating as the implanted material has the potential to ignite and result in pox-like scars after treatment.

Table 1 highlights the factors affecting the number of treatments needed for tattoo removal.

Interval Between Sessions

Treatment should be done at least 6–8 weeks apart. Continued clearance of the lesion occurs due to removal of pigment by macrophages and lymphatics between treatments. Optimal interval between treatments therefore needs to be determined on an individual basis.[20]

Q-switched lasers are very effective for dark-blue, black, and green tattoos, whereas red and yellow tattoos are more difficult to treat as the absorption spectrum for these colors lies in the 500–600 nm spectrum (green light). The QSNY laser has a 532 nm wavelengths (WL) that can be used for red ink but use of high fluence is difficult in Indian patients due to the darker skin types. The QS 660 nm WL can also be used for yellow/red colors. The risk of dyschromias is high with these WLs. Pigments which contain iron oxide tend to darken on exposure to laser; hence a test patch is desirable. While amateur tattoos can be removed in fewer sessions, professional tattoos which are intricate and multicolored may need more sessions. Some professional tattoos may not clear completely, in spite of repeated treatments, and a ghost image of the design may be left behind.[14,21-27]

Figures 11 and 12 show an amateur tattoo on the arm of a young female before and after four 1,064 nm QS Nd:YAG (QSNY) laser sessions. **Figures 13 and 14** show amateur tattoos on the chin before and after 1,064 nm QS Nd:YAG laser treatment.

TABLE 1: Factors affecting number of treatments needed for tattoo removal.

Characteristics	*Less sessions*	*More sessions*
Tattoo type	Amateur, traumatic	Professional, cosmetic
Color	Black	Multicolored
Age	Old	New
Intensity	Faded	Dark
Layering	No	Yes
Skin type	Fairer	Darker
Scarring	No	Yes
Location	Proximal	Distal

Figures 15 to 18 show amateur tattoos before and after QSNY laser demonstrating the excellent response to therapy.

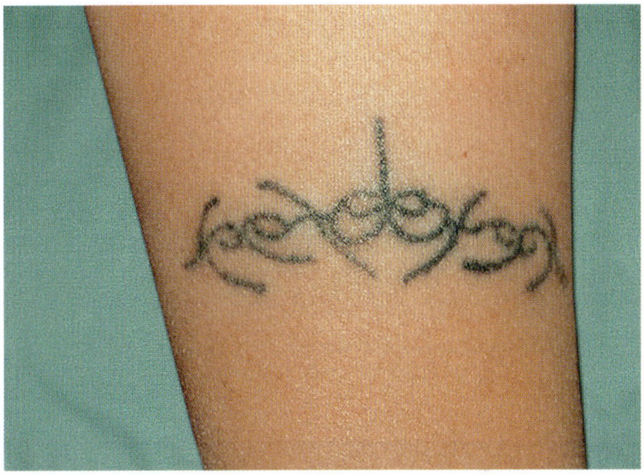

Fig. 11: Amateur tattoo on the arm.

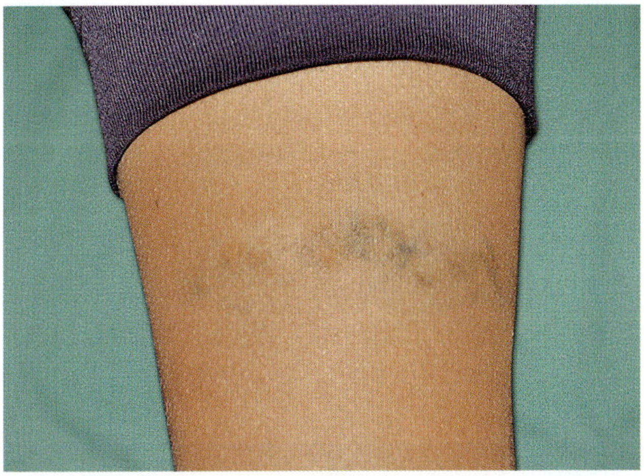

Fig. 12: Amateur tattoo on the arm after four 1,064 nm QS Nd:YAG laser sessions.

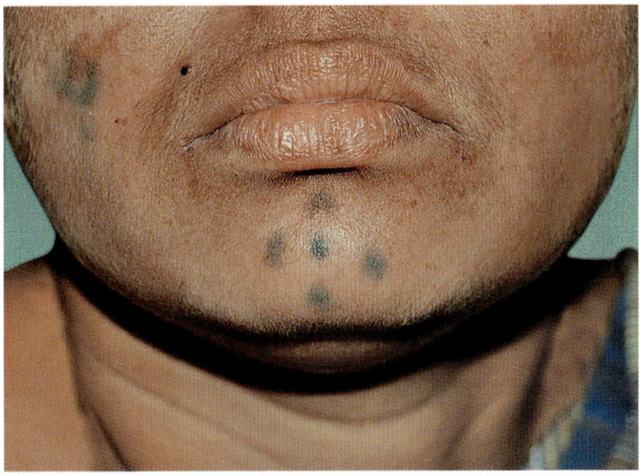

Fig. 13: Amateur tattoos on chin.

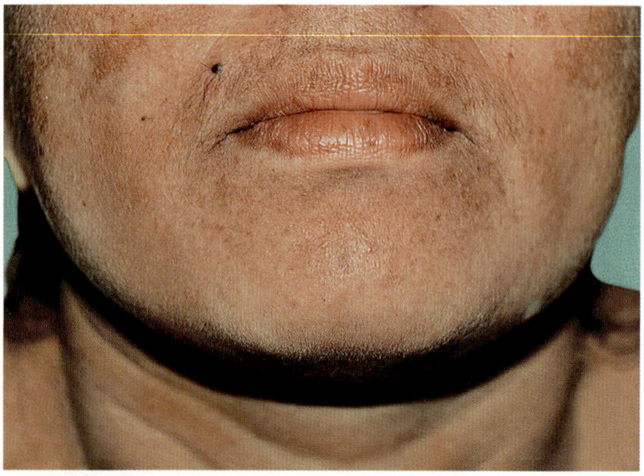

Fig. 14: Amateur tattoos on chin after a single 1,064 nm QS Nd:YAG laser treatment.

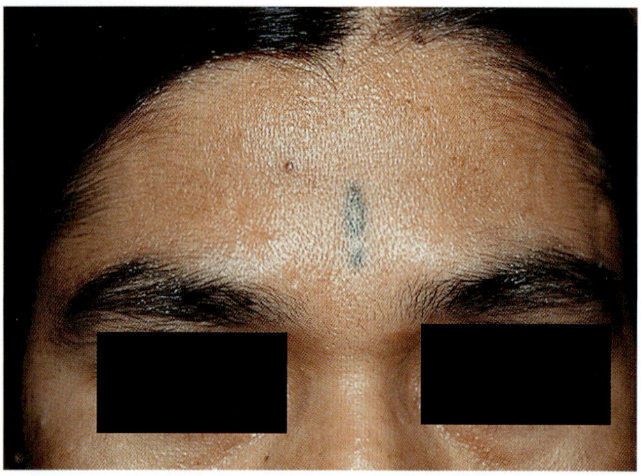

Fig. 15: Amateur tattoo on forehead.

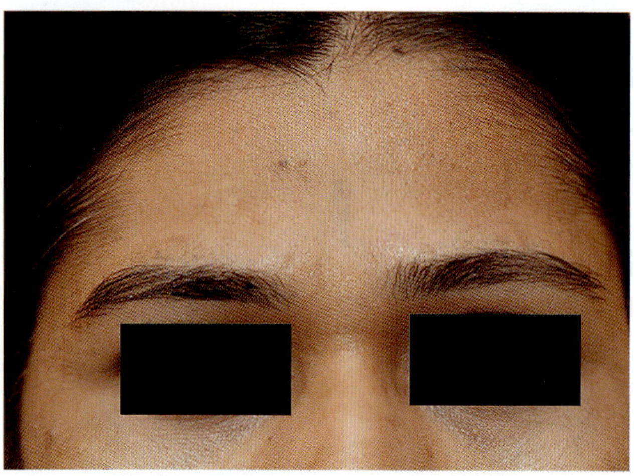

Fig. 16: Amateur tattoo after six QSNY sessions.

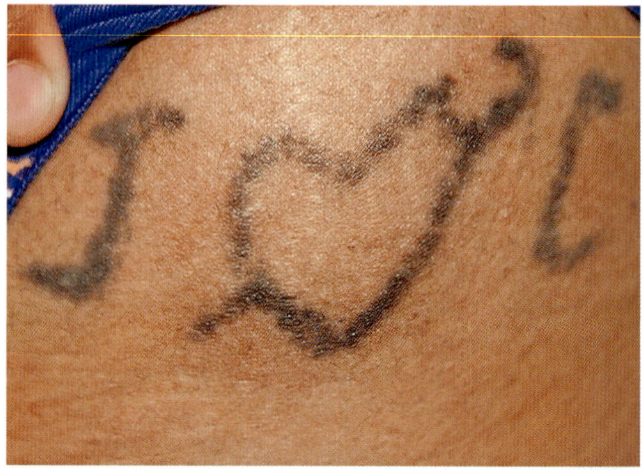

Fig. 17: A faded old amateur tattoo on the hip.

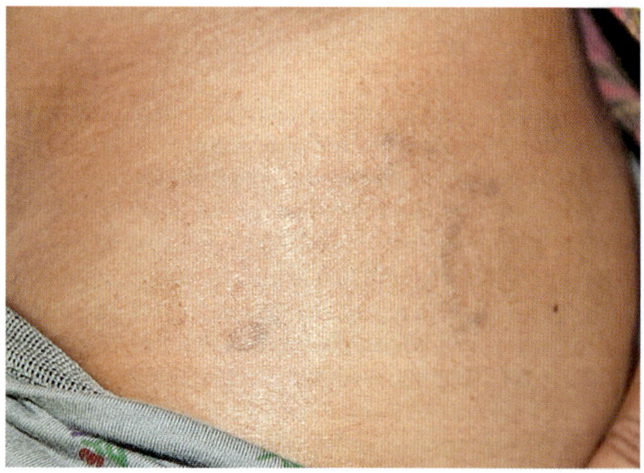

Fig. 18: Excellent response to QSNY laser after five sessions.

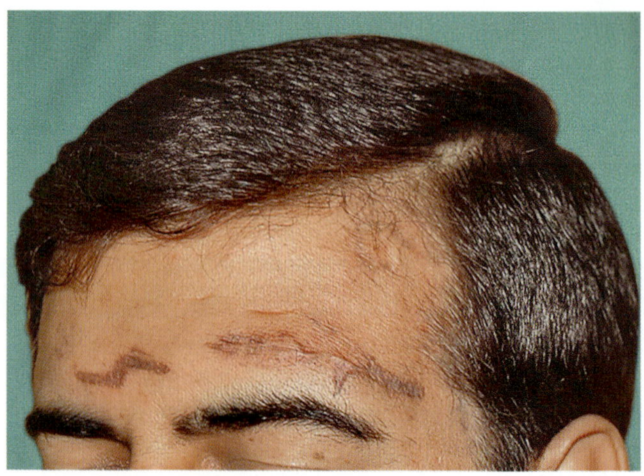

Fig. 19: Traumatic tattoo on the forehead after road traffic accident.

Traumatic tattoos: These tattoos occur after road traffic accidents where asphalt granules may be deposited in the skin. Usually, a small amount of pigment as deposited superficially in the skin and often clears with one or two treatments with 1,064 nm Q-switched Nd:YAG laser.[27,28]

Figure 19 shows a traumatic tattoo on the forehead.

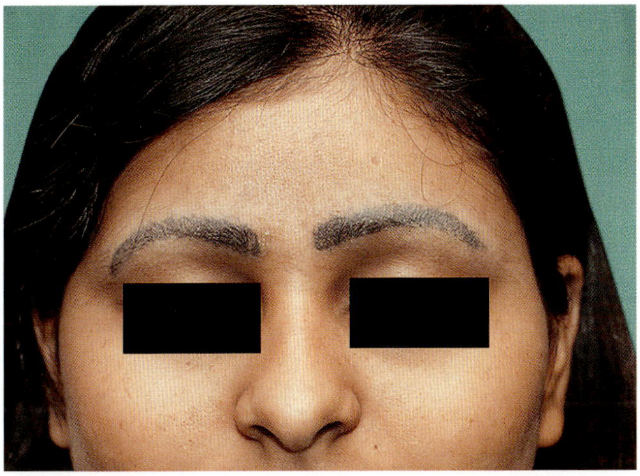

Fig. 20: Cosmetic tattoo permanent make up of eyebrows.

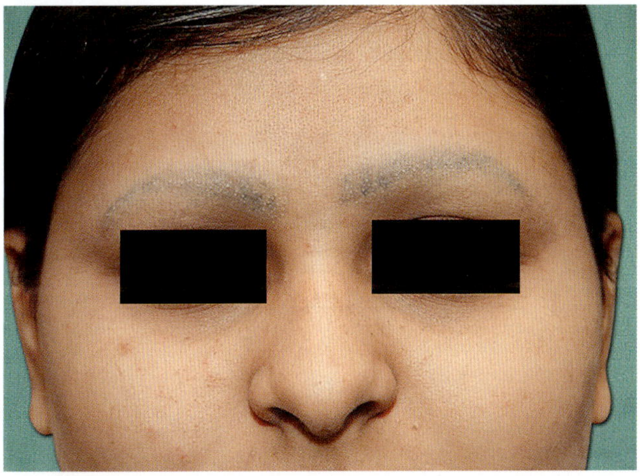

Fig. 21: After four sessions of QSNY laser treatment.

Cosmetic tattoos: These tattoos are usually red, white, or flesh colored. The pigment is placed to create areolae after breast reconstruction surgery or is in the form of lip liner tattoos. Pigment darkening may occur after laser therapy of these tattoos, hence, test patches are recommended. The patients should follow-up for 6–8 weeks after a test patch. If there is no darkening of the test patch and the tattoo lightens or fades, treatment can be undertaken for the rest of the tattoo. However, if the tattoo darkens, it is best to avoid further treatments.[29,30] **Figures 20 and 21** show a case of cosmetic tattoo (permanent eyebrows) before and after QSNY laser treatment.

Gunpowder and firework tattoos: Care should be taken while treating these types of tattoos, as the implanted material has the potential to ignite, and pox-like scars can develop. A test spot is mandatory in such cases and only after evaluating the patient after 6–8 weeks should further treatments be taken up.[31,32]

Figure 22 shows multiple hyperpigmented scattered spots of firework tattoos on the right side of face and eyelid in a male patient.

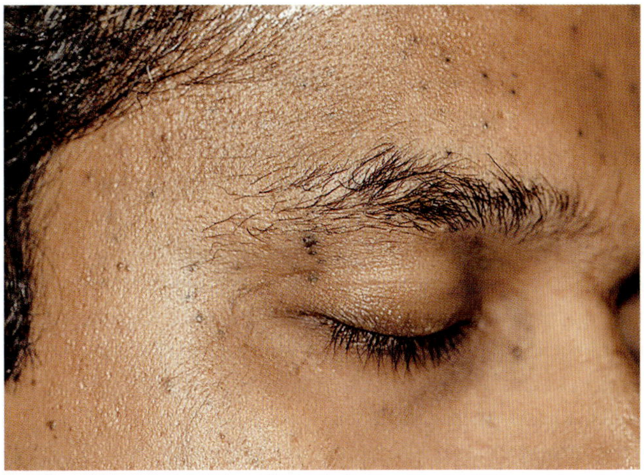

Fig. 22: Firework tattoos on the right side of face and eyelid after a fire cracker injury.

The Kirby-Desai scale: It has been proposed to be used to estimate the approximate number of sessions needed for a given tattoo based on the following factors:[33]

- Fitzpatrick skin type
- Location
- Color
- Amount of ink used
- Scarring and tissue damage
- Ink layering.

Each of these six factors is given numerical score and the total of these will give an estimate of the approximate number of sessions required for tattoo removal.

NEWER TECHNIQUES FOR LASER TATTOO REMOVAL

The limitations of conventional protocol of tattoo removal led to the development of newer techniques.[4] These limitations include a long total duration of treatment (interval of 6–8 weeks between treatments), ink retention despite multiple sessions (which could be due to wrong or ineffective wavelength choice for multicolored tattoos, poor technique, insufficient interval between sessions, etc.), ghosting (shadow or outline of the residual tattoo), and complications such as hyper- and hypopigmentation, blistering, and scarring. The newer protocols attempt to overcome these shortcomings by modifying the technique or combining multiple lasers to achieve optimal results and minimize adverse effects.

The newer techniques for laser tattoo removal are:

- R20 technique
- R0 technique
- Combining fractional lasers with Q-switched lasers.

R20 Method

Tattoo removal in a single laser session, based on method of repeated exposure.[34,35] Four treatment passes are done with an interval of 20 minutes between passes. Immediate whitening is seen on the first pass with little or no whitening on subsequent passes. Kossida et al. in a study found that treatment with the R20 method was much more effective than conventional single-pass laser treatment.[34]

After removing the EMLA cream and cleaning the area, first pass with the QSNY laser at 1,064 nm WL is made. There is immediate whitening of the treated area. This is due to the intracellular steam formation and gas bubble formation. Upon waiting for 20 minutes following the first pass, the gas bubbles are cleared due to absorption of the gases where by the next laser pass can be delivered. This allows further bombardment of the tattoo particles by the QSNY laser pulses. Energy is either constant as the first pass of lowered by 10–20%. A total of four such passes are made. The tattoo clears well after this over time. Based on the response another R20 session can be done after an interval of 6–8 weeks. The drawback of R20 is the long waiting time in the clinic for the patient and physician. The patient will need to be there for over 2 hours. This is a limitation of this technique.

R0 Method

Repeated exposure on same day without waiting period can be performed by applying perfluorodecalin (a perfluorocarbon compound, commercially available as "Zero-W") immediately after lasing **(Fig. 23)**.[36] This compound dissolves the gas bubbles formed upon initial laser exposure thus opening the optical window by reducing scatter. This allows an immediate next pass to be performed without the waiting time of 20 minutes as in the R20 technique.

This method significantly cuts down on the waiting time for the patient in the clinic unlike the R20 method. The only downside is the additional cost of the perfluorodecalin and its availability.

Results are similar to R20 and overall both these techniques score over the standard tattoo removal methods by reducing the length of time taken for fading of the tattoo.

Some examples of improvement with the R0 method can be seen in **Figures 24 to 29**.

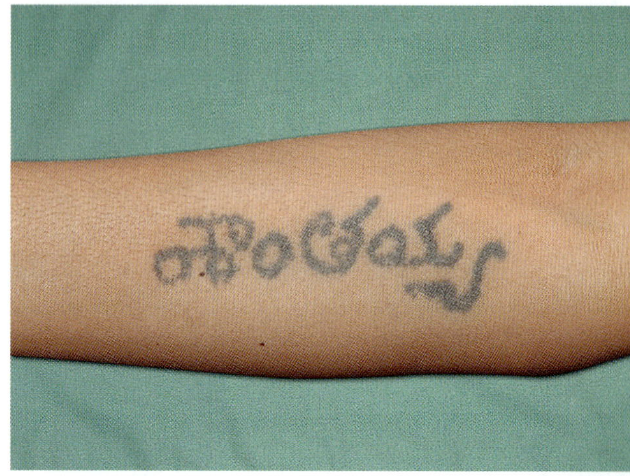

Fig. 24: Amateur tattoo on the forearm.

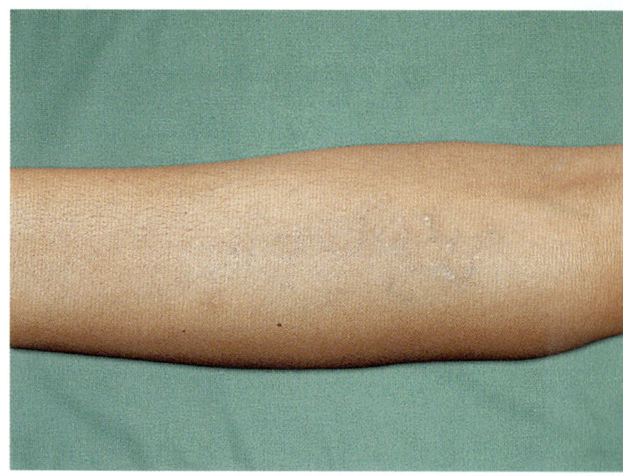

Fig. 25: Amateur tattoo after a single "R0" session with QSNY. (QSNY: QS Nd:YAG)

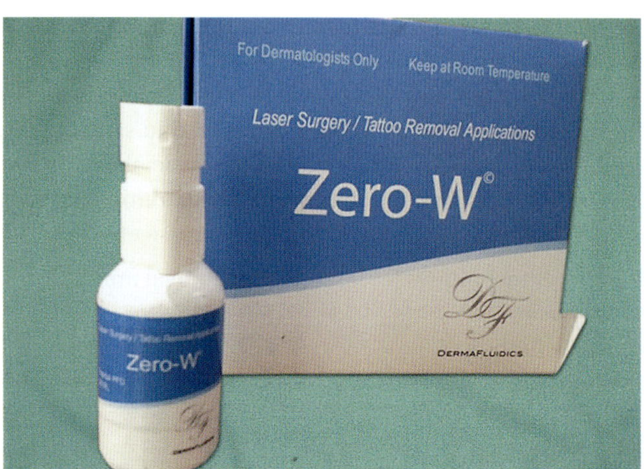

Fig. 23: Perfluorodecalin spray available commercially as Zero-W.

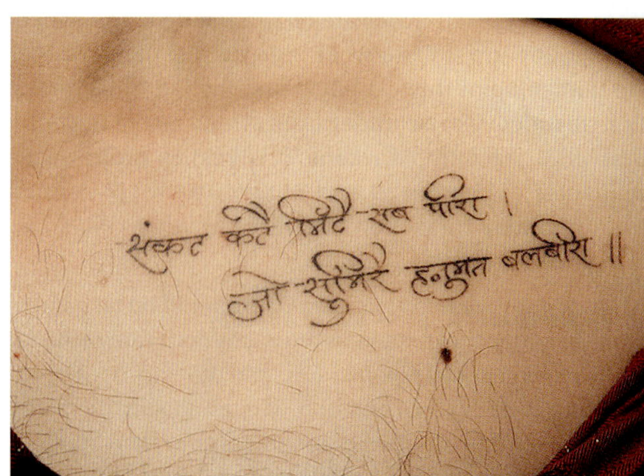

Fig. 26: A fresh tattoo on the chest with well-defined margins and dark color.

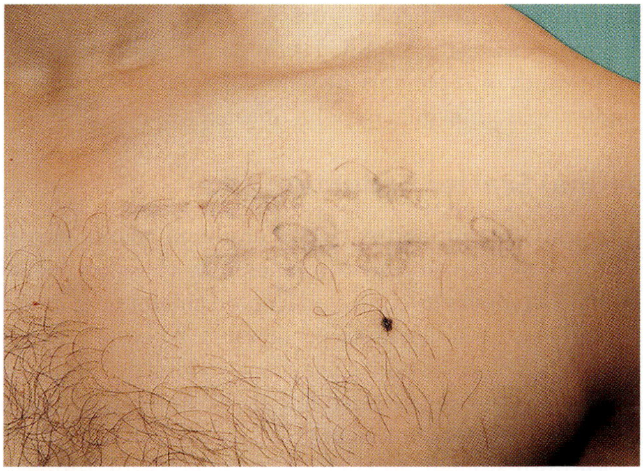

Fig. 27: After two "R0" sessions with QSNY. Excellent clearing of the pigment. (QSNY: QS Nd:YAG)

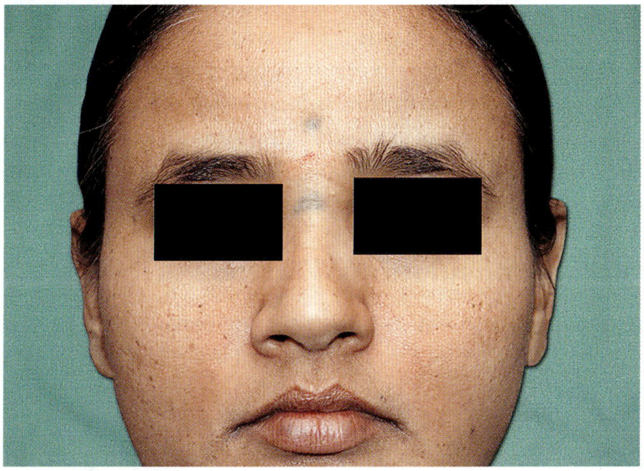

Fig. 28: Amateur tattoo on the nose and glabella.

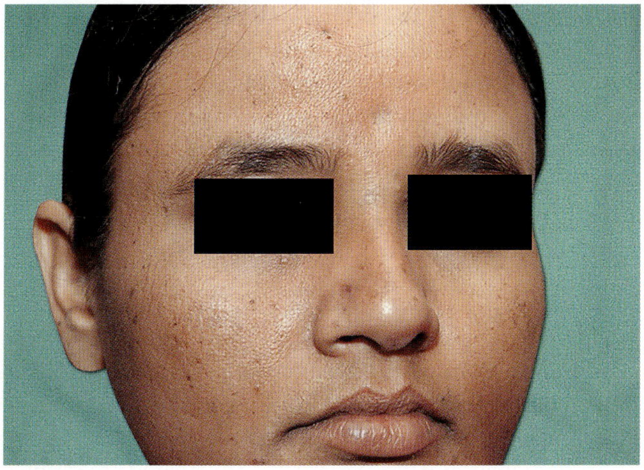

Fig. 29: After single "R0" session with three passes. Note the mild depressed scarring which was unmasked after tattoo removal.

Combining Lasers

Monotherapy with Q-switched laser (QSL) is often effective for tattoo removal but combining QSL with an ablative or nonablative laser may yield faster clearing, minimize number of sessions, and reduce side effects. Combination can be in any order.

Ablative fractional laser followed by QSL helps reduces blister formation. A study by Weiss and Geronemus found that after multiple sessions of QSL followed immediately by either nonablative fractional resurfacing (NAFR) or ablative fractional resurfacing (AFR) increases tattoo clearance, eliminates blistering, shortens recovery, and diminishes treatment-induced hypopigmentation. They noted the addition of AFR to QSL enhances the rate of pigment clearance. Addition of NAFR to QSL may decrease the degree of treatment-induced hypopigmentation.[37]

Marini et al. proposed a combination of fractional Er:YAG laser skin conditioning followed by Q-switched Nd:YAG laser for laser tattoo removal. In their two-step technique, they used a fractional Er:YAG laser to drill microholes into the skin which was followed by QSL treatment. According to the authors, this fractional Er:YAG laser conditioning protects the skin from damages at higher fluences by allowing the escape of gases through these microholes and thus relieving the internal pressure generated by QSL treatment. This also aided in repeating the next pass after 20 minutes. They concluded that this procedure led to a 30% reduction in the number of sessions.[38]

FACTORS AFFECTING TATTOO REMOVAL

Bencini et al. studied the variables influencing the outcomes in QSL tattoo removal. The authors assessed the prognostic factors affecting the outcomes in a large cohort of patients and found that smoking, the presence of colors other than black and red, a tattoo larger than 30 cm^2, a tattoo located on the feet or legs or older than 36 months, high color density, treatment intervals of 8 weeks or less, and development of a darkening phenomenon were associated with a reduced clinical response to treatment.[39]

Picosecond Lasers

Current QSL laser has pulse duration in nanosecond (10^{-9} of a second). If the pulse duration is narrowed further, the peak energy of the laser beam becomes very high. The picosecond lasers have a pulse duration of 10^{-12} of a second. This results in more rapid heating of the tattoos and finer fragmentation.[40] The lymphatic elimination of these finer particles is easier resulting in faster clearing of the tattoos. The picosecond lasers with pulse durations in the range of 450–750 ps were introduced commercially in the early part of 2013. At present, there are three or more systems with a wavelength of 755 nm and 1,064 nm and pulse duration of 450–750 ps.

Au et al. analyzed the incidence of bulla formation after tattoo treatment using the combination of the picoseconds alexandrite laser and a fractionated carbon dioxide (CO_2)

laser ablation.[41] In their study, 32% of patients treated with the picoseconds laser alone experienced blistering, whereas none of the patients treated with the combination developed blistering. The study showed a statistically significant decrease in bulla formation associated with tattoo treatment when fractionated CO_2 ablation was added to the picosecond alexandrite laser.[15]

Because of the shorter WL of the alexandrite and the thermal effects of the fractional CO_2 the risk for hyper- and hypopigmentation is high, caution needs to be exercised while treating dark skin.

Recent studies by Brauer et al. demonstrated the efficacy of 755 nm picosecond laser in treating blue and green tattoos.[42] They demonstrated 75% clearance in just one or two treatment. Saedi et al. also reported similar efficacy. However, they also reported complications such as hypo- and hyperpigmentation at 3 months follow-up in few of their patients.[43] Although effective and safe in white skin, their safety remains to be evaluated in pigmented skin. Furthermore, the cost of these machines is currently very high. Hence they are not yet widely available.

Combination of Imiquimod and Q-switched Laser

Imiquimod is a topical immune response modulator. Topical application of imiquimod alone is known to fade the tattoos to some extent when applied immediately after tattooing. Based on this finding, it was postulated that imiquimod interferes with tattoo pigment phagocytosis and prevents tattoo maturation. Application of laser recreates the biological scene similar to early tattoos. Wherein most of the tattoo pigmented lies freely in the tissue. Thus, it was postulated that combining imiquimod with a laser could increase the efficacy of both modalities.

Elsaie et al. evaluated imiquimod and Q-switched Nd:YAG laser (QSYL) in the treatment of tattoos and reported more favorable outcome in the tattoos treatment with combination than tattoos treated alone or with placebo.[44] However, Ricotti et al. studied 20 patients with daily application of imiquimod cream and 4–6 weekly application of QSYL for five sessions and reported imiquimod as ineffective combination. Furthermore they also reported more complications on imiquimod treated site.[45] Based on the limited studies, the use of imiquimod in combination with QSL remains controversial as of now.

Diascopy in Combination with Q-Switched Nd:YAG Laser

Murphy reported a simple and novel technique to reduce the pain and decrease epidermal damage during laser tattoo removal.[46] The technique consists of application of a glass microscope slide firmly on the treatment area. This applied pressure results in evacuating the blood from capillary plexus. The laser pulse is then applied through the glass slide.

In a study of 31 patients, he reported significantly less pain and less epidermal damage with this technique.

Dermal Scatter Reduction

Light scattering properties of skin and hemoglobin prevent effective penetration of the laser into the skin, which ultimately reduces its clinical efficacy in clearance of deeper tattoos. This becomes more problematic when one tries to remove the colored tattoos since shorter wavelengths (532 nm and 755 nm) are used to treat them. These shorter wavelengths have limited penetration depth.

An optical clearing agent such as glycerol, dimethyl sulfoxide, and glucose is applied to the skin before laser irradiation; because of its high refractive index, hyperosmosis, and biocompatibility into skin, these agents reduce skin scattering of laser beam. This not only allows deeper penetration but also delivery of higher effective energies.

Fox and Diven did the first human study using this concept. They applied glycerol after removing stratum corneum using the low-pressure transdermal delivery device and reported increased efficiency of laser tattoo removal.[47]

Microencapsulation of Tattoo Ink

In recent years, scientists have designed permanent but easily removable ink using a combination of organic and inorganic inks (e.g., β-carotene and iron oxide). This pigment is then stabilized by a transparent microencapsulation technique using polymethylmethacrylate beads.[8] The pigment in this microsphere can easily targeted using a pigment-specific wavelength. This will result in breakage of microspheres and exposing the ink to the body's defense mechanism. In an unpublished data Klitzman et al. demonstrated 80% clearance of tattoo in a single session using microencapsulated tattoo ink in guinea pig and hairless rats.[14] Although promising modality for faster tattoo removal, there are no published data in humans and its safety and efficacy needs further evaluation. Recently one such brand is available in United States as the Infinitink® (Freedom Ink, USA).[48]

POSTOPERATIVE INSTRUCTIONS[20]

- Broad-spectrum sunscreens with good ultraviolet A/ ultraviolet B (UVA/UVB) coverage are recommended before and throughout the treatment period.
- Immediately after laser treatment, the treated area appears abraded, and inflamed. Apply ice packs till burning sensation subsides, then apply a layer of antibiotic such as mupirocin and cover with gauze. Patient is instructed to clean the area with copious amount of water and apply the ointment twice daily till lesions heal. Healing can take around 5–10 days.

- Oral antibiotics may be used, if considered essential, but are not mandatory. Anti-inflammatory agents may be needed while treating large lesions. Patient should be instructed to avoid sun exposure and cosmetics on the treated area. Treatments are scheduled at an interval of 6–8 weeks.
- Patients are instructed to apply an antibiotic ointment or petrolatum ointment for about a week after procedure. Strict sun protection is advised for darker patients. Ice packs may be used after the procedure to minimize discomfort.
- Postprocedure bleaching agents may be used but only after the crust subsides.

COMPLICATIONS AND THEIR MANAGEMENT[20]

Complications may be encountered, especially in darker skin types. These may be minor and transient or major and persistent. The risk of complications increases with more aggressive treatments, poor priming, multiple treatments, choosing inappropriate laser systems, and in unrealistic patients. Some of the complications which demand considerations are:

- Postinflammatory hyperpigmentation resolves with time; some patients may need bleaching agents such as hydroquinone along with sunscreens.
- Postinflammatory hypopigmentation may persist for several weeks to months and may be difficult to treat. Phototherapy may be used to treat the hypopigmentation. Topical immunomodulators such as pimecrolimus and tacrolimus may be tried in these cases. Targeted phototherapy with 308–311 nm UVB excimer light can also be tried, once weekly till improvement is noted. An average of 15–20 sessions is needed to see a good response. If no improvement is seen in 15 odd sessions then it can be considered as treatment failure.
- Textural changes and scarring.
- Darkening of tattoo pigment, especially flesh colored cosmetic tattoos. Red tattoos can turn black, if it occurs, it is difficult to treat.
- Thermal injury and burns.
- As already discussed, localized allergic reactions can occur in tattoos, with almost any color ink and can result in urticaria and granulomatous reactions. Mercury-containing red ink is the commonest cause for allergic tattoo reactions. Other reactions reported include lichenoid and photoallergic reactions. Cadmium in the yellow ink is known to cause photoallergic reactions. After QS laser treatment, the ink particles may get further mobilized, and trigger a severe allergic response. Systemic allergic reactions may also occur in such patients. Hence, if a patient exhibits a cutaneous reaction within a tattoo, the reaction should be treated with steroid creams and only then should one attempt QS laser treatment with caution. A test patch is always recommended. Patients with persistent allergic reactions in tattoos may be treated with CO_2 or Er:YAG laser ablation.

  Anaphylaxis: Anaphylactic reactions are extremely rare but should be kept in mind.
- Scarring may occur if very high fluence is used. A high fluence may result in burns which, if secondarily infected, may lead to scar formation.
- Acute compartment syndrome of the upper extremity has been reported following QS 1,064 nm Nd:YAG laser treatment of a decorative tattoo.
- Infection, though uncommon, may occur. An antibiotic ointment and a nonadherent dressing should be applied upon completion of treatment. Patients should be instructed regarding the proper local wound care.

Figures 30 to 33 show some complications after QSNY laser treatment.

Table 2 shows some currently available QS and PS lasers and their specifications.

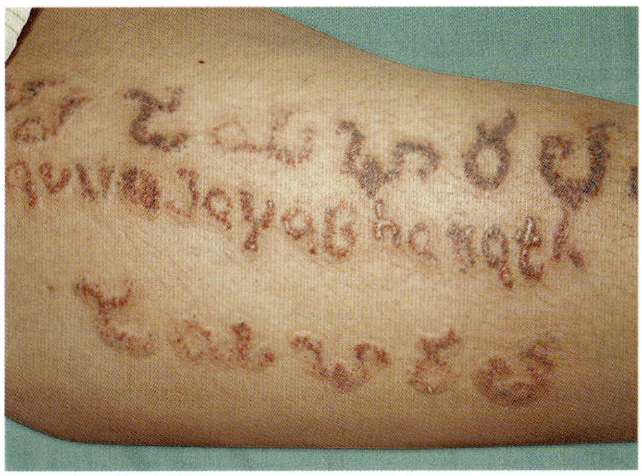

Fig. 30: Purpura and petechiae after QSNY laser treatment. (QSNY: QS Nd:YAG)

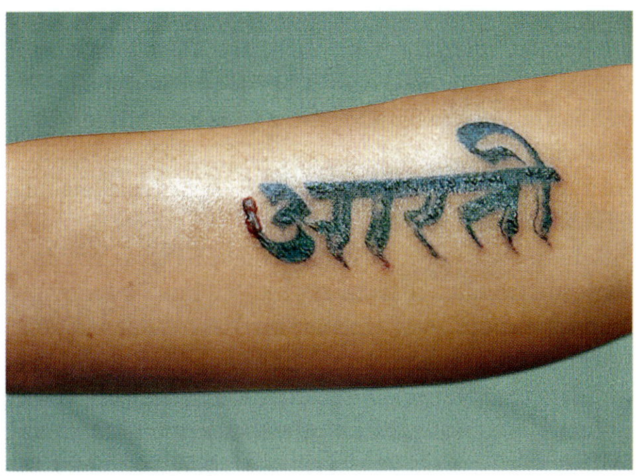

Fig. 31: Blistering following QSNY laser.

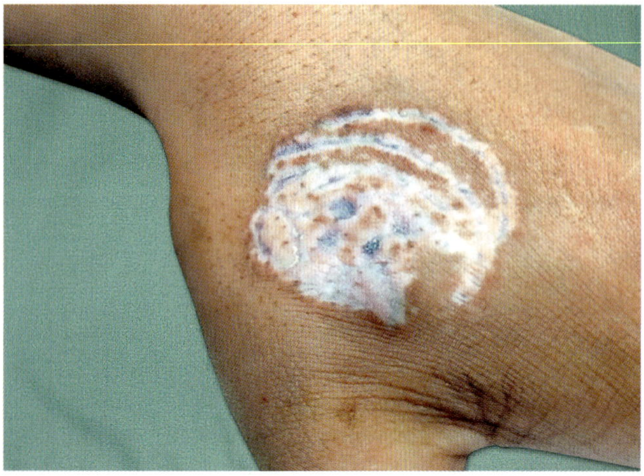

Fig. 32: Hypopigmentation following QSNY laser. (QSNY: QS Nd:YAG)

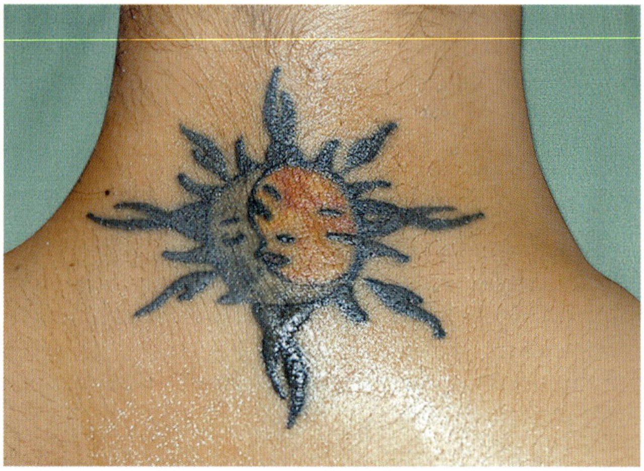

Fig. 33: Allergic reaction to tattoo ink.

TABLE 2: Some available Q-switched lasers and picosecond lasers and their specification.

Laser	*Manufacturer*	*Spot size*	*Fluence*	*Repetition rate*	*Additional features*
Spectra XT-Q-switched Nd:YAG laser	Lutronic	Up to 10 mm variable	2 J @ 1,064 nm	Up to 10 Hz	Extended platform with 4 wavelengths 1,064 nm, 532 nm, 660 nm, and 585 nm
Tribeam	Jeisys	2–10 mm	1–6 J @ 1,064	Up to 20 Hz	• 5–10 ns pulse duration • Dye HP • Zoom HP • Collimated HP • Fractional HP
Helios	Laseroptek	1–7 mm zoom, 8 mm collimated, 4 × 4 and 5 × 5 fractional	• 1.3 J @ 1,064 nm • 0.5 J @ 532 nm	Up to 10 Hz	10 ns pulse duration
Alma-Q	Alma	1–8 mm	• 1,064–1,200 mJ • 532–450 mJ	10 Hz	Triple mode Q-switched, Quasi long pulse and long pulse mode Nd:YAG laser
RevLite and MedLite	Hoya CONBIO-Cynosure	1.2–8.5	Up to 12 J/cm^2	10 Hz	Pulse duration 5–20 ns 1,064, 532, 585, 650 nm wavelengths
Discovery Pico	Quanta	2 × 2; 3 × 3; 4 × 4; 5 × 5; 9 × 9 mm^2; ø 3; 4.5; 6; 7.5; 9; 10.5 mm round; 8 mm fractional round	• Pico 800 mJ @ 1,064 nm • Pico 300 mJ @ 532 nm	Up to 10 Hz	• Q-switched mode pulse duration 6 ns • Photothermal mode 300 microsecond 2 J
PicoPlus	Lutronic	1–10 mm, focused dots hand piece	Up to 2 Joules	Up to 10 Hz	• Pico and nano second range Pico toning • 4 wavelengths 532, 1,064, • 660, 585 nm
PicoSure	Cynosure	2–6 mm zoom HP, fixed HP 6, 8 and 10 mm	Up to 200 mJ	10 Hz	755 nm Alex pico 750 PS pulse duration
PicoWay	Syneron-Candela	2–10 mm	• 400 mJ @ 1,064 nm • 200 mJ @ 532 nm	Up to 10 Hz	375–450 ps pulse duration

TIPS

Tips to avoid complications:
- Avoid tanned patients
- Use of sunscreens every 3 hours if tattoo is on an exposed part
- Avoid excessive overlapping while performing laser
- Avoid pulse stacking
- Use lower repetition rate of say 2–5 Hz (for beginners)
- Use larger spot and lower fluences for dark skin

Tips for approach to laser treatment of tattoos:
- Avoid treating a tanned patient
- Choose appropriate QS laser and do a test area0
- *Red tattoo:* Use 532 nm QS Nd:YAG
- *Dark blue and black tattoo:* Use 1,064 nm QS Nd:YAG
- *Green tattoo:* Use 694 nm QS Ruby, PS Alex or PS Nd:YAG
- Evaluate test spots after 4–8 weeks
- If the test patch lesion clears well, treat the remaining area
- If any worsening or scarring occurs, stop further treatments

CONCLUSION

Tattoo removal with lasers has witnessed a paradigm shift of late. Conventional individual laser sessions are being replaced by multipass techniques delivering the equivalent of 2–3 laser sessions that were spaced over weeks and months. Techniques such as R20 and R0 have proved to be effective yet safe even in darker skin types. Combination protocols such as fractional lasers with Q-switched Nd:YAG lasers and picosecond lasers have shown promise aiding faster clearing and improving the safety profile for patients. The availability of laser responsive inks and picosecond lasers has opened new directions where in some day laser tattoo removal could be possible in a single session!

REFERENCES

1. Buckland AW. On Tattooing, JRAI. 1887;12:318-28.
2. Aurangabadkar SJ. Shifting paradigm in laser tattoo removal. J Cutan Aesthet Surg. 2015;8:3-4.
3. Goldberg DJ. Pigmented lesions, tattoos, and disorders of hypopigmentation. In: Goldberg DJ (Ed). Laser Dermatology Pearls and Problems. 1st edition. Massachusetts: Blackwell Publishing; 2008. pp. 71-114.
4. Shah SD, Aurangabadkar SJ. Newer trends in laser tattoo removal. J Cutan Aesthet Surg. 2015;8:25-9.
5. McClung FJ, Hellwarth RW. Giant optical pulsations from ruby. J Appl Phys. 1962;33:828.
6. Anderson RR, Parrish JA. Selective photothermolysis: precise microsurgery by selective absorption of pulsed radiation. Science. 1983;220:524-7.
7. Polla LL, Margolis RJ, Dover JS, Whitaker D, Murphy GF, Jacques SL, et al. Melanosomes are a primary target of Q-switches ruby laser irradiation in guinea pig skin. J Invest Dermatol. 1987;89(3):281-6.
8. Ho DD, London R, Zimmerman GB, Young DA. Laser-tattoo removal—a study of the mechanism and the optimal treatment strategy via computer simulations. Lasers Surg Med. 2002;30:389-97.
9. Kuperman-Beade M, Levine VJ, Ashinoff R. Laser removal of tattoos. Am J Clin Dermatol. 2001;2:21-5.
10. Kilmer SL. Laser eradication of pigmented lesions and tattoos. Dermatol Clin. 2002;20:37-53.
11. Kilmer SL, Garden JM. Laser treatment of pigmented lesions and tattoos. Semin Cutan Med Surg. 2000;19:232-44.
12. Schmults CD, Wheeland RG. Pigmented lesions and tattoos. In: Goldberg DJ, Dover JS, Alam M (Eds). Procedures in Cosmetic Dermatology: Laser and Lights, 1st edition. Philadelphia: Elsevier; 2005. pp. 41-66.
13. Kilmer SL. Laser treatment of tattoos. Dermatol Clin. 1997; 15:409-17.
14. Grevelink JM, Duke D, van Leeuwen RL, Gonzalez E, DeCoste SD, Anderson RR. Laser treatment of tattoos in darkly pigmented patients: efficacy and side effects. J Am Acad Dermatol. 1996;34(4):653-6.
15. Adrian RM, Griffin L. Laser tattoo removal. Clin Plast Surg. 2000;27:181-92.
16. Barlow RJ, Hruza GJ. Lasers and light tissue interactions. In: Goldberg DJ, Dover JS, Alam M (Eds). Procedures in Cosmetic Dermatology: Laser and Lights, 1st edition. Philadelphia: Elsevier; 2005. pp. 1-11.
17. Koay J, Orengo I. Application of local anesthetics in dermatologic surgery. Dermatol Surg. 2002;28:143-8.
18. Drake LA, Dinehart SM, Goltz RW, Graham GF, Hordinsky MK, Lewis CW, et al. Guidelines of care for local and regional anesthesia in cutaneous surgery. Guidelines/Outcomes Committee: American Academy of Dermatology. J Am Acad Dermatol. 1995;33(3):504-9.
19. Kilmer SL, Lee MS, Grevelink JM, Flotte TJ, Anderson RR. The Q-switched Nd:YAG laser (1,064 nm) effectively treats tattoos. A controlled, dose-response study. Arch Dermatol. 1993;129(8): 971-8.
20. Aurangabadkar S, Mysore V. Standard guidelines of care: lasers for tattoos and pigmented lesions. Indian J Dermatol Venereol Leprol. 2009;75:111-26.
21. Kilmer SL, Anderson RR. Clinical use of Q-switched ruby and Q-switched Nd:YAG (1,064 nm and 532 nm) lasers for treatment of tattoos. J Dermatol Surg Oncol. 1993;19:330-8.
22. Levine VJ, Geronemus RG. Tattoo removal with the Q-switched ruby laser and the Q-switched Nd:YAG laser: a comparative study. Cutis. 1995;55(55):291-6.
23. Leuenberger ML, Mulas MW, Hata TR, Goldman MP, Fitzpatrick RE, Grevelink JM. Comparison of the Q-switched alexandrite, Nd:YAG, and ruby lasers in treating blue-black tattoos. Dermatol Surg. 1999;25(1):10-4.
24. Kilmer SL, Lee MS, Anderson RR. Treatment of multi-coloured tattoos with the Q-switched Nd:YAG laser (532 nm): a dose response study with comparison to the Q-switched ruby laser. Lasers Surg Med Suppl. 1993;5:54.
25. Haedersdal M, Bech-Thomsen N, Wulf HC. Skin reflectance-guided laser selections for treatment of decorative tattoos. Arch Dermatol. 1996;132:403-7.
26. Alster TS. Q-switched alexandrite laser treatment (755 nm) of professional and amateur tattoos. J Am Acad Dermatol. 1995;33:69-73.
27. Moreno-Arias GA, Casals-Andreu M, Camps-Fresneda A. Use of Q-switched alexandrite laser (755 nm, 100 ns) for removal of traumatic tattoo of different origins. Laser Surg Med. 1999;25:445-50.
28. Ashinoff R, Geronemus RG. Rapid response of traumatic and medical tattoos to treatment with the QS Ruby laser. Plast Reconstr Surg. 1993;91:841-5.
29. Anderson RR, Geronemus R, Kilmer SL, Farinelli W, Fitzpatrick RE. Cosmetic tattoo ink darkening. A complication of Q-switched and pulsed-laser treatment. Arch Dermatol. 1993;129(8):1010-4.
30. Ross EV, Yashar S, Michaud N, Fitzpatrick R, Geronemus R, Tope WD, et al. Tattoo darkening and nonresponse after laser treatment: a possible role for titanium dioxide. Arch Dermatol. 2001;137(1):33-7.
31. Fusade T, Toubel G, Grognard C, Mazer JM. Treatment of gunpowder traumatic tattoo by Q-switched Nd:YAG laser: an unusual adverse effect. Dermatol Surg. 2000;26(11):1057-9.
32. Taylor CR. Laser ignition of traumatically embedded firework debris. Lasers Surg Med. 1998;22:157-8.
33. Kirby W, Desai A, Desai T, Kartono F, Geeta P. The Kirby-Desai scale: A proposed scale to assess tattoo-removal treatments. J Clin Aesthet Dermatol. 2009;2:32-7.
34. Kossida T, Rigopoulos D, Katsambas A, Anderson RR. Optimal tattoo removal in a single laser session based on the method of repeated exposures. J Am Acad Dermatol. 2012;66:271-7.
35. Bunert N, Homey B, Gerber PA. Successful treatment of a professional tattoo with the R20 method. Hautarzt 2014;65:853-5.

36. Reddy KK, Brauer JA, Anolik R, Bernstein L, Brightman L, Hale E, et al. Topical perfluorodecalin resolves immediate whitening reactions and allows rapid effective multiple pass treatment of tattoos. Lasers Surg Med. 2013;45:76-80.
37. Weiss ET, Geronemus RG. Combining fractional resurfacing with Q-S ruby laser for tattoos. Dermatol Surg. 2010;36:1-3.
38. Marini L, Kozarev J, Grad L, Jezersek M, Cencic B. Fractional Er:YAG skin conditioning for enhanced efficacy for Nd:YAG Q switched laser tattoo removal. J Laser Health Acad. 2012;1: 35-40.
39. Bencini PL, Cazzaniga S, Tourlaki A, Galimberti MG, Naldi L. Removal of tattoos by Q-switched laser: variables influencing outcome and sequelae in a large cohort of treated patients. Arch Dermatol. 2012;148(12):1364-9.
40. Ross V, Naseef G, Lin G, Kelly M, Michaud N, Flotte TJ, et al. Comparison of responses of tattoos to picosecond and nanosecond Q-switched neodymium: YAG lasers. Arch Dermatol. 1998;134(2):167-71.
41. Au S, Liolios AM, Goldman MP. Analysis of incidence of bulla formation after tattoo treatment using the combination of the picosecond Alexandrite laser and fractionated CO_2 ablation. Dermatol Surg. 2015;41(2):242-5.
42. Brauer JA, Reddy KK, Anolik R, Weiss ET, Karen JK, Hale EK, et al. Successful and rapid treatment of blue and green tattoo pigment with a novel picosecond laser. Arch Dermatol. 2012;148(7):820-3.
43. Saedi N, Metelitsa A, Petrell K, Arndt KA, Dover JS. Treatment of tattoos with a picosecond alexandrite laser: A prospective trial. Arch Dermatol. 2012;148:1360-3.
44. Elsaie ML, Nouri K, Vejjabhinanta V, Rivas MP, Villafradez-Diaz LM, Martins A, et al. Topical imiquimod in conjunction with Nd:YAG laser for tattoo removal. Lasers Med Sci. 2009;24:871-5.
45. Ricotti CA, Colaco SM, Shamma HN, Trevino J, Palmer G, Heaphy MR Jr. Laser-assisted tattoo removal with topical 5% imiquimod cream. Dermatol Surg. 2007;33:1082-91.
46. Murphy MJ. A novel, simple and efficacious technique for tattoo removal resulting in less pain using the Q-switched Nd:YAG laser. Lasers Med Sci. 2014;29:1445-7.
47. Fox MA, Diven DG, Sra K, Boretsky A, Poonawalla T, Readinger A, et al. Dermal scatter reduction in human skin: A method using controlled application of glycerol. Lasers Surg Med. 2009;41:251-5.
48. Luebberding S, Alexiades-Armenakas M. New tattoo approaches in dermatology. Dermatol Clin. 2014;32:91-6.

CHAPTER 111

Lasers for Vascular Lesions

Sujay Khandpur, Sindhuja T

KEY MESSAGES

- The different types of lasers used to treat vascular lesions include: pulse dye laser 585, 595 nm, long-pulsed neodymium-doped yttrium aluminum garnet laser 1064 nm, potassium titanyl phosphate laser 532 nm, argon laser, intense pulsed light, etc. The pulsed dye laser is the most common laser used.
- Port-wine stain is the lesion best treated with vascular lasers. Other vascular lesions responding to lasers include hemangiomas particularly residual lesions, telangiectasias, spider angiomas, pyogenic granulomas, erythematotelangiectatic rosacea, etc.
- The factors affecting treatment response include the caliber of the vessels, size and depth of the lesion, laser parameters used, skin phototype of the patient, site of involvement, age of the patient, etc.
- Adverse effects include purpura, edema, blisters, pigmentary and textural alterations.
- A combination therapy that enhances laser penetration, suppresses residual vessel proliferation and targets deeper vessels increases the efficacy of lasers.

INTRODUCTION

Cutaneous vascular lesions are complicated by pain, bleeding, ulceration, infection, obstruction to vital functions, and psychological stress, especially when present on the face. The introduction of lasers for vascular lesions by Dr Leon Goldman in 1963 has alleviated many of these sequelae and provided more reliable and cosmetically acceptable results than earlier employed treatment methods such as camouflage, radiation, electrotherapy, cryotherapy, excision, and grafting. Since the initial use of ruby, neodymium-doped:yttrium-aluminum-garnet (Nd:YAG), and argon lasers to treat port-wine stains (PWS) and hemangiomas, a variety of laser and light devices were introduced for the treatment of vascular lesions. Lasers can be performed in an outpatient setting, which is convenient and easily accessible to the patient.

PRINCIPLES OF LASER FOR VASCULAR LESIONS

Lasers for vascular lesions work on the principle of selective photothermolysis, a process by which blood vessels are selectively destroyed while causing minimal collateral damage to surrounding tissue. To achieve this, the pulse duration of laser must be shorter than the thermal relaxation time of the target vessel. The thermal relaxation time of vessels with a diameter of 10–50 µm is 0.048–1.2 ms. The target chromophore for treating vascular lesions is intravascular oxyhemoglobin and deoxyhemoglobin, which show absorption peaks in the blue (418 nm), green (542 nm), and yellow (577 nm) bands of light and in the near-infrared part of the spectrum (700–1100 nm).[1] Therefore, lasers with wavelengths between 488 and 600 nm are useful to achieve photomechanical and photothermal damage of the target tissue and treat vascular lesions. When hemoglobin is heated, it also heats up and destroys the endothelial cells of blood vessel walls, resulting in thrombosis of the blood vessels. The process of vascular remodeling with a reduction in the number and size of treated vessels starts after 1–2 weeks postlaser. A laser with the appropriate wavelength and exposure time should be selected to avoid tissue destruction and scarring resulting from excess thermal energy to adjacent tissues. The addition of a cooling device protects the epidermis and allows safe use of higher fluences, particularly on young children's skin.

LASERS COMMONLY USED TO TREAT VASCULAR LESIONS

Flashlamp-pumped Pulsed Dye Laser

Pulsed dye laser (PDL) was the first laser developed, based on the principle of selective photothermolysis. It was first used to treat PWS by Tan et al. in 1989 and is the most common laser used for various vascular lesions to date. PDL, powered by flashlamp, emits a pulsed beam of yellow light at 585–600 nm. A short pulse of this light, with a pulse duration ranging from 450 to 40,000 µs, energizes a fluorescent organic dye (rhodamine) dissolved in a liquid solvent (methanol) within a transparent cell. The machine's operating lifetime depends on the dye's chemical structure, solvent and additives used, as they are prone to decomposition. The PDL light is selectively absorbed by oxyhemoglobin (primary absorption peaks at 577 nm), transforms oxyhemoglobin into methemoglobin, and leads to thrombus formation.[2] It can penetrate up to a depth of 0.75–1.5 mm (papillary and superficial reticular dermis), with little or no damage to the surrounding tissue.[2,3]Optical absorption and scattering in the epidermis and dermis limit the depth of PDL penetration.

Pulsed dye laser has undergone multiple improvements since it was first introduced. Current models use a wavelength of 595 nm and larger spot sizes (up to 10 mm) with higher fluences, allowing the laser to penetrate deeper. The brief pulse duration of 300–500 µs with high peak energy can cause vascular rupture, producing immediate purpura. PDL with a longer pulse duration with lower peak energy applies thermal energy to the blood vessels more slowly, minimizing the photoacoustic effects on the vessel wall, hence reduces RBC leakage and thereby purpura, while maintaining clinical efficacy. Longer pulse durations (1.5–40 ms) facilitate the treatment of larger vessels. The new-generation PDL with six to eight evenly spaced micropulses in each macropulse allows delivery of greater total fluence to tissues in a single-pass treatment. An increase in pulse durations, with a larger number of subpulses, at higher fluences provide better selectivity between large and small vessels and result in a higher purpura threshold. The introduction of dynamic cooling, delivered to the epidermis just before the laser pulse, prevents epidermal damage and reduces pain. The safety profile of PDL is generally excellent in infants, children, and skin types I-III. When treating individuals of Fitzpatrick skin types IV-VI, lower energies, and shorter pulse widths are advised.[4] Increments of 0.5–1 J/cm^2 can be made in subsequent sessions based on the treatment response.

Long-pulsed Neodymium:Yttrium-Aluminum-Garnet Laser

The Nd:YAG laser with a wavelength of 1064 nm penetrates up to a depth of 5–6 mm and is absorbed by methemoglobin and thrombi.[2] Upon compressing the skin while performing the laser, depth can be increased further (1–2 cm).[2] Its wavelength corresponds to one of hemoglobin's smaller absorption peaks in the near-infrared range. Nd:YAG, with its longer wavelength, effectively targets deeper tissue but requires higher energy settings to resolve vascular lesions. The absorption coefficient of blood at 1064 nm is 0.4/mm, which is much higher than that of the surrounding dermis (0.05/mm) at the same wavelength. This difference in absorption coefficients provides treatment selectivity of deep blood vessels. Lower absolute values of blood absorption at 1,064 nm may be compensated by increasing the fluence. The Nd: YAG laser is also absorbed by melanin. Though the absolute absorption of melanin is lower at 1064 nm, epidermal damage such as blistering, crusting or necrosis may occur. Hence epidermal cooling is mandatory with this laser, and it is recommended to increase the energy by only 5 J/cm^2 in subsequent sessions. Pulse durations should be selected according to the estimated vessel size of each lesion, 0.3–5 ms for thin, 10–25 ms for medium, and 25–55 ms for thick vessels.

Multiplex 585/1064 nm Laser

The multiplex 585/1064 nm laser delivers sequential PDL and long pulsed Nd:YAG wavelengths. The rationale behind using this combination is that the 1064 nm targets the deeper blood vessels in the dermis where the 585 nm cannot reach. There is a synergistic effect of the combination on treatment as 585 nm converts hemoglobin into methemoglobin, which has an absorption coefficient close to 1064 nm. The multiplex laser effectively treats lesions with varying vessel sizes, density, color, flow and depth using lower fluences. Energy densities of 6.5 and 35 J/cm^2 with pulse durations of 0.5 and 15 ms for the 585 and 1,064 nm wavelengths, respectively, delivered on a spot size of 7 mm, have been used for the treatment of PWS.[5] For Indian skin, fluence ranging from 4 to 10 J/cm^2 for PDL and 20–50 J/cm^2 for Nd:YAG, with a spot size of 7–10 mm and inter-pulse delay of 1 second for sufficient cooling, have been used for PWS on head and neck. The pulse duration ranged between 0.5 and 40 ms for PDL and 15–40 ms for Nd:YAG. More than 70% improvement was seen after five sessions in 45.45% of patients aged >18 years.[6]

Argon Laser

It emits light with peaked wavelengths at 488 and 514 nm, which is well absorbed by hemoglobin. Due to its relatively shorter wavelength, blood vessels in approximately the upper millimeter of dermis are affected. Adverse effects described include pain during the procedure, epidermal crusting lasting about 2 weeks, dyspigmentation, and post-treatment scarring.[3] PDL and potassium titanyl phosphate (KTP) lasers have primarily replaced argon lasers as they have better side effect profile and longer wavelengths.

Potassium Titanyl Phosphate Laser

Potassium titanyl phosphate lasers use a 1,064-nm Nd:YAG source that is passed through a KTP crystal, resulting in a frequency-doubled 532 nm wavelength that corresponds with one of hemoglobin's absorption peaks. It emits green light with long pulse durations ranging from 1 to 100 ms, which gradually heat the blood vessels without causing vessel wall rupture. Hence, it causes less bruising and has a shorter recovery time compared to PDL. Greater absorption by epidermal melanin in darker skin because of its shorter wavelength limits its use in Fitzpatrick skin types III-VI. It also has limited penetration depth, thereby limiting its efficacy.

Intense Pulsed Light

Intense pulsed light (IPL) systems generate pulsed, polychromatic, noncoherent high-intensity light in a broad wavelength spectrum, ranging from 500 to 1400 nm using flashlamps and cut-off filters. Depending on the cut-off filter used, treatment of various superficial or deeper vascular lesions can be facilitated. Cut-off filters at 515, 550, 570, 590 nm are generally used for vascular lesions. It is not a laser but works on similar principles. Larger areas can be treated efficiently with less discomfort using larger spot sizes. Because of the rapid divergence of the IPL beam, the handpiece must be in contact (or almost in contact) with the skin for effective treatment. The larger spot sizes can lead to greater side effects and compromise maneuvering over concave areas. Treatment efficacy varies between the IPL systems, and all are not equally effective.

INDICATIONS FOR VASCULAR LASERS

The dermatological indications for vascular lasers include:

- *Congenital lesions:*
  - Port wine stain (PWS)
  - Hemangioma
- *Acquired lesions:*
  - Rosacea
  - Facial telangiectasia
  - Telangiectasias associated with other conditions
  - Unilateral nevoid telangiectasia
  - Poikiloderma of Civatte
  - Angiofibroma
  - Angiokeratoma
  - Blue Rubber Bleb Nevus syndrome
  - Campbell de Morgan angiomas
  - Cutaneous lesions of Kaposi sarcoma
  - Pyogenic granuloma
  - Morbus Osler (hereditary hemorrhagic telangiectasia)
  - Nevus araneus (spider angioma)
  - Senile angioma (ruby dot)
  - Venous angiomas
  - Venous lake
  - Leg veins
- *Other skin diseases with vascular alterations:*
  - Acne
  - Early immature striae distensae
  - Inflammatory linear verrucous epidermal nevus
  - Psoriasis
  - Red or hypertrophic scars
  - Viral warts
  - Xanthelasma palpebrarum.

Port Wine Stain

Laser is the treatment of choice for PWS, which are the most common cutaneous vascular malformations of low-flow thin-walled ectatic postcapillary venules, affecting 0.3–0.5% of the population.[2] There is progressive dilatation of immature venule-like vessels. PWS initially appear as sharply demarcated, flat red macules in childhood; lesions tend to darken to purple and become thickened with age due to the development of vascular nodules **(Figs. 1 and 2)**. The most common site affected is the face, followed by the neck, chest, and upper limbs.

Treatment aims to improve skin discoloration and prevent late complications. Pulsed dye laser is considered the gold-standard therapy for PWS. Deeper vessels and nodules can be treated with the help of Nd:YAG laser. Pink/red PWS comprises small-caliber vessels, and purple PWS consists of large caliber and deeper vessels, requiring more energy to damage the vessels. Lesions on the forehead, lateral aspect of cheeks, chin, and anterior neck **(Figs. 3 to 5)** respond faster than those on other parts of the face and body **(Figs. 6A and B)**.[7]

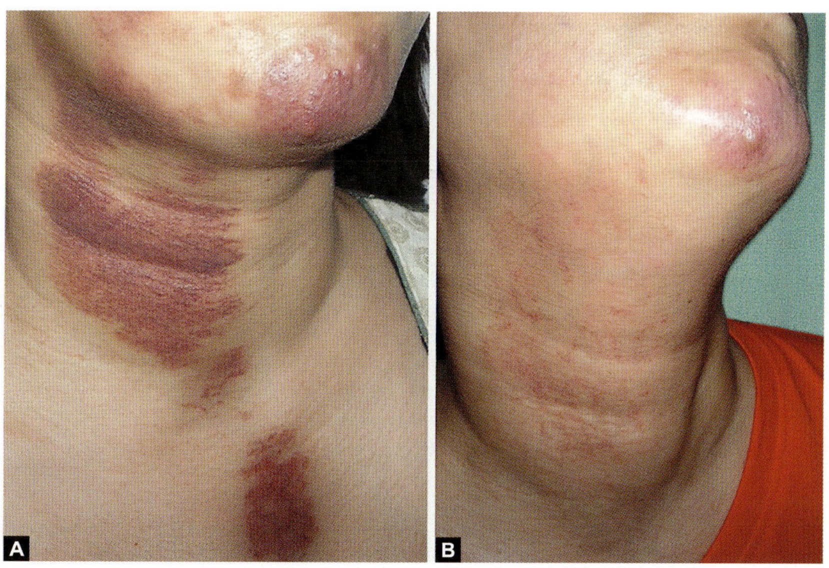

Figs. 1A and B: (A) Red to purple port wine stain over the mandibular area, anterior neck and chest with vascular nodules over the chin; (B) >75% improvement with pulsed dye laser after 10 sessions.

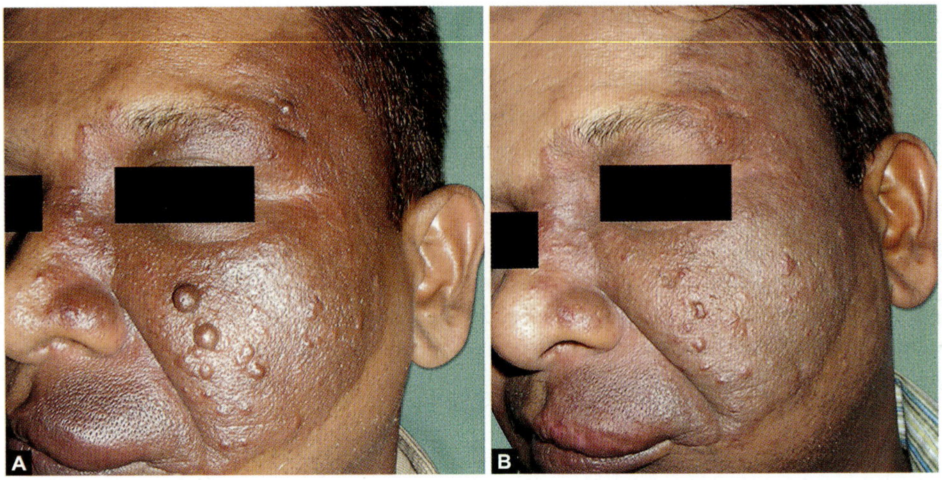

Figs. 2A and B: (A) Hypertrophic port wine stain with vascular nodules over the left side of the face; (B) Around 50% improvement after 10 sessions of pulsed dye laser.

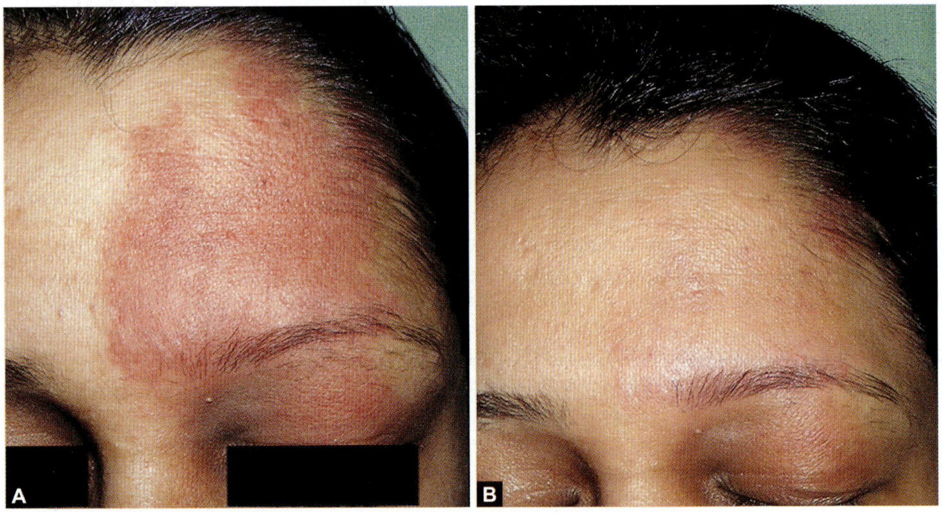

Figs. 3A and B: (A) Red flat port wine stain over left side of forehead and upper eyelid before treatment; (B) >75% lightening after eight sessions of pulsed dye laser.

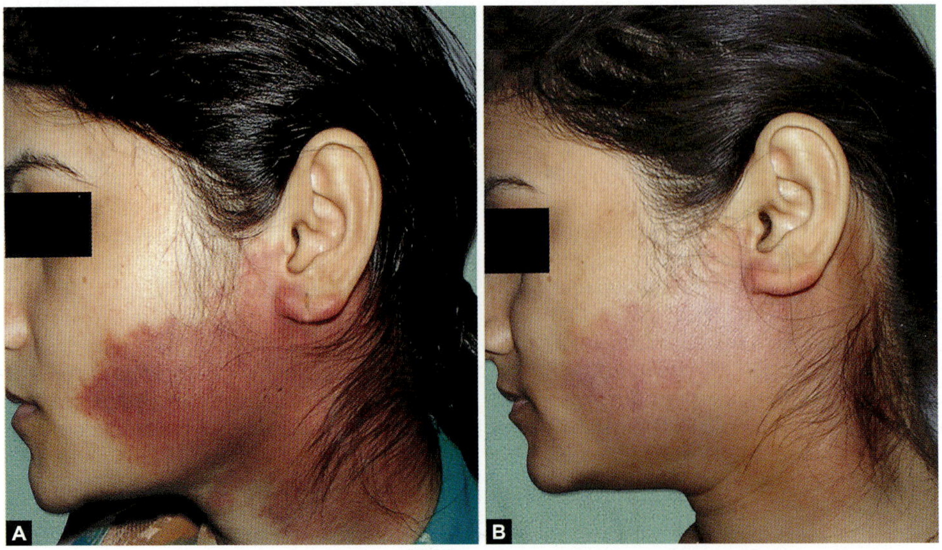

Figs. 4A and B: (A) Red to purple flat port wine stain over left lateral side of the face extending on to the neck and ear; (B) 75% lightening of lesion after pulsed dye laser.

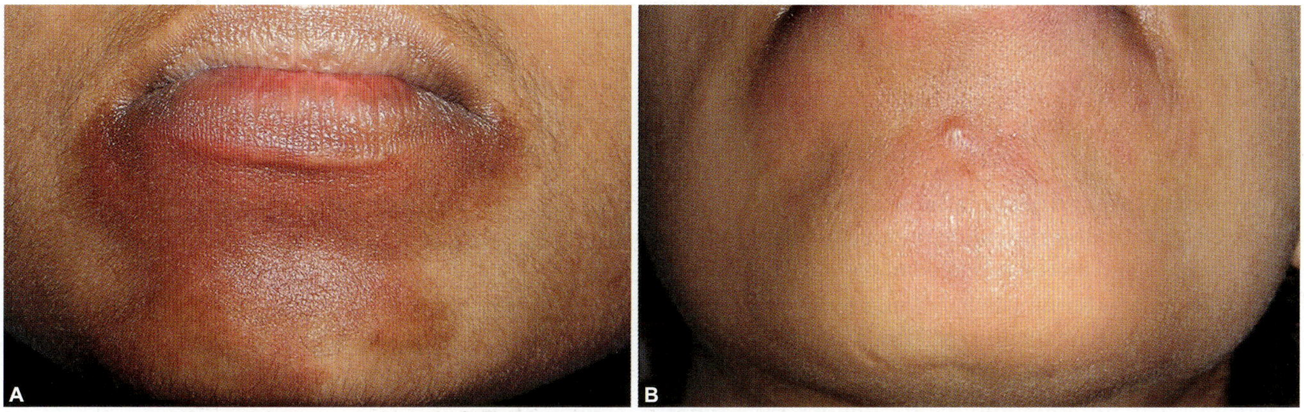

Figs 5A and B: (A) Red flat port wine stain over the chin; (B) >75% lightening after treatment with pulsed dye laser.

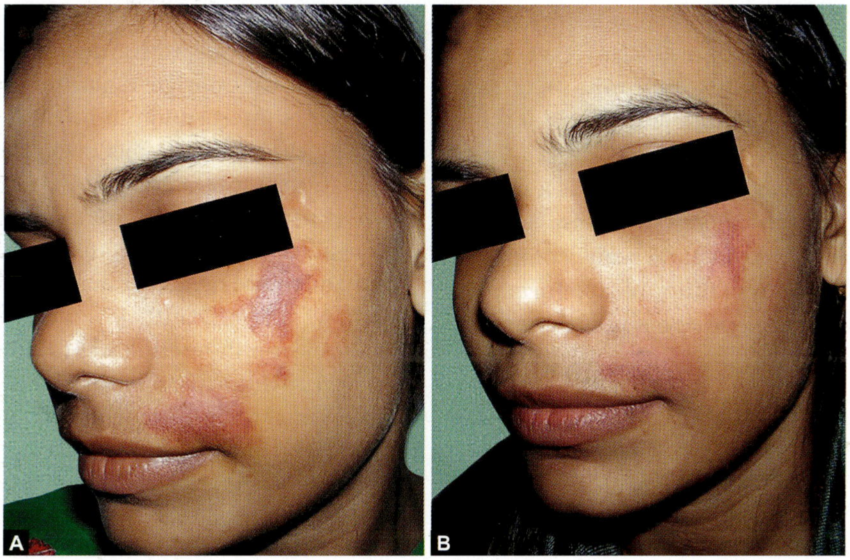

Figs. 6A and B: (A) Port wine stain over the left cheek; (B) 60% lightening after pulsed dye laser.

About 90% of patients with forehead lesions showed grade 3 response (61–80% improvement) after six to eight sessions.[8]

Multiple treatments are required at 4–8 weeks intervals, bringing about interval lightening with each treatment. At least six to eight sessions are needed to achieve 41–60% improvement in adults and 61–80% improvement in children.[8] Several studies have shown that the best results are observed in the first five sittings with plateauing of the response rate with further sessions, probably due to the formation of a fibrous shield in the upper papillary dermis after the destruction of vessels. The fibrosis may obstruct the laser from penetrating the deeper dermis during subsequent sessions.[9] There was 48% lightening of flat PWS and 36.6% improvement in hypertrophic PWS after the first five sessions, with only 10% and 12% further lightening, respectively, in the next five sessions.[9]

Khandpur et al. reported use of PDL in a total of 74 flat and 24 hypertrophic PWS with color ranging from pink to purple in skin types IV and V with a median lesion size of 56 cm^2 and 102 cm^2, respectively. Patients with flat and hypertrophic PWS underwent a mean of 7.3 and 8.5 sessions (range: 4–10 sessions), respectively. A mean lightening of 54% in flat and 40% in hypertrophic PWS was observed. After ten treatments, 46.6% of flat PWS cases showed >75% lightening, and an equal number had 25–75% improvement. More than 75% improvement was observed in 12.5% of hypertrophic PWS, and 75% of cases showed 25% to 75% improvement.[9] Thajudheen et al. demonstrated improvement with PDL in 85.6% of patients after a minimum of eight sessions. Twenty percent of patients had >80% improvement.[8]

Treatment with PDL alone fails to demonstrate significant improvement in nearly 25–50% of PWS lesions even after multiple sessions.[6] In PWS not responding to PDL, an increase in the fluence, spot size, or pulse duration can be tried. Dual 595/1,064-nm wavelength laser was effective in PWS previously recalcitrant to PDL therapy alone, demonstrating moderate improvement in 48% and mild in 52%.[10] Pulse-stacking or applying multiple consecutive pulses has been shown to increase clearance rates by targeting deeper vessels without increasing the risk of side effects. But it is safer to use single pulses with 10% overlap over flat PWS and dual pulses at a higher fluence and pulse durations on hypertrophic PWS, especially in darker skin types.[9]

Complications

- Post-treatment erythema, edema, and occasionally crusting may be observed and are directly related to the fluence used and inversely related to the pulse duration.
- Postlaser pain or burning in 24.3% and 13.5% of patients, respectively.[9] Patients may experience pain over sensitive areas like the upper lip.
- Shorter pulse duration and higher fluence on a dark-skinned individual can induce postinflammatory hyperpigmentation as the competing chromophore is melanin. Postinflammatory hyperpigmentation was observed in 30–40.5% of patients.[8,9] However, this is transient and resolves after 6–9 months with strict photoprotection or in 1–2 months with topical bleaching agents and sunscreen.[8,9]
- Scarring and textural changes rarely occur as a result of inadequate cooling, higher fluences, and pulse-stacking.
- Other minor adverse events include honeycombing of PWS, transient hypopigmentation, blister formation, localized atrophy, and development of vascular nodules over PWS.[9]

Prognostic Factors

The poor prognostic factors include older age at presentation, nonblanching thick PWS, coppery red color, and centrofacial and distal extremity lesions.[8]

- Laser treatment of PWS should be initiated in early childhood to prevent the later sequelae of cutaneous hypertrophy in PWS lesions. The lesions are smaller in early childhood, facilitating faster resolution with fewer treatment sessions. Also, early clearance decreases the psychological effect on the child. Several studies suggest improved results when treatment is started early in life. Compared to adults, a lower fluence and larger spot size are recommended in children. Larger spot sizes prevent cobblestone appearance. Ninety percent of children showed grade 2 improvement (41–60% improvement) as compared to 60% in adults.[8] Although PDL is effective, most PWS gradually redarken after laser treatments are discontinued, necessitating additional treatments in adolescence or adulthood.[11]
- Lin et al. observed that red-hued lesions were more responsive than pink and purple lesions.[7] Lesions on the central face, along V2 dermatome, on the trunk, and limbs responded less favorably than lesions located elsewhere on the face and neck.[7] The upper lip area was observed to be the most recalcitrant area, probably due to the presence of abundant pilosebaceous units.[8]
- The overall response rate of facial PWS to multiplex 585/1064 nm laser was significantly higher than PWS on extremities (84.85% vs. 55.55%, $p < 0.001$).[5] While 9.09% of patients with facial PWS showed complete response, none of the patients with extremity PWS showed complete response. Facial PWS resistant to multiplex laser had higher flow, larger blood vessel diameters and were located deeper in the skin than those that responded to laser, as evaluated by reflectance confocal microscopy.[5] Similarly, laser resistant extremity PWS had higher blood flow, larger diameters, and depth of blood vessels when compared to laser responsive extremity PWS.[5]

Hemangiomas

Infantile hemangiomas (IH) are the most common vascular tumors of childhood, with an incidence of 0.1–1.04% in India.[12] There is no appropriate algorithm to determine the timing and type of intervention in infantile hemangiomas as they are subject to spontaneous involution. The involution time ranges from 3 to 7 years, and IH may resolve with sequelae such as telangiectasia, fibrofatty residue or scars. They can be classified as superficial, deep, and mixed hemangiomas. Deep and mixed hemangiomas occurring in the central facial area have a significantly lower rate of complete regression than those on the peripheral facial sites (33.3% vs. 66.7%, $p = 0.025$).[13] Untreated deep or mixed hemangiomas heal with sequelae including telangiectasia, fibrofatty residue and scars in up to 46% of patients.[13]

The indications for treatment include complications (seen in 20% cases) such as impending obstruction, ulceration, pain, rapid growth, cardiac insufficiency, facial lesions and nonregressing hemangiomas. Lasers can be mainly employed to treat early superficial facial IH, compound IH to preserve overlying skin, IH with refractory ulceration, and significant residual telangiectasia or flat IH persisting after involution.[14] The laser settings commonly used for hemangiomas in various studies are mentioned in **Table 1**. There was no difference observed in the effectiveness of short pulse and longer pulse PDL (0.45 ms vs. 10–20 ms) in the treatment of IH; but, immediate sequelae (edema, erythema and purpura) lasted longer, and postlaser pigmentary and textural changes were more remarkable in the short pulse group.[15] On average, 2–3 treatment sessions per hemangioma are required and are usually repeated every 2–8 weeks. PDL and Nd:YAG demonstrated regression in 89.1% and 87.57% of patients with hemangiomas, respectively.[16,17] Thirty percent of children treated with PDL experienced complete resolution compared to 5% children who did not receive any treatment ($p = 0.001$).[15] Similar number of children (42–44%) experienced near-complete resolution in both the groups, and there was no significant difference in the outcome and residual signs at 5-year follow-up in both the groups. Argon and Nd:YAG lasers showed similar efficacy to PDL laser in terms of excellent or

TABLE 1: Commonly used laser parameters in patients with vascular lesions in various studies.

		Parameters		
Indication	*Laser*	*Fluence (J/cm²)*	*Spot size (mm)*	*Pulse duration (ms)*
Port wine stain Flat Hypertrophic	PDL 595 nm	 8–10 8–15	 7 7	 1.5–3 1.5–6
Hemangioma	PDL 595 nm	7–15	7	0.45–6
	Nd:YAG	25–235	3–7	15–50
Telangiectasia	PDL 595 nm	5–11.5	3–10	0.45–10
Spider nevi	PDL 595 nm	8–15	3–7	1.5–3
Angiokeratoma	Argon	0.5–4 W	0.5–1	0.2–2
	PDL	6.5–15	5–10	0.45–500
	Nd:YAG	30–160	2–7	10–50

Note: Treatment parameters may vary by device.

complete clearance, but Nd:YAG showed superior ability in treating thicker lesions.[15] The use of argon laser in the treatment of hemangiomas is restricted because of its limited penetration (<1 mm) and its tendency to cause hypertrophic scarring due to nonspecific thermal injury. The KTP 532 nm laser demonstrated complete clearance in 30% and marked improvement in 64% of hemangioma patients.[18]

Hemangiomas that take a longer time to involute have a higher incidence of residual changes. Various studies have reported the efficacy of PDL in halting the proliferative phase. Among 100 hemangiomas treated within 12 weeks of their development, 73 lesions required a single treatment and 27 up to five treatments; 23% of lesions showed complete remission, 55% showed partial remission, and 14% stopped growing. Only 8% of lesions continued to grow despite treatment.[19]

Based on the morphology and location, PDL laser demonstrated excellent improvement (75–100% improvement) in 60% segmental-superficial-thick, 66.67% of segmental-superficial-thin, and 100% of segmental-superficial-papular subtypes of hemangioma.[7] In patients with eyelid and perineal hemangiomas associated with complications like visual field defects and ulceration, PDL laser demonstrated excellent improvement in 71.43% and 60%, respectively.[7] Segmental hemangiomas and hemangiomas on extremities have a relatively higher risk of poor outcome and complications than localized hemangiomas. Lesions of the peripheral facial area achieved significantly more volumetric regression than lesions of the central facial ($p < 0.0001$) and chest areas ($p = 0.0002$) and had a considerably higher aesthetic score than those on the central facial site ($p < 0.0001$), chest ($p < 0.0001$), and trunk/extremities ($p = 0.0226$).[20]A retrospective analysis of 60 pediatric patients conducted by Kim et al. showed that in 37% of ulcerated hemangiomas treated with PDL, 50% showed a definite improvement, 18% showed no response, and 5% showed worsening of lesions.[21]

Combination Therapy

The combination of PDL and Nd:YAG laser treatment is considered an effective and safe option. In a retrospective analysis of 149 children, 91.1% and 95.6% of infantile hemangiomas treated with combined Nd:YAG-PDL laser and PDL laser alone, respectively, showed moderate to significant (>50%) improvement.[22] The mean number of laser sessions for each hemangioma were 1.95 for combined Nd:YAG-PDL laser and 1.26 for PDL laser alone.

The oral beta-blocker, propranolol, is a standard treatment of choice for the initial management of infantile hemangiomas. The addition of PDL to propranolol therapy increased treatment effectiveness, significantly lowered the number of days and cumulative dose of propranolol treatment to achieve near-complete clearance.[23] Similarly, addition of PDL laser to topical timolol resulted in more significant improvement in superficial IH. The deeper components of mixed IH responded better to Nd:YAG laser compared to topical timolol.[24]

In a systematic review of studies that used laser for treating ulcerated hemangiomas, all patients achieved re-epithelization of ulcers.[25] The mean healing time was 2.84 ± 0.22 weeks with PDL alone, 1–2 weeks with a combination of PDL and oral propranolol and 13.5 ± 4.5 days with a combination of PDL and Nd:YAG laser.[25]

In 59 patients with infantile hemangiomas with deep and superficial components (thickness >0.6 cm) in Fitzpatrick III or IV skin types, the combination of 1% polidocanol (100 mg in 10 mL) sclerotherapy and multiplex laser resulted in >60% reduction in size and color in 83.1% and 86.5%, respectively.[26]

Complications

Transient blistering is the main side effect seen in around 21.2–55% of the patients.[2] In a meta-analysis, atrophic scarring, ulceration, bleeding, infection, mild textural changes, hyperpigmentation, and hypopigmentation were observed in 6.28% of patients with IH.[16] Treatment of hemangiomas with PDL was associated with more significant scarring than port-wine stains (PWS).[12] The most frequently reported adverse events in one larger Nd:YAG series (684 children) included skin burn (11%), infection (6.6%), and scarring (4.4%). Relapse of hemangiomas was observed in 2% of infants after 3–24 months. Retreatment with combined laser therapy led to satisfactory clinical outcome in these infants.[22]

Telangiectasia

Telangiectasia comprises superficial dilated venules, capillaries or arterioles with an average diameter of 0.1–1.0 mm. Telangiectasias that are arteriolar in origin have a smaller diameter, are bright red, and do not protrude above the skin surface. Those that arise from venules are wider, blue and often protrude above the skin surface. Facial telangiectasias are seen in rosacea, hereditary hemorrhagic telangiectasia, collagen vascular diseases, idiopathic generalized telangiectasia and unilateral nevoid telangiectasia. They are of four types—simple or linear, arborizing, spider and papular, based on clinical appearance.

The laser parameters used to treat telangiectasias are discussed in **Table 1**. Purpura can be minimized by giving two to three pulses over the telangiectasia at lower fluences (stacked pulses), using spot size of 10 mm diameter at 4–5 J/cm^2 using PDL 595 nm laser. This technique provides a more significant benefit in the laser treatment of facial telangiectasias.[7] The dilated telangiectatic vessels in hereditary hemorrhagic telangiectasia respond well to PDL laser, preventing bleeding and significantly improving clinical appearance.[2] Treatment of unilateral nevoid telangiectasia in skin types III and IV using 585 nm PDL has shown a moderate response (26–50% lightening) in 100% of the patients after 2.33 sessions, and an excellent response (>75% lightening) in 33.3% of patients after 3.66 sessions.[27] In another study, 15% of patients with discrete telangiectasia showed complete clearance with KTP 532 nm laser and 77% showed marked improvement, while 93% of patients with matted telangiectasia showed marked improvement.[18]

Rosacea

Rosacea is a chronic inflammatory disorder commonly involving the midfacial region. The four stages of rosacea include:

1. Prerosacea (flushing/easy irritation and erythema)
2. Vascular stage (transient erythema, early telangiectasias)
3. Deeper facial erythema (increased telangiectasias, papules and pustules)
4. Tissue hyperplasia (rhinophyma, ocular inflammation).

Lasers are used to treat persistent facial erythema and telangiectasias (erythematotelangiectatic rosacea). In addition to PDL, other lasers, including 1064-nm Nd:YAG, KTP, and intense pulsed light, have been used to treat facial telangiectasia **(Figs. 7 and 8)**. There is a lack of high-quality studies to support the use of lasers to treat rosacea. From available studies, PDL is more effective than Nd:YAG laser, and as effective as IPL therapy.[28] IPL works better in telangiectasia <1 mm, while Nd:YAG laser in vessels >1 mm. There was improvement in flushing, pruritus and even pustules after 2–3 sessions of PDL therapy in patients with telangiectatic rosacea.[2] Sometimes, IPL can paradoxically aggravate rosacea. In a comparative split-face study, the 532-nm KTP laser had comparable outcomes in the complete clearance of telangiectasias compared to the 595-nm PDL. But, KTP caused more edema, swelling and postlaser erythema.[29] Compared to Nd:YAG laser, KTP laser does not effectively improve either

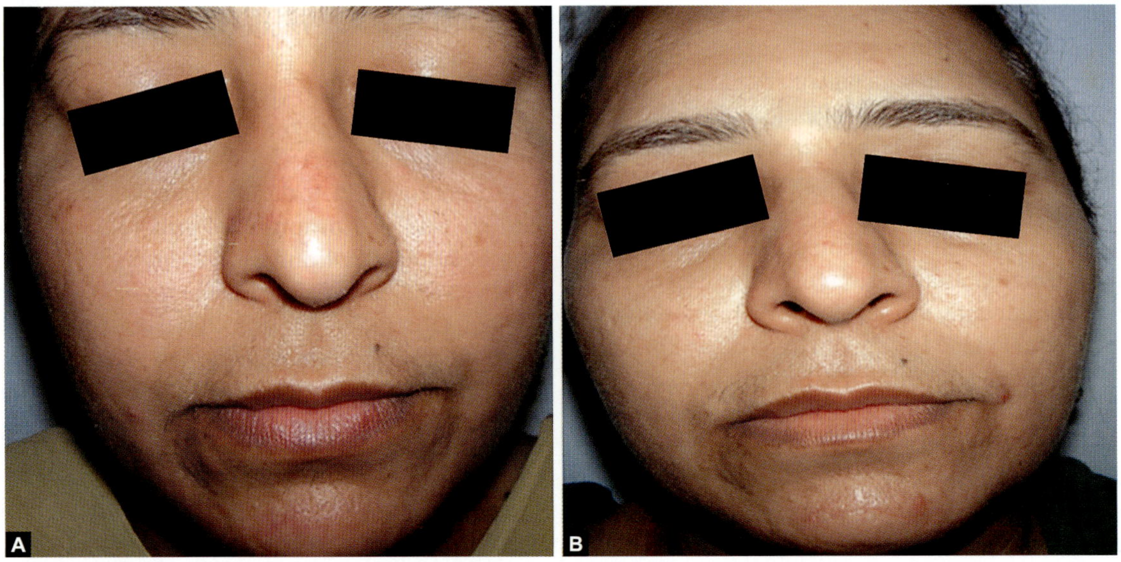

Figs. 7A and B: (A) Erythematotelangiectatic rosacea; (B) >75% improvement after treatment with pulsed dye laser.

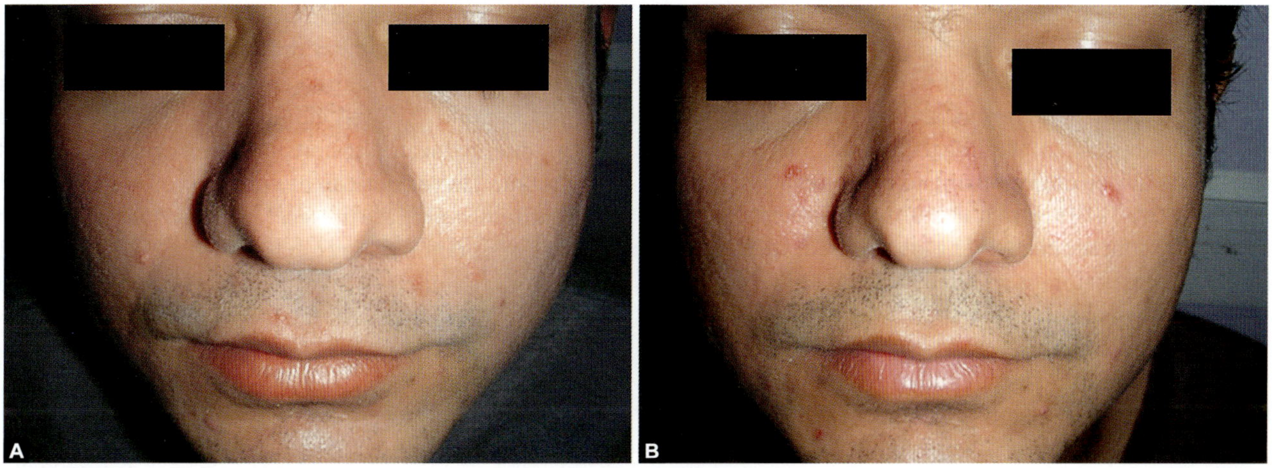

Figs. 8A and B: (A) Facial erythema, telangiectasias, and erythematous papules of rosacea; (B) Improvement in erythema and telangiectasias after five pulsed dye laser sessions.

the inflammatory lesions or the background erythema but has a lower risk of scarring.[30] Telangiectasias over the malar area respond better to Nd:YAG, while those on the ala nasi are most resistant.[31] Nd:YAG laser was also useful in papulopustular rosacea, probably by removing follicular units affected by Demodex mites, which induce perifollicular inflammation.[30]

A combination of 1% topical oxymetazoline, which reduces facial erythema, and PDL, which effectively targets telangiectasias, has been successfully used in patients with erythematotelangiectatic rosacea.[32] Other additions to PDL, such as hydroxychloroquine (200 mg/day), topical retinaldehyde, plus topical tacrolimus, have also resulted in beneficial outcomes.[30] Three consecutive sessions of combined PDL and fractional microneedling radiofrequency has been shown to significantly improve erythema and papulopustular component.[33] There is a theoretical risk of photosensitivity when PDL is combined with doxycycline. However, one retrospective study (PDL plus doxycycline) demonstrated effective control of rosacea with no adverse skin reactions.[34] In one study with 170 participants, the PDL-minocycline combination group showed a 1-year post-treatment recurrence rate of 34.7% compared to 48.3% in the minocycline monotherapy group.[35]

Nevus Araneus (Spider Angioma)

Spider nevi are telangiectasia with a central feeding arterial vessel. They can occur as single or multiple lesions and are found in up to 15% of healthy adults and 47.5% of children.[7,36] PDL, Nd:YAG and KTP lasers have been used to treat spider nevi for cosmetic purposes. Several treatment sessions may be needed because of their high flow. After a single treatment session, 58.87% of patients achieved 50–100% improvement.[37] A small spot size (3 mm) of 595 nm PDL laser can be used to treat the central arterial vessel to achieve good to excellent results instead of large spot sizes covering the whole lesion.[7] The peripheral capillaries disappear after one treatment, but a large central body (diameter >1 mm) may require multiple sessions. A large spot (7 mm) may be used for larger areas outside the 3 mm diameter zone combined with the small spot size for the central spider body to improve the efficacy compared to a small or large spot size alone.[36] Recurrences up to 36% may occur due to the high intravascular pressure.[36] A primary cure rate of 38.5% and 30.8% incidence of adverse reactions were reported with Nd:YAG laser.[38] KTP 532 nm laser showed complete clearance and marked improvement in 51% and 48% of patients with spider nevi, respectively.[18] KTP laser has decreased efficacy in spider nevi in deeper locations and has greater adverse effects in darker skin.

Venous Lakes

A venous lake is usually a solitary, soft, compressible, dark blue to violaceous, 0.2–1 cm sized papule caused by dilatation of venules. These are commonly found on sun-exposed surfaces (face, vermilion border of the lip and ears) in the elderly. Various surgical and laser modalities have been tried for venous lakes. The sequential application of 595 nm PDL (7 mm spot size at 7–11.5 J/cm^2 and 2–10 ms) and 1064 nm Nd:YAG laser (35–40 J/cm^2 at 15–40 ms) resulted in complete resolution of venous lakes in 82.4%of patients after one or two treatment sessions.[39]

Angiokeratomas

Angiokeratomas are benign vascular neoplasms presenting as single or multiple well-defined, hyperkeratotic, red to black papules or plaques. Apart from traditional ablative procedures, which may result in hemorrhage, atrophy, or scarring, several laser modalities like PDL, Nd:YAG, argon, and KTP have been used for their treatment.

Pulsed dye laser resulted in significant improvement (60–100% clearance) in 80% of patients with angiokeratoma of Mibelli.[40] The clearance rate did not depend on lesion size and color of lesions or patient gender. The treatment of genital angiokeratomas resulted in excellent response (75–100% clearance) in 58.3% of patients.[3] PDL treatment decreased the size of the lesions and alleviated symptoms of bleeding and pruritus.[3] Baumgartner et al. demonstrated successful clearance of genital angiokeratomas with PDL in all patients after 1–7 (mean 3.38 ± 2.16) treatment sessions with no permanent sequelae.[41] The long-pulsed Nd:YAG laser for genital angiokeratomas resulted in complete response in 82% of the patients after a mean of 2.2 treatment sessions.[42] In the treatment of genital angiokeratomas, long-pulsed Nd:YAG demonstrated significantly greater improvement than PDL after three sessions (77.6% vs. 61.8% clearance, $p < 0.005$) but was associated with significantly higher pain scores.[43] Long-pulsed Nd:YAG laser is more effective for treating hyperkeratotic angiokeratomas due to its deeper skin penetration. The reported side effects after laser treatment of genital angiokeratomas include transient edema, purpura, bleeding and permanent alteration in skin pigmentation and texture.[3] Several case reports and case series have demonstrated marked resolution of angiokeratomas after 1–3 sessions of argon laser but was associated with post-treatment dyspigmentation and scarring.[3]

Pyogenic Granulomas

Pyogenic granuloma also referred to as lobular capillary hemangioma most commonly develop on exposed areas of skin at sites of trauma including hands, face, and mucous membranes **(Figs. 9A and B).** These are frequently reported in children and pregnant women.

Pulsed dye laser treatment is preferred in children as it is painless and has minimal postoperative recovery. But multiple treatments are required compared to carbon dioxide ablative lasers.[44] Lee et al. reported recurrence rates of 0.43% after PDL and 0.49% after CO_2 laser treatments of pyogenic granulomas.[45] PDL resulted in complete clearance of pyogenic granulomas measuring 2–3 mm after 1–6 sessions in 91% of patients (n = 22). Children having larger (>1 cm) lesions failed to respond.[46] PDL is generally not effective in treating thicker, deeply located lesions due to its minimal depth of penetration. The lesions can be compressed with a glass slide before administering the pulses.[47] Alternate use of 585/595 nm with longer durations using tunable PDL resulted in complete resolution of multiple 1–20 mm sized pyogenic granulomas on the face **(Figs. 10A and B)**. No recurrence was observed during the next 6 months.[47]

Bédard MS et al. reported clearance in 40% patients with pyogenic granulomas (n = 25) after a single session of 1064 nm long-pulsed Nd:YAG laser. They reported complete resolution of lesions after a mean of 2.28 sessions and no recurrence at the end of 2 months. Ninety-six percent of the patients were very satisfied (18/25) or satisfied (6/25) with the treatment and its results. Adverse effects such as induration (13/25), pain during treatment (8/25), transient edema (5/25), hypopigmentation (5/25), and bleeding (4/25) were reported.[48]

In a study, KTP laser resulted in complete clearance of pyogenic granulomas in 96% of patients (n = 28) after an average of 1.1 sessions, but it failed to achieve effective coagulation in three patients. Recurrence was noted in three patients within 7–14 days, which responded to additional KTP laser treatment. Complete healing occurred in 15.8 ± 8.1 days, and slight textural changes were observed in eight patients. No recurrence was seen at the end of 3 months.[49]

Angiofibromas

Angiofibromas are most commonly located on the face and can result in disfigurement and adverse psychosocial outcomes. PDL works by targeting the dilated capillaries. It also affects the fibrous tissue by causing ischemic necrosis

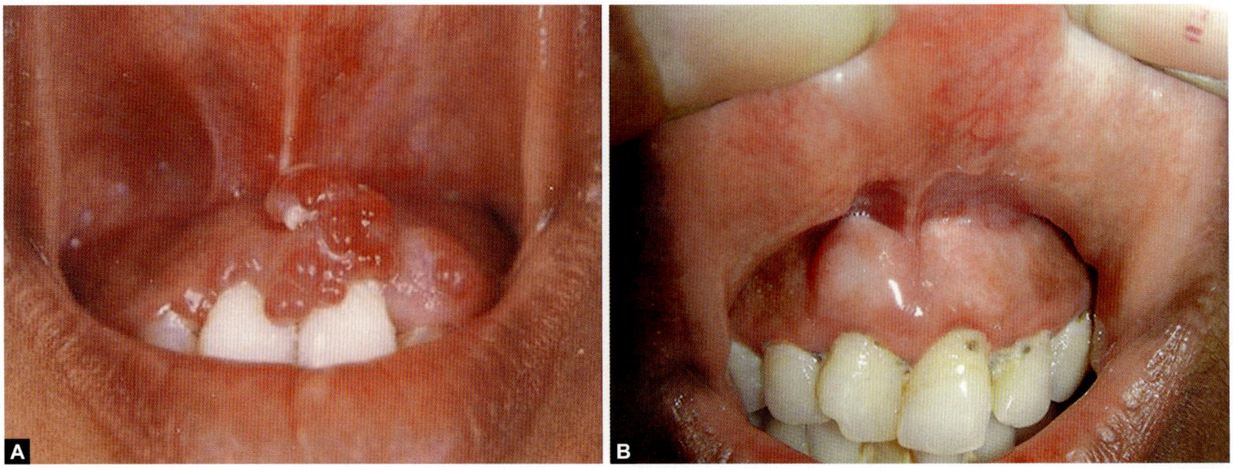

Figs. 9A and B: (A) Multiple 5–10 mm pyogenic granulomas over the upper gingiva; (B) Resolution of all lesions after six pulsed dye laser treatments. *Source:* Khandpur S, Sharma VK. Successful treatment of multiple gingival pyogenic granulomas with pulsed-dye laser. Indian J Dermatol Venereol Leprol. 2008;74(3):275-7.

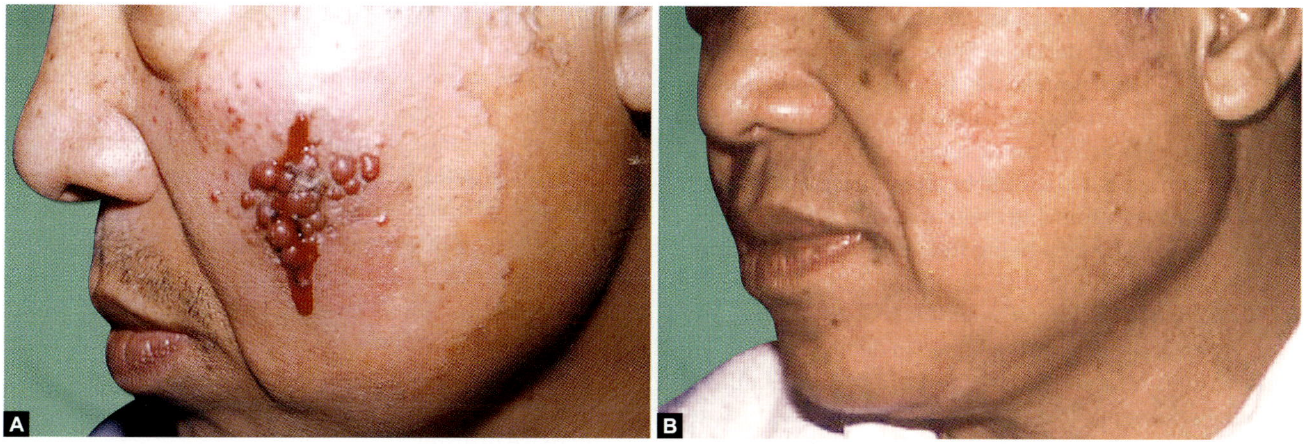

Figs. 10A and B: (A) Multiple 1–20 mm sized pyogenic granulomas over left cheek; (B) Complete subsidence of all pyogenic granulomas after five sessions with the flashlamp pulsed tunable dye laser.
Source: Khandpur S, Sharma VK. Efficacy of pulsed dye laser in cosmetically distressing facial dermatoses in skin types IV and V. Indian J Dermatol. 2008;53(4):186-9.

and through the release of collagenase from fibroblasts in response to thermal injury.[50]

Resolution of unilateral facial angiofibromas was observed after three PDL sessions, with minimal pigmentary and no textural adverse effects.[50] In a study, excellent improvement (76–100%) was observed in 10 patients, and good improvement (51–75%) in two patients after five to eight sessions of PDL. No recurrence was seen after 1 year. After 3 years, five patients had a minimal recurrence, not requiring additional treatments.[51] In another study, 50% and >75% regression was seen with 585 nm PDL after a mean of 2.5 and 5.5 sessions, respectively.[47]

Potassium titanyl phosphate laser resulted in complete flattening of angiofibromas after 1–2 sessions in five patients with Fitzpatrick skin types II-VI. Recurrence was seen after 18–24 months. There were no side effects besides transient hypo- or hyperpigmentation.[52]

Pulsed dye laser has been used in combination with topical sirolimus, electrocautery, ablative fractional lasers and photodynamic therapy with 5-aminolevulinic acid for the treatment of facial angiofibromas.[53-55]

Other Vascular Malformations

Low-flow vascular malformations such as venous malformations (VMs), glomuvenous malformations (GVMs) and verrucous VMs (VVMs) present a therapeutic challenge because of their depth and involvement of large caliber vessels. Laser modalities may be tried in small, accessible, and multifocal lesions or when standard therapies fail or carry significant risk. Long-pulsed Nd:YAG has demonstrated good to excellent results in 66.7% and poor to fair results in 25% of patients (mean age 9.3 years) with VMs, GVMs, or VVMs. Mucosal lesions responded the best. The number of sessions varied between 1 and 16 (mean 4.6), and 27% reported adverse effects, with minor blistering and erosion being the most common.[56]

CONTRAINDICATIONS FOR VASCULAR LASERS

They are absolutely contraindicated in the presence of active local infection and photoaggravated skin diseases or medical conditions. They are relatively contraindicated in patients of unstable vitiligo, psoriasis, keloid or keloidal tendencies, those on isotretinoin, and patients who are not cooperative or have unrealistic expectations.

PATIENT SELECTION

The success rate of lasers depends on the correct diagnosis and indication. All vascular lesions are not amenable to laser treatment. Proper patient selection is vital to achieving favorable results. The goals of laser treatment for vascular lesions are:

- To improve overall appearance, ideally to achieve complete clearance without any permanent complications
- To relieve obstruction and improve the function of an organ
- To prevent disfigurement
- To prevent and treat ulcerated lesions
- To avoid aggressive procedures
- To minimize psychological distress.

PREOPERATIVE CARE AND COUNSELING

- The course of the lesions, including the possibility of natural involution in hemangiomas, different treatment options, need for multiple laser sessions at regular intervals, cost, expected results, and postlaser complications, must be discussed in detail with the patient. The possibility of the persistence of lesions despite treatment should be explained, and any unrealistic expectations of the patient should be actively addressed.

- Patients should be given adequate time and opportunity to make an informed decision. Topical bleaching agents for dark-skinned individuals may be started at least 2 weeks before laser treatment, and a broad-spectrum sunscreen at least 4 weeks before the session.[1]
- The area to be treated should be shaved on the morning of treatment. Hair removing creams should not be used for this purpose. The area being treated should be cleansed with mild soap and alcohol. The patient should not apply any other creams, lotions or sprays.
- The procedure has to be explained in detail to the patient, and written informed consent of the patient should be taken. Prelaser photographs of the lesion should be taken before each session.

ANESTHESIA

Laser treatment is usually well tolerated. Long pulsed Nd:YAG laser is associated with pain while PDL seldom produces pain. Topical anesthetics (such as 2.5% lidocaine + 2.5% prilocaine) should be applied under occlusion for 30–60 minutes to reduce local discomfort. The eutectic mixture of local anesthetics is not recommended for infants below 6 months of age as higher vascular surfaces may cause excessive absorption, which may cause methemoglobinemia.[1] Local anesthesia (or sometimes general anesthesia) is mandatory for Nd:YAG laser treatment as it can cause severe pain. The vasoconstrictor and sympathomimetic effects of topical anesthetics can reduce the effectiveness of vascular lasers. Occlusion by topical anesthetics and plastic film may cause partial vasoconstriction in telangiectasias and spider nevi.[7] Laser treatment of extensive lesions, lesions in very early childhood, and uncooperative children may require short general anesthesia.

INTRAOPERATIVE CARE

- Adequate eye protection of doctor and patient during the procedure should be ensured using glasses or eye shields specific to the laser.
- The correct laser parameters must be selected and recorded. A test shot should be given before the procedure to check for any significant pain. The patient is advised not to move or flinch with each pulse delivered as the machine makes a popping sound.
- The laser is delivered concomitantly with cryogen cooling to prevent thermal damage to the epidermis or surrounding tissue. Cooling can be done by other methods such as cold sapphire contact handpieces or by blowing precooled air across the skin surface. The dynamic cooling device is either an add-on device or integrated within the laser. Epidermal cooling applied with laser enables fewer treatment sessions to achieve more remarkable clearance of lesions compared to no cooling.[15]

POSTOPERATIVE CARE

- The patient is advised to apply cold compresses to the treated side immediately after the procedure. A topical steroid-antibiotic combination cream is applied.
- Patients should be informed about the inevitable side effect of purpura, which will disappear after 1–2 weeks. Cool water compresses may be applied to reduced swelling or discomfort, but direct application of ice should be avoided.
- Postoperative analgesia is usually not indicated. In case of pain and discomfort, acetaminophen is preferred over aspirin or ibuprofen during the healing phase, as they can increase bruising.
- The patient is instructed to follow strict sun protection measures. A broad-spectrum sunscreen with SPF 30 or higher should be used for several months (at least 3 months) to avoid prolonged redness or pigmentary changes.
- Patients should avoid exercise for 3 days; alcohol consumption or blood thinners for 5 days; hot showers, hot tubs, or saunas for 5 days after treatment.
- Showers are permitted, but prolonged hot baths should be avoided for 1–2 weeks. Mild nonirritant soaps may be used to clean the treated site.
- Patients are advised not to rub but dab the area with a towel and avoid picking, scratching, or harsh cleansing of the treated skin.
- Patients should avoid swimming and contact sports during the healing phase (1–2 weeks).
- Cosmetics may be used after laser to cover the purpura if there is no blistering or ulceration.
- An interval of 6–8 weeks should be maintained between subsequent laser sessions. The effectiveness of laser treatment should be evaluated after every session, and the laser parameters should be adapted based on the outcome of the previous treatment.

COMPLICATIONS

- Purpura is commonly seen post-treatment and usually subsides within 1–2 weeks.
- Honey-combing effect if 10–30% overlapping of pulses is not done **(Fig. 11)**.
- Some amount of erythema and edema is expected immediately at the treated site, which subsides by 5–7 days. Appropriate cooling during and after the procedure, sleeping with an extra pillow to augment gravitational clearing of inflammatory fluid, can reduce edema.
- Bleeding can be avoided with proper parameter selection.
- Rare cases of postlaser blistering can be treated with topical fusidic acid cream. They are usually caused by overtreatment, and postinflammatory hypo- or hyperpigmentation may result following blistering.

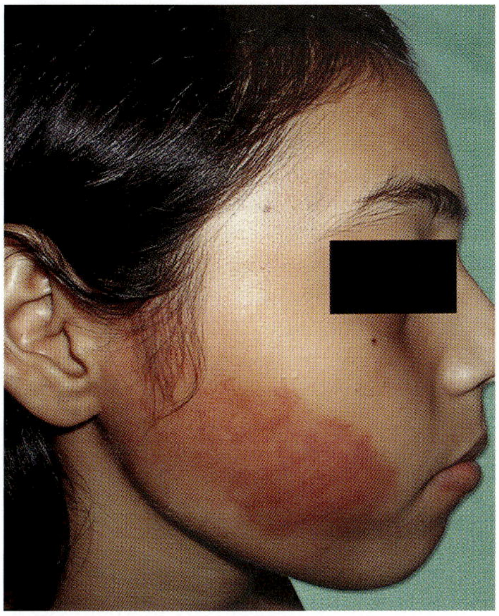

Fig. 11: Honey-combing effect after treatment with pulsed dye laser.

- Similarly, skin texture changes and scarring are caused by over treatment such as excessive fluence or pulse stacking.
- Hyperpigmentation more commonly occurs in darker skin types. Pigmentary changes (hypo- or hyperpigmentation) usually fade in 3–6 months.
- Infection is uncommon and should be suspected in patients with edema, erythema, pain, oozing, crusting, and fever. Reactivation of herpes can occur while treating lesions on the face in patients with a history of herpes.

FACTORS AFFECTING TREATMENT RESPONSE

Age: Young people respond better than the elderly as they have thinner and superficially placed blood vessels.[8] Also, younger children require fewer sessions. In a study on hemangiomas, older children had a more significant response to Nd:YAG laser.[17]

Gender: Female patients with superficial infantile hemangiomas were found to respond better than males to PDL; the difference being statistically significant ($p < 0.001$).[57]

Skin type: Fairer skin types showed better response than darker skin. Darker skin types require longer pulses, longer-pulse intervals, and higher fluence, because epidermal melanin absorbs the laser energy.

Site of lesion: PWS on the face and neck respond the best to laser therapy. Similarly, hemangiomas on the extremities had inadequate response compared to those on the face and trunk (patient satisfaction score 7.25 vs. 4.45, $p < 0.001$).[58]

Size of the lesion: PWS larger than 20 cm^2 respond poorer as compared to smaller lesions.

Depth of the lesion: Lesions with deeper vessels respond poorly. PDL at 585 nm and 6–8 J/cm^2 was found to coagulate the vessels up to 0.65 mm (mean 0.37 mm). Nd:YAG laser was also found to have a greater response in superficial hemangiomas.[17] Dark red and purple PWS (reflecting deeper lesions) are less responsive than red lesions. Pink lesions respond poorly as compared to red lesions as content of oxyhemoglobin is less in pink lesions.

Diameter of vessels: Blood vessels with a diameter greater than 100 μm have a higher thermal relaxation time, and hence require longer-pulse duration. Vessels with higher intravascular pressure (on the nose or legs) require higher fluences to achieve effective thermocoagulation. Also, pink PWS composed of small-caliber vessels does not contain enough blood to be targeted, leading to reduced efficacy.[59]

CONCLUSION

The best therapy for vascular lesions consists of using the most appropriate laser that produces significant clearance of the lesion using minimum treatment sessions with the least morbidity. Because of the variabilities in laser parameters and variations in individual responses, a test spot on a small, representative area may be performed initially before treating the entire lesion. There is robust evidence reporting the efficacy of PDL in the treatment of PWS. But the number of randomized controlled trials comparing laser modalities to each other and evidence regarding the efficacy of different lasers in other vascular lesions is minimal. Lasers may be combined with other modalities to enhance clearance and treat resistant lesions, with enough caution to prevent adverse effects. These modalities enhance laser penetration, destroy deeply situated large-caliber vessels, and prevent residual vessel proliferation.

REFERENCES

1. Srinivas CR, Kumaresan M. Lasers for vascular lesions: standard guidelines of care. Indian J Dermatol Venereol Leprol. 2011;77: 349-68.
2. Zutt M. Laser treatment of vascular dermatological diseases using a pulsed dye laser (595 nm) in combination with a Neodym:YAG-laser (1064 nm). Photochem Photobiol Sci. 2019;18:1660-8.
3. Nguyen J, Chapman LW, Korta DZ, Zachary CB. Laser treatment of cutaneous angiokeratomas: a systematic review. Dermatol Ther. 2017;30(6):1-8.
4. Brauer JA, Geronemus RG. Laser treatment in the management of infantile hemangiomas and capillary vascular malformations. Tech Vasc Interv Radiol. 2013;16:51-4.
5. Fu Z, Huang J, Xiang Y, Huang J, Tang Z, Chen J, et al. Characterization of laser-resistant port wine stain blood vessels using in vivo reflectance confocal microscopy. Lasers Surg Med. 2019;51:841-9.
6. Periyasamy MK, Sekar CS, Rai R. Effectiveness of dual sequential wavelength laser in the treatment of portwine stains – a retrospective study. Indian Dermatol Online J. 2019;10:418-21.

7. Lin MY, Lin CS, Hu S, Chang JM, Chung WH, Zhang ZY, et al. The application of 595-nm pulsed dye laser for vascular anomalies in a Chinese population: a 10-year experience. J Cosmet Laser Ther. 2019;21:171-8.
8. Thajudheen CP, Jyothy K, Priyadarshini A. Treatment of port-wine stains with flash lamp pumped pulsed dye laser on Indian skin: a six year study. J Cutan Aesthetic Surg. 2014;7:32-6.
9. Khandpur S, Sharma VK. Assessment of efficacy of the 595-nm pulsed dye laser in the treatment of facial port-wine stains in Indian patients. Dermatol Surg. 2016;42:717-26.
10. Alster TS, Tanzi EL. Combined 595-nm and 1,064-nm laser irradiation of recalcitrant and hypertrophic port-wine stains in children and adults. Dermatol Surg. 2009;35:914-9.
11. Mann JA. Update on pediatric dermatologic surgery from tots to teens. Curr Opin Pediatr. 2014;26:452-9.
12. Vasani RJ, Khanna D, Singal A. Cutaneous vascular lesions and their management in Indian setting. Dermatol Ther. 2012;25:358-75.
13. Chang SJ, Qiao C, Chang L, Gao W, Jin Y, Ma G, et al. A 7-year follow-up study on untreated deep or mixed facial infantile hemangioma in East-Asian patients: When propranolol was not yet an option. J Dermatol. 2019;46:962-6.
14. Darrow DH, Greene AK, Mancini AJ, Nopper AJ. Section on dermatology, section on otolaryngology–head and neck surgery, and section on plastic surgery. Diagnosis and Management of Infantile Hemangioma. Pediatrics. 2015; 136:e1060-104.
15. Chinnadurai S, Sathe NA, Surawicz T. Laser treatment of infantile hemangioma: a systematic review. Lasers Surg Med. 2016;48:221-33.
16. Shen L, Zhou G, Zhao J, Li P, Xu Q, Dong Y, et al. Pulsed dye laser therapy for infantile hemangiomas: a systemic review and meta-analysis. QJM. 2015;108:473-80.
17. Zhong S, Tao Y, Zhou J, Liu Y, Yao L, Li S. Infantile hemangioma: clinical characteristics and efficacy of treatment with the long-pulsed 1,064-nm neodymium-doped yttrium aluminum garnet laser in 794 Chinese patients. Pediatr Dermatol. 2015;32:495-500.
18. Becher GL, Cameron H, Moseley H. Treatment of superficial vascular lesions with the KTP 532-nm laser: experience with 647 patients. Lasers Med Sci. 2014;29:267-71.
19. Maier H, Neumann R. Treatment of strawberry marks with flashlamp-pumped pulsed dye laser in infancy. Lancet. 1996;347:131-2.
20. Chang SJ, Yu W, Gu Y, Han Y, Shang Y, Chang L, et al. Location of infantile hemangioma is a predictor of volumetric sequelae after involution. J Dermatol 2019;46:371-5.
21. Kim HJ, Colombo M, Frieden IJ. Ulcerated hemangiomas: clinical characteristics and response to therapy. J Am Acad Dermatol. 2001;44:962-72.
22. Hartmann F, Lockmann A, Grönemeyer LL, Haenssle HA, Zutt M, von Fintel H, et al. Nd:YAG and pulsed dye laser therapy in infantile haemangiomas: a retrospective analysis of 271 treated haemangiomas in 149 children. J EurAcad Dermatol Venereol. 2017;31:1372-9.
23. Reddy KK, Blei F, Brauer JA, Waner M, Anolik R, Bernstein L, et al. Retrospective study of the treatment of infantile hemangiomas using a combination of propranolol and pulsed dye laser. Dermatol Surg. 2013;39:923-33.
24. Tawfik AA, Alsharnoubi J. Topical timolol solution versus laser in treatment of infantile hemangioma: a comparative study. Pediatr Dermatol. 2015;32:369-76.
25. Wang JY, Ighani A, Ayala AP, Akita S, Lara-Corrales I, Alavi A. Medical, surgical, and wound care management of ulcerated Infantile hemangiomas: a systematic review [Formula: see text]. J Cutan Med Surg. 2018;22:495-504.
26. Lin L, Guo P, Cao Y, Li Q, Zhang J, Huo R. Combination of sclerotherapy and dual-wavelength laser in the management of infantile hemangiomas in chinese infants. Dermatol Surg. 2019;45:1253-9.
27. Sharma VK, Khandpur S. Unilateral nevoid telangiectasia--response to pulsed dye laser. Int J Dermatol. 2006;45:960-4.
28. van Zuuren EJ, Fedorowicz Z, Carter B, van der Linden MMD, Charland L. Interventions for rosacea. Cochrane Database Syst Rev. 2015;(4):CD003262.
29. Uebelhoer NS, Bogle MA, Stewart B, Arndt KA, Dover JS. A split-face comparison study of pulsed 532-nm KTP laser and 595-nm pulsed dye laser in the treatment of facial telangiectasias and diffuse telangiectatic facial erythema. Dermatol Surg. 2007;33:441-8.
30. Husein-ElAhmed H, Steinhoff M. Laser and light-based therapies in the management of rosacea: an updated systematic review. Lasers Med Sci; 2021.
31. Say EM, Okan G, Gökdemir G. Treatment outcomes of long-pulsed Nd: YAG laser for two different subtypes of rosacea. J Clin Aesthetic Dermatol. 2015;8:16-20.
32. Suggs AK, Macri A, Richmond H, Munavalli G, Friedman PM. Treatment of erythematotelangiectatic rosacea with pulsed-dye laser and oxymetazoline 1.0% cream: a retrospective study. Lasers Surg Med. 2020;52:38-43.
33. Kwon HH, Jung JY, Lee WY, Bae Y, Park GH. Combined treatment of recalcitrant papulopustular rosacea involving pulsed dye laser and fractional microneedling radiofrequency with low-dose isotretinoin. J Cosmet Dermatol. 2020;19:105-11.
34. Schilling LM, Halvorson CR, Weiss RA, Weiss MA, Beasley KL. Safety of combination laser or intense pulsed light therapies and doxycycline for the treatment of rosacea. Dermatol Surg. 2019;45:1401-5.
35. Ko HS, Suh YJ, Byun JW, Choi GS, Shin J. Pulsed dye laser treatment combined with oral minocycline reduces recurrence rate of rosacea. Ann Dermatol. 2017;29:543-7.
36. Zhang C, Ge HS, Yang S, Zhang XJ. Clinical efficacy of 595-nm pulsed-dye laser in treatment of childhood facial spider nevi: a retrospective study of 110 patients. Chin Med J (Engl). 2019;132:2417-22.
37. Yang B, Li L, Zhang L-X, Sun YJ, Ma L. Clinical characteristics and treatment options of infantile vascular anomalies. Medicine (Baltimore). 2015;94:e1717.
38. Ozyurt K, Colgecen E, Baykan H, Ozturk P, Ozkose M. Treatment of superficial cutaneous vascular lesions: experience with the long-pulsed 1064 nm Nd:YAG laser. Sci World J. 2012;2012:197139.
39. Yang J, Guo X, Tong X, Tao J. Treatment of venous lake with multiwavelength 595 and 1064 nm lasers in Asian Fitzpatrick skin type IV patients. Photodermatol Photoimmunol Photomed. 2017;33:267-70.
40. Su Q, Lin T, Wu Q, Wu Y, Guo L, Ge Y. Efficacy of 595 nm pulsed dye laser therapy for Mibelli angiokeratoma. J Cosmet Laser Ther. 2015;17:209-12.
41. Baumgartner J, Šimaljaková M. Genital angiokeratomas of Fordyce 595-nm variable-pulse pulsed dye laser treatment. J Cosmet Laser Ther. 2017;19:459-64.
42. Zeng Y, Zhan K, Xie WL, Lin QZ. Angiokeratoma of Fordyce response to long pulsed Nd:YAG laser treatment. Dermatol Ther. 2016;29:48-51.

43. Ibrahim SM. Pulsed dye laser versus long pulsed Nd:YAG laser in the treatment of angiokeratoma of Fordyce: a randomized, comparative, observer-blinded study. J Dermatol Treat. 2016;27:270-4.
44. Craig LM, Alster TS. Vascular skin lesions in children: a review of laser surgical and medical treatments. Dermatol Surg. 2013;39:1137-46.
45. Lee J, Sinno H, Tahiri Y, Gilardino MS. Treatment options for cutaneous pyogenic granulomas: a review. J Plast Reconstr Aesthetic Surg. 2011;64:1216-20.
46. Tay YK, Weston WL, Morelli JG. Treatment of pyogenic granuloma in children with the flashlamp-pumped pulsed dye laser. Pediatrics. 1997;99:368-70.
47. Khandpur S, Sharma VK. Efficacy of pulsed dye laser in cosmetically distressing facial dermatoses in skin types IV and V. Indian J Dermatol. 2008;53:186-9.
48. Bédard MS, Boulanger J. Treatment of lobular capillary hemangioma with the Nd:YAG laser: retrospective case series of 25 patients. J Cutan Med Surg. 2009;13:181-2.
49. Just U, Hinterhuber G, Knobler R, Neumann R. A potassium-titanyl-phosphate laser is an efficacious tool in the treatment of pyogenic granulomas. A retrospective study in 28 patients. Photochem Photobiol Sci. 2019;18:343-8.
50. Sharma VK, Khandpur S, Khanna N. An interesting case of unilateral angiofibromas successfully treated with pulsed dye laser. J Eur Acad Dermatol Venereol. 2004;18:641-2.
51. Ma G, Wu P, Lin X, Chen H, Li W, Hu X, et al. Nd:YAG laser for "fractional" treatment of angiofibromas. Int J Dermatol. 2014;53:638-42.
52. Tope WD, Kageyama N. "Hot" KTP-laser treatment of facial angiofibromata. Lasers Surg Med. 2001;29:78-81.
53. Bae-Harboe YSC, Geronemus RG. Targeted topical and combination laser surgery for the treatment of angiofibromas. Lasers Surg Med. 2013;45:555-7.
54. Weiss ET, Geronemus RG. New technique using combined pulsed dye laser and fractional resurfacing for treating facial angiofibromas in tuberous sclerosis. Lasers Surg Med. 2010;42:357-60.
55. Weinberger CH, Endrizzi B, Hook KP, Lee PK. Treatment of angiofibromas of tuberous sclerosis with 5-aminolevulinic acid blue light photodynamic therapy followed by immediate pulsed dye laser. Dermatol Surg. 2009;35:1849-51.
56. Murthy AS, Dawson A, Gupta D, Spring S, Cordoro KM. Utility and tolerability of the long-pulsed 1064-nm neodymium:yttrium-aluminum-garnet (LP Nd:YAG) laser for treatment of symptomatic or disfiguring vascular malformations in children and adolescents. J Am Acad Dermatol. 2017;77:473-9.
57. Chen W, Liu S, Yang C, Yang S. Clinical efficacy of the 595 nm pulsed dye laser in the treatment of childhood superficial hemangioma - analysis of 10-year application in Chinese patients. J Dermatol Treat. 2015;26:54-8.
58. Chen W, Yang C, Liu S, Yang S. Curative effect study of pulsed dye laser in the treatment of 43 patients with hand infantile hemangioma. Eur J Dermatol. 2014;24:76-9.
59. Kono T, Sakurai H, Takeuchi M, Yamaki T, Soejima K, Groff WF, et al. Treatment of resistant port-wine stains with a variable-pulse pulsed dye laser. Dermatol Surg. 2007;33:951-6.

CHAPTER 112

Conventional Carbon Dioxide Laser: Indications and Use

Manas Chatterjee, Surbhi Rajput

KEY MESSAGES

- Carbon dioxide (CO_2) lasers are used to ablate a wide range of cutaneous outgrowths with precision. In pulse mode, it works very well as a resurfacing tool for conditions such as acne scars.
- Proper knowledge of the machine is important to obtain desired results and avoid complications.
- Patients need to be properly counseled about the laser and its aspects, especially for aesthetic procedures.

INTRODUCTION

Many advances have been made in the field of laser since 1990. CO_2 laser is the most versatile technology in the field of dermatology as ablative treatment modality in the management of various conditions. It is one of the most widely used lasers with its wavelength, 10,640 nm, being in mid-infrared range. By virtue of this property, it absorbs water which is abundantly present in skin tissues. Hence, this laser is used for ablation of various cutaneous growths with good hemostasis. The laser ensures good recovery with minimal downtime and quick return to daily routine. In addition to that, it is now being used for the management of acne scars and photorejuvenation with fractional mode as the new modality.[1]

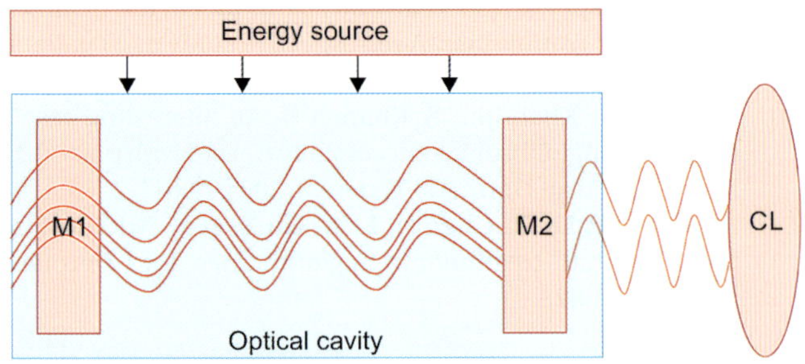

Fig. 1: Illustration of generation of laser. (CL: convex lens; M1: totally reflective mirror; M2: partially transmissive mirror)

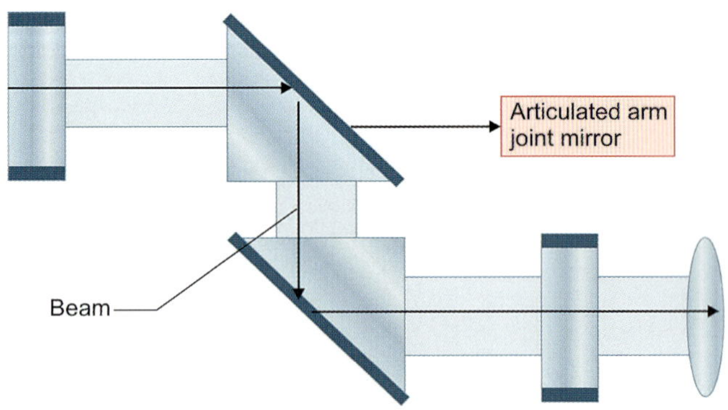

Fig. 2: Schematic illustration of laser articulated arm.

HISTORY

The CO_2 laser was the first laser to be introduced by Indian scientist Kumar Patel in 1964 and was used on the skin by Dr Leon Goldman, and since then it has been extensively used in the dermatological field to remove cutaneous outgrowths. Over the past decade, advances in laser technology have allowed dermatologists to improve the appearance of scars and wrinkles and to remove benign skin growths using CO_2 laser.[2]

COMPONENTS OF CO_2 LASER

- *Energy source:* Electricity
- *Optical cavity* ***(Fig. 1)****:*
  - Active medium
  - Optical resonator—totally reflective (M1) and partially transmissive (M2) mirrors
- *Delivery system* ***(Fig. 2)****:*
  - Articulated arm
  - Hollow tube
  - Mirror joint
  - Lens
  - Handpiece

PRINCIPLES OF CO_2 LASER

The optical cavity contains an active medium comprising gases, predominantly CO_2, along with nitrogen and helium. There are two mirrors on either side of the optical cavity, out of which one is totally reflective and the other is partially reflective. When electric energy is provided to the optical cavity, CO_2 molecules generate photons in mid-infrared range,

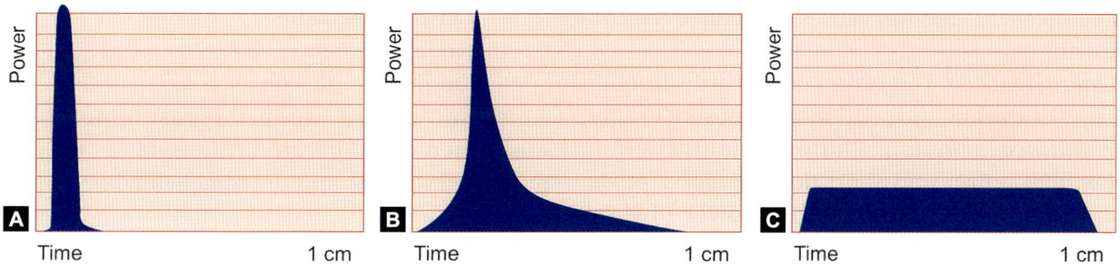

Figs. 3A to C: Modes of CO_2 laser: (A) Ultrapulse; (B) Superpulse; (C) Continuous wave.

which reach a vibratory state, release their energy, and decay to the ground state. The reflective mirror causes the photons to reflect back into the optical cavity to get activated again to a high-energy state, thus causing a state of population inversion. A continuous energy source is required to keep photons in population inversion. Some amount of photons escape through the partially reflective mirror and then converge through a convex lens to the target. The mirror keeps the laser beam collimated. When a focusing lens is attached to the handpiece, it concentrates all the photon energy into a collimated beam, which is then delivered on to the area of interest.[3]

The CO_2 laser is then absorbed by water in skin tissues, which acts as a chromophore. The clinician uses the aiming beam position at the point of focus on the tissue. This amount of laser, on a point of interest, emits an extremely high irradiance converting this energy to heat energy, which is used for ablation. For example, as described by Omi and Numano, a 3 W CO_2 laser light on a spot size of 100 μm will produce a heat energy of 38 W/cm^2 causing precise ablation of the desired tissue. Hence, CO_2 laser is, famously, called the laser scalpel.[3]

As the CO_2 laser emits a high amount of energy, all persons, i.e., the patient, operator, and others in the operating room, are exposed to the laser plume consisting of a high amount of smoke and particulate matter. Hence, a smoke evacuator is mandatory with CO_2 laser to get rid of the side effects of plume.[4]

ENERGY CALCULATIONS

Irradiance is equal to flux per unit area. It is calculated as W/cm^2. Fluence is the total amount of photons pumped into a unit volume of tissues in unit time. The irradiance is inversely proportional to the square ratio of radius or diameter. As the diameter increases, the irradiance decreases. The area is calculated by the formula πr^2. Hence, by simply altering the radius, the operator can drastically increase or decrease the irradiance and can change the mode from excision to vaporization to coagulation.

Calculations:

$$\text{Power} = \text{J/sec (Watts)}$$
$$\text{Spot size} = \pi r^2$$
$$\text{Radius } (r) = \text{Diameter}/2$$
$$\text{Irradiance} = \text{Power/spot size}$$
$$\text{Fluence} = \text{Irradiance} \times \text{Time in seconds}$$

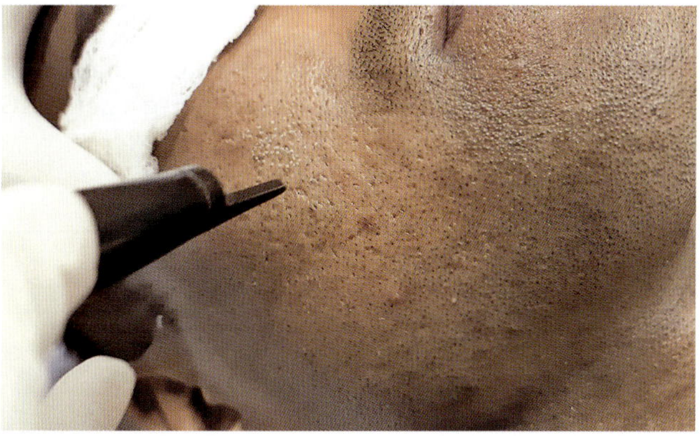

Fig. 4: Delivering pixelated laser energy with conventional CO_2 laser in pulse mode similar to that with fractional laser.

MODES OF CO_2 LASER

There are two modes of CO_2 laser—continuous and pulsed. Continuous mode allows continuous emission of a laser beam as long as the foot pedal is kept pressed. Also, CO_2 laser emits very short high-power outputs with long interpulse intervals. The pulsed mode causes emission of laser radiation at timed intervals through a shutter placed in front of reflection beam. This is referred to as quasi-continuous wave (quasi-CW) laser. It can be short-pulsed or ultrapulsed depending on peak power and interpulse interval. This mode allows precise incision and vaporization with less charring as each pulse duration is shorter than the thermal relaxation time of the tissues. The time can be fixed through a control panel. In pulse mode, one can modify settings to ensure that with free hand, a similar effect to fractional delivery is possible **(Figs. 3 and 4)**.

LASER–TISSUE INTERACTION

The absorption coefficient of 10,640 nm CO_2 laser in water is around 5×10^2/cm. It implies that when a laser beam is incident on tissues, the maximum depth of penetration is 20 μm, hence making this laser a safe modality for ablation of tissue. The various reactions taking place to produce the desired effect are described as follows:

- *Photothermal reaction:* The photothermal reaction occurs at the skin surface where rapid heat emitted by the laser beam is absorbed by water and hence causes vaporization of tissues leading to protein coagulation and cellular necrosis, and this causes immediate removal of the growth.

- *Photochemical reaction:* This causes chemical destruction of the tissues due to low and continuous exposure to light.
- *Photomechanical reaction:* Photomechanical effect requires a high power and short duration laser pulse. When the area is exposed to intense power of short duration, an ionic state of high energy is created, called plasma. When the plasma collides, it disrupts the area of focus of the laser beam with a high amount of energy. There is a threshold energy below which mechanical effect is not seen.
- *Photoacoustic effect:* It is similar to the mechanical effect and is important in yttrium-aluminum-garnet (YAG) lasers.

INDICATIONS

- *Nonaesthetic:*
  - Actinic keratosis and seborrheic keratosis
  - Dermatosis papulosa nigra (DPN)
  - Warts
  - Skin tags and filiform warts
  - Nevi
  - Syringoma and xanthoma
  - Pyogenic granuloma
  - Keratoacanthoma
  - Earlobe keloid and other keloids
  - Sebaceous cyst and mucocele
  - Xanthelasma
  - Dermatofibroma
  - Severe cutaneous photodamage (Favre-Racouchot syndrome)
  - Rhinophyma
  - Actinic cheilitis
  - Sebaceous hyperplasia
  - Pearly penile papule
- *Aesthetic:*
  - Periorbital and perioral wrinkles
  - Facial resurfacing
  - Acne scars
  - Eyelid blepharoplasty

CONTRAINDICATIONS (ALL RELATIVE)

- *Systemic disorders:*
  - Uncontrolled diabetes
  - Uncontrolled hypertension
  - Cardiovascular disorders
  - Bleeding dyscrasias or anticoagulant drugs
  - Collagen vascular disease
- *Local disorders:*
  - Any infection at the site has to be treated
  - History of keloid formation
  - Current ultraviolet radiation and radiation treatment at the site
  - On anticoagulants
  - Chemical peel
  - Dermabrasion

Note: Isotretinoin use in the past 6 months used to be mentioned as a contraindication, but is now no more, as published with the author (cited below).

LASER SETTINGS FOR EACH INDICATION

- *Actinic and seborrheic keratosis:* Topical anesthesia, power: 4–7 W in ultrapulsed mode. Vaporize from top and wipe it with a wet gauze till bleeding points are visible. The ablation should be done till the epidermis only.[5-9]
- *Dermatosis papulosa nigra:* Topical anesthesia, power: 4–8 W. Vaporize from top and wipe it with a wet gauze till it is removed and a clean surface is visible.[10]
- *Warts:*
  - *Verruca vulgaris:* Topical anesthesia for plane warts and local anesthesia (LA) for verruca vulgaris, power: 8–9 W in continuous mode for verruca vulgaris and pulsed mode for flat warts. Vaporize from top with a 2 mm margin to avoid recurrence.[11]
  - *Plantar warts:* Local infiltration, power: 10–12 W with continuous wave mode. Start with vaporizing the wart with a 3 mm margin and then vaporize from top. Wipe the area with a wet gauze piece and the wart will separate. If it does not get removed, repeat the procedure till it happens. Arrest the bleeding by defocusing.[12]
  - *Periungual warts:* Avulse the nail plate to know the extent of the wart. Then, start with a 2 mm margin and vaporize from top. Wipe it with a gauze piece till it is removed.[13]
- *Skin tags, cutaneous horn, and filiform warts:* Topical anesthesia, power: 4–5 W in continuous mode. Avulse the lesion from top and vaporize the base.
- *Nevi—melanocytic nevi, verrucous epidermal nevi, and other dermal and epidermal nevi:* Anesthesia: local infiltration, lase with 4–7.5 W in ultrapulsed mode. Vaporize from top and wipe with a clean gauze piece till a clean base is visible and pigment disappears.[14-20]
- *Syringoma, xanthoma, angiofibroma, and senile comedones:* Topical anesthesia for smaller lesions, local infiltration for larger nodules with power: 4.5–6.5 W. Mark each lesion with a thin surgical pen; vaporize from above till the clear surface is seen. In case of senile comedones, comedone extraction should precede the laser.[21-24]
- *Pyogenic granuloma:* Local infiltration, power: 9–10 W in continuous mode. Vaporize in defocusing mode to avoid torrential bleeding and it is done till hemorrhage is arrested.[25]
- *Keratoacanthoma:* Local infiltration, power: 4–8 W in continuous mode. Vaporize from top and wipe it with a wet gauze piece till the base is clean.[26]

- *Mucocele and pearly penile papules:* Local infiltration, power: 4–4.5 W in ultrapulsed mode with each pulse for 0.1–0.5 seconds. Vaporize till the base is clear.[27]
- *Ear lobe keloid:* Local infiltration, power: 9–15 W in continuous mode and continuous wave. Ablate from the base and inject triamcinolone into the lesion.[28-32]
- *Sebaceous cyst:* Local infiltration, power: 4.5–6 W in continuous mode. A narrow hole is made using the laser followed by squeezing out the sebaceous material and excision of wall through the narrow hole.[33]
- *Actinic cheilitis:* Local infiltration, power: 4–8 W in ultrapulse mode with 0.1–0.5 seconds duration. Vaporize from top with a 2-mm margin and wipe it with a gauze piece till a clear base is visible.[34]
- *Perioral and periorbital rhytides:* Skin resurfacing with conventional CO_2 laser was used for superficial rhytides till the early 90s. The use of a pulsed CO_2 laser was another step forward in skin resurfacing by ablating the superficial epidermis and inducing collagenosis and remodeling. This application, however, came at the cost of unsightly oozing, crusting, and longer patient downtime. For deeper wrinkles, fractional laser and other modalities like fat autologous transplant, thread lift, and dermal fillers are employed. The success of cutaneous resurfacing depends on the number of skin appendages like sweat glands on the skin surface, which act as a source of epithelium required for healing. The more the number of skin appendages, the faster the healing. For this reason, CO_2 laser resurfacing is limited to the face only. Other areas show pigmentation and scarring. Pulsed CO_2 resurfacing has not gained wide acceptance as a resurfacing modality due to thermal damage caused to adjacent tissues. This field is now being taken over by fractional CO_2, Er:YAG, and glass lasers.[35,36]
- *Acne scars:* Pulsed CO_2 laser is used to treat the superficial layer of skin and break the scars. It has been used in the treatment of atrophic scars caused due to acne or trauma. However, the best modality for the treatment of acne scars is fractional CO_2 laser. It helps in the treatment of acne scars with the help of formation of microthermal zones. Candidates for laser treatment should neither have active herpes viral infection 6 months prior to the treatment nor a history of keloids and hypertrophic scars. If there is a history of herpes simplex, prophylactic antivirals are indicated from 3 days prior to laser to 2 days after. Patients with a higher skin phenotype are at a higher risk of hyperpigmentation than patients with a lower phenotype.[37,38] It used to be thought that the use of isotretinoin is a contraindication to the use of ablative lasers but a recent study, which the author was part of and in which all conventional CO_2 laser cases have been those of the author, has debunked this concept.[39] With pulse mode and free hand lasing, one can deliver laser energy in dots leading to untreated tissue in between the pixels, which leads to faster wound healing and lower downtime, almost mirroring that of fractional laser at a much lower cost **(Figs. 5A to D)**.

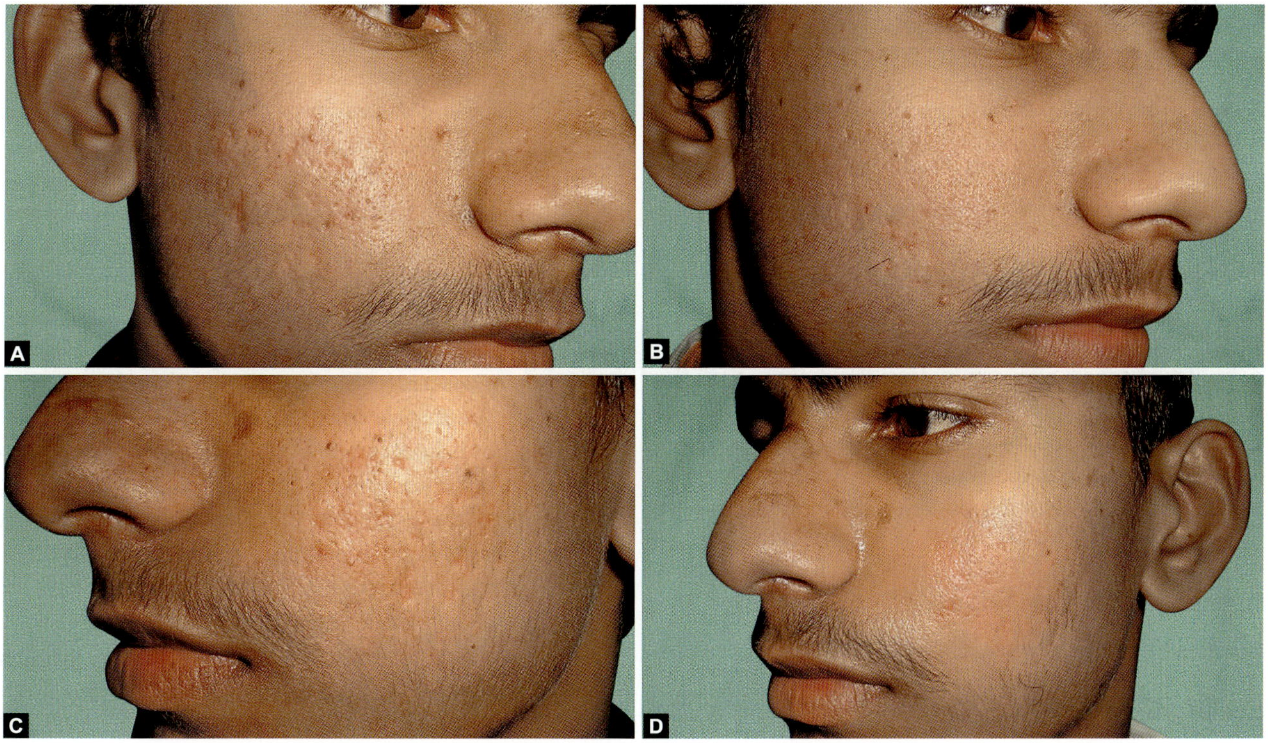

Figs. 5A to D: (A and C) Before; and (B and D) After photographs of both sides of the face with conventional CO_2 laser in pulse mode (5 W, 600 ms on time, 12 ms off time).

MATERIALS NEEDED

- *For surgery:* CO_2 laser, lignocaine as anesthetic agent, physiological saline, needles, syringes, sterile gauze, forceps, suture material, antibiotic cream, and dressing material
- *For safety:* Wavelength-rated spectacles for surgeons and assistants, eye shield for patients, oxygen cylinder, ambu (artificial manual breathing unit) bag, and emergency drug tray
- *Ocular protection:* CO_2 laser which emits wavelength in the mid-infrared range absorbs tissue water, thereby causing damage. Hence, it can absorb tissue water in the cornea and can cause corneal scarring. To prevent this damage, all personnel including the patient and operator should wear wavelength-specific opaque eyewear.
- *Protection from the plume:* The CO_2 laser vaporizes tissues and causes smoke, thus generating tissue debris and various viral particles. Various studies have demonstrated that the laser plume contains human papillomavirus (HPV) DNA. Some reports have shown laryngeal papilloma being caused in patients due to laser plume. Surgical masks should be worn by the operating physician and patient, and smoke evacuators should be kept to remove the viral particles along with smoke.[39,40]
- *Mechanical hazard:* It is essential to know the emergency cutoff switch before using the laser; laser energy can be emitted even without pressing the foot pad. In that case, point the laser beam away from the patient and assistant and press the emergency button to cut the supply.

PREOPERATIVE INVESTIGATIONS

Complete blood picture, random blood sugar, bleeding time, clotting time, viral markers, prothrombin time (PT), activated prothrombin time (APTT) only if indicated, and histopathology (in suspected cutaneous malignancy).

PREOPERATIVE PREPARATION

Written Informed Consent

This should be taken after explaining the disease and the need for procedure, possible postoperative appearance, complications, and need for postoperative care. Selection of a patient is important, and discussing the need for cosmetic surgery and aligning with the patient's expectations should be done in detail.

Control of Systemic Diseases

Diabetes mellitus and hypertension optimization is required.

Local Disease Control

History of previous procedures like dermabrasion, chemical peels, and previous laser resurfacing should be taken. Examination of the skin for dyschromias, elasticity, fibrosis, or scarring should be done. The use of isotretinoin is not a contraindication in pulse mode, but these patients need to be kept under follow-up.

Positioning of Patient

Face, chest, upper limb, abdomen, genitalia, and ventral aspect of lower limb need to be in supine position. Sides of face, neck, and body should be in lateral position. Nape of the neck, back, gluteal region, and dorsal aspect of the lower limb need to be in prone position. Palms should be over the head in supine position. Soles should be in prone position with extended ankles.

Part Preparation

Shave the area minimum 2 cm radius from the lesion. Paint with povidone iodine or other noninflammable agents (spirit should not be used because it is inflammable).

Anesthesia

Depending upon the site and type of lesions, one of the following types of anesthesia can be given:

- *Topical anesthesia:* A eutectic mixture of local anesthesia (EMLA) cream is used. Apply 2 mg/cm^2 topically under occlusion for 60 minutes. The occlusion should be removed just before the procedure.
- *Local infiltration:* Lignocaine 1–2% with or without adrenaline (1:100000) is used. LA is injected as follows: Using 30G needle with a bevel pointing upward, LA is injected immediately below the planned area of the laser. Pinching the lesion before injection will reduce the pain. In case of palms and soles, insert the needle at a 45° angle to the skin surface. Insert the needle at a distance from the lesion such that the tip of the needle is below the lesion after it is pushed into its full length, failing which anesthesia will be deposited distal to the lesion. For the injections near the eyes, always be parallel to the surface to avoid injury to the eyes.
- *Circumferential block:* This block is employed to anesthetize fingers, toes, and penis. It is not deposited as a ring but is injected on both sides at the location of the nerves. In fingers and toes, it is called distal digital block. The needle is inserted at the base of the fingers and toes on either side and anesthetic is deposited on both sides. The LA is injected while withdrawing. In the case of penile region, LA is given at the base of the shaft.
- *Field block:* Local anesthesia is infiltrated circumferentially around the site, blocking the nerve impulse from leaving the area. The actual surgical site is not injected. It is particularly useful when a large area needs to be anesthetized such as a large sebaceous cyst.

GENERAL INSTRUCTIONS FOR THE OPERATION OF LASER

- Hold the handpiece like holding a pen.
- Hold the handpiece perpendicular to the lesion and press the foot pedal to fire the laser. Vaporize the lesion in a coiled, whorled, centrifugal, vertical, or horizontal fashion. Vaporize the flat lesions from the top.
- Pedunculated lesions can be excised by lasing from the base of the lesion. Hold the lesion with toothed forceps on the top and pull it to the side on the top of the wet gauze (to prevent charring of the normal skin). Always use wet gauze as dry gauze can catch fire.
- Wipe the vaporized lesions with wet gauze. Always make sure to dry the area or wipe the water with dry gauze. Look for raw areas. Coagulate the bleeding spots, if any, by defocusing the laser beam.

PRACTICAL TIPS ON USE OF CO_2 LASER

- Always use handpiece pointed on the skin to cut.
- Remember that the lens focuses on the beam and renders it collimated.
- Moving the handpiece away (defocusing) leads to logarithmic fall in irradiance; use it to coagulate.
- Superpulse CO_2 laser reduces dwell time and maximizes power.
- Use continuous wave in highly vascular lesions and areas, debulking, and where aesthetics is not an issue, e.g., foot.
- Undertreat and eschew therapeutic greed.
- Laser settings in texts are often for collimated handpieces; read carefully before applying. One-third to one-fourth of the irradiance suggested in the texts seems to deliver the results.
- The newer CO_2 lasers with advanced output control software when used in the superpulsed mode for carrying out free hand procedures are versatile devices with numerous therapeutic options.

POSTOPERATIVE CARE AND FOLLOW-UP

- For superficial lesions like seborrheic keratosis and DPNs, topical antibiotic cream, bland face wash, and sunscreen will be sufficient and postoperative follow-up is 7th day and 1 month.
- Superficial lesions in covered areas can be treated only with topical antibiotics. For deeper facial lesions like moles, hydrocolloid dressing is important and follow-up is 7 days, 1 month, 3 months, and 1 year.
- Allow the scabs to fall on their own. Avoid picking.
- Emphasize sunscreen application three times a day from day 1 for the lesions on the face and neck.
- Treat for postinflammatory hyperpigmentation, if any, with Kligman's formula.
- Allow occlusive pressure dressing to remain in place for 3–7 days and do not wet the area.
- Look for healthy granulation tissue after removal of the occlusive dressing.
- Avoid contact with dust. Use antibiotic-impregnated premade tapes, if needed, for a couple of days for protection.

COMPLICATIONS[41-43]

Minor Complications

Postoperative edema may occur, which resolves within 2–3 hours with cold compresses. Postinflammatory hyperpigmentation, erythema, milia formation, perioral dermatitis, exacerbation of acne/rosacea, and contact dermatitis are some of the minor complications. Hyperpigmentation or erythema is common in colored skin, which generally resolves within 6 weeks with appropriate treatment.

Major Complications

Viral, bacterial, candidal infection, persistent erythema, hypopigmentation, and delayed wound healing are some common major complications. Scarring, ectropion formation, and disseminated infection are more serious complications.

CONCLUSION

The CO_2 laser is the most widely accepted machine for treating benign cutaneous outgrowths and scars and for skin rejuvenation. It requires proper knowledge about the machine and technique, and if used by a trained physician, it provides the most precise incision and excision. However, its use may be associated with delayed postoperative healing and changes like crusting, oozing, and hyperpigmentation, if not done in the correct manner as described above.

REFERENCES

1. Krupa Shankar D, Chakravarthi M, Shilpakar R. Carbon dioxide laser guidelines. J Cutan Aesthet Surg. 2009;2(2):72-80.
2. Kaplan I. The CO_2 surgical laser. Photomed Laser Surg, 2010;28:847-8.
3. Omi T, Numano K. The Role of the CO_2 Laser and Fractional CO_2 Laser in Dermatology. Laser Ther. 2014;23(1):49-60.
4. Ohshiro T. The laser apple: A new graphic representation of medical laser applications. Laser Therapy. 1996;8:185-90.
5. Trimas SJ, Ellis DA, Metz RD. The carbon dioxide laser: An alternative for the treatment of actinically damaged skin. Dermatol Surg. 1997;23(10):885-9.
6. Phahonthep R, Sindhuphak W, Sriprajittichai P. Lidocaine iontophoresis versus EMLA cream for CO_2 laser treatment in seborrheic keratosis. J Med Assoc Thai. 2004;87:S15-8.
7. Fulton JE, Rahimi AD, Helton P, Dahlberg K, Kelly AG. Disappointing results following resurfacing of facial skin with CO_2 lasers for prophylaxis of keratosis and cancers. Dermatol Surg. 1999;25:729-32.

8. Fitzpatrick RE, Goldman MP, Ruiz-Esparza J. Clinical advantage of the CO_2 laser superpulsed mode. Treatment of verruca vulgaris, seborrheic keratosis, lentigines and actinic cheilitis. J Dermatol Surg Oncol. 1994;20(7):449-56.
9. Quaedvlieg PJ, Ostertag JU, Krekels GA, Neumann HA. Delayed wound healing after three different treatments for widespread actinic keratosis on the atrophic bald scalp. Dermatol Surg. 2003;29(10):1052-6.
10. Furukawa F, Mizawa M, Shimizu T. Treatment of dermatosis papulosa nigra using a carbon dioxide laser. J Cosmet Dermatol. 2020;19(10):2572-5.
11. Takac S. The CO_2 laser and verruca vulgaris. Med pregl. 2000;53(7-8):389-93.
12. Landsman MJ, Mancuso JE, Abramow SP. Carbon dioxide laser treatment of pedal verrucae. Clin Podiatr Med Surg. 1992;9(3):659-69.
13. Lim JT, Goh CL. Carbon dioxide laser treatment of periungual and subungual viral warts. Australas J Dermatol. 1992;33(2): 87-91.
14. Bhat YJ, Hassan I, Sajad P, Yaseen A, Mubashir S, Akhter S, et al. Evaluation of Carbon Dioxide Laser in the Treatment of Epidermal Nevi. J Cutan Aesthet Surg. 2016;9(3): 183-7
15. Hohenleutner U, Wlotzke U, Konz B, Landthaler M. Carbon dioxide laser therapy of a widespread epidermal nevus. Lasers Surg Med. 1995;16(3):288-91.
16. Khoo L. Carbon dioxide laser treatment of benign skin lesions. National Skin Centre Experience. 2001;12:2.
17. Verma KK, Ovung EM. Epidermal and sebaceous nevi treatment with carbon dioxide laser. Indian J Dermatol Venereol Leprol. 2002;68(1):23-4.
18. Ratz JL, Bailin PL, Wheeland RG. Carbon dioxide laser treatment of epidermal nevi. J Dermatol Surg Oncol. 1986; 12:567-70.
19. Boyce S, Alster TS. CO_2 laser treatment of epidermal nevi: Long-term success. Dermatol Surg. 2002;28(7):611-4.
20. Hohenleutner U, Landthaler M. Laser therapy of verrucous epidermal naevi. Clin Exp Dermatol. 1993;18(2):124-7.
21. Wang JI, Roenigk HH Jr. Treatment of multiple facial syringomas with the carbon dioxide laser (CO_2). Dermatol Surg. 1999;25(2):136-9.
22. Wheeland RG, Bailin PL, Reynolds OD, Ratz JL. Carbon dioxide (CO_2) laser vaporization of multiple facial syringomas. J Dermatol Surg Oncol. 1986;12(3):225-8.
23. Belmar P, Boixeda P, Baniandres O, Fernandez-Lorente M, Arrazola JM. [Long-term follow up of angiofibromas treated with CO_2 laser in 23 patients with tuberous sclerosis]. Actas Dermosifiliogr. 2005;96:498-503.
24. Papadavid E, Markey A, Bellaney G, Walker NPJ. Carbon dioxide and pulsed dye laser treatment of angiofibromas in 29 patients with tuberous sclerosis. Br J Dermatol. 2002; 147(2):337-42.
25. Raulin C, Greve B, Hammes S. The combined continuous-wave/pulsed carbon dioxide laser for treatment of pyogenic granuloma. Arch Dermatol. 200;138(1):33-7.
26. Ambur A, Clark A, Nathoo R. An Updated Review of the Therapeutic Management of Keratoacanthomas. J Clin Aesthet Dermatol. 202;15(12 Suppl 1):S16-22.
27. Huang IY, Chen CM, Kao YH, Worthington P. Treatment of mucocele of the lower lip with carbon dioxide laser. J Oral Maxillofac Surg. 2007;65(5):855-8.
28. Nowak KC, McCormack M, Koch RJ. The effect of superpulsed carbon dioxide laser energy on keloid and normal dermal fibroblast secretion of growth factors: A serum-free study. Plast Reconstr Surg. 2000;105(6):2039-48.
29. Garg GA, Sao PP, Khopkar US. Effect of carbon dioxide laser ablation followed by intralesional steroids on keloids. J Cutan Aesthet Surg. 2011;4(1):2-6.
30. Apfelberg DB, Maser MR, Lash H, White D, Weston J. Preliminary results of argon and carbon dioxide laser treatment of keloid scars. Lasers Surg Med. 1984;4(3):283-90.
31. Cheng ET, Pollard JD, Koch RJ. Effect of blended CO_2 and erbium: YAG laser irradiation on normal and keloid fibroblasts: A serum-free study. J Clin Laser Med Surg. 2003; 21(6):337-43.
32. Krupa Shankar DS, Gupta V. Management of ear rim keloid with carbon dioxide laser. Indian J Dermatol Venereol Leprol. 2007;73:445.
33. Wang ZC, Zhao WY, Fang QQ, Wu LH, Tan WQ. CO_2 Laser Punch-Assisted Minimally Invasive Surgery for Sebaceous Cysts. Lasers Surg Med. 2020;52(8):743-6.
34. Ayen-Rodriguez A, Naranjo-Diaz MJ, Ruiz-Villaverde R. Laser Therapy for the Treatment of Actinic Cheilitis: A Systematic Review. Int J Environ Res Public Health. 2022;19(8):4593.
35. Yumeen S, Khan T. Laser Carbon Dioxide Resurfacing. In: StatPearls [Internet]. Treasure Island (FL): StatPearls Publishing; 2024. [online] Available from https://www.ncbi.nlm.nih.gov/books/NBK560544/ [Last accessed February, 2024].
36. Fitzpatrick RE, Goldman MP, Satur NM, Tope WD. Pulsed carbon dioxide laser resurfacing of photo-aged facial skin. Arch Dermatol. 1996;132(4):395-402.
37. Tanzi EL, Alster TS. Single-pass carbon dioxide versus multiple-pass Er:YAG laser skin resurfacing. A comparison of postoperative wound healing and side effect rates. Dermatol Surg. 2003;29(1):80-4.
38. Petrov A, Pljakovska V. Fractional Carbon Dioxide Laser in Treatment of Acne Scars. Open Access Maced J Med Sci. 2016;4(1):38-42.
39. Mahadevappa OH, Mysore V, Viswanath V, Thurakkal S, Majid I, Talwar S, et al. Surgical outcome in patients taking concomitant or recent intake of oral isotretinoin: A Multicentric Study-ISO-AIMS Study. J Cutan Aesthet Surg. 2016;9(2):106-14.
40. Rosio TJ. Basic laser physics. In: Roenigk RK, Ratz JL, Roenigk HH (Eds). Roenigk's Dermatologic Surgery, 3rd edition. New York: Informa Healthcare; 2007. pp. 607-24.
41. Wisniewski PM, Warhol MJ, Rando RF, Sedlacek TV, Kemp JE, Fisher JC. Studies on the transmission of viral disease via CO_2 laser plume and ejecta. J Reprod Med. 1990; 35(12):1117-23.
42. Ramsdell WM. Fractional CO_2 laser resurfacing complications. Semin Plast Surg. 2012;26(3):137-40.
43. Naouri M, Delage M, Khallouf R, Georgesco G, Atlan M. [CO_2 fractional resurfacing: side effects and immediate complications]. Ann Dermatol Venereol. 2011;138(1):7-10.

CHAPTER 113

Er:YAG Laser

Subodh Jane, Mysore Venkataram

KEY MESSAGES

- Ablative erbium-doped yttrium aluminum garnet (Er:YAG) laser resurfacing offers significant improvement with minimal adverse effects and less downtime.
- Tissue water has 12–16 times more absorption coefficient for Er:YAG laser wavelength (2,940 nm) than carbon dioxide (CO_2) laser.
- Higher absorption of laser light in tissue water gives Er:YAG an advantage of precise and controlled depth of ablation and thermal diffusion in skin.
- Ablation and coagulation by Er:YAG laser can be controlled by stacking of pulse and variable pulse width, respectively.
- Ablative laser can be rendered nonablative by using sublative fluence (0.7 J/cm^2) and super long pulse width (200–250 ms).
- Such variable pulse width options give operator ease to use it in multiple skin conditions in an efficient and safe way.

INTRODUCTION

Erbium yttrium aluminum garnet (Er:YAG) was first introduced in 1990s for the resurfacing of photodamaged skin[1] and since then it has been considered as a good alternative modality to the carbon dioxide (CO_2) laser for skin resurfacing. The Er:YAG laser is a flashlamp-pumped yttrium aluminum garnet host crystals laser system, doped with erbium ions. Er:YAG emits light in the infrared range with wavelength of 2,940 nm and its chromophore is water. This wavelength is closer to the peak absorption spectrum of water and therefore has an absorption coefficient 12–16 times higher than CO_2 laser.[2] Since the skin consists of 70% water, the higher absorption in water decreases penetration depth into epidermis by a factor of 10 as compared to the CO_2 laser **(Figs. 1A and B)**.

Therefore, Er:YAG laser can cause precise ablation of the skin tissue with less damage to the surrounding tissue and has been used effectively with fewer adverse effects and faster healing time. A comparison between Er:YAG and CO_2 laser is given in **Table 1**. It is also a versatile laser and can be used in different modes—ablative or fractional ablative and even nonablative modes by varying pulsed delivery.

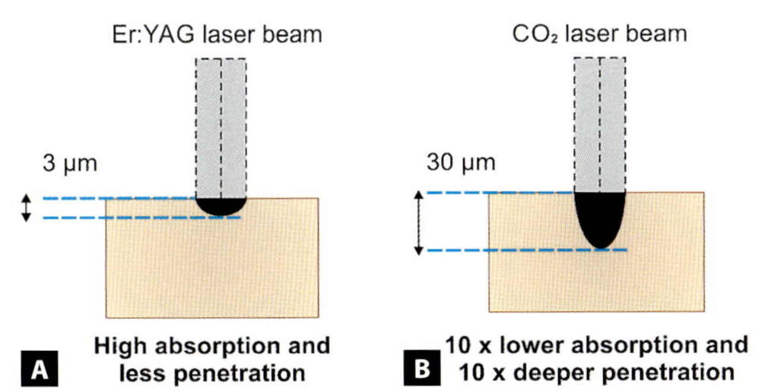

Figs. 1A and B: Depth of penetration of ablative (A) Er:YAG laser beam and (B) CO_2 laser.

Ablation and coagulation: Different laser tissue interactions have been explained in previous chapters. The important types of laser tissue interaction in case of Er:YAG or CO_2 laser include ablation, coagulation, and vaporization. Initially the tissue is heated directly within the optical absorption depth (ablation) followed by indirect heating of deeper tissue by thermal diffusion (coagulation or necrosis).

Stacking of laser pulses: The extent of *direct heating, i.e., ablation* is dependent on the absorption of laser light by

TABLE 1: Comparison of Er:YAG and CO_2 laser.

Parameters	*Er:YAG*	*CO_2*
Wavelength	2,940 nm	10,600 nm
Chromophore	Water	Water
Absorption coefficient	12,000 cm^{-1} (Higher)	800 cm^{-1} (Lesser)
Penetration	Superficial	Deep
Minimum ablation	3 µm	20–30 µm
Coagulation or thermal diffusion	5–50 µm*	80–150 µm*
Energy delivery	Precise	Diffuse
Hemostatic effect	Less	More
Dermal tightening	Less	More
Efficacy	Less	More
Healing time or down time	Short duration	Longer
Treatment specificity	Better for superficial conditions	Better for deeper or dermal conditions
Adverse effects	Less frequent	More frequent

*When short pulsed (250–300 ms) laser is used. Longer pulse width causes deeper thermal diffusion.

the tissue water. As discussed earlier, the coefficient of absorption of water is more with Er:YAG laser wavelength (2,940 nm), so laser light is completely absorbed by the tissue water, limiting its depth of penetration. After the ablation threshold of tissue (1.5 J/cm^2), for every 1 J/cm^2 of fluence the approximate depth of ablation achieved by Er:YAG is 3–5 µm.[3] Thus, we can easily calculate the required fluence to achieve a particular ablation depth. The depth of ablation can be increased by *increasing the repeated delivery of laser (stacking) on the same spot* because of an additive effect. Fluence of 5 J/cm^2 produces depth of 20–40 µm, up to 60 µm and 80–120 µm after 1, 2, and 3 stacking pulses, respectively.[4] In Er:YAG laser, the level of depth achieved is indicated by color change of the tissue after ablation, as mentioned in **Table 2**.[4]

Role of pulse width: Ablation of the tissue is followed by indirect heating or coagulation of deep tissue by heat diffusion, which is totally dependent on the duration of the laser pulse (pulse width). If the pulse width is short then the thermal diffusion will be superficial and if pulse width is long then the heat has enough time to diffuse in the tissue causing deeper coagulation **(Figs. 2A to C)**.

During the past decade, many advances have been made with the Er:YAG laser. Previously, Er:YAG laser had pulse duration in the range of 25–300 microseconds, which produces ablation with minimal or no coagulation.[5] Recently, the pulse duration has been modified (*the so called variable pulse*) by prolonging its duration *up to 250 ms*, producing ablation and more coagulation by deeper heat diffusion.[6] Thus with variable pulse width we get flexibility to adjust the depth of coagulation precisely.

Sublative or nonablative mode of ablative Er:YAG laser: As a result of this modification in pulse width, now one can use Er:YAG laser in "sublative or thermal mode", which means the use of fluence below ablative threshold and pulse duration of 200–250 ms to create heat in upper dermal layer without causing epidermal ablation.[6] If sublative laser fluence (2–3 J/cm^2) with *super long pulse of 200–250 ms* is used, then the epidermis get enough time to cool down by dissipating heat to the deeper tissue. Therefore, the temperature required for ablation will never be achieved and multiple passes of such mode will lead to build-up of heat in deeper tissue causing skin rejuvenation and tightening.[6]

In this way by adjusting pulse width and number of passes (stacking), we can use ablative Er:YAG laser as non-ablative Er:YAG type, as well as erbium-doped yttrium scandium gallium garnet (Er:YSGG) and CO type laser.[3]

TABLE 2: Level of ablation by laser and its external appearance.

Level of ablation	*Indicator*
Epidermis	Yellowish-brown appearance
Epidermal-dermal junction	Pinkish appearance
Papillary dermis	Pinpoint bleeding from small capillaries of the dermis
Upper reticular dermis	More bleeding and transuded as the collateral thermal diffusion by the Er:YAG laser is insufficient to coagulate vessels

INDICATIONS (TABLE 3)

Ablative Er:YAG Laser

- *Facial rhytides:* Er:YAG laser is found to be effective with faster healing time and minimal adverse effects. The parameters used are—fluence of 5–8 J/cm^2 with 2–8 laser passes depending on depth of the rhytides.[7]
- *Lentigines:* Q-switched (QS) frequency doubled Nd:YAG laser (532 nm) followed by low fluence.

  Erbium-doped yttrium aluminum garnet laser has been found to be effective and safe. QS frequency doubled Nd:YAG laser light causes destruction of melanosome containing cells (selective photothermolysis) which results in improvement in the pigmented lesions and ablative Er:YAG helps in transepidermal clearance. The parameters used for Er:YAG laser were—fluence of 0.7 J/cm^2, 12 mm spot size, and 15 Hz frequency with 2–3 passes.[8]
- *Epidermal nevus:* Er:YAG laser is effective in the treatment of superficial and small epidermal nevus, with fluence of 0.45 J/cm^2, 2 mm of spot size, and 4 pulses/second frequency.[9]
- *Vitiligo surgery:*
  - *Er:YAG-assisted punch grafting:* Er:YAG can be used to prepare recipient area 2.25 mm spot size (less than donor punch size), 1,000 mJ/pulse and 10 Hz frequency with 10 passes on hands and 12 passes on legs can be used to create holes for punch grafts. The endpoint

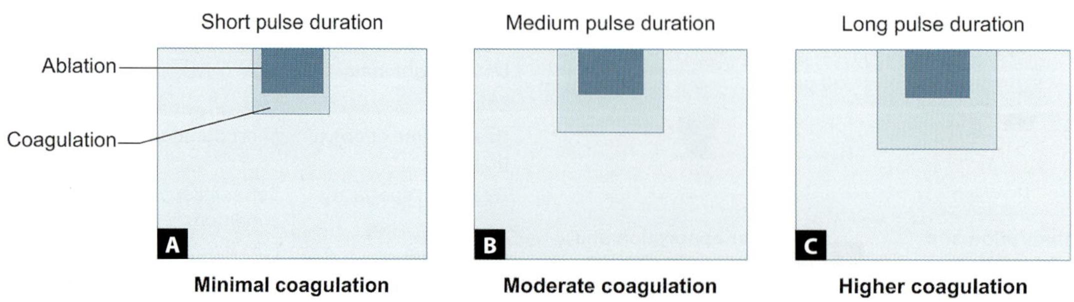

Figs. 2A to C: Influence of laser pulse duration (variable pulse) on heat diffusion.

TABLE 3: Indications of Er:YAG laser.

Category	*Ablative*	*Fractional ablative*
Skin disorders	• Epidermal nevi • Epidermal and benign dermal tumors • Xanthelasma • Lentigines • Verruca vulgaris • Acne keloidalis nuchae • Elevated scar • Rhinophyma • Vitiligo—to prepare recipient area • Seborrheic keratosis • Actinic cheilitis • Vascular growths	• Acne scarring • Melasma • Rhinophyma • Lichen amyloidosis • Drug delivery of drugs • Granuloma annulare • Colloid milium • Porokeratosis
Aesthetics	Deep facial rhytids	• Photoaging • Periorbital wrinkles • Surgical scars • Striae gravidarum • Residual hemangiomas

the procedure is appearance of tiny papillary dermal bleeding. The significance of Er:YAG assisted punch grafting is 2–3 times more perigraft pigmentation and therefore lesser requirement of grafts.[10]

- *Autologous cultured or noncultured melanocyte transfer:* Ablative Er:YAG can be used to prepare recipient area quickly and safely compared to dermabrader. The required depth of ablation is 40–50 µm and 350–450 µm for lips and face or body, respectively. The endpoint is appearance of pinpoint bleeding point which indicates complete removal of epidermis. The benefits of using Er:YAG include fast method, controlled and efficient tissue ablation with minimal risk of thermal injury and scarring.

- *Verruca vulgaris (warts):* Er:YAG laser is found to be a good treatment option for nongenital cutaneous warts especially in case of plantar warts. Er:YAG laser followed after 1 week by podophyllotoxin application (three consecutive days/week for 4–6 weeks) showed good results in plantar wart with lower recurrence compared to Er:YAG alone.[11]

Fractional Ablative Laser

- *Melasma*: Er:YAG can be used in refractory melasma with significant clinical improvement with fluence of 5.1–7.6 J/cm^2.[12]
- *Lichen amyloidosis*: Fractional Er:YAG laser has been found to be effective and well-tolerated modality for the treatment of lichen amyloidosis **(Figs. 3A and B)**. The parameters were: 1,400 mJ of energy with 6–8 stacking of laser pulse at each spot and procedure was done once in 3 weeks.[13]

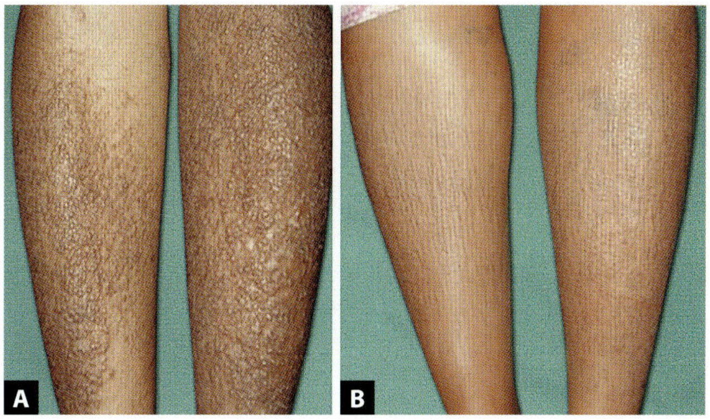

Figs. 3A and B: Lichen amyloidosis (A) before and (B) after six sessions of Er:YAG laser.

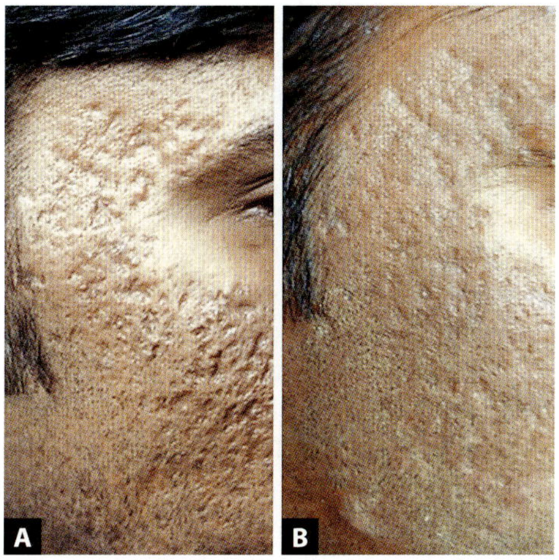

Figs. 4A and B: Grade 4 acne scarring (A) before and (B) after four sessions of Er:YAG laser.

- *Striae distensae:* Fractional Er:YAG laser has been found to be effective in resurfacing of striae distensae with minimal adverse effects.[14]
- *Drug delivery system:* Low fluence ablative or fractional ablative Er:YAG laser can be used to disrupt the stratum corneum and therefore to increase the delivery of drug in the skin. Topical lidocaine or eutectic mixture of local anesthetic cream usually takes long time to act but when used after ablation of stratum corneum by Er:YAG laser, it gives quick and effective local anesthesia. The effect of anesthesia starts within 5 minutes of application and if kept for long time it produces more anesthesia than the topical anesthetic cream alone.[15-17]
- *Other indications*: Atrophic facial acne scars **(Figs. 4A and B)**, rhinophyma, sebaceous hyperplasia, angiofibroma, adenoma sebaceum, hidradenoma, xanthelasma, trichoepithelioma, syringomas, moles, mild dyschromia, Favre–Racouchot disease, and pyogenic granuloma.

ADVANTAGES AND DISADVANTAGES

The advantages and disadvantages of Er:YAG laser have been listed in **Box 1**.

BOX 1: Advantages and disadvantages of Er:YAG laser.

Advantages over CO_2 laser:

- Better control on ablation and thermal diffusion
- Coagulation by thermal diffusion is less and controlled compared to the CO_2 laser
- Less pain, short duration of postprocedure erythema, hyperpigmentation, and recovery[17]

Disadvantages:

- Less efficacy than CO_2 laser
- Less effective in deeper rhytides and severe scar
- Less thermal coagulation of blood vessels so more bleeding compared to CO_2 laser

COMPLICATIONS

The complications of Er:YAG laser depend upon the location being treated and the depth of skin removal. The common, minor, immediate, and predictable complications, which last for few days after therapy include pain, pruritus, swelling, oozing, crusting, postinflammatory hyperpigmentation, and erythema. Less common complications include permanent hyper- or hypopigmentation, milia formation, perioral dermatitis, rosacea exacerbation, contact dermatitis, localized viral, bacterial, candidal infections, hypertrophic scarring, disseminated infection, ectropion, and nail deformity (periungual wart).[18]

Early detection of complications and rapid institution of appropriate therapy are extremely important. Delay in treatment can have severe deleterious consequences including permanent scarring and dyspigmentation.

COMBINATION WITH OTHER TREATMENTS

The Er:YAG laser has been used in combination with other lasers in a number of indications.

- *Hori's nevus or nevus of Ota:* Er:YAG laser with sublative fluence followed by QS Nd:YAG laser has been found to be effective and safe if used in combination. It is postulated that Er:YAG laser with fluence of 0.7 J/cm^2, 12 mm spot size with 2–3 passes partially ablates the epidermis that removes the epidermal melanin. This leads to less scattering and deeper penetration of QS Nd:YAG laser light.[19]
- *Onychomycosis:* Fractional Er:YAG laser followed by application of 5% amorolfine lacquer has been found to be effective and safe treatment method for onychomycosis. Fractional Er:YAG laser treatment was done once in a week for 4 weeks and then once in a month for 2 months and 5% amorolfine was applied twice a week.[20]
- *Palmoplantar warts:* Ablative Er:YAG laser and topical podophyllotoxin has been found to be safe and effective. The laser parameters used were: 5.7-11 J/cm^2 of fluence and 3 mm of spot size. Podophyllum toxin was applied after wound healing for 3 days followed by 4 days of break, 4-6 such cycles were performed.[21]

BOX 2: Practical tips for effective and safe use of Er:YAG laser.

- Proper priming before procedure is very important to avoid post-inflammatory hyperpigmentation (PIH)
- Always consider skin type of patient before setting parameters as patients with skin type IV–VI are prone for development of PIH
- Place the laser handpiece in touch and perpendicular to the focused area
- Use parameters by considering the thickness of treating area, like periorbital skin is thin compared to the face and rest of body
- For pure ablation use shorter pulse width; for less ablation and more heating use longer pulse width
- Depth of ablation can be increased by stacking (multiple passes on same spot) of laser pulses to treat deeper condition
- Higher degree of skills and proper knowledge of laser machine are important to obtain optimum results
- Always undertreat; avoid overtreating

- *CO_2 laser with Er:YAG laser:* Er:YAG laser after CO_2 laser has used to reduce the adverse effects of CO laser.[22]
- *Tattoo removal:* Fractional Er:YAG laser followed by Q switched Nd:YAG laser has been found to enhance the efficacy of laser tattoo removal.[23] This combination of laser appears to prevent blistering by releasing the gases and intercellular fluid through the microchannels. Similarly the combination also enhances pigment clearance through transepidermal elimination. This minimizes number of sessions with faster healing.

OTHER USES

Many in vitro and in vivo studies have been found that fractional ablative Er:YAG laser can be used to increase the transdermal delivery of medications. Singhal M et al. has been found that fractional ablation of Er:YAG laser can be used to enable "needleless" cutaneous deposition of polymeric microparticles containing triamcinolone acetonide (TA). This approach may provide a uniform, effective, targeted, and minimally invasive alternative option to more painful intralesional injections of TA for the treatment of keloid.[24]

Lee WR et al. found that prior use of fractional Er:YAG laser increases imiquimod cream influx by 46–127 fold. Therefore imiquimod concentration of 0.4% cream with Er:YAG laser treatment was sufficient to approximate the flux from the cream with 5% concentration alone, indicating a reduction of the drug dose by 125 fold.[25]

Similarly, Er:YAG laser can be used to increase the penetration of minoxidil and peptides in alopecia;[26] to increase the absorption of narcotic drugs including morphine, nalbuphine, and buprenorphine having low oral bioavailability;[27] and to increase the transdermal flux of vitamin C derivatives.[28]

Recently nonablative mode of Er:YAG laser has found application in vaginal tightening, stress incontinence, and feminine rejuvenation. Here the laser is delivered through a special applicator inserted into the vagina to ensure delivery circumferentially (in 360°) **(Box 2)**.[29,30]

CONCLUSION

The Er:YAG laser is a safe, precise, and versatile laser useful in a number of indications; while its depth of penetration is limited as compared to CO_2 laser. Thorough knowledge of the laser parameters is necessary to ensure optimum and safe results.

REFERENCES

1. Janik JP, Markus JL, Al-Dujaili Z, Markus RF. Laser resurfacing. Semin Plast Surg. 2007;21(3):139-46.
2. Kaufmann R, Hartmann A, Hibst R. Cutting and skin ablative properties of pulsed mid-infrared laser surgery. J Dermatol Surg Oncol. 1994;20:112-8.
3. Sardana K, Ghunawat S. Lasers for lentigines, from Q-switched to erbium-doped yttrium aluminium garnet micropeel, is there a need to reinvent the wheel? J Cutan Aesthet Surg. 2015;8:233-5.
4. Sardana K, Garg VJ. Ablative lasers. In: Sardana K (Ed). Lasers in Dermatological Practice, 1st edition. New Delhi: Jaypee Brothers Medical Publishers; 2014. p. 90.
5. Hibst R, Kaufmann R. Effects of laser parameters on pulsed erbium:YAG laser skin ablation. Lasers Med Sci. 1991;6:391-7.
6. El-Domyati M, El-Ammawi ES, Medhat W, Moawad O, Mahoney MG, Uitto J. Multiple minimally invasive Erbium:YAG laser mini-peels for skin rejuvenation: An objective assessment. J Cosmet Dermatol. 2012;11(2):122-30.
7. Khatri KA, Ross V, Grevelink JM, Magro CM, Anderson RR. Comparison of Erbium:YAG and carbon dioxide lasers in resurfacing of facial rhytides. Arch Dermatol. 1999;135(4): 391-7.
8. Tian BW. Novel low fluence combination laser treatment of solar lentigines in Type III Asian skin. J Cutan Aesthet Surg. 2015;8(4):230-2.
9. Pearson IC, Harland CC. Epidermal naevi treated with pulsed erbium:YAG laser. Clin Exp Dermatol. 2004;29(5):494-6.
10. Pai GS, Vinod V, Joshi A. Efficacy of erbium YAG laser-assisted autologous epidermal grafting in vitiligo. J Eur Acad Dermatol Venereol. 2002;16(6):604-6.
11. Nguyen J, Korta DZ, Chapman LW, Kelly KM. Laser treatment of nongenital verrucae a systematic review. JAMA Dermatol. 2016;152(9):1025-33.
12. Manaloto RM, Alster T. Erbium:YAG laser resurfacing for refractory melasma. Dermatol Surg. 1999;25(2):121-3.
13. Anitha B, Mysore V. Lichen amyloidosis: Novel treatment with fractional ablative 2,940 nm Erbium: YAG laser treatment. J Cutan Aesthet Surg. 2012;5:141-3.
14. Lokhande AJ, Mysore V. Striae distensae treatment review and update. Indian Dermatol Online J. 2019;10(4):380-95.
15. Yun PL, Tachihara R, Anderson RR. Efficacy of erbium:yttrium-aluminum-garnet laser-assisted delivery of topical anesthetic. J Am Acad Dermatol. 2002;47(4):542-7.
16. Tian T, Luo Y1, Jiang T, Dong Y, Yu A, Chen H, et al. Clinical effect of ablative fractional laser-assisted topical anesthesia on human skin: a randomized pilot study. J Cosmet Laser Ther. 2016;18(7):409-12.
17. Oni G, Rasko Y, Kenkel J. Topical lidocaine enhanced by laser pretreatment: a safe and effective method of analgesia for facial rejuvenation. Aesthet Surg J. 2013;33(6):854-61.
18. Jung KE, Jung KH, Park YM, Lee JY, Kim TY, Kim HO, et al. A Split-face comparison of ablative fractional lasers (CO_2 and Er:YAG) in Asian patients; postprocedure erythema, pain and patient's satisfaction. J Cosmet Laser Ther. 2013;15(2): 70-3.
19. Tian BW. Novel treatment of Hori's nevus: a combination of fractional nonablative 2,940-nm Er:YAG and low-fluence 1,064-nm Q-switched Nd:YAG laser. J Cutan Aesthet Surg. 2015;8:227-9.
20. Zhang J, Lu S, Huang H, Li X, Cai W, Ma J, et al. Combination therapy for onychomycosis using a fractional 2940-nm Er:YAG laser and 5 % amorolfine lacquer. Lasers Med Sci. 2016;31(7):1391-6.
21. Wollina U. Er:YAG laser followed by topical podophyllotoxin for hard-to-treat palmoplantar warts. J Cosmet Laser Ther. 2003;5(1):35-7.
22. Goldman MP, Manuskiatti W. Combined laser resurfacing with the 950-microsec pulsed CO_2 + Er:YAG lasers. Dermatol Surg. 1999;25(3):160-3.
23. Shah SD, Aurangabadkar SJ. Newer trends in laser tattoo removal. J Cutan Aesthet Sur. 2015;8(1):25-9.
24. Singhal M, Del Río-Sancho S, Sonaje K, Kalia YN. Fractional laser ablation for the cutaneous delivery of triamcinolone acetonide from cryomilled polymeric microparticles: creating intraepidermal drug depots. Mol Pharm. 2016;13(2): 500-11.
25. Lee WR, Shen SC, Al-Suwayeh SA, Yang HH, Yuan CY, Fang JY. Laser-assisted topical drug delivery by using a low-fluence fractional laser: imiquimod and macromolecules. J Control Release. 2011;153(3):240-8.
26. Lee WR, Shen SC, Aljuffali IA, Li YC, Fang JY. Erbium-yttrium- aluminum-garnet laser irradiation ameliorates skin permeation and follicular delivery of antialopecia drugs. J Pharm Sci. 2014;103(11):3542-52.
27. Lee WR, Shen SC, Fang CL, Liu CR, Fang JY. Skin pretreatment with an Er:YAG laser promotes the transdermal delivery of three narcotic analgesics. Lasers Med Sci. 2007;22(4):271-8.
28. Hsiao CY, Huang CH, Hu S, Ko YS, Sung HC, Huang SY. Skin pretreatment with lasers promotes the transdermal delivery of vitamin C derivatives. Lasers Med Sci. 2011;26(3): 369-76.
29. Lee MS. Treatment of vaginal relaxation syndrome with an erbium:YAG laser using 90° and 360° scanning scopes: a pilot study and short-term results. Laser Ther. 2014;23(2): 129-38.
30. Pardo JI, Solà VR, Morales AA. Treatment of female stress urinary incontinence with Erbium-YAG laser in nonablative mode. Eur J Obstet Gynecol Reprod Biol. 2016;204:1-4.

CHAPTER 114

Fractional Lasers

Anil Ganjoo

KEY MESSAGES

- Fractional laser technology has gained popularity because of its favorable side effect profile, reduced recovery time, and significant clinical outcomes.
- Fractional lasers emit light in a pixilated fashion, which is transmitted to the skin, where they produce small microscopic columns of thermal injury to the skin called the microthermal zones (MTZs).
- The indications include both aesthetic (aging skin, wrinkles, and acne scars), and nonaesthetic (poikiloderma of Civatte, milium, and granuloma annulare).
- While the fractional lasers are generally safe, side effects may occur with aggressive dosage, and hence caution needs to be exercised.

INTRODUCTION

Fractional photothermolysis (FP) is one of the most significant advances that have happened in the world of lasers in the recent past. The idea of treating only a fraction of the affected skin and getting results comparable to conventional therapy is extremely exciting. It cuts down the side effects associated with resurfacing drastically while maintaining the efficacy to a large extent. We have learned a lot since the inception of the technology in 2004. The fractional laser tissue interaction is now better understood and can be applied to get much better outcomes than we used to a decade ago. The future looks bright for this wonderful technology.

Conventional ablative laser skin resurfacing with either the continuous-wave carbon dioxide (CO_2) or erbium:yttrium-aluminum-garnet (Er:YAG) lasers gained popularity in the 1990s as the standard for facial rejuvenation.[1] The suprathreshold fluences result in rapid cellular heating and instant tissue vaporization leading to ablation. Adjacent to the vaporized zone, sublative fluences induce tissue coagulation and protein denaturation through heat transfer.[2] The thermomechanical destruction generally extends 200–300 μm within the dermis and is followed by a predictable and beneficial "skin tightening" through a process of heat-induced shrinkage of collagen and the initiation of new collagen formation.

Traditional ablative laser resurfacing would produce dramatic results, and therefore it remained the gold standard in skin rejuvenation for a long time. A single sitting with a good aftercare would give excellent results as can be seen in **Figures 1 and 2**.

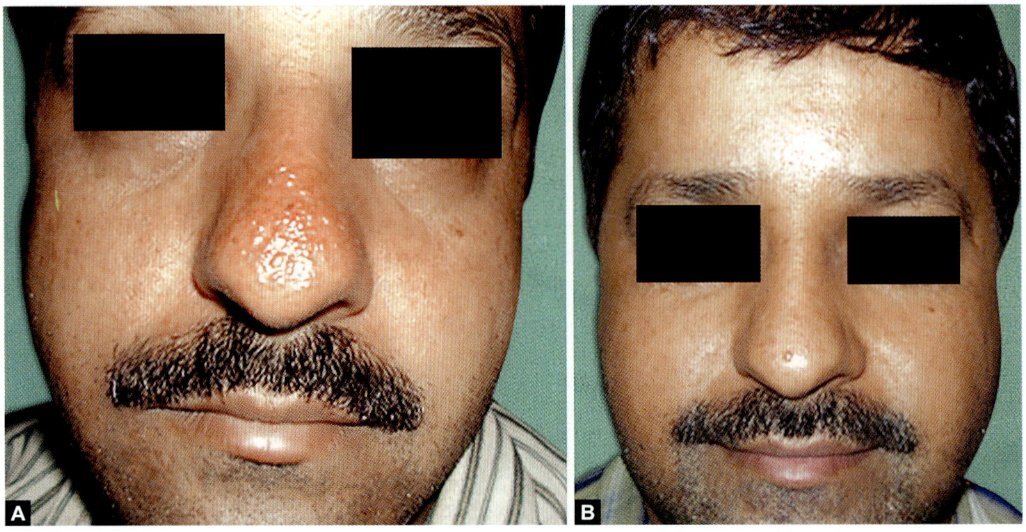

Figs. 1A and B: Trichoepithelioma treated with a single session of conventional CO_2 resurfacing.

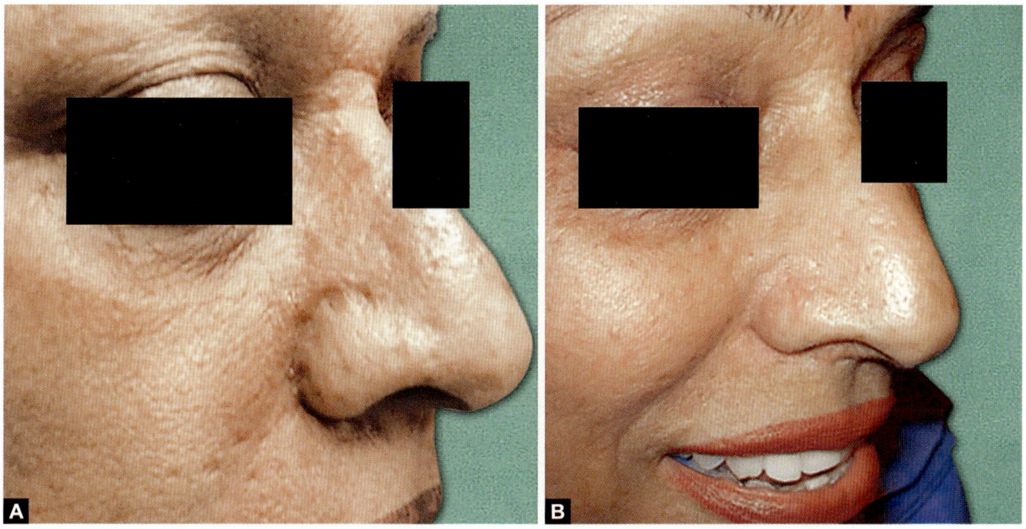

Figs. 2A and B: Postvaricella scars treated with a single session of conventional CO_2 resurfacing.

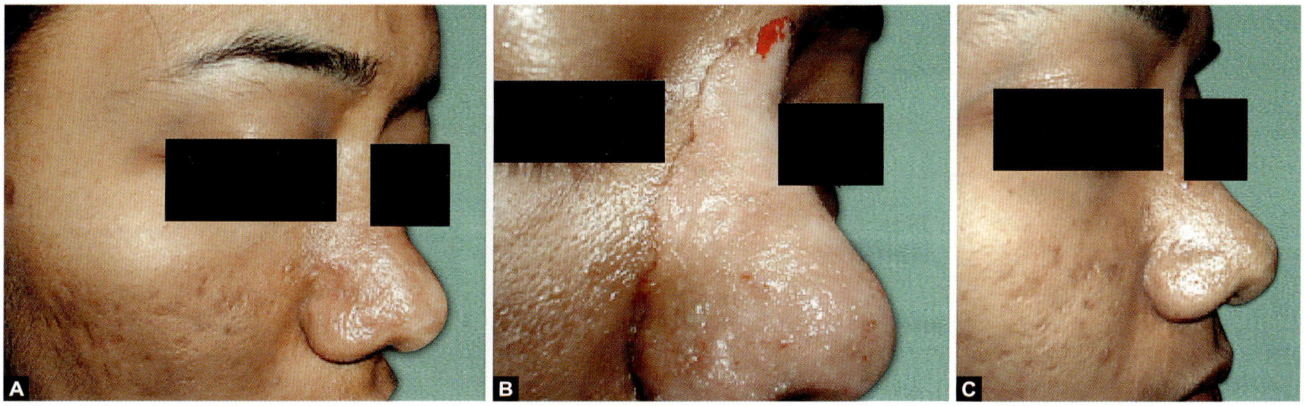

Figs. 3A to C: Increased downtime with risk of scarring, delayed onset hypopigmentation, oozing, and demarcation lines can be seen with conventional ablative CO_2 resurfacing.

However, due to the significant postoperative complications associated with it, conventional resurfacing fell into a lot of disrepute in the 90s, and this led to a reduction in its use. Ablation of the entire epidermis was associated with copious oozing and crusting in the days after the procedure. Delayed healing would often require weeks of curtailment from work or social activities. Postinflammatory hyperpigmentation was a huge risk in dark skin, and erythema would last for up to 3–6 months.[2] The compromised barrier protection significantly increased the risk of infection throughout the recovery period and requires extensive home care. The risk of scarring, delayed onset hypopigmentation, and demarcation lines was significant even in the hands of an experienced operator **(Figs. 3A to C)**.

In an effort to overcome these problems, nonablative dermal remodeling became popular in the ensuing years by using a variety of wavelengths, including near-infrared 1,320, 1,450, or 1,540 nm lasers. Similarly, radiofrequency or intense pulsed light, pulsed dye laser, and high-intensity focused ultrasonography were introduced as they produced selective injury to the dermis with relative or absolute sparing of the epidermis and were termed "nonablative."[3] The theory implied that bulk heating of the dermis without destruction of the epidermis may cause enough protein denaturation to stimulate collagen remodeling and synthesis. Maintaining an intact epidermis using various cooling techniques prevented superficial wounds and lacked the side effects known to occur with the destruction of this layer. Because of these mechanisms, gradual and tentative steps toward nonablative dermal remodeling were achieved. This was much better tolerated than resurfacing with the CO_2 laser, and the downtime was minimal; however, the results were not impressive.

In the quest for the development of safer techniques, came the idea of fractionated laser technology. The concept of fractionated laser surgery was first used in hair transplant surgery, where tiny 1-mm holes were drilled in the bald scalp as recipient sites for hair transplants. Although the transplanted hair looked no better than in conventional hair transplantation, in retrospect, the holes healed up just fine

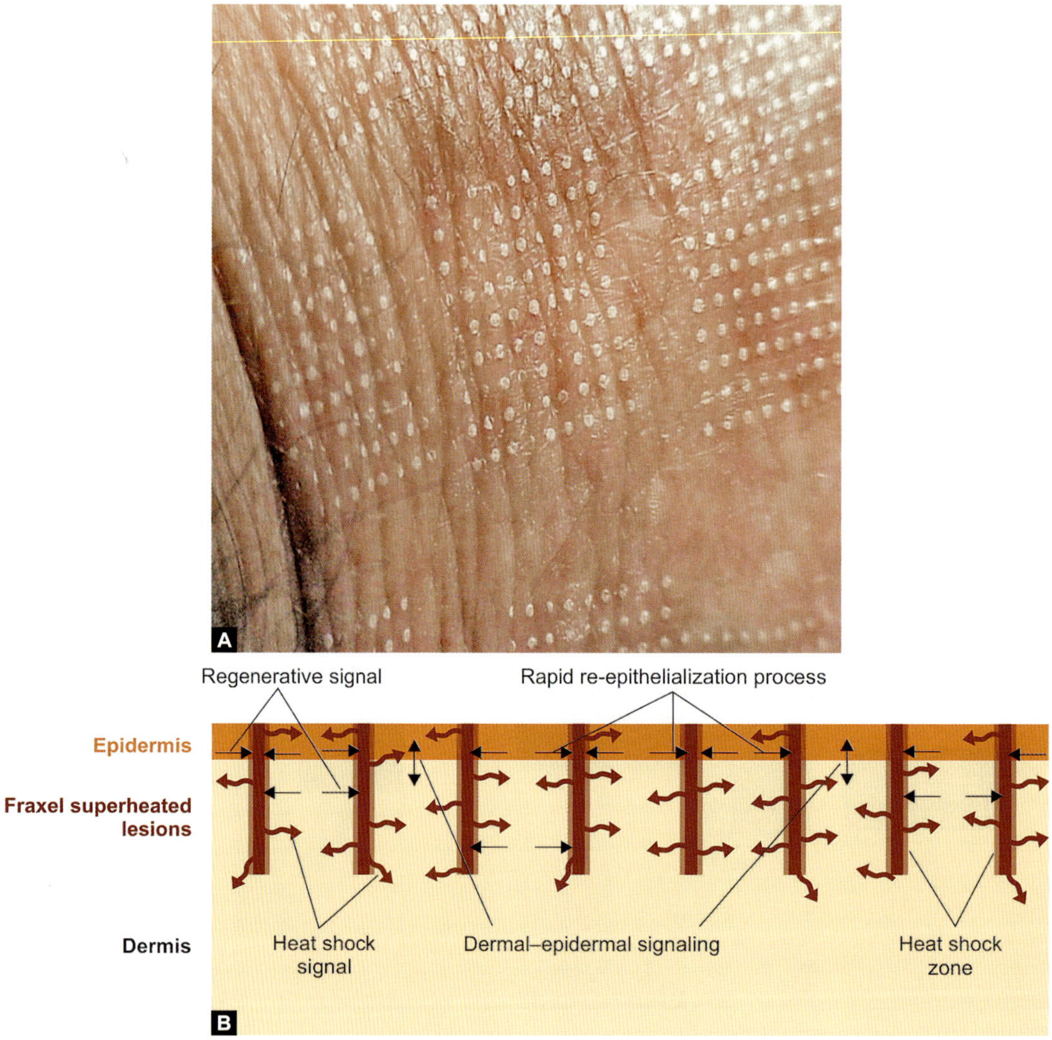

Figs. 4A and B: Concept of fractional resurfacing.

with very limited scarring.[3] This approach was conceptualized by Dr Manstein and Dr Anderson, who first developed the functional concepts of fractionated laser surgery. They published their work in 2004, having used the 1,550-nm nonablative Er:Glass, "Fraxel" laser, now called the Fraxel restore.[3]

Fractional resurfacing evolved as a new technology that could be used in both ablative and nonablative resurfacing lasers by attaching a fractionated scanner device that would treat only a small fraction of skin exposed. The intervening areas are left untouched, which then rapidly repopulate the ablated columns of tissue. Each pass treats only 15–25% of the area exposed. The fractional lasers produce high-precision microbeams that penetrate the skin and produce narrow deep columns of tissue coagulation deep into the dermis. These columns of injury are called the *"Micro thermal zones"* **(Figs. 4A and B)**. The depth of MTZs is proportionate to the energy used. The surrounding tissue is spared. The coagulated tissue then initiates a healing process with the proliferation of myofibroblasts, neovascularization, and neocollagenesis. A mild to moderate improvement is seen after each sitting and about 4–5 sittings done at 4-week interval produces fairly good results.

As fractional lasers enable us to trigger a skin remodeling in both the epidermal and the dermal compartment, they have found a wide acceptance in a rather short time. On a cellular level, the postfractional wound healing is defined by a stereotypical sequence of processes, mainly triggered by the activation of heat shock proteins (HSPs) within the remaining keratinocytes, culminating in an active expulsion of pigmented irreparable tissue parts [microscopic epidermal necrotic debris (MEND)] 3 days later.[2]

Despite a wide use of fractional lasers to treat several skin conditions associated with aging and trauma, the door has just been opened in terms of using this extremely high capacity of self-renewal in the context of treating skin cancers, fibrosing skin diseases, and inflammatory and granulomatous skin conditions, as well as infectious diseases. This review aims at summarizing the current status of fractional lasers in daily clinical routine as well as the underlying technology,

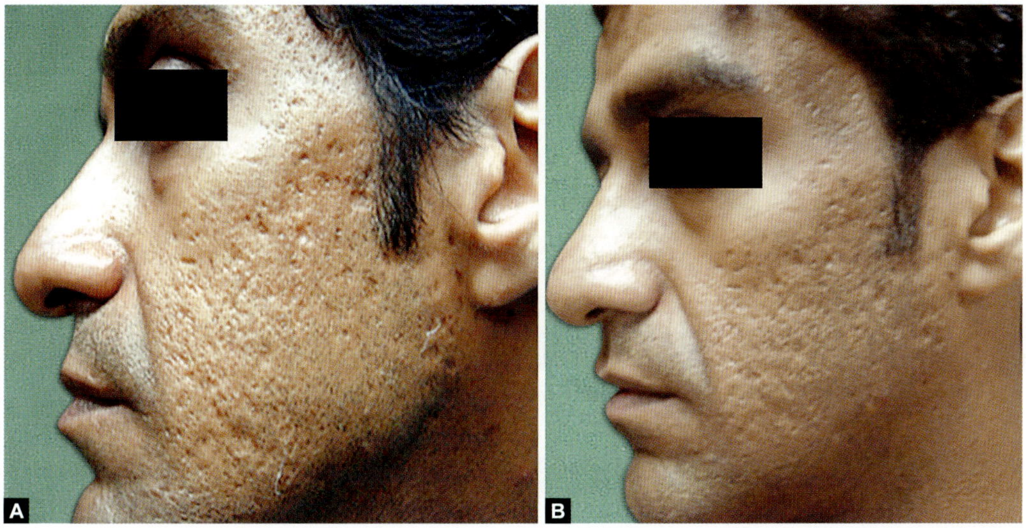

Figs. 5A and B: Subtle improvement in postacne scars after four sessions of fractional Er:Glass laser.

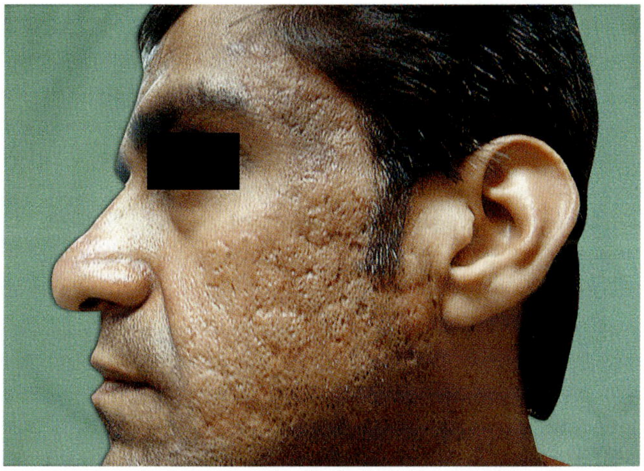

Fig. 6: Minimal downtime after fractional Er:Glass session.

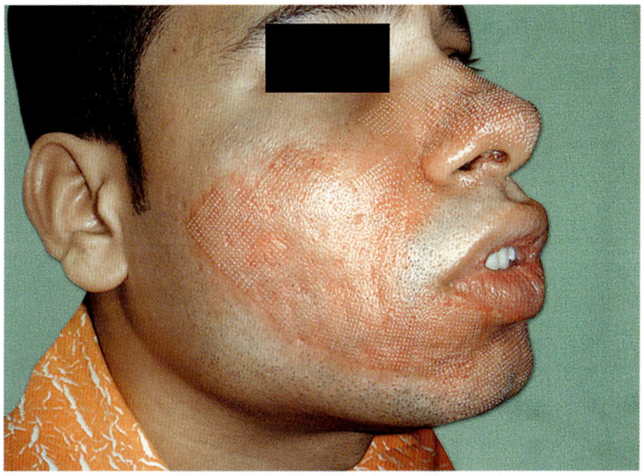

Fig. 7: Long downtime after fractional CO_2 session.

and it provides an outlook for ways in which the as yet unused potential can be transferred to clinics.

The fractional scanner can be attached to any of the resurfacing lasers available:

- *Ablative:*
  - CO_2 laser
  - Er:YAG laser
- *Nonablative:*
  - Mid-infrared lasers
    - 1,320-nm Nd:YAG
    - 1,450-nm diode
    - 1,540-nm Er:Glass

As our knowledge and understanding of fractional resurfacing have improved, we now know that the ablative fractional lasers produce better results than the nonablative ones **(Figs. 5 and 6)**, although the former is associated with greater downtime and a possibility of higher postoperative complications like hyperpigmentation. But this should not deter an experienced laser surgeon to be aggressive and using ablative fractional lasers as we as dermatologists are well equipped to deal with such an eventuality. The superiority of the ablative fractional lasers over the nonablative ones has been proven in a number of studies.

In comparison to nonablative fractional lasers, the downtime with ablative fractional lasers is prolonged and the skin can take 5–7 days to get back to normal, but ablative treatments produce quite desirable results **(Figs. 7 and 8)**.

CHOOSING A MACHINE

In this rapidly improving technology, several machines of nonablative and ablative fractional lasers have become available. The following parameters should be considered while choosing a fractional laser machine:

- Ability to deliver higher fluences per microbeam
- Variable MTZ settings—density of the microbeams
- Variable microbeam sizes
- Ability to choose various shapes for treatment so as to fit properly on the face

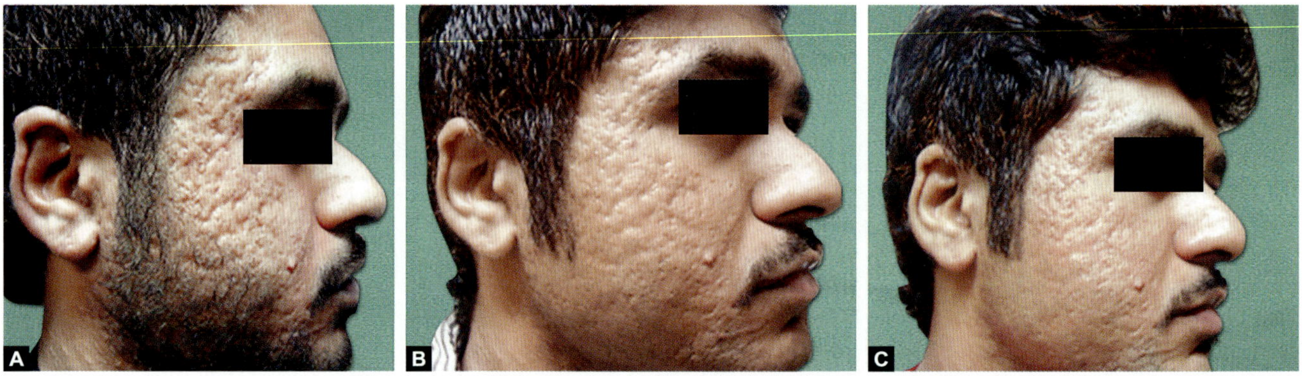

Figs. 8A to C: Major improvement after two and four sessions of fractional CO_2 laser.

TABLE 1: Indications.

Category	*Indications*
Aesthetic	Photoaging, periorbital wrinkles, acne scarring, postburn and surgical scars, stretch marks, melasma, postinflammatory pigmentation, minocycline pigmentation, poikiloderma of Civatte, nevus of Ota, other dyschromias, residual hemangiomas, and telangiectatic matting
Nonaesthetic	Granuloma annulare, colloid milium, disseminated superficial actinic porokeratosis, lichen amyloidosis, Shagreen patch in tuberous sclerosis, and morphea-related contracture

- Easy to use
- Degree of procedural pain or discomfort
- Ability to alter microbeam density, size, and fluence
- Number of treatment sessions required to attain clinical endpoints
- Patient downtime
- Treatment duration
- Clinical validation of the product.

INDICATIONS FOR FRACTIONAL LASERS

Fractional photothermolysis can be used to treat a variety of conditions, including photoaging, pigmentation, superficial or deep rhytids, and scars **(Table 1)**.

Photoaging

In the initial studies using the 1,550-nm nonablative device, Manstein et al.[4] reported significant improvements in periorbital rhytids and skin texture. The authors found a linear pattern of shrinkage related to thermal injury.[4] The initial tissue shrinkage was followed by an apparent relaxation after 1 month, with retightening seen at 3 months.[4]

Since these initial studies, several others, have also shown improvements in photodamaged skin with both ablative and nonablative FP, including improvement of mild-to-moderate rhytids, photoaging of the hand,[5] photoaging of nonfacial skin,[2] and poikiloderma of Civatte.[6]

The newer 1,927-nm fractionated device has been shown to be effective in treating facial actinic keratosis also.[7]

Acne Scarring

The initial studies of fractionated lasers on acne scarring were done with nonablative devices.[2] The nonablative devices have also demonstrated efficacy in atrophic-type acne scars.[8] As already discussed ablative fractional resurfacing has shown much superior results than the nonablative modalities in acne scars.[9] Of note, when treating acne scarring, very high energy in combination with very high density is more efficacious than low energy and low density.

Fractional photothermolysis is becoming increasingly popular in the treatment of darker-skinned patients (Fitzpatrick skin types III–VI) with acne scarring.[10] These skins were considered to be high-risk skins in earlier times. In Korean patients (Fitzpatrick skin types IV and V) with moderate-to-severe scarring, the patients had self-assessed degrees of moderate-to-excellent improvement.[11]

Other Scars

The 1550-nm Fraxel has been shown to be effective in the treatment of hypopigmented facial scars.[12] Tierney et al.[13] compared the efficacy of nonablative FP with that of the pulsed dye laser for the improvement of surgical scars and noted greater improvement with the fractionated device. Hypertrophic scars also seem to improve, but, unlike the treatment of acne scarring, better results are obtained when treated with lower densities **(Figs. 9A and B)**.[14]

Pigmentation

As a matter of fact, the MEND shuttle is characterized by transporting melanin to the epidermal surface. This has created hope to treat dyspigmentations of the skin as well as the specific condition of melasma more effectively. On a cellular level, pigments stored in melanophages will be distributed within the tissue once cells have been disrupted by laser energy. Consequently, the number of melanocytes

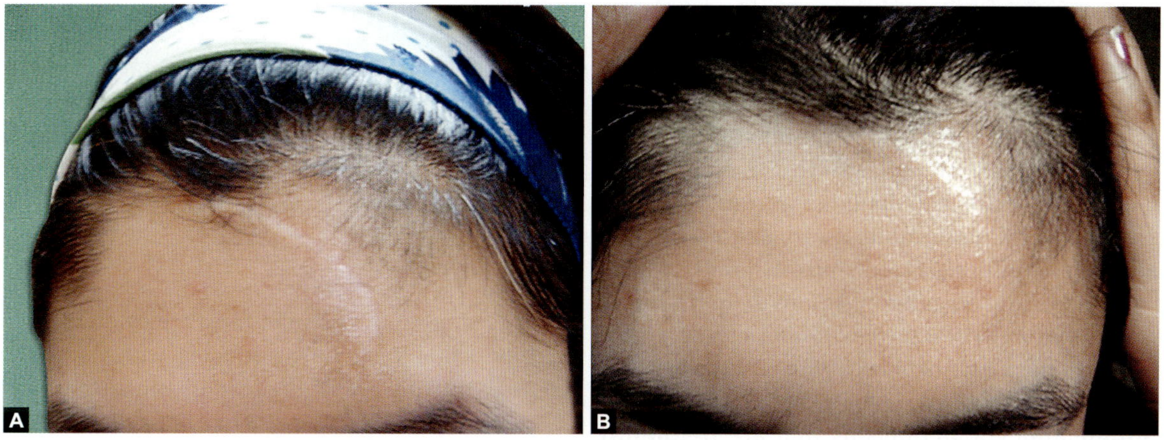

Figs. 9A and B: Improvement in postsurgical scar after two treatments with fractional CO_2 laser.

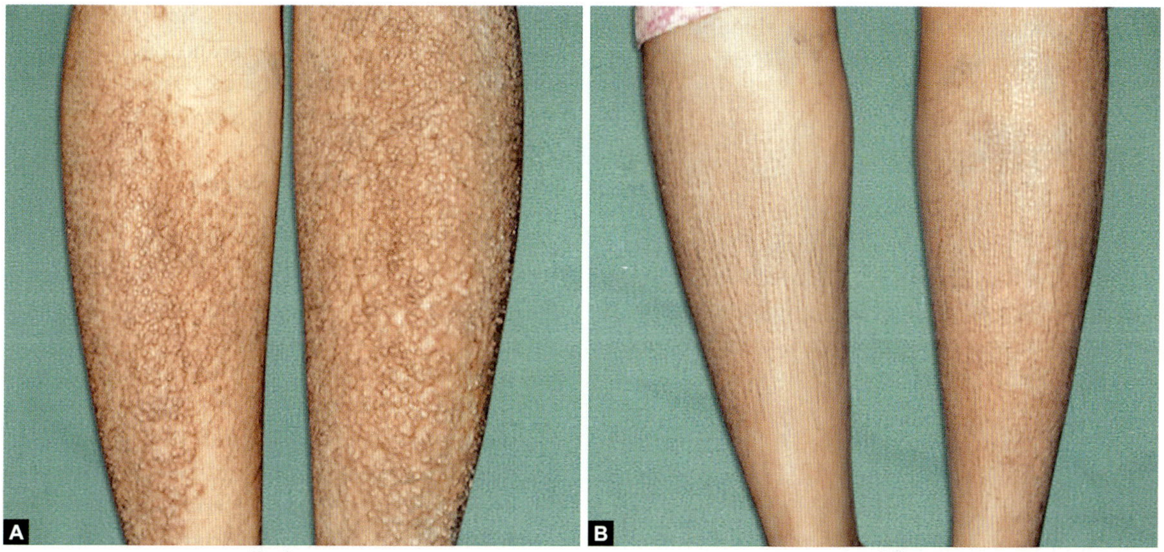

Figs. 10A and B: Lichen amyloidosis successfully treated with erbium:yttrium-aluminum-garnet (Er:YAG) laser.
Courtesy: Dr Venkataram Mysore, Bengaluru.

and the amount of melanin stored in keratinocytes are reduced. Most often, this effect is transient only. In approximately 60% of the patients, improvement is seen in 75–100%, although 30% reported an improvement of 25% only. Low densities and fluences are crucial, especially in darker skin types. It seems that the nonablative fractional laser gives more reliable results; however, it is not rated as a first-line intervention.[14,15]

In the initial reports on the efficacy of nonablative FP in treating melasma, 10 female patients (Fitzpatrick skin types III–V) were treated at 1–2-week intervals with the Fraxel restore.[16] After 4–6 sessions, physician evaluation confirmed that 60% of patients achieved 75–100% clearance.[16] Other conditions that have been successfully treated using FP technology include residual hemangioma,[17] minocycline-induced hyperpigmentation,[18] granuloma annulare,[19] disseminated superficial actinic porokeratosis,[20] and colloid milium.[21] It has also been tried for lichen amyloidosis **(Figs. 10A and B)**. Recently, there is new research on using this technology to improve function in patients with contractures due to sclerosing disorders such as scleroderma.[22]

Vascular Lesions

The efficacy of nonablative fractional lasers to treat hemangiomas, postinflammatory erythema, and telangiectasias has been reported despite the fact that highly selective lasers are available. Histological examination shows that there is a wide intravascular coagulation due to nonablative fractional laser treatment.[14] The ablative fractional laser system seems to be beneficial for atrophic vascular lesions or for those with scar tissue even in children.[23] There is no specific absorbing chromophore other than water. Even lymphangiomas can also be treated using both ablative and nonablative fractional lasers.[24]

Actinic Keratosis and Skin Cancer

A new and very promising treatment modality of fractional lasers has been established in the field of dermatological oncology. The first Food and Drug Administration (FDA) approval of a 1,927-nm thulium laser was based on 83.5% reduction of actinic keratoses (AK) at the face, arms, hands, and on the trunk.[14] Comparable healing rates (86.6%) confirmed this finding during a follow-up of 6 months.[25] With regard to the evidence of other interventions to treat AK [e.g., photodynamic therapy (PDT), topical, and cryotherapy], fractional laser therapy cannot be recommended as first-line intervention.[14]

The nonmelanocytic neoplasms that are frequently associated with chronic actinic skin damage have led to the observation that the use of ablative fractional lasers results in enhanced healing compared with classical ablation of such lesions. However, fractional laser alone is inferior to laser-assisted PDT.[26]

POTENTIAL FUTURE USE

As the MENDs seem to be actively transported, it would be interesting to know if they could be used for other purposes such as removal of foreign bodies (tattoo ink, dirt from traumata, and parasites), granuloma, amyloids, and even localized infectious agents. To some extent, the concept has been proven in cases of tattoo allergy.[27]

The MENDs can also be used for trans-epidermal delivery of large molecules that cannot traverse the intact stratum corneum. Fractionation creates open channels within the stratum corneum, which remain open for some time to allow the application of topical therapies postlaser and effective penetration of these large molecules through the stratum corneum and the epidermis.

COMPLICATIONS

Although FP (ablative and nonablative) is inherently safer because of the pixilated manner of the treatment, complications can happen. These can be prevented by the judicious use of technology. Following complications are however expected.

Infections

Herpes simplex virus is the most common infectious complication after fractional resurfacing, with reported ranges up to 2%.[28] Antiviral prophylaxis can minimize the reactivation to 0.5%.[28] In contrast, the incidence of bacterial infection after FP appears to be extremely low. Occlusive dressings and ointments may be a potential cause of pathogen overgrowth leading to the growth of both *Staphylococcus aureus* and *Pseudomonas aeruginosa,* so they are best avoided.[29] Candidal and pityrosporum infections can also occur, with a recent retrospective study reporting a rate of 1.2%.[30]

Pigmentary Disturbances

Hyperpigmentation is a well-known side effect of both nonablative and ablative fractional resurfacing, particularly in patients with darker skin types (Fitzpatrick skin types III–VI). Hyperpigmentation occurs much less frequently with FP laser skin resurfacing compared with traditional resurfacing. The incidence appears to be dependent on the system used, the parameters applied, and the skin types treated, but can be upward of 12% in certain populations **(Figs. 11A and B)**.[31]

However, we as dermatologists can deal with these minor pigmentary alterations with proper knowledge of dermatological principles.

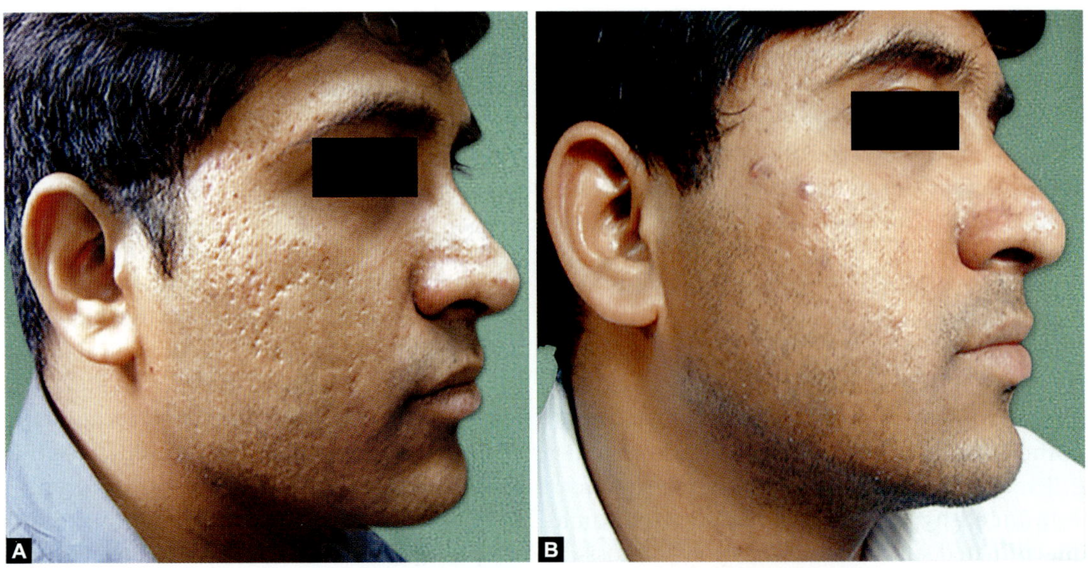

Figs. 11A and B: Postinflammatory hyperpigmentation after successful treatment of postacne scars with fractional CO_2 laser.

Acneiform Eruptions

Milia may occur in nearly 20% of treated patients.[28] The use of occlusive moisturizers and dressings can exacerbate these eruptions, and noncomedogenic equivalents should be used whenever necessary.[32] Acneiform eruptions are common after fractional skin resurfacing, occurring in 2–10%. The rates are significantly lower than that of traditional skin resurfacing.[27] With moderate-to-severe acne flares, a short course of oral antibiotics is often helpful and can even be used before subsequent treatments to prevent outbreaks.[24]

Prolonged Erythema

Immediate posttreatment erythema after nonablative fractional resurfacing is expected and may persist for up to 3 days.[28] About 1% patients may experience prolonged erythema lasting from weeks to months.[28] Prolonged erythema after ablative fractional resurfacing is significant, affecting nearly 12.5% of patients.[33] The erythema typically resolves within 3 months. Although persistent erythema can be concerning, it should be emphasized that erythema is expected and is a sign of continued wound healing and collagen remodeling.

Scarring

Although rare, hypertrophic scarring can be associated with aggressive fractional laser treatments. Vertical and horizontal bands have been described after ablative fractional resurfacing of the neck.[34] This particularly happens in the setting of secondary infection.

Newer Applications of Fractional Lasers

Transepidermal Drug Delivery

Ablative fractional resurfacing creates microscopic vertical holes in tissue, leaving an open channel into which topically applied drugs can migrate. An in vitro study using low-fluence fractionated Er:YAG demonstrated a 125-fold increase in imiquimod delivery.[29,35] Clinical trials are currently underway to determine the feasibility and safety of this enhanced drug delivery in humans. Although far from being optimized, ablative fractional resurfacing may serve as a channel for the delivery of large molecules that are unable to penetrate intact skin. Perhaps ultimately, it may be used for drug delivery, including biological peptides and vaccines.

Tattoo and Pigmented Lesion Treatment

The ablative fractional lasers create small channels that have been postulated to promote transepidermal elimination of tattoo particles and pigment from the dermis. An initial report showed ablative fractional resurfacing in conjunction with Q-switched lasers (QSL) enhanced tattoo removal when compared with tattoo removal alone.[30,36] Ibrahimi et al.[37] reported the use of ablative fractional lasers for the successful treatment of allergic tattoos, in which the use of a QSL can be challenging, given the risk of releasing antigenic proteins into lymphatic circulation. We have seen a significant improvement in the outcome of pigmented lesions and tattoo treatment since we started combining the fractional lasers with the QSL **(Figs. 12A and B)**.

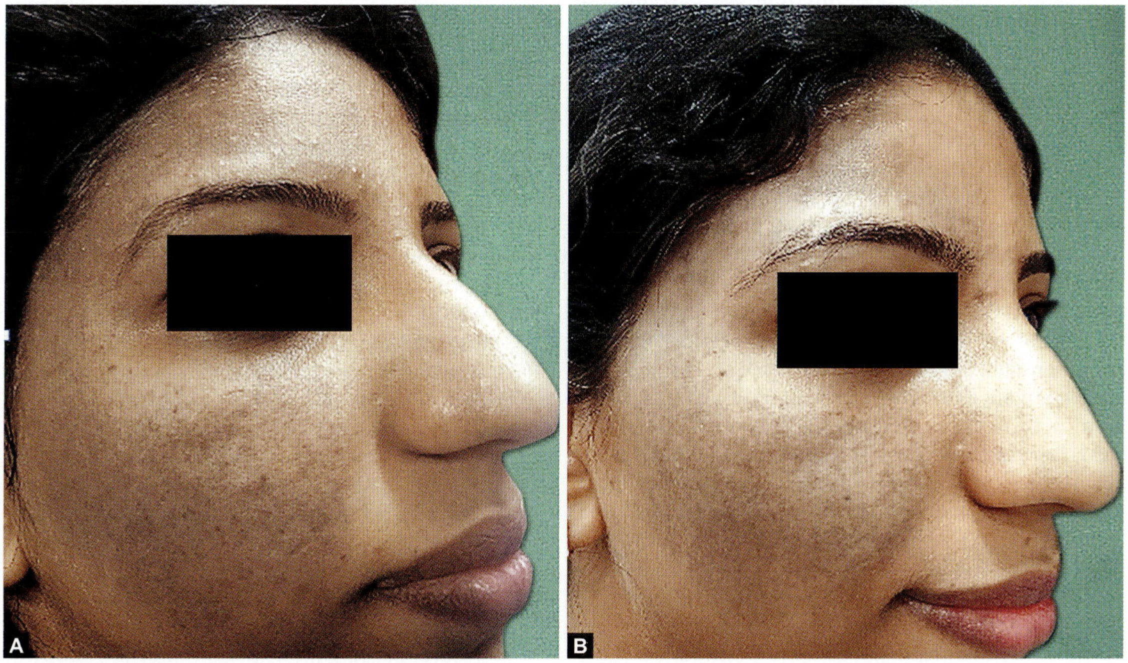

Figs. 12A and B: Rapid clearance of nevus of Ota in just three sittings using a combination of Q-Switched laser (QSL) and fractional CO_2 laser.

CONCLUSION

Fractional lasers are a big leap forward in the world of resurfacing lasers. They have made our job much easier by reducing the likelihood of postlaser complications associated with conventional laser resurfacing. This is particularly true in the case of our kind of skin color where the chances of postoperative complications are really high.

FUNCTIONAL PEARLS

- To get the best out of your fractional laser, combine it with other procedures like in case of acne scars with subcision, chemical reconstruction of skin scars (CROSS) technique, scar revision by punch excision, punch grafting, punch floatation, and also by linear excision.
- Combine the fractional lasers with other lasers like in case of pigmented lesions with QSL.
- Always apply some medication postfractional session as this is the best opportunity for you to deliver the maximum drug into the dermis through the channels created by fractionation. Some large molecules like peptides that do not cross the intact epidermal barrier can be delivered in this way.
- Use low density and high fluence for treating deep scars and high density and low fluence for textural improvement and superficial scars.
- Avoid multiple passes as it increases the density of MTZs, which defeats the idea of fractionation. If you want to be aggressive use higher fluence or multiple stacks.
- More than two stacks are not desirable in CO2 fractional lasers as it leads to high collateral damage. Higher number of stacks can be given in Er:YAG fractional as here the collateral damage is low.

REFERENCES

1. Gold MH. Update on fractional laser technology. J Clin Aesthet Dermatol. 2010;3(1):42-50.
2. Geronemus RG. Fractional photothermolysis: current and future applications. Lasers Surg Med. 2006;38(3):169-76.
3. Saedi N, Petelin A, Zachary C. Fractionation: a new era in laser resurfacing. Clin Plast Surg. 2011;38(3):449-61.
4. Manstein D, Herron GS, Sink RK, Tanner H, Anderson RR. Fractional photothermolysis: a new concept for cutaneous remodeling using microscopic patterns of thermal injury. Lasers Surg Med. 2004;34(5):426-38.
5. Jih MH, Goldberg LH, Kimyai-Asadi A. Fractional photothermolysis for photoaging of hands. Dermatol Surg. 2008; 34(1):73-8.
6. Behroozan DS, Goldberg LH, Glaich AS, Dai T, Friedman PM. Fractional photothermolysis for treatment of poikiloderma of civatte. Dermatol Surg. 2006;32(2):298-301.
7. Weiss E. Nonablative 1927 nm fractional resurfacing effective for facial actinic keratoses. Abstract presented at: The American Dermatologic Surgery Conference; October 2010; Chicago, IL.
8. Alster TS, Tanzi EL, Lazarus M. The use of fractional laser photothermolysis for the treatment of atrophic scars. Dermatol Surg. 2007;33(3):295-99.
9. Ortiz A, Tremaine AM, Zachary CB. Long-term efficacy of a fractional resurfacing device. Abstract presented at: American Society for Laser Medicine and Surgery Conference; April 2009; National Harbor, MD.
10. Tierney EP, Kouba DJ, Hanke CW. Review of fractional photothermolysis: treatment indications and efficacy. Dermatol Surg. 2009;35(10):1445-61.
11. Lee HS, Lee JH, Ahn GY, Lee DH, Shin JW, Kim DH, et al. Fractional photothermolysis for the treatment of acne scars: a report of 27 Korean patients. J Dermatolog Treat. 2008;19(1): 45-9.
12. Glaich AS, Rahman Z, Goldberg LH, Friedman PM. Fractional resurfacing for the treatment of hypopigmented scars: a pilot study. Dermatol Surg. 2007;33(3):289-94.
13. Tierney E, Mahmoud BH, Srivastava D, Ozog DM, Kouba D. Treatment of surgical scars with fractional photothermolysis versus pulse dye laser: randomized control trial. Dermatol Surg. 2009;35:1172-80.
14. Paasch U, Bodendorf MO, Grunewald S. Dermatologische Lasertherapie: Fraktionale Laser. Berlin: KVM Verlag; 2011.
15. Lin JY, Warger WC, Izikson L, Anderson RR, Tannous Z. A prospective, randomized controlled trial on the efficacy of fractional photothermolysis on scar remodeling. Lasers Surg Med. 2011;43(4):265-72.
16. Rokhsar CK, Fitzpatrick RE. The treatment of melasma with fractional photothermolysis: a pilot study. Dermatol Surg. 2005;31(12):1645-50.
17. Blankenship CM, Alster TS. Fractional photothermolysis of residual hemangioma. Dermatol Surg. 2008;34(8):1112-4.
18. Izikson L, Anderson RR. Resolution of blue minocycline pigmentation of the face after fractional photothermolysis. Lasers Surg Med. 2008;40(6):399-401.
19. Karsai S, Hammes S, Rütten A, Raulin C. Fractional photothermolysis for the treatment of granuloma annulare: a case report. Lasers Surg Med. 2008;40(5):319-22.
20. Chrastil B, Glaich AS, Goldberg LH, Friedman PM. Fractional photothermolysis: a novel treatment for disseminated superficial actinic porokeratosis. Arch Dermatol. 2007;143(11): 1450-2.
21. Marra DE, Pourrabbani S, Fincher EF, Moy RL. Fractional photothermolysis for the treatment of adult colloid milium. Arch Dermatol. 2007;143(5):572-4.
22. Kineston D, Kwan JM, Uebelhoer NS, Shumaker PR. Use of a fractional ablative 10.6-μm carbon dioxide laser in the treatment of a morphea-related contracture. Arch Dermatol. 2011;147(10):1148-50.
23. Brauer JA, Geronemus RG. Laser treatment in the management of infantile hemangiomas and capillary vascular malformations. Tech Vasc Interv Radiol. 2013;16(1):51-4
24. Tsilika K, Bahadoran P, Passeron T. Superficial lymphangioma treated with fractional ablative laser: a case report with clinical and reflectance confocal microscopy evaluation. Dermatol Surg. 2013;39(1 Pt 1):141-3
25. Weiss ET, Brauer JA, Anolik R, Reddy KK, Karen JK, Hale EK, et al. 1927-nm fractional resurfacing of facial actinic keratoses: a promising new therapeutic option. J Am Acad Dermatol. 2013;68(1):98-102
26. Helsing P, Togsverd-Bo K, Veierød MB, Mørk G, Haedersdal M. Intensified fractional CO_2 laser-assisted photodynamic therapy vs. laser alone for organ transplant recipients with multiple actinic keratoses and wart-like lesions: a randomized half-side comparative trial on dorsal hands. Br J Dermatol. 2013;169(5):1087-92
27. Ibrahimi OA, Syed Z, Sakamoto FH, Avram MM, Anderson RR. Treatment of tattoo allergy with ablative fractional resurfacing: a novel paradigm for tattoo removal. J Am Acad Dermatol. 2011;64(6):1111-4

28. Graber EM, Tanzi EL, Alster TS. Side effects and complications of fractional laser photothermolysis: Experience with 961 treatments. Dermatol Surg. 2008;34(3):301-5.
29. Metelitsa AI, Alster TS. Fractionated laser skin resurfacing treatment complications: a review. Dermatol Surg. 2010;36(3): 299-306.
30. Shamsaldeen OS, Peterson JD, Goldman MP. The adverse events of deep fractional CO(2): a retrospective study of 490 treatments in 374 patients. Lasers Surg Med. 2011;43(6): 453-6.
31. Chan HH, Manstein D, Yu CS, Shek S, Kono T, Wei WL, et al. The prevalence and risk factors of post-inflammatory hyperpigmentation after fractional resurfacing in Asians. Lasers Surg Med. 2007;39(5):381-5.
32. Tanzi EL, Wanitphakdeedecha R, Alster TS. Fraxel laser indications and long-term follow-up. Aesthet Surg J. 2008; 28(6):675-8.
33. Rahman Z, MacFalls H, Jiang K, Chan KF, Kelly K, Tournas J, et al. Fractional deep dermal ablation induces tissue tightening. Lasers Surg Med. 2009;41(2):78-86.
34. Fife DJ, Fitzpatrick RE, Zachary CB. Complications of fractional CO_2 laser resurfacing: Four cases. Lasers Surg Med. 2009;41(3):179-84.
35. Lee WR, Shen SC, Al-Suwayeh SA, Yang HH, Yuan CY, Fang JY. Laser-assisted topical drug delivery by using a low-fluence fractional laser: imiquimod and macromolecules. J Control Release. 2011;153(3):240-8.
36. Weiss ET, Geronemus RG. Combining fractional resurfacing and Q-switched ruby laser for tattoo removal. Dermatol Surg. 2011;37(1):97-9.
37. Ibrahimi OA, Syed Z, Sakamoto FH, Avram MM, Anderson RR. Treatment of tattoo allergy with ablative fractional resurfacing: a novel paradigm for tattoo removal. J Am Acad Dermatol. 2011;64(6):1111-4.

CHAPTER 115

Nonablative Lasers and Lights Inclusive of Excimer Laser and Intense Pulse Light

BS Chandrashekar

KEY MESSAGES

- Nonablative laser and light treatments are replacing ablative lasers in the treatment of photo rejuvenation, pigmentary and vascular conditions. They are preferred in skin of color for these indications.
- They are associated with faster recovery, minimal complications, less patient discomfort with little to no downtime.
- They can also be used as maintenance procedures following more aggressive ablative treatment.

INTRODUCTION

This chapter covers the nonablative laser excimer laser, intense pulse light (IPL) and other lasers, used in dermatology practice. Although these lasers are less frequently used, choosing the patients wisely and using the appropriate parameters can deliver superlative results.

Nonablative or sub surface remodeling is the latest approach to treat photo damaged skin and signs of aging.

Nonablative resurfacing has evolved from scanning technology to fractional technology. Nonablative lasers do not decisively produce fibroplasia on histologic basis, hence produce poor results with respect to skin tightening. Ablative lasers such as Erbium YAG and CO_2 though gives promising results but have adverse effects virtually experienced by each and every patient such as postprocedure erythema, delayed healing, scarring and postinflammatory hyperpigmentation. When a given indication requires dermal wound and new collagenosis; lasers that do not ablate epidermis but induce collagenosis should be of first choice and this is achieved with ablative lasers.

INDICATIONS

Nonablative procedures are best suited for younger patients who want to improve their skin quality with respect to tone, texture, early rhytides and for ablative laser treated acne scars for saucerization.

Common lasers used for nonablative resurfacing are pulse dye laser (PDL): 585–595 nm, 1,320 mm - Nd:YAG, 1,570/1,450 nm- Diode, 1,064 nm - QS Nd:YAG, 1,540/1,550 nm- Erb glass, and 1,927 nm - Thulium. In addition to above IPL can also be used for nonablative skin rejuvenation. The first nonablative laser introduced was Nd:YAG 1,320 in the year 2001.[1] Over the years new wavelengths have been introduced along with more safety profile, more versatility, and more cooling options. Nonablative lasers can be of additional help when combined with other modalities while treating early aging and photo damaged skin.[2]

The latest innovation in nonablative fractional laser is laser assisted drug delivery (LADD) Erbium doped 1,550 nm laser which is being utilized to treat hypopigmented scars and skin lesions along with topical bimatoprost. Many more such laser assisted drug deliveries are in the pipeline **(Figs. 1 and 2)**.[2,3]

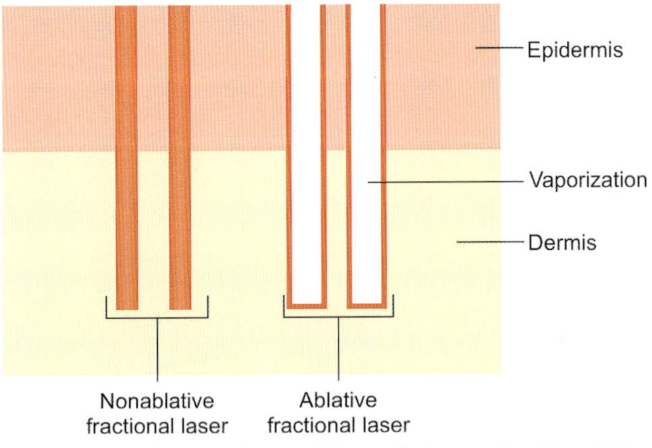

Fig. 1: Creation of microcolumns of thermal injury to the skin, which are known as microthermal zones (MTZs).[3]

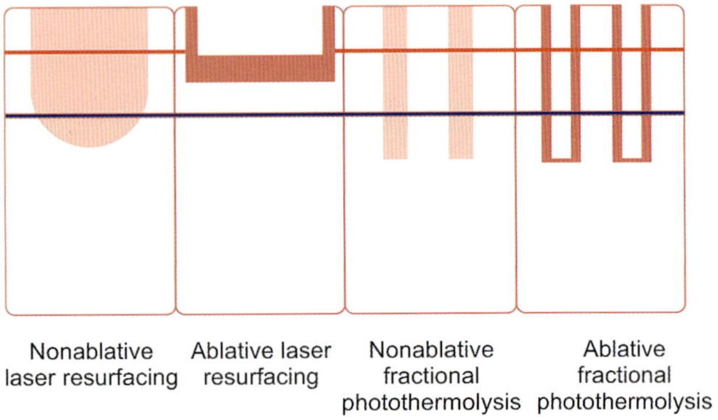

Fig. 2: "Thermal remodeling" techniques in dermatology.[3]

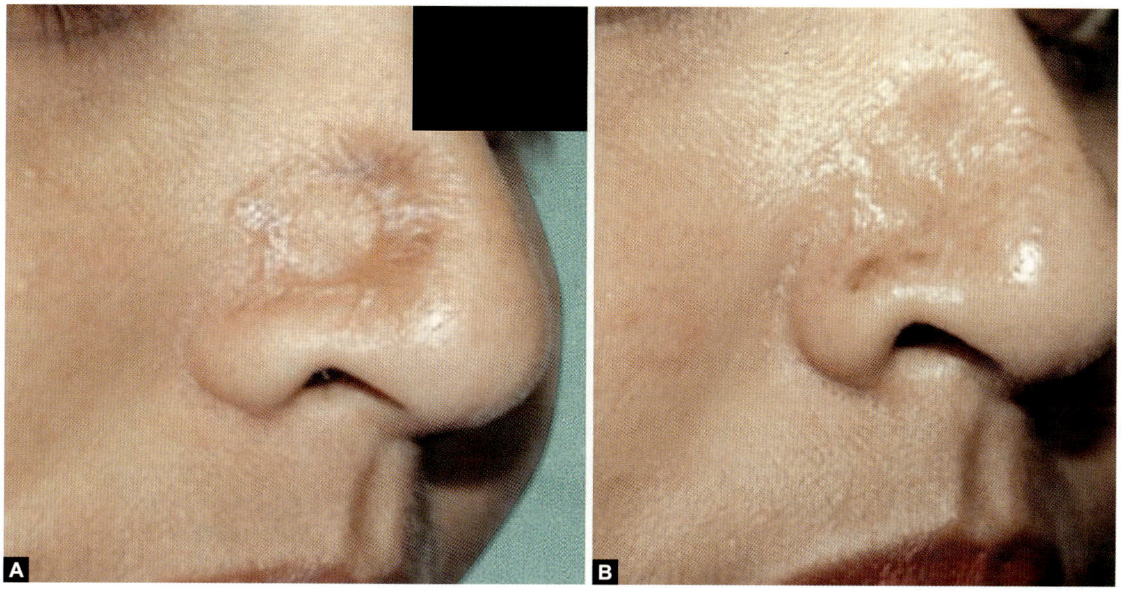

Figs. 3A and B: Erbium glass—for scars. (A) Before; (B) After.

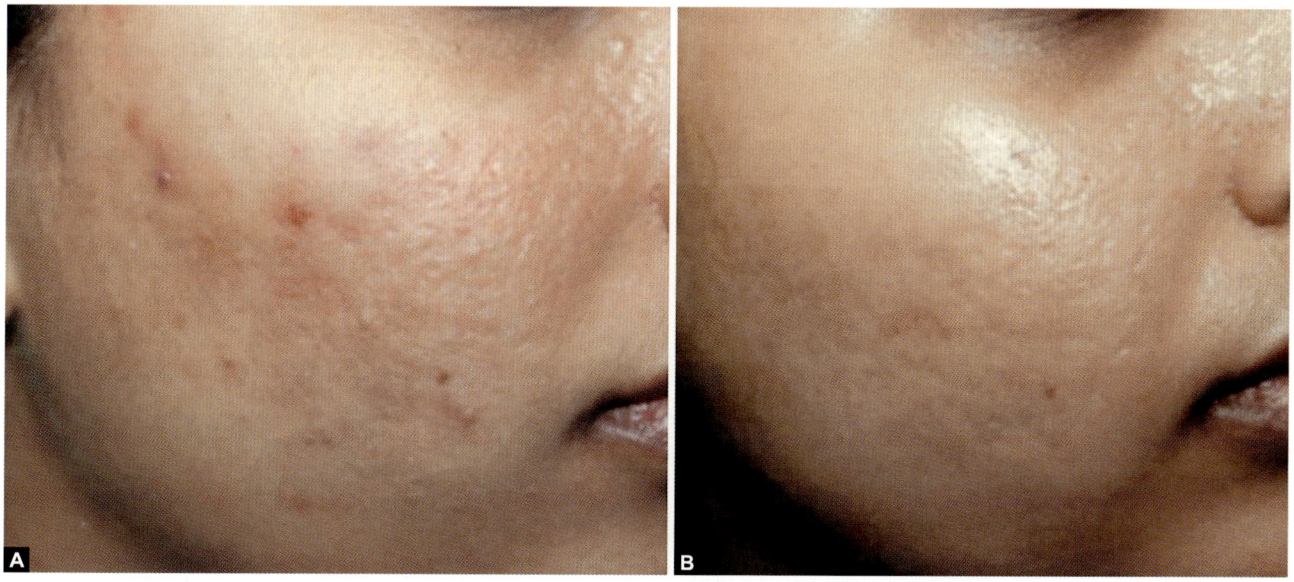

Figs. 4A and B: Erbium glass—for acne and acne scars. (A) Before; (B) After.

ERBIUM GLASS (FIGS. 3 AND 4)

Introduction and Mechanism

Erbium glass is a mid-infrared range (1,540 nm) nonablative laser. The chromophore is intracellular water and the laser reaches to a depth of 0.4–2 mm. It is considered to be relatively safe in darker skin individuals as there is minimal absorption of energy by melanin.[4] Although stratum corneum is intact, epidermal cooling is essential as epidermal necrosis and blistering might happen due to nonspecific absorption of water.[5] The laser induces regulation of matrix metalloproteinases and interleukin expression. Thus it helps in dermal remodeling, anti-inflammatory effects and epidermal differentiation.[6] The mechanism of treatment in hair regrowth is increased blood flow, growth factors, cytokines and direct stimulation of dermal papilla.[7]

Indications[5,7-11]

- Acne scars
- Active acne
- Facial rhytides
- Pores
- Melasma
- Alopecia—male and female pattern hair loss, alopecia areata
- Photoaging
- Striae distensae.

1,320 NM ND: YAG/1,450 nm DIODE LASER

1,320 nm Nd: YAG Laser

This is a nonablative laser which targets the dermal layers to stimulate new collagen growth. It generates controlled thermal damage in the dermis. The water in the skin is the target molecule. It accelerates the production of basic fibroblast growth factor (bFGF) and inhibits transforming growth factor β1 (TGF-β1) production from the fibroblasts. It stimulates collagen types I, III, and VII, and tropoelastin production, thereby reversing visible and histopathological signs of skin aging.[12,13] It is effective for wrinkle reduction and atrophic acne scar improvement.[14] It is effective in the treatment of acne and related scarring, by shrinking sebaceous glands and minimizing sebum production which prevents further acne lesions.[15]

1,450 nm Diode Laser

Water is the principal chromophore for this nonablative laser and the penetration depth of the laser is approximately 200 μm.[16] There is heating of the sebaceous gland and associated structures, leading to the impairment of sebaceous gland activity and associated inflammation. Therefore, it is effective for the treatment of facial acne as well acne scarring.[13] The 1,450 diode laser has also been successfully tried in nonablative dermal remodeling of facial rhytides.[17]

Fractional 1,927 nm Thulium Laser (Figs. 5A and B)

Introduction

Thulium laser is generally known to be a nonablative laser. But it causes minimal disruption of stratum corneum and denaturation in stratum spinosum, along with areas of coagulation in superficial dermis.[18]

Mechanism

Thulium laser (TL) has a wavelength of 1,927 nm which is better absorbed by water as compared to Er:Glass but not as effective as CO_2. TL is therefore used for superficial disorders due to low absorption coefficient.[19]

This controlled injury to the dermis leads to neocollagenesis. Creation of microscopic treatment zones (MTZ) of thermal injury in the dermis leads to rapid healing and reduced downtime as skin surrounding MTZ is left intact. The stimulation of follicular and perifollicular skin along with laser assisted drug delivery could be used in future to promote hair growth.[18]

It also improves pigmentation by extrusion of melanin by the microscopic epidermal necrotic debris (MENDs) which is later exfoliated. Skin tightening is seen after thulium laser when the dermal penetration is more than 1.5 mm with controlled amount of coagulation.[20]

Indication

Indications of thulium laser are given in **Table 1**.[18-21]

585/595 nm Q Switch Laser (Figs. 6 and 7)

Introduction

585/595 nm Q switch laser is a treatment technique for erythema or facial flushing

TABLE 1: Indications of thulium laser.[18-21]

Cosmetic indication	*Therapeutic indication*
Wrinkle reduction	Melasma
Scar reduction	Photoaging
Rejuvenation	Acne
Hair regrowth	Lentigos
	Actinic keratosis
	Laser-assisted drug delivery

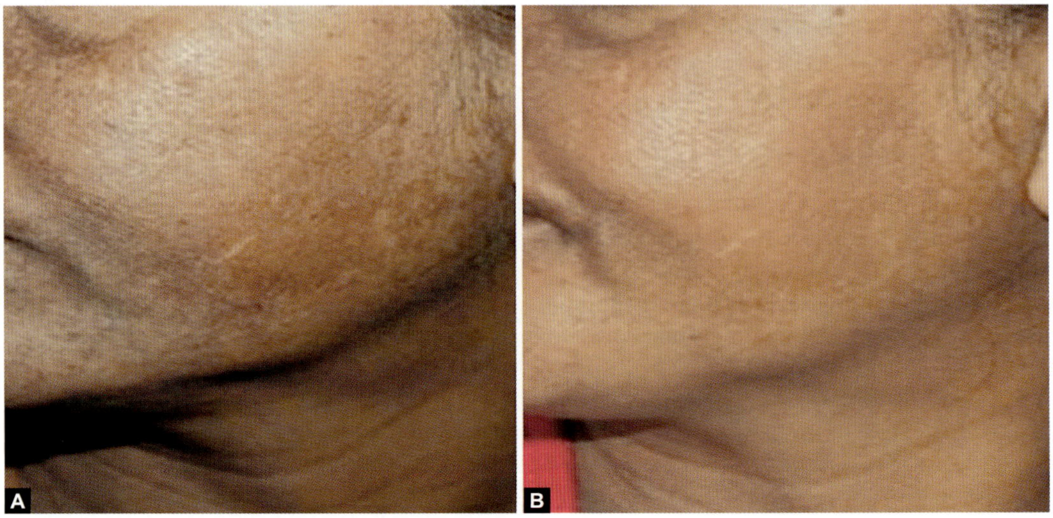

Figs. 5A and B: Thulium laser for melasma. (A) Before; (B) After.

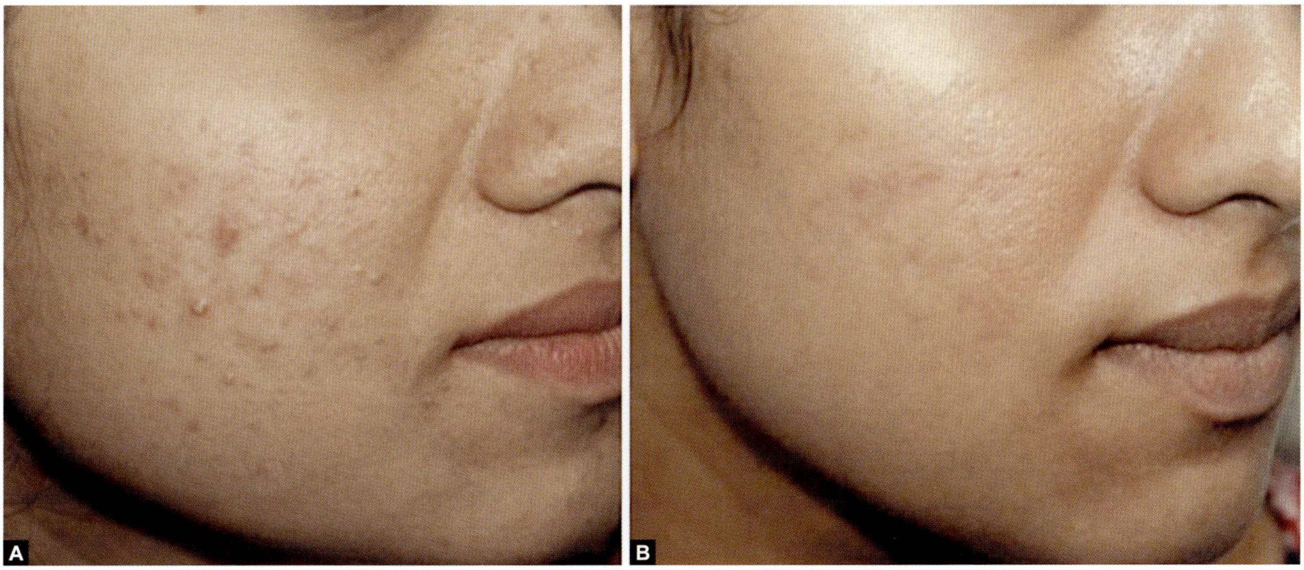

Figs. 6A and B: 595 Q switch laser—for acne. (A) Before; (B) After.

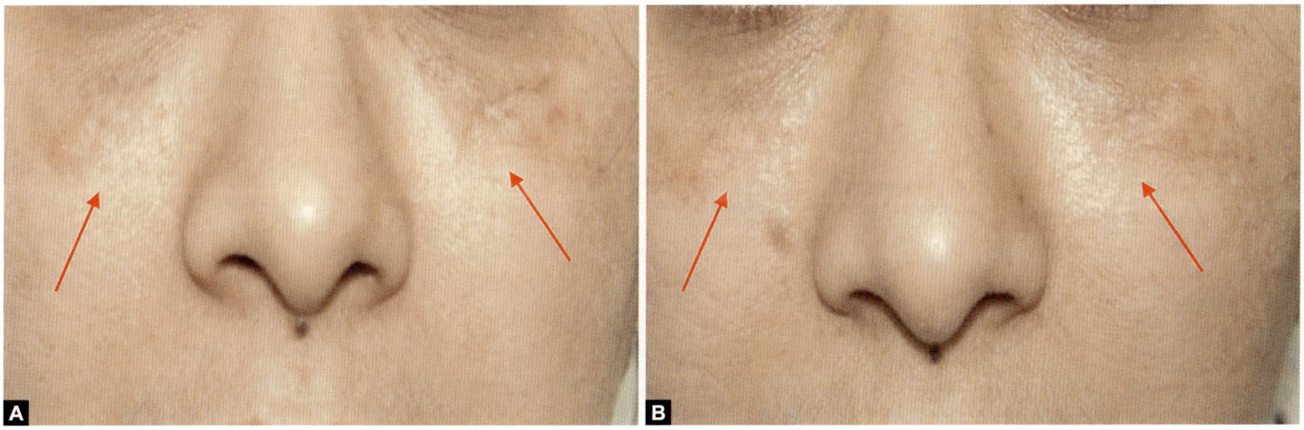

Figs. 7A and B: 595 Q switch laser—for erythematous scar. (A) Before; (B) After.

Mechanism

It has a photoinhibitory effect on endothelial structures and there is photocoagulative destruction of the microvasculature.[22]

Indications[22,23]

It is used for conditions with increased vascularity such as

- Postacne erythema
- Post-traumatic erythema
- Keloid and hypertrophic scar
- Erythematotelangiectatic rosacea
- Facial flushing.
- Melasma and postinflammatory erythema with underlying vascular prominence.

1,319 nm Infrared Laser (Figs. 8A and B)

Introduction

The infrared 1,319 nm laser light is selectively absorbed by water and stimulates the production of collagen and elastin. It also targets the sebaceous glands and improves pores and acne.

Mechanism

The 1,319-nm pulsed energy laser is a member of the mid-infrared laser class. The 1,319 nm laser light is delivered as a continuous wave allowing for controlled, gradual bulk heating of tissue for collagen production and for reduction of sebum production from the sebaceous gland and are not beneficial for treating pigment discolorations or vascular abnormalities.[24]

Indications

- Wrinkles, skin rejuvenation
- Acne scars
- Reduction in the appearance of pores
- Acne vulgaris.

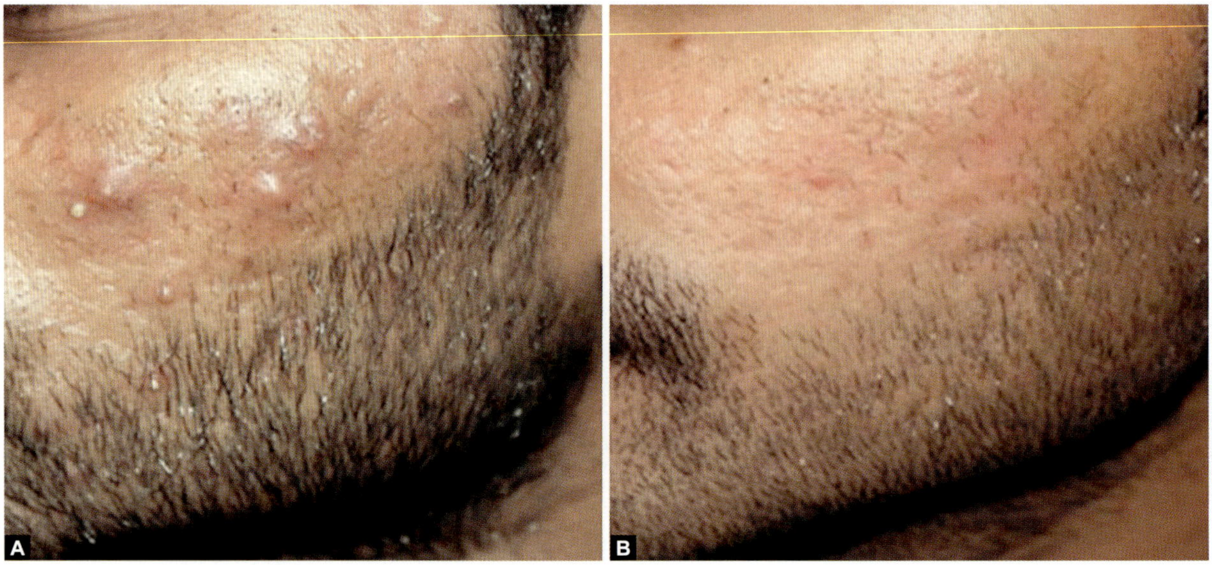

Figs. 8A and B: 1,319 nm laser—for topical steroid damaged face (TSDF) use. (A) Before; (B) After.

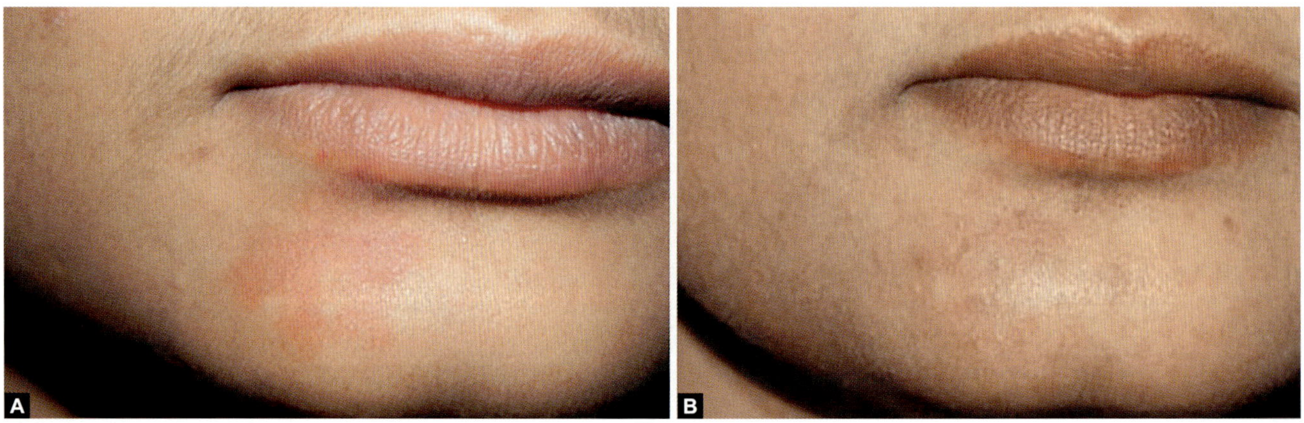

Figs. 9A and B: Intense pulsed light (IPL) for hemangioma. (A) Before; (B) After.

CONTRAINDICATIONS AND COMPLICATIONS OF NONABLATIVE LASERS[25]

Contraindications

- Pregnancy and lactation
- History of recurrent herpes or staphylococcal infections (a course of antiviral/antibacterial prophylaxis is advised)
- Keloidal tendency
- Patients with pacemakers
- Unrealistic expectations.

Complications

- Mild erythema or edema immediately postprocedure, which resolves within several hours
- Tenderness or temporary dysesthesia rarely
- Risk of postinflammatory hyperpigmentation and scarring
- Vesiculation may occur in patients with rosacea or flushing.

INTENSE PULSED LIGHT (FIGS. 9 AND 10)

Introduction

Intense pulsed light is a nonlaser filtered flash lamp device. IPL is a light based device which emits polychromatic, noncoherent, and noncollimated rays (420–1,400 nm). It has a broad spectrum of wavelengths enabling it to be absorbed by a variety of chromophores, making it less selective than laser.[26] Thus second generation devices are developed that use cut off filters to eliminate infrared part of the spectrum making it more selective with optimized treatment and lesser side effects.[27]

The current IPL systems have a versatile action, treating various conditions by targeting multiple chromophores with the same device, using different parameters (wavelength, pulse duration, number of pulses, and interval between pulses).[27]

The advantages and disadvantages of IPL are described in **Table 2**.

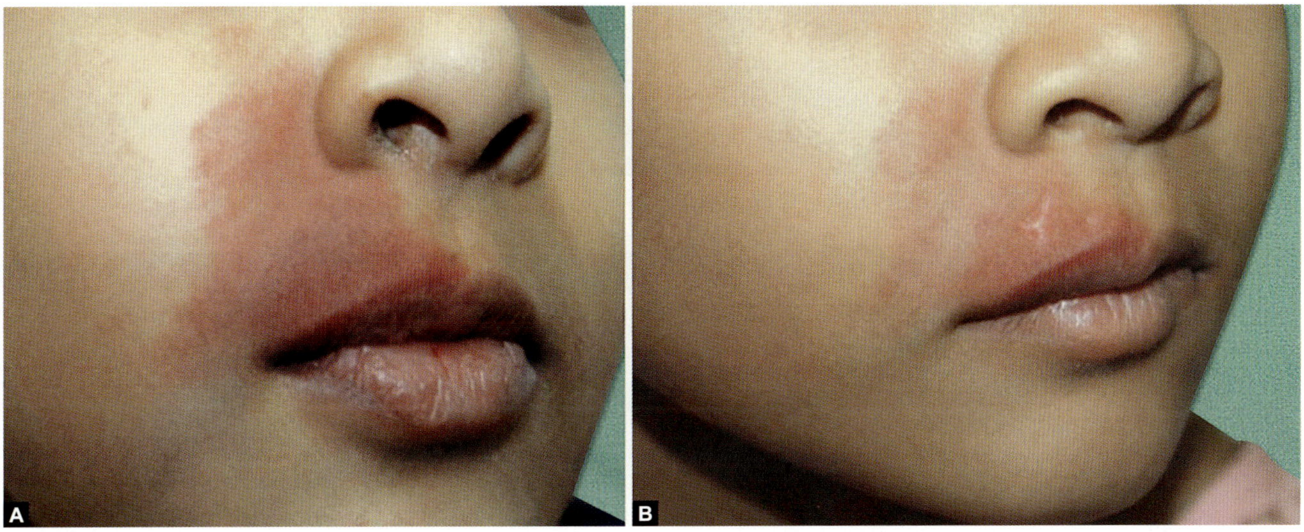

Figs. 10A and B: Intense pulsed light (IPL) for port-wine stain after 8 sessions. (A) Before; (B) After.

TABLE 2: Advantages and disadvantages of intense pulsed light (IPL).[27]

Advantages[27]	*Disadvantages*[27]
• The current IPL systems offer great versatility • Economical • Spot size is large • Time tested technology/ robust technology	• Emits broad wavelength light–nonspecific • Heavy hand piece • Light cannot be focused • Direct observation of treated area is not possible as hand piece has to have full contact with skin

BOX 1: Indications of intense pulsed light.[29,30]

- *Vascular lesions:* Port wine stain, hemangioma, cherry angioma, telangiectasia, spider angioma, angiofibroma, venous lake, etc.
- Rosacea
- Acne vulgaris
- Hair reduction
- Pigmented lesions and dyschromias
- Nonablative skin photo rejuvenation
- Hidradenitis suppurativa
- Hypertrophic/atrophic scar
- Striae
- Photodynamic therapy

Mechanism

Intense pulsed light works on the principle of selective photothermolysis, proposed by Anderson and Parrish in 1983, in which there is controlled destruction of a cutaneous target sparing surrounding tissue.[28]

Chromophores such as hemoglobin, melanin and water, etc., absorb light of a particular wavelength which is then converted to heat energy causing thermal destruction of chosen epidermal and dermal target.[29]

Indications[29,30]

Indications of IPL are given in **Box 1**.

EXCIMER LASER (FIGS. 11A AND B)

Introduction

Since its introduction in 1997,[31] for the treatment of refractory psoriasis, the excimer laser has emerged as an efficacious treatment modality for many dermatologic conditions. It contains a mixture of a noble inert gas (xenon) and a halogen (chloride) that forms unstable "excited dimers" which on dissociation produces a 308 nm ultraviolet (UV) monochromatic coherent wavelength, which lies within the UVB spectrum.[32]

The excimer laser delivers UV light via a hand-held device with a spot diameter of 14–30 mm.[31] As such, it is most appropriate for localized lesions and limited disease. It can also be used to target difficult areas such as the scalp, palms, and soles that would have limited UV exposure with conventional therapy.[33] In comparison to standard NBUVB, the excimer laser requires less treatment sessions, has reduced treatment duration, and requires a lower cumulative dose of UVB, thus reducing the possible side effects associated with UV therapy.[31,34-37]

Mechanism of Action

The major mechanism of its action is that it induces apoptosis of T lymphocytes, which are important in initiating inflammatory skin diseases.[38] The absorption of 308 nm light by T lymphocytes and keratinocytes induces DNA damage,[39] leading to a reduction in T lymphocyte inflammation and keratinocyte proliferation. This leads to upregulation of the tumor suppressor *gene p53*, contributing to cell cycle arrest and apoptosis.[33]

In disorders of depigmentation and hypopigmentation, repigmentation is hypothesized to be due to melanocyte migration and proliferation from increase in peptide ET-1.[40]

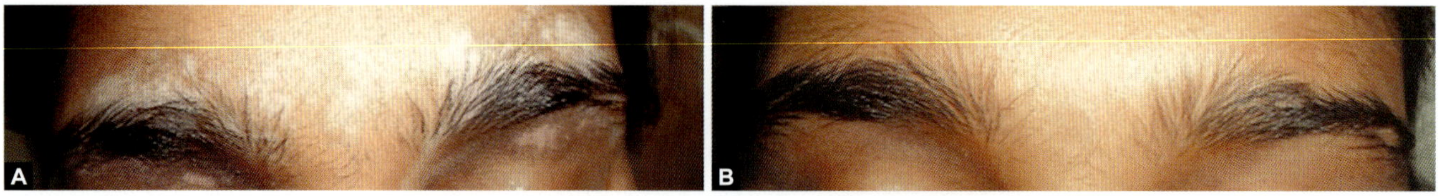

Figs. 11A and B: Excimer laser for vitiligo. (A) Before; (B) After.

Indications of Excimer Light Phototherapy

- Stable localized or recalcitrant plaque psoriasis, with body surface area (BSA) <5% involvement
- Vitiligo with BSA <5% involvement
- Difficult covered anatomical sites such as scalp, axillae, gluteal cleft, inguinal regions, and skin folds
- Other dermatoses responsive to NBUVB, with BSA <5% involvement
- Children who are claustrophobic in the NBUVB phototherapy cabin.

Excimer laser is currently approved by US Food and Drugs Administration (FDA) for the treatment of psoriasis, vitiligo, atopic dermatitis (AD) and leukoderma.[41] In addition to these diseases, the excimer laser has demonstrated efficacy in the treatment of alopecia areata, other hypopigmented disorders, and cutaneous T-cell lymphoma.[34,35]

Other conditions where excimer laser can be used as an adjuvant therapy **(Table 3)**:

- Hypopigmented disorders such as nevus depigmentosus, idiopathic guttate hypomelanosis, lichen striatus and pityriasis alba
- Adult Langerhans cell histiocytosis
- Cutaneous T-Cell lymphoma
- Lichen planus
- Granuloma annulare
- Localized scleroderma.

TABLE 3: Conditions where excimer laser is used.[34,38]

Entity	*Number of sessions*	*Type of disorder*
Psoriasis	18–20	Refractory plaque psoriasis
Vitiligo	30–40	Localized (<10%)
Atopic dermatitis	6–12	Acute exacerbations
Alopecia areata	11–18	Localized

Contraindications of Excimer Light Phototherapy

The contraindications of excimer light phototherapy are given in **Table 4**.

TABLE 4: Contraindications of excimer light phototherapy.[42]

Absolute	*Relative*
• Dermatomyositis, systemic lupus erythematosus • Xeroderma pigmentosum • Photosensitivity • Personal history of melanoma	• Premalignant skin lesions (e.g., actinic keratosis) • Personal history of non-melanoma skin cancer (NMSC) • Family history of skin cancer • Photosensitizing drugs

Adverse Effects of Excimer Laser

The adverse effects of excimer laser are described in **Table 5**.

TABLE 5: Adverse effects of excimer laser.[43]

Acute	*Chronic*
• Erythema, blistering, pain, pruritus • Pigmentation • Aggravation of existing skin disease • Herpes simplex virus reactivation	• Premature photoaging • Skin malignancy (squamous cell carcinoma)

LOW LEVEL LIGHT THERAPY (FIGS. 12A AND B)

Introduction

Low-level laser (or light) therapy (LLLT) is defined as modification of biological activity by using photons. Lasers or noncoherent light sources consisting of filtered lamps or light-emitting diodes (LED) can be used.[44] Other names used include low-intensity laser therapy, soft laser, low-power laser therapy, cold laser, photobiostimulation, and photobiomodulation.[45] The therapeutic applications of LLLT are reduction of pain and inflammation, tissue repair, promoting regeneration of tissues and nerves.[44,46] The properties of LLLT include[47]

- *Wave length:* 600–1070 nm
- *Power output:* 0.001–0.1 Watts
- *Intensity:* 0.01–10 W/cm^2
- *Dose:* 0.01–100 J/ cm^2
- *Pulse rate:* 0–5,000 Hertz (cycles per second)

The laser sources include[44]

- *Ruby:* 694 nm
- *Helium neon (HeNe):* 633 nm
- *Krypton:* 521 nm, 530 nm, 568 nm, 647 nm
- *Argon:* 488 nm and 514 nm
- *Gallium arsenide (GaAs):* > 760 nm (e.g., 904 nm)
- *Gallium aluminum arsenide (Ga-Al-As):* 612–870 nm.

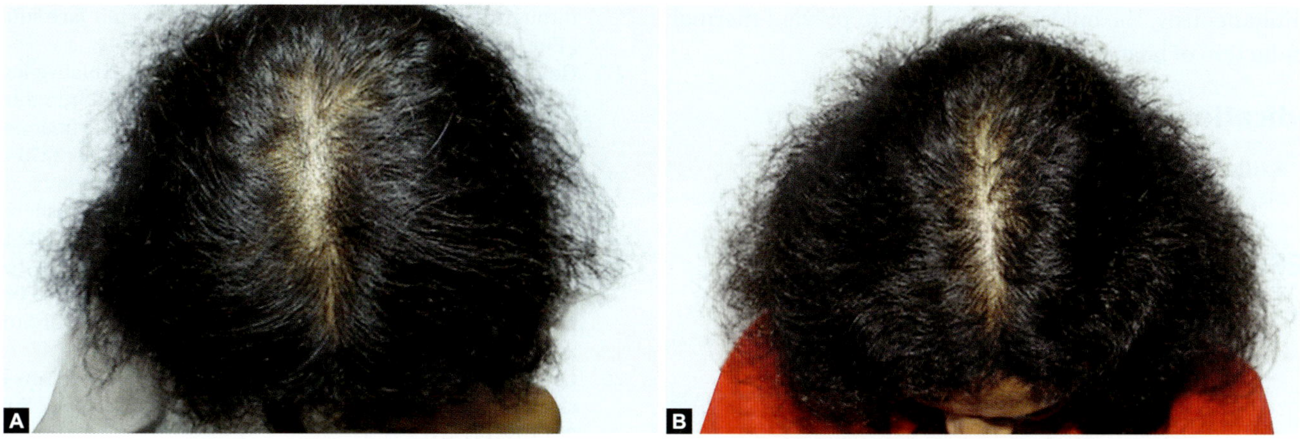

Figs. 12A and B: Low-level laser therapy (LLLT) for female pattern hair loss (FPHL). (A) Before; (B) After.

Mechanism

The mechanism is by absorption of red and near infrared light by mitochondrial chromophores, in particular Cytochrome C oxidase (CCO) which is present in the respiratory chain within the mitochondria. This causes photodissociation of inhibitory nitric oxide from CCO leading to enhancement of enzyme activity, electron transport, mitochondrial respiration and thereby, ATP production. LLLT alters the cellular redox state. It induces activation of various intracellular signaling pathways; alters affinity of transcription factors which is associated with cell proliferation, survival, tissue repair and regeneration.[48]

Indications[44,48-50]

The indications of low-level laser (or light) therapy (LLLT) are given in **Box 2**.

BOX 2: Indications of low-level laser (or light) therapy (LLLT).[44,48-50]

The various uses of LLLT in the field of dermatology include:

- Skin rejuvenation
- Acne vulgaris
- Photoprotection
- Herpes simplex lesions
- Hair loss—male and female pattern hair loss, alopecia areata, chemotherapy induced alopecia
- Vitiligo
- Hypertrophic scars and keloids
- Psoriasis
- Oral lichen planus
- Lichen planopilaris and lichenoid dermatoses
- Wound healing—acute surgical wounds—incisions, excisions, and avulsions, burn wounds, chronic ulcers
- Fat reduction
- Recurrent aphthous ulcers
- Xerostomia
- Burning mouth syndrome
- Mucositis

Contraindications

It is avoided in coagulation disorders since they interfere with blood circulation in a way still unknown. It is also avoided in malignant and precancerous lesions since it stimulates cell growth. Irradiation of endocrine glands, especially thyroid gland should be avoided. During pregnancy, febrile conditions, menstrual cycle, in epilepsy and those who have cochlear implants, the use of lasers is not advised.[47]

Side Effects

Most subjects in the studies reported only mild side effects, commonly pruritus, acne, and scalp tenderness. No studies reported any severe adverse events that lead to discontinuation of treatment, and most of the side effects resolved within 2 weeks.[51]

MICROWAVE LASER

Introduction

Microwaves lie in the electromagnetic spectrum between infrared waves (such as carbon dioxide lasers) and radiowaves (radiofrequency devices) at 104–105 m and travel at the speed of light. Microwaves heat substances through a process called dielectric heating. Electric dipole molecules rotate in response to microwaves in an attempt to align with the alternating electromagnetic field. Rapid movement causes frictional heat. Water has a high dipole moment, which means it is highly absorbent for microwaves, whereas fat has a low dipole moment and absorbs microwaves poorly. As the microwaves are preferentially absorbed by high-water-content tissue, this leads to localized heating.

Mechanism

The microwave energy is concentrated along the dermal-adipose, creating a focal energy zone. At the same time, continuous hydroceramic cooling prevents thermal conduction of heat superficially. The heat at the dermal-adipose energy zone leads to thermolysis of the eccrine glands.

Microwaves are concentrated in this area creating focal energy zone destroying the eccrine and apocrine glands.[52,53]

Simultaneously, the epidermis is cooled to prevent thermal conduction of heat superficially.

Indications

- Axillary hyperhidrosis
- Osmidrosis.

REFERENCES

1. Levy JL, Trelles M, Lagarde JM, Borrel MT, Mordon S. Treatment of wrinkles with the nonablative 1,320-nm Nd:YAG laser. Ann Plast Surg. 2001;47(5):482-8.
2. Freedman J, Greene R, Green J. Histologic effects of resurfacing lasers. Facial Plastic Surgery. 2014;30(01):40-8.
3. Rahman Z, MacFalls H, Jiang K, Chan KF, Kelly K, Tournas J, et al. Fractional deep dermal ablation induces tissue tightening. Lasers Surg Med. 2009;41(2):78-86.
4. Lupton JR, Williams CM, Alster TS. Nonablative laser skin resurfacing using a 1540 nm erbium glass laser: a clinical and histologic analysis. Dermatol Surg. 2002;28(9):833-5.
5. Politi Y, Levi A, Snast I, Ad-EL D, Lapidoth M. Integrated cooling-vacuum-assisted non-fractional 1540-nm erbium: glass laser: a new modality for the simultaneous effective treatment of acne lesions and scars. J Drugs Dermatol. 2018;17(11):1173-6.
6. Amann PM, Marquardt Y, Steiner T, Hölzle F, Skazik-Voogt C, Heise R, et al. Effects of non-ablative fractional erbium glass laser treatment on gene regulation in human three-dimensional skin models. Lasers Med Sci. 2016;31(3):397-404.
7. Alhattab MK, Al Abdullah MJ, Al-Janabi MH, Aljanaby WA, Alwakeel HA. The effect of 1540-nm fractional erbium-glass laser in the treatment of androgenic alopecia. J Cosmet Dermatol. 2020;19(4):878-83.
8. Use of mosaic (erbium glass) laser in treatment of acne scars. J Am Acad Dermatol. 2012;66(4):AB217.
9. Angel S, Boineau D, Dahan S, Mordon S. Treatment of active acne with an Er:Glass (1.54 microm) laser: a 2-year follow-up study. J Cosmet Laser Ther. 2006;8(4):171-6.
10. Al-Dhalimi MA, Al-Janabi MH, Abd Al Hussein RA. The use of a 1,540 nm fractional erbium-glass laser in treatment of alopecia areata. Lasers Surg Med. 2019;51(10):859-65.
11. Puri N. A study on fractional erbium glass laser therapy versus chemical peeling for the treatment of melasma in female patients. J Cutan Aesthetic Surg. 2013;6(3):148-51.
12. El-Domyati M, El-Ammawi TS, Medhat W, Moawad O, Mahoney MG, Uitto J. Effects of the Nd:YAG 1320-nm laser on skin rejuvenation: clinical and histological correlations. J Cosmet Laser Ther. 2011;13(3):98-106.
13. Preissig J, Hamilton K, Markus R. Current laser resurfacing technologies: a review that delves beneath the surface. Semin Plast Surg. 2012;26(3):109-16.
14. Chan HHL, Lam L, Wong DSY, Kono T, Trendell-Smith N. Use of 1,320 nm Nd:YAG laser for wrinkle reduction and the treatment of atrophic acne scarring in Asians. Lasers Surg Med. 2004;34(2):98-103.
15. Yaghmai D, Garden JM, Bakus AD, Massa MC. Comparison of a 1,064 nm laser and a 1,320 nm laser for the nonablative treatment of acne scars. Dermatol Surg. 2005;31(8 Pt 1):903-9.
16. Kwon HH, Park HY, Choi SC, Bae Y, Jung JY, Park GH. Novel device-based acne treatments: comparison of a 1450-nm diode laser and microneedling radiofrequency on mild-to-moderate acne vulgaris and seborrhoea in Korean patients through a 20-week prospective, randomized, split-face study. J Eur Acad Dermatol Venereol. 2018;32(4):639-44.
17. Goldberg DJ, Rogachefsky AS, Silapunt S. Non-ablative laser treatment of facial rhytides: a comparison of 1450-nm diode laser treatment with dynamic cooling as opposed to treatment with dynamic cooling alone. Lasers Surg Med. 2002;30(2):79-81.
18. Chun S. Fractional microneedling radiofrequency and fractional 1927 nm thulium laser treatment offer synergistic skin rejuvenation: a pilot case series. Laser Ther. 2018;27(4):283-91.
19. Lee HM, Haw S, Kim JK, Chang SE, Lee MW. Split-face study using a 1,927-nm thulium fiber fractional laser to treat photoaging and melasma in Asian skin. Dermatol Surg. 2013;39(6):879-88.
20. Ortiz AE, Goldman MP, Fitzpatrick RE. Ablative CO_2 lasers for skin tightening: traditional versus fractional. Dermatol Surg. 2014;12:147-51.
21. Cho SB, Zheng Z, Kang JS, Kim H. Therapeutic efficacy of 1,927-nm fractionated thulium laser energy and polydeoxyribonucleotide on pattern hair loss. Med Laser 2016;5:22-8.
22. Panchaprateep R, Munavalli G. Low-fluence 585 nm Q-switched Nd:YAG laser: a novel laser treatment for post-acne erythema. Lasers Surg Med. 2015;47(2):148-55.
23. Goo BL, Kang JS, Cho SB. Treatment of early-stage erythematotelangiectatic rosacea with a Q-switched 595-nm Nd:YAG laser. J Cosmet Laser Ther. 2015;17(3):139-42.
24. Bogle MA. Fractionated mid-infrared resurfacing. Semin Cutan Med Surg. 2008;27(4):252-8.
25. Sachdev M, Hameed S, Mysore V. Nonablative lasers and nonlaser systems in dermatology: current status. Indian J Dermatol Venereol Leprol. 2011;77:380-8.
26. Husain Z, Alster TS. The role of lasers and intense pulsed light technology in dermatology. Clin Cosmet Investig Dermatol. 2016;9:29-40.
27. Gonzalez-Rodriguez AJ, Lorente-Gual R. Current indications and new applications of intense pulsed light. Actas Dermosifiliogr. 2015;106(5):350-64.
28. Anderson RR, Parrish JA. Selective photothermolysis: precise microsurgery by selective absorption of pulsed radiation. Science. 1983;220:524-7.
29. Goldberg DJ. Current trends in intense pulsed light. J Clin Aesthet Dermatol. 2012;5(6):45-53.
30. Srinivas CR, Kumaresan M. Lasers for vascular lesions: standard guidelines of care. Indian J Dermatol Venereol Leprol. 2011;77(3):349-68.
31. Bonis B, Kemeny L, Dobozy A, Bor Z, Szabó G, Ignácz F. 308 nm UVB excimer laser for psoriasis. Lancet. 1997;350:1522.
32. Spencer JM, Hadi SM. The excimer lasers. J Drugs Dermatol. 2004;3(5):522-5.
33. Ly K, Smith MP, Thibodeaux QG, Beck KM, Liao W, Bhutani T. Beyond the booth: excimer laser for cutaneous conditions. Dermatol Clin. 2020;38(1):157-63.
34. Beggs S, Short J, Rengifo-Pardo M, Ehrlich A. Applications of the excimer laser: a review. Dermatol Surg. 2015;41(11):1201-11.
35. Mehraban S, Feily A. 308 nm excimer laser in dermatology. J Lasers Med Sci. 2014;5(1):8-12.
36. Feldman SR, Mellen BG, Housman TS, Fitzpatrick RE, Geronemus RG, Friedman PM, et al. Efficacy of the 308-nm excimer laser for treatment of psoriasis: results of a multicenter study. J Am Acad Dermatol 2002;46(6):900-6.
37. Trehan M, Taylor CR. Medium-dose 308-nm excimer laser for the treatment of psoriasis. J Am Acad Dermatol. 2002;47(5):701-8.
38. Farkas A, Kemeny L. Applications of the 308-nm excimer laser in dermatology. Laser Phys. 2006;16:876.

39. Wong T, Hsu L, Liao W. Phototherapy in psoriasis: a review of mechanisms of action. J Cutan Med Surg 2013;17(1): 6–12.
40. Pacifico A, Leone G. Photo(chemo)therapy for vitiligo. Photodermatol Photoimmunol Photomed. 2011;27: 261-77.
41. Park KK, Liao W, Murase JE. A review of monochromatic excimer light in vitiligo. Br J Dermatol. 2012;167(3):468-78.
42. Mysore V, Shashikumar BM. Targeted phototherapy. Indian J Dermatol Venereol Leprol. 2016;82(1):1-6.
43. Abrouk M, Levin E, Brodsky M, Gandy JR, Nakamura M, Zhu TH, et al. Excimer laser for the treatment of psoriasis: safety, efficacy, and patient acceptability. Psoriasis (Auckl). 2016;6:165-73.
44. Gupta A, Avci P, Sadasivam M, Chandran R, Parizotto N, Vecchio D, et al. Shining light on nanotechnology to help repair and regeneration. Biotechnol Adv. 2013;31(5): 607-31.
45. Anders JJ, Lanzafame RJ, Arany PR. Low-level light/laser therapy versus photobiomodulation therapy. Photomed Laser Surg. 2015;33(4):183-4.
46. Chung H, Dai T, Sharma SK, Huang YY, Carroll JD, Hamblin MR. The nuts and bolts of low-level laser (light) therapy. Ann Biomed Eng. 2012;40(2):516-33.
47. Posten W, Wrone DA, Dover JS, Arndt KA, Silapunt S, Alam M. Low-level laser therapy for wound healing: mechanism and efficacy. Dermatol Surg. 2005;31(3):334-40.
48. Avci P, Gupta A, Sadasivam M, Vecchio D, Pam Z, Pam N, et al. Low-level laser (light) therapy (LLLT) in skin: stimulating, healing, restoring. Semin Cutan Med Surg. 2013;32(1):41-52.
49. Mahdavi O, Boostani N, Jajarm H, Falaki F, Tabesh A. Use of low level laser therapy for oral lichen planus: report of two cases. J Dent. 2013;14(4):201-4.
50. Randolph MJ, Salhi WA, Tosti A. Lichen planopilaris and low-level light therapy: four case reports and review of the literature about low-level light therapy and lichenoid dermatosis. Dermatol Ther. 2020;10(2):311-9.
51. Egger A, Resnik SR, Aickara D, Maranda E, Kaiser M, Wikramanayake TC, et al. Examining the safety and efficacy of low-level laser therapy for male and female pattern hair loss: a review of the literature. Skin Appendage Disord. 2020;6(5): 259-67.
52. Taylor NAS, Machado-Moreira CA. Regional variations in transepidermal water loss, eccrine sweat gland density, sweat secretion rates and electrolyte composition in resting and exercising humans. Extrem Physiol Med. 2013;2:4.
53. Jacob C. Treatment of hyperhidrosis with microwave technology. Semin Cutan Med Surg. 2013;32:2-8.

CHAPTER 116 Microneedle Radiofrequency

Swapnil Shah, Siddharth Mani

KEY MESSAGES

- Microneedle radiofrequency (MNRF) is a novel energy-based device used for many common aesthetic and dermatological indications.
- Since radiofrequency (RF) energy is colorblind, it can be used safely and effectively in all skin types.
- In comparison with lasers, it is associated with less downtime and is safer in dark-skinned individuals.

INTRODUCTION

Treatment of scars, wrinkles, and skin rejuvenation has always been a special problem in Indian skin. A variety of lasers and light-based technologies are available for the treatment of these common but psychologically disturbing conditions. The risk of pigmentary complications, associated downtime, and mild-to-moderate improvement with these light-based technologies limit their use in the Indian context.

Microneedle radiofrequency (MNRF) is a newer concept where needles are introduced in the skin with a preselected depth and radiofrequency (RF) is delivered through these needles to heat the dermis. Since RF is colorblind, it can be used in any skin type safely with excellent results.

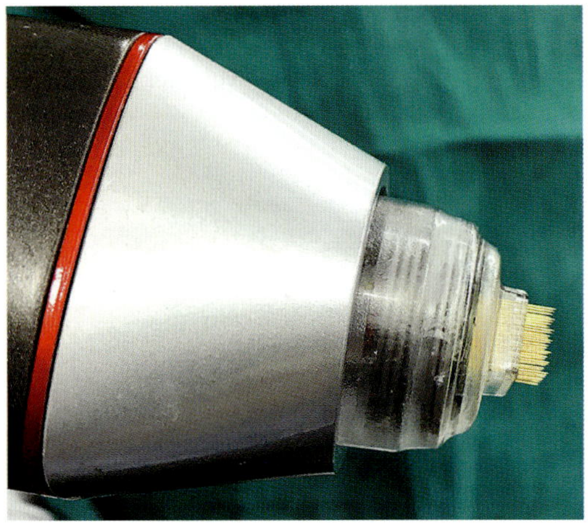

Fig. 1: Microneedle tip.

HISTORY

Radiofrequency is being used in the treatment of dermatological conditions since early 2000.[1]

Hantash et al., in a private study in 2009, proposed the concept of using needles as electrodes, which allowed the RF energy to be delivered into the dermis.[2] Since the RF energy was fractionated among several delivery and return needles **(Fig. 1)**, the terminology became microneedle radiofrequency.

BASIC PHYSICS

Radiofrequency is a high-frequency alternating electric current used traditionally for radiocommunication. Whenever electric current flows through the body, the body offers resistance to its flow. This resistance of the tissue is known as "impedance". According to Joule's law, when electric current meets resistance, it generates heat because of microoscillations of charged particles. When the temperature of the tissues rises to about 60°C, tissues are coagulated. This is the basic mechanism of action of RF. In short, the RF effect is "electrothermal" as against lasers whose effect is photothermal.[2] The depth of penetration of RF is inversely proportional to the frequency of RF. By using a particular frequency, one can target a particular level in the skin.

ADVANTAGES OF RADIOFREQUENCY OVER LIGHT-BASED DEVICES

- Since chromophore is not required for electrothermal effect, RF energy is colorblind and thus can be used to treat any skin type irrespective of the color or tanning.
- Because of the cooling used, it causes no or minimal damage to the epidermis.
- Skin RF energy does not scatter; it offers enhanced tissue penetration independent of skin color.

METHOD OF RADIOFREQUENCY DELIVERY

Radiofrequency can be delivered into the skin noninvasively using monopolar or bipolar RF systems. The monopolar system consists of an active electrode that emits RF and a ground electrode that is in contact with the patient's body. Thus, RF current travels through the patient's body and terminates at the ground electrode to complete the circuit. Monopolar RF penetrates deep into the skin and is very painful. The bipolar systems consist of two active electrodes. RF flows between these two electrodes. The depth of penetration achieved is far less than monopolar RF, since it is directly proportional to the distance between two electrodes. If one of the two electrodes loses contact with the skin, it can cause sparks and result in epidermal burns. Both these RF systems require aggressive skin cooling to protect the epidermis.

These systems have certain limitations such as:

- They are associated with hot spots, so there are chances of epidermal burns.
- Aggressive skin cooling is required to protect the epidermis.
- The monopolar RF causes deep heating and is extremely painful. If used aggressively, it can cause subcutaneous fat necrosis. Often, it is used with less energy to make it tolerable. The tolerable energy used causes partial denaturation and not coagulation collagen.
- In case of bipolar RF, the depth is even lesser since it is proportional to half the distance between the two electrodes.
- There is a high cost of consumables associated with these systems.

Invasive RF systems deliver electromagnetic energy by using electrodes that penetrate the target tissue. MNRF is a novel method that allows nonthermal penetration of the epidermis using needles as electrodes, followed by RF coagulation in a selected depth of the dermis surrounded by a zone of noncoagulative volumetric heating.[3]

MECHANISM OF ACTION OF MICRONEEDLE RADIOFREQUENCY

Water, dermal microvasculature, collagen, and melanin offer resistance to RF energy producing bulk heating of the dermis. This results in the secretion of cellular mediators and growth factors related to wound healing.[3] Following thermal injury, various heat shock proteins (HSPs) are expressed in the dermal dendritic cells.[4] These HSPs including HSP47, HSP70, and HSP72 are thought to be responsible for collagen induction.[5] A marked induction of tropoelastin, fibrillin, and procollagens 1 and 3 is also seen by 4 weeks post-treatment.

The zone of denatured collagen in the RF thermal zones (RTZ) is replaced by newly formed collagen in the next 3 months **(Figs. 2 to 4)**. In addition to collagen, new elastic fibers were also deposited in the skin.[3] The combination of neoelastinogenesis and neocollagenesis induced by treatment with the MNRF system is the basis of providing a reliable treatment option for skin laxity and/or rhytids.

The MNRF also increases the epidermal hyaluronan content,[6] providing an additional mechanism for skin rejuvenation. The simple nonthermal physical needling stimulates the epidermis and restructures it. There is an additional benefit of the mechanical vertical scar disruption because of the needle insertion.[7]

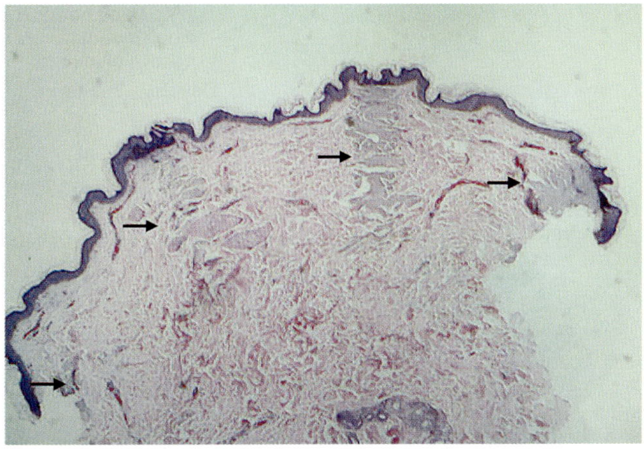

Fig. 2: Histology of human skin after microneedle radiofrequency (MNRF). Scanner view showing four columns of coagulation (Black arrows). *Courtesy:* Slides prepared by Dr Balkrishna Nikam, Karad, Maharashtra.

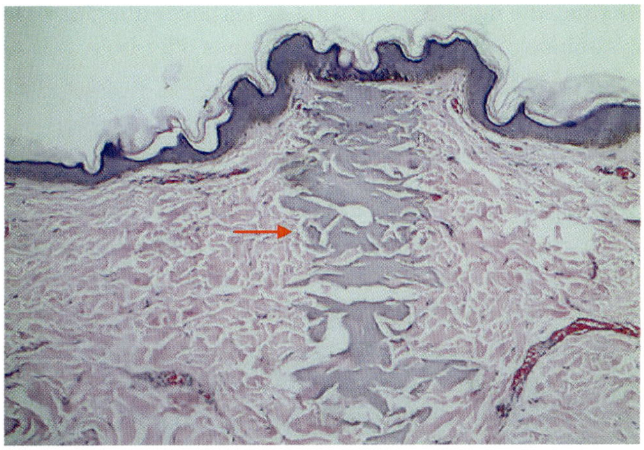

Fig. 3: Close-up of individual zone of coagulation (Red arrow).

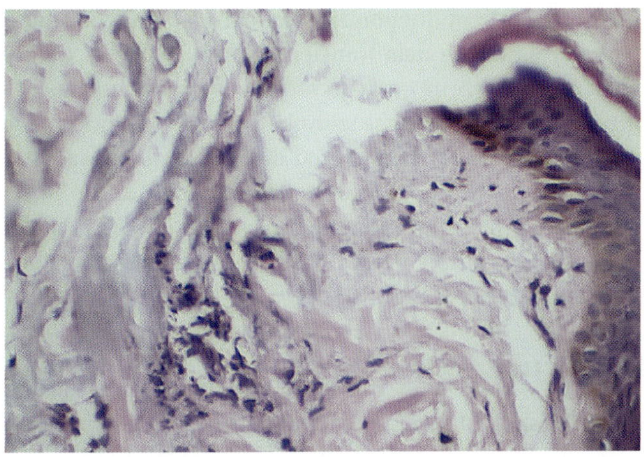

Fig. 4: Zone of coagulation sparing the epidermis.

Since the depth of penetration of these needles can be manually adjusted, it is easy to reach the junction of reticular dermis and subcutaneous fat and nonselectively destroy eccrine sweat glands[8] and inhibit sebaceous glands.[9]

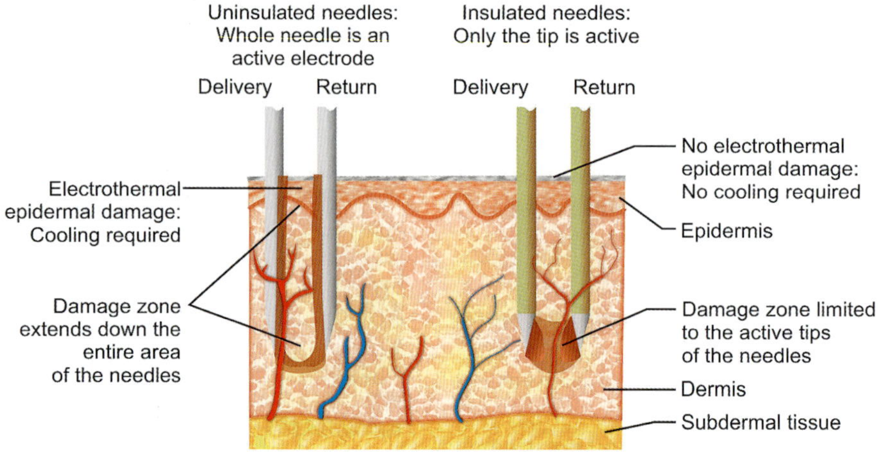

Fig. 5: Difference between insulated and noninsulated microneedle.

TYPES OF NEEDLES

Microneedle radiofrequency machines have either insulated or noninsulated needles. Few machines offer both types of needles **(Fig. 5)**.

Insulated Needles

The microneedles are stainless steel needles of 34G size, which are coated with gold for better conductivity and then double coated with silicone insulation, except for the first 300 μm at the tip **(Fig. 6)**.

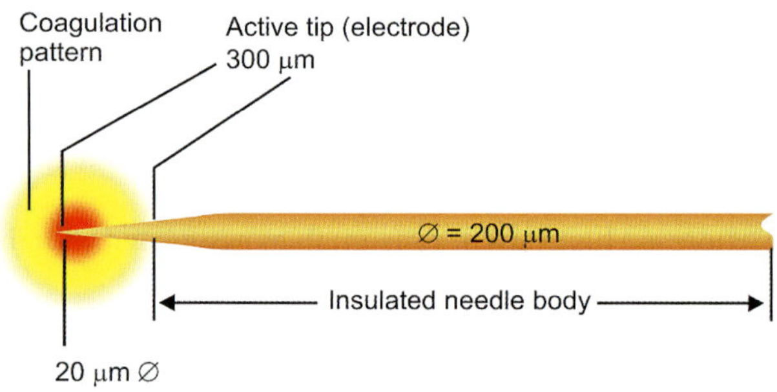

Fig. 6: Schematic diagram showing an insulated microneedle.

Insulation of the needles restricts RF energy delivery to the very tip of the needle. Because of this simple physical needling, damage occurs to the epidermis without any thermal damage **(Fig. 7)**. The RF is delivered into the dermis at a particular depth. However, in real life, there will always be some heat transmitted superficially from the deeper layers just through proximity and conduction as the heat gradually dissipates. Also, there may be heat transferred through the insulation, particularly with more aggressive treatment settings. The physical needling damage stimulates the regeneration of the epidermis over the restructured dermis.[9] Since coagulation occurs only at the tip, it causes lots of oozing and pinpoint bleeding while performing the procedure. The RF has to be delivered in multiple passes, typically three passes, to cover the large part of the dermis.

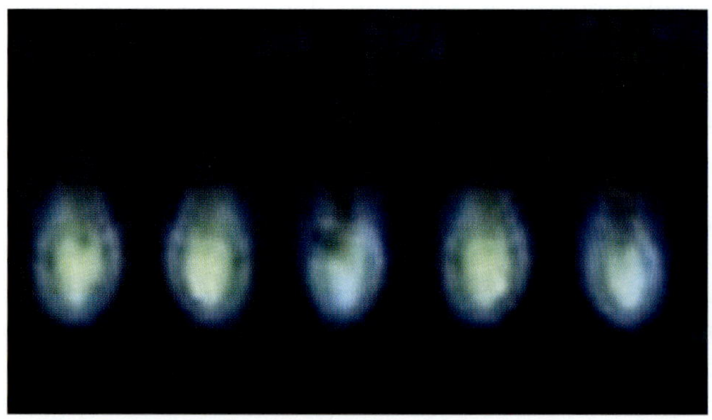

Fig. 7: Thermographic image showing nonthermal ablation of epidermis with dermal coagulation at a selected depth of dermis in case of an insulated microneedle.

Noninsulated Needles

When the shaft of the needles is noninsulated, the needles act as active electrodes all the way from epidermis to the needle tips. Thus, it can cause slight epidermal thermal damage **(Fig. 8)**. They deliver a larger RTZ throughout the entire length of the electrode.

These needles can be more painful, if we use high power. Since RF is delivered throughout the shaft of the needle, it causes more coagulation and no pinpoint bleeding.[7] However, it can be associated with a minimal downtime of 48–72 hours. Epidermal injuries may occur with the noninsulated needles, thus leading to higher risks in darker skin types.

The debate between insulated and noninsulated needles is still inconclusive. In a landmark paper, Na et al. studied noninsulated needles in a micropig skin.[10] In their study, RF was delivered to the skin of a micropig at varying microneedle penetration depths, RF signal amplitudes, and RF conduction times. They have observed the following:

- Coagulation columns of thermal injury were generated separately around each needle tip.

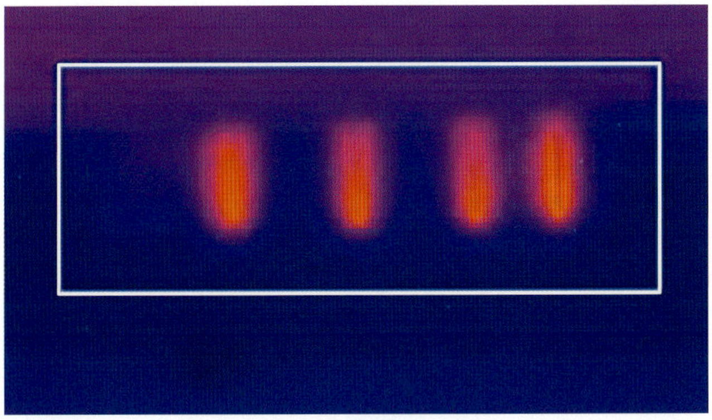

Fig. 8: Thermographic image while using a noninsulated microneedle. The needle is active all along its length.

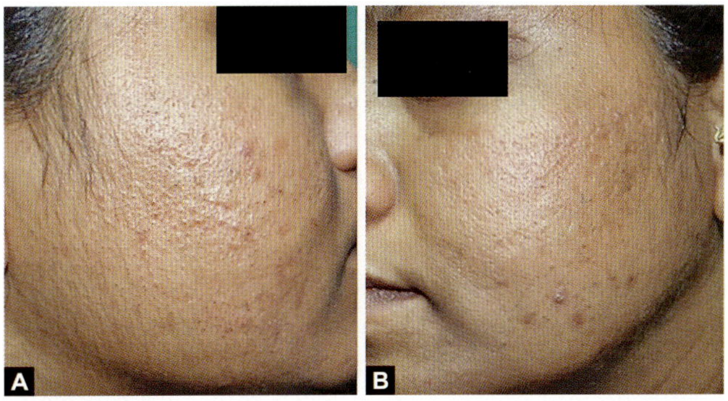

Figs. 10A and B: Image of the same patient 24 hours after the procedure. (A) Microcrusts are visible on noninsulated-treated side; and (B) Complete recovery on insulated-treated side.

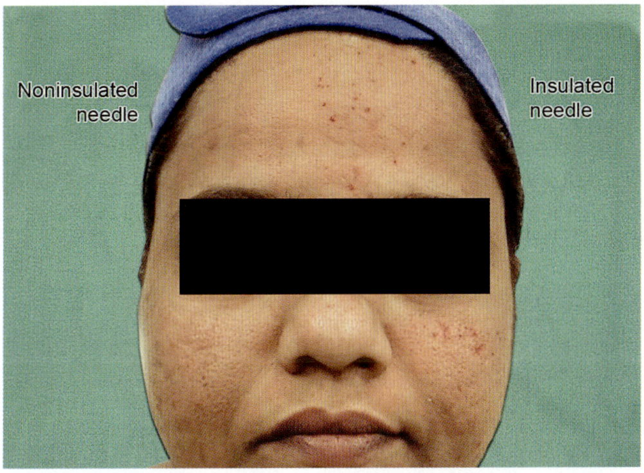

Fig. 9: Split-face image. The side treated with noninsulated microneedles shows erythema and edema but no bleeding. The side treated with insulated needles shows erythema, edema, and pinpoint bleeding.

- No noticeable RF-induced tissue reactions were observed in the epidermis or between the electrodes in the dermis. So, the treatment is essentially fractional.
- Longer RF conduction times created larger areas of coagulation in the dermis while higher RF energy generated greater degrees of tissue destruction and desiccation.
- After 2 seconds of RF conduction time, individual areas of thermal coagulation converged with neighboring RF-induced coagulation columns.
- Deeper penetration with the microneedle electrodes generated larger columns of coagulation at the same RF power and conduction time.
- No epidermal thermal injury was observed even when using noninsulated needles because the electric current follows the path of least resistance and 80% of energy is delivered at the tip of needle.
- By controlling RF conduction times, they showed that the delivery of bipolar RF energy via noninsulated electrodes can induce thermal responses similar to those for insulated electrodes. Thus, practically there is no difference in efficacy whether one uses insulated or noninsulated needles **(Figs. 9 and 10)**.

OTHER VARIABLES AFFECTING MICRONEEDLE RADIOFREQUENCY

Variable versus Fixed-length Needles

Variable length needle allows for more flexibility, which is required as skin thickness and condition vary. Few scars such as acne scars require deeper treatment, with fixed-length devices proving to be more useful. Another thing that is to be kept in mind is that while using the device, if the pressure is not adequate or the needles are not perpendicular, the resistance from the skin might lead to shallower depth than anticipated.

Manual versus Mechanical Insertion

With manual insertion, there is always a possibility of user variation and user fatigue. The mechanical insertion is better; however, in a few cases the poor quality of motor cannot overcome the inherent resistance of the skin and insertion remains superficial. In many cases, due to rapidity of movement, few imperfect impulses exist that may lead to unequal effect.

Temperature and Impedance Feedback

The optimum threshold required to obtain coagulation and maximum neocollagenesis is 65–70°C. Hence, most good machines have temperature and impedance feedback that helps in maintaining the desired temperature. Absence of this monitoring might lead to burns or ineffective results.

PROCEDURE

- Clean the face.
- Apply topical anesthesia.
- Wipe out the anesthetic cream.
- Contact handpiece tip to epidermis.
- The power level, exposure time, and depth of needle insertion are manually set on the machine or handpiece depending on the indication and area to be treated.

- Microneedles automatically penetrate the skin after pressing the foot or finger switch.
- Microfractional holes are created in the epidermis and dermis.
- High RF is emitted in the deep dermis inducing dermal coagulation.
- Microneedles are withdrawn automatically.
- Single or multiple passes are given depending upon the machine used. When multiple passes are used, it is advisable to give the first pass at a deeper level than subsequent passes (e.g., 1.5–2.5 mm) and reduce the exposure time and/or power as one moves up closer to the epidermis.
- After the treatment, the face is cleaned and any oozing or bleeding is controlled with minor pressure. A cooling pack, mask, or cold air is applied to increase the patient's comfort. Antibiotic cream and sunscreen are applied.
- Treatments are done once in 4–12 weeks for a total of three to five sessions depending on improvement.

INDICATIONS OF MICRONEEDLE RADIOFREQUENCY

Different indications of MNRF are listed in **Box 1**.

Acne Scars

Atrophic acne scarring is an unfortunate, permanent complication of acne vulgaris, which may be associated with significant psychological distress. The boxcar and rolling scar **(Figs. 11A and B)** respond well to MNRF. Patient compliance and side effect profile are much better in patients treated with MNRF. MNRF can be combined with various other treatment modalities such as platelet-rich plasma therapy (PRP), sublative RF, or even fractional ablative and nonablative lasers. MNRF also has sebosuppressive effect;[11] therefore, it can be used in patients with active acne **(Figs. 12 to 14)**,[12] open pores, etc. Generally, three to five treatments, placed 4–8 weeks apart, are required to achieve a satisfactory response **(Figs. 15A and B)**.

Various studies demonstrate the efficacy of MNRF in the management of acne scars. Pudukadan[13] studied 19 Indian patients with acne scars. He reported improvement of at least 1 acne-scar grade in 11 out of 19 patients (57.9%) after 1 month and in 9 out of 9 patients (100%) after 3 months. Chandrashekar et al. studied 31 Indian patients with grade 3 and 4 acne scars and found that 80.64% showed improvement by 2 grades and 19.35% showed improvement by 1 grade. Quantitative assessment showed that 58% of the patients had moderate, 29% had minimal, 9% had good, and 3% had very good improvement.[14] Cho et al.[15] and Vejjabhinanta et al.[16] also reported similar findings.

BOX 1: Indications of microneedle radiofrequency (MNRF).

- Acne scars
- Surgical scars
- Photodamaged skin and skin rejuvenation
- Skin laxity and wrinkles
- Seborrhea
- Large/open pores
- Striae
- Axillary hyperhidrosis
- Transepidermal drug delivery

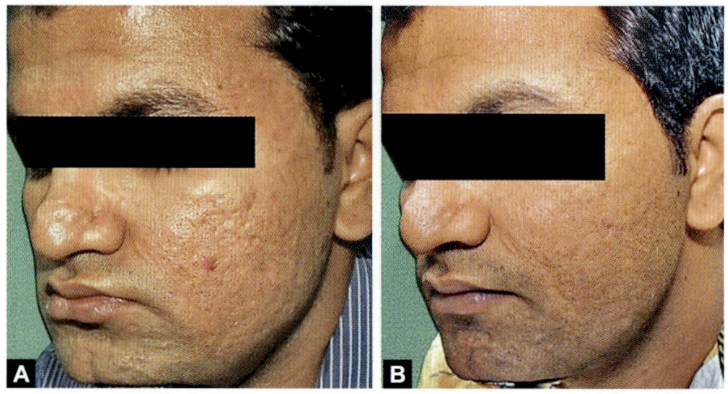

Figs. 11A and B: (A) Grade 4 acne scars; (B) Treated with four sessions of PRP and MNRF. (MNRF: microneedle radiofrequency; PRP: platelet-rich plasma therapy)

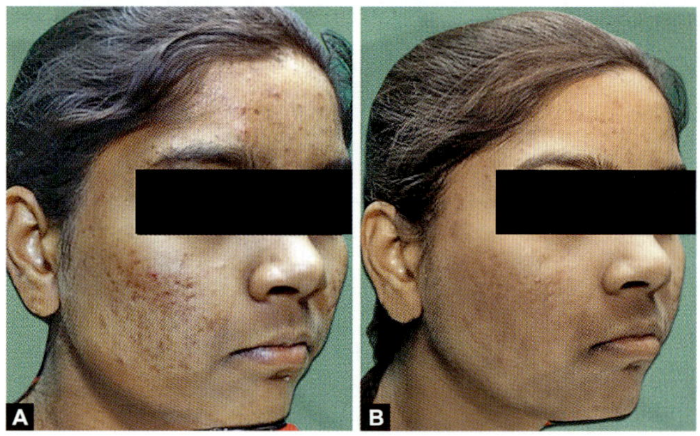

Figs. 12A and B: Acne scar in type V skin. (A) One session; and (B) 3 months after.

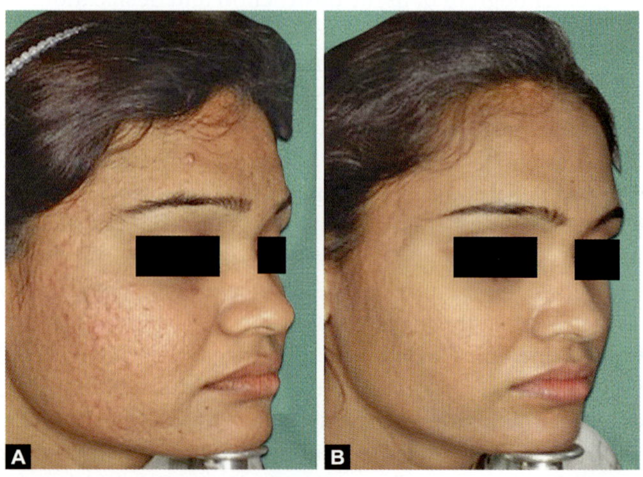

Figs. 13A and B: Acne scars with seborrhea and grade 2 acne. (A) Two sessions; and (B) 1 month apart. Decrease in scars, seborrhea, and acne is observed.

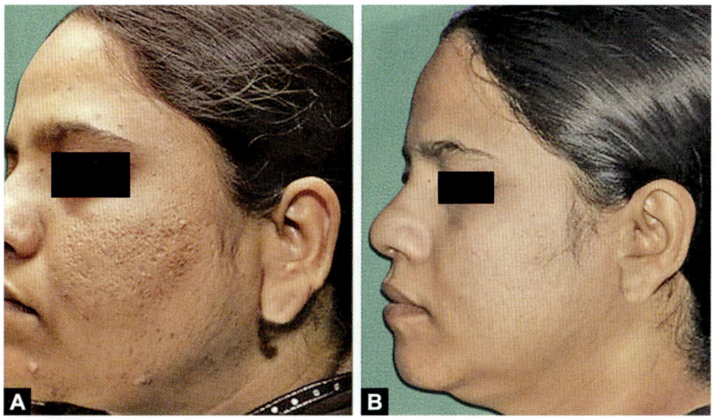

Figs. 14A and B: (A) Grade 3 acne scars with predominantly ice prick scarring; and (B) Treatment after three sessions.

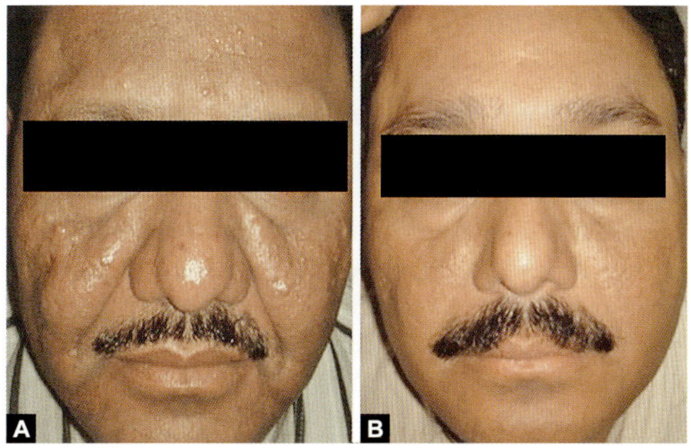

Figs. 16A and B: (A) Marked sebaceous hyperplasia; (B) Treated with MNRF with aggressive settings in two sessions. (MNRF: microneedle radiofrequency)
Courtesy: Dr Jagadish Sakhiya, Surat.

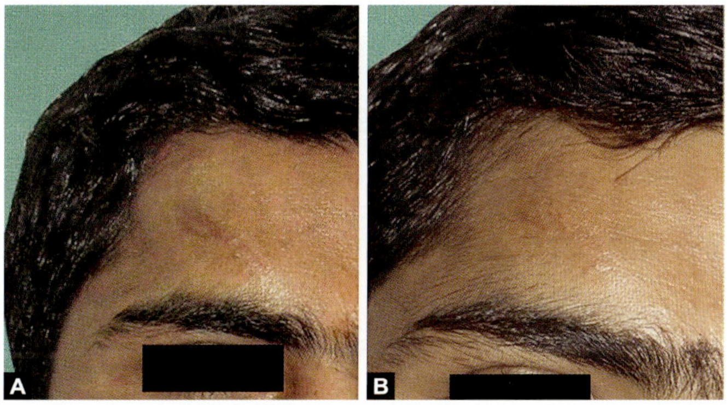

Figs. 15A and B: (A) Traumatic scar on forehead; (B) After three sessions once a month.

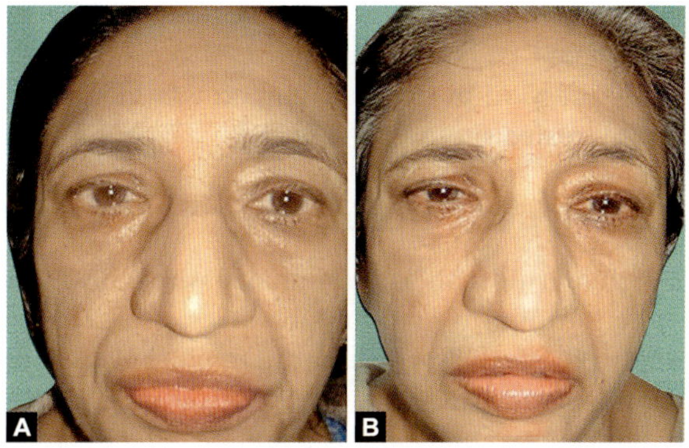

Figs. 17A and B: (A) Before; and (B) After wrinkles and skin tightening.
Courtesy: Dr Jagadish Sakhiya, Surat.

Skin Laxity, Wrinkles, and Photodamaged Skin

Microneedle radiofrequency is an extremely safe and effective treatment for skin laxity, wrinkles, and photodamaged skin **(Figs. 16 to 18)**. Tanaka[17] studied 20 Japanese patients with noninsulated needle MNRF and observed significant skin tightening on the lower two-third of the face with a median volumetric reduction of 12.1 mL at 6 months post-treatment. Lee et al.[18] found MNRF effective and safe for periorbital wrinkles in 20 Korean patients. They found that only 2 out of 20 patients developed mild hyperpigmentation. Jeon et al. compared MNRF against botulinum toxin A in periorbital rejuvenation in a split-face study in 12 Korean patients.[19] They observed that botulinum toxin-treated side showed a superior effect at 3 and 6 weeks. However, MNRF-treated side showed a better effect at 18 weeks. Gold et al.[20] studied MNRF in 49 patients in a multicentric study. They observed improvement in 100% of the patients with 65% of patients having significant improvement in wrinkles, skin tightening, and skin lifting. A similar observation was also reported by Clementoni and Munavalli[21] while studying mild-to-moderate skin laxity in the lower face and neck.

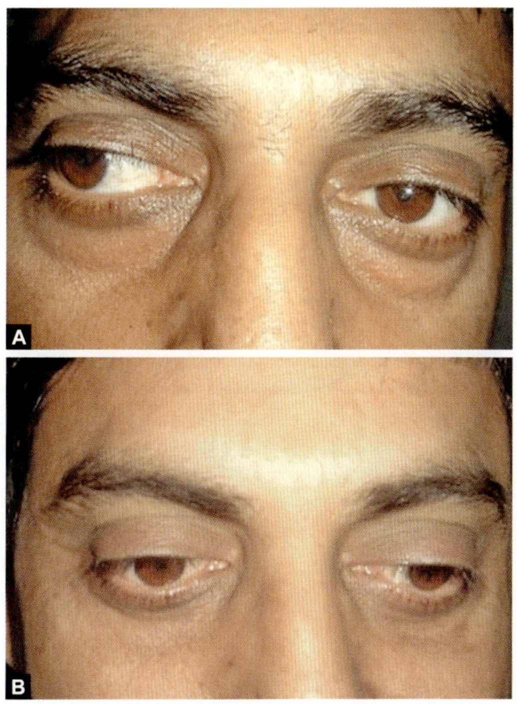

Figs. 18A and B: (A) Periorbital wrinkling and eye bags; (B) After three sessions once a month.
Courtesy: Dr Jagadish Sakhiya, Surat.

Striae/Stretch Marks

Striae distensae are dermal scars with flattening and atrophy of the epidermis **(Figs. 19A and B)**. Striae developed because of pregnancy or other causes are very difficult to treat. While no therapeutic modality can effectively treat striae completely, a combination treatment using MNRF and fractional CO_2 laser with or without platelet-rich plasma therapy often produces cosmetically acceptable improvement in striae. Fatemi et al. compared MNRF and MNRF plus fractional CO_2 in treatment of striae alba in 48 patients in a split-side study.[22] They found that both sides showed significant improvement, but the side treated with combination treatment improved significantly better. Similar findings were also reported by Ryu et al.[23] in 30 Korean patients. They observed a thickened epidermis and a clear increase in the number of collagen fibers in the MNRF and fractional CO_2 combination-treated sites. There is also greater expression of transforming growth factor β-1 and stratifin in treated sites.

Axillary Hyperhidrosis

Axillary hyperhidrosis is an embarrassing condition for patients. Botulinum toxin, microwaves, and surgery are reported to be effective in treating this troublesome condition. MNRF has been tried to treat this condition due to its safety profile and ability to reach and heat the deep dermis easily. Kim et al.[8] studied 20 patients of primary axillary hyperhidrosis with MNRF for two sessions. They found significant improvement in sweating with starch-iodine reactions reduced in 95% patients. Histological examination also showed a decrease in the number and size of both apocrine and eccrine glands 1 month after the final treatment. Fatemi Naeini F et al.[24,25] studied 25 patients for 3 treatments 3 weeks apart in a sham-control study. They found a significant decrease in hyperhidrosis severity score in MNRF-treated site. About 50% of their patients reported a persistent decrease at 1-year follow-up. They also reported a significant correlation between hyperhidrosis disease severity scale (HDSS) changes in relapse and body mass index (BMI). They suggested that MNRF should be repeated at 1 year, particularly in overweight patients with high BMI.

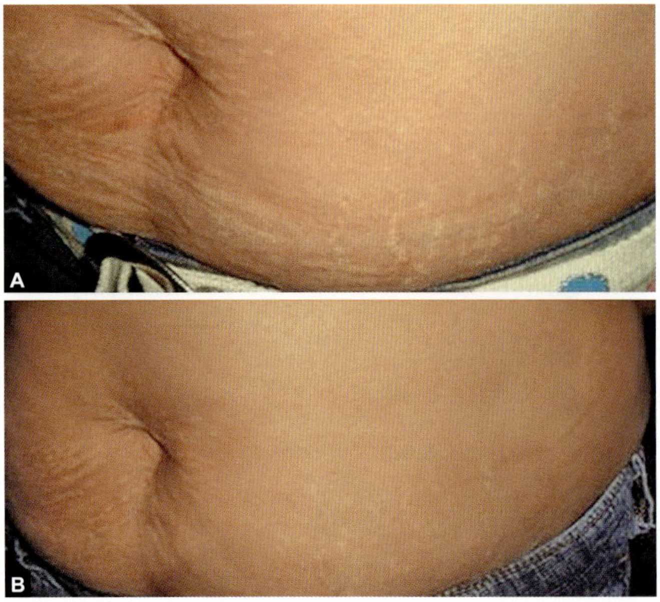

Figs. 19A and B: (A) Striae gravidarum; (B) After five sessions of MNRF.
(MNRF: microneedle radiofrequency)
Courtesy: Dr Jagadish Sakhiya, Surat.

Pigmentary Disorders

Few authors have used MNRF in pigmentary disorders as melasma, Riehl's melanosis and periorbital melanosis with limited success. However, in most of these studies MNRF has been used as adjuvant rather than monotherapy.

CONTRAINDICATIONS

Contraindications for MNRF are shown in **Box 2**.

COMPLICATIONS

Microneedle radiofrequency is generally a safe procedure, but minor complications as shown in **Box 3** can occur.

POSTOPERATIVE INSTRUCTIONS

Postoperative instructions are shown in **Box 4**.

BOX 2: Contraindications.

- Active infections
- Herpes simplex virus infection
- Patients with pacemakers
- Patients with facial metal implants
- Patients with unrealistic expectations

BOX 3: Complications.

- Erythema and crusting
- Pain
- Infections
- Postinflammatory hyperpigmentation **(Figs. 20 and 21)**
- Scarring
- Needle-track marks
- Flare-up of acne
- Milia-like eruptions

BOX 4: Postoperative instructions.

- No sun exposure
- No soaps and pricking or rubbing of skin
- Adequate skin cooling
- No fumes or steam
- No sweating and exercise
- Light makeup can be worn after 72 hours

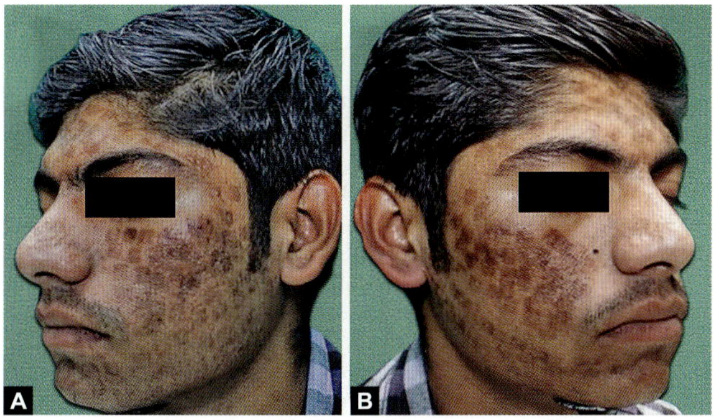

Figs. 20A and B: Postinflammatory hyperpigmentation (PIH) and scarring seen with wrong parameters.

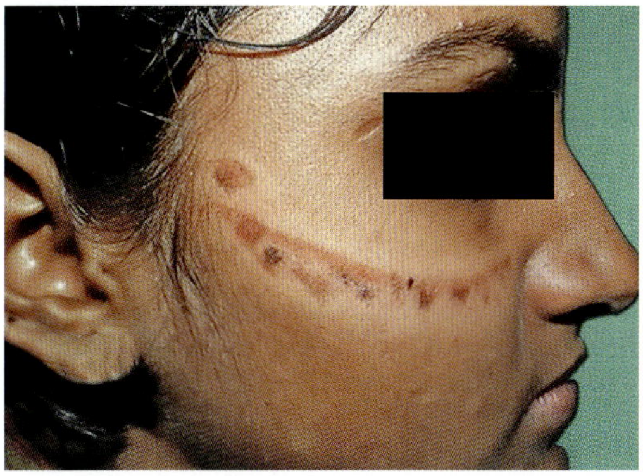

Fig. 21: Linear scar, postinflammatory hyperpigmentation (PIH) and scarring, too superficial needle placement, and aggressive parameters.

TABLE 1: Comparison of different MNRF systems available in the market.

	Infini	*Intensif*	*Ultracel*	*Secret*	*Explore*	*Body shape RF*	*Vivace*	*Scarlet*
FDA approval	Yes	Yes	Yes	Yes	–	–	Yes	Yes
Power	50 W	–	30 W	20 W	60 W	240 W	61 W	20 W
Available needle length	0.1–3.5 mm	–	1.0, 1.5, and 2.0 mm (0.5/unit)	0.5, ~ 3.5 mm (0.1/unit)	0.5–4 mm	• 0.5–1, and 1.5 mm • Different tips for different length	0.5–3.5 mm	0.5–3.5 mm
Needle type	Insulated	Noninsulated	Insulated	Noninsulated	Noninsulated	Both insulated and noninsulated	Both insulated and non-insulated	Noninsulated
Tip life	Unlimited shots	1,000 shots	1,000 shots	1,000 shots	1,200 shots	Limited	Limited	Limited
Number of needles	49	25	49	25	25	36	36	25
Superficial fractional RF	Available	Available	N/A	N/A	Available	N/A	N/A	Available
RF	1 MHz	–	1 MHz	2 MHz	–	6.8 MHz	1 and 2 MHz	1 MHz
Pulse duration	10–2,000 ms	–	40–2,000 ms	50–950 ms	0.1–3.0 s	–	800 ms	–
Microneedle insertion mechanism	Solenoid motor action is like an hammer	Stepping motor	Solenoid motor	Stepping motor	Stepping motor	Stepping motor	Stepping motor	–
Microneedle thickness combination	0.3 mm	0.3 mm	Thicker needles	0.3 mm	0.3 mm	Not mentioned	0.3 mm	–
Combination with other technologies	Nil	Nonablative bipolar RF	HIFU+ stamped monopolar RF	Fractional CO_2	Nil	Nonablative bipolar and quadrapolar RF	Blue and Red LED	–

(HIFU: high-intensity focused ultrasound; LED: light emitting diode; MNRF: multineedle radiofrequency; RF: radiofrequency)

COMPARISON OF DIFFERENT MULTINEEDLE RADIOFREQUENCY SYSTEMS

The MNRF is a rapidly evolving technology and new machines are being developed rapidly. Some commonly used machines and their specifications are shown in **Table 1**. It is recommended that the buyer should study the details carefully before buying a machine.

CONCLUSION

Microneedle radiofrequency is a versatile technology that can be used safely and aggressively in patients with pigmented and tanned skin. It has the advantage of less downtime, which results in better patient compliance. A lot of research is underway to make this technology usable not only in aesthetic medicine but also in treating various dermatological conditions. Practical instructions for better results and minimizing complications are mentioned in Tips given below.

TIPS

For getting better results with MNRF:
- Proper patient selection; e.g., rolling and box scars respond better to MNRF than ice prick scars
- Give good topical anesthesia as MNRF is painful; so, proper anesthesia is a must
- Stretch the skin in bulky areas and pinch the skin near bones; this will reduce oozing and pain
- Sessions should be placed at least 1 month apart
- Tips are disposable and need to be used for a single patient
- Proper postoperative care is necessary
- Combination treatment is the key

To minimize downtime/complications/risks:
- Always keep the handpiece perpendicular in all directions to the skin
- Allow for skin cooling—alternate sides if multiple passes/small areas require breaks before additional passes
- Choose appropriate power settings and depths for the skin condition/area of the body or face/skin type
- Avoid stacking pulses
- Avoid superficial depths in Fitzpatrick skin types IV–VI
- Higher energies should be reserved for deeper passes only
- Maintain firm pressure on the handpiece to ensure the appropriate depth of the needles

REFERENCES

1. Hainer BL. Electrosurgery for the skin. Am Fam Physician. 2002;66:1259-66.
2. Hantash BM, Bedi VP, Kapadia B, Rahman Z, Jiang K, Tanner H, et al. In vivo histological evaluation of a novel ablative fractional resurfacing device. Laser Surg Med. 2007;39(2): 96-107.
3. Hantash BM, Ubeid AA, Chang H, Kafi R, Renton B. Bipolar fractional radiofrequency treatment induces neoelastogenesis and neocollagenesis. Lasers Surg Med. 2009;41(1):1-9.
4. Manuskiatti W, Pattanaprichakul P, Inthasotti S, Sitthinamsuwan P, Hanamornroongruang S, Wanitphakdeedecha R, et al. Thermal response of in vivo human skin to fractional radiofrequency microneedle device. BioMed Research International. 2016;2016.
5. Vidal Magalhães W, Gouveia Nogueira MF, Kaneko TM. Heat shock proteins (HSP): dermatological implications and perspectives. Eur J Dermatol. 2012;22(1):8-13.
6. Lee HJ, Seo SR, Yoon MS, Song JY, Lee EY, Lee SE. Microneedle fractional radiofrequency increases epidermal hyaluronan and reverses age-related epidermal dysfunction. Lasers Surg Med. 2016;48(2):140-9.
7. Harth Y, Elman M, Ackerman E, Frank I. Depressed acne scars—effective, minimal downtime treatment with a novel smooth motion noninsulated microneedle radiofrequency technology. Journal of Cosmetics, Dermatological Sciences and Applications. 2014;4(3):212-18.
8. Kim M, Shin JY, Lee J, Kim JY, Oh SH. Efficacy of fractional microneedle radiofrequency device in the treatment of primary axillary hyperhidrosis: A pilot study. Dermatology. 2013;227(3):243-9.
9. Calderhead RG, Goo BL, Lauro F, Gursoy D, Savant SS, Wronski A. Lutronic. (2013). The clinical efficacy and safety of microneedling fractional radiofrequency in the treatment of facial wrinkles: A multicenter study with the INFINI system in 499 patients. [online] Available from http://ayalasers.com/pdf/INFINI_WP_multicenter_499_cases_20130710.pdf [Last accessed February, 2024].
10. Na J, Zheng Z, Dannaker C, Lee SE, Kang J, Cho SB. Electromagnetic initiation and propagation of bipolar radiofrequency tissue reactions via invasive non-insulated microneedle electrodes. Sci Rep. 2015;5:16735.
11. Lee KR, Lee EG, Lee HJ, Yoon MS. Assessment of treatment efficacy and sebosuppressive effect of fractional radiofrequency microneedle on acne vulgaris. Lasers Surg Med. 2013;45(10):639-47.
12. Kim ST, Lee KH, Sim AJ, Suh KS, Jang MS. Treatment of acne vulgaris with fractional radiofrequency microneedling. J Dermatol. 2014;41(7):586-91.
13. Pudukadan D. Treatment of acne scars on darker skin types using a noninsulated smooth motion, electronically controlled radiofrequency microneedles treatment system. Dermatol Surg. 2017;43(Suppl)1:S64-9.
14. Chandrashekar BS, Sriram R, Mysore R, Bhaskar S, Shetty A. Evaluation of microneedling fractional radiofrequency device for treatment of acne scars. J Cutan Aesthet Surg. 2014; 7(2):93-7.
15. Cho SI, Chung BY, Choi MG, Baek JH, Cho HJ, Park CW, et al. Evaluation of the clinical efficacy of fractional radiofrequency microneedle treatment in acne scars and large facial pores. Dermatol Surg. 2012;38(7 Pt 1):1017-24.
16. Vejjabhinanta V, Wanitphakdeedecha R, Limtanyakul P, Manuskiatti W. The efficacy in treatment of facial atrophic acne scars in Asians with a fractional radiofrequency microneedle system. J Eur Acad Dermatol Venereol. 2014;28(9):1219-25.
17. Tanaka Y. Long-term three-dimensional volumetric assessment of skin tightening using a sharply tapered non-insulated microneedle radiofrequency applicator with novel fractionated pulse mode in Asians. Lasers Surg Med. 2015;47(8):626-33.
18. Lee SJ, Kim JI, Yang YJ, Nam JH, Kim WS. Treatment of periorbital wrinkles with a novel fractional radiofrequency microneedle system in dark-skinned patients. Dermatol Surg. 2015;41(5):615-22.
19. Jeon IK, Chang SE, Park GH, Roh MR. Comparison of microneedle fractional radiofrequency therapy with intradermal botulinum toxin a injection for periorbital rejuvenation. Dermatology. 2013;227(4):367-72.
20. Gold M, Taylor M, Rothaus K, Tanaka Y. Non-insulated smooth motion, micro-needles RF fractional treatment for wrinkle reduction and lifting of the lower face: International study. Lasers Surg Med. 2016;48(8):727-33.
21. Clementoni MT, Munavalli GS. Fractional high intensity focused radiofrequency in the treatment of mild to moderate laxity of the lower face and neck: A pilot study. Lasers Surg Med. 2016;48(5):461-70.
22. Fatemi Naeini F, Behfar S, Abtahi-Naeini B, Keyvan S, Pourazizi M. Promising option for treatment of striae alba: Fractionated microneedle radiofrequency in combination with fractional carbon dioxide laser. Dermatol Res Pract. 2016; 2016:2896345.
23. Ryu HW, Kim SA, Jung HR, Ryoo YW, Lee KS, Cho JW. Clinical improvement of striae distensae in Korean patients using a combination of fractionated microneedle radiofrequency and fractional carbon dioxide laser. Dermatol Surg. 2013;39(10): 1452-8.
24. Fatemi Naeini F, Abtahi-Naeini B, Pourazizi M, Nilforoushzadeh MA, Mirmohammadkhani M. Fractionated microneedle radiofrequency for treatment of primary axillary hyperhidrosis: A sham control study. Australas J Dermatol. 2015;56(4):279-84.
25. Abtahi-Naeini B, Fatemi Naeini F, Saffaei A, Behfar S, Pourazizi M, Mirmohammadkhani M, et al. Treatment of primary axillary hyperhidrosis by fractional microneedle radiofrequency: Is it still effective after long-term follow-up? Indian J Dermatol. 2016;61(2):234.

CHAPTER 117

Noninvasive Body Contouring

Sachin Dhawan, Naina Jain

KEY MESSAGES

- Noninvasive contouring devices improve the body's appearance through the removal of excess adipose tissue, particularly in areas in which fat persists despite optimal diet and exercise routine.
- Various modalities for noninvasive body contouring include: cryolipolysis, laser, high-intensity focused electromagnetic field, radiofrequency and high-intensity focused ultrasound.

INTRODUCTION

Body contouring (or body sculpting or body shaping) refers to alteration of appearance with changes in size and/or shape, primarily through targeting body's fat compartment.[1] It may be achieved through conservative measures (i.e., diet and exercise), invasive procedures (such as liposuction) or through an ever-growing demand for noninvasive technologies in view of shorter recovery time, satisfying results, fewer side effects and lack of anesthesia and surgery-associated complications.

ANATOMY OF BODY FAT

Subcutaneous fat, present below the dermis is composed of two layers, the more superficial mantle layer with vertically oriented, larger fat cells and a deeper fat compartment with horizontally oriented, smaller fat cells. Adipocytes (fat cells), each with a feeding capillary, aggregate to form fat lobules. Each lobule is supplied by a neurovascular bundle of arterioles and venules. Fat lobules constitute fat pearls. Subunits of these pearls organize into fat sections, and further into fat compartments. Each fat section is contained by a thin fibrous membrane, branching into collagenous septae intersecting through the fat substance. Blood vessels, lymphatic channels and sensory nerve elements run along these fibrous sheets.[2]

Obesity is defined by an increase in size and/or number of adipocytes, with a body mass index (BMI) of ≥30 kg/m^2. Whereas, cellulite is noticeable dimpling of the skin (peau d'orange appearance) involving body areas such as thighs, buttocks, breasts, abdomen, and upper arms **(Box 1)**.[3]

Formation of cellulite has been hypothesized to be multifactorial in nature, namely, due to architectural and hormonal differences amongst males and females, thicker fibrous sheets, impaired dermal vasculature and drainage, and variable degree of inflammation.[3] In men, the fibrous septae through fat compartments are obliquely placed to the skin surface, while in women, they are more perpendicularly aligned, facilitating herniation of fat into the undersurface of overlying reticular dermis.[4] Slim women may still present with cellulite, with its absence in obese men.

BOX 1: Classification of cellulite[5,6]

- Grade I (mild)—visible changes with skin clamping or muscle contraction
- Grade II (moderate)—visible changes without manipulation
- Grade III (severe)—visible changes associated with nodules

BOX 2: Noninvasive techniques.[1,7-9]

- *Ultrasound based:* Nonthermal focused ultrasound (low frequency: 17.5 W/cm^2) (NTFU) and thermal focused ultrasound (high frequency: 1000 W/cm^2) [high-intensity focused ultrasound (HIFU)]
- *Radiofrequency*: Unipolar, monopolar, bipolar, tripolar, and multipolar
- Cryolipolysis (fat freezing), contrast cryolipolysis
- *Magnetic resonance:* High-intensity focused electromagnetic (HIFEM) therapy
- *Lasers:* Low-level laser therapy (LLLT) (635–680 nm); Diode (1,064 nm); Infrared (1,210 nm), near IR

Noninvasive body contouring devices result in fat reduction through efflux of triglycerides (TGs), lipolysis and/or apoptosis of desired adipocytes, skin tightening, and lifting, toning and muscular hypertrophy in varying proportions **(Box 2)**.[1,7]

ULTRASOUND

Mechanism of action: Delivery of focused, pulsed ultrasound, with a frequency of >20,000 Hz, may achieve fat reduction in two ways. HIFU with the use of lower frequency of 220 kHz results in mechanical disruption of adhesion between adipocytes forming a cavity. Cavitation ultrasound technologies are nonselective, produce heat and thus, are liable to cause epidermal injury. An ideal ultrasound technology, which will non-thermally and selectively disrupt/destroy adipocyte membrane integrity without causing significant damage to the epidermis or to nearby cells in the adipose layer, such as blood vessels or nerves, is needed.[10-12]

High-intensity focused ultrasound (HIFU), on the other hand, transfers energy at a frequency of 2 MHz, bringing out vibration of fat cells and further raising the temperature of the targeted fat compartment by >56°C leading to cell death. Necrotized adipocytes release TGs into the interstitial space. TGs are then broken down into glycerol and free fatty acids by the tissue lipase and cleared away by the lymphatic and vascular systems to the liver. The adjacent structures such as skin, nerves, blood vessels, and muscles remain unaffected.[10-12] Macro-focused ultrasound technology (MFU) with 8× bigger handpiece and high density of energy is used for body contouring as it is suitable for fat destruction (due to less pain sensitivity of fat tissue) as opposed to micro-focused ultrasound used for the face contouring.

Histopathological changes: Coagulative necrosis of adipocytes in the subcutaneous plane is evident after the procedure with sparing of epidermis and dermis of changes. Localized infiltration by macrophages clearing the cellular debris by phagocytosis follows 2 weeks later.[12]

Indications: Ultrasound-assisted body shaping is indicated for areas with subcutaneous fat of at least 1.5 cm thickness in a healthy individual of 18 years and above, with a BMI of <30. The most commonly treated areas include abdomen, thighs, and flanks.[12]

Contraindications: Pregnancy (in the last 12 months), lactation, in-situ devices, metabolic disorders, liver disease, state of immune dysfunction, connective tissue diseases, bleeding disorders, abdominal hernia, rectus diastasis, aortic aneurysm, open wounds/keloids/hypertrophic/depressed scarring (in the areas to be treated).[11]

Treatment regimen: Multiple sessions are required at an interval of 3–4 weeks. Duration of each session depends on the site treated, lasting from 30–90 minutes, with gradual improvement observed over a course of 2–6 months.[1]

Treatment Details (Fig. 1)

- Assess the treatment area for thickness of subcutaneous fat.
- Photographs and consent form.
- Clean and prepare the treatment area.
- Mark the treatment area with a skin marking pencil and subdivide the area into smaller zones/squares viz. 30 × 30 mm based on the length of the treatment zone of the device.
- Mark out areas of neurovascular bundle and superficial bony areas in order to avoid those areas.
- Choose the transducer and power as recommended by the device manufacturer based on the thickness of skin and fat in the treated area. Many devices have transducers that penetrate to a depth of 6 mm, 9 mm, 11 mm, and 13 mm. Choose the depth based on the location and depth of fat placement.
- Make sure to have complete contact with the skin to prevent epidermal burns and to ensure delivery at the correct depth.
- Place treatment lines 2–3 mm apart.
- Take feedback of the patient regarding pain as acute pain can indicate nerves in the treatment area.
- Avoid moving the handpiece while the shot is being delivered. Glide the handpiece in between shots.
- Advise sun protection. Avoid irritating activities such as exercise and creams for 2–3 days after the treatment.

Results: Shek et al. undertook a single treatment for 12 participants with HIFU at an average energy of 161 J/cm^2 on the anterior abdominal wall. An average reduction of 1 cm in the waist circumference was recorded at a 12-week follow-up.[13] Likewise, a study with 85 individuals treated with HIFU at a mean energy of 134.8 J/cm^2 over 60–90 minutes/session, reports an average reduction of 4–6 cm in the waist circumference.[14]

Studies based on the use of HIFU for body contouring showed that self-reported patient's satisfaction is approximately 47–86%. These treatment effects are not dependent

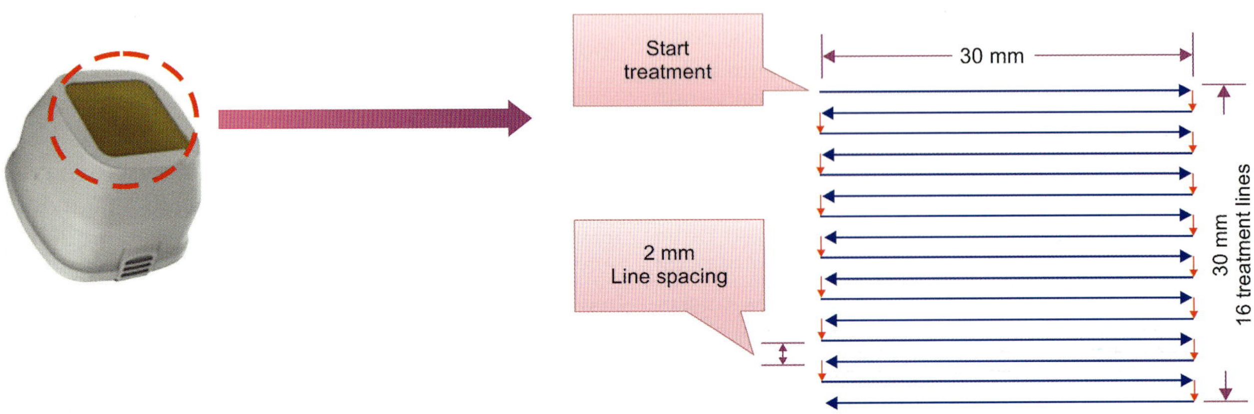

Fig. 1: Placement of treatment lines.

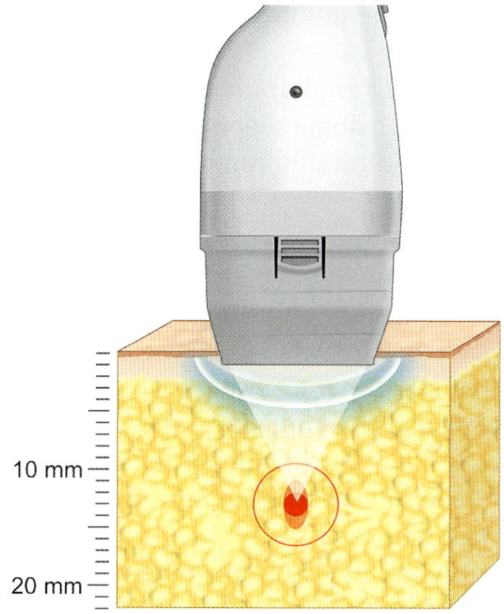

Fig. 2: HIFU with 13-mm transducer. Depth of penetration 1.3 cm (without contact cooling). It can be increased to 2 cm with contact cooling. (HIFU: high-intensity focused ultrasound)

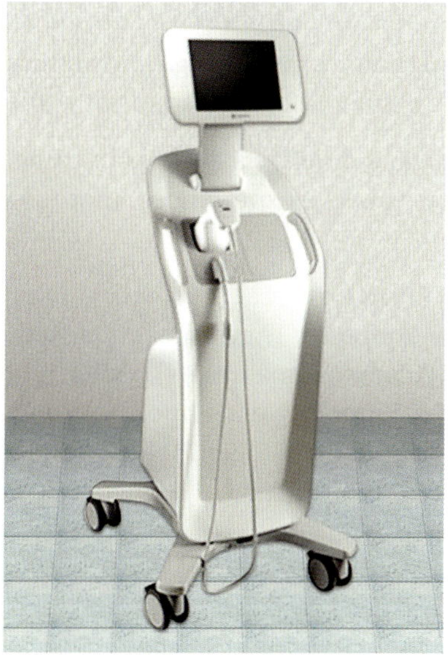

Fig. 3: Liposonix.
Courtesy: Solta Medical.

on diets or daily physical activity. In addition to the abovementioned benefits of HIFU, the recovery time of the procedure is minimal, which can be considered as an important advantage. However, according to available evidences no considerable influence was reported on BMI or body weight.[15]

Side effects: In most cases, the adverse effects are mild, localized, and self-limiting over a few months. These include erythema, pain and tenderness, bruising, blistering, and swelling.

Devices: Liposonix (Solta Medical), UltraShape (UltraShape), VASERShape (Solta Medical), Lipocell (Jeisys, Korea), Ultraformer III (Classys) **(Figs. 2 to 4)**.

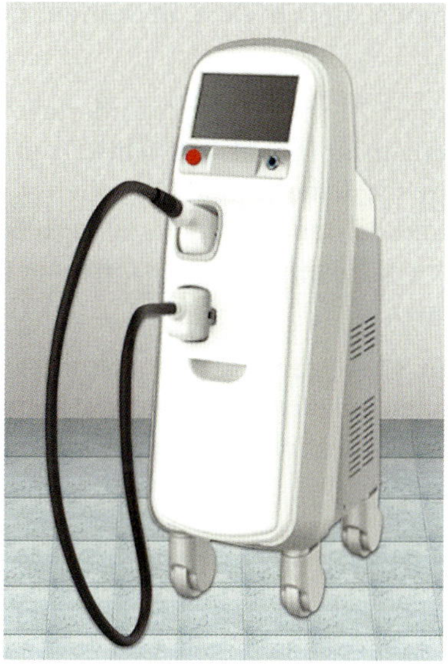

Fig. 4: Lipocell.
Courtesy: Jeisys, Korea.

RADIOFREQUENCY

Mechanism of action: Radiofrequency (RF) based body contouring technologies include application of an electric current ranging from 3 kHz to 300 GHz through the fat layer imposing collisions between the charged molecules. This raises the skin temperature to 40–42°C and fat temperature to 60–68°C. The tissue resistance to the flow of current generates heat which in addition to fat reduction has shown to stimulate collagen and elastin production, and hence, skin tightening. Depending on the electrode used, it may be subcategorized as the following:

- *Unipolar/monopolar:* The RF machine consists of a single electrode and a returning pad, which is to remain in touch with the patient's body to complete the circuit. The flow of current is from the electrode through the tissue to the grounding plate. Monopolar RF devices work on electric current while unipolar RF machines generate heat-induced changes through high frequency electromagnetic radiation.
- *Bipolar:* These devices use two poles, one on either side of the treating site. The depth and rate of penetration into the tissue increase proportionate to the distance between the two electrodes.
- *Tripolar/quadripolar/multipolar:* As the terms suggest, such machines contain three or more electrodes respectively.[16]

Histopathological changes: There is heat-induced apoptosis of the adipocytes, evident by presence of foamy histiocytic infiltrate around the fat cells in the subcutaneous layer and fibrosis in the upper dermis.[14,17]

Indications: Food and Drug Administration (FDA) approved indications include use of RF for skin tightening and fat reduction of sites such as face, abdomen, buttocks, and thighs.[1]

Contraindications: RF should not be undertaken in pregnant or lactating women; individuals with a history of heart disease, thrombosis, cancer, diabetes mellitus, epilepsy, autoimmune diseases or keloidal tendency. It is also to be avoided in patients on anticoagulants, photosensitizers or with implants in the site of interest.[16]

Treatment plan: There standard protocols for the use of RF for body shaping depend on the device used. It may range from 1 to 24 weeks, each session undertaken 7 days apart, lasting over 8–10 minutes.[14]

Treatment Protocol for Monopolar Radiofrequency (Contact Heating)

- Assess and mark the treatment area (standing position).
- Photographs and consent form.
- Remove all jewelry and personal electronics.
- Apply fresh grounding pad on the back or buttock of the patient (opposite side).
- Apply topical ultrasound gel or mineral oil.
- Set energy according to the manufacturer's recommendation.
- Place handpiece firmly in contact with the skin and with uniform gentle movements, achieve a temperature of 40-43°C in 1–2 minutes.
- Advise patient to hydrate the body with water intake, both before and after the treatment.
- Avoid cooling the area for 24 hours after the treatment to avoid heat dissipation.

Treatment with Noncontact Field Radiofrequency Device (Fig. 5)

- Focal point is 10 mm below the surface.
- Device uniformly heats the zone between 5 and 15 mm under the surface.
- Examination of the area and measurements, photograph, and consent form.
- Remove all jewelry and electronic devices.
- Initially place the applicator flaps in contact with the skin.
- Adjust the screws so that the applicator is 10 mm away from the skin in a dome shape.
- Check treatment area temperature with infrared (IR) thermometer.
- Set parameters and start treatment as per the manufacturer's recommendations.
- Keep checking temperature it should not go >43°C.
- Ask the patient to repeatedly rate the discomfort on a scale of 0–4, treatment should always be comfortable.
- Use cooling pads if temperature goes >43°C.
- Skin should reach the therapeutic temperature of 40–43°C after 10–15 minutes of treatment with sweating in the last part of the treatment.
- Total treatment time is 30–45 minutes.
- Four treatments are advised with a 7–10 day interval.

Response: Manuskiatti and colleagues observed appreciable circumferential reduction across the abdomen and thighs using TriPollar RF technology over eight sessions done weekly.[18] A study by Del Pino et al.[19] reports an average reduction of 2.64 and 1.8 mm in thigh and buttocks respectively with only two treatments 2 weeks apart with unipolar RF use.[14]

Side effects: Local side effects such as burning, ecchymosis, pain, tenderness may be experienced, more so with unipolar devices.[14,16]

Devices ***(Figs. 6 to 9)****:*

- *Monopolar/unipolar:* Thermage (Solta Medical, Hayward, CA, USA), Accent (Alma Lasers), Exilis Elite (BTL).
- *Bipolar:* VelaSmooth, VelaShape.
- *Tripolar:* TriPollar (Pollogen, Tel Aviv, Israel),
- *Multipolar:* 4Plus (Q Medical), 3D-skintech (3D-lipo) and iLipo Xcell (Energist).

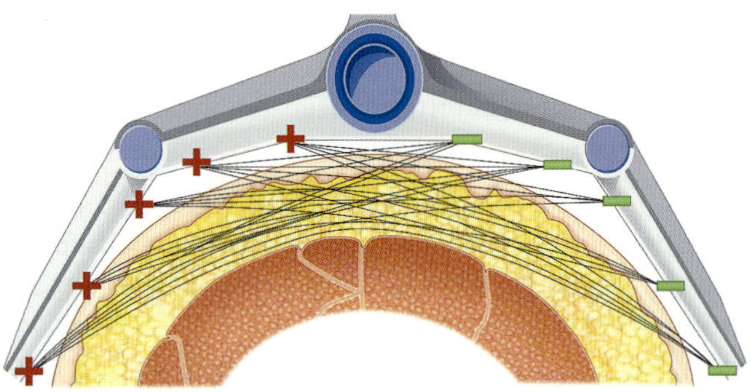

Fig. 5: Field radiofrequency (RF) device.

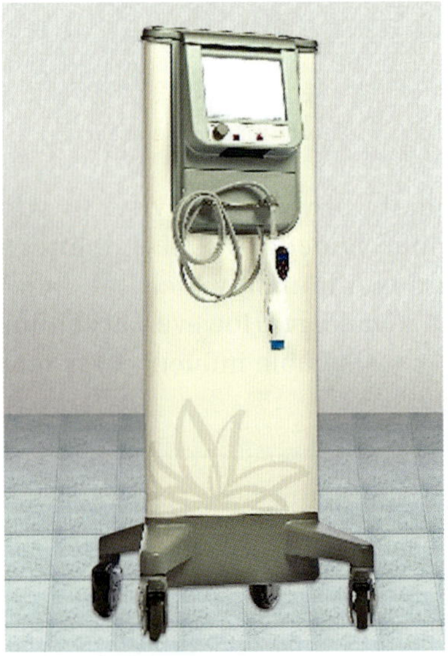

Fig. 6: Thermage.
Courtesy: Solta Medical.

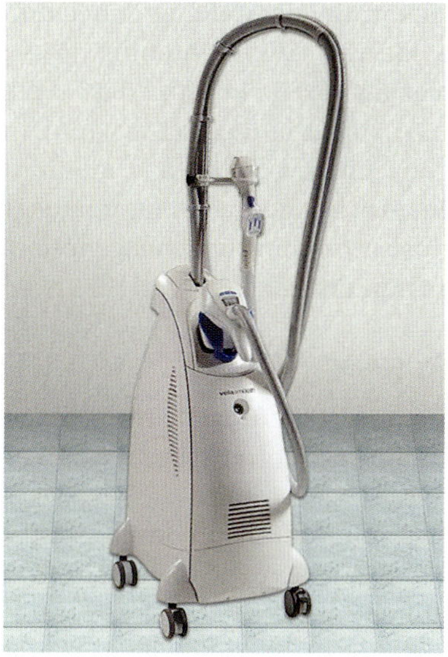

Fig. 7: VelaSmooth.

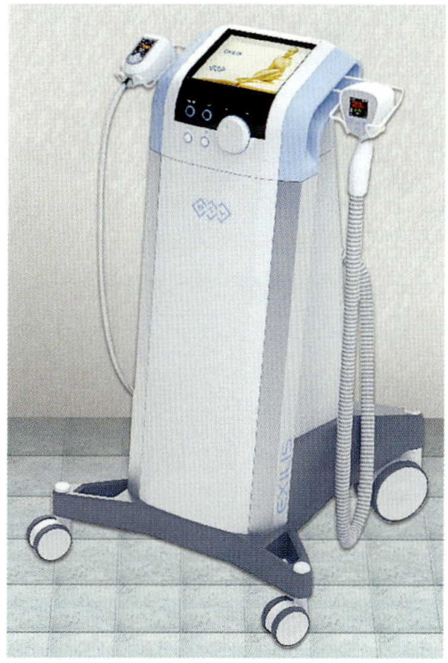

Fig. 8: Exilis Elite.
Courtesy: BTL.

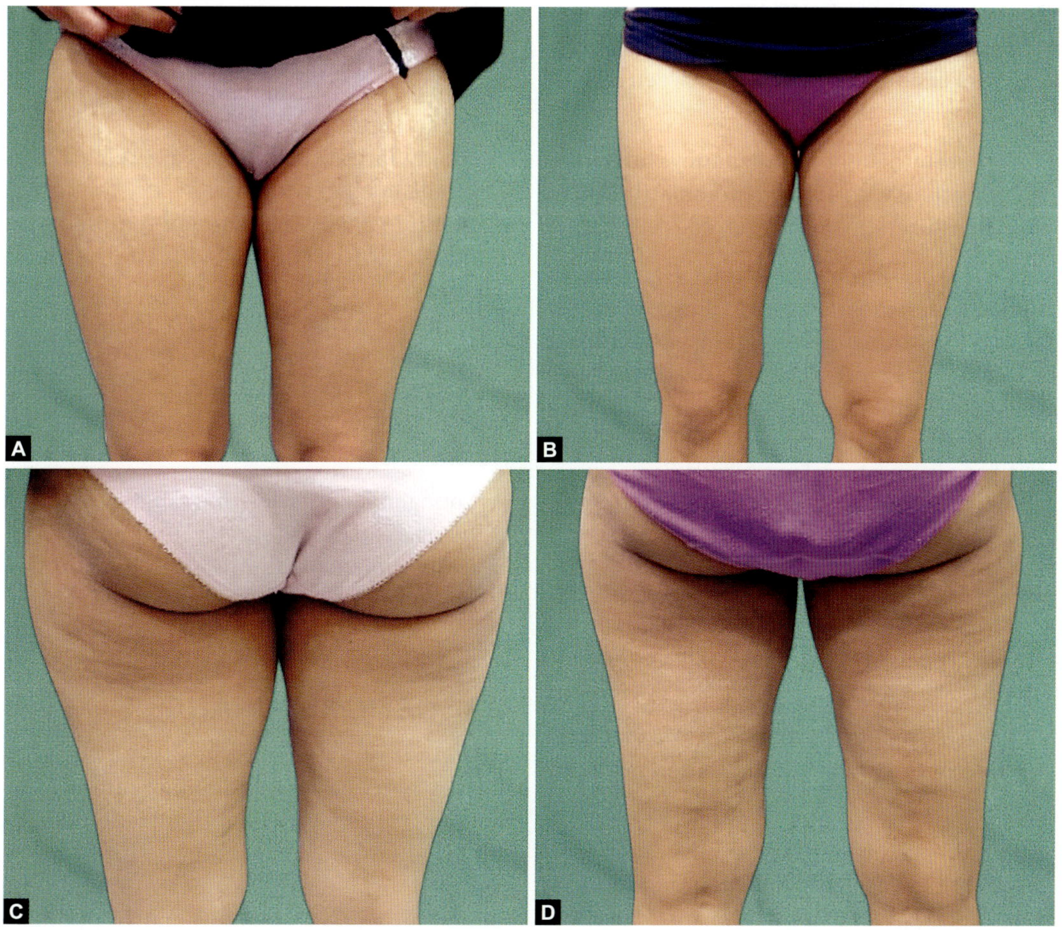

Figs. 9A to D: Before (A and C) and after (B and D) of a participant post four sessions, 15 days apart with Exilis Elite.

LASERS

Mechanism of Action

Low-level laser therapy (LLLT): The underlying mechanism by which LLLT brings about fat reduction remains unclear. However, there have been a few explanations to its action on adipocytes. LLLT leads to lipid peroxidation, wherein there is formation of micropores into the cellular membranes of fat cells by reactive oxygen species, thereby discharging the lipids out of them. Low level laser has also shown to activate

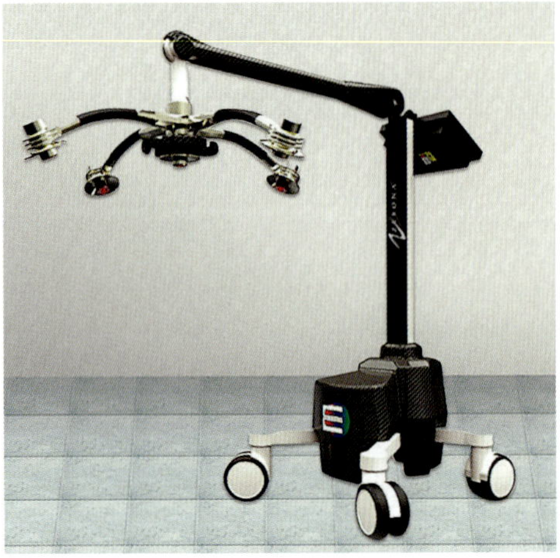

Fig. 10: Zerona Lipolaser.

complement-mediated fat apoptosis with subsequent lipid release.[20,21]

Indications: Zerona Lipolaser is US FDA approved for circumferential reduction of waist, hips, and thighs, in healthy individuals of 18 years or above with a BMI between 25 and 29.9 kg/m^2.

Contraindications: Recent history of pregnancy, infection, surgery, trauma. Individuals with a known psychiatric illness and those on photosensitizers are best deferred.

Procedure and duration of treatment: The device consists of five adjustable diode laser heads. Each head emits 17 mW of 635 nm of laser light. Eight treatment sessions, undertaken twice a week for 4 weeks have most commonly been practiced. Each session lasts 20–25 minutes. Cellulite reduction may require deeper penetration with 660 nm (red) to 950 nm (near infrared) with more number of sessions.[14,22]

Results: Jackson et al. report total fat reduction of 8.91 cm across the hips, waist, and thighs, with maximum benefit observed around the waist of 2.66 cm, with six sessions over 2 weeks.[23] In a study by Caruso-Davis et al., average fat reduction around the waist with a total of eight treatments over a month was 2.15 cm.[14]

Side effects: LLLT has been reported to be better tolerated with only mild pain, tenderness, swelling or induration resolving over 1–3 weeks' duration.[1]

*Devices **(Fig. 10)**:* LLLT—Zerona Lipolaser (FDA approved), Meridian LAPEX 2000 Lipolaser system (Meridian Medical Inc. Anyang, South Korea).[14]

Infrared Lasers

Mechanism of action: Near to mid infrared wavelengths (i.e., 780–1,000 nm) have shown to induce skin tightening by penetrating to about 2.5 mm from the skin surface. This results in deep dermal heating, and less scattering of the incident light due to lower absorption by water and melanin at this depth, sparing the epidermis. Skin tightening takes places in two stages at a molecular level. The immediate tightening effect is the consequence of heat-induced cleavage of hydrogen bonds of tropocollagen, reducing collagen to one-third of its original length. This, in turn, initiates an inflammatory response, and histamine release promoting neocollagenesis responsible for long-term skin tightening.[22]

Treatment Protocol

- Cleanse the treatment area of any residues. Remove any jewelry from the concerned site.
- Shave off any excessive hair.
- Take photographs for future comparison.
- Eye protection goggles to be worn by both the patient and the practitioner.
- Apply a thin layer of cold ultrasonic gel or mineral oil.
- Carry out a skin test on three predetermined sites to assess patient's tolerance to fluence and time exposure settings according to the manufacturer's recommendations.
- The handpiece is placed perpendicular, gently on the skin surface, and activated by pressing the foot switch during the course of the treatment.
- Steady, large brush strokes are utilized in motion, with an inbuilt contact cooling.
- Multiple passes per site are required to reach 40–44°C temperature. (Check with RF thermometer, a well-tolerated, epidermal temperature of 40–44°C or mild erythema as the end point is desired).
- The procedure is repeated at a 2 weekly interval, with a total of 4–6 sessions for body contouring.

Indications

- Younger patients desiring skin tightening, denying or not being able to avail surgical options.
- Older patients with mild-to-moderate skin laxity, not fit or not keen on surgery.

*Devices **(Figs. 11 and 12)**:* Harmony XL Pro (Alma).

MAGNETIC RESONANCE

Mechanism of action: High intensity focused electromagnetic therapy works through depolarization of motor neurons by high frequency oscillating magnetic fields. This causes the targeted tissue to undergo supramaximal muscular contractions, and in turn increasing the muscle tone. Fat reduction is due to local, repetitive, persistent apoptotic reactions, and increased metabolic rate due to an increase in the mass/tone of the muscle, promoting lipid breakdown.[24]

Histopathological changes: Studies suggest apoptosis of adipocytes with subsequent reduction in subcutaneous layer. The inflammatory infiltrate may not be profound as seen with other techniques due to nonthermal nature of HIFEM.

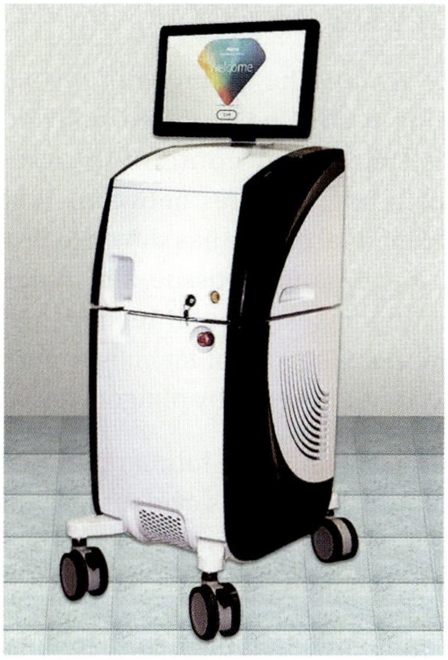

Fig. 11: Harmony XL Pro.
Courtesy: Alma.

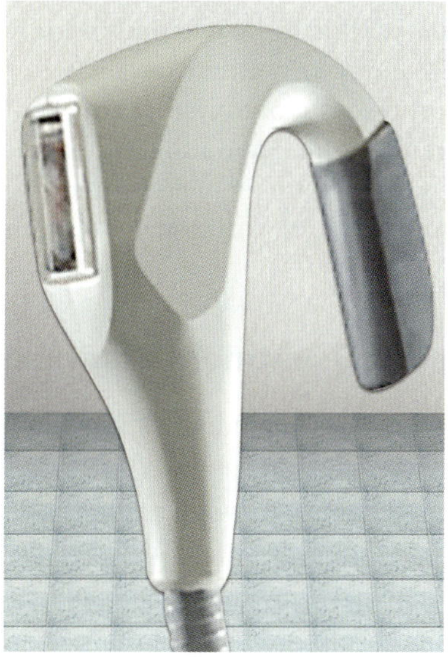

Fig. 12: Skin tightening (ST) Probe.
Courtesy: Alma.

Indications: Areas that have been studied include different parameters of the whole abdomen and the buttocks. Better results have been appreciated in individuals with a lower BMI and targeted subcutaneous thickness of <2.5 cm.[1]

Contraindications: Pregnancy, breastfeeding, history of heart diseases, conditions contraindicating the use of electromagnetic field, and open wounds in the area of concern.

Treatment plan: Studies so far have utilized on an average of four treatment sessions in total, parted by 2–3 days, each lasting for about 30 minutes of duration. The patient is asked to remove all the clothes and jewelry from the concerned site and made to lie comfortably. A coil emitting magnetic fields of intensity up to 1.8 Tesla is placed over the treatment area, with a penetration depth of 7 cm. The intensity is adjusted to patient's tolerance threshold.

Treatment Details

- Patient assessment, photography, and consent form.
- The patient should remove all metallic accessories.
- Place the center of the applicator(s) over the area to be treated with the connective cable(s) facing towards the feet.
- Make sure the applicator(s) are entirely in contact with patient's body.
- Fix the applicator(s) using the fixation belt.
- When using single applicator, the center of the stimulation coil should be positioned over the umbilicus.
- For larger patients, use two applicators.
- Start the therapy according to chosen parameters and adjust the stimulation intensity until the comfortable motor response of the treated area is achieved.
- Increase the intensity until reaching patient's tolerance threshold.
- Keep the treatment intensity at the level which causes the strongest muscle contractions that are comfortable to the patient.
- If the patient reports uncomfortable pain at the site of application during therapy, stop therapy immediately.
- Remove the applicator(s) and the fixation belt when the therapy ends.
- The aim is to achieve 20,000 supramaximal contractions in 20–30 minutes.
- Four treatments, 2–3 days apart are done.
- In addition to abdomen, calves, biceps, triceps, and gluteal muscles can be treated.

Efficacy: Katz B et al. studied the effect of HIFEM on the whole abdomen. They report an overall fat reduction of 19% (4.4 mm), with subumbilical reduction of 26.6% on ultrasound. Similarly, Kinney BM et al. report reduction in abdominal fat thickness by 18.6% or 4.3 mm and increase in the abdominal muscle mass by 15.4%, along with an average reduction of 10.4% in diastasis recti. They also noticed a decrease in the waist circumference by 1.4 inch. Jacob CI and Paskova K claim reduced waist size by about 4.37 cm at 3 month follow-up. 85% of patients studied by Jacob C reported significant improvement in shape, tone, and fullness of their buttocks.[24-30]

Side effects: No significant adverse effects have been noted so far expect mild muscle fatigue lasting for 12–48 hours.

Devices ***(Figs. 13 to 15)****:* Emsculpt (BTL Industries, Inc., Boston, MA, USA).

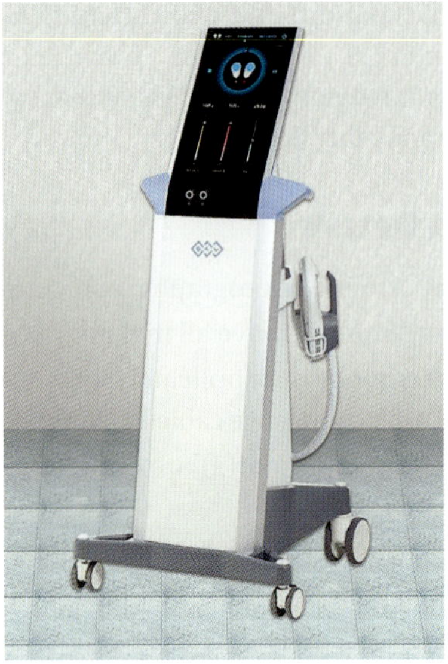

Fig. 13: Emsculpt.
Courtesy: BTL Industries.

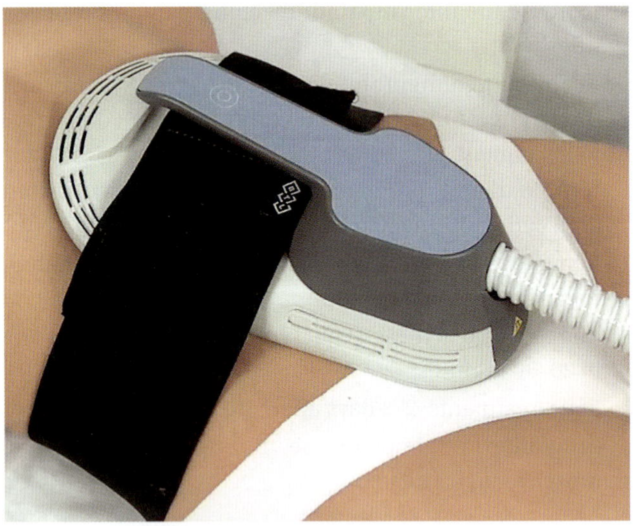

Fig. 14: Applicator of Emsculpt.

CRYOLIPOLYSIS

Mechanism of action: The rationale of cryolipolysis lies in lipid containing tissues being more susceptible to lower temperatures than water containing tissues. Targeted exposure to cold temperatures between -8 and 10°C for a predetermined interval of time has shown to disrupt the blood flow, crystallizing the adipose tissue, and initiating apoptosis of the frozen adipocytes through reactive oxygen species, sparing the dermis. The loss of fat cells is permanent. Body eliminates the apoptotic cells by phagocytosis.[31]

Histopathology: Cold-induced lobular panniculitis followed by an inflammatory infiltrate is evident by a month after the treatment. Cellular debris is cleared away by macrophages within 3 months thereafter.

Indications: Cryolipolysis has been most frequently employed for fat pockets not responding to calorie restriction and physical activity such as abdomen, arms, flanks, thighs and knees, and less often for back fat, bra bulge, gynecomastia.

Contraindications: It is to be avoided in individuals with a history of cold-induced dermatoses such as cold urticaria, cold agglutinin disease, paroxysmal cold hemoglobinuria, cryoglobulinemia, and Raynaud's phenomenon. Others specific to the site of treatment include preexisting or repaired hernia and diastasis recti, varicose veins, dermatitis, or any skin lesions.

Procedure and Treatment Regimen

- Preprocedure assessment and estimation of the number of cycles needed for each area.
- Check for pinchable fat. Avoid treating non-pinchable fat.
- Make the patient stand and mark the peak of the fat bulge.
- Apply gel pad on the treatment area that helps in sealing the vacuum handpiece. Ensure the peak of the bulge is covered.

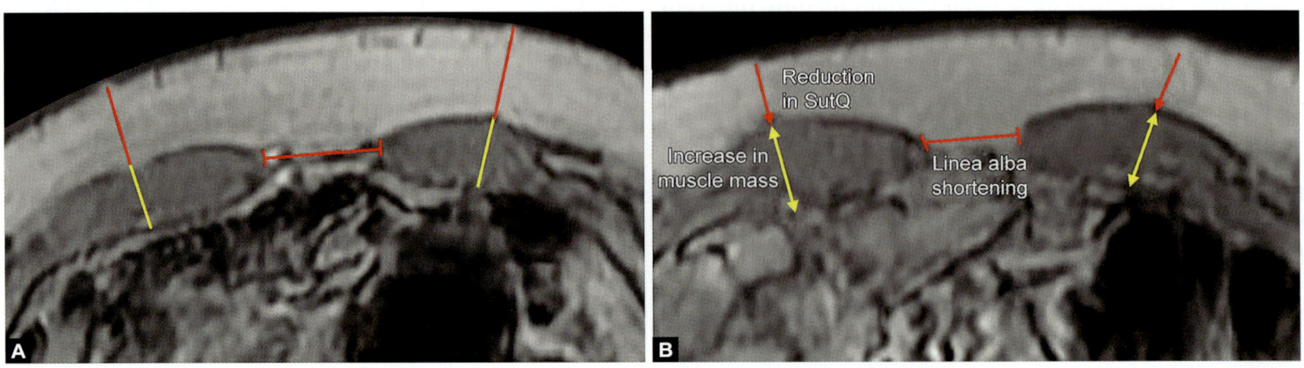

Figs. 15A and B: MRI-assisted documentation of rectus abdominis growth and reduction in diastasis recti 2 months after four treatments.
Courtesy: BTL Industries.

- The device consists of a cup-shaped applicator with two cooling probes designated for application to the treatment site.
- The handpiece sucks the tissue in with the help of an inbuilt vacuum to achieve tissue stability.
- The desired temperature is regulated by the thermoelectric elements with sensors monitoring the amount of heat exiting the tissue.
- Treating each site may last up to 45 minutes and is to be followed by a postprocedural 2-minute massage to augment clinical outcome by facilitating adipocyte damage through tissue reperfusion injury.
- Being a lunch time procedure, the patient can be instructed to return home and resume routine activities immediately after the procedure.
- The number of treatment sessions required depends on the site concerned. For instance, flanks have shown to respond well to a single session while thighs and back may even need >2 sessions, each 8–12 weeks apart.
- Best results are achieved 12 weeks after the treatment. Patient alignment for the same is extremely important.
- To manage initial pain and swelling, nonsteroidal anti-inflammatory drugs (NSAIDs) can be prescribed for 1–3 days.
- Ask the patient to report back in case of intense pain as that may indicate fat necrosis.

Results: Objective outcomes have been studied using fat calipers, ultrasound, and three-dimensional imaging (VECTRA M3; Canfield Scientific, Inc., Fairfield, NJ, USA) in various studies. On an average, fat reduction ranged from 14.67 to 28.5% using calipers and from 10.3 to 25.5% on ultrasound. The response may only be evident after 3 weeks with continued improvement over the following 6 months.[1]

Side effects: Pain due to cold-induced panniculitis, lasting from a few hours to days is commonly reported. Others include bruising as a result of vacuum application, transient numbness, redness, and swelling. A rare but significant risk, the clinician must be aware of is that of paradoxical adipose hyperplasia (PAH) that may develop within 6 months of treatment.[31-33]

Devices ***(Figs. 16 to 18)****:* CoolSculpting (ZELTIQ Aesthetics).

EXTRACORPOREAL SHOCKWAVE THERAPY

This comprises application of defocused, low energy shockwaves for the purpose of body sculpting and cellulite reduction by converting electrical energy to mechanical energy. Angehrn et al. studied the effects of extracorporeal shockwave therapy (ESWT) targeting cellulite on lateral thigh of 21 participants with 12 sessions over a period of 6 weeks while another randomized trial evaluated the response of ESWT in conjunction with physical activity on thighs and buttocks with six sessions, weekly apart.[34]

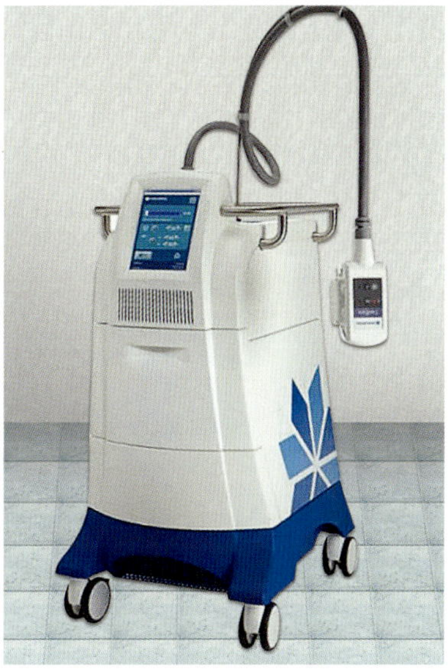

Fig. 16: CoolSculpting.
Courtesy: ZELTIQ Aesthetics.

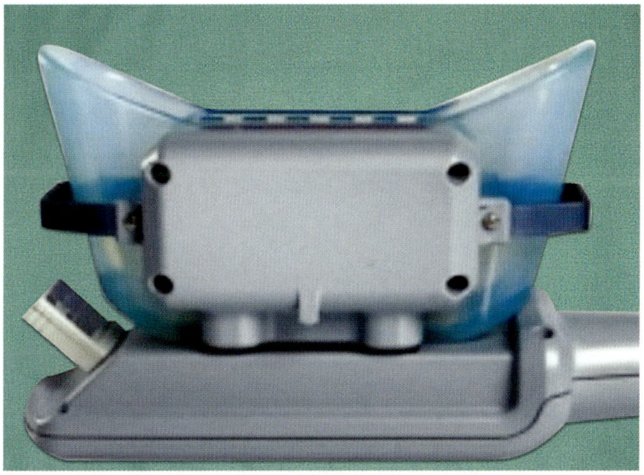

Fig. 17: Cup-shaped applicator for coolsculpting.
Courtesy: ZELTIQ Aesthetics.

ESWT has shown to bring about collagen remodeling, improve skin elasticity, and in turn skin appearance.[14]

EXPECTATION ALIGNMENT

This is of an utmost importance as most patients are looking for an easier means to reduce weight and have unrealistic expectations of losing 6–8 inches around the waist. Various studies and clinical experience reveal an average circumferential reduction of about 1–5 cm across the waistline after completing a series of treatment, which varies from device-to-device and patient-to-patient.

Body contouring devices are a part of larger scheme of things to achieve an attractive physique that includes eating healthy, regular physical activity, stress reduction and identifying, and treating any underlying hormonal and metabolic imbalances.

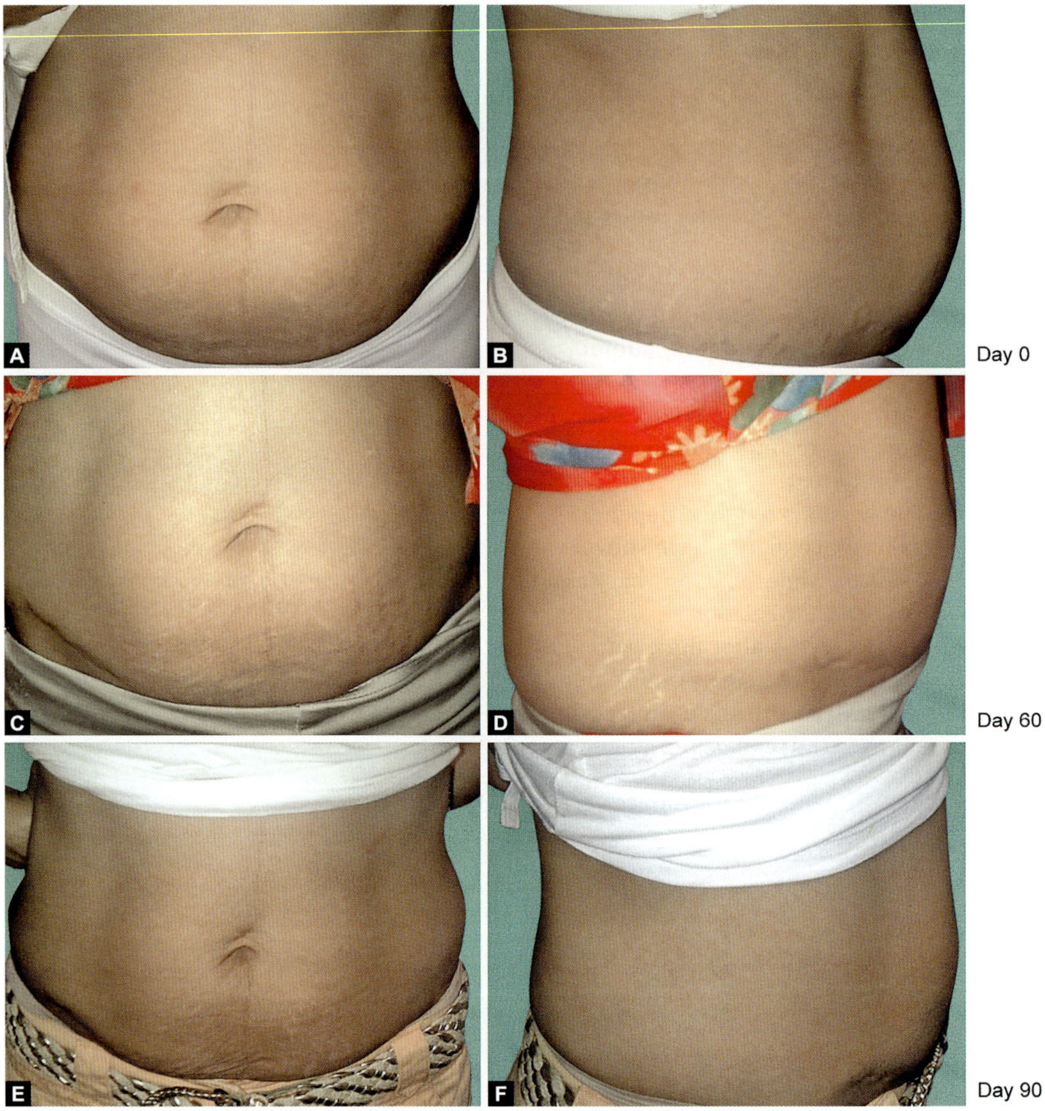

Figs. 18A to F: Pre and postpictures of a candidate treated with CoolSculpting depicting changes over a period of 3 months.

CONCLUSION

Cryolipolysis, laser, high-intensity focused electromagnetic field, radiofrequency, high-intensity focused ultrasound and extracorporeal shockwave therapy are some of the non-invasive techniques available for body contouring. One of the most important aspects of body countering methods is patient satisfaction following treatment, which is not noticeable in most cases because most of the participants expect similar outcomes to surgical procedures. The results vary with every individual patient and every individual technique.

REFERENCES

1. Mazzoni D, Lin MJ, Dubin DP, Khorasani H. Review of non-invasive body contouring devices for fat reduction, skin tightening and muscle definition. Australas J Dermatol. 2019;60(4):278-83.
2. Klein JA. Subcutaneous Fat: Anatomy and Histology. In: Tumescent Technique: Tumescent Anesthesia and Micro-cannular Liposuction. St. Louis: Mosby. 2000.
3. Ortiz AE, Avram MM. The architecture of cellulite. Fat Removal. 2015; 59-67.
4. Querleux B, Cornillon C, Jolivet O, Bittoun J. Anatomy and physiology of subcutaneous adipose tissue by in vivo magnetic resonance imaging and spectroscopy: relationships with sex and presence of cellulite. Skin Res Technol. 2002;8(2):118-24.
5. Soares JL, Miot HA, Sanudo A, Bagatin E. Cellulite: poor correlation between instrumental methods and photograph evaluation for severity classification. Int J Cosmet Sci. 2015;37(1):134-40.
6. Nurnberger F, Muller G. So-called cellulite: an invented disease. J Dermatol Surg Oncol. 1978;4(3):221-9.
7. Kennedy J, Verne S, Griffith R, Falto-Aizpurua L, Nouri K. Non-invasive subcutaneous fat reduction: a review. J Eur Acad Dermatol Venereol. 2015;29(9):1679-88.

8. Zhou B, Leung BYK, Sun L. The effects of low-intensity ultrasound on fat reduction of rat model. BioMed Resh Int. 2017;2017:4701481.
9. Schilling L, Saedi N, Weiss R. 1060 nm diode hyperthermic laser lipolysis: the latest in non-invasive body contouring. J Drugs Dermatol. 2017;16(1):48-52.
10. Jewell ML, Solish NJ, Desilets CS. Non-invasive body sculpting technologies with an emphasis on high-intensity focused ultrasound. Aesthetic Plast Surg. 2011;35:901-12.
11. Moreno-Moraga J, Valero-Altes T, Riquelme AM, Isarria-Marcosy MI, de la Torre JR. Body contouring by non-invasive transdermal focused ultrasound. Lasers Surg Med. 2007;39(4):315-23.
12. Hotta TA. Nonsurgical body contouring with focused ultrasound. Plast Surg Nurs. 2010;30(2):77-82.
13. Shek SY, Yeung CK, Chan JC, Chan HH. Efficacy of high-intensity focused ultrasonography for noninvasive body sculpting in Chinese patients. Lasers Surg Med. 2014;46(4): 263-9. doi: 10.1002/lsm.22232. Epub 2014 Mar 3. PMID: 24585511.
14. Alizadeh Z, Halabchi F, Mazaheri R, Abolhasani M, Tabesh M. Review of the mechanisms and effects of noninvasive body contouring devices on cellulite and subcutaneous fat. Int J Endocrinol Metab. 2016;14(4):e36727.
15. Gadsden E, Aguilar MT, Smoller BR, Jewell ML. Evaluation of a novel high-intensity focused ultrasound device for ablating subcutaneous adipose tissue for noninvasive body contouring: safety studies in human volunteers. Aesthet Surg J. 2011;31(4):401-10.
16. Glancey L. Radiofrequency technologies: applications for body contouring. J Aesthet Nurs. 2019;8(Suppl):12-9.
17. Goldberg D, Fazeli A, Berlin AL. Clinical, laboratory, and MRI analysis of cellulite treatment with a unipolar radiofrequency device. Dermatol Surg. 2008;34:204-9.
18. Manuskiatti W, Wachirakaphan C, Lektrakul N, Varothai S. Circumference reduction and cellulite treatment with a TriPollar radiofrequency device: a pilot study. J Eur Acad Dermatol Venereol. 2009;23(7):820-7.
19. Emilia del Pino M, Rosado RH, Azuela A, Graciela Guzmán M, Argüelles D, Rodríguez C, Rosado GM. Effect of controlled volumetric tissue heating with radiofrequency on cellulite and the subcutaneous tissue of the buttocks and thighs. J Drugs Dermatol. 2006;5(8):714-22.
20. Caruso-Davis MK, Guillot TS, Podichetty VK, Mashtalir N, Dhurandhar NV, Dubuisson O, et al. Efficacy of low-level laser therapy for body contouring and spot fat reduction. Obes Surg. 2011;21(6):722-9.
21. Avci P, Nyame TT, Gupta GK, Sadasivam M, Hamblin MR. Low-level laser therapy for fat layer reduction: a comprehensive review. Lasers Surg Med. 2013;45(6):349-57.
22. Friedmann DP. A review of the aesthetic treatment of abdominal subcutaneous adipose tissue. Dermatol Surg. 2015; 41(1):18-34.
23. Jackson RF, Dedo DD, Roche GC, Turok DI, Maloney RJ. Low-level laser therapy as a non-invasive approach for body contouring: a randomized, controlled study. Lasers Surg Med. 2009;41(10):799-809.
24. Katz B, Bard R, Goldfarb R, Shiloh A, Kenolova D. Ultrasound assessment of subcutaneous abdominal fat thickness after treatments with a high-intensity focused electromagnetic field device: a multicenter study. Dermatol Surg. 2019;45(12): 1542-8.
25. Weiss RA, Bernardy J. Induction of fat apoptosis by a non-thermal device: mechanism of action of non-invasive high-intensity electromagnetic technology in a porcine model. Lasers Surg Med. 2019;51(1):47-53.
26. Busso M, Denkova R. High-Intensity Focused Electromagnetic (HIFEM) field therapy used for non-invasive buttock augmentation and lifting: feasibility study. J Aesthet Reconstr Surg. 2019;5(1):2.
27. Kinney BM, Lozanova P. High intensity focused electromagnetic therapy evaluated by magnetic resonance imaging: safety and efficacy study of a dual tissue effect based non-invasive abdominal body shaping. Lasers Surg Med. 2019;51(1): 40-6.
28. Jacob CI, Paskova K. Safety and efficacy of a novel high-intensity focused electromagnetic technology device for noninvasive abdominal body shaping. J Cosmet Dermatol. 2018;17(5):783-7.
29. Jacob C, Kinney B, Busso M, Chilukuri S, McCoy JD, Bailey C, et al. High Intensity Focused Electro-Magnetic Technology (HIFEM) for non-invasive buttock lifting and toning of gluteal muscles: a multi-center efficacy and safety study. J Drugs Dermatol. 2018;17(11):1229-32.
30. Lewis, J. Cryolipolysis is an effective treatment modality for non-invasive body sculpting. J Aesthet Nurs. 2016;5(7):337-8.
31. Ingargiola MJ, Motakef S, Chung MT, Vasconez HC, Sasaki GH. Cryolipolysis for fat reduction and body contouring: safety and efficacy of current treatment paradigms. Plast Reconstr Surg. 2015;135(6):1581-90.
32. Derrick CD, Shridharani SM, Broyles JM. The safety and efficacy of cryolipolysis: a systematic review of available literature. Aesthet Surg J. 2015;35(7):830-6.
33. Langdon, S. Cryolipolysis and the opportunity for body contouring treatments. J Aesthet Nurs. 2019;8(Suppl):6-11.
34. Angehrn F, Kuhn C, Voss A. Can cellulite be treated with low-energy extracorporeal shock wave therapy Clin Interv Aging. 2007;2(4):623-30.

CHAPTER 118

Picosecond Lasers

Ganesh S Pai, Anusha H Pai

KEY MESSAGES

- Pico lasers have shorter pulse duration then nano lasers.
- Initially approved by FDA for tattoo removal now Pico lasers are used in treatment of acne, acne scars, traumatic scars, photoaging skin rejuvenation.
- Pico laser works by epidermal vesicle formation and dermal hemorrhage bye vessel damage which stimulates growth factors.
- Pico lasers are more effective with fewer side effects.
- Laser downtime and shorter sessions.

INTRODUCTION

Picosecond lasers clinically became available in the late 1990s. Ho and colleagues found an optimal pulse duration range of 10–100 picoseconds for effective pigment destruction and clearance with little collateral damage.[1] In 2012, Picolasers were approved by FDA for tattoo removal and treatment of benign pigmented lesions.[2] They are available in multiple wavelengths, including lasers that emit wavelengths of 755 nm; 532, 680, 1064 nm; and 532, 785, 1064 nm. Picotechnology in neodymium-doped yttrium aluminum garnet (Nd:YAG) (1064 nm and 532 nm) has revolutionized the treatment of tattoos, nevi, scars, stretch marks, rhytides and photoaging with minimum downtime. It is fast, mild and a more efficient way of treating various skin conditions.

Pico pulses have shorter pulse duration than nanopulses and generate more photoacoustic than photothermal effect since the laser pulse duration is less than acoustic stress. Picosecond pulses are produced using a technique called mode locking. The base is a Q-switched system in which the non-linear effects of the Q-switched crystal are stimulated and modulated inside the resonator in order to create faster pulses with a technique in which only they are amplified. The picosecond laser generates very high peak power, making the photomechanical fragmentation of the target tissue and consequently the treatment more effective. Generating very low energy results in milder treatment and faster recovery.[3]

Power (W) = Energy (J)/Duration of the Pulse (s)

Pico pulses are much shorter than nanopulses and generate more photoacoustic than photothermal pulses. That means shorter pulses produce higher power for same energy. This helps in treating various skin conditions without much downtime and post-inflammatory hyperpigmentation as only the target tissue is treated without causing collateral damage to the surrounding tissues. Thereby its efficacy in the treatment of tattoos, melasma, nevi and under eye pigmentation is superior to nanopulse Nd:YAG lasers.[3]

At appropriate energy levels laser induced optic breakdown (LIOB) causes epidermal vesicle formation and dermal hemorrhage by vessel damage. This new injury stimulates growth factors and induces dermal remodeling by increased fragmentation of collagen fibers eventually leading to smoothening of scars **(Figs. 1A and B)**. LIOB may be initiated upon absorption of the picosecond laser energy by a chromophore. Melanosome chromophore emits a free seed electron, resulting in an ionized plasma at focal area and subsequently drives a shockwave that further expands outward to create LIOB. It enhances phagocytic removal of smaller pigment particles by macrophages.[4]

Picosecond lasers minimize unnecessary epidermal injuries as epidermal injury during the laser can increase the risk of post-inflammatory hyperpigmentation which occurs in nanosecond lasers.[5]

The picosecond Nd: YAG laser device has many handpieces-1064 nm fractional, 532 fractional, collimated and zoom. The fractional handpiece fractionates the laser beam and effectively removes the superficial hyperpigmentation. There are three tips available for the fractional handpiece. Focal length of the small tip penetrates the dermal layer, the medium tip penetrates the dermoepidermal layer and the long tip penetrates the epidermal layer. The fractional handpiece is used in the treatment of acne, acne scars, hypertrophic scars, burn scars, chickenpox scars and facial rejuvenation. The collimated handpiece with both 1064 nm and 532 nm is used in the treatment of melasma. The zoom handpiece which can switch wavelengths between 1064 nm and 532 nm is used for tattoos, freckles, lentigines, nevi, drug induced hyperpigmentation, Café-au-lait macules and solar lentigines **(Figs. 2A and B)**. The energy can be raised up to 500 mJ and

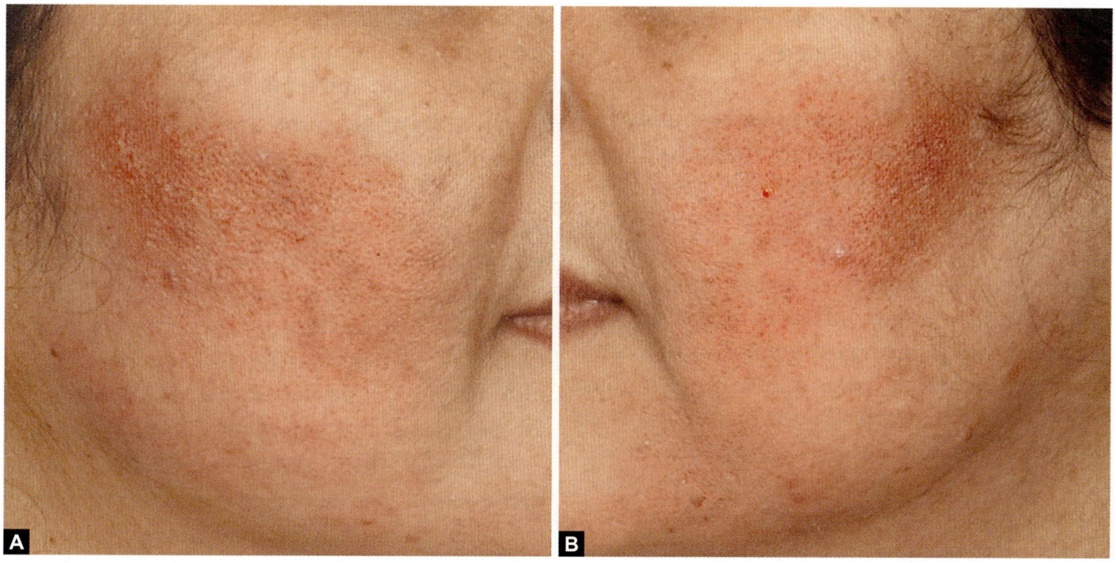

Figs. 1A and B: Observe the redness on the bilateral cheeks immediately post-picosecond laser. This occurs due to laser induced optic breakdown (LIOB).

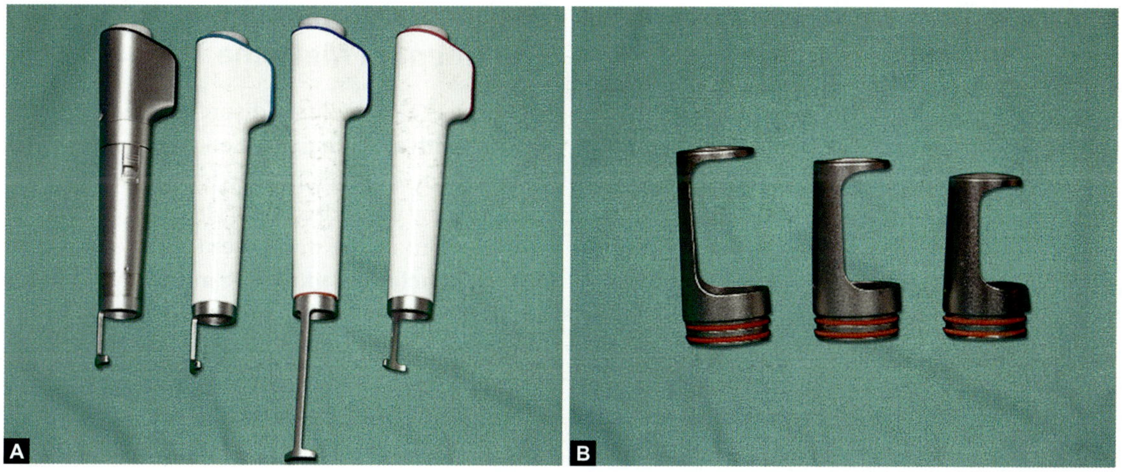

Figs. 2A and B: (A) Zoom handpiece, fractional handpiece, collimated handpiece and fractional handpiece; (B) From left to right - long tip, medium tip and small tip.

with a beam diameter between 1 and 7 mm. The focal length of the handpiece should be at the level of the reticular dermis for the optimum results. For this to be achieved the handpiece is held perpendicular to the skin while operating the laser.

PREPROCEDURE

- An informed consent form from the patient is mandatory. The consent form should mention the risks associated with the procedure such as hypo- or hyperpigmentation and scar formation.
- Take clear preprocedural photographs. The different colors in the tattoos should be clearly visible.
- Anesthesia cream containing lidocaine and prilocaine is applied 45 minutes prior to the procedure. This makes the patient comfortable during the procedure. If the patient has low threshold of pain, local anesthesia injection containing lignocaine is injected locally on the area to be treated.
- The eyes of the patient have to be covered with an external metal eye shields even if the treatment area is away from the eye. The operator has to wear protective eye wear.

USES OF PICOSECOND LASER

There is no single laser for perfect tattoo removal. Q-switched lasers fade most tattoos. Amateur tattoos contain carbon placed superficially and fade easily, but professional tattoos have organic dyes and metallic elements which are placed at mid-dermis and are difficult to remove. Black and blue tattoos are easy to remove whereas red and yellow colors are difficult to remove. Care should be taken while treating tattoos in Fitzpatrick skin types IV-VI as lasers may damage the epidermal pigment during the treatment. The older the tattoo better the response to laser treatment as macrophages are already present in the skin to phagocytose the foreign pigment particles.[6]

Kirby-Desai scoring is used to estimate the number of treatment sessions a patient will require for tattoo removal. It is based on Fitzpatrick skin phototype, location, color, amount of ink used in the tattoo, scarring or tissue change and ink layering.[7]

For tattoo removal we have been using nanosecond Nd: YAG lasers thus far. An average of five to nine sessions is needed in tattoo removal. A variety of chemical compounds can be used for tattoos which make it difficult to predict the treatment outcome. Picosecond laser pulses are more efficient in clearing cosmetic tattoos. Pulse duration was shown to be a significant factor in tattoo removal when other laser parameters are held constant. Pulse duration of picosecond laser is less or equal to that of the thermal and acoustic relaxation time of the tattoo ink. The diameter of the tattoo ink is far less than that of melanosome, the energy delivery in the picosecond range is able to achieve selective photothermolysis while protecting the surrounding normal tissues.[6] Picosecond laser pulses are more efficient in clearing-colored tattoos requiring lesser number of sessions. It produces less damage to the surrounding skin and scarring due to the low fluence level.[8]

Zoom handpiece in the picosecond laser is used to remove the tattoo ink. Since it has both 1064 nm for black ink and 532 nm for red, blue and green inks. Various tattoo inks can be targeted with a single handpiece. The handpiece should be kept in contact with the skin throughout the procedure. The fluence can be increased by reduction of the laser beam to a smaller spot size area. Larger spot sizes enable deeper penetration and more effective treatment of pigments.[9] Immediate whitening or graying of the skin occurs as soon as the laser light falls on the pigmented skin. This suggests the cavitation of the tattoo ink.[10]

Treatment sessions are done at 1-month intervals. Procedure is usually performed with fluence of 0.7–1.3 J/cm^2, spot size of 1–7 mm and a frequency of 5 Hz for 1064 nm. For 532 nm, fluence of 0.8 J/cm^2, frequency of 6 Hz and spot size of 5 Hz is used. During the subsequent sessions, if the improvement is minimal, fluence is increased by 20%. Generally, five sessions show more than 80% clearance of tattoo ink. The patient has to keep the treated area clean, moisturized and protected from sun. It takes around 7 days for the treated area to re-epithelialize and the scabs to fall off.

The side effects which are commonly associated with nanosecond Nd:YAG laser during tattoo removal such as hypopigmentation, hyperpigmentation and depigmentation is less common and scar formation is virtually nil with picosecond laser **(Figs. 3A to C)**.

Picosecond Nd: YAG in Treatment of Melasma

Melasma is a pigmentary disorder, affecting both males and females with a multifactorial etiology and no single modality of treatment is satisfactory. Strict avoidance of sun exposure, stopping any triggering factors like oral contraceptives, using creams containing depigmenting agents such as azelaic acid, kojic acid constitutes the main stay of treatment. Lasers are used with varying degree of success as the risk of post-inflammatory hyperpigmentation is high. The epidermal melasma is easier to treat than the melasma with dermal melanin.

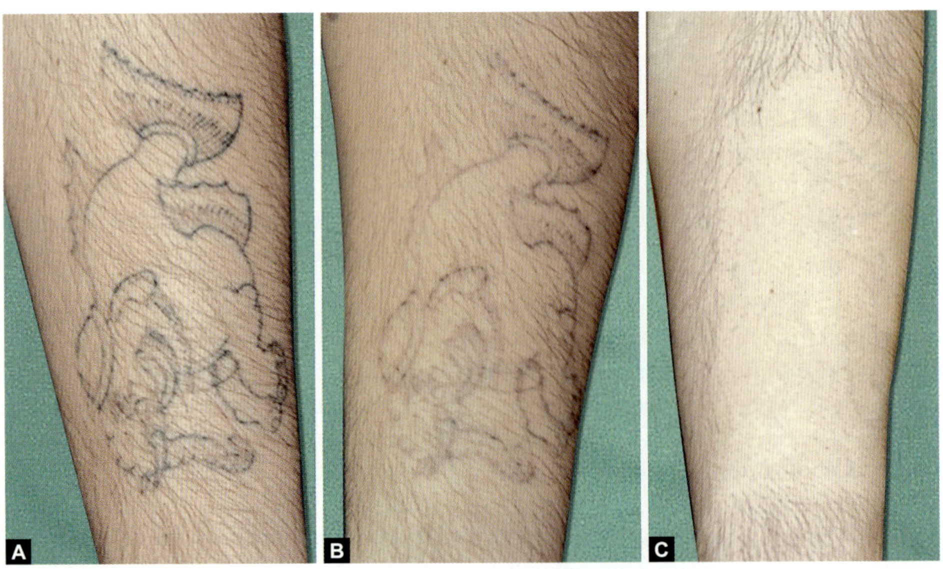

Figs. 3A to C: (A) A 7-year-old tattoo on a 25-year-old male at first visit; (B) Note the incomplete clearance of pigment post-five sessions of nanosecond laser; (C) The pigment was cleared by two sessions of Picosecond laser (PicoLO by Laseroptek, Inc.). Fluence of 1.3 J/cm^2, frequency of 5 Hz and aperture of 5 mm.

Low fluence Q-switched Nd: YAG laser toning has been used so far for the reduction of melasma pigment. Picosecond Nd:YAG laser improves both dermal and epidermal melasma with no post-inflammatory hyperpigmentation. The pulse duration of picosecond laser is much shorter than thermal relaxation time of the melanosomes. More selective subcellular photothermolysis of the melanosomes is achieved with a picosecond laser.[11] The melanogenic activity of the melanocytes is downregulated so that they do not produce fully matured melanosomes.[12] A few sessions of repeated laser treatment utilizing the photoacoustic twin pulse mode is a safe and effective way to treat facial melasma. Photoacoustic twin pulse involves splitting of the laser pulse into two with an interval of 100 microseconds between the two pulses which reduces the energy by half.[11] Patients should be counseled about the number of sessions involved as well as the potential improvement achieved post laser which is normally in the range of 50–60%. This tempers down patient's expectations about unrealistic results before the laser sessions are commenced.

Six sessions are done at weekly intervals. Topical anesthesia is not required pre procedure as the treatment is relatively pain free. Collimated handpiece is used for this procedure. Both 1064 nm and 532 nm are done in the same sitting which are both available in the same handpiece. The procedure involves using a large spot size of 20 mm, fluence of 0.06 J/cm^2, frequency of 10 Hz for 1064 nm. A fluence of 0.02 J/cm^2 with the spot size of 20 mm and frequency of 10 Hz for 532 nm for 2–3 passes **(Figs. 4A and B)**. Mild erythema appears on the skin post laser which is transient and disappears within ten minutes post procedure. Picobeam targets the melanosomes in the melanocytes without affecting the melanocytes with its photoacoustic mechanism thus preventing post inflammatory hyperpigmentation.[3]

Guttate hypomelanosis which is a known risk associated with nanosecond laser is significantly less with picosecond laser. It may occur due to the recovery of downregulated melanocytes. Early discontinuation of laser toning, use of tacrolimus ointment and excimer light targeted phototherapy may therefore help in this situation.[12] Postinflammatory hyperpigmentation (PIH) is rarely observed in melasma treated with picosecond laser.

Less recurrence and prolonged maintenance periods can be achieved with the picosecond laser treatment.[13] Laser treatment for melasma has to be used as an adjunct to topical and oral medication but not as the only modality of treatment. Since melasma can recur it is maintenance session can be done once in 3 months.

Picosecond Nd: YAG Laser in Treatment of Other Pigmented Lesions

Based on the location of the pigment the pigmented lesions are classified as epidermal, dermal and mixed. Common pigmented lesions which we come across in our practice are melasma, lentigines, freckles, post-inflammatory hyperpigmentation, melanocytic nevi, Café-au-lait macule, nevus of Ota, Becker's nevi and drug induced hyperpigmentation. Topical treatment options are ineffective and surgical treatment options produce suboptimal results. Lasers are preferred mode of therapy to diminish the pigmented lesions of the skin.

The lasers with shorter wavelengths are utilized for superficial pigmented lesions and for dermal pigmentation longer wavelength lasers are employed.[12] The pulse duration

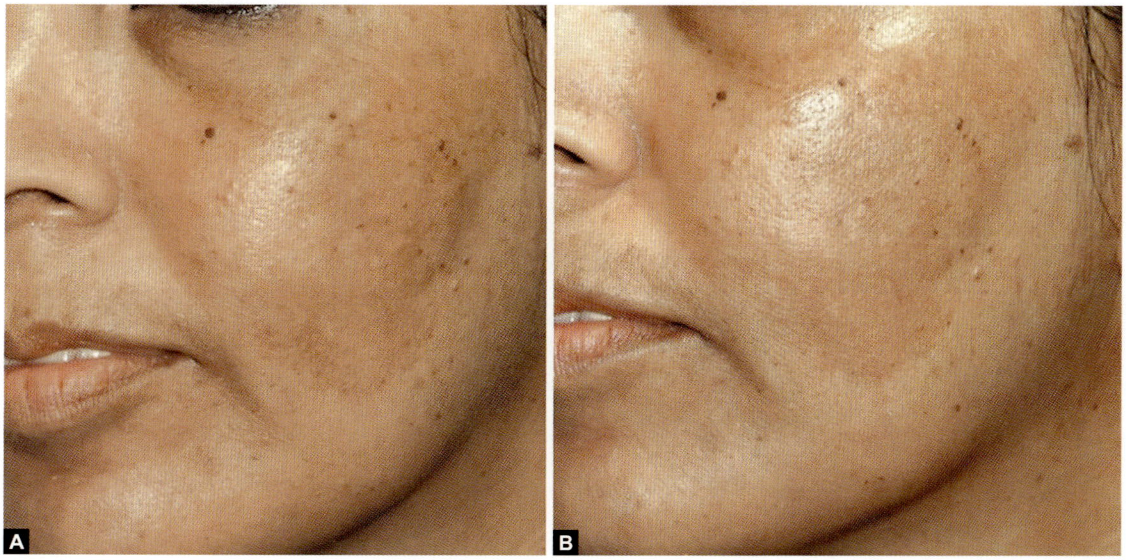

Figs. 4A and B: (A) A 40-year-old lady with melasma present on bilateral cheeks; (B) She underwent three sessions of Picosecond laser (collimated handpiece) at weekly intervals with fluence of 0.02 J/cm^2, spot size of 20 mm, frequency of 10 Hz for 1064 nm and fluence of 0.06 J/cm^2, spot size of 20 mm and frequency of 10 Hz for 532 nm.

of the picosecond laser is shorter than the thermal relaxation time of the melanosomes and pigmented epidermal cells. The melanin containing melanosomes are 1 μm in diameter and have a thermal relaxation time of 50–500 ns.[14] A very high energy laser pulse within a short time span results in rapid heating of the target melanosome causing it to explode leading to LIOB.[15] Destruction of melanocytes and melanized keratinocytes occur due to mechanical damage from acoustic waves that arise from the absorbing melanosome. Following damage, repigmentation results from migration of residual melanocytes from adnexal structures or adjacent untouched skin.[16]

Immediate ash white color at the site of impact is generated while treating pigmented lesions with picosecond laser. This occurs due to heat induced steam cavities in melanosomes which cause scattering of visible light, producing a white color.[10] These appear like gas bubbles within melanosomes when observed under electron microscopy. These gas bubbles gradually disappear in around 20 minutes. If the whitening does not appear that means the exposure dose is insufficient. Darker skin will have lower threshold for whitening due to a higher epidermal melanin content. Subthreshold fluences stimulate melanogenesis due to activation of epidermal melanocytes after nonlethal injury.[17]

Preprocedural topical or local anesthesia is required while treating pigmentary lesions. In case of nevi the degree of lightening is directly proportional to number of sessions performed.[18] With Picosecond Nd:YAG laser 70% lightening of the nevi can be seen within four to five sessions **(Figs. 5A to C)**. Subsequent sessions are performed after a gap of one month each.

Freckles respond well to picosecond laser since in freckles, there is an increase in melanin than the melanocytes. In darker skinned patients it is essential to perform a test spot before treating the entire face. A maximum of two sessions will be required to reduce the number of freckles **(Figs. 6A and B)**. Patients have to be counseled about the recurrence of the freckles after the treatment. Regular use of sunscreen has to be practiced by the patient to prevent recurrence. Lentigines on the other hand have increased melanocytes in the basal layer. 532 nm in picosecond laser is effective in reduction of the lentigines.

The fluence used for reduction of pigmented lesions depends on the whitening of the lesion. If the fluence is high there is likelihood of bleeding, post-inflammatory hypopigmentation or depigmentation. Lower fluences can be used in the patients with type V and type VI skin as the whitening response can occur at lower fluences in these skin types.

Erythema and swelling at the site of treatment is usually seen in the post procedure period. Hyperpigmentation or hypopigmentation, purpura and textural changes are common risks associated with lasers used for treatment of pigmented lesions. Hyperpigmentation is rare with picosecond laser but hypopigmentation is seen with the use of 532 nm especially when used for lentigines. Recurrence of some lesions are seen in both picosecond as well as nanosecond laser.

Pico Nd:YAG in Treatment of Acne and Acne Scars

Acne vulgaris is a common skin condition which commonly affects teenagers though it can affect people of all ages. It is

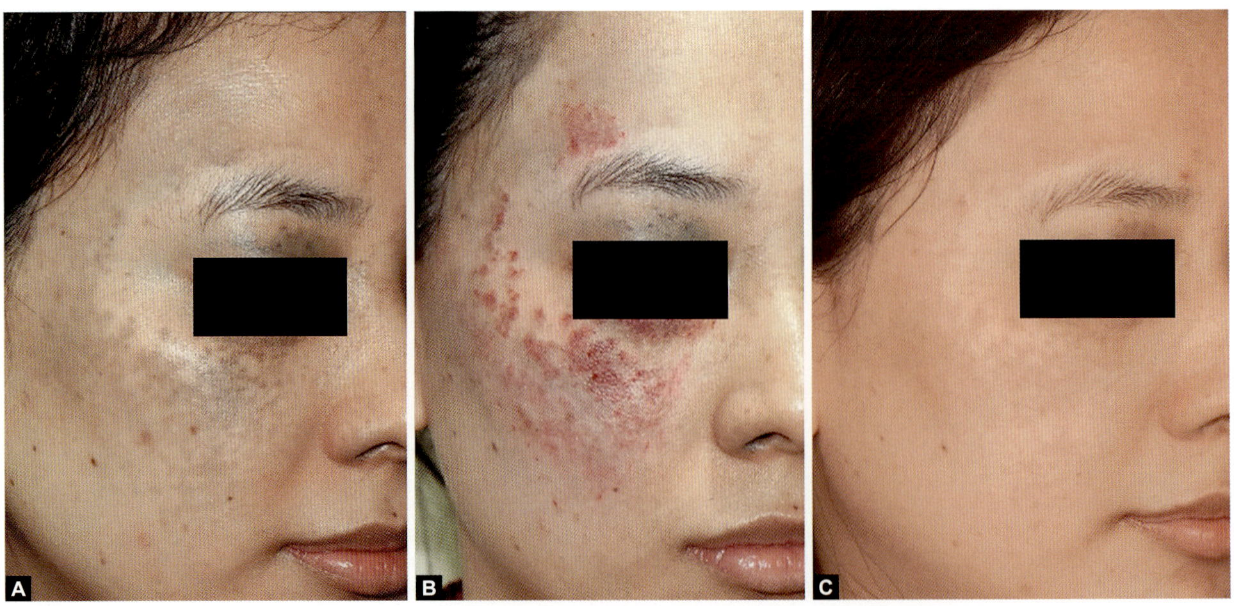

Figs. 5A to C: (A) Nevus of Ota in a young female at first visit; (B) She underwent four sessions of Picosecond laser (zoom handpiece) with the fluence 1.4 J/cm², spot size of 5 mm and frequency 10 Hz. Note the petechiae at the site of treatment; (C) Significant lightening of pigmentation with no textural changes can be noted.

a multifactorial disorder of the pilosebaceous unit that can cause permanent scarring and disfigurement. Four major pathogenic factors causing acne are:

1. Increased sebum production
2. Hypercornification of pilosebaceous duct
3. Follicular colonization by *Cutibacterium acnes*
4. Inflammation.[19]

Acne usually leaves behind scars which may be permanent. Acne scars are of various types. Icepick scars, boxcar scars and the rolling scars. Common therapies used for treatment of acne and acne scars include antibiotics, retinoids, hormonal therapy, peels, radiofrequency microneedling and laser resurfacing. The author has been able to achieve good results in improving acne and acne scars with picosecond Nd:YAG lasers. The picosecond energy when deposited at the dermal level causes dermal remodeling by stimulation of growth factors and collagen. LIOB caused by the picosecond pulses works like subcision of the scars. It reduces acne by reducing the sebum secretion by photoacoustic damage of sebaceous glands.[20]

Acne is treated with small tip of the fractional handpiece. Three passes with the following parameters are used, i.e., wavelength of 1064 nm, fluence of 0.25 J/cm^2, spot size of 10 mm and frequency of 10 Hz. Sessions are performed 2 weeks apart. Improvement is seen within a week of the first session. Mild erythema is observed immediately post laser which lasts for about 2 hours. The active acne reduces within a week post laser **(Figs. 7A and B)**.

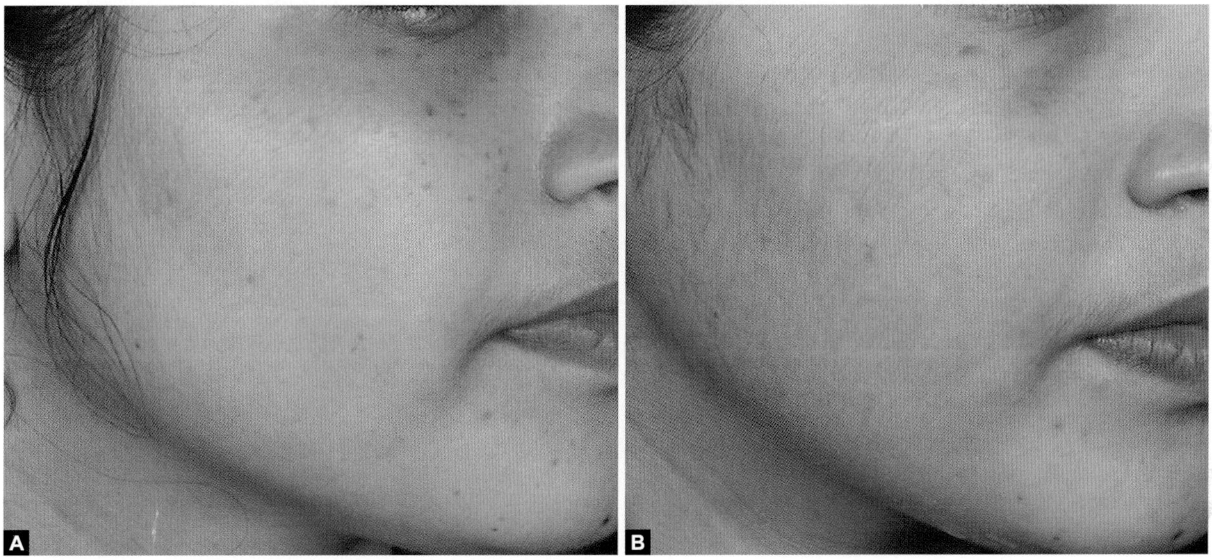

Figs. 6A and B: (A) Freckles on the face at first visit; (B) Patient underwent one session of picosecond laser with zoom handpiece using a fluence of 0.8J/cm^2, spot size of 4 mm and frequency of 3 Hz.

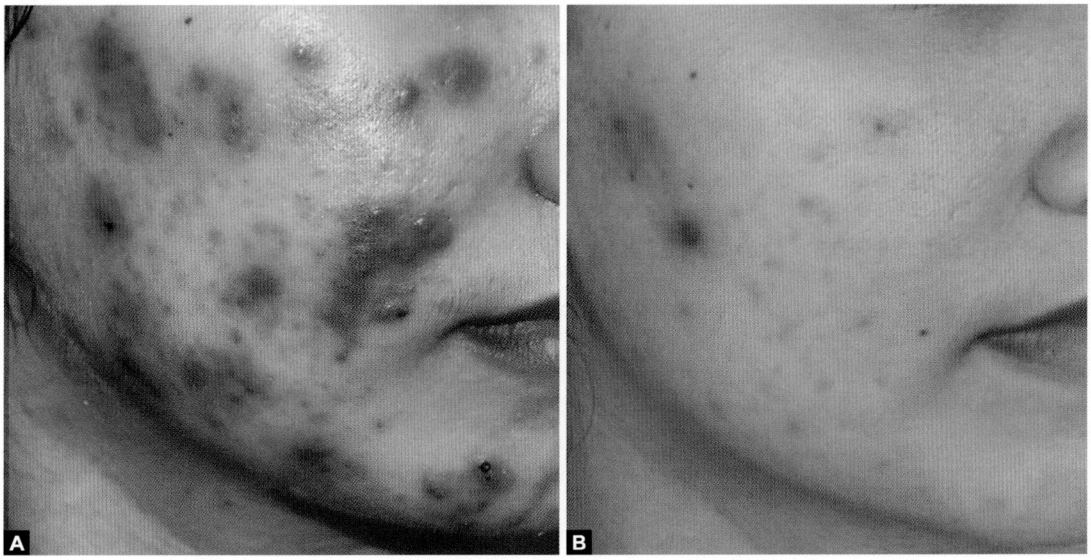

Figs. 7A and B: (A) A 19-year-old girl presented with grade III acne on bilateral cheeks; (B) After three fortnightly sessions of Picosecond laser (fractional handpiece) with a fluence of 0.25 J/cm^2, frequency of 10 Hz and spot size of 10 mm.

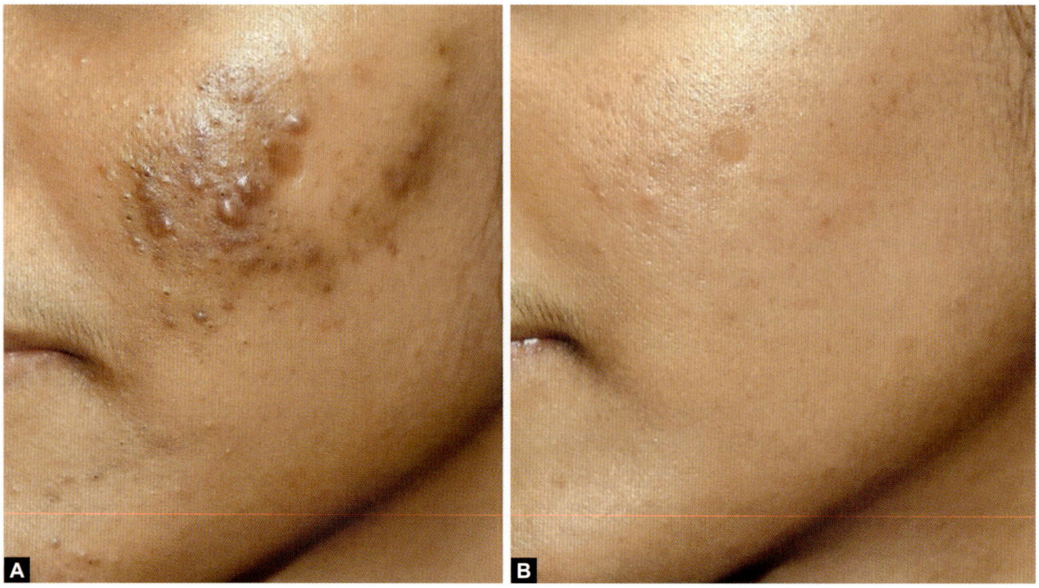

Figs. 8A and B: (A) A 16-year-old girl with grade II acne on face; (B) She underwent three fortnightly sessions of picosecond Nd:YAG laser (fractional handpiece) with fluence of 0.25 J/cm^2, frequency of 10 Hz and spot size of 10 mm. Note the improvement in chickenpox scar.

Fractional handpiece is preferred for acne scars. The surface of the skin need not be anesthetized as the procedure is relatively pain free. All the three tips are used sequentially in the same session. Small tip is used first with the fluence of 0.3–0.5 J/cm^2, frequency of 10 Hz and spot size of 10 mm. The medium tip is used next with a fluence of 0.25–0.35 J/cm^2, frequency of 10 Hz and the spot size of 10 mm. The long tip is used at the end with fluence of 0.13–0.15 J/cm^2, frequency of 10 Hz and spot size of 10 mm is delivered on the skin. 3 passes are performed while using each tip. Use low fluence around the periorbital area. Mild to moderate erythema and petechiae is what we observe immediately post laser. Patient will have mild burning sensation which lasts only for a few minutes post laser. This can further be alleviated by using ice pack on the treated area. Patient should be counseled that the erythema and petechiae may sometimes last for up to 48 hours **(Figs. 8A and B)**. Usually, it takes around two to three sessions to achieve significant improvement. For optimum results picosecond laser can be combined with fractional CO_2 laser simultaneously for the treatment of acne scars.

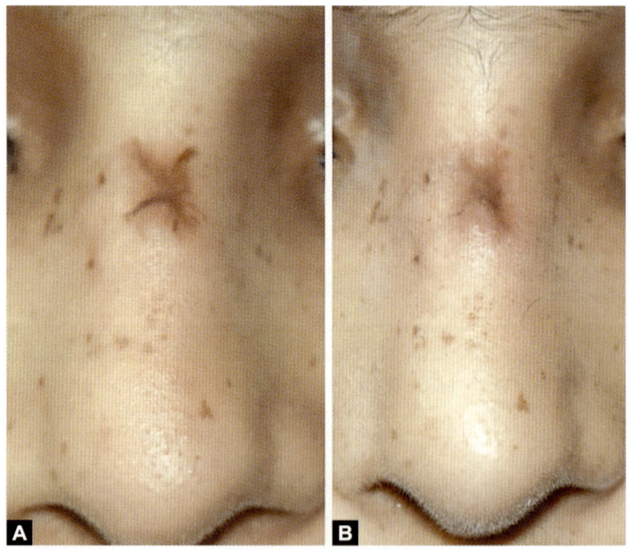

Figs. 9A and B: (A) A 22-year-old female patient presented with hypertrophic scar resulting from accident on the nose; (B) She underwent three sessions of picosecond laser (fractional handpiece) with fluence of 0.20 J/cm^2, spot size of 7 mm and frequency of 10 Hz.

OTHER USES OF PICOSECOND LASER

Picosecond Nd:YAG laser has shown promising results in treatment of hypertrophic scars. Fractional CO_2 laser, long-pulsed 1064 nm Nd:YAG laser, pulsed dye lasers have been commonly used for the improvement in the appearance and texture of hypertrophic scars **(Figs. 9A and B)**. Compared to conventional 1064 nm QS-Nd:YAG laser, picosecond Nd:YAG laser can treat hypertrophic scars more effectively and safely while reducing the adverse effects.[21] Picosecond laser has proven to be safe and effective in improving various photoaging-associated facial pigmentation.[22]

CONCLUSION

To date nano Q-switched lasers have been the preferred laser for treatment of pigmented lesions. Increased efficacy can be expected from the versatile uses of the picosecond Nd:YAG laser which has a wider range from treatment of inflammatory acne, acne scars, injury scars (accident and burns) to wrinkles.

The advantages of picosecond laser are its efficacy in the treatment of all pigmented lesions in a manner which increases reduction of pigment with less side effects and consequently less downtime. Unlike the nanotechnology it can be used to treat all moderate scarring which makes its usage versatile. Picosecond Nd:YAG laser are seen as being more effective with fewer side effects lesser down time and shorter sessions. With improved outcomes and fewer side effects the picosecond laser will be the choice of laser in the years to come.

The future prospects for picosecond lasers are bright as production costs for manufacturers come down because of increased sales. With over half a dozen indications for pico lasers which are not treatable by nano Q-switched lasers and a refinement in tattoo clearance, it will replace the older technology in the next few years, making it a financially sound investment in a multipronged approach while treating various cosmetic disorders.

REFERENCES

1. Ho DD, London R, Zimmerman GB, Young DA. Laser-tattoo removal—a study of the mechanism and the optimal treatment strategy via computer simulations. Lasers Surg Med. 2002;30:389-97.
2. Torbeck RL, Schilling L, Khorasani H, Dover JS, Arndt KA, Saedi N. Evolution of picosecond laser: a review of literature. Dermatol Surg. 2019:45(2):183-94.
3. Kasai K. Picosecond laser treatment for tattoos and benign cutaneous pigmented lesions. Laser Ther. 2017;26(4):274-81.
4. Habbema L, Verhagen R, Van Hal R, Liu Y, Varghese B. Minimally invasive non-thermal laser technology using laser-induced optical breakdown for skin rejuvenation. J Biophotonics. 2012;5(2):194-9.
5. Haimovic A, Brauer JA, Cindy Bae YS, Geronemus RG. Safety of a picosecond laser with diffractive lens array (DLA) in the treatment of Fitzpatrick skin types IV to VI: a retrospective review. J Am Acad Dermatol. 2016;74(5):931-6.
6. Ross V, NAseef G, Lin G, Kelly M, Kelly M, Michaud N, Flotte TJ, et al. Comparison of responses of tattoos to picosecond and nanosecond Q-switched Nd:YAG lasers. Arch Dermatol. 1998;134:167-71.
7. Kirby W, Desai A, Desai T, Kartono F, Geeta P. The Kirby-Desai scale: a proposed scale to assess tattoo removal treatments. J Clin Aesthet Dermatol. 2009;2(3):32-7.
8. Welch AJ, van Gaemert MJC. Optical-Thermal Response of Laser-irradiated Tissue, 2nd edition. Berlin: Springer; 2011. pp. 13.
9. Cencic B, Lukac M, Marincek M, Vizintin Z. High fluence, high beam quality Q-switched Nd:YAG laser with optoflex delivery system for treating benign pigmented lesions and tattoos. J LAHA. 2010;1:9-18.
10. Dover JS, Margolis RJ, Polla LL, Watanabe S, Hruza GJ, Parrish JA, et al. Pigmented guinea pig skin irradiated with Q-switched ruby laser pulses. Arch Dermatol. 1989;125;43-9.
11. Kim JE, Chang SE, Yeo UC, Haw S, Kim IH. Histopathological study of the treatment of melasma lesions using a low-fluence Q-switched 1064-nm neodymium:yttrium-aluminium-garnet laser. Clin Exp Dermatol. 2013;38:167-71.
12. Jang YH, Park JY, Kang HY. Changes in melanin and melanocytes in mottled hypopigmentation after low fluence 1064 nm Q-switched Nd:YAG laser with low pulse energy. Clin Exp Dermatol. 2009;34:e847-50.
13. Tse Y, Levine VJ, McClain SA, Ashinoff R. The removal of cutaneous pigmented lesions with the Q-switched ruby laser and Q-switched neodymium:yttrium-aluminium-garnet laser. A comparative study. J Dermatol Surg Oncol. 1994;20:795-800.
14. Anderson RR, Parish JA. Selective photothermolysis: precise microsurgery by selective absorption of pulsed radiation. Science. 1983;220:524-7.
15. Levins PC, Anderson RR. Q-switched ruby laser for the treatment of pigmented lesions and tattoos. Clin Dermatol. 1995;13:75-9.
16. Taylor CR, Anderson RR, Gange RW, Michaud NA, Flotte TJ. Light and electron microscopic analysis of tattoos treated by Q-switched ruby laser. J Invest Dermatol. 1991;97:131-6.
17. Kossida T, Farinelli W, Flotte T, Anderson RR. Mechanism of immediate whitening during tattoo removal. Lasers Surg Med. 2006;18:70.
18. Watanabe S, Takahashi H. Treatment of nevus of Ota with the Q-switched ruby laser. J Am Acad Dermatol.1993;29;997-1001.
19. Tahir CM. Pathogenesis of acne vulgaris: simplified. J Pak Assoc Dermatol. 2010;20:93-7.
20. Estarabadi AR, Eber AE, Nouri K. Laser and light therapies for acne. In: Nouri K (Ed). Lasers in Dermatology and Medicine, 2nd edition. Switzerland: Springer; 2018. pp. 227-36.
21. Choi YJ, Kim JY, Nam JH, Lee GY, Kim WS. Clinical outcome of 1064-nm picosecond neodymium-doped yttrium aluminum garnet laser for the treatment of hypertrophic scars. J Cosmet Laser Ther. 2019;21(2):91-8.
22. Kim JY, Suh HY, Choi ME, Jung CJ, Chang SE. Clinical improvement of photoaging-associated facial hyperpigmentation in Korean skin with a picosecond 1064-nm neodymium-doped yttrium aluminium garnet laser. Lasers Med Sci. 2020;35(7): 1599-606.

CHAPTER 119

Complications of Lasers

Apratim Goel, Zeba Chhapra

KEY MESSAGES

- Laser and light sources have a particular therapeutic window, narrow or wide, for a particular lesion or condition. In order to avoid complications, fluence in the therapeutic range, called optimal fluence, should be maintained to give predictable and effective clinical outcomes.
- Laser-treated skin requires special care, regardless of the laser used or the lesion treated. As different lasers produce different skin responses, customized posttreatment regimens should be advocated to eliminate adverse after effects.
- During counseling, elicit history of sun exposure, tanning, retinoids, and photosensitizing drugs as they increase the chances of adverse effects.
- Cultivate diligent postprocedure counseling practices. Postprocedure the skin is drier and needs to be protected from heat, sun exposure, handling, and infection. Soothing, moisturizing, and sun-protective preparations should be advised. Also SOPs (standard operating procedures) are a must.
- In laser treatment, complications can be categorized into immediate and late complications; based on whether they occur within a few minutes or hours of laser treatment, or later than 2 days.
- Operator and physician knowledge of device, patient, complication, prevention, and management are keys to deliver results using laser technology.

INTRODUCTION

With the advent of new lasers being used for various indications, the need to understand the possible complications is very important to limit the downtime and increase the efficacy of treatment by preventing damage to the surrounding skin. The use of lasers, lights, and radiofrequency in dermatologic surgery has rapidly advanced since the device was first introduced more than four decades ago.[1] Invention of new devices and upgradation of the existing ones has allowed growth in the field of laser industry. Based on the principle of selective photothermolysis elucidated by Anderson and Parrish in 1983, an entire generation of lasers has been developed to improve tissue specificity.[1]

Selective photothermolysis is accomplished through the use of appropriate wavelength and pulse duration best absorbed by specific chromophores, such as melanin or hemoglobin. However, not all lasers and light sources adhere to this principle. Continuous wave lasers are least selective and may produce unwanted tissue damage and scarring through heat conduction to neighboring normal skin. Quasi-continuous wave lasers limit excessive thermal destruction by delivery of a series of brief laser pulses but still pose a higher risk of nonspecific tissue damage and thermal injury. The pulsed and Q-switched (QS) systems adhere most closely to the principles of selective photothermolysis and result in the highest degree of selective destruction with the lowest risk of scarring from excessive thermal diffusion.[2]

Complications are adverse events or responses to a therapy or procedure. Many complications that can arise are not laser specific; however, there are some complications that are more likely to arise with certain laser and light procedures. Although complication rates reported with cutaneous lasers, light, and radiofrequency are consistently low, potential adverse reactions still do occur, even in the hands of an experienced laser surgeon.

COMPLICATIONS

Various lasers are used in dermatology for diverse indications, associated with their diverse complications **(Box 1)**. The term complication implies the occurrence of undesired effects or outcome of a specific laser intervention and can be immediate or delayed. The only way we can reduce and manage them is by understanding the principles and the science underlying the technology. Many of the complications arise from inadequate knowledge of laser parameters or inappropriate use of the machine. However, darker skin types tend to have more complications due to excess melanin that is a target chromophore in the epidermis for many lasers. Therefore, in such patients priming is of utmost importance. Further, patients have to be counseled that if the post-laser instructions are followed meticulously, several complications may be avoided.[3]

BOX 1: Complications of lasers.

Immediate:
- Postoperative erythema and edema
- Blistering and crusting
- Irritant or allergic contact dermatitis
- Milia
- Acneiform eruptions
- Purpura
- Pain and discomfort
- Delayed wound healing
- Burns

Delayed:
- Hyperpigmentation
- Hypopigmentation
- Scarring
- Demarcation line

Rare:
- Leukotrichia
- Urticaria
- Keloids
- Viral, bacterial, and fungal infections of skin
- Koebnerization
- Tingling sensation or dysesthesias or paresthesias
- Superficial phlebitis

Immediate Complications

These complications occur within 48 hours of laser treatment and primarily include edema, erythema, allergic contact dermatitis (ACD) or irritant contact dermatitis (ICD).

- *Erythema* **(Fig. 1)** usually subsides within few hours of the treatment. Adequate icing of the area along with application of a mild steroid cream will allow it to settle faster. Rarely, the erythema can last longer and may need a potent steroid preparation for it to subside. Exposure of laser-treated skin to topical products that may be a source of irritation should be avoided in order to reduce the risk of prolonged or aggravated erythema. At focal sites of erythema with induration and tenderness signaling early scar formation, topical corticosteroids and/or pulsed dye laser (PDL) is warranted.
- *Blistering* **(Fig. 2)** can be an immediate complication after effect of many lasers. It occurs due to epidermal damage, particularly in patients with a recent tan. Moreover, it can occur with all types of laser procedures. The other causes include high fluence of the laser light and increased absorption through a compromised epidermis. Hence, blisters are common occurrence after laser hair removal associated epidermal injury. Crusting too is caused by laser-induced epidermal damage and is common with QS lasers used for tattoo removal but can also be observed with other lasers, though less often.[3]
- *Contact dermatitis:* During the acute recovery phase before re-epithelialization is completed; barrier function is compromised and facilitates irritant effects of chemicals. An increased susceptibility to fragrances, preservatives, and other allergens found in skin care products and topical antibiotics may also occur postoperatively.

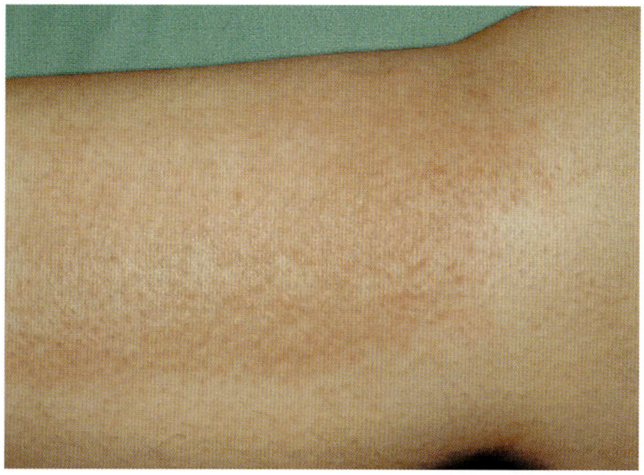

Fig. 1: Laser-induced erythema and edema which generally settles in few minutes to hours.

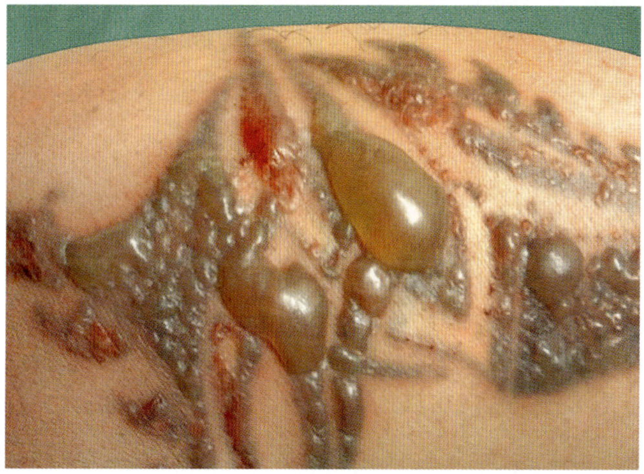

Fig. 2: Blistering post Q-switch laser for tattoo removal.

  - Irritant contact dermatitis **(Figs. 3A and B)** may occur within few hours of contact with any irritant substance limited to the area of contact and associated with erythema, edema, blistering, and crusting.
  - Allergic contact dermatitis **(Figs. 3A and B)** occurs within 24–48 hours of exposure and usually presents with urticarial plaques which tend to extend beyond the exposure sites. In most cases, the reaction develops in response to application of topical antibiotic post-treatment. Topical steroid cream and oral anti-inflammatory agents are hence used to treat the condition.[3]

  Symptomatic management includes the use of potent topical corticosteroids and oral antihistamines. Frequent application of cool compresses can also reduce symptoms and minimize inflammation.
- *Milia* **(Fig. 4)**: It is a type of keratin retention cyst on the skin surface which arises post-laser treatment, while the skin is healing, generally, after a session of carbon dioxide (CO_2) or erbium laser skin resurfacing.[3] They

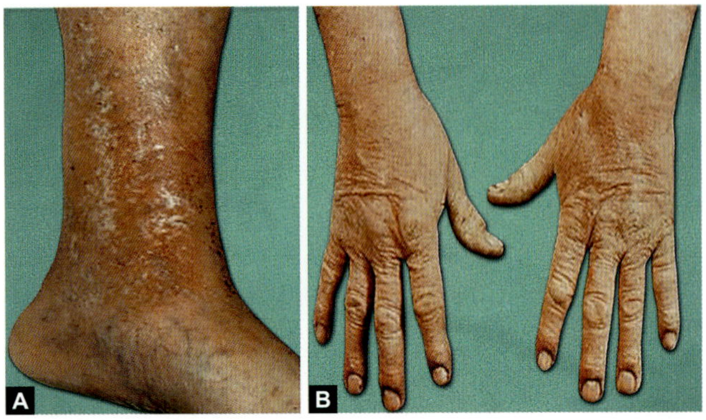

Figs. 3A and B: Contact dermatitis—(A) Allergic contact dermatitis; (B) Irritant contact dermatitis.

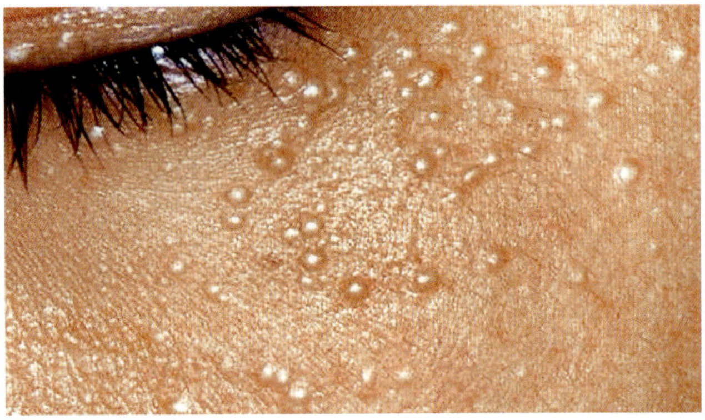

Fig. 4: Multiple milia arising post-laser skin resurfacing using Er:YAG.

occur during the acute recovery period, mainly due to occlusive local anesthetic application and use of occlusive ointments or dressings postprocedure However, it is a minor aftermath of a laser procedure and can easily be extracted using a sterile needle or radiofrequency.[4]

- *Acneiform eruptions:* These are very common with laser exposure as the beam provides heat and leads to activation of sebaceous gland activity leading to breakouts. Higher incidences of acne after ablative laser resurfacing are reported in literature, but it is also frequently seen with other lasers such as QS-Nd:YAG (neodymium-doped yttrium aluminum garnet) and diode. Further, aberrant follicular epithelialization 1–2 weeks postprocedure adds to the acne flare, more so in patients with previous history of acne. Occlusive healing ointments and dressings post-laser also add to the brunt. Mild topical anti-inflammatory agents given topically for 2–3 days take care of the condition. However, patients should be counseled in advance about the possibility of an acne flare and a prophylactic topical preparation can be optionally added postprocedure.[4] A course of oral antibiotics such as doxycycline for moderate to severe acneiform eruptions can be prescribed, particularly in patients who have a history of acne. For inflamed acneiform cysts or nodules, intralesional corticosteroid injections are most effective.

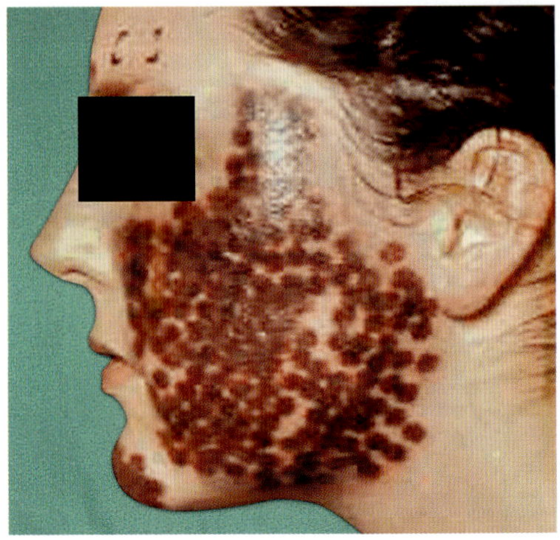

Fig. 5: Purpura post-pulsed dye laser.

- *Purpura:* Purpura is an immediate but transitory phenomenon, generally occurring as an adverse effect post use of lasers such as PDL and long-pulsed Nd:YAG laser or intense pulsed light (IPL), particularly for treatment of vascular lesions, such as port wine stain, cherry hemangioma, etc. It can also occur after the use QS lasers for pigmentary lesions. Pulsed dye laser **(Fig. 5)** treatment is deemed most notorious in causing a purpuric reaction which may last about 7–14 days in most cases but are cosmetically unacceptable while they last.[3] The PDL deposits a large amount of energy in a short period of time, often leading to vessel rupture and purpura formation.

  The first generation PDLs used a small spot size, short pulse duration and wavelengths with high fluence parameters. This combination was associated with high incidences of purpura and other complications such as blistering and scarring. The high peak energy of short pulse duration PDL leads to photoacoustic shattering of capillary walls with resultant extravasation of red blood cells into extravascular tissue, causing purpura.[5] The new generation PDL uses longer pulse duration with increasing number of subpulses; where the slower application of thermal energy minimized any photoacoustic effects and hence risk of purpura is lessened while maintaining clinical efficacy **(Figs. 6A and B)**.[6]

  Transitory purpura has also been reported with IPL-associated treatment of port wine stain and other vascular lesions when high fluence and short pulse duration have been used.[7]

- *Pain and discomfort:* Postprocedure pain was a frequent discomfort associated with the older lasers. The newer lasers, especially those with cooling devices are virtually painless or inflict mild bearable ache. To curb the pain during the procedure, topical anesthetics can be applied to the skin. High intensity focused ultrasound (HIFU) technology for noninvasive facelift and skin tightening can however leave a dull deep pain and discomfort which can take 1–3 weeks or more to resolve.

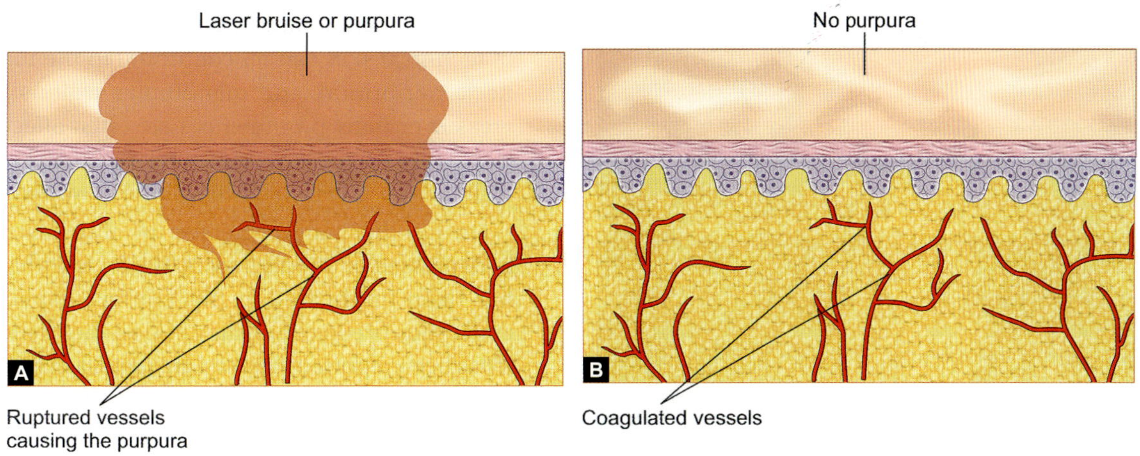

Figs. 6A and B: (A) Purpura caused by short pulse duration; (B) No purpura when longer pulse durations implied by the new generation pulsed dye lasers.

- *Delayed wound healing:* One of the rare dermal adverse effects of laser skin procedures, delayed wound healing is more commonly seen with aggressive CO_2 or erbium laser skin resurfacing. It has been thought to occur more in patients on isotretinoin.[8] In most cases, it occurs secondary to wound infection or due to coexistence of other systemic conditions (e.g., lupus erythematous). In their absence, its idiopathic nature is best managed with conservative wound management. Tissue fibrosis and scarring are expected sequelae.[3]
- *Burn:* It is a common undesirable event with the use of almost any laser. Laser for hair removal **(Fig. 7)**, vascular lesions and nonablative skin rejuvenation or even IPL can lead to a burn if one of the three laser taboos has been committed—high fluence, short pulse duration, and insufficient epidermal cooling. Dark-skinned patients pose a greater risk due to excess melanin in skin and hence it is essential to set the fluence low with high pulse duration while dealing with darker skin tones, in order to allow a longer thermal relaxation time (TRT). Burns characteristically present themselves within 24 hours of the treatment preceded by local warmth, intense burning, and erythema. Though it is temporary, it causes immense physical and physiological discomfort to the patient and may heal with dyspigmentation which in itself is another complication, required to be managed. A mild burn may present with prolonged erythema and will resolve with topical steroids. A moderate to severe burn may lead to blistering and scarring. Fortunately, the emergence of safer new generation lasers has significantly reduced device-associated incidence of burns.[9]

Delayed Complications

They occur after 48 hours of the treatment and can last long if not treated properly. Some of these complications resolve with time.

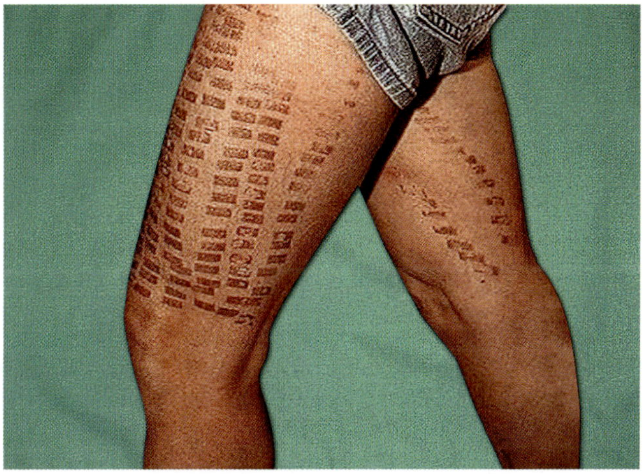

Fig. 7: Burns after laser hair removal.

Hyperpigmentation: This is one of the most frequent complications that are noticed after treatment, commonly seen in Fitzpatrick skin types III to VI because of the presence of excess melanin in the epidermis leading to post-inflammatory hyperpigmentation (PIH). Tanned skin too is susceptible to PIH postprocedure. It is not a permanent effect; instead, it fades with time and responds well to topical depigmenting therapy. It is a particularly common occurrence with laser hair removal **(Fig. 8)** using IPL10 and CO_2 skin resurfacing.

Management strategies for hyperpigmentation include strict photoprotection and use of broad-spectrum sunscreen. The use of topical corticosteroids immediately after ablative skin resurfacing also has been shown to effectively decrease postinflammatory hyperpigmentation, particularly in patients with darker skin tones. Mineral sunblocks containing iron oxide or titanium dioxide would avert potential sensitization effects related to the use of chemical sunscreen filters.

It may take up to 6–18 weeks to achieve clearance and hence patients have to be counseled and reassured.[3,10]

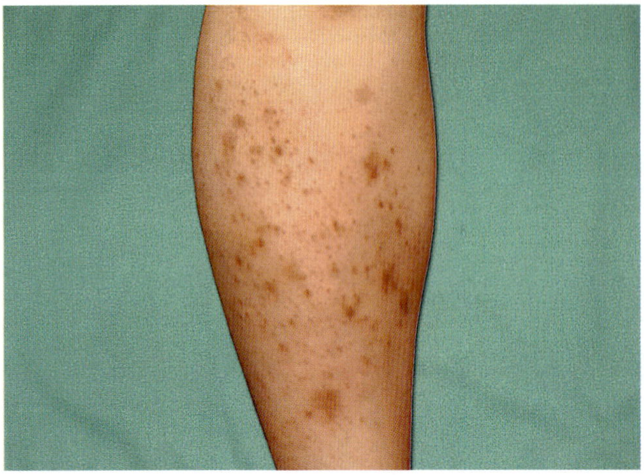

Fig. 8: Postinflammatory hyperpigmentation over leg after laser hair removal.[9]

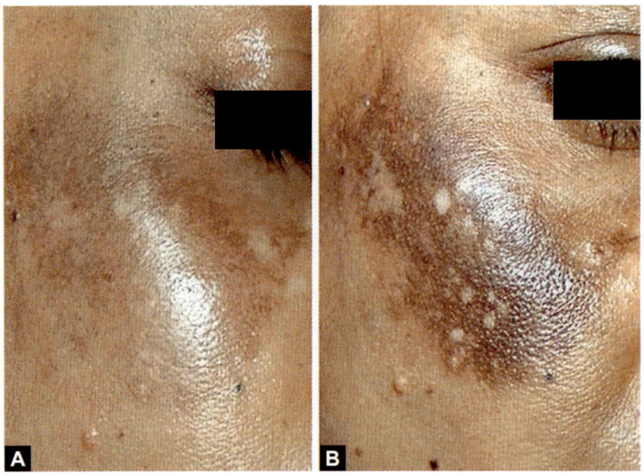

Figs. 9A and B: Mottled hypopigmentation after four sessions of 1,064 nm Q-switched Nd:YAG laser for melasma. The configuration of the lesions corresponds to that of the laser spot.
Courtesy: Dr Apratim Goel, Mumbai.

Hypopigmentation: Another dreaded pigment-related condition experienced post-laser treatment is hypopigmentation **(Figs. 9A and B)** due to the melanin being targeted as a chromophore by the beam while using lasers for tattoo removal, hair removal or for treating pigmentation, such as QS ruby, alexandrite, and Nd:YAG lasers. In case of an epidermal injury, hypopigmentation is a possibility with any laser, usually treated with topical medium potency steroid or immunomodulators such as 1% tacrolimus or 1% pimecrolimus twice daily for 10–16 weeks. Local trichloroacetic acid application has also been used to treat the condition. Coal tar-based preparations, psoralens, targeted phototherapy, and 308 nm excimer laser too show significant improvement when used for the condition.[11]

- *Scars:* Hypertrophic scarring is a well-established yet rare complication of fractional ablative resurfacing, though also commonly seen after QS-Nd:YAG associated tattoo removal. Use of excessively high-energy densities and fluences, postoperative infection of the skin, and lack of technical skill can all contribute to the mishap. The neck, periorbital, and mandibular regions and other areas over bony prominences are often affected due to lesser pilosebaceous units, poor vasculature, and thin architecture, all of which contribute to wound healing.[12]

  On the other hand, aggressive use of any laser can result in depressed or atrophic scars. IPL for laser hair removal has been implicated in this context, especially post application of eutectic mixture of local anesthetics (EMLA). It has been reported to pose a greater risk of burns leading to scarring, possibly by lengthening the IPL exposure time.[13] Interestingly, monopolar radiofrequency for skin tightening also can result in cutaneous depressions, weeks or even months postoperative and seem to result from overheating of adipose tissue and fibrous septae during treatment. Caution must be used when treating over bony prominences or thin skin, such as the forehead and temples. Treating with lower fluences and multiple passes is advisable to avoid such unnecessary adverse events. Mild dermal depressions often resolve spontaneously with time while contour irregularities and scarring may require subcision, autologous fat transfer or dermal fillers.[12]

- *Demarcation line:* It represents an abrupt change in skin color, clearly outlining the boundary between the treated and untreated areas on face or body, as a result of pigment loss in area exposed to laser. As a rule, treatment comprises lightening the untreated constituent to match its counterpart. The neck is the most common area affected. A clear demarcation can be appreciated after CO_2 resurfacing or lower face laser hair reduction in a patient with tanning or other signs of photodamage over the neck region. The patient should be counseled pretreatment and prophylactically primed with topical tretinoin and hydroquinone to match the color of the neck to that of the face. Specifically in the case of CO_2 laser resurfacing, avoid aggressive parameter use close to the mandible. However, once it occurs, superficial chemical peeling, cosmeceuticals for lightening, and cosmetic camouflage render favorable outcomes.[14]

Rare Complications

- *Leukotrichia:* A rare entity generally associated with hair removal with the use of IPL. Leukotrichia represents the destruction of the melanocyte in the follicle sparing the germinative cells. Radmanesh et al. reported an incidence of up to 3.5%, of which 31% patients experienced a temporary change in hair color which reversed by itself in a few months. In temporarily affected cases, the provisional arrest in melanin synthesis due to damaged but not totally destructed melanocytes could be a possible explanation for the phenomenon. Adequate fluences to

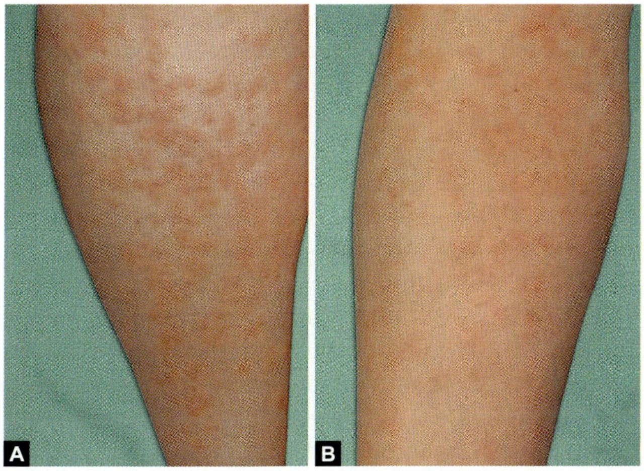

Figs. 10A and B: Urticaria post-laser epilation.[21]

cause concomitant germinative cell death are essential to avoid this adverse effect.[15,16]

- *Urticaria* **(Figs. 10A and B)**: Persistent urticaria is a rare adverse reaction, mainly to laser epilation due to a delayed hypersensitivity reaction in predisposed allergic individuals. Bernstein E reported cases of urticarial rashes in patients treated 810 nm diode, long-pulsed alexandrite laser and long-pulsed Nd:YAG for laser hair reduction. Hence, a preliminary extended laser patch test, re-evaluated 48 hours later, is highly recommended to avoid any serious reactions. Sequentially, prophylactic oral prednisone can be prescribed to patients who develop an urticarial rash on the test area.[17]
- *Keloids:* Keloid formation in association with tattoo removal using 1,064 nm QS-Nd:YAG laser is not an infrequent complication. Specifically, African Americans demonstrate a genetic tendency to scarring with this laser. However, its incidence is as low as 0.28% in some studies and is likely to be secondary to inappropriate selection of treatment devices, aggressive parameters, and inadequate patient aftercare.[18]

It is also well established in literature that patients on oral isotretinoin undergoing invasive laser resurfacing especially with CO_2 laser have a greater risk of developing delay in wound healing, hypertrophic scars, and keloids invasive procedures. Hence, it was previously recommended that these procedures should be opted for 6–12 months after cessation of oral isotretinoin therapy. However, more recently it has been established that isotretinoin does not appear to delay wound healing, and hence invasive procedures can be concomitantly along with it, without any compromise on the outcome.[19] An uncommon type of scarring that may occur is indentations and grooving. The Nd:YAG laser has been shown to create a grooving indentation due to collagen damage from heating. Deep indentations from isolated subcutaneous fat injury or panniculitis-like inflammation can occur. This type of atrophic scarring can be permanent.

BOX 2: Causative agents in CO_2 laser-induced infection.

- *Pseudomonas aeruginosa*
- *Staphylococcus aureus*
- *Streptococcus epidermidis*
- *Candida* spp.
- Herpes simplex virus
- *Enterobacter*
- *Escherichia coli*
- *Proteus*
- *Corynebacterium*
- *Serratia*

- *Viral, bacterial, and fungal infections:* These infections are rare, usually appearing in the first postoperative week. It is important to treat infections immediately to avoid scarring, delayed wound healing, and systemic dissemination. Any laser can precipitate an underlying infection; however laser hair reduction and laser lightening do not generally lead to infections, which are comparatively more common with resurfacing lasers **(Box 2)**.

Reactivation of herpes simplex virus (HSV) infection with the earlier use of traditional resurfacing laser was frequent, with the incidence ranging from 2 to 7%. With the emergence of fractional laser skin resurfacing, incidence has come down to 0.3–2%; however, HSV reactivation still remains the most common associated infection with laser resurfacing. Any previous history of herpes labialis puts the patient at risk of disseminated herpes. Patients may present with classic herpetiform vesicopustules or the preliminary superficial erosions. In either case, antiviral prophylaxis should be administered in all patients with prior history of HSV.[12] Acyclovir, valacyclovir or famciclovir is administered 1–2 days before and about 7 days postprocedure or until re-epithelization is complete.[20]

Bacterial infection has a lower incidence (0.1–4.5%) including *Staphylococcus aureus*, *Pseudomonas aeruginosa*, and *Enterobacter cloacae*-associated infections in patients undergoing laser resurfacing.[12] Increased pain, intense erythema, exudate, erosions with crusting 1–3 days post-laser treatment should caution the physician. Topical such as mupirocin and oral antibiotics such as penicillins, amoxiclav, etc., can be administered. Patients additionally are advised to clean their hands with antiseptic soap prior to application of healing ointments and dressing changes.

Fungal infections are extremely rare. Cutaneous candidiasis due to *Candida albicans* is the most common fungal infection reported after fractional laser skin resurfacing, noticed 1–2 weeks post-session. Topical and oral ketoconazole or fluconazole should be started early to prevent scarring.[12]

- *Koebnerization*: The phenomenon has to be carefully considered in patients opting for ablative laser resurfacing.

Scleroderma, lupus erythematosus, unstable vitiligo, lichen planus, psoriasis, and verrucae may undergo Koebnerization and hence should be identified with a meticulous dermatological history before treatment.[22] Laser hair removal too may rarely be associated with this phenomenon.[23]

Tingling and paresthesia: Mild tingling sensation may be experienced after laser hair removal in the localized area being treated and is considered a mild phenomenon. IPL may present with local persistent heat sensation after procedure which recovers in few days.[24] However, a case of chronic facial pain post-IPL epilation has been recently reported and demands caution in patient selection and procedural protocol.[25] Hyperesthesia and increased sensitivity post-laser resurfacing with lasers such as erbium-doped yttrium aluminum garnet (Er:YAG) is also a possibility, mainly due to loss of epithelial surface. Emollients and sunscreen can alleviate these symptoms.[24]

Perioral tingling and numbness should always raise suspicion of an associated HSV infection and hence history of the same should be taken presession to decipher if the phenomenon is due to the viral pathology or laser induced.[20] Paresthesias, though uncommonly seen, may also occur as a late complication of endovenous laser ablation (EVLA) done for treatment of varicose veins.[26]

Anesthesia toxicity with use of topical anesthesia containing 30% lidocaine gel, not properly removed prior to procedure, presenting with perioral tingling along with agitation, anxiety, palpitations, etc., has been reported in literature. Increased percutaneous absorption of lidocaine by fractional photothermolysis could be a possible explanation.[27]

- *Superficial phlebitis:* Superficial phlebitis or vein inflammation is another infrequent side effect, reported in approximately 5% of EVLA (Endovenous laser ablation) procedures. It may be due to damage to vessel wall, disruption of blood flow or coagulation disorder. Usually transient with favorable prognosis, it presents with slow onset pain, tenderness, erythema, and warmth over skin overlying the course of the affected vein.[27]

COMPLICATIONS RELATED TO SPECIFIC LASERS

- *Resurfacing lasers:* The introduction of ablative laser skin resurfacing techniques with high-energy, pulsed CO_2 and Er:YAG devices in the mid-1990s was met with great enthusiasm. They displayed excellent clinical outcomes in the treatment of atrophic scars and photodamaged facial skin, including rhytides, lentigines, and dermal elastosis. However, the prolonged recovery period and risk of potential side effects made them less attractive treatment options.[4] Ablative laser resurfacing results in complete epidermal ablation and upper papillary dermal destruction with collagen remodeling. As a result, newly resurfaced skin lacks an intact epithelium, producing an exposed weeping wound with copious serous discharge. Complete reepithelialization occurs within an average of 8.5 days for CO_2 laser-resurfaced skin, compared with 5.5 days in case of Er:YAG laser. These complications are much less after fractional mode was introduced. Complications **(Table 1)** of fractional cutaneous laser resurfacing range from transient side effects to permanent disfigurement.[28] Complications of moderate severity include reactivation of HSV, superficial bacterial, and fungal infections, postinflammatory hyperpigmentation, and delayed onset hypopigmentation. The most severe complications associated with resurfacing include hypertrophic scar formation, ectropion, and disseminated infection.[4,28-30]
- *Vascular-specific lasers:* Vascular-specific laser systems target intravascular oxyhemoglobin to effect destruction of various congenital and acquired vascular lesions. Lasers and light sources that have been used to treat vascular lesions include the argon (488/514 nm), argon-pumped tunable dye (577/585 nm), potassium-titanyl-phosphate (KTP; 532 nm), krypton (568 nm), copper vapor/bromide (578 nm), PDL (585–595 nm), and Nd:YAG (532/1064 nm) lasers and the IPL source (515–1200 nm).[2] The most common complications of KTP are linear crusting of skin overlying treated blood vessels, transient pigmentary changes, mild fibrosis, cutaneous depressions, and hypopigmentation.[4,31] The most common complications of PDL include transient purpura, erythema, edema, and dyspigmentation.[4] These complications are typically self-resolving and last days to months.[2,29]
- *Intense pulse light:* It emits noncoherent broadband light in the range of 515–1,200 nm. Indications for IPL treatment are numerous and include pigmented and vascular lesions, photoaging, and photoepilation. Common side effects after treatment with IPL **(Table 2)** include mild postoperative erythema, edema, and ecchymosis more serious superficial burns and scarring can occur with aggressive treatment parameters. Because of the potential for competition between different chromophores with IPL systems, this device should be used cautiously in type III to VI skin and suntanned skin.[2,29,31]

TABLE 1: Complications of fractional laser skin resurfacing based on degree of severity.[27]

Mild	*Moderate*	*Severe*
• Prolonged erythema • Acne and milia • Delayed purpura • Superficial erosions • Contact dermatitis • Recall phenomenon	• Infection • Pigmentary alteration • Anesthesia toxicity • Eruptive kerato-acanthomas	• Hypertrophic scarring • Ectropion • Disseminated infection

Source: With permission of dermatologic surgery.

TABLE 2: Adverse events and their characteristic features that may occur after intense pulsed light treatment.[32]

Adverse event	*Incidence*	*Graveness*	*Surgence*	*Heat damage*
Erythema and edema	Most frequent	Minor	Premature (immediately after treatment)	Yes
Vesicles, blister	Infrequent	Minor	Premature (immediately after treatment)	Yes
Purpura	Rare	Minor	Premature (immediately after treatment)	No
Hematoma	Infrequent	Minor	Premature (immediately after treatment)	No
Scabs	Frequent	Minor	Premature	Yes
Infections	Infrequent	Minor	Premature	No
Zebra appearance	Infrequent	Minor	Premature	Yes
Transitory hyperpigmentation	Frequent	Minor	Tardive	Yes
Temporary hypochromatic variations	Infrequent	Minor	Tardive	Yes/No
Temporary hair discoloration	Rare	Minor	Tardive	No
Permanent pigmentation variations	Infrequent	Major	Tardive	Yes/No
Stimulation to hair growth	infrequent	Major	Tardive	No
Leukotrichia	Infrequent	Major	Tardive	No
Uveitis and iritis	Infrequent	Major	Tardive	No
Scars	Infrequent	Major	Tardive	Yes/No

- *Pigment specific lasers:* The three most common types of pigment specific QS lasers used in practice today are the 694-nm ruby, 755-nm alexandrite, and 532/1,064-nm Nd:YAG. Each produces an immediate ash-white epidermal tissue response when targeting cutaneous pigment or tattoo ink.
  - Possible common treatment side effects include:[29]
    - Punctuate bleeding
    - Tissue splatter
    - Edema
    - Pruritus
    - Vesiculation
    - Textural changes
    - Skin crusting.
- *Laser-induced hypopigmentation:* Small white macules matching the laser spot size and shape occur within weeks of treatment. They may last for a few months or rarely become permanent. Primarily, an adverse effect of the darker skin type, the risk of hypopigmentation appears to be directly proportional to the number of treatment sessions and fluence. Several treatment options are reported to be effective; including topical psoralen with ultraviolet A phototherapy (PUVA), narrow band ultraviolet B (NB-UVB) phototherapy, and 308 nm excimer laser and fractional resurfacing. Recently, targeted phototherapy (TPT) has emerged as a promising option. It induces repigmentation more effectively by delivery of super-erythemogenic doses of radiation, requiring fewer sessions.[33]
  - Potential complications reported from QS laser irradiation of tattoos include the following:[29]
    - Generalized cutaneous allergic reactions—to cadmium—or mercury-containing inks
    - Hemorrhagic bullae—particularly in the distal extremities
    - Irreversible darkening of cosmetic tattoos—particularly white, flesh-tone, pink or red inks due to presence of iron oxide or titanium dioxide pigments that undergo a laser-induced oxidation reduction reaction. Laser conversion of ferric oxide to ferrous oxide in tattoo ink leads to formation of the insoluble black pigment.
    - Scarring and tissue fibrosis—rarely occurring, particularly with inadequate wound management.[31]
    - *Chrysiasis or hyperpigmentation in patients receiving gold therapy:* Patients who have received gold therapy in the past for arthritis or other indications, and undergo QS laser treatment may rarely experience hyperpigmentation due to alteration of gold particles still present in the skin.[34]
- *Laser hair removal:* The most common reactions (**Table 3**) include pain during treatment, transient erythema, and perifollicular edema; vesicle formation, pigmentary alteration, burning, and scarring have also been documented.[35] Less obvious reactions include reticulate erythema and ocular complications. Most of the latter complications have occurred in individuals who are either tanned or have darker skin phototypes (IV to VI).[30,31] Because the 1,064-nm wavelength is less efficiently absorbed by endogenous melanin, significantly fewer incidences of blistering, crusting, and dyspigmentation occur after Nd:YAG laser treatment of patients with darker or tanned skin. Complication rates increase with increase in skin melanin content and fluence. However, even in light-skinned individuals, with proper treatment parameters, complications and side effects can arise.

TABLE 3: Complication and treatment of adverse effects of laser hair reduction.

Complication	*Treatment*
Common:	
1. Mild pain and numbness	• Epidermal-cooling devices (preventive), EMLA
2. Erythema (up to 3 days)	• Ice pack application, topical steroid
3. Edema (up to 2 days)	• Ice pack application, topical steroid • Oral antihistamine
4. Itching (up to 1–2 hours)	• Topical steroid, oral antihistamine
Occasional:	
1. Postinflammatory hyper- or hypopigmentation	• Topical steroid, sun protection • Lightening agents such as kojic acid, azelaic acid • Avoid aggressive parameters (preventive)
2. Acneiform eruption	• Topical antibiotics, tretinoin, and azelaic acid
3. Infection, e.g., reactivation of herpes simplex virus	• Observe aseptic measures • Oral antivirals, antifungals, and antibiotics • If known history—prophylactic treatment from 2 days preprocedure to 5–10 days postprocedure
Rare:	
1. Burn	• Avoid aggressive parameters (preventive) • Immediate-ice application • Topical steroid, topical antibiotic
2. Blistering and crusting	• Do not pop blisters • Topical steroid, topical antibiotic • Oral antibiotics (optional)
3. Laser-induced and paradoxical hypertrichosis	• Laser therapy for area with hair growth
4. Purpura	• Avoid aggressive parameters • Topical arnica montana • Nd:YAG laser, intense pulsed light

(EMLA: eutectic mixture of local anesthetics)
Source: Printed with permission of editor in chief dermatologic surgery.

Paradoxical hair growth is a possible side effect of photoepilation occurring in selected patient populations and body areas, usually located adjacent to an area treated by laser.[4,29,36-38] The phenomenon has been reported when subthreshold fluences are delivered to a susceptible patient, triggering hair induction rather than follicular destruction. Several cases of post-epilation hair growth have been reported with the use of IPL, alexandrite, and 1,064 nm Nd:YAG laser. Interestingly, it occurs more frequently after alexandrite laser and IPL treatments than the later. Further, patients may present with growth of terminal hair in previously treated areas that contained thin hairs.[33]

PREVENTION OF COMPLICATIONS

- *Effective cooling along with application of pressure* on skin with the probe head while doing the procedure, avoids complications like burns in laser hair removal as it protects the surrounding and leads to vasoconstriction of blood vessels, allowing the beam to reach its target chromophore, follicular melanin, more effectively. Cooling can be achieved with icepacks or ice rollers with the cooling starting 10–15 minutes before procedure and continuing during and up to 30–60 minutes after the procedure. Newer LASERs have an efficient cooling attachment to the probes, which can be utilized.
- *Ocular complications:* These can be due to the direct or indirect contact with laser irradiation. Thermal, mechanical, and photochemical damage to ocular structures include corneal burns, uveitis, cataract formation, and retinal burns. Patients presenting with blurred vision, photophobia, pain, and conjunctival hyperemia postprocedure must raise suspicion of ocular damage, the extent of which depends on the wavelength of the laser beam in question.[39] Cases of iris atrophy and post-brows epilation uveitis after the use of diode lasers have been described. Corneal abrasions may occur due to contact with topical numbing preparations, or inadvertent rubbing of the eye by the patient when the eyelid is numb.[12] Therefore, it is mandatory that both, doctor and patient use eye protection throughout the procedure, for all treatments, to avoid any such consequences. To protect the patient's eyes during laser procedures, along with use of intra- or extraocular protectors, care should be taken to direct the laser beam away from the ocular region.[40]

  Ideally eye shielding **(Figs. 11A and B)** should cover bilateral ocular surfaces in its entirety from the superior orbital rim down to the inferior orbital rim as it forms the roof of the maxilla. This includes the caruncle, nasally, zygomatic arch, temporally. In addition, if patients complain of eye pain, then the procedure should be instantly terminated an ophthalmic consultation mandated immediately.[39]
- *Complications related to fire or electric shock:* Chances of fire, such as ignition due to laser beam when it comes in contact with cloth, any flammable material or hair is a major safety issue when handling lasers and has to be addressed with caution.

Medical grade lasers are grade IIIB or IV lasers (emitting >500 mV radiant power). The "fire triangle" including heat, fuel, and oxidizer are required to start a fire. "Heat" represents the flame or spark and is the key in ignition of the fire. The heat source can be an overhead light, electrocautery unit or fiberoptic light. Precautionary measures should comprise discarding the ignitable material and cover the hair completely to avoid further risk, keeping in mind that only trained and informed

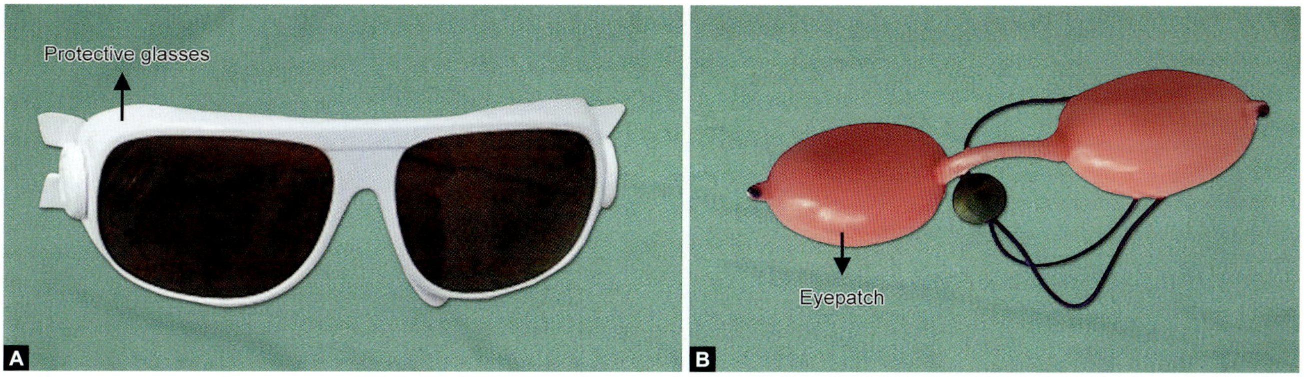

Figs. 11A and B: Protective eye wear used during laser procedure.

personnel enter the laser area. The main risk when handling laser is that when the laser comes in contact with the "fuel" required to ignite the heat source, such as the laser device itself. The oxidizer acts as a catalyst to speeden combustion such as alcohol, oxygen, and methane. Flammable materials on the patient such as hairspray, perfume, mascara should also be covered or removed before procedure.[41]

- *Complications related to infection:* The tissue's interaction with laser can produce smoke plume. It is difficult to determine the risks that can occur, though transmission of HPV and HSV is a possibility. CO_2 laser is most notorious in this context though it may occur with any laser. To ensure safety, a laser mask which is especially made to evacuate smoke must be used.
- *Laser safety in isotretinoin use:* Oral isotretinoin is used very often for moderate-severe grade acne in patients attending an aesthetic clinic. Earlier it was believed that such patients would be at increased risk of scarring post-laser treatment. However multiple studies have established that the risk of performing laser procedures on patients receiving isotretinoin or having recently completed a course is lower than the currently perceived risk.[42] This matter is dealt separately with in another chapter.
- *Postoperative care:* The provision of optimal wound care and maintenance of good wound healing conditions during the initial stage, first 2 weeks, are essential for achieving optimal re-epithelialization.
  - *Posttreatment care in the acute healing stage (0–2 weeks):* The purpose of care during this stage is to shorten the re-epithelialization time, repair the skin barrier function, and engage anti-UV care to prevent hyperpigmentation and reduce inflammation. Modern wound care is focused on moist wound healing which has been demonstrated to be more beneficial than traditional dressings.[43] Occlusive dressings provide a moist wound-healing environment, they may be open or closed. Open dressing refers to the direct application of an ointment or cream alone to the wound. Although inexpensive, convenient and easy for home care, this method may increase the risk of acne, milia, and infection.[44] The goal of wound care in the first week after laser skin resurfacing (LSR) treatment is to prevent infection, avoid environmental irritation and achieve complete and even re-epithelialization. Closed dressings have appeared to offer a superior moist wound environment whereby they facilitate epidermal cell migration more easily than with ointment, accommodate changes in pH, PO_2, and PCO_2, and sequester growth factors and proteinases in the wound area.[45] Topical application of Avène spring water spray had pronounced effects in reducing erythema, improving patient tolerance by hydrating post-laser skin and even reducing itching.[46] Epidermal growth factor (EGF) has been used recently to whiten the skin and prevent postinflammatory hyperpigmentation (PIH).[47] Adipose-derived stem cells (ADSCs) also appear to accelerate wound healing.[48]
  - *Posttreatment care in the chronic recovering stage (3 weeks–1 year):* PIH affects darker patients with greater frequency and severity, despite meticulous laser technique and adequate posttreatment care using the described first-stage measures. Strict sun avoidance and sunscreen for both UVA and UVB should be continued daily to avoid UV aggravation of the apparent PIH. Goldman and colleagues provided the following recommendations regarding preventive and curative measures for PIH after LSR based on their 8-year experience with >3,000 patients.[49]
    - Hydroquinone should be started immediately in patients at the first sign of hyperpigmentation, initially at a concentration of 2% once daily (at night to avoid morning UV radiation) and then increased to 4% as tolerated;
    - The combination of hydroquinone with other depigmenting agents is more effective than hydroquinone alone;

BOX 3: Pearls of precaution for the dermatologist.

The dermatologist must be aware of the following point about the laser:

- Know the laser light's properties
- Know the laser light's characteristics related to each of its wavelength
- Know the laser light's selection for absorption of the chromophores
- Know the laser light's power, power density, pulse parameters, fluence, energy, and density
- Know the spot size of the laser light along with its delivery systems and its equipment
- Know the techniques and its application
- Know the specific complications in skin of color and how to prevent these
- Know the basic maintenance and standard operating procedures of the laser to prevent malfunction and accidents

TABLE 4: Preoperative patient assessment to minimize complications.

Medical history	• Underlying inflammatory or immunosuppressive conditions (e.g., collagen vascular disease) • Excessive scarring (e.g., keloids) • Oral herpes simplex virus (HSV) • Prior aesthetic treatments • Current medications (e.g., anticoagulants, antiplatelet therapy, and gold) • Known allergies
Physical examination	• Skin phototype • Type, depth, and location of lesions • Presence of inflammation/infection (e.g., acne, HSV) • Evidence of recent sun exposure on treatment sites • Baseline standardized photography
Patient education	• Counsel regarding realistic expectations • Ensure post-care compliance (e.g., sunscreen) • Discussion regarding anticipated side effects and potential complications

TABLE 5: Factors affecting the risk of complications secondary to laser treatment.

Patient characteristics	• Patient skin phototype • Individual preprocedure condition • Anatomic location undergoing treatment
Treatment techniques	• Selection of laser parameters (e.g., energy, pulse duration) • Number of laser passes delivered • Degree of pulse or scan overlap

- For PIH accompanied by signs of inflammation, the use of a topical corticosteroid is recommended;
- If the patient experiences inflammation due to the use of certain agents, adjustments to the products may be necessary. These adjustments should be made in accordance with the relative order of these products based on their skin irritation potential, which is as follows: azelaic acid < kojic acid < 2% hydroquinone < tretinoin < 4% hydroquinone **(Box 3, Tables 4 and 5)**.

TIPS

Tips for the dermatologist.[50,51]

- Have smart approach to any problem
- Know the effects of the laser well
- Understand the importance of safety
- Completely analyze the patient including complete history and examination
- Avoid negligence
- Be sure with the problem diagnosed
- Work on the problem and consult the expert beforehand
- Be aware of the setting to do with the wavelength of the laser
- Check for the skin tan of the patient
- Use the appropriate tools before handling the laser
- Know the risks of topical anesthesia28
- In darker patients, keep low fluence and longer pulse duration with effective cooling to prevent burns and ensure effective results (Box 3)
- Address the patient's concerns
- Counsel the patient beforehand regarding the procedure, post-procedure care, and expected side effects
- Plan timely follow-ups: When recognized and managed expeditiously, the severity and duration of side effects and complications will be minimized
- Make them aware of the risks to diagnose them early
- Avoid patients with unrealistic expectations
- Initiate prophylactic therapies as required

CONCLUSION

Whole in whole, lasers work efficiently rendering superior results as monotherapy or as an adjuvant to oral, topical or other procedural management options. However, they also come with a wide range of complications, some mild and others highly notorious. They treat a number of skin conditions and certainly come with their fair share of risks and precautions. Besides running the risk of having to deal with these adverse effects, laser skin procedures are also very expensive. Proper patient selection and adequate pretreatment history of patient, assessment, examination, and counseling may aid in avoiding complications, managing them resourcefully and help the patient maintain realistic expectations, eventually rendering better patient retention. Posttreatment instructions should be provided and its importance emphasized at every session. In conclusion, proper time and steps taken to ensure thorough preprocedure education and counseling with close posttreatment follow-up by the physician will facilitate early recognition and management of potential laser complications.

Cosmetic laser technology has come a long way since the continuous wave argon and traditional ablative CO_2 lasers of the past. The newer generation laser devices are built to protect, with cooling tips, system lock setting until probe is placed in stand, etc. On the part of a skillful and competent dermatologist, updated knowledge on the device and patient characteristics is the primary tool to avoid unwanted events and also to be prepared to effectively manage it, if at all.

REFERENCES

1. Anderson RR, Parrish JA. Selective photothermolysis: precise microsurgery by selective absorption of pulsed radiation. Science. 1983;220:524-7.
2. Alster TS, Khoury RR. Treatment of laser complications. Facial Plast Surg. 2009;25:316-23.
3. Brown CW Jr. (2016). Complications of Dermatologic Laser Surgery: Overview, Laser Surgery Principles and Potential Complications, Introduction to Classification of Dermatologic Laser Complications. [online] Available from Emedicine. medscape.com/article/1120837-overview#a2. [Last accessed August 2023].
4. Tanzi EL, Alster TS. Complications of ablative and nonablative laser and light sources. In: Gloster HM (Ed). Complications in Cutaneous Surgery, 1st edition. USA: Springer Science + Business Media LLC; 2008. pp. 167-83.
5. Jasim ZF, Woo WK, Handley JM. Long-pulsed (6-ms) pulsed dye laser treatment of rosacea-associated telangiectasia using subpurpuric clinical threshold. Dermatol Surg. 2004;30:37-40.
6. Tanghetti E. Pulsed dye laser extended pulse format effect on purpuric threshold. Lasers Surg Med. 2003;15:74.
7. Kalil CL, Curcio BL, Signachi S. Nd:YAG laser and intense pulsed light in the treatment of port wine stains: case report and review of the literature. Surg Cosmet Dermatol. 2009;1(2):95-8.
8. Mahadevappa OH, Mysore V, Viswanath V, Thurakkal S, Majid I, Talwar S, et al. Surgical outcome in patients taking concomitant or recent intake of oral isotretinoin: a multicentric study-ISO-AIMS Study. J Cutan Aesthet Surg. 2016;9(2):106-14.
9. Goldberg DJ, Man J. Complications and legal considerations of laser and light treatments. In: Hruza GJ, Avram M (Eds). Lasers and Lights: Procedures in Cosmetic Dermatology Series (Expert Consult), 3rd edition. Elsevier Health sciences; 2012. pp. 130-5.
10. Lee SJ, Oh WJ, Park KY, Seo SJ, Hong CK, Chung WS. Treatment of epilation-related postinflammatory hyperpigmentation using a 1,927-nm thulium fiber fractional laser. J Clin Investigat Dermatol. 2015;3(1):2.
11. Vachiramon V, Thadanipon K. Postinflammatory hypopigmentation. Clin Exp Dermatol. 2011;36(7):708-14.
12. Al Nomair N, Nazarian R, Marmur E. Complications in lasers, lights, and radiofrequency devices. Facial Plast Surg. 2012;28(3):340-6.
13. Cil Y. Second-degree skin burn after intense pulsed light therapy with EMLA cream for hair removal. Int J Dermatol. 2009;48(2):206-7.
14. Niamtu J. Skin resurfacing. In: Niamtu J III (Ed). Cosmetic Facial Surgery. Missouri: Elsevier Health sciences; 2010. pp. 517-603.
15. Radmanesh M, Mostaghimi M, Yousefi I, Mousavi ZB, Rasai S, Esmaili HR, et al. Leukotrichia developed following application of intense pulsed light for hair removal. Dermatol Surg. 2002;28(7):572-4.
16. Stebbins WG, Tsao SS, Hruza GJ, et al. Laser hair removal. In: Robinson JK, Hanke CK, Siegel DM, Fratila A, Bhatia AC, Rohrer TE (Eds). Surgery of the Skin: Procedural Dermatology, 3rd edition. UK, Mosby: Elsevier Inc.; 2014. pp. 509-23.
17. Bernstein E. Severe urticaria after laser treatment for hair reduction. Dermatol Surg. 2010;36:147-51.
18. Kirby W, Alston DB, Chen AH. The incidence of hypertrophic scarring and keloid formation following laser tattoo removal with a quality-switched Nd:YAG laser. J Clin Aesthet Dermatol. 2016;9(5):43-47.
19. Chandrashekar BS, Varsha DV, Vasanth V, Jagadish P, Madura C, Rajashekar ML, et al. Safety of performing invasive acne scar treatment and laser hair removal in patients on oral isotretinoin: a retrospective study of 110 patients. Int J Dermatol. 2014;53(10):1281-5.
20. Alster TS, Lupton JR. Treatment of complications of laser skin resurfacing. Arch Facial Plast Surg. 2000;2(4):279-84.
21. Landa N, Corrons N, Zabalza I, Azpiazu JL. Urticaria induced by laser epilation: a clinical and histopathological study with extended follow-up in 36 patients. Lasers Surg Med. 2012;44(5):384-9.
22. Ibrahimi OA, Saedi N, Kilmer SL. Laser based treatment of the aging face for skin resurfacing: Ablative and non-ablative lasers. In: Robinson JK, Hanke CK, Siegel DM, Fratila A, Bhatia AC, Rohrer TE (Eds). Surgery of the Skin: Procedural Dermatology, 3rd edition. UK, Mosby: Elsevier Inc.; 2014. pp. 549-60.
23. Doshi SN, Levy ML, Markus R. Koebnerization of reactive perforating collagenosis induced by laser hair removal. Lasers Surg Med. 2003;32(3):177-9.
24. Weiss RA, Munavalli GS, Choudhary S, Leiva A, Nouri K. Intense pulsed light. In: Nouri K (Ed). Lasers in Dermatology and Medicine, illustrated edition. Springer Science and Business Media; 2011. pp. 207-19.
25. Gay-Escoda C, Párraga-Manzol G, Sánchez-Torres A, Moreno-Arias G. Chronic neuropathic facial pain after intense pulsed light hair removal. Clinical features and pharmacological management. J Clin Exp Dent. 2015;7(4):e544-7.
26. Vaz C, Matos A, Pereira M, Nogueira C, Loureiro T, Loureiro L, et al. Iatrogenic complications following laser ablation of varicose vein. In: Yamanouchi D (Ed). Vascular Surgery. Intech; 2012. pp. 151-64.
27. Metelitsa AI, Alster TS. Fractionated laser skin resurfacing treatment complications: A review. Dermatol Surg. 2010;36: 299-306.
28. Alster TS, Lupton JR. Prevention and treatment of side effects and complications of cutaneous laser resurfacing. Plast Reconstr Surg. 2002;109:308-16; discussion 317-8.
29. Willey A, Anderson RR, Azpiazu JL, Bakus AD, Barlow RJ, Dover JS, et al. Complications of laser dermatologic surgery. Lasers Surg Med. 2006;38(1):1-15.
30. Alster TS. Cutaneous resurfacing with CO_2 and erbium: YAG lasers: preoperative, intraoperative, and postoperative considerations. Plast Reconstr Surg. 1999;103:619-32; discussion 633-4.
31. Dawson E, Willey A, Lee K. Adverse events associated with nonablative cutaneous laser, radiofrequency, and light- based devices. Semin Cutan Med Surg. 2007;26:15-21.
32. Amore R, Rauso R. Intense pulsed light. In: Curinga G, Rusiani A (Eds). Minimally Invasive Procedures for Facial Rejuvenation. USA: OMICS Group E-book; 2014. Also [online] Available from: http://www.esciencecentral.org/ebooks/minimally-invasive/intense-pulsed-light.php. [Last accessed August 2023].
33. Ganjoo A. Successful treatment of laser induced hypopigmentation with targeted narrow band UVB therapy. J Cutan Aesthet Surg. 2013;6(2):120.
34. Geist DE, Phillips TJ. Development of chrysiasis after Q-switched ruby laser treatment of solar lentigines. J Am Acad Dermatol. 2006;55(Suppl 2):S59-60.

35. Vano-Galvan S, Jaen P. Complications of nonphysician-supervised laser hair removal: Case report and literature review. Can Fam Physician. 2009;55(1):50-2.
36. Kelly KM, Svaasand LO, Nelson JS. Optimization of laser treatment safety in conjunction with cryogen spray cooling. Arch Dermatol. 2003;139:1372-3.
37. Lolis MS, Marmur ES. Paradoxical effects of hair removal systems: a review. J Cosmetol Dermatol. 2006;5(4):274-6.
38. Weisberg NK, Greenbaum SS. Pigmentary changes after Alexandrite laser hair removal. Dermatol Surg. 2003;29:415-9.
39. Parver DL, Dreher RJ, Kohanim S, Zimmerman P, Garrett G, Devisetty L, et al. Ocular injury after laser hair reduction treatment to the eyebrow. Arch Ophthalmol. 2012;130(10):1330-4.
40. Ammar A, Costa FB, Kalil C, Campos VB. Complications in laser dermatologic surgery Part I: non-fractional non-ablative lasers. Surg Cosmet Dermatol. 2011;3(1):47-53.
41. Beeson W. Laser safety. In: Carniol P, Sadick NS (Eds). Clinical Procedures in Laser Skin Rejuvenation. USA: CRC Press; 2007. pp. 1-10.
42. Prather HB, Alam M, Poon E, Arndt KA. Laser safety in isotretinoin use: a survey of expert opinion and practice. 2017;43(3):357-63.
43. Queen D, Orsted H, Sanada H, Sussman G. A dressing history. Int Wound J. 2004;1(1): 59-77.
44. Weinstein C. Postoperative laser care. Clin Plast Surg. 2000;27(2):251-62.
45. Svensjö T, Pomahac B, Yao F, Slama J, Eriksson E. Accelerated healing of full-thickness skin wounds in a wet environment. Plast Reconstr Surg. 2000;106(3):613-14.
46. Sulimovic L, Licu D, Ledo E, Naeyaert JM, Pigatto P, Tzermias C, et al. Efficacy and safety of a topically applied Avène spring water spray in the healing of facial skin after laser resurfacing. Dermatol Surg. 2002;28(5):415-18.
47. Park GH, Rhee D, Moon HR, Won CH, Lee MW, Choi JH, et al. Effect of an epidermal growth factor-containing cream on postinflammatory hyperpigmentation after Q-switched 532-nm neodymium-doped yttrium aluminum garnet laser treatment. Dermatol Surg. 2015;41(1):131-5.
48. Yang JA, Chung HM, Won CH, Sung JH. Potential application of adipose-derived stem cells and their secretory factors to skin: discussion from both clinical and industrial viewpoints. Expert Opin Biol Ther. 2010;10(4):495-503.
49. Goldman MP. The use of hydroquinone with facial laser resurfacing. J Cutaneous Laser Ther. 2009;2(2):73-7.
50. Omar Ibrahimi. (2016). Lasers: Safety and Complications. [online] Available from MauiDerm website. http:// mauiderm.com/lasers-safety-and-complications. [Last accessed August 2023].
51. Smalley PJ. Laser safety: risks, hazards, and control measures. Laser Ther. 2011;20(2):95-106.

SECTION 16

Procedures for Pigmentation

CHAPTER 120

Periocular and Perioral Melanosis

Manas Chatterjee, Ruchi Hemdani

KEY MESSAGES

- Periocular and perioral darkening are both conditions with multifactorial etiology.
- Constitutional variety of periocular melanosis is more common in Indians.
- There are five main pathophysiologic mechanisms for periocular melanosis: melanin or other sources of pigment, thin skin with visible veins (the latter could occur with venous congestion as well), cutaneous laxity, prominent tear trough, and periorbital edema.
- The stretch test is able to distinguish whether periocular melanosis is due to pigment (no change on stretching the lower eyelid skin downward at the level of the cheek), laxity (improvement), or vascular (worsening).
- In addition to aging and altered subcutaneous fat distribution, sun exposure is a common aggravating factor.
- Treatment of both periocular and perioral melanosis depends primarily on the cause and additionally consists of pigment-lightening agents, chemical peels, lasers, and fillers as and when required as per etiology.

INTRODUCTION

Melanosis anywhere on the body is unacceptable, more so over the face and especially in women. In this chapter, we are going to deal in entirety about two aesthetically concerning conditions: Periocular and perioral melanosis in separate sections.

PERIOCULAR MELANOSIS

Periocular hyperpigmentation (POH) has been known by various names such as periorbital melanosis, dark circles, infraorbital pigmentation, and idiopathic cutaneous hyperchromia of the orbital region. It is defined as bilateral, round, homogeneous pigment macules on the infraorbital regions. It is worsened by generalized fatigue, especially lack of sleep, in which case, it is associated with puffy eyes/eye bags **(Fig. 1)**. It is associated with fluctuation of intensity, which is regarded as physiologic by some. As a matter of fact, this condition is considered a phenomenon within the limit of physiology.

Certain ethnic groups such as mixed races and those with Jewish inheritance are more severely affected. Multiple members of family may be affected, related to anatomic considerations. By definition, it does not include conditions which also cause facial pigmentation.

Patients, especially women, are really concerned about it, relating dark circles with impairment in their quality of life. It interferes with facial appearance, giving a tired, sad, or hangover look.

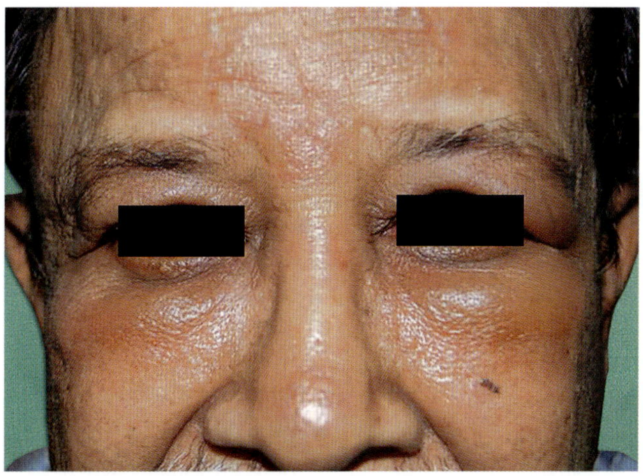

Fig. 1: Puffy eyes leading to periocular darkening.

Epidemiology

There is no available data on prevalence of POH due to it being transitory, with lack of etiological explanations and is considered a cosmetic nuisance. About 9% of American women below 30 years of age are concerned about this condition.[1] There is scarcity of data regarding the incidence and prevalence of POH in India as well due to its transitory nature and lack of reasonable etiological explanation. In an Indian study, it was found that POH was most prevalent in the age group of 16–25 years [i.e., 95 out of 200 patients (47.50%)]. Among the 200 patients studied, it was more prevalent in women [162 (81%)] than men and the majority of the affected women were housewives [91 (45.50%)].[2]

History

One of the first references to this condition was by Touraine in 1937, wherein it was said to be due to prominence of vessels due to loss of subcutaneous fat and muscle tonus in the region. The probable earliest publication dealing exclusively with this condition was by Adlercreutz,[3] where he referred to it being caused by biliary and genitourinary tract diseases. Winkelmann in 1965 attributed this condition to dehydration due to severe systemic disorders. Mark in 1966 associated it to allergic rhinitis.

Etiology and Diagnostic Considerations

Causative factors[4] that are known to play a role in the occurrence of periocular pigmentation **(Table 1)** are as follows:

- Genetic trait
- Sun exposure
- Dermal melanin deposition
- Melanocyte-stimulating hormone-induced melanosis
- Post-traumatic
- Postinflammatory [eczemas: atopic dermatitis **(Fig. 2)**/ allergic contact dermatitis/airborne contact dermatitis **(Fig. 3)**]
- Cosmetics containing phototoxic agents **(Fig. 4)**, usually psoralens, etc.
- Acanthosis nigricans (AN) **(Fig. 5)**
- Seborrheic melanosis **(Fig. 6)**
- Bilateral nevus of Ota[5]
- Fixed drug eruptions[6]
- Macular and systemic amyloidosis[7]

TABLE 1: Specific colors of some causes of periocular pigmentation.

Cause	*Color*	*Associated features*
Mercurial or silver preparation	Blue-gray	Pigmentation of nasolabial and neck folds
Chrysiasis	Mauve	Slate-blue discoloration of sun-exposed skin
Eczema	Brown	Typical eczema changes
Familial	Brown	—
Hormone-induced	Brown	Facial hyperpigmentation
Hypohidrotic ectodermal dysplasia	Dark brown	Frontal bossing, saddle nose, prominent supraorbital ridge, hypohidrosis, dental changes
Lichen planus	Violaceous, sometimes brown	Typical lichen planus changes
Minocycline	Gray	Blue-gray pigmentation within areas of inflammation or scarring, legs, forearms
Nevus of Ota	Blue-gray	Involvement of ocular structures, nasopharynx, auricular mucosa, tympanic membrane, dura mater
Postinflammatory	Brown	—
Post-traumatic	Brown	—
Psoralens	Brown	Sunburn, nausea and vomiting, itching

Source: Adapted from Feletti F et al.[11]

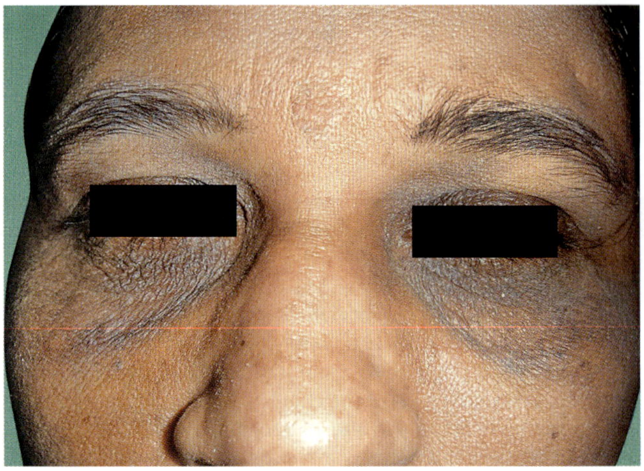

Fig. 2: Postinflammatory periocular pigmentation following atopic dermatitis.

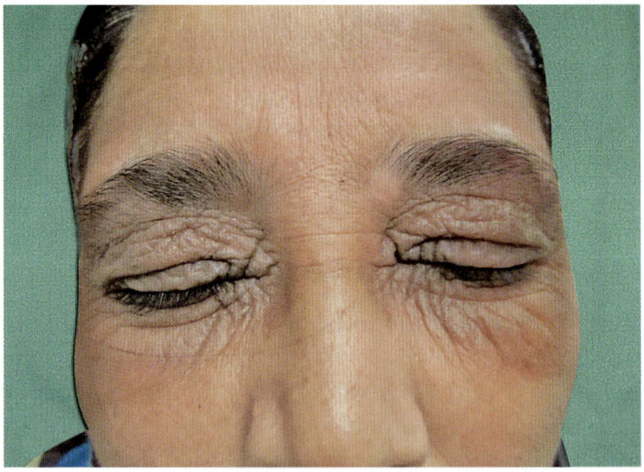

Fig. 3: Inflammatory pigmentation in airborne contact dermatitis.

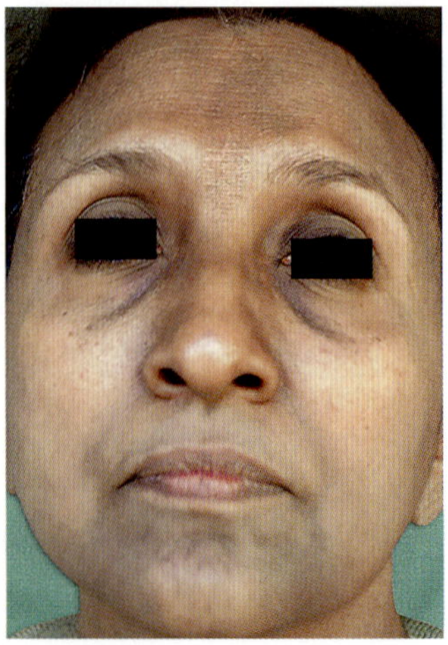

Fig. 4: Pigmented cosmetic contact dermatitis.

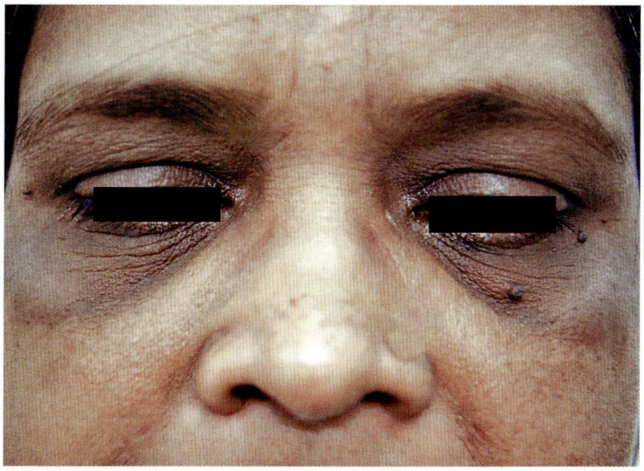

Fig. 5: Periocular acanthosis nigricans with acrochordons.

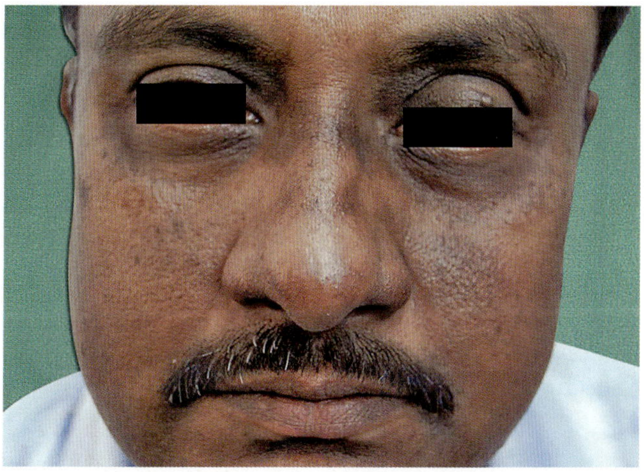

Fig. 6: Periocular and facial seborrheic melanosis.

- *Lead of Kohl pencils:*[8] Originally antimony trisulfide—the ore stibnite, scarce and expensive and replaced by galena (lead sulfide) with same gray-black color and shiny appearance;[9] abnormal pigmentation of eyelid and lacrimal sac seen in patients with eyeliners of lead due to deposition of metal particles in dermis and increased epidermal melanin production; lead may also be tattooed; lead hue with pallor and lividity seen; high blood (twice) and conjunctival (six times) lead levels seen in quoted study; D-penicillamine effective by chelating lead at low dose of 750 mg/day.
- Application of travoprost[10,11] and bimatoprost,[12,13] with the latter available as 0.3% solution; the prescribing information for bimatoprost includes warnings related to skin changes such as possible lid pigmentation of the periorbital tissue; the most common adverse events caused by Latisse's use are described as eye pruritus, conjunctival hyperemia, skin hyperpigmentation, ocular irritation, dry eye symptoms, and erythema of the eyelid; these have been described in <4% of patients:
- Free radical/oxidant damage
- Fatigue
- Periorbital edema, subcutaneous fat herniation, gravitational
- Superficial location of vasculature
- Shadowing due to skin laxity.

Systemic factors that play a role in the etiology of this condition are as follows:

- Prolonged use of mercurial or silver preparation
- Parenteral gold therapy
- Long-term minocycline
- Biliary disease, endocrine disturbances (thyroid and menstrual disturbance/hormonal)
- Pregnancy, breastfeeding
- Lichen planus, especially lichen planus pigmentosus
- Peutz–Jeghers syndrome[14]
- Erythema dyschromicum perstans[15]
- Iron deficiency anemia
- Gastrointestinal diseases
- Renal diseases
- Suprarenal disorders
- Vascular disorder associations.[16]

Aggravating factors in periocular pigmentation:

- Sun exposure
- Aging process of skin sagging
- Altered subcutaneous fat distribution
- Acquired idiopathic patterned facial pigmentation (AIPFP) in periorbital area[17]
- Periorbital acquired macular hyperpigmentation (ADMH).

Recently, the clinical and dermoscopic features of "periorbital ADMH" as a distinct clinical entity have been described. It presents early in age and shows subtle pigmentation on dermoscopy with accentuation of dots and globules at outer corner of eyes (outer corner crease sign).[18]

Pathomechanisms of Periocular Pigmentation[19]

- *Postinflammatory:* It is caused by rubbing or scratching of the skin around the eye or by accumulation of fluid due to facial allergy. It presents with irregular patches of brownish or gray pigmentation on the skin on the upper, lower, or both eyelids with features of lichenification, accentuation of skin creases, and eczematous papules or patches in the surrounding areas. Excessive pigmentation can also be due to postinflammatory hyperpigmentation (PIH) secondary to atopic and allergic contact dermatitis and other dermatological conditions (e.g., lichen planus pigmentosus) and can be drug-induced, such as in the case of fixed drug eruptions and erythema dyschromicum perstans.
- *Periorbital edema:* This worsens in the morning or after a salty meal. It leads to a purplish color and follows the undefined contours of the underlying fat compartments.

- *Increased melanin deposition:* This is caused mainly by dermal melanocytosis and hemosiderin synthesis.
- *Increased visibility of blood vessels:* This is caused by visible prominence of subcutaneous vascular plexus or vasculature contained within the orbicularis muscle which is caused by thin lower eyelid skin overlying the orbicularis oculi muscle. It is associated with erythema, predominantly involving the inner aspect of the lower eyelids, with prominent capillaries or telangiectasia in addition to veins (bluish color).
- *Aging with increased skin laxity (dermatochalasis):* This is caused by combination of dryness of skin and rhytides causing shadowing with overlying pseudoherniation of infraorbital fat. Patients have a dark shadow under an overhanging tarsal muscle, with eye bags.
- *Prominent tear trough:* This is an inherited anatomical deformity causing hollowness of the area immediately above the inferior orbital rim. It disappears on direct lighting.

We shall now elucidate some of these pathomechanisms as described here.

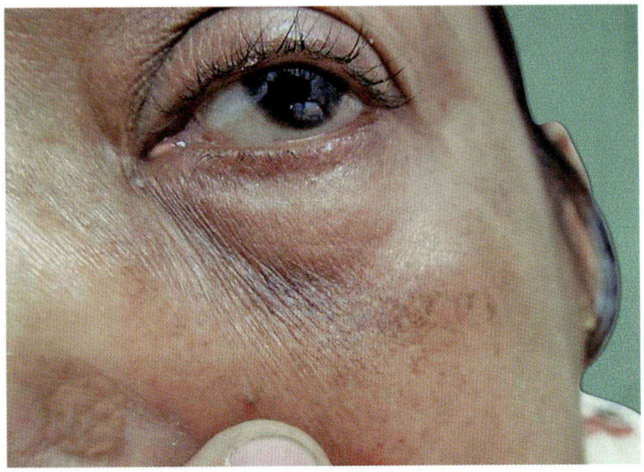

Fig. 7: A curved band of brownish skin approximating shape of underlying inferior orbital rim in periocular pigmentation.

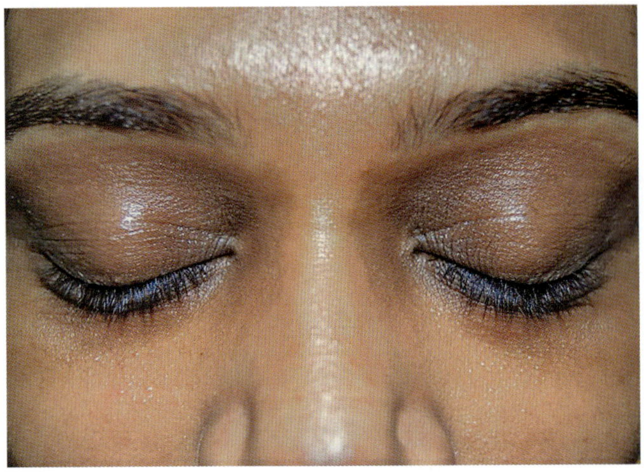

Fig. 8: Autosomal dominant circumocular pigmentation.

Pigmentation

Pigmentation is mostly caused by dermal melanocytosis. It is dark brown to blue-gray in color. The most common causes are excessive sun exposure, postinflammatory due to rubbing, drug ingestion, erythema dyschromicum perstans, fixed drug eruption, familial, and nevus of Ota. It sometimes presents as a slightly curved band of brownish skin approximating shape of underlying inferior orbital rim **(Fig. 7)**. It looks darker when present below the bulging lower eyelids induced by pseudoherniation of orbital fat, leading to shadowing. Stretching of the lower eyelid does not significantly lighten this pigment. This is called the "stretch test" for periocular pigmentation.

Genetic (familial or constitutional) factors play an important role in pigmentation. It is associated with a curved band of brownish-to-black pigmentation on the skin of the lower eyelids with velvety or coarse texture pigment with frequent involvement of the upper eyelids. This form of pigment is most common among Indians. Peters reported a kindred of 20 individuals in five generations and first speculated that this might be an autosomal dominant disorder.[20] Additional large pedigrees have confirmed the heritable nature of this condition. A report in 1969 confirmed that the condition progressed with age.[21] This study stated that it usually starts in the lower eyelid and progresses to around the eye **(Fig. 8)**. Fatigue, worry, anxiety, and illness worsen this condition and good health and rest tends to improve it. Genetic factors affect the sexes equally. There is wide variation in its ultimate extent and intensity and this condition is seen more frequently in individuals with dark complexions.[22] In most of the persons it remains unnoticed from childhood, only to be revealed after any triggering factor(s) such as sun exposure, puberty, pregnancy, use of oral contraceptives, some acute illnesses such as viral hepatitis, typhoid and chickenpox, stress, eye strain, cachexia, etc.[23] In its exaggerated state, it gives the eyes the impression of "raccoon eyes" **(Fig. 9)**.

It is considered that some of these cases may be extensions of pigmentary demarcation line-F (PDL-F) of the face **(Fig. 10)**. In 92 (92%) patients out of 100 in a study, periorbital melanosis was found to be an extension of PDL-F.[24]

Dermatoscopically, pigment may be perifollicular, reticuloglobular similar to melasma (epidermal and dermal), reticulated, or even speckled with dermal granular appearance **(Fig. 11)**. Some cases show blunted reticular appearance similar to erythema dyschromicum perstans (author's observation).

The pigment may be scored as:

- Light brown
- Dark brown
- Brown-black

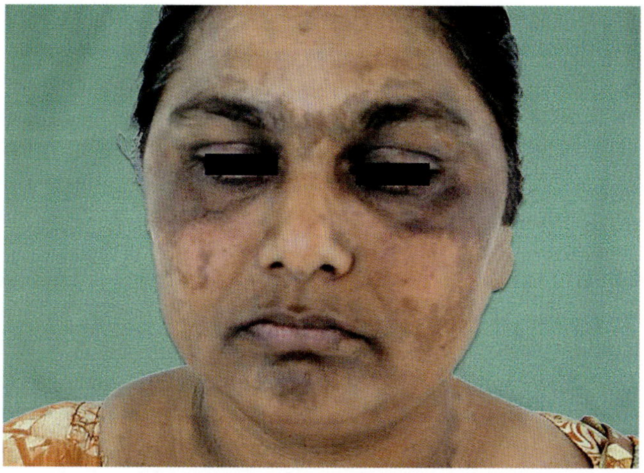

Fig. 9: The raccoon eyes in advanced autosomal dominant periocular pigmentation.

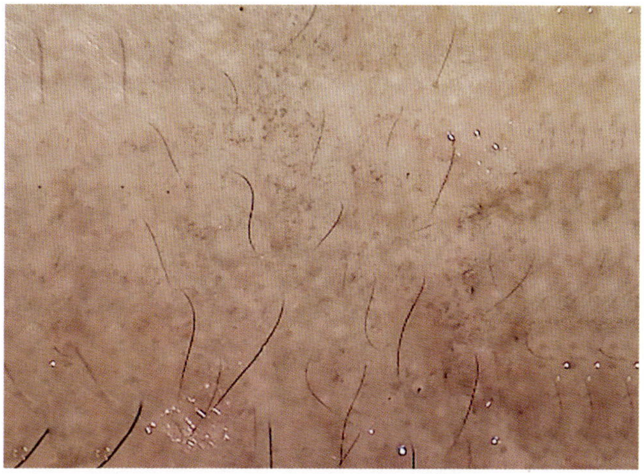

Fig. 11: Dermal granular pigment on dermatoscopy 10X nonpolarized.

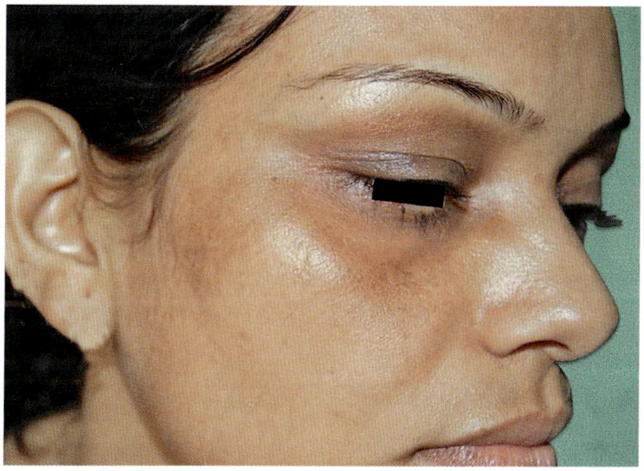

Fig. 10: Periocular pigmentation with pigmentary demarcation line-F.

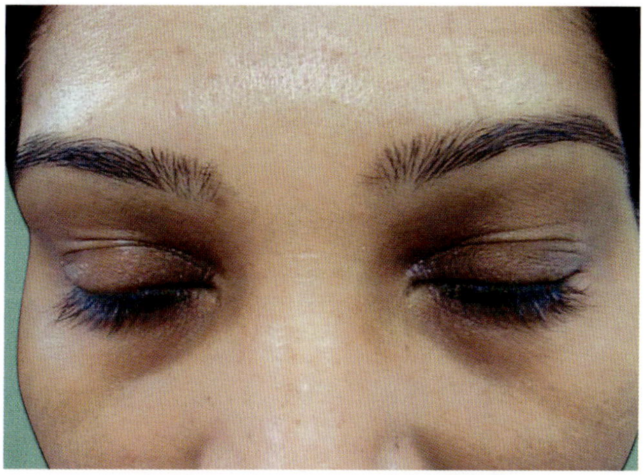

Fig. 12: Periocular edema in a young girl.

If melanocytosis is a fixed finding, what explains the daily fluctuation seen and complained of by patients? Dermal edema leads to Tyndall effect as the eyelid region has a "sponge" property that helps accumulation of fluid in systemic or local edema situations. The evidence for this is the worsening in the morning or after salty meal.[25] A natural corollary is the differentiation of fat and fluid (edema) over the periocular skin. Compared with normal orbital fat, edema is still present in downgaze **(Fig. 12)** and does not change much in upgaze, whereas fat disappears in downgaze and appears in upgaze **(Fig. 13)**. This is due to change in contours of regional fat complements on the face. CO_2 laser causes tightening of dermal tissues and improvement of the skin surface texture in both conditions.

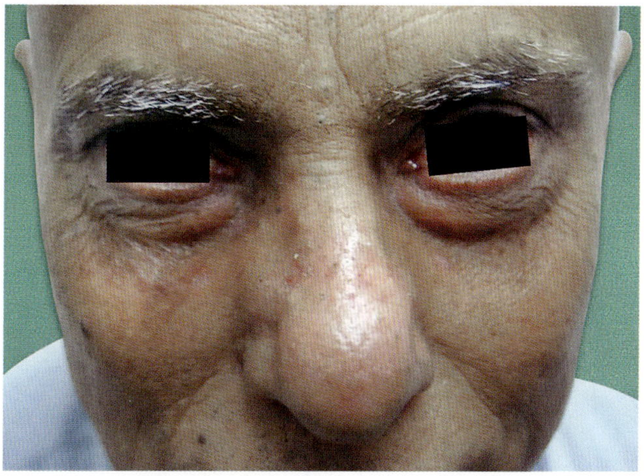

Fig. 13: Periocular fat appears in upgaze.

Translucent Skin

This condition is due to thin, translucent lower eyelid skin overlying the orbicularis oculi muscle, with little or no subcutaneous fat. This leads to a visible prominence of the subcutaneous vascular plexus or vasculature contained within the muscle. There is a violaceous appearance of this color, which is more in the inner aspect **(Fig. 14)**. There is accentuation during menstruation in females. The stretch test deepens the violaceous color **(Figs. 15A and B)**. Improvement with subcutaneous injection of filler/fat indicates that fat is in musculature and not subcutaneous. Associated venous engorgement accentuates this discoloration. Congestion of nasal and paranasal cavities is a common cause of engorgement of these veins. Venous drainage of this area is by branches of sphenopalatine veins passing backward to the pterygoid plexus **(Fig. 16)**. Allergic edema of mucous membrane causes pressure effect on veins, interfering with drainage. This engorgement of lower venous marginal arcades and palpebral veins, which drain via angular and inferior ophthalmic vein to same sphenopalatine vein and pterygoid plexus, causes the effect of eyelid discoloration. This has been studied and an increased amount of hemoglobin and decreased hemoglobin oxygen saturation has been seen with blood flow rate which was found to be slow at dark eye circles (DEC) in comparison with the cheek. Blood flow stagnation seems to be one of the factors that could induce DECs.[26] There are other studies that link periorbital hyperchromia (dark circles) to postinflammatory hemodynamic congestion producing a typical bruising aspect on the lower eyelids.[27] Differentiation between vascular and pigment causes of periorbital pigmentation is also by Wood's lamp and polarized diagnostic light imaging.

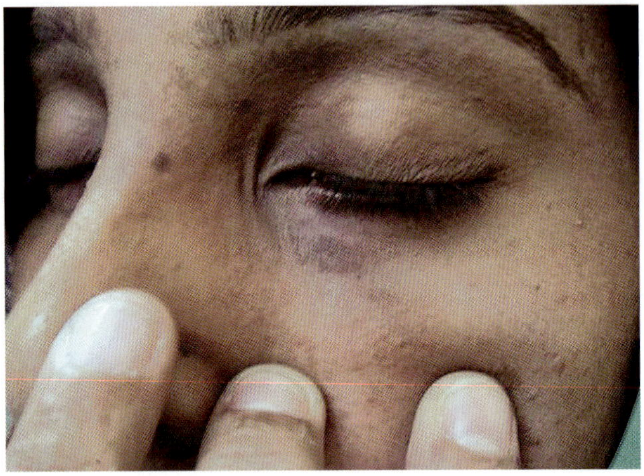

Fig. 14: Violaceous appearance of periocular vasculature, more in the medial aspect.

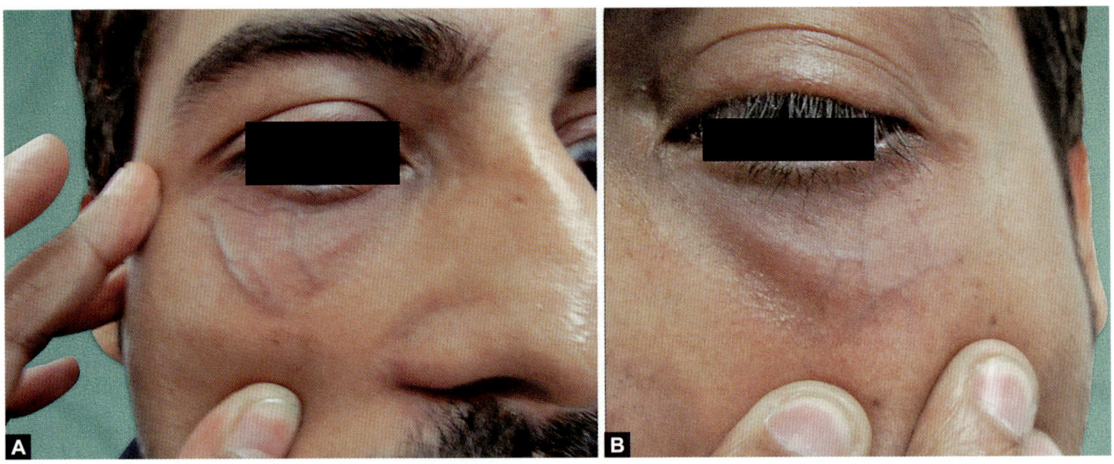

Figs. 15A and B: The stretch test in a patient with thin skin and prominent periocular veins.

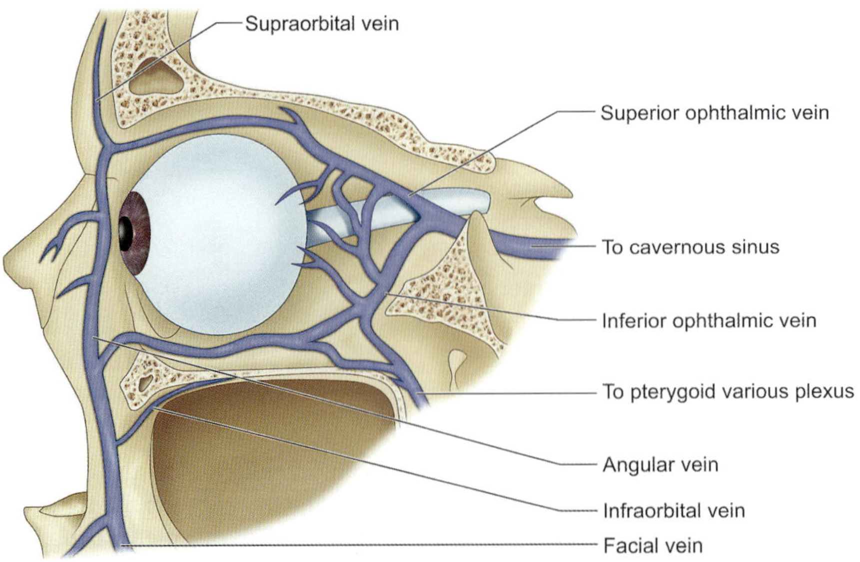

Fig. 16: Venous drainage of the periocular tissues.

Cutaneous Laxity

Collagen and elastin in the thin tissue of the eyelids and periorbital skin undergo ultraviolet (UV)-induced and age-related degeneration. The damaged epidermis releases collagenases, which further contributes to collagen degeneration. This laxity leads to a shadowing appearance on the lower eyelids which can occur as a genetic trait **(Figs. 17A and B)**.

Tear Trough

The tear trough extends from the medial canthus to mid-pupillary line **(Fig. 18)**. It is normally 3 cm or less and continues to the lid–cheek junction (palpebromalar groove). It corresponds to junction of the palpebral and orbital portions of orbicularis oculi muscle. It deepens as patients age because the infraorbital fat is displaced anteriorly, creating shadowing below it, depending on lighting conditions, leading to hollowness; also the orbital bony space increases. The stretch test shows improvement of this condition.[28,29]

Tear trough deformity (TTD) is graded[30] as follows:

- *Class I:* Hollowing in medial one-third of orbital rim
- *Class II:* Defect up to midpupillary line
- *Class III:* Full depression extending circumferentially along orbital rim.

Multiple etiologies may contribute to dark circles in the same patient.[31] Hyperpigmentation, superficial microvasculature due to engorgement or visibility and slackness of periorbital anatomical structures may all be present in one patient **(Fig. 19)**.

In addition, a number of these patients also have xanthelasma associated with this condition, which the author has found to be more than that in age-matched controls (unpublished) **(Fig. 20)**.

Studies on Etiological Factors and Types of Periocular Melanosis

Several studies have analyzed the proportion of the various etiologies in the genesis of periocular pigmentation.

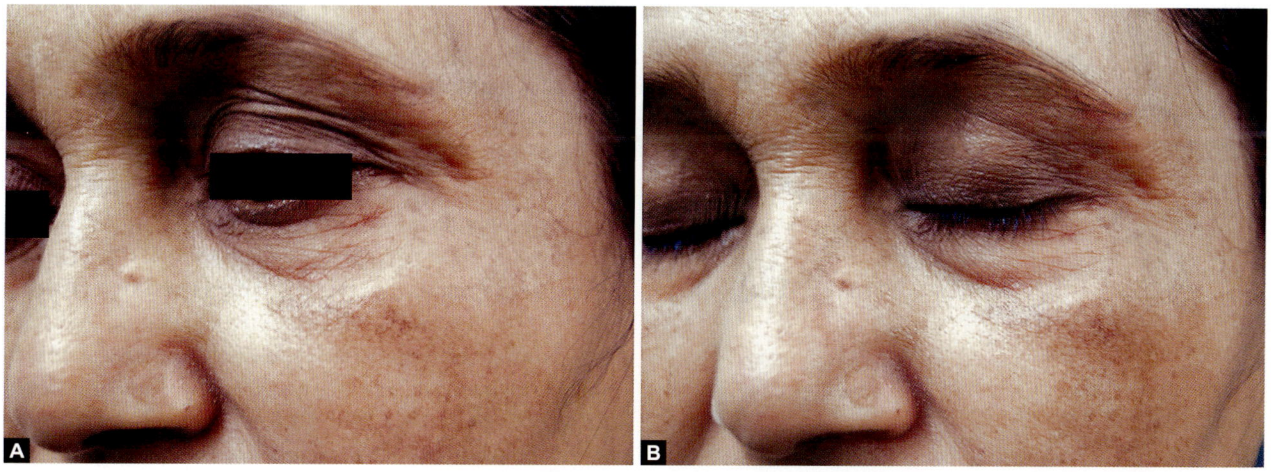

Figs. 17A and B: Shadowing due to skin laxity.

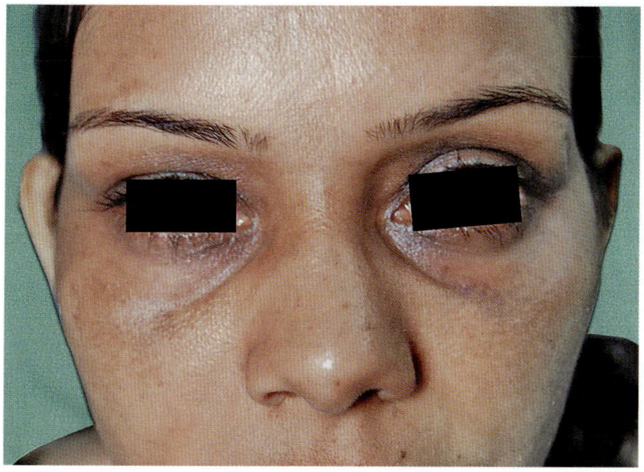

Fig. 18: Class II tear trough.

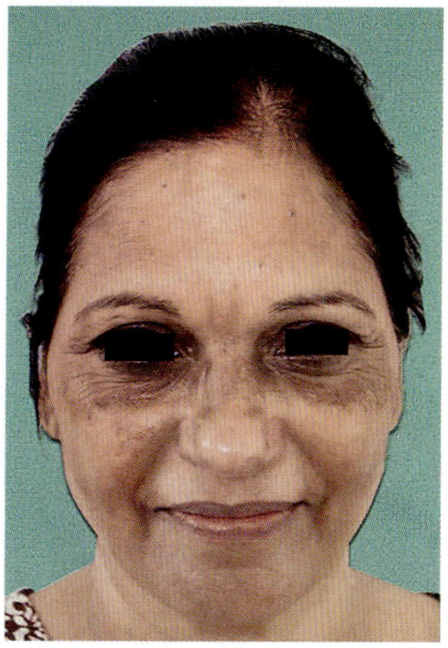

Fig. 19: Hyperpigmentation, cutaneous laxity, and vascular etiologies of periocular darkening in the same patient.

In Asians,[32] in a study of 184 patients, the vascular form of pigmentation was found to be the most common type in 41.8% of patients. The next most common (38.6%) was constitutional, followed by PIH (12%). Shadow effects (11.4%) due to an overhanging tarsal muscle, eye bags, or a deep tear trough was fourth. The rest were due to other causes like skin laxity, dry skin, hormonal disturbances, nutritional deficiencies and other chronic illnesses. No significant correlation was found between sleep deprivation or other aggravating factors and POH.

Other studies have been undertaken to establish the cause of periocular pigmentation. Spectrophotometric intracutaneous analysis (SIA), which is a combination of dermatoscopy, contact remittance spectrophotometry, and hyperspectral imaging, enables concentration and distribution of eumelanin, oxyhemoglobin, and dermal collagen to be measured in vivo.[33] A study to analyze the proportion of hemoglobin and melanin in patients with this condition was conducted with the help of this instrument.[34]

It found no correlation with family history, atopic dermatitis, contact dermatitis, melasma, and hormonal factors in periocular pigmentation. It found that the quantity index of total melanin, dermal melanin, and hemoglobin to be more in dark circles as compared to normal skin.

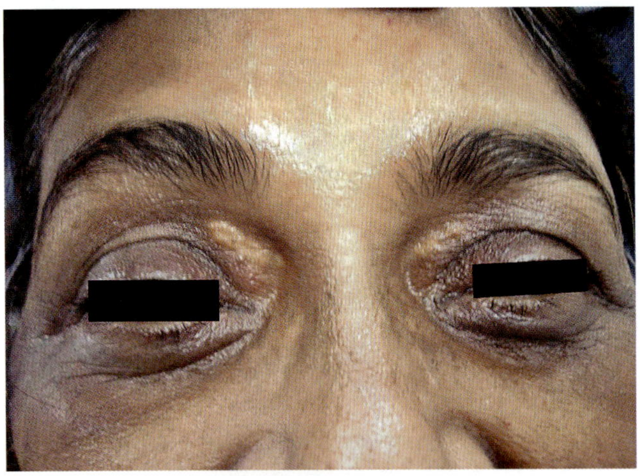

Fig. 20: Periocular pigmentation with associated xanthelasma.

The only histopathological[35] study other than the one conducted by the authors [which also included immunohistochemistry **(Figs. 21A to C)**][36] studied 28 patients with biopsies from the medial lower eyelid with retroauricular skin as control and found that hemosiderin was absent, with increased melanin in papillary dermis correlating with severity of lesions. There was dilatation of blood vessels. Histological characteristics of periorbital hyperpigmentation suggest that it can be both epidermal and dermal in nature. Biopsy specimen must be stained with routine hematoxylin and eosin. Special stains can also be used. Fontana-Masson silver stain can be used to stain melanin. Hemosiderin deposits seen in few cases (resulting from extravasation and superficial location of vasculature) can be stained with Perls' potassium ferrocyanide.

Another clinical analysis[37] reiterated that Wood's lamp can enhance epidermal pigmentation, and established that ultrasonogram can show real-time anatomical structures of eyelids. By ultrasound, the vascular type with periorbital puffiness was found to have increased preseptal thickness of the soft tissue, and infraorbital palpebral bags of the structural type were found to have protruded retroseptal fat pads. It classified POH into pigmented (brown color), vascular (blue/pink/purple color), structural (skin color), and mixed type pigmented-vascular (PV subtype), pigmented-structural (PS subtype), vascular-structural (VS subtype), and the combined three. Structural included infraorbital palpebral bags, infraorbital grooves, blepharoptosis, and loss of fat or soft tissue volume with bony prominence. It scored DEC by means of Wood's lamp and ultrasound. It revealed that pigmented, vascular, structural, and mixed type accounted for 5%, 14%, 3% and 78%, respectively. The mixed type, PV (37%), and three-combined type (26%) were most common. The overall mean POH score was 6.4, while the different types had scores of 4.3, 4.1, 5.0, and 7.0, respectively for pigmented, vascular, structural, and mixed forms showing that mixed form was the most common. Though this was, in essence, what had already been described, this study formalized the essentially different causes of this entity and that treatment would have to be based on the etiology rather than a "one-size-fits-all" kind of therapy.

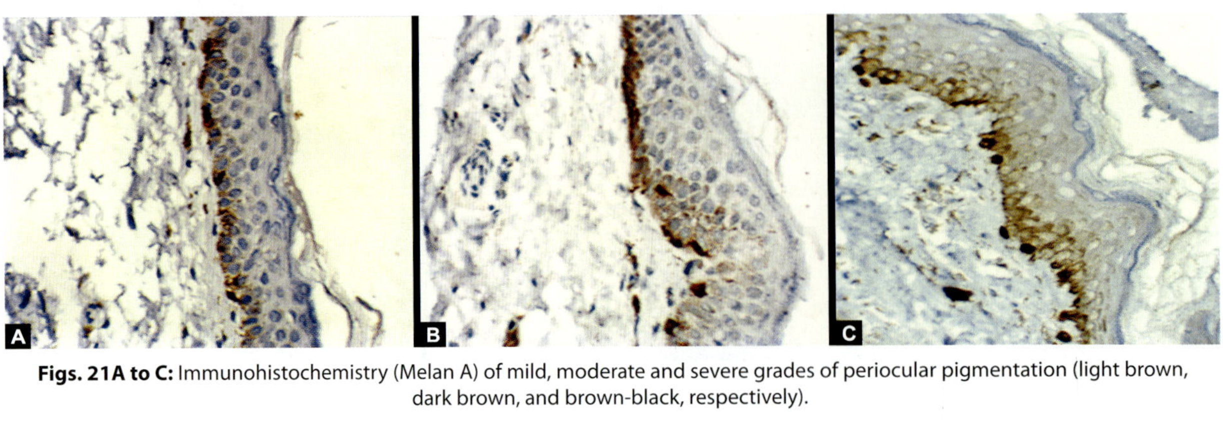

Figs. 21A to C: Immunohistochemistry (Melan A) of mild, moderate and severe grades of periocular pigmentation (light brown, dark brown, and brown-black, respectively).

Treatment

A search of amazon.com revealed 302 products for "dark circles". There are 120,000 videos on YouTube dedicated to this entity. Disguising the lesions is almost mandatory for individuals who depend on a well-cared and positive appearance for work or social activities. As individual anatomical basis for dark circles is not clearly defined, treatments may render suboptimal results. The first step in managing infraorbital dark circles is to identify the specific constellation of etiologic factors present so that a customized therapy can be crafted which tackles the particular etiology. A spectrum of interventions exist, including noninvasive options such as concealment and camouflage, to minimally invasive treatments such as soft-tissue fillers and resurfacing as well as more invasive treatments including surgical intervention. We shall be dealing with the treatment as per the etiology of POH.

Treatment Modalities to Reduce Pigment

- *Topical therapy:* There are multiple treatment modalities for reducing the pigment out of which topical therapies are the most widely used for treatment of POH. The important point to note here is that treatment needs to be continued for several months failing which there is incomplete response or relapse.

  There is a vast range of depigmenting agents available in the market but most work via one or multiple of the following mechanisms: inhibition of tyrosinase activity, inhibition of DNA synthesis in hyperactive melanocytes, reduction of epidermal content of melanin and thickening of epidermis (granular layer), and decreased melanosome transfer to keratinocytes. Out of wide range of topical options, bleaching agents are most effective for targeting excess melanin and both hydroquinone (HQ) and kojic acid have been found to work well.[38]

  Details of these agents are available in relevant chapters of this textbook:
  - HQ is a competitive antagonist for tyrosinase, which plays a critical role in the pigmentation pathway. A range of concentrations of HQ is available, typically through a compounding pharmacy. Using low concentrations such as 2–6% HQ is typically sufficient to achieve melanocyte stabilization as means to decrease the pigment deposition in the periorbital region. Kligman formula and its modifications are used.
  - *Kojic acid* is a naturally occurring fungal derivative produced by *Aspergillus* species and *Penicillium* species. It acts by inhibiting tyrosinase, and is used in a concentration ranging from 1 to 4%. Although there are no studies, kojic acid has been tried anecdotally in the treatment of periorbital hyperpigmentation and has been found to be effective. Side effects of kojic acid include erythema and contact dermatitis.
  - *Retinoids* are vitamin A derivatives that impact multiple pathways to decrease the appearance of dark circles in the infraorbital region. First, they promote collagen synthesis and promote reorganization of collagen bundles to improve skin turgor and quality. They also decrease melanin content and reduce the size of melanocyte Golgi complex and endoplasmic reticulum. The sum of these effects results in increased skin smoothness and decreased discoloration and dyschromia.
  - Azelaic acid (1, 7-heptanedicarboxylic acid) was initially developed as a topical anti-acne agent, but because of its effect on tyrosinase, it has also been used in the treatment of hyperpigmentary disorders such as melasma. Its mechanism of action includes the inhibition of DNA synthesis and mitochondrial enzymes, thereby inducing direct cytotoxic effects on the melanocyte. Since it was found to be effective for facial PIH, it is a potentially promising agent for POH due to PIH.
  - Arbutin is an extract of leaves of bearberry shrub and cranberry, pear, or blueberry plants. It inhibits tyrosinase activity, but also inhibits melanosome maturation. Its effects are dose-dependent, but high concentrations of arbutin can cause hyperpigmentation. It is available in a concentration of 3%.
  - Other agents include azelaic acid, steroids, and pidobenzone. There is increasing collagen with vitamin C which may conceal dark discoloration due to congested blood.[39] Vitamin C, an antioxidant, has also been used for the treatment of hyperpigmentation. Because ascorbic acid is unstable in many topical preparations, esterified derivatives such as L-ascorbic acid 6-palmitate and magnesium ascorbyl phosphate are used in compounds. L-ascorbic acid is the predominant cutaneous antioxidant. It scavenges the free oxygen radicals in the aqueous compartment which trigger melanogenesis. Vitamin C promotes collagen production and conceals color of blood stasis, which could improve appearance of dark circles under the lower eye lid. Some other compounds have been specifically studied for dark circles.
  - *Sunscreens:* Hyperpigmentation can be improved with sunscreen alone. Patients should be cautious while using chemical sunscreen in the delicate eye area. Similarly, broad spectrum sunscreen and UV-coated sunglasses are considered to be beneficial in POH.
  - Optical diffusers are a useful adjunct in the concealment of infraorbital dark circles. These compounds are composed of microionized mineral particles that are designed to reflect light away from the skin. Molecules commonly used as optical diffusers include boron nitride, mica, nylon, polymethyl methacrylate, polyurethane powder, sericite, silica, silicone powder,

talc, Teflon, titanium dioxide, and zinc oxide. Optical diffusers are an important adjunct in the camouflage of dark circles in the periorbital region.
- Several randomized controlled trials (RCTs) exist on the beneficial role of vitamin C serums in increasing dermal thickness, but with less impressive results pertaining to reduction in POH and overall less effective than glycolic acid (GA) and lactic acid (LA) peels.[40]
- The Trifecting Night Cream 1.0 consisting of oligopeptide, Lumixyl, encapsulated retinol, and botanical extracts of bisabolol and bakuchiol. It has a submicron delivery system which ensures the penetration of retinol into the skin and efficacy is reserved until it fully reaches its cellular target. It works by reducing inflammation, neutralizing free radicals, and boost cellular turnover.[41]
- A recent study showed some improvement in POH by twice daily application of a cream containing low-molecular-weight heparin sulfate (LMWH-S) and several naturally derived extracts when applied for 12 weeks.[42]
- *Others:* These include *Pfaffia paniculata/Ptychopetalum olacoides* B/*Lilium candidum* L-associated compound (PPLAC) which is applied as 5% twice a day for 28 days. In a study, 90% patients showed improvement on colorimetric testing.[27] Ingredients such as vitamin K and caffeine have been shown to be effective in improving pigmentation indirectly via thickened capillary walls from vitamin K.[43] Some other products such as Brazilian herbal compound,[27] TriHex peptides and active botanicals,[44] a gel containing phytonadione, retinol, vitamin C, and vitamin E have been found to be fairly or moderately effective. Adverse effects range from limited to mild erythema and contact dermatitis with a serum of phytonadione, retinol, and vitamin C.[45]
- *Combined therapy:* A combination of dermaroller microneedling sessions with an antiaging serum followed by a kojic acid serum showed some benefit as per a case report.[46]

- *Chemical peels for POH:* Peels can be used as less or more intense regimen. Trichloroacetic acid (TCA), other alpha-hydroxy acids stimulate formation of glycosaminoglycans as an additional mechanism of improvement of periocular darkening in addition to causing reduction of pigment per se. Peels can be superficial, medium, or deep. Superficial peeling with TCA is still widely used in concentrations of 15%, 25%, 50%, and even 75%. GA is the most widely used alpha-hydroxy acid. At 50–80% concentrations, GA produces epidermolysis, so physicians should perform the peel only as an office procedure. Salicylic acid 30% has been found to be as effective as 4% HQ pigment reduction as per a study[47] and can thus be useful especially for cases of periorbital hyperpigmentation with coexisting acne.

  The risk of side effects and complications such as dyspigmentation increases according to the depth of the chemical peeling agent and skin type.

  As per a recent systematic review, 20% GA, 15% LA, and 10% TCA peels were found to be effective in combination with microneedling for a reducing pigment albeit less effective than fractional CO_2 laser.[48] In comparative studies, chemical peels (15% LA and 3.75% TCA) was found to be as effective as carboxytherapy and vitamin C mesotherapy when applied weekly for 5 weeks.[49]

  In a similar study, 20% GA peel applied thrice a week was more effective compared to 15% LA peel applied thrice a week or 20% topical vitamin C applied once daily, corollary being its side effects (erythema, burning, irritation, or itching) which made it least tolerable.[40] Topical vitamin C was found to be the least effective in improving POH. Another study showed the combination of 3.75% TCA and 15% LA working with success and as effective as carboxytherapy and vitamin C mesotherapy in improving POH.[49]

- *Lasers:* There have been maximum publications on lasers as treatment modality for POH.

  A recent systematic review on treatment modalities for periocular pigmentation found treatment with 1,064-nm neodymium-doped yttrium aluminum garnet (Nd:YAG) and 694-nm Q-switched ruby lasers (QSRL) to be the most successful modality in reducing melanin pigment despite PIH occurring as a complication with 1,064-/532-nm laser.[38]
  - Q-switched Nd:YAG laser 1,064 nm reduces deep pigment and vascular component of pigment.

    Combination of 1,064-nm Q-switched Nd:YAG laser with a 578-nm copper bromide laser and an invasive pulsed electric signal has been shown to be effective in up to 80% patients a with >50% pigment reduction in POH.[50]

    In a comparative study, a dual wavelength picosecond 1,064-/532-nm Nd:YAG laser was found inferior and caused posttreatment PIH when compared with a picosecond 755-nm alexandrite laser which showed significant improvement without PIH.[51]
  - QSRL have been found to be effective in studies.[4,52] Up to 88.9% of patients have been shown to be improved with two sittings with significant decrease in melanin index (MI) and erythema index.[53] Reduced dermal melanin post treatment has been demonstrated histologically. Adverse effects seen are PIH and hypochromia of the lower eyelid[53]

    A combination of 694-nm QSRL with topical bleaching agents (0.1% tretinoin gel and 5% HQ ointment) has been used in Asians. Initial medical treatment was used to reduce epidermal pigment followed by laser for dermal pigment. Excellent to good response was seen in 15 of 19 patients.

Postinflammatory pigmentation was seen in two patients and reduced dermal pigment in three patients.[31]

- 2,790-nm erbium:yttrium scandium gallium garnet (Er:YSGG) laser, a 1,550-nm fractionated erbium doped fiber laser, and CO_2 lasers have also been shown to be safe and effective in treating POH[38] CO_2 lasers have additionally shown reduction in MI and were found superior to microneedling and TCA peel.[48]

Lasers require metal eye shielding over anterior eye for safe treatment.[54] Because the eye is particularly vulnerable to laser injury. The retina and the choroid contain the highest concentration of melanin in the body, and eye damage is possible even through closed eyelids. Safety must be emphasized upon when treating infraorbital dark circles with lasers which includes use of proper eyewear.

- *Platelet-rich plasma (PRP) therapy:* It involves intradermal placement of autologous concentrated platelet injections in periocular area for treatment of POH. This is considered effective because of intrinsic platelet properties resulting in the release of growth factors after endogenous or exogenous platelet activation, and an increase in expression of Type-1 collagen.[55-57] the resultant action being homogeneity in color and reduction in melanin content[58] along with significant increase in under-eye skin elasticity and firmness.[59] However, owing to its side effect profile (severe pain and ecchymosis), and varying success rate, it is relatively less used in treatment of POH.
- Normobaric oxygen therapy was found to be mildly effective in pigment reduction as per a study wherein POH patients were administered oxygen @ 1 L/min via nasal cannula twice a week for 3 weeks.[60]
- Carboxytherapy has also been anecdotally used. It is a relatively new technique and although the mechanism is not fully clear, it is believed that carbon dioxide gas creates a relative state of hypercapnia which is compensated by vasodilatation and increment in the capillary blood flow to the injected area and reduced cutaneous oxygen consumption along with recruitment of growth factors such as vascular endothelial growth factor (VEGF), leading to neoangiogenesis, improved elasticity, promotion of collagen repair, and lipolysis, ultimately causing dermal rejuvenation.[61,62] The therapy requires subcutaneous administration of weekly injections of CO_2 with durations varying from 7 weeks to 12 months in different studies[38,55] and resulting in reduction of facial fine lines, wrinkles and periorbital hyperpigmentation. Side effects were only transient.[62]

Carboxytherapy was found to be effective and well tolerated in several studies with a superiority over PRP.[49,54] It is considered an effective choice for mixed-type POH.[38]

- Blepharopigmentation is commonly performed to enhance the lower eyelid margin; this tattooing procedure has also been used to smoothen transitions in hyperpigmentation in the lower eyelids.

Treatment Directed at Skin Laxity

Medical therapy has been tried. Human growth factors and cytokines cream, with caffeine, bisabolol and glycyrrhetinic acid and sodium hyaluronate have been used. Wrinkles, lower eyelid bags and sagging, dark circles, skin texture have improved by 14–28% in 6 weeks.[63]

However, the main therapy for these etiologies of periocular darkening is procedural. The basis of these is reversal of age-related changes. They are best treated with ablative and nonablative lasers and surgical methods to improve laxity.

- Blepharoplasty is ideal for periorbital dark circles that are of structural origin, and is well tolerated.[64] Dermatochalasis and periorbital rhytides are significantly improved post blepharoplasty. However, prolonged dyschromia, scarring, infection are possible sequelae.[38]

  In combination with laser resurfacing, blepharoplasty resulted in correction of malar bags and wrinkles, along with pigment reduction:
- Radiofrequency (RF) devices use energy produced by an electric current (as opposed to a light source as in a laser) to create a thermal effect that results in collagen contraction and neocollagenesis while minimizing collateral damage.[65]
- CO_2 laser leads to 50% improvement; however, melanin readings post-treatment is not much different compared to pretreatment. This is explained by tightening of dermal tissues and improvement of the skin surface texture.[38] A multistage treatment of two types of lasers has been described. Shadowing occurs secondary to the bulging contour of the lower eyelid. Bluish color occurs secondary to the visible dermal capillary network, and brown color is caused by dermal melanin. Treatment was undertaken by CO_2 laser followed by Q-switched Alexandrite 755 nm. Results were seen in 6–8 weeks.[66] Other lasers that have been used include fractional lasers, pulsed dye laser, diode laser, 1,320-nm Nd:YAG laser, 1,540-nm erbium: glass laser and intense pulse light. Fractional 1,550-nm erbium-doped fiber laser has been used. It is a single case report of four sessions monthly.[67] It is postulated to eliminate melanin pigment from the epidermis and dermis through "melanin shuttle," which exudes the pigment from the skin through microthermal zones. It causes less PIH and removes dermal melanin as well. It also improves laxity of skin.[68]
- DermaFrac™ is a newer modification of the microneedling technique that utilizes the microconduits created by the microneedling to simultaneously passively diffuse antiaging peptides or other sera with pharmaceutical properties.[69]

Procedures to Correct Tear Trough Depression

These include:

- *Fat transfer:* Although off-label, autologous fat transfer is an effective technique to achieve facial rejuvenation and efface the infraorbital rim hollow. By injecting directly into the orbicularis retaining ligament (ORL), deep volume augmentation is achieved which minimizes superficial irregularity, thereby effacing the facial hollows and yielding a smoother lower eyelid–midface contour. The advantage of using autologous fat is that it can avoid the Tyndall effect which can occur when hyaluronic acid (HA) filler is injected superficially.[70]
- *Fillers:* Hyaluronic acid gel is used as a filler for three-dimensional reshaping of periorbital complex. Patient satisfaction is high, but some patients with dark circles noted darker pigmentation after HA gel. Bosniak et al. treated 12 patients with POH, TTD, or prominent nasojugal groove with the HA push technique. All patients experienced immediate improvement after the procedure. Excellent tear trough contour improvement was achieved in all patients and under-eye dark circle improved. Minor postinjection erythema and edema were observed, which resolved within 72 hours.[71]

In cases of mixed POH wherein TTD is associated with pigmentation, HA can lift and emphasize excess pigmentation thereby giving poor results. Calcium hydroxyapatite filler instead has unique rheological and biostimulatory properties, which effectively lifts and supports the prolapsed tear trough ORL when placed in small quantities beneath it without adding excess volume. It is thus a novel treatment for periorbital pigmentation and/or discoloration associated with the TTD.[72]

The risk for adverse effects with fillers can be reduced by using a cannula, and injecting at the level of the supraperiosteal submuscular fat.[73] Contraindications for volume augmentation are septal fat pad herniation or severe dermatochalasis, as significant structural changes cannot be well corrected by soft-tissue filler and require surgical correction.[74]

Recently recommendations for the treatment of tear trough using crosslinked HA filler have been published.[75]

- *PRP:* Recently, PRP has been used in treating dark circles due to TTD and wrinkles. A single session with intradermal injections of 1.5 mL PRP was given into the tear trough area and wrinkles of crow's feet. Effect was compared 3 months after treatment with baseline. The improvement in infraorbital color homogeneity was statistically significant.
- *Surgery:* Lower eyelid blepharoplasty can be used to address dark circles related to shadowing effects from overhead lighting. Adjuvant chemical peel or laser resurfacing can be used to treat pigmentary causes. A variety of lower eyelid blepharoplasty techniques are available. Transconjunctival fat excision blepharoplasty is an effective means of treating relative volume excess superior to the orbitomalar ligament that, when combined with age-related volume loss in the cheek, contributes to dark circles. When the dense attachments of the orbitomalar ligament prevent fat excision blepharoplasty from smoothing the eyelid–cheek contour, transposition lower eyelid blepharoplasty is an effective means of treating these contour irregularities.

Treatment for Translucent Eyelids and Visible Veins

The vascular subtype of POH is caused by increased visibility of underlying capillaries and veins in subcutaneous vascular plexus within muscle (orbicularis oculi). Therefore, the principles of therapy aim at restoring the volume underneath the eyelid. It has been shown to be most responsive to treatments that increase dermal thickness.[76]

- Vitamin C serums and retinols have been shown to improve POH via increase in collagen synthesis causing increased dermal thickness.[38]
- Pulsed dye lasers are well suited for the treatment of dark circles with a vascular etiology. Pulsed dye lasers use the principle of selective thermolysis with hemoglobin as the chromophore. These lasers produce visible light at a wavelength of 585–595 nm with pulse durations of 0.45–40 ms.

  1,064-nm Nd:YAG laser (both Q-switched and long-pulsed) were found to be successful for vascular POH, with full resolution and high patient satisfaction.[77,78]
- Autologous fat transplantation or soft-tissue fillers are the lines of therapy to create volume between the thin skin and the veins in the musculature. Fat is readily available, safe, noncarcinogenic, easily acquired, and autologous. In a study of autologous fat, patients showed an average of 78% improvement.[19] Other studies have also concluded that autologous fat transplantation is an effective method for the treatment of infraorbital dark circles due to thin and translucent lower eyelid skin over the orbicularis oculi muscle.[70] In addition, HA fillers have been used.[29] Non-crosslinked HA with glycerol has also been used. Three monthly superficial injections using micropuncture technique led to improvement of between 25 and 50% in skin brightness, texture, and turgor. Papules were present after each application, and hematoma was the longest lasting adverse effect.[79]

Issues with the use of injectable fillers in the periorbital tissues include some patients with dark circles noticing dark pigmentation after HA gel filling, palpable nodules with fillers and swelling, bruising, asymmetry, cellulitis, migraine. It is best to use fillers with cannula rather than needles and deposit the filler just above the periosteum. This would ensure less activity of tissue hyaluronidase leading to increased duration of effect of the filler.[80]

- Ablative resurfacing is a powerful means to improve infraorbital dark circles by resurfacing the skin to treat pigmentary irregularity as well as enhancing skin tightness and the collagen and extracellular matrix (ECM) to improve concealment of the underlying orbicularis and vascular network.

PERIORAL MELANOSIS

Perioral area is a part of aesthetic unit comprising lips and mouth and holds a very important place in an individual's attractiveness and beauty. Any unusual pigmentation in this area is of prime concern to the patient as changed facial appearance negatively hampers confidence and beauty. Perioral melanosis can result from a myriad of etiologies primarily postinflammatory in nature and others like structural and functional variations in the skin, or the influence of cultural practices. There are a multitude of causes that can lead to perioral pigmentation as mentioned in etiological classification **(Table 2)** divided into endogenous causes and exogenous causes with further delineation of endogenous causes depending on the nature of deposition which ultimately determines the color of melanosis. Perioral pigmentation can be a part of facial melanosis which has been dealt with effectively in the relevant chapter or occur in conjunction with genodermatoses which are beyond discussion here or less commonly reported as isolated phenomenon or unique entity. Therefore, we aim to provide a comprehensive view on perioral pigmentation through this section of the chapter.

TABLE 2: Etiology of perioral melanosis.

Endogenous	*Exogenous*
• *Melanin-associated:* – Acquired idiopathic patterned facial pigmentation – Familial/constitutional – PDL H – Facial frictional melanosis – Postinflammatory hyperpigmentation (PIH) – *Melasma:* ◆ Seborrheic melanosis ◆ Acanthosis nigricans – *Solar lentigines/ephelides:* ◆ *Genodermatoses:* Lentigines on lips and in perioral area in Laugier–Hunziker syndrome (LHS), Peutz–Jeghers syndrome (PJS), LEOPARD, LAMB, Cronkhite–Canada syndrome (CCS); café-au-lait macules (CALMs) ◆ *Hormonal:* Addison's disease[81] (Cushing's disease, Graves disease) ◆ *Tumors:* Malignant melanoma (MM), nevus, lentigo maligna, seborrheic keratosis – Vitamin B_{12} deficiency	• Cosmetic-induced • Chemical in ointment • *Heavy metals:* Silver, gold, mercury, lead, arsenic • Tattoos • Procedural (laser, chemical peels) • *Drugs:* FDE, antimalarials, TCA, topical steroids
• *Heme-associated:* – Petechiae – Ecchymosis – Hemangioma – Angiosarcoma – Kaposi sarcoma – Hereditary hemorrhagic telangiectasia	
• *Iron-associated:* – Hemochromatosis	

(FDE: Fixed drug eruption; TCA: trichloroacetic acid)

Pathophysiology

Perioral hyperpigmentation is mainly due to an increase in number or activity of melanocytes. Other less common causes are deposition of other substances (heme, iron, carotenes, metals). Specific pathophysiologies are mentioned under each condition.[81]

Investigations

Wood's lamp and dermoscopy may be useful in the evaluation and differentiation of various etiologies especially since skin biopsy in perioral hyperpigmentation is not acceptable to most patients.

Treatment of Perioral Melanosis

Knowledge about normal variations in pigmentation is a prerequisite to discern abnormal pigmentary dermatoses. Having differentiated that, patient needs to be counseled adequately regarding the cause of their pigmentation and thereafter treatment ensues. It mainly revolves around the identification and removal of contributing factors if any, and aesthetic modalities, whenever suitable.

Topical agents include HQ, kojic acid, azelaic acid, arbutin, vitamin C, etc. Like any other facial pigmentary disorder, perioral melanosis responds well to sunscreens, particularly broad-spectrum sunscreen. Chemical peels have been dealt with in the treatment of AN where they are primarily used. Lasers for perioral melanosis are usually employed in treatment of solar lentigines. Most data on lasers pertain to the Western population, and there is a paucity of literature regarding the effectiveness, safety, and tolerability of different lasers in Indian population.

Prevention of Perioral Melanosis

Prevention depends on treating the primary condition at the earliest and effectively along with limiting sun exposure and using sunscreen regularly especially in patients with fair skin (types I–III) and avoiding unnecessary procedures and cosmetic application.

Here, in this chapter we have restricted our focus on conditions causing isolated perioral pigmentation which has not been mentioned exclusively in literature. The individual conditions are as described here.

Postinflammatory Hyperpigmentation

Although it is supposed to be the most common etiology of perioral melanosis, an extensive literature search showed only one case report on isolated perioral PIH.[82] The possible explanation could be that it is usually considered as a part of facial melanosis or is less commonly reported as an individual entity. It is mostly a psychological stressor to patients as it tends to persist for long and affects their appearance. Sometimes it may resolve spontaneously over a long time period.

Epidemiology: It can affect all skin types but is usually seen in dark skin (Fitzpatrick types IV–VI) including African-Americans, Hispanics/Latinos, Asians, Native Americans, Pacific Islanders, and those of Middle-eastern descent.[82]

Clinical features

Postinflammatory hyperpigmentation appears as darkly pigmented irregular macules at sites of previous injury or inflammation. Epidermal hypermelanosis appears as tan, brown, or dark brown and may take months to years to resolve without treatment. Hyperpigmentation within the dermis is due to melanophages and has a bluish-gray clinical appearance due to Tyndall effect. PIH worsens with sun exposure and with persistent or recurrent inflammation.

Etiology

Postinflammatory hyperpigmentation is an acquired hypermelanosis following melanocyte response to cutaneous injury or inflammation in the perioral area **(Box 1)** which causes increased production and/or redistribution of melanin.

Causes of perioral dermatitis are multiple with simplest being contact dermatitis from repeated lip-licking or thumb-sucking, especially during winter, and others being application of cosmetic preparations, topical corticosteroids, tartar control toothpaste, and bubble gum. PIH following herpes simplex virus (HSV) infection is also commonly seen as well as secondary to lesions of seborrheic dermatitis, acne, and rosacea.

*Pathogenesis **(Fig. 22)**:* The exact mechanism of PIH is unknown; however, it is postulated that inflammatory mediators and reactive oxygen species (ROS) released during the inflammatory process stimulate increase in melanocyte activity with studies supporting the theory of melanocyte-stimulating properties of leukotrienes, prostaglandins (PG) E2 and D2, thromboxane A2 (TXA2), interleukin 1 (IL-1), IL-6, tumor necrosis factor alpha (TNF-α), epidermal growth factor (EGF), and nitric oxide (NO).[83]

Treatment: The management of PIH begins with recognizing the underlying inflammatory conditions. Treatment is often difficult requiring prolonged courses of therapy and excellent patient compliance. Treatments with skin-lightening agents, chemical peeling agents, and lasers can be tried; however, these can worsen the lesion and therefore should be used with caution. Available options include HQ 3 or 4%, azelaic acid 20% cream, retinoids, salicylic or GA peels, and laser therapy; monotherapy is often unsatisfactory.[84] Serial GA peels with 2% HQ plus 10% GA combination twice daily application and tretinoin 0.05% applied at bedtime were found to cause lightening without significant adverse effects in a study.[85] Tazarotene has been tolerated and used in reducing pigment and disease severity.[86]

Postinflammatory hyperpigmentation following LASER procedure is a common side effect of therapy which discourages the patient from undergoing an effective therapeutic modality. Pretreatment with topical therapies has been studied in patients with skin types I–III undergoing carbon dioxide laser resurfacing. No conclusive benefit was noted in one limited trial involving patients at the lowest risk

BOX 1: Causes of perioral postinflammatory hyperpigmentation (PIH).

- *Infection:* HSV, varicella, verruca plana, folliculitis/pyodermas, chikungunya, HIV-associated melanosis, tinea faciei, tinea barbae
- *Inflammation:* Acne, rosacea, lip licker's dermatitis, perioral dermatitis, frictional, contact dermatitis, atopic dermatitis, paederus dermatitis, latex syndrome, fixed food eruption, LPP, and EDP
- Postinjury (physical trauma, irritants, burns)
- Post-cosmetic procedures (LASER)
- *Papulosquamous disorders:* Psoriasis, lichen planus
- Hypersensitivity to medication/allergic reaction to insect bites

(EDP: erythema dyschromicum perstans; HIV: human immunodeficiency virus; HSV: herpes simplex virus; LPP: lichen planus pigmentosus)

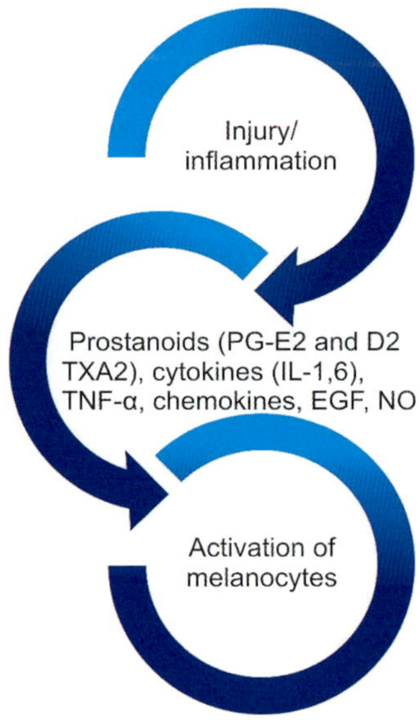

Fig. 22: Pathophysiology of perioral postinflammatory hyperpigmentation (PIH). (EGF: epidermal growth factor; IL-1: interleukin 1; PG-E2: prostaglandin E2; NO: nitric oxide; TNF-α: tumor necrosis factor alpha; TXA2: thromboxane A2)

for PIH.[87] At present, no preventive measures have proven beneficial in any skin type.

Pigmentary Demarcation Line H

Pigmentary demarcation line H is one of the three facial PDLs described in Indians. These appear as two symmetrical linear bands of hyperpigmentation extending from the angle of the mouth to the lateral aspect of chin. An additional band below and parallel to the lower lip, joining the two oro-mental bands thus forming the letter (H) has been seen in some women. Their appearance is distinctive enough to be recognized as a fairly common variant of normal pigmentation in the Indian subpopulation. It commonly coexists with the other facial PDLs.[88] It is more commonly observed in females and this could be related to sex hormones clubbed to the fact that they first appear around puberty.[89] It becomes more apparent with age.[23] There may be a genetic predisposition to these lines and cutaneous mosaicism is implicated in its genesis. Histopathology is usually unremarkable with some cases showing basal and suprabasal pigmentation and mild pigmentary incontinence in the papillary dermis.

Pigmentary demarcation line H is a cosmetic concern to patients and counseling is an important aspect of management here. These are recalcitrant to treatment which has been tried with triple combination cream, serial GA peels, and sunscreen but not to much avail. Minor improvement achieved with these is lost on discontinuation. Therefore, camouflage is the best option available.

Acquired Idiopathic Patterned Facial Pigmentation

It has been described as an acquired idiopathic condition which progresses over time and appears bilaterally as homogenously diffuse gray to dark gray or slate-gray pigmentation. It is believed to occur following genetically determined increased pigmentary functional activity to various factors like UV rays and aging and mosaicism could also be contributory. AIPFP in perioral area rarely exists solo. This pigmentation is said to be akin to PDL.[17]

Peribuccal Pigmentation of Brocq

It is seen in middle-aged women and appears as symmetrical, diffuse brownish-red pigmentation around mouth sparing a narrow perioral ring which may extend up to the forehead. A photodynamic substance in cosmetics is assumed to be the probable cause.[90] Treatment involves avoidance of the implicated cosmetic agent, sun protection, and sequential chemical peels can also be utilized **(Fig. 23)**.

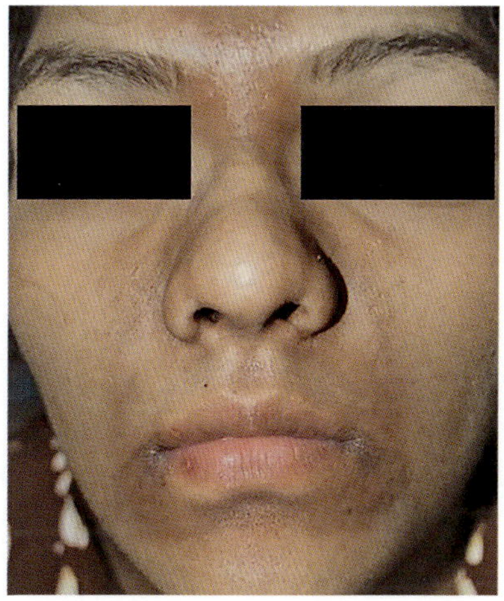

Fig. 23: Erythrose peribuccale of Brocq.

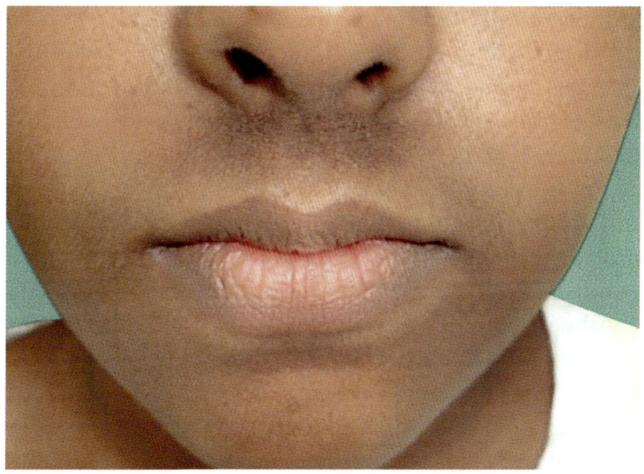

Fig. 24: Frictional hyperpigmentation.

Facial Frictional Melanosis

The common features seen in this type of perioral pigmentation are: Positive history of rubbing, predominantly male gender, associated hyperhidrosis, bilaterally symmetrical uniform deep, dark brown pigmentation.[91] The squeezing of melanocytes against the underlying bony structures releases melanosomes to the dermis seen as melanophages after engulfment by macrophages resulting in the pigmentation seen clinically at sites of friction.

Dermoscopy reveals brownish structureless areas arranged in a reticular fashion.[92] On histopathology, irregular acanthosis of epidermis with antler-like projection of the rete ridges, hypermelanosis of the basal layer, patchy melanin incontinence, a superficial papillary perivascular lymphohistiocytic infiltrate, and vertical banding of the collagen fibers with both epidermal and dermal melanosis are found. Treatment here entails removal of friction by habit changing along with depigmenting and exfoliating agents. Also, patients need to be counseled regarding photoprotection **(Fig. 24)**.

Acanthosis Nigricans

Acanthosis nigricans can be a manifestation of metabolic syndrome or associated with insulin resistance, diabetes

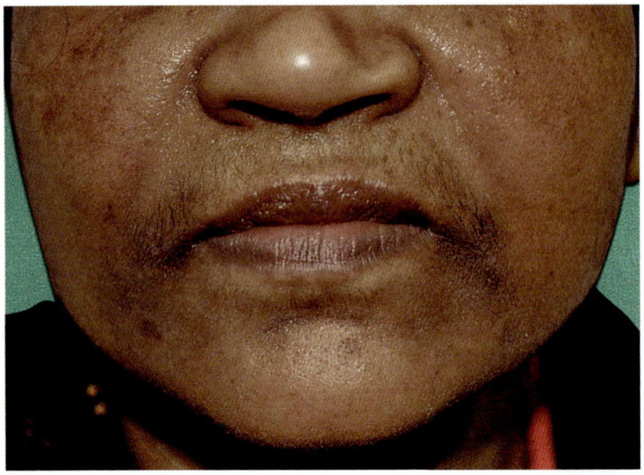

Fig. 25: Perioral acanthosis nigricans.

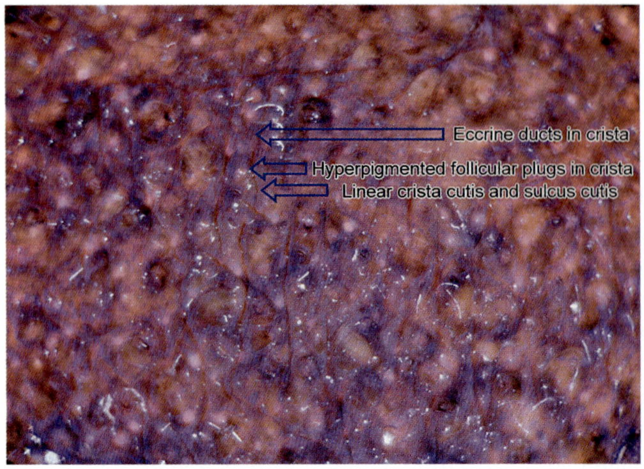

Fig. 26: Dermoscopy of acanthosis nigricans.

mellitus, obesity, internal malignancy, endocrine disorders, and drug reactions. It is characterized by thick velvety hyperpigmented plaques commonly of the intertriginous and flexural areas of the skin. Isolated perioral AN is rarely encountered **(Fig. 25)**. It is usually seen in association with AN at other classical sites.

Dermoscopy shows linear crista cutis and sulcus cutis with focal hyperpigmented dots in the crista cutis seen **(Fig. 26)**. AN on histopathological examination (HPE) shows acanthosis with or without papillomatoses together with dermoepidermal melanosis.

Treatment is multifactorial because of associated underlying disease which requires correction in the form of weight reduction in obesity-related AN, cessation of the causative agent in drug-induced AN, conventional insulin-sensitizing agents such as metformin or thiazolidinediones in AN associated with insulin resistance and surgical removal of tumors in malignancy-associated AN. The therapeutic modalities for AN take into account and go along with cosmetic resolution which is equally important for patients and their quality of life. Existing cosmetic treatment options include retinoids (topical/oral), topical vitamin D analogs and chemical peels.

Retinoids normalize epithelial growth and differentiation. Case reports on successful usage of 0.1% tretinoin and 0.1% adapalene for AN exist.[93-95]

Oral retinoids are also effective but in large doses (3 mg/kg/day of isotretinoin) and extended courses with frequent relapses.[96,97] Combination therapy has also been successful in treating AN. A combination of 0.05% tretinoin cream and 12% ammonium lactate cream resolved obesity-related AN lesions as per one case report.[98] Another case report highlighted the disappearance of perioral AN lesions with topical erythromycin in combination with isotretinoin and metformin along with significant weight reduction.[99]

Vitamin D analogs inhibit keratinocyte proliferation and promote differentiation by increasing keratinocyte intracellular calcium and cyclic guanosine monophosphate (GMP) levels. By reducing the number of keratinocytes, it may minimize the cutaneous effects of insulin. Calcipotriol has been reported to be a safe, effective, and well-tolerated treatment for AN.[100]

Superficial chemical peels primarily TCA are a relatively safe and effective treatment option for AN. TCA is easily accessible, inexpensive, easily prepared, and a stable compound. It causes coagulation and precipitation of skin proteins, leading to necrosis of epidermis which is followed by inflammation and wound repair culminating in re-epithelialization. There are studies reporting improvement in AN with TCA.[96,101]

Dermabrasion and alexandrite lasers are expensive but effective options. As per published case reports, fish oil, podophyllin, and combination therapy with urea, salicylic acid, and triple-combination depigmenting cream have also been seen to improve AN lesions to some extent.[96]

Solar Lentigines

These are hyperpigmented, well-circumscribed macules (1–3 cm) on sun exposed surfaces of the skin including perioral area. They often have a variegated appearance. These are more commonly seen in skin types I–III and frequently coexist with ephelides. These occur due to local proliferation of basal melanocytes resulting in melanization.

Treatment consists of topical therapies and ablative therapies. Available topical therapies for solar lentigines comprise mostly of depigmenting agents. HQ has been used most and is moderately effective but acts slowly and frequent relapse following its discontinuation make it a less favorable option. A combination of mequinol/tretinoin has been shown as safe and effective treatment along with prolonged maintenance.[102]

Chemical peels with 30–35% TCA have shown significant improvement in lentigines but recurrences are common. Cryotherapy with liquid nitrogen is useful but long-term improvement data is lacking.[103]

Laser therapy has superior results than cryotherapy with frequency-doubled Q-switched ND:YAG laser performing optimally.[104]

Ephelides

These are small (1–2 mm), sharply defined macules of uniform color, most often found on the face, neck, chest, and arms. Onset is usually in childhood following sun exposure. Perioral ephelides are commonly seen in beach workers.[105] These are asymptomatic and usually fade during winter months, therefore treatment is not necessary. For cosmesis, these are treated similar to lentigines (cryotherapy, HQ, azelaic acid, GA peels, and laser therapy).

Melasma

Melasma in perioral area may appear under each nostril symmetrically, or on entire upper lip, giving it a darkened, mustache-like appearance. It is seen more commonly in women on oral contraceptive pills or on hormone replacement therapy and usually reverses on stopping the medication. In other cases, it may be resistant to treatment and persist. Patients are advised to change hormonal contraceptive to nonhormonal one. Also avoidance of perfumes, cosmetics, and creams containing photoallergens helps in some cases where a phototoxic reaction is the trigger of melasma. Treatment lasts for quite some time and requires strict compliance in terms of absolute sun protection. Specific treatment modalities are similar to melasma at other sites and have been discussed at length elsewhere.

Seborrheic Melanosis

Seborrheic melanosis is classically seen as localized darkening along with variable erythema of seborrheic areas commonly in Fitzpatrick skin type IV and above along with seborrheic dermatitis. Some consider it to be a PIH secondary to seborrheic dermatitis but in a few cases, isolated perioral involvement may be seen. Seborrhea, greasy appearance of lesions, and dyssebacea are the clinical findings **(Fig. 27)** helping to favor the diagnosis which distinguish it from frictional melanosis.[106]

It is essential to recognize this entity and differentiate from other causes of perioral pigmentation as initial treatment consists of topical antifungal/anti-inflammatory drugs. Topical lightening agents should be used at a later stage. Also role of avoidance of sunlight/rubbing/cosmetics which work as additional components to intensify the pigmentation need to be explained to the patient along with slow treatment response and chronicity of the condition.

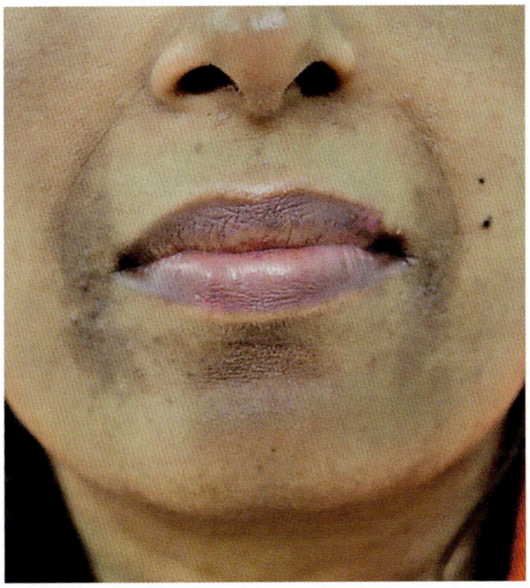

Fig. 27: Seborrheic melanosis.

CONCLUSION

Both periocular and perioral melanosis are important not only for all people irrespective of gender as these are important areas of face that define a person's appearance and can have a lasting effect on confidence and psychology, but also because these require to be dealt with utmost care and precaution by keeping in view the patients' desire along with the degree of improvement that can be achieved and avoiding possible side effects associated with the treatment.

REFERENCES

1. Gupta MA, Gupta AK. Dissatisfaction with skin appearance among patients with eating disorders and non-clinical controls. Br J Dermatol. 2001;145(1):110-3.
2. Sheth PB, Shah HA, Dave JN. Periorbital hyperpigmentation: a study of its prevalence, common causative factors and its association with personal habits and other disorders. Indian J Dermatol. 2014;59(2):151-7.
3. Aldercreutz E. Periocular hyperpigmentation (Masque Biliaire) and its relation to biliary and genito-urinary tract diseases. Acta Medics Scandinavica. 1949;135(1):63-7.
4. Lowe NJ, Wieder JM, Shorr NS, Boxrud C, Saucer D, Chalet M. Infraorbital pigmented skin. Preliminary observations of laser therapy. Dermatol Surg. 1995;21(9):767-70.
5. Kolde G, Schmollack KP, Sterry W. Periorbital hyperpigmentation. Bilateral nevus of Ota. Hautarzt. 2001;52(5):460-3.
6. Rubegni P, Tognetti L, Tosi GM, Flori ML, Fimiani M. Ocular involvement in generalized fixed drug eruption from nimesulide. Clin Experiment Ophthalmol. 2013;41(9):896-8.
7. Barbhuiya JN, Guha PK, Dutta BN. Primary systemic amyloidosis, presenting as periorbital pigmentation. Ind J Dermatol Venereol Leprol. 1994;60:34-6.
8. El Safoury OS, El Fatah DS, Ibrahim M. Treatment of periocular hyperpigmentation due to lead of kohl (surma) by

penicillamine: a single group non-randomized clinical trial. Indian J Dermatol. 2009;54(4):361-3.
9. Omar SS, Inas FG, Laila R, Hany S. Periorbital pigmentation by lead in kohl. J Egypt Womans Dermatol Soc. 2006;3:4-18.
10. Schmutz JL, Barbaud A, Tréchot P. Periocular hyperpigmentation following travoprost application. Ann Dermatol Venereol. 2008;135(6-7):537.
11. Feletti F, Vincenzi C, Pazzaglia M, Tosti M. Periocular pigmentation associated with use of travoprost for the treatment of alopecia areata of the eyelashes. J Eur Acad Dermatol Venereol. 2007;21(3):421-3.
12. Kapur R, Osmanovic S, Toyran S, Edward DP. Bimatoprost-induced periocular skin hyperpigmentation: Histopathological study. Arch Ophthalmol. 2005;123(11):1541-6.
13. Lee DW. Clinical course of bimatoprost-induced periocular skin hyperpigmentation after stopping bimatoprost treatment. J Kor Ophthalmol Soc. 2007;48:1082-7.
14. Traboulsi EI, Maumenee IH. Periocular pigmentation in the Peutz-Jeghers syndrome. Am J Ophthalmol. 1986;102(1):126-7.
15. Sardana K, Rajpal M, Garg V, Mishra D. Periorbital hyperpigmentation mimicking fixed drug eruption: a rare presentation of erythema dyschromicum perstans in a paediatric patient. J Eur Acad Dermatol Venereol. 2006;20(10):1381-3.
16. Sorhage B. Increased pigmentation of the sclera and periorbital region associated with increased cutaneous vascularization of the left arm. J Dtsch Dermatol Ges. 2005;3(4):301-3.
17. Sarma N, Chakraborty S, Bhattacharya SR. Acquired, Idiopathic, Patterned Facial Pigmentation (AIPFP) Including Periorbital Pigmentation and Pigmentary Demarcation Lines on Face Follows the Lines of Blaschko on Face. Indian J Dermatol. 2014;59(1):41-8.
18. Razmi TM, Thakur V, Vinay K, Aggarwal D, Radotra BD, Kumaran MS, et al. Periorbital Acquired Dermal Macular Hyperpigmentation: A Distinctive Clinical Entity in Young Adults-Observational Case-Control Study. Indian Dermatol Online J. 2020;11(4):590-3.
19. Roh MR, Chung KY. Infraorbital dark circles: definition, causes, and treatment options. Dermatol Surg. 2009;35(8):1163-71.
20. Peters R. Auffallende Dunkelfarbung der unteren Lider als erbliche Anomalie. Zbl Prakt Augenheilk. 1918;42:8-11.
21. Goodman RM, Belcher RW. Periorbital hyperpigmentation. An overlooked genetic disorder of pigmentation. Arch Dermatol. 1969;100(2):169-74.
22. Anstey AV. Disorders of skin colour. In: Burns T, Breathnach S, Cox N, Griffiths C (Eds). Rook's Textbook of Dermatology, 8th edition. Oxford: Wiley-Blackwell; 2010. p. 58.19.
23. Somani VK, Razvi F, Sita VNVL. Pigmentary demarcation lines over the face. Indian J Dermatol Venereol Leprol. 2004;70(6):336-41.
24. Malakar S, Lahiri K, Banarjee U, Mondal S, Sarangi S. Periorbital melanosis is an extension of pigmentary demarcation line-F on face. Indian J Dermatol Venoreol Leprol. 2007;73(5):323-5.
25. Freitag FM, Cestari TF. What causes dark circles under the eyes? J Cosmet Dermatol. 2007;6(3):211-5.
26. Masuda Y, Takahashi M, Satou A, Yanai M, Yamashita T, Iikura T, et al. Dermatological study on dark eye circles and their improvement with newly developed cosmetics. Int J Cosmet Sci. 2004;26:315-6.
27. Eberlin S, Del Carmen Velazquez Pereda M, de Campos Dieamant G, Nogueira C, Werka R, Queiroz MLS. Effects of a Brazilian herbal compound as a cosmetic eyecare for periorbital hyperchromia ("dark circles"). J Cosmet Dermatol. 2009;8(2):127-35.
28. Goldberg RA, McCann JD, Fiaschetti D, Ben Simon GJ. What causes eyelid bags? Analysis of 144 consecutive patients. Plast Reconstr Surg. 2005;115(5):1395-402.
29. Kane MA. Treatment of tear trough deformity and lower lid bowing with injectable hyaluronic acid. Aesthetic Plast Surg. 2005;29(5):363-7.
30. Hirmand H. Anatomy and nonsurgical correction of tear trough deformity. Plast Reconstr Surg. 2010;125(2):699-708.
31. Momosawa A, Kurita M, Ozaki M, Miyamoto S, Kobayashi Y, Ban I, et al. Combined therapy using Q-switched ruby laser and bleaching treatment with tretinoin and hydroquinone for periorbital skin hyperpigmentation in Asians. Plast Reconstr Surg. 2008;121(1):282-8.
32. Ranu H, Thng S, Goh BK, Burger A, Goh CL. Periorbital hyperpigmentation in Asians: an epidemiologic study and proposed classification. Dermatol Surg. 2011;37(9):1297-303.
33. Moncrieff M, Cotton SD, Claridge E, Hall P. Spectrophotometric intracutaneous analysis: a new technique for imaging pigmented skin lesions. Br J Dermatol. 2002;146(3):448-57.
34. Verschoore M, Gupta S, Sharma VK, Ortonne JP. Determination of melanin and haemoglobin in the skin of idiopathic cutaneous hyperchromia of the orbital region (ICHOR): a study of Indian patients. J Cutan Aesthet Surg. 2012;5(3):176-82.
35. Graziosi AC, Quaresma MR, Michalany NS, Ferreira LM. Cutaneous idiopathic hyperchromia of the orbital region (CIHOR): a histopathological study. Aesthetic Plast Surg. 2013;37(2):434-8.
36. Chatterjee M, Suwal B, Malik A, Vasudevan B. A study of epidemiological, etiological, and clinicopathological factors in periocular hyperpigmentation. Pigment Int. 2018;5:34-42.
37. Huang YL, Chang SL, Ma L, Lee MC, Hu S. Clinical analysis and classification of dark eye circle. Int J Dermatol. 2014;53(2):164-70.
38. Michelle L, Pouldar Foulad D, Ekelem C, Saedi N, Mesinkovska NA. Treatments of Periorbital Hyperpigmentation: A Systematic Review. Dermatol Surg. 2021;47(1):70-4.
39. Ohshima H, Mizukoshi K, Oyobikawa M, Matsumoto K, Takiwaki H, Kanto H, et al. Effects of vitamin C on dark circles of the lower eyelids: quantitative evaluation using image analysis and echogram. Skin Res Technol. 2009;15(2):214-7.
40. Dayal S, Sahu P, Jain VK, Khetri S. Clinical efficacy and safety of 20% glycolic peel, 15% lactic peel, and topical 20% vitamin C in constitutional type of periorbital melanosis: a comparative study. J Cosmet Dermatol. 2016;15:367-73.
41. Jiang L, Hino PD, Bhatia A, Stephens TJ, Jimenez F. Efficacy of Trifecting Night Cream, a Novel Triple acting Skin Brightening Product: A Double-blind, Placebo-controlled Clinical Study. J Clin Aesthet Dermatol. 2018;11(12):21-5.
42. Colvan L, Fleck T, Vega VL. Global periorbital skin rejuvenation by a topical eye cream containing low molecular weight heparan sulfate (LMW-HS) and a blend of naturally derived extracts. J Cosmet Dermatol. 2019;18:530-8.
43. Ahmadraji F, Shatalebi MA. Evaluation of the clinical efficacy and safety of an eye counter pad containing caffeine and vitamin K in emulsified Emu oil base. Adv Biomed Res. 2015;4:10.
44. Reivitis A, Karimi K, Griffiths C, Banayan A. A single-center, pilot study evaluating a novel TriHex peptide- and botanical-containing eye treatment compared to baseline. J Cosmet Dermatol. 2018;17:467-70.
45. Mitsuishi T, Shimoda T, Mitsui Y, Kuriyama Y, Kawana S. The effects of topical application of phytonadione, retinol and

vitamins C and E on infraorbital dark circles and wrinkles of the lower eyelids. J Cosmet Dermatol. 2004;3(2):73-5.

46. Kassir M, Sahni K. Dermafrac^{TM}: an innovative new treatment for periorbital melanosis in a dark-skinned male patient. J Cutan Aesthet Surg. 2013;6:158.
47. Ranjan R, Sarkar R, Garg VK, Gupta T. A Comparative Study of Two Modalities, 4% Hydroquinone Versus 30% Salicylic Acid in Periorbital Hyperpigmentation and Assessment of Quality of Life Before and After Treatment. Indian J Dermatol. 2006;61(4):413-7.
48. Zamanian A, Azizi M, Ghasemi M, Behrangi E, Naeji S. Comparing the effectiveness of fractional CO_2 laser and the combination therapy with micro-needling and topical 10% trichloroacetic acid to remove infra-orbital dark circles in Tehran women. J Cosmet Laser Ther. 2019;21:61-4.
49. Ahmed NA, Mohammed SS, Fatani MI. Treatment of periorbital dark circles: comparative study of carboxy therapy vs chemical peeling vs mesotherapy. J Cosmet Dermatol. 2019;18:169-75.
50. Jung YS, Bae JM, Kim BJ, Kang JS, Cho SB. Periorbital melasma: hierarchical cluster analysis of clinical features in Asian patients. Ski Res Technol. 2017;23:552-7.
51. Vanaman Wilson MJ, Jones IT, Bolton J, Larsen L, Wu DC, Goldman MP. Prospective studies of the efficacy and safety of the picosecond 755, 1,064, and 532 nm lasers for the treatment of infraorbital dark circles. Lasers Surg Med. 2018;50:45-50.
52. Watanabe S, Nakai K, Ohnishi T. Condition known as "dark rings under the eyes" in the Japanese population is a kind of dermal melanocytosis which can be successfully treated by Q-switched ruby laser. Dermatol Surg. 2006;32(6):785-9.
53. Xu TH, Li YH, Chen JZ, Gao XH, Chen HD. Treatment of infraorbital dark circles using 694-nm fractional Q-switched ruby laser. Lasers Med Sci. 2016;31:1783-7.
54. West TB, Alster TS. Improvement of infraorbital hyperpigmentation following carbon dioxide laser resurfacing. Dermatol Surg. 1998;24(6):615-6.
55. Paolo F, Nefer F, Paola P, Nicolò S. Periorbital area rejuvenation using carbon dioxide therapy. J Cosmet Dermatol. 2012;11(3):223-8.
56. Lee KS, Kim SA, Lee KS. Platelet-rich plasma induces increased expression of G1 cell cycle regulators, type I collagen, and matrix metalloproteinase-1 in human skin fibroblasts. Int J Mol Med. 2011;29:32-6.
57. Leo MS, Kumar AS, Kirit R, Konathan R, Sivamani RK. Systematic review of the use of platelet-rich plasma in aesthetic dermatology. J Cosmet Dermatol. 2015;14:315-23.
58. Mehryan P, Zartab H, Rajabi A, Pazhoohi N, Firooz A. Assessment of efficacy of platelet-rich plasma (PRP) on infraorbital dark circles and crow's feet wrinkles. J Cosmet Dermatol. 2014;13:72-8.
59. Aust M, Pototschnig H, Jamchi S, Busch KH. Platelet-rich plasma for skin rejuvenation and treatment of actinic elastosis in the lower eyelid area. Cureus. 2018;10:e2999.
60. Mostafa WZ, Kadry DM, Mohamed EF. The effects of normobaric oxygen therapy on patients with periorbital darkening: an open, uncontrolled trial. Indian J Dermatol Venereol Leprol. 2015;81:427-9.
61. Nofal E, Elkot R, Nofal A, Eldesoky F, Shehata S, Sami M. Evaluation of carboxytherapy and platelet-rich plasma in treatment of periorbital hyperpigmentation: a comparative clinical trial. J Cosmet Dermatol. 2018;17:1000-7.
62. Lee GSK. Quality survey on efficacy of carboxytherapy for localized lipolysis. J Cosmet Dermatol. 2016;15:484-92.
63. Lupo ML, Cohen JL, Rendon MI. Novel eye cream containing a mixture of human growth factors and cytokines for periorbital skin rejuvenation. J Drugs Dermatol. 2007;6(7):725-9.
64. Epstein JS. Management of infraorbital dark circles. A significant cosmetic concern. Arch Facial Plast Surg. 1999;1:303-7.
65. Gao L, Kang H, Li Y, Lu M, Song W, Wang Y, et al. Clinical Efficacy and Safety of 3DEEP Multisource Radiofrequency Therapy Combined with Fractional Skin Resurfacing for Periocular Skin Aging. J Clin Aesthet Dermatol. 2020;13(3): 41-4.
66. Alster TS, Bellew SG. Improvement of dermatochalasis and periorbital rhytides with a high-energy pulsed CO_2 laser: a retrospective study. Dermatol Surg. 2004;30(4 Pt 1):483-7;discussion 87.
67. Manuskiatti W, Fitzpatrick RE, Goldman MP. Treatment of facial skin using combinations of CO_2, Q-switched alexandrite, flashlamp-pumped pulsed dye, and Er:YAG lasers in the same treatment session. Dermatol Surg. 2000;26(2):114-20.
68. Moody MN, Landau JM, Goldberg LH, Friedman PM. Fractionated 1550-nm erbium-doped fiber laser for the treatment of periorbital hyperpigmentation. Dermatol Surg. 2012;38(1):139-42.
69. Sahni K, Kassir M. Dermafrac^{TM}: An Innovative New Treatment for Periorbital Melanosis in a Dark-Skinned Male Patient. J Cutan Aesthet Surg. 2013;6(3):158-60.
70. Roh MR, Kim TK, Chung KY. Treatment of infraorbital dark circles by autologous fat transplantation: a pilot study. Br J Dermatol. 2009;160(5):1022-5.
71. Bosniak S, Sadick NS, Cantisano-Zilkha M, Glavas IP, Roy D. The hyaluronic acid push technique for the nasojugal groove. Dermatol Surg. 2008;34(1):127-31.
72. Corduff N. An Alternative Periorbital Treatment Option Using Calcium Hydroxyapatite for Hyperpigmentation Associated with the Tear Trough Deformity. Plast Reconstr Surg Glob Open. 2020;8(2):e2633.
73. Lee SK, Kim HS. Recent trend in the choice of fillers and injection techniques in Asia: a questionnaire study based on expert opinion. J Drugs Dermatol. 2014;13:24-31.
74. Sharad J. Dermal fillers for the treatment of tear trough deformity: a review of anatomy, treatment techniques, and their outcomes. J Cutan Aesthet Surg. 2012;5:229.
75. Anido J, Fernández JM, Genol I, Ribé N, Pérez Sevilla G. Recommendations for the treatment of tear trough deformity with cross-linked hyaluronic acid filler. J Cosmet Dermatol. 2021;20:6-17.
76. Park SR, Kim HJ, Park HK, Kim JY, Kim NS, Byun KS, et al. Classification by causes of dark circles and appropriate evaluation method of dark circles. Skin Res Technol. 2016;22:276-83.
77. Xu TH, Yang ZH, Li YH, Chen JZ, Guo S, Wu Y, et al. Treatment of infraorbital dark circles using a low-fluence Q-switched 1,064-nm laser. Dermatol Surg. 2011;37:797-803.
78. Ma G, Lin XX, Hu XJ, Jin YB, Chen H. Treatment of venous infraorbital dark circles using a long-pulsed 1,064-nm neodymium-doped yttrium aluminum garnet laser. Dermatol Surg. 2012;38:1277-82.
79. Succi IB, da Silva RT, Orofino-Costa R. Rejuvenation of periorbital area: treatment with an injectable nonanimal non-crosslinked glycerol added hyaluronic acid preparation. Dermatol Surg. 2012;38:192-8.
80. Goldberg RA, Fiaschetti D. Filling the periorbital hollows with hyaluronic acid gel: initial experience with 244 injections.

Ophthal Plast Reconstr Surg. 2006;22(5):335-41; discussion 41-3.
81. Sreeja C, Ramakrishnan K, Vijayalakshmi D, Devi M, Aesha I, Vijayabanu B. Oral pigmentation: A review. J Pharm Bioallied Sci. 2015;7:S403-8.
82. Baby TK. Isolated postinflammatory perioral hyperpigmentation: A rare case report. Indian J Multidiscip Dent. 2019;9:115.
83. Davis EC, Callender VD. Postinflammatory hyperpigmentation: A review of the epidemiology, clinical features, and treatment options in skin of color. J Clin Aesthet Dermatol. 2010;3:20-31.
84. Plensdorf S, Martinez J. Common pigmentation disorders. Am Fam Physician. 2009;79(2):109-16.
85. Burns RL, Prevost-Blank PL, Lawry MA, Lawry TB, Faria DT, Fivenson DP. Glycolic acid peels for postinflammatory hyperpigmentation in black patients. A comparative study. Dermatol Surg. 1997;23(3):171-5.
86. Grimes P, Callender V. Tazarotene cream for postinflammatory hyperpigmentation and acne vulgaris in darker skin: a double-blind, randomized, vehicle-controlled study. Cutis. 2006;77(1):45-50.
87. West TB, Alster TS. Effect of pretreatment on the incidence of hyperpigmentation following cutaneous CO_2 laser resurfacing. Dermatol Surg. 1999;25(1):15-7.
88. Antony A, Kumar P. Pigmentary demarcation lines: a clinical profile of 50 subjects and report of new pattern of pigmentation observed. Int J Res Dermatol. 2018;4(3):323-7.
89. Kathuria S, Khunger N, Ramesh V. Clinical and hormonal evaluation in facial pigmentary demarcation lines: a pilot study. Indian J Dermatol Venereol Leprol. 2012;78(6):742-4.
90. Khanna N, Rasool S. Facial melanoses: Indian perspective. Indian J Dermatol Venereol Leprol. 2011;77:552-64.
91. Mutalik SD, Pethe SV, Nikam BP, Rasal YD. Facial frictional melanosis in Indian patients: Defining the entity. Clin Dermatol Rev. 2019;3:78-83.
92. Errichetti E, Stinco G. Dermoscopy in general dermatology: a practical overview. Dermatol Ther (Heidelb). 2016;6:471-507.
93. Darmstadt GL, Yokel BK, Horn TD. Treatment of acanthosis nigricans with tretinoin. Arch Dermatol. 1991;127(8):1139-40.
94. Schwartz RA. Efficacy of topical 0.1% adapalene gel for use in the treatment of childhood acanthosis nigricans: a pilot study. Dermatol Ther. 2015;28(4):266.
95. Treesirichod A, Chaithirayanon S, Wongjitrat N, Wattanapan P. The efficacy of topical 0.1% adapalene gel for use in the treatment of childhood acanthosis nigricans: a pilot study. Indian J Dermatol. 2015;60(1):103.
96. Patel NU, Roach C, Alinia H, Huang WW, Feldman SR. Current treatment options for acanthosis nigricans. Clin Cosmet Investig Dermatol. 2018;11:407-13.
97. Phiske MM. An approach to acanthosis nigricans. Indian Dermatol Online J. 2014;5(3):239-49.
98. Blobstein SH. Topical therapy with tretinoin and ammonium lactate for acanthosis nigricans associated with obesity. Cutis. 2003;71(1):33-4.
99. Ozhan B, Yilmaz Agladioglu S, Yuksel S, Sanli B. Perioral Acanthosis nigricans. J Pediatr. 2015;167(6):1453.
100. Gregoriou S, Anyfandakis V, Kontoleon P, Christofidou E, Rigopoulos D, Kontochristopoulos G. Acanthosis nigricans associated with primary hypogonadism: successful treatment with topical calcipotriol. J Dermatolog Treat. 2008;19(6):373-5.
101. Zayed A, Sobhi RM, Abdel Halim DM. Using trichloroacetic acid in the treatment of acanthosis nigricans: a pilot study. J Dermatolog Treat. 2014;25(3):223-5.
102. Jarratt M. Mequinol 2%/tretinoin 0.01% solution: an effective and safe alternative to hydroquinone 3% in the treatment of solar lentigines. Cutis. 2004;74(5):319-22.
103. Almond-Roesler B, Zouboulis CC. Successful treatment of solar lentigines by brief gentle cryosurgery using a Kryomed device. Br J Dermatol. 2000;143(1):216-8.
104. Todd MM, Rallis TM, Gerwels JW, Hata TR. A comparison of 3 lasers and liquid nitrogen in the treatment of solar lentigines: a randomized, controlled, comparative trial. Arch Dermatol. 2000;136(7):841-6.
105. Lucena EE, Castro AC, Farias DB, Lima PT, Silveira EJ, Lima KC. Prevalence of lip and perioral Ephelides in beach workers. An Bras Dermatol. 2013;88(1):56-63.
106. Vashisht KR, Garg S. Seborrheic melanosis: a unique under-recognized entity in Ethnic skin. J Clin Aesthet Dermatol. 2022;15(1):15-6.

CHAPTER 121

Melasma and Its Aesthetic Management

Biju Vasudevan, Indrashis Podder

KEY MESSAGES

- Melasma is a very common cosmetic condition, causing significant morbidity and psychological stress.
- Sun protection and depigmenting agents are mandatory part of treatment.
- Chemical peels, systemic medications, and lasers are adjuncts.
- Newer technologies of lasers especially vascular lasers, fractional lasers, third generation Q-switched lasers have opened new horizons for treatment.
- Proper patient counseling is of utmost importance.

INTRODUCTION

Melasma is a commonly acquired circumscribed hyperpigmentary disorder mainly involving sun exposed areas, especially the face. Its pathogenesis is poorly understood and treatment is challenging. Females in the 3rd and 4th decade are most prone to develop this condition; however, Sarkar et al. have reported a prevalence of 20.5% among Indian males.[1] It is more common in Fitzpatrick skin types IV, V and VI namely the Hispanic, Caribbean and Asian races as they live in areas exposed to intense ultraviolet radiation resulting in larger amounts of melanin production.[2] In India, melasma is the most common pigmentary disorder, with an incidence of approximately 10%,[3] often developing at a younger age having strong correlation with positive family history, thus supporting the role of genetic factors in its development.[4] The significance of this condition is due to the fact that it relapses frequently, is difficult to treat, and it severely affects social and emotional well-being of patients.

HISTORY

Melasma is derived from a Greek word, "*melas*" which means black. It was earlier called chloasma which is derived from a Greek word, "*chloazein*" which means green. Chloasma also means "mask of pregnancy", indicating its high prevalence in pregnant women.

ETIOLOGY

Some of the important risk factors for melasma are mentioned in **Box 1**.

PATHOGENESIS

Although, the exact pathogenesis of melasma is yet to be deciphered, recent and emerging postulates consider two groups of factors to be most instrumental:

1. *Endogenous factors:* Genetic predisposition, cutaneous vasculature, hormonal factors.
2. *Exogenous factors:* Sun exposure (UV radiation, visible light).

The major etiological factors of melasma with their mechanisms are depicted in **Flowchart 1**.[5]

Recently, melasma is being considered a "photoaging" disorder, involving the role of senescent fibroblasts and keratinocytes, possibly accounting for its relapsing nature. It is postulated that senescent fibroblasts and keratinocytes release various growth factors, cytokines and hormones including inducing nitric oxide synthase (iNOS), which subsequently stimulate melanin production. Besides, interaction between keratinocytes, mast cells, neovascularization, p53 genetic alteration, and basement membrane damage is being increasingly reported.[6]

CLINICAL FEATURES

Melasma clinically manifests as symmetrical, hyperpigmented macules with irregular, serrated, geographic or arciform

BOX 1: Risk factors.

- Sun exposure
- Pregnancy
- Hormonal therapy
- Genetic factors
- Thyroid disorders
- Liver dysfunction
- *Drugs:* Oral contraceptive pills (OCPs), phenytoin, spironolactone

Flowchart 1: Major etiological factors in melasma.

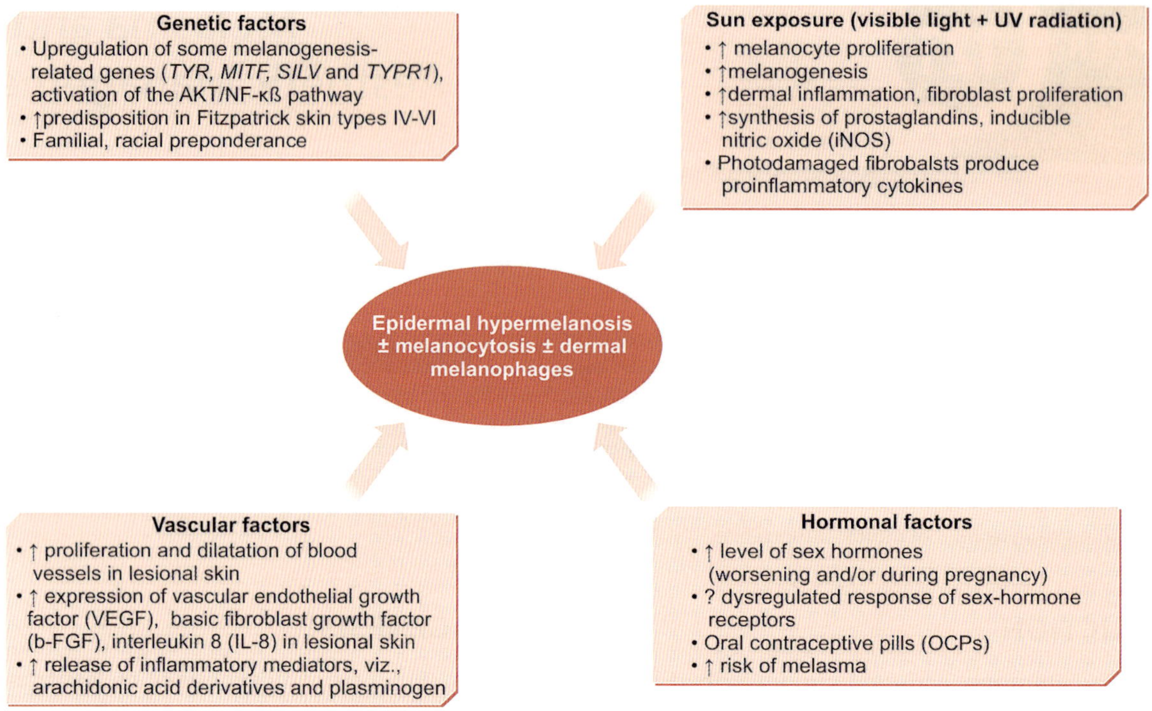

spreading borders. It is classified into three main patterns depending on distribution over the face. These patterns are:

1. *Centrofacial* (63%): This is the most common variant worldwide affecting the cheeks, forehead, upper lip, nose and chin.
2. *Malar pattern* (21%): It involves the cheeks and nose.
3. *Mandibular pattern* (16%): It involves the ramus of mandible. The mandibular region is more affected in older patients and is uncommon.

However, in India the malar region is involved most frequently (73%).[7] Rarely, other sun-exposed regions like extensors of forearm may be involved.

Melasma can also be classified into four histopathological types aided by Wood's lamp examination depending on the depth of pigment deposition.[8]

1. *Epidermal*: This is the most common variant where pigmentation is more intense with Wood's lamp examination. It is described as brown in color. In this type, melanin is present throughout epidermis.
2. *Dermal*: In this variant, there are lots of melanophages inside the dermis and pigmentation is never intensified with Wood's lamp. The color is described as blue gray.
3. *Mixed*: The mixed variant has features of both above types and Wood's lamp intensifies pigmentation at some places and not in others. The color is described as brown gray.
4. *Indeterminate*: In darker skin type, Wood's lamp examination offers no benefit and are classified as indeterminate.[9]

However, a good correlation between Wood's lamp findings and histopathology may not be present at all times. Clinically and histologically, melasma in men is similar to women.[10]

A further classification is as *transient* and *persistent* variants depending on natural history. Lesions disappearing within a year of stopping any risk factors such as oral contraceptives (OCPs) or after pregnancy is classified as transient while lesions present even after 1 year of absence of any risk factors is called persistent, this results from uninterrupted sun-exposure.

DIFFERENTIAL DIAGNOSIS

Differential diagnoses include melanocytic nevus, nevus of Ota, pigmented cosmetic dermatitis (Riehl's melanosis), poikiloderma of Civatte, occupational melanosis, lichen planus pigmentosus, lichen planus actinicus, fixed drug eruption, macular amyloidosis, urticaria pigmentosa, exogenous ochronosis and postinflammatory hyperpigmentation (postinflammatory pigmentary alteration).

ASSESSMENT OF SEVERITY OF MELASMA

It is generally assessed based on melasma area and severity index (MASI).[11] MASI is calculated by considering four regions of the face namely forehead (30%), right malar region (30%), left malar region (30%), and chin (10%). Other than area (A), the two other factors considered are darkness (D) and homogeneity (H). MASI is calculated using the formula $(D + H) \times A$. The score ranges from 0 to 48. A modified MASI has recently been proposed by removing the homogeneity component which is difficult to assess. This has scores ranging from 0 to 24. It is calculated as follows:

0.3 (A × D) Forehead + 0.3 (A × D) Left malar region + 0.3 (A × D) Right malar region + 0.1 (A × D) Chin

Where Area: 0 = absent, 1 = 10%, 2 = 10–29%, 3 = 30–49%, 4 = 50–69%, 5 = 70–89%, 6 = 90–100%, Darkness: 0 = absent, 1 = slight, 2 = mild, 3 = marked, 4 = severe.[12]

Objective measurement of the melanin content can be done with instruments like mexameter and confocal microscopy.

INVESTIGATIONS

A detailed history of precipitating and aggravating factors including use of OCPs, hormonal preparations, phenytoin, photosensitive medications, and cosmetics must be taken. Investigations to diagnose and confirm melasma can be grouped under two heads: (1) noninvasive and (2) invasive.

- *Noninvasive investigations:*
  - *Wood's lamp examination:* Wood's lamp can be used to assess the depth of pigmentation and differentiate the types of melasma, though it is very difficult in skin types V and VI. The epidermal type becomes more prominent with the Wood's lamp, but not so in the dermal variant.
  - *Dermoscopy:* Dermoscopy or epiluminescence microscopy is an evolving investigative tool and some patterns are consistent with this disorder. Dermoscopy is proving to be a superior investigation in comparison with Wood's lamp for diagnosis, assessment and monitoring of melasma.[13] Dermoscopic examination of melasma is based on the following parameters:[14]
    - *Pattern:* Reticuloglobular pattern is the most commonly observed pattern; occasionally blotches and granules may be present. A pseudonetwork pattern with concave borders is often observed due to sparing of sweat glands and follicular openings, called the "jelly sign".[15]
    - *Color:* The color of lesion depends on the amount of pigment, depth and location; ranging from black (localized in the stratum corneum), shades of brown (lower epidermis) to blue or bluish-gray (dermis).
    - *Others:* Dermoscopy is also useful to detect complications arising from overuse of topical medications such as atrophy, telangiectasia, depigmentation, exogenous ochronosis and steroid dermatitis.
  - *In vivo reflectance confocal microscopy (RCM):* Reflectance confocal microscopy is a noninvasive investigation suitable for monitoring the treatment of melasma in addition to aiding in its diagnosis.

    In vivo RCM images of melasma show markedly increased hyper-refractile cobblestone pattern at the basal layer in the lesional skin, compared with perilesional normal skin suggesting epidermal hyperpigmentation.[16] RCM also shows increased number of melanophages in almost 34.5% of these patients having a heterogenous distribution and hyperactive melanocytes in some patients.[17,18]
- *Invasive investigations:*
  - *Histopathological examination:* Histopathological examination (HPE) of the lesional skin is done rarely to confirm the diagnosis as melasma is a well-recognized clinically. The characteristic finding is increased melanin deposition in all the layers of epidermis which may be present in almost 83%of patients.[19] The basement membrane becomes disrupted probably through upregulation of MMP2 resulting from chronic UV irradiation,[16] leading to the leakage of melanin into dermis and formation of dermal melanophages. These findings have doubted the existence of a true dermal type of melasma.[19] The number of melanocytes is normal or slightly increased as detected by NK1 immunostaining, however, Mel-5 or MITF staining failed to corroborate this finding.[19] Recently, Lee et al. have depicted the presence of characteristic pendulous melanocytes in melasma.[20] The dermis also shows increased vascularization compared to perilesional skin[21] due to increased expression of vascular endothelial growth factor (VEGF) by the keratinocytes and increased number of fibroblasts.[22]

TREATMENT MODALITIES

The aims of treatment in melasma are to increase degradation of melanosomes, inhibit melanosome formation, and decrease proliferation of melanocytes. Sunscreen and sun avoidance are primary essential components of melasma therapy. Patients are advised to discontinue OCPs, antiseizure medications and avoid cosmetics. Melasma treatment can be very frustrating as many modalities can turn out to be ineffective. Dermal and mixed variants are quite resistant to therapy. Most patients seek medical help much after the onset of the condition, making treatment even more difficult. Treatment modalities range from various topical bleaching agents to chemical peels and lasers.

Medical Management

Topical Therapy

Medical management of melasma comprises mainly of sunscreens and skin lightening agents. Sunscreens with sun protection factor (SPF) of at least 30 should be used and broad-spectrum sunscreens including a physical agent like zinc oxide and/or titanium oxide are preferred as they provide protection against UV, visible and infrared spectra. Addition of iron-oxide to sunscreens is beneficial as it has maximal blocking effect of visible light. They are opaque, providing a good camouflage effect. Organic sunscreens are also available, viz., p-aminobenzoic acid (PABA), benzophenones and cinnamates; however reports of contact dermatitis and photo-instability have limited their use. Two-four hourly applications between 8 AM and 4 PM are recommended, in generous amount to attain a concentration of 2 mg/cm^2 ("teaspoon rule"- 1 teaspoon→ face/head/neck, 1 teaspoon→ each upper extremity, 2 teaspoons→ total for front and back torso, 2 teaspoons→ each lower extremity). Currently, an oral photoprotective agent called *Polypodium leucotomos* extract is being evaluated as an adjunct to sunscreen in the treatment of melasma.[23,24]

Skin lightening agents take a minimum of 2 months to initiate effect and at least 6 months for removing pigmentation. Dermal melasma does not respond well to topical medications. The various depigmenting agents used are given in **Table 1**.

Tranexamic acid is a new kid on the block for treatment of melasma. It is found to decrease tyrosinase activity in melanocytes by preventing binding of plasminogen to the keratinocytes. This results in reduced prostaglandin and arachidonic acid production which are both inflammatory mediators involved in the melanogenesis. An intralesional preparation is also available and is found to have a better safety profile, temperature stability, UV insensitiveness, and is not easily oxidized.

Newer drug delivery systems such as dissolving microneedle (DMN) patch using 4-n-butylresorcinol, a resorcinol derivative, tranexamic acid either by iontophoresis or liposomal preparation may become future trendsetters.

Combination Topical Therapy

This is based on the principle that different topical agents may act at different stages in the process of melanization, and may offer better efficacy in combination and may reduce side effects of each other. The most common combination is that of topical steroids with hydroquinone and retinoids popularly called the "triple therapy". Topical steroids reduce the inflammation and irritant effects of retinoids and hydroquinone. Retinoids reduce steroid atrophy, help penetration across stratum corneum and also protect hydroquinone from oxidative damage. Kligman and Willis first noticed the better efficacy of this regime and their combination actually had hydroquinone 5%, tretinoin 0.1% and dexamethasone 0.1% which has been referred to as the Kligman's regime ever since.[24] Various modifications of this regime have been formulated over the decades. Triple therapy takes about 4 weeks to show significant improvement and 8 weeks for maximum results **(Figs. 1A and B)**. These combinations are currently considered as the first-line therapies in melasma globally.[25] Serial use of glycolic acid (GA) peels also significantly improves clinical efficacy of modified Kligman's formula. GA in combination with hydroquinone enhances the penetration of hydroquinone. Other combinations include azelaic acid 20% with tretinoin 0.05 or 0.1%, azelaic acid hydroquinone 4% and GA 20%, mequinol 2% with tretinoin 0.01%, hydroquinone 2% and kojic acid 2% with GA 10% and mequinol 2% with 0.01% tretinoin.[26] Combinations of sunscreens with demelanizing agents are also used commonly. Presently, even combination of tyrosinase inhibitors (e.g., alpha-arbutin) + exfoliative agents (e.g., glycolic acid) + melanin transfer blockers (e.g., niacinamide) are available.

TABLE 1: Various skin lightening agents.

Types of agent	*Agents*
Competitive tyrosinase inhibitors	Hydroquinone, Mequinol, N-acetyl-4-S-cysteaminyl phenol, Arbutin, Azelaic acid, Kojic acid
Noncompetitive tyrosinase inhibitors	Haginin A, N-acetylglucosamine, Glabridin, Licorice, Mulberry extract, Polyphenols
Newer tyrosinase inhibitors	Hydroxyphenyl-naphthol, Quinolines (chloroquine, quinine), Diarylpropane, Flavonoids, Aloesin, Rucinol
Serine protease inhibitors	Niacinamide, Soy
Tyrosine oxidation blockers	P-coumaric acid
Copper chelators and antioxidants	Ascorbic acid, ellagic acid
Altering keratinocytes	Glycolic acid, retinoids, liquiritin
Miscellaneous	Dioic acid, magnolignan, undecylenoyl phenylalanine, silymarin, resveratrol, oligopeptides

Adverse Reactions

Although, topical therapy is remarkably safe, some adverse effects such as irritation, erythema, stinging, colloid millia, contact dermatitis, nail discoloration and paradoxical postinflammatory hyperpigmentation have been reported in some patients, especially to the hydroquinone (HQ) component. Prolonged use of HQ may lead to the development

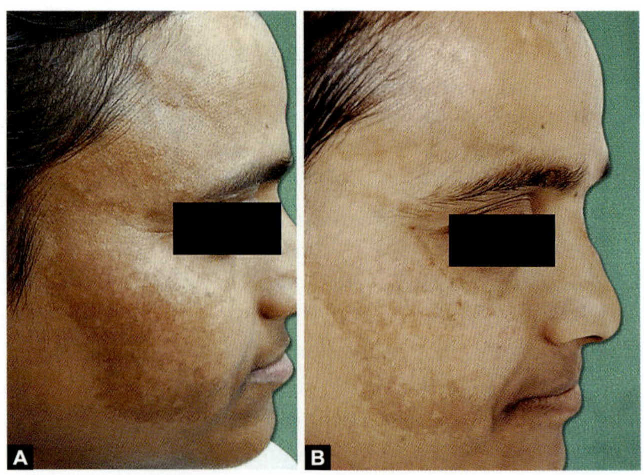

Figs. 1A and B: Pre- and post-photographs after 8 weeks of triple therapy.

of blue-black pigmentation in the affected areas called ochronosis.[27] Some authors have raised concern regarding the carcinogenicity of HQ in rodents; however not a single case of malignancy (cutaneous or internal) has been reported in human beings till date.[28]

There are, however, many issues with the triple combination: Most patients tend to use these formulations for a longer duration than advised. The steroid used in the combination can result in epidermal atrophy, erythema and hypertrichosis. So, dermatologists need to be cautious while prescribing the triple formulations and should stress on the importance of regular follow-up while prescribing them. There is an increasing feeling that the triple combinations should no longer be considered as first-line agents and be used only as third-line management in specific resistant cases. However, it yields excellent results under supervision.

Systemic Medical Therapy

Vitamin C thought to act by inhibiting tyrosinase, has been found to be ineffective. Pycnogenol (25 mg thrice daily for 30 days), obtained from bark of *Pinus pinaster*, a pine tree, is a powerful antioxidant. It is a more powerful antioxidant than vitamin C and E used at 75 mg/day, it protects against harmful effects of sun exposure.[29] Procyanidin is another similar agent with equivalent efficacy. Oral tranexamic acid is the most widely used systemic therapy, showing satisfactory results in most studies though prolonged administration may be required (250 mg twice daily for 6 months). Significant side effects in the form of visceral injury and coagulation problems may prevent its routine use.[30] Recently, glutathione, a potent antioxidant is being evaluated as a skin lightening agent as it has been found to inhibit the tyrosinase enzyme thus blocking melanin synthesis; however, some authorities have expressed doubts regarding its safety and efficacy. Although, intravenous glutathione is more popular, oral administration is being preferred for its better safety profile.[31]

Procedural Management

Chemical Peels

Chemical peels are described in detail in later chapters. What is discussed here is the use of chemical peels with specific reference to melasma. Glycolic acid (GA), salicylic acid (SA), trichloroacetic acid (TCA), lactic acid, mandelic acid, and arginine are the commonly used peeling agents for melasma **(Table 2)**.[32] They can be combined with medical treatment for rapid clearance. They are of definitive use in epidermal melasma. Few medium depth peels also help in dermal melasma by causing inflammation and inducing macrophages to phagocytose stagnant melanin though the chances of pigmentary changes are high. The type of chemical, concentration, the number of coats applied and duration of application are some of the factors which affect efficacy and

TABLE 2: Types of peel based on depth.

Type of peel	*Depth of necrosis*	*Agents used*				
		TCA	*GCA*	*SA*	*JS*	*Others*
Very superficial	Stratum corneum	10%	30–50%	20–30%	1–3 coats	Tretinoin 1–5%
Superficial	Stratum basale	10–30%	50–70%	–	4–7 coats	–
Medium peels	Upper reticular dermis	35–50%	+TCA	+TCA		

(GCA: glycolic acid; JS: Jessner's solution; TCA: trichloroacetic acid; SA: salicylic acid)

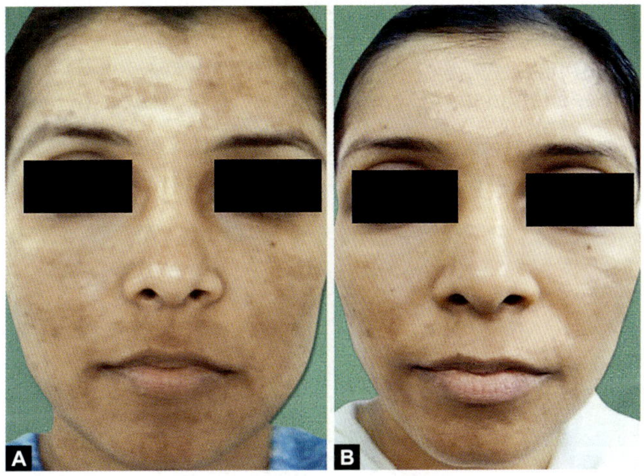

Figs. 2A and B: Pre- and post-photographs after three sessions of glycolic acid peel.

adverse effects.[33] The interpeel interval is dependent on peel depth, duration of contact and concentration of the agent. Proper selection of patients, good counseling, priming of skin, good operative and postoperative care are all essential for good cosmetic results.

Glycolic acid peel: For melasma peeling, 50–70% concentrations are used. They are safe and are repeated once in 3–4 weeks for a minimum of 3–4 peels. Once a month for 3 months, is a minimum requirement for noticing improvement **(Figs. 2A and B)**. Significant reductions in MASI have been achieved in 91% of subjects with epidermal forms responding better than mixed and dermal type not responding at all.[34] Combination with medical therapy enhances depth and penetration while reducing toxicity.[35] Modified Kligman formulation daily plus six serial GA treatments at 3-week intervals showed rapid and better improvements than modified Kligman's alone. Also combinations are useful in resistant cases when faster response is needed **(Figs. 3A and B)**.

Trichloroacetic acid peel: Beginners usually should start at 10–15%. Concentrations up to 20–25% can be safely used. TCA shows rapid but unpredictable response and has significant local reactions and relapse rate **(Figs. 4A and B)**. GA has slower onset, but incidence of local irritant reactions is less frequent. So, TCA is better used initially to get rapid response followed by GA as maintenance.

Salicylic acid peel: Used in concentrations ranging from 15 to 30%, they can be applied at weekly intervals for 6–8 weeks. A lipophilic derivative of the SA namely lipohydroxy acid, has newly been introduced. Used in concentrations of 5–10%, with a pH closer to normal skin pH, it has the advantage of not requiring neutralization.[36]

Jessner's peel: Effects are comparable to 70% GA.

Tretinoin peel: Tretinoin peels used in the strength of 5–10% are newer, slow-release peels found to be useful in melasma by helping to reduce epidermal pigmentation, minimizing photodamage and improving the texture of skin. Tretinoin peel (1% strength) applied for 4 hours once a week, for 12 weeks has been found to show equal efficacy as glycolic acid peel.[37]

Other peels: Arginine, lactic acid, mandelic acid, phytic acid and amino fruit peels are newer peels which have better safety profile and are increasingly being used nowadays, but their superiority is doubtful.

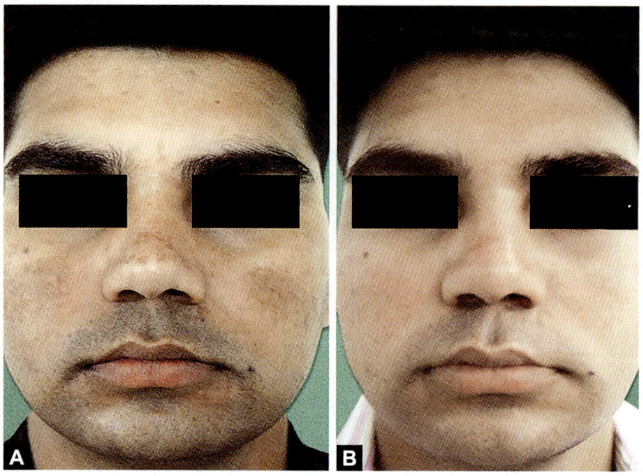

Figs. 3A and B: Pre- and post-photographs after three sessions of glycolic acid peel in addition to triple regime.

COMPLICATIONS

Postprocedure hyperpigmentation is the most common side effect, particularly in darker skin population. Others include: scarring, secondary infection, atrophy, milia and persistent erythema. Proper selection of patients, good counseling, skin priming, and supporting medications along with adequate intrapeeling and postpeel care are all essentials in achieving good cosmetic results. Identifying patients who are at risk and using milder peels can help in reducing complications.

Combination of peels: A combination of peeling agents enhances the depth of the peel without using a higher concentration of the peeling agent. However, these medium depth peels should be used cautiously in darker-skinned patients because of the risk of uneven depth of peeling and increased risk of side effects such as postinflammatory hyperpigmentation and scarring. The combinations include:

- Glycolic acid 70% combined with TCA 35%. In darker skins, lower concentrations of TCA (10–25%) may be used.
- Jessner's solution (JS) with 35% TCA (Monheit's peel).

Dermabrasion

Dermabrasion and microdermabrasion have been tried, but incidence of postprocedure hyperpigmentation precludes routine use, especially in darker skin. They are better utilized in refractory cases. Some reports, however, claim good improvement in dermal melasma treated with this modality.[38]

Laser Therapy

Laser treatment of melasma is usually not recommended as first-line therapy because of the high incidences of relapse,

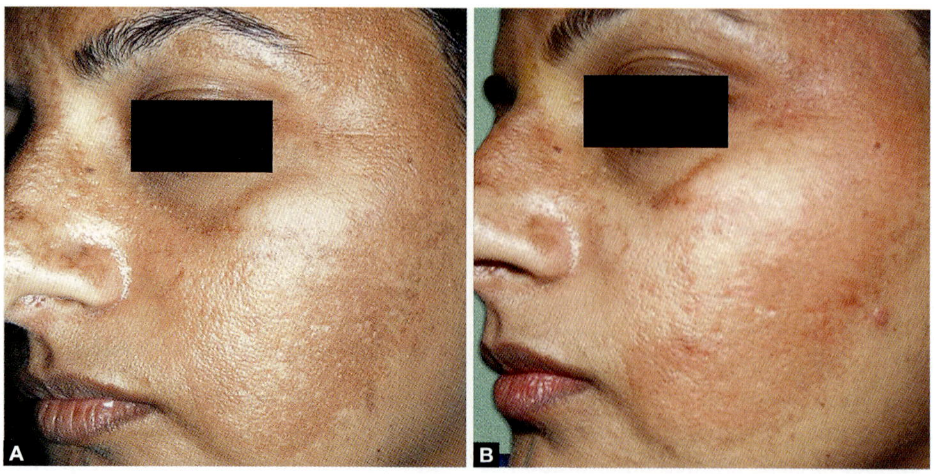

Figs. 4A and B: Pre- and post-photographs after five sessions of trichloroacetic acid peel.

postinflammatory hyperpigmentation, high cost and modest efficacy.[39] The various lasers which are reported to be of benefit are discussed accordingly.

Ablative Lasers

Erbium: YAG and CO_2 lasers are quite effective but not preferable for skin types IV to VI due to higher chances of scarring and pigmentary alteration.[40] Refractory melasma treated with combination of Erbium:YAG laser of 2920 nm wavelength and GA peels has shown significant improvement after 6 months.[41]

Q-switched Laser

- *Ruby*: QS Ruby laser was one of the earliest tried laser in melasma. However, due to severe postinflammatory hyperpigmentation, it is now not considered as a good therapy especially in the darker skin types.
- *Nd:YAG*: Q-switch Nd:YAG in the large spot size with low energy mode is gaining popularity as a new mode of therapy. Spot size of 6–8 mm diameter with energy of 400–900 mJ is ideal. Local weals and tiny purpura are the only transient side effects. By selective photothermolysis, the laser precisely targets lesional melanocytes. Another advantage is that it is effective in dermal melasma due to its deep penetration.[42]
- *Alexandrite*: 755 nm Q-switched Alexandrite laser has also been found to be effective in few cases.

Vascular Lasers

Lasers targeting the vascular component have been found to be recently useful in melasma.

- *Pulsed dye laser (PDL)*: The usage of PDL (585 nm, 595 nm) for the treatment of melasma is based on the rationale that skin vascularization plays an important role in the pathogenesis of melasma.
- *Copper bromide lasers:* Copper bromide lasers emit green beam with wavelength at 511 nm. With fluences ranging from 12 to 14 J/cm2, they can be utilized in treating pigmentary lesions. Spot size of 1 mm with emission time of 50–60 minutes, 7.7–8.3 pulses per second and four passes are the ideal settings. The advantage with green 511 nm wavelength of this laser is that the melanin absorbs this spectrum to greater extents producing a more selective damage. Also thermal destruction is restricted to melanin containing epidermis. It is valuable in cases with associated telangiectasia. Transient hyperpigmentation does occur in approximately 10% of the patients treated.[43] Another wavelength of 578 nm is also being used with some success.
- *1927-nm fractional low-powered diode laser:* It is still under trial and is a new option.

Intense Pulsed Light

Intense pulsed light (IPL) in the wavelength of 515–1,200 nm has shown satisfactory results in epidermal melasma. Cut-off filters can help deliver specific wavelengths depending on skin type. Lower fluences are preferred for preventing side effects.

Nonablative Fractional Resurfacing

It is a new method of treatment in melasma. Improvements to the tune of 80% have been registered 26–28 weeks after one session of fractional photothermolysis. Energy settings between 6 mJ and 8 with a density setting of 250 MTZs/cm^2 with total density of 2,000 MTZ/cm^2 is usually the ideal setting.[44] Three treatment passes are used with one-third horizontal and vertical overlap. It is useful in therapy resistant cases. Sessions can be repeated 3 weekly with improvement marked at 6 months postprocedure. Initial erythema for 2 days, followed by hyperpigmentation of 3–4 days, is the usually observed side effect. About 60%of patients reported 75–100% clearances in a study on fractional lasers in melasma.[45] The limitations are mainly in darker skin where efficacy and improvement is limited and recurrence rates are high.[46]

- *Fractional 1,550 nm erbium-doped fiber restore lasers*: Energy of 6–12 mJ with once in 4-week sessions for four sessions is the average duration of treatment. The wavelength of 1,550 nm allows penetration in dermis up to 300–1,400 mm depth leading to benefits in the treatment of dermal and mixed melasma.[47]
- *Q-switch fractional Ruby laser*: This new modality with wavelength of 692 nm, pulse width of 40 ns and spot size of 7.1 × 7.1 mm is being used successfully in certain centers. Fluences of 2–3 J/cm^2 with six sessions at 2-week intervals covering the whole face three times per session are found ideal for this therapy. This wavelength is more strongly absorbed and is definitely more selective for melanin than the similar Nd:YAG variant and should, therefore, be more useful in the times to come.[48]
- *Fractional thulium 1927 nm nonablative laser*: With its higher water absorption coefficient, lesser down-time, PIH and recurrence is another new laser on the horizon.

Combination lasers may provide better relief. The 950 µsec pulsed CO_2 laser in one pass at 300 mJ/cm^2 decreases the hyperpigmentation by removing the entire epidermis and destroying melanocytes. Following this, the application of Q-switched Alexandrite laser at 6 J/cm^2 can target dermal melanin.[49]

Laser Toning

This is a very recent, promising method wherein collimated, low fluence, Q-switched Nd:YAG 1,064 nm laser is being used with good results in several studies. This treatment reduces thermal damage by using top-hat beam mode, shorter pulse width, higher peak power and lower fluence. About 5–7 ns pulses with 7 mm spot size and 1.6–2.0 J/cm^2 fluences weekly for 8 weeks and two passes per treatment session have been found to be ideal. It works on the principle of *selective subcellular photothermolysis* and claims to damage only subcellular organelles such as melanosomes. Triple cream combination either before or after the laser therapy adds on to the benefits.[50]

Lasers do not alter the basic pathomechanisms of melasma namely genetic influences, sun exposure and hormonal factors. Lasers rarely give reproducible and long-standing improvement and recurrence almost always occurs. The high cost and risk of adverse effects place them as third line therapies for melasma. Medical management and chemical peels should ideally go hand in hand along with the laser therapy.

INVESTIGATIONAL THERAPIES

Recently, several novel/investigational therapies are being tried as none of the conventional therapies are able to secure complete cure and zero recurrence. *Microphthalmia-associated transcription factor-siRNA (small interfering ribonucleic acid) agents* are being tried as transdermal peptide targets which may inhibit the tyrosinase pathway of melanin production, without major side effects. Other novel options being investigated include *Metformin* (oral diabetic drug which may reduce melanin synthesis by reducing cAMP concentration within melanocytes), *topical proton-pump inhibitors like omeprazole* (hypothesized to block the role of copper as cofactor of tyrosinase by interfering with ATP7A) and a *combination topical therapy containing estrogen and VEGF antagonist*, to address both melanogenesis and vasculogenesis.[6]

TREATMENT OF MELASMA IN PREGNANCY

Treating melasma during pregnancy is debatable as the continuous hormonal upsurge would make treatment ineffective. Treatment should be ideally postponed till after delivery and preferably till end of lactation as safety of the drugs if absorbed into systemic circulation are not established. Melasma may regress or reduce spontaneously after delivery.

Quality of Life in Melasma

Quality of life in melasma can be assessed by the MELASQOL, an instrument consisting of a 10 question scale, on which patients are assessed on each question by a rating from 1 to 7 based on the Likert scale. Questions were based on physical, emotional, social and financial well-being. Scores range from 7 to 70 with higher scores indicating worse quality of life.[51] A recent Indian study has delineated the MELASQOL in Hindi for Indian population.[52,53]

Counseling

All patients must be counseled regarding natural course of melasma and necessity to adhere to long-term regimes. Recurrence of melasma occurs on exposure to sunlight and other sources of ultraviolet rays.

TIPS

- Sun protective measures and counseling are the cornerstones of therapy
- Sunscreens are the single most important medications in therapy
- Use medical management alone in epidermal melasma for good results
- Lasers along with bleaching agents and chemical peels are useful options in mixed and dermal melasma
- Even short-term benefits improve quality of life tremendously in melasma. So, therapy is justified, even though recurrence is unavoidable

PITFALLS

- Relapse is inevitable in melasma if strict sun protection is not adhered to
- Medical management cannot treat dermal component
- Lasers have still not proved to be the panacea for dermal melasma
- Pigmentary side effects are high restricting use of newer laser/surgical techniques

CONCLUSION

Treatment of melasma is very challenging due to its relapsing tendency, dermal component which is difficult to treat and emotional swings associated with the condition. Dermal and

TABLE 3: Suggested stepwise approach to management of different types of melasma.

	Epidermal	*Mixed*	*Dermal*
Step 1	Sun avoidance along with hydroquinone and other bleaching agents	Sun avoidance along with hydroquinone and other bleaching agents	Sun avoidance along with hydroquinone and other bleaching agents
Step 2	Superficial peels	Medium depth peels	• Medium depth peels, • Lasers: Q-switch Nd:YAG • Fractional Q-switch Ruby • Fractional erb glass
Step 3	• Q-switch Nd:YAG/IPL • Laser toning • Triple therapy	• Q-switch Nd:YAG • Fractional • Q-switch Ruby • Fractional erb glass • Triple therapy	

(Rider: Medium depth peels are to be done cautiously in darker skin).

mixed melasma are usually resistant to medical therapy. Laser, dermabrasion, chemical peels and camouflage are, therefore, required in such cases. Approach to treatment depends on type and severity of melasma. A stepwise approach which can be adopted based on presently available literature is as given in **Table 3**.

REFERENCES

1. Sarkar R, Puri P, Jain RK, Singh A, Desai A. Melasma in men: a clinical, aetiological and histological study. J Eur Acad Dermatol Venereol. 2010;24:768-72.
2. Al-Hamdi KI, Hasony HJ, Jareh HL. Melasma in Basrah: a clinical and epidemiological study. MJBU. 2008;26:1-5.
3. Pasricha JS, Khaitan BK, Dash S. Pigmentary disorders in India. Dermatol Clin. 2007;25:343-52.
4. Krupashankar DS, Somani VK, Kohli M, Sharad J, Ganjoo A, Kandhari S. A cross-sectional, multicentric clinicoepidemiological study of melasma in India. Dermatol Ther (Heidelb). 2014;4:71-81.
5. Sonthalia S. Pathogenesis of melasma. In: Sarkar R (Ed). Melasma: a monograph, 1st edition. New Delhi: Jaypee Brothers Medical Publications; 2014.
6. Rajanala S, Maymone MBC, Vashi NA. Melasma pathogenesis: a review of the latest research, pathological findings, and investigational therapies. Dermatol Online J. 2019;25:13030.
7. Kanwar AJ, Dhar S, Kaur S. Treatment of melasma with potent topical corticosteroids. Dermatol. 1994;188:170.
8. Katsambas A, Antoniou C. Melasma: classification and treatment. J Eur Acad Dermatol Venereol. 1995;4:217-23.
9. Hann SK, Im S, Chung WS, Kim DY. Pigmentary disorders in the South East. Dermatol Clin. 2007;25:431-8.
10. Vázquez M, Maldonado H, Benmamán C, Sánchez JL. Melasma in men. A clinical and histologic study. Int J Dermatol. 1988; 27:25-7.
11. Pandya AG, Hynan LS, Bhore R, Riley FC, Guevara IL, Grimes P, et al. Reliability assessment and validation of the MELASMA Area and Severity index (MASI) and a new modified MASI scoring method. J Am Acad Dermatol. 2011;64:78-83, 83.e1-2.
12. Jimbow K, Obata H, Pathak MA, Fitzpatrick TB. Mechanism of depigmentation by hydroquinone. J Invest Dermatol. 1974;62:436-49.
13. Talmer C, Fonseca RMR, Pereira FBC, Barcaui CB. Classification of melasma by dermoscopy: comparative study with Wood's lamp. Surg Cosmetic Dermatol. 2009;1:115-9.
14. Katoch S. Investigations in melasma: Dermoscopy in melasma. In: Sarkar R (Ed) Melasma: a monograph. New Delhi: Jaypee Brothers Medical Publishers (P) Ltd.; 2015. pp. 24-6.
15. Mahajan SA. Melasma. In: Khopkar U (Ed). Dermoscopy and trichoscopy in diseases of the brown skin. New Delhi: Jaypee brothers Medical Publishers (P) Ltd; 2012. pp.50-62.
16. Kang HY, Bahadoran P, Suzuki I, Zugaj D, Khemis A, Passeron T, et al. In vivo refelectance confocal microscopy detects pigmentary changes in melasma at a cellular level resolution. Exp Dermatol. 2010;19:e228-33.
17. Longo C, Pellacani G, Tourlaki A, Galimberti M, Bencini PL. Melasma and low-energy Q-switched laser: treatment assessment by means of in-vivo confocal microscopy. Lasers Med Sci. 2014;29:1159-63.
18. Tsilika K, Levy JL, Kang HY, Duteil L, Khemis A, Hughes R, et al. A pilot study using reflectance confocal microscopy (RCM) in the assessment of a novel formulation for the treatment of melasma. J Drugs Dermatol. 2011;10:1260-4.
19. Kang WH, Yoon KH, Lee ES, Kim J, Lee KB, Yim H, et al. Melasma: histopathological characteristics in 56 Korean patients. Br J Dermatol. 2002;146:228-37.
20. Lee DJ, Park KC, Ortonne JP, Kang HY. Pendulous melanocytes: a characteristic feature of melasma and how it may occur. Br J Dermatol. 2012;166:684-6.
21. Kim EH, Kim YC, Lee ES, Kang HY. The vascular characteristics of melasma. J Dermatol Sci. 2007;46:111-6.
22. Kang HY, Hwang JS, Lee ES, Ahn JH, Kim JY, Lee ES, et al. The dermal stem cell factor and c-kit are overexpressed in melasma. Br J Dermatol. 2006;154:1094-9.
23. Sarkar R, Gokhale N, Godse K, Ailawadi P, Arya L, Sarma N, et al. Medical Management of Melasma: A Review with Consensus Recommendations by Indian Pigmentary Expert Group. Indian J Dermatol. 2017;62:558-77.
24. Ahmed AM, Lopez I, Perese F, Vasquez R, Hynan LS, Chong B, et al. A randomized, double-blind, placebo controlled trial of oral Polypodium leucotomos extract as an adjunct to sunscreen in the treatment of melasma. JAMA Dermatology. 2013;149:981-3.
25. Lim JT. Treatment of melasma using kojic acid in a gel containing hydroquinone and glycolic acid. Dermatol Surg. 1999;25:282-4.
26. Kligman AM, Willis I. A new formula for depigmenting human skin. Arch Dermatol. 1975;11:40-8.
27. Rendon M, Berneburg M, Arellano I. Treatment of melasma. J Am Acad Dermatol. 2006;54:S272-81.
28. Sarkar R, Bansal S, Sethi S. Hydroquinone based therapies for melasma. In: Sarkar R (Ed). Melasma: Amonograph. New Delhi: Jaypee Brothers Medical Publishers (P) Ltd.; 2015. pp. 35-43.
29. Nordlund JJ, Grimes PE, Ortonne JP. The safety of hydroquinone. J Eur Acad Dermatol Venereol. 2006;20:781-7.
30. Sarkar R, Bhalla M, Kanwar AJ. A comparative study of 20% azelaic acid cream monotherapy versus a sequential therapy in the treatment of melasma in dark-skinned patients. Dermatol. 2002;205:249-54.
31. Ortonne JP, Passenow T. Melanin pigmentary disorders: treatment update. Dermatol Clin. 2005;23:209-26.
32. Sonthalia S, Daulatabad D, Sarkar R. Glutathione as a skin whitening agent: facts, myths, evidences and controversies. Ind J Dermatol Venereol Leprol. 2016;82:262-72.
33. Cotelessa C, Peris K, Onorati MT. The use of chemical agents in the treatment of different cutaneous hyperpigmentations. J Dermatol Surg. 1999;25:450-4.
34. Resnik SS, Resnik BI. Complications of chemical peeling. Dermatol Clin. 1995;13:309-12.
35. Javaheri SM, Handa S, Kaur I, Kumar B. Safety and efficacy of glycolic acid facial peel in Indian women with melasma. Int J Dermatol. 2001;40:354-7.
36. Kakita LS, Lowe NJ. Azelaic acid and combination therapy of facial hyperpigmentation in darker skinned patients: a clinical comparison with hydroquinone. Clin Ther. 1998;20:960-70.
37. Uhoda E, Pierard-Franchimont C, Pierard GE. Comedolysis by a lipohydroxy acid formulation in acne-prone subjects. Eur J Dermatol. 2003;13:65-8.
38. Khunger N, Sarkar R, Jain RK. Tretinoin peels versus glycolic acid peels in the treatment of melasma in dark-skinned patients. Dermatol Surg. 2004;30:756-60.
39. Kunachak S, Leelaudomlipi P, Wongwaisayawan S. Dermabrasion: a curative treatment for melasma. Aesthetic Plast Surg. 2001;25:114-7.
40. Taylor CR, Anderson RR. Ineffective treatment of refractory melasma and postinflammatory hyperpigmentation by Q-switched Ruby laser. J Dermatol Surg Onco. 1994;20:592-7.

41. Manaloto RM, Alster T. Erbium:YAG laser resurfacing for refractory melasma. Dermatol Surg. 1999;25:121-3.
42. Zhou X, Gold MH, Lu Z. Efficacy and safety of Q-Switched 1,064-nm neodymium-doped yttrium aluminum garnet laser treatment of melasma. Dermatol Surg. 2011;37:962-70.
43. Passeron T, Fontas E, Kang HY, Bahadoran P, Lacour JP, Ortonne JP. Melasma treatment with pulsed dye laser and triple combination cream: a prospective, randomized, single-blind, split-face study. Arch Dermatol. 2011;147:1106-8.
44. Lee HI, Lim YY, Kim BJ. Clinicopathologic efficacy of copper bromide plus/yellow laser (578 nm with 511 nm) for treatment of melasma in Asian patients. Dermatol Surg. 2010;36:885-93.
45. Tannous ZS, Astner S. Utilizing fractional resurfacing in the treatment of therapy-resistant melasma. J Cosmet Laser Ther. 2004;7:39-43.
46. Rokhsar CK, Fitzpatrick RE. The treatment of melasma with fractional photothermolysis: a pilot study. Dermatol Surg. 2005;31:1645-50.
47. Naito SK. Fractional photothermolysis treatment for resistant melasma in Chinese females. J Cosmet Laser Ther. 2007;9: 161-3.
48. Katz TM, Glaich AS, Goldberg LH. Treatment of melasma using fractional photothermolysis: a report of eight cases with long-term follow-up. Dermatol Surg. 2010;36:1273-80.
49. Jang WS, Lee CK, Kim BJ. Efficacy of 694-nm Q-switched Ruby fractional laser treatment of melasma in female Korean patients. Dermatol Surg. 2011;37:1133-40.
50. Nouri K, Bowes L, Chartier T, et al. Combination treatment of melasma with pulsed CO2 laser followed by Q-switched Alexandrite laser: a pilot study. Dermatol Surg. 1999;25:495-7.
51. Jeong SY, Shin JB, Yeo UC. Low-fluence Q-switched neodymium-doped yttrium aluminum garnet laser for melasma with pre- or post-treatment triple combination cream. Dermatol Surg. 2010;36:909-18.
52. Balkrishnan R, McMichael AJ, Camacho FT, Saltzberg F, Housman TS, Grummer S, et al. Development and validation of a health-related quality of life instrument for women with melasma. Br J Dermatol. 2003;149:572-7.
53. Sarkar R, Garg S, Dominguez A, Balkrishnan R, Jain RK, Pandya AG. Development and validation of a Hindi language health-related quality of life questionnaire for melasma in Indian patients. Indian J Dermatol Venereol Leprol. 2016;82:16-22.

CHAPTER 122

Approach to Diffuse Facial Pigmentation

Senkadhir Vendhan, Pankaj Das, Biju Vasudevan

KEY MESSAGES

- Facial pigmentation is a very common and challenging disorder.
- Identifying the etiology is paramount to avail good treatment options.
- Sunscreens and topical depigmenting creams are mainstay of treatment along with topical tacrolimus in a few conditions.
- Lasers, microdermabrasion, chemical peels and PRP also have significant roles in treatment of this group of disorders.

INTRODUCTION

Facial pigmentation disorders represent a significant challenge in dermatological practice, with diffuse facial pigmentation being one of the most common presentations encountered. The etiology of diffuse facial pigmentation is multifactorial, involving complex interactions between genetic predisposition, environmental factors, hormonal influences, and various cellular processes within the skin.[1] Diffuse facial pigmentation poses a significant challenge in dermatological practice, necessitating advanced procedural interventions for effective management. This chapter explores cutting-edge procedures employed in the treatment of diffuse facial pigmentation, focusing on their mechanisms of action, indications, efficacy, and safety profiles.

PATHOPHYSIOLOGY

Diffuse facial pigmentation encompasses a spectrum of conditions characterized by the abnormal accumulation of melanin, the pigment responsible for skin color, within the epidermis, dermis, or both. Melanogenesis, the process by which melanin is synthesized and distributed within the skin, is tightly regulated by a complex interplay of molecular pathways involving melanocytes, keratinocytes, fibroblasts, and various signaling molecules.[2]

DISEASES CAUSING DIFFUSE FACIAL PIGMENTATION[3]

Diseases causing diffuse facial pigmentation are as follows:

- Melasma
- Riehl's melanosis/pigmented cosmetic dermatitis
- Lichen planus pigmentosus (LPP)
- Periorbital melanosis
- Exogenous ochronosis
- Poikiloderma of civatte/erythromelanosis interfollicularis colli
- Erythromelanosis follicularis of the face and neck
- Erythema dyschromicum perstans (EDP)/ashy dermatosis of Ramirez, erythema chronicum figuratum melanodermicum
- Addisonian pigmentation
- Nevus of Ota
- Acanthosis nigricans (AN)
- Drug-induced pigmentation
- Postinflammatory hyperpigmentation
- Human immunodeficiency virus (HIV)
- Seborrheic melanosis

SEVERAL KEY MECHANISMS CONTRIBUTING TO THE DEVELOPMENT OF DIFFUSE FACIAL PIGMENTATION

- *Melanocyte activation and proliferation:* External stimuli such as ultraviolet (UV) radiation, inflammatory mediators, and hormonal fluctuations can stimulate melanocytes residing in the basal layer of the epidermis to increase their activity and proliferation.
- *Hyperpigmentation:* Increased production and transfer of melanin from melanocytes to adjacent keratinocytes result in hyperpigmentation of the epidermis and/or dermis, leading to clinically visible patches of pigmentation.
- *Postinflammatory hyperpigmentation (PIH):* Inflammatory processes, including acne, eczema, and trauma, can trigger the release of cytokines and growth factors that stimulate melanocyte activity, resulting in localized hyperpigmentation at the sites of inflammation.
- *Hormonal influences:* Hormonal changes associated with pregnancy, oral contraceptive use, or endocrine disorders can disrupt melanogenesis, leading to the development of

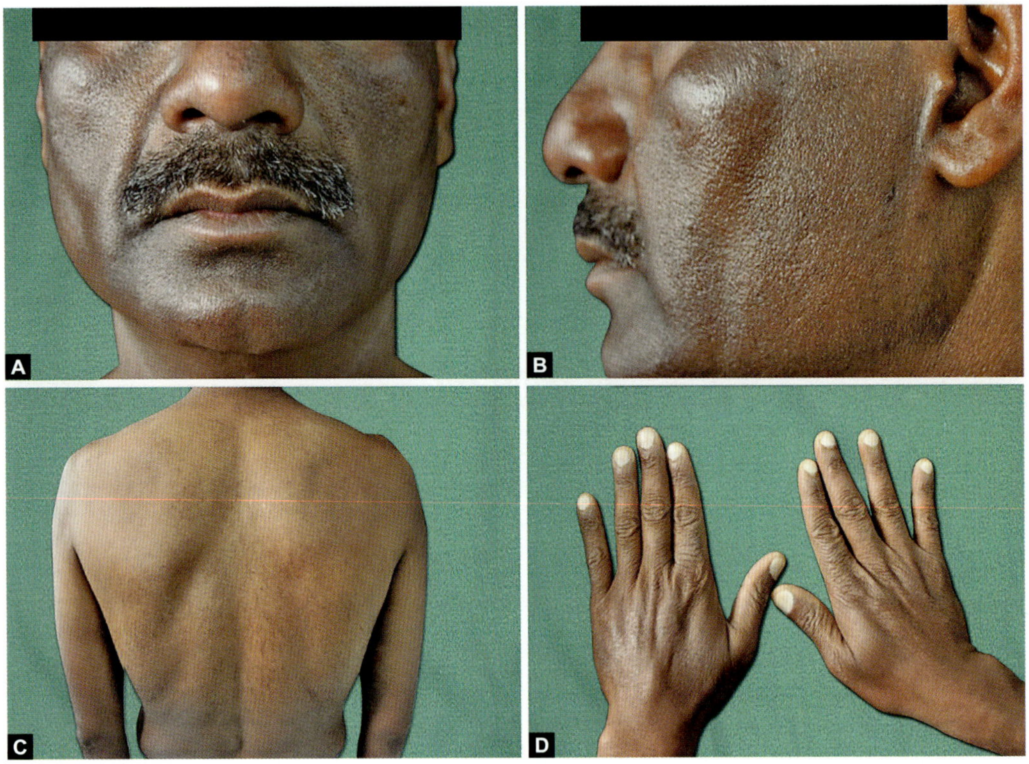

Figs. 1A to D: A patient presenting with diffuse hyperpigmentation of face and body and was found to be human immunodeficiency virus (HIV) positive.

melasma, a common form of diffuse facial pigmentation characterized by symmetric hyperpigmented patches.

- *Genetic factors:* Certain genetic polymorphisms and familial predispositions may increase an individual's susceptibility to developing diffuse facial pigmentation upon exposure to environmental triggers.[4]

APPROACH TO EVALUATION

The evaluation of patients presenting with diffuse facial pigmentation begins with a comprehensive history and physical examination, focusing on identifying potential triggering factors such as sun exposure, hormonal fluctuations, medications, and prior inflammatory skin conditions. History of application of hair dye, cosmetics, and over-the-counter skin lightening formulations containing steroids and hydroquinone must be taken. The body weight, risk of diabetes mellitus, and metabolic syndrome must be taken into account for evaluation of insulin resistance causing AN. Homeostatic model assessment for insulin resistance (HOMA-IR) should be calculated for all patients by assessing serum-fasting insulin and glucose levels. Metformin increases insulin sensitivity and is a preferred therapeutic option in AN.

Addison's disease and sometimes HIV can present with generalized pigmentation of the body, and patients must be investigated for the same **(Figs. 1A to D)**. Wood's lamp examination and dermoscopy may aid in assessing the depth and distribution of pigmentation, while histopathological examination of skin biopsies can provide valuable insights into the underlying pathophysiology.[5] The latter is especially helpful in identifying diseases like exogenous ochronosis, LPP, and EDP.

MANAGEMENT STRATEGIES

Management of diffuse facial pigmentation is tailored to the underlying etiology and may involve a combination of topical agents, procedural interventions, and lifestyle modifications. Sun-protection measures, including broad-spectrum sunscreen use and sun-protective clothing, are fundamental in preventing further pigmentation and minimizing UV-induced damage.

Topical agents such as hydroquinone, retinoids, azelaic acid, kojic acid, tranexamic acid, and corticosteroids can help inhibit melanogenesis, promote epidermal turnover, and reduce inflammation, thereby improving the appearance of hyperpigmented lesions **(Figs. 2A and B)**. Combination therapies utilizing multiple agents with complementary mechanisms of action may enhance treatment efficacy. In cases where diffuse facial pigmentation is refractory to conventional therapies, adjunctive treatments such as oral tranexamic acid, oral antioxidants, or fractional laser resurfacing may be considered under close supervision.[6]

Oral drugs indicated in facial pigmentation: Dapsone, isotretinoin, and oral steroids have been used in the management of LPP. Clofazimine has been reported to be effective in EDP;

however, isolated case reports point to the utility of dapsone as well.

ADVANCED PROCEDURES FOR THE MANAGEMENT OF DIFFUSE FACIAL PIGMENTATION

Chemical Peels

Chemical peels are a versatile modality for the management of diffuse facial pigmentation, offering tailored treatment options based on the depth of exfoliation required and the specific pigmentary concerns of the patient. The choice of peeling agent, concentration, and technique is individualized to optimize outcomes while minimizing adverse effects and downtime[7] **(Table 1)**.

Microdermabrasion

Microdermabrasion is particularly effective in addressing superficial pigmentation concerns by promoting the shedding of hyperpigmented keratinocytes and enhancing the penetration of topical depigmenting agents **(Table 2)**. Multiple sessions are often required for significant improvement, with minimal downtime and risk of complications. Combination therapies with chemical peels or topical agents may further enhance treatment outcomes by targeting multiple pathways involved in melanogenesis and skin remodeling.[8]

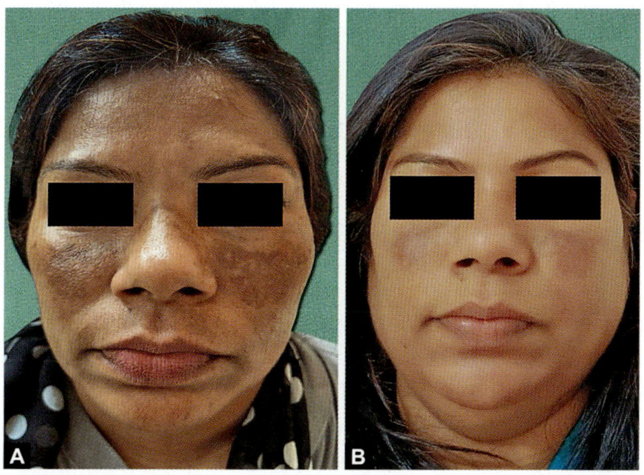

Figs. 2A and B: Melasma treated with kojic acid cream and sunscreen.

Laser Therapy

Laser therapy encompasses a diverse range of devices and modalities utilized in the treatment of diffuse facial pigmentation, offering precise targeting of melanin-rich lesions while sparing surrounding tissues.

- *Q-switched lasers*, including the neodymium-doped yttrium–aluminum–garnet (Nd:YAG) laser and alexandrite laser, emit short pulses of high-energy light at specific wavelengths, selectively targeting melanin within the skin and inducing photothermal destruction of pigmented cells. These lasers are particularly effective in treating melasma, lentigines, and PIH, with minimal risk of scarring or dyspigmentation.
- *Fractional laser resurfacing*, utilizing 1,540 nm/1,550 nm Er:glass laser, 2,940 nm Er:YAG laser, and 10,600 nm CO_2 laser, delivers microscopic columns of laser energy to the skin, promoting epidermal turnover, collagen remodeling, and uniform skin rejuvenation. This approach offers precise control over the depth and density of treatment, making it suitable for patients with diverse skin types and pigmentary concerns with reduced downtime and mostly avoiding adverse effects like PIH.
- *Fractional nonablative laser*, like thulium laser (1,927 nm and 1,550/1,540 nm), has shown promising results. The latter is the only laser treatment for melasma that has been approved by the Food and Drug Administration (FDA).

Combination therapies incorporating laser therapy with topical agents, chemical peels, or oral medications may synergistically enhance treatment efficacy while minimizing adverse effects and downtime. Laser therapy stands as a cornerstone in the management of diffuse facial pigmentation, providing safe and effective options for patients seeking improved skin appearance and texture[9] **(Figs. 3A and B)**.

Intense Pulsed Light Therapy

Intense pulsed light (IPL) therapy utilizes broad-spectrum light energy to target melanin and hemoglobin within the skin, offering a noninvasive approach to treating diffuse facial pigmentation and vascular irregularities. IPL devices emit multiple wavelengths of light, allowing for selective absorption by melanin and subsequent photocoagulation of pigmented lesions. This modality is particularly effective in treating diffuse melasma, solar lentigines, and telangiectasias, with minimal downtime and risk of

TABLE 1: Different peeling agents with depth of exfoliation, mechanism of action, and indications.

Peeling agent	*Depth of exfoliation*	*Mechanism of action*	*Indications*
Alpha-hydroxy acids (AHAs)	Superficial	Promote desquamation of hyperpigmented cells	Mild cases of diffuse facial pigmentation
Beta-hydroxy acids (BHAs)	Superficial	Similar to AHAs, with enhanced lipophilicity	Mild cases of diffuse facial pigmentation
Trichloroacetic acid (TCA)	Medium-depth	Induces collagen remodeling and neocollagenesis	Moderate cases of diffuse facial pigmentation
Phenol	Deep	Penetrates into the reticular dermis, leading to profound skin resurfacing and remodeling	Severe cases of diffuse facial pigmentation

TABLE 2: Microdermabrasion.

Procedure	*Description*	*Indications*
Microdermabrasion	Minimally invasive exfoliation technique utilizing abrasive crystals or a diamond-tipped wand to mechanically remove dead skin cells and stimulate epidermal renewal	Superficial pigmentation, including post-inflammatory hyperpigmentation and solar lentigines

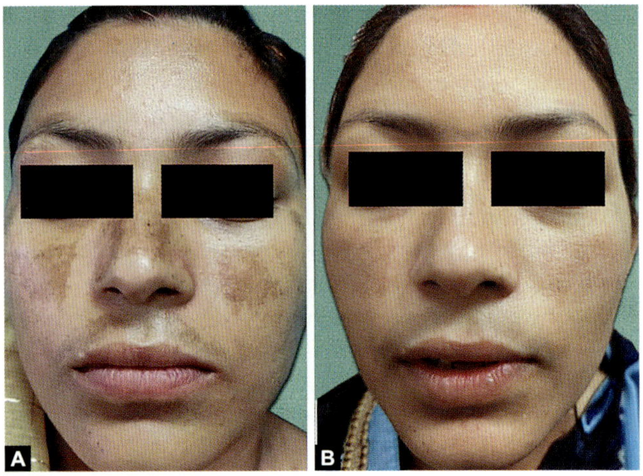

Figs. 3A and B: Improvement in melasma after four sessions of fractional CO_2 laser with platelet-rich plasma (PRP).

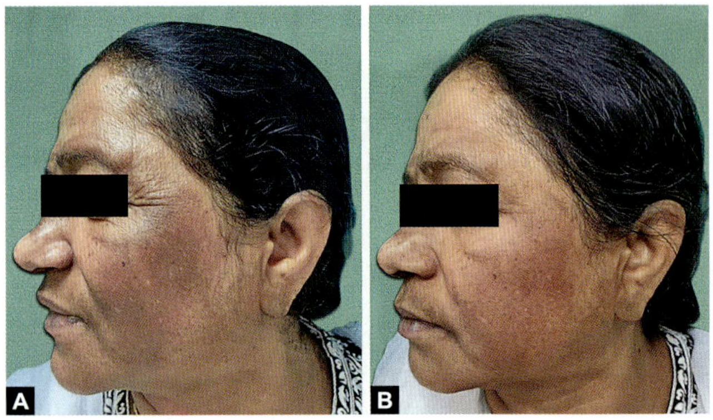

Figs. 4A and B: Improvement in facial hyperpigmentation after three sessions of radiofrequency (RF) microneedling with topical tranexamic acid.

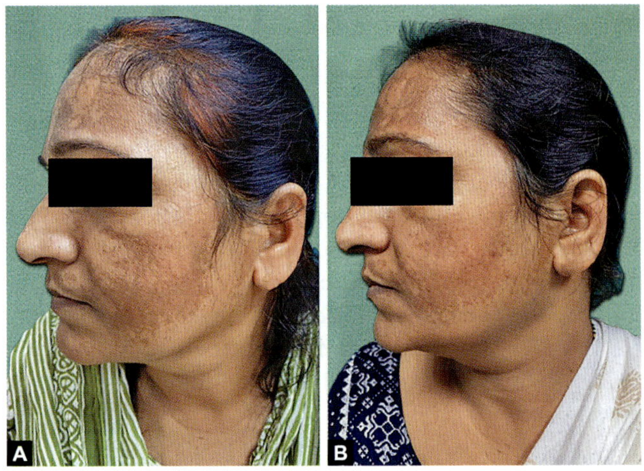

Figs. 5A and B: Improvement in facial hyperpigmentation after three sessions of microneedling with dermaroller, topical platelet-rich plasma (PRP), and topical tranexamic acid.

complications. Optimal treatment parameters, including pulse duration, fluence, and pulse sequence, are determined based on the patient's skin type, pigmentary disorder, and treatment goals. Combination therapies incorporating IPL therapy with topical agents, chemical peels, or laser therapy may further enhance treatment outcomes by targeting multiple components of the pigmentary pathway and vascular abnormalities.[10]

Radiofrequency Microneedling

Radiofrequency microneedling combines the benefits of microneedling with radiofrequency energy to stimulate collagen production, tighten skin, and improve skin texture and tone. This procedure involves the insertion of insulated or noninsulated microneedles into the skin, followed by the delivery of radiofrequency energy to the targeted tissue layers. Radiofrequency microneedling induces controlled thermal injury, leading to collagen remodeling, neocollagenesis, and tissue tightening, while sparing the epidermis and minimizing downtime. This modality is particularly effective in treating pigmentary disorders associated with skin laxity and textural irregularities, such as melasma and atrophic scars. Combination therapies incorporating radiofrequency microneedling with topical agents like tranexamic acid, chemical peels, or laser therapy may synergistically enhance treatment outcomes by addressing both pigmentation and skin aging[11] **(Figs. 4A and B)**.

Platelet-rich Plasma Therapy

Platelet-rich plasma (PRP) therapy involves the collection and concentration of autologous platelets from the patient's blood, followed by the injection or application of PRP into the skin. PRP contains growth factors, cytokines, and bioactive proteins that promote tissue regeneration, angiogenesis, and wound healing. PRP therapy is increasingly utilized in the management of diffuse facial pigmentation, offering a natural and biocompatible approach to skin rejuvenation and pigmentation correction. PRP injections can improve skin texture, tone, and luminosity while reducing the appearance of hyperpigmented lesions and vascular irregularities **(Figs. 5A and B)**. Combination therapies incorporating PRP therapy with microneedling with or without RF, laser therapy, or topical agents may enhance treatment efficacy by promoting collagen remodeling, neovascularization, and melanocyte regulation.[12]

CONCLUSION

Advanced procedural interventions play a pivotal role in the management of diffuse facial pigmentation, offering precise targeting of pigmentary abnormalities while minimizing downtime and risk of complications. Chemical peels, microdermabrasion, laser therapy, IPL therapy, radiofrequency microneedling, and PRP therapy represent versatile modalities that can be tailored to the individual patient's needs, skin type, and pigmentary concerns. By integrating advanced procedures with comprehensive skincare regimens and preventive measures, diffuse facial pigmentation can be effectively managed and enhance the overall health and appearance of the skin. Ongoing research and technological advancements in the field of dermatology continue to expand the armamentarium of procedural options available for the management of pigmentary disorders, offering new opportunities for innovation and improvement in patient care.

REFERENCES

1. Mosca S, Morrone A. Human skin pigmentation: from a biological feature to a social determinant. Healthcare (Basel). 2023;11(14):2091.
2. Videira IF, Moura DF, Magina S. Mechanisms regulating melanogenesis. An Bras Dermatol. 2013;88(1):76-83.
3. Dharman BK, Sridhar S. Diffuse facial melanosis: an overview of etiology and dermoscopic findings. J Skin Sex Transm Dis. 2020;2(2):86-93.
4. Brown DA. Skin pigmentation enhancers. J Photochem Photobiol B. 2001;63(1-3):148-61.
5. Thawabteh AM, Jibreen A, Karaman D, Thawabteh A, Karaman R. Skin pigmentation types, causes and treatment: a review. Molecules. 2023;28(12):4839.
6. Moolla S, Miller-Monthrope Y. Dermatology: how to manage facial hyperpigmentation in skin of colour. Drugs Context. 2022;11:2021-11-2.
7. Samargandy S, Raggio BS. Chemical peels for skin resurfacing. In: StatPearls [Internet]. Treasure Island (FL): StatPearls Publishing; 2024. [online] Available from: https://www.ncbi.nlm.nih.gov/books/NBK547752/ [Last accessed February, 2024].
8. Shah M, Crane JS. Microdermabrasion. In: StatPearls [Internet]. Treasure Island (FL): StatPearls Publishing; 2024. [online] Available from: https://www.ncbi.nlm.nih.gov/books/NBK535383/ [Last accessed February, 2024].
9. Arora P, Sarkar R, Garg VK, Arya L. Lasers for treatment of melasma and post-inflammatory hyperpigmentation. J Cutan Aesthet Surg. 2012;5(2):93-103.
10. Goldberg DJ. Current trends in intense pulsed light. J Clin Aesthet Dermatol. 2012;5(6):45-53.
11. Singh A, Yadav S. Microneedling: advances and widening horizons. Indian Dermatol Online J. 2016;7(4):244-54.
12. Everts P, Onishi K, Jayaram P, Lana JF, Mautner K. Platelet-rich plasma: new performance understandings and therapeutic considerations in 2020. Int J Mol Sci. 2020;21(20):7794.

SECTION 17

Miscellaneous Topics in Aesthetics

CHAPTER 123

Aesthetics of Nail

Soni Nanda, Sonal Bansal

KEY MESSAGES

The number of nail cosmetic procedures being done at the salons are increasing by the day. It is pertinent for the dermatologist to have full knowledge about these in order to identify any side effects caused and guide the patient accordingly. Also the number of patients visiting a dermatologist for nail issues is going up steadily. The aesthetic procedures like chemical peels and gel nails can be integrated in our everyday dermatology practice to increase the patient satisfaction by many folds, for our patients facing difficult to treat nail issues. In the current chapter, we aim to talk about the commonly used nail cosmetics, routinely performed nail procedures in salons and aesthetic procedures done by dermatologists, highlighting the detailed procedure, indications, contraindications and the expected side effects.

INTRODUCTION

Historically nail has been an important tool in protecting terminal phalanx against injury, improving manual dexterity, and the ability to pick up small objects. Ancient civilizations such as Egypt and China have been practicing the art of nail adornment by painting it in various colors. Their increasing demand is indicated by the plethora of nail care products and cosmetics available in the market these days. With an increase in awareness and spending power of today's consumer, the desire for healthy skin and hair has now extended to the nails as well.

Nail care clinics and salons are now seen everywhere. The upward trend of this industry is here to stay and its expansion requires the dermatologist to be aware of the procedures and techniques applied. An aware customer may want to consult a dermatologist to know more about the pros and cons of the nail products and adornment techniques. Complications and side effects associated would invariably be treated by a dermatologist and hence a thorough knowledge of the probable ingredients and processes involved is imperative **(Table 1)**.[1]

A vast medical armamentarium of both topical and systemic drugs is now available for nail disorders. Also, the use of intralesional therapies is increasing by the day. Still due to side effects or associated pain, we often see cases where the severity of nail abnormality may not warrant medical therapy.

TABLE 1: Adverse reactions/complications due to nail cosmetics.[1]

Nail cosmetics—adverse reactions	*Cause*	*Management*
Acute bacterial paronychia	Cutting of skin during pedicure or manicure	Avoid cutting of cuticles and sterilize the equipment properly
Chronic paronychia	Cuticle cutting, irritant contact dermatitis, water exposure	Protect cuticle, if proven yeast infection—antifungal, swollen nail folds—topical corticosteroid
Brittle nails	Dehydration due to solvent exposure	Avoid harsh chemicals. Do not use nail polish remover frequently
Allergy	Acrylates, formaldehyde, TSFR in nail polish	Avoid using cosmetics in known cases of allergy
Fracture of nail plate	Long and rigid extensions	Keep nail enhancements short and thin, enough to be flexible
Infections *Bacterial:* Mycobacterium *Fungal:* Yeast (Candida), dermatophyte *Viral:* Herpetic, verruca, other systemic Viral diseases	Infections caused by improper sanitation of implements used on multiple clients	Antifungal, antibiotic or antiviral as per the nature of infection
Onycholysis	Bond between the artificial nail and the natural nail plate is stronger than the adhesion between the natural nail and the nail bed and minor trauma rips the nail from the nail bed	Rest to nails every 3 months

(TSFR: toluenesulfonamide formaldehyde resin)

In such cases aesthetic procedures such as gel nails and nail peels come to the rescue and prove to be useful treatment modality. While these procedures can be made a part of our treatment armamentarium, they can also cause a variety of side effects if not done properly. The aim of present chapter is to discuss various aesthetic procedures, their uses in a dermatologist's clinic and their side effects.

CHARACTERISTICS OF A HEALTHY NAIL[2]

Healthy nails indicate internal well-being as well as attention to personal hygiene and fashion trends. A nail is considered healthy if it has these features:

- A surface that is smooth and glossy
- A tip extending beyond the nail bed
- When viewed from above—an oval contour; when viewed laterally—a gentle curve
- Healthy periungual tissue with smooth and nonragged cuticle
- Translucent so that pink nail bed is clearly visible.

The fingernails are longer than wide, whereas most toenails are wider than long.

NAIL CARE: NAIL GROOMING AND CONSEQUENCES OF IMPROPER GROOMING

Improper grooming techniques and excess use of cosmetic products lead to discolored and damaged nails which invariably land up in dermatologist's office. An important component of treatment then constitutes educating the patients regarding personal hygiene and nail care. Pertinent pointers are elaborated in **Table 2**.[3]

Manicure and Pedicure

They are most popular grooming procedures for hands and feet.

TABLE 2: Points for patients for nail care and hygiene.

1.	Keep chemicals, soaps and detergents exposure to a minimum
2.	Avoid excessive wetting of nails
3.	Avoid nail biting and picking of periungual skin
4.	Wear gloves while doing gardening, household chores, etc.
5.	Avoid cutting nails too short or pointed, they should always be cut parallel to the free edge of the nail plate
6.	Soaking nails before cutting, decreases the mechanical stress
7.	Be wary of over-aggressive nail technicians; too much cuticle manipulation or over buffing can lead to irreversible nail plate changes
8.	Avoid sharing nail care instruments in a salon
9.	Be cautious with extra-long nails; they may easily result in substantial injury to the nail unit and its components
10.	Filing should be optimally performed in a single direction

Definition: When fingernails or toenails are cleaned, shaped, and sometimes augmented by the application of a nail lacquer or other nail enhancement, it is called a manicure or pedicure. It might also involve the smoothening or filing of any calluses, especially on soles.[4]

There is a plethora of nail lacquers available in the market including the chic looking French manicure nail paint. They look very attractive and hygienic.

Precautions to be Taken During a Manicure/Pedicure[5]

- Distal filing is preferred over clipping of nails and should always be done with a disposable filer.
- Trimming should be done shaping the nail with a very slight curve with corners left untouched to avoid ingrown nails and paronychia. When clipping is necessary, the cutting implement should be held perpendicular to the nail plate to prevent onychoschizia.[6]
- Manipulation of cuticles should be as less as possible as damaged cuticle could lead to bacterial, fungal or viral infections.
- Aggressive buffing should be avoided as it can lead to thinning of nails.

Thus a fairly simple and routine procedure has the potential to sometimes irreversibly damage the cosmesis of the nail unit, or cause chronic infections with a long recovery period **(Boxes 1 and 2)**.

Nail Cosmetics

The most common nail cosmetic being used is the humble nail polish, variously known as nail paint, nail enamel and

BOX 1: Safety concerns regarding nail salons and spas.

- All metal instruments should be sterilized after each use
- Files should be disposable
- Preferably use your own the nail polish
- Pedicure baths should be washed and all suction screens cleaned between nail clients
- Be aware that hepatitis B carriers may be high among nail technicians and that *carriers are* asymptomatic

BOX 2: Patient information on safe use of nail products and salons.

- Use a licensed nail technician and salon
- Wash hands before going to nail salon
- Look for cleanliness in the salon
- Ask about sanitization and sterilization in the salon
- Bring your own instruments, particularly files that cannot be sterilized
- If you experience any itching or burning, inform the staff immediately, it could signal a reaction
- Allergy to nail polish can affect the face, eyelids, and neck
- Keep nail extensions short
- Do not allow the technician to file the surface of the nail excessively
- Do not over buff the nails, which can weaken them
- Wear gloves for all wet work chores to protect the manicure and help prevent infections associated with artificial enhancements
- If you experience a nick or cut during a salon procedure, seek medical attention to avoid infections

nail lacquer. Its primary purpose is beautification of nails. They have also been found to give mechanical protection, improve water binding of the nail and the base coat has been used to fill in fractures and camouflage ridges. Nail polish, once applied, should be removed after 4 days, especially in health care workers and food handlers, else it can harbor microorganisms.[7]

Nail polish remover is another commonly used nail cosmetic. The most common available are acetone based and excess use can lead to nail dryness and irritant reactions in some cases. Acetone-free nail polish removers containing ethyl acetate, butyl acetate, or ethyl lactate are now available. Nail polish remover pads containing gamma-butyrolactone, are safe and convenient to use. Rarely they get converted to GHB (gamma-hydroxybutyrate) resulting in systemic toxicity.[8]

Adverse Reactions to Nail Polish

- *Allergic dermatitis:* Usually sites distant from the fingers develop this dermatitis. It is seen in 1–3% of cases, and the most common presentation is unilateral eyelid dermatitis or linear areas of dermatitis on the face and neck caused by habitual rubbing of these areas with freshly painted fingernails. Rarely generalized eczema or involvement of the genitalia may be seen.

  The most common allergen is 7% thermoplastic resin toluene sulfonamide formaldehyde resin (TSFR) which is the most common adhesive used in nail polish. Hypoallergic nail polishes have alkyl polyester resins instead.
- *Color changes:* Prolonged use can lead to yellow/red discoloration which fades in 14 days. The proximal end of the discoloration is parallel to the proximal nail fold.
- Nail keratin granulations can simulate superficial white onychomycosis. It usually happens when the old nail polish is not removed before applying a fresh coat **(Fig. 1)**.
- Nail polish removers (acetone based) cause dryness and brittleness.

Nail moisturizers, hardeners, and nail Shellacs are also commonly used nail cosmetics **(Table 3)**.

Nail Adornments

- To enhance cosmetic appeal of nail polish, several ready-to-use plastic or metal artifacts are available that have to be applied immediately, after polish application.
- The design pieces are skillfully lifted from a template with forceps and placed on the freshly applied wet nail polish.
- Top coat is applied to prevent dislodgement.

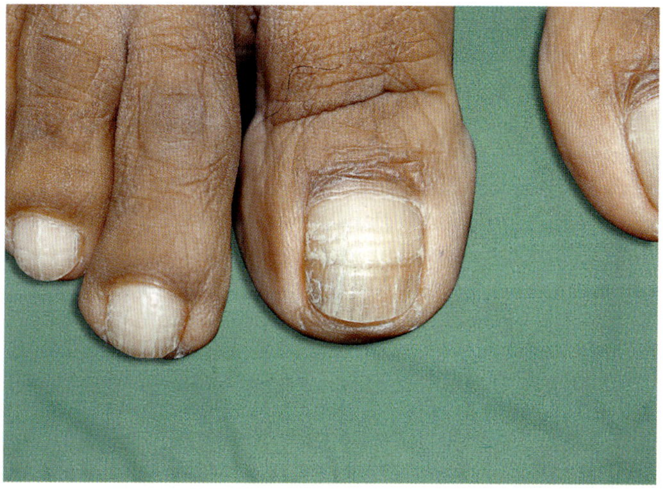

Fig. 1: Superficial white granulations due to prolonged nail paint use.

TABLE 3: Differences between nail moisturizers, hardeners and shellacs

	Nail moisturizers	*Nail hardeners*[9,10]	*Nail shellacs*[11]
Ingredients	Creams/lotions containing occlusives (petrolatum or lanolin), humectants (glycerin, propylene glycol), proteins, fluorides (ammonium hexafluorophosphate) and silicium	Titanium–silicone–zirconium polymers, polyteflon, nylon, calcium, biotin, keratin, vitamins, calcium fluoride, natural oils, nylon fibers, Teflon and silk	Hybrid, meaning half nail polish, half gel
Method of application	Applied under occlusion at bedtime for minimum 3 months	A modification of nail polish that is applied as a base coat for the purpose of strengthening the nail plate	Similar to nail polish on natural nails
Side effects/ Limitations	None	Contact allergic dermatitis, onycholysis and subungual hyperkeratosis	• No lengthening of nails possible • Special removal process • Requires a healthy nail for application • Removal process may weaken the nail plate
Advantages	Moisturizes the nails and periungual area	Strengthens the nail plate	• Natural look and shine • Increases flexibility and durability of nail plate • Lasts up to 14 days
Brands	Si Nails	OPI, Sally Hansen	Patent pending nail product created by creative nail design (CND)

- If one allows the first layer of color polish to dry and then apply a second contrasting color on top that also gives an aesthetic nail design.

Artificial nails are being very commonly used for both medical and cosmetic purposes. These are more durable than nail polish. Preformed nails are useful for breaking the habit of nail biting and also for lengthening/ reinforcing soft, brittle or damaged nails. These can be partially attached as nail tips or used to reinforce the entire length as sculpted nails (acrylic or gel based).

Nail Tips/Nail Extensions

These are plastic plates used to elongate nails and are readily available at nail salons. They are available in a variety of styles: colored-uncolored, precut-uncut, press-on, pre-glued forms and in forms requiring glue application. The nails also come in a variety of sizes and shapes to match the patient's natural nail plate.[12] These are glued to the free edge of the nails after a rough filing with adhesives containing methacrylate or ethyl 2-cyanoacrylate. The glued on tips may then be painted or decorated with nail art and finally coated with acrylic or gel. They can be removed with acetone.

Despite the wide variety of options available, patients do not find a suitable preformed nail, accounting for the increasing popularity of custom-made nail prostheses.

Custom nail prostheses, also known as sculptured nails are an increasingly popular method of obtaining long, hard nails.

Sculptured nails can be *acrylic, gel or nail wraps* (silk, linen, and fiberglass).

Nail wraps[13]*:* These wraps are thin products made from paper, silk, linen, fiberglass, mesh, or other fabrics applied to the nail for extra reinforcement. Developed in the early 1980s, they can be embedded within acrylics and gels or used as a natural nail coating or extension and sealed with resin.

They cannot lengthen the nails, hence someone who is looking to keep their short nails strong, would be an ideal candidate. These are also a possible alternative for those who are allergic to chemicals used in the acrylic or gel process. They are also a viable option for "transitioners", or clients who are giving up acrylics and want to grow out their nails. As these people have weaker nails and are predisposed to a higher chance of breakage, nail wraps are a good way to keep these nails stronger.

Acrylic nails[14]*:* Acrylic nails are a combination of a liquid monomer (ethyl methacrylate) and a powder polymer (polymethacrylate). Hence in common parlance, they were referred to as "liquid and powder" nails. As it hardens on air exposure, a uniform thin layer is applied quickly. It is transparent after setting and provides a robust canvas for further nail adornment. They last long and can be removed easily. Small breaks or fractures can almost always be corrected at home. But they require more care than natural fingernails. They need filling every 2–3 weeks wherein new acrylic is applied proximally and the loose acrylic is clipped from the nail edge. Else a lever arm gets created that predisposes the natural nail plate to traumatic onycholysis. Since they look less natural, especially if applied incorrectly, they are losing popularity. The application involves strong chemicals and fumes which inhibit its use in pregnancy. If they are used continuously for 2–4 months, they also have a real potential to damage the nail bed. The natural nail plate may become yellow, dry, thin with multiple ridges **(Fig. 2)**. It is highly recommended that the patient's natural nail be allowed to grow and act as a support, by stopping the acrylic nail application every 3 months.

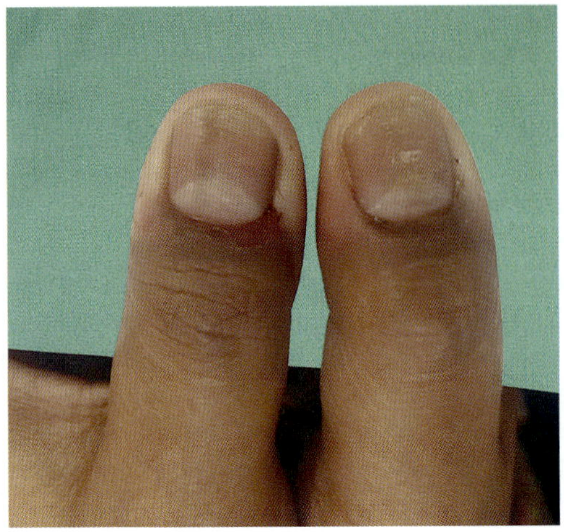

Fig. 2: Damage due to repeated acrylic nail application.

Gel nails: Gel nails, which started with the use of dental porcelain gel, have been around for last four decades. In present time, thin, clear, flexible gel acrylic has become the most popular type of sculptured nails.

Hard gel and soft gel are the available types. Hard gel post curing, is tough enough to be made into a nail extension while soft gels are too soft to create a nail extension. This includes gel polishes and thicker gels meant for gel-overlay services. Soft gels can be easily integrated in dermatologists' practice and will be discussed in this chapter.

Gel nails, has been gaining lot of popularity in the last 10 years but are being done mostly at nail salons. These are primarily being used to enhance the look of natural nails and make the nail polish stay for a longer time **(Figs. 3A and B)**. Gel nails are more natural and glossy, safer, more ecofriendly and procedure causes no fumes. But they are not durable, self-fixing is difficult and are more expensive.

With right patient selection and correct technique, gel nails can be used to improve the appearance of cosmetically disfigured nails where other treatment options are not warranted, either because the condition is self-limiting or irreversible; or to avoid possible drug side effects.[15] Also these can be useful to increase the patient satisfaction while medical treatment takes time to show results.

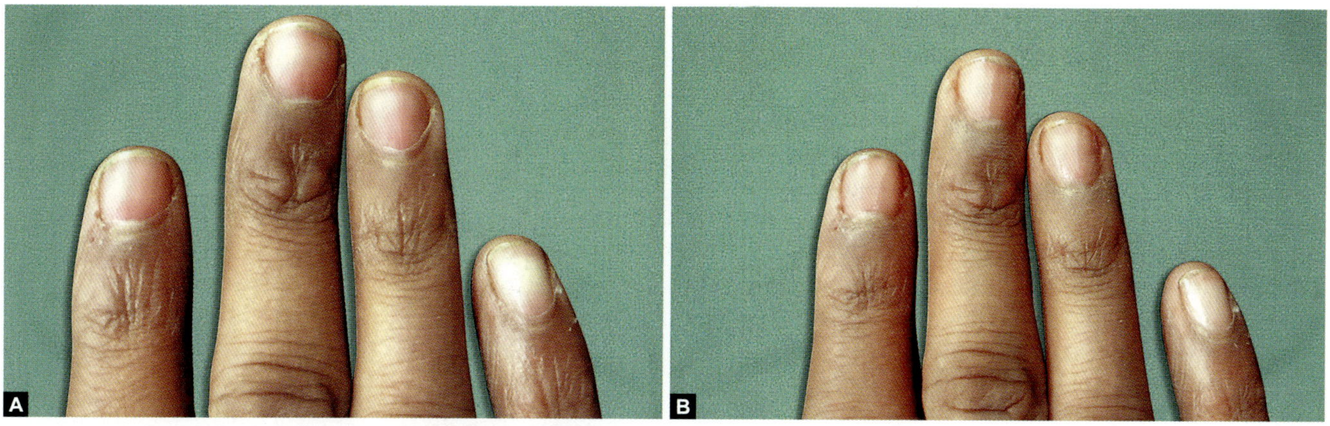

Figs. 3A and B: (A) Normal nail; (B) Gel on normal nail.

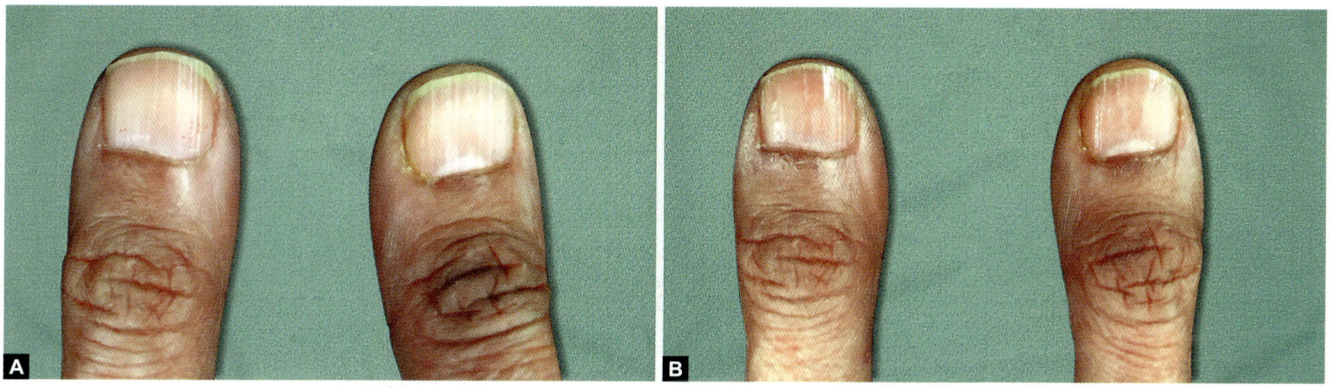

Figs. 4A and B: (A) Pregel onychorrhexis; (B) Postgel onychorrhexis.

Indications[16]

Gel nails have been used to improve the appearance of normal nails and diseased nails. They impart luster and give a shiny look to the nail. They also make the nail polish stay for long. Also, they have camouflaging capability in nails with superficial abnormalities. It has been seen that gel nails improve the patient satisfaction manifold when combined with medical treatment in conditions such as nail lichen planus or psoriasis where treatments takes a long time for nails to improve. Also, gel nails are very useful for conditions such as brittle nails and for breaking the habit of nail biting. These have also been found to be useful in professionals like guitarist who experience damaged nails due to occupational reasons. Gel nails are an excellent option for improving quality of life inventory (QOLI) in patients with self-limiting conditions like trachyonychia or nails with permanent damage like pterygium.

Authors have used gel nails in various conditions such as trachyonychia, nail pitting, onychorrhexis **(Figs. 4A and B)**, onychoschizia, Beau's lines, nail psoriasis, nail lichen planus (even with pterygium), onychophagy (nail biting) and brittle nails with gratifying results. The use of gel nails on cosmetically disfigured nails is also more rewarding as compared to their use over apparently normal nails. This is because, commonly the rate of growth of diseased nails is slower; hence, gel nail lasts longer. The nail plate in most of the disfigured cases is already not smooth; hence minimal, if any, buffing is required. Also where nail plate is thick buffing does not cause damage to the nail plate as opposed to using it on normal nail plate. Also, patient satisfaction is much higher as any improvement in their nail condition is very gratifying to them.

Contraindications

- Infection of the nail plate or surrounding skin like onychomycosis or paronychia.
- Cases of melanonychia
- Known allergy to acetone or any component of gel.

Procedure: Application of gel nails: The nail plate is cleaned and degreased with alcohol. Paraffin ointment should be applied on the nail fold and the cuticle. Careful buffing of the nail plate surface is done to ensure smooth and steady application of primer. A very thin coat of primer (100% methacrylic acid) that acts as a double sticking tape is applied. It helps remove oils and dehydrate the nail plate, ensuring better adhesion of the artificial nails. This is known to be caustic for skin and may cause nail thinning, hence minimal application is advocated. Newer gel nails that do not use primer are in the pipeline.

Subsequently, a single layer of nail gel is applied. This can be used as a double coat if the condition demands; in that case, each layer needs to be cured separately.

The last step is curing, or hardening. This is done under an ultraviolet (UV) light or light emitting diode (LED) lamp. A comparison of both these light sources is given in **Table 4**.

It is seen that the time for curing/hardening with a UV lamp is 2 minutes while LED light cures in 30 seconds. Skin of the hand should be covered with cloth or gloves cut at the tips can be used, when curing is done. Patient is also advised regular use of sunscreens on hands postprocedure. Any remnant of gel that has not been cured is removed with a gel remover.

This procedure should be conducted in a well-ventilated room with exhaust and the operator should wear a mask to minimize the side effects to the operator.

The apparatus required for gel nails is depicted in **Figure 5**.

Removal of gel nails: Removing gel nails by dipping hands in pure acetone for 30 minutes is the normal salon practice that is mostly responsible for the acquired brittleness of nails and contact dermatitis of surrounding skin. These can be safely removed by using nail polish remover-soaked cotton under occlusion on the nail for 5–7 minutes. In some cases, scraping out of gel nail might be required. This might leave the nail looking dry and dull. Some peeling of the surrounding skin may also be seen. The patient is advised to use lots of moisturizer on the nail and skin. At least a 1-week gel nail free period, should be advised to all patients. During this period patient should be advised to extensively use moisturizer on nail and the surrounding skin.

TABLE 4: Comparison of Light Emitting Diode (LED) light and Compact Fluorescent Lamp [CFL (UV)] lamp.

LED	*CFL*
Emits visible light with UV light	Emits UV light
Expensive	Relatively cheap
Long lasting (50,000 hours)	Requires earlier replacement of bulb (5,000 hours)
More efficient (30–60 sec)	Less efficient (2–4 min)
More portable	Less portable
Low UV exposure	Relatively high UV exposure
Does not cure all gel nails	Cures all types of gel nails

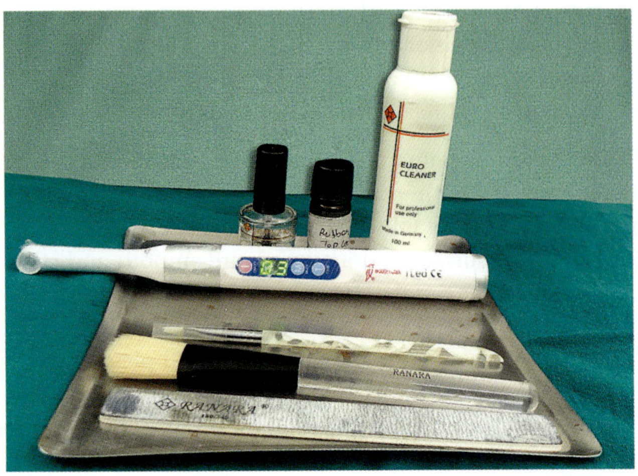

Fig. 5: Apparatus for gel nail.

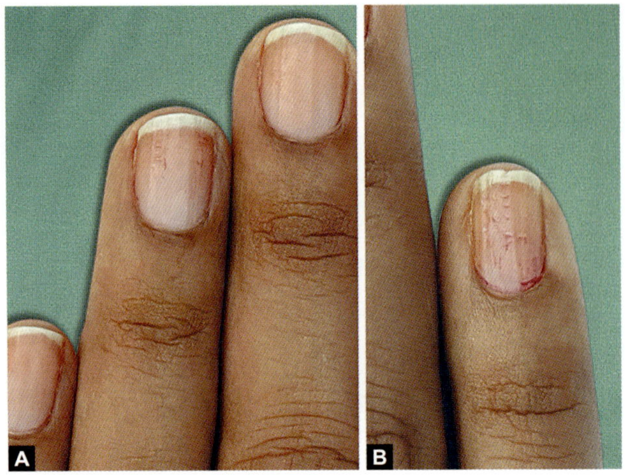

Figs. 6A and B: (A) Dryness postgel nail removal in a nail salon; (B) Damaged nail postgel nail removal in a nail salon.

Side effects: Reported side effects include dryness of nails **(Figs. 6A and B)**, contact allergic dermatitis of surrounding skin, paronychia, brittleness, masking of underlying nail disorders and reported cases of nonmelanoma skin cancer.[17] However, most of these side effects can be avoided by using the proper technique for gel application. Additionally, the initial claims of increased risk of skin cancer due to UV curing have been refuted by subsequent publications. Markova and Weinstock have shown that 250 years of weekly nail treatment is equivalent to a single course of NB UVB.[18] It has been proved that two hands in UV lamp for 10 min, twice/month amounts to 2.7 min in sunlight every day for 1 month. According to Dowdy and Sayer, UV Lamp can be used for 2.8 h/day without additional protective measure,[19] whereas for curing gel nails, the exposure amounts to 2 minutes per curing cycle.

Key points to decrease the side effects of gel nails:

- Choose your patient wisely
- Avoid manipulation of the cuticle
- Do nail buffing only where required
- Avoid doing in-fills (to avoid missing underlying nail disease)
- Advise the patient to apply sunscreen regularly on hands
- While putting the hand in the UV lamp cover the rest of the hand with a white cloth or glove with tips cut
- If the lamp does not cure in 2 minutes, it needs cleaning or the bulbs need to be changed. Normally, the lamp should be cleaned once a week and bulbs need to be replaced after 6 months
- Avoid using acetone for removal of gel nails; use normal nail polish remover.

Limitations: Major limitation of soft gels is that these cannot be used in cases of anonychia. These can be applied only on an existing nail plate.

Reported side effects for the operator:

- Miscarriages in pregnant women
- Cancer [acrylic dusts/additives like dibutylphthalate (DBT)]
- Cataract/macular degeneration.

Nail Peels

- Chemical peels have been an important tool at dermatologists' office for long. Facial and body peels are widely used and most dermatologists have extensive experience; applying that to nails can be very beneficial if the choice of candidate and the peel is correct. They are easily available and do not require any special set up or skill. Peels being cheap and painless, patient acceptance is also high.

An extensive history, including any history of previous nail treatments or cosmetic procedures has to be taken before the peels are started.

CHOICE OF PEELING AGENT

Medium depth chemical peels are preferred keeping in mind the relatively thick structure of the nail plate and limited penetration through the impervious structure and better safety profile.[20] There is no risk of postinflammatory hyperpigmentation, milia formation, excessive itching/ erythema with peels done on nails. The use of both glycolic acid 70% and combination peel of 8% phenol with 15% trichloroacetic acid (TCA) has been described in literature with good results and minimal side effects.[21,22] The primary mechanism of action of peels, in nail disorders is discohesion of corneocytes/onychocytes leading to their shedding.

Indications: Chemical peels can be used as a treatment modality for any nail plate surface abnormality like trachyonychia, pitting, onychorrhexis, and discoloration **(Fig. 7)**. These are also useful in improving the appearance of dry, rough, lusterless nails. These are also a good option for superficial pigmentation of nails.

Contraindications

- Presence of any active infection or inflammation in or around the nails
- Very thin nail plate
- Any history of hypersensitivity to the chemical
- Pregnant or lactating women
- Heavy manual workers
- Patients with unrealistic expectation.

Steps of the Peel

Detailed history of nail treatments/cosmetic procedures done on nails should be taken

- Take consent and prephotographs
- *Apply Vaseline on the cuticles and surrounding skin*
- Clean the affected nail with alcohol/prepeel cleanser
- Apply single coat of the peel with nylon brush/ear bud for rejuvenation for dry and dull nails; for pathological nail conditions presenting as deeper defects, 2–3 coats can be applied
- Ask the patient to wash hands after 10 minutes
- Liberally moisturize the nails in between sessions
- Repeat sessions at 2–4 weeks gap. The peels most commonly used are 70% glycolic acid and phenol.

Nail peels are a very safe treatment option if the surrounding skin and cuticle is effectively protected. Multiple sessions are required and the gap between the sessions should be increased to 4 weeks after the first 2–4 sessions.

ONYCHOCOSMECEUTICALS[23]

Many preparations are available in the market, which claim to be useful for nail disorders. These include combinations

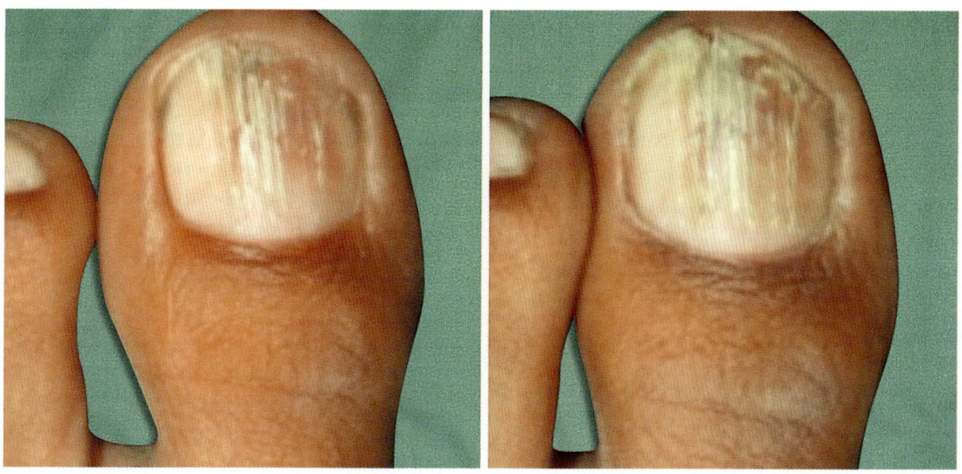

Fig. 7: Pre and post 4 monthly phenol peels.

of several vitamins, minerals, sulfur-containing amino acids or proteins, hormones, medicinal yeast, crushed egg shells, and even organic food. Their effect appears to be mainly psychological as some patients report miraculous improvement within a few days or weeks, whereas most others do not see any effect. Even though some overt deficiency states may cause brittle, fragile, or soft nails, this has not proven that their supplementation might improve the nails of an otherwise healthy person.

Most recent change in the use of onychocosmeceuticals is in the use of biotin, also known as vitamin B_7. Its recommended daily allowance (RDA) is 30 µg. Earlier a daily dose of 2.5–10 mg was recommended for hair and nail health, but recent studies show that this can lead to a reversible dysfunction of thyroid profile. Interference with immunoassays leads to falsely low or high thyroid hormone values if biotin is taken in moderate to high doses. Interference is not limited to thyroid tests and has the potential to affect a wide range of analytes.[24]

Onychocosmeceuticals responsible for nail health are pyridoxine, ascorbic acid, thiamine, calcium D-pantothenate, medicinal yeast, L-cystine, keratin, and p-amino benzoic acid. Both increase and decrease of vitamin A has been implicated in brittleness of nails. Vitamin E, sulfur-containing amino acids and proteins, fluorides, calcium's role is not clear.[25]

Supplementation of Iron[26], Zinc, Selenium, Silica, Rhodanides without manifest deficiency, is known to benefit nail health as there is evidence that their deficiency may result in several nail disorders.

NUTRITION

Malnutrition has a negative effect on nail growth; severe nail dystrophy is observed in kwashiorkor. Soft, brittle, often fissured nails, can be seen in cachexia and bulimia.[27-29] In severe cases in dark-skinned people, multiple longitudinal pigmented bands may occur.[30]

Genetically determined nail consistency does not show any influence with any particular food, even so called organic or biologic.

NAIL CARE OILS

There are a lot of so-called nail oils containing jojoba oil, bisabolol, panthenol, vitamins, and amino acids. Some oils may help to hold humidity. In general, oils as well as creams and ointments make the nail more elastic and thus prevent nail splitting.

CONCLUSION

Beautiful nails have been the privilege of rich and noble people for more than 3000 years. Nowadays, beautiful nails are affordable for almost everybody. Nail cosmetics offer a way to protect weak, brittle, or soft nails from trauma. Techniques such as gel nails and nail peels, if done properly, can help in camouflaging any underlying nail disorder whose treatment is otherwise either futile or does not justify the associated side effects.

The nail cosmetics are in general safe, but wrong practices can promote disease, deformity, and allergic and irritant contact dermatitis. Therefore it is a dermatologist's duty to provide clear recommendations regarding safe nail care practices and to recognize cosmetic causes of nail disease.

REFERENCES

1. Chang RM, Hare AQ, Rich P. Treating cosmetically induced nail problems. Dermatol Ther. 2007;20(1):54-9.
2. Madnani NA, Khan KJ. Nail cosmetics. Indian J Dermatol Venereol Leprol. 2012;78:309-17.
3. Scher RK. Nail cosmetics. Cutis. 2012;89(4):154-5.
4. Lawry M, Rich P. The nail apparatus: a guide for basic and Clinical Science. Curr Probl Dermatol. 1999:11:202-4.
5. Jefferson J, Rich P. Update on nail cosmetics. Dermatol Ther. 2012;25(6):481-90.
6. Rich P, Kwak H. Nail physiology and grooming. In: Draelos ZD (Ed). Cosmetic Dermatology Products and Procedures, 1st edition. Hoboken, NJ: Wiley-Blackwell, 2010. pp. 197-205.
7. Nanda S. Basic Nail Care and Hygiene. In: Textbook of Onychology (Nail Society of India). Nairobi, Kenya: Evangel Publications; 2020.
8. Cosmetics Info. Tosylamide/Formaldehyde Resin. [online] Available from: https://cosmeticsinfo.org/ingredient/tosylamideformaldehyde-resin-0. [Last Accessed May, 2020].
9. Dahdah MJ, Scher RK. Nail diseases related to nail cosmetics. Dermatol Clin. 2006;24:233-9.
10. Lorizzo M, Piraccini BM, Tosti A. Nail cosmetics in nail disorders. J Cosmet Dermatol. 2007;6:53-58.
11. Atelier Emmanuel. The difference between Acrylic, Gel and Shellac Nails. [online] Available from: http://atelieremmanuel.com/the-difference-between-acrylic-gel-and-shellac-nails/. [Last Accessed May, 2020].
12. Brauer EW. Selected prostheses primarily of cosmetic interest. Cutis. 1970;6:521-4.
13. Nails. Return of the Nail Wrap. [online] Available from: http://www.nailsmag.com/article/97861/return-of-the-nail-wrap. [Last Accessed May, 2020].
14. Diffen. Shellac vs. Gel Nails. [online] Available from: http://www.diffen.com/difference/Gel_Nails_vs_Shellac_Nails. [Last Accessed May, 2020].
15. Nanda S, Grover C. Utility of gel nails in improving the appearance of cosmetically disfigured nails: experience with 25 cases. J Cutan Aesthet Surg. 2014;7(1):26-31.
16. Nanda S, Banga G, Bansal S, Patel K. Dermatologist driven aesthetic procedures. In: Textbook of Onychology (Nail Society of India). Nairobi, Kenya: Evangel Publications; 2020.
17. MacFarlane DF, Alonso CA. Occurrence of nonmelanoma skin cancers on the hands after UV nail light exposure. Arch Dermatol. 2009;145:447-9.
18. Markova A, Weinstock MA. Risk of skin cancer associated with the use of UV nail lamp. J Invest Dermatol. 2012;133:1097-9.
19. Dowdy JC, Sayre RM. Photobiological safety evaluation of UV nail lamps. Photochem. Photobiol. 2013;89:961-7.

20. Dewandre L. The chemistry of peels and a hypothesis of action mechanisms. In: Rubin MG (Ed) Chemical Peels: Procedure in Cosmetic Dermatology. New York: Elsevier Inc.; 2006. pp. 1-12.
21. Banga G, Patel K. Glycolic acid peels for nail rejuvenation. J CutanAesthet Surg. 2014;7:198-201.
22. Daulatabad D, Nanda S, and Grover C. Intra-individual right-left comparative study of medium depth peels in superficial nail abnormalities. J Cutan Aesthet Surg. 2017;10(1):28-32.
23. Haneke E. Onychocosmeceuticals. J Cosmet Dermatol 2006;5(1):95-100.
24. Elston MS, Sehgal S, Du Toit S, Yarndley T, Conaglen JV. Factitious Graves' disease due to biotin immunoassay interference: a case and review of the literature. J Clin Endocrinol Metab. 2016;101(9):3251-5.
25. Forslind B. Biophysical studies of the normal nail. Acta Dermato-Venereol. 1970;50:161-8.
26. Djaldetti M, Fishman P, Hart J. The iron content of fingernails in iron deficient patients. Clin Sci. 1987;72:669-72.
27. Daniel CR, Sams WM, Scher RK. Nails in systemic disease. Dermatol Clin. 1985;3:465-83.
28. Hediger C, Rost B, Itin P. Cutaneous manifestations in anorexia nervosa. Schweiz Med Wochenschr. 2000;130:565-75.
29. Ruymann FB. Juvenile polyps with cachexia. Report of an infant and comparison with Cronkhite-Canada syndrome in adults. Gastroenterology. 1969;57:431-8.
30. Bisht DB, Singh SS. Pigmented bands on nails: a new sign in malnutrition. Lancet. 1962;1:507-8.

CHAPTER 124

Threads

Gulhima Arora, Ishmeet Kaur

KEY MESSAGES

- Threads are a versatile tool for lifting, contouring and rejuvenation.
- These are associated with minimal side effects and downtime.
- The success of treatment depends on an ideal patient selection and correct insertion techinques.
- Threads can be used in combination with other aesthetic treatments.

INTRODUCTION

Aging is an inevitable phenomenon associated with loss of tissue elasticity and volume, owing to alterations in the framework of collagen. Facial aging is identified by the presence of wrinkles, folds, loss of volume and ptosis of the tissues. A variety of rejuvenation techniques have been introduced to manage these signs of aging.[1] Most patients desire antiaging procedures with minimal incision, short downtime and less frequent sessions.[2] Use of dermal threads has become a common antiaging procedure that provides rejuvenation and an actual facelift with short recovery time, no scarring and long-lasting effect. Being a safe and semi-invasive procedure, it has gained huge popularity as a "lunch time facelift procedure".[3] This chapter deals with different types of threads, relevant anatomy, techniques, complications and tips and tricks of a threadlift procedure pertaining to the face.

HISTORY

Barbed sutures were first utilized for suturing wounds. The concept was first described by Alcamo in 1961, Fukuda in 1984 and Ruff in 2001 where they were used to suture wounds without any need to tie knots.[4] It was in 1999, when Marlen Sulamanidze et al. described the cosmetic application of barbed threads for the first time with Aptos lift sutures.[5]

Thereafter many other threads and threadlift techniques were described in literature including the Woffles thread utilized in the Woffles Lift, Isse Threadlift, utilizing unidirectional barbed sutures; the contour threads; the silhouette lift, etc.[6]

The polydioxanone (PDO) threads gained popularity in South Korea and a lot of scientific insight into their use has come from there.[7] Various biomaterials were exploited to produce better qualities of threads including PDO threads followed by poly lactic acid (PLA) and polycaprolactone (PCA) threads. Since then, many different types of threads, both absorbable and nonabsorbable with varying efficacy, longevity and side effect profile have been introduced.[8]

TABLE 1: Mechanisms of action of threads.

Immediate lift	*Prolonged lift*
Due to mechanical lifting by the threads	• Stimulation of collagen production • Promotion of local blood microcirculation • Activation of reparative processes

MECHANISMS OF ACTION AND RELEVANT ANATOMY

Mechanisms of action of threads is depicted in **Table 1**.

Relevant Anatomy

It is of utmost importance for a dermatosurgeon to understand the relevant anatomy of the area where the threads have to be inserted, in order to deliver the desirable clinical results, ensure longevity of the procedure and avoid complications.

The two most important anatomical structures that need to be kept in mind with this procedure are the superficial fat pads and the ligaments, true or false, in the surgical area **(Fig. 1)**. All threads, whatever the type or material, should be inserted in the subcutaneous plane for optimum results. Anchoring suspending/lifting threads in an area with a ligament, ensures improved longevity of the clinical results.

The vasculature and nervous network in the area should also be kept in mind in order to avoid a hematoma or nerve injury. This is rare if the plane of insertion is correct, as these structures lie deeper.

TYPES OF THREADS

- *Based on fixation:* Free floating and fixed.[9] The fixed threads are anchored and fixed to a deep structure. They are usually inserted through an incision.

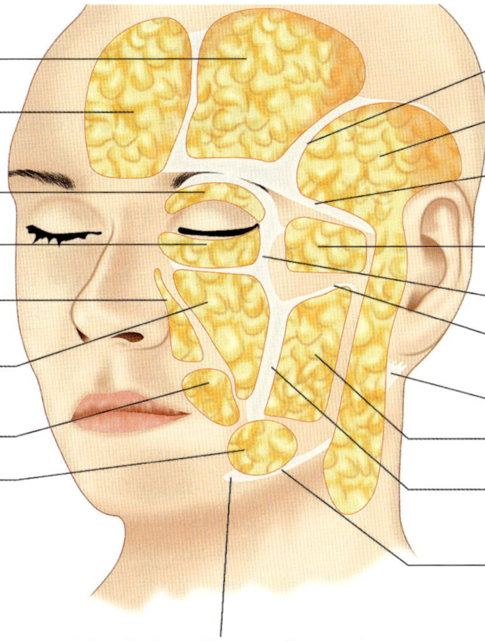

Fig. 1: Anatomy of face with fat pads and ligaments.

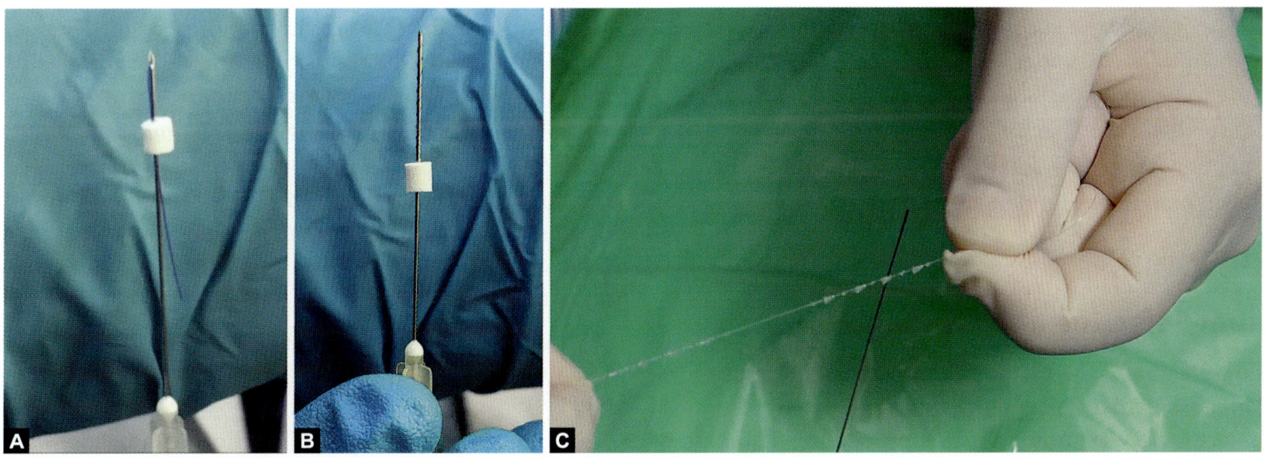

Figs. 2A to C: Types of threads. (A) Monothreads; (B) Screw thread; (C) Silhouette soft.

- *Based on type of main filament:* Barbed, cone and smooth sutures. The number of cones and their direction may vary while barbed sutures may be unidirectional or bidirectional having cogs in one or two directions or may be spirally arranged.
- *Based on the type of material:*
  - *Absorbable:* They may be polydioxanone (PDO), poly L-lactic acid (PLLA) or polycaprolactone (PCL), polycaproamide threads and catgut.[10]
  - *Nonabsorbable:* Polypropylene.
- *Based on the length of the suture:* Long sutures are greater than or equal to 90 mm in length, and short ones are less than 90 mm.
- *Types of threads according to thread structure:*
  - *Monofilaments **(Fig. 2A)**:* Simplest form of thread, with a single length of suture in a needle.
  - *Screw/twin **(Fig. 2B)**:* Threads which are wound around the needle.
  - Double screw is like a double helix wound around the needle.
  - Barbed cog threads where the cogs are cut from the main thread skeleton or are molded out of the main thread. The barbs may be unidirectional or bi-directional.
  - *Cones* ***(Fig. 2C)***: Here there are cones along the main thread. They may be unidirectional or bidirectional.
- *Other types of threads:* Two-needle PDO, PLLA or PCL threads with lengths as much as 42 cm for use along multiple vectors, in 1-0 or 2-0 sizes, usually barbed or with cones. They may be used for the body too.[10,11]

Nose threads are the latest generation barbed threads, used for nonsurgical rhinoplasty.[12,13]

INDICATIONS

Monofilaments

- Tightening
- Glow
- PDO monofilaments cause lipolysis
- Reduction of pores
- Helpers to lifting threads
- Volumizing.

Barbed

- *Upper face:* Forehead, eyebrow, nose
- *Mid-face:* Nasolabial fold, cheeks
- *Lower face:* Marionette line, jowl, jaw
- Neck.

CONTRAINDICATIONS

- Pregnancy
- Keloidal tendency
- On antiseizure medication
- Herpes simplex or any other active infections in any area
- Noncompliance (patients who are unwilling to follow the post-treatment instruction)
- Nonrealistic expectations
- Patient with coagulation disorders
- Permanent fillers/implants in the same region.

PROCEDURE

Patient Selection and Evaluation

Patient selection is the first important step of the procedure. A proper assessment of patient profile and extent of aging is necessary before planning for this procedure. The patient should be counseled well that this is not a substitute to a surgical intervention. An appropriate patient is one who has mild skin laxity, mild fat ptosis and few superficial rhytides.[14] Patients with thin skin may have more chances of sutures showing, rippling effect and bruising.[15] Poor response is observed in obese candidates, severe sagging, old age and therefore should be counseled accordingly. Favorable clinical outcomes have been reported in patients with a low body fat percentage and prominent bony projections.[16] The best results have been reported to be seen involving the malar and nasolabial fat pads.[17] The procedure should be avoided in patients with unrealistic expectations, bleeding disorders, allergic tendencies, permanent facial implants/fillers (silicon, PMMA) immunosuppressive state (HIV/AIDS), systemic infections such as tuberculosis and diabetes. The treating surgeon can offer a combination of aesthetic treatments along with thread lifts to the patient for better clinical outcomes.[18] A proper consent should be obtained from the selected candidate after explaining about the procedure and the possible complications.

Choice of Thread

The choice of the thread in terms of type and material to be used, the size and length of the thread, the types and size of the delivery system have to be planned prior to the procedure after assessment of the patient. All these factors impact the outcome of threadlift procedure.

Before choosing the thread, a proper evaluation of the skin and severity of aging is necessary, taking into consideration the expectations of the patient.

Absorbable PDO threads are the most commonly used threads for the facelift. Monofilament threads can provide a good skin tightening and revitalization, but due to less surface area and because of a more superficial plane of insertion, they fail to give a good lifting effect. They can be used as helper threads along with lifting threads. Barbed/cog threads and cone threads are better lifting threads. They can tighten, contour and reposition volume as well.[19]

The material used depends on the budget of the patient and the desirability of longevity of clinical results. Longer the thread, and greater the resorption time, more long lasting the results with higher collagen production.

The size of the thread when using monofilaments depends on the vectors chosen and the area to be treated. Longer and wider treatment areas need longer threads. When using lifting threads, the length of the thread depends on the length of the tissue to be lifted. The thicker the thread, larger the size and better the lifting power.

For mild lift, PLA threads are preferred. PCA or threads, on the other hand are more beneficial when moderate lifting effect is desired.[20]

The delivery system may be a needle, a needle-cannula or a blunt cannula **(Figs. 3A and B)** the last being the

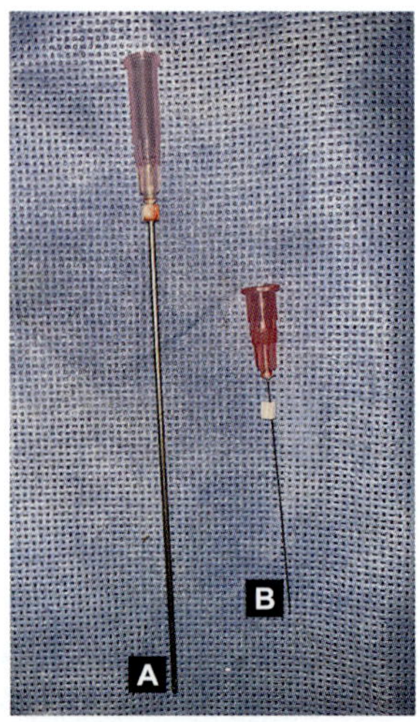

Figs. 3A and B: Thread delivery systems. (A) Cannula; (B) Needle.

least traumatic. A needle and needle-cannula systems do not need an entry port to be made for insertion of the thread. Monofilament threads usually come attached to a needle, and lifting threads are attached to a cannula.

The number of threads per area of indication should not be compromised upon. Using less than adequate number, which can be assessed by the degree of sag, will result in suboptimal and shorter lasting clinical results.

Preparation and Anesthesia

It is of utmost importance that the area to be treated is made sterile with the usual 3-step skin preparation procedure of using betadine, alcohol and betadine, as for any invasive skin procedure. A sterile drape should cover the rest of the face and a sterile cap should be used for the scalp. Anesthesia used for threadlift procedures is local, either topical or injectable.

Mono/Screw or Twin Threads

A topical anesthetic such as eutectic mixture of lidocaine with prilocaine cream, 30–45 minutes prior to the procedure can be used. Usually, while using monofilament threads, since the gauge of the delivery system is very small, patients often tolerate insertion without any form of anesthesia.

Barbed/Cone Threads

Either an injection of 2% xylocaine with 1:10,000 adrenaline can be used at the site of making the entry port or injected in the whole track along the premarked vector. However, the authors have experienced that if the thread is in the right plane, there is very little discomfort felt by the patient, and an entry-point bolus with the anesthetic solution suffices.

Some physicians like to use tumescent anesthesia, infiltrating the entire area to be treated. This is useful when performing a full-face lift with threads, when many threads have to be inserted.

Markings of Vectors

It is always a good idea to design the vectors according to the indication for the procedure **(Figs. 4A to G)**.

Monofilaments

- Cross-hatch
- Parallel
- Random
- Fan.

Barbed Sutures

The face is divided into two functional halves by a vertical line drawn from the lateral canthus to the jaw **(Fig. 5)** area lateral to this is a relatively fixed area, suitable to make the entry ports for lifting threads for better fixation and the area medial to this line is more suitable for mobile, monofilament/screw threads.

The vectors are perpendicular to the area to be lifted.

Technique

Monofilaments/Screw Threads

They are inserted along the marked vectors, bevel up. They are inserted in the deep dermis to superficial fat compartment **(Fig. 6)**. Usually, many threads are needed about 0.5 cm apart **(Fig. 7)**. They are inserted till the full length of the delivery system which is a needle with a small gauge and then placing a finger of the nondominant hand, the needle is slowly withdrawn. There is a white guard present on the needle up to which the thread should be inserted perpendicularly and then its direction changed.

Barbed Threads

These have cogs cut or molded in the length of the thread **(Fig. 8)**. They are usually wound around a blunt cannula. When attached to a needle or sharp cannula, there is no need to make an entry port for insertion.

- Choose a fixed anchor point for the threads, usually a retaining ligament, dense fibrotic tissues, subcutaneous tissue.
- Inject local anesthesia at the site of the entry point and/ along the entire vector.
- Make an entry point with a sharp needle of a size larger than that of the cannula of the thread.
- Insert the thread perpendicularly until there is a feeling of "give away". This indicates the cannula is beyond the dermis. Some threads have a mark on them for the depth they are to be inserted perpendicularly. Alternatively insert the thread vertically until the guard before changing direction.
- Insert the thread smoothly maintaining the same plane. All threads are inserted in the superficial fat compartment above the superficial musculoaponeurotic system (SMAS) except when repositioning volume, when they are to be inserted deeper.
- The end point of insertion depends on the indication. If a fold like the nasolabial has to be softened, the end of the cannula should be advanced beyond the fold for a better lift. If it is an area like the jowl to be lifted, the cannula can stop short and the traction will be enough to lift the area.
- The nondominant hand should be used to hold the end of the thread before rotating the hub while withdrawing the cannula.
- The same entry point is preferred to insert at least two threads. This ensures better anchoring.
- Anchoring can be improved by tying a knot between two threads or twisting them. There are several other forms of

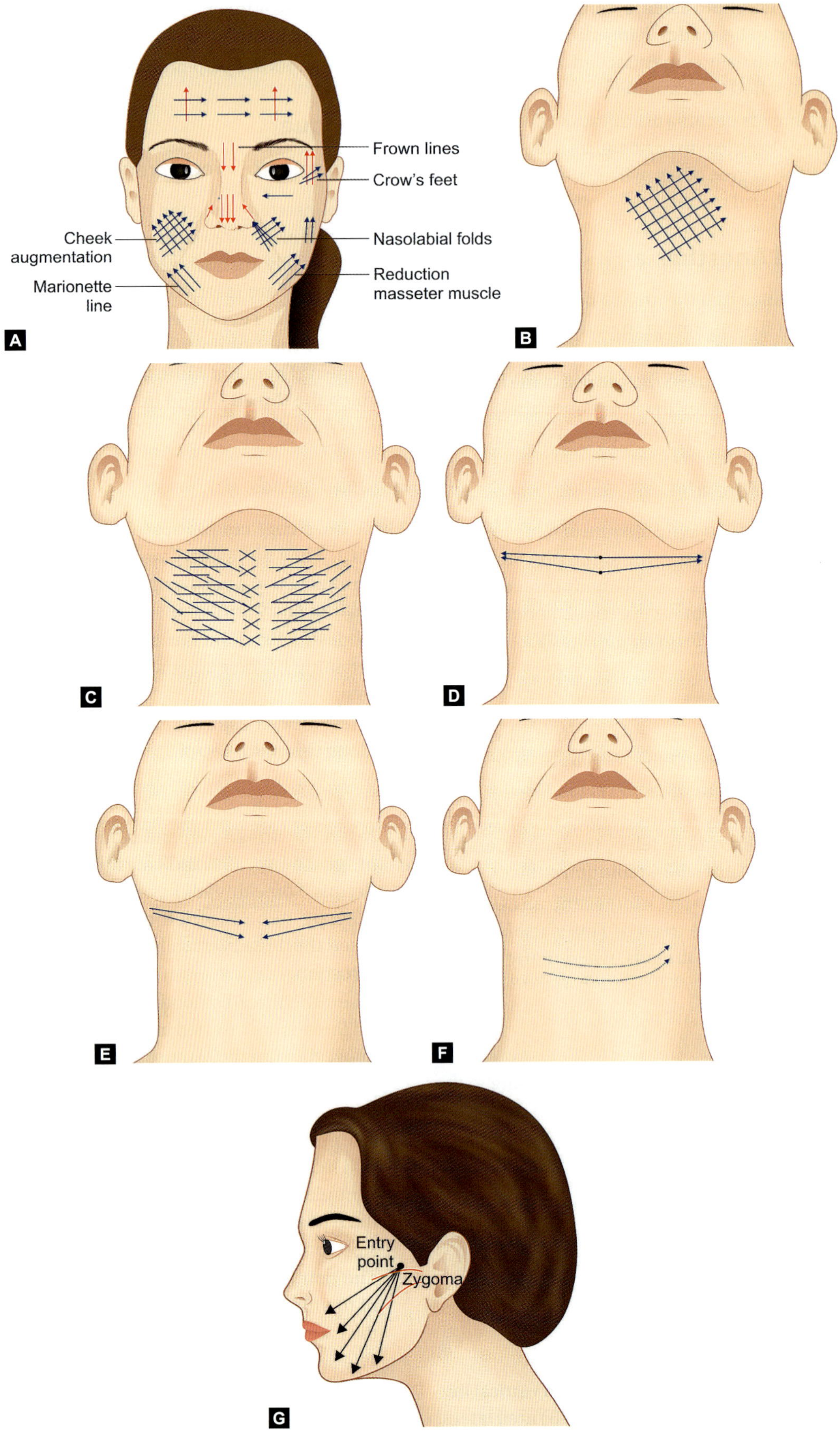

Figs. 4A to G: Vectors for thread insertion. (A) Face; (B to F) Neck; (G) Nasolabial and mentolabial folds.

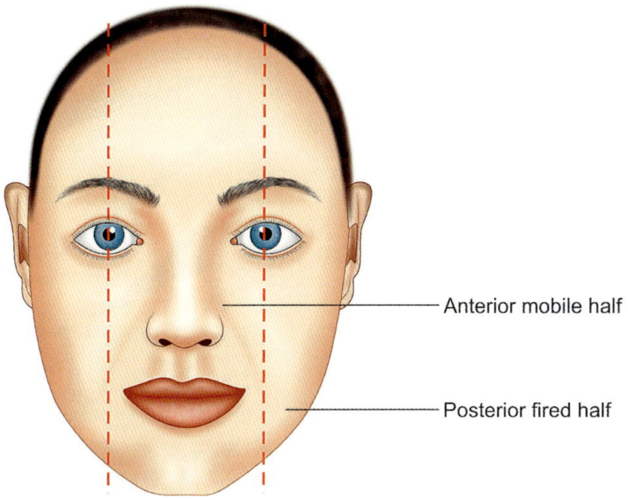

Fig. 5: Schematic diagram of division of face in two vertical halves.

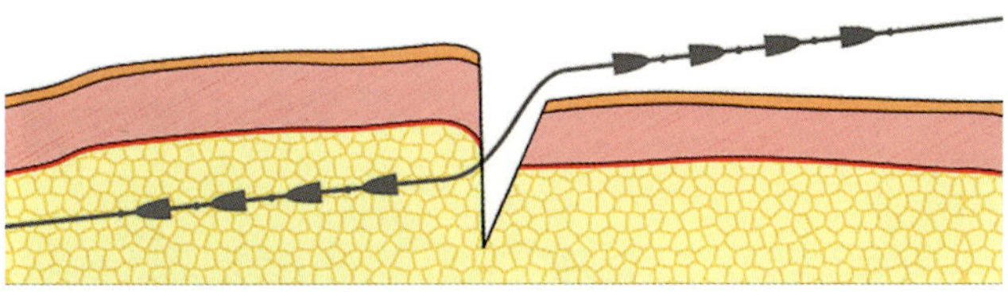

Fig. 6: Correct depth of thread insertion.

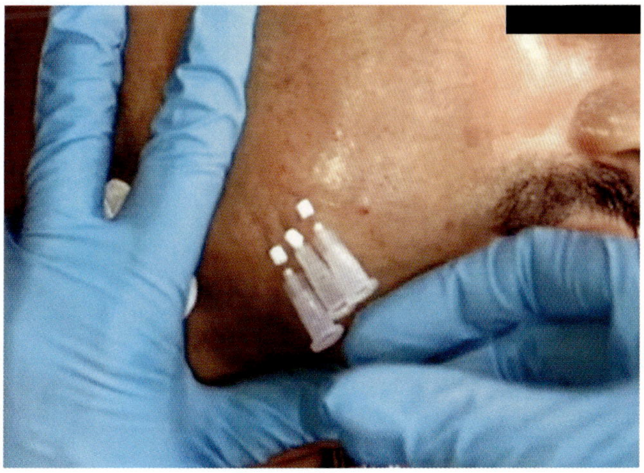

Fig. 7: Multiple polydioxanone (PDO) monothreads inserted along intended vectors.

anchoring like a "U" vector when double needle threads are used.

- The skin should be redraped over the inserted threads. The barbs open and hold the tissue better while massaging the skin. A gritty sensation can be felt when this happens.
- The symmetry should be checked before snipping the threads after burying the knot through the entry port. A forceps or the blunt end of a needle can be used to achieve this. Snipping should be as close to the skin as possible using a Mayo's curved scissors **(Figs. 9A to H)**.

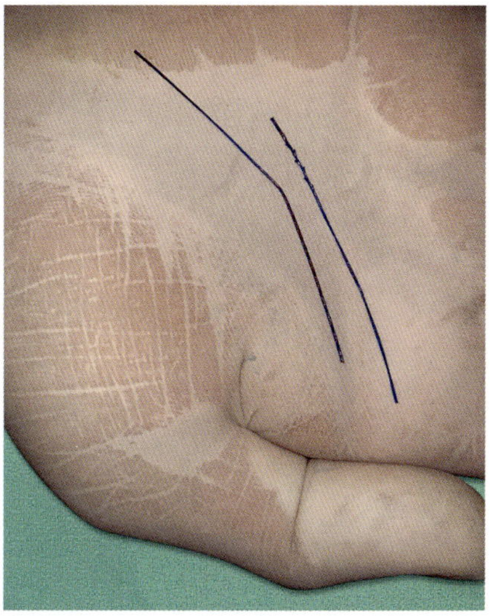

Fig. 8: Barbs on threads.

Postprocedure Care

Topical antibiotics can be prescribed for the next 7 days to prevent infections. Instructions must be given to the patient to avoid heavy strenuous exercise, to take soft food and keep head end elevated for at least 1 day. Patients should also be asked to sleep on their back and not on their sides.[21] For pain, acetaminophen can be prescribed; other non-steroidal anti-inflammatory drugs (NSAIDs) like ibuprofen should be avoided due to risk of bruising.[21] Patient should avoid excessive mouth opening, scrubbing, hot steam, massaging of face for the next 7 days. Procedures like laser or radiofrequency should not be planned for the next 3–4 weeks.

RESULTS

The skin may look uneven for 3–4 days. Some instant effects are seen with monofilament threads because of edema; this effect improves over next 3 weeks to 3 months due to new collagen build-up. Effect of cog threads is also seen instantly because of edema and due to pull of cog threads; additional tissue tightening effect gets added to the initial result as collagen builds up.

SIDE EFFECTS AND COMPLICATIONS

Threadlift is essentially a safe procedure. Complications are usually very mild which can be managed and reversed without leaving behind any permanent sequalae.[22] The risk of complications increases with the number of threads inserted.[22] In one study of 37 thread lifts done with monofilament suspension threads, complication reported were 6% slight asymmetry: small ecchymosis (62%), mild erythema (40%), mild transitory erythema (6%), and swelling (40%). In authors experience edema and swelling followed by ecchymosis and minor asymmetry were the more common complications in

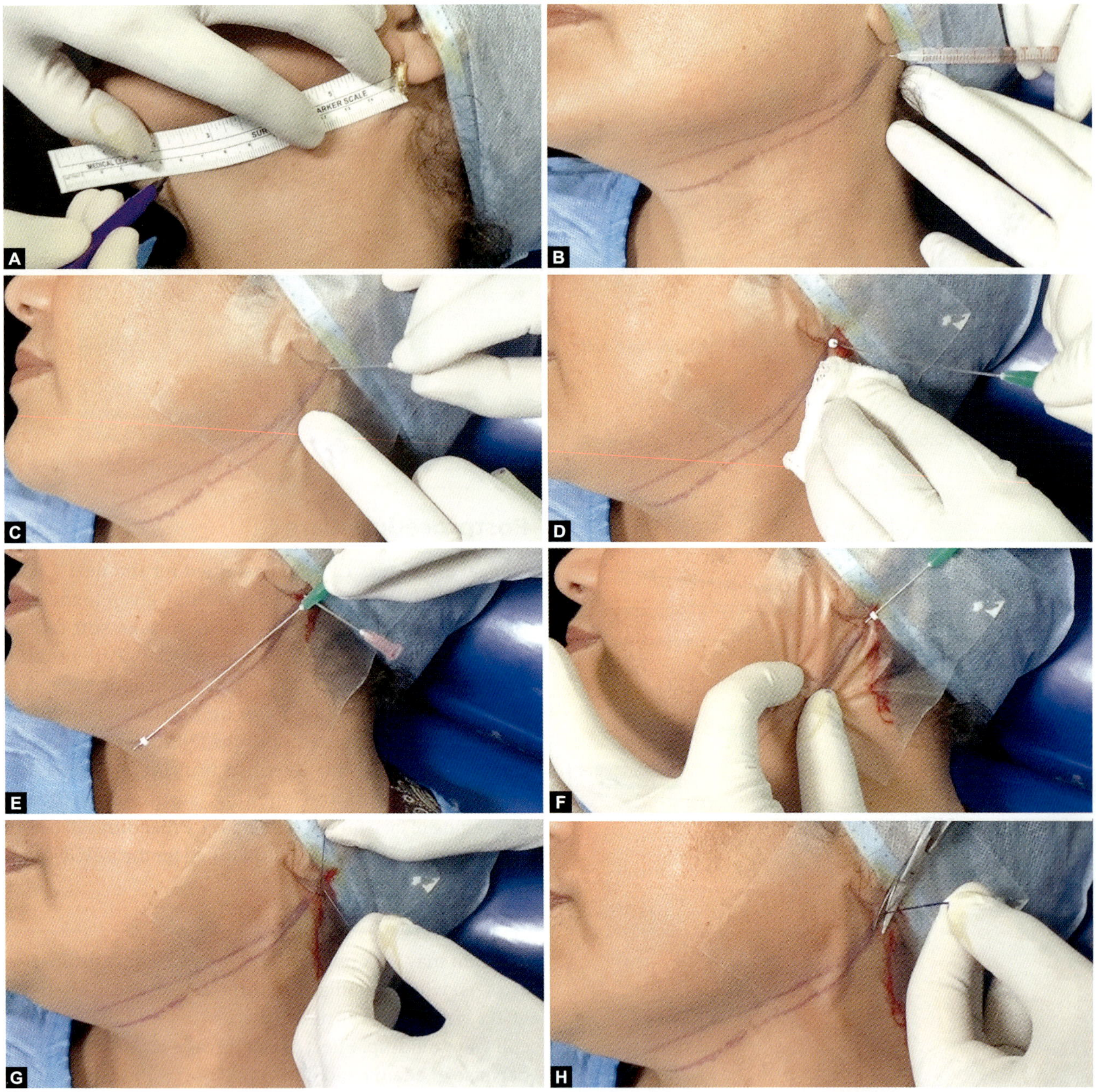

Figs. 9A to H: Steps of barbed thread insertion. (A) Assessment of thread length and point of insertion; (B) Infiltrate local anesthesia; (C) Insertion point; (D) Introduce the cannula/needle and determine depth; (E) Confirm direction, length are in confirmation with the vector; (F) Pinch and introduce cannula/needle; (G) Anchor threads; (H) Snip threads and bury ends.

the earlier stage and puckering or dimpling of skin in the late stage.[23]

Immediate

- Pain, edema and bruising and discomfort are the most common side effects which are usually self-limiting in nature but may prolong the recovery time. Pain and edema can be easily managed with help of NSAIDs. For bruising, ice packs should be gently packed.
- Hematoma or ecchymosis formation.
- Rippling, pricking, puckering, dimpling or visibility of the thread from under the skin may occur due to poor placement or superficial insertion of thread. Dimpling at the exit point can be avoided by ensuring placement of thread within the malar pad and not too superficial in the dermis.[24] Usually it is self-limiting which can be corrected with gentle massaging of the treated area but if persistent, it may necessitate correction with the help of subcision.[10,25]
- Asymmetry of the face may also be observed immediately after the procedure which can be corrected with insertion of one or more threads on the required side of the face.

Early

- Local infection
- Transient sensory impairment
- Ear numbness
- Parotid gland injury
- Partial extrusion of thread (early or late). This can be tackled by pulling out the thread in case of a monofilament or stretching the skin to try to push it back in. In case of barbed threads, a surgical incision may be needed to remove the thread
- Infection may occur if proper sterile precautions are not followed during the procedure. A rare complication of infection with *Mycobacterium massiliense* and *M. abscessus* has recently been reported with threadlift.[26]

Late

- Hair sinus
- Inclusion cysts (mostly with barbed/surgical threads)
- Granulation tissue at entry point
- Cellulitis
- Abscess[22]
- Scar tissue formation at entry or exit points
- Thread migration or expulsion is a complication reported more with nonabsorbable threads and unlikely with absorbable ones.

TIPS AND TRICKS

Monofilaments

- Use narrow gauge delivery systems for better patient comfort, as the number of threads to be inserted are often many.
- In case of a part of the thread remains outside the entry point or gets extruded, stretch the skin with the thumb and index finger to try and push the thread in. If this does not happen, snip the extruded thread close to the skin and then try.

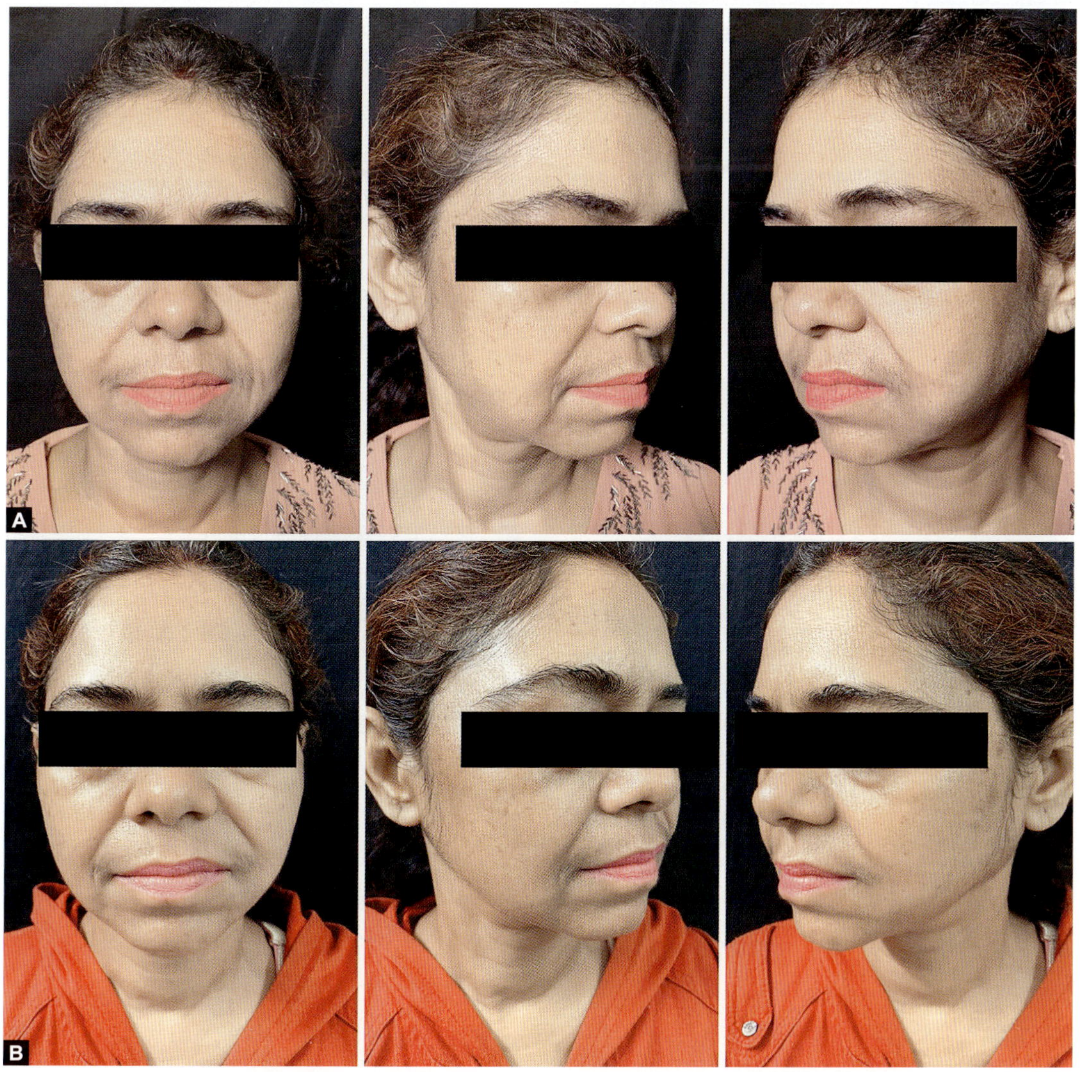

Figs. 10A and B: Facelift with barb threads preprocedure (A) postprocedure (B).

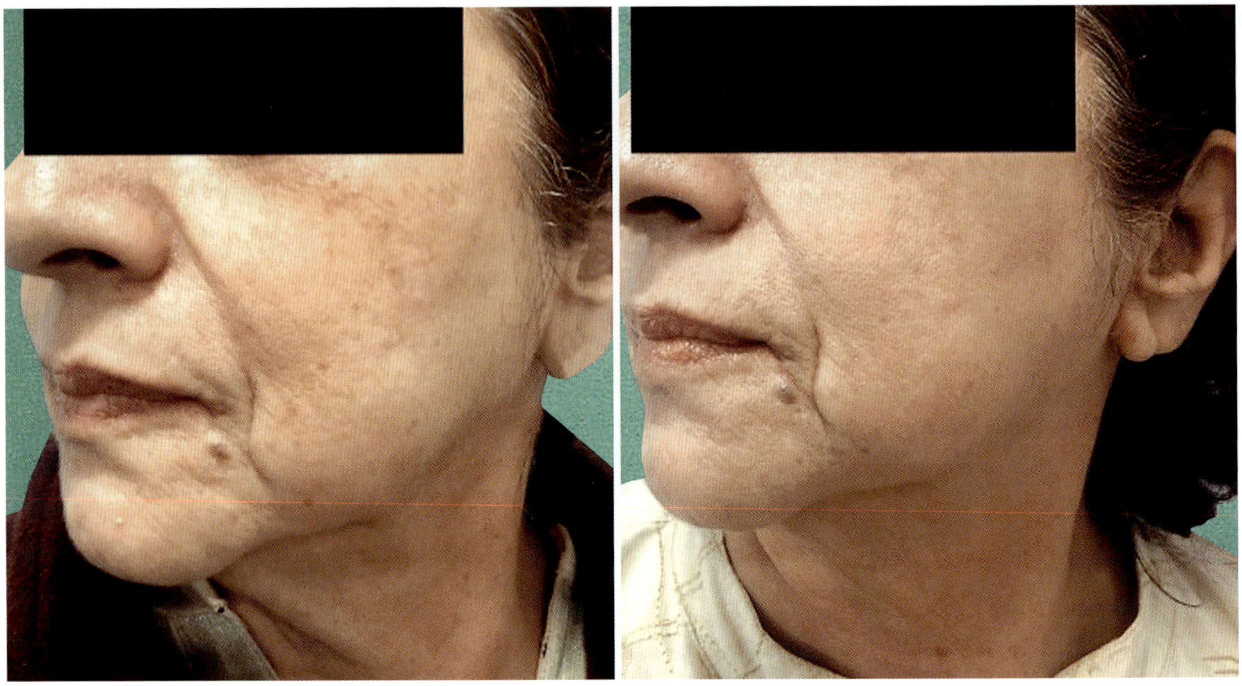

Fig. 11: Lower facelifting with barb threads.

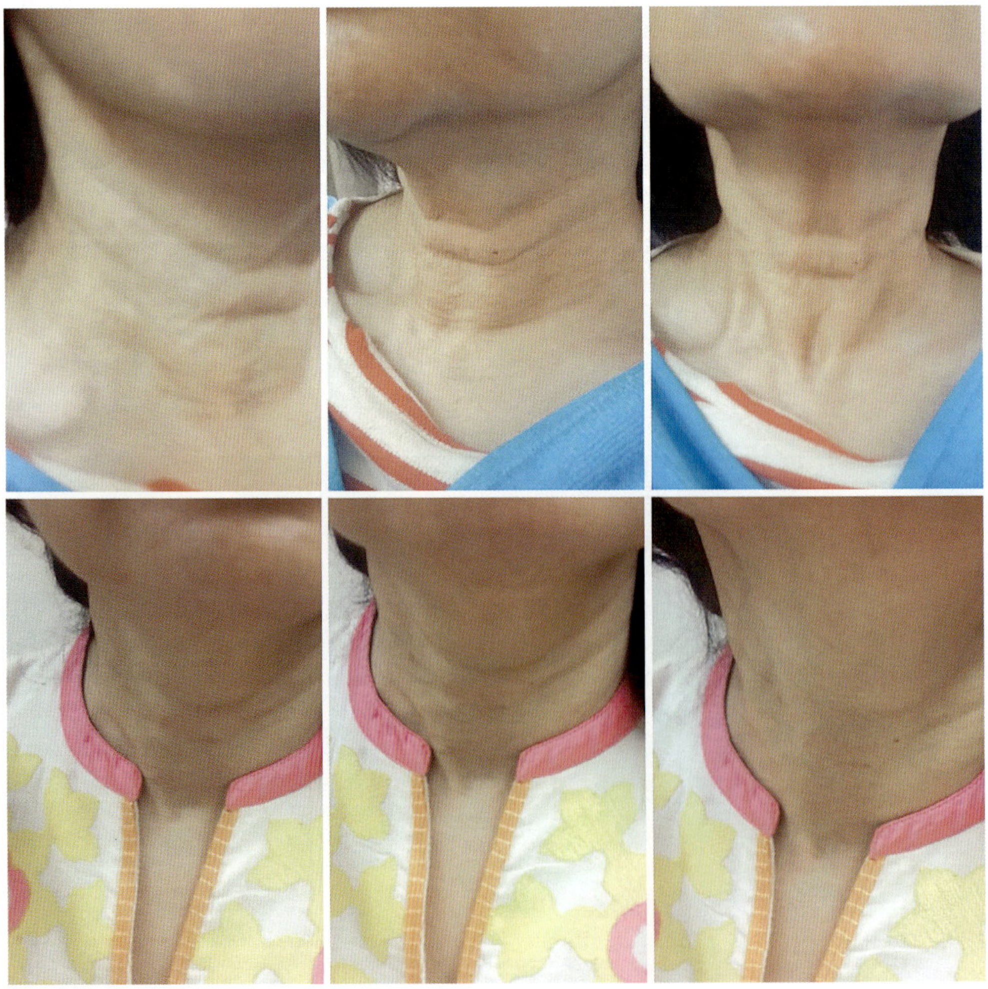

Fig. 12: Neck rejuvenation with combination of threads.

- For rejuvenation, it is best to insert threads in a slightly more superficial plane, the deep dermis.

Barbed/Cone Sutures

- The beginning of the insertion has to perpendicular to the skin, before changing the direction of the thread parallel to the skin surface.
- If the thread needs to be withdrawn a little to maintain the correct plane, the hub of the cannula should be blocked so that the thread does not slip inside and cause bunching.
- Rotate the hub of the cannula while withdrawing to ensure proper attachment of the barbs.
- To reposition volume, the threads should be inserted deeper, in the sub-SMAS layer.
- Always massage and reposition skin prior to snipping the thread, which should be done as close to the skin as possible.
- Check for symmetry in the sitting position before snipping the thread.
- For double needle threads, avoiding dimpling can be done by the blunt end of the cannula by teasing the tissue at the entry point.

NEW ADVANCES

Assessment of the plane of insertion of thread can be challenging. Ultrasound evaluation has been recently utilized to study the insertion level of thread and to detect any displacement of thread. B-mode two-dimensional ultrasonographic analysis can be performed 90 days after the procedure to evaluate successful collagen formation and fibrosis which can be ensured by observing hyperechogenic shadows in the tissue along the thread route.[16,27]

Doppler ultrasound can be used to assess the location of important vascular structures within the target area to avoid vascular complications.[28]

Threadlift has been combined with various other antiaging procedures such as microfocused ultrasound[29] and small incision rhytidectomy[30] to improve the outcomes of face rejuvenation and contouring. A peculiar observation of early biodegradation of PDO threads has been observed in the presence of hyaluronic acid.[31]

CONCLUSION

Threadlift is an increasingly used antiaging procedure due to its semi-invasive nature, less downtime and long-lasting effect **(Figs. 10 to 12)**. It is, however, necessary to understand the physiology of threads and the anatomy of facial planes and vital structures to improve the outcome of the lift with minimal possible complications. With new and better threads being introduced in the market, the desired quality and indication of different types of threads holds great importance in deciding which thread is best suitable for the patient.

REFERENCES

1. Ganceviciene R, Liakou AI, Theodoridis A, Makrantonaki E, Zouboulis CC. Skin anti-aging strategies. Dermatoendocrinol. 2012;4:308-19.
2. Arora G, Arora S. Neck rejuvenation with thread lift. J Cutan Aesthetic Surg. 2019;12:196-200.
3. Atiyeh BS, Dibo SA, Costagliola M, Hayek SN. Barbed sutures "lunch time" lifting: evidence-based efficacy: "lunch time" lifting. J Cosmet Dermatol. 2010;9:132-41.
4. Kress DW. The history of barbed suture suspension: applications, and visions for the future. In: Shiffman MA, Mirrafati SJ, Lam SM (Eds). Simplified Facial Rejuvenation. Berlin, Heidelberg, Germany: Springer-Verlag; 2008. pp. 247-56.
5. Sulamanidze MA, Shiffman MA, Paikidze TG, Sulamanidze GM, Gavasheli LG. Facial lifting with APTOS threads. Int J Cosmetic Surg Aesthetic Dermatol. 2001;3:275-81.
6. Wu WTL. Facial rejuvenation using APTOS and WAPTOS (The Woffles Lift): a novel approach. Sydney, Australia: Paper presented at: the 13th International Congress of the International Confederation of Plastic and Reconstructive Surgery (IPRAS); 2003.
7. Medgadget. (2020). Cosmetic Threads Market is valued at expected to reach USD 151.8 Million by 2025 (CAGR 7.6%). [online] Available from: https://www.medgadget.com/2019/07/cosmetic-threads-market-is-valued-at-expected-to-reach-usd-151-8-million-by-2025-cagr-7-6.html. [Last accessed May, 2020].
8. Shin JJ, Park TJ, Kim BY, Kim CM, Suh DH, Lee SJ, et al. Comparative effects of various absorbable threads in a rat model. J Cosmet Laser Ther. 2019;21:158-62.
9. Han HH, Kim JM, Kim NH, Park RH, Park JB, Ahn TJ. Combined, Minimally Invasive, Thread-based Facelift. Arch Aesthetic Plast Surg. 2014;20:160.
10. Parada MB, Yarak S, Cassiano D. Thread lifting. In: Issa MCA, Tamura B (Eds). Botulinum Toxins, Fillers and Related Substances. Cham: Springer International Publishing; 2019. pp. 381-90.
11. Padin VL. Experience in the use of barbed threads and non-barbed serdev sutures in face and body lift – comparison and combination. In: Serdev N (Ed). Miniinvasive Face and Body Lifts - Closed Suture Lifts or Barbed Thread Lifts. New York: InTech; 2013.
12. Lee HY, Yang HJ. Rhinoplasty with barbed threads. Plast Reconstr Surg Glob Open. 2018;6:e1967.
13. Jaafar AFL. Nose abscess after thread rhinoplasty: a case report. J Cosmet Med. 2018;2:46-51.
14. Halepas S, Chen XJ, Ferneini EM. Thread-lift sutures: anatomy, technique, and review of current literature. J Oral Maxillofac Surg. 2020;78:813-20.
15. Paul MD. Complications of barbed sutures. Aesthetic Plast Surg. 2008;32:149.
16. Suh DH, Jang HW, Lee SJ, Lee WS, Ryu HJ. Outcomes of polydioxanone knotless thread lifting for facial rejuvenation. Dermatol Surg. 2015;41:720-5.
17. Eremia S, Willoughby MA. Novel face-lift suspension suture and inserting instrument: use of large anchors knotted into a suture with attached needle and inserting device allowing for single entry point placement of suspension suture. Preliminary report of 20 cases with 6-to 12-month follow-up. Dermatol Surg. 2006;32:335.
18. Pourang A, Rockwell H, Karimi K. New frontiers in skin rejuvenation, including stem cells and autologous therapies. Facial Plast Surg Clin N Am. 2020;28:101-17.

19. Arora G, Arora S. Thread lift in breast ptosis. J Cutan Aesthetic Surg. 2017;10:228.
20. Wong V, Rafiq N, Kalyan R, Hsenriksen A, Funner R. Hanging by a thread: choosing the right thread for the right patient. J Dermat Cosmetol. 2017;1:86-8.
21. Kalra R. Use of barbed threads in facial rejuvenation. Indian J Plast Surg. 2008;41(Suppl):S93-S100.
22. Ahn SK, Choi HJ. Complication after PDO threads lift. J Craniofac Surg. 2019;30:e467-9.
23. Arora G, Arora S. A study of complications of aesthetic thread lift: a review of 250 cases. ResearchGate; 2018.
24. Hochman M. Midface barbed suture lift. Facial Plast Surg Clin North Am. 2007;15:201-7.
25. Kang SH, Byun EJ, Kim HS. Vertical lifting: a new optimal thread lifting technique for Asians. Dermatol Surg. 2017;43:1263-70.
26. Shin JJ, Park JH, Lee JM, Ryu J. *Mycobacterium massiliense* infection after thread-lift insertion. Dermatol Surg. 2016;42:1219-22.
27. Savoia A, Accardo C, Vannini F, Di Pasquale B, Baldi A. Outcomes in thread lift for facial rejuvenation: a study performed with happy lift TM revitalizing. Dermatol Ther (Heidelb). 2014;4:103-14.
28. Lee W, Moon HJ, Kim JS, Chan BL, Yang EJ. Doppler ultrasound-guided thread lifting. J Cosmet Dermatol. 2020;19:1921-7.
29. Rho NK, Chung ST. Improvement of infraorbital laxity and wrinkles by combined use of microfocused ultrasound and absorbable polydioxanone threads in a post-blepharoplasty patient. Med Lasers. 2018;7:38-40.
30. Tang S, Sun Z, Wu X, Wang YY, Zhang J. An innovative thread-lift technique for facial rejuvenation and complication management: a case report. Medicine (Baltimore). 2018;97:e10547.
31. Suárez-Vega D, Velazco de Maldonado G, García-Guevara V, Miller-Kobisher B, Morena-López K. Microscopic and clinical evidence of the degradation of polydioxanone lifting threads in the presence of hyaluronic acid: a case report. Medwave. 2019;19:e7575.

CHAPTER 125

Microblading

Aseem Sharma, Madhulika Mhatre, Trupti Agrawal, Gunjan Shah

KEY MESSAGES

- Microblading has evolved from early methods of pigment implantation to create hyper-realistic eyebrows. This semipermanent makeup technique involves depositing pigment into the upper-to-mid dermis using needles arranged like a blade, offering a more natural appearance compared to traditional eyebrow tattooing.
- Recent years have seen the development of various eyebrow enhancement techniques such as powder brows, microshading, hair stroke brows, hybrid/fusion brows, and nanoblading. These methods cater to different aesthetic preferences, from creating a gradient effect to achieving hyper-realistic hair strokes, demonstrating the field's innovation beyond simple microblading.
- Successful microblading hinges on thorough preprocedure consultation, precise eyebrow mapping, choice of pigment, and adherence to postprocedure care instructions to ensure optimal healing and pigment retention. Postmicroblading care is crucial for the longevity of the results, emphasizing the need for detailed patient education on maintenance and touch-up sessions.
- Microblading serves both cosmetic and corrective purposes, aiding individuals with scanty eyebrows, hypotrichosis, trichotillomania, alopecia, and other conditions. However, it is not suitable for everyone, with contraindications including pregnancy, certain dermatologic and ophthalmologic conditions, communicable diseases, and patients undergoing specific treatments like chemotherapy.
- While microblading has a low incidence of complications, potential risks include infections, allergic reactions, and unsatisfactory aesthetic outcomes. Techniques for pigment removal, if necessary, include exfoliation, laser treatment, saline, and magnetic removal, highlighting the importance of professional skill and client education in managing expectations and outcomes.

INTRODUCTION

Eyebrows have always been regarded as a form of nonverbal communication and facial expression. They are often the first facial features to get noticed. Few know that they serve a physiological function—that of protecting the orbit (and eye) from sweat, water, and debris to maintain clarity of sight.

Needless to say, eyebrows have gone through many innovative trends from a cosmetic standpoint—thin or bushy, arched or pointed, curved or straight, high set or low set, bold, or even none. It was not long before the realization dawned that the eyebrows needed to be modified, recreated, and not merely shaped. This is where microblading and permanent makeup came into play. In 1979, Dr Linda Dixon coined the term microblading for this process of depositing pigment in the skin, erstwhile called microfeathering, microstroking, eyebrow tattooing, eyebrow embroidery, the Japanese method, and other *de facto* names.

By definition, microblading is a form of permanent makeup wherein inert pigment is deposited in the upper-to-mid dermis with the help of stacked needles arranged on the shape of a blade. It is considered as a superficial form of micropigmentation. From the early days of its inception where blocks of tattoo pigment were used, microblading has evolved to produce hyperrealistic results using a combination of manual and machine pigment implantation.

MICROBLADING VERSUS MACHINE TECHNIQUES

Simple microblading is a manual technique and does not involve any mechanization. It is the oldest technique of eyebrow tattooing, and the equipment and pigments have evolved over time. In the past few years, it has been gradually taken over by more modern eyebrow enhancement techniques, which use an electric motorized machine. The manual technique has also evolved and given rise to nanoblading (explained more in detail under the description of equipment).

NEWER ADVANCES AND TRENDS[1,2]

- *Powder brows:* Synonymous with microshading or ombré powder brows, it is a semipermanent technique for concealing the eyebrows to rectify their shape, fill in scanty areas, and make a gradient-like impact. The procedure entails making pixelated dots that bestow a powder-like, concealed brow, which is lighter at the front of your brows and advances to becoming darker at the finishes. However, many variations of which areas to keep light or dark can be given, based on requirement of the client/patient, and the ongoing fashion trends.
- *Microshading:* This gives a look similar to powder/ombré brows, but uses manual methods such as microblading,

instead of a machine (described more in detail in the equipment section).

- *Hair stroke brows:* Hair strokes are created using a motorized machine. This is a very intricate technique and far more complex than hair strokes with microblading or microdot shading with machine. It looks more natural and creates strokes with much less trauma compared to microblading.
- *Hybrid or fusion brows:* A combination of hair strokes and shading is known as hybrid brow or fusion/combo brow. The techniques are merged together to give a more natural look. Most often, a motorized device is used to treat the tail end and head end of the brow is done manually. The mix of microbladed hair strokes or machine hair strokes and a powder fill gives an extraordinarily common looking brow. It looks well defined and filled in.
- *Nanoblading:* This uses the same technique as microblading, but the needles/pins/projections are of a much smaller diameter compared to a microblade, hence creating less trauma. The duration of nanoblading vis-à-vis conventional microblading is debatable.
- *3D/4D/6D brows:* These are not different techniques, but merely marketing gimmicks employed to distinguish oneself through marketing.

Settling on the choice to do microblading is definitely not a simple one. It is akin to tattooing of the face that will characterize one's face and change it, quite visibly. This needs to be explained in detail to the patient. This semipermanent technique is unique as in this each stroke is drawn on the skin separately, which gives it a more natural appearance; however, if done by an untrained person, it can turn out conversely.

At the point when done appropriately, microblading pigment is deposited in the papillary dermis and will start fading in 6 months to 1 year. However, if the pigment is deposited too deep, it will behave like a permanent tattoo, and hence more likely to appear grayish/ashy in color. Even deeper, and the pigment will leach into the subcutis and be carried away by lymphatic channels. Needless to say, training is of paramount importance, as is true for any aesthetic or dermatosurgical procedure.

From a more functional point of view, there are many indications to do permanent eyebrow makeup (PMU), which are as follows:

- Scanty eyebrows
- Hypotrichosis
- Trichotillomania
- Madarosis
- Alopecia areata, alopecia totalis, and alopecia universalis affecting the brow
- Cosmetic enhancement (with varied phenotypes)
- Cosmetic camouflage in conditions such as brow vitiligo
- Burns and scars
- Short eyebrows
- Drooping eyebrows

In the same breath, there are certain "relative" contraindications for performing microblading, which are as follows:

- Pregnancy/breastfeeding
- Blood-thinning drugs, especially coumarin derivatives
- Ophthalmologic diseases, such as glaucoma
- Dermatologic conditions, such as psoriasis and lichen planus where isomorphic phenomenon can be precipitated
- Communicable diseases, such as human immunodeficiency virus (HIV) or hepatitis B and C
- Epilepsy, hemophilia, or skin malignancy
- Undergoing radiotherapy or chemotherapy
- A pacemaker or any other heart condition
- Organ transplant patients
- Active viral infections
- Known allergies or hypersensitivities.

COMPLICATIONS

The complications of microblading:

- Possibility of infections (low incidence currently with the advent of onetime use, disposable equipment)
- Site pain, edema, and erythema
- Allergic reactions (to pigment/dye)
- Possibility of unnatural look and brow asymmetry
- Koebnerization of other skin diseases
- Fading or spreading of color
- Rarely granulomas
- Anaphylaxis

There are various means and methods by which a microblading methodology can turn out badly, which are as follows:

- Different shape than the patient's expectation
- Pigment fading
- Unnatural looking results
- The outcome is patchy or uneven.

There are different ways by which the pigment can be removed if the outcome does not align. They are as follows:

- Using an exfoliant daily in the treated area
- *Laser removal:* A Q-switched neodymium-doped yttrium–aluminum–garnet (Nd:YAG) laser can be used at a low fluence with 2–3 mm spot size for 4–6 sittings depending on the results. It requires experience to perform this as a higher fluence may cause scarring, infection, and post-inflammatory hypopigmentation or hyperpigmentation, especially when a passive machine is used.[3]
- *Saline removal:* It is not done routinely, possibly for colors that cannot be removed by a laser. It works by promoting desquamation.
- *Magnetic removal:* This rare procedure works only if the pigments contain iron oxide.

Pigments

Microblading professionals are constantly worried about the nature of the color. Low-quality pigment can cause skin sensitivity, blurred eyebrow color, and uneven, unpredictable pigment retention. It is, ergo, important to choose the right sort of good quality pigment for the procedure. Skin tone is an important factor to consider while choosing the same.[4]

There are two types of microblading pigments available in the market, organic and inorganic.

Organic pigments are oil dispersible. This implies that the color will mix in with skin more comprehensively with minimal clumping. These are usually fruit or vegetable based. Organic pigments are less saturated than inorganic ones and may impart a dull look to the brows. Organic color does not change color depending on skin tone, but sun exposure or exposure to chemicals can cause mild fading of the color over time.

Good-quality inorganic pigment is often made up of iron oxides. Lower quality of inorganic pigments is replete with heavy metal impurities such as lead, arsenic, and mercury, which may cause color leaching and a change over a period of time.

Both organic and inorganic pigments may also contain fragrances and additives that may lead to scarring or an allergic reaction/sensitization when applied to skin. All pigments respond and change tone with sun exposure. A reddish tinge is seen with inorganic iron oxide-containing pigments, whereas a blackish tinge is seen with organic pigments in Caucasian skin, but the same cannot be extrapolated to Indian phototypes.[5]

Premixed colors and shades are commercially available as composite pigments. These pigments are known for their solidness, life span, and dependability.

HOW TO START MICROBLADING?

Assessment

The most important part before starting any cosmetic procedure is consultation. A detailed consultation regarding the patient's needs and expectations should be delineated. Expectations and outcomes must be marginalized at this stage. The patient should be explained about the procedure steps, the fading of pigment, as well as the outcome and postprocedure care in great detail. A detailed history of the daily routine of the patient—application of creams, sun exposure, occupation, facial treatments done in recent past, sweating, keloidal or hypertrophic tendencies, and a history of past herpetic infection (*Herpes simplex*) should be taken. A preprocedure examination of skin phototype, color, tone, texture, laxity, and thickness should be carried out and recorded. This helps to determine the duration, the kind of instruments such as blade, number of pins, and the appropriate pigment required for the procedure.

Preprocedure Precautions

To avoid rescheduling of the appointment and to get best results out of the procedure, the following things should be followed:

- Avoidance of swimming or any other form of workout on the day or immediately after procedure for approximately 3–4 weeks.
- Avoid certain medications such as vitamin E, acetylsalicylic acid, and ibuprofen at least 72 hours before the procedure date. Topical retinols, retinoids, and other vitamin A derivatives must be stopped a week prior to the elective date. Also, using retinol (or any other exfoliating creams) on or around the eyebrows can lead to faster fading of the color.
- Avoid scratching or sun exposure.
- Avoid threading or waxing 24 hours prior to the appointment.
- Avoid the procedure during gestation or lactation.
- Avoid soft tissue augmentation such as botulinum toxin, dermal fillers, or laser skin tightening/resurfacing at least 4 weeks prior to the procedure.
- Avoid alcohol or caffeine and tobacco at least 24 hours prior.
- Take in-depth history of medications consumed and procedures performed (if any) in the last few days.

Anesthesia

Anesthesia involves making superficial cuts into the skin, and there is bound to be a fair amount of pain. The pain can be reduced by using topical anesthesia, for patients with a low threshold. Usually, a topical anesthetic cream containing 2.5% of lidocaine and 2.5% of prilocaine is used as a "pre-numb." The topical anesthesia is kept for about 30–45 minutes, preferably under occlusion for better results.

It is important to note that:

- Topical anesthesia should not be used after starting the procedure.
- The numbing gels meant for open skin and mucosae are not effective on intact skin. Instead, a eutectic mixture of local anesthetics (EMLA) should be used.

Procedure

1. *Designing the brow:* The technique is started by checking the surrounding skin for any skin disorders. It is helpful to take photos of patients' eyebrows before—not just for a before photograph to exhibit the scope of work, but also to show the patient the changes that should be made and have been made toward the end. Under aseptic precautions, antiseptic cleansing of the eyebrow and surrounding area is done. The eyebrow shape is drawn utilizing a specific golden mean brow caliper and eyebrow-marking pencil. Since it is a purely cosmetic procedure, it

is necessary to take into consideration what the patient wants and what accommodates their face shape, based on the standard calculations based on their orbital structure and nose. After discussion with the patient about their eyebrow shape, one can duplicate similar extents on the other eyebrow. Mapping the eyebrow has been delineated pictorially as in **Figures 1A and B**.

2. *Instruments:* The microblade is fitted at a point of roughly 155° into the microblading pen to facilitate all needles going into the skin simultaneously at 90° when the pen is held up.[4]
3. *Matching the correct pigment:* It is quintessential to have the perfect matching in terms of pigment, depending on the skin type of the patient and the existing normal hair to avoid any undesirable color change in the final outcome. The skin type, skin tone, and undertone have to be taken into consideration while selecting the pigment. Black colored pigment should be avoided, unless the patient is looking for a gray-haired look.
4. *Method:*
   a. *Stretching the skin:* The skin is stretched in three different directions. The skin in the treatment area should be taut and flat to have better results. The little finger of the hand used for the procedure stretches the skin from one side. The other hand is used to stretch the other two areas. Stretching the skin helps to make even strokes and place the pigment at a uniform depth.
   b. Any side can be begun first.
   c. Place the pigment holder with the pigment on a finger on the nondominant hand. The tip of the blade is dipped into the pigment holder to fetch pigment via capillary action. Excess pigment is wiped off and the first stroke is made.
   d. The most common technique entails drawing the main hair strokes using a blade with a little color on the tip of the blade from the start to end of the brow, mimicking the natural anatomy of the hair strokes.
   e. A depth of 1 mm roughly (papillary dermis) should be maintained per stroke. Deeper strokes result in leaching away of the pigment and the lines may look coarse and smudged. Very superficial may cause loss of pigment during the healing phase with epidermal turnover. The ideal depth also depends on individual thickness of skin and should be confirmed by the

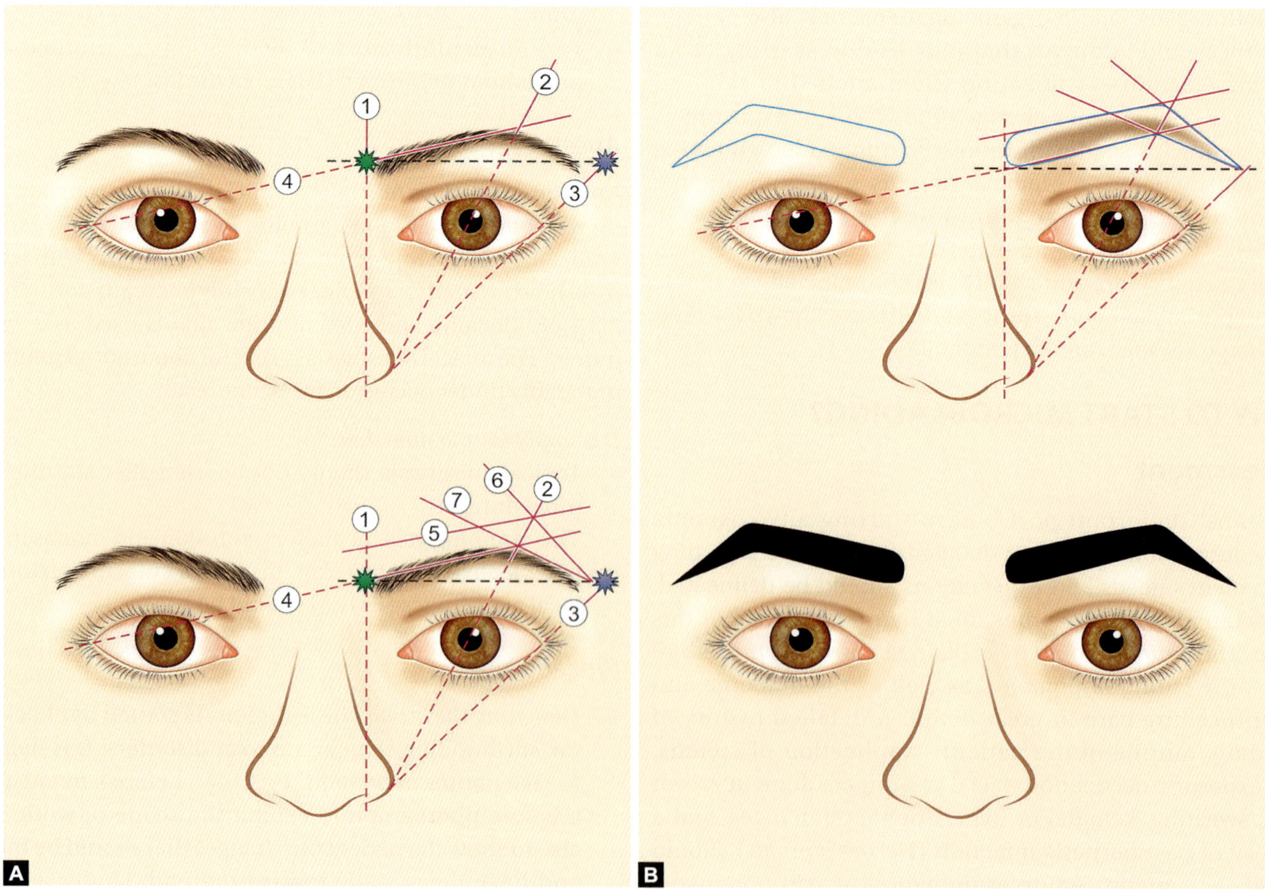

Figs. 1A and B: Represent a schematic diagram of lines which will assist the reader in doing microblading—these can be thought of as a stencil. The numbered lines are lines drawn between two anatomical landmarks to maintain constancy between surface landmarks: (1) Medial most point on brow and nasal bridge-ala junction, (2) Lateral ala and ocular limbus and arch of the brow, (3) Lateral ala and lateral canthus, (4) Cross-section between an imaginary line drawn between the medial and lateral heads of the brow and the contralateral limbus, (5) Cross-section between point 1 and 2 parallel to line 4. (6) Between lateral brow end and cross-section between points 1 and 2. (7) From lateral brow end and line 2 and 4 cross-section.

following three factors—a peculiar grating sound while making the stroke, pinpoint bleeding, and exudation of lymph.

f. *Stroke pattern:* Strokes can be individualized as there are various types. Different areas in the eyebrow have different types of strokes. To get the most natural results, the exact direction of the strokes needs to be studied and trained. The training is done first on paper and then on fake silicone skin. The strokes taken at the medial/head end are usually vertical, whereas laterally at the tail end, an acute angle in an oblique manner. All strokes are made at a point of 45° from their origin point, so that they mimic hair strands. Stroke making has been depicted in **Figures 2A to C**. Marwah et al. have classified the strokes as main strokes and supporting strokes.[1] Some authors prefer beginning the eyebrow with one to three hair strokes inside the brow marking away from the nose and adding extra hair strokes. Strokes are made medial to lateral along the brow and must never be adjacent to each other. In the event that the lines are excessively far separated, they will give a fake/"done-up" appearance. In case the lines are too closely placed, they will cause blurring after healing and look filled up or smudged. Intersecting lines will look unnatural and lead to blotching of pigment, thus cross-hatching should be avoided at all costs.[6]

On completing the microblading, for 5–10 minutes, the pigment is spread over the treated area, commonly known as a pigment bath. This helps in deeper penetration of the pigment and retains pigment in the areas where it is lost due to pinpoint bleeding and exudation. The same has been depicted in **Figure 2C**. The excess pigment is cleaned with normal saline.

Expected Outcome

Inflammation in the form of mild edema and erythema may be seen, which is transient. There can be crusting, flaking, or peeling of skin after a few days. Strokes can be blurry or may fade up to a month. The exact color is seen only after healing. Loss of 10–50% of the pigment is seen during the healing process, and the results vary from person to person.

Expected Timeline of Results

The brows will go through a few stages during the recovery cycle, which are as follows:

Days 1–4: The pigment or color will appear sharp and dark for the first few days. The color will soften progressively thereafter. The brows may expand and seem (disproportionately) bigger during the healing phase, which is an expected outcome.

Days 5–7: Once the healing process begins, the skin will appear flaky (same color as pigment used) or dry. At this stage, the color will seem to blur excessively fast; this is due to the superficial pigment and dry skin being shed off normally from the eyebrows.

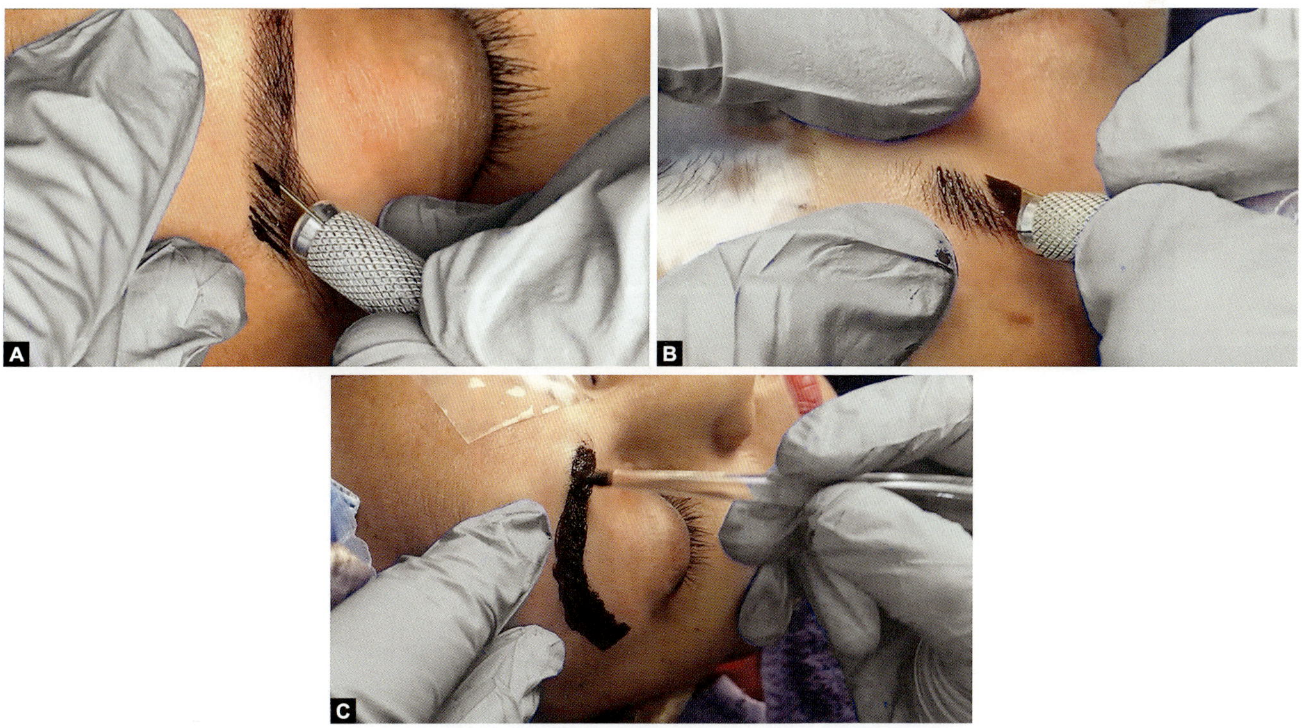

Figs. 2A to C: The procedure being done on the (A) Eyebrow body; (B) Eyebrow tail, and (C) Pigment soak (bath) postprocedure for saturating the skin breach.

Days 8–12: Near-total fading of the pigment by the end of the second week.

Days 14–28: The eyebrow color shade might appear inconsistent or unequal, but the color will begin to "return" as the skin recovers.

Detailed results by the authors with serial photos and all profiles have been appended as **Figures 3 to 5**.

Postprocedure Precautions

Good postmicroblading is essential for the desired outcome and patients' need to be counselled accordingly. A few tips are as follows:

- Apply a small quantity of clear petroleum jelly or virgin coconut oil to keep it hydrated. This may be increased as flaking ensues and healing begins. There are two schools

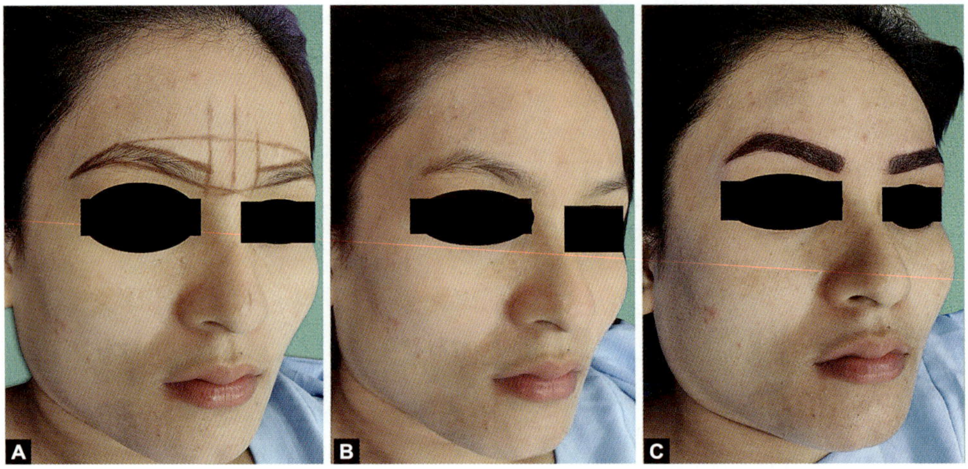

Figs. 3A to C: (A) Eyebrow mapping on a patient; (B) Premicroblading; (C) Postmicroblading.

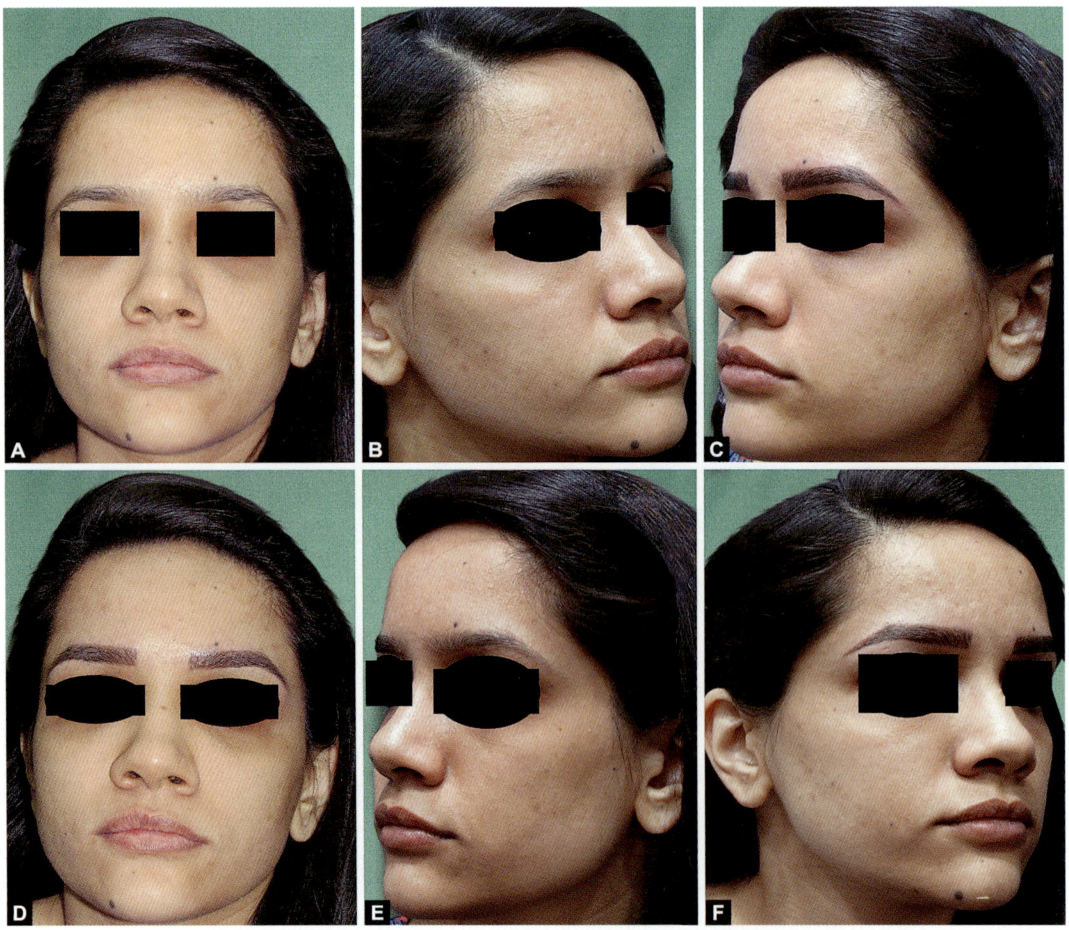

Figs. 4A to F: Before microblading profiles: (A) Front, (B) Right, and (C) Left. Postprocedure profiles: (D) Front, (E) Right, and (F) Left.

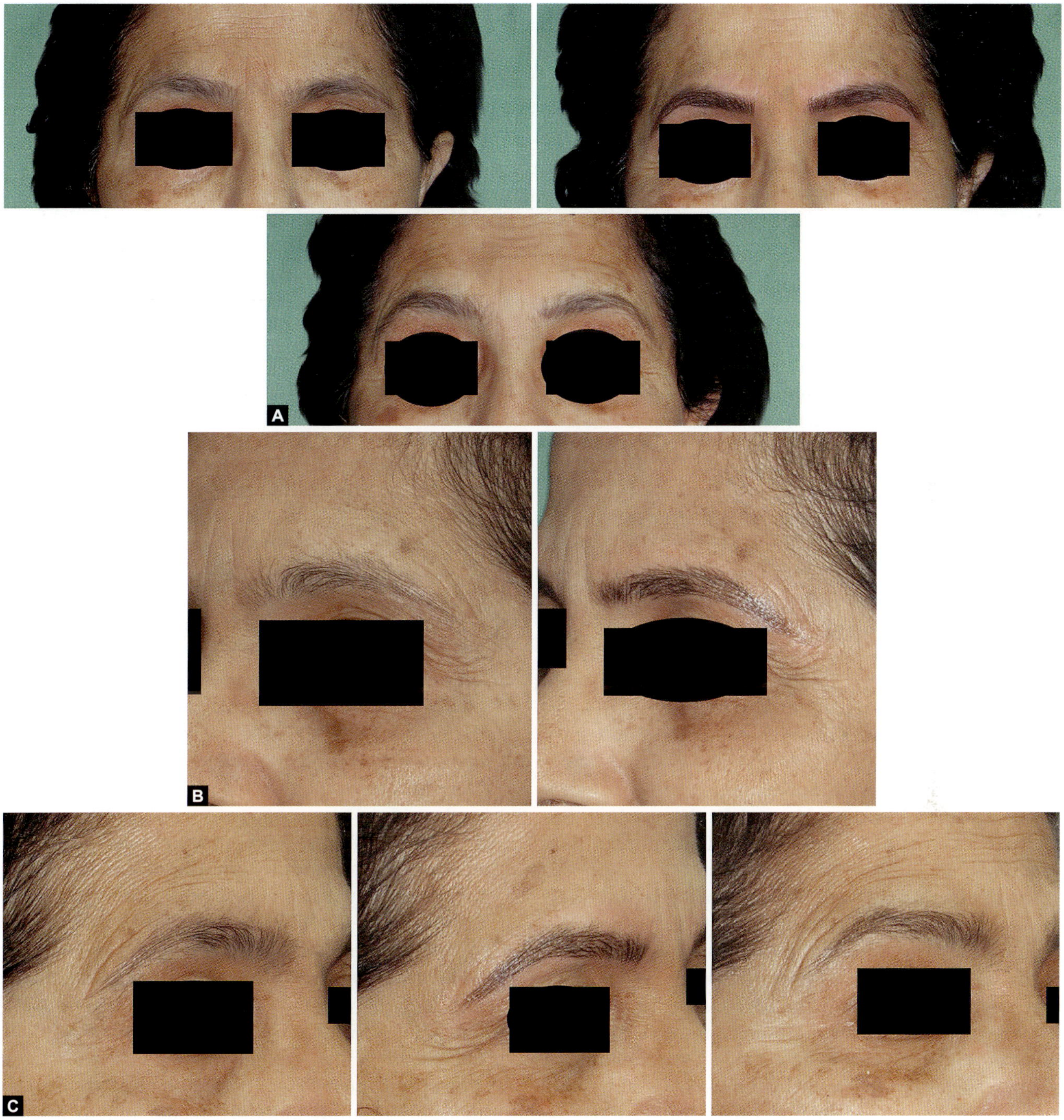

Figs. 5A to C: Serial profiles: Preprocedure, immediate postprocedure and 6 months' follow-up, in a side-by-side comparison. (A) Frontal; (B) Left profile; (C) Right profile.

of thought in terms of postprocedure care—dry healing (no water/petroleum jelly for 2 weeks till crusting is complete) and wet healing (as mentioned). Wet healing is preferred in our setting as it is better for wound healing and may prevent secondary infections. Depending on the micropigmenter and patient profile, either method may be employed.

- *Avoid the following strictly:*
  - Getting the eyebrows wet or touching them for 2 weeks
  - Anti-acne products or lightening creams around your brows
  - Antiaging creams for 4 weeks
  - Makeup for up to 2 weeks
  - Scrubbing, peeling, or picking the treated area
  - Sun exposure
  - Waxing, threading, or any other hair removal procedures
  - Any cosmetic procedure on the face
  - Rigorous physical activity or excessive sweating for 3–4 weeks
  - Swimming/bathing tubs for 3–4 weeks.

Review Session and Touch-up

Review session and touch-up can be done 6–8 weeks after microblading. It is usually required to fill in the gaps that were created due to loss of pigment after healing and to correct aberrant stroking during the session.

Special Precautions (While Doing Other Cosmetic/Dermatological Procedures)

- Use of clear petroleum jelly over the treated area
- Always wear a sunscreen postprocedure
- Avoid direct heat
- A zinc oxide paste can be used as an occlusive prior to doing lasers to prevent fading of the pigment.[1]
- Avoid waxing; threading, plucking, or trimming can be done to remove the extra hair outside the treated area.

ANATOMY OF THE EYEBROWS

The eyebrows are one of most important structures of the upper face and lend a unique quality to the human facial structure. Emotional attributes can easily be judged by the placement of one's brows—anger, surprise, frown, and many others. There is a difference in both shape and placement of brows in males and females. Male eyebrows are thicker, flatter, and grow as the age advances. The female brow is thin and more arched. For microblading, it is important to know the anatomical markers of the eyebrows as these structures change with age.

The eyebrow is a transition zone present in between the eyelid which has thin skin and forehead which has thick skin.[7] The brow has more dermal component than hypodermic.

The three principal types of hair in the eyebrow are: (1) Fine, vellus hair, (2) marginally bigger and faintly pigmented hair, and (3) large terminal hair, otherwise called the supercilia. The supercilia give the eyebrow its obvious tone and configuration. While planning incisions, the flat and vertical eyebrow hair angulations should be remembered.

Both the eyebrows are to be treated as sisters and never as twins. The eyebrows are divided into head, body, arch, and tail.[8] The head is the start or the medial most and the broadest part of the eyebrow. It is important as it has many hairs which are in vertical direction. The body is the center part that extends from the head to the elevation of the arch. A fold of hair in the hair direction is seen in many cases. The arch is the most elevated point at the intersection of the body and tail of the eyebrow; it begins tapering and getting limited toward the tail. The tail extends from the arch in the downward direction with feathering appearance. It is the most lateral part of the eyebrow. Microblading strokes should merge in a line called the "spine" of the eyebrow. There can be various placements of the spine, which will determine the direction of the strokes.

TOOLS USED IN MICROBLADING

The tools commonly required for the procedure include:

- *Microblades:* The process of microblading cannot be completed without a needle. There are numerous variations in the market. These microblades have multiple needles/pins in a row. They are classified depending upon the number of pins, diameter of pins, and how they are arranged and bound. The number of pins might range from 7 to 21 or more, the diameter varies from 0.15 to 0.30 mm. The arrangement can be slanting, U shaped, V shaped, or serrated and binding can be flexible, hard, or combination. For beginners, it is better to use flexi needles as they are bound by a flexible polymer. The experts in the field who are confident of their depth and strokes can safely use hard needles. Semiflexible needles or combination needles possess both features; they are flexible to an extent and also allow deep stroke in a single pass. Single- or double-row needles are also available. For parallel strokes, double-row needles are helpful. They are the extension of your hand and your principal instrument, so pick well.

  Use of multiple needle blade—the needle has to be layered with pigment till it is coated by dipping in the pigment. The longest needle is constantly positioned at the point we need the hair root to begin. For creating an illusion of hair, the maximum pigment is deposited where the longest needle is placed. The amount of pigment taken up by the blade is determined by the number of needles. More needles and bigger blades are required for longer strokes.
- *Measuring calipers:* This instrument is utilized for measuring the eyebrow proportion. It helps to create an ideal brow shape and perfect symmetry between the eyebrows. There are various calipers in the market for assessing the eyebrow, but golden mean brow caliper is used maximum. Few professionals use a combination of T-shaped eyebrow scale along with Vernier caliper. Forehead scales that can be taped to the forehead are also used.
- *Universal holder:* This is a specific manual instrument that holds the microblading needle and, as the name suggests, it can fit any cutting blade. As this instrument is used to take micro cuts on the skin, choose the one with a long life expectancy. It comprises three sections, the immobile handle, the rotating adjuster, and the grooved blade holder. On the tip of the third part is a cross-shaped groove. When turned anticlockwise, it opens to fix the needle. In clockwise direction, it is tightened by screwing after fixing the needle. Single-use, disposable, prefitted microblading pens are also available. There are various types of heavy or light and double-ended pens in different shapes and setups, according to the needle being used. Additionally, the pigment of the material ought to be

appropriate for cleansing, ergonomic, and lightweight so you can utilize it easily.

- *Marking pen:* Marking pen or pencil is utilized for drawing the exact brow shape before the treatment. It gives the plan to both you and your patient about the shape and design of your future eyebrows. While picking your pen, be cautious and pick the one that is exact, lasting, and does not smear.
- *Pigment rings:* Pigment rings, also known as pigment holders, are made up of metal or plastic. The plastic ring goes on your finger and is loaded up with the color. It provides immediate access to the pigment during the process. It also maintains the sanitization by not plunging the microblading pen over and again into the pigment pot. It also helps to wipe off the excess pigment on the walls of the holder.
- *Scissors and tweezers:* These small instruments should consistently be with you. They are used while planning eyebrows for the treatment to accomplish the best look.

FACIAL MORPHOLOGY

The study of shape and form of the face is known as facial morphology. Symmetry is very important when planning to draw eyebrows. So, whenever you plan to draw, proper measurements should be taken. After drawing a template of the eyebrow design and it is approved by the patient, tweeze and shave the extra hair. The patient can also use an eyebrow pencil to design the desired eyebrow shape. In the event that the subject has no current eyebrow, for example, in instances of alopecia totalis, then the cushion of fat on the orbital edge can be taken as the beginning point at the medial side. In patients with a bigger nose, the medial nasal alae are considered for estimations and in patients with a thin nose, the lateral nasal alae are considered for estimations.

The various factors on which the shape of the eyebrows depends include natural growth pattern of hair, symmetry of face, and marking the brows according to the anatomy of face.[9]

To make the template:

- Glabellar line/establishing line
- Make a straight line equidistant from each eye in between the brows. It is important to mark this correctly as all the measurements are taken from here—medial line/brow origin.
- Length of the brow/lateral line—it is a line passing through and that extends upward from nasal alae to lateral canthus and above. The typical thickness of an eyebrow differs from 6 to 9 mm. When deciding the length of the brows, kindly consider the following points:
  - Width of the eyes
  - Natural pattern of hair
  - Face shape of the patient
  - Depth and width of the forehead
  - The brow bone
- *Arch line:* The arch is marked depending upon the length of the eyebrow. The position is marked by dividing the length with the golden caliper or roughly two thirds of the brow length. It is also drawn as a diagonal line passing from the nasal alae to the mid pupillary point extending upward.
- *Baseline:* Mark a straight horizontal line parallel with the eyes from the lowest point of the brows.

When the eyebrow is drawn, the thickness of the eyebrow ought to be reverified with a Vernier caliper for the eyebrow length.

Check all the eyebrows' measurements for symmetry and length to be double sure before proceeding for the actual treatment.

Different Shapes of Eyebrow

There are diverse face structures as per age, sex, and different races. An eyebrow is drawn keeping in mind the regular face and bone construction; consequently, each of these remarkable face structures has a specific eyebrow shape that suits them the best. The eyebrows can be curved, straight, S-shaped, and high or low arched.

The head is the start and an anchor of the brow, the place of the head is the main part as its position will direct the remainder of the eyebrow shape.

The body: Too much arch in this area will give a "McDonalds" eyebrow, so it is better to keep it flat.[10]

The arch: For giving a wider face appearance, the arch is placed further out by drawing a line from the nose through the mid-pupillary line of the eye. For giving a thinner face, the arch is placed further in by drawing a line from the nose through the pupil.

The tail's position is determined by drawing a line from nose to the lateral canthus of the eye.

To get the right eyebrows, do not place the head much lower than the tail and the tail much lower than the arch.

In case of wide faces (e.g., square, round, or heart), a narrower look can be given by widening the brow.

For narrow faces (oval and oblong), a wider appearance can be given by decreasing the length of the brow.

The arch can be more angulated and acute to augment an angular face.

A prominent angular arch is given for very rounded faces to give better definition.

BENEFITS OF MICROBLADING

The benefits are as:

- Hyperrealistic hair strokes rather than block brows
- Individual hair strokes impart a very natural look.
- Fades off naturally
- Less painful and more superficial than a conventional tattoo
- Touch-ups between 1 and 3 years

CONCLUSION

Microblading is a niche procedure that has recently come into the limelight as a part of permanent makeup. Its true indications fall beyond the gambit of superciliary madarosis, alopecia areata, leprosy, and other conditions. It traverses tattooing and surgical restoration of the brow. A microblading setup is easy, but the procedure requires technical skill and a lot of practice, but once mastered, is an indispensable tool in an aesthetic dermatology clinic for a myriad of indications.

REFERENCES

1. Marwah MK, Kerure AS, Marwah GS. Microblading and the science behind it. Indian Dermatol Online J. 2021;12(1):6-11.
2. Pai D. (2021). Microblading Eyebrows, Microshading, and Microfeathering: What's the Difference? [online] Available from: https://www.glamour.com/story/what-is-microblading-microshading-microfeathering [Last accessed August, 2023].
3. Mao JC, DeJoseph LM. Latest innovations for tattoo and permanent makeup removal. Facial Plast Surg Clin North Am. 2012;20:125-34.
4. Price KM, Gupta PK, Woodward JA, Stinnett SS, Murchison AP. Eyebrow and eyelid dimensions: An anthropometric analysis of African Americans and Caucasians. Plast Reconstr Surg. 2009;124:615-23.
5. Høgsberg T, Jacobsen NR, Clausen PA, Serup J. Black tattoo pigments induce reactive oxygen species production correlating with aggregation of pigment nanoparticles and product brand but not with the polycyclic aromatic hydrocarbon content. Exp Dermatol. 2013;22:464-9.
6. Asch C. The procedure. In: Asch C (Ed). The Microblading Bible, 1st edition. USA: Createspace Independent Publishing Platform; 2016.
7. Chokthaweesak W, Annunziata CC, Korn BS, Kikkawa DO. (2016). Eyebrows, Eyelids, and Face: Structure and Function. Available from: https://entokey.com/eyebrows-eyelids-and-face-structure-and-function/ [Last accessed August, 2023].
8. Van der Velden EM, Drost BH, Ijsselmuiden OE, Baruchin AM, Hulsebosch HJ. Dermatography as a new treatment for alopecia areata of the eyebrows. Int J Dermatol. 1998;37:617-21.
9. Hetzler L, Sykes J. The brow and forehead in periocular rejuvenation. Facial Plast Surg Clin North Am. 2010;18:375-84.
10. Scott E. (2017). McDonald's brows are here to save you from the horror of silly makeup trends. [online] Available from: https://metro.co.uk/2017/09/09/mcdonalds-brows-are-here-to-save-you-from-the-horror-of-ridiculous-makeup-trends-6914574/ [Last accessed August, 2023].

CHAPTER 126

Stretch Marks

Vikas Pathania, Reetu Agarwal, Siddharth Mani

KEY MESSAGES

- Management of stretch marks includes both preventive and therapeutic measures.
- The ideal topical agent for prevention of striae is still a mirage. Tretinoin has been used with some success. Its contraindication in pregnancy warrants the search for an ideal agent.
- Hydration of the skin is a key factor in its prevention.
- Fractional nonablative and ablative lasers have been tried, but the results are not fully satisfactory.
- Experimental therapies such as platelet-rich plasma, dermaroller, and microdermabrasion are being tried.

INTRODUCTION

Stretch marks, known as striae distensae, are one of the commonly occurring dermal lesions. They are known to mankind since time immemorial with a specific mention in the 16 century BC by a poet Ovid who mentioned women fearing and aborting pregnancy to prevent stretch marks.[1] Later ancient Egyptians described several formulations for the treatment of stretch marks with special mention of unripe olive oil and sea salt.[2] The significance of stretch marks, even though they are mainly asymptomatic, is due to its prevalence and persistence of the lesion in the population. Their psychological effect on the self-perception of the patient's body image has far-reaching consequences. They are found to be the most common connective tissue changes in pregnancy.[3]

ETIOLOGY

The etiology of striae distensae is poorly understood. The etiopathogenesis involves a combination of genetic[4] and hormonal factors[5,6] causing the predisposition along with various other host and environmental factors that cause dermal connective tissue disruption.[7,8] These factors are enumerated in **Table 1**. There are other anecdotal reports of risk factors, which include reduced blood vitamin C levels, use of indinavir in human immunodeficiency virus (HIV), low serum relaxin level, and alcohol intake.[9,10]

CLINICAL FEATURES

There are two forms of stretch marks found commonly in the clinical practice: (1) striae rubra and (2) striae alba. Striae rubra is considered to be the early form, is erythematous, and may be slightly elevated above the normal skin. It is sometimes associated with symptoms such as itching and irritation. While in the chronic stage, the striae distensae is known as striae alba. They appear wrinkly, faded, and hypopigmented.[11] Hermans et al. have described two newer varieties of stretch marks: (1) striae nigra and (2) striae caerulea, seen in dark-skinned patients, based on objective colorimetric assessments due to an increase in melanogenesis.[12] Striae are predominantly located on the arms, thighs, abdomen, and lumbosacral area, but may involve other regions, including the face, and flexures in case of striae induced by Cushing's syndrome or steroid therapy **(Fig. 1)**.[13] The striae occurring during pregnancy have been named as striae gravidarum.[14] In pregnancy, they occur most commonly on abdomen and breasts.[15] In obese patients, striae are lighter with less atrophy and narrower than those with Cushing's syndrome.[16] In Cushing's syndrome, there is presence of purple (violaceous) striae >1 cm in diameter. Very rarely, severe, extensive striae may ulcerate or tear.[17] Bullous

TABLE 1: Etiology and risk factors for striae.

Etiology	*Risk factors*
Sudden weight loss or weight gain	Previous history of striae gravidarum
Obesity	Family history of striae gravidarum
Pregnancy	Higher body mass index (BMI) before pregnancy
Growth spurt during adolescence	Higher gestational weight gain
Young weightlifters	Younger maternal age
Long-term usage of corticosteroids	
Cushing's syndrome	
Marfan syndrome	
Congenital arachnodactyly	
Idiopathic	

striae have been reported by Gupta et al.[18] in a patient with an anasarca.

HISTOPATHOGENESIS OF STRIAE

Although the exact pathogenesis of striae is still an enigma, various hypotheses have been put forward. Sheu et al.[19] suggested that the mast cells release enzymes, namely elastases, which cause elastolysis in the dermis and are the key initiators of the striae. This is followed by influx of activated macrophages, which engulf these fragmented elastic fibers. They suggested that the elastic fibers were the primary tissue targeted during the formation of stretch marks and found the tissue damage to exist up to 3 cm beyond the clinically obvious stretch marks. A remodeling and reduction of the elastic fiber network of skin in the striae-affected area was reported by Watson et al.[20] They demonstrated looser and more floccular dermal matrix of striae, when compared to the normal skin and elastin and fibrillin fibers in the deeper dermis showed realignment.

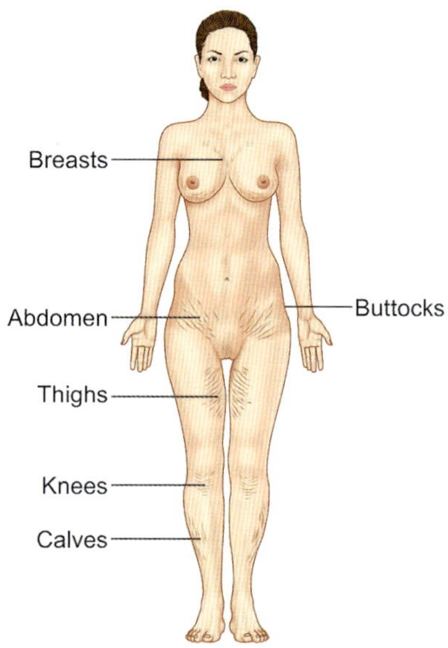

Fig. 1: Common anatomical location of striae.

Striae lesional skin is characterized histologically on light microscopy by thinning of the overlying epidermis, fine dermal collagen bundle with dermal edema, and perivascular lymphocytic cuffing. In later stages, epidermal atrophy and loss of rete ridges are evident.[21] In addition, hair follicles and other appendages are absent.[22] The area of striae is discernible from the surrounding skin by a densely packed area of thin eosinophilic collagen bundles, horizontal to the surface in a parallel fashion. There is a significant reduction in elastin content of papillary dermis and reduced fibrillin microfibrils are seen at dermal-epidermal junction (DEJ) and dermis. There is also an alteration in orientation of elastin and fibrillin microfibrils from the normal pattern (being arranged perpendicular to the DEJ) to an abnormal parallel pattern in which arrangement parallel to DEJ is seen.[20] The transmission electron microscopy and immunofluorescence reveal the primary histopathology of striae to be a diminution of elastin fibers and fibrillin microfibrils in the dermis and increased mucopolysaccharide content in response to hormonal changes and physical factors.[20]

MANAGEMENT OF STRIAE

Flowchart 1 shows different options for the management of stretch marks.

Topical Treatment

Preventive Options

There has been no treatment option shown to consistently resolve the striae completely; hence, great emphasis has been laid upon its prevention, especially during pregnancy. The incidence of striae gravidarum occurring during pregnancy

Flowchart 1: Different options for management of stretch marks.

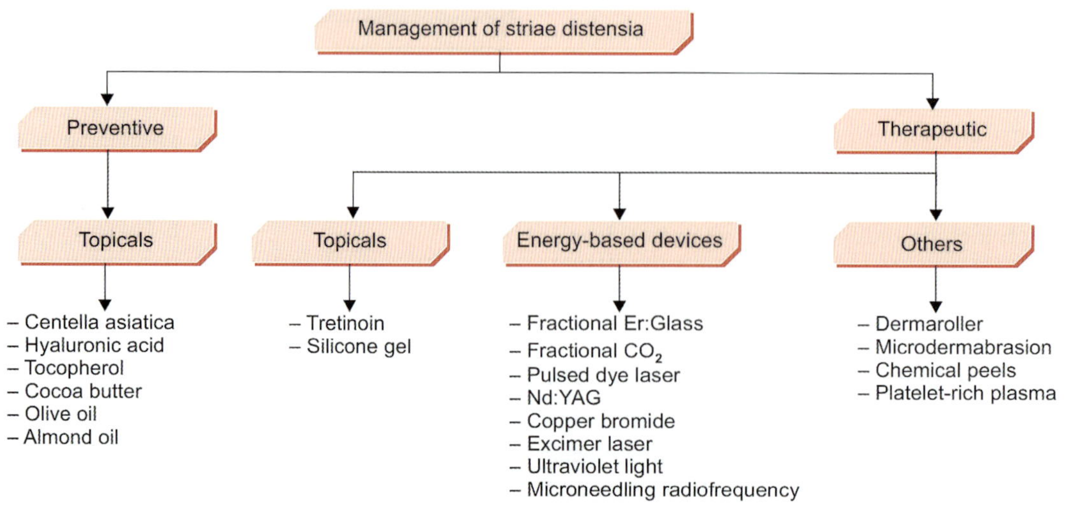

(Nd: YAG: neodymium-doped yttrium aluminum garnet)

is 50–90%. Topical therapy is the mainstay of preventive medications. The efficacy of topicals containing *Centella asiatica*,[23] hyaluronic acid,[24] cocoa butter,[25,26] and olive oil has been evaluated as a randomized control study with level 2 evidence.[27] Topical preparation containing the active ingredients *Centella asiatica*, tocopherol, and collagen-elastin hydrolysate was found to significantly reduce the incidence of striae gravidarum in women, who used it from 12th week of gestation till delivery. *Centella asiatica* is known to stimulate cell production and fibroblasts in striae distensae.[28] In the study conducted by De Buman et al.[24] the incidence of occurrence of striae gravidarum in the group using cream-containing hyaluronic acid as the main ingredient was only 10%, whereas it was 70% in placebo group. Cocoa butter and olive oil application did not seem to have any beneficial effects in comparison to the placebo. Almond oil application, when combined with a gentle massage, has been shown to have a better preventive action than application of almond oil without massage or the placebo.[29] Other ingredients such as coconut oil, licorice extract, marine collagen, marine elastine, panthenol (vitamin B_5), and vitamin E have been used in the stretch marks prevention, although the proof of their efficacy is limited.[27]

Various topical agents and their proposed mechanism of action are as in **Table 2**.

Therapeutic Options

Various studies have shown beneficial action of 0.1% tretinoin in striae rubra.[30,31] Meta-analyses of various studies show improvement seen in 60–80% cases with better results seen with 0.1% tretinoin in comparison to lower concentrations of tretinoin.[30] Treatment duration of 6 months or longer has been described in the studies for the achievement of satisfactory results.[32] Topical tretinoin is a "Category C" drug and has contraindications in pregnancy but thorough literature reviews showed no reported contraindication data regarding usage in lactating mother.[33] Effects with tretinoin are better for striae rubra as compared to striae alba **(Figs. 2A and B)**. Application of tretinoin is followed by a short period of erythema and exfoliation, so it is better to counsel the patients in advance **(Figs. 3A and B)**. Silicone gels applied daily for 6 weeks duration on the other hand helped in increasing the collagen levels and melanin in striae alba.[34]

Lasers and Light-based Devices

Fractional Nonablative Lasers

The most common laser reported in the treatment of stretch marks is fractional erbium:glass (Er:Glass) laser with a wavelength of 1,540, 1,550, and 1,565 nm.[35] In the study done by de Angelis et al.[36] all the 51 patients treated

TABLE 2: Topical agents with mechanism of action.

Agent	*Mechanism of action*
Tretinoin	Increases collagen production
Centella asiatica extract	Stimulates the action of fibroblast thus promoting extracellular matrix formation
Almond oil	Maintains hydration and skin elasticity
Cocoa butter	Moisturizing effect
Chamomile	Decreases skin irritation
Collagen–elastin hydrolysates	Scaffold for tissue regeneration
Hyaluronic acid	Provides hydration
Vitamin B_5 (panthenol)	Promotes cell growth and differentiation
Tocopherol acetate	Antioxidant
Retinyl palmitate	Increases cell proliferation
Resveratrol	Inhibits keratinocyte proliferation
Marine collagen	Improves elasticity
Marine elastine	Improves elasticity
Licorice extract	Mechanism not known
Palm oil	Mechanism not known

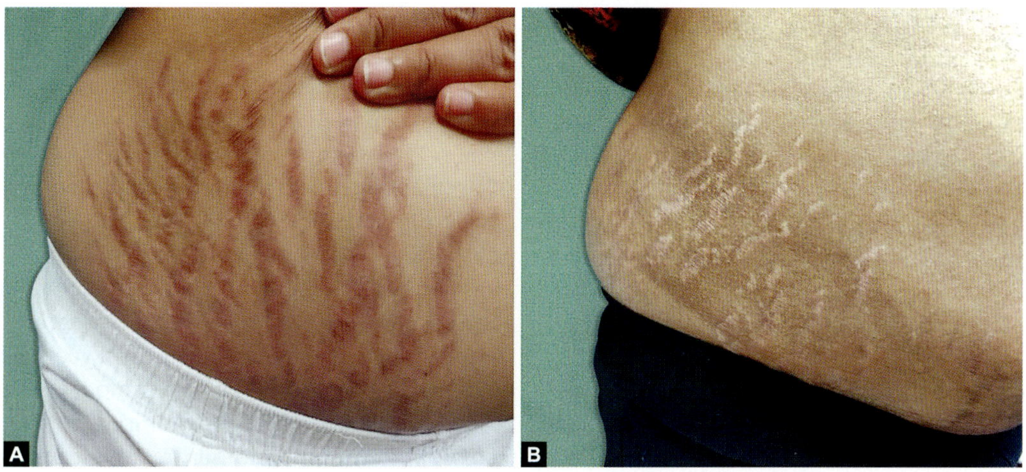

Figs. 2A and B: (A) Before and (B) after 3 months of 0.1% tretinoin.

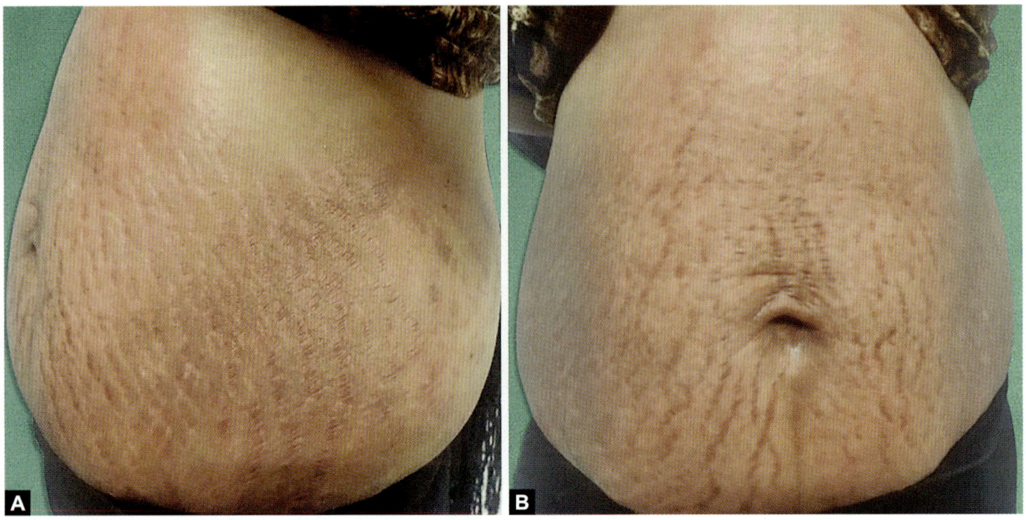

Figs. 3A and B: Erythema and exfoliation after application of 0.1% tretinoin.

with 1,540 nm fractional Er:Glass laser had more than 50% improvement. Neocollagenesis and increase in elastic fibers were demonstrated in the biopsy sections from the treated area. Out of 22 Asian women were treated with two sessions of fractional Er:Glass laser for striae alba, 27% of them had marked (51–75%) improvement after the final session. The authors noted an increase in the thickness of epidermis and dermis as well as an increase in collagen production in the post-treatment biopsy.[37]

Clementoni et al. studied the safety and efficacy of 1,565 nm nonablative fractional laser in striae atrophicans in 12 patients of skin type II and III. They received three sessions at 4 weeks intervals. All the patients had good (51–75%) improvement, along with volume improvement in 91.66% (11 out of 12) and color improvement in 83.33% (10 out of 12) of the striae distensae.[38]

Fractional Carbon Dioxide Laser

Both ablative and nonablative fractional treatments have shown promising results for treating stretch marks, although ablative lasers such as CO_2 have been associated with longer recovery period and more pain.[35]

In the retrospective analysis done by Lee et al.[39] of 27 women of skin type IV with striae alba were treated with a single session of ultrapulsed fractional CO_2 laser. Two patients had excellent improvement (>75%), 51–75% improvement was noted in 14 patients, and a moderate improvement (26–50%) was noted in nine patients, 3 months after the treatment. The common adverse effects reported were transient postinflammatory hyperpigmentation, scaling, and crusting.

Ninety-two striae in six women of skin type III and IV were divided into two groups of 46 matched striae each to be treated with ultrapulsed fractionated CO_2 laser for the first group and topical application of glycolic acid (10%) and tretinoin (0.05%) cream. Statistical analysis demonstrated that the laser treatment was more effective in improving the striae alba appearance and decreasing its surface area, in comparison to topical therapy. Hyperpigmentation was reported in one patient following laser therapy.[40]

Fractional Erbium-doped Yttrium Aluminum Garnet Laser

Split body comparison of fractional erbium-doped yttrium aluminum garnet (Er-YAG) and pulsed dye laser (PDL) on axillary striae by Gauglitz et al.[41] demonstrated beneficial effects of the fractional ablative 2,940 nm Er-YAG fractional laser for the treatment of striae, although the authors state that the risk of associated hyperpigmentation should not be underestimated with this laser, especially in individuals of darker skin type.

Pulsed Dye Laser

Since dilated blood vessels are an important component in striae rubra, it yields to treatment with PDL. Jiménez et al. have noted that the PDL (585 nm) was beneficial in reducing the degree of erythema in striae rubra and clinical change was not apparent in striae alba. They also warned against the use of PDL therapy for patients with phototypes V–VI even in low fluences, due to the higher chances of postinflammatory hyperpigmentation.[42]

McDaniel et al. reported that treatment of striae with four sessions of PDL (585 nm) at low energy densities showed improvement in the appearance of striae, and was associated with an increase in dermal elastin 8 weeks after the therapy. They also concluded that the protocol with a 10-mm spot size using 3.0 J/cm^2 fluence improved the appearance of striae better than the other treatment protocols.[43] Aldahan et al. noted that the microscopic changes observed in the various studies done on striae using PDL are predominantly subclinical and most likely insufficient for noticeable improvement clinically.[35]

Neodymium-doped Yttrium Aluminum Garnet

The neodymium-doped yttrium aluminum garnet (Nd:YAG) laser has affinity for vascular chromophores, thus making it an ideal laser for the treatment of striae and has been known to increase dermal collagen, and hence suitable for striae alba. Goldman et al. used a 1,064-nm long-pulsed laser to treat striae rubra in 20 patients. 55% of the patients considered the results as excellent, whereas 40% of the results were graded as excellent (>75%), and 40% had good (30–70%) improvement on physician assessment. The best results were noted after at least three sessions. The patients received an average of 3.6 sessions once every 3–6 weeks. No major side effects were noted.[44] Elsaie et al.[45] used long-pulsed Nd:YAG laser in the treatment of striae distensae, and found that a fluence of 100 J/cm^2 with a 5-mm spot and 15 ms pulse duration significantly improved the striae alba. All the patients received four treatment sessions at a 3-week interval. They also demonstrated an increase in collagen and elastin fibers histopathologically, 3 months postlaser. The authors stated that treatment with long-pulsed Nd:YAG laser enhances wound contraction, the remodeling of collagen fibers by thermal necrosis, activation of the release of basic fibroblast growth factor (FGF) along with inhibition of transforming growth factor beta-1.[45]

Excimer Laser and Ultraviolet Light Therapy

The excimer laser and the ultraviolet (UV) B light source have been established as excellent, safe treatments for vitiligo and other hypopigmented lesions. Goldberg et al.[46] studied the effect of target phototherapy on the hypopigmentation of striae alba. 10 patients were divided into two groups, 5 were treated with 308 nm excimer laser, and the other 5 with UVB light device for 10 sessions after either full repigmentation or until the subject was noted to have a 75% or greater increase in pigment in the treatment area. 6 months post-treatment electron microscopic biopsies from the treated areas showed the presence of enlarged melanocytes and also increased number of melanosomes. The authors concluded that the excimer and UVB-induced improvement in striae can be long-lasting, but not permanent. Alexiades-Armenakas et al. observed that mean final pigment correction rates were approximately 60–70% by visual assessment and a total correction by colorimetric analysis after nine treatments of 308-nm excimer laser administered biweekly. They observed that maintenance treatment once in every 1–4 months was necessary to sustain the aesthetic benefit. Splaying of pigment onto the normal skin was a commonly noted side effect.[47]

Copper Bromide Laser

A 577-nm copper bromide laser has been studied in 15 women of Fitzpatrick skin type II–III with striae distensae. 5 of the 15 patients had complete resolution of their striae and 8 had modest improvement after five treatment sessions. The results of the treatment were well maintained in 13 patients followed up for 2 years.[48]

Radiofrequency

Fractional radiofrequency (RF) is thought to cause a bulk heating effect on the dermis due to the absorption of energy by water, collagen, melanin, and the dermal microvasculature, which in turn induces growth factor secretion, such as vascular endothelial growth factor (VEGF) and FGF resulting in dermal remodeling.[49] Ryu et al. assessed 30 patients of skin type Fitzpatrick IV with striae distensae. They were divided into three groups randomly: to be treated with fractional CO_2 laser alone, microneedling RF alone, or a combination of both. The improvement was graded by physicians and patients on a scale of 1–4, with 4 standing for near-total improvement. The mean clinical improvement score after three sessions was 2.4 in the fractional CO_2 laser-treated group, 2.0 in the microneedle RF-treated group, and 3.4 in the combination group. The combined therapy of microneedle fractional RF with a fractional CO_2 laser that showed statistically significant improvement in roughness and thinning of the skin, which correlates with the markedly increase in the number and thickness of collagen fibers histologically after treatment. Pain, pregnancy-induced hypertension (PIH), and pruritus were the commonly seen temporary side effects.[49] Naeini et al. supported the findings that microneedling RF in combination with fractional CO_2 laser had more therapeutic effects on striae than microneedling RF alone.[50]

Other Modalities of Treatment

Microdermabrasion

Microdermabrasion has been known to induce epidermal signal transduction pathways, which are associated with remodeling of the dermal matrix.[51] 20 patients with striae distensae underwent a series of five microdermabrasion treatments at weekly intervals. 6 weeks after the treatments, four patients showed less than 25% improvement, six had 25–50% improvement, six had 51–75% improvement, and four had more than 75% improvement. Striae rubra showed better response to treatment than striae alba. PIH and transient erythema were the side effects seen in the study.[52] The authors demonstrated a significant increase in type I procollagen alpha-1 messenger ribonucleic acid in treated area compared to nontreated control area. Further studies on larger number of patients are needed to confirm the efficacy of this procedure.

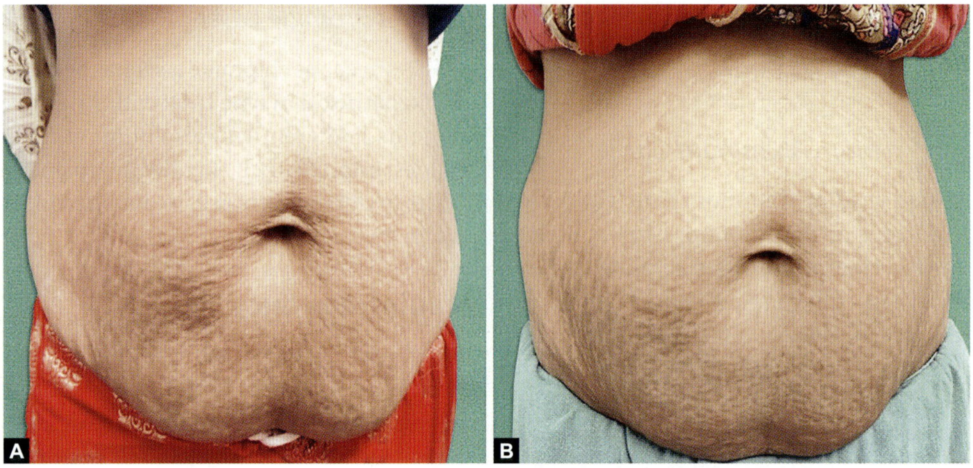

Figs. 4A and B: (A) Before and (B) after six sessions of platelet-rich plasma (PRP).

Chemical Peels

Various studies have used glycolic acid and trichloroacetic acid (TCA) for superficial skin peels as a treatment of striae distensae with inconsistent results. Although anecdotal reports of good resolution with multiple sessions of chemical peeling are present, there is a paucity of controlled studies.[53] Sanad et al.[54] treated 30 women with abdominal striae with a combination of TCA and microdermabrasion on one side and only microdermabrasion on the other side. 63.3% patients showed good to excellent improvement in the striae, on the side of combination in comparison to 33.3% with microdermabrasion alone.

Platelet-rich Plasma

Platelet-rich plasma (PRP) has been demonstrated to increase the length of the dermoepidermal junction, the amount of collagen, and also the number of fibroblasts.[55] Arshdeep et al.[56] have stated that growth factors contained in alpha granules of platelets in the PRP are responsible for the modulation of tissue repair and regeneration, whereas the plasma proteins such as fibronectin, fibrin, and vitronectin act as a scaffold for the bone, connective tissue, and epithelial migration. Furthermore, PRP is known to increase the hyaluronic acid production, which draws water into the matrix causing volume reconstruction and lubrication in atrophic scar tissue. Hyaluronic acid promotes fibroblast proliferation, extracellular matrix synthesis, and modulates collagen fibers diameter proving its role in remodeling. PRP activates matrix metalloproteinases (MMPs), and MMP in the skin facilitates damage collagen fragment resorption leading to efficient new collagen deposition. The concentrate is used as intradermal injections given at an amount of 0.05–0.1 mL/cm^2, in a retrograde fashion from deep to superficial, at every centimeter, throughout the treated site. The author has observed early and fast clinical improvement in PRP group with continuous clinical improvement noticed in successive sittings although the degree of improvement was lower in fifth and sixth sittings **(Figs. 4A and B)**. Ibrahim et al. compared the effect of PRP and microdermabrasion in patients with striae. 68 patients with striae distensae were randomly assigned to three groups: intradermal injection of PRP alone, microdermabrasion alone, and combination of intradermal PRP and microdermabrasion in the same session. The procedures were performed every 2 weeks for six sessions. They concluded that both techniques were equally effective in the treatment of striae distensae, but in microdermabrasion combined with PRP, lesser number of sessions was required.[57]

CONCLUSION

Despite the vast array of treatment options available to treat stretch marks, there is no evidence-based treatment which provides consistent results. Also, there are no standard guidelines or recommendations for any topical or interventional treatment. Tretinoin has shown some benefits; however, it cannot be used in pregnancy. PRP is another unexacting method that has shown promising results. Fractional nonablative and ablative lasers have shown the best results so far, though more evidence is needed to ensure consistent protocols for management. It is the physician's experience and knowledge of the device in hand, which determines that better results can be delivered to the patient with stretch marks.

REFERENCES

1. Rayor DJ, Batstone WW (Ed). Latin Lyric and Elegiac Poetry: An Anthology of New Translations, 1st edition. New York: Garland; 1995.
2. Owsei T (Ed). Soranus' Gynecology, 1st edition. Baltimore: John Hopkins University Press; 1991. p. 42.
3. Brennan M, Clarke M, Devane D. The use of anti stretch marks' products by women in pregnancy: a descriptive, cross-sectional survey. BMC Pregnancy Childbirth. 2016;16(1):276.
4. Di Lernia V, Bonci A, Cattania M, Bisighini G. Striae distensae (rubrae) in monozygotic twins. Pediatr Dermatol. 2001;18(3): 261-2.

5. Cordeiro RC, Zecchin KG, de Moraes AM. Expression of estrogen, androgen, and glucocorticoid receptors in recent striae distensae. Int J Dermatol. 2010;49(1):30-2.
6. Lurie S, Matas Z, Fux A, Golan A, Sadan O. Association of serum relaxin with striae gravidarum in pregnant women. Arch Gynecol Obstet. 2011;283(2):219-22.
7. Fitzpatrick T, Wolff K. Access Medicine: Fitzpatrick's Dermatology in General Medicine. New York: McGraw-Hill Medical; 2008.
8. Tung JY, Kiefer AK, Mullins M, Francke U, Eriksson N. Genome-wide association analysis implicates elastic microfibrils in the development of nonsyndromic striae distensae. J Invest Dermatol. 2013;133(11):2628-31.
9. Farahnik B, Park K, Kroumpouzos G, Murase J. Striae gravidarum: risk factors, prevention, and management. Int J Womens Dermatol. 2016;3(2):77-85.
10. Darvay A, Acland K, Lynn W, Russell-Jones R. Striae formation in two HIV-positive persons receiving protease inhibitors. J Am Acad Dermatol. 1999;41(3):467-9.
11. Singh G, Kumar LP. Striae distensae. Indian J Dermatol Venereol Leprol. 2005;71(5):370-2.
12. Hermanns JF, Pierard GE. High-resolution epiluminescence colorimetry of striae distensae. J Eur Acad Dermatol Venereol. 2006;20(3):282-7.
13. Burrows NP, Lovell CR. Disorders of connective tissue. In: Burns T, Breathnach S, Cox N, Griffith C (Eds). Rook's Textbook of Dermatology, 7th edition. Oxford: Blackwell Science; 2004. pp. 46-7.
14. Osman H, Rubeiz N, Tamim H, Nassar AH. Risk factors for the development of striae gravidarum. Am J Obstet Gynecol. 2007;196(1):62.e1-5.
15. Sparker MK, Garcia-Gonzalez E, Sanchez LT. Sclerosing and atrophying conditions. In: Schachner LA, Hansen RC (Eds). Pediatric Dermatology, 2nd edition. New York: Churchill Livingstone; 1996. p. 897.
16. Garcia Hidalgo L. Dermatological complications of obesity. Am J Clin Dermatol. 2002;3(7):497-506.
17. Sparker MK, Garcia-Gonzalez E, Sanchez LT. Sclerosing and atrophying conditions. In: Schachner LA, Hansen RC (Eds). Pediatric Dermatology, 2nd edition. New York: Churchill Livingstone; 1996. p. 897.
18. Gupta V, Yadav S. Bullous striae distensae. Postgrad Med J. 2017;93(1096):108.
19. Sheu HM, Yu HS, Chang CH. Mast cell degranulation and elastolysis in the early stage of striae distensae. J Cutan Pathol. 1991;18(6):410-6.
20. Watson RE, Parry EJ, Humphries JD, Jones CJ, Polson DW, Kielty CM, et al. Fibrillin microfibrils are reduced in skin exhibiting striae distensae. Br J Dermatol. 1998;138(6):931-7.
21. Korgavkar K, Wang F. Stretch marks during pregnancy: a review of topical prevention. Br J Dermatol. 2015;172(3):606-15.
22. Garcia-Fernandez RA, Perez-Martinez C, Garcia-Iglesias MJ. In vivo long-term effects of retinoic acid exposure in utero on induced tumours in adult mouse skin. Vet Dermatol. 2014;25(6): 538-46, e93-4.
23. Mallol J, Belda MA, Costa D, Noval A, Sola M. Prophylaxis of striae gravidarum with a topical formulation: a double blind trial. Int J Cosmet Sci. 1991;13(1):51-7.
24. De Buman M, Walther M, de Weck R. Effectiveness of Alphastria cream in the prevention of pregnancy stretch marks (striae distensae): results of a double-blind study Gynakol Rundsch. 1987;27(2):79-84.
25. Osman H, Usta IM, Rubeiz N, Abu-Rustum R, Charara I, Nassar AH. Cocoa butter lotion for prevention of striae gravidarum: a double-blind, randomised and placebo-controlled trial. BJOG. 2008;115(9):1138-42.
26. Brennan M, Young G, Devane D. Topical preparations for preventing stretch marks in pregnancy. Cochrane Database Syst Rev. 2012;11(11):CD000066.
27. Ud-Din S, McGeorge D, Bayat A. Topical management of striae distensae (stretch marks): prevention and therapy of striae rubrae and albae. J Eur Acad Dermatol Venereol. 2016;30(2):211-22.
28. Brinkhaus B, Lindner M, Schuppan D, Hahn EG. Chemical, pharmacological and clinical profile of the East Asian medical plant Centella asiatica. Phytomedicine. 2000;7(5):427-48.
29. Timur Tashan S, Kafkasli A. The effect of bitter almond oil and massaging on striae gravidarum in primiparaous women. J Clin Nurs. 2012;21(11-12):1570-6.
30. Kang S, Kim KJ, Griffiths CE, Wong TY, Talwar HS, Fisher GJ, et al. Topical tretinoin (retinoic acid) improves early stretch marks. Arch Dermatol. 1996;132(5):519-26.
31. Rangel O, Arias I, Garcia E, Lopez-Padilla S. Topical tretinoin 0.1% for pregnancy-related abdominal striae: an open-label, multicenter, prospective study. Adv Ther. 2001;18(4):181-6.
32. DeBuman M, Walther M, de Weck R. Effectiveness of Alphastria cream in the prevention of pregnancy stretch marks (striae distensae). Results of a double-blind study. Gynakol Rundsch. 1987;27(2):79-84.
33. Akhavan A, Bershad S. Topical acne drugs: review of clinical properties, systemic exposure, and safety. Am J Clin Dermatol. 2003;4(7):473-92.
34. Ud-Din S, McAnelly SL, Bowring A, Whiteside S, Morris J, Chaudhry I, et al. A double-blind controlled clinical trial assessing the effect of topical gels on striae distensae (stretch marks): a non-invasive imaging, morphological and immunohistochemical study. Arch Dermatol Res. 2013;305(7): 603-17.
35. Aldahan AS, Shah VV, Mlacker S, Samarkandy S, Alsaidan M, Nouri K. Laser and light treatment for striae distensae: a comprehensive review of the literature. Am J Clin Dermatol. 2016;17(3):239-56.
36. de Angelis F, Kolesnikova L, Renato F, Liguori G. Fractional nonablative 1540-nm laser treatment of striae distensae in Fitzpatrick skin types II to IV: clinical and histological results. Aesthet Surg J. 2011;31(4):411-9.
37. Bak H, Kim BJ, Lee WJ, Bang JS, Lee SY, Choi JH, et al. Treatment of striae distensae with fractional photothermolysis. Dermatol Surg. 2009;35(8):1215-20.
38. Clementoni MT, Lavagno R. A novel 1565 nm non-ablative fractional device for stretch marks: A preliminary report. J Cosmet Laser Ther. 2015;17(3):148-55.
39. Lee SE, Kim JH, Lee SJ, Lee JE, Kang JM, Kim YK, et al. Treatment of striae distensae using an ablative 10,600-nm carbon dioxide fractional laser: a retrospective review of 27 participants. Dermatol Surg. 2010;36(11):1683-90.
40. Naein FF, Soghrati M. Fractional CO_2 laser as an effective modality in treatment of striae alba in skin types III and IV. J Res Med Sci. 2012;17(10):928-33.
41. Gauglitz GG, Reinholz M, Kaudewitz P, Schauber J, Ruzicka T. Treatment of striae distensae using an ablative Erbium: YAG fractional laser versus a 585-nm pulsed-dye laser. J Cosmet Laser Ther. 2014;16(3):117-9.
42. Jiménez GP, Flores F, Berman B, Gunja-Smith Z. Treatment of striae rubra and striae alba with the 585-nm pulsed-dye laser. Dermatol Surg. 2003;29(4):362-5.

43. McDaniel DH, Ash K, Zukowski M. Treatment of stretch marks with the 585-nm flashlamp-pumped pulsed dye laser. Dermatol Surg. 1996;22(4):332-7.
44. Goldman A, Rossato F, Prati C. Stretch marks: treatment using the 1,064-nm Nd:YAG laser. Dermatol Surg. 2008;34(5):686-91.
45. Elsaie ML, Hussein MS, Tawfik AA, Emam HM, Badawi MA, Fawzy MM, et al. Comparison of the effectiveness of two fluences using long-pulsed Nd:YAG laser in the treatment of striae distensae. Histological and morphometric evaluation. Lasers Med Sci. 2016;31(9):1845-53.
46. Goldberg DJ, Marmur ES, Schmults C, Hussain M, Phelps R. Histologic and ultrastructural analysis of ultraviolet B laser and light source treatment of leukoderma in striae distensae. Dermatol Surg. 2005;31(4):385-7.
47. Alexiades-Armenakas MR, Bernstein LJ, Friedman PM, Geronemus RG. The safety and efficacy of the 308-nm excimer laser for pigment correction of hypopigmented scars and striae alba. Arch Dermatol. 2004;140(8):955-60.
48. Longo L, Postiglione MG, Marangoni O, Melato M. Two-year follow-up results of copper bromide laser treatment of striae. J Clin Laser Med Surg. 2003;21(3):157-60.
49. Ryu HW, Kim SA, Jung HR, Ryoo YW, Lee KS, Cho JW. Clinical improvement of striae distensae in Korean patients using a combination of fractionated microneedle radiofrequency and fractional carbon dioxide laser. Dermatol Surg. 2013; 39(10):1452-8.
50. Naeini FF, Behfar S, Abtahi-Naeini B, Keyvan S, Pourazizi M. Promising option for treatment of striae alba: fractionated microneedle radiofrequency in combination with fractional carbon dioxide laser. Dermatol Res Pract. 2016:2896345.
51. Karimipour DJ, Kang S, Johnson TM, Orringer JS, Hamilton T, Hammerberg C, et al. Microdermabrasion: a molecular analysis following a single treatment. J Am Acad Dermatol. 2005;52(2):215-23.
52. Abdel-Lati AM, Elbendary AS. Treatment of striae distensae with microdermabrasion: a clinical and molecular study. J Egypt Worn Dermatol Soc. 2008;5:24-30.
53. Elsaie ML, Baumann LS, Elsaaiee LT. Striae distensae (stretch marks) and different modalities of therapy: an update. Dermatol Surg. 2009;35(4):563-73.
54. Sanad EM, Aginaa HA, Sorour NE. Microneedling system alone versus microneedling system with trichloroacetic acid in the management of abdominal striae rubra: a clinical and histopathological study. J Egyp Wom Dermatol Soc. 2015;12:96-101.
55. Shin MK, Lee JH, Lee SJ, Kim NI. Platelet-rich plasma combined with fractional laser therapy for skin rejuvenation. Dermatol Surg. 2012;38(4):623-30.
56. Arshdeep, Kumaran MS. Platelet-rich plasma in dermatology: Boon or a bane? Indian J Dermatol Venereol Leprol. 2014; 80(1): 5-14.
57. Ibrahim ZA, El-Tatawy RA, El-Samongy MA, Ali DA. Comparison between the efficacy and safety of platelet-rich plasma vs. microdermabrasion in the treatment of striae distensae: clinical and histopathological study. J Cosmet Dermatol. 2015;14(4):336-46.

SECTION 18

Interface of Dermatosurgery and Cosmetology with Patents, Legality, Academics, and Market

CHAPTER 127

Patient Satisfaction

Bhanu Prakash

KEY MESSAGES

- It is important to recognize that patient care has moved towards a healthcare industry and patient has evolved to become a consumer.
- Patient satisfaction is the strongest determinant of hospital functioning. Ultimate goal of the hospital is satisfaction of its customers.
- Increased patient satisfaction leads to greater profitability; improved patient retention and patient loyalty; improved productivity; better staff satisfaction; reduced risk of malpractice suit; and finally personal and professional fulfillment.
- Various factors influence patient satisfaction—doctor, staff; services provided and the behavior, etc. play a big role
- Patient satisfaction is a measurable tool and therefore steps can be taken to improve the patient satisfaction.

INTRODUCTION

The practice and system of medicine has evolved over centuries. Significant developments have taken place in the health systems, such as:

- The establishment of corporate hospitals equipped with the latest facilities, thus increasing the cost of health services to a common man.
- The advent of third-party payers (insurance companies, governments, companies, etc.), thus increasing the monitoring of healthcare services provided by the doctors.
- Availability of information through the internet, thus increasing lay knowledge and self-help among patients; the awareness among patients of professional fallibility and diagnostic uncertainty.
- Higher expectations of patient care.
- Pressure to increase accountability and thus increasing litigations for unsatisfying results.

All these factors have resulted in a challenging profile for the healthcare industry—away from the traditional concept of a noble profession and a paternalistic doctor toward a service industry and a demanding patient.

SPECIAL FEATURES OF AESTHETIC PRACTICE

1. Chronicity of skin diseases and poor patient compliance in following instructions given by the dermatologist and aesthetician.
2. Patients are riddled with intense emotions—anxiety, frustration disfigurement, etc., which drives them to come towards dermatologists. Sadly, it also leads to frustration and anger against the doctors they have consulted.
3. High expectations versus low and unpredictable outcome for both aestheticians and patients.
4. Poor communication may lead to wrong understanding.
5. Consumer attitude—demanding, litigant and "I know everything".
6. Ethical practice versus "make hay while the sun shines" practice.
7. Wide and varied perception of job satisfaction perceived by physician and patient satisfaction perceived by patient.

In view of the above issues, it would be more appropriate to address the patients as "consumers". The word "consumer" literally means one who acquires commodities or services. Today, the patient sees himself as a buyer of health services. Once the concept of an industry and a consumer or a customer is accepted, then there is a need to recognize that every patient has certain rights, which puts a special emphasis onto the delivery of quality health care and an attempt made to meet his/her expectations. And one of the key determinants of quality health care is patient satisfaction.

This explains why many hospitals, aesthetic clinics have begun to function like a service industry by employing nonmedical staff such as HR professionals, management graduates, professional front desk operators, etc.

WHAT IS PATIENT SATISFACTION?

Though there is no universally accepted definition, different authors and workers have attempted to define patient satisfaction. Most acceptable are:

- "The patient's opinion of the care received from nursing staff."[1]
- "An expression of patient's judgment on the quality of care in all its aspects, but particularly as concerns the interpersonal process."[2]

Satisfaction is not a phenomenon, which can be defined or measured easily, but an attitude or a judgment, the patient develops over a period, based on past experiences. A simple and practical definition would be the degree to which the desired goals have been achieved. Satisfaction is achieved when the patient's perception of quality of care and services that they receive has been more than their expectations.

The benefits of a high patient satisfaction are manifold[3]

1. *Improved patient royalty and increased referrals:* Thus, we will have more patients repeatedly turning up for procedures such as chemical peels, microdermabrasion, PRP, Lasers and other cosmetic procedures.
2. *Improved patient retention*: According to the Technical Assistant Research Programs (TARPs), if we satisfy one customer, the information reaches four others. If we alienate one customer, it spreads to 10, or even more if the problem is serious. So, if we annoy one customer, we will have to satisfy three other patients just to stay even.[4] Also in this era of Social Media, people's ability to communicate the negative issues rapidly needs to be kept in mind.
3. *Improved compliance:* A satisfied patient understands and is likely to follow the instructions given by the dermatologists. This reduces the chances of complications, side effects and litigations. It also increases the efficiency of the staff.
4. *Improved financial collections:* They are less vulnerable to price wars. There is sufficient evidence to prove that organizations with high customer loyalty can command a higher price without losing their profit or market share. In a study conducted in Voluntary Hospitals of America, nearly 70% of patients were willing to pay more money if they had to consult a quality physician of their choice.[5]
5. *Consistent profitability:* It is estimated in USA, that loss of a patient due to dissatisfaction, can result in the loss of over $200,000 in income over the lifetime of the practice.[6]
6. *Increased staff morale* with reduced staff turnover also leads to increased productivity.
7. *Reduced risk of malpractice suits:* An inverse correlation has been reported for patient satisfaction rates and medical malpractice suits.[7]
8. *Accreditation issues:* It is now universally accepted that various accreditation agencies such as International Organization for Standardization (ISO), National Accreditation Board for Hospitals (NABH), Joint Commission on Accreditation of Healthcare Organizations (JCAHO), etc., all focus on quality service issues.[8]
9. *Increased personal and professional satisfaction:* Patients who improve with our care definitely make us happier.[9] The happier the doctor, the happier will be the patients.

Thus, in total, the process of ensuring patient satisfaction will lead to a total quality improvement in the organization.

SPECIAL FEATURES OF AESTHETIC AND DERMATOSURGERY PRACTICE

- Many dermatological disorders are characterized by chronicity. Thus, adherence to topical and/or systemic therapies for a long period of time is essential for successful management. It is estimated that more than one-third of patients fail to take medications as prescribed, especially for chronic disorders.[10,11] This may lead to poor compliance and further to treatment failure and thereby to poor patient satisfaction.
- People may come to dermatologists with high expectations of a definitive cure for all their skin disorders. Experience tells us that it is not possible for us to guarantee magical solutions. This leads to a huge gap between the service provider and the service seeker, leading to decreased patient satisfaction.
- Poor communication by dermatologist/dermatosurgeon, lack of empathy, and the chronicity of many of the disorders lead to dissatisfaction.
- The patients, particularly the youth, are keen to have quick solutions to their problems and therefore are more likely to be dissatisfied. People aged between 25 and 49 years, who form a major part of the new consumer cohort, have the lowest patient satisfaction scores compared with other age groups.[12]
- Recent fascination for aesthetic treatments has changed the scenario to a large extent. These "patients" who are otherwise healthy have a higher level of expectation. Aesthetic dermatology care is also delivered by other players such as beauty clinics and nonmedical professionals, who may not be necessarily bound by the ethical rules of the medical profession. They often resort to exaggerated claims, prominent advertisements leading to heightened expectations and later disappointments.

A dermatologist's professional job satisfaction and a patient's satisfaction need not necessarily complement each other. We rate our job satisfaction by our professional knowledge, attending CMEs, conferences, mastering new skills, and keeping pace with new technologies. All these factors are not always relevant to the patient. Ultimately however, whether a patient is happy with a doctor's approach depends on different nonclinical factors such as listening to him or her, promptness of services, and how we talk and gesture, etc.

Healthcare service quality indicators:

They can be categorized in three ways:[13]

1. *Technical aspects:* How well clinicians diagnose and treat problems.
2. *Interpersonal component:* Provider responsiveness, friendliness and attentiveness.
3. *Amenities:* Healthcare facility appeal and comfort.

Doctor

Undoubtedly, the physician has the twin responsibilities of giving the best health care to the patient, and leading the team or the organization in attaining the goal of satisfying the patient. Listed here are few "house rules" to handle the patient so as to attain a satisfying and a non-complaining patient:[3]

- *Break the ice*: Make eye contact, smile, call people by name and express with words of concern.
- *Show courtesy*: Kind gestures and polite words make a patient very comfortable.
- *Listen and understand*: Encourage patients to tell their problem. Invite and answer their questions.
- *Inform and explain*: It promotes compliance. People are less anxious when they know what is happening.
- *See the whole person*: See beyond illness the whole person.
- *Share the responsibility*: Risks and uncertainty are facts of life in medical practice. Acknowledging risks builds trust.
- *Pay undivided attention*: This reduces distractions and interruptions as much as possible.
- *Secure confidentiality and privacy*: Watch what you say, where you say, and to whom you say.
- *Preserve dignity*: Treat the patient with respect. Respect modesty.
- *Remember the patient's family*: Families feel protective, anxious, frightened, and insecure. Extend yourself, reassure, and inform.
- *Respond quickly*: Keep appointments, return calls, and apologize for delays.
- *Explain what you are going to do to manage the patient*: Patients feel less anxious if they understand what's being done to them.

Patient

A patient's liking the doctor has a lot to do with the patient getting better. A patient's expectations of a good service depend on age, gender, nature of illness, hour of the day, his/her attitude toward the problem and the circumstances.[14]

In general, patients expect their doctors to keep up the timings, behave cordially, and communicate in their language. They expect care, concern, and courtesy in addition to a good professional job.

Understanding a Patient

Certain tips can help a doctor or a hospital to understand the patients better:

- Recognize that patients expect a personal relationship that shows compassion and care.
- Recognize that the patient has got certain rights. Various regulatory authorities and hospitals have drawn a charter of rights for the patients.[15]
- Make sure a patient has got a good first impression of you and your set up.
- Step into your patients' shoes; see through their eyes and hear through their ears.
- Minimize the patient's waiting time to the least possible.
- Try to make your problem-solving system to be functional.
- Always obtain feedback from your patients and correct shortcomings if any. Always thank your patients for their feedback, even if they are negative.

To conclude a happy patient can do a good job of a highly trained sales force to spread word to their friends and family. This is called as "word-of-mouth" publicity, a very effective method of marketing.

Hospital

Many a times, it happens that with a competent doctor and a compliant patient, the problems persist because of the policies, work culture, and attitude shown by the hospital. Traditionally, hospitals have had discrete functional services such as housekeeping, dietary services, pharmacy, laboratory, etc. Unfortunately, this specialization has led to more fragmentation, costly care, and less than ideal customer service. A study describes that during a typical 3- to 4-day stay in a large hospital, a patient may interact with 50–60 employees.[16] Building and sustaining a service-oriented organizational culture through "lean hospitals"[17] is important for the success of any organization. Several changes are being seen in the management strategies with the goal of serving better and improving the service quality.

Telephone Service

Ensure that a smart, competent, and intelligent person is placed to handle the telephone for he/she will be the voice of the practice. Establish standards to ensure that the telephone is picked within a certain time, mode and tone of speech are cordial, and a triage protocol[18] is followed which helps to ward off the unnecessary calls when the doctor is busy in his/her professional work. Periodically, a survey can be made to monitor how these standards are followed **(Box 1)**:

- *Establishing phone communication protocols:* Train all office staff in telephone etiquette, including how to handle angry or dissatisfied patients. Several authors have highlighted the need for communication skills training in a telephone consultation context that is patient centered and specifically addresses active listening and advising skills, providing guidance on how to structure the call.[19]
- Allow callers to speak first, and ask for and get permission to place them on hold. Monitor calls that are put on hold.
- Conduct telephone conversations out of the hearing range of patients to protect the caller's privacy and to ensure that the patient sitting in the room is not unduly disturbed. When a return call is required, obtain the caller's phone number, set an approximate time for the return call to be made. Then, make return calls as promised.

BOX 1: More tips for using the phone effectively.

- Speak slowly and pace yourself with the other person
- Be polite and friendly
- A smiling face makes your voice warm and friendly and encourages a positive response
- Time your calls to avoid
- Use "please" and "thank you" copiously and "I" sparingly

This conveys a message to patients that you care and are respectful of their time and concerns.

- If you are allowing staff members to give telephonic advice, ensure a protocol manual is in place, which addresses handling routine questions and telephonic assessments. It is better to write down in advance what one has to say and in what order.
- Use a reliable answering service during off-hours. Place test calls regularly to assess the quality of the service. Document all calls/responses in the patient record. Ensure that the after-hours phone message system is in place.

Using Information Technology (Box 2)

New technologies have increased the choice for communication. The personal computers, laptops and android phones all serve as wonderful instruments to improve communication with the patients. Some of the important tools, which can be used, are: e-mails, faxes, digital photography, etc. After the Covid-19 pandemic, the Government of India has given the permission for teleconsultation and has framed guidelines on using this facility. This helps us in giving professional consultation over telephone and reducing face-to-face interaction.

Office Appearance

An aesthetically designed office, which is well-furnished, properly spaced with good interiors, well equipped with lighting, water, furniture, etc., and well-dressed, ever-smiling, and pleasant staff go a long way in bringing the patient to the doctor's office.[17] Patients may not remember what you said to them; patients may not remember what you did to them; but they always remember how you made them feel. You can use office spaces to promote publicity such as education material, newspaper articles, publications, TV and radio interviews, etc., to promote publicity. However, a strict word of caution; keep it within the purview of legal and ethical borders.

Waiting Time (Box 3)

The amount of time the patient spends in the waiting corridor area plays a very important role in determining the outcome of patient satisfaction. With so many choices available, few people will stick to a doctor who has no respect for their time. The waiting time depends on a lot on factors, like the doctor's style of working, the kind of patients he/she sees, the locality where he/she practices, and the efficacy of the supportive staff.

Doctor–Patient Interaction

This is perhaps the most important indicator to determine the patient's satisfaction outcome. Improving the physician's interpersonal skills can increase patient's satisfaction, which is likely to have a positive effect on treatment adherence and health outcomes.[20] Up to 25% of patients have comorbid psychosocial problems.[21] Such patients require more time from the dermatologist. Doctors frequently end up prescribing more and talking less to the patient. In one study, insufficient communication was recognized by psoriasis patients as a major cause of dissatisfaction with treatment.[22]

Not much stress is laid upon in our curriculum regarding the importance of communication in our clinical working. It is important to understand the importance and salient features of communication:

Poor communication is the number one cause of noncompliance and loss of earnings in our practice. Studies have shown nearly half of our patients either leave us or choose us for the way we communicate with the patients. Because of the reasons mentioned elsewhere in this chapter nearly three-fourths of our patients assess hospital quality based on their perception of care rather than other objective measures and communication is the most important factor.

Advantages of Good Communication

- Better health outcomes
- Improved adherence to treatment and instructions
- Highly-satisfied patient
- Decreased liabilities for the physician
- High professional satisfaction.

Guidelines for Good Communication (Box 4)

- Patient first; your entire practice should revolve around your patient's needs. Treat all patients in a courteous manner at all times without exception.
- Listen attentively to the patient avoiding distractions such as handling mobiles, computers, etc.
- Allow patient to talk completely what he wants to say.

BOX 2: Tips for using IT services effectively.

- Try attending classes of using basic IT services
- Use Faxes and e-mails effectively to save time
- Use brief, essential and business-like mails
- Avoid obscene languages, insults, racist and sexist remarks in your mails
- Avoid delays in replying to patients doubts and queries
- Delegate routine mail correspondence to your staff

(IT: information technology)

BOX 3: Tips on reducing waiting time.

- Invest in electronic health records and gather date in advance
- For every hour a physician spends on attending to patients, they spend almost twice as much on paperwork. This can be reduced to a great extent by hiring good support staff to do the paper work
- *Use various appointment systems:* Cluster appointments, unitarian systems, online appointments effectively
- Identify bottlenecks and try reducing them
- Embrace telehealth solutions
- Provide a comfortable reception area

BOX 4: Tips for good communication.

- Dress professionally and elegantly
- Establish good eye-to-eye contact
- Greet the patient formally and smiling
- Start by introducing yourself
- Listen with attention
- Appear unrushed
- Assess the patient's feelings and concerns
- Watch for nonverbal cues of the patient
- Practice nonmedical gestures
- Discuss the plan of management using layman's words

- Provide adequate time during each patient visit, and allow patients to communicate effectively their reasons for visiting without feeling rushed. Studies have shown that about 80% of patients feel the doctor interrupts them within half a minute and does not listen to him completely. More than 50% of the patients have reported that they were not able to talk what they had intended to, and doctor did not either agree or respected his attitudes, beliefs or his feelings during his talk.
- Provide adequate information to the patient, especially regarding diagnosis, the etiology, complications and treatment plan opted. If possible, allow the patient to be a part of the decision-making process.
- Respect patients' modesty, dignity, and confidentiality.
- Document all the information you gave if possible, especially in the prescription. Guidelines for how a rational prescription has to be made are available.[23] Studies point out that nearly 75% of our prescriptions are incomplete prescriptions not fulfilling all the requirements framed in the guidelines. Failure to inform the patient has dangerous consequences like medication errors, etc., thus inviting legal issues.
- To reduce the chance of miscommunication when providing treatment instructions, ask the person with whom you are speaking to repeat what you said, and then repeat it once more.

Patient Education

Typically, today's patients are more educated, computer savvy, and much richer. It is essential to clear all their rightly or wrongly earned doubts with much patience and compassion. According to a National Research Corporation (NRC) survey, on a scale of 10, patients listed willingness to explain things as the most important criterion in selecting a physician. Other factors used in the study were reasonable fees, telephone access, friendly office, convenient appointments, and convenient location; the willingness to explain things was given a rating of 9.6, well above the others.[24] Incomplete, improper, and poor communication may lead to unrealistic goals and expectations which in turn can lead to dissatisfaction especially in cosmetic and chronic disorders.

Successful education increases patient satisfaction and results in improved adherence to treatment and thus to a better outcome. Various methods such as verbal education, written information (handouts, articles in popular magazines, etc.), group-based learning, audiotapes, videotapes, computer-assisted education, and the internet can be used to educate the patient about the disease.[24]

Problem Solving

This is perhaps the most important among all the patient-related issues. To have accreditations to organizations such as Joint Commission on Accreditation of Healthcare Organizations (JCAHO), National Accreditation Board for Hospitals and Healthcare Providers (NABH), ISO, etc., a hospital should have a good system for handling complaints. According to the JCAHO manual:[8]

1. A mechanism must exist for receiving complaints.
2. Patients must be informed of this mechanism and of their right to complain.
3. The organization must respond to significant complaints and take appropriate actions; patients cannot be penalized for complaining.
4. All healthcare facility providers must document patient complaints and their responses to them.

The Technical Assistance Research Project (TARP) has conducted a survey of assessing the loss sustained by an organization to measure the financial consequence of dissatisfied customers. According to the report, if 150 complaints are voiced in a year, for every complaint voiced, an additional 26 complaints are not voiced. That means there are 150 × 26 or 3,900 complaints in that period. Approximately, 1 complaint in 5 is serious. That means of the 3,900 complaints, about 780 are serious. If 50% of the people with serious complaints go elsewhere the next time, they need service that means 390 people will choose another doctor or hospital next time. It is estimated that 40% of these patients or their close family members will need hospitalization in the next 12-month period. Thus, the financial implication will be too heavy for the doctor and the organization.[26]

So, when there is a lapse in the service delivered, one should always try to accept and acknowledge the mistake with grace. While acknowledging the lapse, one is expressing the regret only for the process. Apologizing does not mean that one is accepting the guilt. Steps should be taken to ensure, that such lapses do not recur.

The simple take home message: An existing patient inside is much more valuable than a potential one outside.

Feedback

The feedback given by the patient helps to improve the work of the physician, place, and also the system. Despite the advantages of self-assessment, dermatologists rarely have a system to analyze and evaluate quality of care rendered in the practice. Patient feedback can be obtained by patient questionnaires, follow-up phone calls, suggestion box, referral physician's survey, etc. The Dr Score website (*http://www.drscore.com*) provides an online patient satisfaction survey designed to respond to the needs of dermatologists by providing data to individual dermatologists to help them improve the quality of patient perceptions of physician quality. The data can be used to design effective strategies to improve efficiency of care given to the patients.[6]

Limitations of Patient Satisfaction Surveys

Several questions have been raised regarding the validity of depending on patient's satisfaction as the criteria for the success of the medical intervention done.

Patient feedback may not be credible because patients may not be competent to judge for the medical care provided. Patient's expectations may not be realistic and in fact detrimental to their health, which may have a bearing on their judgment.

Factors such as cost, ambience, etc., may influence their opinion and thus may give more readily negative views. Further to get a favorable opinion, the doctor may resort to populist measures (prescribing particular drugs or resorting to unnecessary procedures), defensive practice and also lead to manipulations to get favorable views.

Therefore, until an alternative, more robust and scientific ways are evolved, the patient satisfaction surveys should be accepted as a reliable guide in planning our practice.

Determinants of Patient Satisfaction

- Generally, patients with poor health, chronic morbid patients and patients needing to make more visits to the hospitals/clinic tend to have more negative satisfaction.
- Young patients, younger parents and educated patients tend to complain more of the services than their older counterparts. Therefore, hospitals need to pay more attention to these "high-risk" groups.
- Sometimes indices of patient dissatisfaction could be factors which are beyond dermatologist's professional aspect - car parking, canteen, cleanliness, noise levels, information, reception and other staff, nursing or ward care, visiting arrangements, etc., which can create a poor patient satisfaction.

Physician's Communication Skills

Tucker states that communication is the degree to which the patient is heard, kept informed through understandable terms, afforded social interaction and time during consultation and provided psychological and non-technical information. He also states that unclear, contradictory and inconclusive relationships exist between: satisfaction and gender; race; marital status; and social class.

BOX 5: Ten pillars of patient satisfaction.*

- *Leadership:* Vision and commitment
- Continuous improvement
- *Employee:* Engagement and empowerment
- Accountability
- Monitoring and feedback
- *Communication:* Both horizontal and vertical
- Staff development and training
- Rewards and recognition
- *Service recovery:* Dissatisfaction to satisfaction
- Patient focus

*(Wendy Leebov 1984, "The Ten Pillars")

CONCLUSION

Patient satisfaction is only an indirect or a proxy indicator of the quality of doctor or hospital.[4] Patient's satisfaction with medical care comprises on two components: (1) how care is delivered–process; and (2) the results of that care-outcome. Aesthetic consumers will demand excellence in process and outcome from care providers. Providing of such high-quality outcomes and consumer satisfaction with services will be a priority and a challenge if the aesthetic clinics have to survive and flourish.

Patient-focused care requires that we do not provide care in a particular way sometimes or usually but we must do it always. It must be every patient every time. It is an ironic fact: the better you are, the better you must become. Quality does not stand still. One should strive to provide better care and soar above each and every patient's expectations.[27] Healthcare service providers must measure and evaluate patient's satisfaction. The results should be used to improve the quality services provided by the organization. Some workers have questioned the merits of the use of patient satisfaction.[28,29] However, till a viable alternative proposal can be constructed, it will continue to be a very important tool for measuring and assessing the quality of health care. The ten pillars of patient satisfaction listed in the **Box 5** should always be borne in mind in any organization for achieving high scores in patient satisfaction.

"A satisfied patient is a practice builder."

REFERENCES

1. Hinshaw AS, Atwood JR. A patient satisfaction instrument: precision by replication. Nurs Res. 1982;31(3):170-5, 91.
2. Donabedian A. Explorations in quality assessment and monitoring, National Center for Health Services Research. Michigan: Health Administration Press; 1980
3. Wendy L, Scott G. Service Quality Improvement. The customer satisfaction strategy for health care. New York: AHA Company; 1994.
4. TARP Technical Assistance Research Programs. Membership services as a revenue centre: cost justification and marketing impact of an aggressive service program. Washington, DC: TARP Working paper; 1986.
5. Voluntary Hospitals of America. Special report: quality care. Market Monitor. 1988;11.

6. Luecke RW, Rosselli VR, Moss JM. The economic ramifications of "client" dissatisfaction. Group Pract J. 1991:8-18.
7. Poulas GA, Brodell RT, Mostow EN. Improving quality and patient satisfaction in dermatology office practice. Arch Dermatol. 2008;144:263-5.
8. Joint Commission Accreditation of Health Care Organizations: Accreditation Manual for Hospitals. Oak Brook Terrace: JCAHO; 1992.
9. Foot F. How to be a happy dermatologist? Dermatol Psychosom. 2004;5:112-3.
10. Berg JS, Dischler J, Wagner DJ, Rias JJ, Palmer-Shevlin N. Medication compliance: a healthcare problem. Ann Pharmacother. 1993;27:S1-24.
11. Serup J, Lindblad AK, Maroti M, Kjellgren KI, Niklasson E, Ring L, et al. To follow or not to follow dermatological treatment—a review of the literature. Acta Derm Venereol. 2006;86:1193-7.
12. Cohen G. Age and health status in a patient satisfaction survey. Soc Sci Med. 1996;42:1085-93.
13. Donabedian A. Criteria and standards for quality assessment and monitoring. Qual Res Bull. 1986;12(3):99-108.
14. Brown SW, Nelson AM, Bronkesh SJ, Wood SD. Quality Service for Practice Success. Maryland: Aspen Publication; 1993.
15. Department of Health, The Patient's Charter. Patient Satisfaction Pays. London: HMSO; 1992.
16. Hein EC. Contemporary Leadership Behaviour, Selected Readings, 5th edition. Philadelphia, New York: Lippincott; 1998.
17. Graban M. Lean Hospitals: Improving Quality, Patient Safety, and Employee Satisfaction. New York: CRC Press, Taylor and Francis Group; 2009.
18. Buppert C. Guidelines for telephone triage. Dermatol Nurs. 2009;21:40-1.
19. Purc-Stephenson RJ, Thrasher C. Patient compliance with telephone triage recommendations: a meta-analytic review. Patient Educ Counsel. 2012;87(2):135-42.
20. Becker F, douglass S. The ecology of the patient visit: physical attractiveness, waiting times, and perceived quality of care. J Ambul Care Manage. 2008;31:128-41.
21. Renzi C, Abeni D, Picardi A, Agostini E, Melchi CF, Pasquini P, et al. Factors associated with patient satisfaction with care among dermatological outpatients. Br J Dermatol. 2001; 145:617-23.
22. Picardsi A, Abeni D, Melchi CF, Puddu P, Pasquini P. Psychiatric morbidity in dermatological outpatients: an issue to be recognised. Br J Dermatol. 2000;14:920-1.
23. Krueger G, Koo J, Lebwohl M, Menter A, Stern RS, Rolstad T. The impact of psoriasis on quality of life: results of a 1998 National Psoriasis Foundation patient-membership survey. Arch Dermatol. 2001;137:280-4.
24. Prakash B, Nadig P, Nayak A. Rational prescription for a dermatologist. Indian J Dermatol. 2016;61(1):32-8.
25. National Research Corporation. Voluntary Hospitals of America. Marketing Monitor. 1998:6.
26. Zirwas MJ, Holder JL. Patient education strategies in dermatology-Part 2: methods. J Clin Aesthet Dermatol. 2009; 2(12):28-34.
27. Tabbish S. Hospital and Health Services Administration Principles and Practice. Oxford: Oxford University Press; 2001. pp. 699.
28. Prakash B. Patient satisfaction. J Cutan Aesthet Surg. 2010;3: 151-5.
29. Vuoiri H. Patient satisfaction—does it matter? Qual Assur Health Care. 1991;3:183-9.

CHAPTER 128

Psychological Issues in Aesthetics and Dermatosurgery

Abdul Latheef EN

KEY MESSAGES

- Skin, being the visible outermost organ of an individual, has a major role in appearance, self-perception, social relation and communication.
- There is an exponential growth in the demand and treatment options in the field of aesthetic medicine to change or improve one's appearance and to attain unreachable standards of the perceived ideal beauty.
- Dermatology is changing from disease-oriented specialty to a desire-satisfying specialty, especially the area of aesthetics.
- One-third of the patients visiting a dermatologist have emotional and associated psychosomatic issues.
- Body dysmorphic disorders, personality disorders, mood disorders and obsessive–compulsive disorders are in the forefront.
- Psychological assessment is a must before selecting any patient for aesthetic procedures, especially body dysmorphic disorder which is a major threat to aesthetic surgeons.

INTRODUCTION

Skin, being the visible outermost organ of an individual, has a major role in appearance, self-perception, social relation, and communication. Now due to the amount of focus and emphasis put by the society on what is perceived as ideal beauty, via advertisements of beauty products, movies or social media, the beauty-related psychological issues are on the increase.[1] There is an exponential growth in the demand and treatment options in the field of aesthetic medicine to change or improve one's appearance and to attain unreachable standards of the perceived ideal beauty. It may be associated with underlying component of stress, depression or obsession, somatoform disorders, compulsive disorders, somatization disorders, personality disorders body dysmorphic disorders (BDDs) or the procedure may be done to please a third party. Request for surgery can be a substitute solution for mental problems, with underlying psychosocial conflicts being suppressed or not readily recognized.[2] If these circumstances are associated with psychiatric morbidities such patients will be a real threat to the aestheticians and cosmetic dermatologists. Clinical studies have shown that 20–48 % of patients presenting for cosmetic surgery have a psychiatric diagnosis.[3] When the emotional disturbance stands in the forefront, even successful procedure can lead to destabilization of the psychological status. Hence, understanding and evaluation of psychology of an aesthetic patient should play a major part in selection of the patients and training of an aesthetician.

CHANGING TRENDS

In recent years, there is drastic change in the trends of cosmetic procedures and a marked hike in demand of aesthetic procedures. Increased awareness, increased longevity of mankind, changing tastes and attitudes, media hype, shift from disease dermatology to desire dermatology, increased affordability, availability of newer treatments, and availability of simple and safe treatments (weekend/lunch time procedures) all contribute the list of contributory reasons.[1]

The statistics shows the changing trend: Dermatologic surgeons performed—nearly 9.5 million procedures in 2014 (ASDS), 6.4 million cosmetic treatments—injectables, wrinkle-relaxers and soft-tissue fillers to laser/light/energy-based procedures and body sculpting.[4] Paradoxically, coinciding with the demand for procedures there is an increase in fear of side effect, an obsessive urge for procedure and a paranoid fear of side effect. The twin demand of providing "guaranteed efficacy with absolutely no side effects" is one of the challenges of aesthetic practice.[5]

Disease Dermatology Versus Desire Dermatology

Dermatology is changing from disease-oriented specialty to a desire-satisfying specialty, especially the area of aesthetics, where a patient demands a procedure for a perceived problem. This has led to a debate as to whether such patients are indeed patients or should be called by the term clients. An aesthetic patient usually has the following emphasis on treatment which should have comfort, results, safety profile, patient satisfaction and that should be a painless joyful experience.[1]

The difference between a dermatology patient and an aesthetic patient is given in **Table 1**.

NEED AND EXPECTATIONS OF THE PATIENT

In an aesthetic clinic, there are different types of patients. They come from different age groups, various social backgrounds, and financial status. Each patient comes with specific complaints and specific expectations. The need and expectation of the patient have to be assessed before doing any procedure. Depending on their expectations, the physician can get a clue toward the psychology of the patient. Patients with unrealistic expectations are one of the warning signs of an underlying psychiatric disorder. **Flowchart 1** simplifies and divides these patients as per their approach to their problems.[5,6]

Patients of the type 1 group are the best candidates. The type 3 patients usually have an insight and on adequate counseling, they may willingly accept them. Types 2 and 4 patients need careful assessment to identify an underlying psychiatric component if present. Most cases of body dysmorphic syndrome fall in type 4 category, and such patients will never be satisfied with the procedures and get repeated surgeries. They will benefit only with adjuvant psychiatric interventions.[6]

UNDERSTANDING THE PSYCHOLOGICAL MOTIVATION BEHIND THE AESTHETIC PROCEDURES

The request for cosmetic procedures is on the increase day by day. Not all patients seeking an aesthetic procedure necessarily have an underlying physiological issue. A significant chunk of patients has some or other form of underlying emotional or psychosomatic morbidities behind seeking an aesthetic surgery. An "Ideal" self-image built by the person is one common motive.[5,7] These psychosomatic disorders include various personality disorders, mood disorders, and obsessive-compulsive disorders (OCDs). These are the patients who need to be identified and segregated before the procedure.

- *Ideal self-image:* Based on sociocultural perception and influence of media, every individual may have formed an ideal self which will be different from actual self. The ideal self-image may affect every sphere of our life. Every decision an individual takes, like the choice of clothes, house or car is based on this. Similarly, patients usually have an ideal self-image in their mind when they approach for an aesthetic procedure. For example, a perfectly good-looking male patient may demand for a cleft in the chin even though it is not required only because he visualizes his ideal self-image with a cleft in the chin.[7] So they may be requesting this procedure for satisfaction of this pseudo self-image which will be difficult to attain. So, after a procedure if that psychological requirement is not fulfilled that may lead to dissatisfaction. But if the patient has realistic expectations and is self-motivated, the procedure is going to benefit the patient not only physically, but emotionally also.
- *Psychosomatic causes:* One third of the patients visiting a dermatologist have associated emotional and psychosomatic factors.[8] Mere treatment of the physical aspect will not be rewarding in these patients. The psychosomatic factor needs to be addressed before any aesthetic procedures. BDD is the most common problem creating condition in an aesthetic practice and a little bit detailed understanding may help in early recognition; however, personality disorders, mood disorders, and OCDs have to be considered.[9] Distinguishing between different mental health disorders is generally difficult for dermatologists than distinguishing between medical conditions. Hence, when there is strong suspicion of an underlying psychiatric disorder, it is preferable to take a psychiatrist's or psychologist opinion before starting any treatment.

TABLE 1: Conventional dermatological patient versus aesthetic patient.

Dermatological patient	*Aesthetic patient*
• Has a disease	• Has a desire
• Mostly needs medical treatment; occasional surgical treatment	• Mostly needs a procedural treatment
• Fear of consequences of disease, infection and spread of the disease	• Well aware; often has read well, knows what treatment is needed
• Accepts treatments willingly	• Wants options—safe options
• Easier to counsel about side effects	• Paranoid about side effects
• Respectful towards doctor; doctor is dominant	• Demands an equal relationship
• Easier to handle if there is a side effect	• Demanding; can be aggressive, more likely for a medicolegal situation
• Treatment result satisfaction good	• Result satisfaction poor

Mental Disorders Associated with Aesthetic Surgery[2]

Primary Psychiatric Disorders

- Body dysmorphic disorder
- Factitious disorders

Flowchart 1: Types of patients based on their demand for surgery and expectations.

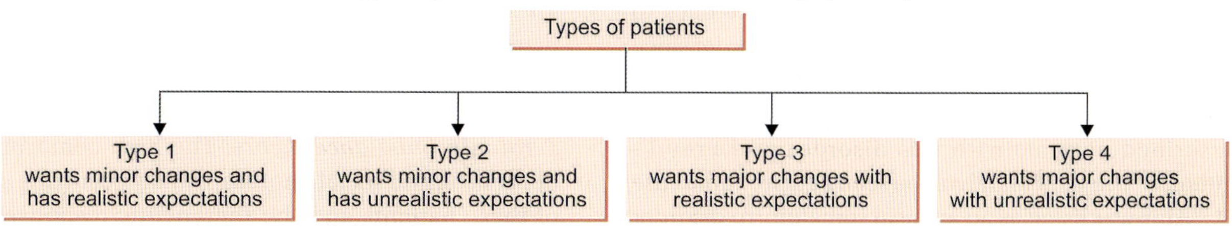

- Munchausen syndrome
- Affective/bipolar disorder
- Intentional self-harm (suicide)
- Social phobia (anxiety disorders)
- Somatoform disorders
- Hypochondriasis
- Somatization disorder (multiple complaints of physical illness).

Secondary Mental Disorders and Comorbidities

- Reactions to severe stress
  - Acute stress reaction
  - Posttraumatic stress disorder
- Adjustment disorder
- Anxiety disorder/social phobia
- Depressive disorder.

Personality Disorder

- Emotionally unstable personality disorder (borderline disorder)
- Obsessive-compulsive personality disorder
- Narcissistic personality disorder.

BODY DYSMORPHIC DISORDER

Introduction

Body dysmorphic disorder consists of an excessive preoccupation with an uncorrectable, imagined deficiency, or disfigurement in the outward appearance.[10] The excessive preoccupation cannot be satisfactorily explained by another psychiatric disorder and deficiency which either does not exist at all or is only very minor. This exaggerated preoccupation may lead to marked limitations in social, professional, and functional areas.[11] Individuals with this disorder express a wide variety of symptoms, generally involving obsessive thoughts and compulsive behaviors relating to physical appearance. Facial features are most commonly the object of dissatisfaction.[10] For dermatologists, cosmetic surgeons, and plastic surgeons, patients with BDD are the most important group of problem patients. The various synonyms used for this condition are dysmorphophobia, disfiguration syndrome, dermatological nondisease,[12] ugliness syndrome, and Thersites complex (Thersites was the ugliest warrior in Odysseus's army, according to Homer's saga).[2]

Even though BDD has only recently been included in diagnostic systems, recognizable descriptions date back to 19th century. It had been recognized as a mental disorder since 1980. The characteristic features of "dysmorphophobia" were first described in 1886 by Morselli.[10] Subsequently, Kraepelin also described patients with this disorder and Freud's description of "the Wolf Man" can be seen as a probable case of BDD.[10] This was listed as an atypical somatoform disorder in the American Psychiatric Association's DSM-III (Diagnostic and Statistical Manual of Mental Disorders) in 1980. No diagnostic criteria were included until the 1987 revision (DSM-III-R), in which it was classified as a separate disorder, with delusional and nondelusional subtypes.[10] It was classified in DSM-IV as a somatoform disorder and in DSM-5 [300.7 (F45.22)-American Psychiatric Association 2013] included in obsessive-compulsive and related disorders. The ICD-10 (10th revision of the International Statistical Classification of Diseases and Related Health Problems) categorizes the illness in the group of somatoform disorders under hypochondria (F45.2)[13] and the draft of ICD-11 lists BDD under the category of obsessive-compulsive or related disorders.[14]

Epidemiology

The prevalence of BDD is cited as approximately 1.8–2.4% in the general population.[15] Among American students, up to 4% meet the criteria of BDD according to DSM-IV.[16] The prevalence in Germany is approximately 1.7%.[16] The prevalence is 9–15% among dermatology patients, 7–8% among US cosmetic surgery patients, 3–16% among international cosmetic surgery patients.[12] The mean age of onset of disorder is 16–17 years, the median age of onset is 15 years, and the most common age at onset is 12–13 years. Two thirds of individuals have disorder onset before the age of 18 years.[12] Subclinical BDD symptoms begin, on an average, at age 12 or 13 years. Subclinical concerns usually evolve gradually to the full disorder, although some individuals experience abrupt onset of BDD.[12] Women between the age of 35 years and 50 years and men younger than 35 years are usually affected.[17]

Theories

Body dysmorphic disorder usually develops in adolescence, the time when people are generally most sensitive about their appearance. Multifactorial etiology is presumed comprising combination of psychological, biological, and environmental factors.[10] Genetic predisposition is suggested by family studies. It has been observed that approximately 20% of people with BDD have at least one first-degree relative with this disorder. No twin studies or genetic studies have been conducted specifically for BDD.[10] A family history of OCD has also been found to exist in those with BDD suggesting a possible shared genetic vulnerability. The various theories regarding the causation of this disorder include:[2,18]

- *The self-discrepancy theory:* According to this theory, the marked discrepancy between the desired ideal image (self-ideal) and the actual (self-actual) image is responsible for it.
- *Serotonin imbalance theory:* The high comorbidity of depression and social phobias, usually occurring in >70% of these patients and the therapeutic response of the

disorder to selective serotonin reuptake inhibitor (SSRIs) are the arguments in favor of this theory.
- *The bonding theory:* Insecure or anxiety-bound individuals during childhood are highly prone.
- Separation and dependency conflicts.
- *Inflammatory process* in the frontotemporal area of the brain.
- *Media-induced factors predispose* individuals to this disorder by ingraining certain ideals of beauty.

Clinical Features

Clinical examination usually does not reveal any pathological findings or only minimum variations from normal. The presumed defects in outward appearance may be either localized or a whole-body complaint, or may be either qualitative or quantitative of skin and its appendages. The localized complaints are mainly focused on the face, breast, and genitalia. Women are usually obsessed with body proportion concerns, while men tend to be preoccupied with the need to be larger and more muscular.[19] The spectrum of presumed deficiencies in outward appearance is endlessly variable. The patients may be preoccupied with asymmetries or disproportionality of the eyebrows, nose, eyelids, lips, teeth, breasts, genitals, hair loss or hair thinning, dyspigmentations, visible blood vessels, pore size, pallor, reddening of the skin, sweating or of any other organs **(Box 1)**.[2]

Common Symptoms[2,20]

Common symptoms are:
- Preoccupation with perceived appearance of defect
- Delusional beliefs and thoughts related to appearance
- Feelings of shame, chronic low self-esteem
- Self-consciousness in social situations; thinking that others notice and mock their perceived defect
- Social and family withdrawal, social phobia, self-imposed social isolation, and loneliness. Overdependence on others such as a partner, friend, or parents
- Inability to work or inability to focus at work due to preoccupation with appearance
- Decreased academic performance (problems with school/ college attendance and in maintaining grades)
- Problems in initiating and maintaining relationships (both intimate relationships and friendships)
- Drug and/ or alcohol misuse (often an attempt to self-medicate)
- Depressive symptoms, anxiety, panic attacks, and suicidal ideation.

Common Compulsive Behaviors[2,20]

Common compulsive behaviors include:
- Mirror checking, glancing in windows, reflective doors, and other reflective surfaces
- Avoidance of one's own reflection or photographs, often the removal of mirrors from the home
- Attempting to camouflage imagined defect (e.g., using cosmetic camouflage, maintaining specific body posture or wearing hats, wearing baggy clothing)
- Excessive grooming behaviors (e.g., skin-picking, combing hair, shaving, and plucking eyebrows)
- Compulsive skin-touching, especially to feel or measure the perceived defect
- Becoming hostile toward people for no known reason, especially those of the opposite gender
- Seeking reassurance from loved ones
- Excessive exercise and dieting
- Comparing appearance or body parts with that of others or obsessive viewing of models or favorite celebrities that the person with BDD wishes to resemble
- *Use of distraction techniques:* An attempt to shift attention away from the person's perceived defect (e.g., wearing extravagant clothing or excessive jewelry)
- *Compulsive information-seeking:* Reading books and articles in newspapers and websites which relate to the person's perceived defect (e.g., hair loss or dieting and exercise)

BOX 1: Common locations and frequency of perceived defects.[2,20]

- Skin (73%)
- Hair (56%)
- Nose (37%)
- Eyes (20%)
- Thighs (20%)
- Teeth (20%)
- Legs (overall) (18%)
- Body build/bone structure (16%)
- Facial features (general) (14%)
- Lips (12% face size/shape) (12%)
- Buttocks (12%)
- Eyebrows (11%)
- Chin (11%)
- Hips (11%)
- Ears (9%)
- Arms/wrists (9%)
- Waist (9%)
- Genitals (8%)
- Cheeks/cheekbones (8%)
- Calves (8%)
- Height (7%)
- Head size/shape (6%)
- Forehead (6%)
- Mouth (6%)
- Back (6%)
- Feet (6%)
- Hands (6%)
- Jaw (6%)
- Fingers (5%)
- Neck (5%)
- Shoulders (3%)
- Knees (3%)
- Toes (3%)
- Ankles (2%)
- Facial muscles (1%)

- Preoccupation with plastic surgery or cosmetic dermatology procedures
- Attempt to perform cosmetic surgery on themselves, including lipolysis or removal of unwanted blemishes
- *Avoidant behavior:* Avoiding leaving the home, or leaving the home at certain times, e.g., at night.

Diagnostic Criteria of Body Dysmorphic Disorders, DSM-5-300.7 (F45.22)[11]

The latest diagnostic criteria of BDD is put forward by DSM-V (Diagnostic and Statistical Manual of Mental Disorders Fifth Edition. American Psychiatric Association, 2013). This is simple and more useful than ICD-10 [World Health Organization (WHO, 2006)], even for those without psychiatric background. The major advantage in the present DSM-V criteria from the previous one is that it gives significance to the preoccupation of body build and the insight of the patient. Based on these criteria, decision of therapeutic approach is also easy.

A. Preoccupation with one or more perceived defects or flaws in physical appearance that are not observable or appear slight to others.
B. At some point during the course of the disorder, the individual has performed repetitive behaviors (e.g., mirror checking, excessive grooming, skin picking, reassurance seeking) or mental acts (e.g., comparing his or her appearance with that of others) in response to the appearance concerns.
C. The preoccupation causes clinically significant distress or impairment in social, occupational, or other important areas of functioning.
D. The appearance preoccupation is not better explained by concerns with body fat or weight in an individual whose symptoms meet diagnostic criteria for an eating disorder.

For the diagnosis, all the four criteria (A, B, C, and D) are needed. In addition, DSM-V suggests to specify whether muscle dysmorphia is present or not and to assess the degree of insight of the patient. This is useful to decide the management strategy.

Specify if:

With muscle dysmorphia: The individual is preoccupied with the idea that his or her body build is too small or insufficiently muscular. This specifier is used even if the individual is preoccupied with other body areas, which is often the case.

Specify if:

Indicate degree of insight regarding BDD beliefs (e.g., "I look ugly" or "I look < deformed").

With good or fair insight: The individual recognizes that the BDD beliefs are definitely or probably not true or that they may or may not be true.

With poor insight: The individual thinks that the BDD beliefs are probably true.

With absent insight/delusional beliefs: The individual is completely convinced that the BDD beliefs are true.[2]

Body Dysmorphic Disorder and Aesthetic Patient

Studies have proven that 3–16% of the patients visiting dermatologist for aesthetic procedures suffer from BDD. This emphasizes the need for aesthetic dermatologists to be aware of this condition and its presentation in the cosmetic population. Patients with BDD are the most problematic patients in aesthetic dermatology. Unless the dermatologists are aware of this problem, they may accept such patients for procedures which may lead to legal suits. New types of BDD continue to be described. Harth et al. described a subtype of BDD known as botulinophilia, characterized by persistent demands of botox injections to treat hyperhidrosis despite absence of symptoms.[1,2]

For easy diagnosis, a screening questionnaire and visual analog scale (VAS) can be used. The first structured interview modules for screening for BDD were developed in the United States and Germany in 1993.[2] Even though different questionnaires are available, only two of them have been validated in a cosmetic dermatology setting: the Body Dysmorphic Disorder Questionnaire-Dermatology Version (BDDQ-DV) and the Dysmorphic Concern Questionnaire (DCQ).[21]

Screening Questionnaire for Body Dysmorphic Disorder[22,23]

Key Questions

1. Do you believe that a part of your body is abnormal?
2. Have you ever been very concerned about your appearance?
3. Do you often and carefully view yourself in the mirror? How much time do you spend doing so?
4. Do you attempt to hide your defect with your hands, cosmetics, or clothes?
5. What effects does your preoccupation with appearance have on your life in the areas of your profession, social contacts, and partnerships? Have you neglected normal activities because of the defect?

   If the answer to these five questions is "yes", it is highly likely that the patient has BDD, and aesthetic surgery should not be performed. But even in milder cases, the answer to the above questions may be yes, where it is very important to assess the insight of the patient. If the insight of the patient is *good or fair,* after proper counseling aesthetic procedure may be considered. But if the insight is *poor or absent*, or *delusional beliefs* are present and the answer to the following additional questions are yes, aesthetic procedures are absolutely contraindicated.

Additional Questions[22,23]

1. Do you expect a radical change in your life as the result of surgery?
2. Are you sometimes so desperate that you wish you were dead or want to harm yourself?
   If the answer to these questions is "yes" aesthetic procedures are absolutely contraindicated.

The Visual Analog Scale[1,2]

It has been found helpful as a simple tool to determine BDD. The doctor and patient independently rate disfigurement and record severity on an optical VAS using value between 0 and 10 (with 0 meaning "no disfigurement" and 10 meaning "most severe disfigurement"). When a discrepancy of more than 4 points on the VAS occurs, BDD is to be suspected.

Comorbidity

About 80% of people with BDD will experience major depressive disorder at some point in their life.[2,20] About 37% have social phobia, 32% fulfill criteria for OCD, and 49% have substance-use disorders.[16] Eating disorders such as anorexia nervosa and bulimia nervosa are also sometimes found in women. Generalized anxiety disorder and trichotillomania also occur as comorbidity.[10] Studies have consistently shown that suicidal ideation and suicide attempts are common in people with BDD. Suicidality may increase when cosmetic surgery is denied.[24] It is found that 25–30% of patients with BDD in a psychiatric clinic have had a history of attempted suicide. About 0.3% per year committed suicide.[10]

Course

The course of the disorder is often chronic, the prognosis usually poor, and complete recovery rare. The recovery process is often long, even with specialized treatment remission and relapse is common.[10,11]

DEPRESSIVE DISORDERS

Affective disorders are particularly prominent in elective surgical treatment, constituting around 20%.[25] The main symptoms of affective disorders are depressed mood, loss of interest or happiness, lack of motivation, and rapid fatigue. The spectrum of depression ranges from mild, temporary disturbances to severe psychotic disorders with suicidal ideation. Additional symptoms of depression, according to the ICD-10, are disturbed sleep, poor concentration or indecisiveness, low self-confidence, poor or increased appetite, suicidal thoughts or acts, bleak and pessimistic view of future, guilt or self-blame present for at least 2 weeks and ideation of or attempted suicide.[13]

ANXIETY DISORDERS

Anxiety before surgery is a common phenomenon. In comparison to patients undergoing plastic reconstructive surgery, patients undergoing elective aesthetic surgery have higher anxiety scores.[2,26] Preoperative panic disorders can occur with clearly demarcated episodes of intensive anxiety or uneasiness with autonomic symptoms such as sweating, trembling, palpitations, rapid pulse, shortness of breath or respiratory distress, fear of death, paresthesia, numbness, hot flushes, or chills. Generalized anxiety disorder has to be differentiated from acute panic disorders.[2,11,13]

OBSESSIVE–COMPULSIVE DISORDERS

In connection with cosmetic surgery, patients often report continual preoccupation with their outward appearance. In OCDs, either obsessive thoughts, compulsive behavior or mixed symptoms exist. Obsessive thoughts can be defined as repeated and continual thoughts and imaginations regarding aesthetic factors that are perceived as obtrusive and inappropriate and cause great discomfort and severe anxiety. Compulsive behavior includes repeated aesthetic procedures, including requested elective surgery, highly repetitive skin care, or control of outward appearance. They may engage in prolonged skin and hair care sitting in front of the mirror.[2,11,13]

SOMATOFORM DISORDERS

By definition, the characteristic of somatoform disorders is the repeated presentation of physical symptoms in connection with the persistent demand for medical diagnosis (therapy) despite repeated negative results and assurance by the physician that symptoms have no organic basis. Among patients that requested cosmetic surgery, the subgroups of somatization disorder and dysmorphophobia as a special hypochondriac disorder are important. Divergent opinions on the question "to operate or not to operate?" may exist here, leading to conflicts in the physician–patient relationship.[2,11,13]

PERSONALITY DISORDERS

Every individual has his own style of thoughts, behaviors, and emotions. Personality disorders are characterized by aberrations in the thoughts, behaviors, and emotions from most other common people. Personality disorders often associated with other psychiatric morbidities such as depression and substance abuse. There are four defining features common to all types of personality disorders. These are:

1. Distorted thinking patterns
2. Problematic emotional responses
3. Over- or under-regulated impulse control
4. Interpersonal difficulties.

Flowchart 2: Classification of personality disorders as per DSM-5.

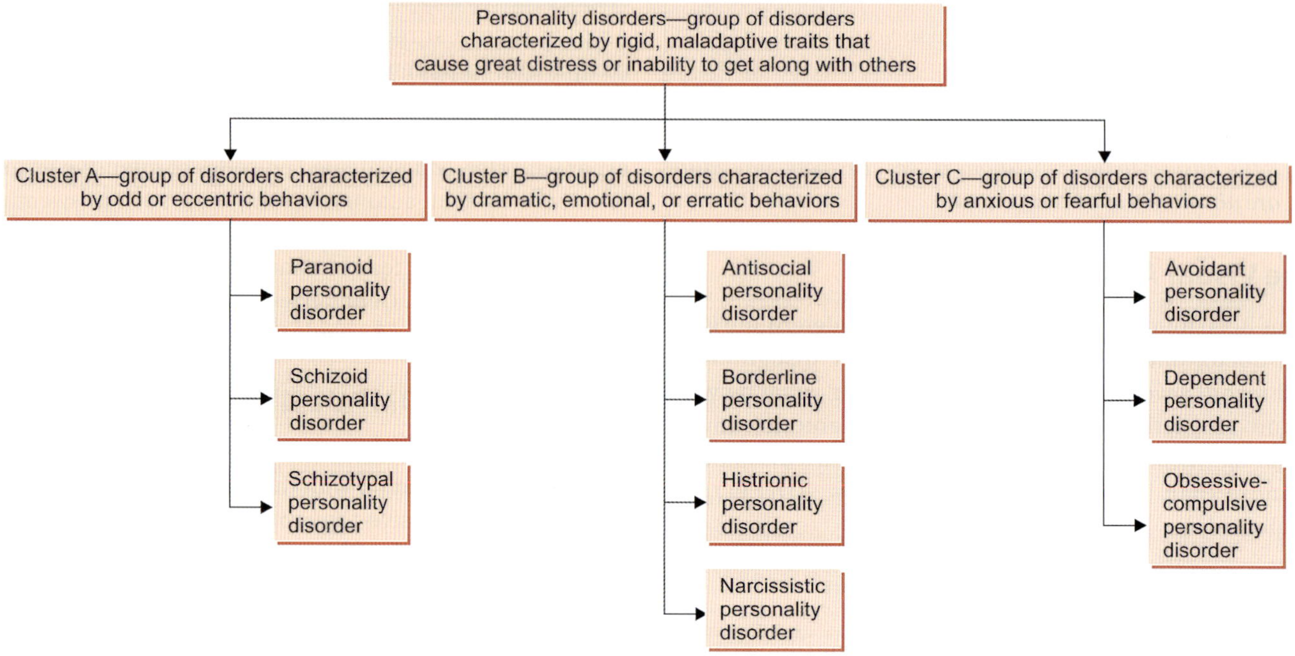

These four key features intermingle in various ways to form ten specific personality disorders identified in DSM-V.[5,11] Furthermore, the ten different personality disorders can be grouped into three clusters based on descriptive similarities within each cluster **(Flowchart 2)**.

Cluster A personality disorders are characterized by the individual's ability to relate to other people, leading to the perception that other people are odd. An example of this is paranoid personality disorder, where the individual is unusually distrustful and suspicious of others. They include schizoidal, paranoid, and schizotypal personalities. These patients usually suffer from social withdrawal and awkwardness and have distorted thinking as a dominant feature. For example, whenever a doctor suggests any treatment to such a patient and the patient consistently doubts the doctor and is apprehensive and requires long hours of counseling.

Cluster B personality disorders: The sufferer struggles to regulate his/her moods, often switching rapidly between feeling very down and very happy, and exhibiting similar variations in his/her view of others. An example is borderline personality disorder, which is characterized by erratic relationships, unstable moods and often self-harm. They include antisocial personality disorder, histrionic personality disorder and narcissistic personality disorder. Such patients can only be detected by careful observation of their body language and accurate history taking, especially of personal relations. Attention-seeking behavior and loud dressing sense is common and is histrionic type of personalities. They may also have multiple body piercings or tattoos as part of their attention seeking behavior.

Cluster C personality disorder: In this group, feelings of fear and anxiety dominate the individual's existence. This leads them to become socially withdrawn. These individuals are often misunderstood, because it is easy to mistake their crippling fear of rejection as a disinterest in social interaction. It includes the avoidant, dependent, and obsessive-compulsive personality disorders. These three personality disorders share a high level of anxiety, e.g., such patients frequently visit an aesthetician, searching for a remedy to be better accepted by the society. They may also have history of recurrent surgeries done in the past, since they consider improving their physical appearance will help better their acceptance in society. The second scenario seen in these patients is that they visit the doctor along with a relative/family and are less talkative during their counseling. It is usually their guardian or caregiver who wants them to undergo the surgery and proper history-taking will help in these cases.

MÜNCHAUSEN SYNDROME AND SURGERY ADDICTION

Münchausen syndrome is characterized by the triad of wandering from hospital to hospital, pseudologia phantastica, and self-inflicted injury.[2,27] In Münchausen syndrome, the physician can be misused as the executor of the manipulation. Some patients seem to like and welcome surgery (formerly termed "mania operativa") and can particularly be observed in elective cosmetic surgery. Patients enjoy the surgery because of the attention they receive from the friends, family, or surgical team. The diagnosis of the wish for nonindicated surgery can be presumed when there is a history of multiple previous surgeries with unclear explanations.[2,27]

History of Suicide

A high risk of suicide with mortal danger must be expected in depressed patients. Suicidal tendencies must be asked about and excluded when planning for surgery or procedures. When appropriate signs of suicidal ideations or attempted suicide with acute suicidal tendencies exist, surgery is absolutely contraindicated, and immediate psychiatric treatment is necessary.[2] In cases with chronic or reactive suicidal tendencies due to disfigurement or when there is a history of attempted suicide, the situation is more difficult, and the indication for cosmetic surgery should be made in an interdisciplinary manner in cooperation with a psychiatrist.[9]

MANAGEMENT OF PSYCHOSOMATIC PATIENTS SEEKING COSMETIC SURGERY

Before considering any procedure, the underlying psychiatric problem should be addressed. Depending upon the clinical severity and psychiatric comorbidity, if the patient is treated in a systematic manner including psychological interventions and psycho pharmacotherapy, chance of recovery and remission is high.[2,9] But there are many obstacles for their effective delivery. Many people with BDD are suffering from depression, making them unmotivated for regular treatment. Others are highly skeptical of accepting that they have a psychological disorder at all and seek cosmetic procedures as an alternative to psychological intervention. Many are house bound and have extreme social phobia, anxiety, embarrassment, or ashamed to seek treatment and even to talk to a therapist.[2] In practice, the first goal is to take the patient's complaints seriously and understand them. Confrontation with the psychiatric disorder too early is not appropriate. Various structured questionnaires are available, such as Minnesota Multiphasic Personality Inventory (MMPI) and California Personality Inventory (CPI).[28] However, these questionnaires have the drawback in that patient can manipulate the results and are time consuming. Most appropriate approach would be thorough evaluation of the patient with suitable history, which should include past and present medical history, detailed psychiatric history, drug history, and family history of psychiatric illness, etc. Four basic information have to be gathered:

1. Specific requirement of patient
2. Why he/she wants to get operated now?
3. Why patient demands specific procedure?
4. Why patient has chosen particular surgeon?[28]

Presence of a family member during psychiatric evaluation and informed consent with pretreatment images form essential component of pretreatment assessment. After establishing a good doctor–patient rapport, psychoeducation regarding the nature of the disease, the psychosocial provocative situations, consequences of the defect, coping with the disease, past experience with disease and the need of psychosomatic care might be helpful. Building a supportive relationship by taking the patient seriously and showing understanding of the complaints is fundamental in basic psychosomatic care.[1] Usually, patients present with external or internal motivations to undergo surgery. *External motivations* include desire to satisfy friend, spouse, or others. They are not good candidates for surgery as their motivations are passive. Other common motivation is to improve their career prospect based on ill-founded notion that good looks can fetch better jobs. Counseling helps these patients to realize the limitations of surgery, so that they accept outcome of procedure. Patients with strong *internal motivation* may be good candidates for surgery. However, there are two conflicting aspects of this. One aspect is, if deficiency is the cause of psychiatric illness, then correction of the defect may relieve their anxiety. However, if defect is the only focus, once the defect is corrected, the patients will come with new defect to perpetuate their neurotic symptoms.[28]

STEPWISE PLAN FOR PSYCHOLOGICAL INTERVENTIONS

That includes:

- Psychoeducation
- Motivation for psychotherapy
- Cognitive behavioral therapy (CBT)
- Behavior therapy
- Psychopharmaceuticals

Psychological Interventions

Psychoeducation

Psychoeducation is very important in the management of psychiatric disorders, especially BDD and somatoform disorders.[1,2] It implies teaching of psychosomatic concepts by providing information and knowledge about the problem, thereby teaching a biopsychosocial model of the disease. Patients are frequently not open to biopsychosocial concepts and are not willing for psychotherapy. These patients usually have a purely somatic concept and a desire for somatic therapy only. There are so many myths, misconceptions, and anxieties regarding the disease. The educator should be able to give them a comprehensive picture of the disease, to help alleviate the anxieties and to cope up with the disease. Thus, "soothing assurances" can contribute to the reduction of anxiety, gain knowledge for self-management, even in unmotivated patients.[9]

Cognitive Behavioral Therapy

Cognitive behavioral therapy is very useful especially in the treatment of BDD. Here the thought of imagined deficiency or disfigurement in the outward appearance is the pathological processes that can be changed by CBT by an experienced therapist. There have been a small number of randomized controlled trials (RCTs) demonstrating the effectiveness of CBT in various conditions.[29]

Exposure and Response Prevention

Exposure and response prevention (a form of behavioral therapy) involve facing anxiety-provoking situations in a graded manner while resisting the typical (reinforcing) response to them.[10] It is often given in conjunction with CBT. A hierarchical list of feared and avoided situations are prepared and then introduced in a graded manner. Repeated exposure will reduce their anxiety and patients may be asked to consider an alternative explanation for their body image problem. They will be encouraged to check their coping level and strengthen it. Gradually, patients are motivated to increase exposure to public and social situations.[9,30]

Relaxation Therapy

When the patient reports of excessive fear, anxiety, and stress which include autonomic arousal, then in such conditions, relaxation procedures can be applied, which help to calm down. These include muscular relaxation training, autogenic training, biofeedback, meditation, imagery, and paced breathing. These techniques basically help the patients to reduce the arousal. Deep state of relaxation could reduce arousal in both central nervous system (CNS) and autonomic nervous system (ANS) and as a result, it could resort or promote psychological and physical well-being.[30]

Pharmacological Treatment[31]

In minor psychiatric morbidity, psychological intervention may be enough but in major problems pharmacotherapy also needed. That include antipsychotics, antidepressants, and anxiolytics. The common antipsychotics are:

- *Typical antipsychotics* (Block dopamine receptors–D2)
  - Chlorpromazine, trifluoperazine, haloperidol, fluphenazine, and pimozide
- *Atypical antipsychotics* (Both dopamine-D_2 and serotonin -5 HT_2 receptor antagonists)
  - Risperidone, ziprasidone, olanzapine, quetiapine, and aripiprazole
  - *Common adverse effects:* Extrapyramidal symptoms, QT prolongation, anticholinergic effects, metabolic syndromes, hyperprolactinemia, sexual dysfunction, sedation, increased risk of seizures, parkinsonism, dystonia, akathisia, neuroleptic malignant syndrome, weight gain, cerebrovascular accidents, and agitation.

Antidepressants

- *Selective serotonin re-uptake inhibitors (SSRI)*:
  - Citalopram, escitalopram, fluoxetine, fluvoxamine, paroxetine, and sertraline
  - *Common adverse events:* Anxiety, irritability, increased suicide rates, sexual dysfunction, akathisia, hypomania/mania, agitation, and weight gain
- *Serotonin-norepinephrine-reuptake inhibitors (SNRIs)*:
  - Venlafaxine, duloxetine
  - *Common adverse events:* Hypertension, tachycardia, anxiety
- Norepinephrine—dopamine reuptake inhibitors
  - Bupropion
  - *Common adverse events:* Seizures; avoid in patients with convulsive history or eating disorders
- *Tricyclic antidepressants:*
  - Amitriptyline, nortriptyline, clomipramine, and doxepin
  - *Common adverse events:* Arrhythmias, hypertension, orthostatic hypotension, dry mouth, constipation, sexual dysfunction, avoid in glaucoma.
- Anxiolytics
- Benzodiazepines
  - Alprazolam, lorazepam, clonazepam, diazepam.
  - *Common adverse events:* Insomnia, sedation, impaired concentration, habituation potential, fatigue, impotence, tremors, impaired orgasm, lower convulsion threshold, psychomotor impairment, and drug dependence.

Moderate-to-severe depression requires medications with psychotherapy. SSRIs—escitalopram, fluoxetine, sertraline—, SNRIs—venlafaxine, desvenlafaxine, duloxetine—and tricyclic antidepressants are used for treatment. Drugs such as mirtazapine and tricyclics have antihistaminergic action as well that may be useful in pruritus.[2,10,31]

Anxiety treatment consists of SSRIs or SNRIs with cognitive behavioral therapy. An episode of acute anxiety may be managed with benzodiazepines; however, they should not be given for long-term due to high risk of dependence. [2,31] A range of antidepressants have been used in BDD, most commonly SSRIs. Higher doses of SSRIs and longer durations of treatment than those used for other psychiatric disorders are often needed. There is a possibility of relapse on discontinuation of SSRIs. Fluoxetine, sertraline, paroxetine, and citalopram generally show good efficacy. Clomipramine is also found to be effective in patients with delusional beliefs.[2,10]

OCDs: Management includes pharmacotherapy with SSRIs, TCAs (tricyclic antidepressants), and low-dose antipsychotics clubbed with cognitive behavioral therapy focusing on exposure and response prevention.[2,10]

Other Medical and Surgical Treatments

Other medical and surgical treatments do not appear to be effective for the majority of people with psychiatric comorbidities. In a study of 200 individuals with the disorder, dermatological and procedural treatment was most frequently sought, followed by surgery (most often rhinoplasty).

TABLE 2: Pros and cons: Aids in decision-making regarding requested surgery.[2,32]

Surgery: Yes—Positive indicators	*Surgery: No—Negative indicators*
• No mental disease • Objective physical defect • Surgery planned with proper consideration and duration • Realistic expectations • Feasibility of surgery • Acceptable risk • Improvement by corrective previous surgeries	• Mental disturbance • No objective physical defect • Body dysmorphic disorder • Suicidal tendencies • Unrealistic expectations • Multiple unsuccessful corrective surgeries • Surgeon shopping • Unacceptable surgical risk • Impending deterioration

But none of these treatments reliably improved the psychiatric morbidity, especially BDD.[10] Aesthetic procedures are rarely helpful and there is a chance for transferring concern to another bodily "abnormality" or increasing focus on the surgically corrected one, seeing it as still ugly and in need of further attention.[10] Cosmetic surgery can lead to never-ending requests for more surgeries and that can lead to financial and legal consequences. So, the aesthetic surgeon should be highly aware of the alarming signals and the possible indications and contraindications in selecting patients for aesthetic procedures.

Alarm Signals in Aesthetic Surgery (Table 2)[2,32]

- Aggression, lack of insight, impulsivity, hostility, self-manipulation
- Idealization of the surgeon
- Life crisis, suicidal tendencies
- Pessimism, anxiety disorders, affective disorder
- Regression and child-like behavior
- Attribution of guilt or charges (toward other therapists)
- Secondary gain due to disease (especially attention by others)
- Somatization of mental problems (multiple complaints of illness)
- Carelessness (side effects), denial of reality
- Lack of independence disturbed compliance
- Disturbed coping with the disease
- Treatment for the sake of another person
- Deep disturbance of self-valuing or self-image
- Over attribution: Exaggeration of the physical defect
- Over identification with the defect
- Unclear motivation
- Unclear previous surgeries
- Expectations of treatment that are too high.

CONCLUSION

- Psychological assessment is a must before selecting any patient for aesthetic procedures
- Out of psychiatric disorders, BDD is the major threat to the aesthetic surgeons.
- Screening questionnaires and VAS are highly useful for easy diagnoses.
- Management of underlying psychopathology is vital in the success of any aesthetic surgery.
- It is important for an aesthetic dermatologist to understand when not to do surgery, particularly in such patients.

REFERENCES

1. Sharma M, Mysore V. Psychology of an aesthetic patient. In: Abdul Latheef EN (Ed). Handbook of Psychodermatology, 1st edition. New Delhi: Jaypee Brothers Medical Publishers; 2016. pp.119-29.
2. Harth W, Gieler W, Kusnir D. Clinical Management in Psychodermatology. Berlin, Heidelberg: Springer Verlag; 2009. pp. 159-67.
3. Napoleon, A. The presentation of personalities in plastic surgery. Ann Plast Surg. 1993;31(3):193-208.
4. American Society for Dermatologic Surgery. New ASDS Survey: 9.5 Million Treatments Performed in 2014. [online] Available from: http://www.prweb.com/releases/2015/05/prweb12746609.htm. [Last accessed August, 2022].
5. Marwah M. Psychology of an aesthetic patient. In: Venkataraman M (Ed). ACS(I) Textbook on Cutaneous and Aesthetic surgery, 2nd edition. New Delhi: Jaypee Brothers Medical Publishers; 2017. pp. 1327-31.
6. Phillips KA, Dufresne RG. Body dysmorphic disorder. A guide for dermatologists and cosmetic surgeons. Am J Clin Dermatol. 2000;1:235-43.
7. Tory HE. Self-discrepancy: a theory relating self and affect. Psychological Review. 1987;94(3):319-40.
8. Gupta MA, Gupta AK. Psychodermatology: an update. J Am Acad Dermatol. 1996;34:1030-46.
9. Latheef A EN. Body dysmorphic disorder. In: Venkataraman M, (Ed). ACS (I) Textbook on Cutaneous and Aesthetic surgery, 2nd edition. New Delhi: Jaypee Brothers Medical Publishers; 2017. pp.1332-37.
10. Ross J, Gowers S. Body dysmorphic disorder. Adv Psychiatr Treat. 2011;17(2):142-9.
11. American Psychiatric Association. Diagnostic and Statistical Manual of Mental Disorders (DSM-5). USA: APA; 2013. pp. 242-47.
12. Cotterill JA. Body dysmorphic disorder. Dermatol Clin. 1996;14(3):457-63.
13. World Health Organization. The International Statistical Classification of Diseases and Health Related Problems, Tenth Revision (ICD-10). [online] Available from: https://www.who.int/standards/classifications/classification-of-diseases. [Last accessed August, 2022].
14. World Health Organization. The International Statistical Classification of Diseases and Health Related Problems, eleventh revision - draft (ICD-11 draft). [online] Available from: https://icd.who.int/en. [Last accessed August, 2022].
15. Thanveer F, Khunger N. Screening for body dysmorphic disorder in a dermatology outpatient setting at a tertiary care centre. J Cutan Aesthet Surg. 2016;9:188-91.
16. Rief W, Buhlmann U, Wilhelm S, Borkenhagen A, Brähler E. The prevalence of body dysmorphic disorder: a population-based survey. Psychol Med. 2006;36:877-85.

17. Phillips KA, Dufresne RG, Wilkel CS, Vittorio CC. Rate of body dysmorphic disorder in dermatology patients. J Am Acad Dermatol. 2000;42:436-41.
18. Veale D, Kinderman P, Riley S, Lambrou C. Self-discrepancy in body dysmorphic disorder. Br J Clin Psychol. 2003;42: 157-69.
19. Phillips KA, Diaz SF. Gender differences in body dysmorphic disorder. J Nervous Mental Disorders. 1997;185:570-7.
20. Phillips KA (Ed). The Broken Mirror Understanding and Treating Body Dysmorphic disorder. Revised and expanded edition. New York: Oxford university press; 2005.
21. Picavet V, Gabriëls L, Jorissen M, Hellings PW. Screening tools for body dysmorphic disorder in a cosmetic surgery setting. Laryngoscope. 2011;121(12):2535-41.
22. Dufresne RG, Phillips KA, Vittorio CC, Wilkel CS. A screening questionnaire for body dysmorphic disorder in a cosmetic dermatologic surgery practice. Dermatol Surg. 2001;27:457-62.
23. Stangier U, Janich C, Adam-Schwebe S, Berger P, Wolter M, et al. Screening for body dysmorphic disorder in dermatological outpatients. Dermatol Psychosom. 2003;4:66-71.
24. Veale D, Gournay K, Dryden W, Boocock A, Shah F, Willson R, et al. Body dysmorphic disorder: a cognitive behavioral model and pilot randomized controlled trial. Behav Res Ther. 1996;34(9):717-29.
25. Meningaud JP, Benadiba L, Servant JM, Herve C, Bertrand JC, Pelicie Y. Depression, anxiety and quality of life among scheduled cosmetic surgery patients: multicentre prospective study. J Craniomaxillofac Surg. 2001;9(3):177.
26. Sonmez A, Biskin N, Bayramicli M, Numanoglu. Comparison of preoperative anxiety in reconstructive and cosmetic surgery. patients. Ann Plast Surg A. 2005;54(2):172-5.
27. Oostendorp I, Rakoski J. Münchhausen syndrome. Artefacts in dermatology. Hautarzt. 1993;44:86-90.
28. Shulman BH. Psychiatric assessment of the candidate for cosmetic surgery. Otolaryngol Clin North Am. 1980;13: 383-9.
29. Rosen JC, Reiter J, Orosan P. Cognitive-behavioral body image therapy for body dysmorphic disorder. J Consult Clin Psychol. 1995;63(2):263-9.
30. Rai S. Psychological intervention in psychodermatological conditions-1.In:Abdul Latheef EN, (Ed). Handbok of Psychodermatology, 1st edition. New Delhi: Jaypee Brothers Medical Publishers; 2016. pp. 93-106.
31. Tharayil HM. Drug treatment of psychodermatological conditions. In: Abdul Latheef EN, (Ed). Handbook of Psychodermatology, 1st edition. New Delhi: Jaypee Brothers Medical Publishers; 2016. pp. 77-92.
32. Latheef A EN, Sangolli PM. Psychological issues in esthetic surgery. In: Mysore Venketaram (Ed). ACS (I) Textbook on Cutaneous and Aesthetic Surgery, 1st edition. New Delhi: Jaypee Brothers Medical Publishers; 2012. pp. 858-62.

CHAPTER 129

Accreditation

Manish Gautam

KEY MESSAGES

- There is a paradigm shift in doctor–patient relationship and it has tilted in favor of the patient, now more a client.
- Good healthcare is not only a right but seen as a status symbol.
- Accreditation proves, sustains and exhibits the standards of quality care.
- NABH accreditation standards are the formal stamp of authenticity and discipline in a healthcare organization.
- Accreditation is not an endpoint, but rather a means to improve quality.

INTRODUCTION

The 21st century has seen a paradigm shift in the doctor-patient relationship among other things. The balance has tilted in favor of the patient, who has evolved into a "consumer" with a myriad of options for approaches and treatment, particularly for surgical, interventional, cosmetic, and aesthetic procedures.

The internet has been repurposed as a teacher, strengthening the consumer's knowledge about his rights, his disease, available treatment options, and even the best centers for treatment. Corporate hospitals and chains of clinics have come up, which follow protocols and standards to woo the patients who are called "clients". Patients too, with this newfound status, look at good health care not only as a right, but also as a status symbol and enjoy the cajoling and mollycoddling.

Social media only adds insult to injury by highlighting even the slightest error or negligence on the part of the treating doctor/clinic or hospital. This change has forced doctors (now healthcare providers or HCPs) and healthcare organizations to look at quality control and establish and implement standards in medical practice.

There is a wide spectrum that links the HCP to the patient. It involves clinics, day care centers, nursing homes, small hospitals, multispecialty hospitals, and corporate hospitals. The increasing instances of poor patient care, lack of communication, medical negligence, unnecessary interventions, and unexpected outcomes call for standardization of healthcare services on top priority.

To raise the bar, a quintessential tool is accreditation—this improves, sustains, and exhibits the standards of quality care that must be provided in a hospital.

DEFINITIONS AND NOMENCLATURE

Accreditation is defined as the action or process of officially recognizing someone (or a body) as having a particular status or being qualified to perform a particular activity in a specified manner.

Hospital accreditation has been defined as "a self-assessment and external peer assessment process used by healthcare organizations to accurately assess their level of performance in relation to established standards and to implement ways to continuously improve."

The primary goal of accreditation is to ensure that the hospitals perform evidence-based practices involving access, affordability, efficiency, quality, and predefined outcomes in health care. Accreditation standards are usually regarded as optimal and achievable and are designed to encourage continuous improvement within organizations that have been accredited.

Healthcare services may acquire accreditation through various national and international bodies such as National Accreditation Board for Hospitals and Healthcare Providers (NABH), Joint Commission International (JCI), International Organization for Standardization (ISO), International Society for Quality in Health Care (ISQua), CRISIL Rating, and so on. Among the various accreditation systems, the NABH accreditation evolved by the Quality Council of India is the most popular, standard, and sound form. It is the principal accreditation system for hospitals in India.

HISTORY

The idea of standardization dates back to 1917 wherein the American College of Surgeons established a set of minimum standards for hospitals. In 1951, the American College of Surgeons collaborated with several other professional associations to form the Joint Commission on Accreditation of Healthcare (JCAH). There are over 70 national healthcare accreditation agencies worldwide that develop or apply standards, or both, specifically for health services and organizations. In India, accreditation has assumed importance only in the last two decades since NABH was established in 2006.

NATIONAL ACCREDITATION BOARD FOR HOSPITALS AND HEALTHCARE PROVIDERS STANDARDS

The first edition of standards was released in the year 2006. Following that, the standards have been revised every 3 years. The 5th edition of NABH standards along with the guidebook was released on 15th February, 2020 and is the latest edition. This was accredited by ISQua on 14th April, 2020.

Over the years, successive NABH standards have brought about a significant change in the approach taken by the healthcare units in managing and delivering standardized, quality healthcare services to the patients. NABH standards focus on patient safety and quality of the healthcare environment.

Without being prescriptive, the objective elements remain informative and guide an accredited organization in conducting its operations with a clear focus on patient safety.

The latest edition of NABH standards has some changes from the previous edition. For the first time, there are core objective elements related to the patient safety goals that have to be complied with mandatorily, irrespective of the compliance to other elements. There are a total of 651 elements, which are assessed at various levels during process of initial accreditation and reaccreditation. This will help the healthcare organization (HCO) in stepwise progression to a mature quality system covering the entire accreditation cycle.

The scoring methodology has also been changed to a graded system to help recognize the progressive efforts by the organization in implementation of the standards. The chapter on "Continuous Quality Improvement" has now been replaced with "Patient Safety and Quality" to increase the focus on this aspect of healthcare.

ACCREDITATION PROCESS

For all practical purposes, the NABH accreditation program is the most popular program for accreditation of healthcare organizations in India. Therefore, it is important for us as medical personnel to understand the process of NABH accreditation, especially so for an exclusive dermatology care center.

National Accreditation Board for Hospitals and Healthcare Providers accredit healthcare organizations by classifying it into 12 different types of healthcare establishments.

In all probabilities, an exclusive dermatology center can be brought under allopathy clinic establishment, as dermatologists usually practice in clinics, polyclinics, or dispensaries.

Accreditation standards for allopathic clinics have *two sections*:

1. *Section 1* deals with standards for accreditation of clinics practicing modern system of medicine (allopathy) and has eight chapters—each having standards and objective elements as given in **Table 1**.
2. *Section 2* serves as a guidebook to standards for accreditation of allopathic clinics. It gives a brief interpretation of the objective elements and methods to achieve the same.

The standards can be divided as patient-centered standards and organization-centered standards. To comply with these standard elements, the hospital will need to implement a process-driven approach in all aspects of hospital activities—from registration, admission, hospitalization, and discharge from the hospital and other areas of activities such as information provided to patients, rights of the patient and family, quality control in investigations, medications, infection control, facility and infrastructure maintenance, and so on. Thus, the NABH aims at not only streamlining the patient care policies, but also the administrative and infrastructural policies.

Since NABH accreditation has grown in popularity across the country, many clinics/nursing homes/hospitals (healthcare setups) are now trying to get themselves accredited and there is also subtle pressure from government agencies for the healthcare provider to be accredited; there is fear now in the industry that too many healthcare centers being NABH accredited will lead to a watering down of the whole purpose. To overcome this fear and to keep a firm grip on the limits of the accreditation process, a new concept called

TABLE 1: Standards for allopathic clinics.

Chapter	*Standards*	*Objective elements*
Chapter 1: Access, Assessment and Continuity of Care (AAC)	7	33
Chapter 2: Care of Patients (COP)	6	27
Chapter 3: Patient Rights and Education (PRE)	5	26
Chapter 4: Infection Control (IC)	2	8
Chapter 5: Continuous Quality Improvement (CQI)	2	8
Chapter 6: Responsibilities of Management (ROM)	4	20
Chapter 7: Facility Management and Safety (FMS)	3	12
Chapter 8: Community Participation and Integration (CPI)	1	5
Total standards/elements	30	139

"entry-level accreditation" has been introduced wherein the healthcare setup will be assessed for the feasibility of accreditation and on satisfaction of the assessors, a temporary entry-level accreditation will be awarded for a period of 2 years during which the standards in the setup are to be raised to the NABH levels.

The establishment should have documented policies/protocols/strategies outlined for each of the 169 standard and objective elements. The following documents are required for accreditation of a clinic:

- General information brochure
- National Accreditation Board for Hospitals and Healthcare Providers standards and elements for allopathic clinics
- Application form
- Matrix for applicant healthcare facilities
- Self-assessment toolkit
- Terms and conditions for maintaining NABH accreditation
- An assess or guidebook
- Policy and guidelines for use of NABH mark
- Procedure on handling complaints and appeals
- National Accreditation Board for Hospitals and Healthcare Providers policies and procedures for dealing with adverse and difficult decisions
- Policies and procedures for assessments, surveillance, and reassessment of HCO.

NATIONAL ACCREDITATION BOARD FOR HOSPITALS AND PATIENT SAFETY

Prime emphasis is laid on patient safety in NABH accreditation program. It is mandatory on the part of the accredited organization to document the occurrence of any safety violation within a reasonable period of time. Failure to do so may result in punishments including temporary disqualification from NABH.

The various steps and stepwise time involved for the accreditation phase are listed in **Table 2**.

Award of Accreditation

To be eligible for certification, the score earned by the hospital should be such that:

- No standard should have >10
- The average of each chapter should be at least 7
- The average of all chapters should be >7
- No tolerance/No zeroes are acceptable against elements related to legal implication.

National Accreditation Board for Hospitals and Healthcare Providers accreditation is not a one-time phenomenon. Once the organization gets accredited, it shall be valid for a defined period, which is usually 3 years. NABH conducts a regular surveillance of all accredited organizations. The surveillance visit will be planned during the second year to confirm compliance of standards and conditional improvement of quality. After 3 years, the certificate requires reassessment and renewal.

TABLE 2: Stepwise time schedule for accreditation of hospital and small healthcare organizations.

Sl No.	*Accreditation steps*	*Approximate time schedule*
1.	Submission of application (along with fee amount) + Self-assessment toolkit + Documents + Signed copy of terms and conditions	
2.	• Registration and acknowledgment to HCO along with unique reference number • Reflect same on website	Within 10 days
3.	Preassessment	Within 3 months of fee deposition
4.	Take corrective action and send report to NABH secretariat	
5.	Final assessment	Within 6 months of preassessment
6	Take corrective action on nonconformities raised during final assessment and send report to NABH secretariat	Within 3 months of final assessment
7	Review by accreditation committee	
8.	Verification assessment (as and if decided by AC)	
9.	Surveillance assessment	Within 18 months of accreditation

(HCO: healthcare organization; NABH: National Accreditation Board for Hospitals and Healthcare Providers)

NATIONAL ACCREDITATION BOARD FOR HOSPITALS AND HEALTHCARE PROFESSIONALS

Benefits of Accreditation

- Demonstrates credibility, reputation, and a commitment to quality and accountability
- Helps organizations create and implement systems and processes that improve operational effectiveness and performance
- Makes quality everyone's responsibility rather than that of an individual or section
- Decreases the costs of liability
- Minimizes the risk of adverse events
- Helps the organizations to utilize resources optimally
- Continued professional upgradation leads to a high degree of professional satisfaction
- Highly standardized patient care, thus improves patient satisfaction, safety, and effective retention
- Improves medical reconciliation
- Provides a competitive edge in the market place for organizations to brand themselves

- Recognized by insurers and other third parties
- Provides a framework for organizational structure and management
- Strengthens interdisciplinary team effectiveness and human resource management
- Promotes medical tourism, helps establish the credibility of the center for international patients, and, thus, generates more revenue
- It can protect against lawsuits.

CRITICISMS AGAINST ACCREDITATION

- Due to accreditation being in its infancy, many of these guidelines are subject to changes, which lead to difficulties, inconveniences, and economic burden on the organization, while implementing the changes required for accreditation.
- For many organizations, there may be a question as to whether accreditation is worth the time, effort, and cost, as the process can be stressful, time-consuming, and may require a significant investment of resources.
- A fear may arise where the company starts manipulating statistics and documentation in view of certification rather than truly interested in improving the quality.
- There are no separate standards for dermatology, dermatosurgery, or aesthetic dermatology clinics. Usually, these come under the category of day care clinics, which, sadly, are excluded as far as NABH accreditation is concerned.
- Very stringent, meticulous, and elaborate standards discourage smaller hospitals and standalone clinics to even consider the accreditation process.

CONCLUSION

Accreditation is based on the premise that adherence to evidence-based standards will reliably produce higher quality health services in a safer environment.

However, accreditation is not an endpoint in itself, but rather a means to improve quality. When implemented appropriately, accreditation can strengthen the quality of health services provided. Accreditation has become a powerful indicator of an organization's commitment to high-quality care and patient safety. Several countries have made accreditation mandatory for all public acute care hospitals. The process has also begun in our country and the government is trying to bring legislation into the matter. In the United States, quality improvement and patient safety have already been introduced into the curriculum of medical students.

The recent circular by the Insurance Regulatory and Development Authority of India (IRDAI) mandating its 33,000 empaneled hospitals to meet NABH preaccreditation entry-level standards that should make the healthcare organizations to take up the accreditation program.

As we look forward for international accreditation for our hospitals, institutes, and medical schools, it is only a matter of time before quality concepts will come in a big way in our country as well. When the time comes, we must be prepared to embrace such a change, no matter what it takes.

PITFALLS

Problems in the process of getting accreditation:

- Lack of commitment on the part of top management
- Inappropriate and incomplete documentation
- Lack of training to the employees
- Resistance to change by employees
- Lack of resources for system development and implementation
- Inadequate internal auditing and lack of corrective action on deficiencies identified.

SALIENT POINTS

- Accreditation is the formal stamp of authenticity and discipline in a healthcare organization.
- In India, NABH under the purview of Quality Control of India (QCI) oversees the accreditation process.
- National Accreditation Board for Hospitals and Healthcare Providers standards focus primarily on patient safety and quality of services rendered by the healthcare organizations in the ever-changing health scenario.
- We need defined exclusive standards for dermatosurgery, aesthetic dermatology clinics, and day care centers.

More information is available with *helpdesk@nabh.co; info@nabh.co*

RECOMMENDED READING

1. Caldwell J, Varkey P. Basics of quality improvement. In: Giardino AP, Riesenberg LA, Varkey P (Eds). Medical Quality Management: Theory and Practice, 2nd edition. Sudbury, MA: Jones and Bartlett Publishers; 2010.
2. Joint Commission on Healthcare Organization (JCAHO). Available from: www.isqua.org.au. [Last accessed on August, 2021].
3. Joshi SK. NABH accreditation. In: Joshi SK (Ed). Quality Management in Hospitals, 2nd edition. New Delhi: Jaypee Brothers Medical (P) Pvt. Ltd.; 2014. pp. 51-65.
4. Mysore V, Bhanuprakash S. Accreditation. In: Mysore V (Ed). Essentials of Practice Management in Dermatology and Plastic Surgery, 1st edition. New Delhi: Jaypee Brothers Medical (P) Pvt. Ltd.; 2020. pp. 44-9.
5. National Accreditation Board for Hospitals and Healthcare Providers (NABH) (2020). Standard Accreditation Agreement between NABH-QCI and Healthcare Organization/Hospital. [online] Available from: https://www.nabh.co/Images/PDF/Agreement_hos.pdf. [Last accessed on August, 2021].
6. Rawlins R. Hospital accreditation is important. BMJ. 2001; 322:674.

CHAPTER 130

Medicolegal Issues in Aesthetic Surgery

KH Satyanarayana Rao

KEY MESSAGES

- Increasing awareness about consumers' rights and unrealistic expectations often result in dissatisfaction among clients, which may end up in litigation. Aesthetic surgeons in their own interest must familiarize themselves with basic legal issues and take preventive steps to avoid allegations of malpractice.
- Issues such as aesthetic surgeon's duties, preoperative counseling, informed consent, standard of care, confidentiality of medical data, medical negligence, and civil, criminal, and professional liabilities need attention.
- Ignorance of law cannot be a defense while facing a case in courts/consumer forums.
- The importance of good doctor–patient relationship, communication skills, and documentation need to be emphasized.

INTRODUCTION

Aesthetic surgery has become very popular over the world as it has become safer and widely available.[1-3] It is being practiced not only by qualified professionals such as plastic surgeons, dermatosurgeons, ophthalmic surgeons, ENT (ear, nose, and throat) surgeons, gynecologists, dental surgeons, but also by self-styled specialists and quacks with considerable competition for wooing clients. Cosmetic procedures are not only being done in hospital settings or clinics or office-based surgeries, but also in medical spas, beauty parlors, massage parlors in malls, etc. Even cosmetic health tourism is being promoted.[4,5] Safety is the casualty in many such situations.[6,7] Demand for aesthetic surgery emanates from peoples' desire to look "normal" or "more attractive", or hope to look like a specific celebrity or to wipe away or camouflage the signs of aging.

Undue importance given by the society to outward appearance of individuals[8-10] and the idealistic images of beauty created by the print and visual media have created unrealistic expectations out of the cosmetic procedures.

When the outcome of aesthetic surgery does not come up to the patient's expectations, resultant patient dissatisfaction may end up in litigation. With the increasing awareness about patient's rights, the number of medical malpractice cases is rising, and this has adversely affected the doctor–patient relationship, which rests on mutual faith.

The enactment of the Consumer Protection Act (CPA)[11] in 1986 and its subsequent interpretation by the Supreme Court that it applies to medical practice[12] has changed the attitude of doctors toward their patients (consumers) and has in a way forced them into defensive practice.

The damages being claimed and awarded in medical malpractice cases are astronomical these days. Compensation of 6.08 crore rupees awarded by the Supreme Court of India in Anuradha Saha case,[13] 76 lakh rupees verdict against Maharaja Agrasen Hospital and Others by the Supreme Court of India,[14] and 1 crore rupees awarded by the Supreme Court of India in a medical negligence case against Nizam's Institute of Medical Sciences[15] are some examples. Hence, it is very important for the aesthetic surgeon to understand the legal issues involved in the practice of aesthetic surgery. Ignorance of legal requirements is not a valid excuse before the court of law.

There is no distinct medical law in Indian legal system. Common laws as applicable to the practice of medicine in general, and aesthetic surgery in particular are of relevance.

HOW IS AESTHETIC SURGERY DIFFERENT FROM OTHER SURGERIES?[16-19]

Aesthetic surgery is different from other surgeries in several ways:

- In case of aesthetic surgery, which is totally elective, there are no patients in the traditional sense of the term, but only clients or consumers who seek a service.
- It is desire- or demand-based rather than need-based.
- There is no ailment or suffering to be relieved but only camouflage, enhancement, or modification of external appearance.
- Unlike medically indicated surgeries, cost is not generally covered by medical insurance and individual has to bear it out of his/her own pocket.
- Patients are usually willing to accept some risk of morbidity in case of regular surgery, and even mortality in case of oncosurgery, neurosurgery, and other high-risk surgeries; whereas in case of aesthetic surgery, there is zero tolerance for complications or mishaps.

- Clients may not appreciate the fact that no aesthetic surgeon can assure 100% success and it is simply not possible in medical field to give any such assurance or guarantee.

The rosy picture of before and after photographs in the file can create an unrealistic imagination in the mind of the individual. Hence, there is need for detailed counseling to explain the realistic results that can be expected out of the procedures. After all, the ultimate test of success of any aesthetic surgery is the satisfaction that it gives to the client.[20]

AESTHETIC SURGEON'S LEGAL DUTIES TO PATIENTS[21,22]

Duty of Care in Deciding Whether to Undertake the Case

Indications for the treatment should be clear, and proper counseling should be performed. One should not undertake a case if it is beyond one's competence. Necessary infrastructure with standard essential equipment and machines must be available and kept in perfect working condition. Essential supplies such as oxygen, resuscitation equipment, and emergency drugs must be available.

Duty of Care in Deciding What Treatment to Give

One should have up-to-date knowledge in the specialty. Evidence-based guidelines[23] and established protocols[24] help to offer standard care. Indian Association of Dermatologists, Venereologists and Leprologists and Association of Cutaneous Surgeons of India have also published dermatosurgery guidelines.[25]

Duty of Care in the Administration of Treatment

One should possess the necessary skill in doing the procedure and the assistant should also be trained in it. One must be competent and possess necessary qualification, experience, and training in the specialty one professes to practice. There is no law, which says which doctor can or cannot practice aesthetic or plastic surgery. If a particular case is beyond the expertise of the aesthetic surgeon to handle or if one feels that another aesthetic surgeon is in a better position or more qualified/experienced to handle the case, one should not hesitate to refer. Surgery should only be undertaken in premises that are fully equipped with resuscitation facilities and staff trained in advanced life support.[26]

New equipment needs careful handling and training provided by the manufacturers in their appropriate usage should be utilized. Keeping medical equipment, such as lasers and lights, in perfect working condition and taking adequate precautions during their usage will help to prevent machine-related mishaps.

A breach of any of these duties gives a right of action for negligence to the patient.

SELECTION OF CLIENTS FOR AESTHETIC SURGERY

Clients for aesthetic surgery must be carefully selected based on various factors such as clients' age, medical condition, history of previous procedures undergone, presence of depression, contraindications, and chances of complications. Psychiatric consultation may be needed in those with suspected body dysmorphic disorder (BDD).[27] There are instances of damages being claimed by patients from surgeons for doing multiple procedures without failing to diagnose BDD.[28]

COUNSELING

Before subjecting a patient to any kind of aesthetic procedure, the patient should be counseled and given adequate information to enable him/her to take a proper decision. How much information is to be given depends upon what a "prudent client" would expect or demand to know. This should include the type of condition that the client has, modes of possible treatment, the procedure proposed, number of sittings, duration and approximate cost of treatment, expected results, need to follow instructions before and after the procedure, possible side effects or complications, etc.[29]

Cosmetic surgery is not without risk.[30-33] Generally in the surgical field, it is felt that very low risk need not be communicated, but it cannot be so in the case of aesthetic surgery. Moreover, even if a specific risk is remote, it may be highly relevant and important in respect of a particular client. For example, even minor pigmentation or scarring on the face may be of high concern to a television news reader, while a home maker may choose to ignore the same.

Good communication skills of the surgeon go a long way in making the client understand things in the proper perspective before they actually decide to undergo the aesthetic procedure and have realistic expectations out of it.[34] Repeated sessions of counseling may be needed in case of adolescents.[35]

WHAT IS CONSENT?

Under Indian Law, consent has not been defined.[36] Consent generally means permission, but legally, it is a *contract.* As per the Indian Contract Act, "two or more persons are said to consent when they agree upon the same thing in the same sense." In the medical field, it can be defined as an instrument of mutual communication between doctor and patient with an expression of authorization or permission or choice by the latter for the doctor to act/not act in a particular way.[37]

Why Should One Take Consent?

In addition to the ethical need to respect the principle of an "individual's autonomy,"[35,37,38] there is the legal concept that no one has the right to even touch, let alone treat another person without obtaining permission. Such unlawful act would be termed "battery" or physical assault and client can claim compensation for damages even when there is no intention to harm.[39] Hence, obtaining consent is a must for doing any aesthetic procedure.

What Constitutes a Valid Consent?

There are three important criteria for consent[40] to be valid:

1. It should be given by an adult or in case of minors by one of the parents. For those, aged between 12 and 18 years, the law is not very clear.[41] Hence, it is better to take assent of the teenager and consent of one parent before subjecting such clients to any aesthetic procedure.
2. It should be fully voluntary and free from any kind of coercion, fraud, pressure, inducement, influence, misrepresentation, or mistake.
3. Consenting person must be of sound mind and in the right state of mind at the time of giving consent.

What is an Appropriate Consent for Aesthetic Surgery?

- It should be a written consent signed by both the client and the doctor.
- It should be signed by a witness, who is preferably an uninterested third party, which does not include a relative or friend.
- Consent should be an informed consent that means it should be preceded by adequate disclosure of relevant information as mentioned earlier. Opportunity should be given to the client to clarify doubts, if any.
- Consent should be obtained a day or two earlier than the day of procedure, not on the day of the surgery or weeks prior to it.
- Consent form should be in patient's own language and without use of technical jargon, so that it is understood properly.
- Consent is procedure specific. So, consent for one procedure does not mean permission to do anything more in addition or in lieu of it.
- Consent is person specific. So, if consent is taken by Dr A, surgery cannot be done by Dr B or by Dr A's assistant.
- Consent is purpose specific. Therefore, specific consent is necessary for photographing the patient for scientific or educational or research purpose or for follow-up. Specific consent must be taken if the identity of the patient is likely to be revealed while publishing.
- Specific mention in the consent form is a must if a new procedure or equipment is being tried out with proper disclosure of risks/benefits involved.
- There is no prescribed or standard format for a consent form. It should be customized or may be even hand-written by the client.

Lack of informed consent is a frequent cause of allegations of medical negligence.[42]

Audio-visual recording of the consent process is increasingly being used as an option, in different surgical procedures such as hair transplantation and liposuction. Draft guidelines for the same applicable in case of clinical trials have been published by the Central Drug Standard Control Organization, Government of India.[43]

A mnemonic—*PARCODE*—can help to remember the important components of an informed consent to be taken before performing any aesthetic surgery.

- *P*rocedural details
- *A*lternatives available
- *R*isks involved
- *C*omplications that can arise
- *O*utcome expected
- *D*uration of treatment
- *E*xpenses involved

> Client's signature, on a dotted line in a printed consent form, obtained casually by a staff cannot constitute a proper consent and can be contested legally by the client.

Importance of Documentation

Medical record is admissible as documentary evidence in a legal suit. So, it is important to maintain meticulous record[42] of clinical details of the client, counseling process, consent taking, preoperative, operative, and postoperative notes and instructions, follow-up visits, etc.

Photographs taken before and after the procedure provide adequate proof of the outcome of the procedure. Client will not be in a position to claim lack of improvement later. Patient's failure to adhere to postprocedure consultations, neglect of precautions, and noncompliance of instructions, if any, should also find a place in the record.

Manual records carry greater evidentiary value, but computerized data is cheaper to maintain, and helps in standardization, storage, and easy retrieval of records.[44] Ministry of Health and Family Welfare, Government of India, has published standards for electronic medical records.[45] Medical records of aesthetic surgery must be preserved for 3 years, but those pertaining to malpractice suits must be preserved till the final settlement of the case. But it must be noted that under CPA, the consumer forums have power to condone delay in filing a case of negligence beyond the prescribed limitation period of 2 years from the date of occurrence of the alleged negligent act.[46] A child can file a case of medical negligence after acquiring the age of majority. Suppose a teenager has undergone tattoo removal procedure and develops unacceptable scarring, aesthetic surgeon must be prepared for a case of negligence after several years!

Custodial ownership of medical records vests with the aesthetic surgeon or the hospital. But on request by the client or an authorized representative, a copy must be provided within 72 hours.[47] Erasing of entries and overwritings are always viewed with suspicion by the courts. Therefore, all corrections must be done by scoring so that the previous entry is still visible, and the rewriting done under signature with date and time. Missing consent papers,[48] tampered medical records, and failure to record the name of the anesthetist[49] may be interpreted as medical negligence.

Proper medical record is the doctor's best defense against charges of medical negligence.

CONFIDENTIALITY OF MEDICAL DATA

Client has the right to confidentiality of medical information. It flows from the Right to Privacy and Autonomy, which in turn emanates from Right to Life and Liberty enshrined in Article 21 of the Indian Constitution.[40] When medical data is computerized, there is risk of unauthorized access and breach of confidentiality of clients' sensitive information. Failure to protect confidential medical data of a patient could lead to civil liability for invasion of privacy, and intentional or negligent infliction of emotional distress. Inadvertent disclosure of HIV positive status of a patient may be held negligent.[50]

Medical information being of personal nature is outside the purview of Right to Information Act unless public interest is involved. But, of late there have been a few contrary decisions by the Information Commissions.[51]

NEGLIGENCE

Negligence per se is defined as "conduct, whether of action or omission, which may be declared and treated as negligence without any argument or proof as to the particular surrounding circumstances, either because it is in violation of statute or because it is so palpably opposed to the dictates of common prudence that it can be said without hesitation or doubt that no careful person would have been guilty of it."

Negligence is the omission to do something which a reasonable man would do or doing something which a prudent and reasonable man would not do. Negligence is culpable rashness and carelessness.

Medical Negligence[46]

Under Indian legal system, there is no separate law to deal with medical negligence. Legally, medical negligence is the lack of reasonable care and skill, or willful negligence on the part of the doctor in respect of acceptance of a patient, history taking, examination, diagnosis, investigation, and treatment—medical or surgical—resulting in injury or damage to the patient. Damage may be physical, mental, or functional injury.

Negligence of an Aesthetic Surgeon

Medical negligence arises from an act of commission or omission by the aesthetic surgeon, which no reasonably competent and careful aesthetic surgeon would have committed. What is expected of an aesthetic surgeon is reasonable skill and care expected from any other similarly qualified aesthetic surgeon acting in similar circumstance and geographic location. The skill need not be of the highest level.[46] When the standard of care falls below the reasonable standard expected, it is liable to be declared deficient service.

What is Standard Care in Aesthetic Surgery?[46,52-56]

There is no set standard of care which is universally applicable or acceptable. One of the yardsticks useful in this regard is the standards established by a professional body of similarly qualified aesthetic surgeons in a country or region. Other resources are also helpful—textbooks, peer-reviewed journals, evidence-based guidelines, etc.

Generally, when the medical care is alleged to be substandard by a client, courts take the opinion of expert aesthetic surgeons. But the stand taken by such an expert is not binding on the court. Court will see whether the deposition of the expert is logical, reasonable, and responsible before taking a decision as to its acceptability.[46]

The standard of care as existent at the time the aesthetic surgery was carried out is taken into consideration and not that at the time of hearing of the case. Suppose laser X was the most preferred choice earlier for a particular condition, and later at the time of the hearing of the case laser Z stands as the gold standard, aesthetic surgeon cannot be held negligent for using the laser X as the standard treatment earlier.

LEGAL LIABILITY OF AN AESTHETIC SURGEON[57-59]

An aesthetic surgeon's liability arises from negligent acts of omission or commission on three fronts: (1) Civil liability to pay damages, (2) criminal liability to be punished when the degree of recklessness and negligence is so gross that it is considered a wrong against the society at large, and (3) professional liability to be penalized by the apex medical professional body, i.e., Medical Council of India. A single act of negligence can lead to independent liabilities on all the three fronts.

It is important to note that an aesthetic surgeon is vicariously liable for the negligent acts of assistants/staff working under him/her. It is therefore important for the aesthetic surgeon to ensure that all staff who perform/assist in procedures are adequately trained.

Consumer forums provide a speedier, simple, and cheap pathway for the aggrieved clients to claim compensation for deficient service in place of prolonged, cumbersome, and expensive Civil Court procedures. Different liabilities and the consequent actions have been summarized in **Table 1**.

TABLE 1: Types of legal liabilities and possible consequential actions.

Law	*Forum*	*Wrong committed*	*Action*
Law of Torts	Civil Courts	Injury or damage	Compensation
Criminal Law	Magistrate Courts	Death, injury, or risk of injury	Punishment—imprisonment or fine or both
MCI Ethical Code	State Medical Council or MCI	Misconduct	Warning or cancellation of license—temporary or permanent
CPA	Consumer forums	Deficiency of service	Compensation

Medical Malpractice[57-59]

The client who comes up with a case of negligence has the burden to prove the following points to establish negligence of the aesthetic surgeon:

- Duty of aesthetic surgeon to provide standard care
- Breach of this duty
- Consequent injury or damage
- Direct cause and effect relation between the breach of duty and injury/damage.

A doctor is not guilty of negligence if he has acted in accordance with a practice accepted as proper by a responsible body of medical men skilled in that particular art. A doctor is not guilty if he is acting in accordance with such a practice, merely because there is a body of opinion that takes a contrary view (Bolam Test).[46,60]

An aesthetic surgeon may be held negligent when he departs from accepted practice and seeks to introduce innovations. Such innovations and departure from approved practice per se may not be held negligent if the surgeon is able to justify his actions. It is recognized that, otherwise there will be no place for innovations, improvements, and refinement of procedures.

Error in judgment per se is not negligence.[61] Supreme Court of India has said "it is wrong to assume negligence on the part of the doctor merely because something went wrong with the patient."

Res Ipsa Loquitur[46]

It is a legal concept which literally means "the thing speaks for itself." Suppose an aesthetic surgeon has operated on a wrong client, wrong part, or wrong side of the body, it will be evident to even a common man that it could have happened only because of negligence. In such a situation, negligence is presumed, and the aesthetic surgeon will have the burden to prove that there was no negligence on his part. Examples of other situations which may fit into such a legal stand include:

- Not giving test dose of a drug which has allergic potential such as penicillin and procaine
- Client experiencing electric shock from equipment during treatment.

Liability of the Healthcare Institution[14,46,62]

The institution is vicariously liable for the negligent acts of medical staff employed by it, as the responsibility to appoint competent persons lies with the institution. In addition, the institution is also directly liable for acts of negligence like not providing safe environment, misleading claims of availability of facilities,[63] not keeping equipment in good working condition,[64] nonavailability of oxygen at times of emergency, etc.

Contributory Negligence[46,57,64]

A patient has certain duties to adhere to. He/she is expected to act like a reasonable patient. Society expects a patient to conduct in such a way that it would not adversely affect his/her own safety. If he fails in this duty and it leads to injuries, then it is said to be contributory negligence of the patient. In such a case, damages payable as compensation by the surgeon get reduced in proportion to the degree of patient's negligence contributing to the injury.

Examples of patient's conduct, which may fall into this category, are:

- Not giving proper past medical history
- Failure to disclose important information like drug allergy in the past
- Not cooperating during administration of treatment
- Not adhering to postoperative advice
- Not coming for follow-up, etc.

Criminal Liability[46]

To fix criminal liability on an aesthetic surgeon, the standard of negligence required to be proved should be so high that it can be described as "gross negligence" or "recklessness", not merely lack of necessary care.

Section 304A of the IPC states "Whoever causes the death of any person by a rash or negligent act not amounting to culpable homicide shall be punished by imprisonment for up to two years, or by fine, or both."

Supreme Court has given the guideline that unless arrest is necessary for furthering the investigation or for collecting evidence or unless the investigating officer feels satisfied that the doctor proceeded against would not make himself available to face the prosecution unless arrested, the arrest may be withheld.[65]

There are two sections in the Indian Penal Code which are helpful. According to Section 80 "when adequate care and caution are exercised, but things go wrong because of accident or misfortune they are not offences" and as per Section 88, "any act done in good faith in the interest of the person is not an offence provided the person has given consent to take the risk associated with the said act."

- Taking informed consent for aesthetic surgery is a preventive step.
- Proving that the alleged injury or damage was due to accident is a legal defense.

LEGAL DEFENSE FOR AESTHETIC SURGEON[46,66,67]

Professional indemnity insurance, which covers cosmetic surgery, may be a prudent step to take. Indian Medical Association and Indian Association of Dermatologists, Venereologists and Leprologists offer such a scheme for its life members. Maintaining cordial relationship with the client and skillful communication go a long way in preventing litigations. Despite sincere professional job being done and all possible precautions being taken, things can go wrong at times. Many times, frank and truthful discussion with the client can prevent unnecessary litigation. A dissatisfied client may still come up with a case of negligence. At such time, aesthetic surgeon should keep his cool and take legal opinion and assistance. Possible defenses available to aesthetic surgeon include the following mentioned here.

Technical Defenses

- *No territorial jurisdiction:* For example, District Forums and State Commissions have fixed jurisdictions.
- *No pecuniary jurisdiction:* For example, District Forums can entertain cases wherein the consideration/fee paid by the consumer to the seller/service provider does not exceed 1 crore rupees, whereas for State Commissions, it is more than 1 crore and up to 10 crore rupees. Only National Commission can handle cases involving amounts beyond rupees 10 crores.[68]
- *Time-barred:* Normally, a case can be filed within 2 years of occurrence of the incident.
- *Totally free service:* In such a case, the client cannot be considered as a consumer.
- *Case involving complex medical issues:* To be handled by Civil Court and not by Consumer Forum.

Factual Defenses

- *Suppression of material facts by patient:* For example, duration of illness, previous illness, or treatment, known drug allergy, etc.
- Known complication, which has been duly brought to the notice of the patient before taking consent and documented accordingly
- Unexpected/unforeseen occurrence for which aesthetic surgeon cannot be held responsible
- *Contributory negligence:* Patients' or attendants' action has resulted in the damage, lack of follow-up, not following instructions, self-medication, etc.
- *Novus Actus Interveniens:* This means a new act or an event occurring in the chain of events between the alleged act of negligence and the resultant damage. For example, simultaneous treatment by another doctor, use of alternative system of medicine

Consumer Protection Act 2019

Consumer Protection Act 1986 has been repealed and CPA 2019[68] has become effective from 24 July 2020. The Act provides for redressal of consumer grievances with a three-tier mechanism:

1. District Consumer Disputes Redressal Commission (DCDRC)
2. State Consumer Disputes Redressal Commission (SCDRC)
3. National Consumer Disputes Redressal Commission NCDRC)

Filing of Complaint by the Client

An aggrieved patient can simply file a complaint on plain paper providing all the details of the grievance along with details of the opposite party and self. Even online mode of registering complaints will be available soon.

Time limit for filing is 2 years from the date of occurrence of the cause of action. But the consumer forums have the power to condone the delay if the complainant can provide convincing reasons for the delay in filing complaint.

It is not mandatory to engage a lawyer for filing a complaint.

Quantum of court fee payable depends upon the consideration paid by the complainant for availing the service. If it is <5 lakh rupees, no court fee is payable at DCDRC.

Where can the Client File a Complaint?

Patient can file a complaint at the district consumer forum of the district in which he/she resides or is gainfully employed. This provision is patient friendly but disadvantageous to the aesthetic surgeon.

Pecuniary jurisdiction of the consumer forums is not dependent on the quantum of compensation claimed, but on the amount of consideration paid by the aggrieved patient to avail the service of the aesthetic surgeon.

- If the consideration paid is up to rupees 1 crore—DCDRC
- If the consideration paid is more than rupees 1 crore up to 10 crores—SCDRC
- If the consideration paid is more than rupees 10 crores—NCDRC.

Nature of Grievances and Reliefs

- *Deficiency of service:* This may be in respect of the treatment given, information provided, or consent obtained before carrying out the treatment or procedure.

Relief in this instance is either removal of the deficiency or refund of the consideration in full or part.

- *Negligence:* Carelessness or indifference resulting in damage or injury. In all cases of negligence, there will be some extent of deficiency of service but in all cases of deficiency of service there may or may not be the element of negligence.
  The degree of carelessness to the extent of being grossly reckless makes it a case of criminal negligence.
  Relief in this instance is the compensation to be determined by the consumer courts. In case of criminal negligence, there will be punishment in the form of fine, imprisonment, or both.
- *Unfair trade practice:* If misleading information or false claims or misrepresentation of facts have been employed in any form to enhance practice, and the complainant finds out later that the claims are untrue, there lies a ground for alleging "unfair practice". For example, if an aesthetic surgeon claims to be using a Food and Drug Administration (FDA)-approved Laser, but later it turns out to be far from truth, patient can file a complaint.

Issue of Notice to the Opposite Party

The consumer courts take a decision about the admissibility of the complaint within 21 days of filing of the complaint. If no action is taken, the complaint is deemed to have been admitted.

Then a notice is sent to the opposite party—that is the aesthetic surgeon in this context.

Reply must be sent by the aesthetic surgeon within 30 days. There is provision for seeking extension of time by another 15 days. In the absence of reply, proceedings may be held *ex-parte.*

While giving the reply, it is very important to counter each point in the complaint along with proper evidence. It is better for the aesthetic surgeon to avail the services of a legal practitioner.

Scope for Settlement by Mediation

Mediation cell will be available at all three tiers of the consumer disputes redressal commissions. If a case is referred for mediation by the forum, a mediator from the panel maintained will conduct the mediation to explore the possibility of reaching an agreement between the opposing parties.

If such an agreement is reached and signed by both the parties, it is forwarded to the concerned commission for passing suitable orders. If no settlement happens, the case is taken up for normal proceedings.

Proceedings of the Consumer Forum

Aesthetic surgeon can present his/her own case, but it is advisable to consult or engage a lawyer to represent and defend before the consumer forum. It is equally important to furnish all the medical records pertaining to the case as well as relevant medical literature in the form of extracts from standard textbooks, peer reviewed medical journals, guidelines issued by professional medical bodies, etc. Producing supporting expert opinion in the form of an affidavit from a colleague with good standing will be helpful.

The forum settles the dispute based on the evidence brought before it by the complainant and the opposing party. It can refer the matter to an expert or a panel of experts to seek opinion whether the treatment provided, or procedure done by the doctor is as per accepted professional practices or not. Disposal of complaint is to be made within 3 months from the date of receipt of notice by the opposite party (5 months in cases requiring testing/analysis of products).

Provision to Challenge the Order

Appellate jurisdiction to contest orders of the District Commission lies with the State Commission, that of State Commission lies with the National Commission and that of National Commission lies with the Supreme Court of India. Such appeals must be filed within 30 days of the communication of the order to be challenged. There is provision for condonation of delay in case the concerned commission/Apex court is convinced that the delay is due to compelling/unavoidable reasons.

Penalty for Noncompliance of Orders

If the order of any consumer disputes redressal commission is not complied with, penalty may be imposed in the form of imprisonment (from 1 month to 3 years) or fine (from rupees 25,000/- to 1 lakh) or both.

Frivolous Complaints

Under Section 26 of the CPA 1986,[11] there was scope to impose penalty on the complainant to the extent of 10,000 rupees to curb the tendency to file false, trivial, or vexatious complaints with the intention to extract money/harass/tarnish the reputation/intimidate. But unfortunately, no such provision appears to be there under the CPA 2019.[68]

CONCLUSION

- Clients going in for aesthetic procedures expect perfect results and show zero tolerance for complications.
- Taking informed consent with full disclosure of all relevant information is of paramount importance.
- Being competent, following standard procedures, and carrying out surgeries with due care in a well-equipped surgical facility go a long way in avoiding mishaps.
- Good communication skills come in handy to build rapport with and make the client understand the realistic outcomes expected out of the aesthetic surgery.

- Cordial doctor–patient relationship helps to avoid dissatisfaction and consequent litigation.
- Notice from a consumer forum should be replied within 30 days, preferably with the help of a lawyer.
- Meticulous documentation and careful preservation of medical records for prescribed periods of time provide best defense in case of alleged medical negligence.

REFERENCES

1. ISAPS Global Statistics. Aesthetic/cosmetic procedures performed in 2018. [online] Available from: https://www.isaps.org/wp-content/uploads/2020/10/ISAPS-Global-Survey-Results-2018-1.pdf. [Last accessed July 2022].
2. Neville JA, Housman TS, Letsinger JA, Fleischer Jr AB, Feldman SR, Williford PM. Increase in procedures performed at dermatology office visits from 1995 to 2001. Dermatol Surg. 2005;31(2):160-2.
3. Cassetta M. Ethics in esthetic nursing, avoiding the ugly side of beauty. Plast Surg Nurs. 2008;28(3):117-20.
4. Gupta AS. Medical tourism in India: winners and losers. [online] Available from: https://www.ijme.in/wp-content/uploads/2016/11/1320-5.pdf. [Last accessed July 2022].
5. Mehta A, Goldstein SD, Makary MA. Global trends in center accreditation by the Joint Commission International: growing patient implications for international medical and surgical care. J Travel Med. 2017;24(5):tax048.
6. The South West's Premier Cosmetic Treatment Centre. BAAPS Consumer Safety Guidelines. [online] Available from: https://www.davidolivercosmeticsurgery.co.uk/wp-content/uploads/2012/09/BAAPS-Consumer-Safety-Guidelines.pdf. [Last accessed July 2022].
7. Byrd HS, Barton FE, Orenstein HH, Rohrich RJ, Burns AJ, Hobar PC, et al. Safety and efficacy in an accredited outpatient plastic surgery facility: a review of 5316 consecutive cases. Plast Reconstr Surg. 2003;112(2):636-41.
8. Stafford BM, La Puma J, Schiedermayer DL. One face of beauty, one picture of health: the hidden esthetic of medical practice. J Med Philos. 1989;14:213-30.
9. Hinderer UT. Indications and significance of esthetic plastic surgery. Handchir Mikrochir Plast Chir. 1984;16:145-50.
10. Alam M, Dover JS. On beauty: evolution, psychosocial considerations, and surgical enhancement. Arch Dermatol. 2001;137:795-807.
11. Gazette of India. The Consumer Protection Act, 1986. Arrangement of Sections. [online] Available from: https://legislative.gov.in/sites/default/files/A1986-68_0.pdf. [Last accessed July 2022].
12. IndianKanoon.org. (1995). Indian Medical Association v V.P. Shanta, AIR 1996 SC 550. [online] Available from: https://www.legalserviceindia.com/legal/article-6010-case-analysis-vp-shanta-v-s-indian-medical-association.html#:~:text=In%201995%2C%20the%20Supreme%20Court,this%20issue%20given%20by%20various. [Last accessed July 2022].
13. IndianKanoon.org. (2013). Balram Prasad vs Kunal Saha & Ors. [online] Available from: https://indiankanoon.org/doc/35346928/ [Last accessed July 2022]
14. LatestLaws.com. (2019). SC awards ₹76 Lakhs compensation in Medical Negligence case. [online] Available from: https://drive.google.com/file/d/195_6ZrloKOX16AmvizmtzrxtyGnVshQ1/view. [Last accessed July 2022].
15. IndianKanoon.org. (2009). [online] Available from Nizam's Institute Of Medical ... vs Prasanth S.Dhananka & Ors. https://indiankanoon.org/doc/1110505/. [Last accessed July 2022].
16. De Sousa A. Concerns about cosmetic surgery. [online] Available from: https://www.ijme.in/wp-content/uploads/2016/11/1304-5.pdf. [Last accessed July 2022].
17. Ito S, Kono H, Why is the take-up of microinsurance so low? Evidence from a health insurance scheme in India. The Developing Economies. 2010;48(1):74-101.
18. Dogra S. Fate of medical dermatology in the era of cosmetic dermatology and dermatosurgery. Indian J Dermatol Venereol Leprol. 2009;75:4-7.
19. Buppert C. Misadventures in cosmetic dermatology. [online] Available from: https://www.medscape.com/viewarticle/708186_1. [Last accessed July 2022].
20. Mody B. Scar revision is a useless operation. Indian J Plast Surg. 2004;37:23-4.
21. Agarwal P. Perception of plastic surgery in the society. Indian J Plast Surg. 2004;37:110-4.
22. Nejadsarvari N, Ebrahimi A, Ebrahimi A, Hashem-Zade H. Medical ethics in plastic surgery: a mini review. World J Plast Surg. 2016;5(3):207-12.
23. Goh CL. The need for evidence-based esthetic dermatology practice. J Cutan Aesthet Surg. 2009;2:65-71.
24. Expert Group on the Regulation of Cosmetic Surgery: Report to the Chief Medical Officer, Department of Health, UK. January 2005.
25. "https://ind01.safelinks.protection.outlook.com/?url=https%3A%2F%2Fijdvl.com%2Fissue%2F2009-75-8%2F&data=05%7C01%7Cnedup.bhutia%40jaypeebrothers.com%7C8834fce98ae34c1dade408dba38c423e%7C9e7fa850 fd9547b7bda2a51c357d60ae%7C0%7C0%7C638283595044499726%7CUnknown%7CTWFpbGZsb3d8eyJWIjoiMC4wLjAwMDAiLCJQIjoiV2luMzIiLCJBTiI6Ik1haWwiLCJXVCI6Mn0%3D%7C3000%7C%7C%7C&sdata=sxE8WK8NE%2FHBlhFpXfWVxarbV%2FrSjMfJci%2FIjHZA1oo%3D&reserved=0" https://ijdvl.com/ issue/2009-75-8/. Accessed on 23rd August 2023.
26. The Ethics of Cosmetic Surgery. [online] Available from: http:// medicalmatrix.blogspot.com/2007/08/ethics-of-cosmetic-surgery.html. [Last accessed July 2022].
27. Ritvo E. Never-ending cosmetic surgeries—the patient with body dysmorphic disorder. [online] Available from: http://www.medscape.com/viewarticle/725216. [Last accessed July 2022].
28. Caselaw Access Project. (2001). Lynn v. Hugo, 96 N.Y.2d 306, 752 N.E.2d 250, 728 N.Y.S.2d 121. [online] Available from: https://cite.case.law/ny2d/96/306/. [Last accessed July 2022].
29. Rao K. Safer practice of dermatosurgery. Indian J Dermatol Venereol Leprol. 2008;74:75-7.
30. American Society for Esthetic Plastic Surgery warns patients to steer clear of injection fat loss treatments. [online] Available from: https://www.cosmeticsurgery-news.com/article3025.html. [Last accessed July 2022].
31. Bradbury E. Clinical risk in cosmetic surgery. Clin Risk. 2009;15(6):227-31.
32. Nahai F. Minimizing risk in esthetic surgery. Clin Risk. 2009;15(6):232-6.
33. Khoo C. Risk reduction in cosmetic surgery. Clin Risk. 2009;15(6):237-40.
34. De U. Genesis and mechanics of malpractice suits—Minimizing the risks. Indian J Surg. 2004;66:301-3.

35. Mousavi SR. The ethics of esthetic surgery. J Cutan Aesthet Surg. 2010;3:38-40.
36. Bastia BK, Kuruvilla A, Saralaya KM. Validity of consent—A review of statutes. Indian J Med Sci. 2005;59:74-8.
37. Satyanarayana Rao KH. Informed consent: an ethical obligation or legal compulsion? J Cutan Aesthet Surg. 2008; 1:33-5.
38. Beauchamp TL, Childress JF. Principles of Biomedical Ethics, 5th edition. Oxford: Oxford University Press; 2001.
39. Legal Match. Medical Battery Definition. [online] Available from: http://www.legalmatch.com/law-library/article/medical-battery.html. [Last accessed July 2022].
40. Trehan SP, Sankhari D. Medical Professional, Patient and the Law: The Institute of Law and Ethics in Medicine, 2nd edition. Bengaluru: National Law School of India University; 2002.
41. Kohli, A. Medical consent in India—Ethical and legal issues. Anil Aggrawals Internet J Forensic Med Toxicol. 2007;8(2).
42. Mavroforou A, Giannoukas A, Michalodimitrakis E. Medical litigation in cosmetic plastic surgery. Med Law. 2004;23(3): 479-88.
43. Central Drugs Standard Control Organisation. [online] Available from: https://cdsco.gov.in/opencms/export/sites/CDSCO_WEB/Pdf-documents/GCT_PDFs/FAQ_CT.pdf [Last accessed July 2022].
44. Nanda L. The need for a computerized patient-record system for the public hospitals in Andhra Pradesh. J Academy of Hosp Administration. 2000;12:7-13.
45. Ministry of Health and Family Welfare, Government of India. [online] Available from: https://main.mohfw.gov.in/sites/default/files/EMR-EHR_Standards_for_India_as_notified_by_MOHFW_2016_0.pdf. [Last accessed July 2022].
46. Satish M, Menon R, Rao KV. Professional Accountability and Patients' Rights, 2nd edition. Bengaluru: The Institute of Law and Ethics in Medicine, National Law School of India University; 2002.
47. Gazette of India. (2002). Indian Medical Council (Professional Conduct, Etiquette and Ethics) Regulations, 2002. [online] Available from: https://wbconsumers.gov.in/writereaddata/ACT%20&%20RULES/Relevant%20Act%20&%20Rules/Code%20of%20Medical%20Ethics%20Regulations.pdf. [Last accessed July 2022].
48. Lawyer Services. (1997). Force v/s. M Ganeswara Rao & others. 1998 (3) CPR 251; 1998 (1) CPJ 413 (AP SCDRC). [online] Available from: https://www.lawyerservices.in/Force-Versus-Dr-M-Ganeswara-Rao-and-Others-1997-08-22. [Last accessed July 2022].
49. Indiankanoon.org. Meenakshi Mission Hospital and Research Centre V. Samuraj and Anr I (2005) CPJ 33 (NC). [online] Available from: https://indiankanoon.org/doc/967273/. [Last accessed July 2022].
50. Lawyer Services. (1998). Dr Tokugha Yeptomi V Apollo Hospital Enterprises Ltd and Anr III (1998) CPJ 132 (SC). [online] Available from: https://www.lawyerservices.in/Dr-Tokugha-Yepthomi-Versus-Apollo-Hospital-Enterprises-Ltd-1998-09-21. [Last accessed July 2022].
51. NAIR, M R Hariharan RTI v medical ethics: some questions arising from the recent decision of the Chief Information Commissioner under the RTI Act. Indian J Med Ethics. 2015;12(3):182-5.
52. Dogra TD, Gupta S. Medico-legal aspect of health care delivery. [online] Available from: https://www.indmedica.com/journals.php?journalid=6&issueid=104&articleid=1441&action=article [Last accessed July 2022].
53. Goldberg DJ. Cosmetic dermatology: legal issues. Dermatol Clin. 2009;27:501-5.
54. Goldberg DJ. Medicolegal issues for the dermatologist. Semin Cutan Med Surg. 2000;19:181-8.
55. Goldberg DJ. Legal issues in dermatology: informed consent, complications and medical malpractice. Semin Cutan Med Surg. 2007;26:2-5.
56. Goldberg DJ. Legal issues in laser operation. Clin Dermatol. 2006;24:56-9.
57. Murthy KKSR. Medical negligence and the law. Indian J Med Ethics. 2007;4(3):116-8.
58. Singh K, Sharma B, Singh A. Legal liabilities and duties of a doctor, Part 1. [online] Available from: https://www.djo.org.in/articles/28/1/legal-liabilities.html. [Last accessed July 2022].
59. Shiffman MA. Medical liability issues in cosmetic and plastic surgery. Med Law. 2005;24(2):211-32.
60. Norrie KM. Medical negligence: who sets the standard?. J Med Ethics. 1985;11(3):135-7.
61. Dr. KunalSaha vs. Dr. Sukumar Mukherjee and Ors. III (2006) CPJ 142 (NC). [online] Available from: https://indiankanoon.org/doc/22051430/. [Last accessed July 2022].
62. Koodamara N, Kumar A. Error of judgment and vicarious liability of the hospitals in case of medical negligence in India. Indian J Public Health Res Dev. 2018;9(12):1642.
63. Meera T, Phanjoubam M, Nabachandra H. Hospital's liability in malpractice suits. J Med Soc. 2016;30:1-2.
64. Satyanarayana Rao KH. Ethics, Etiquettes and Legal Issues, Management Issues for a Dermatologist, 1st edition. New Delhi: Jaypee Brothers Medical Publishers (P) Ltd; 2009.
65. Indiankanoon.org. Jacob Mathew V. State of Punjab AIR 2005 SC 3180. [online] Available from: https://indiankanoon.org/doc/871062/. [Last accessed July 2022].
66. Srinivas P. Consumer Protection Act and Dermatological Practice, a Dermatologists' Perspective of Medical Ethics and Consumer Protection Act: An IADVL Book, 1st edition. 2007.
67. Mathiharan K. Landmark case. [online] Available from: https://www.medindia.net/doctors/cpa/case-1_print.asp. [Last accessed July 2022].
68. The Consumer Protection Act, 2019. [online] Available from: http://egazette.nic.in/WriteReadData/2019/210422.pdf. [Last accessed July 2022].

CHAPTER 131

Clinical Photography in Surgical and Aesthetic Dermatology

Ashique KT, Feroze Kaliyadan

KEY MESSAGES

- A good photograph speaks more than a thousand words.
- While choosing a camera, specific attention should be paid to lens, megapixels, zoom and macromode.
- While taking a photo, depth of field, background, lighting, need to be considered.
- Storage and documentation using specific software need to be addressed.
- Proper consent is a must prior to taking clinical pictures.
- Mobile phones also play a vital role in clinical photography in the present times.

INTRODUCTION

The shift from conventional film photography to digital photography for clinical documentation has been a big milestone in the history of clinical photography. Many limitations associated with film photography have been overcome by shifting to digital imaging. Digital photography also has gradually become cost-effective. The rapid advances in digital imaging technology have thrown up newer opportunities and challenges as far as clinical photography is concerned. The present day dermatosurgeon needs to be very aware of not only what technology has in store for clinical photography but also how well he can utilize the same in his clinical practice.[1,2]

HISTORY OF PHOTOGRAPHIC DOCUMENTATION IN COSMETIC SURGERY

Photographic documentation has always been considered important in cosmetic surgery. Photographic documentation of plastic and cutaneous surgery has been going on for a long time now. Gordon Buck (1807–1877) is considered to be one of the first surgeons to use preoperative patient photographs to communicate his results in 1845. The first use of photography in plastic surgery per se was by James Balossa (1814–1868) of Budapest University for demonstrating a nasal reconstruction.[3,4]

IMPORTANCE OF GOOD IMAGING

A good photograph does speak more than a thousand words. Standardized imaging is an essential part of assessing clinical or cosmetic improvement after medical, surgical or cosmetic dermatology treatment. Imaging can also be invaluable in counseling the patient regarding his or her medical problem and possible results that can be attained post-treatment. This actually saves time for the clinician and also increases the confidence in the patient to undergo the procedure.[5] It goes without saying that good photographs are essential to communicate effectively with the scientific community through presentations and publications, apart from insurance companies and laboratories as and when the need arises. Good images are also essential for making brochures and other marketing tools.

BASIC PRINCIPLE OF A DIGITAL CAMERA (ANATOMY AND PHYSIOLOGY)

Unlike a film camera, a digital camera has a sensor that converts light into electrical charges. The image sensor employed by most digital cameras is a *charge coupled device (CCD)*. Some cameras use *complementary metal oxide semiconductor (CMOS)* technology instead. Both CCD and CMOS image sensors convert light into electrons, which in turn generate the digital images.

Charge coupled device and CMOS have their respective pros and cons:

- CCD sensors create higher-quality images with less noise compared to CMOS sensors. The light sensitivity of a CMOS chip is lower.
- CMOS sensors consume less power compared to CCD sensors.[6]

EQUIPMENT (GEAR)

Camera: Digital Single-lens Reflex versus Point-and-Shoot

One of the questions, which come up quite often in discussions on clinical photography, is whether to go for a digital single-lens reflex (DSLR) or a point-and-shoot camera. As far as the quality of photos is concerned, the DSLRs definitely outscore the common point-and-shoot varieties. SLR stands for single lens reflex, which in simple terms refers to a camera which has lens interchangeability feature and also maximum of manual controls or, in layman's term, "the professional camera". The SLR has the advantage that what we see through the view finder is exactly what we get in the resultant image. For all practical purposes in clinical dermatology, however, including publications and presentations, the image quality of most of the commercially available compact cameras are more than sufficient. Besides, the exorbitant cost of DSLRs especially when going for specialized lenses is another prohibitive factor for an average clinician. The one disadvantage of most compact cameras is a limitation in manual adjustments specifically in relation to controlling factors such as aperture size, shutter speed and flash intensity. There are intermediate, "prosumer" or "bridging" cameras available these days which have functional capabilities between a simple compact camera and a DSLR. Most of these are relatively more affordable compared to a DSLR and less bulky to carry around especially in a doctor's bag. Most compact digitals do not have a fixed focal length, so it is not possible to achieve standardization, unlike SLR cameras. The chances of getting a distorted (blurred) image are high when the subject is approached beyond a certain distance. Generally, it is advisable to maintain the camera more than 1 m away from the patient. This can be done using a zoom lens, preferably a fixed focal length one of 100 mm or 50 mm. A zoom lens increases and reduces the field and angle, allowing optimal capture of details. It is very important that physician should only rely on the optical zoom of the lens.[7] Most point-and-shoot cameras have a specialized mode for close-up photography, otherwise called the "macro" mode (denoted by the symbol). A relatively newer option, which has image quality on par with DSLRs, but is less bulky, is the mirrorless camera. However, as of now these mirrorless cameras are limited by a higher cost and fewer options in terms of lens availability.

Camera Resolution

How many megapixels (MP) do you really need? This is another question which may sound "*Latin and Greek*" for a novice medical photographer. The amount of detail that the camera can capture is called the resolution, and it is measured in pixels (which stands for *picture cells*). Basically, the more pixels a camera has the more detail it can capture. Also, as the pixels increase, larger prints can be made without losing detail.[2,8-10] Earlier studies have suggested that even a resolution of 1.3 MP is sufficient for dermatological photography.[8] All modern dedicated digital cameras, even of the point-and-shoot variety have resolutions upwards of 8 MP, so camera resolution is not really a major concern in terms of choosing a camera for clinical photography. Many mobile phone cameras now come at high resolution ranging from 5 to 12 MP; however, in spite of this high resolution mobile phone cameras have a lot of limitations, especially an absence of dedicated close-up/macro-modes and difficulty in maintaining a standardized/consistent positioning or setting, making them unsuitable for precision clinical photography. Moreover, the reflection of light from the camera flash is an issue with mobile phone cameras too.[11]

OTHER EQUIPMENT AND SETTING

The only variable among photographs taken to show change over time should be the patient. Everything else should stay the same—viewpoint, positioning, lighting, color, magnification, perspective, contrast and background.[12]

Patient Positioning and Preparation

The convention used by most medical photographers is, wherever possible, to photograph the patient in the anatomical position. This works for most views but some parts of the anatomy are best viewed from other angles. The arms are best photographed in extension, and are normally photographed in a horizontal position. However, the palms should still face forward, so the back of the forearm should be photographed with the patient facing away from the photographer **(Fig. 1)**.

Face

Hair should be pulled off the face and placed behind the ears. For facial procedures such as dermabrasion or laser resurfacing, remove all makeup. All distracting jewelry should be removed **(Figs. 2A and B)**.

Torso

All clothing and jewelry should be removed. Patients can wear specific photo-garments (like an operative gown) where indicated.

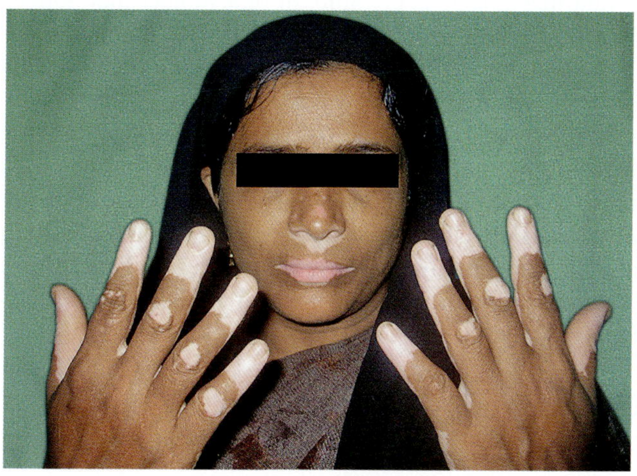

Fig. 1: Acrofacial vitiligo with the positioning of the palms facing away from the camera.

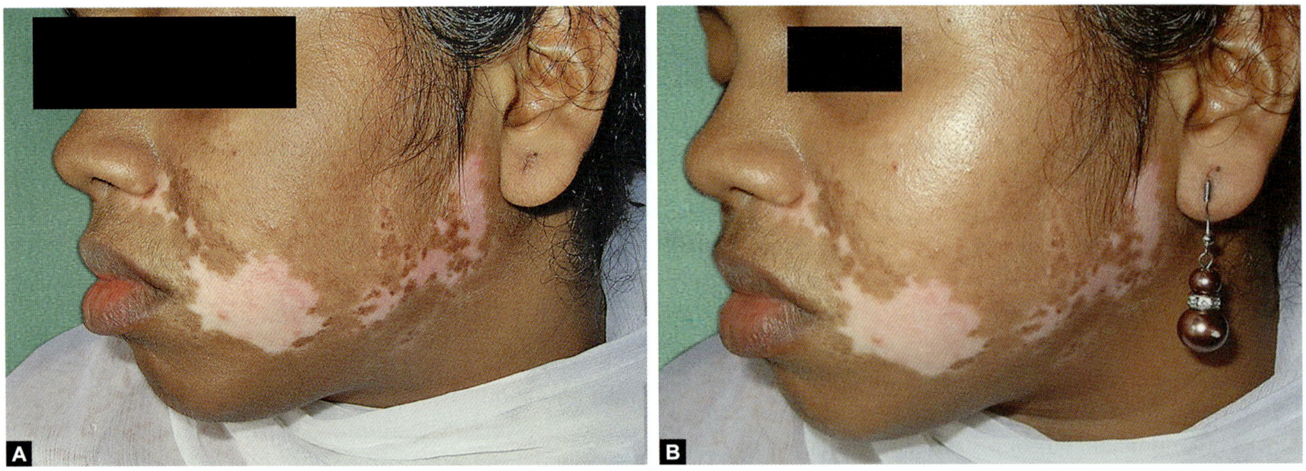

Figs. 2A and B: Distracting jewelry should be removed to increase the attention towards the point of clinical interest: (A) Without ornament; (B) With ornament.

Hands

Hands should be away from the background. Take care to ensure that rings/shirtsleeves are out of the frame.

Lower Extremity

Ensure that the homogeneous background covers the floor also, so that the patient can just step into it[13] **(Fig. 3)**.

Magnification, Perspective and Depth of Field

Magnification

The magnification of clinical photographs should also always be controlled and standardized. Similarly the distance from which a photograph is taken should be standardized.

Depth of Field

Depth of field (DOF) is another parameter which needs to be standardized. DOF is the amount of a subject that appears sharp in front of, and behind, the principal plane of focus. The smaller the lens aperture, the greater the depth of field, and this is particularly critical in close-up work where there is considerable depth, such as when photographing the teeth. Relative aperture size is denoted on a lens by f-numbers—the higher the number, the greater the depth of field, but smaller is the amount of light passed through the lens. Generally, in clinical photography, we need the maximum depth of field so our flash should be bright enough to allow us to use the smallest possible aperture.[12]

Background

The best background would be a plain light blue, black (not suitable for hair photography) or green nonreflective surface like a linen cloth. All accessories like jewelry and hair clips

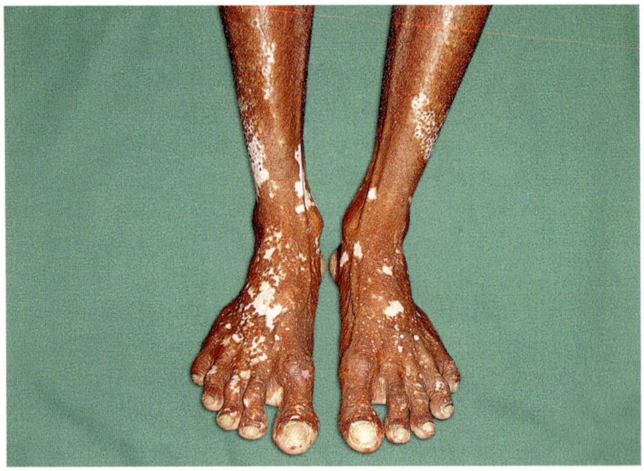

Fig. 3: Photograph of the legs taken with the patient standing on a linen sheet to avoid the distraction from the floor tiles.

tend to unnecessarily divert focus from the lesion of interest and therefore should be removed prior to photographing the patient. Other accessories required are measurement tapes and skin markers.[2,14] When a proper studio setting is not feasible, a staff can hold a black curtain to make it a background and the images captured with the patient positioned comfortably **(Figs. 4A and B)**.

Lighting

Lighting is often a tricky issue in dermatological photography. Ideally broad daylight or a naturally lit room, if available, would be the best; however, many times we have to take our photographs indoors with the use of flashes or other accessory light sources. It should be understood that the aim of clinical photography is to capture the clinical condition and not aesthetics. Inbuilt camera flash units and sharp overhead lamps (as in operation theaters) should be avoided, as they tend to whiten out the area of interest and also produce sharp reflections **(Figs. 5A to D)**. Ideally, you should have two main lights at a 45° angle to the subject on a parallel plane to the frontal plane of the subject. This can be combined with one light from above in a sagittal plane perpendicular to the frontal one aiming downward (or two lights at a 45° angle with respect to the subject) and one light behind the patient on a plane parallel to the frontal one aiming forward and at a distance of 30–60 cm from the background so as to detach the patient from the background, thus highlighting surface details.[7,12] Further soft box lights can be used to balance out reflections, if space is not an issue **(Fig. 6)**. If you are shooting with only the available room lighting, make sure that any lighting that you have is slightly in front and above the area to be photographed and the source of lighting should never be behind the subject. Again the important thing is to ensure that whatever lighting set-up is used it must be consistent.[11] The important thing while using an inbuilt flash is to avoid getting too close, as the distinctive features of the lesion may get washed off. Also it would be advisable to vary the "white balance" on the camera depending on the primary lighting (e.g., adjust the white balance to fluorescent if shooting under predominantly fluorescent light). External light sources can be useful in taking very close shots with the "macro" feature turned on (using the flash while taking extreme close-up tends to cast a shadow of the camera head over the image). Another enhancement which might help for very close shots is a "ring" flash **(Figs. 7A to C)**. However, this too may reflect from the surface of the skin lesion being photographed, particularly if the distance between the camera and the lesion is small, and wash away all the surface details.[2]

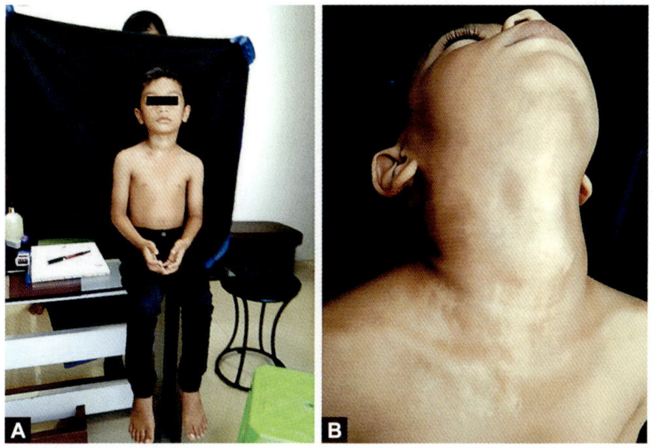

Figs. 4A and B: The child with nevus depigmentosus on the anterior aspect of the neck seated at a height and images shot with the curtain held in the background.

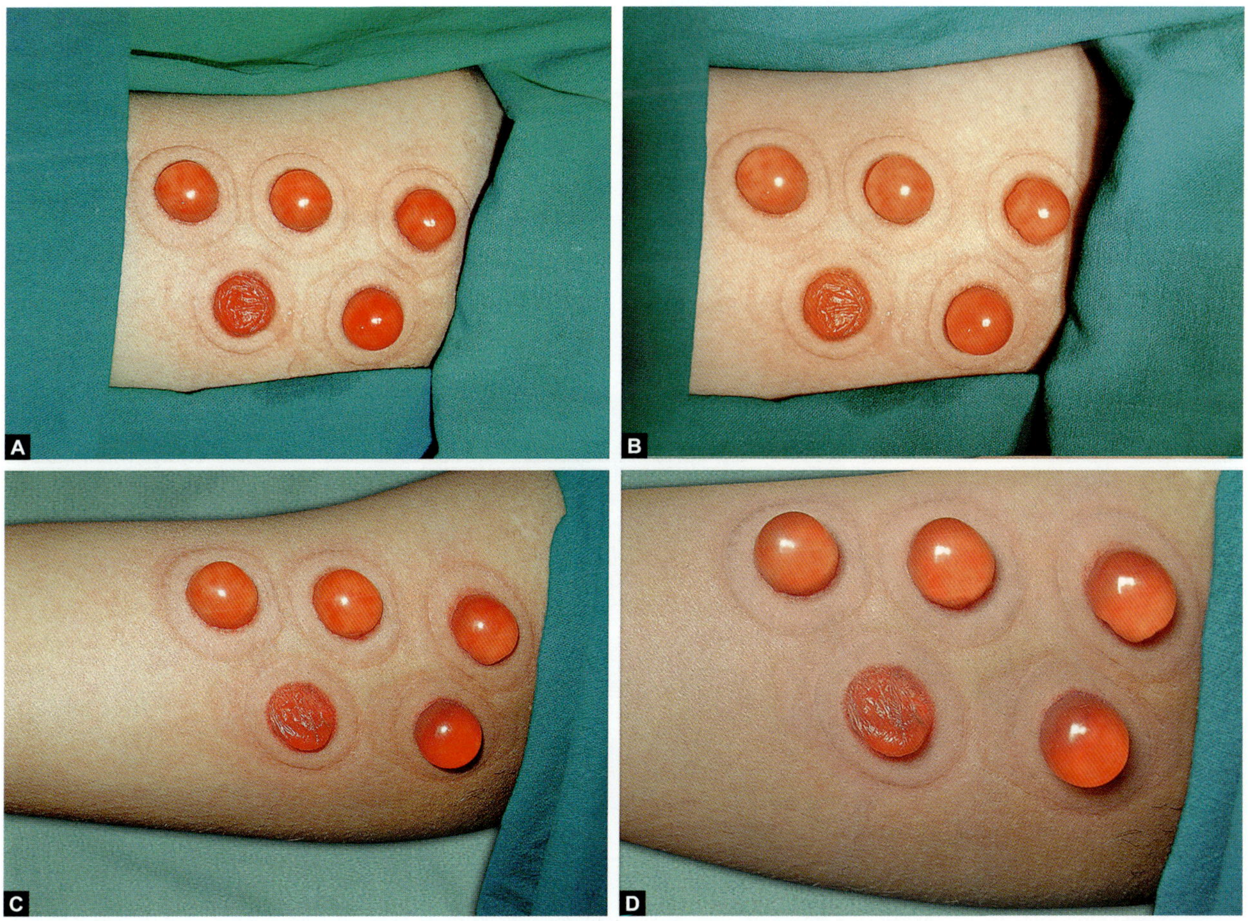

Figs. 5A to D: Effect of lighting in various circumstances: (A) OT lights and autoflash in the camera; (B) Camera flash OFF and OT lights ON; (C) Natural light (most acceptable); (D) Natural light with forced flash.

Other Accessories

A tripod is an essential tool to ensure standardized imaging and is more useful when more than one person operates the camera, especially in a clinical setting. It not only helps us to use a consistent camera position and height, but also helps to prevent blurring of images which might occur when patients are photographed without a flash turned on. Fixed focal length macro-lenses have an edge over conventional lenses in photographing isolated small lesions like nail pits or a subungual fibroma. However, good macro-lenses are costly, and standardization of macro-images is technically more challenging.

Frames

Photographic frames are another essential tool, especially for serial photography. Commercially available frames can be very much handy especially when taking pictures of face and head and neck region. They are very costly and not very easily available in the market **(Fig. 8)**.

Display Devices

A good LCD monitor is a valuable accessory for displaying the clinical images both for subjective assessment by the physician and for patient counseling. Ideally, the patient must be photographed at each visit, with the images being indexed in a slide presentation format or a collage format so that the improvement or changes can be easily visualized on the screen. Larger sized television LCD displays are another option of displaying the images. This can be overcome if a dedicated laptop is spared for this purpose which can also serve as a store house of data.

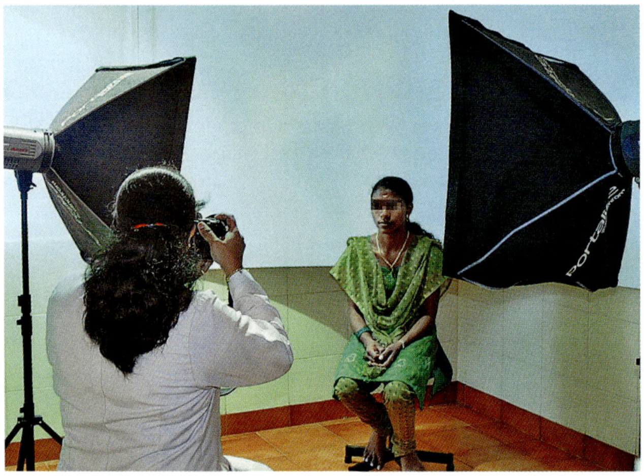

Fig. 6: Studio setting in the clinic with patient positioning and soft box lighting.
Courtesy: Dr Akhter Hussain. MDS, Principal and Professor of Orthodontics. Yenepoya University, Mangaluru.

Framing Tips (Boxes 1 and 2)[2,11,13]

- For different body areas certain standard framing patterns are followed[13]
- For all lesions make it a point to take at least two shots from each point of focus. Minimal blurring may not be obvious in the LCD screen and may be noticeable only after the images are viewed on the monitor.
- It is always better to have an extra copy from every focus point so that the best image can be selected.
- Always try to capture distinctive elements such as typical representative lesions, particular configuration or distribution patterns.

Flash-on-off/Flash Diffuser

One of the most common problems when using an onboard flash in the OPD for taking clinical pictures is the "burnt out" appearance of the images, especially when pictures of face are

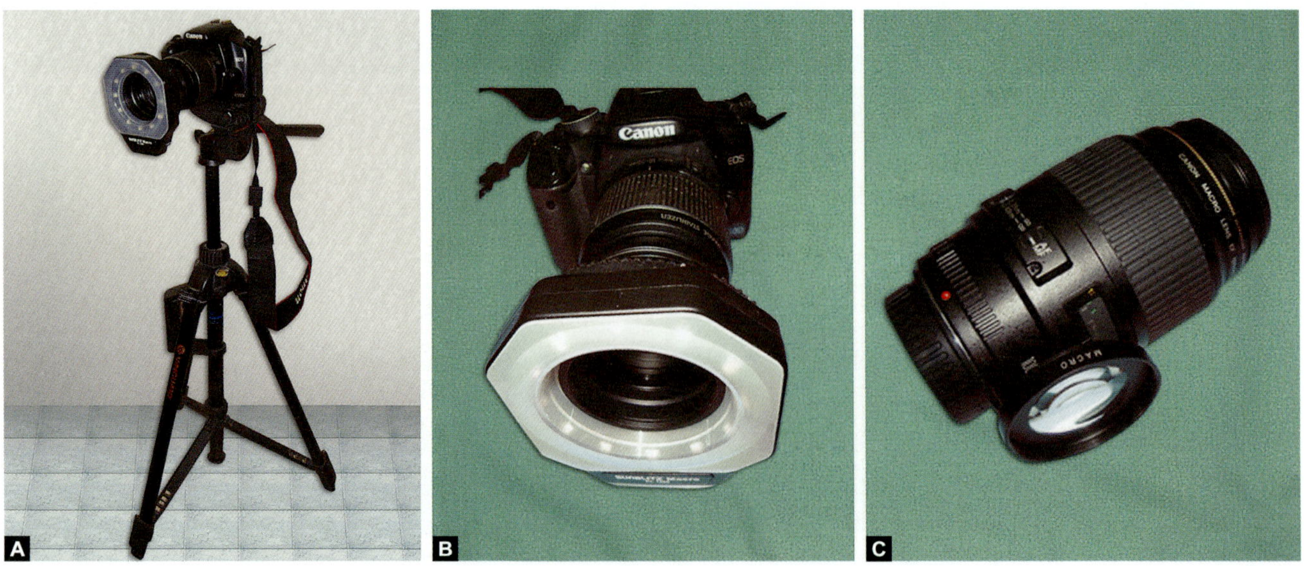

Figs. 7A to C: Some vital accessories in clinical photography: (A) Tripod; (B) Ring flash; (C) Fixed focal length macro-lens and macro-adaptor.

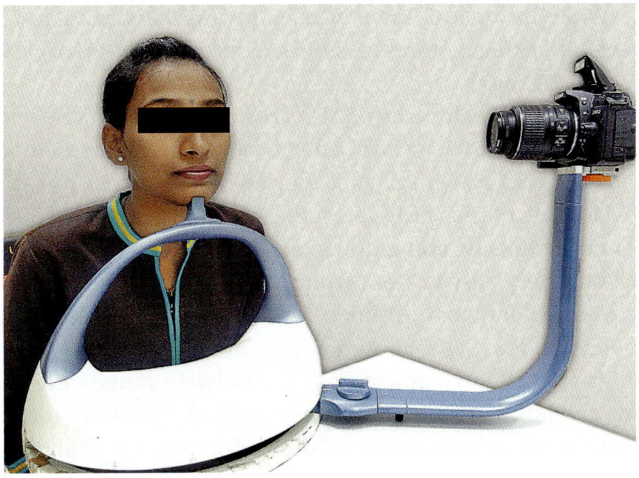

Fig. 8: Omnia Photo Stand® is an excellent tool for aesthetic photography. *Courtesy:* Dr Apratim Goel, Mumbai.

BOX 1: Framing tips for generalized lesions.

Take shots from at least three ranges:
1. A complete vertical view of the patient showing the extent and distribution of the pigmentary change or a rash
2. A medium distance shot showing the arrangement and configuration of the pigmentary change or the rash
3. A close-up view highlighting a representative lesion

BOX 2: Framing tips for localized lesions.

Take shots from at least two points:
1. A medium view showing the rash/lesion with respect to location and configuration (always include a recognizable body landmark so that the location is obvious, e.g., lesions on the chest include the nipples in the medium distance shot) **(Figs. 9A and B)**
2. A close-up view of the representative lesion. For isolated lesions it is also advisable to include a discernible landmark in one of the shots. For the close-up shots use a measuring tape in the frame to demonstrate the size of the lesion. It would be advisable to take the close-up shots from more than one angle and include oblique shots. Shots with or without flash may be taken and the best shot is selected for storage[2,12,14]

taken in close proximity. Most of the commercially available external flash units sport a built-in optional filter to overcome this problem. This can also be done by placing a butter paper or a handkerchief on the flash and taking pictures (this may require expertise and decreasing 1 or 2 f-stops to compensate for the light). A cheaper and handy alternative adopted by the authors is the use of the old 35 mm film case made of plastic with a slit to fit itself on to the onboard camera flash which can act as a diffuser to minimize the intensity of the flash light on the subject's face **(Figs. 10 and 11)**.

Storage[2,15]

Most electronic manuscripts submissions accept the joint photographic expert group (JPEG) format as the standard. The major advantage of the JPEG format is that the image size can be compressed considerably without significant visible loss of resolution and is readable in most software. This ensures ease in online submission as well as PowerPoint presentations. Some journals insist on the tagged image file format (TIFF) images to be sent on CDs as a follow-up to online submission (where digital images are the only source).

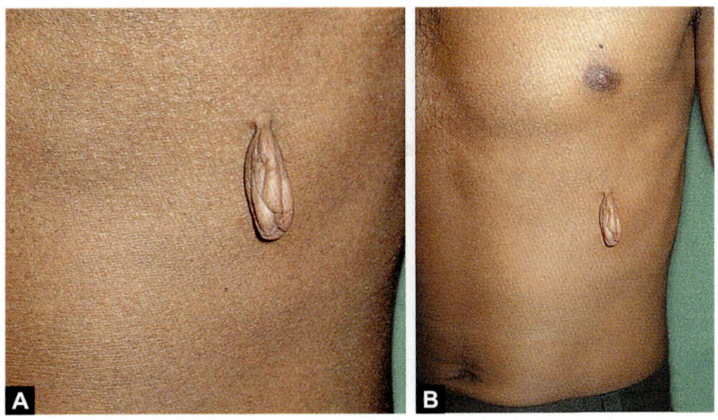

Figs. 9A and B: An anatomical landmark in the frame: (A) Skin tag where the location is not recognizable; (B) The same image with a different view, nipples included in the frame.

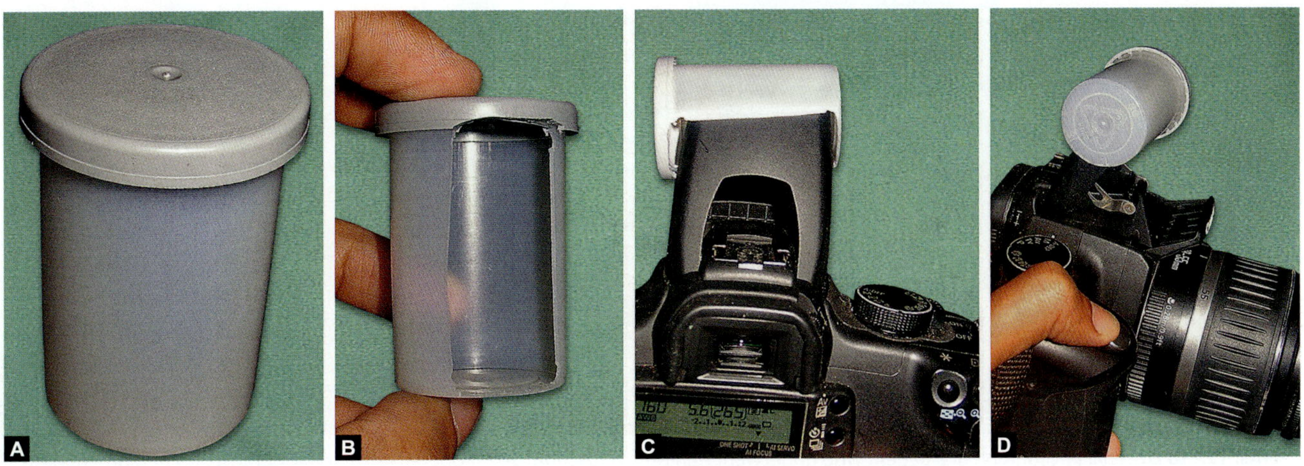

Figs. 10A to D: Diffuser made easy: (A) Film case; (B) An area carved out to accommodate the onboard flash of the SLR; (C) Diffuser affixed; (D) Side view.

TIFF is considered to be the default industry standard for a cross platform image format that can be opened by virtually all graphics applications. The disadvantage of TIFF files vis-à-vis JPEG is a bigger file size.

Other standard formats used for storage include the Photoshop document (PSD), portable network graphics (PNG), Windows bitmap (BMP) and graphics interchange format (GIF). Another file format used in the context of SLRs is that of the RAW files. This refers to the minimally processed data file from the image sensor of a digital camera. The advantage obviously is the markedly higher quality of image as virtually no pixels are lost, as a corollary, the disadvantage is that the files are two to six times larger than JPEG files.

Most digital cameras save the images by default at a resolution of 72 dpi. This can be converted to 300 dpi with the use of basic photo-editing software. The resolution of 300 dpi is the general standard for most journal submissions.

In situations, where the number of images submitted per article has restrictions from the publisher's end, multiple images can be made to one file using the collage tool available in most of the editing software. This can be very useful in taking pictures of serial events or follow-up of cases **(Figs. 12A to D)**.

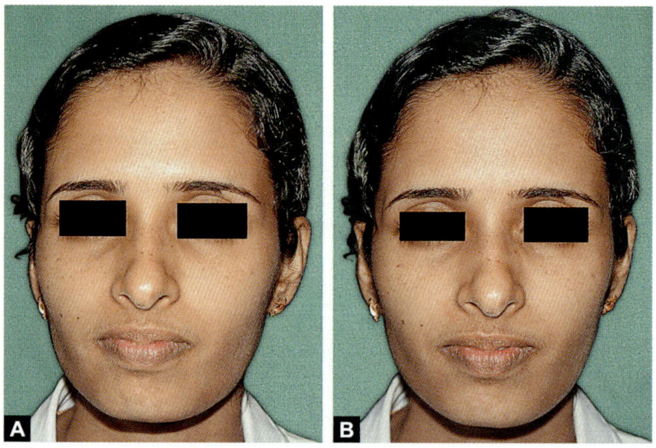

Figs. 11A and B: Diffuser effect to minimize the impact of flash on aesthetic photography of the face: (A) Without diffuser; (B) With diffuser.

Compact flash cards or SD cards are now available with large capacities. It is always better to carry at least two memory cards for your camera, so that you can change the cards easily in case one of the cards gets full. With the cost of hard disks also dramatically going down over the last few years, it has become very easy to store entire image inventories in single spaces. Other than the primary hard disk it is always advisable to keep at least two backup copies of all the images on an additional site like an external hard disk (a range of which are available at very reasonable prices). It always makes sense to delete images that are blurred or found unfit after the shoot as they are unlikely to be useful at a later date and will unnecessarily clutter up the hard disk space.

Cataloging of Clinical Images

This is probably one of the most important and crucial aspects of photography in clinical practice. The method adapted to catalog picture in the system (computer) has to be simple enough to be operated by more than one person without creating any confusion to others who use the system without tampering the files. The image files should also be easily retrievable. This has got extreme importance, especially when assistants or technicians are entrusted the job to shoot and transfer images to the archives especially in big clinics and departments.

It is always advisable to catalog all saved images (or containing folders), tagging them with the patient's name, hospital number, date and even the provisional diagnosis if possible. Meticulous cataloging may seem cumbersome at the beginning but makes future retrieval of imaging very convenient.[15] There are a large number of free and paid software available in the market. Apart from the readymade ones available off the shelf, they could also be tailored to one's

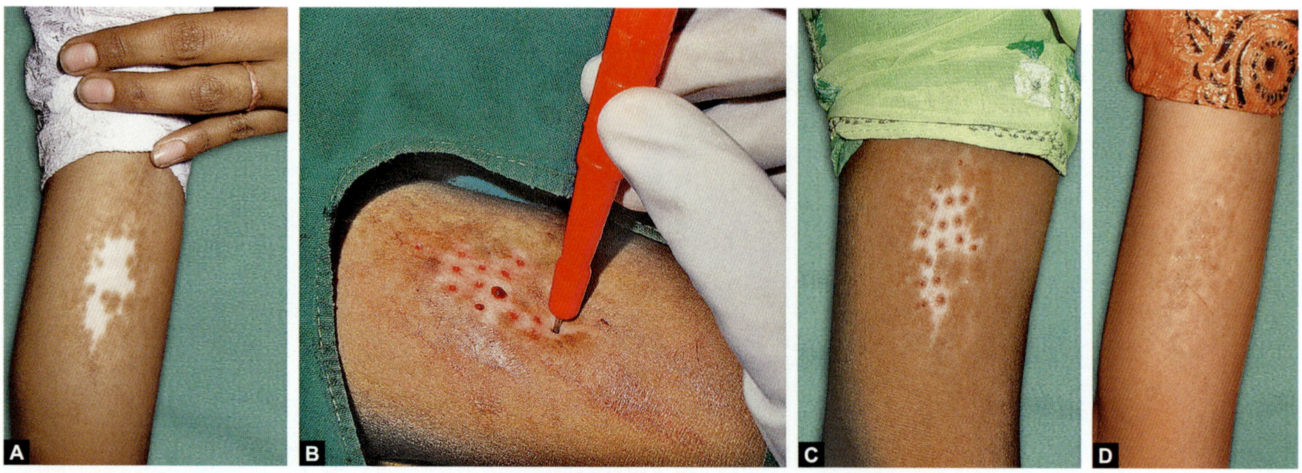

Figs. 12A to D: Serial photograph of a patient who underwent minipunch grafting: (A) Preoperative; (B) Intraoperative; (C) Repigmentation; (D) Complete repigmentation.

requirements for photo cataloging if it so warrants. Of the freely downloadable ones available online, the most popular ones are the Picasa™ (available on *www.picasa.google.com*) and Irfanview™ (available on *http://www.irfanview.com/*). Both of them have an excellent track record of free updates. They also help us to transmit multiple images via email or post online on blogs or websites.

One methodology which the authors follow is to create multiple folders with diagnosis as folder names, and the files are renamed as quoted below. Those pictures without a diagnosis can be grouped under "miscellaneous" or similar titles.

"Name_patient ID_year_month_date_serial number" (The patient ID can be replaced by the patient's mobile number in case the clinic does not have electronic data storage). This helps in sequential arrangement of the files irrespective of the date taken or modified in the folder, when "sort by name" is chosen in "right click" within the folder under consideration. Once done this way, freeware like Picasa™ can be easily used to arrange and retrieve images very quickly from the stored files on the disk by simple search of any of the words or even numbers on the file name as mentioned earlier. It is mandatory *not to use* short forms for year and month (e.g., patient id_2021_01_08_sl.no is the correct form and not patient id_21_1_8_sl.no) to avoid technical confusion on the operating system of the computer.[11]

It would be a good idea to add all relevant images into the same folder, as subfolders as they are obtained (such as dermoscopy, histopathology and radiology images). It would also be ideal to take a photography of the patient notes, hospital id card (or a screenshot, if electronic medical record is functional), to remember the pertinent points in the history on revists. Although the local legal restrictions regarding this should be clearly ascertained.

ETHICS AND LEGAL ISSUES

Consent, Image-tampering and Copyright

It is absolutely essential to have the patient sign an informed consent form for any clinical photography. The consent form should be clear and specific in terms of: (1) confidentiality of the data, (2) protection of patient identity as much as possible but may be revealed inadvertently in some situations, and (3) dissemination of the photographs through print or electronic and social media. This is important because the patient might sometime give consent for photography but not for dissemination of the images for publication or presentation. It should be understood that it is well within the patient's rights to do so and that any violation of the same from the clinician's side may invite punitive measures. The ease of editing digital images opens way to the possibility of unethical manipulation of photographs, especially to demonstrate dramatic cosmetic improvement with specific procedures.[16-18] The question of *"how much is too much?"* of editing a clinical image has been discussed in detail by many authors in the past. Generally, image editing falls under two categories:

1. Improving the visual quality of the image in terms of adjusting sharpness, color, brightness and contrast or editing the image so as to ensure focus on a particular area of interest. For example, changing the background of a patient's photograph to remove distracting elements in the background or cropping the image for the same purpose.
2. Editing the image so as to alter the actual lesion or lesions. For example, airbrushing a postchemical peel picture to give the impression of a better cosmetic result or editing a vitiligo patch to fake response to treatment.

It is obvious that both the above mentioned types of image editing must be avoided as far as possible. Even though the first type of editing mentioned is acceptable to a certain degree, the second category is essentially fraudulent and unethical. Unfortunately, it is often difficult to really say for sure if an image is altered or not. Hence, the onus is on the medical practitioner to avoid unethical tampering with digital images for any purpose. In cases where only minor editing has been done, it is advised that the original nonedited image be retained by the practitioner for legal purposes.[17] Ensure that patient's confidentiality is strictly maintained with regards to the photographs. Use the image for publication, peer-communications and presentations only if clear patient's consent is present. As far as possible, mask the patient's identity even if you have the patient's consent **(Figs. 13A and B)**.

It also makes sense to add a watermark to your photographs in certain instances, like sharing on online discussion forums to convey a message of the ownership and copyrights of the clinical picture. There are a number of software available for doing this, one of the most commonly used is Adobe Photoshop®, where you can simply use the "type" tool and place a text string over the photo after duplicating the initial layer. The watermark can be further edited to increase or decrease its translucency by using "blending option". There are plenty of online tutorials available to understand the creation of more complex watermarks.

PHOTOGRAPHY USING SMARTPHONES

Smartphones with good cameras have come in a big way in the recent times and they are now an indispensable part of a clinician in view of the versatility and ease of use.[19] However certain points have to be kept in mind while opting for photography using smart phones vis-a-vis digital camera. All the basics elements of clinical photography apply the same way to smartphone based photography too. If judiciously used in spite of some limitations, the smartphone camera does most of the job that a clinician needs for his routine photography.

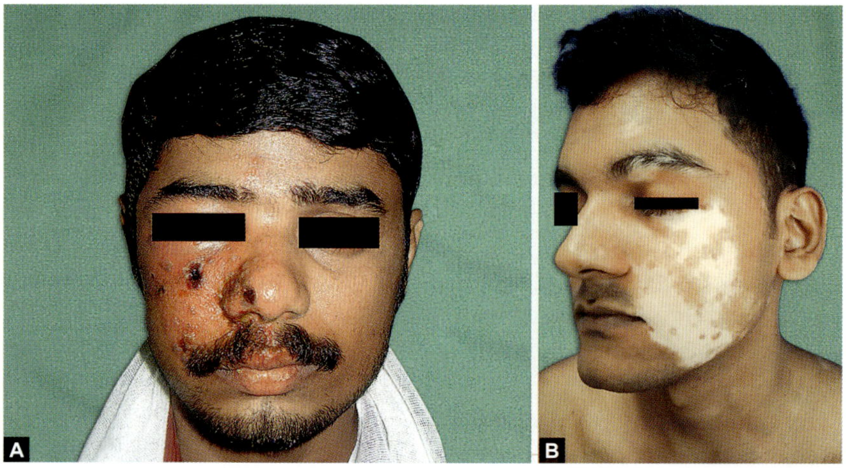

Figs. 13A and B: Masking the patient's identity with a black color on the eyes.

Advantages of smartphone camera over conventional camera

- The smartphone camera is easy-to-use and more operator friendly
- Larger preview and immediate retake are possible
- Battery life is not a major compromise
- Lighting is not a major concern as most of the smartphones have good flash light enough to cover the area of interest
- Video mode is a very good feature especially when procedures are to be recorded for presentation or documentation.

Disadvantages

- The sensor size of the smartphone and that of camera are not the same and pixel elements are different, e.g., a 3MP digital camera can give very good print quality images than a 3MP smartphone camera.
- The display is deceptive and images that look ultra-clear in the smartphone screen may not be that much appealing when viewed on the computer monitor or in print
- The natural tones of the skin may be altered and in situations where the original tone has to be retained smartphone camera may fall short
- Standardization is very difficult and that becomes a limitation in serial photography especially in research where consistent imaging is necessary.

Photography in the Context of Teledermatology

Images captured by ubiquitous smart phones are becoming an integral part of patient initiated teledermatology consultation.[20-22] A study by Mars et al., identified important legal and ethical issues related to the use of self-taken photographs for telemedicine.[22] Besides issues such as consent, data security/confidentiality and patient satisfaction, one important factor that needs adequate attention, is the quality of the image itself (which in turn is directly linked to the strength of diagnosis, especially in a specialty like Dermatology for obvious reasons).[3] In the era of the COVID-19 pandemic, telemedicine is gaining further momentum.[23,24] In the context of dermatology, patient-initiated teledermatology is bound to increase and for dermatologists [service provider] the image quality is vital for effective diagnosis and best line of management.

The common problems, we have seen, in terms of quality of patient self-images include the lesions being out of focus and poor lighting/exposure (and improper use of flash). We would suggest the use of a simple, easy to understand checklist for patients to follow, which will improve diagnostic concordance for patient initiated teledermatology. A point by point checklist as summarized here can serve as a guide document to be sent to any patient seeking a tele-consult with images shot on a smart phone camera.

1. Shoot multiple images—you are more likely to get an image which the dermatologist will find useful for proper assessment and diagnosis (Help them to help you).
2. Shoot images with and without the flash in a clear background without any distractions.
3. Choose a well-lit room to shoot the images.
4. Keep the other settings of the smartphone camera to "default", but for close-up images, use the "macro" mode (symbolized by the "flower" icon).
5. For elevated lesions, shoot the images from different angles. This will give the dermatologist a better perspective of your illness.
6. For lesions distributed over a larger area (or in condition like hair loss), take a video covering the entire area, followed by a close-up shot preferably without flash.
7. Stabilize the affected area and the camera as best as possible to avoid blur incurred due to phone camera shake.
8. Generally photographs shot by another person work better than a selfie. Elderly people, if not familiar with the settings of the smartphone camera, may engage anyone in the family to help them out.

9. Review all photographs and videos before you send, especially if sensitive areas are involved or the identity is revealed as in tattoo (You can black out the eyes, in case of facial images and can watermark images, as long as it does not interfere with viewing the skin lesion itself).
10. For those who might find it difficult or uncomfortable to type in the history on the phone, and for all patients who are comfortable with a video consult, patient history can be conveyed using live videos (ideal) or as an alternative pre-recorded voice messages may be used.

At the dermatologists' end, *it is important to make the patient understand that teledermatology does not substitute for a proper dermatological examination*, especially because of the limitation of not being able to feel the lesions and use additional examination tools such as a hand lens, dermoscope or Wood lamp and also the inability to perform bedside tests to confirm the diagnosis-like smears or biopsies. Teledermatology does help as an instrument of triage to advise an immediate actual examination by a dermatologist in cases that need immediate point of care. It is also important to understand and convey the prevalent local/regional rules related to ethical and legal aspects of online consultation (teledermatology). If the images are not clear, insist upon a clearer image as per the checklist stated above. When giving suggestions, always start with a disclaimer mentioned at the beginning of this paragraph. Err of on the side of caution, especially in the context of conditions like suspected malignancy, scenarios which can lead to serious complications and conditions which can be infectious to other patients.

Finally, while we realize that a more detailed guide with embedded images might help in improving patient self-photos, we are of the opinion that it might seem more daunting for the average patient. The checklist we mention covers the most common issues faced in patient initiated consults and effectively addressing them will help in improving quality of images and corresponding strength of diagnosis and quality of care.

GENERAL RECOMMENDATIONS: SUMMARY AND TIPS[2]

1. Always take the patient's consent before photographing, especially if the shots are taken during a surgical procedure when the patient may not be aware of the same. A written informed consent would be the best, and is a must if one is planning to use the photograph for publications.
2. Include the patient's hospital card, tag or number in all or at least one of the images of a series so as to enable easy identification later.
3. Always try to take before and after photographs in the same settings with respect to patient's positioning, background, lighting and camera settings.
4. Use autofocus as often as possible, use manual controls only if you are well versed with them.
5. Select the "macro" mode for close-up shots.
6. Use flash as often as possible when the available lighting is poor, but avoid getting too close to the lesion as the overexposure may wipe out the details.
7. For very close shots, oblique views may be preferred.
8. Try to add some shots of areas you expect to be involved in some of your differential diagnoses, but are apparently free of involvement in the particular case (e.g., nails in psoriasis).
9. Eliminate distractions from the background. Try to take all photographs with a plain nonreflective blue or green background.
10. Make sure while photographing very young children and infants that the subject is comfortable and not anxious. Children tend to be fidgety, and getting blurred images because of the movement is a common problem. A small toy or a pen would come in handy, although this should not be included in the frame. If your camera has an option of adjusting shutter speeds, a fast shutter speed would be useful in shooting photographs of children. Also, use the flash as often as possible. Avoid pointing the flash directly into the eyes, especially in the case of infants.
11. Many procedures may require videographic documentation. While it is best to have a dedicated video camera for the same, most point-and-shoot cameras, as well as some of the newer DSLRs, now come equipped with good quality video. You can, therefore, combine still images with videos using the same equipment. Better lighting is a necessity for taking the videos.

FUTURE

Many aesthetic procedures require multiple images taken from different angles to assess the treatment plan, as well as to evaluate postprocedure results. Some studies have attempted to combine images taken from different angles to get a three-dimensional (3-D) view of the area of interest (especially facial contours). The software available for such 3-D photography is cumbersome, with a steep learning curve at present, but might well be commonly used in the future.[25,26] Digital image analysis is now being increasingly used to assess clinical improvement, especially in chronic ulcers.[26,27]

For pigmentary problems, reproducibility on different cameras and display devices is a problem. Haeghen et al. have proposed a simple calibration system to overcome this, using a computer algorithm that transforms digital images to the standard sRGB color space. It is based on a card with a number of color squares with known colorimetric properties that is included in the image, thereby removing any ambiguity about the color information in the image.[28] Last but not the least, tamper proof images are a dream which may also come true in the near future.

In Photography: Remember the 3 Ds—Distance, Detail and Development.
- *Distance:* It should be appropriate to the problem. Not too far nor too close. Photographs of periocular CO_2 would not show well in a full face photograph and a facelift photograph would not show well if you could not see the full lower third of face and neck.
- *Detail:* Show the lumps, bumps, lines, creases, hills, and valleys. This is achieved by adjusting focus, change the lighting and change the angle.
- *Development:* Look at the photographs in the imaging program. What looks like a good photograph immediately after it is taken may actually be out of focus when seen on the full screen.

USEFUL WEBSITES AND LINKS

- http://en.wikipedia.org/wiki/Portal:Photography
- www.steves-digicams.com/hardware_reviews.html
- www.dpreview.com/reviews/

REFERENCES

1. MedScape. (2010). Digital photography. [online] Available from: http://emedicine.medscape.com/article/1131303-overview. [Last Accessed May, 2011].
2. Kaliyadan F, Manoj J, Venkitakrishnan S, Dharmaratnam AD. Basic digital photography in dermatology. Indian J Dermatol Venereol Leprol. 2008;74:532-6.
3. Şen Z, Kaya B, Serel S, Sağlam H, Can Z. Photographic standardization in esthetic surgery. Ankara Üniversitesi Tlp Fakültesi Mecmuasl. 2005;58:5-10.
4. Rogers BO. The first pre- and postoperative photographs of plastic and reconstructive surgery: contributions of Gurdon Buck (1807-1877). Aesthetic Plast Surg. 1991;15:19-33.
5. Kaliyadan F. Digital photography for patient counseling in dermatology—a study. J Eur Acad Dermatol Venereol. 2008; 22:1356-8.
6. HowStuffWorks. (2011). How digital cameras work. [online] Available from: http://electronics.howstuffworks.com/digital-camera.htm. [Last Accessed May, 2011].
7. Persichetti P, Simone P, Langella M, Marangi GF, Carusi C. Digital photography in plastic surgery: how to achieve reasonable standardization outside a photographic studio. Aesthetic Plast Surg. 2007;31:194-200.
8. Miot HA, Paixão MP, Paschoal FM. Basics of digital photography in dermatology. An Bras Dermatol. 2006;81:174-80.
9. Siegel DM. Resolution in digital imaging: enough already? Semin Cutan Med Surg. 2002;21:209-15.
10. Mutalik S. Digital clinical photography: practical tips. J Cutan Aesthet Surg. 2010;3:48-51.
11. Ashique KT, Kaliyadan F. Clinical photography for trichology practice: tips and tricks. Int J Trichology. 2011;3:7-13.
12. Nayler JR. Clinical photography: a guide for the clinician. J Postgrad Med. 2003;49:256-62.
13. DiBernardo BE, Adams RL, Krause J, Fiorillo MA, Gheradini G. Photographic standards in plastic surgery. Plast Reconstr Surg. 1998;102:559-68.
14. American Telemedicine Association. (1999) Dermatologic Photography. Available from: http://www.americantelemed.org/files/public/membergroups/teledermatology/telederm_Dermatologic Photography.pdf. [Last Accessed May, 2011].
15. Roach D. Imaging. In: Nouri K, Leal-Khouri S (Eds). Techniques in Dermatological Surgery, 1st edition. St. Louis, Missouri: Mosby Publishers; 2003. pp. 33-42.
16. Cutrone M, Grimalt R. The true and the false: pixel-byte syndrome. Pediatr Dermatol. 2001;18:523-6.
17. Scheinfeld N. Photographic images, digital imaging, dermatology, and the law. Arch Dermatol. 2004;140:473-6.
18. Suvarna SK, Ansary MA. Histopathology and the 'third great lie'. When is an image not a scientifically authentic image? Histopathology. 2001;39:441-6.
19. Ashique KT, Kaliyadan F, Aurangabadkar SJ. Clinical photography in dermatology using smartphones: an overview. Indian Dermatol Online J 2015;6:158-63.
20. Burns K. Digital photography and the medical selfie. J Participat Med. 2015 Feb 11; 7:e3.
21. Tan L, Hu W, Brooker R. Patient-initiated camera phone images in general practice: a qualitative study of illustrated narratives. Br J Gen Pract. 2014;64(622):e290-4.
22. Mars M, Morris C, Scott RE. Selfie Telemedicine - What Are the Legal and Regulatory Issues? Stud Health Technol Inform. 2018;254:53-62.
23. Greenhalgh T, Wherton J, Shaw S, Morrison C. Video consultations for covid-19. BMJ. 2020;368:998.
24. Smith AC, Thomas E, Snoswell CL, Haydon H, Mehrotra A, Clemensen J, et al. Telehealth for global emergencies: implications for coronavirus disease 2019 (COVID-19). J Telemed Telecare. 2020;26(5):309-313.
25. Lee S. Three-dimensional photography and its application to facial plastic surgery. Arch Facial Plast Surg. 2004;6:410-4.
26. Tollefson TT, Sykes JM. Computer imaging software for profile photograph analysis. Arch Facial Plast Surg. 2007;9:113-9.
27. Pressley ZM, Foster JK, Kolm P, Zhao L, Warren F, Weintraub W, et al. Digital image analysis: a reliable tool in the quantitative evaluation of cutaneous lesions and beyond. Arch Dermatol. 2007;143:1331-3.
28. Haeghen YV, Naeyaert JM. Consistent cutaneous imaging with commercial digital cameras. Arch Dermatol. 2006;142: 42-6.

CHAPTER 132

Teledermatology Consultation in Cutaneous and Aesthetic Surgery

Garehatty Rudrappa Kanthraj, Jayadev B Betkerur

KEY MESSAGES

- Dermatosurgery and aesthetic surgery has progressed exponentially. Developments in lasers and other techniques and their application to cutaneous and cosmetics needs is phenomenal.
- Teledermatology consultation (TC) is an effective, safe, and fast medium to reach one who is difficult to reach. Triage, diagnosis, counseling, and postsurgery follow-up care can be provided for the needy patients by virtual means.
- Advances in information technology, innovation in smart phones and various apps as made it convenient for dermatologists and patients to communicate.
- Recent outbreak of Coronavirus disease-2019 (COVID-19), a viral pandemic, has forced the global community for social distancing and enforcement of lockdown. This situation has motivated the dermatologist and patients to adopt TC as a medium to seek and provide patient care.
- A dermatologist has to select appropriate case and define the purpose for TC.
- Common indications of TC in cutaneous and aesthetic surgery are pre-procedure counseling, postsurgery/procedure follow-up care.
- Store-and-forward (SAF) teledermatology and mobile messenger applications (e.g., WhatsApp) are commonly used to perform capture, transfer, and store the clinical images.
- In an Indian scenario, SAF meets the technical requirement, is economical, and easy to practice. TC is followed after observing all conditions as in telemedicine guidelines prepared by the National Medical Council with due caution.

HISTORY OF TELEMEDICINE

The milestones in the developments of telemedicine and its transformation to teledermatology are summarized in **Table 1**. Teledermatology consultation (TC) is performed everywhere.[1-11] Teledermatology is a branch of dermatology involving application of electronics, communications, and information technology to transmit the information between the patient and dermatologist and vice versa for research and practice to cater dermatology care.[4,12]

Similar to radiology, dermatology is a visual specialty; availability of clinical and histopathological images for diagnosis makes it an ideal choice for TC.

TRANSFORMATION/REVOLUTION OF TELEDERMATOLOGY CONSULTATION

Images were captured by ordinary camera, scanned and sent through E-mail. Digitalization across the globe resulted in the transmission of images through E-mail/web and social media. Digital cameras transformed the art of TC. Images were easily transferred between the computers using the Internet. Advances in technology resulted in enhanced speed of the Internet. Transfer of images between mobile phones is made easy. Advent of android technology and mobile messenger applications has revolutionized the TC. Phases of transformation are illustrated in **Figure 1**.

The Need of Teledermatology Consultation in COVID-19 Setting

A TC is provided without exposing staff to viruses/infections in the times of contagious disease outbreaks such as COVID-19. TC can prevent the transmission of infectious diseases, reducing the risks to both healthcare workers and patients. COVID-19, a viral pandemic, is a well-suited scenario, in which dermatologists can evaluate and manage patients on a virtual platform.

TABLE 1: Milestones in telemedicine and its transformation to teledermatology.

Year	*Milestones*
1906	Wilhelm Einthoven discovered telecardiogram[1] successful transmitting electrocardiogram using a telephone network
The Nebraska Project,[2] USA in 1959	Videoconference for psychiatry patients was conducted between two hospitals within a distance of 150 km
1960 and 1970[3]	Research to monitor astronaut's heart rate, blood pressure, and electrocardiogram was conducted
1995	The term teledermatology was introduced by Perednia and Brown[4]
1997	Teledermatology in a nursing home setting was first demonstrated by Zelickson and Homan[5]

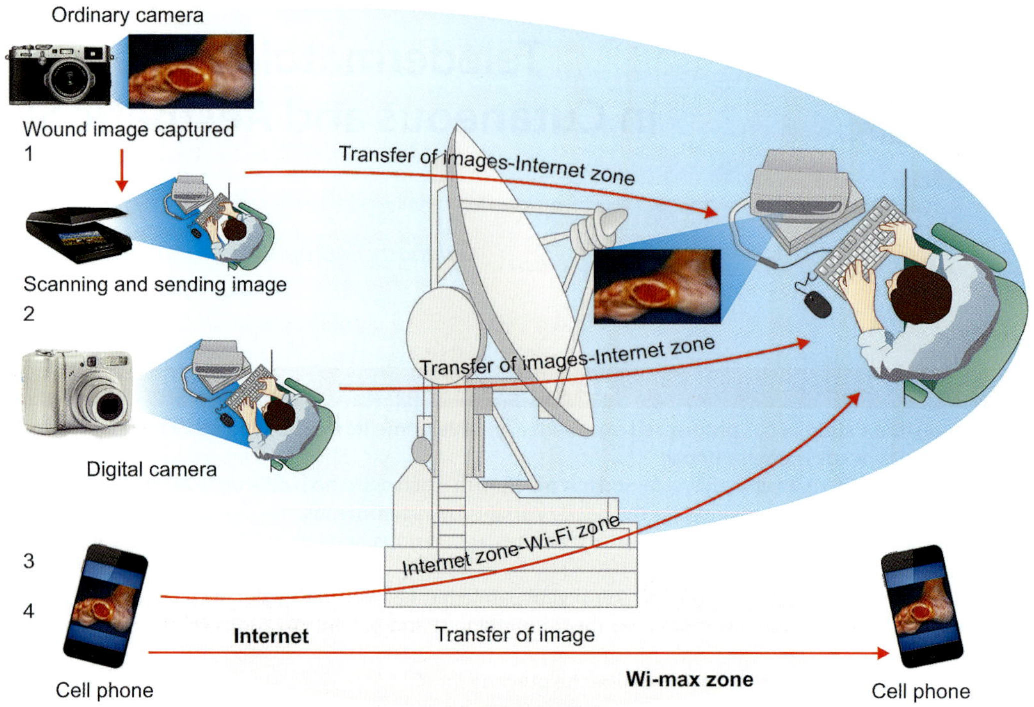

Fig. 1: Transformation/revolution of teledermatology consultation.

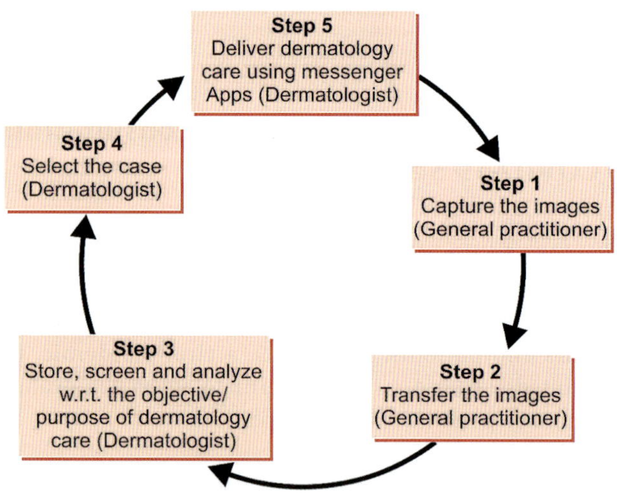

Fig. 2: The steps involved in teledermatology practice.
Source: Reproduced with permission from Kanthraj GR, Betkerur JB. Teledermatology practice in the COVID-19 pandemic. Int J Health Allied Sci. 2020;9(Suppl S1):3-10.

Process involved in teleconsultation: Capture, transfer, and storage of the data are the steps involved between the patient and the dermatologist. It is illustrated in **Figure 2**.

Aim

The aim of TC is to reach the one who is difficult to reach. For dermatology care in remote geographic regions or needy population in situations such as serious pandemics such as COVID-19 where the population is under lockdown, early care is provided and difficult to manage cases that are not neglected.

Scope and Purpose/Indications

The purposes of TC are: (1) diagnosis, (2) triage and counseling, (3) follow-up care, and (4) investigation. A dermatologist should identify the purpose before offering TC. **Table 2** identifies the parameter for the purpose of TC. The various indications[13-26] of TC are summarized in **Box 1**. The various indications[27] of TC in cutaneous and aesthetic surgery are summarized in **Table 3**.

Advantages of Teledermatology Consultation

A TC reduces multiple visits for follow-up care and benefits elderly, especially those coming from far-off places. It saves cost and time. Teledermatology was found to be cost-effective and reliable in reducing in-person visits saves time, and allows for the faster delivery of care. TC provides triage and reduces waiting time. Various advantages of TC are summarized in **Table 4**.

Teledermatology Consultation in Relation to Cutaneous and Aesthetic Surgery

Cases can be triaged for priority in-person examination and posted for investigational procedures such as skin biopsy. Presurgery/procedure counseling can be performed. Follow-up care is easy and feasible in wound care/postchemical peels and vitiligo surgeries. Studies[27] have revealed TC to be useful following post-laser procedures to provide follow-up care.

TABLE 2: Identifying the parameter for the purpose of teledermatology consultation.

	Diagnosis	*Triage/Counseling*	*Follow-up care*	*Investigation*
Parameter	History and case presents with characteristic morphology and distribution pattern	Prioritize the case for face-to-face examination and investigation or both	Chronic disease presents with longer duration with remission and exacerbation	Involves multiple patch test readings in allergic contact dermatitis

BOX 1: The various indications for teledermatology practice.

- *Diagnosis:* Cases that present with characteristic morphology with typical distribution pattern
- *Follow-up care:* Chronic cases that persists for a longer period and are characterized by remissions and exacerbations such as leg ulcer,[13-14] psoriasis,[15-17] leprosy[18] and acne vulgaris[19-20]
- *Investigation procedure:* Patch test in allergic contact dermatitis[21,22]
- Skin cancer triage[23-25]
- *Dermatosurgery/aesthetic care:* Triage and counseling[26]
- Second-opinion for difficult to manage cases
- *Education:* Train residents and update knowledge for dermatologists

TABLE 3: Purpose and indications for teledermatology practice in cutaneous and aesthetic surgery.

Purpose	*Indications*
Triage and counseling	• Cutaneous and aesthetic surgery • Prioritize for in-person examination
Follow-up care*	• Monitoring wound care • Post-cutaneous and aesthetic surgeries • Post-chemical peel Post-acne procedures • Post-skin graft for vitiligo/hair transplant procedures • Post-laser procedures

*Follow-up care is satisfactory provide teledermatology consultation, if it is not satisfactory to the patient call for in-person examination.

TABLE 4: Achievement/advantages in teledermatology consultation.

Diagnosis	Instant diagnosis and treatment for spotters
Triage and counseling	Prioritize for in-person examination
Follow-up care	• Minimizes/eliminates in-person follow-up visits • Saves cost and time
Investigation	• Minimize in-person follow-up visits • Saves cost and time • Convenient to capture the serial images of the upper back and compare

Teledermatology Consultation for Geriatric Care

Store-and-forward (SAF) teledermatology can improve diagnostic and therapeutic care for skin disease in the elderly who lack easy and/or direct access to dermatologists.[28]

Teledermatology Consultation for Pediatric Care

Accurate triage and diagnosis of childhood dermatology cases decrease travel and outpatient clinic visits and provide an avenue for ongoing support and education for primary care physicians.[29]

Teledermatology Consultation for Emergency Conditions[30-32]

The Skin Emergency Telemedicine Service has proved to be a successful, sustainable, and valuable addition to the specialist dermatology services provided across Queensland, Australia.[30] The use of teledermatology within the context of emergency-based care has gained high degree of patient acceptance and confidence.[31] New-generation mobile devices reduce the cost of video-conferencing, increase the adaptability of teledermatology, and decrease general practitioner time.[32]

Teledermatology Consultation and Diagnostic Agreement

Systematic reviews by Levin and Warshaw[33] showed that there is a good diagnostic agreement when comparing a teledermatology diagnosis and in-person clinical diagnosis or histopathology with traditional face-to-face consultations. The diagnosis concordance between dermatologists and teledermatologists increased from 92 to 98% [95% confidence interval (CI): 87–100%] when overlaps between differential diagnoses were considered as partial agreements. The diagnostic accuracy of SAF-TC was good and comparable to videoconference TC. Healthcare providers need to plan for appropriate utility of SAF-TC either alone or in combination with videoconference TC to implement and deliver teledermatology care in India.[34] Messenger Apps (e.g., WhatsApp) are a medium for TC.

Teledermatology Consultation and Patient Satisfaction

One of the main areas of patient dissatisfaction for both live video and SAF teledermatology revolved around the lack of follow-up.[35] Therefore, the referring physician plays a pivotal role in conveying the dermatologist's recommendations to the patient, which can have a major impact on patient satisfaction in the field.[36] Patient satisfaction will play an integral role in the further growth, development, and implementation of teledermatology. Direct consult may increase patient satisfaction.

Teledermatology Consultation and Cost-effectiveness

Teledermatology is cost-effective in terms of significantly decreasing the need for in-person visits.[37] Real-time

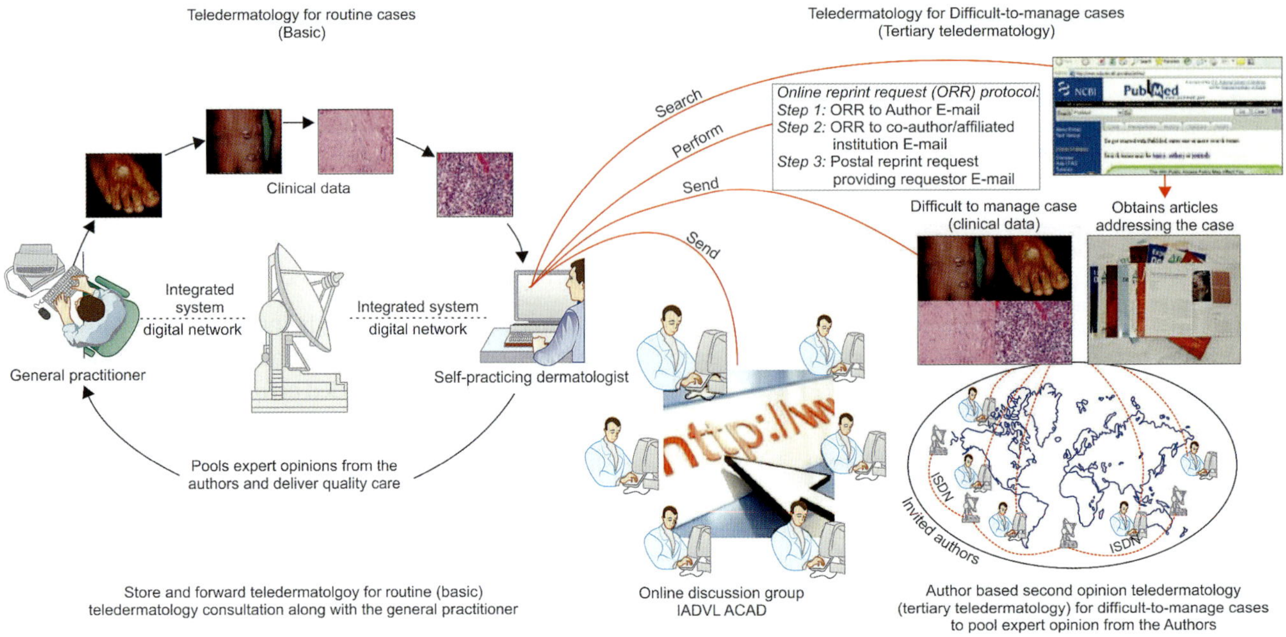

Fig. 3: Illustration of the organization and process involved in of teledermatology practice for a dermatologist to manage regular case (to use Store and forward teledermatology practice) as well as difficult-to-manage cases to use online discussion forum and deliver care.
Source: 1. Modified with permission from Kanthraj GR. Authors' willingness for second-opinion teledermatology in difficult-to-manage cases: An online survey. J Eur Acad Dermatol Venereol. 2010; 24:961-6.
2. Kanthraj GR. Newer insights in teledermatology practice. Indian J Dermatol Venereol Leprol. 2011;77:276-87.

interactive teledermatology has been found to be time-consuming than SAF dermatology.[38] Video call is mostly used to counsel the patient.

Organization of Teledermatology Consultation

The organization of TC for a self-practicing dermatologist is illustrated in **Figure 3**. It comprises a basic model SAF teledermatology where a dermatologist interacts with the patients directly for regular cases (spotters) along with online discussion forum to obtain a second opinion on management of difficult-to-manage cases.[12,39]

Prerequisites for Teledermatology Consultation

- A dermatologist should obtain a proper history
- Patient should be able to provide electronic images of the skin disorder. Landow[37] summarizes the requirements for a successful TP as: (1) image quality; (2) preselection of patients (tumoral conditions are the simplest; nevi evaluation should not exceed 1–2 lesions at most; multiple nevi patients should be excluded; and hair conditions are difficult to photograph and diagnose);[40] and (3) a dermoscopic image is a requirement for pigmented and tumoral lesions; and (4) good Internet connectivity is a necessity.

Patient consent to offer TC is needed. Indian Association of Dermatologists, Venereologists and Leprologists (IADVL) has developed both patient consent form and teledermatology consultation form.[41] The members of IADVL can freely download these forms and utilize for TC **(Annexures 1 and 2)**.

Store-and-Forward Teledermatology Consultation

Static images of clinical and histopathological data are accessed anytime and anywhere. They are transferred from a general practitioner to a specialist to deliver the management **(Fig. 4)**. Dermatology cases that can be diagnosed by face-to-face examinations (spotters) have a good diagnostic accuracy by SAF-TC. A diagnosis agreement of 89%[42] has been documented. SAF-TC is cheap and easy to set up and practice. It is the most common teledermatology tool as most of the cases are dealt and often regarded as a basic model for a TC.[12]

Videoconference

It is a live or interactive teledermatology. General practitioner, patient, and specialist interact with one another using live/motion images. Various feasibility studies[43,44] have confirmed good diagnostic accuracy when videoconference is compared to face-to-face consultation.

Hybrid Teledermatology

This is a combination of both videoconference and SAF-TC to overcome the shortcomings faced when either of them is used individually.[45]

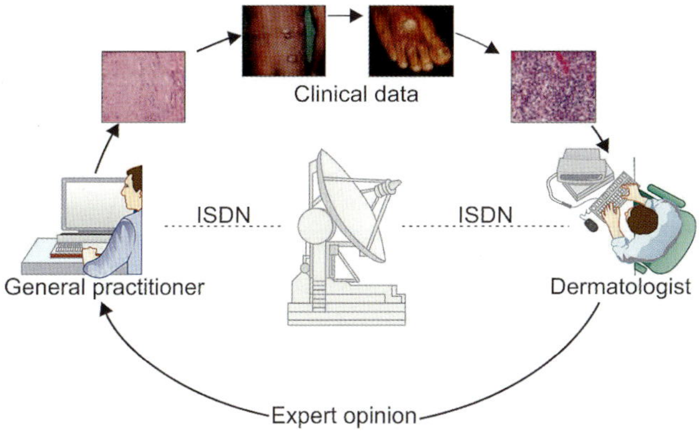

Fig. 4: The steps involved in store and forward teledermatology.

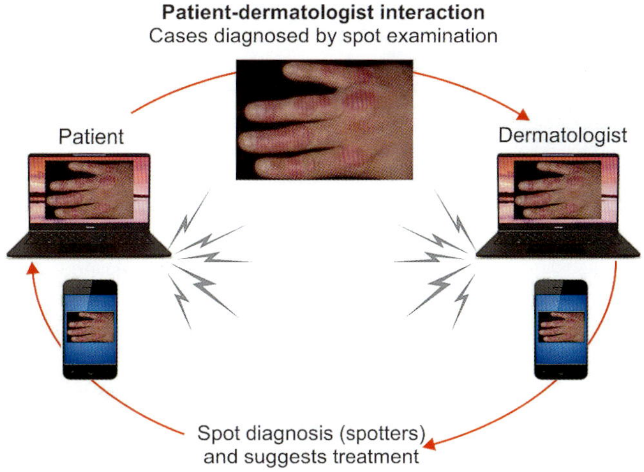

Fig. 5: The process of patient assisted teledermatology consultation.

Store-and-Forward Teledermatology versus Videoconference

Good patient and physician satisfaction along with good diagnostic accuracy is achieved in all. The simultaneous presence of a healthcare professional is required in videoconference and hybrid teledermatology and his or her presence may not be required in SAF-TC. SAF-TC is the most cost-effective and convenient compared to videoconference. The time taken for consultation is least for SAF-TC and more in videoconference and hybrid teledermatology. Motion images are used in videoconference, still images are used in SAF-TC, and both the types of images are used in hybrid teledermatology. A hybrid system with audio is no better than SAF-TC alone.[46] However, in the current context of mobile messenger apps—WhatsApp consultation, for example, still images and videos can be stored and forwarded. It has emerged as a widely used medium for TC.

Mobile Teledermatology

The term mobile teledermatology represents the transmission of images via mobile phones[47,48] as well as through personal digital assistants.[49] Motion and still images are transferred. Advanced network technology along with the mobile messenger Apps has revolutionized TC. Android technology and Apps find an application medium to capture, transfer, and store the images.[50,51]

Patient-assisted teledermatology practice is where in a teledermatology service patient or his attendants participate actively to send images and receive the treatment. **(Fig. 5)**.

Teledermatopathology

Transmission of histopathological images of the skin using information technology for expert opinion is called teledermatopathology.[52] Teledermatopathology is achieved by: (1) video-image (dynamic) analysis; (2) SAF (static); and (3) web-based virtual slide system.[53] A virtual slide system is a recently developed technology where a robotic microscope is used; any field of the specimen is selected for better digitalization at any required magnification at the discretion of the dermatopathologist.

Teledermoscopy[25,54-57]

Pigmented skin lesions and melanoma are analyzed based on the dermoscopic criteria[54] that depend on characteristic changes in the epidermis and dermis. Dermoscopy images[25] are transmitted for expert opinion using routine TC tools such as SAF-TC or tertiary TC for the second opinion. If these images are transferred using mobile technology, it is called mobile teledermoscopy. Pigmentary skin lesions are screened using mobile teledermoscopy.[55]

Online Discussion Forums[39, 58-62]

Difficult to manage cases is a challenge to the healthcare system. An online discussion forum is formed with a group of dermatologists who share constructive suggestions[58-60] for a submitted case. Feasibility studies have confirmed 81% concordance with face-to-face consultation.[58] Members of academic societies such as the IADVL have formed an online discussion forum at ACAD_IADVL@googlegroups.com (an E-mail group) and participate in regular academic discussions **(Fig. 6)**. Telederm.org,[58] Rxderm,[59] Virtual Grand Rounds in Dermatology,[60] and Black Skin Dermatology Online[62] are the examples of online discussion forums. Experts may be unavailable for an instant case or dermatologists and allied research workers who might have carried out research involving an online discussion forum may not have registered at the site and at times consensus may not be reached for a case without these experts are the limitations of online discussion forum.

Author-based teledermatology[39] is one medium where expert opinion is pooled for a difficult to manage cases **(Fig. 6)**. It is a tertiary teledermatology consultation. Various process involved in second opinion teledermatology[39] is illustrated in **Figure 7**.

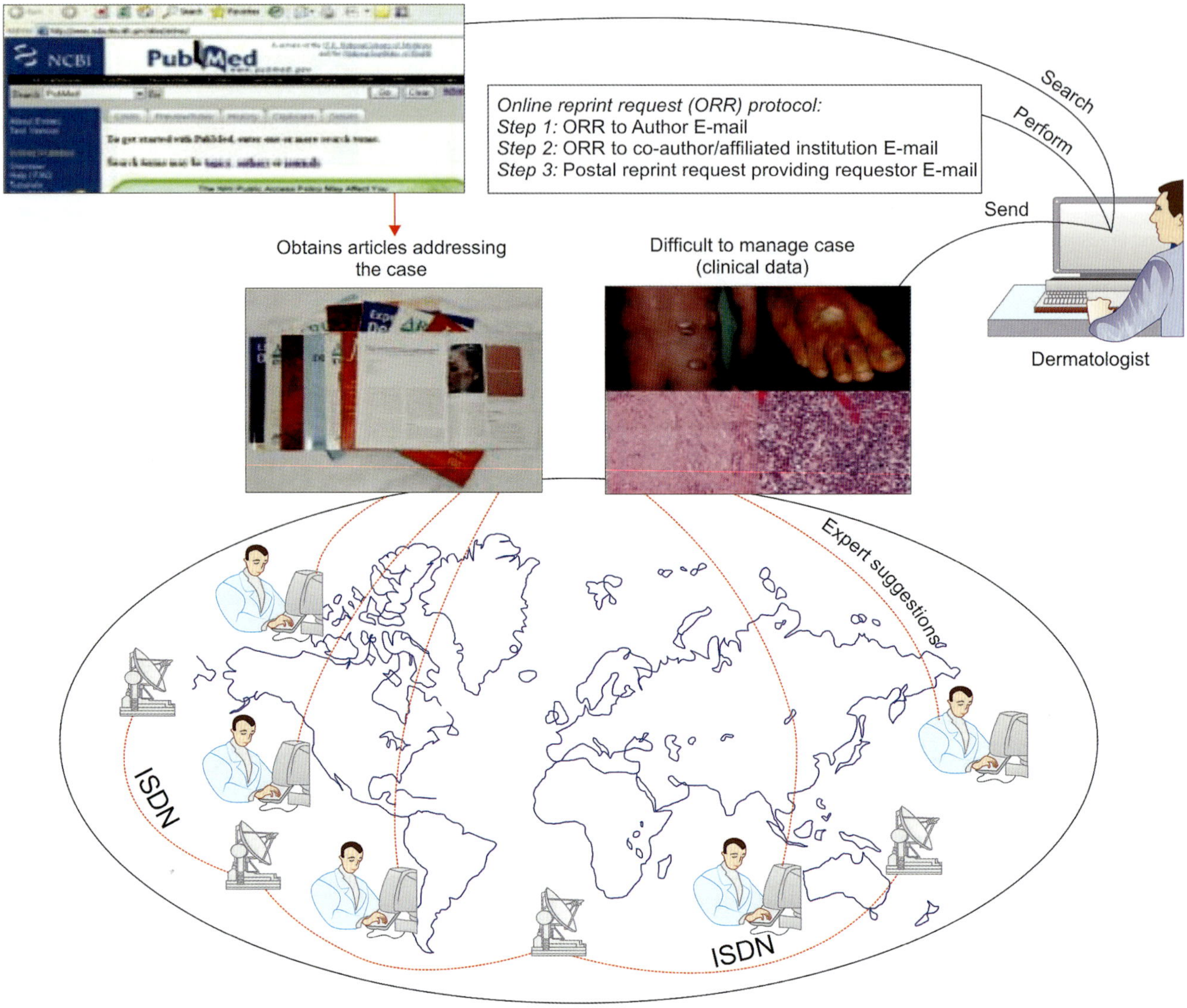

Fig. 6: The Concept of second opinion teledermatology.
Source: Reproduced with permission from Kanthraj GR. Authors' willingness for second-opinion teledermatology in difficult-to-manage cases: an online survey. J Eur Acad Dermatol Venereol. 2010;24:961-6.

The various teledermatology tools and healthcare professionals involved to provide dermatology care are summarized[63] in **Figure 8**.

Approach to a Case for Teledermatology Consultation

Selection of cases for teledermatology practice depends on three of the following criteria **(Fig. 9)**:

1. Type of clinical presentation and distribution pattern
2. Course of the disease
3. Purpose/objective of dermatology care

Parameter and purpose of teledermatology practice are summarized in **Table 2**.

Approach to a case for diagnosis: The salient steps are illustrated in **Figure 10**.

The Need for Teledermatology Consultation in Chronic Dermatology Conditions

The chronic disorders persists for a longer period, may be characterized by remissions and exacerbations. Therefore it requires multiple visits for follow-up care. In chronic disorders, TP has a significant impact in elderly and especially those coming from far-off places. It saves cost and time **(Fig. 11)**. If patient is not satisfied, then he will be called for in-person examination.

LIMITATIONS

Poor net connectivity, poor image quality, and lack of referral pro forma data can limit TC. All cases may not be feasible with an objective of diagnosis in TC. The cases that are not diagnosed by instant/spot examination are summarized

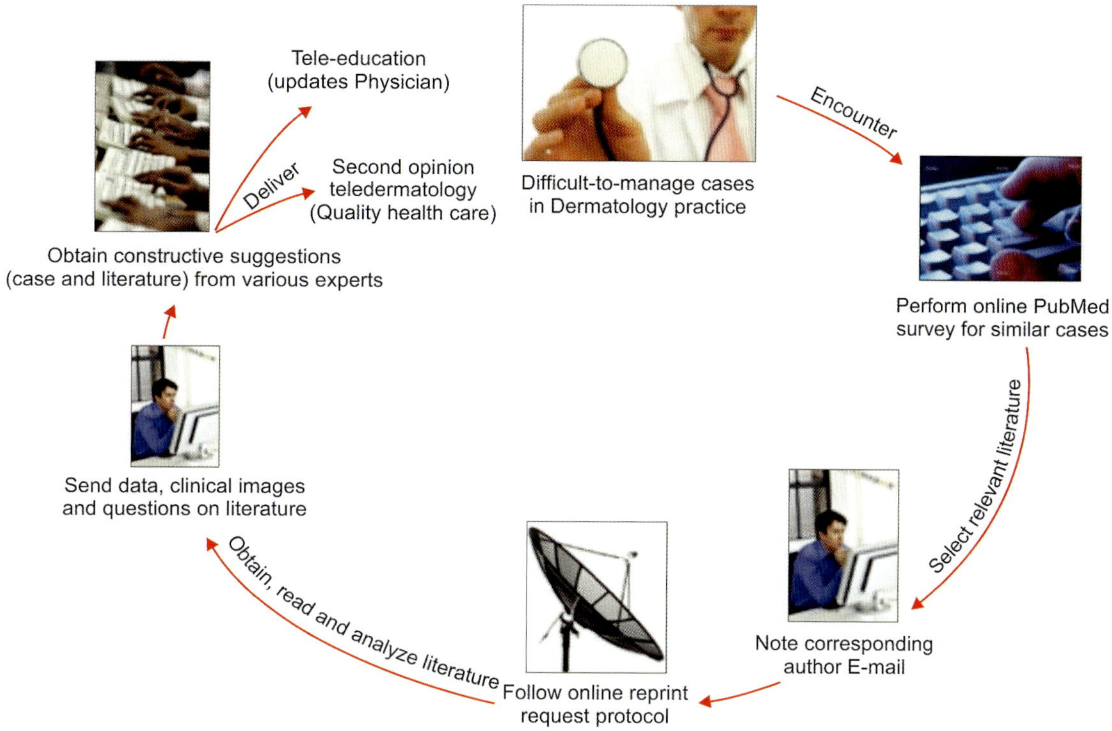

Fig. 7: The process involved in second opinion teledermatology.
Source: Reproduced with permission from Kanthraj GR. Authors' willingness for second-opinion teledermatology in difficult-to-manage cases: an online survey. J Eur Acad Dermatol Venereol. 2010;24:961-6.

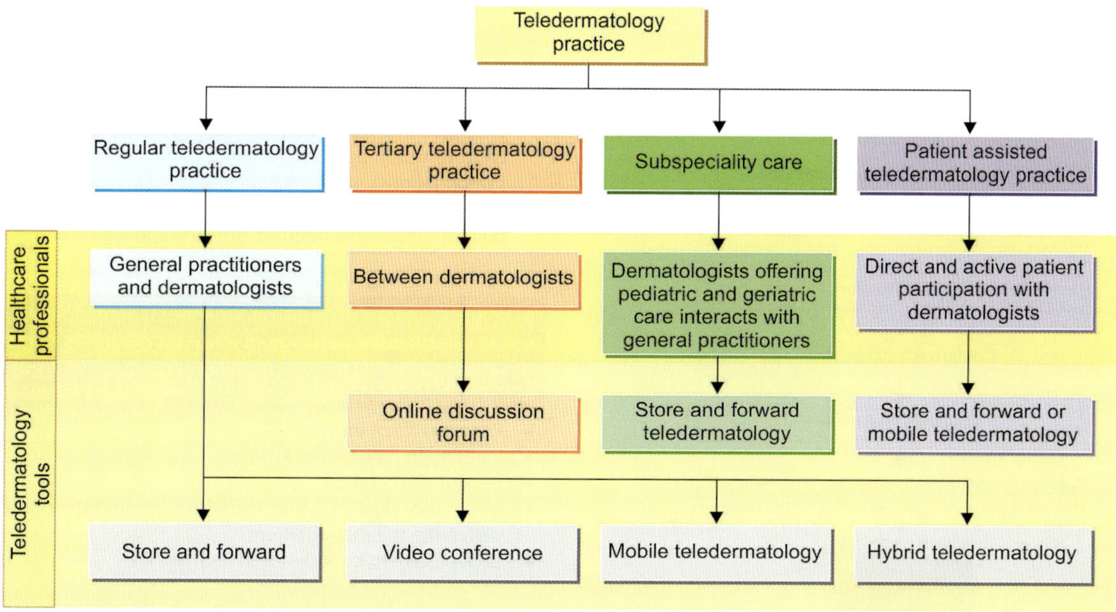

Fig. 8: The various teledermatology tools used for patient care.
Source: Reproduced with permission from Kanthraj GR. Patient-assisted teledermatology practice: what is it? When, where, and how it is applied? Indian J Dermatol Venereol Leprol. 2015;81:136-43.

in **Box 2**. The various technical situations a dermatologist may choose not to offer teledermatology consultation is summarized in **Box 3**.

The requirements for real-time videoconferencing (synchronous encounters) and SAF teledermatology have been specified by the American Telemedicine Association.[64] Monitors for viewing images shall have a minimum of 1024 × 768 pixel resolution, minimum contrast ratio of 500:1, minimum luminance of 250 cd/m^2, and minimum dot pitch of 0.19.[63]

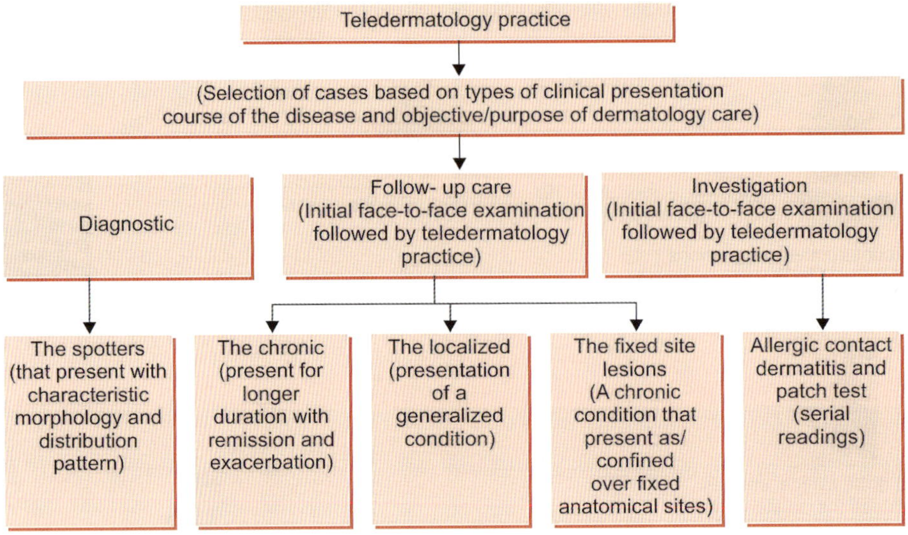

Fig. 9: The criteria for teledermatology consultation.

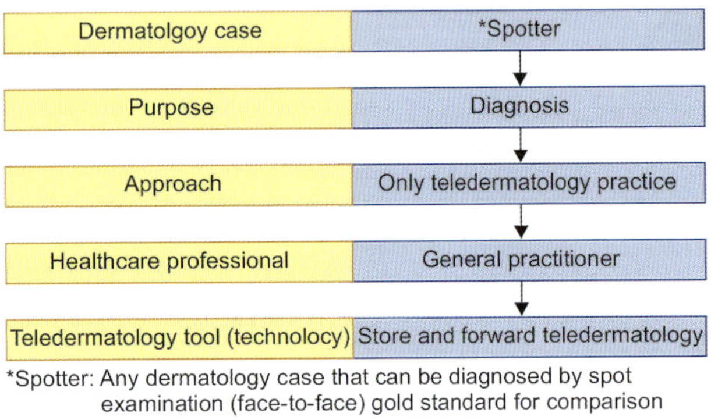

Fig. 10: The steps to approach a case for diagnosis purpose.

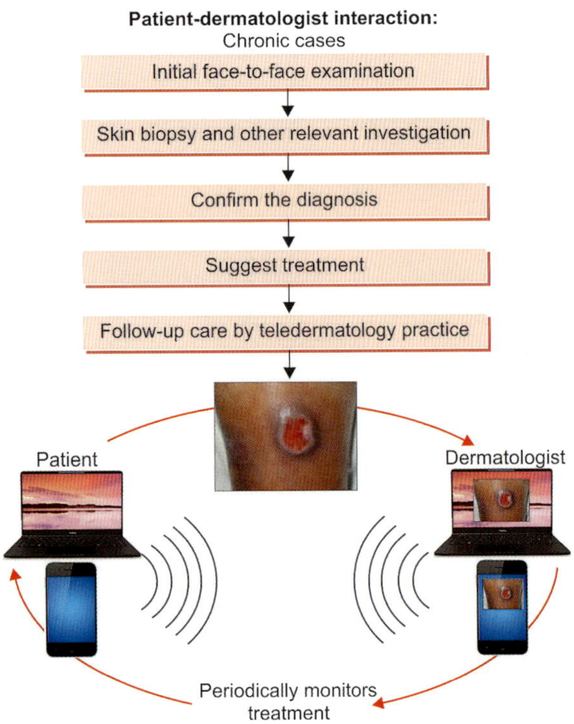

Fig. 11: The steps to approach a chronic case for follow-up care.

BOX 2: The various clinical situations a dermatologist may choose not to offer teledermatology practice for diagnosis purpose. In these situations, initial face-to-face examination needs to be performed followed by teledermatology practice and deliver follow-up care.

- Nonspecific presentation
- Varied morphology
- Requires palpation, e.g., skin tumors
- Multiorgan involvement, e.g., Stevens–Johnson syndrome/toxic epidermo necrolysis
- *Rare diseases:* Syndromes/genodermatoses (apart from skin examination palpation for multisystem involvement may be needed)
- Diseases that requires criteria to diagnose, e.g., atopic dermatitis, systemic lupus erythematosus and Behçet's disease
- Symptomatic presentation, e.g., generalized itching, burning excessive sweating/hyperhidrosis (without any obvious lesions to capture the image and requires evaluation of the symptom(s) by investigations)
- Represent a clinical entity due to various causes, e.g., erythroderma, palmoplantar keratoderma, urticaria and leg ulcer

BOX 3: The various technology situations a dermatologist may choose not to offer teledermatology practice for diagnosis purpose. In these situations, initial face-to-face examination needs to be performed followed by teledermatology practice and deliver follow-up care.

- Poor quality of images
- Inability to palpate the lesions
- Lack of clinical data
- Misinterpretation while transferring the information or while delivering the management
- Lack of patient confidence in technology

In India, till now, there was no legislation or guidelines on the practice of telemedicine through video, phone, and Internet-based platforms (web/chat/Apps, etc.). Recently, the Board of Governors (BoGs) of the Medical Council of India (MCI) along with NITI Aayog have prepared the guidelines for telemedical practice.[65] The detailed guidelines about the role of patient, healthcare provider, and technology platform are highlighted.[65] Each patient will be identified by a unique and universal patient identifier so that one central patient information record can be assimilated, comprehensive medical databases can be built, or if the patient wants, he/she can move across multiple providers without losing data. The same principles apply irrespective of the mode (video, audio, and text) used for a telemedicine consultation.[65]

Guidelines for Technology Platforms Enabling Telemedicine Prepared by the Board of Governors of Medical Council of India along with NITI Aayog[65]

This specifically covers those technology platforms which work across a network of Registered Medical Practitioners (RMPs) and enable patients to consult with RMPs through the platform.

1. Technology platforms (mobile Apps, websites, etc.) providing telemedicine services to consumers shall be obligated to ensure that the consumers are consulting with RMP duly registered with National Medical Councils (NMCs) or respective state medical council and comply with relevant provisions.
2. Technology platforms shall conduct their due diligence before listing any RMP on its online portal. Platform must provide the name, qualification, registration number, and contact details of every RMP listed on the platform.
3. In the event some noncompliance is noted, the technology platform shall be required to report the same to BoGs, in supersession to the MCI who may take appropriate action.
4. Technology platforms based on artificial intelligence/machine learning are not allowed to counsel the patients or prescribe any medicines to a patient. Only a RMP is entitled to counsel or prescribe and has to directly communicate with the patient in this regard. While new technologies such as artificial intelligence, Internet of things, and advanced data science-based decision support systems could assist and support a RMP on patient evaluation, diagnosis, or management, the final prescription or counseling has to be directly delivered by the RMP.
5. Technology platform must ensure that there is a proper mechanism in place to address any queries or grievances that the end-customer may have.
6. In case any specific technology platform is found in violation, BoG, MCI, may designate the technology platform as blacklisted, and no RMP may then use that platform to provide telemedicine.

TELEDERMATOLOGY AND LAW

There is no definite legislation addressing the TP. One cannot take shelter on the pretext of teledermatology consultation. A medicolegal principle of traditional consultation applies to TC.[66,67] All prescriptions need to be signed duly by a RMP as per the Drugs and Cosmetic Rules 1945. The physician is responsible for the issues related to security, privacy, and confidentiality of patient data. The American Telemedicine Association Guidelines[64] recommend that each healthcare provider and patient should have a unique identifier and the images are stored confidentially in secured database. Encryption for storage of patient data and for transmitting medical information should be inbuilt.

MEDICAL ETHICS, DATA PRIVACY, AND CONFIDENTIALITY[65]

Principles of medical ethics including professional norms for protecting patient privacy and confidentiality as per the Indian Medical Council (IMC) Act shall be binding and must be upheld and practiced. RMP would be required to fully abide by the IMC.

Professional conduct, Etiquette, and Ethics (Regulations), 2002, and with the relevant provisions of the IT Act, data protection and privacy laws or any applicable rules notified from time to time for protecting patient privacy and confidentiality and regarding the handling and transfer of such personal information regarding the patient.[68] This shall be binding and must be upheld and practiced.

Registered Medical Practitioners will not be held responsible for breach of confidentiality, if there is a reasonable evidence to believe that patient's privacy and confidentiality has been compromised by a technology breach or by a person other than RMP. The RMPs should ensure that reasonable degree of care is undertaken during hiring such services.

TELEDERMATOLOGY AND EDUCATION[40,69-71]

Teledermatology consultation plays a vital role in education. Resident training, exchange of knowledge and opinion between different dermatologists, and learning of dermatological diseases from different parts of the world are the roles of tele-education.[69]

WhatsApp groups make it possible for dermatologists[69] and other specialties to discuss various dermatological diseases and their appropriate management. It is one of the easiest media to exchange knowledge and experience on a one-on-one basis. It is considered to be one of the safest instant messaging media because of encryption technology.[69] Dermatology residents feel more confident at handling various disorders with additional TC learning.[70] TC can reduce the residents' empathetic nature toward patients and reduce the patient–physician relationship and loss of integral approach rather than focusing on single lesions.[70,71]

TELEDERMATOLOGY AND REIMBURSEMENT

Reimbursement policies for teledermatology services are rather new and vary significantly from place to place.

The Netherlands offers full reimbursement for services and has completely integrated teledermatology into its healthcare system.[72] However, in the United States, reimbursement remains a major challenge in telemedicine and continues to evolve in recent years. Currently, all States and the District of Columbia have defined telemedicine law, regulations, and Medicaid policies. In USA reimbursement varies from state to state.[73] Reimbursement for live-video teledermatology far exceeds the reimbursement for SAF teledermatology. Many states restrict reimbursement coverage to live video teledermatology only and exclude SAF teledermatology.[73]

In the Indian context as per the recent NMC guideline,[65] telemedicine consultations should be treated the same way as in-person consultations from a fee perspective: RMP may charge an appropriate fee for the telemedicine consultation provided.[65] An RMP should also give a receipt/invoice for the fee charged for providing telemedicine-based consultation.

A PROTOCOL FOR TELEDERMATOLOGY PRACTICE

According to a survey completed by Armstrong et al.,[74] most teledermatology programs have shifted from live interaction video to the SAF modality due to its technological flexibility and lower cost of service delivery. A dermatologist should screen the received clinical image from a general practitioner or self-acquired patient images[75,76] (selfies) and define the objective/purpose of dermatology care **(Fig. 2).** If the case suits for diagnostic purpose, a treatment is offered. A clinician should be aware of the dermatological conditions where not to offer consultation for diagnostic purpose **(Boxes 2 and 3)**. In these cases, a dermatologist can perform face-to-face examination, investigate, analyze the case, offer treatment, and provide follow-up care by TC[77] **(Fig. 2).**

CONCLUSION

In an Indian scenario, mobile teledermatology using messenger Apps, e.g., WhatsApp, can be used with good diagnostic accuracy and patient satisfaction. Mobile messenger Apps provide a dermatologist to capture and transfer the clinical images either in still (SAF) and motion (video) or both. Recently, the BoGs (MCI) have proposed guidelines for telemedical practice. In view of COVID-19 situation a dermatologist can perform TC and provide care by observing all conditions as in telemedicine guidelines prepared by NMC with due caution.

REFERENCES

1. Stanberry B. Telemedicine: barriers and opportunities in the 21st century. J Intern Med. 2000;247:615-28.
2. Zundel KM. Telemedicine: history, applications, and impact on librarianship. Bull Med Libr Assoc. 1996;84:71-9.
3. Cipolat C, Geiges M. The history of telemedicine. Curr Probl Dermatol. 2003;32:6-11.
4. Perednia DA, Brown NA. Teledermatology: one application of telemedicine. Bull Med Libr Assoc. 1995;83:42-7.
5. Zelickson BD, Homan L. Teledermatology in the nursing home. Arch Dermatol. 1997;133:171-4.
6. Sun A, Lanier R, Diven D. A review of the practices and results of the UTMB to South Pole teledermatology program over the past six years. Dermatol Online J. 2010;16:16.
7. Jemec GB, Heidenheim M, Dam TN, Vang E. Teledermatology on the Faroe Islands. Int J Dermatol. 2008;47:891-3.
8. Feroze K. Teledermatology in India: practical implications. Indian J Med Sci. 2008;62:208-14.
9. Vallejos QM, Quandt SA, Feldman SR, Fleischer AB Jr., Brooks T, Cabral G, et al. Teledermatology consultations provide specialty care for farmworkers in rural clinics. J Rural Health. 2009;25:198-202.
10. Kaddu S, Soyer HP, Gabler G, Kovarik C. The Africa teledermatology project: preliminary experience with a sub-Saharan teledermatology and e-learning program. J Am Acad Dermatol. 2009;61:155-7.
11. McManus J, Salinas J, Morton M, Lappan C, Poropatich R. Teleconsultation program for deployed soldiers and healthcare professionals in remote and austere environments. Prehosp Disaster Med. 2008;23:210-6.
12. Kanthraj GR. Newer insights in teledermatology practice. Indian J Dermatol Venereol Leprol. 2011;77:276-87.
13. Hofmann-Wellenhof R, Salmhofer W, Binder B, Okcu A, Kerl H, Soyer HP. Feasibility and acceptance of telemedicine for wound care in patients with chronic leg ulcers. J Telemed Telecare. 2006;12(Suppl 1):15-7.
14. Bianciardi Valassina MF, Bella S, Murgia F, Carestia A, Prosseda E. Telemedicine in pediatric wound care. Clin Ter. 2016;167: e21-3.
15. Koller S, Hofmann-Wellenhof R, Hayn D, Weger W, Kastner P, Schreier G, et al. Teledermatological monitoring of psoriasis patients on biologic therapy. Acta Derm Venereol. 2011;91: 680-5.
16. Frühauf J, Schwantzer G, Ambros-Rudolph CM, Weger W, Ahlgrimm-Siess V, Salmhofer W, et al. Pilot study using teledermatology to manage high-need patients with psoriasis. Arch Dermatol. 2010;146:200-1.
17. Armstrong AW, Parsi K, Schupp CW, Mease PJ, Duffin KC. Standardizing training for psoriasis measures: effectiveness of an online training video on Psoriasis Area and Severity Index assessment by physician and patient raters. JAMA Dermatol. 2013;149:577-82.
18. Trindade MA, Wen CL, Neto CF, Escuder MM, Andrade VL, Yamashitafuji TM, et al. Accuracy of store-and-forward diagnosis in leprosy. J Telemed Telecare. 2008;14:208-10.
19. Watson AJ, Bergman H, Williams CM, Kvedar JC. A randomized trial to evaluate the efficacy of online follow-up visits in the management of acne. Arch Dermatol. 2010;146:406-11.
20. Singer HM, Almazan T, Craft N, David CV, Eells S, Erfe C, et al. Using network oriented research assistant (NORA) technology to compare digital photographic with in-person assessment of acne vulgaris. JAMA Dermatol. 2018;154:188-90.
21. Ivens U, Serup J, O'goshi K. Allergy patch test reading from photographic images: disagreement on ICDRG grading but agreement on simplified tripartite reading. Skin Res Technol. 2007;13:110-3.
22. Grey KR, Hagen SL, Hylwa SA, Warshaw EM. Utility of store and forward teledermatology for skin patch test readings. Dermatitis. 2017;28:152-61.

23. Moreno-Ramírez D, Ferrándiz L. A 10-year history of teledermatology for skin cancer management. JAMA Dermatol. 2015;151:1289-90.
24. Massone C, Maak D, Hofmann-Wellenhof R, Soyer HP, Frühauf J. Teledermatology for skin cancer prevention: an experience on 690 Austrian patients. J Eur Acad Dermatol Venereol. 2014;28:1103-8.
25. Moreno-Ramirez D, Ferrandiz L, Nieto-Garcia A, Carrasco R, Moreno-Alvarez P, Galdeano R, et al. Store-and-forward teledermatology in skin cancer triage: experience and evaluation of 2009 teleconsultations. Arch Dermatol. 2007;143:479-84.
26. Kanthraj GR. Teledermatology: its role in dermatosurgery. J Cutan Aesthet Surg. 2008;1:68-74.
27. Chee SN, Lowe P, Lim A. Smartphone patient monitoring post-laser resurfacing. Australas J Dermatol. 2017;58(4):e216-e222.
28. Rubegni P, Nami N, Cevenini G, Poggiali S, Hofmann-Wellenhof R, Massone C, et al. Geriatric teledermatology: store-and-forward vs. face-to-face examination. J Eur Acad Dermatol Venereol. 2011;25:1334-9.
29. Fieleke DR, Edison K, Dyer JA. Pediatric teledermatology: a survey of current use. Pediatr Dermatol. 2008;25:158-62.
30. Finnane A, Siller G, Mujcic R, Soyer HP. The growth of a skin emergency teledermatology service from 2008 to 2014. Australas J Dermatol. 2016;57:14-8.
31. Jünger M, Arnold A, Lutze S. Teledermatology for emergency patient care: two-year experience with teledermatological emergency care. Hautarzt. 2019;70:324-8.
32. Duong TA, Cordoliani F, Julliard C, Bourrat E, Regnier S, de Pontual L, et al. Emergency department diagnosis and management of skin diseases with real-time teledermatologic expertise. JAMA Dermatol. 2014;150:743-7.
33. Levin YS, Warshaw EM. Teledermatology: a review of reliability and accuracy of diagnosis and management. Dermatol Clin. 2009;27:163-76.
34. Kanthraj GR. A longitudinal study of consistency in diagnostic accuracy of teledermatology tools. Indian J Dermatol Venereol Leprol. 2013;79:668-78.
35. Williams TL, Esmail A, May CR, Griffiths CE, Shaw NT, Fitzgerald D, et al. Patient satisfaction with teledermatology is related to perceived quality of life. Br J Dermatol. 2001;145: 911-7.
36. Whited JD. Teledermatology: current status and future directions. Am J Clin Dermatol. 2001;2:59-64.
37. Landow SM, Mateus A, Korgavkar K, Nightingale D, Weinstock MA. Teledermatology: key factors associated with reducing face-to-face dermatology visits. J Am Acad Dermatol. 2014;71:570-6.
38. Loane MA, Bloomer SE, Corbett R, Eedy DJ, Hicks N, Lotery HE, et al. A comparison of real-time and store-and-forward teledermatology: a cost-benefit study. Br J Dermatol. 2000;143:1241-7.
39. Kanthraj GR. Authors' willingness for second-opinion teledermatology in difficult-to-manage cases: an online survey. J Eur Acad Dermatol Venereol. 2010;24:961-6.
40. Pasquali P, Sonthalia S, Moreno-Ramirez D, Sharma P, Agrawal M, Gupta S, et al. Teledermatology and its current perspective. Indian Dermatol Online J. 2020; 11:12-20.
41. The Indian Association of Dermatologists, Venereologists and Leprologists. Teleconsultation consent form and case record form. [online] Available from: https://www.iadvl.org/announcements.php?announcementid=5ed3a6d89f2d292bc3618a54. [Last Accessed May, 2021].
42. High WA, Houston MS, Calobrisi SD, Drage LA, McEvoy MT. Assessment of the accuracy of low-cost store-and-forward teledermatology consultation. J Am Acad Dermatol. 2000;42:776-83.
43. Baba M, Seçkin D, Kapdaği S. A comparison of teledermatology using store-and-forward methodology alone, and in combination with Web camera videoconferencing. J Telemed Telecare. 2005;11:354-60.
44. Wootton R, Bloomer SE, Corbett R, Eedy DJ, Hicks N, Lotery HE, et al. Multicentre randomised control trial comparing real time teledermatology with conventional outpatient dermatological care: societal cost-benefit analysis. BMJ. 2000;320:1252-6.
45. Edison KE, Dyer JA. Teledermatology in Missouri and beyond. Mo Med. 2007;104:139-43.
46. Romero G, Sánchez P, García M, Cortina P, Vera E, Garrido JA. Randomized controlled trial comparing store-and-forward teledermatology alone and in combination with web-camera videoconferencing. Clin Exp Dermatol. 2010;35:311-7.
47. Braun RP, Vecchietti JL, Thomas L, Prins C, French LE, Gewirtzman AJ, et al. Telemedical wound care using a new generation of mobile telephones: a feasibility study. Arch Dermatol. 2005;141:254-8.
48. Massone C, Lozzi GP, Wurm E, Hofmann-Wellenhof R, Schoellnast R, Zalaudek I, et al. Cellular phones in clinical teledermatology. Arch Dermatol. 2005;141:1319-20.
49. Massone C, Lozzi GP, Wurm E, Hofmann-Wellenhof R, Schoellnast R, Zalaudek I, et al. Personal digital assistants in teledermatology. Br J Dermatol. 2006;154:801-2.
50. Pecina JL, Wyatt KD, Comfere NI, Bernard ME, North F. Uses of mobile device digital photography of dermatologic conditions in primary care. JMIR Mhealth Uhealth. 2017;5:e165.
51. Moreno-Ramírez D, Argenziano G. Teledermatology and mobile applications in the management of patients with skin lesions. Acta Derm Venereol. 2017;(Suppl 218):31-5.
52. Massone C, Soyer HP, Lozzi GP, Di Stefani A, Leinweber B, Gabler G, et al. Feasibility and diagnostic agreement in teledermatopathology using a virtual slide system. Hum Pathol. 2007;38:546-54.
53. Massone C, Brunasso AM, Campbell TM, Soyer HP. State-of-the-art of teledermatopathology. Am J Dermatopathol. 2008;30: 446-50.
54. Piccolo D, Smolle J, Argenziano G, Wolf IH, Braun R, Cerroni L, et al. Teledermoscopy – results of a multicentre study on 43 pigmented skin lesions. J Telemed Telecare. 2000;6:132-7.
55. Massone C, Hofmann-Wellenhof R, Ahlgrimm-Siess V, Gabler G, Ebner C, Soyer HP. Melanoma screening with cellular phones. PLoS One. 2007;2:e483.
56. Carli P, de Giorgi V, Chiarugi A, Nardini P, Weinstock MA, Crocetti E, et al. Addition of dermoscopy to conventional naked-eye examination in melanoma screening: a randomized study. J Am Acad Dermatol. 2004;50:683-9.
57. Dahlén Gyllencreutz J, Paoli J, Bjellerup M, Bucharbajeva Z, Gonzalez H, Nielsen K, et al. Diagnostic agreement and interobserver concordance with teledermoscopy referrals. J Eur Acad Dermatol Venereol. 2017;31:898-903.
58. Soyer HP, Hofmann-Wellenhof R, Massone C, Gabler G, Dong H, Ozdemir F, et al. telederm.org: freely available online consultations in dermatology. PLoS Med. 2005;2:e87.
59. Huntley AC, Smith JG. New communication between dermatologists in the age of the Internet. Semin Cutan Med Surg. 2002;21:202-4.

60. Lozzi GP, Soyer HP, Massone C, Micantonio T, Kraenke B, Fargnoli MC, et al. The additive value of second opinion teleconsulting in the management of patients with challenging inflammatory, neoplastic skin diseases: a best practice model in dermatology? J Eur Acad Dermatol Venereol. 2007;21:30-4.
61. Hu SW, Foong HB, Elpern DJ. Virtual grand rounds in dermatology: an 8-year experience in web-based teledermatology. Int J Dermatol. 2009;48:1313-9.
62. Ezzedine K, Amiel A, Vereecken P, Simonart T, Schietse B, Seymons K, et al. Black skin dermatology online, from the project to the website: a needed collaboration between North and South. J Eur Acad Dermatol Venereol. 2008;22:1193-9.
63. Kanthraj GR. Patient-assisted teledermatology practice: what is it? When, where, and how it is applied? Indian J Dermatol Venereol Leprol. 2015;81:136-43.
64. McKoy K, Antoniotti NM, Armstrong A, Bashshur R, Bernard J, Bernstein D, et al. Practice Guidelines for Teledermatology. Telemed J E Health. 2016;22:981-90.
65. Ministry of Health and Family Welfare. Telemedicine Telemedicine Practice Guidelines. Available from: http://www.mohfw.gov.in›pdf›. [Last Accessed May, 2021].
66. Eedy DJ, Wootton R. Teledermatology: a review. Br J Dermatol. 2001;144:696-707.
67. Thomas J, Kumar P. The scope of teledermatology in India. Indian Dermatol Online J. 2013;4:82-9.
68. International Lawyers Network. Lex Counsel Law Offices. Legal Position Concerning Telemedicine in India. [online] Available from: https://www.ilntoday.com/2014/02/legal-position-concerning-telemedicine-in-india/. [Last Accessed May, 2021].
69. Hogan SC, van Hees C, Asiedu KB, Fuller LC. WhatsApp platforms in tropical public health resource-poor settings. Int J Dermatol. 2019;58:228-30.
70. Yeung H, Sargen MR, Luk KM, Berry EG, Gurnee EA, Heuring E, et al. Teledermatology and teledermatopathology as educational tools for international dermatology: a virtual grand rounds pilot curriculum. Int J Dermatol. 2018;57:1358-62.
71. Williams CM, Kedar I, Smith L, Brandling-Bennett HA, Lugn N, Kvedar JC. Teledermatology education for internal medicine residents. J Am Acad Dermatol. 2005;52:1098-9.
72. Tensen E, van der Heijden JP, Jaspers MW, Witkamp L. Two decades of teledermatology: current status and integration in national healthcare systems. Curr Dermatol Rep. 2016;5:96-104.
73. Center for Connected Health Policy. (2016). National Telehealth Policy Resource Center. [online] Available from: http://www.cchpca. org/national-telehealth-policy-resource-center. [Last Accessed May, 2021].
74. Armstrong AW, Wu J, Kovarik CL. State of teledermatology program in the United States. J Am Acad Dermatol. 2012;67:939-44.
75. Hogan K, Cullan J, Patel V, Rajpara A, Aires D. Overcalling a teledermatology selfie: a new twist in a growing field. Dermatol Online J. 2015;21:13030.
76. Damanpour S, Srivastava D, Nijhawan RI. Self-acquired patient images: the promises and the pitfalls. Semin Cutan Med Surg. 2016;35:13-7.
77. Kanthraj GR, Betkerur JB. Teledermatology practice in the COVID-19 pandemic. Int J Health Allied Sci. 2020;9(Suppl S1):3-10.

ANNEXURE 1: Teledermatology Consultation Consent

Authorization and Consent to participate in Teledermatology Consultation

Patient Name:

Gender:

Date of Birth:

Address:

Patient ID number:

Provider name:

I have requested Dr. .... (Degree .. ; MCI/State registration number ......) for teleconsultation for my skin condition by my free will. This consultation is being conducted through Text message/Video consultation/Audio consultation. I have/will provide/d the doctor all necessary clinical history and my clinical images in the prescribed format. I understand that the diagnosis, inference of reports and treatment advised is based on the information provided by me. I agree to abide by the advice given to me explicitly. I will show all the medication advised, to the doctor before starting the medications and in case of doubt will enquire with the doctor immediately. I also understand that there could be some adverse effects due to medications advised or worsening of my skin disease. I undertake that I will inform the doctor without any delay in case of such an event verbally and with images. I undertake that this consultation is/was very much necessary for me and I have initiated the same, with my full knowledge about the limitation of the teleconsultation. I am willing to pay consultation charges, if any, by any mode of payment suggested by the doctor.

My signature below indicates:

I have read and understood the information given in this form.

I had a chance to ask questions about the consultation.

I have received satisfactory answers to my questions.

I understand my medical records and medical information is private and confidential to the extent permitted by law.

I understand that there are no guarantees about the results of the consultation.

I understand that all existing and applicable national & state medical laws regarding patient's access to medical information applies to this telemedicine consultation.

Signed: .... Date: ....

(Patient/legal guardian)
If other than patient: Indicate relationship

Signature of Witness: .... Date: ....

This consent form is part of your medical records. Preserve a copy of this consent form with you for your future reference.

Please Note: **The consent for consultation is already implied when the patient initiates teleconsultation by his/herself. This document may be aimed at familiarizing the patient to the details of teleconsultation. If consultation is by whatsApp for example, take a printout of this form and patient may be asked to sign and then send a scanned document/photograph.**

Source: Reproduced with permission from Indian Association of Dermatologists, Venereologists and Leprologists.

ANNEXURE 2: Teledermatology Consultation Proforma

Tele-dermatology Case Record form:

Please preserve this in your medical records

The consultation outcome depends on the details you provide below

You may be requested to provide further details and a repeat consultation could be required

Name: .... Date: ....

Age: .... Gender: .... Mobile No: ....

Address: ....

Patient identity proof used with details: ....

Weight: ....

Mode of communication: WhatsApp/video call/email/ Telephone ....

Quality of photographs shared: Able to interpret clearly/Need in person examination

---

First consultation/Follow-up consultation

Patient examined in person in the past 6 months- Yes/ No

Presenting for same complaint/New complaint

History & Examination:

Presenting complaints:

Type of Primary lesion: Macule/papule/patch/plaque/vesicle/nodule/erosion/ulcer/other

Sites affected:

BSA(%) Involved:

Duration:

Associated symptoms:

Comorbidities:

History of allergies (including to any medications) including nature, severity ofreaction, and treatment:

Family History of similar complaint:

Patient previous diagnosis, if any:

Medications: A- For present illness

B- Concomitant complaints

Response to previous medications: Very good/satisfactory/Poor/ None

Present consultation Diagnosis/Provisional Diagnosis:

Is it an emergency- Yes/ No

Investigations:

Date:

Drug Name with dosage	*Frequency*	*Instructions regarding intake*

Follow up Consultation on:

Contact in case of Emergency/Adverse effect at:

Doctor's seal/Digital Signature:

MCI Number

Clinic Address:

Contact details:

Patient Privacy Consent:

As per the legal requirements I, as patient or guardian of the patient, hereby authorize and give my consent to the clinic (please strike out if not relevant)

1. To store and process my health records
2. To contact me via email/SMS with respect to transactional messages relevant to me.
3. To use my anonymized records for research and analysis.

Date: .... Signature: ....

Disclaimer: This is an online consultation response. The patient has not been physically examined. The prescription or advice is based on the patient's description of the problem that is stated verbatim above"

Source: Reproduced with permission from Indian Association of Dermatologists, Venereologists and Leprologists.

CHAPTER 133 Social Media and Aesthetics

Rohit Batra, Nitika Nijhara

KEY MESSAGES

- Social media plays an imperative role in marketing for an aesthetic practice. However definite data on its impact is still lacking in literature.
- Exponential rise in the number of aesthetic procedures carried out per year was seen in 2014, hence necessitating the use of social media to reach out to the target population.
- Social media includes websites and applications that enable users to create and share content or to participate in social networking.
- Social media refers to the content you are sharing while social networking is the sharing of that content with the audience you intend to connect with.
- Facebook, Twitter and YouTube are the most popular media, followed by Instagram, Google plus and Pinterest.
- Based on demographics of users such as number, age, gender etc., an informed choice can be made about the social networks that are most beneficial to be used.
- Media posts should be 80% for patient benefit and 20% to boost your practice such as new technologies, offers, etc.
- Remember, consistency is the key!
- Reputation managers can be employed for search engine optimization (SEO) and managing feedbacks.
- Link all media to the motherboard—your website; it holds the most detailed facets about you and your practice.
- Social media use significantly predicts desire for cosmetic surgery.

INTRODUCTION

Pursuit of beauty and aesthetic enhancement is not a novel phenomenon but one which has stood the test of time and will never cease to survive. Practices to enhance beauty date back to the late 20th century were reflected in Cleopatra's milk baths and the use of *kohl* to darken and enhance the eyes. Further, the advent of lasers, light and energy-based devices and an array of injectables flooding the market, have enabled aesthetic practitioners to almost always triumphantly render a *look* their patient desires. Amidst this popularity and novel breakthroughs on a daily basis, how else will an aesthetician educate the patients on newer technologies, noteworthy information, patient experiences and personal expertise; if not for *social media*.

Social media plays an imperative role in marketing for an aesthetic practice. Numerous potential patients can be reached while sitting in the comfort of your home or office, doing the job equally or even more effectively than any advertising or public relation feat. Besides, a fortune can be saved and channeled toward better resources. However, social media trends go through constant changes, which can be quite challenging, time-consuming, and even agonizing for a practitioner. It helps to keep in mind that this strategy works in the long run in terms of cost-effectiveness, outreach, effort and outcome, however definite data on its impact is still lacking in literature.[1,2]

This chapter will help elucidate the salient features of social media per say and that of several popular social media; further expounding their role and application in daily aesthetic practice. Tips, tricks, and pearls to aid the novice and the veteran will be discussed.

AESTHETIC MEDICINE: AN INDIVIDUAL ENTITY

In the present times, beauty is equated with *youth and vitality* unlike the yesteryears where aging gracefully was an accepted notion. This explains the exponential rise in aesthetic procedures with patients chasing surgical and nonsurgical options to reverse signs of aging and restore signs of youth. 2014 was a milestone year; in this sense; as per the International Society of Aesthetic Plastic Surgery (ISAPS), over 20 million people underwent aesthetic procedures, surgical or minimally invasive, worldwide.[3] The even more interesting facet was that these people did not belong to a particular age or gender group; rather people from all ages, locations, genders and economic strata were surprisingly a part of this trend. Further, 2015 witnessed an increase of 1 million procedures over that of 2014,[4] reaffirming the notion that the popularity and demand of the field is multiplying and that all aestheticians need to reach out to the target population.

Nonetheless, while the constant societal pressure to look vivacious, attractive and radiant drives the desires of multiple individuals to invest in cosmetic procedures, to correct bothersome imperfections and modify and enhance their appearance, there has also been emerged a huge section of people with dedicated inclination toward cosmetic treatments in order to improve their career prospects and job competitiveness. Television and media too have had a remarkable effect on the average person's psyche and covet to look good. The ever-growing aspiration to better what they are, in terms of external outlook and confidence, makes every living human a potential patient for an aesthetic practitioner and this is where *social media* pertinently steps in.

UNRAVELING SOCIAL MEDIA

Google defines *social media* as *"websites and applications that enable users to create and share content or to participate in social networking."*

Customarily, *social media is a platform for brands to showcase themselves, whilst bringing their best foot forward.* It enables one to reach his target population, on a personal note, and highlight its most striking aspect. It is a simple tool with complex manipulations and high-yielding results **(Fig. 1)**.

Common Features of Every Social Media Platform

- *User account:* It is mandatory for users to create their own account in order to reach other users and share content.
- *Profile page:* Information about the individual user, such as profile photo, educational and family background can be shared through a personalized page where friends and family can connect and update.
- *News feed:* Users get updated on information in real-time via this option.
- *Notification:* On the user's permission, the portal notifies users about specific information as and when it occurs.

Social Media versus Social Networking[5]

Used interchangeably but are different entities by itself. Social media refer to the content you are actually sharing such as an image, PDF file, article, video or even a mere status update. On the other hand, social networking indicates the sharing of that content with the audience you intend to connect with.

Different Social Media

The social media pandemic encloses infinite options for use and application. In this scenario, opting for the accurate platforms, which will help establish and accentuate your media as well as market presence, is essential. All the options might not be used, but it will be helpful to set-up a profile each on the most popular ones of the bunch. At present, Facebook, YouTube and Twitter are the most accepted media sites, followed by the next wave, including Instagram, Google plus and Pinterest **(Fig. 2)**. The site most popularly used by your patients is the one you should invest most time and resources on. Whichever platforms you finally decide to choose, should be displayed on your website and blog to encourage visitors to share your content.

Further, it is also possible to exactly track where your clicks are coming from and analyze outcomes on a monthly basis. However, accept the fact that this is not an aesthetician's forte, in most cases, and hence do not hesitate to opt for analytics, who are proficient in continually measuring and analyzing the response and are umpteen in number and readily available as well.

Also, social networking and marketing includes discovery of new angles about old services and products on various

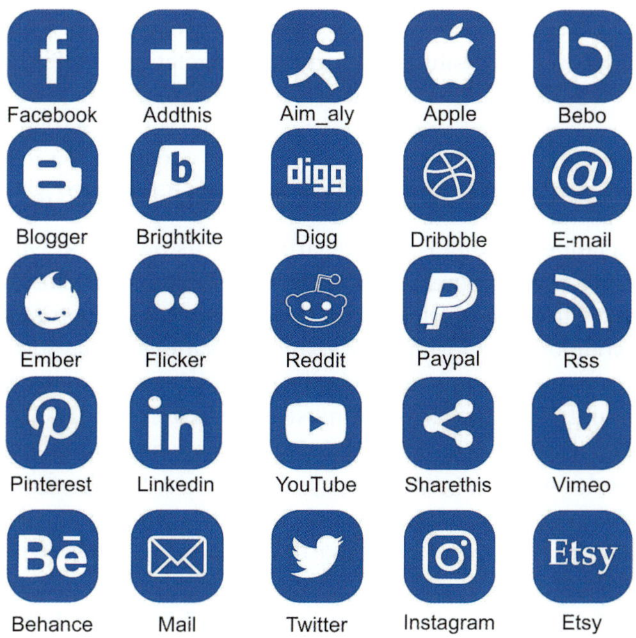

Facebook
Addthis
Aim_aly
Apple
Bebo
Blogger
Brightkite
Digg
Dribbble
E-mail
Ember
Flicker
Reddit
Paypal
Rss
Pinterest
Linkedin
YouTube
Sharethis
Vimeo
Behance
Mail
Twitter
Instagram
Etsy

Fig. 1: Social media icons.

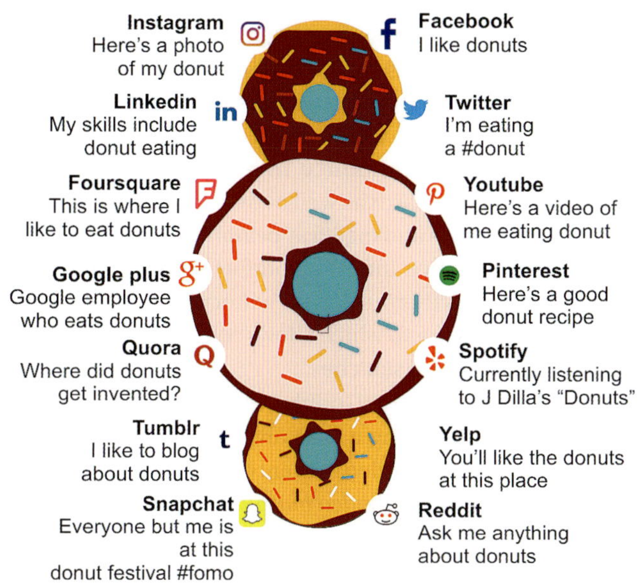

Instagram Here's a photo of my donut
Facebook I like donuts
Linkedin My skills include donut eating
Twitter I'm eating a #donut
Foursquare This is where I like to eat donuts
Youtube Here's a video of me eating donut
Google plus Google employee who eats donuts
Pinterest Here's a good donut recipe
Quora Where did donuts get invented?
Spotify Currently listening to J Dilla's "Donuts"
Tumblr I like to blog about donuts
Yelp You'll like the donuts at this place
Snapchat Everyone but me is at this donut festival #fomo
Reddit Ask me anything about donuts

Fig. 2: Popular social media.

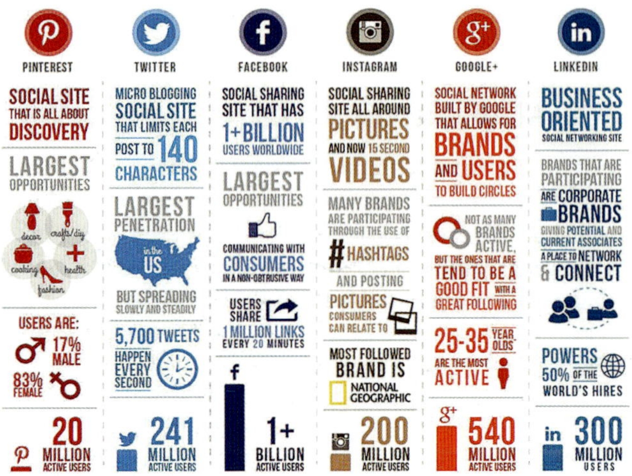

Fig. 3: Salient features of various social media.

platforms, on a continuous basis along with repeated posting of this information, each time in different aspects. The information remains valuable for only a short period after which newer ones replace it. Hiring somebody to maintain your social media image would be a good idea to save time and generate appropriate following.

A brief preview of the most famed media is explained below, from a cosmetologist's point of view **(Fig. 3)**.

- *Facebook:* Pioneer of the social media outburst, a highly connective site, used by solo practitioners, small clinical set-ups and global chain of clinics equally. Maintaining an up-to-date profile on Facebook can help engage patients on a personalized front, erect brand loyalty, boast the expertise—that of yourself, staff and set-up, and most essentially divert the buzz to your website. One of the most user-friendly medium, its apt for beginners. Further, it facilitates your control over your fan base and displayed content. A negative comment may be deleted and the commenter banned from ever posting again.
- *Twitter:* Gaining immense popularity, Twitter's highlights lie in its 140 or less character limit, making the portal precise and portable. It allows users to directly talk to a brand or interact with other users. It may be used by practitioners to announce milestones such as clinic anniversary or awards as well as offers, job openings, new branch openings and media appearances. Twitter will help take your practice into the comfort zone of your target population. Furthermore, it is Twitter which is responsible for the *hashtag* trend which allows content to surface more frequently on web searches.
- *YouTube:* Owned by Google, this platform has taken the trend of blogging a step ahead; when users started uploading original video content over YouTube and called it *vlogging—short for video blogging*. Visual, effective and highly educational and informative, it portrays a virtual picture of how the procedure, clinic, doctor, and result will be in the mind of the patient. Furthermore, actual procedures, doctor commentary, and patient experiences are depicted through this medium.
- *Pinterest:* Images and videos which impress the users are *pinned* to their pin board and displayed to their followers. Images are strong tools, which can be used through this application to engage consumers on your expertise, practice, treatments, products, and staff. Informative images and tips can be uploaded for the benefit of your patients to help them procure the information they need about a procedure and you may also deliver procedural postcare instructions and other treatment options through this portal. About 80% of Pinterest users are women and therefore content can be regulated to match the user population.
- *Instagram:* This platform is growing exponentially as it has comparably younger users at its recipient end and effectively uses photo sharing to employ patients. Great for sharing photos of your office, staff or beauty products and similar to Twitter, you may add relevant *has hashtags* to make your content searchable. It also allows modification and customization of photos which can then be shared with other Instagram, Twitter, or Facebook users.
- *Google+:* It facilitates the formation of *circles* amidst which important content can be shared from time to time. Unlike Pinterest, its major target population is male and hence *lunch time procedures* or treatments or disorders pertaining to males such as laser beard shaping, after shave care, pseudofolliculitis barbae, etc., can more often be discussed over this platform by inviting potential patients to join the circle. Presently, Google+ provides a platform to improve a practice's search results and hence it is imperative for any business clan to highlight themselves through it.
- *LinkedIn:* It is a business-centric networking tool which allows professional interactions and relation building on a broad platform. It makes it easier to connect to people, opportunities and to stay active in your professional circle.

HOW TO CHOOSE WHICH SOCIAL MEDIA?

Social networking is too gregarious for its own good while being highly time-consuming. It reflects your external image to the users and hence has to be accurate, pertinent, revolutionary, and impressive. Once the various media portals are known, an informed choice on which social networks should be invested in is of utmost importance. Demographics **(Fig. 4)** such as number of active monthly users, dominant gender and age group, occupation, etc., can help choose effectively. The value of a social network can be judged by analyzing how well it fits your target audience, content, and strategy.

Facebook is by far the largest network, followed by Twitter, YouTube, and Instagram. A short and simple list of three

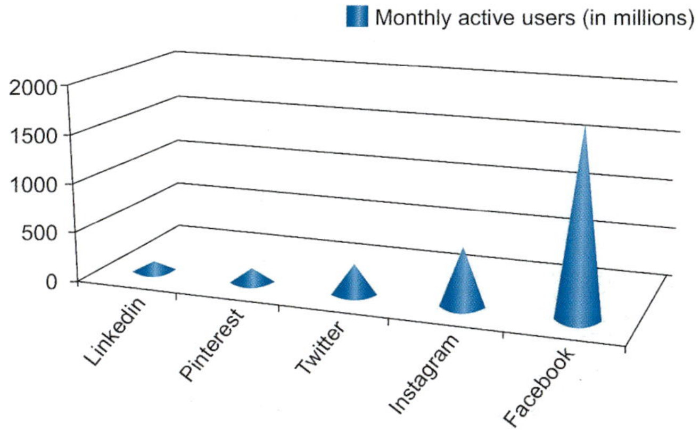

Fig. 4: Social networks infographics for January 2017, ranked by monthly active users: Facebook: 1,871 million, Instagram: 600 million, Twitter: 317 million, Pinterest: 150 million, and LinkedIn: 106 million.[6]

important questions to be considered before choosing a social network may aid in making a decision:

1. Is it appropriate for your content?
2. Are your potential patients primarily using this platform?
3. Is it feasible and appropriate for you in terms of time spent, ease of use and your practice?

SOCIAL MEDIA AND AESTHETICS

Aesthetic practice relies a lot on word of mouth and social media can give you just that. It is not just about a profile page or media account on display, but it is also about reaching out to your patients, educating them, sharing exciting news about your field, practice or yourself. Further, it aids in building relationships with patients, peers, media and vendors, and keeps them updated on what is happening in your practice. However, the most valuable use is that it behaves as a portal for booking consultations and scheduling appointments for procedures as well.

When it comes to marketing via social media platforms, it is important to be clear about the following aspects:

Q.1. How do you wish to portray yourself or your brand? For example, dermatology and aesthetic clinic, laser center, etc.

Q.2. Who are your patients? For example, affluent class, mediocre population, etc.

Q.3. What makes you stand out from your competitors? For example, technology, devices, cost-effectiveness, procedures, products, board certified and experienced doctors, visiting faculty, etc.

Q.4. What are the most effective ways to attract and encourage patients for treatments? For example, broadcasting deals, introductory offers, free consults, etc.

SOCIAL MEDIA IN YOUR PRACTICE

Social media is important to promote your practice but do not use it as a platform to sell products or services as patients do not like to be sold to. Follow the 80:20 rule, which means that 80% posts should be for the benefit of the patient such as skincare tips, nutritional advice, make-up recommendations, etc., while 20% may boost offers, promotions or new technologies and services **(Box 1)**.

Dealing with Media Challenges

Social media is a powerful tool. On one side where a positive review encourages patient engagement and referral, a negative one equally damages your image. Therefore, before indulging understand that social media is challenging, destructive as well as rewarding in equal proportions and requires proper management to maintain its integrity **(Table 1)**. The following points may aid practitioners in managing social media crisis.

Be Prompt to Respond

A negative review is fueled out of an unhappy experience, best consoled at the earliest. When faced with negative posts, respond swiftly, and reassure to consider the matter.

BOX 1: Benefits of social media.

How social media can benefit your aesthetic practice?
- Brings in leads
- Brand exposure
- Patient education
- Improves referral traffic
- Broadcasting of novel technologies and products
- Positive corporate public relation
- Facilitates appointments and feedbacks

TABLE 1: Pros and cons of social media in aesthetics.

Pros	*Cons*
• Most are easy to use • Can be operated via various devices such as laptops, smartphones, tablets, etc. • Allows public and private communication • Real-time communication is possible • Appeals to a wide audience • Enables sharing of knowledge and expertise • Text, images, and videos can be shared through various portals • Prompts direct business relationships • Some integrate with other programs, e.g., Google+ can be synchronized with Gmail and Google docs	• Time-consuming • Information overload may pose difficulty • Uploaded images need to be well-chosen and sharply designed to create appeal, requiring professional expertise • Regular posts are required to create outcomes, posing time and cost concerns • Privacy issues with few media like Facebook • Poor analysis of audience demographics may not yield results • Too many advertisements can deploy users • Handling too many portals can be agonizing and take you off-track • Negative feedbacks or Internet trolls can affect practice • Competitors can too follow your marketing and clinical updates

Later, get back to them with updates and reinstate that you are trying to be of genuine help. In no circumstances, remain silent and let it pass without being effectively tackled or resolved. If it was indeed your fault, tactfully own up, rarely even apologize. Privately, over personal chat or phone call, you may even offer complimentary services to make up for it. However, avoid doing so online as it may attract false complaints from people looking for free treatments.

Be Neutral: Do not Deny or Argue

Social media is open to all, so always beware of who are watching. Do not unduly deny allegations or argue with customers. Set an example and reflect your online image. An uncouth response is worse than no response!

Do not Delete Posts

Deleting posts do not make them vanish. People who have read it before deletion already have set an image and by deleting the comment you have unknowingly deemed yourself *guilty*. Constructive criticism should be taken as a milestone for improvisation. Furthermore, it is insulting to the patient to see his post deleted and may stir up more anger with spiteful consequences.

Push Down Negative Comments

Positive reviews can push down the negative ones. Several reputation management services are present online who aid in improving your rankings and appearance on web search results.

Overall, social media reputation management is tricky and an expert or *reputation manager* may be employed to deal with such situations. Trending nowadays are also *Internet trolls* who discordantly post over media platforms, webpages and blogs to generate negative responses. Reputation managers help deal with these as well. They work on the principle of *search engine optimization (SEO)*. It is the art of designing content that will score high on specific search results, such as your name or the name of your clinic. Their services empower you to control what shows when people search about you or your organization. They suppress negative results from appearing and even prevent future ones from surfacing at all while promoting web content that reflects you in a good light. By improvising search results, they help you stand out from the competition.

TIPS AND TRICKS OF PRACTICE

A Facebook or Linkedin page may sometimes be the only thing the patient knows about you and hence will be the deciding factor to whether he/she approaches you for a consult/treatment or not. Media provides a strong visual impact which will help customers to opt for you as a brand, so make the most of it. Consider the following practice ideas when designing and utilizing your social media image:

Consistency is the Key

Be the sunshine not the rain! A single burst of image upload or blogging will not do much good. Post consistently and innovatively to draw and keep the attention focused on you. Some patients may be considering a particular issue and will be drawn to you at the first post itself. However, majority of them will keep in mind for the future. When an issue arises, regular posts from your side will be an indirect reminder about all that you have to offer. Plan and formulate the content in advance and broadcast on daily or weekly basis. Remember, out of sight is truly out of mind!

Tell Stories

Being a medical practitioner, a personalized approach always adds ethic and trust to your image. Blog regularly about your patients and your experience while treating them. Post before and after pictures with their consent to further add value. This will illustrate how your practice has made a difference in people's lives and will reflect that what you do actually renders results and relief.

Modify according to the Media Platform

Every social media site has its own attributes. Work accordingly to deliver effective posts with maximum impact. For example, Twitter requires short message less than 140 words so use *hashtags* and be precise. In case of Instagram, post high quality pictures with good clarity.

Prioritize and Engage

Your time is valuable! The platform which is most popular with your patients is the one to be mainly focused on. The ability to schedule status updates in advance and use of tools that allow updates through multiple social media sites at once are the key features in this context. Further, you may engage with your patients through live chats, online consults, contests, and promotions to attract them. However, all these activities have to be for a *limited period of time* to retain its worth. Avoid free giveaways as a rule!

Create an Identity and Theme

All your stories, blogs, images and posts at the end should display your logo, location, punch line or website to familiarize your patients with your identity as a practice and finally direct them towards you. For example, *Cutis skin studio* adds its name along with its logo, punch line *skin experts with a difference* and website – www.cutis.in, at the end of all its posts.

Encourage patients to interact on your social media platforms.

Promote patients to post positive reviews, check in at the clinic, post a selfie with the clinic's background or like your posts as this is a personal experience shared with many and draws the most attention. This way others become curious about your practice and are compelled to check out your media page or website.

Link All Media to Your Website

It is of utmost important that all your media pages finally link to your motherboard, your website. Your website should be professionally designed and user-friendly to allow easy browsing. A single click under your post should be able to link them to your webpage which holds detailed information on your experience, services, practice and even new ventures. On your website, there should be provision for entering the patient's name and email id which may win them a free consult or product. This will increase your database and make way for future interaction with the patient.

SOCIAL MEDIA: ITS LINK WITH AESTHETICS AND DERMATOSURGERY

Social media is a blessing for doctors, giving them the option of interacting with patients in public forums. Frequent posts of treatments and procedures serve to teach prospective patients about the treatment options currently available. It is easier to check options available today at the click of a button. Since most patients refer to materials regarding aesthetic procedures online, one great way to find out areas of public interest is by using Google Trends® (GT). Marketing specialists in various fields employ GT to compile data regarding media-related trends in the interest of the customer.[7]

A study published by Hopkins et al. showed the rising popularity of the most "searched" terms on social media platforms such as Dermatologist, Botox, Juvederm, Radiesse, CoolSculpting® and Kybella. This was the combined data of both Instagram and Facebook users. The data suggested that the interest of people lay in minimally invasive procedures.[8]

With the rising trend in the use of social media, a large number of young people are getting cosmetic procedures done. Cosmetic surgery involves maintenance, renewal or improvement of one's physical appearance through surgical and non-surgical techniques.[9]

Alghonaim Y et al. also studied the impact of social media on aesthetic procedures among females in Saudi Arabia.

Out of the 1,449 participants, the majority felt that the cosmetic specialized accounts on social media were useful. The influence of social media upon participants was observed to be 68%. However, 31.9% felt there was no influence of social media. The most influential application was found to be Instagram. Snapchat and Twitter were considered to be equally popular. Half of the participants routinely applied Snapchat filters and 42% decided to undergo facial changes after applying these filters.

Patients browse to get the newest aesthetic treatments from social media influencers such as YouTube stars, Facebook-based gurus, Instagram celebrities and other online personalities having thousands of followers.[10]

In a study by Arab K et al., it shows that those who were influenced by cosmetic advertisements usually had relations or friends who have also undergone cosmetic treatments. Approximately one-third of those who reported being influenced by the advertisements followed plastic surgeons on social media. This was because of the choice of procedural techniques and the illustrations of the procedures from a medical point of view.[11]

Optimal strategies involving social media are considered a "moving target". Such strategies are likely to become even more important in the future.

Some popular ones are before and after photos, success stories, and patient testimonials.

Non-surgical procedures like Hyaluronic acid fillers used in lip injections, CoolSculpting®, which is a fat-cell freezing procedure, and nonsurgical nose jobs, in which a temporary filler such as hyaluronic acid is injected into the nose to subtly change the shape, have shown 20% more interest since 2015.

Open communication and personal sharing of experiences through tools like a "wall post" on Facebook and messaging on Twitter have become a rage. Many people choose to share their aesthetic experience through photos and videos uploaded via smartphones, tablets, and other devices which can instantly post a message on Twitter or load content onto their Facebook pages for others to see.

Even though the social networking outlets, such as Facebook and Twitter, may be replaced by others, but it appears that social media is here to stay.[12]

A study published in the May 2013 issue of Plastic and Reconstructive Surgery based on survey results showed the following trends:

- 50% of the cosmetic surgeons used social media regularly to connect with their patients.
- Facebook was the primary social media tool for surgeons followed by Linkedin, Twitter and YouTube.
- Social media use was considered to be a professional necessity and was important for marketing purposes for attracting new patients.
- Some of the major reasons for the use of social media were patient education about surgical procedures, followed by patient referrals and feedback.

Participants who had viewed images of cosmetically enhanced females showed a preference for an increased desire for cosmetic surgery. The more the participants used social media in their everyday lives, the more likely they were to consider it.

CONCLUSION

Indulgence and sustenance within the social media whirlpool is mandatory for any aesthetic setup as it is a practice of extravagance, self-satisfaction, reassurance, and expectations.

Social media gives an aesthetician an image which a patient can relate to and then connect with. However, managing time and resources around this feat is highly vital and also a challenge for an authentic medical personnel. It does yield long-term benefits, but choosing the right platforms and targeting the right audience in the most effective way is that which finally draws results. The increasing presence of social media in this field has led to fundamental changes in how patients interact with the health care system.

PEARLS

Social media use:
- Keep it simple
- Be innovative and creative
- Be pertinent
- Be useful, no hard selling
- Reflect your brand
- Plan your blogs and posts in advance
- Choose platforms wisely
- Manage time spent on it
- Always link back to your website
- No free giveaways
- Respond with gratitude to positive reviews:
  - Post videos of procedures
  - Make before-after posts
  - Get creative with new marketing strategies

REFERENCES

1. Montemurro P, Porcnik A, Heden P, Otte M. The influence of social media and easily accessible online information on the aesthetic plastic surgery practice: literature review and our own experience. Aesthetic Plast Surg. 2015;39(2): 270-7.
2. Vardanian AJ, Kusnezov N, Im DD, Lee JC, Jarrahy R. Social media use and impact on plastic surgery practice. Plast Reconstr Surg. 2013;131(5):1184-93.
3. International Society of Aesthetic Plastic Surgery. (2015). The International Society of Aesthetic Plastic Surgery Releases Global Statistics on Cosmetic Procedures. [online] Available from: https://www.isaps.org/ Media/Default/global-statistics/July%202015%20ISAPS%20 Global%20Statistics%20Release%20-%20Final.pdf. [Last Accessed May, 2021].
4. International Society of Aesthetic Plastic Surgery. The International Society of Aesthetic Plastic Surgery Releases Global Statistics on Cosmetic Procedures. [online] Available from: https://www.isaps.org/Media/Default/global-statistics/ISAPSQuickFactsMS_V6%20(1). pdf. [Last Accessed May, 2021].
5. Bucher T. Networking or what the social means in social media. Social Med Soc. 2015;1(1):9.
6. The Statistics Portal. Most famous social network sites worldwide as of January 2017, ranked by number of active users (in millions). [online] Available from: https://www.statista.com/statistics/272014/global-social-networks-ranked-by-number-of-users/. [Last Accessed May, 2021].
7. Tijerina JD, Morrison SD, Nolan IT, Vail DG, Nazerali R, Lee GK. Google trends as a tool for evaluating public interest in facial cosmetic procedures. Aesthe Surg J. 2019;39(8):908-18.
8. Hopkins ZH, Moreno C, Secrest AM. Influence of Social Media on Cosmetic Procedure Interest. J Clin Aesthet Dermatol. 2020;13(1):28-31.
9. Walker CE, Krumhuber EG, Dayan S, Furnham A. Effects of social media use on desire for cosmetic surgery among young women. Curr Psychol. (2019).
10. Alghonaim Y, Arafat A, Aldeghaither S, Alsugheir S, Aldekhayel S. Social media impact on aesthetic procedures among females in Riyadh, Saudi Arabia. Cureus. 2019;11(10): e6008.
11. Arab K, Barasain O, Altaweel A, Alkhayyal J, Alshiha L, Barasain R, et al. Influence of social media on the decision to undergo a cosmetic procedure. Plast Reconstr Surg Glob Open. 2019;7(8):e2333.
12. Camp SM, Mills DC. The marriage of plastic surgery and social media: a relationship to last a lifetime. Aesth Surg J. 2012;32(3):349-51.

CHAPTER 134

Establishing and Setting Up a Dermatoaesthetic Practice and Related Marketing

D Dinesh Kumar

KEY MESSAGES

- Aesthetic dermatology and practice is rewarding and is expected to grow further in the coming years.
- Adhere to the legal protocol and clinic establishment guidelines to setup a practice.
- Have a plan of action, financial plan and allocation.
- Patient data management is of paramount importance both legally and also for continuous growth of practice.
- Do not compromise on infrastructure, equipment, and human resources.
- Market your practice well, but always within the framework of the Medical Council.
- Always have an able legal adviser and financial consultant.
- Keep yourself abreast on not only latest developments in your specializations but also financial and legal matters.
- Network with other medical professional and be a part of not only medical associations but also social networks.

INTRODUCTION

In India, dermatology is one of the much sort out fields in healthcare. Currently, India has more than 12,000 qualified dermatologists (Postgraduate, Masters or Diploma in Dermatology).

Aesthetic dermatology practice has been on the forefront and continues to increase and nonsurgical aesthetic procedures constitute a large majority of them.

Growing cosmetic awareness and need among the population have led to an increased demand for aesthetic services. This trend has kindled the interest among dermatologists to start an individual aesthetic practice. Many dermatologists prefer to set up a "comprehensive clinic" as it has the advantage of covering all aspects of dermatology per se, i.e., clinical dermatology, dermatosurgery and aesthetic dermatology.

As per the 2020 statistics from the Annual Aesthetic Plastic Surgery Statistics for 2020 the top nonsurgical procedures are as follows: 2,643,366 Dermal Fillers: 1,313,206 Skin Treatment (Chemical Peels, Hydrofacials, etc.): 1,038,968 Skin Treatment (IPL, Combination LASERs): 280,815 Hair Removal: 271,628. The statistics also reveal that aesthetic practice persisted in popularity even amid the COVID-19 pandemic.[1]

In the year 2015, of the aesthetic procedures performed in the United States 61.9% were in office-based facilities, 26% in freestanding surgicenters and 11.9% in hospital setting.[2] Comparing this to the 2005 data 48.3% were in office-based facilities; 27.9% in freestanding surgicenters and 23.8% in hospitals.[3]

This underlines the need to have a self-sufficient clinic-based aesthetic practice adhering to regulations by budding dermatologists. This chapter aims to outlay the prime considerations on how to kick start an aesthetic practice either as:

- A new comprehensive clinic (dermatoaesthetic clinic) or
- To include an aesthetic component to complement an ongoing dermatology practice.

GUIDELINES TO SET UP A DERMATOAESTHETIC PRACTICE

The sections below covered in this chapter are intended to provide a brief understanding on how to bring about a good aesthetic practice:

- Establishing and setting up a dermatoaesthetic practice
- Standards for setting up an aesthetic clinic
- Marketing dermatoaesthetic practice.

Establishing and Setting up a Dermatoaesthetic Practice

Prior to establishing a clinic, it is important for any dermatologist to abide by the rules and regulations laid down by the Government and Medical Council. An ethical practice is all that makes a difference between a qualified dermatologist and other illegal quacks. Adherence to legal framework is fundamental and assures the confidence of the dermatologist at his/her legal front.

Legal Implications for a Dermatoaesthetic Practice[4]

Registration of the clinic: Legal requirements such as licenses and permissions should be obtained. With the licenses and permissions, registration of the clinic can be applied at the Office of the District Health Officer. Post application process, an inspection team verifies and issues a certificate which bears the registration number with the photograph of the proprietor/dermatologist. As per the Consumer Protection Act 1986, *"A skin clinic, akin to any medical clinic, is regarded as a business or a trade enterprise by government authorities and as a service provider",* hence, registration is compulsory.

It is deemed to be unethical and an act of disrepute to the profession, if the dermatologist practice is not in accordance with the guidelines or the local rules and regulations.[5]

Patient data management: Management and maintenance of proper patient records is of paramount importance for any private practice. Being an aesthetic clinic, preoperative and postoperative photographs have to be maintained, providing information on consultations, consent forms, treatment and procedures, preferably using clinic management software [electronic maintenance records (EMR)] or a patient register. The dermatologist should be able to show all relevant patient documents if checked for legal compliance.

Biomedical waste disposal: Proper disposal of biomedical waste is mandatory. Improper or inadequate waste management against guidelines may be subjected to cancellation of license, penalty or even imprisonment.

Financial accounts and taxation: The income from a dermatoaesthetic practice is considered as a professional income and hence taxable. Maintenance of accounts on a yearly basis is crucial, i.e., 1st April to 31st March. As per Section 36 of the CGST Act, 2017, every registered taxable person must maintain the accounts books and records for at least 72 months (6 years). Break-up of accounts can be stored in the following ways:

- Cash flow details must be stored in the form of cash book/ receipts.
- Bills and registers of stationeries, equipment, and consumables must be preserved.
- A daily case register in form no. 3C as per income tax act must be maintained.
- If there is a pharmacy-generated income, it is considered as a business income. In this case, separate accounting has to be done with the help of inventory registers.

Taxation: GST is applicable. When it comes to a dermatoaesthetic practice, the point to be remembered is inclusion of GST to patient bills. It is important to be aware that GST can be levied only for cosmetic procedures enhancing beauty such as LASERs, cosmetic surgery, hair transplantation, etc. GST returns should be filed every month.

Insurance: On a general note, an aesthetic practice may uncommonly experience worst-case scenarios due to unrealistic expectations, errors, and as the results are seen visibly by the patient. Dissatisfied patients may create bitter experiences, rarely ending up in a legal tangle. Hence, having an insurance cover (professional indemnity cover) is a good practice to protect against any medicolegal litigation filed against the doctor.

Standards for Setting up a Dermatoaesthetic Clinic[6]

Objective (Fig. 1)

The objective is to treat patients of skin, hair, nail disorders with medical line of management and to do aesthetic dermatological procedures such as LASERs, chemical peels, botulinum toxin A injections, dermal fillers and minor dermatosurgical procedures like vitiligo surgeries, scar revisions, excisions, hair transplantation, flaps and grafts, etc., without any inpatient services or day care facilities.

Location of the Clinic

Location should be noticeable and accessible with convenient parking options. The location to some extent determines the demographic profile of the patient base.

Preferable areas would upscale residential areas, vicinity of business center, IT parks, etc. One should also be familiar with nearby hospitals, dermatology and other specialty clinics and also other cosmetic centers.

Clinic Infrastructure and Ambience

Area of 800-1,500-3,000 sq feet and even more sq feet may be required, depending on the clinic load, type of surgeries, the number of laser machines, etc. The infrastructure should have the following areas **(Box 1)**:

Reception-cum-waiting area:

- In the reception area, there should be provision for the secretary's desk and chair with a landline phone.
- The consultant's name and credentials should be displayed prominently in the reception area. The chairs to be arranged in a way that space is utilized adequately at the same time not giving a claustrophobic feeling to the patients.
- Magazines/newspapers, television, background light music will keep the patient engaged during waiting hours.

Consultation room:

- The consultation room should have a comfortable desk and chair for the doctor along with a revolving patient stool and chairs for the patient's attendants.
- There should also be an examination bed with a lamp and separated by a curtain from the consultation desk.

Procedure room: It is better to allocate the procedure rooms for each type of procedure if there is more than one procedure room. There should be a room where exclusively lasers and other similar equipment such as ablative/non-radiofrequency/body contouring machines, etc., may be kept. A room should be allocated for procedures such as chemical

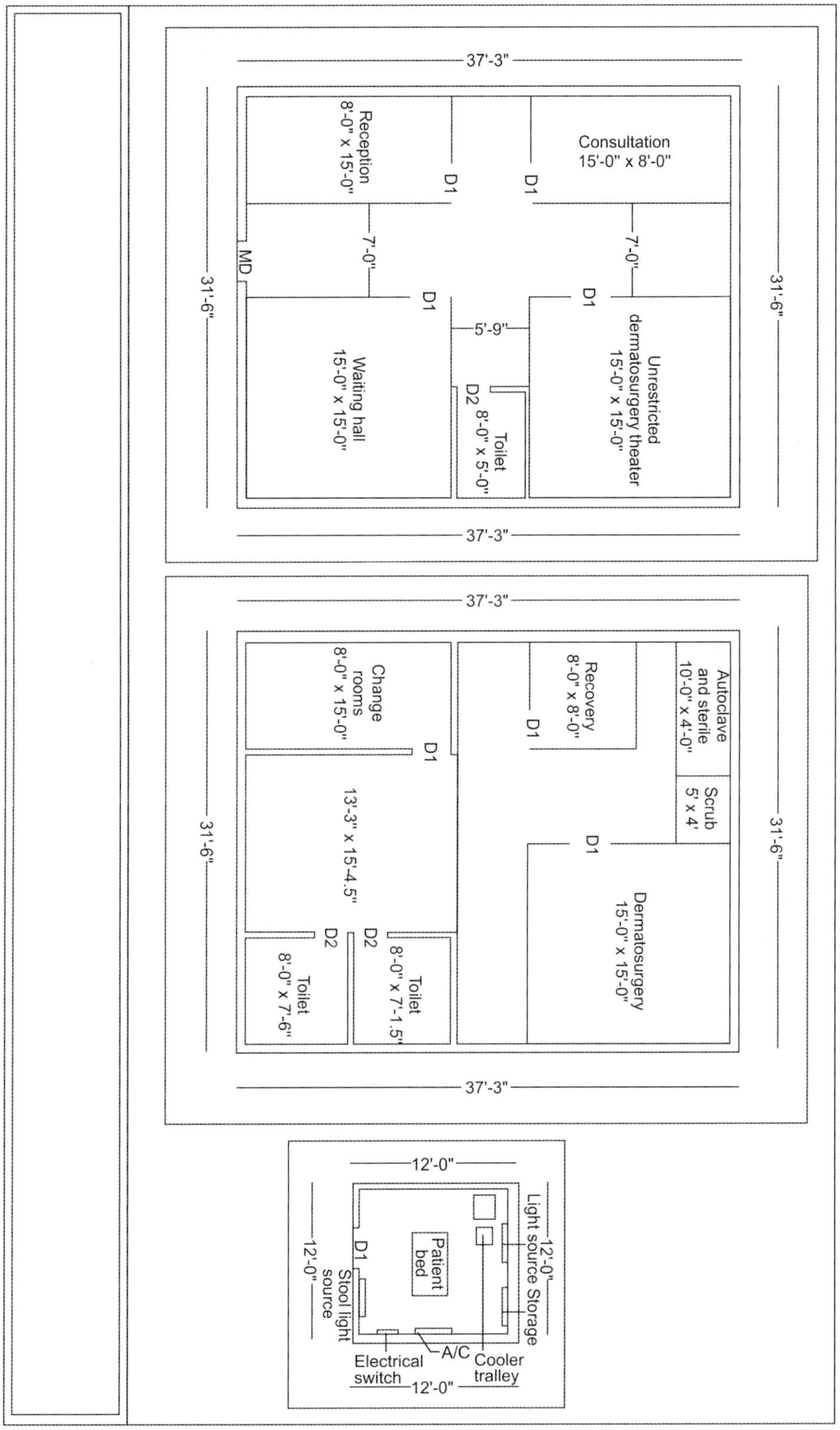

Fig. 1: Floor plan design for a dermatoaesthetic clinic.

peels, microdermabrasion, neurotoxin injections, dermal fillers injections, etc. Similarly a separate room should be labeled as minor OT and used for dermatosurgical procedures such as vitiligo surgeries, scar revisions, excisions, etc. (this room should be periodically fumigated).

Safety and electricity backup: The laser room should have all safety measures implemented along with signage regarding safety precautions and hazards. The access to room should be restricted. It is preferable to have UPS connectivity to the entire center, if not at least there should UPS connectivity only to the laser room. The laser equipment should not be cluttered and placed close to each other. An emergency drug kit along with a resuscitation kit is a must in the procedure room.

Rest rooms and pantry: Rest rooms should be maintained clean and a chart should be drawn to be periodically checked by the housekeeping staff. Trash bins, air fresheners and toiletries should be always available. Continuous water supply should be ensured. If feasible, a pantry should be included in the scheme of the clinic as it would be a place where the staff should relax and also would help in providing refreshments to the patients waiting for longer periods.

BOX 1: Infrastructure plan.

- Reception-cum-waiting area
- Consultation room(s)
- Procedure room(s)
- Minor theater/s
- Rest rooms and pantry
- A counseling room (optional)
- A back-office room (optional)
- Pharmacy (optional)
- Blood collection for laboratory investigations (optional)

Human Resources (Table 1)

Equipment required:

Diagnostic: Magnifying lens, Woods Lamp, dermatoscope, stethoscope, blood pressure apparatus, knee hammer, punch biopsy probes, hand-held torch, thermometer and if affordable imaging systems of the face such as VISIA™.

Therapeutic: Lasers, body contouring equipment, electrocautery, ablative radiofrequency, minor surgical equipment such as forceps, comedone extractors, scissors, etc., are a must. In the field of aesthetic dermatology, it is important to identify what type of procedures or sub specialty dominates your practice and it is wise to invest in LASER equipment accordingly.

TABLE 1: Human resources for dermatoaesthetic practice.

Human resources	*Qualification*	*Roles and responsibilities*
Consultants	• Dermatologist-MD/DNB/DDVL • Plastic surgeons-MCh, DNB	Consultation, treatment and procedures
Secretary-cum-clinic manager	Any basic degree/diploma with good communication skill (Fluency in English and local language, should be able to read and write in English with basic computer skills)	*Clinic management and communication:* • Handle phone enquiries and appointments • Oversee cleanliness of the clinic • Handle other support staff • Maintain stock details in the clinic, utility bills and directly reporting to the consultant who would oversee everything • Counseling patients before and during procedure based on their expectations. Pricing of the procedure, payment options should be handled sensitively
Nursing staff/Practitioners	Nursing (BSc/Diploma) with previous experience in aesthetics	*Assistance and carrying out basic procedures:* • Assist the consultant during the procedures and examination • Collect laboratory samples, sterilize the equipment • If competent enough, can carry out certain procedures such as nonablative RF skin tightening and full body laser, hair removal under the guidance of the dermatologist
Marketing staff	Any basic degree/diploma with previous experience in marketing, fluent in English and local language, should possess social skills	*Marketing the clinic:* • Maintain cordial relationship with the referral sources • Organize camps and educational awareness programs and lectures in corporate companies, hospitals, educational institutions, etc. • Since most of the procedures done in aesthetic dermatology is not covered by insurance companies, the marketing staff should be helpful in identifying corporate companies which provides reimbursement for aesthetic dermatology procedures and further tie up with them
Housekeeping/Support staff	Primary educational level	*Cleanliness and safety:* • Cleaning the clinic regularly and also to run errands • Safety of the clinic • To be courteous with the patients

Emergency drug kit: Consisting of adrenaline, atropine, betamethasone/dexamethasone, hydrocortisone, ranitidine, pheniramine maleate, intravenous (IV) set, syringes and artificial tears eye drops. In procedures where indicated, it is advisable to have a standby anesthetist.

Miscellaneous: Digital Single Lens Reflex and Single Lens Reflex Camera, examination bed, examination/spot light, trolley, refrigerator (to store medicines requiring cold chain), consumables (like slides, gloves, local anesthetic injections, topical anesthetic creams, antibiotic creams, etc.), autoclave, formalin chamber and weighing apparatus are accessories that are necessary in an aesthetic center.

Computer/Laptop: Preferably two, one in the reception and one in the consultant's room. The computer would be invaluable in the modern clinic not only helping in managing the appointment schedules but also in storing the electronic medical record which is the order of the day. The computer can also be used by the staff to send mailers to the patients, email them their laboratory reports. The consultant can have a CCTV camera in the reception and monitor the activities of the reception in his/her computer.

Dermatosurgery theaters: For centers performing surgeries, a separate surgery theater is needed. The reader is referred to the chapters on setting up a theater and hair transplant clinic for details.

Marketing Dermatoaesthetic Practice[7]

In the current competitive world, marketing is important to synergize your practice. In addition to regular patient services, marketing helps to reach out to the community at a larger level within a short period.

Marketing can be done in the following ways:

- *Word of mouth advertising:* This is the most conventional and best of all methods. A satisfied patient may serve as a marketing vehicle that shall bring the desired reputation to you and your clinic. The target is "Give every patient the best of the services". Treat every patient important and equal, irrespective of his/her background and medical condition. A satisfied patient would not hesitate to refer your name, not only to their kith and kin but also to their acquaintances. A "patient referred patient" who is contented with the treatment may further refer your name to another and thus keeps forming a chain of patients. Eventually, a marketing web would have already formed building your credibility. So, update yourself with recent dermatologic advances and practices, and treat every patient with care and respect. A quality practice with the standards mentioned earlier itself is a form of marketing.
- *Name of the clinic:* The name board should be simple and clear giving the necessary details such as the doctor's name, qualification, phone number, etc. In fact, the clinic board may be the first mode which should encourage the patient to visit the clinic. A unique logo is of value; hence, spend some effort in designing a logo to bring in a professional look to the clinic board. Make the color and the dimensions of the name board such that it is visible from a distance. Flashy boards may leave a commercial look; hence, try to keep the board a bit professional adhering to the regulations by the Medical Council.
- *Marketing through staff:* The staff should look professional and neat with a label carrying the clinic logo. They should be courteous, cheerful and friendly to the patients. Good communication is an essential aspect here. Appropriate informal-friendly talk may help reduce patient anxiety and create a "feel at home" atmosphere. It is evident that a clinic with good hospitality is likely to invite patients. The best way to achieve this is to keep the staff happy at your level:
  - Keep motivating the staff at regular intervals. Never stop appreciating/rewarding them whenever a good service is rendered.
  - Give the staff mandatory holidays or compensation. Refrain from correcting them in front of the patients as it not only demotivates them but would also leave a question in the patient's mind on the quality of the treatment.
  - Listen to their problems and take appropriate action as and when required. Make them feel that they play an important role in the success of the practice.
  - Help them upgrade their skills as per the need.
- *Promotions and publicity:* As dermatoaesthetic practice is consumer driven, it has come to rely heavily publicity for promotion. Care should be taken to avoid unethical promotions and to adhere to guidelines laid by State Medical Councils. If utilized ethically, media may take your practice to a different level. So, utilize the opportunities that may be available through television/radio/social media/blogs/webinars. Sharing the right information with the public will give you the desired recognition as the reach via media is infinite. Bear in mind, a good impression induced through media may linger in the patients mind for long and can seek your help even beyond several years.

  In this fast moving world, an online presence is very important as virtual access is convenient to many patients especially the urban working community. Design an attractive and informative website and post regularly on social media to have a better recall value of you. Make the online website interactive answering patient queries. Ensure that the administrators of the website are alert and manage patient testimonials regularly. It should be understood that it may not always be the case of positive reviews from patients; a negative feedback may also arrive. Do not get demotivated by negative comments, instead look at it as a challenge to improve patient services. Negative reviews may be removed if you think they are not genuine. Regularly post videos or pictures giving excellent information related to advancements and current practices in your clinic.

Teledermatology practice has been approved by the Government of India and it would aid in the follow-up of your patients who find it difficult/unable to travel to your clinic.[8] Make sure to store the patient consultation records of Teledermatology.

Finances and Equipment Procurement (Box 2)

- Make up your mind on what you intend to do and analyze on how much finances is possible at your disposal (money on hand, assets, bank loan).
- Create a business plan and budget for setting up the center. Earmark and allocate finances for each quarter. (On how much you would want to spend on buying new equipment, maintenance of clinic, equipment, staff salary, etc.).

BOX 2: Business plan for a dermatoaesthetic practice.

Business plan

Objectives:

Financial:

- *Funds:* Generation and expenditure
- Projected number of patients to be seen in OPD
- Projected number of patients taking up procedures
- Projected revenue generation in first 6 months, at 1 year and thereafter

Nonfinancial:

- Quality of care provided
- Types of procedures

Budget outlay

Start-up expenses:

- Clinic lease and rent, clinic furnishing, staff recruitment and salary, purchase of equipment, beds, medical software or medical record system, housekeeping items and clinic stationery, marketing and branding if any
- Make an inventory of your assets and divide your assets into short-term assets (ones which will depreciate quickly, have not much of resale value and need to be replaced) and long-term assets (ones which do not depreciate much and has a resale value)

Operational expense:

- Clinic rent, clinic maintenance, staff salary, AMC, clinic development
- Always maintain monthly records (Excel sheet and charts) regarding income generation and expenditure and analyze them periodically

Market analysis:

- Existing market scenario
- Current market players
- Current market revenue generation
- Market needs and how many are met satisfactorily
- Markets needs not met in current scenario and their potential
- Future market trends

Procedures or services:

- Procedures to be done initially and their projected usage and income generation
- *Income generation projection:* Find out the depreciation value of your investment in a particular period then plan to recover that amount in that particular period of time
  (for example, If your equipment depreciates by Rs. 200,000 at the end of 2 years, you should have recovered at least Rs. 200,000 in 2 years, for a sustainable business model)
- Future procedures and their projected usage and income generation

Management and administration:

Clinic administration, staff management, marketing, public relations

- Prioritize the purchase/spends according to market demand and then create a timetable on acquiring them with your budget:
  - Ablative radiofrequency (RF) equipment along with good microdermabrasion (MDA) equipment would be good enough to start practice, along with chemical peels, dermarollers and if proficient, neurotoxins and dermal fillers should be practiced.
- One should prioritize the purchase of LASERs in the following order; high to low:
  - Hair reduction LASER,
  - Fractional ablative/nonablative LASER, MNRF
  - Q switch LASER,
  - Skin tightening/contouring equipment (energy based),
  - LASER for vascular lesions.[9]
- After finalizing your potential type of equipment and its allocated budget:
  - Get as many quotations as possible from different people handling that type of equipment.
  - Talk with as many colleagues who have the equipment; ask about cost, efficacy, maintenance, after sales service, depreciation.
  - Shortlist the good ones and ask for demonstration. Initiate discussions with short listed companies regarding the cost, flexibility in pricing, etc.
  - Finalize on the company which satisfies criteria on quality of the equipment, efficacy, cost, after

TIPS AND PEARLS

Tips and pearls for beginners:

- The government regards a dermatology clinic as a business or a trade enterprise and as a service provider
- The first step in setting in a clinic is to familiarize with local rules regulations and the required licenses
- For the location of the center, if possible settle on a location which is noticeable, accessible and with sufficient parking facility nearby. The locality should be preferably not too crowded
- Patient treatment record books have to be diligently maintained. It is preferable to EMR along option for storage of patient's clinical photographs
- Proper biomedical waste disposal (solid as well as liquid) is absolutely mandatory
- Insurance coverage and professional indemnity coverage is mandatory
- Ensure and follow minimum standards of practice as it not only ensures quality of your practice, it also enhances of the practice and this measure by itself can be a great source for word of mouth referrals
- Never ever lose focus of the fact that you are dealing with human beings, and those in distress due to some or the other reason
- The backbone of a successful clinic is a team of assistants, technicians and receptionists who are diligent, courteous and driven to succeed because they have faith in you and your mission
- Ensure that the patient trusts you that it is also paying them in monetary terms to stick with your clinic
- A transparent, honest discussion with the patient by the doctor and staff not only helps to build a good longstanding rapport but also minimizes the unnecessary litigations
- Cornerstones of a successful dermatology practice: Honesty, competence, availability

sales service, AMC charges, and depreciation rate. Also explore the option of buyback or upgradation of the equipment from the company and get an assurance on it.

- Always insist on Certificate of Authenticity and Certificate on Date of manufacture/programming from the parent company.[9]
- Be confident of your equipment but do not oversell your equipment to your patient. Set realistic expectations to the patients and price the services competitively keeping in mind a projected period of recovery of the investment.

- *Insurance:* Always cover yourself and your clinic with insurances (fire, accidents, calamities, burglary malpractice). Profession liability insurance need to be taken. Dermatologists, Venereologists and Leprologists (DVL) Trust of Indian Association of Dermatologists, Venereologists and Leprologist (IADVL) might be helpful. Schemes of IMA also need to be looked into. Insurance for equipment including LASERs can be purchased. It important to an able legal advisor and financial consultant.

ACKNOWLEDGMENT

I would like to acknowledge "RP architects" for their assistance in helping with the floor plan design.

REFERENCES

1. The Aesthetic Society. (2021). Annual Aesthetic Plastic Surgery Statistics for 2020. [online] Available from: https://cdn.surgery.org/media/statistics/aestheticplasticsurgerynationaldatabank-2020stats.pdf. [Last Accessed May, 2021].
2. American Society of Esthetic Plastic Surgery. (2015). Cosmetic Surgery National Data Bank Statistics. [online] Available from: https://www.surgery.org/sites/default/files/ASAPS-Stats2015.pdf. [Last Accessed May, 2021].
3. American Society of Esthetic Plastic Surgery. (2006). 11.5 million cosmetic procedures in 2005. [online] Available from: https://www.surgery.org/sites/default/files/Statistics%20Quick%20Facts.pdf. [Last Accessed May, 2021].
4. Jayanth DP, Mysore V. For the dermatological entrepreneur-regulations setting up a clinic. Dermapractice. 2015;1(1):15-27.
5. Goh C. The need for evidence-based esthetic dermatology practice. J Cutan Aesthet Surg. 2009;2:65-71.
6. Kumar DD. Minimum standards for setting up a clinic. Dermapractice. 2015;1(2):5-13.
7. Sharma OS. Marketing: getting and sustaining the patient to the clinic. Dermapractice. 2015;1(2):14-8.
8. MOHFW. (2020). Telemedicine Practice Guidelines Enabling Registered Medical Practitioners to Provide Healthcare Using Telemedicine. Available from: https://www.mohfw.gov.in/pdf/Telemedicine.pdf. [Last Accessed May, 2020].
9. Aurangabadkar SJ, Mysore V, Ahmed ES. Buying a laser—tips and pearls. J Cutan Aesthet Surg. 2014;7:124-30.

CHAPTER 135

Documentation and Electronic Medical Record, Consent and Counseling

Pradyumna Vaidya, Nitika Deshmukh

DOCUMENTATION AND ELECTRONIC MEDICAL RECORD

KEY MESSAGES

- Medical records are critical part of medical practice.
- Electronic medical record (EMR) is an advancement to simplify the task.
- Accurate and consistent records are important defense in malpractice claims.
- Standardization ensures consistency in quality of record-keeping.
- Standards compliant EMR solution protects against vendor lock-in.
- Data security and safety critical in EMR.
- Internet-based EMR systems are more cost-effective due to benefit of scale.
- EMR system can be integrated with disease surveillance systems for better community health.

INTRODUCTION

While practicing in an era where the aesthetic and trichology practice has commercialized, documentation and accurate medical records are critical in medical practice. While its primary purpose is to help in offering better healthcare service to the patient, it is an indispensable defense against allegations of medical malpractice.[1] Even from the perspective of insurance claim, it is vital to maintain accurate medical records.

Accurately, consistently maintained and accessible medical records of a patient help in making informed decisions about course of treatment, resulting in better success rate of treatment and higher satisfaction ratings by the patient. These in turn result in enhanced practice of the medical practitioner. This is especially true for physicians handling aesthetic patients.

In case of a medicolegal litigation, improperly maintained medical records and documentation can seriously handicap the defense of the physicians and the medical practitioners. In case of a malpractice case, the reviewer will invariably look at the system of record keeping followed by particular practitioner and not focus only on case records of the claimant. This makes it vital that the record-keeping be consistent and accurate.

HISTORY

Early days of the medical science era, when the records were referred to as case books, case records, etc.[2,3] and the computers were not prevalent in the medical practice management, the case histories were recorded in the hard copy format. Such approach led to difficulties in managing the patient information and also sufferings from many issues such as incomplete, illegible records maintained on an offline mode. Offline recording approach limited the feasibility of getting inputs from practitioners across geographies.

With digitization in medical practice, the trend of maintaining medical records on paper is declining in developed countries, but still commonly followed in developing and underdeveloped countries. Also, economies of scale are helping lower down the costs of owning a digital platform, thereby encouraging the need to move toward digitization.

BENEFITS OF ELECTRONIC MEDICAL RECORD

Documentation and medical record in electronic/digital form offers some significant benefits:

- Quality of patient care and treatment plan certainly enhances due easy, concurrent accessibility of patient history, including past treatment and past complaints.
- Electronic records also allow superior visual presentation of medical history. For example, a graphical chart of blood sugar over last 1 year can quickly provide an insight into the patient's diabetes control.
- With enhancements in digital imaging technologies, it is significantly easier to capture patient images, scans, MRI images, etc.
- For frequent follow-up cases, an ability to mark EMR with priority/importance can enhance interaction.

- Electronic records also help in performing group statistical analysis and identifying trends and geographical spread of disease for community health care.
- Advanced data analytics can be utilized for early detection and disease spread pattern.
- EMR eases teledermatology practice in times of pandemics and helps to maintain accuracy in patient management, consulting follow-up patients, saving clinical records including images and their clinical data.
- Electronic records on the other hand require almost no physical space—and with appropriate safety mechanisms in place—can practically be treated as indestructible.[4]
- EMR eases medical referrals to other specialties whenever required.

LIMITATIONS

- While cloud storage offers significant benefits with regards to scalability, accessibility, security and safety, it is important to maintain appropriate contracts for data confidentiality.
- Availability of power supply and appropriate internet connection.
- Cloud setup can be expensive if the requirement is not correctly understood (hybrid, public, private).
- Risk of data loss, data corruption, etc.

DOCUMENTATION STANDARDS

Medical record standardization plays an important role in getting insights into the efficacy of the treatment plan though aggregation and statistical analysis of data sourced from disparate agencies. Further, with increasing need of data exchange between various stakeholders in the patient care (patient, consultant, insurance company, pharmacies), it is necessary to have standardization in medical records.

Standardization helps in:

- Maintaining documents pertaining to patients' identity (ID cards such as Aadhar card, PAN card, etc.)
- Making a good protocol of treatment
- Medical insurance and claims processing
- Identification of trends and spread of diseases
- Availability of real-life data for research studies.

A range of standards have evolved over the years to address different aspects of health care and medical record-keeping. More details of each of these are available on their respective sources provided in the references section **(Box 1)**. In addition to these, patients' government identity documents (Aadhar card, PAN card, etc.) should be also be documented and stored in the software systems.

BOX 1: Commonly used standards.

- Terminology
- Disease classification
- Electronic medical records
- Intervention classification
- e-prescription
- Privacy and security
- SNOMED International
- ICD-10/11
- SOAP, HL7, FHIR
- ICHI
- NCPDP
- HIPAA, ISO 27001

(FHIR: Fast Healthcare Interoperability Resources; HIPAA: Health Insurance Portability and Accountability Act; HL7: Health Level Seven; ICD10: International Statistical Classification of Diseases and Related Health Problems; ICHI: International Classification of Health Interventions; NCPDP: National Council for Prescription Drug Program; SOAP: Subjective, Objective, Assessment, and Plan; SNOMED: Systematized Nomenclature of Medicine)

Terminology Standardization

Standardization of terminology helps in accurately conveying patient disease status across languages and cultures. With globalization and increasing movement of patients, a need for standardization of terminology is imperative. SNOMED-CT standard addresses the need for terminology standardization.

Systematized Nomenclature of Medicine—Clinical Terms (SNOMED-CT)[5] is a standardized, multilingual vocabulary of clinical terminology that is used by physicians and other healthcare providers for the electronic exchange of clinical health information. SNOMED-CT is owned and maintained by International Health Terminology Standards Development Organization (IHTSDO).

Disease Classification Standardization

Disease classification system provides consistent classification of disease across organizations and medical practitioners. A standardized disease classification system not only codifies the disease, it also provides a standard guideline and a criterion for classifying patient condition into a particular category.

International Statistical **C**lassification of **D**iseases and Related Health Problems (ICD)[6] is a medical classification list by the World Health Organization (WHO). It contains codes for diseases, signs and symptoms, abnormal findings, complaints, social circumstances, and external causes of injury or diseases. WHO has released updates of this standard over the years. The latest version of ICD has been released in 2017 and added to the ICD system recently.

A significant feature of ICD is the availability in multiple languages—the ICD codes have been translated in 43 languages, enhancing its application across geographical and cultural boundaries.

Electronic Records Standardization

While the actual storage format for EMRs is bound to vary for vendor to vendor, it is critically important to have a standard for exchange of this information. This protects against vendor lock-in, and health care provider can switch systems without losing fidelity of the medical record created using earlier system. Also, the standardization allows exchange of data between systems created by different vendors for different purposes.

For example, it is vital to allow sharing of treatment plan and diagnosis data with insurance company in electronic form for easier and faster processing of insurance claims.

Subjective, objective, assessment, and plan note (SOAP) is a popular standard for recording patient interaction and treatment plan. It is a method of documentation employed by healthcare providers to write out notes in a patient's chart, along with other common formats, such as the admission note.

Health Level Seven (HL7)[7,8] defines a standard and provides a framework for the exchange, integration, sharing, and retrieval of electronic health information. These standards define how information is packaged and communicated from one party to another, setting the language, structure and data types required for seamless integration between systems. HL7 standards support clinical practice and the management, delivery, and evaluation of health services, and are recognized as the most commonly used in the world.

A newer interoperability standard from the HL7 community is Fast Healthcare Interoperability Resources (FHIR).[9] FHIR is a significantly enhanced standard compared to HL7 and it is more likely to be adapted by the vendors due to its technical superiority and because it is agnostic to the platform/technology used by the vendor.

The actual data exchange mechanisms are covered by various transport protocols. While it is important piece of medical data exchange jigsaw, it does not contribute in actual data format; hence, we are not covering it here.

Intervention Classification

Intervention classification system provides a uniform classification of health intervention allowing comparable reporting and statistical analysis.

The classification focuses on three pillars—target (entity on which the intervention was performed), action (the intervention performed on the target) and means (the processes/methods used to perform the intervention).

The International Classification of Health Interventions (ICHI)[10] defines the standard for this classification. Besides the ICHI codes, it also provides extension code, to allow the actor performing the intervention, to document additional details about the intervention. ICHI is still a draft standard and is yet to be adopted by the healthcare professionals.

e-Prescription

An offshoot of increasing popularity of cloud-based EMR and practice management systems is cloud-based pharmacies that allow online ordering of drugs. Though, the rules for online ordering and dispensation of drugs are dictated by the local government policies—a standard way of exchanging information between the ordering doctor and online pharmacy is desired, and made necessary to ensure controlled dispensing of scheduled drugs. National Council for Prescription Drug Program (NCPDP)[11] is one such body that provides electronic prescribing standards. While NCPDP specified electronic prescription standards, local governing bodies [for example, Medical Council of India (MCI) does provide their own guidelines for prescriptions as well as e-prescriptions]. It is advised that practitioner follows the guidelines of the local governing body wherever there is a conflict in the NCPDP and local body guideline.

Electronic Medical Record Security

Like any other electronic data, increased accessibility also brings in associated threats of unauthorized access. Patient medical record is categorized as personal sensitive information.[12] A breach in privacy of a patient through leakage of his disease condition can result in significant mental, physical and financial trauma to the patient. In order to address these concerns, it is utmost important to follow the guidelines suggested by the legal authorities legislating on these issues. In a large part of the developed world, Health Insurance Portability and Accountability Act (HIPAA)[12] is applicable, and the healthcare provided must ensure that the tools and systems used to manage patient medical data are compliant with the HIPAA requirements. International Organization for Standardization (ISO) 27001 standard is applicable to information security management systems. With increasing trend toward outsourcing and cloud-based EMR systems, it is critical to ensure that the service provider facility is ISO 27001 certified to ensure safety against unauthorized access and cyber-attacks.

ISSUES

Need for Global Involvement

Disease classification systems and other standards have evolved through large volume of medical data. So far, such data have been available only from developed countries; as a result, the disease classification standards required for the conditions prevalent in developing and underdeveloped countries have not received requisite attention. It is of utmost importance for these countries to get involved in standardizing process and ensure inclusion of conditions that impact disease classification in their geographies and cultures.

Multilingual

Multilingual countries, such as India, present a unique challenge to the medical practitioners as the patient may prefer medication instructions in a language that the patient can understand.

Accessibility

Effectiveness of medical record system lies in its ability to provide the information when required. Paper-based systems of medical records often suffered from accessibility issue. A misclassification of record may mean that the record is lost forever.

TECHNOLOGY FOR RESCUE

Without proper tools/processes for documentations, electronic record management can be an overwhelming task. Developing countries with poor doctor-patient ratio find it particularly difficult to maintain proper records due to severe time constraints. While the EMR management practice is very good from patient's perspective, it impacts doctor's efficiency.

The technology can come to the rescue of the doctor as it can help store the medical data in appropriate format, make reference data available at the click of a button. Having said that, it is important to choose appropriate tools for EMR management to ensure doctor's productivity is not impacted.

DATA SECURITY: BEST PRACTICES

With the advent of desktop-based and cloud-based medical record systems, the task of record-keeping has got simplified, but it has opened up the possibility of patient data privacy breach. Practitioners are advised to introduce necessary data protection initiatives.

Here is a nonexhaustive checklist for ready reference:

- Secure socket layer communication for data exchange between client computer and server
- Enforcement of strong passwords
- Nonrepeatability of passwords
- Ability to auto lock-out to protect against cyber attacks
- Force password change at regular intervals
- Vendor policy about access to data in their custody
- Data back-up responsibility and schedule
- Nonreliance on third party identity service.

CHECKLIST FOR ELECTRONIC MEDICAL RECORD SYSTEMS

While the need for documentation and electronic record-keeping is well-understood, selecting an appropriate EMR system can be a daunting task due to large number of options available, each with different capabilities. Hence, it is important to have assess EMR system that suits the clinic/practice's requirements.

Flexibility and Extensibility

Conduct a thorough vendor assessment to meet the EMR management system requirements. In India, support for vernacular prescription could be critical to achieve better treatment compliance resulting in higher success.

Mobile Access

In order to ensure that the EMR is available at point of service, check if the vendor provides mobile applications for accessing the EMR, to increase on-the-go productivity for doctors and patients.

Standards Compliance

Standards compliant system automatically offers an assurance of completeness of the system.

Legal Compliance as per Government Norms

Ensure that the vendor system is compliant with the local rules governing the medical practice.[13]

Easy Data Accessibility

Allow quick and easy audit trail access to previous visits and clinical notes, treatment plan, imaging data, etc. **(Fig. 1)**.[14]

Easy Patient Interaction Capture

Primary source of data into EMR is the interaction between the patient and the treating physician. It is, therefore, vital that the EMR system is flexible enough to allow faithfully capturing all patient inputs, physician's observations in an user friendly way **(Fig. 2)**.[14]

Special features that cater to specific working conditions of the practitioner should also be looked into while selecting a solution. For example, in developing and underdeveloped countries with low internet penetration, a pure cloud-based system may not work efficiently due to lower bandwidth

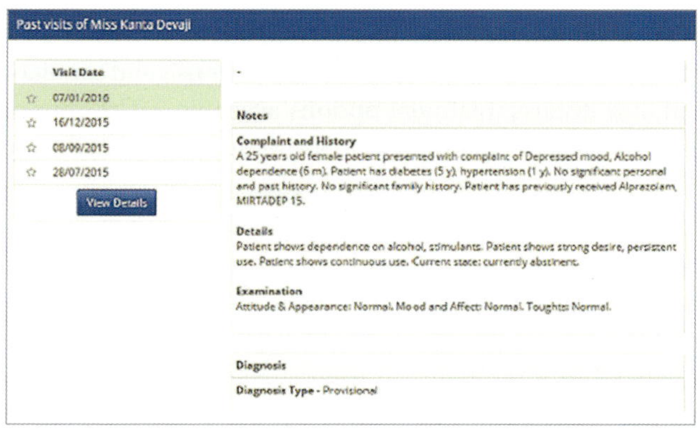

Fig. 1: Easy data accessibility.

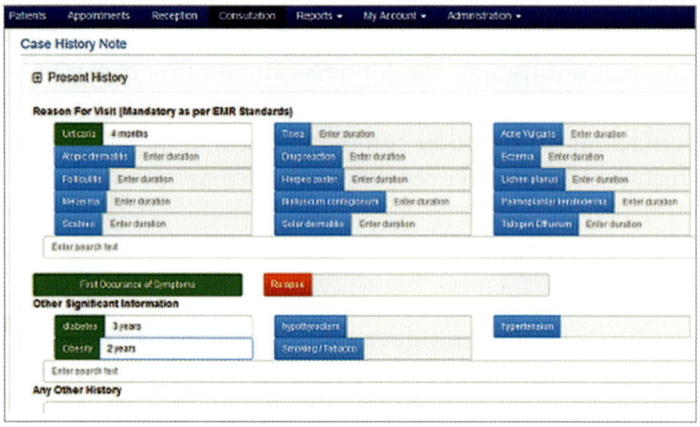

Fig. 2: Easy patient interaction capture.

and intermittent connection availability. In such cases, one should go for hybrid systems that offer online as well as offline operation support.

Safety and Security

It is critical for a health care practitioner, custodian of patient's EMR, to ascertain that the EMR system use has adequate

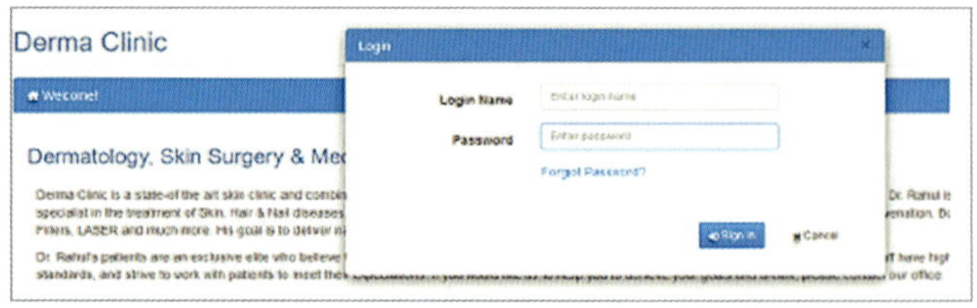

Fig. 3: Authenticated access to EMR system.

measures in place to ensure safety (regular scheduled backup) and access security (against hacking/virus attacks) of patient data. Safety and security of cloud based EMR systems is managed by professionals that ensure the servers are secure, the operating systems are regularly updated, etc.

Privacy and Access Control

An EMR system used by an organization is accessed by multiple users—administrator, medical staff, support staff, etc. Ensure that the EMR system provides appropriate access control mechanisms to limit access to patient data **(Fig. 3)**. There must be a provision to provide appropriate user specific access to the system.[14]

ROLE OF COUNSELORS IN AESTHETIC PRACTICE

KEY MESSAGES

- Good communication between the clinic and patient is the key to good patient education.
- A patient who has been well-educated about medications and procedures is more likely to adhere to treatment, be more punctual with follow-ups and causes less problems in future.
- Good patient education includes giving information about the nature of the condition, use of medication, procedural treatment options, possible complications and need for follow-ups.
- Counselors come in handy to perform the above functions for busy practitioners.
- Front office staff, nurses, technicians, nondermatologists can be trained to be counselors.
- A good counselor can save time and effort of the dermatologist and also help to expand the practice by building a good rapport with the patient and their family.
- Counselors need to be retrained and monitored regularly to avoid complications in the clinic.

CHANGING DOCTOR-PATIENT COMMUNICATION RELATIONSHIP

With advancement of the internet and increase in awareness, patients tend to ask questions about the diagnosis and condition; and also discuss treatment options available.[12] The younger patients ask more questions and are more demanding.[13]

Willingness to listen and answer has been shown to be the most important criteria for selecting the doctor.[14] Redundant questions from patients urges the doctors to dislike the patients with paternalistic belief of doing the best for their patients, time consumed in a busy practice, the efforts needed and a tendency to treat such patients as difficult patients.[12] Also, many patients coming to cosmetic clinics do not suffer from any dermatological disorder but come for an enhancement in their looks.[15,16] Such patients are well read, aware and hence have demands which have to be met and hence need to be handled very carefully **(Box 2)**.

ROLE OF PATIENT EDUCATION: NEED FOR COUNSELORS

Patient education establishing a communication bridge between the health care provider and the patient **(Box 3)**.[12] Communication is also important for compliance and final outcome. A patient, who is well-informed, is more relaxed, feels more in control, has more faith in the doctor and is more adhering to the treatment.

Aesthetic solutions are also provided by beauty parlors and other spas, beauty "clinics", etc. These are not governed by any medical regulating and hence it is important to educate

BOX 2: Doctor-patient communication.

- Merely writing a prescription and naming the procedure is not enough
- Patients like a doctor who listens to them and explains
- Explain nicely to alleviate the feelings of mistrust and skepticism about treatment

BOX 3: Patient education.

- Inform the patient about the condition, the medication and procedures
- Clear myths and doubts
- Set realistic expectations
- Explain the proper method of application
- Good education improves adherence and compliance to treatment
- Compliance to medication also improves outcome of procedures
- An informed patient is more satisfied and less anxious

the patients about the scientifically proven treatments and procedures with realistic expectations.[17]

Since most dermatological conditions require long-term treatment, which lasts for months to years, it is vital to counsel the patient regarding the duration of treatment and the prognosis of the disease.

Dermatological treatments are unique as in they involve usage of a lot of topical medicines. The correct method of application has to be told clearly, so that unwanted side effects and poor effects can be avoided.[18] Prime example of the above is explaining proper application of retinoids to avoid irritation.

Relapse of any condition creates a negative image in the mind of the patient about the doctor. A patient who has been warned about the possibility of relapse is more likely to accept it easily. If a patient has been suggested about ways and means to reduce the chances of relapse, he/she is more likely to adhere to the precautions. As an example, take a patient of acne who has gone into remission. Such a patient should be told about the role of diet and lifestyle and emphasized about the need to apply topical retinoids even when the acne is under-control.

A good communication and rapport with the patient before, during and after the procedure helps if some complication arises.[19,20] A satisfied patient is less likely to go formal practice suits.

Counselors in Aesthetic Skin Clinics

Counselors have an important role to play in aesthetic clinics.

Who can be Counselors?

There is no certifying authority, approved courses or basic qualification requirement for counselors in aesthetic clinics in India. Some clinics do engage MBBS doctors or even doctors of alternative medicine as counselors. Counseling is more of a continuous change management process.

The counselor should be aware of the clinic protocols and precautions to be followed before, during and after the procedure. This helps in quality assistance to the practitioners.

BOX 4: Role of counselors.

- Anyone in the clinic can be counselor, but chose the person carefully
- Counselors should have good communication skills to educate patients
- Train the counselors well
- Every member of the clinic has to chip in
- Counselors save time and energy
- They help to pacify patients and also help in scheduling and ensuring follow-ups

Printed handouts explaining about the do's and don'ts before and after the procedure should be given to patient and explained by the counselors.

The following are the advantages of counselors in aesthetic practice:

- *Time saving:* Because of the lower doctor to patient ratio, most of the doctors in India, it becomes difficult for the doctors to devote enough time total history, explain medication and treatment options available. A counselor helps to fill in this gap so that communication is done effectively between the clinic and the patient.
- *Effort saving:* Aesthetic procedures apart from being time consuming also requires lot of physical and mental efforts. A counselor can provide more effective response to the patients in such cases.
- *Handling common queries:* A well-educated counselor can handle common queries, thereby saving efforts and time of the physician.
- *Patient education:* Many unscientific and false accusations are circulated against cosmetic procedures, in the internet world. A good counselor can fill in the gaps and also politely correct a patient, if he/she is carrying some wrong information or incorrect facts. Counselors can also get involved in discussions on costing of a procedure, as patients tend to negotiate for better prices!
- *Pacifying patients who develop side effects/complications:* Any patient undergoing even a minor aesthetic procedure can develop a complication. It helps if the patient had been well-counseled about the likelihood of minor problems that may develop following the procedure and also remedies for such issues. Also, if minor self-resolving side effects develop, a counselor can effectively suggest ways to minimize it. A very good example is the dryness and peeling that many times develop after a chemical peel. If the patient had been forewarned and a good moisturizer suggested, he/she is not likely to bother the clinic staff or the dermatologist.
- *Follow-up and appointments*: Most procedures are repetitive and optimum results depend on completion of the sessions as per protocols. Counselors can be used to remind patients and ensure proper follow-up **(Box 4)**.

Important Points for a Counselor

- The counselor should have a pleasing appearance, well dressed and be patient.
- The counselor should effectively tell the patient about the treatments available for the particular problem along with the expected results, precautions to be taken and common trivial side effects.
- The ability to explain treatments, medication and procedures is the important for selecting a particular doctor.[21]
- The information provided should be clear and concise.[18]
- Multimedia presentations can promote audiovisual impact which can engage the patient.[22]
- The counselor helps to identify patients with dysmorphophobia or related disorders[23,24] and assist in reducing the distress.
- Counselor must be able to encourage patients on realistic expectations.[23,24]
- The counselor can also help in providing feedback from the patients, which can greatly improve the services of the clinic and increase patient satisfaction[25] **(Box 5)**.

BOX 5: Tips for a counselor.

- Dress neatly, smile, and talk politely
- Make the patient comfortable
- Listen to the patient
- Explain slowly, clearly and in simple language
- Keep cool with a demanding patient
- Learn well about the medicines and procedures
- Educate, inform about treatments pertaining to the patients problems
- Do not over commit
- Do inform about minor post procedure side effects
- When in doubt, check with the doctor
- Watch out for psychologically disturbed patients and those with unrealistic expectations
- Take feedback and inform the dermatologist

BOX 6: Precautions.

- Choose the right person for the job of a counselor
- Do not rely on just one person
- Safeguard patient data
- Keep a tab on the working of all counselors
- Take blinded feedback from the patients on the counselor's performance

PRECAUTIONS TO AVOID PITFALLS

Counselors with a slight medical background and with composure can contribute to patient's comfort to great extent. It is important that the counselor manages to respond to majority of patient's concerns to build the trust relationship. In the authors experience, an over enthusiastic counselor, who wants to "convert" all patients to undergo procedures at any cost is to be watched out for.

Having said that, it is not good for a clinic to overtly depend on one counselor, it is preferable to have multiple counselors, separately for aesthetics, for lasers and for surgery. Doctors can introduce survey/feedback mechanism to gauge counselor's performance **(Box 6)**.

SUMMARY

Counselors are becoming an integral part of aesthetic practices as dermatologists venture into aesthetic procedures which take a lot of time and effort. There is no certifying authority for counselors in dermatology practice, so we have to rely on a well-trained clinic staff to perform this role.

ROLE OF INFORMED CONSENT IN DERMATOLOGY PRACTICE

KEY MESSAGES

- A well written informed consent is a key for a safe and secure practice.
- A consent is medicolegal contract between the doctor and the patient explaining the details of the procedure including the risks involved during and after the procedure.
- A consent should also include details about the success rate and failure rate of the said operation/procedure.
- It is a crucial part of aesthetic dermatology, clinical dermatology and trichology practice.
- Written informed consent form must also include willingness of the patient to under photography and also to publish the clinical data on web or for research purpose.

INTRODUCTION

Dermatology practice has undergone tremendous changes in the last few decades. With the advent of newer lasers, advancements in hair restoration surgeries and much more, the role of written informed consent becomes crucial. As medical practice is also within the limits of Consumer Protection Act (CPA), it is highly important for a dermatologist to enforce informed consent strictly in his day to day practice.[26]

WHAT IS AN INFORMED CONSENT?

It is a voluntary and revocable agreement of a competent individual to participate in a therapeutic, diagnostic or research procedure, based on adequate understanding of its nature, purpose, and implications.[27]

Legal Elements of Informed Consent

It is doctor's legal duty to disclose details in the consent form **(Box 7)**.

BOX 7: Elements of informed consent.

- Diagnosis
- Nature and purpose of the said treatment or procedure
- Risks and benefits of the procedure
- Diagnostic or therapeutic relevance of the procedure
- Alternatives available
- Post procedure side effects (immediate/late; reversible/ irreversible)
- Any unforeseen risks involved (anaphylaxis, physical, psychological, social, sexual, economic harms)
- What will happen if the procedure is not done or delayed
- Special postoperative precautions to be followed by the patient
- What the doctor recommends

Sections Dealing with Informed Consent under Indian Law[28-31]

Indian Penal Code (IPC) sections 87 to 91 deal with consent. As per section 88 IPC, if an act is performed without any intention or not knowing that it would likely cause death, and is done in good faith with his consent in order to benefit the individual, then the act cannot be labeled as offence.

Thus, after a valid consent, if the patient dies on operation table, then the surgeon cannot be held guilty for the patients' death. IPC section 52 states that any act which is done with due care and attention is considered as an act done in good faith. Section 91 of IPC serves as a corollary to sections 87 to 89. It states that the exceptions contained in sections 87 to 89 do not extend to acts, which are offences independently of any harm, which they may cause to the person, giving consent.

Any medical procedure except physical examination requires a written consent.

Importance of Informed Consent

With advent of newer clinical treatments like biologics, it is safe to have a written consent before starting the scheduled treatment explaining in detail about the implications and interactions of the drug with the individual's immunity. It is vital to discuss about the pregnancy category of the drug, its wash out period, any side effects pertaining to sexuality or infertility and its risk/benefit ratio before starting any specific drug for any dermatoses (e.g., Cyclophosphamide, Rituximab, TNFα-antagonists, Secukinumab, etc.). It is crucial to take clinical digital photographs of individual at every visit before and after starting any treatment. Hence, the consent form must include the willingness of the patient for clinical photography and no objection consent for publishing the data on web. In hair restoration surgeries and other aesthetic surgeries, it is of utmost importance to discuss the pros/cons, risks/benefits, unforeseen complications, reversibility of side effects, expected results, failure rates, relapse rates in the consent form.

Types of Consent[32]

- *Implied consent:* It is a verbal consent and displays patient's will to express his clinical problems in front of the doctor which is sufficient for general physical and dermatological examination and routine bedside interventions.
- *Expressed consent:* It is a written consent which is imperative to be signed by both doctor and patient before any minor or major operative or cosmetic procedure.

Components of a Valid Consent Form

- *Patient specific details:* Age, sex, demographic data, and contact details of patient is mandatory. If patient is a minor (<18 years of age), then his/her guardian should sign the consent form.
- *Language:* Consent should be written in the language which is comprehended and known to the patient. It should be in a printed format. Where printing resources are not available, a good hand-written consent form with legible handwriting is acceptable.
- *Information disclosure:* The patient should be well informed about the risks involved, side effects and purpose of undergoing the diagnostic/therapeutic procedure **(Box 7)**.
- Date and time must be mentioned on the signed agreement.
- Signature of doctor and patient is compulsory as it indicates the voluntary free will of the patient to undergo the procedure.
- Details about the place should be mentioned along with contact details where the procedure is conducted.
- Medical registration number of practitioners is also required to be filled in the form.
- *Record keeping:* A signed consent copy in duplicate must be handed over to the patient whereas a scanned copy in EMR and hard copy must be stored for at least 3 years by the doctor.

CONCLUSION

Although, maintaining a good cordial relationship with the patient is important, written informed consent helps a clinician and an aesthetician work in a safe and secure environment. It makes sure that the patient is well informed about the procedure and it further reduces the chances of lawsuits and penalization of doctors.

REFERENCES

1. Swaminath G. Psychoeducation. Indian J Psychiatry. 2009;51:171-2.
2. Brown SW, Nelson A, Bronkesh SJ, Wood SD. Patient Satisfaction Pays: Quality Service for Practice Success. Maryland: Aspen Publication; 1993.
3. National Research Corporation. Voluntary Hospitals of America. Marketing Monitor. 1988. pp. 6.
4. MalickF, Howard J, Koo J. Understanding the psychology of the cosmetic patients. Dermatol Ther. 2008;21:47-53.
5. Elsaie ML. Psychological approach in cosmetic dermatology for optimum patient satisfaction. Indian J Dermatol. 2010; 55:127-9.
6. Prakash B. Patient satisfaction. J Cutan Aesthet Surg. 2010;3: 151-5.
7. Zirwas MJ, Holder JL. Patient education strategies in dermatology-Part 1: benefits and challenges. J Clin Aesthet Dermatol. 2009;2(12):24-7.
8. Goldberg DJ. Cosmetic dermatology: legal issues. Dermatol Clin. 2009;27(4):501-5.
9. Sacchidanand SA, Bhat S. Safe practice of cosmetic dermatology: avoiding legal tangles. J Cutan Aesthet Surg. 2012; 5(3):170-5.
10. Poulas GA, Brodell RT, Mostow EN. Improving quality and patient satisfaction in dermatology office practice. Arch Dermatol. 2008;144:263-5.
11. Zirwas MJ, Holder JL. Patient education strategies in dermatology--Part 2: methods. J Clin Aesthet Dermatol. 2009;2(12):28-34.
12. Thomas J. Medical records and issues in negligence. Indian J Urol. 2009;25(3):384-8.
13. University of Cambridge. History of medical record-keeping. [online] Available from: http://www.magicandmedicine.hps.cam.ac.uk/on-astrological-medicine/further-reading/history- of-medical-record-keeping. [Last Accessed May, 2021].
14. Medical Coding Degree. Medical Records: A Brief History. [online] Available from: http://medicalcodingdegree.org/medical-records-history/. [Last Accessed May, 2021].
15. Bali A, Bali D, Iyer N, Iyer M. Management of medical records: facts and figures for surgeons. J Maxillofac Oral Surg. 2011;10(3):199-202.
16. SNOMED CT. The Global Language of Healthcare. [online] Available from: http://www.snomed.org/snomed-ct. [Last Accessed May. 2021].
17. WHO. Classification of Diseases. [online] Available from: http://www.who.int/classifications/icd/en/. [Last Accessed May, 2021].
18. HL7 International. Health Level Seven International. [online] Available from: http://www.hl7.org/. [Last Accessed May, 2021].
19. HL7 India. Health Level Seven India. [online] Available from: http://www.hl7india.org/. [Last Accessed May, 2021].
20. HL7 International. FHIR DSTU2. [online] Available from: www.hl7.org/fhir. [Last Accessed May, 2021].
21. WHO. International Classification of Health Interventions (ICHI). [online] Available from: http://www.who.int/classifications/ichi/en/. [Last Accessed May, 2021].
22. NCPDP. [online] Available from: http://www.ncpdp.org/. [Last Accessed May, 2021].
23. HHS. Health Information Privacy. [online] Available from: https://www.hhs.gov/hipaa/. [Last Accessed May, 2021].
24. Electronic Medical Records Standards in India. [online] Available from: http://mohfw.nic.in/showfile.php?lid=4138. [Last Accessed May, 2021].
25. Mediverse Technologies LLP. Images. [online] Available from: https://www.mediverse.co.in. [Last Accessed May, 2021].
26. Shrivastava S, Shrivastava P, Ramaswamy J. Scope of consumer protection at in medical profession in India. J Clin Sci. 2014;11(1):25
27. Shaha KK, Patra AP, Das S. The importance of informed consent in medicine. Sch J App Med Sci. 2013;1(5):455-63.
28. Vakilno1. Guardians and Ward Act 1890. [online] Available from: http://www.Vakilno1.com/bareacts/guardiansandwardact/guardianwardsact.htm. [Last Accessed May, 2021].
29. Ratanlal, Dhirajlal. The Law of Torts, 25th edition. Nagpur: Wadhwa and Co.; 2006. pp. 75.
30. Section 9 of the Principal Act, subsection (1B). The Transplantation of Human Organs (Amendment Bill, 2011), Transplantation of Human Organs Act, 1994.
31. Universal Law Series: The Code of Criminal Procedures. Delhi: Universal Law Publishing; 1973. pp. 34-5.
32. Nirmal B, Sachchinadand SA. Informed consent in dermatology: what's known and what's new? Indian J Dermatol Venereol Leprol. 2014;80:58-61

CHAPTER 136

Evidence-based Medicine in Cutaneous and Aesthetic Surgery

Rashmi Sarkar, Suvarna Samudrala, Mysore Venkatram

KEY MESSAGES

- Evidence-based dermatology and dermatosurgery implies the judicious use of current best evidence and its integration with one's clinical expertise to optimize patient outcomes.
- In the hierarchy of evidence-based medicine (EBM), systematic surveys, meta-analyses and randomized controlled clinical trials (RCCTs) remain the gold standards of dependable evidence for therapeutic drugs and procedures.
- There has been a steady increase in the number of cosmetic procedures conducted both in India and worldwide, though many are being done in the absence of reliable scientific data.
- Lack of regulatory control over the standard protocols for procedures and the qualification and experience requirements for professionals offering these services, has resulted in a consumer-driven approach.
- Evidence based medicine helps to choose from a wide range of treatment options, by providing information regarding their scientific basis, efficacy, safety of each procedure.
- The Indian Association of Dermatologists, Venereologists and Leprologists (IADVL) Dermatosurgery Task Force has been instrumental in: (1) evaluation of available evidence for specific dermatosurgical and cosmetic procedures, and (2) formulation of standard guidelines of care for these procedures.

INTRODUCTION

Evidence-based medicine (EBM) is increasingly becoming more relevant in the field of dermatosurgery and aesthetics, due to the recent boom in cosmetic and aesthetic procedures worldwide. The rapid pace of technological advancements in the field, along with the lack of reliable scientific data makes it challenging for dermatologists to decide the appropriate line of management for their patients. Evidence-based medicine plays an important role in dermatosurgery and aesthetics, as it helps the dermatologist choose from a wide range of treatment options, by providing information regarding their scientific basis, efficacy, safety of each procedure. It also helps the patient to make an informed choice about undergoing a particular procedure, thus reducing the incidence of lawsuits filed. Therefore, there is an urgent need to understand and follow evidence-based practice by dermatologists, dermatosurgeons and aestheticians.

EVIDENCE-BASED MEDICINE

The term "evidence-based medicine" or "evidence-based practice" was defined as the conscientious, explicit, and judicious use of current best evidence in making clinical decisions about the care of individual patients".[1] The hierarchy of evidence starts with systematic reviews at the top with anecdotes and case reports at the bottom[2] **(Box 1)**.

The ideal study design depends on the question to be answered. Randomized controlled trials (RCTs), especially double-blind, offer the most reliable way of minimizing bias when trying to answer a question on efficacy of a drug or procedure for a disease.[3] Bias is defined as a systematic error that results in the incorrect interpretation of a study result. It may be deliberate (e.g., using a comparator drug at an inappropriate dose or frequency to make the new drug look better) or unavoidable (e.g., it is impossible to fully blind an RCT of oral retinoids compared to placebo).[5] For assessment of etiological association, cohort or case-control studies are best. Cohort studies are best suited to establishing the long-term outcome of a disease.

The critical steps in the performance of EBM are:[3]

- Generate answerable questions
- Track down the best available evidence
- Critically appraise the evidence for validity and usefulness
- Apply the results in clinical practice
- Evaluate the performance.

Two terms are highly relevant in context of EBM—"levels of evidence", which are based on study design and the methodology used, and "grades of recommendations",

BOX 1: Hierarchy of evidence in evidence-based medicine.

- Systematic reviews and meta-analyses of randomized controlled trials
- Randomized controlled trials
- Nonrandomized intervention studies
- Cohort studies
- Case series
- Case reports and expert opinion

BOX 2: Harbour and Miller's revised grading system for recommendations in evidence-based guidelines.[4]

Levels of evidence

- 1++ High-quality meta-analyses, systematic reviews of randomized controlled trials (RCTs) or RCTs with a very low risk of bias
- 1+ Well-conducted meta-analyses, systematic reviews of RCTs, or RCTs with a low risk of bias
- 1– Meta-analyses, systematic reviews or RCTs, or RCTs with a high risk of bias
- 2++ High-quality systematic reviews of case-control or cohort studies or high-quality case-control or cohort studies with a very low risk of confounding, bias, or chance and a high probability that the relationship is causal
- 2+ Well-conducted case-control or cohort studies with a low risk of confounding, bias, or chance and a moderate probability that the relationship is causal
- 2– Case-control or cohort studies with a high risk of confounding, bias, or chance and a significant risk that the relationship is not causal
- 3 Nonanalytic studies, e.g., case reports, case series
- 4 Expert opinion

Grades of recommendations

A. At least one meta-analysis, systematic review, or RCT rated as 1++ and directly applicable to the target population or a systematic review of RCTs or a body of evidence consisting principally of studies rated as 1+ directly applicable to the target population and demonstrating overall consistency of results
B. A body of evidence including studies rated as 2++ directly applicable to the target population and demonstrating overall consistency of results or extrapolated evidence from studies rated as 1++ or 1+
C. A body of evidence including studies rated as 2+ directly applicable to the target population and demonstrating overall consistency of results or extrapolated evidence from studies rated as 2++
D. Evidence level 3 or 4 or extrapolated evidence from studies rated as 2+

BOX 3: GRADE Working Group definitions in grading the quality of the evidence.[5]

High: Further research is very unlikely to change our confidence in the estimate of effect

Moderate: Further research is likely to have an important impact on our confidence in the estimate of effect and may change the estimate

Low: Further research is very likely to have an important impact on our confidence in the estimate of effect and is likely to change the estimate

Very low: Any estimate of effect is very uncertain

based on the strength of supporting evidence and includes the judgment of guideline developers.[3] Some of the recommendations include: Harbour and Miller's grading recommendations[4] **(Box 2)**, GRADE Working Group Grading System[5] **(Box 3)** and the Cochrane Skin Group.

Research evidence should be reviewed by assessing four key elements:

1. Study design
2. Study quality
3. Consistency
4. Directness.

NEED FOR ETHICAL GUIDELINES FOR AESTHETIC MEDICINE BASED ON EVIDENCE

There is a strong need to formulate and implement guidelines for dermatosurgery and aesthetic procedures. Those procedures which have a strong evidence-based proof of efficacy and safety are likely to be preferred by the practitioners and patients.

Anecdotal testimonials from patients and physicians are commonly used by cosmetic agencies to advertise their products and technologies. Patients surfing the internet often stumble onto websites prompting them to approach their dermatologists and cosmetologists to use the same for them. Enthusiastic dermatosurgeons are likely to give in to the pressure from the patient and often try these advertised products on willing patients. Further, the placebo effect may also convince the doctor and patient about the therapeutic benefit of the technique even though such results may not withstand scientific scrutiny by means of a controlled trial. The results of small poorly-controlled studies are often negated by larger well-planned controlled trials and hence the quality of evidence is of great importance before using these products.[3]

Many procedures such as mesotherapy, skin whitening injections, mechanized massages for cellulite treatment are being offered without any reliable scientific data. The existing large gap between evidence and consumer-driven practice by aestheticians has resulted in a loss of conventional pursuit of excellence and ethical responsibility in the practice of medicine.

This has also led to an alarming number of law-suits filed against medical practitioners by patients dissatisfied due to lack of benefit despite huge expenditures or due to sustenance of significant adverse effects. Therefore, appropriate guidelines are required for aesthetic procedures, based on the current available data and their level of evidence.

INCREASING SCOPE OF AESTHETIC PROCEDURES

According to the statistics collected by the Aesthetic Plastic Surgery National Databank, the overall number of cosmetic procedures performed in 2019 has increased since 2015.[6] Surgical procedures increased by more than 6.2%, and nonsurgical procedures increased by 13.3% in 2019. In 2019, surgical procedures accounted for 25% of the total number of procedures with nonsurgical procedures making up 75% of the total number of procedures.[6]

The top five cosmetic surgical procedures in 2019 were: breast augmentation, liposuction, breast lifts, tummy tuck, and eyelid surgery. The top five nonsurgical cosmetic procedures were: Botulinum toxin type A, hyaluronic acid fillers, laser hair removal, nonsurgical fat reduction, and photorejuvenation. Women contributed to 93% of the total number of cosmetic procedure patients; liposuction was the most commonly performed procedure in men and breast augmentation in women.[6] India ranks fifth in the world in terms of the number of aesthetic procedures performed with almost 900,000 surgical and nonsurgical procedures performed annually.[7] The recent boom in the demand for aesthetic procedures can be attributed to a number of reasons:[8]

- Increasing consciousness about self-image and the desire to prolong youthfulness
- Technological advances in the procedures and equipment resulting in increased safety profile and reduced downtime
- Improved spending capacity
- Peer pressure and the desire to look as good or "better" than contemporaries
- Media influence
- Emulation of celebrities' facial or bodily features
- High-pressure advertising by manufacturers of cosmetic devices and cosmeceuticals
- Aggressive promotion by medical practitioners as well as beauticians and other personnel involved in the cosmetic industry
- Lack of regulatory control over the standard protocols for procedures and the qualification and experience requirements for professionals offering these services.

Thus, unfortunately, dermatosurgical and cosmetic procedures are increasingly becoming consumer-driven. Pressures from the patients (sometimes called "consumers" or "clients" in cosmetic industry) and the profit margins to the practitioners from these procedures are leading to questionable practices and infringement of medical ethics.

COCHRANE COLLABORATION AND COCHRANE SKIN GROUP

The Cochrane Skin Group *(http://skin.cochrane.org)* was formed in 1997, for producing and updating reviews of trials relating to skin conditions and to produce the best possible evidence on the effectiveness of health care interventions for the same. The group has published many full reviews and a similar number of published protocols that have eventually become full reviews. To date, the CSG has over 100 Cochrane reviews covering various topics, ranging from efficacy of interventions to the safety of drugs. Cochrane reviews are published quarterly in an online product called the Cochrane Library *(www.cochranelibrary.com)*. The advantages of Cochrane reviews include: Periodic updating with availability of new evidence, and full and free access to the library in any part of the world including India. While some have criticized Cochrane reviews for always concluding that there is insufficient evidence to recommend anything, such conclusions are also helpful for the clinicians, in that it at least reassures us that we are not missing some new important finding about treatments that we should be using in practice.[2]

APPLICATION OF EBM IN AESTHETIC SURGERY

Cutaneous and aesthetic surgery is an exclusive specialty that links surgical outcomes with patient satisfaction. Dermatosurgeons have encompassed EBM and have conducted various surveys to determine the safety, efficacy and patient satisfaction scores. Questionnaires filled by both the surgeon and the patient about the procedure are evaluated for EBM. Surveys can be used to make descriptive affirmations about a population, employing multivariate analysis, and explorative research can be taken up to further enlighten the research topic.[9] For example, the Owsley Facelift Satisfaction Survey is a four-page survey (14 questions) espoused by Dr John Owsley, aimed at his superficial musculoaponeurotic system (SMAS)—platysma facelift technique. The survey asked patients to rate the improvement of their facial appearance at 1 year and 10–15 years after surgery.[10]

SURGICAL MYTHS AND BELIEFS VERSUS EVIDENCE-BASED MEDICINE: LESSONS LEARNT

History is replete with examples of well-meaning doctors causing harm to their patients because of their failure to conduct RCTs and then summarize those RCTs within systematic reviews. For example, although early reports of intralesional interferon (IFN) in basal cell carcinoma (BCC) were promising, later studies on larger populations showed variable cure results.[3] It was noted that studies reporting high cure rates had small duration of follow-up and excluded the severe varieties of the tumor.[11] Other examples include mutilating surgical excisions for primary cutaneous melanoma and radical vulvectomy for lichen sclerosus, which were practiced for decades, purely on the basis of anecdote and case reports and a failure to question the rationale for the treatments.[5]

Throughout medical training and clinical practice, many of our surgical tenets and practices are deep seated and believed to be evidence-based. It is often assumed that long-standing surgical techniques have been investigated in a controlled study, when they are no more than opinion. For example, it is commonly believed that local anesthetic solution of lidocaine on digits should never contain epinephrine as it will result in necrosis. However, substantial evidence now exists for the safe and more effective use of standard preparations of lidocaine and epinephrine in infiltrative and block anesthesia of the digits.[12,13]

Another example is the preoperative hair removal traditionally done to minimize postoperative surgical site infections (SSIs). However, evidence has shown no significant difference in the incidence of SSIs with or without hair removal. This was therefore dropped from the latest Centers for Disease Control and Prevention (CDC) guidelines.[14]

Similarly, resurfacing procedures were previously contraindicated in patients recently taking systemic retinoids. However, based on the recent evidence, the Association of Cutaneous Surgeons, India, has concluded that isotretinoin can be safely used with the surgical procedures with no effect on healing, although it is still reported in articles and textbooks (based on a very low level of evidence).[12]

FACTORS CONTRIBUTING TO PERCEIVED IMPROVEMENTS

Both physicians and patients can conclude that a treatment has worked for them, even if later it is shown not to be useful. This may be attributed to the following:

- *Natural resolution:* It refers to the natural history of some diseases to fluctuate or improve with time on their own, coinciding with the treatment. For example, treatments for alopecia areata or postsurgery hypertrophic scars may be labeled effective if not compared to a control group without treatment.
- *Regression to the mean:* The tendency of extreme values to move closer to the average on repeated measurement.
- Coincidental effects of treatment.
- *The placebo effect or treatment effect:* It may also be due to additional interventions given in addition to the placebo, observer bias, subsiding toxic effect of previous medication and patient bias (including patient politeness in front of the physician and experimental subordination).

The role of patients' expectations plays a strong role in their perception of treatment outcome, especially in aesthetic procedures.[3]

Few examples can be quoted here. Mesotherapy has continued to be practised despite no established evidence. The position paper by IADVL Task Force recommended that there is lack of evidence in the use of mesotherapy for dermatological indications, and this is true even today.

It has been advised that the length-to-width ratio for an elliptical excision should be at least 3:1 for the best cosmetic results, and to avoid dog ears. However, the current level of evidence shows that circular excisions can be done with smaller scars, and no risk of dog ears, resulting in improved cosmesis.[12]

Platelet rich plasma (PRP) is another modality which has gained popularity for management of hair loss; face lift (popularly known as the vampire lift), scar management and aging skin. While there are several papers that have suggested some efficacy, a recent blinded study suggested that there is no increase in hair counts and density.[15] More details can be found in the chapter on PRP. It is therefore important that this modality be studied properly, evaluated fully, and then adopted into routine practice.

APPLICATION OF EBM IN PRACTICE OF DERMATOSURGERY IN INDIA: IADVL DERMATOSURGERY TASK FORCE

The IADVL instituted the IADVL Dermatosurgery Task Force in 2006, with the objective of evaluating available evidence for the efficacy and safety of specific dermatosurgical or cosmetic procedures as well as publishing recommendations for standard guidelines of care for dermatosurgical procedures.[16-18] The task force framed standard guidelines of care for several dermatosurgical procedures, such as vitiligo surgery, electrosurgery, CO_2 laser, chemical peels, tumescent liposuction, botulinum toxin A, laser hair reduction, etc., and also a position paper that evaluated the available evidence for efficacy of mesotherapy. It concluded that *"acceptable scientific evidence for its (mesotherapy) effectiveness and safety is lacking. IADVL Task Force, therefore, would like to state that the use of this technique remains controversial at present. Further research and well-designed controlled scientific studies are required to substantiate the claims of benefit of this mode of therapy."*[19] Such efforts help in providing the practitioner and also patients an information about evidence available, minimum standards that need to be followed while performing such procedures and finally also provide a minimum reference framework for medicolegal situations.

FURTHER SCOPE

The concept of EBM has grown over the years. The current literature shows general agreement on the hierarchy of clinical trial design and the value of systematic reviews and meta-analysis but a divergence of opinions about optimal EBM rating schemes remains. Research also suggests that clinical practice guideline implementation studies are needed if their content is to be fully appreciated by practicing clinicians. The challenge is to ensure EBM continues to integrate individual clinical expertise with the best available external clinical evidence from high-quality research. Evidence-based dermatology is every clinical dermatologist's business. Patient and surgeon filled proformas and surveys can serve as a useful tool as double-blinded RCTs may be difficult to conduct in the field of dermatosurgery. To optimize treatment outcomes, we should not be afraid of challenging current practices and changing our practice in light of new knowledge, regardless of how experienced we become.

CONCLUSION

With more patients and third-party payers increasingly demanding evidence-based diagnostics and treatments, dermatologists must be aware of EBM, especially in the current era, where medical information is just "a mouse-click away".

Clinical judgment in an individual case management requires careful integration of personal experience, interactions with colleagues, and use of currently available and latest external evidence. The tenets of EBM hold that all evidence is not equal. Systematic surveys, meta-analyses and RCTs remain the gold standards of dependable evidence for therapeutic drugs and procedures. For treatments lacking such levels of evidence, outcome of uncontrolled trials or anecdotal reports may be considered; however, the possibility of instituting a useless or potentially harmful treatment always exists. In the field of cutaneous and aesthetic surgery, it is becoming increasingly difficult to find higher levels of evidence; most are level IV or V evidence, and hence surveys can be used. It is therefore important for physicians to counsel patients properly while adopting such treatments.

Periodically updating one's own knowledge bank through peer-reviewed journals and critical appraisal of medical literature will allow a more balanced use of all the information available to optimize patient care.

REFERENCES

1. Chi C. Evidence-based dermatology. Dermatologica Sin. 2013;31:2-6.
2. Williams H. Why is the center of evidence-based dermatology relevant to Indian dermatology? Indian J Dermatol. 2009;54: 118-23.
3. Berg D, Asgari M. Evidence-based medicine for dermatologic surgeons: concepts in critical appraisal of information. Dermatol Surg. 2001;27:511-4.
4. Harbour R, Miller J. A new system for grading recommendations in evidence-based guidelines. BMJ. 2001;323:334-6.
5. GRADE Working Group. Grading quality of evidence and strength of recommendations. BMJ. 2004;328:1490.
6. The Aesthetic Society. Aesthetic Plastic Surgery National Data Bank Statistics. (2019). [Online] Available from: https://www.surgery.org/sites/default/files/Aesthetic-Society_Stats2019Book_FINAL.pdf. [Last Accessed May, 2021].
7. ISAPS. (2018). Global Survey on Aesthetic/Cosmetic Procedures Performed in 2018. [Online] Available from: https://www.isaps.org/wp-content/uploads/2019/12/ISAPS-Global-Survey-2018-Press-Release-English. [Last Accessed May, 2021].
8. Rana A. 9 cosmetic procedures getting popular in India. The Statesman [Internet]. 2019
9. Alderman AK, Salem B. Survey research. Plast Reconstr Surg. 2010;126(4):1381-9.
10. Pusic A, Klassen AF, Scott AM, Cano SJ. The measure of face-lift patient satisfaction: the Owsley facelift satisfaction survey with a long-term follow-up study. Plast Reconstr Surg. 2010;126(1):258-60.
11. Anasagasti-Angulo L, Garcia-Vega Y, Barcelona-Perez S, Lopez-Saura P, Bello-Rivero I. Treatment of advanced, recurrent, resistant to previous treatments basal and squamous cell skin carcinomas with a synergistic formulation of interferons. Open, prospective study. BMC Cancer. 2009;9:262.
12. Bruce AM, Spencer JM. Surgical myths in dermatology. Dermatol Surg. 2010;36:512-7.
13. Ilicki J. Safety of epinephrine in digital nerve blocks: a literature review. J Emerg Med. 2015;49(5):799-809.
14. Müller CS, Hubner W, Thieme-Ruffing S, Pföhler C, Vogt T, Volk T, et al. Pre- and perioperative aspects of dermatosurgery. J Dtsch Dermatol Ges. 2017;15(2):117-46.
15. Puig CJ, Reese R, Peters M. Double-blind, placebo-controlled pilot study on the use of platelet rich plasma in women with female androgenetic alopecia. Dermatol Surg. 2016;42(11): 1243-7.
16. Sacchidanand S. IADVL dermatosurgery guidelines: charting uncharted territory. Indian J Dermatol Venereol Leprol. 2008;74:4.
17. Mysore V. Guest editor's remarks. Indian J Dermatol Venereol Leprol. 2008;74:3.
18. Mysore V. Guest editor's remarks. Indian J Dermatol Venereol Leprol. 2009;75:65-6.
19. Sarkar R, Garg VK, Mysore V. Position paper on mesotherapy. Indian J Dermatol Venereol Leprol. 2011;77:232-7.

CHAPTER 137

Training Opportunities in Dermatologic Surgery

Kanika Sahni, Nikhil Mehta

KEY MESSAGES

- Dermatosurgery is one of the subspecialties of dermatology which has made great progress and has the potential to become a superspecialty.
- Dermatosurgery is a specialized subject with the need for special skills and overlaps with plastic surgery to an extent. A structured training and certification are therefore highly essential to establish this subject.
- Almost all procedures under dermatosurgery are outpatient-based surgeries. They do not need hospital admissions; hence, they also avoid the stress and infection risk associated with a hospital admission.

INTRODUCTION

For a dermatology resident, the best time to start training in dermatologic surgery is the day of joining the residency. The second best time is perhaps when she/he realizes the importance of this training. To pursue any kind of training beyond residency, it is imperative that the fundamentals of dermatologic surgery are correctly established during the residency itself. This entails correctly imbibing all the teachings during the residency. Before jumping to fillers, botulinum toxin injections, and hair transplants, it is useful to understand the principles of paring, intralesional injections, minor radiofrequency ablations, punch biopsies and excisions, etc. The former might rarely be practiced in universities, while the latter procedures are routinely performed, often by the junior most of the residents, and unfortunately rarely with the due diligence they deserve. Despite having the same duration and workload of posting in minor procedures, a trainee eager to learn will obviously understand procedures significantly more than one biding her/his time. One can maximize benefits from minor procedure postings by reading thoroughly before and after the procedures, planning the procedures adequately, observing experienced seniors performing them, watching videos of ideal procedures, and following up one's own patients. For example, a resident just observing a procedure like injecting triamcinolone intralesionally a few times and then doing it on other patients will definitely be less skilled than another resident, who after observing it reads about the ideal method of performing it, watches videos of ideal procedure and its variations, indications for it, ideal plane of injection and site of insertion, concentration and volume required, expected response from studies using it as monotherapy, suitable procedures to combine it with, modifications for special situations, etc.

When faced with problems like intolerable pain in patients, leakage of triamcinolone solution from the junction of the needle and the syringe tube, difficulty in loading the triamcinolone, etc., a resident who consistently seeks solution to any such problems through searching textbooks, articles, and asking from seniors, and observes for changes after attempting such solution, will learn more than those who do not even think that other people might have faced similar problems or a change in approach might be needed. A problem-solving attitude, analytic mind throughout the procedures, frequent tinkering and observing for the best response, trial of ideas of others and oneself, and an innovative approach are helpful in maximizing the opportunities of training offered during residency. These good practices develop into good habits later on. They build confidence and train to handle and manage patients. They should be adopted with a positive attitude irrespective of the facilities and the quality of training available at the resident's center. Also, institutes need to encourage learning in dermatologic surgery during residency, as it constitutes a significant unmet need in dermatology.[1] A formal practical examination as a part of the residency-qualifying examination is a good way to provide emphasis to dermatologic surgery during residency.[2]

To reiterate, the earliest training opportunity for a resident to learn dermatologic surgery is during the residency itself, by establishing strong fundamentals. Many reasons may preclude a resident to train optimally during the residency, including lack of various facilities, different priorities during residency, lack of focus on procedural dermatology during residency, etc. However, as mentioned before, it is never too late to catch up and learn. The various ways to learn after residency include through various workshops and conferences, resource materials, observerships and fellowships, further training by working under established dermatosurgeons, and obviously through practice. The learning does not stop till the desire for improvement persists.

WORKSHOPS AND CONFERENCES

There are multiple state, regional, national, and international workshops and conferences held regularly on the topic of dermatologic surgery, including a separate domain of aesthetic dermatological surgeries. These yield maximum exposure to procedures in the shortest time. Apart from this, conferences based on specific domains offer training in procedures for diseases in that domain. For example, a conference focused on acne usually has talks and demonstrations of various acne procedures. Similarly, vitiligo conferences include workshops on vitiligo surgeries, and ONYCHOCON has workshops, including cadaveric workshops, on nail surgeries. Apart from this, the broad state, national, and international conferences including state CUTICONs, national DERMACON, World Congress of Dermatology, etc., respectively, have procedural workshops, either on separate days or running parallelly with the rest of the conference. In addition, the Indian Association of Dermatologists, Venereologists and Leprologists (IADVL) Special Interest Groups (SIGs) on dermatosurgery and lasers frequently conduct procedural workshops aimed at teaching postgraduates. Some of these conferences are summarized in **Table 1**. This list is by no means exhaustive and is ever expanding, considering the rapidly evolving field of dermatologic surgery.

Most of them do not offer a hands-on experience but offer good introduction to various procedures which one might not have seen before. For people already performing the procedures, such conferences offer places to finetune and improve the skills, pick up pearls, tips and tricks to improve the procedures, and discuss ways to counter the unique problems faced in special situations.

RESOURCE MATERIALS

While reading this book, you are utilizing a precious well-illustrated resource, well supplemented with step-by-step images and videos of the procedures. Similarly, various other resource materials include videos of various procedures in the Association of Cutaneous Surgeons of India (ACSI) and IADVL websites (accessible only to members), certifiable online courses by SIG Dermatosurgery and SIG Lasers on the IADVL website, various videos by various centers available freely on YouTube or their own websites, social media including IADVL Facebook group, and various interventional

TABLE 1: Various conferences offering workshops and sessions on procedural dermatology.

Conference	*Level*	*Frequency*
Conferences dedicated to procedural dermatology		
ASDS	International	Annual
DASIL World Congress	International	Annual
National Conference of ACSI: ACSICON	National	Annual
Annual Workshop on Aesthetic Procedures by the Delhi Aesthetic Education Group: Aestheticon	National	Annual
Annual Congress of Cosmetic Dermatology Society India: COSDERMINDIA	National	Annual
Broad conferences having surgical workshops		
World Congress of Dermatology	International	Once every 4 years
AAD annual meeting	International	Annual
BAD annual meeting	International	Annual
EADV Congress	International	Annual
DERMACON	National	Annual
MID-DERMACON	National	Annual
CUTICONs of various states	State	Annual
DAAS summit	National	Annual
Stalwarts of Dermatology Congress	Various	–
Domain/disease-specific conferences with related procedural workshops		
Various vitiligo CMEs, conducted around vitiligo day (June 25, 2023), have vitiligo surgery-focused workshops	Various	At least annual
ONYCHOCON—has nail surgery-focused workshops	National	Annual
FUE Asia	International	–

(AAD: American Academy of Dermatology; ACSI: Association of Cutaneous Surgeons of India; ASDS: American Society for Dermatologic Surgery; BAD: British Association of Dermatologists; DAAS: Dermatology and Allied Sciences; DASIL: Dermatology, Aesthetics, and Surgery International League; EADV: European Academy of Dermatology and Venereology; CME: continuous medical education) and procedural dermatology-based WhatsApp and Telegram mobile application-based groups. These resources represent a do-it-yourself (DIY) form of training and cannot replace hands-on training but can definitely supplement it.

OBSERVERSHIPS AND FELLOWSHIPS

Various organizations, including American Society of Dermatologic Surgery (ASDS), the Dermatology, Aesthetics, and Surgery International League (DASIL), IADVL, and individual centers offer preceptorships, observerships, and fellowships. Some of them entail a fee, and only few of them have hands-on training. Some of these are summarized in **Table 2**.

WORKING UNDER/WITH OTHER DERMATOSURGEONS

Many dermatologic surgeons do not offer any formal accredited or certifiable observership program or fellowship course, but frequently work with and train juniors and budding dermatosurgeons in a more informal manner. The dynamics of such an arrangement may range from apprenticeship to partnership. No specific certificate of training is needed over the residency degree to perform most dermatosurgical procedures; rather, it is the skill which matters. Good interpersonal relationship skills are useful to establish these informal arrangements.

TABLE 2: Some of the international and national centers/organizations offering dermatologic surgery and/or aesthetics fellowships.

Sponsoring organization	*Country*	*Centers/Doctors*	*Program and duration*	*Eligibility*
ASDS and DASIL	USA	• Variable • Established through the Lawrence M Field, MD, International Dermatologic Surgery Educational Exchange Fund[3]	International Preceptorship Program (1–3 weeks)	• International dermatologic surgeons (i.e., not American or Canadian, and not residents-in-training) practicing full time in an academic institution or private practice • Current member of the ASDS or another internationally recognized dermatologic surgery organization
	Saudi Arabia	Salman AlSaad, MD	ITMP[4] (Up to 4 weeks)	Considered hosts must be an ASDS or other member. Be in an authoritative position in dermatologic surgery at a hosting institution
	USA	• Brett Coldiron, MD • Terrence Cronin, MD • Roberto L Davila-DePedro, MD • Daniel Eisen, MD • Michael Gold, MD • Patrick Lillis, MD • Peter J Panagotacos, MD • Thomas Rohrer, MD • Christine H Weinberger, MD		
	Indonesia	• Khairuddin Djawad, MD • Moerbono Mochtar, MD • Chadijah Rifai, MD • Indah Julianto, MD, PhD		
	Canada	Sahar Ghannam, MD		
	India	• Somesh Gupta, MD • Nilesh N Goyal, MD,		
	Germany	• Michael Haeberle, MD • Eckart Haneke, MD, PhD • Mark Tanner, MD		
	Hungary	Istvan Juhász, MD		
	Netherlands	Gertruud Kreckels, MD		
	Israel	• Marina Landau, MD • Isaac Zilinsky, MD		
	Romania	Mihaela Leventer, MD		

Contd...

Contd...

Sponsoring organization	*Country*	*Centers/Doctors*	*Program and Duration*	*Eligibility*
	Dubai	• Mahaveer Mehta, MD • Syed AA Shah, FRCP (UK), CCST (UK)		
	UK	Richard J Motley, FRCP		
	Greece	Constantine Noutsis, MD, PhD		
	South Africa	Derek Odendaal, MD Marc B Roscher, MD		
	Brazil	Ramos-e-Silva, MD, PhD		
	Philippines	Manalo-Manuel Remedios, MD		
	South Korea	Ki Hoon Song, MD		
	Thailand	C Treewittayapoom, MD		
NYU Langone's Health	USA	Skin and Cancer Unit of the Ronald O Perelman, Department of Dermatology at NYU Langone Ambulatory Care Center, and faculty practice of Jerry Shapiro, MD[5]	International Observership Program in Dermatology (1 month)	Completed documented formal training in dermatology at least equivalent to a residency or in another subspecialty or area of interest relevant to the practice of dermatology, such as public health or infectious disease
Cleveland clinic	USA	Dermatology and Plastic Surgery Institute, Center for International Medical Education[6]	International Physician Observership Program (1 month)	• Fully trained international practicing physicians and specialists • International residents, fellows, and medical students currently enrolled in a residency/fellowship program at a foreign institution and who are expected to graduate from that same school/institution
MD2B Connect	USA	St Louis, Missouri[7]	Outpatient Externship in Dermatology	IMGs and students seeking hands-on patient care experience in dermatology
Massachusetts General Hospital	USA	International Patient Center at Massachusetts General Hospital[8]	International Observership Program (1–3 months)	Practicing physicians with MD, PhD, or MBBS degree. Medical students or graduates are not eligible to apply
Wake Forest School of Medicine	USA	Dr Rita Pichardo-Geisinger, MD, Department of Dermatology[9]	International Dermatology Fellowship Program (6 months to 1 year)	International dermatology residents or dermatology graduates
National Skin Centre	Singapore	National Skin Centre[10]	Clinical Hands-On Fellowship (3–12 months)	A recognized basic degree in medicine and traineeship or specialist degree in dermatology
Seoul National University Hospital	Korea	Dr Dong Hun Lee, Department of Dermatology[11]	Short-term Visiting Fellowship Program (2–4 weeks)	Dermatologists
Mahidol University	Thailand	Department of Dermatology at Faculty of Medicine, Siriraj Hospital[12]	Clinical fellowship in dermatologic surgery (1 year)	Dermatologist, MSc in Dermatology
Rajiv Gandhi University of Health Sciences	India (Bengaluru)	• Bangalore Medical College and Research Institute[13] • Cutis Academy of Cutaneous Sciences[14] • Kempegowda Institute of Medical Sciences • St John's Medical College[15] • Venkat Charmalaya[16]	Dermatosurgery, Aesthetic Dermatology, Lasers (6 months to 1 year); Hair Transplantation (1–2 weeks)	• MD/DVD/DNB in Dermatology • 3 years' experience • DM/MCH/DNB in concerned specialty • Plastic surgeons (preferably with 2 years of professional experience after postgraduation)
Maharashtra University of Health Sciences	India	Institute of Skin Cosmetology and Lasers, Solapur	Basic Phototherapy and Lasers (1 year)	MD, DNB, or DVD in Dermatology, Venereology, and Leprosy

Contd...

Contd...

Sponsoring organization	*Country*	*Centers/Doctors*	*Program and Duration*	*Eligibility*
DY Patil University	India	Dr Shrilata Suresh Trasi, Dr Pradeep Sethi, Mumbai[17]	Fellowship in Cosmetology (6 months), Hair Transplant (1 year)	MD or Diploma in Dermatology
Datta Meghe Institute of Medical Sciences	India	Jawaharlal Nehru Medical College and AVBRH	Fellowship in Dermatosurgery	MD/DNB in Dermatology
JIPMER	India	JIPMER[18]	Lasers and Dermatosurgery (1 year)	MD/DNB in Dermatology
Christian Medical College	India	Department of Dermatology[19]	Postdoctoral Fellowship in Dermatosurgery (1 year)	MD/DNB in Dermatology
IADVL	India	• Dr Chiranjiv Chhabra and Dr Kavish Chouhan, New Delhi • Dr Dasika Subba Rao, Eluru • Dr Sachin Varma, Kolkata • Dr Sumit Sharma, Panipat	Training course in procedural dermatology (3 months)[20]	Candidates who have obtained their MD or Diploma or DNB in Dermatology
IADVL	India	• Dr Yogesh M, Surat • Dr Suruchi Garg, Chandigarh • Dr Parmjit Singh Walia, Mohali • Dr Muhammed Razmi, Calicut • Dr Debjit Kar, Odisha • Dr Mahendra Deora, Pune • Dr Sumit Gupta, Lucknow • Dr Koushik Lahiri, Kolkata • Dr Vishalakshi Viswanath, Thane • Dr Subrata Malakar, Kolkata • Dr Rohit Bansal, Chandigarh • Dr Madhavi Pudi, Hyderabad • Dr JK Sadana, Patiala • Dr Sachin Varma, Kolkata • Dr Sumit Sharma, Panipat • Dr Imran Majid, Srinagar	Dermatosurgery, Aesthetic Dermatology, Lasers, Phototherapy, Phlebology, Hair Transplant (2–4 weeks)[21]	Candidates who have obtained their MD or Diploma or DNB in Dermatology
ACS(I)	India	• Dr Dhanashree Bhide, Dr Pradyumna Vaidhya, Pune • Dr Imran Majid, Srinagar • Dr Jaishree Sharad, Mumbai • Dr Koushik Lahiri, Kolkata • Dr Niteen Dhepe, Pune • Dr Niti Khunger, New Delhi • Dr Raj Kirit, Dr Rajyalakshmi, Hyderabad • Dr Venkataram Mysore, Bengaluru	Training Observerships in Dermatosurgery, Laser Surgery, and Cosmetic Dermatology (2–4 weeks)[22]	Life members of the ACS(I) who are not working in the same institution and who have completed their degree or diploma

(ACS(I): Association of Cutaneous Surgeons of India; ASDS: American Society of Dermatologic Surgery; AVBRH: Acharya Vinoba Bhave Rural Hospital; CCST: Certificate of Completion of Specialty Training; DASIL: Dermatologic, Aesthetics, and Surgery International League; FRCP: Fellowship of the Royal College of Physicians; IADVL: Indian Association of Dermatologists, Venereologists, and Leprologists; IMG: International Medical Graduate; ITMP: International Traveling Mentorship Program; JIPMER: Jawaharlal Institute of Postgraduate Medical Education and Research; NYU: New York University)

CONCLUSION

Many ways and opportunities exist for training in dermatologic surgery, and their number is slowly increasing, along with the realization of the unmet need of dermatologic surgery in India and the world. They exist for all stages of a dermatosurgeon's career, from the residency level to consultants wanting to upskill. We hope that this chapter will serve as a ready reckoner for anyone needing information about various workshops and conferences, resource materials, and observerships and fellowships available for training in dermatologic surgery.

REFERENCES

1. Mehta N, Sharma A, Sindhuja T, Dudani P, Sahni K, Khanna N, et al. Procedural dermatology and its unmet need. Indian J Dermatol Venereol Leprol. 2023;89(6):807-18.
2. Mehta N, Dudani P, Sahni K, Gupta S. Procedural dermatology evaluation for residents: A system in progress. Indian J Dermatol Venereol Leprol. 2023;89(4):640-2.
3. American Society for Dermatologic Surgery. International Preceptorship Program. [online] Available from https://www.asds.net/medical-professionals/education/international-dermatologists/international-preceptorship-program [Last accessed March, 2024].

4. American Society for Dermatologic Surgery. International Traveling Mentorship Program. [online] Available from https://www.asds.net/medical-professionals/education/international-dermatologists/international-traveling-mentorship-program [Last accessed March, 2024].
5. NYU Langone Health. International Observership Program in Dermatology. [online] Available from https://med.nyu.edu/departments-institutes/dermatology/education/international-observership [Last accessed March, 2024].
6. Cleveland Clinic Center for International Medical Education. International Physician Observership Program. [online] Available from https://my.clevelandclinic.org/departments/international-medical-education/international-programs/physician-observer [Last accessed March, 2024].
7. MD2B Connect Dr Samir Desai [Internet]. Outpatient externship in dermatology. [online] Available from https://www.md2bconnect.com/st-louis-dermatology [Last accessed March, 2024].
8. Massachusetts General Hospital. International Observership Program. [online] Available from https://www.massgeneral.org/education/international-observership [Last accessed March, 2024].
9. Wake Forest School of Medicine. International Dermatology Fellowship Program. [online] Available from https://school.wakehealth.edu/education-and-training/residencies-and-fellowships/international-dermatology-fellowship#:~:text=A%20six%2Dmonth%20or%20one,the%20needs%20of%20the%20fellow [Last accessed March, 2024].
10. National Skin Centre. Clinical Hands On. [online] Available from https://www.nsc.com.sg/Education-Training/Doctors-Attachment/Overseas-Doctors/Pages/default.aspx.
11. Seoul National University Hospital. Department of Dermatology. [online] Available from http://www.snuh.org/upload/global/common/Dermatology.pdf.
12. Mahidol University, Faculty of Medicine, Siriraj Hospital. Applying for Clinical Fellowship in Dermatologic Surgery. [online] Available from https://www2.si.mahidol.ac.th/en/dermatology/clinical_fellowship_training_program_in_dermatologic_surgery/ [Last accessed March, 2024].
13. Bangalore Medical College and Research Institute. Fellowship Programme. [online] Available from https://bmcribengaluru.karnataka.gov.in/storage/pdf-files/OfficialMemorandumregardingSelectionofVariousFellowshipCoursesfortheacademicyear 2023-24.pdf [Last accessed March, 2024].
14. Cutis. Fellowship. Available from https://www.cutis.org.in/fellowship/[Last accessed March, 2024].
15. St. John's National Academy of Health Sciences. Fellowship Programmes for Post Graduates. [online] Available from https://stjohnsadmissions.in/fellowship-courses [Last accessed March, 2024].
16. The Venkat Center. Training At the Venkat Center. [online] Available from https://www.venkatcenter.com/?s=Training+At+The+Venkat+Center [Last accessed March. 2024].
17. DY Patil University. Fellowship in Cosmetology. [online] Available from https://dypatil.edu/programs/fellowship-programs/medicine/school-of-medicine/fellowship-in-cosmetology [Last accessed March, 2024].
18. Jawaharlal Institute of Postgraduate Medical Education and Research. (2019). The post doctoral fellowship (PDF) course. [online] Available from https://jipmer.edu.in/sites/default/files/Fellowship%20Prospectus%202019%20final_0.pdf [Last accessed March, 2024].
19. Christian Medical College. Prospectus Admissions 2021-2022. [online] Available from https://www.cmcludhiana.in/REGISTRAR_UG/Files/BPT/BPTProspectus2022.pdf [Last accessed [March, 24].
20. Indian Association of Dermatologists Venereologists and Leprologists. Announcement inviting applications for IADVL Training Course- 2024. [online] Available from https://www.iadvl.org/announcements.php?AnnouncementId=6555a4f8efa07007d15ca612[Last accessed March, 2024].
21. Indian Association of Dermatologists Venereologists and Leprologists. Announcement inviting applications for IADVL Observerships 2023. [online] Available from https://www.iadvl.org/announcements.php?AnnouncementId=637b0ddeefa07022c13ece92 [Last accessed March, 2024].
22. Association of Cutaneous Surgeons. Training Observerships. [online] Available from https://www.acsinet.net/observership.php#:~:text=Applicants%20above%2045%20years%20can,from%20the%20association%20to%20candidates. [Last accessed March, 2024].

CHAPTER 138 Suppliers' Details for Laser Machines, Dermatosurgical, and Aesthetic Equipment/Products

Ankur Talwar, Kshama Talwar, Suresh Talwar, Rachita Talwar

KEY MESSAGES

- Supplier details for commonly used products in aesthetic dermatology like botulinum toxin, dermal fillers, skin boosters, chemical peels, lipolytic agents and polydioxanone (PDO) threads.
- Distributors of different models of dermoscopes in India.
- Supplier of different dermatosurgical instruments in India.
- Different models of laser machines and their suppliers for India.

INTRODUCTION

Details of various companies supplying laser machines, surgical equipment, and aesthetic machines/products are appended below. This may not be a complete list; however, it will serve as a guideline for procuring various equipment and instruments.

DISTRIBUTORS OF BOTULINUM TOXIN

Allergan, Inc., USA: Brand name: BOTOX

- Onabotulinum toxin
- 900 kD molecular weight
- 24–36 months shelf life
- Spray-dried powder
- 7.4 pH

Galderma: Brand name: DYSPORT

- Abobotulinum toxin
- 500–900 kD molecular weight
- 24 months shelf life
- Freeze-dried powder
- 7.4 pH

Merz Pharma: Brand name: XEOMIN

- Incobotulinum toxin
- 150 kD molecular weight
- 36 months shelf life
- Freeze-dried powder
- 7.4 pH

Dr Reddy's Laboratories: Brand name: Nabota

- Prabotulinum toxin
- 900 kD molecular weight
- 36 months shelf life
- Vacuum-dried powder

Gufic Biosciences: Brand name: STUNNOX

- This product has been indigenously developed in India.
- Manufactured in collaboration with the United States (US)-based Prime Bio
- Also available under the brand name ZARBOT, marketed to neurologists

Aakaar Medical Technologies: Brand name: SIAX

- Botulinum toxin type A—product of Medy-Tox Inc., South Korea
- Lyophilized white powder for injection in a colorless transparent vial
- Store at –15 ~ –5°C or at 2 ~ 8°C in a refrigerator.

SKIN BOOSTERS IN DERMATOLOGY

JUVÉDERM VOLITE: Product of Allergan Inc.

- Cross-linked injectable HA (hyaluronic acid) developed using Vycross technology
- Containing butanediol diglycidyl ether (BDDE) as a cross-linker
- HA concentration (mg mL^{-1}): 12 mg/mL
- 1 mL prefilled syringe; 0.05 mL per injection is given.

RESTYLANE-VITAL: Product of Galderma Inc.

- Non-animal stabilized HA (NASHA) technology
- HA concentration (mg mL^{-1}): 20 mg/mL

RESTYLANE-VITAL LIGHT: Product of Galderma Inc.

- Contains lower concentration of HA
- HA concentration (mg mL^{-1}): 12 mg/mL

PROFILHO: Product of Alma Medicals

- Made using hybrid NAHYCO Technology
- Mix of both high molecular weight and low molecular weight HA
- HA concentration (mg mL^{-1}): 32 mg/mL
- Prefilled syringe of 2 mL

PRINCESS RICH/SAYPHA RICH: Marketed by Aakaar Medical Technologies

- Contains 18 mg/mL of hyaluronic acid and 20 mg/mL of glycerol
- Available as one syringe of 1 mL

BELOTERO HYDRO: Marketed by Merz Aesthetics

- Combines non-crosslinked HA with glycerol
- Highly concentrated hyaluronic acid in the amount of 18 mg/mL.

DEFINISSE HYDROBOOSTER: Marketed by Menarini

- Non-crosslinked HA with glycerol
- 18 mg/mL HA+ 20 mg/mL glycerol
- 1 mL glass syringe

DISTRIBUTORS OF DERMAL FILLERS

Restylane range of dermal fillers: Product of Galderma Inc.

- *Restylane® LYFT:* Suited for lifting the cheeks, enhancing the jawline or chin
- *Restylane® DEFYNE:* Preferred for thinner tissue coverage as it is slightly softer and more flexible.
- *Restylane® REFYNE:* Softer and more flexible dermal filler for treatment of more dynamic areas of your face, like around the lips, the nasolabial folds and the marionette lines.
- *Restylane® VOLYME:* Create volume and softness in your face, to enhance your cheeks or lips, or to regain volume lost with age.
- *Restylane® KYSSE:* Create perfect and full lips.
- *Restylane® EYELIGHT:* Targeted filler for the treatment of the tear trough area.

JUVÉDERM range of dermal Fillers: Product of Allergan Inc.

- *JUVÉDERM VOLUX XC* injectable gel is for deep injection to improve moderate-to-severe loss of jawline definition in adults.
- *JUVÉDERM VOLUMA XC* injectable gel is for deep injection in the cheek area to correct age-related volume loss and for augmentation of the chin region.
- *JUVÉDERM VOLLURE XC, JUVÉDERM® Ultra Plus XC, and JUVÉDERM Ultra XC* injectable gels are for injection into the facial tissue for the correction of moderate-to-severe facial wrinkles and folds, such as nasolabial folds.
- *JUVÉDERM Ultra XC* injectable gel is also for injection into the lips and perioral area for lip augmentation.
- *JUVÉDERM VOLBELLA XC* injectable gel is for injection into the lips for lip augmentation and correction of perioral lines, and for injection into the under-eye hollows to improve the appearance of under-eye hollows.

BELOTERO range of Dermal Fillers: Product of Merz Aesthetics Inc.

- *BELOTERO SOFT:* Belotero Soft ensures the optimal correction and smoothening of fine lines due to its excellent cohesivity.
- *BELOTERO BALANCE:* Belotero Balance integrates seamless into the skin and is designed for the correction of moderate lines and wrinkles.
- *BELOTERO INTENSE:* Belotero Intense fills deep lines and is optimal for lip augmentation treatments.
- *BELOTERO VOLUME:* Belotero Volume models and restores facial volumes through its outstanding malleability and powerful volumizing capacity.

DEFINISSE range of Dermal Fillers: Marketed by Menarini

- *DEFINISSE TOUCH filler:* Indicated to correct moderate-to-severe facial wrinkles and folds. It can also be used to increase lip volume.
- *DEFINISSE RESTORE:* Indicated for correction of deeper wrinkles and folds, increase or restore facial volume and remodel facial contours.
- *DEFINISSE CORE* filler is intended for facial tissue augmentation in order to correct midface volume deficit, for restoring facial volume and shaping the contours of the face.

SAYPHA (FORMERLY PRINCESS) Range of Fillers: Marketed by Aakaar Medical Technologies

- SAYPHA FILLER
- SAYPHA VOLUME
- SAYPHA VOLUME PLUS

ART FILLER: By FILLMED LABORATORIES. Marketed by Aesthetics Zone Inc., New Delhi in India

- *ART FILLER® FINE LINES:* Fine lines
- *ART FILLER® UNIVERSAL:* Medium to deep wrinkles, lips
- *ART FILLER® VOLUME:* Volume

MONALISA range of Fillers

- *SOFT:* Facial wrinkles, Tear trough
- *MILD:* Perioral lines, Cheek volume, Forehead lines
- *HARD:* Forehead volume, Nasolabial fold, Chin and Facial oval
- *ULTRA:* Nasal augmentation, Chin and Facial oval

POLYDIOXANONE THREADS SUPPLIERS IN INDIA

- *AESTHETICS ZONE, New Delhi:* Supplier of Mint polydioxanone (PDO) threads:
- *UNITY DERMA, Bengaluru:* Supplier of Honey Derma Thread
- *MENARINI DERM:* Definisse Threads/Happy Lift
- *AAKAAR MEDICAL TECHNOLOGIES:* Alfa Aqulift Threads

LIPOLYTIC AGENTS SUPPLIERS IN INDIA

GEOLYSIS: Marketed by Geosmatic Cosmeceuticals

- Contains deoxycholic acid
- 3 vials × 5 mL

INNO TDS DRAINING PPC: Marketed by Aakaar Medical Technologies

- Made from phosphatidylcholine
- Comes in a 25-mL vial

CHEMICAL PEELS DISTRIBUTORS IN INDIA

Sesderma

Sesderma range of chemical peels

Dolphin Skin Solutions

Chemical peels

Spectra Medical India Private Limited

- Chemical peels from MESOESTETIC, Spain.
- *Dermamelan:* Dermamelan mask, Dermamelan treatment, degreasing lotion.
- *Cosmelan:* Cosmelan-1 cream, Cosmelan-2 cream, degreasing lotion, and hydrovital factor K.

Ethicare Remedies

- IPEEL
- IPEEL Enhancer

Geosmatic Cosmeceuticals and Cosmocare

Chemical peels from SIMILDIET Laboratories

ASAP Medical, New Delhi

- DERMAQUEST range of chemical peels
- BIOREE Peel (TCA) from CMED aesthetics

Aakaar Medical Technologies

- Inno Exfo Lightening Yellow Peel: Made in Spain by Innoaesthetics
- THERADERM range of chemical peels

DERMAINDIA/LAZHORA Inc.
Zhora range of chemical peels

COSDERMA PRIVATE LIMITED, MUMBAI
Cosderma melano pack, melano pack yellow peel cream exfoliating lightening cream, carbon gel Nd:YAG laser carbon peel, Cosderma black peel for acne, Cosderma melano pack yellow peel retinol peel, and retinol yellow peel

SOL DERMA PHARMACEUTICALS PRIVATE LIMITED

Chemical peels range from Amaira Aesthetics

RADIUS HEALTHCARE PRIVATE LIMITED, AHMEDABAD
Le Dore range of chemical peels

DERMATOSCOPE DISTRIBUTORS IN INDIA

DERMLITE RANGE: Distributed by Timpac Healthcare

- DermLite Cam
- DermLite DL1, DermLite DL200, DermLite DL3/DL4
- DermLite FOTO System, DermLite Foto II Pro

HEINE RANGE: Distributed by Timpac Healthcare

- DELTA 20T
- NC2 Dermatoscope
- iC1

CANFIELD RANGE: Distributed by Spectra Medical India Private Limited

- VEOS HD1/HD2
- VEOS SLR

DERMOSCAN/ILLUCO DERMOSCOPE: Distributed by JP Esthetics Private Limited
Illuco IDS-1100

DINO-LITE EDGE SERIES, DINO-LITE PREMIER SERIES
Distributed by Kontrelek Instruments, Pune

FIREFLY DE300, FIREFLY DE350
Distributed in India by Collateral Medical Private Limited.

SURGICAL INSTRUMENTS SUPPLIERS IN INDIA

Parulekar Surgical Industries, Mumbai

All types of instruments and equipment for dermatosurgery, nail surgery, hair transplant surgery, and cosmetosurgery.

All India Surgical Manufacturing Company, Mumbai

- For all surgical instruments.
- http://www.allindiasurgical.com

Basco India, Chennai

- Cryogun, cautery machine, tattoo pencil, biopsy punches, magnifying lens
- www.bascoindia.com

Delta Scientific, Mumbai

- CAFLON range of ear piercing equipment and consumables imported from England
- OPTIVISOR stereoscopic headband magnifying visors
- THERMOPAD flexible heating pads for medical use

Norma DND Products, Delhi

- *Silicone gel sheet*—for the effective prevention and treatment of hypertrophic scarring and keloids
- *NORMA pressure garments*—for taking care of postburn hypertrophic scarring, keloids.

- *NORMA Compression Stockings*—for varicose veins, DVT.
- *NORMA post-liposuction garments*
- *NORMA Pneumatic Ripple Beds*—to prevent and manage pressure sores.

Tejco Vision

- Hair transplantation equipment and accessories
- Threads, peels, hair fibers, SCALP micropigmentation device, optics, masks.

Rajdhani Surgicals, Delhi

- Dermatosurgery and liposuction cold steel instruments
- Hair transplantation equipment
- www.rajdhanisurgicals.co.in

ALPHA Surgicals

- All surgical instruments
- www.fueinstrument.in

LASER MACHINES

Mikro Scientific Instruments Private Limited

- *FOTONA SP SPECTRO/DYNAMIS:* Nd:YAG and Er:YAG platform lasers and aesthetic work station for hair removal, acne, vascular lesions, rejuvenation, antiaging, laser lipolysis, endovascular surgery, 4D noninvasive facelift, noninvasive body sculpting, and feminine rejuvenation.
- *Fotona Q-Switched Nd:YAG laser (FOTONA Star Walker)* for pigmented lesions and tattoos.
- *UM-L25 developed by Union Medical:* CO_2 surgical laser. Super pulse CO_2 - Normal: 0.1 - 25 W, Super: 0.5–10 W.
- *UNIXEL RF (Union Medical):* CO_2 fractional laser
- *DE ORO Dual* is a fractional dual wavelength (1550 Erbium Glass and 1927 Thulium) laser. Peak power 1550: 1–15 W. 1927: 1–10 W.

Lumenis India Private Limited

- *ResurFX™*—ResurFX™ is an advanced 1,565 nm fiber laser system for true fractional nonablative skin resurfacing.
- *AcuPulse*—MultiMode, SuperPulse fractional CO_2 laser.
- *UltraPulse* - Fractional CO_2 laser technology
- *LightSheer® DESIRE™*—Diode laser for hair reduction. Three handpieces with various spot sizes. The LightSheer DESIRE combines two advanced technologies—high-speed integrated technology (HIT™) and ChillTip™ Technology.
- *LightSheer DUET™*—advanced form of LightSheer with vacuum-assist technology and by dramatically increased spot size of 22 × 35 mm.
- *M22™*—M22 is a modular multi-application platform. It can be upgraded to include the following technologies: Universal IPL, ResurFX™, Multi-Spot™ Nd:YAG, and Q-Switched Nd:YAG.
- *NuEra® Tight:* Noninvasive, radio frequency body sculpting treatment treating fat reduction, skin tightening, wrinkle, and cellulite reduction.
- *FemTouch:* CO_2 laser technology which enables precise and controlled fractional laser microbeams to be applied to the vaginal lining for vaginal tightening.
- *SPLENDOR X:* Nd:YAG and Alexandrite laser system to be powered by BLEND X™ technology

Alma Medical Private Limited

- *Harmony-XL Pro:* IPL based multi technology platform with various US FDA indication
- *Soprano Ice Platinum:* The hair reduction platform with Alex + Diode + Nd:YAG wavelength for all hair types and skin types.
- *Soprano ICE:* This features Alma's unique Alex technology which combines the high absorption benefits of the Alexandrite 755 nm wavelength with the treatment coverage, comfort, and low maintenance of the diode laser.
- *Soprano Pro:* Gold Standard 810-nm laser diode provides reliable results. Features SHR + HR technology. Sapphire Dual Chill tip
- *Alma Q:* The Triple Mode Latest Generation Q-Switch Nd:YAG system with q-switched mode, quasi mode and long pulsed mode for pigmentation, tattoos, vascular, skin rejuvenation, etc.
- *Alma Hybrid:* It combines the power of three core energies—CO_2 laser, 1,570 nm laser, IMPACT for TransEpidermal Delivery (TED)
- *PICO CLEAR:* Q-Switched Nd:YAG laser with shortest pulse duration of 300–350 picoseconds.
- *Pixel CO_2:* The US FDA approved fractional CO_2 lasers system with multiple attachments for aesthetic, surgery, gynecology, and ENT.
- *Accent prime:* Selective lipolysis ultrasound and RF for body countering and skin tightening
- *Excimer 308:* The Excimer 308 nm system for treatment of psoriasis, vitiligo, etc.

Aakaar Medical Technologies

- *EpiSheer Platina Diode Laser System*—diode laser for laser hair removal
- *Platina Pro system*—trio clustered diode technology for laser hair removal (Classic - 808 nm, Alex - 755 nm, YAG - 1,064 nm)
- *REX-CO fractional CO_2 Laser system*—CO_2 metal tube to improve the effects of treatment
- *Q5 Nano* is a high fluence, high beam quality Q-Switched Nd:YAG laser
- *VIORA V10* multi technology platform is a powerful RF and fractional RF-based technology.

- *FREEZE SCULPT* involves the incorporation of three technologies—cryolipolysis, radiofrequency, and cavitation.

Timpac Healthcare Products, Delhi

- *Ellman's radiofrequency and Kentamed radiofrequency:* Radiofrequency surgery machine.
- *Mediostar Next Diode Laser:* From Asclepion Laser Technologies, Germany.
- *MultiPulse CO_2 Laser:* From Asclepion Laser Technologies, Germany.
- *Photomedex Vtrac excimer lamp and laser systems.*
- *Dermatoscope:* DERMLITE and HEINE range of dermatoscopes.
- *FREEZPEN 8G and 16G:* Powerful yet simple cryosurgery instrument
- *Laser accessories:* To protect the patient and personnel from the laser and IPL, Oculo-Plastik offers many stainless steel laser shields and instruments.
- *Peels:* Neostrata.

G3 Medical Systems Private Limited

- *ARTAS:* ARTAS® Robotic Hair Transplant System
- *Thermi RF:* Temperature Controlled RF Device
- *Cryo 6 - Zimmer:* Cold air device from the world leader - Zimmer.
- *Elite+, Cynosure:* Alexandrite 755 and Long Pulse Nd:YAG 1,064 nm wavelengths
- *Medlite C6, Cynosure:* Q-Switched Technology—four different wavelengths— MultiLite handpieces, 585 nm (yellow), and 650 nm (red)
- *Picosure, Cynosure:* World's first and only Picosecond laser using 755 nm Alexandrite laser
- *Surgitron Dual RF 120, Ellman:* Surgical RF System
- *Cynergy Vascular Workstation:* 585 nm pulse dye and 1,064 nm Nd:YAG laser system.
- *Elite + Aesthetic Workstation:* Hair removal laser with a combination of classic 755 nm Alexandrite wavelength and high-powered 1,064 nm Nd:YAG wavelength.
- *Multixel CO_2 Laser:* Hi-tech UltraPulse Fractional CO_2 Laser.
- *Imaging Solutions from Canfield Scientific USA.*
- *ZO (Zein Obagi) range of cosmeceuticals*

BTL India Private Limited

- *BTL Vanquish ME:* Lipolysis
- *BTL Exilis Elite*—combination of l 3.2 MHz Monopolar RF with 3 MHz of ultrasound—fat lipolysis with skin tightening.
- *BTL Exilite*—intense pulse light.
- *BTL Lymphastim*—for enhancement of lymphatic drainage and skin tightening on body areas.
- *BTL Intima*—for gynecological cosmetic solution (labia tightening).

Skinnovation

- *Ultracel:* Ultracel is a revolutionary no downtime, triple face-lifting technology which uses the powerful but focused ultrasound, radiofrequency, and fractionalized microneedling radiofrequency.
- *VIKINI:* VIKINI is a high powered 808 nm diode laser for permanent hair reduction. In addition, there is a 940 nm handpiece for facial rejuvenation.
- *Primelase HR:* Combined wavelengths (810 nm, 940 nm, 1,060 nm) for complete hair reduction.
- *EXSYS 308:* The EPL® (Excimer Pulsed Light) technology, optimized by GME.
- *Fraxis:* CO_2 microfocusing conventional laser with scanner fractional laser.
- *Fraxis Duo:* The Fraxis Duo is a combining CO_2 laser and microneedle fractional RF technology for optimal result of scars, photoaging, and striae distensae.
- *Intragen:* Noninvasive RF system
- *EnerJet 2.0:* EnerJet uses Jet Volumetric Remodeling (JVR) technology—a high-pressure jet technology to laterally introduce healing agents deep into the dermal layer of the skin.
- *ACURE:* Acure is 1,450 nm high performance diode laser system in acne therapy.
- *Cool shaping:* Cryolipolysis device for local reduction of fat cells to reshape body contours.
- *Tribeam premium:* Q-Switched Nd:YAG laser. Includes rich—PTP™ (photoacoustic toning pulse) technology for subcellular selective photothermolysis.

Stellar Medical

- *Platinum Pro:* Triple-wave platinum pro laser combines 755 nm + 810 nm + 1,064 nm into a single handpiece.
- *EM Shape:* Using electromagnetic energy, noninvasive technology for burning fat, and building muscle at the same time.
- *VERVE HIPRO-V:* HIFU technology

IN MODE Laser

- *TRITON:* It combines the three most popular wavelengths in one platform, using Fusion Technology, for hair removal
- *MORPHEUS 8:* Morpheus 8 is a minimally invasive bipolar radiofrequency (RF) tissue treatment.
- *EMPOWER RF:* It provides neuromuscular re-education for weak pelvic floor muscles, relief from stress, urge, and mixed urinary incontinence.
- *EMBRACE RF:* Subdermal adipose coagulation resulting in targeted tissue treatments.

Spectra Medical India Private Limited

- *CoolSculpt from Zeltiq, USA*—cryolipolysis system.
- *HYDRAFACIAL ELITE:* Patented hydrafacial system
- *Gentlemax Pro Series, Candela*—Single lightweight ergonomic handpiece delivering both 755 nm and 1,064 nm wavelengths.
- *VBEAM*—VBEAM Perfecta is the gold standard pulsed-dye laser.
- *ELASE*—ELASE is a diode laser platform.
- *EPLUS*—EPLUS work station combines optical energy and bipolar radiofrequency with 10 treatment applicators.
- *Velashape, Velasmooth Pro*— ELOS technology-based noninvasive class II system for effective treatment of cellulite and circumferential reduction.
- *Chemical Peels from Mesoestetic, SPAIN*— Cosmelan, Dermamelan.
- Home care and professional products from mesoestetic, Spain.
- Imaging solutions from Canfield Scientific, USA.

Geosmatic Cosmeceuticals and Cosmocare, Pune

- *Spectra XT, Spectra Gold:* With four distinct Q-switched mode wavelengths—1,064 nm, 532 nm, 585 nm, and 650 nm
- *EXCIPLEX 308 NM:* Excimer lamp system
- *Ultraformer II and Ultraformer III:* HIFU system
- Hair removal (LinScan 808) and Magma IPL + 810 Diode.
- *Endymed Pro, Endymed Pure 2.0:* RF based device that allows for skin tightening and microneedling RF. Utilizes EndyMed's proprietary 3DEEP technology which employs a multisource, phase-controlled radiofrequency energy source.
- *ECO2:* Fractional CO_2 device. Features the patented Controlled Chaos Technology.
- *Infini:* From Lutronics Private Limited. Microneedle RF-based device.
- *Fotofinder:* For facial analysis, hair analysis and full body analysis.
- *Forma Light:* IPL working under TRT with unique square pulse technology.

Derma India, Chennai

- *Whole body phototherapy Chamber (UVA and NB-UVB), Hand, and Foot Units*
- *Lasers*
- *Radiofrequency (RF)*
- *Iontophoresis*
- *Microdermabrasion machine*
- *MRF premier*
- *Fractional RF excited CO_2 laser*
- *Tixel*
- *Conmed Hyfrecator*
- *Brymill LN2 Cryo*
- *Dermachairs*

Unity Derma

- *Finebeam Dual:* Q-switched and long-pulsed Nd:YAG laser
- *Finebeam Q plus:* Q-switched Nd:YAG laser
- *Finebeam Max:* Long-pulsed Alexandrite and Nd:YAG laser
- *Finexel:* All-in-one CO_2 laser
- *Selriah:* 808 nm diode laser
- *EVE Ace:* Electrical Muscle Stimulation (EMS) function delivers low voltage (1–1.5 mA) electric pulses (47–2,000 Hz) to the face and neck muscles.

CHAPTER 139

Dermatologic and Cosmetic Procedures in Pregnancy

Adit Mohan Garg, Mysore Venkataram

KEY MESSAGES

- Procedures in pregnancy can be categorized as urgent, nonurgent and elective and also as procedures for dermatologic, cosmetic and surgical indications.
- Understanding the physiologic changes of pregnancy helps a dermatosurgeon in deciding safety of a procedure.
- Preprocedural care in the form of anesthetics and postprocedural in the form of analgesics and antibiotics is crucial to decide the outcome of procedure.

INTRODUCTION

Dermatologic surgery includes a variety of procedures such as essential and cosmetic procedures, lasers, and surgical procedures. Undertaking them requires the dermatosurgeon to take into account the risk/benefit analysis for every patient. This is particularly so in a pregnant woman. Patients may seek treatment for skin changes that occur in pregnancy, such as melasma, striae, varicose veins, hirsutism and increased skin growths. In such situations, it is for the physician to evaluate advantages and disadvantages of such an intervention. The ethics of performing such procedures in pregnancy needs very careful consideration.

While a lot of data pertaining to the safety of drugs in pregnancy is available, data on different dermatologic procedures in pregnancy is lacking as it is ethically problematic to perform large scale randomized trials in pregnant women. In this chapter, we outline the latest information on safety and necessity of different procedures pertaining to aesthetics and dermatological diseases.

CATEGORIZATION OF PROCEDURES

Dermatologic procedures during pregnancy can be divided into three categories: (1) *urgent, (2) nonurgent, and (3) elective. Urgent* procedures include taking a biopsy and/or treating a lesion suspicious of melanoma or an aggressive nonmelanoma skin cancer. A friable, bleeding pyogenic granuloma also needs to be managed promptly. *Nonurgent* procedures include procedures such as treating a nodular basal cell carcinoma (BCC), which may be undertaken during second trimester. Lastly, *elective* procedures are those which can be deferred until after delivery, such as scar excision, chemical peeling and other cosmetic procedures.[1]

PHYSIOLOGICAL SKIN CHANGES IN PREGNANCY

Pregnancy induced physiological and hormonal changes in the body can alter a dermatosurgeon's approach to undertake different procedures during that period. Increase in circulating blood volume, decreased hematocrit, increased flushing, increased melanocyte stimulation (risk of hyperpigmentation), altered wound healing (increased tendency to develop hypertrophic scars and keloids) are among the few.[2-4] The hormonal fluctuations can induce other skin manifestations such as melasma (or the mask of pregnancy, which is the second most common complaint after striae and may resolve within 1 year of delivery in 70% women without taking any treatment),[5,6] hypertrichosis, striae and certain growths over the skin such as acrochordons, angiomas, nevi and warts. These may increase in number, grow in size or even darken.[5,7]

Pregnancy is associated with physiological immunosuppression, which can be a cause of multiple warts and may increase the risk of bacterial and viral infections during and after the procedures.[5] The systemic physiologic changes relevant to a dermatosurgeon that occur in pregnancy are summarized in **Table 1**.

LOCAL ANESTHESIA

Local anesthesia is needed for most dermatological procedures and includes topical, infiltration, blocks and tumescent anesthesia.

Injectable Local Anesthetics

The commonly used injectable anesthetics are: Lidocaine, prilocaine, etidocaine (pregnancy category B); Bupivacaine and mepivacaine (pregnancy category category C).[8]

TABLE 1: The systemic physiologic changes relevant to a dermatosurgeon that occur in pregnancy.

System	*Physiologic changes*	*Implication*
Cardiovascular system	• Hemodilution due to proportional increase of plasma volume compared to red cell volume[8] • *BP:* Decreases and remains low up to week 24; returns to prepregnancy levels in 3rd trimester[8,9] • Uterus causes compression of abdominal vessels resulting in decreased venous return[8,10] • WBCs increase[2] • Platelets reduce, but aggregation coupled with reduced vascular resistance and increased production of coagulation factors may occur[2]	• Monitor BP regularly • False impression of infection[2] • Increased risk of thromboembolic events late in gestation[2]
Gastrointestinal	Decreased tone of GE sphincter due to progesterone[8,10]	• Reflux symptoms during supine position • Head elevation advised
Renal	Urinary volume and frequency increases because of high renal blood flow with increased GFR and pressure effect by uterus[10]	Frequency of micturition should be taken into consideration during a procedure
Endocrine	• Insulin antagonists such as estrogen, progestin, adrenocorticoids and human placental lactogen progressively increase • Fasting sugar levels decrease 10–15 mg/dL compared to nonpregnant levels as there is transplacental drainage of glucose to the fetus[2,11] • Progesterone mediated vasodilatation may predispose a pregnant woman to postural hypotension and fainting[1]	• Starvation may predispose woman to ketosis, relevant during a dermatological procedure • Ensure adequate hydration along with slow movement in getting on and off the procedure table[1]
Musculoskeletal	Muscular cramps and pelvic discomfort can occur due to ligament laxity caused by progesterone and relaxin[2,4,8]	Frequent repositioning with or without pillow support may be required to relieve this discomfort
Miscellaneous	*Compression syndrome:* After 20 weeks of gestation, the growing uterus can cause aortocaval compression leading to delirium, cephalea, nausea, vomiting, intense sweating, hypotension and tachycardia[8,10,12]	Adjust the patient in a left lateral decubitus position with the support of a pillow beneath her hip or between the knees.[8,10,12]

Bupivacaine and mepivacaine are not indicated in pregnancy unless potential benefits outweigh the risks. Mepivacaine is associated with fetal bradycardia, preterm labor and twice the incidence of congenital abnormalities.[8-13]

What is the risk?

Local injectable anesthetic (predominantly lignocaine) usage during pregnancy leads to an estimated 11–23% exposure to the fetus.[8] A relative acidosis with poor protein binding increases the free drug exposure to the fetus.[14] However, this exposure may not always cause toxicity as the fetal liver is well capable of metabolizing lignocaine.[15]

Pregnancy induced rise in progesterone enhances the membrane sensitivity of nerves to local anesthetics, thereby lessening the required anesthetic dosage in early pregnancy.[14] Rarely, lignocaine toxicity arises when there is accidental arterial injection or excessive high doses being used (>4.5 mg/kg upto a maximum of 300 mg, which is rare in dermatologic procedures).[8,10,13,16] The symptoms of lignocaine toxicity mimic aortocaval compression syndrome such as dizziness, tachycardia, agitation, headaches, sweating and headache.[2,4,10]

Once these symptoms appear in the mother, chances of fetal exposure increase in the form of cardiac or CNS toxicity.[7,8] There is a theoretical risk of inhibiting neutrophil chemotaxis, cell division and neural development in the newborn when local anesthetic (LA) concentration exceeds 100 µg/mL.[17,18] Adverse fetal outcomes such as septal cardiac anomalies, cerebral palsy, twin-to-twin transfusion syndrome, Turner syndrome, cleft lip and palate, umbilical hernia have been mentioned in literature.[19-22]

To decrease systemic spread of LA, adrenaline (Category C) is used alongside lignocaine. Although this increases the safety profile of LA, inadvertent intra-arterial absorption of high doses of adrenaline could lead to uterine artery spasms resulting in fetal compromise and prematurity. Thankfully, the doses used in dermatologic indications are very low with a high dilution of 1:200,000 which negates this risk.[8,10,19,20]

Therefore, lignocaine with or without adrenaline is considered the safest option to provide local injectable anesthesia.

Topical Anesthesia

Different forms of topical anesthetics are available such as EMLA cream (lidocaine 2.5% + prilocaine 2.5%), EMLA anesthetic disk (lidocaine 2.5% + prilocaine 2.5%), ELA-Max topical anesthetic cream (lidocaine 4% cream) and Lidoderm (lidocaine 5% patch).[23] Unlike injectable forms, topical creams are considered much safer. Still we need to be vigilant with some topical agents as follows:

1. Prilocaine in high doses holds a risk of methemoglobinemia in the fetus, because of which, lidocaine-prilocaine (both Category B) cream should be used in moderation.[24] Occlusion should be avoided as should the use near periocular and mucosal surfaces, as this can increase systemic absorption and irritation.[16,25,26] Tetracaine is the preferred topical anesthetic (in nonpregnant patients) for periocular procedures because of its low risk of irritation.[25,26]
2. Tetracaine and benzocaine (both Category C) are associated with fetal methemoglobinemia.[25,27]

Therefore, a lidocaine/prilocaine mixture (in moderation) is the preferred choice for topical anesthesia and for those concerned about its safety profile, liposomal lidocaine can be used as it provides a longer duration of anesthesia than nonliposomal preparations.[16,26]

PROCEDURES FOR DERMATOLOGIC CONDITIONS

Certain infective conditions such as warts and other benign growths such as acrochordons, seborrheic keratoses, pyogenic granulomas, hemangiomas, keloids and nevi can be removed via different procedures such as electrocautery, laser ablation, cryotherapy, intralesional steroid and minor surgical procedures under LA. Available data about their safety in pregnancy is limited and is summarized in **Table 2**.

TABLE 2: List of procedures and their safety in pregnancy.

S. No.	*Procedure*	*Safety profile*
Procedures for dermatologic conditions		
1.	Electrocautery and radiofrequency	Safe *Note:* Smoke plume can be carcinogenic, use smoke evacuators
2.	Intralesional steroid injection	Indicated only if benefits outweigh risk
3.	Lasers (CO_2, Nd:YAG, PDL, etc.)	Safe
4.	Cryotherapy	Safe
Procedures for aesthetic indications		
5.	Chemical peeling	Safe *Note:* Caution with salicylic acid (SA) and trichloroacetic acid (TCA) peel. Not to be used over large areas, under occlusion or over very thin skin
6.	Lasers, intense pulsed light (IPL), electroepilation	Not indicated (due to lack of satisfactory safety data) *Note:* Hormonal changes stimulate new hair growth, hence hair removal should be done only via depilation
7.	Platelet-rich plasma (PRP) therapy	Safe, but benefits should outweigh risk of anesthesia, pain and the fact that hairfall may normalize 6–12 months post delivery
8.	Botulinum toxin	Safe (warrants more research)
9.	Fillers	Relative contraindication
10.	Sclerotherapy	Contraindicated
11.	Microdermabrasion	Safe
Dermatosurgical procedures		
12.	Surgical resection of neoplasms	See Text
13.	Vitiligo surgery	Inadequate data to comment
14.	Liposuction and fat grafting	Contraindicated
15.	Suturing and suture removal	Leave sutures for 5–7 days longer than normal

Electrocautery and Radiofrequency

Electrocautery is considered harmless to the fetus when used in the mother. However, measures should be taken to reduce smoke plume exposure which can be mutagenic and carcinogenic.[28] This risk is same for both nonpregnant and pregnant patients by extension to the fetus.[8,26] Masks are considered poor barriers for this plume, therefore a smoke evacuator is preferred for reducing smoke exposure.[4]

Intralesional Steroid Injections

Intralesional steroid in hypertrophic scars, keloids and alopecia areata is not recommended until benefits outweigh risk, as corticosteroids are considered category C and have been reported to cause cleft lip and palate, along with risk of hypoadrenalism in newborns.[29]

Lasers

The limited data available suggest safe use of most lasers in pregnancy:

CO_2 laser: CO_2 lasers have a good efficacy and low complication rate for treatment of HPV genital condyloma and verrucous carcinoma in pregnant females.[30-33] Since this laser has only limited penetration into the skin with added advantage of bloodless destruction due to coagulation property, no harmful effects on the fetus are reported unless a direct exposure occurs.[30,32]

Some concern arises regarding exposure of mother to possibly mutagenic aerial particles generated as a result of vaporization by the laser, which can be eliminated using aspirators, smoke evacuators and masks used both by the patient and doctor.[10] Er:YAG laser is even more limited in penetration in to skin and hence can be considered safe.

Nd:YAG laser: Nd:YAG laser can be considered safe for dermatological indications in pregnancy. Genital condylomas have also been treated successfully with Nd:YAG laser therapy without any maternal or fetal complications.[34] For nongenital indications, Nd:YAG laser has been used for severe inflammatory acne and pyogenic granuloma during gestation without any adverse effects.[35,36]

PDL: Pulsed dye laser (585 nm) specifically targets hemoglobin within a lesion, therefore it has been used for variety of indications.[37] In a study, PDL was used to treat pyogenic granulomas and warts during pregnancy and reported a good safety profile with this laser.

Among nondermatologic indications, few authors have used PDL to treat symptomatic urolithiasis, without any reported adverse events.[38,39]

Therefore, the available medical evidence suggests good safety profile for PDL in pregnancy except for few minimal side effects such as mild erythema and pain.[40]

Other lasers: Compelling medical evidence in pregnancy for use of lasers such as other nonablative lasers, intense pulsed light (IPL), etc., is not available.[41,42]

PROCEDURES FOR AESTHETIC INDICATIONS

Generally, the advice is to postpone all aesthetic procedures in pregnancy. However, aesthetic concerns in a patient, although not an urgent indication during pregnancy, can be quite distressing in a female patient, especially if she is from the entertainment industry or show business. Ethically, thorough counseling should be done by explaining to the patient all the risks involved in writing as well as receiving an informed consent from her. A video consent is also recommended in selected cases. It should be noted that the principle of "cause no harm" applies to the pregnancy situation more than any other situation.

Different facial pigmentations, acne scars, aging changes of the face such as rhytids or wrinkles, unwanted facial hair, visible veins, etc., are some of the common indications for which cosmetic procedures are sought for. Their safety during gestation is discussed as under.

Chemical Peeling

Glycolic acid (GA) peel: Glycolic acid induces epidermolysis and exfoliation of the skin. It is a superficial peel and is considered safe in pregnancy due to negligible dermal penetration.[7,43,44]

Lactic acid (LA) peel: Lactic acid induces keratolysis. 2% LA peel has been used for gestational acne without any fetal risks as there is negligible dermal penetration.[7]

Salicylic acid (SA) peel: Salicylic acid is a β-hydroxy acid with comedolytic and keratolytic properties. It is classified as pregnancy category C (Fabbrocini et al., 2009). Up to a 25% dermal penetration is reported with usage of SA peel for large areas or when applied under occlusion.[25] However, low doses of acetylsalicylic acid (aspirin) have been studied for their safety profile in gestational indications such as preeclampsia, and there was no increase in adverse effects noted in the fetus.[34,45] Therefore, it is recommended that if SA peels are used in a pregnant patient, the area of application should be limited.

Jessner's peel: It is a combination of SA, LA and resorcinol. Because of the presence of salicylic acid, it should be used with caution.

Trichloroacetic acid (TCA) peel: TCA peels can act both as superficial as well as medium depth peel. There is a possibility of dermal penetration when used in and around ocular and oral mucosal surfaces.[25] High doses of TCA (i.e., >1,000 mg/kg/day) found in drinking water disinfection-by-products (DBPs) has been associated with fetal growth retardation and low birth weight; however, such high concentrations are not attained in dermatologic surgery procedures.[46] TCA has been safely used in pregnancy to treat genital condylomata.[25,47]

Energy-based Devices (Lasers, IPL and Electrosurgery)

As already mentioned earlier, theoretically, lasers for cosmetic purposes act on the very principle of selective photothermolysis, which prevents their action to go beyond deep dermis, thereby precluding any harm to the fetus. Still, due to a lack of satisfactory safety data, cosmetic lasers should be avoided until after the delivery.

Hair removal by means of laser, IPL or electrolysis is not recommended due to unavailability of safety data. The hormonal changes continue to stimulate new hair growth, leading to unsatisfactory treatment response.[6] Also, amniotic fluid is considered to be a good conductor of galvanic current, which poses risk to the fetus during electroepilation.[7] Women are recommended to treat excess hair by means of waxing, shaving, threading, and chemical depilation.[6,7]

Treatment of striae: PDL has shown some promising results, but it is recommended to wait until postpartum period to start any treatment.[48,49] After delivery, different ablative (CO_2 fractional laser)[50] and nonablative (1540 nm Er doped glass fractional nonablative,[51] PDL,[48,49] Nd:YAG[52] and Copper bromide[53]) lasers have been tried with varying results.

Platelet Rich Plasma Therapy for Hair Loss

The hormonal fluctuations during gestation causes anagen phase of hair cycle to be prolonged leading to hair looking fuller and healthy. Upon childbirth, there is a major shift to telogen phase causing increased hair fall and thinning. In maximum cases, the hair cycle normalizes within about a year. Therefore, platelet rich plasma therapy which involves extracting and concentrating platelets from whole blood and injecting into the scalp is only beneficial post delivery and not indicated in pregnancy, with an added risk of sepsis, putting the fetus at risk.[54,55]

Botulinum Toxin

Botulinum toxin type A has been used for both cosmetic and medical indications.[56] Correct intramuscular or intradermal administration of botulinum toxin does not lead to significant systemic concentrations.[56] Furthermore, the size of the toxin molecule prevents it from crossing the placental barrier.[56,57] The doses used in aesthetic purposes (up to 100 U) is significantly lower than the hazardous doses of 600 U.[57]

Botulinum toxin has been used for medical indications such as achalasia, cervical dystonia and migraine prophylaxis during pregnancy.[16] No complications (such as infant neuromuscular blockade or weakness)[25] have been noted in the delivery or health of the infants born to these mothers even after few years.[58-60] A single case of a 39-year-old pregnant woman who had a twin pregnancy miscarriage at 10 weeks is reported. She received 500 U of onabotulinum toxin at 4 weeks of gestation for cervical dystonia. The woman was on concomitant benztropine (Category C), clonazepam (Category D) and fluoxetine (Category C) during the toxin injection. She also had a history of one miscarriage prior to this episode. It is difficult to determine whether the toxin had any role to play in the fetal demise, as she had many collateral risk factors associated for the same.[61]

To conclude, although botulinum toxin may be safe in pregnancy, ethical considerations, possible medicolegal issues and the cosmetic nature of the use necessitate serious considerations regarding its use. A detailed discussion about the use with the patient is necessary. Proper psychological assessment of the patient and her need for the procedure needs to be understood. Botulinum toxin type A is a category C drug and demands more research to make concrete recommendations on its usage in pregnancy.

Fillers

Most commonly used cosmetic filler is hyaluronic acid, which has much similarity with the intrinsic hyaluronic acid of the human body. This property makes it a safe compound to be injected into the skin during pregnancy. However lignocaine (the amount used is far lower than recommended maximum dosage), is generally mixed with the filler, and this needs to be taken into consideration, as discussed previously.[62,63]

Theoretically, fillers rarely may cause hypersensitivity or injection site infection.[64] So, after injecting a filler, there is some local inflammation followed by collagen remodeling. Vascularity is also increased and there is increased susceptibility to hyperpigmentation encountered in pregnancy.[4] Looking upon these issues, manufacturer recommendations include fillers in pregnancy as a relative contraindication.

Sclerotherapy

Varicose veins that develop during pregnancy, have high chances of resolving within 6 to 12 months postpartum.[65] A divided opinion exists in the literature, where the German Society of Phlebology and Rabe et al. suggested that sclerosants can cross the placenta and are absolutely contraindicated in pregnancy.[65,66] On the other hand, Abramowitz and Reich-Schupke et al showed that sclerotherapy is a safe procedure in pregnancy and no complications were observed in either the mother or the baby.[67,68] Of all the commonly used agents (i.e., sodium tetra decyl sulfate, polydocanol, hypertonic saline, etc.), hypertonic saline is considered to have the lowest risk of causing adverse reactions.[25] Very limited data over safety of sclerosants in pregnancy prevents us from making a concrete statement whether they can be used during gestation or not.

Miscellaneous

Microdermabrasion: It is a safe procedure to perform during pregnancy as it is a physical noninvasive procedure.[69]

Cryotherapy: It is considered safe during pregnancy[62] and may be the preferred treatment of genital warts. Cryotherapy or electrocautery is preferred over chemical treatments for removal of acrochordons, angiomas, nevi and warts.[5]

When to perform a procedure?

Dermatological procedures, in general, should be conducted preferably during second trimester or the postpartum period, because first 12 weeks of gestation are critical for organogenesis and increases the risk of spontaneous abortion, whereas surgery during the third trimester may predispose to premature delivery.[1,10]

POSTPROCEDURAL CARE

Most dermatological procedures warrant postprocedural care in the form of antibiotics, analgesics or cleaning of the wound with antiseptics. Safety in pregnancy has to be looked into to attain an optimum benefit. An overview of these medications is provided as under.

Antibiotics

The antibiotics (pregnancy category) used during dermatological procedures are given in **Table 3**.

Topical Antiseptics

Alcohol preparations and chlorhexidine gluconate are not associated with any risk to the fetus, however should be avoided in periocular region in general (risk of keratitis and corneal opacity).[2,72] Povidone-iodine is contraindicated as it can be absorbed through mucous membranes and is associated with fetal hypothyroidism.[8,10] Hexachlorophene is associated with CNS toxicity in fetuses and is avoided.[8,10,20] Therefore, alcohol or chlorhexidine solutions should be preferred for sterility purposes in pregnant patients.

TABLE 3: Antibiotics.

S. No.	*Antibiotic (pregnancy category)*	*Safety profile*	*Risk*	*Special points*	*Reference*
1.	Penicillin (B)	Safe	-	-	[1,13,70]
2.	Cephalosporin (B)	Safe	-	-	[1,13,70]
3.	Azithromycin (B)	Safe	-	Used when penicillin allergy suspected	[1,13,70]
4.	Erythromycin base (B)	Safe	Estolate form association with risk of cholestatic jaundice in mother	Used when penicillin allergy suspected	[1,13,70,71]
5.	Metronidazole (B)	Safe	-	-	[13]
5.	Cotrimoxazole (D)	Unsafe	Fetal hyperbilirubinemia	Especially in 2nd Trimester	[1]
6.	Doxycycline (D)	Unsafe	Brown discoloration of teeth	-	[1]
7.	Tetracycline (D)	Unsafe	Brown discoloration of teeth, enamel toxicity, decreased bone development in infant	-	[1,8,13]
8.	Fluoroquinolones (C)	Unsafe	Cartilage defects	-	[1,8]
9.	Clindamycin (B)	Avoided	Abnormal LFT, pseudomembranous colitis in mother	-	[8]
10.	Sulfonamides (C)	Unsafe	Fetal hyperbilirubinemia with kernicterus	Especially during 3rd Trimester	[8]
11.	Aminoglycosides (D)	Unsafe	Fetal ototoxicity	-	[8,13]
12.	Chloramphenicol (C)	Unsafe	Gray baby syndrome, fetal death, maternal blood dyscrasias	-	[8]

Analgesics

Acetaminophen (Category B) is a safe option. Although it can cross the placenta, limited usage has negligible risk. Prolonged or high dosage can lead to hemolytic anemia in the new born and/or renal toxicity in the mother as well as the fetus.[1,2]

Short term use of opioids is considered safe for intense pain. Larger doses are associated with neonatal respiratory depression.[1,8,10]

Ibuprofen and salicylates are known to cause platelet dysfunction, leading to increased risk of postpartum hemorrhage in the third trimester. They can also cause a delay in the onset of labor, abruptio placenta and/or a premature closure of ductus arteriosus.[1,8] Additionally, salicylates are known to occasionally cause birth defects and delayed fetal growth.[10] Therefore, ibuprofen and salicylates are contraindicated in pregnancy.

DERMATOSURGICAL PROCEDURES IN PREGNANCY

Surgical Resection of Tumors and Malignant Lesions

Commonly seen tumors and malignant lesions in pregnancy are nevi, pyogenic granuloma, dermatofibroma/dermatofibrosarcoma, melanoma, BCC, and squamous cell carcinoma (SCC).[4,21]

During pregnancy, surgical intervention for malignant lesions is most likely to be performed for melanoma (95%), followed by SCC (67%) and least likely for BCC (45%).[21] Second trimester is considered to be the optimal period for surgical intervention, however, under local anesthesia, surgery can be performed in any trimester.[21]

Benign nevi my undergo morphological changes in gestation such as increase in size and/or pigmentation[73] along with dermoscopic alterations such as new dot formation (6%), thicker pigment network, dark globules, and increase in vascularity which may revert to normal post delivery. These changes, regardless of pregnancy state, warrant immediate biopsy.[4,74]

Melanoma accounts for 8% of all malignancies diagnosed in pregnancy and have a poor prognosis.[1,21,75] Although transplacental transmission is unusual, melanoma represents 31% of metastases to placenta and 58% of those involve the fetus.[1,75] Fetal involvement is always associated with placental involvement, but vice versa may not be true.[76] Treatment of cutaneous melanoma is primarily surgical and is similar in both pregnant and nonpregnant patients. Early diagnosis and thickness of the lesion are the predictors of therapeutic prognosis.[4] Lesions 1 mm or less in thickness should be excised with a 1 cm margin; intermediate lesions (1–4 mm thickness) should be excised with a 2 cm margin and lesions which warrant lymph node dissection, should be operated under GA, preferably in the 2nd trimester.[77]

Staging of melanoma in a pregnant woman has enormous importance, as less thick lesions can be excised under LA. Biopsy of sentinel lymph node during gestation is subjected to a debate among various authors, as some advocate for delay until the postpartum period in view of risk to the fetus,[78] whereas majority recommend that sentinel lymph node biopsy can be conducted any time after the 1st trimester to avoid complications during organogenesis.[76,79,80]

Basocellular carcinoma (if not growing) in the thorax or abdomen can be removed after delivery whereas an aggressive SCC on the nose may require urgent micrographic surgery.[10]

Vascular tumors: Hormonal status in pregnancy has a stimulant effect on vascular structures, which may cause growth in pyogenic granulomas, glomus tumors and hemangioendotheliomas.[81] Pyogenic granulomas can be very symptomatic in a pregnant woman, and necessitates treatment through shave removal with cauterization of the feeder vessel. Lasers such as nonablative Nd:YAG and PDL can also be used.[4,36,82,83]

Therefore, when a suspicious lesion is detected which shows signs of malignancy such as bleeding, change in size and pigmentation, most dermatologists prefer a biopsy followed with necessary intervention such as an excision. The risk of leaving such a lesion untouched is greater than that of conducting a procedure for its removal.[2]

Vitiligo Surgery

The course of vitiligo during pregnancy is variable and unpredictable and hence surgery is not recommended.

Hair Transplantation

Generally, hair loss tends to improve during pregnancy. Thus, the cosmetic nature of the surgery and the prolonged duration of surgery necessitate any consideration of HT only after pregnancy.

Liposuction and Fat Grafting

Since the fetus places increased nutritional demand on the mother, liposuction and fat grafting may compromise the fetus' nutritional requirements. Risk of fat embolism and occlusion also cannot be ruled out. Therefore fat transfer surgery is not recommended during pregnancy and it is advised that the woman waits until her weight stabilizes after delivery.[25]

Suturing and Suture Removal

Due to delayed cicatrization in pregnant women, it is advised to use longer lasting absorbable sutures or nonabsorbable sutures with high tensile strength, especially over the trunk and abdomen. They should be left 5–7 days longer than usual.[1] Also, removal of sutures should be in stages to prevent any chances of dehiscence.[10]

CONCLUSION

It is important to understand that only procedures which are safe and necessary should be performed in a pregnant woman. These may include electrocautery, radiofrequency or cryotherapy for warts, surgical intervention for skin malignancies and lasers such as CO_2 and Nd:YAG for verrucae and other small growths. Procedures which are safe but need caution along with proper risk assessment include intralesional steroid injections, aesthetic procedures such as chemical peeling, botulinum toxin, microdermabrasion and biopsies for suspicious lesions. Finally, some procedures which are contraindicated include fillers, sclerotherapy and liposuction including adipocyte transfer.

An assessment of the patient, both medical and psychological needs to be carried out. Patients need to be counseled about the procedures and the concerned gynecologist may be involved in decision where necessary. As stated earlier, the principle of malfeasance *"Above all, do no harm"* applies in pregnancy more than any other situation.

REFERENCES

1. MDedge. (2017). Pregnancy not a barrier to providing cutaneous surgery. [online] Available from: https://www.mdedge.com/dermatology/article/144443/dermatologic-surgery/pregnancy-not-barrier-providing-cutaneous-surgery. [Last Accessed May, 2021].
2. Gontijo G, Gualberto GV, Madureira NA. Dermatologic surgery and cosmetic procedures during pregnancy - a systematic review. Surg Cosmet Dermatol. 2010;2(1):39-45.
3. MDedge. (2015). Cosmetic procedures in pregnancy. [online] Available from: https://www.mdedge.com/obgyn/article/98661/aesthetic-dermatology/cosmetic-procedures-pregnancy. [Last Accessed May, 2021].
4. Goldberg D, Maloney M. Dermatologic surgery and cosmetic procedures during pregnancy and the post-partum period. Dermatol Ther. 2013;26(4):30-2.
5. The Dermatologist. (2010). When the Patient is Pregnant. [online]. Available from: https://www.the-dermatologist.com/content/when-patient-pregnant. [Last Accessed May, 2021].
6. Nussbaum R, Benedetto A. Cosmetic aspects of pregnancy. Clin Dermatol. 2006;24(2):133-41.
7. Trivedi M, Kroumpouzos G, Murase J. A review of the safety of cosmetic procedures during pregnancy and lactation. Int J Womens Dermatol. 2017;3(1):6-10.
8. Richards K, Stasko T. Dermatologic surgery and the pregnant patient. Dermatol Surg. 2002;28(3):248-56.
9. O'Day M. Cardio-respiratory physiological adaptation of pregnancy. Semin Perinatol. 1997;21(4):268-75.
10. Sweeney SM, Maloney ME. Pregnancy and dermatologic surgery. Dermatol Clin. 2006;24(2):205-14.
11. Rudolf MC, Sherwin RS. Maternal ketosis and its effects on the fetus. Clin Endocrinol Metab. 1983;12(2):413-28.

12. Gianopoulos JG. Establishing the criteria for anesthesia and other precautions for surgery during pregnancy. Surg Clin N Am. 1995;75(1):33-45.
13. Moore PA. Selecting drugs for the pregnant dental patient. J Am Dent Assoc. 1998;129(9):1281-6.
14. Steinberg ES, Santos AC. Surgical anesthesia during pregnancy. Int Anesthesiol Clin. 1990;28(1):58-66.
15. Kuhnert BR, Knapp DR, Kuhnert PM, Prochaska AL. Maternal, fetal, and neonatal metabolism of lidocaine. Clin Pharmacol Ther. 1979;26(2):213-20.
16. Jakharia-Shah N, Chadha P, Watson L. A review of the safety of common aesthetic procedures during pregnancy. J Plast Reconstr Aesthet Surg. 2018;71(9):1362-80.
17. Gasparoni A, De Amici D, Ciardeli L, Autelli M, Regazzi-Bonora M, Bartoli A, et al. Effect of lidocaine on neutrophil chemotaxis in newborn infants. J Clin Immunol. 1990;18(3):210-3.
18. Fujinaga M, Mazze RI. Reproductive and teratogenic effects of lidocaine in Sprague-Dawley rats. Anesthesiology. 1986;65(6):626-32.
19. Fayans EP, Stuart HR, Carsten D, Ly Q, Kim H. Local anesthetic use in the pregnant and postpartum patient. Dent Clin North Am. 2010;54(4):697-713.
20. Gormley DE. Cutaneous surgery and the pregnant patient. J Am Acad Dermatol. 1990;23(2):269-79.
21. Dermatology Times. (2018). Surgeons defer procedures during early stage pregnancy. [online] Available from: https://www.dermatologytimes.com/view/surgeons-defer-procedures-during-early-stage-pregnancy. [Last Accessed May, 2021].
22. Hagai A, Diav-Citrin O, Shechtman S, Ornoy A. Pregnancy outcome after in utero exposure to local anesthetics as part of dental treatment: a prospective comparative cohort study. J Am Dent Assoc. 2015;146(8):572-80.
23. Physicians' Desk Reference. 50th Edition Medical Consultant: Ronald Arky. Medical Economics Co., Montvale, NJ. J Med Chemistr. 1996;39(11):2278.
24. Chen BK, Eichenfield LF. Pediatric anesthesia in dermatologic surgery: when hand-holding is not enough. Dermatol Surg. 2001;27(12):1010-8.
25. Lee KC, Korgavkar K, Dufresne RG, Higgins HW. Safety of cosmetic dermatologic procedures during pregnancy. Dermatol Surg. 2013;39:1573-86.
26. Friedman PM, Mafong EA, Friedman ES, Geronemus RG. Topical Anesthetics Update: EMLA and Beyond. Dermatol Surg. 2001;27(12):1019-26.
27. Guay J. Methemoglobinemia related to local anesthetics: a summary of 242 episodes. Anesth Analg. 2009;108(3):837-45.
28. Gatti JE, Bryant CJ, Noone RB, Murphy JB. The mutagenicity of electrocautery smoke. Plast Reconstr Surg. 1992;89(5):781-4.
29. Drugs. Triamcinolone use during pregnancy. [online] Available from: https://www.drugs.com/pregnancy/triamcinolone.html. [Last Accessed May, 2021].
30. Adelson MD, Semo R, Baggish MS, Osborne NG. Laser vaporization of genital condylomata in pregnancy. J Gynecol Surg. 1990;6(4):257-62.
31. Hsu CK, Lee JYY, Yu CH, Hsu MML, Wong TW. Lip verrucous carcinoma in a pregnant woman successfully treated with carbon dioxide laser surgery. Br J Dermatol. 2007;157(4):813-5.
32. Arena S, Marconi M, Frega A, Villani C. Pregnancy and condyloma. Evaluation about therapeutic effectiveness of laser CO_2 on 115 pregnant women. Minerva Ginecol. 2001; 53(6):389-96.
33. Ferenczy A. Treating genital condyloma during pregnancy with the carbon dioxide laser. Am J Obstet Gynecol. 1984; 148(1):9-12.
34. Buzalov S, Khristakieva E. The treatment of neglected cases of condylomata acuminata in pregnant women with the Nd:Yag laser. Akush Ginekol (Sofiia). 1995;34(2):38-9.
35. Ballin JS, Uebelhoer NS. The use of the low-fluence 1064 nm Nd:YAG laser in a female with contraindications to systemic antiacne therapy. J Drugs Dermatol. 2009;8(11):1025-6.
36. Powell JL, Bailey CL, Coopland AT, Otis CN, Frank JL, Meyer I. Nd:YAG laser excision of a giant gingival pyogenic granuloma of pregnancy. Lasers Surg Med. 1994;14(2):178-83.
37. Richards KA, Garden JM. The pulsed dye laser for cutaneous vascular and nonvascular lesions. Semin Cutan Med Surg. 2000;19(4):276-86.
38. Carlan SJ, Schorr SJ, Ebenger MF, Danna PA, Anibarro GB. Laser lithotripsy in pregnancy. A case report. J Reprod Med. 1995;40(1):74-6.
39. Scarpa RM, De Lisa A, Usai E. Diagnosis and treatment of ureteral calculi during pregnancy with rigid ureteroscopes. J Urol. 1996;155(3):875-7.
40. Erceg A, Bovenschen HJ, van de Kerkhof PC, de Jong EM, Seyger MM. Efficacy and safety of pulsed dye laser treatment for cutaneous discoid lupus erythematosus. J Am Acad Dermatol. 2009;60(4):626-32.
41. Kim SG, Kim EY, Kim YJ, Lee SI. The efficacy and safety of ablative fractional resurfacing using a 2,940-Nm Er:YAG laser for traumatic scars in the early posttraumatic period. Arch Plast Surg. 2012;39(3):232-7.
42. Hasegawa T, Matsukura T, Mizuno Y, Sugo Y, Ogawa H, Ikeda S. Clinical trial of a laser device called fractional photothermolysis system for acne scars. J Dermatol. 2006;33(9):623-7.
43. Andersen FE. Final report on the safety assessment of glycolic acid, ammonium, calcium, potassium, and sodium glycolates, methyl, ethyl, propyl, and butyl glycolates, and lactic acid, ammonium, calcium, potassium, sodium, and TEA-lactates, methyl, ethyl, isopropyl, and butyl lactates, and lauryl, myristyl, and cetyl lactates. Int J Toxicol. 1998;17(1):1-241.
44. Grimes PE. Microdermabrasion. Dermatol Surg. 2005; 31(9 Pt 2):1160-5.
45. James AH, Brancazio LR, Price T. Aspirin and reproductive outcomes. Obstet Gynecol Surv. 2008;63(1):49-57.
46. Costet N, Garlantezec R, Monfort C, Rouget F. Environmental and urinary markers of prenatal exposure to drinking water disinfection by-products, fetal growth, and duration of gestation in the PELAGIE birth cohort (Brittany, France, 2002–2006). Am J Epidemiol, 2012;175(4):263-75.
47. Schwartz DB, Greenberg MD, Daoud Y, Reid R. Genital condylomas in pregnancy: use of trichloroacetic acid and laser therapy. Am J Obstet Gynecol. 1988;158(6 Pt 1):1407-16.
48. McDaniel DH, Ash K, Zukowski M. Treatment of stretch marks with the 585-nm flashlamp-pumped pulsed dye laser. Dermatol Surg. 1996;22(4):332-7.
49. Jimenez GP, Flores F, Berman B, Gunja-Smith Z. Treatment of striae rubra and striae alba with the 585-nm pulsed-dye laser. Dermatol Surg. 2003;29(4):362-5.
50. Yang YJ, Lee GY. Treatment of striae distensae with nonablative fractional laser versus ablative CO(2) fractional laser: a randomized controlled trial. Ann Dermatol. 2011;23(4):481-9.
51. de Angelis F, Kolesnikova L, Renato F, Liguori G. Fractional nonablative 1540-nm laser treatment of striae distensae in Fitzpatrick skin types II to IV: clinical and histological results. Aesthet Surg J. 2011;31(4):411-9.
52. Goldman A, Rossato F, Prati C. Stretch marks: treatment using the 1,064-nm Nd:YAG laser. Dermatol Surg. 2008;34(5):6.

53. Longo L, Postiglione MG, Marangoni O, Melato M. Two-year follow-up results of copper bromide laser treatment of striae. J Clin Laser Med Surg. 2003;21(3):157-60.
54. Belgravia Centre. (2020). Can you have PRP hair loss treatment whilst pregnant? [online] Available from: https://www.belgraviacentre.com/blog/can-you-have-prp-hair-loss-treatment-whilst-pregnant/. [Last Accessed May, 2021].
55. Cosmetic M D. (2020). Platelet Rich Plasmafor Skin Rejuvenation. [online] Available from: http://cosmeticmd.com.au/Treatments/PRP-FAQ.php. [Last Accessed May, 2021].
56. Tan M, Kim E, Koren G, Bozzo P. Botulinum toxin type A in pregnancy. Can Fam Physician. 2013;59(11):1183-4.
57. Morgan JC, Iyer SS, Moser ET, Singer C, Sethi KD. Botulinum toxin A during pregnancy: a survey of treating physicians. J Neurol Neurosurg Psychiatry. 2006;77(1):117-9.
58. Wataganara T, Leelakusolvong S, Sunsaneevithayakul P, Vantanasiri C. Treatment of severe achalasia during pregnancy with esophagoscopic injection of botulinum toxin A: a case report. J Perinatol. 2009;29(9):637-9.
59. Robinson AY, Grogan PM. Onabotulinum toxin A successfully used as migraine prophylaxis during pregnancy: a case report. Mil Med. 2014;179(6):e703-4.
60. Newman WJ, Davis TL, Padaliya BB, Covington CD, Gill CE, Abramovitch AI, et al. Botulinum toxin type A therapy during pregnancy. Mov Disord. 2004;19(11):1384-5.
61. Bodkin CL, Maurer KB, Wszolek ZK. Botulinum toxin type A therapy during pregnancy. Mov Disord. 2005;20(8):1081-2.
62. Manela-Azulay M, Issa MCA, Tamler C, Pinheiro AMC, Costa A. Procedimentos esteticos. In: Costa A, Alves G, Azulay L (Eds). Dermatologia e gravidez. Rio de Janeiro: Elsevier; 2009. pp. 449-53.
63. Dix SK, Rosner GF, Nayar M, Haris JJ, Guglin ME, Winterfield JR, et al. Intractable cardiac arrest due to lidocaine toxicity successfully resuscitated with lipid emulsion. Crit Care Med. 2011;39(4):872-4.
64. Lolis M, Dunbar SW, Goldberg DJ, Hansen TJ, MacFarlane DF. Patient safety in procedural dermatology: Part II. Safety related to cosmetic procedures. J Am Acad Dermatol. 2015;73(1):15-24.
65. Rabe E, Pannier F. Sclerotherapy of varicose veins with polidocanol based on the guidelines of the german society of phlebology. Dermatol Surg. 2010;36(Suppl 2):968-75.
66. Rabe E, Pannier-Fischer F, Gerlach H, Breu FX, Guggenbichler S, Zabel M. Guidelines for sclerotherapy of varicose veins (ICD 10: I83.0, I83.1, I83.2,and I83.9). Dermatol Surg. 2004;30(5):687-93.
67. Abramowitz I. The treatment of varicose veins in pregnancy by empty vein compressive sclerotherapy. S Afr Med J. 1973;47(14):607-10.
68. Reich-Schupke S, Leiste A, Moritz R, Altmeyer P, Stücker M. Sclerotherapy in an undetected pregnancy - a catastrophe? Vasa. 2012;41(4):243-7.
69. Bhalla M, Thami GP. Microdermabrasion: reappraisal and brief review of literature. Dermatol Surg. 2006;32(6):809-14.
70. Babcock MD, Grekin RC. Antibiotic use in dermatologic surgery. Dermatol Clin. 2003;21(2):337-48.
71. Garland SM, O'Reilly MA. The risks and benefits of antimicrobial therapy in pregnancy. Drug Saf. 1995;13(3):188-205.
72. Stott WG. Antiseptic (hibiclens) and eye injuries. Med J Aust. 1980;2(8):456.
73. Driscoll MS, Grant-Kels JM. Nevi and melanoma in the pregnant woman. Clin Dermatol. 2009;27(1):116-21.
74. Hu W, Nelson JE, Mohney CA, et al. Malignant melanoma arising in a pregnant African American woman with a congenital blue nevus. Dermatol Surg. 2004;30(12 pt 2):1530–2.
75. Baergen RN, Johnson D, Moore T, Benirschke K. Maternal melanoma metastatic to the placenta: a case report and review of the literature. Arch Pathol Lab Med. 1997;121(5):508-11.
76. Jhaveri MB, Driscoll MS, Grant-Kels JM. Melanoma in pregnancy. Clin Obstet Gynecol. 2011;54(4):537-45.
77. Teplitzky S, Sabates B, Yu K, Beech DJ. Melanoma during pregnancy: a case report and review of the literature. J La State Med Soc. 1998;150(11):539-43.
78. Broer N, Buonocore S, Goldberg C, Truini C, Faries MB, Narayan D, et al. A proposal for the timing of management of patients with melanoma presenting during pregnancy. J Surg Oncol. 2012;106(1):36-40.
79. Pagès C, Robert C, Thomas L, Maubec E, Sassolas B, Granel Brocard F, et al. Management and outcome of metastatic melanoma during pregnancy. Br J Dermatol. 2010;162(2):274-81.
80. Schwartz JL, Mozurkewich EL, Johnson TM. Current management of patients with melanoma who are pregnant, want to get pregnant or do not want to get pregnant. Cancer. 2003;97(9):2130-3.
81. Kroumpouzos G, Cohen LM. Dermatoses of pregnancy. J Am Acad Dermatol. 2001;45(1):1-19.
82. Ballin JS, Uebelhoer NS. The use of the low-fluence 1064 nm Nd: YAG laser in a female with contraindications to systemic antiacne therapy. J Drugs Dermatol. 2009;8(11):1025-6.
83. Alexander A, Samlowski WE, Grossman D. Metastatic melanoma in pregnancy: risk of transplacental metastases in the infant. J Clin Oncol. 2003;21(11):2179-86.

CHAPTER 140

Dermatosurgery in Pediatric Population

Shristi Shrestha, Arpita Arghya, Mysore Venkataram

KEY MESSAGES

- Insights into the procedures done on pediatric population, what needs to be done and what can wait.
- How to deal with the children, parents, guardian during the surgery.
- Prevention of complication is better than managing them.
- Try to incorporate all the relevant procedures under one roof.

INTRODUCTION

Over the last decade dermatologic and aesthetic procedures have dramatically increased in popularity in all ages. The reasons for this are:

- Simpler procedures under local anesthesia
- Minimum downtime
- Safety of these procedures
- Increasing awareness
- Affluence and affordability
- Increasing desire.

Correspondingly many procedures are sought to be performed in children. Performing surgeries in younger age may have some benefits such as:

- Easier removal when lesions are small
- Better cosmetic results due to increased skin elasticity
- Excellent tissue regeneration.

However, performing dermatologic procedures in infants and children present with various challenges such as:

- Local anesthesia in children is challenging as children may not cooperate
- General anesthesia (GA) has its own risks
- Medicolegal issues
- Ethical concerns in case of cosmetic treatments, which are being sought for children because of the awareness of self, changing attitudes about beauty and influence of social media.

This chapter deals with this complex issue of dermatosurgical and aesthetic procedures in children.

Skin conditions requiring procedural interventions in children can be classified as in **Box 1**.

TIMING OF SURGERY/PROCEDURE

The timing of surgical intervention is a key aspect in optimizing surgical outcome and needs to be decided; taking in to account nature of the lesion, nature of the procedure/surgery physical and psychological health of the child and is typically a joint decision between the parents of the patients and the physician. Benefits should always outweigh the risk. Few examples to illustrate the timing of surgical intervention are:

- During infancy large lesions present over the back are much easier to excise in children due to the presence of "baby fat" which is much less in a teenager and hence creates tension on the wound as the wound is more likely to stretch due to muscular presence.
- In children the scalp is much thinner so nevus sebaceous can be excised easily than during adolescence, which might require staged procedure or a flap.
- A congenital nevus can be removed if the parents desire it before the preschool age because child become aware and may suffer loss of self-esteem.

Based on the above classification, recommended age for different procedures and their considerations are given in **Table 1**.

APPROACH TO MANAGING A PEDIATRIC PATIENT

After deciding what procedure is indicated, various age groups have to be dealt differently. A child's developmental age should be considered while considering and executing

BOX 1: Skin conditions requiring procedural interventions.

- Lesions with active symptoms, signs and possible complications and hence need removal for medical reason, e.g., hemangiomas, malignancies such as BCC in xeroderma pigmentosum, nevoid BCC syndrome
- Lesions having potential for disfigurement, e.g., scars, vitiligo
- Lesions having potential for the spread and health risk, e.g, viral warts, Molluscum contagiosum
- Lesions with impact on psychosocial development, e.g., hypertrichosis
- Lesions best removed early for superior cosmetic outcome, e.g., PWS[1]

(BCC: basal cell carcinoma; PWS: port-wine stains)

TABLE 1: Recommended age for different dermatosurgical procedures.

Indications	*Recommended age*
Infective lesions; Warts, molluscum	As early as possible
Malignancies in xeroderma pigmentosum	As early as possible
Port wine stains, angiofibromas	Earlier the better
Nevus of Ota, lentigines and freckles	As per parents' desire
Hirsutism	Minimum 2 years after menarche
Facial hyperhidrosis	Adolescent
Vitiligo surgery	Adolescent in stable lesions
Comedonal and cystic acne	16–18 years
Acne scars	16–18 years and above
Scars	16–18 years
Masseter hypertrophy, gummy smile	18 years and above
Non-surgical rhinoplasty, lip augmentation	18 years and above
Tattoo removal	18 years and above
Excess skin after bariatric surgery	18 years and above
Autologous fat transfer	Performed in childern above 6 years of age
Liposuction for gynecomastia	18 years and above if unresponsive to diet and exercise
Hair transplantation for scars	Above 16 years
Chin augmentation	18 years and above[2]

TABLE 2: Developmental stage and its effects on surgical approach.

Patient age range	*Expected behavior*	*Possible accommodations*
Neonate (0–4 week)	Crying with adverse/ unfamiliar stimuli	Reassurance from physician and caregiver(s); swaddle
Infant (2–12 months)	Crying with adverse/ unfamiliar stimuli	Reassurance from physician and caregiver(s); swaddle
Toddler (12–36 months)	Active resistance to restriction	Consider sedation if high anxiety; secure all limbs to minimize injury or involve caregiver in positioning
Early childhood (4–7 years)	Variable anxiety, poor understanding of the procedure	Consider sedation if high anxiety; secure all limbs to minimize injury or involve caregiver in positioning
Late childhood (8–10 years)	Variable anxiety, open to negotiation	Consider sedation if anxiety is high; explain procedure clearly, offer reward
Pre-teen (11–13 years)	Variable anxiety, communicates needs clearly	Obtain assent, address questions directly, reassure, offer personalized comfort measures
Teenage (13 years)	May demonstrate angst, indifference, withdrawal, resistance to or minimization of discomfort	Obtain assent, address questions directly, reassure, offer personalized comfort measures[1]

the procedure.[3] The Bayley Scales of infant development initially published in 1969 by Nancy Bayley, and standardized to the Baley-III in 2006, is an example of a tool for reference. Assessment is aimed at children of 16 days to 42 months corrected age, the caveat being that each child progresses through development at their unique rate.[1] The **Table 2** shows the developmental stage and its effects on surgical approach.

Developmental testing of infants and young children is difficult and time-consuming task. Through **Table 2** the authors have tried to educate the surgeons what to expect at a particular age. **Table 2** has also provided few accommodations as in how to handle a particular age group during surgery.

Counseling

The aims of counseling in a pediatric patient are as follows:

- Understanding the needs of the child—medical, psychological and anesthetic needs—is of priority and often difficult
- Social and educational impact of the condition and also the treatment needs to be assessed. In particular, interference with social and extracurricular activities in school, educational need to be discussed in detail to time the treatment appropriately
- Counseling should also aim at understanding the concerns of the parents. Particular attention needs to be given to whether patients are pushing for procedures. Individuals accompanying the patients are not always parents and it is important to determine, who is the authorized person to provide the consent
- Detailed explanation of the procedure, its impact of performing the procedure versus postponing the procedure need to be determined and then explained to the parents
- More than one consultation is advised
- Proper documentation of counseling sessions is mandatory

Role of Parental Presence

Conflicting views and practices exist regarding whether parents should be present at the time of their child's medical procedure **(Box 2)**. A systemic review revealed no evidence of technical complications when a parent was present.[4]

The authors feel that, in procedures where there is no blood involved, it is helpful to let the parents stay in the room

BOX 2: Advantages and disadvantages of parental presence.

Advantages:
- Decreased anxiety in child
- Elimination of separation anxiety (which begins to develop around 9 months of age)
- Parental satisfaction

Disadvantages:
- Increased physician anxiety
- Increased parental anxiety

BOX 3: Techniques that help to make children comfortable both before and during dermatologic procedures.

- Sit at or below the level of the child; this is less intimidating than having a physician standing or sitting
- Indulge the child in having conversation with you. The child is more likely to believe and trust what is being said
- The child has to be explained the procedure in an unthreatening manner. It is important to use the words carefully while avoiding words that spell painful images, such as "shot", "needle", or "prick"
- Try to describe what the procedure will feel like; for instance, with injections a "pinch can be felt associated with warmth and it will get over immediately and nothing will be felt after". There should be no surprises
- Do not lie to the child. If a child is told that a procedure will not hurt and it does, trust of that physician will be compromised in the future[4]

of the procedure as it reduces the anxiety in the children as well as the parents. The children are less cranky and more supportive. However, where there is excision and likely bleeding, it is preferable for parents to be in the waiting room.

Handling children during procedures: This is a matter of challenge and needs training, patience, and skill. **Box 3** lists some easy techniques that can help to make children more comfortable both before and during dermatologic procedures.

IMPORTANCE OF ADDRESSING ANXIETY IN CHILDREN

This can be done by distraction techniques and also drug administration.

Distraction techniques: Distraction diverts attention from painful stimuli and is most effective in children younger than 7 years old.[5] Placing a television with some cartoon channels is a simple and inexpensive way to provide distraction during procedures. If children begin watching a movie before the procedure, they tend to be less nervous about the procedure. Another trick is to provide a hand-held gaming device, before the procedure.

Drugs: However, the older pediatric group sometimes may need to be treated with anxiolytic.[6] Chloral hydrate and diphenhydramine are commonly used for this purpose. Oral benzodiazepines are not preferred drugs.

Anesthesia in Children

Local and general anesthesia are used for skin procedures. Topical anesthesia is particularly suitable for children.

Topical Anesthesia

In children, a topical anesthetic is preferable over an injectable anesthetic in most situations. Eutectic mixture of lidocaine + prilocaine (EMLA) is preferred and must be applied under an occlusive dressing for at least 1 hour before a procedure. Longer application times increase effectiveness and depth of anesthesia. Over the denuded and mucous membranes only 5–30 min are needed.[7] Depth of penetration after 60 minutes application, is 3 mm and 5 mm after 120 minutes.[8] Caution should be used when applying EMLA to large areas because children have larger surface area in relation to weight and increased absorption of lidocaine and prilocaine may lead to methemoglobinemia.[9] Infants 0–3 months of age have lower levels of erythrocyte methemoglobin reductase than adults rendering red blood cells and more susceptible to the oxidative stress that leads to methemoglobinemia.[10]

Local Anesthesia

The most commonly used anesthetic is the amide lidocaine which has the advantage of rapid onset of action and moderate duration of activity. It can cause allergic reactions, both immediate and delayed. Toxicity may result from large dose, rapid administration, intravenous administration or slow elimination and biotransformation.[8] Details of local anesthesia are dealt with in a separate chapter.

Most frequently used infiltration anesthetics in children: time of onset, duration and dosage recommendations are shown in **Table 3**.[11]

Iontophoresis: Iontophoresis, for drug delivery through the use of an electric current, is another method of providing local anesthesia painlessly.[8] Iontophoresis takes advantage of lidocaine and epinephrine existing as positively charged their ions in solution. When in positive mode, the positive charged electrode repels the positively charged drug, forcing it through the skin. Anesthesia occurs in 10–30 min. The bulkiness of the machine is a disadvantage and electrochemical burns may result from the application of DC current to the skin.[12]

Sedation: Conscious sedation is defined as pharmacologically induced state of decreased consciousness that does not compromise the patient's ability to maintain protective respiratory reflexes and a secure airway, allows the patient to have purposeful and appropriate reactions to physical or verbal stimuli.[13,14] IV Codeine, Ketamine and midazolam can be quite effective and hence used. However, this administration needs to be performed only in set up with proper protocols and in presence of a trained person as mentioned in **Box 4**.

Regional Anesthesia

Nerve blocks in children avoid multiple injections and minimize dosage of lignocaine and can be used for large lesions.

TABLE 3: Time of onset, duration and dosage recommendations of a local anesthesia in children.

Anesthetic Drug	*Time of onset*	*Duration*	*Maximal recommended dose without epinephrine*	*Maximal recommended dose with epinephrine*
Lidocaine 1%	<2 min	30–60 min	1.5–3 mg/kg	4.5–7 mg/kg children
Prilocaine 1%	10–15 min	3–4 hour	6 mg/kg	10 mg/kg
Bupivacaine 0.25%	2–10 min	3–7 hour	0.5–2 mg/kg	2 mg/kg
Ropivacaine 0.2%	5–15 min	2–6 hour	3 mg/kg: Maximum 225 mg from age 12	-
Articaine 4%	2–4 min	1–3 hour	5 mg/kg from age 4	7 mg/kg from age 4

BOX 4: Equipment for procedural sedation and analgesia.

- High flow oxygen and delivery device
- Suction and large bore catheters
- Vascular access materials
- Airway management supplies: endotracheal tubes, bag valve masks, and laryngoscopes
- Pulse oximetry, blood pressure device, electrocardiography*, Capnography*
- Resuscitation drugs, including intravenous fluids
- Reversal agents, including flumazenil and naloxone

*May be optional devices[15]

Performing nerve blocks requires thorough knowledge of the anatomy of the surgical field.[11]

Tumescent Anesthesia

Tumescent local anesthesia (TLA) uses the subcutaneous infiltration of large volumes of dilute anesthetic to produce swelling and firmness of the targeted areas[15,16] and has been used in children. TLA is discussed in detail in a separate chapter. Heister et al. demonstrated that TLA is a suitable treatment option also in infants under the age of six months, without major complications.[17] It has been seen that TLA induces long lasting analgesia in pediatric patients reducing the need for additional analgesic drugs postoperatively, thereby reducing the risk of drug-induced side effects.[18] There is no general recommendation for the dosing of TLA, different formulations are utilized in different settings and centres.[18] Roerden A et al. recommend a formulation of 10 mL lidocaine 2%, 10 mL ropivacaine 1% and 0.5 mg epinephrine 1:1,000 in 500 mL of balanced electrolyte solution in infants[18] without adverse effects.

Precautionary and emergency measures for TLA are discussed in **Table 4**.

TABLE 4: Precautionary and emergency measures for tumescent local anesthesia (TLA).

Side effects	*Precautionary and emergency measures*
Local anesthesia systemic toxicity (LAST)	Discontinue application of TLA Oxygenation, seizure management (benzodiazepines), advanced cardiac life support, administration of 20% lipid emulsion, continuous monitoring of vital signs
Neurologic symptoms (convulsions, loss of consciousness, agitation)	Discontinue application of TLA Oxygenation, airway management, seizure management (benzodiazepines), consider EEG, ECG monitoring
Apnea following cerebral toxicity	Discontinue application of TLA, Oxygenation, advanced cardiac life support, continuous monitoring of vital signs
Cardiovascular symptoms (bradycardia, hypotension, cardiac arrhythmias)	Discontinue application of TLA, Oxygenation, ECG monitoring, epinephrine and/or atropine for bradycardia, consider cardiac pacing for severe bradycardia, IV-fluids for hypotension, advanced cardiac life support in case of cardiac arrest, specific treatment according to ECG findings
Methemoglobinemia	Discontinue application of TLA, Oxygenation, administer methylene blue in symptomatic acute toxicity (or ascorbic acid in individuals with G6PD deficiency or on serotonergic medication), seizure management (benzodiazepines) if needed, consider blood transfusions in anemic patients
Allergic reactions	Discontinue application of TLA, ECG monitoring, IV-fluids, H1-receptor antagonist, consider corticosteroids (IV) and epinephrine (IM or IV) in severe cases, advanced cardiac life support in case of bradycardia[18]

General Anesthesia

It is performed in the following instances in children:

- Who are too young for administration of a local anesthetic,
- In case of large skin lesions that require excision, or
- In cases of multiple lesions
- Laser treatments, such as for hemangiomas that would otherwise expose the child to several painful interventions.

The risk of complications following general anesthesia in children is usually low because most patients are healthy and the dermatosurgical procedures are usually short. Recent published data showed that there were no statistically significant differences in neurodevelopmental outcomes in children who had undergone general anesthesia for inguinal surgery before the age of 3 in comparison to siblings who had not undergone anesthesia.[19] However, this decision to administer general anesthesia should be taken after careful consideration of all factors and with specific prior informed consent, in a facility that has all infrastructure necessary for GA.

Analgesia: Ensuring proper analgesia is essential post-surgery. Most commonly used analgesics in children with route of administration are shown in **Table 5**.

PLANNING THE PROCEDURE

Role of treatment team: Proper training of the support staff is of utmost importance while executing any procedure in a pediatric patient. Their contribution to the overall plan will minimize the pain and anxiety of the patient/caregiver. They can also help by engaging the patient and family in pleasant conversation. Nurses or medical assistants can apply topical anesthesia, supervise the surgical tray, and educate the family regarding wound care instructions. They can also assist in postoperative instructions and care.

Procedure room environment: It is important to provide a familiar environment to a pediatric patient in the treatment room. Appropriate position of the patient with respect to the body area to be operated gives comfort to the patient and helps improve procedure efficiency. Usage of gel bars/donuts to cushion pressure point, safety straps, and arm boards further ensures security and prevents any fall or injury to the patient. Distraction devices as mentioned earlier can be used to create a calming environment. The following are recommended to maintain a low-anxiety environment during the procedure:

- Soiled gauze should be discarded discretely as soon as generated and should not be visible
- Sharp instruments should remain out of the line of sight when not in use
- Conversation should be maintained throughout the procedure
- If the table is raised, it should be lowered before the patient gets up to avoid falls
- Always congratulate parent and child participating in the procedure. Younger children readily accept small inexpensive gifts such as toys or chocolates as reward for their bravery
- Review restrictions and wound care instructions verbally.

TABLE 5: Most commonly used analgesics in children.

Route of administration	*Drug*	*Dosage*	*Maximum dose per day*
Oral	Ibuprofen	5–10 mg/kg	40 mg/kg/day
	Metamizole	10 mg/kg	74 mg/kg/day[20]
	Acetaminophen	10–15 mg/kg	30 mg/kg/day if <10 kg; 60 mg/kg/day >10 kg[21]
	Diclofenac drops	0.5 mg/kg	1.5 mg/kg[22]
Intravenous	Paracetamol	20 mg/kg	60 mg/kg[22]
	Nalbuphine	0.1–0.2 mg/kg	160 mg[23]

Recommendations for Specific Dermatosurgical and Cosmetic Conditions and their Procedures in Pediatric and Adolescent Age-group

1. *Nevi:* Procedural intervention may be indicated for certain conditions such as melanocytic nevi, nevus sebaceous, and spitz nevi. Recent advances in the pathogenesis of these conditions have allowed more precise recommendations for when and if intervention is necessary.
   a. *Congenital melanocytic nevi (CMN):* There is 2% risk of melanoma among patients with CMN larger than 20 cm and a 12% risk with CMN larger than 60 cm.[24] The highest risk of melanoma has been observed during childhood (mean age 12.6 years), emphasizing the need for close follow-up from an early age.[25,26] Most pediatric dermatologists recommend clinical monitoring of CMN and satellite nevi (including serial photography and dermatoscopy), monitoring of central nervous system in case of large CMN (LCMN) **(Table 6)**, with excisional biopsy for new concerning papules or nodules that appear within the nevus.[27] Excision may be prudent for small CMN in locations that can cause psychosocial distress (e.g., face) or are difficult to monitor (e.g., scalp and buttocks).
   Excision of LCMN is usually performed by plastic surgeons involving multiple surgeries with tissue flaps, tissue expanders, skin grafting, or skin substitutes. Curettage or dermabrasion of the epidermis and superficial dermis may reduce pigmentation in LCMN. This technique must be performed in the first 8 weeks of life.[28]
   For small and medium CMN, it is at the parents' discretion whether to proceed with excision in the first few years of life, before the child develops self-consciousness or let the child decide during adolescence, during which time the nevi can be excised under local anesthesia. It is important to inform the parents that spontaneous lightening of the nevi may occur over time.[27]
   b. *Spitz nevi:* Although Spitz nevi are benign, they share histologic features with melanoma, making accurate

TABLE 6: Ruiz-Maldonado's classification of congenital melanocytic nevi (CMN).[29]

Small	*<1.5 cm in diameter*
Medium	1.5–10 cm
Large	11–20 cm
Giant	>20 cm

diagnosis and proper management challenging and controversial. It is recommended to do excisional biopsy for suspected Spitz nevi in postpubertal patients and in a child of any age with atypical features (size larger than 1 cm, rapid evolution, asymmetry, pain, or ulceration).[27,30]

c. *Nevus sebaceous:* Although nevus sebaceous is a benign hamartoma, because of the appearance and perceived risk of basal cell carcinoma (<1% risk)[31,32] in adulthood, dermatologists recommend excision. This can be done during adolescence under local anesthesia for most of the lesions, unless there are any compelling factors to excise during childhood including cosmesis and avoidance of trauma especially in case of large lesions.[33]

d. *Acquired melanocytic nevi:* The onset of common acquired melanocytic nevi (CAMN) usually occurs during childhood or adolescence which goes through various stages from junctional to compound to intradermal nevus. Although the treatment of CAMN is in most scenarios dictated by cosmetic necessity,[34] the dermatologist should always keep in mind the possibility of melanoma or dysplasia particularly in white skin patients. Though dermoscopy[35,36] is a good noninvasive choice in trained hands, in doubtful cases, a biopsy is probably the only way of confirming dysplasia. Surgical excision is probably the oldest technique, and involves various techniques such as shave excision, scoop-shave excision, round excision, deep excision, punch excision and razor-blade excision.[34,37-40] Although radiofrequency and electrocautery are commonly used for managing CAMN, they cause nonspecific thermal damage and the consequent cosmetic results do not justify their use in CAMN, removal of which is largely a cosmetic concern.[34] The spectrum of lasers used ranges from the green lasers [pulsed dye, Q-switched (Qsw), and neodymium (Nd):yttrium aluminum garnet (YAG) 532] to the far-infrared lasers [CO_2 10,600 nm and erbium (Er):YAG 2,940 nm]. Laser treatment is more effective for smaller and thinner lesions (junctional nevus) while recurrence is common with deeper lesions (compound and dermal nevus).[41] However, laser removal of CAMN is itself controversial since no specimen is submitted for tissue diagnosis and margin assessment. Additionally, the possibility of laser irradiation having the potential to induce malignant change in nevus cells is to be considered. Studies on recurrent nevus previously treated with Q-switched lasers have found changes in cell surface integrin expression, alteration of cell migration, an increase in p16INK4a in p16 positive cell lines. Benign appearing nevi that recur following laser treatment may show new found clinical and histologic atypia, referred to as pseudomelanoma. However, there has never been a report of true malignant transformation following laser treatment. This is epidemiologically low in the Asian skin type even without any intervention.[34]

BOX 5: Indications for scar treatment in children and adolescents.

- Conspicuous scars
- Contracted scars causing functional impairment
- Local or regional lymphedema suggestive of outflow obstruction
- Scars causing severe psychosocial distress
- Symptomatic scars causing pruritus, pain, and tenderness
- Scars located over high-tension areas leading to keloids
- Recurrent infections in the scars
- Recurrent ulcerations within the scars

2. *Scar management:* The necessity to actively treat scars in children and adolescents depends on many factors **(Box 5)**.[2]

While each scar will need specific planning and management, some general principles are stated here:

a. For fresh scars, appropriate topical therapy is recommended as most scars will improve over time.[2]

b. For hypertrophic scars, intralesional corticosteroids remain a mainstay in the treatment of hypertrophic scars and keloids. However, children and adolescents may not tolerate the pain and the procedure should be performed under topical anesthesia. Intralesional 5-FU is considered "off-label" for scars, and its safety and effectiveness in children have not been established.[42]

c. Earlobe keloids are common and also particularly problematic in teenagers who go in for multiple ear piercings. They can be managed with pressure therapy, intralesional steroid, cryotherapy or surgery. One prospective pediatric study involving 15 patients with earlobe keloids included aggressive treatment regimen with a single recurrence noted at 18 months of follow-up.[43] Patients were treated with a preoperative intralesional injection of 0.5 mL triamcinolone 0.5% at their initial visit followed by surgical excision in 4 weeks, where the lesion was injected again intraoperatively. Care was taken to approximate skin edges without tension. Sutures were removed within 10–14 days. The area of their lesion was injected again after 4 weeks. The injections were given again at any sign of abnormal scar formation and repeated every 6 weeks until complete resolution of the lesion.

d. Laser resurfacing with nonablative and ablative fractional lasers (Erbium glass laser 1,550 nm, CO_2 laser 10,600 nm, erbium yttrium-aluminum-garnet laser 2,940 nm) or pulsed dye laser (585 nm) can improve the scars. Anecdotal evidence shows that fractional laser therapy is well tolerated with a low rate of complications in children, although relatively few safety reports in pediatric population are available.[42] To avoid discomfort, appropriate anesthesia should be used in laser therapy for this population. Laser-assisted drug delivery, using a fractional laser followed by topical steroid/PRP, can also be used.[2]

e. Postacne scarring is of concern especially in adolescents. They suffer from lower self-esteem, and lower quality of life when compared to adolescents without acne.[44] These scars should be treated in a similar manner as in adults and treatment should be tailored for each patient. Reader is referred to the chapter on *Management of Post-acne Scar.*

It needs to be emphasized that multimodal approach is required for management of most scars[42]

3. *Laser hair reduction:*[2,45] Laser hair reduction (LHR) in pediatric age group can be done for either hypertrichosis or hirsutism. Hypertrichosis may be congenital or acquired, localized or generalized, and can be a cosmetic or psychosocial problem for the patient. Laser hair reduction for hirsutism is a common cosmetic procedure sought by adolescent girls. The etiology should be first identified and treated before attempting laser hair removal for hirsutism. Patients with polycystic ovarian syndrome should be motivated to make lifestyle changes such as dietary restrictions on unhealthy junk food, weight loss, exercise, and medical therapy if necessary. While laser hair removal is a simple procedure without any significant complications, in view of evolving hormonal status during puberty, it is recommended that the procedure be delayed till about 15–16 years of age. The minimum age of LHR is 2 years post menarche or 15 years of age as per the Indian Association of Dermatologists, Venereologists and Leprologists (IADVL) guidelines on LHR.[46] Though it can be done in younger age group if absolutely necessary particularly for noncosmetic indications. Many teenagers also opt for underarms, arms, legs or a full-body LHR. This gives freedom from frequent temporary hair removal methods. Boys also opt for beard shaping and LHR of the chest, back, and arms. The expectation in boys is to have a well-defined beard line and reduced density of coarse hair on the body. Apart from cosmetic concerns, LHR is sometimes required to treat conditions such as Becker's nevus, acquired compound melanocytic nevus, pilonidal sinus, hidradenitis suppurativa, pseudofolliculitis barbae, trichostasis spinulosa and hair-bearing flaps or grafts after reconstructive surgeries.
4. *Pigmentary lasers:* A number of pigmented lesions in childhood including lentigines, nevus of Ota, congenital melanocytic nevi, café-au-lait macules, and nevus spilus, can be treated with pigment-specific lasers.[45] Q-switched neodymium-doped YAG (Nd:YAG) laser 1,064 nm and KTP (Potassium Titanyl Phosphate laser 532 nm) are most commonly used. It is recommended that treatment should begin early in childhood to prevent darkening and worsening.[2] In a retrospective study on laser treatment of 104 cases of nevus of Ota, it was seen that the younger the first treating age, the lesser the treatment sessions were required. At the same time, earlier treatment leads to less psychological impact on children during their growth. There was no correlation between first treating age and recurrence of the lesion.[47]

Table 7 summarizes the common indications for pigmentary lasers in pediatric population.[45]

TABLE 7: Common indications for pigmentary lasers in pediatric population.

Lesion	*Laser treatment*	*Comment*
Lentigines	All pigment-specific lasers Qs-Nd:YAG in ethnic skin	Most common on lips in child
Nevus of Ota	Q-switched ruby, Q-switched alexandrite, Q-switched Nd:YAG 1,064 nm Qw ND:YAG-(Most commonly used)	Brown lesions with best result; rare recurrence
Congenital melanocytic nevi	Normal ruby, Q-switched ruby, Q-switched Nd:YAG 532 nm and 1064 nm	Controversial; biopsy prior to laser therapy; laser therapy not definitive
Café-au-lait macules	Q-switched ruby, Q-switched Nd:YAG 532 nm, copper vapor	Variability in response
Nevus spilus	Normal ruby, Normal alexandrite, Q-switched ruby, Q-switched Nd:YAG 532 nm	Variability in response; biopsy prior to laser therapy (in case of atypical lesions)

5. *Tattoo removal:* There has been a trend of tattooing in teenagers both in boys and girls. They often think it is trendy and glamorous and do not understand the risks involved in tattooing and then seek its removal. In an Indian study, the mean age of doing tattoos was 15.8 ± 3 years. For cultural reasons, tattooing is done even in early childhood. The most common reason for doing a tattoo was for fashion in 87.7%, fun in 6.6%, and peer pressure in 4.7%. The most common reason for tattoo removal in this study was eligibility for jobs (49.5%); regret (21.7%); social reasons, such as elder or school pressure (14.2%); personal (12.7%); and unsightly appearance and complications such as hypertrophic scarring in tattoo (1.9%).[48] Tattoo removal is done by the Q-switched Nd:YAG laser, picoseconds laser, or combination techniques including fractional lasers. Despite advances in technology, it requires several treatments, is painful and is rarely complete, without scarring. Teenagers should be made aware of the consequences of tattooing as well as tattoo removal.

Indications for tattoo removal in children and adolescents include:

1. Patient planning a career/job which requires no tattoos on the body, e.g., Armed forces

2. Complications of tattooing, e.g., infections, granulomatous reactions
3. Tattoos causing psychological stress
4. Social and religious obligations

6. *Vascular lasers:* Although initially developed for the treatment of port-wine stains, vascular lasers are now being used for the treatment of multiple types of vascular lesions in the pediatric patient including hemangiomas, pyogenic granulomas, telangiectases, spider telangiectases, and angiofibromas, straie distensae in early stages, erythematous scars and keloids.[2,45,49]

   According to current literature, there is evidence of a marked reduction in port-wine stains in children whose treatments begin at less than 1 year to prevent progression and thus increase the likelihood of complete removal.[50] Detailed discussion on this topic is found in the chapter on vascular lesions and a summary is provided in **Table 8**.[45]
7. *Chemical peels, microdermabrasion (MDA) and microneedling:* Today's tech savvy teenagers demand procedures such as chemical peels, MDA and microneedling after reading from the internet and following their role models such as actors, bloggers and models. These procedures, while being safe, should not be encouraged as a first-line therapy.

   Salicylic acid, mandelic acid, lactic acid and glycolic acid are common peels used for acne and dyspigmentation. Similarly, MDA and microneedling (dermaroller) should be done only when absolutely indicated. They believe that these procedures can magically improve acne, pigmentation or scarring. Therefore, it is important to discuss with teenagers the outcomes, number of sessions required and risk of PIH especially in dark skinned individuals. They should be motivated enough to follow proper home care regimens and be regular with their treatment.
8. *Vitiligo surgery **(Box 6)**:* Autologous grafting should be reserved to stable vitiligo lesions (i.e., lesions with no progression for at least 1 year). The best indication for grafting is stable segmental vitiligo.[51] Different grafting techniques have been described, including punch grafting, split-thickness skin graft, suction blister grafting and the most recent is melanocyte transfer grafting. Grafting techniques have shown great results, although there is a concern about the long-term maintenance of these results in non-segmental vitiligo (NSV).[52] Therefore, in NSV, other therapies should be offered along with camouflage till the child grows and vitiligo becomes stable. An important step for success of vitiligo surgery is immobilization of the recipient area, and this should be emphasized to the child and the parents. All possible outcomes, possibility of incomplete/mottled pigmentation, scarring/pigmentation of donor area, unpredictability of results over large areas, and likely complications should be discussed. Gupta and Kumar[53] reported more than 75% repigmentation with suction blister grafting in 80% of children and adolescents with vitiligo. The results were better in children as compared to adults. However, it should be kept in mind that suction blister technique requires prolonged immobility for the formation of blisters, particularly in children because they have strong dermoepidermal adherence and keeping them in restricted posture for a long time requires a high level of motivation.

   Sahni et al.[54] used noncultured autologous epidermal cell transplantation technique in 13 children and adolescents with stable vitiligo with 75–90% repigmentation at the end of 1 year. Microdermabrasion with pimecrolimus cream (1%) in childhood nonsegmental vitiligo showed more than 50% repigmentation after 3 months in 60.4% of patches versus pimecrolimus alone (32.1%) and placebo (1.7%).[55]

TABLE 8: Treatment of different vascular lesions.

Lesion	*Laser treatment*	*Comment*
Port wine stain	Flash lamp-pumped pulsed dye 585 nm, 595 nm	Start >1 year; edge effect: Edge of the lesion responds better, larger circumference has better response; central forehead most responsive
Hemangiomas	Flash lamp-pumped pulsed dye	Controversial for superficial lesions; used if compromise vital structures or cosmetic morbidity; used for ulcerated hemangiomas
Telangiectasias	Flash lamp-pumped pulsed dye Green light lasers	Good response in spider telangiectasia and large facial venules
Pyogenic granuloma	Flash lamp-pumped pulsed dye 585 nm Carbon-dioxide laser, combined continuous-wave/pulsed	Small, flat lesions respond better
Angiofibromas	Carbon dioxide, copper vapor KTP, flash lamp-pumped pulsed dye	Facial angiofibromas Early, small lesions respond better

BOX 6: IADVL guidelines on vitiligo surgery.[56]

Age Considerations for Surgery and Patient Selection

As such, no uniformly accepted opinion exists concerning the minimum age for surgery. Vitiligo surgery is generally performed under local anesthesia, which would be difficult in children. General anesthesia for vitiligo surgery in a young child poses unacceptable risks and the progress of the disease is difficult to predict in children. Hence, many dermatologists feel that surgical procedures should not be performed in children. However, studies have suggested that results of transplantation procedures were better in younger individuals than in older ones. Thus, no consensus exists in this aspect and physicians should exercise their judgment after taking all aspects of the individual patient into consideration.

9. *Injectables:* Botulinum toxin injection has been used for various cosmetic indications such as masseter hypertrophy, brow lift, bunny lines, gummy smile, and chin reshaping. However, it should be discouraged in children and adolescents. Similarly, hyaluronic acid fillers have been extensively used for facial reshaping and asymmetry, nose or chin reshaping, and under-eye dark circles. These too should be strongly discouraged, till they are 18 years.[2] It is of extreme importance to counsel them and their parents, and repeatedly emphasize that the effects are temporary and the risks and complications involved in these procedures. Psychotherapy may be of great help in overcoming their distress. However, the use of botulinum toxin for non-cosmetic indication such as hyperhidrosis (facial, axillary, palmoplantar) is of great benefit in school going children and adolescents. It has been found to greatly improve the quality of life, social skills, and day-to-day activities.[57-59]

Considerations for Cosmetic Procedures and Surgery

While considerations for procedures in medical reasons are clear and easy to decide, decisions for cosmetic procedures are more difficult and need to address below issues:

- *Physical aspects:* It should be remembered that children's bodies continue to develop well into their mid-20s. This is also the age group when opinions change quickly.
- *Social aspects:* In the society with continuous change and development, adolescents have an idea of beauty which mirrors the current trends, which are influenced by social media and magazines.[2] These change with time as fashions and trends become obsolete.
- *Psychological factors:* Adolescent age is a susceptible age for different influences. Body image is important during adolescents during development as it is an important contributor to adolescent's self-esteem, and negative body image leading to anxiety, depression, anxiety and fear of negative evaluation.[60] Hence, it is not surprising that most cases of body dysmorphic disorders (BDD) develop initially during adolescence as they get obsessed with the body image eventually leading to depression and even suicidal tendencies. It has been reported that 5–15% of patients who present with cosmetic disorders, may meet the diagnostic need for BDD.[60,61] Body dysmorphic disorder undermines whatever capacity for autonomy the adolescent has and even if there is valid parental consent, the presence of BDD means that cosmetic surgery will fail in its aims.[62] Some studies have shown that repeated surgeries do not improve BDD.[63] Thus, screening for BDD should be done in teenagers who are obsessed with their body image and such patients referred to a psychologist who is well versed in dealing with adolescents.[64]
- *Emotional:* Adolescence phase is a time where the peer pressure is usually very dominant; such pressure can lead to body shaming and these emotional aspects need to be handled carefully.
- *Ethical:* Beneficence (best interest), nonmaleficence (principle of no harm) and autonomy are the key ethical aspects of medical practice.[65] A child is not in a position to decide on any procedure and patients may bring in their own external influences in decision making. Careful analysis is therefore essential.[65]
- *Legal aspects:* Informed consent of adolescents is a complex issue as the age is 18 years to give consent for any procedure. In any cosmetic surgery on teenagers, it is safer to have informed consent of the parents.[2] The parents and patients both must be given enough time to assess the risks of the procedure and ask all the questions they wish to ask. It should be understood that consent should be documented in detail, and all documents need to be preserved until patient becomes an adult. *In a child, medicolegal liability lasts not just for a limited period of 5 years post-procedure, but until patient becomes an adult.*

COMPLICATIONS AND RISKS

There is paucity of literature regarding the safety and complications of dermatosurgical and cosmetic procedures in pediatric population. A study comparing the complication rates of cosmetic procedures between adolescents and older adults showed a lower incidence of major complications in adolescents (0.71% in adolescents vs. 1.99% in adults, $P < 0.01$).[66]

General complications, which should be kept in mind, are complications due to anesthesia bleeding, hematoma, edema, Infections, poor esthetic outcome and scarring.

CONCLUSION

Performance of dermatosurgical and cosmetic procedures in children and adolescents is complicated and needs thorough understanding of all aspects. It is important to consider the safety, age of the patient, indications, psychological and legal aspects before performing a procedure in pediatric patient. Only procedures which are safe and necessary should be performed, e.g., treatment of port-wine stains, hemangiomas compromising vital structures, large congenital melanocytic nevi, warts and molluscum (surgical or energy based procedures). Procedures which are safe but need caution along with proper risk assessment include aesthetic procedures like chemical peels, microdermabrasion, microneedling, LHR, tattoo removal, vitiligo surgery, treatment of freckles and lentigines, scar revision and botulinum toxin for hyperhidrosis. Finally, some procedures should be strongly discouraged until adulthood, e.g., injectables for aesthetic indications, plastic surgery procedures such as liposuction, breast augmentation and rhinoplasty.

Parents and pediatrician/pediatric surgeon should be involved in decision making when necessary. Involvement of a psychiatrist may be necessary particularly when dealing with adolescents for aesthetic indications. Dermatosurgical procedures in children should be performed in a set-up where all the necessary equipment and emergency facilities are available.

REFERENCES

1. Agim NG, Shah KM. Pearls for Dermatologic surgery in pediatric patients. Dermatol Clin. 2019;37(3):387-95.
2. Khunger N, Pant H. Cosmetic procedures in adolescents: what's safe and what can wait. Indian J Paediatr Dermatol. 2020;22:12-20.
3. Sharp M, DeMauro SB. Counterbalanced comparison of the BSID-II and Bayley-III at eighteen to twenty-two months corrected age. J Dev Behav Pediatr 2017;38(5):322-9.
4. Metz BJ. Procedural pediatric dermatology. Dermatol Clin. 2013;31(2):337-46.
5. Kleiber C, Harper DC. Effects of distraction on children's pain and distress during medical procedures: a meta-analysis. Nurs Res. 1999;48(1):44-9.
6. Otley CC, Nguyen TH. Conscious sedation of pediatric patients with combination oral benzodiazepines and inhaled nitrous oxide. Dermatol Surg. 2000;26(11):1041-4.
7. Babich D, Crollick JS. Pediatric dermatologic surgery for the primary care pediatrician. Pediatr Clin North Am. 1998; 45(6):1437-53.
8. Lener EV, Bucalo BD, Kist DA, Moy RL. Topical anesthetic agents in dermatologic surgery: a review. Dermatol Surg. 1997;23(8):673-83.
9. Taddio A, Stevens B, Craig K, Rastogi P, Ben-David S, Shennan A, et al. Efficacy and safety of lidocaine-prilocaine cream for pain during circumcision. N Engl J Med. 1997;336(17): 1197-201.
10. Kumar AR, Dunn N, Naqvi M. Methemoglobinemia associated with a prilocaine-lidocaine cream. Clin Pediatr (Phila). 1997; 36(4):239-40.
11. Crisan D, Scharffetter-Kochanek K, Kastler S, Crisan M, Manea A, Wagner K, et al. Dermatologic surgery in children: an update on indication, anesthesia, analgesia and potential perioperative complications. J Dtsch Dermatol Ges. 2018; 16(3):268-276.
12. Greenbaum SS, Bernstein EF. Comparison of iontophoresis of lidocaine with a eutectic mixture of lidocaine and prilocaine (EMLA) for topically administered local anesthesia. J Dermatol Surg Oncol. 1994;20:579-83.
13. American Academy of Pediatrics, American Academy of Pediatric Dentistry, Coté CJ, Wilson S, Work Group on Sedation. Guidelines for monitoring and management of pediatric patients during and after sedation for diagnostic and therapeutic procedures: an update. Pediatrics. 2006; 118(6):2587-602.
14. Guidelines of care for office surgical facilities. Part I. J Am Acad Dermatol. 1992;26(5 Pt 1):763-5.
15. Meredith JR, O'Keefe KP, Galwankar S. Pediatric procedural sedation and analgesia. J Emerg Trauma Shock. 2008;1(2): 88-96.
16. Klein JA. Tumescent technique for regional anesthesia permits lidocaine doses of 35 mg/kg for liposuction. J Dermatol Surg Oncol. 1990;16:248-63.
17. Heister M, Häfner H, Breuninger H, Schulz C, Meier K, Kofler L, et al. Tumescent local anaesthesia for early dermatosurgery in infants. J Eur Acad Dermatol Venereol. 2017;31:2077-82.
18. Roerden A, Neunhoeffer F, Götz A, Häfner HM, Kofler L. Benefits, safety and side effects of tumescent local anesthesia in dermatologic surgery in infants. J Dtsch Dermatol Ges. 2021;19(3):352-7.
19. Sun LS, Li G, Miller TL, Salorio C, Byrne MW, Bellinger DC, et al. Association between a single general anesthesia exposure before age 36 months and neurocognitive outcomes in later childhood. JAMA. 2016;315(21):2312-20.
20. Fieler M, Eich C, Becke K, Badelt G, Leimkühler K, Messroghli L, et al. Metamizole for postoperative pain therapy in 1,177 children: a prospective, multicentre, observational, postauthorisation safety study. Eur J Anaesthesiol. 2015;32(12):839-43.
21. Verghese ST, Hannallah RS. Acute pain management in children. J Pain Res. 2010;3:105-23.
22. Diedericks J. Postoperative pain management in the paediatric patient. South African Fam Pract. 2006;48(3):37-42.
23. Schultz-Machata AM, Becke K, Weiss M. Nalbuphine in pediatric anesthesia. Anaesthesist. 2014;63(2):135-43.
24. Vourc'h-Jourdain M, Martin L, Barbarot S. Large congenital melanocytic nevi: therapeutic management and melanoma risk: a systematic review. J Am Acad Dermatol. 2013;68:493-8.
25. Krengel S, Hauschild A, Schäfer T. Melanoma risk in congenital melanocytic naevi: a systematic review. Br J Dermatol. 2006; 155:1-8.
26. Watt AJ, Kotsis SV, Chung KC. Risk of melanoma arising in large congenital melanocytic nevi: a systematic review. Plast Reconstr Surg. 2004;113:1968-74.
27. Mann JA. Update on pediatric dermatologic surgery from tots to teens. Curr Opin Pediatr. 2014;26(4):452-9.
28. Rasmussen BS, Henriksen TF, Kølle S-FT, Schmidt G. Giant congenital melanocytic nevus: report from 30 years of experience in a single department. Ann Plast Surg. 2015; 74(2):223-9.
29. Ruiz-Maldonado R. Measuring congenital melanocytic nevi. Pediatr Dermatol. 2004;21:178-9.
30. Metzger AT, Kane AA, Bayliss SJ. Differences in treatment of Spitz nevi and atypical Spitz tumors in pediatric patients among dermatologists and plastic surgeons. JAMA Dermatol. 2013;149(11):1348-50.
31. Idriss MH, Elston DM. Secondary neoplasms associated with nevus sebaceous of Jadassohn: a study of 707 cases. J Am Acad Dermatol. 2014;70:332-7.
32. Chepla KJ, Gosain AK. Giant nevus sebaceus: definition, surgical techniques, and rationale for treatment. Plast Reconstr Surg. 2012;130:296e-304e.
33. Correale D, Ringpfeil F, Rogers M. Large, papillomatous, pedunculated nevus sebaceus: a new phenotype. Pediatr Dermatol. 2008;25(3):355-8.
34. Sardana K, Chakravarty P, Goel K. Optimal management of common acquired melanocytic nevi (moles): current perspectives. Clin Cosmet Investig Dermatol. 2014;7:89-103.
35. Zalaudek I, Grinschgl S, Argenziano G, Marghoob AA, Blum A, Richtig E, et al. Age-related prevalence of dermoscopy patterns in acquired melanocytic naevi. Br J Dermatol. 2006;154:299-304.
36. De Giorgi V, Massi D, Salvini C, Trez E, Mannone F, Carli P. Dermoscopic features of combined melanocytic nevi. J Cutan Pathol. 2004;31:600-4.

37. Ferrandiz L, Moreno-Ramirez D, Camacho FM. Shave excision of common acquired melanocytic nevi: cosmetic outcome, recurrences, and complications. Dermatol Surg. 2005; 31(9 Pt 1):1112-5.
38. Gambichler T, Senger E, Rapp S, Alamouti D, Altmeyer P, Hoffmann K. Deep shave excision of macular melanocytic nevi with the razor blade biopsy technique. Dermatol Surg. 2000;26(7):662-6.
39. Tursen U, Kaya TI, Ikizoglu G. Round excision of small, benign, papular and dome-shaped melanocytic nevi on the face. Int J Dermatol. 2004;43(11):844-6.
40. Breuninger H, Garbe C, Rassner G. Shave excision of melanocytic nevi of the skin: indications, technique, results. Hautarzt. 2000;51(8):575-80.
41. Sardana K. The science, reality, and ethics of treating common acquired melanocytic nevi (moles) with lasers. J Cutan Aesthet Surg. 2013;6(1):27-9.
42. Krakowski AC, Totri CR, Donelan MB, Shumaker PR. Scar management in the pediatric and adolescent populations. Pediatrics. 2016;137:e20142065.
43. Hamrick M, Boswell W, Carney D. Successful treatment of earlobe keloids in the pediatric population. J Pediatr Surg. 2009;44(1):286-8.
44. Halvorsen JA, Stern RS, Dalgard F, Thoresen M, Bjertness E, Lien L. Suicidal ideation, mental health problems, and social impairment are increased in adolescents with acne: a population-based study. J Invest Dermatol. 2011;131:363-70.
45. Cantatore JL, Kriegel DA. Laser surgery: an approach to the pediatric patient. J Am Acad Dermatol. 2004;50(2):165-84.
46. Buddhadev RM. Standard guidelines of care: laser and IPL hair reduction. Indian J Dermatol Venereol Leprol. 2008;74:68-74.
47. Zong W, Lin T. A retrospective study on laser treatment of nevus of Ota in Chinese children--a seven-year follow-up. J Cosmet Laser Ther. 2014;16(4):156-60.
48. Thakur BK, Verma S. Tattoo practices in North-East India: a hospital-based cross-sectional study. J Cutan Aesthet Surg. 2016;9:172-6.
49. Shokeir H, El Bedewi A, Sayed S, El Khalafawy G. Efficacy of pulsed dye laser versus intense pulsed light in the treatment of striae distensae. Dermatol Surg. 2014;40:632-40.
50. Nguyen CM, Yohn JJ, Weston WL. Facial port wine stains in childhood: prediction of the rate of improvement as a function of the age of the patient, size and location of the port wine stain and the number of treatments with the pulsed dye (585nm) laser. Br J Dermatol. 1998;38:821-5.
51. Ezzedine K, Silverberg N. A Practical approach to the diagnosis and treatment of vitiligo in children. Pediatrics. 2016;138(1):e20154126.
52. Parsad D, Pandhi R, Dogra S, Kanwar AJ, Kumar B. Dermatology Life Quality Index score in vitiligo and its impact on the treatment outcome. Br J Dermatol. 2003;148(2):373-4.
53. Gupta S, Kumar B. Epidermal grafting for vitiligo in adolescents. Pediatr Dermatol. 2002;19:159-62.
54. Sahni K, Parsad D, Kanwar AJ. Noncultured epidermal suspension transplantation for the treatment of stable vitiligo in children and adolescents. Clin Exp Dermatol. 2011; 36:607-12.
55. Farajzadeh S, Daraei Z, Esfandirpour I, Hosseini SH. The efficacy of pimecrolimus 1% cream combined with microdermabrasion in the treatment of non-segmental childhood vitiligo: a randomized placebo-controlled study. Pediatr Dermatol. 2009;26:286-91.
56. Parsad D, Gupta S. Standard guidelines of care for vitiligo surgery. Indian J Dermatol Venereol Leprol. 2008;74:37-45.
57. Glaser DA, Pariser DM, Hebert AA, Landells I, Somogyi C, Weng E, et al. A prospective, nonrandomized, open-label study of the efficacy and safety of Onabotulinum toxin A in adolescents with primary axillary hyperhidrosis. Pediatr Dermatol. 2015;32:609-17.
58. Kouris A, Armyra K, Stefanaki C, Christodoulou C, Karimali P, Kontochristopoulos G. Quality of life and social isolation in Greek adolescents with primary focal hyperhidrosis treated with botulinum toxin type A: a case series. Pediatr Dermatol. 2015;32:226-30.
59. Bohaty BR, Hebert AA. Special considerations for children with hyperhidrosis. Dermatol Clin 2014;32:477-84.
60. Phillips KA, Didie ER, Menard W, Pagano ME, Fay C, Weisberg RB. Clinical features of body dysmorphic disorder in adolescents and adults. Psychiatry Res. 2006 30;141(3): 305-14.
61. Crerand CE, Franklin ME, Sarwer DB. Patient safety and body dysmorphic disorder in cosmetic surgery patients. Plast Reconstr Surg 2008;122:1-15.
62. Spriggs M, Gillam L. Body dysmorphic disorder: contra-indication or ethical justification for female genital cosmetic surgery in adolescents. Bioethics. 2016;30(9):706-13.
63. Veale D, Gournay K, Dryden W, Boocock A. Body dysmorphic disorder: a cognitive-behavioral model and a pilot randomized controlled trial. Behav Res Ther. 1996;34:717-29.
64. Higgins S, Wysong A. Cosmetic surgery and body dysmorphic disorder - an update. Int J Womens Dermatol. 2018;4:43-8.
65. Desousa A. Concerns about cosmetic surgery. Indian J Med Ethics. 2007;4:171-3.
66. Yeslev M, Gupta V, Winocour J, Shack RB, Grotting JC, Higdon KK. Safety of cosmetic surgery in adolescent patients. Aesthet Surg J. 2017;37(9):1051-9.

Index

Page numbers followed by *b* refer to box, *f* refer to figure, *fc* refer to flowchart, and *t* refer to table.

B

D

E

G

I

J

K

N

O

P

Q

T

U

V

W

X

Y

Z